P9-DNS-790

Nelson TEXTBOOK OF PEDIATRICS

TENTH EDITION

Edited by

VICTOR C. VAUGHAN, III, M.D.

Professor and Chairman, Department of Pediatrics,
Temple University School of Medicine;
Medical Director, St. Christopher's Hospital
for Children, Philadelphia

R. JAMES McKAY, M.D.

Professor and Chairman, Department of Pediatrics,
The University of Vermont College of Medicine;
Chief of Pediatric Service, Medical Center Hospital
of Vermont, Burlington

Consulting Editor

WALDO E. NELSON, M.D.

Professor of Pediatrics, Temple University School of
Medicine and Medical College of Pennsylvania;
Attending Pediatrician, St. Christopher's Hospital
for Children; Editor, Journal of Pediatrics

WITH THE COLLABORATION OF 101 CONTRIBUTORS

W. B. SAUNDERS COMPANY *Philadelphia • London • Toronto*

W. B. Saunders Company: West Washington Square
Philadelphia, PA 19105

1 St. Anne's Road
Eastbourne, East Sussex BN21 3UN, England

1 Goldthorne Avenue
Toronto, Ontario M8Z 5T9, Canada

Listed here is the latest translated edition of this book together with the language of the translation and the publisher.

Portuguese—Editora Interamericana Ltda.,
Rio de Janeiro, Brazil

Nelson Textbook of Pediatrics ISBN 0–7216–9018–1

©1975 by W. B. Saunders Company. Copyright 1933, 1937, 1941, 1945, 1950, 1954, 1959, 1964 and 1969 by W. B. Saunders Company. Copyright under the International Copyright Union. All rights reserved. This book is protected by copyright. No part of it may be reproduced, stored in a retrieval system, or transmitted in any form or by any means, electronic, mechanical, photocopying, recording, or otherwise, without written permission from the publisher. Made in the United States of America. Press of W. B. Saunders Company. Library of Congress catalog card number 73-77943.

Print No.: 9 8 7 6

Dedicated
to
All Children Everywhere

CONTRIBUTORS

MARVIN EARL AMENT, M.D. Assistant Professor of Pediatrics and Medicine, UCLA Center for Health Sciences, Los Angeles, California

JOHN A. ANDERSON, M.D., Ph.D. Professor of Pediatrics, School of Medicine of the University of Minnesota; Attending Pediatrician, University of Minnesota Hospital, Minneapolis, Minnesota

JAMES B. AREY, M.D., Ph.D. Professor of Pathology, Temple University School of Medicine; Pathologist, St. Christopher's Hospital for Children, Philadelphia, Pennsylvania

VICTOR H. AUERBACH, Ph.D. Research Professor in Pediatrics (Biochemistry), Temple University School of Medicine; Director, Research Chemistry, St. Christopher's Hospital for Children, Philadelphia, Pennsylvania

HENRY W. BAIRD, III, M.D. Professor of Pediatrics, Temple University School of Medicine; Attending Physician, St. Christopher's Hospital for Children, Philadelphia, Pennsylvania

GIULIO J. BARBERO, M.D. Professor and Chairman of Child Health, Department of Child Health School of Medicine of the University of Missouri, Columbia, Missouri

LEWIS A. BARNESS, M.D. Professor and Chairman, Department of Pediatrics, University of South Florida College of Medicine, Tampa, Florida

JOHN B. BARTRAM, M.D. Professor of Pediatrics, Temple University School of Medicine; Senior Attending Pediatrician, St. Christopher's Hospital for Children, Philadelphia, Pennsylvania

PAUL C. BEAVER, Ph.D. William Vincent Professor of Tropical Diseases and Hygiene, Tulane University School of Public Health and Tropical Medicine, New Orleans, Louisiana

RICHARD E. BEHRMAN, M.D. Professor and Chairman, Department of Pediatrics, Columbia University College of Physicians and Surgeons; Director, Pediatrics, Babies Hospital, New York, New York

WILLIAM H. BERGSTROM, M.D. Professor of Pediatrics, State University of New York at Syracuse; Attending Pediatrician, University Hospital, Syracuse, New York

JOSEPH B. BILDERBACK, M.D. Late Clinical Professor of Pediatrics, University of Oregon Medical School, Portland, Oregon

RUSSELL JOHN BLATTNER, M.D. Professor and Chairman, Department of Pediatrics, Baylor College of Medicine; Physician-in-Chief, Texas Children's Hospital, Houston, Texas

CARROLL F. BURGOON, JR., M.D. Professor of Dermatology, Temple University School of Medicine; Chief Attending Pediatrician, Skin and Cancer Hospital, Philadelphia, Pennsylvania

ELSIE R. CARRINGTON, M.D. Professor and Chairman, Department of Obstetrics and Gynecology, The Medical College of Pennsylvania, Philadelphia, Pennsylvania

HUGO F. CARVAJAL, M.D. Assistant Professor, Department of Pediatrics, Shriner's Burns Institute and the University of Texas Medical Branch, Galveston, Texas

ESTHER LADEN CAVA, Ph.D. Assistant Professor of Psychology, Temple University School of Medicine; Psychologist, St. Christopher's Hospital for Children, Philadelphia, Pennsylvania

J. JULIAN CHISOLM, JR., M.D. Assistant Professor of Pediatrics, Johns Hopkins University School of Medicine; Associate Chief Pediatrician, Baltimore City Hospital, Baltimore, Maryland

AMOS CHRISTIE, M.D. Professor of Pediatrics Emeritus, Vanderbilt University School of Medicine; Emeritus Staff, Vanderbilt University Hospital, Nashville, Tennessee

DAVID F. CLYDE, M.D., Ph.D., D.T.M.&H. Professor of International Medicine, University of Maryland School of Medicine, Baltimore, Maryland; Member, Expert Advisory Panel on Malaria of the World Health Organization, Geneva, Switzerland

CHARLES DAVENPORT COOK, M.D. Professor of Pediatrics, Columbia University College of Physicians and Surgeons; Director, Department of Pediatrics, Harlem Hospital, New York, New York

ALLEN C. CROCKER, M.D. Associate Professor of Pediatrics, Harvard Medical School; Senior Associate in Medicine, Children's Hospital Medical Center, Boston, Massachusetts

EDWARD C. CURNEN, M.D. Carpentier Professor of Pediatrics Emeritus, Columbia University College of Physicians and Surgeons; Consultant in Pediatrics, Columbia, Presbyterian and St. Luke's Medical Centers and Attending Pediatrician, Harlem Hospital Center, New York, New York

F. L. DEBUSK, M.D. Professor of Pediatrics, University of Florida College of Medicine, Gainesville, Florida

FLOYD W. DENNY, M.D. Professor and Chairman, Department of Pediatrics, University of North Carolina School of Medicine; Medical Staff, North Carolina Memorial Hospital, Chapel Hill, North Carolina

ANGELO M. DIGEORGE, M.D., M.S.(Ped.) Professor of Pediatrics, Temple University School of Medicine; Senior Attending Pediatrician and Director, Section of Endocrine and Metabolic Disorders, St. Christopher's Hospital for Children, Philadelphia, Pennsylvania

PAUL A. DI SANT'AGNESE, M.D., Sc.D. (Med.), Dr. Med. (Hon.) Clinical Professor of Pediatrics, Georgetown University School of Medicine, Washington, D.C.; Chief of Pediatric Metabolism Branch, National Institutes of Health, Bethesda, Maryland

JOHN J. DOWNES, M.D. Professor of Anesthesiology and Pediatrics, University of Pennsylvania School of Medicine; Director, Department of Anesthesiology, Children's Hospital of Philadelphia, Philadelphia, Pennsylvania

ALLAN L. DRASH, M.D. Associate Professor of Pediatrics, University of Pittsburgh School of Medicine; Director, Clinical Research Center, Children's Hospital of Pittsburgh, Pittsburgh, Pennsylvania

KEITH N. DRUMMOND, M.D., C.M., F.R.C.P.(C) Professor and Chairman, Department of Pediatrics, McGill University; Physician-in-Chief and Director, Department of Nephrology, Montreal Children's Hospital, Montreal, Canada

JOHN MALCOLM DUNN, M.D. Clinical Associate Professor of Psychiatry (Child Psychiatry), Temple University School of Medicine; Attending Psychiatrist, St. Christopher's Hospital for Children, Philadelphia, Pennsylvania

HEINZ F. EICHENWALD, M.D. Professor and Chairman, Department of Pediatrics, University of Texas, Southwestern Medical School; Chief of Staff and Director of Pediatrics, Children's Medical Center, Chief of Pediatrics, Parkland Memorial Hospital, Dallas, Texas

ELLIOT F. ELLIS, M.D. Professor of Pediatrics, University of New York at Buffalo; Director, Clinical Research Center and Division of Allergy, Children's Hospital, Buffalo, New York

ERNEST CARROLL FAUST, Ph.D. Emeritus Professor of Parasitology, Tulane University School of Public Health and Tropical Medicine, New Orleans, Louisiana

HARRY A. FELDMAN, M.D. Professor and Chairman, Department of Preventive Medicine, State University of New York, Upstate Medical Center, Syracuse; Attending Physician, State University and Silverman Hospitals, Consultant, Syracuse V. A. and Syracuse Psychiatric Hospital, Syracuse, and Chenango Memorial Hospital, Norwich, New York

MARC A. FORMAN, M.D. Associate Professor of Psychiatry (Child Psychiatry) and Associate Professor in Pediatrics, Temple University School of Medicine; Medical Director, Child Psychiatry Center at St. Christopher's Hospital for Children, Philadelphia, Pennsylvania

F. CLARKE FRASER, Ph.D., M.D., C.M., D.Sc. (Acadia), F.R.S.C. Professor of Human Genetics, McGill University; Director of Department of Medical Genetics, Montreal Children's Hospital, Montreal, Canada

VINCENT A. FULGINITI, M.D. Professor and Head, Department of Pediatrics, University of Arizona; Chief of Pediatrics, University Hospital, Medical Staff Tucson Medical Center, Pima County General Hospital, Tucson, Arizona

LYTT I. GARDNER, M.D. Professor of Pediatrics, State University of New York, Upstate Medical Center at Syracuse; Attending Pediatrician, State University Hospital, Syracuse, New York

SYDNEY S. GELLIS, M.D. Professor and Chairman, Department of Pediatrics, Tufts University School of Medicine, Pediatrician-in-Chief, Boston Floating Hospital for Infants and Children (New England Medical Center Hospital), Boston, Massachusetts

ELI GOLD, M.D. Professor and Chairman, Department of Pediatrics, University of California at Davis, Director of Pediatrics, Sacramento Medical Center, Sacramento, California

ARMOND S. GOLDMAN, M.D. Professor, Department of Pediatrics, Shriners Burns Institute, The University of Texas Medical Branch, Galveston, Texas

SHIRLEY A. GRAVES, M.D. Assistant Professor of Anesthesiology and Pediatrics, University of Florida College of Medicine; Medical Director, Pediatric Intensive Care Unit, Shands Teaching Hospital, Gainesville, Florida

ROBERT J. HAGGERTY, M.D. Professor and Chairman, Department of Pediatrics, University of Rochester School of Medicine and Dentistry; Pediatrician-in-Chief, Strong Memorial Hospital, Rochester, New York

SCOTT BARKER HALSTEAD, M.D. Professor and Chairman, Department of Tropical Medicine and Medical Microbiology, University of Hawaii School of Medicine, Honolulu, Hawaii

ROBISON D. HARLEY, M.D., Ph.D. Professor and Chairman, Department of Ophthalmology, Temple University Health Science Center; Attending Surgeon, Wills Eye and St. Christopher's Hospitals for Children, Philadelphia, Pennsylvania

JEROME SYLVAN HARRIS, M.D. Professor of Pediatrics and Biochemistry, Duke University; Assistant Pediatrician, Duke Hospital, Durham, North Carolina

HAROLD EDWARD HARRISON, M.D. Professor of Pediatrics, Johns Hopkins University School of Medicine; Chief of Pediatrics, Baltimore City Hospital and Pediatrician, Johns Hopkins Hospital, Baltimore, Maryland

WILLIAM H. HETZNECKER, M.D. Associate Professor of Psychiatry and Pediatrics, Temple University School of Medicine; Staff Psychiatrist, Chief Psychiatry Center at St. Christopher's Hospital for Children, Philadelphia, Pennsylvania

ROBERT H. HIGH, M.D. Clinical Professor of Pediatrics, University of Michigan Medical School, Ann Arbor; Former Chairman, Department of Pediatrics, Henry Ford Hospital, Detroit, Michigan

PAUL H. HOLINGER, M.D. Professor of Bronchoesophagology, Department of Otolaryngology, University of Illinois College of Medicine; Attending Bronchoesophagologist and Laryngologist, Children's Memorial Hospital, University of Illinois Research and Education Hospital, Illinois Eye and Ear Infirmary, Chicago, Illinois

PHILIP G. HOLTZAPPLE, M.D. Assistant Professor of Pediatrics and Medicine, University of Pennsylvania School of Medicine; Chief, Gastroenterology Section, Children's Hospital of Philadelphia, Philadelphia, Pennsylvania

PETER R. HUTTENLOCHER, M.D. Professor of Pediatrics (Neurology), University of Chicago; Attending Physician, Wyler Childrens' Hospital, Chicago, Illinois

JOHN B. ISOM, M.D. Professor of Pediatrics and Associate Professor of Neurology, University of Oregon Medical School; Pediatric Neurologist, University of Oregon Medical School Hospital, Portland, Oregon

CHARLES ALDERSON JANEWAY, M.D., A.M. (hon), M.D. (hon.), Dr. (hon.) Thomas Morgan Rotch Professor of Pediatrics, Harvard Medical School; Physician-in-Chief Emeritus and Senior Associate in Medicine and Immunology, Children's Hospital Medical Center, Boston, Massachusetts

MARY JANE JESSE, M.D. Berenson Professor of Pediatric Cardiology, University of Miami School of Medicine; Director, Pediatric Cardiology, University of Miami Medical Center, Miami, Florida

SAMUEL KAPLAN, M.D. Professor of Pediatrics and Associate Professor of Medicine, The University of Cincinnati College of Medicine; Director, Division of Cardiology, Children's Hospital, Cincinnati, Ohio

ROBERT KAYE, M.D. Professor and Chairman, Department of Pediatrics, Hahnemann Medical School College; Pediatrician-in-Chief, Hahnemann Hospital, Philadelphia, Pennsylvania

C. HENRY KEMPE, M.D. Professor of Pediatrics, University of Colorado School of Medicine; Attending Pediatrician, Colorado General Hospital, Denver, Colorado

JOHN A. KIRKPATRICK, JR., M.D. Professor of Radiology, Harvard Medical School; Radiologist-in-Chief, Children's Hospital Medical Center, Boston, Massachusetts

ROBERT A. KRAMER, M.D. Professor of Pediatrics and Director, Division of Child and Adolescent Behavior, University of Connecticut School of Medicine; Chief of Pediatrics, Mount Sinai Hospital, Hartford, Connecticut

JOHN W. LACHMAN, M.D. Professor of Orthopedic Surgery, Temple University School of Medicine; Chairman of Orthopedics Temple University Hospital, Attending Surgeon, St. Christopher's Hospital for Children, Assistant Chief Surgeon, Shriners' Hospital for Crippled Children, Philadelphia, Pennsylvania

WILLIAM E. LAUPUS, M.D. Professor and Chairman, Department of Pediatrics, Medical College of Virginia Sciences Division of the Virginia Commonwealth University; Pediatrician-in-Chief, Medical College of Virginia Hospital, Richmond, Virginia

HEROLD LILLYWHITE, Ph.D. Professor Emeritus of Speech Pathology, Department of Pediatrics University of Oregon Medical School, Portland, Oregon

JENNIFER M. H. LOGGIE, M.B., B.Ch. Associate Professor of Pediatrics and Pharmacology, University of Cincinnati School of Medicine; Attending Pediatrician, Children's Hospital Medical Center, Cincinnati, Ohio

C. CHARLTON MABRY, M.D. Professor of Pediatrics, Department of Pediatrics, University of Kentucky Medical Center, College of Medicine; Attending Pediatrician, University Hospital, Lexington, Kentucky

GEORGE H. MCCRACKEN, JR., M.D. Associate Professor of Pediatrics, University of Texas Southwestern Medical School; Attending Physician, Parkland Memorial Hospital and Children's Medical Center, Dallas, Texas

R. JAMES MCKAY, M.D. Professor and Chairman, Department of Pediatrics, University of Vermont College of Medicine; Chief of Pediatric Service, Medical Center Hospital of Vermont

ALBERT MILLER, Ph.D. Associate Professor of Medical Entomology, Tulane University School of Public Health and Tropical Medicine, New Orleans, Louisiana

ROBERT W. MILLER, M.D. Clinical Professor of Pediatrics, Georgetown University School of Medicine, Washington, D.C.; Chief, Epidemiology Branch, National Cancer Institute, Bethesda, Maryland

MANDAYAM J. NARISIMHAN, JR., M.D. Ph.D. Scientist, University of Minnesota School of Medicine, Minneapolis, Minnesota

JOHN D. NELSON, M.D. Professor of Pediatrics, University of Texas, Southwestern Medical School; Attending Physician, Children's Medical Center, Senior Attending Physician, Parkland Memorial Hospital, Dallas, Texas

CHARLES M. NORRIS, M.D., F.A.C.S. Professor and Chairman of Department of Laryngology and Broncho-esophagology (Chevalier Jackson Clinic), Temple University School of Medicine; Chief, Chevalier Jackson Clinic, Temple University Hospital and Consultant in Otolaryngology, Lankenau Hospital, Philadelphia, Pennsylvania

RICHARD W. OLMSTED, M.D. Formerly Professor and Chairman, Department of Pediatrics, University of Oregon Medical School, Portland, Oregon; Associate Executive Director, American Academy of Pediatrics, Evanston, Illinois

DEMOSTHENES PAPPAGIANIS, M.D., Ph.D. Professor and Chairman, Department of Medical Microbiology, School of Medicine of the University of California, Davis, California

FREDERICK M. PARKINS, D.D.S., M.S.D., Ph.D. Professor and Head, Department of Pedodontics, College of Dentistry, University of Iowa, Iowa City, Iowa

HOWARD A. PEARSON, M.D. Professor and Chairman, Department of Pediatrics, Yale University School of Medicine; Attending Pediatrician, Yale-New Haven Hospital, New Haven, Connecticut

CAROL FENTON PHILLIPS, M.D. Associate Professor of Pediatrics at University of Vermont College of Medicine; Associate Attending Pediatrician, Medical Center Hospital of Vermont, Burlington, Vermont

LAWRENCE K. PICKETT, M.D. Professor of Surgery and Pediatrics and Associate Dean, Clinical Affairs, Yale University School of Medicine; Attending Surgeon, Yale-New Haven Hospital, New Haven, Connecticut

STANLEY A. PLOTKIN, M.D. Professor, Department of Pediatrics, University of Pennsylvania School of Medicine; Member, The Wistar Institute, and Director, Infectious Disease Service, Children's Hospital of Philadelphia, Philadelphia, Pennsylvania

V. BALAGOPAL RAJU, M.D. Professor of Pediatrics, Madras Medical College, Madras; Director and Superintendent, Institute of Child Health and Hospital for Children, Egmore, Madras, India

RUSSELL C. RAPHAELY, M.D. Assistant Professor of Anesthesia, University of Pennsylvania School of Medicine; Director, Pediatric Intensive Care Unit, Children's Hospital of Philadelphia, Philadelphia, Pennsylvania

FREDERICK C. ROBBINS, M.D. Professor of Pediatrics and Dean, Case Western Reserve University School of Medicine; Associate Pediatrician, University Hospital, and Pediatrician, Cleveland Metropolitan General Hospital, Cleveland, Ohio

ALAN M. ROBSON, M.D., M.R.C.P. Associate Professor of Pediatrics, Washington University School of Medicine; Associate Pediatrician, St. Louis Children's Hospital, St. Louis, Missouri

JOHN H. SEASHORE, M.D. Assistant Professor of Surgery and Pediatrics, Yale University School of Medicine; Attending Pediatric Surgeon, Yale-New Haven Hospital, New Haven, Connecticut

JANE GREEN SCHALLER, M.D. Associate Professor, Department of Pediatrics, University of Washington School of Medicine, Seattle; Attending Pediatrician, University Hospital (Director, Pediatric Arthritis Clinic, Attending Pediatrician, Immunology Clinic); Attending Pediatrician, Children's Orthopedic Hospital (Director, Rheumatoid Arthritis Clinic), Attending Physician, Arthritis Clinic (Department of Medicine), University Hospital, and Attending Physician, Harborview Medical Center, Seattle, Washington

BARTON D. SCHMITT, M.D. Assistant Professor of Pediatrics, University of Colorado Medical Center; Pediatric Consultant, National Center for the Prevention and Treatment of Child Abuse and Neglect, and Attending Pediatrician, Denver General and Children's Hospitals, Denver, Colorado

SARAH H. W. SELL, M.D. Associate Professor of Pediatrics, Vanderbilt University School of Medicine; Visiting Physician, Vanderbilt University Hospital and Consultant in Infectious Diseases, St. Thomas, Baptist, and Metropolitan General Hospitals, Nashville, Tennessee

CALVIN F. SETTLAGE, M.D., M.S. Director of Child Psychiatry, Staff Psychiatrist and Associate Chief, Department of Psychiatry, Mt. Zion Hospital and Medical Center; San Francisco, California

HARRY C. SHIRKEY, M.D. Professor and Chairman, Department of Pediatrics, Tulane University School of Medicine; Senior Visiting Physician and Director, Tulane Pediatric Service, The Charity Hospital of Louisiana, New Orleans, Louisiana

OTTO F. SIEBER, JR., M.D. Assistant Professor, Department of Pediatrics, University of Arizona; Head, Infectious Disease Section, University Hospital and Medical Staff, Tucson Medical Center and Pima County General Hospital, Tucson, Arizona

DAVID H. SMITH, M.D. Associate Professor, Department of Pediatrics, Harvard Medical School; Chief, Division of Infectious Diseases, Children's Hospital Medical Center, Boston, Massachusetts

DAVID W. SMITH, M.D. Professor of Pediatrics, University of Washington School of Medicine, Seattle, Washington

ALEX J. STEIGMAN M.D. D.Sc.(hon.) Professor of Pediatrics, Mt. Sinai School of Medicine; Attending Pediatrician, Mt. Sinai Hospital, New York, New York

ROBERT J. TOULOUKIAN, M.D. Associate Professor of Surgery and Pediatrics, Yale-New Haven Hospital, New Haven, Connecticut

IRENE A. UCHIDA, Ph.D. Professor of Pediatrics (Genetics), McMaster University; Director, Regional Cytogenetics Laboratory McMaster University Medical Centre, Hamilton, Ontario, Canada

P. M. UDANI, M.D., D.C.H., F.A.M.S.(hon.), F.A.A.P. (USA) Director and Professor, Institute of Child

Health, J. J. Group of Hospitals, and Grant Medical College, Byculla, Bombay; Visiting Pediatrician, Institute of Child Health, J. J. Group of Hospitals, Grant Medical College and Bombay Hospital, Bombay, India

MARIE A. VALDES-DAPENA Professor of Pathology and Professor in Pediatrics, Temple University School of Medicine; Associate Pathologist, St. Christopher's Hospital for Children, and Consultant in Pediatric Pathology, Lankenau Hospital and Philadelphia Naval Hospital, Philadelphia, Pennsylvania

VICTOR C. VAUGHAN, III, M.D. Professor and Chairman, Department of Pediatrics, Temple University School of Medicine; Medical Director, St. Christopher's Hospital for Children, Philadelphia, Pennsylvania

LEWIS W. WANNAMAKER, M.D. Professor of Pediatrics and Microbiology, University of Minnesota; Consultant, St. Paul Children's Hospital, and Career Investigator, American Heart Association and University Hospitals, Minneapolis, Minnesota

JOSEF WARKANY, M.D. Professor of Research Pediatrics Emeritus, University of Cincinnati Medical College; Fellow, Children's Hospital Research Foundation, and Director of Mental Retardation Research, Institute for Developmental Research, Cincinnati, Ohio

RALPH J. WEDGWOOD, M.D. Professor, Department of Pediatrics, University of Washington School of Medicine; Attending Physician, Children's Orthopedic Hospital and Medical Center, Harborview Medical Center, and University Hospital, Co-Director, Pediatric Arthritis Clinics, University Hospital and Children's Orthopedic Hospital and Medical Center, Associate Chief, Pediatric Services, University Hospital and Children's Hospital and Medical Center, Seattle, Washington

WARREN E. WHEELER, M.D. Professor of Pediatrics Emeritus, University of Kentucky College of Medicine; Senior Pediatrician, University Hospital, Lexington, Kentucky

PREFACE

Thirty-four years ago the editorship of the Textbook of Pediatrics, which had been earlier edited by Griffith and Mitchell, was assumed as an obligation of friendship by Waldo E. Nelson after the death of A. Graeme Mitchell. The Fourth and subsequent editions, first as "Mitchell-Nelson" and then as "Nelson," have thrived, with the indispensable help of a host of contributors and under the gifted leadership and editorial direction of Dr. Nelson.

It is with some trepidation and a sense of somewhat awesome responsibility that we have taken on the job of editing the Tenth edition of the Nelson Textbook of Pediatrics. As contributors since the Sixth (VCV) and Seventh (RJM) editions we have been taught and had our writing and editorial skills sharpened by a master of the art, in whose tradition of excellence we hope to follow; we cannot expect to equal Dr. Nelson's incredible capacity for sustained hard work devoted to "the book." We can appreciate and are thankful for the fact that the editorial burden is shared between us.

Unlike the Fourth (Dr. Nelson's first) edition, which was published 30 years ago, this Tenth edition is not a "new" book. It has, however, been extensively revised and is as close to current knowledge and practice as we have been able to achieve. It is larger than the last edition, in response to the continued rapid expansion of pediatric knowledge; we have attempted to balance the needs to keep this edition both comprehensive and not unwieldy in size.

With Dr. Nelson, we subscribe to the idea of a book that will meet the needs both of medical students and of practicing physicians. In addition, we hope that it may be of use to nurses and to pediatric nurse practitioners, to child health associates, to family physicians' assistants and other "new" health professionals who now participate in the delivery of health care to children.

We have lost three contributors through death since the last edition. They are Joseph B. Bilderback, M.D., Howard W. Robinson, Ph.D., and Stanley W. Wright, M.D. We should like to record our indebtedness to these men for their help with previous editions.

We would like to thank our contributors not only for their help but for their forbearance at what must have, at times, seemed ruthless editing. The job could not have been accomplished without the patience and support, both direct and indirect, of Deborah Vaughan and Elizabeth McKay and of the members of the Departments of Pediatrics of Temple University and of the University of Vermont. Particular thanks must go to Mrs. Billie Brick of the editorial staff of W. B. Saunders Company; to Mrs. Marion Canedy, and Doctors Stephen V. Cantrill, Joseph D. Dickerman, and Carol F. Phillips of the University of Vermont; and to Mrs. Michiko Claflin and Doctors Mary L. Coté, Harold W. Lischner, and Myles G. Turtz of Temple University and St. Christopher's Hospital for Children. A host of others have contributed in countless ways to making the task both easier and more rewarding.

Finally we must acknowledge our very special debt to Dr. Waldo E. Nelson, who calls himself and is known affectionately as "the old man." He has continued as our mentor, model and guide, and has participated energetically in the preparation of this Tenth edition. Where the editorial touch has special merit, the achievement is likely his, one way or another.

VICTOR C. VAUGHAN III, M.D.
R. JAMES MCKAY

CONTENTS

9. THE IMMUNOLOGIC SYSTEM, ALLERGY AND RELATED DISEASES

10. INFECTIOUS DISEASES

12. THE RESPIRATORY SYSTEM

14. DISEASES OF THE BLOOD

23. THE SKIN

24. PEDIATRIC OPHTHALMOLOGY

25. NEOPLASMS AND NEOPLASTIC-LIKE LESIONS

26. UNCLASSIFIED DISEASES

27. RADIATION INJURY

28. POISONING FROM FOOD, CHEMICALS, DRUGS AND METALS

29. MORPHOLOGIC SYNDROMES

30. APPENDIX

1
THE FIELD OF PEDIATRICS

Pediatrics differs from most other medical specialties in that it is not oriented to an organ system, to a category of diseases, to a biologic process, or to a method or system of care, but rather toward the comprehensive and continuing health care of the people it serves. Most of those who choose the field of pediatrics do so because they like children and they enjoy working with children and their parents to help them to achieve their maximum potential as individuals and as families. The scientific and special interests of pediatric investigators and subspecialists may closely resemble the traditional orientations of other medical specialists, but are still secondary to a love of children shared by all pediatricians.

The broad mandate and developmental orientation of pediatricians have given them a community of interests and goals and a fellowship which other physicians tend to find both baffling and admirable. Because pediatricians have these characteristics, pediatrics has since its inception been identified as being in the vanguard of social concern in the medical profession, the future of any society being inextricably bound to the welfare of its children.

History of Pediatrics

Historically, pediatrics became differentiated as a medical specialty about a century ago in response to a growing appreciation and acceptance that the problems of children are different in kind from those of adults and that the prevalence of those problems varies with age, as does the child's reaction to them. From the beginning there has been a continual revision of the focus and scope of the field of pediatrics.

The health and the health problems of children vary widely among the nations of the earth, in accordance with a variety of factors, which include: (1) the prevalence and ecology of infectious agents and their hosts, (2) climate and geography, (3) agricultural resources and practices, (4) educational and economic and sociocultural considerations, and (5) in many instances, the gene frequencies for some disorders. These factors are often interrelated; for example, the frequency of the gene for sickle cell hemoglobin may reflect the historic impact of the prevalence of the malarial parasite in many areas, this prevalence being dependent in turn upon the climatic and geographic considerations favoring the growth of certain mosquitos.

Not only do problems differ in certain parts of the world, but priorities also, since they must reflect local concerns, resources and needs. The assessment of the state of health of any community must begin with epidemiologic and other studies which describe the prevalence of illness and must continue with studies which show the changes that occur with time and in response to programs of prevention, case finding, therapy and adequate surveillance. As contemporary problems in any community have yielded to study and to improved management, new problems are recognized, or arise de novo, to attract the attention and efforts of pediatric clinicians and research workers. Accordingly, with time, there may be major changes in the relative importance of the various causes of childhood morbidity and mortality.

In the late 19th century in the United States, of every 1000 children born alive as many as 200 might be expected to die before the age of 1 year of such conditions as dysentery, pneumonia, measles, diphtheria, whooping cough, and the like. Efforts of the pioneers among microbiologists and immunologists helped to change this expectation.

The early and continuing efforts of the young specialty of pediatrics, combined with those of the early immunologists and pioneers in public health have led to such better understanding of the origin and management of many problems of infants that in the past half century the infant mortality in the United States has fallen to the point where in 1970 it was at 20.01 deaths per 1000 live births. The data from which Figure 1–1 was constructed indicate that of all deaths of infants under 1 year of age three quarters now occur within the first 28 days of life, 90 per cent of these within the first 7 days of life, and that more than one half of those within the first 7 days occur within the first day (35 per cent of all deaths in the first year of life). The distribution of ages of infants at the time of death in earlier years was vastly different, and the growing science and subspecialty of neonatology responds to this change. Early in the 20th century the efforts of those who contributed to the control of infectious disease began to be complemented by those of nutritionists. New and continuing discoveries were translated into effective practice by those with an interest in public health who set up the earliest well-child clinics. Acute infections and the chronic disturbances associated with deficits of calories, vitamins, minerals or proteins were studied intensively, and the acute nutritional and metabolic disturbances such as the disorders of fluid and electrolyte balance which accompany acute diarrhea also received attention. The growing understanding of infant nutrition led to the evolution of a scientific basis for infant feeding, and for a period of time, in applying it, to a degree of rigidity and artificiality now seen to be excessive.

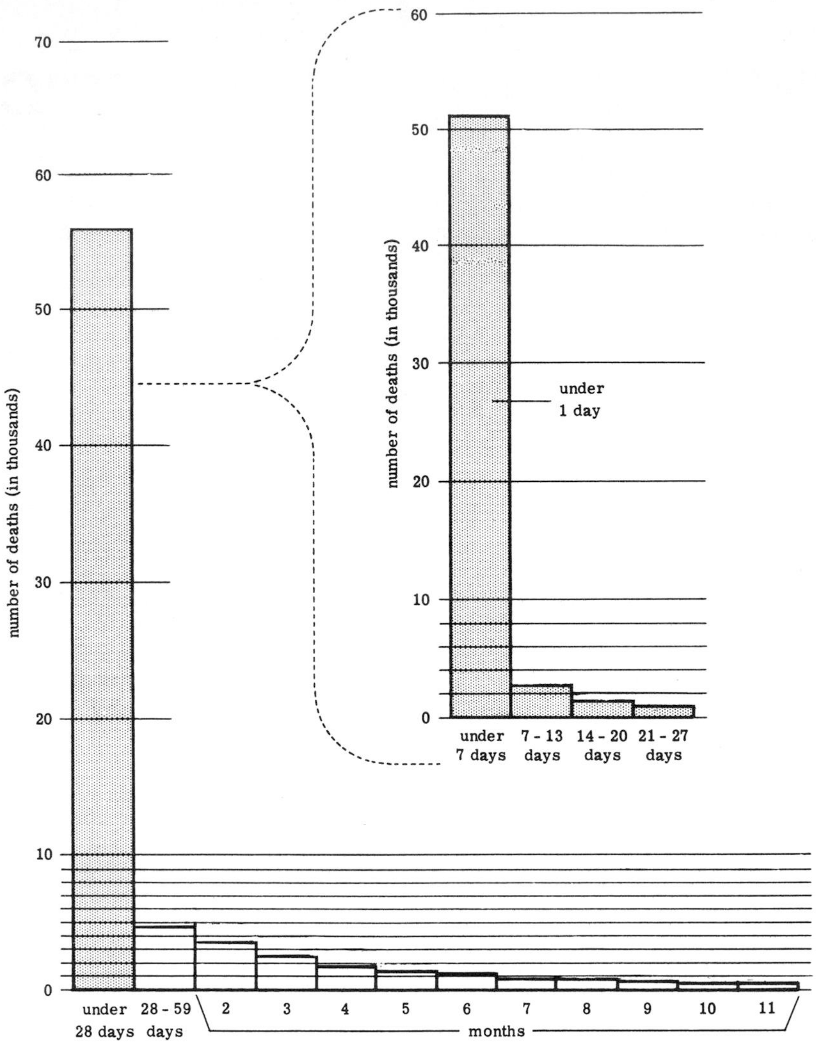

Figure 1-1 Infant mortality by age, United States, 1970. (United States Department of Health, Education, and Welfare, Social and Rehabilitation Service, Children's Bureau. Data from United States Public Health Service, National Center for Health Statistics.)

In the middle years of the 20th century, a profound revolution in child health was brought about by the introduction of antibacterial chemicals and antibiotic agents. With improved control of infectious disease through both prevention and treatment, and with other concurrent scientific and technical advances, pediatric medicine turned its attention to the conditions affecting relatively small numbers of children. These included both lethal conditions, such as leukemia and cystic fibrosis, and temporarily or permanently handicapping conditions, such as congenital heart disease, mental retardation, genetic defects, rheumatic diseases, renal diseases and metabolic and endocrine disorders.

Changing Mortality and Morbidity

Tables 1-1 and 1-2 show how problems of older children have changed in the United States over a half century; the implications for priorities are evident. These tables list the 10 leading causes of death for children aged 1 to 4 years and 5 to 14 years of age for each 10th year from 1920 to 1970. Table 1-1 shows that the mortality of children 1 to 4 years old in 1970 from all causes was less than that from either enteritis, lower respiratory disease, or diphtheria in 1920, and less in 1970 than the sum of the mortalities in 1920 of any pair among measles, whooping cough or tuberculosis. The record with respect to accidents has improved in both age groups, except that motor vehicle accidents remain close to early levels, while accidents as a whole have moved from fourth place to first among the causes of death and in 1970 amounted to more than a third of deaths in the younger age group and (with homicide) to more than half of all deaths in children 5 to 14 years of age. In neither age group do the next nine causes of death contain clearly preventable conditions, ex-

TABLE 1-1. MAIN CAUSES OF DEATH AMONG CHILDREN 1–4 YEARS OF AGE: UNITED STATES, 1970 AND SPECIFIED YEARS

CAUSE OF DEATH*	EIGHTH REVISION CATEGORY NUMBERS IN USE 1968 TO DATE	YEAR 1970	1965	1960	1950	1940	1930	1920	SIXTH AND SEVENTH REVISION CATEGORY NUMBERS IN USE 1949–67	COMPARABILITY RATIO†
		Rate per 100,000 children 1–4 years								
All causes	000–E999	84.5	92.9	108.8	139.4	289.6	563.6	987.2	001–E999	1.000
Main causes		64.4	72.3	83.5	98.0	198.4	409.7	794.4		— — —
Accidents	E800–E949	31.5	31.8	31.5	36.8	48.7	61.2	80.2	E800–E962	0.957
Accidents, except motor vehicles	E800–E807, E825–E949	20.0	21.3	21.5	25.3	36.3	46.7	71.1	E800–E802, E840–E962	0.925
Motor vehicle accidents	E810–E823	11.5	10.5	10.0	11.5	12.4	14.5	—	E810–E835	0.992
Congenital anomalies	740–759	9.7	10.2	12.8	11.1	10.3	—	—	750–759	1.020
Influenza and pneumonia	470–474, 480–486	7.6	11.4	16.2	18.9	62.5	123.1	283.7	480–483, 490–493, 763	0.993
Malignant neoplasms, including neoplasms of lymphatic and hematopoietic tissues	140–209	7.5	8.6	10.8	11.7	—	—	—	140–205	1.002
Symptoms and ill defined conditions	780–796	2.1	2.4	2.8	—	—	—	—	780–795	0.994
Meningitis	320	1.9	2.6	2.8	2.8	—	—	—	340	0.959‡
Acute respiratory infections, including acute bronchitis (except influenza)	460–466	1.7	—	—	—	8.9	15.2	12.3	470–475, 500	— — —
Enteritis and other diarrheal diseases	008, 009	1.4	2.3‡	3.2§	— — —	30.2	95.6	141.3	571, 764	1.185‡
Meningococcal infections	036	1.0	1.8	1.4	2.6	—	—	—	057	— — —
Gastritis, duodenitis, diverticula of intestine, chronic enteritis and ulcerative colitis	535, 562, 563	—	0.1	0.1	— — —	—	—	—	543, 572	— — —
Bronchitis	490, 491	—	1.1	2.1	2.5	—	—	—	501, 502	1.062
Measles	055	—	—	—	—	—	21.9	56.4	085	— — —
Tuberculosis, all forms	010–019	—	—	—	6.3	12.3	25.9	45.4	001–019	0.950‡
Whooping cough	033	—	—	—	—	9.7	23.4	57.7	056	— — —
Diphtheria	032	—	—	—	—	9.0	33.5	90.5	055	— — —
Appendicitis	540–543	—	—	—	—	6.8	—	—	550–553	— — —
Streptococcal sore throat and scarlet fever	034	—	—	—	—	—	9.9	23.2	050, 051	— — —
Dysentery	004, 006, 007	—	—	—	—	—	—	12.8	045–048	— — —
All other causes	Residual	20.1	20.6	25.3	41.4	91.2	153.9	192.8	Residual	— — —

*Causes of death listed each year are the 10 main causes in that year. For 1970, titles of the causes listed, and inclusions in each cause group, are those of the Eighth Revision, International Classification of Diseases; for 1960 and 1965, inclusions are those of the Seventh Revision; for 1950 and 1955, inclusions are those of the Sixth Revision; for 1940, inclusions are according to the Fifth Revision; for 1930, according to the Fourth Revision; and for 1920, according to the Second Revision. Rates are unadjusted for changes in the classification of causes of death in successive revisions of the lists. In 1950 and later years, "Diarrhea of the newborn" was included in Enteritis and other diarrheal diseases (ICDA Nos. 008, 009). Based on data from the National Center for Health Statistics, Public Health Service, Department of Health, Education, and Welfare.

Symbol: —Class or item not applicable.
— — —Class or item not available.

†Ratio of estimated total deaths assigned according to the Eighth Revision to total deaths assigned according to the Seventh Revision. Ratios by age are not available.

‡These ratios may be slightly underestimated because of the method of computation.

§These figures revised to correspond to the category numbers shown for the Sixth and Seventh Revisions.

TABLE 1–2 MAIN CAUSES OF DEATH AMONG CHILDREN 5–14 YEARS OF AGE: UNITED STATES, 1970 AND SPECIFIED YEARS

CAUSE OF DEATH*	EIGHTH REVISION CATEGORY NUMBERS IN USE 1968 TO DATE	YEAR 1970	1965	1960	1950	1940	1930	1920	SIXTH AND SEVENTH REVISION CATEGORY NUMBERS IN USE 1949–67	COMPARABILITY RATIO†
		Rate per 100,000 children 5–14 years								
All causes	000–E999	41.3	42.2	46.6	59.8	103.7	171.7	263.9	001–E999	1.000
Main causes		33.2	32.8	35.9	44.7	67.6	111.8	196.3		– – –
Accidents	E800–E949	20.1	18.7	19.2	22.6	28.6	36.1	44.3	E800–E962	0.957
Motor vehicle accidents	E810–E823	10.2	8.9	7.9	8.8	11.5	14.7	13.0	E810–E835	0.992
Accidents, except motor vehicle	E800–E807, E825–E949	9.9	9.8	11.3	13.8	17.1	21.4	31.3	E800–E802, E840–E962	0.925
Malignant neoplasms, including neoplasms of lymphatic and hematopoietic tissues	140–209	6.0	6.5	6.8	6.7	3.0	–	–	140–205	1.002
Congenital anomalies	740–759	2.2	2.8	3.6	2.4	2.1	–	–	750–759	1.020
Influenza and pneumonia	470–474, 480–486	1.6	2.1	2.6	3.2	9.0	18.8	45.1	480–483, 490–493, 763	0.993
Homicide	E960–E978	0.9	0.6	–	–	–	–	–	E964, E980–E985	0.997
Diseases of the heart	390–398, 402, 404, 410–429	0.8	0.4	1.3	3.9	10.6	15.1	21.8	400–402, 410–443	1.004
Cerebrovascular diseases	430–438	0.7	0.7	0.7	–	–	–	–	330–334	0.990
Symptoms and ill defined conditions	780–796	0.5	–	0.5	0.8	–	–	–	780–795	0.994‡
Benign neoplasms and neoplasms of unspecified nature	210–239	0.4	0.6	0.7	0.8	–	–	–	210–239	0.968‡
Anemias	280–285	–	0.4	0.5	–	–	–	–	290–293	0.944‡
Acute poliomyelitis	040–043	–	–	–	2.5	–	–	–	080	– – –
Appendicitis	540–543	–	–	–	–	0.8	13.1	–	550–553	– – –
Tuberculosis, all forms	010–019	–	–	–	1.8	5.5	11.9	22.4	001–019	0.950‡
Nephritis and nephrosis	580–584	–	–	–	–	1.7	–	3.5	590–594	0.886
Diphtheria	032	–	–	–	–	1.7	8.1	28.0	055	– – –
Typhoid fever	001	–	–	–	–	–	4.4	7.1	040	– – –
Meningococcal infections	036	–	–	–	–	–	4.3	–	057	– – –
Enteritis and other diarrheal diseases	008, 009	–	–	–	–	–	3.0	4.1	571, 764	1.185‡
Diabetes mellitus	250	–	–	–	–	–	–	3.5	260	0.997
All other causes	Residual	8.1	9.4	10.7	15.1	36.1	59.9	67.6	Residual	– – –

*Causes of death listed each year are the 10 main causes in that year. For 1970, titles of the causes listed, and inclusions in each cause group, are those of the Eighth Revision of the International Classification of Diseases; for 1960 and 1965, inclusions are those of the Seventh Revision; for 1950 and 1955, inclusions are those of the Sixth Revision; for 1940, inclusions are according to the Fifth Revision; for 1930, according to the Fourth Revision; and for 1920, according to the Second Revision. Rates are unadjusted for changes in the classification of causes of death in successive revisions of the lists, but the category "Diseases of the heart" was adjusted to include rheumatic fever for each year specified. Based on data from the National Center for Health Statistics, Public Health Service, Department of Health, Education and Welfare.

Symbol – Class or item not applicable.

– – – Class or item not available.

†Ratio of estimated total deaths assigned according to the Eighth Revision to total deaths assigned according to the Seventh Revision. Ratios by age are not available.

‡These ratios may be slightly underestimated because of the method of computation.

cept that influenza and pneumonia and meningitis might be so construed if their occurrence could be anticipated in the individual instance.

The data of Table 1-2 not only reflect the general improvement in health of children 5 to 14 years of age in half a century, but show that specific diseases once highly prevalent (tuberculosis, diphtheria, typhoid fever) have disappeared from among the leading causes of death, that others have appeared (benign or malignant neoplasms, cerebral vascular diseases and, rather recently, homicide), and that poliomyelitis was only once among the 10 leading causes of death (in 1950).

These tables further reflect (see their footnotes) the difficulties in interpretation of comparable statistics over extended periods of time. Criteria for diagnoses change with growing knowledge and sophistication, and changes in diagnostic categories render comparison difficult between successive revisions of the official International Classification of Diseases (ICD). The National Center for Health Statistics, which produced these tables, has calculated "comparability ratios" for the changes in diagnostic categories which took place between the Seventh (1960) and Eighth (1968) Revisions of the ICD.

Changes may occur relatively rapidly. Tables 1-3 and 1-4 record the changes in 10 leading categories of disease causing mortality within the first year of life between the years 1965 and 1970, in terms both of numbers of infants (Table 1-3) and infant mortality rates (Table 1-4). The importance of changes in designation of diagnostic categories is again evident, the most relevant figures being those given for the "adjusted percentage change." Table 1-5 gives similar data for changes in the causes of death between 1965 and 1970 for older children.

Death rates and mortality figures give only a partial view of the health problems of children. Tables 1-6 and 1-7 show how hospitals are used for children, the most common admission by far in 1967 being for "hypertrophied tonsils and adenoids," Table 1-7 indicating that virtually all such children were managed by removal of tonsils, usually no doubt with adenoids as well. In view of the controversy which surrounds this procedure, these figures must stand as testimony to the inertia with which the health system confronts a need to re-examine precepts perhaps honored only with time or tradition.

It is relatively easy to count the numbers of infants born, deaths, admissions to hospitals, surgical procedures, numbers of immunizations, occurrences of certain reportable diseases, and the like (though the reporting of preventable diseases is far from complete). It is more difficult to assess such essential features of the health of the community as its nutritional status, or the prevalence of emotional, behavioral, family or social problems which the pediatrician may have the opportunity to prevent, to anticipate or to manage through his own efforts or in cooperation with others. The National Center for Health Statistics has in the past decade mounted a number of studies aimed at assessing the prevalence of certain problems in substantial samples of children and of adults in the United States. Attention has been given to nutritional problems and needs, to physical growth and development, to the prevalence of such potentially handicapping conditions as visual or auditory impairment, and to the dental health of children. Surveys have also touched on the intellectual development of children, their levels of school achievement, and the prevalence of behavioral disorders. Some investigations have been carried out as yet only in restricted age groups; further studies are planned. The effect of these studies and others like them is to help the nation to identify its needs, and ultimately to set appropriate priorities for meeting them.

Planning a System of Care

In an era when both health care and the research capable of improving it have become increasingly expensive it is unlikely that the further evolution of a health system for children and their families will be as spontaneous or unregulated as it has been in the past. Pediatricians and others caring for children have a considerable opportunity and a heavy responsibility to see that the needs of children are given appropriate weight in whatever planning is to take place.

In this context, the physician caring for children has become increasingly involved with aspects of the health of children having to do with the *quality of the child's life.* A growing science of child development, nourished by new insights from developmental neurologists and psychologists and from psychoanalytic schools, has given us new ways of looking at the behavior problems of children and at normal growth and development as well. Pediatricians find themselves increasingly called upon to advise in the management of disturbances of behavior or of relationships between child and parent, child and school, or child and community; and pediatricians are increasingly concerned with problems having impact on broader aspects of mental and social and even societal health. There is, moreover, an increasing concern with disparities in how the benefits of what we know about child health reach various groups of children. In many developing countries the health of children lags far behind what it could be if the means and will to apply current knowledge could be brought to bear, and even in such an economically privileged country as the United States there are many children growing up under socioeconomically disadvantaged conditions which impair their health. Lead poisoning, for example, and iron deficiency are largely problems of the socioeconomically disadvantaged in the United States, and these medical problems are intimately related to problems of mental and social health. The children most at risk in American communities often belong to ethnic minority groups.

TABLE 1-3 LIST OF COMPARABLE CATEGORY NUMBERS FOR SELECTED CAUSES OF INFANT DEATHS ACCORDING TO THE EIGHTH AND SEVENTH REVISIONS, AND NUMBER OF DEATHS: UNITED STATES, 1965 AND 1970

LIST TITLE ACCORDING TO THE EIGHTH REVISION OF THE INTERNATIONAL CLASSIFICATION OF DISEASES, 1965	CATEGORY NUMBERS ACCORDING TO THE EIGHTH REVISION, 1965	CATEGORY NUMBERS ACCORDING TO THE SEVENTH REVISION, 1955	NUMBER OF DEATHS IN 1970	NUMBER OF DEATHS IN 1965
All causes	000–E999	001–E999	74,667	92,866
Certain gastrointestinal diseases	004, 006–009, 535, 561, 563	045–048, 543, 571, 572, 764	900	2,161
Influenza and pneumonia	470–474, 480–486	480–483, 490–493, 763	6,303	10,809
Congenital anomalies	740–759	750–759	11,259	13,443
Birth injuries	764–768 (.0–.3), 772	760, 761	2,395	7,018
Blood dyscrasias	774, 775, 778.2	770, 771	1,322	1,952
Asphyxia of newborn, unspecified	776.9	762	9,438	15,429
Immaturity unqualified	777	776	8,752	14,431
Other diseases of early infancy	Remainder of 760–778*	Remainder of 765–774	21,630	12,705
Accidents	E800–E949	E800–E962	2,294	3,316
Homicide	E960–E978	E964, E980–E985	150	213
All other external causes	E980–E999	– – –	126†	– – –
All other causes (residual)	By subtraction	By subtraction	10,458	11,409

*Assumes the value of 773 will be zero.

†A total of 93 of these 126 deaths was assigned to Injury by other and unspecified means, undetermined whether accidentally or purposely inflicted (ICDA No. E988). The recorded homicides (150 deaths) together with the deaths for which it was undetermined whether the injury was accidentally or purposely inflicted (126) gives a total of 276 deaths.

Figures 1–2 and 1–3, for example, show that the use of physician's health services is unevenly distributed among the children of the United States with respect to white or nonwhite ethnicity, urban or rural residence, financial income of the family and educational level of the head of the family. Figure 1–4 shows that these and other impairments to access by a disadvantaged group (nonwhite in this instance) to the benefits of modern health practices are reflected in continuing disparities in infant mortality between white and other groups of citizens. Pediatricians have a responsibility to address themselves aggressively to problems such as these.

Linked to the broader notion of health implicit in these views of the scope of pediatric concern is the concept that health and health services are a right of the individual, to be maintained in aspects ranging from the molecular to the social by the commitments and efforts of the community or society to which the individual belongs. The failure of health services and health benefits to reach all who need them has led to re-examination of the design of the health care system in many countries; but problems such as the maldistribution of physicians, institutional unresponsiveness to the perceived needs of the individual, and the failure of medical services to be adapted to the convenience of the patient remain unsolved in most systems. Efforts to make the delivery of health care more efficient and effective have led imaginative pediatricians into the creation of new categories of health care providers who can magnify and multiply the effectiveness of the individual physician. We may expect the pediatric nurse associate and other allied professional persons increasingly to find productive roles in the health care of children which supplement or complement the work of the pediatrician.

New insights into the needs of children have pointed the way toward reshaping the child care system in other ways. Growing understanding of the need of the infant for certain qualities of stimulation and care has led to restudy and revision of the care of the newborn infant and of procedures leading to adoption or to foster care. Institutions for handicapped children have also been reexamined, and it seems likely that the massive centralized institutions of past years will be replaced by community-centered arrangements offering a better opportunity for these children to achieve their maximal potential. The pediatrician has been involved in shaping these institutions and his insights and active contributions will continue to be needed.

Evaluation of Health Care

Akin to the growing concern with the design of the health care system for children, and with its ability to distribute the benefits of creative child health programs, is a more intense preoccupation with the *quality of health care,* and with how care of the highest quality can be made both efficient and effective. There is increasing public and political pressure for explicit, continuing evaluation of care in terms of what actually takes place rather than in terms of what modern medical knowledge has made possible. In this connection, two new developments deserve mention: these are the introduction of the problem-oriented system of keeping of health care records (see Section 5), and in the United States, the introduction of methods of as-

TABLE 1-4 INFANT MORTALITY RATES AND COMPARABILITY RATIOS* FOR SELECTED CAUSES OF INFANT DEATHS: UNITED STATES, 1965 AND 1970

CAUSE OF DEATH		DEATHS AT AGES UNDER 1 YEAR PER 100,000 LIVE BIRTHS		PER CENT CHANGE BETWEEN 1965 AND 1970	PROVISIONAL COMPARABILITY RATIO¶	95 PER CENT CONFIDENCE LIMITS‡		ADJUSTED PERCENTAGE CHANGE‡
		1970	1965			Upper	Lower	
All causes		2,001.1	2,469.6	−19.0	1.000	— — —	— — —	−19.0
Certain gastrointestinal diseases	004, 006–009, 535, 561, 563	24.1	57.5	−58.1	1.075	1.113	1.038	−61.0
Influenza and pneumonia	470–474, 480–486	168.9	287.4	−41.2	1.075	1.137	1.014	−45.3
Congenital anomalies	740–759	301.7	357.5	−15.6	1.036	1.073	1.000	−18.5
Birth injuries	764–768(.0–.3), 772	64.2	205.2	−68.7	0.330	0.391	0.269	− 5.2
Blood dyscrasias	774, 775, 778.2	35.4	51.9	−31.8	— — —	— — —	— — —	— — —
Asphyxia of newborn, unspecified	776.9	252.9	410.3	−38.4	0.871	0.893	0.849	−29.2
Immaturity unqualified	777	234.6	383.8	−38.9	0.868	0.912	0.824	−29.6
Other diseases of early infancy	Remainder of 760–778	579.7	337.9	+71.6	1.477‖	1.505‖	1.448‖	+16.2‖
Accidents	E800–E949	61.5	88.2	−30.3	— — —	— — —	— — —	— — —
Homicide	E960–E978	4.0	5.7	−29.8	— — —	— — —	— — —	— — —
All other external causes	E980–E999	3.4	— — —	— — —	— — —	— — —	— — —	— — —
All other causes	Residual	280.3	303.4	− 7.6	1.004	1.025	0.984	— — —

*The comparability ratios are based on a stratified random sample of 1966 infant deaths assigned according to the Eighth Revision and on all infant deaths in 1966 assigned according to the Seventh Revision of the International Classification of Diseases. Numbers after causes of death are category numbers of the Eighth Revision of the International Classification of Diseases.

†Ratio of deaths assigned according to the Eighth Revision to deaths assigned according to the Seventh Revision.

‡The probability is 95 per cent that the true comparability ratio will have a value between the upper and lower limits shown.

§Percentage change after adjusting 1965 rate to level it would have been if Eighth instead of Seventh Revision had been in use.

‖Based on a comparability ratio that included Blood dyscrasias (ICDA Nos. 774, 775, 778.2).

TABLE 1-5 DEATH RATES FOR CHILDREN 1–14 YEARS OF AGE FOR MAIN CAUSES: UNITED STATES, 1965 AND 1970*

CAUSE OF DEATH	DEATHS AT AGES 1–14 YEARS PER 100,000 POPULATION 1970	1965	PER CENT CHANGE BETWEEN 1965 AND 1970	PROVISIONAL COMPARABILITY RATIO†
All causes.....000–E999	52.2	57.2	− 8.7	1.00
Accidents, except motor vehicle.....E800–E807, E825–E949	12.4	13.2	− 6.1	0.925
Motor vehicle accidents.....E810–E823	10.5	9.4	+11.7	0.992
Malignant neoplasms.....140–209	6.4	7.1	− 9.9	1.002
Congenital anomalies.....740–759	4.1	5.0	−18.0	1.020
Influenza and pneumonia.....470–474, 480–486	3.1	4.8	−35.4	0.993
Diseases of the heart.....390–398, 402, 404, 410–429	1.1	1.0	+10.0	1.004
Meningitis.....320	0.7	1.0	−30.0	0.959‡
Symptoms and ill defined conditions.....780–796	0.9	1.0	−10.0	0.994‡
Enteritis and other diarrheal diseases.....008, 009	0.5	0.8	−37.5	1.185‡
Gastritis, duodenitis, diverticula of intestine, chronic enteritis and ulcerative colitis.....535, 562, 563	0.0	0.1	−100.0	— — —
Homicide.....E960–E978	1.1	0.8	+37.5	0.997
All other causes.....Residual	11.4	13.0	−12.3	— — —

*Numbers after causes of death are category numbers of the Eighth Revision of the International Classification of Diseases. Deaths for 1970 are classified according to the Eighth Revision of the International Classification of Diseases; and for 1965 are classified according to the Seventh Revision of the International Classification of Diseases.

†Ratio of estimated total deaths assigned according to the Eighth Revision to total deaths assigned according to the Seventh Revision. Ratios by ages are not available.

‡These ratios may be slightly underestimated because of the method of computation.

Data from the National Center for Health Statistics, United States Public Health Service, Department of Health, Education, and Welfare.

TABLE 1–6 NUMBER AND RATE OF DISCHARGES FROM HOSPITALS AND AVERAGE LENGTH OF STAY, FOR CHILDREN UNDER AGE 15, BY THE LEADING CAUSES OF HOSPITALIZATION: UNITED STATES, 1967

CAUSE OF HOSPITALIZATION	NUMBER OF DISCHARGES (1000's)	DISCHARGE RATE PER 10,000 CHILDREN*	AVERAGE LENGTH OF STAY IN DAYS
Respiratory diseases:			
Acute upper respiratory infections	233	39	4.6
Pneumonia, all forms	289	48	7.8
Acute bronchitis	81	14	6.0
Hypertrophy of tonsils and adenoids	859	144	2.0
Appendicitis	123	21	5.8
Inguinal hernia	111	19	3.4
Gastroenteritis	184	31	4.3
Congenital malformations	126	21	8.4
Fractures, all sites	201	34	6.7
Head injury (excluding skull fracture)	85	14	3.5

*Based on estimated noninstitutional population of 59,812,000.

NOTE: Excludes newborn infants. Includes noninstitutional, short-stay hospitals exclusive of Veterans Administration and military hospitals.

surance of quality through peer review, a process through which the quality of the work of a physician or other provider of health care can be examined objectively by fellow professionals on behalf of the community. The problem-oriented system, or something like it, seems likely to make peer review more feasible, when it is compared to the traditional manner of keeping medical records.

Growth of Specialization

In the past quarter-century the growth of specialization within the field has had a major impact upon pediatrics. Specialization has taken a number of different forms: interests in particular *age groups* of children have created neonatology and adolescent medicine; interests in *organ systems* have created pediatric cardiology, allergy, hematology, nephrology, gastroenterology, chest disease, and endocrinology, and pediatricians with interests in metabolism and genetics; interests in *the care system* have created pediatricians primarily devoted to ambulatory care on the one hand, and those specializing in intensive care on the other hand; and finally, multidisciplinary subspecialties have grown up around the problems of *handicapped children,* to which pediatrics, neurology, psychiatry, psychology, nursing, physical and occupational therapy, special education, speech and hearing, and nutrition all make essential contributions to the care of children with chronic disabilities. This growth of specialization has been such that the role of the pediatric generalist or "primary care pediatrician" may now be regarded as a subspecialty.

The rapid growth of specialization has responded to the fact that the amount of information relevant to child health care doubles about every 10 years now, and to the fact that no person can make herself or himself master of all this information. Physicians are more and more dependent upon one another for assurance of the highest quality of care

TABLE 1–7 NUMBER AND RATE OF DISCHARGES FROM HOSPITALS FOR CHILDREN UNDER AGE 15, BY THE LEADING SURGICAL PROCEDURES, BY SEX: UNITED STATES, 1967

SURGICAL PROCEDURE	NUMBER OF DISCHARGES (1000's)			RATE OF DISCHARGES PER 100,000 CHILDREN*	
	Both sexes	*Boys*	*Girls*	*Boys*	*Girls*
Tonsillectomy with or without adenoidectomy	853	441	408	1449.1	1388.7
Appendectomy	145	77	67	253.0	228.0
Operations on tympanum	130	72	57	236.6	194.0
Reduction of fracture without internal fixation	129	84	45	276.0	153.2
Repair of inguinal hernia	121	107	14	351.6	47.7

*Based on estimated noninstitutional population of 30,432,000 for boys and 29,380,000 for girls.

NOTE:Excludes newborn infants. Includes noninstitutional, short-stay hospitals exclusive of Veterans Administration and military hospitals.

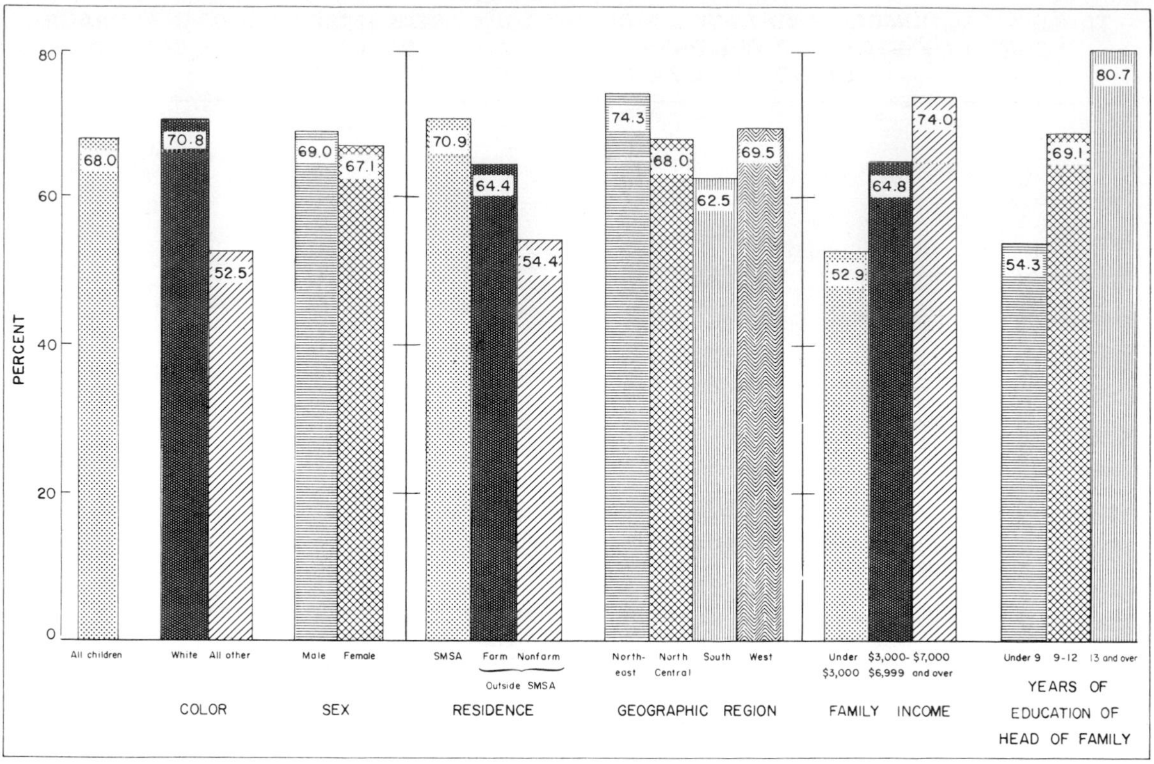

Figure 1-2 *Per cent of children under age 17 who saw a physician within 1 year of interview, by color, sex, place of residence, geographic region, family income, and education of head of family: United States, July 1966–June 1967. SMSA = Standard Metropolitan Statistical Area. (From The Health of Children–1970: Selected Data from the National Center for Health Statistics, Washington, D.C., U.S. Government Printing Office, Public Health Service Publication No. 2121, 1970.)*

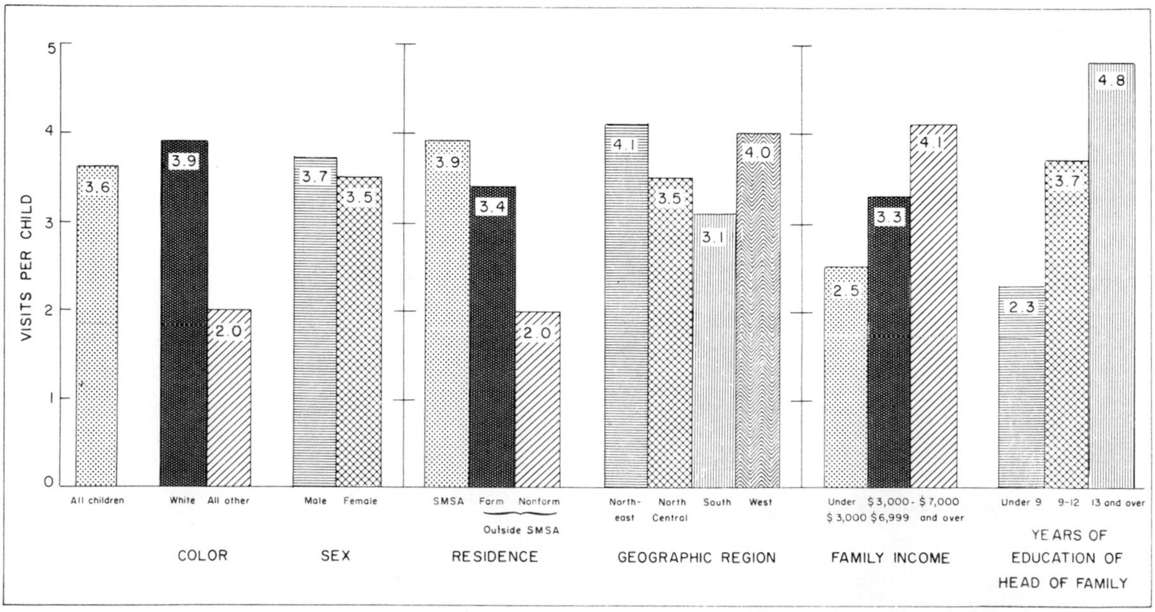

Figure 1-3 *Number of physician visits per year per child under age 17 by color, sex, place of residence, geographic region, family income, and education of head of family: United States, July 1966–June 1967. SMSA = Standard Metropolitan Statistical Area. (From The Health of Children–1970: Selected Data from the National Center for Health Statistics, Washington, D.C., U.S. Government Printing Office, Public Health Service Publication No. 2121, 1970.)*

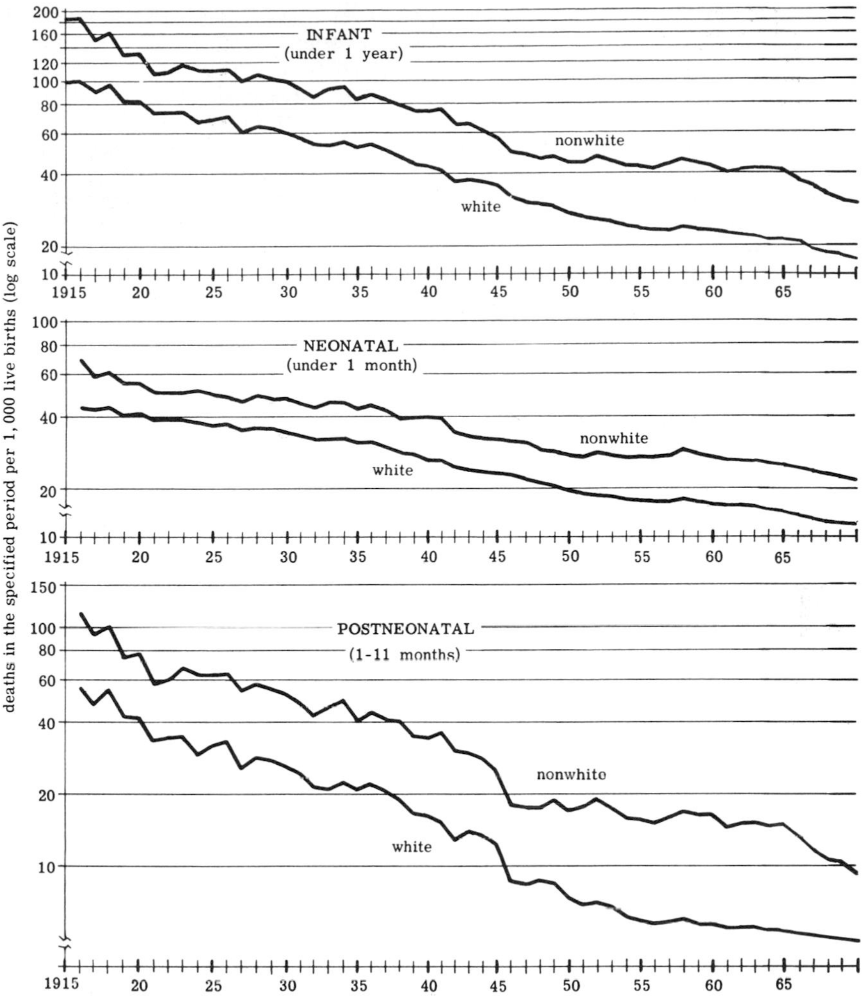

Figure 1–4 *Mortality rate of white and of nonwhite infants by age, United States, 1915-1970 (birth registration area). (United States Department of Health, Education, and Welfare, Social and Rehabilitation Service, Children's Bureau. Data from United States Public Health Service, National Center for Health Statistics.)*

for their patients; practitioners of pediatrics are increasingly gathering themselves into groups within which each physician may play in some measure the role of subspecialist.

The Need for Continuing Self-Education

The explosion of information has also created a need for continuing education, which was much less keenly felt in earlier years, when the relevant new information in any field of medicine was likely to be easily accessible through the reading of a relatively small number of journals, texts or monographs. Now, relevant information is so widely scattered among the many journals published that elaborate electronic data systems have been proposed and implemented to facilitate the dissemination of new knowledge, and new auditory and visual aids to learning abound, as well as postgraduate courses through which the participating physician can be brought up to date on various aspects of child health care. It also seems likely that examinations for certification and recertification in medicine or pediatrics, or in medical or pediatric subspecialties, will ultimately, in the United States, be linked to medical licensure, which is the process through which the public assures itself of the presumptive fitness of the physician to carry his responsibilities for the care of patients.

There is no touchstone through which the physician can assure that the process of his own continuing education will keep him abreast of advancing knowledge in his field, but he must find a way if he is to discharge his responsibility to his patients. An essential element of this process of continuing education may be that the physician take an *active* role in it. The passive role, reading or listening or watching, is far less effective than an active one in which the physician translates what he reads, sees or hears into some action of his own. His efforts in continuing self-education will be fostered, for example, if he can use them to teach, and particularly if they are relevant to the problems he actually encounters in his practice. He will learn best if he makes each clinical conundrum or problem a stimulus for a thorough review of standard literature, alone or in consultation with an appropriate colleague. This continuing review will do much to assure that he will find those inconsistencies or contradictions which will indicate, in the ultimate best interest of his patients, that things are not what they seem or have been said to be. Physicians still learn most from their patients, but not if they fall into the easy habit of accepting their patients' problems casually or at face value because they appear to be simple.

The tools which the physician must use in dealing with the problems of children and their families fall into three main categories: *cognitive* (up-to-date factual information regarding diagnostic and therapeutic issues, available on recall or easily found in readily accessible sources known to the physician); *interpersonal or manual skills* (the ability to carry out a productive interview, execute a reliable physical examination, perform a deft venipuncture, or manage cardiac arrest or the resuscitation of a depressed newborn infant, for example); and *attitudinal* (the physician's commitment to fullest possible implementation of his knowledge and skills on behalf of children and their families, in a climate of empathetic sensitivity to their needs and of concern for their welfare in the largest sense in which health can be construed). It scarcely needs saying that the workaday needs of professional persons for knowledge and skills in care of children will vary widely in depth in various areas of concern. The primary care physician needs depth in developmental concepts and in the ability to organize an effective system for achieving quality and continuity in assessing and planning for health care during the entire growing period of his patients; he may have little need for immediate recall of esoterica. On the other hand, the consultant or subspecialist not only needs a comfortable grasp of esoterica within his field of interest and responsibility, and perhaps within related fields, but he must also be able to cope with controversial issues in his field, and he may need the flexibility which will let him adapt the most relevant aspects of a variety of points of view to the best interest of his unique patient.

At whatever level of care (primary, secondary or tertiary), or in whatever role (as student, as pediatric nurse practitioner, as resident pediatrician, as a practitioner of pediatrics or of family medicine, or as a pediatric or other subspecialist), professional persons dealing with children must be able appropriately to identify their roles of the moment and their levels of engagement with a child's problem; and each must determine whether his experience and other resources at hand are adequate to deal with this problem and must be ready to seek other help when they are not. Among the resources to be kept at hand or called upon will be general textbooks, more detailed monographs in subspecialty areas, selected journals, audiovisual materials, and above all the human resources represented by colleagues with exceptional or complementary experience and expertise. The intercommunication of all these levels of interest in and engagement with medical and health problems of children offers the best hope that each generation may more closely approximate the goal of maximum achievement of the innate potential of every child.

ACKNOWLEDGMENT

We are indebted to the National Center for Health Statistics, Department of Health, Education, and Welfare for Tables 1-1, 1-2, 1-3, 1-4 and 1-5, and for the data from which Figures 1-1 and 1-4 were prepared. Tables 1-6 and 1-7 and Figures 1-2 and 1-3 were taken from *The Health of Children—1970: Selected Data from The National Center for Health Statistics.* Washington, D.C., U.S. Government Printing Office, Public Health Service Publication No. 2121, 1970.

VICTOR C. VAUGHAN, III, M.D.
R. JAMES MCKAY, M.D.

National Center for Health Statistics. *Current Listing and Topical Index to the Vital and Health Statistics Series (1962–1972),* publication No. (HSM)73-1301 (Revised). Department of Health, Education, and Welfare, Washington, 1973.

A catalog of studies (all are from Series 11):

Height and Weight of Children—United States (No. 104)
Height and Weight of Children: Socioeconomic Status—United States (No. 119)
Visual Acuity of Children—United States (No. 101)
Binocular Visual Acuity of Children: Demographic and Socioeconomic Characteristics—United States (No. 112)
Eye Examination Findings Among Children—United States (No. 115)
Hearing Levels of Children by Age and Sex—United States (No. 102)
Hearing Levels of Children by Demographic and Socioeconomic Characteristics—United States (No. 111)
Hearing Sensitivity and Related Medical Findings Among Children—United States (No. 114)
Hearing and Related Medical Findings Among Children: Race, Area, and Socioeconomic Differentials—United States (No. 122)
Decayed, Missing and Filled Teeth Among Children—United States (No. 106)
Periodontal Disease and Oral Hygiene Among Children—United States (No. 117)
Intellectual Development of Children as Measured by the Wechsler Intelligence Scale—United States (No. 107)
Intellectual Development of Children by Demographic and Socioeconomic Factors—United States (No. 110)
Intellectual Maturity of Children as Measured by the Goodenough-Harris Drawing Test—United States (No. 105)
Intellectual Maturity of Children: Demographic and Socioeconomic Factors—United States (No. 116)
School Achievement of Children by Demographic and Socioeconomic Factors—United States (No. 109)
Behavior Patterns of Children in School—United States (No. 113)
Parent Ratings of Behavioral Patterns of Children—United States (No. 108)
Relationships Among Parent Ratings of Behavioral Characteristics of Children—United States (No. 121)

National Center for Health Statistics. Provisional Estimates of Selected Comparability Ratios Based on Dual Coding of 1966 Death Certificates by the Seventh and Eighth Revisions of the International Classification of Diseases. *Monthly Vital Statistics Report,* Vol. 17, No. 8, supplement, October 25, 1968.

2
DEVELOPMENTAL PEDIATRICS

GROWTH AND DEVELOPMENT

The ripening of a fertilized human ovum through the stages of embryonic and fetal life, infancy, childhood and adolescence has physical, behavioral, intellectual, emotional, social and cultural aspects. Each aspect is the focal point of a growing body of knowledge. Growth and development do not take place independently in discrete areas or systems, but represent a continuum of interactions between innate genetic potential on the one hand and the environment on the other. The potentialities of each individual reside in a unique manner in the genetic substance of the fertilized ovum.

The degree of realization of biologic potential in the individual is the product of many interrelated factors or forces. *Genetic* factors, which are often thought of as establishing final limits to biologic potential, are inextricably interwoven with the environment. For example, in galactosemia the deleterious effect of abnormal genes may be aborted if the diet of the newborn infant does not contain lactose. *Trauma* may be prenatal or postnatal; it may be chemical as in the distortion of growth by drugs such as thalidomide and abortifacients, or it may be physical, radiant, immunologic, or residual from infection. *Nutritional* factors are fundamental to optimal growth, both prenatally and postnatally. Nutritional and *socioeconomic* factors are closely interwoven. *Social and emotional* factors are important modifiers of growth potential. The position of the child in the family, the quality of interaction between child and parent within the first few days or weeks of life, the child-rearing patterns and the personal concerns and needs of the parents are profoundly important to the degree of self-realization achieved by the growing child. *Cultural* considerations may limit the child by establishing conventional expectations as to what his behavior will be throughout his life, and may conspicuously alter the time scale for acquisition of skills such as sitting, creeping, standing or walking, which were once thought to be almost entirely maturationally determined. Further study is needed to determine the degrees to which developmental patterns depend upon genetic, nutritional, emotional, socioeconomic and cultural determinants.

SOME ASPECTS OF GROWTH AND DEVELOPMENT

The term *growth* has commonly been used for those aspects of maturation which can be described by a measurement of size; the term *development* refers to changes in the function of the organism. Because these two aspects cannot be sharply differentiated, the term *growth and development* is generally given a unitary meaning implying both the magnitude and quality of maturational changes.

Physical growth and development encompasses changes in the size and function of the organism. Changes in function range from those at the molecular level in fetal life through the activation of enzyme systems in the neonatal period to the complex metabolic changes associated with puberty and adolescence.

Intellectual growth and development is difficult to differentiate from neurologic and behavioral maturation in early infancy. In later infancy or early childhood, intellectual function is increasingly measured by communicative skills and the ability of the child to handle abstract and symbolic material.

Emotional growth and development depends upon the infant's ability to establish effective bonds of feeling with persons who have the greatest meaning for him. The capacity for love and affection, the ability to handle anxieties arising out of frustrations, and the ability to control aggressive impulses are aspects of the emotional life which each child needs opportunities to develop.

Closely related to emotional growth and development are social and cultural patterns of maturation which, in the final analysis, prove to be the strongest determinants of emotional maturity. The earliest and most basic factors are the relations with parents. These relations are extended during childhood to familial and extrafamilial contacts. As early as 4 to 6 months of age one may expect imitation of a primitive sort, at 8 or 9 months the beginnings of imitative play, and by 3 to 5 years creative play which includes the playing of adult roles.

Learning is an essential aspect of acculturation. Current learning theory suggests that the behavior of the infant is modified both by inner needs and tensions and by contingencies in the environment. If a pattern of behavior is reliably followed by pleasant circumstances such as reduction of need or by intrinsically satisfying stimuli, then that pattern of behavior will tend to occur with increasing probability; if by unpleasant circumstances, then with decreasing probability.

In the process of acculturation, and in many other areas of their lives, the behavior of children is very responsive to the manner in which it is rewarded, and this relationship exists both for desirable behavior and for undesirable behavior, viewed in parental or social perspective. The *reinforcement* of behavior may be *positive* or *negative*, in accordance with whether it consists of a pleasant or rewarding experience or the termination of some uncomfortable, unpleasant or aversive situation. In contrast to negative reinforcement, *punishment* implies the creation of an unpleasant situation upon the exhibition of undesirable behavior.

There is a need to set limits to the behavior of children from time to time through restraint or other measures which might be construed as punishment. The evidence is good that punishment or reprimand is maximally effective when it takes place immediately upon exhibition of undesirable behavior, and that the likelihood of repetition of this behavior increases with delays between its manifestation and evidence of disapproval. There is evidence also that positive reinforcement is a generally more effective way than punishment to elicit desirable behavior from children. (See Discipline.)

The techniques of *behavior modification* and *behavior shaping* have broad implications for socialization and discipline in childhood. The shaping of behavior begins with giving positive reinforcement to elements of behavior that move a child in a desired direction, undesirable behavior to be *extinguished* through being for the most part not responded to. As behavior approaches in quality the desired goal, rewards are increasingly limited to behavior representative of goal conditions, which can be maintained, once achieved, through occasional further positive reinforcement.

A further consideration in the socialization and acculturation of children is the important role which *models* play, children even in the first year of life having a tendency to imitate the behavior of those around them. As the child grows older, he is able to draw lessons and inferences not only from experiencing the consequences of his own behavior, but from seeing that certain forms of behavior have predictable consequences for other children or adults. The importance of models to the child can scarcely be overemphasized. There is no doubt that what the child sees about him in reality or what he experiences through mass media, such as television, newspapers, literature and the like, may profoundly affect his system of values and his notions as to what is to be expected of him. The importance for the child of essential congruity between his parents' value systems and their behavior is discussed elsewhere. The same considerations will, of course, prevail with respect to other significant persons in the child's world.

The broad picture of growth and development, then, is an intricate pattern of genetic, nutritional, traumatic, social and cultural forces dynamically affecting the child from conception to adulthood. The pattern is unique for each child and may be profoundly different for individual children within the broad limits which designate "normality." The most obvious differences are those which distinguish male and female. Beyond these the patterns of growth and development may have such variability that they can be adequately expressed only in statistical terms.

VARIABILITY IN HUMAN GROWTH PATTERNS

In biologic data which vary over a range of normal values the largest number tend to cluster about a mean value. When data are plotted on a graph in the manner indicated in Figure 2–1, the resultant curve is often a close approximation of the theoretic bell-shaped curve (Fig. 2–2) which describes the ideal or equal distribution of continuously variable values about a population mean. Statistical treatment of data so arranged may give a number of useful concepts, the most important of which are the *mean* or *average* and the *standard deviation* from the mean.

In a theoretically perfect distribution the average value will be the one most commonly found, i.e., the *modal* or *normal* value (mode or norm) for the population under study. If, on the other hand, a distribution includes a larger number of high values than low, or vice versa, the average value may not be the most representative or modal value for the population studied. Asymmetrical curves of this sort are said to be *skewed*. Figure 2–3, which presents the weights of a group of children, is an example of such a skewed curve.

Occasionally a bimodal curve is found. Under these circumstances it may generally be inferred that not one but two groups are being studied, which have some feature differentiating one from the other. When two different samples or populations vary with respect to average values for some biologic trait, it is often difficult to evaluate this difference unless the distribution or dispersion of values in each sample is known. When the *standard deviations* of two samples are available, then the likelihood can be calculated whether an observed difference between them may have occurred solely as the result of randomly distributed values or whether the variable is a significant differential factor between the two groups.

The *standard deviation* (root mean square or quadratic mean) describes the degree of dispersion of observed values as they deviate from the mean

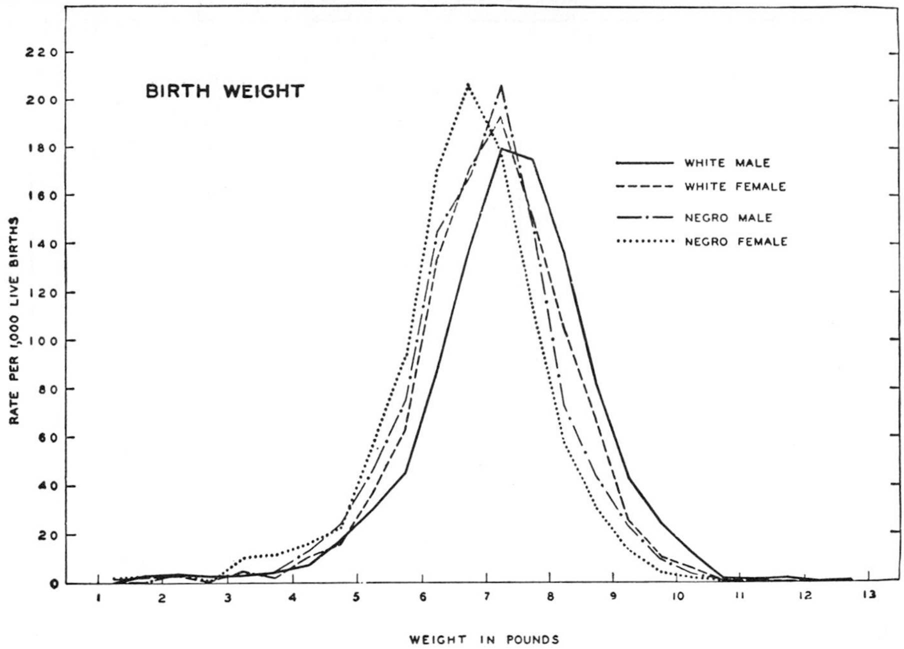

Figure 2–1 *Weight at birth; rates by color and sex per 1000 live births. (After Anderson, Brown and Lyon: Causes of prematurity. III. Influence of race and sex on duration of gestation and weight at birth. Am. J. Dis. Child. 65:523, 1943.*

value. The range of values lying between the points one standard deviation below and one standard deviation above the mean value will include about 68 per cent of all values on a theoretic distribution about this mean. The range, *mean plus or minus 2 standard deviations,* will include about 95 per cent of values distributed about this mean, and the range, *mean plus or minus 3 standard deviations,* will include about 99.7 per cent of such values. Such measurements of dispersion are commonly used to locate an individual member of a population with respect to the average member. The growth charts in common use for following the physical development of children make this location easy by showing developmental lines at a number of different positions corresponding to deviations from average values above and below the mean. These are often expressed in terms not of

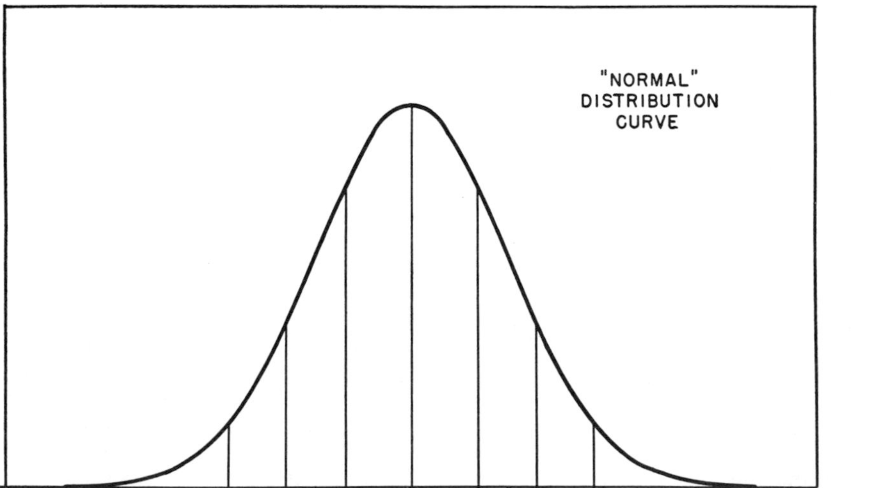

Figure 2–2 *"Normal" distribution curve. This theoretical curve represents a type of distribution characteristic of the range of variability between values for many measurements obtained from groups of children at a given age. The percentiles indicate certain positions within this distribution, as do the standard deviations from the mean. Samples of actual distributions of values obtained from children are shown for comparison with this curve in Figures 2–1 and 2–3.*

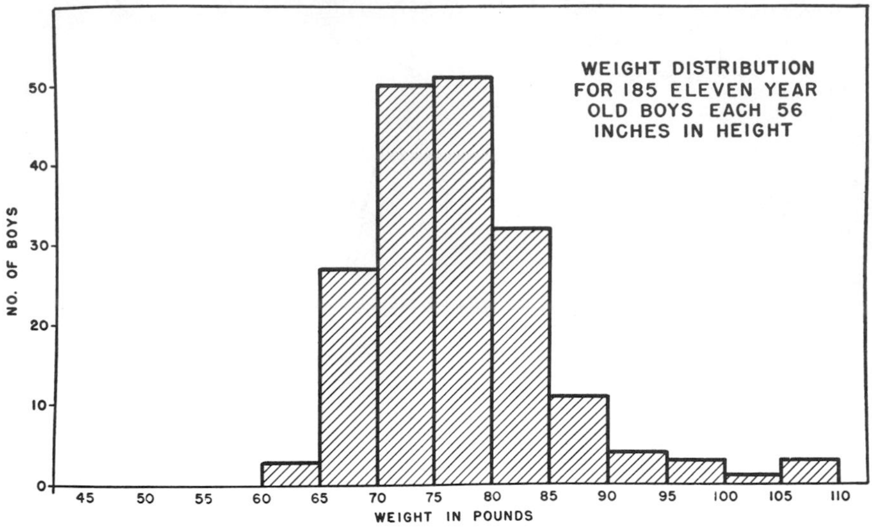

Figure 2–3 *Weight distribution of 185 boys. The mean for the distribution of weights is 77.2 pounds, within the range of the column of greatest concentration of values. There is a slight skew to the right of this curve, suggesting the inclusion of a few obese subjects. (Values from Franzen: School Health Research Monograph No. II. New York, American Child Health Association, 1929.)*

standard deviation, but of *percentile* location in the distribution pattern.

When the items in a set of quantitative data are arranged in order of ascending or descending magnitude, a value can be found which is called the *median,* above and below which lie half the observed values. In the distribution described by the symmetrical normal curve, the median, the mode and the average fall at the same point. Values may also be designated which divide the data into two groups at the *first quartile point,* below which will lie one quarter of the values, the *second quartile point* (which corresponds to median), and the *third quartile point,* below which lie three quarters of the observed values. The *percentile* points in a distribution of ordered data have similar meaning, one tenth of observations falling below the tenth percentile, three tenths below the thirtieth percentile, nine tenths below the ninetieth percentile, and so on.

Although such measures of growth as weight, height, and circumference of head at a particular time do indicate the status of a given child in relation to other children of the same age, only sequential measurements for some months or even years will indicate whether the child is achieving his growth potential. For example, a child below the tenth percentile point in weight for age might be thought of as undernourished, but one in 10 normal children will be below this level. If such a child continues to grow in height and weight within expected limits, he may be considered to be within the normal range in respect to his physical growth status. On the other hand, another child whose height and weight at a given time might approximate the fiftieth percentiles for his age might be significantly below his ideal levels. Only the repeated recording of growth measurements throughout infancy and childhood will provide a certain means to demonstrate the adequacy of physical growth.

Whenever one aspect of growth differs significantly from other aspects, possible reasons should be sought. For example, if a child's height and bone age place him at the fiftieth percentile for age, one would be concerned to find his weight at the third or ninety-seventh percentile. The differences in *physique* which would be represented by such findings can be readily imagined.

In evaluating the possibility that a growth pattern is deviant, it may also be helpful to examine the physical patterns of other members of the child's family. The small child of small but normal parents seems less out of place than the conspicuously small child of average or large parents.

It may be helpful at any age to be able to suggest what the approximate adult height of a child may be. Bayer and Bayley developed predictive standards corrected in some measure for the relative rapidity with which the child was maturing (as indicated by bone age), but these predictions did not take into account parental heights. More recently Tanner and coworkers have developed for children between the ages of 2 and 9 years standards for height which are appropriately adjusted for the parents' heights. Wingert and coworkers have also indicated how an appraisal of the preadolescent child's height can account for parental height; they found that the correlation of child's with parents' heights increases with age.

With allowance for normal influences which may put it at a given percentile at a particular time, the growth curve of each healthy child is sufficiently smooth so that any substantial perturbations of the growth line are likely to reflect physical illness, nutritional disturbances or psychosocial difficulties. The possibilities for early intervention will be maximized when appropriate records are kept of the careful measurements made during infancy and early childhood.

The setting in which apparent growth failure or such growth excess as obesity occurs may give clues to its meaning. The tensions, anxieties and cultural goals of parents and children may be intimately involved in potential or actual disturbances of growth. Before such causal relations are assumed, however, the child must be adequately studied clinically to ensure that no disturbance such as chronic renal disease or metabolic disorder is responsible for an abnormal growth pattern.

FETAL GROWTH AND DEVELOPMENT

The period of intrauterine life may be divided into two principal phases, the *embryonic* and the *fetal*. The dividing line is not sharp, but the embryonic period is usually considered to be the first 8 weeks of growth, during which the fertilized ovum differentiates rapidly into an organism which has most of the gross anatomic features which distinguish the human form. Organogenesis does continue beyond 8 weeks in some systems, so that some prefer to designate the embryonic period as the first trimester of pregnancy, or the first 12 weeks. The period after the twelfth week of gestation and through the fortieth week is distinguished by rapid growth and elaboration of function. Before the twenty-eighth week of gestation the fetus is generally considered *previable;* from 28 to about 38 weeks the infant is considered *viable,* with decreasing degrees of prematurity.

Many abnormalities of children have their origins in abnormal genes or chromosomes or derive from disturbances in growth during the embryonic period. During this period the mortality rate is probably higher than at any other time of life. Causes of mortality include abnormalities of genes and chromosomes and alterations of maternal health, and these may at times be interrelated. Advanced maternal age, for example, seems to dispose to chromosomal abnormalities which may give rise to Down syndrome, Klinefelter syndrome or other conditions. Maternal infection during the first trimester of pregnancy may alter the differentiation of the fetus in such a way as to produce congenital anomalies, e.g., those resulting from rubella in the mother during the first 8 weeks of pregnancy. In general, intrauterine environmental factors responsible for defects in differentiation of the newborn infant exert their effects within the first trimester of pregnancy.

Morbidity during the fetal period may result from a variety of intrauterine factors. These include interference with *oxygenation* of the fetus through disturbances of the placenta or umbilical cord, *infections* such as syphilis, toxoplasmosis, cytomegalic inclusion disease and other viral or bacterial conditions, *injury* by radiation, trauma or noxious chemicals, by *immunologic* disorders in which erythrocytes, white blood cells or platelets are altered by isoantibodies or by maternal *nutritional* disturbances.

Deficiencies in the maternal diet seem more apt to affect the weight and general condition of the human infant than to produce such specific anatomic defects as occur in certain animals. Malnutrition in the pregnant woman leads to a high incidence of stillbirths or premature births, and deficiencies of calcium and of protein in the maternal diet seem to be clearly related to osseous structure and muscular mass in the newborn infant. Recent studies suggest that the life-long undernutrition of the mother, extended into pregnancy, may be more serious for the baby than an acute nutritional disturbance during pregnancy in the previously well nourished mother. The long-term effects on the child are more severe and may be devastating when intrauterine malnutrition is followed by malnutrition in the first months of life. The size and number of cells in the brain may be diminished and ultimate intellectual capacity compromised.

FETAL DEVELOPMENT

The embryo is grossly inert during the first 7 weeks of development, except for the heart beat, which begins by about 4 weeks. The first week of embryologic life is germinal, consisting of active cell division. During the second week the tissues differentiate into two layers, entoderm and ectoderm, and during the third week the third layer, mesoderm, is added. During the fourth week the growing organism elaborates the somites and between the fourth and eighth weeks undergoes rapid differentiation into an essentially human form. At 8 weeks of age the fetus weighs approximately 1 gm and is about 2.5 cm in length; at 12 weeks it weighs about 14 gm and is about 7.5 cm long. By the end of the *first trimester of pregnancy* the sex of the fetus can be distinguished by external examination.

The *second trimester of pregnancy,* ending by about 28 weeks, is characterized by rapid growth in size of the fetus, especially in linear dimensions, and by rapid acquisition of new functions. By the end of the second trimester the fetus weighs approximately 1000 gm and is about 35 cm (14 inches) in length. During the *third trimester* the further increase in size of the now viable fetus involves especially subcutaneous tissue and muscle mass.

The *circulatory* system of the fetus attains its final form between the eighth and twelfth weeks of gestation. Blood returning to the fetus from the placenta through the umbilical vein enters the inferior vena cava through the ductus venosus. As it enters the right atrium, this blood tends to be preferentially shunted through the patent foramen ovale into the left atrium. From the left ventricle this blood then enters the ascending aorta and is distributed to the head and the brain. Blood returning from the head by way of the superior vena cava tends to move across the right atrium into the right ventricle, and through the pulmonary artery and ductus arteriosus into the descending aorta, whence it is returned to the placenta by way of the umbilical arteries. In this way the head and brain receive proportionately more oxygenated blood than other parts of the body.

At birth, or shortly thereafter, there is closure of the ductus venosus, the ductus arteriosus, the foramen ovale and the umbilical arteries and vein. Closure of the foramen ovale is very likely functionally complete within the first few minutes after birth, owing to establishment of a lower pressure on the right side of the heart than on the left, after aeration of the lungs. Temporary reversal of flow through the foramen ovale may occur with crying and lead to mild cyanosis during the first few days of life. Closure of the ductus arteriosus probably occurs somewhat later, though usually within the first 2 or 3 days of life. The stimulus for this closure is very likely the establishment of a high oxygen level in the arterial blood. Umbilical arteries undergo spasm with the cutting of the umbilical cord, and are reduced ultimately to fibrous cords. The changes in blood flow with birth of the infant have the effect of transforming the circulatory system from the fetal one in which the two ventricles act in parallel, with shunts adjusting possible unequal outputs, to a system in which the two pumps act in series, which requires that the outputs of the right and left sides of the heart be equal.

Although *respiratory* movements of the fetus may be seen as early as the eighteenth week of gestation, the development of the alveolar structures of the lung will not generally be sufficient to permit survival until the twenty-seventh or twenty-eighth week. The respiratory movements of the fetus result in a tidal flow of amniotic fluid into and out of the developing lung and may contribute to pulmonary arborization. Respiratory movements may be intensified by anoxia. Late in pregnancy, when amniotic fluid contains a larger number of cells than earlier and may contain meconium and other debris, aspiration may lead to deposition of these materials in the alveoli and to consequent respiratory embarrassment at delivery.

The hemoglobin of the fetus is predominantly fetal in type (hemoglobin F) and differs from that of adults (hemoglobin A) in its greater resistance to alkaline denaturation. Fetal hemoglobin carries more oxygen at a given oxygen tension than adult hemoglobin, which begins to be produced late in fetal life and represents about 30 per cent of the hemoglobin of the mature newborn infant.

The fetus makes swallowing movements as early as the fourteenth week of gestation; at 17 weeks it may protrude the upper lip on stimulation in the oral area, and by 20 weeks it may protrude both lips on stimulation. At 22 weeks the lips are pursed upon stimulation, and by 28 to 29 weeks the fetus may actively suck in an attempt to gain nourishment.

Bile begins to be formed by about 12 weeks of gestation, and digestive enzymes appear soon thereafter. Meconium, the distinctive intestinal content of the fetus, is present by 16 weeks; it consists of desquamated intestinal cells and intestinal juices, and of squamous cells and lanugo hair swallowed by the fetus in amniotic fluid. Meconium is typically dark green to black and is gelatinous and sticky in consistency.

Neurologic activity in the fetus is first manifest by about 8 weeks of gestation, when isolated local muscular reactions may be seen in response to stimulation. By 9 weeks contralateral flexion may be followed by ipsilateral flexion (swimming motions), and some spontaneous movements may be seen. In the fetus of 9 weeks' gestation the palms and soles have become reflexogenic; by 13 to 14 weeks graceful flowing movements may be produced by stimulation of all areas except the back, the back of the head and the vertex. At this time the movement of the fetus may first begin to be perceptible to the mother. The grasp reflex is evident by 17 weeks and is generally well developed by 27 weeks. Respiration may occur in the fetus delivered at 18 weeks; at 22 weeks respiratory activity may be accompanied by weak phonation. By 25 weeks the earliest signs of the Moro response can be elicited.

After the fifteenth to seventeenth week of gestation there is apparently some decrease of fetal activity, the fetus being somewhat sluggish until the time of birth.

It seems clear that the amount of activity differs among fetuses, and there is evidence that fetal activity may be responsive to maternal emotions, possibly as a result of placental transfer of epinephrine or other humoral concomitants of strong feelings. Virtually nothing is known as to how the activity of newborn infants or the quality of the infant's demands during the first few weeks of life may reflect aspects of his gestation which were dependent upon maternal emotional states. The fetus is capable of being conditioned to certain sensory stimuli; e.g., changes in the fetal pulse rate in response to noise transmitted through the mother's abdomen are blunted by repetition of the noise. The comfort derived by some newborn infants from rhythmic motion or rhythmic sound may stem from similar sensations imparted in utero by maternal respiration or heart sounds.

The placenta is the principal avenue of metabolic interchange between mother and fetus. Its most urgent function is to provide for gas exchange between mother and fetus, which requires adequate perfusion on both sides. The placenta is a complex organ, elaborating hormones and enzymes which participate in the regulation of pregnancy, and effecting the selective transfer of nutrients and metabolites between mother and infant. Placental permeability is selective even for such closely related substances as antibodies against viruses and bacteria, the former being more readily transmitted than the latter. Much of the transfer of calcium, iron and gamma globulins to the infant occurs in the last trimester of pregnancy, with the result that the infant born prematurely may have unusual needs for calcium and iron and an unusual susceptibility to infection.

THE NEWBORN INFANT

(See also Section 7)

The general physical features of the newborn infant differentiate him sharply from the older infant, child or adult in respect to body proportions (Fig. 2–4). The head is relatively large, the face round and the mandible relatively small. The chest tends to be rounded rather than flattened anteroposteriorly; the abdomen is relatively prominent, and the extremities are relatively short. The midpoint of the stature of the newborn infant is approximately at the level of the umbilicus, whereas in the adult it is at the symphysis pubis.

At birth the infant is generally covered with vernix caseosa, a cheesy white substance adherent to the skin. There may be edema of the vertex or other presenting part, or an abnormal shape to the head molded by the forces of labor, with overriding of the bones of the cranial vault.

The predominant posture of the newborn infant is one of partial flexion. It is often possible to establish what the predominant intrauterine position of the infant was by determining the most comfortable pattern into which the extremities can be flexed and adjusted to each other ("folded") so as to make the infant assume a more or less ovoid shape. Sometimes minor, and occasionally major orthopedic abnormalities reflect the effect of intrauterine posture upon the growing fetus. (See also Section 22.)

Localized anatomic variants which may be observed in the newborn infant include telangiectases of the eyelids and of the nape, mongolian spot, milia, phimosis, and epithelial pearls of the oral mucous membrane. The external auditory canal of the newborn infant is short, and the drum is placed obliquely across the canal. The eustachian tube is short and broad. There is usually a single mastoid cell in the antrum; maxillary and ethmoid sinuses are small, and the frontal and sphenoidal ones undeveloped. The liver and spleen are commonly felt at or just below the costal margins, and the kidneys are often palpable.

An average newborn infant weights approximately 3.4 kg ($7^1/_2$ pounds), boys being slightly heavier than girls. Approximately 95 per cent of full-term newborn infants weigh between 2.5 kg ($5^1/_2$ pounds) and 4.6 kg (10 pounds). The length averages about 50 cm (20 inches), approximately 95 per cent of infants being between 45 and 55 cm (18 and 22 inches). The head circumference averages about 35 cm (14 inches).

The most critical need of the newborn infant is for the establishment of adequate respiratory activity with effective exchange of gases. The rate of established respirations averages 30 to 40 per minute. Other activity useful in respiration includes crying, sneezing, coughing, yawning and stretching.

The cardiac adjustments of the neonatal period are often associated with transient cardiac murmurs. The heart rate ranges from 120 to 160 per minute. The heart of the newborn infant often seems large with respect to the size of the chest when measured by adult standards.

The activity of the newborn infant directed toward meeting his nutritional needs includes crying when hungry, a tendency when hungry to turn his head toward and to "root" about for the nipple or other stimulus placed close to his oral area (rooting reflex) and sucking, gagging and swallowing reflexes. The newborn infant is capable of manifesting nausea and of vomiting.

Breast feeding of the newborn infant will be facilitated if the mother is instructed as to the nature and meaning of the rooting reflex and if she knows that in nursing the infant will draw an unexpectedly large amount of nipple and areola into his mouth and that there will be rhythmic closure of the jaw upon the nipple in such a manner as to empty the postareolar sinus located at the point of confluence of lacteal vessels. Most failures of

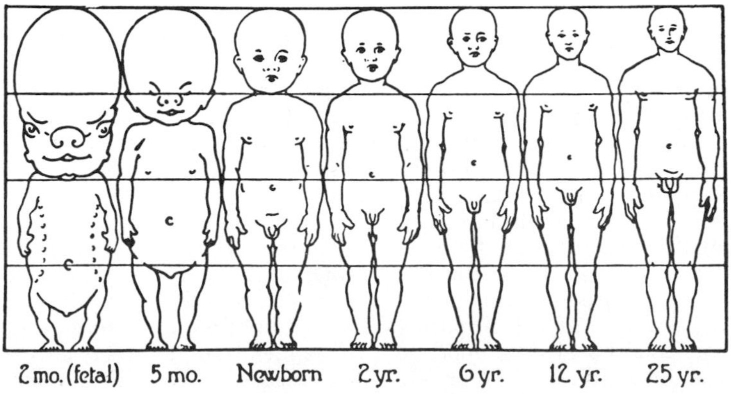

Figure 2–4 *Changes in body proportions from second fetal month to adulthood. (From Robbins et al.: Growth. New Haven, Yale University Press. By permission of publisher.)*

breast feeding are the result of errors in technique or of an emotional set against breast feeding.

The infant initially expresses his hunger at irregular intervals, but during the first week he will fall reasonably comfortably into patterns of feeding at intervals ranging from 2 to 4 or 5 hours. No schedule of feedings will meet the demands or needs of all infants; if infant and mother are close to each other during the immediate postnatal period, as in a rooming-in arrangement, the opportunities for comfortable meeting of the baby's needs are optimal.

The first stools will generally be passed within 24 hours and will consist of meconium. With the establishment of milk feedings, the meconium stools begin to be replaced on the third or fourth day by *transitional* stools, which are greenish brown and may contain milk curds. The typical milk stool of the older infant follows after an interval of 3 or 4 days. The frequency of stools in the newborn infant seems closely related to the frequency with which he is fed and the amount of food obtained, averaging between 3 and 5 stools a day by the end of the first week of life. On any given day during the first week about one infant in 50 will have no stool at all; it is unusual for an infant to have as many as 6 or 7 stools after the second day.

At delivery the infant's body temperature is likely to be virtually the same as his mother's. After delivery there is a transient fall in temperature, which is usually restored within 4 to 8 hours. Under usual environmental circumstances the daily caloric need of the infant to maintain body heat and basal activity is about 55 calories per kg. By the end of the first week the caloric needs will be approximately 110 calories per kg, of which 50 per cent supplies basal metabolic needs, 40 per cent is invested in growth and in activity, 5 per cent is for the specific dynamic action of protein, and 5 per cent is lost in urine and feces or as other caloric loss in excreta.

The newborn infant is well supplied with body water; that in the extracellular compartment may constitute up to 35 per cent of body weight. During the first few days of life there is a loss of excess fluid which, in the absence of unusual oral intake, generally averages about 6 per cent of body weight and may occasionally exceed 10 per cent. When this loss is excessive, there may be so-called dehydration or inanition fever on the third or fourth day.

After the first week of life the need for water will be in the range of 120 to 150 ml per kg. Approximately half of this will be devoted to formation of urine and the rest to insensible loss by lungs and skin and to other losses. The insensible loss is in a relatively fixed relation to the calories metabolized by the infant (about 40 ml per 100 calories). Losses in stool are variable; those in sweat, minimal.

The metabolism of the newborn infant favors the anaerobic or glycolytic pathway, so that he is more tolerant of periods of deprivation of oxygen than is the older infant, child or adult. This tolerance for anoxia is only relative, however. If oxygenation of the newborn infant is not quickly established, there may be a rapidly developing metabolic acidosis (owing to the accumulation of lactic acid) and respiratory acidosis (owing to rapid accumulation of carbon dioxide).

Renal function in the newborn infant does not meet the standards of later life. Urine often contains protein in small amounts and during the first week of life may contain an abundance of urates, which may give the diaper a pink stain. Urea clearance is low, and the ability to concentrate urine is limited. There is limited production of ammonium ion and relatively limited clearance of phosphate ion. There may be a transient, slight rise in the blood urea nitrogen level during the first days.

The hemoglobin level of the newborn infant averages around 17 to 19 gm/dl; mild reticulocytosis and normoblastemia may be observed for the first day or two of life. Leukocytes number about 10,000/mm^3 at birth and generally increase in number for the first 24 hours, with a relative neutrophilia. Occasionally counts as high as 25,000 to 35,000 are encountered. After the first week the white cell count is likely to be below 14,000, with the characteristic relative lymphocytosis of infancy and early childhood. Stressful situations in the newborn infant, including overwhelming infection, may on occasion be associated with little or no leukocytosis and even with leukopenia.

The transition from intrauterine to extrauterine life imposes upon the infant the need to activate a number of functions which have been dormant. Some of them, such as respiratory activity and the maintenance of body temperature, are under usual circumstances quickly achieved. By contrast, there are delays in the development of certain enzymatic, hemostatic and immunologic functions, so that the infant may temporarily be subject to increased risk when exposed to infection or when given certain drugs which he is able to metabolize adequately only some weeks after birth.

There appears to be little or no passive transfer of certain clotting factors from mother to infant. Establishment of normal hemostatic mechanisms depends upon early establishment of normal intestinal flora and elaboration of vitamin K.

Placentally transmitted maternal hormones are responsible for temporary changes in the breasts (enlargement, and production of milk), uterus and possibly other tissues, and the withdrawal of maternal hormones or other metabolites may contribute to temporary hypofunction of the fetal parathyroid. Blood levels of sugar and calcium are normally relatively low in the newborn infant, and further decreases (below about 20 mg/dl of sugar or about 7.5 mg/dl of calcium) may be responsible for convulsions.

Adjustment to extrauterine life is likely to be prolonged in respect to resistance to infection. The gamma globulin level of the newborn infant (almost entirely IgG) is slightly higher than that of his mother, a fact which suggests that there is an active transport mechanism for gamma globulin. Protection is afforded in some measure against many viral and some bacterial diseases by antibodies of the IgG variety transferred from mother to infant. Antibodies against certain antigens of gram-negative enterobacteria, on the other hand, like isohemagglutinins, are found in the IgM fraction of immune globulins, which do not cross the placenta in large amounts. IgM antibodies may be formed, however, by the fetus in response to intrauterine infection. IgA antibodies and IgE (reagins) do not generally cross the placenta.

The gamma globulin level of the infant falls to a low level by about 3 months of age, with a subsequent rise to those levels which characterize the older child and the adult. The responses of the newborn infant to immunization are relatively sluggish by the standards of older infants; this sluggishness is accentuated in premature infants. Antibodies belonging to the major blood group system usually appear by the end of the first month of life.

The secretory enzymes of the digestive tract are usually adequate for the diet of the newborn infant, though fat is handled somewhat less well than protein or carbohydrate. At the cellular level, however, a number of deficiencies may have important clinical consequences. The red blood cells of the newborn infant have a relatively low level of reduced glutathione, which may contribute to increased hemolysis of red blood cells under a variety of circumstances. A deficiency in capacity of the liver to conjugate bilirubin with glucuronic acid leads to hyperbilirubinemia, often with no evidence of abnormal hemolysis. When hyperbilirubinemia is severe, kernicterus becomes a threat.

These evidences of metabolic immaturity generally do not persist beyond the first week of life; they may persist longer in premature than in full-term infants.

The repertory of behavior of the infant at birth is limited. Tensions arising from hunger, cold, pain or other discomfort lead to restlessness or crying. Prompt satisfaction of indicated needs will usually restore the infant's composure. Some infants seem to need more than the usual amount of "mothering" and are comforted by gentle handling, rocking and the like.

Recent work has emphasized the importance of the early emotional and social attachment of the infant to his mother in determining some future aspects of his personality or of the relationship that he will have with his mother and other people. Klaus and Kennell have shown how the effects of as little as 16 hours of contact between mother and infant in the first three days of life can modify the emotional quality of the relationship between them in ways which can be detected as long as a year later. Some aspects of the manner in which emotional bonds are set between newborn infants and their mothers seem to represent analogues of *imprinting*, the process through which the young of many vertebrate species identify the social milieu to which they belong and to which they will turn as a refuge or for social interaction. *Critical periods* exist for some aspects of imprinting in certain species; it is not clear what critical periods exist in man, but it is certain that increasing attention to the circumstances surrounding the delivery of the infant, his care in the hospital, and the early weeks at home will lead to substantial revision of some current practices of care. In particular, there is a need for greater involvement of both mothers and fathers in prenatal activities oriented to education for childbirth and child rearing, for further encouragement of breastfeeding and of the rooming-in arrangements in the neonatal period which make this most physiologic, and for greater restraint in the use of analgesic and anesthetic agents in labor.

GROWTH AND DEVELOPMENT OF THE INFANT BORN PREMATURELY

(See also Section 7)

The fetus born prematurely has some chance of survival by about 28 weeks' gestation, at which time its weight is about 1000 gm and its length approximately 35 cm. The specific areas in which the premature infant faces difficulties owing to failure of adequate maturation of enzymatic, renal, metabolic, hematologic and immunologic mechanisms are discussed elsewhere.

The behavioral characteristics of premature infants vary with their gestational age. The heads of infants whose birth weights are 1000 to 1500 gm tend to be rounded, and large in relation to body size; the skin appears transparent. They tend to be predominantly atonic and to lie in a tonic neck attitude, often with little motion of the extremities. Vocalization is weak, as are the grasp and Moro responses. The sucking responses may also be weak, and these infants may show little evidence of hunger on deprivation of food. It is difficult to tell when they are awake and when asleep, though they can be stimulated to greater alertness.

Somewhat larger infants, those from 1500 to 2000 gm, have more subcutaneous tissue and relatively less enlargement of the head. These infants have good muscle tone when stimulated, more vigorous grasp and complete Moro responses. A sleep pattern is easily discernible, and they are able to fixate visually some objects in their environment. The more vigorous of these babies are able to manage breast feeding.

Infants weighing between 2000 and 2500 gm at birth generally have the appearance of small full-term infants, from which they cannot usually be differentiated by developmental examination. They have a good cry and sustained muscle tone.

The average premature infant is likely to gain 6 to 7 kg (13 to 15 pounds) in the first year, which is the average gain for the full-term infant. Although a small premature infant, by the time he reaches his expected date of delivery, may seem more alert and active than a full-term baby born on that day, the actual developmental level which is reached later in the first year will generally be lower than that indicated by his chronologic age. The deficit in attained level tends to correspond to the degree of prematurity. These differences become less conspicuous and will generally have disappeared by the end of the second year of life, so long as no complicating factors occur. Developmental defects are more common in premature infants than in full-term infants and often include impairment of intellectual or motor function.

The premature infant is particularly sensitive to the effects of sensory and social deprivation in the neonatal period, owing to the circumstances of his care and the sometimes prolonged period in which he remains in relative isolation. Recent studies emphasize the importance of involving the mothers of even the smallest babies in some aspects of their care as early as possible, in order to familiarize the mothers with their infants and their care and to enhance the opportunities for their mutual emotional attachment.

GROWTH DURING THE FIRST YEAR

Most full-term infants regain their birth weight by the age of 10 days. After this, weight gain averages approximately 20 gm per day for the first 5 months of life and approximately 15 gm per day for the remainder of the first year. The full-term infant will generally double his birth weight by 5 months and triple it in 1 year. The length of the normal infant increases during the first year by 25 to 30 cm or 10 to 12 inches. (The average length at birth is 50 cm, or 20 inches.) There is a conspicuous increase of subcutaneous tissue in the early months of life, which reaches its peak by about 9 months.

The anterior fontanel of the newborn infant may increase in size for several months after birth, but generally diminishes in size after 6 months and may become effectively closed at any time from 9 to 18 months. The posterior fontanel is generally closed to palpation by 4 months.

The circumference of the head, which is 34 to 35 cm at birth, increases to approximately 44 cm by 6 months and to 47 cm by 1 year (Table 2–1). The circumference of the head is somewhat larger than that of the chest at birth, but the two become approximately equal at 1 year.

Deciduous teeth appear in most infants between 5 and 9 months. The first to erupt are the lower central incisors, followed by the upper central and then the upper lateral incisors. The lower lateral incisors follow, the first deciduous molars, canines and second deciduous molars appearing in that order. By the age of 1 year most children have 6 to 8 teeth. Occasionally an infant has as few as 2 teeth at 1 year without other evidence of growth disturbance.

TABLE 2–1 MEDIAN VALUES FOR CIRCUMFERENCE OF HEAD AND OF THORAX BY AGE IN THE FIRST 5 YEARS OF LIFE

AGE	HEAD CIRCUMFERENCE		CHEST CIRCUMFERENCE	
Yr. Mo.	In.	Cm.	In.	Cm.
Birth	13.8	35.0	13.0	33.0
3	15.9	40.4	15.8	40.2
6	17.1	43.4	17.1	43.4
9	17.8	45.3	18.0	45.7
1–0	18.3	46.6	18.6	47.3
1–6	18.9	47.9	19.4	49.2
2–0	19.3	48.9	19.8	50.4
2–6	19.5	49.5	20.2	51.4
3–0	19.6	49.8	20.6	52.2
3–6	–	–	20.8	52.8
4–0	19.8	50.4	21.0	53.4
5–0	20.0	50.8	21.5	54.6

From studies at Harvard School of Public Health. For percentile distributions of these measurements by sex, see Table 2–7.

THE FIRST THREE MONTHS OF LIFE
(Table 2–5)

With adequate nutrition and mothering the infant will make rapid developmental progress during the first 3 months of life, his principal achievement being an appreciation of and relation to persons and objects in his environment. The newborn infant's range of behavior is limited, but there are qualities of excitation and inhibition and, even at this early age, differences among infants in levels of activity and in intensity of reactivity.

Recent studies emphasize that a major part of the interaction between mother and infant is initiated by the infant, not just as an expression of immediate need, but as a pattern of development in which the infant appears to be seeking an object (the mother) upon which to place certain responses. The newborn infant, for example, has complicated visual and visuomotor mechanisms which permit him not only to fixate points of contrast, movement or changing intensity of light within his visual fields but to maintain these fixations against passive movement of his own body during the first week or so of life; responses originally partly vestibular become increasingly oculomotor alone. The steady gaze of the newborn infant into the eyes of his mother is often felt by her as a powerful stimulus to emotional attachment.

The infant is generally able to fixate a light or bright object in the first hours or days of life, and will be able to follow it with his eyes for a few degrees away from the line of vision. He should be able to follow it through an arc of 180 degrees by the end of the second month.

When the newborn infant is placed prone upon a firm surface, he is able to avoid suffocation by turning his face from side to side. By 4 weeks of age he is able to lift his head above the surface. By 4 weeks the stiff and rather symmetrical flexed posture of the infant has become more relaxed, and he is likely to lie, when supine, in a tonic neck posture (head turned to one side).

When the infant within the first 4 to 8 weeks of life is pulled from a supine to a sitting position, the head lags, and with the infant in the upright position, head control is absent. By 12 weeks of age he has some control of his head as he is drawn to a sitting position, but holds the head forward when he is upright; irregular head control results in a bobbing motion.

The grasp reflex persists until the age of about 8 weeks, after which, with growing eye and hand coordination, active grasp becomes more evident; by 12 weeks the infant attempts to make contact with an offered object and will hold it briefly if appropriate contact is made. The coordination of eye and hand implicit in this activity seems to arise in some measure out of the tonic neck attitude. After 8 to 12 weeks the visual patterns in the environment which hold the attention of the infant are no longer dominated by contrast, movement or changes of intensity, but now by their resemblance to the human face.

By 8 weeks most infants will smile when social contact is made with them. The infant who at 4 weeks was able to vocalize small throaty noises and at 8 weeks to produce some vowel sounds will at 12 weeks produce these sounds with evident pleasure on social contact.

The 3 month old infant is still relatively undiscriminating as to persons in his environment; there is little evidence that various persons are differentiated as individuals. These social responses are important milestones, and the infant who does not have a social smile at the age of 12 weeks should be regarded as deviant with respect either to developmental potential or to quality of antecedent experiences.

Child-rearing practices differ widely in various parts of the world with respect to the attention accorded this age period. Little is known about the specific ways in which differing practices may modify the quality of socialization of the infant in these early months. There is reason, however, to feel that his sense of security will be optimally fostered when he is given care by a mother or mother-figure during this period in a prompt, confident and loving manner.

Both consistency and promptness seem important in the responses of the caretakers to the behavior of infant or child. The timing and quality of maternal responses to the infant, for example, may have powerful motivational impact. In instances of defective mothering the infant's normal or appropriate behavior may not be consistently or reliably rewarded by reduction of tension, or an effective maternal response may come so late and after so much anxiety or hostility, that the infant cannot associate any specific action of his own with relief of tension. Such infants may come to feel that they have no way to affect their environment through their own actions. Life-long retreat, anxiety or hostility may be the consequence.

THREE TO SIX MONTHS

(Table 2–5)

By the age of 3 months the infant placed prone upon a firm surface is generally able to raise his head and chest from the surface, with his arms extended before him. By 4 months he is able in this position to raise his head to a vertical position, and it can be turned easily from side to side. At 5 to 6 months of age the infant begins purposefully to roll over, at first from the prone to the supine position and then in the reverse direction.

Between 3 and 4 months of age the infant gradually abandons the tonic neck posture as his predominant posture, and the head becomes generally maintained in the midline, with the arms and legs in more or less symmetrical positions, and the hands often brought together in the midline or at the mouth. In this position the 4 to 6 month old infant often develops a bald spot over the occiput. By 4 months the infant becomes more adept in making contact with objects brought within reach and will often bring these to the midline and to the mouth for oral exploration.

When the infant of 4 months is pulled to a sitting position, the head is brought up without lag; in the upright position the head tilts a little forward, but is held steadily without bobbing. The head will be maintained erect and steady by 5 months of age.

By 4 to 5 months the infant will enjoy being supported in an upright posture and becomes increasingly attracted to objects presented on a plane surface. By 6 months of age he is able to change the orientation of the entire body in order to extend a hand toward a desired large object such as a rattle or ring.

At 4 months of age the infant will be able to grasp an object of moderate size, but will have difficulty in visualizing such a small object as a pellet. By 7 months the pellet is promptly seen and may be vigorously pursued by raking motions of the fingers, but the infant is not apt to be able to pick it up.

After 6 months the functions of the hand are increasingly lodged in the structures on the radial side, the thumb being used in conjunction with the palm. By 6 to 6½ months most infants can grasp a large object, such as a rattle, and transfer it from hand to hand.

At 6 to 6½ months the infant is often able to sit alone, leaning forward upon his hands, or with slight support; he will not yet have developed a lumbar lordosis, and the spine will have a gentle kyphotic curve from sacrum to cervical region. At 5 to 6 months the infant can often be pulled from a sitting to a standing position and will support his weight upon extended legs. At 6 to 6½ months, in this same position, he will often flex the knees momentarily and return to a standing posture.

By 3 to 4 months of age the infant ought to have

become clearly related to *objects* in his environment and to persons who give him care. By 4 months he is able to *laugh* aloud at pleasurable social contact. Moreover, if a pleasant contact is terminated, he may show displeasure by change of expression, fussing or crying. Between 4 and 7 months the infant begins to be responsive to the emotional tone of his social contacts, and by 7 months he will respond to changes in the facial expressions of those having close rapport with him. There is evidence that as early as 4 months of age the infant may be able to discriminate between the face of his mother and other faces in the environment; and by the end of the sixth month the normal infant will show a preference for contact with the person giving him most of his care.

SIX TO TWELVE MONTHS

(Table 2–5)

By 7 months the infant in the prone position is able to *pivot* in pursuit of an object, but if it is not within his reach, he may be unable to attain it. By 9 to 10 months most infants have learned to *creep* or to *crawl.*

The supine infant is able by 6 months or so to lift his head up and becomes increasingly interested in his legs. By 8 to 9 months he is able to assume a sitting position without help and soon is able to maintain this with the back straight. He is often able at 8 months to stand steady for a short while so long as his hands are held, and by 9 months may be able to take some steps with both hands held.

Between 6 and 9 months the radial palmar grasp becomes clearly elaborated into movements involving thumb and forefinger. The index finger is used to poke at objects by 9 months, and at this time the thumb and forefinger can be brought into sufficiently accurate apposition to permit a pellet to be picked up with a pincer motion. This movement is apt to be made with the ulnar surface of the hand supported on the same surface upon which the pellet lies. By 12 months the pincer movement will be executed without this ulnar support.

The infant is able to make repetitive vowel sounds at 6½ months and by 8 months is likely to execute repetitive consonant sounds, such as ba-ba, ma-ma, da-da, although not necessarily associating these sounds with objects. The child of 8 or 9 months becomes attentive at the sound of his own name. He may knowingly use 1 word besides ma-ma or da-da by the age of 1 year and may show by his behavior that he knows the names of some objects.

The preference for his mother which was manifested by the 6-month-old infant may, by 8 months, have evolved into a complaint when his mother leaves the room. About this same time a mother may experience difficulty in putting a baby to sleep who always went willingly before. Sometimes a mother whose child is fretful when she leaves the room can comfort him by maintaining vocal contact with him. By 9 to 10 months the infant begins to be less dependent upon the physical presence of his mother, partly because he is increasingly able to follow her around. It can be demonstrated also at this time that, if an object which has attracted his attention is covered with a cloth before he has an opportunity to grasp it, he is able to uncover it and grasp it with the apparent sure knowledge that its being out of sight did not mean that it was not available. Peek-a-boo often becomes a pleasant game about this time.

Between 6 and 12 months one sees the earliest beginnings of imitative behavior. At 6 months, if shown how to tap a table with a pencil, he may crudely imitate this behavior. At 9 months he will wave bye-bye or bring the hands together imitatively; at 12 months a child may enter into very simple games with a toy such as a ball.

At 9 months an infant may be able to release an object upon request, if the object is grasped as the request is made. By 1 year most infants will extend the object and release it into an offered hand.

The demands on mother and infant during the first year are for the development of comfortable interactions which will lead to the infant's movement from a position of dependency to one of independent activity. The satisfactions of the first year of life are gained in large measure through *oral* activity and through bodily contacts of feeding and other care. Failure of achievement of the developmental goals of the first year leads to emotional dissatisfaction or to chronic anxieties on the part of the infant, which may be the root of life-long personality disorders.

GROWTH AND DEVELOPMENT IN THE SECOND YEAR

During the second year of life there is a further deceleration in the rate of growth; the average child will gain about 2.5 kg (5 to 6 pounds) and about 12 cm (5 inches). (See Tables 2–5 and 2–7.) After 10 months of age there is often a decrease in appetite extending well into the second year. The result is a loss during the second year of some of the subcutaneous tissue which reached its maximal development around 9 months; the plump infant begins to change gradually to the lean and muscular child. The mild lordosis and protuberant abdomen appear which are characteristic of the second and third years of life.

The growth of the brain decelerates during the second year; head circumference, which increased approximately 12 cm (4+ inches) during the first year, will increase only 2 cm during the second year. By the end of the first year the brain has reached approximately two thirds, and at the end of the second year four fifths, of its adult size.

Weech suggested a useful set of mnemonics for recalling the height and weight of children during the preschool and school years; a slight modification is given in Table 2–2.

During the second year 8 more teeth erupt, mak-

TABLE 2–2 MNEMONICS (WEECH) FOR APPROXIMATE HEIGHT AND WEIGHT OF INFANTS AND CHILDREN

(a) At birth:	Weight (W) in lb	= 7 lb 6 oz (7.35 lb)
(b) From 3 to 12 months:	W (lb)	= age (mo) plus 11
(c) From 1 to 6 years:	W (lb)	= (age [yr] × 5) plus 17
(d) From 6 to 12 years:	W (lb)	= (age [yr] × 7) plus 5

Note: (c) and (d) give the same value (47 lb) at 6 years. 48 lb is a closer approximation of average. The following mnemonic is suggested: "Up to 5: 5A plus 17. From 7 on: 7A plus 5. At 6: use either one, but add 1."

(e) At birth:	*Length* = 20 in
(f) At one year:	*Length* = 30 in
(g) From 2 to 14 years:	*Height* (in) = (age [yr] × 2½) plus 30

ing a total of 14 to 16, including the first deciduous molars and the cuspids. The order of eruption may be irregular; the cuspids commonly appear after the first molars have erupted.

During the second year the infant moves from an awkward upright stance in which he could walk with support to a high degree of locomotor control. By 15 months he is generally able to walk alone, and by 18 months he may run stiffly. At this time he is able to sit down upon a chair of proper height.

At 18 months the infant can climb stairs, with one hand held, going one step at a time. By 20 months he is able to go downstairs, one hand held, and may be able to climb stairs holding to the stair railing. By 24 months he is able to run well and has generally outgrown the tendency to fall. Between 18 and 24 months the child normally enters the "run about" age. He is able to move quickly from a safe or protected environment into danger and will need constant surveillance.

With the second year the infant enters a period when he will vigorously and imitatively exploit the objects in his environment. He can empty waste baskets, drawers and shelves and may try to examine everything within his reach. Fragile objects and certainly all household poisons, drugs and chemicals must be kept in places inaccessible to him.

The child who at 12 months was able to release a pellet into the hand of a person requesting it will at 15 months generally be able to put the pellet into a small bottle. He may attempt to remove the pellet from the bottle by inserting his finger; by 18 months he will be able to dump a pellet from a glass bottle.

By 15 months the child is able to put a 1-inch cube on top of another in response to a demonstration; by 18 months he is able to make a tower of 3 cubes and by 24 months a tower of 6 cubes. Imitative behavior and conceptual behavior continue to evolve, with spontaneous scribbling and with imitation of vertical lines at 18 months; by 24 months the child imitates circular strokes and can make a horizontal line.

The normal infant, who often has 1 word besides ma-ma or da-da by the end of the first year, commonly has a vocabulary of 10 words by 18 months. There is wide variation in the times at which words begin to flow readily; it is not unusual for an entirely normal child to have few or no sounds conveying a definite meaning until 18 months or later. Some children with delay in development of recognizable speech have a rich jargon before communicative sounds appear; this jargon often has many of the intonations and punctuations of human speech, but the sounds otherwise convey no meaning. In those normal children in whom speech is delayed to 18 or 20 months, there is often rapid acquisition of words and meaning after this time, with the result that most normal children by their second birthday are able to put 3 words together.

The 3 words which the child puts together at the end of the second year are likely to be subject, verb and object. This ability appears to reflect the growing awareness in the child of his individuality, so that the subject of the short sentence is often "me." Shortly thereafter he is able to use the nominative "I" in an appropriate manner.

During the second year the child becomes highly imitative. He becomes increasingly aware of and responsive to other persons, including siblings. Until the end of the second year, however, the infant's play is generally solitary and consists in active manipulation of objects available to him. During the third year of life he moves increasingly into play activities in which other children are involved. By the end of the fourth year the child is increasingly engaged in activity with other children in which the group begins to enact imaginative roles and activities. This tendency to role-playing will increase into the school years.

By 18 to 24 months most children are able to verbalize their toilet needs and can be helped at this time to follow acceptable social patterns in meeting them. In settings in which the young child has adequate models to follow it seems increasingly evident that toilet training need not become the focus of either emotion-laden educational activity on the part of parents or disciplinary concern.

The need for the child to submit his growing control of his body and of his environment to social and cultural pressures often produces frustration and anger in him. Temper tantrums, breath-holding spells and less dramatic outbursts are common consequences. These episodes respond best to management by a firm and loving parent who is able to set the necessary limits for the child.

GROWTH AND DEVELOPMENT DURING THE PRESCHOOL YEARS

During the third, fourth and fifth years of life gains in weight and height are relatively steady at approximately 2.0 kg (4.5 pounds) and about 8 to 6 cm ($3\frac{1}{2}$ to $2\frac{1}{2}$ inches) per year, respectively (see Table 2–5). Most children are lean relative to their earlier body configuration. The lordosis and protuberant abdomen of late infancy tend to disappear by the fourth year along with the pads of fat which underlie the normal arches of the feet during the earlier years.

By $2\frac{1}{2}$ years the 20 deciduous teeth have usually erupted. During the rest of the preschool period the face tends to grow proportionately more than the cranial cavity and the jaw to widen preparatory to the eruption of permanent teeth.

The refinement of motor skills includes alternation of the feet in ascending stairs by 3 years and alternation in descending stairs by 4 years. By 3 years most children can stand for a short period on 1 foot; by 5 years they are generally able to hop on 1 foot and soon to skip.

By 3 years an infant may be able to imitate crudely the drawing of a cross. By 4 years the cross figure may be copied without previous demonstration, possibly as a 4-element figure. By 5 years the child can make correctly proportionate copies of the figures and for the first time becomes able to handle figures with slanting lines, such as triangles. A diamond-shaped figure may not be accurately and proportionately reproduced until the sixth year.

By 3 years the child is able to count three objects correctly; a 4 year old, four; a 5 year old, 10 or more.

By 3 years most children can state their ages and whether they are boys or girls. With the increasing awareness that they are destined to become larger children and adults, children in the later preschool period begin to seek adequate models by which to learn and play their future roles. The most accessible models are, of course, the parents and other members of the immediate family. The child's imperfect perception of the realities of his future often engenders conflicting pressures and anxieties. The so-called Oedipus situation may be regarded as the natural setting in which a child of 4, 5 or 6 years assumes those habits of thought, feeling and action which surround his growing perception or fantasy as to his future life. Inside the home the child's fantasies about his future role include playing the part of the parent of the same sex, and he may have an increasing curiosity and concern as to what the realities of this role may be, along with more general questions and fantasies as to the origin of babies, differences between boys and girls, and the like.

Outside the home, concerns and fantasies about future roles are likely to be expressed in play, children assuming the parts of exciting figures ranging in immediate knowledge of them from milkman to jet pilot. The interest of children of this age in sex differences, which often appears as questions inside the home, may appear in the form of sex play among children of each sex. This is so common as to appear to be entirely normal, although neither questions about reproductive or sexual matters nor sex play among small children is likely to be received with equanimity by parents in Western culture.

This is a time when the changing pattern of parent-child interaction and of other relations in and out of the home often leaves elements of hostility or aggression in the child's behavior, thoughts and fantasies. Anxieties may be expressed as nightmares or as fears of separation, death or bodily injury. Children with serious problems may display bedwetting or thumb-sucking, speech or learning difficulties, inability to enter into a comfortable sharing relation with others, temper tantrums or other behavior appropriate to earlier developmental levels.

With the development of the child's ability to translate his conception of abstract forms into figures and structures, by the age of 6 he should be ready for formal education.

GROWTH AND DEVELOPMENT DURING THE EARLY SCHOOL YEARS

The early school years are a period of relatively steady growth beginning by about the age of 6 years and ending in a preadolescent growth spurt by about the age of 10 in girls and about 12 in boys. The average gain in weight during these years is about 3 to 3.5 kg (7 pounds) per year, and that in height approximately 6 cm ($2\frac{1}{2}$ inches) per year. Growth in head circumference is much slower than earlier, the circumference increasing from about 51 cm (20 inches) to 53 to 54 cm (21 inches) between the ages of 5 and 12 years. At the end of this period the brain has reached virtually adult size.

The school years are a time of vigorous physical activity. The spine becomes straighter, but the child's body is supple, and postural attitudes may be assumed which are often disturbing to parents and to teachers. Mild degrees of knock-knee or flatfoot which may be apparent in the late preschool years tend to correct during the first year or two of the school years. The crude motor activities, such as running and climbing of the earlier years, become increasingly directed to more specialized activities and games requiring particular motor and muscular skills.

The development of the facial bones continues actively during the school years, particularly with enlargement of the sinuses. The frontal sinus has usually made its appearance by the seventh year.

The first permanent teeth, the first molars, most often erupt during the seventh year of life. With these so-called 6-year molars in place, the shedding of deciduous teeth begins, following approximately the same sequence as their acquisition. They are replaced at a rate of about 4 teeth a year over the next 7 years. The second permanent molars are commonly erupted by the fourteenth year; the third molars are irregular in their occurrence and time of eruption and may not appear until the early twenties.

Lymphatic tissues are at the peak of their development during these years and generally exceed the amount of such tissue in the normal adult. The abundance of lymphoid tissue during this time of life bears some relation to the frequency with which tonsillectomy and adenoidectomy are incorrectly recommended. Respiratory infections are common during these years, and the response of the child to infection begins to be more like that of the adult than of the infant or young child. The usual number of respiratory infections during the school years is high; as many as 6 or 7 illnesses a year is not uncommon.

With the removal of a large portion of the child's life from the home to the school environment, children begin increasingly to live independently and to look outside the home for goals and for standards of behavior. This shifting of interests is often anxiety-provoking for parents. Needless to say, if earlier problems between parent and child have not been adequately resolved, adjustments to forces outside the home are apt to be difficult.

A large responsibility of the school years is the creation in the child of the senses of duty, of responsibility and of accomplishment. There is a possibility of great frustration for parents and children when the child's achievement does not measure up to parental hopes or expectations. The child unable to meet adequate standards may learn for the first time the sense of *failure* and may react with anxiety and hostility to the school situation or to specific persons. Antisocial behavior may develop through which the child attempts to gain recognition which he cannot attain otherwise.

GROWTH AND DEVELOPMENT IN ADOLESCENCE

Adolescence comprises nearly half of the growing period in man. It has its beginning by about the age of 10 years in girls and 12 in boys. The end of adolescence is not clearly delineated and varies with the physical, emotional, mental, social or cultural criteria which define the adult. The word *puberty* is used to designate an arbitrary point in the continuum of maturation: the menarche in girls, and some less clearly defined event occurring approximately 2 years later in boys. *Pubescence,* which is the time during which secondary changes such as pubic hair are appearing, is not clearly demarcated as to length, but it seems to be about 2 to 3 years. *Prepubescent* changes precede the first secondary sex changes of adolescence and are integral elements of maturation.

Growth and development in adolescence must be considered separately for boys and girls. Some parameters of growth differ in boys and girls from early infancy. Boys on the average are larger than girls from birth to the prepubescent period, and their deciduous teeth erupt somewhat earlier. They have slightly less subcutaneous fat during the middle years of childhood and a slightly higher basal metabolic rate when referred to body surface. Boys and girls have much the same degree of motor activity and coordination until the age of 7 or 8 years, but by 9 years, while still preadolescent, boys move ahead of girls in some motor skills. By contrast, the acquisition of permanent dentition, another preadolescent growth feature, is earlier in girls than in boys.

For both boys and girls there is wide individual variability in the time of onset and rate of acquisition of adolescent changes. Not all the factors are known which contribute to this variability; some certainly are genetic, some nutritional and others socioeconomic. Neither climatic nor racial differences in average rates of adolescent growth seem well established. Growth in height occurs at an accelerated rate in the spring months, growth in weight in the fall of the year.

Individual variability in the progress of events in adolescence is best documented in longitudinal studies which indicate that growth patterns are established early in life and tend to follow a consistent course within set limits for each child. It has been shown, for example, that as early as 2 years of age those children who will be slow to mature at adolescence are smaller than their contemporaries. Girls in whom the menarche occurs early have a greater velocity of growth, but a shorter growth period, during adolescence. Girls who mature early continue to have an increased ratio of weight to height in adult life when compared to those who mature more slowly.

A trend toward increasing height and weight of adults has been evident over the past 100 years and probably longer. This trend can be observed in heights and weights of children as early as the seventh year of life. Concurrently there has been a tendency to earlier appearance of the menarche; in the United States the average age at menarche is now 1 year earlier (just under 13 years) than it was 50 years ago.

PREPUBESCENT AND POSTPUBESCENT PHASES OF MATURATION

The earliest indications of specific preparatory change for adolescence seem to occur by about 7 years of age in both boys and girls; at this time there is an increased production of adrenal steroids. Shortly afterward there is a gradual increase in production of estrogen and a little later of androgen in each sex. At the onset of pubescent changes in girls (9 to 11 years) estrogen production becomes greatly increased, attaining the levels for normal adults; similarly, increased androgen production occurs in boys between the ages of 12 and 14 years. The differences between male and female adult output of 17-ketosteroids become established after 14 to 16 years of age.

The fat in subcutaneous tissue, which showed a steady proportionate decrease in amount from the ages of 1 to 6 years in both sexes, begins to reaccumulate as early as 8 years in girls and 10 years in boys. This reaccumulation will be clinically apparent as a filling out of subcutaneous tissue in most girls and in about two thirds of boys. This increase in fat content will tend to remain in girls, but will be a temporary feature of most boys, much being lost during the adolescent growth spurts in height and weight.

About a year after the increase in fat is first apparent the general growth spurt is initiated; it is concomitant in both sexes with the first signs of secondary sex maturation. Urinary gonadotropins may generally be detected by this time.

The earliest secondary sex changes observed in boys are usually an increase in the size of the testes and scrotum and later of the penis. About a third of boys have some conspicuous swelling of the breasts, often unilateral, and commonly with a small, sometimes tender, lump of tissue centrally located behind the nipple. This may persist for several months. Pubic, axillary and facial hair appears in that order, a sparse growth of downy pubic hair occurring close to the time of early enlargement of the testes and penis, becoming darker and more heavily pigmented within a year's time and, over the next 2 or 3 years, more curly and more extensive until the adult distribution is reached. Axillary hair usually appears about 2 years after pubic hair, along with facial hair. The change of voice occurs gradually, beginning with the early pubescent phase, and nocturnal emissions occur for the first time about a year after the beginning of secondary sex changes. There is some uncertainty as to when fully competent spermatozoa begin to be produced; relative infertility may extend in males to the fifteenth or sixteenth year or later.

In girls the secondary sex changes of pubescence have their onset on the average 2 years earlier than in boys. An increase in the width of the pelvis follows shortly upon the establishment of the secretion of estrogen and is most pronounced during the year of most rapid growth which just precedes the menarche. The first overt sign of pubescence is generally development of the breasts. Occasionally pubic hair will appear first, by as much as a year, and rarely the development of either breasts or pubic hair may anticipate true pubescence by a number of years—premature thelarche or pubarche. Axillary hair appears approximately a year after pubic hair. Along with early breast development, the vaginal secretion changes from alkaline to acid, and Doederlein's bacillus becomes established as the predominant flora.

About 2 years after the first evident pubescent change in the breasts the menarche is likely to occur. It is commonly preceded for several months by a regularly recurrent, clear vaginal discharge. The first few menstrual periods may be anovular, and irregularity is not unusual; this irregularity, sometimes with mild menorrhagia, is sufficiently common to be a normal variant, and generally subsides within a year after menarche. Irregularities after this time will be related more often to factors of general health, such as nutrition, fatigue or emotional tensions, than to primary endocrine or glandular abnormalities.

In both boys and girls the order of events in adolescence is subject to some variability and the time of onset to wide variability. The generally acceptable range of onset of pubescent changes in boys is from 10 to 14 years of age and in girls from 8 to 13 years. The earlier onset of the prepubescent growth spurt in girls decrees that, though boys are generally larger than girls of the same age for the first 11 years of life, between 11 and 13 years they will generally be smaller. The maximum increase in physical growth in girls occurs just before the menarche, at an average age of just under 13 years, with a range from 10 to 16 years. In boys the maximum increase occurs at a less well defined point with respect to the beginning of pubescent changes, about 2 years after the first change.

Radiographic examination of the epiphyses (bone age) gives the best indication of physiologic maturity in adolescence. For example, the standard deviation of chronologic age at menarche in relation to the mean age at menarche is 0.94 year, whereas the standard deviation of osseous age at menarche in relation to the mean chronologic age is only 0.44 year. The closure of the epiphyses occurs rapidly as the general growth spurt subsides.

In the period of rapid growth just preceding the menarche in girls or in the corresponding period in boys, there are increased retentions of nitrogen and calcium which fall to substantially lower levels in the following period of deceleration of growth. The slipped capital femoral epiphysis is particularly likely to appear in tall, heavy children during the active growth period, and vertebral epiphysitis during the following period, when growth of extremities has ceased, but vertebral growth continues a while longer.

The tendency of girls to retain fat accumulated during the prepubescent phase is matched by a tendency on the part of boys and a few girls to expand muscle mass in the later adolescent period. Boys grow rapidly in muscular strength and coordination after the average age of 13 years.

Other differentials between male and female become established during adolescence; these include the lower red blood cell counts and hemoglobin levels characteristic of women, the increased creatinine output in males, stabilization of basal body temperature at a level somewhat higher in females than in males, and a possibly related increased heart rate in girls. The blood pressure and pulse pressure attain normal adult values during adolescence, being slightly higher in boys than in girls. Respiratory rate and volume are higher for boys, as are maximal breathing capacity and alveolar carbon dioxide. This last appears related to the large muscle mass in males and is accompanied by a slightly higher average plasma bicarbonate level.

Social and educational activities for adolescents are set at levels determined by school achievement or chronologic age, rather than by physiologic maturity. The peak of physical differential between the sexes is reached in the eighth grade, when most girls are larger than their male classmates, a fact which gives the school dance and other social activities a mildly grotesque air. The slowly maturing child is often left out of social activities and team sports. By the time he or she matures physically the opportunity may have been lost for self-realization in some of these areas. The emotional integrity of adolescents is threatened by physical and sensory changes, by their changing status at home and in the community and by anxious preoccupation as to the meaning or adequacy of these changes and of their relation to their future roles in society. The physician can often be of great help to the adolescent in interpreting these changes in a friendly and casual way, with reassurance that physical changes are following normal and expected pathways.

The physician will often find himself under pressure to relieve anxiety through action other than reassurance. He may be urged, for example, to give hormones to the small boy to make him larger or to the tall girl to limit her ultimate height. An adequate assessment of growth records and of the present developmental status of the child in respect to chronologic age will generally permit reasonable predictions to be made. A slowly maturing boy of 16 or 17 may need study for hypogenitalism *(q.v.)*, and sometimes a trial of therapy. The long-range effects of using estrogen in tall girls to reduce ultimate height by hastening epiphyseal closure have not yet been assessed adequately.

Medical problems of adolescence include overnutrition and undernutrition, sometimes related to dietary habits determined by social pressure rather than by absence of adequate diet at home. Fatigue is common in adolescence and may be related to protein or iron deficiency, the latter sometimes expressed not so much by anemia as by lessened optimal function of enzyme systems using heme prosthetic groups. During adolescence there is heightened susceptibility to some illnesses and heightened reactivity to others. Myopia commonly has its onset during adolescence, as may some orthopedic conditions leading to kyphosis or scoliosis.

Acne adds to the physical and emotional burden of adolescents, leading as it does to some disfigurement and accompanied as it is by a complex folklore. Adolescents are often reluctant to discuss their acne with the physician, who often must initiate its management.

The most significant health problem of adolescence is the frequency with which serious accidents occur. These are often directly related to the intense physical activity and emotional strivings of this age, particularly in boys. In the accident-prone child repeated accidents may be related to poorly solved problems of earlier life.

The hallmark of adolescence Erikson refers to as the *identity crisis,* a crisis because the increasing emotional tension and pressure of biologic drives must meet and ultimately accommodate to increased demands and expectations from the environment. The process of attaining one's own *identity* or "finding oneself" in adolescence and early adulthood has become prolonged in Western culture as the duration of formal education and dependency increases, and has become complicated by the breakdown of traditional patterns of family life and social class. The quest for one's own set of values involves gender identity, social class identity and vocational and avocational identity, and takes place increasingly in the community outside the home.

A further stage in development Erikson calls *intimacy,* which is being able to avoid emotional isolation, or an inability to relate to others, in favor of skill and comfort in shared close experiences. Intimacy requires facing the fear of rejection in shared physical activities such as sports, in close friendships and in sexual experiences. Intimacy is a private affair, not usually shared with parents. Intimacy implies the sharing of feelings, which is the essential quality of empathy, the ability to know how others feel and to respond understandingly.

Erikson's next stage he calls *generativity,* "the interest in establishing and guiding the next generation or whatever in any given case may become the absorbing object of a parental kind of responsibility." Generativity involves the commitments of persons to each other in love affairs, courtship or marriage, or to other accepted responsibilities or tasks.

The final stage of growth is *ego integrity.* Erikson visualizes this as the ability "to accept one's individual life cycle and the people who have become significant to it as meaningful within the segment of history in which one lives.... Integrity thus means a new and different love of one's parents, free of the wish that they should have been different and an acceptance of the fact that one's life is one's own responsibility. It is a sense of comradeship with men and women of distant times and of different pursuits, who have created orders and objects and sayings conveying human dignity and love."

SPECIAL ASPECTS OF GROWTH

Many structural and functional details of growth and development are inconspicuous for the broad pattern outlined above, but take on significance as they become foci of clinical concern or contribute to the evaluation or management of a clinical problem. The physician who monitors the growth and development of the child will need to know or find the limits of normal variability in these details, not only quantitatively and qualitatively, but also with respect to their interrelations.

VARIABILITY IN BODY PROPORTIONS

Besides the profound changes in general body proportions between fetal life and adult life (Fig. 2–5), there are also individual differences which seem to be the expression of innate growth potential and environmental modifications. These variations in body forms of normal persons may be designated as differences in *physique.* The term *constitution* connotes loosely the potentialities inherent in the individual at the time of birth for the development of a particular physique. Sheldon classified the physical types of man into three broad groups: the ectomorphic, the mesomorphic and the endomorphic (Fig. 2–6). The ectomorphic group is characterized principally by relative linearity, relatively light bone structure and relatively small mass in respect to body length. The endomorphic group is characterized by relatively stocky build and relatively large amounts of soft tissue. The pattern of the mesomorph is between that of the ectomorph and the endomorph. A variety of psychic and other functional attributes may be loosely related to constitution and to body type.

Somatotype is sometimes evident in early childhood, and at other times becomes clear only with the termination of the growth period. Somatotype does not seem to be closely related to the ultimate height or weight achieved, but the endomorph appears to mature earlier than the ectomorph. As a result of this early maturation the endomorphic child may have a tendency to be taller than the ectomorphic one in late childhood, the differences being reduced as the ectomorph completes his growth.

Other changes in bodily proportions depend not upon constitution or somatotype, but on different rates of growth of various body parts. The most conspicuous changes are in head size relative to body length, and length of the extremities relative to total body length. The size of the brain and cranial cavity approaches adult levels much more rapidly than the size of the face or the length of the legs. This relative preponderance of growth at the cephalad part of the body in fetal life, infancy and early childhood, with corresponding early elaboration of function, followed by the growth of trunk and extremities, has been termed the cephalocaudad progression. One of the last consequences of this for man is that the adolescent may find the extremities growing more rapidly than skills can be developed in their utilization.

Alterations in proportionate sizes of trunk, extremities and head are characteristic of certain disturbances of growth, and may give insight as to the underlying pathophysiologic process. The measurements which are usually most helpful will be

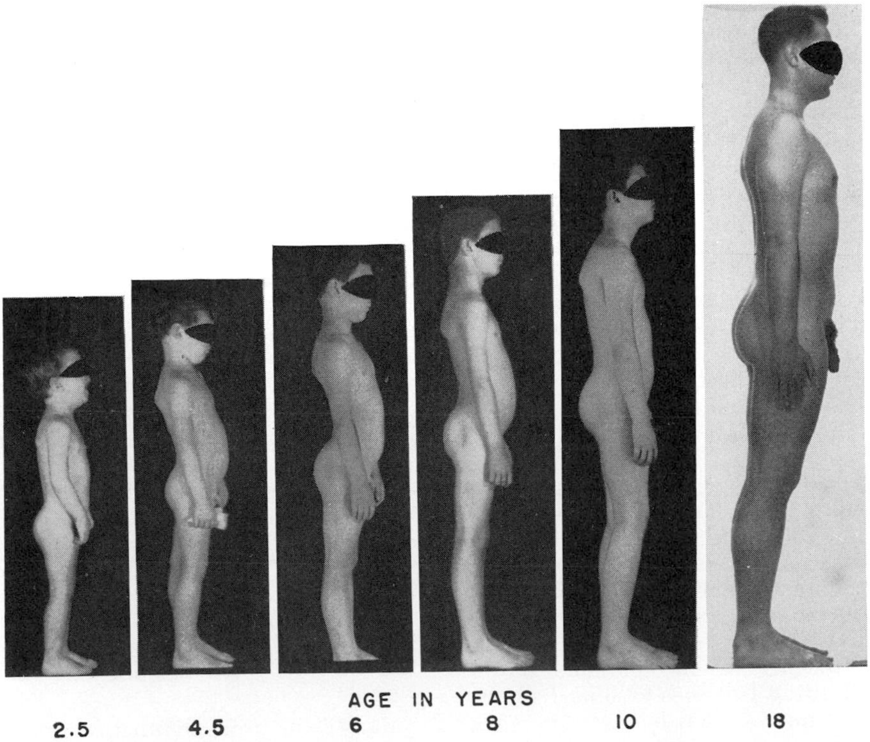

Figure 2–5 *Lateral photographs which show characteristic developmental changes in body proportions and in erect posture. (From unpublished studies at Harvard School of Public Health.)*

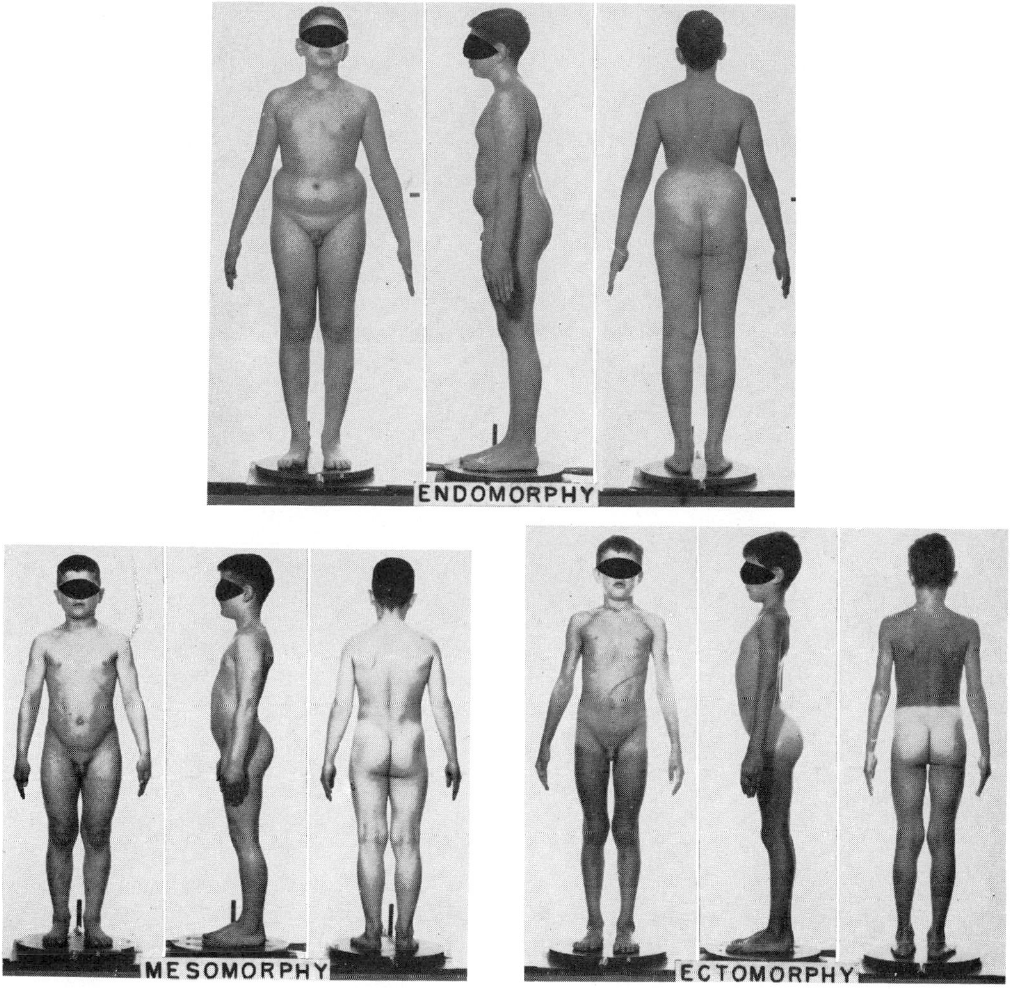

Figure 2–6 *Examples of dominance of the three types of body build according to somatotype classification of Sheldon.* (Photos provided by E. E. Hunt, Forsyth Dental Infirmary, Boston.)*

The principal characteristics of each of the three components of bodily constitution, some of which may be recognized in these photographs, are as follows:

Endomorphy—*relative preponderance of soft roundness throughout the body, with large digestive viscera and accumulations of fat, usually large trunk and thighs and tapering extremities.*

Mesomorphy—*relative preponderance of muscle, bone and connective tissue, with heavy, hard physique of rectangular outline.*

Ectomorphy—*relative preponderance of linearity and fragility, with large surface area and thin muscles and subcutaneous tissue.*

**Sheldon: The Varieties of Human Physique, New York, Harper & Brothers, 1940.*

sitting and standing heights, span, body weight, and circumference of head. Normally the sitting height represents about 70 per cent of body length in the newborn infant, but only 57 per cent at 3 years, and about 52 per cent at the time of the menarche in girls and about 15 years in boys. Following this lowest ratio, there is a slight increase of 1 or 2 percentage points, as the trunk continues and the extremities have ceased their growth in the postpubescent period.

Other variations in rapid growth, again correlated with function, are distinctive for a number of body systems. Figure 2–7 illustrates the proportionate rates of growth for several body systems. Standards are available for the weights of organs at various ages, which indicate that organs follow characteristic patterns which may be designated as lymphoid, neural, general and genital. There are a number of deviations. For example, although the ovary and testes follow the designated genital pattern, the uterus and adrenals are relatively large at birth, and show involution in the early weeks of life. The spleen appears to follow the lymphoid pattern, and the liver the general growth pattern. Skeletal muscle follows the general pattern, but is slow to achieve its ultimate mass. Cardiac muscle is initially proportionately large to body size and thereafter follows the general growth curve.

The weight of the thymus is labile in childhood,

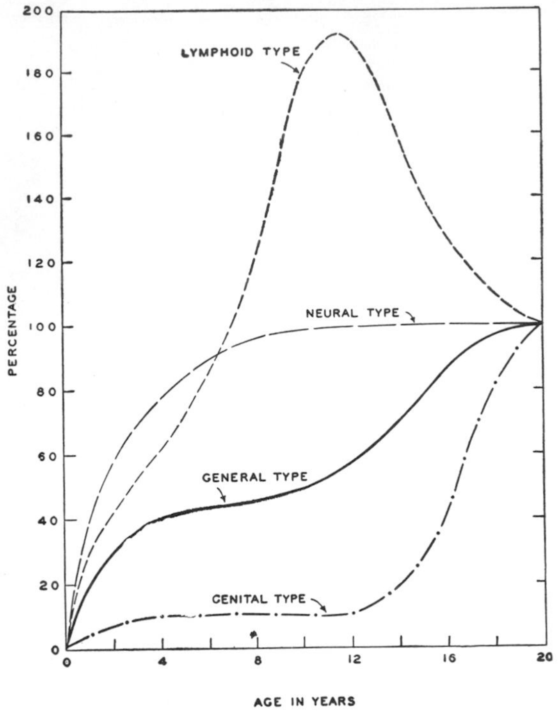

Figure 2–7 *Main types of postnatal growth of the various parts and organs of the body. (After Scammon: The measurement of the body in childhood. In Harris et al.: The Measurement of Man. Minneapolis, University of Minnesota Press, 1930.)*

decreasing rapidly during illness. It appears to follow the general pattern of growth during the first 5 years of life, then maintains a relatively steady state, with involution at adolescence.

As indicated earlier, the proportionate mass of subcutaneous tissue is greatest by about 9 months; it then decreases steadily to about 6 years, when the increase begins which presages the "fat spurt" in preadolescence, at which time sex differences become apparent (Fig. 2–8).

EVALUATION OF OSSEOUS MATURATION

The ossification of the skeleton of the fetus begins by about the fifth month and from that time makes considerable demands upon the maternal supply of bone-forming substances. Ossification occurs earliest in the clavicles and membranous bone of the skull, and follows rapidly in long bones and spine. The distal femoral and proximal tibial epiphyses are usually ossified in the normal full-term infant. The fusion of the humeral capitellum with the shaft is said to mark the end of the period of most rapid growth in girls and to predict the menarche within the next year.

There is no better index of general growth than bone age as determined from roentgenograms. This is based (1) on the number and size of epiphyseal centers at a given chronologic age, (2) on the size, shape, density, and sharpness of outline of the ends of bones, and (3) on the distance separating epiphyseal center and zone of provisional calcification or the degree of fusion between these 2 elements. The information gained from the various epiphyseal areas varies with chronologic age. The hand and wrist are useful at all ages of childhood; useful information can also be derived from the lower extremity, especially in early infancy. The most widely used standards are those of Todd, of Greulich and Pyle, and of Vogt and Vickers for the hand. Reynolds and Asakawa have provided useful standards for the lower extremity, head of the

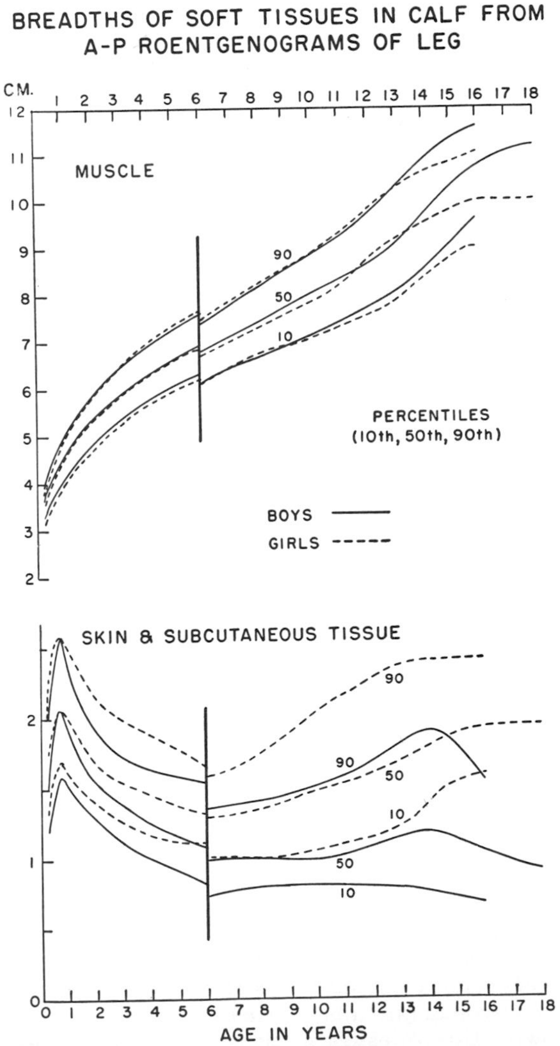

Figure 2–8 *Breadths of muscle and of double layers of skin and subcutaneous tissue at greatest width of calf by age and sex from 3 months to 18 years of age. The graphs reveal the close similarity in pattern of the curves for muscle to those of general growth, but a unique pattern of increase and decrease and a sex difference in the skin and subcutaneous tissue. (For details, see Stuart and Sobel: J. Pediatr., 28:637, 1946, and Lombard: Child Dev., Vol. 21, 1950. For distribution of subcutaneous fat in childhood and adolescence, see Reynolds: Monographs Soc. Res. Child Dev., Vol. 15, 1950.)*

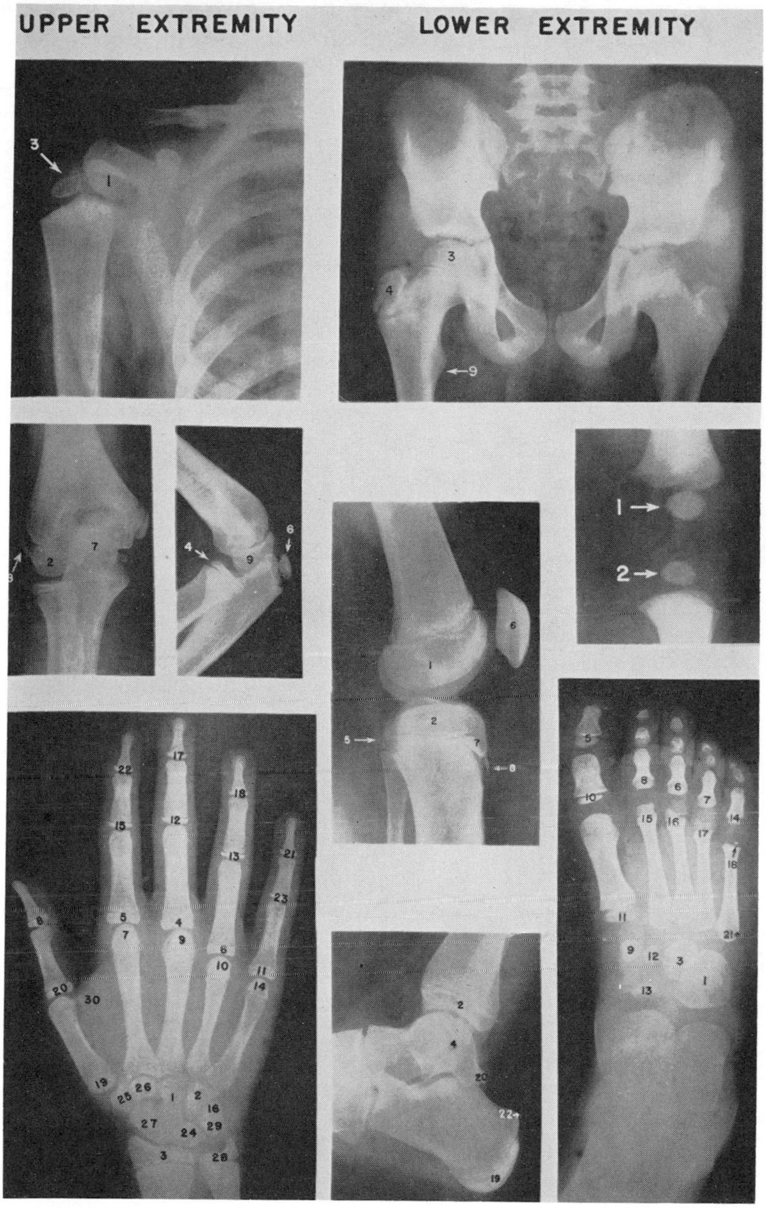

Figure 2–9 *Centers of ossification in the extremities for use in referring to Table 2–3. Roentgenograms of children of different ages selected to show as clearly as possible the epiphyseal centers of interest in each view and to identify them by the numbers which correspond to those in Table 2–3. (Figure prepared by I. Pyle, D. G. Shields, and W. H. Golden.)*

humerus, and capitellum in early infancy. Figure 2–9 and Table 2–3 show expected times of appearance of various ossification centers, with normal variabilities for each. Since girls are more advanced than boys in skeletal development at all ages, separate standards are necessary.

No interpretation of skeletal age should fail to take into account that 1 normal child in 20 can be expected to have a skeletal age either advanced or retarded by 2 standard deviations from the mean for his chronologic age. Data of Pyle, Reed and Stuart indicate that in boys the standard deviation of bone age (given by the norms of Greulich and Pyle) around chronologic age is about 2 months in the first year of life, and increases to 4 months during the second year, to 6 months during the third year, and to 10 months by the seventh year. Thereafter, for the rest of the growth period, the standard deviation is about 12 to 15 months. The variability is less for girls than for boys, especially in later childhood. The theoretical percentile points corresponding to such variability can be calculated.

EVALUATION OF DENTAL DEVELOPMENT

The calcification of teeth begins in fetal life about the seventh month. This calcification involves principally deciduous teeth, but shortly before term calcification begins in the permanent teeth which will be first to erupt. Nutritional dis-

TABLE 2–3 AGES AT ONSET OF OSSIFICATION, RECOGNIZED BY APPEARANCE OF CENTERS IN ROENTGENOGRAMS, USEFUL AS MATURITY INDICATORS DURING INFANCY AND CHILDHOOD

BOYS			NO. CORRESPONDING TO CENTER IN FIG. 2-9	BONE AND OSSIFICATION CENTER	GIRLS		
Mean		*Standard Deviation**			*Mean*		*Standard Deviation**
Yrs	*Mos*	*Mos*			*Yrs*	*Mos*	*Mos*
				Shoulder and Elbow			
3 weeks		—	1	Humerus, head	3 weeks		—
0	7	4	2	Humerus, capitellum	0	4	2
1	1	7	3	Humerus, greater tuberosity	0	6	3
5	5	15	4	Radius, proximal epiphysis	4	1	14
6	1	15	5	Humerus, medial epicondyle	3	7	12
—	—	—	6	Ulna, olecranon, 1	—	—	—
—	—	—	7	Humerus, trochlea	—	—	—
—	—	—	8	Humerus, lateral epicondyle	—	—	—
—	—	—	9	Ulna, olecranon, 2	—	—	—
				Hand and Wrist			
0	2	2	1	Capitate	0	2	2
0	3	2	2	Hamate	0	2	2
1	1	5	3	Distal epiphysis, radius	0	10	4
1	4	4	4	Proximal epiphysis, 3rd finger	0	10	3
1	4	4	5	Proximal epiphysis, 2nd finger	0	11	3
1	5	5	6	Proximal epiphysis, 4th finger	0	11	3
1	6	5	7	Epiphysis of metacarpal II	1	0	3
1	7	7	8	Distal epiphysis, 1st finger	1	0	4
1	8	5	9	Epiphysis of metacarpal III	1	1	3
1	11	6	10	Epiphysis of metacarpal IV	1	3	4
1	9	5	11	Proximal epiphysis, 5th finger	1	2	4
2	0	6	12	Middle epiphysis, 3rd finger	1	3	5
2	0	6	13	Middle epiphysis, 4th finger	1	3	5
2	2	7	14	Epiphysis of metacarpal V	1	4	5
2	2	6	15	Middle epiphysis, 2nd finger	1	4	5
2	6	16	16	Triquetral	1	9	14
2	4	6	17	Distal epiphysis, 3rd finger	1	6	4
2	4	6	18	Distal epiphysis, 4th finger	1	6	15
2	8	9	19	Epiphysis of metacarpal I	1	6	5
2	8	7	20	Proximal epiphysis, 1st finger	1	8	5
3	1	9	21	Distal epiphysis, 5th finger	1	11	6
3	1	8	22	Distal epiphysis, 2nd finger	1	11	6
3	3	10	23	Middle epiphysis, 5th finger	1	10	7
3	6	19	24	Lunate	2	10	13
5	7	19	25	Greater multangular	3	11	14
5	9	15	26	Lesser multangular	4	1	12
5	6	15	27	Navicular (hand)	4	3	12
6	10	14	28	Distal epiphysis of ulna	5	9	13
—	—	—	29	Pisiform	—	—	—
12	8	18	30	Sesamoid in adductor pollicis	10	1	13
				Hip and Knee			
(Usually at birth)			1	Femur, distal epiphysis	(Usually at birth)		
(Usually at birth)			2	Tibia, proximal epiphysis	(Usually at birth)		
0	4	2	3	Femur, head	0	4	2
3	6	10	4	Femur, greater trochanter	2	5	5
3	9	12	5	Fibula, proximal epiphysis	2	9	11
3	10	11	6	Patella	2	5	7
—	—	—	7	Tibia, tuberosity, 1	—	—	—
—	—	—	8	Tibia, tuberosity, 2	—	—	—

* *Standard deviation* adjusted to nearest month. The range included between minus 1 and plus 1 standard deviation from the mean for any center will usually include about 68 per cent of a population of healthy children.

TABLE 2-3 *(Continued)*

BOYS			NO. CORRESPONDING TO CENTER IN FIG. 2-9	BONE AND OSSIFICATION CENTER	GIRLS		
Mean		*Standard Deviation**			*Mean*		*Standard Deviation**
Yrs	*Mos*	*Mos*			*Yrs*	*Mos*	*Mos*
				Foot and Ankle			
2 weeks		—	1	Cuboid	2 weeks		—
0	4	2	2	Tibia, distal epiphysis	0	4	1
0	4	4	3	Lateral cuneiform	0	4	4
1	1	4	4	Fibula, distal epiphysis	0	9	3
1	4	6	5	Distal epiphysis, great toe	0	9	3
1	7	5	6	Proximal epiphysis, 3rd toe	0	11	4
1	8	5	7	Proximal epiphysis, 4th toe	1	1	4
1	9	5	8	Proximal epiphysis, 2nd toe	1	1	4
2	1	10	9	Medial cuneiform	1	4	7
2	4	5	10	Proximal epiphysis, great toe	1	6	4
2	5	5	11	Metatarsal I	1	7	3
2	5	9	12	Middle cuneiform	1	7	7
2	7	13	13	Navicular (foot)	1	9	10
2	7	7	14	Proximal epiphysis, 5th toe	1	8	5
2	10	7	15	Metatarsal II	2	0	5
3	5	8	16	Metatarsal III	2	5	5
3	11	8	17	Metatarsal IV	2	9	7
4	5	10	18	Distal epiphysis, metatarsal V	3	2	8
7	5	11	19	Calcaneus, epiphysis, 1	5	0	11
—	—	—	20	Accessory talus	—	—	—
—	—	—	21	Proximal epiphysis, metatarsal V	—	—	—
—	—	—	22	Calcaneus, epiphysis, 2	—	—	—

AGE AT ONSET OF FUSION IN SKELETAL REGIONS USEFUL AS MATURITY INDICATORS DURING ADOLESCENCE

BOYS	SKELETAL REGION	GIRLS
*Modal Skeletal Age in Years**		*Modal Skeletal Age in Years**
	Elbow	
13.0 — 13.5	Begins in humerus	11.0 — 11.5
15.0 — 15.5	Completed in ulna	12.5 — 13.0
	Foot and ankle	
14.0 — 14.5	Begins in great toe	12.5 — 13.0
15.5 — 16.0	Completed in tibia and fibula	14.0 — 14.5
	Hand and wrist	
15.0 — 15.5	Begins in distal phalanges	13.0 — 13.5
17.5 — 18.0	Completed in radius	16.0 — 16.5
	Knee	
15.0 — 15.5	Begins in tibial tuberosity	13.5 — 14.0
17.5 — 18.0	Completed in fibula	16.0 — 16.5
	Hip and pelvis	
15.5 — 16.0	Begins in greater trochanter	14.0 — 14.5
after 18.0	Completed in symphysis	17.5 — 18.0
	Shoulder and shoulder girdle	
15.5 — 16.0	Begins in greater tuberosity	14.0 — 14.5
after 18.0	Completed in clavicle	17.5 — 18.0

* Modal skeletal age is given for onset of fusion because satisfactory means and standard deviations are not available for these ages.

Note. The norms in this table present a composite of published data from the Fels Research Institute, Yellow Springs, Ohio (Pyle and Sontag: *Am. J. Roentgenol.*, Vol. 19), and unpublished data from the Brush Foundation, Western Reserve University, Cleveland, Ohio, and the Harvard School of Public Health, Boston, Massachusetts. Compiled by Lieb, Buehl and Pyle.

orders and prolonged illness in infancy may interfere with calcification of deciduous and permanent teeth.

Such nutritional disturbances, if temporary, may leave defects in the enamel ranging from a line of small pits across the tooth to a broader band of hypoplasia. It is possible at times to date a nutritional disturbance by these bands of hypoplasia.

The formation of healthy tooth structure is fostered by a diet adequate in protein, calcium, phosphate and vitamins, especially C and D, and depends further upon an adequate supply of thyroid hormone. The resistance of teeth to dental caries is significantly increased when fluoride is available in optimal quantities.

Table 2–4 lists the times of eruption of the deciduous and permanent teeth. Delay in eruption of deciduous teeth occurs in hypothyroidism and in other nutritional and growth disturbances, but the normal variability in eruption prevents such delay from being useful as an index of a growth disorder. In some families the children have conspicuously

TABLE 2–4 CHRONOLOGY OF HUMAN DENTITION

Primary or Deciduous Teeth

	CALCIFICATION		ERUPTION		SHEDDING	
	Begins at	*Complete at*	*Maxillary*	*Mandibular*	*Maxillary*	*Mandibular*
Central incisors	5th fetal month	18–24 months	6–8 months	5–7 months	7–8 years	6–7 years
Lateral incisors	5th fetal month	18–24 months	8–11 months	7–10 months	8–9 years	7–8 years
Cuspids (canines)	6th fetal month	30–36 months	16–20 months	16–20 months	11–12 years	9–11 years
First molars	5th fetal month	24–30 months	10–16 months	10–16 months	10–11 years	10–12 years
Second molars	6th fetal month	36 months	20–30 months	20–30 months	10–12 years	11–13 years

Secondary or Permanent Teeth

	CALCIFICATION		ERUPTION	
	Begins at	*Complete at*	*Maxillary*	*Mandibular*
Central incisors	3–4 months	9–10 years	7–8 years	6–7 years
Lateral incisors	Max., 10–12 months Mand., 3–4 months	10–11 years	8–9 years	7–8 years
Cuspids (canines)	4–5 months	12–15 years	11–12 years	9–11 years
First premolars	18–21 months	12–13 years	10–11 years	10–12 years
Second premolars	24–30 months	12–14 years	10–12 years	11–13 years
First molars	Birth	9–10 years	6–7 years	6–7 years
Second molars	30–36 months	14–16 years	12–13 years	12–13 years
Third molars	Max., 7–9 years Mand., 8–10 years	18–25 years	17–22 years	17–22 years

Adapted from chart prepared by P. K. Losch, who carried out roentgenographic assays of the jaws of 1000 children in metropolitan Boston in 1942 at the Harvard School of Dental Medicine and provided the data for this chart.

early or late dentition without other signs of retardation or acceleration of growth.

The first permanent teeth to erupt are the 6-year molars; they are often mistaken for deciduous teeth by the uninformed. The first permanent molars serve as focal points in the dental arch and so have a great deal to do with the ultimate shape of the jaw and the orderly arrangement of teeth. Caries or other defects in them should receive prompt attention; these teeth should not be extracted.

SPECIAL ASPECTS OF GROWTH IN THE RESPIRATORY TRACT

Anatomically the respiratory tract of the newborn infant is distinguished by the lack of well developed accessory sinuses, by the close relation of the nasopharynx to the middle ear through a eustachian tube which is relatively short and broad, and by the absence of well developed mastoid air cells. The maxillary sinus at this time consists of a single cell, the ethmoid sinus of a few cells, and the mastoid only of an antrum. The sphenoidal sinuses appear by about the age of 3 years, and the frontal sinuses between 3 and 7 years of age.

The tympanic membrane in the newborn infant has a more oblique position with respect to the external auditory canal than it will have in later life, and the drum is somewhat thicker and more opaque. The middle ear at birth is filled with a mucoid substance which may be mistaken for exudate of infection if the ear is opened. The shortness and relative wideness of the eustachian tube contribute to the high incidence of otitis media in infancy.

DEVELOPMENTAL ASPECTS OF THE CARDIOVASCULAR SYSTEM

Figures 2–10 and 2–11 show the pulse and respiratory rates for children of various ages and indicate the distinctive differences between boys and girls which become evident at adolescence. See Section 13 for other aspects of development of the cardiovascular system.

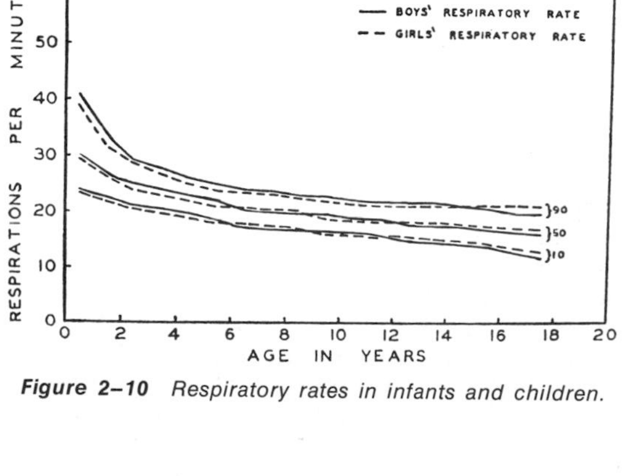

Figure 2–10 Respiratory rates in infants and children.

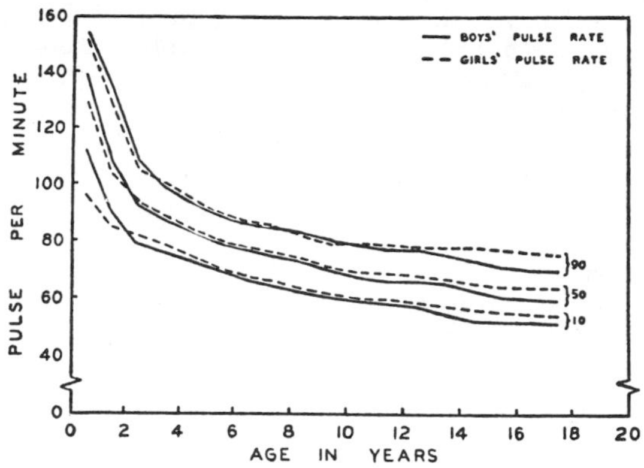

Figure 2–11 Pulse rates in infants and children.

DEVELOPMENTAL ASPECTS OF NUTRITION AND METABOLISM

The infant's and child's nutritional requirements increase with growth in size. The parameter of growth with which many of the nutritional factors bear the most nearly constant relation is body surface, which appears to be as closely related to the body's mass of metabolically active tissue as any other simple measurement. Owing, however, to fundamental differences in the metabolic activity of infants and children at various ages, adjustments may be necessary. This is particularly evident with respect to administration of drugs in the neonatal period.

Measurements of body surface which correspond to given heights and weights are available; reasonably accurate estimates of body surface can be obtained from nomograms (Section 30). Cruder estimates of body surface from weight only can be made for children whose physique is average; Lowe's formula is:

$$\text{surface area } (M^2) = \sqrt[3]{Wt^2 \text{ (kg)}} \times 0.1$$

Another crude estimate for children of average physique is given by the simpler formulas:

Approximation of Surface Area (M²) to Weight (kg)

WEIGHT RANGE	APPROXIMATE SURFACE AREA
1 to *5* kg	$M^2 = (0.05 \times kg) + 0.05$
6 to *10* kg	$M^2 = (0.04 \times kg) + 0.10$
11 to *20* kg	$M^2 = (0.03 \times kg) + 0.20$
21 to *40* kg	$M^2 = (0.02 \times kg) + 0.40$

(The figures 5, 10, 20 and 40 are given in italics to indicate a simple mnemonic.)

Examples:
for 7-kg infant, area $(M^2) = (0.04 \times 7) + 0.10 = 0.38\ M^2$
for 17-kg infant, area $(M^2) = (0.03 \times 17) + 0.20 = 0.71\ M^2$
(estimates of 0.4 M^2 and 0.7 M^2, respectively, would be reasonable)

(The formula $M^2 = (0.02 \times kg) + 40$ is reasonably accurate from 21 to 70 kg)

Basal caloric needs, when referred to body surface, appear to be somewhat lower in premature infants than in full-term ones. They increase during the first year of life from approximately 30 calories per square meter per hour to about 50 by the second year, with a subsequent fall to adult levels of 35 to 40 calories per square meter per hour. The data of Lewis indicate that the rate of fall is slowed during prepubertal and adolescent years, owing to the need for additional energy for accelerated growth.

Needs for water and electrolytes remain roughly constant in their proportion to body surface through most of the growing period; the inevitable variations in intake are met by the capacity of homeostatic mechanisms to adjust to varying conditions of supply and demand. Talbot, Richie and Crawford have outlined the limits within which the body is equipped to adjust to variations in intake and output.

ASSESSMENT OF PHYSICAL GROWTH AND DEVELOPMENT

Appraisal of growth and development in the infant and the child has its greatest usefulness only if it is accurate and continuous in each of the areas in which changes can be observed. In the infant the most useful physical measurements are head circumference, length and weight (Fig. 2–12 and Tables 2–5, 2–6 and 2–7). Note should also be made of the nutritional state, dentition, and the size or patency of fontanels. In selected instances measurements of the thickness of subcutaneous tissue or the lengths of body segments may be appropriate.

The record of the child's growth can be kept in a number of ways and according to various standards. This information will be most useful if it is recorded at serial examinations on charts permitting comparisons with standards for each age. The Harvard charts (Fig. 2–12), Iowa charts (Fig. 2–13) and Wetzel grids offer ways in which this may be accomplished. The standards used for these charts reflect the achievement of Caucasian children of predominantly middle class origin and may need revision for other socioeconomic, ethnic or racial stocks. There is growing evidence that ethnic differences depend in largest measure upon differences in prevalence of malnutrition and infectious diseases in different parts of the world. Accuracy of measurement is essential to the reliable interpretation of growth data; slight variations in technique may result in significantly large errors in the placement of children according to percentile rank.

TECHNIQUES OF MEASUREMENT

HEIGHT. *Recumbent length* can be more accurately measured than standing height in children under the age of 5 years, after which measurement of standing height is generally more convenient. Recumbent length is measured as the child lies on a firm table which has a measuring stick at least 125 cm or 50 inches long inserted along one edge. The soles of the feet are held firmly against a fixed upright placed at the zero mark. A movable upright crosses the table above the head and is brought firmly against the vertex. If recumbent length is used after 5 years of age, the value obtained may be reduced by 1 cm and then considered against the scale for standing height.

Standing height is measured as the child stands erect, his heels, buttocks, upper part of the back and occiput against a vertical upright; the heels should be close together, and the arms should hang naturally at the sides. The external auditory meatus and the lower border of the orbit should lie in a plane parallel with the floor. A wooden head piece having two faces at right angles may be placed firmly on the head against a 2-meter or 6-foot measuring scale attached to the vertical surface against which the child is positioned.

HEAD CIRCUMFERENCE. This measurement is particularly valuable in infants; it need not be taken routinely after 3 years of age. The tape is applied firmly over the glabella and supraorbital ridges anteriorly and that part of the occiput posteriorly which gives the maximal circumference. Difficulties with measurement of head circumference will sometimes arise when the head has an abnormal shape, as in hydrocephalus. Under these circumstances serial measurements of the changing size of the head may best be made through positioning the tape over whatever points on the forehead and occiput give the *maximal* circumference.

Measurements of circumference should be made with steel, cloth or disposable paper tapes. Cloth tapes may stretch with aging and will need to be checked frequently against wooden or steel standards.

CHEST CIRCUMFERENCE. Measurement of chest circumference is made in midrespiration, at the level of the xiphoid cartilage or substernal notch, in a plane at right angles to the vertebral column. Measurement is made recumbent up to the age of 5 years, the child standing thereafter.

ABDOMINAL CIRCUMFERENCE. This measurement is taken to 3 years only and will be of value principally in recognizing and following the course of chronic intestinal disturbances. Measurement is made in the plane of the umbilicus when the infant is recumbent.

OTHER MEASUREMENTS. Studies of nutritional status or of specific growth problems will often require other measurements, such as skinfold thickness or circumference of calf (in nutritional assessment), relationship of sitting height to length or span (in growth disturbances), pelvic breadth (in adolescence), and the like. Standards exist for these in various reference works; tables of pelvic breadth, leg circumference and stem length (sitting height) have been given in earlier editions of this text, from studies carried out under direction of Howard V. Meredith, Iowa Child Welfare Research Station, The State University of Iowa.

(Text continued on page 50)

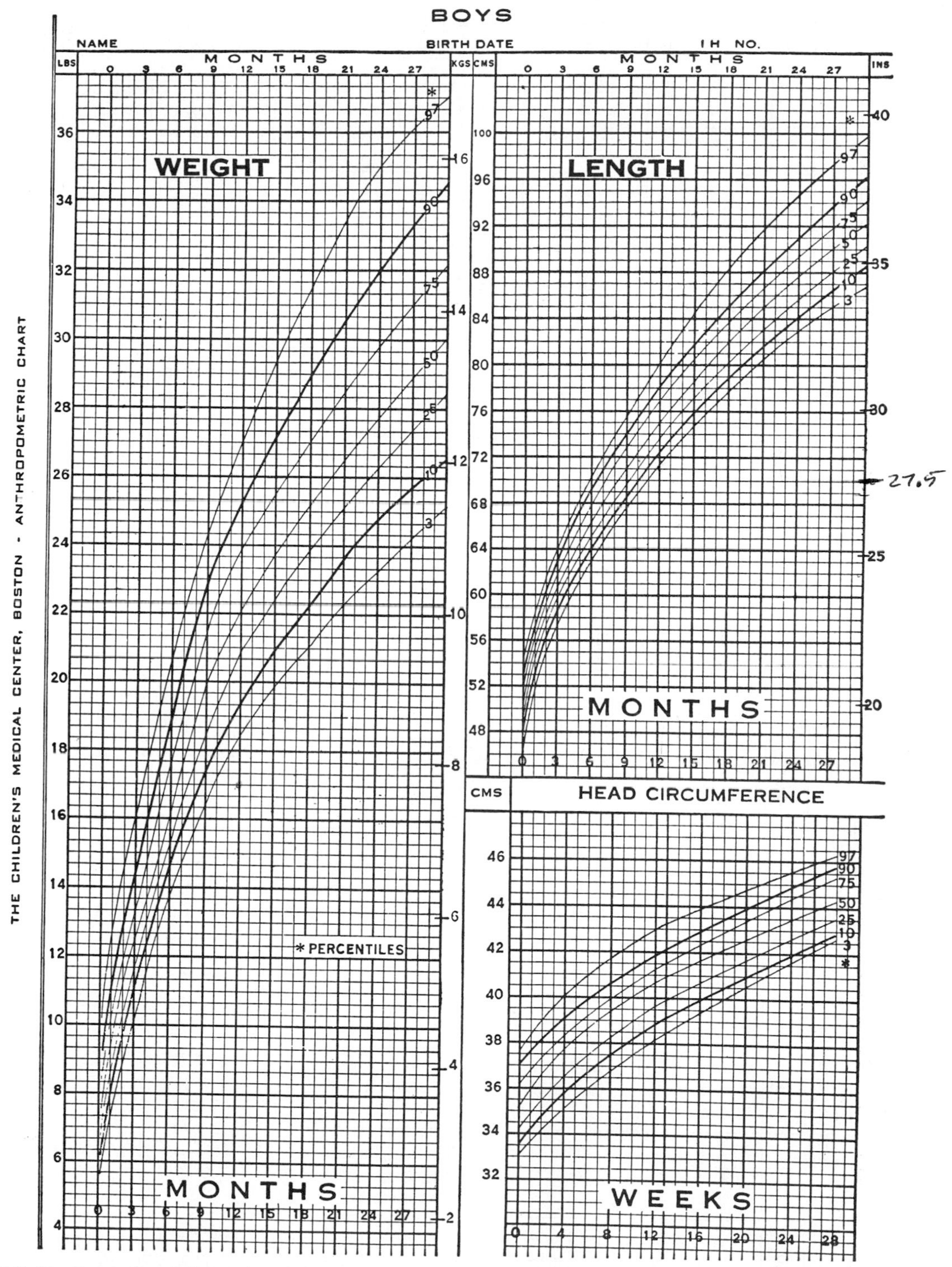

Figure 2–12 Graphs for plotting selected measurements in infancy. These graphs as well as those in Figure 2–13 are based on studies conducted by the Harvard School of Public Health of white children in Boston of predominantly north European stock. Separate charts are used for girls, since norms for the two sexes differ appreciably.

These graphs serve for plotting weight and height measurements up to 30 months and head circumference up to 30 weeks. The percentile values on which they are based are given in Tables 2–5 and 2–7.

TABLE 2–5 PERCENTILES FOR WEIGHT AND LENGTH–BIRTH TO 5 YEARS

PERCENTILES (BOYS)								PERCENTILES (GIRLS)						
3	10	25	50	75	90	97		3	10	25	50	75	90	97
							Birth							
5.8	6.3	6.9	7.5	8.3	9.1	10.1	Weight in Pounds	5.8	6.2	6.9	7.4	8.1	8.6	9.4
2.63	2.86	3.13	3.4	3.76	4.13	4.58	Weight in Kg.	2.63	2.81	3.13	3.36	3.67	3.9	4.26
18.2	18.9	19.4	19.9	20.5	21.0	21.5	Length in Inches	18.5	18.8	19.3	19.8	20.1	20.4	21.1
46.3	48.1	49.3	50.6	52.0	53.3	54.6	Length in Cm.	47.1	47.8	49.0	50.2	51.0	51.9	53.6
							3 Months							
10.6	11.1	11.8	12.6	13.6	14.5	16.4	Weight in Pounds	9.8	10.7	11.4	12.4	13.2	14.0	14.9
4.81	5.03	5.35	5.72	6.17	6.58	7.44	Weight in Kg.	4.45	4.85	5.17	5.62	5.99	6.35	6.76
22.4	22.8	23.3	23.8	24.3	24.7	25.1	Length in Inches	22.0	22.4	22.8	23.4	23.9	24.3	24.8
56.8	57.8	59.3	60.4	61.8	62.8	63.7	Length in Cm.	55.8	56.9	57.9	59.5	60.7	61.7	63.1
							6 Months							
14.0	14.8	15.6	16.7	18.0	19.2	20.8	Weight in Pounds	12.7	14.1	15.0	16.0	17.5	18.6	20.0
6.35	6.71	7.08	7.58	8.16	8.71	9.43	Weight in Kg.	5.76	6.4	6.8	7.26	7.94	8.44	9.07
24.8	25.2	25.7	26.1	26.7	27.3	27.7	Length in Inches	24.0	24.6	25.1	25.7	26.2	26.7	27.1
63.0	63.9	65.2	66.4	67.8	69.3	70.4	Length in Cm.	61.1	62.5	63.7	65.2	66.6	67.8	68.8
							9 Months							
16.6	17.8	18.7	20.0	21.5	22.9	24.4	Weight in Pounds	15.1	16.6	17.8	19.2	20.8	22.4	24.2
7.53	8.07	8.48	9.07	9.75	10.39	11.07	Weight in Kg.	6.85	7.53	8.03	8.71	9.43	10.16	10.98
26.6	27.0	27.5	28.0	28.7	29.2	29.9	Length in Inches	25.7	26.4	26.9	27.6	28.2	28.7	29.2
67.7	68.6	69.8	71.2	72.9	74.2	75.9	Length in Cm.	65.4	67.0	68.4	70.1	71.7	72.9	74.1
							12 Months							
18.5	19.6	20.9	22.2	23.8	25.4	27.3	Weight in Pounds	16.8	18.4	19.8	21.5	23.0	24.8	27.1
8.39	8.89	9.48	10.07	10.8	11.52	12.38	Weight in Kg.	7.62	8.35	8.98	9.75	10.43	11.25	12.29
28.1	28.5	29.0	29.6	30.3	30.7	31.6	Length in Inches	27.1	27.8	28.5	29.2	29.9	30.3	31.0
71.3	72.4	73.7	75.2	76.9	78.1	80.3	Length in Cm.	68.9	70.6	72.3	74.2	75.9	77.1	78.8
							15 Months							
19.8	21.0	22.4	23.7	25.4	27.2	29.4	Weight in Pounds	18.1	19.8	21.3	23.0	24.6	26.6	29.0
8.98	9.53	10.16	10.75	11.52	12.34	13.33	Weight in Kg.	8.21	8.98	9.66	10.43	11.16	12.07	13.15
29.3	29.8	30.3	30.9	31.6	32.1	33.1	Length in Inches	28.3	29.0	29.8	30.5	31.3	31.8	32.6
74.4	75.6	77.0	78.5	80.3	81.5	84.2	Length in Cm.	71.9	73.7	75.6	77.6	79.4	80.8	82.8
							18 Months							
21.1	22.3	23.8	25.2	26.9	29.0	31.5	Weight in Pounds	19.4	21.2	22.7	24.5	26.2	28.3	30.9
9.57	10.12	10.8	11.43	12.2	13.15	14.29	Weight in Kg.	8.8	9.62	10.3	11.11	11.88	12.84	14.02

30.5	31.0	31.6	32.2	32.9	33.5	34.7	Length in Inches	29.5	30.2	31.1	31.8	32.6	33.3	34.1
77.5	78.8	80.3	81.8	83.7	85.0	88.2	Length in Cm.	74.9	76.8	79.0	80.9	82.9	84.5	86.7
							2 Years							
23.3	24.7	26.3	27.7	29.7	31.9	34.9	Weight in Pounds	21.6	23.5	25.3	27.1	29.2	31.7	34.4
10.57	11.2	11.93	12.56	13.47	14.47	15.83	Weight in Kg.	9.8	10.66	11.48	12.29	13.25	14.38	15.6
32.6	33.1	33.8	34.4	35.2	35.9	37.2	Length in Inches	31.5	32.3	33.3	34.1	35.0	35.8	36.7
82.7	84.2	85.8	87.5	89.4	91.1	94.6	Length in Cm.	80.1	82.0	84.7	86.6	88.9	91.0	93.3
							2½ Years							
25.2	26.6	28.4	30.0	32.2	34.5	37.0	Weight in Pounds	23.6	25.5	27.4	29.6	31.9	34.6	38.2
11.43	12.07	12.88	13.61	14.61	15.65	16.78	Weight in Kg.	10.7	11.57	12.43	13.43	14.47	15.69	17.33
34.2	34.8	35.5	36.3	37.0	37.9	39.2	Length in Inches	33.3	34.0	35.2	36.0	36.9	37.9	38.9
86.9	88.5	90.2	92.1	94.1	96.2	99.5	Length in Cm.	84.5	86.3	89.3	91.4	93.8	96.4	98.7
							3 Years							
27.0	28.7	30.3	32.2	34.5	36.8	39.2	Weight in Pounds	25.6	27.6	29.6	31.8	34.6	37.4	41.8
12.25	13.02	13.74	14.61	15.65	16.69	17.73	Weight in Kg.	11.61	12.52	13.43	14.42	15.69	16.96	18.96
35.7	36.3	37.0	37.9	38.8	39.6	40.5	Length in Inches	34.8	35.6	36.8	37.7	38.6	39.8	40.7
90.6	92.3	93.9	96.2	98.5	100.5	102.8	Length in Cm.	88.4	90.5	93.4	95.7	98.1	101.1	103.5
							3½ Years							
28.5	30.4	32.3	34.3	36.7	39.1	41.5	Weight in Pounds	27.5	29.5	31.5	33.9	37.0	40.4	45.3
12.93	13.79	14.65	15.56	16.65	17.74	18.82	Weight in Kg.	12.47	13.38	14.29	15.38	16.78	18.33	20.55
37.1	37.8	38.4	39.3	40.3	41.1	41.9	Length in Inches	36.2	37.1	38.1	39.2	40.2	41.5	42.5
94.3	96.0	97.5	99.8	102.5	104.5	106.5	Length in Cm.	92.0	94.2	96.9	99.5	102.0	105.4	108.0
							4 Years							
30.1	32.1	34.0	36.4	39.0	41.4	44.3	Weight in Pounds	29.2	31.2	33.5	36.2	39.6	43.5	48.2
13.65	14.56	15.42	16.51	17.69	18.78	20.09	Weight in Kg.	13.25	14.15	15.2	16.42	17.96	19.73	21.86
38.4	39.1	39.7	40.7	41.9	42.7	43.5	Length in Inches	37.5	38.4	39.5	40.6	41.6	43.1	44.2
97.5	99.3	100.8	103.4	106.5	108.5	110.4	Length in Cm.	95.2	97.6	100.3	103.2	105.8	109.6	112.3
							4½ Years							
31.6	33.8	35.7	38.4	41.4	43.9	47.4	Weight in Pounds	30.7	32.9	35.3	38.5	42.1	46.7	50.9
14.33	15.33	16.19	17.42	18.78	19.91	21.5	Weight in Kg.	13.93	14.92	16.01	17.46	19.1	21.18	23.09
39.6	40.3	40.9	42.0	43.3	44.2	45.0	Length in Inches	38.6	39.7	40.8	42.0	43.0	44.7	45.7
100.6	102.4	104.0	106.7	109.9	112.3	114.3	Length in Cm.	98.1	100.9	103.6	106.8	109.3	113.5	116.2
							5 Years*							
33.6	35.5	37.5	40.5	44.1	46.7	50.4	Weight in Pounds	32.1	34.8	37.4	40.5	44.8	49.2	52.8
15.24	16.1	17.01	18.37	20.0	21.18	22.86	Weight in Kg.	14.56	15.79	16.96	18.37	20.32	22.32	23.95
40.2	40.8	41.7	42.8	44.2	45.2	46.1	Length in Inches	39.4	40.5	41.6	42.9	44.0	45.4	46.8
102.0	103.7	105.9	108.7	112.3	114.7	117.1	Length in Cm.	100.0	103.0	105.7	109.1	111.7	115.4	118.8

From Studies of Child Health and Development, Department of Maternal and Child Health, Harvard School of Public Health.

*The figures for the several percentiles of each measurement at 5 years differ slightly from those given in Table 2–6 for this age because they were obtained from a different population of children.

TABLE 2-6 PERCENTILES FOR WEIGHT AND HEIGHT—5 TO 18 YEARS

PERCENTILES (BOYS)								PERCENTILES (GIRLS)						
3	10	25	50	75	90	97		3	10	25	50	75	90	97
							5 Years*							
34.5	36.6	39.6	42.8	46.5	49.7	53.2	Weight in Pounds	33.7	36.1	38.6	41.4	44.2	48.2	51.8
15.65	16.6	17.96	19.41	21.09	22.54	24.13	Weight in Kg.	15.29	16.37	17.51	18.78	20.05	21.86	23.5
40.2	41.5	42.6	43.8	45.0	45.9	47.0	Height in Inches	40.4	41.3	42.2	43.2	44.4	45.4	46.5
102.1	105.3	108.3	111.3	114.2	116.7	119.5	Height in Cm.	102.6	105.0	107.2	109.7	112.9	115.4	118.0
							$5\frac{1}{2}$ Years							
	38.8	42.0	45.6	49.3	53.1		Weight in Pounds		38.0	40.8	44.0	47.2	51.2	
	17.6	19.05	20.68	22.36	24.09		Weight in Kg.		17.24	18.51	19.96	21.41	23.22	
	42.6	43.8	45.0	46.3	47.3		Height in Inches		42.4	43.4	44.4	45.7	46.8	
	108.3	111.2	114.4	117.5	120.1		Height in Cm.		107.8	110.2	112.8	116.1	118.9	
							6 Years							
38.5	40.9	44.4	48.3	52.1	56.4	61.1	Weight in Pounds	37.2	39.6	42.9	46.5	50.2	54.2	58.7
17.46	18.55	20.14	21.91	23.63	25.58	27.71	Weight in Kg.	16.87	17.96	19.46	21.09	22.77	24.58	26.63
42.7	43.8	44.9	46.3	47.6	48.6	49.7	Height in Inches	42.5	43.5	44.6	45.6	47.0	48.1	49.4
108.5	111.2	114.1	117.5	120.8	123.5	126.2	Height in Cm.	108.0	110.6	113.2	115.9	119.3	122.3	125.4
							$6\frac{1}{2}$ Years							
	43.4	47.1	51.2	55.4	60.4		Weight in Pounds		42.2	45.5	49.4	53.3	57.7	
	19.69	21.36	23.22	25.13	27.4		Weight in Kg.		19.14	20.64	22.41	24.18	26.17	
	44.9	46.1	47.6	48.9	50.0		Height in Inches		44.8	45.7	46.9	48.3	49.4	
	114.1	117.2	120.8	124.2	127.0		Height in Cm.		113.7	116.2	119.1	122.6	125.6	
							7 Years							
43.0	45.8	49.7	54.1	58.7	64.4	69.9	Weight in Pounds	41.3	44.5	48.1	52.2	56.3	61.2	67.3
19.5	20.77	22.54	24.54	26.63	29.21	31.71	Weight in Kg.	18.73	20.19	21.82	23.68	25.54	27.76	30.53
44.9	46.0	47.4	48.9	50.2	51.4	52.5	Height in Inches	44.9	46.0	46.9	48.1	49.6	50.7	51.9
114.0	116.9	120.3	124.1	127.6	130.5	133.4	Height in Cm.	114.0	116.8	119.2	122.3	125.9	128.9	131.7
							$7\frac{1}{2}$ Years							
	48.5	52.6	57.1	62.1	68.7		Weight in Pounds		46.6	50.6	55.2	59.8	65.6	
	22.0	23.86	25.9	28.17	31.16		Weight in Kg.		21.14	22.95	25.04	27.13	29.76	
	47.2	48.6	50.0	51.5	52.7		Height in Inches		47.0	48.0	49.3	50.7	51.9	
	120.0	123.5	127.1	130.9	133.9		Height in Cm.		119.5	122.0	125.2	128.8	131.8	

							8 Years							
48.0	51.2	55.5	60.1	65.5	73.0	79.4	Weight in Pounds	45.3	48.6	53.1	58.1	63.3	69.9	78.9
21.77	23.22	25.17	27.26	29.71	33.11	36.02	Weight in Kg.	20.55	22.04	24.09	26.35	28.71	31.71	35.79
47.1	48.5	49.8	51.2	52.8	54.0	55.2	Height in Inches	46.9	18.1	49.1	50.4	51.8	53.0	54.1
119.6	123.1	126.6	130.0	134.2	137.3	140.2	Height in Cm.	119.1	122.1	124.8	128.0	131.6	134.6	137.4
							8½ Years							
	53.8	58.3	63.1	68.9	77.0		Weight in Pounds		50.6	55.5	61.0	66.9	74.5	
	24.4	26.44	28.62	31.25	34.93		Weight in Kg.		22.95	25.17	27.67	30.35	33.79	
	49.5	50.8	52.3	53.9	55.1		Height in Inches		49.0	50.1	51.4	52.9	54.1	
	125.7	129.1	132.8	137.0	140.0		Height in Cm.		124.6	127.3	130.5	134.4	137.5	
							9 Years							
52.5	56.3	61.1	66.0	72.3	81.0	89.8	Weight in Pounds	49.1	52.6	57.9	63.8	70.5	79.1	89.9
23.81	25.54	27.71	29.94	32.8	36.74	40.73	Weight in Kg.	22.27	23.86	26.26	28.94	31.98	35.88	40.78
48.9	50.5	51.8	53.3	55.0	56.1	57.2	Height in Inches	48.7	50.0	51.1	52.3	54.0	55.3	56.5
124.2	128.3	131.6	135.5	139.8	142.6	145.3	Height in Cm.	123.6	127.0	129.7	132.9	137.1	140.4	143.4
							9½ Years							
	58.7	63.7	69.0	76.0	85.5		Weight in Pounds		54.9	60.4	67.1	74.8	84.4	
	26.63	28.89	31.3	34.47	38.78		Weight in Kg.		24.9	27.4	30.44	33.93	38.28	
	51.4	52.7	54.3	55.9	57.1		Height in Inches		50.9	52.0	53.5	55.1	56.4	
	130.6	134.0	137.9	142.1	145.1		Height in Cm.		129.4	132.2	135.8	139.9	143.2	
							10 Years							
56.8	61.1	66.3	71.9	79.6	89.9	100.0	Weight in Pounds	53.2	57.1	62.8	70.3	79.1	89.7	101.9
25.76	27.71	30.07	32.61	36.11	40.78	45.36	Weight in Kg.	24.13	25.9	28.49	31.89	35.88	40.69	46.22
50.7	52.3	53.7	55.2	56.8	58.1	59.2	Height in Inches	50.3	51.8	53.0	54.6	56.1	57.5	58.8
128.7	132.8	136.3	140.3	144.4	147.5	150.3	Height in Cm.	127.7	131.7	134.6	138.6	142.6	146.0	149.3
							10½ Years							
	63.7	69.0	74.8	83.4	94.6		Weight in Pounds		59.9	66.4	74.6	84.1	95.1	
	28.89	31.3	33.93	37.83	42.91		Weight in Kg.		27.17	30.12	33.79	38.15	43.14	
	53.2	54.5	56.0	57.8	58.9		Height in Inches		52.9	54.1	55.8	57.4	58.9	
	135.1	138.4	142.3	146.8	149.7		Height in Cm.		134.4	137.5	141.7	145.9	149.7	
							11 Years							
61.8	66.3	71.6	77.6	87.2	99.3	111.7	Weight in Pounds	57.9	62.6	69.9	78.8	89.1	100.4	112.9
28.03	30.07	32.48	35.2	39.55	45.04	50.67	Weight in Kg.	26.26	28.4	31.71	35.74	40.42	45.54	51.21
52.5	54.0	55.3	56.8	58.7	59.8	60.8	Height in Inches	52.1	53.9	55.2	57.0	58.7	60.4	62.0
133.4	137.3	140.5	144.2	149.2	151.8	154.4	Height in Cm.	132.3	137.0	140.3	144.7	149.2	153.4	157.4
							11½ Years							
	69.2	74.6	81.0	91.6	104.5		Weight in Pounds		66.1	74.0	83.2	94.0	106.0	
	31.39	33.84	36.74	41.55	47.4		Weight in Kg.		29.98	33.57	37.74	42.64	48.08	
	55.0	56.3	57.8	59.6	60.9		Height in Inches		55.0	56.3	58.3	60.2	61.8	
	139.8	142.9	146.9	151.4	154.8		Height in Cm.		139.8	143.1	148.1	152.9	157.0	

Table 2-6 continued on following page.

TABLE 2–6 PERCENTILES FOR WEIGHT AND HEIGHT–5 TO 18 YEARS *(Continued)*

3	10	25	50	75	90	97		3	10	25	50	75	90	97
							12 Years							
67.2	72.0	77.5	84.4	96.0	109.6	124.2	Weight in Pounds	63.6	69.5	78.0	87.6	98.8	111.5	127.7
30.48	32.66	35.15	38.28	43.55	49.71	56.34	Weight in Kg.	28.85	31.52	35.38	39.74	44.82	50.58	57.92
54.4	56.1	57.2	58.9	60.4	62.2	63.7	Height in Inches	54.3	56.1	57.4	59.8	61.6	63.2	64.8
138.1	142.4	145.2	149.6	153.5	157.9	161.9	Height in Cm.	137.8	142.6	145.9	151.9	156.6	160.6	164.6
							12½ Years							
	74.6	80.6	88.7	102.0	116.4		Weight in Pounds		74.7	83.7	93.4	104.9	118.0	
	33.84	36.56	40.23	46.27	52.8		Weight in Kg.		33.88	37.97	42.37	47.58	53.52	
	56.9	58.1	60.0	61.9	63.6		Height in Inches		57.4	58.8	60.7	62.6	64.0	
	144.5	147.5	152.3	157.2	161.6		Height in Cm.		145.9	149.3	154.3	159.1	162.7	
							13 Years							
72.0	77.1	83.7	93.0	107.9	123.2	138.0	Weight in Pounds	72.2	79.9	89.4	99.1	111.0	124.5	142.3
32.66	34.97	37.97	42.18	48.94	55.88	62.6	Weight in Kg.	32.75	36.24	40.55	44.95	50.35	56.47	64.55
56.0	57.7	58.9	61.0	63.3	65.1	66.7	Height in Inches	56.6	58.7	60.1	61.8	63.6	64.9	66.3
142.2	146.6	149.7	155.0	160.8	165.3	169.5	Height in Cm.	143.7	149.1	152.6	157.1	161.5	164.8	168.4
							13½ Years							
	82.2	89.6	100.3	115.5	130.1		Weight in Pounds		85.5	94.6	103.7	115.4	128.9	
	37.29	40.64	45.5	52.39	59.01		Weight in Kg.		38.78	42.91	47.04	52.35	58.47	
	58.8	60.3	62.6	64.8	66.5		Height in Inches		59.5	60.8	62.4	64.0	65.3	
	149.4	153.1	158.9	164.6	168.9		Height in Cm.		151.1	154.4	158.4	162.6	165.9	
							14 Years							
79.8	87.2	95.5	107.6	123.1	136.9	150.6	Weight in Pounds	83.1	91.0	99.8	108.4	119.7	133.3	150.8
36.2	39.55	43.32	48.81	55.84	62.1	68.31	Weight in Kg.	37.69	41.28	45.27	49.17	54.29	60.46	68.4
57.6	59.9	61.6	64.0	66.3	67.9	69.7	Height in Inches	58.3	60.2	61.5	62.8	64.4	65.7	67.2
146.4	152.1	156.5	162.7	168.4	172.4	177.1	Height in Cm.	148.2	153.0	156.1	159.6	163.7	167.0	170.7
							14½ Years							
	93.3	101.9	113.9	129.1	142.4		Weight in Pounds		94.2	102.5	111.0	121.8	135.7	
	42.32	46.22	51.66	58.56	64.59		Weight in Kg.		42.73	46.49	50.35	55.25	61.55	
	61.0	62.7	65.1	67.2	68.7		Height in Inches		60.7	61.8	63.1	64.7	66.0	
	155.0	159.4	165.3	170.7	174.6		Height in Cm.		154.1	156.9	160.4	164.3	167.6	

							15 Years							
91.3	99.4	108.2	120.1	135.0	147.8	161.6	Weight in Pounds	89.0	97.4	105.1	113.5	123.9	138.1	155.2
41.41	45.09	49.08	54.48	61.23	67.04	73.3	Weight in Kg.	40.37	44.18	47.67	51.48	56.2	62.64	70.4
59.7	62.1	63.9	66.1	68.1	69.6	71.6	Height in Inches	59.1	61.1	62.1	63.4	64.9	66.2	67.6
151.7	157.8	162.3	167.8	173.0	176.7	181.8	Height in Cm.	150.2	155.2	157.7	161.1	164.9	168.1	171.6
							15½ Years							
	105.2	113.5	124.9	139.7	152.6		Weight in Pounds		99.2	106.8	115.3	125.6	139.6	
	47.72	51.48	56.65	63.37	69.22		Weight in Kg.		45.0	48.44	52.3	56.97	63.32	
	63.1	64.8	66.8	68.8	70.2		Height in Inches		61.3	62.3	63.7	65.1	66.4	
	160.3	164.7	169.7	174.8	178.2		Height in Cm.		155.7	158.2	161.7	165.3	168.6	
							16 Years							
103.4	111.0	118.7	129.7	144.4	157.3	170.5	Weight in Pounds	91.8	100.9	108.4	117.0	127.2	141.1	157.7
46.9	50.35	53.84	58.83	65.5	71.35	77.34	Weight in Kg.	41.64	45.77	49.17	53.07	57.7	64.0	71.53
61.6	64.1	65.8	67.8	69.5	70.7	73.1	Height in Inches	59.4	61.5	62.4	63.9	65.2	66.5	67.7
156.5	162.8	167.1	171.6	176.6	179.7	185.6	Height in Cm.	150.8	156.1	158.6	162.2	165.7	169.0	172.0
							16½ Years							
	114.3	121.6	133.0	147.9	161.0		Weight in Pounds		101.9	109.4	118.1	128.4	142.2	
	51.85	55.16	60.33	67.09	73.03		Weight in Kg.		46.22	49.62	53.57	58.24	64.5	
	64.6	66.3	68.0	69.8	71.1		Height in Inches		61.5	62.5	63.9	65.3	66.6	
	164.2	168.4	172.7	177.4	180.7		Height in Cm.		156.2	158.8	162.4	165.9	169.2	
							17 Years							
110.5	117.5	124.5	136.2	151.4	164.6	175.6	Weight in Pounds	93.9	102.8	110.4	119.1	129.6	143.3	159.5
50.12	53.3	56.47	61.78	68.67	74.66	79.65	Weight in Kg.	42.59	46.63	50.08	54.02	58.79	65.0	72.35
62.6	65.2	66.8	68.4	70.1	71.5	73.5	Height in Inches	59.4	61.5	62.6	64.0	65.4	66.7	67.8
159.0	165.5	169.7	173.7	178.1	181.6	186.6	Height in Cm.	151.0	156.3	159.0	162.5	166.1	169.4	172.2
							17½ Years							
	118.8	125.8	137.6	153.6	166.8		Weight in Pounds		103.2	110.8	119.5	130.2	143.9	
	53.89	57.06	62.41	69.67	75.66		Weight in Kg.		46.81	50.26	54.2	59.06	65.27	
	65.3	67.0	68.5	70.3	71.6		Height in Inches		61.5	62.6	64.0	65.4	66.7	
	165.9	170.1	174.1	178.5	182.0		Height in Cm.		156.3	159.0	162.5	166.1	169.4	
							18 Years							
113.0	120.0	127.1	139.0	155.7	169.0	179.0	Weight in Pounds	94.5	103.5	111.2	119.9	130.8	144.5	160.7
51.26	54.43	57.65	63.05	70.62	76.66	81.19	Weight in Kg.	42.87	46.95	50.44	54.39	59.33	65.54	72.89
62.8	65.5	67.0	68.7	70.4	71.8	73.9	Height in Inches	59.4	61.5	62.6	64.0	65.4	66.7	67.8
159.6	166.3	170.5	174.5	178.9	182.4	187.6	Height in Cm.	151.0	156.3	159.0	162.5	166.1	169.4	172.2

*The figures for the several percentiles of each measurement at 5 years differ slightly from those in Table 2–5 for this age because they were obtained from a different population of children.

The measurements in this table are from studies by and are reproduced by courtesy of Howard V. Meredith, Iowa Child Welfare Research Station, The State University of Iowa.

TABLE 2-7 PERCENTILES FOR SELECTED MEASUREMENTS—BIRTH TO 3 YEARS—IN CENTIMETERS

PERCENTILES (BOYS)								PERCENTILES (GIRLS)						
3	10	25	50	75	90	97		3	10	25	50	75	90	97
							Birth							
33.0	33.5	34.4	35.3	36.2	37.0	37.5	Head Circ.	32.5	33.4	33.9	34.7	35.4	36.0	36.6
29.8	30.6	31.8	33.2	34.4	35.7	36.8	Chest Circ.	30.0	30.8	31.8	32.9	34.0	35.0	36.0
							3 Months							
38.7	39.2	40.0	40.9	41.5	42.1	43.2	Head Circ.	37.9	38.5	39.2	40.0	40.8	41.7	42.3
37.6	38.3	39.3	40.6	41.6	42.9	44.1	Chest Circ.	36.5	37.6	38.8	39.8	40.9	42.0	43.0
33.6	35.5	36.8	38.5	39.8	41.4	43.5	Abd. Circ.	32.3	34.4	36.8	38.4	40.4	41.7	42.7
							6 Months							
42.1	42.7	43.3	43.9	44.8	45.4	45.9	Head Circ.	40.9	41.4	42.0	42.8	43.6	44.5	45.4
40.1	41.6	42.5	43.7	45.0	46.3	47.2	Chest Circ.	39.4	40.6	41.8	43.0	44.2	45.4	46.6
36.4	38.4	39.8	41.4	43.2	45.0	46.0	Abd. Circ.	36.2	37.9	39.5	41.4	43.5	45.0	46.2
							9 Months							
43.8	44.5	45.1	46.0	46.5	47.1	47.8	Head Circ.	42.6	43.2	43.8	44.6	45.4	46.3	47.2
42.0	43.7	44.8	46.0	47.5	48.9	49.9	Chest Circ.	41.7	42.7	44.0	45.4	46.6	47.9	49.2
38.1	40.1	41.7	43.4	45.6	47.6	48.4	Abd. Circ.	38.0	39.9	41.3	43.4	45.7	47.7	49.2
							12 Months							
44.9	45.5	46.5	47.3	47.8	48.4	48.9	Head Circ.	43.6	44.3	45.0	45.8	46.7	47.7	48.4
43.5	45.1	46.3	47.6	49.3	50.7	51.9	Chest Circ.	43.1	44.2	45.6	47.0	48.2	49.5	50.9
39.3	41.1	42.9	44.6	47.0	48.9	50.0	Abd. Circ.	38.7	40.9	42.4	44.5	46.9	49.2	51.1

							15 Months							
45.6	46.3	47.1	48.0	48.5	49.2	49.8	Head Circ.	44.3	44.9	45.6	46.5	47.4	48.4	49.1
44.7	46.1	47.3	48.6	50.1	51.7	52.8	Chest Circ.	44.1	45.1	46.5	47.9	49.2	50.5	51.9
40.0	41.7	43.5	45.1	47.4	49.3	50.5	Abd. Circ.	39.3	41.5	43.0	45.0	47.3	49.8	51.8
							18 Months							
46.2	47.0	47.7	48.7	49.2	49.9	50.6	Head Circ.	44.9	45.5	46.2	47.1	48.0	49.0	49.8
45.9	47.0	48.2	49.5	50.9	52.6	53.7	Chest Circ.	45.0	46.0	47.3	48.8	50.2	51.4	52.9
40.6	42.2	44.0	45.5	47.8	49.6	50.9	Abd. Circ.	39.8	42.1	43.6	45.5	47.6	50.3	52.5
							2 Years							
47.0	48.0	48.2	49.7	50.2	51.0	51.7	Head Circ.	45.8	46.4	47.2	48.1	49.1	50.1	50.9
47.4	48.4	49.5	50.8	52.2	53.9	54.9	Chest Circ.	46.3	47.4	48.6	50.1	51.8	53.0	54.2
41.6	43.4	44.8	46.2	48.4	50.2	51.5	Abd. Circ.	40.7	42.8	44.4	46.3	48.5	51.4	53.5
							2½ Years							
47.5	48.5	49.2	50.2	50.9	51.6	52.3	Head Circ.	46.3	47.0	47.8	48.8	49.8	50.8	51.5
48.2	49.3	50.3	51.7	53.2	54.9	55.8	Chest Circ.	47.3	48.4	49.7	51.2	52.8	54.3	55.5
42.0	44.0	45.5	46.7	49.1	50.7	52.0	Abd. Circ.	41.7	43.6	45.2	47.0	49.4	52.6	54.7
							3 Years							
47.9	48.9	49.6	50.4	51.3	51.9	52.7	Head Circ.	46.8	47.5	48.4	49.3	50.3	51.1	52.0
48.9	49.9	51.0	52.4	54.1	55.8	57.0	Chest Circ.	47.9	49.3	50.5	51.9	53.5	55.1	56.7
42.1	44.6	46.0	47.2	49.6	51.1	52.7	Abd. Circ.	42.7	44.5	46.0	47.7	50.2	53.6	55.8

From Studies of Child Health and Development, Department of Maternal and Child Health, Harvard School of Public Health.

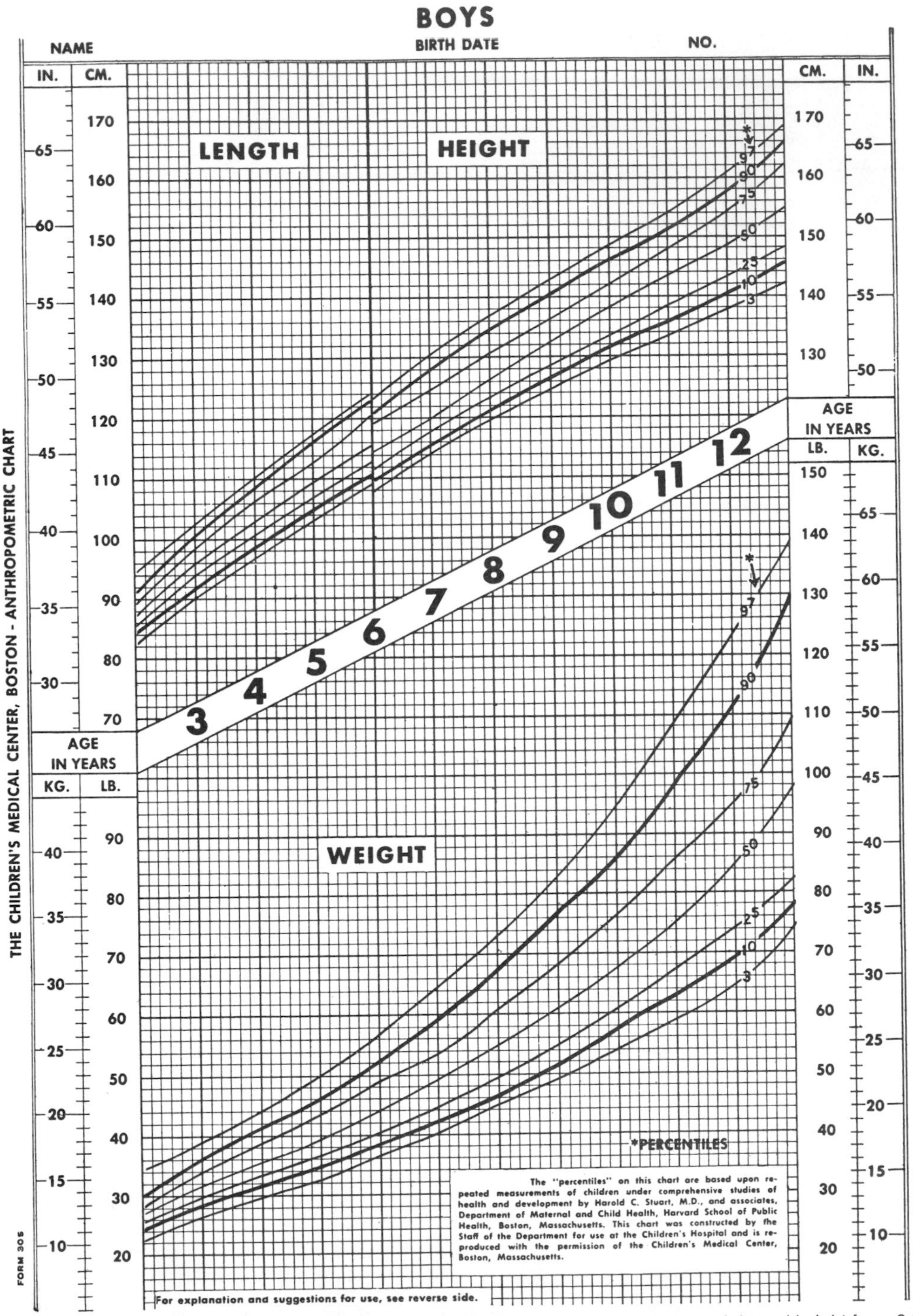

Figure 2–13 *Graphs for plotting weight and height in childhood. This graph serves to plot weight and height from 2 to 13 years of age (height is measured in recumbent position to 6 years of age).*

Percentile graphs for plotting measurements against chronologic age are not as satisfactory for use after 13 years, owing to the wide age variability in the timing of maximum growth during adolescence. For graphs which extend to 18 years based on the percentile values given in Tables 2–6 and 2–8, see Stuart and Meredith: Am. J. Pub. Health, Vol. 36, 1946. Other percentile graphs covering various age periods are available from the Iowa Child Welfare Research Station, University of Iowa.

In evaluation of the measurements of the 13 year old child it is usually possible to recognize by the appearance of secondary sex characters those children who deviate from expected percentile positions because of early or late pubescence.

TABLE 2–8 EMERGING PATTERNS OF BEHAVIOR DURING THE FIRST YEAR OF LIFE

NEONATAL PERIOD (FIRST 4 WEEKS)	
Prone:	Lies in flexed attitude; turns head from side to side; head sags on ventral suspension
Supine:	Generally flexed and a little stiff
Visual:	May fixate face or light in line of vision; "doll's-eye" movement of eyes on turning of the body
Reflex:	Moro response active; stepping and placing reflexes; grasp reflex active
AT 4 WEEKS	
Prone:	Legs more extended; holds chin up; turns head; head lifted momentarily to plane of body on ventral suspension
Supine:	Tonic neck posture predominates; supple and relaxed; head lags on pull to sitting position
Visual:	Watches person; follows moving object a few degrees
AT 8 WEEKS	
Prone:	Raises head slightly farther; head sustained in plane of body on ventral suspension
Supine:	Tonic neck posture predominates; head lags on pull to sitting position
Visual:	Follows moving object 180 degrees
Social:	Smiles on social contact; listens to voice and coos
AT 12 WEEKS	
Prone:	Lifts head and chest, arms extended; head above plane of body on ventral suspension
Supine:	*Tonic neck posture predominates*; reaches toward and misses objects; waves at toy
Sitting:	Head lag partially compensated on pull to sitting position; early head control with bobbing motion; back rounded
Reflex:	Typical Moro response has not persisted; makes defense movements or selective withdrawal reactions
Social:	Sustained social contact; listens to music; says "aah, ngah"
AT 16 WEEKS	
Prone:	Lifts head and chest, head in approximately vertical axis; legs extended
Supine:	*Symmetrical posture predominates,* hands in midline; reaches and grasps objects and brings them to mouth
Sitting:	No head lag on pull to sitting position; head steady, held forward; enjoys sitting with full truncal support
Standing:	When held erect, pushes with feet
Adaptive:	Sees pellet, but makes no move to it
Social:	Laughs out loud; may show displeasure if social contact is broken; excited at sight of food
AT 28 WEEKS	
Prone:	Rolls over; may pivot
Supine:	Lifts head; rolls over; squirming movements
Sitting:	Sits briefly, with support of pelvis; leans forward on hands; back rounded
Standing:	May support most of weight; bounces actively
Adaptive:	Reaches out for and grasps large object; *transfers* objects from hand to hand; grasp uses radial palm; rakes at pellet
Language:	Polysyllabic vowel sounds formed
Social:	Prefers mother; babbles; enjoys mirror; responds to changes in emotional content of social contact
AT 40 WEEKS	
Sitting:	Sits up alone and indefinitely without support, back straight
Standing:	Pulls to standing position
Motor:	Creeps or crawls
Adaptive:	Grasps objects with *thumb and forefinger*; pokes at things with forefinger; picks up pellet with assisted pincer movement; uncovers hidden toy; attempts to retrieve dropped object; releases object grasped by other person
Language:	Repetitive consonant sounds (mama, dada)
Social:	Responds to sound of name; plays peek-a-boo or pat-a-cake; waves bye-bye
AT 52 WEEKS (1 YEAR)	
Motor:	Walks with one hand held; "cruises" or walks holding on to furniture
Adaptive:	Picks up pellet with unassisted pincer movement of forefinger and thumb; releases object to other person on request or gesture
Language:	2 "words" besides mama, dada
Social:	Plays simple ball game; makes postural adjustment to dressing

GROWTH MEAS.

TABLE 2-9 EMERGING PATTERNS OF BEHAVIOR FROM 1 TO 5 YEARS OF AGE

	15 MONTHS
Motor:	Walks alone; crawls up stairs
Adaptive:	Makes tower of 2 cubes; makes a line with crayon; inserts pellet in bottle
Language:	Jargon; follows simple commands; may name a familiar object (ball)
Social:	Indicates some desires or needs by pointing
	18 MONTHS
Motor:	Runs stiffly; sits on small chair; walks up stairs with one hand held; explores drawers and waste baskets
Adaptive:	Piles 3 cubes; imitates scribbling; imitates vertical stroke; dumps pellet from bottle
Language:	10 words (average); names pictures
Social:	Feeds self; seeks help when in trouble; may complain when wet or soiled
	24 MONTHS
Motor:	Runs well; walks up and down stairs, one step at a time; opens doors; climbs on furniture
Adaptive:	Tower of 6 cubes; circular scribbling; imitates horizontal stroke; folds paper once imitatively
Language:	Puts 3 words together (pronoun, verb, object)
Social:	Handles spoon well; often tells immediate experiences; helps to undress; listens to stories with pictures
	30 MONTHS
Motor:	Jumps
Adaptive:	Tower of 8 cubes; makes vertical and horizontal strokes, but generally will not join them to make a cross; imitates circular stroke, forming closed figure
Language:	Refers to self by pronoun "I"; knows full name
Social:	Helps put things away
	36 MONTHS
Motor:	Goes up stairs alternating feet; rides tricycle; stands momentarily on one foot
Adaptive:	Tower of 9 cubes; imitates construction of "bridge" of 3 cubes; copies a circle; imitates a cross
Language:	Knows age and sex; counts 3 objects correctly; repeats 3 numbers or a sentence of 6 syllables
Social:	Plays simple games (in "parallel" with other children); helps in dressing (unbuttons clothing and puts on shoes); washes hands
	48 MONTHS
Motor:	Hops on one foot; throws ball overhand; uses scissors to cut out pictures; climbs well
Adaptive:	Copies bridge from model; imitates construction of "gate" of 5 cubes; copies cross and square; draws a man with 2 to 4 parts besides head; names longer of 2 lines
Language:	Counts 4 pennies accurately; tells a story
Social:	Plays with several children with beginning of social interaction and role-playing; goes to toilet alone
	60 MONTHS
Motor:	Skips
Adaptive:	Draws triangle from copy; names heavier of 2 weights
Language:	Names 4 colors; repeats sentence of 10 syllables; counts 10 pennies correctly
Social:	Dresses and undresses; asks questions about meaning of words; domestic role-playing

After 5 years the Stanford-Binet, Wechsler-Bellevue and other scales offer the most precise estimates of developmental level. In order to have their greatest value, they should be administered only by an experienced and qualified person.

ASSESSMENT OF NEUROLOGIC AND PSYCHOLOGIC DEVELOPMENT

(See also page 66 and Section 20)

The assessment of the functional status of the infant or child is an essential part of each examination, but is all too often uncritical. Only with some knowledge of developmental standards can the physician caring for children be adequately sensitive to deviations which indicate slight or early impairment of development. Moreover, only if he can quickly and confidently compare his observations with the normal developmental schedule will he be able to handle the questions of parents or make appropriate suggestions for further study.

In making the developmental examination an integral part of the routine office visit, the observations made and the techniques used must be appropriate to the age of the infant or child. The physician will often use readily available materials which have not been standardized, but which will usually reveal whether a more comprehensive developmental evaluation is indicated, possibly by a psychologist. The casual examination should be interpreted with caution, particularly when an infant or child who is irritable, hungry or ill fails to perform at his chronologic level. For such patients a future reassessment is in order. For the premature infant an adjustment in chronologic age will need to be made for the degree of prematurity.

In the young infant the examination may begin by observation of the child in the prone and supine positions, note being taken of his spontaneous activity in each position, and then of the manner in which he adjusts to being pulled from a supine to a sitting position and being held in ventral suspension *(Landau response)*. His reaction to moving persons or to objects brought within his sight or grasp can be determined, both for relatively large objects such as a rattle or stethoscope and for such small objects as a pellet. His behavior when standing with support should also be observed.

After the first year of life the child may be given blocks as well as a pencil and paper and his ability observed to mimic or copy the scribblings or figures of the physician. The standard blocks used in construction of various figures are 1-inch red cubes. After 3 years the child can be asked to "draw a man," to draw figures and to count pennies.

Tables 2–8 and 2–9 list expected behavior of infants and children of various ages and circumstances. The data are derived from those of Gesell, Shirley, Provence, Wolf, and others.

A number of relatively simple tests permit the physician or his assistant to make helpful assessments of the intellectual level of older children as part of normal office practice. Such tests include the Peabody Picture Vocabulary Test, the Quick Test, the Raven Matrices, the Thorpe Developmental Inventory, and the Denver Developmental Screening Test.* Occasional or casual testing may be misleading. In using these or other tools for evaluation of performance the tester should become thoroughly familiar with the procedures, their rules for administration, and their limitations. The Draw-a-Man Test, for example, should be given to a child who is comfortably seated; he is given a plain piece of white paper 8½ by 11 inches and a pencil with an eraser, and should be left undisturbed for as long as he needs to complete his drawing. The test may have grossly distorted values when the child uses a ball-point pen to put a hasty drawing on a prescription pad, while he stands at a corner of the physician's desk. When doubt exists as to the interpretation of any of these tests, the child should be referred to a qualified psychologist.

*See Appendix for description of Denver Developmental Screening Test.

VICTOR C. VAUGHAN, III

Barnett, C. R., Leiderman, P. H., Grobstein, R., and Klaus, M.: Neonatal separation: Maternal side of the interaction. Pediatrics *45*:197, 1970.

Bayer, L. M., and Bayley, N.: Growth Diagnosis. Chicago, University of Chicago Press, 1959.

Erikson, E. H.: Childhood and Society. New York, W. W. Norton and Co., 1950.

Falkner, F. (ed.): Human Development. Philadelphia, W. B. Saunders Company, 1966.

Frankenburg, W. K., and Dodds, J. B.: The Denver Developmental Screening Test. J. Pediatr. *71*:181, 1967.

Gesell, A., and Amatruda, C. S.: Developmental Diagnosis. 2nd ed. New York, Paul B. Hoeber, Inc., 1947.

Greulich, W. W., and Pyle, S. I.: Radiographic Atlas of Skeletal Development of the Hand and Wrist. Stanford, Calif., Stanford University Press, 1950; 2nd ed., 1959.

Iliff, A., and Lee, V. A.: Pulse rate, respiratory rate, and body temperature of children between two months and eighteen years of age. Child Develop. *23*:237, 1952.

Illingworth, R. S.: The Development of the Infant and Young Child, Normal and Abnormal. Edinburgh, E. & S. Livingstone, 1960.

Klaus, M. H., and Kennell, J. H.: Mothers separated from their newborn infants. Pediatr. Clin. N. Amer. *17*:1015, 1970.

Klaus, M. H., Jerauld, R., Kreger, N. C., McAlpine, W., Steffa, M., and Kennell, J. H.: Maternal attachment: Importance of the first post-partum days. New Engl. J. Med. *286*:460, 1972.

Lewis, R. C., Duval, A. M., and Iliff, A.: Standards for the basal metabolism of children from 2 to 15 years of age, inclusive. J. Pediatr. *23*:1, 1943.

Meiks, L. T., and Green, M. (eds.): Symposium on Adolescence. Pediat. Clin. N. Amer. *7*:1–226, 1960.

Munn, N. L.: The Evolution and Growth of Human Behavior. Boston, Houghton-Mifflin Co., 1955.

Pyle, S. I., Reed, R. B., and Stuart, H. C.: Patterns of skeletal development in the hand. Pediatrics *24*:886, 1959.

Reynolds, E. L., and Asakawa, T.: Skeletal development in infancy: Standards for clinical use. Am. J. Roentgenol. & Radium Ther. *65*:403, 1951.

Root, A. W.: Endocrinology of puberty. J. Pediatr. *83*:1, 187, 1973.

Stuart, H. C.: Normal growth and development during adolescence. New Engl. J. Med. *234*:666, 693, 732, 1946.

Talbot, N. B., Richie, R. H., and Crawford, J. D.: Metabolic Homeostasis: A Syllabus for Those Concerned with the Care of Patients. Cambridge, Mass., Harvard University Press, 1959.

Tanner, J. M.: Growth at Adolescence. Springfield, Ill. Charles C Thomas, 1956.

Tanner, J. M., Goldstein, H., and Whitehouse, R. H.: Standards for children's height at 2–9 years allowing for height of parents. Arch. Dis. Child. *45*:755, 1970.

Todd, T. W.: Atlas of Skeletal Maturation (Hand). St. Louis, The C. V. Mosby Company, 1937.

Vaughan, V. C., III: New insights in social behavior. J.A.M.A. *198*:46, 1966.

Vaughan, V. C., III (ed.): Issues in Human Development. Washington, Government Printing Office, 1971.

Vogt, E. C., and Vickers, V. S.: Osseous growth and development. Radiology, *31*:441, 1938.

Watson, E. H., and Lowrey, G. H.: Growth and Development of Children. 5th ed. Chicago, Year Book Publishers, Inc., 1967.

Watson, R. I.: Psychology of the Child. New York, John Wiley & Sons, 1959.

Weech, A. A.: Signposts on highway of growth. Am. J. Dis. Child. *88*:452, 1954.

Wingert, J., Solomon, I. L., and Schoen, E. J.: Parent-specific height standards for preadolescent children of three racial groups, with method for rapid determination. Pediatrics *52*:555, 1973.

PSYCHOLOGIC DEVELOPMENT

At birth only a few of the inherited patterns of adaptive behavior of the human infant are sufficiently mature to contribute to his survival. He has inherent rooting, sucking and swallowing reflexes which enable him to find and take nourishment, provided the breast or bottle is within the range of his head movements. He is capable of vocalizing relatively undifferentiated cries of distress, signalling that he is in need. Within a period of days he can make cooing noises and winsome facial expressions which, importantly, evoke feelings of tenderness and warmth in his mother. Except for these rather primitive patterns and certain automatic and homeostatic regulative functions, he is helpless and, unless cared for, will die.

The infant's prolonged dependency and vulnerability are, however, well compensated by his ultimate capacity for the higher mental abilities such as conscious memory, anticipation, speech, abstract reasoning, and communication by spoken and written language. The fact that he inherits few automatic, autonomous and complex patterns of behavior means that he is much less bound to automatic and rigid ways of adaptation. His inherited abilities mature slowly and they are subject to influence; full realization of the child's skills, the effectiveness with which he uses them, and the use to which they are put are determined by interaction with his environment.

Out of this interaction the mind or psyche develops, which takes over the management of the inherited patterns of behavior and the higher mental abilities. The result is man's capacity to alter his environment and adapt it to his needs. On the other hand, the fact that his development is so much shaped by experience allows for the possibility of unfavorable influences and accounts in large measure for his susceptibility to emotional and mental illness.

Since psychic or personality development, or *psychologic development* (in accordance with the terminology used here), takes place after birth, postnatal experiences are of great importance. The capacity for memory and the related faculty of anticipation have their beginnings in the first months of life; they make it possible for earlier experiences to influence the response to situations encountered subsequently. Significant experiences in the first days, weeks, months and years of life are especially important because they affect the very foundations of psychologic development.

Psychologic development can be appraised in terms of the interaction of the child's *natural endowment* and *environmental factors.*

BIOLOGIC FACTORS

The role of the child's innate potential in his development can be discussed in terms of three different but closely interrelated factors: (1) *endowment,* (2) the predetermined pattern and schedule of *biologic maturation,* and (3) the *energy* necessary for growth, development and functioning.

ENDOWMENT. The term endowment refers to inherited or constitutional patterns; basic elements are the physical and physiologic make-up of the individual, his potential for intelligence, and his more specific potentials such as talents for music or mathematics.*

In the first months of life a predominant temperament or behavioral pattern is observed in some infants which may persist relatively unchanged through childhood into adulthood. Temperament or personality in infants and children stems from such relatively independent qualities of behavior as activity level, rhythmicity, adaptability, the tendency to approach or withdraw from new stimuli, intensity of reaction to stimuli, mood, sensory threshold, distractibility and attention spans. The qualities of feeling in mother-infant relations are also vital to personality development and have early impact on the infant. The relative importances of heredity or endowment and of environmental-social factors in forming temperament or personality have not been clearly delineated; but it is clear that degrees of compatibility or incompatibility may exist between the temperament of the child and the attitudes and expectations he meets in his environment which may contribute either to healthy development and adaptation or to disturbances in behavior.

Endowment is shaped not only by heredity, but also by postconceptional factors. Untoward events during the intrauterine, parturient or postnatal periods, for example, may produce conditions such as cerebral palsy, which may determine that the constitution of the child at birth differs from what was intended by heredity. The motor defect in cerebral palsy is usually readily perceived, and parents and physicians will make allowance for this handicap when evaluating the development of the child. When alterations in innate endowment have no clearly demonstrable clinical manifestations, the child is not likely to be recognized as constitutionally handicapped, and appropriate allowances will not be made. This situation may cause problems in development when the child fails to measure up to expectations. Subtle handicaps may result either from structural damage or from physiologic malfunctioning. The consequent impairments or delays in development may produce anxiety in parents, frustration and anxiety in the child,

*Evidence suggests that such talents may reflect not only endowment, but also such factors as early exposure to specific kinds of stimulation and unusually strong interest and motivation, which result in greater development of potential in particular areas of capability.

and a disturbed relationship between child and parents.

Optimum development requires that the child's endowment and parental expectations be in accord. It is important to make careful and continuing appraisals of constitutional as well as environmental factors.

BIOLOGIC MATURATION. Innate factors largely determine not only the physical characteristics of the infant and child but such features as the times of emergence of the capacity to walk, of puberty and of the ability for abstract reasoning. The time of appearance of each of these various capacities and functions is fairly predictable, but there is considerable individual variation; as with organic or constitutional differences, it is important that the environmental expectations be in keeping with the time schedule of the individual child.

The child's psychologic and personality development is closely related to the development of his mental abilities. The biologically predetermined maturation of nervous system pathways proceeds sequentially from the autonomic level to the spinal cord level of the sensory and lower motor neuron reflex arc, to a subcortical level, and to the level of the upper motor neuron and cerebral cortex. At birth (except in some cases of prematurity) the autonomic nervous system, which participates importantly in the homeostatic regulative functions, is normally reasonably well functioning and integrated, as are the lower motor neuron reflex arcs.

The further integration of sensorimotor reflex pathways with other sensory and motor pathways and with the higher centers is dependent upon continuing maturation of the central nervous system and upon experience. For example, the retina and oculomotor apparatus are at birth capable of receiving light stimuli and transmitting nerve impulses to the brain which indicate a response to patterns of light, but a preferential response to a pattern resembling the human face will be delayed for 2 to 3 months and will be dependent upon exposure to the face or to such facial patterns. Both maturation and practice are required before the various sensorimotor pathways involved in walking are sufficiently functional and integrated for the child to be able to walk. On a less observable level, there is evidence to suggest that the capability for abstract reasoning appears by about the age of 12 years, when there is further maturation of the endocrine and possibly of the central nervous systems.

The innately predetermined timing of sensorimotor maturation may itself be affected by experience. For example, serious nutritional deficiency can impair physiologic functioning and the rate and ultimate quality of physical growth. Under such conditions delay in onset of puberty might have important implications for psychologic development. Studies of emotional deprivation during infancy suggest that certain optimal amounts and qualities of stimulation are necessary to bring forth innate patterns. It has not been established that the biologic mechanisms responsible for imprinting (see p. 21) in lower animals also exist in man, but it does seem reasonable to draw certain analogies, at least in the sense that healthy development may depend upon certain kinds of stimulation and experience at certain critical periods in the course of human development. As a rather extreme illustration, the continuous bandaging of the eyes of chimpanzees during a critical period of visual development results in blindness. Similarly, work with psychotic children suggests that the development of language may be seriously impaired in the child whose mother was essentially nonvocal while caring for him in his infancy.

ENERGY. The third biologic factor, energy of life, is utilized in two related but different ways. On the one hand, energy is invested in the growth of the child and in the physiologic functions necessary for sustaining and ultimately for reproducing life. On the other hand, it is used for mental and physical activities which are not immediately and directly related to the viability of the individual or to the survival of the species.

Fundamentally the biologic destiny of man is to reproduce his kind. The capacity for procreation does not appear until puberty, but the developmental years are largely concerned with helping the child, first, to become a social being able to get along with others and, ultimately, to marry, to function sexually and to rear children. In this context, though much of the activity and behavior of man are not directly sexual, the energy used in other activities serves or is derived from the sexual drive. It is from this viewpoint that Freud described the sexual drive as the central factor in human behavior. His original conceptualizations were misunderstood and met with much resistance, but his ideas, in their intended meaning, are essential to an understanding of child development.

In the foregoing sense, energy derived from chemical processes is utilized by and channeled through the sexual drive. Qualities of pleasure, affection, and satisfaction are normal characteristics of behavioral manifestations of the sexual drive, which tend to relate the individual to other people. There are other feelings, however, of different quality which are associated with the overcoming of obstacles and the solution of problems. The behavioral manifestations of these activities have been summed up under the term "aggression." There continue to be differences of opinion about the number and nature of basic life drives, but for practical purposes child development can be adequately understood in terms of these two qualitatively different drives: *the sexual drive* and *the aggressive drive.*

Observation of the infant in the neonatal period tends to support this formulation of drives. When the healthy infant has recovered from the effects of birth, and is receiving care appropriate to his needs, the observable evidence as to a non-neutral emotional state suggests pleasure and satisfaction; normally he is relaxed, he coos, he smiles. With frustration of his needs, which is inevitable in spite of the best possible care, evidence of aggression is observed. If he is hungry, restrained or hurt, he cries in a way which suggests anger, and he shows increasingly vigorous, uncoordinated movements which at a later age, directed and coordinated, would undoubtedly aim at avoidance of or coping with the cause of his discomfort.

If the infant's first aggressive actions call forth an environmental response which relieves his frustration, he does not become unduly distressed; it is reasonable, therefore, to think of a capacity for aggression as normal and constructive. On the other hand, if his discomfort continues and his tension increases, his behavior takes on a destructive quality. In acute distress he shows the equivalent of rage and hostility. If he does not have the means for directing his aggression toward solving the problem, with continuing neglect of his needs the rage subsides, and the aggression is contained and expressed internally. In moderate situations this internalized aggression may become manifest in various kinds of physiologic disturbance. In extreme cases of deprivation of emotional needs the infant exhibits a clinical picture analogous to depression; without proper treatment there ensues a progressive decline of emotional tone and physiologic functioning.

The developing personality of the child increasingly shapes subsequent development. In early infancy the sexual and aggressive drives readily gain expression, owing to the relative lack of internal organization and means of control. Initially the energy of these drives is utilized largely for physical purposes. As the mind develops, it is directed also to mental activities and is identified as psychic energy.

The psychic energy derived from the sexual drive is termed *libido*. Libido is conceived of as a force or flow of psychic energy which can be controlled and directed toward or away from parts of oneself, other people and tangible or abstract goals, in dynamic and constantly changing ways and amounts. For example, normal stimulation of the sensory endings of the skin of the infant is viewed as causing libido to be invested in this body area. In this experience the anatomic limits of the body are defined, the development of the body image promoted, and the child helped to demarcate himself from the rest of the world. Later, as relationships are increasingly established with other human beings, certain amounts of libido must be directed toward or invested in other persons.

The supply of psychic energy varies with physiologic changes in different stages of development or in physical illness, but the total amount available at any given time is limited. If too much energy is expended in emotional conflicts rather than in effective action, the individual has a problem. For example, the child whose mental energy is consumed by a conflict between an intense desire to excel and an equally strong fear of failure may not invest sufficient libido in the task of learning, and he may fail in school for this reason rather than because of deficiency in intelligence.

The choice as to investment of libido will primarily determine the basic pattern of the child's development and behavior. The psychic energy of the aggressive drive is secondary to libido, being used to implement or fulfill libidinal choices or aims. In a sense, life is a succession of patterns of tension and relief-of-tension. The expression of sexual and aggressive drives in overt behavior can be temporarily held in check, but inevitably they will gain expression, in ways which may be either healthy or abnormal.

One way to evaluate a child's development is to study his use of libido and of aggression in relation to others and to himself, comparing his current use with that of his earlier development and with that of the average child of his age and social group.

ENVIRONMENTAL FACTORS

The work of Freud demonstrated that experiences retained outside of conscious awareness can significantly influence behavior. The age at which the human organism is first able to retain impressions at conscious or unconscious* levels is largely speculative. Nevertheless the question needs consideration in view of growing concern that certain clinical practices applied to the infant may have psychologic impact contrary to past interpretations. For example, there is considerable concern that various aspects of the care of premature infants, including their isolation, may impair subsequent personality and cognitive functions. More concretely, circumcision shortly after birth without adequate anesthesia has been justified on the assumption that the painful experience has no untoward psychologic influence.

The conditioned reflex offers data relevant to the question of retention of impressions. Conditioning outside of conscious awareness can take place even in the human fetus during the last trimester of pregnancy, with persistence after birth. Studies have indicated that the restlessness of infants can be lessened by an instrument reproducing the sound of the mother's heartbeat. And at a few weeks of age infants have been observed to respond to their mother's voice with a lessening of distress and tension, even though the mother was not in direct contact with them, and in spite of simultaneous exposure to the sounds of other voices. It seems probable that impressions can be retained before conscious memory is possible.

One cannot fail to be impressed with the tremendous capacity of the human being to absorb trauma and survive. Perhaps it is only this capacity, at least in part, which has permitted us inappropriately to discount the significance of untoward events in the earliest period of life.

---

*The term *unconscious* as used in psychology is equivalent to the lay term *subconscious*, and means outside of conscious awareness. It is not to be confused with the physical state of being unconscious or in coma.

Concern for the psychologic development and future mental health of the child requires that events in the neonatal as well as in any later stage of development be managed in such a way as to keep tension in the child within tolerable limits.

PRENATAL ENVIRONMENTAL INFLUENCES. Physicians do not attribute birthmarks and other physical characteristics of infants and children to acute or chronic emotional upsets in the mother during pregnancy. The probability of such a cause and effect is exceedingly unlikely. On the other hand, one cannot be certain that the mental and emotional state or physical activity of the mother during pregnancy is not reflected in some way in the personality of the child. One may speculate that hormonal influences associated with acute or chronic states of tension in the mother can be passed through the placental barrier to the fetus. Such effects might be only temporary, but the possibility must be considered that they may have a continuing effect.

POSTNATAL ENVIRONMENTAL INFLUENCES. The emotional and attitudinal climate into which a child is born has its beginnings long before his arrival. Even the fantasies about babies and motherhood which the mother had as a little girl and as an adolescent play a role in her functioning as an adult. The extent to which husband and wife agree as to when to have and how to rear children also is important. The experience of the mother during pregnancy, labor and delivery is particularly significant; an earlier fantasy may now be fulfilled or contradicted by reality. A woman who feels that her husband has faltered in his love and emotional support during her pregnancy may feel conscious or unconscious resentment toward the still unborn child. Or, when the child is born, she may "love" it too much, trying to recover from the child the love which she normally should be receiving from her husband. During the infant's first months of life any overt or subclinical depressive reaction in the mother may produce an infant-mother relationship that is unnatural and lacking in warmth and spontaneity.

A clear need for emotional satisfaction exists in the neonate. This is seen in his pleasure in sucking and clinging, and in "following" his mother with sight and hearing, as well as in the various sensory experiences provided through his mother's ministrations, such as body warmth, cuddling, rocking, bathing, anointing the skin, and her soothing voice. These needs become increasingly strong and meaningful during the first year of life, and ultimately are subsumed under what we call the need for love.

The crowded hospital nursery cannot provide the kind of infant-mother interaction described above. It is difficult even for a trained mother-substitute to give the unique care provided by the infant's own mother. Placement of the infant in the mother's hospital room most or all of the time ("rooming-in") provides opportunities for the establishment of better mother-infant relations. There is no substantiated indication of risk in such arrangements to the physical health of normal infants.

It seems reasonable to generalize that, whenever possible, the newborn infant as well as the sick infant or young child should have a close and continuing relation with his parents.

Owing to the immaturity of the infant's perceptual and motor apparatus, the mother must supplement his undeveloped functions and must meet his needs. This places the mother in a unique position which may explain the tendency for some mothers to feel unduly guilty when problems arise in their child's physical or emotional development and for the physician to look particularly to the child-mother relationship in an attempt to understand emotional imbalance in a child. Objectivity requires, however, that one neither excuse the parents from responsibility for the child's psychologic development nor hold them entirely responsible. The physician should attempt to convey an understanding of this to parents.

The infant also needs an optimal amount of frustration and opportunities to learn to tolerate tension. These needs, although less well recognized, are as important as the need for satisfaction. Mothers and fathers play both roles, satisfier and frustrator, giving on the one hand, as they meet the child's needs, but also confronting him with the realities of physical and social living. In the first weeks and months of life the primary needs of the infant are satisfaction and relief of tension. It is generally the mother who must decide how much the infant should be held, whether he should be permitted to cry himself to sleep, whether he should be fed on "demand" or according to schedule, and a host of other common but important matters. She is influenced both by her own needs and the needs of other people, particularly of the father, the immediate family and other relatives. As the infant approaches the end of his first year, both father and mother are expected to begin to present the culturally prescribed limits upon his behavior which will assure him an adequate personality and character structure.

The sine qua non *of successful child rearing is the achievement of an optimal balance between satisfying the child's needs on the one hand and frustrating and challenging him on the other, so as to stimulate the development of his latent abilities and potentialities.*

PSYCHOLOGIC FACTORS

THE ID. The normal state of the infant is a dynamic one in which tensions are constantly being built up and relieved. At the beginning the tensions are largely due to internal, physiologic processes necessary for the sustenance of life, e.g., the hunger tension. Very early, however, the infant becomes more wakeful, and this presages the beginning of mental development. The only element of psychic structure present at this time is the id. *The id can be defined as the inherited reservoir of unorganized drives. It is mostly unconscious, is governed by the pleasure-pain principle, aims at immediate satisfaction of libidinal urges, is unmoral, is illogical and lacks unity of purpose.*

THE EGO. Out of the interaction between mother and infant with its repetition of stimulation, tension and relief-of-tension, the mental organization and ego of the infant begin to develop. As his personality and capacities gradually emerge, more is expected of him, and the mother begins to introduce the previously referred to limits and frustrations. The infant responds with his biologically innate tendency to strive for mastery. For example, though the potential for walking is biologically provided, the development of the capacity to walk is ascribed to the ego as part of psychologic development.

The ego can be defined as the integrating or mediating part of personality, which develops out of the interaction of id and environment and controls the tendencies of the id, excluding or modifying those tendencies which are in conflict with reality. It is predominantly conscious or preconscious, and has perception both of the internal self and of the external world.

The ego of the mother complements and supplements the ego of the child. As the child's ego and initiative develop, however, she must gradually turn over to the child an increasing amount of responsibility for himself until he is able to function relatively autonomously and independently.

The skills acquired by the ego and used in the solution of problems and conflicts can be referred to as *ego defenses.* An individual's ego defenses serve the purposes of adaptation and survival and of productive and creative functioning. Certain defenses deal mostly with the external world, e.g., the ability to perceive, to walk and to talk. Other defenses deal more with the internal world of drive, conflict, tension and emotion.

SUPEREGO. As we ascend the phylogenetic scale, an increasing amount of energy becomes available for activities other than those directly concerned with sustaining life. Purely pleasurable or play activity is more characteristic of mammals than of other animals. Man not only plays, but is also uniquely capable of creative activity. As a social being he has had to develop a system of values for guiding behavior. He makes laws and concerns himself with religion and philosophy. In so doing he develops a conscience or superego. The behavior of man without a conscience does not differ materially from the behavior of the lower animals.

The child is born without a superego. This element of personality structure, like the ego, is developed under the training and influence of the environment. The superego normally develops under the aegis of love. As the child's urges and behavior bring him into conflict with his parents, it is his need to continue receiving their love and approval which causes him to accept their judgments and disciplinary actions, and to internalize their values to form his own superego.

The superego makes value judgments about the individual's urges, impulses and activities, and can be defined as the latest development of the mind (both phylogenetically and ontogenetically), embodying the code of society and including concepts of right and wrong, the value system, and the ideals.

CONSCIOUS, PRECONSCIOUS AND UNCONSCIOUS AREAS OF THE MIND. It appears that conscious perception at birth is exceedingly limited. Even when fully awake, the newborn infant is thought to have no awareness of himself as separate from the rest of the world. As his various sensory systems mature and are repeatedly stimulated, impressions are received and integrated on a cortical level. Conscious awareness is thought to develop gradually during the first year of life.

The conscious mind is defined as that relatively small part of mental life of which the individual is aware at any given time. Although conscious awareness is a continuum during normal waking life, its content is transitory and constantly changing. On the other hand, there is a great deal of the mental life which is available to consciousness through recall or association of ideas. *For purposes of definition, this material, which is readily available to consciousness, is referred to as being preconscious.*

There is still another significant body of material which is *unconscious* and either not available to consciousness at all, or available to it only with special techniques such as the free association technique of psychoanalytic treatment or hypnosis. Certain experiences may be unconscious because their engrams were established before the development of the capacity for conscious memory. One evidence in support of this idea is the "screen" or false memory observed in psychoanalytic treatment, wherein a patient claims to have a memory of some experience occurring in the first year or two of life, at a time for which conscious memory normally is not functional. The proposed explanation is that the patient did have an experience which was stored in the nervous system, most likely more in terms of feelings or emotions than in terms of visual or verbal images, and that the patient now fabricates visual and verbal imagery to suit the experience he is attempting to recall.

Experiences may be unconscious for another reason. One of the ways in which the mind attempts to protect itself from unpleasant or intolerable tension is to eliminate the memory of the experience and the associated feelings from conscious awareness. This is known as *repression.* Though the painful thoughts or feelings are no longer in conscious awareness, they are nevertheless still a part of mental life. Within certain limits repression can be a normal and successful way of dealing with tension and conflict. On the other hand, repression may be the basis for development of emotional disturbance, since the repressed material is invested with psychic energy and can influence behavior in spite of the person's having no conscious awareness that this is the case. A primary goal in the consideration of normal child development should be the prevention of pathologic repression, with its ensuing development of emotional problems.

GENERAL PRINCIPLES GOVERNING CHILD DEVELOPMENT

The sexual drive and aggressive drives may be increased or decreased by changing conditions of stimulation, physical health, and environment, but they demand fulfillment. The child needs to develop a personality which can exercise these drives in sufficiently satisfying ways and at the same time keep their exercise within the requirements of social living. The sexual curiosity of a 6 year old child at times will be satisfied with direct information about sexual matters, for example, but much of the time will be sublimated, his energy being used in the classroom to learn subjects far removed from sex, which prepare him, nonetheless, at least in principle for his adult role.

As a result of progressive biologic maturation and cultural conditioning the aims of the sexual and aggressive drives are constantly changing. Freud proposed the term *psychosexual development* to characterize the child's progress through what he called oral, anal, phallic, latency and adolescent stages (see Table 2–10).

EGO MASTERY. Erikson has clarified the importance of ego development as the counterpart of the changing focus of sexual and aggressive drives. He lists for each stage of development of the child a certain predominant *ego quality* which is normally acquired during that stage, out of mastery of the challenges presented and from resolution of the resulting conflicts. For example, at the close of the oral phase the infant normally should have acquired a feeling of trust as a result of his various experiences with his mother, including the experience of being weaned. The infant should derive ego strength from having been able to give up pleasure in sucking the breast or bottle in return for maternal approval.

The experience of surmounting the various challenges and conflicts presented to him by his own biologic maturation and by his environment is important to the child's development of a sense of ego mastery.

MATURATION-DEVELOPMENT. The infant is usually ready for weaning toward the end of the first year of life, when the need for sucking seems to have been sufficiently satisfied and erupted teeth provide the ability and the motivation for chewing food. Weaning at either 6 or 18 months of age may be out of step with biologic maturation, and may create an unnecessarily intense conflict over an inevitable step in development. Similarly, an unexpected biologic deviation may cause difficulty such as onset of puberty and menstruation in a 9 year old girl whose environment is understandably not prepared for this event and has not prepared her.

Biologic maturation and psychologic development should optimally progress hand in hand and complement each other.

PLEASURE-PAIN VERSUS REALITY PRINCIPLE. Early in life the child is governed by what Freud called *the pleasure-pain principle:* he seeks that which is pleasurable and avoids or rejects that which is unpleasurable. At first this behavior is essentially reflexive, but as conscious awareness increases, the infant becomes more discerning and his behavior becomes increasingly purposeful. His parents first, and then society, take cognizance of his increasing ability to understand and to exercise self-control and begin to present various demands which intrude upon his pleasure. These demands gradually increase throughout the child's development and require him to take on increasing amounts of responsibility for himself and finally for others.

During the course of his development the child learns to postpone and moderate his needs, wants and pleasures in order to function as a responsible member of a society; thus the pleasure-pain principle gradually yields to the reality principle.

PROGRESSION-REGRESSION. The child does not find the demands of reality always to his liking, nor is he able to meet and master them easily. In spite of the inevitability of his biologic maturation and the strength of his innate tendency toward achievement and mastery, the child will at times retreat temporarily in the face of difficult problems and tension-creating conflicts. Within certain limits regression is not only normal but may be essential and helpful, since the child may need the opportunity to replenish his emotional energy and to prepare himself once again to forge ahead.

Child development is normally characterized by a pattern of progression and regression.

LOVE AND LIMITS. The early training of the child and his later education constitute his acculturation, which is achieved through the judicious use of approval and disapproval by parents and teachers. Generally speaking, parents readily voice approval and disapproval, but they frequently have difficulty in backing up these attitudes with convincing firmness and consistency. Words alone are not always enough. For example, if a 7 year old child who is having difficulty learning in school feels that his relation to his parents is superficial and lacking in emotional support, their verbal encouragement may have little motivating force. The toddler who does not respond to repeated verbal admonishments against touching and playing with a forbidden object will have more convincing evidence of the parent's intent when the object is removed.

Just as the use of aggression in overcoming obstacles is normal in the child, the use of aggression in training the child is normal in the parent. Difficulties arise when parents do not have sufficient conviction about the values they present to their child, or when for other reasons they fail to take action sufficiently early. If they permit their anger to mount before taking some effective actions, their aggression often bursts out of control in the form of

(Text continued on page 65)

TABLE 2–10 STAGES OF PSYCHOLOGIC DEVELOPMENT

1. STAGE. Both pediatric and psychoanalytic terminologies are used to designate the successive stages of development.

2. AGE. The years of growth and development are divided into periods based on both physical and psychologic characteristics. These periods are not sharply demarcated, but each blends imperceptibly into the following one, and there are wide normal variations in the rates of transition.

3. BIOLOGIC MATURATION. Each stage is characterized by the appearance of certain physical and mental abilities which are innately predetermined.

4. LIBIDO. As the predetermined abilities mature, their proper functioning requires that they become invested with psychic energy (libido).

5. BIOLOGIC AND CULTURAL CHALLENGES. Each new capacity arising out of biologic maturation presents the child with a challenge requiring mastery. Concurrently, certain cultural and familial attitudes insist that he give up early forms of gratification and assume gradually increasing responsibility. As he responds to and masters these challenges, his unique physical and psychologic development takes place, and he becomes a social being able to function in his particular culture or subculture.

6. AGGRESSION. Under normal circumstances aggression arises and is expressed in response to the challenges and insistences on renunciation of gratification and as an aid in facing and mastering them.

7. OBJECT RELATIONSHIP. In psychoanalytic psychology the term "object" includes inanimate and animate objects, human and nonhuman, but most commonly refers to people. The establishment and maintenance of relationship require that the object be invested with libido (see 4, above).

8. EGO AND IDENTITY. The ego is that part of personality structure which serves an integrating function in relation to the self and a mediating function between the self and the environment. An important aspect of the ego is the concept of self or of one's own identity which develops gradually throughout childhood. Attention will be called to the *ego qualities* and to the development of the *sense of reality.*

9. SUPEREGO (CONSCIENCE AND IDEALS). The superego arises out of the ego and embodies the code of the parents and of society or, more specifically, concepts of right and wrong and the individual's ideals and aspirations.

10. TYPICAL NORMAL BEHAVIOR. The composite of all aspects of development in any given stage should result in behavior characteristic and normal for that age period.

TABLE 2–10 STAGES OF PSYCHOLOGIC DEVELOPMENT *(Continued)*

NEONATAL AND EARLY INFANCY

1. STAGE. Oral stage: Normal autistic phase.

2. AGE. Birth to 3 or 4 months.

3. BIOLOGIC MATURATION. After birth the infant must adjust immediately to extrauterine existence. Normally, the basic autonomic and subcortical homeostatic functions are operative at birth, as are the less automatic, sensorimotor reflexes responsible for sucking and crying. Crying is initially an unrefined signal to the mother. The newborn infant is ill equipped to bear tension and has a stimulus barrier, which functions to avoid excessive stress.

4. LIBIDO. Because the infant at birth lacks both conscious awareness and a concept of self, it is conceived that investment of libido in his biologic functions takes place automatically and unconsciously, as each of the various systems is activated. As conscious awareness increases, libidinization becomes increasingly volitional. In the first months of life libidinal investment proceeds sequentially from the internal visceral systems, to the respiratory function, to the oral zone involved in sucking and ingestion, and then to the surface of the body, as the various sensory end-organs mature and receive stimuli from the general physical environment and through the ministrations of the mother.

5. BIOLOGIC AND CULTURAL CHALLENGES. The primary challenges to the infant are the biologic requirements of shifting from intrauterine to extrauterine existence.

   Culture generally makes no additional demands upon the infant. It influences this transition, however, through customs and practices such as whether the infant is with the mother from birth or is put in a nursery, whether feeding is by breast or bottle, whether the bottle-fed infant is held by the mother during feeding, and by the amount and kinds of exposure to light, sound, tactile and other stimuli. Such considerations as how long the baby is permitted to cry, how he is comforted or when, and how he is dressed, swaddled, or carried may modify developing patterns of personality.

6. AGGRESSION. The newborn infant lacks sufficient coordination and ability for effective aggressive acts. But with frustration of his needs and any undue disturbance in his homeostasis, aggression is evidenced in crying and aimless motor activity. The most severe state of distress has been termed infantile rage. Gradually, as a result of the mother-infant interaction, aggressive responses become more purposeful; e.g.,the hunger cry has a different quality from the cry of pain.

7. OBJECT RELATIONSHIP. In the same way that he unconsciously and automatically libidinizes his body systems, the infant also libidinizes the mother. During these first few months, while the perceptual-conscious system is still developing, he does not discern his mother as separate from himself, and his experience is truly autistic, as if everything arose from and took place within him. It is necessary also that the mother properly invest her newborn child with her libido.

8. EGO AND IDENTITY. Such functions as sucking and crying can be regarded as rudiments of the ego, since they function to mediate the needs of the infant in relation to the environment. Those ego functions which are not yet developed are provided by the mother (maternal auxiliary ego). The task of the combined mother-infant ego is to meet the needs of the infant, keeping his tensions within tolerable limits.

   There is no concept of the self and therefore no identity, but the experiences in these first months presumably are recorded on an unconscious level and can give a feeling of well-being and contribute to the development of feelings of security, confidence and integration.

9. SUPEREGO (CONSCIENCE AND IDEALS). Superego as such does not exist. The pleasure-pain principle is the basis for the later development of concepts of good and bad and of right and wrong.

10. TYPICAL NORMAL BEHAVIOR. The infant functions in close union with the mother, manifesting an alternation of tension, gratification and relief of tension. At the beginning of this stage the most characteristic behavior is brief wakefulness and restlessness, and then sleeping after eating. Gradually, as the periods of wakefulness increase, personality begins to develop.

Table 2–10 continued on following page.

TABLE 2–10 STAGES OF PSYCHOLOGIC DEVELOPMENT *(Continued)*

INFANCY PERIOD

1. STAGE. Oral stage: Symbiotic phase.

2. AGE. 3 to 4 months until 12 to 18 months. The *separation-individuation phase* of ego development begins in the latter part of the oral stage and continues through the phallic stage (3 to 6 or 7 years), as the child gradually separates from his mother and becomes increasingly autonomous.

3. BIOLOGIC MATURATION. There is continuing maturation of the end-organs of taste, smell, touch, vision and hearing, and of the nervous pathways permitting development of the first coordinated movements, such as binocular vision and hand-to-mouth integration, and walking begins.

4. LIBIDO. Libidinization of these various organ systems is contributed to by the mother through nursing, skin contact, being held and rocked, and seeing her facial expressions and hearing her voice. Evidence of the infant's precise identification of his own mother among other faces begins to be found by 4 months, should be secure by 6 months.

5. BIOLOGIC AND CULTURAL CHALLENGES. Biologic maturation presents the challenge of coordinated movement and the purposeful use of the perceptual-conscious system, and also the discomfort associated with the eruption of teeth, and subsequently the use of teeth and jaws in mastication.

   Partly in relation to the appearance of teeth, but also partly as a cultural attitude, the infant is weaned from the breast or bottle near the end of the first year of life. The mother allows the infant to bear tension for increasing periods of time; when he is hungry, she will not feed him so promptly as in the first few weeks of life.

6. AGGRESSION. Aggression is manifest in proportion to unpleasant or frustrating experiences such as interference with feeding, excessive stimulation, painful dentition, too early or too abrupt weaning, or separations from the mother.

7. OBJECT RELATIONSHIP. The infant gradually becomes aware of his close relationship with his mother. As his abilities to perceive and to remember develop, he begins to distinguish himself from his mother. Evidence of awareness of separateness from his mother appears by about 8 months of age; he may have severe anxiety when separated. Investment of libido in relationships becomes increasingly volitional and under the control of the ego.

8. EGO AND IDENTITY. The infant's behavior has gradually become more purposeful. His vocal signals are more purposeful, and his mother responds more specifically. His first coordinated movements allow him to begin to do for himself, e.g. to convey food to his mouth. Repeated sensory experiences have enabled him to begin to define the boundaries of his body, laying the foundation for his body-image concept and the feeling of identity. As his ego develops, his mother is able to relinquish some of the ego functions she had to provide for him.

   As a result of optimum experiences in the oral stage, including a satisfactory weaning experience, the infant should have gained the *ego quality* of a feeling of *trust* (Erikson) in his mother and a good feeling about life.

   The infant's *sense of reality* is beginning to develop. Ferenczi postulated that the infant (if he had any concept of self) would have a feeling of *"unconditional omnipotence,"* everything seeming to be self-contained and under his control. In the latter part of the first year the infant begins to be aware that this is not the case, and he attempts to manage his mother and maintain his feeling of omnipotence with *"magical gestures,"* e.g., a smile, a cry or a reaching out with his hand.

9. SUPEREGO (CONSCIENCE AND IDEALS). In many little ways, both verbal and nonverbal, the mother conveys attitudes of approval and disapproval to the infant. The first renunciation is weaning, which requires that the infant give up the pleasure of sucking the breast or bottle and substitute drinking from a glass and eating solid food. This is a precursor of superego, since it implies a value judgment and introduces the idea that one's drives or impulses are to be controlled.

10. TYPICAL NORMAL BEHAVIOR. Throughout the first year of life the infant is dependent, demanding and mostly oral in his orientation. He responds positively to experiences of pleasure or manifestations of love. He normally suffers relatively little hurt or frustration during his first year and therefore has not yet reacted with hostility and other defenses which serve a protective function. As his wakefulness, coordination and motility gradually increase, he explores his own body, parts of his mother, and the environment, using all his sensory organs, but mostly his mouth.

TABLE 2–10 STAGES OF PSYCHOLOGIC DEVELOPMENT *(Continued)*

TODDLER YEARS

1. STAGE. Anal stage.

2. AGE. 12 to 36 months

3. BIOLOGIC MATURATION. Maturation of nerve pathways from the cerebral cortex to the external sphincters of the bowel and bladder occurs by about 18 months of age and allows for the possibility of volitional control of these organs. There is heightened awareness of pleasurable sensations from the mucosa, skin and musculature of the anal zone, and continuing maturation of neuromuscular systems, most importantly the locomotor system and the speech apparatus.

4. LIBIDO. A principal libidinal investment of a sensual or erotic quality is in the anal (perineal) area. Additionally, and importantly, the speech apparatus, with beginning language formation, and the locomotor and other neuromuscular functions are libidinized.

5. BIOLOGIC AND CULTURAL CHALLENGES. Biologic maturation presents the challenges of sphincter control and such neuromuscular coordination as that involved in walking, running, talking and manipulating objects. Culture requires the child to gain control of evacuation of his bladder and bowel, and to control himself in the pleasure of uninhibited motility and physical exploration of the environment. This last demand typically is conveyed by his mother's oft-repeated "No! no!"

6. AGGRESSION. Aggression increases considerably in response to the first disciplinary experiences. The toddler meets the mother's attempts at training with vocal and physical resistance. He may lash out against his mother or other frustrating objects, or may vent his feelings in a temper tantrum.

7. OBJECT RELATIONSHIP. The child-parent relationship undergoes a decided change. The child's feeling of power and sense of omnipotence are disabused by increasing parental demands and by his ability to recognize his dependence and relative helplessness. His aggressive urges and his need for love and approval are in conflict with each other. He is ambivalent, aggressive, independent, negativistic, and helpless and clinging. From the parental point of view, the child, who has been enjoyable during the oral stage, is now becoming difficult; their concept of him as they fantasied and wished him to be is disturbed. With increasing awareness of himself as a separate being, he is more discerning of people, and begins to exercise choice as to relationships and their intensity.

8. EGO AND IDENTITY. Ego growth is rapid. Control of bowel and bladder and of various motility patterns and learning defensive techniques for managing feelings and impulses are achieved. Locomotion permits active rather than passive separation. The toddler masters his anxiety as he experiments with separation. His motility increases his sphere of contact, and he learns about physical and social realities. His intellect is sufficiently developed that he can learn his language. He plays and fantasies with much trial-acting and make-believe, these being the forerunners of thinking.

   He gains the *ego quality* of a feeling of *autonomy* (Erikson), rather than excessive feelings of shame or doubt. His body-image concept becomes more clearly defined. His identity takes on more meaning in terms of *his* name and *his* family. Parental attitudes convey that he is good or bad, or clean or dirty. He identifies himself as a boy or girl, although the anatomic basis for this differentiation is not entirely clear to him.

   This stage is characterized by a tendency to view all objects as alive and animate. In his fantasy play, animals, plants, trucks and blocks of wood are imbued with qualities of people.

9. SUPEREGO (CONSCIENCE AND IDEALS). Toilet training and the "No! no!" admonitions contribute to superego formation. Value judgments and character traits of giving and taking, responsibility, self-control, cleanliness, orderliness, punctuality, property rights, and right and wrong begin to develop.

10. TYPICAL NORMAL BEHAVIOR. Behavior is characterized by great energy and a desire to be constantly on the go. Interference is resisted to the point of obstinacy, negativism or temper tantrums. Ambivalence with rapidly oscillating feelings of love and anger is characteristic of relationships with people. A concern about power and control, and who bosses whom, is manifest in play activities.

Table 2–10 continued on following page.

TABLE 2–10 STAGES OF PSYCHOLOGIC DEVELOPMENT *(Continued)*

PRESCHOOL YEARS.

1. STAGE. Phallic stage.

2. AGE. From 3 to 4 until 5 to 7 years.

3. BIOLOGIC MATURATION. Continuing maturation allows for increased pleasurable sensation in the penis and clitoris. General physical and intellectual maturation continues, but the pace is slackened.

4. LIBIDO. The predominant investment of libido, psychologically, is in the phallic area, i.e. the penis or clitoris.

5. BIOLOGIC AND CULTURAL CHALLENGES. The new biologic challenge is control and moderation of the urge for enjoyment in stimulation of the penis or clitoris. The broader challenge of mastery of the maturing neuromuscular and intellectual systems continues.

   Cultural attitudes focus on phallic pleasure and on sexualized or eroticized play. The incest prohibition is mostly implicit, but may be explicit, e.g. parental interdictions against brother and sister continuing to bathe together or against body-contact play. This same sensual quality enters into the child-parent relationship. A parent feels uncomfortable about close physical contact with the child, and previous practices of hugging, kissing and holding the child upon the lap usually are curtailed or modified. Parents generally react with discomfort and disapproval to masturbatory activity. Even when the parent intellectually regards masturbation as a normal phenomenon of development, he still is likely to *feel* disapproving, and the child, consciously or unconsciously, perceives this disapproval. Fear of injury to the penis or clitoris, or a fantasy that these organs may already have been damaged (particularly in the female), is a universal concern at this age, and is referred to as *castration anxiety.*

6. AGGRESSION. As the previously comfortable, affectionate relation with the parent of the opposite sex is interfered with by genital sexual feelings, the child is confronted with the necessity of giving up the close physical attachment. This mobilizes feelings of resentment and aggression which normally are directed most strongly toward the parent of the same sex. Frequently the aggression is displaced to siblings, teachers or other objects where the fear of the loss of love is less important.

7. OBJECT RELATIONSHIP. Sexual feelings threaten to disrupt the child-parent relationship. As the boy feels or imagines disapproval from the parent, his urges and fears conflict with each other. He feels that his father is a competitor for his mother's love, and his aggressive fantasies and impulses are directed toward his father. In consequence, he fears punishment or retaliation from his father, usually in the form of injury to the penis. But the boy also loves his father, and needs him and his approval. The conflict is resolved when the boy gives up his sexual urges toward his mother (later directing them toward females outside his own family) and contents himself with tender but asexual feelings toward her. At the same time he identifies more strongly with his father, thus affirming his identity as a male. He thus yields much of his former dependency, particularly upon his mother. The child normally is ready for school by about 5 or 6 years of age.

   The girl too finds her dependent relationship with mother threatened by sexual feelings. Additionally, she may resent having been somehow deprived by her mother of the seemingly more desirable male genital organ. Her initial reaction of envy of the penis is due in part to the fact that the girl at this age is comparing external genitalia only. Both she and the boy have little or no knowledge of the vagina and its significance in relation to internal sexual organs and the childbearing potentiality. The little girl shifts her sexual feelings from mother to father, and then is in a position comparable to that of the boy in relation to his mother. Ultimately she yields her sexualized feelings for her father, retaining feelings of tenderness for him, and identifies with her mother.

   These conflicts, which stem from the triangular relationship of the child and the parents, are known as the *oedipal conflict.*

8. EGO AND IDENTITY. The ego is strengthened by consolidation of the physical skills and intellectual capabilities which have been developing in the preceding stages. Control of sexual urges and repression of incestuous feelings and fantasies also add an increment of ego strength, provided this is achieved with real mastery rather than as a hasty solution amounting only to an avoidance of the conflict. In the latter instance an excessively defensive repression may form the basis for subsequent development of a neurosis.

   The ego quality of *initiative* (Erikson) derives from resolution of the oedipal conflict—guilt and inertia from its persistence. Identity as a male or female is strengthened by identification with the parent of the same sex. Through this identification the child takes on personality traits of the parent of the same sex; the child also identifies with and acquires some of the qualities and traits of the parent of the opposite sex.

   Because of the child's rapidly changing situation and its attendant anxieties, the development of the *sense of reality* again is characterized by a resort to magic for reassurance. This may take the form of *magical words, thoughts and fantasies,* e.g., the game-like compulsion of touching every pale of a fence, or avoiding the cracks in the sidewalk in order to prevent unforeseen disaster.

9. SUPEREGO (CONSCIENCE AND IDEALS). With resolution of the oedipal conflict, the superego is crystallized into a definite structural component in the psyche. The impetus for this crystallization comes from the urgent necessity of controlling incestuous feelings and from attitudes and value judgments derived from the preceding stages of development.

10. TYPICAL NORMAL BEHAVIOR. Ambivalence toward both parents is common as the child shifts back and forth from one side of his conflicts to the other. Characteristically there is an alternation of displays of aggressive and regressive behavior. Much of the time the boy appears confident and self-assured, and the girl appears coy and flirtatious. This bold front collapses, however, suddenly and frequently, and the child is easily "crushed." The boy, in particular, is physically active, with much aggressive play and fantasy, the latter sometimes cruel and violent in its content.

TABLE 2–10 STAGES OF PSYCHOLOGIC DEVELOPMENT *(Continued)*

MIDCHILDHOOD YEARS

1. STAGE. Latency stage.

2. AGE. From 5 to 7 until 8 to 10 years.

3. BIOLOGIC MATURATION. There is a continuing, gradual maturation of central nervous system pathways, permitting increasingly skillful and coordinated physical movements and providing greater intellectual capacity.

4. LIBIDO. Some libidinal energy continues to be invested in the phallic zone. Masturbatory activity and conflict and an interest in sexual matters persist to a greater or less degree throughout the latency stage. A large share of libidinal energy, however, is channeled into intellectual curiosity and the development of mental abilities and physical skills.

5. BIOLOGIC AND CULTURAL CHALLENGES. The child is challenged to develop his physical and intellectual skills, even more than in the phallic stage. Culture first of all asks the child to renounce his interest and pleasure in direct sexual activity. Secondly, he is introduced to the requirement of work. This is presented in the home by giving small responsibilities such as picking up his clothes or helping with the dishes, and in school by being expected to give proof of his learning.

6. AGGRESSION. Aggression is mobilized and (hopefully) constructively used to meet the frustrations and challenges of healthy competition in scholastic and physical activities.

7. OBJECT RELATIONSHIP. The pattern of identification with the parent of the same sex, and feelings of tenderness for the parent of the opposite sex, reached at the end of the phallic stage continue. Additionally, the child increasingly turns to other people, particularly to the teacher, as a model for identification.

   Children of latency age tend to form groups and clubs, this being their first experience in a kind of society of their own making. These groups characteristically are limited to members of the same sex.

8. EGO AND IDENTITY. The ego consolidates the technique of sublimation which is so important in learning and in the development of the capacity for thinking.

   The important *ego quality* of *industry* (Erikson) is acquired, rather than the undesirable trait of feelings of inadequacy. Physical and intellectual abilities are further refined.

   Although a certain amount of magical and wishful thinking persists, and likely will persist even in the adult, the child of latency age is capable of *reality adaptation.* His increasing powers of perception and evaluation of what he perceives allow him to test reality. As his dependency on his parents lessens, he begins to see them more realistically. They are no longer seen as "God-like" figures, all-powerful and all-knowing. The child's disillusionment in his parents is compensated, however, by the satisfaction he gains from pointing out to them their inconsistencies and ineptitudes.

9. SUPEREGO (CONSCIENCE AND IDEALS). The superego becomes more firmly established and serves in aiding adaptation to the external world and in controlling and redirecting the instinctual drives. The superego may be modified if the child discerns that the cultural values of society differ greatly from the values taught him by his parents.

10. TYPICAL NORMAL BEHAVIOR. Continuing concern about controlling sexual and aggressive drives causes sleep disturbances in the latency stage. The nightmares of the phallic stage are likely to be replaced by insomnia, often in association with a conscious fear of death.

    The clubs, with boys, may take on qualities of a "gang" if the aggressive feelings and destructive fantasies get out of hand. This activity is part of the attempt to master and control the sexual and aggressive drives. The girl of latency age is likely to be a year or two ahead of the boy in social and emotional maturity, and perhaps in the capacity to use intellectual abilities.

Table 2–10 continued on following page.

TABLE 2–10 STAGES OF PSYCHOLOGIC DEVELOPMENT *(Concluded)*

ADOLESCENCE

1. STAGE. Puberty and adolescence.

2. AGE. From 10 to 12 until 16 to 18 years.

3. BIOLOGIC MATURATION. During the prepubertal and early adolescent years there is a sharp increase in general body growth; increase in the size of the genital organs; change in body configuration with the development of the secondary sex characteristics; the appearance of menstruation in the female and ejaculation in the male; and the emergence of the capacity for the highest form of abstract thinking and reasoning.

4. LIBIDO. Libido is concentrated in the various changes occurring in the body, particularly in the sexual parts. At the same time there is an actual increase in total energy available, with a resultant strengthening of the sexual and aggressive drives. The greater mental capacity also is highly libidinized.

5. BIOLOGIC AND CULTURAL CHALLENGES. The tremendous physical and physiologic changes of puberty tend to disturb the child. The sexual and aggressive drives pose the threat of inadequate control over impulses. The changes in body size and configuration disturb the body-image concept and require that it be revised. The sexual changes confront the child with the fact that he will shortly be capable of adult sexual functioning. The biologic changes challenge him to accept himself in his new form and to become master of himself.

   The rapid changes and increase in energy and activity of the adolescent cause society to regard him with mixed feelings. Normally he is given greater responsibility, but he is also expected to control his sexual and aggressive impulses and to continue in the role of a child subject to adult authority.

6. AGGRESSION. Aggression is mobilized by the frustrations experienced by the adolescent as he seeks to fulfill his destiny of adulthood under the controls exercised by his parents and society. A certain amount of rebellion is inevitable, but hopefully the aggression is channeled into constructive attempts to gain independence, as well as into healthy competitive activity and productivity.

7. OBJECT RELATIONSHIP. The increased strength of sexual drives causes the adolescent to withdraw even further from parental relationships than was the case in the phallic stage of development. Temporarily and characteristically the adolescent seeks relationship with other adolescents. He and his peer group stand apart from adult society, and to some extent are in conflict with it. The adolescent often finds satisfactory relationship with adults younger than his parents. His interest in these persons is often intense and may amount to hero worship. If the hero is a good leader and socially responsible, the adolescent is led in the right direction. On the other hand, identification with the wrong kind of hero can result in antisocial behavior, which may become serious because the adolescent is endowed with physical strength and sexual capacity which permit him to carry his thoughts and fantasies into action.

   Also characteristic of adolescence, particularly in the latter half, is the experience of falling in love (normally at least several times) as a preliminary to the eventual choice of a marital partner.

   As the adolescent masters the biologic and cultural challenges, he once again draws closer to his parents. Ultimately he normally takes his place in society as a cooperative and constructive young adult.

8. EGO AND IDENTITY. The increase in sexual and aggressive drives reawakens the conflicts of earlier stages and presents new conflicts. The id-ego-superego equilibrium which had attained a fair degree of stability in the latency stage is disturbed. There is a renewed struggle on the part of the ego to gain mastery over the disturbing forces. In this struggle the ego may run the gamut of its defensive techniques. At times the ego is in alliance with the superego, and its inner needs and impulses are denied and inhibited to the point of asceticism. At other times the superego is ignored, and urges are permitted immediate satisfaction. Temporary regressions to behavior associated with earlier stages of development are common.

   As the revived conflicts are reworked and again solved, and as the adolescent comes to terms with his new sexual and aggressive capacities, the equilibrium is reinstated. The final outcome of the adolescent stage is the attainment of a reasonably clear and stable *identity* (Erikson) which permits the pursuit of educational, occupational and marital goals.

   The *capacity for self-evaluation and introspection increases,* and ideally culminates in a capacity for *insight,* or understanding of oneself.

9. SUPEREGO (CONSCIENCE AND IDEALS). Withdrawal from dependency on the parents results in a weakening of the superego, since originally it is derived largely from the parents. In consequence, the adolescent, more or less consciously, is able to examine and decide for himself about many of the value judgments put forth by his parents. Much of the time it appears as though he had completely rejected everything the parents stand for. This is part of the assessment process, and normally the adolescent returns to the parental value system.

10. TYPICAL NORMAL BEHAVIOR. Particularly in the first half of adolescence, the adolescent is in turmoil with rapidly changing moods and behavior. The feelings of internal disorganization and inadequacy for the most part are denied and covered up by bravado, loudness and expansiveness. The problem of control of drives and feelings is evidenced in unpredictability and impulsiveness. The intense interest in the peer group is evidenced by clothing fads, teen-age heroes, and a taste for a kind of music which generally is abhorrent to the parents. There tends to be considerable falling in and out of love, and much experimenting with extrafamilial relationships, most of which serves the purpose of aiding the definition of the self. As equilibrium is regained, there is a turning toward more intellectual and philosophical interests. The grasp on the peer group is loosened, and the adolescent moves toward taking his place in adult society.

hostility, and their effectiveness is thereby diminished. Many parents feel that love and aggression are mutually exclusive and fear that a consequence of aggression toward their child will be the loss of his love. Firmness on the part of the parent does not alienate the child; after his temporary negative response to frustration the child tends to identify with the parent, gaining a feeling of confidence and strength from the experience of having his drives controlled. While he is learning to control his drives, the child is acquiring a sense of values. These values come to make up the bulk of his superego, or conscience. Following through on attitudes of approval and disapproval is essential to the development of ego and superego.

Actually, love requires that the parents do what is best for the child; only by their setting and holding limits on the child's behavior will the child develop into a reasonably controlled and social human being.

AIMS IN CHILD DEVELOPMENT

According to the principles stated above, the broad aims in any given stage of child development can be stated as follows: (1) sufficient gratification of the child's basic needs, both physiologic and emotional, so as to provide feelings of well-being, satisfaction, security and self-esteem; (2) the gradual presentation of the inevitable and essential frustrating parental and societal demands, properly timed in accord with the child's rate of biologic maturation and ego development; (3) mastery by the child of these demands and of the accompanying feelings and conflicts, with the twofold result of learning new techniques of managing himself and of gaining feelings of competence and self-confidence.

As the above process unfolds, the basic child-parent love bond, however strained, should not be broken. The inevitable incidences of resentment and hostility should be temporary, and the desired relation should be re-established before the limits of the child's tolerance of the threat of loss of love are exceeded.

As the child is called upon to yield gradually his earlier modes of satisfaction and his dependency, he is helped to redirect or rechannel his drives into socially approved, preferably constructive and creative outlets.

STAGES OF PSYCHOLOGIC DEVELOPMENT

The format of Table 2–10 facilitates the understanding of sequential psychologic development during infancy and childhood. A longitudinal view of child development as a continuum is gained by tracing an aspect of development from page to page through the successive stages; a cross-sectional view of development at a particular age or stage is gained by reading in a vertical direction on each page. Evaluation of the development of a particular child at a particular time requires careful study of all available data, current and past, using and correlating the cross-sectional and longitudinal points of view. Sources listed in the bibliography provide more detailed information.

CALVIN F. SETTLAGE

Aldrich, C. A., and Aldrich, M. M.: Babies Are Human Beings. New York, The Macmillan Company, 1938.

Bateson, G.: Cultural Determinants of Behavior; in J. McV. Hunt (ed.): Personality and the Behavior Disorders. New York, Ronald Press, 1944, Vol. II, pp. 714–33.

Benedict, R.: Patterns of Culture. Boston, Houghton Mifflin Company, 1934.

Bowlby, J.: Maternal Care and Mental Health. Geneva, World Health Organization, 1951.

Brazelton, T. B.: Observations of the neonate. J. Am. Acad. Child Psychiat. *1*:38, 1962.

Brenner, C.: An Elementary Textbook of Psychoanalysis. New York, International Universities Press, 1955.

Chess, S., Thomas, T., and Birch, H. G.: Behavior problems revisited. J. Am. Acad. Child Psychiat. *6*:321, 1967.

English, O. S., and Pearson, G. H. J.: Emotional Problems of Living, New York, W. W. Norton & Co., 1945.

Erikson, E. H.: Childhood and Society. New York, W. W. Norton & Co., 1950, pp. 219–34.

Escalona, S.: Emotional Development in the First Year of Life; in M. J. E. Senn (ed.): Problems of Infancy and Childhood. New York, Josiah Macy, Jr. Foundation, 1949, pp. 30–51.

Ferenczi, S.: Stages in the Development of the Sense of Reality; in Contributions to Psychoanalysis. Boston, Richard C. Badger, 1916.

Freud, A.: The Ego and the Mechanisms of Defense. New York, International Universities Press, 1946.

Freud, A.: Some Remarks on Infant Observation; in Psychoanalytic Study of the Child. New York, International Universities Press, 1953, Vol. 8.

Freud, A.: Adolescence; in Psychoanalytic Study of the Child. New York, International Universities Press, 1958, Vol. 13.

Freud, S.: Three Contributions to the Theory of Sex (1905); in A. A. Brill (Ed.): The Basic Writings of Sigmund Freud. New York, Random House (Modern Library), 1938.

Josselyn, I.: Psychosocial Development of Children. New York, Family Service Association of America, 1948.

Josselyn, I.: The Adolescent and His World. New York, Family Service Association of America, 1952.

La Barre, W.: The Human Animal. Chicago, University of Chicago Press, 1954.

Mahler, M. S., and Gosliner, B.: On Symbiotic Child Psychosis; in Psychoanalytic Study of the Child, New York, International Universities Press, 1955, Vol. 10, pp. 195–212.

Newton, N., and Newton, M.: Mothers' reaction to their newborn babies. J.A.M.A., *181*:122, 1962.

Ribble, M. A.: Infantile Experience in Relation to Personality Development; in J. McV. Hunt (Ed.): Personality and Behavior Disorders. New York, Ronald Press, 1944.

Settlage, C.: Values of Limits in Child Rearing. Children, 5: No. 5, September-October, 1958.

Spitz, R.: The Psychogenic Diseases in Infancy; in Psychoanalytic Study of the Child. New York, International Universities Press, 1951, Vol. 6.

Waelder, R.: Basic Theory of Psychoanalysis. New York, International Universities Press, 1960.

Psychologic Assessment of the Child

SOURCES OF DATA. The information needed for psychologic assessment is often interwoven with that required for physical assessment. Both assessments begin with the initial contact with patient and parents; final assessment may require a number of visits, as well as supplementary information from other physicians, hospitals, schools, or other agencies. Usually it is the concerns of the parents which will be most useful in evaluation. There is an advantage in interviewing the parents together: to get both points of view, to learn details that may be known to only one, and especially to observe how they relate to each other in discussing problems with and about their child and to determine their capacities for solving problems together.

In the initial interview it is generally wise to encourage the parents to present the problem as they understand it in as much detail as possible, more or less without interruption. On the other hand, if their dissertation strays from the child's problem or deals with irrelevancies or reflects an obsessive need to talk, the physician must impose gentle but firm limits and refocus attention upon the child. The key concerns will be the parents' views of how their child is behaving or adjusting within the family, at school if he is of school age, with peers and adults outside the home, and so on. The physician will search for points of stress in the child's life, both currently and in the past, and for the parents' evaluation of the child's ability to cope with stress. Areas of possible influence which the parents avoid may justify the physician's active guidance in developing the history. For example, if the parents do not volunteer comment on how a child reacted to the birth of a sibling or to the death of a grandparent, the physician must explore the reactions to such situations.

In analyzing the data the physician is influenced by several factors: First, if the history develops consistently and clearly, the physician is likely to accept the data as relatively reliable. However, if certain pertinent information was exposed only through the physician's questioning, it may be particularly heavily weighted. Certain activities of the child take on more weight if, as the parents describe them, they seem not to conform to expected behavioral patterns. For example, discovery that a child of 5 or 6 years is sleeping with his mother while his father sleeps elsewhere would lead to further questions which might reveal qualities of the parents' relationship with each other. Whenever the parents demand inappropriately that the physician find immediate answers or prescriptions, the physician should look behind these defensive maneuvers for their emotional source.

One of the purposes of the interview is to help the parents to bring some order into their thinking about their problem. The child's own contributions may be verbal or nonverbal. If the child is present at the interview it will be important to note his reactions to the discussion. If he is old enough to make significant contributions, the physician should encourage his participation by direct questions to him. This diversion permits observation of interplay between child and parents, supports the child's ego, and often results in the parents' contributions becoming more spontaneous and less defensive. There are times, particularly with children of school age, when the physician will find it helpful to interview the child alone, to get "his side of the story." In the case of adolescents it may be important that the patient have the opportunity of talking with the physician before the parents are seen, so that an understanding can be reached concerning the confidentiality of the physician-patient relationship.

Previous health records including those from other physicians or agencies who have cared for the patient may provide essential information such as that of acute or chronic illness, of a pattern of unusually frequent visits to the physician's office for relatively minor problems, or of an obsessive focus on certain areas of the body.

Relatively simple *screening tests* such as the Peabody Picture Vocabulary Test, the Denver Developmental Screening Test, the Thorpe Developmental Inventory, and others, may be administered by the trained pediatrician or by his assistant; they may reveal areas of intellectual or perceptive function which deserve further study. The major danger of these tests is that they may be relied upon too heavily and not used purely as screening tests.

School reports are important to the psychologic assessment of children of school age, especially if they include in addition to academic assessment, a description of the child's relations with schoolmates and teachers. School reports should be requested only with the written permission of the child's parents or legal guardian.

Reports from *child care agencies* may be helpful, especially in the case of adoptive children or children in foster care. Such agencies often have intensive and extensive histories and sometimes reports of earlier psychologic examinations.

Birth records help to explore questions of injury at the time of birth, as raised in the physician's mind or as presented by parents. Such records are often deficient, but may provide the only objective view of the events of the patient's birth and early days.

Formal psychologic testing will be described in more detail later. It is important that the physician know what kinds of psychologic tests are available, what they can reveal, and what questions they may answer. If the patient has had psychologic testing at school, the results should be examined before expensive new tests are requested that may be unnecessary. As much as possible, tests should be chosen to assess specific problems, rather than as a comprehensive battery of multiple, though standard, tests.

Occasionally genetic, endocrine, and/or neurologic studies will be required to determine whether organic problems may contribute to or be responsible for any psychologic disorder.

ASSESSMENT OF DATA. The physician must avoid early diagnostic closure, even when the parents' initial description of their problem gives the physician a reasonably clear idea of what is going on. So long as he remains a receptive and perceptive listener, new and important information will emerge as parents and perhaps patient begin to feel more trusting and are in fact educated by the physician's questions. Furthermore, the weighing of data must be done in the context of the age and developmental stage of the patient, as well as in the context of the family's sociocultural patterns. It is important that the physician not use his personal value system or style of living as a yardstick against which to measure the family's behavior, or their success or failure in coping with their life situation. Their own feelings of anger, frustration, anxiety, failure or depression are the more valid indicators of where they need help.

The next important point is to identify the principal item of concern. Many times parents present as the immediate prime concern a problem such as bed wetting, which may have existed for many years. Why then have they come now? It is important to determine whether there may, in fact, be more important hidden issues not recognized or acknowledged or able to be faced by the parents.

CONCEPTUAL MODELS. There are five basic conceptual frameworks or models within which the basic problem and the accompanying data can be analyzed. A physician may generally be more partial to one conceptual model than another, but there are certain problems for which a particular model is more appropriate than the others; in some instances several models may be utilized in a complementary manner.

The *first model* is that of the *physiologic state* of the child. An asthmatic child, for instance, needs to be understood in terms of his general state of health, his immunologic status, his exposure to allergens, and the possibility of infection, in addition to his needing assessment of psychic factors which may be contributing to his discomfort.

The *second model* sees the *behavioral* pattern of the child as a reflection of the rewards and punishments experienced in his environment. A behavioral analysis may indicate what to suggest as suitable rewards for desired performances and otherwise how to help the parents and the child extinguish undesirable behavior. A simple example is a system prescribed for enuretic children, wherein the parents reward the child with a gold star on a chart for those nights on which the bed has been dry. Stars may be converted to more tangible rewards.

The *third model* deals with the child's *intrapsychic conflict.* In this case the data obtained are examined in terms of trying to understand what the child is trying to achieve, how he is being thwarted, and how frustration of his goals results in symptomatic behavior. The same enuretic child, angry at his parents, may for a variety of reasons have found no other way to express his anger except through wetting of the bed. Punishment for this has the effect of maintaining anger, in a circular reaction. The intrapsychic approach in such a case might emphasize the child's need to be able to express his angry feelings in words or in other acceptable ways.

A concept useful in the intrapsychic model is that of "developmental lines." Anna Freud pointed out that instead of thinking of or sampling the child's psychologic development in a cross-sectional way, it makes more sense to think of the longitudinal development of certain functions. For example, a child of 3 or 4 years who is physically and even socially ready to be involved with other children of similar age may not be emotionally ready because he is still struggling with his parents over dependency problems. The parents of such a child can be helped to understand that, while the child's behavior is appropriate to his age in many areas, he is not ready for independence in certain areas or to have it thrust upon him. This type of developmental conflict must be worked through by the child himself and its resolution may require only patience on the part of the parents. Parents who can understand and accept appropriate differentials in rates of development often gain a marked sense of relief.

The *fourth model* is that of the *family as a dynamic unit.* The data from the parents and the symptomatic child can be supplemented by seeing the family as a whole. Psychologic problems may be the result of events and relationships in the family. For example, the birth of a new baby might pre-empt the mother's interest and time, impose new functions on an unwilling father, and leave a 2 or 3 year old child wondering why her mother was so much less attentive and her father so irritable. Her regressive behavior can be fully understood only in the context of the interaction of the whole family.

The *fifth model* is the *social* one and takes into consideration both the family interaction and the child's relation to his social milieu. This model has more relevance to school age than to younger children. Problems may occur in response to stressful situations between the patient and other children in the school or between patient and teacher. The child's reactions are influenced, in turn, by the support, or lack of it, he receives from his family. The physician's efforts to manage this sort of problem may lead him to intervention or counseling with teachers or other school personnel and/or to help the child and family to understand the school's role in the child's life and to understand what they can do to improve the situation. A child with a conversion hysteria evidenced by pain in the leg may have developed this symptom following some precipitating stressful episode of rejection by peers or teachers in school, only to maintain it in response to family interactional problems, perhaps of long standing.

When problems have not been internalized by the child, it may be sufficient simply to counsel parents and/or the school personnel. If this has been done and the child continues to present problems, and if parents seem unable to make appropriate changes in their approach to the maladaptive child, the child will probably require more intensive or extensive help and should be referred to a child psychiatrist or to a psychiatric clinic.

Finally, it must be understood that the parents' assessment of the problem is critical for the child. There will be occasions when the physician, having collected and assessed appropriate data, can only conclude that the child is functioning within normal limits. In such a case, it must be determined what personal, familial, social or cultural considerations caused the parents to see the child's behavior as a major problem; it must then be determined what kind of re-education they may need in order to feel reassured and not be left with the impression that their anxieties or concerns have been discounted or casually dismissed.

J. M. DUNN

Finch, S. M., and McDermott, J. F.: Psychiatry for the Pediatrician. New York, W. W. Norton & Co., 1970.

Kessler, J. W.: Psychopathology of Childhood. Englewood Cliffs, N. J., Prentice-Hall, Inc., 1966.

Freud, A.: Normality and Pathology in Childhood: Assessments of Development. New York, International Universities Press, 1965.

PREVENTION OF PSYCHOLOGIC DISORDERS

Role of the Physician in Prevention of Psychologic Disorders in the Well Child

GENERAL DEVELOPMENTAL ISSUES

One of the ways in which the physician can help to prevent psychologic disorders in the well child is to identify for parents those issues within the normal range of life's vicissitudes which seem to be related to psychologic problems and which most parents, with assistance, can control to an appreciable extent. Many parents look to physicians for this kind of help.

Factors which are likely to contribute to psychologic disorders in children and which are manageable by most parents include: (1) innate temperamental differences in infants; (2) temperamental differences in parents; (3) differences of style in filling the role of parent; (4) techniques used to control the child's behavior; (5) handling the child's (or parents') expression of feelings; (6) preparation of the child for stressful encounters; (7) interpretation of normal landmarks in child development; and (8) the degree to which the home is child-centered.

It can be pointed out to parents of a very active infant, for instance, that such a child will probably need a highly structured and consistent environment. Such a child may feel more secure when mealtimes, bedtimes and waking times are kept relatively constant and predictable from day to day. This pattern of basic security appears to be a necessary foundation for the confidence with which he can later cope with unexpected and unpredictable events. All parents should be advised that this kind of orderly environment is generally conducive to the psychologic well-being of children, but it is the relatively active child who is most likely to develop psychologic and behavioral problems if reared in an unstructured, inconsistent setting.

Problems which can be generated by temperamental differences in parents are related to those that may arise from innate temperamental differences in infants. The temperamentally somewhat passive parent may, for example, find it difficult to cope with a very active child. The physician can help to alleviate conflicts between parent and child and perhaps prevent psychologic problems in the child if he advises that the early imposition of firm and consistent behavioral controls will lead to the development of internalized control in the child which will make him less impulsive. In this kind of situation parents can be encouraged to set clear limits on the amount of random activity and noise permitted within the house. If the child then consistently experiences the consequences when these limits are exceeded, he should be able to learn to harness his activity to within acceptable limits of noise level or other physical activity. It is important in this context that the nature of desirable or acceptable behavior be made clear to the child and that he be consistently rewarded, most often simply with an expression of approval or other signs of affection, for performance which meets the family standard. (See p. 14 and below.) When confrontations between parent and child seem to reflect innate temperamental differences, the simple pointing out to parents that these differences play an important part in child-parent relationships may help to prevent later friction.

There is evidence to suggest that a warm and accepting style in the rearing of children is superior to parental behavior which the child, and perhaps others, perceive as aloof, cold or rejecting. The physician can to some extent help parents who exhibit the latter characteristics by encouraging them to accept behavior in the child which cannot result in harmful consequences for the child or others, and by advising them in the use of nonpunitive disciplinary measures, such as deprivation of privileges in or out of the home. The temporary loss of clearly defined privileges is less likely than some sort of physical punishment to be perceived by the child as the hostile act of a rejecting parent.

Consistency in parental standards and behavior may be more important than differences in styles of parenting. For instance, a child will find it easier to cope with a parent who tends to appear somewhat cold and even rejecting if the parent's response can be predicted, than with a parent who is warm and accepting one moment and, for no consistent reason, cold and rejecting the next moment. In preventing psychologic disorders, the importance of consistency in parental style extends to the area of communication. The parent who tells the child one thing in words while communicating the opposite nonverbally may render the child confused and anxious. For instance, the child who is told to play outside because exercise in fresh air will be good for him may perceive the reality that his mother may want him out of the house for her own comfort or relief; he will be confused because he cannot be sure which message is valid, the one which expresses concern for his welfare or the one expressing possible rejection.

The importance of consistency in parental styles to the prevention of psychologic disorders is particularly crucial in respect to *discipline.* Children who can predict the consequences of their unacceptable actions are less likely to choose such behavior and will tend to learn more easily to take responsibility for their behavior. It is not always possible to devise consequences of an item of misbehavior which logically follow the nature of that particular behavior, but if parents are taught the value of utilizing logical consequences wherever possible, they will have a tool which will tend to render them more effective in their parental roles. It is probably more effective to deprive a child temporarily of his bicycle, for instance, if he has ridden it beyond prescribed limits, than to deprive him of watching television. When clear-cut, logical consequences are not available, isolation for antisocial behavior can be construed as logical: if the child cannot get along with others, perhaps he should remain by himself for a period of time.

Helping children to cope effectively with intense feelings can prevent serious psychologic disorders. Acceptable modes of expression for such feelings should be encouraged. Parents can be advised to help a child to verbalize his anger, for instance, by asking him an appropriate question, such as why he is angry. If this fails to elicit a verbal expression of anger, the parent himself can, if he is certain that the child is angry and suspects the reason, verbalize the anger for the child by saying something like, "You are probably angry because Johnny won't play with you." This often elicits a response from the child, in addition to communicating to him that it is acceptable for him to have feelings and to express them verbally, even to discuss them. Affect that is not ventilated verbally tends to be expressed in other, often maladaptive ways, such as, in the case of anger, general misbehavior, poor performance in school or other behavior that will elicit anger in others.

Verbalization is also important in preparing a child for future events which may be stressful, such as going to school for the first time, a trip to the dentist or to the doctor, or entering the hospital. The parent can be advised first to explain to the child in simple, concrete terms the actual conditions he will encounter. The child can then be encouraged to verbalize his feelings concerning the event: his anxiety or fear, his conceptions of what is to occur and the like. Finally, the parent indicates that he accepts the child's feelings while correcting his misconceptions. In this way, the intensity of the stress encountered during the actual event is reduced.

The physician can help to prevent childhood psychopathology if he can prepare the parents for the normal landmarks or pivotal periods in their child's development. The parent who knows what his child can be expected to do at various stages in development is less likely to make unrealistic demands of the child than if he were not so aware. Some of this awareness can be imparted to the parent through developmentally oriented questions as part of the routine assessment of the infant or young child. The parent of the 6 month old infant can be told, for example, that it is relatively normal for children around 8 months of age to be fearful of strangers; and the parents of the 10 month old that the apparent appetite of many infants seems to decline surprisingly after 10 months as their rate of gain in weight declines sharply.

In general, the physician will be most effective in giving child-rearing advice if he can supplement his suggestions with specific, concrete examples of technical maneuvers reflecting sound basic principles, but he should be careful in counseling parents lest he inadvertently encourage the parents to be overly child-centered. They should be encouraged to see that their own valid needs as individuals are met, and should be cautioned that anxiety about and overconcern with technical details of child rearing can result in a manipulative overprotectiveness which may increase rather than decrease the likelihood of psychologic disorders.

ESTHER L. CAVA

CRITICAL DEVELOPMENTAL ISSUES

PRENATAL ATTITUDES. Even in utero the infant has become the object of a set of parental attitudes and expectations, albeit in various degrees of formulation. The content and quality of the prenatal psychologic influence depend on many factors, including the adequacy of the marriage, the couple's feelings about each other, the economic circumstances of the family and the unmet emotional needs of the parents as individuals. The unborn child may be viewed as a "mistake" or as a "saviour." He may represent an unconscious or deliberate attempt to hold a shaky marriage together or a compensatory substitute for an ungratifying partner. In more normal circumstances we tend to view our children as extensions of ourselves, and we see in them our genetic legacy and certain aspects of our own personalities. Even such a perspective can become pathologic if parents expect their children to fulfill all their own unrealized dreams and ambitions, rather than to lead their own lives.

The child who is planned as a replacement for one who has recently died is particularly at risk. From his birth he may be treated as a fragile child, with considerable overindulgence, as though he were especially vulnerable to the same fate which befell the previous child. The firstborn child after several miscarriages may be viewed similarly. Anticipatory guidance and counseling by the physician can be of considerable benefit in these instances.

ADOPTION. Most adopted children and their families handle the matter of adoption with considerable common sense and sensitivity, but there are some issues concerning adoption which require comment.

Adoptions accomplished through approved agencies are preferred over independent adoptions since they tend to have more adequate assessment of the psychosocial setting of the prospective adoptive family and perhaps better safeguards for the physical condition of the infant. Adoptive placement should be made as soon after birth as possible in order to foster a firm attachment and bonding of infant to the adoptive mother. Adoptions across religious and ethnic lines and by single parents are, in appropriate instances, reasonable alternatives to having large numbers of potentially adopted children languish in institutions or temporary foster homes, but adoption of older children presents distinct risks in some situations. When a family seeks to rescue a 4 or 5 year old child who has a history of severe emotional deprivation and multiple foster home replacements, they may find that the child has already been severely traumatized and will display major psychologic disturbances in later life, even when the adoptive parents offer very acceptable homes.

The adopted child should be told of his adoption as soon as he has achieved reasonably good verbal facility and comprehension, by the age of 3 or at the latest 4 years. The explanation can be repeated at intervals when circumstances are appropriate, such as during a family discussion about the birth of a neighbor's baby. Explanations should not become a ritualized treatise. Children's books on adoption can be read to young children; later they can read them themselves.

Controversy continues as to whether adopted children are at increased risk for development of emotional problems. If they are, it is likely to reflect problems of parental adjustment or management. Since the adopted child generally arrives in the context of marital infertility, he may be treated with considerable overindulgence as a "special child." His adoption need not be perceived by the child as a threat to his self-esteem, but in the case of individual and family problems, the child's adoptive status may reinforce his otherwise existing doubts about his competence and worth. It is not infrequent following an adoption that a natural child is born to previously "infertile" parents. For the adopted child the event may initiate a competitive struggle requiring both understanding and firmness on the part of the parents.

ATTACHMENT BEHAVIOR. The importance of the experience of the first days of life in determining the quality of attachment of mother and infant has been discussed elsewhere (page 21), along with implications for management of prenatal and postnatal care.

The continuing support of a nurturant family is vital for a child in all stages of his development. When social and emotional deprivation fail to provide a nurturant environment or when severe disruption occurs in the early mutual bonding of infant and mother within the first two years of life, there may be psychologic and cognitive sequelae. While there is evidence that some deleterious effects may be reversible, there is little doubt that children may experience lasting damage to social development, especially when deprivation occurs within the context of major familial conflict, psychotic illness in one or both parents, prolonged separation or abandonment. "Failure to thrive" in infancy is frequently a subacute manifestation of maternal depression and reflects the inability of the mother to give her child adequate psychologic warmth and care; it is occasionally confused with hypopituitarism. For treatment to be effective, the mother must be helped to emerge from her withdrawn or depressive state toward more active involvement with her child. Chronic social deprivation has been shown to contribute to intellectual retardation and to major emotional disturbances.

In the case of working mothers who see their children daily and who have arranged for adequate daytime care, there is little risk of psychic harm to the child. A mother who is to be separated from her child for a prolonged period of time should find a single consistent and stable surrogate, rather than a series of caretakers. Hospitalization of children under the age of 5 or 6 years should, wherever possible, involve the rooming-in of the mother, in order to minimize the child's anxiety and to prevent subsequent maladaptive emotional responses. The normal child demonstrates separation anxiety at the age of 7 to 9 months, the onset of this phenomenon being an important step in the evolution of attachment behavior of mother and infant. The child becomes fretful when his mother leaves the room and fearful when persons outside the family attempt to remove him from his mother's arms. His parents can be reassured that he has simply begun to recognize his separateness from and dependence upon his mother, and that after a few more months he will have a better understanding of her permanence, and separation anxiety will diminish.

Maternal care during the first two years should be sufficiently reliable, predictable and warm to give the child a sense of basic trust about the world, but not overindulgent. The infant's learning to tolerate some frustrations that he can survive, as well as inevitable or appropriate delays in the satisfaction of his wishes, probably contributes positively to the quality of his social development and the strength and health of mother-child attachment.

Parents of infants handicapped by physical abnormality may, owing to feelings of depression or shame, maintain an emotional distance from the child and create a situation of relative deprivation. Blind, deaf and physically disabled infants and children require considerable interaction and stimulation to reach their full potential; a diminution of parental contact compounds their difficulties.

The role of the mother is vital in early infant-parent attachment. Less is known of the role of fathers, which may be quite variable, but there is little doubt that the participation of fathers and siblings in the care and stimulation of infants may be of paramount importance in their emotional development.

SIBLING RELATIONSHIPS. The impact of a new sibling upon a young child can be felt very early. As soon as she knows herself to be pregnant the mother may alter her attitudes toward her other children and sometimes begin to intensify her concern with activities such as feeding, toilet training and the like, which she wants to have under a different level of control by the time the new baby is born. The physician will properly show an interest in such areas of family dynamics, and may well caution mothers against letting the deadline of the date of expected delivery provoke conflict in these areas. With the birth of a new sibling, the older child may show a variety of responses, ranging from denial of the sibling's birth through regressive behavior, such as wetting and soiling, to happy acceptance of the event. The older child requires such preparation for the sibling's birth as will impart the reassurance that he remains loved, and some involvement, even if minor, in caretaking responsibilities for the new sibling. His questions regarding babies, hospitals and birth should be answered as factually and comfortably as possible.

Spacing of siblings two to three years apart is felt to represent an optimal interval; with the trend to smaller families this is less of an issue than a few years ago. There is no conclusive evidence that the ordinal position of siblings has any predictable effect on their individual development of personality. Firstborn children are not necessarily more neurotic or more gifted, and there is little evidence that they are reared essentially differently from subsequent children. The so-called middle child syndrome probably does not exist, though it may be used to rationalize other problems which bear no relationship to ordinal position.

Bickering and competition among siblings are normal and serve the purpose of developing interpersonal skills. Rough and tumble play is probably beneficial to such growth. Severe problems, however, in sibling relationship frequently reflect marital difficulties or inadequacies in parental management. Sometimes one of several siblings may be unconsciously assigned a role by one or both parents which involves him in a conflict between them, and such a child may be implicitly encouraged by one parent to be an ally against the other. In a similar vein, a sibling may serve as a scapegoat for other family psychopathology, owing to the timing of his birth, a birth defect, his temperament, his sex, or his resemblance to or identification with a particular parent or grandparent. At other times a child may unconsciously fall into the role of scapegoat in order to maintain family psychopathology at such a level of homeostasis that more serious or threatening disintegration in family interaction is held off.

Parents frequently complain about sibling jealousies as one of the problems inherent in raising more than one child, but it is evident that older siblings are important in the education, socialization and support of younger ones, and that siblings may sometimes be the closest of friends.

TOILET TRAINING. The impact of conflicts around toilet training on the child's later emotional development has been exaggerated. There is little to indicate that the usual experiences involved in the toilet training of most children are of major psychologic consequence. Only when toilet training is allowed to become a field of battle between overdemanding parents and the child, or where it is pursued unrealistically early or overzealously, would one expect conflict over toilet training to have any lasting effect on personality development.

Parents may wish to start toilet training when the child is old enough to verbalize his need for care after wetting or soiling, and when he can appreciate a simple reward system. The substitution of training pants for diapers is an important step in the toilet training process, though it is to be expected that accidents will occur. If resistance is significant, parents should not make toileting a battleground but merely postpone further efforts in the area for several weeks or months. Though it may be disappointing, annoying or irritating to parents, it is neither uncommon nor harmful for toilet training to be achieved even as late as the third year. Many children, by tuning in on the parents' implicit or gently expressed wishes, appear to train themselves; some are trained by the encouragement of siblings.

LOCOMOTION. The beginning of locomotor ability brings rewards and risks to the child. Mobile exploration is a vital step in his acquisition of knowledge and of a sense of initiative, but adequate parental supervision is necessary to minimize the risk of accidents. Stairways must be barred, poisonous substances removed from reach, electrical outlets plugged, and the handles of gas burners kept out of reach or removed. The physician is required to see that parents receive careful instruction on safety measures; at the same time, he must encourage parents to allow the child considerable freedom to move about in safe places.

Recent data indicate that restraint of the child's mobility by surgical and medical procedures involving splints or casts, oxygen or mist tents, prolonged intravenous feedings, dressings for burns, and the like, may contribute to the development of subsequent emotional or personality problems or to speech or learning difficulties. When such procedures as restraint of the child's locomotor function are necessary, they should be complemented by considerable emotional support in the form of rooming-in parents, close contact with medical and other supportive staff, and by diversions such as appropriate games, television, and so on.

Excessive motor activity in the toddler may be an early warning sign of the *hyperkinetic syndrome.* Involved children may be reported by their mothers to have many accidents, "to get into things," to wander away from home, "not to understand the meaning of the word *NO*," and to be "always on the go." Except where there is evidence of a constitutionally based hyperkinetic syndrome, difficulties in managing the active toddler mostly reflect inconsistent discipline by the parents. This particular period can be a difficult one, the toddler "feeling his oats," exercising newly developed skills and testing limits. Occasionally the setting is complicated by the birth of a new sibling. Parents must know what they want, mean what they say, use a firm approach and follow through in a consistent fashion. Usually a parental reproach, sometimes repeated, and removal of the child from an undesired activity will be sufficient. Temper tantrums will be common, with a peak incidence in the child around $2^1/_2$ years of age. They are an excellent attention-getting device and should generally be accepted by the parent as an understandable expression of the child's frustration that has no power to change the rules; when the tantrum proves useless, the child tends to give up this unprofitable behavior.

PRESCHOOL AND SCHOOL. Preschool experiences can be of considerable value to the young child, enhancing socialization, peer group interaction and perhaps even learning. Four year olds should be enrolled in nursery school and, in selected instances, 3 year olds who appear to be mature enough to spend a half day away from home. Even at 18 months of age some children may benefit from a half day or two or more each week in a supervised setting where they may interact with other children. The evidence is not conclusive regarding the impact on infants and toddlers of care outside the home during the working hours of their parents, but there has been no documentation of deleterious effects in well staffed programs of high quality. On the contrary, in such programs beneficial results have been demonstrated. If there is to be a truly national commitment to day care, however, it must be safeguarded by provision for a large pool of competent and dedicated personnel.

The refusal of a child to go to school (*school phobia*) is not common in kindergarten, first or second grade children. The children involved are generally good students with obsessive traits, who have tended to have previous problems in separating from parents or from home. Somatic complaints may accompany the refusal to attend school. The physician should help parents to insist upon the child's prompt return to school and continued attendance; otherwise, early and transient school refusal may evolve into an ingrained and chronic difficulty. In preadolescence and adolescence, an episode of school refusal may indicate rather serious underlying psychopathology, and it is wise not to push for a return to school until psychiatric assessment has been made.

Poor school performance in an intellectually able child may be the result of emotional problems, sensory deficits, other physical illness or inadequate teaching. Boys may be less ready developmentally than girls to assume the passive role of student, and the normally exuberant activity of young grade school boys may present problems for teachers in the early school years, most of whom are women. As a general principle, it may be wise not to have boys begin their first grade experience before the age of 6, or at times closer to 7 years. Referrals of schoolchildren to mental health agencies may be for evaluation of either academic or disciplinary problems, or may cloak the school's desire to exclude a troublesome pupil; alternatively, the school's concerned referral may reflect the inability of parents to perceive or come to grips with poor adjustment or deviant behavior. Despite some dangers of mislabeling and inaccurate diagnoses, the early school years do provide a good setting for identifying a number of health, psychologic and educational problems, including mental retardation, reading disorders, hyperkinesis, sensory deficits and emotional difficulties. Identification is of value, however, only if schools and community agencies can provide the appropriate remedial programs. In recent years schools have been experimenting with a variety of new educational techniques, including "open classrooms," programmed learning, "family" groupings and operant conditioning. These approaches may be more valid for some children than others. For example, a withdrawn and inhibited child may function quite well in an open setting; an overactive child may require a more structured educational program. Most children, however, do well in school, and schools do well by most children. Wherever possible, it makes good sense for those who are interested in children to work closely with schools, not only around individual children who present problems but in a variety of collaborative efforts which will strengthen the ability of schools to foster the child's emotional development. Together with the family, the school is a social institution of major force in the transmission of our cultural values, and schools will raise our children in a manner reflective of our value system.

NORMAL FEARS OF CHILDREN. Fears are normal and perhaps a necessary part of psychologic development. To be realistically afraid of real danger and to take steps to avoid it or to minimize its effects are necessary for adaptation and survival. Fear is the perception of an external threat, real or possible. Anxiety implies the feelings associated with fear in the absence of any immediate perception of external threat. It may be the result of fantasies reflecting internal conflicts. Though the object of fear or anxiety may be imaginary or fictitious, the sensation itself is, of course, not and has familiar physiologic components. The distinction between fear and phobia is essentially that between normal and pathologic, phobia being defined within a psychoanalytic framework as involving certain mechanisms of defense, such as repression, projection or displacement.

The things which children are likely to fear change with age, becoming more specific to the child's environment and experience as he grows older. Studies of childhood fears show that the younger child's fears are centered on basic conditions or situations such as darkness, or being left alone or abandoned, or upon cultural stereotypes of fear-inducing objects, such as wild animals, monsters, ghosts and goblins. The preverbal and even school-age child does not necessarily have a fear that corresponds to the concerns which adults may have for him or may try to inculcate. He may not, for example, be concerned about fire, traffic or the friendly stranger who may spirit him away. As the child becomes older, his fears become more oriented toward specific culturally appropriate threats in his environment and toward specific past experiences of his own. He may generalize isolated experiences of his own that were threatening or fear-inducing, sometimes appropriately, sometimes not. The cosmologic threats which adults feel, such as the threat of destruction from atomic or nuclear weapons, the threat of war, or the threat of flood or hurricane, are not particularly fearful for the preadolescent child and may be of no major concern even to the adolescent.

Children's fears may readily reflect those of their parents, and these fears may be transmitted from parent to child explicitly, or more often implicitly and somewhat vaguely. Among the culturally approved fears that preschool and young school-age children may have are those of thunder and lightning, punishment, pain, hospitals, and such people as physicians or dentists. Parents also may be feared objects for the child. Even when parents are not punitive, cruel or harsh, most children are afraid of them under some situations. The anger of a parent is particularly frightening for the child, even though the parent refrains from any physical contact with the child.

Children manifest their fears in various ways, depending upon age and sophistication and upon ability to verbalize and willingness to do so. The preverbal child may cling, cry, scream and try to escape from a situation that frightens him, and it may be very difficult at times to identify the specific fear-provoking stimulus. The older child may be hesitant to name what he is afraid of, or to discuss it in any detail, owing to the additional fantasy and fear that talking about it will make it come true, the words being given magical powers.

The physician can help parents to be patient with their children's fears. Even very intense fears are not necessarily a sign of emotional disturbance in the child, still less of cowardice. For the preverbal and young verbal child, the parents can be encouraged to give physical and emotional support through hugging, holding and physical comforting, conveying reassurance through their availability and presence that the feared object or condition has no power actually to hurt. In such young children logical explanation is of little or no value and is incomprehensible to the anxious and excited child. Cold, rational, logical explanations without other support can at times be rather cruel to a fearful young child. For the child of school age and older, verbal reassurance should supplement physical and emotional support, for the child can respond to the logic and reason of his parents in terms both of its tone and of its realism. Simple, direct explanations oftentimes require repetition each time the feared situation or object is encountered, and the child may gain strength and support even as the formula is repeated in the same way each time. After a while he may internalize the formula and be heard saying it to himself or to his younger brothers and sisters when they show concern with the same object or situation. The child becomes able to distinguish between the feeling of fear and the fact that the feared situation, object or condition really has no actual power to harm him. Parents should be advised neither to shame nor to demean the child, nor to try to force him into feared situations, hoping that in surviving them without support or in crying it out, he will overcome fear. This procedure induces terror in some children and complicates subsequent management of fears.

The unrealistically feared situation needs eventually to be faced by the child, with parental support. Parents may need advice in devising appropriate ways to help children to master specific fears. The child afraid to be separated from the parents at night may be allowed to stay outside their bedroom sleeping on the hall floor, to be gradually moved into his own bedroom or into the bedroom of a sibling as he becomes more secure. It is helpful if he is given some power over his situation, such as being able to turn on or keep a light on if he is afraid of the dark, being able to reach his parents by telephone when they have left him for an evening, or having contact with a nonthreatening puppy or kitten if his fear is centered on dogs and cats. Whatever is done, the parents' own capacity to be calm, reassuring, encouraging and supportive is essential. Each time the child masters even in a slight way the fearful situation, he should be given praise and encouragement.

Parents whose own fears of the dark, of being alone, of thunder or lightning or of dentist or doctor give models to their children's fears, have the responsibility to underplay those threatening situations, if possible, and to exert self-control. When their children ask them if they are afraid, it is important that the parents be able to acknowledge their own fears, since to deny them is to deny the child's perception and recognition of what is going on, and this denial could confuse him. Parents do not have to be fearless nor to appear fearless to the child in all situations. Parents should be able to say, "Yes, I have the same fear and I know it is not sensible, but I have learned to live with it." They may then be able to give the child some advice about how to handle fears and may encourage the child to feel that he does not have to be burdened with the same fears that his parent has. With this approach some children may learn to cope with fears with more success than their parents.

When fears last an inordinately long time, when one set of fears is replaced by another, or when fears become increasingly incapacitating to the child or to parental or family function, a more definitive psychologic and psychiatric evaluation will be needed.

REACTION TO SEPARATION AND DEATH. The younger the child, the more likely he will respond to the loss of a parent through separation or death in a typical way. In the older child the reaction is more individualized and reflects the differential characteristics of his own experience. Relatively brief separations and reunions usually produce rather transient effects, either in response to the separation or to the reunion. Such generally benign brief separations might include travel away from home, by one or both parents, a visit of the child to the grandparents' home, a short stay of the child in a hospital, or the brief hospitalization of a parent. The potential impact of each event must be considered in the light of the age and stage of development of the child and the particular relationship with the absent person, as well as the nature of the separation. It is more frightening for a child to be taken to the hospital and to be left by his parents than to have his parent leave for the hospital while he stays at home in familiar surroundings with his other parent and siblings.

Initial reaction to separation may involve crying, either of a tantrum-like, protesting type or of a quieter, sadder type. After a few hours or a day or so of separation, the child may appear more subdued, withdrawn, quiet or irritable, fussy, moody, and resistant to authority. He may repeatedly ask where his parent is and when he or she will return home, or he may not refer to parental absence at all. Young children may go to the window or door or out into the neighborhood looking for the absent parent; a few may even leave home or their places of temporary placement to try to find the hospital or place where their parents are. This last rather unusual response needs to be considered when a child cannot be found for a while shortly after the separation or departure of a parent. Disturbance of appetite may occur, and there may be special difficulties at bedtime, such as reluctance in going to bed and problems in getting to sleep, with a resurgence of old fears, and in the younger child perhaps regressive behavior such as a return to bed-wetting.

The child's response to reunion may surprise or alarm the parent who is not prepared. The parent who returns to the family enthusiastic, joyful and exuberant in greeting the child or children may be met by wary or cautious children, who, after a brief interchange of affection, may move away from the parent and seem indifferent to his or her return and presence. The interpretation of this response will depend on the child and his style; it may indicate his anger at being left and his wariness that the event will happen again, or since children tend to personalize, the child may have felt he caused the parent's departure for the hospital. For instance, if the mother who frequently says, "Stop it, or you'll give me a headache," is hospitalized, the child may unrealistically feel at fault and guilty. As a result of these feelings the child may seem to be more closely attached to the other parent than the absent one, or even to the grandparent or babysitter who cared for him during his parent's absence. Immediately after the reunion or after a few days, other children, particularly younger ones, may become more clinging and dependent than they were prior to separation, with continuation of any regressive behavior which had occurred during separation. Such behavior may engage the returned parent more closely and help to re-establish the bond that the child felt was broken. Usually such reactions are transient; within a week or two the child will have recovered his usual behavior and equilibrium. Recurrent separations can have more prolonged effects and may tend to make the child more wary and guarded about re-establishing the relationship with the repeatedly absent parent, and may generalize to other personal relationships.

Permanent or semipermanent loss such as divorce or placement in foster care can give rise to the same kinds of reactions listed above but more intense and possibly more permanent. School-age children may respond with obvious depression; some children manifest indifference and others are markedly angry. Other children appear to deny the fact or avoid the issue, either behaviorally or verbally. Most children may cling to the hope or fantasy that the actual placement or separation is not real. Guilt may be generated by the child's feeling that his loss, separation or placement represents rejection and perhaps punishment for his misbehavior. In other instances he may feel that it was his misbehavior that caused his parents to separate or become divorced. In this case he may exaggerate the significance of some very trivial behaviors or recurrent behavioral patterns of his own as having caused his parents to become angry with each other.

Beneath many of the above reactions to loss or separation lies the egocentricity of the young child, who sees himself as the causative agent, and holds the magical wish for the reappearance of the lost parent. He may protect his parents at his own expense, believing and asserting that he must have been bad and that this caused the parent to leave him or place him, rather than that the parent has been bad or irresponsible. Besides his own feeling of guilt, the child cannot blame the parent because he senses it may be fairly risky. The parent who found out that the child harbored resentment might punish him further for these thoughts or feelings.

The school-age or adolescent child may understand the explanations of parents as to divorce or the child's placement outside the home, but emotionally the event is felt as rejection, for which in perhaps some unknown manner he is to blame.

As to the ultimate separation, death of a parent, there seems to be agreement that most preadolescent children do not go through a true mourning period as defined in psychoanalytic concepts. Others feel that the child's mourning is masked by behavior not typically seen in adults. In 42 children ranging in age from about 5 or 6 years to adolescence who had lost a parent through death Wolfenstein found that immediately after the loss sad feelings were not markedly evident, nor was there much crying. The children continued in everyday activities, the child's major mechanism in dealing with this catastrophe being denial, both overt and unconscious, and maintained by the magical wish and hope for reunion and reappearance. Any depressed moods which occurred were not connected with thoughts of the parent's death, which could be acknowledged intellectually as a fact but was isolated in the emotionally nurtured expectation of return. Some children seemed to maintain remarkably good moods; some were more active than usual. These good moods were seen as an effective accompaniment of denial, as ways of avoiding the feelings of loss. As Wolfenstein described it, "If one does not feel bad, then nothing bad has happened." Some children show hostile and angry feelings toward their surviving parent and tend to identify with and idealize the lost parent, sometimes engaging in reunion fantasies along with denial. Guilt may be present, which points up the child's tendency toward egocentricity: An orphan of the Hiroshima bomb said, "We did nothing bad—and still our parents died."

Bowlby has described the sequence of events in very young children after separation from or loss of a parent; first, angry protest, which is essentially an expectation and demand that the mother return; then withdrawal and apathy; and, finally, a recovery period in which the child attempts to establish new relationships or strengthen older ones, often with an impairment of ability to risk really close and warm attachment in the future.

The physician can help the child and those who remain as his caretakers through a period of separation or adjustment to death of parent or sibling; he should recognize that the adults themselves may be going through a period of grief and mourning. It is not unhealthy for children to see their surviving or remaining parent mourn the loss of a dead mate or grieve for a divorced or separated spouse. In the case of a dead parent the child needs the support and reassurance of having the remaining parent or other important caretakers available to him. Close physical contact and emotional exchange, with verbal explanations and reassurance for those children who can understand are important aspects of support. The child should not be expected or forced to discuss all his feelings or to put into words his reactions to a parent's death, but he should be helped to continue to function in his everyday activities. He should not be expected to interrupt his usual social or recreational activities for weeks or months after death of a parent, neither out of respect for that parent nor in recognition of the remaining parent's sorrow or grief. Life's usual activities are the greatest healer and help the child to use denial in a healthy way to effect a healing process. Evidence of this process should not be interpreted by adults or older children as callousness or indifference. It should rather be recognized as the child's way of dealing at his stage of cognitive and emotional development with what is as much a catastrophe for him as it is for the adult. It is also important that the child not be expected to serve as a primary comforter or support to the remaining parent or others in their grief or mourning.

In most cases it seems helpful for the child to participate in an appropriate way in the rituals which generally surround the death and burial of a parent. A young child can attend a funeral, viewing, or wake so long as there is no morbid preoccupation or demand that the child remain a long time or be involved in prolonged religious ceremonies. To keep the young child away from some participation in the burial rituals, whatever they are, will be a misguided effort to protect, and more confusing and isolating than helpful.

GENDER ROLE IDENTITY. Sex typing, or the establishment of a gender identity, is a complicated process which begins before the birth of the child on at least two different levels. At the biologic level the sex chromosomes determine the structures and hormonal elaborations which lead to the development of gonads and sex organs of the appropriate sex, normally with congruence between genotype and phenotype. At the psychologic level the gender of the child plays a part in the wishes, hopes, expectations, anxieties and projections of the expectant parents. Their levels of satisfaction in their own gender identities and their previous experiences as parents of boys or girls will establish certain gender expectations or wishes. The genital organs are the single most important psychosocial cue to gender-specific responses for persons in the infant's environment. The psychosocial aspects of gender role identification complement the more exclusively intrapsychic processes.

The study of psychologic aspects of sexual anomalies and other investigations emphasize social determinants of sexual identification, arising both from within the family and from the larger social and cultural environment. The work of Money and coworkers indicates that by 18 months of age the child may have a firm grasp on his or her gender role. Others feel that sexual self-identification takes place between 2½ and 3 years. Among the determining factors in molding gender role identification are those standards, expectations and behaviors of parents and others which have sex role implications for the child, and the child's imitation and identification of others whom he will use as models. Study of children born with incongruity between genotypic and phenotypic sex (hermaphrodites, pseudohermaphrodites, and the like) suggests that it is the *social* determinants of sex which are crucial. If parents and others important in the child's environment label, raise and treat the child consistently as belonging to one sex, then that is the sex identity which the child will internalize and act upon, without regard to gonads possessed. (The rare phenomenon of the true transsexual may be an exception. This person has congruent chromosomal and physical sex characteristics and is raised socially in accord with anatomic phenotype, but such an individual declares that from earliest recollections he or she has felt, thought and believed himself or herself to be of the opposite sex. The common and revealing statement is, "I'm a woman imprisoned in a man's body," or vice versa. Adult transsexuals do not consider their sexual desires as being homosexually oriented.)

Sex role *standards* are beliefs as to the behaviors or attitudes appropriate to a given sex role, and serve as an internal guide as to what is male and what is female. Standards grow out of identification with important models in the environment, especially parents, and out of expectations of approval of certain behaviors or attitudes (or disapproval of others). By the age of 7 years the child's notion of sex role as a dichotomous concept has been established. Physical attributes perceived by the child as determining sexual role are fairly clear and direct; cultural standards are somewhat vaguer. Traditional Western cultural standards rate aggressive, assertive behavior as masculine, and dependent, passive, socially compliant and emotionally labile behavior as more in keeping with a female gender. The cultural stereotype has boys more dominant in interpersonal relationships, more interested in mechanical things, more interested and active in sports, developing greater skill in use of large muscles, and more independent. Girls are typified as more expressive emotionally, more concerned and skilled in interpersonal relationships, and more nurturant, with athletic prowess limited to certain sports. For the boy the mastery of games and skills is more important than how he relates to others in the process of achieving this mastery. For girls many of the critical gender role behaviors depend upon interpersonal feedback.

Sexual role *identity* is an individual's belief as to his own appropriate gender traits, and is very emotionally laden. There is never perfect correspondence between sexual standards and sexual identity, but some congruity is necessary to emotional health. A child who has many standard traits may not necessarily be psychologically secure in his or her sex role; children with weak or vague traits may have great difficulty in identifying themselves as female or male. Seeing oneself as similar to a parent of the same sex and different in critical ways from the other parent is important, as are the availability and adoption of activities, games and interests, and the acquiring of skills associated with one's own gender. Upon entry into school the child's comparison of self with peers may either strengthen or threaten his conviction about his own gender.

Academic achievement is not specifically sex typed, but our culture tends to stress academic success for boys, particularly in adolescence, in pursuit of vocational success. Girls in the elementary school years generally outperform boys academically except in mathematics, and learning disabilities are three to six times more frequent in boys than girls. By adolescence, however, boys have generally caught up with and at times surpass girls in many areas of academic achievement. Possible explanations include the fact that striving for excellence in intellectual achievement may be viewed by girls as a form of aggressive or assertive behavior in conflict with traditional sex role standards. Alternatively, such competition may put the girl in a position of besting boys, in conflict with that component of her sex role that stresses her ability to attract and hold a loved one. Such attitudes represent a cultural prescription designed to maintain psychologic and economic domination of women by men and to make the female attractive as a marital candidate. These attitudes also support the female role of being loved and provided for, protect her future role fulfillment in motherhood, and assume that her economic security will come through her husband's efforts to maintain her and their children.

In the past 10 years an important social and cultural phenomenon, the Women's Liberation Movement, has challenged the cultural stereotypes of gender roles, both for adults and for children. This movement has questioned the child-rearing techniques and sex role standards which mold girls into passive, nonassertive, noncompetitive adults, emphasizing exclusively nurturant and expressive roles; it challenges the cultural assumption that the main task of little girls' childhoods is preparation for the adult role of wife-mother. It is felt that it is concern with the security of the male ego and protection of the dominant socioeconomic position of men that wittingly and unwittingly supports traditional gender role standards and behaviors. The Women's Liberation Movement has tapped a very responsive chord among a broad range of women in the United States. The more vocal leaders and most of their followers have been mainly upper and middle class women, but the impact will probably be felt among all classes.

Pediatricians and other physicians can expect some problems of child behavior and child rearing to reflect this new attitude toward behaviors, games, interests and activities heretofore assigned to one gender or the other. Moreover, the way in which parents serve as sexual role models may undergo some marked shifts. All this may proceed smoothly and agreeably, or be marked with conflict and strife. Among middle class couples gender roles have become blurred in respect to many household activities, but the primary responsibility for day-to-day care of children has generally continued to be the mother's or that of her female surrogate (grandmother, babysitter, and the like). There is now greater pressure on the husband and father to assume or share more direct child-rearing responsibilities, and conflict may occur over what is suitable. Neither the immediate nor the long-term effects of these new life styles on children and families are as yet known.

The physician who is consulted regarding appropriate parental roles or who finds children caught in a struggle between parents over such roles can help parents to see that they are engaged in a renegotiation of the terms of their relationship (or social contract). He can help to promote an atmosphere for this negotiation in which each party states his or her terms and expectations and both then decide which conflictual areas or issues can be compromised or traded off. The physician must also help parents to avoid dragging their children into a power struggle, generating conflicting loyalties and possibly confusing the children as to their own roles. Children are very vulnerable when caught in struggles for their loyalty and affection, and one of their typical responses to such situations is to develop symptoms—behavioral, emotional or physical.

PUBERTY AND ADOLESCENCE. Adolescence is a physical and psychosocial process of long duration, lasting in Western society from the age of 12 or 13 years to the late teens or even the early 20's. Uncertainty as to the termination point of adolescence reflects whether one is measuring it by relatively internalized psychologic processes or by more social benchmarks such as economic and social emancipation from the parental family.

The notion of adolescence as a period of crisis has dominated much of the writing about adolescence in the past 20 years. The major contributors to this notion have been psychoanalytically oriented practicing clinicians (Erikson, Blos, Deutsch, and Josselyn). They have all tended to generalize a normative theory of general adolescent development out of clinical data dealing with sick and disturbed patients. In brief, adolescence has been seen as a time of marked upsurge in sexual and aggressive drives. Biologic maturation and social opportunity have combined to increase the occasions for expression of these drives. At the same time, it has been held that a re-emergence of earlier conflicts of a preoedipal and oedipal period centering on parent-child relationships has increased the instability of the adolescent psychic structure (pp. 64, 91). These biologic and intrapsychic factors, coupled with cultural demands for academic and social success and choice of vocation, have added to the storm and stress of the period. This somewhat vague notion of "adolescent turmoil" has been considered more or less normative. Fluctuating clinical symptoms, sometimes of a fairly serious nature, have been held to be part and parcel of the turmoil state, and a more or less successful adaptive outcome has been predicted, with appropriate support, reassurance and sometimes therapy.

More recent longitudinal studies of normal adolescents (Offer and Offer) and comparisons of patients and controls (Masterson) and examination of a large population of boys and girls (Douvan and Adelson) provide a less conflict-ridden picture of the adolescent experience, and the notion has gained currency that conspicuous adolescent turmoil is likely to have psychiatric implications.

Sexual attitudes and behavior become important developmental issues in adolescence, and in recent years standards of sexual conduct have been openly challenged among many ages and social groups. The impact upon sexual behavior has been difficult to assess. In a survey of normal English adolescents aged 15 to 19 years during 1962-63, Schofield found that 20 per cent of the boys and 12 per cent of the girls had experienced sexual intercourse. Ten years later Sorenson made a national survey of United States adolescents aged 13 to 19 years, through a probability sample of households, and found in the total group that 50 per cent of boys and 45 per cent of girls had had sexual intercourse; among 13 to 15 year olds, the corresponding percentages were 44 per cent for boys and 30 per cent for girls. In both surveys a majority of both sexes had had initial sexual intercourse with a "steady" or a close friend. The markedly different results of these two surveys of normal adolescents conducted 10 years apart may reflect rapid social change in the decade between the surveys, the increased availability of a variety of contraceptives, and/or intrinsic cultural differences between the two countries.

In any case, even among presumptively experienced adolescents there is still much ignorance about basic sexual and reproductive physiology and much less sophistication in knowledge and use of contraceptive devices than one might expect.

The physician who deals with adolescents, even those who may be sexually active, should not assume that their theoretical knowledge, particularly in the area of contraception, is measured by their practical experience in sexual intercourse. Many sexually active adolescents find it difficult to admit ignorance about sexual matters, since bravado, an air of sophistication and saving face at any cost is for them a highly invested coping style. Accordingly it becomes the physician's responsibility to take the initiative in providing instruction and guidance.

The failure of some adolescents to use contraceptives involves motivational factors as well as ignorance. Obtaining and using contraceptives makes the intention to have intercourse explicit. By not being prepared in advance, the adolescent attempts to avoid guilt through maintaining the fiction that intercourse resulted from overwhelming passion or a miscalculation. For some adolescent girls pregnancy fulfills conscious or unconscious needs; it can boost self-esteem, provide reassurance of femininity, or become an act of defiance or of self-denigration, or be used as a weapon against family, boyfriend or self. For some boys, successfully impregnating their girlfriend serves as a proof of their virility.

In guiding the adolescent, the physician needs to take into account two other crucial and related issues in adolescent development: the relationships between adolescents and parents and between adolescents and their peers. The young adolescent may vacillate between extreme attempts at independence and sudden reversions to overt or camouflaged dependence. The adolescent is trying out new ideas and new relationships and is trying to renegotiate the old relationship with parents to win somewhat new and different terms. Since adolescence in Western society can be viewed as a time of rehearsal for a variety of adult roles, it is natural to expect that early attempts at adult performance will be clumsy, overdone, exaggerated and not satisfactory either to the adolescent or to those around him. One of the most important roles of the physician is to point out to both the adolescent and his parents, but particularly to the parents, that parents and child are entering upon a new phase of relationship. Both parents and adolescent must get used to the idea that they are in the process of separating from each other, reaching the final stage of a process that began in the first year of life. Anxiety and depression are to be expected at times, on the part either of the child or of the parent, as they modify their earlier closer bond. Behind a facade of negativism, indifference, scoffing and demeaning of parental values or beliefs, the adolescent is frequently asking, albeit unconsciously, for guidance, advice and explicit statements of values or standards, and at times for firmly stated limits. The parental attitudes most threatening to the adolescent may be either premature total emancipation on the one hand or a resort to physical coercion on the other. Parental indifference might be equally threatening. In ordinary activities the adolescent fears most and does his best to avoid loss of face, the appearance of being a fool to himself or to his peers, siblings or parents. The physician can be most helpful to parents if, as a semi-objective outsider, he can help them to avoid power struggles in which the loss of face by child or parent is a frequent outcome.

The normative studies cited above indicate that for many families adolescent-parent relationships are not particularly crisis-laden or filled with conflict. Bickerings or disagreement about use of the family automobile, curfew, companions, school effort and achievement, and the verbal challenging and defending of cherished values, are the usual kinds of confrontations that most families experience.

Marijuana has come to be the symbol of differences between the generations. It seems likely that most high school students have had an opportunity for or some experience with marijuana, but the frequency of heavy use, daily to several times a week, is low. The use of alcohol seems to be increasing among adolescents in the middle classes. There is some evidence that heroin usage and addiction are decreasing, both among high school students and among those young people who have left high school. Lysergic acid diethylamide (LSD) was in the 1960's used by many older adolescents and college students, but its use is in decline among both groups. The use of barbiturates, of other sedatives such as methaqualone and of amphetamines is still frequent enough among high school students and older adolescents to constitute a serious psychosocial issue. What physicians need most is accurate and adequate information about the current practices and trends in use of drugs among the subcultures from which their patients come. The physician must know such things as types of drugs, frequency of use, among which age groups, and whether the use is distinctive by social class, by school, or by local community; they must be aware of what parental, school and other community resources are doing to cope with the problems. Only if he is adequately informed can he be helpful to his adolescent patients or their families who face problems of drug abuse (See later, this Section).

The choice of future career, whether it follows immediately upon high school or after college and postgraduate work, is an important preoccupation of adolescents. The physician can be helpful to the adolescent in knowing what resources are available for vocational training, for advice regarding choice of possible colleges, or regarding requirements and preparation needed for a career in which the adolescent is interested. The adolescent frequently needs an opportunity to discuss with an experienced adult his concerns about his future. As someone outside the family the physician can provide a realistic and acceptable assessment of career possibilities and expectations.

The adolescent in America is today under great pressure to succeed both academically and vocationally. A salient psychosocial factor in the counterculture movement is the reaction of individuals and groups to the premium put upon competitive achievement, both in the lives of parents and in parents' expectations of their children. The adolescent is likely to expect too much of himself, to become discouraged and give up, or to strive inordinately hard, paying a high price emotionally and socially, and sometimes with respect to health. Suicide attempts are at peak incidence in the age group between 15 and 25 years; suicide is the second most frequent cause of death in this age group, following accidents.

Jean Piaget and other investigators have indicated that it is in the adolescent period that the final stage is reached in development of abstract reasoning and facility with logic and other symbolic forms of thought. Along with this comes increased sophistication in moral reasoning. Recent studies indicate that traditional notions that adult-level ideas of right and wrong were established by the age of latency are in error. Just as with physical and emotional development, maturity in cognitive and moral reasoning is achieved in adolescence. Only then does the maturing individual become capable of the most highly developed form of moral reasoning: the formulation of abstract principles based upon notions of justice, from which are derived ethical guides to action. Not all adolescents reach full maturity in cognitive or moral development; some achieve full integrity only as adults, some never.

The physician can be helpful to the adolescent and his parents in providing developmental interpretations of behavior which increase the adolescent's understanding of himself as well as his parents' understanding of him. The propensity of some adolescents for discussion and arguments around such issues as religion, philosophy, politics, social concerns and ethical questions is one way in which they develop and test their new cognitive and logical skills.

The normative studies cited above show the average adolescent to be subject to anxiety and to episodes of depression. Among the fairly effective strategies usually developed for dealing with stress and avoiding too much self-preoccupation are goal-directed academic or extracurricular or social activities. Discussions with their peers support adolescents in coping with the stresses and strains of everyday life. Humor is a major coping strategy, the butts of which may be parents and adult-dominated institutions, but also themselves, and often each other in terms of kidding and clowning.

Anxiety may be generated by threats either to academic achievement or to social success, and frequently signals increased effort in goal-directed, productive activities. A relationship with a significant adult outside the family, such as teacher, coach, youth leader, clergyman, collateral relative or older sibling, often gives important support to the adolescent which he may use in solving some of his problems. The physician may serve as a source of this kind of support and help, particularly if he has established a significant relationship with the child as a preadolescent.

It should be underscored that one must view with skepticism the idea that what appears to be "adolescent turmoil" can be dismissed as normal stresses and strains, particularly if someone is clearly unhappy or if recurrent crises suggest serious conflicts. An adolescent who presents symptoms suggestive of an emotional disturbance requires careful and complete evaluation. Among signs requiring attention will be sudden declines in scholastic achievement, choices of new companions with whom parents are uncomfortable or of whom they disapprove, or evidence of a preference almost exclusively for activities outside the home, especially when there appears to be a breakdown in communication within the home. The latter may occur not only between adolescent and parents but also between parents. When such signs appear, it is well for the family physician, pediatrician or generalist to have a high index of suspicion of serious illness, such as may well warrant psychiatric referral. Masterson arrived at the following conclusions from study of adolescents in difficulty: "The symptomatic adolescent is believed to step to a different drummer, only temporarily under the surge of the adolescent growth process. However, the music to which these adolescents stepped was not a transient malady orchestrated by growth and development but a persistent and a pervasive symphony arranged by psychiatric illness. Somber cadence pursued these patients through their adolescent years into adulthood." Masterson found that many of his patients had a long history of psychiatric illness that began in childhood and was only temporarily colored by the developmental stage of adolescence.

MARC A. FORMAN
WILLIAM H. HETZNECKER

Bowlby, J.: Attachment and Loss. Vol. II, Separation. New York, Basic Books, Inc., 1973.

Douvan, E., and Adelson, Y.: The Adolescent Experience. New York, John Wiley & Sons, Inc., 1966.

Masterson, J. F.: The psychiatric significance of adolescent turmoil. Am. J. Psychiat., *124*:107, 1968.

Miller, J. B. M.: Children's reaction to the death of a parent: A review of the psychoanalytic literature. J. Am. Psychoanal. Ass. *19*:697, 1971.

Money, J.: Psychosexual differentiation. *In* Money, J. (ed.): Sex Research, New Developments. New York, Holt, Rinehart and Winston, 1965.

Offer, D.: The Psychological World of the Teenager: A study of Normal Adolescent Boys. New York, Basic Books, Inc., 1969.

Offer, D., and Offer, J. L.: Profiles of normal adolescent girls. A.M.A. Arch. Gen. Psychiat. *19*:513, 1968.

Reiss, I. L.: The Social Context of Premarital Sexual Permissiveness. New York, Holt, Rinehart and Winston, 1967.

Schofield, M.: The Sexual Behavior of Young People. Boston, Little, Brown and Company, 1965.

Sorenson, R. C.: Adolescent Sexuality in Contemporary America. New York, World Publishing Co., 1972.

Wolfenstein, M.: How is mourning possible? *In* The Psychoanalytic Study of the Child. New York, International Universities Press, 1966.

Role of the Physician in Prevention of Psychologic Disorders in the Sick Child

Whenever an illness alters the child's functions, or changes the way in which his parents or others feel about him, there may be psychologic disturbances. These effects can be minimized and fixed psychogenic disease may be prevented through anticipatory guidance. An upper respiratory infection may make a child feel miserable. Prompt and confident handling by parents and physicians will give appropriate emphasis to fluids, rest and other treatment if needed, and will reduce regression by not overdramatizing the illness through requirement of strict bedrest, excessive laboratory studies or unnecessarily prolonged absence from school. A poorly handled trivial illness in a child with other problems might set the stage for a fixed school phobia, through the arousal of anxiety at separation from protection of home and mother.

Psychologic impact of illness may derive from discomfort, anxiety and changes of sensorium (clouding of consciousness, hallucinations, delusions and disorientation) and may be manifest as withdrawal, depression, irritability and regression. Regression is a psychologic state which should be regarded as normal for ill children and for ill adults as well. The caretaking process reinforces regression and can lead to prolongation of illness if excessive and inappropriate. The sick child withdraws his interest from the outside world and invests it in himself and his hurt. This is normal for a while, but the parents should be advised by the physician to increase their expectations of the patient as clinical signs of illness subside.

PSYCHOSOMATIC INTERPLAY. We have also become increasingly aware of the ways in which psychogenic factors modify responses to experiences, including illnesses. Every clinical phenomenon has reverberations at all organizational levels: molecular, anatomic, physiologic, intrapsychic, interpersonal, family and social. For instance, the wish to avoid a stressful interpersonal situation may have for the child a concomitant autonomic nervous system response, mediated through the hypothalamus and reticular activating system, which leads to abdominal pain, diarrhea, and so on, with changes in personal and social state.

There are three important implications for the physician of the above considerations. First, he must maintain an open attitude toward the cause of the child patient's discomforts, rather than a position that symptoms are *either* organic *or* psychologically determined. A laceration, for example, may occur in an accident-prone child whose parents may need preventive guidance. On the other hand, while the parents of a stubborn, retentive, encopretic child may need insightful psychotherapeutic guidance, the child may need an enema just as much, for relief of his own distress. Second, the psychosocial aspects of the spectrum of potential etiologies of illness should be examined along with the physiologic aspects from the outset of consideration of a clinical problem with parents and child. This early interest and attention will prevent the impression later that interest in psychogenic factors has been aroused because the "doctor can't find anything wrong" or that the child is "just faking" an illness. Third, the physician has the opportunity to act as a model for the parents and the child by making explicit his interest in the child's feelings. When he asks about the child's feelings, both child and parents may learn that it is possible and appropriate to communicate discomfort in verbal, symbolic language, and not just in somatic language. A good opening question is "How are you feeling?" rather than "Where does it hurt?" The latter will come out soon enough.

The sick child who reaches the *hospital* is faced with a number of potential challenges. These include coping with separation, adaptation to a new environment, adjustment to multiple caretakers, often association with very sick children, sometimes care in an intensive care unit, submission to machines, to anesthesia or to surgery, and possibly other strange experiences. The psychologic stages of adapting to the hospital have been outlined for different ages in previous sections. The most intense hospital fears for the infant and young child are generated by separation from and loss of parent, often equated in the mind of the young child with loss of love and/or abandonment; the school-age child may be more concerned with painful procedures, some of which carry the threat of bodily mutilation; the adolescent most fears the loss of control and of options implicit in the use of anesthesia involved with surgery. Preventive measures can ease the child's adaptation to the hospital and lessen the psychologic and behavioral after-reactions.

For the child under the age of 3 or 4 years, the rooming-in of a parent is basic, if it is at all feasible. Verbal explanations are of little value to such children. For the older child whose admission is to be arranged for a future date an earlier visit to the hospital is crucial. He should be given the opportunity of seeing where he will be, meeting the people who will be caring for him, and receiving answers to his questions as to what will happen. A creative and active recreational or socialization program, liberal or open visiting hours, and a chance himself to act out feared procedures in play with dolls or mannequins are all helpful. Needless to say, the staff must maintain a sensitive, sympathetic and accepting attitude toward child and parents. Some nurses or physicians at times find themselves at odds with parents, toward whom they take condescending or critical attitudes, overtly or unconsciously. Such nurses or physicians may feel, for example, that they are better able to meet the child's needs than the parents, who may appear to be anxious or distraught or, alternatively, less concerned than circumstances seem to warrant. At these times such nurses or physicians may convey to the parents an "I-am-the-good-parent-you-must-be-a-bad-parent" feeling which may greatly impair the adjustment of parents and child to hospitalization. Parents are often already, though irrationally, feeling guilty enough that their child became ill; they may act in a hostile manner to compensate for their own feelings of guilt, or they may not be able to ask crucial questions for fear of "sounding stupid." Physician and nurse and other professional persons all need to help to establish and to maintain effective communication in a climate of interest and affection for the child and family, in whatever degree this climate can be created.

Ambulatory care presents particular problems in clinics in which patients receive discontinuous care from a series of physicians whose intercommunication is often negligible, whether it takes place verbally or through the hospital record or chart. When continuity of interest and care are compounded with language and intercultural barriers to communication, the parents of children are often unable to verbalize their major concerns about their child to the doctor or other professional personnel. Recommendations for care are inappropriate or irrelevant, and the compliance with which parents follow the physician's advice or directions, such as in taking prescribed medication, is poor. At the end of any initial diagnostic or management activity, the physician should have the habit of inquiring as to whether there are other things parents or children may wish to ask or talk about during this visit to the clinic. Medical care will be improved, and preventive measures taken against medical or emotional problems arising out of feelings of loneliness, inadequacy, frustration and anger if paramedical personnel can be used who are familiar with the language and culture of the patient's family and who can convey the concerns of parents and physicians reliably to each other. In bilingual communities, bilingual employees and signs are essential. Visits to such clinics should be followed up by telephone, or by visits on the part of health aides or public health nurses to the home.

In the increasingly busy "emergency rooms" of hospitals in urban centers conflicting expectations exist between how the house staff or emergency room staff expect the emergency room to be used (for trauma or for acute and serious illness of recent onset) and what the patients seeking care there actually need, which is a medical agency offering the services of a local family physician. These differing expectations are often frustrating to house staff waiting for the drama of a "real" emergency, or to staff whose ability to care for any real emergency is blunted by the less urgent but insistent demands of large numbers of patients with relatively minor complaints, as seen from the staff's (but not the patient's or parents') point of view. When these different expectations are faced and clarified, a way may be found to deal differently with the patients' patterns of use at the point of entry. Triage and true emergency care may be accurately identified early, and appropriately assigned; with these roles clarified, house staff often feel they have clearer goals and can be more comfortable in doing what they are expected to do.

The employment of ombudsmen in emergency rooms, to whom patients and parents can turn for help, has often been shown to clarify and resolve individual, social and cultural differences and conflicts.

The chronically or fatally ill child presents special problems to the physician in private practice, to the specialist and his team in a regional hospital, and to the general staff of any hospital. Some of these issues are discussed elsewhere (pp. 139–144). Here we shall touch those issues in which certain preventive measures can lessen the psychologic discomfort of the child and parents during illness, and prevent psychologic problems for surviving parents and siblings.

Every symptom experienced by a child is vaguely or perhaps unconsciously perceived by him and by his parents as a threat to his physical integrity and, when carried to its extreme, as a threat to his life and as a reminder of his mortality. The more serious and potentially lethal the clinical state, the greater the intensity of emotions aroused. The young child experiences this primarily as discomfort, as increased ministrations, and perhaps as an anxiety, often reflecting parental anxiety, and so on. By the age of 9 years, however, children begin to conceive of death in the abstract as a state that means more than just going away. By adolescence they can think of death in philosophic terms much like an adult, albeit with limited experience.

In chronic illnesses which shorten life, such as cystic fibrosis, parents need the physician's early support in developing a relatively guilt-free understanding of the disease process and in learning how to help to ameliorate it. In addition, they need guidance in developing a comfortable approach to the child's questions about his disease. The young child will take most cues from the parents. With the older child, and especially the adolescent, the parents must be prepared for the anger of the child at his fate. This will be less in degree and easier to accept if the child has been given at each phase of illness such relatively consistent, accurate and simple information as is needed and can be assimilated. The success of this process depends not only on the parents' psychologic strength and resources but also on the physician's availability and objectivity. The role of the physician is difficult. He must stand for hope and for amelioration of discomfort. He must also be ready to help parents and child to avoid emotionally crippling psychologic handicaps. Parents need, for example, to be encouraged to meet their own needs, even when this requires temporary and perhaps recurrent separation from the child; at times this may help the child to learn to tolerate frustration. Experiences with groups of parents of chronically or fatally ill children indicate that parents may creatively support each other, under professional guidance of physician, psychologist or social worker.

In less chronic, more fulminating lethal processes, such as leukemia, the intensity of anxiety, guilt and despair may be greater than in more chronic illnesses. An index of the intensity of family stress in coping with fatal illness in children is that the divorce rate among parents of leukemic children is significantly higher than that in unaffected families. With most children over 9 or 10 years of age it has been found most supportive to treat fatal illnesses such as leukemia factually with the child, so far as diagnosis and prognosis are concerned. Children do not usually ask the physician if or when they are going to die, though they may reveal their fears to others in the hospital. The young child primarily wants to be reassured that his parents will not desert him and that he is loved. Both in and outside the hospital the development of a supportive team representing medical, nursing, psychologic and social work disciplines, and perhaps others, can help to assure that the agonizing experiences surrounding the illness and death of a child retain as much growth-promoting power as possible for patient and survivors. The primary physician also needs to stay involved and close to the child and the clinical situation; he often knows the child and family best and can be most supportive. The hospital team needs frequent conferences for their own mutual support in the difficult situation of losing a patient. If objectivity is lost, the physician who feels he has failed may himself become anxious or depressed and lose his supportive role toward the patient and family.

After the death of a fatally ill child the parents need a chance to talk out their feelings with the physician, one of whose goals should be to help them psychologically not to encapsulate the lost child in an unmourned state. Here, too, groups of parents who have gone through the same experience may provide help.

Organ transplant in the child has so far been largely restricted to the kidney. Hemodialysis precedes renal transplant for many children for varying lengths of time. Dialysis begins in the hospital, but parents are often expected to learn to carry out this procedure at home. They are often ambivalent about being given control of a life-threatening process. The child receiving dialysis becomes psychologically dependent and often withdrawn. It helps if the shunt is placed in the leg rather than the arm; this allows the child to be more active during the long periods of dialysis.

Family problems multiply with the question of donor of the transplanted organ. If a live related donor is available, there may be tension between possible donors as to who should "make the sacrifice." In some cases it may relieve guilt if the physician arbitrarily (but thoughtfully) makes this decision. Here, as in the case of other children with chronic or fatal illness, a medical support team of carefully chosen staff is essential to decision-making and continuing care. There is a high suicide rate among adults on hemodialysis, but it appears less traumatic to children, probably owing to the younger child's greater capacities for denial and for acceptance of a support system (including parents) which prolongs his dependence. Adolescents are concerned with distortions of body image, which they cannot always express verbally. The physician needs the patience to listen (to both the stated and the implied questions and misconceptions), to interpret, to set appropriate limits and to help families and patients with technical details and with decision-making.

J. M. Dunn

PREVENTION

Well Child

A. General Comments

Cava, E.: Questions and Answers in Child Rearing. New York, Hawthorn Books, Inc., 1972.

Ginott, H.: Between Parent and Child. New York, The Macmillan Company, 1965.

Dodson, F.: How to Parent. Los Angeles, Nash Publishing Corporation, 1970.

Thomas, A., Chess, S., and Birch, H. G.: Temperament and Behavior Disorders in Children. New York, New York University Press, 1968.

Work, H., and McCall, J. D.: A Guide to Preventive Child Psychiatry; The Art of Parenthood. New York, McGraw-Hill Book Company, Inc., 1965.

B. Critical Issues

Berlin, I.: Learning and Its Disorders. Palo Alto, California, Science and Behavior Books, 1966.

Blos, P.: On Adolescence: A Psychoanalytic Interpretation. New York, Free Press, 1962.

Bowlby, J.: Attachment. New York, Basic Books, Inc., 1969.

Gardiner, R. A.: The Boys and Girls Book About Divorce with an Introduction to Parents. New York, Science House, 1970.

Group for Advancement of Psychiatry Committee on Adolescence: Normal Adolescence: Its Dynamics and Import. New York, G.A.P., 1968.

Sabinga, M. S., and Friedman, C. J.: Restraint and speech. Pediatrics *48*(No. 1):116–122, 1971.

Schofield, M. G.: The Sexual Behavior of Young People. London, Longmans, Green & Co., 1965.

Schooler, C.: Birth order effects: Not here, not now. Psychol. Bull. *78*(No. 3):161–175, 1972.

Spitz, R.: The First Year of Life; A Psychoanalytic Study of Normal and Deviant Development of Object Relations. New York, International Universities Press, 1965.

Stoller, R. J.: Sex and Gender. New York, Science House, 1968.

Sick Child

Bergman, T.: Children in the Hospital. New York, International Universities Press, 1966.

Movie, "You See, I Had a Life.": The Eccentric Circle, Cinema Workshop. P.O. Box 1981, Evanston, Ill. 60204.

Prugh, D. G.: Toward an understanding of psychosomatic concepts in relation to illness in children. *In* Solnit, A. J., and Provence, S. A. (eds.): Modern Perspectives in Child Development in Honor of Milton J. E. Senn. New York, International Universities Press, 1963, pp. 246–370.

Robertson, J.: Young Children in Hospitals. New York, Basic Books, Inc., 1958.

Solnit, A. J., and Green, M.: Psychologic considerations in the management of deaths on pediatric hospital services. 1. The doctor and the child's family. Pediatrics *24*(No. 1):106–112, 1959.

Vernon, D.: The Psychological Responses of Children to Hospital and Illness: A Review of the Literature. Springfield, Illinois, Charles C Thomas, 1965.

THE PHYSICIAN'S ROLE IN ESTABLISHED PSYCHOLOGIC DISORDERS

Balint, M.: The Doctor, His Patient and the Illness. New York, International Universities Press, 1957.
Levine, M.: Psychotherapy in Medical Practice. New York, The Macmillan Company, 1942.
Proskauer, S., and Rolland, R.: Youth who use drugs: Psychodynamic diagnostic and treatment planning. J. Am. Acad. Child Psychiat. *12*(No. 2): Jan., 1973.
Schneiderman and Swenson: Suicide Among Youth. A supplement to the bulletin of suicidology, NIMH. Washington, D.C., U.S Government Printing Office, 1969.
Wolberg, L. R.: The technique of short term psychotherapy. In Wolberg, L. R. (ed.): Short Term Psychotherapy. New York, Grune & Stratton, 1965.

PSYCHOLOGIC DISORDERS

Man's great adaptive capacity and developmental flexibility account in part for his susceptibility to emotional and mental illness. Since psychic development takes place after birth and is determined by the interaction of the child with his environment, there are possibilities for unfavorable as well as favorable experiences.

PSYCHOPATHOLOGY

TRAUMATIC EXPERIENCES. Psychopathology may result from physical or emotional traumatic experiences. It may be evident immediately, or it may remain latent and become manifest under sufficiently stressful conditions. Even optimal parental care and rearing cannot foresee or prevent such severely disturbing events as physical illness or injury, hospitalization, loss of or separation from loved ones or other emotional disturbances. Whether such experiences have lasting psychopathologic effects depends essentially upon the degree to which the child is able to gain mastery over them.

A particular traumatic experience can be viewed as having three phases: preparation for the untoward event, management of it, and subsequent attempts at mastery of the unfavorable psychologic effects.

Preparation. No preparation can be made for a truly accidental traumatic experience, but the way in which previous experiences have been handled by parents or pediatrician can be helpful to the child in unanticipated circumstances. Adults should be honest with a child about the nature and meaning of unpleasant experiences and give attention to the child's emotional needs at those times so that he comes to have confidence in adults.

Whenever possible, the child should be forewarned of an unpleasant experience in keeping with his understanding and his ability to bear tension. These capacities change as the child develops. A 4 year old child is not helped by long and detailed discussion of the anxiety-creating aspects of a forthcoming tonsillectomy; nor is it wise to tell him about it more than a day or so in advance; otherwise, his apprehension causes too much tension which must be borne too long. On the other hand, an 11 year old child is capable of understanding a good deal about such things, and a carefully considered explanation, avoiding discussion of the more dire possibilities, can be extremely helpful in preventing psychologic trauma. He can be told about the event considerably in advance, and he will likely use the intervening time to think and to ask questions and to prepare himself.

Parents and physicians may overidentify with the child in his fear of pain and become distressed by his crying and protests in anticipation of the frightening event. For this reason they often rationalize that the child is better off not knowing what is coming. Although this plan may spare both the child and the adults some moments of distress in advance of the event, its consequences are highly undesirable. The child feels betrayed by those whom he must trust and depend upon and is deprived of the opportunity to prepare himself for what is to come. The crying and protests of the child at such a time are needed and healthy expressions of feeling and relief of tension.

Management of the Threatening Event. It is important to try to keep the tension within the child's limits of tolerance. Physical pain and psychological fright should be kept to a minimum, and the child's relation to his parents should be maintained as the principal source of emotional support and security so far as is possible. If the parents cannot be close and supportive enough to meet the child's needs, a parent-substitute should be provided. The parents should ensure that the child understands that this person is acting on their behalf. Proper explanation to the child of the nature and meaning of happenings and procedures is important.

"Working Through" or Mastery. Children universally and spontaneously re-enact threatening experiences in their play and fantasy. For example, a 3 year old girl given an enema will subsequently administer enemas to her dolls in her play; or, after a visit to the pediatrician for a routine physical examination, the young child will most likely play doctor. This normal, innate response helps the child to come to terms with the experience and to master the feelings associated with it. Perhaps the most helpful factor is the change in role from passive recipient to active doer.

This natural tendency in the child, even when

minimally evident, can and should be called forth and utilized, just as the child psychiatrist uses the spontaneous play of the child as a means of understanding and helping him. Unfortunately, both the laity and the medical profession commonly think that the best remedy for the distress of the child who has undergone a threatening experience is to "help him to forget it." But to pretend that an unpleasant experience has not occurred deprives the child of the opportunity of playing out and mastering the experience; if fantasies and tensions persist, repression may take place. Because the repressed experience continues to be invested with psychic energy (libido), it persists as an active but unconscious force in the psychologic equilibrium, and may provide a basis for subsequent psychologic disorder.

A traumatic experience may leave a psychopathologic imprint for three general reasons: (1) the experience may be overwhelming, e.g., loss of the mother to a 6 month old infant, without replacement with a mother-substitute (René Spitz); (2) the child may be given inadequate help through the three phases described above; or (3) the child may be unable to cope with the experience owing to his own deficiencies.

The Child's Ability to Cope. In order to understand the child's ability to cope with inside and outside forces, it may be helpful to view the progress of his psychic development from the standpoint of homeostasis. This term was originally used by Cannon to designate the tendency of the physiologic bodily processes to maintain a state of equilibrium. Neither physical nor psychologic homeostasis implies a completely stable state, but rather an equilibrium of constantly varying and changing forces. In a state of absolute stability there would be no growth or development, either physical or psychologic.

A parallel can be drawn between physiologic homeostasis and the structural components of personality. Thus, the basic biochemical and biophysiologic processes can be conceived of as the prototype of the id; the innate mechanisms which regulate these physiologic processes are the prototype of the ego; and the limits within which, for example, the pH of body fluids and the body temperatures may vary constitute physiologic laws which bear similarity to the attitudes and value judgments which come to compose the child's superego, or conscience.

In the normal autistic stage of psychologic development the neonate is functioning essentially on a physiologic level. In the symbiotic stage the situation changes with beginning maturation and the emotional alliance of mother and infant. The gradual organization of biochemical processes into sexual and aggressive drives, seen only indirectly through manifestations in tension and behavior, begins to give the id some meaning on a psychologic level. The physiologic regulatory mechanisms persist and are supplemented on a psychologic level by the combination of the "rudimentary" ego of the infant and the ego of the mother (maternal auxiliary ego). The superego, at this stage, is represented by the maternal-familial or cultural value system. Because of the lack of ego capacity in the infant, his mother does most of his coping. He tends to fare well in proportion to her ability to understand and meet his needs for gratification, stimulation and frustration. If the mother misinterprets his needs, or if other circumstances such as illness and hospitalization of the infant or prolonged separation from his mother prevent her from helping him, psychopathology is likely to result.

As the infant begins to separate from his mother and progresses through the successive stages of psychosexual development, the id drives become more clearly focused in their aims, and the functions provided by the maternal auxiliary ego are gradually taken over by the child's own ego. Similarly, the external value system gradually becomes internalized to form the child's superego.

As the child develops, he acquires an increasing array of skills and ego defensive and adaptive techniques, and his psychologic and mental functioning becomes increasingly complex. His first attempts at mastery of a bad experience through play must be fairly primitive, amounting only to a re-enactment on the basis of memory, with little or no elaboration in imagination or fantasy. By the age of 2 or 3 years the child is capable of fantasy which makes his play more varied, but still rather literal and lacking in make-believe. Once he has gained the rudiments of language and is able to distinguish between what is real and what is pretended, his play begins to serve the purpose of trial-acting. Ultimately, in the mastery and working through of bad experiences, play activity tends to be replaced by verbalization, or "talking it out."

Although fantasy and imagination play important roles in the mastery of bad experiences, they can also contribute to the development of psychopathology. Through them a child may so distort reality that fears and conflicts develop which contribute to the development of a psychologic disorder. For example, if a child who has been repeatedly warned not to play in the street is struck by a car while playing there, he may interpret the injury as severe punishment for his disobedience. Such a fantasy could excessively reinforce his developing conscience and lead him unduly to inhibit his aggression in order to avoid an even worse fate. Such a child might become passive and conforming.

If the child's attempt to master a threatening experience through re-enactment does not succeed, the tendency toward re-enactment persists in the form of disturbed behavior. The term "repetition-compulsion" has been used to characterize this pathologic re-enactment. Thus, a child who continues to feel or fantasy himself to be rejected by his parents may be repetitiously provocative to them, as well as to other adults, such as teachers. His underlying wish or goal is that he should not be rejected, but be loved in spite of his provocativeness; naturally, the adult response is likely to be to the provocativeness rather than to the underlying aim. Accordingly he undergoes further rejection and additional reinforcement of his feeling of being unloved.

In the light of this understanding of the roles of reality-distorting fantasy, of anxiety, of repression and of unconscious mental life in the causation of psychopathology, one can appreciate the importance for the developing child of adequate explanations, of permitting re-enactment in play, of inviting questions and of appropriate discussion.

Another concept pertaining to the child's ability to cope with traumatic experiences is that of "phase-specificity" (Hartmann). This concept holds that an experience will be particularly traumatic if it happens to impinge on those developing functions which characteristically are most heavily libidinized in the particular stage during which the child suffers the experience (see under Libido in Table 2–10). For example, a fracture of the jaw in an 11 month old infant at the time he is being weaned which forces him abruptly to give up his oral gratification could be severely traumatic. On the other hand, the same injury in a child 3 years of age is not likely to have the same effect because he is beyond the oral stage of development. Similarly, an operation performed on a child 5 or 6 years of age, who at that age is normally greatly concerned about injury to his body or his genitals, is likely to have threatening implications which it might not have at the age of 9 or 10 years. The concept of phase-specificity of trauma may lead the psychologically oriented physician to advise postponement of certain surgical or medical procedures (provided postponement is not detrimental to health) until the child has entered another stage of development.

In summary, the ability of the child to cope with experience is influenced (1) by the constitutional adequacy of the ego apparatus and functions, (2) by the adequacy of the care provided in support of the child's ego functions by the mother or mother-substitute, (3) by the level of psychologic development and the adequacy of the ego defensive and adaptive techniques available at the time of a traumatic experience, and (4) by how the nature of the trauma relates to the particular stage of development in accordance with the concept of phase-specificity.

KINDS OF PSYCHOPATHOLOGY. It is important to understand that a child may have a psychologic disorder without psychopathology having been firmly established within him. Conflict usually begins and exists for a time outside the child's basic psychic structure before it becomes internalized. Conflict between the child and his environment can cause psychologic disorders which symptomatically appear to be the same as disorders resulting from internal psychopathology. Such situational disorders, however, respond to early correction of the circumstances causing conflict, and direct treatment of the child is usually not necessary. The potential of many situations for producing psychologic difficulties is well known, and they can be anticipated or managed with preventive or corrective measures which have a high probability of preventing lasting disability in most children.

Psychologic disorders which are manifestations of internal psychopathology are serious and difficult to treat. Conflicts exist within the personality structure that has developed out of the interaction of the child and his environment. Through the mental mechanisms of introjection and identification, the attitudes and traits of the parents and other significant persons in the child's life normally become internalized to form parts of the ego and superego. This internalization tends to take place gradually and results in a reasonably harmonious internal personality structure so long as the state of tension or the psychologic equilibrium of the child is kept within reasonable limits and he gains mastery over the disturbing experiences which inevitably occur in the course of development.

If the infant or young child experiences too much tension, he internalizes the images derived from his tension-provoking experiences too quickly and unselectively. This internalization is aimed protectively at regaining psychologic equilibrium, but it tends to set up conflicts between the id drives and needs, the ego, and the superego, in various combinations. For example, a child who experiences his mother as unduly harsh during toilet training may internalize her restrictive or punitive attitudes to avoid further conflict with her. These attitudes now become a part of his superego, which is, as a result, set at odds with his normal aggressive drives and his normal id needs for pleasure and gratification; these features are damaging to his developing self-image and self-esteem, which are in the realm of the ego. Thus, what was formerly a conflict with the external world (his mother) has now become an internal or intrapsychic conflict.

It is possible to distinguish two major kinds of internal psychopathology. These are designated: *psychoses,* which appear to have their origin from constitutional deficiencies, or from traumatic experiences occurring in the first 2 years or so of life; and *neuroses,* which have their origin from traumatic experiences occurring, for the most part, in the age range from 2 to 6 or 7 years.

The basic images—those of the mother and the self—begin to be established gradually during the symbiotic phase of development. The acute anxiety occurring normally by about 8 or 9 months of age is presumed to be due to the infant's acquisition of sufficiently clear images of mother and self that he realizes that his mother is not part of him. It seems probable that it takes a further period, extending well into the period between 12 and 24 months of age, until these first images (both perceptual and emotional) have become sufficiently stable so that the child can call forth a memory of his mother as a kind of reassurance when she is absent from him. At this point he has attained an important step in his psychologic independence. Before these images of mother are available from memory, traumatic experiences tend to be felt as a *threat or fear of abandonment by or of loss of the love object,* i.e., the mother. If the traumatic experiences during this period are severe, or if there is unduly prolonged or too frequent separation from the mother, the effect on the child is proportionately severe.

Severe traumatic experiences occurring in this early period of development may cause a psychosis at the time of the trauma, or can predispose the infant to the development of a psychotic disorder at a later age.

After the establishment of reasonably stable and constant images of the mother, traumatic experiences cause *fear of loss of her love.* This is a lesser threat than the threat of losing the love object itself. Ego development and the establishment of basic identity have had a good beginning; the developing personality is well integrated; the child has confidence in people and seeks to continue receiving love from them; and his good relations with the outside world facilitate his adaptation. If now he and his environment come into conflict, his wish to continue receiving love causes him to attempt to control and modify the impulses and feelings which are bringing him into conflict with his parents. But if the traumatic experience has caused an excessive amount of conflict and tension, he cannot manage himself by normal defensive and adaptive techniques, and he will exhibit symptoms.

Traumatic experiences occurring after the establishment of stable images and reasonably adequate relations with people may either cause neurosis at the time of the trauma, or predispose to the development of a neurotic disorder at a later age.

GENERAL CONSIDERATIONS IN DIAGNOSIS AND TREATMENT

DIAGNOSIS

Diagnostic evaluation requires careful study both of the child and of the persons in his environment. The evaluation of the role of the environment in the child's disorder will be concerned largely with his relation to his mother in the neonatal and infancy periods; it extends to the father and other members of the family during the preschool years and to persons outside the family during the middle years and adolescence. Most discussion of normal child development and of the genesis of psychologic disorders centers about the child's relation with his mother, since his life begins in closeness with her, and since she is most directly concerned with his care and rearing during the early years. This situation does not discount the importance of the father. Even if he has little to do with the care of his infant or young child in a direct way, his influence is felt indirectly in terms of emotional support of the mother. In our present culture the father shares increasingly in the care of the infant and figures importantly in the life of the young child.

An important concept relevant to the study of the environment is that of *family dynamics.* The family is conceived to be a social unit with its dynamic equilibrium determined by the interaction of all the members of the family. Particular children may acquire certain roles which are important to the equilibrium of the family group, e.g., the good child or the bad child, or the smart child or the dull child. This concept rejects the notion that members of a family function only as individuals. Family dynamics is being increasingly studied by child psychiatrists through the technique of bringing all the members of the family together in a discussion with the psychiatrist. The ways in which they relate to each other and the roles they play in the family equilibrium can be observed for diagnostic purposes, and in some instances the observations can be discussed with the family with therapeutic benefit.

In general terms, the kinds of environmental influences to be considered are (1) understimulation, (2) overstimulation, (3) emotional deprivation, (4) overindulgence, (5) overprotection, (6) too little challenge, (7) undue pressure, (8) inconsistency, in either parent or between the parents, (9) excessive conflict and tension in the home atmosphere, and (10) unconscious consent by the parents to behavior of which they consciously disapprove (the child acting in accordance with the unconscious or true attitude of the parents).

In the study of the child the history of his earlier development is obtained from his parents. The neonatal and infancy periods are carefully reviewed and an attempt is made to evaluate the role of environmental factors as opposed to factors in the constitutional make-up of the child. Evaluation may be difficult, since environmental influences begin so early that responses to them in the child may be misattributed to his innate endowment and since, conversely, subtle innate factors may be the cause of environmental responses or attitudes which are falsely viewed as primary and etiologic. The latter possibility needs especially to be weighed when the possibility of incompatibility between the child's temperament or behavior style and the mother's ministrations or expectations is considered.

The most crucial qualities in the make-up of the child are the following, as suggested by Anna Freud. These important qualities are determined both by constitution and by environmental influence and experience.

INTENSITY OF DRIVES AND NEEDS. The needs of the undemanding child may go unrecognized and therefore unmet. The overdemanding child, on the other hand, because he is difficult to satisfy and to manage, may cause anxiety or other feelings in the parent, which will secondarily disturb the parent-child relation.

ABILITY TO TOLERATE FRUSTRATION. The child who can tolerate frustration has less need to resort to the use of pathologic defenses.

WILLINGNESS TO ACCEPT SUBSTITUTES. The child who cannot accept a substitute, whether this is a substitute parent such as a baby-sitter, or substituted food, toys or activities, remains tied to the frustration, and tensions increase.

ABILITY TO TOLERATE ANXIETY. The ability to tolerate tension and anxiety and to control urges and feelings without repressing them into the unconscious enables the child to face difficulties, to learn to interpose thought between the urge to act and action, to give and take and to negotiate with his parents and other people.

Evaluation of the child by means of historical review is followed by appraisal of his current functioning and behavior. This is done through information gathered from parents, school or other sources and through direct observation and study of the child. The young child will reveal something of his ability to relate to others, his anxiety level, self-control, spontaneity, and the like during the course of physical examination or other procedures or in a play situation. Such information about the older child and adolescent can sometimes be gained through conversation with him. Whether one observes the child at play or engages him in conversation, the information is gained through study of his ego defensive and adaptive behavior. Understanding of other facets of his personality such as his drives (id) or his conscience (superego) is deduced from their apparent effect upon the ego. The inner conflicts and outer reality problems which motivate his defenses and behavior are reflected in the defenses and can be inferred from them.

An evaluation of a child and his disorder adequate for diagnosis and prognosis requires consideration of all aspects of each of the stages of psychologic development (Table 2–10).

TREATMENT

Treatment must be based upon an adequate diagnosis of the underlying psychopathology. Confronted with a patient whose primary symptom is headache, no physician would regard the headache as an entity. He would feel that he must diagnose the underlying cause of the headache, and treat this basic cause to gain relief of the headache. Possible treatments would differ considerably, depending upon whether the headache was caused by tension, fatigue, systemic infection or brain tumor.

The same principle holds in the treatment of psychologic disorders. *It is fallacious to regard such concerns as thumb-sucking, temper tantrums, enuresis, masturbation and social ineptitude as anything other than symptoms, or to expect them to be treatable in specific ways as diagnostic entities.* Suggestions can be made for the management of symptomatic behavior (in the same way that one can prescribe aspirin for a headache of undetermined origin), but *the real diagnostic and treatment effort must be directed at determining and remedying the underlying cause.*

If a disorder has its basis in internal psychopathology, its remedy almost always requires psychotherapy with the child. The aim is to help him uncover, understand and work through his inner conflicts and the experiences which produced them. In order to do this effectively, the physician as a rule needs to undergo special training in the theory and technique of psychotherapy. He also must be able to offer an amount of time and a regularity of appointment schedule which is difficult for the pediatrician or general physician to provide. Unless a pediatrician has had special training in psychotherapy with children, he may find it difficult to treat a child with a neurosis or any of the more severe disorders. On the other hand, the child's physician can and should provide support to the child and parents while arrangements are being made for further evaluation or psychotherapy, as well as during psychotherapy. This support may be primarily verbal, or it may include the judicious use of sedative or tranquilizer drugs. The pediatrician's responsibility for the general well-being of the child continues during psychiatric treatment; optimum for the child and parents is a truly cooperative liaison between pediatrician and child psychiatrist.

The pediatrician is in an ideal position to help children with psychologic disorders by recognizing potential illness early and by directing therapeutic efforts to the incipient or less severe *developmental* and *situational* disorders. (See below and pp. 68 to 79.) With these conditions he may with relatively little special training and relatively small demands upon his time be quite effective, since the treatment is directed at resolving conflict between the child and his environment. The child's contribution to the conflict needs to be understood, but the task consists for the most part in working with the parents. They need to be aided initially to see how their attitudes, wishes, fears, resentments or guilt feelings relate to their child and how these attitudes are affecting him. Then they need emotional support and guidance in changing their attitudes and practices and in helping each other and their child to resolve the undesirable conflicts.

NOSOLOGY

Most attempts at classification of psychologic disorders in children have been based upon descriptions of clinical manifestations and upon similarities in mode of expression of symptoms. In such systems a clinical pattern may be falsely regarded as a clinical entity. For example, persistent thumb-sucking, nail-biting and masturbation are recognized as habits and are classed as habit disorders. Stealing, lying and destructiveness of property are antisocial acts and are categorized as conduct disorders. Asthma, neurodermatitis and ulcerative colitis are modes of expression of dysfunction of the autonomic nervous system and are grouped together as psychophysiologic disorders.

Although a nosologic system can be constructed on this basis, it is unsatisfactory. Clinical manifestations and modes of expression of symptoms are superficial variables which do not permit valid assessment of prognosis or requirements for treatment.

The ideal nosologic system would be based primarily upon the underlying psychopathology as determined by psychogenesis (etiology) and psychodynamics, as well as upon the capacity for adaptation. The categories presented here are based upon these more fundamental considerations and are felt to be both simple and understandable. They do not correspond exactly to other nomenclatures.

CATEGORIES OF PSYCHOLOGIC DISORDERS

Categories of psychologic disorders are listed in order of their increasing severity, which is measured by their intensity of psychopathology, their prognosis, and their potential for reversibility with treatment:

1. Developmental disorders
2. Situational disorders
3. Neurotic disorders
4. Neurotic character disorders
5. Psychotic character disorders
6. Psychotic disorders
7. Psychologic disorders associated with organic brain damage

The basic characteristics of the disorders in each category will be considered under the headings of *psychopathology* and *adaptability*. *Psychopathology* will deal with the internal condition of the child. This will be viewed primarily in terms of the child's psychologic equilibrium. *Adaptability* will deal with the child's functioning in relation to his environment. The main subjects commented upon are his relations with people (object relations), his ability to perceive and evaluate the world of external reality, and his performance.

DEVELOPMENTAL DISORDERS

Developmental disorders are due to the inevitable and characteristic conflicts associated with the successive stages of psychologic development. They are usually transitory and within certain limits are to be regarded as phenomena of normal development. They will be discussed in general terms and in relation to the stages of psychologic development. (See Table 2–10 and pp. 52–65.)

PSYCHOPATHOLOGY. In normal development the conflicts between the child and his environment lead to the establishment of normal adaptive and defensive techniques. A certain amount of conflict results within the child between his drives and his methods of self-control. Under usual circumstances the conflict is readily managed by the child and should not be regarded as psychopathologic. If circumstances cause the conflicts to be unduly intense or to persist unduly long, they tend to take on psychopathologic significance. Hence, the importance of anticipatory guidance in the prevention of developmental disorders and their proper management should be apparent (pp. 68–79).

ADAPTABILITY. Disturbance in functioning or relationship is minimal, temporary and usually limited to a particular aspect of the total personality.

TREATMENT. If the conflict and the resulting symptoms become too severe and it is felt that help is needed, the therapeutic effort is directed mainly to the environment. If the parents can be helped to understand the conflict situation, and to modify those demands and attitudes which exceed the child's capacity, the disorder in the child is indirectly alleviated.

Developmental Disorders in the Neonatal Period (Oral Stage: Normal Autistic Phase)

CLINICAL MANIFESTATIONS. The first signs of distress are likely to be excessive crying, disturbance in function of the alimentary tract, such as refusal to suck, excessive sucking, excessive regurgitation or vomiting, constipation or diarrhea, and disturbance in the sleep pattern. The intensity and duration of symptoms vary with the severity of the environmental situation.

DIFFERENTIAL DIAGNOSIS. The same symptoms may also be caused by temporary disturbances related to the trauma of birth and to postnatal infectious or organic factors.

TREATMENT. When constitutional or organic factors in the infant have been ruled out, attention must be focused on the environment. Developmental disorders occurring in this period suggest that the mother or mother-surrogate is deficient in meeting the infant's physiologic or emotional needs. The infant needs protection from changes in body temperature and from excessive stimulation by light, sound and handling. On the other hand, as he matures he has a gradually increasing need for an optimal amount of gentle stimulation of his various sensory end-organs, e.g., through body contact, through bathing and anointing the skin, through being held and rocked, through the sound of mother's voice, and through various objects which he can see, particularly the mother's face. Anxiety or other emotional difficulty in the mother is the most common reason for her inability to meet the child's needs in a reasonably adequate manner.

Developmental Disorders in the Infancy Period (Oral Stage: Symbiotic Phase)

CLINICAL MANIFESTATIONS. During the latter part of infancy the same kinds of symptoms may occur as were described in the neonatal phase. The manifestations may become more patterned, however, as psychologic development permits more specific expression. Thus, crying may occur in relation to a particular experience, or sleep disturbance may be linked to a particular time of day. The observant mother may have noted a cause and effect relation between events and the infant's symptom pattern.

When the infant is capable of distinguishing

himself from his mother, he becomes aware of his dependence upon her. A need for love has been added to his physical and physiologic needs. Toward the end of this phase the infant is prone to greater conflict, tension and anxiety because of his awareness that his mother is separate from him, and because of the frustration of weaning. Severe crying at separation and various disturbances in feeding and bowel function are common.

DIFFERENTIAL DIAGNOSIS. It is necessary to distinguish the causes of these clinical manifestations from those in situational disorders, and also to rule out organic causes.

TREATMENT. Treatment usually consists in working with the parents to help them to perceive and to change those attitudes or reactions which the child finds threatening in his relations with them. If, for example, a child has the symptom of excessive thumb-sucking as a response to being weaned too quickly, the remedy is to persuade the mother that the weaning should be more gradual.

Developmental Disorders in the Toddler Years (Anal Stage)

CLINICAL MANIFESTATIONS. With the advent of locomotion the child's sphere of contact with his environment is greatly increased. At the same time his parents note his developing coordination and control and his increasing ability to understand, and begin to expect more of him. He is subjected to his first disciplinary experiences. This usually causes a good deal of conflict between the child and his parents.

The child has difficulty in managing his increased aggression. Tantrums are frequent, sometimes severe. On the other hand, some children may curb their aggression to the point at which they become unduly passive.

Because speech is developing during this stage, conflicts are not uncommonly reflected in a transient stutter. Sleep disturbances commonly take the form of resistance to going to bed and to sleep or of night terrors. As the child is falling asleep, ego control over aggressive impulses diminishes, and he is frightened by the feeling that his aggressive fantasies and impulses may be expressed in action. Fear and anxiety on separation from the parents at bedtime or when left with a baby-sitter also are common.

Coercive or even normal toilet training tends to produce problems at this stage. Frustration or anxiety may give rise to symptoms such as messing with food, temporary food dislikes, smearing feces, constipation or diarrhea. Directing aggression toward playmates, siblings, pets or inanimate objects is also common. Thumb-sucking and eating disturbances may be seen in this stage as a consequence of regression to the previous stage with the aim of easing tension through oral gratification.

DIFFERENTIAL DIAGNOSIS. The same kinds of problems may also be seen in situational disorders, but usually with greater intensity and persistence. As the child approaches the end of this stage, he is normally beginning to develop some of the precursors of superego. This allows for the possibility of internal conflicts between his impulses and his developing superego. Neurotic disorders therefore may be seen in children at 2 to 3 years of age, but are relatively rare. This diagnosis is suggested by unusually severe or persistent symptoms of the type mentioned above, particularly in a child with precocious psychologic development as evidenced, for example, by unusually good language development.

TREATMENT. Treatment is aimed at helping the parents to be kindly and sympathetic, but also to be sufficiently firm and controlling so that the child feels protected from external dangers and from his own impulses. The experience of being controlled by his parents, even though he protests it, is reassuring and provides the model for development of self-control. The child may have considerable difficulty if he is given too much freedom in making decisions. The parents must be able to use their own aggression in a healthy way in the management of the child. On the other hand, if the parents are too strict and too demanding, this tends to increase the strength of the child's impulses, poses a problem in control, and tends to make him feel unloved. The parents are encouraged to ease up and give the child more time to meet their requirements.

Developmental Disorders in the Preschool Years (Phallic Stage)

CLINICAL MANIFESTATIONS. The problem of control of aggressive impulses continues. There is a heightened awareness of pleasurable sensations in the genital area, and sexual feelings are now added to and complicate the love feelings toward the parents. Fear of loss of love and of punishment persists and tends to be expressed in fantasies of injury to the penis or clitoris. Because of the diminution of ego control during sleep, the intensified sexual aggressive urges and fantasies cause sleep disturbances. At times a nightmare may continue into a semiwakeful state, and the child may be delirious. Phobias also are common, particularly of destructive animals or "bad" men, such as robbers who will break into the house at night. These are the result of an unconscious mental mechanism whereby the child tries to escape his frightening impulses and fantasies by projecting them outside of himself and attributing them to external objects; but this is only a partial solution, for he now fears them as external dangers.

As a result of regression there may be lapses in bladder and bowel control, and various oral symptoms. Some children become excessively clinging and dependent. Symptoms of passivity and conformity in the boy may be the unconscious defensive means of avoiding transgression, which would bring punishment or the imagined threat of castration. The girl may reject her femaleness and behave like a tomboy.

DIFFERENTIAL DIAGNOSIS. In addition to distinguishing between developmental and situational disorders, a neurotic disorder must be considered, since its likelihood increases with increases in age and psychic development. There is also the possibility that some of the defenses the child is using are becoming habitual and that he is developing a neurotic character disorder.

TREATMENT. One of the best guarantees that the child will successfully resolve the conflicts of this stage is a good sexual and social relationship between the parents. Conversely, if the parents are at odds with each other, the child's fantasies of maintaining intimate relations with the parent of the opposite sex are encouraged.

The child continues to need firmness in controlling his impulses, but without excessive threat at this age. It is helpful if the parents begin to introduce the concept of modesty and to exercise more restraint in dressing and undressing and in the use of the bathroom.

For the child with temporary sleep difficulties a small night light, or the parent staying with the child until he goes to sleep, may be helpful. These aids, however, should be regarded as temporary measures; the child's continued requirement of them may indicate a more serious disorder.

The child who awakens frightened from a bad dream should be comforted and returned to his own bed. He often wishes to sleep with one or both of his parents, but this is not to be encouraged. Not only would he literally come between his parents, but also the physical proximity to the parent stimulates his sexual feelings and fantasies. These factors can aggravate his oedipal conflict and delay its resolution.

Owing to the child's preoccupation with sexual difference and its implications, it is reassuring to children to know that in contrast to the externally evident sexual organs of the male, the sexual organs of the female are concealed and internal, and that the female is not simply a damaged or defective male. A specific case requiring help is the boy with an undescended testis. If his condition and the fact that it can be remedied are explained to him, he will be spared much worry as well as potential psychopathology resulting from his own distorted, imaginary explanations.

Developmental Disorders in the Midchildhood Years (Latency Stage)

CLINICAL MANIFESTATIONS. The most common cause of problems in these years is failure of resolution of the oedipal conflict. As a result, the dependency-independency conflict is unduly troublesome, and the anxieties of the phallic stage persist; symptoms disappear and change as the child tries out different defensive solutions. At one extreme a child may become withdrawn and excessively shy and passive; at the other extreme a child who is unable to ease his tensions and maintain control over his impulses may "act-out" his feelings and conflicts. The latter solution results in a behavior problem, with such symptoms as destructiveness, bullying or stealing.

As in the phallic stage, the child may seek solution by temporarily reversing his identification, so that the boy identifies with the mother, the girl with the father. Phobias, sleep disturbances and problems of bladder control may persist.

The disturbed child often has difficulty in learning in school. His mental energies may be tied up in his internal conflicts to such a point that he has little energy left for concentration; he may have curbed his aggression so thoroughly that he is unable to use it in a healthy way in asking questions and seeking knowledge; or the fears and fantasies associated with his sexual curiosity may have caused him to inhibit his curiosity.

DIFFERENTIAL DIAGNOSIS. As in earlier age periods, developmental disorders must be distinguished from situational ones. The possibility that symptoms may reflect a more serious neurotic disorder or a neurotic character disorder must also be kept in mind.

TREATMENT. The aims of treatment are essentially the same as in the phallic stage. The child is helped indirectly if the parents can be guided to modify their attitudes and improve their relations with each other. In addition, as the child grows older, healthy identifications may stem from contacts with other adults such as teachers and scout leaders, and from supervised group activities with children.

Developmental Disorders in the Adolescent Years

CLINICAL MANIFESTATIONS. Owing to the tremendous physiologic and psychologic upheaval during these years, problems occur frequently and in great variety. Like the child in the phallic stage, the adolescent struggles with strong sexual and aggressive impulses, but now with the advent of physical and sexual maturity. Loss of self-control with acting-out of conflicts can result either in antisocial behavior or in behavior detrimental to himself. At the other extreme, control gained by severe inhibition may result in pathologic withdrawal from relations with people. Urges and desires may be so much denied that the adolescent becomes an ascetic. Overintellectualization is resorted to in an attempt to manage feelings and impulses by thought. Overcompensation for feelings of inferiority and inadequacy results in false bravado and acts of daring. Some adolescents remain too dependent and too attached to their parents; others break away too completely.

Commonly the adolescent is upset over sexual and aggressive feelings and fantasies which he feels to be abnormal, since he may not have discussed them with anyone and does not know that they are universal. The great turmoil and feeling of disorganization and the poor self-control are responsible for the common fear of becoming insane.

Precocious puberty is likely to cause at least a

developmental disorder, since biologic maturation is ahead of the child's emotional readiness for this event. Some children react to an early onset of puberty by attempting to grow up quickly. These children have a façade of sophistication and a pseudomaturity. Since they have been deprived of some of their childhood years, there may be a more serious disorder later. Other children react to early puberty by regression to an earlier stage of development. If they are subsequently able to face and deal with the changes caused by puberty, their adolescence may be fairly normal.

Psychologic problems also result from a delayed onset of puberty. The child begins to worry about his physical normality and feels undesirably different from his peers. If he is helped to verbalize his fears and is reassured, the development of feelings of inferiority and inadequacy, as well as of social estrangement, may be prevented.

DIFFERENTIAL DIAGNOSIS. The average adolescent can temporarily assume rather extreme positions of defense, such as withdrawal, asceticism, overindulgence in oral or other pleasures, or antisocial acting-out. The total personality and functioning of the adolescent therefore must be carefully evaluated before concluding that the behavior pattern is normal and need cause no concern, or that the adolescent is mentally ill. Because similar clinical patterns may be based upon different underlying psychopathologic disturbances, one must consider the possibility of any category of psychologic disorder, including psychotic ones.

TREATMENT. The adolescent is likely to engender anxiety in his parents, causing them to lose the objectivity and the stability which he so much needs. If this happens, confusion is compounded, tensions rise, and problems increase. It is important that the parents understand the nature of normal adolescence and do not overreact to the typical adolescent behavior with its wide mood swings and changeability.

In making the transition from childhood to adulthood the adolescent needs opportunities for independent action and decision, and for assuming an increasing amount of responsibility for himself. On the other hand, he is in such inner turmoil and so much at the mercy of his impulses that he also continues to need the guidance and support of his parents, particularly in the setting of limits on his behavior. Characteristically the adolescent complains that his parents do not care about him if they give him too much freedom, but he resents and rebels against too much restriction.

It is important that adolescents have accurate factual knowledge about the changes in growth and physiologic functions which are occurring in their bodies, particularly those having to do with sexual functioning such as nocturnal emissions and menstruation. Ejaculatory or orgastic experiences associated with masturbation or sexual arousal, although pleasurable, can be frightening and may cause severe guilt feelings. The adolescent needs to know that sexual and aggressive fantasies are common at his age and are a normal part of his attempt to gain mastery over his new capabilities and newly strengthened drives. The physician may be able to help by discussing these matters with the adolescent. Such discussion frequently has not taken place in the family because of mutual embarrassment and discomfiture between parent and adolescent.

SITUATIONAL DISORDERS

Situational disorders stem from environmental situations which are abnormal for a given child at a given age, and with which he is unable to cope. Any of the problems which occur as developmental disorders may also be seen in situational disorders. The latter diagnosis is to be suspected whenever symptoms are severe, persistent and especially clearly defined.

PSYCHOPATHOLOGY. As in developmental disorders, the conflict is initially between the child and his environment; if this is resolved in time, internal psychopathology can be prevented. Because the abnormal environmental situation interferes with satisfaction of the child's needs, his sexual and aggressive drives are likely to be increased. Regressively, he may attempt to ease his tension through indulgence in libidinal pleasure or self-gratification. The form of indulgence will vary with the age of the child. For example, the 2 year old who is frustrated by coercive toilet training may turn to excessive thumb-sucking, and the adolescent whose strivings for independence are unduly frustrated may turn to excessive masturbation. Aggression may also be displayed in severe temper tantrums or in verbal rebelliousness.

ADAPTABILITY. The child may evidence difficulty in relations with people by being withdrawn or excessively aggressive toward them. His usual level of mental performance may be lowered.

ENVIRONMENTAL FACTORS. Determination of the pathologic environmental situation is essential to the diagnosis of a situational disorder. Table 2–11 lists situations which can be of etiologic significance.

TREATMENT. Treatment for the most part consists in alleviation of the unhealthy interaction between the child and his environment. It may be helpful to discuss the problem with the older child or adolescent with the aim of increasing his understanding, easing his anxiety and giving him emotional support. The extent to which discussion with the parents will be helpful is determined by their ability to gain understanding and to change. If there is significant psychopathology in the parents, it may be necessary to refer them for additional psychotherapeutic help.

Clinical Patterns

CONFLICTS BETWEEN TEMPERAMENT (PERSONALITY) AND ENVIRONMENT. Some behavioral patterns can be understood as deriving from incompatibility between the temperament or personality of the infant and those of one or both parents. Tem-

TABLE 2–11. FACTORS OF ETIOLOGIC SIGNIFICANCE IN SITUATIONAL DISORDERS

Rough handling, excessive handling or differences in handling of the neonate by the mother and father, or by the mother and a nursemaid or babysitter

Too little handling and stimulation of an infant by a mother who for neurotic reasons fears that her ministrations may be harmful

Incompatibility between the temperament or personality of the infant or young child and that of the parent

Excessive or irritating stimulation from inanimate sources, e.g., from rough fabrics next to the infant's skin

A feeding schedule out of phase with the infant's desires

Self-demand feeding when the mother is unable to distinguish between the various causes of tension and crying and gives the bottle not only for relief of hunger, but also as a panacea for distress of all kinds

Insufficient kinesthetic stimulation as evidenced by the infant who rocks in bed (the rocking chair may be helpful)

Postpartum depression in the mother

Maternal anxiety about breast feeding communicated to the child (breast feeding may be unwise in such a case)

Inconsistent and uncertain care of an infant by a mother who feels unsure of herself and unconsciously avoids responsibility by attempting to follow the advice of other people (the infant may be helped if the pediatrician authoritatively insists that the mother follow only his advice)

Detrimental attitudes in a mother who feels guilty because her child was conceived before marriage, or in a mother who strongly wished that the child be of the other sex. Illness or death of close relatives during the pregnancy or postnatally may upset the mother and make her unable to adequately invest herself emotionally in the relationship with the child. Sometimes she unconsciously may feel that the child's birth was in some way responsible for the death of the loved one

Maternal worry about her own health, the health or the welfare of another child, or about her relationship with her husband

Leaving the infant alone too much of the time

Overeagerness of the parent to get the child to bed and to sleep; the child senses that the parent is pulling away, and resists separation

Attempts to create a favorable situation for sleep by making the child's room quiet and dark; this may be distressing to the infant who finds familiar sounds and objects reassuring, even if they are only in the background

Failure of parents to say goodbye when they are leaving temporarily, because they feel that they are sparing the child distress if they slip away while he is awake or leave after he is asleep

Difficulty of some mothers in letting the child separate and become more independent. Such mothers may either prolong the child's infancy by overprotecting him and meeting his needs too well, or may deal with their anxiety by pulling away too completely too soon

Too little maternal attention after the next child is born; the child should not be neglected in favor of the new baby, nor should he be overindulged in an attempt to prevent a normal amount of envy

Competition of one parent with the child for the attention of the other parent; this is usually not recognized by the parents

Too early toilet training

A mother who is rejecting of her role as a female, or a father who is passive and not sufficiently masculine; the child has difficulty in development of appropriate identity or gender role.

Teasing, threatening and lecturing to the child

An immature parent who may be unconsciously sexually seductive to the child, overstimulating him and encouraging unhealthy fantasies with ensuing fears

Parental separation or divorce, particularly during the preschool and middle years; the child uses his fantasy ability to give himself explanations which create anxiety or a sense of guilt

High parental expectations for the child with relatively little support in helping him to measure up to the expectations. The parental expectations may be implicit rather than openly expressed. This is a common cause of learning difficulty

Significant differences in the child's family and cultural background from those of most of the other children in his school

Alcoholism in a parent

Too little contact with the father, who is important for the development of both boy and girl; also, the mother may not feel sufficiently supported in the task of rearing the children, and they sense her resentment

The mother who is a slave to her children and home; entanglements with the children usually develop

Too many outside interests and activities by the mother

---

perament or personality may be partly innate or in part shaped by the earliest life experiences. Parent-child interaction should be studied both for parental influences on the child, and for the influence of the child's personal characteristics on the parent. With the identification of the pertinent temperamental and environmental issues, the parents can be guided toward modifying their interactive pattern with the child in a healthy direction.

A temperamental pattern in the infant or child which carries a high risk for the development of behavior problems combines irregularity in biologic functions, predominantly negative (withdrawal) responses to new stimuli, nonadaptability or slow adaptability to change, frequent negative moods and predominantly intense reactions. As infants, children with this pattern have irregular sleep and feeding patterns, slow acceptance of new foods, prolonged adjustment periods to new routines, and frequent periods of loud crying. They are not easy to feed, to put to sleep, to bathe, or to dress. They respond to new places, to new activities or to strange faces with initial loud protest or with crying, and frustration characteristically produces a violent tantrum. These children experience as stressful the demands of socialization, such as the demands to conform to the usual patterns of family, school or peer group. Yet, once they learn the rules, they may function easily, consistently and energetically.

The care of these infants makes special demands upon the parents for unusually firm, patient, consistent and tolerant handling. If new demands are presented inconsistently, impatiently or punitively, negativism is a frequent outcome.

At the opposite end of the temperamental spectrum from the "difficult" child is the child who is regular, responds positively to new stimuli, adapts quickly and easily to change, and shows a predominantly positive mood of mild or moderate intensity. As infants, they develop regular sleep and feeding schedules easily, smile at strangers, and later, as children, they adapt quickly to a new school, accept most frustrations with a minimum of fuss, and learn the rules of new games quickly. The "easy" child, in short, confronts his parents with few if any problems in handling. Although these children do, as a rule, develop significantly fewer behavior problems than do the difficult infants, their very ease of adaptability may under certain circumstances be the basis for a psychologic disorder. If problems develop, they may occur most typically when there is severe dissonance between the expectations and demands of the family and of the community. When the child is engaged in situations outside the home, such as in peer play and school activities, stress and malfunction may develop if the extrafamilial standards and demands conflict sharply with the patterns learned in the home. For example, pressures for conformity and attentiveness to rule may conflict with need for individuality and freedom of expression. Such conflicts are relatively easily resolved if the parents are willing to modify their attitudes to be more in keeping with the realities of the external world.

Another important temperamental pattern combines negative responses of mild intensity to new stimuli with slow adaptability after repeated contact. These children usually do not have irregularity of function, frequent negative moods, nor intense reactions, and their withdrawal from the new is quiet rather than loud. With the first bath the child lies still and fusses mildly, with a new food he turns his head away quietly and lets the food dribble from his mouth, and when a stranger greets him loudly, he clings to his mother. If given the opportunity to re-experience new situations without pressure, such a child gradually comes to show quiet and positive interest and involvement. A key issue, therefore, is whether parents and teachers allow this child to make an adaptation to the new at his own tempo or insist on immediate positive involvement.

In contrast to the child who is slow to respond is the very persistent child who is most likely to experience stress, not with his initial contact with a situation, but whose persistence after the first positive adaptation has been made leads him to resist interference or attempts at subsequent diversion. If the parent or adult interferes arbitrarily or forcefully, tension and frustration tend to mount quickly in these children and may reach explosive proportions.

The foregoing samples of temperamental patterns are not exhaustive. Further careful observation and study will permit other maladaptive interactions to be identified and appropriate management to be determined.

EATING OR OTHER ORAL DISORDERS

Infantile Colic. Colic may be caused by various factors singly or in combination; one of the possible causes is an environmental situation which creates tension in the infant.

Pica. Perverted appetite occurs most often in the first 3 years of life. A child may ingest any of a large variety of unsuitable substances, such as sand, earth, grass, wool from blankets, broken glass, animal droppings, paint from furniture, coal, ashes, or plaster from the wall. Lead poisoning is a hazard.

The crawling infant and the toddler normally put foreign objects into their mouths, partly for exploration of the outside world and partly to satisfy a craving for mouthing experiences and sucking. This behavior often accompanies messy play and interest in dirt and feces.

This activity may also be seen in neurotic children, and it is common in mentally defective ones. The possibility of an underlying physiologic or nutritional disturbance must also be considered; the behavior may indicate mineral, vitamin or other deficiency.

Provision for the child to have adequate sucking, biting, chewing and other mouth, lip and tongue pleasures during the oral stage of development may eliminate the need for abnormal continuation of these activities.

Obesity. (See also Section 3.) A child who is unhappy or under tension because of a difficult situation may seek to ease his tensions and give himself pleasure by overeating, consequently becoming obese. If the situation can be changed, the abnormal eating usually subsides. Attention should be directed primarily at the psychologic disorder.

Thumb-sucking. Thumb-sucking and its equivalents, such as sucking of the tongue, fingers, toes, lips, a rubber nipple, pacifier or the corner of a blanket, are common and normal in infancy. Thumb-sucking is one of the first coordinated acts through which the infant can give himself pleasure and become somewhat less dependent upon the environment.

Thumb-sucking that persists beyond infancy, particularly into the preschool years, suggests the possibility of a situational disorder. It is most likely to occur when the child is about to go to sleep, when he is watching television or when he is hungry, sleepless or ill. It may occur if the child feels displaced by a younger child or otherwise senses withdrawal of parental interest from him. In most instances the habit is given up spontaneously, particularly if it has not become an issue between child and parents. If it persists continuously and intensely, it may cause malpositioning of the teeth and require orthodontia.

In the case of the infant it is important to reassure the parents that the activity is normal. If the infant is taking his feedings too rapidly and has too little sucking pleasure, it is desirable to lengthen the feeding periods.

In older children threats of punishment, shaming and reminders to remove the thumb from the mouth are usually of no avail and tend to reinforce the activity. Applying bad-tasting substances to the thumb and using thumb covers, metal mittens or elbow splints are equally ineffective and may cause additional emotional trauma. Effective treatment is indirect, consisting in correcting an unfavorable situation or, when thumb-sucking is a symptom in a neurotic child, alleviation of his internalized conflicts.

Nail-biting. Whereas thumb-sucking is primarily a pleasurable and comforting activity, nail-biting is more a manifestation of aggression. It is seen more commonly in the older child and may be an unconscious means of controlling aggressive urges. Nagging and scolding should be avoided. Treatment is aimed at correcting the underlying cause.

ECZEMA. (See also Section 9.) Emotional conflict and tension may be important aggravating factors in infants with eczematous lesions. Treatment for emotional factors is directed at remedying the environmental causes of tension and improving parent-child relations.

SLEEP DISORDERS. In early childhood sleep disturbances are usually a manifestation of separation anxiety, in later childhood more likely fear of loss of control over aggressive impulses. In mid-childhood, fear of aggressive impulses in combination with awareness of the reality of death may cause insomnia. The pathologic environmental situation has the effect of increasing the child's impulses and fears, thereby causing more severe sleep disturbance.

A child needs to be reassured verbally, and at times by the physical presence of the parent. If movies or television shows with a frightening content are connected with a sleep disturbance, they should be eliminated. Effective treatment requires alleviation of the disturbing situation.

RHYTHMIC MOVEMENTS. These may be seen in normal, emotionally disturbed or mentally retarded infants.

Head-rolling. Head-rolling by the infant lying in bed may be continued until the hair is almost completely worn away from the back of the head. This behavior is most likely in the very young infant. When determined by situational factors, it is usually due to emotional deprivation and may also be seen in undernourished or chronically ill children.

Head-nodding. This is relatively rare and is the equivalent of head-rolling. It occurs with the child in a sitting position and consists of either a vigorous nodding, or a lateral shaking movement. Head-rolling and nodding may also be seen in spasmus nutans.

Body-rocking. Body-rocking may take place in a sitting position or in a semikneeling position, resting on the elbows and knees. It is fairly common in infancy and usually occurs before going to sleep. It usually disappears spontaneously, but may persist into later childhood.

In the severe forms it may occur frequently during the day and may continue for hours at a time. In such instances emotional deprivation is suggested, e.g., inadequate satisfaction of the need for stimulation of kinesthetic sensations through the normal experiences of being held, carried or rocked by the mother.

Head-banging. This appears to be an extension of rocking, usually in the knee-elbow position. It usually occurs in the latter half of the first year of life. The infant does not seem to experience pain or discomfort; bruising and callus formation may occur. Head-banging suggests a greater amount of tension in the infant, since the aim has shifted from pleasurable self-stimulation (autoerotism) to unpleasant or painful self-stimulation (autoaggression).

Treatment of these symptom patterns consists in helping the parents to meet the unfulfilled needs. The parent most able to give, or a mother-surrogate, is encouraged to spend more time holding or rocking the infant, or staying with him and soothing him at bedtime. Gentle vocal stimulation through talking or singing and stroking or rubbing the skin may also be helpful. In the more severe cases, there may be serious emotional difficulty in the mother or tension in the home environment.

PICKING, PULLING, AND RUBBING HABITS. These are similar to rhythmic movements, but involve more specific coordination patterns in respect to a particular part of the body. A child may pick at his nose, lips or scabs, or he may pull at his penis or the lobe of an ear. An infant may repetitiously pull his hair (trichotillomania) until large areas of the scalp become bare. In some cases swallowed hair may produce a hairball in the stomach (see *Bezoar*). These activities may be seen in any category of disorder, including psychoses. Contributory factors such as local irritation, fatigue and malnutrition need to be considered.

Nagging or shaming the child is of no avail, and treatment is directed at remedy of the underlying cause.

BREATH-HOLDING. Breath-holding usually occurs in response to frustration and is similar to a temper tantrum. It may be seen in the young infant when he is startled. He cries, hyperventilates and has a sudden cessation of respiration, followed by cyanosis and rigidity. In severe cases there may be momentary loss of consciousness (syncope), possibly convulsive twitching, pallor or cyanosis, and finally, general relaxation. Presumably this series of symptoms results from hypoxia.

As with a temper tantrum, the child cannot be dealt with during the height of an attack, owing to the temporary loss of object relationship. Understanding and kindness are most effective. Punishing the child is not helpful, and in some instances may precipitate an attack. Measures should be taken to avoid precipitating conditions and to correct faults in the environment.

TEETH-GRINDING. Bruxism is observed chiefly during sleep; it may be associated with various acute and chronic disturbances, including disturbing dreams. When determined by emotional or environmental factors, it suggests that the child is having difficulty managing his aggression. It may occur in mental deficiency, and is fairly common in unconscious states due to disease, especially of intracranial origin, e.g., meningitis.

There is no treatment other than to improve the environmental situation which is creating the conflict and tension in the child.

BOWEL AND BLADDER DISORDERS. In a child beyond 2½ or 3 years of age, symptoms such as diurnal or nocturnal enuresis, fecal smearing, defecation elsewhere than in the toilet, and fecal soiling suggest a situational disorder. The most common cause is excessive pressure from the parents during toilet training, with resultant resentment and rebellion on the part of the child. Occasionally these symptoms indicate that toilet training has not been seriously attempted, usually because the mother cannot manage her own or her child's aggression.

These same symptoms in midchildhood or adolescence suggest a neurotic or more severe disorder. Treatment is directed at correcting the environmental situation.

MASTURBATION. This may be performed by manipulation of the genitals, by movement of the thighs or contraction of the perineal musculature, by copulatory movements sometimes with an object such as a pillow between the legs; or an equivalent sensation may be derived from tight clothing or activities such as horseback riding, straddling rails and climbing trees. In the younger child who is not aware of the cultural taboo against masturbation, the parents may observe the activity or the associated signs of intense concentration and excitement. Most children sense parental disapproval, however, and the activity is carried out in privacy. Rarely the child may masturbate openly, an act which suggests poor awareness of social reality by the child or lack of censorship by the parents. Some well-meaning parents who know that masturbation is a normal activity may inadvisedly encourage it.

Masturbation is normal. In the young child it presents a self-gratification analogous to thumb-sucking. In the older child, particularly the adolescent, it serves the purpose of exploring and experimenting with newly developing sexual capacities and feelings and may aid in gaining control over the sexual urges and becoming less afraid of them.

Masturbation occurs most commonly at bedtime when anxiety is increased, owing to separation or fear of loss of control over sexual and aggressive impulses. For the same reasons the child is most likely to masturbate when he is alone and lonely. This fact leads to the usually mistaken assumption on the part of parents and others that the urge to masturbate is the motive for being alone, rather than its consequence. Masturbation may also be performed, sometimes repetitiously and compulsively, as a reassurance against fear of injury to the genitalia. Excessive masturbation suggests some problem or deficiency in object relationships. In some instances it is a symptom of a neurotic or more severe disorder.

It is appropriate for the parent to censor open masturbation and to be concerned about excessive masturbation; but to forbid it absolutely, to shame the child, to threaten punishment or to suggest injury to the genitals is not only ineffective, but also tends to create guilt and additional anxiety which may even increase the activity. The most helpful treatment is to remedy any environmental situation which is interfering with gratification of the child's needs or is causing tension and anxiety. It is important that the child be reassured that masturbation does not cause physical or mental deterioration. The adolescent should be given an explanation of ejaculation, orgasm and menstruation, so that he or she can understand them as normal body functions.

ACTING-OUT BEHAVIOR. During the course of growing up some children act out those tensions and impulses which stem from conflicts in their relations with other people. This acting-out most commonly takes the form of antisocial or "delinquent" behavior which expresses aggressive or sexual urges or admixtures of both. More common manifestations are cruelty to animals, fighting, stealing, destroying property, and sexual activity such as mutual examination of the genitals or mutual masturbation. Such activities may be normal in the early years of childhood, but indicate developmental or situational problems in the later years. In some instances the child may not feel sufficiently loved. If so, the main reason for exercise of self-control and restraint is lacking. In other instances the child may be acting out unconscious wishes or urges in the parents.

In most instances firmness and protection of the child from his impulses by adequate supervision are indicated. Severe punishment or threats do not help, since they tend to increase the strength of the child's impulses and create a greater problem in ego control. Effective treatment requires determination of the underlying cause and correction of the environmental situation.

NEUROTIC DISORDERS (NEUROSES)

Developmental, situational and neurotic disorders can present the same or similar clinical manifestations, and differential diagnosis may be difficult. The child is more likely to suffer a situational disorder when faced with a situation in which the parental problem is gross and can be perceived and identified as such by the child; he is more likely to suffer a neurotic disorder when the parental disorder is less obvious, as when unconscious parental attitudes are masked by seemingly benign conscious attitudes and behavior. The child has difficulty in coping with what is outside his conscious awareness.

If the history indicates severe environmental disruption, the likelihood of a neurotic disorder is increased. The longer the duration of symptoms, the greater the likelihood of a neurosis. A neurotic disorder is seen only infrequently in a child under the age of 4 or 5 years, since the psychic structure before this age is usually not sufficiently developed to permit internal conflict of pathologic significance.

If treatment measures appropriate to developmental and situational disorders do not succeed, or if there is uncertainty about the diagnosis, it is wise to seek psychiatric consultation.

PSYCHOPATHOLOGY. In neurotic disorders the conflicts are internalized and constitute a definite psychopathologic situation in the child.

It is essential to the definition of neurosis that the internalized conflict, either entirely or in part, be outside the child's conscious awareness. Repression is an automatic and unconscious defense mechanism whereby there is an attempt to escape unpleasant feeling, fantasy or tension by making it unconscious. At times this may be successful, but in a neurosis it fails, and symptoms and difficulty in adaptation result.

Because the trauma occurs after basic ego development has taken place, the personality disturbance in neurotic disorders is only partial, and with proper treatment the child can come to function normally. The earlier the neurotic disorder is diagnosed, the more facilitated will be the treatment.

ADAPTABILITY. As is true of the child with a developmental or situational disorder, the child with a neurotic disorder is able to relate well. The fact that his first experiences with people have been reasonably good causes him to value them and seek to continue receiving their love and approval. His perception of the world of external reality, on the whole, is good, although at times it may be distorted by his fantasies or through the use of defense mechanisms such as projection or displacement. His disorder usually interferes with only a relatively small part of his total functioning.

TREATMENT. Treatment of neurotic disorders requires work with the parents to allay their anxiety, to give them understanding, to gain their cooperation, to acquire additional information about the child's disorder and to alleviate current environmental difficulties. At the same time it is necessary to engage the child in psychotherapy. This is done through regular appointments, usually at no less than weekly intervals, in a setting which offers play or other activity appropriate to the child's age. The aim of the treatment is to ascertain and help the child to understand his anxieties and unconscious conflicts, thereby permitting him to re-experience and gain mastery over them.

In successful treatment the child comes to trust the therapist, has some temporary dependence upon him and becomes involved in the treatment both intellectually and emotionally. The unresolved conflicts and problems from the past are transferred into the treatment situation. The conflicts increase in intensity, and if they are not understood and dealt with in an adequate way, symptoms may become aggravated, and the neurotic disorder may be reinforced rather than eliminated. Therapeutic competence based upon adequate theoretical knowledge, and training and supervision in technique are essential.

Clinical Patterns

Neurotic conflicts may be expressed at various levels: (1) at an ideational level in the form of conscious worries, guilt feelings, irrational fears, or of disturbing wishes, thoughts and fantasies; (2) at the level of sensory or motor functions by either inhibition or exaggeration of activity, such as functional aphonia or blindness, enuresis, disturbance in physiologic functioning; and (3) at the level of disturbance in physiologic function, such as peptic ulcer.

ANXIETY NEUROSIS. This is the simplest form of neurosis. The impulses and fantasies which were disturbing when in the child's conscious awareness have been dealt with by repression, without the use of other mental mechanisms. Anxiety is the ego's reaction to the danger that those things which are repressed may re-enter conscious awareness. Technically, anxiety is defined as a state of tension and apprehension wherein the cause is not discerned by the patient. This is in contrast to fear, wherein the danger is consciously recognized. Secondary symptoms may develop as a result of the anxiety, e.g., repression with thumb-sucking, overeating with consequent obesity, nail-biting, various fears, and sleep disturbances.

Neurotic anxiety must be differentiated from similar tension resulting from organic causes such as hypoglycemia, hyperthyroidism and Sydenham's chorea.

PHOBIA. In a phobia diffuse anxiety is replaced by fear of a specific thing or situation. The fear, although real to the child, is not rational, since it is caused by unconscious factors rather than by that to which he attributes his fear. The child, for example, may be preoccupied with a fear of tigers or of robbers in his bedroom at night. In phobia, repression is supplemented by the mechanism *displacement,* whereby fear of a real object, e.g., of the father, is shifted away from the father to another object, or by *projection,* whereby anxiety-creating impulses are falsely attributed to an external object or situation.

Phobias occur normally at certain stages in childhood, and may also be a manifestation of a situational disorder.

In *school phobia* the child appears to be irrationally afraid of going to school. He may say that he is afraid of the teacher or of other students in the school. In some instances what at first appears to be a phobia can be described more accurately as a refusal of school. The real cause of school phobia is fear of leaving home, or separation anxiety. Careful study, as a rule, will reveal that the parent also fears separation or is abnormally fearful that something will happen to the child when he is away.

OBSESSIVE-COMPULSIVE DISORDER. An obsession is a persistent and repetitious thought, usually recognized by the child as having little or no basis in reality. As an example, a child may be obsessed with the idea that his parent is going to die. A compulsion is a persistent and repetitious act, also recognized as being unrealistic and serving no constructive purpose. For example, a child may not be able to go to sleep unless he first closes the closet door, carefully aligns his shoes, putting the ends of his shoelaces inside of them, and tucks loose ends of the covers beneath the mattress. Obsessive-compulsive behavior is most likely to be seen during the middle years or adolescence. The obsessive-compulsive activity keeps the repressed thoughts and feelings from entering conscious awareness. At times a compulsion becomes ritualistic and serves magically to forestall dangers which usually are not consciously discerned.

CONVERSION DISORDER. In this disorder repressed conflicts are prevented from entering consciousness in recognizable form by being converted to symptoms such as blindness, deafness, paralysis of the arm or leg or various somatic complaints. There is no physiologic disturbance in the affected part. Psychosomatic symptoms due to conversion take place on a psychologic level; these differ from psychophysiologic disturbances, which take place at the level of the autonomic nervous system.

Conversion symptoms are relatively rare in children and are most likely to be seen in the adolescent. Differential diagnosis requires consideration of organic causes.

DISSOCIATIVE DISORDER. This condition is a functional disturbance of consciousness, usually short-lived. It is relatively rare in children. It may be manifest as sleepwalking, amnesia or states of confusion resembling delirium. The alteration of consciousness maintains repression and in some instances enables the child to do something which he would not do if he were fully conscious. For example, a child in a confused state may express aggression in some destructive activity or may express forbidden thoughts.

It is necessary to rule out the possibility of organic causes such as infectious illness, drug intoxication and cerebral injury.

Somnambulism. Sleepwalking occurs mainly in midchildhood and in adolescence. The child, although not fully conscious, is able to get out of bed and walk about the house. On occasion he may leave the house or climb out on a roof or window ledge. The eyes are open, but the child either is unresponsive to questions or answers them briefly in a voice devoid of normal modulation and inflection. He usually returns to bed by himself and resumes sleep. Characteristically there is amnesia for the sleepwalking. If awakened during this state, the child is sometimes frightened, but more usually is puzzled and at a loss to understand his behavior.

Sometimes the activities during sleepwalking may give indication of the underlying problem. For example, the child may walk into the parents' bedroom, thus revealing a desire to be with the parents or perhaps a repressed curiosity as to their activities in the bedroom.

DEPRESSION. Neurotic depression is seen most frequently in the adolescent. This in part is due to the fact that depressive feelings in the younger child may be masked by activity or regression.

A fully developed and strict superego is usually a requisite for depression. Most commonly angry feelings and hostile impulses cannot be expressed toward the person causing them because the superego prohibits this. In consequence they are turned toward the self. In other instances the child has a superego or ego ideal which requires him to achieve in accordance with unrealistically high standards. When he does not measure up to these standards, he feels that he has failed and becomes depressed. At the same time he may also have feelings of frustration and anger which are blocked from expression.

Aggression turned toward the self sometimes causes a child to have an unusual number of accidents. Suicidal thoughts are rare in young children, but common in adolescents. Thoughts of suicide are far more numerous than suicidal attempts, but accidents and suicide rank high among the causes of death in adolescents, particularly during late adolescence. Accident proneness and persistent or severe depression require careful evaluation and merit psychiatric consultation.

ACTING-OUT DISORDER. In this disorder the child acts out unconscious conflicts and impulses without awareness of the meaning of his behavior. Stealing, for example, may be an unconscious expression of feelings of rejection and a need for love. Aggressive or sexual impulses are expressed outwardly in destructive or sexual behavior. The impulses may gain expression because they temporarily override the ego controls, or because, although prohibited, they are felt to be justified. Some children may act out repetitiously because the punishment for the misdeeds brings temporary relief from unconscious guilt feelings. Antisocial behavior of this type can be termed neurotic delinquency.

ACCIDENT PRONENESS. One cause of accident proneness is masked depression as described above. Another cause is acting-out behavior. This behavior is sometimes described as counterphobic, because the child attempts to cope with his unconsciously determined fear by exposing himself to the very danger he is afraid of. This child is the type who must take the dare, or who rushes headlong into situations without considering the risks. He often is a tense, high-strung child who seems to be under pressure to be active. In some instances, however, particularly in the older child, the activity may be deliberate, as for example in carrying out a dangerous chemical experiment or making an explosive device.

LEARNING PROBLEMS. As in developmental and situational disorders, problems in learning may be caused by a severe inhibition of aggression and curiosity, owing to unconscious fear of the consequences.

Another cause of learning difficulty is excessively high standards. The child characteristically begins each school term with enthusiasm and high ambition. Because he expects so much of himself, however, even a slight or moderate amount of dropping away from "perfect" performance is painful. He becomes unwilling to risk further effort and further investment of libidinal energy because of the blow to self-esteem which he experiences with failure. He finds it much less painful to fail without having put forth effort, since this kind of failure is not so disappointing and he can rationalize that he could have succeeded if he had wanted to do so.

A child also may have difficulty in learning because of inability to concentrate, owing to the distraction of daydreams. Children with this kind of difficulty sometimes are better able to study with background noise from a radio, which seemingly serves to screen out the fantasies from within.

A child may have a pattern of repeated failures because successful achievement is equated at an unconscious level with the attainment of a forbidden goal. For example, the child who has not resolved his oedipal conflict may unconsciously equate success in school with success in winning his mother's affection from the father.

These are examples of learning difficulties on a neurotic basis. Organically caused intellectual deficiency and inability to acquire basic skills need to be ruled out.

ENURESIS. (See also Section 15.) Enuresis is defined as an involuntary discharge of urine occurring beyond the age when control of the urinary bladder should have been acquired. A few children achieve voluntary control as early as 1 year of age. The majority do not begin to gain control before 15 to 18 months of age, and nocturnal control is usually not established until 2 or 3 years of age. Some children may not be dry at night until 4 to 6 years of age. In children who have acquired good control there still may be, for several years, occasional lapses in nighttime control associated with fatigue or emotional turmoil, or even in daytime control at times of excitement, extreme urgency or engrossment in play. In some cases development of bladder control may be delayed because the parent has made no reasonable attempt at toilet training.

Before 5 or 6 years of age, enuresis is usually a manifestation of a developmental or situational disorder. Enuresis as a symptom of neurosis is most likely to be seen in midchildhood (the latency years) or in adolescence. Whereas nocturnal enuresis is fairly common, diurnal enuresis, in the absence of an organic lesion, is rare and usually indicates a more severe pathologic disturbance. Enuresis may be a symptom of nocturnal epilepsy or of lesions of part of the spinal cord or of the genitourinary system. It may also be a symptom of diabetes mellitus or diabetes insipidus.

The most common cause of persistent bedwetting extending from infancy is too vigorous and too early attempts at toilet training, before the age of physiologic readiness (usually 15 to 18 months). The same conflicts which cause enuresis in developmental and situational disorders become established internally and persist as a basis for neurotic enuresis. Enuresis may express (1) a desire to regress and receive the care and attentions associated with earlier childhood, (2) unconscious resentment of the parents, or (3) anxiety caused by an unconscious fear of injury to the genitals. This last fear is frequently associated with feelings of guilt due to sexual fantasies or activities, such as masturbation.

Occasional lapses are indicative of temporarily aggravated emotional conflicts and need cause little concern. If the child sleeps deeply, it is possible that signals from the bladder indicating that it needs to be emptied may not reach consciousness in time for the child to get out of bed and go to the bathroom. The child may be given a little more time to see whether control ultimately is gained. On the other hand, both the deep sleep and the enuresis may be determined by emotional factors.

The primary treatment is psychotherapy for the underlying neurotic disorder. Shaming, nagging and punitive actions by the parents do not help and may aggravate the problem. Contrariwise, if the parents can be helped to become less concerned, this may help the child to gain mastery over the problem. The older child may sometimes gain control as he becomes increasingly fearful of humiliation if the condition comes to the attention of his friends, e.g., when he visits at someone's home or goes to summer camp. Disappearance of the symptom under these circumstances does not necessarily mean that the neurotic problem is solved; it may still persist and show itself in another form.

Limiting fluids for a few hours before bedtime and waking the child up so that he may void before he has wet the bed are sometimes helpful. These measures should not be a substitute, however, for direction of attention to the emotional causes.

The use of drugs such as tincture of belladonna, ephedrine, dextroamphetamine or tranquilizers is of doubtful value. Their effectiveness, if any, is often only temporary, and may be more on a psychologic than pharmacologic basis.

It has been assumed by some that the enuretic child has a smaller than average bladder capacity. It is proposed that bladder capacity may be increased by increasing the intake of fluids during the daytime and encouraging the child to suppress the urge to void. This may be worthy of trial. On the other hand, the small bladder capacity and frequent urination may both be a manifestation of tension and anxiety.

Some success is claimed for the conditioning type

of treatment wherein a bell rings and wakens the child when the voided urine completes an electrical circuit in a pad placed beneath the child. This generally is not effective, however, particularly if the enuresis is a symptom of neurosis.

ENCOPRESIS. Fecal soiling in a child beyond the age of 4 or 5 years may be a manifestation of a neurotic disorder as well as of more severe psychopathologic disturbances. There usually has been serious difficulty in the parent-child relations, most likely having its beginnings during bowel training. Treatment is aimed at remedying the underlying psychopathology.

PEPTIC ULCER. Gastric and duodenal ulcers may occur at all ages of infancy and childhood. In the young child the cause is more likely to be organic, but a severe pathogenic environmental situation should be considered. Chronic peptic ulcers occur more frequently after infancy, the incidence being highest in late childhood. The symptoms are similar to those in adults, and range from vague digestive complaints to severe pain, vomiting and blood in the stools.

The neurotic child with ulcer often presents an external appearance of competence and self-sufficiency, while denying strong dependent and regressive urges. There may be tension, compulsiveness or other signs of maladjustment. Psychiatric evaluation and psychotherapy should be considered.

Peptic ulcer may also be a manifestation of neurotic character disorder.

NEUROTIC CHARACTER DISORDERS

Because the young child is rapidly changing and is in a continuing process of development, his behavior patterns are usually not stabilized or ingrained in his personality. Therefore, character disorders are seldom seen in children under 10 years of age. The developmental history of the child with a neurotic character disorder includes traumatic experiences which for the most part are equivalent to those of the neurotic child. Differentiation is made on the basis of the psychopathology and adaptability described below.

PSYCHOPATHOLOGY. The child with a neurotic character disorder attempts to maintain psychologic equilibrium by using certain defenses in a habitual way. His equilibrium is somewhat more unstable than that of the neurotic child because early relations with people have had a more adverse effect on his psychic development. Owing to greater frustrations, the strength of the drives and impulses is increased. Parental disciplinary attitudes are prematurely internalized in an attempt to control the impulses and to achieve more comfortable relations with the parents. The superego is thus likely to be excessively harsh and incompatible with the drives. For these reasons the ego, which has the task of mediating between the child's needs and the demands of his conscience and external reality, is hard pressed and is relatively weaker than that of the neurotic child.

Because strong aggressive and sexual feelings and fantasies are disturbing, the child with a neurotic character disorder eliminates them from his conscious awareness. He is then cut off from his feelings and fantasies, and because they normally are important to thought and action, this internal isolation has the consequence of further limiting his flexibility, creativity and adaptability.

Another result of this defense is a lack of awareness of anxiety and a lack of insight. Although he may acknowledge that he is having trouble learning in school, the child with a neurotic character disorder is unable to see that this is a consequence of difficulty within himself. He lacks the capacity for self-observation and self-evaluation.

ADAPTABILITY. The child with a neurotic character disorder has had more difficulty in his relations with people during the earlier developmental years than has the neurotic or normal child. He values relations with people, but has difficulty in relating to them and they to him. He may be described as excessively shy or quiet or "hard to get to know."

His perception of external reality is fairly adequate, although less so than that of the child with a neurotic disorder. His adaptation is usually considerably more impaired than that of the neurotic child, owing largely to the rigidity of his character structure.

TREATMENT. The same general considerations described under treatment of neurotic disorders apply to treatment of neurotic character disorders. The treatment is more difficult, however, because of the rigidity of the character structure and the lack of awareness of anxiety and the lack of capacity for self-observation and for insight. The first phase of treatment is concerned with establishing a working relationship and making the child aware that he does in fact have internal conflicts, feelings and fantasies which are interfering with his adaptation.

Clinical Patterns

Many of the clinical patterns discussed under neurotic disorders also occur as neurotic character disorders, but with the differences described above; problems discussed previously will not be taken up under this category.

PASSIVE-AGGRESSIVE CHARACTER DISORDER. The passive-aggressive child is outwardly passive and conforming; he does not display aggression toward others in a direct way. Aggression, when evident, takes the form of such symptoms as uncooperativeness, stubbornness, pouting, procrastination and "passive" obstructionism. Passivity and passive resistance are rigidly used as defenses against aggression.

IMPULSE-RIDDEN CHARACTER DISORDER. This child is almost the direct opposite of the passive-aggressive child. He seemingly makes little or no attempt to control his impulses, and there is no apparent anxiety or appropriate concern when the impulsive actions get him into trouble. The causes of this problem are much the same as those discussed in connection with neurotic acting-out.

ANTISOCIAL CHARACTER DISORDER. This condition is analogous to neurotic delinquency, but the child has little or no anxiety and on the surface appears relatively unconcerned about his deeds.

In some of the more severe cases the child may have had good or reasonably adequate relations with people in infancy, but subsequently may have suffered severe deprivation and abuse. Characteristically this type of child is "tough," aloof and seemingly disinterested in receiving help. Yet he may be reached through strenuous therapeutic efforts.

SEXUAL CHARACTER PROBLEMS

Reversed Sexual Identification. Effeminate tendencies in the boy and tomboyishness in the girl may become habitual patterns of adaptation.

Sexual Maladjustments. Persistent homosexual activity must be considered dysfunctional and most likely indicates a character disorder. The same is true for persistent transvestism, i.e., dressing up in the clothing of the opposite sex. This is more common in boys and is usually done covertly because of the awareness that the behavior is disapproved.

STUTTERING. Stuttering may persist into the later years of childhood and become habitual, being a part of everyday speech or appearing at times of stress. Although stuttering may occur transiently and normally in the toddler, it is a serious problem at later ages and often is exceedingly difficult to resolve, even with thorough treatment of the underlying psychopathology.

TICS. Tics are spasmodic, irregular movements of isolated groups of muscles not associated with organic disease. They occur most often in later childhood, but may be seen during the preschool years. On occasion the origin of a tic may be traced to interference with normal motility during early childhood due to illness or artificial restraint such as that imposed by casts or elbow splints.

Tics are of various types and degrees of severity. The movements may be occasional or frequent. They are performed unconsciously, although the child is sometimes able to restrain them for a time. They generally are increased when the child is excited or under stress. The majority of tics involve the facial muscles and consist of twitching or distortion of the mouth, wrinkling of the forehead or winking and blinking of the eyes. Sighing, coughing, sniffling, or jerking movements of the head may be seen. Less often there are jerking movements of the body which may be localized in the hands, arms or shoulders.

Tics also may be seen in neurotic disorders, but when well established they suggest psychopathology more in keeping with neurotic character disorders.

Gilles de la Tourette Syndrome. This relatively uncommon syndrome occurs most often in late childhood or in adolescence. The symptoms are violent twitching or convulsive movements, usually of the muscles of the face and arms, but sometimes of other parts of the body. With the movements there are associated explosive sounds, such as a loud barking cough or indistinct vocal sounds. At times these sounds are enunciated more clearly, and then are discerned to be obscene words.

Since the tic is of unconscious origin, it is of no avail to call attention to it or to pressure the child to control it. Treatment needs to be directed toward the underlying psychopathology.

ANOREXIA NERVOSA. (See also Section 11.) This syndrome, more common in girls than in boys, is most frequent in adolescence. It is characterized by intense self-starvation, severe loss of weight, and at times amenorrhea in the female.

The condition may be precipitated by a relatively small criticism or confrontation with imperfection, such as being called fat or being unable to achieve in some athletic endeavor. The anorexia may be preceded by a conscious and deliberate refusal of food.

These children usually have strict superegos and very high standards for themselves. Distorted fantasies about conception and pregnancy may enter into the determination of the condition. There may be the fear, for example, that impregnation takes place through the mouth and can occur after kissing. In other children the ingestion of food may be associated with frightening aggressive fantasies of devouring or being devoured. These fantasies are usually revealed only during psychotherapy.

The more severe cases may be confused with Simmonds's cachexia, and with malnutrition due to other organic causes. Although the onset of the anorexia may be acute, the associated underlying character disorder develops over a relatively long time.

Treatment consists initially in correction of any electrolyte imbalance and in establishing minimally adequate nutrition. This may require hospitalization and parenteral therapy. Immediate psychiatric consultation should be requested in order to begin psychotherapy promptly. The condition is difficult to treat, and the prognosis is often grave.

PSYCHOTIC CHARACTER DISORDERS

Like neurotic character disorders, psychotic character disorders are seen mostly in the older child and adolescent. In contrast to neurotic character disorders, which are based upon psychopathology similar to that of neuroses, psychotic character disorders are based upon a kind of psychopathology similar to that of psychoses. (See below.)

PSYCHOPATHOLOGY. The psychotic character disorder is manifest in habitual patterns of behavior which are even more rigid and less varied than those in neurotic character disorders. The child has had serious difficulty during his early psychologic development, so that his equilibrium is easily disturbed. In his attempt at maintenance of equilibrium he isolates and distorts his perception of his own feelings and fantasies. Because unexpected events or experiences are very disturbing, he avoids them by limiting his activities and contacts with people. Thus, his perception of the world around him becomes constricted and his character make-up increasingly rigid. His ability to deal with his drives and impulses, with the demands of his conscience and with external reality is inadequate.

ADAPTABILITY. The child with a psychotic character disorder appears to place relatively little value on relations with people. Nevertheless, he does not withdraw completely. He fails in his adaptation to an even greater extent than does the child with neurotic character disorder, and he is often regarded as "peculiar" or eccentric. He does not adjust well with his peer group, and he has a tendency to isolate himself, either alone or with one or two friends whose make-up is similar to his own. He is likely to perform poorly. He has had difficulty in most aspects of psychologic development. Although his general performance is poor, he may do well in a specific area. For example, an adolescent may be outstanding in academic learning, while failing to achieve in social and physical skills.

TREATMENT. The psychotherapy is difficult and delicate. Although the patient wishes for relationships, he is afraid of them. The therapist must proceed slowly and cautiously lest he disturb the precarious psychologic equilibrium.

Clinical Patterns

Psychotic character disorders usually bear little resemblance to neuroses or neurotic character disorders, the symptoms and behavior being more akin to those of psychotic disorders.

INADEQUATE CHARACTER DISORDER. A child with an inadequate character is unable to respond adequately to intellectual, emotional, social and physical demands. Although children with this disorder are not mentally or physically defective, they function so inadequately as to suggest that they are. This condition may be due in part to constitutional inadequacy. It can result from severe emotional deprivation with an attempt at adaptation through withdrawal and passivity.

SCHIZOID CHARACTER DISORDER. The symptoms and behavior in the schizoid character disorder resemble those seen in schizophrenia. The child is unable to form close relations or to express aggression; his awareness of reality is much constricted. He lives mainly in a fantasy world of his own creating. He may have sufficient capacity to fit into the family routine and to carry out certain specific tasks and activities. In the more serious cases the child may avoid speaking for periods of time, since relationship with people is disturbing to his equilibrium.

PARANOID CHARACTER DISORDER. This disorder, rare in children, is also characterized by a schizoid type of behavior in which the child's own feelings of inadequacy and hostility are projected onto other people and then are felt to be directed toward himself as accusations from them. This kind of child is excessively suspicious, envious, jealous and prone to project the blame for his failures upon other people or upon inanimate factors.

DYSSOCIAL CHARACTER DISORDER. The term "dyssocial" connotes a lack of social values and is to be distinguished from the term "antisocial," which suggests values which are against those of society. Although the dyssocial child may have a generally good sense of reality, he lacks conscience and appreciation of social reality. This can result from his having been brought up in a morally abnormal environment or in a subcultural group with values very much different from those of society in general. His dyssocial behavior is based not upon emotional conflicts or traumatic experiences, but upon a difference in his character structure, specifically in the content of his superego. Because he comes into sharp conflict with society and in effect has a character defect, he is viewed, somewhat inappropriately, as having a psychotic character disorder.

ULCERATIVE COLITIS. Ulcerative colitis is characterized by recurrent episodes of diarrhea with loss of appetite, malnutrition and bleeding due to ulceration of the lower bowel. (See also Section 11.) In some instances psychologic factors may play a large role in the illness. The child usually has had difficulty in managing his hostility and aggression since early childhood. Although he relates to people, he prefers to be by himself and is not comfortable with other children. He has ambivalent feelings toward everyone in his environment, and particularly toward his parents. Eating and elimination usually have become very much involved in the child's emotional conflicts. Characteristically he has a strict, punitive superego which forbids the expression of his strong oral needs and of aggression. Outwardly he may appear to be calm, but inwardly he seethes with tension. During the course of psychotherapy primitive and distorted oral and anal fantasies are likely to be revealed. They usually include fantasies of destruction as well as of procreation.

Intense psychotherapy of long duration is usually required to improve the severe psychopathology.

PSYCHOTIC DISORDERS (PSYCHOSES)

Psychotic disorders are the most serious of the psychologic disorders, having comparability to "insanity" in the adult.

PSYCHOPATHOLOGY. In psychotic disorders difficulty in early psychologic development has resulted in deficiencies in personality development and integration. The young psychotic child often has defects in coordination which are difficult to distinguish from those caused by organic lesions. Language development may be grossly impaired or completely lacking. Thought processes are disorganized, and social reality either is not perceived or is ignored.

ADAPTABILITY. Owing to insurmountable difficulties in the early relations with the parents or other adults, the psychotic child has little or no interest in relating to people. He is withdrawn, preferring to live in a fantasy world of his own creation, and usually fails completely in his adaptation.

TREATMENT. Children with psychotic disorders, particularly in early childhood, are among the most difficult to treat. Even with intensive and prolonged efforts, utilizing individual psychotherapy, supervised group experience, special education, treatment of the parents, and the use of parent substitutes with or without institutionalization, most of these children are unable to achieve a level of functioning anywhere near that of the normal child.

CLINICAL PATTERNS IN EARLY CHILDHOOD

ANACLITIC DEPRESSION. The term "anaclitic" connotes dependence or leaning upon. This disorder is seen in infants at 4 to 6 months of age after complete separation from the mother. Initially the infant reacts with crying and apprehension, and then by withdrawal of interest in people. Over a period of weeks psychologic development becomes retarded, and there is decreased motility and responsiveness to stimuli (Spitz).

AUTISTIC CHILDHOOD PSYCHOSIS (AUTISM). This disorder, originally described by Kanner, is characterized by profound withdrawal from contact with people, including the parents, an obsessive desire for preservation of sameness, a skillful and even affectionate relation to inanimate objects, retention of an intelligent, pensive physiognomy, and mutism or a kind of language development which is not understandable. In rare instances the diagnosis has been made as early as 18 months of age. More often the symptoms, although present, go unrecognized until the age of 4 or 5 years. Parents frequently minimize signs of the condition until the child goes to nursery school or kindergarten, where his difficulties become clearly evident.

In the more severe cases the child may appear extremely regressed. He may sit and rock back and forth incessantly; he may drool, and his only vocalizations may be grunts or other animal-like sounds. Although he may seem aware of people, he makes no attempt to relate to them. He may scratch his skin to the point of excoriation and bite or slap himself when frustrated or intruded upon, without evident awareness of pain. Physical coordination may be poor.

In the less severe cases the child has good physical coordination and sometimes may be skillful in handling his body or manipulating objects. He uses words and on occasion may verbalize a request, but sentence formation and language development are inadequate for his age. He has the capacity for memory, sometimes to a remarkable degree. His level of intelligence is difficult to gauge, but his activities suggest ability to reason and to understand cause-and-effect relations. He is interested in and sometimes intensely preoccupied with inanimate objects. Intrusions of other people into his autism are resented, and at first will be ignored or brushed aside. If one persists in the intrusion or attempts to establish a relationship, he becomes upset and has a severe temper tantrum in which he may break things or display aggression toward himself.

In some instances the disorder is felt to be due to constitutional deficiencies, as suggested, for example, by the history of absence of a smiling response or acceptance of cuddling as early as the neonatal period. In other instances the history indicates that the child most likely was severely traumatized through environmental experiences in infancy, when serious physical problems in the infant or serious emotional problems in the mother may have interfered with adequate maternal care. There is often a combination of constitutional and environmental factors.

Differential diagnosis includes consideration of mental retardation, brain injury causing interference with mental functioning, e.g., agnosia or aphasia, deafness and Heller's disease. Heller's disease is a rare progressive degeneration of the central nervous system. It has an acute onset between 18 months and 4 years of age and is characterized by progressive deterioration of all aspects of mental functioning.

SYMBIOTIC CHILDHOOD PSYCHOSIS. This disorder, described by Mahler, is frequently precipitated by separation or threat of separation from the mother. The child at first may protest with severe crying and then by regression, with bizarre behavior such as attempting to climb into the toilet bowl, taking off all clothing and going out of doors naked, eating in an animal-like fashion, talking or singing in an endless and singsong fashion, and staying awake and moving about aimlessly through the night. During such behavior the child is withdrawn and is unamenable to management by reason or persuasion. The possible causes are similar to those of the autistic childhood psychosis. Careful consideration should be given to the possibility of organic factors.

The acute phase may last for hours or days. It is followed by a chronic phase which may last for months or years. In the chronic phase the child seeks to relate to people, but in an abnormal way. He lacks normal reticence, and family and complete strangers are approached without discrimination. Frequently the child seeks close physical contact, and in some instances behaves as if he would wish to merge with or burrow into the other person. He may be uncommunicative; or language development may appear to be normal, and the child may engage in conversation, but its content is disorganized or monothematic.

Clinical Patterns in Later Childhood

Whereas the psychoses of early childhood represent failure to achieve psychologic development, the psychoses of later childhood result from a breakdown in personality integration and ego functioning. This type of psychotic disorder is seen occasionally in the prepuberty period, but more often in adolescence. These children usually have had traumatic experiences during their early psychologic development, with a resulting predisposition to psychotic disorder at a later date. Nevertheless, they were able to progress in their development, functioning sufficiently well to cause no great concern and to attend school. In some instances the personality of the child before the collapse in functioning resembles that of the child with a psychotic character disorder. The combination of predisposition and the increased emotional stress normally associated with puberty accounts for the onset of psychotic disorder in adolescence. On the other hand, inasmuch as emotional stress is normally increased at this age, a psychosis in adolescence often has a less serious prognosis than the same condition occurring either in midchildhood or in adulthood.

The psychoses of later childhood are characterized by (1) withdrawal from relations with people, (2) distorted perception and evaluation of reality, (3) disordered thinking which may include delusions and hallucinations, and (4) general disorganization and regression resulting in bizarre behavior. In some instances the child may be completely withdrawn, uncommunicative and essentially immobile (catatonic). In other instances he may behave in an infantile manner, seemingly without awareness of the cultural mores which he previously had accepted. For example, he may eat messily with his fingers, be careless about his personal appearance and body hygiene, soil and wet himself, masturbate openly, or simply be silly (hebephrenic). In some instances aggressive impulses are expressed in destructive behavior or in serious assault on people. Psychotic disorders in adolescents are similar to schizophrenic and manic-depressive psychoses in adults. The schizophrenic reactions are not sufficiently differentiated in their symptoms to warrant classifying them in the adult subtypes of simple (inadequate), hebephrenic, catatonic and paranoid schizophrenia. Psychotic clinical patterns may also be caused by organic brain lesions, such as brain tumor, and by toxic effects of an infectious illness.

When the diagnosis of psychotic disorder has been made or is suspected, immediate psychiatric consultation is indicated. Hospitalization is usually necessary both for the protection of the child and of the family and in order to carry out treatment measures.

PSYCHOLOGIC DISORDERS ASSOCIATED WITH ORGANIC BRAIN DAMAGE

An organic disorder (see also Section 20) may be the principal cause of a psychologic disorder in some instances, whereas in others organic and psychologic disorders may exist in the same child with little or no relation in terms of cause and effect. The basis for a diagnosis of a psychologic disorder in this category therefore is the same as in each of the six preceding categories, but is complicated by the necessity of having to evaluate the significance of the organic problem as to its possible causative role in the psychologic disorder and its current influence on the child's adaptation and behavior.

An organic defect or problem in the child is likely to stir up latent guilt feelings and neurotic conflicts in otherwise well adjusted parents. They may lose their objectivity and behave unrealistically in their attempt to meet the needs of the child. They may be unnecessarily overprotective and overindulgent, thus interfering with maximum development of the child's potentialities. At the other extreme they tend to deny the reality of the limitations which the organic problem poses and expect of the child achievement which is impossible.

The parents need to have an opportunity to discuss their reactions, feelings and concerns about the child. The perceptive physician can serve an important role in preventing the parents from repressing their feelings and denying reality.

CALVIN F. SETTLAGE

Burks, H. L., and Harrison, S. I.: Aggressive behavior as a means of avoiding depression. Am. J. Orthopsychiat., *32*:416, 1962.

Chess, S., Thomas, T., and Birch, H. G: Behavior problems revisited. J. Am. Acad. Child Psychiat. *6*:321, 1967.

Cramer, J. B. Common neuroses of childhood. *In* Arieti, S. (ed.): American Handbook of Psychiatry. New York, Basic Books, Inc., 1959, Vol. 1, p. 797.

Cutter, A. V., and Hallowitz, D.: Diagnosis and treatment of the family unit with respect to the character-disordered youngster. J. Am. Acad. Child Psychiat. *1*:605, 1962.

Finch, S. M.: Fundamentals of Child Psychiatry. New York, W. W. Norton & Co., 1960.

Finch, S. M., and Hess, J. H.: Ulcerative colitis in children. Am. J. Psychiat. *118*:819, 1962.

Freud, A.: Assessment of childhood disturbances. *In* Psychoanalytic Study of the Child. New York, International Universities Press, 1962, Vol. XVII, pp. 149–58.

Hartmann, H.: Psychoanalysis and developmental psychology. *In* Psychoanalytic Study of the Child. New York, International Universities Press, 1950, Vol. V, pp. 7–17.

Johnson, A. M.: Juvenile delinquency. *In* Arieti, S. (ed.): American Handbook of Psychiatry. New York, Basic Books, Inc., 1959, Vol. 1, p. 840.

Kahn, J. H., and Nursten, J. P.: School refusal: A comprehensive view of school phobia and other failures of school attendance. Am. J. Orthopsychiat., *32*:707, 1962.

Kanner, L.: Child Psychiatry. 2nd ed. Springfield, Ill., Charles C Thomas, 1948.

Kanner, L.: Early infantile autism. Am. J. Orthopsychiat., *19*:416, 1949.

MacKeith, R., and Sandler, J. (eds.): Psychosomatic Aspects of Paediatrics. Pergamon Press, 1961.

Mahler, M. S.: Ego psychology applied to behavior problems. *In* Lewis, N. D. C., and Pacella, B. L.; Modern Trends in Child Psychiatry. New York, International Universities Press, 1949, pp. 43–56.

Mahler, M. S., Furer, M., and Settlage, C. F.: Severe emotional disturbances in childhood psychoses. *In* Arieti, S. (ed.): American Handbook of Psychiatry. New York, Basic Books, Inc., 1959, Vol. 1, pp. 821–4.

Meyer, R., Levitt, M., Falick, M., and Rubenstein, B.: Essentials of Pediatric Psychiatry. New York, Appleton-Century-Crofts, Inc., 1962.

Pearson, G. H. J.: Emotional Disorders of Children. New York, W. W. Norton & Co., 1949.

Prugh, D. G.: Investigations dealing with the reactions of chil-

dren and families to hospitalization in illness: Problems and potentialities. *In* Caplan, G. (ed.): Emotional Problems of Early Childhood. New York, Basic Books, Inc., 1955.
Ribble, M. A.: Rights of Infants. New York, Columbia University Press, 1943.
Settlage, C. F.: Psychoanalytic theory in relation to the nosology of childhood psychic disorders. J. Am. Psychoanal. Assn., *12*:776–801.
Spitz, R.: Anaclitic depression. *In* Psychoanalytic Study of the Child. New York, International Universities Press, 1946, Vol. II, pp. 313–42.
Spitz, R.: Hospitalism. *In* Psychoanalytic Study of the Child. New York, International Universities Press, 1945–46, Vols. I and II, Parts I and II.
Toolan, J. M.: Depression in children and adolescents. Am. J. Orthopsychiat., *32*:404, 1962.
Toolan, J. M.: Suicide and suicidal attempts in children and adolescents. Am. J. Psychiat., *118*:719, 1961.

Role of the Physician in Management of Established Psychologic Disorders

ASSESSMENT. When it has been determined that there is psychopathology in a child and/or his family which requires intervention, the physician must develop the therapeutic plan. When the primary physician, family practitioner or pediatrician decides that he understands the problem and feels that he can comfortably manage it, he should proceed to do so. This decision need not be final. If improvement does not seem adequate, or if some unresolved issues remain, referral to a more specialized level of care may be appropriate. Depending on the nature of the problem, such referral may be to pediatrician, pediatric subspecialist, child psychologist or psychiatrist. Referral should not, however, end the role of the primary physician as the ongoing medical caretaker. He will need to assess the psychiatric intervention being offered and what the child or family eventually gain from it. His positive and expectant attitude and his continuing interest in what is happening to his patient will do much to ensure that he obtains helpful feedback from his consultants.

Assessment at each level of care should build on the studies of previous assessors. The physician of primary contact often depends mostly on screening tests. He can take responsibility for the evaluation in greater depth if he is interested in doing so and adequately experienced. In certain instances he may arrange with the psychologist for certain tests, but retain the initiative of primary caretaker until he has information to indicate what treatment is needed and who will carry it out.

Psychologic tests are generally of four types: The *first* type of test is concerned with perceptuomotor integrity; these tests are felt to be especially sensitive to "organicity," or to reflect structural or physiologic abnormalities in the central nervous system. The Bender-Gestalt test is probably the best known in this category. In the *second* category are "intelligence" tests, such as the Stanford-Binet or Wechsler Intelligence Scale for Children (WISC). The WISC is a 10-category test which gives both verbal and performance IQ scores. The Peabody Picture Vocabulary Test, easily administered in the office, can give a limited and rough estimate of verbal ability. The *third* type of test is usually administered in schools. These are achievement tests (like the Wide Ranging Achievement Test, or WRAT) which report the grade level of achievement in various subject areas, such as reading, spelling or mathematics. A score of 4.5 in mathematics would indicate, for example, that a child's level of mathematic achievement corresponded to that of the average child at the fifth month of the fourth year of school. The *fourth* type of test includes the projective tests, such as the Rorschach test (ink blots) or the thematic apperception test (TAT). These give some indication of the fantasy life of the child, as well as of his reality testing and personality characteristics. Final choice of tests to be made should be left to the psychologist, after the physician has communicated the nature of the problem and the reasons for consultation. If these tests and their interpretation are not well and confidently understood by the physician, he should arrange to have the psychologist meet with him together with the parents for an interpretive interview. Otherwise, costly tests may be ordered, the results of which are never adequately communicated to the parents or child.

When *referral* of a child for psychotherapy is considered, it is important first to know the resources in the community. These include not only private practitioners in child psychiatry, social work or psychology, but child guidance agencies, child welfare and family service agencies, and children's psychiatric wards or hospitals. Some school districts have both psychologic evaluative services and treatment facilities, as well as special classes. The physician is well advised to become personally acquainted with some knowledgeable person in one or in each category of resource, through whom he can gain a broad picture of the services and special skills available in his or her community.

Among factors to be considered in referral of the child or family are the nature of the problem, the abilities of the consultant or agency insofar as they are known, financial and geographic feasibility of a treatment program, and the quality of the referring physician's communication with the referral resource. In justifying referral to the child or to the parents, the simplest statement is the best. The most reassuring factor will be the physician's own conviction and confidence that this is a necessary step. If he is uncertain as to the wisdom or value of referral, it should be deferred until he has had a chance to resolve his doubts in further discussion with a psychiatric or psychologic consultant. The choice of treatment should be left up to the consultant, with reassurance to the family and patient by the referring physician that he will be in close communication with the consultant. The referring physician should ordinarily retain interest in and plan actively for the continuing care of his patient within those areas of preventive practice and episodic illness which demand his attention. He should not leave child or parents with the feeling that "there is nothing he can do" or that his reluctant referral constitutes an admission of failure on his part or on the parents' part or an abandonment by him to another system of care.

MODES OF TREATMENT. Some treatment modalities are currently used virtually exclusively by the mental health professional; others may be employed successfully by the nonpsychiatric physician. Most mental health workers use combinations of various methods. Some nonpsychiatric physicians with special interests or formal training are competent at psychologic treatment, which may differ very little from that of the formally trained psychiatrist, but their activities generally represent some subspecialization in their roles as generalists or pediatricians.

Treatment methods used by the psychiatrist can be divided roughly into two categories, which are not mutually exclusive. The first category emphasizes the resolution of the problem through involvement of the patient in a process of change. The second category stresses an educative and directive approach to the patient through the use of explanation, demonstration and encouragement; these are sometimes supplemented by drug therapy, hopefully temporary.

The second way of categorizing treatment is in terms of *systems.* (See also pp. 67–68.) A rather classic arrangement for psychotherapy with the child has the therapist working directly with the patient in the task of resolving intrapsychic conflict. If this is done intensively, it is called child psychoanalysis; if less intensively, it is termed child psychotherapy. Efforts may range from specific requests of the child for alteration of behavior to interpretive therapy aimed at giving the child an opportunity to change his intrapsychic structure and coping behavior. Both require some allegiance on the part of the child to the therapeutic effort. Parents may be involved in concurrent casework with social worker or psychologist, may be seen occasionally by the therapist, and are sometimes not involved at all by the therapist in the treatment process.

A second therapeutic system involves working with the family as a group, in part or in whole. This approach gives most attention to the relationships between family members, rather than to what goes on inside the emotional life of each individual family member. There is heavy stress on mending communication difficulties between family members, and upon having each member learn what his healthy role is, accept it and gain acceptance for it, and function effectively within it.

A third system involves group therapy for children, which is particularly helpful to the child who has problems in development of social skills. Group therapy for preadolescent children tends to emphasize physical and other structured activities through which therapist and children alike can discover how they relate to each other and find ways to change, as indicated.

Still another way of classifying psychotherapeutic approaches depends on the importance of the verbal expressivity and fantasy life of the child. The *psychodynamic* approach stresses the importance of having child and parents come to understand how past patterns of behavior have influenced current feelings and function. The *behavioral modification* approach stresses a complete analysis of the behavior of the child, in terms of the current behavior's immediate antecedents and consequences. Desirable behavioral changes are then brought about by changing the reward system, with the goal of modifying activities and attitudes that perpetuate undesirable behavior or fail to reinforce desired behavior. Expressions of approval and other emotional support will also be used to reinforce desired responses or activities of the child. Insofar as possible, undesired behavior is responded to with as little behavior as possible that might tend to reward it.

Psychotherapy by the Nonpsychiatric Physician. Time is a very frequently cited barrier to the generalist's or pediatrician's becoming involved in the behavioral or emotional components of a child's problem (i.e., in psychotherapeutic activity). The physician is inclined to wonder whether his other professional responsibilities will permit him to do justice to severe emotional problems. Another basic roadblock is the lack of an adequate conceptual background. Only with the experience of successfully grappling with and ultimately finding that he *can* treat many of these problems will the physician accept responsibility and function with confidence in this area.

The first therapeutic impact, and a major one, is conveyed by the interest of the physician, as expressed both in acceptant listening and in directing probing questions that evoke new thoughts in parents or children. In exposing and allaying the anxieties of the parents and their child, the physician helps parents to gain a more objective view of how they and their child or children function as a family unit, and may be able to put the child's symptoms into larger perspective.

When assessment has reached certain nodal points, the physician may wish to synthesize those data and impressions that appear to be helpful or relevant into a diagnosis or a hypothesis, which he shares with the parents, or into a further set of questions. A diagnosis can be stated at various levels of certainty; or a hypothesis can be presented as a possibility worthy of consideration, often with a question appended, such as "Do you think (or feel) that that might be the case?" or "Is there anything else you can think of which might guide our thoughts along these lines?" A thoughtful initial statement or formulation may be both diagnostic and therapeutic. Even if not exactly on the mark, it will often help parents to think about their child's problems in new terms.

The physician must expect that parents or families will vary in readiness to take the next step. If an initial formulation or a probing question draws blank looks or open resistance, the initiative can be given to the parents at their level of understanding by asking them how *they* see the problem at this point. Depending upon the response, it may be appropriate to re-explain, in hope of clearing up minor misunderstandings, or to give some immediate, concrete advice which seems likely to help lower tension, and to set a time for a next visit. At a next visit in a few days it may be found that the parents have begun to see their child's or the family problem in different perspective; a new review of the situation may indicate whether further explanations and suggestions are needed, or are advisable, or will be effective.

In the case of a trusting and well established relationship between physician and family, it may be appropriate to convey directly and simply the diagnostic impressions and suggestions for management. In less predictable situations the physician may wish to be more tentative. His suggestions might include recommending that the parents talk with their child about their feelings about the problem and encourage the child to express his own. In giving suggestions to parents as to how they may alter their behavior in order to help a child to cope with a problem, it is best to focus upon one issue and upon one change at a time. If parents can deal effectively with this change, the positive effect will often generalize to other problems and reduce their importance.

An adolescent should usually be included in the discussion which formulates the problem and suggests changes. For the younger child it is often enough that change occurs at the parental level of feeling and action without involving the child in the planning process. If, for example, a problem in a young child is seen as reflecting maternal anxieties, loneliness or fears, then the mother must be given counsel and support before direct manipulation of the child is considered. The psychologic management of the child demands being in tune with parental needs.

Much supportive therapy of this kind can be viewed as representing a contract between physician, parents and child, which on formulation of the problem indicates actions to be taken by each party with respect to the focal point of concern. Progress toward solution of the problem is reviewed at successive visits, with a set of questions to be answered at each one. How effectively has each party been able to do his or her part in meeting defined goals? What resistances have become apparent? Has there been improvement or general relief? Does the problem need refocusing? What new problems have come up? The physician examines the new data with parents and child and continues the visits as long as there is progress. If little or no improvement occurs, the physician may wish to seek the advice of a psychiatrist as to what may be happening or as to what avenues he might explore next, or to refer the patient for more intensive study or therapy.

An important aspect of the psychotherapeutic process is that patients or parents often do not "hear" or cannot assimilate or follow the physician's explanations or advice. It is important for the physician not to let his own frustration be expressed in ways which increase the parents' resistance, by accusing them implicitly or explicitly of ignorance, of not caring, or of uncooperativeness. It is appropriate for him, however, to give the parents a simple, gentle and unemotional analysis of the problem as he sees it, have the parents reply, and examine with them the areas in which they have misunderstood each other or have different goals. When the question of continuation of psychotherapeutic discussion arises, it must be the parents' decision whether they will continue with the physician to seek some resolution or will seek some other recourse.

Patients will usually seek out the physician whose personality best meets their needs. Sometimes, however, physicians have found that helping a parent with one child-rearing problem only leads to another problem's being presented. In this case it may be that the relationship of the parent to the physician has become more central to the parent's needs than the child's problem. The parent will most likely be unaware of this; the physician will need to confront the parent with the possibility gently and gradually, indicating that a reformulation of the emotional problem is necessary.

In summary, the process of psychotherapy with the nonpsychiatric physician emphasizes effective listening and interviewing, conceptualization of the problem, first to self and then to parents, exploration of problem-solving techniques with parents in one or more conferences, a willingness to stay involved as long as needed, and a readiness to accept limitations and to make appropriate referrals when these are indicated.

Hospitalization. At times hospitalization of the disturbed or emotionally ill child in a general or pediatric hospital will be helpful or necessary, and may serve a number of functions. In the case of many psychosomatic disorders or of a suicidal or drugged adolescent, indications may be medical as well as psychiatric. Sometimes adolescents who talk of suicide, of feeling depressed, or of being cut off from family or peer group can be supported by a relatively brief hospitalization. Hospitalization, with appropriate studies, permits observation of behavior in a structured setting, away from the family. If parents can see their child's behavior as different in the hospital, they may be helped to a more objective look at the problem than was earlier possible. The changing perceptions which parents may have of the behavior of the child must be handled delicately by the physician, so as not to arouse parental guilt or anger, which might threaten the therapeutic process.

If residential treatment of a child in a psychiatric hospital is thought to be necessary, consultation with a psychiatrist and/or a social agency will be helpful in decision-making and planning. Admission to residential treatment indicates the family's decompensation as often as the child's. Whenever the physician feels that child care at home is grossly inadequate or involves physical abuse, he must, in most communities, report this fact to some public authority, and in any case should consult with an appropriate social agency.

Psychopharmacology. The use of drugs in modifying behavior of children is controversial; the effectiveness of drugs appears to depend not only on pharmacodynamics but also on the personality or charisma of the physician prescribing them, and upon the problem, the patient, the parents, the time of day given, and so on. The specific mode of action on the central nervous system of the drugs commonly used is generally unclear and their effects on behavior are influenced by the maturity of the central nervous system, as well as by intrapsychic and estrapsychic factors. Barbiturates will often make an overly excited young child paradoxically more so. Many studies of the use of dextroamphetamine and methylphenidate for the "hyperkinetic" child provide no clear conclusion, although many physicians and parents feel these drugs produce definite improvement in some children. Other children do not improve, and there is no way to predict which hyperkinetic child will benefit. Beneficial effects of these drugs are seen only in preadolescents; adolescents have sympathomimetic responses more like those of adults; they should not receive these drugs for hyperkinesis. Recent studies indicate growth retardation in young children who have received large doses of these drugs for several years.

Major and minor "tranquilizing" drugs have been used in children, in doses proportional to those given to adults. Indications for their use are not well established, however, especially in young children. In disturbed adolescents these drugs may be used much as in young adults. In any case, the use of drugs may be contraindicated if they are perceived or grasped as alternatives to the establishment of the kind of psychotherapeutic relationship which has been discussed above.

Recent studies indicate that childhood depression is much more common than has been supposed in the past. With the exception of imipramine, which has been extensively used in the management of enuresis, antidepressant drugs have been given little trial in children. There is as yet no evidence that drugs have any important part to play in the initiation or maintenance of a therapeutic regimen in childhood depression.

The physician contemplating use of psychotropic drugs in children should make sure he knows the parental attitudes toward such drugs. Some parents are adamantly opposed, and it is inappropriate as well as useless to prescribe drugs for their children. If drugs are to be used, it is to be hoped that it will be only for as short a period as possible.

J. M. Dunn

For references, see p. 83.

NEGLECT AND ABUSE OF CHILDREN

The term "battered child syndrome" was coined for an American Academy of Pediatrics Symposium in 1961, a symposium that focused the concern of physicians on unexplained fractures and other forms of severe physical abuse of children. Since that time the definition of "child abuse" has been broadened to include any problem resulting from the lack of reasonable care and protection of children by their parents, guardians or other caretakers.

The physician has two main responsibilities toward abused children: detection and reporting. He must be able to identify this entity in his own patients and in patients brought to him by other professional persons. Case finding is especially important in the first six months of the child's life, because the risk of a fatal outcome is high if the diagnosis is missed during this period. In all 50 states the physician must report suspected cases of child abuse and/or neglect to a local agency providing protective services. Reluctance to report can lead to recurrence of injuries or even to death. The laws protect the physician from liability if his suspicion should prove to be wrong.

THE SPECTRUM OF CHILD ABUSE AND NEGLECT

PHYSICAL ABUSE. This can be defined as nonaccidental trauma inflicted by a caretaker. Such injuries may include bruises, burns, head injuries, fractures, and the like, and their severity can range from minor bruises to fatal subdural hematomas. Since physical punishment is acceptable in our society, physicians must develop guidelines as to when it is excessive or unduly severe and represents physical abuse. Corporal punishment that causes bruises or leads to an injury that requires medical treatment is outside the range of normal punishment.

NUTRITIONAL NEGLECT. Caloric deprivation is the most common cause of underweight in infancy. Over half of cases of failure to thrive are due to this single cause. Water deprivation has also been described as a form of child abuse.

SEXUAL ABUSE. *Sexual* exploitation of children is probably the most underdiagnosed type of child abuse. In most cases the victimized child is a girl. Vulvitis, vaginitis, or venereal disease in the prepubertal child must make the physician suspicious of sexual abuse. The main goal of therapy is to separate the child from the offending adult.

EMOTIONAL ABUSE. This occurs when children are abandoned in public places or left at home locked in a cellar, closet or small room while the adults are elsewhere. Protective service agencies usually remove children from such emotionally destructive environments. There is more subtle emotional abuse in the continual or chronic scapegoating, terrorizing, berating and rejection of a child; such treatment mutilates the developing personality. This type of child abuse is difficult to prove; affected children may gain relief only when they come to attention through eventual physical abuse of some degree or through abandonment.

NEGLECT OF MEDICAL CARE. Neglect of the treatment recommended for a child with a treatable chronic disease may lead to serious deterioration of his condition. Such cases may require reporting to gain court-enforced supervision or foster placement. Examples would be the young asthmatic not given his aminophylline, or the diabetic child not given his insulin. Court orders to hospitalize and treat are also needed in situations in which an emergency exists which the parents will not acknowledge, such as a needed blood transfusion that is refused, or a child with meningitis whom the parents refuse to hospitalize.

EPIDEMIOLOGY

Physical abuse involves about six of every thousand children born. Episodes of abuse number approximately 300 cases per million population per year. In hospital emergency rooms approximately 10 per cent of injuries seen in children under 5 years of age are inflicted, with a mortality of about 1 per cent, leading to 600 deaths per year in this country. Failure to thrive is reported with one quarter the frequency of physical abuse.

The victims of physical abuse are estimated to be one third under 6 months of age, one third from 6 months to 3 years of age, and one third over 3 years. Premature infants have a threefold greater risk. Stepchildren are also at increased risk.

The child with failure to thrive is usually less than 2 years of age, because he can usually obtain food for himself after that age. In bizarre circumstances an older child may be confined to his room and slowly starved.

Parents who abuse their children come from all ethnic, geographic, religious, educational, occupational and socioeconomic groups. The socioeconomically disadvantaged may have an increased incidence of child abuse, owing to increased numbers of crises and their limited material and emotional resources. Women are more often involved in abuse than are men, because mothers spend more time with their children. This difference does not occur when fathers are unemployed.

ETIOLOGY

For physical abuse to occur it requires not only the right parent but also the right child and the right day. The right child has characteristics that make him demanding; the right day usually is a day of crisis. The most common crises include losing a job, being evicted, having the car break down, birth of a sibling, or an acute illness of the child which leads to intractable crying.

Over 90 per cent of abusing parents are neither psychotic nor sociopathic. They have injured their children in anger after being provoked by some misbehavior or other behavior they could not control. They often have experienced physical abuse themselves when they were children, and their poor impulse control is a re-enactment of what happened to them.

The main cause of failure to thrive in infancy is that the baby is not fed enough. Factors in the mother, in the baby and in the environment contribute to this failure. Most mothers involved in maternal deprivation feel themselves to be deprived and unloved. In the majority of cases the baby was unwanted. Multiple ongoing crises commonly overwhelm the mother. Crises frequently involve the physical absence of the father, who may be in the armed forces, a truck driver, a merchant seaman, or a traveling salesman.

CLINICAL HISTORY

Many cases of physical abuse are first suspected because an *implausible history* is offered to explain a child's injury. Some parents will be reluctant to elaborate on how the injury might have happened, and others might say they have no idea about it. Some will give a vague explanation such as, "He might have fallen down." These explanations are self-incriminating. Normal parents usually know to the minute where and when their child was hurt.

Sometimes there is a *discrepancy* between the histories offered by the two parents or between the histories offered two interviewers. Another common contradiction occurs between the history offered of a minor accident and the physical findings of a major injury. Sometimes a discrepancy exists between the history given and the child's developmental age. The child under 6 months of age is unlikely to induce an accident. Stories of babies rolling over on their arms and breaking them or getting their heads caught in the crib and fracturing the skull are fabrications. Allegations that older children deliberately injure themselves are also usually false.

There is often delay in seeking medical help for abused children. Normal parents bring their injured children immediately for examination. Some abused children are not brought in for a considerable period of time despite major injuries. Smith found that 40 per cent of children did not come to medical attention until the morning after the injury; another 40 per cent came in one to four days after the injury.

The *diet history* in caloric deprivation is not usually helpful because the parent reports that her baby consumes an abundance of calories; but about 20 per cent of cases of failure to thrive are due to errors in preparation of formula or errors in frequency or amount of feedings rather than maternal deprivation, and these cases are diagnosed by a detailed diet history. Errors in formula preparation are especially likely with powdered milk. Breastfed babies occasionally fail to thrive because their mother has been advised never to supplement.

PHYSICAL EXAMINATION

Bruises, welts and scars identify physical abuse. Bruises confined to the buttocks and lower back are almost always related to punishment. Finger and thumb prints may be found on the arms where a child was grabbed. Attempts to silence a screaming child with impatient, forced feedings may lead to bruising of the upper lip and frenulum. Human bite marks are distinctive, crescent-shaped areas of hyperpigmentation with light centers. When a blunt instrument is used in punishment, a bruise or welt will often resemble it in shape. Loop marks on the skin are secondary to a doubled-over cord or rope. Lash marks are seen after beating with a belt, tree branch or hard-edged ruler. Choke marks may be seen on the neck, and circumferential tie marks on the ankles or wrists. Bruises and scars may be found at multiple stages of healing. A mongolian spot may be mistaken for a bruise.

Approximately 10 per cent of cases of physical abuse involve *burns*. The commonest inflicted burn is from a cigarette. These are circular, punched-out areas of similar size. These lesions are often found on the palms or soles.

Dry contact burns can occur when the child is forcibly held against a radiator. These are usually second-degree burns without blister formation. They usually involve only one surface of the body or both palms.

Hot water burns are of several types. A dunking burn occurs when a parent holds the thighs against the abdomen and dunks the buttocks and perineum in scalding water as punishment for enuresis or resistance to toilet training. This results in a circular burn of the buttocks with a clear-cut water level on the thighs and waist. The hands and feet are spared, which is incompatible with falling into a tub or turning the hot water on while in the bathtub. Forcible immersion of a hand or foot as punishment can be suspected when a burn goes well above the wrist or ankle.

Ocular damage in the battered child syndrome may include acute hyphema, dislocated lens and detached retina. Over half of these injuries result in permanent impairment of vision in one or both eyes.

The most serious injury in terms of death and serious sequelae is a *subdural hematoma*. These children often present with coma and convulsions. Some have multiple skull fractures after being hit against a wall or door; over half have no fracture. Subdural hematomas without fracture used to be called spontaneous, but recent studies prove that the hematoma is due to violent shaking. The rapid acceleration and deceleration of the head as it bobs about leads to tearing of the bridging veins, with bleeding into the subdural space, usually bilaterally. Retinal hemorrhages are nearly always present and help to establish this diagnosis.

Intra-abdominal injuries are the second most common cause of death in battered children. These children present with recurrent vomiting, abdominal distention, absent bowel sounds or localized tenderness. The most common findings are tears of the mesentery or tears of the small intestine at sites of ligamental support such as the duodenum and proximal jejunum. Chylous ascites has been observed.

The child with failure to thrive usually has a weight that is below the third percentile and a height that is above the third percentile. Although growth curves help, failure to thrive is diagnosed mainly by the paucity of subcutaneous tissue. Reduction in subcutaneous tissue leads to a pinched face from lack of buccal fat pads, prominent ribs, wasted buttocks with much redundant skin, and spindly extremities. A common error is mistaking short stature for failure to thrive; of the 3 per cent of children who are under the third percentile in height, the majority are short but well nourished.

LABORATORY DATA

The diagnosis of inflicted bruises requires a demonstration of normal bleeding time, platelet count, partial thromboplastin time and prothrombin time. These can quickly determine whether the patient actually "bruises easily."

A child with failure to thrive and an otherwise normal physical examination requires very few baseline laboratory tests. A complete blood count, erythrocyte sedimentation rate, urine analysis, urine culture, stool pH, serum electrolyte determination, calcium level and BUN are adequate.

RADIOLOGIC FINDINGS

A radiologic survey for trauma consists of examination of the long bones, skull, ribs and pelvis, and should be obtained on all patients with suspected physical abuse or confirmed nutritional neglect. Usually no major fracture is present, but grasping, wrenching, twisting and jerking injuries to the long bones usually dislodge the periosteum and a corner of metaphysis. The chip fracture or corner fracture is visible immediately after the injury. From 10 to 14 days after injury the subperiosteal bleeding that has occurred will begin to calcify at the periphery and appear on the roentgenogram as an involucrum. The most diagnostic findings include multiple bone injuries at different stages of healing; these imply repeated assaults.

Rare bone disorders such as osteogenesis imperfecta, infantile cortical hyperostosis, scurvy, syphilis and neoplasms may resemble inflicted trauma, but a skilled radiologist can easily differentiate these entities.

DIAGNOSIS

DIAGNOSIS OF PHYSICAL ABUSE

Physical abuse may be diagnosed if an injury is unexplained or inadequately explained. Certain bruises, burns and scars are pathognomonic. Subdural hematomas do not occur spontaneously and are often secondary to violent shaking. Radiographic findings of chip fractures or multiple bony injuries at different stages of healing are also diagnostic.

DIAGNOSIS OF FAILURE TO THRIVE SECONDARY TO CALORIC DEPRIVATION

An attempt at nutritional rehabilitation is the starting point for reaching a definitive diagnosis in infants with failure to thrive. The child should be placed on unlimited feedings of a regular diet for age. A milk formula should be identical to the one used at home, since rapid weight gain on a formula free of cow's milk protein or lactose might have other causes than relief of caloric deprivation. The daily caloric intake should approach 150–200 cal/kg/day. This therapeutic trial of feeding should last a maximum of two weeks. The underweight infant who gains rapidly and easily in the hospital is a victim of underfeeding at home. A rapid weight gain of greater than 45 gm/day sustained for two weeks, or a gain of over 60 gm/day in a one-week period is diagnostic. In any case, the weight gain is significantly greater than it was during a similar period at home.

TREATMENT

When a physician sees a child whom he suspects of being abused or neglected, a logical plan of action should be initiated. The following steps are recommended:

Hospitalize Child. Any child suspected of having been abused requires hospitalization to protect him until evaluations regarding the safety of the home are completed. The reason given to the parents for the hospitalization is that his "injuries need to be watched." Potentially incriminating questions should be kept to a minimum in the outpatient setting. A more detailed history can be pursued once the child is safely admitted to the ward. If the parents refuse hospitalization, a court order can be obtained.

Treat Injuries or Malnutrition. Once the child is in the hospital, medical and surgical problems should be cared for in the usual manner. The primary physician will often require consultation from orthopedists, ophthalmologists, neurologists, neurosurgeons and plastic surgeons. Nutritional rehabilitation has already been described.

Maintain a Helping Approach to the Parents. This is the hardest step. Feeling angry with abusing parents is natural, but expressing this anger is very damaging to the establishment of a cooperative relationship. The physician should keep in mind that the injury occurred in a moment of anger, that it was not deliberate, and that abusing parents already feel inadequate and unloved. Confrontation, accusation and repeated interrogation must be avoided.

Tell Parents Diagnosis and Need to Report It. The parents must hear the diagnosis before it is reported. The physician can say: "I am obligated by state law to report any injury that is hard to explain." It is the physician's responsibility to do this, since the case is reported on the basis of his medical findings. He can add that a protective agency will be involved (not the police), that the matter will be kept confidential (not publicized in the newspaper), and that everyone's goal is to help the parents find better ways of dealing with their child (not to punish *them*).

Report to Protective Agency. A telephone call goes to the agency charged with children's protective services in the patient's county of residence within 24 hours of the child's admission.

Complete Official Written Report. The official medical report should be written by a physician within 48 hours and contain the following: (1) a concise history—the alleged cause of the injury (with dates and times), or of malnutrition; (2) results of physical examination—description of the injury (use nontechnical terms), or of the weight gain before and during hospitalization (in ounces per day, not in kilograms); (3) results of laboratory tests performed—e.g., blood studies and roentgenograms; and (4) a concluding statement as to why the findings represent nonaccidental trauma or severe underfeeding, as well as any special concerns regarding the child's safety.

Obtain Hospital Social Service Consultation. Within 72 hours the social worker should evaluate the safety of the home, how disturbed the parents are, how likely they are to accept therapy, the marital relationship and the totality of family problems. Occasionally the social worker will need assistance from a psychiatrist.

Attend Disposition Meeting. The hospital social worker, pediatrician, protective agency worker, occasionally a psychiatrist, and any other community agencies involved with the family should meet within three working days of the child's admission. All evaluations should have been completed. At this multidisciplinary, interagency meeting the best immediate and long-range plans for the patient should be decided.

Discharge Patient When Protective Agency Authorizes It. The protective agency decides whether the child needs court-enforced follow-up in the home, voluntary follow-up in the home or foster home placement. The pediatrician is obligated to keep the child in a protected environment until the safest course of action is determined.

Provide Medical Follow-up. The battered child needs more frequent well child care than the average child. Following discharge, he should be seen weekly for a while. He needs follow-up to detect any recurrence of abuse and to monitor weight gain. If he has sustained head injury, he needs follow-up for possible retardation, spasticity or subdural hematoma.

Functions of Protective Agency. The protective agency will provide psychosocial follow-up and treatment. Some innovative types of therapy that have been successful when designed for individual cases involve lay therapists or mothering aides, homemakers, parents' anonymous groups, telephone hotlines, day care centers, crisis nurseries, psychotherapy for the child, marital counseling, vocational rehabilitation, and others. The protective agency also makes home visits and locates the patient who becomes "lost to follow-up."

Testify in Court If This Is Needed. Most cases of child abuse are heard in Juvenile Court rather than in a criminal court. Petitions in the Juvenile Court are sustained on the basis of a "preponderance of evidence." The physician's statement that it is highly unlikely that the injury was due to an accident puts the burden on the parents to prove that they did not cause the accident. The purpose of the adjudicatory hearing is to sustain a dependency petition which will make the child a ward of the state for the next 6 to 12 months.

PROGNOSIS

If the child who has been physically abused is returned to his parents without any intervention, 5 per cent are killed and 35 per cent are seriously reinjured. Moreover, the untreated families tend to produce children who grow up to be juvenile delinquents and murderers, as well as the child batterers of the next generation.

Although weight loss and lack of stature from malnutrition are retrievable, brain growth and head circumference may not be. The child with nutritional neglect usually suffers from prolonged emotional deprivation and subsequent emotional problems. Some die from starvation; others sustain superimposed physical abuse.

BARTON D. SCHMITT
C. HENRY KEMPE

Abbott, S. L.: Gonococcal tonsillitis-pharyngitis in a 5-year-old girl. Pediatrics *52*:287, 1973.

Adelson, L.: Homicide by starvation. J.A.M.A. *186*:458, 1963.

Caffey, J.: Some traumatic lesions in growing bones other than fractures and dislocation: Clinical and radiological features. Brit. J. Radiol. *30*:225, 1957.

Caffey, J.: On the theory and practice of shaking infants. Am. J. Dis. Child. *127*:161, 1972.

Chase, H. P., and Martin, H. P.: Undernutrition and child development. New Engl. J. Med. *282*:933, 1970.

Fischhoff, J., Whitten, C. F., and Pettit, M. G.: A psychiatric study of mothers of infants with growth failure secondary to maternal deprivation. J. Pediatr. *79*:209, 1971.

Gillespie, R. W.: The battered child syndrome: Thermal and caustic manifestations. J. Trauma *5*:523, 1965.

Guthkelch, A. N.: Infantile subdural hematoma and its relationship to whiplash injuries. Brit. M. J. *3*:402, 1971.

Helfer, R. E., and Kempe, C. H.: The Battered Child. 2nd ed. University of Chicago, Chicago Press, 1973.

Hertzig, M. E., et al.: Intellectual levels of school children severely malnourished during the first two years of life. Pediatrics *49*:814, 1972.

Holter, J. C., and Friedman, S. B.: Child abuse: Early case finding in the emergency department. Pediatrics *42*:128, 1968.

Kempe, C. H.: Pediatric implications of the battered baby syndrome. Arch. Dis. Child. *46*:28, 1971.

Kempe, C. H., and Helfer, R. E.: Helping the Battered Child and His Family. Philadelphia, J. B. Lippincott Company, 1972.

Kempe, C. H., et al.: The battered child syndrome. J.A.M.A. *181*:14, 1962.

Klein, M., and Stern, L.: Low birth weight and the battered child syndrome. Am. J. Dis. Child. *122*:15, 1971.

Koel, B. S.: Failure to thrive and fatal injury as a continuum. Am. J. Dis. Child. *118*:565, 1969.

Kohler, E. E., and Good, T. A.: The infant who fails to thrive. Hosp. Pract. *4*(7):54, 1969.

Leonard, M. F., Rhymes, J. P., and Solnit, A. J.: Failure to thrive in infants. Am. J. Dis. Child. *111*:600, 1966.

Mushin, A. S.: Ocular damage in the battered-baby syndrome. Brit. M. J. *3*:402, 1971.

Pickel, S., Anderson, C., and Holiday, M. A.: Thirsting and hypernatremic dehydration—a form of child abuse. Pediatrics *45*:54, 1970.

Silverman, F. N.: Radiologic aspects of the battered child syndrome. *In* Helfer, R. E., and Kempe, C. H.: The Battered Child. Chicago, University of Chicago Press, 1968, p. 59.

Smith, S. M.: Child abuse syndrome. Brit. M. J. *3*:113, 1972.

Sussman, S. J.: Skin manifestations of the battered-child syndrome. J. Pediatr. *72*:99, 1968.

Touloukian, R. J.: Abdominal visceral injuries in battered children. Pediatrics *42*:642, 1968.

Whitten, C. F., Pettit, M. G., and Fischhoff, J.: Evidence that growth failure from maternal deprivation is secondary to undereating. J.A.M.A. *209*:1675, 1969.

DRUG ABUSE BY ADOLESCENTS

The abuse of drugs in adolescence can be considered an indication of the level of social and personal stress in current society. The abuse of drugs generates secondary problems ranging from innate toxicity to socially destructive behavior, and it is essential that the physician have a clear understanding of the *personality and motivation* of the drug-abusing youth, the *pharmacology and toxicology* of the major classes of drugs abused, and the *methods and resources for treatment and rehabilitation.* It is appropriate to ask how the use of drugs came to be perceived by adolescents as problem-solving behavior, and it may be of equal importance to be able to deal effectively with society's responses to the drug issue. The knowledgeable professional person can emphasize that youthful drug abuse is a behavioral disorder and should be managed in this perspective, and that inappropriate or regressive reactions on the part of the community through educational, governmental or law enforcement agencies ought to be avoided.

DEFINITIONS. The National Commission on Marihuana and Drug Abuse has listed the following drugs as subject to popular abuse: alcohol, marihuana, barbiturates, amphetamines, opiates, cocaine, hallucinogens and "others."

Public law and public discussion tend to regard alcohol (ethanol) as a beverage, food or relaxant rather than as a drug. A survey of American youth sponsored by the National Commission on Marihuana and Drug Abuse in 1973 revealed that 80 to 96 per cent considered barbiturates, amphetamines, and heroin to be drugs, whereas only 34 per cent so identified alcohol; but alcohol is a psychoactive substance like other drugs, with pharmacologic, toxic and lethal doses. American youth are apparently using alcohol in increasing numbers, owing possibly to the relative acceptance of its use by parents and public authorities.

The use of opiates chiefly involves heroin, which has been used in recent years by an increasingly young group of adolescents. The experiential reward of opiates seems to exceed that of other drugs, and physical dependency is most likely to follow continued use.

The adolescent drug user may be concerned with two types of stimulants today, cocaine and the amphetamines. Cocaine is one of the most expensive "street" drugs; it is often combined with heroin and rarely used as the primary drug. During the 1960's and early 1970's amphetamines have come to rate among the most popular drugs used by youth and young adults.

Natural hallucinogens include mescaline (peyote), psilocybin (mushroom), and datura (jimson weed). Street drugs sold as either mescaline or psilocybin rarely contain the stated drug (Table 2–12).

The synthetic hallucinogens were discovered accidentally, when ingestion of LSD (lysergic acid diethylamide) produced its hallucinogenic effect in an investigator. LSD has been joined by dimethyltryptamine (DMT), dimethoxymethyl amphetamine (DOM or "STP") and others. The ease of synthesis of LSD led in the 1960's to its wide dispersion among college youth and then among adolescents. Research has continued on such medical applications of LSD as the treatment of depression in terminal cancer, but most LSD usage has been self-administered for hallucinatory experiences. Scientific study of LSD usage has suggested chromosomal damage, congenital malformations, postingestion psychoses and mental deterioration, but proof of cause and effect relationships is not convincing in these respects. Clinical experience does indicate, however, that prolonged or recurrent use of LSD can in some individuals produce a syndrome of dissociative behavior that outlasts the immediate pharmacologic phase of action.

The Marihuana Tax Act of 1937 made possession of marihuana a criminal act. In spite of this prohibition, marihuana has become almost universally available. In January, 1972, the National Commission on Marihuana and Drug Abuse reported that 24,600,000 Americans had reported using marihuana and 8,340,000 were admitted current users. This survey revealed that 14 per cent of American youth had used marihuana and 7 per cent were regular users. It is probable that the single greatest problem of marihuana use in the United States has been the contradiction between the experience of marihuana use and the dangers advertised and purported by law enforcement agencies. There appears to be a trend now to a more liberal legal position toward use of marihuana and toward a more objec-

TABLE 2–12 ANALYSES OF "STREET" DRUGS*

PURPORTED CONTENT	NUMBER OF SAMPLES	ACTUAL CONTENT†
Mescaline	163	LSD – 114 LSD & PCP – 16 STP (DOM) – 4 PCP – 6 Mescaline – 1 No drug – 10
Psilocybin	56	LSD – 41 LSD & PCP – 6 LSD & PCP & amphetamine – 1 PCP – 2 No drug – 6
Tetrahydrocannabinol (THC)	29	PCP – 26 Librium – 1 THC – 1

†STP = dimethoxymethylamphetamine (DOM); PCP = phencyclidine; THC = tetrahydrocannabinol; LSD = lysergic acid diethyamide.

*Compiled and abstracted from: (1) Maryland Anonymous Drug Testing Service, University of Maryland School of Pharmacy; Pharm-Chem Analysis; (2) Anonymous, in Phar-Chem Newsletter, Vol. 1, No. 7, 1972; and (3) Bulletin of Pacific Information Services on Street Drugs, University of the Pacific School of Pharmacy, 1969–1972.

tive consideration of its medical as well as recreational potential.

Numerous other psychoactive substances have been used by young people in their search for recreation, status and relief from stress, including solvents, hairsprays, deodorants, fuels, cleaning fluids, and many stimulants, sedatives and analgesics available without prescription or not under legal control. The ultimate game of the drug user is a form of pharmacologic "roulette," in which pills of unknown or untried effect are taken just to see what will happen.

The hydrocarbon and fluorocarbon inhalants deserve special consideration. These compounds are exemplified by the toluene used in model airplane glue and the freon in aerosol spray products, and can produce significant intoxication and hallucinogenic experiences. Rebreathing them in paper or plastic bags may produce anoxia, cardiac arrhythmias and death.

The efficiency is remarkable with which information is transmitted through the youth subculture as new psychoactive substances are identified. An example of this is the rapid recognition and adoption of methaqualone (Quaalude and other brands) in the early 1970's as a "safe" and preferred intoxicant. At first promoted as an innocuous nonbarbiturate sedative, the adoption of this drug led rapidly to a new vocabulary ("luding out," "sopors"), and in a period of one to two years to a special act of Congress which added it to the list of controlled substances (Methaqualone Act of 1973, S-1253).

CLINICAL FEATURES. In 1964 the WHO Expert Committee on Addiction-producing Drugs refined the nomenclature of drug abuse, recommending that the term "drug dependence" replace the terms "drug addiction" and "drug habituation," which had failed to make clear distinctions. Drug dependence was defined as a "state arising from repeated administration of a drug on a periodic or continuing basis. Its characteristics will vary with the agent involved, and this must be made clear by designating the particular type of drug dependence in each specific case; i.e., drug dependence of the morphine type, of cocaine type, etc."

Drug dependency as defined by the WHO includes one or more of the following:

1. A desire or need to continue taking the drug, which may vary in intensity from a simple desire for the subjective effects to an overpowering desire to obtain the drug by any means; the degree of desire is related to the specific physical and psychologic effects of the drug used.
2. A tendency to increase the dose owing to the development of tolerance.
3. A psychic dependence on the effects of the drug, related to a subjective and individual appreciation of those effects.
4. A physical dependence on the effects of the drug, requiring its presence for maintenance of homeostasis and resulting in a definite, characteristic and self-limited abstinence syndrome when the drug is withdrawn.

Adolescents may achieve drug dependency comparable to that of adults in respect to the duration of use, drug-seeking behavior and resistance to giving up drugs. Adolescents are distinguished from adults in their choice of multiple drugs (polypharmacy), in their sense of invulnerability and in their delay in psychosocial maturation with chronic drug use. They respond less well than adults to the intense confrontations and pressures to achieve independence which are typical of some adult rehabilitation programs.

Data regarding adolescent drug dependence are contaminated by folklore, misconceptions and unsubstantiated theory; and the testimony of drug-dependent adults has been applied to youth without taking into account developmental differences. A study of the behavioral characteristics of drug-dependent adolescents at the University of Connecticut Health Center's Adolescent Drug Dependency Program may provide perspective: among drug users ranging in age from 10 to 17 years 60 per cent were boys, and the drugs purportedly used were heroin, LSD, phencyclidine (PCP), peyote, mescaline, "STP," tetrahydrocannabinol (THC), hashish (HASH), amphetamines (including methamphetamine, or "speed"), barbiturates, alcohol, cocaine, methaqualone, gasoline, various cleaning fluids, aerosol deodorants (freon), glue (toluene), methylchloroform, and an assortment of tranquilizers and unidentified compounds; the duration of drug use was over six months in 85 per cent of the patients, over one year in 65 per cent, and over two years in 45 per cent.

Many of the youngsters in the Connecticut study claimed to be taking peyote, mescaline, psilocybin or pure THC, but what users report they use and actually buy may be quite different. Analyses indicate that there is little mescaline, psilocybin or pure THC among "street" drugs in the United States. Table 2–12 summarizes three studies which showed that drugs sold as mescaline, psilocybin or THC were far more likely to contain LSD (sometimes with PCP), or PCP alone, or other substitutes. Heroin, amphetamine, cocaine, LSD and marihuana are less subject to misrepresentation, according to the same studies.

Drug-seeking behavior includes stealing, trafficking in drugs ("dealing") and prostitution. Fifty-five per cent of the Connecticut study group acknowledged theft in order to obtain funds for their drugs, with the heroin-dependent youth most committed to this behavior. Shoplifting is common.

Prostitution was generally limited to heroin-dependent girls. Sexual promiscuity was common among users of all classes of drugs; the sexual activity of users increases their exposure to venereal disease.

As among adults, dealing in drugs may be for adolescents the safest and most lucrative means of maintaining one's own supply. The market is active, the overhead is low, and the risk of detection may be less than that of being caught at petty theft or burglary.

Sociocultural factors appear to influence the choice of drugs. Inner city youth tend to use three or fewer drugs, often developing dependency on opiates and/or cocaine; alcohol and barbiturates are becoming more popular. Among suburban youth polypharmacy is more the rule, the typical suburban youth using more than six or seven different compounds, the choice of drugs largely reflecting their availability. It is not uncommon to find heroin, "speed," a hallucinogen, and barbiturates all used within one week's time. This pattern is quite different from the drug abuse behavior of adults.

The class of drugs used influences the drug-seeking behavior. Dependency on opiates is as much as thirty times more expensive than dependency on hallucinogens, stimulants or hypnotic-sedatives. As a result, there is greater risk-taking among opiate-dependent youth; this generates patterns of exploitive behavior which might otherwise be rejected. Stealing from friends and family, deceit and prostitution are accepted by these users as necessary to support their "habit"; but in periods of remission, when these adolescents are concerned about their damaged self-image or self-esteem, these activities are perceived as unacceptable. Recidivism is as high as with adults.

Many youth in the subculture using nonopiate drugs are in rebellion against adult and societal standards and will display a sense of invulnerability both in their indiscriminate use of intoxicants and in provocative antisocial behavior ranging from petty theft to running away from home. This sense of invulnerability is comparable to that of the adolescent diabetic who denies his need for insulin or of the sexually active girl who denies the need for contraception. This behavior tends to be more self-destructive than exploitive in character, and this feature is important in planning rehabilitation programs.

An abstinence syndrome due to physiologic dependence occurs with opiates, barbiturates and alcohol. A limited form is observed in chronic amphetamine dependency. Table 2–13 lists the characteristic symptoms.

Among adolescents who use opiates, the abstinence syndrome is notorious, fear and anxiety being generated by folklore. There is no evidence that adolescents experience withdrawal any differently from adults, but the syndrome tends to be milder because duration of dependency and the dose levels tend to be less. The symptoms of withdrawal can be severe, but death is not likely. The barbiturate abstinence syndrome may result in convulsions and death unless either the primary drug or an analog is given in gradually decreasing doses. Since the barbiturate withdrawal syndrome generally requires a barbiturate intake of over 200 mg/day for more than three to four weeks, it is rarely encountered in adolescents. The alcohol withdrawal syndrome is also unusual in adolescents, again as a function of dose and duration of use.

Among youth who have prolonged regular use of the hallucinogens and stimulants, there is a syndrome which they describe as having one's "mind messed up." Characteristics include poor interpersonal relationships, distortions of time and place, and dissociative behavior. These symptoms persist in the intervals between drug ingestion. With sustained abstinence the syndrome appears to be self-limited, but flashbacks (brief dissociative or hallucinatory experiences without further drug ingestion) may continue to occur for many months.

TABLE 2–13 ABSTINENCE SYNDROMES

Opiates:	Onset 4 to 8 hours after last dose; yawning, lacrimation, rhinorrhea, agitation, mydriasis, insomnia, piloerection, abdominal cramps, diarrhea, systolic hypertension, tachycardia
Barbiturates:	Onset 12 to 16 hours after last dose; anxiety, twitching, tremor, weakness, vertigo, visual distortions, nausea, vomiting, postural hypotension, convulsions, delirium, death
Alcohol:	Tremor, hallucinations, delirium tremens
Amphetamines:	Apathy, psychomotor retardation, sleep disturbance

Physical dependency may be feared among adolescents using hallucinogens, stimulants or sedatives, but it is rarely a problem. Psychologic dependency, on the other hand, may produce as intense a craving as opiate dependency. High recidivism is related to persistent or recurrent stress and to specific rebellion against controls. Sometimes the return to drugs represents the adolescent's testing of the commitment of the therapeutic team to his help and support.

TREATMENT. The treatment of drug abuse behavior has three phases: acute (withdrawal), short term (motivation to change) and long term (rehabilitation).

The acute phase involves not only coping with physical and psychologic effects of the drug, possibly in overdose, but also decision-making regarding and in anticipation of withdrawal. It may include separation of the adolescent from the environment in which drug-taking behavior is generated.

Table 2–14 summarizes the typical behavioral and physical signs of acute drug reactions. It is important to identify accurately the precise drug taken when there is evidence of overdose, of abstinence syndrome or of psychologic decompensation; but the history is often unreliable and the content of street drugs uncertain. Careful inquiry as to the patient's behavior after ingestion or injection of the drug is often more valuable than the report of the patient or his colleagues as to the agent taken. Inappropriate or even dangerous potentiation of pharmacologic responses may occur if treatment is instituted on the basis of testimony alone.

TABLE 2–14 CHARACTERISTICS OF ABUSED DRUGS AND THEIR ACUTE REACTIONS IN ADOLESCENTS

CLASS	EXAMPLE	ROUTE	BEHAVIORAL SIGNS	PHYSICAL SIGNS	MEDICAL COMPLICATIONS
Opiates	Heroin, methadone morphine	Subcutaneous, intranasal, intravenous	Euphoria, lethargy to coma	Constricted pupils, respiratory depression, cyanosis, rales	Injection site infection, hepatitis, bacterial endocarditis, amenorrhea, peptic ulcer, pulmonary edema, tetanus
Hypnotic-sedatives	Barbiturates, glutethimide	Oral, intravenous	Slurred speech, ataxia, short attention span, drowsiness, combative, violent	Constricted pupils (barbiturates), dilated pupils (glutethimide), needle marks	Injection site infection, hepatitis, endocarditis
	Alcohol	Oral	As above		Gastritis, CNS depression
Stimulants	Amphetamines	Oral, subcutaneous, intravenous	Hyperactive, insomnia, anorexic paranoia, personality change, irritability	Hypertension, weight loss, dilated pupils	Injection site infections, hepatitis, endocarditis, psychosis, depression
	Cocaine	Intravenous, intranasal	Restless, hyperactive, occ. depression or paranoia	Hypertension, tachycardia	Nausea, vomiting, inflammation or perforation of nasal septum
Hallucinogens	LSD, THC, PCP, STP (DOM), mescaline, DMT*	Oral	Euphoria, dysphoria, hallucinations, confusion, paranoia	Dilated pupils, occ. hypertension, hyperthermia, piloerection	Primarily psychiatric with high risk to individuals with unrecognized or previous psychiatric disorder
Hydrocarbons, fluorocarbons	Glue (toluene)	Inhalant	Euphoria, confusion, general intoxication	Nonspecific	Secondary trauma, asphyxiation from plastic bag used to inhale fumes
	Cleaning fluid (trichloroethylene)	Inhalant	Euphoria, confusion, general intoxication, vomiting, abdominal pain	Oliguria, jaundice	Hepatitis, renal injury
	Aerosol sprays (freon)	Inhalant	Euphoria, dysphoria, slurred speech, hallucinations	Nonspecific	Psychiatric
Cannabis	Marihuana, hashish, THC	Smoke, oral	Mild intoxication and simple euphoria to hallucination (dose-related)	Occ. tachycardia, delayed response time, poor coordination	Occ. psychiatric, with depressive or anxiety reactions

*For abbreviations, see Table 2–12.

Acute therapy requires individualization of management, focused upon evolving symptoms. In the treatment of an acute drug reaction it is rarely necessary to use medication, except in the case of the respiratory depression of opiate overdose, when nalorphine or naloxone may be required, and in the case of barbiturate dependency, when there is a need for gradual lowering of the dose of the drug.

The use of methadone in detoxification of youthful opiate users may be necessary if they have acquired adult levels of use; it is more common, however, to find that adolescent opiate users are receiving low doses of heroin and that their withdrawal from the drug involves relatively mild symptoms. The time needed for detoxification varies with the dose generally taken, and may be from three to eight days. Severe anxiety may exist about the horrors of the abstinence syndrome; in such cases chlorpromazine or diazepam may be useful.

In the case of stimulants, hallucinogens, inhalant hydrocarbons or fluorocarbons, or cannabis, the primary treatment for an acute drug reaction is psychologic support, which should include close and sympathetic human contact in a nonthreatening environment.

In the case of primarily psychologic dependency, withdrawal from the environment is as important as withdrawal from the drug itself. Either an acute reaction or an attempt at termination of chronic intake requires an environment with low levels of stimulation that provides human contacts conveying understanding and a wish to be helpful without condescension or censure.

In some adult treatment programs, the "ex-addict" has played a useful role in therapy through his having shared a common experience, the latter purported to give him superior ability to understand and to relate to the patient. Among adolescents, a young adult or older adolescent who is warm, accepting and flexible is preferable to an ex-addict as a therapist or paraprofessional. Adolescents tend to respect a contemporary's success in personal and social adjustment.

The second or *motivation* phase of treatment has the goal of establishing in the adolescent both a sense of self-worth and a commitment to self-help. The philosophy is basically the same without regard to the drug used, so long as one recognizes and adjusts for the different urgencies of craving and drug-seeking behavior with different past experiences.

The motivation phase begins with a relationship of acceptance and trust between patient and professional staff, or with the youthful paraprofessional who may be part of the team. A thorough evaluation is made of the adolescent's physical, psychologic, educational and vocational status, culminating in an assessment of his assets and deficits. The goal is a realistic appraisal of his potential, from which attainable alternative objectives can be identified. Most drug-dependent youth have a long history of maladaptive experiences, often including family conflict, school failure and legal entanglements or delinquency. Many also have significant psychiatric symptoms, such as depression or passive-aggressive behavior patterns, and a few will be so severely disabled as to require formal psychiatric intervention.

The *rehabilitative phase* can begin when the drug-dependent youth has decided with the concurrence of supportive adults that he wants to change and can change. This requires him to be ready to substitute dependency on people for dependency on chemicals. Rehabilitation may proceed either in a residential or in an ambulatory setting, depending on the suitability of the patient's natural environment and the current strength of his own commitment. Alternative educational models, work-study programs, vocational education, group homes, group and individual therapy, and family therapy offer a variety of modalities for the rehabilitation process.

Psychologic dependency and craving must be accounted for in designing a rehabilitation program. For this reason the reaching out to the rebellious youth with understanding, the setting of clear limits and firm discipline are essential. In whatever phase of treatment, both the adolescent and the adults constituting his support system must be prepared for recidivism and have a plan for reentry into the treatment process. The return to drug dependency must be understood as a failure in treatment of a behavioral disorder and not as a disciplinary failure.

In dealing with drug-related behavior of youth it is important that the physician examine his own philosophy of use of drugs, that he be able to define and distinguish between their use and abuse, that he understand the difference between physical dependency and psychologic dependency, that he be able to differentiate self-determination from exploitation in his patient, and that he be able to separate the personal danger to his patient from the legal danger.

ROBERT A. KRAMER

Blum, R. H., et al.: Society and Drugs. Vol. I. San Francisco, Jossey-Bass, 1969, pp. 98–114.

Brill, L., and Lieberman, L.: Major Modalities in the Treatment of Drug Abuse. New York, Behavioral Publications, 1972.

Drug Use in America: Problem in Perspective. Second Report of the National Commission on Marihuana and Drug Abuse. Washington, D.C., U.S. Government Printing Office, March, 1973.

Kramer, J. C.: Controlling narcotics in America. Drug Forum *1*:51, 1971.

Kramer, R. A.: Behavioral characteristics of drug dependency in the young adolescent. Proceedings of the 30th International Congress on Alcoholism and Drug Dependence. Amsterdam, 1972.

Kramer, R. A., and Pierpoli, P.: Hallucinogenic effect of propellant components of deodorant sprays. Pediatrics *48*:322–323, 1971.

Kupperstein, L. R., and Susman, R. M.: A bibliography on the inhalation of glue fumes and other toxic vapors—A substance abuse practice among adolescents. Int. J. Addictions *3*:177–197, 1968.

Snyder, S.: Uses of Marijuana. New York, Oxford University Press, 1971.

WHO Expert Committee on Addiction Producing Drugs, Thirteenth Report. Geneva, Wld. Hlth. Org. Techn. Rep. Series, Publication 273, 1964.

DISORDERS OF COMMUNICATION

HEARING DISORDERS

Hearing is the principal sensory pathway through which speech and verbal communication develop. Learning and other aspects of maturation are also influenced by hearing. Since even mild impairment of hearing may significantly hinder the development of the child, early diagnosis is essential. Impaired hearing may not be obvious, however, and the child may not sense or express his difficulty; accordingly, diagnosis is often delayed.

GENERAL CONSIDERATIONS. The human ear responds to frequencies of sound ranging from 20 to 20,000 Hertz (cycles per second), but receives speech and most environmental sounds in the frequency range of 400 to 3000 Hertz, at varying levels of intensity (loudness). Impairments of hearing affect perception of both the intensity and the frequency of sound.

In some hearing impairments the main deficiency is a reduction in the loudness of sound. If a moderate reduction is even or nearly even throughout the frequency range, speech sounds are muffled but not otherwise distorted in clarity, and there is little difficulty in discrimination of their meaning.

The clarity of sounds is determined by both their intensity and their frequency spectrum. If certain frequencies are perceived less perfectly than others, speech sounds may be distorted and the discrimination of their meaning is difficult.

The severity of the handicap imposed by a hearing impairment depends upon which components of sound are primarily affected and to what degree. In general the younger the child affected, the greater the functional disability.

MEASUREMENT OF HEARING AND CLASSIFICATION OF HEARING DISORDERS. The measurement of hearing acuity is concerned with (1) the intensity level at which sounds are perceived and (2) the ability of the person to discriminate and recognize the meaning of complex sounds, particularly those of speech.

Hearing acuity is measured by delivery to the auditory apparatus of pure tones at specific frequencies from a standardized audiometer. Level of intensity is measured in decibel units. The tone is delivered to the external auditory canal to measure air conduction and to the mastoid tip to measure bone conduction. Normally the levels of perception by the two routes are equal, as measured by the audiometer. In certain instances, such as when disease involves the middle ear, air conduction will be diminished in comparison with bone conduction. Whenever the air conduction and bone conduction are about equally involved in hearing loss, this finding is suggestive of a sensorineural defect.

For measurement of discrimination between individual sounds, techniques other than pure-tone audiometry must be used. A variety of tests have been developed to measure speech reception threshold (the least intensity level at which words are heard) and speech discrimination (the ability to make fine phonetic discriminations). Other types of hearing tests have been developed to aid in delineation of the exact nature and severity of hearing impairments.

Impairments of hearing are difficult to classify, since many variables are involved. Designations such as "hard of hearing" or "deaf" have led to confusion, both among the public and among physicians. The important consideration must be the effect of a hearing impairment on the functioning of the child as a whole.

If a person perceives sound at levels between 0 and 20 decibels at all the frequencies commonly tested in the human speech range, hearing is considered to be normal. If greater than 20 decibels intensity is required for perception of sound at any frequency in the speech range (400 to 3000 Hertz) or if there is any difficulty in discrimination of sound, hearing is considered abnormal. With losses between 20 and 30 decibels (mild loss), speech reception becomes difficult, and the person must strain to hear. With losses of 40 decibels (moderate) or more, only the peaks of loudness of conversational speech can be heard, and speech reception becomes very difficult without amplification or lip reading.

Hearing acuity cannot be classified in terms of decibels alone. If certain frequencies are affected more than others, speech sounds are distorted, and misunderstanding of words results. The problem becomes not so much that speech cannot be heard, but that it cannot be translated. The high-frequency sounds of speech are most commonly affected.

Even in the so-called deaf child with the most profound impairment of hearing, some residual hearing is generally present, particularly in the low frequencies. This fact has important implications for the use of amplification and in the education of these children.

TYPES OF HEARING DEFECTS

Conductive Defects. Conductive defects result most commonly from pathologic changes in the middle ear. These include congenital or acquired abnormalities of the ossicles, the presence of fluid, adhesions, or other material in the middle ear, and congenital atresia or other obstructions of the external canal. Conductive defects are the most common of hearing impairments in children. They are most often of mild degree and are amenable to medical or surgical therapy.

In conductive defects, reception of sound at most frequencies is affected to essentially the same degree. The main effect on sound is a reduction in loudness, but clarity is not distorted. Mild conductive losses frequently remain undetected, particularly when the loss is unilateral.

Sensorineural Defects. Sensorineural defects result from abnormalities of the inner ear or the auditory nerve. High frequencies tend to be more affected than low tones, but with more severe involvement acuity for both high and low tones is impaired. In any event, sounds appear distorted and discrimination is made difficult.

Sensorineural defects generally result in a greater handicap to communication than do conductive losses. They are rarely amenable to medical or surgical therapy.

Central Auditory Defects. Central auditory defects are extremely complex, and their cause and pathogenesis poorly understood. The peripheral auditory apparatus appears to convey stimuli adequately, and the affected child seems to be aware of sound but unable to discriminate its meaning.

The incidence of central auditory dysfunction may be increasing as more children survive formerly fatal conditions of early infancy with impairment of certain sensory functions. Moreover, certain lifesaving drugs may affect the auditory system. Central auditory defects cause severe problems in communication.

Psychogenic Loss of Hearing. Apparent loss of hearing of psychogenic origin is not uncommon and is often difficult to differentiate from that due to organic causes. The patient commonly presents exaggerated symptoms of hearing impairment, which may be unilateral or bilateral. There is often a history of prior ear infections or of preexisting organic loss of hearing; the ear thus appears to act as a "shock organ" for localization of the psychic symptoms. It is important that malingering be distinguished from pure psychogenic impairment. Appropriate specialized audiologic techniques combined with careful clinical appraisal can usually make the differentiation possible.

ETIOLOGY OF HEARING DEFECTS. Hearing defects may be *congenital,* including heritable types, or *acquired.* The conductive and the sensorineural defects have, for the most part, different causations.

Inherited Defects. An increasing number of hearing defects, particularly of the sensorineural type, are known to be genetically determined. Despite genetic transmission, the defect may not express itself until late in life. Thorough investigation of families with history of hearing defects is essential. Many defects are associated with other disorders, such as pigmentary defects, or renal or thyroid disease. Some heritable disorders may be associated with abnormalities of the external ear or ear canal which lead to conductive losses.

Prenatal or Perinatal Factors. Rubella in the early months of pregnancy, and possibly other maternal infections of viral or other origins, may affect the auditory system of the fetus. Bilirubin encephalopathy (kernicterus) has a predilection for damage to the auditory system. Premature and other low-birth-weight infants and infants suffering from trauma or hypoxia at birth are at high risk for the development of hearing defects.

Acquired Defects. Most conductive defects are acquired, most commonly from the accumulation of fluid in the middle ear. This fluid may result from repeated infections of the middle ear, may be associated with respiratory allergy, or may stem from other causes. It may lead to adhesions or even to destruction of the ossicular chain.

Sensorineural defects also may be acquired. Hearing impairment may be a sequel of meningitis, of certain viral infections, and of mumps in particular.

Certain drugs such as streptomycin, kanamycin, and possibly gentamicin, have specific ototoxic effects, which may be greater in infants than in older children owing to increased susceptibility of the developing auditory system.

DIAGNOSIS OF HEARING IMPAIRMENTS. The diagnosis of impaired hearing may be difficult. Children rarely complain of difficulty in hearing, and even those with the most profound impairments compensate for their defects in many ways. Essential to the diagnosis are a high degree of suspicion on the part of the physician, and an awareness that certain children are at high risk for the development of hearing disorders.

In addition to clinical evaluation, the detection of impaired hearing is aided by audiometric screening techniques. The definitive diagnosis of the exact nature and severity of a hearing defect is dependent upon the use of specialized audiologic procedures.

Clinical Diagnosis. Conductive defects may be present in infancy, but most commonly they are not manifested until the child is older. The loss of hearing is usually of mild to moderate degree.

In the younger child the presenting complaint is often that the child pays little attention to the parents' commands. Parents frequently feel or may be told that such a child is stubborn or that he is "normal and will outgrow it." Conductive defects in the younger age group are undoubtedly more common than is recognized.

In the older child hearing difficulty may first be suspected by the parents or detected by audiometric screening examination at school or in the physician's office. The signs of a hearing defect are, however, frequently unrecognized by parents or by others. Even on direct questioning the child with a hearing loss may deny difficulty. The presenting symptoms may be scholastic difficulty, inattentiveness, or change in personality. If the loss of hearing remains unrecognized, the symptoms will become more severe, with distressing consequences to the child.

Speech disturbances due to conductive defects are less common than those due to sensorineural losses, but if such a hearing loss has existed from infancy, a speech disorder may result.

Detection of mild to moderate conductive losses by clinical evaluation alone is difficult. The child's ability to hear speech at close range does not rule out a handicapping hearing loss. For example, a child with only a 20- to 25-decibel loss is able to hear conversational voice in a face-to-face situation. Under other conditions, as in a large classroom, this same degree of loss will prevent him from hearing adequately. Furthermore, the loss of hearing may be unilateral, making its detection even more difficult.

A history of chronic nasal obstruction, of recurrent otitis media, or of persistently abnormal appearance of the tympanic membranes suggests the possibility of a conductive defect.

Since sensorineural defects, in general, produce more severe impairment of hearing function than do the conductive ones, it would seem that they should persist in some more obvious way, but this is not the case. The sensorineural defects may be of mild to moderate degree and may be unilateral; in such instances the symptomatology and the differential diagnostic considerations are similar to those of the conductive defects.

Because sensorineural losses of hearing may involve only certain frequencies, the child may respond to most sounds at ordinary levels of loudness. He may fail to hear only high-pitched sounds. This kind of loss is least appreciated by parents and teachers, and it is not uncommon to find high-frequency losses in children previously thought to have normal hearing.

A most important factor in diagnosis of a hearing defect, besides its severity, is its time of onset. If hearing loss of moderate to profound degree is present before the normal time for acquisition of speech, the presenting symptom will likely be failure to speak, or delayed or distorted speech. If the loss occurs after acquisition of speech, other symptoms will predominate. In any instance of delayed or distorted speech, however, the presence of an auditory defect must be considered.

A common pitfall in evaluation of losses of hearing in infants is the history that the child said words at one time. Even the deaf child may babble in the first months of life, and may produce such sounds as ma-ma, da-da and ba, which may be interpreted as meaningful words. Babbling tends to decrease if the hearing defect is marked, and the deaf child tends to be relatively silent after the first year of life. There is, however, variability in the amount of sound an individual deaf child makes and in the time at which he becomes more silent. The presence or absence of vocalizations or sound production is not, therefore, an infallible indicator of deafness.

In the older child the onset of a sensorineural defect may present as an obvious decrease in auditory acuity. Commonly, however, the presenting symptoms are a decrease in scholastic achievement or change in personality. Older children with organic defects are frequently considered to be malingerers.

The clinical manifestations of the central auditory disorders may be variable. In general, they are similar to those of the child with a severe sensorineural defect.

Screening Audiometry. With increasing frequency mass surveys of hearing are being instituted in the schools of the United States. These surveys utilize audiometers which deliver pure tones under standardized conditions. Children found to have losses of 20 decibels or more in one or more frequencies tested should be suspected of having a significant hearing impairment and be referred for further otologic and audiologic evaluation. Though some of these children prove to have only transient or insignificant hearing losses, these screening programs detect many children with significant losses who otherwise would have remained undetected.

Screening audiometry is also being used with increasing frequency in physicians' offices. It is of particular value in determining whether or for how long hearing loss follows otitis media and for the detection of otherwise unsuspected hearing impairment.

Pure-tone audiometry can be used with relative reliability in children from about the age of 3 years. For screening of younger children, procedures have been developed which use such sound generators as tissue paper for high tones and other appropriate noise-makers for lower tones. These procedures require that the infant's attention be first directed away from the sound source, and then the sound delivered. The infant's response is observed, such as quieting, turning toward the sound, or eye blinking. With experience the physician or a trained assistant can perform these tests with considerable reliability, even for infants under 1 year of age. If obvious responses are repeatedly obtained, it can be assumed that there is no loss of hearing sufficient to interfere with function. If the infant fails to respond, if his responses are variable, or if there is any doubt on the part of the examiner, the patient should be referred for more thorough evaluation.

Owing to the importance of early detection of hearing loss, auditory screening of newborn infants has been recommended; but the results of mass screening programs of newborns have been inconsistent and possibly misleading. Further research is required to determine the reliability and validity of available techniques. At the present time routine auditory screening of newborn infants is not recommended. In newborn and other young infants, however, the responses produced in the electroencephalogram by sound stimuli may be a valuable means for detection of hearing impairment. This procedure has its greatest value in testing of newborn infants who are at high risk of hearing impairment, such as those born to mothers who have had rubella or other infections during pregnancy.

Definitive audiologic evaluation utilizes, besides pure-tone audiometry, speech reception and speech discrimination tests and a variety of other specialized techniques. These procedures require the services of a skilled audiologist.

TREATMENT. Conductive defects are due mainly to disturbances within the middle ear, and most of them are amenable to medical or surgical therapy. Appropriate treatment of acute infections of the middle ear and the prevention of chronic infections will greatly reduce the incidence of impaired hearing. Serous otitis media is probably the single most common cause. Though its etiology may be imperfectly understood, its impairment of hearing can be ameliorated. Appropriate therapy of respiratory allergy will also reduce the incidence of conductive hearing impairments. Other causes of eustachian tube obstruction, such as hypertrophied adenoids or anatomic abnormalities, are less common causes of conductive defects.

For children with sensorineural defects the principal modes of therapy are audiologic and educational. The management of these children requires the services of skilled specialists in many disciplines, particularly in otology, audiology, psychology, and special education. Management extends over a long time, and it is essential that someone be identified who will coordinate the efforts of the various specialists involved; preferably this should be the child's physician.

Most children with moderate sensorineural defects will probably need a hearing aid, auditory training, lip reading instruction, and language training. The type of amplification required can be determined only after precise audiologic evaluation, best conducted by an audiologist skilled with children. Special educational adjustments will also be required in most instances. Most affected children will be able to attend regular schools, so long as they may have continued access to such supplementary speech, language, and auditory training as is necessary.

For children with more profound hearing defects special schooling may be required, but even children with profound losses, so-called "deaf" children, may have reasonable expectation for achievement of normal education. Full development of this potential, however, is almost totally dependent upon early diagnosis of the hearing defect.

The management of children with central auditory dysfunctions is extremely difficult and requires extensive and prolonged individual therapy with persons especially trained to work with these problems. The prognosis for the development of adequate communication is generally guarded.

Richard W. Olmsted

SPEECH AND LANGUAGE DEVELOPMENT AND DISORDERS

Disorders of speech and language in childhood are not uncommon. Therapy for them requires understanding of those processes involved in the normal development of speech and language function.

DEVELOPMENT OF SPEECH AND LANGUAGE. Development of speech and language skills depends upon a broad range of activities of many organ systems. The first stage, audition, requires an intact peripheral auditory mechanism. The second stage is the transmission of sound from the organs of hearing to the brain and the organization of the transmitted impulses for a response. The third stage, the verbal response, involves respiration, phonation, resonation, and articulation. A high degree of intricate cortical and neuromuscular integration is required for all these activities.

The processes involved in development of speech and language are highly vulnerable, since the organ systems on which they depend have more urgent biologic functions to serve than communication. For example, the basic function of the respiratory apparatus is gas exchange; of the larynx, air control; and of the articulators, mastication of food. These functions take precedence over those of communication, since man can function, albeit inadequately, without being able to hear or speak. Thus illness, trauma, and other factors may result in disruption of the "unnecessary" function of communication, either temporarily or permanently. Awareness of this instability of the process of communication is essential to the understanding of speech and language disorders.

Normal Speech and Language Development. Maturation of a child's speech and language normally keeps pace with the maturation of the total organism, and follows a fairly predictable pattern up to the age of about 6 years.

The early stages of speech and language development reflect the child's reception of speech sounds and are revealed by his responses to them. By 4 to 6 months the infant normally demonstrates ability to discriminate among speech sounds by beginning to babble close approximations of a number of the early consonant sounds, principally *m, n, p, b, k, g, t* and *d*. By 6 to 8 months he has learned to enjoy making these sounds and should exhibit a rather wide repertory of babbling combinations of these consonants with a few vowels such as *ba-ba, ma-ma, da-da, goo,* and so on.

By about 9 months the child further demonstrates his ability to discriminate among various inputs by imitating changes of pitch he hears in voices around him. At the same time he also begins to attempt to imitate facial expressions and formation of sounds on the lips of people who talk to him.

At 10 to 12 months, through these processes of discriminative babbling, changes of pitch and imitation of visual and auditory sound combinations, the child begins to discover that particular combinations repeated often enough will bring about certain desirable ends. Usually among the earliest discoveries is that the combination *ma-ma* will bring his mother to pay some attention to him or to administer to some want.

By 12 months he should be using at least one to three such combinations meaningfully; i.e., he uses them to gain some specific end—usually food or attention. He will not develop meaningful use of these early combinations, however, unless they have been observed and repeatedly reinforced by responses from someone near him, usually his mother.

The entire first year is ideally a "vocal play" period in which the child learns to enjoy making vocal noises, has them pleasantly reinforced, and eventually becomes able to discriminate among and make use of particular combinations for his own benefit. From these early few meaningful combinations vocabulary develops by extension of the process, new meanings being associated with the repetition of other combinations which lead to fulfillment of other needs.

Between 12 and 18 months there is relatively little demonstrated increase in the expressive vocabulary, although the child continues with a great deal of vocal play, and he may learn to use with considerable effectiveness perhaps a dozen more words by the time he is 18 months of age. During this period he is preoccupied with learning to walk and exploring his physical environment and seems not to have much time to devote to the intricacies of language production. He is, however, rapidly expanding his comprehension vocabulary and the number and variety of his responses to meaningful vocalizations of others.

By about 18 months the child has considerable mastery of locomotion and other physical activities, and there is now likely to be an acceleration of the development of speech and language. Between 18 and 24 months he begins to try to put together many of the combinations he has been hearing, and to make some sort of organized system of responses. At this time the relation of meaning to sound symbols begins to become important. Frequently what he utters during the early part of this period is a complicated, largely unintelligible jargon—sometimes so bizarre that parents are frightened by it. If all goes well, however, out of this jargon will develop two- and three-word phrases by the age of about 24 months. At this age the child should begin to use connected speech for a purpose, such as *go bye-bye, want cookie,* and so forth.

Comprehension of language develops more rapidly than the ability to verbalize; almost from the very beginning the child is able to understand many more words and more complicated combinations than he can use. This remains true until his adult speech pattern is established.

At the time the child begins to use connected speech, intelligibility becomes important. At 2 years 50 to 60 per cent of his words and phrases should be understood, so long as the general context of his speech effort is known.

Between the second and third birthdays, owing to his limited expressive ability and vocabulary, the child often has difficulty trying to express complicated ideas. During this period he is trying also to develop fluency and some rhythm to his speaking; but so many children are not capable of a stable rhythm until 4 or 5 that the period from 2 to 5 years has been called the nonfluent period. It is during this time that the child, particularly the boy, may begin to say something and cannot find a word for it, so that he searches for the word, and while doing so repeats effortlessly, "I - I - I - I," or uses some other verbal stopgap. This nonfluency period may last only a few months or it may continue to about the age of 5, but it normally disappears as the child increases his vocabulary and masters syntax, general language structure and rhythm.

Between the ages of 3 and 4 years the child becomes very conscious of the importance of speech and the power it gives him. Because his speech and language are unstable and he is nonfluent, the process of communicating easily can be interfered with, and speech troubles may have their origin during this period.

By age 3 years the child should have mastered the use of all vowels, and the consonants *w, m, n, p, b, k, g, t* and *d.* At this age he generally is 70 to 80 per cent intelligible, and uses an average of three words per speech attempt. At the age of 4 he should be 100 per cent intelligible and use an average of four words per response. At 5 years of age he should use an average of five words. At 5, also, he should be using some blends, such as *tr, bl, pr, gr,* and use *f, v, r* and *l,* generally without error; but these may not be mastered until age 6.

At 4 years the child uses some adjectives, adverbs, prepositions and simple sentences. Articles begin to appear, and he recognizes plurals and sex differences. He generally replaces the pronoun *me* with nominative *I,* when appropriate, and uses a few other personal pronouns.

By age 6 the child's general language structure is stable, the nonfluency has passed, and he has mastered all the consonant sounds with the exception perhaps of the sibilants and sibilant combinations, primarily *s* and *z.* After 6 years, school and other social influences play such a large part in shaping the child's speech and language that it becomes increasingly difficult to relate his performance to innate developmental aspects.

It has become obvious that the preschool years are extremely important to the development of speech and language in the child, *especially the first year.* Many speech and language problems can be prevented if deviations are detected and treated early. Abnormal development of speech and language in the first year or two, moreover, may be the first clue to other developmental deviations.

CONDITIONS WHICH MAY INTERFERE WITH DEVELOPMENT OF SPEECH AND LANGUAGE. Any condition which seriously impairs or disrupts the normal development of the child, physically, psychologically or socially, may disrupt the development of his speech and language skills. Among such conditions are the following:

1. *Mental retardation* is by far the most frequently associated factor in the child's failure to develop speech and language normally. The child with either generalized or specialized areas of retardation is almost certain to have a delay in

achievement of speech and language skills; moreover, when these skills do develop, they may be faulty from a symbolic, structural and articulatory point of view. The degree of delay or distortion in speech and language will generally correlate with the amount of mental retardation. Even the "educable" retarded child (IQ 50 to 70) exhibits relatively severe speech and language deficiencies when compared with children of normal intelligence.

2. *Prematurity* may sometimes affect preverbal achievement levels during the first year of life; but the prematurely born child of normal mentality and without organic injury generally begins to attain normal developmental landmarks in speech and language by the age of about 2 years.

3. *Abnormalities of neuromuscular function,* such as cerebral palsy, or *structural inadequacies,* such as cleft palate, may also profoundly distort development of language. Children with cerebral palsy and those with cleft palate are almost universally delayed rather markedly (for the first 2 or 3 years) in speech and language development, even when they have normal mentality. They also may have associated problems of hypernasality, articulation and inadequate voice.

4. *Serious illness or injury* to the child, especially during the first year, may delay or severely distort the development of speech or language. This is especially true of illnesses which require prolonged hospitalization and extensive treatment procedures, including physical restraint.

5. *Neurologic dysfunctions,* even when unassociated with the motor disabilities of cerebral palsy, may be associated with retardation in the development of speech and language. When these skills do develop, they may be distorted by disorders of symbolic language of an aphasic nature and also by severe articulatory disorders or by inadequate voice production. The so-called congenital aphasia is typical of this kind of interference with speech and language development, but the deficiencies are likely to be more limited and localized than with the congenitally affected child.

6. Profound *deafness* always causes communication disorders, but much more frequent and more elusive than severe deafness is mild to moderate hearing loss; it is difficult to recognize, but often results in distortions of both receptive and expressive communicative skills. The child's hearing should always be investigated if there is a problem in the development of speech and language.

7. Some *dysfunction of the tongue* is commonly blamed for speech which is distorted or does not develop. The tongue is rarely responsible, however, unless there is some actual structural damage or paralysis. Tongue-tie accounts only rarely for problems of speech unless there is so much restriction of the tongue-tip that adequate articulation is not possible. In those rare instances in which the tongue, when protruded slightly beyond the lower incisors, is grooved in the middle by a tight frenulum, it may be necessary to free the tip surgically before adequate articulation can be achieved.

8. *Tongue-thrust* is a cause of articulatory problems when the thrust is strong or when the pattern is not reversed by the age of 7 or 8 years. This occurs when the tip of the tongue is forced strongly between the teeth or against the upper incisors during speaking and swallowing. This results in a forward displacement of the upper incisors, causing an interference with sibilant sounds, principally *s* and *z*. The condition can be corrected if detected before the child reaches the age of 7 or 8 years.

9. *Excessive adenoid tissue* may cause a hyponasal quality of the voice, but only rarely interferes with the development of vocabulary and intelligible speech. Equally rarely will the removal of adenoids result in improvement of the child's speech. In fact, removal occasionally may result in hypernasal speech.

10. *Social, psychologic and environmental conditions,* if severe, may interfere with speech or language development. Serious communicative and emotional disturbances such as autism or schizophrenia may result, or less severe adjustment problems involving primarily the child's inability or unwillingness to use ordinary communicative skills. Environmental stresses must be severe to interfere with language development; it is likely that well intentioned parents have often been made to feel unnecessarily guilty by professional persons who blamed them for children's communication problems lying outside their power to influence.

11. The common scapegoats of baby-talk, position in the family, "only" children, sibling rivalry, parental anxiety, or interference with speech, and the child's "not being required to talk" rarely create severe disturbances in the development of speech and language. Parental anxiety and interference may, however, contribute significantly to stuttering.

STUTTERING. Stuttering certainly relates to environmental and psychosocial factors, but there are many aspects of stuttering which are not understood. There are strong emotional components in secondary stuttering, but it is not clear that these are basic causes. There is some evidence to suggest that the child who develops stuttering has a less well integrated nervous system, to which are added environmental factors with which he is unable to cope.

Stuttering often begins during the nonfluent period, between the ages of 2 and 5 years, especially in the male. Adverse psychosocial and environmental factors during this period can prolong the nonfluency until it becomes a real dysfluency, and eventually secondary stuttering.

The physician's advice to parents of the preschool child who is said to be stuttering is often to ignore it. This good advice may not be adequate, however, since it may also be necessary to instruct the parents as to *how* to ignore the speech. They must be helped to treat the child as normal, to understand that nonfluency is a normal developmental stage, and to accept the child's speech without hurrying him, without demanding repetition, and without showing concern. They must give the child full attention during his speech attempts. Approximately 99 per cent of children pass through this nonfluency period to develop stable, nonstuttering speech; many who do not would develop adequate speech if handled as described.

When the older child with strong secondary stuttering is presented to the physician, the same kind of help should be given to the parents, but every effort should be made also to refer the child to a speech pathologist or speech clinic.

ASSESSMENT AND TREATMENT OF DEVIATIONS IN DEVELOPMENT OF SPEECH AND LANGUAGE. When speech or language disorder is suspected, the physician must answer such questions as, "Are the speech and language skills of this child developing within the range of normal? If not, what further studies will disclose the nature of the disorder? What therapy may be needed?" To answer such questions the physician will need to take the following steps: (1) obtain an accurate history of the child's acquisition of developmental landmarks of speech and language; (2) ascertain through tests whether hearing is normal or defective; (3) estimate the child's levels of development in the areas of verbal comprehension, expression, articulation and intelligibility; (4) form an estimate of the child's level of intellectual function; (5) determine through careful physical and neurologic evaluation whether any organic defects are present; (6) make an assessment of the environment to discover any major psychosocial factors which might interfere with the development of communication skills.

In addition to the foregoing rather general screening procedures, the physician may find the following 20 conditions of speech and language development useful as rough guidelines in determining whether a child has a problem, what its nature may be, and whether he should be referred to a speech pathologist or audiologist for more detailed evaluation. If any of the following conditions exist, the child should be referred:

1. If the child is not producing any intelligible speech by age 2
2. If speech is largely unintelligible after age 3
3. If there are many omissions of initial consonants after age 3
4. If there are no sentences by age 3
5. If sounds are more than a year late in appearing, according to expected developmental sequence
6. If there is an excessive amount of indiscriminate, irrelevant verbalizing after 18 months
7. If there is consistent and frequent omission of initial consonants at any age
8. If there are many substitutions of easy sounds for difficult ones after age 5
9. If the amount of vocalizing decreases rather than steadily increases at any period up to age 7
10. If the child uses mostly vowel sounds in his speech at any age after 1 year
11. If word endings are consistently dropped after age 5
12. If sentence structure is consistently faulty after age 5
13. If the child is embarrassed and disturbed by his speech at any age
14. If the child is noticeably nonfluent (stuttering) after age 5
15. If the child is distorting, omitting or substituting any sounds after age 7
16. If the voice is a monotone, extremely loud, largely inaudible, or of poor quality
17. If the pitch is not appropriate to the child's age and sex
18. If there is noticeable hypernasality or lack of nasal resonance
19. If there are unusual confusions, reversals or telescoping in connected speech
20. If there are abnormal rhythm, rate and inflection after age 5.

For children with communication disorders, help may be found in university or college speech and hearing clinics, in community speech and hearing centers, and with certified speech pathologists or audiologists in private practice or in the special education departments of the public schools. Speech and hearing specialists also may be found in medical schools, child development programs, rehabilitation centers, mental health clinics and child guidance centers. The speech and hearing specialist should hold the Certificate of Clinical Competence in the American Speech and Hearing Association as assurance that he is adequately trained and experienced.

HEROLD LILLYWHITE

PARENT EDUCATION

Van Riper, C.: Helping Children Talk Better. Chicago, Science Research Associates, 1951.
(A pamphlet [about 80 cents] available from Science Research Associates, Inc., 259 East Erie Street, Chicago, 60611).

READING DISABILITIES

Extraction of meaning from written symbols is the unique feature of reading. Facility with spoken language ordinarily precedes acquisition of reading skill. This facility is not a necessary antecedent, but its absence, as in the deaf person, is ordinarily a serious handicap.

Learning to read can be considered a two-stage process. The first stage consists in perceiving written symbols in their proper spatial and temporal sequence. The second stage is the obtaining of meaning from these written words. Children with reading disabilities generally have more difficulty with the first stage than the second. This simplistic description of reading does not deny the importance of linguistic analysis, perception of grammar and sensitivity to semantics to the reading process; it recognizes that present knowledge does not permit precise definition of the influence of these processes.

There is variability in the rates at which normal children mature in certain basic functions required for reading. These functions include differential perception of various letter and syllabic forms, the ability to associate these symbols with their sounds, and short-term memory sufficient for correct sequential representation of them. Fluency in speech and in reading support each other. A critical listening ability is necessary for the development of vocabulary, proper pronunciation, and the rules of grammar and spelling.

A minimal level of visual acuity is necessary for reading, but striking reduction in acuity need not prevent effective reading.

Intellectual capacity is a principal determinant of reading ability, but the educational categories of *overachiever* or *underachiever* indicate that there are other influences. In the range of IQ's from 80 to 130 there is some correlation between IQ and reading ability, particularly in the early grades of school. This correlation diminishes in the higher grades and is much less in college. Children who score below 80 in IQ tests generally do not read well; poor readers are distinctly uncommon among those with IQ's greater than 130.

The child's general motivation and his interest in the content of the material being read are powerful determinants of his reading achievement. The attitudes of peers, family members and others also exert profound influences.

A few children can read at 3½ to 4 years of age; most can learn to read easily at 5 to 6 years of age. A few are not ready for reading until 9 or 10 years; an unknown number never acquire functional reading skill.

It is generally considered that a child with normal or superior intelligence and without significant sensory deficit who cannot learn to read at his age level in an ordinary school setting has a reading disability or "developmental dyslexia" or "specific reading disability." Children in the primary grades may be considered retarded readers if they are 6 to 12 months below grade placement; at higher grade levels a criterion of 24 months or more below grade placement defines the poor reader.

The term "reading disability" is not limited to a single clinical entity. Among poor readers are children and adults who from their earliest encounters with reading have had difficulties; others have mastered the fundamental skills, but through lack of motivation or opportunity, or because of emotional or socioeconomic stresses, have failed to mature in reading skills to the point at which reading has become an effective tool for them.

The literature on reading disability contains many apparent inconsistencies and mutually exclusive statements with respect to etiology, clinical manifestations, diagnosis and prognosis. These reflect differences in populations studied, in methods of analysis, in judgments regarding what is fundamental and what fortuitous, and in personal experiences and philosophies.

ETIOLOGY. The causes suggested for reading retardation reflect the prevalent confusion about definitions and gaps in understanding. Because so many affected children appear to be unable to master the most elementary reading skills in spite of normal intelligence, and because impairment of the ability to perceive or register items in an orderly sequence seems to lie at the root of much disability, attention has been focused upon central nervous system dysfunction. Reading disability has been ascribed to brain damage or "minimal cerebral dysfunction," to inheritance of a specific reading disability, to incomplete or crossed or mixed laterality or cerebral dominance, to defects in visuomotor coordination, and to deficits in spatial perception or directional orientation, as well as to such peripheral defects as abnormalities of ocular structure or movement. The notion of central defect gains support from the fact that affected children commonly display "soft neurologic signs," such as generalized motor awkwardness, "overflow" of voluntary muscle activity, inability to concentrate, short attention span, hyperactivity and easy distractibility. But these signs are not precisely defined or quantitated, nor is it clear whether they represent organic or functional disorders. Moreover, it is difficult in this context to explain how children with such central disabilities as severe athetosis, spastic paraplegia or congenital nystagmus may learn to read well so long as general intelligence is preserved.

Some children with reading disabilities show spontaneous improvement late in the first decade of life or early in the second; it is difficult to reconcile this finding with the notion of an organic defect. Such improvement may follow change of residence, of teacher or of system of reading instruction, whether in a regular school program or in remedial work.

So far as poor sequencing and visuomotor coordination are concerned, one finds poor readers who read music well, or who can follow diagrammatic outlines to assemble intricate models or devices. The importance of failure of binocular vision, of refractive errors, or of oculomotor imbalance as causes of reading disability has been exaggerated. These conditions may discourage reading because of fatigue, but they do not prevent children from developing reading skills.

Many children will not learn to read if presented with dull or difficult reading materials, if they live in home environments which do not encourage or which actively discourage reading, or if they have no opportunity to acquire an adequate vocabulary. These factors may prove stronger than the influence of the school. The poor reader often comes from a disorganized family setting.

The literature on reading disability contains limited reference to the influence of the teacher in acquisition of reading skills. Some recent studies suggest that although the nature of a particular system or technique of teaching reading is of little influence on acquisition of reading skills, there are obvious variations in reading achievement from classroom to classroom and from school to school. The teacher's influence is a cardinal one, but how she exercises it and the weight of its impact cannot be described with precision.

Some observers feel that if a teacher or teaching staff considers learning to read a matter of high priority, children learn to read early and well. Conversely, if the teacher believes that reading is learned spontaneously or that its teaching can be postponed or delayed, the children exhibit a slower and less complete acquisition of reading skills. These attitudes of the teacher appear to operate almost irrespective of the methods, materials, media, techniques, procedures or systems she uses to teach reading and can override other influences, such as IQ, socioeconomic status or family background. On the other hand, social or cultural factors may be sufficiently influential to reduce the importance of orthography, sequencing ability, IQ, and the like to very low levels.

CLINICAL MANIFESTATIONS. Reading difficulties may come to the physician's attention because of academic failure or for less clearly related reasons such as psychosomatic complaints or behavioral disturbances.

Contrary to widely held opinion, the poor reader does not generally do well in arithmetic, sciences or other fields of study. He has particular difficulty with spelling, with grammar and with rapid retrieval of words required for precise description and exposition. Even if he can learn through audition and perform adequately orally through bypassing reading and writing, he will be increasingly unable to keep up with his classmates, particularly after the third grade. The effectiveness of his style will vary with his intelligence, motivation and emotional strengths.

Observation of the child in the act of reading may show that he does not persevere unless prodded, or that he may lose interest rapidly. Embarrassed by his poor performance, he may try to hide it by dropping his voice, turning his head or covering his mouth. His impairment is magnified by anxiety or fatigue, with pressure of time or with fear of failure. He may brighten perceptibly with encouragement.

Some poor readers do not pause at words they cannot correctly pronounce, nor attempt to phoneticize them. As if to terminate a painful process as quickly as possible, they produce words variously comparable to the one read, which may have a common initial letter or syllable but disparate meaning (*course* for *cause*), different spellings but related meaning (*mother* for *father* or *brother* for *sister*), minor perceptual differences which produce major semantic changes (*humidity* for *humility*), or no relationship, representing blind guesses.

Errors which demonstrate disturbances of serial order or temporospatial sequence are substitutions, deletions, additions and faulty juxtaposition of letters, especially consonants. Reversals are common (strophic errors, or strephosymbolia); *was* for *saw* and *left* for *felt* are two familiar examples. The equivalent of strophic errors in arithmetic can alter the written sequence of digits or lead to the "carrying" of the wrong digit in addition. Studies of reversals of individual letters and of the position of letters within words have indicated that these two phenomena are discrete, rather than variations of the same process, and that they occur much less frequently when an individual is reading familiar, as opposed to novel, material. These and other considerations cast doubt upon the existence of a defined process called strephosymbolia and particularly upon its role, if any, in the production of reading disability.

Phonic errors include confusion of two or more sound values corresponding to the same symbol, such as *kity* for *city* or *seize* for *size*. Other less common errors include inappropriate use of clues from context or accompanying pictures, mispronunciation of words, and incorrect intonation of phrases and sentences. These latter errors are considered secondary results of imperfect reading.

Some poor readers may have poorly performed diadochokinetic movements, clumsy voluntary acts, impaired right-left orientations and other equivocal neurologic signs. These do not correlate closely with the severity of the impairment nor with the success of treatment.

After years of scholastic difficulty, repeating of grades, and perhaps much fruitless remedial instruction, the poor reader may progressively restrict his social contacts and extracurricular activities, manifest behavioral and disciplinary difficulties and be intractable to help, unwilling to undertake new ventures because of the fear of failure and the pain of expected frustration.

Many more boys than girls have reading disabilities, for reasons not yet established.

DIAGNOSIS. The adequate assessment of reading disabilities may require neurologic and psychologic examination as well as review by someone with experience in reading disorders. Only rarely does a discrete diagnostic entity account for a relatively isolated reading problem, but the exclusion of organic disease may allay parental fears of some more serious deficit.

Appropriate studies must determine: (1) whether a disability actually exists in perceptual abilities, in developing meaningful sequential order from items of sensory input, or in the level of reading achievement by a child with adequate perceptual skills; (2) whether emotional problems may have been responsible for the development of reading difficulties; (3) whether spontaneous improvement can be anticipated or treatment will be needed; and (4) what treatment may be appropriate, if any, and where it can be obtained.

It is usually more difficult to evaluate children in the primary grades than in subsequent ones. Performance tests exploring short-term memory for serial items are particularly useful and relatively reliable in children by their tenth year. These include the span of retention of memory for a succession of digits, or the ability to reproduce such items of "automatic" memory as one's birth date, name, address, telephone number, days of the week and months of the year. From the age of 9 through 15 years there are an increasing number of children who can perform on these tests at levels comparable to those of normal adults. Children with reading disabilities generally do poorly at these tasks; a good performance casts doubt on the diagnosis of reading disability.

On the whole, poor readers have lower IQ's than average or good readers, though most fall within the normal range. It is characteristic of these children that their scores on the performance items of an intelligence scale, such as the Wechsler (WISC), tend to be substantially higher than their verbal scores. When the verbal score is relatively high, the child's difficulty may more likely be the result of emotional problems, of lack of motivation, or of a nonliterary milieu in the home than the result of a "primary" reading disability. Such interpretations become unreliable when the child's IQ approaches or is in the retarded range.

If a child has attained the fifth grade in school and his reading achievement tests indicate that he is functioning below a third or early fourth grade level, he will generally not have mastered basic reading skills. These will be the children considered to have "dyslexia," "primary reading retardation" or "specific language disorder." They present a different problem from children in the higher grades whose reading ability is considered to be retarded about 2 years. The latter children have clearly mastered the basic mechanics of reading. Their low levels of achievement are usually attributable to lack of motivation, to culturally impoverished home environments, to limited educational opportunities, and the like. These two groups will require different approaches to improvement of reading skills.

DIFFERENTIAL DIAGNOSIS. Consultants in problems of "dyslexia" must make sure that the child has a reading problem. In children with learning problems of whatever sort, reading is likely to be involved, but it may not be the primary problem. Children may be referred for reading or language problems because their styles in reading or in other academic functions are out of step, or because their classroom behavior is unacceptable. Such children may be awkward, ungainly, slow, socially immature, inattentive or distractible. Careful evaluation may detect causes other than reading disability for their behavior.

PROGNOSIS. It is doubtful whether there are any children with reading disabilities in the context used here who remain totally unable to read, but the degree of impairment may be severe. It is not presently possible to distinguish the relatively small percentage of children with reading disability who will improve spontaneously from those who will not. Well motivated children who are not overwhelmed by their difficulties and who have only mild deficiencies may improve gradually or suddenly and have no lasting impairment. Many remedial programs can be expected to benefit the poor reader, whether they are devoted exclusively to the teaching of reading or coupled with visuomotor and perceptual training procedures. There are, however, no programs of remedial reading which, with high probability and efficiency, will lead to development of normal reading skills in those with significant difficulty. If in the early years of school the reactions of those close to the child are unsympathetic to his poor performance, he may remain a poor reader for emotional reasons.

Poor readers usually have little or no gross motor disability as adults. They tend to seek occupations which require minimal verbal but high mechanical skills. Their imperfections of speech tend to improve. Their ability to reproduce familiar items (names, days of the week, alphabet, and the like) also improves, but difficulty remains for newly presented items (e.g., series of random digits, unrelated words).

TREATMENT. Two broad categories of therapy are available for children with reading disabilities: **remedial reading** for the child with decoding difficulties due to faulty sequencing or other visuoperceptual or integrative disabilities, and **corrective instruction** or exercises for the child or adult whose basic equipment and reading skills may be adequate, but who has lacked motivation to read or has had an arrest in reading development.

The plan for remedial reading should be individually designed for a child after careful analysis by appropriately trained specialists. In corrective instruction or exercises the primary purpose is to induce greater interest, attention and diligence in school tasks. The child's self-confidence, willingness to risk failure, and motivation for self-directed achievement must be assessed. It is important that the older retarded reader achieve some success, however limited, quickly and easily upon beginning remedial work or instruction. The resulting self-esteem enhances interest and creates a desire for further progress.

Finally, the child's unique or idiosyncratic approach to learning should be accounted for in the instructional setting. Some children are rash and impulsive, others reflective and systematic in a learning situation; some prefer longer, uninterrupted periods of instruction, others shorter periods; some respond better when errors are pointed out, others when accomplishments are emphasized. All these aspects of the child's learning may be subsumed under the descriptive term "cognitive style." It is, perhaps, the effectiveness of incorporation of the pupil's cognitive style into the instructional setting, with an individual or a group, that best reflects the art, skill and influence of the teacher.

JOHN B. ISOM

CEREBRAL DYSFUNCTION
(Learning Disorders)

A number of children, estimated to be greater than 10 per cent of the school population, though they are not mentally retarded or defective or do not have readily detectable neurologic defects, have problems in learning and in behaving like other children. They seem to represent not a clear-cut syndrome, but a continuum of developmental difficulties in respect to certain learning abilities. Although some children with demonstrable organic changes present the symptoms to be described, experience has shown that it is rarely to the child's advantage (except as a prerequisite for admission to a special educational class) to label him "organic" or to imply that he has a disease. This is a heterogeneous group, and there is no single or clear-cut cause of the behavioral deviations, many of which are similar in the affected children.

During the past decade a variety of categorical terms has been proposed for these disorders, based on assumed cause, either intrinsic or environmental, or on manifestations, symptoms or consequences of an apparent learning and behavior disorder. Of the many terms proposed or used, "children with learning disorders" and "minimal cerebral dysfunction syndrome" seem to be least objectionable. To some, minimal brain dysfunction is an unproved presumptive diagnosis without demonstrable physiologic, biochemical or structural alteration in the brain. To others, deviate behavior, developmental lags, learning disabilities and various perceptual irregularities, including visual and auditory, are valid indices of altered brain functions. It seems reasonable to accept as a working basis that these children have some disorganization of their central nervous system and that this factor in some way adversely affects their capacities to learn at the usual developmental rate and manner.

The term "cerebral dysfunction" is currently used to identify some children who, in spite of average or nearly average intellectual ability, have learning or behavioral disabilities ranging from mild to moderately severe, which are attributable to such deviations of cerebral function as impairment in perception, conceptualization, language comprehension or expression, memory, or control of attention, impulse or some motor functions. Similar deviations may at times complicate the more obvious disorders of the central nervous system such as mental retardation, seizures, cerebral palsy, behavioral disorders, blindness or deafness, which are discussed elsewhere. There are many who feel that some hyperkinetic children and most who have reading disabilities, dyslexia, aphasia, and so forth, represent a delay in mental maturation. See the pages above (this section) on Disorders of Communication and on Reading Disabilities.

In the majority of instances no specific cause can be determined for the syndrome of minimal cerebral dysfunction, but in some there is an apparent relation with a genetic disorder, birth injury, or prenatal or postnatal illness or injury of the central nervous system. In any event, it is helpful for one who is familiar with variations of developmental rates in normal children to think of this group as evidencing, as they grow, a variety of problems associated with delayed or arrested development. When a particular skill is gained late, the child behaves like a normal younger child in respect to that skill. Such a concept helps to shift the focus from cause and categorization, which is usually imprecise, to rational and effective methods of helping the child, which are more readily available.

CLINICAL MANIFESTATIONS. In the preschool child the symptoms may include a variety of relatively minor deviations in behavioral development or in motor development. Among the characteristic manifestations are unpredictable variations of behavior, distractibility, short attention span for the age (or the converse—perseveration), hyperactivity, impulsiveness, irritability, low frustration level, perceptual and conceptual difficulties, poor motor coordination, sleep disorders, and abnormal reactions to environmental stimuli.

The school child exhibits unreadiness to learn reading, and frequently in addition, difficulties in organizing and finishing his work, in comprehending and following instructions, in learning, particularly in the communication skills, and in memory and abstract thinking. All these contribute to some degree of school failure. Throughout childhood there is usually increasing emotional reaction in being different from one's peers.

None of these variations of integrated behavior by itself is of major significance, but when several are manifest by a child, they suggest a disturbance in cerebral function. The child's behavior may vary from day to day without relation to any recognizable factor and is apparently as unpredictable to himself as to others. His restlessness is frequently marked by running to and fro, by constant physical activity, and by a briefer interest for any one activity than is appropriate for his chronologic age. His enthusiasms may be intense but short. Many of his acts appear to follow no pattern of thought. He tends to react violently to frustration and to other stimuli, and he may be a constant storm center in the family, at play or at school. Although by many tests he has normal, superior or borderline intelligence, he usually has difficulty in numeral concepts, in associating the particular with the general, and in drawing logical conclusions from abstract material. He can think in concrete terms much better than in abstract ones, so that he may do well in rote memory subjects, such as spelling and multiplication tables, as opposed to reading and other areas in which symbols and their orientation to each other are important. Allied to the problem of handling abstract concepts are deficiencies in perception of environmental situations in their entirety; rather he is apt to direct his attention only to a minimally important part of what he sees or hears, with a reaction as confusing and disturbing to others as to himself.

As the child grows older, secondary behavioral manifestations related to his frustrations with how he feels about himself and to his contacts with people may obscure the earlier pattern. In many instances the secondary symptoms are manifest as emotional immaturity, anxieties and fears, inattention, school failure and the like. The results of his impulsive behavior may lead to severe remorse, and he frequently shows an inappropriate display of affection.

The syndrome might well be suspected in any child with several of the above-mentioned symptoms, particularly if there is clinical evidence or a history of brain damage. There may be a history of some delay in motor development, and there may be considerable variation from time to time in the reported hyperactivity or hypoactivity.

In many instances no abnormalities can be demonstrated by conventional neurologic examination; however, many "soft neurologic signs" significant of inappropriate response or failure to function appropriately for age may be found. Many affected children exhibit clumsiness in gross or fine motor activities or poorer coordination than expected for their chronologic age. There may be poor or tardy development of skill in use of scissors or pencil, in bouncing or catching a ball, in hopping or in jumping rope. Handedness may develop late, and there is frequently mixed or confused laterality. Abnormalities may or may not be detected by electroencephalography. Pneumoencephalography and cerebral arteriography usually give normal results, and no laboratory test is specific for the syndrome. Some of the children have mild visual or hearing impairment in addition to the evidence of disorganization and of tardy neurosensory development.

Psychologic testing will frequently provide clues to and sometimes pinpoint the special learning disabilities of the child with minimal cerebral dysfunction. There are often great variations in performance and specific deficits in conceptual thinking. There also may be problems of perceptual motor adequacy, so that tasks such as copying geometric forms are characterized by particular distortions and other evidences of inadequacy of coordinated function. There may be evidence of impaired discrimination of size, of right to left, of up to down, and of impaired tactile discrimination in children of an age at which such skills are expected. There may be evidence of poor spatial orientation, impaired understanding of time and distorted concept of body image. Perceptual reversals in reading and in writing letters and in numbers may persist longer than normal. There may be difficulty in fusing sensory impressions into meaningful entities. Projective tests, such as the Rorschach, may disclose inadequate emotional controls, excessive impulsivity or impotence, and failure in perception. Intelligence quotients alone often tend to obscure more than they reveal, since these children may have a normal or even superior performance in some areas of functioning, but the overall score may be low as a result of excessively poor ratings in verbal areas. Such scatter is the rule rather than the exception. It is important for the psychologist to define as accurately as possible the specific assets and liabilities of the child and to define his optimal method of learning. Without such specific help for the child's parents and for his teacher, the diagnosis of this syndrome is a handicap rather than an aid in planning a constructive learning program.

DIFFERENTIAL DIAGNOSIS. This syndrome of poorly integrated behavior associated with learning disabilities should be distinguished from mental retardation or mental deficiency, from hearing loss, from behavioral disorders arising principally on an emotional basis, and from developmental delay due to socioeconomic or environmental factors. A careful history of events in the prenatal and perinatal periods and a detailed developmental history will frequently give clues that lead to an understanding of the basic problem and to the separation of the primary manifestations from the secondary behavior or emotional ones. The child with cerebral dysfunction is likely to have a history of slow motor development, such as difficulty in self-feeding, in manipulating buttons, tying shoelaces, or in balancing, whereas the retarded child is more likely to be slow in all achievements. The deprived child may start out with a normal developmental pattern, and at some later time manifest delay in achievement, particularly in language and social skills. Primary delay in speech should suggest a hearing loss.

TREATMENT. Although the educational psychologist and the teacher in special education have the principal responsibility to develop a program for specific management and treatment, the pediatrician is in a position to help in identifying the child with a learning disability, in explaining the problems to the parents, and in assisting them in developing an atmosphere at home that supports the child's best development. He should identify and secure corrections of visual and auditory defects, if any; should plan and manage the therapy if the child has seizures; and should supervise the general mental and physical health program. Such children are frequently characterized as "bad" or "lazy" or "nervous," and an explanation of the real problem should relieve pressures and aid in the achievement of academic success and in effective living with others. Parents are frequently put at ease if behavior is explained on the basis of a physical factor or developmental delay rather than as a result of parental incompetence. Since behavior appropriate to the age usually cannot be expected in these children, their erratic behavior and lack of self-control point to the need for establishment of definite limits of conduct and for consistent controls and establishment of self-discipline. Firm, constructive guidance is indicated rather than permissiveness. It is most important that the child be given goals that are obtainable so that he may profit by the feeling of success rather than of continuing frustration and disappointment.

Giving recognition for what he does accomplish is crucial. It is also important for the parents to recognize and support those coping strategies that the child has discovered that work for him. For example, some find that it is helpful to work in a small enclosed space where there are fewer distractions. The child who needs to move around may be able to cope by carrying out rather short-term tasks, receive recognition for all he has accomplished, and then move on to another activity. Many children seem to benefit from using different or additional sensory inputs. These are some of the principles of special education, but the parents should benefit by having them discussed in simple specific ways by the physician.

Medication may at times be a helpful adjunct in the management of children with learning disabilities. A drug should be used as a tool to help the child to control his behavior, have an increased feeling of self-esteem and be more attentive. The greatest success can generally be anticipated in the smaller group of children whose hyperactivity appears to be constitutional in nature rather than related to stress, such as that from inappropriate competition and expectations at school or at home. Medication does not seem to make children learn better or faster but does appear to aid children whose control of impulse, attention, and focus of interest is immature or delayed, helping them to control behavior as they wish and not be at the mercy of every sensory stimulation. The drugs of choice are dextroamphetamine (Dexedrine) and methylphenidate (Ritalin). The initial dose of each is 5 mg in the morning; this may be increased to 20 mg or given as needed in divided doses. Smaller amounts are usually effective, and if benefit is to result, it should be apparent within a day or two. Both drugs may inhibit physical growth, but neither appears to be habit forming. Chlorpromazine (Thorazine), thioridazine (Mellaril) and diphenhydramine (Benadryl) are occasionally of value. Anticonvulsive drugs should not be used unless the child also has seizures; phenobarbital in the usual doses may have an undesirable stimulating effect on children with constitutional hyperactivity.

It is important that any medication be seen as an agent to help the child to change his behavior and that any positive change be reinforced by parents and teachers and attributed to action of the child; the drug itself should not be seen as the controlling factor.

The physician should give teachers and others concerned with the child all the information about his behavior and learning that will be helpful in developing an appropriate program for him. An increasing number of private and public schools are providing special classes for children with learning disabilities. Modification of curricula and techniques by placement in smaller classes, by individualized attention, by use of concrete materials in teaching abstractions, by minimizing competition, and by the use of multisensory approaches to reinforce perception is frequently helpful. The curriculum at school and the expectations at home should be such that the child must succeed. Diagnostic teaching which encourages a flexible approach in the classroom should be encouraged, with ongoing trial of varying techniques to discover and then to reinforce the child's strengths in learning. Since each child's problems, both in behavior and in learning, are individual, ideally the psychologist, the parent, the physician and the teacher should work together in developing a program individualized for this child and taking into account all facets of his growth and development: physical, mental and social, as they relate to his learning ability.

Richardson and Ozer have developed in conjunction with a public school system an economical approach, bypassing the traditional consultant role of professionals. They emphasize "collaborative diagnosis as a problem-solving rather than a labeling process, active and meaningful participation of parents and teachers at each step of the program, and ongoing low-cost evaluation of the effectiveness of the program," and demonstrate that if the teacher, parent and child are brought together, with help by consultants a brief series of observations can be made from which the child's optimal method of learning can be established and his success anticipated. The system appears to have beneficial fallout to other children in the class, multiplying the effectiveness of the consultant's time.

PROGNOSIS. The outlook for such children appears to be dependent in part on the attitude and guidance of those who deal with them, on the age at which effective intervention is initiated, and on the degree of success which can be achieved in family living. In conjunction with a planned educational program, desired achievement depends on the extent to which the child develops a feeling of competency within himself. Some children unfortunately become delinquent or are labeled mentally defective or psychotic. Most, however, who can be helped to feel confident in themselves are able to attain a reasonable level of adjustment during adolescence and eventually to achieve a comfortable way of life in relatively competitive activities.

PATIENT EDUCATION

Becker, W.: Parents Are Teachers: Urbana, Illinois, Research Press, 1971, ($3.75) Write to: Association for Children with Learning Disabilities, 5225 Grace Street, Pittsburgh, Pa. 15236

Birch, H. G.: Brain Damage in Children: The Biological and Social Aspects. Baltimore, Williams & Wilkins Company, 1964.
Clements, S. D.: Minimal Brain Dysfunction in Children. Washington, D.C., United States Department of Health, Education and Welfare, Public Health Service. Publication #1415, 1966.
Golick, M.: A Parents' Guide to Learning Problems. Quebec Association for Children with Learning Disabilities, P. O. Box 22, Montreal 29, P.Q. (50 cents.)
Learning Disabilities, A Practical Office Manual and History and Exam Supplement. Victoria, B.C., Canadian Paediatric Society, Morris Printing Co.
Ozer, M. N.: Diagnosis of the Child with Learning Problems: A Child Development Approach. Clinical Proceedings of the Children's Hospital National Medical Center, Vol. XXVIII, No. 6, June, 1972.
Paine, R. S.: Syndromes of "minimal cerebral damage." Pediat. Clin. N. Amer., 15:779, 1968.

MENTAL RETARDATION

Mental retardation, as the term is used diagnostically, implies impairment in intelligence from early in life and inadequate mental development throughout the growth period; it is manifest by slow and incomplete maturation, impaired learning ability and poor social adjustment. In the minority of cases, mental retardation is primarily a medical problem. As a significant cause of lifetime disability and as a complex medical, social, educational and economic problem, mental retardation currently presents a strong challenge to science and society, and defies easy solution.

Mental retardation may well be the most handicapping of all childhood disorders. There are only 4 other significantly disabling conditions – mental illness, cancer, heart disease and arthritis – that have a higher prevalence, but each of these is in greatest measure a problem of adult life. It is estimated that 3 per cent of the population may be identified as mentally retarded at some point in their lives. Of preschool children, approximately 0.5 per cent are retarded. The peak period of recognition is between 6 and 16 years of age, when the pressures of formal schooling seem to identify a larger number, that may reach 10 per cent or more of the school population in some urban deprived areas. Only approximately 1 per cent of adults are considered to be retarded, the percentage having been reduced by death and by successful assimilation of some of the survivors into the general population. Mental retardation appears to be more frequent in boys than in girls: 55 per cent to 45 per cent. This disparity may in part be related to biologic factors (sex-linked genetic disorders) and in part to differences in social expectations for the sexes. At least 75 per cent of the retarded have no obvious physical stigma, although the group as a whole has a higher percentage of sensory defects, language disorders, neuromuscular impairment, seizures and physical anomalies than the general population. The retarded, like other children with handicapping defects, are more vulnerable to emotional problems; conversely, children with emotional problems frequently function at a retarded level.

At present it is estimated that of the probable six million mentally retarded persons in the United States, 200,000 are in institutions, 300,000 are on waiting lists for such care, and an equal number are in general or special hospitals or prisons. More than 85 per cent live at home. Seven out of 10 of these are of school age, and it is estimated that the majority receive only minimal medical care and guidance.

Intelligence is not the result of a single mental process, but includes abstract thinking, visual and auditory memory, causal reasoning, verbal expression, manipulative capacities and spatial comprehension. This multifactor concept is taken into account in the development of mental and psychologic tests. The current inadequate practice of quantitatively identifying intelligence in terms of mental age or of intelligence quotient (IQ), which is the ratio of mental age to chronologic age, supplies only averages of the composite attainments in some of these mental abilities. Since it also reflects in part the experience and cultural background of the subject tested, the IQ may conceal more than it reveals. The IQ is not fixed and may be modified by a number of factors, largely environmental. This method of grading intelligence apparently depicts the status of persons of average or better than average mental ability more accurately than it does that of those of lesser ability. Arrested or inadequate mental development is only rarely equally manifest in the various intellectual spheres. Frequently some mental functions are within normal limits in moderately retarded children.

The importance of this concept in relation to diagnosis of mental deficiency becomes apparent when it is realized that the various mental abilities do not play equal roles in influencing subsequent social or vocational adjustment. Acceptable progress in academic schooling in the main depends on adequate development of such factors as visual and auditory memory, verbal facility, abstract reasoning, and creativity, as well as conformity to existing social standards. Other aspects of intelligence also play a role in school progress, but in general not to the extent as do those mentioned. In contrast, reasonable success in adjusting to many of the simple industrial disciplines in later life depends much more on such aspects of intelligence as those related to visual-manual coordination, spatial relations, and causal reasoning, as well as on acceptable personality characteristics. The relative value of comprehensive psychologic examination is dependent more on these broader concepts of multiple factors in intelligence and their interaction in terms of potential social adaptability than simply on estimates of average mental age. Unfortunately, there is no objective measure or scientific standard of adaptive behavior to differentiate which behavior is a function of inherent or organic inferiority and which is a function of cultural background. This becomes a subjective judgment.

For academic and administrative purposes the intelligence quotient, though inadequate and not infrequently misleading, does help to classify mentally subnormal children in regard to the degree of defect.

Persons with an IQ between 50 and 75 are considered to be mildly retarded and "educable." This group comprises 85 to 90 per cent of the total. They are usually capable of reaching the fourth or fifth grade level in a conventional school system and can generally make a moderately satisfactory social adjustment. In general, they are self-supporting in times of high employment, particularly in jobs not requiring abstract thought. The majority of this group are recognized in the early school years through their poor academic achievement.

Moderately retarded children have an IQ approximately in the range of 35 to 50. They are considered "trainable" and can be capable of their own physical self-care. They also, if accepted, can make an adequate social adjustment in the home and the neighborhood, and some will achieve some degree of economic usefulness at home or in a sheltered type of occupation. This group comprises 5 to 10 per cent of the total. They are usually identified during preschool years because of significantly delayed developmental milestones, and many have physical defects.

Persons with an IQ below 35 are classified as severely retarded, and those below 20 are considered to be profoundly retarded. They have minimal response to their environment, are generally considered to be "nontrainable," and are usually dependent on others for most of their care. They constitute approximately 5 per cent of the total retarded group. The majority are identified during infancy and have multiple disabilities requiring medical diagnosis and special care.

More than 100 different factors have been identified as being closely or causally related to mental retardation; yet there is not an identifiable biologic or organic cause for 65 to 75 per cent of retarded children. This largest segment of the retarded is probably caused by sociocultural or environmental deprivation and is often a byproduct of poverty. The majority of the mildly retarded children come from the more disadvantaged classes of society, characterized by low income, limited educational achievement, unskilled occupations and generally impoverished environment. These children are, in general, poorly nourished, subject to more acute and chronic illness, and receive less medical and dental care than do those from the middle and upper income groups. Children of migrant farm workers and from the ghetto are rarely brought up in homes where there is stimulating conversation, where books are read, where there is an opportunity for good education, or where the intellectual and cultural advantages taken for granted by the children of middle and upper income groups are available. Many come from disadvantaged and broken homes. Many are born to mothers who are poorly nourished and who receive little prenatal, perinatal or postnatal care. Many are unplanned and unwanted children; they are frequently born out of wedlock and grow up in homes with absent fathers and with an inconstant or unstable mother figure. They learn to survive, but not to thrive. The premature rate in such environments is two to three times that of the national average. Retardation in these underprivileged children is largely acquired, possibly beginning in utero in many instances, and becomes apparent during the second or third year of life, probably as a consequence of lack of healthy interpersonal relations, the absence of psychologic stimulation, and an overall sensory, emotional, environmental and nutritional deprivation. In most instances the way of life is inherited, rather than genes that are associated with or create mental retardation. The cycle of dependency, poverty and frustration of many welfare recipients is a typical example.

Children reared in significantly deprived circumstances arrive at school age equipped with neither experience, skills, nor motivation necessary for formal learning. They are, in general, behind age level in language development and in ability for abstract thinking necessary for success at school. They perform poorly; this results in negative feelings toward the learning process, and continued failure follows. Frustration, anxiety, low motivation, lack of opportunity and unstimulating school curricula lead to lack of self-respect, to truancy, to dropouts, and may predispose to delinquency. Many, as young adults, are unemployed and are unable to meet minimum mental or health standards for military service. This large group of the poor whose cultural and psychologic background simply prevents them from performing competitively in middle-class society constitutes 75 to 80 per cent of those considered mentally retarded. In a more fortunate environment this group would probably approach the same range of intellectual ability and performance as that shown by the more favored groups. It is frequently difficult to distinguish objectively between the child who functions at a retarded level because of environment and the one who suffers from prematurity, nutritional deprivation or a variety of medical problems associated with neglect, since both are frequently children of poverty.

In contrast to the finding that mild retardation is often associated with disadvantaged socioeconomic groups, the more severe degrees of retardation appear to be more evenly distributed throughout the population. Some of the medical and biologic causative factors which can be identified as significant in over 25 per cent of the cases appear to be increasing. More low-birth-weight babies live because of somewhat better medical care. More infants with intracranial trauma during the perinatal period and more of those with serious infections or poisoning during early childhood survive. Nonfatal accidents in and out of the home are increasing.

The **etiologic classification** which follows includes only the major causes, which account for approximately 25 per cent of the retarded. Children with these disorders, in general, are the more severely retarded and can usually be identified early in life by the physician. Most of the children so affected have other manifestations of central nervous system defect or damage such as motor handicaps, seizures, sensory defects and learning disabilities, and many have involvement of skeletal, circulatory, endocrine and other systems. Many developmental syndromes are consistently, and others only rarely, associated with mental retardation.

I. Prenatal
   A. Genetically determined
      1. Disorders of protein, carbohydrate or fat metabolism, e.g., histidinemia, homocystinuria, maple syrup urine disease, phenylketonuria, galactosemia and the cerebral lipidoses
      2. Cerebral demyelinating diseases
      3. Mucopolysaccharidoses
      4. Cranial anomalies: primary microcephaly, craniostenosis and congenital hydrocephalus
      5. Congenital ectodermoses: tuberous sclerosis, neurofibromatosis, cerebral angiomatosis
      6. Chromosomal abnormalities: Down syndrome, Klinefelter syndrome, triple X syndrome, hermaphroditism, *cri du chat* syndrome, trisomy-18, trisomy-D_1 and others
   B. Maternal and fetal infections: syphilis, rubella, toxoplasmosis, cytomegalic inclusion disease
   C. Fetal irradiation
   D. Kernicterus (bilirubin encephalopathy)
   E. Cretinism
   F. Prenatal unknown or indefinite causes associated with placental abnormality, toxemia of pregnancy, prematurity, maternal medication, poisoning, nutritional deficiency, infection or trauma
II. Natal
   A. Birth injuries, infection, cerebral trauma, hemorrhage, anoxia, hypoglycemia
III. Postnatal
   A. Cerebral infections: meningitis, encephalitis, abscess
   B. Cerebral trauma
   C. Poisoning (lead, carbon monoxide, and others)
   D. Cerebral vascular accidents, occlusion and hemorrhage from congenital defects, deficiency diseases, or unknown cause
   E. Postimmunization encephalopathy: pertussis, smallpox, rabies and others

Most of these conditions are discussed elsewhere, and reference should be made to discussions of symptoms, differential diagnosis and specific treatment.

PHENYLKETONURIA

Phenylketonuria is a genetic defect of phenylalanine metabolism, in which mental retardation is the most serious manifestation. It occurs once in approximately 10,000 births in the United States. The disorder was identified by Følling in 1934 and named phenylpyruvic oligophrenia, a term no longer used. Phenylalanine, which is present in all natural proteins, accumulates in the blood at abnormal concentrations in the absence of the enzyme phenylalanine hydroxylase, which normally converts it to tyrosine. Damage to the developing brain almost always results when these abnormal concentrations of phenylalanine and other metabolites persist in the blood. The biochemical mechanism by which this occurs is not clearly understood.

GENETICS. Phenylketonuria is transmitted by an autosomal recessive gene. Approximately 1 in 50 persons is an asymptomatic heterozygous carrier, who cannot be identified with certainty, though phenylalanine loading tests may be suggestive.

CLINICAL FEATURES. The untreated affected child may have clinical evidence of arrested brain development by 4 months of age, and eventually the typical "classic" picture of a moderate to severely retarded child with schizoid behavior evolves. Such children are blonder than unaffected siblings, have blue eyes, a musty odor and a tendency to seborrheic eczematous skin lesions. Many have abnormal electroencephalographic patterns, and approximately one third have seizures. There are no consistent neurologic abnormalities, although many of these children are hypertonic or hyperactive and have unsocial behavior.

Infants with phenylketonuria appear to be normal at birth and during the perinatal period. Plasma phenylalanine levels are normal at delivery (0.4 to 2.0 mg/dl), and phenylalanine does not appear in the urine until plasma phenylalanine levels rise to about 30 mg/dl or higher during the neonatal period. During late infancy and thereafter phenylpyruvic acid may appear in the urine when plasma phenylalanine levels are over 15 mg/dl. By this time cerebral damage has begun, which probably reaches its maximum at 2 to 3 years of age. Hence dietary treatment should be begun as soon after birth as the diagnosis can be established. Though the blood level of phenylalanine rapidly rises to significant values within a few days after birth, the appearance of phenylpyruvic acid in the urine of an affected infant may be delayed for a somewhat longer time.

DIAGNOSIS. A screening test, the bacterial inhibition assay method of Guthrie, is widely used for detection of abnormal levels of serum phenylalanine in newborn infants. Most states mandate screening at birth for phenylketonuria, and many health departments provide consultation through medical centers in the diagnosis and management of this relatively rare disease.

The Guthrie test requires several drops of capillary blood; plasma concentrations of phenylalanine may not be significantly elevated until the third to sixth day of life or until the infant has had dietary protein for 24 to 48 hours. When this test indicates an elevated level or when the urine reaction is positive at any age, the phenylalanine concentration of the plasma should be determined chemically before the diagnosis of phenylketonuria is considered to be established. Newborn infants whose results are negative should be reappraised with a urine test within 4 to 6 weeks after birth.

The amount of phenylpyruvic acid excreted in the urine varies with the protein intake; on an ordinary diet it is in the range of 0.5 to 2.5 gm/day. For preliminary diagnostic or screening purposes after the neonatal period, a random urine specimen is usually satisfactory. Phenylpyruvic acid is indicated by the deep bluish green color produced by a few drops of 10 per cent ferric chloride solution in about 5 ml of urine or by the use of Phenistix. This color fades within seconds or minutes, depending on the urinary concentration of phenylpyruvic acid. Color changes are also produced by ferric chloride in the urines of patients with other types of aminoaciduria and of those who have ingested aspirin or one of the phenothiazine derivatives. A few drops of this solution on a urine-wet diaper of an affected infant will yield the characteristic color.

The finding through screening programs of transient, slightly elevated serum levels of phenylalanine in some infants has led, in a few cases, to the diagnosis of maternal phenylketonuria. Some of these infants with transient elevations of serum phenylalanine are believed to be heterozygous carriers for the phenylketonuria trait.

Owing to the delayed maturation of the tyrosine oxidizing system, many premature infants and occasionally full-term ones have slightly elevated serum values for phenylalanine, usually in the range of 5 to 15 mg/dl. These infants also have elevated serum and urinary concentrations of tyrosine and elevated urinary values for parahydroxyphenylacetic acid. The oral administration of ascorbic acid usually corrects this defect promptly. There is no similar effect from ascorbic acid on tyrosinosis, which is an inherited metabolic disorder of tyrosine metabolism.

TREATMENT. As a rule, increased concentrations of phenylalanine in the blood of children or adults are associated with mental retardation. There are, however, several documented instances in which persons with persistently high serum levels of phenylalanine have had normal intelligence. Systematic controlled studies of children in whom phenylalaninemia was demonstrated in early infancy have not yet permitted definitive evaluation of the effects of dietary treatment upon subsequent physical and mental status.

At present, restriction of phenylalanine in the diet appears to be indicated for infants with persistent serum phenylalanine concentrations over 20 mg/dl and normal concentrations of tyrosine in serum and with phenylketones in the urine. Those with transient hyperphenylalaninemia probably do not require treatment. Infants with serum phenylalanine concentrations in the range of 10 to 20 mg/dl, and with normal serum tyrosine values and no phenylketonuria while they are receiving a normal diet, probably need not be treated. If reduction of dietary protein intake to 1.2 to 2.0 gm/kg/day is not effective in significantly reducing serum concentrations of phenylalanine, restriction of phenylalanine in the diet is indicated. All infants for whom dietary restriction of phenylalanine is prescribed should be placed on a regular diet for 2 to 3 days at periodic intervals to determine whether the metabolic abnormality has persisted and whether there is a need for continued dietary treatment to maintain the plasma phenylalanine level within the desired range. All infants for whom dietary restriction is not undertaken should be followed systematically with developmental evaluations and repeated urine or blood tests to establish the safety of continuing with a nontreatment regimen.

The purpose of the diet is to prevent or minimize brain damage in susceptible children. A milk substitute has been prepared, especially for use in infants, but its use is continued for a variable time into childhood. It is an enzymatic hydrolysate of casein, which contains a very small amount of phenylalanine, but normal amounts of other amino acids, and has added carbohydrate and fat.* Other natural foods which are calculated for their phenylalanine equivalents are added gradually after an initial period of feeding limited to this milk substitute. The optimal serum level to be maintained probably lies between 3 and 7 mg/dl. Since most natural food proteins contain approximately 5 per cent of phenylalanine, their intake must be limited. The administration of the low phenylalanine diet demands close nutritional supervision of the child and frequent monitoring of the serum concentration of phenylalanine. Phenylalanine is not synthesized in the body; hence "overtreatment," particularly in rapidly growing infants, may lead to phenylalanine deficiency, which is manifest by lethargy, anorexia, anemia, skin rashes and diarrhea.

Initiation of dietary treatment at a later age, but before the age of 2 or 3 years, may limit the progress of the brain damage. It does not, however, appear to reverse the process. In older phenylketonuric children there is no apparent improvement of mental capacity from the use of such diets. Low-

*Dietary management with this milk substitute is described in a pamphlet: Phenylketonuria—Low Phenylalanine Dietary Management with Lofenalac, available from Mead Johnson Laboratories, Evansville, Indiana 47721. (Other similar products have been produced; Lofenalac appears to be optimal for use in the United States.)

ering of the high concentration of phenylalanine or its metabolites in these children by dietary measures, however, frequently results in improved attention span, less hyperactive behavior, diminution of the number of seizures or changes in the electroencephalographic pattern.

More difficult than the dietary management is the prevention of emotional problems resulting from dietary restriction and abnormal eating habits. The parents have obvious difficulty in controlling the diets of ambulatory children, and they become disturbed by the realization that ingestion of normal amounts of usual foods may increase the mental retardation. The maintenance of such dietary control without psychologic difficulties is attained with difficulty, and it is understandable that parents of these children will need continuous support and guidance.

The birth of mentally retarded children without phenylketonuria to phenylketonuric mothers suggests that cerebral damage of the fetus may be caused by placental transfer of increased amounts of phenylalanine from the maternal circulation. This observation is an indication for identifying the pregnant phenylketonuric woman and for maintaining her on a low phenylalanine diet during gestation; unfortunately, however, a suitable diet has not been devised.

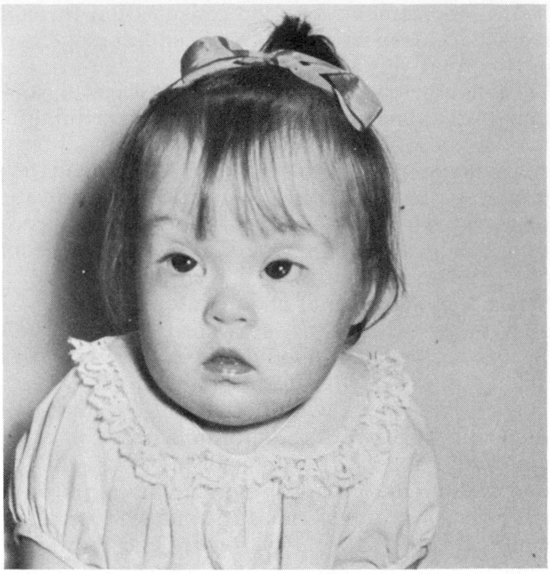

Figure 2–14 *Typical facial appearance of young child with Down syndrome.*

DOWN SYNDROME

(Mongolism)

See also *Chromosomal Abberations.*

Down syndrome is one of the most common of the clinically classifiable categories of mental retardation. The incidence is estimated at 1.5 per 1000 births. It accounts, frequently inappropriately, for approximately 10 per cent of retarded individuals in institutions. The majority have trisomy-21; a small percentage have partial translocation of chromosomes in the D group with 21. The chromosomal abnormality is the most consistent finding and is essential for the definitive diagnosis.

The clinical diagnosis depends on the presence of mental retardation in association with a variety of manifestations of disordered growth of the skeletal system, particularly of the skull and long bones. Evidence of defective development of other tissues is also usually manifest.

The abnormal development of the skull is responsible for the characteristic facies. The circumference of the head is usually in the third to twentieth percentile, and the head tends to be flattened anteriorly and posteriorly. The bony orbits are smaller than normal. There is a lateral upward slope of the eyes, and an epicanthic fold is present in the younger child which differs from that of Asiatic races by being confined to the inner angle rather than including most of the upper lid. The epicanthus tends to disappear during puberty. Chronic inflammatory changes involving the conjunctivae and lid margins are common. Cataracts are occasionally present; strabismus is common, as are speckling of the iris (Brushfield spots) and sparse, thin eyelashes. The external ears are usually small, and there may be cartilaginous anomalies. The tongue is usually protuded as a result of the smallness of the oral cavity and hypoplasia of the mandible. The surface may be fissured and furrowed (scrotal tongue) as the result of sucking and mouth-breathing. The nose is short with a flat bridge, resulting from underdevelopment of the nasal bone. The teeth are usually delayed in eruption; they are small and frequently abnormally aligned.

The neck is short and broad, and there is laxity of the skin on the lateral aspects. Generalized hypotonia is usually evident in infancy and becomes less apparent as the child becomes older. In the young child the abdomen is prominent, owing to hypotonia of the abdominal muscles, and there are frequently associated diastasis recti and umbilical hernia.

The extremities are shortened, especially the phalanges, so that the hands and feet tend to be broad, flat and square. The fifth finger is proportionately small and tends to curve inward. The second phalanx of the fifth finger is rudimentary in about 40 per cent of affected children. The spaces between the first and second fingers and toes are increased; in the foot this is frequently associated with a prominent skin crease and with partial syndactyly. The dermal ridge pattern in the hands and feet is frequently abnormal. Frequently there is a single transverse palmar crease instead of the two normally present.

Alterations in the bony pelvis recognizable radiographically in early infancy consist of broad ilia, small acetabular angles and elongated ischia.

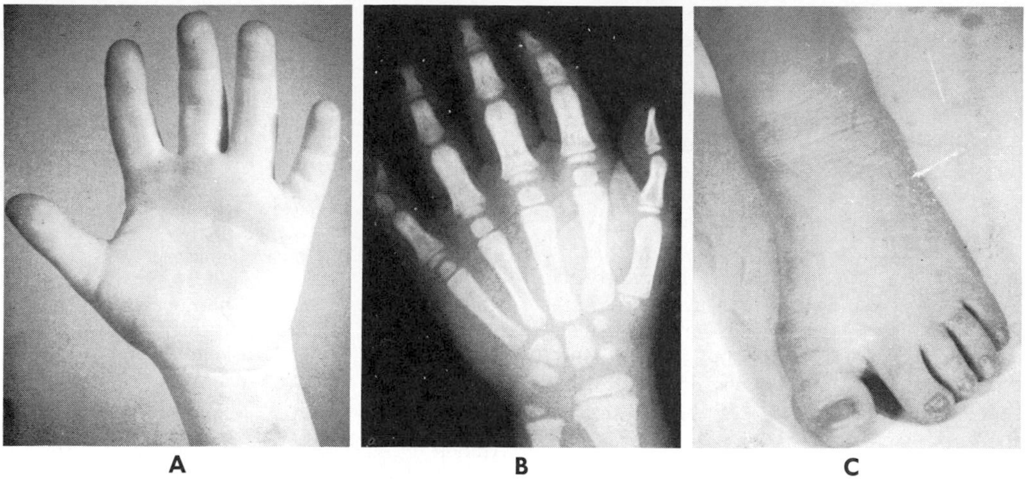

Figure 2–15 A, *The typical broad, spadelike hand of Down syndrome in a 12-year-old boy. Note the shortness of all fingers, especially the fifth. The presence of a single transverse palmar crease, instead of the 2 creases normally seen, is well shown.* B, *Roentgenogram of the hand of a 7-year-old girl with Down syndrome. Note the maldevelopment of the second phalanx of the fifth finger responsible for the shortening and incurving. The metacarpal bones and remaining phalanges also tend to be short and broad.* C, *The typical broad flat foot of Down syndrome in a 12-year-old boy. Note the wide space between the first and second toes.*

Cardiac anomalies are more common than in the general population, most often involving the atrioventricular structure. Duodenal atresia is also relatively common. The genitalia are usually poorly developed; secondary sex characteristics are delayed in their appearance, and the pubic hair tends to be straight and to have a silky quality. There are frequently abnormalities of the white blood cells, and the incidence of leukemia in Down syndrome is 10 to 20 times greater than in the general population. An increase in some of the gamma globulin fractions has also been observed. There have been reported decreased levels of serotonin in serum, increased levels of acid and alkaline phosphatase in white blood cells, and increased levels of G-6-PD in red blood cells.

There are no pathognomonic changes in the brain or spinal cord. Minor fissural and gyral deviations have been described, and histologically there are minor changes in the ganglion cells, as well as areas of defective myelin formation.

The mental status is usually in the moderately to severely retarded range, though in some instances the rate of development may approach normal for the first 3 or 4 years of life and then decelerate. In the absence of serious associated congenital defects, and when the child is given good medical care, the life span can be expected to approach normal.

Probably owing to the dryness of the skin, with frequent fissuring and cracking during cold weather, furunculosis and other skin infections are more common than in normal children. The patient is also more susceptible to acute and chronic infections of the upper respiratory tract, perhaps owing to the decreased anteroposterior diameter of the nasopharynx, which contributes to inadequate drainage.

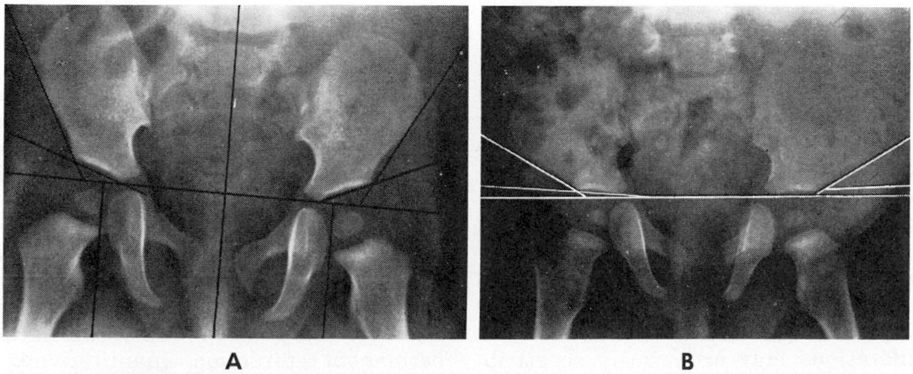

Figure 2–16 A, *Roentgenogram of pelvis and hips of a normal infant at 9 months of age.* B, *Roentgenogram of pelvis and hips of an infant with Down syndrome at 7 months of age. The acetabular roofs are almost horizontal, and there is flaring of the ilia. These abnormalities may be measured as illustrated and as described by Caffey.*

The diagnosis of Down syndrome in the older child is relatively simple, being based on the combination of the characteristic physical pattern and mental retardation. In the early weeks of life, however, when most of the signs are not so obvious, it may be less certain. The typical facies, generalized muscular hypotonia, and the dermatoglyphic changes are the most common early findings; the diagnosis is confirmed by chromosomal analysis.

Cretinism, which is not usually manifest at birth, may cause some difficulty in the differential diagnosis. The child with Down syndrome may, however, also be a cretin. There is no evidence that the overall course of mongolism is significantly benefited in any way by the use of hormonal or other types of medication, though the physical appearance may be altered.

TABLE 2–15 DIFFERENTIAL FACTORS IN DOWN SYNDROME AND CRETINISM

FACTOR	DOWN SYNDROME	CRETINISM
Recognizable	At birth	After 2–3 months
Body growth	Retarded	Retarded
Head	Brachycephalic	Normal size
Eyes	Upward, outward slant	Puffy
Osseous orbits	Smaller than normal	Normal
Epicanthus	Present at inner angle	Not present
Nose	Small; bridge underdeveloped	Normal
Tongue	Scrotal; may protrude	Thick, large; protrudes
Hands	Short; incurved 5th finger; single palmar crease; dermatoglyphic changes	Short; square
Feet	1st and 2nd toes widely spaced	Short; square
Skin	Occasionally dry	Very dry, pale, coarse
Hair	Variable	Very dry and coarse
Muscle tone	Poor; joint laxity	Unchanged
Constipation	Uncommon	Common
Congenital anomalies	Frequent: heart; eyes; duodenum; leukocytes	Umbilical hernia
Ossification	Slight or no delay	Considerable delay
Tests of thyroid function	Normal	Decreased
Chromosomal pattern	Abnormal	Normal

DIFFERENTIAL DIAGNOSIS OF MENTAL RETARDATION

Diagnosis involves consideration of the most common conditions which may be mistaken for mental retardation or which may so interfere with the capacity to learn as to result in a clinical picture characterized by depressed intellectual function. A critical use of psychologic tests, evaluation of the physical status, and knowledge and understanding of the family and the social background are essential for the diagnosis and an appreciation of the complex contributory factors. Since psychologic tests are, as a general rule, based on the acquisition of learned experiences, the following conditions, by impairing the learning process, may also adversely affect the results of these tests and add to the diagnostic difficulty.

DELAYED EDUCATIONAL MATURATION. This is a normal variation in the development of motivation or readiness to partake in organized learning experiences, especially those involving academic schooling. It usually becomes evident as a diagnostic problem when the child enters school if the immaturity is great. Some of these children will catch up and do well if academic competition with their peers is temporarily modified.

PERIPHERAL SENSORY DEFECTS. Screening tests for visual and hearing acuity should be done on all children before 3 or 4 years of age, particularly if there is any developmental delay. Irreversible changes affecting the learning capacity take place very early in children with critical defects in these sensory mechanisms.

CEREBRAL PALSY. In infancy assessment of development is in great part dependent on such motor achievements as holding up the head, sitting, hand manipulations, crawling, standing, walking, and the like. Low developmental quotients based on these considerations may erroneously be attributed to mental retardation in the presence of motor defects such as cerebral palsy. Such motor defects not only interfere with learning opportunities, but also, particularly when language function is involved, prevent effective functioning of the intellectual capacity.

LANGUAGE AND SPEECH DISORDERS. These include disturbances of the cortical mechanisms that control expressive, central and receptive language which, when severely impaired, are manifest clinically as aphasia. Lesser degrees of difficulty may show up as reading disorders, speech disabilities, visual motor or space discrimination disorders, or a variety of learning disabilities involving only one or two of the processes of intelligence. All can seriously affect the learning potential and create diagnostic problems which will require psychologic testing and evaluation of language development in support of the clinical appraisal.

ENVIRONMENTAL DEPRIVATION. The absence of adequate learning opportunities, the lack of emotional stimulation, and other environmental factors prevent development of intellectual potential and, if not corrected early in life, result in functional or permanent retardation. Quantitatively, within the total population, deprivation factors are largely related to poverty, although broken homes, inadequate parent-child relations, unsatisfactory social environment and lack of motivation are not restricted to any geographic, social, racial or economic group. Emotional disorders may block normal intellectual functioning and may interfere with the learning process.

PRIMARY PERSONALITY DISORDERS. These include basic personality defects which are believed to be the result of faulty cerebral development; some may be genetically determined. The basic clinical manifestations are failure to relate appropriately to the environment and failure in the development of normal interpersonal relations. There is a spectrum of disorder which has at one extreme the complete failure of personality development sometimes called infantile autism, and at the other extreme the minor variations in personality structure that blend with normal behavior. Childhood schizophrenia fits into this scheme. Such defects seriously impair the learning capacity and are frequently mistaken for or are associated with mental retardation.

Other factors to be considered in the differential diagnosis include seizure disorders, drug-induced states, some allergies, and nutritional deprivation.

PREVENTION

The complexity of mental retardation defies a single approach to any phase of its management. The prevention of mental retardation in the large group of children who are deprived of the opportunity for optimal development requires a broad, community-wide social, educational, cultural and economic approach. The relatively smaller group of children with associated organic and physical defects tends to be more severely retarded, but fortunately it seems that many of these disorders could be prevented by application of existing biomedical knowledge. The physician must be involved with both groups; in the case of the first group he must support and participate in community activities designed to provide appropriate living, educational and health opportunities for all children. In the latter group he must provide or secure early diagnostic evaluation and a suitable plan of management for the child and general support for the parents, including, when indicated, genetic counseling.

The most important aspects in the prevention of mental retardation are centered in preconceptional and prenatal factors. The best insurance for a healthy physical and mental life is to be born after a wanted pregnancy at term to healthy parents and to be reared in a stable, responsible home. Such a wide variety of factors—genetic, chromosomal, and intrauterine environmental—can interfere with mental as well as physical development that they cannot be enumerated here, but they are discussed in the sections on Developmental Pediatrics, Prenatal Disturbances, Inborn Errors of Metabolism, The Fetus and the Newborn Infant, and Infectious Disease.

An increasing number of disorders related to mental retardation and other disabling conditions that are associated with chromosomal abnormalities are identifiable; a few of these are transmitted. Many of the metabolic disorders are of genetic origin, and in some, such as galactosemia and phenylketonuria, mental retardation can be avoided or lessened by early diagnosis and appropriate management. In some disorders heterozygote carriers can be identified, and genetic counseling, if accepted, can be highly effective in limiting the production of probable defectives. An increasing number of medical conditions which may lead to fetal damage of the nervous system are becoming identifiable through maternal or fetal diagnostic procedures, such as amniocentesis. In such circumstances the advisability of therapeutic abortion must be judiciously considered (see below).

Appropriate use of available immunologic agents to prevent infectious and contagious diseases, prevention and adequate treatment of infections, prevention of poisoning, accidents and child abuse, and an early intervention in the lives of sensorially and otherwise deprived children by provision of appropriate learning experience would eliminate many instances of retardation.

PROGNOSIS

When he has reached his fifth birthday, a retarded child has as good a chance of growing up and probably has about the same life expectancy as do others who receive good medical care, an adequate diet, early and adequate treatment of infections, and the like. For severe and profoundly retarded children with multiple defects the life expectancy is substantially less, though with appropriate care it can be significantly extended.

It must be remembered that intelligence is not a fixed factor and that modification of environment, with improvement in learning opportunities and in social acceptance, will bring about some improvement in all retarded children. The degree of improvement is predictably less in the more severely involved child and in the one with multiple handicaps.

TREATMENT AND MANAGEMENT

See also the next subsection, The Physician and the Child with a Permanent Handicap.

The effective management of a retarded child is a complex problem requiring the physician to become involved as a compassionate, understanding, resourceful person who treats the child, supports the family, and communicates effectively with others in the community over a considerable period of time.

As a physician, he is daily involved in the prevention and early recognition of the infant and child with a developmental disability. Frequently with the help of other professional persons and parents, he establishes the fact of the child's slow intellectual development. He should particularly avoid such categorizing or labeling as may stigmatize the child, but rather should encourage an approach that emphasizes assets and capabilities rather than defects and limitations. He identifies and secures treatment, if any is established as effective, for conditions that cause or are associated with decreased effectiveness of learning capacity, such as motor, visual and hearing disorders. These include metabolic disorders of protein, such as phenylketonuria, maple syrup urine disease, hyperglycinuria, leucine intolerance, tyrosinosis and Hartnup disease; abnormal carbohydrate metabolism, such as galactosemia, fructose intolerance and hypoglycemia; pyridoxine dependency; hyperbilirubinemia; plumbism; hypercalcemia; hypothyroidism; hypoparathyroidism; hydrocephalus; craniostenosis; and subdural accumulations. For many identifiable syndromes there is still only symptomatic and supportive treatment.

Unless a specific defect is identified, there is no generally accepted evidence to support the efficacy of a variety of therapies recommended at one time or another, which include the use of glutamic acid, vitamins, hormones, tissue extracts, minerals, drugs of various kinds, surgical procedures, or manipulations to increase cerebral blood flow or to improve neurologic organization.

Retarded children require the same general pediatric care which is desirable for all children. If a good parent-child relation early in life and a home environment providing adequate learning experiences, relative security, love and acceptance as an individual are essential for development of the inherent potential of the normal infant, these factors are even more essential for the development of the retarded child. Efforts to decrease disability and to increase functional capacity are essential at all ages, but are most effective early in life when the child is developing and is most actively using his learning capacity. Developmental gains by the retarded child should be assessed on the basis of his potential and estimated ability to approximate relative independence. During the pediatric age the specific amount of knowledge acquired is perhaps less important than is the development of effective work habits, of sustained interest in an activity, of satisfaction from attainable goals, and of personality factors that make for successful relations with family, with social contacts, and with potential employers. It is as essential for the retarded boy or girl to be provided an ongoing and appropriate health and sex educational experience at home as it is for the brighter sibling.

The family of a retarded child needs support, particularly in the interpretation of the child's problems, in the daily management, in developing and carrying out long-term plans, in the use of community resources, in self-understanding, in the understanding of genetic factors if present, and at times of crisis (see below). The physician must share these responsibilities with the family, the school, the community and the government.

Others may make a greater contribution to the ultimate adjustment of the retarded child than the physician. His ability, however, to understand growing children, to communicate his knowledge to others, and to be realistic in helping set goals may be critical factors. As family advisor, the physician must know what resources are available in the community, help the family to use the services which are appropriate, and perhaps help to develop services not available in the community. These may include specialized diagnostic facilities, home nursing programs, genetic counseling, specialized nursery and day-care centers, special classes in public and other day schools, religious nurture, camping and other recreational programs, vocational training, sheltered workshops, specialized employment services, income maintenance when necessary, foster homes and emergency or respite care facilities, as well as longer term residential homes in the community.

Great strides have been made in the field of special education in helping children who have special learning problems. Special classes are becoming available in greater number, and curricula are being developed on an individual basis. Formal and informal learning experiences are being developed for younger children such as the Head Start, Get Set, and day care developmental programs.

It is generally agreed that most children with mild to moderate retardation should be kept and cared for within their own homes. Serious emotional and behavior disorders may arise, but the use of behavior modification techniques is frequently helpful in bringing about more acceptable behavior. Foster home care or group living in the community may be considered. Supportive care away from home for the more severely retarded should be considered only when home care is completely impossible or has proved unsuccessful. The decision for removal of the child from the home is a parental responsibility, but parents should be guided and supported by the physician. The decision depends less on the economic status of the family than on the availability of space and an appropriate program in a state-supported or private institution, on reaction of other children in the family, and on the emotional stability of the parents, particularly the mother.

There are certainly defendable medical, genetic, social, economic and moral indications for the voluntary limitation of the number of children in certain families, and for therapeutic abortion under certain circumstances. Sterilization of certain individuals can be supported for genetic reasons or because of poor potential for undertaking responsibilities of parenthood. The legal status, personal rights, moral and social acceptability, and practical indications for these procedures are undergoing debate and rapid change. The physician has a large responsibility in discussing and influencing such changes within the community, and in implementing the intent of "informed consent."

Both government and private citizen organizations have accomplished much in developing better services for the retarded. The physician should give guidance and perspective in the areas of his competence to both groups so that realistic programs are developed with appropriate priorities to meet the extensive needs of the retarded, and to provide as normal a life for every individual as is possible.

JOHN B. BARTRAM

American Academy of Pediatrics: The Pediatrician and the Child with Mental Retardation. 1972. Box 1034, Evanston, Illinois 60204.

Bibliography for Parents: Write to National Association for Retarded Citizens., 2709 Avenue E East, Arlington, Texas 76011.

Committee on the Handicapped Child: Selected References on Mental Retardation: An Annotated Bibliography. Evanston, Ill., American Academy of Pediatrics, 1967.

Hurley, R. L.: Poverty and Mental Retardation: A Causal Relationship. State of New Jersey, Department of Institutions and Agencies, Trenton, N.J., 1968.

Mental Retardation: A Family Crisis—The Therapeutic Role of the Physician. New York Group for the Advancement of Psychiatry, Report No. 56, 1963.

Mental Retardation Abstracts. Washington, D.C., United States Department of Health, Education, and Welfare, Public Health Service, National Institutes of Health, annually, starting 1964.

Mild Mental Retardation: A Growing Challenge to the Physician. New York, Group for the Advancement of Psychiatry, Report No. 66, 1967.

THE PHYSICIAN AND THE CHILD WITH A PERMANENT HANDICAP

It is increasingly important for the physician who cares for children to become familiar with the special problems of the child who chronically and perhaps permanently deviates from normal because of some congenital or acquired disability. The successful management of such a child depends as often on the social, academic and home adjustments that can be achieved as it does on purely technical and medical procedures.

THE PHYSICIAN. Some physicians are not suited by temperament or training to provide adequate management for the handicapped child and his family. The comprehensive care required is time-consuming, and many of the children as well as their parents are uncooperative. They may disrupt a busy appointment schedule, and much time must be spent with parents whose emotional reactions frequently present greater problems than do those of the child. The physician who extends his responsibility beyond the treatment of the "chief complaint," however, will find rewards in helping the young handicapped patient and his family to live more comfortably and effectively with a long-term disability.

The physician may feel inadequate because the complexity of the problems makes them appear unsolvable or beyond means at his immediate command. He must be aware of his own possible negative attitudes, prejudices and limitations, or these will be reflected in his poor relationships with the child and the family. He must, above all, be able to utilize other professional disciplines to make appropriate referrals and to use other resources in the community while he maintains his own professional relationship as primary physician to the family. Abandonment or rejection of the handicapped child and his family by a physician, through his failing to provide good pediatric care, ignoring the real problem, giving the family false assurances, or not seeking and using help which is available in the community, only compounds everyone's difficulties. The physician may feel inadequate if a specific diagnosis cannot be made or if the evaluation cannot be completed at one visit. Intelligent management should begin at the first meeting with the family with a simple functional appraisal of the child and a simple explanation to the parents.

The physician who cannot be a patient, uncritical listener, who cannot be satisfied with small gains, who cannot project himself into the child's and the parents' position sufficiently to offer intelligent support when a cure or complete recovery is not possible, who clings to outmoded concepts and is not realistically aware of both the possibilities and limitations of habilitation, who cannot communicate and work effectively with others in the community, and who does not provide adequate general pediatric care for the child and support an acceptable role for the parents at all times should not complain if others take over where he has failed.

MANAGEMENT OF THE CHILD. The child with a handicap should receive the same comprehensive health care that is available to all children in the community. Through continuing contacts and interest in the child and the family the physician can help in developing and periodically revising a plan that is realistic for all concerned. He should help the child to make use of his abilities as effectively as possible and become as socially acceptable and self-sufficient as his limitations permit. Immediate goals should be realistic so that success is possible and likely, since failure discourages further effort.

The physician who is aware that the child with single or multiple handicaps has limited opportunities for normal learning and development will make particular efforts to see that a variety of experiences are available at appropriate ages. Opportunities for learning, for social and group experiences, and for the achievement of self-discipline should be provided. A balance between overprotection and overstimulation must be sought. The child with multiple handicaps is rarely capable of achieving a high degree of independence, so that the physician must interpret the child and his behavior to those who are in regular or occasional contact with him. Every effort should be made to minimize secondary handicaps in personality development so that they do not become more serious than the primary defect. The physician should above all else try to help the child lead a happy life, in which the perhaps limited ways in which the child can be useful or contribute to the comfort of others are appropriately rewarded in a manner which leaves him or her with a healthy degree of self-esteem.

THE FAMILY'S PROBLEMS. Since the child's environment and the emotional climate of the home are of equal and sometimes of greater importance than the medical care for the child's eventual adjustment, every effort must be made to assist the family to understand their own feelings and to fulfill their own needs. They must always be given something constructive to do. Parents' reactions to a defective child depend on the extent to which they feel their competency, social standing and anticipated way of life to be threatened by the handicap. Most parents initially attempt to deny the reality of the defect, particularly if it is not obvious physically. This stage is usually followed by one of frustration and disorganization and of self-accusation and questioning in which fears and anxieties about the future become overwhelming. Simple explanation, support and guidance for the family are particularly necessary during this stage. As parents' defenses become organized, denial, hostility and shifting of responsibility take place. If communication and counseling with the mother and father are not effective, the "no one ever told me anything" reaction sets in and "shopping around" ensues. Establishment of support by communicating a genuine professional interest and concern in the child often spells the difference between active family involvement and rejection of help, with subsequent poor adjustment and failure to achieve the maximum potential in the child. Depending on the degree of maturity and emotional resources of the family, they can be helped to accept their problems realistically and to plan constructively for the long-term needs of the child.

The problems are as varied as the people involved. Most parents, regardless of their background, have feelings of guilt which must be resolved lest attitudes of self-sacrifice, excessive overprotection or rejection of the child develop. Most families have ambivalent feelings about the child, varying from overt hostility to gross overindulgence. The child may actually become deprived of normal experiences because of overindulgence or, because of his neglect and deprivation, be inadequately stimulated. The establishment of limits of acceptable behavior and the consistent teaching of discipline which are so important to a child's emotional development may thus be lacking. The handicapped child frequently may be the precipitating factor in marital difficulties which are not basically related to him.

As the child grows older the parents have to accept many roles, and make psychologic adaptations which would otherwise not be necessary, because of the child's prolonged dependency upon them. The problems of social isolation, sexual development and unpleasant behavior become increasingly important to the family as the child grows older.

The principles of behavior modification should be discussed with the family, and on occasion help in establishing and maintaining an appropriate program of conditioning for acceptable behavior should be provided. Since most parents are less than adept at providing ongoing health and sex education for their children, they should be given support and acceptable materials for such use. Appropriately modified material is available for the child with a handicap. (See references below.)

FAMILY THERAPY. Parents in retrospect often complain that the status of the child was not made clear to them, that the diagnosis was based on an incomplete examination or hasty judgment, that poor prognosis was not justified or that their part in helping the child was not explained. It must be remembered that many parents hear, retain and comprehend only in part, and that various interpretations and suggestions must be given *and repeated* in an acceptable and understandable way to those concerned. Reinforcement of information given the family may be made by other members of the physician's staff or by members of various other disciplines if consultation services are available through a clinic or other community agency.

The initial explanation of the facts about a child with a handicap should be made to the parents *together* in as simple a way as possible. Technical explanations are usually only confusing. Long-term prognosis and planning should be left for a later interview, but emphasis should be on management of immediate problems and symptoms. Questions should be answered simply, reassurance be given to minimize guilt feelings, and the importance of time in determining the developmental ability of the child should be stressed. Attention cannot be given too early to the avoidance of secondary emotional problems in the child and his family. The practical problems of carrying out a reasonable home program can best be appreciated by a visit to the home. Grandparents and other relatives who may be involved in family affairs should be brought into explanations as necessary in order that the parents' efforts with the child will not be negated. The time, expense and effort involved in the evaluation of the handicapped child may be largely wasted if explanation and interpretation to all concerned is not simply and effectively carried out.

A physician who is not aware that the parents' feelings of guilt about the child may be projected to him will be unprepared to act with the necessary understanding and patience and will emerge with a bruised ego. Guidance and support to the family are a continuing affair, and acceptance of the handicapped child is probably never fully accomplished by the parents because the problems change with advancing age.

Care should be taken to assure the siblings an equal share of the parents' time, attention and interest. With inadvertent or intentional neglect their problems may become greater than those of the affected child. Their questions about the abnormal child should be answered simply and honestly. The experience of living with a seriously handicapped brother or sister may be used constructively to teach tolerance, patience and understanding of others. If parents openly accept the child as an individual despite his limitations, and if they accept his failures as inevitably as they do his more limited successes, a good example is set for others in the community. This is the best method of "public education." The converse is also true.

The question of the probable outcome of future pregnancies is frequently raised by parents. If the cause of the disability is clearly an accidental one, it is easy to be reassuring. If it is known to be genetically determined or to arise as a result of circumstances that might be repeated, the physician should explain the facts as simply and clearly as possible and help the parents to make their own decision based on available evidence. When the family has made its decision on grounds that for them are valid, the physician should support them in it.

INSTITUTIONAL CARE. With a seriously involved child who will always be completely or partially dependent on others for his care, the question of support away from home will arise. The physician should help the family to make their own decision about this by objectively discussing with them the advantages and disadvantages of such care. The decision is the family's and not the physician's, though he may diplomatically initiate the discussion if the family appears reluctant to open the question and if he is convinced that such a solution might be beneficial to all.

The potential value of home care during infancy and early childhood, not only for the child's subsequent development but also for the family's sense of participation and accomplishment, is emphasized. Even seriously handicapped children can profit by tender loving care at home; it has been shown that children with Down syndrome have a much greater potential if given good care in the average home than if placed in an institution at birth.

It is sometimes said that defective children should be placed away from home at birth lest the parents become abnormally devoted to them. This is unlikely, and the average family with guidance can handle such children to advantage at home for a few years. Parents, in general, feel more comfortable about later placement if they gradually gain acceptance of the child's limitations by normally fulfilling their role as parents. Too early placement may lead to doubts and greater feelings of guilt. The physician should be aware of the appropriateness, the cost and the availability of supportive or educational facilities away from home before advising their use.

Temporary placement away from home is indicated when the child himself can profit by greater opportunities in a different environment or for a short term when inevitable family emergencies arise or when a vacation is needed by all. Relatively short-term living away from home with concurrent support and instructions to the family may permit effective modification of disturbing or unacceptable behavior. If the defective child becomes a serious burden to the physical or emotional health of the parents and siblings, the change should be made. Placement is wrongly used as an escape from the physician's or the family's responsibility. It is usually not wise to encourage brothers and sisters to assume the permanent care of a dependent child.

USE OF COMMUNITY RESOURCES. The physician should help to develop and make effective use of local community resources such as public health nurses, baby-sitters, "home-maker" services, day-care centers, special schools, social agencies, voluntary health agencies and temporary boarding homes to give the family a vacation or to tide them over emergencies. The physician often overlooks the support which the church can give to families in time of stress. A religiously oriented parent is better able to accept the burden of a handicapped child than one without such a resource. Better communication between the clergy and the medical profession can lead to more effective family counseling and support. With the family's consent the physician may properly take the initiative by informing the designated priest, rabbi or minister of the child's problems, the plan proposed and the family's reaction and needs.

For less severely affected children the physician should assist the family to get appropriate help from public or private schools that may offer programs for exceptional children. An increasing number of special classes for orthopedically, mentally and emotionally handicapped children, as well as for those with visual, hearing, language and learning defects, is being provided by the public school systems in many areas. The physician is in a unique position to interpret to others in the school, the church and the community center the special problems presented by the child with a handicap. It is incumbent on him to take leadership in this area.

Fortunately, the rationale of supplying comprehensive services for children with problems and disabilities is gradually being accepted and implemented as a substitute for inadequate support of piecemeal programs for categorical disease entities, and most communities, encouraged by voluntary health agencies and by parents' organizations, are developing services for children with handicaps. These include medical facilities for early diagnosis, evaluation and treatment, social casework, genetic counseling, home care by nurses, psychologic evaluation and counseling, babysitting or temporary home care, educational and recreational facilities, occupational training and vocational placement, sheltered workshops as well as smaller local residential programs and supportive care. Community centers for mental health and mental retardation are being developed in many areas, and such centers can provide many of the services needed by children with multiple handicaps. Greater use is being made of volunteers and of nonprofessional workers to provide services in a variety of areas. The physician can contribute significantly to the training and orientation of such personnel as well as help in planning community service centers.

PARENTS' ORGANIZATIONS. Parents' organizations have been outstandingly successful in affording those with common problems an opportunity to share their anxieties, to gain strength and hope through identification with a group, and to bring about effective changes in legislative and community health and educational programs, and in support of legal and civil rights of the handicapped. Efforts in behalf of community education, support of research and voluntary participation in a variety of services are psychologically important to the families of children with handicaps and are constructively helpful to the community.

JOHN B. BARTRAM

Battle, C. U.: Pediatrician as ombudsman for handicapped child. Pediatrics *50*:6, 1972.

Gordon, S.: Facts about Sex for Exceptional Youth: New Jersey Association for Brain Injured Children, 61 Lincoln Street, East Orange, New Jersey 07017 ($2.95).

Kempton, W. et al.: Guide for Parents; Love, Sex and Birth Control for Mentally Retarded. Planned Parenthood Association of Southeastern Pennsylvania, 1402 Spruce Street, Philadelphia 19102.

Pattullo, A.: Puberty in the Girl Who is Retarded: National Association for Retarded Citizens, 2709 Avenue E East, Arlington, Texas 76010 ($1.00).

THE CARE OF THE CHILD WITH A FATAL ILLNESS

From time to time every physician has the painful duty of caring for a child with a fatal illness. It is then his responsibility to help the family cope with *their* pain and grief in such ways that the experience may have the best possibility of being growth-promoting, rather than destructive of family integrity or of the emotional well-being of the family members. The physician's acceptance of these goals as realistic and urgently in need of his professional skills will help to blunt his own sense of frustration, grief or professional inadequacy.

When the physician is certain of a fatal outcome, there should ordinarily be no equivocation in conveying the diagnosis to the family in a frank, direct and empathic way. If both parents are available, the fact that their child has an illness from which recovery is not expected should be conveyed to them when they are together. The words chosen and the manner of the physician should be gentle and honest, and he should be prepared to meet the parents' anguish or disbelief with answers to their questions and with information as to what measures will be taken to try to forestall what seems to be inevitable.

The place in which this conversation occurs should be carefully chosen. It should be apart from the other activities of the hospital or office, and should be available for an adequate, uninterrupted time. The physician should understand that much of the conversation at this time will not be truly heard or registered by the parents of the sick child, and he should plan another session later in the day or on the next day when he can review the information he has given and answer new or recurring questions.

Ordinarily the physician should avoid taking the stand that nothing can be done in a situation which the parents sense as a disaster, but should emphasize the positive steps which he and the parents can take together to surmount the difficulties ahead. He should generally avoid detailed predictions of the course of the illness, emphasizing that in such situations one generally lives from day to day, and that it is usually possible to avoid undue suffering or pain. When the illness may endure for months or years, it may not be inappropriate to hold out the hope that medical research may provide methods of control which are not currently available.

Parents are often reluctant to ask whether some other physician or the resources of some other medical center may offer more hope, or even whether the diagnosis may be in doubt. They will need help in expressing these concerns and should be encouraged and helped to seek additional medical opinions if they wish. These matters should be discussed in such a way that the family should feel no embarrassment, and they should know that they are causing none. They can be helped to understand that medical communication is generally good enough to provide prompt dissemination of any real break-through in the management of the otherwise fatal illness of their child. It is also reasonable to advise them that they may do the ill child and the rest of the family a disservice if they dissipate the family's emotional and other resources in a frantic search for something that is not available.

It is natural and inevitable that parents will ask themselves whether the fatal illness of their child was not in some measure avoidable. Some will seek causes in inadequate medical care, in incompetent physicians or in other environmental circumstances; others will assume a burden of guilt at their own failure to recognize the symptoms of illness or to take action quickly enough so that a cure could have been effected. Each of these reactions may be irrational. When these feelings are implicit in questions or responses of parents, the physician should often make them explicit; he should point out the inevitability of such feelings, and when he can honestly do so, he should reassure the parents that there are no grounds for their shouldering blame for a situation which no one could say might have been averted. The feeling of guilt, or the sense of punishment, may be particularly strong in genetic disorders. Here it may be helpful to encourage the family to regard genetic mutations as tragic accidents, most often beyond the ability of man to avoid.

In the management of the affected child, parents should be encouraged to handle the life situation of the child as normally as possible. This may be difficult for parents, who may think that their usual disciplinary activities may make the child's pain or illness worse. These feelings should be allayed, and the parents should be encouraged to maintain the child in his normal place in the family hierarchy. Special arrangements, such as the celebration of Christmas in the summertime, or other public dramatizations of the child's illness should be discouraged; they may be more anxiety-provoking for the child than fulfilling of some special need. As much as possible, the parents should be encouraged to participate in the care of the child in the hospital, so long as their responsibilities to other children at home are adequately met. They may also need encouragement to take adequate respite from the care of the ill child.

As the physician follows the evolution of a fatal illness in a child, he should observe the manner in which the parents are coping with the situation. He may, for example, see that the parents are increasingly turning their attention to other sick children in the hospital. This is a healthy sign if it is not premature; if it comes too early, it may represent the parents' unresolved burden of guilt or their pain in facing the ill child. This turning away to help other children is healthy, so long as the parents still have adequate resources and strength for the sometimes increasing or diminishing needs of the patient.

At times the guilt of parents is intensified by a wish that the illness were all over, or by an unexpected sense of relief or release at the terminal event itself. The considerate and skillful physician will be on the watch for signs of these reactions and find the right words of reassurance or encouragement that such feelings are normal and that the parents have given everything that could have been expected of them in a situation which they have found very trying and toward which they will forever have sensitive and tender feelings.

What to tell the child who has a fatal illness about his future will vary with the condition and circumstances. Most young children do not ask whether they are going to die. They can often be told that they have an illness which may last for some time and which has ups and downs, and that it is important for them to get adequate rest and to be active when they feel up to it. Unrealistic reassurances that they look well and are doing fine will be less helpful than the frank recognition of the child's feeling that being ill is no fun and that having it going on so long is discouraging. This can be accompanied by assurances that the physician will get the child back to school or whatever activity is normal for him as soon as possible. Meanwhile it is supportive, when appropriate, for the child to receive attention from schoolteachers and play therapists in the hospital, who will help blunt the sense of inevitability of worsening illness.

In the case of preadolescent or adolescent children with chronic and fatal illness, the plan for care may often include sharing the diagnosis with the child and examining with parents and child together the implications of diagnosis and prognosis, answering their questions, and laying out with them a program of action and support which will have as its goal keeping the patient as comfortable as possible and forestalling any conclusion to the effort as long as possible. In this atmosphere of frankness, trust, and cooperation, free of secrets or evasions, many families and patients will find an unexpectedly healthy climate for the expression of tenderness and love toward each other, and the physician may find his own work easier. As a chronic illness becomes terminal, this climate makes it easier to meet the needs of the patient for a sense of not being abandoned, for assurances of the continuing love and affection of those about him, and for reasonably prompt responses to his needs for care. Needless to say, such a plan as that outlined must have the full understanding and cooperation of parents before the decision is made as to when or how the diagnosis of a potentially fatal illness is to be shared with the child, and the parents will need to have given some thought to how the news of the child's illness is to be handled with siblings, relatives and neighbors.

In dealing with the problems of patient and family around a fatal illness, the physician will often call upon other professional persons for help. The family s minister or other spiritual advisor can often be of immense comfort. When family problems are likely to be ameliorated by the use of community resources, the help of skilled social workers may be extremely important. When the family is not intact, owing to the death or previous separation of a parent, the likelihood of emotional difficulties complicating the management of the illness is sufficiently great that social service resources should probably be involved from the time when the diagnosis is known.

In the management of terminal illness the physician should not leave decisions about what is to be done for the child to the parents, but should give positive advice as to what he plans to do. He should be responsive, however, to the suggestions of parents when these represent a helpful and realistic appraisal of the child's needs.

When death is imminent, the patient should be kept comfortable and the parents, as much as possible, should be close at hand. The physician should be available to both parents and the patient. Control of his own feelings is important; if he allows his own distress to let him become less involved, the anger of the child or parents at what may be perceived as abandonment of them may make terminal care much more difficult. The continued interest and concern of the physician are important in preventing the emotional situation from deteriorating at this time.

As the moment of death approaches, the child should be in a room where he can be alone, his parents at the bedside or nearby. The sensitive physician will see that the occasion is accorded appropriate dignity and not rendered more frustrating or agonizing by fruitless efforts to prolong vital functions in a climate of purposeless hyperactivity.

When death has occurred, the patient, bed and room should be made neat, and the paraphernalia of illness removed. If the parents are not at hand, they should be asked to come to the hospital and be informed of the circumstances. Parents should be given the opportunity to be with the child a little while in the relatively peaceful and uncluttered setting which has been created. A brief and tender parting may help the parents in the adjustments which they must ultimately make. In the case of a newborn infant, the body can often be taken to the mother or both parents at her bedside or some other point in the hospital, where this contact with her baby may be the mother's only opportunity to establish for herself the reality of the birth and death of her infant, and to adjust toward reality her current or future fantasies as to what might *really* have happened.

A request for postmortem examination should be made by the responsible physician who knows the family best. This is often not the house officer, but the attending physician. The need for postmortem examination should be urged as strongly as conviction permits. It can be emphasized that such examinations are always helpful, that information is gathered and saved which may be extremely useful in years to come in solving similar problems of other children, or in providing definitive answers to questions which other children in the family or their relatives or descendants may have concerning the patient's illness, now or in the future.

Later the physician should describe the important and relevant findings of the gross postmortem examination for the parents in simple terms, and they should be permitted to discuss them as freely as they desire.

VICTOR C. VAUGHAN, III

Evans, A. E.: If a child must die...New Engl. J. Med. 278:138, 1968.
Hamovitch, M. B.: The Parent and the Fatally Ill Child. City of Hope Medical Center, Duarte, California, 1964.
Howell, D. A.: A child dies. J. Pediatr. Surg. 1:2, 1966.
Kübler-Ross, E.: On Death and Dying. New York, The Macmillan Co., 1969. (Available also in paperback.)

DIFFICULT DECISIONS IN PEDIATRICS

Among the more difficult decisions faced by the physician caring for children and their families are those which involve a variety of moral or ethical judgments with respect to which the community has no uniformity of feeling or of standards. Among these are: informed consent for surgery or other procedures or for the enlistment of a child in an experimental procedure; decisions regarding organ transplantation; genetic counseling; amniocentesis; abortion or other interruption of pregnancy; euthanasia; and determination of the point at which the potential has been passed for vital processes to be restored and the patient who still has a beating heart is effectively dead.

Among the factors which may influence or ultimately determine the responses of physicians to such problems are such considerations as the educational level, culture and religion of the involved families, such larger social issues as eugenics or overpopulation or other interests of the community, and in many instances legal constraints. In some instances the rights of parents and the rights of their children may appear to be in conflict. There is a growing feeling in the United States that the child deserves his or her own advocacy before the law. The rights of adolescents to receive medical care without the consent or knowledge of their parents has been recognized in a number of states through legislation aimed particularly at helping the adolescent in difficulties with sexual problems or with drug abuse. The physician who deals with adolescents will need to be well informed as to local statutes governing the rights of minors to confidentiality in their relationship with him.

Physicians who find themselves faced with difficult decisions involving moral or ethical judgment will generally assume positions which they regard as appropriate and rational, sometimes with the support of notions borrowed from the physiologic or psychologic substrates of medicine. But they must accept that their own logical, scientific, intellectual and satisfying positions or attitudes may not at all be so construed by others. The investment of emotions on both sides may be very great, with feelings of fear, guilt, anger and anxiety very close to the surface.

In dealing with these matters, an overriding principle ought to be that the issues must be examined in the context of the value system of the *patient* and of the *patient's family,* not that of the physician. The goal is to help the family to find a solution to their problem with which they can most comfortably live. With an assessment of the needs and resources of his patients and their families, the physician serves as a catalyst through which the most satisfying or least damaging solutions of difficult problems may be found. Occasionally the decisions are of such difficulty that they must be made by the physician on behalf of the family, but he must be as sure as circumstances permit that his decision is one which the family can accept in terms of *their* system of values, not his.

If a physician becomes involved in moral or ethical issues concerning which the family cannot accept his judgment, then he should make clear to the family that they should feel free to seek advice from another consultant.

It is tempting to provide guidelines and examples as to how specific problems ought to be handled. But there are often no specific guidelines, and each occasion must be evaluated on its own merits. The skills most useful to the physician will be in the psychotherapeutic realm, and will involve skillful listening, gentle and sensitive probing, and compassionate help in decision-making.

VICTOR C. VAUGHAN, III

3
NUTRITION AND NUTRITIONAL DISORDERS

NUTRITIONAL REQUIREMENTS

A clear understanding of the fundamentals of nutrition is required for skillful supervision of the health of children. The Food and Nutrition Board of the National Research Council has established a table of Recommended Dietary Allowances as a guide to the attainment of good nutritional status for healthy persons of all ages. In most instances these recommendations include a safety factor of 50 to 100 per cent, providing a margin of sufficiency above minimal needs as compensation for individual variations in utilization and for needs arising from unanticipated daily stresses. Nutrition studies in children are even more complex to perform and interpret than those with adults, and much remains to be learned about human metabolism. It is best to consider the Recommended Dietary Allowances as "educated guesses"; they are not *a priori* optimal levels of intake. Fomon has used the designation "advisable intake" for normal infants to indicate an adequate amount which is greater than the requirement to prevent deficiencies, but less than the Allowances.

Although the range for good nutrition must be accorded considerable variability, it is well to remember that mild excesses of caloric intake may prove to be as undesirable as mild deficiencies. The present evidence is insufficient to permit final conclusions as to the influence of diet in infancy and childhood upon the aging process, atherosclerosis or longevity in adult life, but avoidance of excessive caloric and fat intake would appear to be wise at any age.

WATER

Water is second only to oxygen as an essential for existence; lack of it results in death in a matter of days. The water content of infants is relatively higher (70 to 75 per cent of the body weight) than of adults (60 to 65 per cent). Assuming that water comprises 70 per cent of the body weight, 5 per cent is blood plasma, 15 per cent is interstitial fluid, and 50 per cent is intracellular fluid. Fluids provide the principal source of water; some is obtained from the oxidation of foods (mixed diets yield about 12 gm of water per 100 calories) as well as of body tissues.

Requirements for water are related to caloric consumption and to the specific gravity of the urine. The infant must consume much larger amounts of water per unit of body weight than the adult, but when calculated per 100 calories of intake, the amounts required are practically the same (Table 3–1). The daily consumption of fluid by the healthy infant is equivalent to 10 to 15 per cent of his body weight, whereas it is only 2 to 4 per cent in the adult. The natural food of infants and children is high in water content, most of the solid food in the child's diet containing 60 to 70 per cent water, and many of the fruits and vegetables, 90 per cent.

Little if any water is absorbed directly from the stomach; absorption is through the entire intestinal tract. Some water may go directly into the lymph stream, but most is taken into the blood stream. The quantity of water in the interstitial compartment changes considerably in order to maintain homeostatic balance within the intracellular and vascular compartments. The interchange of water among these compartments is dependent on their respective protein and electrolyte concentrations. Depending upon the rate of growth, about 0.5 to 3 per cent of the fluid intake will be retained. Fomon has calculated water retentions of the order of 13 to 9 ml per day for the "male reference infant" in the first year of life.

TABLE 3–1 WATER REQUIREMENTS

	INFANT—3 KG 300 CALORIES* INTAKE			ADULT—70 KG 3000 CALORIES* INTAKE		
URINE SP.GR.	WATER INTAKE			WATER INTAKE		
	Gm	Gm/100 Cal	Gm / Kg	Gm	Gm/100 Cal	Gm / Kg
1.005	650	217	220	6300	210	90
1.015	339	113	116	3180	106	45
1.020	300	100	100	2790	93	40
1.030	264	88	91	2430	81	35

*In this sense calorie = large calorie = 1 kcal = 1 Cal (see text).

TABLE 3-2 RANGE OF AVERAGE WATER REQUIREMENT OF CHILDREN AT DIFFERENT AGES UNDER ORDINARY CONDITIONS

AGE	AVERAGE BODY WEIGHT IN KG	TOTAL WATER IN 24 HOURS, ML	WATER PER KG BODY WT IN 24 HOURS, ML
3 days	3.0	250- 300	80-100
10 days	3.2	400- 500	125-150
3 months	5.4	750- 850	140-160
6 months	7.3	950-1100	130-155
9 months	8.6	1100-1250	125-145
1 year	9.5	1150-1300	120-135
2 years	11.8	1350-1500	115-125
4 years	16.2	1600-1800	100-110
6 years	20.0	1800-2000	90-100
10 years	28.7	2000-2500	70- 85
14 years	45.0	2200-2700	50- 60
18 years	54.0	2200-2700	40- 50

Water balance depends on such variables as fluid intake, protein and mineral content of diet, solute load presented for renal excretion, metabolic and respiratory rates and body temperature. Fecal losses are small (3 to 10 per cent of intake). Evaporation from lungs and skin accounts for 40 to 50 per cent of intake (sometimes more), and renal excretion for 40 to 50 per cent or more. The kidney preserves the fluid and electrolyte equilibrium of the body by varying the osmolar content and volume of urine. Urine usually has a greater osmotic pressure (300-1000 mosm/l) than the internal environment (293 mosm/l).

CALORIES

The unit of heat in metabolism is the **large calorie** or **kilocalorie** (kcal.). The large calorie is the same unit (abbreviated Cal) with which the literature of dietetics and nutrition has traditionally referred to the energy content of foods (1 Cal = 1 kcal.). Most references in this volume to the energy of foodstuffs will be expressed as large calories (e.g., in the tables). A kilocalorie is defined as the amount of heat necessary to raise the temperature of 1 kg of water from 14.5 to 15.5° C.

The production of heat varies with the oxidation of different foods, so that measuring the amount of oxygen consumed is an indirect method for measuring the amount of food oxidized and the heat produced. Estimates of heat production obtained from measurements of the end-products of oxidation, carbon dioxide and water, approximate those obtained by direct calorimetry.

There is great variation in the energy needs of children at different ages and under various conditions (Fig. 3-1 and Table 3-3). The average expenditure of energy by the child of 6 to 12 years of age is approximately as follows: maintenance of basal metabolism, 50 per cent; specific dynamic action of food, 5 per cent; growth, 12 per cent; physical activity, 25 per cent; and loss by way of feces, about 8 per cent, mainly as unabsorbed fat.

Basal metabolism is measured at room temperature (20° C) 10 to 14 hours after a meal, with the patient physically and emotionally quiet. For each degree centigrade of fever the basal metabolism is increased approximately 10 per cent. The basal requirement in infants is about 55 kcal/kg/day and decreases to 25 to 30 kcal/kg/day at maturity. The term *specific dynamic action* (SDA) refers to the

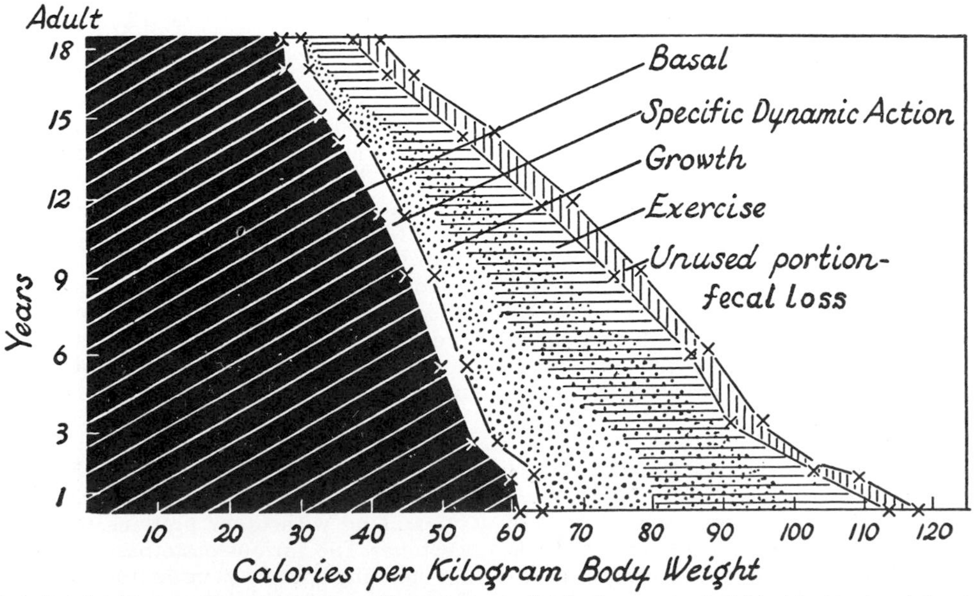

Figure 3-1 Total daily expenditure of calories with approximate distribution among individual factors in relation to age and weight (calorie = large calorie = 1 kcal = 1 Cal).

TABLE 3-3 APPROXIMATE DAILY REQUIREMENTS OF CHILDREN FOR CALORIES,* PROTEIN AND WATER

AGE IN YEARS	CALORIES†		PROTEIN	WATER	
	Per Kg	Per Lb	Gm/Kg‡	Ml /Kg	Oz /Lb
Infancy§	110	50	3.5-2.0	150	2 1/4
1-3	100	45	2.5-2.0	125	2-
4-6	90	41	3.0	100	1 1/2
7-9	80	36	2.8	75	1.0+
10-12	70	32	2.0	75	1.0+
13-15	60	27	1.7	50	3/4
16-19	50	23	1.5+	50	3/4
Adult	40	18	0.8	50	3/4

*Calorie = large calorie = 1 kcal = 1 Cal (see text).
†At least 10 per cent variation.
‡To convert gm/kg to gm/lb, divide by 2 and subtract 10 per cent of the quotient. Thus 4 gm/kg is equivalent to 1.8 gm/lb.
§First weeks lower; first 6 months relatively higher than last 6 months.

increase in metabolism over the basal rate brought about by the ingestion and assimilation of food. Protein may increase the metabolism as much as 30 per cent above the basal level, except when it is being deposited in tissues, whereas fat and carbohydrate, which have a "sparing" effect on the specific dynamic action of protein and upon each other, cause increases of only 4 to 6 per cent, respectively. Practically, the theoretic specific dynamic action is probably never attained. In infants about 7 to 8 per cent of the total caloric intake goes to specific dynamic action, whereas in older children on an ordinary mixed diet it is not likely to be more than about 5 per cent of total intake. The energy necessary to build body tissue *(growth)* is estimated to be the difference between the calories ingested and those expended for other purposes. The average requirement for *physical activity* is 15 to 25 kcal/kg/day, peak utilizations being as high as 50 to 80 kcal/kg/day for short periods of time. The amount of energy-producing food lost in the stools *(unused portion)*, except when absorption is impaired, is not more than 10 per cent of the intake.

Although caloric requirements can best be predicted from the surface area rather than from age or weight, the final criteria for meeting the child's needs depend upon the growth pattern, the sense of well-being and satiety. As indicated in Figure 3–3, the daily requirement is approximately 100 to 120 kcal/kg for the first year of life, with subsequent decreases of about 10 kcal/kg for each succeeding 3-year period. Periods of rapid growth and development near puberty require increased caloric consumption. The average distribution of calories in a well balanced diet is as follows: protein, 15 per cent; fat, 35 per cent; carbohydrates, 50 per cent.

Each gram of ingested protein or carbohydrate provides 4 kilocalories and 1 gram of fat, 9 kilocalories. A continued caloric intake greater or less than the body expenditure will result in an increase or decrease in body fat. Abnormalities or adjustments in body weight will not be discussed here, but, in general, a consistent caloric imbalance of 500 kcal/day results in a body weight change of about 1 pound per week.

PROTEINS

Protein, the predominant solid structure of the body, constitutes about 20 per cent of the body weight of the adult. Its amino acids are essential nutrients in the formation of cell protoplasm. It is found principally in the muscular and nervous systems and in the visceral and glandular tissues. Protein is an integral part of most body fluids and secretions.

The kind, number and arrangement of the amino acids in a protein molecule determine the characteristics of the protein. Twenty-four amino acids have been identified; nine have been found to be essential for infants: threonine, valine, leucine, isoleucine, lysine, tryptophan, phenylalanine, methionine and histidine (necessary only for young infants). New tissue cannot be formed unless all the essential amino acids are present in the diet simultaneously; hence the absence of only one essential amino acid will result in a negative nitrogen balance. The requirements for the individual amino acids are considerably smaller for the school child than for the infant.

Complex protein structures are broken down to proteoses, peptones, simple peptides and finally to α-amino acids in the digestive process. The hydrochloric acid of the stomach provides the optimum pH for peptide cleavage by pepsin. Rennin changes casein of milk to paracasein, which pepsin hydrolyzes along with other proteins to proteoses and peptones. The various proteinases show preference for splitting specific peptide linkages, some cleaving linkages in the interior of the peptide chain and others acting at more terminal junctures. In the alkaline medium of the intestine, trypsin, chymotrypsin and carboxypeptidase from the pancreas hydrolyze these proteoses and peptones to dipeptides, tripeptides and tetrapeptides and to some amino acids; other peptidases from the intestinal juices carry digestion of these to the amino acid stage.

Minute amounts of certain proteins may be absorbed unchanged, as evidenced by immunologic reactions, but it is the hydrolytic products, the amino acids, which are normally absorbed through the intestinal mucosa. The amino acids are carried to the liver by the portal circulation and from there distributed by the systemic circulation and taken up rapidly by the tissues. Excess amino acids undergo deamination, and the nitrogenous portions are converted to urea in the liver and excreted by the kidneys. The carbon from amino acids is oxidized much as that of carbohydrate or fat, some amino acids being glycogenic, others ketogenic. The absorption of protein is so efficient that little nitrogen is found in the stools.

The total plasma protein in the normal child ranges from 6 to 7.5 gm/dl, with somewhat lower values in newborn and premature infants. The albumin-globulin ratio is usually 2:1, fibrinogen varying from 0.1 to 0.4 gm/dl.

Aberrations in the metabolism of protein and the amino acids constitute a significant portion of the disease entities known as inborn errors of metabolism. Important among these are phenylketonuria, leucine-induced hypoglycemia, maple syrup urine disease, histidinemia, hyperglycinemia, argininosuccinic aciduria and other aminoacidurias.

There is an abundant protein supply available for infants and children in the United States. But neither the minimal nor the optimal intake is actually known, despite the fact that the supply of protein in many countries is so limited that the greatest need of infants throughout the world is for this nutrient.

CARBOHYDRATES

The greatest portion of the caloric needs of the body is supplied by carbohydrates, which also supply the necessary bulk of the diet. Carbohydrates are stored chiefly as glycogen in the liver and muscles, but probably make up no more than 1 per cent of the body weight. The infant's liver is one tenth that of the adult and the muscle mass one fiftieth; hence, the infant has only a small fraction (approximately one twenty-sixth) of the glycogen reserve of the adult.

Carbohydrate is oxidized as glucose (dextrose), but is consumed in various forms: the monosaccharides (glucose, fructose, galactose), the disaccharides (lactose, sucrose, maltose, isomaltose) and the polysaccharides (starches, dextrins, glycogen, gums, cellulose). Pentoses are poorly absorbed.

Through a series of enzymatic and chemical reactions in the digestive tract, complex carbohydrates are split into simpler structures. Salivary and pancreatic amylases are primarily concerned in the breakdown of starch to oligosaccharides (dextrins) and disaccharides, primarily maltose. The disaccharides are absorbed intact into the intestinal brush border cells, where the various disaccharidases in the membrane fraction of the microvilli complete the hydrolysis to the monosaccharides: maltose to two molecules of glucose; sucrose to glucose and fructose; lactose to glucose and galactose. The monosaccharides are rapidly absorbed, glucose and galactose being actively taken up against concentration gradients, whereas fructose absorption is passive. During absorption phosphoric acid "carrier" radicals combine with hexose sugars in the intestinal mucosa for transport across the cell membrane. Sodium must be present for absorption to continue when the intra-intestinal sugar concentration is low. These hexose-phosphates separate again into their component parts, permitting the sugar to diffuse into the portal blood stream.

Some glucose may be oxidized directly, as in the brain and heart. Most of the absorbed sugar is converted to glycogen in the liver, though glycogenesis also occurs in other tissues of the body. Up to 15 per cent of of the weight of the liver and 3 per cent of the muscle may be glycogen; small amounts are also found in the skin and in practically all other organs. Glycogenolysis in the liver yields glucose as the chief product, whereas glycogen breakdown in the muscle yields lactic acid. The overall oxidation of glucose has two phases, the anaerobic (glycolysis) and the aerobic (tricarboxylic acid cycle). In the former, glucose is broken down to pyruvic acid; in the aerobic cycle pyruvic acid is completely oxidized to carbon dioxide and water. Insulin and the pituitary and adrenal hormones are involved in these processes, and nicotinic acid, thiamine, riboflavin and pantothenic acid take part in the enzymatic reactions. Carbohydrate which is not oxidized or stored as glycogen is converted to fat.

The principal carbohydrate metabolic disorders are diabetes mellitus, glycogen storage disease, galactosemia, fructose intolerance and glucose intolerance; deficiencies of sugar-splitting enzymes in the intestines (lactase, invertase, maltase) are associated with diarrhea and malabsorption resulting from the osmotic effect of the unabsorbed sugar and from fermentation of the carbohydrate by intestinal bacteria.

FATS

Simple lipids are esters of fatty acids with various alcohols. They are the most abundant fats in the body and in food, the most common being triglycerides. *Compound lipids* (lecithin, cephalin, sphingomyelin, cerebrosides, sulfa and amino lipids) contain nitrogen bases, phosphoric acid, sugar, sulfur or amino groups with fatty acids and

TABLE 3–4 FUNCTION, EFFECTS OF DEFICIENCY AND EXCESS, REQUIREMENTS AND SOURCES OF WATER, PROTEINS, CARBOHYDRATES AND FATS

FOODSTUFFS	FUNCTIONS	EFFECTS OF DEFICIENCY	EFFECTS OF EXCESS	REQUIREMENTS	SOURCES
Water	Structure of cells; solvent for cellular changes; medium for ions; transport of nutrients and waste products; regulation of body temperature	Thirst, dryness of tongue, dehydration, anhydremia, high sp. gr. of urine, loss of kidney function (acidosis, oliguria, uremia, death)	Abdominal discomfort, headache, cramps (water without salt), intoxication, convulsions, edema and circulatory failure	See Tables 3-1, 3-2 and 3-3 Related to calories consumed; greater in hot weather	Water as such All foods
Proteins	Supply amino acids for growth and repair of tissue cells; sols for osmotic equilibrium; ions in acid-base balance. With prosthetic groups to form hemoglobin, nucleoproteins, glycoprotein and lipoproteins. Enzymes, hormones, cellular respiratory substance, antibodies. Protective structures (nails and hair). Source of energy	Lassitude, abdominal enlargement, edema; depletion of plasma proteins, negative nitrogen balance; (no clinical syndrome due to lack of specific amino acid); kwashiorkor (protein malnutrition); marasmus (protein-calorie malnutrition)	Prolonged high protein intake probably not harmful. Important in certain anomalies involving amino acid and protein metabolism	See Table 3-3	Milk, eggs, meat, fish, poultry, cheese, soybeans, peas, beans, cereals, nuts, lentils
Carbohydrates	Readily available source of energy, antiketogenic, structure of cells, antibodies, source of stored calories (glycogen and fat), conversion to fat, resynthesis of amino acids, roughage	Ketosis if protein intake is less than 15% of calories or in starvation; underweight if total calories are low	Overweight if total calories are high. Various syndromes due to inborn errors of sugar metabolism.	To supply 25 to 55% of calories	Milk, cereals, fruits, sucrose, syrups, starches, vegetables
Fats	Concentrated source of energy; physical protection for vessels, nerves, organs: insulation against changes in temperature; structure of body tissues, cell membranes and nuclei; vehicle for absorption of vitamins (A, D, E and K); appetite appeal; aids satiety (delays emptying time of stomach); avoids necessity of ingestion of large bulk of foods; spares protein, vitamin A and thiamine; supplies linoleic acid	Lack of satiety (craving for fat); underweight; skin changes with intakes very low in linoleic acid	Overweight; abdominal symptoms in familial hyperlipidemia; high cholesterol intakes may be harmful to selected populations.	Minimal not known; usually supplies 35% of calories Probably 1-2% of calories as linoleic acid	Milk, butter, egg yolk, lard, bacon, meat, fish, cheese, nuts, vegetable oils Breast milk usually supplies 4-5% of calories as linoleic acid; vegetable oils vary greatly, safflower, corn, soy and others being especially rich

alcohol. *Derived lipids* from these two groups are separated out by hydrolysis; they include cholesterol and saturated and unsaturated fatty acids.

Naturally occurring fats contain straight-chain fatty acids, both saturated and unsaturated, varying in length from 4 to 24 carbon atoms, most of them containing 16 or 18. The degree of absorption varies in general with the melting point and the degree of unsaturation.

Ingested triglycerides are emulsified in the stomach by the continuous shearing action of the gastric muscular contractions. This emulsion passes into the duodenum, where pancreatic lipase hydrolyzes the triglycerides to monoglycerides and fatty acids. Intraluminal solubility is greatly enhanced by the presence of bile salts, which form polymolecular micelles with the monoglycerides and fatty acids; the remaining unsplit diglycerides and triglycerides are insoluble even in the presence of bile salts.

Long-chain fatty acids and monoglycerides (those with more than 10 carbon atoms) are presumably absorbed into the mucosal cell by diffusion. Transport across the cell involves re-esterification of these fatty acids and monoglycerides to triglycerides, which are then "coated" with lipoprotein to form the moiety known as the chylomicron, in which the fat is transported in the lymph system to the venous circulation via the thoracic duct.

Short and medium-chain triglycerides are handled differently; they are readily hydrolyzed by pancreatic lipase to free fatty acids which are transported through the cell. Even when intraluminal hydrolysis is inadequate because of pancreatic lipase or bile salt deficiency, these fats will be absorbed and will be hydrolyzed to free fatty acids within the cell by mucosal lipase. With neither esterification to triglycerides nor subsequent chylomicron formation, these free fatty acids directly enter the intestinal veins and pass to the liver via the portal system. This alternate pathway for short- and medium-chain triglycerides is utilized in many of the newer nutritional formulations for children with severe absorptive problems.

LINOLEIC AND ARACHIDONIC ACIDS. Human beings do not synthesize lineolic acid, an 18-carbon atom chain with 2 double bonds (dienoic acid); hence, it must be supplied in the diet. Rapidly growing young infants maintained on diets very low in linoleic acid undergo dryness and thickening of the skin with desquamation and intertrigo. These clinical symptoms disappear readily when the diet contains 1 to 2 per cent of the calories as linoleic acid. In healthy infants the serum levels for unsaturated fatty acids depend upon the amount of linoleic acid in the diet.

Arachidonic acid, which can be synthesized readily if the diet contains linoleic acid, is much less efficient in alleviating the clinical and chemical manifestations of fat deficiency. Diets extremely low in linoleic acid require greater caloric consumption for comparable growth in both experimental animals and in infants.

The relation of dietary fat intake in infancy and childhood to the intimal fat streaking which begins in the major arterial vessels early in life remains to be clarified. Reduction of total fat intake and an increase in the ratio of unsaturated to saturated fats is associated with significant reduction in serum cholesterol levels in adults with hyperlipidemia, particularly those with the type II form. In the United States polyunsaturated vegetable fats have been widely substituted for the more saturated butterfats in commercial milk formulas for many years; it has not yet been established whether atheromatous changes in young human subjects or in other primates are lessened by such substitutions.

MINERALS

Table 3–5 summarizes the physiologic aspects and dietary sources of the principal mineral elements which have nutritional significance.

The ash content of the fetus is low, constituting only about 3 per cent of the body weight at birth. It increases continuously throughout childhood, both absolutely and relatively, so that in the adult the mineral content is 40 times greater than in the newborn, whereas the body weight is but 23 times greater. In the adult the ash content is 4.35 per cent of the body weight, 83 per cent of which is in the skeleton and 10 per cent in the muscle. It has been estimated that for each gram of protein retained, 0.3 gm of mineral matter is deposited. The important electropositive elements (cations) are calcium, magnesium, potassium and sodium; the important electronegative ones (anions) are phosphorus, sulfur and chloride. Iron, iodine and cobalt appear in important organic complexes. The trace elements fluorine, copper, zinc and manganese have known metabolic roles; selenium, silicon, boron, nickel, aluminum, arsenic, bromine, molybdenum and strontium are present in the diet and in the body, but their functions have not been clarified.

SELENIUM. In areas where there is a high concentration of selenium in the soil and food, animals have severe nutritional disturbances. The significance in man is not known; however, in children in certain parts of Oregon where a high content of selenium has been found in soil and water, the incidence of dental caries and the urinary excretion of selenium are greater than in areas where exposure to selenium is known to be not as great.

SILICON. Silicon is present in all tissues, constituting as much as one ninth of the total ash. Because the amount in the skin decreases with age, it is believed to be related to its elasticity. Blood levels in man are as high as 16 mg/dl. Some silicon is excreted in the urine, but most in the feces. Silicosis has not been known to result from a dietary source.

BORON, NICKEL, ALUMINUM, BROMINE, ARSENIC. These elements exist in minute traces in man, but have not thus far been shown to be signif-

(*Text continued on page 155.*)

TABLE 3–5 PHYSIOLOGY AND SOURCES OF NUTRITIONALLY IMPORTANT MINERALS

MINERAL	FUNCTION	PHYSIOLOGY	EFFECTS OF DEFICIENCY	EFFECTS OF EXCESS	DAILY ALLOWANCE	SOURCES
Calcium	Structure of bone and teeth, muscle contraction, nerve irritability, coagulation of blood, cardiac action, production of milk	Absorbed from upper small intestine: aided by vitamin D, ascorbic acid, lactose, acid reaction; hindered by excesses of dietary oxalic acid, phytic acid, fat, fiber, phosphate. Deposited in bone trabeculae and maintained in dynamic equilibrium with body tissues through action of parathyroid hormone. About 70% excreted in feces, 10% in urine; 15-25% retained, depending on growth rate. Serum level 9–11 mg/dl, 60% ionized.	Poor mineralization of bones and teeth; osteomalacia; osteoporosis; tetany; rickets; impairment of growth	Unknown	Infants: 0.4-0.6 gm Children under 10 years, 0.7-1.0 gm, depending on size and age; over 10 years, 1.2-1.4 gm, depending on vitamin D and sunlight. FAO-WHO* allowances less (0.5-0.7 gm)	Milk, cheese, green leafy vegetables, canned salmon, clams, oysters
Chloride	Osmotic pressure; acid-base balance; HCl in gastric juice	Readily absorbed; about 92% of intake is excreted, mainly in the urine, some in feces and sweat; comprises about 2/3 of the blood plasma anions; blood serum level, 99-106 mEq/L; in intracellular and extracellular fluids; parallels sodium intake and output	Hypochloremic alkalosis may occur in prolonged vomiting or excessive sweating, with the use of parenteral fluids (glucose) without saline; with excessive ACTH therapy and in congenital alkalosis (rare)	Unknown	Probably 0.5 gm; average diet contains 3-9 gm as NaCl	Table salt, meat, milk, eggs
Cobalt	Part of vitamin B_{12} (cobalamin) molecule; contained in erythropoietin	Not utilized for synthesis of cobalamin by man; readily absorbed and excreted	None known	None (dietary); taken medicinally, may be goitrogenic, may produce cardiomyopathy	None	Widely distributed
Copper	Essential for production of red blood cells; catalyst in hemoglobin formation; absorption of iron. Associated with activity of tyrosinase, catalase, uricase, cytochrome C oxidase, delta-aminolevulinic acid dehydrase (porphyrin formation)	Little information on factors affecting absorption; transported in plasma bound to plasma proteins and in ceruloplasmin; present in erythrocytes in a labile form and the more stable hemocuprein; highest concentration in liver and central nervous system (cerebrocuprein); excretion is mainly via the intestinal wall and bile; deranged metabolism in Wilson's disease (hepatolenticular degeneration)	Not established but may be cause of refractory anemia during recovery from kwashiorkor	None (dietary)	Estimated for children, 0.05-0.1 mg/kg	Liver, oysters, meats, fish, whole grains, nuts, legumes
Fluorine	Tooth and bone structure	Retained when intake above 0.6 mg/day; excreted in urine and sweat; deposited in bones as fluorapatite (dynamic equilibrium)	Tendency to dental caries	Fluorosis: mottling of teeth with intake of more than 4-8 mg./day	0.5-1 mg; recommended that community water supply contain 1 ppm fluorine	Water, sea foods, plant and animal foods, depending upon content in soil and water

*Food and Agricultural Organization of United Nations.

TABLE 3–5 PHYSIOLOGY AND SOURCES OF NUTRITIONALLY IMPORTANT MINERALS (*Continued*)

MINERAL	FUNCTION	PHYSIOLOGY	EFFECTS OF DEFICIENCY	EFFECTS OF EXCESS	DAILY ALLOWANCE	SOURCES
Iodine	Constituent of thyroxine (T_4) and triiodothyronine (T_3)	Readily absorbed from intestine; circulates as inorganic and organic iodide; selectively concentrated about 25:1 in the thyroid gland, quickly iodized and incorporated into a complex known as thyroglobulin; proteolytic enzymes release thyroxine and triiodothyronine into the blood. Excretion mainly in urine. Antithyroid compounds interfere with iodine metabolism: goitrin of Brassicae; certain drugs	Simple goiter, endemic cretinism	Not harmful (less than 1 mg / day); medicinally may cause iodism	Infants: 25-45 micrograms Children: ages 1-10, 55-110 micrograms; ages 10-18, 125-150 micrograms for males, 110-125 mg. for females	Iodized salt, sea food, food grown in nongoitrous areas
Iron	Structure of hemoglobin and myoglobin for O_2 and CO_2 transport; oxidative enzymes: cytochrome C and catalase	Absorbed in ferrous form according to body need, aided by gastric juice and ascorbic acid; hindered by fiber, phytic acid, steatorrhea. Transported in plasma in ferric state bound to transferrin (a beta-1 globulin); stored in liver, spleen, bone marrow and kidney as ferritin and hemosiderin; carefully conserved and reused; minimal losses in urine and sweat; about 90% of intake excreted in the stool	Anemia: hypochromic, microcytic	Hemosiderosis in Bantu people of Africa due to low phosphorus and high iron contents of diet Poisoning by medicinal iron	Infants: 6-15 mg or 1 mg /kg Children: ages 1-3, 15 mg ; ages 3-12, 10 mg ; ages 12-18, 18 mg	Liver, meat, egg yolk, green vegetables, whole grains, legumes, nuts
Magnesium	Structure of bones and teeth; activation of enzymes in carbohydrate metabolism; muscle and nerve irritability. Important intracellular cation, essential to all metabolic processes	Principal cation of soft tissue; location chiefly intracellular; absorption from small intestine varies with level of intake; some urinary excretion, but excellent renal conservation; antagonist to calcium action	Not adequately understood; occurs in malabsorption and deficiency states; may be expressed clinically as tetany; associated frequently with hypocalcemia.	None (dietary); toxicity from intravenous medication	Infants: 40-70 mg Children: ages 1-3, 100-150 mg ; ages 3-12, 200-300 mg ; ages 12-18, 350-400 mg	Cereals, legumes, nuts, meat, milk
Manganese	Enzyme activation, especially in mitochondria; normal bone structure	Poor absorption from intestine; transported in plasma; particularly high turnover rate in mitochondria; excretion mainly via the intestine in the bile	Not known	None (dietary); toxicity from chronic inhalation (encephalopathy and extrapyramidal disease)	Unknown	Legumes, nuts, whole grain cereals, green leafy vegetables
Molybdenum	Component of enzymes: xanthine oxidase for conversion to uric acid and mobilization of ferritin iron in liver, liver aldehyde oxidase	Readily absorbed from intestine; excreted chiefly in urine, some in bile	Not observed in man	Not established	Unknown	Legumes. grains, dark green leafy vegetables, animal organs

Table 3–5 continued on following page.

TABLE 3–5 PHYSIOLOGY AND SOURCES OF NUTRITIONALLY IMPORTANT MINERALS (*Continued*)

MINERAL	FUNCTION	PHYSIOLOGY	EFFECTS OF DEFICIENCY	EFFECTS OF EXCESS	DAILY ALLOWANCE	SOURCES
Phosphorus	Constituent of bones and teeth; structure of nucleus and cytoplasm of all cells; acid-base balance; key position in energy transformations and transmission of nerve impulses; metabolism of carbohydrate, protein and fat	About 70% of intake absorbed as free phosphates from intestine; vitamin D implicated in intestinal absorption and kidney retention; excreted in urine and feces; occurs in blood as phospholipids, organic esters and inorganic phosphates; inorganic phosphates in blood serum of infants and children, 4-7 mg/dl; ratio of inorganic-organic phosphates in whole blood is about 1:20	Not established; rickets may develop in rapidly growing, very low-birth-weight babies with low intakes of both P and Ca; muscle weakness	Possibility of tetany during recovery from rickets or in newborn on formula with low Ca: P (1:1) ratio	Infants: 0.2-0.5 gm Children under 10, 0.7-1.0 gm; ages 10-18, 1.2-1.4 gm	Milk, milk products, egg yolk, flesh foods, legumes, nuts, whole grains
Potassium	Muscle contraction; nerve impulse conduction; intracellular osmotic pressure and fluid balance; heart rhythm	Primarily intracellular; absorption via intestine; excretion 80% in urine—some in sweat and feces; about 8% retained by growing child; blood serum level 4.0-5.6 mEq /L	In starvation or in such pathologic conditions as diarrhea, diabetic acidosis, ACTH excess: muscle weakness, anorexia, nausea, abdominal distention, nervous irritability, drowsiness, confusion, tachycardia; deficiency exaggerates effects of sodium	Heart block at serum levels of 10 mEq./L.; important in Addison's disease, renal failure or administration of K-containing salts	1-2 gm or 1.5 mEq /kg or 40 mEq /M^2	All foods
Sodium	Osmotic pressure; acid-base balance; water balance; muscle and nerve irritability	Readily absorbed from intestine; excreted chiefly in urine (98%); parallels intake; renal excretion controlled by adrenal cortical hormone; extracellular cation, but small amount in muscle and cartilage; blood serum level, 135-145 mEq /L	Nausea; diarrhea, muscle cramps, dehydration	Edema if inadequate excretion or excessive parenteral fluids	2.0 mEq /kg or 50 mEq /M^2 (newborn and prematures less)	Table salt, flesh foods, milk, eggs, sodium compounds as baking soda and powder, glutamate, seasonings and preservatives
Sulfur	Constituent of all cellular protein; cocarboxylase; melanin; mucopolysaccharides of mucous secretions, vitreous humor, synovial fluid, connective tissues, cartilage, heparin; insulin; metabolism of nerve tissue; detoxification mechanisms; tissue metabolism as SH group in coenzyme A, cystathionine and glutathione	Only sources utilized are cystine and methionine; inorganic forms unavailable to body; excreted as inorganic sulfate or ethereal sulfate via urine and bile	Not known; growth failure from protein deficiency may be due in part to deficiency of S-containing amino acids	Not harmful; excreted in urine as sulfates	Not known; average intake 0.5-1.0 gm	Protein foods contain about 1%

TABLE 3–5 PHYSIOLOGY AND SOURCES OF NUTRITIONALLY IMPORTANT MINERALS (*Continued*)

MINERAL	FUNCTION	PHYSIOLOGY	EFFECTS OF DEFICIENCY	EFFECTS OF EXCESS	DAILY ALLOWANCE	SOURCES
Zinc	Constituent of several enzymes: carbonic anhydrase (in erythrocytes) which is essential for CO_2 exchange; carboxypeptidase of intestine for hydrolysis of protein; dehydrogenase of liver	Found in liver and organs, muscles, bones, red and white cells; higher tissue concentration in young subjects; excreted chiefly from intestine	Dwarfism, iron deficiency anemia, hepatosplenomegaly, hyperpigmentation and hypogonadism in young males in Egypt (Nile Valley) and Iran is probably zinc deficiency state	Gastrointestinal upsets (from galvanized iron cooking utensils)	Not known; estimated intake 0.3 or more mg /kg body weight; slight retention by children, therefore may be required	All foods

icant in either human or animal nutrition. Boron is essential for plants; nickel delays insulin hypoglycemia; aluminum in excess may interfere with absorption of phosphorus; and bromine and arsenic are important pharmacologically.

STRONTIUM-90. This and other radioactive isotopes are of increasing concern owing to their potential for radiation injury. They should also be studied in respect to their effects on nutrition.

VITAMINS

The word "vitamin" refers to organic compounds which are required in minute amounts to catalyze cellular metabolism essential for maintenance or growth of the organism. They must be supplied wholly or in part exogenously. In general, the B-complex vitamins function as coenzymes in a variety of specific biochemical reactions, whereas the exact modes of action of ascorbic acid and vitamins A, D, E and K are still obscure. Table 3–7 outlines aspects of the individual vitamins pertinent to human metabolism.

The physician should be aware that both vitamin deficiencies and excesses may exist. Hypervitaminosis A and hypervitaminosis D have been recognized for many years. Toxicity from vitamin A has been associated with treatment of acne in adolescents and with dietary faddisms in which doses of 25,000 to 50,000 units per day are ingested; increased intracranial pressure mimicking brain tumor, dry skin, sparse hair, irritability and anorexia are the most common manifestations. An increased incidence of idiopathic hypercalcemia of infancy in Great Britain was traced to the vitamin D enrichment of cereals and dried milks in addition to normal prophylactic vitamin supplementation. Daily intakes of up to 3000 to 4000 IU of vitamin D became common; this is 7 to 10 times the currently recommended allowance of 400 I.U. per day.

TABLE 3–6 RECOMMENDATIONS FOR DAILY INTAKE OF MINERALS AND VITAMINS

AGE	MINERALS			VITAMINS						
	Ca*	P	Fe	A	Thiamine	Riboflavin	Niacin	Ascorbic Acid	D	B_6
	gm	gm	mg	I U	mg	mg	mg	mg	I U	mg
Infancy	0.6	0.5	15†	1500	0.5	0.6	8	35	400	0.4
1 to 3 years	0.8	0.8	15	2000	0.6	0.7	8	40	400	0.8
4 to 6 years	0.8	0.8	10	2500	0.8	0.8	11	40	400	0.8
7 to 9 years	1.0	1.0	10	3500	1.1	1.1	15	40	400	1.0
10 to 12 years	1.2	1.2	10	4500	1.3	1.3	17	40	400	1.2
13 to 15 years	1.4	1.4	18	5000	1.5	1.5	20	55	400	1.4
16 to 19 years	1.4	1.4	18	5000	1.5	1.5	20	60	400	1.4

Adapted from recommendations by the Food and Nutrition Board of the National Research Council. Slight variations were made in order to state the amounts necessary for each 3-year period after infancy in direct arithmetic progression. Values in adolescent years are for males.

*Food and Agricultural Organization of United Nations recommends somewhat lower intakes for calcium than those of the National Research Council: e.g. 0-12 mo., 500-600; 1-9 yrs., 400-500; 10-15 yrs., 600-700; 16-19 yrs., 500-600; adults, 400-500; with pregnancy, 1000-1200, and lactation, 1500-2000 mg /day.

†Or 1 mg /kg.

TABLE 3–7 PHYSICAL AND METABOLIC PROPERTIES AND FOOD SOURCES OF THE VITAMINS

NAME AND SYNONYMS	CHARACTERISTICS	METABOLISM	BIOCHEMICAL ACTION	EFFECTS OF DEFICIENCY	EFFECTS OF EXCESS	RECOMMENDED ALLOWANCES	SOURCES
VITAMIN A: Retinol (Vitamin A_1) is an alcohol of high molecular weight *Provitamin A:* The plant pigments, alpha-, beta- and gamma-carotenes and cryptoxanthin	Fat-soluble; water-insoluble; heat-stable at usual cooking temperatures; destroyed by oxidation, drying and very high temperatures	Bile is necessary for absorption of the provitamins. Conversion of provitamins takes place primarily in the walls of the intestine, to some extent in the liver. Vitamin A and provitamins stored in liver. Absorption of both facilitated by the presence of fat, impaired by intake of mineral oil or by defect in fat absorption. Vitamin E minimizes oxidation of both in the intestine	Vitamin A aldehyde is retinal, which combines with specific proteins to form the retinal pigments, rhodopsin and iodopsin, for vision in dim light; bone and tooth development; formation and maturation of epithelia of skin, eye, digestive, respiratory, urinary and reproductive tracts	Nyctalopia, photophobia, xerophthalmia, conjunctivitis, keratomalacia leading to blindness; faulty epiphyseal bone formation; defective tooth enamel; keratinization of mucous membranes and skin; retarded growth	Dietary excess of vitamin A unlikely. Excessive carotene intake may produce carotenemia with xanthosis cutis. Individual variation in sensitivity to high intakes of vitamin A concentrates; 50,000 I U taken daily for prolonged periods may be toxic and cause anorexia, slow growth, drying and cracking of skin, enlargement of liver and spleen, swelling and pain of long bones, bone fragility, increased intracranial pressure	Up to 1 year, 1500 I U/day; 1 to 12 years, 2000 I U increasing to 4500 I U with age; over 12 years, 5000 I U/day. These amounts assume that 2/3 comes from the provitamins, which are less efficiently utilized than the vitamin. If only vitamin A is taken, then 900 to 3000 I U would suffice	Liver, fish-liver oils, whole milk, milk fat products, egg yolk, fortified margarines. Carotenoids from plants—green vegetables, yellow fruits and vegetables
VITAMIN B COMPLEX: *Cobalamin:* Group of complex coordination compounds of cobalt-vitamin B_{12}; antipernicious anemia factor; Castle's extrinsic factor; animal protein factor (APF)	Slightly soluble in water; stable to heat in neutral solution; labile in acid or alkaline ones; destroyed by light	Castle's intrinsic factor of the stomach required for absorption	Transfer of one-carbon units in purine and labile-methyl group metabolism; essential for maturation of red blood cells in bone marrow; metabolism of nervous tissue	Juvenile pernicious anemia, due to defect in absorption rather than to dietary lack; also secondary to gastrectomy, celiac disease, inflammatory lesions of small bowel, long term drug therapy (PAS, neomycin)	Unknown	Infants: 1-2 micrograms; children: ages 1-18, 2-5 micrograms, from exogenous sources, depending on age	Muscle and organ meats, fish, eggs, milk, cheese
Vitamin B_6 3 active forms: pyridoxine, pyridoxal, pyridoxamine	Water-soluble; destroyed by ultraviolet light and by heat	Readily absorbed; phosphorylated in tissue to form coenzyme; intestinal synthesis important	Constituent of coenzymes for amino acid metabolism: decarboxylation, transamination, transsulfuration, conversion of tryptophan to niacin; fatty acid metabolism	Infants: irritability, convulsions, hypochromic anemia; peripheral neuritis in patients receiving isoniazid, a vitamin B_6 antagonist	Unknown	Infants: 0.2-0.4 mg; children: ages 1-10, 0.5-1.2 mg; ages 10-18, 1.4-1.8 mg If abnormal B_6 metabolic state exists, 5-10 mg	Meat, liver, kidney, whole grains, peanuts, soybeans
Folacin: Group of related compounds containing pteridine ring, para-amino benzoic acid and glutamic acid. Pteroylglutamic acid (PGA); folinic acid; citrovorum factor; leucovorin	Slightly soluble in water; labile to heat, light, acid	Excreted in both urine and feces in amounts in excess of intake (intestinal bacterial synthesis).	Concerned with formation and metabolism of one-carbon units; hence participates in synthesis of purines, pyrimidines, nucleoproteins and methyl groups	Megaloblastic anemia (infancy, pregnancy); usually occurs secondary to malabsorption disease	Unknown	Infants: 1-2 micrograms; children: ages 1-18, 2-5 micrograms from exogenous sources, depending on age	Liver, green vegetables, nuts, cereals, cheese

TABLE 3-7 PHYSICAL AND METABOLIC PROPERTIES AND FOOD SOURCES OF THE VITAMINS (*Continued*)

NAME AND SYNONYMS	CHARACTERISTICS	METABOLISM	BIOCHEMICAL ACTION	EFFECTS OF DEFICIENCY	EFFECTS OF EXCESS	RECOMMENDED ALLOWANCES	SOURCES
Niacin: Nicotinamide; nicotinic acid; antipellagra vitamin	Water- and alcohol-soluble; stable to acid, alkali, light, heat, oxidation	Readily absorbed from small intestine; limited storage; excess excreted in urine as several metabolites; synthesized in the body from tryptophan; vitamin B_6 is essential for conversion	Active constituent of coenzymes I and II, cofactors in a number of dehydrogenase systems	Pellagra: multiple B-vitamin deficiency syndrome. Early symptoms: fatigue, anorexia. weight loss, headache	Nicotinic acid (not the amide) is vasodilator; reactions include skin flushing and itching, circulatory disturbances, increased peristalsis	6.6 mg /1000 calories; infants: 5-8 mg. children 2-10 years, 8 to 15 mg ; over 10 years, 15 to 20 mg /day, depending on caloric intake	Meat, fish, poultry, liver, whole-grain and enriched cereals, green vegetables, peanuts. Protein foods in general, from conversion of tryptophan (60 mg. forms 1 mg. of niacin)
Riboflavin: Vitamin B_2	Sparingly soluble in water; sensitive to light and alkali; stable to heat, oxidation, acid	Absorbed from the intestines; limited storage in tissues; excess excreted in urine; careful economy when intake is low and rapid excretion when intake is high. Absorption impaired in achlorhydria, diarrhea, vomiting. Utilization greater with increased metabolism	Constituent of 2 coenzymes which are components of a number of flavoprotein enzymes important in hydrogen transfer in a variety of reactions: amino acid, fatty acid and carbohydrate metabolism and cellular respiration. Retinal pigment of eye for light adaptation	Ariboflavinosis; early symptoms: photophobia, blurred vision, burning and itching of eyes, corneal vascularization, poor growth. One of the most common dietary inadequacies, often accompanying other B-vitamin deficiencies	Not harmful	0.025 mg /gm of dietary protein; infants: 0.4-0.6 mg ; children 2-10 years, 0.6 to 1.2 mg ; over 10 years, 1.3 to 1.5 mg /day, depending on food intake and age	Milk, cheese, liver and other organs, meats, eggs, fish, green leafy vegetables, whole or enriched grains
Thiamine: Vitamin B_1; antiberiberi vitamin; aneurin	Water- and alcohol-soluble; fat-insoluble; stable in slightly acid solution; labile to heat, alkali, sulfites	Readily absorbed from small and large intestines; combines with phosphate in all cells to form thiamine pyrophosphate (cocarboxylase); limited body stores; excess excreted in urine; destroyed in body by intake of raw fish or clams which contain thiaminases. Poor absorption in persistent GI disturbances	Component of carboxylases, which act in various oxidative decarboxylations, including that of pyruvic acid	Beriberi—early stages: easily fatigued, irritable, emotional instability, anorexia. Later: indigestion, constipation, headache, insomnia, tachycardia after exercise. Late stage: polyneuritis, cardiac failure, edema. Diagnosis: elevated pyruvic acid in the blood after exercise or after intake of standard amount of glucose, in conjunction with low urinary thiamine	None from oral intake	0.4 mg /1000 kcal; infants: 0.2-0.5 mg ; children 2-10 years, 0.6 increasing to 1.1 mg ; over 10 years, 1.2 to 1.5 mg / day, increasing with caloric requirement	Liver, meats, especially pork, milk, whole-grain or enriched cereals, wheat germ, legumes, nuts
VITAMIN C: *Ascorbic acid:* Vitamin C; antiscorbutic vitamin	Water-soluble; easily oxidized; oxidation is accelerated by heat, light, alkali, oxidative enzymes, traces of copper or iron; fairly stable in acid solution at low temperature	Readily absorbed; blood plasma levels reflect daily intake, whereas concentration in leukocytes reflects tissue level; excess excreted in urine; little tissue storage, but high concentrations in glandular tissues; man, monkeys, guinea pigs cannot synthesize it from glucose; dehydroascorbic acid, first oxidation product, is biologically active	Mechanism of action not known; structure and maintenance of intercellular material in all tissues; facilitates absorption of iron, conversion of folic acid to folinic acid; probably coenzyme in the metabolism of tyrosine and phenylalanine. Contributes to activity of succinic dehydrogenase and serum phosphatase in infants, not in adults	Scurvy: early symptoms are irritability and slow growth; susceptibility to infection; hemorrhagic manifestations; poor wound healing	Not harmful	First year, 35 mg ; 1 to 12 years, 40 mg ; 10-18 years, 40-60 mg depending on age and sex	Citrus fruits, tomatoes, berries, cantaloupe, cabbage, green vegetables. Cooking has deleterious effect

Table 3-7 continued on following page.

TABLE 3–7 PHYSICAL AND METABOLIC PROPERTIES AND FOOD SOURCES OF THE VITAMINS (*Continued*)

NAME AND SYNONYMS	CHARACTERISTICS	METABOLISM	BIOCHEMICAL ACTION	EFFECTS OF DEFICIENCY	EFFECTS OF EXCESS	RECOMMENDED ALLOWANCES	SOURCES
VITAMIN D: Group of sterols having similar physiologic activity. D_2-calciferol is activated ergosterol. D_3 is activated 7-dehydrocholesterol	Fat-soluble; stable to heat, acid, alkali and oxidation	Absorbed from intestine with fat, bile salts being required. Provitamin D_3 is synthesized in the skin and is converted to the vitamin by ultraviolet irradiation and absorbed. Calciferol is converted to 25-HCC (25-hydroxcalciferol) in liver, 25-HCC is an intermediary of most potent metabolite, 1,25-dihydroxycholecalciferol which is secreted in manner of hormone by kidney.	Mechanism of action not known. Regulates absorption and deposition of calcium and phosphorus, presumably by affecting permeability of intestinal membrane. Regulation of level of serum alkaline phosphatase, which is believed to be concerned with calcium phosphate deposition in bones and teeth	Rickets (high serum phosphatase level appears before bone deformities); infantile tetany, poor growth, osteomalacia	Wide variation in tolerance; in general, 20,000 to 50,000 I U /day is toxic when continued for weeks (prolonged administration of 1800 I U /day may be toxic (see Hypercalcemia, Section 22). Manifestations are nausea, diarrhea, weight loss, polyuria, nocturia, eventually calcification of soft tissues, including heart, renal tubules, blood vessels, bronchi, stomach	400 I U /day	Vitamin D-fortified milk and margarine, fish liver oils, exposure to sunlight or other ultraviolet sources
VITAMIN E: Group of related chemical compounds — tocopherols — having similar biologic activity	Fat-soluble; heat-stable in absence of oxygen; unstable to ultraviolet light, alkali; readily oxidized by oxygen, iron, lead, rancid fats. Antioxidant in foods and the body	Absorption may be affected by fat digestion. Some storage in fatty tissues, but not in liver	Mechanism of action unknown (cell maturation and differentiation). Minimizes oxidation of carotene, vitamin A and linoleic acid in the intestine. Possibly related to muscle metabolism and to erythrocyte fragility	Anti-oxidant; important to cell membrane integrity, endoplasmic reticulum and mitochondrial oxidative functions; requirements related to polyunsaturated fat intake; may be involved in red blood cell hemolysis in premature infants	Unknown	Infants: 5 I U children: ages 1-6, 10 I U ; ages 6-10, 15 I U ; ages 10-14, 20 I U ; ages 14-18, 25 I U	Germ oils of various seeds, green leafy vegetables, nuts, legumes
VITAMIN K: Group of compounds: naphthoquinones, with similar biologic activity K_1 is phylioquinone	Natural compounds are fat-soluble, but several water-soluble products have been developed (menadione). Stable to heat and reducing agents; labile to oxidizing agents, strong acids, alcoholic alkali, light	Bile salts necessary for intestinal absorption of fat-soluble forms. Limited storage in liver; synthesized by intestinal microorganisms	Mechanism of action unknown; necessary for prothrombin formation, hence normal blood clotting; coagulation factors II, VII, IX, X are K-dependent	Hemorrhagic manifestations: result of faulty intestinal synthesis of vitamin K (newborn, prolonged use of sulfonamides and antibiotics), faulty intestinal absorption, or inability to synthesize prothrombin (hepatic damage). Except in the last condition, menadione and bile salts effective. Dicumarol and salicylates act as vitamin K antimetabolites	Not established. Medicinally may produce hyperbilirubinemia in prematures	Not a dietary problem. 1 to 2 mg./day appear to be adequate	Green leafy vegetables, pork liver. Widely distributed

MISCELLANEOUS FACTORS

ROUGHAGE. Roughage is indigestible vegetable fiber. Amounts as high as 170 to 300 mg/kg/day appear to cause no difficulty. Most children who receive average, well balanced diets obtain sufficient amounts of roughage.

DIGESTIBILITY. The relative amount of a given food available for assimilation is high in most of the common food classes: carbohydrate is 97 per cent; fat, 95 per cent; protein, 92 per cent. Cooking is a factor in digestibility. For example, the boiling of milk reduces the size of the curd and renders it more digestible for infants; by contrast, heating destroys vitamin C activity.

SATIETY. The ingestion of a meal should provide a sense of well-being. Whole milk, cream, eggs and fatty foods have a high satiety value; sugar increases the flow of gastric juice and delays emptying of the stomach, thus increasing satiety. Bread and potatoes have relatively low satiety values, as do lean fish, vegetables and many fruits.

AVAILABILITY. Poverty, ignorance and lack of practical education in food buying and preparation, and sometimes illness leading to parental neglect, are the main causes of malnutrition in children. Diets of families in the lower income brackets are likely to be deficient in milk, fruits, fresh vegetables and meats. A suggested method for planning low-cost meals is to divide the money available for food into fifths: one fifth each for vegetables and fruits; milk and cheese; meats, fish and eggs; bread and cereals; and fats, sugar and other food adjuncts.

Geographic distribution also influences the availability of foods, the tendency being for a population to consume foods indigenous to its own area. The effect of geographic factors on deficiency diseases is evidenced in the high incidence of goiter owing to a deficiency of iodine in certain areas and by the relation between dental caries and fluoride in communal water supplies.

BACTERIAL SYNTHESIS. Certain vitamins are synthesized in the human gastrointestinal tract; however, the extent to which they can meet the body needs is uncertain. Once the bacterial flora of the intestinal tract has been established, vitamin K is readily available to the body. Pantothenic acid and biotin play essential roles in human metabolism; bacterial synthesis alone is sufficient to meet the body needs for them. Thiamine, riboflavin, niacin, vitamin B_6, vitamin B_{12} and folic acid are synthesized in some species, but synthesis is limited or does not exist at all in man. The kind of

TABLE 3–8 RECOMMENDED FOOD INTAKE FOR GOOD NUTRITION ACCORDING TO FOOD GROUPS AND THE AVERAGE SIZE OF SERVINGS AT DIFFERENT AGE LEVELS

FOOD GROUP	SERVINGS PER DAY	AVERAGE SIZE OF SERVINGS					
		1 year	2-3 years	4-5 years	6-9 years	10-12 years	13-15 years
Milk and cheese (1.5 oz cheese = 1 C milk) (C = 1 cup – 8 oz or 240 gm)	4	1/2 C	1/2-3/4 C	3/4 C	3/4-1 C	1 C	1 C
Meat group (protein foods)	3 or more						
Egg		1	1	1	1	1	1 or more
Lean meat, fish, poultry (liver once a week)		2 Tbsp	2 Tbsp	4 Tbsp	2-3 oz (4-6 Tbsp)	3-4 oz	4 oz. or more
Peanut butter			1 Tbsp	2 Tbsp	2-3 Tbsp	3 Tbsp	3 Tbsp
Fruits and vegetables	At least 4, including:						
Vitamin C source (citrus fruits, berries, tomato, cabbage, cantaloupe)	1 or more (twice as much tomato as citrus)	1/3 C citrus	1/2 C	1/2 C	1 medium orange	1 medium orange	1 medium orange
Vitamin A source (green or yellow fruits and vegetables)	1 or more	2 Tbsp	3 Tbsp	4 Tbsp (1/4 C)	1/4 C	1/3 C	1/2 C
Other vegetables (potato and legumes, etc.) *or*	2	2 Tbsp	3 Tbsp	4 Tbsp (1/4 C)	1/3 C	1/2 C	3/4 C
Other fruits (apple, banana, etc.)		1/4 C	1/3 C	1/2 C	1 medium	1 medium	1 medium
Cereals (whole-grain or enriched)	At least 4						
Bread		1/2 slice	1 slice	1 1/2 slices	1-2 slices	2 slices	2 slices
Ready-to-eat cereals		1/2 oz	3/4 oz	1 oz	1 oz	1 oz	1 oz
Cooked cereal (including macaroni, spaghetti, rice, etc.)		1/4 C	1/3 C	1/2 C	1/2 C	3/4 C	1 C or more
Fats and carbohydrates	To meet caloric needs						
Butter, margarine, mayonnaise, oils: 1 Tbsp = 100 calories (kcal)		1 Tbsp	1 Tbsp	1 Tbsp	2 Tbsp	2 Tbsp	2-4 Tbsp
Desserts and sweets: 100-calorie portions as follows: 1/3 C pudding or ice cream 2-3" cookies, 1 oz cake, 1 1/3 oz pie, 2 tbsp jelly, jam, honey, sugar		1 portion	1 1/2 portions	1 1/2 portions	3 portions	3 portions	3-6 portions

Prepared in collaboration with Mildred J. Bennett, Ph.D., from "Four Food Groups of the Daily Food Guide," Institute of Home Economics, U.S.D.A., and Publication #30, Children's Bureau of the United States Department of Health, Education, and Welfare.

food or nature of intestinal flora may affect vitamin production or availability. For instance, 3 per cent of the population in Kobe, Japan, were found to harbor intestinal bacteria which split thiamine, and evidences of beriberi appeared in these persons.

ANTIMICROBIAL AGENTS. Administration of antimicrobial agents may influence the nutritional status. Sometimes appetite is impaired sufficiently to precipitate borderline deficiency states. Several antibiotics are known to produce steatorrhea; penicillin and sulfonamides seem to provoke the syndrome only when used together. Neomycin has been shown to produce malabsorption in adults. Orally administered broad-spectrum antibiotics decrease nitrogen balance. Isoniazid combines with pyridoxal phosphate and may produce symptoms of vitamin B_6 deficiency. Antimicrobial compounds may be transmitted in breast milk and may be ingested in foods from animals which have been fed these compounds.

ENDOCRINE FACTORS. Antithyroid substances (goitrogens) have been found in turnips, rutabagas, cabbage, soybeans, cobalt-containing foods, food additives and medications; they increase the requirement for iodine. Administration of ACTH or corticosteroids necessitates an increase in protein and calcium and a decrease in sodium intake. Relative hypoparathyroidism with tetany has been observed in the neonatal period after excessive intakes of vitamin D and phosphates.

RADIOACTIVITY. Apparently there is little danger from carbon-14, owing to its low activity. Iodine-131 is removed from milk by aeration or storage. Cesium-137 may be found in meat and milk products and can be counteracted by a high potassium intake or by the use of Diamox. Strontium-90 is filtered out to a large extent by the mammary gland, and only 10 per cent of ingested strontium-90 is found in milk.

EMOTIONAL FACTORS. Along with increased knowledge of the significance of various nutrients there has developed excessive parental and professional concern over the food intake of the individual infant or child. The mother may become so impressed with statements of so-called experts in nutrition that she develops a sense of fear, even guilt, about her child's eating habits. The result is a battle of wits between mother and child which may have far-reaching effects. The physician who sees children in his practice must be well informed in the fundamentals of nutrition in order to recognize and manage emotional and behavioral problems arising from undesirable dietary practices.

EVALUATION OF DIET

The physician who sees children should have a reasonable knowledge of the properties of various foods so as to be able to take and evaluate a meaningful dietary history, to know which laboratory tests have value for diagnosis, and to be able to interpret therapeutic responses. (See Tables 3–8, 3–9, and 3–10).

The recall-interview for determining food habits of children is satisfactory under usual circum-

TABLE 3–9 COMPARISON OF NUTRIENT VALUES OF THE DIETS PRESENTED IN TABLE 3–8 WITH THE RECOMMENDED DIETARY ALLOWANCES [FIGURES IN ( )]

AGE AND WEIGHT (Boys and Girls 25-75th percentiles)	CALORIES*	PROTEIN gm	CALCIUM gm	IRON mg	VITAMIN A IU	THIAMINE† mg	RIBOFLAVIN† mg	NIACIN† mg	ASCORBIC ACID mg	VITAMIN D IU
1 year (22 ± 2 lb)	1020 (1000)	42 (25)	0.6 (0.7)	5.4 (15.0)	2325 (2000)	0.47 (0.6)	1.0 (0.6)	3.4 (8.0)	40 (40)	300 (400)
2-3 years (30 ± 5 lb)	1320 (1250)	48 (25)	0.8 (0.8)	6.1 (15.0)	3225 (2000)	0.64 (0.6)	1.0 (0.7)	7.3 (8.0)	51 (40)	400 (400)
4-5 years (39 ± 6 lb)	1720 (1600)	67	1.0 (0.8)	8.4 (10.0)	4270 (2500)	0.85 (0.8)	1.5 (0.9)	11.7 (11.0)	60 (40)	500 (400)
6-9 years (56 ± 15 lb)	2130 (2100)	76 (35)	1.1 (0.9)	11.4 (10.0)	5140 (3500)	1.2 (1.0)	2.0 (1.1)	19.3 (13.0)	88 (40)	600 (400)
10-12 years (81 ± 20 lb)	2480 (2500)	93 (45)	1.4 (1.2)	13.0 (10.0)	4590 (4500)	1.4 (1.3)	2.5 (1.3)	23.0 (17.0)	102 (40)	600 (400)
13-15 years (108 ± 27 lb)	2580-3080 (2500-3000)	100 (50-60)	1.4 (1.4)	14.4 (18.0)	5540 (5000)	1.5 (1.3)	2.5 (1.5)	23.7 (20.0)	107 (50)	600 (400)

Recommended Dietary Allowances, Revised 1968, National Research Council, National Academy of Sciences, and FAO recommendations for calcium requirements.

*Selections from fats and carbohydrate group included for caloric values, but not for other nutrients. Calorie = large calorie = kcal = Cal. (See text.)

†Based on the following: thiamine, 0.4 mg /1000 calories; riboflavin, 0.025 mg /gm of protein; niacin, 6.6 mg /1000 calories.

TABLE 3–10 DIETARY HISTORY

Food Record of ______________________

Age ________ Sex ________ Height ________ in. (________ %ile) Weight ________ lb. (________ %ile)

FOOD GROUP	AM'T/WK.	AM'T/DAY	SERVINGS/DAY PER GROUP* ACTUAL	SERVINGS/DAY PER GROUP* RECOMMENDED
Milk and cheese (1.5 oz. cheese = 1 C milk)				
Milk (indicate whole or skim; include that taken as beverage, on cereal, in cooked foods)	______	______		
Cheese	______	______		
Total milk equivalents			______	(4)
Meat group (protein foods)				
Eggs (cooked any way, in custards, etc.)	______	______		
Lean meat (beef, veal, pork, ham, lamb, poultry, fish)	______	______		
Liver	______	______		
Peanut butter	______	______		
Total			______	(3)
Fruits and vegetables				
Vitamin C (orange, grapefruit, berries, tomato, cantaloupe, etc.)	______	______		
Green or yellow (leafy vegetables, peas, green beans, carrots, yellow squash, peaches, apricots, etc.)	______	______		
Other vegetables (potato, beans, parsnips, turnips, etc.)	______	______		
Other fruits (apple, banana, pear, etc.)	______	______		
Total			______	(4)
Cereal group (whole grain or enriched)				
Bread	______	______		
Cooked cereal (farina, oatmeal, macaroni, rice, spaghetti, etc.)	______	______		
Ready-to-eat	______	______		
Total			______	(4)
Miscellaneous (for calories and satiety)				
Fats—Butter and margarine	______	______		
Mayonnaise	______	______		
Oils and salad dressing	______	______		
Sweets (cake, pie, cookies, candy, soft drinks, sugar, etc.)	______	______		
Total			______	

*See Table 3-8 for sizes of servings for the different ages.

Evaluation and/or recommendations ______________________

stances, but for more accurate accounting of food consumption the mother should be instructed to observe the actual food intake. It is best to report the *amount* and *frequency* of food intake in terms of the standard measuring cup or tablespoon, weight or size of pieces. The data may then be converted to "servings" appropriate to the age of the child (Table 3–8). It is important to include items such as liver, cake and eggs, which may not be consumed daily.

The dietary guide according to food groups (Table 3–8) provides flexibility according to cultural, religious and personal preferences and seasonal, regional and economic availability. The food intake record (Table 3–10), based on selections from the food groups, is helpful in indicating possible nutritional imbalances. An excessive intake of foods of one group may result in a high caloric level and, hence, overweight and may lead to a dangerously low intake of other essential nutrients. A notable example is the overconsumption of milk and the underconsumption of meat and eggs, with the resultant danger of iron deficiency anemia. When certain key foods, such as milk, eggs and citrus fruits, are eliminated for personal or medical reasons, the deficiencies imposed may be compensated by judicious substitutions. Following is a list of the primary nutrient contributions, besides calories, of the food groups:

Milk: high-quality protein, calcium and phosphorus; riboflavin; vitamin A; vitamin D (if fortified)

Meat and eggs: high-quality protein, iron, B vitamins; vitamin A from liver and eggs

Fruits and vegetables: vitamin C; provitamin A from green and yellow ones; trace elements; fiber

Cereals: less expensive and supplementary amounts of protein, minerals, fiber, B vitamins

Suspected dietary insufficiencies may be corroborated by appropriate laboratory tests and clinical evaluation. When malnutrition, either as dietary deficiency or excess, or failure to thrive exists in spite of what appears to be a satisfactory food intake, intense efforts must be made to detect evidences of infection, malignancy, faulty absorption, excretion or utilization, endocrine disorders, parasitic infestation, degenerative disease and especially errors in metabolism.

This section originally prepared for this textbook by Arild E. Hansen and Mildred J. Bennett.

WILLIAM E. LAUPUS

GENERAL

Bondy, P. K., and Rosenberg, L. E.: Duncan's Diseases of Metabolism. 7th ed. Philadelphia, W. B. Saunders Company, 1974.

Burton, B. T.: The Heinz Handbook of Nutrition. Published for H. J. Heinz Co. Inc., New York, Blakiston Division, McGraw-Hill Book Company, Inc. 1965.

Cheek, D. B.: Human Growth. Philadelphia, Lea & Febiger, 1968.

Committee on Nutrition, American Academy of Pediatrics: Water requirement in relation to osmolar load as it applies to infant feeding. Pediatrics *19*:339, 1957.

On the feeding of solid foods to infants. Pediatrics *21*:685, 1958.

Trace elements in infant nutrition. Pediatrics *26*:715, 1960.

Composition of milks. Pediatrics *26*:1039, 1960.

Appraisal of nutritional adequacy of infant formulas used as cow's milk substitutes. Pediatrics *31*:329, 1963.

Factors affecting food intake. Pediatrics *33*:135, 1964.

Protection of the infant diet: Government and industry. Pediatrics *36*:648, 1965.

Nutritional Management in hereditary metabolic disease. Pediatrics *40*:290, 1967.

Obesity in childhood. Pediatrics *40*:455, 1967.

Iron balance and requirements in infancy. Pediatrics *43*:134, 1969.

Filled milks, imitation milks, and coffee whiteners. Pediatrics *49*:770, 1972.

Everson, G. J.: Bases for concern about teenagers' diets. J. Am. Diet. A. *36*:17, 1960.

Goodhart, R. S., and Shils, M. E. (eds.): Modern Nutrition in Health and Disease. Philadelphia. Lea & Febiger, 1973.

Falkner, F. (ed.): Human Development. Philadelphia, W. B. Saunders Company, 1966.

Fomon, S. J.: Infant Nutrition. Philadelphia, W. B. Saunders Company, 1967.

Food and Nutrition Board: Recommended Dietary Allowances. Washington, D.C. National Research Council, 1972.

Hansen, A. E.: Symposium on nutrition and nutritional problems. Pediat. Clin. N. Amer. *9*:877–1045, 1962.

Mitchell, H. S., Rynbergen, H. J., Anderson, L., and Dibble, M. V.: Cooper's Nutrition in Health and Disease. 15th ed. Philadelphia, J. B. Lippincott Company, 1968.

Stanbury, J. B., Wyngaarden, J. B., and Frederickson, D. S. (eds.): The Metabolic Basis of Inherited Disease. 2nd ed., New York, McGraw-Hill Book Company, Inc., 1966.

Turner, D. (ed.): Handbook of Diet Therapy. 4th ed. Chicago, University of Chicago Press (American Dietetic Association), 1965.

White, A., Handler, P., and Smith, E. L.: Principles of Biochemistry. 4th ed., New York, Blakiston Division, McGraw-Hill Book Company, Inc., 1968.

Protein, Fat and Carbohydrate

Albanese, A. A. (ed.): Protein and Amino Acid Metabolism. New York, Academic Press, Inc., 1959.

Cornblath, M., and Schwartz, R.: Disorders of Carbohydrate Metabolism in Infancy. Philadelphia, W. B. Saunders Company, 1966.

Flodin, N. W. (ed.): Protein nutrition. Ann. New York Acad. Sc. *69*:855, 1958.

Food and Nutrition Board, Division of Biology and Agriculture: Evaluation of Protein Nutrition. Washington, D.C., National Research Council, Committee on Amino Acids, 1959.

Garonger, J. D., Brown, M. S., and Laster, L.: The columnar epithelial cell of the small intestine: digestion and transport. N. Engl. J. Med. *283*:1196; 1264; 1317, 1970.

Hansen, A. E., Stewart, R. A., Hughes, G., and Soderhjelm, L.: The relation of linoleic acid to infant feeding: A review. Acta Pediatr. *51*:Suppl., 1962.

Holt, L. E., Jr., Gyorgy, P., Pratt, E. L., Snyderman, S. E., and Wallace, W. M.: Protein and Amino Acid Requirements in Early Life. New York, New Press, 1960.

Isselbacher, K.: Biochemical aspects of fat absorption. Gastroenterology, *50*:78, 1966.

Sargent, D. W.: An Evaluation of Basal Metabolic Data for Infants in the United States. United States Department of Agriculture. Home Economics Research Report No. 18, 1962.

Vitamins

Committee on Nutrition, American Academy of Pediatrics: Appraisal of the use of vitamin B_1 and B_{12} as supplements promoted for the stimulation of growth and appetite in children. Pediatrics *21*:860, 1958.

Vitamin K. Compounds and the water-soluble analogues. Pediatrics *28*:501, 1961.

Infantile Scurvy and Nutritional Rickets in the United States. Pediatrics *29*:646, 1962.

Vitamin E in human nutrition. Pediatrics *31*:324, 1963.

The prophylactic requirement and the toxicity of vitamin D. Pediatrics *31*:512, 1963.

Vitamin B_6 requirements in man. Pediatrics *38*:1068, 1966.

DeLuca, H. F.: Vitamin D: A new look at an old vitamin. Nutr. Rev. *29*:179, 1971.

FEEDING OF INFANTS

Successful infant feeding requires *cooperative* functioning between the mother and her baby, commencing with the initial feeding experience and continuing throughout the child's period of dependency. Prompt establishment of comfortable, satisfying feeding practices contributes greatly to the infant's emotional well-being. Feeding time should be a pleasant and pleasurable period for both mother and child. Maternal feelings are readily transmitted to the baby and, in large measure, determine the emotional setting in which feeding takes place. Mothers who are tense, anxious, irritable, easily upset or emotionally labile are more likely to experience difficulty in the feeding relationship; frequently they become more comfortable and confident with appropriate guidance and support from an empathetic and experienced relative or friend.

The feeding of infants requires practical interpretation of specific nutritional needs and of the widely varying limits of the normal baby's appetite and behavior with regard to food. The emptying time of the infant's stomach may vary from 1 to 4 or more hours; thus, considerable difference in desire for food may be expected in the infant at different times of the day, and ideally the feeding schedule should be based on reasonable "self-regulation" by the infant. Variation in the time between feedings and in the amount taken per feeding is to be expected in the first few weeks with such a plan of "self-regulation," but by the end of the first month more than 90 per cent of infants will have established a suitable and reasonably regular schedule.

Most healthy infants will want 6 to 8 feedings a day by the end of the first week of life. The majority will take enough at one feeding to satisfy them for approximately 4 hours; some who are smaller or whose gastric emptying time is more rapid will want milk about every 3 hours; breast-fed infants often prefer 3-hour or shorter intervals. Many infants will not awaken for the middle-of-the-night feeding after 3 to 6 weeks of age; some may never want it. The majority will omit the late evening feeding between 4 and 8 months of age and will be satisfied with three meals a day by 9 to 12 months.

In helping to fashion a schedule guided by the infant's needs and behavior, it is important to establish that he may cry for reasons other than hunger and that *he need not be fed every time he cries;* some infants are placid, some unusually active, some irritable; sick infants are often disinterested in food. Babies who awaken and cry consistently at short intervals may not be receiving enough milk or may have discomfort from some cause other than hunger. Included in the last category are too much clothing; soiled, wet or uncomfortable diapers and clothing; colic; swallowed air ("gas"); uncomfortably hot or cold environment; and illness. Some babies cry to gain sufficient or additional attention, whereas others deprived of adequate mothering become disinterested. Some infants simply need to be held; those who stop crying when they are picked up or held do not usually need food; those who continue to cry when held and when food is offered should be carefully evaluated for other causes of distress. The habit of offering frequent, small feedings or of holding and feeding to pacify all crying should not be cultivated.

The advantages to the infant in supplying his needs as they are expressed are several: his physiologic requirements are met promptly; he does not learn to associate prolonged crying and discomfort with feeding; and he is less likely to develop poor eating practices such as gulping his feedings or taking small amounts too frequently. He soon establishes a regular schedule which permits the family to resume normal function. If he does not, individual feedings or the whole day's schedule can be moved ahead or delayed sufficiently to avoid conflicts with necessary family activities.

Some mothers will not understand the goals of "self-regulation" by the infant; some will misinterpret the physician's instructions, and others may not have the capacity to adjust themselves to the regimen of the infant. *The orderly, overanxious and compulsive parent will do better with a more specific outline for the infant's activities.*

The postpartum period is often a time of great anxiety and insecurity for the first-time mother, who may be temporarily overwhelmed by the reality of the responsibilities of motherhood. It is important that the hospital setting and the attitude of the hospital personnel be comforting and supporting while the mother finds and develops confidence in her maternal abilities. Time is rewardingly spent in conferences at the hospital or in the home, where simple procedures are explained and potential problem areas are discussed. *The questions of inexperienced or uncertain mothers will frequently go unanswered unless time is set aside to consider them.*

Fathers and other members of the household should not be neglected by physicians in these anticipatory guidance sessions. Knowledge of the personalities and expectations of both parents is invaluable in helping to avert physical and psychologic problems centered around feeding. Parental misconceptions and confusion concerning the dietary and satiety needs of infants and children are often the bases for abnormal parent-child relations which can be avoided by appropriate counseling. The experienced physician will utilize similar general principles pertaining to infant feeding practices whether the infant is breast- or bottle-fed.

BREAST FEEDING

Breast feeding continues to have practical and psychologic advantages which should be considered when the mother selects the way in which she will feed her baby. Milks produced by the various mammals are uniquely adapted to the needs of offspring of the particular species. Human milk appears to be the most appropriate of all available milks for the human infant.

ADVANTAGES OF BREAST FEEDING. Human milk is always readily available at the proper temperature wherever the mother may be. No time is required in preparation of the feeding. The milk is fresh and free of contaminating bacteria, so that the chances of gastrointestinal disturbances are lessened. Although there is little if any difference in mortality rates in formula-fed and breast-fed infants receiving good care, among the lower socioeconomic groups and where sanitary conditions are poor the breast-fed infant continues to have a much greater likelihood of survival.

Allergy and intolerance to cow's milk are responsible for significant disturbances and feeding difficulties not seen in breast-fed infants. The list now includes diarrhea, intestinal bleeding and occult melena as well as the more commonly accepted manifestations of milk allergy. "Spitting," colic and atopic eczema are less common in infants receiving human milk. Heiner and others have correlated chronic pulmonary hemosiderosis with the presence of precipitins to milk proteins in the serum of infants and have described improvement when cow's milk is removed from the diet.

The influence of the various bacterial and viral antibodies in human milk on resistance to infection in the infant is not clear. Stevenson noted a slightly higher incidence of respiratory infections during the second 6 months of life in formula-fed babies. Human milk contains relatively high concentrations of secretory IgA antibodies, but its meaning has not yet been clarified in terms of immunity for the infant. Breast-fed infants of mothers with high antipoliomyelitis titers are relatively resistant to infection by the attenuated live poliomyelitis vaccine viruses. The effect may be pronounced in the neonatal period, but does not seem to interfere with active immunization at 2, 4 and 6 months of age. It has also been shown that growth of the mumps, influenza, vaccinia and Japanese B encephalitis viruses can be inhibited by substances in human milk. These ingested antibodies from human colostrum and milk may afford local gastrointestinal immunity against organisms which enter the body via this route.

The stool of the breast-fed infant has a lower pH than that of the infant fed cow's milk, and its bacterial content is predominantly of the lactobacillus group in contrast to preponderance of the coliform group in artificially fed infants. Many believe that the intestinal flora of infants fed human milk endows special benefits, particularly against infections caused by species of *E. coli.* Gyorgy demonstrated that a fastidious strain of *Lactobacillus bifidus* require a "growth factor" contained in human milk for its propagation; no human nutritional advantage has been attributed to this substance other than facilitation of intestinal colonization by lactobacilli rather than coliform organisms.

Breast milk is the natural food for full-term infants during the first months of life. Milk from the mother whose diet is quantitatively adequate and properly balanced will supply the necessary nutrients with the exception of vitamin D, fluoride and iron. Iron stores will be sufficient for the first 3 or 4 months in term infants, but should be supplemented after 3 months of age by the addition of cereal and meat to the diet or by administration of one of the ferrous iron preparations. Although the community water supply contains adequate amounts of fluoride, the breast-fed infant may receive little of it, and fluoride should be supplied during the first months of life. Human milk contains sufficient vitamin C for the infant's needs, provided the mother's intake of it is adequate.

The psychologic advantages of breast feeding for the infant and for the mother have been widely proclaimed. Certainly successful breast feeding is a satisfying experience for both. The mother is personally involved in the nurturing of her baby, gaining both a feeling of essentialness and a sense of great accomplishment. The infant is afforded a close and comfortable physical relationship with his mother. Breast feeding offers increased opportunity for close sensual contact between mother and infant; studies in other mammals suggest that tactile contact and stimulation may be of considerable importance in the "imprinting process" and in determining the quality of mothering which is provided the infant.

The mother who wishes but is unable to nurse her infant need have no less sense of affection for him. Though it has been suggested that the breast-fed infant will be emotionally more stable than the bottle-fed infant, it would seem that the latter, provided he is a "wanted baby," would have adequate contact and affection from his mother. Speculation that emotional instability is likely to be an aftermath of bottle feeding requires confirmation which is not available; until it is, the prevailing impression that adequate security and affection can be given to the bottle-fed infant deserves strong emphasis.

DISADVANTAGES OF AND CONTRAINDICATIONS TO BREAST FEEDING. For the average healthy full-term infant there are no disadvantages to breast feeding, provided the mother's milk supply is ample and her diet contains sufficient amounts of protein and vitamins. Infrequently, allergens to which the infant is sensitized may be conveyed in the milk. In such instances an attempt should be made to find the specific allergen and to remove it from the mother's diet; the presence of such allergens rarely becomes a valid reason for weaning the baby.

From the standpoint of the mother, there are few contraindications to breast feeding. Markedly inverted nipples may be troublesome, but most respond to exercise during pregnancy. Fissuring or cracking of the nipples rarely necessitates cessation of nursing, but does require special attention such as exposure to air and application of pure lanolin. Mastitis was formerly considered to call for discontinuance of nursing, but Newton and many others now recommend continued and frequent nursing on the affected breast to keep it from becoming engorged, in addition to local heat applications and antibiotics. Acute illness in the mother may be considered a contraindication to breast feeding, if the infant does not have the same infection; otherwise there is no need for cessation of nursing unless the condition of either makes it mandatory. When the infant is not affected and the mother's condition permits, the breast may be emptied and the milk given to the infant after sterilization.

Several disturbances such as septicemia, nephritis, eclampsia, profuse hemorrhage, active tuberculosis, typhoid fever or malaria are permanent contraindications to nursing, as are chronic poor nutrition, debility, convulsive disorders, severe neuroses and postpartum psychoses.

The resumption of menstruation should not be a deterrent to continued nursing, although temporary changes in the behavior of mother or baby may call for reassurance. Pregnancy does not necessitate immediate cessation of nursing, but the combined demands of supplying milk to the infant and nutrients to the fetus are formidable and require special attention to maternal diet and nutrition; breast feeding probably should not be continued beyond the first 20 weeks of gestation.

Prematurely born infants weighing 2000 gm (4½ pounds) or more usually thrive well on breast milk. But infants of lesser birth weight (1000 to 2000 gm) may have such rapid rates of growth that human milk alone cannot provide quantities of phosphorus and protein, and possibly of calcium, sufficient for normal growth.

Breast feeding, inadequate maternal nutrition or deprived socioeconomic circumstances, alone or more often in combination, have long been cited in the development of the vitamin K-dependent hypoprothrombinemic variety of hemorrhagic disease of the newborn. The studies of Jewett and Sutherland strongly suggest that the initial period of relative starvation in breast-fed infants and the low vitamin K content of human milk are the important features in this disorder, which they find confined to breast-fed infants receiving no vitamin K prophylaxis. *Administration of 1 mg of vitamin K_1 parenterally at birth is recommended for all infants and appears to be mandantory for those who will be breast-fed.*

Sporadic occurrence of prolonged unconjugated hyperbilirubinemia has been reported by Gartner, Arias and others in breast-fed infants. An unusual steroid metabolite of progesterone, pregnane-3 alpha, 20 beta-diol, which inhibits glucuronyl transferase activity in vitro, has been isolated from the milk of mothers of infants with this problem. Breast feeding is very unlikely to be responsible for hyperbilirubinemia within the first 4 days of life. In the rare instance in which hyperbilirubinemia is due to this, cessation of breast feeding leads to prompt decline in the bilirubin level, which reaches normal in 4 to 6 days. Interruption of nursing for 2 to 3 days will usually provide sufficient lowering of the serum bilirubin value to permit safe resumption of breast feeding.

Hemolytic disease of the newborn (erythroblastosis fetalis) is not a contraindication to breast feeding if the infant's general condition warrants it, since antibodies in the mother's milk are inactivated in the intestinal tract and do not contribute to further hemolysis of the infant's red blood cells.

PREPARATION OF THE PROSPECTIVE MOTHER. Despite the fact that breast milk is the natural food for infants, many receive little or none of it. Few mothers are such poor producers of milk that they are unable to provide an amount sufficient for partial feeding of their infants (combined breast and supplemental milk feedings). Most women are physically capable of breast feeding, provided they receive sufficient encouragement and are protected from dispiriting experiences and comments while the secretion of breast milk is becoming established.

The physician interested in aiding the prospective mother to breast feed will discuss the advantages of breast feeding during the midtrimester of pregnancy or whenever the mother becomes naturally concerned with the planning for her baby. Many mothers whose feelings toward breast feeding are ambivalent will be able to nurse successfully if they are given reassurance and support by physicians whose own convictions accord breast feeding a natural and logical place in childbearing and child-rearing. If the mother rejects the suggestion that she nurse her infant, it is probably wise to avoid overpersuasion, which might distort mother-infant relations.

Physical factors conducive to breast feeding include establishing and maintaining a state of good health: proper balance of rest and exercise, freedom from worry, early and sufficient treatment of any intercurrent disease and adequate nutrition. Nutritional deficiencies are contributory factors to inadequate lactation and to infant morbidity.

Nipple care should begin during pregnancy. La Leche League recommends conditioning the nipples by pulling on them firmly several times once or twice daily, preferably after application of an oily lubricant (pure lanolin, cold cream, or baby oil), beginning in midpregnancy. During the last 6 weeks the manual expression of colostrum may be helpful in reducing the discomfort of postnatal engorgement. Retracted nipples are usually benefited by daily manual or breast pump traction during the latter weeks of pregnancy; truly inverted nipples may be helped by the use of Woolwich Breast Shields, starting as early as the third month of pregnancy.

The mother may be confidently told that she need not gain or lose weight if her diet is adequate. Both mother and father should be reassured that breast tone will be preserved by the use of a properly fitted brassiere to support the breast, especially before delivery and during the nursing period.

To permit the mother greater freedom of activity outside the home, an occasional relief bottle of formula can be substituted for one of the breast feedings, once the milk supply is well established 6 weeks or so post partum.

ESTABLISHMENT AND MAINTENANCE OF MILK SUPPLY

The only known satisfactory stimulus to the secretion of human milk is regular and complete emptying of the breasts; milk production is reduced when the secreted milk is not drained. Once lactation is well established, mothers are capable of producing far more milk than their infants will need. There are many reasons for incomplete nursing, but the principal ones are weakness of the infant and failure of initiation of a natural hunger cycle. When the breasts are not emptied by the infant during the early days of nursing, they should be emptied regularly by artificial means. This is sometimes necessary on the fifth day to relieve lacteal overdistension of the breast, so that the infant is able to grasp the mother's nipple. An electric breast pump may be used, or the mother may be taught manual expression. Water suction and hand breast pumps are less satisfactory. Every effort should be directed toward the early establishment of normal, vigorous nursing by letting the infant empty the breast frequently during the time when colostrum is being formed. The infant should be allowed to nurse when he is hungry whether or not there appears to be any milk.

Breast feeding should be begun as soon after delivery as the condition of the mother and of the baby permits, preferably within 6 to 12 hours. If the infant cannot be fed on demand, he should be brought to the mother for feeding about every 3 hours during the day and every 4 hours during the night. He should be fed from both breasts at each feeding until the supply from one breast is sufficient for his needs. Breast feeding can be successful when delayed for 24 hours or more, but, barring maternal conditions which necessitate such delay, a sufficient supply of milk will generally appear earlier in the mother whose milk supply is stimulated by frequent suckling as soon after birth as is feasible. There is no justification for routine use of prelacteal feedings of sugar water or formula. To minimize nipple trauma the nursing time is limited initially and gradually increased as the milk supply increases. In the period before the appearance of colostrum, 5 minutes' suckling at both breasts at each feeding is usually well tolerated and stimulates early milk production. As the condition of the breasts and the supply of milk permit, the nursing time can be gradually increased to 20 minutes, or even longer, if the baby insists. In beginning to nurse, almost all mothers experience some nipple tenderness, discomfort or pain which is greatest during the first part of the feeding. When expected and accepted as an unavoidable but temporary difficulty, anxiety is lessened and milk production is little affected.

Appropriate care for tender or sore nipples should be instituted before severe pain from abrasions and cracking develops. Exposure of the nipples to air; application of pure lanolin; avoidance of soap, alcohol and tincture of benzoin; frequent changes of disposable nursing pads lining the brassiere cups; and 1- to 3-minute daily exposures to ultraviolet rays have all been recommended. Nursing more frequently, at 2- or 3-hour intervals, may be more helpful than nursing less often. When the tenderness causes apprehension in the mother, the "let-down" reflex may be delayed, leading to frustration in the baby and to increasingly vigorous nursing, which further injures the nipple and alveolar area. Manual expression of milk to start the flow will be helpful in reestablishing normal feeding relationships.

The first 2 weeks of the neonatal period are the crucial time for the establishment of breast feeding. Lactogenic hormones have not been shown to be effective in the stimulation of breast secretion of the human being. Too much emphasis has been put on daily weight gains. When early supplemental milk feedings are given to achieve this false goal, attempts at breast feeding are doomed to failure; usually the infant finds that it is easier to get milk from a bottle than from a breast. An exception may be made on the day the mother is discharged from the hospital, particularly if her confinement is limited to 4 or 5 days. By this time lactation may not be well established, and the excitement of going home may not be conducive to an initially successful nursing experience there. A wise physician will anticipate this experience and discuss it with the mother. In some instances, providing the mother with enough isocaloric formula for one or two complementary feedings may prevent discouragement, which might prejudice further nursing.

PSYCHOLOGIC FACTORS. Attention to the details of maternal hygiene is paramount. No factor is more important than a happy, carefree state of mind; worry and unhappiness are the most effective means for decreasing or abolishing breast secretions.

Mothers worry that their babies are abnormal when they cry, are drowsy, sneeze or regurgitate milk. Mothers are upset by any suggestion that their milk may be lacking in quantity or quality. They are disturbed at the scanty supply of colostrum, at tenderness of the nipples and at the fullness of the breasts on the fourth or fifth day. Many mothers cannot feel comfortable when trying to nurse in an open ward or with another person in the room. Mothers worry about what is going on at home while they are hospitalized and about what is going to happen when they arrive home. An alert physician is conscious of these worries, particularly if the baby is a first-born, and by tactful reassurance and explanation he can help prevent or minimize worry, thus contributing to successful breast feeding.

FATIGUE. Avoidance of fatigue is important, but the mother should have sufficient exercise to promote a sense of physical well-being.

HYGIENE. Once a day the breasts should be washed as part of the daily shower. If soap is drying to the nipple and alveolar area, it should be discontinued. The nipple area should be kept dry. Pure lanolin may be helpful in reducing soreness and healing minor abrasions from sucking. *Boric acid must not be used.* Care should be taken to prevent irritation and infection of the nipples by prolonged initial nursing, maceration from wetness of the nipple, irritation of clothing, or difficult nursing associated with engorged or overdistended breasts. Engorgement difficulties can usually be avoided by feeding more frequently from the affected breast and by expressing the milk manually. Occasionally nipple shields may be of temporary help.

The mother will be more comfortable if a properly fitted brassiere is worn day and night. Plastic liners should be removed. An absorbent pad (commercially available) or a clean cloth or handkerchief may be placed inside the brassiere to absorb any milk which leaks out. Change to a clean brassiere should be made at least daily.

DIET. The diet should contain enough calories to compensate for those contained in the secreted milk as well as those required for its production. A diet adequate to maintain weight and relatively high in protein, fluid, vitamins and minerals will suffice, but the mother should have the benefit of more specific instruction in composing her diet. Weight reduction diets should be avoided by the nursing mother. Milk is important, but should not replace other essential foods. When the mother is allergic or has an aversion to milk, 1 gm of calcium may be added to her daily diet. The fluid intake should approximate 3 quarts daily; urinary output is a good measure of the adequacy of fluid in the daily diet.

There are mistaken ideas that such substances as milk, beer, oatmeal and tea are galactogenic. There is no objection to small amounts of alcoholic beverages if they contribute to the mother's peace of mind. Smoking of cigarettes should be discouraged. Particular foods in the mother's diet seldom have a disturbing influence on the breast-fed infant. Occasionally, however, maternal ingestion of certain berries, tomatoes, onions, members of the cabbage family, chocolate, spices and condiments may cause gastric distress or loose stools in the infant. No food need be withheld from the mother's diet unless it causes distress to the infant. It is better to control maternal constipation by inclusion in the diet of raw and cooked fruits and vegetables, whole wheat bread and an adequate amount of water than by use of laxatives. Certain substances, such as the arsenicals, barbiturates, bromides, iodides, lead, mercurials, salicylates, opium, atropine, sulfonamides, most antimicrobial agents and cascara may be transmitted through the milk and exert an effect on the infant.

TECHNIQUE OF BREAST FEEDING

The technical aspects of breast feeding require careful consideration. It is not unusual for breast feeding to be deemed impossible simply because the attending physician fails to recognize that the difficulties are related to the manner of feeding and not to qualitative or quantitative inadequacy of the milk.

The infant should be hungry at feeding time, dry and neither too cold nor too warm. He should be held in a comfortable, semisitting position for his enjoyment and for facilitation of eructation without vomiting. The mother, too, must be comfortable and completely at ease. When she is able to be out of bed, a moderately low chair with armrest is preferable, and a low stool is advantageous for resting her foot and raising her knee on the nursing side. The baby is supported comfortably with his face close to the breast by one arm and hand while the other hand supports the breast so that the nipple is easily accessible to the infant's mouth and yet does not obstruct his nasal breathing. The baby's lips should be expected to engage considerable areola, as well as nipple.

Success in infant feeding depends to a great extent upon the adjustments during the first few days of life. Difficulties are likely to result when attempts are made to adapt the infant to the nursing procedure rather than to try to satisfy his natural desires. Rigid adherence to clock schedules and the "assembly line" manner in which babies are handled in many nurseries may contribute to the baby's confusion. Most of the trouble can be avoided by conforming to the infant's spontaneous pattern. If he is put at the breast when there is normal hunger crying and if his appetite is satisfied, the fundamental requirements are met. Aldrich emphasized the natural initial responses to hunger; his account of one of them, the rooting reflex, is so well phrased that we have taken the liberty of reproducing it here.

> At the time he is born, the normal infant is equipped with several reflexes, or behavior patterns, which are designed to make him a successful feeder from the breast. The most obvious of these reflexes are those concerned with the actual getting of food—rooting, sucking, swallowing, and satiety reflexes.
>
> The *rooting reflex* is the first one of these to come into play. When a baby smells milk, he moves his head around and attempts to find its source. If one cheek is touched by a smooth object, he will turn his mouth toward that object and open it in anticipation of grasping the nipple. This obviously gives a clue as to how milk should be given to the baby. His cheek applied to his mother's breast will start him rooting with his mouth for the nipple.
>
> I can illustrate a mistake made in this regard by telling the . . . experience of a patient in one of our best hospitals. As I was making daily rounds, she said to me: "Your nurses don't know their stuff! . . . They don't know anything about the rooting reflex. They bring my baby in, place her beside me and with their hand on the baby's cheek try to push her head around to meet the nipple. The baby, feeling the pressure of the hand, tries to turn toward the nurse's palm instead of toward my breast. A fight ensues, and usually the natural response is prevented. I always tell the girls to go out of the room; that I can handle this myself if they just lay the baby down beside me. I touch her cheek with my breast and let her do the rest." This experienced mother had learned to respect her baby's ability in these basic matters. This is a highly important lesson for anybody to learn.

Mothers should know that if the infant is not hungry, he will not search for the nipple or suck. Infants are usually sleepy for several days, and most are not initially avid suckers. Particularly on the third day, when there has been some weight loss, mothers are anxious about infants who do not seem particularly interested in eating. It is reassuring for them to know that most healthy babies "wake up" and become good eaters on the fourth day. Kron and Brazleton have reported that infants whose mothers received obstetric sedation during labor sucked at lower rates and pressures and consumed less milk than comparable infants from mothers given no sedation.

Some infants will empty a breast in 5 minutes; others will be more leisurely and nurse well for 20 minutes. The baby should be permitted to suck until he is satisfied unless the mother has sore nipples. Efforts to wake up a sleepy baby and to "make him" nurse by snapping his feet, pinching or shaking him are rarely successful.

At the end of the nursing period the infant should be held erect over the mother's shoulder or on her lap to eructate swallowed air; often this "burping" procedure is necessary one or more times during the feeding as well as 5 to 10 minutes after the infant has been put into the crib. It is an essential procedure during the early months, but should not be overdone. When nursing is completed, the infant should be placed in the crib on his abdomen or on his right side to facilitate emptying of the stomach into the intestines and to lessen the chances of regurgitation.

ONE OR BOTH BREASTS PER FEEDING. The infant should empty at least one breast at each feeding; otherwise it will not be stimulated to refill. Both breasts should be used in the early weeks at each feeding to encourage maximal production of milk. After the milk supply has been established the breasts may be alternated at successive feedings, and the baby will usually be satisfied with the amount obtained from one. If the secretion of milk becomes too great, both breasts may again be offered at each feeding and incompletely emptied with the intent of securing a partial decrease in lactation.

DETERMINATION OF ADEQUACY OF BREAST SUPPLY. If the infant is satisfied at the completion of the nursing periods, sleeps 2 to 4 hours and gains weight adequately, it can be assumed that the milk supply is sufficient; weighing of the infant at other than weekly to monthly intervals is neither necessary nor desirable. Some babies are "light sleepers" and require a lot of body contact with the mother during the first months. Wakefulness in these babies should not be interpreted as poor milk supply. If the infant nurses avidly and is not satisfied after completely emptying both breasts, does not go to sleep or sleeps fitfully and awakens after an hour or two, and fails to gain weight satisfactorily, the milk supply is probably inadequate. The program of La Leche League* which establishes close relationships between successful nursing mothers and mothers needing assistance, is often helpful in such circumstances.

The "let-down" or milk-ejection reflex is an important sign of successful nursing. Sucking or often psychologic stimuli associated with nursing, leads to secretion of the oxytocic principle by the posterior pituitary. As a result, the smooth muscle fibers surrounding the alveoli deep in the breast contract, expelling milk into the larger ducts, where it is more easily available to the sucking infant. When this reflex is functioning well, milk will flow from the opposite breast as the baby begins to nurse. It is frequently absent or erratic during the periods of emotional distress, and its malfunction is thought to be responsible for retention of milk in women who are unsuccessful in breast feeding.

Having the mother weigh her baby before and after nursing is a generally unsatisfactory way of judging the adequacy of milk supply. It wrongly focuses attention on how much the infant takes at a given time (normally there may be variations of one to several ounces in the various feedings in a 24-hour period), and the results obtained are readily misinterpreted. Small gains may cause the mother additional worry, and, in turn, her milk supply may diminish. She may soon find it urgent to give the baby a bottle to assure herself that he is getting enough and to see how many ounces he will take. The result of the "test bottle" may so discourage her that subsequent breast feeding becomes impossible, even when she has an adequate supply of milk. Before it is assumed that the mother is unable to produce sufficient milk, 3 possibilities should be excluded: (1) errors in feeding technique responsible for the infant's inadequate progress; (2) remediable maternal factors related to diet, rest or emotional distress; or (3) physical disturbances in the infant which interfere with eating or otherwise with gain in weight.

SUPPLEMENTARY FEEDINGS. An occasional replacement feeding, after the first 6 weeks when the mother's milk supply has been adequately established, has the advantage of permitting the mother greater freedom in her activities. For the otherwise normal and healthy baby who is getting insufficient breast milk, artificial feeding may be offered either immediately after or in place of one or more breast feedings. Any of the milk formulas described under Formula Feeding may be offered to the baby in amounts sufficient to satisfy him. If formula is to be given after the baby has completed a breast feeding, the bottle should be warmed and handy so that it can be offered immediately after the infant has been given an opportunity to eructate any swallowed air. The holes in the nipples should not be so large that the baby gets this portion of his food without any effort, or he will quickly abandon any efforts to suck adequately at his mother's breast.

MANUAL EXPRESSION OF BREAST MILK. This is achieved by two movements: The first is compression of the whole breast between the hands, starting at the base and continuing toward the areola. Firm pressure is maintained throughout the movement, which is repeated several times. The purpose is to impel milk to the lacteal sinuses. The second movement empties the sinuses. The breast is supported with one hand while the tissue just behind the areola is repeatedly compressed between the thumb and first finger of the other hand. The direction of the force is backward toward the center of

*La Leche League International, 9616 Minneapolis Avenue, Franklin Park, Illinois 60131, has many local affiliates composed of successful nursing mothers who are willing to assist other mothers desiring to nurse.

the breast rather than toward the nipple. The fingers are not moved from this initial position, nor is the skin rubbed over the breast tissue. The procedure should not be painful even though the nipples are sore and cracked.

MECHANICAL EXPRESSION OF BREAST MILK. Hand pumps are often ineffectual and may increase the irritation and pain in congested breast and nipple tissues. Many prefer to use an electric breast pump such as the Egnall Electric Breast Pump (Pilling Co.), which is more comfortable and effective than hand expression when repeated drainage of milk is required.

WEANING. The breast-feeding infant and his mother have a close relationship based upon mutual needs and satisfactions. This relationship changes as the baby grows and develops independence. Most infants will have voluntarily reduced the number of breast feedings as they become accustomed to solid foods, usually between 6 and 9 months of age, and many will wean themselves at this time; some will need to continue the nursing relationship beyond the first birthday.

When a bottle feeding per day has been substituted for one of the breast feedings, as suggested previously, there is no difficulty in weaning. If the infant is not acquainted with the bottle, cup feeding may be tried. Not infrequently the cup is taken as readily as the bottle and the intermediate transfer to cup from bottle feeding is avoided. In any event, when the mother's milk is abundant, the process of weaning should be sufficiently gradual to avoid causing her unnecessary discomfort and to let the baby learn to accept milk from a new source. Initially, one of the breast feedings is replaced by a bottle feeding. After several days another breast feeding is replaced, and so on, until the baby is weaned completely. The total time required is governed by the status of the maternal milk supply.

When cessation of nursing is necessary at an earlier age because of illness of the mother or prolonged illness or death of the infant, a tight breast binder may be used and ice bags applied for a day or so. Restriction of the mother's fluid intake is also helpful in decreasing milk production rapidly.

FORMULA FEEDING

Artificial feeding is now viewed as a simple procedure in which complicated calculations and elaborate preparations are not necessary. Cow's milk in the whole state or some modified form is the basis for most formulas. Other milks and milk substitutes are available for infants who cannot tolerate cow's milk. Drastic reduction in the morbidity and mortality from gastrointestinal infections has resulted from sterilization of the formula and refrigeration of it until used. Milk processing (varying from simple boiling in the home to commercial pasteurization, homogenization and evaporation) has so altered the casein that small and readily digestible curds are formed in the stomach, thereby eliminating the principal cause for indigestibility of cow's milk protein.

Though breast feeding is considered superior to formula feeding for normal infants, surveys indicate that more than 80 per cent of infants in the United States receive formula from birth. Changing social and cultural patterns have contributed in largest measure to this increased reliance on formulas. Many mothers are reluctant to nurse their infants because of employment outside the home or implied limitations on social activities; others refuse because of fear of failure or of worry that loss of physical attractiveness will ensue from gain of weight and loss of breast tone; some do not consider breast feeding socially acceptable. Whatever the mother's reason or combination of reasons, the present popularity of artificial feeding could not have been reached without prior improvements in the safety and quality of the substitute milks.

The superiority of breast milk (as distinct from breast feeding) over the present-day artificial feedings derived from cow's milk has become less critical with better understanding of milk processing and food chemistry. Objective studies of the state of nutrition in growing infants (rate of growth in weight and length, normality of various constituents in blood, performance in metabolic studies, body composition, and the like) show relatively small differences between infants fed human milk and a variety of cow's milk feedings. Such techniques* may not be sufficiently sensitive to record small but important variations. Nonetheless, these investigations attest to the ability of the normal infant to thrive by making satisfactory physiologic adjustments to relatively wide ranges of intake of protein, fat, carbohydrate and minerals.

Conventional whole and evaporated cow's milk formulas provide approximately 3 to 4 gm of protein per kg per day ("high protein" intake with a relatively large excess above basic need), whereas breast milk and many commercially prepared feedings simulating the composition of breast milk supply 2.0 to 2.5 gm/kg/day ("low protein" intake supplying a smaller margin of excess). Other milk products which furnish a protein intake intermediate between the "high" and "low" levels are also marketed.

The basic question as to whether the formula-fed infant should be provided with a higher allowance of protein than the breast-fed one has not been completely resolved. The available evidence, although lacking in many essential details, may be summarized as follows: (1) only minor differences in the nutritional values of protein from human and cow's milk have been demonstrated; (2) the

*For example, the commonly used gain in weight does not differentiate between accumulations in lean body mass and fat stores and includes increases in body water due to excess solute retention under certain circumstances, as has been demonstrated by Kagan's studies in the nutrition of premature infants.

natural and commercial milks for which analyses are available contain at least the minimal amounts, and usually a surplus, of the essential amino acids; (3) the existence of a "protein reserve" similar to that for glycogen and fat, implying the storage of proteins in the body in excess of current requirements and available to meet stressful situations, is open to question; (4) protein metabolism ("turnover") is closely related to and conditioned by the level of intake: (5) studies relating high and low intakes of protein to resistance to infection are inconclusive; and (6) normal infants receiving low, intermediate or high intakes of protein appear to do equally well clinically.

Fomon has calculated the rate of increase in total body protein mass in the "male reference" term infant to average approximately 3.5 gm per day in the first 4 months of life. Assuming 0.5 gm per day nitrogen loss from the skin, total protein need is estimated to be about 4.0 gm per day during the first 4 months and slightly less during the remainder of the first year.

It seems reasonable to conclude that normal infants can be expected to thrive on dietary intakes within the wide range of protein (2.0 to 3.5 or 4.0 gm/kg/day) and of minerals which are provided by the usual daily ingestion of human milk, of the whole and evaporated cow's milk formulas in common use, and of the commercially prepared feedings of low, intermediate and high protein content.

TECHNIQUE OF ARTIFICIAL FEEDING

The setting is similar to that for breast feeding, with the mother in a comfortable position, pleasant, unhurried and free from distractions. The infant should be hungry, fully awake, warm and dry; he should be held as though he were being nursed. The bottle should be held so that milk, not air, is channeled through the nipple. Bottle propping, even with a "safe" holder, should be avoided; propping not only deprives the infant of the physical contact, comfort and security of being held, but may also be dangerous to small infants, who may aspirate if unattended.

The bottle of milk is customarily warmed to body temperature, though no harmful effects have been demonstrated from feedings at room temperature or cooler, even when the bottle is taken directly from the refrigerator. The temperature may be tested by dropping milk on the wrist. The nipple holes should be of such size that milk will drop slowly.

Especially during the first 6 or 7 months of life, the eructation of air swallowed during feeding is important for avoidance of abdominal discomfort and of regurgitation. Holding the infant upright over the shoulder with or without gently rubbing or patting the back assists in expelling the air. A few babies relieve themselves best after being replaced in the crib. All babies will, at times, regurgitate or "spit up" a small amount of milk after feeding, a fact the mother should know. "Spitting" occurs more often in the artificially fed than in the breast-fed infants. Aspiration of this milk is less likely if the infant lies on his right side or abdomen, rather than on his back.

A feeding may require from 5 to 25 minutes, depending on the vigor and the age of the infant. Since the appetite varies from feeding to feeding, each bottle should contain more than the average amount taken per feeding. In no instance should the baby be urged to take more than he desires. The excess milk should be discarded, and the bottle and nipple rinsed with cool water.

COMPARISON OF HUMAN AND COW'S MILKS

Average values for the various constituents of human milk and whole fresh and evaporated cow's milk are listed in Table 3–11. Human milk and cow's milk differ during the various stages of lactation, and there are some differences between milks of individual women as well as of cows. The differences in milks from women whose diets are adequate are insignificant.

COLOSTRUM. The secretion of the breasts for the first 2 to 4 days after delivery is termed "colostrum." It has a deep lemon yellow color, its reaction is alkaline, and its specific gravity is 1.040 to 1.060, in contrast to the average specific gravity of 1.030 for fresh breast milk. The total amount of colostrum secreted daily is not large (10 to 40 ml.). Colostrum contains several times as much protein as breast milk and more minerals, but less carbohydrate and fat. After the first few days of lactation, colostrum is replaced by secretion of a transitional form of milk which gradually assumes the characteristics of mature breast milk by the third or fourth week.

WATER. The relative amounts of water and solids in human and cow's milks are about the same, each having a water content of about 87 to 87.5 per cent; the specific gravity of each is in the range of 1.030 to 1.032.

CALORIES. The energy value of each milk may vary slightly, but for practical purposes each may be assumed to contain 20 kilocalories per ounce or 0.67 kcal/ml.

PROTEIN. There are both qualitative and quantitative differences between the proteins of the two milks. Human milk contains only 1.0 to 1.5 (average 1.1) per cent protein in contrast to about 3.3 per cent in cow's milk. The increased protein of cow's milk is almost entirely accounted for by the sixfold higher content of casein. The principal quantitative differences are in the relative amounts of whey proteins and casein. In human milk the protein consists of approximately 60 per cent whey proteins, largely lactalbumins and lactoglobulins, and 40 per cent casein; whereas in cow's milk the ratio is reversed, to 18:82. The proteins of the two milks are essentially equivalent for infant nutrition.

CARBOHYDRATE. The sugar of the two milks differs only quantitatively, both containing lac-

TABLE 3–11 COMPARISON OF HUMAN AND COW'S MILKS

	REPRESENTATIVE COMPOSITION OF MATURE MILKS			VARIATIONS IN COMPOSITION OF UNPOOLED MILK SAMPLES*	
	HUMAN	COW'S	COW'S EVAP.	HUMAN	COW'S
Components (per cent):					
Water	87.6	87.3	73.0	87.0 - 89.0	83.0 - 88.0
Total solids	12.4	12.7	27.0	8.5 - 15.0	8.5 - 19.0
Proteins	1.2	3.3	7.3	0.7 - 2.0	2.8 - 3.6
Casein	0.4	2.8	6.2	0.14- 0.68	2.1 - 2.8
Whey	0.6	0.6	1.3	0.5 - 1.1	0.3 - 0.6
Lactalbumin	0.3	0.4	0.88	0.14- 0.6	0.27- 0.57
Lactoglobulin	0.2	0.2	0.44		0.14- 0.42
Lactose	7.0	4.8	10.6	5.0 - 9.2	4.0 - 5.5
Fat	3.8	3.7	8.2	1.3 - 8.3	3.1 - 5.2
Minerals (ash)	0.21	0.72	1.6	0.16- 0.27	0.64- 0.75
Minerals (per liter):					
Sodium (mEq)	7.0	25.0	55.0	2.0 - 13.0	13.5 - 93.0
Potassium (mEq)	14.0	35.0	77.0	9.5 - 17.5	9.7 - 74.0
Chloride (mEq)	12.0	29.0	46.0	2.6 - 21.0	27.0 - 40.0
Calcium (mg)	330.0	1250.0	2750.0	170.0 - 610.0	560.0 -3810.0
Phosphorus (mg)	150.0	960.0	2112.0	70.0 - 270.0	560.0 -1120.0
Magnesium (mg)	40.0	120.0	264.0	20.0 - 60.0	70.0 - 220.0
Sulfur (mg)	140.0	300.0	660.0	50.0 - 300.0	240.0 - 360.0
Iron (mg)	1.5	1.0	2.2	0.2 - 1.8	0.2 - 1.4
Zinc (mg)	1.2	3.8	8.4	0.17- 3.02	1.9 - 6.6
Copper (mg)	0.4	0.3	0.66	0.1 - 0.7	0.2 - 0.8
Iodine (mg)	0.07	0.21	0.46	0.05- 0.09	0.13- 1.8
Amino Acids (mg/liter):					
Histidine	230.0	800.0	1760.0	160.0 - 340.0	700.0 -1300.0
Isoleucine	860.0	2120.0	4664.0	460.0 -1020.0	1800.0 -2900.0
Leucine	1610.0	3560.0	7832.0	720.0 -1590.0	2400.0 -3900.0
Lysine	790.0	2570.0	5654.0	530.0 -1040.0	2200.0 -3100.0
Methionine	230.0	870.0	1914.0	90.0 - 210.0	600.0 - 900.0
Phenylalanine	640.0	1730.0	3860.0	300.0 - 580.0	1400.0 -2200.0
Threonine	620.0	1520.0	3344.0	400.0 - 760.0	1200.0 -2200.0
Tryptophan	220.0	500.0	1100.0	130.0 - 260.0	400.0 - 800.0
Valine	900.0	2280.0	4956.0	480.0 -1140.0	2100.0 -2800.0
Calories† (approximate):					
Per fluid ounce	20.0	20.0	44.0‡	18.0 - 24.0	17.0 - 25.0
Per liter	710.0	690.0	1520.0	600.0 - 790.0	570.0 - 850.0

*Values are taken from several studies; agreement is approximate, but not all components were evaluated in each.
†Calorie = large calorie = kcal = Cal. (See text.)
‡In practice, commonly regarded as 40 calories (40 kcal).
The data are assembled from a number of sources.

tose. Human milk contains 6.5 to 7.0 per cent, and cow's milk about 4.5 per cent.

FAT. The fat content of milks is more variable than any other constituent, but the average content is about 3.5 per cent. The amount in human milk varies somewhat with maternal diet; the fat content of milk obtained during a single nursing is higher in the latter portion of the feeding.

The milks of different breeds of cattle vary in fat content. Most market milk in urban areas, however, is pooled, and the fat content is adjusted to a standard level, generally from 3.25 to 4 per cent.

There are qualitative differences between the fats of human and cow's milks. The fats of each are composed principally of the triglycerides, olein, palmitin and stearin. Human milk, however, contains twice as much of the more readily absorbed olein. The volatile fatty acids (butyric, capric, caproic and caprylic) account for only about 1.3 per cent of the fat of human milk, in contrast to about 9 per cent in cow's milk. Hansen called attention to the need for linoleic acid, a dienoic fat, in infant nutrition. Babies fed fat-poor diets deficient in this substance develop thickened, dry and scaly skin and fail to grow normally; the small amount of linoleic acid in most milks is sufficient to prevent deficiency. The normal infant has no difficulty in digesting the fat of cow's milk, whereas the premature or debilitated infant may have steatorrhea after ingesting it. For such infants it is wise to keep the fat content of the milk formula relatively low or to substitute a more readily assimilated vegetable fat.

MINERALS. The total mineral content of human

milk (0.15 to 0.25 per cent) is considerably less than that of cow's milk (0.7 to 0.75 per cent). With the exception of iron and copper, cow's milk contains considerably more of all the minerals. Neither milk contains an adequate amount of iron; the deficiency is compensated for in the first 4 months or so of life by iron stored in fetal life. Although the need for calcium and phosphorus is relatively great during periods of rapid growth, adequate balances are maintained on breast milk in spite of its comparatively low content of these minerals.

VITAMINS. The vitamin content of each milk varies with the maternal intake. Each has relatively large amounts of vitamin A and small amounts of vitamin D. Human milk has more vitamin C except when the maternal intake is deficient in vitamin C-containing foods. Cow's milk contains more thiamine and riboflavin than human milk and about an equal quantity of niacin. It is assumed that each milk contains adequate amounts of vitamin A and the B-complex vitamins and inadequate amounts of vitamins C and D for the nutritional needs of infants in the first months of life.

BACTERIAL CONTENT. Human milk is essentially free from bacterial contamination. Pathogenic organisms in significant numbers may gain access to the milk from mastitis. Both tubercle bacilli and typhoid bacilli may be found at times in the milk of women infected with these organisms. Cow's milk is regularly contaminated, but in most instances the bacteria are not harmful to man. Milk, however, is a good culture medium for pathogenic bacteria, and many infections are milkborne. Such infections include streptococcal diseases, diphtheria, typhoid fever, salmonellosis, tuberculosis and brucellosis. Furthermore, certain bacteria which may not affect older children or adults may cause diarrhea in infants. For this reason, in most cities, pasteurization of all marketed whole milk is required. In addition, boiling the milk immediately before mixing the infant's formula or terminal sterilization is advisable.

DIGESTIBILITY. The emptying time of the stomach is more rapid for human than for whole cow's milk; however, there is no appreciable difference in gastrointestinal passage time during the first 45 days of life between human milk and processed milk formulas. The curd of cow's milk is reduced in size by boiling and is made considerably less tough and much smaller by the heating required in evaporation, by the addition of acid or alkali and by homogenization. In contrast, the curd of breast milk is fine and flocculent and readily broken down in the stomach. The fat of cow's milk is less readily digested than that of breast milk.

FORMS OF COW'S MILK USED IN FORMULAS

RAW MILK. This milk is not advised for infant feeding; it forms large curds in the stomach, is slowly digested, and is easily contaminated with pathogenic organisms. Its sale is forbidden in most urban communities.

PASTEURIZED MILK. Pasteurization destroys pathogenic bacteria and modifies the casein so that smaller and less tough curds are produced in the stomach. It is accomplished by holding heated milk at a specified temperature for a specific length of time, e.g., at 145° F (63° C) for 30 minutes or, more commonly, at 161° F (72° C) for 15 seconds followed by rapid cooling to 148° F (65° C) or lower (60° C). Standards for the bacterial content of pasteurized milk vary in different cities, tolerable counts ranging as high as 50,000 nonpathogenic bacteria per ml.; average counts in many cities, however, are as low as 5000 to 10,000. Pasteurized milk should be boiled when used for infant feeding. If allowed to stand in the refrigerator for as long as 48 hours, a significant increase in bacterial count may occur.

HOMOGENIZED MILK. The processing of milk so that the fat globules are broken into a homogeneous emulsion of minute particles is termed homogenization. Owing to the decrease in size and dispersion of the fat molecules, the cream does not separate. The principal advantage of homogenized milk lies in the smaller and less tough curd produced in the stomach.

EVAPORATED MILK. Evaporated milk has many advantages, including almost universal availability. In the unopened can it will keep for months without refrigeration. The casein curd produced in the stomach is softer and smaller than that of boiled whole milk; homogenization of the fat also contributes to smaller curd formation. The lactalbumin appears to be less allergenic than that of fresh milk. The sugar is unchanged. When necessary, evaporated milk can be fed in higher concentrations than whole milk formulas. The standard can contains 14.5 ounces avoirdupois or 13 fluid ounces* (384 ml.). Each fluid ounce is equal to about 44 kilocalories; in practice the value is generally considered to be 40 kilocalories. Whether diluted with an equal quantity of water (13 ounces or 384 ml) or reconstituted at a ratio of 1:1.2 (15½ ounces or 458 ml), one can is equivalent to only about 28 ounces (or 828 ml) of whole milk. Vitamin D is usually added in the processing so that each reconstituted quart contains 400 IU.

CONDENSED MILK. About 45 per cent cane sugar has been added in sweetened condensed milk, making the carbohydrate content approximately 60 per cent in the evaporated form before dilution. The usual dilutions (1:10 to 1:4) are disproportionately high in sugar and low in fat and protein. Although readily digestible, it has no use in infant feeding for more than short periods when a high caloric diet is desired.

DRIED WHOLE MILK. Standard regulations govern the production of dried milk. The fat content of fluid milk is adjusted to 3.5 per cent, and the milk is evaporated with extreme rapidity to powder

*One fluid ounce is equivalent to approximately 29.57 ml.

form by spray-, freeze- or roller-drying. Reconstituted dried milk has most of the advantages of evaporated milk, but does not keep well when exposed to air.

DRIED SKIM MILK. Available as either nonfat skim milk (fat content 0.05 per cent) or half-skim milk (fat content 1.5 per cent), these milks have limited usefulness: (1) for infants with fat intolerance; (2) for infants convalescing from diarrheal diseases; and (3) for premature infants when diets high in protein and low in fat are prescribed. Many of these products do not contain added vitamin D.

ACID AND FERMENTED MILKS. So-called acid milks are prepared by addition of acid or are fermented by bacterial action. Acid milk may be prepared by the addition of lactic acid, U.S.P. (or other acids), to previously boiled and cooled cow's milk formulas; the amount required varies with the fat content, those with higher concentrations requiring more acid. Milks containing 3.5 to 4 per cent fat require about 1½ fluid drams (6 ml) to the quart. Reconstituted evaporated milk requires about the same amount. The acid is added drop by drop to the cooled milk formula with constant stirring with a wooden spoon to avoid curd formation. Several commercial preparations of dried lactic acid whole and skim milk are also available. Most fermented milks (i.e., buttermilks) are acidified by the addition of lactic acid-producing organisms *(Lactobacillus acidophilus and L. bulgaricus).*

These milks require less hydrochloric acid for gastric digestion. The casein is altered so that smaller and less tough curds are formed in the stomach. Their use appears to be limited to the feeding of infants with digestive disturbances and those convalescing from diarrheal disease; currently they are rarely used in infant feeding.

OTHER MILKS USED IN FORMULAS

GOAT'S MILK. In many countries goat's milk is used extensively for infant feeding; its use in this country is limited to management of cow's milk allergies; because of inconsistent antigenic cross-reaction between cow's and goat's milks it is less popular than the soya "milks" or the formulas derived from lamb and beef and from casein hydrolysis.

Goat's milk is similar in composition to cow's milk; it contains less sodium, more potassium and chloride, and more of the essential linoleic and arachidonic acids; its fat may be more digestible and its curd tension is lower than cow's milk. It is low in vitamin D, iron and folic acid; infants fed exclusively on goat's milk are prone to megaloblastic anemia due to folate deficiency. The goat is especially susceptible to brucellosis; the milk should be boiled before use. It is commercially available in evaporated and powdered forms.

PREPARED MILKS. Numerous commercially prepared premodified milks which require only the addition of water are widely used in infant feeding. They are derived basically from cow's milk, and many are available in both liquid and powder forms. The majority have compositions which simulate breast milk in one or more ways: reduced protein contents, which vary from 1.5 to 2.8 gm/dl of reconstituted milk; reduced mineral salts (sodium, potassium, chloride, calcium, phosphorus); fat modification by substitution of vegetable fat for butterfat; and addition of carbohydrate (lactose or dextrin-maltose). All are fortified with vitamin D; many contain other vitamins, and some have added iron. In the recommended 1:1 dilution of most of the liquid forms, each can provides 26 ounces (768 ml) of formula. Table 3–12 lists the varieties of milks and milk substitutes available for infant feeding.

These milks are nutritionally adequate for normal infants, simple to prepare and convenient to use. Their cost is somewhat greater than evaporated milk-carbohydrate-water formulas.

Other prepared milks which may have virtue for special circumstances are now available. Those with very low electrolyte content (mineral content similar to human milk) may be helpful in infants with congestive heart failure, nephrogenic diabetes insipidus and marginal renal function. A low sodium milk, containing about 1 mEq of sodium per reconstituted quart, is commercially available for use in the management of infants with congestive heart failure. Milks low in phenylalanine content are useful in the management of infants and children with phenylketonuria.

MILK PROTEIN. Powdered protein is used chiefly for increasing the protein content of dilute skim milk or other formulas for feeding during diarrheal conditions, or to premature or debilitated infants.

MILK SUBSTITUTES AND HYPOALLERGENIC MILKS. There are a number of milks and milk substitutes for infants allergic to cow's milk. These include evaporated goat's milk, a preparation in which nutrient nitrogen is supplied as an amino acid mixture (casein hydrolysate), nonmilk foods in which the protein is derived from soybeans, and meat-base formulas (beef and lamb sources). All appear to be nutritionally satisfactory and to have a place in the management of infants who cannot tolerate cow's milk; those which do not contain lactose are useful for infants with galactosemia.

MILKS, FILLED AND IMITATION. Imitation milk products and nondairy "white" beverages are being developed and tested for use in countries where milk and other high quality protein sources are in short supply. Many of these products lack the full nutritional benefits of fluid milk; they are not intended as formula for infants nor as a substitute for breast milk; when they are used for older children, the physician should be aware of the qualitative and quantitative composition, including the limitations of the product.

ELEMENTAL DIETARY SUBSTITUTES FOR MILK. A number of specialty products have been developed to meet complicated dietary and nutritional problems in children and adults with malabsorption on the basis of primary disease or extensive surgical resection of small bowel. These include diets prepared with known quantities of purified chemical

TABLE 3–12 NATURAL MILKS, PREPARED MILKS AND MILK SUBSTITUTES USED IN INFANT FEEDING

	NORMAL DILUTION		APPROXIMATE PERCENTAGE COMPOSITION IN NORMAL DILUTION (Grams per 100 ml.)				APPROXIMATE ELECTROLYTE COMPOSITION IN NORMAL DILUTION (Milliequivalents per liter)					MILLIGRAMS PER LITER
	*Ratio**	*Cal/oz (kcal/oz)*	*Protein*	*Carbohydrate*	*Fat*	*Minerals*	*Na*	*K*	*Cl*	*Ca*	*P†*	*Fe*
Human milk, mature, average	Undiluted	20	1.2	7.0	3.8	0.21	7	14	12	17	9	1.5
Cow's milk, market, average	Undiluted	20	3.3	4.8	3.7	0.72	25	35	29	62	53	1.0
Cow's milk, evaporated, many brands	1:1	22	3.8	5.4	4.0	0.8	28	39	32	65	59	1.0
Cow's milk, powdered:												
Klim, Borden	1:7	20	3.3	4.7	3.5	0.7	22	35	28	58	48	1.0
Commercial premodified milks:												
Infant Formula, Baker‡	1:1	20	2.2	7.0	3.3	0.6	17	23	19	42	37	7.9
Bremil with Iron, Borden	1:1	20	1.5	7.0	3.5	0.5	11	16	13	35	18	8.5
Bremil Powder, Borden	1:8	20	1.5	7.1	3.5	0.4	16	36	13	35	18	8.5
Modilac, Gerber	1:1	20	2.2	7.8	2.7	0.4	17	27	19	42	37	10.6
Enfamil, Mead‡	1:1	20	1.5	7.0	3.7	0.3	11	19	12	32	32	8.5
Olac, Mead‡	1:1	20	3.4	7.5	2.7	0.7	22	41	29	60	58	tr.
Nan Powder, Nestlé	1:7	20	1.6	7.3	3.4	0.3	10	19	12	22	23	7
Lactogen Powder, Nestlé	1:6	20	2.4	7.6	3.5	0.5	13	27	17	42	37	7
Lactogen Powder, Full Protein, Nestlé	1:5.5	20	3.4	7.9	2.9	0.7	19	38	24	61	53	7
Pelargon Powder, Nestlé	1:5	22	28	9.7	2.9	0.6	16	32	20	52	45	7
Similac with Iron, Ross§	1:1	20	1.8	6.6	3.4	0.4	12	26	18	34	30	12
Similac Powder with Iron, Ross§	1:8	20	1.8	6.6	3.4	0.5	17	31	17	41	30	12
Similac PM 60/40 Powder, Ross	1:8	20	1.5	7.2	3.4	0.2	7	14	12	17	10	–
SMA S-26, Wyeth*	1:1	20	1.5	7.2	3.6	0.25	7	14	12	21	21	8
Goat's milk, powdered:												
Dale's, Cutter	1:6	20	3.3	4.7	4.1	0.77	18	46	45	61	55	tr.
High protein, low fat powdered milks:												
Dryco, Borden	1:8	16	4.0	5.7	1.5	0.9	27	38	32	65	57	1.0
Alacta, Mead	1:7	14	4.2	5.9	1.5	0.9	26	75	36	75	65	1.2
Probana, Mead	1:7	20	3.9	7.3	2.0	0.6	26	31	28	100	58	3.0
Protein Milk, Mead	1:10	14	3.8	2.7	2.7	0.7	30	30	29	63	57	1.3
Eledon, Nestlé	1:8	14	3.7	4.8	1.6	0.8	20	40	25	66	54	7
Nestogen, Half-Skimmed, Nestlé	1:5	21	3.4	10.1	2.0	0.8	20	39	26	64	52	7
Skim milk, many brands	1:10	10	3.5	4.8	0.2	0.7	26	34	32	62	56	0.5
Hypoallergenic milk substitutes:												
Mullsoy Liquid, Borden (Soya)	1:1	20	3.1	5.2	3.6	0.8	16	40	16	60	46	5
Mullsoy Powder, Borden (Soya)	1:8	20	3.1	4.5	4.0	0.7	26	35	13	65	58	4
Neo-Mullsoy, Borden (Soya)	1:1	20	1.8	6.4	3.5	0.5	17	25	6	42	24	8.4
Nursoy, Wyeth	1:1	20	2.3	6.8	3.6	0.4	9	15	15	31	32	12
Lambase, Gerber	1:1	20	2.4	7.9	2.4	0.3	24	28	7	46	45	7.9
Meat-base, Gerber (Requires added carbohydrate)	13:19.5	17.4	2.7	4.0	3.1	0.33	12	12	17	52	40	9.7
Soyalac Liquid, Loma Linda (Soya)	1:1	20	2.1	5.9	4.0	0.3	14	23	10	21	21	10
Soyalac Powder, Loma Linda (Soya)	1:8	20	2.9	5.9	3.5	0.45	14	34	15	42	21	10
Nutramigen Powder, Mead	1:6	20	2.2	8.5	2.6	0.6	17	26	23	50	52	10
Pro-Sobee, Mead (Soya)	1:1	20	2.5	6.8	3.4	0.5	24	28	7	47	42	8.5
Sobee, Mead (Soya)	1:1	20	3.2	7.7	2.6	0.5	22	33	14	50	32	8.5
Isomil, Ross (Soya)	1:1	20	2.0	6.8	3.6	0.4	13	16	15	35	28	12
Milk substitutes, specialty products												
Cho-Free Formula Base, Borden (12.5% dextrose added)	1:1	20	1.8	6.4	3.5	0.5	17	25	6	47	47	8.4
Flexical, Mead	1:45	30	2.2	15.5	3.4		15	38	34	25	43	5.0
Jejunal Beverage, Johnson and Johnson‖		27.3	1.9	19.7	0.08		34	21	57	31	59	4.9
Jejunal Broth, Johnson and Johnson‖		27.3	1.9	19.7	0.08		98	21	131	31	59	4.9
Lofenalac, Mead	1:6	20	2.2	8.5	2.7	0.75	26	38	23	47	47	1.6
Lonalac, Mead	1:6	20	3.4	4.8	3.5	0.6	1.1	27	14	56	57	2.1
Portagen, Mead	1:6	20	2.7	7.7	3.2	0.7	17	33	23	48	46	11.3
Pregestimil, Mead	1:7	20	2.1	8.7	2.5		18	24	23	47	24	12.1
Vivonex Standard, Eaton¶	#	30	2.0	23.9	.15		37	30	51	22	43	5.5
Vivonex HN, Eaton¶	#	30	4.2	21.1	.07		34	18	52	13	26	3.3
W-T Low Residue, Warren-Teed¶	#	30	2.2	22.7	.07		56#	30#	84	28	31	10
W-T Peptide L4, Warren-Teed¶	#	30	2.6	22.2	.08		39#	33#	69#	28	31	10
W-T Protein L4, Warren-Teed¶	#	30	2.6	22.2	.11		42#	33#	60#	28	31	10
Similac Advance, Ross	1:1	16.5	3.6	6.6	1.6		17	36	24	50	26	18

Data supplied by processors or assembled from other sources.

*Number of ounces of milk to number of ounces of water. (Most powdered milks may also be prepared by adding 1 level tablespoonful or special measuring spoonful of powder to each 2 ounces of water.)

†Calculated for valence of 1.8.

‡Also available in powdered form with similar composition.

§Also available without iron supplementation.

‖Dilution ratio 60-gm package: 210 ml – 240 ml

¶Dilution ratio 80-gm package: 255 ml – 300 ml

#Varies with flavoring.

elements (free glucose, amino acids and essential fatty acids). Thus far, none of the marketed products are truly "elemental"; all are low residue, chemically defined and nutritionally adequate, at least for short-term use. They have been most useful in severely ill infants with intractable diarrhea, through reducing stooling and/or "resting" the colon in inflammatory bowel disease, in making maximum use of short bowel segments after surgery, and in maintaining very ill patients in positive nitrogen balance while decreasing the bulk and bacterial content of the colon prior to and after major bowel surgery. (See Milk Substitutes, Specialty Products in Tables 3–12 and 3–15.)

MILK FORMULAS

Most methods for calculating milk formulas result in somewhat similar combinations of milk, water and sugar. No method stands out as definitely superior. Although there has been increasing simplification in the construction of formulas, understanding of the nutritional requirements and eating habits of infants is fundamental for proper guidance of mothers in the feeding of infants and children.

The ingredients of the formula are milk, water and sugar. Some modification of the milk which results in smaller curd formation in the stomach is desirable and is achieved to some extent by boiling raw milk and to a greater extent by boiling previously pasteurized milk. Homogenization and evaporation further alter the milk curd; the addition of acids or alkalis has a similar effect. The choice of milk depends somewhat upon available supplies and upon individual preferences. The formula should contain approximately 20 kilocalories per ounce.

CALORIC REQUIREMENTS. (See also above.) The average caloric requirements of full-term infants are about 50 to 55 kilocalories per pound or 110 to 120 kilocalories per kg during the first few months of life; and about 45 kilocalories per pound, or 100 per kg (or slightly less), by 1 year of age; individual variations are significant, and for many infants intakes of this order are in excess of caloric need.

FLUID REQUIREMENTS. (See also above.) Fluid requirements are high during infancy. During the first 6 months of life they range from 2 to 3 oz/lb/day, or 130 to 190 ml/kg/day. The requirements may be increased during hot weather. As a rule, the infant will regulate his own fluid intake, provided adequate amounts are offered. Most of the fluid requirement is in the formula, but some is supplied in orange juice and other foods and by water between feedings.

NUMBER OF FEEDINGS DAILY. The number of feedings required per day decreases throughout the first year so that by 1 year of age most infants are satisfied with 3 meals a day (Table 3-13). The interval between feedings differs considerably among infants, but, in general, ranges from 3 to 5 hours during the first year of life, with an average of 4 hours for full-term, healthy infants. Small and weak infants may prefer feedings at 2- to 3-hour intervals. For the first month or two, feedings are taken throughout the 24-hour period, but thereafter the infant will usually sleep from 10 or 12 P.M. to 6 or 7 A.M. Time of omission of the late evening feeding (10 to 12 P.M.) varies from the third to the eighth month.

TABLE 3–13 AVERAGE NUMBER OF FEEDINGS PER 24 HOURS

AGE	AVERAGE NUMBER OF FEEDINGS IN 24 HOURS
Birth-1 week	6-10
1 week-1 month	6-8
1-3 months	5-6
3-7 months	4-5
4-9 months	3-4
8-12 months	3

QUANTITY OF FORMULA PER FEEDING. Although the quantity taken at a feeding will vary with different infants of the same age and with the same infant at different feedings, it is necessary to know the average amounts taken at various ages. A general rule for the estimation of the quantity of the individual feeding to be offered during the first half year of life is to add 3 to the age in months. It is good practice to put more in each bottle than the infant is expected to take. Estimates which more nearly reflect the average infant's intake are shown above. The "rules of thumb" are, at best, guides; each infant must be given the primary responsibility in determining the quantity of his intake. Rarely will an infant want to take more than 7 or 8 ounces of milk at one feeding if his caloric and nutritional needs are adequately supplemented by other foods.

AGE	AVERAGE QUANTITY TAKEN IN INDIVIDUAL FEEDINGS
1st and 2nd weeks	2–3 ounces (60– 90 ml)
3 weeks–2 months	4–5 ounces (120–150 ml)
2–3 months	5–6 ounces (150–180 ml)
3–4 months	6–7 ounces (180–210 ml)
5–12 months	7–8 ounces (210–240 ml)

QUANTITY OF MILK. The amount of whole milk usually taken daily in the first 6 months of life varies from 1¾ to 2 ounces per pound (115–130 ml/kg) of body weight (evaporated milk, approximately 1 oz/lb, or 65 ml/kg). The relative requirements are somewhat less in the first 2 weeks than in the succeeding 5 or 6 months. After this time milk, though still of great value, has diminishing importance in meeting total nutritional requirements.

Rarely is it necessary to use more than one can (13 fluid ounces) of evaporated milk or a quart of whole milk per day. By the time the infant is taking these quantities, other foods will be added to the diet in increasing amounts.

WATER. It is common practice to dilute cow's milk with water for the feeding of infants during the first few months of life. In the 2 weeks or so after birth, dilution of cow's milk will lessen the possibility of tetany by reducing the amount of phosphorus to be excreted. Although it has been demonstrated that infants will tolerate undiluted cow's milk or fully reconstituted (ratio 1:1) evaporated milk after the first few days of life, infants so fed tend to have a moderate elevation of the blood urea nitrogen level and to obligate a large proportion of the ingested water for renal solute excretion. Increased insensible water loss with fever or high environmental temperatures may exceed the narrow margin of safety provided in the solute-to-water ratio of these formulas. Therefore, it is helpful to add water and sugar to milk for infants up to 4 or 6 months of age in order to reduce the renal solute load with respect to ingested protein and minerals. With whole and evaporated cow s milk feedings, water should be offered between feedings during periods of high environmental temperature, and additional water will be needed when there are unusual losses as with vomiting or diarrhea.

SUGAR. A number of carbohydrates are used in infant feeding, and all seem to be satisfactory. Theoretically it might seem that lactose, the sugar of milk, would be the one of choice; it appears to have little advantage, however, over the others and may even cause an increased amount of flatulence, owing to a greater degree of fermentation. Cane sugar has advantages of universal availability and low cost. Its only apparent disadvantage is a greater sweetness than the others. There are a number of popular dextrin-maltose preparations whose principal advantages are a slower rate of digestion and absorption and a less sweet taste. Honey is also used, but has no particular advantages. There are several rules for estimating the quantity of sugar. In our clinic 1/2 ounce of sugar is added to the daily formula during the first week or so of life, and then 1 ounce until about 4 to 6 months, when it is discontinued, usually in two equal steps with an interval of a week or so. (See Table 3–14).

EXAMPLE OF FORMULA CALCULATION. The following are formulas for an infant 3 months of age weighing 11 pounds:

			KCAL*
1. Total fluid per 24 hours	(11 × 2–3)	= 28 oz	
2. Total **whole milk**	(11 × 1 3/4–2)	= 21 oz	420
3. Water	(28 − 21)	= 7 oz	
4. Carbohydrate		1 oz	120
			540

(kcal per oz = 540 ÷ 28 = 19+)
(kcal per lb = 540 ÷ 11 = 49+)

1. Total fluid per 24 hours	(11 × 2–3)	= 28 oz	
2. Total **evaporated milk**	(11 × 1)	= 11 oz	440
3. Water	(23 − 11)	= 17 oz	
4. Carbohydrate		1 oz	120
			560

(kcal per oz = 560 ÷ 28 = 20)
(kcal per lb = 560 ÷ 11 = 51)

5 bottles of 5 1/2 oz each

*kcal = large calorie = Cal (see text).

These formulas are satisfactory for an initial prescription. Subsequent adjustments of milk and water should be made in accordance with the infant's satiety and the growth curve.

TABLE 3–14 HOUSEHOLD MEASURES OF SOME COMMONLY USED SUGARS*

	TABLESPOONFULS PER OUNCE
Lactose	3
Sucrose (cane)	2
Dextrin-maltose preparations:	
Mead's Dextri-Maltose	4
Karo	2
Cartose	2
Dexin	6

*Caloric value of each is 120 calories per ounce, except Dexin, 115.

Preparation of Formula

Utensils. Several more bottles than the required number for feedings are needed for water and orange juice. Bottles should be made of heat-resistant glass, be smooth inside and marked in ounces. A wide-mouthed bottle is preferable because it is more easily cleaned, and those with adequate protection of the nipple are preferable if the baby is to be fed away from home. There should be several more nipples than the number required for feedings. Rubber caps or a plastic such as Pliofilm held in place by cardboard retainers may be used as bottle covers. The graduate should be made of heat-resistant glass and marked in ounces. A saucepan for heating and mixing the formula, a container for nipples, a glass funnel if narrow-mouthed bottles are used, a large kettle or special bottle sterilizer, a measuring spoon, a can opener, a knife, a standard tablespoon and a strainer complete the list of utensils.

CLEANSING OF UTENSILS. All utensils required for the mixing and storing of the formula should be sterilized by boiling for 5 to 10 minutes. The rubber nipples and caps should not be boiled more than 5 minutes. After each feeding the bottle and nipple should be thoroughly flushed and the bottle filled with water until washed with water and a detergent.

Method. The hands should be thoroughly scrubbed and the sterilized bottles and utensils arranged on a clean table. If whole milk is used, the bottle is shaken so that the contents are mixed, and the top is washed with hot water before the cap is removed. The water for the formula (it is necessary to allow for a slight loss in boiling) is brought to the boiling point in a saucepan; the amount of whole milk ordered is added; and the whole is boiled for 5 minutes. Constant stirring is necessary. The sugar is added while the milk is still warm.

If evaporated milk is used, the top of the can is washed with soap and hot water, rinsed with hot water, and two holes punctured in it. The water for the formula is boiled for 5 minutes, and the evaporated milk and sugar are added to it. No further boiling is necessary.

The freshly prepared and sterile formula is poured in appropriate amounts into sterilized nursing bottles. The bottles are capped by aseptic technique and stored in the refrigerator until time for the feedings.

TERMINAL HEATING. This method has practical advantages and does not require presterilization of bottles or utensils. The formula is poured into clean nursing bottles, and the nipples are applied. The nipples are then loosely covered with glass, metal or paper caps and placed in a container with a rack on the bottom and tall enough to prevent the bottles from touching the lid. The container is filled with water to about the midpoint of the bottles, covered and placed over a moderate flame. The water is allowed to boil gently for 25 minutes. The bottles are then removed with tongs and placed in a container of cold water for 10 minutes. The caps are then tightened and the bottles stored in a refrigerator.

WHOLE MILK. Whole milk or a reconstructed evaporated milk without added carbohydrate may be substituted for the formula when the infant is 4 to 6 months of age. Subsequently most infants will take 1½ pints to a quart of milk a day. There is no advantage in the ingestion of more, and there is the possible disadvantage that other essential foods may be displaced. Some of the milk may be incorporated in the cereal and in the preparation of such foods as custards, soups and sauces.

OTHER FOODS

VITAMINS. The diets of breast-fed babies should be supplemented from early in the neonatal period by vitamins C and D and possibly by vitamin A. Almost all artificial milk feedings are fortified with 400 IU of vitamin D and often with other vitamins as well. Hence, it is essential to know the vitamin content of the milk before prescribing additional vitamins for the bottle-fed baby. (See Table 3–15.)

Orange and other citrus fruit juices are natural sources of *vitamin C,* but since many young infants do not seem to tolerate them in amounts large enough to supply an adequate vitamin intake, it is preferable to give 25 to 50 mg of ascorbic acid initially. During the second month of life orange juice diluted with water may be offered; when at least 2 ounces of fresh, frozen or canned orange juice (or equivalent amounts of other sources of vitamin C) are taken daily, the ascorbic acid may be discontinued.

Vitamin D should be started early in the neonatal period with a daily intake of approximately 400 IU only if the baby is breast-fed or is taking a formula which does *not* contain vitamin D. A number of preparations are available which in recommended doses contain this amount of vitamin D, 50 mg of ascorbic acid and 3000 to 5000 IU of vitamin A. Concentrates in water-miscible vehicles are desirable to avoid aspiration of oil.

IRON. Foods rich in iron tend to be restricted in the diet of the least affluent groups in the population. The most effective way to prevent iron deficiency is to provide iron supplementation in the form of iron-fortified milk formula or medicinal iron (2 mg/kg up to a total of 15 mg/day) beginning at 6 weeks of age. It is doubtful that iron-supplemented cereals can provide sufficient supplementation for infants with reduced iron stores.

"SOLID" FOODS. The caloric contents of the various prepared baby foods differ widely. Egg yolk, cereals with added milk, meats and puddings have greater caloric density than milk, whereas vegetables and fruits have a similar or lower energy value than milk. Food selection by many mothers tends to be poorly discriminating without good advice and supervision and plays a significant role in the caloric intake of infants receiving "solid" foods, thus contributing to obesity in infancy.

Cereal is an excellent food to offer the baby who has a large appetite early in life and is not satisfied with the calories provided by his intake of milk; it will also add significant amounts of iron to the infant's diet. Fruits, especially bananas and applesauce, are usually well tolerated and may be offered first. There is little evidence that the addition of any of these foods to the normal infant's diet before 3 or 4 months of age contributes in any significant way to his well-being, although many physicians are advocating the introduction of "solid" foods at 3 to 6 weeks of age.

Any new food should be offered initially once a day in small amounts (1 to 2 teaspoonfuls). A demitasse spoon that easily fits the baby's mouth may be used. New foods are generally best accepted if fairly thin or dilute. Food is frequently pushed out rather than back by the tongue because the baby does not yet know how to swallow efficiently. This possibility should be mentioned to the mother, who might otherwise interpret the "spitting-back" of new foods as an idiosyncrasy or dislike. It is usually wise to offer the same food daily until the baby becomes accustomed to it and not to introduce new foods more often than every week or two.

The feeding at which these foods are offered is not particularly important. They should be given when the baby's hunger is no longer satisfied by milk alone and when they logically fit into the daily schedule. There is no reason for persisting with or forcing a particular food that is definitely disliked. The family's dislikes and prejudices for particular foods are contagious and should not be displayed before the infant. The physician should avoid prescribing a definite amount of a given food lest the mother interpret the suggestion too literally. *Many infants are overfed by overzealous parents who mistake acceptance of food for appetite.* The infant's appetite is the best index of the proper amount, and respect for his wishes will avoid many problems.

Cereal. The various precooked cereals on the market provide in a convenient form a variety of grains excellent for infants. Most contain iron and factors of the vitamin B complex. They are easily prepared by adding boiled milk or formula.

Fruits. Strained or puréed cooked fruits furnish minerals and some water-soluble vitamins and usually have a mildly laxative effect. Raw ripe banana is readily digested and enjoyed by most

TABLE 3–15 VITAMIN CONTENT OF NATURAL MILKS, PREPARED MILKS AND MILK SUBSTITUTES

	VITAMIN CONCENTRATION PER LITER IN NORMAL DILUTION								
	A (IU)	D (IU)	E (IU)	C (mg)	THIAMINE (μg)	NIACIN (μg)	PYRIDOXINE (μg)	PANTOTHENATE (μg)	RIBOFLAVIN (μg)
Human milk, mature, average	1898	21	6.6	43	160	1470	100	1840	360
Cow's milk, market, average	1025	13	1.0	11	440	940	640	3460	1750
Cow's milk, evaporated, many brands	1850	420	1.3	5.5	280	1000	370	3500	1900
Cow's milk, powdered:									
Klim, Borden	1850	423	–	1.9	380	1300	–	–	1900
Commercial premodified milks:									
Infant Formula, Baker	1782	423	–	35	446	7400	297		1102
Bremil with Iron, Borden	2640	423	5.3	53	420	6340	420	–	1060
Bremil Powder, with Iron, Borden	2640	423	5.3	53	420	6340	420		1060
Modilac, Gerber	1585	423	–	48	528	5300	740		740
Enfamil, Mead	1586	423	–	53	423	4200	317	2100	1000
Olac, Mead	2643	423	–	tr.	–	–	–	–	–
Similac with Iron, Ross	2640	423	5	53	700	6000	240	2000	1100
Similac Powder with Iron, Ross	2640	423	5	53	700	6000	220	2000	1100
Similac PM 60/40, Ross	2640	423	5	53	700	5300	220	–	1100
SMA S-26, Wyeth	2650	423	8.5	53	710	5300	420	2100	1100
Goat's milk, Powdered:									
Dale's, Cutter		–	–	14	480	2700	70	2900	1140
High protein, low fat powdered milks:									
Dryco, Borden	2640	423	–		500	220			2000
Alacta, Mead		–	3.7						230
Probana, Mead	5285	1057	11	–	–	–	–	–	–
Protein Milk, Mead	–	–	–	–	–	–	–	–	–
Skim milk, many brands	–	None	4.8	–	360	1060	450	3880	1890
Hypoallergenic milk substitutes:									
Mullsoy Liquid, Borden (Soya)	2100	423	10.6	42	530	9500	420	1000	845
Mullsoy Powder, Borden (Soya)	–	None	4		80	3500	235	1000	260
Neo-Mullsoy, Borden (Soya)	2110	423	10.6	53	530	7390	420	2640	1060
Nursoy, Wyeth	2500	400	9	58	700	10000	400	3000	1000
Lambase, Gerber	1585	423	5.3	48	420	5300	630		1050
Meat-Base, Gerber	1585	423	5.3	42	420	10600	507		1370
Soyalac Liquid, Loma Linda (Soya)	1584	423	5	32	422	6000	422	–	634
Soyalac Powder, Loma Linda (Soya)	1584	423	5	32	422	6000	422	–	634
Nutramigen, Powder, Mead	1586	423	5.3	32	486	4200	529	3400	1903
Pro-Sobee, Mead (Soya)	1586	423	5	53	530	7400	427	2600	1057
Sobee, Mead (Soya)	1586	423	5	53	530	7400	427	2600	1057
Isomil, Ross (Soya)	1500	423	5	50	600	6000	400	5000	600
Milk substitutes, specialty products									
Cho-free Formula Base, Borden	2110	423	10.6	53	530	7390	420	2640	1060
Flexical, Mead	2500	200	15	50	700	9000	1000	5000	850
Jejunal Beverage, Johnson and Johnson	2500	200	15	30	700	9000	1000	5000	850
Jejunal Broth, Johnson and Johnson	2500	200	15	30	700	9000	1000	5000	850
Lofenalac, Mead	1586	423	5.3	32	486	4200	529	3400	
Lonalac, Mead	1015	–	–	–	423	900	–	–	1800
Portagen, Mead	3540	284	7	57	850	1140	830	7100	1135
Pregestimil, Mead	2000	400	10	52	600	8000	500	3000	1000
Vivonex Standard, Eaton	2778	223	17	39	667	7222	1111	5555	666
Vivonex HN, Eaton	1666	133	10	23	389	4444	667	3333	389
W-T Low Residue, Warren-Teed	2778	223	17	39	778	11111	1111	5555	944
W-T Peptide L4, Warren-Teed	2778	223	17	33	833	11111	1111	5555	944
W-T Protein L4, Warren-Teed	2778	223	17	33	833	11111	1111	5555	944
Similac Advance, Ross	3000	400	6.25	50	750	10000	700	5000	900

babies. It should be mashed with a fork. Many infants who are slow in accepting new foods seem to prefer fruits.

Vegetables. The various "colored" vegetables are moderately good sources of iron and other minerals and of the vitamins of the B complex. They may be freshly cooked and strained, but many mothers prefer the commercially prepared vegetables because of their convenience. "Colored" vegetables are usually added to the infant's diet by about 4 months of age.

Meats, Eggs and Starchy Foods. Eggs and starchy foods are usually introduced during the second 6 months of life, although some physicians offer egg yolk at an earlier age. The yolk of the egg is used initially and is preferably hard-cooked and then added to cereal or other food. As with all new foods, a small amount (pea-sized) is offered at first, with gradual increases up to a whole yolk 2 or 3 times a week. Egg white should be introduced with equal caution to minimize any possible allergic manifestations.

Potatoes, rice, spaghetti, bread and similar starchy foods have principally a caloric value. As a rule, they are not included in the infant's diet until the more essential foods mentioned above are being taken regularly. Baked potato, mashed with milk and butter, is a favorite. Zwieback, toast or graham crackers may be offered to the infant when he shows an interest in "gumming" on coarser foods (usually 6 to 8 months of age). It is with such foods that he learns to chew and to feed himself.

Meat is an excellent source of protein as well as of iron and vitamins. Ground fresh beef or liver or the strained canned meats may be used initially by about 4 months of age. Meats may be more readily accepted when mixed with another food.

The commercial "soups" and meat and vegetable mixtures are relatively high in carbohydrate and are not considered optimal sources of iron or protein. Many home-prepared soups are bulky out of proportion to their food value, and much of the vitamin content is lost by overcooking.

Desserts. Puddings, junkets and custards are good foods for older infants, particularly if they temporarily prefer milk in that form. If, however, such foods are given as a bribe or reward or only after other foods have been finished, poor eating habits are apt to be established. Sweet foods should be offered as casually as the rest of the meal and at any place in the meal that the child desires.

SALT INTAKE. To increase their palatability, particularly for the parent, salt has been added to commercially prepared baby foods; soups, cereals, meats, and meat with vegetable mixtures have contained unexpectedly large amounts of salt. In 1966 Puyau calculated the sodium intake of 11- to 13-month-old infants to be approximately 60 mEq per day, equivalent to a daily salt intake of 20 or more gm in the adult. Fortunately, the practice of adding salt and other additives has been modified by the processors, so that the salt content of commercial baby foods is now much lower. The significance of large intakes of sodium, which are in the ranges seen in populations with a high incidence of hypertension, is not clear, but the possibility that they might contribute to the development of hypertension later in life cannot be ignored.

FOOD ADDITIVES. Both naturally occurring chemicals and food additives, particularly the artificial flavors and colors, have been implicated in the health and behavior of man. It has been estimated that more than 3000 flavors are currently being used, and few children are spared exposure to many of them in their daily diet. Artificial flavors and colors have been associated with respiratory allergic disorders, with urticaria and angioedema, with lesions of tongue and buccal mucosa, with digestive disturbances, with arthralgia and hydrarthroses and with headache and behavioral disturbances, including hyperkinesis in childhood. Many of the additives contain salicylates or tartrazine radicals, substances which have been associated with restlessness and hyperactivity of the degree seen in schoolchildren with learning difficulty. Salicylate-free diets should exclude foods and products which contain artificial flavors and colors.

FIRST-YEAR FEEDING PROBLEMS

UNDERFEEDING. Underfeeding is suggested by restlessness and crying, and by failure to gain weight adequately in spite of complete emptying of the breast or bottle. Underfeeding may also result from the infant's failure to take a sufficient quantity of food even when offered. In these instances the frequency of feedings, the mechanics of nursing, the size of the holes in the nipple, the adequacy of eructation of air, and the possibility of systemic disease in the baby should be investigated. The extent and duration of underfeeding determine the clinical manifestations. Constipation, failure to sleep, irritability and excessive crying are to be expected. There may be poor gain in weight or an actual loss. In the last instance the skin becomes dry and wrinkled, subcutaneous tissue disappears, and the infant assumes the appearance of an "old man." Deficiencies of vitamins A, B, C and D and of iron and protein may be responsible for characteristic clinical manifestations.

Treatment consists in increasing the fluid and caloric intake, correcting deficiencies in vitamin and mineral intake, and instructing the mother in the art of infant feeding. The physician should anticipate the possibility that some infants will fail to thrive despite the institution of all the recognized corrective measures. In such instances careful clinical search is indicated to determine whether some underlying disorder is responsible for the failure to thrive.

OVERFEEDING. Overfeeding may be quantitative or qualitative. Regurgitation and vomiting are frequent symptoms of overfeeding. As a rule, infants can be depended upon not to take excessive quantities; but occasionally an infant who has postprandial discomfort from eating too much may nonetheless gain weight excessively. Diets too high in fat delay gastric emptying, cause distention and abdominal discomfort and may cause excessive gain in weight. Diets too high in carbohydrate are likely to cause undue fermentation in the intestine, resulting in distention and flatulence and in too rapid gain in weight. Such diets may be deficient in essential protein, vitamins and minerals. Formulas too high in caloric content in the first week or two of life are likely to result in loose or diarrheal stools. Obesity is undesirable at any time in life; all too frequently the excessively fed infant becomes the obese child and adult.

REGURGITATION AND VOMITING. The return of of small amounts of swallowed food during or shortly after eating is termed "regurgitation" or "spitting up." More complete emptying of the stomach, especially when it occurs some time after feeding, is termed "vomiting." Within limits, regurgitation is a natural occurrence, especially during the first half-year or so of life. It can be reduced to a negligible amount, however, by adequate eructation of swallowed air during and after eating, by gentle handling, by avoidance of emotional conflicts and by placing the infant on his right side or abdomen for a nap immediately after eating. One should also ensure that the head is not lower than the rest of the body during the rest period.

Vomiting is one of the most common symptoms in infancy and may be associated with a wide variety of disturbances, both trivial and serious. Its cause should always be investigated. (See Section 11.)

LOOSE OR DIARRHEAL STOOLS. Acute infectious diarrhea and chronic diarrheal conditions are discussed elsewhere; only milk disturbances of dietary origin will be considered here.

The stool of the breast-fed infant is naturally softer than that of the infant fed cow's milk. From about the fourth to the sixth day of life the stools go through a transitional stage in which they are rather loose and greenish yellow and contain mucus; within a few days the typical "milk stool" appears. Subsequently the use of laxatives or the ingestion of certain foods by the mother may be temporarily responsible for an infant's loose stools. Excessive intake of breast milk may also increase the frequency and the water content of the stool. Actual diarrhea in a breast-fed infant is unusual and should be considered infectious until proved otherwise.

Though the stools of artificially fed infants tend to be firmer than those of breast-fed infants, under certain circumstances loose stools may result from artificial feeding. In the first 2 weeks or so of life, overfeeding is likely to cause loose, frequent stools. Later, formulas which are too concentrated or whose sugar content is too high, especially in lactose, may be responsible for loose, frequent stools. Many of the temporary diarrheal disturbances in artificially fed infants are the result of contaminations of food which would not disturb an older child and are not serious enough to cause prolonged difficulty for the infant. The ease with which artificially fed infants acquire diarrheal disturbances and the potential seriousness of them are strong arguments for extreme care in providing a food supply free of pathogenic bacteria.

Mild diarrheal disturbances due to overfeeding respond quickly to temporary decrease or cessation of feeding. The withholding of all solid food and of one or several milk feedings, with the substitution of boiled water or 5 per cent glucose in water or in a balanced electrolyte solution, is usually all that is required.

CONSTIPATION. (See also Section 11.) Constipation is practically unknown in breast-fed infants who receive an adequate amount of milk, and is rare in artificially fed infants receiving an adequate diet. The nature of the stool, and not its frequency, is the criterion of constipation. Although most infants have one or more stools daily, an occasional infant will have a stool of normal consistency only at intervals of 36 to 48 hours. Whenever constipation or obstipation is present from birth or shortly thereafter, a rectal examination should be performed. Tight or spastic anal sphincters may occasionally be responsible for obstipation, and correction usually follows finger dilatation performed daily. Anal fissures or cracks may also cause constipation. If irritation is removed, healing usually occurs quickly. Aganglionic megacolon may be manifest by constipation in early infancy; the absence of stool in the rectum on digital examination suggests this possibility.

Constipation in the artificially fed infant may be due to an insufficient amount of food or fluid. In other instances it may result from diets too high in fat or protein or deficient in bulk. Simply increasing the amount of fluid or sugar in the formula may be corrective in the first few months of life. After this age better results are obtained by adding or increasing the amounts of cereal, vegetables and fruits. Prune juice (1/2 to 1 ounce) may be given as a temporary measure, but it is better to add foods with some bulk. Enemas and suppositories should never be more than temporary measures. Milk of magnesia may be given in doses of 1 or 2 teaspoonfuls, but should be reserved for unresponsive or severe constipation.

COLIC. The term "colic" describes a frequent symptom complex of paroxysmal abdominal pain, presumably of intestinal origin, and of severe crying. It usually occurs in infants under 3 months of age.

The clinical pattern is characteristic. The attack usually begins suddenly; the cry is loud and more or less continuous; so-called paroxysms may persist for several hours; the face may be flushed, or there may be circumoral pallor; the abdomen is distended and tense; the legs are drawn up on the abdomen, though they may be momentarily extended; the feet are often cold; the hands are clenched. The attack may terminate only when the infant is completely exhausted, but often there is relief with the passage of feces or flatus.

Certain infants seem to be peculiarly susceptible to colic. The cause of recurrent attacks is usually not apparent, though they may be associated with hunger and with swallowed air which has passed into the intestine. Overfeeding may also cause discomfort and distention, but rarely to the degree seen in colic. Certain foods, especially those of high carbohydrate content, may be responsible for excessive fermentation in the intestines, but only occasionally does a change in diet prevent further attacks of colic. Crying from intestinal discomfort is seen in infants with intestinal allergy, but colic is not limited to this group. Intestinal obstruction or peritoneal infection may mimic an attack of colic. Recurrent attacks commonly occur late in the afternoon or evening, suggesting that events in the household routine may serve as possible causes. Worry, fear, anger or excitement may cause vomiting in an older child, and may result in colic in an infant. Certainly no single causative factor consistently accounts for colic, nor does any method of treatment consistently provide satisfactory relief.

Holding the baby upright or permitting him to lie prone across the lap or on a hot water bottle or heating pad is occasionally helpful. Passage of flatus or fecal material spontaneously or with expulsion of a suppository or enema sometimes affords relief. Carminatives before feedings are ineffective in preventing the attacks. Sedation is occasionally indicated for a prolonged attack, and sometimes may be given to parent or child for a period of time if other measures fail. Temporary hospitalization of the infant, often without resorting to more than a change in the infant's feeding routine and providing a period of rest for his mother, may be helpful in extreme cases. The prevention of attacks should be sought through adequate feeding techniques, including burping, the provision of a stable emotional environment, identification of possibly allergenic foods in the infant's or nursing mother's diet and avoidance of underfeeding. The condition rarely persists after 3 months of age.

FEEDING DURING THE SECOND YEAR OF LIFE

Most infants naturally adapt themselves to a schedule of three meals a day by about the end of the first year of life. Though considerable latitude in the diet of the individual infant must be permitted to allow for personal idiosyncrasies and family habits, the mother should be given an outline of the daily basic dietary needs.

REDUCED CALORIC INTAKE. Toward the end of the first year of life and during the second year, owing to the constantly decelerating rate of growth, there is a gradual reduction in the infant's caloric intake per unit of body weight. In addition, it is not unusual for him to have temporary periods of disinterest in food in general or in certain articles of it. Failure to recognize these features, especially the decreasing caloric needs, results in attempts to force feeding. The natural reaction of the child is rebellion, and feeding problems ensue. Prevention is much more effective than are methods of correction, and the changing pattern of the infant's food habits during the second year of life should be explained to the mother before its appearance.

SELF-SELECTION OF DIET. Though a great variety of foods is not possible at each meal, strong likes or dislikes of children for particular foods should be respected. Spinach is an example of a nonessential food whose virtues have been overemphasized, conceivably to the point of causing feeding difficulties. When rejected foods consistently include such basic dietary staples as milk and eggs, the possibility of food allergy should be given consideration.

Children, including infants, tend to select diets which over a period of several days assume a balanced nature. Thus, the child may be permitted a rather wide choice of foods without concern so long as the eating performance is adequate over the longer period. Under normal circumstances the child should determine the quantity to be eaten with respect to both a given food and to the entire meal. At this age the development of his eating habits may be strongly influenced by older children in the family, particularly in respect to food likes and dislikes. Eating patterns and habits developed in the first 2 years of life are likely to persist for several years.

SELF-FEEDING BY INFANTS. Before the infant is a year of age he should be permitted to participate in the act of feeding himself. By 6 months or so he can hold his bottle. Within another 2 or 3 months he can hold a cup. The introduction of zwieback, graham crackers and bacon by the time he is 7 to 8 months of age gives the infant something which he can hold and thus learn one of the principles of self-feeding. He may use a spoon for feeding himself as soon as he can hold and direct it to his mouth, possibly by 10 to 12 months of age. Mothers often inhibit this learning process because of their objection to the messiness incident to the learning of adequate control.

Acquisition of the ability to feed himself is an important step in the infant's development of self-reliance and of a sense of responsibility. By the end of the second year of life the infant should be largely responsible for his own feeding.

The practice of permitting infants and children to go to sleep while holding and sucking intermittently from a bottle of formula, whole milk, sweetened fruit juice or water should be discouraged. Pedodontists have called attention to the correlation of this habit with enamel erosion in deciduous teeth, terming it "the baby bottle syndrome." Bacterial action upon dissolved carbohydrate provides increased formation of lactic and other acids which are harmful to dental enamel, especially that of the young child.

In comparison with the supervision commonly maintained over the feeding of infants, the diets of children beyond the age of 2 years are badly neglected. Though it is desirable that children should not be aware of constant supervision of their dietary habits and that they should be given every opportunity to form eating habits naturally, the diets of all children should be supervised. Surveys of dietary habits of children in various economic groups reveal a high incidence of inadequate diets and of malnutrition. Although the nutritional requirements per unit of body weight are constantly decreasing with increasing age (110 kcal/kg in infancy; 50 kcal/kg at 15 years), at all times the need for calories as well as for protein, vitamins and minerals is relatively greater than it is in the adult.

DAILY BASIC DIET. Parents should be given a daily basic diet for the child from which the family menu can be prepared. The quantity of the intake after the basic requirements have been met can in most instances be determined by the healthy growing child; the obese child is an exception. A history of the dietary habits of the child is essential for evaluation of his nutritive intake, but such histories are often unreliable unless an accurate dietary diary is kept for several days. From such information, corrections in the diet may be made more effectively. The recommended daily dietary intake is shown in Table 3–8.

Adequate quantities of all the essential classes of foods must be provided in order to avoid specific nutritional deficiencies. The child should know the content of a basic diet and its importance to proper growth and good health, but this information should never be presented as a threat to enforce rigid feeding practices.

The following is a daily menu which will provide all the essential nutrients:

Breakfast: Citrus fruit or tomato juice
Cereal—whole grain or enriched
Egg
Whole-wheat toast
Butter
Milk

Lunch: Sandwich with whole-wheat bread or
Casserole dish—containing meat or meat substitute and starchy vegetable
Green vegetable, raw
Milk
Custard, pudding, cake, ice cream or gelatin dessert

Dinner: Meat—fish—liver
Potatoes, rice or spaghetti
Green vegetable
Whole-wheat bread, butter
Milk
Fruit

Vitamin D (throughout childhood)

EATING HABITS. As stated previously, eating habits formed in the first year or two of life have a distinct effect upon those of subsequent years. Feeding difficulties between the ages of 2 and 5 years frequently result from excessive parental insistence on eating, with excessive anxiety when the child does not conform to some arbitrary standard. Negativistic reactions by the child are natural consequences of undue stress at mealtime, and correction requires improvement in parent-child relations. Other factors which disturb eating are too much confusion at mealtime, insufficient time for eating, either on the part of the adult or of the child, food dislikes of other members of the family, and poorly prepared and unattractively served food. A comfortable chair of proper height with a foot-rest is important for a child's ease at the table.

It is good practice to call the child from play 15 to 20 minutes before mealtimes, allowing time for going to the toilet and washing the hands and face and cooling off from strenuous activity. This is an excellent time, especially for younger children, to spend with the father, reading or playing quiet games. Mealtimes should be happy. Discussion about the food, except for occasional favorable comments, should be avoided, and the conversation should be on subjects of interest to the entire family. The child should feel that he is part of the family group. The child's appetite should be respected; if his desire for food at times is below average, there should be no persuasion to eat more. Adults should realize that eating habits are taught better by example than by formal explanation.

LUNCHES BETWEEN MEALS. During the second year and even for several years thereafter, orange juice or other fruit juice or fruit together with a cracker may be given in either or both of the midmeal periods. For older children midmeal nourishment should be avoided if it reduces the appetite for the following meal. When a snack after school results in greater enthusiasm and energy for play and does not reduce the appetite for the evening meal, it should be encouraged. Fruits are especially recommended for such lunches.

There are differences of opinion about midsession lunches in school. In general they are just as well omitted, but when a session is relatively long, fruit juice may be advantageous, especially for the younger child.

WILLIAM E. LAUPUS

Aldrich, C. A.: Ancient processes in scientific age; Feeding aspects. Am. J. Dis. Child. *64*:714, 1942.

Applebaum, R. M.: The modern management of successful breast feeding. Pediat. Clin. N. Am. *17*:203, 1970.

Call, J. D.: Emotional factors favoring successful breast feeding of infants. J. Pediatr. *55*:485, 1959.

Committee on Nutrition, American Academy of Pediatrics: Composition of milks. Pediatrics *26*:1039, 1960.

Committee on Nutrition, American Academy of Pediatrics: Proposed changes in food and drug administration regulations concerning formula products and vitamin-mineral supplements for infants. Pediatrics *40*:916, 1967.

Feingold, B. F.: Food additives and child development. Hosp. Prac. (No. 10)*8*:11, 1973.

Fomon, S. J., Thomas, L. N., Filer, L. J., Jr., Anderson, T. A., and Bergman, K. E.: Requirements for protein and essential amino acids in early infancy. Acta Paediat. Scand. *62*:33, 1973.

Fomon, S. J.: Comparative study of protein from human milk and cow's milk in promoting nitrogen retention by normal full-term infants. Pediatrics *26*:51, 1960.

Fomon, S. J.: Body composition of the male reference infant. Pediatrics *40*:863, 1967.

Fomon, S. J.: Infant Nutrition. Philadelphia, W. B. Saunders Company, 1967.

Gartner, L. M., and Arias, I. M.: Studies of prolonged neonatal jaundice in the breast-fed infant. J. Pediatr. *68*:54, 1966.

Gordon, H. H., and Ganzon, A. F.: On the protein allowances for young infants. J. Pediatr. *54*:503, 1959.

Holt, L. E., Jr.: The protein requirement of infants. J. Pediatr. *54*:496, 1959.

Holt, L. E., Jr., and Snyderman, S. E.: The amino acid requirements of infants. J.A.M.A. *175*:100, 1961.

Hytten, F. E., and Thomson, A. M.: Clinical and chemical studies in human lactation. X. The maintenance of breast feeding. Brit. M. J. *2*:232, 1955.

Jelliffe, D. B., and Jelliffe E. F. P. (eds.): The uniqueness of human milk. Am. J. Clin. Nutr. *24*:463, 1971.

Kagan, B. M., Stanincova, V., Felix, N. S., Hodeman, J., and Kalman, K.: Body composition of premature infants: Relation to nutrition. Am. J. Clin. Nutr. *25*:1153, 1973.

La Leche League International: The Womanly Art of Breast Feeding. Interstate Printers and Publishers, Inc., 1963. Available through La Leche League International, Inc., 9616 Minneapolis Ave., Franklin Park, Illinois 60131.

Macy, I. G., Kelly, H. J., and Sloan, R. E.: The Composition of Milks. A Compilation of the Comparative Composition and Properties of Human, Cow and Goat Milk, Colostrum and Transitional Milk. Washington, D.C., Publication 254, National Academy of Science—National Research Council, 1953.

Newton, M.: Mammary effects. Am. J. Clin. Nutr. *24*:987, 1971.

Newton, M., and Newton, N.: The normal course and management of lactation. Clin. Obstet. Gynec. *5*:44, 1962.

Newton, N., and Newton, M.: Psychologic aspects of lactation. New Engl. J. Med. *277*:1179, 1967.

Omans, W. B., Barness, L. A., Rose, C. S., and Gyorgy, P.: Prolonged feeding studies in premature infants. J. Pediatr. *59*:951, 1961.

Powers, G. F.: Infant feeding: Historical background and modern practice. J.A.M.A. *105*:753, 1935.

Puyau, F. A., and Hampton, L. P.: Infant feeding practices, 1966. Salt content of the modern diet. Am. J. Dis. Child. *111*:370, 1966.

Spock, B.: Baby and Child Care. New York, Pocket Books, Inc., 1962.

Sutherland, J. M., Glueck, H. I., and Gleser, G.: Hemorrhagic disease of the newborn: Breast feeding as a necessary factor in the pathogenesis. Am. J. Dis. Child. *113*:524, 1967.

Von Sydow, G.: Study of development of rickets in premature infants. Acta Paediat. Scand. *33* (Suppl. 2.):3, 1946.

Woodruff, C. W.: Protein requirements of full-term infants. J.A.M.A. *175*:114, 1961.

NUTRITIONAL DISORDERS

MALNUTRITION

Malnutrition may be due to improper or inadequate food intake or may result from inadequate absorption of food. Deficient supply of food, poor dietary habits, food faddism and emotional factors may limit intake. Certain metabolic abnormalities may also cause malnutrition. Requirements for essential nutrients may be increased during stress and disease and during the administration of antibiotics or of catabolic or anabolic drugs. Malnutrition may be acute or chronic, reversible or irreversible.

Precise evaluation of nutritional status is difficult. Severe disturbances are readily apparent, but mild disturbances may be overlooked, even after careful physical and laboratory examinations. The diagnosis of malnutrition rests on an accurate dietary history, upon evaluation of present deviations from average height and weight and of past rates of growth in height and weight or of certain organs, and upon evidence of specific clinical deficiencies. Deficiencies of some nutrients may be revealed by low blood levels of them or their metabolites, by observing biochemical or clinical effects of administration of the nutrient or its products, or by giving the patient substantial amounts of appropriate nutrients and noting the rate at which they are excreted.

The most acute nutritional disturbances are those which involve water and electrolytes, especially sodium, potassium, chloride and hydrogen ions. These are discussed in Section 5. The more chronic conditions, involving deficits of calories, proteins and vitamins, are discussed here. Clinical malnutrition usually involves deficits of more than a single nutrient.

MARASMUS

(Infantile Atrophy; Inanition; Athrepsia)

Severe malnutrition in infants is common in areas with insufficient food, inadequate knowledge of feeding techniques or poor hygiene. The synonyms listed above have been applied to patterns of clinical illness emphasizing one or more features of protein and calorie deficiency.

ETIOLOGY. The clinical picture of marasmus is due to general starvation. It stems from an inadequate caloric intake due to insufficiency of the diet, to improper feeding habits such as those of disturbed parent-child relations, or to metabolic abnormalities or congenital malformations. Severe impairment of any body system may result in malnutrition.

CLINICAL MANIFESTATIONS. In marasmus there is failure to gain weight, followed by loss of weight until emaciation results, with loss of turgor in skin and subcutaneous tissue; the skin becomes wrinkled and loose as subcutaneous fat disappears. Because fat is lost last from the sucking pads of the cheeks, the face may retain a relatively normal appearance for some time before becoming shrunken and wizened. The abdomen may be distended or thin. The intestinal pattern becomes readily visible. Atrophy of muscles occurs, with resultant hypotonia. Edema may be present.

The temperature is usually subnormal, the pulse may be slow, and the basal metabolic rate tends to be reduced. At first the infant may be fretful, but later he becomes listless and his appetite diminishes. The infant is usually constipated, but the so-called starvation type of diarrhea may appear, with frequent, small stools containing mucus. Terminally, frank diarrhea is common.

PROTEIN MALNUTRITION

(Hypoproteinemia; Kwashiorkor; Third-degree Malnutrition [Gómez]; Plundeficiency Syndrome)

During the period of growth enough nitrogenous food must be consumed to maintain a positive nitrogen balance, whereas adults need only maintain nitrogen equilibrium. Not all protein is equally efficient in the maintenance of nitrogen equilibrium or in the establishment of nitrogen retention. When the diet does not contain adequate amounts of the essential amino acids, nitrogen equilibrium is not maintained, irrespective of the total quantity of protein in the diet. Adequate caloric intake as carbohydrate or fat helps to minimize protein requirements.

Adequate intake and metabolism of protein serve multiple functions. Among these are the maintenance of levels of serum protein, particularly of serum albumin, the formation of globin for heme, the production of enzymes and hormones, and the preservation of cellular structure and integrity. Measurable effects on serum proteins, hemoglobin and body chemical processes occur only after prolonged malnutrition. Attempts to detect early chemical evidence of protein malnutrition have been inconclusive; they have included examination of levels of essential as compared to nonessential amino acids in the serum, study of hydroxyproline excretion, measurement of serum transferrin, examination of defective hair formation and other tests.

ETIOLOGY. Protein malnutrition may follow deprivation of sufficient quantity or quality of protein foods. It may also be due to impaired absorption of protein, as in chronic diarrheal states. Abnormal losses of protein in proteinuria (nephrosis), infection, hemorrhage or burns, or failure of protein synthesis, as in chronic liver disease, may also result in protein malnutrition.

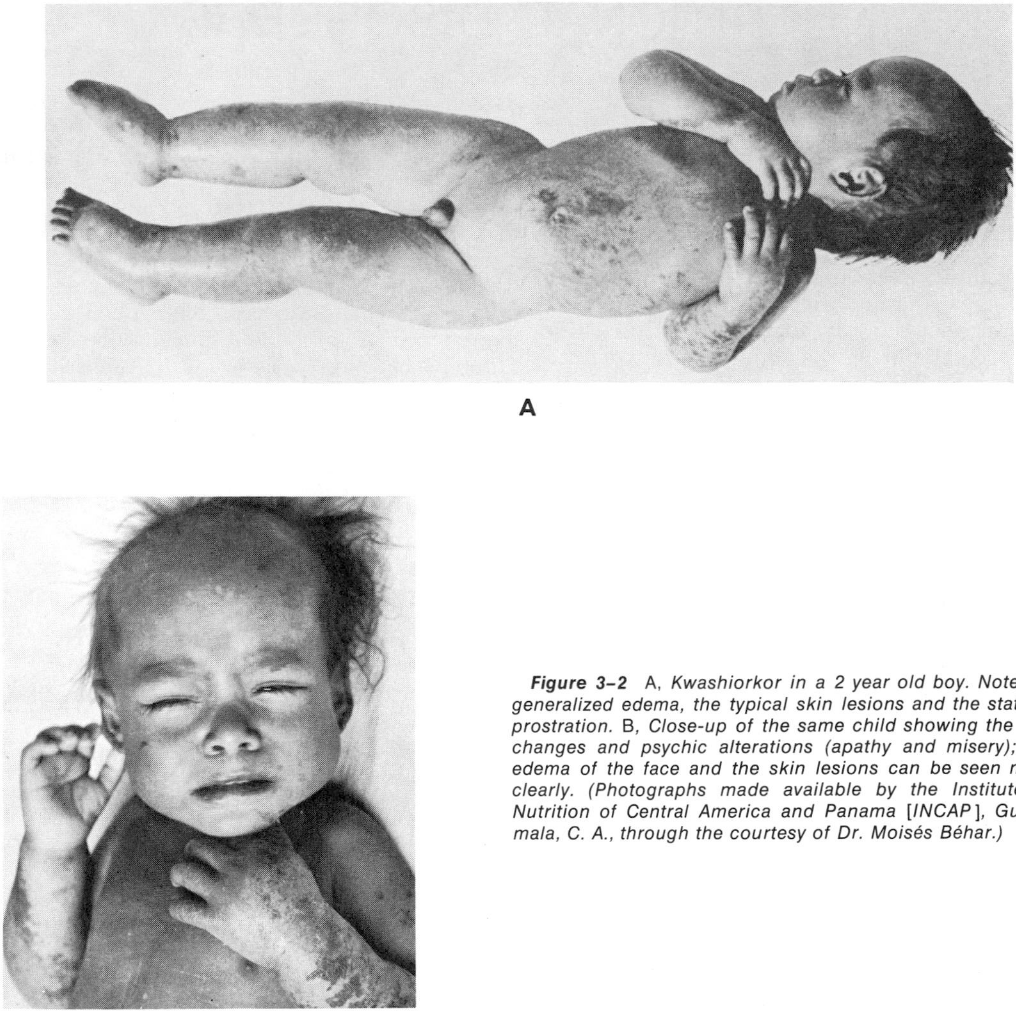

A

B

Figure 3–2 A, *Kwashiorkor in a 2 year old boy. Note the generalized edema, the typical skin lesions and the state of prostration.* B, *Close-up of the same child showing the hair changes and psychic alterations (apathy and misery); the edema of the face and the skin lesions can be seen more clearly. (Photographs made available by the Institute of Nutrition of Central America and Panama [INCAP], Guatemala, C. A., through the courtesy of Dr. Moisés Béhar.)*

Kwashiorkor is a clinical syndrome which results from a severe deficiency of protein with adequate or almost adequate caloric intake. It is the most serious and prevalent form of malnutrition in the world today, especially in technically undeveloped areas. Although deficiencies of calories and other nutrients may complicate the clinical and chemical patterns, the principal symptoms are due to deficiency of protein of good biologic value.

Kwashiorkor refers to the "deposed child," i.e., the child who is no longer suckled; it occurs in children from 4 months to 5 years of age. In areas where kwashiorkor is common the height and weight curves of infants and young children after weaning are below those of children of similar ages in areas where good nutrition is available. Although gains in height and weight are accelerated with treatment, these attainments never equal those of consistently well nourished children.

CLINICAL MANIFESTATIONS. Early clinical evidence of protein malnutrition is vague and includes lethargy, apathy, or irritability. When well advanced it results in inadequate growth, lack of stamina, loss of muscular tissue, increased susceptibility to infections, and edema.

The infant may develop anorexia, flabbiness of subcutaneous tissues, and loss of muscle tone. Enlarged liver may be an early or late sign. Edema usually develops early, not necessarily in those receiving the poorest basic diet, but more often in those in whom an added stress has occurred. Infection constitutes the most important added stress, and diarrhea may occur shortly before the onset of edema. Ascites and pleural effusions are unusual. Failure to gain weight may be masked by edema, which is often present in internal organs before it can be recognized in the face and limbs. Renal plasma flow, glomerular filtration rate, and renal tubular function are decreased.

Dermatitis is common. Darkening of the skin appears in areas of irritation, but not in those exposed to sunlight, in contrast to the situation in pellagra. Dyspigmentation may occur in these areas after desquamation; vitiligo may occur elsewhere. The hair is often sparse and thin and loses

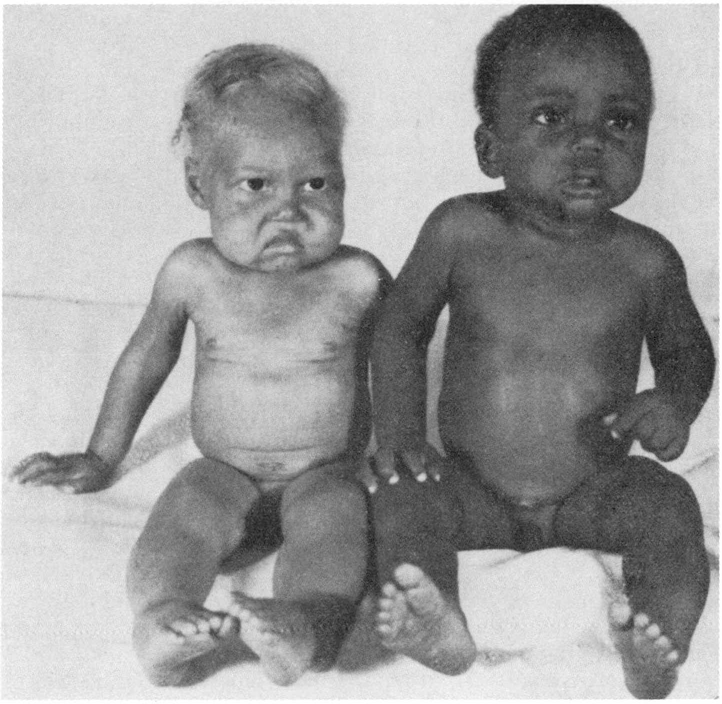

Figure 3–3 Jamaican infants of predominantly African stock. Left, *Infant with "sugar-baby" kwashiorkor, showing stunting, edema of feet and hands, hepatomegaly with fatty infiltration, moon face, misery and extreme dyspigmentation of the hair (hypochromotrichia) and of the skin generally.* Right, *Normal infant of same racial group. (N.B. The hypochromotrichia here is one of the most extreme examples seen in Jamaica.) (From D. B. Jelliffe: Hypochromotrichia and malnutrition in Jamaican infants. J. Trop. Pediat., Vol. 1.)*

its elasticity. In dark-haired children, dyspigmentation may result in a streaky red or gray color of the hair. Hair texture becomes coarse in chronic disease.

Infections and parasitic infestations are common, as are anorexia, vomiting, and continued diarrhea. The muscles are weak, thin, and atrophic, but there may be an excess of subcutaneous fat. Mental changes, especially irritability and apathy, are common. Stupor, coma, and death may follow.

Liver enlargement is common; biopsy usually reveals fatty infiltration. Necrosis or fibrosis may occur, but cirrhosis is rare. The heart may be small in the early stages of the disease, but is usually enlarged later.

LABORATORY DATA. The most significant index of protein malnutrition is the lowering of the serum albumin level. In early stages the albumin level may be only slightly reduced; severe lowering of the albumin concentration is one of the factors responsible for nutritional edema.

Ketonuria is common in the early stage of inanition, but frequently disappears in the later stages. Blood glucose is low. Glucose tolerance curves may be diabetic in type. Urinary excretion of hydroxyproline relative to creatinine may be decreased. Levels of essential amino acids in plasma may be decreased relative to unessential amino acids, and there may be increased aminoaciduria. Potassium and magnesium deficiencies are frequently present. The serum cholesterol level is low; it returns to normal after a few days of treatment. The serum values of amylase, esterase, cholinesterase, transaminase, lipase and alkaline phosphatase are decreased. There is diminished activity of the pancreatic enzymes and of xanthine oxidase. Enzyme values return to normal shortly after the onset of treatment. Anemia may be normocytic, microcytic or macrocytic. Other deficiencies, as of vitamins and minerals, are usually evident. In addition to general slowing of development, bone growth is usually delayed. Growth hormone secretion may be increased.

DIFFERENTIAL DIAGNOSIS. Differential diagnosis of protein deprivation includes chronic infections, diseases in which there is an excessive loss of protein through urine or stools, and conditions with a metabolic inability to make protein.

PREVENTION. This requires a diet containing an adequate quantity of protein of good biologic quality. Since kwashiorkor has not only a serious and often fatal course, but often permanent and devastating aftereffects in recovered children and their offspring, adequate dietary instruction and food distribution are urgently needed in endemic areas.

TREATMENT. Treatment of kwashiorkor requires immediate management of any acute problems presented by diarrhea or shock (see Section 5 for their management) and ultimately the replacement of missing nutrients. Shock should be treated as an emergency; renal function must be re-established. Gradual increases in the dietary intake of calories and protein should follow. Skim milk, casein hydrolysates or synthetic amino acid mixtures may be used. When high calorie and high protein diets are given too early and rapidly, the liver may become enlarged, and the child improves slowly. Protein hydrolysates, when used alone, may result in hypoglycemia. Vegetable fat is better absorbed than cow's milk fat. Disaccharidase levels are low in intestinal biopsies; lactose particularly should be limited in early treatment. Impaired glucose tolerance has been improved in some affected children by the administration of 250 μg of chromium chloride. Vitamins and minerals, especially vitamin A, potassium, and magnesium, are necessary from the outset of treatment. Iron and folic acid usually correct the anemia.

Infections must be treated concomitantly with the dietary therapy, whereas treatment of parasitic infestation, if not severe, may be postponed until recovery is under way.

After treatment has been initiated the patient may lose weight for a few weeks, owing to loss of edema. Weight loss may occur even when edema was not previously obvious and will reflect inapparent edema or unusual distribution of water within body fluid compartments. During recovery, serum and intestinal enzymes return to normal, and intestinal absorption of fat and protein improves.

If impairment of growth and development has been extensive, mental and physical retardation may be permanent. Apparently the younger the infant at the time of deprivation, the more devastating are the long-term effects. Deficits in perceptual and abstract abilities are especially long-lasting.

MALNUTRITION IN CHILDREN BEYOND INFANCY

ETIOLOGY. Malnutrition in older infants and children may be a continuation of an undernourished state begun in infancy, or it may stem from factors which become operative during childhood. In general, the causes are the same as those responsible for malnutrition in infants. The problem may be complex. Poor dietary habits may be associated with a generally poor hygienic situation, with chronic disease, with finical eating habits of other members of the family, or with disturbed parent-child relations, especially with overanxiety about eating habits.

Poor eating habits in children under the age of 5 or 6 years can often be traced directly to parental factors, of which overconcern about the quantity or quality of the diet is a common one. In children of all ages inadequate rest, insufficient sleep, and too much emotional excitement, such as that associated with the movies, radio, and television, are important factors. In older children schoolwork and social activities may interfere with securing adequate rest. School-age children often develop irregular or inappropriate eating habits, especially at breakfast and lunch, because sufficient time is not allotted or because the meals may be poorly balanced. During adolescence girls frequently restrict their dietary intake for esthetic reasons. Eating between meals, especially of such items as candy, ice cream, and snack foods, is likely to reduce the appetite at mealtime.

CLINICAL MANIFESTATIONS. Malnutrition does not invariably result in underweight. Fatigue, lassitude, restlessness, and irritability are frequent manifestations. Restlessness and overactivity are frequently misinterpreted by parents as evidences of lack of fatigue. Anorexia, easily induced digestive disturbances, and constipation are common complaints, and even in older children the starvation type of mucoid diarrheal stool may be observed. Malnourished children often have a limited span of attention and do poorly in schoolwork. They have increased susceptibility to infections, especially of the gastrointestinal and respiratory tracts. Muscular development is inadequate, and the poor tone of the flabby muscles results in a posture of fatigue, with rounded shoulders, flat chest and protuberant abdomen. Such children often look tired; the face is pale, the complexion is "muddy," and the eyes lack luster. Hypochromic anemia is common. In protracted cases there may be delayed epiphyseal development, irregularities in dentition, and delayed puberty.

Evaluation should always include a careful history of dietary habits, physical hygiene, and illness, a thorough physical examination, and such laboratory examinations as will establish, whenever possible, the cause or causes of malnutrition.

TREATMENT. There is a great need for individualization of treatment aimed at correction of the underlying psychologic and physical disturbances. An adequate diet (p. 159) should be outlined; vitamin concentrates may be added and continued for a time after the dietary intake has become adequate. When anorexia is a problem, the essential items of the diet should be provided in as concentrated a form as possible, and the fat content should be low. Between-meal snacks need not be prohibited if they do not interfere with the appetite for the next meal; milk and candy should not be given at such times, but fruit or fruit juices provided. Re-education of the whole family in respect to eating habits may be necessary.

Reasonable regularity in habits without regimentation should be encouraged. Quiet periods of 15 to 20 minutes before meals may abolish the tension which at times interferes with the appetite. Bedtime should be sufficiently early to ensure a full night's sleep, and a nap during the daytime may be helpful. Exciting stories, movies, radio, and television should be avoided before bedtime. Outdoor activity is to be encouraged in sedentary children, and group play for those who tend to be seclusive. Every attempt should be made to permit the child to develop natural interests.

Caddell, J. L., and Goddard, D. R.: Studies in protein-calorie malnutrition. I. Chemical evidence for magnesium deficiency. New Eng. J. Med. *276*:533, 1967.

Cravioto, J., and Delicardie, E. R.: Mental performance in school age children. Am. J. Dis. Child. *120*:404, 1970.

Graham, G. C., Cordano, A., and Baertl, J. M.: Studies in infantile malnutrition. IV. The effect of protein and calorie intake on serum proteins. Am. J. Clin. Nutr. *18*:11, 1966.

Hopkins, L. L., Ransome-Kuti, O., and Majaj, A. S.: Improvement of impaired carbohydrate metabolism by chromium (III) in malnourished infants. Am. J. Clin. Nutr. *21*:203, 1968.

James, W. P. T.: Intestinal absorption in protein-calorie malnutrition. Lancet *1*:333, 1968.

Metcoff, J.: Biochemical effects of protein-calorie malnutrition in man. Ann. Rev. Med. *18*:377, 1967.

Pimstone, B. L., Barbezat, G., Hansen, J. D. L., and Murray, P.:

Studies on growth hormone secretion in protein-calorie malnutrition. Am. J. Clin. Nutr. *21*:482, 1968.
Saunders, S. J., Truswell, A. S., Barbezat, G. O., Wittman, W., and Hansen, J. D. L.: Plasma free amino acid pattern in protein-calorie malnutrition. Lancet *2*:795, 1967.
Wharton, B. A., Jelliffe, D. B., and Stanfield, J. P.: Do we know how to treat kwashiorkor? J. Pediat. *72*:721, 1968.

PROTEIN EXCESS

Excessive protein intake, especially in the absence of sufficient water, may lead to signs of dehydration—protein fever. Signs of protein excess are rare, but premature infants fed a high protein diet have an increased morbidity and mortality. Marasmic infants fed high protein diets during the recovery phase may develop hyperammonemia and large livers, with irritability or lethargy. Signs of protein intoxication have also been noted in children with liver disease. Some weight reducing diets with high protein content may be responsible for protein intoxication.

Barness, L. A., Omans, W. B., Rose, C. S., and Gyorgy, P.: Progress of premature infants fed a formula containing demineralized whey. Pediatrics *32*:52, 1963.

OBESITY

There is no exact line of demarcation between normal nutrition and overnutrition; practically, the diagnosis is made from the appearance of the child rather than from an arbitrary excess in weight. Children of the stocky type may have relatively large skeletal frames and more than the average amount of muscular tissue, so that their weight and height as well as their appearance of bigness exceed those of the average child of their age, but they are not to be considered obese. Obesity or overnutrition is a generalized excessive accumulation of fat in subcutaneous and other tissues.

ETIOLOGY. Obesity is usually due to an excessive intake of food compared with its utilization. Concepts of desirable body proportions vary with family, social and cultural factors. Food intake may be responsive to these considerations or to psychic disturbances; or hypothalamic, pituitary or other brain lesions or hyperinsulinism may be responsible for hyperphagia.

In 1901 Fröhlich reported a boy with a tumor at the base of the brain who presented a picture of obesity accompanied by physical and sexual infantilism. Since then the term "Fröhlich's syndrome" has been loosely applied, and many preadolescent obese boys are erroneously labeled with this diagnosis. (See Section 17.)

Endocrine and metabolic disturbances are rare causes of obesity, though disorders of the thyroid, adrenals, pituitary, and gonads may occur in obese persons. Genetic predisposition to obesity occurs in certain animals and may occur in man. In a study of adults, obesity was found to be seven times more common in the lowest than in the highest social class. Lack of activity causes obesity in some children whose intake of food may not be unusual. Inherited syndromes such as the Laurence-Moon-Biedl, Prader-Willi, or Cushing usually include obesity, either on an endocrine or inactivity basis.

Obesity results from increases either in numbers or in size of fat cells, adipocytes. Adipocytes appear to increase in number when caloric intake is increased, especially in the 6th to 9th gestational months and during the first year of life; this stimulus to increased numbers operates at a reduced intensity through puberty. During periods of weight reduction, the size but not the number of adipocytes decreases.

The obese and lean respond differently to insulin. Resistance to insulin may occur in the obese, with increases in levels of circulating insulin. Insulin decreases lipolysis and increases fat synthesis and uptake. The obese have an increased insulin response to a carbohydrate meal, and a decreased utilization of free fatty acids. On weight reduction regimens, the obese deliver less food to their cells than the lean, owing to decreased mobilization of free fatty acids. In starvation after obesity, fat is mobilized as serum insulin decreases. Protein conservation is facilitated as the brain utilizes ketones for energy. During starvation, serum alanine levels decrease and glycine levels rise.

Purified sugars cause greater insulin secretion than complex carbohydrates, and a high protein diet increases insulin secretion.

The chronic and uncritical offering of a bottle as a means of dealing with a fretful or crying infant may lead to the development of a habit pattern, so that for any frustration the infant may expect or seek food. If obesity were initiated early, it would be likely to persist. Similarly, the uncritical early introduction of solid food of high caloric density into the diet of the infant may lead to rapid weight gain and to obesity.

CLINICAL MANIFESTATIONS. Obesity may become evident at any age, but makes its appearance most frequently in the first year of life, at 5 to 6 years of age, and during adolescence. The child whose obesity is due to excessively high caloric intake is usually not only heavier than his cohorts, but also taller, and bone age is advanced. The facial features often appear disproportionately fine, the nose and mouth being small; there is often a double chin. The adiposity in the mammary regions is often suggestive of breast development, a feature usually embarrassing to the boy. The abdomen tends to be pendulous, and white or purple striae are often present. The external genitalia of boys appear disproportionately small, but actually are of average size; the penis is often deeply imbedded in the pubic fat. Puberty may occur early, with the result that the ultimate height of the obese may be less than that of their slower maturing peers. In only a few instances are the genitalia smaller than would be expected for age, with delayed puberty. The development of the external genitalia is normal in the majority of girls, and menarche is usually not delayed. The obesity of the extremities is usually greater in the upper arm and thigh and is at times limited to them. The hands may be relatively small, and the fingers tapering. Genu valgum is common, and coxa vara and slipping of the epiphysis of the head of the femur may occur. Skinfold measurements with calipers placed over the triceps muscle, at the midpoint of the back of the right upper arm flexed at 90 degrees, have been found useful in assessing fatness of children.

Psychologic disturbances are common in obese children. Even in the apparently well adjusted child adequate psychologic evaluation often discloses significant underlying emotional problems. These may have contributed initially to the causes of obesity, and in any event are usually an additive factor.

PREVENTION AND TREATMENT. Because obesity may be self-perpetuating for psychologic or perhaps physiologic reasons, children of obese parents or obese siblings should be encouraged to adhere to a systematic program of energetic exercise and a balanced diet reduced in calories. Idealized weight is desirable not only for esthetic reasons, but also to prevent such complications of obesity as dislocated hips, diabetes, shortness of breath, and early death. Untreated overweight infants almost always remain overweight as adults.

In planning the diet, the basic nutritional needs must be met (see above). All the essential dietary needs may be included in a 1000- to 1200-Calorie diet for children 10 to 14 years of age for several months. Some children avoid excessive eating after they have been allowed to return to a free choice of diet. The diet should contain as much bulk as possible. At times greater cooperation is secured if small portions of the diet are permitted between meals, especially in the afternoon. If there is doubt that the daily vitamin intake is adequate, vitamin concentrates may be prescribed. Vitamin D should be included, as for all growing children. Too rapid decreases in weight should not be attempted, and medical supervision should be maintained. There is at best a limited place for drug therapy. A trial with amphetamine in conjunction with dietary restriction and psychotherapy may be justified for children whose habits are sedentary or who have frequent states of depression. Psychologic support is often an essential element in management, and both dietary and psychologic treatment should involve the entire family.

The *Pickwickian syndrome* is a rare complication of extreme exogenous obesity, in which there is severe cardiorespiratory distress. It is termed "Pickwickian" for the fat boy, Joe, in Dickens's *Pickwick Papers*. The extreme obesity causes alveolar hypoventilation, with a decrease in pulmonary, tidal, and expiratory reserve volumes. The manifestations include polycythemia, hypoxemia, cyanosis, cardiac enlargement, congestive cardiac failure, and somnolence. High concentrations of oxygen may be dangerous in the treatment of the cyanosis, since respiration may depend solely on the stimulatory effect of hypoxia. Reduction in weight is extremely important and should be accomplished as rapidly as feasible.

TABLE 3-16 1200-1400 CALORIE DIET

Breakfast

1 orange, 1/2 grapefruit or 1 cup of tomato juice
1 egg
1 slice of whole-wheat bread or 1 serving of cereal without sugar
1 teaspoonful of butter
1 cup of whole milk

Lunch

2 ounces of lean meat, 1 egg or 1/2 cup of cottage cheese
1 serving of raw vegetable as salad—no dressing
1 slice of whole-wheat bread
1 teaspoonful of butter
1 serving of fresh or unsweetened fruit
1 cup of whole milk

Dinner

2 ounces of lean meat (liver once a week), poultry or fish
2 servings of green, yellow or red vegetables*
1 serving of fresh or unsweetened fruit
1 cup of whole milk
(Part or all of bread and butter from one of the other meals may be included here)

A 1000-calorie diet may be obtained by eliminating the butter or cream from milk. In this case it becomes especially important to add vitamin A to the daily diet.

*Does not include Irish or sweet potatoes, parsnips, dried peas or beans, lima beans or corn.

Felig, P., Owen, O. E., Morgan, A. P., and Cahill, G. F.: Utilization of metabolic fuels in obese subjects. Am. J. Clin. Nutr. *21*:1429, 1968.
Para, A., Schultz, R. B., Graystone, J. E., and Cheek, D. B.: Correlative studies in obese children and adolescents concerning body composition and plasma insulin and growth hormone levels. Pediat. Res. *5*:605, 1971.
Salans, L. B., Horton, E. S., and Sims, E. A. H.: Experimental obesity in man: Cellular character of the adipose tissue. J. Clin. Invest. *50*:1005, 1971.
Wilson, N. L. (ed.): Obesity. Philadelphia, F. A. Davis Co., 1969.

VITAMIN A DEFICIENCY

The term "vitamin A" is a generic label for all β-ionone derivatives other than provitamin A carotenoids. Retinol signifies vitamin A alcohol; retinyl ester, vitamin A ester; retinal, vitamin A aldehyde; and retinoic acid, vitamin A acid. "Provitamin A carotenoids" is the generic descriptor for all carotenoids exhibiting the biologic activity of β-carotene.

Provitamin A carotenoids or their derivatives with vitamin A activity are required in the diets of infants and children.

Beta-carotene is partly absorbed by the intestinal lymphatics and partly cleaved into two molecules of retinol. Dietary retinyl ester is hydrolyzed to retinol in the intestine. Retinol is esterified inside the mucosal cell with palmitic acid. Retinyl palmitate is stored in the liver. It is hydrolyzed in the liver to free retinol, which is transported to its site of action bound to a specific transport protein in human plasma. The lower limit of normal levels of retinol in the blood is uncertain. In normal infants, levels of 20 to 50 μg/dl and in older children and adults levels of 30 to 225 μg/dl are considered normal.

In children with congenital absence of enzymes necessary to convert provitamin A carotenoids, in those with liver disease, diabetes mellitus, or hypothyroidism, or in those ingesting unusual quantities of carotenoids, carotene may appear in unusual amounts in the blood (carotenemia). In children with carotenemia the skin shows a yellow discoloration, but the color of the scleras remains unchanged.

ETIOLOGY. The liver at birth has a low vitamin A content which is rapidly augmented, since colostrum and the initial breast milk furnish large amounts of the vitamin. Breast milk and whole cow's milk are satisfactory sources of vitamin A. Other foods (vegetables, fruits, eggs, butter, liver) or vitamin supplements provide vitamin A as the infant's diet is expanded. The loss in cooking is small, and canning and freezing of foodstuffs do not appreciably affect their vitamin A content. Oxidizing agents, however, destroy this vitamin.

The danger of vitamin A deficiency is small in healthy children with varied diets. Deficient diets commonly cause disease by 2 to 3 years of age. Vitamin A deficiency also results from inadequate intestinal absorption or from metabolic disorders; these include chronic intestinal disorders, celiac disease, hepatic and pancreatic diseases, iron deficiency anemia, chronic infectious diseases, or chronic ingestion of mineral oil. Low intake of dietary fat results in low vitamin A absorption. Vitamin A excretion is increased in cancer, urinary tract disease, and chronic infectious diseases. Low protein intake results in deficient carrier protein and decrease in serum levels of vitamin A.

PATHOLOGY. The human retina contains two distinct photoreceptor systems: the rods are sensitive to light of low intensity, the cones to colors and to light of high intensity. Retinal is the prosthetic group of photosensitive pigment in both rods and cones. The major difference between the visual pigment in rods (rhodopsin) and cones (iodopsin) is the nature of the protein bound to retinal. All-*trans*-retinol isomerizes in the dark to the 11-*cis*-form. This combines with opsin to form rhodopsin. Energy from light quanta reconverts 11-*cis*-retinal back to the all-*trans* form; this energy exchange produces excitation transmitted via the optic nerves to the brain, resulting in visual sensation. This energy can also be measured by an electroretinograph to assess vitamin A status.

Vitamin A is apparently necessary for membrane stability. Large doses lead to rupture of lysosomal membranes, with release of hydrolases; deficiency may result in a similar phenomenon. The vitamin plays a role in keratinization, cornification and mucus formation.

Characteristic changes in epithelium occur in vitamin A deficiency, including proliferation of basal cells, hyperkeratosis, and the formation of stratified, cornified, squamous epithelium. Epithelial changes may also occur in the respiratory system, causing bronchiolar obstruction. Squamous metaplasia of the renal pelves, ureters, urinary bladder, enamel organs, and pancreatic and salivary ducts may lead to increase in infections in these areas. In a group of children dying of protein malnutrition 80 per cent had evidence of severe vitamin A deficiency.

CLINICAL MANIFESTATIONS. Ocular lesions develop insidiously. First the posterior segment of the eye is affected, with impairment of dark adaptation and night blindness. Later the anterior segment is affected, with drying of the conjunctiva (xerosis conjunctivae) and of the cornea (xerosis corneae), followed by wrinkling and cloudiness of the cornea (keratomalacia) (Fig. 3–4). Dry, silver-gray plaques may appear on the bulbar conjunctiva (Bitot's spots), with follicular hyperkeratosis and photophobia.

Symptoms of vitamin A deficiency include retardation of mental and physical growth, and apathy. Anemia with or without hepatosplenomegaly is usually present. Night blindness, or loss of visual acuity in dim light, may be due to vitamin A deficiency.

The skin is dry and scaly, and at times follicular hyperkeratosis may be found on the shoulders, buttocks, and extensor surfaces of the extremities. The vaginal epithelium may become cornified, and

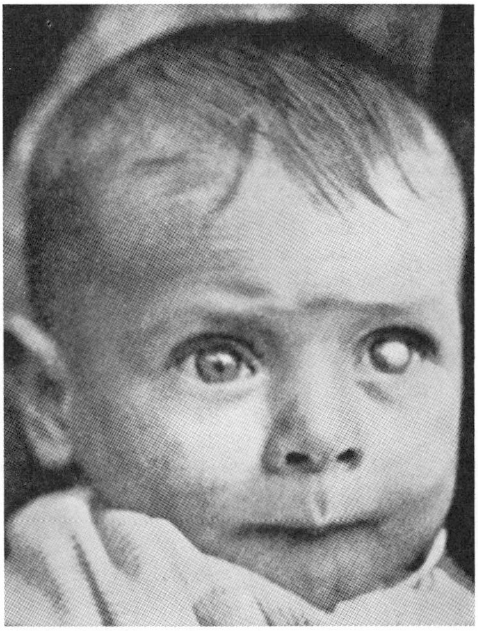

Figure 3–4 Recovery from xerophthalmia, showing permanent eye lesion. (Bloch: Am. J. Dis. Child., Vol. 27.)

epithelial metaplasia of the urinary tract may contribute to pyuria and hematuria. Increased intracranial pressure with wide separation of cranial bones at the sutures may occur. Hydrocephalus, with or without paralyses of the cranial nerves, is an infrequent manifestation.

DIAGNOSIS. Dark adaptation tests, made carefully and under strictly standardized conditions, may be helpful, but the method is not adaptable to routine clinical practice. If xerosis conjunctivae precedes night blindness, it can be detected by biomicroscopic examination of the conjunctiva. Examination of the scrapings from the eye and vagina has also been recommended as a diagnostic aid. The plasma carotene level falls quickly, but the vitamin A concentration decreases more slowly. A standard absorption test for vitamin A is available. Low absorption curves are obtained in children with cystic fibrosis, celiac disease, obliteration of the bile ducts, and cretinism. (See Section 11.)

PREVENTION. Infants should receive at least 1500 I.U. daily, older children 2000 to 4500 IU of vitamin A or carotene, and adults, 5000 IU.* The average diets of infants and children in this country supply enough vitamin A to prevent symptoms of deficiency. If children receive, in addition, one of the vitamin A and D concentrates or a multiple vitamin preparation, most of which contain 3000 to 5000 IU of vitamin A per recommended dose, their requirements are more than adequately covered.

Children on a low fat diet for therapeutic reasons should receive supplementary vitamin A. In disorders which result in poor absorption of fat or increased excretion of vitamin A, water-miscible preparations of vitamin A should be administered in amounts equivalent to several times the usual daily requirement. Premature infants, who absorb fats and vitamin A less efficiently than do full-term infants, should also receive water-miscible preparations. The World Health Organization recommends that, in areas of the world where vitamin A deficiency occurs, 100,000 IU of vitamin A be given orally in a water-miscible base four times yearly, and the same dose post partum to the mothers of breast-fed infants.

TREATMENT. In cases of latent vitamin A deficiency a daily supplement of 5000 IU of vitamin A to the diet is all that is required. For xerophthalmia 5000 IU per kg per day is given orally for 5 days, and then combined with intramuscular injection of 25,000 IU of vitamin A per kg in oil daily until recovery occurs.

HYPERVITAMINOSIS A. Acute hypervitaminosis A may occur in infants after the ingestion of 300,000 IU or more. The symptoms are nausea, vomiting, drowsiness, and bulging of the fontanel. Diplopia, papilledema, and other symptoms suggesting brain tumor (pseudotumor cerebri) may also occur.

*One international unit (IU) of vitamin A is equivalent to 0.3 μg of vitamin A alcohol.

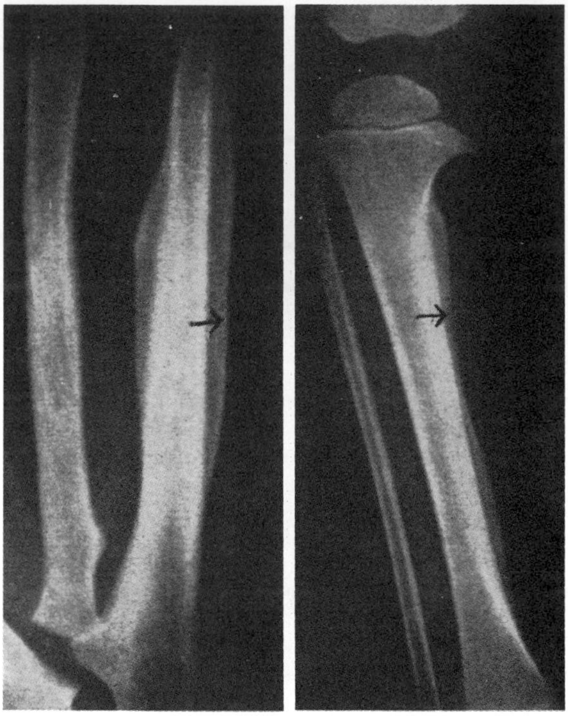

A B

Figure 3–5 Hyperostosis of the ulna and the tibia in an infant 21 months of age, resulting from vitamin A poisoning. A, *Long, wavy cortical hyperostosis of ulna.* B, *Long, wavy cortical hyperostosis of right tibia; striking absence of metaphyseal changes. Caffey, J. (PEDIATRICS. Vol. 5. Courtesy of Charles C Thomas, Publisher, Springfield, Ill.)*

Chronic hypervitaminosis A appears after ingestion of excessive doses for several weeks or months. The initial manifestations are not specific. The child has anorexia, pruritus, and a lack of gain in weight. There are increasing irritability, limitation of motion, and tender swelling of the bones. Alopecia, seborrheic cutaneous lesions, fissuring of the corners of the mouth, and hepatomegaly may develop. Craniotabes and desquamation of the palms and soles are common. Roentgenograms reveal hyperostosis affecting several long bones; it is most notable at the middle of the shafts. A history of excessive ingestion of vitamin A is helpful in the differentiation from cortical hyperostosis (Caffey's disease). The serum vitamin A level is elevated. Electron microscopic study of the liver of a child who had received 60,000 to 90,000 IU daily for 4 years showed increased lysosomes, focal cytoplasmic degradation and other storage material. Hypercalcemia occasionally occurs.

Fisher, K. D., Carr, C. J., Huff, J. E., and Huber, T. E.: Dark adaptation and night vision. Fed. Proc. *29*:1605, 1970.
Hayes, K. C.: On the pathophysiology of vitamin A deficiency. Nutr. Rev. *29*:3, 1971.
Keating, J. P., and Feigin, R. D.: Increased intracranial pressure associated with probable vitamin A deficiency in cystic fibrosis. Pediatrics *46*:41, 1970.
McLaren, D. S., Shirajain, E., Tchallian, M., and Khoury, G.: Xerophthalmia in Jordan. Am. J. Clin. Nutr. *17*:117, 1965.
Roels, O. A.: Vitamin A physiology. J.A.M.A. *214*:1097, 1970.
Rubin, E., Florman, A. L., Degnan, T., and Diaz, J.: Hepatic in-

jury in chronic hypervitaminosis A. Am. J. Dis. Child. *119*:132, 1970.
Wald, G.: Molecular basis of visual excitation. Science *162*:230, 1968.

VITAMIN B COMPLEX DEFICIENCY

Vitamin B complex includes a number of factors which vary greatly in chemical composition and function. Several members of the B complex are important constituents of enzyme systems. Since many of these enzymes are closely related functionally, lack of a single factor can interrupt an entire chain of normal chemical processes and produce diversified clinical manifestations.

Diets deficient in any one factor of the B complex are frequently poor sources of other B vitamins. It is therefore not unusual to find manifestations of several B deficiencies in one patient, and sharp separation of the symptoms caused by deficiencies of the single factors may be impossible. It is usually advantageous to treat with the entire B complex.

Factors such as pantothenic acid, choline, biotin, and inositol are of importance for the normal function of the human organism, but at present no specific deficiency syndromes can be ascribed to lack of them in the diets of children.

THIAMINE DEFICIENCY

(Beriberi)

ETIOLOGY. Vitamin B_1 (thiamine) is one of the water-soluble vitamins and, as thiamine pyrophosphate or cocarboxylase, functions as a coenzyme in carbohydrate metabolism. Thiamine is required for the synthesis of acetylcholine, and deficiency results in impaired nerve conduction. It is the coenzyme in transketolation and in decarboxylation of α-keto acids. Transketolase participates in the hexose monophosphate shunt which generates NADPH and pentose.

The foods usually given to infants—breast milk or cow's milk, vegetables, cereals, fruits, eggs—are fair sources of thiamine. Mothers with thiamine deficiency produce a milk deficient in thiamine, and infants fed their milk may acquire beriberi. Older children whose diet contains such good sources of thiamine as meats and legumes do not require supplements of this vitamin.

Thiamine is easily destroyed by heat in neutral or alkaline media and is readily extracted from foodstuffs by cooking water. The presence of a destructive enzymatic factor in certain types of fish explains why a diet low in thiamine induces beriberi rapidly when it is supplemented by such fish. Since the covering of grains of cereals contains most of the vitamin, polishing reduces its availability.

Thiamine absorption is decreased with gastrointestinal or liver disease. Requirements are increased with fever, surgery, or stress. Thiamine dependency has been described in an 11 year old with megaloblastic anemia and in an infant with otherwise typical maple syrup urine disease.

PATHOLOGY. In fatal cases of beriberi, lesions are located especially in the heart, peripheral nerves, subcutaneous tissue, and serous cavities. The heart is dilated, particularly the right side; the interstitial tissue is edematous; and fatty degeneration of the myocardium is commonly present. Generalized edema or edema of the legs, serous effusions, and venous engorgement of the viscera may be present. The peripheral nerves undergo varying degrees of degeneration of myelin and axon cylinders, with wallerian degeneration, beginning in the distal locations. The nerves of the lower extremities are affected first. Lesions in the brain include vascular dilatation, hemorrhage, and proliferation similar to that associated with superior hemorrhagic polioencephalitis (Wernicke's disease). These changes are more likely to be found in chronic deficiency states.

CLINICAL MANIFESTATIONS. The effects of deficiency are peripheral neuritis, congestive heart failure, and psychic disturbances, commonly recognized as beriberi. Infantile beriberi is rare in the United States. Congenital beriberi in infants of mothers with a severe deficiency has been observed, usually within the first 3 months of life. The vague initial symptoms are restlessness, anorexia, vomiting, and constipation.

In *dry* beriberi the infant may appear plump, but is pale, flabby, listless, and dyspneic; the heart rate is rapid and the liver enlarged. In *wet* beriberi the infants are undernourished, pale, and edematous, and have dyspnea, vomiting, and tachycardia. Knee and ankle jerks are absent in each type. There is no gain in weight except in infants who have edema, which is usually restricted to the distal parts of the extremities. The skin appears waxy. The urine may be scanty and contain albumin and casts.

The cardiac signs at first are slight cyanosis and dyspnea. Tachycardia, enlargement of the liver, loss of consciousness, and convulsions may develop rapidly. The heart is enlarged, especially to the right. The heart sounds are rapid, and the second pulmonic sound is accentuated. Gallop rhythm may be present. The roentgenogram shows cardiac dilatation, and the electrocardiogram shows increased Q-T interval, inversion of T waves, and low voltage, changes which rapidly revert to normal with treatment. Circulation time is decreased. Pulse pressure is increased. Cardiac failure may lead to death in either chronic or acute beriberi. In the latter it may occur with dramatic suddenness in infants previously considered healthy.

Apathy and drowsiness are common. There may be ptosis of the eyelids and atrophy of the optic nerve. Hoarseness due to paralysis of the laryngeal nerves is a characteristic sign. Paralytic symptoms are rare in infants. Paresthesias, hyperesthesias, and pain and burning of the feet are more common in adults than in children. Muscle atrophy and tenderness of nerve trunks are followed by ataxia, loss of coordination, and loss of deep sensation. Later, signs of increased intracranial pressure, meningismus and coma occur.

DIAGNOSIS. The early symptoms, such as restlessness, anorexia, gastrointestinal disturbances, and pallor, are encountered in many types of nutritional disturbances which are not necessarily caused by thiamine deficiency. Since blood lactic and pyruvic acid levels rise in thiamine deficiency, these may be measured after oral administration of glucose or after exercise. The levels should return to normal after ingestion of thiamine. Demonstration of decreased red cell transketolase and increased blood or urinary glyoxylate has been proposed as a diagnostic test of thiamine deficiency. Excretion after an oral loading dose of thiamine or its metabolites, thiazole or pyrimidine, may help to determine the deficiency state. Clinical response to administration of thiamine remains the best test for thiamine deficiency.

PREVENTION. Thiamine deficiency in breast-fed infants is prevented by a maternal diet which contains sufficient amounts of this vitamin. The recommended daily dietary allowances of thiamine are 1.7 mg during pregnancy and during lactation. The recommended daily dietary allowance of thiamine is 0.5 mg for infants and 0.7 to 1.5 mg for older children. Thiamine requirements are increased with a high carbohydrate diet. Excessive cooking of vegetables or the refining of cereal grains destroys available thiamine.

TREATMENT. If beriberi occurs in a breast-fed infant, both mother and child should be treated with thiamine. The daily dose for adults is 50 mg, and for children 10 mg or more. Oral administration is effective unless gastrointestinal disturbances prevent absorption. Thiamine should be given intramuscularly or intravenously to children with cardiac failure. Such treatment is followed by dramatic improvement within 2 hours. Complete cure requires several weeks; the beriberi heart is not permanently damaged. There is often deficiency of other B vitamins in patients with beriberi; for this reason all the vitamins of the B complex should be administered in addition to large doses of thiamine chloride.

RIBOFLAVIN DEFICIENCY
(Ariboflavinosis)

Riboflavin deficiency is rarely encountered without manifestations of other deficiencies of the B complex. Riboflavin is a water-soluble, yellow, fluorescent substance, stable to heat and acids, but destroyed by light and alkalis. The coenzymes flavin mononucleotide (FMN) and flavin adenine dinucleotide (FAD) are synthesized from riboflavin and form the prosthetic groups of several enzymes important in electron transport. The vitamin occurs in large amounts in liver, kidney, brewer's yeast, milk, cheese, eggs, and leafy vegetables. Cow's milk contains about five times as much riboflavin as human milk.

Riboflavin deficiency is usually due to inadequate intake, but faulty absorption may be a contributory factor in those with biliary atresia or hepatitis, or in patients receiving probenecid.

CLINICAL MANIFESTATIONS. Signs of riboflavin deficiency include cheilosis, glossitis, keratitis, conjunctivitis, photophobia, lacrimation, marked corneal vascularization and seborrheic dermatitis. Cheilosis begins with pallor at the angles of the mouth, followed by thinning and maceration of the epithelium. Superficial fissures often covered by yellow crusts develop in the angles of the mouth and extend radially into the skin for distances of 1 to 2 cm. Cheilosis (*perlèche*) occurs in epidemics in institutions and in families in which the diet is inadequate. In ariboflavinosis the tongue is smooth and shows loss of papillary structure. A normocytic, normochromic anemia with bone marrow hypoplasia can occur.

DIAGNOSIS. Urinary excretion of riboflavin below 30 μg/day is abnormally low. Levels of erythrocyte glutathionine reductase, a flavoprotein requiring FAD, may reflect the stores of riboflavin.

PREVENTION. The daily amount of riboflavin recommended for infants is 0.6 mg; for children and adults, 1 to 2 mg. Riboflavin deficiency is usually prevented by a diet which contains adequate amounts of milk, eggs, leafy vegetables, and lean meats.

TREATMENT. Treatment consists in the oral administration of 3 to 10 mg of riboflavin daily. If no response is obtained within a few days, intramuscular injections of 2 mg of riboflavin in saline solution may be made 3 times daily. The child should also be given a well balanced diet and, temporarily at least, more than the usual requirements of the B complex.

NIACIN DEFICIENCY
(Pellagra)

Pellagra (*pellis,* skin; *agra,* rough) probably has existed under certain unfavorable conditions at all times in all parts of the world.

ETIOLOGY. Pellagra is a deficiency disease which affects all the tissues of the body. Although it is doubtful whether all its manifestations can be attributed to the deficiency of a single vitamin, the lack of niacin (nicotinic acid) is presumably responsible for most of them.

Niacin forms part of 2 enzymes important in electron transfer and glycolysis: diphosphopyridine nucleotide, or nicotinamide adenine dinucleotide (DPN, NAD); and triphosphopyridine nucleotide, or nicotinamide adenine dinucleotide phosphate (TPN, NADP). Although 60 mg of tryptophan can be utilized in place of 1 mg of niacin, exogenous sources of niacin are necessary. Liver, lean pork, salmon, poultry, and red meat are good sources of niacin, but most cereals contain only small amounts of it. Pellagra occurs chiefly in countries where corn (maize), a poor source of tryptophan, is used as a basic foodstuff. Milk and eggs, which contain little niacin, are good pellagra-preventive foods because of their high content of tryptophan. Because niacin is a stable compound, there are only small losses in cooking if the cooking water is not excessive and not discarded.

The incidence of pellagra is increased in spring and early summer months. This disorder is frequent in women in the postpartum period, since pregnancy and lactation increase the niacin requirement. Pellagra usually does not occur in breast-fed infants.

PATHOLOGY. Histologically there is edema and degeneration of the superficial collagen of the dermis. The papillary vessels are engorged, and there is perivascular lymphocytic infiltration in the dermis. The epidermis is hyperkeratotic and later becomes atrophic.

Changes comparable to those in the skin are present in the tongue, buccal mucous membranes and vagina. These changes may be associated with secondary infection and ulceration. The walls of the colon are thickened and inflamed, with patches of pseudomembrane; later the mucosa atrophies. Changes in the nervous system occur relatively late in the disease and consist of patchy areas of demyelinization and degeneration of ganglion cells; demyelinization in the spinal cord may involve the posterior and lateral columns.

CLINICAL MANIFESTATIONS. The early symptoms of pellagra are vague. Anorexia, lassitude, weakness, burning sensations, numbness, and dizziness may be prodromal symptoms. After a long period of niacin deficiency the characteristic symptoms of pellagra appear. The classic triad consists of dermatitis, diarrhea, and dementia. Manifestations in children who have parasites or chronic disorders may be especially severe.

The most characteristic manifestations are the cutaneous ones, which may develop suddenly or insidiously and may be elicited by irritants, particularly by intensive sunlight. They first appear as a symmetrically developed erythema of the exposed surfaces. The erythema resembles sunburn and in mild cases, especially in young children, may easily escape recognition. The lesions are usually sharply demarcated from the healthy skin around them, and their distribution may change frequently. The lesions on the hands sometimes have the appearance of a glove (pellagrous glove) (Fig. 3–6), and similar demarcations are occasionally seen on the foot and leg (pellagrous boot) or around the neck (Casal's necklace). In some instances vesicles and bullae develop (wet type), or there may be suppuration beneath the scaly, crusted epidermis; in others the swelling disappears after a short time and desquamation begins. The healed parts of the skin may remain pigmented.

The cutaneous lesions are sometimes preceded by symptoms in the alimentary tract, such as stomatitis, glossitis, vomiting, and diarrhea. Swelling and redness of the tip of the tongue and its lateral margins appear relatively early. Later there may be intense redness of the entire tongue with swelling of the papillae and even ulceration.

Nervous symptoms include depression, disorientation, insomnia, and delirium.

The classic symptoms of pellagra are usually not well developed in infants and children. Anorexia, irritability, anxiety, and apathy are observed frequently in young children of "pellagra families." They may also have sore tongues and lips, and the skin is usually dry and scaly. Diarrhea and constipation may alternate and a moderate secondary anemia may occur. Children who have pellagra often have evidences of other nutritional deficiency diseases.

DIAGNOSIS. Diagnosis is usually made from the physical signs of glossitis, gastrointestinal symptoms and a symmetrical dermatitis. Rapid clinical response to niacin is an important confirming test. Urinary levels of N-methyl-nicotinamide, a normal metabolite of niacin, are almost undetectable in niacin deficiency.

PREVENTION. The recommended daily allowance of niacin is 8 mg for infants and 9 to 20 mg for older children. A well balanced diet containing meat, vegetables, eggs and milk meets this requirement, so that supplements of niacin are

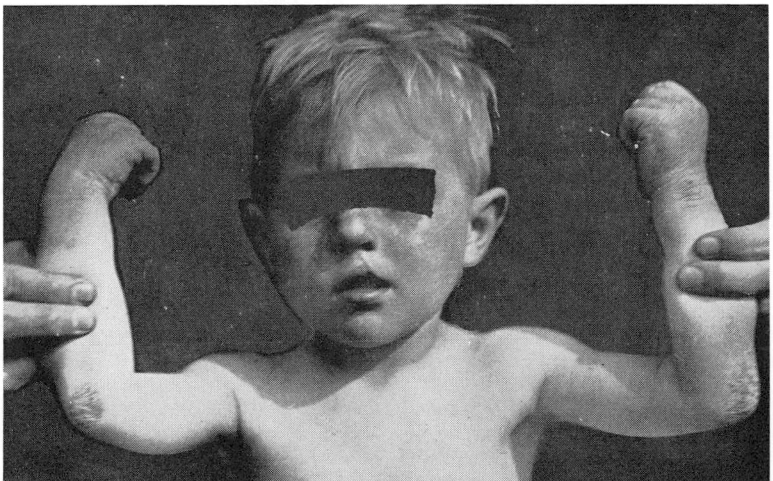

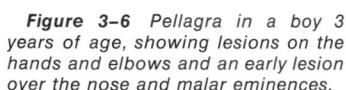

Figure 3–6 *Pellagra in a boy 3 years of age, showing lesions on the hands and elbows and an early lesion over the nose and malar eminences.*

necessary only in breast-fed infants whose mothers suffer from pellagra or in children on restricted diets.

TREATMENT. Children respond rapidly to antipellagral therapy. A liberal and well balanced diet should be supplemented with 50 to 300 mg of niacin daily; a smaller amount may be given intravenously, or approximately 100 mg by hypodermoclysis in severe cases or in those patients in whom intestinal absorption is poor. The administration of large doses of niacin is often followed within a half hour by a sensation of increased local heat and flushing and burning of the skin. These unpleasant effects are not produced by niacinamide.

Since vitamin deficiencies are rarely single, it is good practice to supplement the diet with other vitamins, especially with the other members of the B complex. Sunshine should be avoided during the active phase, and the skin lesions may be covered with soothing applications. A blood transfusion may be helpful in cases of severe anemia; the less severe hypochromic ones should be treated with iron. The diet of the cured pellagrin should be continuously supervised to prevent recurrence.

Thiamine Deficiency

Brin, M.: Erythrocyte as a biopsy tissue for functional evaluation of thiamin adequacy. J.A.M.A. *187*:762, 1964.

McCandless, D. W., and Schenker, S.: Neurologic disorders of thiamine deficiency. Nutr. Rev. *27*:213, 1969.

Porter, F. S., Rogers, L. E., and Sidbury, J. B., Jr.: Thiamin responsive megaloblastic anemia. J. Pediatr. *74*:494, 1969.

Scriver, C. R., Mackenzie, S., Clow, C. L., and Delvin, E.: Thiamine-responsive maple-syrup-urine disease. Lancet *1*:310, 1971.

Riboflavin Deficiency

Rillotson, J. A., and Baker, E. M.: An enzymatic measurement of the riboflavin status in man. Am. J. Clin. Nutr. *25*:425, 1972.

Rivlin, R. S.: Riboflavin metabolism. New Engl. J. Med. *283*:463, 1970.

Niacin Deficiency

Goldsmith, G. A.: Niacin-tryptophan relationships in man, and niacin requirements. Am. J. Clin. Nutr. *6*:479, 1958.

PYRIDOXINE (VITAMIN B_6) DEFICIENCY

Vitamin B_6 includes pyridoxal, pyridoxine, and pyridoxamine. These are converted to pyridoxal-5-phosphate (or pyridoxamine-5-phosphate), which acts as a coenzyme in decarboxylation and transamination of amino acids, e.g., in the decarboxylation of 5-hydroxytryptophan in the formation of serotonin, and in the metabolism of glycogen and fatty acids. Vitamin B_6 is also essential for the breakdown of kynurenine. When this does not occur, xanthurenic acid appears in the urine. Adequate functioning of the nervous system is dependent on pyridoxine; its deficiency results in seizures in man and in peripheral neuropathy. Pyridoxal phosphate is the coenzyme for both glutamic decarboxylase and gamma aminobutyric acid transaminase, both necessary for normal brain metabolism. It participates in active transport of amino acids across cell membranes, chelates metals, and participates in the synthesis of arachidonic acid from linoleic acid. If it is lacking, glycine metabolism may lead to oxaluria. It is excreted largely as 4-pyridoxic acid.

ETIOLOGY. Pyridoxine deficiency was first recognized in infants fed a proprietary formula which had been processed several times. Pyridoxine is adequately available in human and cow's milk and in cereals, but prolonged heat processing of the latter two may alter its availability. Diseases with malabsorption, such as celiac syndrome, may contribute to vitamin B_6 deficiency.

There are several types of vitamin B_6 dependency syndromes, presumably the result of errors of enzyme structure or function, in which the patient responds to very large amounts of pyridoxine. These syndromes include B_6-dependent convulsions, a B_6-responsive anemia, xanthurenic aciduria, cystathioninuria, and some patients with homocystinuria.

Pyridoxine antagonists, such as isonicotinic acid hydrazide (isoniazid), which is used in the treatment of tuberculosis, increase the requirement for pyridoxine; deficiency symptoms are not so readily produced in children as in adults. Other drugs, such as penicillamine and the oral progesterone-estrogen contraceptives, increase pyridoxine requirements, as does pregnancy.

CLINICAL MANIFESTATIONS. Four clinical disturbances due to vitamin B_6 deficiency have been described in man; convulsions in infants, peripheral neuritis, dermatitis, and anemia.

A small percentage of infants fed a formula deficient in vitamin B_6 for 1 to 6 months may exhibit irritability and generalized seizures. Gastrointestinal distress and an aggravated startle response are common.

Peripheral neuropathy may occur during treatment of tuberculosis with isonicotinic acid hydrazide. The neuropathy responds to administration of pyridoxine or to a decrease in the dose of the drug. Administration of isonicotinic acid also may be followed by manifestations of pellagra.

Skin lesions include cheilosis, glossitis, and seborrhea around the eyes, nose, and mouth. Microcytic anemia, oxaluria, oxalic acid bladder stones, hyperglycinemia, lymphopenia, decreased antibody formation and infections occur.

Convulsions from B_6 dependency occur 3 hours to 2 weeks after birth. In several cases the mothers had received large doses of pyridoxine during pregnancy for control of emesis.

In B_6-dependent anemia the red cells are microcytic and hypochromic. There are increased serum iron concentration, increased saturation of iron-binding protein and markedly increased hemosiderin deposits in bone marrow and liver, with failure of iron utilization for hemoglobin synthesis.

Xanthurenic aciduria following tryptophan load tests is an apparently benign occurrence in some families. Xanthurenic acid excretion becomes normal following large doses of vitamin B_6. Cystathioninuria is similarly not accompanied by any clear clinical disturbance. Cystathioninase is vitamin B_6 dependent. (See also Section 8.)

In some patients with homocystinuria serum levels of homocysteine will fall following B_6 administration. Cystathionine synthetase is B_6 dependent. (See also Section 8.)

LABORATORY DATA. Anemia is not common in affected infants. After administration of 100 mg per kg of tryptophan, large amounts of xanthurenic acid will be found in the urine of patients with pyridoxine deficiency; in normal persons none is detected. This test result may be normal in patients with "pyridoxine dependency." Serum and red blood cell glutamic oxalacetic transaminase is decreased in experimental B_6 deficiency.

DIAGNOSIS. Infants with seizures should be suspected of having vitamin B_6 deficiency or dependency. If commoner causes of infantile seizures such as hypocalcemia, hypoglycemia and infection can be eliminated as causative factors, 100 mg of pyridoxine should be injected. If the seizure stops, B_6 deficiency should be suspected, and a tryptophan loading test is indicated. Similarly, in older children with seizure disorders, 100 mg of pyridoxine may be injected intramuscularly while the electroencephalogram is being recorded; a favorable response of the EEG suggests pyridoxine deficiency.

Erythrocyte glutamic pyruvic transaminase is reduced in pyridoxine deficiency; its level may be used as an indicator of vitamin B_6 status.

PREVENTION. Balanced diets usually contain enough pyridoxine so that deficiency is rare. Children receiving high protein diets should have vitamin B_6 added. Infants whose mothers have received large doses of pyridoxine during pregnancy are at increased risk of seizures due to pyridoxine dependency. Any child receiving a pyridoxine antagonist such as isoniazid should be carefully observed for neurologic manifestations. If these develop, either pyridoxine should be administered or the dose of the antagonist decreased. Daily intake of 0.1 to 0.5 mg in the infant, 0.5 to 1.5 mg in the child, or 1.5 to 2.0 mg in the adult prevents deficiency states.

TREATMENT. For convulsions possibly due to pyridoxine deficiency 100 mg of the vitamin should be given intramuscularly. One dose should suffice if the diet is adequate. For "pyridoxine-dependent" children 2 to 10 mg intramuscularly or 10 to 100 mg by mouth daily may be necessary.

Aly, H. E., Donald, E. A., and Simpson, M. H. W.: Oral contraceptives and vitamin B_6 metabolism. Am. J. Clin. Nutr. *24*:297, 1971.

Cinnamon, A. D., and Beaton, J. R.: Biochemical assessment of vitamin B_6 status in man. Am. J. Clin. Nutr. *23*:696, 1970.

Frimpter, G. W., Andelman, R. J., and George, W. F.: Vitamin B_6-dependency syndromes. Am. J. Clin. Nutr. *22*:794, 1969.

Hansson, O., and Hagberg, B.: Effect of pyridoxine treatment in children with epilepsy. Acta Soc. Med. Upsal. *73*:35, 1968.

Scriver, C. R.: Vitamin B_6 deficiency and dependency in man. Am. J. Dis. Child. *113*:109, 1967.

SCURVY

Scurvy is a manifestation of deficiency of vitamin C (ascorbic acid). Ascorbic acid is a dietary essential for primates, guinea pigs, the Indian fruit bat, and the red-vented bulbul. It is a potent reducing agent, easily oxidized and destroyed by heating.

Premature infants fed high protein diets which contain large amounts of tyrosine excrete p-hydroxyphenyllactic and p-hydroxyphenylpyruvic acids unless given increased quantities of ascorbate. The reduction of folic acid to its tetrahydro derivative apparently requires ascorbate. (See also Megaloblastic Anemias, Section 14.)

Defects in collagen formation explain most of the abnormalities in vitamin C deficiency. Ingested hydroxyproline is not used in building collagen, but proline is built into a protein unit by cellular ribosomes. Ascorbate and oxygen are then essential for addition of a hydroxy group to form normal collagen. Similar mechanisms direct the formation of hydroxylysine and hydroxytryptophan. The adrenals and lenses have particularly high content of vitamin C.

ETIOLOGY. The infant is born with adequate stores of vitamin C if the mother's intake has been adequate. The vitamin C content of cord blood plasma is 2 to 4 times greater than that of maternal plasma. As a rule, breast milk contains about 4 to 7 mg of ascorbic acid per dl and is an adequate source of vitamin C. A deficiency of vitamin C in the mother's diet may result in scurvy in her breast-fed infant. Infants fed artificially must receive vitamin C supplements; such supplements will provide additional protection for the breast-fed infant.

Scurvy may occur at any age, but is extremely rare in the newborn infant. The majority of cases are seen in the latter half of the first and in the second year of life. The need for vitamin C is increased by febrile illnesses, particularly infectious and diarrheal diseases, and by iron deficiency, cold exposure, protein depletion or smoking by children or their mothers.

PATHOLOGY. Collagen formed during vitamin C deficiency is said to be low in hydroxyproline, and formation of collagen and chondroitin sulfate is impaired. The tendencies to hemorrhage, to defective tooth dentin and to loosening of the teeth are due to deficient collagen. Since osteoblasts no longer form their normal intercellular substance (osteoid), endochondral bone formation ceases. The bony trabeculae which have been formed continue to be calcified, but become brittle and fracture easily. The periosteum becomes loosened, and subperiosteal hemorrhages occur, especially at the ends of the femur and tibia. In severe scurvy there may be degeneration in skeletal muscles, cardiac hypertrophy, bone marrow depression and adrenal atrophy.

CLINICAL MANIFESTATIONS. Scurvy requires time for its development; after a variable period of vitamin C depletion vague symptoms of irritability, tachypnea, digestive disturbances, and loss of appetite appear. The irritability becomes progressively greater, and there is evidence of general tenderness, especially noticeable in the legs when the infant is picked up or when the diaper is changed.

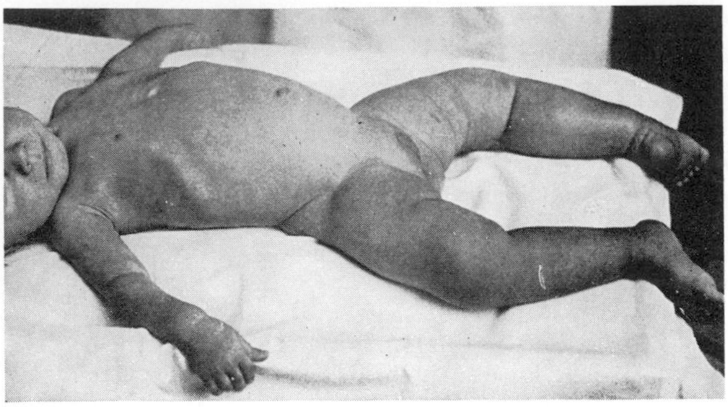

Figure 3–7 Scorbutic rosary, depression of sternum and the so-called frog position.

The pain causes pseudoparalysis, and the legs assume the typical "frog position" (Fig. 3–7), which consists in semiflexion of the hips and knees with the feet rotated outward. Edematous swelling along the shafts of the legs may be present, and in some cases a subperiosteal hemorrhage can be palpated at the end of the femur. The facial expression is apprehensive. Changes of the gums, most noticeable when the teeth are erupted, are characterized by bluish purple, spongy swellings of the mucous membrane, usually over the upper incisors. The swollen gums sometimes completely conceal the teeth. There may be a "rosary" at the costochondral junctions and a depression of the sternum. The angulation of the "scorbutic beads" is usually sharper than that in the rachitic rosary, since it is produced by a subluxation of the sternal plate at the costochondral junction (Fig. 3–7) rather than by widening of the softened epiphyses as occurs in rickets (see below, this Section).

Petechial hemorrhages may occur in the skin and mucous membranes. Hematuria, melena, or orbital or subdural hemorrhages may be found. Low-grade fever is usually present. Anemia may reflect inability to utilize iron or impaired folic acid metabolism (Section 14). Wound healing is delayed, and healed wounds may break down. Swollen joints and follicular hyperkeratosis may develop, as well as the "sicca" syndrome of Sjögren, which is usually associated with collagen disorders and includes xerostomia, keratoconjunctivitis sicca and enlargement of the salivary glands.

ROENTGENOGRAPHIC MANIFESTATIONS. The diagnosis of scurvy is usually based on roentgenographic changes in the long bones, especially of their distal ends. Changes are greatest, as a rule, in the area of the knee. In the early stages the appearance resembles that of simple atrophy of the bone. In the shaft the trabeculae cannot be discerned, and the bone assumes a "ground-glass" appearance. The cortex is reduced to "pencil-point thinness," and the epiphyseal ends are sharply outlined. The white line of Fraenkel, which represents the zone of well calcified cartilage, can be clearly discerned as an irregular but thickened white line at the metaphysis. The epiphyseal centers of ossification also have a ground-glass appearance and are surrounded by a white ring corresponding to the white line of the shaft (Fig. 3–8). At this stage scurvy cannot be diagnosed with certainty from the roentgenogram; if, however, under the white line at the metaphysis the zone of rarefaction becomes apparent, the roentgenogram is diagnostic. The zone of rarefaction is a linear break in the bone proximal and parallel to the white line. It often does not traverse the shaft in its entire width and may be seen only in its lateral parts as a triangular defect (Fig. 3–8, *B*). A spur, as lateral prolongation of the white line, may be present. Epiphyseal separation may occur along the line of destruction, with linear displacement (Fig. 3–9) or compression of the epiphysis against the shaft. Subperiosteal hemorrhages are not visible roentgenographically in active scurvy. During healing, however, the elevated periosteum becomes calcified and presents a striking picture. The affected bone assumes a dumbbell or club shape, since the hemorrhage occurs at the ends of the bone and elevates the periosteum more at this site than in the middle of the shaft (Fig. 3–8, *C*). As healing progresses, the shadow of the hemorrhage becomes more intense, but diminishes in width; the rings around the epiphyseal centers of ossification become more distinct, and the zone of destruction disappears and is replaced by calcified tissue.

DIAGNOSIS. Diagnosis is based mainly on the characteristic clinical picture, the roentgenographic appearance of the long bones, and history of poor intake of vitamin C. Occasionally a mother will have been boiling the infant's fruit juices.

Laboratory tests for scurvy are unsatisfactory. A fasting vitamin C level of the blood plasma of over 0.6 mg/dl aids in the exclusion of scurvy, but a lower vitamin C level does not prove its presence. A better index of vitamin C deficiency is furnished by the ascorbic acid concentration of the white cell-platelet layer (buffy layer) of centrifuged oxalated blood. A level of zero in this layer indicates latent scurvy, even in the absence of clinical signs of deficiency. The saturation of the tissues with vitamin C can be estimated from the amount of urinary excretion of the vitamin after a test dose of ascorbic acid. During the 3 to 5 hours after the parenteral administration of the test dose, 80 per cent of the total 24-hour excretion can be found in the urine. Children with vitamin C deficiency excrete less ascorbic acid under these conditions than normal children with well saturated tissues. A

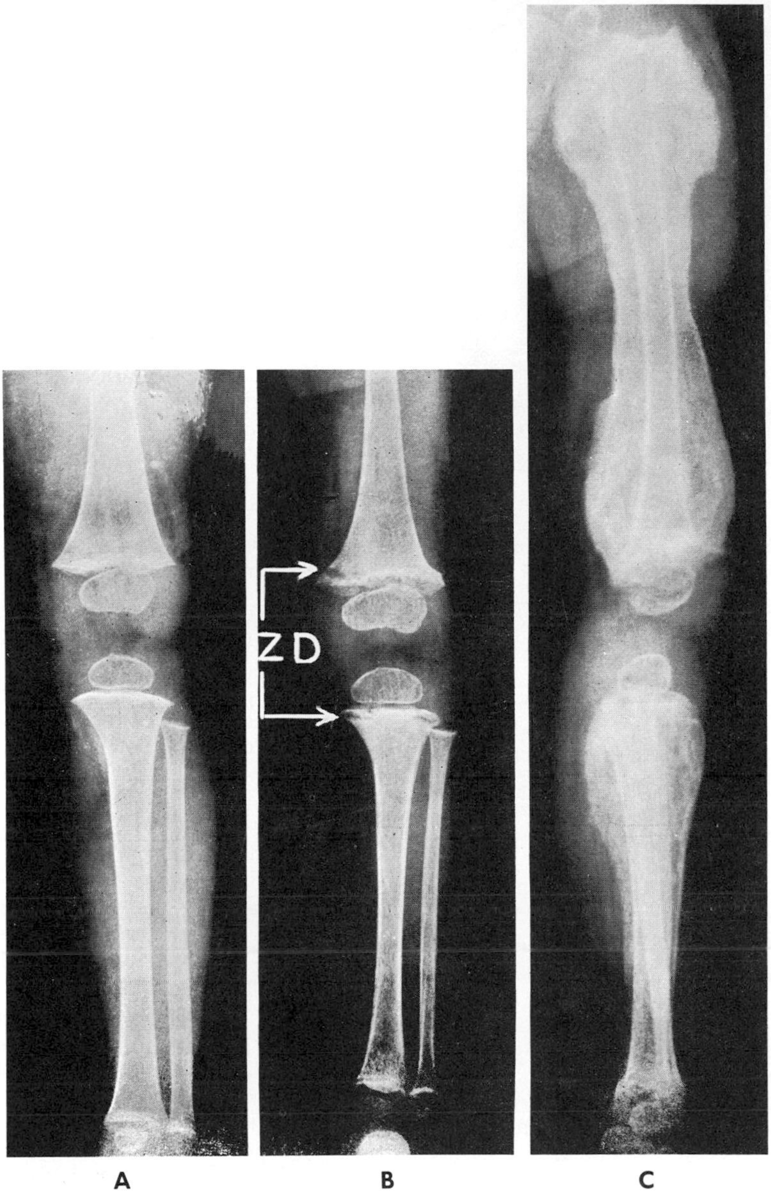

Figure 3–8 *Roentgenograms of leg.* A, *Early scurvy: "white line" is visible on the ends of the shafts of the tibia and fibula; rings around epiphyses of femur and tibia.* B, *More advanced scorbutic changes; zones of destruction (*ZD*) in femur and tibia.* C, *Healing scurvy; calcification of subperiosteal hemorrhages.*

generalized, nonspecific amino-aciduria occurs in children with scurvy, while blood values of amino acids remain normal. After a tyrosine load the scorbutic infant excretes metabolites similar to those of the premature one. These may be detected with Millon's reagent. Tests for capillary fragility, almost always with positive results in scurvy, may give negative results in latent scurvy. Prothrombin time may be markedly increased.

DIFFERENTIAL DIAGNOSIS. The tenderness of the limbs and the pain elicited by movement have often led to a false diagnosis of arthritis or acrodynia. The patient's age aids in differentiating scurvy from rheumatic fever, since rheumatic fever is rare in children under 2 years of age. Suppurative arthritis and osteomyelitis occur in young children and infants and should be considered in the differential diagnosis. The pseudoparalysis of syphilis usually occurs at an earlier age than does that of scurvy and is often accompanied by other signs of syphilis. A roentgenogram aids in the diagnosis. Poliomyelitis causes a true flaccid paralysis, and in infants the exquisite tenderness present in the limbs in scurvy is absent. Henoch-Schönlein purpura, thrombocytopenic purpura, leukemia, meningococcemia, or nephritis may be suspected.

PROGNOSIS. Recovery occurs rapidly in cases

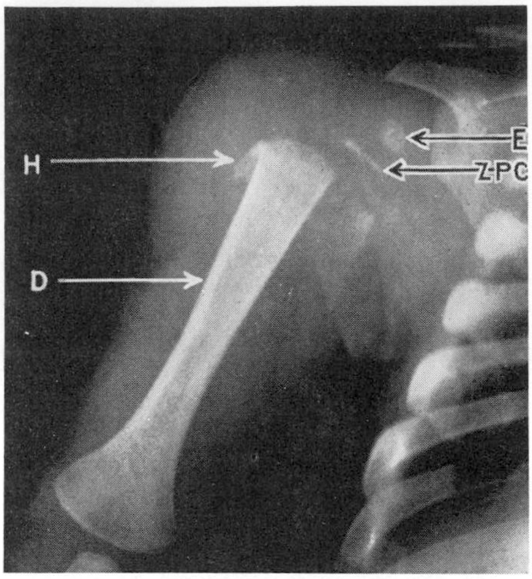

Figure 3-9 *"Slipped diaphysis" in scurvy. The epiphysis (E) of the humerus and calcified cartilage of the zone of primary calcification (ZPC) remained in place and in contact with the glenoid fossa. The diaphysis (D) was displaced laterally and separated from the epiphysis. The shadow (H) at the proximal end of the diaphysis represents beginning calcification of a subperiosteal hemorrhage.*

correctly treated. Pain ceases in a few days, but the swelling caused by subperiosteal hemorrhage may require months to disappear. Body growth is usually quickly resumed. In unrecognized and untreated cases death is likely to occur after a few months from malnutrition, exhaustion, some complication, or intercurrent disease. Permanent deformity from scorbutic lesions is uncommon; even when there has been metaphyseal separation, reconstruction is usually good without orthopedic treatment.

PREVENTION. Scurvy may be prevented by a diet adequate in vitamin C. All infants, even breast-fed ones, should receive ascorbic acid (25 to 50 mg), orange juice (1 to 2 ounces) or fresh or canned tomato juice (2 to 3 ounces) daily, beginning at 2 to 4 weeks of age. Lactating mothers should take generous amounts of vitamin C; a minimum daily intake equal to 150 mg of ascorbic acid has been recommended. A daily intake of 25 to 50 mg of ascorbic acid for infants, 50 mg for children, and 75 mg for adults is considered adequate.

Infections are common in scorbutics, but evidence that unusual intake of vitamin C (1 to 3 gm daily) prevents upper respiratory infections is too tenuous to warrant its use for this purpose.

TREATMENT. The administration of 3 to 4 ounces of orange juice or tomato juice daily will quickly produce healing, but ascorbic acid is preferable. The daily therapeutic dose is 100 to 200 mg or more, orally or parenterally.

Hodges, R. E., Hood, J., Canham, J. E., Sanberlich, H. E., and Baker, E. M.: Clinical manifestations of ascorbic acid deficiency in man. Am. J. Clin. Nutr. *24*:432, 1971.

King, C. G.: Present knowledge of ascorbic acid (vitamin C). Nutr. Rev. *26*:33, 1968.

RICKETS OF VITAMIN D DEFICIENCY*

Rickets is a metabolic disorder of growing bone resulting in bony deformities. In contrast to scurvy, in which the connective tissue is defective but calcification proceeds, rickets is characterized by formation of normal collagen and matrix and of osteoid, with defective mineralization. When ossification improves with administration of vitamin D, the rickets is termed vitamin D-deficient; if no improvement occurs after conventional administration of usual doses of vitamin D, the condition is called vitamin D-resistant or refractory rickets. Vitamin D deficiency produces osteomalacia in nongrowing bone.

ETIOLOGY. Appropriate concentrations of calcium and phosphorus in serum are essential for mineralization of osteoid. Vitamin D participates in both the absorption of calcium from the intestine and the mobilization of calcium from bone. Two forms of vitamin D are active in man: vitamin D_2 (calciferol); and vitamin D_3 (activated 7-dehydrocholesterol or cholecalciferol). There is no vitamin D_1.

Secretions of the human skin contain 7-dehydrocholesterol (provitamin D_3). Under natural living conditions this provitamin is activated by ultraviolet rays of sunlight (296 to 310 nm) and converted into vitamin D, which is absorbed into the blood.

Sunlight which has passed through ordinary window glass is deprived of its antirachitic potency. As a rule, infants in the temperate and arctic zones escape rickets only when they receive a protective amount of vitamin D in their diet.

Dietary vitamin D is absorbed through the lymphatics in the presence of bile and, bound to an alpha-2 globulin, is transported to the liver, where it is stored. In the liver vitamin D_3 is hydroxylated to 25-OH cholecalciferol, which circulates in the plasma and is effective in curing rickets. 25-OH cholecalciferol is converted in the kidney to 1,25- or 24,25-dihydroxycholecalciferol, which acts to initiate both intestinal calcium transport and bone mineral mobilization. Other hydroxylated calciferols may also be active.

Many sterol derivatives have antirachitic value, but only two of them, 7-dehydrocholesterol and ergosterol, are of practical importance. The biologic properties of activated 7-dehydrocholesterol resemble those exhibited by vitamin D preparations of animal origin. Ergosterol is of plant origin and is the sterol found in fungi. Irradiation transforms ergosterol into vitamin D_2 (calciferol), with certain by-products such as tachysterol and lumisterol.

The natural diet of infants contains only small

*Vitamin D-refractory rickets, vitamin D dependency, familial hypophosphatemia, renal osteodystrophy, vitamin D resistant hypoparathyroidism, and metabolic bone disorders simulating rickets are described elsewhere. (See Section 22.)

amounts of vitamin D; breast milk is a poor source and cow's milk contains only 5 to 40 IU per quart. Sugar, cereals, vegetables, and fruits contain only negligible amounts. Egg yolk contains 140 to 390 IU per gm.

Besides lack of vitamin D in the diet or lack of access of skin to ultraviolet irradiation, several factors may predispose to vitamin D deficiency. Rickets or epiphyseal dysplasia may develop during rapid growth, as occurs in premature infants and adolescents.

Black children are singularly susceptible to rickets. Whether this is due to the pigmentation of their skin or to their living conditions has not been determined. Genetic factors are responsible for vitamin D-refractory rickets (Section 22), but there is no evidence that they have any role in vitamin D-deficient rickets.

Children with disorders of absorption, such as celiac disease, steatorrhea, pancreatitis, or cystic fibrosis, may acquire rickets because of failure to absorb vitamin D or calcium, or both. In children with hepatic disease, rickets may develop because of an inability to absorb vitamin D or calcium or because of inability to hydroxylate cholecalciferol. In those with kidney diseases, defective formation or increased destruction of 1,25-dihydroxycholecalciferol may be responsible for defective bone metabolism. Glucocorticoid administration appears to be antagonistic to vitamin D in calcium transport, but the mechanism is independent of vitamin D.

PATHOLOGY. New bone formation is initiated by the osteoblast, which is responsible for matrix deposition and its subsequent mineralization. Osteoblasts secrete collagen, and changes in polysaccharides, phospholipids, alkaline phosphatase and pyrophosphatase follow until mineralization occurs in the presence of adequate calcium and phosphorus. Resorption of bone occurs when osteoclasts secrete enzymes on the bone surface, dissolving and removing matrix and mineral. Osteocytes covered by bone both resorb and redeposit bone. Factors affecting bone growth are poorly understood; phosphorus, calcium, and growth hormone all have some influence on bone growth. Fluoride, which acts on the osteoblastic cell to increase collagen synthesis, promotes bone growth, but the new bone formed is often excessively calcified and irregularly formed.

Defective growth of bone in rickets results from retardation or suppression of normal growth of epiphyseal cartilage and of normal calcification. These changes are dependent upon a decrease in the calcium and phosphorus salts available in the serum for mineralization. Cartilage cells fail to complete their normal cycle of proliferation and degeneration, and subsequent failure of capillary penetration occurs in a patchy manner. The result is a frayed, irregular epiphyseal line at the end of the shaft.

There is also failure of mineralization of osseous and cartilaginous matrix. The zone of preparatory calcification fails to mineralize, and newly formed uncalcified osteoid is deposited. As a result a wide, irregular, frayed zone of nonrigid tissue (the rachitic metaphysis) is produced, composed of noncalcified cartilage and osteoid tissue. This zone is responsible for many of the skeletal deformities. It becomes compressed and bulges laterally, producing flaring of the ends of the bones and the rachitic rosary.

Changes also occur in bone at sites other than the epiphyseal-metaphyseal region. Mineralization is lacking in subperiosteal bone, and a shell of osteoid tissue is formed which surrounds the shaft over its entire length. Pre-existing cortical bone is resorbed in a normal manner, but is replaced by osteoid tissue which fails to mineralize. If this process continues, the shaft loses its rigidity, and the resulting softened and rarefied cortical bone is readily distorted by stress; deformities and fractures result.

Healing Rickets. With healing, degeneration of cartilage cells occurs along the diaphyseal border of the cartilage, capillary penetration of the resultant spaces is resumed, and calcification takes place in the zone of preparatory calcification. This calcification occurs approximately at the line at which normal calcification would have occurred had the rachitic process not supervened, and produces a line clearly demonstrable in roentgen films. As healing progresses, the osteoid tissue between this line of preparatory calcification and the diaphysis also becomes mineralized (Fig. 3–10). Osteoid tissue in the cortex and about the trabeculae in the shaft rapidly becomes mineralized. Months or years may be required to repair the deformities, and in extreme instances complete repair may be impossible.

Chemical Pathology. In healthy infants the inorganic serum phosphorus concentration is 4.5 to 6.5 mg/dl, whereas in rachitic infants it is usually reduced to 1.5 to 3.5 mg. The serum calcium level is usually normal, but under certain conditions it too is reduced, and tetany may develop.

Rickets can be understood if one assumes it to be an attempt of the body to maintain normal serum calcium levels, presumably because calcium is necessary for normal function of nerve, muscle and endocrine glands, and for intercellular bridging. In the absence of vitamin D, less calcium is absorbed from the intestine. With slightly lowered serum calcium, parathormone is secreted. This leads to mobilization of calcium and phosphorus from the bone. The serum calcium is thus maintained, but secondary effects occur, which include the changes of rickets in bone, the lowered serum phosphorus (because parathormone decreases phosphorus reabsorption in the kidney) and the elevated serum phosphatase (from increased osteoblastic activity).

The alkaline phosphatase of serum, which in normal children ranges between 5 and 15 Bodansky units/dl, is elevated in mild rickets to 20 to 30 units/dl and to 60 units or more in severe cases. (For International or other units, see Section 30.) As rickets heals, the phosphatase level returns slowly to normal levels. Serum alkaline phosphatase may be normal in infants with rickets who are

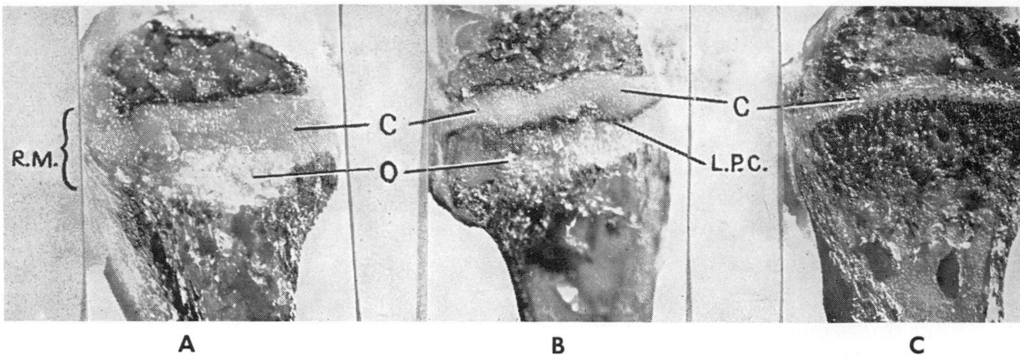

Figure 3–10 Line tests in rats (proximal end of tibia) (calcified tissue stained with silver appears black.) A, Active rickets. The light broad zone between epiphysis and shaft represents the rachitic metaphysis (R.M.); C, cartilage; O, osteoid. B, Healing rickets. Line of preparatory calcification (L.P.C.) between zone of cartilage (C) and osteoid (O). C, Healed rickets. Cartilaginous disk (C) between epiphysis and normal shaft.

protein depleted. With protein repletion, the alkaline phosphatase rises.

Calcium and phosphorus homeostasis depends on dietary calcium and phosphorus. Maximum calcium absorption occurs in man when the ratio of calcium to phosphorus in the diet is about 2:1; increase in phosphate decreases absorption of calcium. Acidity of intestinal contents increases absorption of calcium. An increase in calcium absorption occurs with lactose as the dietary sugar. Chelating agents such as ethylenediaminetetraacetic acid (EDTA) or the phytates of cereals may decrease calcium absorption, and dietary iron may decrease absorption of phosphate. High dietary levels of stearic and palmitic acids, which are poorly absorbed, decrease calcium absorption.

Calcium absorption is facilitated by 1,25-dihydroxycholecalciferol or similar hydroxylated forms of vitamin D. Calcium deficiency alone, however, does not lead to the failure of calcification seen in rickets and osteomalacia; it results only in a diminished amount of bone.

When there is a low serum calcium, owing to deficient absorption of vitamin D or other causes, negative feedback to the parathyroid is lessened and parathormone secretion is increased. Parathormone lowers tubular reabsorption of phosphorus, resulting in hypophosphatemia and hyperphosphaturia. In addition, parathormone mobilizes calcium from the bone through an effect on osteocytes, leading to calcium release from mature bone crystals and a slower effect on bone turnover. It also acts on the kidney to reduce calcium clearance and on the gut to increase calcium absorption. These actions of parathormone involve increased formation of cyclic AMP. The action of parathormone on the bone and gut is enhanced by 1,25-hydroxycholecalciferol. Remodeling of bone occurs continuously. Accordingly, vitamin D is required at all ages.

When serum magnesium is increased, serum calcium is usually increased. Magnesium is necessary for parathormone secretion. Magnesium deficiency may be accompanied by a decreased intestinal response to vitamin D. In magnesium deficiency, increased calcium excretion may lead to renal stone formation.

Calcitonin, which is secreted by the thyroid, inhibits bone resorption and lowers serum calcium in hypercalcemia. Calcitonin activity increases with increasing levels of serum phosphate.

Hyperthyroidism leads to increased release of calcium from bone, secondary to increased remodeling, with variable elevations of serum calcium, phosphorus and alkaline phosphatase. Gonadal hormones depress bone resorption.

Bone resorption is increased in acidosis and decreased in alkalosis. Conversely, when bone is formed from circulating calcium and phosphate, hydrogen ions are released, and when bone is resorbed, calcium and phosphorus buffer hydrogen ions. Carbonate removed from bone during resorption provides further buffering. During resorption the levels of pyrophosphate and of hydroxyproline rise in serum and in urine.

Normal serum calcium levels vary from 9 to 11 mg/dl, but only 5 to 6 mg is ionic; the remainder is nondiffusible and bound to protein. Both neuromuscular irritability and bone metabolism are related more closely to ionic than to total calcium. Acidosis increases ionic calcium. Decreased levels of serum proteins are accompanied by low levels of serum calcium, but ionic calcium may be normal. Normally, levels of serum calcium and phosphorus have an inverse relation. In hyperparathyroidism, however, both may be elevated, and in rickets, depressed. Calcitonin, citrate, and tartrate decrease serum calcium, probably through its deposition in bone. Heparin chelates serum calcium, and its administration may be followed by osteoporosis. Immobilization of the child is followed by mobilization of calcium from the bone and by osteoporosis and hypercalcemia. Osteoporosis may also follow the administration of adrenal cortical steroids; the mechanism is unclear. Magnesium may replace calcium in some biochemical reactions and compete with it in others.

Vitamin D has three probable sites of action in the regulation of calcium and phosphorus metabolism: it increases renal tubular reabsorption of phosphate; it increases intestinal absorption of both calcium and phosphorus; and it has a direct effect on deposition in bone.

Vitamin D deficiency is also accompanied by generalized aminoaciduria, a decrease of citrate in bone and increased urinary excretion of it, decreased ability of the kidneys to make an acid urine, phosphaturia, and occasionally mellituria. The parathyroid glands hypertrophy in rickets. Hemolytic anemia has been associated.

CLINICAL MANIFESTATIONS. After several months of vitamin D deficiency osseous changes of rickets can be recognized. Breast-fed infants whose mothers have osteomalacia may have rickets develop within 2 months. Florid rickets becomes apparent toward the end of the first and during the second year of life. In later childhood clinical rickets is rare.

One of the early signs of rickets is craniotabes. Craniotabes is due to thinning of the inner table of the skull and is detected by pressing firmly over the occiput or posterior parietal bones. A ping-pong ball sensation will be felt. Craniotabes near the suture lines is a normal variant. Premature infants are particularly prone to rickets and to craniotabes. Palpable enlargement of the costochondral junctions (the "rachitic rosary") and thickening of the wrists and ankles are other early evidences of osseous changes. Increased sweating, particularly around the head, may be present.

Advanced Rickets. Signs of advanced rickets are easily recognized.

Head. Craniotabes may disappear before the end of the first year, though the rachitic process continues. The softness of the skull may result in flattening and, at times, permanent asymmetry of the head. The anterior fontanel is larger than normal; its closure may be delayed until after the second year of life. The central parts of the parietal and frontal bones are often thickened, forming prominences or bosses, which give the head a boxlike appearance *(caput quadratum)*. The head may be larger than normal and may remain so throughout life. Eruption of the temporary teeth is sometimes delayed and out of the normal order. There may be defects of the enamel and extensive caries. The permanent teeth which are calcifying may be affected; usually the permanent incisors, canines and first molars show defects of the enamel, especially on the distal portion.

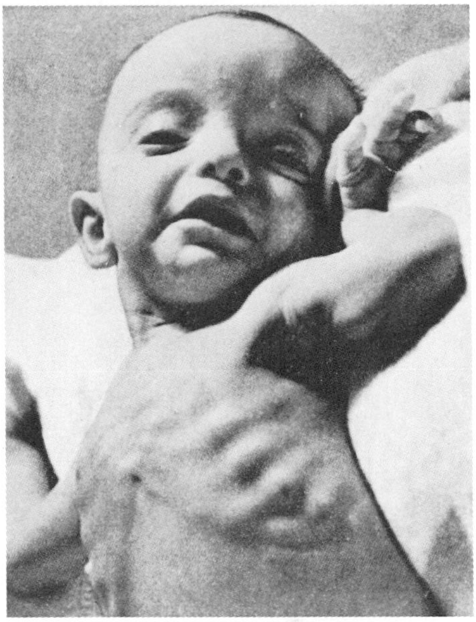

Figure 3–11 Rachitic rosary in a young infant. (Lyons and Wallinger: (Pediatrics and Pediatric Nursing.)

Thorax. In advanced rickets the enlargement of the costochondral junctions may become prominent; in many cases the beading of the ribs is not only palpable, but also visible (Fig. 3–11). The sides of the thorax become flattened, and longitudinal grooves develop posterior to the rosary. The sternum with its adjacent cartilages appears to be projected forward, producing the so-called pigeon breast deformity. Along the lower border of the chest there develops a horizontal depression, Harrison's groove (Fig. 3–12), which corresponds to the costal insertions of the diaphragm. The chest may show a variety of other deformities, and the bones of the shoulder girdle may also be involved.

Spinal Column. Slight to moderate degrees of lateral curvature (scoliosis) are common, and a kyphosis may appear in the dorsolumbar region in rachitic children who sit up (Fig. 3–13). Lordosis of the lumbar region may be seen in the erect position.

Pelvis. In children with lordosis there is

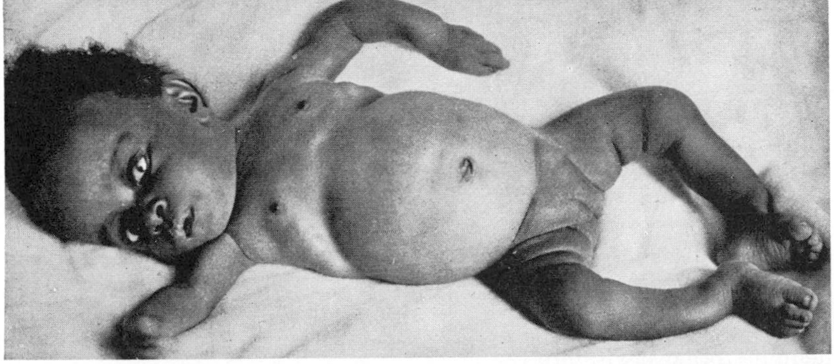

Figure 3–12 Deformities in rickets, showing curvature of the limbs, potbelly and Harrison's groove.

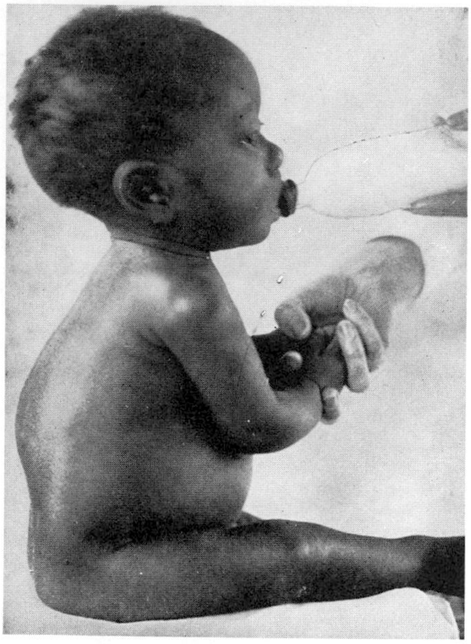

Figure 3–13 Rachitic spinal curvature, well marked when the child is sitting.

frequently a concomitant deformity of the pelvis. The pelvis in rickets is small and continues to be retarded in growth. The pelvic entrance is narrowed by a forward projection of the promontory, and the exit by a forward displacement of the caudal part of the sacrum and the coccyx. In the female these changes, if they become permanent, add to the hazards of childbirth and may necessitate cesarean section.

Extremities. As the rachitic process continues, the epiphyseal enlargements at the wrists and ankles become more noticeable. The enlarged epiphyses can be seen (Fig. 3–14) or palpated, but are not distinct in roentgenograms, since they consist of cartilage and uncalcified osteoid tissue. Bending of the softened shafts of the femur, tibia, and fibula results in bowlegs or knock knees; the femur and the tibia may also show an anterior convexity. Coxa vara is sometimes the result of rickets. Greenstick fractures occur in the long bones, but seldom cause clinical symptoms.

Deformities of the spine, pelvis, and legs result in reduction in height of the body, *rachitic dwarfism.*

Ligaments. Relaxation of ligaments aids in producing deformities. It partly accounts for the production of knock knees, overextension of the knee joints, weak ankles, kyphosis, and scoliosis.

Muscles. The muscles are poorly developed and lacking in tone. As a result, children with moderately severe rickets are late in standing and walking. The common condition of potbelly (Figs. 3–12 and 3–14) depends to a large extent upon weakness of the abdominal muscles; weakness of the gastric and intestinal walls aids in its production.

DIAGNOSIS. The diagnosis of rickets is based on a history of inadequate intake of vitamin D and on clinical observation and is confirmed by serum chemical determinations and roentgenographic examination. The serum calcium level may be normal or low, the serum phosphorus level is below 4 mg/dl, and the serum alkaline phosphatase is usually elevated.

Roentgenographic Changes. *Active Rickets.* A roentgenogram of the wrist is best for early diagnosis, since characteristic changes of the ulna and the radius occur at an early stage. The distal ends of the radius and the ulna appear widened, concave (cupping), and frayed, in contrast to the normally sharply demarcated and slightly convex ends. The distance between the distal ends of the ulna and the radius and the metacarpal bones is increased, since the large rachitic metaphysis, which is not calcified, does not appear on the roentgenogram. The density of the shafts is decreased, but the trabeculae are unusually prominent. In Figure 3–15, *A*, two dense areas are seen in the ulna and represent callus formation at sites of healing fractures. The outer contour of the radius appears double and could be mistaken for "periostitis." The double contour represents, however, the layer of osteoid tissue formed by the periosteum, and not an inflammatory process.

Healing Rickets. Beginning healing is indicated by the appearance of the line of preparatory calcification (Fig. 3–15, *B*). This line is separated from the distal end of the shaft by a zone of decreased calcification, the zone of the osteoid tissue. As healing progresses and the osteoid tissue becomes calcified, the shaft "grows" toward the line of preparatory calcification (Fig. 3–15, *C*) until it becomes united with it (Fig. 3–15, *D*).

DIFFERENTIAL DIAGNOSIS. Nonrachitic craniotabes is sometimes present in the immediate postnatal period, but it tends to disappear before rachitic softening of the skull would become manifest

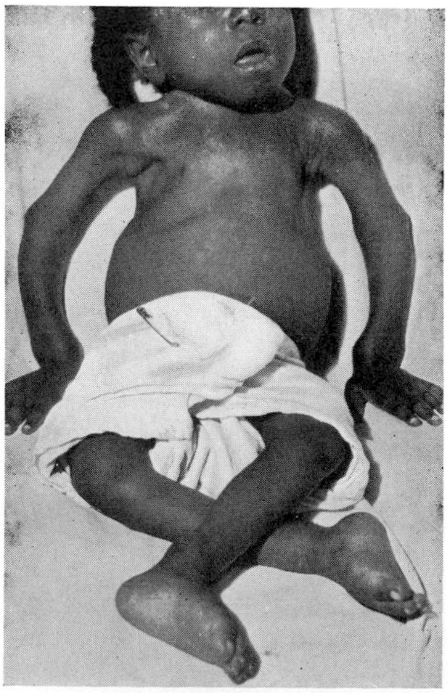

Figure 3–14 Curvature of arms, deformed "violin-shaped" chest, potbelly, enlarged epiphyses in a child 3 years of age.

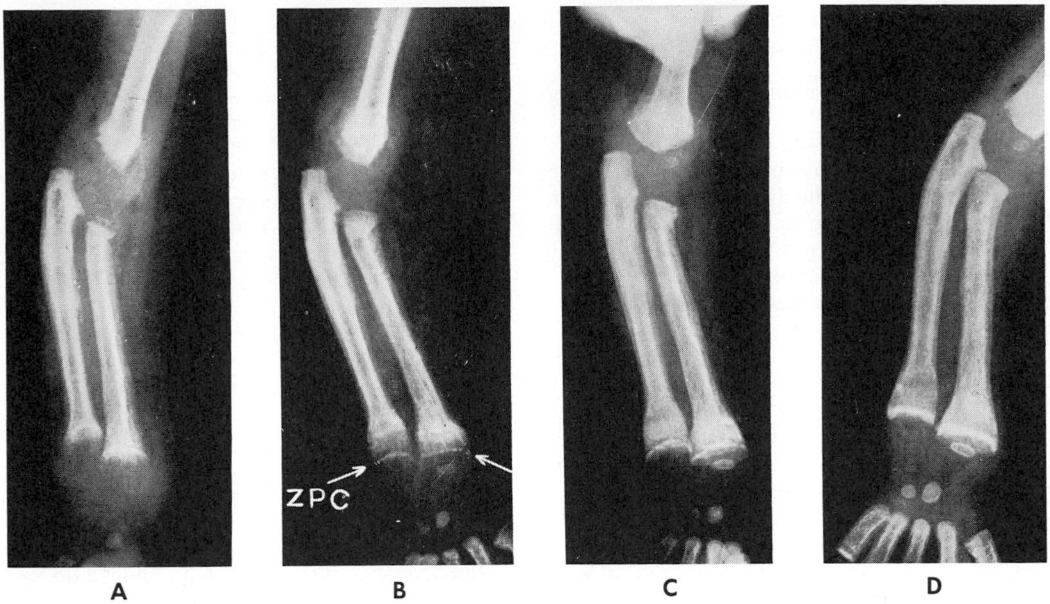

Figure 3–15 A, *Active rickets; cupping and fraying of distal ends of radius and ulna; double contour along lateral outline of radius (periosteal osteoid). The 2 dense zones in the shaft of the ulna are calluses of greenstick fractures.* B, *Healing rickets after 12 days of treatment with vitamin D. Zones of preparatory calcification (ZPC); above them in the rachitic metaphyses there is beginning calcification.* C, *Healing rickets after 18 days of treatment. The zones of preparatory calcification are well defined, and the rachitic metaphyses appear well calcified. The epiphysis of the radius has become visible.* D, *Healing rickets after 29 days of treatment. Zones of preparatory calcification, rachitic metaphyses and shafts have become united.*

(second to fourth months of life). Craniotabes also occurs in hydrocephalus and osteogenesis imperfecta, but it is not difficult to differentiate these conditions from rickets.

Enlargement of the costochondral junctions occurs in rickets, scurvy, and chondrodystrophy. The enlargements in rickets are rounded knobs, whereas in scurvy there is a ledgelike depression with the chondral or sternal portion lower than the osseous. In chondrodystrophy there may be irregular concave outlines of the distal ends of the bones, but there is no roentgenographic evidence of fraying. It is sometimes difficult to distinguish rachitic deformities of the chest from congenital deformities. Bowlegs can be the result of rickets, but may be a familial characteristic. Vitamin D-resistant rickets and other metabolic disturbances with osseous lesions resembling rickets must be differentiated. (See Section 22.)

COMPLICATIONS. Respiratory infections such as bronchitis and bronchopneumonia are common in rachitic infants. Pulmonary atelectasis is not infrequently associated with severe deformities of the chest.

Chronic gastroenteric disturbances are common; there may be diarrhea or constipation, or the two may alternate.

Anemia due to iron deficiency or accompanying infections often develops in severe rickets.

PROGNOSIS. Though "spontaneous" healing of mild rickets often occurs from exposure to sunshine, severe cases require more energetic treatment. If sufficient amounts of vitamin D are administered, healing begins within a few days and progresses until the normal bony structure is restored. Recovery, however, from the bony deformities is slow; in many instances the enlargement of the epiphyses and of the rosary and the deformities of the skull disappear only after months or years of treatment. Even rather severe bowing of the legs may correct itself after several years of vitamin treatment, without osteotomies. In advanced cases there may be permanent osseous alterations in the form of bowlegs, knock knees, curvature of the upper arms, deformities of the chest and spine, rachitic pelvis, rachitic coxa vara, and even dwarfism.

Rickets in itself is not a fatal disease, but complications and intercurrent infections such as tetany, pneumonia, tuberculosis, and enteritis are more likely to cause death in rachitic than in normal children.

PREVENTION. Rickets can be prevented by exposure to ultraviolet light or by oral administration of vitamin D. Sunlight, as a prophylactic agent, can be considered effective in the temperate zones only during the summer months in haze-free areas.

The daily requirement of vitamin D is estimated to be 400 IU per day. Much of the whole milk available in urban areas and evaporated milk are fortified by the addition of vitamin D concentrate, so that 1 quart of fresh, whole milk or a can of evaporated milk contains 400 IU of vitamin D. It would seem reasonable not to rely upon vitamin D milk alone, but to provide added protection by the administration of 400 IU of vitamin D in a concentrate. Vitamin D should be given to breast-fed as well as bottle-fed infants, and full-term as well as premature infants, beginning at about 5 to 10 days of age.

Vitamin D should be administered to the pregnant or lactating mother.

TREATMENT. Natural and artificial light are effective therapeutically, but oral administration of vitamin D is preferred. The daily administration of 1500 to 5000 IU (6 to 20 drops of a preparation containing 10,000 units per gm) will produce healing demonstrable on roentgenograms within 2 to 4 weeks except in the unusual cases of vitamin D-refractory rickets.

The feeding of 600,000 units of vitamin D in a single dose, and no further vitamin for several months, may be advantageous. This is followed by more rapid healing, possibly prompt differential diagnosis from resistant rickets, and less dependence on the parents. If no healing occurs within 2 weeks, the dose may be repeated once. If still no healing occurs, the rickets is resistant to vitamin D. After healing is complete the dose of vitamin D should be lowered to 400 units daily.

Aurbach, G. D., and Chase, L. R.: Cyclic 3,5′-adenylic acid in bone and the mechanism of action of parathyroid hormone. Fed. Proc. *29*:1179, 1970.

DeLuca, H. F.: Vitamin D: A new look at an old vitamin. Nutr. Rev. *29*:179, 1971.

Harris, W. H., and Heaney, R. P.: Skeletal renewal and metabolic bone disease. New Engl. J. Med. *280*:193, 253, 1969.

Lapatsanis, P., Deliyanni, V., and Doxiadis, S.: Vitamin D deficiency rickets in Greece. J. Pediatr. *73*:195, 1968.

Raisz, L. G.: Physiologic and pharmacologic regulations of bone resorption. New Engl. J. Med. *282*:909, 1970.

Rasmussen, H.: Cell communication, calcium ion, and cyclic adenosine monophosphate. Science *170*:404, 1970.

TETANY OF VITAMIN D DEFICIENCY
(Infantile Tetany)

Tetany due to deficiency of vitamin D is an occasional accompaniment of rickets. Formerly relatively common, it is now rare, owing to the widespread prophylactic use of vitamin D. Tetany is also an infrequent manifestation of vitamin D-refractory rickets. Occasionally it is observed in association with celiac disease, probably as a result of deficient absorption of both vitamin D and calcium. Tetany of vitamin D deficiency occurs most frequently between the ages of 4 months and 3 years; rarely is it observed before 3 months of age. Acute infections or hepatitis may precipitate an attack of tetany.

CHEMICAL PATHOLOGY. When the serum calcium level falls below 7 to 7.5 mg/dl there is muscular irritability, apparently due to the loss of the inhibitory control which the ionized calcium of the serum exerts upon the neuromuscular junctions. Why serum calcium is decreased in some infants or children with rickets is not clear; failure of the parathyroids to compensate for the low serum calcium level may occur. Tetany also occasionally occurs in infants with rickets shortly after vitamin D treatment has been started. This is assumed to be due to a rapid depletion of serum calcium secondary to increased deposition of calcium in the rachitic osteoid tissue and perhaps also to a decrease in parathyroid activity.

CLINICAL MANIFESTATIONS. The symptoms are those of tetany, irrespective of the cause. (See Section 19.) Vitamin D-deficient tetany may exist in either a latent or a clinically manifest stage. In practically all instances there are manifestations of rickets.

Latent Tetany. There are no evident symptoms, but they can be elicited by means of the Chvostek, Trousseau and Erb procedures. (See Section 19.) The serum calcium level is less than 7 to 7.5 mg/dl.

Manifest Tetany. Spontaneous clinical manifestations include carpopedal spasm, laryngospasm, and convulsions. The serum calcium level is often well under 7mg/dl.

DIAGNOSIS. The diagnosis is based on the combination of rickets, low serum calcium level, and the symptoms of tetany. The serum phosphorus level may be low, normal or elevated; the serum phosphatase level is increased. In the differential diagnosis other causes of tetany must be eliminated.

PROGNOSIS. The prognosis is good unless treatment is delayed. Death rarely occurs in tetany, though it may result from laryngospasm and possibly from cardiac dilatation, as so-called cardiac tetany.

PREVENTION. Prophylactic treatment is identical to that for rickets (see above).

TREATMENT. Active treatment is designed to raise the serum calcium above the tetany level. This level may be attained by administration of calcium chloride in 1 or 2 per cent solution in milk. For the first day or two, 4 to 6 gm daily may be given in 1-gm doses, the initial dose being 2 or 3 gm; smaller doses of 1 to 3 gm a day should then be continued for a week or two. Calcium chloride in more concentrated solution may cause severe gastric ulceration. Large doses of calcium chloride may cause acidosis. Calcium lactate may be added to milk in doses of 10 to 12 gm a day for 10 days. When oral medication is impractical, calcium gluconate (5 to 10 ml of a 10 per cent solution) can be administered intravenously, but not subcutaneously or intramuscularly because of the dangers of local necrosis.

Oxygen inhalation is indicated during convulsive seizures. When intravenous administration of calcium gluconate does not quickly control the attacks, sodium phenobarbital may be given intramuscularly. (For dosage see Convulsive Disorders, Section 19.) Prolonged attacks of laryngospasm are usually controlled by sedation and the administration of calcium salts. Intubation is only occasionally necessary. After the acute manifestations have been controlled, administration of vitamin D in daily doses of 2000 to 5000 IU should be started and the oral administration of calcium continued (see above). When the rickets is healed, the dose of vitamin D should be decreased to the usual prophylactic one.

Fraser, D., Kook, S. W., and Scriver, C. R.: Hyperparathyroidism as the cause of hyperaminoaciduria and phosphaturia in human vitamin D deficiency. Pediat. Res. *1*:425, 1967.

HYPERVITAMINOSIS D

Ingestion of excessive amounts of vitamin D results in signs and symptoms similar to those of idiopathic hypercalcemia (Section 22), which may be due to hypersensitivity to vitamin D. Symptoms develop after 1 to 3 months of large intakes of vitamin D; they include hypotonia, anorexia, irritability, constipation, polydipsia, polyuria, and pallor. Hypercalcemia and hypercalciuria are notable. Evidences of dehydration are usually present. Aortic valvular stenosis, vomiting, hypertension, retinopathy, and clouding of the cornea and conjunctiva may occur.

The urine may contain albumin. With continued excessive intake, renal damage and metastatic calcification occur. Roentgenograms of the long bones reveal metastatic calcification and generalized osteoporosis.

Excessive intake of vitamin D may result from inadvertently substituting a concentrated form of vitamin D for a more dilute preparation, from increase of a prescribed dose by a parent ("if a little is good, a lot is better") and from inadequate control of dosage in children receiving large amounts of vitamin D for chronic hypophosphatemic states. (See Section 22.)

DIFFERENTIAL DIAGNOSIS. This includes chronic nephritis, hyperparathyroidism and idiopathic hypercalcemia. All may cause metastatic calcifications, and the latter two are accompanied by hypercalcemia.

PREVENTION. Prevention consists in careful evaluation of vitamin D dosage.

TREATMENT. This includes discontinuance of vitamin D intake and a decrease in intake of calcium. For severely involved infants, aluminum hydroxide by mouth, cortisone, or sodium versenate may be used.

Forbes, G. B., Cafarelli, C., and Manning, J.: Vitamin D and infantile hypercalcemia. Pediatrics *42*:203, 1968.

VITAMIN E DEFICIENCY

Vitamin E deficiency leads to varied effects in different animal species. It is a fat-soluble antioxidant and may be involved in nucleic acid metabolism. No precise biochemical action of vitamin E (α-tocopherol) has been found; it resembles in many of its actions ubiquinone (coenzyme Q), but is structurally unrelated. Vitamin E is widely present in foods.

Deficiency may occur in malabsorption states such as cystic fibrosis or acanthocytosis. Diets with a high unsaturated fatty acid content increase the vitamin E requirement in premature infants. Premature infants absorb vitamin E poorly. Excess iron administration exaggerates signs of vitamin E deficiency.

Vitamin E serum levels are low in patients with biliary atresia. This has been used as a presumptive test for biliary atresia.

Some patients deficient in vitamin E have creatinuria, ceroid deposition in smooth muscle, focal necrosis of striated muscle, and muscle weakness. Some improvement may occur after administration of vitamin E. Vitamin E deficiency has been suggested as a causative factor in the anemia of kwashiorkor. Premature infants may have low serum levels of tocopherol, with development of a hemolytic anemia at 6 to 10 weeks of age which is corrected by administration of vitamin E.

DIAGNOSIS. Blood levels of vitamin E reflect vitamin E status. If vitamin E has recently been administered, three days should elapse before determining blood levels, as oral vitamin E may circulate for one to two days. An in vitro hemolysis test adds peroxide to the patient's erythrocytes, the peroxidizability of the red cells reflecting the vitamin E status.

PREVENTION. Minimal daily requirements of vitamin E are not known; 1 mg per 0.6 gm of unsaturated fat in the diet appears adequate. Intake should be increased in children with deficient fat absorption. Premature infants should receive at least 5 mg daily.

Melhorn, D. K., and Gross, S.: Vitamin E-dependent anemia in the premature infant. I. Effects of large doses of medicinal iron. J. Pediatr. *79*:569, 1971.
Oski, F. A., and Barness, L. A.: Vitamin E deficiency: A previously unrecognized cause of hemolytic anemia in the premature infant. J. Pediatr. *70*:211, 1967.

VITAMIN K DEFICIENCY

Vitamin K is a naphthoquinone which participates in oxidative phosphorylation. The exact function of vitamin K is uncertain; absence of the vitamin or failure of its absorption from the intestinal tract results in hypoprothrombinemia and decreased hepatic synthesis of proconvertin. Prothrombin (factor II) and proconvertin (factor VII) are important to the second stage of coagulation. (See Section 14.) The second stage of coagulation is studied by the one-stage prothrombin time (Quick). Administration of vitamin K to the newborn infant increases levels of prothrombin, proconvertin, plasma thromboplastin component (factor IX, PTC), and Stuart-Prower factor (factor X).

SOURCES OF VITAMIN K. Naturally occurring vitamin K is fat-soluble and found in high concentrations in hog's liver, soybeans, and alfalfa, and in smaller amounts in some vegetables such as spinach, tomatoes, and kale. The natural vitamin, whose formula is 2-methyl-3-phytyl-1,4-

naphthoquinone, has been labeled vitamin K_1 to distinguish it from synthetic naphthoquinones with vitamin K activity.

Many bacteria, including normal intestinal flora, are capable of synthesizing quinones with vitamin K activity. Suppression of intestinal bacteria by various antibiotics may be responsible for vitamin K deficiency, with resultant diminution of prothrombin. Radiated foods have been related to vitamin K deficiency in animals. Cow's milk has more vitamin K than human milk.

CLINICAL MANIFESTATIONS. Deficiency of vitamin K, or hypoprothrombinemia, should be considered in all patients with a hemorrhagic disturbance. The incidence of hemorrhagic disease of the newborn (q. v.) has been markedly decreased by the prophylactic administration of vitamin K. Vitamin K deficiency in childhood is usually due to factors affecting absorption or utilization of fat, or to factors limiting synthesis of vitamin K in the intestine, such as prolonged use of antibiotics. Diseases of the liver may lead to hypoprothrombinemia; in these cases hypoprothrombinemia does not usually respond to administration of vitamin K.

Hypoprothrombinemia may also result from administration of certain drugs. Dicumarol, obtained from spoiled sweet clover, is used specifically for the production of hypoprothrombinemia in the prevention and treatment of venous thrombosis. Bishydroxycoumarin (Dicumarol) is thought to prevent the liver from utilizing vitamin K and to have no direct effect on prothrombin. Blood prothrombin is continually destroyed in the body; since Dicumarol prevents its replacement, a fall in prothrombin occurs. If a dangerously low level results, massive doses of vitamin K_1 may be necessary to restore the prothrombin to the normal level; whole blood transfusions may be necessary.

Salicylic acid, a degradation product of Dicumarol, produces hypoprothrombinemia by similar action. The fall in prothrombin resulting from the use of salicylates, however, is only mild as compared with that brought about by Dicumarol. The hemorrhagic manifestations in acute rheumatic fever may be due in some instances to large doses of salicylates. Vitamin K is effective in neutralizing this action of salicylates, and its routine use in children receiving large doses of salicylates is recommended.

TREATMENT. Mild prothrombin deficiency may be corrected by oral administration of vitamin K. One to 2 mg daily for an infant will usually suffice. If prothrombin deficiency is severe and hemorrhagic manifestations have appeared, vitamin K_1, 5 mg daily, should be given parenterally. Large doses of synthetic vitamin K analogues, but not of vitamin K_1, may result in hyperbilirubinemia and kernicterus in the glucose-6-phosphate dehydrogenase (G-6-PD) deficient newborn, and in the premature infant. When hypoprothrombinemia is due to liver damage, vitamin K_1 may be given, but whole blood is usually necessary.

LEWIS A. BARNESS

Babior, B. M.: Role of vitamin K in clotting factor synthesis. Biochim. Biophys. Acta *123*:606, 1966.

4

PREVENTIVE PEDIATRICS AND HYGIENE

PREVENTIVE PEDIATRICS

Organization of preventive services for children began in the late nineteenth century with attention to provision of bacteriologically safe cow's milk to combat the most serious health problem of childhood at that time—infantile diarrhea. Early in the twentieth century the development of immunization procedures gave further impetus to preventive services. Today the scope of preventive pediatrics embraces whatever will enable each child to reach his full physical, emotional, and intellectual potential. Pediatrics has been more concerned with preventive services than any other clinical specialty; today over 50 per cent of the time of most practicing pediatricians is spent in preventive services.

DEFINITION. Prevention of illness in children occurs at five levels: (1) promotion of general health (e.g., nutrition, hygiene); (2) prevention of specific diseases (e.g., immunizations); (3) early diagnosis of asymptomatic disease, so as to permit early therapy and prevent sequelae (e.g., screening tests for vision and hearing); (4) early diagnosis and appropriate therapy of symptomatic disease to prevent sequelae (e.g., diagnosis and therapy of streptococcal infections to prevent rheumatic fever); and (5) prevention of unnecessary disability due to established symptomatic disease (e.g., rehabilitation to prevent contractures or emotional crippling in cerebral palsy). In addition to providing such preventive services for the individual child, the pediatrician should work as an advocate for all children, to see that the community provides an environment for optimal development of children. The preventive point of view in pediatrics should embrace all of health care; its impact should be felt not only at those visits to the physician for which the main purpose is a preventive service, such as the so-called well-child visit, but at every medical contact with a child. For example, if parents are alerted to hazards observed during a home visit for an acute illness, more can often be done to prevent accidents than by exhortation in the office.

SCOPE AND GOALS. To have significant impact, preventive services must be related to the health problems most prevalent in the community. Specific programs will therefore vary from place to place, population to population, and time to time. Health problems include those that cause death, acute or chronic disease, functional disabilities of emotional or social nature, or other kinds of distress and dissatisfaction. The principal causes of death and of acute and chronic diseases are listed in Tables 1–1 to 1–5. Table 4–1 indicates how common the conditions may be which underlie emotional, social, and intrafamilial disability and distress. To promote the optimal functioning of each child, the physician will need to "help parents become capable and self confident, to build good parent relations, and to promote family well being" (Standards of Child Health Care, 1972).

Not all preventive health services are best administered by the physician. Many, such as provision of safe water and milk, are community responsibilities. Other preventive services first introduced at the personal level have with time been transferred to the community level (e.g.,

TABLE 4–1 SOCIAL ENVIRONMENT OF CHILDREN (NEWCASTLE 1000 FAMILY STUDY: BIRTH TO 4 YEARS)

	PER 1000 CHILDREN	
Deprivation of Parental Care	452	
Permanent loss of one or both parents		74
Temporary loss of one or both parents		105
Mothers working full-time		142
Parents incapacitated by illness		121
Marital instability		137
Deficiency of Care		
Defective diet, cleanliness, supervision	160	
Social Dependence	202	
Unemployment for more than 3 months		153
National assistance		70
Crime		23
Delinquency, truancy, corrective supervision		53

From Miller, F. J. W., Court, S. D. M., Walton, W. S., and Knox, E. G.: Growing up in Newcastle-upon-Tyne. Oxford, Nuffield Press, 1960.

fluoridation of water supplies) because they can be safely and more efficiently implemented in this way. Some personal preventive services are best provided by pediatric nurse practitioners and other health workers.

Since pediatrics is concerned with the well-being of all children, not just those who readily come to physicians, it is appropriate to lodge responsibility for certain preventive services with community agencies, especially those services that do not depend upon an established professional relation between physician and patient for their success. At certain periods in their life children represent captive populations (e.g., in the neonatal period and in school); at these times all can be relatively easily reached for certain technical procedures. The individual physician should not devote his time to tasks that others can perform more efficiently, but should seek to use his specialized or unique skills or his particular professional relationships to individual patients where they are most needed and can be most productive. The allocation of responsibility for defined groups of children will help to ensure that all children in specified groups receive preventive services, not only those who voluntarily come to the physician.

Since not all children have the same risk of development of any given disease, to deliver all preventive services at the same level of intensity to all children is inefficient. For instance, the mother of a third child in an upper middle-class family, who has successfully reared previous children and whose infant is the result of a normal pregnancy and delivery with no evidence of congenital disease by 6 months of age, will have considerably less need for certain aspects of counseling during the so-called well-child visits than would the mother of a first-born premature infant of a lower socioeconomic class. The shortage of health personnel, their inefficient distribution and concern for rising costs of care demand that we be more discriminating in our use of preventive services.

This concept of varying degrees of vulnerability has led to the development of "high-risk registries" in certain areas. These are usually developed at a community level and identify children who at birth have a high risk of disease in subsequent months or years (e.g., premature infants of mothers with unfavorable obstetric history, children with anomalies or defects detected during the neonatal period). The physician should build his own high-risk registry in order to give such children more careful attention and to be certain that they are receiving preventive or remedial care.

CONDUCT OF PREVENTIVE CHILD HEALTH SERVICES

Visits for preventive services (so-called well-child visits) constitute 40 to 60 per cent of all visits to pediatricians in the United States. In most other countries these preventive services are carried out at physical locations and by personnel both different from those concerned with treatment of acute or chronic illness. There is no evidence that the American pattern is more effective; on the other hand, since 10 to 30 per cent of children who come for well-child visits are actually sick, it seems potentially useful to have both curative and preventive services centralized and supervised by a single person or team. Knowledge of the whole child and his family is more comfortably gained in this setting, which may be the office of the private physician, of a group practice, or of a clinic providing comprehensive care. There are many preventive services which should be given by others than physician members of the health team, and certain screening tests which should be utilized with large groups of children when possible; these considerations do not deny the advantages of and need for a central responsible source of coordinated medical care for each child.

The American Academy of Pediatrics has recommended the following schedule of well-child visits:

Prenatal—Initial contact with pediatrician urged.

Birth—At least two examinations in the hospital: one within the first 24 hours, the second just before discharge.

First 6 months—Monthly visits.

Second 6 months—Visits every 2 months.

Second year of life—Four visits.

Two to 6 years—One or two visits a year.

After 6 years—Annual visits.

For many children the most vulnerable period is the first 4 to 6 weeks of life, and more frequent contact may be necessary than recommended above, at least by telephone. Many later visits will be for immunizations and simple screening tests that can be accomplished in the low-risk patient by the physician's assistant. There is increasing skepticism that all infants need as many visits as previously recommended; low-risk populations may need less, and high-risk populations more. The "routine" physical examination at each visit has also been shown to yield very few new diagnoses and need be performed only two to three times in the first year unless family history, symptoms, or screening tests suggest possible emerging abnormalities. Aggressive follow-up of patients, or outreach, is often needed to reach those most in need. A commitment to a community or population approach should ensure that all children are reached and that effective services are given, rather than that ineffective services are wasted on the few.

For some disorders (e.g., those of vision or hearing) diagnosis should be made long before entry into school if developmental problems such as amblyopia or speech problems (see pp. 1576 and 120) are to be prevented. The physician is principally responsible for such detection in the preschool period, and his preventive services may be critical. The screening of school-age children for defects of vision or hearing, and group psychologic testing, can be done best in the school; but communication must be maintained and treatment coordinated between the school and the child's physician.

SCREENING TESTS. Screening tests should separate from groups of apparently healthy persons those with a high probability of having defects. Such tests should be simple to perform, inexpensive, and yield few false negative or false positive responses. In addition, they should identify health problems for which effective prevention or therapy exists.

The accurate recording of *height* and *weight* on a growth chart (p. 39) constitutes the most important screening procedure. Since growth rate is most rapid in the first year and during preadolescence, the frequency of measurements should be greatest at these times, but they should be recorded at least annually through the rest of childhood. During the first year head circumference should be recorded at each visit.

Screening for visual acuity (p. 1570) can be done from approximately 3 years of age; for squint, much earlier. Between 5 and 10 per cent of preschool children have some visual impairment; the number increases to 30 per cent at school age. The illiterate E charts, Allen cards* or the "Stycar" set are adequate to screen for visual acuity in the preschool period. After 5 to 6 years of age an ordinary Snellen chart can be used. Good lighting, a 20-foot distance, and proper cover for the occluded eye are important technical points. Difficulty in completing a screening test for visual acuity in the child 3 to 6 years of age should suggest behavior problems, perceptual problems, or developmental retardation. Latent squint should be looked for by cover tests.

Screening tests for *hearing* (p. 119) are difficult, but since about 1 per cent of young school children have hearing impairments, such screening is important. At 4 to 6 months of age hearing can be tested by having the child sit on his mother's lap, facing another person. The examiner stands behind the child and crackles tissue paper, spins a rattle, or utters k-k-k, s-s-s or buh-buh sounds. The child who hears will turn toward this sound. After this age the most useful screening tests are the mother's suspicion of hearing loss, a family history of hearing loss, or in the older child the repeated turning up in volume of radio or television. Retardation or defects in speech or repeated ear infections always call for evaluation of hearing. Since most offices and clinics are too noisy for confident use of the three-tone screening audiometer, most audiologists recommend formal hearing tests.

Developmental assessment and diagnosis can be carried out by a variety of tests. The most useful for the pediatrician are the Denver Developmental Screening Test (Section 30) and the Knobloch Developmental Test. After the age of 5 years the Draw-a-Man Test is a useful screening test, as are the Amman's Quick Test and the Sprigle School Readiness Test. Behavior problems are best identified through an adequate history from the mother or teacher; a simple questionnaire is useful (Standards of Child Health Care, 1972). Early assessment of maternal competence is most important for those children likely to suffer neglect or child abuse. No good standards exist as yet for this assessment, but some historical facts (frequent accidents, use of multiple sources of health care) and clinical assessment of the mother's feelings and attitudes allow the experienced physician or nurse to identify some high-risk families.

Urinalysis is a traditional screening test, but the number of treatable conditions detected by routine test is low. The "dip stick" tests for protein and glucose are simple and adequate. The justification for a screening microscopic examination is debatable; in girls it seems wise at least once during the school years to perform a *quantitative urine culture,* rather than to rely on microscopic examination for white blood cells to exclude bacteriuria. The treatment of girls with significant bacteriuria seems wise, but the benefits or long-term results are not yet clear.

Tuberculin tests give increasingly fewer positive reactions, so that a positive test is likely to identify significantly infected children; their early detection and identification of their contacts are important both for therapy and prophylaxis. Positive reactors today in suburban areas number under 1 per cent even by high school age, but the test is so simple and reliable that it should be done yearly. In groups of children at high risk (low income, disadvantaged) vigorous efforts should be made to see that all are screened. Mantoux tests using O.T. or P.P.D. or tine tests are very effective. The Vollmer patch test is not reliable.

Either the microhematocrit or the falling-drop copper sulfate method is an adequate screening test for *anemia* and should be performed in high-risk infants at 9 to 12 months and 2 years of age.

The only *biochemical abnormality* that is presently tested for routinely is phenylketonuria, through examination of blood of the newborn infant after milk feedings are begun. In the future considerable numbers of other screening tests may become available; if several screening tests for rare diseases with potential for successful treatment (galactosemia, Wilson's disease, etc.) could be done on single samples, the yield might become high enough to generate more enthusiasm for such methods.

Screening for *lead poisoning* is recommended for children of 18 months to 5 years of age living in old or dilapidated housing, where 5 to 10 per cent of children will have abnormally high blood levels of lead. There is no entirely satisfactory screening test; children living in "lead belts" must have blood lead levels determined. No other test is sufficiently reliable. Recent development of micromethods for blood lead will make this more feasible.

Sickle cell trait and *G6PD* (glucose 6-phosphate dehydrogenase) deficiency are much more common in black populations than other biochemical abnormalities. Reliable micromethods for screening tests are now available. Detection of G6PD defi-

---

*Available from Ophthalmic Corporation, LaGrange, Illinois.

ciency is especially important for prevention of hemolytic anemia on administration of certain drugs. All black children should be screened once for each of these conditions, the results recorded in their medical records, and their parents informed and counseled.

PREVENTIVE MEASURES AT DIFFERENT AGE PERIODS

There are general features of preventive services appropriate to each age period of childhood. (See also sections 2 and 7.)

PRENATAL AND NEONATAL PERIODS

No greater benefit to children could occur than the development of effective methods to prevent prematurity (low birth weight) and congenital malformations. Effective prevention starts before conception; there is evidence that the early life of the mother, her childhood nutrition, and her pattern of living are related to her reproductive efficiency. Preventive services to children may do much to prevent problems of the perinatal period for the next generation, including genetic counseling of adolescents and young adults. (See page 317.)

During pregnancy the maintenance of good maternal nutrition, the early diagnosis and adequate management of maternal infections, the cautious use of drugs and the minimal use of radiation, along with identification of the high-risk mother (blood group incompatibility, maternal diabetes, etc.), and a safe, atraumatic delivery are largely in the hands of the obstetrician; yet these things may have great impact upon the child's subsequent health. Pediatrician and obstetrician should encompass the field of perinatology as a joint enterprise. Many pediatricians meet prospective parents at a prenatal visit in order to ultimately establish better physician-patient relations, to promote attitudes favoring the mental health of the child, to determine any potentiality for genetic disease, and to help the family to prepare physically and emotionally for the new baby.

Amniocentesis can detect some congenital and genetic abnormalities as early as the 13th to 15th week of gestation. If it is acceptable, therapeutic abortion can then prevent the birth of severely damaged babies. Most work in this field has involved rare inborn errors of metabolism, but greater benefits to the affected family and to the community may come from routine search by this method for trisomy-21 in pregnancies in women over 35 or 40 years of age, where the risk of Down's syndrome is 1 to 2 per cent. Prevention of abnormal births by contraception and abortion may accomplish greater reduction of infant mortality than the delivery of very sophisticated postnatal care. These considerations are consistent with the goal of both obstetric and pediatric prenatal care: that every baby be well born.

The pediatrician should carry out a careful physical examination of the newborn infant within 24 hours of delivery, or in the delivery room in the case of high-risk mothers or infants, in whom complications are expected or may develop; a second examination is made before the baby is discharged from the hospital. Such examinations aim at early detection of anomalies, such as congenital heart disease, hip dysplasia, and neurologic disorders. Other aspects of medical care at this time, such as initiation of feeding, prevention of infection, screening tests, and promotion of a healthy mother-child relation, are described elsewhere (p. 330).

INFANCY

The main problems for which some measure of success of preventive measures can be expected during the first year of life are nutritional disorders, infections, developmental problems, and deficiencies of maternal care. The physician also seeks to make early diagnosis of congenital anomalies and hereditary metabolic disturbances.

At each visit an assessment of *nutrition* should be made. The chart of height and weight, the dietary history, and the physical assessment of the child constitute adequate screening for malnutrition. The scientific basis for nutritional advice is given elsewhere (pp. 146–162). Among the well educated in the United States general affluence and simplified nutrients make this advice relatively easy to follow, but among migrant workers, the rural poor, and the disadvantaged of the inner city, deficiencies in calories, vitamins, and protein continue to be seen.

All the dietary essentials can be obtained from natural foods except vitamin D, which must be given as a supplement, either in a separate vehicle or in fortified foods, such as cow's milk. Occasionally supplementation of the diet with other vitamins is necessary to prevent the development of specific deficiencies (p. 155).

In many localities the problem of undernutrition is less common than that of *obesity.* The prevention of overnutrition is properly an objective of preventive pediatrics because of the high morbidity and mortality attributable to this condition in later years. The causes of obesity are many, but the common denominator is the intake of more calories than are needed to balance energy output. Prevention is far easier than cure, and is dependent upon *early* detection of those factors in the infant's or child's environment or personality which might predispose to obesity (p. 187).

The principal nutritional deficiency of infancy is *iron deficiency,* which has its peak incidence in the last half of the first year of life. This is preventable if solid foods, and especially the infant cereals which contain added iron, are introduced between 3 and 6 months of age, when most children accept these additions willingly. Infant formulas with iron supplements are now accepted and will prevent iron deficiency, but inasmuch as iron deficiency anemia is common mainly in socioeconomically disadvantaged groups (10 to 20 per cent compared to only about 1 per cent in better advantaged children), there is still controversy over their routine or universal use. Weaning from bottle to cup between 6 and 12 months of age will lessen the intake of milk and increase that of solid food, much of which contains iron. A screening test for anemia should be done on infants at 6 months and at 1 and 2 years of age if they are socioeconomically deprived or if they may have a poor dietary intake of iron.

Fluorine can now be considered an essential element in prevention of *dental caries.* It is easiest and best given in the public water supply; where this is not yet available, sodium fluoride drops containing 0.5 mg of fluoride should be given daily from birth until 10 to 12 years of age. Good dental hygiene and restriction of sugar intake are also important in prevention of caries.

The other large area of nutritional difficulty during this period involves conflicts between mother and child over weaning and feeding. Almost all babies have a decrease in appetite around 1 year of age as their growth rate slows; in some it appears marked. Anticipatory guidance beginning at about 10 months should prepare parents for this and will prevent many feeding problems.

INFECTIONS. Table 4–2 summarizes the schedule recommended in the definitive booklet published by the American Academy of Pediatrics (the Red Book, 1974) for immunizations against infectious diseases. This booklet should be immediately available to all physicians who treat children. Details of the techniques of administration of the various immunizing agents are given, as are the contraindications to and complications of their use. It is more important that all children receive immunizations than that an arbitrary schedule be followed. Parents should be given a record of the child's immunization, and the physician should also keep a record.

All children should receive immunization during the first year of life against diphtheria, pertussis, tetanus, measles, rubella, poliomyelitis, and probably mumps. Smallpox vaccination should *not* be given routinely to children in the United States, but should or must be given before travel to certain areas where smallpox is endemic. If all children were to receive smallpox vaccination, the risks of vaccination would be considerably higher than the risks of smallpox in most areas of the world today; and the worldwide eradication of smallpox by a concerted effort of the World Health Organization now appears possible.

Active immunization against diphtheria (p. 613), *pertussis* (p. 589) and *tetanus* (p. 619) is accomplished by use of a mixture of killed pertussis organisms with alum-precipitated or aluminum hydroxide-adsorbed diphtheria and tetanus toxoids (DPT). Most 0.5 ml preparations contain adequate amounts of diphtheria and tetanus toxoids and 4 N.I.H. units of pertussis vaccine. The minimal course is three injections of 0.5 ml at about monthly intervals, usually starting at about 2 months of age.

Injections are given intramuscularly into the lateral thigh of infants or into the deltoid or triceps muscles of older children. It is best to use a different site for each injection. Deep injection and massage after injection reduce the incidence of so-called antigenic cysts.

Mild fever often occurs within 12 to 24 hours and is not a contraindication to further injections. Administration of aspirin may make an irritable child more comfortable. *When a convulsion occurs as part of a reaction, further administration of pertussis vaccine is contraindicated.* Subsequent immunization may be carried out with diphtheria and tetanus toxoids alone (DT), beginning with reduced doses (0.05 to 0.1 ml).

After 6 years of age children should not receive pertussis vaccine; booster immunizations should then consist of "adult" diphtheria and tetanus toxoids (DT) to reduce reactions. A Schick test is no longer used routinely, since reactions to "adult" DT are so uncommon or mild that it is simpler to give a booster injection than a Schick test. Booster doses are important to maintain immunity and should be kept up for diphtheria and tetanus throughout life. There appears to be no need for tetanus boosters at a greater frequency than every 5 to 10 years after primary immunization.

It is usually unwise to give any immunization during an acute illness, because the fever from the injection may confuse the picture of the illness. Some children who have frequent upper respiratory tract infections may have long delays in completion of immunizations if this policy is over-rigidly followed; mild convalescent or healing

TABLE 4–2 RECOMMENDED SCHEDULE FOR ACTIVE IMMUNIZATION OF NORMAL INFANTS AND CHILDREN

2 mo	DTP[1]	TOPV[2]
4 mo	DTP	TOPV
6 mo	DTP	TOPV
1 yr	Measles[3]	Tuberculin Test[4]
	Rubella[3]	(Mumps[3])
1½ yr	DTP	TOPV
4–6 yr	DTP	TOPV
14–16 yr	Td[5]	and thereafter every 10 years

[1] DTP. Diphtheria and tetanus toxoids conbined with pertussis vaccine.

[2] TOPV. Trivalent oral polio virus vaccine. This recommendation is suitable for breast-fed as well as bottle-fed infants.

[3] May be given at 1 year as measles-rubella or measles-mumps-rubella combined vaccines. See Rubella, p. 661, and Mumps, p. 681 for further discussion of age of administration.

[4] Frequency of repeated tuberculin tests depends on risk of exposure of the child and on the prevalence of tuberculosis in the population group. The initial one should be at the time of, or preceding, the measles immunization.

[5] Td. Combined tetanus and diphtheria toxoids (adult type) for those over 6 years of age in contrast to diphtheria and tetanus (DT) containing a larger amount of diphtheria antigen. Tetanus toxoid at time of injury: For clean, minor wounds, no booster dose is needed by a fully immunized child unless more than 10 years have elapsed since the last dose. For contaminated wounds, a booster dose should be given if more than 5 years have elapsed since the last dose.

infections should not be an absolute contraindication to immunization.

Administration of oral live attenuated *poliomyelitis vaccine* (p. 721) containing the three types of virus (OPV) is the safest of all immunization procedures. There may during the summer be some competition with other enteric viral infections, but poliomyelitis vaccination need not be deferred. It may be wise in the breast-fed infant to defer polio immunization until weaning, since protective antibodies in breast milk may reduce somewhat the effectiveness of oral polio vaccine.

Vaccination against measles (p. 658), using an attenuated strain of virus, should be initiated after 12 months of age. Booster doses of this vaccine are not recommended.

Other active immunizations are recommended for various parts of the world. Information on these can be found in the Red Book and in publications of the United States Public Health Service.*

Passive immunization is possible against measles, rubella, infectious hepatitis, varicella, and poliomyelitis through the use of gamma globulin, but except for infectious hepatitis and occasionally varicella *(q.v.)*, the use of active immunization is far preferable, even in an epidemic situation.

Quarantine is not generally effective for the control of the contagious diseases of childhood.

Parents commonly seek advice about prevention of other infections for which no specific immunization is available. It is wise not to invite exposure of children to such bacterial infections as impetigo, salmonellosis or shigellosis, but it is hardly practical and may even be unwise to try to prevent contact of normal children with the common epidemic viral upper respiratory and gastrointestinal tract infections. Since many asymptomatic children excrete the viruses of these diseases, prevention of contact with only symptomatic children will not be very effective. Moreover, after the first few months of life it is part of the process of growing up to develop immunity to a wide variety of agents through being infected with them. Even if we could prevent such infections through isolation techniques, it is questionable whether we should postpone for the healthy child the development of this normal immunity against common infections.

OTHER PREVENTIVE MEASURES. There is no evidence that a physical examination is necessary at each well-child visit, unless there are new symptoms. Perhaps the most useful procedure for each visit is a developmental examination, such as the Denver Developmental Screening Test (Section 30), which will find that 3 to 5 per cent of children need further or continuing study.

Special mention should be made of the principle of *anticipatory guidance*, which aims to prevent problems through application of knowledge of normal growth and development. Some examples: (1) Normal children begin to roll over by 4 to 5 months of age; anticipatory guidance alerts parents to this possibility by about 2 to 3 months of age and suggests that infants should not be left unprotected on a bassinet or bed. (2) The normal child's growth rate decelerates markedly at about 10 to 12 months of age, with reduction of appetite; if parents know this, they are unlikely to be alarmed, less likely to force their children to eat, and may thus avoid a common type of feeding problem. (3) Most children are not ready for toilet training until after 18 months; informing parents of this within the first 6 months of life may prevent much anxiety or guilt over early failures of training.

The following is a general guide to the scheduling and conduct of health visits during the first 2 years of life, and assumes that much preventive care is shared by the physician with a nurse as the other prime member of a health team. In this program the child health nurse is given more initiative and responsibility than has been customary. Controlled study has shown this expanded coprofessional role of the nurse to be acceptable to patients and their families, to be financially feasible, and to render care of at least as high quality as the physician can deliver alone (Charney and Kitzman, 1970). Neither schedule nor content need be followed rigidly: for some children more frequent visits are essential; for others less frequent ones are adequate.

AGE AT CONTACT	SERVICES AND CONCERNS
1 to 3 weeks	A telephone contact is made with the mother. Questions are asked about feeding, stools, color, skin, urinary stream (boys), sleep, and mother's health and concerns. A home visit at about 3 weeks of age is one of the most useful.
4 to 6 weeks	Office visit with physician. History as above; complete physical examination, with special attention to weight, length, head circumference, nervous system, vision, heart, abdominal masses (especially kidneys), and hips for dislocation. Immunizations started by nurse, with first DPT and OPV.
8 to 10 weeks	Office visit. History, which may be taken by nurse, includes illnesses since last visit and any pertinent events in family; length, weight, head circumference, and developmental assessment by nurse are adequate screening if no symptoms or complaints. Second DPT and OPV given by nurse. Introduction of solid food, with cereal as tolerated.
14 to 16 weeks	Office visit, as at 10 weeks. Same screening examination as at 10 weeks. Observe for strabismus. Third DPT and OPV. Begin to add other baby foods.
5 to 6 months	Office visit with physician. History and physical examination; hearing screening; developmental appraisal. Weaning from bottle or breast to cup may begin for some.
9 months	Office visit with nurse. History, length, weight, developmental appraisal. Hematocrit determination if diet doubtful or poor. Anticipatory guidance about change of appetite.

*Superintendent of Documents, Government Printing Office, Washington, D.C. 20402.

12 months	Office visit with physician. Weaning from bottle should be complete. Breast-fed babies may continue longer since this does not interfere with intake of solids. Tine test; measles vaccine. Accident prevention discussed.
15 months	Office visit with nurse. Height, weight, developmental appraisal. Accident prevention discussed.
18 months	Office visit with nurse. DPT booster, OPV booster. Toilet training may be begun. Accident prevention precautions reinforced.
24 months	Office visit with physician. Toilet training is reviewed. Accident prevention again stressed. Urinary test for coproporphyrins in population susceptible to lead ingestion.

At each visit inquiry is made into the health of other family members, any family changes such as job changes of father, illness or death of grandparents, and mother's feelings. Perhaps the most useful guide to preventive services which the health team has to offer during this period comes through assessment of the mother's skills and problems in child care. The key processes during the first year of life are the development in the mother of a sense of self-confidence and in the child, of a sense of trust of the mother, along with a readiness on the part of the child to risk some separation from the mother during the second year, in the service of his own developing identity and autonomy. The physician should assess the progress of these developments and assist the mother in achieving them. Praise for the mother, especially for skills shown in care of her first child, is a valuable way to build her confidence. Since there are many different successful techniques for rearing children, the pediatrician will be wise to refrain from intervention unless he is sure that deleterious effects are evident or can be expected. Mothers receive bewilderingly different kinds of advice; it is generally better to support and praise a mother for what she is doing well and naturally and to foster her self-confidence than to try to cast her into one's own image of what a proper mother should be.

PRESCHOOL PERIOD

The health problems of the preschool child consist principally of morbidity from acute infections and accidents and of the development of chronic diseases. Deaths are rare; most are due to accidents.

ACCIDENT PREVENTION. The magnitude of this problem demands that physicians and others educate parents about the hazards to children, aiming their efforts particularly at high-risk groups. Age is an important risk factor. Most accidental poisonings occur in children 1 to 4 years of age, whereas injuries from firearms occur mostly in school-age children. Boys have more accidents than girls, and recurrent accidents are more likely in impulsive, acting-out, attention-seeking children. Some parents are too anxious about the risk of accidents; they must be reoriented toward the fostering of self-confidence and responsibility in their children. The mildly painful experience of a fall may be far more effective in prevention of future accidents than attempts at complete protection of the child from all hazards. Table 4–3 outlines the kinds of accidents that are most likely at various ages and the precautions that can be taken. It is useful to have pamphlets or printed sheets for parents to remind them of these hazards, but these cannot substitute for personal discussions.

OTHER PREVENTIVE MEASURES. *Malignant neoplasms,* including *leukemia,* are the second cause of death in this age period. Aside from a few tumors which follow radiation (thyroid carcinoma, etc.), a few associated with congenital defects (e.g., aniridia, etc.) (p. 1601) and a few solid tumors which can be detected early enough to allow successful treatment, no anticipatory measures are now available.

Most *congenital anomalies* will have been detected by this age, so that it cannot be expected that physical examinations will identify many unrecognized ones.

Of the acute *infections* common in this period, primary prevention is possible for only a few. Immunization should have been completed by 2 years of age against diphtheria, tetanus, pertussis, poliomyelitis, measles, rubella, and probably mumps. Prevention of other infections is by avoidance of children with severe infections, such as shigellosis and salmonellosis, the protection of food and public water supplies, and early detection and treatment of complications of the common respiratory infections, such as otitis media, pneumonia, and meningitis.

The early discovery of chronic disabilities not threatening to life, such as impairment of vision, hearing, and development, and the promotion of an emotionally satisfying pattern of living are the main goals of prevention in the preschool period. A simple behavior questionnaire can help to select those parents who have most need to discuss problems in these areas.

The following is a guide to preventive measures during this age period.

chart

AGE AT CONTACT	SERVICES AND CONCERNS
2½ to 3 years	Office visit. History of behavior, illnesses, and accidents, eating, sleeping, elimination, toilet training, current family situation. Examination: height, weight, development, hearing, vision test. Tuberculin test. Discussion of accident prevention and nursery school. Dental referral.
4 years	Office visit. History as for 3 year old. Examination: height, weight, development. Tuberculin test. Discussion of accident prevention.
5 years	Office visit, as for 4 year old. School readiness screening tests (Sprigle or Frostig) and discussion with parents about child's behavior and development. D–T and OPV booster.

TABLE 4–3 ACCIDENT PREVENTION AT VARIOUS AGE LEVELS

TYPICAL ACCIDENTS	NORMAL BEHAVIOR CHARACTERISTICS	PRECAUTIONS
	First year	
Falls Inhalation of foreign objects Poisoning Burns Drowning	After several months of age can squirm and roll, and later creeps and pulls self erect Places anything and everything in mouth Helpless in water	Do not leave alone on tables, etc., from which falls can occur Keep crib sides up Keep small objects and harmful substances out of reach Do not leave alone in tub of water
	Second year	
Falls Drowning Motor vehicles Ingestion of poisonous substances Burns	Able to roam about in erect posture Goes up and down stairs Has great curiosity Puts almost everything in mouth Helpless in water	Keep screens in windows Place gate at top of stairs Cover unused electrical outlets; keep electric cords out of easy reach Keep in enclosed space when outdoors and not in company of an adult Keep medicines, household poisons and small sharp objects out of sight and reach Keep handles of pots and pans on stove out of reach and containers of hot foods away from edge of table Protect from water in tub and in pools
	2-4 years	
Falls Drowning Motor vehicles Ingestion of poisonous substances Burns	Able to open doors Runs and climbs Can ride tricycle Investigates closets and drawers Plays with mechanical gadgets Can throw ball and other objects	Keep doors locked when there is danger of falls Place screen or guards in windows Teach about watching for automobiles in driveways and in streets Keep firearms locked up Keep knives, electrical equipment out of reach Teach about risks of throwing sharp objects and about danger of following ball into street
	5-9 years	
Motor vehicles Bicycle accidents Drowning Burns Firearms	Daring and adventurous Control over large muscles more advanced than control over small muscles Has increasing interest in group play; loyalty to group makes him willing to follow suggestions of leaders	Teach techniques and traffic rules for bicycling Encourage skills in swimming Keep firearms locked up except when adults can supervise their use
	10-14 years	
Motor vehicles Drowning Burns Firearms Falls Bicycle accidents	There is a need for strenuous physical activity Plays in hazardous places (street, railroad tracks, near rivers) unless facilities for supervised, adequate recreation are provided Need for approval of age-mates leads to daring or hazardous feats	Teach the rules of pedestrian safety Teach bicycling safety Instruct in safe use of firearms Provide safe and acceptable facilities for recreation and social activities Prepare for automobile driving by good example on part of adults and by closely supervised instruction

Adapted from Shaffer, T. E.: Pediat. Clin. N. Amer., *1*:426, 427, 1954.

SCHOOL AGE

School health programs have come under criticism as too often isolated from other medical activities, such as the care of the child's illnesses, and even from the educational process and from problems related to school activities. Much of this criticism is justified; on the other hand, there are ways in which the school can contribute uniquely to the health care system for children. Some screening tests, such as those for visual acuity and hearing, and group psychologic tests are most efficiently performed in the school. Moreover, the quality of the child's relationships with peers and teachers and his performance in school are as good a screening assessment for psychologic problems as there is. The child's physician should receive appropriate information regarding these matters from the school and should remain the focal point for medical care. The physician should, in turn, transmit to the school pertinent medical information about the child, with appropriate recommendations for individualized attention.

The important role of the school physician is not to perform periodic physical examinations on children who have a family physician, but to participate in conferences with teachers and school nurses about children with physical or emotional problems, to help in planning of curricula in health (including sex education and drug problems) and in biology, and to interpret health matters to school boards and school administrators. Some physicians serve as part- or full-time consultants to schools to promote the health of this defined population.

CONDUCT OF PREVENTIVE SERVICES FOR SCHOOL-AGE CHILDREN. It is customary to recommend yearly visits of the child to the physician in the interest of maintaining an active relationship among physician, patient, and family, but every two years is sufficient for most children. Developmental problems are best indicated by school performance; emotional and learning problems are frequent. The child's physician will be asked for advice on child rearing, discipline, summer camps, sleep, the viewing of television, sports, sex education, dating, school performance, and a host of other matters. He must be interested in these matters and learn as much as possible about them, including controversial aspects. He should avoid ex cathedra advice, preferring to foster a feeling of confidence in parents so that they can make their own wise decisions. For the physician to assume he knows the answers to all these problems of growing up is presumptuous and does a disservice to patients, who should be helped to make healthy but independent decisions in the context of their own lives, experience, and value systems.

The periodic physical examination provides an opportunity to anticipate or answer some of the questions which all children have about their developing bodies, and as adolescence approaches, to help the youngster to realize and accept that his body is normal and can be examined without discomfort or shame. Height and weight remain useful screening tests for significant occult illnesses and should be recorded yearly. Vision and hearing should be tested and development assessed. The school may be equipped and able to do this through group testing. It is important that innocent heart murmurs and other minor self-correcting problems be recognized, and that children having them not be referred for unnecessary and potentially anxiety-provoking diagnostic studies.

Learning disabilities, reading problems, and the so-called minimal brain dysfunction syndrome are most important and difficult areas. Reading readiness and school readiness tests are available which may forestall some of these problems through identifying them before they become much overlaid by anxiety, anger, and a sense of failure on the part of child and family (see p. 7). Progress in school should be under continuous review, and if trouble occurs, an early, full investigation should be made under the direction of the child's regular physician; he should be best able to put together the family history, perinatal experiences, and emotional climate of the home in such a way as to make sensible recommendations to the family and school regarding need for further evaluation or treatment. Prevention lies in helping parents and children as early as possible to have realistic expectations for achievement.

PREVENTION IN THE FUTURE

The major efforts of the pediatrician of the future will be to initiate measures in early childhood that will not have their effects in prevention of illness until decades later. Atherosclerosis, arterial hypertension with associated coronary heart disease and cerebrovascular disease, cancer (especially cancer of the lung), chronic urinary tract infection leading to renal failure, accidents, and mental illness are now rarely the target of the pediatrician's preventive approach. It would seem prudent at this time not to initiate vigorous measures whose efficacy is not known and whose side effects and costs could be great and are certainly unknown. Yet to ignore the potential for prevention of premature death and disability in adult years is to deny the essential role of the pediatrician. The great potential of this activity can be illustrated by the following brief summary.

ATHEROSCLEROSIS. The best hope at present of preventing the early serious complications of this nearly universal process lies in identifying those children with the familial type II hyperlipoproteinemia, which occurs in about 2 per cent of the population (Drash, 1972). Perhaps these children can be detected at birth (from analysis of cord blood), but in childhood any child from a family with a history of atherosclerosis of early onset should have his serum cholesterol measured in the fasting state. Levels above 235 mg./dl. all have a heavy beta pattern on lipoprotein electrophoresis. Whether other children besides those from high-risk families should have screening tests of cholesterol levels performed is questionable. Diets low in cholesterol and in saturated fat will lower serum cholesterol, but whether early atherosclerosis is prevented has not been proved. Drug therapy with cholestyramine in children is still investigational.

Arterial hypertension is clearly one of the predisposing factors in coronary heart disease. It too is familial, and elevation can be detected in childhood (Zinner et al., 1971). But the usual methods of measurement of blood pressure in ordinary practice are unreliable, variable, and time consuming, and normal ranges for children need to be established more clearly. Careful measurement of blood pressure with proper size cuff (covering two thirds of arm) should be done as part of the physical examination in childhood, and if significant elevation is found, diagnostic studies should be initiated. The danger of raising needless anxieties is high;

borderline elevations should simply be monitored until their significance can be established. The prolonged prophylactic use of antihypertensive drugs does not seem warranted in childhood. Excess salt in the diet seems related to development of hypertension in some persons. It seems wise to keep the salt content of all diets lower than is now customary in the United States and to work for elimination of the added salt in infant foods (it is put there by the manufacturer only to make them more palatable to the mother!).

CANCER. The major known cause of human adult cancer is cigarette smoking in cancer of the lung. The habit is clearly established in late childhood and adolescence. Effective methods to prevent the habit have not been demonstrated, but physicians should provide a positive role model by not smoking in their offices and by giving their patients the facts. Group approaches through public advertising and involvement of groups in operant conditioning may well be the most effective antismoking measures.

Other human cancers may also yield to prevention in the future. Cancer of the cervix seems associated with infection with herpes simplex type II virus and with early sexual activity. Prevention might be achieved by appropriate sex education. Cancer of the skin is associated with excessive solar radiation; excess tanning should be discouraged.

Where will preventive measures go in the future? The physical function of adults is more clearly related to patterns of living than other factors; lack of sleep, excessive use of alcohol, lack of exercise, obesity and smoking of cigarettes are known to correlate most closely with poor function. Added to the effects of these are the strong effects of psychologic stress as causes of many diseases. No reliable measures are now available which will significantly change these habits, but it may be that in the future pediatricians will spend more time promoting healthy patterns of living and successful strategies for coping with stress than they now spend immunizing children against common contagious diseases. It should be clear that in the future prevention of childhood diseases and distress will come more from social progress than from individual medical contacts or procedures. More may be done to improve the health of the community through full employment, improvement of housing, quality education for all, development of recreational facilities, strengthening of the family, and the development of community and societal goals for all citizens than through traditional individual curative or preventive medicine.

ROBERT J. HAGGERTY

Charney, E., and Kitzman, H.: The child health nurse (pediatric nurse practitioner) in private pediatric practice: A controlled trial. New Engl. J. Med. *285*:1353–1358, 1971.

Drash, A.: Atherosclerosis, cholesterol, and the pediatrician. J. Pediatr. *80*:693–696, 1972.

Frankenburg, W. K., and Dodds, J. B.: The Denver Developmental Screening Test. J. Pediatr. *71*:181, 1967.

Harper, P. A.: Preventive Pediatrics: Child Health and Development. New York, Appleton-Century Crofts, Inc., 1962, p. 798.

Health Supervision of Young Children: A Guide for Practicing Physicians and Child Health Conference Personnel. Revised edition. New York, American Public Health Association, 1960.

Immunization Information for International Travel. Washington, D.C., U.S. Department of Health, Education, and Welfare, Public Health Service Publication No. 384.

Report of the Committee on the Control of Infectious Diseases (Red Book). Evanston, Ill., American Academy of Pediatrics, P. O. Box 1034, 1972.

Report of the Committee on School Health. Evanston, Ill., American Academy of Pediatrics, 1966.

Standards of Child Health Care. Evanston, Ill., Council on Pediatric Practice, American Academy of Pediatrics, 1972.

Wallace, H. M.: Health Services for Mothers and Children. Philadelphia, W. B. Saunders Company, 1962, p. 466.

Zinner, S. H., Levy, P. S., and Kass, E. H.: Familial aggregation of blood pressure in children. New Engl. J. Med. *284*:401, 1971.

HYGIENE

Parents are sometimes overwhelmed by advice on the bringing up of children. Magazine articles, syndicated columns in the daily press, advertising and radio and television commentaries all bring information to this receptive group. Most of the advice is good, but some is contradictory and much is subject to misinterpretation; undue emphasis on minor and unimportant detail is a common failing. Well meant suggestions from family and friends frequently add to the parents' difficulties in selecting proper courses of action. Child health supervision at selected intervals offers the physician ample opportunity to give meaningful guidance, and the role of the physician in health education will usually include interpretation of conflicting recommendations and opinions as well as direct instruction on child rearing or on the place of health practices in the home.

HABITS. The daily practices which promote good health and personal well-being, usually referred to as personal hygiene, are facilitated by the development of habits which begin at birth and continue throughout life. They usually arise from conscious acts reinforced by repetition and frequent use until they function as patterned reactions requiring little or no thought. Generally, habits are considered to be good when they conform to acceptable behavior and bad when they do not. Praise, encouragement, attention and personal satisfaction strengthen them, whereas lack of attention and parental displeasure discourage them; they are easily formed and much less easily changed or eliminated.

Although children appear to do equally well with strict or *laissez-faire* discipline, reasonable expectations and acceptable limits to behavior need to be defined and upheld. When parents appreciate that their responsibility in guiding habit formation is to help the child to gain increasing independence at his own optimal rate, much concern over trivia is avoided. *Consistency of action by both parents is essential if children are to be helped rather than confused.* Personal examples are more important in promoting good habits than what is said, especially when parents do not "practice what they preach." Comparison with others, the setting of too rigid standards and impatience with lack of success lead to frustrations and tensions in both children and their parents. When demands made by the family exceed the ability or readiness of the child, conflicts result which the physician may help to resolve and explain. Children want to conform to what is expected of them, and their well intended efforts toward a goal, as well as successful achievement, merit praise. (See also comments on Discipline and Learning, Section 2.)

Habit formation is usually thought of in relation to establishment of eating, sleeping, and bowel and bladder patterns. Regularity and relatively automatic functioning in these fields are necessary before children are free to progress to more complicated learning.

EATING. Eating habits of infants are discussed in Section 3.

SLEEP. There is considerable variation in the amount of sleep required by different children. Many children get too little rest, and often the symptoms of irritability, lethargy, anorexia, temper tantrums and perhaps increased susceptibility to infection result. Many behavior problems are precipitated by fatigue.

Most infants sleep 15 to 20 hours a day during the first half year; by 6 months of age they sleep through the night and are awake for periods totaling 6 to 8 hours. By 1 year of age the child sleeps an hour or two less and by 2 years of age averages 12 to 14 hours a day. The need for sleep gradually decreases, but rarely becomes less than 10 hours during childhood. A nap during the day is desirable until school interferes with this routine, and rest periods should have an important place in kindergarten and first and second grade schedules.

Early establishment of regularity of bedtime is most important; nowhere in the field of habit formation is consistency more important. The presleep period should be free of excitement, rushing, scolding and physical activity. Stimulation of children by exciting stories, radio, television, active play or a battle of wills should be avoided. A familiar story, quiet discussion of happy events of the day, a warm bath and reassurance of love and affection are conducive to easy sleep. Children, even when sleepy, normally do not want to stop doing something interesting. The habit of going to bed on schedule and to sleep promptly can be established and maintained by a consistent and understanding approach.

Infants and children should have their own beds and, if possible, their own rooms. The sleeping room should be ventilated, but free of drafts. Bed clothing is frequently too heavy and should be varied with the temperature. Overall sleeping garments for infants who may get uncovered in cold weather are useful. Although position during sleep is relatively unimportant, the position of infants, especially of premature ones, should be changed often enough to prevent moulding of the cranium from constant pressure on one area.

Disturbances of sleep are discussed in Section 2.

ELIMINATION. Control of the anal and bladder sphincters is naturally acquired by most children during the second or third year of life. Efforts to "train" a baby before he is ready for voluntary control of his sphincters are usually disastrous and frequently lead to unhappy parent-child relations. He is not ready to use the toilet until he is old enough to understand what it is for and to let his mother know of his needs, until his bowel movements come at fairly regular times, and until he is willing to sit on the toilet. A comfortable seat with a rest for the feet and a strap for safety should be provided. Suppositories or soap sticks have no place in the establishment of regular bowel habits, and coercive methods of any sort are contraindicated.

By about 18 months of age most toddlers have acquired enough bladder control to retain urine for 2 hours or so. At this age they may be encouraged to sit on the toilet and void. It is best to make initial efforts just after meals or naps and when the child is dry and likely to void readily. Other routines or interesting play should not be interrupted for this purpose. Nocturnal control of urination is not usually attained until the third year of life or later.

EXERCISE. The normal infant or child, in a reasonable environment, will have sufficient muscular activity for good growth and development. The young infant begins to develop his large muscles by kicking, stretching, crying and squirming. He should be allowed to do so several times a day on a safe flat surface, unencumbered by clothes. He should be provided with easily grasped toys to develop hand use. Limits for safety's sake must be provided when he crawls and begins to walk. His activities at this stage should not be limited to a playpen—a piece of furniture designed for adult convenience, not to aid the child's development. Toddlers should be provided with safe areas both indoors and outdoors in which to run, climb and explore. They need large blocks, push and pull toys, materials for imitative play, and the privilege of getting dirty and playing with water. Children's toys should, in general, be washable, not easily broken and free of sharp edges and splinters and of removable parts that can be swallowed or aspirated.

Schools should provide an opportunity for universal participation in organized sports. Intramural teams can offer the less well coordinated boy or girl an opportunity to take part in group sports.

SUNLIGHT AND FRESH AIR. Sunshine and fresh air are essential for the development and maintenance of sound health. Dependence is no longer placed on sunlight for the prevention of rickets, but many other benefits accrue from it. There is no reason, however, to justify making a fetish of exposure of young infants to the sun, particularly in cold weather. Care should always be taken to avoid sunburn. Outdoor play should be encouraged at all ages when the weather permits and clothing is adequate. Fresh air should be provided indoors by adequate ventilation.

CLOTHING. Tremendous improvements have been made in the functional design and in the materials of infants' and children's clothing. The diaper is still standard equipment, but tapes, drawstrings, many tiny buttons, frilly dresses and bulky winter clothes have largely been replaced by elastic materials, grippers, zippers, a few large buttons, slip-on shirts and pants and by new materials of lighter weight for cold weather. The principles guiding the choice of good clothing for children are attractiveness and color, simplicity in design, ease of use, softness of texture, lightness of weight, washability, relative looseness of fit and freedom from irritation to the skin. Knitted cotton is usually best next to the body. Children should be dressed appropriately for the environment. The universal tendency to overdress children in the winter frequently results in excessive perspiration. Extra water-repellent garments are easily put on a child to secure the warmth and protection needed for outdoor activities, and they should be removed as soon as he re-enters the warm house or schoolroom. The legs should be covered in cold weather.

Layettes are usually too elaborate. Infants need shirts with and without sleeves, nightgowns, diapers, socks or booties, a sweater and an outer garment with a hood for outdoor winter use. Rubber or plastic pants should be loose enough to permit evaporation, and should not be used except for relatively short periods to avoid otherwise troublesome situations; they are a prime cause of diaper eruptions. Lightweight cotton blankets are generally preferable to heavy woolen ones; a well made sleeping bag is satisfactory for cold weather.

Children's shoes are discussed in Section 22.

CLEANLINESS. Certain aspects of cleanliness such as the bath, washing at mealtimes and at toilet time, the use of a handkerchief and of a napkin, brushing the teeth and some responsibility in caring for clothing are essentials that should be reduced to the level of habitual reactions as early in life as possible. Formation of habits of personal cleanliness is encouraged, like all other habits, by the examples of parents, by praise and recognition of effort, by pleasant rather than unpleasant experiences, by consistency and by gradually decreasing assistance on the parents' part. Many parents need help in achieving a perspective on healthy cleanliness, which lies somewhere between asepsis and filth.

A daily bath for infants is a good rule. In warm weather more frequent sponging may be necessary. As soon as the umbilicus has healed, the infant may be immersed in a basin or tub. The room should be comfortably warm; supplies should be ready at hand; a safe flat working surface must be available; care must be taken not to let the infant slip or fall; and the experience should be made a happy, playful one. A regular time for bathing as well as for other routine activities should be established. A nonirritating soap is lathered over the trunk and extremities, with care to avoid the eyes and mouth, and the baby is then rinsed with fresh, comfortably warm water. The scalp should be washed as needed. The skin is patted dry, with special attention to the creases.

Oil, powder or lotion is usually not necessary, although their use is sometimes helpful for dry skins and in the diaper area. Caution should be used to avoid inhalation of any powder, and zinc stearate should not be permitted in the nursery.

The face is washed with clear water, except when soap or oil is necessary to remove dried excretions or vomitus.

The external ear may be washed with a soft cloth; dried accretions in the creases may be removed with a cotton-tipped applicator moistened with oil. The ear canal, except at its opening, should not be cleaned by an untrained person.

The eyes usually require no special care. Accumulated secretions in the corner of the eye should be wiped out with a piece of cotton saturated with clear water.

The nose does not need cleaning unless there are dried secretions at the openings of the external nares. Secretions may be removed with a dry or moistened cotton-tipped applicator. Oil should not be used.

Under no circumstances should attempts be made to clean the mouth, since the mucous membrane is easily damaged and is then especially susceptible to infection.

Brushing the teeth is not advised until the third year of life. Before this time they may be cleaned occasionally with a cotton-tipped applicator saturated with saline or sodium bicarbonate solution.

Nails need trimming when they protrude beyond the ends of the fingers or toes. Toenails should be cut straight across without rounding the corners so that ingrowing toenails may be prevented.

The bathing of older children requires no special consideration. In summertime there should be daily baths; in the winter months this is not necessary and, in children with dry skins, should be avoided. In the latter instance 2 to 4 baths a week are adequate, depending on the state of cleanliness. Baths should be taken preferably at night to lessen the degree of chafing, which is reduced significantly by thorough drying (dry towels and warm air). Anointing the skin with oil or skin lotion helps to avoid chafing of dry and sensitive skins.

The genitals should be washed at bath time. In the uncircumcised male infant the foreskin may be retracted as far as possible without trauma. Adhesions will usually be broken as the child grows older, and no strenuous effort need be made to break them. Smegma may be removed from the vulva with a soft cloth or a cotton pledget saturated with oil. Genitalia of both sexes should be rinsed with clean water at the end of the bath to prevent irritation from soap, which otherwise might dry on the mucous membranes.

WILLIAM E. LAUPUS

5
GENERAL CONSIDERATIONS IN THE CARE OF SICK CHILDREN

CLINICAL EVALUATION OF INFANTS AND CHILDREN

Whether the immediate purpose is the diagnosis of illness or the maintenance of health, the evaluation of the infant, child or adolescent should be comprehensive and continuing, and should embrace psychologic and environmental as well as somatic factors. Careful and complete ascertainment of history and performance of a physical examination are generally more informative than are laboratory tests. The latter should be used (1) as screening procedures when direct observation is impossible or when specific and otherwise hidden conditions are being sought, (2) to confirm or further define conditions suspected on the basis of history and observation, (3) as a guide to complex therapy or (4) to gather data for purposes of research.

Children and their parents should be approached with gentleness, respect, empathetic understanding, sympathetic warmth and thoughtful kindness. These qualities in the physician are appreciated by patients large and small, and will enhance effective gathering of data, ensure greater therapeutic compliance and increase mutual satisfaction in the doctor-patient relationship.

GENTLENESS. The touch of the physician should be gentle, both literally and figuratively. Roughness, rudeness or crudeness in manner, speech or handling of the patient should be scrupulously avoided; they usually lead to resistance (conscious or unconscious) on the part of the patient, especially of an infant or child. On the other hand, the approach of the gentle physician is generally welcomed.

RESPECT. Self-respect is essential to the healthy psyche and therefore to each healthy person. The child evaluates himself in the mirror through which he sees how he and his parents are treated by others. Each time a child witnesses disrespect shown to either or both of his parents, he loses some of his own self-respect; when he sees himself and them handled with respect, his self-esteem is confirmed and reinforced.

The most basic form of respect is to care enough to learn and to use a person's name. Inquiry as to the name the child prefers should be made at the first encounter and consistently remembered and used thereafter. It is an unhappy common practice of many physicians and other medical personnel to address minority group parents or others whom they feel to be socially, educationally or mentally inferior (including the aged) by their first names in the absence of previous first-name familiarity; this is an overt sign of disrespect. A parent, Mrs. Jane Doe, should be addressed as "Mrs. Doe," not as "Jane" or "Mother." In like manner, the common practice of referring to boys as "males" and girls as "females" tends to depersonalize the individual, whether child or parent, and to create or widen gaps in communication or feeling.

UNDERSTANDING. The physician is often faced by behavior or actions on the part of children or parents which he may regard as uncooperative, hostile, reprehensible or distasteful. In order to deal with them with an appropriate degree of professional equanimity he must learn to recognize, understand and accept that such behavior or actions may be dictated by forces beyond the control of the individuals concerned. Efforts to understand why parents are angry, demanding, depressed or withdrawn usually improve the doctor-patient relationship and the care of the child.

SYMPATHY. The warm expression of concern or of sympathy by word or touch relieves the uncomfortable child or troubled parent of the feeling that they are alone with pain or worry. It is much appreciated and adds to the rapport between physician and parent. The empathetic physician has the capacity to recognize and respond to negative feelings and behavior with therapeutic rather than countervailing utterances and behavior. Likewise, when sympathetic feelings of his own (e.g., of grief or depression) are aroused, he is able to rally his professional skills to provide the needed support to the patient (child or parent) rather than to terminate as quickly as possible an unhappy or unpleasant encounter.

KINDNESS. The physician who willingly seeks small ways of making his patient feel more comfortable in mind or body increases the trust placed in him, and he himself finds an emotional reward in the patient's reaction to the thoughtful, considerate and giving attitude expressed.

INITIAL CONTACT

With the initial contact the physician should identify himself in a friendly manner to both parents and child, even if the latter is a small infant. In subsequent encounters a friendly greeting to both is always in order. The establishment of a relaxed and friendly atmosphere will facilitate the elucidation of history and the performance of physical examination. Expressions of concern for the comfort of both parent and child ("Is the room too cold?", "Would she like to have her diaper changed?") increase confidence in the physician, as they reveal the degree of his personal interest and sensitivity. The *infant* will usually remain in the parent's arms during an interview. The *small child,* if ill, may do the same, but should otherwise be provided with a box of toys or other distraction to prevent boredom. On the other hand, if sensitive areas of the child's own behavior and management are going to be discussed, it may be better to arrange to talk with the parent or parents alone; the same should be done when discussing serious prognoses. As a rule, such discussions should not be held in the presence of the child until some decision has been reached as to how his possible or probable questions are to be answered.

The child of *school age* is usually self-sufficient enough to remain quiet during an interview, and should be included from time to time in the questioning. Interviews with parents alone may alarm excluded children of this age with the implication that something serious is being kept from them. Opinions differ as to the degree to which the older child should be included in the discussion of serious illness and prognosis; it is probably best to make individual judgments in this regard (see Fatal Illness, Section 2). Speaking with parents alone is important when discussing behavior disorders. It is often possible to find some activity for the child elsewhere in such instances; in any case, it is wise to afford the child "equal time," during which, with the parents' knowledge and concurrence, the physician can and should be frank with the child about the subject, if not the content, of the earlier conversation with the parents.

The parents of *adolescents* often need opportunities to express their concerns about their children to the physician without the child present, but the physician should always make it clear both to them and to the adolescent that the basic relationship is between the physician and the adolescent, not the physician and the parents; the interviewing procedures should be arranged accordingly.

HISTORY

The traditional initial medical history is made up of the following components:

Chief Complaint (C.C.), i.e., the chief reason for the visit.

Present Illness (P.I.), i.e., all details of and bearing directly on the chief complaint.

Past History (P.H.), including previous illnesses, a systems review and data concerning prophylactic or screening measures, such as immunizations, and the like.

Family History (F.H.), i.e., all medical conditions present in blood relatives which may by their presence or absence have a bearing on the health of the patient.

Social History (S.H.), i.e., relation of environmental circumstances which may bear on the physical or emotional well-being of the patient.

The history obtained at subsequent contacts is usually limited to a C.C. and P.I.; new items of P.H., F.H. and S.H. are added as they come to light.

In eliciting the medical history of a child, the parent or patient should initially be asked the reason for the visit or hospitalization. With acutely ill patients the reason may be obvious and may be better regarded as implicit. In other situations, simple questions such as "Would you tell me what the problem is from your point of view?" are appropriate for opening communication. The physician should listen carefully and respectfully to what follows, and should not initially interrupt with questions. At the end of the parent's or the child's free recital, the physician should recapitulate what he has understood from the story in order to make certain that all are in agreement as to what has been said and what it means. Often a number of problems other than the chief complaint are touched upon. They should be noted as they emerge for specific pursuit later (the "problem-oriented" approach). During the recital the observant physician may gain important clues from parent-child and parent-parent interactions, as he may from near-tearfulness, blushing, disordered hair, nail-biting, changes in tone of voice and neuromuscular tension during the telling or discussion of specific items of the history.

Particular care should be taken to allow the informant to answer each of his questions fully before going on to another. Failure to do so implies impatience or disrespect, and carries the impression to the parent or child that the interviewer is not really interested in or listening to what is being related. It is important also to *avoid leading questions,* which may result in an inaccurate history. Sympathetic remarks (e.g., "All that activity must really tire you out at times") or oblique questions (e.g., "Does your husband's job often keep him away on weekends?") are often more effective than direct or blunt questions in eliciting data in sensitive areas. Material in sensitive areas (family relations, sexual information or behavior) may be withheld by parents until one or more visits have reassured them as to the physician's interest, concern, empathy and discretion.

At the conclusion of many interviews, it is well to formulate some such question as "I want to be sure that I have answered all your questions; can you tell me just what you expected or wanted to get from this visit?" Sometimes only in this way will the physician discover such things as that the prime concern of the mother of an obvious cretin may be his constipation rather than his endocrine status; compliance in management of the latter may only be obtained after her concerns with the former have been adequately attended to.

PHYSICAL EXAMINATION

SETTING. The room in which a child is examined contributes to the emotional climate. White is cold, and buff impersonal, to the small child; pastel walls achieve a cheerful and familiar effect, as do bright colors, comfortable furniture and pictures, which may be of familiar things and characters such as "Snoopy" or "Mickey Mouse" or of unfamiliar but attractive and recognizable objects. Glaring lights and unfamiliar equipment may be frightening. The latter should be introduced in familiar terms; the blood pressure cuff may be called a "special" or a "funny" balloon, and the otoscope and ophthalmoscope "funny" or "special" flashlights. The warmth and texture of cotton flannel sheets instead of paper or regular woven sheets will make lying on the examining table more comfortable for the unclothed infant or child.

APPROACH. The approach to physical examination of the infant and child should be unhurried and not structured according to preconceived notions. The anxieties of even 6- or 8-week old infants may be allayed and their "cooperation" obtained by getting them to smile in response to friendly voice sounds before beginning the examination. Such an approach is also reassuring to parents, whose anxiety at brusque manipulation may otherwise be transmitted to the infant by vocal or neuromuscular tension. Small children usually profit from having a little time to get used to the place where they are to be examined and to the examiner. This is best afforded by allowing the child freedom to explore while the history is being obtained. They should then be told ("I want you"), not asked ("Will you please?"), to remove all their clothes, specifically excepting underpants, since the latter seem to represent a last bastion of self-respect and protection against assault. At the end of the examination, when the child has confidence that the examiner does not intend to hurt him, the underpants can usually be lowered or removed without objection. The physical examination can be performed on an examining table or on the mother's lap, whichever seems more opportune. Some children are very comfortable if examined standing. Small children are reassured if they are not required to be supine until the end of the examination, when they have gained confidence in the examiner's gentleness and good intentions. The older the child the more he can be treated like an adult; this implies no less gentleness, respect and consideration for feelings of privacy or anxiety. The least threatening order of examination is usually inspection, palpation, percussion, auscultation, ophthalmoscopy (children 2½ years or older will usually cooperate if not mentally retarded or emotionally disturbed) and otoscopy. Examination of the pharynx is left for last with small children since it is usually the most uncomfortable. On the other hand, many children of 3 years and older are quite comfortable standing, with an examination "to look you over from tip to toe" that begins with "shining a light in your ear" and moves easily to nose, mouth, teeth, pharynx, retina, and so on to the soles.

CONTENT. The content and order of recording of the physical examination should be reasonably standardized for ease of review and should differ little from those used in adult medicine except for: (1) the inclusion of head circumference as a standard measurement for children under 2 years; (2) the use of a growth chart (Figs. 2–12 and 2–13); (3) the inclusion of a developmental evaluation, especially for small children; and (4) an assessment of speech. This emphasis on developmental data is the major difference between the physical examinations of the child and of the adult. This developmental orientation is essential to the interpretation of data in health and in disease, since many physical signs (e.g., blood pressure, pulse, heart sounds, breath sounds, organ size, neurologic signs) are influenced by the developmental process.

THE PROBLEM-ORIENTED MEDICAL RECORD

The problem-oriented medical record formalizes and gives structure to some time-honored principles of medical record-keeping in a way which discourages oversight, simplifies audit of performance in regard to management of individual conditions, reinforces logical thought, makes explicit the process followed, and adapts the medical record for computerization. Problem-oriented record-keeping is the cornerstone of "problem-oriented medical practice," which consists of (1) establishment and use of a defined *data base*; (2) formulation and maintenance of a *problem list*; (3) a *plan for man-*

agement of each appropriate problem; (4) *education of the patient* in regard to appropriate items in the data base, problem list, plans and their implementation, and (5) establishment and maintenance of some form of continuing audit. Other important components are an expanded role for allied health personnel, especially in gathering data, and the use of algorithms.*

DATA BASE. The data base is the result of the registration in the medical record of a defined store of information pertinent to the patient and his problem(s). It may be general and comprehensive (for new or continuing patients) or limited to the problem of immediate concern (for new patients with acute, minor problems or those on whom a general data base has already been gathered and is up-to-date and available). The *basic components* of the pediatric data base are:

Presenting Problem(s) or Concern(s)
Patient Profile (identifying, demographic and social information)
Present Illness or Illnesses (history relevant to presenting problem(s) and concern(s))
Past History
Previous Illnesses
Systems Review
Family History
Physical Examination
Growth Charts
Developmental Flow Sheet or Screening Test
Defined Baseline *Laboratory Data*

The content of the data base will vary with the *age* of the patient (e.g., the menstrual history should be a routine part of the work-up of an adolescent girl but not of that of an infant girl); with the *population* from which the patient is drawn, (e.g., routine screening for sickle cell trait might be appropriate for a black but not for a white population); and with the *reason* for any specific patient-physician encounter (e.g., the data base for the problems of cough and fever will differ from that for vomiting and diarrhea). Other factors affecting the content of the data base include the ability and willingness of the patient or others to pay for its development (the less the ability or willingness to pay, the fewer components of low benefit or high cost can be included); the interests or concerns of individual physicians or health agencies initiating the collection of the data (these may reflect professional anxieties, confusions or research interests, for example); and changes in medical practice or knowledge.

Ideally the standard or general data base should be completely defined and uniform; in practice it varies with the factors listed above. The additional data bases for individual patients, diseases or circumstances (e.g., a defined data base for a specific complaint such as diarrhea and vomiting) are added only as necessary. *Flow sheets* are a form of continuing data base which may be standard, as for health supervision (Table 5–1) or diabetes, or which may be tailored to the needs of an individual with a rare disease or complication. The self-discipline and potential anguish involved in the definition of a data base is usually more than repaid in professional satisfaction that nothing important has been overlooked, and often in the long-term saving of professional time.

The initial defined data base is often best obtained or facilitated through use of a screening questionnaire appropriate to the age and environment of the patient. Table 5–2 represents such a questionnaire for parents to complete which has been found useful for both hospital and ambulatory pediatric care. The questionnaire is designed so that all answers circled in the right hand column represent actual or potential problems; this simplifies their identification. From it and the rest of the data base a problem list is developed. Answers circled in the right hand columns usually indicate a need for specific actions, such as obtaining more detailed information, obtaining a roentgenographic study or laboratory test, or carrying out an appropriate educational activity for parent or child. This questionnaire is designed for use with infants, children or adolescents; accordingly, it contains for each group some inappropriate questions. In practice, four or five blank lines are left at the end of each section for the entering by the physician of details (coded by the appropriate numbers) relevant to answers circled in the right hand column. The questionnaire may provide the historical part of a defined data base, serving as a screening instrument and as the patient profile, past history, systems review and family history in most cases. Most literate parents need about 20 minutes to complete it.

Certain laboratory tests (e.g., urinalysis, hematocrit, skin test for tuberculosis, serum cholesterol) may be included as part of the data base. The initial data base may also be obtained and recorded in the traditional manner under the headings of presenting problem (or chief complaint), present illness, past history, family history, physical examination and routine initial laboratory tests. It is a convention of the problem-oriented record that all data be recorded under the headings of "*Subjective*" (related by the patient or other lay person) or "*Objective*" (observed directly by the physician or his delegate or reported by another physician or a laboratory). Distinctions between "subjective" and "objective" sometimes become blurred under this convention, but it is generally useful, particularly in the recording of progress notes.

Once the initial data base has been recorded, further data are recorded in relation to specific, named and numbered problems. The *number* of the problem is entered in the left-hand margin of the page for easy reference and the *name* of the prob-

*An **algorithm** is defined as a step-by-step plan for proceeding from a clearly identifiable point in diagnosis or management to another identified point at which an objective is achieved or at which clinical judgment or a new algorithm must be applied. Algorithms are of particular value in directing the clinical activities of allied health personnel and of physicians or student physicians dealing with situations which are unfamiliar to them but well known to and defined logically by others.

TABLE 5–1 FLOW SHEET FOR HEALTH SUPERVISION

WELL CHILD FLOW SHEET NAME:______________ DOB:________

Age	Immunizations	HGB	U/A	P/R BP	Hearing	Vision	Health Education: Guidance	Health Education: Diet	Comments
1 mo.			PKU				Clothes, Travel, Infant Seat, Sleep, Thermometer, Father, Mother, Observation, Vitamins, Fluoride	Bottle in bed, Solids	
2 mos.	DPT TOPV			◤			Pain, Fever, ASA, Sibling Rivalry, Mother	Quant. Formula	
4 mos.	DPT TOPV		◤				Observation, Toys, URI, Foreign Objects, Car Seat, Discipline, Toilet Training	Milk, Vitamins, Solids	
6 mos.	DPT TOPV				◤		Crawler, Poisons, Ipecac, Strangers	Peanuts	
9 mos.	Tine	◤					Climber, Accidents, Temper Tantrums Masturbation	Cup	
1 yr.	Measles Rubella			◤	◤	◤	Family play, Dental Care, Matches, Appetite	Candy	
1 1/2 yr.	DPT TOPV						Streets, Cars, Seat Belts	Soft Drinks	
2 yr.	Tine Mumps						Bed Wetting, Peers, Independence, Manners		
3 yr.			◤	◤	◤	◤	Strangers		
4 yr.	Tine			◤			Water Safety		
5 yr.	DPT TOPV	◤		◤	◤	◤	School, Bike		
6 yr.	Tine			◤			Chores, Money		
7 yr.				◤					
8 yr.	Tine			◤			Drugs, Alcohol, Tobacco		
9 yr.	Rh HAI			◤			Menstruation, Sex		
10 yr.	Tine			◤			Guns, Rh		
11 yr.				◤		◤	Limits		
12 yr.	DT Tine			◤			Drugs, Alcohol, Tobacco, Sex		
13 yr.				◤			Freedom, Parents		
14 yr.	Tine			◤			Cars, Sex		
15 yr.				◤			Education		
16 yr.				◤			Future plans		
17 yr.	DT			◤			Marriage		
18 yr.	Tine			◤			Children		

◤=mandatory

DEVELOPMENT

Milestone	Age
Smile	
Grasp & Reach	
Sit Alone	
Walk Alone	
Words	
Bowel Control	
Urine Control	

PREVIOUS IMMUNIZATIONS

DPT					
OPV					
Tetanus					
Smallpox					
Measles					
Rubella					
Mumps					
Tine					
Other					

Abbreviations: DOB=Date of Birth, Hgb= Hemoglobin, U/A=Urinalysis, P/R=Pulse/Respiratory rate, PKU=urine test for phenylketonuria, DPT=Diphtheria-Pertussis-Tetanus vaccine, TOPV=Trivalent oral poliomyelitis vaccine, ASA=aspirin, Tine=skin test for tuberculosis, Rh=Rh blood typing (girls), HAI=Hemagglutination inhibition test for rubella antibodies (girls), DT=Diphtheria-Tetanus toxoid.

lem is the first part of the entry. A more detailed data base is obtained and recorded for each problem if all relevant data are not already contained in the initial data base. In many instances it is convenient to develop defined data bases for specific illnesses or categories of illnesses. Table 5–3 shows a check-off form for acute respiratory infections. Such forms save time and help ensure completeness through indicating gaps or incompletions. They may be color-coded to render them easy to locate and file. Flow sheets are useful in defining the continuing data base for specific patients or conditions.

PROBLEM LIST. The problem list is developed from information obtained from the data base. It should include any medical, social, developmental, psychologic, economic or environmental problems which have been identified, to each of which is assigned a number and a name. Each subsequent entry in the record, including those on the hospital order sheet, is identified with the number and name of the problem to which it refers. This form of record-keeping makes it easier to locate all entries relating to a single problem, simplifies an *audit* (critical review) of the record, and is ideally adapted to computerization, with easy ultimate retrieval of the data, notes and orders referable to specific problems.

An essential feature of the problem list is that it remain intellectually honest; that is to say, each problem should be expressed only at a level of understanding or confidence which can be substantiated by objective evidence, including the course of the illness. This consideration helps the formulator of the problem list to keep an open mind about diagnostic possibilities and to avoid jumping to potentially erroneous diagnostic conclusions. For example, the initial entry on the problem list

(Text continued on page 231)

TABLE 5–2 PEDIATRIC DATA BASE QUESTIONNAIRE

Date __________ NAME OF CHILD ______________________ Birthdate __________

Instructions:

This questionnaire is designed to help obtain some idea about the health of your child. Together with a physical examination and suitable laboratory tests, it will help to determine what health or medical problems, if any, your child may have. Since this questionnaire is used for children of all ages, some of the questions are bound to be inappropriate for this child and may be left unanswered.

Please answer the questions by circling the "yes" or "no," or by writing in the requested information. If you are not sure of the answer, please *circle the response on the outer right* so the doctor will discuss it with you. If there are questions you prefer not to answer, leave them blank. All information is, of course, confidential.

Filled out by: ______________________ Relationship to child: __________

I. CHIEF COMPLAINT AND GENERAL HEALTH

1. What is (are) the chief reason(s) that your child is being seen in the office or admitted to the hospital today?

____
____
____

2. Are there other problems that you are concerned about or questions you would like to have answered? — No Yes

   If yes, please list them:

   a. __________ e. __________
   b. __________ f. __________
   c. __________ g. __________
   d. __________ h. __________

3. How would you describe your child's general health?

   (Please check one) excellent ______
   good ______
   fair ______
   poor ______

4. In the past year has your child
   a. missed more than 7 days of school because of illness? — No Yes
   b. taken any medications for more than two weeks? — No Yes

5. Has your child ever
   a. been hospitalized? (If yes please list below:) — No Yes
   b. had an operation? — No Yes

Hospital	City	Problem	Date

6. Has your child ever been involved in a serious accident? — No Yes

____
____
____
____

II. FAMILY PROFILE

7. Years at present address? __________
8. Type of dwelling? __________
9. Owned or rented? __________
10. Father's age? __________
    11. Education __________
    12. Employment __________ How long? __________
    13. Previous Marriages __________
14. Mother's Maiden Name __________

TABLE 5–2 (Continued)

15. Age ______
16. Education ______
17. Employment ______ How long? ______
18. Previous Marriages ______

19. Brothers and Sisters:

Name	Sex	Age	Name	Sex	Age

20. Other People Living with Family:

Name	Relationship	Age

21. Do any people living in the home have persistent medical problems? ______ No Yes
22. How many years have the parents been married? ______
23. Are you separated? ______ No Yes
24. Are there any problems in your present marriage that you feel you would like help with? ______ No Yes
25. Are you satisfied with your present living conditions? ______ Yes No
26. Are you satisfied with your work? ______ Yes No
27. Is your husband (wife) satisfied with his (her) work? ______ Yes No
28. Does your health interfere with your ability to perform your work? ______ No Yes
29. Does your husband's (wife's) health interfere with his (her) ability to perform his (her) work? ______ No Yes
30. Do any of the following interfere with any member of your family receiving medical care?
    - Can't pay for it ______ No Yes
    - Hard to pay for it ______ No Yes
    - Transportation problems ______ No Yes
    - No babysitter ______ No Yes
    - No appointments at convenient times ______ No Yes
    - Don't like doctors ______ No Yes
    - Don't like hospitals ______ No Yes
    - Any other reasons? ______ No Yes

III. PATIENT PROFILE

31. Is this child adopted? ______ No Yes
32. How would you describe this child? (personality, interests, likes and dislikes, etc.)
______
______
______
______
______
______
______
33. If this child goes to school, please give
    - Name of school ______
    - Town ______
    - Grade ______
    - Teacher's name ______
    - Grades at last marking period ______

IV. PREGNANCY

34. Are you Rh negative? ______ No Yes
35. How many times have you been pregnant? ______
36. How many living children do you have? ______
37. Did you have regular medical care while pregnant with this child? ______ Yes No
38. Did you have any problems while pregnant with this child (such as excessive

(Table continued on following page)

TABLE 5–2 PEDIATRIC DATA BASE QUESTIONNAIRE (Continued)

bleeding, kidney or bladder infection, high blood pressure, diabetes or high blood sugar, any operations, convulsions, weight gain over 30 lbs, German (3-day) measles, x-rays during the first 3 months, any other illnesses)? ________ No Yes

39. Did you take iron or vitamins during this pregnancy? ________ Yes No
40. Did you take any medications during this pregnancy (such as fluoride, antibiotics, birth control pills, fertility pills, pills to prevent miscarriage, aspirin, laxatives, any other medicines)? ________ No Yes
41. Did you have an unusually long or difficult labor with this child? ________ No Yes
42. Were any of your babies born more than 2 weeks early? ________ No Yes
43. Were any of your babies born more than 2 weeks late? ________ No Yes
44. Did any of your babies weigh more than 10 lbs? ________ No Yes
45. Did any of your babies weigh less than 5 lbs? ________ No Yes
46. Did any of your babies receive a blood transfusion in the first month of life? ________ No Yes

V. BIRTH

47. Was this child born in a hospital? ________ Yes No
48. Was this child born feet first? ________ No Yes
49. Was this child born by cesarian section? ________ No Yes
50. How much did this child weigh at birth? ________ lbs. ________ oz.
51. Were there any problems with this child's delivery? ________ No Yes
52. Was this child normal at birth? ________ Yes No
53. Did this child go home from the hospital at the same time you did? ________ Yes No
54. Did this child have any unusual problems in the hospital (such as blue spells (cyanosis), yellow jaundice, trouble breathing, trouble feeding, infection, convulsions, or any other illness)? ________ No Yes
55. Did this child need any special treatment while in the hospital (such as incubator, oxygen, blood transfusion, medicines, feeding with a tube, or any other unusual treatment)? ________ No Yes

VI. HEALTH MAINTENANCE

56. Where does this child usually go for medical care? ________
57. When was this child's last complete checkup and who performed it? ________
58. What did this child eat yesterday (or the last day he (she) was well)?
    breakfast ________
    lunch ________
    dinner ________
    snacks ________
59. Was (Is) this child breast-fed? ________ Yes No
60. Does this child take vitamins? ________ No Yes
61. Does this child take iron medicine? ________ No Yes
62. Does this child drink more than a quart of milk per day? ________ No Yes
63. Does this child brush his/her teeth regularly? ________ Yes No
64. Does this child use dental floss regularly? ________ Yes No
65. Does this child drink fluoridated water or take fluoride supplements? ________ Yes No
66. Does this child, if under 4, ride in a safe car seat? ________ Yes No
67. Do you and your children over 4 use seat belts in the car? ________ Yes No
68. Do you have a supply of syrup of ipecac in your home to be used in case of an accidental poisoning? ________ Yes No

TABLE 5-2 (Continued)

69. Does this child use a lifejacket when boating? ________ Yes No
70. Does this child know how to swim? ________ Yes No
71. Does this child know how to handle a gun safely? ________ Yes No
72. Does this child operate, play or work around farm machinery? ________ No Yes
73. Do you have a record of this child's immunizations? ________ Yes No
74. Please list the dates or approximate ages at which this child received the following immunizations:
    - DPT 1 ____ 2 ____ 3 ____ 4 ____ 5 ____
    - Oral Polio 1 ____ 2 ____ 3 ____ 4 ____ 5 ____
    - Measles ________
    - Mumps ________
    - Rubella ________ (German measles)
    - Smallpox ________
    - Others ________
75. Please check any of the following diseases that this child has had.
    - Chickenpox ________
    - Mumps ________
    - Measles ________
    - Hepatitis ________
    - Whooping Cough ________
    - Rubella (3-day or German measles) ________
76. Has this child been to the dentist in the past 2 years? ________ Yes No
77. Does this child get regular physical exercise? ________ Yes No

VII. GROWTH—ENDOCRINE

78. Was this child born—on time? ________ Yes No
    —more than 2 weeks early? ________ No Yes
    —more than 2 weeks late? ________ No Yes
79. Have you ever thought that this child was growing too slowly? ________ No Yes
    —too rapidly? ________ No Yes
80. Have you ever thought that this child was —too fat? ________ No Yes
    —too thin? ________ No Yes
81. Has this child lost weight that he/she has not regained? ________ No Yes
82. Do you think that this child's sex organs are developing—too slowly? ________ No Yes
    —too rapidly? ________ No Yes
83. Has this child ever had trouble with the thyroid gland? ________ No Yes
84. Has this child ever taken a thyroid drug? ________ No Yes
85. Does this child have a blood relative with thyroid trouble? ________ No Yes
86. Does a tendency for obesity (being overweight) run in this child's family? ________ No Yes
87. Do any of this child's parents, grandparents, sisters or brothers have diabetes? No Yes
88. Does this child have a blood relative with a sex abnormality? ________ No Yes

VIII. DEVELOPMENT

89. Do you think that this child's mental development is normal? ________ Yes No
90. If in school, has this child had trouble keeping up with his/her classmates? ________ No Yes
91. Do you think that this child is too clumsy? ________ No Yes
92. Did this child a. smile by 6 weeks of age? ________ Yes No
    b. sit alone by 7 months? ________ Yes No
    c. walk alone by 14 months? ________ Yes No
    d. say simple sentences by age 2 years? ________ Yes No
    e. ride a tricycle by age 3 years? ________ Yes No
    f. tie his own shoelaces by age 6 years? ________ Yes No
93. Has this child ever had to repeat a school grade? ________ No Yes
94. Does this child have a blood relative who is mentally retarded? ________ No Yes

IX. SPEECH AND HEARING

In the past year has this child

95. —had more than 3 ear infections? ________ No Yes
96. —spoken as well as other children who are his/her age? ________ Yes No
97. —had trouble hearing? ________ No Yes
98. Has this child ever had any difficulty with speech? ________ No Yes
99. Was this child's speech understood by neighbors by 5 years of age? ________ Yes No
100. Does this child have any blood relatives who are deaf? ________ No Yes
101. Are this child's ears cleaned with sharp objects or Q-tips? ________ No Yes

(Table continued on following page)

TABLE 5–2 PEDIATRIC DATA BASE QUESTIONNAIRE (Continued)

X. VISION		
Has this child ever		
102. –had trouble seeing?	No	Yes
103. –worn glasses?	No	Yes
104. –had an eye which turned in or out?	No	Yes
Does this child have a blood relative with		
105. –*blindness* developing before age 50?	No	Yes
106. –*cataracts* developing before age 50?	No	Yes
107. –*glaucoma* before age 50?	No	Yes
108. –*detached retina?*	No	Yes
109. –*color blindness?*	No	Yes
XI. RESPIRATORY		
In the past year has this child had		
110. –more than 6 colds?	No	Yes
111. –a persistent runny nose?	No	Yes
112. –a cough that hangs on?	No	Yes
113. –pneumonia?	No	Yes
114. –an asthma attack?	No	Yes
115. –wheezing?	No	Yes
116. –shortness of breath?	No	Yes
117. –frequent sore throats?	No	Yes
Has this child ever		
118. –had asthma?	No	Yes
119. –had a positive skin test for tuberculosis (tuberculin or tine test)?	No	Yes
120. –been around a person with tuberculosis?	No	Yes
121. Does this child have a blood relative with cystic fibrosis?	No	Yes
122. Does this child have a blood relative with emphysema that developed before age 40?	No	Yes
123. Does anyone in the household smoke?	No	Yes
XII. CARDIOVASCULAR		
Has this child ever had		
124. –a heart murmur?	No	Yes
125. –cyanosis (blue spells)?	No	Yes
126. –an extremely rapid or irregular heart beat?	No	Yes
127. –rheumatic fever?	No	Yes
128. Has this child had a blood relative with		
a heart attack under age 50?	No	Yes
a heart attack over age 50?	No	Yes
elevated blood fats (cholesterol or triglycerides)?	No	Yes
high blood pressure?	No	Yes
diabetes?	No	Yes
obesity (overweight)?	No	Yes
a stroke under age 60?	No	Yes
a stroke over age 60?	No	Yes
129. Does this child have a throat culture taken when he/she has a sore throat to check for a "strep throat"?	Yes	No
XIII. GASTROINTESTINAL		
Has this child ever had		
130. –recurrent stomachaches?	No	Yes
131. –recurrent vomiting?	No	Yes
132. –recurrent diarrhea?	No	Yes
133. –recurrent constipation?	No	Yes
134. –blood in his/her bowel movements?	No	Yes
135. –medicine for stomachaches or constipation?	No	Yes
136. Has this child ever had x-rays of the stomach or intestines?	No	Yes
Does this child have a blood relative with		
137. –intestinal or rectal polyps?	No	Yes
138. –Wilson's disease?	No	Yes
139. Has a member of the household had hepatitis (yellow jaundice) in the past 6 months?	No	Yes

TABLE 5–2 (Continued)

XIV. GENITOURINARY

Has this child ever

140. —had a bladder or kidney infection? ______ No Yes
141. —had trouble with pain on urination, increased urinary frequency or loss of control? ______ No Yes
142. —had trouble with bedwetting? ______ No Yes
143. —had bloody or smoky-colored urine? ______ No Yes
144. —had x-rays of the kidney or bladder? ______ No Yes
145. Does this child have a blood relative with nephritis, kidney failure, kidney cysts, kidney stones, or other kidney problems? ______ No Yes

Girls 10 years or older—

146. Does this girl have an excessive vaginal discharge? ______ No Yes
147. Is this girl having menstrual periods? ______ No Yes
148. Are there problems with her periods? ______ No Yes
149. Does this girl understand menstruation? ______ Yes No
150. Does this girl understand contraception? ______ Yes No
151. Do you want this girl to receive education in contraception? ______ No Yes
152. Does this girl know her Rh blood type? ______ Yes No

XV. HEMATOLOGIC

Has this child ever

153. —been anemic? ______ No Yes
154. —taken iron medicine? ______ No Yes
155. —seemed to bruise or bleed excessively? ______ No Yes
156. —had a blood transfusion? ______ No Yes
157. —had an operation to remove the spleen? ______ No Yes
158. —had blood destroyed by a medicine he (she) took? ______ No Yes

Do any of this child's blood relatives have

159. —hemophilia or other bleeding disorders? ______ No Yes
160. —spherocytosis or other hemolytic anemia? ______ No Yes
161. —sickle cell anemia? ______ No Yes
162. —any other kind of anemia? ______ No Yes

XVI. SKIN

163. Has this child ever had any skin disease or skin problem? ______ No Yes

XVII. MUSCULOSKELETAL

Has this child ever had

164. —painful or swollen joints? ______ No Yes
165. —a broken bone? ______ No Yes
166. —a limp that persisted for more than a week? ______ No Yes
167. —to wear corrective shoes, splints or braces for a foot, leg or back problem? ______ No Yes
168. —other treatment for a bone, joint or muscle problem? ______ No Yes

Does this child have a blood relative with

169. —muscular dystrophy or other muscle disease? ______ No Yes

XVIII. NEUROLOGIC

Has this child ever had

170. —troublesome headaches? ______ No Yes
171. —a head injury that caused unconsciousness? ______ No Yes
172. —a seizure or convulsion? ______ No Yes

Does this child have a blood relative with

173. —seizures, convulsions or epilepsy? ______ No Yes
174. —Huntington's chorea? ______ No Yes
175. —a disease that affected the brain or nervous system? ______ No Yes
176. Does this child eat paint chips, plaster or putty? ______ No Yes

XIX. PERSONALITY

177. How would you describe your child?

happy ______	Yes	No	irritable ______	No	Yes
cooperative ______	Yes	No	too active ______	No	Yes
usually obedient ______	Yes	No	too lazy ______	No	Yes
fearful ______	No	Yes	shy ______	No	Yes
destructive ______	No	Yes	nervous ______	No	Yes
difficult ______	No	Yes			

(Table continued on following page)

TABLE 5–2 PEDIATRIC DATA BASE QUESTIONNAIRE (Continued)

178. Does this child
act babyish ______ No Yes
have temper tantrums ______ No Yes
rock back and forth ______ No Yes
have nightmares ______ No Yes
have any sleep problem ______ No Yes
soil pants with stool ______ No Yes
fight excessively ______ No Yes
steal ______ No Yes
have a fear of school ______ No Yes
eat dirt or plaster ______ No Yes
stutter ______ No Yes
bite his (her) nails ______ No Yes
suck his (her) thumb ______ No Yes

179. Are you concerned about any of the following:
bedwetting? ______ No Yes
thumbsucking? ______ No Yes
masturbation (playing with himself/herself)? ______ No Yes
biting? ______ No Yes
lying? ______ No Yes
fire setting? ______ No Yes
other? ______ No Yes

Has this child ever had
180. –problems making friends? ______ No Yes
181. –complaints about his/her behavior in school? ______ No Yes
182. –medicines to "calm him/her down"? ______ No Yes
183. Has a blood relative or member of the household of this child had mental illness, "nervous breakdowns" or emotional problems? ______ No Yes
184. Are there marriage, drug, drinking or other problems in the family? ______ No Yes
185. Are you prepared to discuss with this child now or in the future: sex, drugs, smoking, drinking, venereal disease, contraception, marriage, divorce and death? ______ Yes No
186. Would *you* like to know how to find out more about any of these? ______ No Yes

XX. ALLERGY

Has this child ever had
187. –allergy testing? ______ No Yes
188. –allergy shots? ______ No Yes
189. –a reaction to a medicine or shot? ______ No Yes
190. –a reaction to bee or wasp stings? ______ No Yes
191. –an allergic reaction to a food? ______ No Yes
192. –hives? ______ No Yes
193. If this child has an allergy to a medicine, does he/she wear a tag or carry a card which states this? ______ Yes No
194. Does this child have blood relatives with allergies? ______ No Yes

XXI. MEDICATIONS

195. Please list all medicines, prescription and nonprescription, that this child takes regularly. ______
a) ______
b) ______
c) ______
196. Has this child received any medications, shots or immunizations in the past two months? ______ No Yes
______

XXII. MISCELLANEOUS

Does this child have any blood relatives
197. –with congenital malformations? ______ No Yes
198. –who died in infancy or childhood? ______ No Yes
199. –who are crippled? ______ No Yes
200. –who have had cancer? ______ No Yes
201. Did you take any hormone pills or shots before or during this pregnancy (birth control pills, stilbestrol, fertility pills, pills to stop bleeding, pills to control menstruation, menopause pills)? ______ No Yes
202. Has this child ever had x-ray or radium treatments? ______ No Yes

TABLE 5–2 (Continued)

203. Is there any disease or condition which runs on either side of this child's family?__ No Yes

____

____

204. Are there any other problems not covered in the questionnaire or any general comments that you would like to make?__________ No Yes

____

____

____

of a child with suspected meningitis would be "Fever, vomiting and stiff neck." If a spinal tap shows purulent fluid, an arrow is drawn and the problem updated to "meningitis." If the cerebrospinal fluid culture grows out *Hemophilus influenzae* two days later, the problem is again updated to the final diagnosis of "*H. influenzae* meningitis." Each time an arrow is drawn to update a problem, the date or time of the updating is indicated over the shaft of the arrow (Table 5–4). The problem list thus encourages logical rather than intuitive thinking in the clinical appraisal of the patient.

Generally speaking, a problem is entered into the problem list and given a number when it requires specific and separate attention or action; naturally, what this means will vary with the individual physician in accordance with his level of concern, experience, and the like. Several conventions may be employed to keep the problem list from becoming unwieldy. For children, *health supervision* may be entered as Problem No. 1 routinely and all items relating to the observation of normal development, anticipatory guidance and immunization referred to it. If a developmental abnormality of major or continuing importance (such as enuresis or mental retardation) becomes apparent, it is then listed as a separate problem with a separate number. Minor or transient complaints without sequelae are often listed as "Temporary Problems." These are listed separately, with space to indicate the dates of recurrences; if the latter are frequent, transfer to the main problem list may be justified. Certain problems may be critical at the time they occur but of little long-term significance. This is particularly likely with problems leading to hospitalization. Take, for example, the case of a child whose appendicitis is complicated by wound infection and dehiscence, bacteremia, penicillin reaction, water intoxication with convulsions, hypokalemia and a near-fatal accidental overdose of morphine. Each of these is a major problem at some time, but only appendicitis, appendectomy and penicillin reaction would be appropriate for inclusion in the permanent problem list. This situation may be handled either (1) by entering the associated problems as subproblems, e.g.,

No. 2 Right lower quadrant pain ⟶ appendicitis ⟶ appendectomy

a. Convulsions ⟶ water intoxication
b. Wound infection
c. *E. coli* bacteremia
d. Hypokalemia
e. Wound dehiscence
f. Morphine overdose
g. Penicillin reaction

TABLE 5–3 DATA BASE AND RECORD FOR ACUTE RESPIRATORY ILLNESS

SUBJ: DURATION	OBJ:	NAME ___ AGE ___ DATE ___
SORE THROAT	TOXIC?	DX:
EAR ACHE/DRAINAGE	TEMP.	THROAT CULTURE
COUGH	RESP. RATE PULSE	WBC
RUNNY NOSE	THROAT	DIFF
CROUP	TONSILS	X-RAY
TROUBLE BREATHING	EXUDATE	LP
CHEST PAIN	MOUTH/GUMS	
WHEEZING	NOSE	
FEVER	EAR DRUMS	RX + Ed: DOSE/FREQ/COURSE
HEADACHE	RALES	
STOMACHACHE	WHEEZES	
STIFF NECK	RHONCHI	
SWOLLEN GLANDS	RETRACTIONS	
ANOREXOA	FLARING	
MALAISE	BRUDZINSKI/KERNIG	
MYALGIA	NODES	
	RASH	FOLLOW-UP: (OVER)
	SPLEEN	
		PROBLEM:
	SIGNED:	

or (2) by listing each complication as a separate problem on a "single-admission problem list" and transcribing only "appendicitis ⟶ status postappendectomy" and "penicillin reaction" onto the permanent problem list, which remains separate from the single-admission problem list.

Ideally there should be only one problem list for a patient and it should be continuous from birth to death, but in practice this may become cumbersome. As a result, problem lists may have to be revised from time to time. Moreover, other persons who see patients (including nurses, dietitians, social workers or other allied health professionals) may need their own problem lists to guide them; and even patients themselves may need their own problem lists, which are sometimes surprisingly different in orientation from those of the physician. In any event, the primary physician should be responsible for keeping a "permanent" or "master" problem list which is shared with patient or parent and which can serve as a guide to maintaining perspective and to ensuring that individual problems are not forgotten.

It is to be expected that disagreements will arise as to what should be entered as separate problems, but the principle is sound and should be implemented so that all perceived problems be specifically identified and that management efforts be specifically directed in accordance. So long as the list helps the physician to deliver comprehensive and auditable care, its purpose is accomplished.

ASSESSMENT. Ordinarily, regular assessments should be made of each problem, including in each instance a direct or implied statement of the goal of the *plan* which is to be followed. For instance, if the assessment is "Probable febrile convulsion, r/o (rule out) meningitis," the implied goal of the initial plan is the elimination of meningitis as a diagnostic possibility. Once that has been done, the fever may become a problem separate from the convulsion, each requiring its own assessment and plan (which may be merely that certain possibilities should be diagnostically eliminated). In each instance, the assessment should place in perspective a reasonable, explicit or implicit goal and a logical plan of action which will achieve that goal; accordingly, the assessment might be not to work up a problem at all, or it might define the extent of therapeutic effort to be expended.

PLAN. The plan should consist of four parts: (1) information related to diagnosis, (2) treatment, (3) patient or parent education, and (4) follow-up; in order to save time, the headings are usually abbreviated respectively to "Dx," "Rx," "Ed," and "F-U." Each plan, whether initial or subsequent, should contain these components in a clearly stated manner, including "none" if no plan is being made under that heading.

PROGRESS NOTES. Progress notes should be identified by the number and name of the problem to which they refer. Each note should contain four sections: (1) *subjective* for "hearsay" data, usually supplied by the patient or parent; (2) *objective* for directly ascertained data such as a new physical or laboratory finding; (3) *assessment* for a statement of the significance of the data, including an explicit or implied goal for the following plan; and (4) a *plan* which follows logically from the content of (1), (2) and (3). The plan should contain *specific* statements regarding (1) information related to diagnosis, (2) treatment, (3) patient education, and (4) follow-up.

FLOW SHEETS. Most good plans for continuing problems require flow sheets which list the appropriate parameters to be followed, thus serving as both simplified progress notes and reminders that certain items should be and/or have been checked periodically. Table 5–1, for example, is a flow sheet for health supervision. It serves both as a reminder and a checklist (the guidance items, for instance, may be checked off on the sheet as they are carried out, thus providing a handy record of what has and has not been done in this regard). The use of flow sheets increases the efficiency of the physician; once they have been prepared, most of the data can be gathered by an assistant, for review and decision-making by the physician.

AUDIT. Audit of the problem-oriented record consists of two phases: nonprofessional and professional. *Nonprofessional audit* can be done by other than a physician through use of a checklist. It concerns chiefly elemental aspects of thoroughness, such as:

Was a data base obtained?
Are all the components of the data base contained in the record?
Are the components completed as defined?
Is there a problem list?
Are all entries in the progress notes referred to specific problems?
Were plans carried out?
Was patient education done?
Was planned follow-up carried out?

Professional audit is for quality of care; it includes: (1) review of the nonprofessional audit, if that has been done; (2) review of the data base to see if all problems have been identified and entered on the problem list; and (3) general review of the record for thoroughness, efficiency, analytic sense, reliability and professional knowledge and competence.

ADVANTAGES OF THE PROBLEM-ORIENTED RECORD. The problem-oriented record (POR) incorporates most of the elements and principles traditionally held important to medical care and record keeping. Its logically structured form makes it more suitable than traditional records for audit, education, research and computerization. The problem list can be initiated as a routine and formal part of every record; when initiated at birth it provides a complete and terse history of the patient's medical and social problems, facilitates the location of all entries in the record which relate to specific problems, and encourages thoroughness, efficiency, analytic sense and reliability.

TABLE 5–4 SAMPLE MASTER PROBLEM LIST

MASTER PROBLEM LIST

NAME: Margaret B. (Peggy) Doe
BIRTH DATE: 8 October 1967
IDENTIFYING NUMBER: 009-00-0000
DATE INITIATED: 12 December 1970

Date: Onset	Date: Noted	Active Problems	Date Resolved	Inactive/Resolved Problems
10-8-67		1. HEALTH SUPERVISION		
10-67		2.		OPHTHALMIA NEONATORUM
	12-12-70	3. MOTHER UNMARRIED	6/6/71	
10-30-71		4. FUO —11/20/71→ RHEUMATOID ARTHRITIS		
	11-7-72	5. STEROID TOXICITY	12/73	
6-20-73		6. HYPERSENSITIVITY TO BEE STING		
10-12-73		7. PENICILLIN REACTION		
	12-10-73	8. SCHOOL PROBLEM		
	2-14-74	9. RECURRENT PNEUMONIA —6/74→ ASTHMA		
		10.		
		11.		
		12.		
		13.		
		14.		
		15.		
		16.		

Temporary Problems (w/date of occurrence)	1	2	3	4
A. PNEUMONIA	1/68	4/71	10/73	2/74
B. OTITIS MEDIA	11/68	12/69	4/73	
C. STREP THROAT	12/71	1/73		
D. FRACTURE, L. RADIUS	7/72			
E.				
F.				
G.				

MASTER PROBLEM LIST
Medical Center Hospital of Vermont
Page 2

Date: Onset Noted	Active Problems	Date Resolved	Inactive/Resolved Problems
	17.		
	18.		
	19.		
	20.		
	21.		
	22.		
	23.		
	24.		
	25.		
	26.		
	27.		
	28.		

Temporary Problems (continued)					Admission Dates	For Probs.	Attending
H.							
J.							
K.							
L.							
M.							
N.							
P.							
Q.							
R.							

Copy Date:

Resident's initials for approval of Problem List at discharge.

Physician's signature for final approval of discharge Problem List.

DISADVANTAGES. The relatively rigid and detailed structure of the problem-oriented record can result, when improperly and overcompulsively used, in a greatly increased expenditure of time and paper. The method is still undergoing modification to meet unanticipated problems which have arisen in the course of its use. Some fear that it will foster medical care by rote, and that it may lead to depersonalization of care or to an educational overemphasis on structure rather than substance. Problems encountered in its implementation and use are more easily handled if users recognize and can agree that arbitrary judgments must be made in the adaptation of any new system to local conditions and that they must remain the masters and the system the tool.

R. JAMES MCKAY

Barness, L. A.: Manual of Pediatric Physical Diagnosis. 4th ed. Chicago, Year Book Medical Publishers, Inc., 1972.
Korsch, B. M.: The pediatrician's approach to his patient. Am. J. Dis. Child. *126*:146, 1973.
Walker, H. K., Hurst, J. W., and Woody, M. F. (eds.): Applying the Problem-Oriented System. New York, MEDCOM Press, 1973.

THE PATHOPHYSIOLOGY OF BODY FLUIDS

Clinically the physiology of body fluids must be considered from three standpoints: (1) the amounts of water and solutes such as electrolytes in the body as a whole; (2) the distribution of these materials in the various compartments of the body; and (3) the concentration of the solutes within each compartment.

The body content of individual substances is the result of the balance between intake and output which, for materials of physiologic significance, is under careful regulation. Many of these controlling mechanisms are extremely complex, and only those of particular or special importance to the clinician will be discussed in detail. The distribution of water and solutes within body compartments is also of critical importance, and considerable energy is required to maintain steady states, since relatively few materials are kept in simple equilibrium, free of energy-requiring processes. Alterations in concentrations of substances within the body may lead to profound changes in function; the percentage and rate of change in concentrations, rather than the absolute change, are of maximal physiologic importance. Thus, small absolute changes in the concentration of a substance normally present in low concentration are usually of more clinical significance than a similar change in concentration of a substance present in high concentration. For example, an alteration in the extracellular fluid concentration of potassium of 2.5 mEq/l from normal represents a change of approximately 60 per cent and may result in profound physiologic effects, whereas a similar change in extracellular sodium concentration amounts to a change of less than 2 per cent and is of little clinical significance.

Changes in volume are relatively well tolerated, but here, too, percentage and rate of change are more critical than absolute change. Thus, the loss of 100 ml of blood in a few minutes in a large adolescent would produce a negligible disturbance; in a newborn infant it would result in shock. The same hemorrhage in the infant extended over days could be fairly well compensated.

WATER

FLUID COMPARTMENTS. Total body water is comprised of intracellular, extracellular and transcellular components (Fig. 5–1). As a percentage of body weight, total body water decreases with age from 78 per cent at birth to the adult value of approximately 60 per cent at 1 year of age. As shown in Figure 5–2 there is a linear relationship between total body water (TBW) and body weight (wt), the equation describing this relationship being TBW (liters) $= 0.611$ wt (kg) ± 0.251. Thus, approximate estimates of total body water can be obtained from body weight alone. However, fat is low in water content, so that total body water represents a smaller percentage of body weight in an obese than in a normal person. A more exact estimate of total body water can be obtained from lean body mass (LBM), where the relationship is TBW (liters) $= 0.72$ LBM (kg).

Extracellular fluid volume (ECF) is larger than the intracellular space in the fetus, but the ratio of extracellular water to intracellular water falls to the adult level by 9 months of postnatal life. This relative loss of ECF is presumably the result of the increasing growth of cellular tissue and the decreasing rate of growth of collagen relative to muscle during the early months of life. Thereafter, ECF bears a fairly straight-line relation to weight

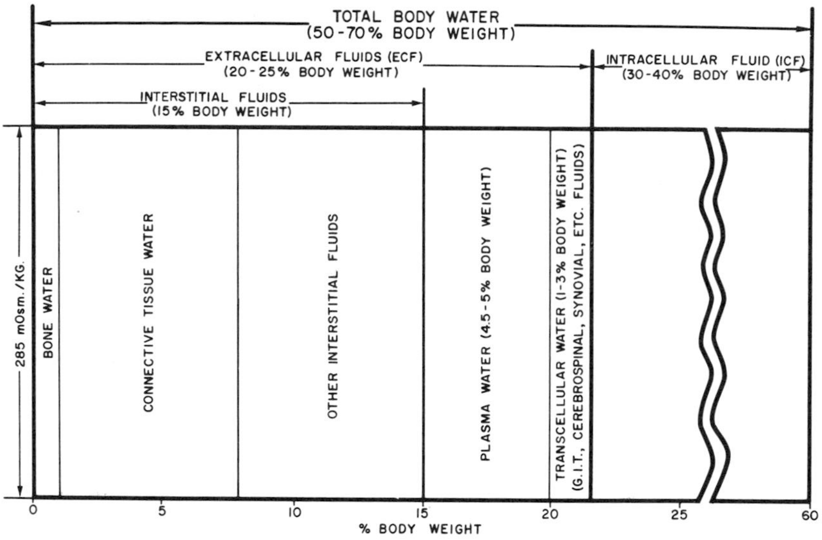

Figure 5–1 *A schematic representation of the distribution of water in the body. Percentages = per cent of body weight; G.I.T. = gastrointestinal tract.*

(ECF = 0.239 wt (kg) + 0.325) and to total body water in normal infants and children. Under conditions of normal hydration in the older child (Fig. 5–1) ECF can be assumed to equal 20 per cent of body weight and is comprised of plasma water (5 per cent of body weight) and interstitial water (15 per cent of body weight).

The **transcellular water** compartment is composed primarily of gastrointestinal secretions plus cerebrospinal, intraocular, pleural, peritoneal and synovial fluids. Transcellular fluid is usually considered as a specialized fraction of extracellular fluid, although it is probably more correct to consider fluid in the gastrointestinal tract as being extracorporeal. The volume of the transcellular compartment is highly variable, depending on the absorptive and secretory activities of the intestine; during the fasting state it represents about 1 to 3 per cent of body weight.

Intracellular fluid volume (ICF) is calculated as the difference between total body water and extracellular water. It approximates 30 to 40 per cent of body weight. Although frequently considered as a homogeneous phase, it is important to remember that it represents the sum of fluids from cells in different locations and with varying functions and intracellular composition.

REGULATION OF BODY WATER

To maintain a constant state, the amount of body water derived from intake and from oxidation of carbohydrate, fat and protein of both exogenous and endogenous origin must equal losses from the kidneys, lungs, skin and gastrointestinal tract. Precise control of the amount of water in the body is dependent upon a finely regulated feedback system involving the hypothalamus, posterior pituitary and collecting ducts of the nephrons.

Thirst, regulated by a center in the midhypothalamus, determines water intake under normal circumstances. Elevation of extracellular fluid osmolality, such as is seen with the infusion of a hypertonic saline solution, increases thirst. The infusion of urea, which diffuses rapidly into both intracellular and extracellular water, is, in contrast, a weak stimulus to thirst and produces little sustained change in water intake. A sensation of thirst may also result from reduction in volume of

Figure 5–2 *Total body water in boys plotted against body weight. The relevant equation is given in the text. The data of Cheek are indicated by X; those of Friis Hansen, by ⊗. (From D. B. Cheek: Human Growth. Philadelphia, Lea & Febiger, 1968; and B. Friis Hansen: Changes in body water compartments during growth. Acta Paediat., 1957.)*

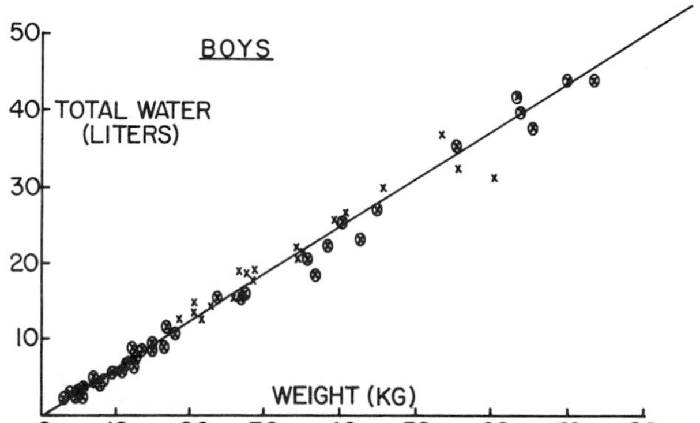

body fluids. When hypotonicity and decreased volume occur simultaneously, as is the case in some clinical situations, the volume signal is dominant, and thirst causes increased water intake, restoring volume at the expense of tonicity. The thirst mechanism and antidiuretic hormone (ADH) release may be interrelated.

Disorders of the thirst mechanism may be seen with diseases of the central nervous system, potassium deficiency and malnutrition and may lead to increased drinking, even though the content of body water is greater than usual and osmolality is decreased.

Absorption of water from the gastrointestinal tract takes place by passive diffusion in response to active solute transport from intestinal lumen to interstitial fluid and plasma. The active transport of sodium is the bulk process responsible for generating the osmotic gradient leading to movement of water. Any inhibition of sodium transport or failure of reabsorption of solute, as in disaccharidase deficiency, can lead to large volumes of unabsorbed intestinal water and result in diarrhea.

Losses of water occur from the lungs, skin, gastrointestinal tract and kidney. Evaporative water losses from the lungs and skin and that part of urine necessary to excrete the urinary solute load are obligatory losses; they represent the minimum volume of fluid a person must ingest each day to maintain balance. Evaporative water losses are proportionate to body surface and are influenced by body and environmental temperature, respiratory rate and the partial pressure of water vapor in the environment. Sweating is controlled by the autonomic nervous system and may be reduced in heat stress, by severe deficits in volume of body fluids or by concentration of electrolytes.

Urine volume can be reduced only to that necessary to excrete the solute load and is thus influenced by diet. Other factors which influence urine flow include glomerular filtration rate (GFR), the state of the renal tubular epithelium, concentrations of adrenal steroids and levels of ADH. In man changes in GFR are of little importance as a regulatory mechanism for water excretion; ADH is the principal effector.

ANTIDIURETIC HORMONE (ADH). The primary action of ADH is to increase the permeability of the renal collecting ducts to water. This allows water to diffuse into the hypertonic interstitium of the renal medulla, which has an osmolality of up to 1200 mOsm/kg, generated in large part as a result of the countercurrent multiplier and exchange systems of the loops of Henle and blood vessels of the medulla—the vasa recta.

Secretion of ADH has been localized to the supraoptic-hypophyseal system, interruption of which results in diabetes insipidus and an inability to concentrate the urine. The axons which descend through the infundibular stem from the supraoptic and paraventricular nuclei to the pars nervosa of the posterior pituitary carry a neurosecretory substance which is stored in and released from the terminal arborizations in the posterior pituitary. This material is probably ADH itself; depletion occurs in animals deprived of water, and storage occurs when water loads are administered.

Secretion of ADH is regulated in part by the relationship of ECF to ICF osmolality. This is probably monitored by vesicles in the supraoptic nuclei which act as osmoreceptors, swelling when ICF becomes hypertonic and shrinking when it becomes hypotonic in relation to ECF. The absolute level of osmolality appears to have no effect on ADH release or inhibition. Thus, the administration of urea, which increases both ECF and ICF osmolality, produces little shift of water between cells and interstitial fluid and does not evoke consistent antidiuresis. However, the intravenous injection of hypertonic saline solution evokes intense antidiuresis, since the sodium remains predominantly in the ECF, increasing its osmolality in relation to that of ICF. Conversely, the administration of water inhibits release of ADH. ADH secretion may also be modified by volume and distribution of body fluids, a decrease in effective arterial blood volume appearing to stimulate secretion.

Release of ADH may be stimulated or inhibited by emotional factors. Stressful stimuli such as pain or the mass discharge of peripheral receptors resulting from trauma, burns or surgery increase ADH output and are important considerations in fluid therapy. Nicotine is a potent stimulator of ADH output, but most other drugs producing antidiuresis do so by affecting glomerular filtration rate. Morphine and barbiturates are probably antidiuretic in this way, although the results of some experiments are interpreted to the contrary. Anesthesia also reduces urinary flow, probably by altering renal hemodynamics. Alcohol is a potent inhibitor of ADH release, with a consistent dose-response relation.

MECHANISMS OF DISTRIBUTION OF FLUID IN THE BODY. The distribution of water between intracellular and extracellular spaces is determined by physical factors. Intracellular volume is maintained relatively constant by osmotic forces operating across membranes freely permeable to water. The maintenance of these forces is dependent upon active transport of potassium into and sodium out of cells by energy-requiring processes. There is no evidence to support the concept of active transport or secretion of water per se. A rise in extracellular osmolality (e.g., with a sodium load) results in a fall in cell water. Conversely, with water intoxication a decrease in extracellular osmolality leads to an increase in cell volume. Disturbances in cellular function may also result in an increase in the fluid content of cells.

The volume of fluid in the intravascular space (plasma water) is maintained in a steady state by a balance between filtration and oncotic (effective osmotic) forces at the capillary level. A net loss of plasma ultrafiltrate occurs at the arteriolar end of the capillaries as a result of the dominant effect of hydrostatic pressure at this site. In health, oncotic pressure results in the net return of an equivalent amount of fluid and electrolytes at the venous end. Oncotic pressure (colloid osmotic pressure) is equal to only a small fraction of total osmotic pressure* but results in an effective osmotic gradient across capillary walls since it represents the osmotic pressure exerted by protein molecules, primarily albumin, that do not readily pass through the capillary pores. Decreases in protein concentration (as in the nephrotic syndrome) or acidosis (which alters the association of proteins with cations through the Donnan effect) leads to reduction in plasma volume with an equivalent increase in interstitial volume. Because plasma volume is only one third of interstitial volume, its reduction through shifts of water to the interstitial space may not be observed clinically as edema, even though circulating volume may be compromised enough to reduce glomerular filtration rate (GFR) and blood flow to other vital organs. Any increase in capillary permeability to protein, as in angioneurotic edema, leads to a rise in protein concentration of the interstitial fluid, with a reduction in the oncotic pressure and an increase in interstitial fluid. The increase may be localized, appearing as a wheal or urticaria, or may be generalized. Interstitial fluid volume may also be increased by an increase in the capillary filtration pressure due to increased venous pressure associated with heart failure or to retention of sodium and resultant hypervolemia as seen in glomerulonephritis.

The volume of the transcellular space may increase markedly in inflammatory bowel disease, e.g., eosinophilic gastroenteropathy, in early and severe diarrhea or in ileus with multiple fluid levels.

The concentrations of individual solutes of the extracellular and intracellular fluids vary (Fig. 5–3). However, the concentration of solute particles (osmoles) in each compartment is the same (Fig. 5–1), so that the chemical activity of water (i.e., the tendency of molecules to escape to another compartment) is the same in each compartment. Despite this, the volume of water in various spaces or tissues differs considerably. These variations are of clinical significance only in regard to large changes in plasma water. When serum solids, i.e., the proteins and lipids, are elevated, as may occur in diabetic ketosis with hyperlipemia, the content of water in the serum, expressed per liter of serum, is markedly decreased as a result of volume displacement of water by lipids. *Since electrolytes are dissolved in the aqueous phase of serum, electrolyte concentrations determined and expressed in the usual way (as mEq per liter of serum) will appear decreased even though their concentration per liter of serum water will be normal.* Apparent hyponatremia is most often noted in this circumstance;

*The plasma proteins exert an osmotic pressure of approximately 28 mm Hg compared to 5100 mm Hg exerted by the crystalloidal solutes of plasma. However, the capillary walls are very permeable to water and the crystalloidal solutes, which therefore exert no osmotic force across the capillary walls. Albumin, being the most abundant plasma protein and the one with the lowest molecular weight, is the principal solute responsible for colloid osmotic pressure.

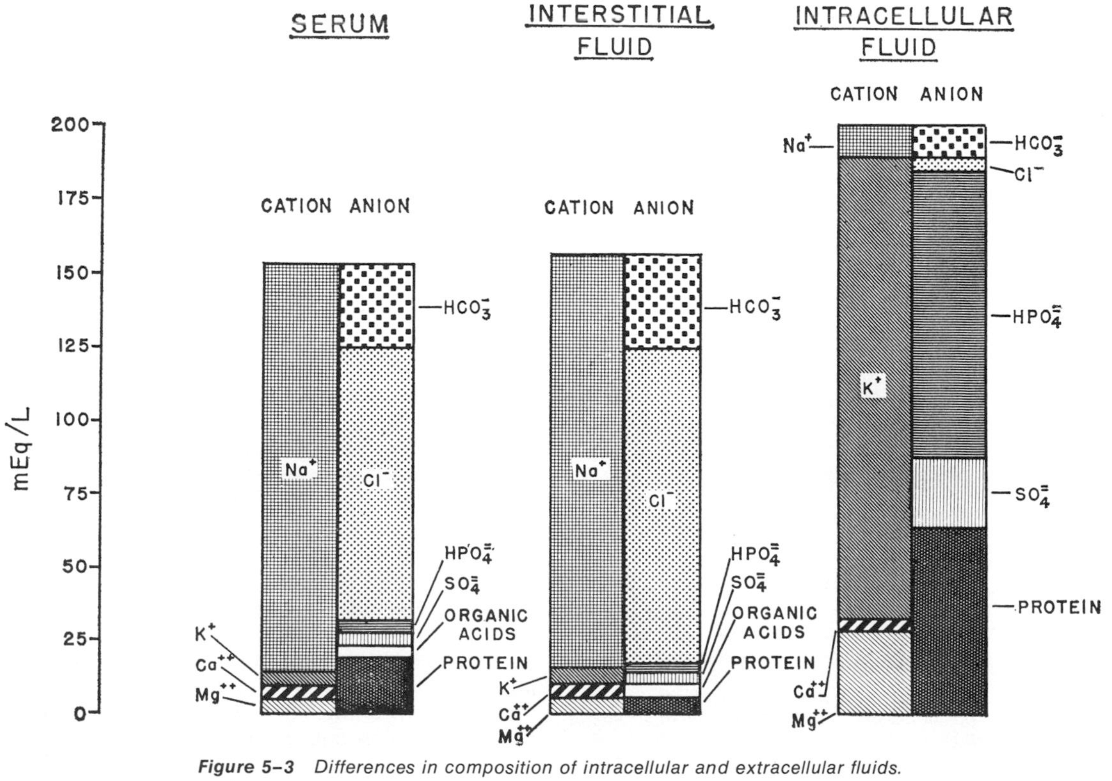

Figure 5–3 Differences in composition of intracellular and extracellular fluids.

treatment of such a patient on the basis of hyponatremic dehydration could be disastrous. Measurement of osmolality by freezing point depression (osmometry) provides true values, since this determination measures solute content as related to the water fraction of serum only.

SODIUM

BODY CONTENT OF SODIUM. Sodium is the bulk cation of the extracellular fluid and is the principal osmotically active solute responsible for the maintenance of intravascular and interstitial volumes. The quantity of sodium in the body approximates 58 mEq/kg body weight. Of this, 6.5 mEq/kg is in the plasma sodium pool, 16.8 mEq/kg is in the interstitial fluid and 1.4 mEq/kg is in the intracellular fluid. About 25 mEq/kg body weight (43 per cent of total body sodium) is present in bone, radioisotope studies indicating that much of it is either slowly exchangeable or completely nonexchangeable. Figure 5–4 indicates the percentage distribution of sodium in the body.

The **sodium content of the fetus** is relatively higher than that of the adult, exchangeable sodium averaging approximately 85 mEq/kg body weight compared to the adult value of 40 mEq/kg. This is due to the fetus's relatively large amounts of cartilage, connective tissue and extracellular fluid (all of which contain considerable amounts of sodium) and the relatively small mass of muscle cells with their low sodium content.

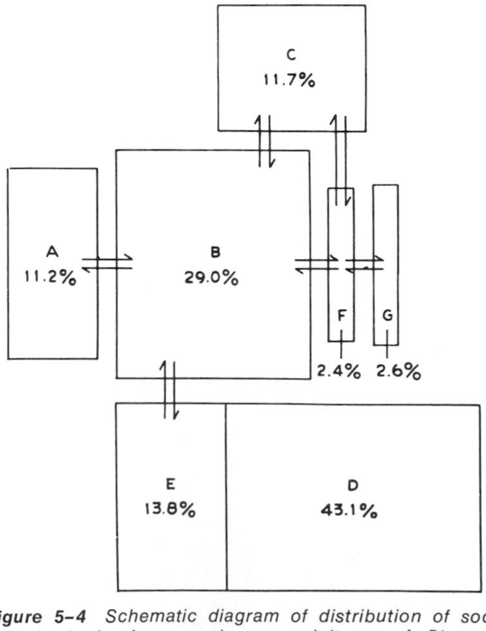

Figure 5–4 Schematic diagram of distribution of sodium within the body of a normal young adult man. A, Plasma sodium; B, interstitial-lymph sodium; C, Dense connective tissue and cartilage sodium; D, total bone sodium (including E); E, exchangeable bone sodium; F, intracellular sodium; G, transcellular sodium. (From Edelman, I. S., and Liebman, J: Am. J. Med. 27:256, 1959.)

REGULATION OF SODIUM. The amount of sodium in the body is determined by the balance between intake and output. In the average adult, dietary intake of sodium usually varies between 100 and 170 mEq per day (equivalent to between 6 and 10 gm of salt), depending on the cultural characteristics of the person. In children sodium intake is less, in proportion to their smaller intake of food. Infants generally have a relatively high sodium intake, because of the high sodium content of milk.

When compared to the thirst mechanism for water, the regulatory mechanism for **sodium intake** is poorly developed but may respond to gross changes, e.g., salt craving may occur in some patients with salt-wasting disorders. Absorption of sodium occurs throughout the gastrointestinal tract, minimally in the stomach and maximally in the jejunum, probably by way of a sodium-potassium activated ATPase (adenosine triphosphatase) system. This transport mechanism is augmented by aldosterone or desoxycorticosterone acetate (DCA). Excretion of sodium occurs in urine, sweat and feces, the kidney being the principal organ for the facultative regulation of sodium output.

Sweat sodium concentrations normally range roughly between 5 and 40 mEq/liter. Higher values are seen in cystic fibrosis and Addison's disease, lower ones in sodium depletion, acclimatization and hyperaldosteronism. However, there is little evidence to indicate that changes in sweat sodium levels are responsible for regulating sodium excretion.

Renal regulation of sodium excretion is dependent on a balance between glomerular and tubular functions. Under normal conditions the amount of sodium filtered daily by the kidneys is more than 100 times that ingested in the diet, but less than 1 per cent of the filtered sodium is excreted in the urine, the remaining 99 per cent being reabsorbed along the length of the nephron. The three principal areas of reabsorption are the proximal and distal convoluted tubules and the loop of Henle.

Approximately two thirds of the filtered sodium is reabsorbed by the proximal convoluted tubule. Experimentally induced changes in glomerular filtration rate over a wide range are accompanied by proportional changes of sodium reabsorption in the proximal tubules, resulting in glomerulotubular balance; the mechanisms responsible have yet to be fully defined. One hypothesis suggests that glomerulotubular balance may be maintained by peritubular oncotic pressure. According to this theory, an increase in glomerular filtration rate, without a change in renal plasma flow, results in an increased filtration fraction and a decrease in blood volume in the glomerular efferent arterioles. In consequence, the concentration of protein in the efferent arterioles and the peritubular oncotic pressure is increased, thus facilitating increased proximal tubular reabsorption of salt and water and the maintenance of glomerulotubular balance. It has also been suggested that sodium reabsorption in the proximal tubule may be regulated by a natriuretic hormone secreted from the midbrain or hypothalamic region. Although there is considerable indirect evidence to support this latter hypothesis, such a hormone has yet to be isolated.

The mechanism responsible for the reabsorption of sodium from the loop of Henle has been studied extensively; evidence suggests that sodium reabsorption here may be secondary to the active transport of chloride, a system which may be unique to Henle's loop. A maximal rate for sodium transport at this site has not been demonstrated, nor has any precise mechanism for regulation been delineated.

The fine regulation of sodium balance probably occurs in the distal nephron. Reabsorption of sodium in the distal convoluted tubule is stimulated by aldosterone, secretion of this hormone apparently being governed both by the renin-angiotensin system and by some aspect of potassium balance (Fig. 5–5). Renin release from the cells of the juxtaglomerular apparatus results in the conversion in the plasma of angiotensinogen into angiotensin I and in the production of angiotensin II; this latter compound stimulates aldosterone secretion from the adrenal. The stimulus for renin release may be a decrease in renal perfusion pressure or a change in the sodium concentration (or delivery) in the distal tubule at the level of the macula densa, either system providing a "servomechanism" to prevent excessive changes in sodium balance.

Additional mechanisms may be responsible for the renal regulation of sodium. It has been postulated that the cortical nephrons with their short loops of Henle may be sodium-losing nephrons, the juxtamedullary nephrons with long loops of Henle being sodium-retaining nephrons. Sodium balance could be accomplished by altering the proportion of renal blood flow directed to these two nephron populations. Such a regulatory mechanism could be intrarenal and could respond to local renin release.

In health, 1 per cent or less of filtered sodium is normally excreted in the urine to maintain sodium balance. This may increase to 10 per cent or higher with a high sodium intake or decrease to very low levels in response to a reduced dietary sodium intake in order to maintain sodium balance. This allows considerable flexibility in sodium intake without causing a significant positive or negative sodium balance, thus preventing the development in health of either edema or significant volume contraction.

In many disease states ability to maintain body sodium at normal levels is lost. Patients with chronic renal disease usually can modify sodium excretion rates, but upper and lower limits of tolerance for sodium are characteristically limited; exceeding the upper limit results in positive sodium balance and edema. However, patients with chronic renal disease in the absence of nephrotic syndrome frequently do not develop positive sodium balance until their GFR falls to levels of below 10 or even 5 per cent of normal. Some renal diseases, especially those affecting renal tubules, are associated with a limited renal ability to conserve sodium. In such patients the unnecessary restriction of sodium will result in volume contraction and a further reduction in renal function.

Positive sodium balance may be seen in association with acute decreases in glomerular filtration rate, such as those seen in acute glomerulonephritis, unless tubular reabsorption of sodium is equally depressed. It may also result from a decrease in plasma oncotic pressure (e.g., with the nephrotic syndrome), from a decrease in effective arterial volume (e.g., with congestive heart failure) or from the administration or increased secretion of steroids with mineralocorticoid effects.

Negative salt balance with inappropriately elevated urine sodium is seen in Addison's disease

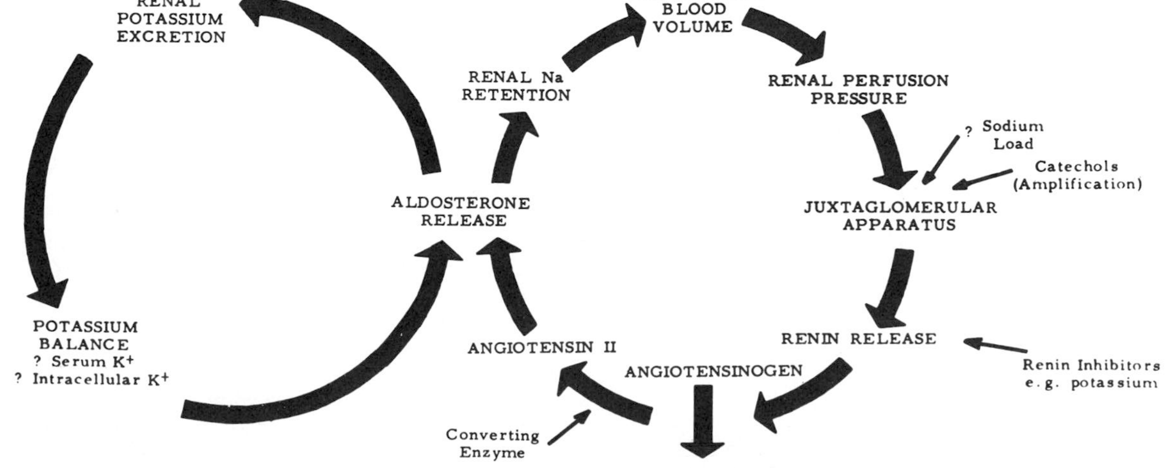

Figure 5–5 The interrelationship of the volume and potassium feedback loops with aldosterone secretion. Integration of signals from each loop determines the level of aldosterone secretion. (From Williams, G. H., and Dluhy, R. G.: Am. J. Med. 53:595, 1972.)

and in some patients with neurologic lesions, but more frequently results from extrarenal losses of sodium such as are seen with severe or protracted diarrhea.

Although cell membranes are relatively permeable to sodium, it is predominantly extracellular in distribution; intracellular concentrations are maintained at levels of approximately 10 mEq/l and extracellular ones at approximately 140 mEq/l. The low intracellular sodium concentration is achieved by the active extrusion of sodium from cells by the sodium-potassium activated ATPase system; an additional component of this system is stimulated by magnesium. No other cation can replace sodium stimulation of the enzyme but potassium can be replaced by ammonium, rubidium, cesium and lithium. Calcium inhibits the enzyme, as do ouabain and related cardiac glycosides.

Although intracellular sodium concentrations are low and represent a small part of total body sodium, they may be critical in modifying certain intracellular enzyme activities. In general, changes in total body sodium reflect changes in extracellular sodium, but redistribution of sodium between the intracellular and extracellular compartments may occur in the absence of significant changes in total body sodium. Such a change may be observed in the severely ill patient and is sometimes referred to as the "sick cell syndrome."

Sodium concentration in interstitial fluid is approximately 97 per cent that of the serum sodium value as the result of the Donnan distribution of anionic proteins; changes in the serum sodium concentrations are reflected by proportional changes in the concentration in the interstitial fluid. Transcellular sodium concentrations vary considerably, indicating that such fluids are not in simple diffusion equilibrium with plasma (Table 5–5). Changes in composition of these fluids may occur and may necessitate the changing of therapeutic regimens designed to replace abnormal losses of such fluids.

TABLE 5–5 SODIUM, POTASSIUM AND CHLORIDE CONCENTRATIONS IN TRANSCELLULAR FLUIDS

FLUID	SODIUM (MEQ/L)	POTASSIUM (MEQ/L)	CHLORIDE (MEQ/L)
Saliva	33.1 ± 13.4	19.5 ± 3.4	33.9 ± 10.2
Gastric juice	60.4 (9-116)	9.2 (0.5-32.5)	84.0 (7.8-154.5)
Ileal fluid	129.4 (105.4-143.7)	11.2 (5.9-29.3)	116.2 (90-136.4)
Cecal fluid	52.5	7.9	42.5
Pancreatic juice	141.1 (113-153)	4.6 (2.6-7.4)	76.6 (54.1-95.2)
Bile	148.9 (131-164)	4.98 (2.6-12)	100.6 (89-117.6)
Cerebrospinal fluid	140.0 (130-150)	3.3 (2.7-3.9)	126.8 (115.5-132.4)
Aqueous humor (rabbits)	143.0 (141.7-145.0)	4.7	107.9 (106.2-109.5)
Sweat	45.0 (18-97)	4.5 (1-15)	57.5 (18-97)

From Edelman, I. S., and Liebman, J.: Am. J. Med. 27:256, 1959.

POTASSIUM

BODY CONTENT OF POTASSIUM. The potassium content of the adult approximates 50 mEq/kg of body weight; isotope dilution techniques indicate that 95 per cent is exchangeable. The bulk of body potassium is intracellular (Fig. 5–6), amounting to about 48 mEq/kg. Extracellular potassium comprises only 5.5 mEq/kg, of which 4 mEq/kg is in bone. Because potassium is principally intracellular, the change in total potassium content with age and growth is an index of cellular mass, total body potassium being highly correlated with body weight and height.

Intracellular concentrations of potassium approximate 146 mEq/l of cell water; extracellular concentration is 4 to 5 mEq/l. Most intracellular potassium is unbound and osmotically active, but sequestration by active transport in subcellular particles such as mitochondria is likely. Intake of potassium varies with the quantity of food ingested; it is present in remarkably constant quantities in almost all animal and vegetable tissues.

REGULATION OF POTASSIUM. Absorption of potassium is fairly complete in the upper gastrointestinal tract, but in the lower tract potassium from the plasma is exchanged for sodium from the lumen. In this manner sodium is conserved, but large losses of potassium may occur with diarrhea, with chronic catharsis and with frequent enemas.

Potassium is lost in both sweat and urine. The concentration in sweat varies from 10 to 25 mEq/l. It may be higher in aldosteronism and cystic fibrosis, but losses are not significant. *Excretion by the kidney* provides the primary means for regulation of the body's potassium content. Under normal conditions the rate of urine potassium excretion approximates 15 per cent of the rate at which it is filtered. With the administration of large amounts of potassium, urinary excretion may be more than twice the amount filtered at the glomerulus, indicating the ability of the tubules to add potassium to the urine. Indeed, most of the potassium in the final urine probably results from tubular secretion rather than glomerular filtration.

Potassium is freely filtered at the glomerulus. Its concentration along the length of the proximal tubule is similar to that of plasma, indicating that 60 to 80 per cent is reabsorbed at this site. Concentrations of potassium increase in the loop of Henle but are decreased to below plasma levels in the early distal tubular fluid. As the fluid traverses the distal tubule, both the concentration and the abso-

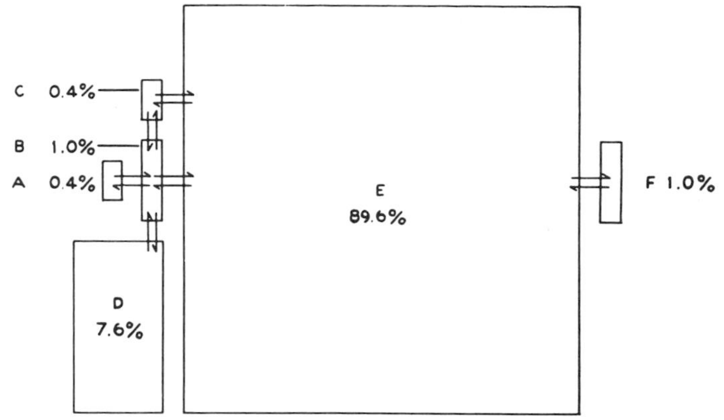

Figure 5–6 *Schematic diagram of distribution of potassium within the body of a normal young adult man. A, Plasma potassium; B, interstitial-lymph potassium; C, dense connective tissue and cartilage potassium; D, bone potassium; E, intracellular potassium; F, transcellular potassium. (From Edelman, I. S., and Liebman, J.: Am. J. Med. 27:256, 1959.)*

lute amount of potassium present increase progressively. This secretion of potassium is thought to be driven by an electrical gradient generated by the reabsorption of sodium. Although potassium secretion is dependent on sodium reabsorption, movement of these two cations across the luminal membrane in the distal tubular cell is not on an ion for ion basis, since hydrogen ion is also excreted into the distal tubule in exchange for sodium. Evidence indicates that potassium, in addition to being secreted into the distal tubule, is also reabsorbed at this site, the net amount excreted depending on a balance between the amounts secreted and reabsorbed.

Potassium excretion frequently cannot be correlated with serum potassium levels but may be correlated with intracellular potassium concentrations. Regulation probably occurs by the modification of potassium exchange in the distal tubule in response to changes in potassium concentration of the distal tubular cells. Potassium excretion may also be modified by delivery of sodium to the distal tubule, a low rate of delivery minimizing potassium excretion, an increased sodium delivery augmenting it. In addition, since both potassium and hydrogen ions are exchanged for sodium in the distal tubule, hydrogen ion balance may modify potassium excretion. Thus, a kaliuresis and hypokalemia are frequently seen with systemic alkalosis.

Aldosterone plays a large role in potassium regulation in the kidney as well as in other tissues. Injected intravenously into a patient with Addison's disease it reduces urinary excretion of sodium and increases the excretion of potassium. It acts at the level of the distal tubule, possibly by altering permeability of the luminal membrane to sodium, thus allowing increased exchange between luminal sodium and intracellular potassium. Aldosterone secretion appears to be affected by both sodium and potassium balance (Fig. 5–5).

Abnormally low amounts of total body potassium have been demonstrated in a variety of disease states characterized, in general, by a decrease in muscle mass or by renal potassium "wasting." They include muscular dystrophy, myotonic dystrophy, renal tubular disease and such endocrinopathies as Cushing's disease, aldosteronism and thyrotoxicosis. External losses of potassium result in a shift of intracellular potassium to the extracellular phase. Intracellular potassium is replaced in part by sodium, hydrogen ions and dibasic amino acids. If these changes become severe, intracellular acidosis in the renal tubular cells may result in the excessive exchange of intracellular hydrogen for sodium in the distal tubular fluid to cause a paradoxical aciduria with the excretion of ammonia, and systemic alkalosis of the extracellular fluid.

The relation of extracellular to intracellular potassium concentration is of vital importance to cell function. Hypokalemia produces functional alterations in the heart, skeletal muscle, smooth muscle, kidney and possibly the brain. The effects on muscle are probably dependent on the rate of change on a percentage basis and are manifested by weakness and characteristic electrocardiographic changes. In the kidney, potassium deficiency leads to vacuolar change in the tubular epithelium. If maintained for a long time it contributes to nephrosclerosis, interstitial fibrosis and a pathologic lesion indistinguishable from that of pyelonephritis. Functionally, nephropathy associated with potassium deficiency is characterized by reduced clearance of free water, marked reduction of concentrating ability and some reduction in diluting capability, with a net result of polyuria and polydipsia; bicarbonate reabsorption and hydrogen ion secretion are increased and lead to systemic alkalosis.

Increase of total body potassium has not been described but would probably be lethal. Except in the newborn, elevations of serum potassium lead to alterations in cardiac function with characteristic changes in the electrocardiogram.

Extracellular fluid potassium concentration may be modified by acidosis (lowered pH) which leads to extracellular movement of potassium as a consequence of the intracellular movement of hydrogen ions, and to a decrease in urine potassium excretion and a rise in serum potassium. Conversely, alkalosis decreases serum potassium and is usually associated with a kaliuresis. Alterations in cellular metabolism or in oxygenation may also result in a shift of intracellular potassium to the plasma.

CALCIUM

The metabolism of this divalent ion is discussed in other sections. (See Tetany, Rickets, and Metabolic Disorders of Bone.) It is considered here briefly because of its interrelations with other electrolytes.

At all ages 99 per cent of the body's calcium is in bone, but the bones of infants are less densely mineralized than those of adults, there being approximately 400 mEq of calcium per kilogram of body weight in the infant and about 950 mEq in the adult. In health the extracellular and plasma calcium pools and the serum calcium concentration remain remarkably constant despite fairly free exchange with the enormous reservoir in bone. The concentration of serum calcium is maintained at 2.5 mM/l (10 mg/dl), with 40 to 45 per cent of this calcium bound to protein, so that the calcium level of the protein-free interstitial fluid is about 1.5 mM/l (6 mg/dl).

The regulation of body calcium content is primarily by way of the gastrointestinal tract. Through an obscure feedback mechanism, shortage of bone minerals elicits an increase in intestinal absorption of calcium in the presence of vitamin D. It has been shown that vitamin D_3 is converted in the liver to 25-hydroxycholecalciferol, which in turn is converted to 1,25-dihydroxycholecalciferol by the kidney. This latter compound stimulates the gastrointestinal uptake of calcium and this is probably the pathway by which vitamin D increases calcium absorption. Low calcium intake, pregnancy, vitamin D administration and parathormone (PTH) also lead to increased intestinal absorption of ingested calcium. Alterations leading to hypercalcemia occur in sarcoidosis, carcinomatosis and multiple myeloma.

Renal excretion is a small factor in the maintenance of calcium balance. Maneuvers designed to modify urinary sodium excretion are usually accompanied by changes in the clearance of calcium that are in proportion to, and in the same direction as, the changes in the clearance of sodium. Urinary output of calcium increases during hypercalcemia and during chronic acidosis, at which time bone calcium is lost. Parathyroid hormone increases calcium reabsorption by the renal tubules, but this effect may be masked by the concomitant hypercalcemia and resultant increase in the glomerular filtered load of calcium seen in hyperparathyroidism.

The balance between deposition and mobilization of calcium in bone determines to a large extent the concentration of calcium in the blood. Parathyroid (PTH) hormone and thyrocalcitonin play opposing roles in modulating changes in the concentration of extracellular calcium, PTH promoting increased calcium resorption from bone and elevation of the serum calcium. Calcium is partially bound to protein; calcium levels vary directly with the level of serum albumin. However, ionized calcium levels remain normal in hypoalbuminemia, so that symptoms and signs of hypocalcemia do not develop. The level of ionized calcium is influenced by changes in hydrogen ion activity in the plasma, a pH change of 1.0 unit altering the ionized calcium concentration by 10 per cent. Acidosis increases the proportion of calcium ionized, alkalosis decreases it, so that symptomatic hypocalcemia may be seen during the rapid or overcorrection of acidosis.

In addition, the serum concentrations of sodium and potassium may play some role in the balance between deposition and mobilization of bone calcium, so that treatment of hypernatremia with fluids low in potassium content may result in hypocalcemia. Concentrated calcium solutions should always be administered cautiously, with monitoring of the electrocardiograph whenever possible. Calcium loading increases renal excretion of sodium and potassium and produces a profound reduction in ability to concentrate the urine, an effect which may explain the polyuria and polydipsia seen clinically in patients with hypercalcemia due to hypervitaminosis D.

MAGNESIUM

Magnesium is the fourth most abundant cation in the body and plays a major role in affecting cellular enzymatic activity, especially glycolysis. The total body content of magnesium is about 2000 mEq in a 70-kg man. (The contents of calcium, sodium and potassium are approximately 60,000, 5500 and 3000 mEq, respectively). The infant contains approximately 22 mEq of magnesium per kg body weight, the adult 28 mEq. Sixty per cent of the body's magnesium is in bone; most of the remainder is intracellular. Extracellular magnesium accounts for only 1 per cent of the total.

Serum magnesium is normally maintained at 1.5 to 1.8 mEq per liter, of which 60 to 85 per cent is ultrafilterable. Much of the intracellular magnesium is not free for exchange with magnesium in the blood, whereas bone magnesium is.

The intake of magnesium ranges from 10 to 25 mEq per day, depending on age; more is required during periods of rapid growth. Approximately 70 per cent of the intake is lost in the feces. Vitamin D increases, and increased calcium intake tends to decrease, absorption of magnesium. Increased intestinal motility increases stool losses of magnesium.

Serum magnesium levels are maintained largely through renal regulation. Urinary excretion amounts to about one third of the intake and is increased by calcium loading. Parathyroid hormone increases tubular reabsorption of filtered magnesium, which can be almost complete when the intake of magnesium is very low. Low concentrations of serum magnesium increase the release of parathyroid hormone, which decreases urinary losses of magnesium and elevates serum calcium. Unfortunately the serum magnesium is not a reliable indicator of magnesium depletion. Reduction in serum magnesium may occur in the absence of appreciable losses and, conversely, may be normal during magnesium depletion.

Experimental magnesium deficiency leads to hypercalcemia, slight reduction in muscle magnesium (in growing animals the deficiency is severe) and a reduction in muscle potassium. The most prominent pathologic change is calcification of the kidney. Clinically, intense vasodilatation occurs, and audiogenic seizures result. In human magnesium deficiency, particularly in severe nutritional insufficiency such as kwashiorkor, the content of magnesium in muscle is decreased.

Hypomagnesemia occurs in a variety of clinical states, especially in adults with alcoholism, malabsorption syndromes, hypoparathyroidism, diuretic therapy, hypercalcemia, renal tubular acidosis, primary aldosteronism and prolonged fluid therapy. The symptoms are primarily those of increased neuromuscular irritability, tetany, severe seizures, tremors and, occasionally, electrocardiographic alterations and changes in cardiac function.

Hypermagnesemia, with serum levels in excess of 5 mEq per liter, occurs rarely in Addison's disease and in acute renal failure; it is usually iatrogenic in origin from treatment of hypertension or toxemia of pregnancy with magnesium sulfate or from the use of magnesium sulfate orally or in enemas for megacolon. Depression of deep tendon reflexes usually antedates respiratory depression, drowsiness and coma. Symptoms are rapidly reversed by intravenous administration of calcium.

HYDROGEN ION (ACID-BASE BALANCE)

The availability of apparatus for determination of the blood gases in small samples of blood and the demonstration of the clinical significance of acidosis in both respiratory distress of the newborn and in cardiovascular surgery have led to increased awareness of clinical problems related to hydrogen ion activity of body fluids. The subject has been obscured over the years by a confusion of terminologies, each with a reasonable but conflicting approach. The older terminology which referred to fixed cations such as sodium and potassium as bases, and chloride and phosphate as anions had value in clinical thought, but alienated students of modern chemistry. The terminology used here is that agreed upon under the auspices of the New York Academy of Sciences.

Emphasis is placed on the *hydrogen ion*, which is a hydrogen atom with its neutralizing electron removed. An acid is a proton (hydrogen ion) donor; a base, a hydrogen ion acceptor. Hydrochloric, sulfuric, phosphoric and carbonic acids are *conventional acids,* each with dissociating hydrogen ions. A *strong acid* is one which is highly dissociated and therefore presents a high concentration of hydrogen ions; a *weak acid* is one which is poorly dissociated. Hydroxyl ions, ammonia and the anions of the salts of weak acids can bind free H+ ions and are *bases.* Anions and cations such as chloride, sodium, potassium, magnesium and calcium are neither acids, bases nor buffers and have been termed "*aprotes.*" A *buffer* is defined as a substance which reduces the change in free hydrogen ion concentration of a solution upon the addition of an acid or base. The presence of a buffer in a solution increases the amount of acid or alkali that must be added to cause unit change in pH. The addition of a strong acid to one of these buffer systems results in the production of a neutral salt and a weak acid. By generating a poorly dissociated acid the increment in free hydrogen ion concentration is considerably reduced in comparison to the change that would have been observed in the absence of a buffer.

REGULATING MECHANISMS. The amount of potential hydrogen ion in the body is very large, but most is buffered and is therefore not in free form. Indeed, at a blood pH of 7.40 free hydrogen ion concentration in the plasma is only 0.0000398 mEq per liter (or 3.98×10^{-8} Eq per liter). pH is determined as the negative logarithm of free hydrogen ion concentration. Thus, in normal plasma:

$$\begin{aligned} pH &= -\log (H+) = -\log (3.98 \times 10^{-8}) \\ &= -(0.60 - 8.0) = 7.4 \end{aligned}$$

pH is kept relatively constant by the presence in both the ECF and ICF of buffer systems. The principal buffer of the extracellular fluid is the bicarbonate–carbonic acid system. Intracellular buffers include various proteins and organic phosphates; in the urine, phosphate in its mono- and dihydrogen forms acts as the principal buffering mechanism. Despite the presence of buffer systems the increased production of hydrogen ion and its addition to the plasma will increase hydrogen ion concentration, decrease pH and result in acidosis. Conversely, the addition of base may produce alkalosis, with a decrease in hydrogen ion concentration and an increase in pH.

Buffer systems alone could not maintain normal acid-base balance for prolonged periods of time. They must be supplemented by physiologic adjustments in the lungs and kidneys. For example, under conditions associated with increased hydrogen ion production, the hydrogen ion added to the plasma is buffered in large part by bicarbonate, the principal buffer in plasma, with the generation of a neutral salt and carbonic acid.

$$H\,A + B\,HCO_3 \longrightarrow B\,A + H.HCO_3$$

Carbonic acid is a weak acid with a relatively low solubility coefficient and is in equilibrium with dissolved carbon dioxide as follows:

$$H.\,HCO_3 \rightleftharpoons H_2CO_3 \rightleftharpoons CO_2 + H_2O$$

Thus, hydrogen ion added to the plasma is buffered; in consequence its concentration there (and thus pH) is changed relatively little. However, to achieve this, plasma bicarbonate levels are reduced and carbon dioxide levels (pCO_2) increased.

From the Henderson-Hasselbalch equation:

$$pH = pK + \log \frac{Base}{Acid}$$

where pK is a constant calculated from the dissociation of the base/acid pair. In the case of the bicarbonate/carbonic acid system

$$pH = 6.1 + \log \frac{Bicarbonate}{Carbonic\ acid}$$

(Equation A)

Since carbonic acid is in equilibrium with dissolved carbon dioxide, measurement of the partial pressure of carbon dioxide (pCO_2) can be used as a clinical estimate of carbonic acid concentration in equation A. Thus, despite the presence of buffers, the addition of hydrogen ion to the plasma will decrease pH by decreasing bicarbonate concentration and increasing pCO_2.

However, it is apparent from equation A that pH is dependent not on absolute levels of bicarbonate and carbonic acid, but rather on the *ratio* of bicarbonate to carbonic acid (pCO_2) levels in the plasma. A decrease or increase in bicarbonate concentration will not modify pH if the pCO_2 is lowered or increased in proportion. Thus, the lungs can modify pH by altering the rate at which carbon dioxide is excreted. Although enormous quantities of carbon dioxide are produced from normal metabolic activity (Table 5–6), little change in pH results because of the unique properties of the bicarbonate-carbonic acid buffer system and a highly developed respiratory control mechanism. An increased respiratory rate, stimulated by increased levels of carbon dioxide, increases the excretion of carbon dioxide, decreases pCO_2 and thus increases pH (see equation A). Conversely, a decreased respiratory rate will result in an increase in pCO_2 and a decrease in pH.

Although the lungs modify pH by changing pCO_2 and altering the ratio of carbonic acid to bicarbonate, changes in respiratory rate do not result in any net loss (or gain) in hydrogen ion from the body. The excretion of hydrogen ions and the generation of new bicarbonate is the responsibility of the kidneys. The mechanisms for this are highly developed, energy-requiring, active transport processes, in contrast to the pulmonary excretion of carbon dioxide, which results from simple passive diffusion. Under the influence of carbonic anhydrase, proximal renal tubular cells generate hydrogen ions by the conversion of carbon dioxide and water initially to carbonic acid and then to bicarbonate and hydrogen ions (Fig. 5–7). These hydrogen ions are transported into the proximal tubule and exchanged for filtered sodium, which is reabsorbed into the peritubular capillaries with the bicarbonate generated from the formation of the hydrogen ion. In the lumen of the proximal tubule the hydrogen ion combines with filtered bicarbonate to form carbon dioxide and water. The net result is that virtually no bicarbonate passes to more distal segments of the nephron and that an amount of bicarbonate equal to the amount filtered is returned to the peritubular capillaries with an equivalent amount of sodium. This process is responsible for the reclamation of up to 5000 mEq per day of bicarbonate filtered through the glomeruli but does not result in net loss of hydrogen ion from the body.

In the distal tubular cells hydrogen ion is generated by the same process as that described for the proximal tubular cells. It is also excreted into the lumen in exchange for sodium, probably by an active process. The transport of hydrogen ion at this site appears to be gradient limited, the distal tubule being able to generate a gradient for free hydrogen ion from tubular lumen to tubular cell of only 1000:1. Transport is thus facilitated by the presence in the tubular fluid of buffers which decrease free hydrogen ion concentration and permit increased movement of hydrogen ion from cells into the tubular fluid. The principal buffers at this site are phosphate and ammonia.

Under most conditions large amounts of phosphate are present in the distal tubular fluid. In the presence of a high free hydrogen ion concentration the phosphate is converted from a monohydrogen to a dihydrogen form, reducing the free hydrogen ion concentration in the tubular fluid. The amount of hydrogen ion excreted in the urine in this form can be measured by determining the amount of alkali required to bring the urine to a neutral pH and is termed *titratable acidity.*

Ammonia, a hydrogen ion acceptor, is synthesized in tubular cells from the deamidation and deamination of glutamine in the presence of glutaminase, this reaction being stimulated by systemic acidosis. Ammonia diffuses through the lipid membrane of the cells into the tubular fluid, where it reacts with hydrogen ion to form ammonium ion, NH_4^+. This charged cation cannot readily diffuse back from luminal fluid.

These two processes, by reducing free hydrogen ion concentration in the tubular fluid, enable an increased rate of transport of hydrogen ion into the distal renal tubule and allow the generation of new

TABLE 5–6 APPROXIMATE ORDER OF MAGNITUDE OF CERTAIN FACTORS IN HYDROGEN ION METABOLISM IN STANDARD MAN OF 1.73 M²

Total CO_2 turnover	24,000 mM /24 hr
Total hydrogen turnover	69 mEq /24 hr
Total buffer in body	2100 mEq
Total hydrogen in buffer (max. capacity)	700 mEq
Total hydrogen in buffer (normal amount)	105 mEq
Total free H^+ in body fluids	0.0021 mEq

From Elkington, J. R.: Ann. Intern. Med. 57:660, 1962.

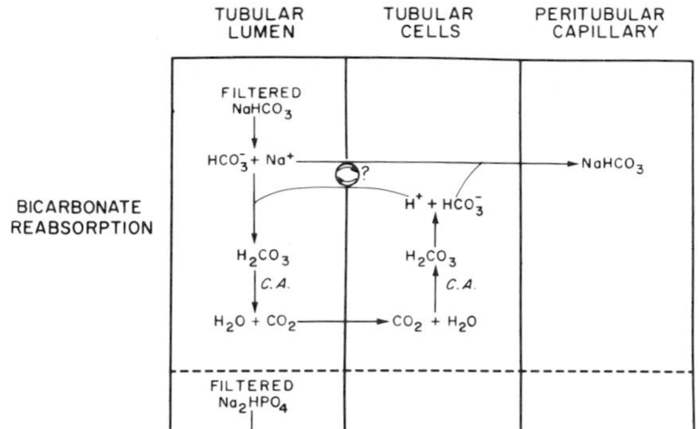

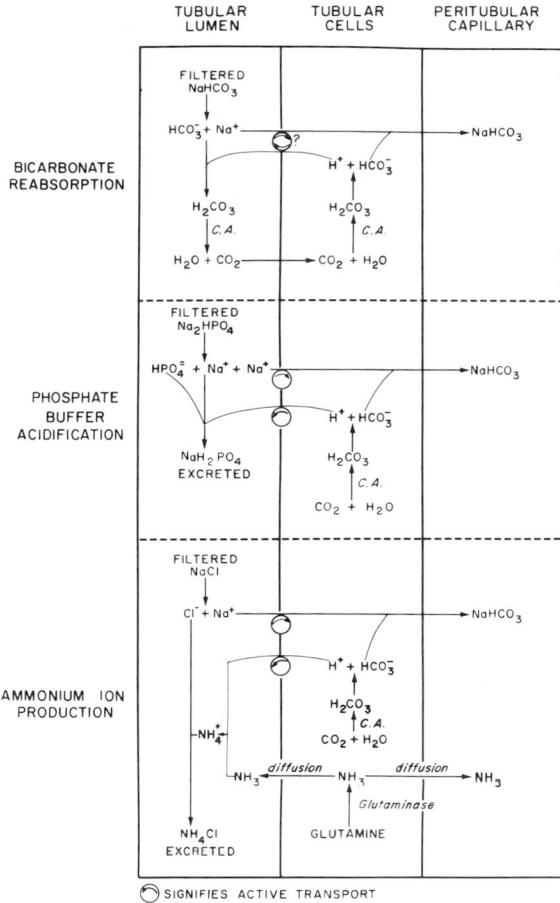

Figure 5–7 *A summary of the renal mechanisms involved in acid-base homeostasis. Bicarbonate reabsorption normally occurs in the proximal tubule where the presence of carbonic anhydrase on the luminal brush border facilitates the conversion of bicarbonate to carbon dioxide and water. This mechanism does not effect any net excretion of hydrogen ion from the body but results in the reclamation of bicarbonate in an amount equal to that lost from the plasma into the glomerular filtrate. Incomplete reabsorption of bicarbonate in the proximal tubule results in bicarbonate entering the distal nephron, where it decreases the amount of hydrogen ion available for the production of ammonium and the titration of phosphate to sodium dehydrogen phosphate and thus reduces net acid excretion. It is still uncertain whether the movement of sodium and hydrogen ions across the luminal border of the proximal tubular cell occurs by an active linked-transport mechanism.*

bicarbonate which can enter the plasma and replenish depleted levels of plasma bicarbonate (Fig. 5–7).

The absolute net rate of excretion of hydrogen ions by the kidney is calculated as the sum of the excretion rates in the urine of titratable acid and ammonium ion minus urine bicarbonate. On an average diet about one third of the hydrogen ion excreted in the urine is in the form of titratable acid, the remaining two thirds is ammonium.

The buffer, pulmonary and renal systems are not independent of one another, but act in concert. Thus, a hydrogen ion load administered to a patient would initially be buffered in the ECF by the bicarbonate system. Serum bicarbonate would fall, pCO_2 increase and serum pH would fall (but to a lesser extent than if no buffering mechanism was available). The resulting systemic acidosis and increased pCO_2 would stimulate the respiratory center to increase the respiratory rate, thus increasing the rate of excretion of carbon dioxide. Plasma pCO_2 (and thus carbonic acid levels) would fall, partially or totally correcting the acidosis but at the expense of a decrease in both plasma bicarbonate and pCO_2. The acidosis would also stimulate the kidney to increase ammonia production and hydrogen ion excretion into the urine. As a result, there would be an increased generation of new bicarbonate, returning plasma bicarbonate to normal. In turn, respiratory rate would then decrease, with the pCO_2 returning to normal. At this point the patient's acid-base status would have returned to the normal state in existence before the hydrogen ion load was administered.

The daily turnover of hydrogen ions is large, amounting to more than half of the hydrogen ion usually present in the body buffers and one tenth the maximum storage capacity of the buffer (Table 5–6). Most diets result in the production of hydrogen ions. The metabolism of protein is the largest source, accounting for approximately 65 per cent of the total. Hydrogen ion derived from protein is generated primarily from the oxidation of sulfur-containing amino acids to yield sulfuric acid, and from the oxidation and hydrolysis of phosphoproteins to yield phosphoric acid. The remainder of the hydrogen ion comes from the incomplete catabolism of carbohydrates, fats and organic acids such as pyruvic, lactic, acetoacetic and citric acids. Complete oxidation of these compounds does not produce excess hydrogen ions, since water and carbon dioxide are the final reaction products; incomplete metabolism results in the formation of organic acids and adds hydrogen ions. Thus, milk and meat diets generate about 70 mEq of hydrogen ion per day and require the daily excretion by the kidney of an equal amount to maintain a normal blood pH of between 7.35 and 7.45.

DISTURBANCES OF ACID-BASE BALANCE

Systemic acidosis may result from increased production or inadequate excretion of hydrogen ions, or from excessive loss of bicarbonate in the stools or urine. It may result from either metabolic or respiratory causes, as may systemic alkalosis.

METABOLIC ACIDOSIS

Renal Causes. With *chronic renal insufficiency* the reduced tubular mass limits the capacity of the kidney to generate ammonia and thus to secrete hydrogen ions. Diseases involving the proximal tubules may limit the ability of this segment of the nephron to secrete hydrogen ions. In consequence there may be incomplete bicarbonate reabsorption at this site and bicarbonate may be present in the distal tubular fluid, resulting in the proximal form of renal tubular acidosis. In distal renal tubular acidosis the distal tubule is unable to maintain a normal hydrogen ion gradient, so that urine pH remains relatively alkaline, rarely falling below 5.5. This results in a reduction of titratable acid, a decreased hydrogen ion secretion and systemic acidosis. A low glomerular filtration rate, such as that seen in the newborn, limits the renal capacity to excrete hydrogen ion. In addition, the filtered load of phosphate is reduced, with the bulk of it being reabsorbed in the proximal tubule; little is left for buffering of added hydrogen ion in the distal tubule. Hydrogen ion transport is thus reduced by rapid attainment of a maximal concentration gradient in the absence of buffer. Rarely, reduction in ammonia synthesis, as in the cerebro-oculo-renal syndrome of Lowe, occurs.

Other Causes. Metabolic acidosis may also develop in *diabetic ketoacidosis*. Here it results from incomplete metabolism of body lipids and catabolism of body proteins, with the production of large amounts of acetoacetic, β-hydroxybutyric, phosphoric and sulfuric acids. In *salicylism*, metabolic acidosis results not only from hydrogen ion derived from the salicylic acid, but also from the uncoupling of oxidative phosphorylation by salicylates. Metabolic acidosis is also seen in severe *diarrhea* as a result of increased losses of bicarbonate in diarrhea fluid and possibly from the formation of organic acids from incomplete breakdown of carbohydrates in the stools; in certain of the inherited aminoacidurias, e.g., methylmalonicaciduria; and in hypoxemia and shock.

In each of the preceding examples the excess hydrogen ion is buffered by both extracellular and intracellular buffers. In addition, respiratory rate is stimulated, so that the blood chemistries are characterized by a decrease in both plasma bicarbonate and pCO_2. Blood pH is decreased but rarely is as low as might be predicted from the low plasma bicarbonate level, since the increased respiratory loss of CO_2 lowers pCO_2 and partially compensates the reduction in plasma bicarbonate (Fig. 5–8).

RESPIRATORY ACIDOSIS. Respiratory acidosis results from the inadequate pulmonary excretion of carbon dioxide. It usually occurs with hypoventilation of all or a major portion of the lung or with uneven ventilation in relation to blood perfusion. Blood pCO_2 and, thus, carbonic acid concentration rise, pH falls. Initially the retained hydrogen ions are buffered, but the acidosis stimulates the kidney to increase hydrogen ion excretion as ammonium and titratable acidity, and to generate and to reabsorb more bicarbonate, so that plasma bicarbonate levels may be increased somewhat above normal. At this stage the respiratory acidosis has been "compensated" by renal mechanisms.

METABOLIC ALKALOSIS. Metabolic alkalosis usually results either from excessive loss of hydrogen ion such as is seen with prolonged gastric aspiration or persistent vomiting associated with pyloric stenosis, or from excess administration of base. The buffer systems minimize pH change, but both plasma bicarbonate and pH values are increased. Respiration may be depressed with some increase in plasma pCO_2, but this response is limited by increasing hypoxia. The renal threshold for bicarbonate is exceeded and bicarbonate appears in the urine, which may have a pH as high as 8.5 or 9.0.

RESPIRATORY ALKALOSIS. Respiratory alkalosis results from excessive pulmonary loss of carbon dioxide. It may be observed with hyperventilation of psychogenic origin, from overventilation with mechanically assisted ventilation, or in the early stages of salicylate overdosage due to stimulation of the respiratory center by salicylate or to increased sensitivity of the respiratory center to pCO_2. Plasma pCO_2 falls and pH rises. The renal excretion of bicarbonate increases slowly to reduce plasma bicarbonate levels and to compensate for the excessive loss of carbon dioxide.

INTERRELATIONSHIPS OF HYDROGEN ION DISTURBANCES

It is apparent from the foregoing discussion that acid-base disturbances of respiratory etiology may have partial or almost complete compensation by renal mechanisms. Similarly, abnormalities induced by metabolic diseases may be partially compensated by respiratory changes modifying pCO_2. Mixed disturbances can occur, as in respiratory distress syndrome, in which metabolic and respiratory acidosis often coexist. In such a situation pH changes are usually of greater magnitude than those seen when only a single disturbance exists.

Clinically, acid-base status can be determined from serum pH, pCO_2 and bicarbonate levels (Fig. 5–8). If only two of these values are known, the

	pH	pCO_2	Bicarbonate
Metabolic acidosis	↓	↓	↓
Respiratory acidosis	↓	↑	↑
Metabolic alkalosis	↑	↑	↑
Respiratory alkalosis	↑	↓	↓

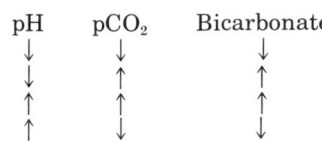

Figure 5–8 *Summary of typical serum findings in clinical disturbances of acid-base balance. It has been assumed that the primary acid-base disturbance has been partially compensated. (See text for details.)*

third can be calculated.* True bicarbonate ion concentration in the plasma can be measured and this value is used in physiologic studies. For clinical purposes the precision of this determination is not required and it is customary to determine total carbon dioxide concentration of the serum as an estimate of bicarbonate level. This value is obtained either by titration or by generation of carbon dioxide from serum with a strong acid. The carbon dioxide is derived principally from bicarbonate but also from dissolved carbon dioxide, carbonic acid, carbonate ion and carbamine compounds. The normal value is 25 to 28 millimoles (mM) per liter, except in the first year of life when values are lower, often being between 20 to 23 mM, probably owing to low renal threshold for bicarbonate. The concentration of carbonic acid (H_2CO_3) in biologic fluids is quantitatively negligible in comparison with dissolved carbon dioxide. The latter is measured as the partial pressure of carbon dioxide (pCO_2) in a gas phase in equilibrium with the biologic fluid. The normal value approximates 40 mm Hg. Normal blood pH is between 7.35 and 7.45 and can be measured accurately even on small samples of blood.†

The *hydrogen ion concentration of the cerebrospinal fluid* does not change instantaneously with change in extracellular pH. Increases or decreases in carbon dioxide tension of blood are reflected in similar changes in cerebrospinal fluid. Increases or decreases in bicarbonate concentration in blood lead to only small and delayed changes in the concentration in cerebrospinal fluid, so that the pH of each fluid at times may differ significantly, particularly if active respiratory compensation of a metabolic disturbance of acid-base balance has occurred. In acute situations, these alterations in cerebrospinal fluid concentration of free hydrogen ion may lead occasionally to abnormalities in respiration.

Intracellular pH has been estimated to be 6.8 by the DMO (5,5-dimethyl-2, 4-oxazolidinedione) method; values as low as 6.0 have been obtained using microelectrodes. Thus, intracellular pH appears to be maintained at a lower level than that of extracellular fluid. Mitochondrial pH may be even lower, since intracellular pH is probably inhomogeneous.

Carbon dioxide diffuses readily across cell membranes, so that intracellular and extracellular values for pCO_2 are similar. Thus, intracellular

*pCO_2 may be estimated from the equation

$$pCO_2 = \frac{[H^+] \times [\text{total } CO_2 \text{ content}]}{25}$$

$[H^+]$ expressed as nanoequivalents per liter (nEq/l) can easily be estimated from serum pH. At a pH of 7.40 $[H^+]$ is approximately 40 nEq/l (see Regulating Mechanisms). Each decrease in pH of 0.01 unit is associated with an increased $[H^+]$ of 1 nEq/l. Conversely, each increase in pH of 0.01 unit is associated with a decreased $[H^+]$ of 1 nEq/l. Thus, $[H^+]$ at a pH of 7.30 is 50 nEq/l and at 7.45 is 35 nEq/l. The maximum error in pCO_2 calculated by this simple formula is 7 per cent for pH values between 7.10 and 7.50 and even less in the pH range 7.28 to 7.45. (See New Engl. J. Med. *272*:1067, 1965.)

†In this discussion clinical disturbances in acid-base balance have been described in relation to changes in bicarbonate concentration and pCO_2, since this is the least misleading system for the interpretation of physiologic processes. An alternate system (Fig. 5-9) uses measurement of base excess or deficit. For this system buffer base is, in Brønsted terminology, the sum of concentrations of the buffer anions of whole blood, i.e., bicarbonate, plasma proteins and hemoglobin. Base excess is measured by titration of whole blood with a strong acid to pH 7.40 at a pCO_2 of 40 mm Hg at 37° C. For negative values of base excess the titration is carried out with base. Negative values can be denoted by the term *base deficit.* Values are expressed as mEq per liter.

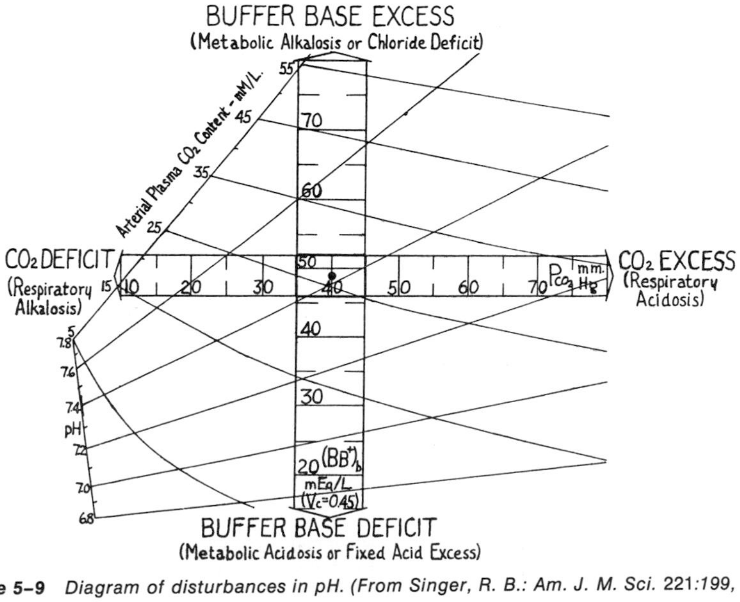

Figure 5–9 *Diagram of disturbances in pH. (From Singer, R. B.: Am. J. M. Sci. 221:199, 1951.)*

changes in hydrogen ion concentration may occur as a result of either hypocapnia or hypercapnia. With *hypo*capnia intracellular alkalosis as measured by the DMO method is proportional to the degree of extracellular alkalosis. However, with *hyper*capnia intracellular or CSF bicarbonate concentrations cannot be adjusted so rapidly as those in the ECF, so that intracellular acidosis may be proportionally greater than that seen in the extracellular fluid. In contrast to the situation in respiratory acidosis, intracellular pH may be maintained in the face of severe metabolic acidosis until extracellular pH drops below 7.0.

The effects of extracellular acidosis and alkalosis on cellular functions are not yet fully understood. A low pH produces a slight change in the Donnan distribution across the capillary membrane, so that some decrease in oncotic pressure results in a reduced plasma volume. Low pH also seems to reduce myocardial contractility, impair catecholamine action and increases the likelihood of arrhythmia, particularly with hypoxia. Moreover, if hydrogen ion concentration rises rapidly it may inhibit further transport of the ion in the kidney. Metabolic disturbances also lead to an alteration in exchange of sodium and potassium for hydrogen ion; deficiency of potassium may result in a decrease in the intracellular pH at the same time that extracellular pH is elevated.

Changes in intracellular pH probably affect the activities of many enzymes. Decrease in carbohydrate tolerance has been observed in acidosis, and increase in neuromuscular irritability (latent or manifest tetany) occurs in alkalosis. Hypocapnia leads to an increase in blood lactic acid, with a decrease in bicarbonate concentration and production of acidosis of metabolic origin.

CHLORIDE

Chloride is the bulk anion of extracellular fluid. It is not directly involved in the regulation of free hydrogen ion concentration; nevertheless, as metabolic adjustments within the kidney are made and plasma levels of bicarbonate change as a result of secretion of hydrogen ions, reciprocal changes in the concentration of chloride generally occur.

Total body chloride amounts to 33 mEq/kg of body weight. Most of it is in the extracellular and transcellular fluid, except for small quantities in red blood cells and connective tissue (Fig. 5–10). Exchangeable chloride as determined by isotope dilution or with bromide is in a fairly straight-line relation to age.

The intake and output of chloride parallel those of sodium. In general, the transport of chloride is to a large extent passive and down an electrochemical gradient created in part by sodium transport. However, recent evidence suggests that sodium transport out of the thick ascending limb of the loop of Henle in the kidney may be secondary to the active transport of chloride. This mechanism appears to be inhibited specifically by the diuretic furosemide (Lasix) and by ouabain.

Chloride may be lost in excess of sodium and potassium in vomitus or gastric drainage. It may be conserved in excess of sodium and potassium by the kidney, with the formation of alkaline urine during the renal correction of alkalosis. Conversely, it may be excreted in excess of sodium and potassium through the substitution of hydrogen ion and ammonium ion for fixed cations in the renal correction of acidosis.

Although chloride is described as playing a sec-

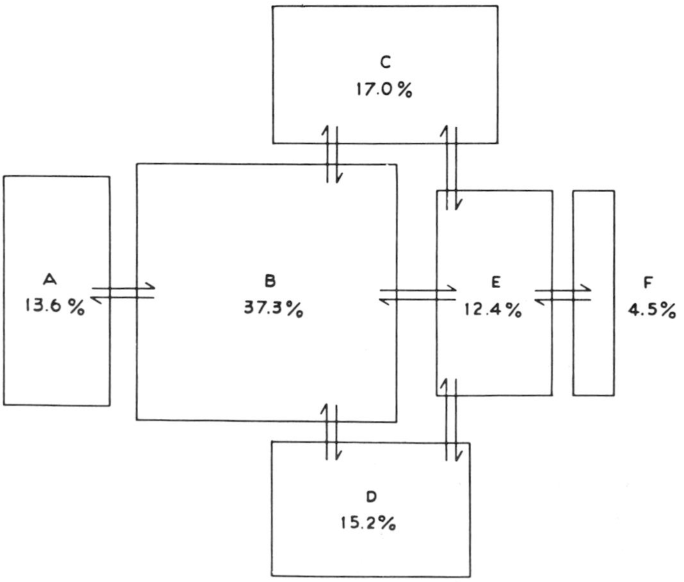

Figure 5–10 Schematic diagram of distribution of chloride within the body of a normal young adult man. A, Plasma chloride; B, interstitial-lymph chloride; C, dense connective tissue and cartilage chloride; D, bone chloride; E, intracellular chloride; F, transcellular chloride. (From Edelman, I. S., and Liebman, J.: Am. J. Med. *27:256, 1959.)*

ondary role in body physiology, ample evidence exists that correction of alkalosis with or without potassium deficiency cannot be achieved without the administration of adequate amounts of chloride. Under such circumstances the administration of either potassium or sodium chloride results in the prompt excretion of bicarbonate into the urine and correction of the alkalosis. Renal chloride wasting is excessive in potassium deficiency, and both potassium and chloride should be given in correction of deficits of each. Early amino acid solutions used in parenteral alimentation contained excessive chloride ion in the form of salts of the amino acids. Their administration resulted in hyperchloremic acidosis. Substitution of acetate has largely solved this problem.

PHOSPHORUS

Inorganic phosphate is present at relatively low concentrations in extracellular fluids and is even lower in intracellular fluid despite massive quantities of it in bone salts. Organic phosphates exist as sources of energy in all cells of the body. The largest quantities exist in muscle with creatine phosphate, ATP and glucose. The principal sources of phosphorus are milk and meat products. Excessive quantities of calcium interfere with intestinal absorption of phosphorus, forming insoluble complexes; likewise, large amounts of phosphorus interfere with absorption of calcium.

The excretion of phosphorus is by glomerular filtration, with facultative reabsorption by the proximal tubule. Recent evidence suggests that phosphate may also be added to the urine in the distal tubules. *Parathyroid hormone* reduces tubular reabsorption of phosphorus and is associated with phosphaturia. Thus, hyperparathyroidism is associated with hypophosphatemia and hypoparathyroidism with hyperphosphatemia. *Vitamin D* may be necessary for appropriate renal tubular transport of phosphorus, so that hypophosphatemia is characteristic of both vitamin D deficiency and vitamin D-resistant rickets; the role of parathyroid hormone in the genesis of this hypophosphatemia has yet to be fully delineated.

Reduction in the glomerular filtration rate below 25 per cent leads to an elevation of serum inorganic phosphate and to reciprocal changes in serum calcium, resulting in secondary hyperparathyroidism. This process begins with small decreases in GFR but usually does not become clinically apparent until GFR has fallen to low levels. Hyperparathyroidism may persist for weeks or months after successful renal transplantation.

In the young infant glomerular filtration (GFR) is low in relation to active cell mass and the dietary phosphorus intake is high; consequently, serum inorganic phosphorus is high. The premature infant has serum concentrations ranging from 2.5 to 3.0 mM/l (7.5 to 9.0 mg/dl), whereas in the adult the concentration is 1.0 to 1.3 mM/l (3 to 4 mg/dl). Hence, reduction in GFR or relative hypoparathyroidism in infants rapidly leads to very high serum values of phosphate, with depression of calcium concentration and latent or manifest tetany as a consequence. The deficit of calcium results from its formation into bone salts.

Inorganic phosphorus serves a critical function as the principal urinary buffer in the regulation of free hydrogen ions (see above). Intracellularly it serves as the source of phosphorus for high-energy synthesis of ATP. Lowering of serum phosphorus is observed in the treatment of *diabetic ketosis,* as carbohydrate is phosphorylated in the formation of glycogen. The clinical significance of this phenomenon is not known, but efforts should probably be made in therapy to minimize this decrease by administering some phosphate as part of the therapeutic regimen. Low serum and urinary phosphorus levels may occur in protein calorie malnutrition, explaining in part the inability of such patients to excrete an acid load.

Ad Hoc Committee on Acid-Base Terminology: Report. Ann. N.Y. Acad. Sci. *133*:25, 1966.

Cheek, D. B. (ed.): Human growth. Philadelphia, Lea & Febiger, 1968.

Cooke, R. E. (ed.): The Biologic Basis of Pediatric Practice. New York, McGraw-Hill Book Company, Inc., 1968.

Earley, L. E., and Daugharty, T. M. Sodium metabolism. New Engl. J. Med. *281*:72, 1969.

Edelman, I. S., and Liebman, J.: Anatomy of body water and electrolytes. Am. J. Med. *27*:256, 1959.

Elkinton, J. R.: Hydrogen ion turnover in health and in renal disease. Ann. Intern. Med. *57*:660, 1962.

Kassirer, J. P., Berkman, P. M., Lawrenz, D. R., and Schwartz, W. B.: The critical role of chloride in the correction of hypokalemic alkalosis in man. Am. J. Med. *38*:172, 1965.

Katz, A. I., and Epstein, F. H.: Physiologic role of sodium-potassium-activated adenosine triphosphatase in the transport of cations across biologic membranes. New Engl. J. Med. *278*:253, 1968.

Klahr, S., and Slatopolsky, E.: Renal regulation of sodium excretion. Arch. Intern. Med. *131*:780, 1973.

Leaf, A.: The clinical and physiologic significance of the serum sodium concentration. New Engl. J. Med. *267*:24, 1962.

Omdahl, J. L., and DeLuca, H. F.: Regulation of vitamin D metabolism and function. Physiol. Rev. *53*:327, 1973.

Pitts, R. F.: Physiology of the Kidney and Body Fluids. 2nd ed. Chicago, Year Book Medical Publisher, 1968.

Rector, F. C., Jr. (ed.): Symposium on acid-base homeostasis. Kidney Int. *1*:273, 1972.

Rocha, A. S., and Kokko, J. P.: Sodium chloride and water transport in the medullary thick ascending limb of Henle. Evidence for active chloride transport. J. Clin. Invest. *52*:612, 1973.

Schwartz, W. B., and Relman, A. S.: A critique of the parameters used in the evaluation of acid-base disorders. New Engl. J. Med. *268*:1382, 1963.

Schwartz, W. B., and Relman, A. S.: Effects of electrolyte disorders on renal structure and function. New Engl. J. Med. *276*:383, 452, 1967.

Walser, M.: Magnesium Metabolism. Reviews of Physiology, Biochemistry and Experimental Pharmacology. Berlin, Springer-Verlag, 1967.

Williams, G. H., and Dluhy, R. G.: Aldosterone biosynthesis: Interrelationship of regulatory factors. Am. J. Med. *53*:595, 1972.

Winters, R. W. (ed): The Body Fluids in Pediatrics. Boston, Little, Brown and Company, 1973.

PARENTERAL FLUID THERAPY

The daily turnover of water in the 3-kg infant is equal to almost 25 per cent of his total body water compared to the daily turnover of only 6 per cent of total body water in the 70-kg adult. As a result of this, the infant is especially susceptible to illnesses affecting fluid balance. The consequences of vomiting (with reduction of intake) or diarrhea (with increased losses) appear much more rapidly in the infant than in the adult. Thus, the correct management of fluid and electrolyte therapy deserves special emphasis in pediatric practice. This will be considered in three separate phases.

DEFICIT THERAPY. Dehydration, with deficits of total body fluids and electrolytes, may result either from inadequate intake, as seen in thirsting or fasting, or from excessive losses, as seen in diarrhea or diabetic acidosis. Deficit therapy is designed to replace such deficiencies, the aim of this phase of therapy being to return volume and composition of body compartments to normal in a dehydrated patient.

MAINTENANCE THERAPY. Any patient deprived of a normal oral intake will continue to lose basal amounts of fluids and electrolytes from the body as urine, sweat and feces and will have additional losses of water from the lungs as a result of moisturizing inhaled air. The presence of disease states may modify the amount and type of these losses. For example, pyrexia may be associated with increased sweating; renal disease may result in either oliguria or polyuria; both diarrhea and gastric suction will result in increased losses from the gastrointestinal tract. Finally, less easily recognized but equally important losses are those that may result from sequestration of fluid in a body space, e.g., a patient with paralytic ileus may have pooling of fluid in the gastrointestinal tract. Even though total body fluid and electrolyte content may not be changed, this pooled fluid may not be in equilibrium with the vascular compartment and may cause a functional deficit. Failure to replace these losses would result in the development of fluid and electrolyte deficits. Maintenance therapy is designed to replace ongoing normal and abnormal losses of fluids and electrolytes. It is required by any previously healthy patient unable to take a normal oral intake, as well as by previously dehydrated patients who have continuing normal or abnormal losses. The aim of this phase of therapy is to maintain patients in normal balance and to prevent deficits from developing.

SUPPLEMENTAL THERAPY. Specific fluid and electrolyte therapies may be required for treatment of certain disease states. For example, in salicylate intoxication, alkalinization and the induction of a diuresis are frequently employed as therapeutic measures to increase salicylate excretion in the urine.

The division of fluid and electrolyte therapy into deficit and maintenance phases is rather artificial but assists in the understanding of the principles involved. In practice, total fluid and electrolyte requirements in any individual patient are calculated as the sum of each of the components appropriate for that individual. Thus, a patient after uncomplicated surgery may require only "normal" maintenance therapy. A postoperative patient with gastric drainage will require normal maintenance therapy plus replacement of the water and electrolytes lost in the gastric fluid, whereas a dehydrated patient with severe diarrhea will require replacement of the deficits that have resulted from the diarrhea, the replacement of continuing abnormal stool losses (for as long as the diarrhea persists) and the replacement of normal fluid and electrolyte losses.

Finally, it must be emphasized that regardless of the accuracy of planning a therapeutic regimen, a patient's response to treatment is not always as predicted. In consequence, the patient must be assessed frequently so that, if he is not following an optimal course, appropriate modifications of therapy can be instituted promptly. Such evaluation usually consists of frequent physical examinations to determine clinical status, regular weighing to determine changes in body weight, frequent review of intake and output charts and regular monitoring of blood chemistries. Serial measurements of the blood urea nitrogen, serum creatinine and serum electrolytes may also be essential, the interval between determinations depending on the clinical status of the patient.

MAINTENANCE THERAPY

REPLACEMENT OF NORMAL LOSSES. As already outlined, any patient deprived of normal dietary intake requires water and electrolytes to replace obligatory losses in urine, sweat, feces and water of evaporation in exhaled air. Protein and calories are also required, but complete parenteral replacement is difficult and is not essential if therapy is required for a limited period of time. It is now well established that normal fluid and electrolyte requirements are directly related to metabolic rate. An increase in metabolic rate requires an increase in catabolism of metabolic fuels and has three effects: (1) it increases the rate of endogenous water production from the oxidation of carbohydrate, fats and protein; (2) it increases urinary solute excretion which, in turn, increases obligatory urine flow rates and urinary water losses; and (3) it increases heat production, which increases water loss as sweat and as water lost through respiration. Thus, water requirements are directly related to metabolic rate. Similarly the turnover rates of electrolytes are related to water loss and to metabolic rate.

In consequence, if a patient's caloric expenditure can be estimated, his normal maintenance requirements of fluid and electrolytes can be calculated, water, sodium and potassium requirements per unit of metabolic rate (e.g., per 100 calories metabolized) having been well established from numerous observations.

Calculation of Caloric Expenditure. Metabolic rate is dependent on age and body weight and is modified by several factors, the principal ones being degree of activity and body temperature. Values for basal metabolic rates have been well established; representative values for male and female children of different body weights are shown in Table 5–7. When calculating caloric expenditure and maintenance requirements, the basal values should be adjusted for the patient's activity, body temperature and any pathologic state present to derive an estimate of the patient's caloric expenditure. Adjustments for activity are made from observation of the patient. No increments are needed for patients in coma or under anesthesia. Usual bed activity rarely increases basal expenditure by more than 30 per cent. Caloric expenditure is increased by fever (12 per cent per ° C rise in body temperature) and by hypermetabolic states such as salicylism and hyperthyroidism (by 25 to 75 per cent). It is decreased by hypothermia (12 per cent per ° C fall in body temperature) and by hypometabolic states such as hypothyroidism (by 10 to 25 per cent).

Using these calculations a good estimate of caloric expenditure can be obtained in all but the obese and the very young infant. To calculate caloric requirements for obese infants and children

TABLE 5–7 STANDARD BASAL CALORIES

WEIGHT (KG)	CALORIES/24 HOURS MALE AND FEMALE	
3	140	
5	270	
7	400	
9	500	
11	600	
13	650	
15	710	
17	780	
19	830	
21	880	
25	1020	960
29	1120	1040
33	1210	1120
37	1300	1190
41	1350	1260
45	1410	1320
49	1470	1380
53	1530	1440
57	1590	1500
61	1640	1560

Modified from Talbot.

Increments or decrements:

1. Add or subtract 12% of above for each degree C (8% for each degree F) above or below rectal temperature of 37.8° C (100°F)
2. Add 0 to 30% increments for activity.

TABLE 5–8 WATER AND ELECTROLYTE LOSSES PER 100 CALORIES METABOLIZED UNDER NORMAL CONDITIONS AND IN DISEASE STATES

	USUAL LOSS			RANGE OBSERVED IN DISEASE STATES		
ROUTE OF LOSS	H_2O (ml)	Na (mEq)	K (mEq)	H_2O (ml)	Na (mEq)	K (mEq)
Evaporative						
Lungs	15	0	0	10–60	0	0
Skin	40	0.1	0.2	20–100	0.1– 3.0	0.2– 1.5
Stool	5	0.1	0.2	0–50	0.1– 4.0	0.2– 3.0
Urine	65	3.0	2.0	0–400	0 –30.0	0 –30.0
Total	125	3.2	2.4			

"ideal" weight (fiftieth percentiles for age and height) should be used. In the neonate, activity during the first 3 to 5 days of life is low. Total caloric expenditure does not usually exceed 50/kg of body weight per day; this figure should be used when calculating requirements for such infants.

Water and Electrolyte Requirements. Having estimated caloric expenditure, water and electrolyte requirements are then easily determined. The usual losses of water and electrolytes from the lungs, the skin, in the stool and in the urine have been well documented and are related to caloric expenditure. Table 5–8 shows that for every 100 calories metabolized the patient requires approximately 125 ml of water, 3 mEq of sodium and 2.5 mEq of potassium. Maintenance requirements for water should be reduced by 10 to 15 ml/100 calories, to approximately 115 ml/100 calories metabolized, to allow for the release of an equivalent volume of water during oxidation of endogenous and exogenous carbohydrate, fat and protein. This recommended fluid requirement is less than that prescribed in usual oral infant feeding, in which the recommended fluid intake is 140 ml per 100 calories of food; milk and other protein-containing diets increase the solute load to be excreted by the kidney, increase the obligatory water loss by this route, and thus increase fluid requirements. Thus (for every 100 calories metabolized) water, sodium and potassium requirements for normal maintenance therapy are 115 ml, 3 mEq and 2.5 mEq, respectively, and total daily requirements of water and electrolytes can easily be calculated from an estimate of daily caloric expenditure.

In health the kidney can adjust urine flow and electrolyte excretion rates over wide ranges. The maintenance requirements as calculated above do not require maximal renal concentration or dilution of urine and do not exceed the solute load which can be excreted by the kidney nor its ability to conserve electrolytes. The designated requirements thus provide some latitude in the amounts of fluids and electrolytes which can be safely administered. With renal damage or in other disease states this is frequently not the case, and maintenance requirements must be modified precisely, as outlined below.

Caloric Intake. In a patient receiving maintenance fluids by the parenteral route, it is difficult to match caloric expenditure with adequate caloric intake. Fortunately this is unnecessary if maintenance therapy is to be administered for only short periods of time. However, administration of maintenance electrolytes in a 5 per cent dextrose solution is desirable. This provides approximately 20 per cent of the calories metabolized and results in a decreased catabolism of endogenous protein and a decreased solute load to be excreted by the kidney.

Concentrations of dextrose above 5 per cent when administered at infusion rates sufficient to meet the requirement of water frequently result only in loss of dextrose in the urine. This may actually increase water requirements through an osmotic diuretic effect. At slower infusion rates such as those used in the anuric patient or the neonate, higher concentrations may be effectively used but increase the risk of intravenous thrombosis and infection.

Alternate Methods to Compute Normal Maintenance Requirements. The procedure outlined above for the calculation of maintenance requirements from caloric expenditure is derived from first principles and is accurate. However, difficulty may be experienced in calculating caloric expenditure without the availability of appropriate reference tables. To overcome this problem several simpler methods have been devised. Most are derived from the principles already outlined but relate maintenance requirements either to body weight or to body surface area. They result in values for maintenance therapy that are similar to those derived from the basic method already presented.

An example of a suitable alternate method which has appeal because of its simplicity is shown in Table 5–9. Caloric expenditure can thus be obtained from an easily remembered formula. The values depicted are for the average hospitalized patient and allow for usual activity in bed. Although values for caloric expenditure obtained by this method are slightly higher than those using the basic system, the derived values for maintenance requirements are identical, since it is recommended that for every 100 calories expended, only 100 ml of fluid should be administered (compared to 115 ml with the basic system); this solution should contain 25 mEq of sodium and 20 mEq of potassium per liter, and 5 per cent dextrose. Appropriate commercially prepared solutions with this composition are readily available (Table 30–15) and have the advantages of providing magnesium (3 mEq/l) and giving some of the anion as phosphate (3 mEq/l) and either lactate or acetate (23 mEq/l). If such a solution is not readily available, an appropriate solution can easily be prepared from standard intravenous preparations.

TABLE 5–9 A SIMPLIFIED ALTERNATE METHOD TO CALCULATE CALORIC EXPENDITURE FROM BODY WEIGHT

BODY WEIGHT (KG)	CALORIC EXPENDITURE PER DAY
Up to 10	100 Cal/kg
11–20	1000 Cal + 50 Cal/kg for each kg above 10 kg
Above 20	1500 Cal + 20 Cal/kg for each kg above 20 kg

Modified from Holliday and Segar.

Maintenance requirements calculated by this system are virtually identical to those calculated by the basic method presented earlier. For example, to calculate daily maintenance requirements for an afebrile previously healthy male child weighing 45 kg, basic caloric expenditure obtained from Table 5–7 would be 1410. Allowing a 20 per cent increment for physical activity, the estimated expenditure of calories would be 1692. Based on this figure, daily water requirements would be $16.92 \times 115 = 1946$ ml; sodium requirements, $16.92 \times 3 = 51$ mEq (equivalent to 26 mEq/l of administered solution) and potassium requirements, $16.92 \times 2.5 = 42$ mEq (or 21 mEq/l of administered solution). The administered fluid should contain 5 per cent dextrose. Using the alternate system presented in Table 5–9 caloric expenditure would be estimated as 2000 calories, which would indicate the need to administer 2000 ml of the maintenance solution containing 5 per cent dextrose, 25 mEq/l of sodium and 20 mEq/l of potassium.

MODIFICATION OF MAINTENANCE REQUIREMENTS BY DISEASE STATES. In the presence of certain disease states water and electrolyte losses may be markedly abnormal, and maintenance requirements may have to be modified considerably. Some idea of the magnitude of such modifications can be obtained from Table 5–8.

In anuria or extreme oliguria (urine flow of less than 10 ml/100 calories metabolized), only about 45 ml of exogenous water per 100 calories are required, since only evaporative and stool losses occur. Appropriate reductions in electrolyte administration should also be made. Excessive or inappropriate release of antidiuretic hormone, as in some acute infections (particularly meningitis), results in a markedly reduced urine flow rate, so that fluid intake should not exceed 80 to 90 ml/100 calories. When renal concentrating and diluting ability is lost, as in chronic renal disease, water requirements may rise to 150 ml/100 calories, and in diabetes insipidus of nephrogenic or hypothalamic origin to as high as 400 ml/100 calories. In such instances, the thirst of the patient, changes in his body weight, and an awareness of the urinary output are usually more reliable indicators of the patient's needs than are the physician's estimates. As an additional precaution, oral feedings should be used whenever possible.

Usually, but not always, urinary losses of water should be replaced on a volume-for-volume basis. For example, in acute tubular necrosis the increased urine output seen in the diuretic phase may eliminate fluid retained during the oliguric phase; these increased losses are not replaced, since such therapy would only perpetuate the presence of edema.

In hyperventilation and in heat stress, evaporative losses of water may increase as much as 90 and 120 ml per 100 calories, respectively. Increments in fluid intake should be made accordingly. High humidity, as in incubators, may reduce evaporative losses of water by 20 to 50 per cent; appropriate decrements in intake should be made.

Just as intake of water must be adjusted to meet specific alterations in body functions in the presence of disease, so must intakes of electrolytes be individualized. For example, in anuria or severe oliguria, it is ideal if no electrolytes are administered for maintenance. In congestive heart failure, limitation of sodium intake is as important in parenteral as in oral therapy. Reduction of sodium intake during fluid therapy of a patient with cardiac failure also demands some limitation of water, since renal ability to excrete a solute load is decreased and retention of water may occur.

REPLACEMENT OF ABNORMAL LOSSES. The principles underlying the concomitant replacement of abnormal losses of fluids and electrolytes require little explanation. Such losses depend on the specific clinical disturbance (Table 5–10). Considerable variation in the composition of abnormal losses exists from patient to patient and from time to time in the same patient. Although only an approximation can be made, these losses must be replaced as nearly as possible, volume for volume, as they occur in order to prevent physiologic readjustment which may further deplete the body of water and electrolytes. On occasion it is necessary to measure the electrolyte concentrations in the fluid being lost from the body so that a more exact determination of replacement needs can be made. Losses in gastric or intestinal drainage can be replaced satisfactorily by isotonic or somewhat hypotonic solutions that contain more chloride than sodium for gastric replacement and more sodium than chloride for intestinal replacement. Although gastric fluid contains relatively little potassium, the alkalosis that develops from the loss of significant quantities of hydrogen ion usually results in an increased urinary potassium loss, so that replacement fluid for a patient with gastric drainage should contain 10 to 20 mEq of potassium per liter (providing renal function is well maintained). Losses of sodium chloride in sweat are of little significance except in adrenal insufficiency and cystic fibrosis; heat stress should be avoided in such patients.

TABLE 5–10 COMPOSITION OF EXTERNAL ABNORMAL LOSSES

FLUID	NA (mEq/L)	K (mEq/L)	CL (mEq/L)	PROTEIN GM %
Gastric	20-80	5-20	100-150	–
Pancreatic	120-140	5-15	90-120	–
Small intestine	100-140	5-15	90-130	–
Bile	120-140	5-15	80-120	–
Ileostomy	45-135	3-15	20-115	–
Diarrheal	10-90	10-80	10-110	–
Sweat:*				
Normal	10-30	3-10	10-35	–
Cystic fibrosis	50-130	5-25	50-110	–
Burns	140	5	110	3-5

*Sweat sodium concentrations progressively increase with increasing sweat flow rates.

TABLE 5–11 COMPOSITION OF TYPICAL INFUSATE USED IN INTRAVENOUS ALIMENTATION

CONSTITUENT	CONCENTRATION (PER LITER)	APPROXIMATE INFUSION RATE (PER KG/DAY)
Amino acids*	25 gm	3.6 gm
Glucose	200 gm	27 gm
Sodium†	Up to 40 mEq	2-3 mEq
Potassium†	Up to 30 mEq	2-3 mEq
Chloride†	Up to 45 mEq	4-5 mEq
Acetate	15 mEq	2 mEq
Calcium	9.3 mEq	1-2 mEq
Magnesium	2.5 mEq	1 mEq
Phosphate	67 mEq	
Multivitamin	5.0 ml	
Folic acid	0.45 mg	

*Derived from an amino acid preparation Neoaminosol (Abbott Laboratories) or FreAmine (McGaw). Alternate sources of amino acids – 5 per cent beef fibrin hydrolysate (Aminosol:Abbott Laboratories) or casein hydrolysate (Amigen:Baxter Laboratories) – should be present in a higher concentration of 33 gm protein/l.

†Adjusted to meet individual patient's needs.

ADMINISTRATION OF MAINTENANCE REQUIREMENTS. Maintenance therapy may be given by either oral or parenteral routes until the usual dietary intake is reinstituted. When oral fluid administration is not possible, it is preferable to give maintenance solutions intravenously. If, owing to technical difficulties, therapy must be conducted by subcutaneous administration, glucose in water or in a very dilute electrolyte solution should not be given since diffusion of sodium chloride into such an extravascular pool and the subsequent loss of fluid from the ECF may acutely reduce plasma volume and precipitate shock.

INTRAVENOUS ALIMENTATION. The regimens for fluid and electrolyte replacement and maintenance already discussed will not sustain growth and are therefore suitable only for relatively short periods of time. In some infants and children, especially newborns undergoing major surgery and children with protracted diarrhea, it is necessary to provide parenteral nutrition for prolonged periods. Regimens have now been developed to meet this need and have been shown to be effective in maintaining positive nitrogen balance and growth for periods of 60 days or longer. The infusion solution is prepared from an amino acid preparation, and contains 20 per cent glucose, sodium, potassium, calcium, magnesium, phosphorus, chloride and vitamins (Table 5–11) and is infused at a rate of 135 ml/kg/day. In this dose it provides 122 calories per kilogram per day. Essential fatty acids and trace metals are provided by the twice weekly administration of plasma (10 ml/kg); vitamin K (5.0 mg) is given by intramuscular injection at weekly intervals; and a single intramuscular injection of vitamin B_{12} (500 μg) is also administered.

The solution is delivered by a constant speed infusion pump into the superior vena cava through a long catheter. In an attempt to minimize the risk of infection, the catheter is tunneled subcutaneously for a considerable distance before entering the vein and a millipore filter is inserted in the circuit just before the place the tubing enters the patient.

Complications from this procedure are common and include sepsis, severe hyperglycemia and marked electrolyte disturbances, including acidosis. Currently the technique is probably better performed only in those centers with experience in the method and with the necessary intensive monitoring facilities.

DEFICIT THERAPY

Deficits in body water and electrolytes may result either from reduced intake in the presence of usual losses or from excessive losses occurring either in the presence or absence of the usual intake. The severity of the clinical disturbance depends not only on the magnitude of the deficit in relation to the body reserves, but also on the rate at which the deficit developed.

TYPES OF DEHYDRATION

Deficits usually result from the loss of fluids that are *hyponatremic* in relation to the serum (Table 5–10). However, it is important to remember that body composition of dehydrated patients is influenced not only by losses but also by concomitant intake and thus reflects the relative *net* losses of both electrolytes and water. For example, a patient with severe diarrhea, losing fluid with a sodium concentration of as low as 40 mEq/l, may continue to drink tap water containing virtually no sodium. His water losses will be partially compensated for by the water intake but his sodium losses will not be replaced; despite the excess loss of a hyponatremic fluid, the patient may still present with hyponatremia.

Thus, the serum sodium in dehydrated patients may be normal, low or high, depending on the relative losses of water and electrolytes. Dehydration is classified on this basis, being termed *isonatremic* when serum sodium levels are between 130 and 150 mEq/l, *hyponatremic* when serum sodium levels are less than 130 mEq/l and *hypernatremic* when serum sodium levels are above 150 mEq/l. Since plasma osmolality in large part reflects sodium concentrations, these forms of dehydration are usually *isotonic, hypotonic* and *hypertonic,* respectively. However, there are exceptions. For example, in diabetic ketoacidosis serum sodium may be low but the plasma is hypertonic as a result of elevated plasma glucose levels. Classification of dehydration into these three types is of practical importance since each form of dehydration is associated with different relative losses of fluid from intracellular (ICF) and extracellular (ECF) compartments and each requires appropriate modifications in therapeutic approach.

In **isonatremic dehydration** the initial fluid and electrolyte loss is from the ECF. This fluid compartment remains isotonic and there is no osmotic gradient across cell walls, so that ICF volume remains virtually constant; thus, the majority of the fluid loss is borne by the ECF. In **hyponatremic dehydration** the hypotonicity of the ECF results in the osmotically induced movement of fluid from the ECF into cells, resulting in further depletion of ECF and some increase in ICF. Conversely, in **hypernatremic dehydration** the increase in ECF osmolality results in movement of fluid out of the cells, so that ICF volume is depleted and ECF depletion is less than expected. These changes are reflected by differences in physical findings and clinical presentation. These differences are outlined below.

ESTIMATION OF DEFICITS

The magnitude or severity of a deficit can be gauged from change in body weight. Losses of body weight in excess of 1 per cent per day represent loss of body water. In young infants a weight loss of up to 5 per cent is considered to indicate a mild deficit. A 5 to 10 per cent loss represents moderate dehydration; a 10 to 15 per cent loss is severe and is frequently associated with peripheral circulatory failure. Deficits in excess of 15 per cent of body weight are rarely compatible with life. In older children and adults total body water and ECF volume represent a smaller percentage of body weight than they do in the infant, so that any given percentage loss of body weight resulting from fluid and electrolyte deficits indicates a more severe depletion of fluid compartments in these age groups. Thus, comparable figures for severity of the deficit in these age groups are 3 per cent (mild), 6 per cent (moderate) and 9 per cent (severe).

Most errors in fluid management occur in the initial stages of rehydration. In some dehydrated patients the administration of appropriate fluids must be treated as a medical emergency. However, it is frequently not necessary to administer fluids until the patient's state of hydration has been assessed clinically and the type and amounts of fluids to be given for initial resuscitation have been determined carefully. A more complete assessment can be undertaken after fluid therapy has begun and consists of a detailed history and a thorough physical examination, often augmented by appropriate laboratory studies.

HISTORY. Some important aspects are shown in Table 5-12. Infants or children may have had their weight determined prior to the illness, the difference in weight at this time and when seen with dehydration giving an accurate estimate of the magnitude of fluid losses. In the absence of such information a detailed analysis estimating losses and the exact quantities and composition of the infant's feedings prior to being seen may permit a less exact estimate of the magnitude of the deficit and indicate the type of dehydration. Homemade electrolyte mixtures used for the oral treatment of diarrhea are often responsible for severe hypernatremia, especially if the solution has been prepared with excessive amounts of salt or sodium bicarbonate. Urine output characteristically decreases with dehydration; thus, the time and frequency of recent urinations, whether excessive or suppressed, may provide some appreciation of the severity of dehydration. Continued frequent and excessive urination in the face of dehydration is suggestive of diabetes mellitus, diabetes insipidus and nephrogenic diabetes insipidus. Usual output of urine without increased intake of water in association with physical signs of dehydration indicates a loss in the capacity of the kidney to conserve water and suggests the presence of renal disease.

PHYSICAL EXAMINATION. Table 5-13 lists signs of dehydration and of resulting shock. As suggested by the table, physical examination may help to differentiate the type of dehydration. Patients with hyponatremic dehydration have increased losses of fluid from the ECF and are more likely to develop shock; conversely, evidence of ICF volume depletion may be apparent in patients with hypernatremic dehydration. Most infants and children appear unwell when dehydrated. Frequently the eyes appear sunken and the skin around them dark. Intraocular pressure, as elicited by pressing with the fingers over the closed eyes, is low. The mucous membranes of the mouth are usually dry, although prolonged mouth breathing or the tachypnea of acidosis may mimic this finding in the absence of dehydration. Tissue turgor may be reduced. Normally when the skin and subcutaneous tissue are pinched between the thumb and first finger and then released they return to position immediately. Delay in return ("tenting") indicates dehydration. Skin and subcutaneous tissue must be tested together or else laxity of skin may be misinterpreted as dehydration. Skin over the abdominal and chest walls as well as on the thigh should be tested, since abdominal distention may mask loss of turgor at this site. It should also be

TABLE 5-12 HISTORICAL DATA REQUIRED IN ESTIMATING MAGNITUDE AND TYPES OF DEFICIT AND IN PLANNING DEFICIT THERAPY

Intake—during period of illness
Quantity and how given
Kind: water, electrolyte, protein, drugs

Output—during period of illness
Quantity
Kind: urine, vomiting, diarrhea, sweat, drainage

Balance
Weight change

General medical
Age
Cardiovascular, respiratory, renal or central nervous system disease

TABLE 5-13 EFFECTS AND PHYSICAL SIGNS OF DEHYDRATION

	ISONATREMIC DEHYDRATION (PROPORTIONATE LOSS OF WATER AND SODIUM)	HYPONATREMIC DEHYDRATION (LOSS OF SODIUM IN EXCESS OF WATER)	HYPERNATREMIC DEHYDRATION (LOSS OF WATER IN EXCESS OF SODIUM)
ECF Volume	Marked decrease	Severely decreased	Decreased
ICF Volume	Maintained	Increased	Decreased
Physical Signs			
Skin			
Color*	Gray	Gray	Gray
Temperature	Cold	Cold	Cold or hot
Turgor†	Poor	Very poor	Fair
Feel	Dry	Clammy	Thickened
Mucous membrane	Dry	Slightly moist	Parched‡
Eyeball	Sunken and soft	Sunken and soft	Sunken
Fontanel	Sunken	Sunken	Sunken
Psyche	Lethargic	Coma	Hyperirritable
Pulse*	Rapid	Rapid	Moderately rapid
Blood pressure*	Low	Very low	Moderately low

*Signs of shock rather than of dehydration itself.
†Reflects magnitude of fluid loss from ECF.
‡Tongue often has shriveled appearance due to loss of cellular fluid.

remembered that in the well nourished infant or child, skin turgor may remain fairly normal in the presence of dehydration. Depression of the anterior fontanelle in the infant is often an accurate indication of dehydration.

Shock may supervene with severe dehydration. This is manifested by tachycardia, a thin and thready pulse, cyanosis and a low blood pressure. Blood pressure is frequently hard to determine, but even an estimate of only systolic pressure obtained by palpation is useful. Alternately, the use of the Doppler technique may enable an accurate measurement of blood pressure to be made. The state of the peripheral circulation can be assessed by the warmth and color of the skin and by the rapidity of filling of the cutaneous capillary bed after pressure over the ear lobe, the nail bed or the dorsum of the hand or the foot. However, peripheral circulation can be affected by local factors such as ambient temperature, and care must be taken when evaluating these signs.

LABORATORY DATA (Table 5–14). These are helpful in the initial planning of therapy as well as in the determination of the type of dehydration. None is so essential that adequate therapy cannot be initiated without it; the laboratory is of greater importance in assessing the results of deficit therapy and in guiding subsequent maintenance therapy.

An indication of the severity of dehydration may also be obtained from the presence of hemoconcentration (increase in hemoglobin, hematocrit and plasma proteins). However, with a pre-existing anemia, hemoglobin and hematocrit may be normal even in the presence of severe dehydration. Similarly, the measurement of plasma proteins may have limited usefulness at the beginning of therapy. Despite such limitations, these measurements when correlated with physical findings may be useful in planning therapy, and serial determinations are of considerable help in assessing its effectiveness.

Dehydration may result in a decrease in glomerular filtration rate, so that both blood urea nitrogen and creatinine levels will increase. Such elevations may also result from intrinsic renal disease. Measurement of urine concentration may help to separate these two entities; a specific gravity of less than 1.020 in the face of dehydration indicates the presence of a defect in urinary concentrating mechanisms and suggests intrinsic renal disease. With dehydration there may be mild to moderate proteinuria and the urine may contain hyaline and granular casts, a few or many white blood cells and, occasionally, red blood cells. Such findings do not necessarily indicate intrinsic renal disease. However, urinalysis should be repeated after recovery from the dehydration. Serial measurements of urinary output and specific gravity are of value in assessing the degree of renal compensation which may be expected during therapy, as well as in guiding therapy.

TABLE 5–14 LABORATORY DATA USEFUL IN PLANNING THERAPY

Serum or plasma
- Carbon dioxide content and chloride concentration
- Sodium, potassium and magnesium concentration
- Serum osmolality (freezing point depression)
- Protein concentration
- Serum solids (refractometer)

Whole blood
- pH, pCO_2 and standard HCO_3^- (Astrup)
- Hematocrit
- BUN or SUN or NPN

Urine
- Volume and specific gravity (or osmolality)
- Albumin, sugar, acetone
- Sediment

Electrocardiogram

Serum (or plasma) electrolyte values indicate the relative losses of water and electrolytes, the serum sodium indicating the type of dehydration. Total body sodium is depleted *in all three forms* of dehydration, even in the presence of hypernatremia. Serum potassium concentrations are usually not helpful at the beginning of therapy. Values may be elevated because of anoxia, diminished renal function or acidosis, even when there are significant cellular deficits. Serial electrocardiograms may provide clues to disturbances of intracellular potassium levels as well as to those of calcium. The difference between the sum of cation (sodium and potassium) and that of anion (chloride and bicarbonate) concentrations is usually 15 ± 5 mEq/l. This value is increased in renal disease resulting from retention of phosphate and other unmeasured anions as well as in ketosis and in lactic acidosis. The difference may also be useful in indicating the possibility of laboratory error in electrolyte determinations. Determinations of blood pH, pCO_2 and bicarbonate levels are particularly valuable as guides to the severity of metabolic disorders or in patients receiving assisted or artificial respiration.

TYPE AND AMOUNT OF LOSSES. As outlined below, the losses of water, sodium and potassium are similar for many disease states which result in dehydration. Other deficits may be more specific for individual disease states. Thus, severe diarrhea is associated with marked losses of bicarbonate and results in systemic acidosis. Conversely, with pyloric stenosis, major losses of both hydrogen and chloride ions result in **hypochloremic alkalosis.** In chronic diarrhea, continuing losses of magnesium may result in hypomagnesemia. The findings on physical examination that may indicate such deficits are summarized in Table 5–15. It should be emphasized that the characteristic signs of acidosis (increased depth and rate of respiration) may be less in the presence of severe circulatory insufficiency, and that the compensatory diminution in breathing associated with alkalosis, though usually absent in adults, may be seen in infants with pyloric stenosis. Deficiencies of potassium, calcium or

TABLE 5-15 PHYSICAL SIGNS OF VARIATIONS IN CONCENTRATION OF SPECIFIC IONS

Acidosis
Respiration: increased depth and rate
Alkalosis
Respiration: decreased depth and rate
Latent or manifest tetany
Hypopotassemia
Heart: fast or slow; poor quality to heart sounds
Skeletal muscle: weakness or paralyses; diminished reflexes
Smooth muscle: abdominal distention; ileus
Hyperpotassemia
Heart: slow or fast; poor quality to heart sounds
Skeletal muscle: fibrillation; paralyses
Hypocalcemia
Latent tetany (Section 19)
Manifest tetany (Section 19)
Hypercalcemia
Gastrointestinal: fecal masses
Hypotonia
Hypomagnesemia
Latent or manifest tetany
Muscular twitching
Hypermagnesemia
Decreased deep tendon reflexes
Central nervous system depression

magnesium may exist with obvious physical findings. Hypokalemia may not always be present even when cells are depleted of potassium, so that such deficits may have to be inferred from history alone.

The **absolute deficits** of water and electrolytes observed in dehydration produced by different disease states have been estimated by a variety of methods. Representative values are shown in Table 5-16. These figures give only an order of magnitude and are intended to serve as a partially quantitative guide rather than as a precise determinant of therapy. They illustrate that there is a decided similarity in the magnitudes of deficits, irrespective of the precipitating condition. This is not surprising, since deficits reflect not only the results of direct losses, but also the physiologic readjustments by the patient. Thus, when planning therapy for the dehydrated patient, the important considerations are the magnitude of the deficits and the qualitative changes in body composition that have resulted from relative losses of electrolytes in relation to water. Similar basic therapeutic approaches with only minor modifications may be utilized for patients with dehydration that has resulted from widely differing etiologies.

TABLE 5-16 PROBABLE DEFICITS OF WATER AND ELECTROLYTES IN INFANTS WITH MODERATELY SEVERE DEHYDRATION

CONDITION	H_2O (ml)	Na (mEq)	K* (mEq)	Cl (mEq)
	Per Kg of Body Weight			
Fasting and thirsting	100–120	5–7	1–2	4–6
Diarrhea				
Isonatremic	100–120	8–10	8–10	8–10
Hypernatremic	100–120	2–4	0–4	−2–−6†
Hyponatremic	100–120	10–12	8–10	10–12
Pyloric stenosis	100–120	8–10	10–12	10–12
Diabetic acidosis	100–120	8–10	5–7	6–8

*Converted for breakdown of tissue cells: −1 gm N = 3 mEq of K.
†Negative balance of chloride indicates excess at beginning of therapy.

PRINCIPLES OF THERAPY

Deficit therapy is influenced by the magnitudes of deficits of sodium and water, by the type of dehydration and by the status of both potassium and hydrogen ion balance. As has already been stressed, there is a similarity in the magnitudes of deficits resulting from different diseases, so that a single basic approach to therapy can be applied to dehydration from a number of causes.

With mild dehydration it may be possible to administer adequate fluids orally, but usually parenteral administration is required, with the intravenous route being preferred. As with maintenance therapy, if fluids have to be administered subcutaneously, they should not consist of glucose in water or in dilute saline solution, since shock can be precipitated by the rapid migration of salt into the subcutaneous pool with subsequent contraction of the ECF.

Therapy can be considered in several phases. The initial phase is designed to improve circulatory dynamics and renal function, these being of primary importance in the morbidity and mortality of dehydration. In essence, it consists of rapid expansion of extracellular fluid volume. Subsequent therapy is aimed at replacing the remaining intracellular and extracellular deficits of water and electrolytes but at a slower rate, sodium replacement preceding potassium replacement. The final phase consists of the return of the patient's state of nutrition to normal and is usually begun when the patient is able to return to oral feedings.

INITIAL THERAPY. Initial therapy is aimed at rapid expansion of the ECF volume and more specifically the plasma volume, either to treat shock or to prevent its occurrence. Ideally, the entire fluid used for the initial treatment of dehydration should remain in the vascular space. Although the administration of whole blood would appear to be the treatment of choice, this is not so, since needless delays may result during the typing and cross-matching of the blood and since there is a considerable risk of thrombosis accompanying the administration of blood in this circumstance. Similarly, the risk of hepatitis makes the use of pooled plasma undesirable. The use of a sodium-containing fluid with an osmolality and sodium concentration similar to that of normal blood is recommended. Sodium chloride solution 0.9 per cent (Na 154 and Cl 154 mEq/l) is one alternative especially useful in patients with metabolic alkalosis (e.g., with dehydration resulting from pyloric stenosis). In a patient who may be acidotic a solution containing bicarbonate or a bicarbonate precursor is preferable, since the use of sodium chloride alone would not correct acidosis and might even aggravate it by further diluting the plasma bicarbonate. A suitable solution containing bicarbonate is not commercially available, but can easily be made by adding 28 ml of 7.5 per cent sodium bicarbonate solution to 750 ml of 0.9 per cent sodium chloride solution, making the final volume to 1 liter with 5 per cent dextrose in water. This solution contains 140 mEq of sodium, 115 mEq of chloride and 25 mEq of bicarbonate per liter. Similar commercial solutions containing lactate or acetate instead of bicarbonate are available, but have the disadvantage that in severely dehydrated patients with impaired circulation the bicarbonate precursor may not be readily metabolized to bicarbonate, so that therapy with these solutions may aggravate the existing acidosis.

The solution chosen for the initial phase of therapy can be started immediately even though serum electrolyte values are not known. The volume given should equal 20 to 30 ml/kg of body weight and should be given rapidly. If clinical signs of extracellular fluid and blood volume deficit persist, a second and, rarely, a third infusion of 20 to 30 ml/kg may be necessary to restore circulation. Monitoring central venous pressure to minimize the danger of volume overload is sometimes possible. This therapy is equally appropriate in hypo-, iso- and hypernatremic dehydration, the administered fluid tending to return the serum sodium toward normal in each instance. In some patients with hypernatremic dehydration serum sodium may increase even further with the administration of isotonic saline, the mechanism for this being unclear. However, this increase in serum sodium is usually 5 mEq/l or less and does not appear to affect the clinical course adversely.

Potassium should not be administered at this stage of therapy unless the patient is known to be severely hypokalemic; it should be given only after it is established that the patient has functioning kidneys.

Glucose should be included in all fluids, since the sick infant is susceptible to hypoglycemia.

Occasionally the therapy outlined above is inadequate to reverse shock, and under such circumstances blood (10 ml/kg) or other plasma volume expander is required.

SUBSEQUENT THERAPY. Once circulation has been restored, therapy during the remainder of the first 24 hours is aimed at more complete correction of the sodium, water and other deficits. Replacement of potassium losses may be started during this phase of therapy but is not essential and frequently is not attempted until after the first 24 hours of treatment.

By the time this phase of therapy is reached the patient's serum electrolytes should be known and therapy is modified, depending on the presenting serum sodium level.

Isonatremic Dehydration. In isonatremic dehydration there are not only external losses of sodium from the ECF, but there is movement of sodium into the ICF to compensate for intracellular potassium losses. If one were to administer sodium ion in an amount equal to the total loss from the ECF, it would result in an increase in the patient's total body sodium; the increment of sodium in the ICF would later return to the ECF when potassium was administered, resulting in expansion of the ECF. To avoid this, therapy is planned so that only two thirds of the approximate ECF sodium and water losses are replaced during the first 24 hours of therapy. For example, in a patient with severe isonatremic dehydration (15 per cent of body weight) the fluid deficit would be 150 ml/kg of body weight and the sodium deficit 21 mEq/kg (assuming a serum sodium concentration of 140 mEq/l). In the first 24 hours of therapy only 100 ml/kg water and 14 mEq/kg sodium should be administered. Of this, 20 to 30 ml/kg of fluid and 3 to 4 mEq/kg of sodium should be administered in the first 2 to 3 hours in order to expand the ECF. The remaining 70 to 80 ml/kg of water and 10 to 11 mEq/kg of sodium would then be given between the third and the 24th hours of treatment. The fluid used for this phase of therapy should be similar to that used in the first 2 or 3 hours, i.e., 0.9 per cent saline or its equivalent, and is aimed at replacing the bulk of the deficits of water and sodium. However, total fluid and electrolyte administration during this and subsequent phases of treatment should include not only amounts sufficient to replace deficits but also to replace ongoing normal losses and any ongoing abnormal losses from diarrhea, intestinal suction, and so forth. Calculation of these latter components of fluid therapy has been outlined in the earlier section on Maintenance Therapy.

After the first 24 hours the objective is to achieve repletion of sodium and water losses and to start replacing potassium losses. The sodium and water requirements at this point can be estimated by adding 25 per cent to estimated normal maintenance requirements.

Although potassium losses in dehydration may equal sodium losses, potassium is lost almost exclusively from the ICF, but has to be replaced by administration into the ECF. If potassium were replaced at a rate equal to that used to replace sodium, severe hyperkalemia would almost certainly result. Thus, potassium losses are usually replaced over a three- to four-day period. To minimize the risk of inducing severe hyperkalemia, potassium should not be administered if the serum potassium is elevated *and* until it is established that the kidneys are functioning. Moreover, it should be administered cautiously in the presence of severe acidosis. Except under unusual circumstances, the concentration of potassium in the administered fluid should not exceed 40 mEq/l and the rate of potassium administration should not exceed 3 mEq/kg of body weight per day.

Hyponatremic Dehydration. This condition results from relatively greater losses of sodium than of water. The extra sodium loss can be calculated from the formula:

$$\text{Extra sodium loss (mEq)} = 135 - S_{Na} \times \text{total body water (in liters)}$$

where S_{Na} represents the serum sodium observed on admission (135 is a low normal value for serum sodium). Because the patient is dehydrated, total body water should be estimated as between 50 and 55 per cent of admission body weight rather than the usual value of 60 per cent. Even though sodium is principally an extracellular cation, total body water is used for the calculation of sodium deficit. This allows for repletion of sodium lost from the ECF and any expansion of the ECF that occurs with repletion, and for repletion of sodium lost from other exchangeable sodium pools, such as that in the bone. Treatment of hyponatremic dehydration is similar to that of isonatremic dehydration, with the exception that when calculating sodium administration the extra losses of that ion should be taken into account. Administration of the extra amounts of sodium needed to replace the additional losses can be spread over several days, so that gradual correction of the hyponatremia is accomplished as volume is expanded. No attempt is made to elevate sodium concentrations abruptly by the administration of hypertonic saline solutions unless symptoms of water intoxication, such as convulsions, are present. Such symptoms rarely occur unless serum sodium levels fall below 120 mEq/l. In such circumstances symptoms are usually rapidly controlled by the administration of a 3 per cent solution of sodium chloride given intravenously at a rate of 1 ml/minute up to a maximum of 12 ml/kg of body weight. *Hypotonic solutions should be avoided, especially in the initial phase of treatment, because of the risk of inducing symptomatic hyponatremia.*

Hypernatremic Dehydration. Severe hypernatremic dehydration presents one of the more difficult problems in fluid therapy. Too rapid correction of the serum sodium frequently results in convulsions. Therefore, therapy is adjusted to return serum sodium levels toward normal by not more than 10 mEq/l/day. The sodium deficit in hypernatremic dehydration is relatively small and the ECF volume relatively well-maintained, so that the amounts of both sodium and water to be administered in this phase of therapy are reduced compared to those in hypo- or isonatremic dehydration. A suitable regimen would be to administer 60 to 75 ml/kg/day of a 5 per cent dextrose solution containing 25 mEq/l of sodium as a combination of the bicarbonate and chloride.

Amounts of maintenance fluid and sodium should be reduced by about 25 per cent during this phase of therapy because the hypernatremic patient has high ADH levels resulting in low urine volumes. Replacement of ongoing abnormal losses does not require modification.

If seizures do occur they may often be controlled by the intravenous administration of 3 to 5 ml/kg of a 3 per cent sodium chloride solution or the administration of hypertonic mannitol.

Although hypernatremic dehydration can be successfully treated, treatment is difficult and seizures frequently occur even with the best-designed regimens. It is better to emphasize prevention, since this particularly dangerous form of dehydration is frequently iatrogenic in etiology. (See Acute Diarrhea in following pages.)

CORRECTION OF NUTRITIONAL DEFICIENCIES. Although parenteral fluid therapy results in the administration of inadequate calories to meet the patient's needs, this is rarely a cause for concern because of the short periods of time usually involved. When the patient is able to return to a normal diet, he will soon correct any deficits in body fat and protein that may have occurred.

Should parenteral fluid therapy be required for prolonged periods of time, e.g., the patient is unable to eat or develops severe diarrhea whenever oral feeding is restarted, increased caloric and nutritional intake may be required to prevent the development of serious malnourishment. This is best accomplished by using the technique of intravenous alimentation already outlined.

ASSESSMENT OF RESPONSE. Many factors modify the amounts and types of fluids to be administered. Thus, it is of vital importance that the clinician monitor the patient's response to therapy. This should include frequent clinical observation with special emphasis on the child's cry, his degree of activity, skin turgor and blood pressure. In addition, the careful charting of intake and output with stool and urine volumes recorded separately is of value in assessing response to therapy, as is frequent measurement of the patient's body weight. Under certain circumstances serial measurements of serum and urine electrolytes and osmolality and central venous pressure as well as EKG monitoring may be appropriate. In the severely ill child the use of a carefully maintained flow sheet (on which these serial determinations are recorded) as a guide to adjustment of therapy may be lifesaving. Should a patient's response to therapy not be as predicted, appropriate modifications of the regimen must be instituted promptly.

OTHER METHODS TO CALCULATE REQUIREMENTS

Alternate systems to estimate fluid and electrolyte requirements have been developed using the principles already outlined. They combine deficit and maintenance needs. One method (Table 5–17) presents a suggested outline for the management of specific disease entities.

Another method which is in widespread use expresses fluid and electrolyte requirements per unit of the patient's surface area and frequently is referred to as the meter-squared system. The basic principles of this system are shown in Table 5–18. The ability of the kidneys to regulate and to alter markedly the excretion of water and electrolytes ensures that in health a patient can tolerate the administration of fluid and electrolytes over wide ranges. As shown in the table, various disease states may reduce the maximum (ceiling) or increase the minimum (floor) amounts of water or electrolytes that can be tolerated. However, the average dehydrated child with functioning kidneys still has relatively large ranges of tolerance. If water and electrolytes are provided in adequate quantities within the limits of tolerance, the patient will cure himself, renal function providing final regulation.

According to this system, normal *maintenance* of water and electrolytes in older infants and children is provided by 1500 ml/M²/24 hr of a solution containing 5 per cent dextrose, 25 mEq/l of sodium and 20 mEq/l of potassium.

With experience the clinician can determine fluid and electrolyte requirements using these guidelines and does not necessarily go through the several stages of calculations presented earlier. The important exceptions to this generalization are patients with marked renal insufficiency, cran-

TABLE 5–17 DEFICIT THERAPY OF INFANTS WITH MODERATELY SEVERE DEHYDRATION AND ELECTROLYTE DISTURBANCES

CLINICAL CONDITION	SOLUTION	ML/KG	TIME SCHEDULE IN HOURS FROM ONSET OF THERAPY	ROUTE
Fasting and thirsting	Ringer's lactate	20	0-1	IV
	5% or 10% invert sugar or glucose in H_2O	60	1-8	IV
	Darrow's K lactate*	20		
Diarrhea				
Isotonic dehydration	Ringer's lactate	20	0-1	IV
	Blood or plasminate†	10	1-2	IV
	5% or 10% invert sugar or glucose in H_2O	40	2-8	IV
	Darrow's K lactate*	60		
Hypotonic dehydration	Ringer's lactate	20	0-1	IV
	Blood or plasminate†	10	1-2	
	5% invert sugar or glucose in Ringer's lactate	40	2-8	IV
	Darrow's K lactate*	60		
Dehydration in malnourished infants	5% invert sugar or glucose in Ringer's lactate	40	0-1	IV
	Blood or plasminate†	10	1-2	IV
	5% invert sugar or glucose in Ringer's lactate	40	2-8	IV
	Darrow's K lactate*	60		IM
	$MgSO_4 \cdot 7H_2O \cdot 50\%$	0.1		
Hypertonic dehydration	Ringer's lactate	20	0-1	IV
	Blood or plasminate†	10	1-2	IV
	5% or 10% invert sugar or glucose in H_2O	60	2-10	IV
	M/6 Na lactate	20		
	K acetate concentrate§	0.5		
	Calcium gluconate‖			
Pyloric stenosis	Isotonic NaCl	20	0-1	IV
	Blood or plasminate†	10	1-2	IV
	5% or 10% invert sugar or glucose in H_2O	40	2-8	IV
	Isotonic NaCl*	40		
	Isotonic KCl*	20		
Diabetic acidosis	Ringer's lactate	20	0-1	IV
	Blood or plasminate†	10	1-2	IV
	5% or 10% invert sugar or glucose in H_2O	50	2-8	IV
	KPO_4 concentrate‡	0.5		
	Darrow's K lactate*	50		

All of above to be followed by maintenance therapy.
*May be given separately subcutaneously.
†For shock not responding to Ringer's lactate.
‡Phosphate concentrate contains 2 mEq of K per ml.
§K acetate concentrate (Cutter) contains 4 mEq of K per ml.
‖Total dose, 10 ml of 10% solution slowly IV.

TABLE 5–18 PRINCIPLES OF METER SQUARED SYSTEM FOR DETERMINING FLUID AND ELECTROLYTE THERAPY

SUBSTANCE	RANGE OF TOLERANCE (IN HEALTH)	CEILING LOWERED	FLOOR RAISED
Water	1–13 l/m²/24 hr (1–5 in first week of life)	General anesthesia Morphine and related drugs "Nephritis" Hypothalamic lesions Circulatory failure Neonatal period	Diabetes insipidus Nephrogenic diabetes insipidus Cellular K deficiency Na intoxication
Sodium	5–250 mEq/m²/24 hr	Zero potassium intake Hypoalbuminemia Cardiac failure Severe stress Corticosteroid therapy Cushing's syndrome Renal disease	Hypoadrenocorticism Abnormal loss of GI fluids Extensive burns Renal tubular disease (diuretic therapy)
Potassium	10–250 mEq/m²/24 hr	Marked dehydration Circulatory failure Low Na intake Reduced GFR Hypoadrenocorticism Congenital adrenal hyperplasia	Diarrhea GI drainage High Na intake Corticosteroid therapy
Phosphorus	0–4000 mg/m²/24 hr (expressed as phosphorus)	Normal newborn Reduced GFR Hypoparathyroidism Pseudohypoparathyroidism Circulatory failure	Vitamin D intoxication Hyperparathyroidism
Chloride	0–250 mEq/m²/24 hr		
Bicarbonate	5–250 mEq/m²/24 hr		
Glucose	50–300 gm/m²/24 hr		

iopharyngioma, adrenal insufficiency or other defects in the homeostatic mechanisms responsible for regulation of water and sodium metabolism. In such patients severe impairment of renal or other regulatory mechanisms severely limits the ranges of tolerance and requires that each component of fluid and electrolyte be carefully calculated for the individual patient on a daily or even more frequent basis.

THERAPY IN SPECIFIC DISEASE STATES

ACUTE DIARRHEA. Despite improved infant care, diarrhea continues to be a serious problem in many areas of the world. As indicated in Table 5–16, it results in large losses of both water and electrolytes. The proportions of losses vary in different situations.

In approximately 70 per cent of patients the losses of water and electrolytes are proportionate, *isonatremic dehydration* developing. In such patients total solute concentration in body fluids remains relatively normal even though there may be severe acidosis and significant absolute deficits. *Hyponatremic dehydration* with serum sodium levels below 130 mEq/l is seen in approximately 10 per cent of all patients with diarrhea. Sodium losses are increased out of proportion to fluid losses. It is seen when large amounts of electrolytes are lost in the stool, as with bacillary dysentery or cholera in older infants and young children, and may be accentuated or produced if, during the period of diarrhea, a considerable oral intake consisting of low electrolyte or electrolyte-free fluids is continued.

Disproportionately large net losses of water compared to electrolytes result in *hypernatremic dehydration,* with serum sodium levels increased above 150 mEq/l in approximately 20 per cent of patients with diarrhea. Hypernatremia may also result from the oral administration of homemade solutions with too high concentrations of salt, and from the mistaken preparation of formulas with condensed instead of evaporated milk or with heaped or packed instead of level measures of milk powder, all of which increase the renal solute relative to the water load. Indeed, "epidemics" of hypernatremic dehydration resulting from faulty instructions by physicians or failure of mothers to follow instructions exactly have been seen periodically. Hypernatremic dehydration may also occur in young infants with diarrhea in whom renal ability to conserve water is limited, especially if the renal solute load is increased by feeding boiled skim milk. Such factors may be potentiated by high environmental temperatures or hyperventilation, both of which significantly increase evaporative water loss.

Severe hyperosmolality may result in cerebral damage with widespread cerebral hemorrhages and cerebral thromboses or subdural effusions. The cerebrospinal fluid protein level is usually elevated. Cerebral injury may result in permanent neurologic deficit, e.g., cerebral palsy. Seizures are a common clinical manifestation of hypertonicity. They are often seen when the serum sodium is returning to normal after therapy has been instituted. It has been postulated that the seizures may occur at this time because of an increase in the sodium chloride and potassium content of cerebral cells during the period of dehydration, resulting in an excessive movement of water into these cells during rehydration and before excess sodium is eventually extruded. Although the mechanism by which this water movement may result in seizures is still uncertain, it has been amply demonstrated that the incidence of seizures may be reduced by correcting hypernatremia slowly over a period of days.

Treatment of hypernatremic dehydration with large amounts of water, with or without salt, frequently results in expansion of the extracellular fluid volume before there is any notable excretion of chloride or correction of the acidosis. As a consequence, edema and cardiac failure may develop, necessitating treatment with digoxin. Hypocalcemia is also seen occasionally during treatment of hypernatremic dehydration; it may be prevented by the administration of appropriate amounts of potassium during therapy. Once developed, it may require the intravenous administration of calcium. Another complication is renal tubular injury with azotemia and loss of concentrating ability; this may necessitate modification of the therapeutic regimen.

The physical signs of moderate or severe dehydration secondary to diarrhea have been listed in Tables 5–13 and 5–15 and the principles of replacement therapy already outlined. It should be emphasized that persisting diarrhea may cause continuing large losses of fluid. These and the concomitant losses of electrolytes (Table 5–16) must be replaced.

Many infants and children with mild diarrhea do not require parenteral fluid therapy; the decision to use such therapy rests on clinical appraisal of the patient and the circumstances. Intravenous therapy must be given if there are signs of circulatory insufficiency, lethargy, vomiting or gastric distention; or in infants in whom large amounts of fluid are required to meet continued stool losses. In the absence of these indications and with evidence of only mild dehydration, solutions containing carbohydrate and electrolytes may be given orally. Commercial mixtures, such as Pedialyte or Lytren, are available in the U.S., or a similar, less expensive mixture may be prescribed.* Any such mixture must be made exactly as prescribed, since hypernatremia and hyperosmolality may result from more concentrated solutions (see above). An occasional infant receiving 2 to 3 liters of carbohydrate and electrolyte mixtures per day orally may have an apparently related increase in the volume of stools, but such instances are sufficiently rare that they do not contraindicate an initial trial.

In infants with moderate or severe diarrhea it is preferable to give intravenous therapy and to omit oral feedings initially. Although the net absorption of carbohydrate, fats and proteins may be increased by feeding large amounts of milk during diarrhea, there is unquestionably an increase in the volume of stool. This makes the replacement of water and electrolytes exceedingly complicated and extends the need for parenteral fluids by several days. Frequency and volume of stools will usually subside rapidly within 48 hours of starting therapy. When this occurs, and if gastric distention and vomiting are absent, oral feeding of one of the carbohydrate and electrolyte mixtures may be initiated. As soon as the infant tolerates the carbohydrate and electrolyte mixture by mouth without exacerbation of the diarrhea, the caloric intake may be increased gradually by the substitution of mixtures which also contain fat and protein until the usual dietary intake is achieved, usually in 6 to 8 days. Premature administration of large numbers of calories in the form of milk may induce exacerbation of the diarrhea. In the young infant with a family history of allergy the use of a hypoallergenic feeding mixture is recommended for the recovery phase, since permeability of the gastrointestinal tract to whole protein may be increased during this time.

In addition to replacement of the deficits of water and electrolytes, efforts must be made to obtain an etiologic diagnosis so that specific antimicrobial

*Example of a sugar and electrolyte mixture for oral administration:

Sucrose	50.0 gm
NaCl	1.7 gm
$KHCO_3$	2.0 gm

Dissolve in 1 liter (1 quart) of water.

Final concentration	
Sucrose	5 gm%
NaCl	30 mM/l
$KHCO_3$	20 mM/l

therapy may be given if indicated. Such treatment does not modify fluid therapy, except that during the administration of sulfonamides adequate amounts of fluid must be provided for urine formation.

Drugs which inhibit peristaltic activity, or methylcellulose derivatives which absorb intestinal contents and produce a more bulky stool, have relatively little effect on the course of infantile diarrhea.

Dehydration from Diarrhea in Chronically Malnourished Children. Severe malnutrition complicated by diarrheal dehydration is a common problem in subtropical countries, and an occasional one in the temperate zones. Therapy must be adapted to meet the specific disturbances in body composition characteristic of the dehydrated malnourished infant. There appears to be an overexpansion of the intracellular space, with extracellular and presumably intracellular hypo-osmolality. Serum sodium, potassium and magnesium levels tend to be low, and tetany may occasionally result from magnesium deficiency. Serum proteins are frequently below 3.6 gm/dl. The sodium content of muscle is high; potassium and magnesium contents are low. The electrocardiogram frequently shows tachycardia, low amplitude and flat or inverted T waves. Cardiac reserve seems lowered, and heart failure is a common complication.

Despite clinical signs of dehydration and reduced body water, urinary osmolality may be low in the chronically malnourished child. This renal concentrating defect may result from the failure of urea to contribute to a hypertonic fluid in the renal papillae, a defect associated with a low dietary protein intake and resulting in a failure of tubular water conservation. However, the glomerular filtration rate is low, resulting in a smaller loss of water than would otherwise be expected, and renal concentrating ability returns after several days of high protein feedings.

Survival of the malnourished infant with diarrhea is limited by caloric deficit to a greater extent than by water and electrolyte deficit. Reparative calories can be given by slow drip through an indwelling nasogastric tube while electrolyte and water are given parenterally. If appetite is poor and vomiting and gastric distention are absent, feeding is begun early at the level of 30 to 40 Cal/kg/day, given by slow intragastric drip. Increases to 50 to 100 Cal/kg/day and 1 to 2 gm of protein/kg/day are made in a few days. Ad libitum intake should be permitted in the succeeding weeks, up to 250 to 300 Cal/day, and should include an adequate supply of iron and copper.

Initial parenteral therapy is designed to improve the circulation and to expand extracellular volume. The repair solutions recommended resemble those for hyponatremic dehydration. If edema is present, rate of administration and quantity of fluid should be reduced from recommended levels in order to avoid pulmonary edema. Blood should be given if the patient is in shock, severely ill or anemic. Potassium salts can be given early if urine output is good. Controlled trials suggest that survival can be improved by the intramuscular injection of 1.0 to 1.5 ml of a 50 per cent solution of magnesium sulfate (4.0 mEq/ml) every 12 hours for 1 to 3 days. Clinical and electrocardiographic improvement may be more rapid with magnesium therapy, and seizures occurring during recovery from diarrhea complicating severe malnutrition may respond to magnesium.

CHRONIC DIARRHEA. When diarrhea is severe and prolonged, intravenous administration of amino acids, divalent cations, vitamins and additional calories is required in addition to carbohydrate and electrolytes to sustain body reserves. The technique of parenteral alimentation, already described, has been shown to be effective in this respect.

Occasionally full oral feedings are required during chronic diarrhea in addition to parenteral fluid therapy, especially in severe malnutrition as noted above. Allergy to milk protein or specific disaccharidase deficiencies should be suspected in infants with persistent diarrhea. Acquired disaccharidase deficiency (especially for lactose) may develop as a complication of many chronic disorders of the gastrointestinal or other systems. Hypoallergenic feeding mixtures containing monosaccharides as the sole carbohydrate should be administered until cessation of the diarrhea and improvement in nutrition have occurred. Specific tests of carbohydrate (disaccharide) splitting and absorption and of milk protein sensitivity can then be carried out but can be potentially dangerous, sometimes resulting in severe diarrhea with marked fluid and electrolyte losses.

CONGENITAL ALKALOSIS OF GASTROINTESTINAL ORIGIN. Rarely, chronic diarrhea may be the result of a congenital defect in the transport of water and electrolytes across the intestinal wall. In addition to the usual losses of potassium, the watery stools of such patients have a high content of chloride, and alkalosis results. The deficit therapy is analogous to that of pyloric stenosis, but must be on a continuing basis and planned in conjunction with an adequate dietary intake of potassium and chloride.

PYLORIC STENOSIS. This condition exemplifies the correction of deficits associated with alkalosis. The therapy differs little from that of diarrhea, except that potassium repletion should begin early, as soon as the child has urinated (see Section 11), and that relatively more of the sodium and potassium replacement therapy should be given as the chloride, partly because of the larger deficit of chloride seen in pyloric stenosis, and partly because this results in some correction of the alkalosis as volume is expanded. *Correction of the hypochloremia by administration of ammonium chloride without correction of the deficit of potassium results in continued dysfunction of renal tubular cells as well as of other cells and is not recommended.* Severe depletion of intracellular potassium will result in increased exchange of hydrogen ion for sodium in the distal tubules of the kidney. Thus, the paradoxical presence of an acid urine in the face of systemic alkalosis should be interpreted as signifying a marked potassium deficit and the need to increase the amount of potassium used for repletion.

Although deficits may be replaced and serum levels returned to normal within 12 hours, operation should not be performed for at least 36 to 48 hours to permit optimal readjustment of body functions. Such a delay may not be required in mildly ill infants with no signs of dehydration. Adequate fluid therapy prevents deterioration during this period of preparation, and the stomach may be decompressed by gentle suction. (See Preoperative, Paraoperative and Postoperative Care in following pages.)

FASTING AND THIRSTING. Parenteral fluid therapy is usually required in the initial treatment of the infant or child who has taken little or no water and food for 1 to 5 days. Such infants are deficient not only in water, which has evaporated from the lungs and skin, but also in electrolytes, particularly sodium and chloride, which have been excreted in the urine (Table 5–16). The administration of electrolyte-free solutions under such circumstances leads only to an increase in urine volume, with possible increased losses of electrolytes, and may actually increase the dehydration. If fasting and thirsting continue beyond 4 or 5 days, urinary output will fall to such a low level that there will be no significant continued loss of electrolytes, and further severe deficiency of water alone will result.

Therapy is begun with an isonatremic solution to produce rapid and safe expansion of extracellular volume and improvement in renal function. A large part of the remaining deficiency of water and electrolytes may be made up by a solution containing carbohydrate, sodium chloride, some potassium and bicarbonate, and a bicarbonate precursor such as lactate or acetate. Owing to the relatively smaller extracellular reservoirs with increasing age, children and adults should be given approximately one fourth to one third less water and sodium per kg than infants for a given degree of clinical dehydration. Potassium deficits are relatively the same in infants, children and adults, since they have approximately the same quantity of potassium per kg of body weight. Water, carbohydrate and electrolytes may be administered to the mildly ill patient by mouth. Infants, however, often vomit when they are dehydrated, and for this reason initial therapy is usually given parenterally.

DIABETIC ACIDOSIS. (See also Section 16.) The deficit therapy of diabetic acidosis approximates that of diarrhea. Initially extracellular volume is expanded rapidly with Ringer's lactate or an equivalent solution. The balance of the replacement therapy is carried out slowly over the remainder of the first 24 hours. The administration of carbohydrate fairly early in therapy permits glycogenation of the liver after response to insulin and reduces the danger of hypoglycemia.

In the appraisal of deficits in patients with diabetic ketosis, laboratory studies may be misinterpreted. Hypo-osmolality may be assumed erroneously on the basis of measurement of the serum sodium concentration alone; if there is a high concentration of blood glucose, extracellular osmolality may be normal or high even with a low serum sodium concentration. Blood sugar levels of 1800 mg/dl increase plasma osmolality by 100 mOsm/l – equivalent to an additional 50 mEq/l of sodium with an attendant anion. Elevations of serum lipid and protein concentrations in diabetic acidosis may also reduce the water content of the serum, so that sodium concentrations expressed per liter of serum are low, even though the sodium concentration of extracellular water is normal or high.

Administration of potassium early in therapy of these patients is essential. A rapid fall in extracellular potassium concentration occurs shortly after administration of insulin. Untreated, such changes may produce alterations in the functioning of the heart, liver, brain and kidneys, contribute to gastric distention and even lead to respiratory paralysis. Changes in serum inorganic phosphate concentration during therapy are likewise striking, and parallel those in potassium concentration. This fall is due primarily to cellular uptake of phosphorus as glycogen is formed. Although the clinical significance of such changes has not been established, it is probable that serum inorganic phosphorus should be sustained at low normal levels. For this reason some potassium should be administered as the phosphate salt. Magnesium levels may be elevated at the beginning of therapy and fall rapidly to below normal in a manner similar to those of potassium; no clinical significance has been attributed to these changes. No specific attempts are made initially to elevate the low carbon dioxide content and pH; rapid correction of the systemic acidosis with bicarbonate may paradoxically increase the degree of acidosis in the cerebrospinal fluid. Rather, therapy is directed to expansion of the extracellular volume, using a fluid that resembles an ultrafiltrate of normal plasma, such as Ringer's lactate; this frequently results in a significant reduction in acidosis with symptomatic improvement. If extreme respiratory distress persists, the administration of sodium bicarbonate may be indicated. The dose required may be calculated from the formula given under Acidosis in the following pages. There is, however, a large reservoir of potential bicarbonate in the form of ketone acids which are metabolized with improvement in carbohydrate utilization after administration of insulin. Therefore, bicarbonate concentration of the serum should not be elevated abruptly to more than 12 to 15 mEq/l.

The amount of insulin which can be safely administered during this time varies considerably from patient to patient. Enough crystalline zinc insulin to effect clearing of the ketosis by accelerating the utilization of carbohydrate should be given, along with adequate carbohydrate to prevent development of hypoglycemia. An initial dose of approximately 2 units/kg for severe diabetic ketosis, followed by doses of 1/2 to 1 unit/kg at 1- to 3-hour intervals, is usually appropriate. Half of the initial dose of insulin should be given intravenously. Approximately 1 to 2 gm of carbohydrate per unit of insulin may be necessary to prevent hypoglycemia. (In a normal person up to 5 gm of carbohydrate are required per unit of insulin to prevent hypoglycemia.) The aim of therapy should be the elimination of ketonemia and ketonuria, since persistence of acetoacetic acid and betahydroxybutyric acid indicates diminished operation of the Krebs cycle. The patient's response to therapy should be closely monitored. Collection of urine at hourly intervals, preferably without resort to catheterization, is essential for modifying the dosage of insulin and carbohydrate as therapy progresses; only rarely in children will ketones be absent from the urine when the serum level is significantly elevated. Reduction of the blood sugar to a level which avoids excessive glycosuria prevents unusual loss of water in the urine, but reduction of the blood sugar to excessively low levels by administration of insulin without adequate carbohydrate leads rapidly not only to hypoglycemia but to a return or exacerbation of ketosis. During the early stages of treatment of children with severe ketoacidosis serum electrolytes, pH and blood sugar may have to be monitored at regular 4-hour intervals. Blood gas determinations may also be of assistance in monitoring response. Dextrostix give a rapid estimate of blood sugar but are of more benefit in detecting hypoglycemia than in determining the precise value of an elevated blood sugar level.

BURNS. Unless unusual delay has occurred before a burned child is brought to the hospital, preexisting deficits are minimal, and significant deficits result solely from inadequate or delayed fluid therapy after admission.

Maintenance requirements for water are diminished when a large surface area of skin is covered by wet dressings which limit evaporative losses from this site; evaporation from the lungs is normal or increased. Urinary output of water is probably limited by some antidiuresis which results from massive stimulation of nerve receptors. Thus, the fluid therapy of burns is concerned principally with the replacement of abnormal losses. Some of these losses are external, such as oozing of plasma from the burned surface, but the largest part of the abnormal loss is *internal* in the form of plasma and plasma ultrafiltrate sequestered around the burn site. The magnitude of this sequestration has been approximated by measurements of the extracellular space in patients with severe burns. Such measurements are partially invalidated, however, by the fact that large amounts of saline solution have usually been administered therapeutically prior to the determination of extracellular space, and true obligatory losses can only be approximated. In addition to these losses, a significant number of erythrocytes are destroyed or their survival time is shortened by exposure to heat.

Losses of fluids are proportional, not to the weight or metabolism of the patient, but to the surface area of the second- or third-degree burn. This area can be approximated by the "rule of nine"* or from appropriate charts of the body surface.

The composition of an ideal replacement solution cannot be fixed. A mixture of 3 parts of plasma, 1 part of blood and 3 parts of a balanced saline solution† is a reasonable replacement fluid which may be given at a rate of 10 liters per square meter of second- or third-degree burned surface area per 48 hours. One third of this fluid is administered in the first 6 hours, a third in the next 12 hours and a third in the next 30 hours. Such a program can only approximate the actual needs; the patient's progress must be monitored at 1- to 2-hour intervals by the determination of hematocrit values of capillary blood and of plasma protein levels and by careful measurements of the volume and concentration of urine, which may have to be obtained by an indwelling catheter. Urine volume should be held at 30 to 50 ml per 100 calories metabolized. A rising hematocrit and falling urine volume usually indicate an inadequate rate of replacement of fluids. After 48 hours, fluid therapy should be sharply limited; the sequestered fluid may return at this time to the vascular compartment and produce acute pulmonary edema, particularly if there has been thermal injury to the lungs. Digitalis and diuretics, if there has been no renal injury, or even phlebotomy with removal of plasma and replacement of red blood cells may be helpful at this stage. See also section on Burns at end of this Section.

SALICYLATE POISONING. In fluid therapy it is sometimes necessary to supply an excess of certain substances to effect a particular change in physiologic function or to facilitate excretion of a particular substance. In such instances water and electrolytes are given in the absence of specific deficits and above the usual needs. A good example of this form of therapy is the treatment of salicylate intoxication, in which supplemental therapy is of particular importance.

The initial effect of a high concentration of salicylate is to sensitize the respiratory center to carbon dioxide. The resultant hyperventilation, with its characteristic marked prolongation of the expiratory phase of respiration, leads to increased evaporative losses of water and to respiratory alkalosis. The renal compensation for respiratory alkalosis consists in the excretion of large amounts of

---

*Head, arm, one quarter of trunk, one half of leg; each equals 9 per cent of the body surface. The sum of the percentages times total surface area given by nomogram (see section on Drug Therapy which follows) equals the area used in calculating requirements. Infants and small children, owing to relatively larger heads and trunks and smaller extremities, fit more exactly to a "rule of sixes." Arm, one half of head or leg and one eighth of trunk, each equals 6 per cent of the body surface.

†Two parts isotonic saline to 1 part sixth-molar sodium lactate solution.

sodium and potassium bicarbonate. In addition, toxic levels of salicylate uncouple oxidative phosphorylation and may reduce hepatic glycogen, with ketonemia and ketonuria usually resulting. Occasionally hypoglycemia may be seen, but hyperglycemia and glycosuria are common. The loss of sodium and potassium in excess of chloride and the accumulation of acetoacetic and beta-hydroxybutyric acids eventually produce severe metabolic acidosis, which is aggravated by the release of 2 moles of free hydrogen ion from each mole of aspirin absorbed and hydrolyzed. Thus, a dose of salicylate of 200 mg/kg adds an acute hydrogen ion load of 2 mEq/kg. Transition from respiratory alkalosis to a mixed disturbance of acid-base balance with severe metabolic acidosis complicated by respiratory alkalosis may be relatively rapid, and therapy must be followed by periodic evaluation of the serum carbon dioxide content and the pH of the blood and urine.

Except in poisoning due to repeated therapeutic administration of salicylates, the significance of an isolated blood salicylate level depends in part on the interval between the time the drug was ingested and the time the blood sample was obtained; a level of 35 mg/dl 12 hours after an acute ingestion or after the start of aspirin therapy may be more significant than a level of 60 mg/dl two hours after acute ingestion when peak levels may be expected. Active treatment should be considered in any child with a blood level above 30 mg/dl, especially if significant time has elapsed since ingestion or the start of salicylate therapy. Early therapy must supply adequate amounts of water, carbohydrate and electrolytes to meet the increased evaporative losses and to permit maximal renal compensation. Maintenance therapy should provide 200 to 250 ml of water, 15 to 20 gm glucose, 6 to 8 mEq of sodium and 3 to 4 mEq of potassium per 100 calories metabolized. The early administration of sodium bicarbonate and potassium acetate or glutamate to maintain an alkaline urine (pH higher than 7.5) will facilitate excretion of salicylate by reducing the back-diffusion of salicylate in ionized form from tubular urine through the lipid membranes of the renal tubular cells. Indeed, the clearance of salicylate with a urine pH greater than 8.0 is twenty times that at a urine pH of 6.0. The maintenance of a brisk diuresis is also important in increasing salicylate clearance. The dose of bicarbonate necessary to alkalinize the urine is approximately 2 mEq/kg, given over 1 hour. An additional 2 mEq/kg of sodium bicarbonate should be given if urine pH does not reach 7.0. The urinary pH should then be checked every 30 minutes. If the pH falls below 7.0, additional sodium bicarbonate should be given with appropriate amounts of potassium to avoid renal tubular potassium depletion and paradoxical aciduria. The additional administration of acetazolamide (5 mg/kg repeated 2 or 3 times in 24 hours) also increases salicylate excretion and should be a part of the management of all seriously ill patients. Peritoneal dialysis or dialysis by means of the artificial kidney should be considered as a means to remove additional amounts of salicylate loosely bound to plasma proteins of severely ill patients, especially those with very high blood levels of salicylate, those with an elevated pCO_2, those with severe acidosis or those who have failed to respond adequately to alkalinization. The efficiency of dialysis in such patients is increased by the addition of albumin to the dialysis fluid. Exchange transfusion is a relatively inefficient means of removing salicylate in the critically ill patient. If done, heparinized blood should be used because of the often lethal exacerbation of acidosis if citrated blood is used.

In addition, vitamin K_1 oxide (Konakion) should be given intramuscularly to offset possible prothrombin deficiency.

ELECTROLYTE DISTURBANCES ASSOCIATED WITH CENTRAL NERVOUS SYSTEM DISEASES. Of particular pediatric interest are the disturbances in sodium concentration related to diseases of the central nervous system. Three types of changes have been described:

1. Patients with diverse lesions such as surgical or traumatic damage to the brain, encephalitis, bulbar poliomyelitis, cerebrovascular accidents, tumors of the fourth ventricle and subdural hematomas may lose large amounts of sodium in the urine. Dehydration, hypotension and azotemia result unless large amounts of salt are administered and the intake of water is limited.
2. Patients with tuberculous meningitis who are severely ill and comatose are frequently hyponatremic, but exhibit no symptoms which can be attributed to hyponatremia. This situation may be analogous to the asymptomatic hyponatremia of severe malnutrition or pulmonary disease. Relatively large amounts of salt may be lost in the urine when attempts are made to correct the hyponatremia by salt loading. Careful clinical and laboratory observations are essential to ensure that salt depletion and water intoxication do not occur. Potassium should be administered in amounts at least 50 per cent greater than with usual maintenance therapy.
3. Patients with acute infections of the central nervous system occasionally have symptoms of acute water intoxication, with a rapid fall in serum sodium concentration. These patients retain an excessive amount of water and have excessive thirst. Convulsions are severe and resistant to drug therapy, but respond to the intravenous administration of hypertonic saline solution and subsequent restriction of fluid administration.

Convulsions or other symptoms from cerebral edema may respond to hypertonic mannitol solution, although care in its administration should be taken in patients with impaired renal function.

PREOPERATIVE, PARAOPERATIVE AND POSTOPERATIVE CARE. Preoperative preparation of a patient who has no pre-existing deficit or in whom the deficit has been repaired consists mainly in the supply of carbohydrate to ensure adequate storage of glycogen in the liver. Usual maintenance requirements of water and electrolytes are appro-

TABLE 5–19 APPROXIMATE REQUIREMENTS OF WATER WITHOUT ELECTROLYTES DURING OPERATION

WEIGHT KG.	BASAL CAL/24 HOURS	EVAP. WATER, ML/HR (90 ML/100 CAL/24 HOURS)*	URINE WATER, ML/HR (30 ML/100 CAL/24 HOURS)†	TOTAL‡ ML/HOUR
3	150	6	2	8
5	270	10	3	13
7	410	15	5	20
10	550	21	7	28
20	850	32	10	42
30	1100	41	14	55
40	1300	49	16	65

From Harned, H. S., Jr., and Cooke, R. E.: Surg., Gynec. Obst. *104*:543, 1957. By permission.
*This value is assumed to be high because of possible sweating and hyperventilation.
†This value is assumed to be low because of probable antidiuresis.
‡Does not include abnormal losses of fluid (hemorrhage, wound edema, suction) which must be replaced by appropriate electrolyte-containing fluids.

priate. Small infants who are not vomiting should receive carbohydrate and sodium chloride mixtures by mouth until 3 hours before operation. Such fluids are readily absorbed from the gastrointestinal tract and will not produce aspiration pneumonitis if vomited and aspirated.

The most common error in parenteral fluid administration during and after surgery is overadministration, particularly of dextrose in water. Table 5–19 lists water maintenance requirements during surgery.

Preoperative preparation of the newborn involves certain unique hazards. Deficits of water and electrolytes from vomiting or from stasis owing to intestinal obstruction should be replaced before operation. If aspiration pneumonitis is suspected, it should be treated with antibiotics. Nasogastric suction may be inadequate. If so, gastrostomy should be performed to aid in decompression and in postoperative feeding. In intestinal obstruction conjugated bilirubin may be deglucuronidated by intestinal enzymes; an enterohepatic circulation of unconjugated bilirubin can then lead to high serum levels and kernicterus. Hypoprothrombinemia should be prevented by administration of 1.0 mg of vitamin K_1 oxide.

The water requirements during operation are given in Table 5–19. Additional amounts of blood, plasma, saline, or other volume expander must be given if blood loss or tissue trauma is significant. The magnitude of such losses is judged best by the experienced surgeon as he operates. Owing to the danger of anoxia and shock, no potassium should be administered during these periods.

Postoperatively, intake should be limited for 24 hours. Thereafter, usual maintenance therapy is gradually resumed. The water intake should not exceed 85 ml/100 calories metabolized, because of antidiuresis resulting from trauma or circulatory readjustment, unless renal capacity to concentrate the urine is limited (e.g., in sickle cell anemia). If the intake of water is not limited, whether given parenterally or by mouth, water intoxication may result. Sodium intake for maintenance should also be low, owing to the low caloric expenditure during anesthesia and postoperatively.

THERAPY OF ISOLATED DISTURBANCES IN CONCENTRATIONS OF ELECTROLYTES

Acidosis. *Respiratory acidosis* may be seen in the newborn infant with respiratory distress syndrome and in patients receiving assisted ventilation for any reason. Measurements of blood pH and blood gases facilitate correction of acidosis in such patients. With severe respiratory insufficiency, pH may be markedly lowered, primarily as a result of carbon dioxide retention. Mild metabolic acidosis may also exist because hypoxia leads to the accumulation of lactic and other organic acids in the extracellular fluid. The appropriate treatment of such disturbances is improvement of ventilation by assisted respiration rather than by large amounts of sodium bicarbonate, which may produce hyperosmolality and cardiac failure.

Metabolic acidosis, resulting, for example, from renal tubular acidosis or from accumulation of organic acids, may require the administration of alkalinizing agents, especially if symptoms are evident. In lactic acidosis, in glycogen disorders or in circulatory insufficiency and hypoxia, sodium lactate may not be adequately metabolized, so that in these situations sodium bicarbonate is the preferred agent. The dosage required is given by the following general formula:

$(C_d - C_a) \times f_d \times$ body weight in kg = mEq required

where C_d and C_a represent, respectively, the serum bicarbonate concentration desired and the one actually present expressed as mEq/1; f_d represents that fraction of the total body weight in which the administered material is apparently (not actually) distributed. This value varies with the substance administered. The apparent distribution factor for bicarbonate or potential bicarbonate approximates one half to six tenths of the body weight ($f_d = 0.5$ or 0.6). Such calculations indicate that 0.5 ml/kg of a molar solution of sodium bicarbonate would raise the serum bicarbonate concentration approximately 1 mEq/l. There are, however, wide variations in the responses to administered bicarbonate, since it may be sequestered in bone or muscle or lost in urine.

With glomerular insufficiency, caution must be exercised in correcting acidosis because the sodium administered with bicarbonate may result in further expansion of the extracellular fluid volume. In practice it is rarely necessary to attempt to increase serum bicarbonate levels above 15 mEq/l unless the patient is markedly symptomatic from the acidosis. In addition, correction of acidosis in such patients may be complicated by the development of tetany. If hyperphosphatemia coexists with acidosis it should be treated simultaneously by the use of low phosphate diets and aluminum gels given orally.

The use of sodium bicarbonate in the treatment of metabolic acidosis should always be considered as a temporizing measure, and every attempt should be made to treat the underlying cause of the acidosis, e.g., the use of glucose and insulin in diabetic keto-acidosis, improving circulation in shock or the elimination of salicylates, methanol or other toxins.

Alkalosis. Under normal circumstances the kidney has an enormous capacity to excrete bicarbonate, and increased amounts of bicarbonate which gain access to the blood are promptly excreted. However, under certain circumstances, such as the coexistence of volume contraction or the presence of severe potassium or chloride depletion, metabolic alkalosis may be maintained. Rarely, respiration may be so depressed in infants with severe hypochloremic alkalosis that oxygenation of the blood is diminished. Severe alkalotic tetany may also occur. In such instances the administration of ammonium chloride may effect symptomatic improvement. The dose of ammonium chloride may be calculated from the general formula presented above, the probable f_d being 0.2 to 0.3. Such therapy is for relief of symptoms only and must not be used in place of correction of volume concentration or in place of administration of potassium chloride for repair of intracellular deficits; the importance of potassium and chloride administration in the reversal of metabolic alkalosis has been emphasized already.

Hyponatremia. Serum sodium is most commonly reduced as a result of either sodium depletion or water "intoxication" (Table 5–20). A low serum sodium, thought to be due to redistribution of total body sodium, may also be seen in association with severe illnesses or in the terminally ill patient. In addition, apparent hyponatremia may be observed as an artifact; for example, in diabetic ketoacidosis when the water content of plasma is reduced by the presence of increased quantities of lipids.

Patients with a serum sodium below 120 mEq/l are usually symptomatic; those with lesser degrees of hyponatremia are frequently asymptomatic. Treatment of asymptomatic hyponatremia depends on its cause. With water overload, fluid restriction is the appropriate measure. Serum sodium may return to normal rapidly in a patient with good renal function who has been given too much fluid. Conversely, it may take several days or weeks, for example, with the inappropriate ADH syndrome. When sodium deficits are present, addition of extra salt to the diet or increasing the sodium concentration of parenterally administered fluid will often be adequate to correct the deficit. Before starting therapy, care must be taken to determine the cause of hyponatremia, since the wrong therapy will not correct the defect. For example, the administration of sodium to a patient with hyponatremia due to water excess such as that seen with the chronic edema of

TABLE 5–20 CLINICAL STATES COMPLICATED BY HYPONATREMIA

I. Expansion of extracellular space by water
  A. Excessive intake
    1. Parenteral fluid therapy – glucose in water
    2. Oral (with diminished output)
    3. Tap water enemas
    4. Allergy to cow's milk (very rare)
  B. Diminished output (usual intake)
    1. Renal
      a. Intrinsic: nephritis, nephrotic syndrome, tubular necrosis, prematurity
      b. Extrinsic
        (1) Excess of antidiuretic hormone: acute and chronic central nervous system disease, Pitressin therapy, surgery, pulmonary disease
        (2) Circulatory: heart failure, cardiovascular surgery, malnutrition
    2. Skin: premature infant in high humidity
II. Deficiency of extracellular sodium
  A. Inadequate intake
    1. Low salt diet
    2. Parenteral therapy with glucose in water
  B. Excessive losses
    1. Gastrointestinal: vomiting, salivary, gastric, biliary, pancreatic drainage, diarrhea, resin therapy, tap water enemas (especially in megacolon)
    2. Genitourinary
      a. Intrinsic renal disease: chronic nephritis, acute tubular necrosis (recovery phase), nephrotic syndrome (diuresis)
      b. Extrinsic influences: diuretics, Diamox, hypoadrenalism, central nervous system disease (rare), expanded volume (Pitressin, excessive water therapy)
      c. Arachno-ureterostomy
    3. Skin
      a. Normal sweat
      b. Abnormal sweat: cystic fibrosis, adrenal insufficiency
      c. Burn therapy with silver nitrate (hypochloremia)
    4. Parenteral: thoracentesis, paracentesis, burns
  C. Redistribution
    1. Severe malnutrition
    2. Potassium deficiency
    3. Trauma

heart failure, nephrotic syndrome or cirrhosis may only result in further expansion of the extracellular fluid without correction of the serum sodium.

Treatment of symptomatic hyponatremia consists of the administration of a hypertonic saline solution. The dose may be calculated according to the formula in the preceding section on metabolic acidosis, except that C represents serum sodium rather than bicarbonate. Since there is osmotic equilibrium between cells and extracellular water, changes in osmolality are distributed over total body water; when correcting hyponatremia, the value for f_d should be 0.6 to 0.7. A dose of 12 ml/kg of body weight of 3 per cent sodium chloride solution (6 mEq sodium/kg) usually raises the concentration of serum sodium approximately 10 mEq/l.

Elevation of the sodium concentration should be effected in small increments (5 to 10 mEq/l) over 1 to 4 hours.

Hypernatremia (Salt Poisoning). The accidental ingestion of excessive amounts of sodium chloride leads to such serious residuals that special attention is warranted. The accidental substitution of salt for cane sugar in private homes as well as in institutions occurs with sufficient frequency to justify the routine use of liquid sugars in infant feeding. Hypernatremia resulting from the excessive intake of sodium, in contrast to hypernatremic dehydration resulting from diarrhea, is accompanied by increases in total body sodium and in the volume of extracellular water. Severe acidosis results from a shift of organic acids and free hydrogen ions to extracellular fluid. With shift of water from brain cells, distention of cerebral vessels occurs, leading to subdural, subarachnoid and intracerebral hemorrhage. The complications and residuals of salt poisoning are similar to, but may be more severe than, those seen with hypernatremic dehydration. In the former the rapid removal of excess sodium from the body is the principal goal of treatment.

Intravenous fluids should consist of glucose in water, potassium acetate and calcium as needed. Intermittent peritoneal dialysis with glucose solutions can remove large quantities of sodium, correcting the hyperosmolality without the danger of pulmonary edema and heart failure. Approximately 40 ml/kg of 7 per cent glucose solutions in water can be injected intraperitoneally for severe hypernatremia (serum sodium concentration more than 200 mEq/l) and withdrawn 1 hour later. Subsequent dialysis may be carried out using 5 per cent glucose in water as the serum sodium level falls. Exchange transfusion is not a desirable substitute for dialysis because enormous quantities of blood would be required to effect a change in osmolality of total body water. Phenobarbital should be administered to prevent or control seizures. Digitalization may be necessary to counteract heart failure.

Hypokalemia. Disturbances in the concentration of potassium in the absence of disturbances of volume of body fluids have been described in primary hyperaldosteronism and in a syndrome characterized by hypokalemic alkalosis and high plasma renin levels but normal blood pressure (Bartter syndrome). (See Excess Mineralocorticoid Secretion, Section 17.) In these disturbances large amounts of potassium are lost in the urine, resulting in low serum potassium and high serum bicarbonate concentrations. Congenital alkalosis of gastrointestinal origin is associated with large amounts of potassium and chloride being lost in the stools. Severe hypokalemia may result in weakness of skeletal muscles, in decreased peristalsis or ileus and in an inability of the kidney to concentrate the urine. Prolonged hypokalemia results in characteristic pathologic changes in the kidney and a decrease in function which may persist even after potassium repletion.

Treatment of hypokalemia consists of the administration of large amounts of potassium (usually up to 3 mEq/kg of body weight per day); in Bartter syndrome up to 10 mEq/kg may have to be given orally and, if associated with restriction of sodium intake, there may be some clinical as well as biochemical improvement.

Hyperkalemia. Marked elevation of the serum potassium results in ventricular fibrillation and death. In consequence, levels above 6.5 mEq/l should be treated promptly. The oral or parenteral administration of excessive amounts of potassium should be looked for and all potassium intake discontinued. The rapid intravenous administration of sodium bicarbonate (up to 2 mEq/kg of body weight over a 5- to 10-minute period) or glucose and insulin (0.5 gm glucose per kg with 0.3 unit crystalline insulin per gram of glucose, given over a 2-hour period) will result in the intracellular movement of potassium and will lower serum potassium. Intravenous calcium gluconate (up to 0.5 ml of a 10 per cent solution per kg body weight given over 2 to 4 minutes) will counter the cardiac toxicity of potassium, but the EKG should be monitored while it is being administered. None of these measures removes significant quantities of potassium from the patient; they should be considered as temporizing measures until negative potassium balance is established either by the use of ion exchange resins (Kayexalate 1 gm/kg/24 hr in divided oral doses twice daily or as a retention enema) or by hemodialysis or peritoneal dialysis.

Hypocalcemia and Hypercalcemia are discussed in Sections 3, 17 and 19.

Hypomagnesemia. The importance of magnesium in fluid and electrolyte therapy has been reviewed earlier. The only definitive symptom complex associated with hypomagnesemia (serum magnesium less than 1.8 mEq/l) is that of latent or manifest tetany. Convulsions, muscular twitching, disorientation, athetoid movements, carpopedal spasm, and hyperreactivity to mechanical and auditory stimulation have been observed. Lowered serum concentrations and whole body deficits of magnesium are found in chronic diarrhea or vomiting, sprue, celiac disease, prolonged parenteral fluid therapy and hyperaldosteronism. Harrison observed low serum magnesium levels in infantile tetany, presumably on the basis of transient hypoparathyroidism. The intramuscular injection of 0.1 ml of a 25 per cent solution of $MgSO_4 \cdot 7\ H_2O$ (0.2 mEq/kg) repeated every 6 hours for 3 to 4 doses produces symptomatic and biochemical improvement. The addition of 3 mEq of magnesium per liter to maintenance fluids for patients requiring long-term therapy may decrease the chance of serious deficiency. See also Metabolic Disturbances in Section 7.

Hypermagnesemia. Levels of serum magnesium in excess of 10 mEq/l are accompanied by drowsiness and occasionally coma. Deep tendon reflexes may also be abolished along with respiratory depression at higher concentrations. Disturbances in atrioventricular and intraventricular conduction may be detected at levels of 5 mEq/l. Acute renal failure and Addison's disease are accompanied by significant elevations in magnesium concentrations. Iatrogenic magnesium poisoning can result from its use in the treatment of hypertension or toxemia of pregnancy; deaths have been reported from the use of magnesium sulfate enemas in megacolon and from oral administration for purging.

The administration of calcium gluconate intravenously, as in the treatment of tetany, rapidly reverses the depressant effects of magnesium as well as the cardiac abnormalities.

PARENTERAL SOLUTIONS

Table 30–15 lists some solutions commercially available for use in fluid therapy. The large number of carbohydrate and electrolyte mixtures available permits great flexibility and individualization of therapy.

ALAN M. ROBSON

Calcagno, P. L., Rubin, M. I., and Singh, N. S. A.: The influence of surgery on renal function in infancy: The effect of surgery on the postoperative renal excretion of water—The influence of dehydration. Pediatr. *16*:619, 1955.

Colle, E., and Paulsen, E. P.: The responses of the newborn to major surgery: Urinary electrolyte, water and nitrogen losses. Pediatr. *23*:1063, 1959.

Cooke, R. E.: Contributions of the laboratory to the practical management of disorders of body water and electrolyte. Pediatr. *16*:555, 1955.

Cooke, R. E., and Ottenheimer, E. J.: Clinical and experimental interrelations of sodium and the central nervous system. Adv. Pediatr. XI:81, 1960.

Darrow, D. C.: Congenital alkalosis with diarrhea. J. Pediatr. *25*:519, 1945.

Darrow, D. C., and Pratt, E. L.: Fluid therapy: Relation to tissue composition and expenditure of water and electrolyte. J.A.M.A. *143*:365, 432, 1950.

Darrow, D. C., Pratt, E. L., Flett, J., Jr., Gamble, A. H., and Wiese, H. F.: Disturbances in water and electrolyte in infantile diarrhea. Pediatr. *3*:129, 1949.

Finberg, L.: Experimental studies of the mechanisms producing hypocalcemia in hypernatremic states. J. Clin. Invest. *36*:434, 1957.

Finberg, L.: Pathogenesis of lesions in nervous system in hypernatremic states. I. Clinical observations of infants. Pediatr. *23*:40, 1959.

Finberg, L.: Dehydration in infants and children. New Engl. J. Med. *276*:458, 1967.

Harris, F.: Pediatric Fluid Therapy. Philadelphia, F. A. Davis Company, 1972.

Heird, W. C., Driscoll, J. M., Jr., Schullinger, J. N., Grebin, B., and Winters, R. W.: Intravenous alimentation in pediatric patients. J. Pediatr. *80*:351, 1972.

Hinton, P., Allison, S. P., Littlejohn, S., and Lloyd, J. Electrolyte changes after burn injury and effect of treatment. Lancet *2*:218, 1973.

Hirschhorn, N., McCarthy, B. J., Ranney, B., Hirschhorn, M. A., Woodward, S. T., Lacapa, A., Cash, R. A., and Woodward, W. E.: Ad libitum oral glucose-electrolyte therapy for acute diarrhea in Apache children. J. Pediatr. *83*:562, 1973.

Hogan, G. R., Dodge, P. R., Gill, S. R., Master, S., and Sotos, J. F.: Pathogenesis of seizures occurring during restoration of plasma tonicity to normal in animals previously chronically hypernatremic. Pediatr. *43*:54, 1969.

Klahr, S., and Alleyne, G.A.O.: Effects of protein-calorie malnutrition on the kidney. Kidney Int. *3*:129, 1973.

Miller, N. L., and Finberg, L.: Peritoneal dialysis for salt poisoning. New Engl. J. Med. *263*:1347, 1960.

Segar, W. E.: Parenteral Fluid Therapy. Current Problems in Pediatrics. Chicago, Year Book Medical Publishers, 1972.

Smith, M.J.H., and Smith, P. K. (eds.). The Salicylates. A Critical Bibliographic Review. New York. John Wiley & Sons, Inc., 1966.

Weil, W. B.: A unified guide to parenteral fluid therapy. J. Pediatr. *75*:1, 1969.

Winters, R. W. (ed.): The Body Fluids in Pediatrics. Boston, Little, Brown and Company, 1973.

PREOPERATIVE AND POSTOPERATIVE CARE AND CARDIOPULMONARY RESUSCITATION

Pediatric anesthesiology encompasses not only the administration of anesthesia to children, but also the closely related areas of intensive care, cardiopulmonary resuscitation, and other uses of modern respiratory equipment for infants and children.

To provide safe and effective anesthesia for infants and children, a physician must thoroughly understand the basic principles of modern anesthetic practice and the pharmacology of the drugs given. He must recognize the ways in which pediatric patients differ from adults in anatomy, physiology, and response to drugs; he must understand the emotional reactions to anesthesia and surgery encountered in the various pediatric age groups; and in each instance he must be thoroughly familiar with and understand the physical status of the patient, the surgical lesion, and the operation to be performed.

With these factors in mind, the anesthesiologist can make a preoperative evaluation, produce the desired degree of preanesthetic sedation, and select the least hazardous anesthetic agents and techniques that will produce satisfactory operating conditions. He should determine the appropriate modes of monitoring various vital functions and provide for maintenance of an adequate circulating blood volume as well as fluid, electrolyte, and acid-base equilibrium.

PREOPERATIVE EVALUATION

Information provided by the parents and the child's physician enables the anesthesiologist to plan the management of anesthesia and the post-anesthetic period with greater effectiveness. The parents must be questioned about the following:

- Recent upper respiratory tract infection
- Exposure to the exanthems
- Previous laryngotracheobronchitis (croup)
- History of asthma or wheezing during respiratory infections
- Bleeding tendencies
- Abnormal weight loss
- Exercise tolerance
- Reactions to drugs
- Blood transfusion reactions
- Prior administration of corticosteroids
- Medications currently being given
- Emotional reactions of the child to the proposed operation
- When and what the child last ate

A history of frequent croup will require special airway management during anesthesia; a familial history of abnormal response to muscle relaxants might indicate a genetically abnormal pseudocholinesterase which the anesthesiologist must take into consideration when selecting a muscle relaxant; infants and children receiving cortisone, antiepileptic or sedative drugs may have altered responses to anesthetic agents; a patient with a full stomach risks aspiration during induction of anesthesia.

The physical examination should emphasize the heart, the lungs and the upper airways. The presence of heart murmurs, rales in the chest or wheezing requires careful cardiac or pulmonary evaluation before the anesthesiologist proceeds. Small, narrow nares filled with secretions, loose teeth, tonsils and adenoids large enough to cause mouthbreathing, or a small, underdeveloped mandible with a protruding maxilla predispose to upper airway obstruction after sedation or induction of anesthesia. Tracheal intubation may be difficult if the larynx lies anterior to its normal position.

Laboratory tests desirable before anesthesia include hemoglobin or hematocrit determination, white cell count and urinalysis. In patients with serious systemic disease or those about to undergo extensive surgery, a preoperative roentgenogram of the chest, arterial PaO_2 and $PaCO_2$, pH, serum electrolytes and blood urea nitrogen will provide essential data.

The American Society of Anesthesiologists' classification provides a useful numerical scale of physical status:

Class 1. No organic, physiologic, biochemical or psychiatric disturbance.
Class 2. Mild to moderate systemic abnormalities caused either by the disease to be treated surgically or by another pathophysiologic process.
Class 3. Severe systemic abnormality from any cause.
Class 4. Immediately life-threatening, severe systemic disorder.
Class 5. Moribund patient who is submitted to operation in desperation.
Emergency Operation (E). Any patient in one of the classes listed above who is operated upon as an emergency receives the letter "E" beside the numerical classification, such as "2E."

PREOPERATIVE PREPARATION AND SEDATION

Children are frightened by leaving the security and familiarity of home, especially those between 1 and 4 years of age who are unable to understand the purpose of hospitalization. Terrifying experiences during induction of anesthesia or in the immediate postoperative period can produce disabling psychologic changes such as night terrors, enuresis and temper tantrums. Certain steps will minimize the psychologic trauma: (1) For the child over 3 years of age, the parents should explain the purpose of the proposed operation in simple terms, and inform him of the probable sequence of events and discomfort involved. (2) Parents must be encouraged to display confidence and cheerfulness; their tension and anxiety are readily transmitted to the child. (3) The anesthesiologist should visit the child prior to operation, in the presence of the parents whenever possible, so that the child will regard the anesthesiologist as a sympathetic friend who will be caring for him. (4) Preanesthetic sedation should permit the child to be transported to the operating room lightly asleep, allow induction of anesthesia without awakening, and provide some analgesia during postanesthetic recovery.

A wide variety of drugs are used for preanesthetic sedation. Studies have shown that a barbiturate in combination with an opiate and belladonna alkaloid produces suitable preanesthetic sedation in most children. Table 5–21 lists appropriate drugs and dosages for various age groups. Atropine provides more effective abolition of vagal reflexes than does scopolamine and, therefore, is preferred

TABLE 5–21 PREOPERATIVE MEDICATION

AGE (MONTHS)	DRUGS
0-6	Atropine only
6-12	Atropine + pentobarbital
Over 12	Atropine (or scopolamine) + pentobarbital + morphine (or meperidine)

Dosage:

Atropine or scopolamine:	0.02 mg/kg – minimum 0.15 mg, maximum 0.60 mg
Pentobarbital:	3.0-4.0 mg/kg – maximum 120 mg
Morphine:	0.05-0.10 mg/kg – maximum 10 mg
Meperidine:	1.0-2.0 mg/kg – maximum 100 mg

in infants under 1 year of age, in whom vagal reflexes tend to be more active. Scopolamine provides better drying of airway secretions in addition to a sedative effect, and may be used in patients over 1 year of age.

Although the child's stomach should be free of solids prior to anesthesia, it is important not to interrupt fluid intake longer than necessary. No milk or solids should be given less than 12 hours prior to anesthesia. Clear fluids with glucose should be given up to 4 hours prior to induction of anesthesia in infants and up to 6 or 8 hours prior to induction in older children. Since this preoperative oral fluid regimen may not prevent mild dehydration, intravenous balanced electrolyte solution with glucose may be warranted in instances where full hydration is desired.

Before proceeding with an operation the physician should correct dehydration, decrease excessive fever, compensate for acidosis and restore a depleted blood volume.

The febrile, dehydrated child who requires emergency surgery, such as appendectomy, should receive at least partial rehydration rapidly, along with correction of any concomitant metabolic acidosis by intravenous sodium bicarbonate (2.0 to 3.0 mEq/kg). General endotracheal anesthesia with neuromuscular blockade and controlled ventilation followed by surface cooling with water mattresses on the anterior and posterior body surfaces can then be instituted. Cooling should be continued until the colonic or esophageal temperature is under 38° C. The anterior water mattress can be removed when the body temperature is below 39° C (102.2° F), and the operation safely started.

Newborn infants who require immediate operation and who have made little or no recovery from birth asphyxia or who have a body temperature below 35° C (95° F) require oxygen, intravenous sodium bicarbonate (3 to 5 mEq per kg) and elevation of body temperature toward 37° C (98.6° F). Analysis of arterial blood for pH, $PaCO_2$, PaO_2, electrolytes, glucose, osmolality and hematocrit eliminates the guesswork inherent in clinical estimates of ventilation and metabolic status and should be regarded as essential initial monitoring.

INTRAOPERATIVE MANAGEMENT

All the common inhalation agents have been used in children, but in recent years halothane, cyclopropane, and nitrous oxide with *d*-tubocurarine for neuromuscular blockade have replaced diethyl ether as the preferred agent. For induction, most anesthesiologists prefer to use gravity flow of cyclopropane or nitrous oxide over the face, with application of a face mask only after the child has lost consciousness. Regional anesthesia has limited application in infants and small children because of their fears and apprehension.

Experience has shown that the nondepolarizing muscle relaxants, especially *d*-tubocurarine, can be used with effectiveness and safety even in the newborn infant. Tracheal intubation and controlled ventilation provide optimal gas exchange, and neostigmine restores neuromuscular transmission at the conclusion of anesthesia.

Tracheal intubation is indicated in (1) operations about the head and neck, (2) intrathoracic and intraperitoneal procedures, (3) operations in the prone position, (4) most procedures in infants under 1 year of age, and (5) emergency procedures when there is some uncertainty about the contents of the stomach. Ventilation should be controlled manually or mechanically in all intrathoracic procedures and intraperitoneal operations, and when the patient is in the prone position.

During anesthesia, monitoring of heart tones with a precordial stethoscope, continuous measurement of rectal temperature with a thermistor probe and assessment of arterial pressure by the Riva-Rocci or ultrasonic Doppler method or oscillotonometry are mandatory in all age groups. For children in poor physical condition (classes 3 to 5) or when extensive surgery is required, a lead II electrocardiogram should be displayed on an oscilloscope, and continuous direct measurement of intra-arterial and right atrial pressures may be indicated.

Although the infant's heart and peripheral vasculature adapt remarkably to hypovolemia, decompensation may occur suddenly and cardiac arrest ensue rapidly. Awareness of the infant's approximate blood volume (90 ml per kg in the newborn, 75 ml per kg in the older infant) and immediate replacement of losses exceeding 10 to 15 per cent of that volume can prevent hypovolemic shock. Blood for rapid infusion should be warmed to 37° C immediately before use; rapid infusion of cold blood may produce cardiac arrest. When the anticipated losses exceed one third of the patient's estimated blood volume, blood less than 4 days old should be used because older blood becomes extremely acidotic (pH 6.5 to 6.7), hyperkalemic (K– 15 to 25 mEq per liter) and depleted of clotting factors. Serial arterial pH, pCO_2 and electrolyte determinations will detect the acidosis and hyperkalemia that may be associated with rapid, massive blood replacement. Selection of the appropriate blood products and balanced electrolyte solutions in many instances permits restoration of intravascular volume without the use of whole blood.

Continuous monitoring of body temperature is essential during general anesthesia. In modern air-conditioned operating rooms inadvertent hypothermia (colonic temperature under 35° C, 95° F) develops frequently in small infants undergoing laparotomy or thoracotomy and is associated with ventilatory depression, peripheral vasoconstriction and a moderate metabolic acidosis in the immediate postanesthetic period. Overhead radiant heaters and circulating warm water mattresses can minimize this thermal stress. Malignant hyperpyrexia, the abrupt and unexplained rise in body temperature above 41° C (105.8° F) during inhalation anesthesia, occurs in children over 2 years and in young adults. The overall mortality rate exceeds 75 per cent. Successful management demands immediate recognition of a rapid rise in temperature, cessation of anesthesia, and hyperventilation with oxygen. Treatment also includes packing the patient in ice, ice-water gastric lavage, rapid infusion of intravenous fluids at 5 to 10 times the maintenance rate until adequate urine output is established, intravenous administration of sodium bicarbonate (4 to 7 mEq per kg) and peripheral vasodilatation with chlorpromazine by intermittent injection (up to a total of 0.2 mg per kg).

POSTANESTHETIC RECOVERY

Recovery room facilities and nursing must be available to provide constant surveillance of airway patency, adequacy of ventilation and circulatory stability. Following tracheal intubation, patients between 6 months and 6 years of age may develop subglottic edema, especially if there is a history of croup or recent upper respiratory infection. This can often be relieved by intermittent positive pressure breathing with aerosolized racemic epinephrine (0.2 per cent) in addition to supportive measures, including humidified oxygen and intravenous fluids. Intravenous corticosteroids appear to have no beneficial effect. Rarely, orotracheal intubation followed by tracheostomy may be required to guarantee an adequate airway. Malignant hyperpyrexia may also occur in the immediate postanesthetic period, so that careful monitoring of temperature remains important.

INTENSIVE CARE. Necessary elements of intensive care are: (1) nursing and paramedical personnel specially trained in the care of the critically ill; (2) monitoring and alarm systems for continuous assessment of vital functions; (3) respiratory therapy and resuscitation equipment and drugs; (4) immediately available physician specialists in anesthesiology, pediatrics and surgery; and (5) 24-hour laboratory service for routine hematologic studies and rapid, precise determination of blood pH and gas tensions. The objective is to provide maximal surveillance and care to patients with acute, temporary, life-threatening impairment of pulmonary, cardiovascular, renal or nervous system functions.

Commercially available systems are adequate for continuous monitoring and have appropriate alarms for respiratory rate (impedance pneumograph), heart rate, arterial and central venous pressures and body temperature (thermistor probes) in small infants and children. Umbilical artery catheterization in the critically ill newborn infant permits continuous pressure monitoring and frequent blood sampling for pH and gas tensions. In older infants and children, cannulation of a peripheral artery can be utilized. Continuous measurement of ambient oxygen concentrations with high and low alarm devices represents a major advance in oxygen therapy of the small infant. Incubators equipped with servo-controlled heating units regulated by the infant's surface temperature enable the physician to prevent thermal stress.

Patients with existing or impending respiratory failure require intensive respiratory therapy. Respiratory failure exists when the impairment of ventilation poses an immediate threat to life. An acute rise in $PaCO_2$ over 65 mm Hg or PaO_2 under 100 mm Hg at an inspired oxygen concentration over 95 per cent (except in cyanotic heart disease) indicates life-threatening impairment of ventilatory function. Successful therapy usually requires an artificial airway (nasotracheal intubation or tracheostomy) (Table 5–22), mechanical ventilation, continuous humidification of inspired gases, and sterile tracheobronchial toilet at 1- to 3-hour intervals. Infants and children with severe acute lung disease can recover good pulmonary function in a minimum of time when chest percussion, vibration, and postural drainage are also utilized.

Precise administration of intravenous fluids can be provided by mechanical syringe pumps. Total or partial caloric requirements may be infused parenterally in infants able to tolerate a hyperosmolar infusion into a major vein.

CARDIOPULMONARY RESUSCITATION. Cessation of *effective* ventilation or circulation calls for immediate treatment. The cardinal signs of respiratory arrest are apnea and cyanosis. Absence of heart tones and of carotid and femoral pulses denotes circulatory arrest. Primary respiratory arrest can be caused by airway obstruction, central nervous system depression, or neuromuscular paralysis. The 3 types of circulatory arrest that occur are asystole, ventricular fibrillation, and cardiovascular collapse associated with extreme arterial hypotension. If cardiopulmonary arrest is suspected, one should proceed with artificial ventilation and closed-chest massage even if in doubt.

Successful resuscitation must progress in a rapid but orderly sequence, with priority given to coordinated ventilation of the lungs and compression of the heart.

TABLE 5–22 PEDIATRIC OROTRACHEAL TUBE SPECIFICATIONS*

AGE	FRENCH SIZE	INTERNAL DIAMETER (ID in mm)	LENGTH (cm)	15 mm MALE CONNECTOR SIZE (mm ID)
Newborn (<1.0 kg)	11-12	2.5	10	3
Newborn (>1.0 kg)	13-14	3.0	11	3
1-6 months	15-16	3.5	11	4
6-12 months	17-18	4.0	12	4
12-18 months	19-20	4.5	13	5
18-36 months	21-22	5.0	14	5
3-4 years	23-24	5.5	16	6
5-6 years	25	6.0	18	6
6-7 years	26	6.5	18	7
8-9 years	27-28	7.0	20	7
10-11 years	29-30	7.5	22	8
12-14 years	32-34	8.0	24	8

*Clear polyvinyl-chloride endotracheal tubes which satisfy the Armed Forces standard tissue implant test and the American National Standards Institute specifications will be labeled "I.T.-Z 79" and are recommended. Connectors should be of lightweight plastic material.

Airway. A clear airway must be obtained immediately. Vomitus and secretions should be aspirated or removed with fingers and a handkerchief. Soft tissue obstruction can be overcome by extension of the occipito-atlantal joint and forward displacement of the mandible.

Ventilation. Inflation of the lungs with air or oxygen can be accomplished effectively by mouth-to-mouth or mouth-to-nose insufflation, or by bag and mask devices. A good fit of the mask on the face with minimal or no leaks is essential. The hallmark of adequate lung inflation is thoraco-abdominal motion. The lungs should be inflated rapidly, with a breath interposed between each three or four cardiac compressions.

Circulation. An effective cardiac output in the newborn or small infant can be produced by applying maximum pressure with the tips of two fingers over the middle third of the sternum while the vertebral column is firmly supported. In larger infants and children the pressure is applied by the heel of one hand over the sternum opposite the fourth interspace. In large children the heel of the left hand is placed over the right hand to provide the strength of both arms and shoulders. If the maximum compression is held for a fraction of a second, a larger stroke volume will be ejected. The usual rate in infants is approximately 80 per minute, and 60 per minute in older patients.

When ventilation and massage are effective, carotid and femoral pulses become palpable, pupils constrict, and the color of the mucous membranes improves.

Open thoracotomy and direct cardiac massage are not indicated outside the operating room.

Drugs. As soon as artificial ventilation and cardiac massage are effectively established, sodium bicarbonate and epinephrine should be administered (Table 5–23). They may be given intravenously or directly into the heart. Epinephrine may also be instilled intratracheally until an intravenous route can be established. Sodium bicarbonate compensates for the extreme metabolic acidosis which develops rapidly after cessation of circulation. Epinephrine, which increases myocardial contraction force without decreasing the sys-

TABLE 5–23 DRUGS FOR RESUSCITATION

DRUG	CONCENTRATION USED	INTRAVENOUS DOSE	INTRACARDIAC DOSE	FREQUENCY OF DOSE
Sodium bicarbonate	1 mEq/ml	2.0-4.0 mEq/kg, up to 200 mEq	1.0-2.0 mEq/kg, up to 20 mEq	5-10 minutes
Epinephrine	1:10,000 (0.1 mg/ml)	0.01 mg/kg, up to 0.5 mg	0.05-0.01 mg/kg, up to 0.5 mg	3-5 minutes
Isoproterenol	0.2-0.4 mg in 100 ml of isotonic saline solution	Continuous infusion		Continuous infusion
Calcium chloride	10% (100 mg/ml)	0.2 ml/kg–minimum, 1.0 ml, maximum, 10.0 ml	Same as intravenous	10 minutes (if effective)

TABLE 5–24 PEDIATRIC RESUSCITATION KIT: RECOMMENDED CONTENTS

Airway equipment

1. Bag and masks (infant, child, adult) with nonrebreathing valve that has universal 15-mm female adaptor for male 15-mm endotracheal tube connectors
2. Oropharyngeal airways (Guedel sizes 0, 1, 2, 3, 4)
3. Orotracheal tubes (complete sterile set with connectors) (see Table 5–22)
4. Aspiration equipment:
   Metal tonsil suction tip
   Disposable sterile plastic suction catheters sizes (Fr.) 5, 8, 10, 14
5. Laryngoscope:
   Standard handle
   Blades: Miller – newborn
   Wis-Forreger – 1½
   Flagg – child
   Macintosh – adult (no. 3)
   2 extra batteries
   1 extra light bulb for each blade

Drugs

Sodium bicarbonate	1 mEq /ml	4 50-ml vials
Epinephrine	1 mg /ml	4 1-ml vials
Isoproterenol	0.2 mg /ml	2 2-ml vials
Calcium chloride	100 mg /ml (10%)	2 10-ml vials
Dextrose	500 mg /ml (50%)	1 20-ml vial
Pentobarbital	50 mg /ml	1 30-ml vial
Heparin	1000 u /ml	1 10-ml vial
Saline (for dilution)	0.9%	2 30-ml vials

Miscellaneous

Intracardiac needles: 20- and 22-gauge, 6–8 cm. length
Syringes (plastic disposable): 2, 5, 10 ml, 2 each
Needles: 3 each, 18-, 20-, 22-, 25-gauge regular
2 each, 19-, 21-, 23-, 25-gauge scalp vein

Other:

Tongue blades
Sterile 4 × 4 gauze sponges
Alcohol swabs (packaged individually)
Sterile hemostat
Sterile scissors

temic vascular resistance, should be given if artificial ventilation, cardiac massage and sodium bicarbonate have not restored spontaneous, effective circulation within 3 minutes.

Defibrillation. An electrocardiogram should be obtained and run continuously as soon as possible after the diagnosis of circulatory arrest to detect ventricular fibrillation. External defibrillation can be achieved with an appropriate electric shock (100 watt-seconds in infants, 200 to 300 watt-seconds in older children, and 400 watt-seconds in adults) applied through paddles of appropriate size to skin surfaces covered locally with a conductive electrode jelly or saline-soaked pads.

Post-resuscitation care includes vigorous treatment of the cause of the collapse and monitoring and regulation of the electrocardiogram, arterial pressure and arterial pH and gas tensions.

Successful resuscitation cannot be achieved without careful preplanning and a coordinated team effort (Table 5–24).

JOHN J. DOWNES
RUSSELL C. RAPHAELY

GENERAL

Dripps, R. D., Eckenhoff, J. D., and Vandam, L. D.: Introduction to Anesthesia. 4th ed. Philadelphia, W. B. Saunders Company, 1972.

Smith, R. M.: Anesthesia for Infants and Children. 3rd ed. St. Louis, The C. V. Mosby Company, 1968.

Downes, J. J., and Nicodemus, H.: Preparation for and recovery from anesthesia. Pediat. Clin. N. Amer. *16*:601, 1969.

Jordan, W. S., Graves, C. L., and Elwyn, R. A.: New therapy for post-intubation laryngeal edema and tracheitis in children. J.A.M.A. *212*:585, 1970.

Intensive Care

Klaus, M. H., and Fanaroff, A. A.: Care of the High-Risk Neonate. Philadelphia, W. B. Saunders Company, 1973.

Downes, J. J., Fulgencio, T., and Raphaely, R. D.: Acute respiratory failure in children. Pediat. Clin. N. Amer. *19*:425, 1972.

Resuscitation

Avery, M. E., and Fletcher, B. D.: The Lung and Its Disorders in the Newborn Infant. 3rd ed. Philadelphia, W. B. Saunders Company, 1974.

Ehrlich, R., Emmett, S. M., and Rodriguez-Torres, R.: Pediatric cardiac resuscitation team: A 6-year study. J. Pediatr. *84*:152, 1974.

Standards for cardiopulmonary resuscitation (CPR) and emergency cardiac care (ECC). J.A.M.A. *227* (suppl.):833, 1974.

DROWNING AND NEAR-DROWNING

To drown signifies death. "Near-drowning" denotes survival from an aquatic catastrophe. To clarify terminology, Modell has proposed the following definitions:

Drowning without aspiration: To die from respiratory obstruction and asphyxia while submerged in a fluid medium.

Drowning with aspiration: To die from the combined effects of asphyxia and changes secondary to aspiration of fluid while submerged.

Near-drowning without aspiration: To survive, at least temporarily, following asphyxia due to submersion in a fluid medium.

Near-drowning with aspiration: To survive, at least temporarily, following aspiration of fluid while submerged.

Delayed death subsequent to near-drowning: To succumb after apparently successful rescue or resuscitation from near-drowning.

Drowning causes 5000 to 6000 deaths per year in the United States; the highest incidence is in children between 10 and 19 years of age. Most drownings are accidental: inadequately attended infants drown in swimming pools and bathtubs; even accomplished swimmers overestimate their endurance; occupants of pleasure boats fail to wear life jackets; small children fall into ponds, streams and flooded excavations; and the incautious of all ages plunge through thin ice. Particular mention should be made of infants drowned, usually in bathtubs, after being left alone with (not always obviously) jealous older siblings.

The pathophysiologic changes observed following experimental drowning in animals frequently seem to conflict with the clinical picture observed in human victims of near-drowning. For example, in Swann's studies, dogs died of ventricular fibrillation after total immersion in fresh water. More recent experiments by Modell and his associates have demonstrated that the discrepancies arise when experimental drowning of animals by total immersion is compared with near-drowning in human victims.

PATHOLOGY. Postmortem changes after drowning are nonspecific. Cutis anserina (goose flesh), water-wrinkling of the skin of the hands and feet, pale or sanguineous watery foam from the nose and mouth, and vomitus and aquatic debris in the respiratory tract are common. The lungs are hyperinflated and irregularly congested, with pink-to-red mottling. On cutting, the lungs of a drowned child may appear unusually dry, but pressure produces fine bubbling of sanguineous, watery foam from the cut surface. Microscopic sections show varying degrees of alveolar distention, edematous protein precipitate and focal intra-alveolar hemorrhage. The liver, spleen and kidneys appear congested. The stomach may contain swallowed fluid, and the brain appears swollen.

The microscopic appearance of the brain in near-drowning with delayed death varies with the degree and duration of anoxia. With early death, edema and anoxic perivascular hemorrhages may be the only changes. With prolonged and severe hypoxia, the changes may progress to cystic degeneration of the basal ganglia or midbrain. The alterations in the lung vary also according to (1) the duration of survival, (2) whether there has been aspiration of water and/or gastric contents, and (3) whether secondary infection is present.

BLOOD GASES AND ACID-BASE ALTERATIONS. *Hypoxemia* is the most serious consequence of near-drowning, either with or without aspiration. It is accompanied by metabolic acidosis and transient hypercarbia. The severity depends on the duration of submersion, whether aspiration has occurred and the amount of water aspirated.

It is estimated that approximately 10 per cent of drowning victims do not aspirate, but die acutely of laryngospasm or breathholding. If these patients are rescued and given artificial ventilation before the occurrence of circulatory arrest and permanent damage to the central nervous system, recovery is complete.

The picture after near-drowning with aspiration is significantly different from that of submersion without aspiration. In an effort to define the pathophysiology of drowning, Modell and his associates have studied the effects on dogs of aspiration of various quantities of fluid (normal saline, distilled water, chlorinated distilled water, and sea water). Aspiration of as little as 2.2 ml/kg of water produced profound changes in arterial oxygen tension. After aspiration of 11 ml/kg of fresh or sea water, the PaO_2 consistently dropped to values of 30 to 40 mm Hg, and remained depressed for at least 72 hours in survivors. The arterial oxygen tension was lower one hour after sea water aspiration than one hour after aspiration of an equal quantity of fresh water. Immediately after aspiration of either fluid, a *large absolute intrapulmonary shunt* was present (absolute shunt = per cent of cardiac output perfusing nonventilated alveoli, measured with the animal breathing 100 per cent O_2). After fresh water aspiration, the total shunt was significantly greater while the animal breathed room air than while breathing 100 per cent O_2, indicating that, in addition to the absolute shunt seen after either sea or fresh water aspiration, after the latter there is also a greater relative shunt resulting from inequality of ventilation/perfusion. These findings suggest that although hypoxia occurs after aspiration of either fresh or sea water, the mechanisms may be different. Other findings which support a multifaceted etiology of the hypoxia are:

1. Hyperinflation of the lungs after fresh water aspiration increases the arterial oxygen tension and decreases the shunt significantly and for a greater duration than after sea water aspiration,

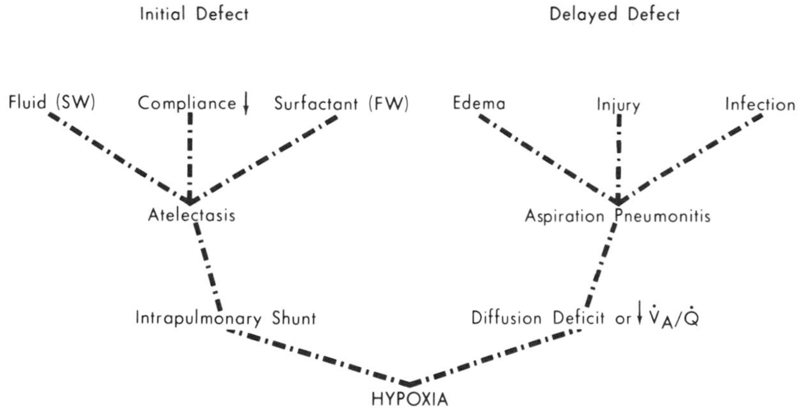

Figure 5–11 *Factors contributing to hypoxia in near-drowning. SW = sea water; FW = fresh water;* $\dot{V}_A/\dot{Q}$ *= ventilation/perfusion ratio.*

suggesting that alveolar collapse or atelectasis is the cause of hypoxia. After fresh water aspiration, surfactant activity is abnormal, predisposing to alveolar collapse. After sea water aspiration surfactant activity is normal.

2. After instillation of sea water into the trachea, a greater volume of fluid than that which has been instilled can be aspirated, supporting the hypothesis of fluid-filled alveoli as the initial defect after sea water aspiration. After fresh water instillation suctioning of the trachea produces little or no return of fluid.

3. In addition to the contribution of surfactant instability and fluid-filled alveoli to hypoxemia, there are a decrease in lung compliance and an increase in airway resistance after aspiration of either fluid. There appears, however, to be no long-term abnormality of pulmonary function.

During the recovery phase, there may be hypoxia during breathing of room air, even after a shunt is no longer demonstrable during breathing of 100 per cent O_2, again suggesting uneven ventilation/perfusion. This may be related to pulmonary edema fluid (interstitial or alveolar), alveolar capillary membrane damage or infection. Figure 5–11 summarizes the possible etiologic factors contributing to the hypoxia seen in near-drowning.

Arterial carbon dioxide tension ($PaCO_2$) initially increases with aspiration, but rapidly returns to normal as experimental animals begin to hyperventilate. Measurements of $PaCO_2$ in human near-drowning victims are variable. They may be elevated owing to hypoventilation but rapidly return to normal with increased spontaneous or mechanical ventilation, indicating that there is no barrier to the elimination of carbon dioxide.

Experimental animals also develop significant acidosis after aspiration of fluid. Initially this may be attributed in part to elevation of the $PaCO_2$, but the acidosis persists in spite of a return to normal carbon dioxide tension. It is, therefore, reasonable to assume that the remaining and persistent metabolic acidosis is primarily due to tissue hypoxia. Modell has found significant acidosis in 78 per cent of human near-drowning victims when the pH was measured in the emergency room; Hasan has reported an incidence of 81 per cent.

SERUM ELECTROLYTE CHANGES. In the past, much emphasis was placed on electrolyte imbalance as the cause of morbidity and mortality from near-drowning. Modell and Davis, however, have found that 85 per cent of such victims died of other factors, presumably anoxia and acidosis. The electrolyte changes in both animals and humans are dependent on the type and volume of water aspirated. The survivor who arrives for treatment after an episode of near-drowning will likely manifest only transient electrolyte changes, which will revert to normal without specific fluid and electrolyte therapy. In human data compiled by Fuller (retrospective) and Modell (prospective), all the serum sodium and chloride values were within 20 mEq/l of normal. None of the values were life-threatening, including the serum potassium concentration, after near-drowning in either sea water or fresh water.

In animal studies, 80 per cent of dogs aspirating 22 ml/kg or less of fresh water survived without therapy; 80 per cent aspirating 44 ml/kg of fresh water died of ventricular fibrillation. Animals aspirating 22 ml/kg of fresh water showed a *drop* in serum sodium and chloride of 10 to 20 mEq/l, but 30 minutes later these values had returned to normal. After aspiration of 22 ml/kg of sea water, these values *rose* 20 to 30 mEq/l. Potassium concentration rose acutely after aspiration of both distilled water and sea water, but not to life-threatening levels, and returned to normal within 30 minutes. On the basis of clinical experience, these data appear to be applicable to humans; after near-drowning with aspiration of as much as 22 ml/kg, there are no significant, persistent changes in serum electrolyte concentrations.

BLOOD VOLUME. Changes in blood volume are dependent upon the tonicity and quantity of fluid aspirated. After fresh water aspiration, there is rapid absorption from the lungs into the circulation, with a transient increase in blood volume. In dogs, the blood volume increases 1.4 per cent for each ml/kg of fresh water aspirated. After sea water aspiration, fluid is lost from the circulation into the lungs owing to the hypertonicity of the fluid aspirated; the resultant hypovolemia may persist as long as 48 hours. Since the amount of fluid the near-drowned patient aspirates is variable, no prediction as to changes in blood volume can be made, except to say that the changes depend on the volume and type of fluid aspirated, and that they are transient.

HEMOGLOBIN AND HEMATOCRIT. Hemoglobin and hematocrit are usually within normal ranges in victims of near-drowning in either fresh or sea water. Hemolysis does occur after aspiration of large quantities of fresh water, but it is seldom of a degree that necessitates specific therapy.

EMERGENCY TREATMENT. Immediate therapy at the scene is imperative for survival. As hypoxia and acidosis are the critical problems, management consists of immediate ventilation, oxygenation and circulatory support. If the victim is apneic when rescued, mouth-to-mouth ventilation should begin at once and be replaced as soon as possible with positive pressure ventilation capable of supplying maximum oxygen concentrations. Closed chest cardiac massage must be added to ventilatory support if effective circulation is not present. All victims of near-drowning should be admitted to a hospital, with maximum support continued during transport to the institution.

HOSPITAL THERAPY. The hallmark of therapy of near-drowning is intensive pulmonary care. This should be suited to the condition of the patient, and will vary from supplying a spontaneously breathing patient with an oxygen-enriched atmosphere to endotracheal intubation and mechanical ventilation. Intravenous administration of sodium bicarbonate seems empirically justified, since hypoxia and severe metabolic acidosis commonly occur in the near-drowned patient. One hundred per cent oxygen should be continued until the patient's arterial pH, pO_2 and pCO_2 are determined. Further adjustments of bicarbonate administration, ventilatory support and inspired oxygen concentration will depend on the condition of the patient and these blood values. Inability of the patient to maintain an adequate arterial oxygen tension at nontoxic concentrations of inspired O_2 (usually considered as less than 50 per cent), or inability to perform the work of breathing without progressive acidosis, is an indication for mechanical ventilation. Since atelectasis occurs following near-drowning, particularly after fresh water aspiration, hyperinflation of the lungs by positive pressure is beneficial. When adequate oxygenation cannot be maintained with intermittent positive pressure ventilation, positive end-expiratory pressure (PEEP) is a useful tool. With PEEP, the airway pressure is maintained at greater than atmospheric levels. This tends to increase functional residual capacity (FRC) and prevent the alveoli from collapsing to the completely airless state. The net result is an improvement in ventilation/perfusion ratios. PEEP is particularly effective after fresh water aspiration, in which the surface tension of the surfactant film is altered and the alveoli tend to collapse. After sea water aspiration PEEP results in significant improvement of PaO_2 with either spontaneous or mechanical ventilation. After fresh water aspiration PEEP combined with mechanical ventilation results in a significantly higher PaO_2 than does intermittent positive pressure ventilation alone. The level of PEEP must be titrated carefully to achieve an optimal PaO_2 with the least deleterious effect on cardiovascular function. Hypothermia to decrease oxygen consumption is worthy of consideration only if intensive pulmonary care fails to maintain the PaO_2 at adequate levels.

If bronchospasm is present, nebulized isoproterenol or racemic epinephrine may be useful. In the presence of intra-alveolar pulmonary edema and froth, inhalation of aerosolized 20 per cent ethyl alcohol acts as an antifoaming agent. Diuretics may also be beneficial in treating interstitial pulmonary edema. With sea water aspiration, colloid loss via the lungs must be taken into consideration, and it may be necessary to give serum albumin or plasma. Bronchoscopy is indicated only if food or solid material has been aspirated. Decompression of gastric dilatation with a nasogastric tube may improve ventilation by decreasing intra-abdominal pressure. Prophylactic use of steroids and antibiotics has been recommended by some for aspiration pneumonitis associated with near-drowning, but their usefulness has yet to be documented by controlled study. Tracheal secretions should be stained and cultured prior to instituting the use of antibiotics, and daily thereafter, so that therapy may be appropriately adjusted if necessary.

FLUIDS. The concept of using hypotonic fluid to treat all sea water and hypertonic fluid to treat all fresh water victims of near-drowning is obsolete and without scientific rationale. Only normal maintenance fluids are ordinarily required, except that with sea water aspiration large amounts of protein may be lost via the lungs, and colloid replacement may be required. As stated previously, electrolyte changes are transient and generally not life-threatening. If significant imbalances are found and persist, however, appropriate therapy should be instituted.

MONITORING. The most important tests in assessing the patient's condition and response to therapy are determinations of arterial blood gas tensions and acid-base status. Other tests of lesser importance include: routine urinalysis, serum electrolyte concentrations, whole blood hemoglobin and hematocrit, plasma hemoglobin and chest x-ray. It is important to remember that the initial chest x-ray may be clear even in the face of extreme hypoxia, particularly after aspiration of fresh water. In addition to determining arterial blood gases, monitoring should include arterial blood pressure, pulse rate and intensity, respiratory rate and pattern, electrocardiogram, body temperature, intake and output, and, in certain patients, central venous pressure and indirect left atrial pressure. With the use of a flow-directed Swan-Ganz catheter, the pulmonary wedge pressure can be measured; this reflects left atrial pressure. This determination is useful in distinguishing left ventricular failure from hypovolemia. This may be of particular importance in cases of near-drowning, because fulminating pulmonary edema can occur secondary to pulmonary injury, despite an adequate cardiac output and hypovolemia. In the small child, usable catheter size limits the use of this technique.

ACKNOWLEDGMENT: This work supported in part by NIH Grant GM17246-04. The author also thanks J. H. Modell, M.D., for his help in preparing the manuscript.

SHIRLEY A. GRAVES

Downs, J. B., Klein, E. F., Jr., and Modell, J. H.: The effect of incremental PEEP on PaO_2 in patients with respiratory failure. Anesth. Analg. *52*:210, 1973.

Giammona, S. T., and Modell, J. H.: Drowning by total immersion. Effects on pulmonary surfactant of distilled water, isotonic saline, and sea water. Am. J. Dis. Child. *114*:612, 1967.

Hasan, S., Avery, W. G., Fabian, C., and Sackner, M. A.: Near-drowning in humans. A report of 36 patients. Chest *59*:191, 1971.

Modell, J. H. (ed.): The Pathophysiology and Treatment of Drowning and Near-Drowning. Springfield, Ill., Charles C Thomas, 1971.

Modell, J. H., Calderwood, H. W., Ruiz, B. C., Downs, J. B., and Chapman, R., Jr.: Effects of ventilatory patterns on arterial oxygenation after near-drowning in sea water. Anesthesiology *40*:376, 1974.

Ruiz, B. C., Calderwood, H. W., Modell, J. H., and Brogdon, J. E.: Effect of ventilatory patterns on arterial oxygenation after near-drowning with fresh water: A comparative study in dogs. Anesth. Analg. *52*:570, 1973.

BURNS

Burns are due to the effects of thermal energy upon skin and other tissues. Tissue damage begins when the temperature reaches 44° C, and the rate of injury increases logarithmically as the tissue temperature rises. Burns are classified as first, second or third degree according to the depth of tissue injured. First degree burns, such as sunburns, involve only the epithelium. Second degree burns destroy the epithelium and part of the corium but spare dermal appendages, from which re-epithelialization may occur. In third degree burns the entire thickness of the dermis is destroyed; re-epithelialization is consequently restricted to the periphery of the lesions. Burns comprising less than 15 per cent of the body surface may be of no major consequence, unless they involve such areas as the hands or face or flexural areas. As the extent of burns increases, the medical consequences increase and the mortality rate rises.

INCIDENCE. It is estimated that approximately two million people receive medical attention, 100,000 are hospitalized, and 7800 die each year in the United States because of burn injuries. The death rate from fire in this country is the second highest in the world, and by far the highest among industrialized nations. Burns are the second leading cause of nonvehicular accidental deaths; 30 per cent of these deaths are among children who are under 15 years of age. Among children aged 1 to 4 years, burns are the leading cause of accidental death in the home, and second only to vehicular injuries overall. Among children 5 to 14 years old, burns are the third leading cause of accidental deaths.

ETIOLOGY. The young, the elderly and those in disadvantaged socioeconomic groups are particularly vulnerable to burns. Nearly all burns in children occur in the home during waking hours. The major vectors of heat energy are hot liquids and solids, and combustible materials such as flammable fabrics, volatile flammable liquids, and domestic dwellings. Combustible materials are most commonly ignited by matches, poorly guarded space heaters, kitchen ranges or water heaters.

Scalds predominate as burn injuries occurring in the first three years of life, and these injuries are usually limited to small areas. Chemical burns are rare and usually benign, with the exception of esophageal burns. Electrical burns are uncommon, but may be devastating. Burns due to the ignition of combustible materials are most common after infancy, and the resultant injuries are commonly large and life-threatening.

PREVENTION. Appropriate strategies to prevent all types of trauma by controlling the sources and expenditure of energy have been outlined by Haddon. We have adapted these principles to the prevention of burns (Table 5–25). The realization of these preventive measures requires: (1) education of the public regarding the potential risks and their avoidance; (2) government regulation of product safety; and (3) technologic advances in the attenuation of the vectors of heat energy and their ignitors. In this regard, the physician has a major responsibility in educating parents and in encouraging appropriate legislative controls.

PATHOPHYSIOLOGY. Hemodynamic, autonomic, cardiopulmonary, renal and metabolic disturbances develop rapidly following severe thermal injury. Within seconds of the burn, cardiac output falls, presumably because of exaggerated reflex responses and decreased venous return. Myocardial contractility does not seem to be affected at this time. A plasma factor which depresses myocardial contractility has been isolated during the

TABLE 5–25 PREVENTION OF TRAUMA, ADAPTED TO BURN INJURIES

GENERAL PRINCIPLES	EXAMPLES OF APPLICATION TO BURNS
Prevent marshaling of latent energy	Do not store gasoline in the home
Reduce the amount of marshaled energy	Reduce temperature of bath or shower water
Modify the rate at which energy can propagate	Use flame-retardant fabrics
Separate in time or space the energy from the susceptible structure	Locate water heaters away from flammable liquids
Separate by interposition of a barrier	Use safeguards for space heaters
Strengthen the structure that might be damaged by energy	Apply more stringent building and fireproofing codes
Detect the danger and counter its rapid continuation and extension	Use fire alarms, sprinkler systems, fire extinguishers

latter stages of shock from severely burned animals and humans, but its nature and its role are poorly understood.

Soon after the injury the permeability of the entire vascular tree increases; as a result, water, electrolytes and proteins are lost from the vascular compartment into interstitial tissues of injured and noninjured sites. These losses are maximal during the first 18 hours after injury and may amount to as much as one third of the blood volume. During the first four days as much as two plasma pools of albumin may be lost; accordingly, deficiencies of albumin and other plasma proteins are common.

Within minutes following a substantial burn, renal plasma flow and glomerular filtration rate are decreased. Severe oliguria may develop, and tubular function is at least transiently compromised. Increased secretion of antidiuretic hormone and aldosterone further contributes to the reduction in urine formation; tubular sodium reabsorption is stimulated, potassium excretion is enhanced, and the urine is maximally concentrated. This antidiuresis is most prominent during the first 12 to 24 hours after the burn, but it may persist for several days thereafter.

Destruction of red blood cells in the period immediately after a burn seldom exceeds 10 per cent of circulating erythrocytes. Additional losses may occur, however, in the ensuing days, as partly damaged cells are lysed and blood is lost from granulation tissues. For these and other reasons, anemia is likely to develop within 4 to 7 days of major burn injuries.

EMERGENCY MANAGEMENT OF SEVERE BURNS. It is imperative that care be administered in an orderly fashion (Table 5–26). First, the adequacy of the airway must be established, especially in a child with facial burns or one who has inhaled smoke. Then, a rapid assessment is made which includes: (1) inspection of wounds, (2) evaluation of the cardiorespiratory status, and (3) determination of previously unrecognized injuries. An intravenous infusion is established through which isotonic fluids are given to expand the blood volume. Lactated Ringer's solution, isotonic saline or plasma may be infused at a rate of 20 ml/kg/hour until more accurate estimates of fluid requirements are made.

The stomach is emptied with a nasogastric tube to prevent gastric dilatation or vomiting. Before the tube is withdrawn, a small quantity of antacid is instilled to retard the development of stress ulcers. Directly thereafter a urinary catheter is inserted so that urinary output can be monitored.

Since the quantities of fluids and medications to be administered depend upon the size of the patient and the extent of injury, the weight and length should be measured carefully, and the areas of the total body surface and of the surface which is

TABLE 5–26 PRIORITIES OF MEDICAL PROCEDURES IN THE EMERGENCY PHASE OF BURN INJURIES

PROCEDURE	INDICATION	COMMENT
1. Establish an adequate airway	Burns of the face Laryngeal edema Smoke inhalation	Avoid emergency tracheostomy
2. Examine for trauma to head, skeleton, or nervous system	Explosions	Remove clothing; radiologic examination helpful
3. Begin intravenous infusion	To prevent intravascular dehydration	Use isotonic fluids
4. Empty stomach through a nasogastric tube	To prevent gastric dilatation, vomiting or aspiration	Antacids may be helpful
5. Insert an indwelling urinary catheter	To monitor hourly urine output	Use a closed drainage system
6. Examine the burn wound	To estimate depth and extent	Use burn charts corrected for age
7. Clean, debride and dress the burn area	To minimize microbial colonization	Use topical antimicrobial therapy
8. Medications	To treat infections; to prevent tetanus; for sedation	Use intravenous route for sedation
9. Begin fluid, electrolyte and protein replacement	To correct antecedent deficits and concurrent losses	Use appropriate formula to estimate requirements

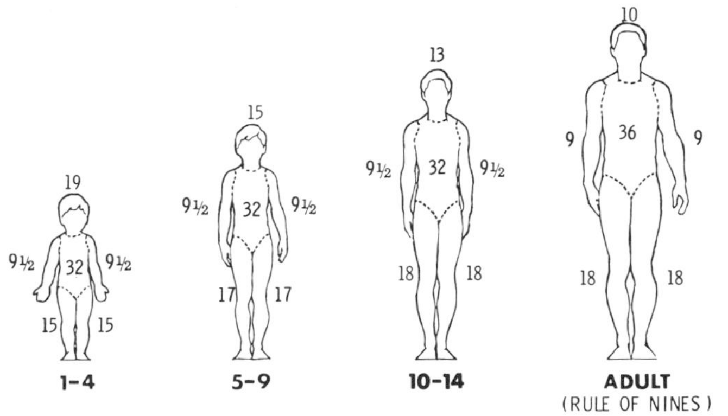

Figure 5–12 Burn assessment chart. (Body proportions modified from Lund and Brower.)

burned should be ascertained. Weight is measured before bedclothing, restraints or dressings are applied, and afterward as well. The wounds are cleansed and debrided, their depth assessed, and the extent of second and third degree burns estimated by using body surface charts corrected for age (Fig. 5–12). Then the wounds are covered with dressings saturated with an antimicrobial agent. In addition, circumferential third degree burns must be recognized and escharotomies performed to prevent ischemia of extremities or respiratory embarrassment resulting from chest wall involvement.

Sedatives may be given if there are no injuries to the central nervous system. The intravenous route is preferred; respiratory depressants should be avoided. Tetanus prophylaxis is given and penicillin administered parenterally to prevent β-hemolytic streptococcal infections.

FLUID, ELECTROLYTE AND COLLOID THERAPY. During the first 24 hours after a burn, the objectives of fluid therapy are: (1) to correct hypovolemia, (2) to maintain the vascular volume, (3) to prevent abnormalities in plasma electrolytes, protein or pH, and (4) to minimize edema.

Fluid therapy in burns, however, remains quite controversial. In adults fluid requirements are estimated commonly by the Brooke or the Evans formula. According to the former, fluid requirements for the first 24 hours are calculated as follows:

1. Burns greater than 50 per cent are calculated as 50 per cent.
2. Colloid (blood, plasma or dextran): Body weight (kg) × (per cent of surface area burned) × (0.5 ml).
3. Electrolyte solutions (lactated Ringer's solution): Body weight (kg) × (per cent of surface area burned) × (1.5 ml).
4. Water (5 per cent dextrose in water): 2000 ml for adults; correspondingly less for children.

The amount of fluids to hydrate small children may be inappropriate if the quantity is estimated by the Brooke formula or a similar method. This is because fluid estimates are based solely on body weight and extent of burn. In this regard, children, particularly infants, have high rates of heat exchange relative to size and weight, high rates of water exchange in relation to their total body water, and somewhat immature renal function. Insensible water losses are proportionally greater, and large volumes of urine are required for excretion of wastes.

Artz has proposed that free water requirements in the Brooke formula (see 4, above) be calculated for children according to body weight:

Age	*ml H_2O/kg*
0–2 years	150
2–5 years	100
5–8 years	75
8 years or older	50

This modification makes the Brooke formula more suitable for children, but it may still be inappropriate for the very young or the obese child.

Another way to estimate fluid requirements in burned children depends upon the use of surface area for most calculations (Eagle, 1956). Though this appeared to be more accurate than programs based on weight alone, Eagle's regimen was complex, difficult to use and not entirely based on surface area. Therefore, we have developed a simplified formula based solely upon surface area. With this formula, the first 24-hour fluid requirements are estimated as follows:

2000 ml/M^2 of body surface/24 hours

plus

50 ml/M^2 of body surface/each 1% burned/24 hours

Burns of greater than 60 per cent of body surface are calculated as 60 per cent in this formula.

Fluids received prior to arrival at a center for definitive care must be reviewed and the amounts to be given adjusted accordingly.

Example: A 4 year old child with a body surface area of 0.68 M^2 sustained third degree burns to approximately 40 per cent of his body surface. Despite having received 200 ml of lactated Ringer's during the first hour, on admission he appeared dehydrated.

1. Fluids received during the initial evaluation period (lactated Ringer's, saline and plasma) need not be included in the calculation of 24-hour requirements. These fluids may be given at a rate of approximately 20 ml/kg body weight/hour for 1 to 2 hours.
2. Calculation of first 24-hour requirements: Maintenance fluid requirement = 2000 ml/M^2 of surface area/24 hours.
   Example: 2000 × 0.68 = 1360 ml/24 hours
   Antecedent deficit and concurrent losses = 50 ml/M^2 of surface area/each 1 per cent burned/24 hours.
   Example: 50 × 0.68 × 40 = 1360 ml
   Total first 24-hour requirement (maintenance + replacement or 1360 ml + 1360 ml) = 2720 ml

Half of the estimated amount is administered during the first 8 hours and half during the subsequent 16 hours.

Example:	First 8 hours	=	170 ml/hour
	Second 8 hours	=	85 ml/hour
	Third 8 hours	=	85 ml/hour

The composition of fluids to be used for resuscitation of the burned child remains controversial. There are those who recommend protein-free electrolyte solutions; we recommend, however, the use of isotonic solutions containing albumin and either lactate or bicarbonate. An electrolyte-protein mixture, similar to the one proposed by Stone, appears to be well suited for this purpose. One liter of the solution is prepared by mixing 920 ml of 5 per cent glucose in 0.45 per cent sodium chloride solution (77 mEq/l); 10 ml of hypertonic sodium chloride (3 mEq/ml); 20 ml of $NaHCO_3$ (1 mEq/ml); and 50 ml of 25 per cent human serum albumin (salt poor). The final composition of the mixture is as follows:

Na	127 mEq/l
Cl	107 mEq/l
HCO_3	20 mEq/l
Glucose	44 gm/l
Albumin	1.25 gm/100 ml

Potassium is not added during the first 24 hours, since large amounts of this ion are released from injured cells into extracellular fluids and renal function may be compromised at that time.

The advantages of using a composite solution are as follows: (1) only one type of solution is required; (2) fluid, electrolyte and proteins are administered simultaneously; and (3) only the rate of the infusion may need adjustment.

No one criterion suffices to guide adjustment of fluid therapy. The state of hydration should be evaluated by assessment of: the sensorium, pulse, blood pressure, peripheral circulation, body weight, urine volume, BUN, and serum and urine electrolytes and osmolarity. In burns of greater than 50 per cent of the body surface, additional information regarding the state of hydration may be derived by monitoring central venous pressure and cardiac output.

Since renal function in severely burned patients is modified by factors other than blood volume, urine output may not adequately reflect the state of hydration. Extreme oliguria, however, is not to be expected unless there is renal damage or severe dehydration. The urine output may vary considerably from hour to hour, but a reasonable output should average to between 25 and 30 ml/M^2 body surface/hour. Greater outputs do not seem necessary.

Fluid requirements for the second 24 hours usually average two thirds to three fourths of the first day's allowance. Intravenous fluids of the same composition are continued and oral feedings are begun. Unless there is extreme oliguria, potassium (20 to 30 mEq/l) should be added to the intravenous fluids; if intravenous fluids are no longer necessary, oral potassium supplements should be considered.

Oral feedings are usually begun with milk offered in small amounts at one- to two-hour intervals. If this is tolerated, the quantity of oral fluid is increased progressively and intravenous fluids are reduced correspondingly. A soft diet is usually tolerated by the second to third day.

During the next several weeks *(subacute phase)*, the child is supported medically to facilitate the healing of second degree burns and the autografting of third degree burns. Management includes daily irrigation of wounds with antiseptic solutions, debridement of the wounds, topical antimicrobial therapy, splinting of affected parts and other surgical procedures. During this period, body weight, serum electrolytes, plasma proteins, hematocrit and hemoglobin should be monitored to detect a developing fluid-electrolyte disturbance, hypoalbuminemia or anemia. Albumin levels should be maintained above 2 gm/100 ml to prevent edema. This may be accomplished by infusing salt poor albumin (1 gm/kg/day) as a 2.5 to 5.0 per cent solution in saline over a 12- to 24-hour period. Blood transfusions are often required to maintain normal hemoglobin levels.

CALORIC REQUIREMENTS. Trauma usually increases basal energy expenditures. In burns this is accentuated by the calories spent in the evaporation of water from the wounds. Evaporative water losses may be estimated as 4000 ml/M^2 of burn area, and the caloric expenditure may be calculated by multiplying the evaporative water loss by 0.576, the number of calories required to evaporate 1 ml of water. These increased caloric demands are usually met by oral feedings of milk and a well balanced diet, but nasogastric feedings may be necessary.

Example: A 4 year old child has a surface area of 0.68 M^2 and third degree burns over 40 per cent of the body surface. The daily caloric requirements are estimated as follows: Surface area burned $= 0.68\ M^2 \times 0.40 = 0.27\ M^2$
Evaporative water loss $= 4\ l/M_2$ burn/24 hr $= 4000 \times 0.27 = 1080$ ml/24 hr
Calories for evaporation $= 0.576$ cal/ml $\times$ 1080 ml/24 hr $= 622$ cal/24 hr
Daily caloric requirement for age = 1400 cal
Calories required for evaporation = 622 cal
Total daily caloric requirement = 2022 cal

CARDIOVASCULAR COMPLICATIONS. With appropriate fluid therapy, cardiac output usually returns to normal in 24 to 48 hours. The cause of persistent cardiac dysfunction in burns is unknown. Burned children are prone to congestive failure and pulmonary edema during septic shock or renal failure. In addition to digitalis, diuretic agents (e.g., furosemide) may be required, and in extreme cases phlebotomy or peritoneal dialysis may be necessary.

PULMONARY COMPLICATIONS. Respiratory problems are common, particularly with smoke inhalation or facial burns. Phillips and Cope found that pulmonary lesions contributed to or were directly responsible for 80 per cent of burn deaths. The most common respiratory problems are pulmonary edema, tracheobronchitis, bronchopneumonia and the alveolar-capillary block syndrome. Moreover, poisoning by inhalation of toxic gases, such as carbon monoxide, may occur in burns. The management of these problems may require the participation of an expert respiratory therapist.

RENAL COMPLICATIONS. Severe oliguria during the immediate postburn period is most likely the result of a reduction in glomerular filtration rate and of ADH secretion; but the possibility of renal damage should not be discarded until normal renal function is evidenced. For example, in the presence of oliguria, the failure of the urine to become concentrated or to show conservation of sodium is indicative of renal dysfunction.

Renal failure in burns may be transient in association with acute hypovolemia or shock, or persistent. With persistent azotemia the patient may or may not be oliguric. The prognosis for oliguric azotemia is extremely poor, but with adequate support recovery may occur. Recognition of nonoliguric renal failure is important since an adequate urine output may mask the fact that the urine volume is fixed; water and sodium are retained and hypervolemia and congestive heart failure may develop. If, on the other hand, the condition is promptly recognized, appropriate restrictions of water, salt and protein intake will usually sustain relatively normal fluid balance and allow for recovery of renal function. When renal failure, particularly of the oliguric type, complicates burns, peritoneal dialysis or hemodialysis is often required.

INFECTION. Sepsis is a leading cause of death in burned children. Besides the loss of the protective skin barrier, additional defects in host resistance such as deficiencies in thymic-dependent lymphocytes, in phagocytic function, in complement and in macrophage activation may predispose the patient to infection for some weeks. Serum levels of immunoglobulins fall in the first week because of loss of plasma into the interstitium, but antibody formation is spared. The infecting organisms vary with exposure, but the principal pathogens are *Staphylococcus aureus* and gram-negative bacteria such as *Pseudomonas aeruginosa.* The main portals of entry are the wound, the respiratory tract, the urinary tract, intravenous catheters and possibly the gastrointestinal tract. Successful treatment of sepsis depends upon early diagnosis and prompt use of parenteral antibiotic therapy. No clinical signs are pathognomonic of sepsis. The diagnosis must be suspected when there are: (1) wound infections, (2) hyper- or hypothermia, (3) tachypnea, (4) conspicuous leukocytosis or leukopenia, (5) thrombocytopenia, (6) sudden change in sensorium, (7) ileus, or (8) arterial hypotension. With such findings, blood and other appropriate cultures are obtained and antibiotic therapy is begun. A broad spectrum antimicrobial agent, such as gentamicin, may be used initially until the responsible pathogen is identified. Then, if necessary, the antibiotic therapy is adjusted and treatment is continued for 3 to 5 weeks.

REHABILITATION. Since the physical and psychologic effects of burns are potentially crippling, a vigorous rehabilitation program to counter these effects should be instituted as soon as possible. Residual deformities or loss of function may greatly impair the child's body image and self-esteem, and prolonged hospitalization may lead to a dependency reaction which extends beyond the period of confinement. The child or parents may harbor guilt feelings about the injury. In the parents such feelings tend to interfere with their ability to cope with the illness of the child; the early facing of these issues with the child and family may therefore be essential. This may require the efforts of a mental health professional and social worker. To be effective any program of emotional support should be closely coordinated with medical, nursing and surgical procedures and other essential rehabilitative measures, including physical therapy, play therapy and continuation of schoolwork.

Plans should be made to return the child to as normal a home life as possible. The parents and the child are instructed in home care procedures such as wound dressing, splints, pressure dressings and physical therapy. These measures are particularly important in reducing hypertrophic scars. The child should return to school and other social activities as soon as possible. In most circumstances this is feasible within the first week after the end of the hospitalization. The continuing rehabilitation of the child will involve the cooperative efforts of the family physician, physical therapist, mental health professional and reconstructive surgeon. Their procedures should be planned so that they will interfere as little as possible with the child's schoolwork and other normal social development.

Hugo F. Carvajal
Armond S. Goldman

Artz, C. P.: The Brooke Formula. *In* Contemporary Burn Mangement. Boston, Little, Brown and Company, 1971, pp. 43–51.
Artz, C. P., and Moncrief, J. A.: The Treatment of Burns. 2nd ed. Philadelphia, W. B. Saunders Company, 1969.
Baxter, C. R., Moncrief, J. A., Prager, M. H., et al.: A circulating myocardial depressant factor in burn shock. *In* Matter, P., Barclay, T. L., and Kowicfova, S. (eds.): Research in Burns. Transactions of Third International Congress on Research in Burns, Prague. Bern, Hans Huber Publishers, 1971, pp. 499–503.
Berman, W., Jr., Goldman, A. S., Reichelderfer, T., and Mofenson, H. C.: Childhood burn injuries and deaths. Pediatrics *51*:1069, 1973.
Eagle, J. F.: Parenteral fluid therapy of burns during the first 48 hours. N. Y. J. Med. *66*:1613, 1956.
Haddon, W., Jr.: On the escape of tigers: An ecologic note. Technology Review *72*(No. 7), May, 1970.
Hutcher, N., and Haynes, B. W., Jr.: The Evans formula revisited. J. Trauma *12*:453, 1972.
Innes, R. L., Goldman, A. S., Schmitt, R., McKinley, A., and Dobrkovsky, M.: A study of the etiology and epidemiology of burn injuries in children. *In* Matter, P., Barclay, T. L., and Kowicfova, S. (eds.): Research in Burns. Transactions of Third International Congress on Research in Burns, Prague, Bern, Hans Huber Publishers, 1971, pp. 437–442.
Metcoff, J., et al.: Losses and physiologic requirements for water and electrolytes after extensive burns in children. New Engl. J. Med. *265*:101, 1961.
Monafo, W. W.: The treatment of burn shock by the intravenous and oral administration of hypertonic lactated saline solution. J. Trauma *10*:575, 1970.
Moncrief, J. A.: Burns. New Engl. J. Med. *288*:444, 1973.
Phillips, A. W., and Cope, O.: The revelation of respiratory tract damage as a principal killer of the burned patient. Ann. Surg. *155*:1, 1962.
Shook, C. W., MacMillan, B. C., and Altemeier, W. A.: Pulmonary complications of the burned patient. Arch. Surg. *97*:215, 1968.
Stoll, A. M., and Chianta, M. A.: Heat transfer through fabrics as related to thermal injury. Trans. New York Acad. Sci. *33*:649, 1971.
Stone, H. H.: The composite burn solution: *In* Polk, H. C., Jr., and Stone, H. H. (eds.): Contemporary Burn Management. Boston, Little, Brown and Company, 1971, pp. 93–104.

DRUG THERAPY

GENERAL CONSIDERATIONS

The physician's diagnostic ability and skills are ultimately expressed in his ability to treat his patient. Treatment may or may not include drug therapy. The decision as to the form of therapy to be used is the responsibility of the physician and should not be relegated to or dictated by parents or others. Confidence in the physician is an essential part of a successful therapeutic program, and the development of this confidence will depend on the physician's attitude and actions. A resourceful physician will adjust his approach and therapy to each patient as seen in different families and under different circumstances. One mother may be overwhelmed by the problem of caring for the first coryza of her first infant, whereas the veteran mother of 6 children may take the sixth case of gastroenteritis too lightly.

Rational therapy depends on (1) precise diagnosis, (2) an understanding of the normal metabolic and emotional processes peculiar to children of different ages, and how these are affected by the disease, (3) knowledge of socioeconomic factors involved, and (4) the therapeutic means available. When a drug is part of the treatment, the physician must know the pharmacologic action and metabolism of the drug in the patient. Improper therapy may be due to inadequate diagnosis, poor choice of drug, improper directions for dispensing or administration, failure of compliance in administration, variable bioavailability of the drug, faulty storage of the drug, or inadequate evaluation of the total situation.

"Self"-medication with drugs available without prescription ("over-the-counter" drugs) may have occurred before, during or after a physician's orders for drugs. He must assess the possible effect.

ADVERSE DRUG REACTIONS

Any active drug may cause an undesirable reaction in addition to or instead of the desired action. The risk of an undesired reaction must be evaluated against the potential benefit. Undesirable reactions may include:

REACTION TO OVERDOSE. Large amounts of most drugs will usually cause toxic manifestations. Some drugs will cause toxic manifestations in amounts taken representing only small excesses over therapeutic amounts.

SIDE EFFECTS. Undesirable pharmacologic effects can be expected with predictable frequency with the *usual* doses of certain drugs. Moreover, such drugs as antibiotics or immunosuppressants may so alter the bacterial flora or the body's resistance that new infections (superinfections) occur, sometimes with organisms (Pseudomonas, *P. carinii,* or fungi) which are not normally pathogenic.

ALLERGIC OR HYPERSENSITIVE REACTIONS AND IDIOSYNCRASY. These are abnormal reactions of the host and are not exclusively related to the dose or to the pharmacologic action of the drug. These responses may be the first manifestations of an immunologic, metabolic, genetic or environmental abnormality.

DEVELOPMENTAL ASPECTS OF ADVERSE DRUG REACTIONS. The above-mentioned reactions may be expected in persons of any age; certain other reactions are intimately or uniquely related to stages of growth and development. The intensity of such reactions is often dependent on the rapidity of the growth process.

During the *embryonic period* (first 8 to 12 weeks of gestation) certain drugs taken by the mother may prove to be teratogenic and produce structural malformations. Among these are: thalidomide, which produces phocomelia and other anomalies; some cancer therapeutic agents, such as methotrexate, which profoundly distort the growth pattern; and progestins, testosterone, other androgenic agents, and even diethylstilbestrol, which may cause masculinization of the female fetus. The teratogenic effects of drugs are likely to be both time- and dose-related.

The European epidemic of phocomelia resulting from the use of thalidomide in pregnant women precipitated world-wide reaction; in the United States this included the passage of Federal amendments in 1962 which require proof of efficacy of drugs as well as of safety.

During the *fetal period*, drugs administered to the mother may be responsible for modification of growth of a structurally intact fetus. For example, goitrogens, such as the iodides, radioactive iodine, thiouracils and perchlorates, or lithium may cause goiters, which may be so large as to interfere with respiration and delivery; tetracyclines may, when deposited in bones and teeth, cause discoloration and distortion of growth; and cancer therapeutic agents may suppress growth and cause congenital anomalies. Administration of diethylstilbestrol during pregnancy may give rise years later to genital cancer in female offspring.

Some drugs administered during or shortly before labor may have little effect on the newborn infant; others may cause serious problems. Among the latter are acidifying and adrenergic agents, analgesics (both narcotic and non-narcotic), anesthetics, antibiotics and chemotherapeutic agents, antihypertensives, endocrine products, hypnotics and sedatives, muscle relaxants, tranquilizers, vitamin K and xanthines (aminophylline or theophylline). Neonatal narcotic addiction may follow heroin, morphine or methadone addiction of the mother. The injudicious use of hypotonic or hypertonic electrolyte solutions in the mother may produce serious disturbances in the newborn infant.

Drugs which can cause difficulty on reaching the fetus through the placenta may cause similar difficulties when administered to the newborn infant, particularly in large or frequent doses.

Drugs may also be secreted into breast milk, but the amounts are seldom sufficient to yield activity in the infant.

Certain drugs which will be tolerated in later infancy may cause serious reactions in the neonatal period. Chloramphenicol, for example, is poorly conjugated and excreted, especially by the premature infant, and may cause the "gray syndrome" in infants less than a week of age. The same dosage may at 3 weeks be insufficient to produce effective blood levels.

Whenever the use of a drug is considered, its potential for harm must be carefully weighed against its potential value, but primum non nocere should not be interpreted to mean "do nothing for fear of doing harm"; difficult decisions are the heart of medicine.

TYPES OF DRUG THERAPY

SPECIFIC THERAPY. The action of a drug is said to be specific when it is capable of combating a specific causative agent (e.g. penicillin versus the beta hemolytic streptococcus) or of alleviating a specific problem for which the pathophysiology is understood (e.g. digitalis for cardiac failure).

EMPIRIC THERAPY. When a drug apparently alleviates symptoms or exerts a beneficial effect on a disease process, but the mode of action is not understood, the effect is termed empiric. Such therapy is based on prior experience, which has established the value and hazards involved. In many instances further study will establish whether the value observed is a true pharmacologic effect or a placebo effect.

THERAPEUTIC TRIAL. Drug therapy may on occasion be diagnostic. The response of rheumatic arthritis to therapy with a salicylate is an example.

SUPPORTIVE AND SYMPTOMATIC THERAPY. Supportive therapy includes palliative and corrective measures which do not directly attack the disease agent or process. Supportive and symptomatic measures may, however, be as important as specific medication, even when the latter is also available. They include correction of fluid and electrolyte imbalance, alleviation of pain, sedation, inhalation of oxygen, and other therapy. Adequate skill in administering such therapy is less readily attained than is competence in the prescription of specific therapy.

PLACEBO THERAPY. There is a place for placebo therapy in the practice of pediatrics, if it is used thoughtfully. *All* drugs have some placebo effect added to their pharmacologic activity. The placebo effect is much stronger in some patients and in some families than in others. The physician's attitude can greatly enhance or minimize this effect; it is essential that when he uses a placebo, he keep its true nature in mind. The physician caring for growing children should feel a responsibility towards education of them and their families to rational attitudes toward drug therapy.

PSYCHOTHERAPY. Though not drug therapy, psychotherapy is in varying degree an essential part of the care of all patients. The physician must be able to deal with anxiety and guilt in parents or child, able to know when emotional entanglements complicate administration of drug or other therapy, and able to assist parents in reaching a realistic assessment of their child's illness which will permit an adequate therapeutic program. Not only what he does but how is important. Attention to small details to facilitate home care or to make hospital care more pleasant is essential: the kindly smile, the unhurried attitude and, above all, the time for explanation.

INITIATION OF DRUG THERAPY

One of the most severe tests of clinical judgment is selection of the proper time to institute drug therapy. Most diseases of infancy and childhood are self-limited. A few are rapidly fatal if proper therapy is not instituted immediately. If a precise diagnosis can be made, the choice of therapy is apt to be obvious. If it cannot be made, the physician must decide either to withhold therapy until the diagnosis can be made or to institute therapy for selected diagnostic possibilities while waiting for information essential to a precise diagnosis. At times such blind therapy may be lifesaving; at other times it may obscure the true diagnosis, with serious consequences. In some instances, when an illness has not responded to a therapeutic program, it will be wise to suspend treatment in order to re-evaluate the initial diagnosis.

CHOICE OF DRUG

If the decision has been made that drug therapy is indicated, several factors should influence choice of the specific drug or drugs. Of equally effective drugs, the least toxic one should be selected; of equally effective and toxic drugs the least expensive should be chosen. No drug should be prescribed except as there is a reason for it. The more drugs used, the greater the chance for undesirable reactions which may confuse the clinical course of the patient. In general, mixtures of several drugs in one vehicle should be avoided, since dosage and periodicity of administration are better controlled when drugs are given separately. Attention must be given to the synergistic or antagonistic effects of drugs given together, which may occur at any of several sites during absorption or transport, within the reactive cell, or on excretion.

For any drug prescribed, the physician should know the route and rate of absorption; the rate, method and organ of excretion or detoxification; the pharmacologic action expected and any possible undesirable reactions. It is desirable for a physican to select one or two drugs from each class of drugs so that he can gain from personal experience the necessary familiarity with the variable reactions expected in different patients. It is not possible to acquire such knowledge for a large number of drugs.

THERAPEUTIC ORPHANS

The "package insert" is a quasi-legal document which accompanies most prescription drugs, and which carries instructions for the use of the drug. Physicians treating children must be familiar with *current* package inserts for the drugs they prescribe. Because the safety and efficacy in children have not, for many drugs, been adequately established, the insert will often carry clear admonitions contraindicating their use in childhood. Physicians are faced with a difficult decision: whether or not to prescribe drugs which may be valuable, but which have been adequately studied and released for use *only* in adults. Children deprived of the use of such drugs have been called "therapeutic orphans," and the term has been applied also to the drugs themselves, as lacking sponsorship for use with children. These drugs may be considered investigational for children.

ADMINISTRATION OF DRUGS

Clear and explicit directions should be written for the administration of drugs. Both the name of the drug and these directions should generally appear on the label of the container. The route of administration and the prepared form of the drug should be chosen with the age and symptoms of the patient clearly in mind. The drug must be in a form that the attendant can administer to an infant or child. The parenteral administration of drugs is the most reliable route, but it is generally not practical for home use. Table 30–1 lists the possible routes of administration, the different prepared forms and doses of many drugs.

The *oral route* can be utilized for many drugs unless refusal or nausea, vomiting or other disorders of the gastrointestinal tract make their use impossible. Children vary in their ability to swallow tablets and capsules. As a rule, liquids should be prescribed for children under 5 years of age. Forced administration of solids or liquids to a struggling child may result in aspiration. If liquid preparations are not available, tablets can often be mashed, or capsules emptied, and the drug mixed with syrups, jams, honey or other vehicles. Unpleasant-tasting drugs should not be put in food that is or should be frequently eaten by the child.

Standardized measuring devices are preferred for measuring dosage. The volumes contained by household teaspoons and droppers vary greatly. Calibrated droppers can be obtained for the measurement of smaller doses. The volume prescribed should always be large enough so that minor errors in measurement will not significantly alter the administered dose. When prescribing for infants and children, the physician must keep in mind all possible factors that may interfere with the drug arriving at the desired place in the recommended dose.

The *rectal route* cannot be expected to provide reliable absorption. If this route is chosen for reasons which seem appropriate in a particular situation, the rectum should be prepared by cleansing with an enema of isotonic saline solution. Multiple enemas may create fluid and electrolyte disturbances. The medication should be dissolved or suspended in 10 to 30 ml of water and gently injected through a catheter or bulb syringe. Then the buttocks should be held together with tape and the catheter withdrawn. Some drugs are incorporated in suppositories; they are poorly absorbed by the dehydrated patient or from a stool-filled rectum (the usual circumstance).

The *parenteral routes* are the most reliable ones for the administration of drugs. In severe or potentially severe illness or when vomiting is a factor, parenteral therapy should be utilized. The rate of absorption varies with the site of administration (subcutaneous, intramuscular or intravenous), with the absorbability of the drug or its vehicle and with the adequacy of the circulation. The objections to the parenteral route include the unavoidable trauma of administration, a greater risk of sensitization, and local or systemic reactions. Especially in infants there is a risk of sciatic palsy when intramuscular injections are given in the gluteal area.

Physicians must know which drugs cannot be given together or with glucose or other substances in parenteral fluids.

Necrotizing or sclerosing drugs should be avoided, if at all possible; when necessary, they should be given intravenously with great caution.

Intrathecal therapy is rarely indicated.

The *sublingual* and *buccal* routes can be utilized for certain drugs, but only older children are able to cooperate with this type of therapy.

Topical therapy is often of great value, but requires careful direction and supervision if it is to be effective. Many parents and nurses have difficulty instilling medication in the eyes, ears, noses or mouths of infants and young children. Solutions are usually easier to handle than ointments for use in the eye or ear. The attendant should be instructed to rest the hand holding the dropper on the head, so that it moves with the head. The dose should be expelled rapidly, not by drops. Plastic droppers should be used rather than glass, and should often be calibrated.

Generally, ointments and creams are ineffective when applied to an oozing surface. Topical medication which is toxic when ingested or rubbed in the eyes should be covered. As a rule, drugs that are commonly used for systemic therapy, such as certain antibiotics or antihistamines, should not be used topically, in order that the possibility of sensitization may be lessened. Some drugs are absorbed in dangerous quantity from large denuded areas.

Inhalation therapy utilizing aerosol medication is practical only for cooperative older children. With younger children, the aerosol must be given in a small tent, and dosage control is uncertain with most drugs.

THE DOSE OF DRUGS

The proper dose of a drug is the amount required to effect safely the desired pharmacologic action. As patients vary in their responses, the average recommended dose may have to be increased to accomplish the purpose or decreased to avoid undesirable reactions. Careful observation of the patient and individualization of therapy are essential. In some instances the dosage should be controlled by serial determinations of the concentration in the blood. Clinical observation and often laboratory measurements are essential to detect early evidence of toxicity, indicating the need to decrease the dose or to discontinue therapy.

Table 30–1 lists the average recommended dose of many drugs. When only the adult dose is known, there are many formulas to calculate the dose for a child. None is entirely satisfactory. Since many physiologic phenomena are more closely related to body surface area than to age, height or weight, the formula utilizing surface area* may be more accurate than others. The West nomogram (Fig. 30–1) can be used to calculate surface area.

Figure 30–2 permits calculation of surface area and the percentage of the adult dose from body weight.

$$^{*}\frac{\text{Surface area of patient (in square meters)}}{1.7} \times \text{Adult dose} = \text{Approximate dose for patient}$$

In Table 30-1 the doses of many drugs are related to surface area (M^2) as well as to body weight. The dose for a given patient based on his surface area can be determined as follows:

Surface area of patient (in M^2) × dose per M^2 = approximate dose for patient.

*Clark's Rule** may be used to estimate dosage on the basis of the child's weight in respect to the adult dose of the drug.

These formulas are highly unreliable when applied to newborn infants, more reliable with children over 2 years of age. Careful clinical observation, or chemical, electronic or other monitoring may be necessary for correct titration of the drug for a particular patient.

HARRY C. SHIRKEY

*Clark's rule:

$$\frac{\text{Patient's weight in pounds}}{150} \times \text{Adult dose} = \text{Approximate dose for patient}$$

Done, A. K.: Developmental pharmacology, Clin. Pharmacol. Ther. *5*:432, 1964.

Done, A. K. (ed.): Problems of drug evaluation in infants and children. Ross Conferences on Pediatric Research *58*, 1968.

Editorial: Diethylstilbestrol contraindicated in pregnancy. FDA Bulletin, November, 1971.

Editorial: Hexachlorophene and newborns. FDA Drug Bulletin, December, 1971.

Editorial: The evaluation of drugs: Whose responsibility? Bull. WHO *68*:256, 1968.

Gellis, S. S., and Kagan, B. M. (eds.): Current Pediatric Therapy. 6th ed. Philadelphia, W. B. Saunders Company, 1973.

Leitman, P. S.: Pharmacologic effects on developing enzyme systems. Fed. Proc. *31*:62, 1972.

Martin, C. M., and Jeghers, H. (eds.): Clinical investigation as an integral feature of medical residency training. J. Med. Educ. *40*:75, 1965.

Mirkin, B. L.: Ontogenesis of the adrenergic nervous system: Functional and pharmacologic implications. Fed. Proc. *31*:65, 1972.

Preliminary Report, Conference on Pediatric Clinical Pharmacology. Washington, D.C., National Academy of Sciences, November 8–9, 1971.

Report of the Conference on Clinical Pharmacology. Washington, D. C., National Academy of Sciences, December 3–4, 1970.

Shirkey, H. C.: Clinical evaluation of drugs used in premature infants, normal infants, and children. South. Med. J. *51*:24, 1963.

Shirkey, H. C.: Clinical pharmacology with ambulatory children. Clin. Pediat. *7*:639, 1968.

Shirkey, H. C. (ed.): Pediatric Therapy, 5th ed. St. Louis, The C. V. Mosby Co., 1975.

Sparber, S. B.: Effects of drugs on the biochemical and behavioral responses of developing organisms. Fed. Proc. *31*:74, 1972.

Symposium on Pediatric Pharmacology. Washington, D. C., Food and Drug Administration, 1970.

Waddell, W. J.: Localization and metabolism of drugs in the fetus. Fed. Proc. *31*:52, 1972.

Wilson, J. T.: Pediatric pharmacology: Who will test the drugs? J. Pediat. *80*:855, 1972.

Yaffe, S. J.: Symposium on pediatric pharmacology. Pediat. Clin. N. Amer. *19*:1–256, 1972.

HARRY C. SHIRKEY

6
PRENATAL DISTURBANCES

PRENATAL FACTORS IN DISEASES OF CHILDREN

Genetic Factors

The interplay of many factors determines health or disease of children. The physician who observes various persons notices that they react differently to traumas, infections or deficiencies of the same type and intensity. Such differences are conveniently explained as being the result of varying "constitutions." It may be useful to attempt an analysis of latent or remote factors underlying this differential behavior. Some of these factors were at work before the child was born, and obviously it is difficult to study them. Nevertheless their remoteness or latency does not make them less real, and they deserve as much study and, if possible, treatment as the factors which finally elicit the disease.

THE FERTILIZED OVUM. The child's development begins with fertilization of the ovum. The genetic composition of the fertilized egg (zygote) determines the potential somatic and mental traits of the new individual, but a favorable environment is also indispensable for coordinated embryonic differentiation and growth. Abnormalities of the elements of the zygote as well as prenatal environmental disturbances may result in congenital defects or "points of minor resistance" in the new organism. Congenital deviations are often at the root of chronic and intractable diseases of children.

Abnormalities of the chromosomes and genes, contained in the nucleus of the fertilized ovum, cause many defects in children. In addition, injurious environmental factors are capable of altering the development of an otherwise healthy zygote and are thus responsible for the production of abnormalities. Such factors should be more accessible to preventive measures than are other prenatal pathogenic factors.

INJURIOUS FACTORS. Injurious genetic and prenatal environmental factors will be discussed separately, although they are often difficult to distinguish in practice. Prenatal development is regulated by a continuous interaction of genes with their surrounding cytoplasm, the latter reacting in turn with the intramaternal and extramaternal environments. This continuous process is a chain of complicated physicochemical reactions, which may be interrupted or diverted by genetic or environmental interference. Genetically determined abnormalities may be imitated by environmental disturbances and result in nonhereditary "phenocopies" of hereditary defects.

CHROMOSOMES. The essential genetic material of the chromosomes is the threadlike intranuclear structures which carry the genes, deoxyribonucleic acid, or DNA. In man the sperm and the egg (gametes) each carry a set of 23 chromosomes; the fertilized egg and the somatic cells derived from it by mitosis therefore contain two such sets, or a total of 46 (44 somatic and 2 sex) chromosomes. The gametes are thus said to be *haploid,* and the somatic cells *diploid.*

The haploid gametes for the next generation are derived from the diploid cells of the gonad by a reduction division, or *meiosis,* in which the homologous chromosomes pair and then separate, one member of the pair going to one pole of the dividing cell, and the other to the opposite pole. Thus the two new cells each have a set of 23 chromosomes to contribute to the next generation. When the homologues separate, it is a matter of chance whether the maternal or the paternal member of the pair goes to a particular pole, so that any germ cell contains a random mixture of maternal and paternal chromosomes. This provides the physical basis for the segregation of genes.

GENES. Protein structure and function are genetically determined. A protein is composed of polypeptides, which are chains of amino acids. The sequence of amino acids in the polypeptides determines the shape, and therefore the physicochemical properties, of the protein. For each polypeptide being synthesized there is a corresponding region of a chromosome in which the structure of the DNA determines the amino acid sequence. That particular area of the DNA is said to be the gene for the corresponding polypeptide. This concept was first suggested by observations in sickle cell anemia, where a single gene difference was shown to be associated with a difference in the beta chain of the hemoglobin molecule; the sixth amino acid from the C-terminal end is glutamic acid in the normal beta chain, whereas it is valine in the sickle cell beta chain. This and other evidence led to the concept of a gene that determines the amino acid sequence of the beta chain, another for the alpha chain, and in fact one gene for every kind of polypeptide chain.

The basic structure of the DNA molecule can be likened to a rope ladder, in which the ropes are made up of alternating deoxyribose and phosphate molecules, and each rung consists of two of four nucleotide bases: guanine *(G)*, cytosine *(C)*, adenine *(A)*, and thymine *(T)*—the whole structure being twisted into a double helix. The physicochemical requirements are such that guanine always pairs with cytosine, and adenine with thymine.

The sequence of bases in the DNA constitutes a code that determines the amino acid sequence of the corresponding protein, a triplet of three bases corresponding to one amino acid. For instance, it appears that the triplet CTT, at a particular place in the DNA, determines that there will be a glutamic acid molecule at a particular place on the corresponding polypeptide.

The genetic information is carried from the chromosomal gene to the cytoplasmic protein-synthesizing site, the ribosome, by a labile type of RNA called messenger RNA. (RNA is like a single-stranded rope with ribose instead of deoxyribose, and uracil instead of thymine.) The messenger RNA is synthesized on the DNA strand, with the same requirements of complementary pairing as the two DNA strands; thus, a CTT triplet of the DNA will result in a GAA triplet in the RNA. The messenger RNA migrates from the nucleus to the ribosomes, where it acts as a mold, or template, on which the amino acids are assembled into polypeptide chains in the following way:

A third type of RNA, the transfer RNA, exists in the cytoplasm in 20 different varieties, one for each amino acid. Each type is characterized by a specific base triplet, which corresponds in some still unknown way to its particular amino acid. Thus, a variety of transfer RNA, with a specific triplet, CUU, at a specific attachment site on the molecule, can attach itself (with the aid of a specific enzyme) to a glutamic acid molecule at the other end. This is an oversimplification; the code is redundant, and several different transfer RNA's may code for the same amino acid.

If the transfer RNA-amino acid complex approaches the messenger RNA template, it can attach itself to the template at any point where there is a triplet corresponding to its own specific triplet. Thus, a transfer RNA carrying glutamic acid at one end and a CUU triplet at the attachment site will fit in wherever there is a GAA triplet in the messenger RNA. Similarly, a transfer RNA carrying valine has a specific CAU triplet and will fit in anywhere where there is a GUA triplet on the template. In this way the amino acids are lined up on the template in an order specified by the sequence of triplets in the messenger RNA, which in turn was specified by the sequence of triplets in the DNA. These findings, coming mainly from microbial genetics, are the basis for the modern concept of a gene—a sequence of base pairs in the chromosomal DNA which determines the sequence of amino acids in a polypeptide.

An alteration in a gene will result in an alteration in the corresponding polypeptide and in the protein of which the polypeptide is a part. This change may lead to altered function of the protein and to a corresponding variation in the development or function of the organism, as in persons with sickle cell hemoglobin.

Since each cell carries the genes for all peptides, but only synthesizes some of them, it follows that a given gene is active only in certain cells. Evidence from microorganisms shows that the activity of groups of functionally related genes is regulated by other genes through the production of cytoplasmic repressors. Systems of genetically controlled regulation of gene activity are being demonstrated in mammals.

For most genetically controlled variations in man the underlying biochemical change has not been identified, and one may think of the gene simply as a locus on a chromosome that carries an instruction regarding a particular characteristic or trait of the organism. Since the chromosomes are paired, the genes also are paired, and the two members of a pair may carry similar or different instructions regarding the trait which they determine, such as five or six fingers, presence or absence of melanin, or presence or absence of red-cell antigen A or B. If the members of a gene pair are the same, the person is said to be **homozygous** for the gene pair. If the members of a gene pair carry different instructions, the person is **heterozygous.** In this case the resulting trait may be determined by only one member of the pair, in which case the gene that is expressed is said to be **dominant,** and the one that is not manifested is **recessive.** The outward appearance, or array of physical traits, is called the **phenotype,** and the underlying genetic constitution is called the **genotype.** Because of recessive genes, as well as other irregularities to be mentioned later, one cannot always deduce the genotype from the phenotype.

It now appears that in the normal female one X chromosome replicates its DNA during mitosis later than the other chromosomes, remains condensed and physiologically inactive in the interphase cell, and forms the sex-chromatin body (**Barr body**) characteristic of female somatic nuclei. Thus the female, like the male, has only one functioning X chromosome. If more than 2 X chromosomes are present, as in the XXX female, or XXXY male, the extra X's are also inactivated; thus the number of Barr bodies is always one less than the number of X chromosomes in the diploid complement (the **Lyon hypothesis**).

Either the maternal or the paternal X may be inactivated in different cells of the same female, so that a woman who is heterozygous for any gene on the X chromosome will be mosaic, with one allele active in some cells and the other allele in other cells.

DOMINANT PATHOLOGIC TRAITS

Because dominant abnormal traits are relatively rare, a person who has such a trait is usually heterozygous. The heterozygote has one dominant, pathologic gene (*P*) and one recessive, normal gene (*p*) for the trait in question. The person shows the pathologic trait, since the abnormal gene expresses itself (*Pp*). The heterozygote usually marries a person who is free of the same pathologic trait and has two normal recessive genes (*pp*) for the character in question. The abnormal person forms two kinds of germ cells in equal numbers, those containing the gene *P* and those containing the gene *p*. All the germ cells of the normal mate contain the gene *p*. Figure 6–1 illustrates the results to be expected from such a mating: half of the offspring (*Pp*) can be expected to exhibit the pathologic trait, but the other half (*pp*) will be entirely free of it. Unless it represents a new mutation, a dominant abnormality appears in every previous generation of a kinship, and each offspring of an affected parent has an equal chance of being affected or unaffected. If one of these affected children marries a normal person, he must expect to see the trait in about half of his offspring. Those children who do not show the trait will have entirely normal offspring if their mates are normal.

Figure 6–2 presents a pedigree in which a pathologic trait, multiple exostoses, is inherited as a dominant factor. The abnormal trait is transmitted from affected parents to approximately half of their children, while the other members who are free of the trait have only healthy offspring. Although each child of an affected parent has exactly a 1:1 chance of inheriting the abnormal gene, the proportion of affected to nonaffected children in any one family may deviate from the 1:1 ratio, within the limits of random variation.

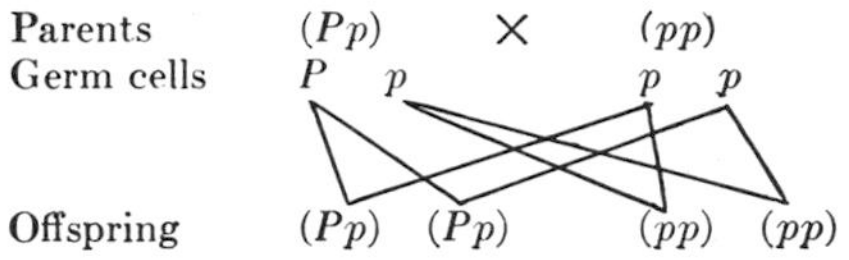

Figure 6–1

A number of pathologic conditions may be inherited as dominant traits. These include achondroplasia, aniridia, diabetes insipidus (ADH-deficient), ectodermal dysplasia (hydrotic), elliptocytosis, epidermolysis bullosa simplex, hemorrhagic telangiectasia, Huntington's chorea, hyperelastosis cutis, keratosis follicularis, multiple exostoses, multiple polyposis, muscular dystrophy (facioscapulohumeral), myotonia congenita, myotonia dystrophica, neurofibromatosis, night blindness (without myopia), osteogenesis imperfecta, peroneal atrophy, polycystic kidney disease (adult type), sicklemia, spherocytosis, split hands or feet, thalassemia minor and tuberous sclerosis. (See McKusick for a more complete list.) It should be emphasized that in some instances the same clinical pattern may be produced in more than one way, e.g. by a mutant gene or an environmental agent; thus, inheritance of a pathologic trait in one or several pedigrees does not imply that the trait in question is always hereditary, nor that it is always inherited in the same manner (Fig. 6–3).

MODIFICATION OF HEREDITARY TRAITS

Skipping of a Generation. Contrary to the rule developed, a dominant trait may occasionally skip a generation. Thus, the abnormal trait may not appear in a person who has inherited the abnormal gene and transmits it to half of his offspring. This behavior may be due to reduced *expressivity* of the gene, which may result in only a slight abnormality not obvious to the casual observer. In some instances the abnormality may be found in a mild form (microform, forme fruste). In some cases of hereditary malformations, such as brachydactyly or exostoses, apparent skipping can be explained by roentgenographic demonstration of the abnormality in a mild form in an apparently

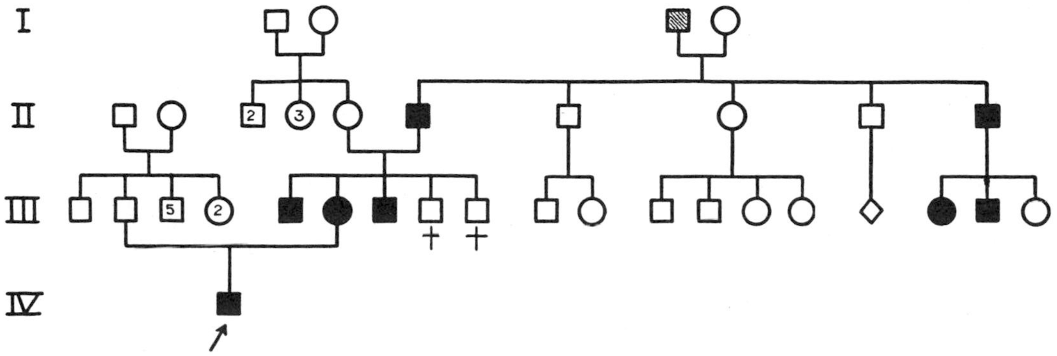

Figure 6–2 *Pedigree of a sibship in which multiple exostoses occurred in several members. The abnormal condition was transmitted by the affected members to part of their offspring, but the children of the unaffected members remained free. This suggests a dominant mode of inheritance. The pedigree was drawn according to the report of the mother of the propositus (↗), a 4-year-old patient of the Children's Hospital, Cincinnati, Ohio.*

■ ● Male and female with multiple exostoses.

▧ Man with a "bone disease" considered tuberculosus(?).

See Figure 6–3 for explanation of other symbols.

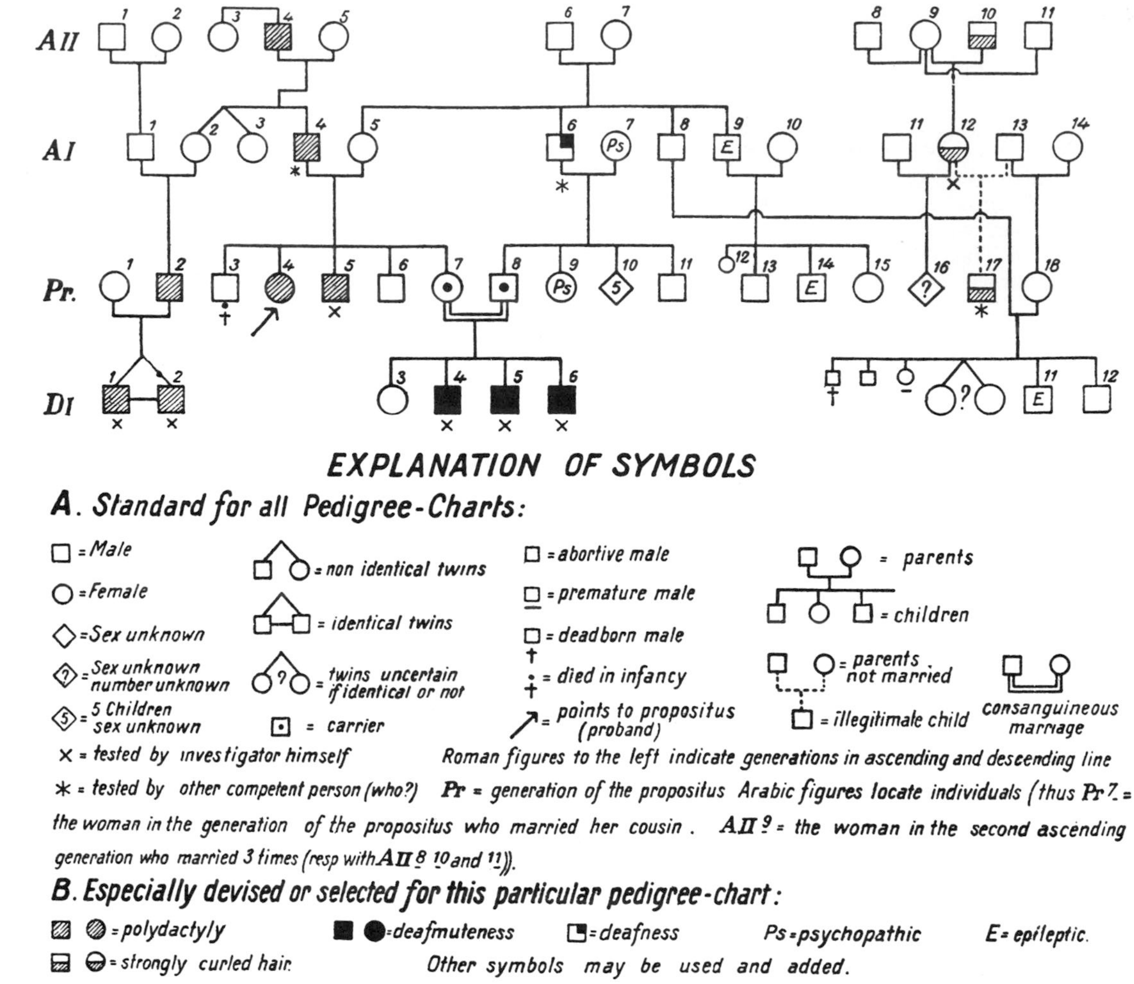

Figure 6–3 *Standard symbols for pedigree charts. (Bureau of Human Heredity, London.)*

normal parent who transmitted the anomaly to some of his children. In other instances chemical or hematologic methods reveal that the transmitting person carries the basic hereditary anomaly (hyperuricemia, spherocytosis) without clinical manifestations (gout, hemolytic jaundice).

In other instances no expression of the abnormal gene can be detected. Skipping of a generation in this manner is attributed to reduced *penetrance* (the percentual frequency with which a heterozygous dominant or a homozygous recessive gene manifests itself). Other genetic or environmental factors may be responsible for the varied expression of the abnormal trait.

Environmental Effects. Environment plays an important role in the prenatal or postnatal manifestation of hereditary disease, in which often only a "tendency" is genetically transmitted. The disease may be manifest in a person with the abnormal tendency only if he encounters certain environmental conditions. Thus the inherited deficiency in glucose 6-phosphate dehydrogenase in red blood cells produces a hemolytic anemia only if the affected person ingests substances which have oxidant properties, such as fava beans, primaquine or sulfonamides.

The basis for such pathologic tendencies may be anatomic, histologic or functional deviations from the normal which often are not manifest clinically. Thus, reduced diameter and spherical shape of the red blood corpuscles (spherocytosis) can be observed in certain families as a dominant hereditary trait. Some carriers of spherocytes are completely unaware of their abnormal trait, whereas in others there is an increased hemolysis of the abnormal cells, with resultant anemia, jaundice, splenomegaly and other manifestations. The clinical patterns of those with manifest disease vary, and occasionally members of an affected family may have no symptoms in common. Spherocytosis, inherited as a simple dominant, may cause a confusing variety of clinical features (**pleiotropism**), which may not be recognized as being related without hematologic studies. Patients with hemolytic jaundice can be freed of their disturbing symptoms by splenectomy. This shows that a hereditary disease can be effectively treated postnatally and refutes the false but widely accepted

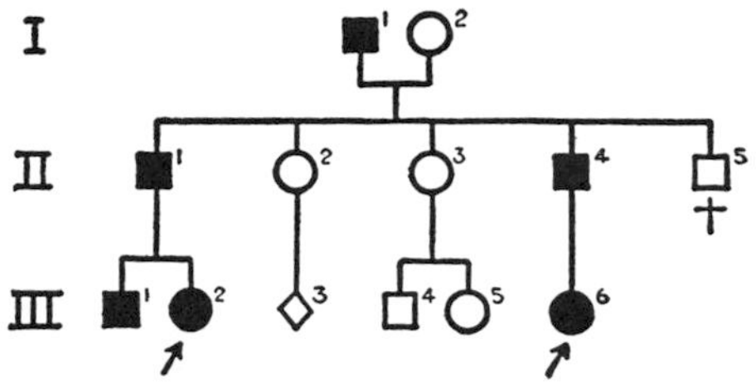

■ ● Persons with blue scleras.

Figure 6–4 Pedigree of a family in which blue scleras occurred in several members. In addition, the following associated symptoms were seen by the recorder or reported by a member of the family (II_4): III_1: long, gracile bones in roentgenograms; III_2: multiple fractures (osteopsathyrosis); III_6: multiple fractures; II_1: multiple fractures; II_4: multiple dislocations, otosclerosis.

The abnormal condition which manifested itself in various symptoms was transmitted as a dominant trait.

opinion that "nothing can be done about hereditary diseases." Splenectomy, however, does not change the patient's genetic make-up, and he can transmit the abnormal trait to half of his offspring.

Another example of multiple symptoms of one dominant hereditary trait is represented by a *mesenchymal dysplasia*, which manifests itself in bluish scleras and long, gracile bones. Such bones may fracture with the slightest trauma. Some affected persons have a tendency to dislocations of joints, some to otosclerosis. In taking a history of the sibship of an affected person one may learn that one member suffered from deafness and multiple dislocations, and that other members were subject to multiple fractures (Fig. 6–4). Unless the observer knows the disease entity, he will not recognize the dominant inheritance of the underlying trait.

INCOMPATIBILITY OF PARENTAL GENETIC FACTORS. The degree of complexity with which genetic factors may interact with other factors in the causa-

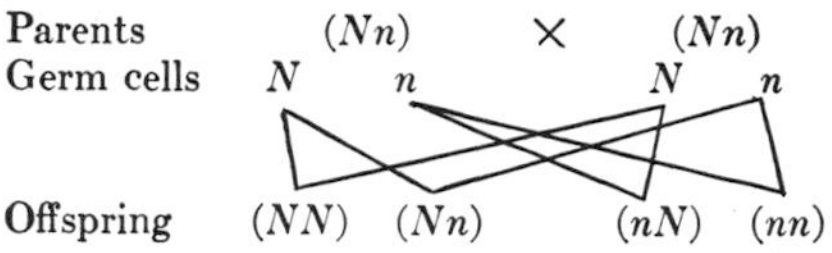

Figure 6–5

tion of disease is well illustrated in erythroblastosis fetalis (hemolytic disease of the newborn, Section 7). In this condition the interaction of *normal* genes of parents and child is associated with a pathologic condition in the fetus or newborn infant which stems directly from these normal genes.

RECESSIVE PATHOLOGIC TRAITS

A person with an abnormal recessive gene paired with a normal dominant gene appears normal and produces normal offspring with a mate who has two normal genes for the trait in question. If, however, such a heterozygous person marries a person who is similarly heterozygous, then each child has one chance in four of being homozygous and of having the pathologic trait. In Figure 6–5 the two apparently normal but actually heterozygous parents are represented by (*Nn*), *N* representing the normal dominant and *n* the pathologic, recessive gene.

The abnormal offspring has the genetic constitution (*nn*). Three fourths of the offspring appear phenotypically normal, but only one fourth (*NN*) are genotypically normal. One half of the children (*Nn*) are heterozygous, like the parents; they appear normal, but carry the pathologic gene. Since such carriers of one recessive abnormal gene appear normal, there is the possibility that they may marry unknowingly a carrier of the same pathologic trait. The chances of such a mating are re-

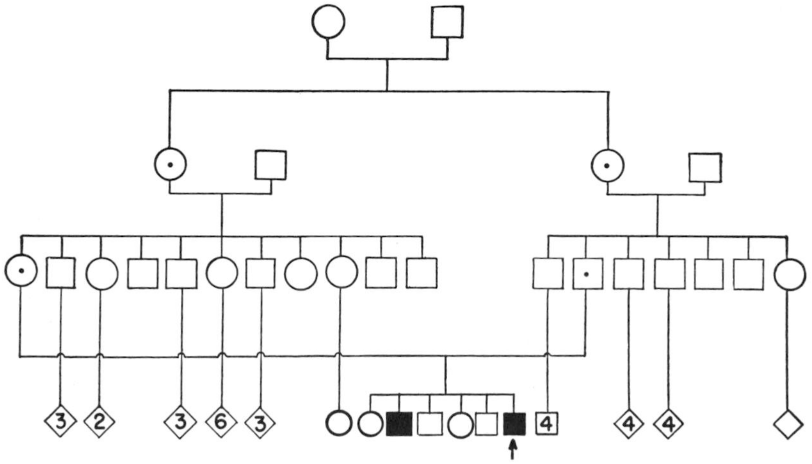

Figure 6–6 Transmission of a recessive pathologic gene by heterozygote parents. Werdnig-Hoffman muscular atrophy (■) occurring in offspring of a consanguineous marriage. The disease does not appear in the collateral close relatives, but because the recessive disease-producing gene was received by both parents from one of their common ancestors, each of their offspring has one chance in four of being homozygous (nn) for it and having the disease.

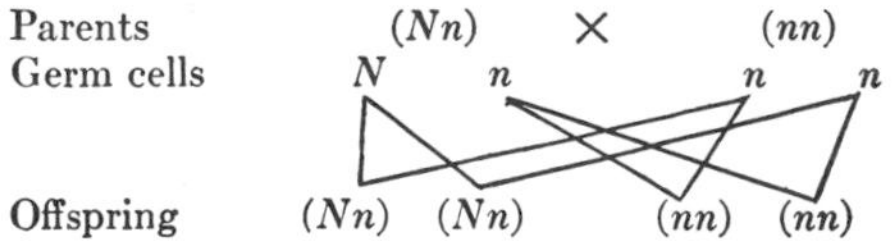

Figure 6–7

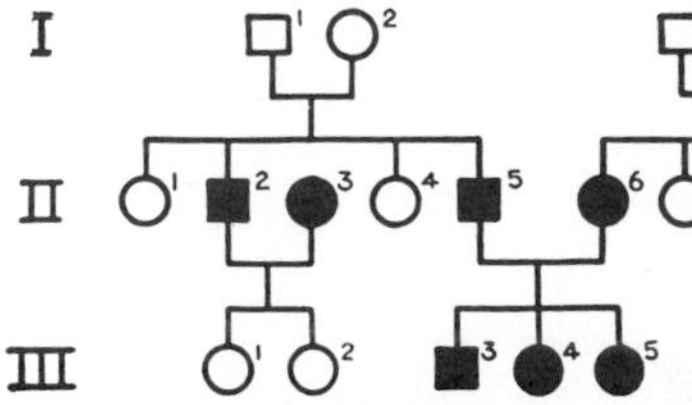

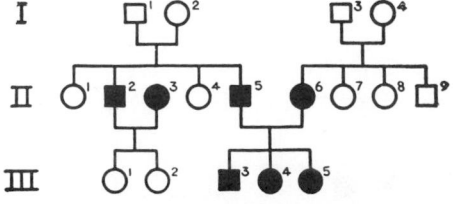

Figure 6–9 Deaf-mutism (■ ●) in a pedigree recorded by Albrecht, inherited as a recessive trait. The deaf-mutism of all the affected persons is genetically determined with the exception of that of II_3, who acquired deafness as a sequel of scarlet fever in infancy. (After Blacker.)

lated to the frequency of the pathologic gene in the general population. Consanguineous marriages favor the appearance of recessive traits. If a recessive gene is rare in a population, a homozygous, affected person may appear only once in a pedigree. *Thus, the lack of a pathologic trait in the traceable genealogy does not exclude its genetic determination* (Fig. 6–6).

If a homozygous person with a pathologic trait caused by recessive genes (*nn*) marries an apparently normal person who is actually a heterozygous carrier of the same pathologic gene (*Nn*) (Fig. 6–7), half of the children will appear normal and the other half will exhibit the pathologic trait. To the observer such a family will appear like the one represented in Figure 6–1, where an abnormal person, heterozygous for a dominant pathologic gene (*Pp*), married a normal person (*pp*). In both cases one of the parents and half of the children show the defect, but the genetic make-up of the children is different. In the case of the dominant pathologic trait the unaffected children are genetically normal. They neither show nor carry the abnormal gene. In the case of the recessive abnormal character the children who appear normal carry the pathologic gene and transmit it to half of their children, who will also appear normal.

Thus, a family history which includes only the parents and their children is insufficient to determine whether an inherited pathologic trait is dominant or recessive.

If two persons who exhibit an abnormal recessive trait and are therefore homozygous (*nn*) marry, the expectation is that all their offspring will be abnormal (Fig. 6–8). Such matings occur sometimes with deleterious effects among hereditary deaf-mutes. On the other hand, there is no objection to the marriage of persons whose deaf-mutism is acquired and not genetically determined. Figure 6–9 presents a pedigree in which two marriages of deaf-mutes occurred: II_5 and II_6 suffered from hereditary deaf-mutism, and all children were deaf-mutes. The marriage of II_2 and II_3 resulted in the birth of two normal children. Though II_2 was genetically a deaf-mute, II_3 was genetically normal and acquired deafness as a sequel of scarlet fever in infancy. Only normal children, all carriers of the pathologic trait, will be expected from such a marriage (Fig. 6–10). It is also possible that two deaf-mute parents who are affected by different genes for deaf-mutism may have normal children.

Pathologic conditions that may show autosomal recessive inheritance include the adrenogenital syndrome, albinism, alkaptonuria, amaurotic idiocy (Tay-Sachs), chondrodystrophia calcificans congenita, chondroectodermal dysplasia, cystinuria, cystinosis, dysautonomia (Riley's), deaf-mutism (several types), epidermolysis bullosa (severe type), familial goitrous cretinism (several types), Friedreich's ataxia, cystic fibrosis, galactosemia, gargoylism, glycogen storage disease (several types), Hartnup disease, hepatolenticular degeneration (Wilson's disease), hereditary spastic paraplegia, hypophosphatasia, Laurence-Moon-Biedl syndrome, microcephaly, Morquio's disease, muscular dystrophy (limb girdle and occasionally Duchenne), progressive spinal muscular atrophy (Werdnig-Hoffmann), Niemann-Pick disease, peroneal atrophy, phenylketonuria, retinitis pigmentosa, sickle cell anemia, thalassemia major and xeroderma pigmentosum. (See McKusick for a more complete list.) Again it is emphasized that the same clinical disease may result from different mutant genes and may therefore show different patterns of inheritance in different families. Thus, a number of clinical entities may be inherited as either dominant or recessive traits.

X-LINKED RECESSIVE PATHOLOGIC TRAITS

Of the 46 chromosomes of human cells, only 44, the somatic ones, can be arranged in 22 homologous pairs. The remaining pair are the sex chromosomes. In males this pair consists of 2 chromo-

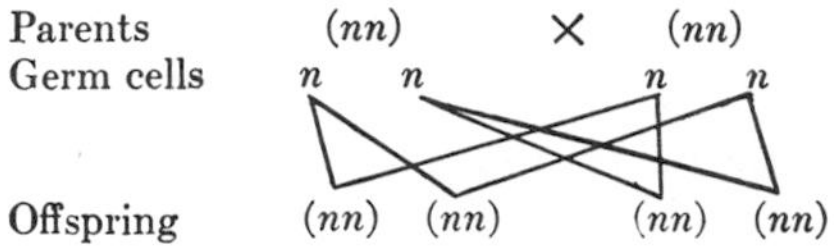

Figure 6–8

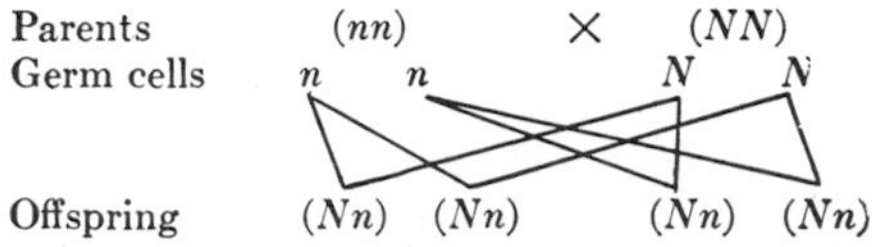

Figure 6–10

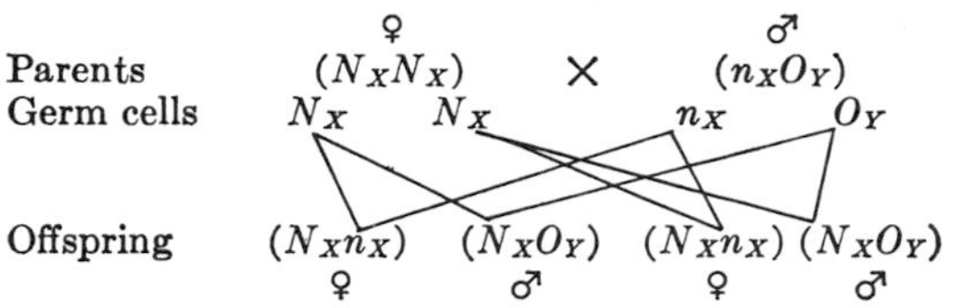

Figure 6–11

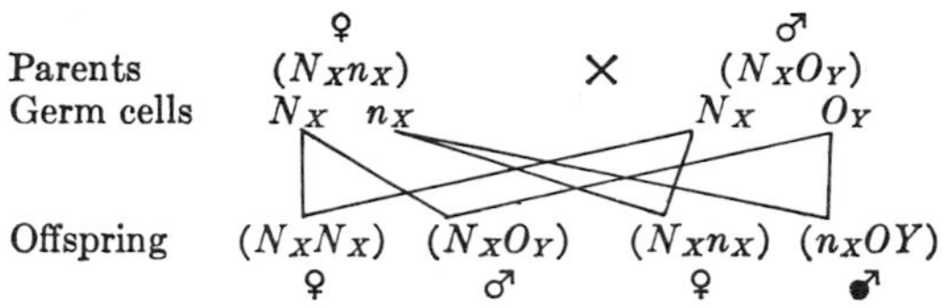

Figure 6–12

somes of unequal size: a large submetacentric X chromosome and a small acrocentric Y chromosome. In females there are 2 X chromosomes. Thus, every somatic cell of the male organism contains 22 pairs of homologous chromosomes (autosomes) plus one X and one Y chromosome, and every somatic cell of the female organism contains 22 pairs of autosomes and 2 X chromosomes. Reduction division, which leads to the formation of germ cells, produces two types of sperm cells: one containing 22 autosomes and a Y chromosome and another containing 22 autosomes and an X chromosome. All the germ cells produced by the female contain 22 autosomes and an X chromosome. Fertilization may result, therefore, in the formation of one of two types of zygotes: one which receives an X chromosome from both father and mother, the resulting offspring being female (XX), and another which receives a Y chromosome from the father and an X chromosome from the mother, the offspring being male (XY). The X chromosome carries many genes; the Y chromosome appears to be mainly concerned with determining maleness. The genes of the X chromosome of the male are, therefore, in an exceptional position because they are not matched by corresponding genes of the Y chromosome. If a mutant gene is located in the X chromosome of the male, it can manifest itself even if it is recessive, since its effects are not masked by a normal gene of the homologous chromosome. A similar recessive mutant gene in the X chromosome of a female may be kept in check, however, by a normal gene in the other X chromosome. In this manner certain hereditary pathologic traits may appear in the males of a family without becoming manifest in the females. Hemophilia A, Christmas disease, color blindness, Hunter type of gargoylism, progressive muscular dystrophy (Duchenne type), peroneal atrophy, night blindness with myopia, and the anhidrotic type of ectodermal dysplasia are such sex-linked traits. (See McKusick for a more complete list.)

Figure 6–11 illustrates the transmission of a recessive pathologic gene located in an X chromosome (n_X). There is no corresponding gene in the Y chromosome (O_Y). The affected father's pair of genes is represented by the formula $(n_X\ O_Y)$. If the mother has two normal dominant genes in her X chromosomes $(N_X\ N_X)$, the following results are to be expected: The sons $(N_X\ O_Y)$ are all normal, having received their normal X chromosome from their mother. All the daughters $(N_X\ n_X)$ appear normal, but carry a recessive pathologic gene (n_X) in one of their X chromosomes. If such a carrier-daughter marries a normal man $(N_X\ O_Y)$, half of her sons $(n_X\ O_Y)$ will show the abnormal trait of the maternal grandfather, and half will be genetically normal $(N_X\ O_Y)$. Half of her daughters will be genetically normal $(N_X\ N_X)$, and half $(N_X\ n_X)$ will carry the pathologic trait in one X chromosome (Fig. 6–12).

Figure 6–13 shows the sex-linked recessive inheritance of progressive muscular dystrophy in a sibship. This type of pathologic trait appears chiefly in males, but in rare cases females will also have it. If an affected man $(n_X\ O_Y)$ marries a carrier $(N_X\ n_X)$, half their daughters $(n_X\ n_X)$ will have the disease and half will be carriers $(N_X\ n_X)$; half their sons will be affected $(n_X\ O_Y)$, and half will be genetically normal $(N_X\ O_Y)$ (Fig. 6–14).

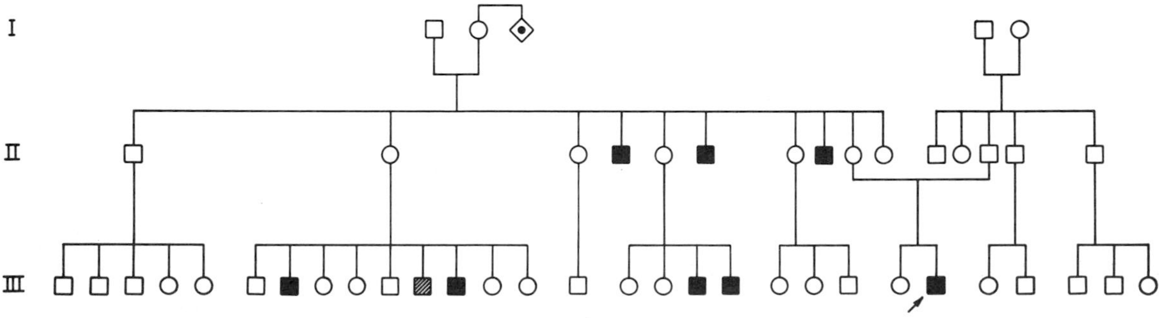

Figure 6–13 *Pedigree in which progressive pseudohypertrophic muscular dystrophy was transmitted as a sex-linked recessive trait. The pedigree was drawn according to the report of the mother of the propositus (↗), a 5-year-old patient in the Children's Hospital, Cincinnati, Ohio.*

The maternal grandmother of the patient was obviously a carrier of the abnormal trait, which was transmitted to 3 of her sons. A fourth son, who did not inherit the disorder, had 5 normal children. Of 5 daughters (generation II), 2 transmitted the muscular disorder to a part of their sons.

■ *Patients with progressive muscular dystrophy.*

▨ *Patient with a mild case of muscular dystrophy who recovered, according to the reporter.*

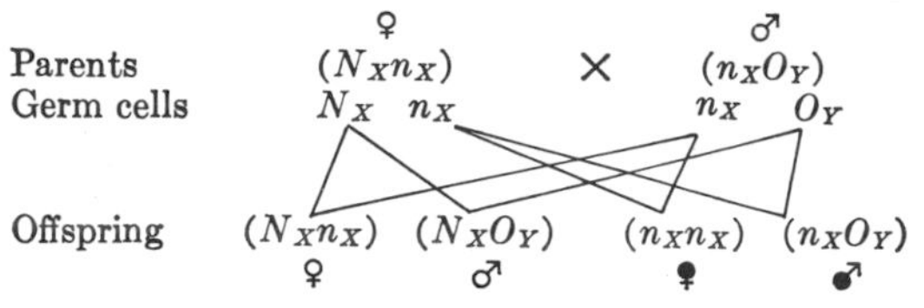

Figure 6–14

PATHOLOGIC TRAITS WHICH DEPEND ON MULTIPLE GENETIC FACTORS

The hereditary traits discussed so far are attributable to one gene or one pair of genes. Hereditary characters, however, may depend on the combined action of several genes. If these genes are located in different chromosomes, they associate and dissociate in different matings according to the laws of chance. Obviously the greater the number of independent genes involved in determining a given trait, the more complicated the pattern of inheritance will be, and the less it will resemble the mendelian patterns described above. Furthermore, such a group of genes may determine only a predisposition, which may or may not produce a clinical disease or defect, depending on the environment in which the individual develops. There is evidence that a number of familial conditions that do not conform to the mendelian patterns of inheritance, such as cleft lip and cleft palate, congenital hypertrophic pyloric stenosis and congenital dislocation of the hip, may fall into this category.

LETHAL TRAITS

A gene or a combination of genes may lead to developmental defects incompatible with life. Severe defects cause intrauterine death; the responsible genes are called "lethal genes." Milder defects may cause death soon after birth; responsible genes are termed "sublethal."

Lethal genes may produce only slight effects, or none at all, in a heterozygous person, but may cause death in the homozygote. For example, a dominant gene is known which, in heterozygous subjects, leads to brachyphalangia, a shortening of the second phalanx of the second fingers and toes. Such a defect is of no practical importance to the affected person. If, however, 2 heterozygous persons with this defect marry, one fourth of their offspring may be homozygous. Such a homozygous person may have no fingers and toes and may have other defects incompatible with postnatal life.

Congenital ichthyosis is an example of a disorder which appears in children homozygous for a recessive sublethal gene. The parents of such children appear normal, but carry the abnormal gene, and some of their offspring have hyperkeratosis incompatible with life.

JOSEF WARKANY
F. CLARKE FRASER

Carter, C. O.: An ABC of Medical Genetics, Boston, Little, Brown and Company, 1969.
McKusick, V.: Mendelian Inheritance in Man. 3rd ed. Baltimore, The Johns Hopkins Press, 1972.
Nora, J. J., and Fraser, F. C.: Medical Genetics – Principles and Practice. Philadelphia, Lea & Febiger, 1974.
Stent, G.: Molecular Genetics. An Introductory Narrative. San Francisco, W. H. Freeman, 1971.

Chromosomal Abnormalities in Man: The Autosomes

(Abnormalities of the sex chromosomes are described in Section 17.)

It was not until 1956 that the correct number of chromosomes in the human karyotype was determined. In 1959 the first evidence for the chromosomal basis for a human disease (the Down syndrome) was demonstrated. It took 10 years more to develop techniques that enabled every chromosome to be identified accurately and small morphologic aberrations to be revealed. Recent advances have seen the successful culture of amniotic fluid cells for prenatal diagnosis, and rapid strides are being made in studies of human meiosis. These techniques, along with somatic cell hybridization studies, have given an impetus to the mapping of human chromosomes and are leading the way to more accurate clinical diagnosis and genetic counseling.

These new developments have led to an increased demand for chromosomal analyses. However, since this is a complicated and expensive laboratory test, discrimination must be exercised in identifying candidates for chromosomal studies. The two most important clinical traits are congenital malformations, especially if more than one system of the body is involved, and mental retardation of unknown origin. Some of the more common features are odd facies, abnormal ears, heart and kidney malformations, abnormal hands and feet, simian creases, single crease on the fifth finger and low birth weight. It has been estimated that one in 150 newborn infants has a chromosomal abnormality. This frequency may be expected to increase as more accurate detection of minor structural changes becomes possible.

METHODOLOGY

CULTURING OF CELLS. The most commonly used cell for the determination of a karyotype is the small lymphocyte, which is readily transformed by stimulation with the plant mitogen, phytohemagglutinin (PHA). Optimum yield of lymphocytes in mitosis is obtained after 72 hours in culture. The dividing cells are arrested in metaphase by exposure to demecolcine (Colcemid) and the chromosomes are dispersed with hypotonic solution. Preparation of chromosome spreads by air-drying is the simplest and most successful procedure.

Cultures of fibroblasts, which involve more sophisticated long-term treatment, are needed for additional studies of mosaicism and biochemical defects. For the diagnosis of blood dyscrasias, bone marrow cell preparations are best, but chromosomes of myelocytes can be prepared from peripheral blood leukocytes after 24 hours in culture if stimulation of lymphocytes is avoided. The methodology for culture of amniotic fluid cells is similar to that for fibroblasts; the cells are usually ready for cytogenetic analysis in two to three weeks.

STAINING. With conventional stains, e.g., Giemsa and orcein, it is possible to identify with certainty only the Y chromosome and six of the 22 pairs of autosomes. Several more pairs of autosomes and all X chromosomes in excess of one can usually be identified with autoradiography, but labeling with tritiated thymidine is a long and cumbersome procedure.

Caspersson and his associates have recently developed a new staining technique utilizing quinacrine fluorescence. When stained with fluorochromes and viewed under the ultraviolet (UV) light of a fluorescence microscope, each chromosome produces its own distinctive banding pattern. Bands corresponding to the fluorescence patterns can also be produced by pretreating the slide preparations with salt solutions or trypsin and varying the pH of Giemsa stain. This Giemsa banding technique, although simpler, is less reliable than fluorescence, but will probably become the routine diagnostic procedure if and when reliability can be assured. Bands produced by quinacrine fluorescence are called *Q bands* and those by modified Giemsa techniques *G bands.*

KARYOTYPING. The chromosomes from photographed mitotic spreads are cut out, arranged in pairs and numbered from 1 to 22 plus the sex chromosomes. The systematized arrangement from a single cell is referred to as a karyotype. Most laboratories routinely analyze 10 to 40 cells per subject; if mosaicism is suspected, more cells may need to be analyzed.

THE NORMAL KARYOTYPE

Man is a diploid creature with a complement of 46 chromosomes consisting of 23 pairs. Thus, 23 is

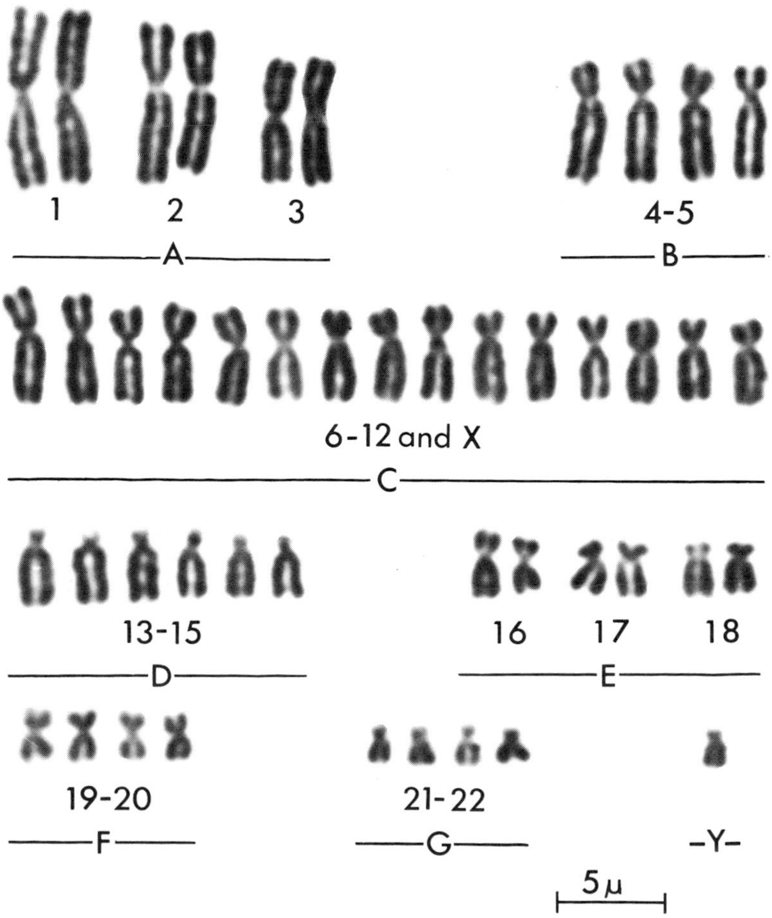

Figure 6–15 Chromosomes of normal male stained with aceto-orcein. Only Nos. 1, 2, 3, 16, 17, 18 and Y can be identified with certainty.

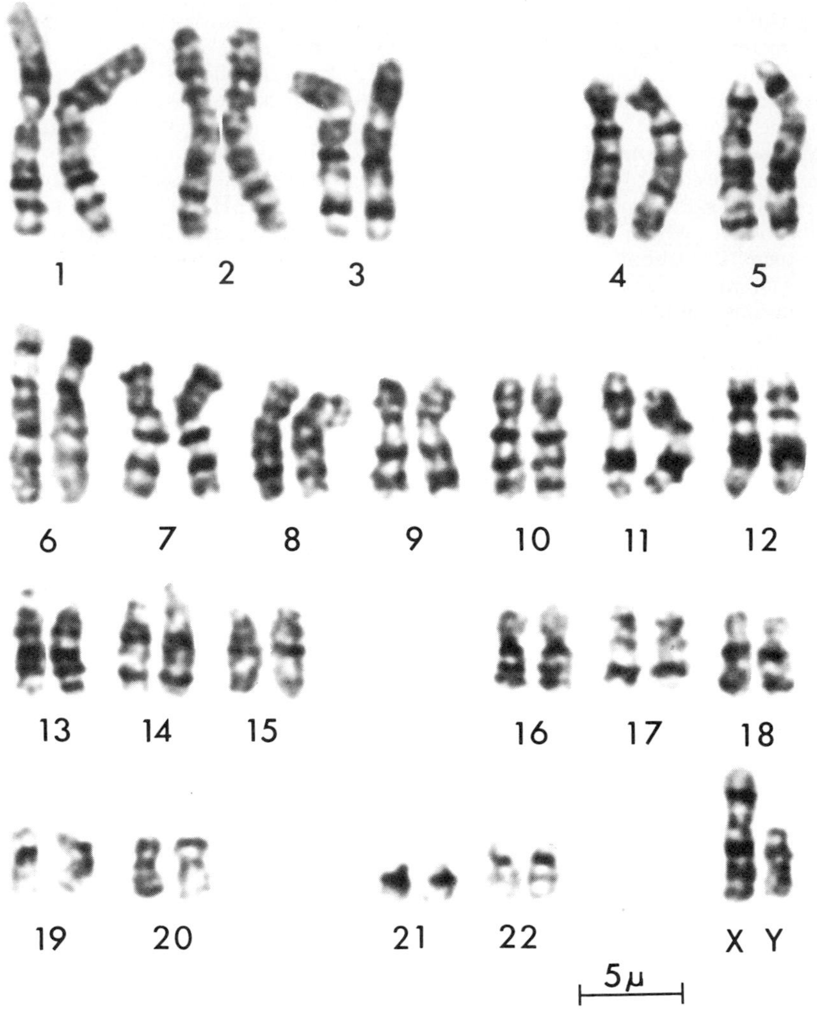

Figure 6–16 *Karyotype of normal male. All chromosomes, pretreated with trypsin and stained with Giemsa, can be positively identified by characteristic banding patterns.*

the haploid number, the complement found in the gametes. The 23 pairs are divided into seven major groups from A to G according to similarity in size and shape (Fig. 6–15). Chromosome shape is determined by the position of the centromere: metacentric (Nos. 1 and 3), submetacentric (B and C groups) and acrocentric (D and G groups). The short arm of an acrocentric chromosome usually has a secondary constriction and satellite.

After the new staining techniques permitted accurate chromosome identification, the numbering of all chromosomes was agreed upon at the Paris Conference in 1971 (Fig. 6–16). The previous decision to arrange the chromosomes in descending order of size raised a problem when the chromosome involved in mongolism, i.e., 21-trisomy syndrome, was found to be the smaller of the two acrocentrics of the G group. It should be No. 22 but, because of the confusion that would be created by a change in nomenclature, a consensus was reached that the smaller chromosome should remain No. 21.

Morphologic variants have been found in the normal karyotype and are usually referred to as *"marker chromosomes."* Best known are elongation of the centromere region of Nos. 1, 9 and 16, extended or deleted short arms or enlarged satellites of acrocentric chromosomes and a satellite on the short arm of No. 17 (Fig. 6–17*A*). The Y chromosome also may vary in length and shape. Other variants have been found with fluorescent stains, e.g., variation in intensity of fluorescent bands and/or satellites on chromosomes Nos. 3, 4 and the acrocentric D and G chromosomes (Fig. 6–17*B*). Such morphologic variants were first observed in abnormal individuals and thought to be associated with disease, but it soon became obvious that they were merely inherited variants which occur frequently in normal subjects. They are useful as genetic markers and are one of the key factors used to localize genes to specific chromosomes. The possibility that they represent interference with normal chromosome division has been raised but not proved.

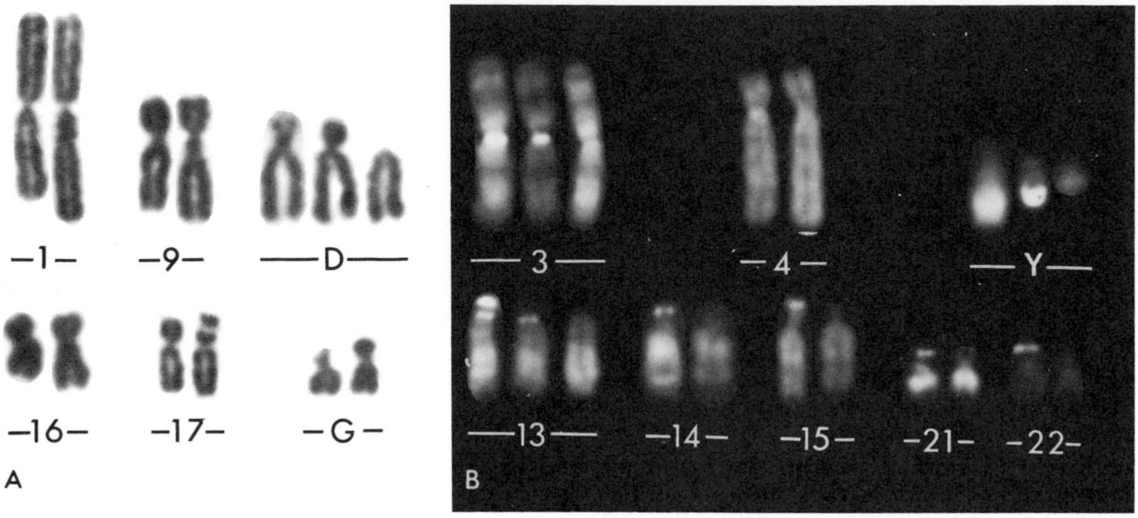

Figure 6–17 Some morphologic variants found in normal subjects. A, Chromosomes stained with aceto-orcein. B, Chromosomes stained with quinacrine dihydrochloride showing differences in intensity of fluorescent bands among homologues. The left-hand chromosome of each pair or triad is a usual or "nonmarker" chromosome.

Cell-to-cell variation in chromosome number has been found in older people. There is a tendency for loss of an X chromosome in women 55 years and over and loss of a Y chromosome in men over 65 years.

ABNORMAL KARYOTYPES

NUMERICAL ABNORMALITIES. Chromosomal aberrations may be divided into two major types: numerical and structural. A cell with the exact multiple of the haploid number, e.g., 46, 69, 92, etc., is referred to as *euploid.* Euploid cells with more than the normal *diploid* number of 46 chromosomes are termed *polyploid.* Cells with any deviation from one of the euploid numbers are termed *aneuploid.*

The most common type of aneuploidy is **trisomy**, i.e., three homologous chromosomes being present instead of the pair normally present. Lack of a chromosome is called **monosomy** (of the affected pair). Aneuploid individuals may be trisomic for more than one pair of chromosomes or may even combine trisomy and monosomy. During meiosis, synapsis occurs between each chromosome and its homologue; after separation each proceeds to an opposite pole of the dividing cell. Failure of synapsis or failure to separate (nondisjunction) interferes with orderly segregation and may result in aneuploidy (Fig. 6–18). Monosomy can result from chromosome loss or anaphase lag, i.e., failure of a chromosome to reach either pole during anaphase. Nondisjunction occurring during mitotic division results in mosaicism, i.e., the presence of more than one chromosomal type of cell population in one individual. The older the mother the greater appears the likelihood of nondisjunction and chromosomal trisomy.

Pure polyploidy appears to be lethal in humans, but individuals with mosaicism have been known to survive. **Triploidy** (three haploid sets, totalling 69 chromosomes) has been found most frequently among abortuses and stillbirths. It arises by fertilization of the ovum by two spermatozoa or by the union of a haploid with a diploid gamete. Tetraploid cells have been found in aborted material and in persons with malignant disease. **Tetraploidy** occurs occasionally in cultured cells, particularly amniotic fluid cells, and appears to arise during the culturing procedure.

STRUCTURAL ABERRATIONS. Structural abnormalities of chromosomes arise from breaks. **Simple deletions** result from a single break, with loss of the broken end of a chromosome. *Deletion syndromes*, such as cri-du-chat (5p–) may result either from a simple deletion or from the inheritance of a chromosome left deleted by a translocation (see below). An isochromosome is formed by misdivision of the centromere. Instead of splitting along the longitudinal axis to produce two normal chromosomes, the centromere may divide transversely to produce two chromosomes, each with duplication of one arm (Fig. 6–19). Isochromosomes are formed most frequently from the X chromosome.

All other structural aberrations result from two chromosome breaks followed by fusion of the broken ends. Most common are **translocations**, which may be inherited or arise de novo. **Reciprocal translocations** result when two nonhomologous chromosomes break and exchange segments. Carriers of reciprocal translocations are normal since they have a full complement of genes. Children of such "**translocation carriers**" will be abnormal if they receive only one of the translocation chromosomes, thus giving rise to "*duplication-deficiency syndromes.*" Depending upon the amount of material duplicated or deficient, the aberration is referred to as partial trisomy or partial monosomy. A special type of translocation is the centric fusion or Robertsonian translocation, in which the breaks

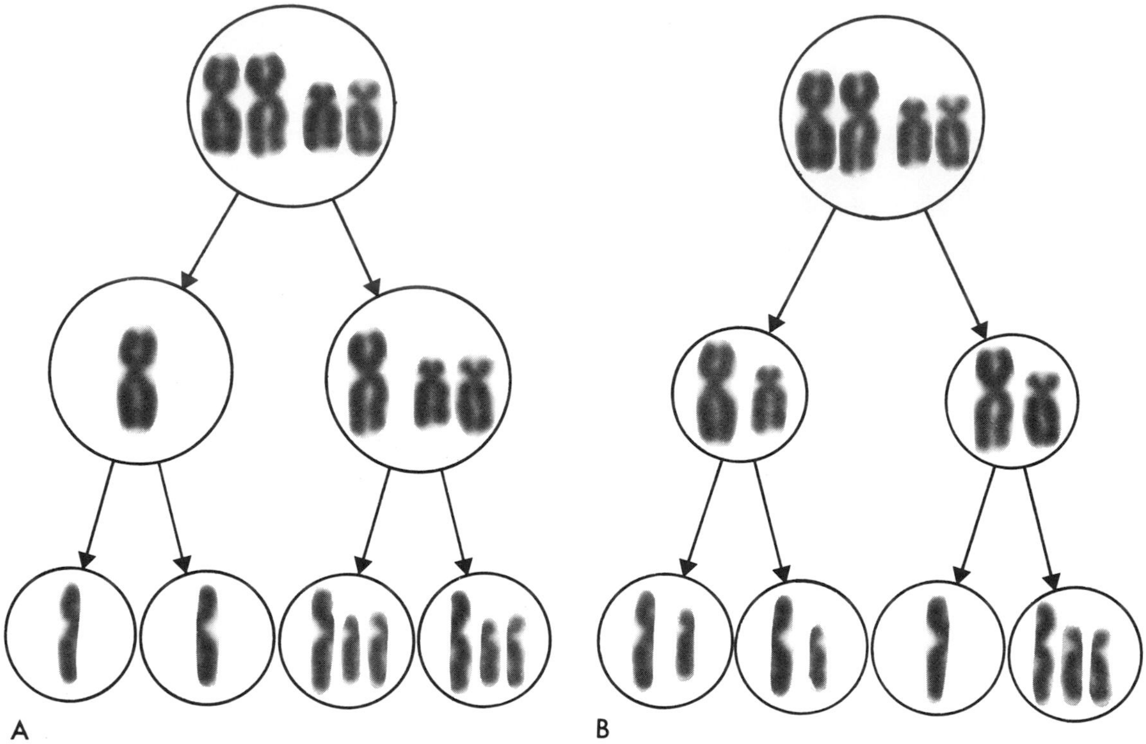

Figure 6–18 *Nondisjunction during meiosis illustrated with two pairs of chromosomes.* A, *First division nondisjunction with failure of smaller homologues to separate gives rise to gametes with no small chromosome or an extra one.* B, *Second division nondisjunction following centromere division. Two newly formed chromosomes fail to separate in cell on the right.*

occur adjacent to the centromere in the short arm of the "recipient" chromosome and in the long arm of the "donor" chromosome. The centromere of the "donor" chromosome and the short arms of both chromosomes are usually lost. Centric fusion most commonly involves D and G group chromosomes and therefore may result in the Down syndrome or 13-trisomy syndrome. Since the short arms of acrocentric chromosomes appear to be genetically inactive, loss of this material in such translocations has no apparent phenotypic effect on carriers.

Ring chromosomes are formed when both tips of a chromosome are broken off and the ends fuse together. They are, therefore, a form of deletion syndrome. *Inversions* result when the section between two breaks in a single chromosome is inverted and the order of the genes reversed. Since an inversion may cause difficulty in synapsis, it may increase the risk of nondisjunction.

Quadriradial configurations are found in breakage syndromes (see below) and in cells exposed to mutagenic agents. They arise from exchanges between two chromatids after replication has taken place. These exchanges may involve the chromatids of two homologous or nonhomologous chromosomes. Since in metaphase the two chromatids have not yet separated, such exchanges result in configurations that resemble crossroads.

With one possible exception, the 18p– syndrome, maternal age has not been found to be an etiologic factor in structural aberrations.

NOMENCLATURE

The nomenclature for describing a karyotype has been standardized to avoid confusion. First, the total number of chromosomes is recorded, then the sex chromosome complement followed by a description of any aberration (Table 6–1). The short arm is referred to as *p* (easily remembered by "petite") and the long arm as *q*. Any addition or loss of chromosomal material is denoted by a plus (+) or minus (–) sign. Chromosomes involved in a translocation are written in brackets preceded by a *t*; e.g., t(14q21q) denotes the translocation most frequently found in mongolism. (Most children with the Down syndrome, however, have three No. 21 chromosomes, the extra denoted as +21).

At the Paris Conference the first attempts were made to standardize the nomenclature describing the regions within the chromosomes delineated by the bands identifiable through the new staining techniques. This nomenclature is complicated, but allows for the anticipated discovery of additional bands and for future adaptation to computer analysis.

DERMATOGLYPHICS

Before the advent of human cytogenetics, analysis of hand and footprints was a fairly reliable test

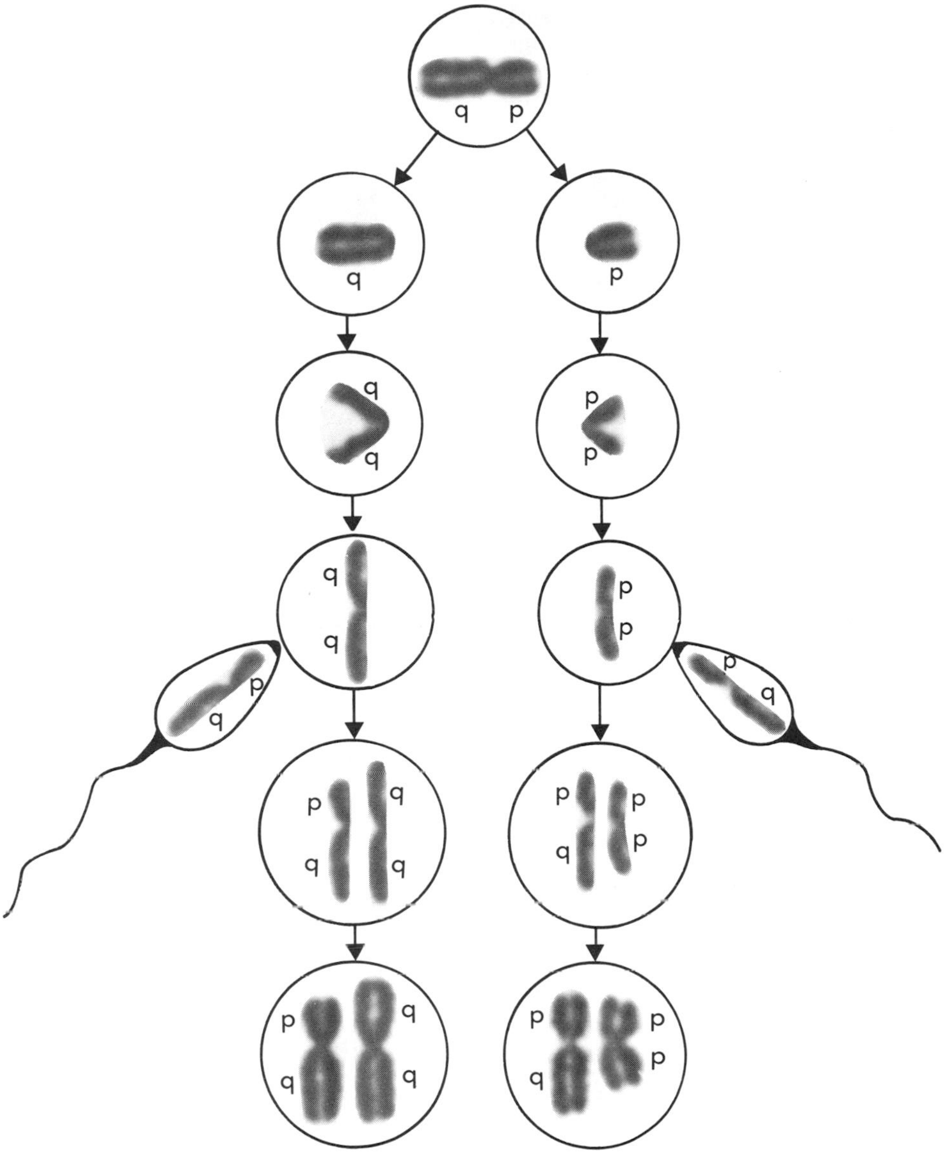

Figure 6–19 Formation of isochromosomes. Misdivision of centromere results in two chromosomes, each with two genotypically identical arms. Fertilization by normal gametes will produce one cell with a pair of chromosomes with one short and three long arms and the other with one long and three short arms.
p = short arm, q = long arm.

TABLE 6–1. SOME REPRESENTATIVE KARYOTYPE NOTATIONS

46,XY	Normal male karyotype
47,XX,+13	Female with 13-trisomy: D-trisomy syndrome
46,XY,–21,+t 21q21q)	Mongoloid with centric fusion translocation replacing one No. 21 chromosome
45,XX,–14,–21,+t(14q21q)	Normal carrier of centric fusion translocation replacing two chromosomes, Nos. 14 and 21
46,XY,5p–	Cri-du-chat syndrome; partial deletion of short arm of No. 5
46,XX,18q–	Partial deletion of long arm of No. 18
46,XY,r(19)	Ring chromosome No. 19
45,X	Turner syndrome
46,X,i(Xq)	Female with isochromosome for long arm of one X
47,XXY/46,XY	Mosaic Klinefelter syndrome

for the diagnosis of mongolism. Subsequently, chromosomal analysis has replaced dermatoglyphics as the definitive diagnostic test. However, examination of dermal patterns remains interesting and useful in instances when the diagnosis remains in doubt despite chromosomal analysis or when cytogenetic studies are not available.

Dermatoglyphics refers to those configurations formed by the dermal ridges, not by the flexion creases. The most important landmarks are the patterns on the distal phalanges of the digits, the position of the triradius in the axis of the palm (Figs. 6–20 and 6–21) and the pattern in the hallucal area of the soles. The patterns themselves are not abnormal, but certain configurations, while not in themselves abnormal, occur with greater than usual frequency in specific syndromes. Some representative patterns are shown in Figure 6–20.

The size of a pattern is estimated by counting the number of ridges needed in its formation, whorls usually having the largest counts, while arches have a count of zero. Digital pattern size is important in certain syndromes. In general, males have higher counts than females but this is reversed in the Klinefelter and Turner syndromes.

A strong correlation between dermatoglyphics and chromosomes was noted soon after the chromosomal basis for many congenital malformations was established. Characteristic dermal patterns are now well known diagnostic criteria for the three trisomies 13, 18, and 21 and in 18 and G deficiency syndromes. They are described under the respective syndromes.

Dermatoglyphic indices have been developed to assist in the diagnosis of the Down syndrome. Walker's method, based on 16 patterns present on the 10 digits, the third interdigital patterns, the positions of the axial triradii of both hands and the hallucal patterns of both feet, makes use of the relative frequencies of these patterns among mongoloids and nonmongoloids to arrive at a probability index. A simpler method, Reed et al.'s *Dermatogram* (Fig. 6–22), uses only four landmarks and appears to be just as informative.

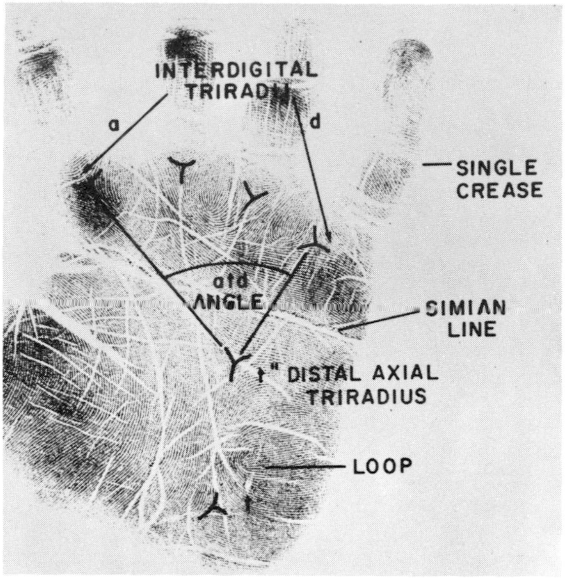

Figure 6–21 *Palm print of child with the Down syndrome, showing typical dermatoglyphic features.*

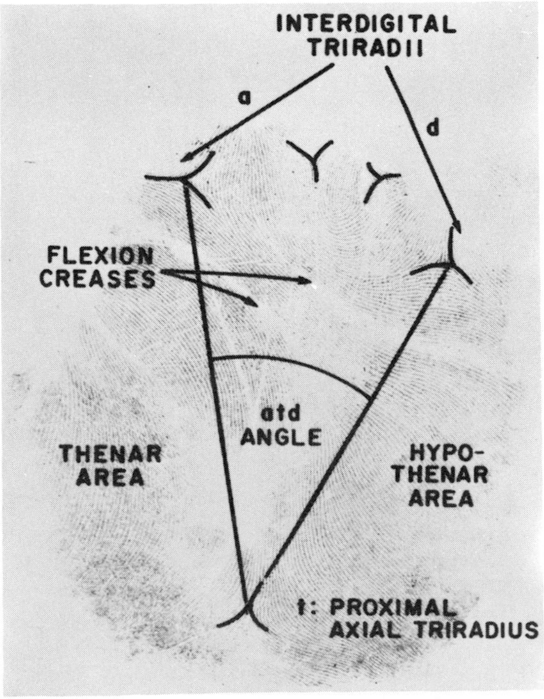

Figure 6–20 *Normal palm print showing principal areas.*

CLINICAL ABNORMALITIES

ANEUPLOIDY

21-Trisomy Syndrome (Mongolism, Down Syndrome). The presence of an extra chromosome No. 21 results in this, the most common and best known chromosomal syndrome (Fig. 6–23*A*). The important clinical features and dermal patterns are listed in Tables 6–2 and 6–3. The incidence in the general population is 1 in 600 to 700 births and rises to a high of 1 in 50 births at maternal ages of 45 years and over (Table 6–4).

Most investigations into the etiology of nondisjunction have centered around 21-trisomics because of their high frequency, but the same principles generally hold true for all autosomal trisomies. Fluorescent markers have furnished cytologic proof for the parental origin of nondisjunction (Fig. 6–23*B*). It is also possible in some cases to tell whether the nondisjunction occurred during first or second meiotic division; if at first division, all three No. 21 chromosomes will have different markers, but if the aberration occurred during second division, two should be identical (Fig. 6–23*B*).

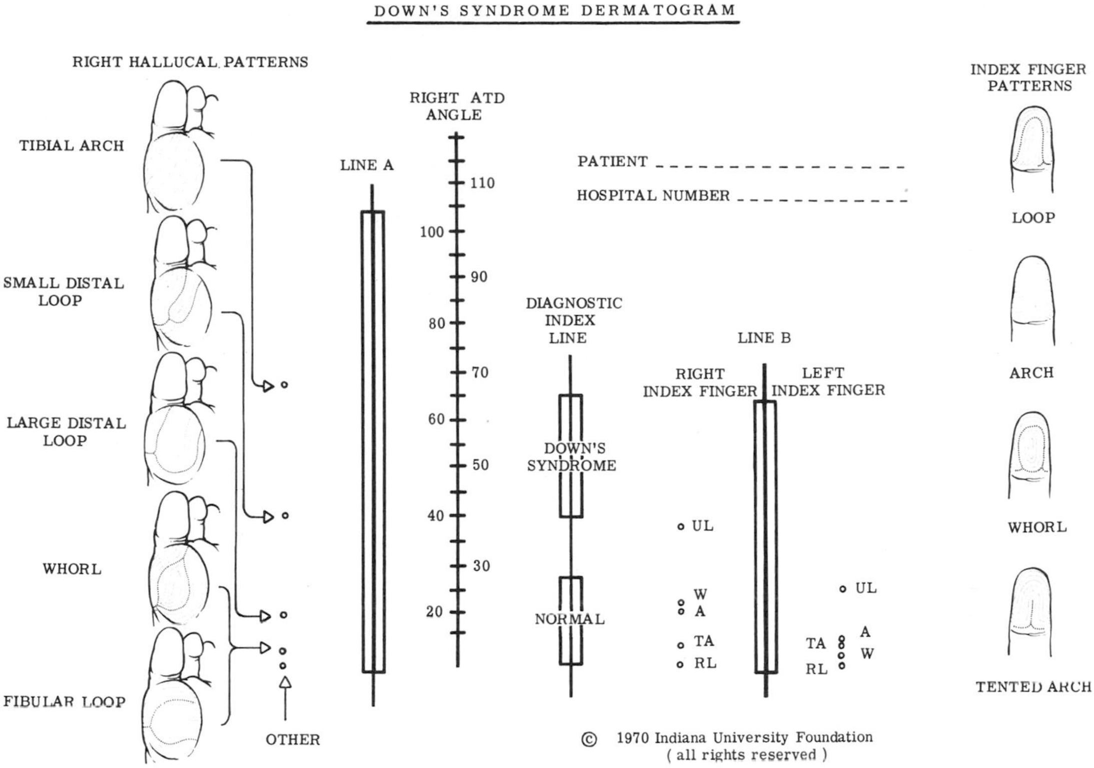

Figure 6–22 Dermatoglyphic nomogram for the diagnosis of mongolism. (Courtesy of T. E. Reed.) Three lines are drawn in the following manner:

Line 1: Connect the point for the pattern type found on the right hallucal area with the size of the right atd *angle.*

Line 2: Connect the points for the types of patterns on the right and left index fingers.

Line 3: Connect the points where the first two lines have crossed Lines A and B.

The point where Line 3 crosses the Diagnostic Index Line gives the diagnosis. If the line passes between the two blocks, the diagnosis is indeterminate.

UL = ulnar loop, RL = radial loop, W = whorl, A = arch, TA = tented arch. A loop is open toward the side away from its triradius; the triradius is indicated on the right side of the top (loop) finger pattern in the figure. For atd *angle, see Figures 6–20 and 6–21. (© 1970 Indiana University Foundation. All rights reserved.)*

Mothers of children with the Down syndrome fall into two age curves. One, which includes the cases due to chromosomal translocations, has the same distribution as the normal population, with a mean of 28 years. The second has a mean of 34 years, and includes the cases dependent on maternal age.

The reason for the correlation between late maternal age and nondisjunction is still a matter of debate. The incidences of both mongolism and maternal exposure to diagnostic x-rays of the abdomen seem to correlate with maternal age. Virus-induced disturbance of chromosomal segregation has been suggested to account for the clustering of births of 21-trisomic infants following epidemics of infectious hepatitis. "Over-ripeness" of the ovum due to delayed fertilization because of decreased frequency of coitus with age has also been suggested. Significant increases in the frequency of thyroid autoantibodies have been observed in patients and mothers, but the mechanism behind this correlation is not known. Finally, a genetic predisposition to nondisjunction could account for the observed repetition not only of 21-trisomics but also of different aneuploids, including those of the sex chromosomes, within the same sibship.

The risk of repetition following the birth of one trisomic child to chromosomally normal parents has yet to be clarified. Figures range from no greater risk to a fiftyfold increase in young mothers. Some suggest a threefold increase in each maternal age group. Analysis of data using only chromosomally proved trisomics indicates that the risk of recurrence, regardless of maternal age, appears to be about the same as that for a mother who is over the age of 45 years (Table 6-5). This increased risk may be due to undetected mosaicism in a parent or exposure to the same environmental insult.

"Regular" trisomics comprise some 95 per cent of patients with mongolism. Approximately 1 per cent are mosaic (this is doubtless a minimum since some mosaics probably remain undetected, particularly among phenotypically normal parents of trisomic offspring); the remainder are translocations. Mosaic patients are less severely affected both in physical appearance and in intelligence, but there is a wide range of variation in phenotype which does not always correlate with the proportion of trisomic cells. This inconsistency may depend on the source of the cells examined; the frequency of trisomic cells tends to vary in different tissues of mosaic individuals.

The majority of translocations giving rise to the

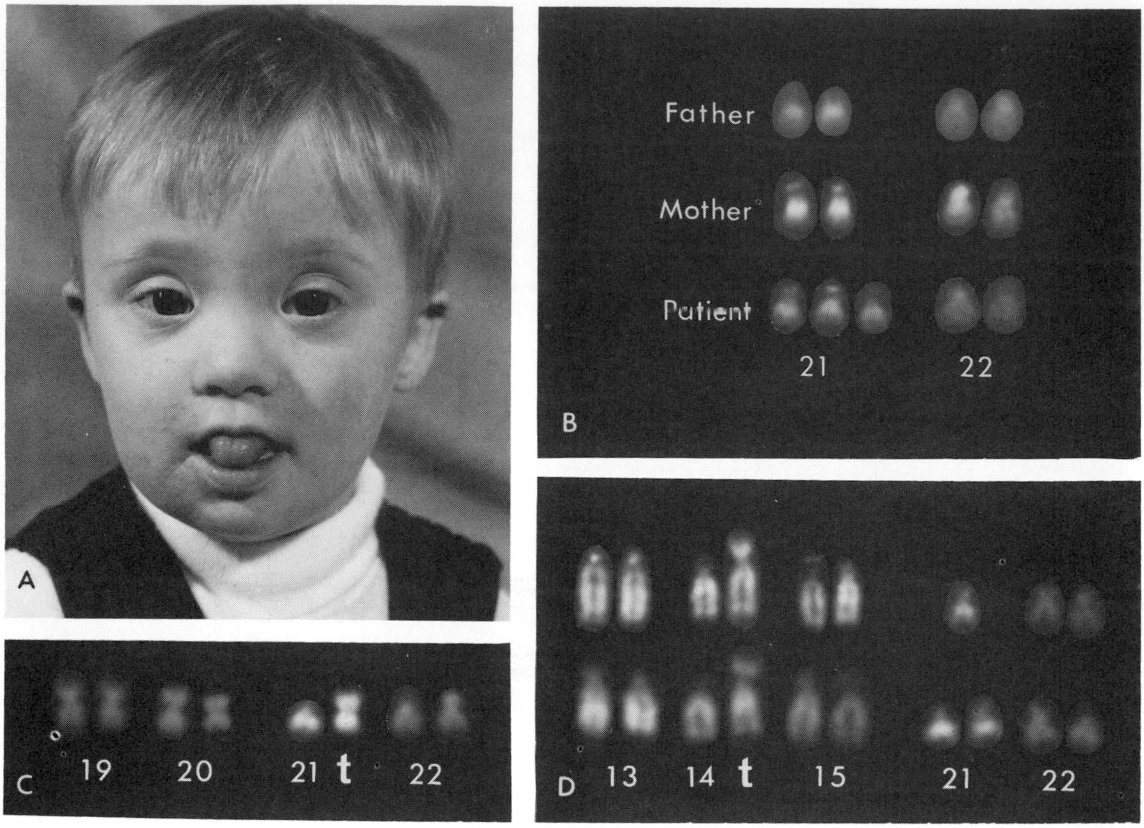

Figure 6–23 *Partial karyotypes from patients with mongolism.*
A, Patient with trisomy-21.
B, G group chromosomes from a patient and her parents. The intensely fluorescent satellites on two No. 21 chromosomes of the patient as well as her mother's indicate that the extra chromosome is maternal in origin.
C, 21q21q translocation.
D, 14q21q translocation in the mother (above) and her affected child (below).

Down syndrome are of the centric fusion type between No. 21 and one D chromosome; approximately half of these are inherited. The vast majority are t(14q21q) (Fig. 6–23*D*) and a few are t(15q21q); t(13q21q) is rare. This probably accounts for the absence of 13-trisomy syndrome, which would be expected to occur among the offspring of phenotypically normal carriers of the Dq21q translocation. Carrier mothers produce three types of offspring: normal phenotype and karyotype, phenotypically normal translocation carrier, and translocation mongoloid. They should, theoretically, occur with equal frequency but only 10 per cent have been abnormal, possibly because of an increased lethality to the zygote or fetus of an abnormal amount of genetically active chromosomal material. The expected frequency of one third affected has been observed, however, among fetuses studied early in gestation. Rarely does a carrier father have affected offspring, though he does produce both normals and carriers.

Only 5 per cent of cases of translocation mongolism involving two G chromosomes are inherited from a carrier parent. The small metacentric translocation chromosome may represent centric fusion of chromosomes Nos. 21 and 22, of two No. 21 chromosomes (Fig. 6–23*C*), or misdivision of the centromere to form an iso-21 chromosome (Fig. 6–19). The low frequency of inherited cases suggests that most of these metacentrics are of the latter two types. Production of a normal carrier with the latter complement would involve translocation in one parent with an unlikely coincidental loss of chromosome 21 either in the gamete of the other parent or after fertilization. All viable offspring from a t(21q21q) carrier would be translocation mongoloids (with the possible exception of 21-monosomics). A t(21q22q) carrier, on the other hand, can produce carrier and normal, as well as mongoloid offspring.

Not all translocations producing the Down syndrome are of the centric fusion type. Some have been reported with increased length of the long arm of one chromosome No. 21. Other patients with the Down syndrome and apparently normal karyotypes may have hidden translocations, i.e., part of No. 21 attached to a larger chromosome and not distinguishable. This type of translocation can be demonstrated with the new staining techniques. However, most children with the Down syndrome and apparently normal karyotypes are probably mosaics with low frequencies of trisomic cells.

The frequency of acute leukemia among patients with mongolism is higher than the incidence in the

TABLE 6–2. MAJOR CLINICAL FEATURES OF THE THREE MOST COMMON AUTOSOMAL TRISOMIES

CHARACTERISTIC FEATURES	21-TRISOMY	18-TRISOMY	13-TRISOMY
General	Mental retardation; hypotonia	Mental retardation; hypertonia; failure to thrive; preponderance of females; low birth weight	Mental retardation; failure to thrive; capillary hemangiomas; increased nuclear projections in neutrophils; persistent fetal hemoglobin; seizures
Craniofacies	Flat occiput; oblique palpebral fissures; epicanthic folds; speckled irides (Brushfield spots); protruding tongue; prominent, malformed ears; flat nasal bridge	Prominent occiput; small features; micrognathia; low-set, malformed ears	Microcephaly; cleft lip ± palate; midline scalp defects; microphthalmia, colobomata; low-set malformed ears; apparent deafness
Thorax	Congenital heart disease, mainly septal defects, especially of the endocardial cushion	Congenital heart disease, mainly V.S.D. and P.D.A.;* short sternum	Congenital heart disease, mainly septal defects, P.D.A.
Abdomen and pelvis	Decreased acetabular and iliac angles; small penis; cryptorchidism	Horseshoe kidney; small pelvis; cryptorchidism; limited hip abduction; inguinal or umbilical hernia	Polycystic kidneys; bicornuate uterus; cryptorchidism
Hands and feet	Simian crease; short, broad hands; hypoplasia of middle phalanx of 5th finger; gap between 1st and 2nd toes	Flexion deformity of fingers; short, dorsiflexed big toes; rockerbottom feet or equinovarus	Polydactyly; hyperconvex fingernails; simian crease
Other features observed with significant frequency	High-arched palate; strabismus; broad, short neck; small teeth; furrowed tongue; intestinal atresia; imperforate anus	Cleft lip ± palate; ocular anomalies; simian crease; hypoplasia of fingernails; widely spaced nipples; webbed neck; single umbilical artery	Flexion deformity of fingers; single umbilical artery; shallow supraorbital ridges; micrognathia; retroflexible thumb; rockerbottom feet

*V.S.D.=ventricular septal defect; P.D.A.=patent ductus arteriosus.

general population, the majority being of the lymphoblastic type. When the Philadelphia (Ph′) chromosome was found in patients with chronic myeloid leukemia, it was thought to be a deleted No. 21; it has now been proved that the Ph′ chromosome is a deleted No. 22, and the broken end has been shown to be translocated to the long arm of chromosome No. 9 (Fig. 6–24).

Biochemical alterations in patients with mongolism (Section 2) have been too inconsistent to provide useful genetic information.

18-Trisomy Syndrome (E Syndrome, Edwards Syndrome). This is the second most common autosomal aberration (Fig. 6–25), originally referred to as the E syndrome until improved techniques permitted distinction between chromosomes Nos. 17 and 18.

Small, delicate facial features serve to distinguish children with 18-trisomy from other trisomics. The principal clinical characteristics are listed in Tables 6–2 and 6–3. Incidence is about 1 in 4000 births. Although usually born post-term,

TABLE 6–3. IMPORTANT DERMATOGLYPHIC PATTERNS AND FLEXION CREASES FOUND IN THE THREE COMMON AUTOSOMAL TRISOMY SYNDROMES*

AREAS	21-TRISOMY	18-TRISOMY	13-TRISOMY
Digits	Ulnar loops on most fingers; radial loops on fingers 4 and 5	Arches on fingers and toes	–
Palms	Distal axial triradius or large *atd* angle	–	Distal axial triradius or large *atd* angle
Soles	Arch tibial or small loop distal in hallucal area	–	Arch fibular or arch fibular-S in hallucal area
Flexion creases	Simian crease; single crease on finger 5	Single crease on finger 5 or on all fingers	Simian crease

*See also Figures 6–20, 6–21 and 6–22.

TABLE 6–4. INCIDENCE OF THE DOWN SYNDROME ACCORDING TO MATERNAL AGE, ESTIMATED FROM FIVE SURVEYS IN ENGLAND, AUSTRALIA AND CANADA

MATERNAL AGE	INCIDENCE
<25	1/2000
25 – 29	1/1800
30 – 34	1/900
35 – 39	1/300
40 – 44	1/100
45+	1/50
Total	1/700

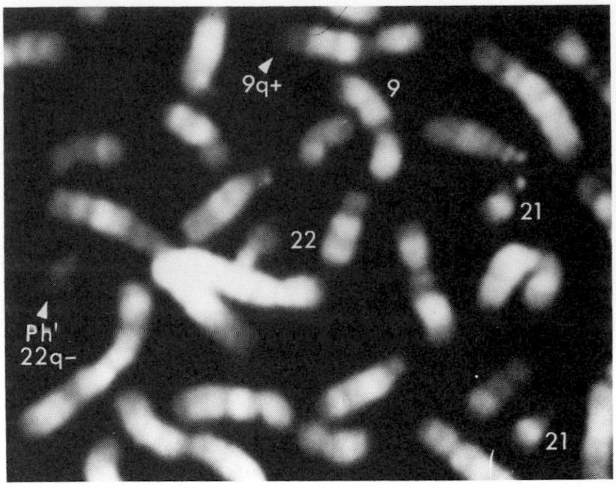

Figure 6–24 Partial spread showing small Ph' chromosome (deleted No. 22) formed by translocation of distal portion of long arm of No. 22 to long arm of No. 9, seen as a band of pale fluorescence.

the birth weight is low. There is a preponderance of females, the sex ratio being one male to four females. Almost all have a cardiac malformation which is a major factor leading to early demise, most frequently within the first three months of life. Exceptional, long-lived cases have been reported, the oldest known patient being 15 years of age. As with 21-trisomy, late maternal age is etiologically important.

Translocations of chromosome 18, though rare, have given rise to partial 18-trisomy syndromes, i.e., only part of one No. 18 chromosome is duplicated either by elongation of its long arm or by translocation to another chromosome. The diagnosis of partial trisomy has generally been based on the clinical picture, since in the absence of a reciprocal translocation in one parent, it has not been possible to confirm cytologically the origin of the extra chromosomal material. As with translocation mongolism, offspring of six different chromosomal types can result from segregation of the chromosomes of a carrier parent, but probably only three are viable: normal karyotype, balanced translocation carrier, and partial 18-trisomy, theoretically in equal proportions. Mosaics and double trisomics have also been reported.

13-Trisomy Syndrome (D Syndrome, Patau Syndrome). Because the three chromosome pairs of the D group were indistinguishable from one another by conventional stains, patients with an extra D chromosome were called D_1 trisomics in anticipation of the future identification of trisomies involving the other two pairs. When autoradiographic techniques were developed, the three pairs could be distinguished by differential labeling. The most heavily labeled of the three was designated No. 13, and it is this chromosome that is found in triplicate in this syndrome. Trisomies for the other two pairs have not been found and are probably lethal. All three pairs can now be more easily identified by differences in fluorescent and Giemsa banding patterns (Fig. 6–26).

Although, in general, virtually the same clinical signs are found in both 13- and 18-trisomics, the constant features of each are different enough that discrimination between the two is usually not difficult. Moreover, the facies are quite different, 13-trisomics having coarser features. The prognosis for 13-trisomics appears to be slightly better than for 18-trisomics, but most patients with either syndrome die in the first year of life; at least one is known to be alive at the age of 10. The incidence is in the range of 1 in 5000 or less. There is no significant difference in the sex ratio and there is an elevation of the average maternal age.

Translocations of chromosome 13 have been more frequently reported than have those of No. 18, probably because of the greater affinity of acrocentric chromosomes for each other and the

TABLE 6–5. RISK OF RECURRENCE OF 21-TRISOMY ACCORDING TO MATERNAL AGE AT BIRTH OF PROBAND (MOSAICS AND TRANSLOCATIONS EXCLUDED)*

MATERNAL AGE	TRISOMY BIRTH RATE (*Manitoba 1960–68*)	CHILDREN BORN AFTER PROBAND *Total Sibs*	*21-Trisomy*	RECURRENCE RISK
< 25	1/2000	181	2	1/90
25 – 34	1/1300	254	5	1/50
35 – 44	1/250	94	1	1/90
45+	1/80	0	0	–
Totals	1/900	529	8	1/65

*Combined data from Manitoba study and Carter, C. O., and Evans, K. A.: Lancet *2*:785, 1961.

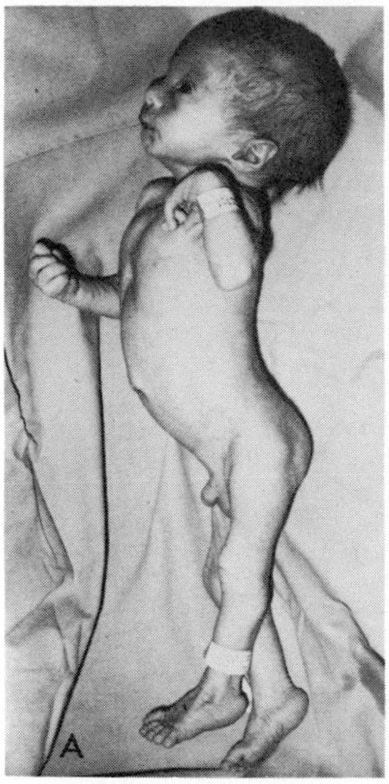

Figure 6–25 *A, Photograph of male infant with trisomy-18, age 4 days. There are prominent occiput, micrognathia, low-set ears, short sternum, narrow pelvis, prominent calcaneus, and flexion abnormalities of the fingers. (Courtesy of Robert E. Carrel.) B, Several of the common anomalies in the 18 trisomy syndrome, including the unusual position of the fingers with hypoplasia of fifth fingernail; the simple arch pattern on the fingers; and the dorsiflexed hallux with hypoplasia of toenails. (From D. W. Smith: Am. J. Obstet. Gynec., 90:1055, 1964.) C, Partial karyotype of trisomy-18 prepared with modified Giemsa stain. (Courtesy of R. L. Summitt and Paula R. Martens.)*

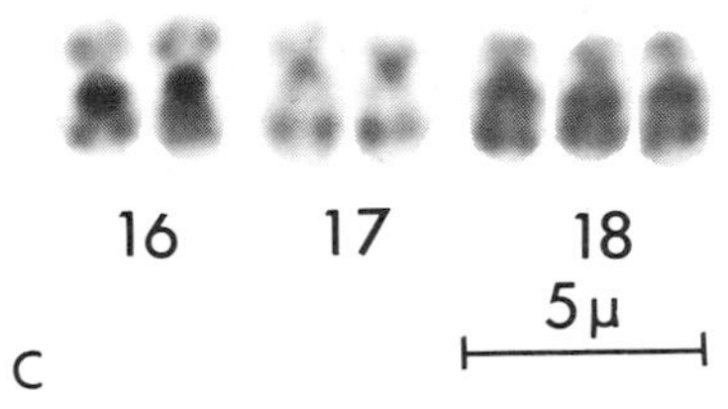

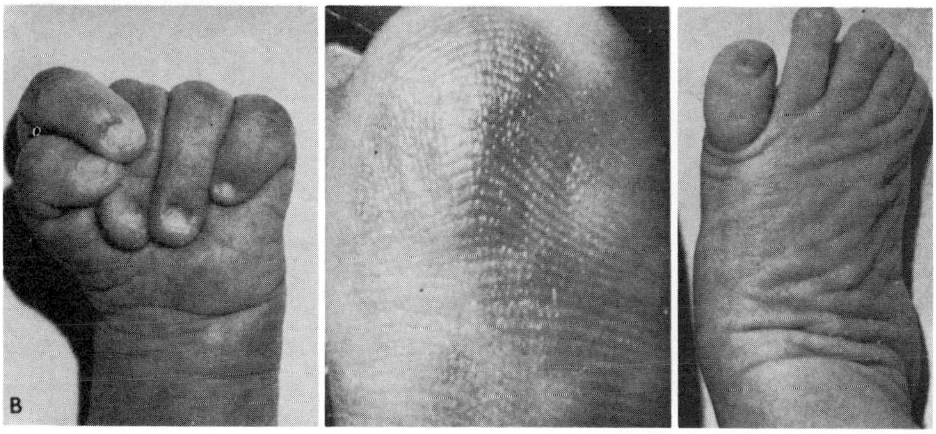

ease of identification due to chromosome length. Most are formed by centric fusion, but some consist of two D chromosomes attached in tandem to form a very long acrocentric chromosome. The pattern of inheritance is similar to that of the 21qGq translocation discussed under 21-trisomy.

There are many large pedigrees with phenotypically normal subjects who have 45 chromosomes, including a centric fusion t(DqDq), but rarely does such a carrier have abnormal offspring. It appears that larger chromosomes with symmetrical arm lengths tend to segregate in an orderly fashion, giving rise to karyotypically normal or balanced carriers. However, increased frequencies of spontaneous abortions or 21-trisomics have been noted. Since the chromosomes forming these translocations are usually Nos. 13 and 14, the abortions are probably effective trisomics for No. 14.

22-Trisomy Syndrome. Karyotypes of patients with none of the clinical signs of mongolism but with an extra small acrocentric were variously interpreted as 22-trisomy, XYY or partial trisomy resulting from deletions of larger chromosomes. However, by using marker chromosomes, autoradiography and fluorescent banding it has been possible to identify three No. 22 chromosomes in some of these patients. A clinical syndrome has now begun to emerge; its characteristics are mental and growth retardation, microcephaly, micrognathia, preauricular skin tags, appendages and/or sinuses, low-set and/or malformed ears, cleft palate, congenital heart disease and deformed lower extremities.

22-trisomics occur with a lesser frequency than 21-trisomics in spite of the similarity in size and shape of the two pairs of G chromosomes. The reason may be a lesser susceptibility to nondisjunction of chromosome No. 22 compared with No. 21. G-trisomy has been observed with a relatively high frequency among abortuses, and these have recently been shown by banding studies to be mainly 21-trisomics.

G-Monosomy. A few cases of apparent monosomy for one of the small acrocentric chromosomes have been reported. Since many of the clinical signs appeared to be the opposite of those found in mongolism, the term "*antimongolism*" was coined to describe these patients. However, there has been

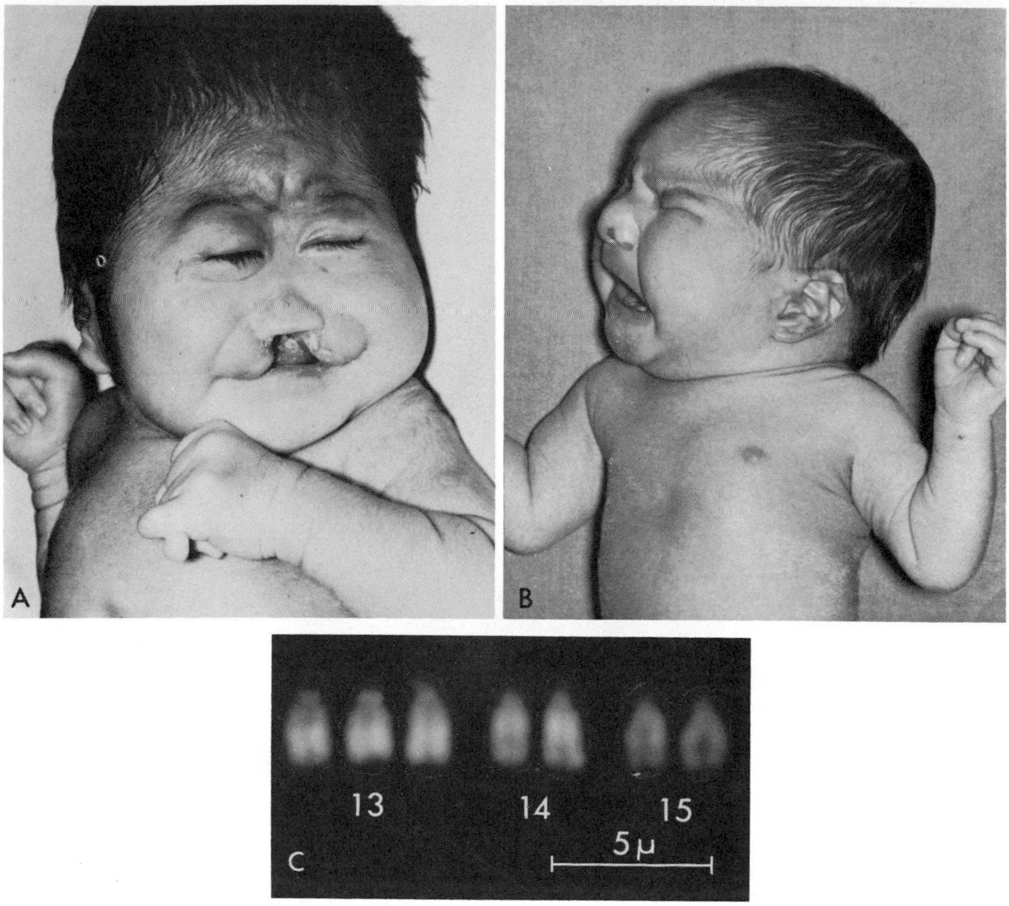

Figure 6–26 A, *Female infant with trisomy-13 syndrome. There is a midline cleft of the lip and palate, microcephaly, hypotelorism, microphthalmus and polydactyly.* B, *Female infant with trisomy-13 syndrome. There are microcephaly, microphthalmus, bulbous nose, overlapping of fingers and scalp defects (not shown). (Courtesy of Miriam G. Wilson.)* C, *Partial karyotype showing D-group chromosomes stained with quinacrine hydrochloride.*

some reluctance to accept a diagnosis of complete monosomy mainly because it has not been possible to rule out with certainty the presence of mosaicism or an undetectable translocation; even fluorescent staining techniques may not be refined enough to detect a translocation of a small nonfluorescent segment. Proof of G-monosomy could be obtained from among the offspring of the rare parent carrying a 21q21q or 22q22q translocation. (See discussion on 21-trisomy.) An infant with 45 chromosomes but lacking the translocation would be monosomic for the missing G chromosome. Since monosomy is an extreme form of deletion, the clinical signs are similar to those of deletions.

Aneuploidy of Other Autosomes. Trisomies of other autosomes have involved mainly the C group; most have been mosaics. Now that each chromosome of this group can be identified, new syndromes may soon be delineated. In a few instances the aberration has been identified as trisomy for chromosome No. 8. Trisomies of other groups have also been reported, but documentation is lacking. Probably most are lethal when normal cell lines are lacking.

STRUCTURAL ABERRATIONS

Translocations. These are the most common structural aberrations. Exchange of segments between two nonhomologous chromosomes is known as a *reciprocal* or *balanced translocation.* The first descriptions were of *simple translocations,* i.e., a piece of one chromosome is broken off and attached to the end of another. However, cross-shaped configurations observed during meiosis indicated that apparently simple translocations were actually interchanges between the terminal segments of two chromosomes. Moreover, loss of genes located on the tip of a recipient chromosome indicated that two broken ends were required for a translocation to occur. It is now generally accepted that simple translocations occur rarely, if at all.

In phenotypically normal individuals translocations are assumed to be *reciprocal* or *balanced,* since loss or gain of chromatin material usually results in an abnormal phenotype. An exception is the balanced (Robertsonian) translocation discussed above. Among the offspring of such subjects can be found unbalanced karyotypes associated with *duplication-deficiency syndromes.* Whether a syndrome is due to partial monosomy or partial trisomy will be determined by which interchange chromosome is transmitted.

Except for those resulting in well known clinical syndromes, it is not possible to identify with certainty the origin of excess chromosomal material in the absence of a reciprocal translocation in a parent, even with the aid of banding patterns. An exception is the translocation of a large segment of the X chromosome that can be positively identified by the X chromatin or thymidine-labeling pattern. When a parent is a translocation heterozygote, the partial trisomy can be accurately determined, making possible the delineation of new clinical syndromes. Small duplications and deletions can now be identified in karyotypes that were thought to be normal with conventional stains.

Although all chromosomes are subject to breaks that result in structural aberrations, the chromosomes most frequently involved in translocations appear to be the acrocentrics of the D and G groups, probably because of their close association as nucleolar organizers. Translocations and their mode of transmission have been discussed in the respective sections under *Aneuploidy.*

Deletions. Deletions were thought at first to be lethal in man, but several clinical syndromes caused by them have now been documented. Some lead to a less severely affected phenotype than do the trisomies. Clinical features of the more common deletions are listed in Table 6–6. It is interesting to note that both trisomies and deletions involve mainly chromosomes 13, 18, 21 and 22.

Chromosomes Nos. 4 and 5 (4p– and 5p– Syndromes). Clinical syndromes have been described as the result of deletion of part of the short arm of either of the B group chromosomes. Best known is the **cri-du-chat syndrome** (5p–) (Fig. 6–27*A*), so named because the cry of affected infants resembles that of a kitten and is characterized by high-pitched, tense phonation. The facilitation of diagnosis by this distinguishing trait probably accounts for the apparent greater frequency of 5p– as compared to other deletions. However, the typical cry tends to disappear in late infancy and a similar cry has been noted on occasion in other retarded infants. Most cases arise sporadically, but a few reports of reciprocal translocation in a parent have been observed. Ring chromosomes with loss of material from both ends also produce the same syndrome.

TABLE 6–6. IMPORTANT CLINICAL FEATURES OF THE DELETION SYNDROMES

FEATURE	4p–	5p–	18p–	18q–	13q–
General	LBW; severe MR; delayed ossification	LBW; MR; cat-like cry	LBW; variable MR; short stature; Turner syndrome-like stigmata	LBW; severe MR; seizures; hypotonia	LBW; severe MR; failure to thrive
Craniofacies	Microcephaly; hypertelorism; epicanthus; ptosis, colobomata; beaked nose, short broad philtrum; cleft palate; micrognathia; simple ears	Microcephaly; round face; hypertelorism; epicanthus; antimongoloid palpebral fissure; micrognathia; low-set malformed ears, preauricular tags	Hypertelorism; epicanthus; flat nasal bridge; micrognathia; low-set, large floppy ears	Microcephaly; ophthalmologic defects; carp-shaped mouth; apparent protruding mandible; atretic ear canals	Microcephaly; trigonocephaly; flat, wide nasal bridge; hypertelorism; ptosis, epicanthus, microphthalmia, colobomata; retinoblastoma; micrognathia
Thorax		CHD (occasional)		CHD (occasional); supernumerary ribs	CHD
Pelvis and abdomen	Inguinal hernia; sacral dimples; hypospadias; cryptorchidism	Inguinal hernia; diastasis recti; small iliac wings		Small penis; cryptorchidism; hypoplastic genitalia in females	Hip dysplasia; cryptorchidism
Hands and feet		Short metacarpals or metatarsals; partial syndactyly; pes planus; simian crease	Stubby hands with high-set thumbs; partial webbing of toes; large digital patterns with high TRC	Long tapering fingers; abnormal implantation of toes; large digital patterns with high TRC	Hypoplastic or absent thumbs; clinodactyly of 5th fingers; syndactyly of toes

LBW = Low birth weight; MR = Mental retardation; CHD = Congenital heart disease; TRC = Total ridge count.

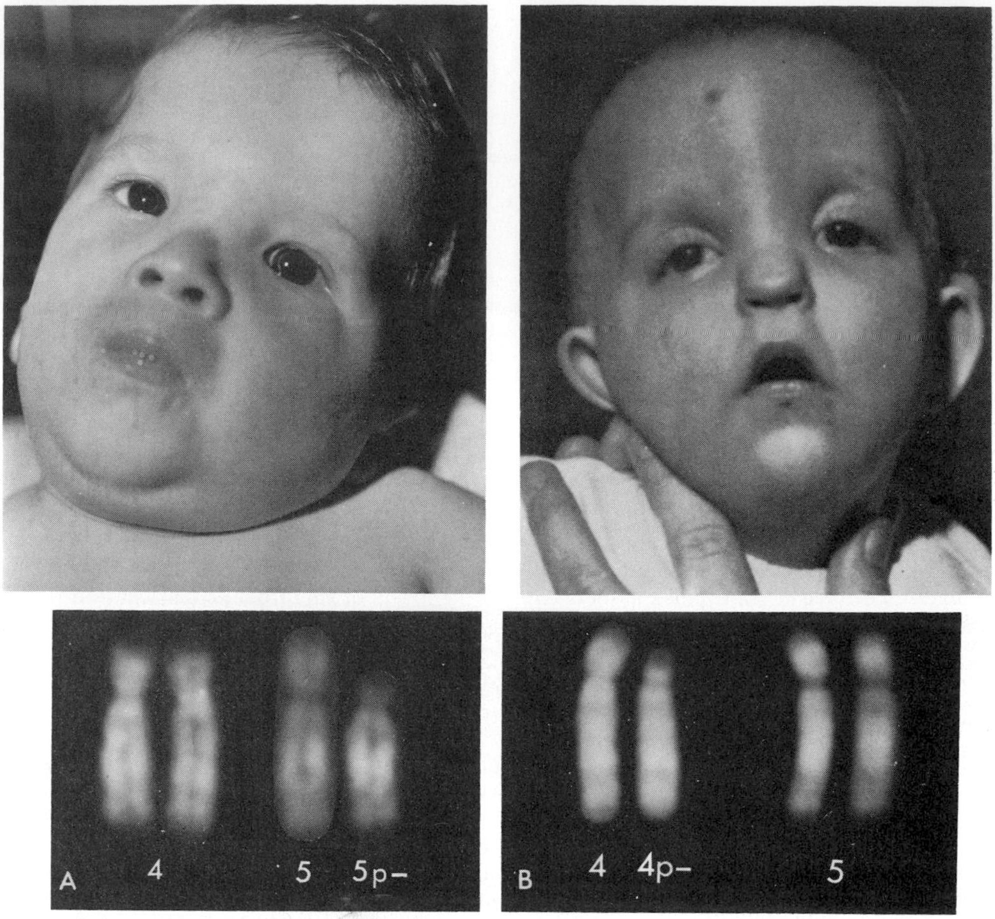

Figure 6–27 Patients with partial deletion of short arm of B group chromosomes. A, An 8 month old boy with cri-du-chat syndrome and deletion of part of the short arms of one chromosome No. 5 (5 p–). B, 1 year old boy with partial deletion of the short arms of one chromosome No. 4. (Courtesy of W. R. Breg.)

Some patients with a B deletion are much more severely malformed and retarded and do not have the typical cry. The suspicion that these were deletions of chromosome No. 4 was confirmed with autoradiography. The clinical signs are listed in Table 6–6. (Also see Figure 6–27*b*.)

Chromosome No. 18 (18p– and 18q– Syndromes). Deletions of chromosome No. 18 take three forms: loss of the entire short arm, 18p–, loss of part of the long arm, 18q–, and deletions of both ends to form a ring, r(18). Patients with 18p– are phenotypically extremely variable. A few have been severely affected, with arhinencephaly, cyclopia or cleft lip and palate, but most have only minor congenital anomalies and are only moderately retarded (Table 6–6 and Fig. 6–28). A diagnosis of the Turner syndrome is often suspected, making ascertainment somewhat difficult. On the other hand, children with 18q– are severely retarded and have more characteristic malformations (Fig. 6–29). Children with a ring chromosome 18 have phenotypic features of both short and long arm deletions since the tips of both ends of the chromosome are lost during ring formation. The 18p– syndrome is the only structural abnormality of the chromosomes in which late maternal age appears to be important.

A number of characteristics are common to the three types of deletion. Prognosis for survival seems to be good. IgA deficiency has been noted in some patients. Large dermal patterns are present on the digits, mainly whorls, giving a very high total ridge count similar to that seen in the Turner syndrome. This is in sharp contrast to 18-trisomy syndrome, in which the presence of arches results in a very low ridge count.

Chromosomes of the D Group. Loss of part of the long arm of a D chromosome has been reported in a few patients. It has not yet been definitely established that the same one is deficient in all cases, but the phenotypic similarities are such that involvement of the same chromosome (13q–) is suspected (Table 6–6).

Chromosomes of the F and G Groups. Deficiencies in these two groups have resulted mainly in ring formation. Loss of material from the long arm has occurred in some subjects, but deletions compatible with life may often be too small to identify unless a ring is formed. *F group aberrations* were first reported only in studies of aborted material and patients with blood dyscrasias. A few patients with severe mental retardation and F group deletions have now been described; others, with F group deletions in only part of their cells (mosaics), appear to be phenotypically normal.

Because many more cases have been described with *G deletions,* two syndromes are beginning to emerge. Common clinical signs are retarded development, hypertonia, epicanthic folds, large and low-set ears, broad and prominent nasal bridge, high-arched palate, micrognathia and microcephaly or dolichocephaly. Since some of the clinical signs of 21 deletions, like those of G-monosomy, are the opposite of those of mongolism, this syndrome has also been referred to as "antimongolism." Patients with r(22) appear to be more severely retarded than those with r(21), but the former have fewer physical signs. Differences in dermatoglyphics have been noted and may be of diagnostic value.

Miscellaneous Aberrations. Several sporadic reports of a variety of chromosomal aberrations have been published. Among the more frequently noted is the **"cat-eye"** or **coloboma and anal atresia syndrome**, most cases of which have an additional tiny satellited chromosome of unknown origin. Chromosomal aberrations have been observed in some 10 per cent of patients with Cornelia de Lange syndrome (Appendix). Since a variety of structural aberrations of different chromosomes as well as apparently normal karyotypes have been

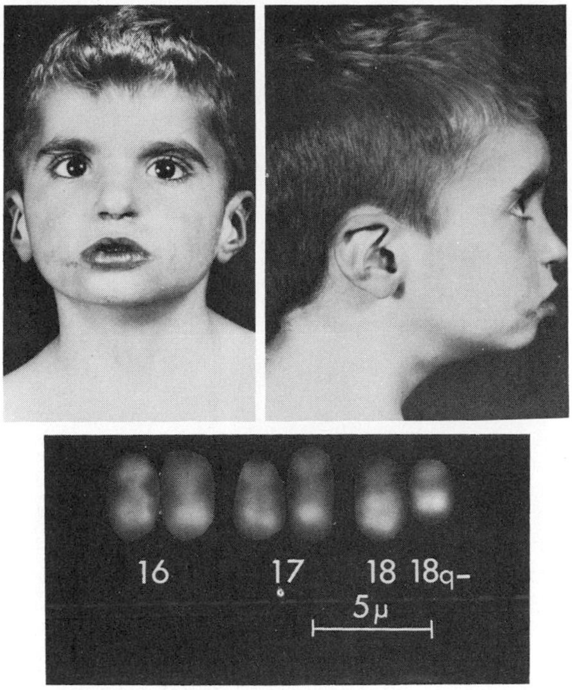

Figure 6–29 *Patient with partial deletion of long arm of chromosome No. 18. (Courtesy of P. S. Gerald and W. Wertelecki.) Partial karyotype showing 18q– stained with quinacrine dihydrochloride.*

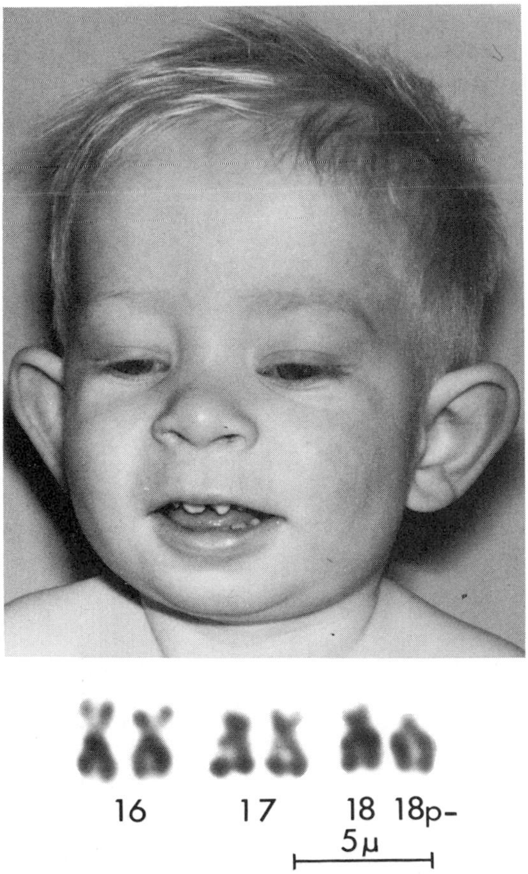

Figure 6–28 *Patient with 18 short arm deletion, 18p–. Chromosomes of E group showing Giemsa banding. (Courtesy of R. L. Summitt and Paula R. Martens.)*

reported, this association may be more apparent than real. It is possible that several clinically similar but etiologically different disorders have been grouped together.

Breakage Syndromes. Chromosomal breakage, structural rearrangements and aneuploidy have been reported in some patients during viral diseases such as measles, chickenpox and infectious hepatitis, but this has not been a consistent finding. Similar aberrations have been observed in both chronic and acute leukemia, but, except for the Ph′ chromosome, there is no karyotypic change of diagnostic value. There are, however, a group of familial (autosomal recessive) diseases with high frequencies of chromosome breaks and rearrangements and increased risk of leukemia: Bloom syndrome (congenital telangiectatic erythema with dwarfism), constitutional aplastic pancytopenia (Section 14), and ataxia telangiectasia (Louis-Bar syndrome). One distinctive cytogenetic feature is characteristic of the Bloom syndrome: the quadriradial configurations formed by chromatid exchanges almost always involve homologous chromosomes (Fig. 6–30); in the other two disorders, exchanges and rearrangements are random and not so informative as the increased frequency of chromatid breaks, gaps and fragments.

SPONTANEOUS ABORTIONS

Some 20 per cent of all conceptions are spontaneously aborted and among these about one quarter

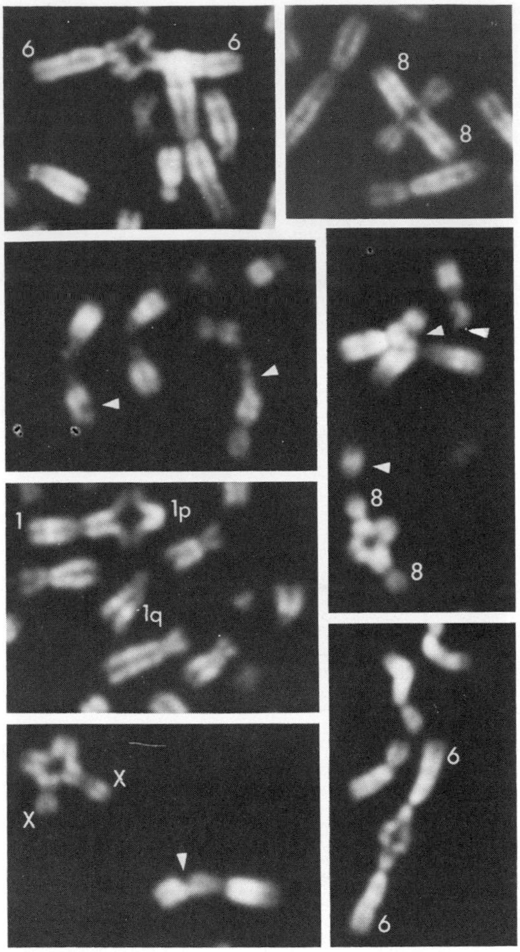

Figure 6–30 *Partial spreads of fluorescent chromosomes prepared from patient with Bloom syndrome. Note quadriradials involving homologous chromosomes as well as several breaks and fragments.*

are caused by chromosomal aberrations, the most common being aneuploidy. Loss of a sex chromosome has been found most frequently. Chromosome banding techniques have resulted in the identification of trisomies for almost all the 23 pairs of chromosomes. Trisomy 16 is by far the most common, followed by trisomies of Nos. 21, 14 and 15. Polyploidy is frequent if conception has occurred within the seven-month period after termination of oral contraceptives. Other types of aberrations have not been associated with birth control pills.

GENETIC COUNSELING IN CHROMOSOMAL DISORDERS

With the many advances in cytogenetic procedures, counseling is becoming more precise. The faulty chromosome can usually be identified, small translocations, deletions and inversions can be distinguished, and with the anticipation of more rapid improvements the outlook is optimistic. Fairly accurate risk figures can be given for inherited translocations. But the risk of repetition following aneuploidy or sporadic deletions and translocations is still based on empirical values.

Amniocentesis, with culture and karyotyping of cells obtained from the fluid, has provided a practical tool to identify chromosomal defects in utero and prevent the birth of chromosomally abnormal offspring. Because of the risks involved in this procedure, though apparently slight, a list of priorities has been suggested and generally accepted. Top priority is given to situations in which there is an inherited translocation, maternal age over 40 years or previous trisomic child. Determination of fetal sex from amniotic fluid cells is also important in the prevention of X-linked recessive disorders.

Gene mapping of chromosomes is a field of investigation which eventually should produce valuable information for genetic counseling. If the locus of a gene is known to be on a specific chromosome and this chromosome can be distinguished from its homologue by differences in structure or banding pattern, it will be possible to trace the transmission of an abnormal gene.

Major advances in chromosome mapping have been made with new research tools. At least one gene has been provisionally assigned to 15 of the 23 pairs of chromosomes. The autosome with the largest number of identified genes is No. 1. Mapping in this instance was facilitated by the recognition of a marker chromosome. Genes located on the X chromosome have been known for some time and the order in which they are linked together is rapidly becoming clear.

ACKNOWLEDGMENTS

Acknowledgment is made to Mrs. Elizabeth Byrnes for preparing the fluorescence and trypsin-Giemsa karyotypes and to Dr. R. L. Summitt for his critical review of this manuscript. The tables of clinical descriptions were prepared by Dr. Celinda del Solar.

IRENE A. UCHIDA

PATIENT EDUCATION

Apgar, V., and Beck, J.: Is My Baby All Right? New York, Simon & Schuster, 1973.

Smith, D. W., and Wilson, A. A.: The Child with Down's Syndrome (Mongolism). Philadelphia, W. B. Saunders Company, 1973.

GENERAL

Apgar, V. (ed.): Down's Syndrome (Mongolism) Annals of the New York Academy of Sciences. Volume 171, No. 2. New York, New York Academy of Sciences, 1970.

Bergsma, D. (ed.): Birth Defects–Atlas and Compendium. Baltimore, The Williams & Wilkins Company, 1972.

Court-Brown, W. M.: Frontiers of Biology. Volume 5, Human Population Cytogenetics. New York, John Wiley & Sons, Inc., 1967.

Freedom, R. M., and Gerald, P. S.: Congenital cardiac disease and the "cat eye" syndrome. Am. J. Dis. Child. *126*:16, 1973.

Hamerton, J. L.: Human Cytogenetics. Volumes I and II. New York, Academic Press, Inc., 1971.

Hsu, L. Y. F., Shapiro, L. R., Gertner, M., Lieber, E., and Hirschhorn, K.: Trisomy 22: A clinical entity. J. Pediatr. *79*:12, 1971.

Intrauterine Diagnosis. Birth Defects–Original Article Series. Volume VII, No. 5. New York, The National Foundation–March of Dimes, 1971.

Kajii, T., Ohama, K., Niikawa, N., Ferrier, A., and Avirachan, S.: Banding analysis of abnormal karyotypes in spontaneous abortion. Am. J. Hum. Genet. *25*:539, 1973.

Levine, H.: Clinical Cytogenetics. Boston, Little, Brown and Company, 1971.
Paris Conference: Standardization in Human Cytogenetics. New York, The National Foundation—March of Dimes, 1971.
Preus, M., and Fraser, F. C.: Dermatoglyphics and syndromes. Am. J. Dis. Child. *124*:933, 1972.
Reed, T. E., Borgaonkar, D. S., Conneally, P. M., Yu, P-L., Nance, W. E., and Christian, J. C.: Dermatoglyphic nomogram for the diagnosis of Down's syndrome. J. Pediatr. *77*:1024, 1970.
Robinson, J. A.: Origin of extra chromosome in trisomy 21. Lancet *1*:131, 1973.
Rowley, J. D.: A new consistent chromosomal abnormality in chronic myelogenous leukemia identified by quinacrine fluorescence and Giemsa staining. Nature (London) *243*:290, 1973.
Warren, R. J., Rimoin, D. L., and Summitt, R. L.: Identification by fluorescent microscopy of the abnormal chromosomes associated with the G-deletion syndromes. Am. J. Hum. Genet. *25*:77, 1973.
Wright, S. W., Crandall, B. F., and Boyer, L. (eds.): Perspectives in Cytogenetics. Springfield, Illinois, Charles C Thomas, 1972.
Yunis, J. J. (ed.): Human Chromosome Methodology. New York, Academic Press, Inc., 1965.

Intrauterine and Environmental Factors

In mammals prenatal development is protected, since it takes place in the uterus, but this protection is not complete. Mechanical, actinic, chemical, nutritional and infectious agents may cause prenatal injury. Such agents are called *teratogens.*

Intrauterine life may be divided into an *embryonic period* (approximately the first trimester) and a *fetal period* (from the twelfth week to birth). This division is arbitrary, but it distinguishes the period in which organogenesis takes place from the period which is devoted chiefly to growth. Severe injuries lead to prenatal death; milder injuries may result in changes compatible with life. Environmental interference during the embryonic period leads to arrest of development and to malformations. A noxious agent may be harmless at certain stages of this period and deleterious at others, since the various organs are sensitive to noxious agents at periods of rapid differentiation and less sensitive in resting stages. Since biochemical differentiation precedes morphologic differentiation, the period sensitive to interference by a teratogen may precede the stage of visible change. It can be assumed that agents responsible for malformations act early in prenatal life, probably within the first two or three months of gestation. Later, during the fetal period, injuries result in changes which more closely resemble those of postnatal damage, such as scars and mutilations.

MECHANICAL INJURIES. Mechanical injuries may result in fetal death. External, intra-abdominal or intrauterine pressure has been said to lead to malformations, but only a few specific possibilities are seriously considered. In extrauterine pregnancies the fetus is often deformed. The deformity cannot be attributed to mechanical causes alone, however, since an ectopic embryo is embedded in an abnormal decidua, and faulty nutrition may be the cause. Malformations in a twin have been attributed to pressure exerted by the other twin. It is often asserted that intrauterine malposition of the fetus leads to malformations; it seems just as reasonable, however, to consider malposition secondary to the malformation. There is a possibility that a deformed fetal part which assumes an abnormal position impairs the normal development of another part and thus causes secondary deformities (mutilations). Amniotic bands are sometimes associated with malformations, but there is no proof that they are the cause of the deformities. Rupture of the amnion has also been considered a cause of fetal malformations.

CHEMICAL INJURIES. Certain chemicals are capable of destroying the embryo, and malformations can be produced in animals by adding toxic substances to the environment. Alcohol, benzol, nicotine, lead and iodine have been suspected as injurious agents, but experimental results have been contradictory. Organic mercury compounds can cause prenatal brain damage (Minamata disease). Quinine taken by the mother during pregnancy may cause congenital deafness in her child.

A number of drugs have been found to be teratogenic in animals. Antimetabolites such as galactoflavin or α-methyl-folic acid have been used successfully to induce congenital malformations in rodents. The folic acid antagonist 4-amino-folic acid (aminopterin) has caused congenital malformations in human embryos whose mothers used the drug in attempted abortion. Thalidomide, alpha (N-phthalimido) glutarimide, a hypnotic and antiemetic, can induce severe malformations in human embryos if ingested by the mother in the first weeks of pregnancy. The incidence of malformations is highest if the drug is taken between the thirty-fifth and fiftieth days after the last menstrual period. Amelia, phocomelia, acheiria (Section 22) and other limb defects may result from the embryo's exposure to this drug. In addition, congenital hemangiomas, ear and eye defects, cardiac malformations and atresias of the gastrointestinal tract have been caused by this chemical compound. These observations have demonstrated that the embryos of man are just as susceptible as other mammalian embryos to chemical injurious agents. Other drugs which may damage the embryo or fetus are dicumarol (fetal bleeding); progestational agents, estrogens and androgens (masculinization of female fetus); thiouracil derivatives, iodine and iodides (goiter). Since it is difficult to be sure that any drug is not harmful to an embryo, drug intake during pregnancy should be restricted to those clearly necessary to the mother's health.

NUTRITIONAL DISTURBANCES. Nutritional disturbances may adversely influence the embryo. Faulty implantation of the ovum and degeneration of the chorion may interrupt the nutrition of the embryo and disturb its development. Malformation in fetuses derived from ectopic pregnancies is mentioned above. Deficiencies of nutritional constituents of the maternal diet and deficiency of oxygen have been responsible for defective offspring in animal experiments, but there is no proof that these observations can be applied to human beings. In many regions of Europe, Asia and South America endemic goiter of the parents is associated with endemic cretinism of the children. The serious mental and physical retardation of the offspring is usually attributed to a lack of iodine in the maternal diet.

Extensive studies have shown a relation between the diet of pregnant women and the physical condition of newborn infants. Stillborn, premature and functionally immature children are born more often to mothers whose diet is poor prior to or during pregnancy than to mothers whose diet is adequate. General starvation, as in war or famine, leads to a sharp fall in the conception rate, associated with amenorrhea.

INJURIES FROM INFECTION. Severe maternal infections during early pregnancy often result in abortion. Mothers who have had German measles during the first two or three months of pregnancy may give birth to infants with a variety of defects and widely disseminated infection (Section 10). Cytomegalic inclusion disease and toxoplasmosis are examples of inapparent maternal infections which can cause extensive damage in the fetus; each may be responsible for microcephaly and hydrocephalus as well as widespread disease.

Infections of the fetus during the latter stages of prenatal life cause manifestations which more closely resemble those of postnatal life. Smallpox has been observed in fetuses older than 3 months; the fetus may recover and be born with scars. Rare cases of fetal measles and scarlet fever have been reported. Placental transmission of typhoid and tubercle bacilli occurs occasionally, and that of *Treponema pallidum* is common in infected, untreated mothers.

ACTINIC INJURIES. Roentgen rays and radium rays are capable of arresting embryonic development and producing malformations. Microcephaly, microphthalmia, mental retardation, and deformities of the extremities have been ascribed to such intrauterine injuries.

OTHER FACTORS. In addition to the pathogenic environmental factors considered, there may be others still unrecognized. The possibility that abnormal endocrine factors influence the development of the embryo deserves consideration. Diabetic mothers treated with insulin often have abortions and stillbirths, and the neonatal death rate of their infants is high. Some children of treated diabetic mothers are born with defects of the sacrum or femora. Administration of progestins to a woman during pregnancy can result in masculinization of a female fetus.

Advanced paternal age may play a role in the origin of congenital defects such as achondroplasia. Advanced maternal age is a factor in the Down syndrome.

CONGENITAL MALFORMATIONS

More deaths occur in the first month of life than in the remaining months of the first year. This is not surprising if neonatal mortality is regarded in part as a continuation of the process of "natural selection" which eliminates defective embryos and fetuses throughout the preceding intrauterine period.

Structural anomalies of the embryo play a leading role in the mortality of the first trimester of intrauterine life. Most abnormal embryos die early, but structural anomalies may be compatible with intrauterine life. Shortly before and after birth (perinatal period) the fetus must adjust to the profound physiologic changes associated with the onset of extrauterine life. Many abnormal fetuses are incapable of doing so and die. They contribute considerably to the peak of mortality, which occurs in the perinatal period. About 20 per cent of deaths in the third trimester of gestation and about 15 per cent in the neonatal period are attributed to gross congenital malformations. Although the elimination of deformed children decreases after the first month of postnatal life, the process of natural selection continues throughout infancy and childhood. The relative importance of congenital malformations as a cause of death is depicted graphically and numerically in the introductory section, The Field of Pediatrics.

Many children with congenital malformations are permanently disabled. Malformations such as clubfoot, dislocation of the hip and spina bifida are among the leading causes of crippling in childhood.

The role of congenital malformations in the causation of diseases of children is difficult to evaluate. Some defects, such as those of the osseous system, the heart and the intestinal tract, are well recognized, but many malformations may go unnoticed for years. The affected organs, e.g., malformed kidneys, may function for some time, but fail when faced with increased demands. Congenital malformations are often predisposing factors to disease because they represent points of inadequate resistance; organs can be damaged by minor infections, toxins or traumas which are usually tolerated by the normal organism without serious consequences. Diseases resulting from such a combination of circumstances may be attributed to the eliciting factor, while the underlying malformation is overlooked.

For example, the primary cause of so-called renal rickets may be a congenital obstruction of the urinary tract. Dwarfism, malnutrition, osseous changes, polyuria, polydipsia, renal insufficiency, chemical changes of the blood, infections of the urinary tract or other symptoms may dominate the clinical picture. Obviously treatment of the symptoms enumerated will not meet with success, whereas early detection and removal of the congenital obstruction may lead to permanent cure.

Congenital defects need not be grossly demonstrable, but may be anomalies of histologic structure. The role of misplaced cells in the genesis of certain tumors is well known. Some disorders of the nervous system or the endocrine glands must be attributed to histologic congenital defects. Spherocytosis is a congenital anomaly. The intimate relation of certain forms of anemia to malformations is indicated by their association in syndromes. For example, in some forms of aplastic anemia, association with congenital defects of the skeleton, heart and genital tract points to the developmental origin of the disorder (e.g., Fanconi's anemia).

ETIOLOGY AND PATHOGENESIS. With respect to etiology, congenital malformations can be considered in four major categories: gene mutations, chromosomal aberrations, adverse intrauterine environmental factors, and a group in which the malformation results from a combination of many factors, both genetic and environmental, no single one of which may be detectable.

It has been roughly estimated that about 10 per cent of congenital malformations result from mutant genes. These are inherited according to mendelian laws, and relatively precise predictions can be made about the probability of occurrence in the patient's sibs, his offspring, and other relatives. Theoretically such malformations should have an underlying biochemical defect. In a few cases structural malformations are associated with inborn errors of metabolism, e.g., adrenogenital syndrome, but in most congenital malformations transmitted by mendelian inheritance no biochemical defect has been identified.

Animals often inherit congenital malformations with great regularity of pattern, and it is possible by systematic examination of their embryos of different ages to ascertain step by step the deviations from normal development. In this way the action and mechanism of the abnormal gene can be investigated and the development of the finished character observed.

Perhaps about 1 per cent of malformations present at birth and 20 per cent or more of early spontaneous abortions have abnormal chromosomal constitutions. (See section on chromosomal abnormalities.) Relatively few congenital malformations can be attributed to the specific environmental teratogens which have been mentioned elsewhere in this section.

Perhaps the majority of congenital malformations are the result of a combination of genetic and environmental factors. Malformations such as congenital hypertrophic pyloric stenosis, cleft lip and cleft palate, congenital dislocation of the hip and talipes equinovarus probably fall into this group. They tend to be familial, but do not have mendelian patterns of inheritance. Most have no demonstrable chromosomal anomaly and no identifiable abnormal prenatal environmental factors. Probabilities of recurrence can be estimated empirically from observation of affected families, and used for counseling.

Teratogenic factors are not specific, and the lack of specificity manifests itself in two ways. An injurious agent may cause various abnormalities, according to the time or intensity of its action, as illustrated by the wide variety of congenital anomalies induced by maternal rubella. Maternal roentgen-ray irradiation results in abnormalities in the offspring which vary with the dose applied and the gestational period in which the exposure took place. An abnormal gene may manifest itself in various abnormalities and exercise a pleiotropic effect. Conversely, a specific type of malformation may be caused by different etiologic factors, and hereditary anomalies may resemble each other. For example, each of the three pathologic conditions illustrated in Figures 6–31, 6–32 and 6–33 can be attributed to three different causes.

SYNDROMES. In spite of the variability of syndromes, it is of definite value to study and record combinations of defects frequently encountered. A

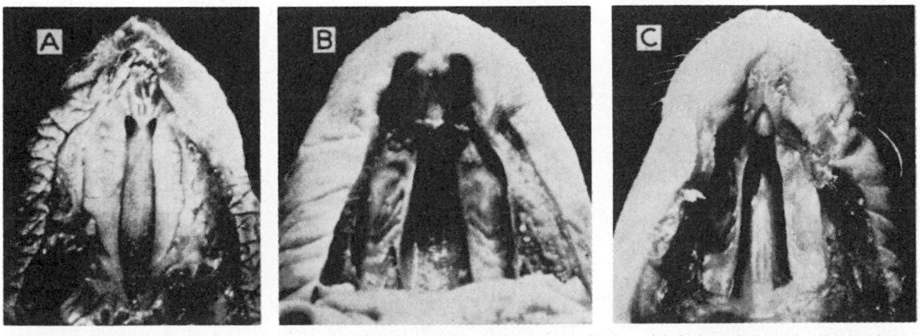

Figure 6–31 *Cleft palates of different etiology. A, Mouse, derived from strain in which harelip and cleft palate were hereditary (Steiniger: Menschl. Vererb. Konstit., Vol. 23); B, rat whose mother was deficient in riboflavin; C, rat whose mother was exposed to roentgen rays on day 15 of gestation.*

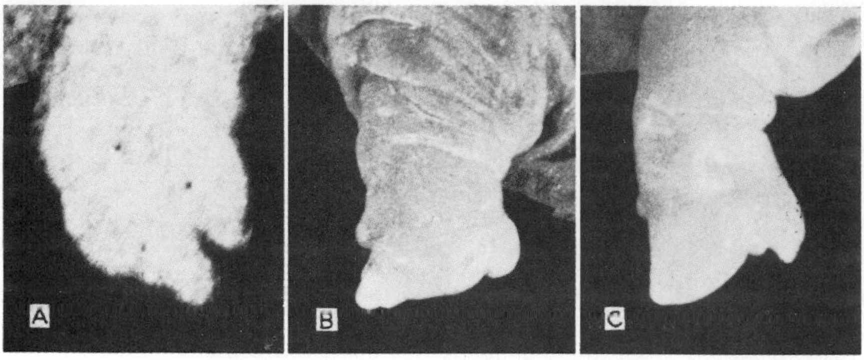

Figure 6–32 *Syndactylism of different etiology.* A, *Mouse, derived from strain with hereditary congenital defects (Bagg: Am. J. Anat., Vol. 43);* B, *rat whose mother was deficient in riboflavin;* C, *rat whose mother was exposed to roentgen rays on day 13 of gestation.*

knowledge of such syndromes is an aid in diagnosis and prognosis, particularly if one keeps in mind that the association of defects may vary. Two examples will suffice: Night blindness may be due to a deficiency of vitamin A, but it is also a symptom of retinitis pigmentosa, a degenerative process of the retina which is a constituent of the Laurence-Moon-Biedl syndrome. Night blindness in a child with polydactylism, obesity and mental retardation assumes, therefore, a different aspect from that in an otherwise normal child. The diagnosis of mental retardation is difficult in the neonatal period. The presence of epicanthal folds, slanting eyes and other somatic anomalies makes possible, however, the diagnosis of the Down syndrome, with all its prognostic implications, immediately after birth.

Besides such well established syndromes, many combinations of congenital defects are encountered which have not been described or named. Thus, in children with congenital heart disease, conditions such as cleft palate, polydactylism, malformations of the kidney, atresia ani, encephalocele and hydrocephalus are more frequent than in the average child population. The occurrence of external and skeletal defects in children with mental deficiency is well known. Such visible defects have been considered "stigmata of degeneration." Though this term is ill chosen, it is correct that malformations are found more often in patients with mental deficiency of prenatal origin than in mentally normal children. It is useful to keep this principle of multiplicity of malformations in mind when there is doubt whether one is dealing with a congenital or a postnatally acquired disorder. The finding of one or several additional malformations makes prenatal origin of the disorder more likely.

Malformations may occur sporadically or repeatedly in a sibship. Identical malformations, such as cleft palate, may be found in several members of a pedigree. Entire syndromes may recur in families, e.g., gargoylism or the Laurence-Moon-Biedl syndrome. But the various symptoms of a syndrome may also be dissociated in a family; one member may have one abnormal manifestation or one group of anomalies, and other members may have another part of the syndrome. Thus, one child may have the entire Laurence-Moon-Biedl syndrome, while another child of the same family is mentally retarded and obese and a third child has mental retardation and polydactylism. In spite of such irregularities, the family history is often a great aid in the diagnosis and prognosis of the disease of an individual patient.

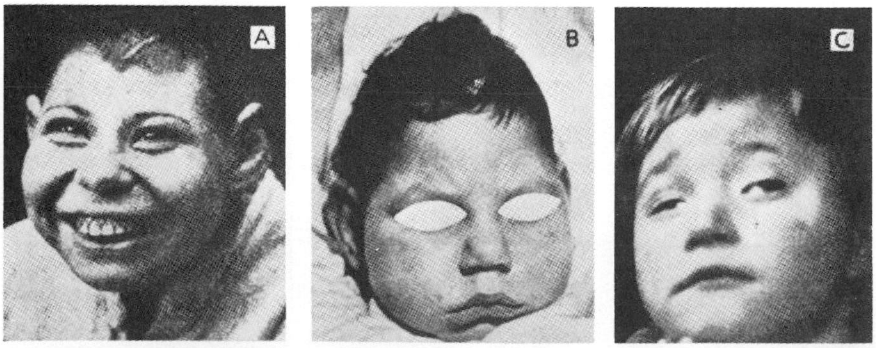

Figure 6–33 *Microcephaly of different etiology.* A, *In a child who had 2 siblings with microcephaly and 3 normal siblings and a paternal granduncle who was mentally deficient (Goldblatt: Arch. f. Psych., Vol. 70);* B, *in a child with toxoplasmosis (Levin and Moore: J. Pediat., Vol. 21);* C, *child of a mother irradiated with roentgen rays during the second and third months of pregnancy (Engelking: Klin. Monatschr. Augenh., Vol. 94).*

(Figures 6–31, 6–32 and 6–33 from Warkany: In Advances in Pediatrics. New York, Interscience Publishers, Inc., Vol. 2.)

Whenever environmental or genetic factors are unfavorable for reproduction, various manifestations of reproductive failure are observed; there may be sterility, abortion, stillbirth, premature birth or neonatal death. Malformations contribute to all degrees of reproductive failure and are a substantial cause of abortions in the first trimester. Thus, the true incidence of malformations cannot be estimated without a thorough examination of aborted and stillborn fetuses.

Ballantyne, J. W.: Manual of Antenatal Pathology and Hygiene, The Embryo. Edinburgh, W. Green & Sons, Ltd., 1904.
Fraser, F. C., and McKusick, V. A. (eds.): Congenital Malformations. New York, Excerpta Medica, 1970.
Gregg, N.: Congenital cataract following German measles in mother. Trans. Ophthalmol. Soc. Aust. *3*:35, 1942.
Mellin, G. W., and Katzenstein, M.: The saga of thalidomide: Neuropathy to embryopathy with case reports of congenital anomalies. New Engl. J. Med. *267*:1184; 1238, 1962.
Pedersen, J.: The Pregnant Diabetic and Her Newborn. Baltimore, The Williams & Wilkins Company, 1967.
Warkany, J.: Congenital Malformations. Notes and Comments. Chicago, Year Book Medical Publishers, Inc., 1971.
Weller, T. H., and Hanshaw, J. B.: Virologic and clinical observations on cytomegalic inclusion disease. New Engl. J. Med. *266*:1233, 1962.
Wolf, A., Cowen, D., and Paige, B. H.: Toxoplasmic encephalomyelitis: New case of granulomatous encephalomyelitis due to a protozoan. Am. J. Pathol. *15*:657, 1939.

GENETIC COUNSELING

If a person or one of his close relatives suffers from a congenital defect, he may ask his physician whether he should have children; or parents who have had a defective child may ask whether they should have more offspring. Such questions can rarely be answered adequately, but a knowledge of the facts discussed in the foregoing pages may serve as a guide.

In general it is preferable to give the parents all the available facts about the cause, the theoretical chance of transmission of the disorder, and its clinical course rather than advise them whether or not to have children. Many nonmedical factors enter into such a decision, such as the parents' desire to have children, the size of the family, economic circumstances and religious convictions.

It is important to ascertain whether a given defect or disorder is hereditary, since the prognosis will differ greatly in cases of genetic origin from those of postconceptional damage. In certain instances such a differentiation can be made without difficulty; in many it may not be possible. Before a statement is made about the heredity of a trait the following considerations should be taken into account:

Not all congenital anomalies and defects are hereditary, and not all hereditary anomalies are congenital. The defects produced in the fetus by maternal rubella or toxoplasmosis are congenital, but not genetically determined and, therefore, not hereditary. On the other hand, hereditary traits such as Friedreich's ataxia, Huntington's chorea, diabetes mellitus, retinitis pigmentosa and many others are not congenital, but develop in postnatal life. The terms "congenital" and "hereditary" are not synonymous.

The widespread belief that anomalies which occur repeatedly in a family are hereditary, whereas those which appear sporadically are not, is not necessarily correct. A defect may be genetically determined, although only one known member of the kindred shows the trait. The defective person may be the first to manifest a genic mutation. In the case of a dominant hereditary trait, his ancestors and siblings are free of the trait, but each of his children has a 1:1 chance to have the anomaly and to pass it on to half of his or her children. This illustrates that sporadic occurrence of a congenital anomaly does not assure normal offspring to the (first) affected member. Similarly, genetically determined defects may appear sporadically if they depend upon recessive factors or if a limited pedigree does not include other defective members. The repeated occurrence of a defect in a pedigree does not prove, however, that it is genetically determined, since several members of a sibship may be exposed to the same pathogenic environmental factors. Thus, endemic goiter, rickets, pellagra, and the like, are often familial, but they are usually not hereditary and may be prevented by a change of dietary habits. "Familial" and "hereditary" are not synonymous terms.

Differentiation between hereditary and nonhereditary anomalies is further complicated by the fact that the clinical picture of a nonhereditary modification may resemble closely that of a hereditary mutation. Thus, congenital cataract is hereditary in some families, but cataract in an infant whose mother had German measles during the first two months of pregnancy is of environmental origin. Similarly, syndactyly, cleft palate, microcephaly, microphthalmus and many other congenital defects may be due to genetic mutation, to environmental modification, or to a combination of the two.

The history of pregnancy should include a description of the mother's state of health during the early weeks of pregnancy and of any roentgen-ray or drug therapy. Organogenesis is finished at approximately 12 weeks of gestation, and most structural anomalies such as congenital heart disease, spina bifida, colobomas of the eye and cleft palate are determined by that time. Anomalies arising during the remaining six months represent trauma, disease or interference with growth of structurally complete organs. Hydrocephalus, microphthalmus, chorioretinitis and malposition of the extremities are examples. Threatened abortions, diseases and traumas of the mother should be recorded.

The birth history may indicate that physical and mental anomalies can be attributed to injuries received during delivery.

Taking the family history is a time-consuming but necessary procedure. The mother's and the father's ages should be recorded, and the parents should be asked whether they are blood-related (consanguineous). It is sometimes useful to make a pedigree chart, but this is usually impractical in a busy clinic. At least there should be a statement whether there is any condition similar to the patient's disease or defect in other members of the family. If there is, and a pedigree is to be constructed, the medical history of the patient (propositus) is recorded, then that of his brothers and sisters. Miscarriages, stillbirths and causes of deaths of siblings are also recorded. Healthy persons as well as defective ones must be included in the family history. Next, the medical histories of the grandparents, parents, their siblings and siblings' offspring, and so on, are obtained until the pedigree is traced backward and collaterally as far as the information is reasonably reliable.

If a pathologic trait known to be usually dominant appears in a family, and if the pedigree of that family suggests dominant inheritance, it is possible to give a genetic prognosis. An affected parent who marries a mate normal for the character in question can be told that his children have a 1:1 chance to be normal. But if the parent comes from a family affected by a dominant pathologic trait, but does not have it he can be assured that he will not transmit the trait to his offspring. Before such assurance is given it should be established that the inherited trait has complete penetrance and expressivity, since otherwise a person may appear normal, but transmit the trait. In case of variable expressivity a person may appear normal on superficial examination, but reveal the abnormal trait in a mild form when subjected to special examinations.

For example, multiple exostoses (Section 22) are usually well developed in affected males, but in affected females may be so small that the carriers may not be conscious of them. If roentgenograms of the prospective mother reveal slight osseous excrescences in places where exostoses usually occur, she is likely to transmit the disorder, and her sons could be severely affected.

At times laboratory tests can aid in detecting carriers of an abnormal trait with low expressivity. A member of a family affected with hemolytic jaundice may be clinically well, but have spherocytosis and increased fragility of the red cells which is revealed only by special tests. "Carriers" of gout can be discovered by chemical demonstration of hyperuricemia. In addition, before a member of an affected family is declared free, one must be sure that he has reached an age after which the onset of the disease is unlikely. Since cerebellar ataxia may not begin before the fourth decade, no member of an affected family should be considered normal before reaching the age of 40 years. These examples demonstrate that even in dominant inheritance a genetic prognosis must be made with caution.

Analysis and prognosis of a recessive trait are more difficult. A recessive gene can be carried in the heterozygous form through many generations without causing visible effects, and then the abnormal trait can appear in about one fourth of the children of normal parents who are both heterozygous carriers. Such traits are sometimes so sporadic that their distinction from nonhereditary similar conditions (phenocopies) may be impossible.

If two carriers who have an abnormal (homozygous) child ask about the chances of a second child, they must be told that the following child has again one chance in four to be affected. The chances that two heterozygous carriers of the same recessive mutant gene will meet are increased by consanguineous marriages. Heterozygous carriers of the abnormal recessive gene for a number of inborn errors of metabolism can be identified by appropriate biochemical tests. (See Section 8, Inborn Errors of Metabolism.)

A man who manifests an X-linked recessive trait will—with a normal wife—have sons who neither show nor transmit the trait, but all his daughters will be carriers. The sons of such female carriers will have a 1:1 chance of showing the abnormal trait; those sons who do not manifest the disorder do not transmit it. All the daughters will appear normal, but have a 1:1 chance of being carriers like their mother. There is usually no way to distinguish the carrier daughters from their normal sisters unless their offspring reveal their heterozygous state.

CALCULATION OF CARRIER STATE (GENE FREQUENCY). It is sometimes useful, in the case of recessively inherited diseases, to know the frequency of heterozygous carriers of the gene. Consider the case of an albino man *(aa)* who wants to know what the probability is that his children will be albinos. The possibility of procreating an albino child depends on the chance of marrying a heterozygote, *Aa*, which (provided he does not marry a relative) depends on the frequency of heterozygotes *(Aa)* in the population.

To estimate this frequency, one must think of the genes on a population, rather than a family, basis. If one in every 100 genes at the "A" locus is *a*, and the other ninety-nine are *A*, and if mating is at random, the probability that one individual will draw 2 *a* genes and be an albino is $1/100 \times 1/100$, or 1/10,000; that is, the frequency of homozygotes in the population is the square of the frequency of the gene. In practice, the known quantity is the frequency of the disease, 1/10,000, and one can estimate the frequency of the gene as the square root of this number, or 1/100.

The probability that a person will be a heterozygote is dependent on obtaining an *a* gene from one parent and an *A* from the other, which, based on the incidence of albinism, is $1/100 \times 99/100$ plus $99/100 \times 1/100$, or roughly 2/100. Thus, there is a 2 per cent probability that the albino's (unrelated) wife will be a heterozygote; the probability that the first child will be albino is half of this rate, or 1 per cent.

Formally stated, the relation between gene frequencies and genotype frequencies is known as the **Hardy-Weinberg rule,** which states that, if mating is random with respect to genotype, and if p is the frequency of an allele *A* and q the frequency of *a*, the frequency of genotypes *AA*, *Aa* and *aa* will be p^2, 2 pq, and q^2, respectively. The relation is also useful in calculations involving the effects of selection, mutation, and the like, on gene frequencies.

Hereditary traits may be transmitted differently in different sibships, as pointed out previously.

If a congenital anomaly was caused by an environmental accident, the prognosis for a subsequent pregnancy will depend upon the kind of interfering agent. If the child's anomalies are due to maternal rubella or toxoplasmosis, to administration of therapeutic doses of roentgen rays or toxic drugs, and a repetition of the faulty treatment can be avoided, the prognosis for a second child is good.

When neither a definite genetic nor a known environmental factor can be shown to be responsible for a congenital defect, the chances for the outcome of a subsequent pregnancy cannot be stated precisely.

When possible, it is helpful to indicate to parents the approximate chances for normal or abnormal children. Such empirical risk figures have been worked out for congenital disorders such as epilepsy, diabetes mellitus, cardiac malformations, facial clefts, clubfoot and others. Since such disorders are of heterogeneous origin, empirical risk figures represent merely average risks for the disorder, which should be used only when actual risk figures cannot be had.

If, for instance, normal parents have a child with harelip (with or without cleft palate), the average risk for another child having a similar malformation is about 5 per cent. If the parents have had two affected children, the risk of having still another is about 10 per cent. If one parent has the anomaly, the average risk for a child is 5 per cent. If, however, one parent and one child of a family are affected, the risk for other children being affected is about 15 per cent. The risk figures are fairly similar for cleft palate without harelip. If the parents are unaffected, but one child has cleft palate, the risk of having this malformation is about 3 per cent for subsequent children. If one parent has the anomaly, the risk for a child is said to be 7 per cent, but this estimate is questionable, since it is derived from a small sample. If one parent and one child are affected, the risk for other children is said to be 17 per cent.

Such risk figures are better than none at all, but they should be considered merely provisional estimates. Table 6–7 provides such estimates for several common congenital malformations.

FETAL DIAGNOSIS OF HERITABLE DISEASE. Currently available techniques of amniocentesis, tissue culture, biochemical analysis and chromosomal analysis make it possible to determine the presence or absence of many heritable defects in the fetus. (See also The Fetus, Section 7.) Many chromosomal disorders are potentially diagnosable in this manner, as are many enzymatic deficiencies and disorders in which abnormal substances are excreted in the fetal urine. Table 6–8 lists some of the conditions which have actually been accurately diagnosed by appropriate analysis of amniotic fluid; this list is constantly being added to. Amniocentesis is usually performed about the 14th week of gestation, when sufficient fluid is present to be withdrawn with relative ease and safety. Amniocentesis should be considered and an appropriate genetic counseling center consulted in any instance

TABLE 6–7. RECURRENCE RISKS FOR SIBLINGS OF CHILDREN WITH VARIOUS COMMON CONGENITAL MALFORMATIONS*

	ANENCEPHALY	SPINA BIFIDA	CLEFT LIP ± CLEFT PALATE	CLEFT PALATE	TALIPES EQUINOVARUS	DISLOCATED HIPS† NEONATAL DIAGNOSIS	HIRSCHSPRUNG'S DISEASE	LEGG-PERTHES DISEASE	PYLORIC STENOSIS
Population frequency/1000	0.2–5	0.2–4	1	0.4	1.2	4	0.2	0.7‡	3
Sex ratio (male/female)	0.5	0.8	1.6	0.7	2.0	0.31	3.7	5.2	5
% risk for sib after 1 affected sib – parents normal	4	6	4	3	3	14	4	4	3
% risk for sib after 2 affected sibs	10		9						

*Risks for offspring are expected to be of similar magnitude.
†An unknown proportion of these would not progress to overt dislocation.
‡Attack rate to age 15 years.
§Risk for either anencephaly or spina bifida.

TABLE 6–8. CONDITIONS IN WHICH ANTENATAL DIAGNOSIS BY AMNIOCENTESIS HAS BEEN MADE

Adrenal cortical hyperplasia
Chromosomal translocations
Down dyndrome
Fabry's disease
Galactosemia
Gaucher's disease
Glycogen-storage disease (type II)
G_{M1} gangliosidosis, Type I
G_{M1} gangliosidosis, Type II
Hunter syndrome
Hurler syndrome
Krabbe's disease
Lesch-Nyhan syndrome
Lysosomal acid phosphatase deficiency
Maple syrup urine disease
Methylmalonic acidemia
Metachromatic leukodystrophy
Niemann-Pick disease
Sex determination
Tay-Sachs disease (G_{M2} gangliosidosis)

in which there is intense parental concern over a known possibility of occurrence of a serious genetic abnormality in a fetus. (A list of centers in the United States may be obtained from The National Foundation, 1275 Mamaroneck Ave., White Plains, N.Y. 10605.)

Amnioscopy is a potential tool in the antenatal diagnosis of congenital malformations but remains experimental. The diagnosis of anencephaly and of spina bifida (with an open neural tube) by the demonstration of increased amounts of alpha-fetoprotein in amniotic fluid also shows some promise. Some current attempts to develop a reliable method of identifying the presence of the gene for cystic fibrosis in the fetus are promising but still in the investigational stage.

PROTECTION OF THE MOTHER. Eugenic measures and advice are not restricted to the genetic aspects of prenatal life. The normal development of the fetus should be assured as far as possible by protection of the expectant mother from adverse environmental influences. Immunization against rubella prior to childbearing should eliminate rubella embryopathy. Exposure to teratogenic chemicals, drugs, and roentgen-ray treatment must be avoided whenever there is the possibility of a pregnancy. It is of great importance to point out that the first three months of pregnancy are decisive in the formation of organs of the child, and that the embryo in its early stages is more vulnerable than the fetus.

JOSEF WARKANY
F. CLARKE FRASER

Beratis, N. G., Conover, J. H., Conod, E. J., Bonforte, R. J., and Hirschhorn, K.: Studies on ciliary dyskinesia factor in cystic fibrosis: Skin fibroblasts and cultured amniotic fluid cells. Pediat. Res. 7:958, 1973.

Carter, C. O.: Genetics of common disorders. Brit. Med. Bull. *25*:52, 1969.

Fraser, F. C.: Counseling in genetics. Its intent and scope. Birth Defects: Original Article Series *6*:7, 1970.

Gardner, D. M.: Antenatal diagnosis of genetic defects. J. Reprod. Med. *10*:261, 1973.

Murphy, E. A.: The rationale of genetic counselling. J. Pediatr., *62*:121, 1968.

7

THE FETUS AND THE NEWBORN INFANT

The neonatal period is defined as the first 4 weeks of life. However, fetal and neonatal life is a continuum during which the growth and development of the human organism are affected by genetic and by intrauterine and extrauterine environmental factors; the latter are modified by social, economic, and cultural influences. For example, low economic status is one of the factors most frequently associated with low birth weight (premature birth), which in turn is associated with high rates of morbidity and mortality, not only in the neonatal period, but also throughout infancy. Social as well as economic factors are reflected in the much higher (50 per cent) neonatal mortality rate in the United States of nonwhite infants than of white ones. The difference in the mortality rates of these groups is even more impressive for the entire first year of life (Table 7–1). Although social influences such as the unwillingness of physicians and their families to live in areas of social and economic poverty affect the availability of medical care to those most in need of it, the failure of many mothers in these areas to make effective use of prenatal and other preventive medical care, even when it is available to them, also contributes to fetal and infant morbidity and mortality. Social factors leading to illegitimate births, and cultural practices, including the use of drugs which may damage the fetus, also increase the incidence of fetal and neonatal death and disease.

Neonatal mortality is highest during the first 24 hours of life, accounting for about 40 per cent of deaths under 1 year of age, and has shown little change in rate in the United States since 1955. The lack of success in combating diseases which result from factors acting during gestation and at delivery, as opposed to diseases arising as a result of postnatal factors, has led to an increasing interest in fetal and neonatal physiology and in the noxious factors which influence them. The term *perinatal mortality* designates fetal and neonatal deaths influenced by prenatal conditions and circumstances surrounding delivery. It is most often defined as deaths of fetuses and infants from the twentieth week of gestational life through the twenty-eighth day after birth. Some of the available perinatal mortality statistics, however, are based on more restrictive definitions and may exclude infants weighing under 1000 gm or infants born before 28 weeks of fetal life, or deaths after 7 days of neonatal life.

Emphasis on perinatal mortality and morbidity has been the greatest single factor in bringing about a team approach, involving obstetricians, pathologists, pediatricians, public health officials and nurses, to the interrelated problems of fetal and neonatal life. Fetal and neonatal deaths contribute about equally to perinatal mortality. When a comparison is made, however, between fetal and neonatal deaths in different weight categories, fetal deaths make up a greater proportion of the perinatal mortality than neonatal deaths in the group of infants weighing over 2500 gm (Fig. 7–1). The key position of the obstetrician in the reduc-

TABLE 7–1 DEATH RATES PER 1000 LIVE BIRTHS FOR INFANTS IN THE UNITED STATES IN 1971 (est), ACCORDING TO COLOR

AGE	WHITE	NONWHITE
Less than 28 days	12.9	20.8
Under 1 year	16.8	30.2

Vital Statistics of the U.S. 1971, Wegman, M. E.: Annual Summary of Vital Statistics. Pediatrics *50*:956, 1972.

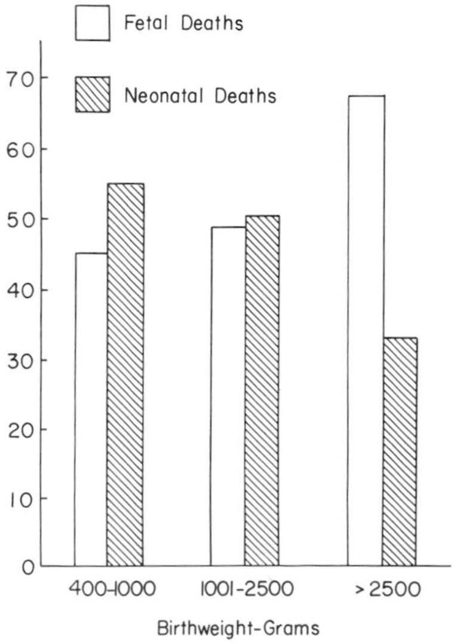

Figure 7–1 *Per cent distribution by weight of fetal and neonatal deaths. (From Behrman, R. E. (ed.): Neonatology. St. Louis, The C. V. Mosby Company, 1973.)*

TABLE 7–2 MAJOR AUTOPSY FINDINGS ON 501 NEWBORN INFANTS (1960-1966)*

	110–1000 gm.	1001–2500 gm.	2501 gm. +	TOTAL
Number of Infants	253	192	56	501
Pulmonary hyaline membrane	59	106	9	174
Inflammatory lesions (infection)	66	50	17	133
Intraventricular hemorrhage	86	43	1	130
Undetermined (over 500 gm)	35	14	3	52
Congenital anomalies	1	28	20	49
Immaturity (less than 500 gm)	47	0	0	47
Fetal anoxia	13	6	6	25
Trauma	0	3	4	7
Hemolytic disease of the newborn	1	2	4	7
Infants of diabetic mothers	2	1	3	6
Idiopathic hydrops	0	1	1	2
Tumor	0	0	1 (thyroid)	1
Totals	310	254	69	633†

*Valdes-Dapena, M. A., and Arey, J. B.: J. Pediatr. 77:366, 1970.
†Some infants had more than one major finding at autopsy.

tion of perinatal mortality and morbidity is obvious. Further, in recent years intrapartum fetal deaths have declined more than antepartum fetal deaths. This may reflect an increasing utilization of fetal monitoring during labor and a more liberal use of cesarean section for fetal distress, breech delivery, and other obstetric complications. It also emphasizes the need to be able to predict the maturity and functional reserve of the fetus prior to the onset of labor. Because of the high incidence of permanent handicaps, especially neurologic ones, among surviving infants with a history of low birth weight, anoxia, birth injury or malformations, research and public health efforts should be directed primarily at determination and elimination of the causes of these problems.

Perinatal and infant mortality rates vary from country to country; they are lowest in the Scandinavian countries and The Netherlands and highest in the so-called developing countries. Even though socioeconomic, cultural and perhaps geographic factors may be the most important influences which determine perinatal mortality, autopsy findings on liveborn infants indicate that there are potentials for further reductions in perinatal mortality by prophylactic health measures (Table 7–2).

The high incidence of disease and excessive mortality rate during the first few days of life emphasize the need to identify as early as possible those fetuses and infants who are at greatest risk. The obstetrician and pediatrician must maintain effective communication so that prenatal and natal problems may be anticipated and preventive and therapeutic measures taken promptly.

Of equal importance with the need to lower perinatal mortality rates is the need to lower the incidence of handicapping conditions resulting from untoward prenatal and natal factors. Since both mortality and permanent neurologic sequelae are in large measure caused by the same or similar disturbances, measures directed at reduction in perinatal mortality should also reduce the incidence of handicapping conditions. That this assumption has limitations is illustrated by the high incidence of mental retardation among infants who required vigorous and prolonged resuscitation at birth and of retinal and pulmonary damage among those who had prolonged exposure to high concentrations of oxygen in the immediate postnatal period.

The regulation of population growth will make it even more critical to combat diseases which may limit the biologic potential of the individual newborn infant. The urgency and importance of the need to diagnose, prevent and treat fetal and neonatal disease increases with a decreasing birth rate. The establishment of regional referral centers to provide appropriate facilities, personnel and equipment for intrauterine diagnosis and for intensive obstetric and neonatal care and observation should help to meet those needs.

THE FETUS

See also Section 2.

Fetal life as differentiated from embryonic life begins with the completion of organogenesis, which is about the twelfth week of gestation. Genetic and environmental influences that affect the fetus are at work even before conception. The genetic material contained in the chromosomes from each parent plays an important role not only in fetal development, but even in fetal survival; recognizable chromosomal abnormalities are 20 to 30 times more frequent among spontaneously aborted embryos and fetuses than among liveborn infants. Environmental factors may influence the selection and propagation of genes transmitted to the infant, as well as be responsible for mutations of parental genes.

The father's health may affect the motility of the spermatozoon and its ability to penetrate the ovum. Likewise the mother's health and state of nutrition may affect ovulation, the viability of the ovum and the zygote, and the availability of an adequate site for implantation; women who suffer from malnutrition or debilitating illness have diminished fertility and often diminished frequency of menstruation. Exposure of the zygote or embryo to drugs, chemicals, infectious diseases and other noxious influences may affect cell division and result in structural malformations. The general health and nutrition of the mother, and possibly her emotional health, during pregnancy also affect the fetus; the infants of malnourished mothers weigh less and are somewhat shorter at birth than those of mothers with adequate nutrition. Illness of the mother during pregnancy may result in fetal death, abortion or premature delivery.

The major emphases in fetal medicine are in four directions: (1) fetal effects of maternal disease; (2) fetal effects of drugs administered to the mother; (3) identification of fetal disease, particularly that of genetic origin; and (4) treatment of fetal disease. In time, increasing knowledge of fetal physiology may pave the way for practical approaches to problems of adaptation of the newborn infant, particularly of the premature one. Unfortunately much of our knowledge of fetal physiology has been obtained from animals and often is not directly applicable to man; the increasing use of primates for fetal studies provides physiologic information more applicable to the human fetus. A number of the known aspects of human fetal growth and development are summarized in Section 2.

MATERNAL DISEASE AND THE FETUS. Infections. Almost any maternal infection with severe systemic manifestations may result in abortion, stillbirth or premature labor. Whether these results are due to infection of the fetus or are secondary to the stress imposed on the mother by the infection is not always clear. Certain agents, however, do infect the fetus more or less regularly without relation to the severity of the maternal infection, and frequently with a disastrous effect on life or development. Such fetuses are frequently of low weight for their gestational age. Some infections, such as rubella, may also produce congenital malformations if they occur during the period of organogenesis. Infections which are known to cause disease in the fetus or newborn infant include *chickenpox* or *herpes zoster, Coxsackie* B *viruses, cytomegalovirus, hepatitis, herpes simplex, listeriosis, malaria* (abortion, premature delivery), *mumps* (fetal death and possibly endocardial fibroelastosis), *poliomyelitis* (abortion, congenital paralysis or poliomyelitis), *rubella, rubeola* (abortion, prematurity, fetal measles, ? congenital malformations), *smallpox* (fetal smallpox), *syphilis, toxoplasmosis, tuberculosis* (congenital tuberculosis), *vaccinia or vaccination* (fetal vaccinia), *vibrio fetus* (abortion, prematurity, meningitis) and *Western equine encephalitis* (encephalitis).

Noninfectious Diseases. *Maternal diabetes* usually results in hypertrophy and hyperplasia of the islets of Langerhans of the fetus, a finding also present in erythroblastosis fetalis. Most of the increase is due to increase in number and size of the beta cells. There is a high incidence of intrauterine death after the thirty-sixth week of gestation (see also disturbances of newborn infants of diabetic mothers, p. 395). *Toxemia* of pregnancy results in small size of the fetus for gestational age or in intrauterine death. These effects are probably due to placental insufficiency secondary to infarction. Uncontrolled *hypothyroidism* or *hyperthyroidism* in the mother is responsible for relative infertility, a tendency to abortion, premature labor and fetal death. The offspring even of treated hypothyroid mothers frequently have low intelligence quotients. Untreated maternal *phenylketonuria* results in abortion, congenital malformations and injury to the brain of the nonphenylketonuric fetus. *Placental tumors* may interfere with placental function and result in low birth weight for gestational age.

MATERNAL MEDICATION AND THE FETUS. The effects of drugs taken by the mother vary considerably, especially in relation to the time in pregnancy when they are taken. Abortion or congenital malformations result from maternal ingestion of teratogenic drugs during the period of organogenesis. Maternal medications taken later, especially during the last few weeks of gestation or during labor, tend to affect the function of specific organs or enzyme systems and to exert their chief adverse function on the neonate rather than on the fetus (Tables 7–3, 7–4). The teratogenic effects of drugs on the embryo may be limited to a specific period of gestation (40 to 60 days after the last menstrual period for thalidomide), and there may be genetically determined differences in susceptibility to some drugs. It is also conceivable that some drugs may be synergistic with others in their teratogenic effects. Nevertheless, exposure to drugs in pregnancy continues to be frequent. Surveys indicate that 90 per cent of pregnant patients have taken at least one drug. The average mother has taken four drugs other than vitamins or iron during pregnancy; 4 per cent have taken 10 or more drugs.

In view of the limited current knowledge of fetal effects from maternal medication, no drugs should be prescribed during pregnancy without weighing the maternal need against the risk of fetal damage.

IDENTIFICATION OF FETAL DISEASE (INTRAUTERINE DIAGNOSIS). The term "intrauterine diagnosis" applies to diagnostic procedures employed for the identification of disease in the fetus when interruption of the pregnancy is under consideration in the interest of the mother or of the baby, and in instances in which direct treatment of the fetus may be possible. In a broader context it might

TABLE 7–3 MATERNAL MEDICATIONS WHICH MAY ADVERSELY AFFECT THE FETUS AND NEWBORN INFANT

DRUG	EFFECT ON FETUS	DEPENDABILITY OF EVIDENCE
Adrenal corticosteroids	Cleft palate	Suggestive
Amphetamines	Congenital heart disease, transposition of the great vessels	Conclusive
Aminopterin	Abortion, malformations	Conclusive
Azathioprine	Abortion	Suggestive
Busulfan (Myleran)	Stunted growth, corneal opacities, cleft palate, hypoplasia of ovaries, thyroid and parathyroids	Doubtful
Chlorambucil	Renal agenesis	Suggestive
Chloroquine	Deafness	Doubtful
Chlorothiazide	Thrombocytopenia	Conclusive
Cigarette smoking	Low birth weight for gestational age	Suggestive
Cyclophosphamide	Multiple malformations	Suggestive
Dicumarol	Fetal bleeding and death, hypoplastic nasal structures	Conclusive
Insulin shock	Death	Conclusive
Lysergic acid diethylamide (LSD) or impurities in commercial preparations	Skeletal defects	Doubtful
	Chromosome damage	Suggestive
Meclizine (Bonine)	Congenital malformations	Doubtful
Mepivacaine	Bradycardia, death	Conclusive
6-Mercaptopurine	Abortion	Suggestive
Methimazole	Goiter	Conclusive
Methyltestosterone	Masculinization of female fetus	Conclusive
17-Alpha-ethinyl-19-nortestosterone (Norlutin)	Masculinization of female fetus	Conclusive
Phenmetrazine (Preludin)	Defect of diaphragm	Doubtful
Potassium iodide	Goiter	Conclusive
Progesterone	Masculinization of female fetus	Suggestive
17-Alpha-ethinyl testosterone (Progestoral)	Masculinization of female fetus	Conclusive
Propylthiouracil	Goiter	Conclusive
Quinine	Abortion, thrombocytopenia	Conclusive
	Deafness	Doubtful
Radioactive iodine (^{131}I)	Destruction of fetal thyroid	Conclusive
Stilbestrol	Masculinization of female fetus	Suggestive
	Vaginal adenocarcinoma in adolescence	Conclusive
Streptomycin	Deafness	Suggestive
Tetracycline	Retarded skeletal growth	Suggestive
	Pigmentation of teeth, hypoplasia of enamel	Conclusive
	Cataract, limb malformations	Doubtful
Thalidomide	Phocomelia, other malformations	Conclusive
Trimethadione and Paramethadione	Abortion, multiple malformations, mental retardation	Conclusive
Tolbutamide	Congenital malformations	Doubtful
Vitamin D	Supravalvular aortic stenosis, hypercalcemia	Doubtful

be applied also to those aspects of the family history, reproductive history of the mother, and course of the pregnancy which lead to the nonspecific diagnoses of "high-risk pregnancy" or "high-risk infant." (See later sections so named.)

Amniocentesis, the withdrawal of amniotic fluid during pregnancy for diagnostic purposes (Table 7–5), is most frequently done to determine the need for fetal transfusion or timing the delivery of fetuses with erythroblastosis fetalis. It is also done to determine the sex of the baby when the mother is known to carry a severe X-linked recessive trait such as hemophilia or progressive muscular dystrophy. Cells from the amniotic fluid can be stained and examined for the presence or absence of the sex chromatin (Barr) body; absence of Barr bodies in the stained nuclei indicates male sex and a child with a 50 per cent chance of having the disease in question. Cells from the amniotic fluid withdrawn as early as the tenth to fourteenth weeks of gestation may be grown in tissue culture and used for chromosomal or biochemical analysis. This technique has been successfully applied in pregnant women to identify normal karyotypes and fetuses with suspected genetic defects (see Table 6–8). Adrenal cortical hyperplasia has been diagnosed before birth through demonstration of higher than normal levels of pregnanetriol and 17-ketosteroids in amniotic fluid. Decreased function of the fetal-placental unit measured by low levels of estriol in amniotic fluid has been correlated with decreased maternal urinary estriol and with chronic fetal

TABLE 7–4 MATERNAL MEDICATIONS WHICH MAY ADVERSELY AFFECT THE NEWBORN INFANT

DRUG	EFFECT ON NEWBORN
Anesthetic agents (volatile)	Central nervous system depression
Adrenal corticosteroids	Adrenocortical failure
Ammonium chloride	Acidosis (clinically inapparent)
Caudal anesthesia with mepivacaine (accidental introduction of anesthetic into scalp of baby)	Bradypnea, apnea, bradycardia, convulsions
CNS depressants (narcotics, barbiturates, tranquilizers) during labor	Central nervous system depression
Cephalothin	Positive direct Coombs test reaction
Coumarin derivatives	High perinatal mortality
Hexamethonium bromide	Paralytic ileus
Intravenous fluids during labor, e.g. salt-free solutions	Electrolyte disturbances Hyponatremia
Lysergic acid diethylamide (LSD) or impurities in commercial preparations	Convulsions (?) Chromosome damage (?)
Morphine and its derivatives (addiction)	Withdrawal symptoms (poor feeding, vomiting, diarrhea, restlessness, yawning and stretching, dyspnea and cyanosis, fever and sweating, pallor, tremors, convulsions)
Naphthalene	Hemolytic anemia (in glucose-6-phosphate dehydrogenase [G-6-PD]-deficient infants)
Nitrofurantoin	Hemolytic anemia (in G-6-PD-deficient infants)
Primaquine	Hemolytic anemia (in G-6-PD-deficient infants)
Reserpine	Drowsiness, nasal congestion
Sulfonamides (long acting)	Interfere with protein binding of bilirubin: kernicterus at low levels of serum bilirubin
Thiazides	Neonatal thrombocytopenia
Vitamin K (excessive amounts)	Hyperbilirubinemia

distress in toxemia, severe maternal diabetes, prolonged gestation, maternal pyelitis and hemolytic disease of the newborn (erythroblastosis fetalis).

The best available chemical indices of fetal maturity are provided by determinations of amniotic fluid creatinine and lecithin, which reflect the maturity of fetal kidney and lung, respectively; after 36 weeks of gestation the creatinine concentration is at least 1.8 mg/dl of amniotic fluid in 98 per cent of pregnancies, with an amniotic fluid/maternal plasma creatinine ratio of 3:1 or greater. The lecithin concentration is usually at least 2 mg/dl, with an amniotic fluid lecithin/sphingomyelin ratio of at least 2.0.

Although amniotic puncture can be carried out with little discomfort to the mother, there is, even in experienced hands, a small risk of direct damage to the fetus, of placental puncture and bleeding with secondary damage to the fetus, of stimulating premature labor, of amnionitis, and of maternal sensitization to fetal blood. The earlier in gestation amniotic puncture is done, the greater the risk to the fetus. Therefore the procedure should be limited to those cases in which it is estimated that the value of the findings will outweigh the risk.

Ultrasonography, employing pulsed sound of short wavelength above the audible limit for man and of high resolution, is used to obtain serial, ac-

TABLE 7–5 APPLICATIONS OF AMNIOCENTESIS DURING PREGNANCY

Biochemical and cytogenetic studies in early pregnancy
Diagnosis and prognosis of erythroblastosis fetalis
Induction of abortion by intra-amniotic injection of hypertonic solutions or drugs
Treatment of polyhydramnios
Injection of radiopaque contrast material for amniography (amniotic fluid volume, hydatidiform mole, multiple gestation, fetal gestational age, fetal deformities, hydrops fetalis, placental localization, fetal function, e. g., swallowing)
Determination of amniotic fluid volume (indicator dilution)
Studies of amniotic fluid circulation
Determinations of fetal maturity
Fetal and placental function study (clearance of injected substances, hormones, etc.)
Induction of labor
Evaluation of amniotic fluid pressure and uterine contractility in labor
Instillation of pharmacologic agents for inhibition of uterine contractions or treatment of the fetus

curately measurable images of the fetus. More than 90 per cent of fetuses whose biparietal diameters measure 9.5 cm or more by ultrasonography weigh over 2500 gm. Fetal gestational age can be predicted between 20 weeks (biparietal diameter equals 5 cm) and 34 weeks (biparietal diameter equals 8.7 cm) with an accuracy of plus or minus 8 to 10 days in 95 per cent of instances. Ultrasonography has been successfully used to diagnose cranial malformations, multiple pregnancies after the sixteenth week, fetal death in utero, hydatidiform mole, and placenta previa; it is also used to locate the placenta prior to amniocentesis.

Continuous wave ultrasound is used for automatic simultaneous counting of fetal heart rate and uterine contractions to determine their relationship to each other. Deceleration in fetal heart rate, which occurs after the peak of uterine contraction (late deceleration or Type II dips), measured by amniotic fluid pressures, and a pattern of deceleration, which occurs irregularly both before uterine contraction starts and after it stops (variable deceleration), correlate with fetal distress, low Apgar score and fetal death. Cardiac arrhythmias have also been diagnosed by fetal electrocardiography, but changes in QRS complexes have not been correlated with fetal hypoxia. No injury to maternal or fetal tissues from pulsed or continuous ultrasound has been demonstrated to date.

Roentgenologic examination is rarely the diagnostic procedure of choice to estimate fetal maturity or to establish fetal diagnoses. If ultrasonography is available, it is substantially more accurate before 36 weeks of gestation and avoids the risks of genetic or developmental injury from diagnostic radiation. Roentgenograms are necessary, however, to detect bony or calcific abnormalities such as achondroplasia, infantile cortical hyperostosis, osteogenesis imperfecta or meconium peritonitis. The edema of fetal hydrops can be detected roentgenographically by edematous thickening of the fetal scalp ("halo sign"), absence of black "fat line" outlining fetal subcutaneous tissues, froglike position of legs, and abducted arms; the ribs may be elevated by enlargement of liver and spleen. Lipid-soluble contrast medium injected into the amniotic fluid (amniography) can be used to outline the fetal soft tissues to identify fetal hydrops and meningomyelocele, or to diagnose upper intestinal atresias through failure of the radiopaque material to traverse the gastrointestinal tract within 12 to 24 hours after injection.

Fetal scalp blood sampling during labor through a slightly dilated cervix may aid in establishing or confirming fetal distress suspected on the basis of variations in fetal heart rate or the presence of meconium in the amniotic fluid. Fetal hypoxia and circulatory insufficiency result in a mixed placental "respiratory" and metabolic acidosis which often, but not invariably, can be detected by the determination of pH, base deficit, and carbon dioxide tension in blood obtained from the fetal scalp. A pH less than 7.25 and base deficit greater than 10 mEq/l strongly suggest fetal distress. Such data may be used to determine whether operative delivery is indicated. Endoscopic examination of the amniotic cavity (*amnioscopy*) has also been employed prior to rupture of the membranes or amniocentesis to detect the presence of meconium in the amniotic fluid in severe toxemia and in abnormally prolonged gestations.

The *excretion of estriol in maternal urine* usually rises to 12 to 50 mg per 24 hours during the third trimester of pregnancy. Serial values between 4 and 12 mg per 24 hours may indicate fetal jeopardy in cases of maternal diabetes, hypertension or toxemia. Values below 4 mg have usually been associated with fetal death, particularly when they represent a documented fall from the normal range. Nevertheless the reliability of maternal estriol excretion as a guide in making decisions about operative intervention during pregnancy remains to be proved. Single or serial determinations of maternal plasma estriol, human placental lactogen, heat-stable alkaline phosphatase, diamine oxidase and oxytocinase have not been demonstrated to be clinically useful in evaluating the fetus; nor have single or serial determinations of maternal urinary excretion of pregnanediol, human chorionic thyrotropin, human chorionic gonadotropin or human chorionic somatomammotropin.

TREATMENT OF FETAL DISEASE. The treatment of diseases of the fetus continues to depend upon coordinated advances in accuracy of diagnosis, in understanding of fetal pathophysiology, pharmacology and immunology, in the availability of antimicrobial and especially antiviral drugs, and in therapeutic procedures. Progress in providing specific treatments for accurately diagnosed diseases has been limited.

Fetal syphilis is nearly always present in untreated maternal disease and can be specifically and safely treated. Fetal mortality associated with maternal bacterial urinary tract infections can be reduced with appropriate antibiotic treatment of the mother. Immunization has effectively reduced fetal mortality and morbidity from rubella.

The incidence of sensitization of Rh negative women by Rh positive fetuses has been reduced by the prophylactic administration of Rh(D) immune globulin to mothers after each delivery or abortion, thus reducing the frequency of hemolytic disease in their subsequent offspring. Fetal erythroblastosis fetalis may now be accurately diagnosed by amniotic fluid analysis and treated with induced premature delivery, which may be combined with intrauterine intraperitoneal transfusions of packed Rh negative blood cells to maintain the fetus until mature enough to have a reasonable chance of survival.

Fetal asphyxia or distress may now be diagnosed with moderate success through monitoring the fetal heart rate and through blood samples obtained by the scalp technique. Treatment, however, remains limited to supplying the mother with high concentrations of oxygen, positioning the uterus to avoid vascular compression, and operative delivery. Pharmacologic approaches to fetal asphyxia and immaturity (e.g., administration of oxygen and glucose to the mother, injection of sodium bicarbonate into the amniotic fluid) are still in an experimental stage. At present the treatment of definitively diagnosed genetic disease in a fetus consists of preventive genetic counseling and/or abortion. The nature of the genetic defect and its consequences as well as ethical concerns of parents, society and the physician must be taken into consideration.

HIGH-RISK PREGNANCIES

See also The High-Risk Infant. Pregnancies in which factors exist that increase the likelihood of abortion, fetal death, premature delivery, low birth weight, disease, congenital malformations, mental retardation or other handicapping conditions are termed high-risk pregnancies (Table 7–6). Some of these factors, such as ingestion of a teratogenic drug in the first trimester, bear a causal relation to the risk; others, such as hydramnios, are associations which merely serve to alert the physician to the existence of the risk or risks. Ten to 20 per cent of pregnant patients can be identified as "high risk" on the basis of their medical history, and over half of all perinatal mortality and morbidity is associated with these pregnancies.

The identification of high-risk pregnancies is important not only because it is the first step toward prevention, but also because in many instances therapeutic steps may be taken to reduce the risks to the fetus or to the neonate, if the physician is alerted to the increased possibility of difficulty. A decreased incidence of low-birth-weight infants correlates with the provision to and the acceptance of good prenatal care by indigent women. Identification and optimum management of high-risk pregnancies are dependent on careful attention to the family history, reproductive history of the mother, course of the pregnancy, and the delivery, *together with close and continuing personal communication between the physician caring for mother and fetus and the physician who will care for the infant after birth.*

GENETIC FACTORS. The occurrence of chromosomal abnormalities, congenital anomalies, inborn errors of metabolism, mental retardation or indeed of any familial disease in blood relatives increases the risk of the same condition in the infant. Because many parents are not aware of the name or existence of these genetically determined diseases, but only of one or more of their manifestations, specific inquiry should be made about any disease affecting more than one blood relative. (See the following sections: Prenatal Factors in Disease; Inborn Errors of Metabolism; Jaundice in the Newborn; Metabolic Disorders; Diseases of the Blood; Mental Retardation; The Bones and Joints; The Muscles; The Skin; The Eye; Allergy; Abnormalities of the Chromosomes; and the sections on each of the systems of the body.)

MATERNAL FACTORS. The lowest neonatal mortality rate (about 2 per cent) occurs in infants of mothers 20 to 30 years of age; it is almost doubled if the mother is 40 to 45 years, and quadrupled if she is 45 or over. The neonatal mortality rate is also high if the mother is less than 15 years of age.

Maternal illness increases the risk to a pregnancy; the degree varies with the illness and its severity. The dangers of incompatibility between maternal and fetal blood groups are discussed in Section 14. Certain diseases in the mother may be transiently manifest in and constitute a risk to her newborn infant. Platelet antibodies may be transferred across the placental membrane to cause temporary platelet deficiency in the infant. Likewise myasthenia gravis and hyperthyroidism may be manifest for a few weeks in the infants of mothers with these diseases. Maternal hyperparathyroidism may result in tetany of the newborn. Certain drugs (Tables 7–3, 7–4) increase the risk to the pregnancy when administered to the mother during its course. Maternal toxemia, diabetes mellitus and blood group incompatibilities may increase the risk to the pregnancy by influencing obstetric management as well as through direct effects on the fetus. Lactation tends to be less successful in the toxemic woman. Prematurity, stillbirth and neonatal death are twice as frequent in infants born to toxemic mothers as in those born to healthy ones. Maternal malnutrition may lead to small size of the baby for gestational age. Multiple pregnancies, particularly those involving monochorionic twinning, are at risk when compared to single pregnancies.

Polyhydramnios is associated with various congenital malformations (Table 7–7) and is present in approximately 80 per cent of infants with trisomy 18 (Section 6). Atresias of the upper intestinal tract presumably interfere with the reabsorption into the circulation of swallowed amniotic fluid; faulty fetal formation or release of antidiuretic hormone is postulated as the mechanism of hydramnios in fetuses with anomalies of the central nervous system. Conversely, congenital aplasia or hypoplasia of the fetal kidneys is often accompanied by a reduced amount of amniotic fluid *(oligohydramnios)*, presumably because fetal urine has not been formed (Table 7–7). Oligohydramnios from whatever cause before the last few weeks of pregnancy may result in mechanically induced abnormalities of the fetal limbs, such as genu recurvatum (Section 22). Intrauterine amputations or

TABLE 7–6 FACTORS ASSOCIATED WITH HIGH-RISK PREGNANCY

A. Demographic Factors
   1. Lower socioeconomic status
   2. Disadvantaged ethnic groups
   3. Marital status: unwed mothers
   4. Maternal age
      a. Gravida less than 16 years of age
      b. Primigravida 35 years of age or older
      c. Gravida 40 years of age or older
   5. Maternal weight: nonpregnant weight less than 100 pounds or more than 200 pounds
   6. Stature: height less than 62 inches (1.57 m)
   7. Malnutrition
   8. Poor physical fitness
B. Past Pregnancy History
   1. Grand multiparity: 6 previous pregnancies terminating beyond 20 weeks' gestation
   2. Antepartum bleeding after 12 weeks of gestation
   3. Premature rupture of membranes, premature onset of labor, premature delivery
   4. Previous cesarean section or mid- or high-forceps delivery
   5. Prolonged labor
   6. Infant with cerebral palsy, mental retardation, birth trauma, central nervous system disorder or congenital anomaly
   7. Reproductive failure: infertility, repetitive abortion, fetal loss, stillbirth, or neonatal death
   8. Delivery of preterm (less than 37 weeks) or post-term (more than 42 weeks) infant
C. Past or Present Medical History
   1. Hypertension or renal disease or both
   2. Diabetes mellitus (overt or gestational)
   3. Cardiovascular disease (rheumatic, congenital, or peripheral vascular)
   4. Pulmonary disease producing hypoxemia and hypercapnia
   5. Thyroid, parathyroid, and endocrine disorders
   6. Idiopathic thrombocytopenic purpura
   7. Neoplastic disease
   8. Hereditary disorders
   9. Collagen diseases
   10. Epilepsy
D. Additional Obstetric and Medical Conditions
   1. Toxemia
   2. Asymptomatic bacteriuria
   3. Anemia or hemoglobinopathy
   4. Rh sensitization
   5. Habitual smoking
   6. Drug addiction or habituation
   7. Chronic exposure to any pharmacologic or chemical agent
   8. Multiple pregnancy
   9. Rubella or other viral infection
   10. Intercurrent surgery and anesthesia
   11. Placental abnormalities and uterine bleeding
   12. Abnormal fetal lie or presentation, fetal anomalies, oligohydramnios, polyhydramnios
   13. Abnormalities of fetal or uterine growth or both
   14. Maternal trauma during pregnancy
   15. Maternal emotional crisis during pregnancy

other malformations due to local constriction during fetal growth may result from amniotic bands or fibrous strings, presumably formed as a result of rupture of the fetal membranes early in gestation.

Obstetric factors are of understandable importance when one considers that neonatal mortality is greatest during the first 24 hours after delivery. A pregnancy should be considered high risk when the uterus is inappropriately large or small. A uterus that is large for the estimated stage of gestation suggests multiple fetuses, hydramnios, or an excessively large infant; an inappropriately small one suggests retardation of intrauterine growth. Rupture of membranes earlier than 24 hours before delivery carries a risk of infection of the intrauterine contents and increased perinatal mortality. Prolonged and difficult labors increase the risks of mechanical and hypoxic damage. The risk of neonatal deaths in uncomplicated labors lasting 24 hours or less is approximately 0.3 per cent; it increases sixfold in labors lasting over 24 hours, and to 6 per cent (twentyfold) in those over 30 hours. A tumultuous short labor, with a precipitate delivery, increases the risk of intracranial hemorrhage. Placental separation at any time prior to delivery, and abnormal implantation or compression of the cord increase the possibility of brain damage from fetal anoxia; brown or muddy amniotic fluid at the time of rupture of the membranes or of prior endoscopic examination suggests that meconium has been passed during an episode of fetal anoxia. Likewise, the occurrence of a transient unusual increase of fetal movement suggests fetal distress due to anoxia.

Although the relative danger of any type of delivery depends upon the skill of the obstetrician, an increased hazard accompanies certain methods (Table 7–8). Obviously this results not only from the method, but also from the circumstances which dictated its use. Neonatal deaths following deliveries by mid and high forceps, breech extraction and version are likely to be related to intracranial injury; those following other forms of delivery are more apt to be due to anoxic disturbances.

Infants born by cesarean section present problems which may be related to the unfavorable obstetric circumstance which necessitated the operation, or to prolonged maternal anesthesia. The impression prevails, however, that even in the absence of these factors, delivery through the abdomen carries a greater risk than delivery through the birth canal. Though the neonatal mortality

TABLE 7–7 FETAL MALFORMATIONS FREQUENTLY ASSOCIATED WITH POLYHYDRAMNIOS OR OLIGOHYDRAMNIOS

POLYHYDRAMNIOS	OLIGOHYDRAMNIOS
Anencephaly (in approximately 20 per cent of cases)	Renal agenesis
Meningocele and encephalocele	Ureteral dysplasia
Esophageal or duodenal atresia	Urethral atresia
Pyloric stenosis	Pulmonary hypoplasia
Klippel-Feil syndrome	Amnion nodosum
Cleft palate and harelip	
Achondroplasia	
Diaphragmatic defects	
Multiple anomalies (not central nervous system)	

TABLE 7–8 MORTALITY RATES PER 1000 BIRTHS BY VARIOUS METHODS OF DELIVERY

	WHITE			BLACK		
METHOD OF DELIVERY	*No. Births*	*Perinatal Death Rate*	*Neonatal Death Rate*	*No. Births*	*Perinatal Death Rate*	*Neonatal Death Rate*
Spontaneous vertex vaginal	7108	31.1	13.7	12135	31.4	17.0
Outlet forceps	4017	6.5	3.2	2594	12.3	8.1
Low forceps	3308	11.8	5.8	2166	10.6	5.6
Mid forceps	2009	14.4	8.0	964	15.6	10.4
High forceps	4	250.0	250.0	7	142.9	142.9
Breech (Total)	626	207.7	104.7	519	314.1	168.2
Spontaneous	69	550.7	295.5	98	459.2	209.0
Internal version	7	1000.0	1000.0	4	750.0	500.0
Partial extraction	287	146.3	82.4	283	229.7	131.5
Total extraction	245	175.5	86.0	111	360.4	211.1
Cesarean section	921	66.2	46.6	992	62.5	41.2

Adapted from The Collaborative Perinatal Study of the National Institute of Neurologic Disease and Stroke: The Women and Their Pregnancies. U.S. Department of Health, Education, and Welfare Publication No. (NIH) 73-379, 1973.

rate from elective cesarean section performed at term by a skilled obstetrician with an experienced anesthetist is extremely low, occasional deaths do occur. A small number of infants so delivered have some degree of respiratory difficulty for a day or two after birth, and idiopathic respiratory distress syndrome is the condition most frequently associated with an unfavorable outcome.

Anesthesia and analgesia affect the fetus as well as the mother; mild maternal hypoxemia or hypotension may result in severe fetal hypoxia and shock. Skilled use of medication consists in avoiding severe fetal narcosis while securing the benefits of gentle and unhurried delivery. Even skilled use often results in a mildly depressed infant whose crying and breathing may be delayed a minute or two and who may be somewhat inactive for several hours. Such infants are of less concern than those in whom an apparently similar status has been produced by anoxia or trauma. When anesthesia and analgesia are carelessly used, or when their milder effects are added to already unfavorable fetal circumstances such as prematurity, anoxia or trauma, the result may be catastrophic.

THE NEWBORN INFANT

See also Section 2.

The *newborn* or *neonatal* period, the first 28 days of life, is a highly vulnerable time during which many of the physiological adjustments required for extrauterine existence are completed. Its importance is attested by the high morbidity and mortality rates; in the United States over two thirds of the deaths in the first year of life occur in the first 28 days after birth. In turn, deaths during the first year of life occur at an annual rate not again reached until the seventh decade.

The transition from intrauterine to extrauterine life requires many biochemical and physiologic changes. Removal from dependence on the maternal circulation via the placenta imposes the necessity of activation of pulmonary function for purposes of exchange of oxygen and carbon dioxide, of gastrointestinal function for absorption of food, of renal function for excretion of wastes and maintenance of chemical homeostasis, of liver function for neutralization and excretion of toxic substances, and of function of the immunologic system for protection against infection. The cardiovascular and endocrine systems also undergo adaptations necessitated by removal from maternal and placental support. Many of the special problems of the newborn infant are related to interference with or failure of these biochemical and physiologic adjustments, owing to premature birth, anatomic abnormalities or adverse environmental influences, either intrauterine or arising at or after birth.

THE HISTORY IN NEONATAL PEDIATRICS

The medical history of the neonatal infant should (1) be aimed at early identification of diseases in which disability or mortality may be prevented by prompt treatment, (2) lead to anticipation of conditions which may be of later importance, and (3) uncover possible causative factors which may help to explain any pathologic condition regardless of its immediate or future significance. Ideally, a detailed family history, including the mother's current and past pregnancies, should be elicited and recorded for every newborn infant (see also High-Risk Pregnancy).

PHYSICAL EXAMINATION OF THE NEWBORN INFANT

The purposes of the initial examination of the newborn infant as soon as possible after delivery are twofold: to detect abnormalities, and to establish a baseline for subsequent examinations. Since examination in the mother's presence affords an ideal opportunity for initiating the anticipatory guidance which should be an integral part of all periodic health examinations, a second one should be performed when she has had a chance to rest from the rigors of her labor. At this time even minor anatomic variations which seem insignificant should be explained, because the mother may be disturbed if she has to point them out or if the physician does not appear to give them adequate consideration. This procedure carries the possibility of unduly alarming otherwise unworried parents unless it is carefully and skillfully done. No infant should be discharged from the hospital without a final examination, since certain abnormalities, particularly heart murmurs, frequently appear or disappear in the immediate neonatal period, or there may be evidence of acquired disease. Pulse and respiratory rates, weight, length, head circumference, and dimensions of any visible or palpable structural abnormality should be recorded.

Many of the physical and behavioral characteristics of the newborn infant are described in Section 2; that section should be consulted before reading this.

The examination of the newborn infant requires patience, gentleness and flexibility in routines of procedure. Thus, if the infant is quiet and relaxed when first approached, palpation of the abdomen or auscultation of the heart should be performed before other, more disturbing manipulations.

General Appearance. Physical activity may be absent in the relaxation of normal sleep or depressed by illness or drugs; the infant may be lying with motionless extremities because all his energies are conserved for the effort of difficult breathing, or he may be vigorously crying with accompanying activity of arms and legs. Coarse, tremulous movements with ankle or jaw clonus are more common and of less significance in newborn infants than at any other age. Such movements tend to occur when the infant is active, whereas convulsive twitching usually occurs in an otherwise quiet state. Nutritional status is evidenced by weight and length and by wrinkling or smoothness of the body surfaces. An appearance superficially suggesting good nutrition may be produced by edema. There may or may not be pitting after pressure, but the fingers and toes will lack the normal fine wrinkles over the knuckles because they are puffed out with fluid. Edema of the eyelids is a common result of irritation from silver nitrate. Generalized edema may be an accompaniment of prematurity. It may also result from hypoproteinemia secondary to severe erythroblastosis fetalis (hydrops fetalis), congenital nephrosis, Hurler's syndrome or unknown cause. Localized edema suggests a congenital malformation of the lymphatic system; when confined to one or more extremities of a female infant, it may be the presenting sign of Turner's syndrome (Section 17).

Skin. Vasomotor instability and sluggishness of peripheral circulation are revealed by deep redness or purple lividity in the crying infant, whose color may darken profoundly with closure of the glottis preceding a vigorous cry, and by harmless cyanosis of the hands and feet, especially when these are cool. Mottling is another example of general circulatory instability. An extraordinary division of the body from forehead to pubis into a red half and a pale half has been aptly named a **harlequin color change**. This is transient, apparently harmless, and inadequately explained. Significant cyanosis may be masked by pallor in circulatory failure; on the other hand, the relatively high hemoglobin content of the first few days and the thin skin may combine to produce an appearance of cyanosis when the arterial oxygen saturation is adequate. Localized cyanosis is differentiated from ecchymosis by the momentary pallor which follows pressure. The same maneuver is also helpful in demonstrating icterus, which may be of considerable degree, but pass unnoticed if the skin is suffused with blood. *Pallor* may represent anoxia, anemia, shock or edema. Early recognition of anemia may lead to a lifesaving diagnosis of erythroblastosis fetalis, rupture of the liver, subdural hemorrhage, or fetal-maternal or inter-twin transfusion. Postmature infants tend to have whiter skin than do term or premature ones.

The vernix is described in Section 23, as are the common transitory capillary hemangiomas of the eyelids and neck. Slate-blue, well demarcated areas of pigmentation are seen over the buttocks and back and sometimes other parts of the body in about half of black infants and occasionally in white ones. These have no known anthropologic significance in spite of their designation as **mongolian spots;** they tend to disappear within the first year. The vernix, skin and, especially, the cord may be stained a brownish yellow if the amniotic fluid has been colored by passage of meconium during or before birth, usually because of intrauterine anoxia. The skin of the premature infant is thin and delicate and tends to be deep red; in extreme degrees of prematurity the appearance is almost gelatinous. Fine, soft, immature hair, lanugo hair, frequently covers the scalp and brow in the premature infant; it may also cover the face. Lanugo hair has usually been lost or replaced by vellus hair in the term infant. The nails are rudimentary at very premature birth; conversely, they may protrude beyond the fingertips in infants born past term. Such infants also tend to have a peeling, parchment-like skin (Fig. 7–8); a severe degree of parchment-like skin suggests ichthyosis congenita (Section 23).

The **skull** may be molded, particularly if the infant is the firstborn and if the head has been engaged for a considerable time. The parietal bones tend to override the occipital and the frontal bones. The head of an infant born by cesarean section or from a breech presentation is identified by its characteristic roundness. The suture lines and the size and tension of the anterior and posterior fontanels should be determined digitally. There is much variation in the size of the fontanels at birth; if small, the anterior fontanel usually tends to increase during the first few months of life. Persistence of excessively large anterior and posterior fontanels has been associated with hypothyroidism. Soft areas **(craniotabes)** are occasionally found in the parietal bones at the vertex near the saggital suture; they are usually inconsequential, but, if they persist, should be differentiated from other causes of craniotabes. Soft areas in the occipital region suggest the irregular calcification and **wormian bone** formation associated with osteogenesis imperfecta, cleidocranial dysostosis, cretinism and occasionally Down's syndrome. Transillumination of the skull in a dark room will rule out hydranencephaly or porencephaly (Section 20).

The **face** may be asymmetric from fetal posture (Section 11); when the jaw has been held against a shoulder or an extremity during the intrauterine period, the mandible may deviate strikingly from the midline. The skull of the premature infant may suggest hydrocephalus because of the relatively larger brain growth as compared to that of other organs. The **eyes** are often opened spontaneously if the infant is held up and tipped gently forward and backward. This is undoubtedly a result of labyrinthine and neck reflexes. This maneuver is more successful than that of forcing the lids apart to inspect the eyes. Focus and equality of pupils are normally established some weeks after birth. Conjunctival and retinal hemorrhages do not by themselves have serious significance. Deformities of the pinnae of the **ears** are seen occasionally. Unilateral or bilateral preauricular papillomas occur fairly frequently; if pedunculated, they can be ligated tightly at the base, and dry gangrene and slough will result. The tympanic membrane is easily visualized otoscopically through the short, straight external auditory canal and is normally dull in appearance. There may be a slight obstruction of the *nose* from an accumulation of mucus in the narrow nostrils. The **mouth** rarely may show precocious dentition, with supernumerary teeth in the lower incisor position or aberrantly placed; these teeth are shed before the deciduous ones erupt. Premature eruption of deciduous teeth is even more unusual.

On the hard palate on either side of the raphe may be temporary accumulations of epithelial cells called **Epstein's pearls.** Retention cysts of similar appearance may also be seen on the gums. Both disappear spontaneously, usually within a few weeks of birth. Clusters of small white or yellow follicles or ulcers on an erythematous base may be found on the anterior tonsillar pillars, most frequently on the second or third day of life. Their cause is unknown, and they clear without treatment in 2 to 4 days. There is no active salivation. The **tongue** appears relatively large; the frenulum may be short, but rarely, if ever, is this a reason for cutting it. Occasionally, the sublingual mucous membrane forms a prominent fold. The *cheeks* have a fullness on both the buccal and the external aspects due to the accumulation of fat which makes up the sucking pads. These pads, as well as the labial tubercle on the upper lip, disappear when the suckling days are over.

The **throat** of the newborn infant is hard to see because of the arch of the palate; this, however, should be clearly visualized because of the possibility of easily missed clefts of the posterior palate or uvula. The small tonsils give no clue to the size to be attained during later lymphoid tissue growth.

The **neck** appears relatively short. Abnormalities are not common; they include goiter, cystic hygroma, branchial cleft rests and lesions of the sternocleidomastoid muscle, which are presumably traumatic (Section 21). Redundant skin or webbing in a female infant suggests Turner's syndrome (Section 17).

Almost as much can be learned about the **lungs** by observation of breathing as by auscultation and percussion. Variations in rate and rhythm are characteristic. The rate may vary from 20 to 100 per minute in normal infants, fluctuating according to physical activity, state of wakefulness or presence of crying. Because fluctuations are rapid, counting of the respiratory rate should be done for a full minute with the infant in the resting state, preferably asleep. Under these circumstances the usual rates for normal term infants are 30 to 40 per minute; for premature infants they are higher and fluctuate more widely. Rates that are consistently over 60 per minute during periods of regular breathing usually indicate cardiac or pulmonary insufficiency. Miller divides newborn infants into three groups, depending on the trend of their resting respiratory rates (Table 7–9). The premature infant may normally breathe with a Cheyne-Stokes rhythm, known as periodic respiration, or with complete irregularity. Periodic respiration is rare in the first 24 hours of life. At any stage of maturity irregular gasping, sometimes accompanied by spasmodic movements of the mouth and chin, strongly indicates serious impairment of respiratory centers.

The breathing of newborn infants is almost entirely diaphragmatic, with the result that the soft front of the thorax is commonly drawn inward during inspiration and the abdomen simultaneously protruded. If the baby is quiet, relaxed and of good color, this "paradoxical movement" is not necessarily a sign or an evidence of insufficient ventilation. On the other hand, labored respiration is important evidence of abnormal pulmonary ventilation,

TABLE 7–9 FIRST-WEEK DEATHS ACCORDING TO BIRTH WEIGHT AND RESPIRATORY GROUP

RESPIRATORY GROUP	BIRTH WEIGHT—(GM) 1001–1500		1501–2000		2001–2500		TOTAL	
	BORN	DIED	BORN	DIED	BORN	DIED	BORN	DIED
I	2	0	20	0	104	0	126	0
II	2	0	30	0	90	0	122	0
III	31	11	42	10	29	2	102	23

Group I: Infants who, while quiet, breathe approximately 40 times per minute from birth on without fluctuations greater than 15 per minute.

Group II: Infants whose respiratory rates are high (usually over 60 per minute) the first hour, show no significant increase after the first hour and subsequently decrease to normal levels, usually within 4 to 48 hours after birth.

Group III: Infants whose respiratory rates show a significant increase (15 per minute or more over the mean for the first hour) during the first 48 hours.

Infants with major anomalies or with hemolytic disease of the newborn were excluded.

Adapted from Miller, H. C.: *Pediatrics 20*:817, 1957.

pneumonia or other mechanical disturbance of the lungs. The intercostal tissues are usually drawn in during respiration when the mechanical difficulty is either too much or too little air in the lungs, so that the differentiation between atelectasis and emphysema must be made from the size and shape of the chest, the percussion note and roentgenographically. The weak groaning or whining cry which often accompanies expiration in severe disturbances of respiration is a most unfavorable prognostic sign. A method of "retraction scoring" which, along with the respiratory rate and the presence or absence of cyanosis, affords a convenient gauge of respiratory difficulty in newborn infants is illustrated in Figure 7–2. This method, which is applicable an hour or two after birth, should not be confused with the Apgar scoring system, which is used to evaluate the infant in the minutes immediately after birth.

Percussion may be more informative than auscultation, because in the small total area of the lungs breath sounds from an adjoining region may be heard as though directly under the stethoscope. Normally the breath sounds are bronchovesicular. Suspicion of diminished breath sounds should always be verified by inducing deeper breathing and, if a local area is suspicious, altering the position of the infant's head and body before final decision. This latter maneuver also applies to suspected percussion dullness. The fine, crackling rales of early pneumonia in the newborn may at times be heard only at the end of the deep inspirations induced by crying.

The size of the **heart** is estimated with some difficulty, owing to normal variations in the size and shape of the chest. There may be transitory murmurs; conversely, congenital malformations may not at once produce the murmur which will be present later. According to Richards, there is only a 1:12 chance that a murmur heard at birth represents congenital heart disease. Evaluation of the heart by roentgenogram and electrocardiogram is desirable when the possibility of significant lesions exists. The pulse may vary normally from 70 per minute in relaxed sleep to 180 during activity. The still higher rate of paroxysmal tachycardia may be counted better on an electrocardiogram than by ear. Premature infants, whose resting heart rate is

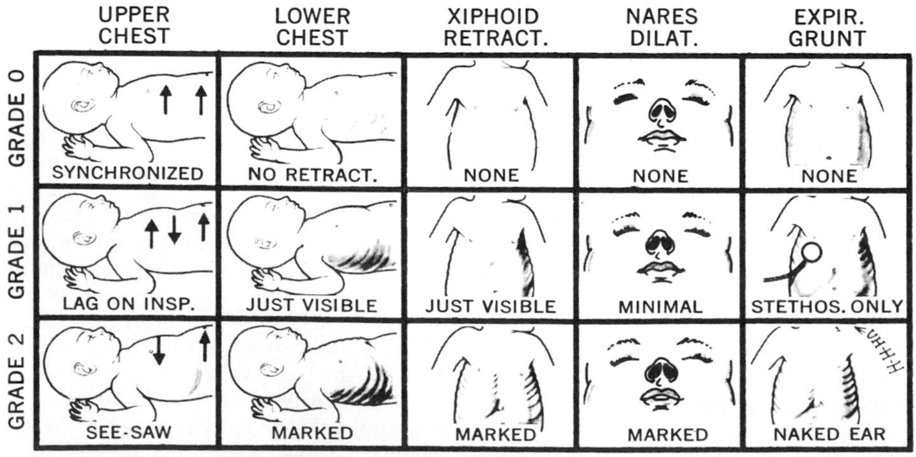

Figure 7–2 Criteria of respiratory distress. Grade 0 for each criterion indicates no respiratory distress; grade 2 for each criterion indicates severe respiratory distress. Abbreviations: *DILAT., dilatation; EXPIR., expiratory; INSP., inspiratory; RETRACT., retraction; STETHOS., stethoscope. (Courtesy of Mead Johnson & Company, Evansville, Ind.; adapted from Silverman and Andersen: Pediatrics, 17:1, 1956.)*

usually 140 to 150, may have a sudden onset of sinus bradycardia, not infrequently associated with nodal escape. The rate may fall as low as 32 beats per minute. Extrasystoles also occur with some frequency, and sinus arrest with nodal escape may be observed during continuous electrocardiographic monitoring. These arrhythmias are most frequently observed during drowsiness or deep sleep, but a significant number occur during gastrointestinal stimulation (defecation, regurgitation, insertion of a rectal thermometer, insertion of a gavage tube). Many are accompanied by a "startle" reaction. Immaturity of the autonomic nervous system has been postulated as the basic reason for the occurrence of these arrhythmias; a causative relation to sudden unexpected death among premature infants has also been proposed.

Blood pressure measurements may be a valuable diagnostic aid. (See Section 13). The *auscultatory method* can often be used satisfactorily, provided the stethoscope head is small enough. The *Doppler method* utilizes a transducer in the cuff to transmit and receive ultrasound waves. It detects movements of the arterial wall to provide a more accurate measure of systolic and diastolic pressures. Other methods are the *palpatory method*, in which the systolic blood pressure is taken to be the point at which the pulse distal to the cuff becomes palpable in the course of deflation, and the *flush method*, in which the extremity is first compressed to render it relatively bloodless below the cuff followed by deflation of the cuff, with the systolic pressure recorded at the point flushing appears in the arm and hand below the cuff. Each has the disadvantage that the pulse pressure is not obtained and that the reading lies between the systolic and diastolic pressures obtained by the auscultatory method. Continuous or intermittent direct measurement of blood pressure using an umbilical artery catheter may be indicated under special circumstances for infants under close observation in an intensive care unit.

In the **abdomen** the liver is usually palpable, sometimes as much as 2 cm below the rib margin. Less commonly the spleen and kidneys may be felt. The approximate size and location of each kidney can usually be determined on deep palpation when this is indicated. Unusual masses should be investigated immediately by "flat film" and cross-table lateral film of the abdomen, followed by intravenous pyelography and exploratory laparotomy if their innocent nature cannot be established. Urinary tract anomalies, renal embryoma, ovarian cysts and intestinal duplications are the commonest masses encountered. Abdominal distention at or shortly after birth suggests perforation of the gastrointestinal tract, which is often due to meconium ileus. Later it suggests lower bowel obstruction or peritonitis. Scaphoid abdomen in the newborn suggests diaphragmatic hernia. At no other period of life is the air content of the gastrointestinal tract so varied in amount, nor may it be so relatively great under normal circumstances. The abdominal wall is normally weak (especially in premature infants), and diastasis recti and umbilical hernias are common, particularly among black infants.

The **genitalia** and **mammary glands** normally respond to transplacentally obtained maternal hormones to produce enlargement and secretion of the breasts in both sexes and prominence of the female genitalia, often with considerable nonpurulent secretion. These are transitory manifestations requiring observation but no interference. The scrotum is relatively large; its size may be increased by the trauma of breech delivery and also by a transitory hydrocele, which is distinguished from a hernia by palpation and transillumination. The testes may be in the scrotum or palpable in the canals, or may not be felt until they descend spontaneously, which may not occur until later infancy. The male black infant usually has dark pigmentation of the scrotum before the rest of the skin assumes its permanent color.

The prepuce of the newborn infant is normally so tight and adherent that no information can be obtained as to later need for circumcision. Apparent hypospadias or epispadias should always arouse suspicion of abnormality of the sex chromosomes (Section 17) or that the infant is actually a masculinized female with enlarged clitoris, since this may be the first evidence of the adrenogenital syndrome (Section 17). Erection of the penis is common and has no significance. Urine is usually passed during or immediately after birth; there may then normally follow a period without voiding, unusually as long as 24 hours.

Some passage of *meconium* usually occurs within the first 12 hours after birth, but may be delayed until the third or fourth day. Imperforate **anus** is not always visible and may require evidence obtained by the gentle insertion of the examiner's little finger or a rectal tube. Roentgenographic study is required. The dimple or irregularity of skinfold often normally present in the sacrococcygeal midline may be mistaken for an actual or potential pilonidal sinus.

In examining the **extremities** the effects of fetal posture (Section 22) should be noted if for no other reason than that their cause and usual transitoriness can be explained to the mother. The suspicion of a fracture or nerve injury associated with delivery is more commonly aroused by observing the extremities in spontaneous or stimulated activity than by any other means.

Neurologic Examination. See Section 19.

ORDINARY CARE OF THE NEWBORN INFANT

The basic requirements of the newborn infant are immediate assistance at birth, when needed, for the *establishment of respiration* and subsequent assistance in obtaining *adequate nutrition,* in maintaining a *normal body temperature* and in *avoiding contact with infection.* These require-

TABLE 7–10 EVALUATION OF THE NEWBORN INFANT

SIGN	0	1	2
Heart rate	Absent	Below 100	Over 100
Respiratory effort	Absent	Slow, irregular	Good, crying
Muscle tone	Limp	Some flexion of extremities	Active motion
Response to catheter in nostril (tested after oropharynx is clear)	No response	Grimace	Cough or sneeze
Color	Blue, pale	Body pink, extremities blue	Completely pink

Sixty seconds after the complete birth of the infant (disregarding the cord and placenta) the 5 objective signs above are evaluated, and each is given a score of 0, 1 or 2. A total score of 10 indicates an infant in the best possible condition.

Modified from Apgar, V.: *Current Res. Anesth. & Analg. 32*:260, 1953.

ments should be met in an environment which not only provides constant nursing and medical alertness for any sign of specific illness, but also reduces separation of the infant from his mother to a necessary minimum. The care of full-term and premature infants differs only in the degree of emphasis on each of the three general factors just listed.

CARE IN THE DELIVERY ROOM. The infant should be suspended head downward immediately after delivery until the mouth, pharynx and nose have been cleared of fluid, mucus, blood, and amniotic debris by gravity and gentle suction with a bulb syringe or soft rubber catheter. Wiping the palate and pharynx with gauze may lead to abrasions and the development of thrush, pterygoid ulcers (Bednar's aphthae) or, rarely, to tooth bud infection with maxillary osteomyelitis and retrobulbar abscess formation. If the infant appears to be in satisfactory condition, he should then be placed on his side, head downward, in a bassinet tilted at an angle of about 30 degrees to promote drainage from the respiratory tract for 4 to 8 hours. When there is a possibility of intracranial hemorrhage following difficult delivery, the reverse position may be indicated. As a guide to prognosis and the need for particularly close observation or care in the delivery room and nursery, the 1- and 5-minute Apgar method of scoring is of practical value (Table 7-10). *It should be taken at 1 minute as an index of asphyxia and of the need for assisted ventilation;* the 5-minute score is a more accurate index of likelihood of death (Figs. 7–3 and 7–4) or neurologic residual (Table 7–11). Infants with prolapsed cord or delayed delivery and evidence of intrauterine asphyxia should receive prompt resuscitation (see later). For reasons not clear, the stomachs of infants delivered by cesarean section may contain more fluid than those of infants delivered normally. It is recommended that the stomach be emptied, preferably before the first breath is taken, in order to prevent possible aspiration of gastric contents.

Maintenance of Body Heat. Relative to body weight, the body surface of the newborn infant is approximately three times that of the adult, and the insulating layer of subcutaneous fat is thinner, particularly in infants of low birth weight. The

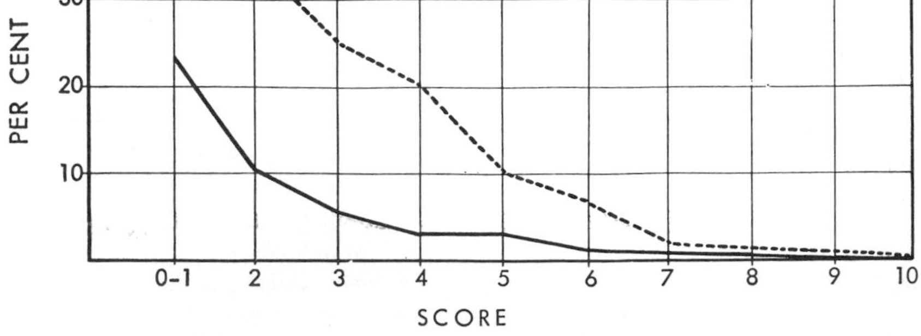

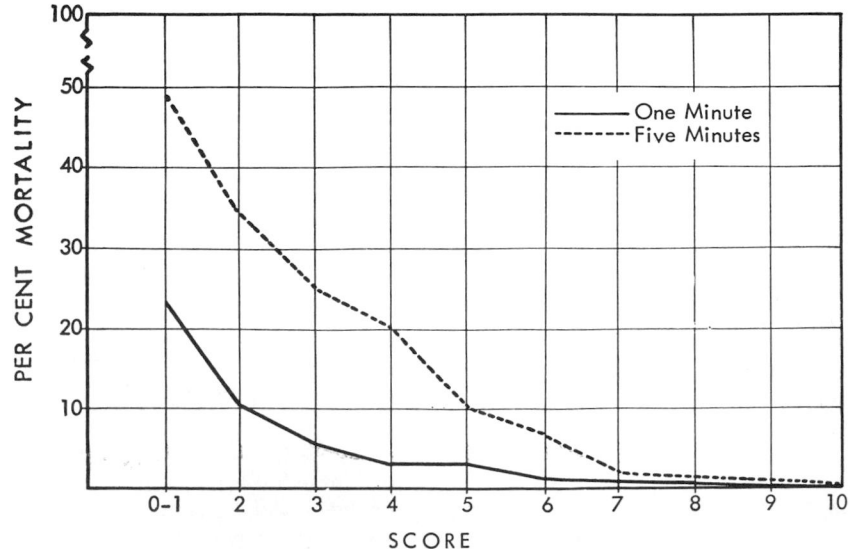

Figure 7–3 *Percentage of infants with various Apgar scores dying during first 28 days of life: comparison of outcome according to scores recorded at 1 minute and at 5 minutes. (From Drage, J. S., and Berendes, H.: Pediat. Clin. N. Amer., 13:635, 1966.)*

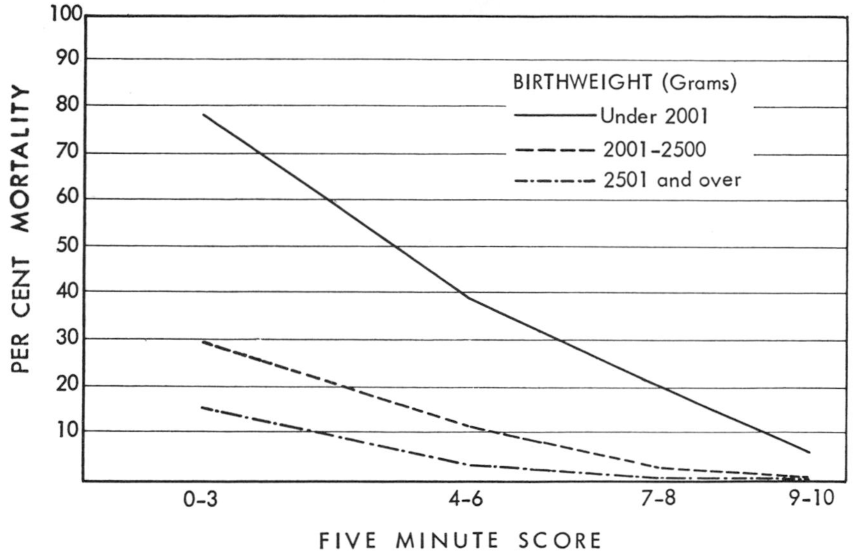

Figure 7–4 *Mortality (percentage) during first 28 days of life of infants with various Apgar scores recorded at 5 minutes, arranged according to birth weight. (From Drage, J. S., and Berendes, J.: Pediat. Clin. N. Amer., 13:635, 1966.)*

rate of heat loss in the newborn is estimated to be approximately four times that of an adult. Under conditions usual in hospital delivery rooms skin temperature falls approximately 0.3°C and deep body temperature approximately 0.1°C per minute during the period immediately after delivery, resulting usually in a cumulative loss of 2 to 3°C in deep body temperature (corresponding to a heat loss of approximately 200 calories per kg). Oxygen consumption in the newborn infant correlates with the gradient between skin and environmental temperatures; it is least when the gradient is less than 1.5°C. Conversely, even slight increases in body temperature of the infant increase oxygen consumption. After labor and vaginal delivery many newborn infants have a mild to moderate metabolic acidosis which is compensated by elimination of carbon dioxide; this compensation is more difficult for depressed infants, and progressive metabolic and respiratory acidosis may result from prolonged exposure to usual room temperatures. Likewise, lower levels of blood glucose are associated with hypothermia. In view of these factors it is desirable to protect the infant from heat loss immediately after birth. This is traditionally done by drying the infant and wrapping him or her with blankets, procedures which are frequently overlooked in the bustle of the delivery room, especially during resuscitation. Since placement of the infant in a preheated closed incubator makes it difficult to carry out resuscitative measures, an open-ended incubator or a heating pad with a protective covering and/or a radiant heat light suspended above the bassinet for immediate reception of the baby may be used.

Antiseptic Skin and Cord Care. In order to reduce the incidence of skin and periumbilical infection, the entire skin and cord should be cleansed in the delivery room, or upon admission to the nursery, with sterile cotton soaked in warm water and/or a detergent solution. A cotton-tipped applicator can be used to cleanse thoroughly the creases where the cord meets the umbilicus. The infant may be rinsed with water at body temperature, if care is taken to avoid chilling. The baby is then dried and wrapped in sterile blankets and taken to the nursery. To lessen the chance of carrying pathogenic organisms into the nursery, the outer blanket can be discarded at the nursery door. Subsequent daily bathing in the nursery or any other necessary washing should be done in a similar manner. Total body exposure to repeated bathing with detergent solutions containing 3 per cent hexachlorophene over prolonged periods may be neurotoxic. Therefore, frequent bathing with such solutions is no longer recommended. A single bath with a 3 per cent hexachlorophene solution at 2 to 4 hours of life, followed by an immediate, thorough rinse, significantly reduces the rate of colonization by *Staphylococcus aureus*. Judicious use of such baths may be indicated where there is a high risk of staphylococcal colonization in a particular nur-

TABLE 7–11 NEUROLOGIC ABNORMALITY AT 1 YEAR OF AGE, BY BIRTH WEIGHT AND 5-MINUTE APGAR SCORE

FIVE-MINUTE APGAR SCORE	BIRTH WEIGHT		
	1001–2000 gm	*2001–2500 gm*	*2501 gm or Over*
0–3	19%	13%	4%
4–6	14%	5%	4%
7–10	9%	4%	1%

Adapted from Drage, J. S., and Berendes, H.: *Pediat. Clin. N. Amer 13*:635, 1966.

sery or when there is a minor skin infection. Nursery personnel should continue to use hexachlorophene-containing detergents or similar effective agents for routine handwashing. Rigid enforcement of hand-to-elbow washing by staff and visitors entering the nursery for 2 minutes in the initial wash and 15 to 30 seconds in the second wash is recommended. Shorter but equally thorough washes between infants also should be required. Initial and daily painting of the umbilical cord stump with a bactericidal dye also may be used until hospital discharge in an attempt to reduce bacterial colonization.

Other Measures. The *eyes* of all infants must be protected against gonorrheal infection. The instillation of 1 per cent silver nitrate drops is the best-proved and only universally lawful method. Prompt subsequent irrigation of the eyes with isotonic saline solution reduces the incidence of chemical conjunctivitis without affecting the prophylactic efficacy.

Though hemorrhage in the newborn may be due to factors other than vitamin K deficiency, an intramuscular injection of 1.0 mg of water-soluble vitamin K_1 is recommended for all infants immediately after birth in order to correct any coagulation defect related to vitamin K deficiency and to prevent the usual neonatal decrease in plasma prothrombin level. Larger amounts may predispose to the development of hyperbilirubinemia and kernicterus and should be avoided. Administration of vitamin K to the mother during labor is less dependable.

NURSERY CARE. Infants not in the "high-risk" category may be taken after examination in the delivery room to the "regular" newborn nursery, or may be placed in the mother's room if the hospital has a rooming-in arrangement.

The bassinet should be easily and frequently cleaned and preferably be of clear plastic material to allow easy visibility. All care should be given in the bassinet; this includes physical examination, change of clothing, temperature-taking, skin cleansing and other procedures which, if performed elsewhere, establish a common point of contact and provide a channel for cross infection. The clothing and bedding should be the minimum needed for the infant's comfort; a constant temperature of approximately 75°F in the nursery simplifies problems of clothing. The temperature of the infant may be taken by rectum or, if properly done, in the axilla. The interval depends on many circumstances, but need not be less than 4 hours during the first 2 or 3 days and 8 hours thereafter. Axillary temperatures of 96 to 99°F are considered within normal limits.

Skin care has been described previously. Clothing can be put on the bathed or unbathed baby. Vernix is spontaneously shed within 2 to 3 days; much of it will adhere to the clothing, which should be completely changed daily. The diaper should be checked before and after feeding and when the baby cries. When wet or soiled, it should be changed. Meconium or feces should be cleansed from the buttocks with sterile cotton moistened with sterile water. The foreskin of the male infant should not be retracted.

Little is gained by frequent *weighing* of the healthy infant. Weighing at birth and on alternate days thereafter is sufficient, and even less frequent weighing is satisfactory for the majority of infants.

The problems of staphylococcal infections in the nursery are discussed near the end of Section 7.

FEEDING. Only the initiation of feeding will be considered here (See Section 3 for other details). More mistakes are made by feeding the infant too much or too early than too little or too late. Inadequate fluid intake, particularly in hot weather, may, however, result in "dehydration fever"; feedings are customarily instituted gradually, beginning 6 to 12 hours after birth. Satisfactory progress is being made if the infant is no longer losing weight by the seventh day and is gaining by the fourteenth. Many infants are unnecessarily fed artificially merely because the physician did not acquaint the mother with the delays normally encountered in establishing breast feeding.

If the principles of feeding are understood by the mother and the nursery staff, fixed routines will have little applicability. The schedule is less important than the principle of unhurried beginning and patient assistance and support by the nurse who takes the infant to the mother. But since some general plan may be useful from the standpoint of the hospital, the following is suggested: During the first 6 to 12 hours after birth no feeding is given. The infant is taken to the mother for the first feeding at 10 A.M. or 6 P.M., whichever is nearer the end of the 12-hour period of postnatal rest. Subsequent feedings are given every 4 hours day and night except for the first two nights, when no 2 A.M. feeding is given. Artificially fed infants should receive 5 per cent glucose or water for the first feeding, since regurgitation and aspiration of these liquids are not likely to cause significant irritation of the respiratory tract. There is no clear need for complicating neonatal care by the addition of vitamins until the infant is about 2 weeks of age.

The High-Risk Infant

(See also High-Risk Pregnancies.)

In order to improve care and to decrease neonatal morbidity and mortality, it is useful to single out those liveborn infants who are at particular risk during the first few days and weeks of life. The term "high-risk infant" has come into common usage to designate infants who should be under close observation by the most interested and experienced nurses available and visited frequently by a physician until such time as complications arising from the circumstances leading to the increased risk may no longer reasonably be expected. The duration of such observation is usually a few days, but may be only a few hours or several weeks. Large institutions may find it advantageous to provide a special nursery for the care of high-risk infants in the hospital.

Infants considered to be in the high-risk category include those (1) born before 37 or after 42 weeks of gestation; (2) weighing less than 2500 grams; (3) who are disparate from expected size or development, e.g., low or very high weight for gestational age determined either by the date of the mother's last menstrual period, by physical examination or by intrauterine evaluation (Fig. 7–5); (4) with a history of serious neonatal illness or death of a sibling, or of more than two fetal deaths of siblings; (5) in poor condition at delivery (Apgar 0 to 4 at 1 minute) or requiring resuscitation in the delivery room or subsequently in the nursery; (6) born to mothers with infections or with a history of any illness during pregnancy, with premature rupture of the membranes, with toxemia, diabetes mellitus or other metabolic disease, with a history

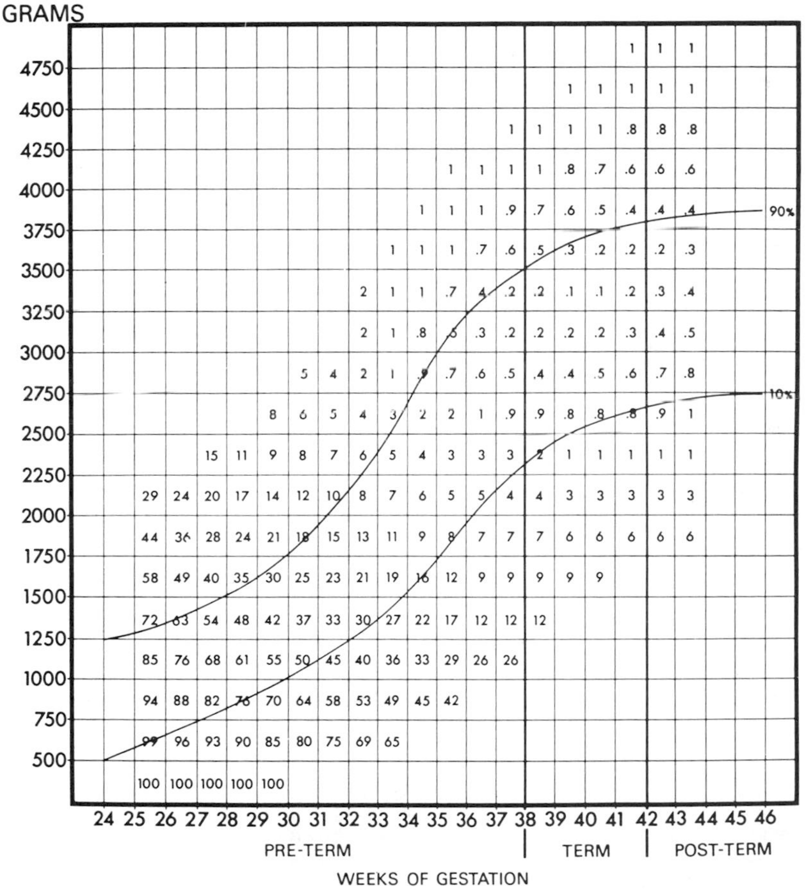

Figure 7–5 *Curvilinear zones of mortality rates obtained by connecting blocks having similar mortality rates. Numbers indicate mortality rate per 100 newborn infants. Infants below the 10th percentile are small for gestational age (SGA), and those above the 90th percentile are large for gestational age (LGA). Those infants between the 10th and 90th percentiles have weights appropriate for gestational age (AGA). Different shades indicate zones of risk, from lowest (white) to highest (gray). (From Lubchenco, L. O., Searls, D. T., and Brazie, J. V.: Neonatal mortality rate: Relationship to birth weight and gestational age. J. Pediatr. 81:814, 1972.)*

of a severe social problem such as teen-age pregnancy, drug addiction or absence of mate, with absent or long-delayed prenatal care, with minimal or no weight gain during pregnancy, with prolonged infertility, with four or more previous pregnancies, who are 35 years or more of age, or who have a history of taking any of the medications listed in Tables 7–3 and 7–4 during pregnancy; (7) of multiple pregnancy or of a gestation commencing within 3 months of a previous pregnancy; (8) delivered operatively or with any unusual obstetric complication, including hydramnios; (9) having a single umbilical artery, or any important malformation or suspicion of one; (10) being observed for anemia or blood group incompatibility; and (11) born to mothers who have had stressful events during gestation, such as severe emotional problems, hyperemesis gravidarum, serious accidents or general anesthesia.

With or without the other conditions mentioned, the majority of high-risk infants are either born prematurely or have low weight for gestational age. Generally speaking, for any given duration of gestation, the lower the birth weight, the higher the neonatal mortality, and, for any given weight, the shorter the duration of gestation, the higher the neonatal mortality (Table 7–12). The highest risk of neonatal mortality is among infants who weigh less than 1000 gm at birth and whose gestation was less than 30 weeks. The lowest risk of neonatal mortality is among infants with birth weights of 3000 to 4000 gm and whose gestational age was 38 to 42 weeks. Nevertheless, approximately 40 per cent of all perinatal deaths occur after 37 weeks of gestation in infants whose weights are 2500 gm or greater; many of these deaths occur in the period immediately before birth, and are more readily preventable than those of smaller and more immature infants. In addition, neonatal mortality rates rise sharply for infants whose birth weight is over 4000 gm and for those whose gestational period is 42 weeks or more

Figure 7–5 is useful for rapid identification of high-risk infants according to birth weight and gestational age.

MULTIPLE PREGNANCIES

INCIDENCE. The reported incidence of twins is highest among blacks and East Indians, followed by whites of northern European extraction, and lowest among the Mongolian races. In the United States twins occur in approximately 1 of 86 pregnancies; some other ratios are: Belgium, 1:56; United States blacks, 1:70; United States whites, 1:88; Italy, 1:86; Greece, 1:130; Japan, 1:150; China, 1:300. Differences in the incidence of twins exist mainly in fraternal (polyovular) twins. Identical (monovular) twins constitute 25 to 33 per cent of twins in all racial and ethnic groups. It is roughly estimated that triplets occur in 1 of 86^2 pregnancies and quadruplets in 1 of 86^3 pregnancies in the United States. Quintuplets, sextuplets and septuplets are rare. The incidence of females increases with the number of fetal products of a multiple pregnancy, reaching approximately 53.5 per cent for quadruplets, as opposed to approximately 48.5 per cent among single births.

CAUSES. The occurrence of monovular twins appears to be independent of genetic or environmental influences. Polyovular pregnancies are more frequent beyond the second pregnancy, in

TABLE 7–12 NEONATAL MORTALITY RATES BY BIRTH WEIGHT AND GESTATIONAL AGE, NEW YORK CITY, 1957-1959 (SINGLE WHITE LIVEBORN INFANTS)

GESTATION (WEEKS)	BIRTH WEIGHT (GM) ≤ 1000	1001–1250	1251–1500	1501–1750	1751–2000	2001–2250	2251–2500	2501–3000	3001–3500	3501+	TOTAL
0-27	944.8	800.0	615.9	305.6	147.1	219.5	111.1	73.2	41.7	83.3	674.2
28	887.3	645.6	594.3	517.2	218.8	74.1	58.8	34.5	20.0	–	400.0
29	833.3	476.9	471.7	442.3	160.7	161.3	68.2	12.0	22.2	27.8	291.0
30	862.1	526.3	474.5	407.4	383.7	137.3	39.0	25.4	–	15.2	207.1
31	772.7	518.5	362.6	274.0	375.0	179.5	73.7	16.7	4.1	20.6	166.9
32	866.7	590.9	400.0	252.3	190.3	109.9	98.7	25.2	23.7	6.1	112.6
33	800.0	294.1	509.4	287.7	142.9	102.6	92.5	16.4	5.0	4.3	70.6
34	750.0	400.0	342.1	205.9	128.3	63.8	46.7	24.5	11.4	13.6	41.6
35	777.8	333.3	285.7	250.0	107.0	57.3	28.1	20.6	10.8	13.0	28.4
36	777.8	125.0	416.7	127.7	84.1	47.3	23.8	13.8	5.0	7.7	17.1
37	714.3	333.3	360.0	156.9	91.8	56.6	18.9	9.3	5.4	9.2	12.0
38	666.7	666.7	71.4	239.1	111.1	39.0	12.2	6.0	4.1	5.0	6.7
39	500.0	400.0	277.8	303.0	68.8	37.0	19.0	4.3	3.3	3.6	4.8
40	428.6	500.0	222.2	178.6	76.3	49.0	16.0	5.8	4.0	3.1	4.7
41–42	714.3	333.3	476.2	350.0	149.1	47.9	21.1	9.6	3.6	4.0	5.7
43+	1000.0	666.7	500.0	230.8	139.5	77.8	41.3	12.3	7.6	8.0	10.4
Total	917.0	613.9	464.8	283.4	151.9	61.6	24.8	8.1	4.3	4.5	14.1

From Yerushalmy, J.: *J. Pediatr. 71*:164, 1967.

older women and in families with a history of polyovular twins. They may result from simultaneous maturation of multiple ovarian follicles, but follicles containing two ova have been described as a genetic trait leading to twin pregnancies. Polyovular pregnancies occur in many women treated for infertility with human pituitary or menopausal urinary gonadotropins or other experimental drugs.

Conjoined twins (Siamese twins) are probably the result of relatively late monovular twinning, as is the presence of two embryos in one amniotic sac. The latter condition has a high fatality rate, owing to obstruction of the circulation secondary to intertwining of the umbilical cords. The prognosis for conjoined twins depends on the possibility of surgical separation.

Superfecundation, the fertilization of an ovum by an insemination which takes place after one ovum has already been fertilized, has occasionally been advanced as the cause of differences in size and appearance of twins. *Superfetation,* the fertilization and subsequent development of an ovum when a fetus is already present in the uterus, has been proposed as a reason for differences in size of certain twins at birth, but evidence to support this theory is lacking.

MONOZYGOTIC VERSUS DIZYGOTIC TWINS. The identification of twins as monozygotic or dizygotic (monovular or polyovular) is important because the study of monozygotic twins is useful to determine the relative influence of heredity and environment on human development and disease. Twins who are not of the same sex are dizygotic. Among twins of the same sex, zygosity should be determined and recorded at birth through careful examination of the placenta, or later through comparison of physical characteristics, detailed blood typing or even trial of tissue transplant from twin to twin, if the determination is of critical importance. It is desirable to furnish the parents with a written report of the results of such examinations.

EXAMINATION OF THE PLACENTA. An *accurate, carefully recorded* examination of the placenta is the simplest and best way of differentiating between monovular and polyovular twins. It may also reveal information of more immediate clinical importance.

Inspection of the placenta is carried out with knowledge of the sex and birth of the twins and with identification of the cords as belonging to twin 1 or to twin 2. If the placentas are separate, they are always dichorionic, but the twins are not necessarily dizygotic, since initiation of monovular twinning at the first cell division or during the morula stage may result in two amnions, two chorions, and even two placentas. Therefore twins of the same sex, if not monochorionic, should be reevaluated between the ages of 2 and 4 years, when physical criteria for identification of monovular twins tend to be most valid. At this time differences caused by inequalities of intrauterine existence have been largely erased and differences created by extrauterine environmental factors have not yet become notable. If there are important physical differences by 2 to 4 years of age, dichorionic twins may be presumed to be dizygotic. If they are physically identical, detailed blood grouping studies should be carried out in an attempt to determine their zygosity.

An apparently single placenta may be present with either monovular or polyovular twins. Yet inspection of the polyovular placenta reveals for each fetus a separate chorion which crosses the placenta between the attachments of the cords. Separate or fused dichorionic placentas may be disproportionate in size. The fetus attached to the smaller placenta or portion of placenta is then usually smaller than its twin, or is malformed. Monochorionic twins may be presumed to be monovular. They are usually diamnionic. Monoamnionic twins have a high rate of stillbirth of one or both twins because of interference with one or both fetal circulations because of extensive intertwining of the umbilical cords.

Placental vascular anastomoses are seen with high frequency in monochorionic twins, and the resulting exchange of blood proteins and cells may have as much to do with later homograft tolerance between monovular twins as does their common genetic make-up. Vascular anastomoses between dichorionic twins have not been described, although the possibility may be inferred from the reported existence of blood group chimeras in heterosexual twins. The female members of such human twin pairs are reproductively competent, phenotypically normal women rather than freemartins as seen in bovine heterosexual twin pairs. Such twins also appear to tolerate reciprocal skin homografts almost as if they were autografts.

The vascular anastomoses in monochorionic placentas may be artery-to-artery, vein-to-vein or artery-to-vein. Usually they are fairly well balanced, so that neither twin suffers. In rare cases one umbilical cord may arise from the other after leaving the placenta. In such instances the twin attached to the secondary cord is usually malformed or dies in utero. Table 7–13 lists the more frequent

TABLE 7–13 CHARACTERISTIC CHANGES IN MONOCHORIONIC TWINS WITH UNCOMPENSATED PLACENTAL ARTERIOVENOUS SHUNTS

TWIN ON ARTERIAL SIDE	TWIN ON VENOUS SIDE
Oligohydramnios	Polyhydramnios
Small premature	Large premature
Malnourished	Well nourished
Pale	Plethoric
Anemic	Polycythemic
Hypovolemic	Hypervolemic
Shock	Cardiac failure
Microcardia	Cardiac hypertrophy
Glomeruli small or normal	Glomeruli large
Arterioles thin-walled	Arterioles thick-walled

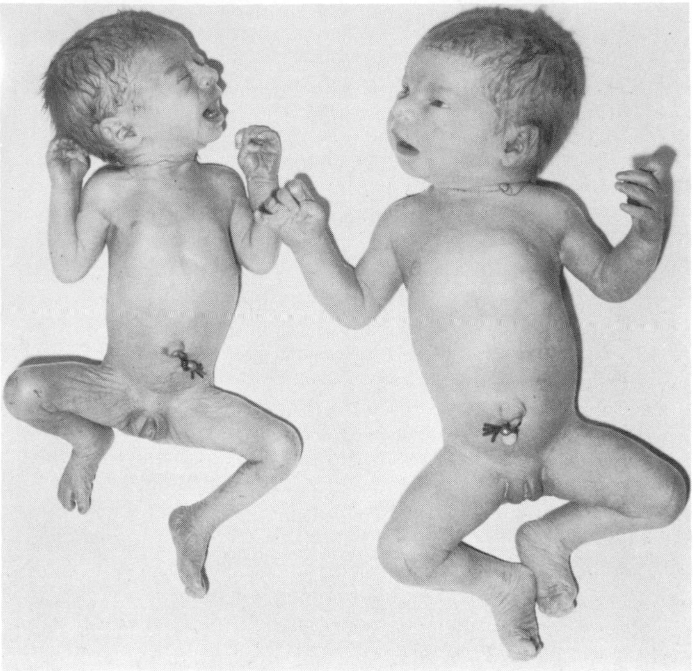

Figure 7–6 *Slightly premature monochorionic "identical" twins at birth. Twin 1 at left weighed 3 pounds 12 ounces, and twin 2 at right weighed 5 pounds 15 ounces. Note appearance of dehydration in groin of smaller twin. (From Benirschke, K.: New York State J. Med., 61:1499–1508, 1961.)*

changes associated with a large uncompensated arteriovenous shunt from the placenta of one twin to that of the other (Fig. 7–6); twins of widely discrepant size are usually monochorionic.

Maternal hydramnios in a twin pregnancy should always lead to suspicion of the "fetal transfusion syndrome." Anticipation of this possibility may lead to lifesaving readiness to give a transfusion to the donor twin or to bleed the recipient twin. The additional cardiac load as evidenced by arteriolar hypertrophy in a distressed recipient twin suggests that digitalization might be indicated. Death of the donor twin in utero may result in generalized fibrin thrombi in the smaller arterioles of the recipient twin, possibly as the result of transfusion of thromboplastin-rich blood from the macerating donor fetus.

POSTNATAL IDENTIFICATION. *Physical criteria* for determining monovular twins are as follows: (1) both must be of the same sex; (2) their features, including ears and teeth, must be obviously alike (but they need not resemble one another more than the lateral halves of one individual); (3) their hair must be identical in color, texture, natural curl and distribution; (4) their eyes must be of the same color and shade; (5) their skin must be of the same texture and color (nevi may be differently apportioned and distributed); (6) their hands and feet must be of the same conformation and of similar size; and (7) their anthropometric values must show close agreement. Dermatoglyphics are of limited use in the diagnosis of zygosity; though prints of monozygous twins may have similar patterns, they are not identical and may be quite dissimilar.

Although *detailed blood typing* can offer absolute proof only that twins are dizygotic, with currently available methods a reasonable presumption of monozygosity may be made if no blood group discrepancies can be demonstrated between twins. Smith and Penrose calculated that in twins who are alike in sex, and in ABO, MNSs, P, Rh, Lutheran, Kell, Lewis, Duffy and Kidd factors, the chance of dizygosity is 0.0116.

PROGNOSIS. Most twins are born prematurely, and maternal complications of pregnancy are more common than with single pregnancies. There is no significant difference between the neonatal mortality rates of twin and single births in comparable weight groups. Yet since most twins are premature by weight, their overall mortality is higher than that of single births. The perinatal mortality of twins is about fourfold that of singletons. The incidence of malformations incompatible with life is greater in multiple than in single pregnancies. There is also an increased incidence of velamentous insertion of the umbilical cord, with an associated higher risk of bleeding during labor. Monoamniotic twins have an increased likelihood of entangling their cords, which may lead to asphyxia. In general, mortality rates of twins do not vary with order of birth if macerated fetuses are excluded. If one of the fetuses is macerated, the live twin is usually delivered first. Theoretically the second twin is more subject to anoxia than is the first because of the possibility that the placenta may separate after the birth of the first twin and before the birth of the second. Notable differences in size at birth of monovular twins usually disappear by the time the infants are 6 months of age. In contrast to the aforementioned lack of statistically significant difference in the mortality of liveborn twins when compared with liveborn single births in comparable weight groups, Benirschke has

TABLE 7–14 PERINATAL MORTALITY OF TWINS ACCORDING TO PLACENTATION

TYPE	BABIES	DEATHS	%
Monoamnionic-monochorionic	6	3	50
Diamnionic-monochorionic	120	28	23
Diamnionic-dichorionic, fused	126	6	5
Diamnionic-dichorionic, separated	148	14	9
Total monochorionic	126	31	25
Total dichorionic	274	20	7

Adapted from Benirschke, K.: *New York State J. Med. 61*:1499, 1961.

shown (Table 7–14) that there appears to be a significant increase in perinatal mortality among monochorionic twins.

MANAGEMENT. Prenatal diagnosis enables the obstetrician and the pediatrician to anticipate the birth of infants who are at high risk because of twinning. Close observation is indicated during labor and in the immediate neonatal period, so that prompt treatment of asphyxia or "fetal transfusion syndrome" can be initiated. The decision to perform an immediate blood transfusion in a severely anemic "donor twin" or to bleed or perform a partial exchange transfusion of a "recipient twin" must be based on clinical judgment.

PREMATURITY AND LOW BIRTH WEIGHT

DEFINITION. Liveborn* infants delivered before 37 weeks from the first day of the last menstrual period are considered to have a shortened gestational period and are termed *premature.* Infants who weigh 2500 gm or less at birth are considered to have had either a shortened gestational period, a less than expected rate of intrauterine growth, or both, and are termed *infants of low birth weight.* Prematurity and low birth weight are usually concomitant, particularly among infants weighing 1500 gm or less at birth, and both are associated with increased neonatal morbidity and mortality. (See High-Risk Infant.)

Since the length of the normal gestational period is essentially the same for all human populations, the foregoing definition of prematurity is considered to be universally applicable. Yet the range of birth weights of infants born at each gestational age varies from one population group to another. Hence, ideally the definition of low birth weight should be set for individual populations which are genetically and environmentally as homogeneous as possible.

HISTORY. For statistical purposes in the United States, since 1935 a premature infant has been defined as a liveborn infant weighing 2500 gm (5 pounds 8 ounces) or less at birth. This definition was also adopted by the World Health Organization in 1950, but its Expert Committee on Maternal and Child Health in 1961 recommended that the term "premature" be replaced by the more appropriate term "low birth weight" and that the term "premature" be used only for infants born less than 37 weeks after the beginning of the mother's last menstrual period. The American Academy of Pediatrics has adopted these recommendations.

Since most of the statistical data of the last 30 years have not related low birth weight to gestational age, many concepts about "prematurity" may have to be changed as statistics based on this relationship are evaluated. Figure 7–5 and Table 7–12 indicate observed variations in neonatal mortality based on birth weight in respect to gestational age.

INCIDENCE OF PREMATURITY. Because statistical emphasis on gestational age as well as on birth weight is recent, the incidence of prematurity (short gestation) has not been adequately determined. Nevertheless, in a largely Caucasian population with a 6.7 per cent incidence of low-birth-weight infants (1000 to 2500 gm), Usher found that approximately half of the low-birth-weight infants had a gestational age of 37 weeks or more. About 4 per cent of the infants who weighed over 2500 gm had gestational ages less than 37 weeks, and the number of premature births among the larger infants was greater than in the low-weight group.

INCIDENCE OF LOW BIRTH WEIGHT. In the United States (1965) 7.2 per cent of white liveborn infants and nearly 14 per cent of nonwhite ones weighed 2500 gm or less (Table 7–15); the incidence varies from 6 to 16 per cent in different areas and populations. In the United States there are approximately twice as many infants born weighing less than 1500 gm than in Sweden; the mortality of this group is about 50 per cent. Since such variability exists throughout the world (Table 7–16), it will be necessary to develop for individual countries and population groups correlations of birth weight and gestational age with risks of neonatal morbidity and mortality. Black, Indian and other South Asian infants tend to weigh less at birth than white and North Asian infants of the same gestational ages; the incidence of birth weight of 2500 gm or less is greater among blacks than among whites in the United States. The perinatal and neonatal mortality rates in each low-weight group, however, are lower for black infants than for white ones.

FACTORS RELATED TO PREMATURE BIRTH OR LOW BIRTH WEIGHT. Because of failure until recently to record both gestational age and low birth weight in the compilation of birth statistics, it is rarely possible to separate completely factors associated with prematurity from those associated

*Live birth is defined by the World Health Assembly (1950) as "the complete expulsion or extraction from its mother of a product of conception . . . which, after such separation, breathes or shows any other evidence of life such as beating of the heart, pulsation of the umbilical cord, or definite movement of the voluntary muscles, whether or not the umbilical cord has been cut or the placenta is attached." This definition is approved by the American Public Health Association.

TABLE 7–15 PERCENTAGE DISTRIBUTION OF LIVE BIRTHS BY BIRTH WEIGHT GROUP AND COLOR, UNITED STATES, 1967*

	500 GM OR LESS	501–1000	1001–1500	1501–2000	2001–2500	2501–3000	3001–3500	3501–4000	4001–4500	4501–5000	OVER 5001 GM
White	0.1	0.4	0.5	1.3	4.6	17.6	38.6	27.8	7.7	1.3	0.2
Nonwhite	0.2	0.9	1.2	2.6	8.4	25.9	38.1	18.1	3.8	0.7	0.1
Total	0.1	0.4	0.6	1.5	5.3	19.0	38.5	26.1	7.0	1.2	0.2

*From Chase, H. C.: Am. J. Pub. Health *60*:1967, 1970.

with low birth weight. In about one third of low-birth-weight infants the birth weight is less than would be expected for gestational age calculated from the mother's last menstrual period. Thus, the small size is due primarily to a retarded rate of intrauterine growth; in the remainder the low weight is appropriate for the early date of delivery (Table 7–17). In general, *premature birth* is associated with conditions in which there is inability of the uterus to retain the fetus, artificial interference with the course of the pregnancy, premature separation of the placenta, or a stimulus to effective uterine contractions prior to term. *Low birth weight for gestational age* is associated with conditions which interfere with the circulation and efficiency of the placenta, with the development or growth of the fetus, or with the general health and nutrition of the mother.

There is a positive correlation of both premature birth and low birth weight with low socioeconomic status. In such families there are relatively high incidences of maternal undernutrition, anemia and illness, inadequate prenatal care, drug addiction, obstetric complications, and maternal histories of reproductive inefficiency (relative infertility, abortions, stillbirths, premature or low-weight infants). Other less clearly associated factors such as illegitimacy, teen-age pregnancies, close spacing of pregnancies, working mothers and mothers who have borne more than four previous children are also encountered more frequently in families living in poor economic conditions. Owing to the difficulties in assigning cause and effect in most instances of premature birth or of low birth weight, it would seem logical in planning studies to determine causes to approach the problems in population groups of low economic status through evaluation of general health measures such as nutrition, infection, housing, overwork, fatigue and family planning. By contrast, such studies in population groups of better socioeconomic status in which the incidence of low-birth-weight infants is relatively low (5 to 6 per cent) would be directed at the presumed specific causes of reproductive inefficiency which appear to exist in spite of good general health measures.

TABLE 7–16 COMPARATIVE PERCENTAGES OF INFANTS WEIGHING LESS THAN 2500 GRAMS AMONG LIVE BIRTHS IN VARIOUS POPULATIONS

POPULATION	PER CENT WEIGHING LESS THAN 2500 GM.
Netherlands	3.5
Denmark	4.6
New Zealand	5.6
Norway	5.7
United States (white)	7.2
Bantu (South Africa)	11.6
United States (nonwhite)	13.8
Indian (South Africa)	18.3
Indian (Calcutta)	34.7

From Verhoestrate, L. J., and Puffer, R. R.: *J.A.M.A. 167*:950, 1958; U.S. Vital Statistics, 1965; and others. (This table is a composite. Data for the United States are for the year 1965, others chiefly from figures gathered in the early 1950's. Despite some variations in the reporting of live births, the basic comparisons seem valid.)

ASSESSMENT OF GESTATIONAL AGE AT BIRTH. Certain physical and neurologic signs may be useful in distinguishing infants under 2500 gm who are of appropriate weight for their gestational age from those with retarded growth. Although infants of either group may lack subcutaneous fat, the infant with retarded growth is likely to be shorter than expected for gestational age and to appear to have a disproportionately larger head relative to body size than the premature infant of appropriate weight. Brain growth is generally less affected than linear or other organ growth by factors that adversely influence intrauterine growth; chronic fetal nonbacterial infections and certain chromosomal anomalies are exceptions. Similarly, the functional development of the fetal nervous system continues to correlate with gestational age, and this may be used to assess gestational age as indicated in Table 7–18. Physical signs may be useful in estimating gestational age at birth. Until 36 weeks of gestation there are only one or two transverse skin *creases on the sole of the foot* anteriorly. By 37 or 38 weeks more creases have appeared, and by 40 weeks there is a complex series of criss-crossed creases covering the entire sole. The *size of the breast nodule* correlates generally with gestational age. It is usually not palpable at 33 or 34 weeks, is usually not over 3 mm in diameter at 36 weeks, and is usually 4 to 10 mm in term infants. The scalp hair tends to be short and fuzzy up to 37 weeks, but to consist mainly of coarse and silky in-

TABLE 7–17 FACTORS IMPLICATED IN THE ETIOLOGY OF INTRAUTERINE FETAL GROWTH RETARDATION

Fetal Factors
- Chromosomal disorders (e.g., autosomal trisomies)
- Chronic fetal infections (e.g., cytomegalic inclusion disease, congenital rubella, syphilis)
- Radiation injury
- Multiple gestation
- Pituitary failure (?)

Placental Factors
- Decreased placental weight or cellularity or both
- Decrease in surface area
- Villous placentitis (bacterial, viral, parasitic)
- Infarction
- Tumor (chorioangioma, hydatidiform mole)
- Placental separation
- Twin transfusion syndrome (parabiotic syndrome)
- Localized transfer lesions (?)

Maternal Factors
- Toxemia
- Hypertensive or renal disease or both
- Hypoxemia (high altitude, cyanotic, cardiac, or pulmonary disease)
- Malnutrition or chronic illness
- Sickle cell anemia

Experimental Factors
- Maternal uterine ischemia—rat
- Fetal placental ischemia—sheep and monkey
- Maternal protein deprivation—rat, guinea pig, and pig

dividual strands by 40 weeks. The *cartilaginous development of the ear lobe* which makes the folds of the helix and antihelix stand out occurs chiefly between 36 and 40 weeks. At 36 weeks the testes are usually not completely descended, and the scrotal rugae are few and limited to the anterior and inferior aspects of the small scrotum; by 40 weeks the testes are usually descended, and rugae cover the entire scrotal surface. Table 7–18 lists some measures for neurologic assessment of fetal age. An infant should be presumed to be at high risk of mortality or morbidity if there is a discrepancy between estimation of gestational age by physical examination, mother's estimated date of last menstrual period or fetal evaluation.

PATHOLOGY IN LOW-BIRTH-WEIGHT INFANTS. Neonatal deaths among premature and term infants of low or normal birth weights for gestational age result from the same general group of pathologic disturbances (Table 7–2), the principal differences being in the distribution of the causes of death. When the cause of death is sought by careful macroscopic postmortem examination, it is found in a high percentage of instances. Prematurity itself should not be considered a cause of death in an infant born alive. The principal causes of death among premature as well as term infants are anoxia, birth injuries (principally cerebral), malformations, idiopathic respiratory distress syndrome (hyaline membrane disease), bronchopneumonia, septicemia and other infections.

Pulmonary hyaline membranes associated with resorption atelectasis are found at autopsy in 40 to 50 per cent of low-birth-weight infants dying 1 hour to 4 days after birth, and rarely in larger infants born at or near term except those delivered by cesarean section or born to diabetic mothers.

Hemorrhage, whether associated with trauma, anoxia, infection, or defect of clotting mechanism, is frequent and often severe. Subcutaneous ecchymoses, bleeding into the choroid plexus, and subependymal and intraventricular hemorrhages are frequent in premature infants of low birth weight and are presumably related to increased capillary fragility. Sudden shock and collapse during the first few days of life are often due to intraventricular hemorrhage. Fatal hemorrhage into the lungs may also occur without identifiable cause.

Retrolental fibroplasia occurs in premature infants treated with oxygen at concentrations above ambient air levels. The increased arterial oxygen tensions which result are believed to lead to severe arterial vasoconstriction with subsequent hypoxic damage to the immature retina. The vasoconstriction stimulates proliferation of vascular tissue and subsequent leakage, hemorrhage and fibrous pro-

TABLE 7–18 REFLEXES OF VALUE IN ASSESSING GESTATIONAL AGE

REFLEX	STIMULUS	POSITIVE RESPONSE	WEEKS OF GESTATION IF REFLEX IS: *Absent*	*Present*
Sucking	Nipple	Strong and synchronized suck with deglutition	Feeble, inconstant < 31	33 or more
Rooting	Touch cheek with finger	Positioning head to maintain contact with finger	< 31	33 or more
Moro	See Neurologic exam (Section 20)	See Neurologic exam (Section 20)	< 28	31 or more
Pupillary reaction	Light	Contraction	< 26	31 or more
Glabellar tap	Tap on glabella	Blink	< 31	31 or more
Neck flexion	Pulled by wrists from supine to sitting	Flexion of neck	< 33	33 or more
Forearm flexion	Extend forearm	Strong return to flexion after extension	< 35	35 or more

liferation. Initial ophthalmologic examination during the period of oxygen administration may reveal vasoconstriction; subsequently the vessels are noted to be dilated and tortuous. Later, the areas of incompletely formed retina develop tufts or arcades of newly formed, thin-walled anastomosing vessels. Small retinal hemorrhages develop from these neovascular sites which then become fibrotic; massive hemorrhage may also occur in these areas. Retinal detachment follows; tearing of the neovascular tissue produces further retinal and vitreous hemorrhages. As the disease advances the entire retina and its fibroblastic and vascular tissue become detached and are pulled forward to lie just posterior to the lens. Spontaneous regression may occur at any time during this process up to the point of fibrosis and extensive vitreous clot formation and retraction. The retina may be left with mild to severe scarring, distortion and detachment, depending on the extent of the active process. The eyes of premature infants exposed to oxygen should be examined after recovery from the illness requiring oxygen therapy, before discharge and at 3 months after discharge; retinal surgery has been proposed for severe detachment. Before this effect of oxygen administration was appreciated 5 to 25 per cent of surviving infants whose birth weights were below 1800 gm (4 lb) became partially or completely blind because of retrolental fibroplasia. The practice of administering oxygen only in such amounts and for such periods of time as are absolutely necessary for the relief of respiratory distress, apnea and cyanosis, along with the frequent monitoring of arterial oxygen tensions, has significantly reduced the incidence of this disease. The exact level or duration of elevated arterial pO_2 which results in injury is unknown, but arterial oxygen tensions should be kept below 100 mm Hg insofar as possible; current practice is to maintain them between 50 and 80 mm Hg.

Kernicterus associated with hyperbilirubinemia is seen in 2 to 20 per cent of autopsies of premature infants. (See section on Kernicterus later in this Section.) Incidences of kernicterus approaching the latter figure are probably the result of inappropriate treatments such as administration of large amounts of vitamin K analogues to mothers in labor or to newborn infants, and use of sulfisoxazole as chemoprophylaxis.

Immaturity of anatomic, physiologic and biochemical functions is an index of the relative inability of the preterm and low-birth-weight infant to survive. Deficiencies in these functions affect the infant's ability to withstand demands that do not exist for him in the protective environment of intrauterine life, such as control of body heat, pulmonary function, nutrition, disposal of metabolic waste, immunologic function, and detoxification and excretion of toxic substances. The immature infant's respiratory function is limited by the underventilation of perfused alveoli, decreased surface for gas exchange and insufficient surface-active lipid surfactant to prevent collapse of alveoli. Underdeveloped airways and pulmonary tissue and persistence of fluid in the lung result in increased resistance to air flow. The ability to minimize heat loss in response to cold stress is proportional to body size and there is a decreased capacity for nonshivering thermogenesis. There are decreased stores of hepatic and myocardial glycogen, which compromises the immature infant's ability to withstand a moderate degree of asphyxia. Renal blood flow, glomerular filtration and tubular functions are decreased. The cardiopulmonary circulation is transitional between that of a fetus and that of an adult; increased shunting through the ductus arteriosus and foramen ovale may occur in response to stress and result in circulatory insufficiency or underperfusion of vital organs.

The shorter the period of gestation, the more likely is the infant to be unprepared to meet the rigors of extrauterine life. Though general immaturity may not permit survival in some very small newborn infants, it is desirable that it not be considered a cause of death since such a designation may detract from a careful search for explicit causes of all prenatal and postnatal deaths. When cause of death is not identified, it should be listed as *undetermined* (see Table 7–2).

Naeye has described two groups of infants of low birth weight for gestational age on the basis of pathologic observations:

One group has anatomic changes similar to those found in infants with postnatal alimentary malnutrition: diminished subcutaneous fat and small organs, particularly the adrenals, liver, spleen and thymus. The small size of organs is due chiefly to a subnormal amount of cytoplasm in individual cells rather than to a diminished number of cells. This group of infants with apparent fetal malnutrition includes infants of toxemic mothers, multiple pregnancies and prolonged pregnancies, or with placental abnormalities which might interfere with intrauterine nutrition.

The other group of infants of low birth weight for gestational age has a reduced number of cells in various body organs, but with a normal amount of cytoplasm per cell. This "hypoplastic" group includes infants with chromosomal abnormalities, congenital heart disease (except transposition of the great arteries), congenital rubella and cytomegalovirus infection.

COMPLICATIONS. Problems of major clinical significance associated with prematurity and/or infants of low birth weight include respiratory distress (hyaline membrane disease, pulmonary hemorrhage, aspiration syndrome, congenital pneumonia, pneumothorax), recurrent apnea, hypoglycemia, hypocalcemia, hyperbilirubinemia, anemia, edema, neurologic signs related to cerebral anoxia, circulatory instability, hypothermia, bacterial sepsis, intrauterine infection syndromes with congenital anomalies, persistent viremia with organ localization, and disseminated intravascular coagulopathies. The morbidity of term infants who are small for gestational age is often the result of fetal distress and central nervous system depression, meconium aspiration, hypoglycemia, chronic intrauterine infections, pulmonary hemorrhage, polycythemia or congenital anomalies. In contrast, preterm infants whose weight is appropriate for their gestational age have a higher incidence of hyaline membrane disease, nonhemolytic hyperbilirubinemia, neonatal bacterial infections, thermal instability, poor feeding and prolonged failure to gain, apnea, cardiac arrhythmias, anemia, bleeding (especially intraventricular hemorrhage in infants less than 1200 gm) and late metabolic acidosis.

CARE. At birth the same measures for clearing of airway, initiation of breathing, and care of the cord and of the eyes are required as for infants of normal birth weight or maturity. Additional considerations are (1) need for incubator care and monitoring, (2) need for increased oxygen, and (3) need for special attention to the details of feeding. Safeguards against infection and against careless or inefficient nursing can never be relaxed. Finally, the need to have the mother participate in the infant's care in the nursery, the need of instructing the mother for the care of the infant at home, and the question of prognosis for later growth and development require special consideration. There can be significant untoward effects on the development of a normal mother-infant relationship as a consequence of separation during the neonatal period; these effects may contribute to subsequent behavioral and physical abnormalities, e.g., failure-to-thrive and deprivation syndromes, child neglect and abuse.

Incubator Care. Modern incubators conserve body heat through provision of a warm atmospheric environment and standard conditions of humidity. They also provide a regulated oxygen supply and reduced atmospheric contamination. The latter aim is accomplished only if they are scrupulously cleaned. On the basis of current experience the optimal incubator temperature for minimum heat loss and oxygen consumption for the unclothed infant is that which will maintain the skin temperature of the infant at approximately 36 to 37°C (97 to 98°F). This is usually an air temperature of approximately 32 to 36°C (90 to 97°F), depending on an infant's size and maturity; infants of 1000 gm or less usually require incubator temperatures in the upper part of this range.

Maintenance of a relative humidity of 40 to 60 per cent aids in stabilizing body temperature by reducing heat loss at lower environmental temperatures, as well as preventing drying and irritation of the lining of respiratory passages, especially during the administration of oxygen and following or during endotracheal or nasotracheal intubation, and in thinning viscid secretions and reducing insensible water loss from the lungs. High humidity, ultrasonic nebulization and the addition of agents to reduce surface tension has not proved to offer additional advantages.

The administration of oxygen to reduce the risk of injury from hypoxia and circulatory insufficiency must be balanced against the risks of hyperoxia for the eyes (retrolental fibroplasia) and oxygen injury to the lungs. Although the presence of cyanosis, dyspnea and apnea are definite clinical indications for treating with only as much oxygen as needed to eliminate these signs, the potential harm from hypoxia and hyperoxia cannot be minimized without monitoring the oxygen tension (pO_2) of arterial blood and continuously readjusting the concentration of oxygen administered on the basis of this laboratory analysis. Lankowski has demonstrated that significant limitations of the ability and reliability of experienced observers to diagnose cyanosis clinically may result in errors of administering too little or too much oxygen unless both clinical and laboratory data are taken into consideration.

If an incubator is not available, the general conditions of temperature and humidity control outlined above can be attained by the intelligent use of blankets, heating lamps, heating pads, and warm water bottles, and by control of the temperature and humidity of the room. It may be necessary to administer oxygen temporarily by face mask or through an intubation tube.

The infant should be removed from the incubator only when the gradual change to the atmosphere of the nursery is not accompanied by a significant change of his temperature, color or activity. The removal may be only a day or two after birth for some infants, or at more than a month of age for less mature ones.

FEEDING. There are a variety of techniques for the feeding of premature infants. It is important to avoid fatigue and the aspiration of food during feeding or by regurgitation. No method of feeding will avoid these risks unless the person using it has been well trained in the process. Oral feedings should not be initiated or should be discontinued in infants with respiratory distress, hypoxia, circulatory insufficiency, excessive secretions, gagging, sepsis, or signs of serious illness. These infants will require parenteral therapy to supply calories, fluid and electrolytes.

Large premature infants can often be fed by bottle or at the breast. Since the effort of sucking is usually the limiting factor, breast feeding is least likely to be successful. In bottle feeding, effort may be reduced by use of special small, soft nipples with large holes. Infants as small as 3 pounds at birth are occasionally vigorous enough for bottle feedings. Smaller or less vigorous infants should be fed by gavage; a soft plastic tube of No. 5 French external and approximately 0.05 cm internal diameters with a rounded atraumatic tip and two holes on alternate sides is preferable. The tube is passed through the nose until approximately 1 inch of the lower end should be in the stomach. The free end of the tube is then placed under water. If bubbles appear with each expiration, the catheter is in the trachea and must be reinserted into the proper position. The free end of the tube has an adapter into which the tip of a glass syringe is fitted, and the measured amount of feeding is allowed to flow in slowly by gravity. Such tubes may be left in place for 3 to 7 days before replacement by a similar tube through the alternate nostril. The tubes may be cleaned, sterilized and reused, but are usually discarded after one use. An occasional infant has enough local irritation from an indwelling tube that troublesome secretions gather around it in the nasopharynx, or there may be gagging. In such instances a sterile No. 10 French rubber catheter may be passed through the mouth by a skilled person and removed at the end of each feeding. Change to bottle or breast feeding may be instituted gradually as soon as the infant displays general vigor adequate for oral feeding without fatigue.

The so-called Breck feeder, with which food is forced into the infant's mouth, is unsafe. Premature infants can be fed successfully and safely with a rubber-tipped medicine dropper by a nurse skilled in the procedure.

Gastrostomy feeding is contraindicated in premature infants, because of an associated increase in mortality, except as an adjunct to the surgical management of specific gastrointestinal conditions. The routine use of partial or total intravenous alimentation for premature infants has not been established to be a substitute for oral or gavage feedings.

Initiation of Feeding. The main principle in the feeding of premature infants is to proceed cautiously and gradually. Comparative inactivity, low heat production if body heat is artificially conserved, and relatively large body water content at birth all reduce the immediate need for calories, water and electrolytes. However, careful early feeding of glucose or saline solutions tends to reduce the incidence of hypoglycemia and hyperbilirubinemia without added risk of aspiration, provided the presence of respiratory distress or other disorder is considered an indication for withholding oral feedings and administering electrolytes, fluids and calories intravenously.

As soon as the infant has recovered from the stress of delivery and appears active and in no distress, oral feedings may be instituted. This interval is usually 2 to 12 hours, but may be 5 to 7 days in sick infants, who will require intravenous feeding in this interim. If the infant is vigorous and making sucking movements, oral feeding may be attempted, though most infants under 1500 gm and many larger ones require initial tube feeding. A suggested schedule is to begin with 1 ml of a sterile solution of 5 per cent glucose in water for infants under 1000 gm; 2 to 4 ml for infants between 1000 and 1500 gm; and 5 to 10 ml for infants over 1500 gm. If the beginning amount is 1 ml, feedings may be given hourly for the first 8 hours, increasing the amount by 1 ml at every other feeding. Feedings may then be given every 2 hours, with an increment of 2 ml at every other feeding until 12 ml is reached. This amount may be continued every 2 to 3 hours for 24 to 48 hours, at which time a mixture of 8 ml of 5 per cent glucose in water and 4 ml of a half-skim milk formula containing 0.67 calorie per ml (20 calories per ounce) may be substituted for two feedings, then 4 ml of 5 per cent glucose in water and 8 ml of formula for two feedings, and then the full strength formula. Amounts of formula may then be gradually increased so that the intake is approximately 150 ml per kg per 24 hours. If the infant still seems hungry or fails to gain weight, the amounts should be further increased. The expected weight increments for infants of various birth weights can be projected from Figure 7–7. Certain infants with small gastric capacities fail to gain on tolerated amounts of formula containing 0.67 calorie per ml. In such instances more frequent feedings may be given in order to increase the total daily intake, or the caloric content may be increased to as high as 1 calorie per ml (30 calories per ounce).

To infants of 1000 to 1500 gm the glucose and water feedings may be given every 2 to 3 hours, with 4-ml increments at every other feeding until feedings of 16 ml are reached, at which point formula may be substituted gradually. With infants over 1500 gm the interval may be 3 to 4 hours with 8-ml increments up to 32 ml, at which point formula is substituted gradually.

The occurrence of regurgitation or vomiting in the early stages of the feeding schedule should arouse suspicion of intestinal obstruction; later it is an indication to drop back in the schedule and increase subsequent feedings slowly. Gain in weight may not be achieved for 10 or 12 days, and a daily intake as high as 130 to 150 calories per kg may be necessary for some infants.

When tube feeding is used, the contents of the stomach should be aspirated before each feeding. If only air or small amounts of mucus are obtained, the feeding is given as planned. If any of the previous feeding is obtained, it is a signal to reduce the amount of the feeding and to proceed more gradually with subsequent increases.

The digestive enzyme systems of premature in-

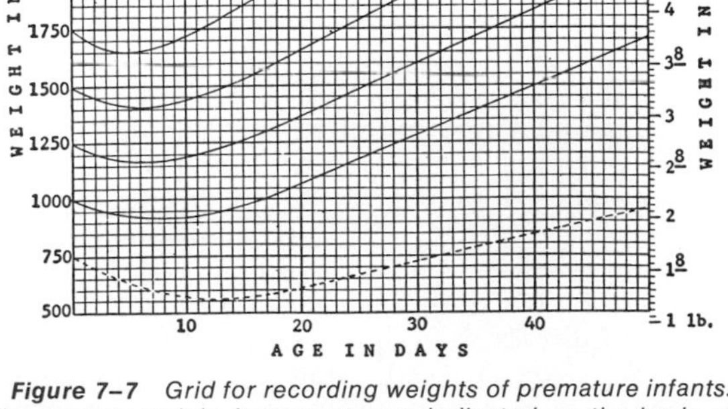

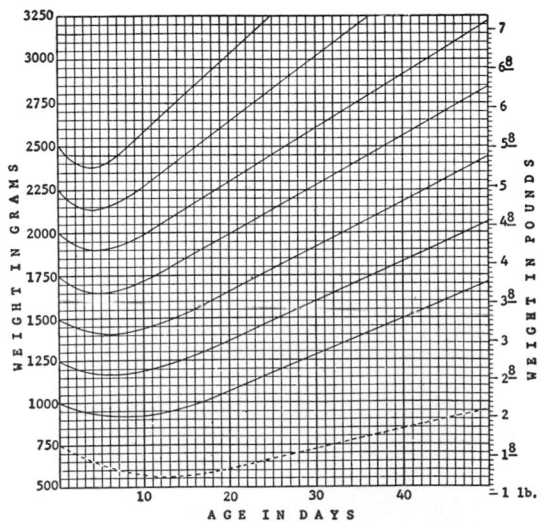

Figure 7–7 Grid for recording weights of premature infants. The average weight increments are indicated on the basis of weight at birth. (From Dancis, J., et al.: J. Pediatr. Vol 33.)

fants seem to be mature enough to permit efficient absorption of protein and carbohydrate. Fat is less well absorbed; unsaturated fats and the fat of human milk are absorbed better than that of cow's milk. Weight gain of infants weighing 1500 gm or more at birth is adequate with a protein intake of 2 gm per kg, but some smaller infants require 3 or 4 gm. Levine and Gordon have shown that better weight gain can be achieved with formulas made with half-skim milk than with human milk, which has a higher fat and lower protein and mineral content. Nitrogen retention of premature infants can be increased by feeding large amounts of protein. The high protein and mineral contents of balanced cow's milk formulas of high caloric content, however, constitute a large solute load for the kidney, a fact which is important in the maintenance of water balance especially in the infant with diarrhea or fever. The exact benefit to the premature or term infant of the secretory immunoglobulins contained in human milk remains to be evaluated.

There is need for an increased intake of vitamins C and D. Intermediary metabolism of phenylalanine and tyrosine depends in part upon ascorbic acid. Moreover, any tendency to loss of fecal fat involves loss of fat-soluble vitamins and calcium. Approximately 50 mg of ascorbic acid and 1000 I. U. of vitamin D daily begun during the second and third weeks, respectively, is ample. Since intakes of vitamin D in excess of 1500 I. U. per day may cause the syndrome of idiopathic hypercalcemia in certain infants (Section 22), the total intake of vitamin D from all sources should not exceed that amount. Supplementation with other vitamins has not been shown to be necessary, though anemia may develop in premature infants severely deficient in vitamin E.

In the low-birth-weight infant, physiologic anemia owing to postnatal suppression of erythropoiesis is exacerbated by smaller fetal iron stores and greater expansion of blood volume as a result of more rapid growth as compared to the term-weight infant, so that the anemia develops earlier and reaches a lower ultimate level. Fetal or neonatal blood loss accentuates this problem. In the premature infant dietary iron is virtually never adequate to supply the iron needed in the course of rapid growth during infancy. Thus, iron supplementation is indicated: 6 mg/kg/day of elementary iron, p.o., starting at about 8 weeks of age, and the early introduction of iron-containing milk and foods rich in iron. The addition of iron to the diet is discussed in Section 14.

The properly fed premature infant may have from one to six stools of semisolid consistency daily; sudden increase in number or a change to a watery consistency is reason for more concern than any arbitrarily stated frequency. Over 50 per cent of preterm low-birth-weight infants pass their first stool within 12 hours of birth and approximately 80 per cent by 24 hours. The premature infant should not vomit or regurgitate. He should be satisfied and relaxed after a feeding, but may normally show the activity of hunger shortly before the next one.

Total Intravenous Alimentation. When oral feeding is impossible for prolonged periods of time, total intravenous alimentation may provide sufficient fluid, calories, electrolytes and vitamins to sustain growth. This technique has been lifesaving in neonatal infants who have had extensive resection of the bowel.

Under sterile conditions a Silastic catheter is usually placed through the internal or external jugular vein so that its tip is proximal to the right atrium. The catheter is carefully secured in place and tunneled to exit in the posterior occipital region in order to avoid dislodgment and to minimize the hazard of infection. A millipore filter is interposed to minimize contamination from microorganisms or particulate matter, and the catheter is attached to a constant infusion pump for accurate control of the flow of the hypertonic acid infusate. The catheter is used only for the infusate in order to decrease the risks of infection.

The infusate should contain a protein equivalent (beef fibrin and casein hydrolysates and synthetic amino acids are available) of 2.5 gm/dl and hypertonic glucose in the range of 10 to 25 gm/dl in addition to appropriate quantities of electrolytes and vitamins. The biochemical limitations of each and the needs of the particular patient should be studied before selection of the appropriate protein source. All solutions should be mixed by a well trained pharmacist using a laminar flow hood.

The complications of intravenous alimentation are related to both the catheter and the metabolism of the infusate. Sepsis is the most important problem and can be avoided only by meticulous catheter care and aseptic preparation of the infusate. Thrombosis, extravasation of fluid and accidental dislodgment of catheters have also occurred. The *metabolic complications* include hyperglycemia from the high glucose concentration of the infusate, which may lead to an osmotic diuresis and dehydration, hypoglycemia from a sudden accidental cessation of the infusate, and hyperammonemia, which may be due to high levels of ammonia in beef fibrin hydrolysates or the lack of arginine in casein hydrolysates. Abnormal liver chemistries have also been noted with beef fibrin hydrolysates. Hyperchloremic acidosis is a rare complication with protein hydrolysates, but a common problem in infants receiving synthetic amino acids. Continuous chemical and physiologic monitoring of infants receiving intravenous alimentation is indicated because of the frequency and seriousness of complications.

PREVENTION OF INFECTION. Premature infants have an increased susceptibility to infection which can be safeguarded against by requiring rigorous hand-to-elbow washing by personnel before and after handling the infant, by taking measures to reduce contamination of the infant's food and the objects that come in contact with him, by preventing contamination of the air he breathes, and by limiting his direct and indirect contacts with nursery personnel (including other infants). No one with an infection should be permitted in the nursery. The risks of infection must be balanced against the disadvantages of limiting the infant's contacts with his mother, which may be detrimental to the infant's ultimate development; early and frequent participation by a mother in the nursery care of her infant may not increase the incidence of infection when appropriate preventive precautions are maintained.

Prevention of transmission of infection from infant to infant is difficult because frequently neither term nor premature newborn infants manifest clear clinical evidence of an infection early in its course. If the unit admits infants born outside the hospital, it should be assumed that they are infected until a week or more of observation in a special nursery or an incubator with an individual air supply proves otherwise.

The most important factor in the successful care of premature infants is the skill, experience and number of the *nursing* staff. It is the responsibility of the physician to insist upon an optimal amount of expert nursing.

GENERAL CONSIDERATIONS OF DISEASE. Prematurity tends to increase the severity and to reduce the clinical manifestations of all neonatal diseases. Subcutaneous and intracranial hemorrhage, "primary" atelectasis, respiratory distress syndrome, pneumonia, bacteremia, hypoglycemia and hyperbilirubinemia occur more frequently among premature than among term infants. Retrolental fibroplasia is seen almost exclusively in premature infants.

Drugs. Renal clearances for almost all substances excreted in the urine are diminished in all newborn infants, but more so in premature ones. Half or less of the customary dose of any drug excreted chiefly by the kidney is usually adequate to maintain a therapeutic level, even when given at longer than the customary interval between doses. For instance, highly satisfactory levels of penicillin, streptomycin and kanamycin are maintained on doses given at 12-hour intervals. Drugs detoxified in the liver or requiring chemical conjugation before renal excretion should also be given with caution and in smaller than usual doses. Decision as to the choice, dose and route of administration of antibacterial agents to possibly infected infants should be made on an individual rather than on a routine basis, owing to the dangers of (1) development of infections with organisms resistant to antibacterial agents, (2) destruction or inhibition of intestinal bacteria which manufacture significant amounts of essential vitamins (e.g., vitamin K and thiamine), and (3) possible deleterious interference in important metabolic processes (e.g., the role of sulfisoxazole in hyperbilirubinemia).

Since pure food and drug laws and regulations are based largely on toxicity studies on adult animals and human beings, apparently "safe" drugs may not be so for newborn infants, especially premature ones. Oxygen, vitamin K analogues, sulfisoxazole (Gantrisin), chloramphenicol and novobiocin, all presumably "safe" drugs, have proved to be toxic to newborn premature infants in amounts not harmful to term infants. Thus, administration of any drug to newborn infants, particularly in large doses, should be done with care and with risk weighed against potential benefit.

The levels of some immunoglobulins of premature infants at birth are significantly lower than those of their mothers at the time of delivery or of those of term infants and they undergo further decrease during the first months of life. However, the routine or prophylactic administration of gamma globulin has not been proved to be of benefit.

PROGNOSIS. Neonatal mortality rates for low-birth-weight infants are shown in Figure 7–5 and Table 7–12, and causes of death in Table 7–2. The mortality rate of low-birth-weight infants who survive to be discharged from the hospital is approximately three times that of full-term infants during the first two years of life. Many of these deaths are attributable to infection and are, therefore, at least theoretically preventable. There is also an increased incidence of the sudden infant death syndrome among premature infants. The possible roles of defects in the regulation of the cardiorespiratory system secondary to immaturity and of high environmental risk factors secondary to low socioeconomic status in increasing the mortality rate have not been fully delineated.

Congenital anatomic anomalies are present in approximately 25 per cent of liveborn infants with birth weights less than 1500 gm, in approximately 12 per cent with birth weights between 1500 and 2500 gm, but in only 6 per cent with birth weights of 2500 gm or more. There is a slight increase in the incidence of congenital anomalies in infants with birth weights above the 90th percentile. They are also more common among low-birth-weight infants who are small for gestational age than among those whose weight is appropriate for gestational age.

In the absence of congenital abnormalities, central nervous system injury or a marked reduction in birth weight for gestational age (intrauterine growth retardation), physical growth tends to overtake that of term infants during the second year; this occurs earlier in premature infants of larger size at birth. Premature birth in itself may prejudice later development. In general, the greater the immaturity and the lower the birth weight, the greater the likelihood of intellectual and neurologic deficit. Follow-up studies of surviving premature infants reveal a discouragingly high incidence of handicaps among the smaller ones (Table 7–19). There is also a greater frequency of other obstetric factors, such as intrauterine anoxia and intracranial hemorrhage, and socioeconomic factors, such as drug addiction and poor nutrition, in these infants than would occur in infants born at term.

TABLE 7-19 OBSERVATIONS ON 72 INFANTS WITH BIRTH WEIGHTS OF 3 LBS. (1360 GM) OR LESS FOLLOWED UP 5 YEARS OR MORE

	CHILDREN
Below 5th percentile in weight	25 (35%)
Below 5th percentile in height	33 (46%)
Below 5th percentile in weight and height	20 (28%)
I.Q. under 100 (66 tested)	60 (91%)
Uneducable in normal school because of physical or mental handicap	26 (36%)
Require special treatment in normal school	25 (35%)
Slower than all siblings (51 had sibs)	39 (76%)
Behavior problem present	51 (71%)
Physical defect	38 (53%)
Physical defect and/or mental retardation	55 (76%)

Data drawn from Drillien, C. M.: The Growth and Development of the Prematurely Born Infant. London, E. & S. Livingstone, Ltd., 1964.

Drillien has also shown the double role played by socioeconomic factors: mothers of low socioeconomic status are more apt to have low-birth-weight babies, and such infants reared under low socioeconomic conditions tend to develop less well than do those in better environments. On the other hand, recent studies evaluating very-low-birth-weight (under 1000 gm) survivors of intensive care nurseries indicate relatively low morbidity in this group. Similarly, major neurologic defects were found to be uncommon in a prospective study of full-term small-for-dates infants, although there was a significant incidence of minimal cerebral dysfunction (hyperactivity, short attention span, learning difficulties), electroencephalographic abnormalities and speech defects.

Behavior and personality problems appear to be common in children born prematurely. The circumstances of isolated nursery care in early infancy and of home care thereafter conspire against a normal relation between the prematurely born infant and his family. The extent to which a defect in the development of the normal maternal-infant "mothering" relationship and understandable parental anxiety and overprotectiveness may foster an abnormal emotional environment for the growing infant should be greatly reduced by avoiding unnecessarily prolonged hospitalization and by encouraging parental visiting and participation in the care of the infant while in the nursery.

HOME CARE. While the infant is in the hospital the mother should be instructed about her responsibilities when the baby is discharged. This program should include at least one visit to her home by a person capable of evaluating domestic arrangements and of advising as to any needed improvements. Premature infants are usually sent home when they reach 5½ pounds (2500 gm) in weight. Many may go before that time, whereas others should be kept longer.

POST-TERM INFANTS

Post-term infants are defined as those born after 42 weeks of gestation, calculated from the mother's last menstrual period, irrespective of weight at birth. This designation is often used synonymously with the term "postmature" for infants whose gestation exceeds the normal 280 days by 7 days or more. Approximately 25 per cent of all pregnancies end on or after the 287th day of gestation, 12 per cent on or after the 294th day, and 5 per cent on or after the 301st day. The cause of post-term birth or postmaturity will presumably remain unknown until the mechanisms determining the onset of labor are fully understood. Large size of the infant correlates poorly with late delivery, but it does correlate with large size of either parent, multigravidity, or a prediabetic or diabetic state in the mother.

CLINICAL MANIFESTATIONS. Post-term infants may be clinically indistinguishable from term infants, but some have received the designation postmature because of appearance and behavior suggesting those of an infant 1 to 3 weeks of age. These post-term, postmature infants are characterized by the absence of lanugo, decreased or absent vernix caseosa, long nails, abundant scalp hair, white skin, parchment-like or desquamating skin, and increased alertness. Occasionally some of these clinical manifestations of postmaturity are observed in term and preterm infants.

PROGNOSIS. When delivery is delayed 3 or more weeks beyond term, there is a significant increase in mortality, which in some series has approximated three times that of a control group of infants born at term; the fetal mortality exceeds that of the neonatal period. Each has been lowered markedly through improved obstetric management. Primiparity and maternal age over 25 years appear to increase the mortality rates.

TREATMENT. The induction of labor before the cervix is soft and dilated is felt by most obstetricians to be a greater risk than postmaturity itself. A possible exception is the performance of cesarean section on elderly primigravidas who go more than a week or two beyond term, particularly if there is evidence of fetal distress.

PLACENTAL DYSFUNCTION SYNDROME

INCIDENCE AND ETIOLOGY. The incidence of some clinically recognizable form of placental dysfunction (abnormal fetal heart rate pattern, retarded intrauterine growth, low maternal levels of estriol, contamination of amniotic fluid by meconium) has been estimated to be as high as 12 per cent of all births. The incidence of the clearly recognizable form of the syndrome, with yellow staining of the vernix and skin, is approximately 1.2 per cent of all births. Although this syndrome is frequently confused with postmaturity, *only about 20 per cent of infants with placental dysfunction syndrome are post-term.* The majority affected are term and preterm infants, particularly those of low birth weight for gestational age who are infants of toxemic mothers, elderly primigravidas and women with "reproductive inefficiency." The placentas are often small or poorly attached. This syndrome has been postulated to be the result of degenerative changes in the placenta resulting in progressive reduction of oxygen and nourishment for the fetus.

CLINICAL MANIFESTATIONS. Infants who are born prematurely at weights lower than expected for gestational age have been discussed previously. Those who are born past term in association with presumed placental dysfunction have been categorized in three groups by Clifford: *stage I*–infants with the usual signs of postmaturity, which are desquamation, long nails, abundant hair, white skin, alert facies and loose skin, especially around the thighs and buttocks, giving the appearance of recent loss of weight; *stage II*–infants with the changes of stage I plus meconium-stained amniotic fluid, skin, vernix, umbilical cord and placental membranes, possibly a manifestation of fetal anoxia; *stage III* (Fig. 7–8)–infants with the signs of stages I and II, except that their nails and skin are stained a bright yellow and the umbilical cord yellow-green.

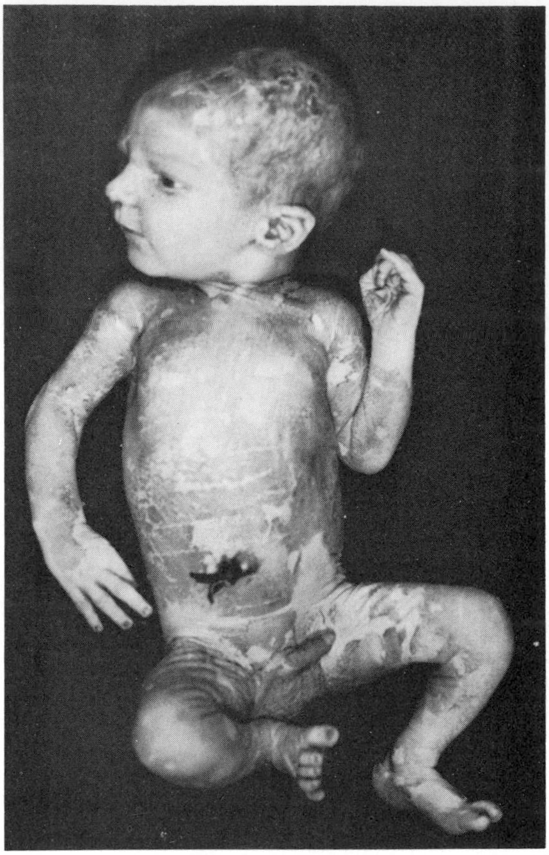

Figure 7–8 *Placental dysfunction syndrome, stage III. Note long, thin infant with loose, peeling, parchment-like skin, alert expression, staining of skin and nails. (From Clifford: Advances in Pediatrics. Vol. 9. Chicago, Year Book Medical Publishers, Inc.)*

PROGNOSIS. Stage I infants have no known mortality associated with the syndrome itself, but they have an increased general mortality which correlates with prolonged gestation, and up to one third of them have been reported as showing some evidence of respiratory distress or central nervous system irritation. Stage II infants are born at the height of intrauterine anoxia or after a moderate to severe hypoxic episode. About two thirds of them have severe respiratory symptoms, apparently resulting from the aspiration of meconium-containing amniotic fluid. A smaller number have clinical signs of anoxic cerebral damage. The overall mortality rate is estimated to be about 35 per cent. Liveborn stage III infants have presumably survived the acute anoxic phase of stage II; they have the same clinical problems, but with a lower morbidity, and a mortality rate of approximately 15 per cent. See also Figure 7–5 and Table 7–2.

TREATMENT. (See also Prematurity and Low Birth Weight.) The treatment of placental dysfunction lies chiefly in preventing the conditions which predispose to it and in alleviating episodes of acute fetal distress which occur during labor. It therefore constitutes an obstetric and perhaps a genetic and social problem. Aspiration pneumonia and cerebral anoxia are treated symptomatically.

HIGH BIRTH WEIGHT

Perinatal and neonatal mortality rates decrease with increasing birth weight until approximately 4000 gm. Over this weight mortality increases with birth weight. These oversized infants are usually born at term, but preterm infants with weights high for gestational age also have a significantly higher mortality than infants of the same size born at term. Infants who are very large, regardless of their gestational age, have a higher incidence of birth injuries, such as cervical and brachial plexus injuries, phrenic nerve damage with paralysis of the diaphragm, fractured clavicles, cephalhematomas and ecchymoses of the head and face. The incidence of congenital anomalies is also higher than in term infants of normal weight. Statistically significant evidence for intellectual and developmental retardation has been observed in high-birth-weight term and preterm infants on subsequent evaluation at school age, as compared to babies of appropriate weight for gestational age. See also discussion of Infants of Diabetic Mothers.

Diseases of the Newborn Infant: Premature and Full Term

It is essential that the child's physician have an appreciation of the wide variety of disorders which may have their origin in utero, during birth or in the immediate postnatal period, and of the need to distinguish them etiologically in respect to their time and place of origin.

Disorders which have their origin in utero may represent genetic mutations, chromosomal aberrations or acquired diseases. Some of these disorders are described in this section under Birth Injury, Disturbances of Organ Systems, Metabolic Disturbances and Infections; others are described in other sections, and include Prenatal Disturbances, Inborn Errors of Metabolism, Immunologic Deficiency Disorders, Nutritional Disorders, Infectious Diseases, and the various systems of the body.

CLINICAL MANIFESTATIONS OF DISEASE DURING THE NEONATAL PERIOD

Recognition of disease in the newborn infant is dependent upon knowledge and appraisal of a limited number of relatively nonspecific clinical signs and symptoms.

Cyanosis usually indicates respiratory insufficiency, which may be due to pulmonary conditions or may be secondary to intracranial hemorrhage or anoxic injury to the brain. If it is due to the former, respirations tend to be rapid and may be accompanied by retraction of the thoracic cage. If it is due to the latter, respirations tend to be irregular and weak and often slow. Cyanosis persisting for several days, when unaccompanied by obvious signs of respiratory difficulty, is suggestive of cyanotic congenital heart disease or methemoglobinemia. Cyanosis from congenital heart disease may, however, on occasion be difficult to distinguish from cyanosis caused by respiratory disease in the first few days of life. Episodes of cyanosis may be the presenting sign of hypoglycemia, bacteremia or meningitis.

In addition to anemia or hemorrhage, *pallor* should suggest hypoxia, hypoglycemia, sepsis, shock or adrenal failure.

Convulsions (see also Section 19) usually point to a disorder of the central nervous system and suggest anoxic brain damage, intracranial hemorrhage, cerebral anomaly, subdural effusion, meningitis, tetany or, rarely, pyridoxine dependency, hypoglycemia, hyponatremia or hypernatremia. They may also be the first sign of bacteremia or other severe infection and may occur as a nonspecific sign in any severe illness, particularly if there is circulatory insufficiency. Infants of mothers addicted to narcotics may also develop seizures as part of their withdrawal syndrome. *Apnea* may be the first manifestation of seizure activity, particularly in a premature infant.

Lethargy may be a manifestation of anoxia, of sedation from maternal analgesia or anesthesia, of cerebral defect, of severe infection and, indeed, of almost any severe disease. Lethargy appearing after the second day should, in particular, suggest infection.

Irritability may be a sign of discomfort accompanying intra-abdominal conditions, meningeal irritation, infections, or any condition producing pain. As in later infancy, the eardrums should always be examined as a possible source of pain.

Hyperactivity, especially of the premature infant, may be a sign of hypoxia, pneumothorax, emphysema, hypoglycemia, hypocalcemia or central nervous system damage.

Failure to feed well is seen in most sick newborn infants and should always occasion a careful search for infection and other abnormal conditions.

Fever may be the result of too high an environmental temperature due to hot weather, overheated nurseries or incubators, or too many clothes or bedclothes. It is also seen in "dehydration fever" of newborn infants. If these causes of fever can be eliminated, serious infection (pneumonia, bacteremia, viremia, meningitis) must be ruled out. On the other hand, serious infections often occur without provoking any febrile response in newborn infants; an unexplained *fall in body temperature* may accompany infection or other serious disturbance of the metabolic processes of the neonatal infant.

Periods of *apnea*, particularly in the premature infant, suggest metabolic as well as respiratory or central nervous system disturbance. They have been described in association with hyponatremia and hypoglycemia.

Jaundice during the first 24 hours of life should be considered due to erythroblastosis fetalis until proved otherwise. Septicemia, cytomegalic inclusion disease, the congenital rubella syndrome and toxoplasmosis should also be considered. *Jaundice after the first 24 hours* may be "physiologic," due to any of the foregoing causes (but especially to *septicemia*), or to hemolytic anemia, galactosemia, hepatitis, congenital atresia of the bile ducts, inspissated bile syndrome following erythroblastosis fetalis, syphilis or herpes simplex.

Vomiting during the first day of life suggests obstruction in the upper digestive tract or increased intracranial pressure. Anteroposterior and lateral *upright* films of the abdomen are indicated, followed by barium studies if the diagnosis remains in doubt. Vomiting also may be a nonspecific symptom of an illness such as septicemia. It is a common manifestation of overfeeding, pyloric stenosis, milk allergy, duodenal ulcer, stress ulcer, adrenal insufficiency and a reflection of a "nervous" or apprehensive mother, or of an emotional upset in the parents. Infants placed in body casts for orthopedic treatment often vomit transiently, apparently as a manifestation of frustration of physical movement. Vomitus containing dark blood is usually a sign of life-threatening illness, whatever the cause. Bile-stained vomitus suggests obstruction below the ampulla of Vater.

Diarrhea may be a symptom of overfeeding, acute gastroenteritis or a nonspecific symptom of infection *(parenteral diarrhea)*. It may be seen in conditions accompanied by compromised circulation of part of the intestinal or genital tract such as mesenteric thrombosis, strangulated hernia, intussusception, and torsion of the ovary or testis.

Abdominal distention, usually a sign of intestinal obstruction or an intra-abdominal mass, may also be seen in infants with enteritis or with temporary ileus accompanying sepsis, respiratory distress, or hypokalemia.

Failure to move an extremity or part of it suggests fracture, dislocation or nerve injury. It is also seen in osteomyelitis and other infections which cause pain on movement of the affected part.

CONGENITAL ANOMALIES

Congenital anomalies are important as a cause of stillbirths and neonatal deaths, but are perhaps even more important as causes of physical defects and metabolic disorders. (Anomalies are discussed in general in Section 6 and specifically in the sections on the various systems of the body. For congenital mental defects, see Section 2; for congenital metabolic and chemical disorders, see Section 8; and for immunologic deficiency disorders, see Section 9). Recognition of anomalies as early as possible is desirable. For some, such as tracheoesophageal fistula or intestinal obstruction, immediate medical and surgical therapy is mandatory for survival. In all instances, early diagnosis permits a planned approach and an explanation to parents, who are likely to be assailed by anxiety and guilt when they become aware of the existence of a congenital anomaly.

BIRTH INJURY

The term *birth injury* is used to denote avoidable and unavoidable mechanical and anoxic trauma incurred by the infant during labor and delivery. These injuries may result from inappropriate or deficient medical skill or attention, or they may occur despite skilled and competent obstetric care and independent of any acts or omissions of the parents. In order to avoid later misunderstandings, recriminations or parental guilt, it is important to counsel parents who have a child with a residuum from birth trauma or anoxia about this broad use of the term "birth injury." The definition does not include injury from amniocentesis, intrauterine transfusion, scalp vein sampling or resuscitation procedures.

The incidence of birth injuries has been estimated at 2 to 7 per 1000 live births. Predisposing factors include macrosomia, prematurity, cephalopelvic disproportion, dystocia, prolonged labor and breech presentation. Although the incidence has decreased in recent years, in part owing to refinement in obstetric techniques and judgment, birth injuries still represent an important problem for the clinician, because even transient problems are frequently readily apparent to the parents and result in anxiety and questions that require supportive and informative counseling. Some injuries may be latent initially, but later result in severe illness or sequelae.

CRANIAL INJURIES

Caput succedaneum is a diffuse, edematous swelling of the soft tissues of the scalp involving the portion presenting during vertex delivery. It may extend across the midline and across suture lines. General or localized ecchymotic discoloration or petechiae may be present at birth. The edema disappears within the first few days of life. Analogous swelling, discoloration and distortion of the face are seen in face presentations. No specific treatment is needed for either, but if there are extensive ecchymoses, early phototherapy for hyperbilirubinemia may be indicated. *Molding* of the head and overriding of the parietal bones are frequently associated with caput succedaneum and become more evident after the caput has receded, but disappear during the first weeks of life.

Erythema, abrasions, ecchymoses and *subcutaneous fat necrosis* (Section 23) may be seen after forceps deliveries. Their location depends upon the area of application of the forceps. Ecchymoses may be seen after manipulative deliveries and occasionally in premature infants for no discernible reason.

Subconjunctival hemorrhages are frequent, and *petechiae* of the skin of the head and neck are not uncommon. Generalized ecchymotic suffusion of the head and neck is rare. All are probably secondary to a sudden increase in intrathoracic pressure during passage of the chest through the birth canal. Parents should be assured that they are temporary and the result of *normal* hazards of delivery.

Cephalhematoma (Fig. 7–9) is a subperiosteal hemorrhage, hence always limited to the surface of one cranial bone. There is no discoloration of the overlying scalp due to subcutaneous hemorrhage and swelling is usually not visible until several hours after birth, since subperiosteal bleeding is a slow process. In approximately 25 per cent of cephalhematomas there is an underlying skull fracture, which is usually linear and not depressed. A sensation of central depression suggesting underlying fracture or bony defect is usually encountered on palpation of the organized rim of a ce-

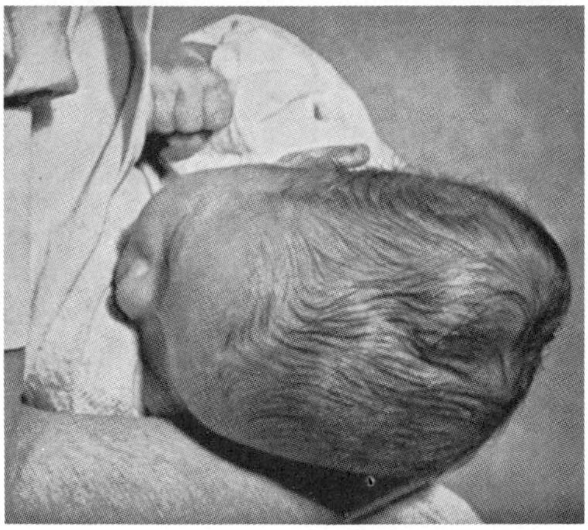

Figure 7–9 *Cephalhematoma of the right parietal bone.*

phalhematoma. Cranial meningocele may be differentiated from cephalhematoma by pulsation, increased pressure on crying and the roentgenographic evidence of bony defect. Most cephalhematomas are resorbed within two weeks to three months, depending upon their size. They may begin to calcify by the end of the second week. A few remain as bony protuberances for years and are detectable roentgenographically as widening of the diploic space; cystlike defects may persist for months or years. Despite these residuals, cephalhematomas require no treatment. Since the introduction of infection is the only serious complication, incision or aspiration is contraindicated.

Fractures of the skull may occur as a result of pressure from forceps or against the maternal symphysis pubis, sacral promontory or ischial spines. Linear fractures are the most common. They cause no symptoms and require no treatment. Depressed fractures are usually indentations of the calvarium similar to a dent in a Ping-Pong ball; usually they are a complication of forceps delivery. It is advisable to elevate such depressions surgically to prevent cortical injury from sustained pressure. Fracture of the occipital bone with separation of the basal and squamous portions almost invariably causes fatal hemorrhage, owing to disruption of the underlying sinuses. It may result from traction on the hyperextended spine of the infant with the head fixed in the maternal pelvis during breech deliveries.

Intracranial Hemorrhage

Intracranial hemorrhage may result from trauma or anoxia and, rarely, from a primary hemorrhagic disturbance or congenital vascular anomaly. Traumatic hemorrhage is especially likely when the fetal head is large in proportion to the size of the mother's pelvic outlet; when for other reasons the labor is prolonged; in breech deliveries; in precipitate deliveries; or when there is injudicious mechanical interference with delivery. The proper use of forceps may decrease the incidence of intracranial bleeding in prolonged hard labors. Intracranial hemorrhages may occur in infants, especially premature ones, delivered spontaneously without apparent trauma. In premature infants subependymal, subarachnoid, intracerebral and intraventricular hemorrhages are common (Fig. 7–10). Spontaneous intraventricular hemorrhage in which no physical damage to the tentorium, falx or other structures is found at autopsy is practically limited to premature infants. Conversely, massive subdural hemorrhages, often associated with tears in the tentorium cerebelli or less frequently in the falx cerebri, are encountered more often in full-term than in premature infants.

Hemorrhage due to anoxia tends to be petechial, and subarachnoid and intracerebral in distribution. There is usually only mild extravasation of

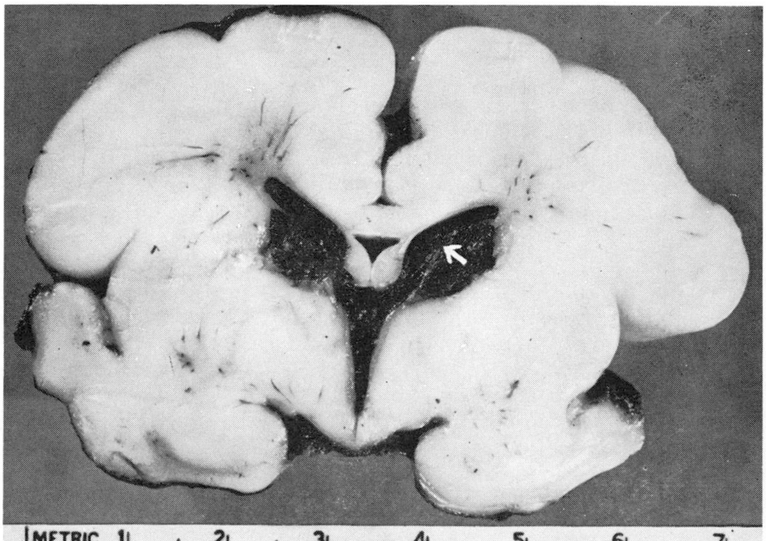

Figure 7–10 *Bilateral subependymal and intraventricular hemorrhage in a premature infant. The floor of the lateral ventricle is marked by an arrow, outside of which is a large subependymal hemorrhage. (From Arey and Dent.: J. Pediatr. Vol. 42.)*

erythrocytes, and symptoms and sequelae are dependent more on anoxia than on hemorrhage. Primary hemorrhagic disturbances usually give rise to subarachnoid hemorrhage, and vascular anomaly to subarachnoid or intracerebral hemorrhage. Rarely, intracranial bleeding may be associated with disseminated intravascular coagulopathy.

CLINICAL MANIFESTATIONS. Symptoms of intracranial hemorrhage may be present at birth or may not appear for a variable time after delivery. The commonest symptoms soon after birth are a general failure to move normally, diminished or absent Moro reflex, lethargy and somnolence. Irregularity of respirations in the absence of other signs of respiratory distress is often a sign of severe hemorrhage. Periods of apnea, pallor, cyanosis or cyanotic attacks, failure to suck well, forceful vomiting, anxiety and restlessness, a high-pitched, shrill cry, muscular twitchings, convulsions or paralyses may be the first indications that intracranial hemorrhage is present. The fontanel *may* be tense and bulging, and an adder-like protrusion of the tongue may be seen. Retinal hemorrhage, ocular palsies, inequality in size and failure of the pupils to react to light, or nystagmus may be observed.

DIAGNOSIS. This is based chiefly on the history of delivery, the clinical manifestations and the course. Since nonlocalizing signs of intracranial hemorrhage are identical with those caused by cerebral edema or anoxia, before carrying out any diagnostic procedure the chance of helping the patient should be weighed against the risk. In the absence of an obstetric history of intrapartum hemorrhage, of other signs of bleeding or extensive bruising in the infant, or of iatrogenic removal of large quantities of blood, a significant fall in hematocrit should suggest the diagnosis of intracranial hemorrhage, as well as that of subcapsular hemorrhage of the liver. Subdural taps are usually unrewarding, even in the presence of subdural hemorrhage, since it is likely that the blood will have clotted; on the other hand, they may on rare occasions be lifesaving. Ventricular taps are rarely done even when there is suspicion of intraventricular hemorrhage, owing to the remoteness of the possibility that it will be either diagnostically or therapeutically efficacious. Lumbar puncture is indicated in the presence of signs of increased intracranial pressure or deteriorating clinical condition to identify gross subarachnoid hemorrhage or to rule out the possibility of bacterial meningitis. Occasionally an infant is too ill to tolerate the physical manipulation implicit in performing lumbar puncture; critically ill premature infants are particularly prone to develop apnea, bradycardia or circulatory insufficiency when positioned for the procedure.

Since a small amount of bleeding often occurs in the course of normal and even cesarean deliveries, small numbers of red blood cells or slight xanthochromia in subarachnoid fluid is not necessarily indicative of significant intracranial hemorrhage. Bilirubin may produce a yellowish discoloration of the cerebrospinal fluid in jaundiced infants; conversely, the subarachnoid fluid may be absolutely clear with severe subdural or intracerebral hemorrhage when there is no communication with the subarachnoid space.

PROGNOSIS. Intrapartum death may occur in the more severe cases; postnatally, fatalities usually occur within the first 3 days and result from respiratory failure. If an infant survives, recovery may be complete, or there may be permanent residuals, mainly in the category of cerebral palsy. Some of the membrane-enclosed subdural effusions observed in later infancy may have their origin in subdural hemorrhage at birth. Statistics on incidence and prognosis of intracranial hemorrhage in the newborn are not available, since autopsy material is the only source and since one can rarely be certain of the diagnosis in the surviving patient.

Because the majority of parents are aware of and fear the possibility of cerebral residuals following intracranial hemorrhage or cerebral anoxia, it is probably wisest to give them an opportunity to air their anxiety in a frank discussion of the problem, during which their questions should be invited rather than suppressed or evaded. As optimistic an attitude as possible, consistent with the physician's opinion of the prognosis of the individual case, should be maintained.

PREVENTION. Prophylactic measures include continuing improvements in obstetric management; many instances of intracranial hemorrhage are avoidable.

TREATMENT. The infant should be handled as little and as gently as possible. He is best kept in an incubator which allows good temperature control, continuous observation, and easy administration of oxygen for cyanosis. Phenobarbital or other anticonvulsant drugs in appropriate doses may be used to control convulsive movement. A small dose of vitamin K_1 oxide should be administered. (See Jaundice and Hyperbilirubinemia in the Newborn Infant later in this Section.) A small (5 ml per pound) transfusion of fresh blood is indicated in the presence of hemorrhagic disease of the newborn. The management of disseminated intravascular coagulopathy is discussed in Section 14. There is lack of agreement about the advisability of spinal punctures for the relief of increased intracranial pressure and to remove gross blood in order to reduce its irritant effect on the cerebral cortex and to prevent possible interference with the normal resorptive mechanisms for cerebrospinal fluid. In our opinion such punctures are indicated if they can be well tolerated, particularly in the presence of grossly bloody spinal subarachnoid fluid. Neurosurgical procedures are not indicated.

Cerebral edema may result in any or all of the clinical signs produced by intracranial hemorrhage. Trauma and anoxia are the commonest causes. It is not usually possible to establish this diagnosis during life except by implication from the obstetric history. Treatment includes avoidance or correction of dilutional hyponatremia and restriction of fluid intake to create a negative water balance (total water intake less than estimated insensible water loss plus urine volume). This is usually accomplished with a fluid intake of 50 to 75 ml/100 calories expended. The indications for and benefits of reducing increased intracranial pressure from edema by removal of cerebral spinal fluid or by the parenteral administration of dexamethasone (10 mg/m^2 initially, then 5 mg/m^2 every 6 hours) have not been established. They may be indicated if an infant's condition is deteriorating with rapidly progressing neurologic signs; mannitol may also be used intravenously with caution, if necessary.

SPINE AND SPINAL CORD

Strong traction exerted when the spine is hyperextended or when the direction of pull is lateral, or forceful longitudinal traction on the trunk while the head is still firmly engaged in the pelvis, especially when combined with flexion and torsion of the vertical axis, may produce fracture and separation of the vertebrae. Such injuries are rare and are most likely to occur when difficulty is encountered in delivering the shoulders in cephalic presentations and the head in breech presentations. The injury is most commonly at the level of the seventh cervical and first thoracic vertebrae. Transection of the cord may occur, but hemorrhage and edema may produce neurologic signs indistinguishable from those of transection, except that they are not permanent. There is complete paralysis of voluntary motion below the level of injury, though the persistence of a withdrawal reflex mediated through spinal centers distal to the area of injury is frequently misinterpreted as representing voluntary motion. The differential diagnosis should include amyotonia congenita and myelodysplasia associated with spina bifida occulta. Severe spinal cord injuries usually cause death soon after birth. In the survivors treatment is supportive and there is often permanent injury. In the compression from a fracture or dislocation the prognosis is related to the time elapsing before the compression is removed.

PERIPHERAL NERVE INJURIES

BRACHIAL PALSY. Injury to the brachial plexus may cause paralysis of the upper arm with or without paralysis of the forearm or hand. Such an injury occurs when lateral traction is exerted on the head and neck during delivery of the shoulder in a vertex presentation or in a breech presentation when the arms are extended over the head or there is excessive traction on the shoulders.

In **Erb-Duchenne paralysis** the injury is limited to the fifth and sixth cervical nerves. The infant loses the power to abduct the arm from the shoulder, to rotate the arm externally and to supinate the forearm. The characteristic position consists of adduction and internal rotation of the arm with pronation of the forearm. The power of extension of the forearm is retained, but the biceps reflex is absent. The Moro reflex is absent on the affected side (Fig. 7–11). There may be some sensory impairment on the outer aspect of the arm. The power in the forearm and the hand grasp are preserved unless the lower part of the plexus is also injured; the presence of the hand grasp is a favorable prognostic sign. When the injury includes the phrenic nerve, alteration of the diaphragmatic excursion may be observed fluoroscopically.

Klumpke's paralysis is a rarer form of brachial palsy; injury to the seventh and eighth cervical nerves and the first thoracic nerve produces a paralyzed hand, and ipsilateral ptosis and miosis if the sympathetic fibers of the first thoracic root are also injured.

The mild cases may not be detected immediately after birth. The paralysis from an injury to the brachial plexus may involve the entire arm. Differentiation must be made from cerebral injury, from fracture, dislocation or epiphyseal separation of the humerus, and from fracture of the clavicle.

The **prognosis** depends upon whether the nerve was merely injured or was lacerated. If the paralysis was due to edema and hemorrhage about the nerve fibers, there should be a return of function within a few months; if due to laceration, permanent damage may result. The involvement of the deltoid is usually the most serious; dropping of the shoulder may result from muscular atrophy. In

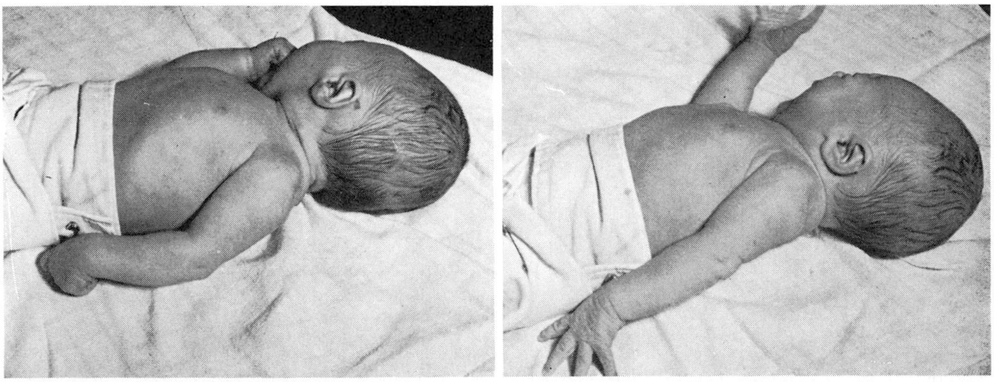

Figure 7–11 Brachial palsy of the left arm (asymmetric Moro reflex).

general, paralysis of the upper arm has a better prognosis than paralysis of the lower arm.

Treatment consists of partial immobilization and appropriate positioning to prevent the antagonistic pull of the nonparalyzed muscles. In upper arm paralysis, the arm should be abducted 90 degrees, with external rotation at the shoulder and with full supination of the forearm and slight extension at the wrist with the palm turned toward the face. This may be done by pinning the sleeve of the infant's garment at the wrist to the undersheet. The restraint should be maintained for 2 to 3 hours at a time, alternating with shorter periods when the arm is free. In lower arm or hand paralysis, the wrist should be splinted in a neutral position and padding placed in the fist. Physical therapy is a necessary adjunct to the treatment. If the paralysis persists, because of laceration of the nerve fibers, for 3 to 6 months, neuroplasty offers hope for partial recovery.

PHRENIC NERVE PARALYSIS. Phrenic nerve injury with diaphragmatic paralysis must be considered when cyanosis and irregular and labored respirations develop. Such injuries are usually unilateral and associated with homolateral upper brachial palsy. Breathing is thoracic in type, so that there is no bulging of the abdomen with inspiration. Breath sounds are diminished on the affected side. The thrust of the diaphragm, which often may be felt just under the costal margin on the normal side, is absent on the affected side. The *diagnosis* is established by fluoroscopic examination, which reveals the elevation of the diaphragm on the paralyzed side (Fig. 7–12) and seesaw movements of the two sides of the diaphragm during respiration.

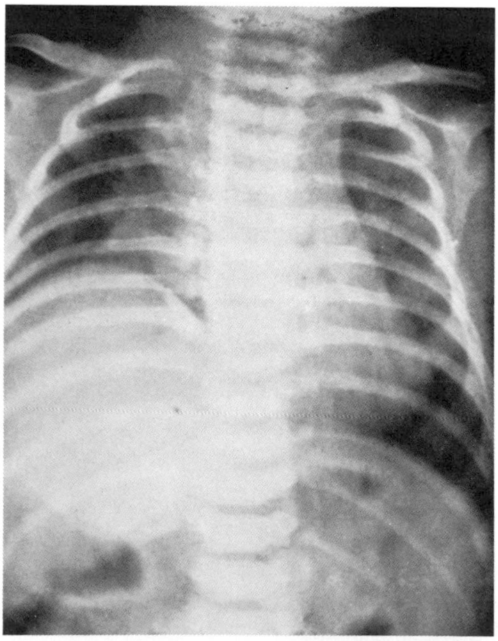

Figure 7–12 Phrenic paralysis in a newborn infant. The right leaf of the diaphragm is elevated, owing to injury to the right phrenic nerve. Fluoroscopically, the right and left leaves of the diaphragm moved in a seesaw manner. There were also fractures of both clavicles and a right brachial palsy.

There is no specific *treatment;* the infant should be placed on the involved side; oxygen therapy may be necessary. Initially, intravenous feedings may be necessary; later, progressive gavage or oral feedings may be started, depending on the infant's condition. Pulmonary infections are a serious complication. Recovery usually occurs spontaneously; rarely, surgical plication of the diaphragm may be indicated.

FACIAL NERVE PALSY. Usually, facial palsy is a peripheral paralysis that results from pressure over the facial nerve in utero, during labor, or from forceps during delivery. Rarely it is nonobstetric, resulting from nuclear agenesis of the facial nerve. When the infant cries, there is movement on only the nonparalyzed side of the face, and the mouth is drawn to that side. On the affected side the eye cannot be closed, the nasolabial fold is absent and the corner of the mouth droops. The forehead will wrinkle on the affected side with central paralysis, since only the lower two thirds of the face is involved. The *prognosis* depends upon whether the nerve was injured by pressure or whether the nerve fibers were torn. Improvement will occur within a few weeks in the former instance. Care of the exposed eye is essential. Neuroplasty may be indicated when the paralysis is persistent.

OTHER PERIPHERAL NERVES. Other nerves are seldom injured at birth, except as they are involved in fractures or hemorrhages.

VISCERA

The **liver** is the only internal organ other than the brain injured with any frequency during birth. The damage usually occurs from pressure on the liver during delivery of the head in breech presentations. Large infant size, intrauterine asphyxia, coagulation disorders and hepatomegaly are other contributing factors. Overzealous manual attempts to apply artificial respiration or extrathoracic cardiac massage are less frequent causes. The injury is rupture of the liver with formation of a subcapsular hematoma. The hematoma may be large enough to cause anemia. Shock and death occur if the hematoma breaks through the capsule, reducing pressure and allowing fresh hemorrhage. Early suspicion and diagnosis, and prompt supportive therapy, can decrease the mortality of this disorder. Surgical repair of a laceration may be required.

Rupture of the spleen may occur in association with rupture of the liver. The causes, complications, treatment and prevention are similar.

Although **adrenal hemorrhage** occurs with some frequency, especially after breech delivery, it is not known whether it is due to trauma, anoxia or severe stress, as in overwhelming infections. Calcified central hematomas of the adrenal have been identified roentgenologically or at autopsy in older infants and children, suggesting that not all adrenal hemorrhages are fatal. The diagnosis is usually made at postmortem examination. The symptoms are profound shock and cyanosis. There may be a mass in the flank with overlying skin discoloration. If adrenal hemorrhage is suspected, the treatment is the same as for acute adrenal failure (Section 17).

INJURY OF THE STERNOCLEIDOMASTOID

A firm mass 1 to 2 cm in diameter is occasionally noted in the midportion of the sternocleidomastoid muscle about the second week of life, although it may be present shortly after birth. See Torticollis, Section 21.

FRACTURES

CLAVICLE. The clavicle is fractured more frequently than any other bone during labor and delivery and is particularly vulnerable when there is difficulty in delivery of the shoulder in vertex presentations and of the extended arms in breech deliveries. The infant characteristically fails to move, or to move freely, the arm on the affected side; crepitus and bony irregularity may be palpated, and occasionally discoloration is visible over the fracture site. The Moro reflex is absent on the affected side, and there is spasm of the sternocleidomastoid muscle with obliteration of the supraclavicular depression at the site of the fracture. In greenstick fractures there may be no limitation of movement and the Moro reflex may be present. Fracture of the humerus or brachial palsy may also be responsible for limitation of movement of an arm and the absence of a Moro reflex on the affected side. The *prognosis* is excellent. *Treatment,* if any, consists in immobilization of the arm and shoulder on the affected side. A remarkable degree of callus develops within a week at the site and may be the first evidence of the fracture.

EXTREMITIES. In fractures of the long bones spontaneous movement of the extremity is usually absent. The Moro reflex is absent from the involved extremity. The possibility of associated nerve involvement must be considered. Satisfactory results for a fractured humerus are obtained by strapping the arm to the chest or applying a Velpeau bandage, and later an airplane splint or a shell cast. For fracture of the femur, good results are obtained with traction-suspension of both lower extremities, even if the fracture is unilateral; the legs are immobilized in a spica cast and the infant suspended by the legs from an overhead frame. Splints are effective for treatment of fractures of the forearm or leg. Healing is usually accompanied by excess callus formation.

Dislocations and *epiphyseal separations* rarely result from birth trauma. The upper femoral epiphysis may be separated by forcible manipulation of the infant's leg as, for example, in breech extraction or after version. There is swelling, slight shortening, limitation of active motion, painful passive motion, and external rotation of the leg. The diagnosis is established roentgenographically. The prognosis is good for the milder injuries, but coxa vara frequently results from extensive displacement.

NOSE. The most prevalent injury of the nose is a dislocation of the cartilaginous portion of the septum from the vomerine groove and the columella. The infant may have difficulty in nursing and some impairment in nasal respiration. Treatment should be instituted immediately.

ANOXIA

Anoxia is not a clinical entity, but a term used to indicate the end-result of lack of oxygen from a number of primary causes. It requires separate consideration, however, since it is the leading immediate cause of perinatal death or of permanent damage to central nervous system cells which is manifest later as cerebral palsy or mental deficiency. Its prevention and treatment are essentially those of the basic conditions which cause it, although death and disability may sometimes be prevented through symptomatic treatment with oxygen or artificial respiration and the correction of associated metabolic acidosis with sodium bicarbonate.

Fetal anoxia may result from (1) inadequate oxygenation of maternal blood as in hypoventilation during anesthesia, cardiac failure or carbon monoxide poisoning; (2) low maternal blood pressure as in the hypotension that may complicate spinal anesthesia or that may result from compression of the vena cava and aorta by the gravid uterus; (3) inadequate relaxation of the uterus to permit placental filling as in uterine tetany caused by administration of oxytocin; (4) inadequate attachment of the placenta as in premature separation of the placenta; (5) impedance to the circulation of blood through the umbilical cord as in compression or knotting of the cord; and (6) placental inadequacy from numerous causes, including toxemia and postmaturity. (See High-Risk Pregnancies.)

After birth, anoxia may result from (1) anemia severe enough to lower the oxygen content of the blood to a critical level as in severe hemorrhage or hemolytic disease; (2) shock severe enough to interfere with the transport of oxygen to vital cells as in adrenal hemorrhage, ventricular hemorrhage, overwhelming infection or massive blood loss; (3) a deficit in arterial oxygen saturation from failure to breathe adequately postnatally, owing to narcosis or cerebral defect or injury; and (4) failure of oxygenation of an adequate amount of blood as in severe forms of cyanotic congenital heart disease or deficient pulmonary ventilation.

Most of the deaths and cerebral damage which result from anoxia are probably related to fetal or postnatal periods of anoxia. Early detection of signs of fetal distress by continuous monitoring of the fetal heart rate and serial determinations of acid-base balance on fetal scalp blood samples dur-

TABLE 7–20 CLASSIFICATION OF FETAL HEART RATE PATTERNS*

Baseline Fetal Heart Rate

The average rate recorded between uterine contractions. Sustained changes of at least 10 minutes' duration are classified as follows:

- Normal: 120–160 beats per minute
- Moderate tachycardia: 181 or more beats per minute
- Moderate bradycardia: 100–119 beats per minute
- Marked bradycardia: 99 or fewer beats per minute

Baseline Fetal Heart Irregularity

This refers to recurrent beat to beat variations or oscillations about the baseline rate, of less than 20 seconds' duration but persisting for 10 minutes or longer:

- Minimal (silent or flat) irregularity: oscillations of 0–5 beats per minute
- Average (narrowed undulatory) irregularity: oscillations of 6–16 beats per minute.
- Moderate (undulatory) irregularity: oscillations of 11–25 beats per minute
- Marked (saltatory) irregularity: oscillations of 25 or more beats per minute

Periodic Fetal Heart Rate Changes

These are deviations in the baseline fetal heart rate which persist for more than 20 seconds but less than 10 minutes, and are either more than 30 beats per minute above or below the baseline or are outside the normal range of 120 to 160 beats per minute. Periodic changes in fetal heart rate (FHR) may occur in relation to fetal movements or during or after uterine contractions.

- Acceleration (periodic tachycardia)
  - Moderate: 161–180 beats per minute
  - Marked: 181 or more beats per minute
- Deceleration (periodic bradycardia or dip)
  - Moderate: 100–119 beats per minute
  - Marked: 99 or fewer beats per minute

Early Deceleration

Begins with the onset of a uterine contraction and returns to the baseline near the end of the contraction (Type I dip)

Late Deceleration

Begins later in the uterine contraction cycle, usually 20 seconds or more after the onset, and persists for a variable time after the contraction has subsided (Type II dip)

Variable Deceleration

Bears no consistent temporal relationship to the onset or duration of the uterine contraction (Type 0 dip)

*The definitions and nomenclature used for fetal heart patterns follow those of Hon and Caldeyro-Barcia (1968), Hammacher (1969), and Huntingford (1969). From Behrman R. E.: Neonatology. St. Louis, The C. V. Mosby Company, 1973.

ing labor holds promise of significantly decreasing the morbidity and mortality associated with anoxia by providing improved criteria for obstetric intervention in labor (Table 7–20). The initial circulatory response of the fetus to anoxia is preferential maintenance of perfusion of the brain, heart and adrenals.

CLINICAL MANIFESTATIONS. The signs of anoxia in the *fetus* are usually noted a few minutes to a few days before delivery. There is sudden increase in activity as if the baby were struggling in utero; this may be followed by diminished activity. The fetal heart rate slows, and the beat may become weak and irregular. Continuous heart rate recording may reveal a variable or late (Type II Dips) deceleration pattern, and scalp blood analysis may show a pH less than 7.20. The acidosis is made up of varying degrees of metabolic and/or respiratory components. Particularly in the infant near term, these are signs which should lead to the administration of high concentrations of oxygen to the mother and to immediate delivery to avoid death or central nervous system damage.

At *delivery* the presence of yellow, meconium-stained amniotic fluid and vernix caseosa is a warning that there has been fetal distress, probably anoxic. Pallor, cyanosis, apnea, slow heart rate, unresponsiveness to stimulation, and muscular flaccidity are definite signs of anoxia.

After delivery anoxia is due to respiratory failure and circulatory insufficiency. Treatment is discussed under respiratory distress and failure and intensive care.

PATHOLOGY. The pathologic changes that result from anoxia are principally those caused by congestion and increased capillary permeability. Congestion and petechiae are found in all organs, but are especially noticeable in the pleura, pericardium, thymus, adrenals, brain and meninges. Cerebral edema is common. Gross subarachnoid, intraventricular or adrenal hemorrhage may be present without demonstrable tear of blood vessels. Histologic study of the brain and liver, particularly the right lobe, may reveal cellular degenerative changes similar to those produced experimentally by anoxia. Fetal anoxia is characterized pathologically by the additional finding of large amounts of amniotic debris in the respiratory passages. Pathophysiologically, within minutes of the onset of total anoxia there are bradycardia, hypotension, severe metabolic as well as respiratory acidosis and marked alterations in regional circulation, such as severe pulmonary vasoconstriction and, often, increased shunting through the ductus arteriosus and the foramen ovale.

PEDIATRIC EMERGENCIES IN THE DELIVERY ROOM

The most common and immediately most important emergencies related to the newborn infant in the delivery room are failure to initiate respiration and to maintain satisfactory respirations. Less frequent, but having potentially serious import, are shock, severe anemia, plethora and convulsions.

RESPIRATORY DISTRESS AND FAILURE. Disorders of respiration in the newborn infant can be categorized in two general groups (Table 7–21), one representing failure or depression of the respiratory center (central nervous system failure) and the other interference with the alveolar exchange of oxygen and carbon dioxide (peripheral respira-

TABLE 7-21 RESPIRATORY DISTRESS AND FAILURE IN NEWBORN INFANTS

TYPE	MANIFESTATIONS	CLINICAL ENTITY
Central nervous system failure	Apnea Slow, irregular, gasping respiratory efforts	Narcosis Prenatal or perinatal anoxia Intracranial hemorrhage or trauma CNS anomalies
Peripheral respiratory difficulty	Rapid respiratory rate Increasing respiratory rate Chest lag Intercostal retraction Subcostal retraction Xiphoid retraction Chin tug Expiratory grunt Frothing at lips	Primary atelectasis Congestive pulmonary failure Idiopathic respiratory distress (hyaline membrane) syndrome Aspiration of amniotic fluid containing formed elements Pneumonia Diaphragmatic hernia Lung cysts Lobar emphysema Pneumothorax Aspiration of food or mucus

tory difficulty). Cyanosis occurs in both groups. The respiratory problems encountered in the delivery room are most frequently those of airway obstruction and of depression of the central nervous system, with the absence of adequate respiratory effort.

Respiratory distress in the presence of good respiratory effort should lead to an immediate consideration of peripheral causes; *respiratory distress is an indication for a roentgenographic examination of the chest* if this is at all possible without undue risk for the infant.

If respiratory movements are made with the mouth closed, but the infant fails to move air in and out of the lungs, bilateral *choanal atresia* (Section 12) or other obstruction of the upper respiratory tract should be suspected. The mouth should be opened and the mouth and posterior pharynx cleared of secretions by gentle suction. Nasal obstruction or hypoplasia of the mandible can be identified and relieved by pulling the tongue forward to allow air exchange. An oropharyngeal airway should be inserted and the source of the obstruction sought immediately, but in an unhurried manner. If effective respiratory flow is not produced by opening the infant's mouth and clearing the airway, laryngoscopy is indicated. With obstructive malformations of the epiglottis, larynx or trachea, an endotracheal tube should be inserted; prolonged nasotracheal intubation or tracheotomy may be required. Respiratory failure from depression or injury of the central nervous system may require continuous artificial ventilation with a face mask and bag, or through an endotracheal or nasotracheal tube.

Hypoplasia of the mandible (Section 11) with posterior displacement of the tongue may result in symptoms similar to those of choanal atresia; they may be temporarily relieved by pulling the tongue forward. A scaphoid abdomen suggests *hernia or eventration of the diaphragm*, as does asymmetry of contour or movement of the chest or shift of the apical impulse of the heart; these latter manifestations are also compatible with tension pneumothorax.

Causes of peripheral respiratory difficulty are discussed below under Disturbances of the Respiratory Tract.

FAILURE TO INITIATE OR SUSTAIN RESPIRATION. Failure to initiate or sustain respiratory effort originates in the central nervous system; immaturity in itself is seldom a causative factor.

Narcosis results from heavy doses of morphine, Demerol, barbiturates, reserpine or tranquilizers administered to the mother shortly before delivery, or from maternal anesthesia, especially if prolonged, during delivery. The infant is cyanotic at birth and slow to cry or breathe; when respiration is established, it is extremely slow.

Narcosis is rarely excusable and should be avoided by appropriate analgesic and anesthetic practices.

Treatment consists of physical stimulants such as frequent snapping of the soles of the feet to stimulate crying and deeper breathing, or insertion of a catheter through the nostril into the nasopharynx to produce reflex irritation and breathing. The efficacy of stimulants of the central nervous system in the initiation of respiratory efforts has not been established. If narcosis is due to morphine or its derivatives, naloxone hydrochloride (Narcan), 0.01 mg per kg, should be injected intravenously. Although this drug has not yet been approved in the United States for use in children, the overdose depressant effect associated with nalorphine (Nalline) has not been reported. Oxygen should be administered as long as cyanosis is present; some form of artificial respiration is necessary until a regular and adequate respiratory pattern is established.

Prenatal or *perinatal anoxia,* whatever the cause, if sufficiently severe, will produce a central nervous system type of respiratory failure, secondary apnea, which does not respond to sensory stimulation. Death is due to apnea and may be prevented by resuscitation, provided the basic cause of the anoxia can be eliminated within a reasonable time and while artificial respiration, if necessary, is being carried out. External cardiac massage, correction of acidosis, and circulatory support may be important adjuncts to ventilation. Hypothermia as a means of temporarily reducing metabolic needs for oxygen during the period of oxygen want has not proved to be of practical value and is contraindicated.

Intracranial hemorrhage and trauma were discussed earlier.

Central nervous system anomalies may be responsible for respiratory failure.

Resuscitation. Failure to breathe spontaneously within 1 minute of birth is an indication for some method of resuscitation. If the central mechanism can be revived, the infant will be more effective in ventilating his lungs safely than will any available artificial technique.

After the upper and central airway has been cleared as adequately as possible by removal of accumulated liquid contents, resuscitation should start with some method of simple, gentle physical stimulation such as snapping the soles of the feet with a finger or repeatedly passing a nasal catheter. If this is unsuccessful in initiating satisfactory respiration, the upper respiratory passage should be suctioned again and a small plastic or metal airway inserted to lift the tongue off the posterior pharyngeal wall. If the infant has an Apgar score of 3 or less, or if the pulse rate is less than 80 beats a minute, some method of artificial respiration or pulmonary inflation is usually indicated. If a gentle flow of oxygen at pressures up to 25 cm of water, administered either steadily or in puffs through a small mask, does not produce improved color and tone followed by spontaneous respiratory movements, direct laryngoscopy or direct endotracheal intubation with suctioning of the lower respiratory passages and an attempt to inflate the lungs through the application of short bursts of oxygen at higher pressures is indicated.

Maintenance of the circulation through closed cardiac massage at a rate of 100 or more per minute is an important adjunct to artificial respiration in infants in circulatory collapse with slow, weak heart beats. This must be synchronized with ventilation (4:1 ratio). Laryngoscopy, intubation and cardiac massage should be carried out by personnel skilled in the techniques, of whom there should be one (usually the anesthetist) in every delivery room. Negative intrathoracic pressures between 20 and 70 cm of water have been recorded during the first few breaths; positive pressure much lower than 20 cm of water is unlikely to introduce oxygen into the lungs. Pressures of 25 cm may rupture the lung if only a small area is being expanded. On the other hand, positive pressures of 40 cm have been safely applied by using a resuscitator which automatically limits the inspiratory phase to 0.1 second and provides an expiratory phase of 5.9 seconds.

Mouth-to-mouth breathing has been successful in resuscitating some infants, but may have been harmful to others by introducing infection or alveolar rupture from uncontrolled pressures.

If the infant is making feeble but spontaneous respiratory movements, their effectiveness will be increased by raising the partial pressure of oxygen at the nose and mouth, even without any change in atmospheric pressure. Oxygen administration, particularly to premature infants, should be at the lowest effective concentration, while monitoring arterial blood levels. It should always be discontinued as soon as the baby can get along without it.

After the airway has been cleared and adequate ventilation provided, severely asphyxiated and acidotic infants often require the slow (1 ml/min) administration of sodium bicarbonate (3-4 mEq/kg) through an umbilical catheter to correct the associated metabolic acidosis; a solution containing 0.5 to 1 mEq of sodium bicarbonate per ml is used. It may also be necessary to administer epinephrine (0.1 ml/kg of a 1:10,000 solution) via catheter or intracardiac injection to combat hypotension.

No drug advocated as a respiratory stimulant has proved to be of definite value; moreover, most of them may be convulsant if given in doses slightly greater than those supposed to stimulate breathing.

SHOCK. Circulatory insufficiency may present at birth as a result of intracranial or other internal hemorrhage; fetal bleeding during gestation, labor or delivery (e.g., fetal-fetal transfusion syndrome); bleeding from the fetal circulation secondary to a placental tear; excessive bleeding from a severed or torn umbilical cord; or severe hemolytic anemia from erythroblastosis fetalis. Clinical manifestations include signs of respiratory distress; cyanosis; pallor; flaccidity; cold, mottled skin; tachypnea or bradycardia; hepatosplenomegaly; and, rarely, convulsions. *Edema* and hepatosplenomegaly also may present in erythroblastosis fetalis or congestive heart failure without shock; severe intrauterine viral infections may also present with organomegaly. Edema and convulsions may result from the administration of large amounts of hypotonic fluids to the mother shortly before and during delivery, with subsequent hyponatremia and water intoxication in the infant.

Supportive treatment with type O, Rh-negative blood or electrolyte solutions is indicated for hypovolemia. Oxygen should be administered, and correction of metabolic acidosis with sodium bicarbonate may also be indicated. Seizures secondary to dilutional hyponatremia may require prompt administration of appropriate amounts of 3 per cent sodium chloride solution by vein, followed by temporary restriction of water. The diagnosis and treatment of erythroblastosis fetalis is discussed in Section 14.

As soon as supportive measures have stabilized the infant's condition, a specific diagnosis should be established and appropriate continuing treatment instituted.

DISTURBANCES OF ORGAN SYSTEMS

DISTURBANCES OF THE RESPIRATORY TRACT

Disturbances of respiration manifested in the immediate postnatal period may have had their origin in utero, in the delivery room or in the nursery. A wide variety of pathologic lesions may be responsible. They are manifested by one or more of the signs of respiratory distress (Table 7–21 and Fig. 7–2); if respiratory embarrassment is severe, pallor or cyanosis may also be present, and it is occasionally difficult to distinguish cardiovascular from respiratory disturbances on the basis of clinical signs alone. The differential diagnosis of signs of respiratory distress in the newborn infant includes the idiopathic respiratory distress syndrome, aspiration syndrome, pneumonia, congenital heart disease, choanal atresia, hypoplasia of the mandible with posterior displacement of the tongue, macroglossia, malformation of the epiglottis, malformation or injury of the larynx, cysts or neoplasms of the larynx or chest, pneumothorax, lobar emphysema, pulmonary agenesis or hypoplasia, congenital pulmonary lymphangiectasia, Wilson-Mikity syndrome, tracheo-esophageal fistula, evulsion of the phrenic nerve, hernia or eventration of the diaphragm, intracranial lesions and metabolic disturbances. (See Table 7–21 for a listing of intracranial and pulmonary lesions.) *Any sign of postnatal respiratory distress* (Fig. 7–2; Tables 7–9 and 7–21) *is an indication for a roentgenogram of the chest.*

ATELECTASIS

Atelectasis, the incomplete expansion of a lung or a portion of a lung, is almost constantly present in infants dying shortly after delivery. The first few breaths taken by a vigorous newborn infant usually produce complete expansion of all parts of the lung with air; accordingly, careful postmortem examination usually reveals a cause for persistent atelectasis.

Primary atelectasis (failure of initial alveolar expansion), common among premature infants without other apparent abnormality at autopsy, is regarded as due to immaturity of the diaphragm and other respiratory muscles, to hypermobility of the thoracic cage, to other defects of the peripheral respiratory mechanism or to severe illness. It is also seen as a result of brain injury with damage to the respiratory center, or of maternal oversedation prior to delivery. Incomplete initial expansion may also result from a relative inability to expand the thick-walled bronchioles, alveolar ducts lined with columnar epithelium and thick-walled alveoli which are characteristic of the immature fetus.

Secondary atelectasis (alveolar collapse after initial expansion by air) may occur as a gross or microscopic lesion in all types of pulmonary disease in the newborn.

PATHOLOGY. In the stillborn infant the lungs have a uniformly beefy red appearance. Histologically the interstitial tissues are congested, and the alveoli present the appearance of a crumpled sac. The degree of crumpling varies inversely with the amount of expansion of the alveoli by fluid formed in the lung, as well as by aspirated amniotic fluid. With sudden anoxia in utero there may be more vigorous inspiratory movements than usual, with an increase in aspiration of amniotic fluid and its contents. The later in pregnancy this takes place, the more likely it is that squamous epithelial cells and debris will be found in the alveolar spaces.

If an infant has breathed, the lungs may show beefy red areas alternating with lighter, aerated, raised portions. Histologically the red areas are congested, and the alveolar spaces may be filled with varying amounts of blood or fluid. In lighter, aerated portions there are varying degrees of alveolar distention. If there has been vigorous inspiration, either natural or artificial, irregular areas of alveolar overdistention may be found. Rupture of distended alveoli may result in interstitial emphysema and, at times, pneumomediastinum and pneumothorax.

CLINICAL MANIFESTATIONS. Persistent cyanosis with poor respiratory effort and air exchange are cardinal signs of primary atelectasis. Respiration may be irregular, with periods of apnea and intermittent cyanosis, especially when there is injury to or depression of the central nervous system. Auld has designated a group of small (800 to 1200 gm) premature infants with extensive atelectasis as having chronic pulmonary insufficiency. These infants are often well, with minimal signs of respiratory distress until the second or third day, when they develop frequent episodes of prolonged apnea and cyanosis that may become progressively severe and terminate in death or may gradually resolve over the ensuing two to three weeks.

The signs of secondary atelectasis usually merge with those of the underlying pulmonary problem. The infant with obstructive atelectasis may make vigorous efforts to breathe; there may be respiratory distress, cyanosis when out of oxygen, rapid deep breathing with retractions, and grunting. A roentgenogram is indicated to diagnose the underlying pulmonary disease and to distinguish lobar or segmental from lobular or patchy atelectasis.

PREVENTION AND TREATMENT. Prevention of premature labor, fetal and neonatal anoxia, intracranial hemorrhage, the respiratory distress syndrome and pneumonia would presumably eliminate most of the causes of atelectasis. Treatment should be aimed at early recognition and proper management of underlying conditions.

IDIOPATHIC RESPIRATORY DISTRESS SYNDROME

(Hyaline Membrane Disease)

This condition is the major cause of death in the newborn period; hyaline membranes with atelectasis are found at autopsy in 20 to 30 per cent of all liveborn infants dying within the first week of life. The highest incidence is in infants weighing less than 2500 gm (70 to 80 per cent), especially those weighing 1000 to 1500 gm. An increased frequency is also observed among infants of diabetic mothers delivered before 37 weeks of gestation, among infants delivered by cesarean section, and when there has been antepartum vaginal bleeding. The disease rarely occurs in full-term infants. It has been estimated to account for 25,000 to 40,000 deaths each year. The clinical incidence is difficult to determine because of differing diagnostic criteria; 10 per cent of all premature infants may have the disease.

ETIOLOGY AND PATHOPHYSIOLOGY. The cause of hyaline membrane disease is unknown, but several mechanisms appear to be central to its development and have been incorporated into two leading hypotheses. The first is that the disorder results from a deficiency of *surfactin*, a surface-tension lowering lipid formed in the walls of alveoli and present in term infants but deficient in premature infants; the tendency of the lungs of affected infants to collapse is correlated with a high surface tension and the absence of surfactin. The precise chemical composition and concentration of surfactin is unknown, but the most likely major constituent is dipalmityl phosphatidyl choline (choline phosphoglyceride), commonly referred to as *lecithin.* Gluck found little synthesis of lecithin in fetuses prior to 20 weeks of gestation. In those of 22 to 24 weeks he identified active synthesis via a methylation pathway involving phosphatidyl ethanolamine and after 35 weeks an active phosphatidyl choline pathway combining cystidine diphosphocholine with diglyceride. These pathways are thus an index of lung maturity. Their absence, presumably indicative of deficient synthesis, degradation or alteration of lecithin, could result in atelectasis, decreased lung compliance, increased work of breathing and eventually insufficient ventilation with asphyxia, hypoxia and acidosis. These latter events can produce pulmonary arterial vasoconstriction, with increased vascular resistance and shunting through the foramen ovale and ductus arteriosus. Pulmonary blood flow would thus be reduced, with ischemic injury to cells producing lecithin and injury to the vascular bed resulting in an effusion of proteinaceous material into the alveolar spaces.

The second, closely related, *"hypoperfusion" hypothesis* is that intrauterine or neonatal asphyxia with hypoxia and mixed respiratory (placental) and metabolic acidosis leads to increased pulmonary vascular resistance and systemic hypotension. As a result, venous blood bypasses the lungs through the foramen ovale and ductus arteriosus. This leads to ischemia of the alveolar lining cells that produce surfactin and/or lecithin, further compromising surfactin production, with resultant atelectasis and hypercarbia from a deficiency of surface-tension lowering lipids and with effusion of plasma and red cells from injured capillaries, leading to formation of fibrin in the air spaces.

PATHOLOGY. The lungs appear deep purplish red and are liver-like in consistency. Microscopically there is extensive atelectasis, with engorgement of the interalveolar capillaries and lymphatics. A number of the alveolar ducts, alveoli and respiratory bronchioles are lined with acidophilic, homogeneous or granular membranes. The presence of osmophilic inclusion bodies, characteristic of phospholipid storage, in type II alveolar lining cells correlates with the time of appearance of surfactant. Amniotic debris, intra-alveolar hemorrhage, pneumonia and interstitial emphysema are additional but inconstant findings (Fig. 7–13); interstitial emphysema may be marked when an infant has been ventilated with a method which employs increased end-expiratory pressure. The characteristic hyaline membranes are rarely seen in infants dying earlier than 6 to 8 hours after birth. Intracranial hemorrhages are common in infants of very low birth weight (less than 1250 gm), but are probably associated with anoxia or prematurity rather than the idiopathic respiratory distress syndrome.

CLINICAL MANIFESTATIONS. The idiopathic respiratory distress syndrome begins with rapid, shallow respirations which usually increase to 60 or more per minute within 2 hours of birth. It is often preceded by a need for resuscitation at birth. Rapid breathing beginning later suggests conditions other than hyaline membrane disease. Other symptoms are listed in Table 7–21 and illustrated in Figure 7–2. Intercostal, subcostal or sternal re-

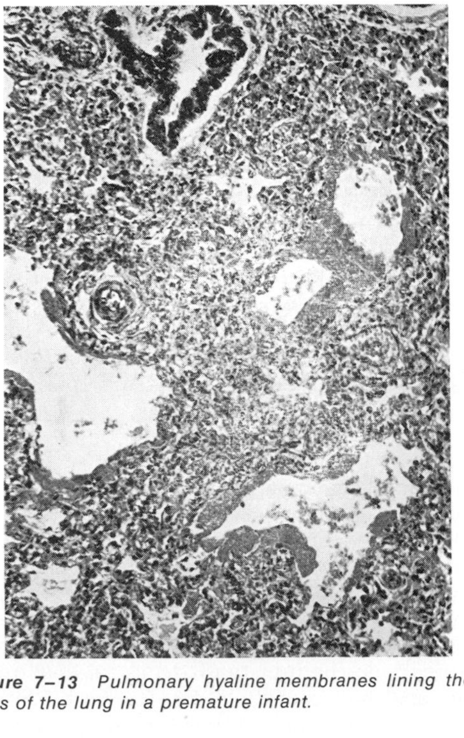

Figure 7–13 *Pulmonary hyaline membranes lining the air spaces of the lung in a premature infant.*

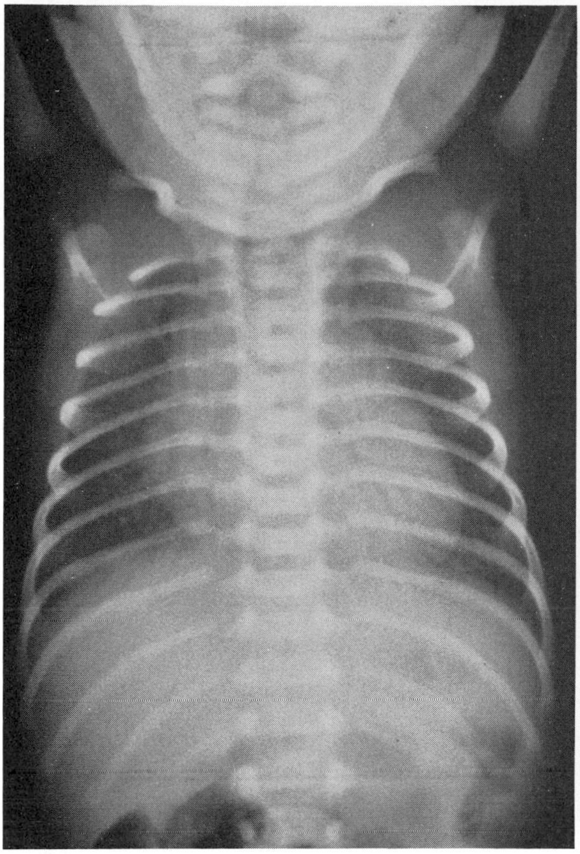

Fig. 7–14

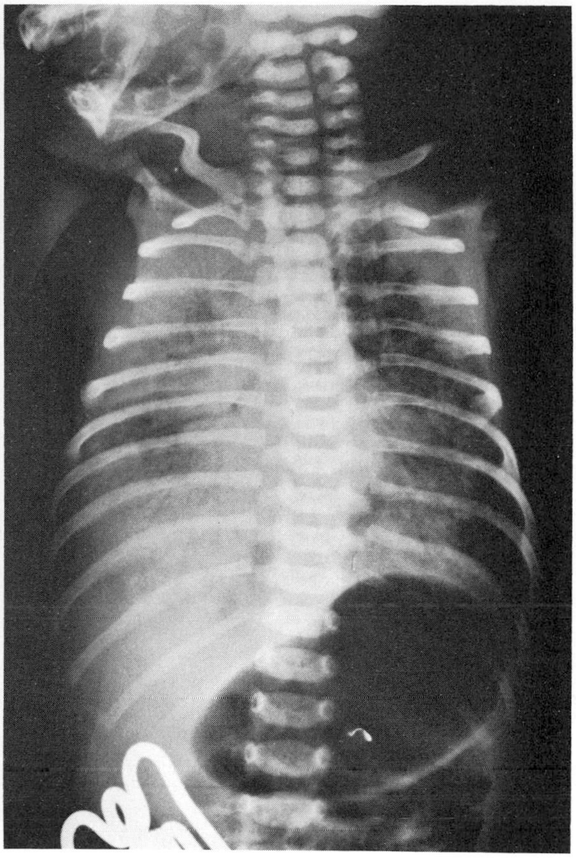

Fig. 7–15

Figure 7–14 *Respiratory distress syndrome. A diffuse reticulogranular pattern is evident throughout the lungs. The air-containing bronchi are visible by virtue of surrounding nonaerated lung, particularly on the left.*

Figure 7–15 *Fetal distress syndrome (aspiration syndrome, aspiration pneumonia).*

Figures 7–14 and 7–15 show the contrasting radiographic pictures seen in infants with neonatal respiratory distress. Figure 7–14 shows the uniform reticulogranular pattern consistently seen in, but not pathognomonic of, the respiratory distress syndrome (hyaline membrane disease). The apparent cardiac enlargement is also characteristic. Figure 7–15 shows the coarsely granular pattern with irregular aeration typical of fetal distress from aspiration of materials such as vernix caseosa, epithelial cells and meconium contained in amniotic fluid.

tractions, and expiratory grunt or whining, and nasal flaring are prominent symptoms. The course is characterized by increasing evidence of air hunger and fatigue from excessive respiratory effort. Body temperature is often low, and dyspnea, pallor and cyanosis increase as the condition worsens. On auscultation, air exchange may seem to be normal or diminished. On deep inspiration fine rales are often heard, especially over the lung bases, posteriorly. There may be hypotension, edema, ileus and oliguria. Roentgenographically (Figs. 7–14 and 7–15) the lungs have a reticulogranular appearance which is characteristic but not pathognomonic. The condition may progress to death within a few hours, but in milder cases the symptoms reach a peak within 3 days, after which gradual improvement sets in. Signs of asphyxia secondary to periods of apnea or partial respiratory failure occur when there is rapid progression of the disease. Death is rare after 3 days, except among infants in whom the natural course of the disease has been altered by the use of a respirator.

PROGNOSIS. Although the diagnosis is established with certainty only at autopsy, there is a high correlation between the clinical diagnosis and the postmortem determination of hyaline membrane disease. This provides a basis for estimating that there is a 20 to 30 per cent mortality. The death rate is lower among more mature and heavier infants. Most deaths occur within 72 hours of birth, with the smallest infants dying within 24 hours unless artificial respiration and intensive care are employed, under which circumstances death may occur much later. When recovery occurs, the prognosis is generally good, although persistent pulmonary disease with fibrosis, and recurrent pulmonary infections do occur in a small percentage of infants. The chronic pulmonary changes may be related to oxygen therapy (see below). Neurologic residuals are probably related more to intracranial hemorrhage, anoxia, hypoglycemia, hyperbilirubinemia and other complications of immaturity than to the respiratory distress syndrome. Long-term follow-up of infants receiving vigorous intensive care suggests that these infants do not have an increased incidence of mental disabilities when compared to infants of similar weight and gestational age without the disease.

PREVENTION. The prevention of prematurity, avoidance of unnecessary cesarean section, and careful management of the diabetic mother and the erythroblastotic fetus are the most important factors in the prevention of the respiratory distress syndrome. In timing cesarean section, the use of estimation of the fetal head circumference by ultrasound and of the lecithin concentration, the lecithin to sphingomyelin (L/S) ratio (see Fig. 7–16) and the creatine concentration in the amniotic fluid decreases the likelihood of delivering a premature infant. A high L/S ratio usually signifies a low risk that the fetus is premature and will develop hyaline membrane disease after delivery; ratios of 1.5 or less represent an increased risk of prematurity and hyaline membrane disease. Avoidance of maternal hypoxia, acidemia and systemic hypotension (with decreased uterine blood flow) is indicated, and intervals of diminished umbilical blood flow should be minimized so far as possible. Chilling, as well as hypoxia, of the newborn infant results in acidemia and pulmonary vasoconstriction; both should be avoided. Prompt treatment or prevention of severe acidemia through intravenous administration of sodium bicarbonate solution may be helpful in reducing the severity of respiratory distress, although there is no evidence that the incidence or mortality is altered.

Attempts to prevent hyaline membrane disease have led to investigation of the effect of corticosteroids in accelerating maturation of the lung, possibly through a beneficial effect on surfactant metabolism. In a recent study betamethasone was administered in conjunction with labor-retarding agents to mothers threatening premature delivery. An injection of 6 mg betamethasone phosphate and 6 mg betamethasone acetate was given and repeated once 24 hours later. In gestations under 32 weeks, and in the absence of maternal edema, hypertension or proteinuria, there appeared to be a decrease in the incidence of hyaline membrane disease and in the mortality from hyaline membrane disease and intraventricular hemorrhage among infants delivered between 24 hours and 7 days after the first dose.

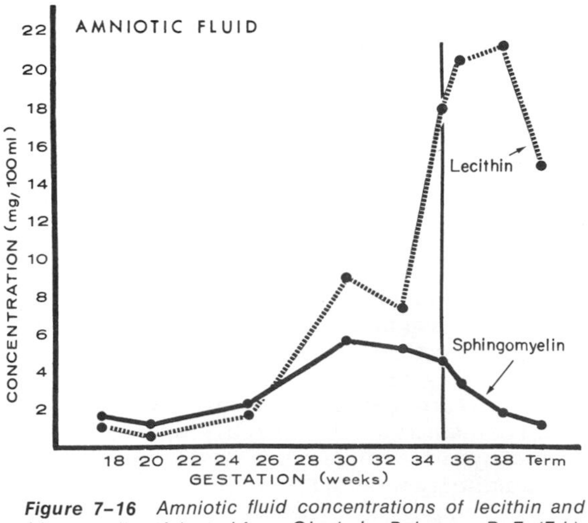

Figure 7–16 Amniotic fluid concentrations of lecithin and sphingomyelin. (Adapted from Gluck, L.: Behrman, R. E. (Ed.): Neonatology. St. Louis, The C. V. Mosby Company, 1973.)

TREATMENT. Regardless of the etiology, the basic defect that requires treatment is inadequate pulmonary exchange of oxygen and carbon dioxide; metabolic acidosis is a secondary manifestation. The infant tries to overcome his ventilatory problem by increasing the rate and depth of respiration. Expiratory grunting, usually an early feature in the clinical course, may serve the physiologic purpose of increasing alveolar ventilation by decreasing the tendency for alveoli to collapse from high intrathoracic pressure transmitted to compliant airways at the beginning of expiration. The mechanical provision of positive end-expiratory pressure serves the same purpose. Grunting decreases or disappears as the disease worsens. It is impossible with an endotracheal tube in place, which may result in decreased arterial oxygen tension unless positive end-expiratory pressure is provided artificially. During spontaneous respirations this may be accomplished by delivering *continuous positive airway pressure* (CPAP) through the tube or *continuous negative pressure* (CNP) by reducing the air pressure surrounding the lung and thorax. CNP and oxygen are more effective than the administration of oxygen alone in improving oxygenation and in reducing the duration of exposure to high oxygen concentrations and the need for respirator therapy in infants with severe hyaline membrane disease. An increase in end-expiratory transpulmonary pressure may also be achieved during artificial ventilation by providing *positive end-expiratory pressure* (PEEP) or *continuous positive pressure ventilation* (CPPV).

Chilling should be avoided. It causes pulmonary vasoconstriction and increases the metabolic need for oxygen and the production of carbon dioxide. Since hypoxia and acidemia both result from and cause pulmonary vasoconstriction, the administration of oxygen and a buffer constitutes rational treatment. Intravenous feeding is a convenient way to administer the buffer solution and also allows the infant to receive fluid and calories without fatigue from oral feeding. Mechanical assistance in breathing *may* be required in order to increase alveolar ventilation directly. The application of these methods is best carried out in a specially staffed and equipped hospital unit, the *intensive care nursery*. The facilities of the intensive care nursery may also appropriately be used for the care of other sick newborn infants and for the initial observation of high-risk infants.

Chilling is avoided and oxygen consumption of premature infants is minimal when abdominal skin temperature is kept between 36 and 37°C. Temperature control is best accomplished by special thermoregulating equipment controlled by a thermistor taped to the skin of the abdomen. If such equipment is not available, an incubator temperature between 32 and 34°C at a relative humidity of 80 to 90 per cent is usually necessary to maintain thermal stability of the infant. Relative humidity of 30 to 60 per cent is adequate when special thermoregulating equipment is being used, but in its absence heat loss is less at a relative humidity of 80 to 90 per cent. *Nebulized water mist* offers no advantage over proper humidification, except when the nose is bypassed, as with the use of tracheal intubation or tracheostomy. In such instances, if an ultrasonic nebulizer is used, care must be taken lest too much water be inhaled into the lungs. The temperature of the nebulized water should be near that of the ambient air in the incubator.

Periodic monitoring of oxygen and carbon dioxide tension and of the pH of arterial or arterialized (by wrapping in a warm, wet compress for 5 minutes) capillary blood is an important part of the management; if assisted ventilation is being used, it is essential. Arterial oxygen tension is conveniently measured in blood drawn from the temporal artery or from an indwelling plastic catheter threaded through one of the umbilical arteries so that its tip lies just above the bifurcation of the aorta or above the celiac axis (Fig. 7–17); the position should be confirmed radiographically (Fig. 7–18). Carbon dioxide tension and pH may also be measured from arterial blood obtained by these methods, and the umbilical arterial catheter may be used for administration of fluids and drugs.

In order to attain an environment with a high, constant oxygen content, it is necessary to use a plastic hood constructed so that it is just large enough to accommodate the infant's head, and through which oxygen flow can be maintained and adjusted on the basis of periodic measurements of the oxygen content of the atmosphere within the box. The air flow in commercially available incubators is such that it is impossible to maintain a high or constant atmosphere of oxygen, particularly when the infant is receiving direct care by nurse or physician.

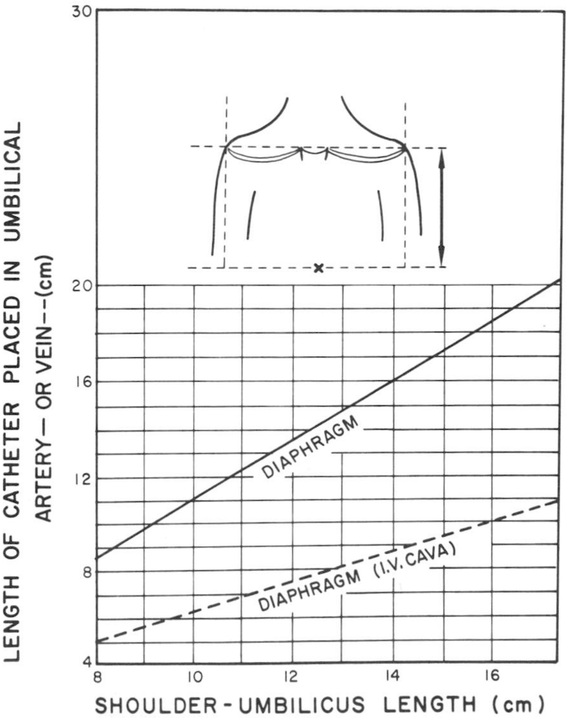

Figure 7–17 Determination of depth of insertion of umbilical catheter to reach level of diaphragm via umbilical artery (——) or umbilical vein (----). (Adapted from Dunn, P. M.: Arch. Dis. Child., 41:69, 1966.)

I.V. Cava = inferior vena cava.

Reasonable indications for *assisted ventilation* are (1) failure to maintain respiration without assistance, (2) persistent cyanosis or arterial oxygen tension under 50 mm Hg while breathing 100 per cent oxygen, or (3) arterial carbon dioxide tension over 70 mm Hg when measured after the infant has breathed 100 per cent oxygen for 15 minutes. In a group of infants who did not receive assisted ventilation and who had arterial oxygen tensions below 100 mm Hg during the first 10 hours of life while breathing 100 per cent oxygen, Boston noted a case fatality rate of 80 per cent.

The simplest method of assisted ventilation is intermittent use of a mask and bag resuscitator for 5 minutes out of every 20 minutes, or another time regimen adapted to the needs of the individual infant. A patient-cycled positive-pressure or controlled volume respirator with a nasotracheal tube in place is widely used, but its use has been accompanied by serious upper airway complications, especially when nursery personnel are inexperienced or are not continually providing respirator care. Fitted plastic nasal prongs are now being used successfully to administer oxygen under pressure early in the course, thus avoiding in some infants the need for the more traumatic method of endotracheal intubation. Trauma from the intratracheal tube may also be avoided in some cases by substituting a well-fitting anesthetic gas mask. Negative-pressure respirators have the advantage of requiring neither a mask nor endotracheal tube. However, negative pressure respirators are not usually effective with infants weighing less than 1500 gm. In general, the extent to which the morbidity and mortality of severe hyaline membrane disease can be reduced with mechanical ventilation and the frequency of complications secondary to the use of respirators can be minimized is directly related to constant maintenance of a high level of experience and skill by an intensive care team that regularly cares for critically ill newborn infants.

Monitoring of *aortic blood pressure* through an umbilical arterial catheter and *central venous pressure* by a catheter passed through the umbilical vein may provide useful guides to management of the shocklike state which may occur during the first hour or so after premature birth of an infant who has been asphyxiated or who has developed respiratory distress.

Owing to the frequency of pneumonia accompanying the respiratory distress syndrome and of infection complicating assisted ventilation and indwelling vascular catheters, the routine administration of antibacterial agents is advocated by

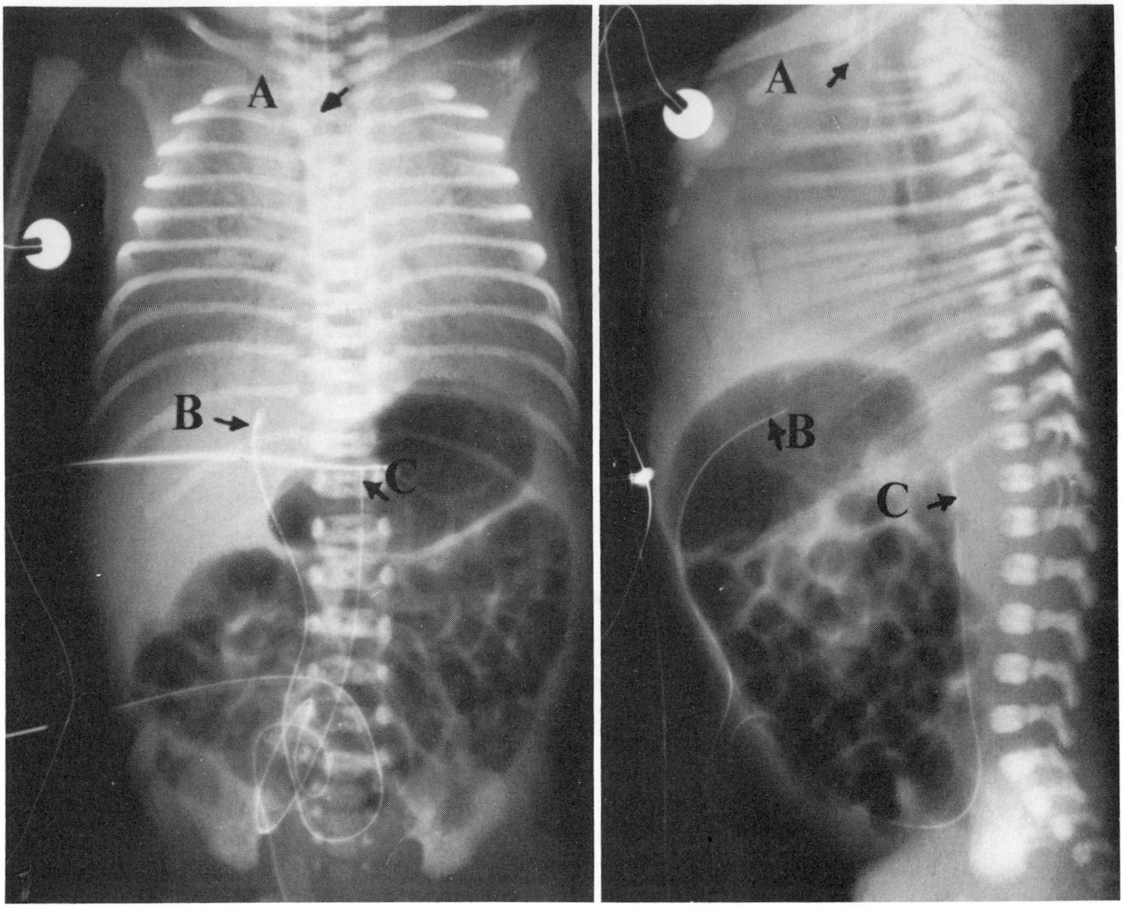

A B

Figure 7–18 Infant with RDS. Note granular lungs, air bronchogram and air filled esophagus. Anteroposterior (A) and lateral (B) roentgenograms are needed to distinguish umbilical artery from vein catheter and to determine appropriate level of insertion. The lateral view clearly identifies that the catheter has been inserted into an umbilical vein and is lying in the portal system of the liver. A, endotracheal tube; B, umbilical venous catheter at the junction of the umbilical vein, ductus venosus and portal vein; C, umbilical artery catheter passed up the aorta to T-12. (Courtesy Walter E. Berdon, Babies Hospital.)

some, but rejected by those who are more fearful of upsetting bacterial ecology. If they are to be used, penicillin or ampicillin with kanamycin or gentamicin is suggested, depending upon the recent pattern of bacterial sensitivities in the hospital where the infant is being treated. Appropriate doses are 25,000 units of penicillin or 50 mg of ampicillin, and 7.5 mg of kanamycin or 2.5 mg of gentamicin per kg every 12 hours until recovery seems assured.

The use of acetylcholine or adrenergic inhibitors, though a logical approach to the problem of pulmonary vasoconstriction, has not been shown to be therapeutically effective and is contraindicated because of the risk of systemic hypotension.

Acidosis during hyaline membrane disease was first noted by Reardon and by Usher. Subsequent studies have indicated the need for serial monitoring of pH, pCO_2, pO_2, bicarbonate, base deficit and electrolytes, and for correction of observed abnormalities. The heart rate and/or electrocardiogram should be continuously recorded in order to identify arrhythmias if they occur. Although no controlled study has established a decrease in mortality or morbidity as a result of correcting the acidosis with sodium bicarbonate, the severity of the disease appears to be lessened and the risks of pulmonary vasoconstriction, untoward cardiovascular shunting, arrhythmias and hypotension diminished. Parenteral buffer therapy may be needed temporarily in addition to ventilatory assistance for profound respiratory acidosis, even when the base deficit from accumulated lactic acidosis is of minor significance.

The metabolic acidosis of hyaline membrane disease is corrected in a similar manner to that of diarrheal dehydration or diabetes mellitus. With respiratory acidosis or a substantial respiratory component in a mixed acidosis, sodium bicarbonate is usually infused in 5 or 10 per cent glucose at an initial rate of 65 ml/kg/24 hours as follows:

pH ARTERIAL OR ARTERIALIZED CAPILLARY BLOOD	CONCENTRATION OF SODIUM BICARBONATE
7.10–7.20	10 mEq or 0.83 gm per 100 ml
<7.10	15 mEq or 1.25 gm per 100 ml

It may be necessary to infuse sodium bicarbonate more rapidly when respiratory distress is severe, especially when there is impending shock; 3–4 mEq/kg of a solution containing 0.5 mEq/ml may be infused over a 20- to 30-minute period. A pH, pCO_2, bicarbonate concentration and estimation of the base deficit should be obtained immediately after such infusions and subsequently at intervals. In the presence of hypernatremia with edema, oliguria, or congestive heart failure, an infusion of 0.3 molar tris-hydroxymethyl aminomethane (THAM), infused at a rate of 1 ml/min to provide 1.0 ml/kg for each pH unit below 7.40, may be preferred to bicarbonate. More than 12 mEq/kg/24 hours of sodium bicarbonate should rarely be given unless the serum sodium is documented to be normal and the output of urine adequate.

Liver necrosis may be caused by rapid infusion of concentrated solutions of sodium bicarbonate or THAM through an umbilical catheter into a portal vein. Since circulatory stasis at the time of rapid infusion of concentrated solutions seems to contribute to their toxicity, caution should be taken to maintain an adequate blood pressure, by careful external cardiac massage if necessary, while they are being given.

It may be necessary, on occasion, to increase the rate of water and glucose infusion substantially above 65 ml/kg/24 hours to avoid dehydration due to water loss from tachypnea and diuresis. Parenteral fluids should be given through a superficial vein in an extremity, as this route results in the fewest complications, but an umbilical catheter already in place for purposes of monitoring may be used occasionally in the severely ill infant. In an emergency, such as acute asphyxia in the delivery room, if an umbilical arterial catheter cannot be inserted, an umbilical vein catheter should be placed to obtain venous blood and to infuse drugs and fluids. Radiopaque catheters should always be used and their position checked roentgenographically after insertion. Placement and supervision should be by skilled and experienced personnel. Catheters should be removed as soon as there is no indication for their continued use.

COMPLICATIONS OF INTENSIVE CARE. The most serious complication of nasotracheal intubation is cardiac arrest during intubation or suctioning. Other complications include bleeding from trauma during intubation, difficult extubation requiring tracheotomy, ulceration of the nares due to pressure from the tube, permanent narrowing of the nostril due to tissue damage and scarring from irritation of infection around the tube, evulsion of a vocal cord, laryngeal ulcer, papilloma of a vocal cord, subglottic stenosis, and persistent hoarseness, stridor or edema of the larynx.

Measures to reduce the incidence of these complications include use of polyvinyl endotracheal tubes that do not contain tin, which is toxic to cells; use of a tube of the smallest practicable size in order to reduce local ischemia and necrosis; avoidance of frequent changes of the tube; avoidance of motion of the tube in situ; avoidance of too frequent or vigorous suctioning; and avoidance of infection through meticulous cleanliness and frequent sterilization of all apparatus attached to or passed through the tube. The personnel inserting and caring for the endotracheal tube should be experienced and skilled. The use of a specially fitted anesthetic gas mask instead of an endotracheal tube has been shown to be practical for selected patients, and to avoid the foregoing complications; care must be taken to avoid damage to the eyes and skin from pressure if a mask is used. The use of a negative-pressure respirator eliminates the need for either tube or mask, but may be less desirable than a patient-cycled positive-pressure machine, especially for infants who require assisted ventilation only; negative-pressure respirators are often difficult to use or ineffective for infants under 1500 gm.

The risks of umbilical vessel catheterization include vascular embolization, thrombosis, spasm and perforation; ischemic and/or chemical necrosis of abdominal viscera; infection; accidental hemorrhage; and impaired circulation to a leg with subsequent gangrene. At necropsy the reported incidence of complications varies from less than 1 per cent to 23 per cent, although most investigators find 3 to 5 per cent. Aortography has demonstrated that clots form in or about the tips of 95 per cent of catheters placed in an umbilical artery. The risk of a serious clinical complication from umbilical catheterization is probably between 2 and 5 per cent and may be slightly greater with venous than with arterial placement.

Transient blanching of the leg may occur during catheterization of the umbilical artery. It is usually due to reflex arterial spasm. The incidence is lessened by use of the smallest available catheters, particularly in very small infants. The catheter should be removed immediately; catheterization of the other artery may then be attempted. Persistent spasm after removal of the catheter may be relieved by warming the opposite leg. Intermittent severe spasm or unrelieved spasm may respond to the cautious intravenous infusion of tolazoline (Priscoline), 10 to 25 mg injected intra-arterially over 5 minutes, or less if vasodilatation occurs. Accidental lodgment of the catheter in a smaller artery so as to block it completely or cause unrecognized local vascular spasm may result in gangrene of the organ or area supplied by the vessel. To prevent this complication the catheter should be removed promptly if blood cannot be obtained through it.

Serious hemorrhage on removal of the catheter is rare; its incidence may be reduced by not removing the catheter for 6 hours after any heparin has been infused through it. Thrombi may form in the artery or in the catheter; their incidence is lowered by use of a smooth-tipped catheter with a hole only at its end, and by rinsing the catheter with a small amount of saline solution containing 10 units of heparin per ml, or by continuously infusing a solution containing 1 unit/ml of heparin. The risks of thrombus formation with potential vascular occlusion can also be reduced by removing the catheter when there are early signs of thrombosis, such as narrowing of pulse pressure and disappearance of the dicrotic notch. Some prefer to use the umbilical artery for blood sampling only, leaving the catheter filled with heparinized saline between samplings. The later hazards of catheterization of the umbilical artery or umbilical vein, particularly when it has been traumatic, are as yet unknown, but may well exist.

The toxicity to the retina of high concentrations of oxygen administered for prolonged periods has been amply demonstrated; retrolental fibroplasia is probably secondary to partial pressures of oxygen above the normal range in the blood and the risk probably varies inversely with the maturity and weight of the infant; it occurs, but it is rare with oxygen concentrations of less than 40 per cent in the inspired air. The blood of a healthy fetus or newborn infant can be 80 to 90 per cent saturated at oxygen tensions of about 35 mm Hg and a pH of 7.4. The oxygen tension of the blood under normal circumstances while breathing air progressively increases in the newborn period from fetal levels to 80 to 100 mm Hg; while breathing 40 per cent oxygen it is usually 140 to 150 mm. Therefore the partial pressures of oxygen in the arterial blood should be monitored in the pink infant receiving oxygen and kept below 80 mm Hg and above 50 mm Hg; the oxygen tensions in cyanotic infants are well below 80 mm Hg.

Oxygen has been demonstrated to be toxic to the lung, particularly if administered by means of a positive pressure respirator. Instead of showing improvement on the third or fourth day, consistent with the natural course of the disease in survivors, some infants who have been on prolonged intermittent positive pressure breathing using high concentrations of oxygen have roentgenographic evidence of worsening of their pulmonary condition (Fig. 7–19, *A*), and they continue to be cyanotic without oxygen in high concentration. The chest roentgenogram is described as gradually changing from a picture of almost complete opacification with air bronchogram to one of small, round, lucent areas alternating with areas of irregular den-

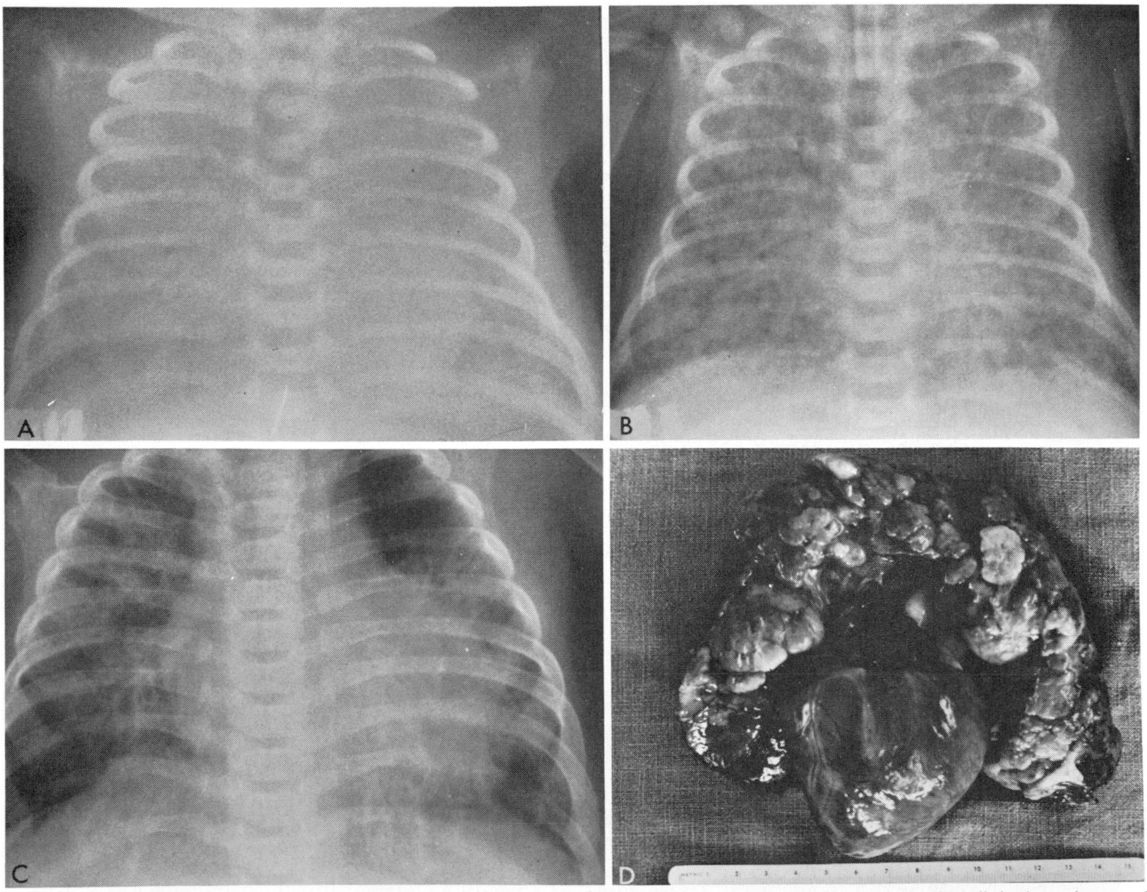

Figure 7–19 *Pulmonary changes in infants who were treated in the immediate postnatal period for the clinical syndrome of idiopathic respiratory distress with prolonged, intermittent positive-pressure breathing with air containing 80 to 100 per cent oxygen. In all infants there was persistent respiratory disease. Nine of 13 infants lived beyond 2 weeks of age; 5 of the 9 died, and all had right-sided congestive heart failure. The remaining were described as having chronic pulmonary disease.* A, *A 5 day old infant with nearly complete opacification of lungs.* B, *A 13 day old infant with "bubbly lungs" simulating the roentgenographic appearance of the Wilson-Mikity syndrome.* C, *A 7 month old infant with irregular, dense strands in both lungs, and cardiomegaly.* D, *Large right ventricle and cobbly, irregularly aerated lung of an infant who died at 11 months of age; this infant also had a patent ductus arteriosus. (From Northway, W. H., Jr., Rosan, R. C., and Porter, D. Y.: New Engl. J. Med., 276:357, 1967.)*

sity resembling a sponge (Fig. 7–19, *B*). This picture is similar to that seen in the "bubbly-lung syndrome' of Wilson and Mikity. In the histologic picture at this stage (10 to 20 days after beginning oxygen therapy) there is less evidence of hyaline membrane formation, progressive alveolar coalescence with atelectasis of surrounding alveoli, interstitial edema, coarse focal thickening of the basement membranes and widespread bronchial and bronchiolar mucosal metaplasia and hyperplasia. In the series studied, respiratory difficulty persisted in the 4 of 13 infants who survived (see legend of Fig. 7–19). Postmortem studies in those who died revealed cardiac enlargement and pulmonary changes consisting of focal areas of emphysematous alveoli with hypertrophy of the peribronchial smooth muscle of the tributary bronchioles, some perimucosal fibrosis and widespread metaplasia of the bronchiolar mucosa, and thickening of basement membranes and separation of the capillaries from the alveolar epithelial cells.

It is suggested that oxygen tension in the arterial blood be kept in the range of 50 to 80 mm Hg when assisted ventilation is being used. A question has also recently been posed regarding the possible toxicity of oxygen for cerebral blood vessels. *The principle of using as little oxygen as possible for the shortest possible time must be rigidly adhered to in the therapy of infants.*

Another iatrogenic complication of intensive care is *anemia secondary to frequent withdrawal of blood samples.* The cumulative amount of blood withdrawn should be carefully recorded. Replacement by transfusion is indicated if more than 10 to 15 per cent of estimated total blood volume is removed.

RESULTS OF INTENSIVE CARE. There is increasing evidence from short- and long-term studies of individual nursery populations and state and regional surveys that early provision of intensive observation and care to high-risk newborn infants can significantly reduce morbidity and mortality due to hyaline membrane disease and other acute neonatal illnesses. However, the results are critically dependent on the existence of a team of experienced and skilled personnel in specially designed and organized hospital units. In contrast, the beneficial effect of intensive care is questionable if respiratory disease is complicated by severe fetal or birth asphyxia, intracranial hemorrhage or irremediable congenital malformation.

OTHER ASPECTS OF INTENSIVE CARE. The concept of intensive care of the newborn implies attention to problems other than respiratory ones. Many of these, such as hypoglycemia and hyperbilirubinemia, are common among infants who are candidates for intensive care because of respiratory difficulties associated with asphyxia or prematurity. The satisfactory management of these problems, like those of respiratory distress, requires a high degree of mutual interest and coordination among anesthetist, obstetrician, pediatrician and pathologist. The continuous night and day availability of interested and skilled clinical and laboratory personnel is essential.

TRANSIENT TACHYPNEA OF THE NEWBORN

Transient tachypnea lasting 24 to 36 hours has been described following uneventful normal or elective cesarean delivery at term. Air exchange is good and there is no cyanosis or acidosis. Roentgenograms of the chest may reveal central perihilar streaking and fluid in the interlobar fissures, suggesting that the syndrome is secondary to slow absorption of lung fluid. The increased respiratory rate may require discontinuance of oral feeding to avoid the risk of aspiration.

PNEUMONIA

Histologic evidence of pneumonia is a frequent finding at autopsy in newborn infants, particularly among those who die after signs of respiratory distress of whatever cause. Its role as a cause of death is not always clear in such instances, and the clinical manifestations may merge indistinguishably with those of the primary disturbance. Perhaps 10 per cent of neonatal deaths are primarily attributable to pneumonia.

ETIOLOGY. There are two main types of neonatal pneumonia. The first, sometimes termed **congenital pneumonia**, occurs during the first few days of life. It is particularly common when there has been premature rupture of the membranes, prolonged labor, premature labor, maternal fever or fetal distress. The presence of chorioamnionitis in most instances suggests aspiration of infected amniotic fluid as its cause. Aspiration of vaginal secretions during delivery may also be a cause. The second type of pneumonia, beginning after the first few days of life, is usually acquired through contact with adults or children with respiratory infections, or through bacteremia. Coliform organisms, nonhemolytic streptococci and *Staphylococcus aureus* (Fig. 7–20) are the most frequent causative organisms for either type of pneumonia. Enterococci, Klebsiella, Pseudomonas, Proteus and Salmonella also tend to be more frequent pathogens in the newborn than are Pneumococcus, *Haemophilus influenzae* and beta-hemolytic streptococcus, the commonest acute pulmonary pathogens of older infants and children. Group B beta-hemolytic streptococci and *Streptococcus agalactiae* may also be associated with early septicemia and pneumonia. The relative incidence of viral pneumonitis in the neonatal period is not adequately defined.

PATHOLOGY. Pneumonia in early infancy is usually bronchopneumonic in type, occasionally interstitial or lobar.

CLINICAL MANIFESTATIONS. The first signs of pneumonia in the newborn are usually nonspecific. They include loss of appetite, listlessness, poor color which may or may not be definable as cyanosis, a rise or sudden fall in body temperature, abdominal distention, sudden loss or gain in weight, tachycardia, and a general impression on the part of the nurse or mother that the baby is doing less well. Cough is inconstant, but almost always

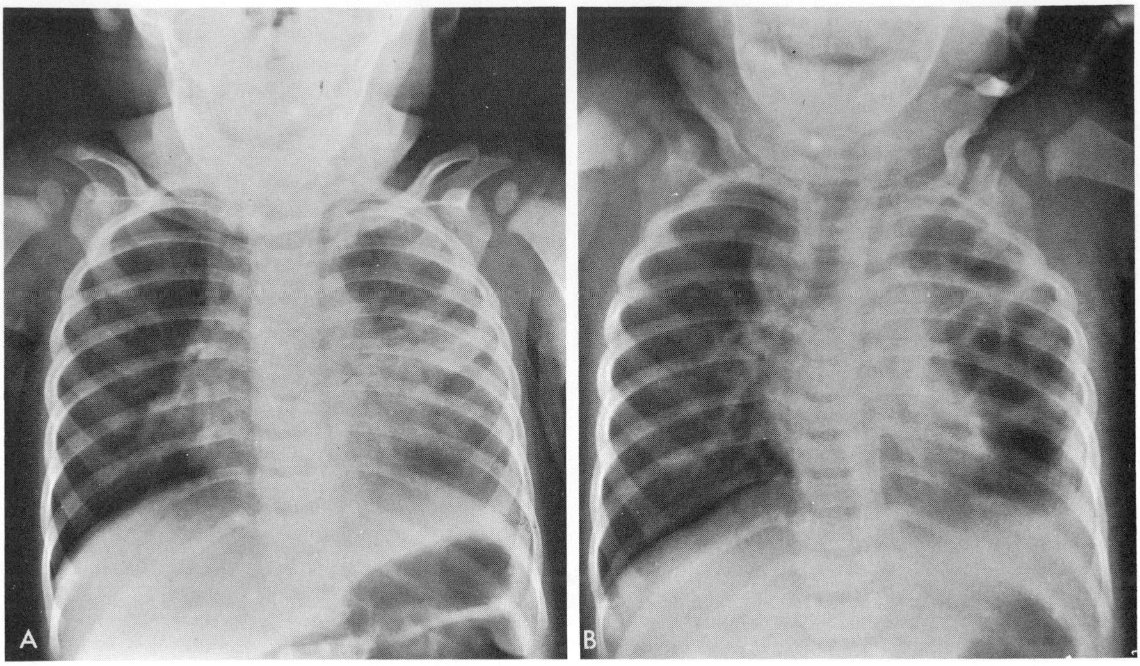

Figure 7–20 Staphylococcal pneumonia in an infant 7 months of age. A, The diffuse inflammatory process involving the left lung and pleura is evident. B, Five days later, just before death, there are multiple air-containing cavities in the lung and pleura.

means pneumonia when present. A significant increase in respiratory rate, usually to about 80, is a constant and early finding. Flaring of the alae nasi, accentuation of the normal irregularity of breathing, and respiratory distress may be present.

DIAGNOSIS. Often no physical signs are elicited; although careful auscultation may reveal fine, crackling rales, most commonly in the perihilar areas posteriorly, they may be localized in any portion of the lungs. It is important to auscultate the chest with the baby crying as well as quiet, since frequently rales are heard only at the end of the deep inspirations which come only with crying in the newborn. Areas of hyperresonance may indicate compensatory emphysema. Roentgenograms of the chest are often helpful and are essential to distinguish pneumonia from other causes of respiratory distress. Nasopharyngeal and blood cultures are helpful in making an etiologic diagnosis.

ASPIRATION OF FOREIGN MATERIAL ("FETAL ANOXIA"; "FETAL DISTRESS SYNDROME"; "ASPIRATION PNEUMONIA"). (See also Section 12.) During prolonged labors and difficult deliveries infants often attempt to breathe in utero, owing to interference with the supply of oxygen via the placenta. Under such circumstances the infant aspirates amniotic fluid containing such debris as vernix caseosa, epithelial cells, meconium or material from the birth canal. This debris blocks the smallest airways and interferes with alveolar exchange of oxygen and carbon dioxide. Pathologic bacteria frequently accompany the aspirated material. When this is the case, pneumonia is apt to ensue, but even in the noninfected cases there are respiratory distress and usually roentgenographic evidences of aspiration (Fig. 7–15).

Other situations in which pulmonary aspiration of foreign material may contribute to serious consequences in the newborn infant include tracheoesophageal fistula, esophageal and duodenal obstructions, improper feeding practices, the administration of medicines and improper handling and placement of infants in their cribs.

The contents of the stomach should always be aspirated through a soft rubber catheter just before operation or other procedures requiring anesthesia. Procedures which may significantly disturb the infant, and particularly those which interfere with changing the infant to the head-down position, such as jugular and femoral punctures, lumbar puncture and subdural taps, should be performed at least 2 hours after a feeding.

STAPHYLOCOCCAL PNEUMONIA. This should be suspected in any infant who shows even slight and nonspecific untoward signs and who has been exposed to staphylococcal skin infections. Empyema and pneumothorax are frequent complications. The latter constitutes such an immediate threat to life that infants with staphylococcal pneumonia must be watched closely for acute onset of respiratory distress, so that treatment by closed thoracotomy drainage can be carried out without delay.

TREATMENT. See Infections of the Newborn later in this Section, and Section 12.

PNEUMOTHORAX AND PNEUMOMEDIASTINUM

Asymptomatic pneumothorax, either unilateral or bilateral, is estimated to occur in 1 to 2 per cent of all newborn infants; symptomatic pneumothorax and pneumomediastinum are less common. The mortality for this disorder is approximately 20 per cent. It is more common in males than in females and in term and post-term infants than in premature ones. The incidence is increased, however, among infants with hyaline membrane disease and those who are receiving artificial ventilation, especially if a continuous elevation of end-expiratory pressure is maintained.

ETIOLOGY AND PATHOPHYSIOLOGY. The most common cause of pneumothorax is overinflation and resulting alveolar rupture. It may be "spontaneous" or idiopathic, or be secondary to resuscitation, to mechanically assisted ventilation, to underlying pulmonary disease such as lobar emphysema or rupture of a congenital or a pneumonic cyst, to trauma, or to a "ball-valve" type of bronchial or bronchiolar obstruction resulting from aspiration. If the ruptured alveoli are on the pleural surface, pneumothorax without pneumomediastinum occurs; if not, pulmonary interstitial emphysema occurs. Air in the interstitial spaces of the lung dissects along the peribronchial and perivascular connective tissue sheaths to the root of the lung. The pulmonary veins may be compressed at the hilum and cardiac output severely reduced with bilateral compression. If the volume of escaped air is great enough, it may follow the vascular sheaths to cause mediastinal emphysema or a rupture with subsequent pneumomediastinum, pneumothorax and subcutaneous emphysema. Rarely, there may be increased mediastinal pressure and interference with venous return to the heart.

Tension pneumothorax occurs if an accumulation of air within the pleural space is sufficient to elevate intrapleural pressure above atmospheric pressure. Not only is ventilation impaired in the collapsed lung by a unilateral tension pneumothorax, but that in the normal lung may be compromised by mediastinal shift to the other side. Compression of the vena cava and torsion of the great vessels may interfere with venous return.

CLINICAL MANIFESTATIONS. The physical findings of asymptomatic pneumothorax are hyperresonance and diminished breath sounds over the involved side of the chest.

Symptomatic *pneumothorax* is characterized by respiratory distress which varies from only an increased respiratory rate to severe dyspnea and cyanosis. Alternatively, irritability and restlessness, or apnea, may be the earliest signs. The onset may be sudden or gradual; an infant may rapidly become critically ill. The chest may appear asymmetric with increased anteroposterior diameter and bulging of the intercostal spaces on the affected side, and there are hyperresonance and diminished or absent breath sounds. The heart is displaced toward the unaffected side, and the diaphragm is displaced downward, as is the liver with right-sided pneumothorax. Since both sides are affected in approximately 10 per cent of patients, symmetry of findings does not rule out pneumothorax.

With *pneumomediastinum,* which occurs in at least 25 per cent of patients, the degree of respiratory distress is again dependent on the amount of trapped air. If it is great, there is bulging of the midthoracic area, the neck veins are distended, and the blood pressure is low. The last two findings are the result of blockage of the circulation by compression of the systemic and pulmonary veins. Subcutaneous emphysema in the newborn infant is almost pathognomonic of pneumomediastinum.

DIAGNOSIS. Pneumothorax and pneumomediastinum should be suspected in any newborn infant with respiratory signs, or who displays restlessness or irritability. The diagnosis is established roentgenographically (Fig. 7–21).

TREATMENT. Without a continued air leak, asymptomatic and mildly symptomatic small pneumothoraces require only close observation. Frequent small feedings may prevent gastric dilatation and minimize crying, which can further compromise ventilation and worsen the pneumothorax. Breathing 100 per cent oxygen accelerates the resorption of free pleural air into the blood by reducing the nitrogen tension in blood with a resultant nitrogen pressure gradient from the trapped air into the blood. With severe respiratory or circulatory embarrassment, emergency needle aspiration may be indicated. If this is unsuccessful in maintaining relief of distress or if there is adequate time, closed thoracotomy is indicated, with the tube connected to a water trap so that air may escape, but not enter the chest.

INTERSTITIAL PULMONARY FIBROSIS OF PREMATURITY

(Wilson-Mikity Syndrome; Bubbly-Lung Syndrome; Pulmonary Dysmaturity; Bronchopulmonary Dysplasia)

Wilson and Mikity described a pulmonary syndrome of premature infants, usually of less than 32 weeks' gestation, and birth weights below 1500 gm, characterized by insidious onset of dyspnea, tachypnea, retractions and cyanosis during the first month of life. Rarely, cases have been reported in full-term infants, usually with a history of meconium aspiration or oxygen administration.

The etiology is unknown. Several variations on the clinical presentation have been described with similar radiographic findings; it is uncertain whether they represent separate entities. Some infants have respiratory distress at birth which is occasionally severe, resembles hyaline membrane disease and requires oxygen. Others have no early respiratory symptoms or history of exposure to oxygen and the onset of symptoms is at several weeks

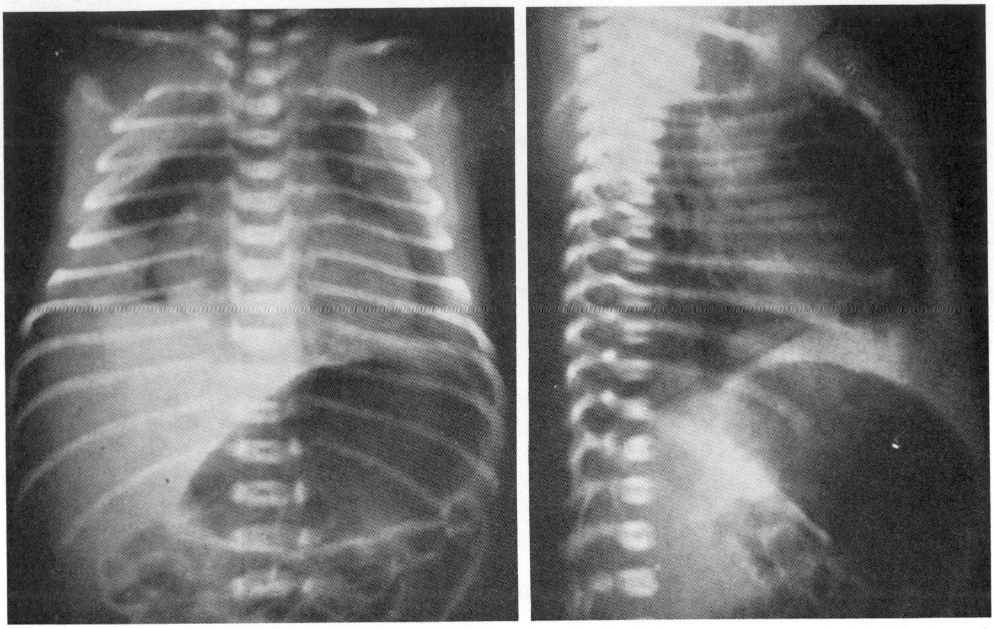

Figure 7–21 Penumomediastinum in a newborn infant. Anteroposterior view demonstrates compression of lungs and the lateral view bulging of the sternum, each resulting from distention of the mediastinum by trapped air.

of life. Northway et al. have reported similar clinical, radiologic and pathologic findings, designated *bronchopulmonary dysplasia,* in infants who developed pulmonary disease following respirator therapy and oxygen for hyaline membrane disease (Fig. 7–19 *B* and *C*).

Cough, wheezing and rales may develop, but fever occurs only with concomitant infection. There may be collapse of a lobe or lung; other complications are right-sided heart failure and osteoporosis and rib fractures. The symptoms usually increase over two to six weeks with increasing oxygen dependency persisting for several months, followed by gradual resolution or progressive respiratory and cardiac failure. The most characteristic features of this syndrome are roentgenographic. Early, they include bilateral coarse reticular streaky infiltrates, and often overexpansion of the lungs with small areas of emphysema which develop into multicystic lesions. Subsequently the cysts enlarge and coalesce to give a hyperlucent, bubbly appearance (Fig. 7–19, *B*). The roentgenograms tend to clear gradually over months to several years. At autopsy in fatal cases, the lungs have a "hobnail" appearance, with cystic and emphysematous areas in the parenchyma and thickened fibrous septa. Microscopically the alveolar walls are thickened, with proliferation of capillaries and infiltration of mononuclear cells.

The syndrome must be differentiated from pneumonia due to *Pneumocystis carinii* and cystic fibrosis. Treatment consists of supportive measures: oxygen for cyanosis, digitalization and diuretics for cardiac failure, acid-base correction, and assisted ventilation when indicated. The mortality is approximately 25 per cent.

LOBAR EMPHYSEMA

See Section 12.

LUNG CYSTS

Most lung cysts observed during the neonatal period are acquired as the result of rupture of alveoli by overinflation or infection, often staphylococcal; congenital cysts are rare. They may be solitary or multiple, air-containing or filled with fluid, and are believed to result as a developmental anomaly of the bronchial buds (see Section 12). Infants with congenital or acquired cysts may be asymptomatic or present with tachypnea and dyspnea at birth or any time thereafter, or with recurrent or persistent pneumonia. Air-filled cysts on the surface of the lung, whatever their origin, sometimes rupture and cause pneumothorax. This is particularly true of multicystic disease. Since most cystic areas discovered by roentgenologic examination will disappear spontaneously, treatment, which is surgical removal, should be reserved for those which cause severe respiratory distress.

PULMONARY HEMORRHAGE

Massive pulmonary hemorrhage is present in about 15 per cent of premature infants and 45 per cent of mature infants who come to autopsy in the first two weeks of life. The reported incidence at autopsy varies from about 1 to 4 per thousand live births. About three fourths of the patients weigh less than 2500 gm at birth.

Most infants in whom pulmonary hemorrhage is demonstrated at autopsy have had symptoms of respiratory distress that are indistinguishable from those of hyaline membrane disease. The onset may be at birth or delayed several days. One fourth to one half of affected infants cough up or regurgitate material containing old or fresh blood from the nose or mouth. Roentgenographic findings are varied and nonspecific, ranging from minor streaking or patchy infiltrates to massive consolidation.

The cause of massive pulmonary hemorrhage is unknown; the incidence is increased in association with acute pulmonary infection, severe anoxia, hyaline membrane disease, hemorrhagic disease of the newborn, kernicterus, and cold injury. Although in the majority of instances bleeding into other organs is observed at autopsy, bleeding other than through the nostrils and mouth is relatively rare during life and should suggest the possibility of an additional bleeding diathesis such as disseminated intravascular coagulation (Section 14). Bleeding is predominantly alveolar in about two thirds of cases, and interstitial in the rest.

Since most of the available knowledge about pulmonary hemorrhage in the newborn has been obtained by retrospective study of the records of patients in whom the diagnosis has been made at autopsy, there is little information about the prognosis of infants who bleed through the mouth or nostrils, except that it is extremely poor. Death occurs in the first 48 hours of life in two thirds of the infants who come to autopsy. Treatment is supportive.

CONGENITAL PULMONARY LYMPANGIECTASIA

This disorder is a rare occurrence among full-term infants with respiratory distress at birth. Cyanosis is marked and generally rapidly progressive. Death is usual during the first month of life, often within hours of birth. Rarely, symptoms abate, and survival up to four years has been noted; an asymptomatic variant has been recognized later in childhood. The chest roentgenogram usually shows a general haziness or diffuse reticulogranular pattern with hyperaeration, prominent fissures and occasionally pleural effusion.

CHYLOTHORAX

This rare condition presents usually in the first days of life with cyanosis and signs of unilateral or bilateral pleural effusion. The fluid is clear initially, becoming opalescent due to fat globules after milk feeding is established. The etiology is unclear, but the condition may occasionally be associated with chylous ascites and/or lymphedema elsewhere, presumably due to congenital malformations of the lymphatic system. *Treatment* is by thoracentesis repeated as necessary, or by continuous drainage of the affected pleural space. About half the patients recover within 30 days. Protein depletion may be a problem if large amounts of the fluid (protein content = 2-4 gm/dl) must be removed.

DISTURBANCES OF THE DIGESTIVE SYSTEM

VOMITING. Infants at times vomit mucus, often blood-streaked, in the first few hours after birth. This vomiting infrequently persists after the first few feedings; it may be due to irritation of the gastric mucosa by material swallowed during delivery. If the vomiting is protracted, gastric lavage with physiologic saline solution may relieve it.

Vomiting is a relatively frequent symptom during the neonatal period. In the majority of instances it is simply regurgitation from overfeeding or from failure to permit the infant to eructate swallowed air. When vomiting occurs shortly after birth and is persistent, the possibilities of increased intracranial pressure and of intestinal obstruction must be considered. An accompanying history of maternal hydramnios suggests upper intestinal atresia.

Obstructive lesions of the digestive tract occur most frequently in the esophagus and intestines (Section 11). Vomiting from esophageal obstruction occurs with the first feeding. The diagnosis of *esophageal atresia* can be suspected if there is unusual drooling from the mouth and if resistance is encountered in the attempt to pass a catheter into the stomach. There is considerable advantage in establishing the diagnosis before the infant chokes on oral feedings and risks aspiration pneumonia. **Cardiospasm** is a rare cause of vomiting in the newborn infant; it is demonstrable roentgenographically by obstruction at the cardiac end of the esophagus, without organic stenosis. Regurgitation of feedings due to continuous relaxation of the esophageal-gastric sphincter, **chalasia,** is an infrequent cause of vomiting, which can be controlled by keeping the infant in a semi-upright position. Vomiting from obstruction of the small intestine usually begins on the first day of life and is frequent, persistent, usually nonprojectile, copious and, unless the obstruction is above the ampulla of Vater, bile-stained; it is associated with abdominal distention, visible deep peristaltic waves, and reduced or absent bowel movements. Upright roentgenographic films of the abdomen will show the distribution of air in the intestine and often aid in locating the site of the obstruction; the use of contrast material for these studies is usually unnecessary. Normally, air can be demonstrated roentgenographically in the jejunum by 15 to 60 minutes, in the ileum by 2 to 3 hours, and in the colon by 3 hours after birth. Persistent vomiting may occur with congenital hernia of the diaphragm (Section 11) when the viscera are crowded. The vomiting of *pyloric stenosis* may begin any time after birth, but does not assume its characteristic pattern before the second or third week. Vomiting may occur with many other disturbances which do not obstruct the digestive tract, such as celiac disease, milk allergy, adrenal hyperplasia of the salt-losing variety, septicemia, meningitis and other infections. It is common with urinary tract infections.

THRUSH (ORAL MONILIASIS). Thrush of the mouth (Section 11) is mentioned here to emphasize its importance in newborn infants. At this age it occurs in healthy infants; later, it is rare except in debilitated infants and children and those receiving antibiotic or immunosuppressive therapy.

There is a positive correlation between maternal vaginal and infantile oral moniliasis. The maternal source appears to be the principal primary means of infection in healthy newborns. Secondary cases develop in the hospital nursery, presumably by contact with infected infants and contaminated supplies or caretakers.

Occasionally a heavy coat forms on the tongue, but its appearance is not that of thrush, nor do cultures from it reveal *Candida albicans.* It can be removed by 1 or 2 applications of a 1 per cent aqueous solution of gentian violet.

Oral thrush in an otherwise healthy infant is usually a self-limited infection, but treatment is advised (Section 11).

DIARRHEA. See Diarrhea in the Newborn later in this Section and Enteropathogenic Escherichia Coli in Section 10.

CONSTIPATION. More than 90 per cent of newborn infants pass meconium within the first 24 hours, and most of the remainder do so within 36 hours. The possibility of intestinal obstruction should be considered in any infant who does not pass meconium within that time. Intestinal atresia or stenosis (Section 11), congenital aganglionic megacolon (Section 11), meconium ileus or meconium plugs should be suspected. Constipation not present from birth, but appearing during the first month of life, suggests congenital aganglionic megacolon, cretinism or anal stenosis. It must be kept in mind that infrequent bowel movements do not necessarily mean constipation. Breast-fed infants may rarely go 7 to 10 days without a bowel movement and without evidence of discomfort, and then pass a large but otherwise normal stool.

MECONIUM PLUGS. Anorectal plugs (Fig. 7–22) of lower water content than normal may be a cause of intestinal obstruction in newborn infants. Rarely a firm mass of meconium may form elsewhere in the intestine and cause intrauterine intestinal obstruction and meconium peritonitis unrelated to cystic fibrosis. Likewise, anorectal plugs may cause intestinal ulceration and perforation. The plug may require irrigation with isotonic sodium chloride solution or half-strength hydrogen peroxide for evacuation. More consistently good results have recently been reported with enemas of the iodinated contrast medium, *Gastrografin.* Such enemas will usually cause passage of the plug, presumably because the high osmolality (1900 mOsm/l) of the medium draws fluid rapidly into the intestinal lumen and loosens inspissated material. Since this rapid loss of fluid into the bowel may result in acute dehydration and shock, it is advisable to dilute the contrast material with an equal amount of water, to correct any existing dehydration with an intravenous infusion of 5 per cent dextrose in 0.2 per cent sodium chloride solution to bring the serum osmolality to about 290 mOsm/l, and to continue the same infusion during and for several hours after the procedure, adjusting the rate of flow to maintain the serum osmolality at about 290 mOsm/l. Approximately 50 to 60 ml of diluted contrast medium usually suffices to fill the colon and distal ileum to the point of a high obstruction, as in meconium ileus. *After removal of a meconium plug the infant should be observed closely for the possible presence of congenital aganglionic megacolon.*

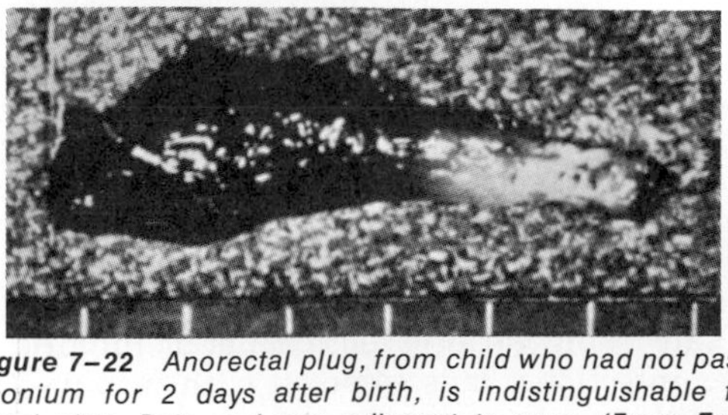

Figure 7–22 Anorectal plug, from child who had not passed meconium for 2 days after birth, is indistinguishable from normal plug. Pale end was adjacent to anus. (From Emery, J. L.: Arch. Dis. Child., Vol. 32.)

MECONIUM BODIES. These light yellow particles are usually no more than 1 mm in diameter, but may rarely be large enough to cause distortion of the intestine. They are occasionally associated with intestinal atresia.

MECONIUM ILEUS. Impaction of meconium is a relatively rare cause of intestinal obstruction in the newborn infant. It is associated with cystic fibrosis. The depletion or absence of pancreatic enzymes limits normal digestive activities in the intestine, and meconium is left in a viscid, mucilaginous state. It clings to the intestinal wall and is moved with difficulty or not at all by intestinal peristalsis. The inspissated and impacted meconium fills the intestinal canal, but is most concentrated in the lower ileum.

Clinically the pattern is that of congenital intestinal obstruction with or without intestinal perforation (see Meconium Peritonitis). Abdominal distention is prominent, and persistent vomiting soon occurs. Infrequently one or more inspissated meconium stools may be passed shortly after birth.

The *differential diagnosis* involves other causes of intestinal obstruction; an exact diagnosis cannot be made except by laparotomy. A presumptive diagnosis can be made on the basis of a history of cystic fibrosis in a sibling, by palpation of doughy or cordlike masses of intestines through the abdominal wall, and by the roentgenographic appearance. Roentgenographically in contrast to the generally evenly distended intestinal loops above an atresia, the loops may vary in width and not be as evenly filled with gas. At points of heaviest meconium concentration the infiltrated gas may create a granular appearance (Figs. 7–23 and 7–24). A negative sweat test in the neonatal period may not rule out cystic fibrosis.

The case fatality rate is high, but a number of infants have survived the neonatal period; their subsequent *prognosis* is dependent upon the basic disturbance, cystic fibrosis.

Treatment is with high Gastrografin enemas as described under meconium plugs above. If this is unsuccessful or if there is reason to suspect a perforation of the bowel wall, laparotomy is performed and the ileum opened at the point of greatest diameter of the impaction. The inspissated meconium is removed by gentle and patient irrigation with warm isotonic sodium chloride solution introduced through a fine catheter which may be passed between the impaction and the bowel wall.

MECONIUM PERITONITIS. Perforation of the intestine may occur in utero or shortly after birth. The tear may be sealed by natural processes relatively quickly, with only a small amount of meconium escaping, or the meconial contents may largely be emptied into the peritoneal cavity. Such perforations occur most often as a complication of meconium ileus in infants with cystic fibrosis, but occasionally the perforation is due to a meconium plug, meconium bodies or intestinal obstruction of whatever cause.

When the intestinal perforation is spontaneously sealed and only a small amount of meconium has escaped, the event may never be known, except as some of the meconial particles become calcified and are subsequently discovered fortuitously on roentgenograms of the abdomen. Otherwise the clinical picture is dominated by the signs of intestinal obstruction or peritonitis. Characteristically there are abdominal distention, vomiting and absence of stools. The treatment is primarily elimination of the intestinal obstruction and drainage of the peritoneal cavity.

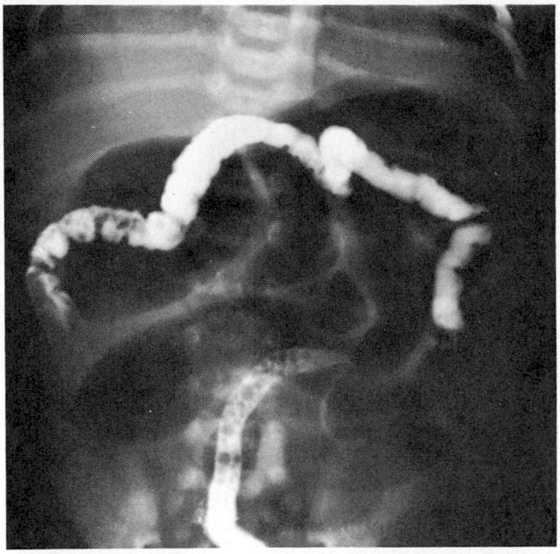

Figure 7–24 Meconium ileus. The colon, outlined by contrast material, is small because meconium has not reached it. The small, circumscribed radiolucencies in the colon represent air injected with the contrast material and mucus present in the colon.

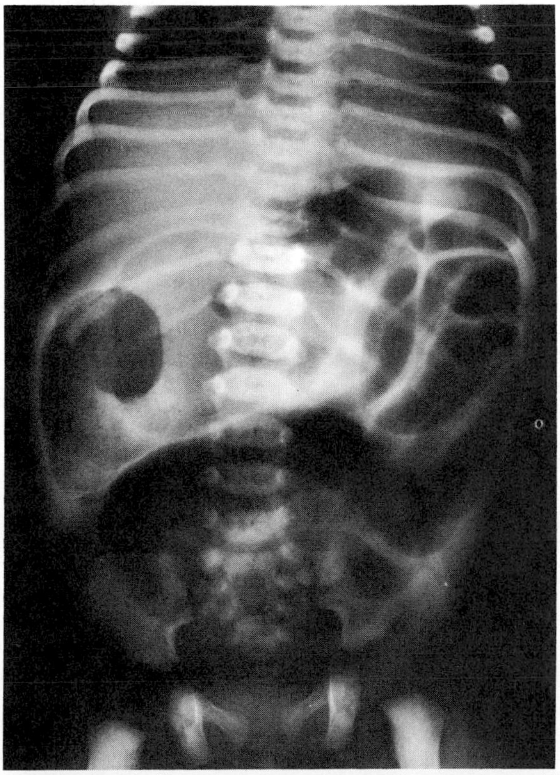

Figure 7–23 Meconium ileus. Impacted meconium with small amounts of air interspersed throughout it in loops of intestine on the right side of abdomen; intestinal loops above this impaction are greatly distended.

JAUNDICE AND HYPERBILIRUBINEMIA IN THE NEWBORN INFANT

Under usual nursery conditions jaundice is observed during the first week of life in approximately 60 per cent of term infants and 80 per cent of preterm infants. The color usually results from the accumulation in the skin of unconjugated, nonpolar, lipid-soluble bilirubin pigment (indirect-reacting) formed from hemoglobin by the action of hemoxygenase and bilirubin reductase; it may also be due, in part, to the deposition of the pigment after it has been converted in the liver cell microsome by the enzyme bilirubin glucuronyl transferase to the polar, water-soluble ester glucuronide of bilirubin (direct-reacting). The unconjugated form is neurotoxic for infants at certain concentrations and under various conditions.

Whether jaundice is considered to be a sign of illness in the infant and the degree of danger that it may represent depend upon factors that affect the production, metabolism, excretion and distribution of bilirubin after birth.

ETIOLOGY. The newborn infant's metabolism of bilirubin is in transition from the fetal stage, when the placenta is the principal route of elimination of the lipid-soluble bilirubin, to the adult stage, when the water-soluble conjugated form is excreted from the hepatic cell into the biliary system and then into the gastrointestinal tract. Any factor which increases the load of bilirubin to be metabolized by the liver (erythroblastosis fetalis, other hemolytic anemias, shortened red cell life owing to immaturity or to transfused cells, infection), any factor which may damage or reduce the activity of the enzyme (anoxia, infection, possibly hypothermia and thyroid deficiency), any factor which may compete for or block the enzyme (drugs and other substances requiring glucuronic acid conjugation for excretion), or any factor leading to absence or decreased amounts of the enzyme (genetic defect, prematurity) may be expected to cause or increase the degree of jaundice. The risk of toxic effects from elevated levels of bilirubin in the serum are increased by factors which reduce the retention of bilirubin in the circulation (hypoproteinemia, displacement of bilirubin from its binding sites on albumin by competitive binding of drugs such as sulfisoxazole, acidosis, hyperosmolality, increased free fatty acid concentration secondary to hypoglycemia, starvation or hypothermia), or by factors which increase the permeability of nerve cell membranes to free bilirubin or the susceptibility of brain cells to its toxicity. (See Table 7-25.) Early feeding decreases and dehydration increases the serum levels of bilirubin. Oral administration of substances such as agar to the newborn infant may bind conjugated bilirubin and prevent its deconjugation and resorption in the intestine.

CLINICAL MANIFESTATIONS. Jaundice may be present at birth or may appear at any time during the neonatal period, depending on the condition responsible for it. *Its intensity bears no dependable relation to the degree of hyperbilirubinemia,* particularly in infants receiving phototherapy. Jaundice resulting from deposition of indirect bilirubin in the skin tends to appear bright yellow or orange; jaundice of the obstructive type (direct bilirubin), a greenish or muddy yellow. This difference is usually apparent only in severe jaundice. The infant may be lethargic, feed poorly and become dehydrated. Signs of kernicterus rarely appear on the first day of jaundice.

DIFFERENTIAL DIAGNOSIS. Jaundice present at birth or appearing within the first 24 hours of life should be considered due to erythroblastosis fetalis (see later section) until proved otherwise; sepsis, cytomegalic inclusion disease, rubella and congenital toxoplasmosis are less frequent possibilities. Jaundice in infants who have received intrauterine transfusions may be characterized by an unusually high level of direct-reacting bilirubin. Jaundice which first appears on the second or third day is usually "physiologic," but may represent the more severe form now called hyperbilirubinemia of the newborn. Familial nonhemolytic icterus (Crigler-Najjar syndrome) also is seen initially on the second or third day. *Jaundice appearing after the third day and within the first week should suggest septicemia as the most likely cause;* it may be due to other infections, notably syphilis, toxoplasmosis and cytomegalic inclusion disease. Jaundice secondary to extensive ecchymosis or hematomas may occur during the first week, especially in premature infants; it may also occur in the second week of life. Polycythemia may lead to early jaundice.

Jaundice initially noted after the first week of life suggests septicemia, congenital atresia of the bile ducts, homologous serum hepatitis, rubella, herpetic hepatitis, idiopathic dilatation of the common bile duct, galactosemia, congenital hemolytic anemia (spherocytosis) or possibly the crises of other hemolytic anemias such as pyruvate kinase and other glycolytic enzyme deficiencies, thalassemia, sickle cell disease, hereditary nonspherocytic anemia or hemolytic anemia due to idiosyncrasy to drugs or other substances, as in congenital deficiencies of the enzymes glucose-6-phosphate dehydrogenase, and glutathione synthetase, reductase and peroxidase. Hemolytic anemia has also been associated with vitamin E deficiency in premature infants.

Persistent jaundice during the first month of life suggests the so-called inspissated bile syndrome, which may follow hemolytic disease of the newborn, hepatitis, cytomegalic inclusion disease, syphilis, toxoplasmosis, familial nonhemolytic icterus, congenital atresia of the bile ducts, idiopathic dilatation of the common bile duct, or galactosemia. Rarely, physiologic jaundice may be prolonged for several weeks, as in infants with hypothyroidism or pyloric stenosis.

PHYSIOLOGIC JAUNDICE (ICTERUS NEONATORUM). Under normal circumstances, the level of indirect-reacting bilirubin in umbilical cord serum is 1 to 3 mg/dl and rises at a rate of less than 5 mg/dl/24 hours; thus, jaundice becomes visible on the second or third day, usually peaking between the second and fourth days at 5 to 6 mg/dl, and decreasing to below 2 mg/dl between the fifth and seventh days of life. Jaundice resulting from these changes is designated "physiologic" and is believed to be the result of breakdown of fetal red cells combined with transient limitation in the conjugation and excretion of bilirubin by the liver. Among premature infants the rise in serum bilirubin tends to be the same or a little slower but of longer duration, generally resulting in higher levels, the peak being reached between the fourth and sev-

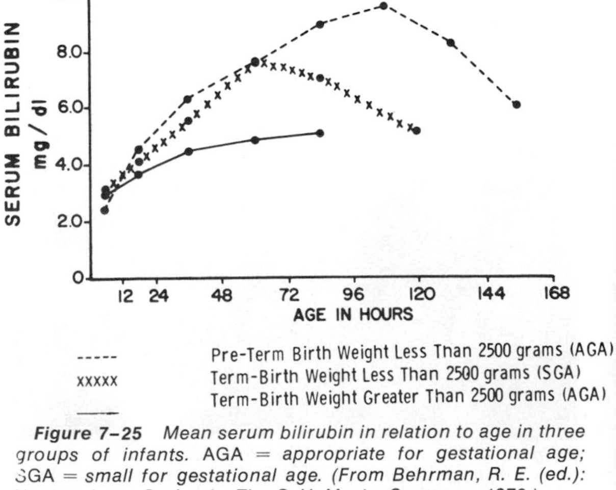

Figure 7-25 Mean serum bilirubin in relation to age in three groups of infants. AGA = *appropriate for gestational age;* SGA = *small for gestational age. (From Behrman, R. E. (ed.):* Neonatology. *St. Louis, The C. V. Mosby Company, 1973.)*

TABLE 7–22 INCIDENCE OF VARIOUS PEAK TOTAL SERUM BILIRUBIN LEVELS AMONG NEWBORN INFANTS ACCORDING TO BIRTH WEIGHT*

SERUM BILIRUBIN LEVEL mg/dl	INFANTS UNDER 2500 GMS		INFANTS OVER 2500 GMS		ALL INFANTS	
	White (1142)†	*Black (2261)*†	*White (17,292)*†	*Black (18,015)*†	*White*	*Black*
0–7	42.7%	50.3%	73.7%	74.5%	71.7%	71.5%
8–12	29.4%	31.8%	20.1%	21.6%	20.7%	22.4%
13–15	11.2%	10.0%	3.3%	2.6%	3.8%	3.5%
16–19	10.0%	5.0%	2.0%	1.3%	2.5%	1.6%
20+	6.7%	3.0%	1.0%	0.6%	1.3%	0.9%

*Data obtained from the Collaborative Perinatal Study of The National Institute of Neurologic Disease and Stroke: The Women and Their Pregnancies. U.S. Department of Health, Education, and Welfare, Publication No. (NIH) 73-379, 1973.

†Numbers in parentheses represent number of infants observed in each category.

enth days (Fig. 7–25 and Table 7–22); the pattern depends upon the time required for the preterm infant to achieve mature mechanisms for the metabolism and excretion of bilirubin. Usually peak levels of 8 to 12 mg/dl are not reached until the fifth to seventh day and jaundice is rarely observed after the tenth day. The diagnosis of physiologic jaundice in term or preterm infants can be established only by excluding known causes of jaundice on the basis of history and clinical and laboratory findings (Table 7–23). In general, a search to determine the cause of jaundice should be made if (1) it appears in the first 24 hours of life; (2) serum bilirubin is rising at a rate greater than 5 mg/dl/day; (3) serum bilirubin is greater than 12 mg/dl in full-term or 15 mg/dl in preterm infants; (4) jaundice persists after the first week of life; or (5) direct-reacting bilirubin is greater than 1 mg/dl at any time.

Pathologic Hyperbilirubinemia. Jaundice and its underlying hyperbilirubinemia are considered pathologic if their time of appearance, duration or pattern of serially determined serum bilirubin concentrations varies significantly from that of physiologic jaundice, or if the course is compatible with physiologic jaundice but there are other reasons to suspect that the infant is at special risk from the neurotoxicity of unconjugated bilirubin. It may not be possible to determine precisely the etiology for abnormal elevation of unconjugated bilirubin, especially in premature infants, and this has led to the use of the term **hyperbilirubinemia of the newborn** for those infants whose primary problem is probably a deficiency or inactivity of

TABLE 7–23 DIAGNOSTIC FEATURES OF THE VARIOUS TYPES OF NEONATAL JAUNDICE*

DIAGNOSIS	NATURE OF VAN DEN BERGH REACTION	JAUNDICE		PEAK BILIRUBIN CONC.		BILIRUBIN RATE OF ACCUMULATION *mg/dl/day*	REMARKS
		Appears	*Disappears*	*mg/dl*	*Age in Days*		
1. **"Physiologic jaundice":**							1. Usually relates to degree of maturity
Full-term	Indirect	2–3 days	4–5 days	10–12	2–3	<5	
Premature	Indirect	3–4 days	7–9 days	15	6–8	<5	
2. **Hyperbilirubinemia due to metabolic factors, etc.:**							2. Metabolic factors: hypoxia, respiratory distress, lack of carbohydrate
Full-term	Indirect	2–3 days	Variable	>12	1st wk.	<5	Hormonal influences: cretinism, hormones
Premature	Indirect	3–4 days	Variable	>15	1st wk.	<5	Genetic factors: Crigler-Najjar syndrome, transient familial hyperbilirubinemia. Drugs: vitamin K, novobiocin
3. **Hemolytic states and hematoma**	Indirect	May appear in 1st 24 hours	Variable	Unlimited	Variable	Usually >5	3. Erythroblastosis: Rh, ABO. Congenital hemolytic states: spherocytic, nonspherocytic. Infantile pyknocytosis. Drugs: vitamin K. Enclosed hemorrhage—hematoma
4. **Mixed hemolytic and hepatotoxic factors**	Indirect and direct	May appear in 1st 24 hours	Variable	Unlimited	Variable	Usually >5	4. Infection: bacterial sepsis, pyelonephritis, hepatitis, toxoplasmosis, cytomegalic inclusion disease, rubella. Drugs: vitamin K
5. **Hepatocellular damage**	Indirect and direct	Usually 2–3 days	Variable	Unlimited	Variable	Variable: can be >5	5. Biliary atresia; galactosemia; hepatitis and infection as in (4)

*From Brown, A. K.: Pediat. Clin. N. Amer. *9*(No. 3):589, 1962.

TABLE 7–24 RELATION OF MAXIMUM TOTAL SERUM BILIRUBIN CONCENTRATION TO INCIDENCE OF KERNICTERUS

MAXIMUM BILIRUBIN CONCENTRATION (mg/dl)	KERNICTERUS
10-18	0
19-24	7%
25-29	30%
30-40	70%

Adapted from Mollison and Cutbush: Recent Advances in Paediatrics. London, J. & A. Churchill, Ltd., 1954, p. 112.

bilirubin glucuronyl transferase rather than an excessive load of bilirubin for excretion.

The *significance* of hyperbilirubinemia lies in the high incidence of kernicterus associated with serum bilirubin levels over 18 to 20 mg per dl. The correlation between serum bilirubin levels and kernicterus or milder forms of brain injury in infants with erythroblastosis fetalis (Table 7–24) probably holds for all newborn infants who develop bilirubin concentrations beyond the physiologic range for their weight and gestational age, independent of the etiology of the jaundice, Low-birth-weight infants have been reported to develop kernicterus at lower levels in association with asphyxia, respiratory distress syndrome, hypoglycemia, acidosis, sepsis and meningitis. Sulfisoxazole also increases susceptibility to kernicterus at relatively low levels (12–15 mg/dl) of serum bilirubin.

Less than 3 per cent of term infants without blood group incompatibility develop bilirubin levels greater than 15 mg/dl. Sixteen per cent of white and 8 per cent of black infants of low birth weight (presumedly preterm) achieve these levels (Table 7–22). Unconjugated hyperbilirubinemia has also been associated with the administration of vitamin K_3 or novobiocin and with the presence of pyloric stenosis, congenital hypothyroidism, mongolism and maternal diabetes.

Jaundice Associated with Breast Feeding. A small number of breast-fed infants develop significant elevations in unconjugated bilirubin between the fourth and seventh days of life, reaching maximum concentrations as high as 15 to 25 mg/dl during the second and third weeks. If breast feeding is continued, the hyperbilirubinemia gradually decreases and then may persist for 3 to 10 weeks at lower levels. If nursing is discontinued, the serum bilirubin level falls rapidly, usually reaching normal levels in 6 to 10 days. Cessation of breast feeding for 3 to 4 days results in a rapid decline in serum bilirubin, after which nursing can be resumed without a return of the hyperbilirubinemia to its previously high levels. These infants have no other sign of illness and kernicterus has not been reported. The milk contains pregnane-3 α, 20 β-diol, which competitively inhibits glucuronyl transferase conjugating activity in approximately 75 per cent of the infants nursed by these mothers.

Transient Familial Neonatal Hyperbilirubinemia. Severe unconjugated hyperbilirubinemia may occur rarely in the first four days of life because of a glucuronyl transferase-inhibiting factor present in the serum of mother and infant. These babies may develop kernicterus unless repeated exchange transfusions are performed. The jaundice subsides spontaneously during the second or third week.

NEONATAL HEPATITIS. See Section 11.

CONGENITAL ATRESIA OF THE BILE DUCTS. See Section 11.

INSPISSATED BILE SYNDROME. See Kernicterus, Late Complications, below.

KERNICTERUS

Kernicterus is a neurologic syndrome resulting from the deposition of unconjugated bilirubin in brain cells. The risk in infants with erythroblastosis fetalis is directly related to serum bilirubin levels (Table 7–24). It is probably similar for infants with hyperbilirubinemia of whatever cause.

The precise blood level above which indirect-reacting bilirubin will be toxic for an individual infant is unpredictable, but kernicterus is rare with serum levels under 18 to 20 mg/dl. The duration of exposure necessary to produce toxic effects is also unknown. There is some evidence that motor disturbances in later childhood are more common among newborn infants whose total serum bilirubin rises above 15 mg/dl. The less mature the infant, the greater the susceptibility to kernicterus. Factors which potentiate the movement of bilirubin into brain cells and its adverse effects on them are listed in Table 7–25. Kernicterus in premature infants has resulted from therapy with sulfisoxazole and from administration of excessive doses of vitamin K analogues to the infants or their mothers. In exceptional circumstances kernicterus in premature infants with serum bilirubin concentrations as low as 9 to 12 mg/dl has been associated with an apparently cumulative effect of a number of the factors listed in Table 7–25.

CLINICAL MANIFESTATIONS. Signs and symptoms of kernicterus usually appear 2 to 5 days after birth in term infants and as late as the seventh day in premature ones, but hyperbilirubinemia may lead to the syndrome at any time during the neonatal period and, very rarely, later in childhood. The early signs may be subtle and indistinguishable from those of sepsis, asphyxia, hypoglycemia, intracranial hemorrhage and other acute systemic illnesses in the neonatal infant. Lethargy, poor feeding and loss of the Moro reflex are common initial signs. Subsequently the infant may appear gravely ill and prostrated, with diminished Moro and tendon reflexes, respiratory distress and failure to suck. Opisthotonos, with bulging fontanel, twitching of face or limbs and a shrill high-pitched cry may follow. In advanced

TABLE 7–25 FACTORS INCREASING THE RISK OF KERNICTERUS*

	MECHANISM OF ACTION		
FACTORS	*Reduced Albumin Binding Capacity*	*Competition for Binding Sites*	*Increased Cell Susceptibility to Toxicity*
Prematurity	+	–	?
Hemolysis	–	+	?
Asphyxia	+	–	+
Acidosis	+	–	?
↑ Nonesterified fatty acids (NEFA)	–	+	–
Hyperosmolality	+	–	?
Cold stress	–	+	–
↓ Serum albumin	+	–	+
Hypoglycemia	–	+	?
Infection	+	–	?
Drugs	–	+	–
Male sex	–	–	?

*Modified from Brown, A. K. *In* Behrman, R. E. (ed.): Neonatology. St. Louis, The C. V. Mosby Company, 1973, and *Birth Defects Series,* New York, The National Foundation, June 1972, Vol. VI, No. 2.

cases convulsions and spasms occur, with the infant stiffly extending his arms in inward rotation with fists clenched. Rigidity is rare at this late stage. Many infants who progress to these severe neurologic signs die; the survivors are usually seriously damaged, but may appear to recover and for two to three months manifest few abnormalities. Later in the first year of life opisthotonos, muscular rigidity, irregular movements and convulsions tend to recur. In the second year opisthotonos and seizures abate but irregular, involuntary movements, muscular rigidity or, in some infants, hypotonia increase steadily. By 3 years of age the complete neurologic syndrome is often apparent, consisting of bilateral choreo-athetosis with involuntary muscle spasm, extrapyramidal signs, seizures, mental deficiency, dysarthric speech, high-frequency hearing loss, and squints and defective upward movement of the eyes. Pyramidal signs, hypotonia and ataxia occur in a few infants. In mildly affected infants the syndrome may be characterized only by mild to moderate neuromuscular incoordination, partial deafness and "minimal brain dysfunction," occurring singly or in combination; these problems may be inapparent until the child enters school.

PATHOLOGY. The surface of the brain is usually pale yellow. On cutting, certain regions are characteristically stained yellow by unconjugated bilirubin, particularly the corpus subthalamicum, hippocampus and adjacent olfactory areas, striate bodies, thalamus, globus pallidus, putamen, inferior clivus, cerebellar nuclei and cranial nerve nuclei. Nonpigmented areas may also be damaged. Large, phylogenetically older cells are usually involved. Loss of neurons, reactive gliosis and atrophy of involved fiber systems are found in late disease. The pattern of injury has been related to the development of oxidative enzyme systems in various regions of the brain and overlaps with that found in anoxic brain damage. Evidence favors the hypothesis that bilirubin interferes with oxygen utilization by cerebral tissue; antecedent hypoxic injury increases the susceptibility of brain cells to injury.

INCIDENCE AND PROGNOSIS. One third of infants with untreated hemolytic disease and bilirubin levels in excess of 20 mg/dl will develop kernicterus. The incidence at autopsy of hyperbilirubinemic premature infants is 2 to 16 per cent, and is related to presence of factors listed in Table 7–25. Reliable estimates of the frequency of the clinical syndrome are not available because of the wide spectrum of manifestations. Overt neurologic signs have a grave prognosis; 75 per cent or more of such infants die and 80 per cent of affected survivors have bilateral choreo-athetosis with involuntary muscle spasm. Mental retardation, deafness and spastic quadriplegia are common.

TREATMENT OF HYPERBILIRUBINEMIA. Irrespective of etiology, the goal of therapy of jaundice is to prevent the concentration of indirect-reacting bilirubin in the blood from reaching levels at which neurotoxicity and kernicterus may occur; exchange transfusion and/or phototherapy may be indicated. The risk of injury to the central nervous system from bilirubin must be balanced against the risk inherent in the treatment for each infant. When identified, the underlying cause of the icterus should be treated, e.g., antibiotics for septicemia. Physiologic factors that increase the risk of neurologic damage should also be treated, e.g., correction of acidosis.

Exchange Transfusion. Exchange tranfusion, repeated as frequently as necessary to keep indirect bilirubin levels in the serum under 20 mg/dl in full-term infants, is a widely accepted treatment. A variety of factors may alter this criterion in either direction in an individual patient. Appearance of clinical signs suggesting kernicterus is indication for exchange transfusion at any level of serum bilirubin. A healthy full-term infant may tolerate a bilirubin concentration slightly higher than 20 mg/dl with no apparent ill effect, whereas a sick premature infant may acquire kernicterus at a significantly lower level. A level approaching that considered critical for the individual infant may indicate exchange transfusion during the first day or two of life when a further rise is anticipated, but not on the fourth day in term infants or on the seventh day in premature infants, when an imminent fall may be anticipated as the conjugating mechanism becomes more effective.

Phototherapy. Clinical jaundice and hyperbilirubinemia are reduced on exposure to a high intensity of light in the visible spectrum. The mode of action is poorly understood, but alteration of the bilirubin molecule in vivo has been hypothesized to occur principally in peripheral tissues and to involve photo-oxidation and the induction of an excited state of molecular oxygen (singlet oxygen). Biliary excretion of indirect-reacting bilirubin is increased during phototherapy.

The use of phototherapy with fluorescent light bulbs has decreased the incidence of exchange transfusion in low-birth-weight infants without hemolytic disease, and has probably decreased the need for exchange transfusion in infants with mild hemolysis and also for repeated exchange transfusion of infants with hemolytic disease. However, whenever there are indications for exchange transfusion (Fig. 7–26), phototherapy should not be used as a substitute.

Phototherapy should be used only after establishment of the presence of pathologic hyperbilirubinemia. The basic cause(s) of the jaundice should be treated concomitantly (e.g., antibiotics for septicemia). The criteria for initiating phototherapy are not generally agreed upon. However, Figure 7–26 presents reasonable guidelines for phototherapy and exchange transfusion. The success of phototherapy in lowering serum bilirubin levels varies inversely with the rate and degree of hemolysis, if present, and varies directly with the often unpredictable degree of absence or inhibition of activity of glucuronyl transferase.

In premature infants without significant hemolysis, serum bilirubin usually declines 1-2 mg/dl after 8 to 12 hours of exposure, and peak levels attained may be decreased by 3-6 mg/dl. The exact dosage and type of light needed to produce a desired therapeutic effect has not been determined; the dosage of light can be estimated from the

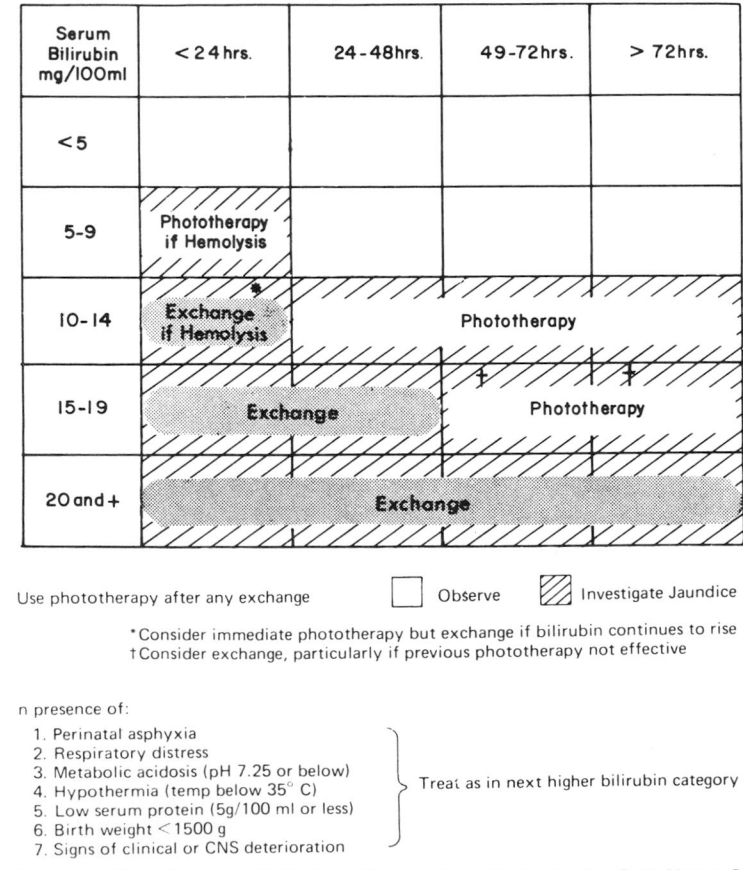

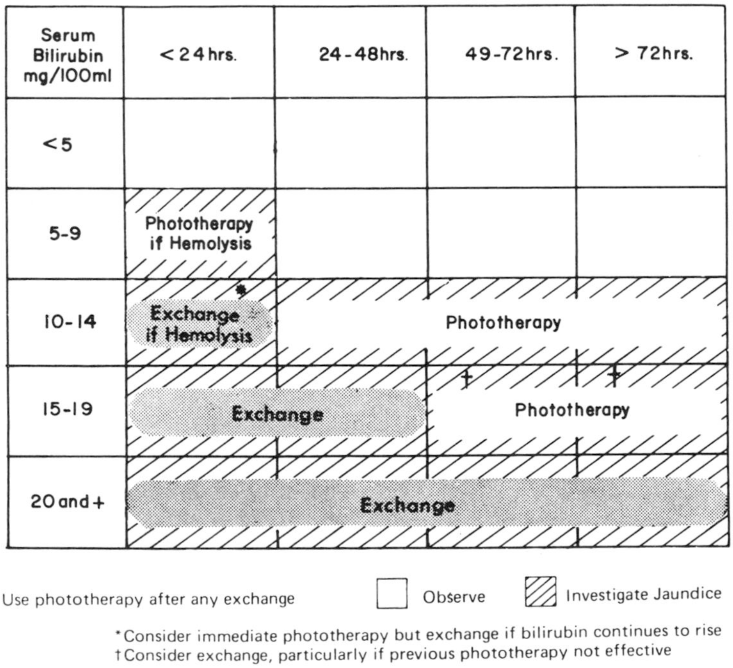
Serum Bilirubin mg/100ml
< 24 hrs.
24-48 hrs.
49-72 hrs.
> 72 hrs.
< 5
5-9
Phototherapy if Hemolysis
10-14
Exchange if Hemolysis
*
Phototherapy
15-19
Exchange
†
†
Phototherapy
20 and +
Exchange
Use phototherapy after any exchange
Observe
Investigate Jaundice
*Consider immediate phototherapy but exchange if bilirubin continues to rise
†Consider exchange, particularly if previous phototherapy not effective

n presence of:

1. Perinatal asphyxia
2. Respiratory distress
3. Metabolic acidosis (pH 7.25 or below)
4. Hypothermia (temp below 35° C)
5. Low serum protein (5g/100 ml or less)
6. Birth weight < 1500 g
7. Signs of clinical or CNS deterioration

} Treat as in next higher bilirubin category

Figure 7–26 *(From Brown, A. K., In Behrman, R. E., (ed.): Neonatology. St. Louis, The C. V. Mosby Company, 1973.)*

product of irradiance at a given wavelength (watts/cm^2/nanometer) × the duration of exposure. Available commercial phototherapy units vary considerably in the spectral output and intensity of radiation emitted, so that the dose can be accurately measured only at the skin surface. Dark skin does not reduce the efficacy of phototherapy.

Phototherapy is applied continuously to the unclothed infant, who is turned frequently for maximal skin exposure. It should be discontinued as soon as the indirect bilirubin concentration has been reduced to levels (usually 10–12 mg/dl) considered safe in view of the infant's age and condition. Serum bilirubin levels and hematocrits should be monitored every 4 to 8 hours in infants with hemolytic disease or those with bilirubin levels near the range considered toxic for the individual infant. Other, particularly older, infants may be monitored at 12- to 24-hour intervals. Monitoring should continue for at least 24 hours after cessation of phototherapy, since unexpected rises of serum bilirubin sometimes occur and require further treatment. Skin color cannot be relied upon for evaluating the effectiveness of phototherapy; the skin of babies exposed to light may appear almost without jaundice in the presence of marked hyperbilirubinemia. The infant's eyes should be closed and adequately covered to prevent exposure to light (excessive pressure from an eye bandage may injure the eyes and, alternatively, the corneas may be excoriated if the infant can open his eyes under the bandage). Body temperature should be monitored, and the infant should be shielded from bulb breakage. If feasible, irradiance should be measured directly, and details of the exposure should be recorded (type and age of bulbs, duration of exposure, distance from light source to infant, etc.). *In the infant with hemolytic disease, care must be taken that focus on the treatment of hyperbilirubinemia does not lead to overlooking developing anemia which may require transfusion; a hematocrit should be obtained with each bilirubin determination.*

Complications of phototherapy include loose stools, skin rashes, overheating from the lights, chilling from exposure of the infant, and "bronze baby syndrome." Animal experiments suggest the possibility of eye injury from light, but it has not been observed in humans, perhaps because it has been routine to cover the eyes since phototherapy was first attempted. Eye injury from the bandages is uncommon.

The term **"bronze baby syndrome"** refers to a dark, grayish brown discoloration of the skin sometimes noted in infants undergoing phototherapy. Almost all infants observed with this syndrome have had a mixed type of hyperbilirubinemia, with significant elevation of direct-reacting bilirubin in the serum and often with other evidence of obstructive liver disease. Once present, the discoloration may last for many months. No permanent adverse effects have been reported.

The question of long-term or hidden adverse effects from the photo-breakdown products of bilirubin or from other as yet unknown biologic effects of phototherapy has been raised strongly. Wide clinical experience to date suggests that such effects are absent, minimal or unrecognized. However, those employing phototherapy should remain alert to the possibility of injury from exposure to light and avoid its unnecessary use.

Results similar to those obtained with fluorescent electric bulbs may be obtained with exposure of jaundiced infants to window-filtered (removes ultraviolet light) daylight. Its use has been hampered by its limited availability in many nurseries, seasons and climates, and by the difficulty of delivering any type of measurable dose.

Phenobarbital. Phenobarbital enhances the conjugation and excretion of bilirubin. Its administration will limit the development of physiologic jaundice in the newborn infant when administered to mothers in a dose of 90 mg/day prior to delivery, or to infants at birth in a dose of 5 mg/kg/day. Since its effect on bilirubin metabolism is usually not manifest until after several days of administration, and since it is less effective than phototherapy in lowering serum bilirubin concentrations and is not additive to the response to phototherapy, it is of little practical value in treating jaundice in the neonatal infant. Its variable excretion in the first weeks of life also leads to unpredictable variations in the hypnotic effects of a standard dose on the individual infant. Phenobarbital probably also affects the metabolism of steroids and of a variety of other metabolites and drugs.

DISTURBANCES OF THE BLOOD

ANEMIA IN THE NEWBORN INFANT

Anemia at birth is manifest by pallor or shock. It is usually caused by hemolytic disease of the newborn, but may also be the result of tearing or cutting of the umbilical cord during delivery or of hemorrhage from the fetal side of the placenta. The last may be caused by accidental incision of the placenta in the course of cesarean section or by so-called transplacental hemorrhage. Anemia at birth may alse be seen in one of twins with conjoined placental circulation, in which case the anemic twin "bleeds into" the other twin. Rarely, scalp blood sampling for fetal distress may result in anemia.

Transplacental hemorrhage, with bleeding from the fetal into the maternal circulation, is probably more common than is generally recognized, but is usually not sufficient to cause clinically apparent anemia at birth. The cause of transplacental hemorrhage is not clear, but its occurrence has been proved by demonstration of significant amounts of fetal hemoglobin and red cells in the maternal blood on the day of delivery.

Anemia appearing in the first few days after birth is also most frequently the result of hemolytic disease of the newborn. Other causes are hemorrhagic disease of the newborn, bleeding from an improperly tied or clamped umbilical cord, large cephalhematomas, intracranial hemorrhage or subcapsular bleeding from rupture of the liver. Rapid decreases in hemoglobin or hematocrit values during the first few days of life may be the initial clue to either of the two last-named conditions.

Later in the neonatal period delayed anemia from hemolytic disease of the newborn, with or without exchange transfusion, may be seen. Vitamin K (as Synkayvite) in large doses may cause anemia in premature infants characterized by inclusion bodies (Heinz bodies) in the erythrocytes. Congenital hemolytic anemia (spherocytosis) occasionally makes its appearance during the first month of life, and hereditary nonspherocytic hemolytic anemia has been described during the neonatal period secondary to deficiency of such enzymes as glucose 6-phosphate dehydrogenase and pyruvate kinase. Bleeding from hemangiomas of the upper gastrointestinal tract or from ulcers caused by aberrant gastric mucosa in a Meckel's diverticulum or duplication is a rare source of anemia in the newborn. Repeated blood sampling of infants requiring frequent monitoring of blood gases and chemistries may also produce anemia.

Since a further "physiologic" decrease in erythrocytes and in hemoglobin content is to be expected in all newborn infants (Table 14–3), treatment of any significant anemia (less than 8 gm of hemoglobin per dl) present at or shortly after birth consists not only in eliminating its cause, if it is still present, but also in small transfusions of packed red blood cells (10 to 15 ml per kg; 2 ml per kg raises hemoglobin about 1 gm per dl). There is inconclusive evidence that early feeding of red meats or intramuscular administration of iron is effective in enabling anemic infants to increase rather than decrease their erythrocyte and hemoglobin concentrations before the second or third month of life.

HEMOLYTIC DISEASE OF THE NEWBORN

(Erythroblastosis Fetalis)

Erythroblastosis fetalis results from the transplacental passage of maternal antibody active against red cell antigens of the infant, leading to an increased rate of red cell destruction. It continues to be an important cause of anemia and jaundice in newborn infants despite the development of a method of prevention of maternal iso-immunization by Rh antigens. Although more than 60 different red cell antigens capable of eliciting an antibody response in a suitable recipient have been identified, significant disease is associated primarily with the D (Rh_0) antigen and its allele d(rh_0) of the Rh group and with incompatibility of ABO factors. Rarely hemolytic disease may be caused by C or E antigens or by other red cell antigens such as K(Kell), Lewis, M, Duffy, S and Kidd.

Hemolytic Disease of the Newborn Due to Rh Incompatibility

The Rh antigenic determinants are genetically transmitted from each parent either as a single gene which determines the Rh type and directs the production of a number of blood group factors, or as a group of closely linked genes, each of which determines an individual Rh blood group factor (C, c, D, d, E and e). Each factor can elicit a specific antibody response under suitable conditions.

PATHOGENESIS. Approximately 15 per cent of Caucasians and 7 per cent of blacks do not have the D antigen and are designated Rh negative (d/d). As a consequence, iso-immune hemolytic disease from this antigen is approximately three times more frequent in whites than in blacks. When Rh-positive blood is infused into an Rh-negative woman through error or when small quantities (usually more than 1 ml) of Rh-positive fetal blood containing D antigen inherited from an Rh-positive father enter the maternal circulation during pregnancy, spontaneous or induced abortion, or at delivery, antibody formation against D may be induced in the unsensitized Rh-negative recipient mother. Once immunization has occurred, considerably smaller doses of antigen can stimulate an increase in antibody titer. Initially there is a rise of maternal IgM antibody that does not cross the placenta; this response is superseded by a rise in IgG antibody which readily crosses the placenta to agglutinate the infant's red blood cells, causing hemolytic manifestations.

Hemolytic disease rarely occurs during a first pregnancy, since transfusions of Rh-positive fetal blood into an Rh-negative mother tend to occur near the time of delivery, too late for the mother to become sensitized in time to transmit antibody to the infant before delivery. The fact that 55 per cent of Rh-positive fathers are heterozygous (D/d) and may have Rh-negative offspring reduces the chance of sensitization, as does small family size, in which there are fewer opportunities for it to occur. Finally, the capacity of Rh-negative women to form antibodies is variable, some producing low titers even after adequate antigenic challenge. Thus, the overall incidence of iso-immunization of Rh-negative mothers at risk is low, with antibody to D detected in less than 10 per cent of those studied, even after five or more pregnancies; only about 5 per cent ever have babies with hemolytic disease.

The risk of sensitization of the Rh-negative woman is variable. Some sensitize easily, with the first pregnancy at risk; others have many Rh-positive infants without producing antibodies. The woman whose husband is heterozygous will not be influenced by an Rh-negative fetus. When mother and fetus are incompatible with respect to groups A or B, the mother is protected to a degree against sensitization by the rapid removal of Rh-positive cells from her circulation by her anti-A or anti-B. Once the mother is sensitized, the infant is likely to have hemolytic disease. There is a tendency in some families for the severity of the illness to worsen with successive pregnancies, but in others there will be many infants mildly affected, whereas in still others there will occur only the most severe forms of illness, which may include the hydropic stillbirth of the first-affected infant. The possibility that the first-affected infant after sensitization may represent the end of the mother's child-bearing potential for Rh-positive infants argues urgently for the prevention of sensitization when this is possible. Such prevention takes advantage of the observation that A or B incompatibility has a protective effect against sensitization, and employs injection into the mother of anti-D gamma globulin (RhoGam) immediately following the delivery of each Rh-positive infant (see below).

CLINICAL MANIFESTATIONS. A wide spectrum of hemolytic disease occurs in affected infants born to sensitized mothers, depending on the nature of the individual immune response. The severity of the disease may range from only laboratory evidence of mild hemolysis (15 per cent of cases) to severe anemia with compensatory hyperplasia of erythropoietic tissue, especially at extramedullary sites, leading to massive enlargement of the liver and spleen. When the compensatory capacity of the hematopoietic system is exceeded, profound anemia results in pallor, signs of cardiac decompensation (hepatosplenomegaly, respiratory distress), massive anasarca and circulatory collapse. This clinical picture, termed **hydrops fetalis,** frequently results in death in utero or shortly after birth. Petechiae, purpura and thrombocytopenia may also be present in severe cases and should suggest the presence of concurrent disseminated intravascular coagulation.

Jaundice is usually absent at birth owing to placental clearance of lipid-soluble unconjugated bilirubin, but in severe cases bilirubin pigments stain the amniotic fluid and vernix caseosa yellow. Icterus is generally evident within the first day of life, as the infant's bilirubin conjugating and excretory systems are unable to cope with the load resulting from massive hemolysis. Indirect-reacting bilirubin therefore accumulates postnatally and may rapidly reach extemely high levels (20 to 50 mg/dl), with a significant risk of bilirubin encephalopathy. There may be a greater risk of developing kernicterus from hemolytic disease than from comparable nonhemolytic hyperbilirubinemia, although some think that the risk in an individual patient is only a function of the severity of illness (anoxia, acidosis, etc.). Hypoglycemia occurs frequently in infants with severe iso-immune hemolytic disease and may be related to hyperinsulinism and hypertrophy of the pancreatic islet cells in these infants.

The availability of techniques for improved intrauterine diagnosis of the severity of disease in an affected fetus has led to the development of obstetric criteria for induced premature delivery. This has decreased the incidence of fetal death for the disease and increased the frequency of premature infants with clinical erythroblastosis, with the added risk of neurologic damage from the combination of immaturity and hyperbilirubinemia.

Infants born after intrauterine transfusion for prenatally diagnosed erythroblastosis are generally severely affected, since the indications for the transfusion are evidences of already severe disease in utero. Such infants usually have very high (but this is extremely variable) cord levels of bilirubin with significant fractions of conjugated bilirubin, reflecting the severity of hemolysis and its effects upon hepatic function. Anemia from continuing hemolysis may be masked by the prior intrauterine transfusion, and the clinical manifestations of erythroblastosis may be superimposed upon various degrees of immaturity owing to spontaneous or induced premature delivery.

LABORATORY DATA. Prior to treatment, the direct Coombs test* is usually positive. Anemia is usual. The cord blood hemoglobin varies, usually proportionally to the severity of the disease; with hydrops fetalis it may be as low as 3-4 gm/dl. Alternatively, despite hemolysis, it may be within the normal range owing to compensatory bone marrow activity. The red blood cells are macrocytic and normochromic. The blood smear usually shows polychromasia and a marked increase in nucleated red blood cells. The reticulocyte count is increased. The white blood cell count is usually normal but may be elevated, and there may be thrombocytopenia in severe cases. The cord bilirubin is usually between 3 and 5 mg/dl; only rarely is there a substantial elevation of direct-reacting (conjugated) bilirubin. The indirect-reacting bilirubin rises rapidly to extremely high levels in the first 6 hours of life.

After intrauterine transfusions the cord blood may show a normal hemoglobin concentration, negative direct Coombs test, predominantly adult red cells, and a relatively normal smear. Marked elevation of both indirect- and direct-reacting bilirubin levels have been reported in these infants; the direct fraction may be equal to or greater than the indirect fraction.

DIAGNOSIS. The definitive diagnosis of erythroblastosis fetalis requires demonstration of blood group incompatibility and the presence of Rh antibody bound to the infant's red cells.

ANTENATAL DIAGNOSIS. In the unsensitized Rh negative primigravida a history of previous trans-

---

*The **Coombs test** detects the presence of antibody globulin attached to red blood cells. In the **direct** Coombs test antiserum against human gamma globulin (Coombs serum) causes agglutination of the red cells of an affected infant. The term "**indirect**" Coombs test refers to a technique that is used to detect antibody in plasma or serum: normal red cells are exposed first to the suspected serum and then to Coombs serum, at which point agglutination occurs if antibody present in the suspected serum has attached itself to the red cells.

fusions or abortion may suggest the possibility of sensitization. The expectant parents' blood types should be tested for potential incompatibility and the maternal titer of albumin-active IgG antibodies to D should be assayed at 12 to 16, 28 to 32, and 36 weeks. The presence of measurable antibody titer in albumin at the beginning of pregnancy, a rapid rise in titer or a titer of 1:64 or greater suggests significant hemolytic disease, although the exact titer correlates poorly with the severity of disease. If a mother is found to have antibody against D at a titer of 1:32 or greater at any time during the first pregnancy in which antibody is found, or 1:16 or greater in a subsequent pregnancy, the severity of fetal disease should be monitored by amniocentesis. In the first sensitized pregnancy, if the indirect Coombs antibody is less than 1:64, the likelihood of serious fetal involvement is small and the first amniocentesis can be deferred until 28 to 29 weeks of gestation. Higher titers suggest a more severely affected fetus and the need for earlier amniocentesis. If there is a history of a previously affected infant and/or a stillbirth and the father is Rh-positive, the infant is usually equally or more severely affected than the previous infant, and the severity of disease in the fetus should be followed by serial amniocenteses.

Amniocentesis. Spectrophotometric analysis of bile pigments in amniotic fluid obtained by direct transabdominal uterine aspiration has proved to be a generally safe and reliable way of predicting the severity and progress of fetal hemolysis. In the affected fetus there is a positive deviation from the normal straight line curve of optical density of the amniotic fluid, measured at wavelengths from 350 to 700 millimicrons and plotted on semilogarithmic paper (Fig. 7–27). The peak of density occurs at 450 millimicrons (ΔOD450) and is used as an index of the risk of intrauterine death when plotted against gestational age and compared to a zoned nomogram devised on the basis of experience with the outcome of a population of affected infants (Fig. 7–28).

POSTNATAL DIAGNOSIS. Immediately after the birth of any infant to an Rh-negative woman, blood from the umbilical cord or from the infant should be examined for ABO blood group, Rh type, hematocrit *and* hemoglobin (as a cross-check), and reaction on the direct Coombs test. If the Coombs test is positive, a serum bilirubin should be done as a baseline, and a commercially available red cell panel (such as Selectogen, Hemantigen or Panocell) should be used to identify as many as possible of the specific red cell antibodies which are present in the mother's serum. This is done not only to identify antibody against the D antigen but against a broad group of other antigens as well, and will help to ensure the selection of the most compatible blood for exchange transfusion, should it be necessary. Although these other antigens may rarely be responsible for clinical erythroblastosis in the infants of Rh-positive as well as Rh-negative mothers, it is not considered cost-effective to perform routine Coombs testing on all newborn infants.

The (direct) Coombs test is usually strongly positive in clinically affected infants and may remain so for a few days up to several months. However, it may be negative at birth in infants who have received intrauterine transfusions.

TREATMENT. The two main goals of therapy are: first, to prevent intrauterine or extrauterine death from severe anemia and its complications, and second, to avoid neurotoxicity from hyperbilirubinemia.

Treatment of the Unborn Infant. The survival of moderately and severely affected fetuses has been markedly improved by inducing labor between 34 and 35 weeks when repeated amniocenteses show flat or rising ΔOD450's in high zone 2

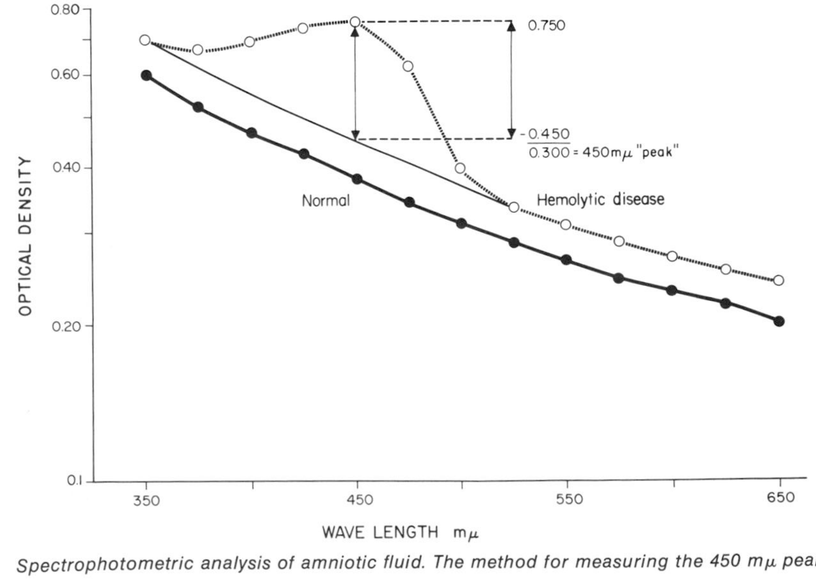

Figure 7–27 *Spectrophotometric analysis of amniotic fluid. The method for measuring the 450 mμ peak is indicated.*

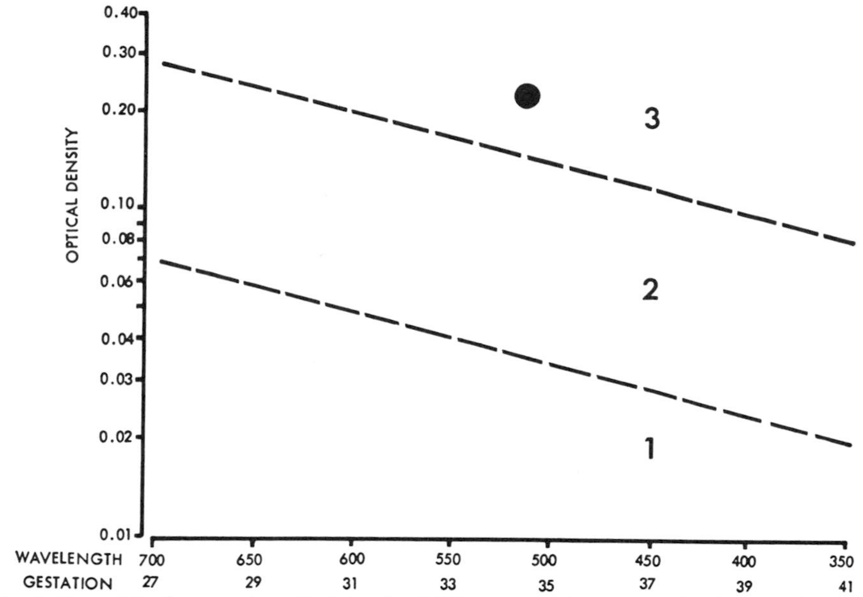

Figure 7–28 *Plotting of the increase in optical density at 450 mμ according to gestational age, and zoning of the increase in optical density according to Liley's data. Zone 3, Severe disease; impending fetal death. Zone 2, Indeterminate disease. Zone 1, Rh-negative infant or mildly affected Rh-positive infant. Predictions should be based on the trend of readings from two or three amniotic fluid specimens serially obtained at 1- to 2-week intervals beginning no later than about 10 weeks before the gestational time at which the previous pregnancy ended. A high reading that remains flat or rises on serial determinations suggests the need for intrauterine transfusion and/or early delivery; a fall in serial readings suggests a good prognosis without interference. (From Bowman, J. M., and Pollock, J. M.: Pediatrics, 35:815, 1965.)*

or in zone 3 (Fig. 7–28). When the chance that a severely affected fetus will survive to a gestational age compatible with early delivery and neonatal survival is small, an intrauterine intraperitoneal transfusion of erythrocytes compatible with the mother's blood may be indicated. A judgment must be made as to whether at a particular gestational age the risk of dying from erythroblastosis or from premature delivery is greater than the risk of dying during or immediately following the procedure. At 34 weeks or more of gestation, delivery should be induced since the risk of intrauterine transfusion is usually greater. Between 30 and 34 weeks of gestation the decision should be based upon a comparison of the mortality rates of the transfusing team and of the premature intensive care unit where the newborn infant will be treated. Additional indications for intrauterine transfusion include several optical density readings in zone 3, especially if the trend is increasing and there is a family history of stillbirths, hydrops fetalis or severely affected infants. Bowman considers radiologic evidence of hydrops fetalis to be an indication for intrauterine transfusion.

Treatment of the Liveborn Infant. The birth should be attended by the physician who will care for the affected infant afterward. Fresh, low-titer, group O, Rh-negative blood, carefully crossmatched against the maternal serum using an indirect Coombs technique, should be immediately available. If clinical signs of severe hemolytic anemia (pallor, hepatosplenomegaly, edema, petechiae or ascites) are evident at birth, supportive measures and exchange transfusion should be instituted at once. Immediate therapy and temperature stabilization before proceeding with exchange transfusion may save some severely affected infants, though hydropic babies rarely survive. Such therapy should include correction of acidosis with 2-3 mEq/kg of sodium bicarbonate and a small transfusion of compatible packed red cells to correct anemia. Correction of acidosis usually reduces central venous pressure, and an apparent need for bleeding to reduce the cardiac load may be obviated. Digitalization, though recommended by some, probably does not act rapidly enough to be effective.

Exchange Transfusion. When the clinical condition of the infant at birth does not indicate immediate exchange transfusion, the decision to do it must be based on a judgment that there is a high risk of a rapidly developing dangerous degree of anemia or of hyperbilirubinemia. The criteria for this judgment include a cord blood hemoglobin of 12 mg/dl or less, verified by an equally low capillary blood hemoglobin (which tends to be higher than that of cord or venous blood), or a cord bilirubin of 5 mg/dl or greater. Some physicians consider previous kernicterus or severe erythroblastosis in a sibling, reticulocyte counts greater than 15 per cent, and prematurity to be further factors supporting a decision for early exchange transfusion. In any case, exchange transfusions in the period shortly after birth should be initiated only after the infant's clinical condition has stabilized following appropriate supportive therapy and monitoring.

If immediate or very early exchange transfusion is not necessary to correct life-threatening anemia the hemoglobin and serum bilirubin levels must be followed carefully. The decision to perform an exchange transfusion is based upon the likelihood that the trend of bilirubin levels plotted against hours of age indicates that the serum bilirubin will reach 20 mg/dl within 72 to 76 hours in a full-term infant, or 16 to 18 mg/dl in a premature infant.

In deciding whether immediate or early exchange transfusion is necessary to correct life-threatening anemia, hemoglobin or hematocrit and serum bilirubin levels must be followed carefully. This should be done at 4- to 6-hour intervals at first, with extension to 8-, 12- or 24-hour intervals if and as the rate of change diminishes. Although most exchange transfusions are performed to prevent or reduce hyperbilirubinemia, one may be indicated as the simplest and most effective way of dealing with rapidly developing anemia. Ordinary transfusions of compatible Rh-negative red cells may be necessary to correct anemia at any stage of the disease up to 6 or 8 weeks of age when the infant's own blood-forming mechanism may be expected to take over. Weekly determinations of hemoglobin or hematocrit should be done until a spontaneous rise has been demonstrated.

Careful monitoring of the serum bilirubin level is essential until a falling trend has been demonstrated in the absence of phototherapy or administration of phenobarbital. Even then an occasional infant, particularly if premature, may experience an unpredicted significant rise in serum bilirubin as late as the seventh day of life. On the other hand, although frequently advocated, predictions of the achievement of a dangerously high level of serum bilirubin based on observed levels exceeding 6 mg/dl in the first 6 hours or 10 mg/dl in the second 6 hours of life, are also uncertain, as are predictions based on a rate of rise exceeding 0.5 to 1.0 mg/dl/hour.

Kernicterus can be eliminated by keeping the serum bilirubin of otherwise well infants below 20 mg/dl by the use of exchange transfusions. Respiratory distress, sepsis, hypoglycemia, or the presence of hypoxia, acidosis, hypoalbuminemia or marked immaturity are indications for exchange transfusion at a lower level of bilirubin. Various indices of bilirubin have not been shown to be reliable aids in this decision.

Blood for exchange transfusion should be as fresh as possible. Heparin, acid-citrate-dextrose (ACD) or citrate-phosphate-dextrose (CPD) may be used as anticoagulants. If the blood is obtained before delivery, it should be from a Type O, Rh-negative donor with a low titer of anti-A and Anti-B, and compatible with the mother's serum by indirect Coombs test. After delivery blood should be obtained from an Rh-negative donor whose cells are compatible with both the infant's and mother's serum; when possible, type O donor cells are usually employed but cells of the infant's blood type may be used. A complete crossmatch, including indirect Coombs test, should be performed prior to the second and subsequent transfusions. Blood should be gradually warmed to and maintained at a temperature between 22 and 37° C throughout the exchange transfusion. It should be kept well mixed by gentle squeezing or agitation of the bag to avoid sedimentation; otherwise, the use of supernatant serum with a low red cell count at the end of the exchange will leave the infant anemic. Whole blood should be used rather than packed red cells, except when venous pressure is persistently high and impending heart failure is suspected. However, an elevated venous pressure probably reflects severe peripheral and pulmonary vasoconstriction which will respond to the intravenous administration of 2-3 mEq/kg of sodium bicarbonate. The infant's stomach should be emptied prior to transfusion in order to prevent aspiration during the procedure, which should be performed under conditions that permit maintenance of body temperature and monitoring of vital signs. A competent medical or nursing assistant should be present with the physician to help monitor the baby, tally the volume of blood exchanged, and perform emergency procedures.

The umbilical vein is cannulated, using strict aseptic technique, with a polyvinyl end-hole catheter to a distance no greater than 7 cm in a full-term infant. When free flow of blood is obtained, the catheter is usually in a large hepatic vein or the inferior vena cava. The venous pressure should be measured intermittently and may be falsely elevated as a result of faulty catheter placement. Exchange should be carried out over a 45- to 60-minute period, alternating aspirations of 20 ml of infant blood and infusions of 20 ml of donor blood. Smaller aliquots (10 ml) may be indicated for sick and premature infants. An initial withdrawal of 10 to 20 ml of the infant's blood without replacement may be indicated when venous pressure is high. The goal should be an exchange of approximately two blood volumes of the infant (2×85 ml per kg.). Some operators advise injection of 0.5 to 2 ml of 10 per cent calcium gluconate after each dl of exchanged citrated blood in order to avoid the reduction of ionized calcium which has been observed during the procedure. If heparinized blood is used, 0.45 ml (4.5 mg) of a 1 per cent solution of protamine sulfate should be injected intravenously at the conclusion of the transfusion for each dl of blood exchanged.

The efficiency of bilirubin removal during an exchange transfusion can be increased 25 to 40 per cent by the intravenous injection of 1 gm per kg of human albumin in a 25 per cent salt-free solution one hour before exchange, or by replacing 50 ml of donor plasma from the bag or bottle of blood with an equal volume of 25 per cent albumin.

Binding of bilirubin by albumin temporarily prevents deposition of indirect-reacting bilirubin in tissues, but because it is not possible to predict the pattern of eventual disposition of the increased circulating bilirubin that occurs subsequently, the administration of albumin should always be followed promptly by exchange transfusion. Albumin should not be given during exchange transfusions immediately after birth or when there is elevated venous pressure, severe anemia or evidence of congestive heart failure or cardiovascular instability. The binding effect makes it difficult to evaluate the significance of bilirubin levels after the administration of albumin.

Elevated umbilical venous pressure (higher than 10 cm of water) is common among infants with severe hemolytic disease and hydrops fetalis or born after intrauterine transfusions. This may represent hypervolemic congestive heart failure and indicate the need for the initial withdrawal of blood (usually 40 to 50 ml) sufficient to reduce the venous pressure to normal levels (5 to 7 cm of water). Digitalization is not indicated. Alternatively, these infants may be hypovolemic and require expansion of the vascular space and correction of acidosis. Measurement of umbilical artery blood pressure may be of value in these instances. These infants and others with acidosis and hypoxia from respiratory distress, sepsis, hypothermia or shock may be further compromised by the significant acid load contained in citrated (ACD) blood, which usually has a pH between 6 and 7. Sodium bicarbonate or THAM should be administered in appropriate dosages to raise the pH of this blood to 7.3 to 7.4, or to maintain continuous correction of the pH of the infant's blood. The subsequent metabolism of citrate may result in a later metabolic alkalosis if ACD blood is used. Fresh heparinized blood or blood anticoagulated with citrate-phosphate-dextrose usually avoids this problem. Symptomatic hypoglycemia may occur before exchange transfusion in moderately to severely affected infants; it may be seen 1 to 3 hours after exchange in any infant subjected to the procedure. Prophylactic antibiotics are not indicated as a routine; sulfonamides and other drugs that may bind to albumin competitively with bilirubin are contraindicated.

After exchange transfusion the bilirubin level must be determined at frequent intervals (every 4 to 8 hours), and second or repeated exchange transfusions should be carried out to keep the indirect fraction from exceeding 20 mg/dl. Symptoms suggestive of kernicterus are mandatory indications for exchange transfusion at any time. Phototherapy appears to have reduced the need for repeated exchange transfusions in infants with mild to moderate hemolysis.

The risk of death from exchange transfusion carried out by skilled and experienced physicians is less than 1 per cent. However, with the decreasing use of this procedure owing to the use of phototherapy and the prevention of sensitization, the general level of competence is likely to decrease. Thus, it may be best to concentrate this mode of treatment in special referral centers.

Late Complications. The infant with hemolytic disease and/or who has had an exchange transfusion must be observed carefully during the first 6 to 8 weeks of life for the development of potentially lethal anemia. Infants who received intrauterine transfusions are at special risk. Treatment with supplemental iron and/or blood transfusion may be indicated.

"*Inspissated bile syndrome*" refers to the rare occurrence of persistent icterus in association with significant elevations of direct as well as indirect bilirubin in infants with hemolytic disease. The cause is unclear, but the jaundice clears spontaneously within a few weeks or months.

Portal vein thrombosis is seen with increasing frequency among children who have been subjected to exchange transfusion as newborn infants. It is probably associated with prolonged, traumatic or septic umbilical vein catheterization.

Prevention of Rh Sensitization. The risk of initial sensitization of Rh-negative mothers has been reduced from between 10 and 20 per cent to less than 1 per cent by intramuscular injection of 300 μg of human anti-D globulin (1 ml of RhoGAM) within 72 hours of delivery or abortion. This quantity is sufficient to eliminate approximately 10 ml of potentially antigenic fetal cells from the maternal circulation. Large fetal-to-maternal transfer of blood may require proportionately more RhoGAM. The use of this technique, combined with improved methods of detecting maternal sensitization and quantitating the extent of the fetal to maternal transfusion, plus the use of fewer obstetric procedures that increase the risk of such fetal to maternal bleeding (versions, manual separation of the placenta, etc.) should eventually almost eliminate erythroblastosis fetalis.

Hemolytic Disease of the Newborn Due to A and B Incompatibility

Major blood group incompatibility between mother and fetus usually results in milder disease than does Rh incompatibility. Maternal antibody may be formed against B cells if the mother is type A, or against A cells if the mother is type B. However, usually the mother is type O and the infant is A or B. Although ABO incompatibility occurs in 20 to 25 per cent of pregnancies, hemolytic disease develops in only 1 in 10 of such offspring and usually the infants are of Type A_1 which is more antigenic than A_2 or B. Low antigenicity of the ABO factors in the fetus and newborn infant may account for the low incidence of severe ABO hemolytic disease relative to the incidence of incompatibility between the blood groups of mother and child. Although antibodies against A and B factors occur without prior immunization ("natural" antibodies), these are ordinarily present in the 19S (IgM) fraction of gamma globulin, which does not cross the placenta. However, antibodies to A antigen may be present in the 7S (IgG) fraction, which does cross the placenta, so that A-O iso-immune hemolytic disease may be seen in first-born infants; when high antibody levels are present an infant may be severely affected.

CLINICAL MANIFESTATIONS. Most cases are mild, with jaundice as the only clinical manifestation. The infant is not generally severely affected at birth; pallor is not present and hydrops fetalis is extremely rare. Liver and spleen are not greatly enlarged, if at all. Jaundice usually appears during the first 24 hours. Rarely it may become severe, and symptoms and signs of kernicterus rapidly develop.

DIAGNOSIS. A presumptive diagnosis is based on the presence of ABO incompatibility, a weakly to moderately positive direct Coombs test, and spherocytes in the blood smear; the latter may at times suggest the presence of hereditary spherocytosis. Hyperbilirubinemia is often the only other laboratory abnormality. The hemoglobin level is usually normal, but may be as low as 10 to 12 gm per dl. Reticulocytes may be increased to 10 to 15 per cent, with extensive spherocytosis, polychromasia and increased numbers of nucleated red cells. In 10 to 20 per cent of affected infants the unconjugated serum bilirubin level may reach 20 mg/dl or more unless phototherapy is employed.

TREATMENT. Phototherapy is effective in lowering serum bilirubin levels when hemolysis is mild. Otherwise, treatment is directed at correcting dangerous degrees of anemia or hyperbilirubinemia by exchange transfusion with blood of the same group and Rh type as that of the mother. The indications for this procedure are similar to those previously described for hemolytic disease due to Rh incompatibility.

Other Forms of Hemolytic Disease

Blood group incompatibilities other than Rh or ABO (c, E, Kell (K), etc.) account for less than 5 per cent of hemolytic disease of the newborn. The direct Coombs test is invariably positive, and exchange transfusion may be indicated for hyperbilirubinemia and anemia. Congenital infections, such as cytomegalic inclusion disease, toxoplasmosis, rubella and syphilis, may present with hemolytic anemia, jaundice, hepatosplenomegaly and thrombocytopenia, but the direct Coombs test is negative and there are usually other distinguishing clinical findings. Homozygous α-thalassemia may present with severe hemolytic anemia and a clinical picture resembling hydrops fetalis; it can be distinguished by a negative direct Coombs test and characteristic clinical and laboratory findings. Anemia and jaundice may occur in infancy from hereditary spherocytosis and, if untreated, can result in kernicterus. Hemolytic anemia producing jaundice in the first week of life has also been reported secondary to congenital deficiencies in red cell enzymes, such as glucose 6-phosphate dehydrogenase (G-6-PD).

PLETHORA IN THE NEWBORN INFANT

See also Polycythemia, Section 14.

Plethora or apparent cyanosis associated with abnormally high erythrocyte, hemoglobin and hematocrit values has been reported in association with and without clinical findings suggestive of placental dysfunction syndrome, plus anorexia, lethargy, cyanosis and convulsions appearing on the second and third days of life. The pathophysiology of the condition is not clear but may, in part, be related to the increased viscosity of the blood. Plethora may also be due to a "placental transfusion" in the recipient twin of monozygotic twins with parabiotic placental circulations. Plethora as the result of transfusion from the maternal to the fetal circulation has also been described. It is also observed in large "cushingoid" infants of diabetic mothers.

The *treatment* of symptomatic plethora of the newborn has been by bleeding and replacement with plasma. A partial exchange transfusion would appear to be a technically simpler and therapeutically more effective approach.

HEMORRHAGE IN THE NEWBORN INFANT

Hemorrhagic Disease of the Newborn. A moderate decrease of prothrombin and factors VII, IX and X normally occurs in all newborn infants by 48 to 72 hours after birth, with a gradual return to birth levels by 7 to 10 days of age. This transient deficiency of vitamin K-dependent factors probably results from a lack of vitamin K in the mother, immaturity of the infant's liver and absence of bacterial intestinal flora normally responsible for synthesis of vitamin K. Rarely among term infants and more frequently among premature infants there is an accentuation and prolongation of this deficiency between the second and fifth days of life, resulting in spontaneous and prolonged bleeding. This form of hemorrhagic disease of the newborn, which is responsive to vitamin K therapy, must be distinguished from disseminated intravascular coagulopathy and from rarer congenital deficiencies of one or more of the other vitamin K-dependent factors or factor V, which are unresponsive to vitamin K. (See also Section 14.)

Hemorrhagic disease of the newborn resulting from severe transient deficiencies of vitamin K-dependent factors is characterized by bleeding which tends to be gastrointestinal, nasal, subgaleal or intracranial. The prothrombin time, blood coagulation time and plasma recalcification time are prolonged and the levels of prothrombin and factors VIII, IX and X are significantly decreased. Bleeding time, fibrinogen, factors V and VIII, platelets, capillary fragility and clot retraction are normal for age and maturity. The administration of 1 mg of natural oil-soluble vitamin K, either intramuscularly or orally, at the time of birth prevents the fall in vitamin K-dependent factors in full-term infants but is not uniformly effective in the prophylaxis of hemorrhagic disease of the newborn in premature infants. The disease may be effectively treated with an intravenous infusion of 5 mg of vitamin K_1, with improvement of coagulation defects and cessation of bleeding within a few hours. However, serious bleeding may require a transfusion of fresh whole blood. The mortality rate is low among treated patients.

Other forms of bleeding may be clinically indistinguishable from hemorrhagic disease of the newborn responsive to vitamin K, but are neither prevented nor successfully treated with it. Treatment of the rare congenital deficiencies of prothrombin and factors V, VII and X requires fresh whole blood or specific factor replacement.

Disseminated intravascular coagulopathy in the newborn infant results in consumption of coagulation factors and bleeding. The infants are often premature; the clinical course is frequently characterized by hypoxia, acidosis, shock or infection. The most frequent sites of bleeding are the skin, lungs and central nervous system. Factors V and VIII and fibrinogen are usually decreased and there is severe thrombocytopenia. Prothrombin time and partial thromboplastin time (PTT) are prolonged even in the absence of marked fibrinolysis. Treatment is directed at correction of the primary clinical problem, such as infection, and at interruption of consumption and replacement of clotting factors. The prognosis is poor regardless of therapy.

Since a clinical pattern identical to that of hemorrhagic disease of the newborn may result from any of the congenital defects in blood coagulation or a consumption coagulopathy (Section 14), infants with central nervous system or other bleeding constituting an immediate threat to life should receive a small transfusion of fresh, compatible whole blood or plasma, as well as vitamin K, as soon as possible after blood has been drawn for coagulation studies, including determination of the number of platelets.

The so-called **swallowed blood syndrome,** in which blood or bloody stools are passed, usually on the second or third day of life, may be confused with hemorrhage from the gastrointestinal tract. The blood may be swallowed during delivery or from a fissure in the mother's nipple. Differentiation from gastrointestinal hemorrhage is based on the fact that the infant's blood contains mostly fetal hemoglobin, which is alkali-resistant, whereas swallowed blood from a maternal source contains adult hemoglobin, which is promptly changed to alkaline hematin upon the addition of alkali. Apt devised the following test for this differentiation:

(1) Rinse a bloodstained diaper or some grossly bloody stool with a suitable amount of water to obtain a distinctly pink supernatant hemoglobin solution. (2) Centrifuge the mixture. Decant the supernatant solution. (3) To 5 parts of the supernatant fluid add 1 part of 0.25 normal (1 per cent) sodium hydroxide. Within 1 to 2 minutes a color reaction takes place: a yellow-brown color indicates that the blood is maternal in origin; a persistent pink, that it is from the infant. A control test with known adult or fetal blood, or both, is advisable.

Widespread **subcutaneous ecchymoses** in premature infants at or immediately after birth are apparently a result of fragile superficial blood vessels rather than of a coagulation defect. In any event, vitamin K administration to the mother during labor seems to have little effect on their incidence. An occasional infant is born with petechiae or a generalized bluish suffusion limited to the face, head and neck. These are probably the result of venous obstruction caused by sudden increases in intrathoracic pressure during delivery. It may take 2 to 3 weeks for such suffusions to disappear.

Neonatal Thrombocytopenic Purpura. See Section 14.

DISTURBANCES OF THE GENITOURINARY SYSTEM

See also Section 15, The Urinary System.

One or both kidneys are often easily palpable in the newborn infant. When both are palpable, there is usually no particular diagnostic problem, but when only one kidney can be felt, it frequently gives the impression that it is larger than normal or represents or is displaced by an intrinsic or extrinsic mass. Fetal lobulation may contribute to the impression of abnormality. Usually the problem resolves itself as the kidney becomes progressively less easily palpable during the early months of life. Since palpable enlargement or displacement of the kidney in the newborn may rarely be due to hydronephrosis, an embryoma or a cystic malformation, an abdominal scout film or intravenous urograms are indicated if there is serious question about the palpable mass. Owing to the poor concentrating ability of the neonatal kidney, relatively large amounts of contrast material (10 to 20 ml of Diodrast) must be injected to get satisfactory films. Elevations of blood urea nitrogen may occur during the neonatal period in association with polycystic disease and hydronephrosis without necessarily implying a poor prognosis.

During the neonatal period moderate elevation of the blood urea nitrogen does not necessarily signify renal disease. The urine may also contain casts and cellular elements simply as a manifestation of dehydration.

BILATERAL RENAL AGENESIS. Infants with bilateral renal agenesis have a characteristic facies: a general appearance of premature senility, a mild increase in width between the eyes, with a prominent fold of skin arising at the inner canthus and extending downward and laterally below the eyes to form a wide semicircle, and unusual flattening and slight broadening of the nose, a recession of the chin, and large, low-lying ears with incomplete cartilaginous development. There is usually a diminished quantity of amniotic fluid, presumably owing to lack of urine formation. At autopsy there is no evidence of the ureters or kidneys. Pulmonary hypoplasia has also been observed. The anomaly has occurred predominantly in male infants. In some of the female infants there has been failure of development of the uterus and the vagina, the gonads and the fallopian tubes being present. In male infants the prostate, seminal vesicles, ductus deferens and testes are normally formed. The bladder is a tubelike structure with little musculature. The rudimentary adrenal glands are normal. The outlook is hopeless, the infant dying during labor or shortly after birth.

URINARY TRACT INFECTION. In contrast to the sex distribution in later infancy, pyuria may occur as frequently in the male as in the female newborn infant. The causative agent is usually the colon bacillus, although it may be any of the urinary tract pathogens.

The symptoms may be vague; on occasion they are predominantly gastrointestinal. Fever, difficulty in feeding and failure to gain weight are commonly encountered; jaundice and meningismus are occasional features. There may be oliguria.

For diagnosis and treatment see Section 15.

THROMBOSIS OF THE RENAL VEIN. See Section 15.

DISTURBANCES OF THE CRANIUM

See also Anencephaly, Microcephaly, Craniosynostosis and Hydrocephalus, Section 20.

CRANIOTABES (CONGENITAL CRANIAL OSTEOPOROSIS). Palpation of the skull of the newborn infant may reveal areas of softening along the suture lines, especially in the parietal area, which indent from pressure of the fingers with the resilience of a Ping-Pong ball. This phenomenon is demonstrated more frequently in premature infants, but occurs in 10 to 35 per cent of all newborn infants. Failure to observe it in breech presentations has led to an assumption that it may be the result of intrauterine pressure against the maternal pelvis. This condition is a harmless and physiologic result of incoordination between the rapid growth of the brain and the calcification processes in the vertex in the last month of gestation and is associated with a generalized osteoporotic process in the newborn infant. Differentiation must be made from the craniotabes of rickets, from lacunar skull, in which honeycombed areas of porotic bone create a characteristic appearance in the roentgenogram of the skull, and from osteogenesis imperfecta.

DISORDERS OF THE SKIN

See Section 23, The Skin.

MASTITIS NEONATORUM. Engorgement of the breasts is physiologic in newborn infants. Infection may be abetted by undue manipulation of the breasts and is manifest by redness, local heat, swelling and pain. Fever and other general symptoms may also be present. The prognosis is favorable unless septicemia develops. Prophylaxis consists in avoidance of manipulation or other trauma of the engorged breasts. Treatment includes systemic antibiotic therapy and hot compresses applied locally. If an abscess develops, it should be incised and drained.

Scar formation after infection may distort the nipple and impair the secreting power of the mammary gland in a female in later life.

DISTURBANCES OF THE EYE

See Section 24.

THE UMBILICUS

UMBILICAL CORD. The cord contains the two umbilical arteries, the vein, the rudimentary allantois, the remnant of the omphalomesenteric duct and a gelatinous substance called the jelly of Wharton. The sheath of the umbilical cord is derived from the amnion. The arteries have a strong contractile capacity; that of the vein is less, so that it retains a fairly large lumen after birth. When the cord sloughs, portions of these structures remain in the base. The blood vessels are functionally closed, but are patent anatomically for 20 to 25 days. The arteries become the lateral umbilical ligaments; the vein, the ligamentum teres; and the ductus venosus, the ligamentum venosum. During this interval the umbilical vessels are potential portals of entry for infection.

Only a **single umbilical artery** is present in about 5 of 1000 births; the frequency is about 35 per 1000 infants born of twin births. Approximately one third of infants with a single umbilical artery have congenital abnormalities, usually more than one, and many such infants are born dead or die shortly after birth. Trisomy of chromosome 18 is one of the more frequent abnormalities associated with single umbilical artery. The defects tend to involve the genitourinary tract, the gastrointestinal tract, the skeleton, the cardiovascular system and the central nervous system. Since many of these abnormalities are not apparent on gross physical examination, it is important that at every delivery the cut cord and the maternal and fetal surfaces of the placenta be inspected. The number of arteries present should be recorded as an aid to the early suspicion and identification of abnormalities in such infants.

TYPES OF NAVEL. There are three types of navels: normal, amniotic, and the skin or cutis navel. When the skin of the abdominal wall meets the umbilical cord at the level of the abdomen, there remains only a small amount of skin at the base when the cord sloughs, and a *normal* umbilical cicatrix results. If the skin does not extend to the base of the cord and the amniotic membrane must cover the skin surface adjacent to the base, a small superficial ulcer will result which closes in by granulation and leaves the flat scar of the *amniotic* navel. When the skin extends up the sides of the cord, a protruding stump, the *skin* navel, remains after the cord has sloughed. The protrusion of the skin or cutis navel must be differentiated from a postnatal hernia, with which, of course, it can be associated; a skin navel does not have a defect in the abdominal wall and therefore is not exaggerated when the infant strains or cries. Usually the skin navel becomes less prominent with age.

ANOMALIES. *Patency of the omphalomesenteric duct* may be responsible for an intestinal fistula, prolapse of the bowel, polyp or a Meckel's diverticulum (Section 11).

A *persistent urachus* (urachal cyst) is due to failure of closure of the allantoic duct. Patency should be suspected if there is a clear, light yellow, urine-like discharge from the umbilicus (Section 15).

CONGENITAL OMPHALOCELE. An omphalocele is a herniation or protrusion of abdominal contents into the base of the umbilical cord. In contrast to the more common umbilical hernia, the sac is covered merely with peritoneum without overlying skin. The size of the sac which lies outside the abdominal cavity depends upon its contents. It has been estimated that there is herniation of intestines into the cord in about 1 of 5000 births and of liver and intestines in 1 of 10,000 births. The abdominal cavity is proportionately small, owing to deficient impulse to grow and develop. Immediate surgical repair, before infection has taken place and before the tissues have been damaged by drying or the sac has ruptured, has been generally considered to be essential for survival. Silastic, Mersilene or similar synthetic material may be used to cover the viscera if the sac has ruptured or if excessive mobilization of the skin would be necessary to cover the mass and its intact sac. Nonoperative treatment of giant omphaloceles occasionally may be successful through "tanning" the sac with a 2 per cent aqueous solution of Merthiolate, applied 2 or 3 times daily. Epithelialization as well as intra-abdominal containment of the viscera has been attained by this method, which, under special circumstances, may also be applied to smaller lesions.

TUMORS. Tumors of the umbilicus are rare; they include angioma, enteroteratoma, dermoid cyst, myxosarcoma and cysts of urachal or omphalomesenteric duct remnants.

HEMMORHAGE. Hemorrhage from the umbilical cord may be due to trauma, to inadequate ligation of the cord or to failure of normal thrombus formation. Hemorrhage may also be an evidence of hemorrhagic disease of the newborn, septicemia or local infection. The infant should be observed frequently during the first few days of life so that, if hemorrhage does occur, it will be detected promptly.

GRANULOMA. The umbilical cord usually dries and separates within 6 to 8 days after birth. The raw surface becomes covered by a thin layer of skin, scar tissue forms, and the wound is usually healed within 12 to 15 days. The presence of saprophytic organisms delays separation of the cord and increases the possibility of invasion by pathogenic organisms. Mild infection may result in a moist granulating area at the base of the cord with a slight mucoid or mucopurulent discharge. Good results are usually obtained by cleansing with alcohol several times daily.

The persistence of exuberant granulation tissue at the base of the umbilicus is common. The tissue is soft, vascular and granular, dull red or pink, and may have a seropurulent secretion. The *treatment* is cauterization with silver nitrate; it should be repeated at intervals of several days until the base is dry.

Umbilical granuloma must be differentiated from **umbilical polyp,** a rare anomaly resulting from persistence of all or part of the omphalomesenteric duct or the urachus. The tissue of the polyp is firm and resistant and bright red, and has a mucoid secretion. If there is a communication with the ileum or bladder, small amounts of fecal material or urine may be discharged intermittently. Histologically the polyp consists of intestinal or urinary tract mucosa. Treatment is surgical excision of the *entire* omphalomesenteric or urachal remnant.

INFECTIONS. Inflammation in the umbilical region, which may be caused by any of the pyogenic bacteria, is especially serious because of the danger of hematogenous spread or extension to the liver or peritoneum. The general manifestations may be minimal even when septicemia or hepatitis has resulted. Prevention of infection depends upon maintenance of a clean umbilical field. Daily baths or daily application of triple dye to the umbilical stump and surrounding skin may reduce the incidence of umbilical infection. *Treatment* includes prompt antibacterial therapy and, if there is abscess formation, surgical incision and drainage.

UMBILICAL HERNIA

Umbilical hernia is due to an imperfect closure or weakness of the umbilical ring and is often associated with diastasis recti. It is common, especially in black infants. It appears as a soft swelling covered by skin which protrudes during crying, coughing or straining and can be reduced easily through the fibrous ring at the umbilicus. The hernia consists of omentum or portions of the small intestine. The size of the defect varies from less than a centimeter in diameter to as much as 5 cm, but large ones are rare.

TREATMENT. Few medical problems have given rise to more contradictory opinions and practices than has the management of umbilical hernia in infancy. Most umbilical hernias which appear before the age of 6 months will disappear spontaneously by 1 year of age. Even large hernias (5 to 6 cm in all dimensions) have been known to disappear spontaneously by 5 or 6 years of age. Strangulation is extemely rare. There is considerable agreement that "strapping" is ineffective as usually practiced. At least one study indicates that any form of strapping has a deleterious rather than a beneficial effect. Another study suggests that careful strapping, in which the hernia is reduced by finger pressure and the defect closed by drawing each side of the adjacent abdominal wall toward the midline by means of interlocking straps of broad adhesive tape, increases the incidence of closure of hernias over 6 mm in diameter or in protrusion. Unfortunately, lack of comparability of data between various studies and, particularly, lack of a careful, long-term study of the natural history of umbilical hernias do not permit establishment of a logical basis for either strapping or surgery. Avoidance of surgery is advised unless the hernia persists to the age of 3 to 5 years, causes symptoms, becomes strangulated, or becomes progressively larger after the age of 1 or 2 years.

METABOLIC DISTURBANCES

HYPERTHERMIA IN THE NEWBORN (TRANSITORY FEVER OF THE NEWBORN: DEHYDRATION FEVER)

Elevations of temperature (100 to 104°F) are occasionally noted on the second or third day of life in infants whose clinical course has been otherwise satisfactory. This disturbance is especially likely to occur in breast-fed infants whose intake of supplementary fluid has been particularly low or in infants exposed to high environmental temperatures, either in the nursery or in a bassinet near a radiator or in the sun. The lack of consistent relation to the extent of weight loss or inadequacy of fluid intake may be a reflection of variation in initial stores of body water. The rise in temperature is associated with an increase in concentration of the serum protein and sodium. The rapid alleviation of symptoms by oral or parenteral administration of fluids can leave no doubt as to the cause.

The infant may be restless, and there may be a precipitous drop in weight. The urinary output and frequency of voiding diminish. The skin may lose some of its elasticity, and the fontanel may be depressed. The infant appears unhappy and takes fluids avidly. The usual apparent vigor of the infant is in contrast to the usual appearance of "being sick" in the presence of infection. Rarely there may be marked tachypnea and tachycardia as the infant attempts to increase heat loss by way of the respiratory tract to compensate for a sudden increase in environmental temperature.

Oral administration of fluids leads to prompt reduction of the fever.

A *more severe form of neonatal hyperthermia* occurs among both newborn and older infants when they are bundled up against an outside low temperature which does not exist in their immediate indoor environment. The diminished sweating capacity of the newborn infant is a contributing factor. Bundled-up infants left near stoves or radiators, traveling in well heated automobiles or left with bright sunlight shining directly on them through the windows of a closed room or automobile are likely victims. Overclothing in hot weather, especially when the infant is left in the sun, is a less common cause. Body temperature is often as high as 106 to 111° F (41 to 44° C). The skin is hot and dry, and initially the infant usually appears flushed and apathetic. This stage may be followed by stupor, grayish pallor, coma and convulsions. Hyperelectrolytemia may contribute to the convulsions. The mortality and morbidity rates (brain damage) are high. Prevention is by provision of clothing suitable for the temperature of the *immediate* environment. In the newborn infant exposure of the body to usual room temperature or immersion in tepid water usually suffices to bring the temperature back to normal levels. Older infants may require cooling for a longer time by repeated immersions or by use of a water-cooled mattress or other apparatus for induction of hypothermia. Attention to possible fluid and electrolyte disturbance is essential.

NEONATAL COLD INJURY

Neonatal cold injury usually occurs among infants in inadequately heated homes during damp cold spells when the outside temperature is in the range of freezing. The presenting features are apathy, refusal of food, oliguria and coldness to touch. The body temperature is usually between 85 and 94° F (29.5 and 35° C), and there are immobility, edema and redness of the extremities, especially of the hands, feet and face. The facial erythema frequently gives a false impression of health, delaying recognition that the infant is ill. Local hardening over areas of edema may lead to confusion with scleredema. Rhinitis is common, as are serious metabolic disturbances, particularly hypoglycemia and acidosis. Hemorrhagic manifestations are frequent; massive pulmonary hemorrhage is a common finding at autopsy. Treatment consists in *gradual* warming with scrupulous attention to recognition and correction of metabolic imbalances, particularly hypoglycemia. Prevention consists in provision of adequate environmental heat. The mortality rate is about 25 per cent; about 10 per cent of the survivors have evidence of brain damage.

EDEMA

Generalized edema occurs in association with the most severe forms of Rh iso-immunization, with homozygous alpha thalassemia, and in the offspring of diabetic mothers. Some premature infants may have considerable edema without identifiable reason; those with hyaline membrane disease may become edematous even without congestive heart failure. Edema of the face and scalp may result from pressure from the umbilical cord around the neck, and transient localized swellings of the hands or feet may similarly be due to intrauterine pressures. Edema may be present with heart failure due to congenital cardiac lesions, even in the absence of a murmur; a lag in renal excretion of electrolytes and water may result in edema when there has been a sudden large increase in intake of electrolytes, particularly with feeding of concentrated mixtures of cow's milk. It is difficult to show a relation between low serum protein or low hemoglobin and the occurrence of edema in older premature infants, but occasionally the therapeutic response to plasma or blood transfusion is prompt. Edema has also been observed in association with anemia and vitamin E deficiency in premature infants. Rarely *"idiopathic hypoproteinemia"* with edema lasting weeks or months is observed in term infants. The cause is unclear, and the disturbance is benign. Persistent edema of one or more extremities may represent congenital lymphedema (Milroy's disease) or, in females, *Turner's syndrome.* Generalized edema with hypoproteinemia may be seen in the neonatal period with congenital nephrosis and, rarely, with Hurler's syndrome or after feeding hypoallergenic formulas to infants with cystic fibrosis of the pancreas. Scleredema is described in Section 23.

TETANY

Hypocalcemic tetany occurs occasionally in neonatal infants. In infants of diabetic mothers, low-birth-weight infants and those born after a high-risk pregnancy or difficult labor and delivery, signs of tetany or hypocalcemia usually become evident within the first 24 hours of life. The etiology is unknown. The onset of tetany after the third or fourth day, but usually within the first few weeks of life, in otherwise normal infants has been associated with transient physiologic hypoparathyroidism, diminished ability of the kidney to excrete phosphate owing to a relatively low filtration rate and a high tubular reabsorption of phosphate, and a high phosphate load from undiluted cow's milk formulas. In both forms of tetany the serum phosphate is elevated and the calcium depressed, resulting in neuromuscular irritability. The serum phosphatase is normal.

Irritability, muscular twitchings, tremors and convulsions are the symptoms. Laryngospasm and carpopedal spasm are less common. Since a positive Chvostek's sign is common in normal newborn infants, it cannot be interpreted as a sign of tetany of the newborn. The serum calcium is below 7 or 8 mg/dl and the serum phosphate is elevated; an absolute diagnosis cannot be made in the absence of these chemical findings. A favorable response to administration of calcium is not sufficient in itself to make the diagnosis, since calcium may act nonspecifically. Furthermore, symptoms such as irritability and tremors may subside spontaneously, and convulsions resulting from cerebral edema, anoxia or injury may not be repeated during the neonatal period. The good prognosis of hypocalcemic convulsions and the guarded to poor prognosis for convulsions from other causes in the neonatal period make establishment of the diagnosis by lumbar puncture (meningitis, intracranial hemorrhage) and by chemical examination of the blood (tetany) desirable. When there is associated proteinuria, pyuria or a persistently high blood urea level not associated with dehydration, urologic studies are indicated.

The response to calcium therapy is dramatic, convulsions being controlled by the intravenous administration of 5 to 10 ml of calcium gluconate in 10 per cent solution. Intramuscular injection of calcium is contraindicated because local induration and necrosis may occur. Calcium should be given orally for approximately a week, preferably as calcium chloride (1.0 gm a day, divided in 3 or more doses) or calcium lactate (2 to 3 gm a day, divided in 3 or more doses) in 10 per cent solution. The hypocalcemia is usually self-limited, as spontaneous improvement occurs in the physiologic functions regulating calcium homeostasis. The use of parathyroid extract or of dihydrotachysterol is not indicated; vitamin D is not effective. (See Section 19.)

Rarely, persistent hypoparathyroidism with hypocalcemia may first present in the neonatal period; it is unresponsive to dietary management. There have also been reports of hypoparathyroidism in infants of hyperparathyroid, hypercalcemic mothers, presumably owing to suppression of the functional development of the fetal parathyroids. The DiGeorge syndrome of incomplete development of the thymus and parathyroids may also present with neonatal tetany as well as an increased susceptibility to infections because of defective cellular immunity.

HYPOMAGNESEMIA

Rarely, hypomagnesemia of unknown etiology may occur in the newborn infant, usually in association with hypocalcemia. This may result from insufficient stores of skeletal magnesium, decreased intestinal absorption, renal loss, a defect in magnesium and calcium homeostasis or an iatrogenic deficiency due to loss during exchange transfusion or insufficient replacement during total intravenous alimentation. It has also been observed in uremic infants. Infants of diabetic mothers tend to have serum magnesium levels which are lower than the normal mean. The clinical manifestations of hypomagnesemia are indistinguishable from those of tetany and may, in fact, be secondary to the accompanying hypocalcemia.

The normal range of serum magnesium levels in the newborn infant is 1.2 to 1.8 mEq/liter, with a mean of 1.5 mEq/liter. During exchange transfusion with citrated blood which is low in magnesium ion, owing to binding by citrate, the serum magnesium drops about 0.5 mEq/liter; approximately 10 days are required for a return to normal. In noniatrogenic hypomagnesemia the serum magnesium may be less than 0.5 mEq per liter. The serum calcium in either instance is usually at levels seen in hypocalcemic tetany, but the serum phosphorus value is normal. *Hypomagnesemia should, therefore, be suspected in any infant with tetany and a normal level of phosphorus in the serum.* Since the hypocalcemia accompanying hypomagnesemia is inadequately corrected by administration of calcium, hypomagnesemia should also be suspected in any patient with tetany not responding to calcium therapy. Almost all the spontaneously occurring cases thus far reported have been in males.

Immediate *treatment* consists in the intramuscular injection of magnesium sulfate. For newborn infants 0.2 ml/kg of a 50 per cent solution daily usually suffices. The accompanying hypocalcemia usually corrects itself as the hypomagnesemia is relieved. In most cases the metabolic defect is transient and treatment can be discontinued after 2 to 3 weeks. A few patients appear to have a permanent form of the disease which requires continuous oral supplementation with magnesium in order to prevent the recurrence of hypomagnesemia.* As with hypocalcemic tetany, there appears to be no residual damage to the central nervous system after prompt treatment.

HYPERMAGNESEMIA

Hypermagnesemia with serum levels as high as 15 mEq/liter may occur in newborn infants of mothers treated with magnesium sulfate for eclampsia. At these levels there is depression of the central nervous system and total paralysis of the skeletal musculature, so that artificial respiration is required to maintain life. Lower levels may result in hypoventilation, lethargy, flaccidity and hyporeflexia. This syndrome may last several days. Rarely, it may be associated with failure to pass meconium (meconium plug syndrome). Exchange transfusion has been used as a means of rapid removal of magnesium ion from the blood. Recovery appears to be complete.

OTHER METABOLIC DISEASES

A number of inborn errors of metabolism may be manifest during the neonatal period; these include phenylketonuria, galactosemia and hyperglycemia. Pyridoxine deficiency and dependency are considered in Section 3.

NARCOTIC ADDICTION AND WITHDRAWALS

Physiologic addiction to narcotics exists in most infants born to actively addicted mothers since many opiates cross the placenta. It may be manifest even before birth by increased activity of the fetus at times when the mother feels the need for the drug or develops withdrawal symptoms. Morphine and its derivatives are the drugs most frequently involved.

A gestation in an addict is a high-risk pregnancy. Prenatal care is usually inadequate and there is a higher incidence of venereal disease, toxemia, premature rupture of the membranes, breech presentations, prolapsed cords and limbs, preterm and low-birth-weight infants, and prenatal morbidity and mortality. The incidence of hyaline membrane disease may be less in low-birth-weight infants of addicts; hyperventilation leading to respiratory alkalosis also has been reported.

For populations with high rates of addiction, the incidence of symptoms of heroin withdrawal in newborn infants has been estimated at 5 per cent. Addiction to methadone or cocaine may produce a similar syndrome. *Withdrawal symptoms* usually appear within 24 hours after birth but may be delayed until the second or third day; there have been reports of symptoms appearing as late as 4 to 6 weeks of life in infants of mothers addicted to or treated with methadone. Infants of mothers taking 2 or 3 "bags" of heroin (5 to 10 mg active ingredient per bag) or 100 mg of methadone per day usually develop symptoms, but the severity and time of onset often correlate poorly with the alleged dose. Coarse tremors and hyperirritability are the most prominent symptoms. The tremors may be fine and indistinguishable from those of hypoglycemia, but are more often coarse, "flapping" and bilateral; the limbs are often rigid, hyperreflexic and resistant to flexion and extension. Irritability and hyperactivity are generally marked and may lead to skin abrasions. Other signs include tachypnea, diarrhea, vomiting, high-pitched cry and fever. Sneezing, yawning, myoclonic jerks, convulsions, nasal stuffiness, respiratory depression or apneic attacks, flushing alternating rapidly with pallor and lacrimation are less common. The *diagnosis* is generally established by the history and clinical presentation. Chromatographic examination of the urine for opiates may reveal only low levels during withdrawal, but quinine, which is often mixed with heroin, may be present in higher concentrations. Hypoglycemia and hypocalcemia should be excluded by blood glucose and calcium determinations.

Treatment has been successful using various combinations of narcotics, sedatives and hypnotics. Phenobarbital, 8 to 10 mg/kg/day in 4 divided doses can effectively reduce irritability and prevent seizures. It is as effective as chlorpromazine, 2.8 mg/kg/24 hours, divided into 3 or 4 doses. It is rarely necessary to administer either drug for more than 5 days. Patients with severe autonomic symptoms may require gradually diminishing doses of morphine, paregoric or chloral hydrate for 2 to 10 weeks. Paregoric at a beginning dose of 3 to 5 drops every 3 to 6 hours, increased to 5 to 10 drops every 4 hours if necessary, depending on the size and response of the infant, is an acceptable al-

---

*Four milliliters per kg per day of the following solution:
Magnesium chloride ($MgCl_2 \cdot 6\ H_2O$) 4.0 gm (39.6 mEq)
Magnesium citrate ($MgHC_6H_5O_7 \cdot 5\ H_2O$) 6.0 gm (39.6 mEq)
Water to 100 ml
Solution provides approximately 0.8 mEq of magnesium per ml.

ternative and will abolish most withdrawal symptoms. The dose and duration of therapy may be adjusted according to the clinical response. Methadone and diazepam have also been used successfully. Parenteral administration of fluids may be necessary to prevent aspiration or dehydration until the symptoms are brought under control. Current mortality is not over 10 per cent and with early recognition and treatment may be negligible. *Prognosis* for normal development is probably good, except as affected by the adverse circumstances of high-risk pregnancy and delivery, and by the environment to which the infant is returned after recovery.

DISTURBANCES OF THE ENDOCRINE SYSTEM

Details of diagnosis and management of the endocrinopathies are covered in the section on The Endocrine System. The purpose of this section is merely to call attention to those endocrine disturbances which may be identified at birth or during the first month of life.

Pituitary dwarfism is usually inapparent at birth, the infant being of normal size. Conversely, constitutional dwarfs usually demonstrate length and weight consistent with prematurity when they are born after a normal gestational period and otherwise have the physical appearance of infants born at term.

Thyroid deficiency may be apparent at birth in genetically determined cretinism or in infants of mothers treated with thiouracil or its derivatives during pregnancy. Constipation, prolonged jaundice, lethargy or poor peripheral circulation as manifested by persistently mottled skin or cold extremities should always rouse suspicion of *cretinism.* Temporary *hyperthyroidism* may be seen at birth in the infants of mothers with hyperthyroidism or of those who have been receiving thyroid medication. *Congenital goiter* is discussed in Section 17.

Transient *hypoparathyroidism* may be manifest as tetany of the newborn.

The *adrenal gland* is subject to numerous disturbances which may be manifest and require lifesaving treatment during the neonatal period. Acute adrenal *hemorrhage* and failure may be seen after breech or other traumatic deliveries or in association with overwhelming infection. Phallic or clitoral enlargement apparent at or soon after birth suggests *adrenocortical hyperplasia.* Signs of deficiency of salt and water hormone are vomiting, diarrhea, dehydration, convulsions or shock. Since the condition is genetically determined, newborn siblings of patients with the salt-losing variety of adrenocortical hyperplasia should be observed closely for manifestations of adrenal insufficiency. *Congenitally hypoplastic adrenal glands* may also give rise to adrenal insufficiency during the first few weeks of life. A syndrome clinically indistinguishable from adrenal insufficiency has been identified as a rare manifestation of cow's milk allergy in the first month of life.

Anomalies of the *gonads* may be apparent at birth. Of particular interest is gonadal dysgenesis (Turner's syndrome). Female infants with webbing of the neck, lymphangiectatic edema, hypoplasia of the nipples, cutis laxa, low hairline at the nape of the neck, deep-set ears, high-arched palate, deformities of the nails, cubitus valgus and other anomalies should be suspected of having gonadal dysgenesis (Section 17).

Transient *diabetes mellitus* (Section 16) of unknown origin is occasionally and only seen in the newborn. It usually presents as dehydration, loss of weight or acidosis. *Hypoglycemic convulsions* may occur during the first few days of life in infants of diabetic mothers, or in low-birth-weight infants.

INFANTS OF DIABETIC MOTHERS

The successful control of diabetes with insulin has led to the survival of increasing numbers of diabetic women who bear children. Their infants and the infants of women who later develop diabetes share certain morphologic characteristics. In addition to distinctive physical characteristics of macrosomia, which may be diagnosed prior to birth, infants of diabetic mothers have a high incidence of associated hydramnios and of intrauterine deaths after the thirty-sixth week of gestation, and high neonatal mortality and morbidity rates. Fetal wastage throughout pregnancy is associated with poorly controlled maternal diabetes, especially keto-acidosis. Perinatal mortality and morbidity is proportional to severity of maternal diabetes, but may also be increased with mild gestational diabetes.

PATHOPHYSIOLOGY. The etiology of this intrauterine metabolic disorder is unknown. With severe maternal vascular disease both the placenta and infant may be of low weight, but usually the weight of each is increased. DNA in proportion to placental weight, maternal plasma lactogenic hormone levels and villous surface area are increased. Weights of the infant's organs, except for the brain, are also increased. Neurologic development and ossification centers tend to correlate with brain size and gestational age rather than total body weight. There is also hypertrophy of pancreatic islets and their beta cells, with an increased insulin content and secretion, leading to elevated blood levels. The rate of disposal of exogenous glucose is increased, and during hypoglycemia free fatty acid levels are decreased. Although fetal hyperinsulinism in response to maternal hyperglycemia has been postulated as the cause of the macrosomia and postnatal hypoglycemia, this does not explain the large size of infants of *pre*diabetic mothers. Also the "cushioned," plethoric appearance is not associated with an elevation of serum 17-hydroxycorticoids in the blood of infants of diabetic mothers as would be anticipated if there were increased secretion of maternal or fetal corticotropin. In addition, there is an increase in total body fat rather than fluid and electrolytes; total body water, particularly extracellular water as a percentage of body weight, is decreased. A central role for fetal pituitary growth hormone in the pathophysiology of this syndrome has also been proposed.

CLINICAL MANIFESTATIONS. The infants of diabetic and prediabetic mothers bear a surprising resemblance to each other (Fig. 7–29). They tend to be large and plump, with a puffy, plethoric facies resembling those of patients who have been receiving corticotropin or a corticosteroid. They have a bloated appearance. These infants may, however, also be of normal or low birth weight, particularly if delivered before term or if there is associated maternal vascular disease. It has also been suggested that macrosomia may be less likely when the maternal diabetes is well controlled.

The infants tend to be "jumpy" or "trembly" during the first three days of life and may have any of the diverse manifestations of hypoglycemia. Early appearance of these signs is more likely to be related to hypoglycemia and later appearance to hypocalcemia; these abnormalities also may occur together. Perinatal asphyxia or hyperbilirubinemia may produce similar signs. Rarely, hypomagnesemia may be associated with the hypocalcemia.

Many infants of diabetic mothers develop tachypnea during the first five days of life. This may be a transient manifestation of hypoglycemia, hypothermia, polycythemia or cerebral edema from birth trauma or asphyxia, or it may represent early hyaline membrane disease. There is also an increased incidence of renal vein thrombosis, which should be suspected in the presence of a mass in the flank, hematuria and thrombocytopenia. The incidence of congenital anomalies is increased, particularly if there is polyhydramnios.

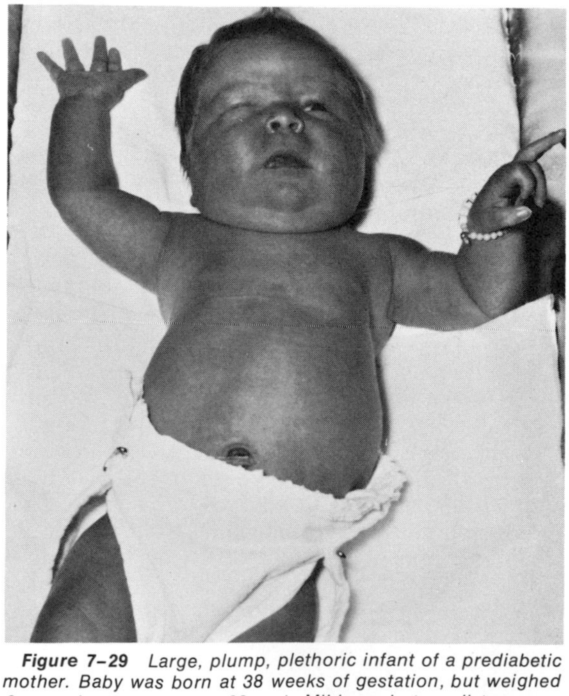

Figure 7–29 Large, plump, plethoric infant of a prediabetic mother. Baby was born at 38 weeks of gestation, but weighed 9 pounds 11 ounces (4408 gm). Mild respiratory distress was the only symptom other than appearance.

PROGNOSIS. The subsequent incidence of diabetes mellitus in infants of diabetic mothers is slightly higher than in the general population. There is also some evidence that the oversized infants have a predilection to obesity in childhood that may extend into adult life. Disagreement persists about whether there is a slightly increased risk of impaired intellectual development unrelated to hypoglycemia.

TREATMENT. Management of these infants should be initiated before birth by frequent prenatal evaluation of all pregnant women with overt or gestational diabetes and by delivering their infants in hospitals where expert obstetric and pediatric care are continuously available. Since there is no predictable relationship between the clinical course of the infant and the severity of maternal disease, all the infants of diabetic mothers, regardless of size, should initially receive intensive observation and care. Asymptomatic infants should have a blood sugar determination within 1 hour of birth and then every hour or 2 for the next 6 to 8 hours; if clinically well and normoglycemic, oral or gavage feedings with 10 to 20 per cent glucose water, or milk formula, should be started at 2 to 3 hours of age and continued at 2-hour intervals. If there is any question about an infant's ability to tolerate oral feeding, it should be discontinued and 10 to 15 per cent glucose given by peripheral intravenous infusion. Blood glucose values under 30 mg/dl should be treated, even in asymptomatic infants, with intravenous infusions of glucose sufficient to keep the blood levels well above this level. A single intramuscular injection of glucagon (300 μg/kg) has been proposed but not generally accepted as treatment, in addition to the administration of glucose, in asymptomatic large hypoglycemic infants who otherwise appear well. The management of hypoglycemia in sick or symptomatic infants is discussed in the following section. For treatment of *hypocalcemia* see Tetany; for that of *hypomagnesemia* and for that of *hyaline membrane disease* see the corresponding preceding sections.

Infants with symptoms pointing to the central nervous system should have diagnostic lumbar puncture to rule out meningitis, cerebral hemorrhage or cerebral edema.

HYPOGLYCEMIA

Hypoglycemia is present when the infant's blood glucose concentration is significantly lower than the mean for a population of infants of similar age and weight. The fetal blood glucose level is substantially lower than and varies directly with that of the mother. After their abrupt removal from the constant placental infusion of glucose, full-term infants usually stabilize their blood levels above 30 mg/dl during the first 72 hours of life, and low-birth-weight infants, above 20 mg/dl. Lower concentrations are considered hypoglycemic.

Four pathophysiologic groups of neonatal infants are at high risk of developing hypoglycemia: (1) Infants of mothers with diabetes mellitus or gestational diabetes and infants with severe erythroblastosis fetalis seem to suffer from hyperinsulinism. (2) Infants of low birth weight may have experienced intrauterine malnutrition resulting in reduced hepatic glycogen stores; those who are small for their gestational age, the smallest of discordant twins, polycythemic infants, infants of toxemic mothers and infants with placental abnormalities are particularly vulnerable. (Other factors in the development of hypoglycemia in this group include increased insulin responsiveness, low cortisol production rates, and possibly increased insulin levels and decreased output of epinephrine in response to hypoglycemia.) (3) Very immature or severely ill infants may develop hypoglycemia owing to increased metabolic needs out of proportion to substrate stores and calories supplied: low-birth-weight infants with respiratory distress syndrome, anoxic injury, hypothermia and systemic infections, as well as infants in heart failure with cyanotic congenital heart disease, are at increased risk. The interruption of intravenous infusions, particularly those with high glucose concentrations, may also result in the precipitous onset of hypoglycemia. (4) Rare infants with genetic or primary metabolic defects, such as galactosemia, glycogen storage disease, maple syrup urine disease, leucine sensitivity, insulinomas or Beckwith syndrome (see below), are also susceptible.

The overall frequency of hypoglycemia is 2 to 3 per 1000 live births but appears to be significantly higher among infants of low birth weight for gestational age, especially those with a complicated prenatal history or severe illness. The incidence among infants of diabetic mothers may be as high as 50 per cent. It is lower in infants of gestationally diabetic mothers and lower but still elevated among infants of low birth weight.

CLINICAL MANIFESTATIONS. In contrast to the frequency of chemical hypoglycemia, the incidence of symptomatic hypoglycemia is highest in low-birth-weight infants. Because many of the symptoms also occur with other conditions such as infections, central nervous system anomalies, meningitis, hypocalcemia, hypomagnesemia and asphyxia, and because some may be seen in normoglycemic well infants, the exact incidence of symptomatic hypoglycemia has been difficult to establish.

The onset of symptoms has been observed from a few hours to a week after birth. In approximate order of frequency there are jitteriness or tremors, episodes of cyanosis, apathy, convulsions, intermittent apneic spells or tachypnea, weak or high-pitched cry, limpness, difficulty in feeding and eye-rolling. Episodes of sweating, sudden pallor and hypothermia also occur. Because these clinical manifestations may result from a variety of causes, it is critical to determine if they disappear with the administration of sufficient glucose to raise the blood sugar to normal levels; if they do not, other diagnoses must be considered.

TREATMENT. This consists in administration through a peripheral vein of 1 to 2 ml per kg of 50 per cent glucose solution for immediate relief of symptoms, followed by continuous intravenous infusion of 10 to 15 per cent glucose solution until blood glucose levels have stabilized within the normal range and the infant can tolerate oral feedings, when it should be discontinued.

If intravenous infusions of glucose in concentrations up to 20 per cent are inadequate to eliminate symptoms and maintain constant normal blood glucose concentrations, hydrocortisone (2.5 mg/kg every 12 hours) or prednisone (1 mg/kg/day) should be administered. Blood glucose should be measured every 2 hours after initiating therapy until several determinations are above 40 mg/dl. Subsequently levels should be obtained every 4 to 6 hours and the treatment gradually reduced and finally discontinued when the blood glucose has been in the normal range and the baby asymptomatic for 24 to 48 hours. Treatment is usually necessary for a few days to a week, rarely for several weeks. Diazoxide, epinephrine and fructose are not of established benefit. Epinephrine may produce lactic acidosis. Glucagon has been advocated for use with glucose in asymptomatic infants of diabetic mothers, but its value has not been established. Infants who are at increased risk of developing hypoglycemia should have their blood glucose measured within 1 hour of birth and subsequently every 1 to 2 hours for the first 6 to 8 hours and every 4 to 6 hours until 24 hours of life. Normoglycemic high-risk infants should receive oral or gavage feedings with 10 to 20 per cent glucose water or with milk formula started at 2 to 3 hours of age and continued at 2-hour intervals for 24 to 48 hours. An intravenous infusion of 10 to 15 per cent glucose should be provided if oral feedings are poorly tolerated or if asymptomatic hypoglycemia develops.

PROGNOSIS. Prognosis for life is good in the absence of congenital anomalies severe enough in themselves to be lethal. Recurrences of hypoglycemia are relatively rare after adequate treatment, but have been reported as late as the age of 8 months. Prognosis for normal intellectual function must be guarded, since prolonged and severe hypoglycemia may be associated with neurologic sequelae and death. Symptomatic infants with hypoglycemia, particularly low-birth-weight infants and large-sized infants of overtly diabetic mothers, have a worse prognosis for subsequent normal intellectual development than asymptomatic infants.

HYPOGLYCEMIA WITH MACROGLOSSIA
(Beckwith Syndrome)

Beckwith and Combs and their co-workers described a syndrome of intractable neonatal hypoglycemia occurring in infants with macroglossia, large size, visceromegaly, mild microcephaly and umbilical abnormalities. The visceromegaly involves chiefly the liver and the kidneys, in which there is a noncystic hyperplasia. Some of the infants are also polycythemic. Treatment is that of hypoglycemia, as described above. The prognosis is poor.

INFECTIONS OF THE NEWBORN

Infections in the neonatal infant are caused by a variety of bacterial, viral, fungal and parasitic organisms. Some of the diseases of special importance to the newborn infant are discussed in other sections. See, in particular, congenital rubella syndrome, syphilis, tetanus, cytomegalic inclusion disease, toxoplasmosis, fungal infections and tuberculosis.

Many immunologic responses of the newborn infant are less developed than those of the older child and adult, and the newborn is particularly susceptible to some organisms that are usually nonpathogenic after the neonatal period until geriatric age, when such infections are again seen with relatively greater frequency. The clinical manifestations of infection in the neonatal infant vary according to the etiologic agent, localization or organ involvement, duration, severity and individual immunologic responsiveness (Table 7–26). The course is often but not invariably fulminant, with high mortality, especially in low-birth-weight infants.

The pneumococcus, beta hemolytic streptococcus and *H. influenzae,* common pathogenic agents in later infancy, are relatively uncommon causes of infection in the first few weeks of life. At this time coliform organisms and *S. aureus* are the most frequent causes of severe infections; *E. coli* is the commonest etiologic agent in pneumonia, septicemia, meningitis and diarrhea of the newborn. Other relatively common bacterial pathogens are enterococci, Klebsiella, Pseudomonas, Proteus and Salmonella. The incidence of group A and group B streptococcal infections is increased among the socioeconomically disadvantaged. Infections may occur periodically in waves, in micro-epidemics, or as sporadic individual episodes. Nursery epidemics caused by any organism with antibiotic susceptibility may be managed in a manner similar to that to be described for the prevention of epidemics of staphylococcal infection (see below).

The most frequent serious infections of the newborn are *pneumonia, septicemia, diarrhea, meningitis* and *peritonitis.* Of these, pneumonia and septicemia are common; diarrhea has become rela-

TABLE 7–26 EPIDEMIOLOGIC AND CLINICAL DATA WHICH SUGGEST OR SUPPORT A DIAGNOSIS OF NEONATAL SEPTICEMIA*

HISTORY	SIGNS	
	General	*Respiratory System*
Low birth weight	Fever or hypothermia	Tachypnea
Amniotic infection, e.g., foul-smelling, cloudy, or purulent amniotic fluid	Scleredema	Dyspnea
Premature rupture of membranes (>24 hours)	Poor feeding	Cyanosis
Resuscitation especially if accompanied by intubation and umbilical vessel catheterization		Apnea
Meconium staining of skin	*Circulatory System*	*Gastrointestinal System*
Congenital abnormality of urinary tract, CNS, lungs, or heart	Pallor/cyanosis/mottling	Abdominal distention
Bloody secretions in upper airway suggesting aspiration of maternal blood or vaginal secretions	Abnormal respirations	Hepatomegaly
Lethargy; "not doing well"; poor feeding	Cold, clammy skin	Vomiting
	Hypotension	Diarrhea
		Decreased stooling
	Central Nervous System	*Hematologic System*
	Lethargy or irritability	Jaundice
	Hyporeflexia	Splenomegaly
	Irregular respirations	Pallor
	Tremors or convulsions	Purpura
	Full fontanel	Petechiae
	Apnea	Bleeding

*Adapted from Gotoff, S. *In* Behrman, R. E. (ed.): Neonatology. St. Louis, The C. V. Mosby Company, 1973.

tively uncommon in the United States, but has a high incidence in individual epidemics; meningitis is present in approximately 25 per cent of cases of septicemia; and peritonitis is relatively rare as a well developed clinical entity. Although relatively less common, otitis media, ophthalmitis, arthritis, osteomyelitis and infections of the urinary tract, skin and mucous membranes can result in the rapid onset of serious illness during the neonatal period. Early diagnosis is often difficult owing to the infant's limited capacity to respond to infection in classic fashion.

In pneumonia, septicemia, meningitis, and other bacterial infections the prognosis is heavily influenced by early diagnosis and institution of specific treatment with appropriate antibacterial agents. *All are distinguished by their lack of specific signs or symptoms in the early stages.* (See earlier discussions of Clinical Manifestations of Disease in the Newborn, and Pneumonia. In the absence of dehydration or high environmental temperature they are the commonest causes of body temperatures over 100°F in the newborn infant. Frequently, however, there is no elevation of temperature, or the temperature may be subnormal, and failure to feed well, lethargy, vasomotor instability, abdominal distention, irritability, vomiting or episodes of cyanosis may be the only evidence of any one of these major infections. The onset of icterus after the second or third day of life is especially suggestive of septicemia. These signs may also be related, however, to noninfectious processes such as intracranial hemorrhage, anoxia, intracranial malformations, hypoglycemia, and gastrointestinal or hematologic disease. The classic signs of meningitis in the small infant (bulging fontanel, high-pitched cry, vomiting and convulsions) are late signs, and the diagnosis must be made before they appear in order to reduce the mortality of the disease. Apnea and tremors may be early signs. Acute meningitis caused by gram-negative bacilli, in particular, frequently becomes chronic, with a high incidence of permanent residuals. Clinical detection of pneumonia, septicemia or meningitis is dependent on liberal indications for securing a roentgenogram of the chest and blood and urine cultures, and for performing a spinal puncture in infants who "are not doing well." Premature or low-birth-weight infants are especially prone to serious infections with few or no clinical manifestations.

EPIDEMIOLOGY. Infections which may be responsible for neonatal morbidity and mortality may be acquired during the embryonic, fetal or neonatal period. From the standpoints of prevention, recognition and management, it is helpful to know as much as possible of the pathogenesis of each of these diseases; one important aspect is knowledge of the time of acquisition. The following tabulation lists the more important infections which may occur during the perinatal period. They are arranged on the basis of preventability in relation to current knowledge. It is important to recognize that a number of these infections may be transmitted by the mother even though she has had no clinical evidence that she is a carrier. Prior to birth, freedom from infection depends on sterile amniotic fluid, the integrity of the placenta and the absence of maternal bacteremia or viremia. Although transplacental infections are relatively uncommon, viral, bacterial and parasitic agents may cross the placenta from an infected mother and cause lethal or crippling disease in a newborn infant. Amniotic infection associated with premature rupture of the fetal membranes, prolonged labor and excessive manipulation during labor may lead to infection in the neonate. Infections may also be acquired in the delivery room or nursery through airborne and contact routes. Resuscitation equipment, respirators, incubators, bassinets, umbilical catheters and central venous catheters may all be sources of contamination.

Infections acquired during gestation

Preventable	*Nonpreventable**
Syphilis	Toxoplasmosis
Tuberculosis	Cytomegalic inclusion disease
Residuals of rubella	Listeriosis
Vaccinia	Myocarditis, viral
Poliomyelitis	Hepatitis, homologous serum
Pneumonia†	Varicella
Sepsis†	Herpes simplex
	Vibrio fetus infection

Infections acquired during birth‡

Preventable	*Nonpreventable*
Gonorrheal ophthalmia	Herpes simplex
Oral moniliasis	Listeriosis
Salmonellosis	Group B streptococcus
Pneumonia§	
Sepsis§	

Infections acquired after birth in the neonatal period

Staphylococcal infections
  Carrier state, skin lesions, pneumonia, otitis media, meningitis, osteomyelitis, diarrhea, generalized sepsis
E. coli infections
  Septicemia, omphalitis, pneumonia, diarrhea, and others
Salmonella infections
  Septicemia, meningitis, osteomyelitis, and others
Beta hemolytic streptococcal infections
  Occasionally responsible for disease in this age period
Pneumococcal and *H. influenzae* infections
  Less frequent pathogenic agents than in subsequent months
Tetanus
Tuberculosis

*On basis of current knowledge.

†Usually secondary to premature rupture of membranes or to interference with placental circulation.

‡Most often from the mother, who may be infected or may be a carrier.

§Usually secondary to premature rupture of membranes, to interference with placental circulation, or to prolonged or traumatic delivery.

Viral infections
 Upper respiratory tract infections, pneumonitis, myocarditis, generalized infections

LABORATORY FINDINGS. Leukopenia (< 4000 white blood cells per cu mm) or leukocytosis (> 25000 white blood cells per cu mm) supports the diagnosis of infection. Hemolytic anemia and thrombocytopenia may accompany systemic infections. IgM concentrations are usually elevated above 17 mg/dl during the first week of life in infants with chronic intrauterine infections and in some infants with perinatal infections. Serologic studies of mother as well as infant may be helpful in the diagnosis of syphilis, toxoplasmosis, rubella, and cytomegalovirus, arbovirus, enterovirus and fungal infections.

DIAGNOSIS AND TREATMENT. A presumptive diagnosis of neonatal septicemia should be made when, in the absence of another diagnosis, the possibility is suggested by the clinical and epidemiologic evidence. After obtaining appropriate cultures, antibiotic therapy should be immediately started because of the potentially rapid course and high mortality. The choice of antibiotic should depend upon what is considered to be the most likely pathogen, the potential effectiveness of the antimicrobial agent against the presumed bacteria, the site of infection, the metabolism of the drug and possible adverse side effects from its use under the circumstances. The antibiotic sensitivity pattern of most bacteria varies with time, place and the local pattern of use of antimicrobial agents. These factors must all be taken into consideration in choosing therapeutic agents prior to availability of the results of cultures and tests of antibiotic sensitivity. Septicemia of unknown etiology occurring within 72 hours of birth is usually treated with parenteral ampicillin or penicillin G and kanamycin or gentamicin. After 72 hours of life a penicillinase-resistant penicillin may be substituted for ampicillin or penicillin G. Antimicrobial therapy for bacterial meningitis is similar to that for septicemia, with the addition of intrathecal therapy with gentamicin (0.5 to 1.0 mg in 1 ml isotonic sodium chloride solution daily for 3 to 5 days) for pseudomonas and unresponsive gram-negative enteric bacteria.

Sepsis, meningitis, pneumonia or other infections usually require intensive observation and supportive management of the sick neonatal infant. Adequate isolation can usually be obtained by use of an incubator and adequate handwashing technique; more elaborate isolation measures may be required for highly contagious diseases like gastroenteritis or varicella. Complications of severe neonatal infections include shock, adrenal insufficiency, consumptive coagulopathy, congestive heart failure and hyponatremia. Circulatory support, correction of acidosis and treatment with steroids (10 mg per kg of hydrocortisone) may be required for shock secondary to septicemia due to gram-negative bacteria.

STAPHYLOCOCCAL INFECTIONS

Staphylococcus aureus is second in frequency to *E. coli* as a cause of infection in the newborn. Strains resistant to many of the commonly used antibacterial agents have been responsible for epidemic nursery infections.

Although staphylococcal pneumonia, septicemia or enteritis may occur without warning in the newborn infant, each is frequently preceded by apparent skin infections of the infant or of contacts. These may consist of small pustules or furuncles, or of large furuncles, cellulitis, bullous impetigo, omphalitis, or breast abscess. Osteomyelitis and meningitis are relatively frequent complications of septicemia. Staphylococcal meningitis without bacteremia suggests the presence of a communication (dermal sinus) between the skin and the subarachnoid space. A leaking meningocele is an obvious portal of entry. The umbilicus, a circumcision wound or other surgical incision may serve as a route for staphylococci to reach the bloodstream, as may any abrasion of the skin.

Nursery epidemics of staphylococcal infection usually begin with increasingly frequent appearance of small pustules. More severe infections of the skin, septicemia or enteritis are usually seen next. Although the initial infection is acquired in the nursery, these and other serious manifestations may not make their appearance for weeks or even months after the baby has been discharged. Therefore the existence of an epidemic of serious proportions may not be suspected unless the infants are followed up carefully after discharge and unless all cases of furuncles, breast abscess, pneumonia and other less frequent staphylococcal infections during the first months of life are reported to the nursery where the infants were born. A high incidence of small pustules may be the only evidence in the nursery of an epidemic which is resulting in major staphylococcal infections among discharged infants and members of their families.

Investigations suggest that epidemics are due to certain strains of hemolytic *S. aureus* which appear to have unusual pathogenicity. Phage type 80/81 has been the most frequently identified in severe hospital epidemics; phage types 2, 55/71 and 71 have been associated with Ritter's disease (scalded skin syndrome) (Section 23). The pathogen is undoubtedly introduced initially into the nursery by personnel or by an infant who acquires it through contact with his mother. Once the organism has been introduced, the infants in the nursery, as well as adult carriers, constitute the reservoir of infection, and it spreads from baby to baby. Anatomic areas of the infant which constitute particular reservoirs are the skin, the anterior nares and the umbilical cord stump.

PREVENTION. All persons with skin infections should be excluded from the nursery and from contact with the infant after discharge. Mothers with staphylococcal infections should be isolated and treated while their infants remain in an isolation nursery out of contact with them or with other newborn infants. Use of soap or detergent containing a low concentration of hexachlorophene tends to reduce the bacterial population on the skin of nursery personnel. The latter should also be specifically instructed that the anterior nares constitute the chief reservoir in carriers. Initial and daily bathing of the infants with a soap or detergent reduces the incidence of skin infection with staphylococci and *E. coli.* Daily painting of the umbilical cord stump with bactericidal dyes* reduces the incidence of nasal and skin colonization of staphylococci, provided all infants in the nursery are so treated. Avoidance of overcrowding in the nursery is important. Since the infants themselves appear to be the chief reservoir of staphylococcal infection in nursery epidemics, it is desirable to place a suspect infant in an incubator of a type which can serve as an individual isolation unit or to have multiple nurseries, each accommodating 4 to 6 infants, so that, once a nursery is filled, no new babies need be admitted until all its previous occupants have been discharged and the nursery has been cleaned. These measures will serve to break any baby-to-baby cycle of infection.

Once an *epidemic* of staphylococcal infection has started, there appear to be only two effective ways of stopping it. The preferable method is to admit all new babies to newly established nurseries staffed by separate, uninfected personnel in a different area of the hospital. Admission of new infants to the regular nurseries is resumed only after all the infant occupants have been discharged, after any staphylococcal carriers have been identified and excluded, and after the nurseries have been thoroughly cleaned and disinfected. An initial bath of all new admissions to the nursery with a soap or detergent containing a low concentration of hexachlorophene (3 per cent or less) or a similar agent may also aid in interrupting the epidemic. *Repeated bathing of infants with hexachlorophene-containing compounds is not advised at any time because of the recently raised possibility of hexachlorophene-induced brain damage.* The second and less preferable method is the routine administration to each infant in the nursery from the day of admission through the day of discharge of full therapeutic doses of an antibiotic effective against the strain of staphylococci responsible for the epidemic. For this purpose erythromycin or one of the synthetic penicillins is usually the drug of choice, owing to the greater potential toxicity of chloramphenicol, novobiocin, bacitracin or kanamycin. Maintenance of this regimen for 3 weeks is ordinarily sufficient to control an epidemic, provided the usual measures of tightening up on nursery techniques in general and the exclusion of personnel who are carriers of the pathogenic strain are also taken.

Artificial colonization of the nose and umbilical cord stump with a nonpathogenic strain of coagulase-positive *S. aureus* has been demonstrated to interfere with colonization by pathogenic strains. The application of this phenomenon to the prevention and interruption of nursery epidemics of staphylococcal infection is in the experimental stage and should be done only by experienced investigators under carefully controlled conditions.

TREATMENT. The treatment of staphylococcal infections is best accomplished by systemic administration of an antibiotic effective against the particular strain of the organism involved.

Because many strains of staphylococci infecting newborn infants produce penicillinase, the drug used should be effective against such strains; if the organism is isolated, it should be tested for its in vitro susceptibility to several of the synthetic penicillins and other antibiotics effective against penicillin-resistant staphylococci. Methicillin, oxacillin or nafcillin may be used for severe staphylococcal infections prior to receipt of information from the laboratory of the in vitro susceptibilities of the bacterium. For the first 5 days of life the dose of these drugs for either premature or term infants is 50 mg/kg given parenterally every 12 hours. After 5 days increased renal clearance in term infants requires an increase to 50 mg/kg every 6 hours. If the organism is sensitive to penicillin G, it is the drug of choice in a dose of 50,000 units per kg every 12 hours for the first 5 days of life and every 6 hours thereafter. The combination of penicillin G or ampicillin (50 mg per kg every 12 hours for the first 5 days and every 6 hours thereafter) and kanamycin in a dose of 7.5 mg per kg, or gentamicin 2.5 mg per kg every 12 hours by the intramuscular route has been effective against many strains of staphylococci and has the advantage, in cases in which the organism is presumed, but not proved, of effectiveness against *E. coli* and a number of other gram-negative organisms. Cephalothin is also effective against penicillinase-producing staphylococci and some gram-negative bacteria, but it has not had adequate trial in newborn infants and has an irritating effect on veins.

Tests of antibiotic sensitivity in vitro should always be done and the medication changed accordingly if the drug being used is not producing a satisfactory clinical response. In the presence of an obviously good clinical response a shift of medication on the basis of the results of sensitivity tests in vitro should be questioned.

In addition to systemic therapy, bathing with soaps or detergents containing a low concentration of hexachlorophene and the local application of bacitracin ointment will aid in eradicating skin lesions. Accumulations of pus, wherever encountered, should be drained surgically.

---

*"Triple-dye": Acriflavine, 1.14 gm.
Gentian violet, 2.29 gm.
Brilliant green, 2.29 gm.
Distilled water, 1000 ml.

PSEUDOMONAS INFECTIONS

See also Section 10.

Perhaps owing to several factors such as measures to eliminate staphylococci from hospital nurseries and the common use of complicated equipment that is difficult to sterilize or that includes water reservoirs, gram-negative and ordinarily nonpathogenic bacteria have become increasingly important as a cause of infections acquired in the newborn nursery. Recent restrictions on the use of hexachlorophene may reverse this trend.

The pseudomonas group of organisms, which are normal inhabitants of water and soil, are important causes of nursery infections; klebsiella, aerobacter and proteus groups are also significant pathogens. Pseudomonas contributes to the mortality from bacteremia, pneumonia and meningitis in premature and intensive care nurseries, where the debilitated infant population is particularly susceptible to infection. The organisms are constantly reintroduced from the skins of nursery personnel, and the use of such equipment as endotracheal and nasopharyngeal tubes promotes their proliferation through interference with clearance of respiratory secretions. Indwelling catheters and excoriation of the skin also favor the growth of these organisms.

Preventive measures include careful and frequent cleansing and sterilization of equipment used for respiratory therapy, avoidance of equipment or procedures which promote stasis of respiratory secretions, and use of a bactericidal agent effective against pseudomonas in the humidification pans of incubators. Meticulous, continuing attention to cleaning and drying the skin and to avoiding trauma or irritation is also important in prevention of infections due to pseudomonas.

Water in humidification pans of incubators may be sterilized by the addition of 50 micrograms of silver nitrate per liter. Distilled water must be used, since chlorine in water will precipitate the silver out as the insoluble and nonbactericidal chloride. Plastic pans should be used, because silver nitrate disappears rapidly from solution in metal pans. The bacterial population in the reservoirs of nebulizers may be kept down by frequent changes of *sterile* distilled water; mist from ultrasonic nebulizers tends to be less contaminated than mist from mechanical nebulizers.

Treatment of infections with the pseudomonas group of bacteria is often unsatisfactory; the infections are rarely rapidly controlled. Prior to determining the pattern of antibiotic sensitivities gentamicin is recommended in a dose of 2.5 mg/kg every 12 hours. If clinical response is good, this treatment should be maintained for a total of 10 days; in term infants the dose is increased to a frequency of every 8 hours after the first 5 days. The addition of carbenicillin may be useful. If response is inadequate, the in vitro sensitivities should be used to pick another drug, usually polymyxin B (1.5 to 2.5 mg/kg every 12 hours intravenously) or colistin (polymyxin E) in a dose of 2 to 4 mg/kg every 12 hours intramuscularly. Colistin should not be administered intrathecally, but intrathecal treatment with gentamicin or polymyxin B is indicated for pseudomonas meningitis.

DIARRHEA IN THE NEWBORN

A scourge because of its great contagiousness and high morbidity and mortality rates, epidemic diarrhea of the newborn is now a relatively infrequent but still serious problem in the United States.

Etiologically it is not an entity. A number of bacterial and viral agents have been identified as the causative or probable causative agents. With the exception of enteropathogenic strains of *E. coli* and occasional viruses causing respiratory or oral infections in adults, they do not differ significantly from the usual causative agents of diarrhea (Section 11). The serologic types of *E. coli* that are associated with diarrheal disease in infancy have been designated enteropathogenic *E. coli*; types 055:B5, 0111:B4 and 0127:B8 have been most frequently identified in epidemics. Enteropathic *E. coli* may be present in the gastrointestinal tract of asymptomatic infants. Enteropathogenic *E. coli,* salmonella and shigellae isolated from newborn infants with diarrhea are usually assumed to be etiologically significant. Recent reports suggest that there may also be cholera-like, enterotoxin-producing strains of *E. coli* other than the usual enteropathogenic serotypes. Rarely, *Pseudomonas aeruginosa*, *S. aureus* (Phage group III), or *Candida albicans* may produce enterocolitis.

The specificity and severity of the disease are related principally to host factors of low immunity, small reserve of water and electrolytes, and poorly developed homeostatic mechanisms. The large, changing, crowded and susceptible population in almost any newborn nursery is also an ideal environmental situation for a contagious disease to become epidemic. Premature or debilitated infants are especially susceptible. Sporadic cases are also seen; they usually occur in the home after exposure to an older sibling or adult with an enteric infection.

CLINICAL MANIFESTATIONS. The incubation period is most commonly 1 to 3 days. At onset the infant usually becomes listless or fretful, nurses less well than usual, fails to gain or may actually lose weight. Vomiting is an inconstant symptom, as is abdominal distention. The temperature is usually normal, but may rise to 100 to 104 F. When the diarrhea starts, the stools tend to be watery, yellowish (later greenish) and acid enough to produce irritation of the skin of the buttocks within a few hours. They are usually frequent and passed explosively. On the other hand, an occasional infant may go into shock and die from water and electrolyte loss into the intestinal lumen before a diarrheal stool is passed. Mucus, pus and macroscopic blood are usually not evident or at least not prominent. As the diarrhea progresses the infant becomes increasingly restless with a frequent, short and feeble cry. With progressive dehydration, thirst may give way to refusal to feed, and the infant becomes drowsy and, finally, comatose. In the final stages of dehydration the eyes are deep-sunken, the skin takes on a grayish cast, and there is circumoral cyanosis and an apparent state of shock. Hyperpnea is frequently absent in spite of acidosis with carbon dioxide levels as low as 2 mEq. per liter. There is hemoconcentration, and protein, white cells and casts are found in the urine in considerable quantities. The severity and the clinical manifestations vary greatly from patient to patient; in every outbreak there are asymptomatic carriers.

The clinical course varies from a few days to several weeks. Exacerbations are common. Complications include otitis media, bronchopneumonia, bacteremia, peritonitis from perforation of an intestinal ulcer, and renal vein and cerebral sinus thrombosis.

PREVENTION. Hospital nursery routines should be designed to eliminate chances of infection or cross infection among the infants. This means adequate floor area to avoid overcrowding, complete individual bassinet units and equipment for each infant, careful supervision of the preparation of formulas, and well trained, conscientious personnel who are numerically adequate.

Any direct or indirect contact with persons with intestinal disease or direct contact with any with respiratory infections must be avoided. This means the exclusion from the nursery of all personnel who have had even mild diarrhea or vomiting within 48 to 72 hours, and of all personnel having more than the most fleeting contact with active cases of diarrhea either professionally or at home. In nurseries a high index of suspicion must be maintained, especially since the onset of an epidemic may be so insidious that the possibility is not considered until several infants have diarrhea. A frequent cause of this situation is the discharge from the nursery of the initial case or cases before definite signs of the disease have appeared, but after the contagious state is already present. Therefore it is essential that the development of diarrhea in an infant after discharge be reported immediately to the person in charge of the newborn nursery. Immediate reporting to local or state health officials is equally important.

Nursery personnel must be constantly on the alert for abnormal stools among their charges. Differentiation must be made between diarrhea and the loose and frequent movements characteristic of transitional stools. The breast-fed infant may have more frequent and more liquid stools than the bottle-fed infant, and may be affected by the dietary or medicinal intake of his mother. Overfeeding, high carbohydrate content of the formula, intestinal intolerance to cow's milk or the use of soybean or protein hydrolysate formulas may be responsible for loose stools in the bottle-fed infant. Aganglionic megacolon may be manifest initially as diarrhea. Once a baby in a nursery for newborns is identified as having diarrhea, he or she should be isolated in a separate nursery and cared for by personnel who do not have contact with the remaining infants. The latter and those discharged from the exposed nursery must be watched closely for untoward signs. New infants should not be admitted to the nursery from the time of recognition of the second case until it has been cleared of its current population. It should then be thoroughly scrubbed and aired before admissions are resumed.

PROGNOSIS. The fatality rate in epidemics of recent years has been about 40 per cent. With presently available treatment it should be lower; in a few epidemics all affected infants have survived. The subsequent course of surviving infants is, in general, uneventful, although chronic intestinal disturbances are an uncommon sequel.

TREATMENT. Except for those epidemics due to bacteria against which effective specific antibacterial agents are available, treatment is symptomatic and supportive. It does not differ from that of diarrheal disturbances in later infancy (Sections 5 and 11). Neomycin has been effective in breaking nursery epidemics due to most of the enteropathogenic types of *E. coli.* For this purpose 50 to 100 mg of neomycin per kg per day may be administered orally in divided doses to all infants in the nursery up to the time of discharge of the last infant present at the time the medication is started. In the unusual event that the causative strain of *E. coli* is resistant to neomycin, oral polymyxin B or colistin sulfate may be substituted. Mild salmonella gastroenteritis does not require antibiotic treatment, but severe infections may require ampicillin or chloramphenicol. Nursery personnel should be cultured, since they may be asymptomatic carriers of enteropathogenic strains of *E. coli.* Any carriers discovered should be relieved of duty and treated with neomycin until the organism has been eradicated from their intestinal tracts.

INFECTION DUE TO LISTERIA MONOCYTOGENES

Of the human infections caused by *Listeria monocytogenes,* purulent meningitis is the most commonly recognized (Section 10) and has constituted as high as 10 per cent of some reported series of cases of neonatal meningitis. A generalized *miliary granulomatosis* in stillborn fetuses and newborn infants also occurs. In some series of cases of neonatal meningitis the incidence of infection with listeria has been as high as 10 per cent.

The fetus is apparently infected transplacentally and usually dies before birth. In those born alive manifestations may be apparent from the time of birth or may be delayed a week or so. The clinical pattern is not characteristic. There is often brownish discoloration of the amniotic fluid. When the onset is shortly after birth, the principal signs are those of cardiorespiratory distress. Diarrhea and vomiting are common. Poor feeding, lethargy, petechiae, jaundice, and vasomotor instability may also be observed. Mortality is close to 100 per cent when symptoms appear during the first 4 days of life. When the onset is delayed, the course may be gradual, but is progressive and is usually characterized by bronchopneumonia. Meningitis is not uncommon. Granulomas appearing as dark red or livid papules are infrequently present on the oropharynx and the skin.

Pathologically there are microscopic to pinhead-sized nodules in many organs, viz., liver, spleen, adrenals, lungs, pharynx, gastrointestinal tract, brain and meninges and skin. This infiltrate is predominantly neutrophilic.

The diagnosis is established by identification of the organism in the urine or blood of the infant, and suggested by similar identification in the mother. High agglutinative titers may be observed for a short time after the infection.

Most of the available antibiotic agents are effective against *L. monocytogenes*; penicillin is probably the agent of choice.

GROUP B STREPTOCOCCAL INFECTION

Group B beta-hemolytic streptococcus (*Streptococcus agalactiae*) may give rise to severe septicemia with pneumonia, with symptoms of respiratory distress and shock present at birth or within the first day of life. The course is often fulminant, the majority of infants dying within 48 hours of life. The organisms are probably acquired in utero or during delivery from aspiration of infected amniotic fluid or vaginal discharge. Abortion may also be caused by this agent and venereal transmission has been postulated. A second clinical syndrome of insidious meningitis may also occur after the first week and as late as 12 weeks of life. A majority of these infants survive, but there may be neurologic or mental abnormalities. The infection is probably acquired postnatally. Penicillin is the treatment of choice.

VIBRIO FETUS INFECTION

Vibrio fetus, a small, gram-negative motile rod with frequent spiral forms, which grows best in an anaerobic medium, is a leading cause of abortion in sheep and cattle. A number of human infections have been identified in pregnant women, suggesting venereal transmission, as is the case in animals. In man the infection is believed to be acquired largely through contact with infected animal tissue.

The usual clinical picture of infection of the newborn infant with *Vibrio fetus* is one of fulminating meningoencephalitis. The placenta often has a necrotic appearance; abortion and premature delivery are common and suggest transplacental infection of the fetus. "Related vibrios" have been isolated from stools and blood of older infants with a relatively mild diarrheal illness in which the stools contain blood and mucus. The bacterium may be *Vibrio jejuni,* the causative agent of winter dysentery in cattle.

Treatment of infections with *Vibrio fetus* in the newborn has not been satisfactory. Chloramphenicol and streptomycin have been suggested as drugs of choice. Data on the use of ampicillin are not available.

VIRUS INFECTIONS

An acute, fulminating febrile illness may result from infection of newborn infants with **Coxsackievirus group B.** It may be associated with minor respiratory or other infection in the mother shortly before delivery or be contracted after birth. Care should be exercised to prevent exposure of neonatal infants to individuals with known or suspected infection with Coxsackievirus. At autopsy the characteristic finding is diffuse myocarditis; other organs, especially the central nervous system, may be involved (Section 10).

Severe and usually fatal generalized infection of the newborn infant may be caused by the virus of **herpes simplex** (Section 10).

RICHARD E. BEHRMAN

Alden, E. R., Mandelkorn, T., Woodrum, D. E., Wennberg, R. P., Parks, C. R., and Hodson, W. A.: Morbidity and mortality of infants weighing less than 1000 grams in an intensive care nursery. Pediatrics *50*:40, 1972.

Avery, M. E.: *The Lung and Its Disorders in the Newborn Infant.* 2nd ed. Philadelphia, W. B. Saunders Company, 1968.

Auld, P., Hodson, A., and Usher, R.: Hyaline membrane disease: A discussion. J. Pediat. *80*:129, 1972.

Baden, M., Bauer, C. R., Colle, E., Klein, G., Taeusch, H. W., Jr., and Stern, L.: A controlled trial of hydrocortisone therapy in infants with respiratory distress syndrome. Pediatrics *50*:526, 1972.

Baker, D. H., Berdon, W. E., and James, L. S.: Proper localization of umbilical arterial and venous catheters by lateral roentgenograms. Pediatrics *43*:34, 1969.

Balagtas, R. C., Bell, C. E., Edwards, L. D., and Levin, S.: Risk of local and systemic infections associated with umbilical vein catheterization: A prospective study of 86 newborn patients. Pediatrics *48*:359, 1971.

Beard, A., Cornblath, M., Gentz, J., Kellum, M., Person, B., Zetterstrom, R., and Haworth, I. C. Neonatal hypoglycemia: A discussion. J. Pediatr. *79*:314, 1971.

Behrman, R. E.: The use of acid-base measurements in the clinical evaluation and treatment of the sick neonate. J. Pediatr. *74*:632, 1969.

Behrman, R. E. (ed.): The Newborn. Pediat. Clin. N. Amer. *17* (No. 4). Nov., 1970.

Behrman, R. E. (ed.): Neonatology. St. Louis, The C. V. Mosby Company, 1973.

Behrman, R. E., Babson, S. G., and Lessel, R.: Fetal and neonatal mortality in white middle class infants. Am. J. Dis. Child. *121*:486, 1971.

Behrman, R. E., Fisher, D., Paton, J. B., and Keller, J.: In utero disease and the newborn infant. *In* I. Schulman (ed.): Advances in Pediatrics; Vol. XVII, p. 13. Chicago, Year Book Medical Publishers, Inc., 1970.

Behrman, R. E., James, L. S., Klaus, M. H., Nelson, N., and Oliver, T. K.: Treatment of the asphyxiated newborn infant. J. Pediatr. *79*:981, 1969.

Bergsma, D., and Hsia, D. Y-Y: Bilirubin metabolism in the newborn. *In* Birth Defects: Original Article Series. Vol. 6. Baltimore, The Williams & Wilkins Co., 1970.

Bernstein, J., Braylon, R., and Brough, A.: Bile plug syndrome. Pediatrics *43*:273, 1969.

Capitanio, M. A., and Kirkpatrick, J. A.: Roentgen examination in the evaluation of the newborn infant with respiratory distress. J. Pediatr. *75*:896, 1969.

Drage, J. S., Kennedy, C., Berendes, H., Schwarz, B. K., and Weiss, W.: The Apgar Score as an index of infant morbidity. A report from the collaborative study of cerebral palsy. Develop. Med. Child Neurol., *8*:141, 1966.

Driscoll, J. M., Heird, W. C., Schullinger, J. N., Gongaware, R. D., and Winters, R. W.: Total intravenous alimentation in low birth weight infants: A preliminary report. J. Pediatr. *81*:145, 1972.

Edelman, C. M., Ogwo, J. E., Fine, B. P., and Martinez, A. B.: The prevalence of bacteruria in full term and premature newborn infants. J. Pediatr. *82*:125, 1973.

Eisenach, K. D., Reber, R. M., Eitzman, D. V. and Baer, H.: Nosocomial infections due to kanamycin-resistant [R]-factor carrying enteric organisms in an intensive care nursery. Pediatrics *50*:395, 1972.

Esterly, N. B., and Solomon, L. M.: Neonatal dermatology. II. Blistering and scaling dermatosis. J. Pediatr. *77*:1075, 1970.

Esterly, N. B., and Solomon, L. M.: Neonatal dermatology. III. Pigmentary lesions and hemangiomas. J. Pediatr. *81*:1003, 1972.

Fanaroff, A. A., Cha, C. C., Sosa, R., Crumrine, R. S., and Klaus, M. H.: Controlled trial of continuous negative external pressure in the treatment of severe respiratory distress syndrome. J. Pediatr. *82*:921, 1973.

Fitzhardinge, P. M., and Steven, E. M.: The small-for-date infant. II. Neurological and intellectual sequelae. Pediatrics *50*:50, 1972.

Freeman, J.: Neonatal seizures—Diagnosis and management. J. Pediatr. *77*:701, 1970.

Gandy, G. N., Adamsons, K., Cunningham, N., Silverman, W. A., and James, L. S.: Thermal environment and acid-base homeostasis in human infants during the first few hours of life. J. Clin. Invest. *43*:751, 1964.

Gluck, L., Kulovich, M. U., Borer, R. C., Jr., Brenner, P. H., Anderson, G. G., and Spellacy, W. N.: Diagnosis of the respiratory distress syndrome by amniocentesis. Am. J. Obstet. Gynec. *109*:440, 1971.

Gotoff, S. P., and Behrman, R. E.: Neonatal septicemia. J. Pediatr. *76*:142, 1970.

Graham, C. G., Barness, L. A., and Gyorgy, P.: Serum calcium and inorganic phosphate in the newborn infant, and their relation to different feedings. J. Pediatr. *42*:401, 1953.

Harche, H. T., Jr., Naeye, R. L., Storch, A., and Blanc, W. A.: Perinatal cerebral intraventricular hemorrhage. J. Pediatr. *80*:37, 1972.

Harrison, V. C., Heese, H. de V., and Klein, M.: The significance of grunting in hyaline membrane disease. Pediatrics *41*:549, 1968.

Hobel, C. J., Oh, W., Hyvarinen, M. A., and Emmanouilides, G. C.: Early versus late treatment of neonatal acidosis in low-birth-weight infants: Relating to respiratory distress syndrome. J. Pediatr. *81*:1178, 1972.

Hon, E. H. G.: Direct monitoring of the fetal heart. Hosp. Pract. *5*:91, 1970.

Huang, P. W., Rozdulsky, B., Garrard, J. W., Geluboff, N., and Golman, G. H.: Crigler-Najjar syndrome in 4 of 5 siblings with postmortem findings in one. Arch. Path. *90*:536, 1970.

Keenan, W. J., Jowett, T., and Glueck, H. I.: Role of feeding and vitamin K in hypoprothrombinemia of the newborn. Am. J. Dis. Child. *121*:271, 1971.

Klaus, M. H., and Kennell, J.: Mothers separated from their newborn infants. Pediat. Clin. N. Amer. *17*:1017, 1970.

Kubli, F. W., Hon, E. H., Khazin, A. F., and Takemura, H.: Observations on heart rate and pH in the human fetus during labor. Am. J. Obstet. Gynec. *104*:1190,1969.

Laya, E. M., Driscoll, S. G., and Munro, H. N.: Comparison of placentas from two socioeconomic groups. Pediatrics *50*:24, 1972.

Lees, M. H.: Cyanosis of the newborn infant. J. Pediatr. *77*:484, 1970.

Levine, S. Z., and Gordon, H. H.: Physiologic handicaps of the premature infant. I. Their pathogenesis. II. Clinical applications. Am. J. Dis. Child. *64*:274, 1942.

Liggins, G. C., and Howie, R. N.: A controlled trial of antepartum glucocorticoid treatment for prevention of the respiratory distress syndrome in premature infants. Pediatrics *50*:515, 1972.

Lockhart, J. D.: How toxic is hexachlorophene? Pediatrics *50*:229, 1972.

Lubchenco, L. O.: Assessment of gestational age and development at birth. Pediat. Clin. N. Amer. *17*:125, 1970.

Lubchenco, L. O., Searls, D. T., and Brazie, J. V.: Neonatal mortality rate: Relationship to birth weight and gestational age. J. Pediatr. *81*:814, 1972.

Lucey, J. F.: Current indications and results of fetal transfusions. Pediatrics *41*:139, 1968.

Maurer, H. M., Shumway, C. N., Draper, D. A., and Hossaini, A. A.: Controlled trial comparing agar, intermittent phototherapy and continuous phototherapy for reducing neonatal hyperbilirubinemia. J. Pediatr. *82*:73, 1973.

McCracken, G. H., Jr.: Group B streptococci: The new challenge in neonatal infections. J. Pediatr. *82*:703, 1973.

Melish, M. E., and Glasgow, L. A.: The staphylococcal scalded-skin syndrome: The expanded clinical syndrome. J. Pediatr. *78*:958, 1971.

Moffett, H. L., Allan, D., and Williams, T.: Survival and dissemination of bacteria in nebulizers and incubators. Am. J. Dis. Child. *114*:13, 1967.

Nadler, H. L.: In utero detection of familial metabolic disorders. Pediatrics *49*:329, 1972.

Naeye, R. L., Dellinger, W. S., and Blanc, W. A.: Fetal and maternal features of antenatal bacterial infections. J. Pediatr. *79*: 733, 1971.

Northway, W. H., Jr., Rosan, R. C., and Porter, D. Y.: Pulmonary disease following respirator therapy of hyaline-membrane disease. Bronchopulmonary dysplasia. New Engl. J. Med. *276*:357, 1967.

Oliver, T. K., Jr., Demis, J. A., and Bates, G. D.: Serial blood-gas tensions and acid-base balance during the first hour of life in human infants. Acta Paediatr. *50*:346, 1961.

Oski, F. A., and Naiman, J. L.: Hematologic Problems in the Newborn. 2nd ed. Philadelphia, W. B. Saunders Company, 1972.

Overall, J. C., Jr., and Glasgow, L. A.: Virus infections of the fetus and newborn infant. J. Pediatr. *77*:315, 1970.

Poland, R. L., and Odell, G. B.: Physiologic jaundice: The enterohepatic circulation of bilirubin. New Engl. J. Med. *284*:1, 1971.

Raivio, K. O., and Osterlund, K.: Hypoglycemia and hyperinsulinemia associated with erythroblastosis fetalis. Pediatrics *43*:217, 1969.

Rajegowda, B. K., Glass, L., Evans, H. E., Maso, G., Swartz, D. P., and Leblanc, W.: Methadone withdrawal in newborn infants. J. Pediatr. *81*:532, 1972.

Rausen, A. R., Seki, M., and Strauss, L.: Twin transfusion syndrome. A review of 19 cases studied at our institution. J. Pediatr. *66*:613, 1965.

Ray, C. G., and Wedgewood, R. J.: Neonatal listeriosis. Pediatrics *34*:378, 1964.

Robinson, R. C. V.: Congenital syphilis. Arch Derm. *99*:599, 1969.

Schmid, R.: Bilirubin metabolism in man. New Engl. J. Med. *287*:703, 1972.

Sinclair, J. C., Driscoll, J. M., Jr., Heird, W. C, and Winters, R. W.: Supportive management of the sick neonate: Parenteral calories, water and electrolytes. Pediat. Clin. N. Amer. *17*:863, 1970.

Solomon, L. M., and Esterly, N. B.: Neonatal dermatology. I. The newborn skin. J. Pediatr. *77*:888, 1970.
Standards and Recommendations for Hospital Care for Newborn Infants, Full-Term and Premature. Evanston, Ill., American Academy of Pediatrics, Committee on Fetus and Newborn, 1971.
Swyer, P. R.: The regional organization of special care for the neonate. Pediat. Clin. N. Amer. *17*:761, 1970.
Tabb, P. A., Savage, D. C. L., Inglis, J., and Walker, C. H. M.: Controlled trial of phototherapy of limited duration in the treatment of physiological hyperbilirubinemia in low-birth-weight infants. Lancet *2*:1211, 1972.
Talbert, J. L., Felman, A. H., and DeBusk, F. L.: Gastrointestinal surgical emergencies in the newborn infant. J. Pediatr. *76*:783, 1970.
Takeuchi, A., and Benirschke, K.: Renal venous thrombosis of the newborn and its relation to maternal diabetes. Report of 16 cases. Biol. Neonat. *3*:237, 1961.
Thaler, M. M.: Perinatal bilirubin metabolism. Vol. XIX, p. 215. In Schulman I. (ed.): Advances in Pediatrics. Chicago, Year Book Medical Publishers, Inc., 1972.
Weiner, A. S.: Diagnosis and treatment of anemia of the newborn caused by occult placental hemorrhage. Am. J. Obstet. Gynec. *56*:717, 1948.
Wennberg, R. P., Schwartz, R., and Sweet, A. Y.: Early versus delayed feeding of low birth weight infants; Effects on physiologic jaundice. J. Pediatr. *68*:860, 1966.
Wilson, M. G., and Mikity, V. G.: A new form of respiratory disease in premature infants. Am. J. Dis. Child. *99*:489, 1960.
Wood, J. L.: Plethora in the newborn infant associated with cyanosis and convulsions. J. Pediatr. *54*:143, 1959.

8

INBORN ERRORS OF METABOLISM

Many disorders have their origin in mutational events which alter the genetic constitution of an individual and disrupt normal function. The number of human hereditary biochemical disorders, named "inborn errors of metabolism" by Garrod at the turn of the century, has grown from the four originally described by him into hundreds. New ones, and variations of old ones, are being discovered at an ever-increasing rate.

Modern biochemical genetics has provided a conceptual scheme to describe how genetic information is translated into the synthesis of proteins with specific metabolic or structural properties. Within the nucleus of each cell, genetic information resides in the chromosomes, encoded in deoxyribonucleic acid (DNA) molecules. The code is made up of combinations of 2 purine and 2 pyrimidine bases arranged on the DNA helix. The genetic information contained in DNA is transcribed to messenger ribonucleic acid (m-RNA), which is free to leave the nucleus. Proteins are synthesized from individual amino acids in the cytoplasm, where the information carried by the m-RNA is translated into the linear array of amino acids comprising the polypeptide chain.

A mutation may alter the structure of a protein by introducing an error into the sequence of amino acids through substitution of one amino acid for another. If the integrity of the region of substitution is necessary for function, then, depending on the nature of the alteration, part or all of the normal function of this protein may be lost. Alternatively, an amino acid substitution may render the protein very labile, and it may be destroyed as rapidly as it is synthesized. Another mutation might affect another set of genes which control the rate of synthesis of a normally structured protein. Such a mutation can result either in lowered rate of synthesis of an enzyme or in its complete lack. In drug-induced hemolytic anemia, for example, a structurally altered form of erythrocyte glucose-6-phosphate dehydrogenase is synthesized, which cannot carry out its normal function, whereas, in analbuminemia, plasma albumin is either not synthesized at all or is made in an altered and unstable form.

Much of what is known of human biochemical genetics has been garnered from studies of the hemoglobin molecule and the genetic factors which determine its chemical and physical properties. Information so obtained has been applied to the study of many other proteins and of the disease processes caused by their malfunction. Hemoglobin serves as a model substance because, unlike most enzymes, it is freely obtainable and can be separated from other protein contaminants with ease. Certain changes in structure are revealed by alteration of electrophoretic mobility, and other analytic techniques can reveal the exact amino acid sequence of the polypeptide chain.

The predominant normal hemoglobin is hemoglobin A, which consists of 2 pairs of polypeptide chains (alpha and beta). Alpha and beta chains, as well as the less common delta and gamma chains (Section 14), differ only slightly in the composition or sequential arrangement of their component aminoacids. The composition of each polypeptide chain is under genetic control, and the sequential arrangement of the amino acids corresponds to the order of bases on the deoxyribonucleic acid molecule.

Studies of many varieties of hemoglobin, some of which are discussed elsewhere (Section 14), indicate that approximately half of the alpha chains and half of the beta chains are synthesized under the control of a gene obtained from the father, and the other half by a gene obtained from the mother. If a gene for an abnormal hemoglobin is obtained from only one parent, then only half of the hemoglobin molecules will be affected (heterozygous). For all the hemoglobin to be affected (homozygous), the same gene must be obtained from each parent.

More than one defect can occur within the same polypeptide chain; there can be at least as many defects as there are positions for amino acids in the molecule. Within the same chain, different defects may occur at the same amino acid locus; in the beta chain of hemoglobin at a point which is normally occupied by glutamic acid, one mutation results in its replacement by valine (hemoglobin S), and another mutation results in replacement by lysine (hemoglobin C). Accordingly, if parents carry different abnormal genes at the same locus, e.g., one parent hemoglobin S, the other hemoglobin C, then all the hemoglobin in the offspring inheriting each parent's abnormal gene will be abnormal. Approximately half of this child's hemoglobin will be hemoglobin S, and the other half, hemoglobin C (hemoglobin SC disease).

A genetic defect in hemoglobin structure may or may not have clinical significance, depending on how it affects the function of the hemoglobin molecule. As indicated, each mutation of a gene manifests itself as a chemically unique structure.

Among persons with sickle cell hemoglobin (hemoglobin S), the heterozygote (hemoglobin A plus hemoglobin S) is identified clinically as having the sickle cell trait, but may have little or no clinical disorder, whereas the homozygote (all hemoglobin S) has sickle cell disease and is seriously affected. In certain types of methemoglobinemia, on the other hand, the heterozygote (hemoglobin A plus hemoglobin M) has a significant clinical disorder. At the other extreme of the spectrum of hemoglobinopathies, alterations in hemoglobin structure are not reflected in functional disorders. For example, the homozygote for hemoglobin G is clinically normal.

Although the terms "recessive" and "dominant," as well as "incompletely recessive," "incompletely dominant," "penetrance" and "expressivity," describe the patterns of inheritance (Section 6), it should be understood that alteration of a structural gene always leads to abnormal protein formation, even in the heterozygote without evidence of clinical disorder.

The mutations just described predominantly affect the amino acid composition of protein; other mutations alter the rate at which protein will be synthesized. Mutations of the second type may be responsible for the thalassemias (Section 14). In these anemias there may be decreased synthesis of either alpha or beta chains of hemoglobin A. In the latter instance, synthesis of fetal hemoglobin (2 alpha plus 2 gamma chains) and hemoglobin A_2 (2 alpha plus 2 delta chains) may continue; when synthesis of the alpha chain is not possible, hemoglobin molecules with only beta chains (4 beta, hemoglobin H) or only gamma chains (4 gamma, Bart's hemoglobin) may appear.

Although hemoglobin has been used as a model for the discussion of genic action, the principles apply to all proteins, including enzymes. In evaluating enzyme function, the biochemist usually measures only the activity of the enzyme. For many enzymatic defects it is not known whether the enzyme is altered in such a way as to have no activity, or is not synthesized in normal quantities.

Other generalizations are germane to a discussion of hereditary defects. It should be appreciated that the absence of activity of a specific enzyme may have one or more of several effects.

1. The end-product is not made. If this is a substance essential to life, the result is lethal.
2. Precursor substances may accumulate. If they are toxic, specific dysfunction results.
3. Minor metabolic pathways may become manifest or more heavily utilized, and normal metabolites may accumulate or be excreted in unusual quantities.

Some enzyme functions may not be fully developed at birth, but mature later, e.g., glucuronide transferase (Section 11). These delays are not to be confused with true enzymopathies in which function will never develop, e.g., Crigler-Najjar disease (Section 11).

The tools of modern biochemistry have revealed that some disorders, such as the abnormal accumulation of glycogen in glycogen storage disease, once thought to be due to the absence of a single enzyme (glucose-6-phosphatase), are in fact a number of different entities, each associated with dysfunction of a different enzyme. All the involved enzymes, however, have roles in glycogen and glucose metabolism.

Even in those disorders in which only one enzyme is involved there is evidence that different mutations result in different degrees of enzyme activity which, in turn, result in a spectrum of phenotypic effects. The possibility exists that for a given enzyme protein at least as many different abnormalities may exist as there are amino acids in the protein chain. The potential number may be large, but only mutations which affect enzyme activity sufficiently to produce clinical disease need be of concern.

Inborn errors of metabolism may have their important clinical effects in almost any body system and be manifest in most aspects of pediatric medicine. A listing of the various inborn errors of metabolism appears in Table 8–1. Discussions of the following defects will be found in other sections of this book where the clinical considerations are germane to the system being discussed: the hemoglobinopathies (Section 14), disorders of clotting mechanisms (Section 14), the lipidoses and disorders of pigment metabolism (this Section), the mucopolysaccharidoses (Section 12), defects of cellular transport (Section 15), defects of hormone synthesis (Section 17), and defects of immunoglobulin synthesis (Section 9). In general, the disorders listed in Table 8–1 and *not* printed in italics will be discussed in this section; these are mainly the disorders associated with defects of metabolism of amino acids, carbohydrates, purines and pyrimidine, and other disorders not easily categorized. Attention is given only to those which have clinical significance.

(Text continued on page 412)

TABLE 8–1 INBORN ERRORS OF METABOLISM*

I. DEFECTS OF AMINO ACID METABOLISM
- A. *Phenylalanine*
  1. Phenylketonuria (PKU)
  2. Phenylalaninemia
  3. Methylmandelic aciduria
  4. Para-hydroxyphenylacetic aciduria
- B. *Tyrosine*
  1. p-Hydroxyphenylpyruvic acid oxidase
     - a. Delayed maturation
     - b. Tyrosinosis (Medes)
     - c. Tyrosinosis (Sakai)
  2. Tyrosine transaminase
     - a. Tyrosinemia
  3. Richner-Hanhart syndrome
  4. Albinism
     - a. Generalized
       1. Tyrosinase negative
       2. Tyrosinase positive
       3. Amish type
     - b. Partial (dominant)
     - c. Ocular (X-linked)
     - d. Waardenburg syndrome (dominant)
     - e. Chediak-Higashi syndrome
     - f. Hermansky-Pudlak syndrome
  5. Alcaptonuria
  6. Parkinsonism
  7. Goitrous cretinism
- C. *Methionine*
  1. Methioninemia
  2. Methionine malabsorption
     - a. Oasthouse disease
  3. Homocystinemia
     - a. Vitamin B_6 responsive
     - b. Vitamin B_6 unresponsive
     - c. Methyltransferase defect
     - d. $^{5\text{-}10}$N-methylene-tetrahydrofolate reductase defect
  4. Cystathioninemia
     - a. Vitamin B_6 responsive
     - b. Vitamin B_6 unresponsive
     - c. Latent cystathioninuria
- D. *Cysteine*
  1. Cystinurias
  2. Cystinosis*
  3. Sulfite oxidase deficiency
  4. β-Mercaptolactate-cysteine disulfiduria
  5. Taurinuria
- E. *Tryptophan*
  1. Hartnup disease
  2. Tryptophanemia
  3. Kynureninuria
  4. Kynureninase defects
     - a. Hydroxykynureninuria
     - b. Pyridoxine dependency (xanthurenic aciduria)
  5. Indicanuria
  6. Hydrindicuria
  7. Indolylacrolylglycinuria
  8. Glutaric acidemia
- F. *Valine, leucine, isoleucine*
  1. Maple syrup urine disease
     - a. Classic form*
     - b. Intermittent form
     - c. Mild variant
     - d. Thiamine-responsive form
  2. Valinemia
  3. Isoleucine-leucinemia
  4. Isovaleric acidemia
  5. β-Methylcrotonyl-CoA carboxylase deficiency
     - a. Vitamin B_{12} responsive
     - b. Vitamin B_{12} unresponsive
  6. Acetoacetyl-CoA thiolase deficiency
  7. Propionic acidemia
     - a. Biotin responsive
     - b. Biotin unresponsive
  8. Methylmalonic acidemia*
     - a. Methylmalonyl-CoA carbonylmutase deficiency
       1. Vitamin B_{12} responsive
       2. Vitamin B_{12} unresponsive
     - b. Defect of B_{12} cofactor formation
     - c. Methylmalonyl-CoA racemase deficiency
- G. *Glycine*
  1. Nonketotic glycinemia
  2. Sarcosinemia
  3. Trimethylaminuria
  4. Glycinuria
  5. Glucoglycinuria
  6. Primary oxaluria and oxalosis
     - a. L-Glyceric aciduria
     - b. Glycolic aciduria
- H. *Proline and hydroxyproline*
  1. Prolinuria
  2. Prolinemia
     - a. Proline oxidase deficiency
     - b. Pyrroline 5-carboxylic acid dehydrogenase deficiency
  3. Hydroxyprolinemia
  4. Glycylprolinuria
- I. *Glutamic acid*
  1. γ-Glutamyl transpeptidase deficiency
  2. γ-Glutamyl cysteine synthetase deficiency
  3. Pyroglutamic aciduria
- J. *Urea cycle*
  1. Carbamyl phosphate synthetase deficiency
  2. Ornithine transcarbamylase deficiency (X-linked)
  3. Citrullinemia
  4. Argininosuccinase deficiency
  5. Arginase deficiency (argininemia)
  6. Ornithinemia
- K. *Histidine*
  1. Histidinemia
  2. Histidine and folic acid metabolism
     - a. Formiminotransferase defect
     - b. Cyclohydrolase defect
     - c. Methyltransferase defect
  3. Histidinuria
  4. Imidazole aciduria
  5. Carnosinemia
- L. *Beta amino acids*
  1. β-Alaninemia
  2. β-Aminoisobutyric aciduria
- M. *Lysine and hydroxylysine*
  1. Lysinemia
  2. Saccharopinemia
  3. Gluturic acidemia
  4. Lysine intolerance
  5. Lysinuria (hyperdibasicaminoaciduria)

*Unless otherwise indicated, an autosomal recessive form of inheritance is assumed. Many of the disorders listed are discussed in this Section and also may be discussed elsewhere in the text. Discussions of those disorders set in italics may be found by consulting the index. Disorders followed by an asterisk (*) are those which have been detected prenatally by culture of aspirated amniotic fluid cells.

(Table 8–1 continued on following page.)

TABLE 8–1 INBORN ERRORS OF METABOLISM* *(Continued)*

- 6. Familial protein intolerance
- 7. Hydroxylysinemia
- 8. Hydroxylysine deficient collagen
  - a. Lysyl-protocollagen hydroxylase defect
  - b. Procollagen peptidase defect

II. DEFECTS OF CARBOHYDRATE METABOLISM

A. Defects in absorption
1. Lactose
   - a. Lactosuria (lactose intolerance)
   - b. Malabsorption of lactose (alactasia)
   - c. Malabsorption of glucose and galactose
2. Malabsorption of sucrose and isomaltose
3. *Renal glycosuria* (Sections 15 and 22)

B. Defects in monosaccharide metabolism
1. *Diabetes mellitus* (Section 16)
2. Scurvy
3. Essential benign pentosuria (L-xylosuria)
4. Essential benign fructosuria
5. Fructosemia (fructose intolerance)
6. Fructose-galactose intolerance
7. Fructose-1,6-diphosphatase deficiency
8. Galactosemia
   - a. Uridyltransferase defects*
   - b. Galactokinase defect
   - c. Epimerase defect

C. Miscellaneous aspects of carbohydrate metabolism
1. Blood group substances
   - a. N-acetylgalactosamine transferase (absent in non-A group)
   - b. Galactose transferase (absent in non-B group)
   - c. Fucose transferase (absent in nonsecretors)
2. Fucosidosis
3. Mannosidosis
4. β-Xylosidase deficiency
5. Aspartylglycosaminuria
6. Sialic acidemia
7. Glycoprotein storage disease
8. Leigh's encephalomyelopathy
   - a. Pyruvate carboxylase deficiency
   - b. Pyruvate carboxylase mutation
9. Lactic acidosis
10. Pyruvate decarboxylase deficiency

D. The mucopolysaccharidoses (Section 22)
1. Hurler syndrome (α-L-iduronidase defect)*
2. Scheie syndrome (α-L-iduronidase defect)*
3. Hurler-Scheie syndrome (α-L-iduronidase defect)*
4. Hunter syndrome (X-linked)
5. Sanfilippo syndromes
   - a. Heparan sulfate sulfatase defect
   - b. N-acetyl-α-D-glucosamidase defect
6. Morquio syndrome
7. Maroteaux-Lamy syndrome
8. β-Glucuronidase defect

E. The glycogenoses
1. Involving principally liver
   - a. Type I (von Gierke, glucose-6-phosphatase)
   - b. Type III (Forbes, Cori, amylo-1,6-glucosidase and/or amylo-1,4→1,4-transglucosidase)
   - c. Type IV (Andersen, amylo-1,4→1,6-transglucosidase)
   - d. Type VI (Hers, phosphorylase)
   - e. Type IXa (Hug, phosphorylase kinase)
   - f. Type IXb (Huijing, phosphorylase kinase, X-linked)
   - g. Type VIII (Hug)
   - h. Type X (Hug, phosphorylase kinase kinase)
   - i. Type O (Lewis, glycogen synthetase)
   - j. Edstrom (low molecular weight glycogen)
2. Involving principally heart
   - a. Type IIa (Pompe, acid and neutral maltase)*
3. Involving principally muscle
   - a. Type V (McArdle, myophosphorylase)
   - b. Type VII (Tarui, phosphofructokinase)
   - c. Thomson (phosphoglucomutase)
   - d. Satoyoshi (phosphohexose isomerase)
   - e. Rosenberg (intramitochondrial glycogen storage, autosomal dominant)
   - f. Type IIb (Pompe, acid maltase and in some instances neutral maltase)
   - g. Type III (Forbes, Cori, amylo-1,6-glucosidase)

III. DEFECTS OF PYRIMIDINE AND PURINE METABOLISM
1. Orotic aciduria
   - a. Orotidylate phosphoribosyl transferase and orotidylate decarboxylase
   - b. Orotidylate decarboxylase only
2. Xanthinuria (xanthine oxidase)
3. Hyperuricemia (gout)
   - a. Hypoxanthine-guanine phosphoribosyltransferase (X-linked)
   - b. Increased phosphoribosylpyrophosphate synthetase activity (X-linked)
   - c. Increased adenine phosphoribosyl-transferase activity
   - d. Increased glutathione reductase activity
   - e. In Type I glycogenosis
4. Lesch-Nyhan disease (hypoxanthine-guanine phosphoribosyl transferase)*
   - a. X-linked form (absent enzyme activity)
   - b. Possible autosomal form
   - c. Altered enzyme kinetics
5. Adenosine-deaminase deficiency (combined immunodeficiency syndrome)
6. Miscellaneous
   - a. Pseudouridinuria
   - b. Renal tubular glutaminase defect
   - c. Hypouricemia
   - d. Possible adenine phosphoribosyl-transferase defect

IV. OTHER DEFECTS OF ENZYMES AND PROTEINS

A. Defects in plasma proteins
1. *Factors associated with clotting of blood* (Section 14)
2. *Immunoproteins* (Section 9)
3. Other plasma proteins
   - a. Analbuminemia
   - b. Haptoglobin deficiency
   - c. Abeta-lipoproteinemia
   - d. Analpha-lipoproteinemia
   - e. Absence of transferrin
   - f. C′-1 esterase inhibitor deficiency
   - g. Alpha-antitrypsin protein deficiency
   - h. Transcobalamine II deficiency

B. Defects in plasma enzymes
1. Pseudocholinesterase
2. Lecithin-cholesterol acyltransferase deficiency
3. Carnosinase deficiency
4. Gamma-glutanyl transpeptidase deficiency
5. Hypophosphatasia

C. Defects of proteins of other tissues

TABLE 8–1 INBORN ERRORS OF METABOLISM* *(Continued)*

1. Ceruloplasmin deficiency (Wilson's disease, copperthionein defect)
2. Menkes kinky hair syndrome (X-linked)
3. Myoglobin
   a. Variants
   b. Duchenne muscular dystrophy (X-linked)
4. Xeroderma pigmentosum
5. Pancreatic enzyme deficiencies
   a. Lipase deficiency
   b. Trypsinogen deficiency
   c. Amylase deficiency
6. Intestinal enterokinase deficiency
7. Lysosomal acid phosphatase deficiency*
8. Procollagen peptidase deficiency
9. Carnitine deficiency
10. Succinyl-CoA,3-keto and CoA transferase deficiency

V. DEFECTS IN ERYTHROCYTE METABOLISM (SECTION 14)

A. *Hereditary methemoglobinemia*
1. Methemoglobin reductase
2. Hemoglobin M diseases

B. *Drug-induced hemolytic anemia*
1. Glucose-6-phosphate dehydrogenase

C. *Hereditary hemolytic anemias*
1. Glucose-6-phosphate dehydrogenase (X-linked)
2. 6-Phosphogluconate dehydrogenase
3. Hexokinase
4. Glucose phosphate isomerase
5. Aldolase
6. Triosephosphate isomerase
7. Phosphoglyceric acid kinase
8. 2,3-Diphosphoglyceric acid mutase
9. Phosphofructose kinase
10. Phosphoglycerate enolase
11. Pyruvate kinase
12. Lactate dehydrogenase
13. PRPP synthetase
14. Glutathione reductase
15. Glutathione peroxidase
16. Glutathione synthetase
17. Adenylate kinase
18. Adenosine triphosphatase

D. *Other erythrocyte enzymes*
1. Catalase (acatalasia)
2. True cholinesterase
3. Elevated ATP production
4. Carbonic anhydrase deficiency
5. Nicotinamide adenine dinucleotide nucleosidase deficiency
6. Glutathione reductase (increased activity—gout)

VI. DEFECTS IN OTHER FORMED ELEMENTS OF BLOOD (SECTION 14)

A. *Platelet defects (several thrombocytopathies and thrombocytasthenias involving metabolic or membrane defects)*

B. *Granulocyte defects (defective oxidation following phagocytosis) (chronic granulomatous disease)*

VII. DEFECTS OF LIPID METABOLISM

A. *The hyperlipoproteinemias*

B. *Lecithin-cholesterol acyltransferase deficiency*

C. *The hypolipoproteinemias*
1. Abeta-lipoproteinemia (acanthocytosis)
2. Analpha-lipoproteinemia (Tangier disease)

D. *Steroid metabolism*
1. Congenital adrenal hyperplasia
   a. Defect of desmolase
   b. Defect of 3-beta-hydroxydehydrogenase
   c. Defect of 21-hydroxylase
   d. Defect of 11-hydroxylase
   e. Defect of 17-hydroxylase
2. Selective defects of aldosterone synthesis
   a. Defect of 18-hydroxylase
   b. Defect of 18-OH-corticosterone dehydrogenase

E. *The lipidoses*
1. Gaucher disease (glucocerebrosidase)*
2. Niemann-Pick disease (sphingomyelinase)*
3. Tay-Sachs disease (hexosaminidase A)*
4. Sandhoff disease (hexosaminidases A and B)*
5. Norman disease (B-galactosidase)
6. Metachromatic leukodystrophy (arylsulfatase A)*
7. Krabbe disease (ceramide B-galactosidase)*
8. Wolman disease (acid lipase)
9. Refsum disease (phytanic acid α-hydroxylase)
10. Fabry disease (X-linked, ceramide trihexogidase)*
11. Farber disease
12. I cell disease
13. Fucosidosis
14. Mannosidosis
15. Sea blue histiocyte disease

VIII. DEFECTS OF PIGMENT METABOLISM

A. *Porphyrin metabolism*
1. Congenital erythropoietic porphyria
2. Intermittent acute porphyria
3. Prophyria variegata
4. Erythropoietic protoporphyria
5. Erythropoietic coproporphyria

B. *Methemoglobinemias*
1. Methemoglobin reductase
2. Hemoglobin M disease

C. *Primary hemochromatosis*

D. *Glucuronide conjugation*
1. Crigler-Najjar disease
2. Dubin-Johnson disease
3. Gilbert disease
4. Rotor syndrome

E. *Melanin metabolism*
1. Albinism
2. Chediak-Higashi syndrome
3. Waardenburg syndrome

IX. DEFECTS OF VITAMIN METABOLISM

A. *Ascorbic acid*

B. *Folic acid*
1. Formiminotransferase defect
2. Cyclohydrolase defect
3. N^5-methyltransferase defects

C. *Niacin*
1. Hartnup disease
2. Tryptophanemia
3. 3-Hydroxykynureninuria

D. *Vitamin B_{12}*
1. Methylmalonic acidemia and homocystinemia

E. *Vitamin D*
1. Vitamin D dependent rickets (1-hydroxylase deficiency)

F. *Thiamine*
1. Thiamine pyrophosphate kinase defect (Leigh disease)

X. PRIMARY DEFECTS OF RENAL TUBULAR TRANSPORT

(Table 8–1 continued on following page.)

TABLE 8–1 INBORN ERRORS OF METABOLISM *(Continued)*

MECHANISM (SECTIONS 15 AND 22)
Many different disorders, e.g., nephrogenic diabetes insipidus, renal glycosuria, Fanconi syndrome

XI. GENETIC DEFECTS RESULTING IN INTESTINAL MALABSORPTION (SECTION 11)
- A. *Carbohydrates*
- B. *Amino acids*
- C. *Lipids*
- D. *Proteins*
  1. Cystic fibrosis
  2. Pancreatic enzyme defects
  3. Gluten-induced enteropathy

XII. DEFECTS INVOLVING MINERAL METABOLISM
- A. *Copper*
  1. Wilson disease (this Section and Sections 11 and 20)
  2. Menkes kinky hair disease (X-linked) (Section 20)
- B. *Iron* (this Section and Section 11)
  1. Hemochromatosis
  2. Absence of transferrin
- C. *Potassium* (Section 21)
  1. Periodic paralysis
- D. *Phosphorus* (Section 22)
  1. Hypophosphatemic-resistant rickets (X-linked)
- E. *Iodine* (Section 17)
  1. Defects of iodine transport
  2. Defects of thyroid hormone formation
- F. *Magnesium* (Section 19)
  1. Hypomagnesemic tetany of infancy
- G. *Cobalt*
  1. Transcobalamin II deficiency

XIII. DEFECTS ABOUT WHICH THE BIOCHEMICAL ABERRATION IS UNKNOWN
Many different disorders, e.g., achondroplasia, Marfan syndrome, Ehlers-Danlos disease and osteogenesis imperfecta.

DEFECTS IN METABOLISM OF AMINO ACIDS

Disorders are considered here which are produced by defects in enzymes responsible for steps in the catabolism of amino acids, the so-called aminoacidopathies. Disorders of cellular transport of amino acids by intestinal mucosa or renal tubule are discussed elsewhere (e.g., methionine malabsorption, Hartnup disease, cystinuria). Aminoaciduria secondary to some other genetic defect is also considered elsewhere (e.g., Wilson's disease, galactosemia). Aminoacidopathies are usually characterized by elevated levels in plasma of the involved amino acid, with overflow into the urine of the amino acid or related metabolites.

PHENYLALANINE

PHENYLKETONURIA (PKU). Phenylketonuria (see also Section 2) is a disorder of metabolism resulting from absence of activity of the hepatic enzyme, phenylalanine hydroxylase, which converts phenylalanine to tyrosine. The dietary phenylalanine, which is not required for protein synthesis, is degraded via the tyrosine pathway (see Fig. 8–1). In phenylketonuria, owing to the enzymatic defect in this pathway, phenylalanine accumulates and is transaminated to phenylpyruvic acid, which can then be converted to other metabolites. These metabolites and the excess phenylalanine are excreted in the urine.

In untreated phenylketonuria, blood levels of phenylalanine rise rapidly in the neonatal period and may reach 60 to 80 mg/dl. In most patients these levels of phenylalanine lead to urinary excretion of large amounts of phenylpyruvic acid and its metabolites. The peculiar musty or mouselike odor characteristic of untreated patients has been attributed to the presence of phenylacetic acid. The frequency with which persons with this disorder are fair-skinned, blue-eyed blondes is due in part to inhibition of the enzyme responsible for melanin formation (tyrosinase) by phenylalanine or its metabolites. The mechanism of the mental retardation, the most important consequence of phenylketonuria, is not known. An occasional patient escapes mental retardation for reasons equally obscure. Dietary management of this condition has been more extensive and successful than with any of the other aminoacidopathies and allows for nearly normal mental development in many affected subjects when instituted early in life; on the other hand, long-term follow-up tends to indicate that even well-managed children with PKU may have persistent psychologic and learning difficulties.

Restriction of dietary phenylalanine to maintain blood levels between 5 and 10 mg/dl and augmentation of the diet with tyrosine, which for these patients becomes an essential amino acid, is necessary for at least the first five years of life.

Infants born to mothers with phenylketonuria may be mentally retarded, even though only heterozygous for the defect, owing to damage sustained in utero. Women with PKU require treatment during pregnancy in order to keep their blood levels of phenylalanine within reasonable bounds, taking into account that the amino acid is necessary for fetal growth and development. The incidence of mental retardation in the offspring seems

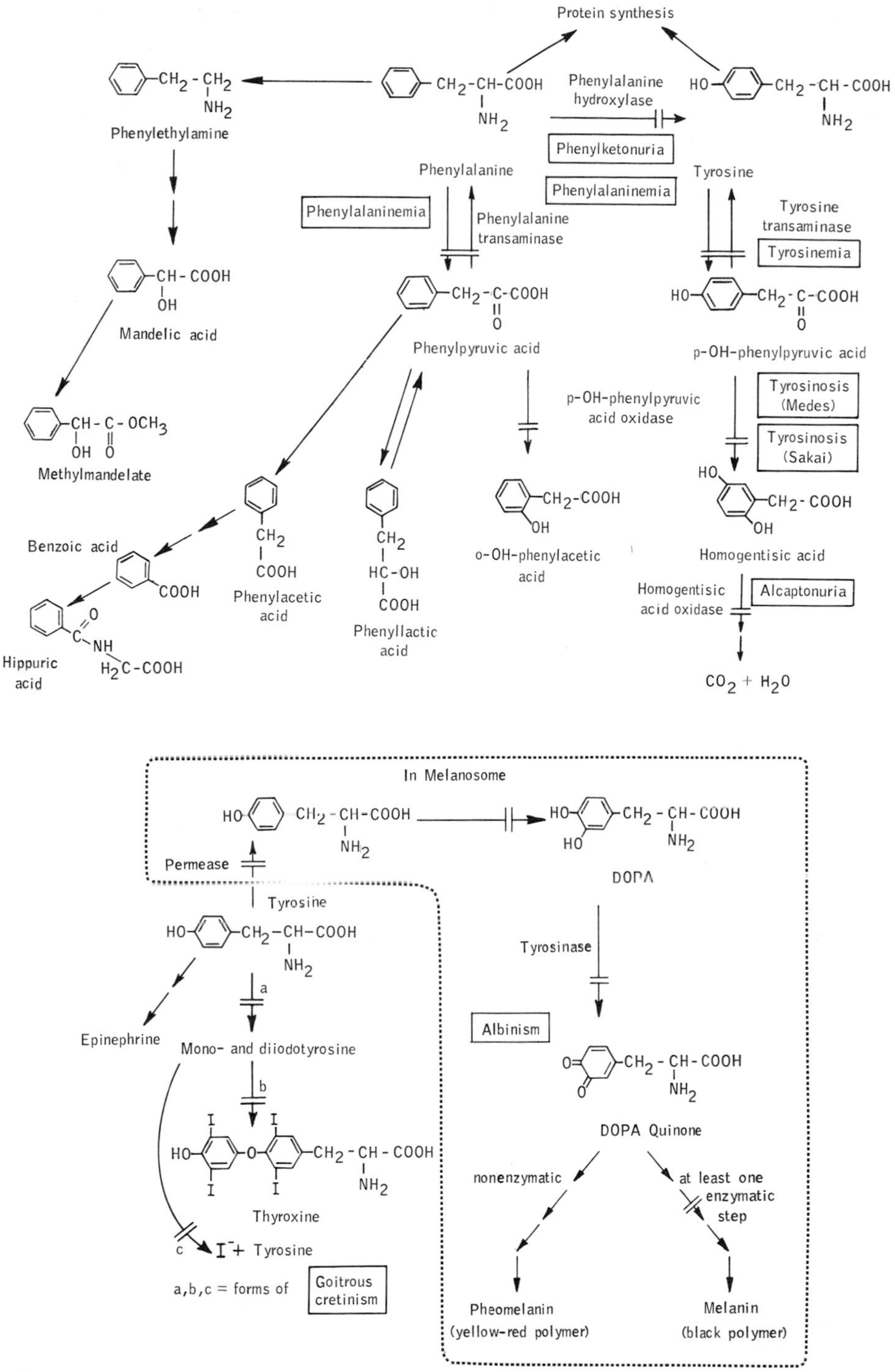

Figure 8–1 *Pathways in the metabolism of phenylalanine and tyrosine. In this and subsequent figures the structural formulas and the names of various metabolites are shown. Inborn errors are depicted as bars crossing the reaction arrow or arrows, and the name of the associated defect or defects is given within the nearest box. In some figures the name of the enzyme is given in association with the reaction arrow. Some of the intermediates shown in some of the figures are metabolized via their coenzyme A (CoA) derivatives. For the sake of simplicity, this is not indicated.*

to be correlated with the degree of elevation of phenylalanine (and of phenylpyruvate excretion) in the mother.

Atypical Phenylketonuria. Whereas classic phenylketonuria is caused by the *absence* of phenylalanine hydroxylase activity in affected persons, atypical phenylketonuria occurs when the genetic mutation produces an altered phenylalanine hydroxylase with substantially *reduced* activity. Although such infants are detected by the Guthrie bacterial inhibition assay, levels of phenylalanine in the blood are not so high as in the usual phenylketonuric child. Phenylpyruvic acid is present in urine. Treatment is the same as for the child with classic phenylketonuria.

OTHER PHENYLALANINEMIAS. Occasionally in affected infants the blood levels of phenylalanine are only slightly elevated and are insufficient (less than 15 to 20 mg/dl) to result in the excretion of phenylpyruvic acid. These infants presumably also have an altered phenylalanine hydroxylase enzyme, but one which has retained much of its activity. Such infants are detected by screening tests in the neonatal period and usually appear to develop normally without special dietary treatment.

Moderately elevated levels of phenylalanine occur secondarily to the transient tyrosinemia in the newborn infant (see below). When the infant's ability to oxidize tyrosine matures, the elevated levels of tyrosine and phenylalanine return to normal.

Absence of or delayed maturation of the enzyme phenylalanine transaminase can also produce phenylalaninemia if the infant is being fed milk with a high protein content. Such infants cannot produce much phenylpyruvic acid even when their blood levels of phenylalanine approach 30 mg/dl; they have normal blood levels when fed milks with the protein content of human milk.

Delayed maturation of phenylalanine hydroxylase activity has been observed on a few occasions. It is recommended that infants on a restricted phenylalanine diet be tested periodically (every 3 months) to examine this possibility. Delayed maturation of phenylalanine transaminase can occur concurrently with classic or atypical phenylketonuria. The absence of phenylpyruvic acid in the urine of such patients presents difficulty in the diagnosis of phenylketonuria. Phenylalanine tolerance tests are rarely of value in the differential diagnosis of the various conditions causing elevated levels of phenylanine.

Methylmandelic Aciduria. Two siblings with ataxia, convulsions and mental retardation have been shown to excrete large amounts of methylmandelic acid. This compound results from the further oxidation of phenylethylamine, the decarboxylated product of phenylalanine. Symptoms could be produced by high protein feeding and abated by the restriction of protein to 0.5 gm/kg/day.

Para-hydroxyphenylacetic Aciduria. In a $3\frac{1}{2}$ month old girl with cardiomegaly, hepatomegaly, hypotonia and anemia, a defect has been postulated in the conversion of phenylacetic acid to benzoic acid, thence to hippuric acid. The patient excreted no appreciable amounts of hippurate but excessive p-hydroxyphenylacetate. Excretion of the latter compound was influenced directly by the injection of phenylalanine but was independent of tyrosine intake. Hippurate could be formed if benzoate was fed. Pathways are indicated in Figure 8–1.

TYROSINE

The hepatic enzyme para-hydroxyphenylpyruvic acid oxidase is necessary for the conversion of parahydroxyphenylpyruvic acid to homogentisic acid (Fig. 8–1). The excretion of tyrosine and parahydroxyphenylpyruvic, -lactic and -acetic acids in patients with deficiency of this enzyme is referred to as *tyrosyluria.* Deficiency of this pivotal enzyme occurs in a variety of clinical conditions. The deficiency is most often transitory, owing to delayed maturation of the enzyme, and occurs commonly in premature infants and occasionally in full-term infants. The levels of tyrosine in the blood (normally less than 2 mg/dl) may be as high as 40 mg/dl.

A secondary increase in the plasma level of phenylalanine is a common occurrence in neonatal tyrosyluria and must be taken into account in the differential diagnosis of causes for phenylalaninemia.

The defect is promptly corrected by the administration of vitamin C. Since vitamin C is necessary for optimal functioning of para-hydroxyphenylpyruvic acid oxidase, it is not surprising that tyrosyluria occurs in scurvy. Deficiency of the enzyme also may occur because of malnutrition or hepatic disease.

TYROSINOSIS (MEDES). In 1932 Medes reported studies of an adult male who had a defect in tyrosine metabolism. No symptoms could be related to the metabolic defect. The presence of parahydroxyphenylpyruvic acid in urine (greater than 1 gm/day) and the excretion of other oxidation products of tyrosine indicated that catabolism of tyrosine was blocked at the level of its keto-acid derivative. Medes proposed that the tyrosyluria was due to virtual absence of activity of parahydroxyphenylpyruvic acid oxidase (Fig. 8–1).

TYROSINOSIS (SAKAI). Another clinical disorder associated with a defect in para-hydroxyphenylpyruvic acid oxidase and occurring in infants and children was first described by Sakai.

Clinical Manifestations. The onset is usually between 1 and 6 months of age. Failure to thrive, irritability, fever and hepatomegaly are the most frequent manifestations. Anorexia, vomiting, diarrhea and abdominal distention are common. Bleeding manifestations such as melena, hematemesis, hematuria and ecchymoses occur early and may be serious. Ascites, jaundice, lethargy, coma and death ensue soon thereafter. Some patients appear to survive the acute hepatic decompensation and undergo chronic hepatic and renal disease. In such children hepatoma may be found at autopsy. The urine has the peculiar odor of methionine.

Laboratory Data. Glycosuria may be present. Generalized aminoaciduria and tyrosyluria are constant findings. Plasma amino acids are elevated, particularly tyrosine and methionine, which may be 5 to 10 times normal levels. Tyrosine crystals have been found in bone marrow. Direct and indirect serum bilirubin levels are increased; those of alkaline phosphatase and total cholesterol are markedly decreased. Hypoproteinemia and hypoprothrombinemia are common; transaminases (SGOT and SGPT) are only slightly increased. Variable degrees of hypoglycemia and rachitic changes are common. Pathologically the principal findings are cirrhosis, and dilation of the renal tubules.

Although para-hydroxyphenylpyruvic acid oxidase activity is absent in this disorder, it is still not clear whether this is the primary defect. Reasons for doubt are based upon the following considerations: (1) Patients with delayed maturation of this enzyme or with isolated defect of it (Medes type) have no clinical manifestations. (2) Levels of another enzyme in the tyrosine pathway (tyrosine transaminase) are also low in this disorder. (3) Elevated levels of methionine in plasma indicate defective methionine metabolism and, indeed, methionine-activating enzyme and cystathionine synthetase levels in liver are low. Whether these findings are caused by a primary defect in amino acid metabolism (tyrosine or methionine) or whether they are secondary to an undefined hepatic disorder is unsettled.

It has not been convincingly demonstrated that all patients with tyrosinosis have the same disorder. The disorder (or disorders) is inherited in an autosomal recessive manner. Large genetic isolates with tyrosinosis have been identified, especially among French Canadians. Early results with diet therapy indicate that the restriction of phenylalanine and tyrosine (and perhaps also of methionine) intake is beneficial.

Most reported cases of tyrosinosis have hepatorenal damage and absence of p-hydroxyphenylpyruvic acid oxidase activity. In some of the involved children derangements of pyrrole metabolism have been noted, with increased excretion of δ-aminolevulinic acid in the urine, with increased activity of δ-aminolevulinic acid synthetase activity in the liver or in hepatoma tissue, and with clinical symptoms of acute intermittent porphyria.

At least two children are known who have tyrosinemia and tyrosyluria without renal, hepatic, methionine, δ-aminolevulinic acid and catecholamine abnormalities, and who are mentally retarded. The relationship of the disorders described above is not known. (See also Section 11.)

TYROSINEMIA. Blood levels of tyrosine as high as 70 mg/dl and excretion of para-hydroxyphenylpyruvic acid have been reported in a child with congenital malformations and mental retardation. In this instance the defect was shown to be the absence of the soluble fraction of tyrosine transaminase. Mitochondrial tyrosine transaminase is present and produces the para-hydroxyphenylpyruvic acid found in urine. Presumably para-hydroxyphenylpyruvic acid oxidase is inhibited by the high levels of tyrosine.

RICHNER-HANHART SYNDROME. This autosomal recessive genetic disorder results in mental retardation, palmar and plantar punctate hyperkeratosis, and herpetiform corneal ulcers. It has recently been shown that a patient with this syndrome had tyrosinemia and tyrosyluria. Treatment with a diet low in tyrosine not only corrected the biochemical abnormalities but also resulted in dramatic healing of the skin and eye lesions.

ALBINISM. Generalized albinism (see also Section 23), one of Garrod's four inborn errors of metabolism, is a defect in the formation of the pigment melanin. There are at least three forms, as shown in Figure 8–1. In the first, the enzyme tyrosinase is not active. In the second type, tyrosinase is present in the melanosome, so that tyrosine can be converted to DOPA and then to DOPA quinone, but the permease for the transport of tyrosine into the melanosome is presumably absent. In both the tyrosinase positive and the tyrosinase negative types of albinism neither melanin nor pheomelanin can be formed. The third type, found among the Amish, is due to a defect in an unidentified enzymatic step between DOPA quinone and melanin. These individuals can produce pheomelanin, a yellowish pigment, from DOPA quinone; they develop normal skin color, but their ocular signs persist through life.

Albinism occurs in all races, varying in incidence from 0.7 per cent in the San Blas Indians of Panama to one in 100,000 in France. In the United States the rate is approximately one in 20,000. It is transmitted as an autosomal recessive characteristic. Normal children have been born to a couple, both of whom had generalized albinism, but of different allelic forms.

In addition to the extremely fair skin and fine silky hair, albinos have numerous ocular abnormalities. Although traces of pigment may occur on the uveal borders, it is absent from the iris, sclera and fundus, and the iris appears gray or blue. Refractive errors, strabismus, nystagmus and photophobia are common. Persistent loss of visual acuity and a red reflex are present in all tyrosinase-negative individuals. In tyrosinase-positive persons, the poor visual acuity may improve with age; the red reflex is found in children and in Caucasian but not black adults.

Other Forms of Albinism. Partial albinism is characterized by localized areas of skin and hair devoid of pigment. In some instances a white forelock or a patch of depigmented hair elsewhere may be the sole manifestation. This form of albinism is inherited as a dominant trait.

In albinism limited to the eye, the depigmentation may be limited to the retina or may also involve the iris. Visual acuity is decreased, and there is nystagmus. This defect is sex-linked, and it follows that the biochemical defect must be different from those occurring in generalized or oculocutaneous albinism.

In Waardenburg syndrome (Section 24) and in the Chediak-Higashi syndrome (Section 14) defective pigment metabolism contributes to the clinical pattern, and each must be taken into account in the differential diagnosis of partial albinism. Hermansky-Pudlak syndrome is an autosomal recessive disorder characterized by oculocutaneous albinism and a hemorrhagic diathesis, in which there appears to be defective glutathione peroxidase activity.

ALCAPTONURIA. Alcaptonuria is a disorder of phenylalanine-tyrosine metabolism characterized by accumulation in the body and excretion in the urine of homogentisic acid (2,5-dihydroxyphenylacetic acid) (Fig. 8–1) and its oxidation products. This disorder was one of four inborn errors of metabolism described by Garrod. More than 600 cases have been recorded. The disorder is transmitted by an autosomal recessive gene. It is estimated that there are about five alcaptonuric persons per million population, and that one person in 200 is a heterozygous carrier of the recessive gene. Defective activity of the enzyme, homogentisic acid oxidase, arrests the catabolism of tyrosine, and large amounts of homogentisic acid are excreted in the urine.

Urine from affected patients becomes black on standing, owing to oxidation and polymerization of the homogentisic acid. In infants, staining of the diaper may lead to detection of the defect. The darkness of the stain increases with continued exposure to air, a dried diaper having a pitch-black stain. Although the abnormality is usually noted in infancy, in some instances the dark urine has not been observed until the second or third decade of life. The slow accumulation of the black polymer of homogentisic acid in cartilage and other mesenchymal tissues produces a black discoloration *(alcaptonuric ochronosis)* of the cheeks, nose, sclerae and ears which becomes evident by mid-adult life. Degeneration of pigmented cartilage leads to arthritis in about half the older patients with alcaptonuria. These changes are sufficiently characteristic to have once suggested the diagnosis of alcaptonuria in an ancient Egyptian mummy. Recent evidence indicates that this may have been an artifact of a particular mummification process. The defect is otherwise asymptomatic.

The urine has reducing properties; it produces a positive reaction with Fehling's or Benedict's reagent and reduces an ammoniacal solution of silver nitrate in the cold. Homogentisic acid does not react with glucose oxidase. The dark urine of phenol poisoning and that associated with melanotic tumors do not have reducing properties. Hyperaminoaciduria is found in phenol intoxication, but not in alcaptonuria.

There is no effective treatment for the disorder.

PARKINSONISM. Another defect in tyrosine metabolism may occur in parkinsonism. The tyrosine hydroxylase of brain is distinct from the tyrosinase of melanocytes; both convert tyrosine to DOPA. Treatment with DOPA has been found to be efficacious. Patients with parkinsonism and some with schizophrenia excrete a compound, once thought to be β-3, 4-dimethoxyphenylethylamine, which has now been shown to be p-tyramine, or decarboxylated tyrosine. Tyramine may accumulate in the brain in excessive amounts if the reaction from tyrosine to DOPA is blocked.

METHIONINE

METHIONINEMIA. Abnormally elevated levels of methionine in plasma are observed in a number of disorders, including liver disease, tyrosinosis and homocystinemia. Some believe that a disturbance of methionine metabolism may be the primary defect in one form of tyrosinosis; others that it is not responsible for any clinical manifestations. Transient methioninemia, presumably due to delayed maturation of an enzyme, has also been reported in an otherwise healthy premature infant. Infants on high protein feedings also show marked elevations of serum methionine levels which revert to normal when protein intake is adjusted to 4 gm/kg/day.

MALABSORPTION OF METHIONINE. A mentally retarded girl with diarrhea, convulsions, tachypnea and a peculiar odor has been found to have a defect in the intestinal absorption of methionine and of other amino acids. Methionine is fermented by intestinal bacteria to alpha-hydroxybutyric, alpha-ketobutyric and alpha-aminobutyric acids, which are absorbed and excreted in urine, where they produce the unusual odor. Alpha-hydroxybutyric acid was demonstrated in urine and/or stools of both parents and of three siblings after methionine loading, which indicates autosomal recessive inheritance. Treatment with a diet low in methionine has shown promise. Alpha-hydroxybutyric acid has been found also in the urine of a child with phenylketonuria; this combination of findings is referred to as *oasthouse disease,* the name suggested by the odor of urine.

HOMOCYSTINEMIA. Homocysteine, an intermediary in the production of cysteine, results when the methyl group of methionine is removed (Fig. 8–2). It is ordinarily not found in plasma or urine. Many patients have been reported who excrete large amounts of homocystine (the dithiol of homocysteine) in the urine and have detectable amounts of both homocysteine and homocystine in the blood. The methionine level of plasma is often elevated, and other unusual thiol compounds are excreted. The biochemical defect has been shown to be a deficiency of the enzyme cystathionine synthetase, which condenses homocysteine with serine to form cystathionine. Normal brain contains large amounts of cystathionine; the brain of a patient who died with homocystinuria was shown to be devoid of this compound, indicating a possible causal relation to the patient's mental retardation.

Many of the patients originally described were mentally retarded, but approximately half the newly found affected persons are intellectually normal. The disease, or at least the principal variant form, is characterized clinically by ectopia lentis, an appearance resembling the Marfan syndrome, malar flush, osteoporosis, and sticky platelets which lead to thromboembolic episodes. Homocystine can be readily detected in urine by the use of the cyanide-nitroprusside reagent. The effect of dietary restriction of methionine has not been adequately assessed. Some patients with defects of cystathionine synthetase respond clinically to large doses of vitamin B_6. In some instances, but not in others, of the B_6-dependent form of the disorder, it has been shown in vitro that pyridoxal phosphate can enhance the activity of the genetically altered cystathionine synthetase. In those instances in which the defect is not at the coenzyme binding site, the administration of pharmacologic doses of B_6 may have enhanced alternate pathways for the removal of homocysteine.

In two other, rarer forms of homocystinuria there is no elevation of blood methionine levels. In both forms there is an ability to remethylate homocysteine to methionine. The first involves the enzyme ^{5}N-methyltetrahydrofolate methyltransferase, which requires B_{12} for activity. A genetic defect impairing the formation of active coenzyme hampers methyltransferase activity as well as the conversion of methylmalonate to succinate. A child with this defect had low blood levels of methionine and increased excretion of homocystine, cystathionine and methylmalonate. Methyltransferase activity, measured post mortem at seven weeks of age, was 2 per cent of normal in the liver and 4 per cent of normal in the kidney. Mental retardation and megaloblastic anemia have been reported in a child with one third of normal hepatic activity of ^{5}N-methyltetrahydrofolate methyltransferase, with no mention of blood levels of methionine or of urinary excretion of homocystine.

In the second rare type the defect is in the enzyme $^{5\text{-}10}$N-methylene-tetrahydrofolate reductase, which is necessary for the production of the ^{5}N-methyltetrahydrofolate, which the transferase uses as a methyl donor for the formation of methionine from homocysteine. The patient with the reductase deficiency (as measured in cultured fibroblasts) at 16 years of age had proximal muscle weakness and other neurologic signs.

CYSTATHIONINEMIA. Cystathionine is an intermediate in the conversion of methionine to cysteine; it is not normally found in plasma or urine. Cystathioninuria occurs in patients with neuroblastoma, other neural tumors, hepatoblastoma or with liver disease, particularly when due to galactosemia. Cystathioninuria in association with cystathioninemia is inherited in an autosomal recessive manner; affected persons have an aberrant form of the enzyme cystathioninase which normally splits cystathionine to homoserine and cysteine (see Fig. 8–2). The binding site for its coenzyme, pyridoxal phosphate, is altered on the affected enzyme molecule. It has been shown both in vitro and in vivo that an increase in function of the enzyme occurs on addition of vitamin B_6 or of its coenzyme form.

About a dozen patients with the disease have been studied, one of whom also had phenylketonuria. Clinical manifestations have been variable and perhaps coincidental; one patient had convulsions; two sisters had mitral regurgitation, and one had thrombocytopenic purpura and renal calculi. Mental retardation has occurred in less than one half of known cases. The association of retardation with this disorder may be a result of selection due to ascertainment. Therapy with vitamin B_6 has led to decreased urinary and blood levels of cystathionine, but its further clinical effects are unknown.

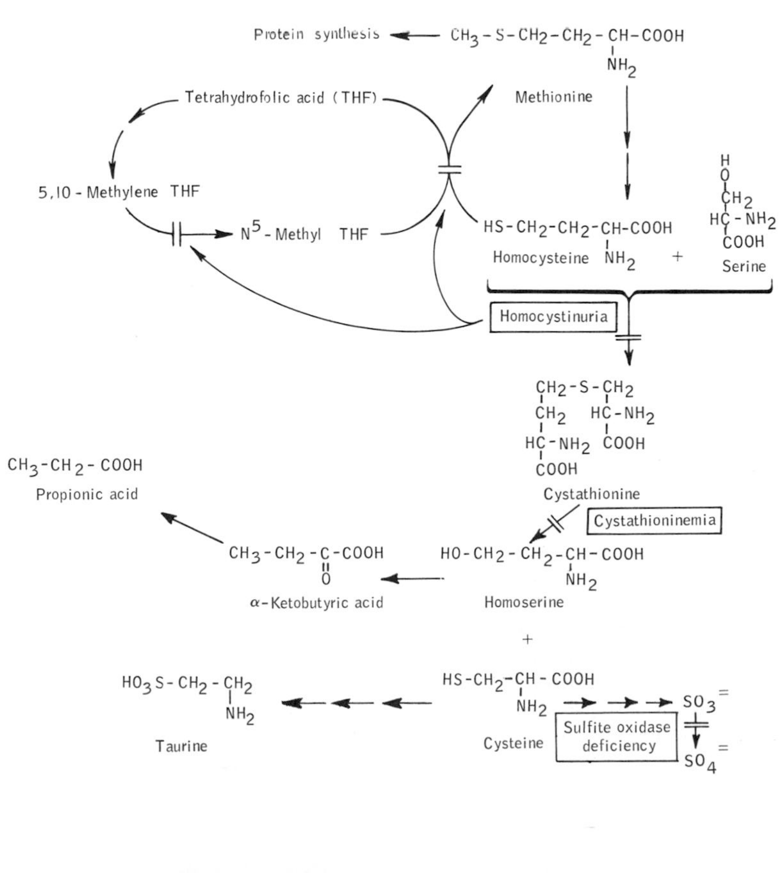

Figure 8–2 Pathways in the metabolism of the sulfur-containing amino acids. See also legend for Figure 8–1.

Two patients with cystathioninemia unresponsive to B_6 are known; one is retarded, the other normal. This form of the disorder is clearly different from the more common B_6 responsive variety.

Cystathioninase is not present in normal fetal liver before birth; therefore, diagnosis of this inborn error of metabolism is not likely to be made in utero.

Latent cystathioninuria has been described in two mentally retarded brothers who excreted large amounts of cystathionine only when loaded with excess methionine, but not when fed normal diets. They do not appear to be heterozygotes for the usual form of cystathioninemia, since another sibling and their mother excreted small amounts of cystathionine after methionine loading. Transient cystathioninuria has also been observed secondary to hepatic disease in a patient later proved to be a heterozygous carrier for cystathioninemia.

A 2 year old boy and his 8 year old sister have been found by chance to be homozygous for cystathioninemia. Both were clinically normal. These observations again point out that abnormal clinical manifestations observed in the first few cases of a newly discovered inborn error of metabolism may or may not be related to the enzymatic defect.

CYSTINE

CYSTINURIA. The term "cystinuria" (see Section 15) is applied to at least three closely related disorders, all of which are inherited in an autosomal recessive manner. The homozygotes all have excessive urinary loss of cystine and of three other dibasic amino acids: arginine, lysine and ornithine. The urinary loss of cystine has been recognized for many years through the formation of renal calculi. This defect was one of the four disorders on which Garrod based his hypothesis of inborn errors of metabolism.

Recently the three forms have been distinguished from each other on the basis of (1) the pattern of excretion of dibasic amino acids in the clinically normal heterozygote, and (2) the nature of the defect in active intestinal transport in affected homozygous persons. The disorder is more fully described elsewhere with other disorders of the renal tubules.

Isolated cystinuria has been reported in a brother and a sister and appears to be inherited as an autosomal recessive.

CYSTINOSIS. In this syndrome (see Section 22) there is excessive storage of cystine crystals in the reticuloendothelial system and parenchymatous organs. The enzymatic defect is unknown. The disorder is transmitted as an autosomal recessive, and heterozygous carriers can be detected by the elevation of intracellular free cystine in peripheral leukocytes or in fibroblasts grown in tissue culture.

SULFITE OXIDASE DEFICIENCY. In the final step of cystine catabolism, inorganic sulfate is formed and excreted in the urine. Absence of inorganic sulfate in the urine has been reported in a mentally retarded child with dislocated lenses who died at 3 years of age. Three siblings (out of seven) died in infancy with neurologic abnormalities. It was proved that the patient lacked sulfite oxidase activity. As a consequence, he excreted large amounts of sulfite, thiosulfate and S-sulfo-L-cysteine in his urine. The defect (Fig. 8–2) is presumably inherited as an autosomal recessive.

β-MERCAPTOLACTATE-CYSTEINE DISULFIDURIA. β-Mercaptolactate-cysteine disulfide is a derivative of cystine in which one of the two amino groups is replaced by a hydroxyl group. This substance has been found in high concentration in the urine of a mentally retarded patient who was the product of a sibling mating. There were no other amino acid abnormalities. It was detected by the nitroprusside test while screening for cystinuria.

TAURINURIA. Taurine is normally excreted in the urine as an intermediate in the oxidation of cysteine. Seventeen persons (in four families) who have camptodactyly (flexion contractures of the fingers) due to a dominant gene have been shown to also excrete excess taurine (Fig. 8–2).

TRYPTOPHAN

HARTNUP DISEASE. Hartnup disease, an eponymic reminder of the affected English family in whom the disease was discovered, is a rare hereditary molecular disease in which there is a defect in the transport of tryptophan by intestinal mucosa and renal tubules.

There is massive aminoaciduria. Plasma amino acid concentrations are normal, so that the aminoaciduria must be due to faulty tubular reabsorption. The single exception to this generalization is the amino acid tryptophan; characteristically, levels in plasma are abnormally low. Impaired intestinal absorption of tryptophan results in its bacterial decomposition to various indole and indoxyl derivatives which are absorbed, detoxified, and excreted in the urine in abnormally large amounts.

Cutaneous photosensitivity is seen early in most affected children. Unprotected areas of skin become rough and red after moderate exposure to the sun. With greater exposure, a rash identical with that of pellagra develops. Patients with Hartnup disease may also have cerebellar ataxia with evidences of involvement of the pyramidal tracts. During febrile illnesses, ataxia may develop without a rash. The clinical course is variable; severe cutaneous and nervous disturbances may alternate with periods of complete remission over many years. Mental deficiency was apparently an incidental finding in the original kindred and has not been observed in other cases. The disease is transmitted by an autosomal recessive gene. Hartnup disease must be considered in the differential diagnosis of pellagra.

The impaired intestinal absorption and urinary loss of tryptophan result in decreased synthesis of nicotinic acid. It is not surprising, therefore, that large doses of nicotinamide may cause sustained remission of the neurologic and cutaneous aspects of the disorder. Such remissions, however, may occur without therapy. The aminoaciduria and urinary excretion of indole compounds are not suppressed by such therapy, nor do they decrease during spontaneous remissions. It has been suggested that high protein diets compensate for the loss of amino acids.

TRYPTOPHANEMIA. In contrast to Hartnup disease, in which there is impaired absorption of tryptophan, the catabolism of tryptophan (presumably in its conversion to kynurenine) is involved in this disorder (Fig. 8–3). The patient was a mentally retarded child with dwarfism who had the same pellagra-like rash seen in Hartnup disease. There were tryptophanemia and tryptophanuria without generalized aminoaciduria or indicanuria. Parental consanguinity and the suspicion of a similar disorder in two cousins indicate autosomal recessive inheritance.

KYNURENINURIA. An abnormality of tryptophan metabolism consistent with a partial block of the enzyme kynurenine hydroxylase has been reported in four generations of a family. Although the propositus had scleroderma, the other members of the kindred were healthy. Abnormal amounts of kynurenine and other tryptophan metabolites proximal to hydroxykynurenine (Fig. 8–3) are excreted in the urine both before and after administration of tryptophan. Pyridoxine did not affect the excretion pattern of tryptophan metabolites. The affected persons appear to be heterozygous for the condition.

KYNURENINASE DEFECTS

Hydroxykynureninuria. A defect has been described in the tryptophan pathway which is consistent with lack of activity of the enzyme kynureninase. In this disorder large amounts of kynurenine, 3-hydroxy-kynurenine and xanthurenic acid are excreted (Fig. 8–3). Signs and symptoms of nicotinic acid deficiency develop in the absence of added dietary nicotinic acid; affected persons cannot synthesize it from tryptophan. A patient was mildly mentally retarded and had

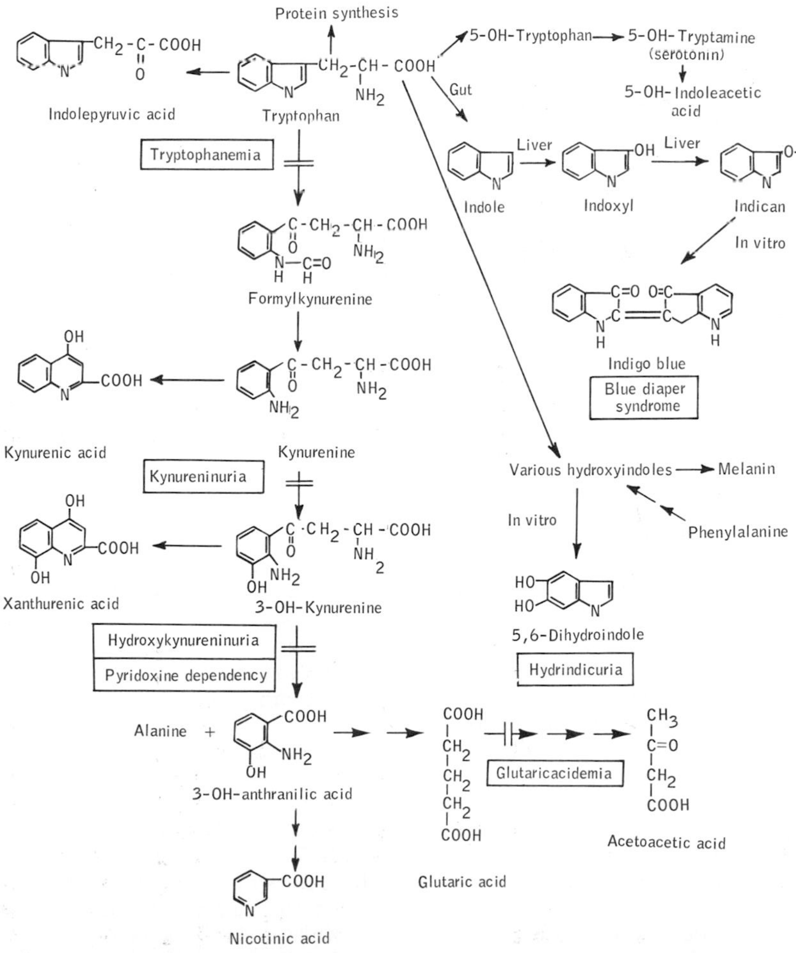

Figure 8–3 *Pathways in the metabolism of tryptophan. See also legend for Figure 8–1.*

migraine-like headaches. Treatment with pyridoxine did not alter the excretion pattern of the tryptophan metabolites, but did relieve the headaches.

Pyridoxine Dependency (Xanthurenic Aciduria). Children with pyridoxine dependency have convulsions and are mentally retarded (Section 3). After tryptophan loading they excrete the same metabolites of tryptophan, mainly xanthurenic acid, as are seen without tryptophan loading in hydroxykynureninuria. These metabolites are also excreted by persons who are deficient in pyridoxine. Pyridoxal phosphate is the coenzyme for many enzymes involved in amino acid metabolism, including kynureninase. Whereas low doses of the vitamin correct the abnormalities in the deficiency state, high doses are required to treat the dependent state. In pyridoxine dependency it has been shown in vitro that there is a defect of the enzyme kynureninase which affects its ability to bind with the coenzyme form of the vitamin.

Excessive excretion of hydroxykynurenine, kynurenine and xanthurenic acid, corrected by pyridoxine, has been observed in five unrelated patients with chronic granulomatous disease.

INDICANURIA. Indicanuria arises when tryptophan is poorly absorbed from the gastrointestinal tract and is converted there by bacterial action to indole. Indole is absorbed, oxidized, sulfated and excreted as an indican (Fig. 8–3). Indicanuria is commonly observed whenever there is stasis in the bowels, such as in constipation or the "blind loop syndrome"; it also occurs in Hartnup disease, in which tryptophan is poorly absorbed, and in phenylketonuria. The *blue diaper syndrome,* a familial disorder characterized by hypercalcemia, nephrocalcinosis and indicanuria, derives its name from the fact that indican is oxidized to indican blue on exposure to air.

HYDRINDICURIA. Indole pigments related to both tryptophan and phenylalanine metabolism have been found in the urine of a mentally retarded child who had a persistent metabolic acidosis, presumably caused by carboxyindole derivatives. Laboratory manipulation of urine containing abnormal urinary indoles converts them to 5,6-dihydroxyindole (hydrindic acid); hence the name of the disorder (Fig. 8–3). Prolonged administration of antibiotics in an effort to halt indole formation in the gut had no effect upon indole excretion, and loading tests showed an increase in urinary hydrindic acid after administration of phenylalanine and tryptophan, but not of tyrosine.

INDOLYLACROYLGLYCINURIA. Indolylacroylglycine is formed by the conjugation of glycine with a molecule of tryptophan from which a molecule of ammonia has been removed to form a double bond. It is one of the many tryptophan metabolites excreted in Hartnup disease, and has been found alone in a family with mental retardation. In all but one member of the family, administration of neomycin temporarily eliminated the indolylacroylglycinuria.

GLUTARIC ACIDEMIA. See below, this Section.

VALINE, LEUCINE, ISOLEUCINE

MAPLE SYRUP URINE DISEASE. This recessive disorder is characterized by the excretion of urine with an odor of maple syrup and by central nervous system manifestations appearing within the first weeks of life. In the neonatal period there is difficulty in feeding, and the beginning of progressive neurologic and mental deterioration. Death usually occurs in untreated patients within the first few months of life.

The blood and urine contain increased amounts of the three branched-chain amino acids, valine, leucine and isoleucine. The urine characteristically also contains increased amounts of the keto-acid derivatives of these amino acids. The defect is known to be in oxidative decarboxylation of the keto-acids (Fig. 8–4). There is some disagreement at present whether each keto-acid is decarboxylated by its specific decarboxylase. It appears, in any case, that the carboxylase has two binding sites for the substrate; the higher affinity site is nonfunctional in maple syrup urine disease. Alloisoleucine, a stereo-isomer of isoleucine formed by way of the keto-acid, and not normally found in blood, becomes readily detectable.

The enzymatic defect can be demonstrated in leukocytes in vitro; this method also serves to detect heterozygotes. Treatment with a diet low in the branched-chain amino acids has been successfully used to arrest the progressively downhill course of the disease. Variable degrees of central nervous system manifestations may persist, depending upon adequacy of treatment and amount of damage present prior to its institution. During treatment it is necessary to monitor the blood levels of leucine and isoleucine carefully. When the ratio of leucine to isoleucine exceeds normal values, a condition resembling acrodermatitis enteropathica results. The rash abates when the isoleucine level of the diet is increased.

Intermittent Branched-chain Ketonuria. This is a variant of maple syrup urine disease. Children who are apparently healthy suddenly become ill, develop the odor of maple syrup, exhibit neurologic symptoms, and excrete leucine, isoleucine and valine and the corresponding keto-acids in urine. The disorder is genetically transmitted as an autosomal recessive. Activity of branched-chain decarboxylase is reduced in leukocytes, but not so much as in the more common form of the disorder.

Mild Variant. In a third form of the disorder the symptomatology is less severe than in the classic form. Elevations of the branched-chain amino and keto-acids persist, and the odor of maple syrup may or may not be present. There is moderate mental retardation. In vivo assay of branched-chain decarboxylase activity yields results which are intermediate between those of the classic type and the intermittent type. Still another form of the disorder may have been observed in an 8 year old boy, who at birth was thought to have classic maple syrup urine disease but who is no longer on dietary control and whose branched-chain amino acid levels are reverting to normal.

Thiamine-responsive Form. In another variant the defect is at the binding site of the enzyme for the cofactor, thiamine pyrophosphate, the coenzyme form of the vitamin thiamine, which is involved in the oxidative decarboxylation of all α-keto-acids. A patient with the odor of maple syrup, moderate elevation of blood levels of leucine, isoleucine, alloisoleucine and valine, and with no excretion of the keto-acid derivatives had a mild clinical course. The biochemical abnormalities responded completely to 10 mg/day of thiamine hydrochloride.

VALINEMIA. A child has been observed with elevated levels of valine in plasma and urine, and with mental deficiency and growth failure, but without the characteristic urinary odor or excretion of keto-acids of maple syrup urine disease. Transamination of valine is impaired; the defect can be demonstrated in leukocytes in vitro.

ISOLEUCINE-LEUCINEMIA. Two siblings with severe neurologic symptoms, mental retardation and failure to thrive have been reported to have unusual biochemical findings. Both had type II prolinemia (see below) and mild (twice normal) to marked (eight times normal) elevations of blood valine, isoleucine and leucine levels, with the latter two predominating. Assays using leukocytes revealed no abnormalities of any of the three branched-chain keto-acid decarboxylase activities or of valine transaminase, but a 50 per cent reduction of isoleucine and leucine transaminase.

ISOVALERIC ACIDEMIA. This condition was first described in two siblings with mild retardation, vomiting, severe acidosis and coma. A more severe form of the disorder was reported in an infant who died in acidosis within a week of birth. The odor of short chain fatty acids led to the biochemical elucidation of the defect, and has been described as the odor of sweaty feet. The defect is in the oxidation of isovaleryl CoA to β-methylcrotonyl CoA (See Fig. 8–4), and has been demonstrated in leukocytes and in cultured fibroblasts.

Patients with isovaleric acidosis do not always

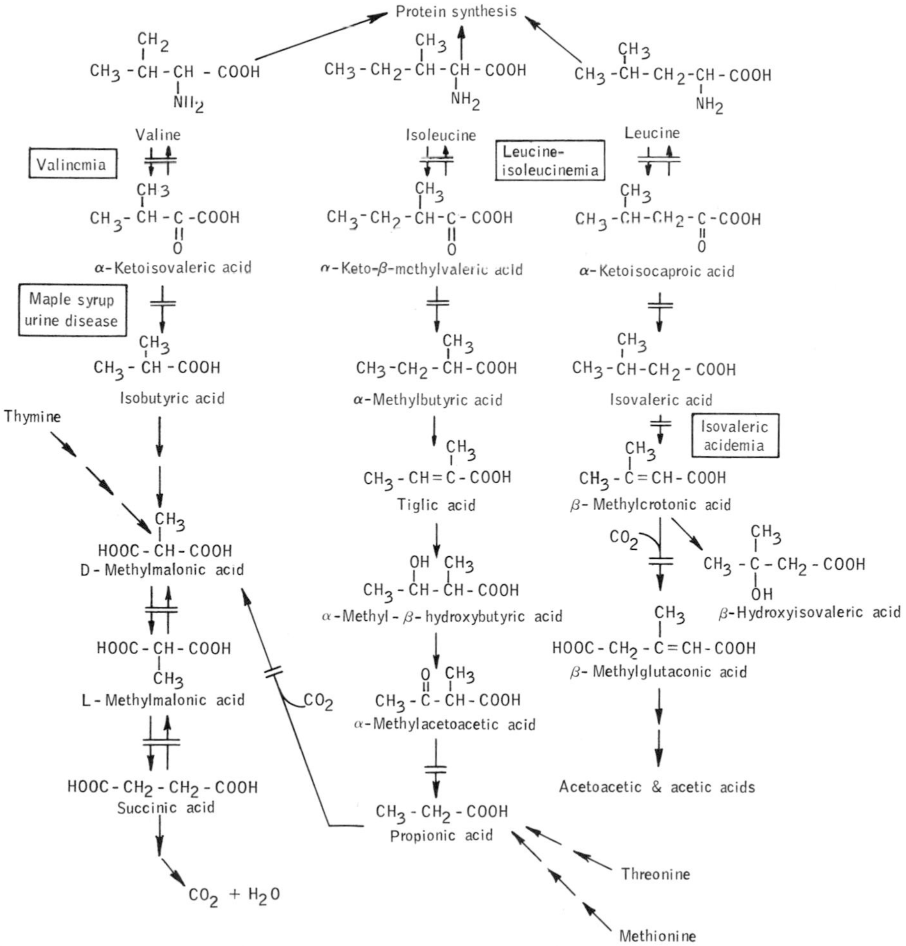

Figure 8–4 Pathways in the metabolism of the branched chain amino acids. (See also legend for Figure 8–1.) Owing to lack of space, some of the defects depicted are not named. In each case, the defect is called by the name of the substrate accumulating (e.g., Methylmalonic acidemia. Propionic acidemia, etc.).

have the odor of sweaty feet. One patient with periodic acidemia, lethargy and coma had elevated plasma levels of glycine and excreted large amounts of isovalerylglycine and lesser amounts of isovalerate during her episodes of acidosis. Isovalerylglycine can be demonstrated easily in thin-layer chromatography.

Another patient with the odor of sweaty feet thought originally to have a defect of the enzyme green acyldehydrogenase has, with gas chromatographic techniques, been shown to have isovaleric acidemia. Patients with the green acyldehydrogenase defect do excrete butanoic and hexanoic acid, but do not smell of sweaty feet.

BETA-METHYLCROTONYL CoA CARBOXYLASE DEFICIENCY. Another condition involving leucine degradation gives rise to a peculiar odor which resembles that of tom cat's urine. The enzyme β-methylcrotonyl CoA carboxylase fixes CO_2 and has biotin as a cofactor (Fig. 8–4). Two errors of metabolism have been recognized here which illustrate that when specific cofactors of metabolic reactions are involved, genetic alterations may affect the protein either at the substrate binding site or at the cofactor binding site: if it is ability to bind cofactor that is reduced (but not abolished), then the in vitro or in vivo addition of massive amounts of cofactor can overcome the effects of the mutation. In both forms of this disorder, β-methylcrotonyl CoA cannot be converted to β-hydroxy, β-methylglutaryl CoA and large amounts of β-methylcrotonic acid are excreted, conjugated with glycine. A patient with the form of the disease unresponsive to B_{12} had neurologic symptoms at 4½ months of age similar to those of Werdnig-Hoffman disease, without acidosis. A patient with the biotin-responsive form presented with severe acidosis and ketosis, and an erythematous rash of the buttocks and joint flexures. Treatment with 10 mg of biotin per day completely eliminated the acidosis, the ketosis and the rash, as well as the excretion of leucine metabolites. Prior to the administration of biotin, this patient also excreted tiglylglycine, the glycine conjugate of an intermediate of isoleucine metabolism, which is thought to accumulate as a result of competitive inhibition of its further degradation by β-methylcrotonate, which is an isomer of tiglic acid. Hydroxyisovaleric aciduria also occurs in this condition, and in biotin-deficient rats.

ACETOACETYL CoA THIOLASE DEFICIENCY. In the normal pathway for isoleucine degradation, the compound α-methylacetoacetyl CoA is converted to acetyl CoA and propionyl CoA (Fig. 8–4). Three children have been found in whom it appears the thiolase responsible for this conversion is deficient, inasmuch as they excrete large amounts of α-methylacetoacetate, α-methyl-β-hydroxybutyrate and the glycine conjugate of tiglic acid. The children had intermittent acidosis, vomiting, lethargy and coma, usually brought on by intercurrent infection. One child died during such an episode. The feeding of additional isoleucine aggravated the condition, whereas reduction of protein intake to 2 gm/kg/day appeared to ameliorate the clinical course. There was no peculiar odor or elevation of amino acid or propionate levels in blood or urine. A defect in isoleucine oxidation was demonstrated in cultured skin fibroblasts.

A defect of β-ketothiolase activity has been reported in an infant with ketotic glycinemia and hyperammonemia but no methylmalonic or propionic acidemia, though the clinical symptoms were those associated with the latter two findings. Treatment with a low protein diet (1.5 gm/kg/day) seemed advantageous.

PROPIONIC ACIDEMIA. The defect in this disorder has been established only recently; formerly the disorder was known as "ketotic glycinemia." The manifestations are severe acidosis and ketosis beginning within the first few days of life and recur later. Mental and physical retardation, osteoporosis and periodic thrombocytopenia and neutropenia follow. The episodes of vomiting, ketosis and acidosis appear to be related to the quantity of protein in the diet; reduction in dietary protein has led to decreased frequency and severity of the clinical attacks and to an increase in circulating neutrophils. Administration of methionine, of threonine, of valine, of leucine, or of isoleucine produces ketosis. Of these, isoleucine, methionine and threonine produce propionic acid, which is normally converted to methylmalonate and subsequently to succinic acid. (See Fig. 8–4.) In the absence of activity of the enzyme, propionyl CoA carboxylase, propionic acid accumulates, and ketones such as 2-butanone, presumably derived from isoleucine, appear in the urine during episodes of ketosis. Tiglic acid and tiglylglycine have also been found in the urine in patients with propionic acidemia.

Treatment consists of careful reduction of the dietary intake of offending amino acids. The defect in propionate metabolism can be demonstrated in leukocytes.

Since propionyl CoA carboxylase requires biotin, it is not surprising that a *variant* form of propionic acidemia has been observed. Treatment of a 2 year old boy with signs and symptoms of "ketotic glycinemia" with 5 mg/day of biotin has eliminated all the biochemical abnormalities. It is too early to assess any clinical improvement. New patients with the biotin-responsive form of propionic acidemia would presumably do well with treatment initiated in the neonatal period.

The majority of patients with propionic acidemia have ketotic glycinemia, but a 10 month old patient with mental retardation and seizures and proven propionyl-CoA carboxylase deficiency had ketoacidosis only when challenged with an isoleucine load. This girl and two other patients with propionic acidemia have responded to an isoleucine or valine load with hyperammonemia, an unusual finding in classic propionic acidemia. Before the nature of the defect in propionic acidemia was defined, an infant with ketotic glycinemia and severe hyperammonemia was found to have decreased activity of hepatic carbamyl phosphate synthetase, an established defect of urea synthesis. Depression of all five enzymes of the urea cycle (q.v.) has been found in one of the proven cases of propionic acidemia with ketotic glycinemia; accordingly, this earlier observation may have been coincidental.

METHYLMALONIC ACIDEMIA. Methylmalonic acid is a structural isomer of succinic acid. The two are normally readily interconvertible in their coenzyme A forms with the aid of the enzyme methylmalonyl CoA isomerase, which requires cobamide. With vitamin B_{12} deficiency, increased amounts of methylmalonic acid are excreted in urine. Methylmalonic acid is normally derived from propionic acid and therefore from the catabolism of isoleucine, methionine and threonine and directly from valine (Fig. 8–2). It is probably by way of these routes that methylmalonic acid appears in excessive amounts in one form of propionic acidemia.

Methylmalonic acidemia and massive methylmalonic aciduria were first described in two unrelated children who failed to thrive and exhibited bouts of severe metabolic acidosis from the time of birth. One died at 2 years of age in acute acidosis; the other, a 6 year old girl, was treated with alkalinization and, despite episodes of vomiting and acidosis, had normal physical and mental development. She had had a brother who died in infancy after vomiting and failure to thrive. Loading tests with protein, valine or propionic acid led to hypoglycemia and ketosis as well as to slight increases in the excretion of methylmalonic acid. A moderate number of additional patients with this disorder are now known; in each of these patients in whom glycinemia was looked for, it also was present (see below).

There are four forms of methylmalonic acidemia. The two most common varieties involve the enzyme methylmalonyl CoA carbonylmutase, which converts L-methylmalonyl CoA to succinyl CoA. Since this enzyme requires 5′-deoxyadenosylcobalamine for full activity, it is not surprising that both B_{12}-responsive and B_{12}-unresponsive forms of the disorder have been identified. The third form is due to a defect in the metabolism of vitamin B_{12} wherein cobalamine cannot be converted into either the deoxyadenosyl form or the methyl form. In this instance, homocysteine (q.v.) is affected, as well as methylmalonate metabolism. The fourth form involves the enzyme methylmalonyl CoA racemase, which interconverts the D and L forms of methylmalonate, and has been observed in an infant who died on the 11th day of life after a stormy course involving severe acidosis, hyperammonemia and coma.

GLYCINE

GLYCINEMIA WITH KETOSIS. Abnormal elevations of plasma glycine levels and episodes of ketosis are found in patients with a number of inborn errors of metabolism, such as methylmalonic acidemia or propionic acidemia or some other defect of metabolism of leucine and isoleucine below the level of the block which occurs in maple syrup urine disease. The metabolic events producing high levels of glycine are not known, but many of the metabolites that accumulate are excreted for the most part as glycine conjugates. Glycinemia may be an adaptive response to an increased need for detoxification of these acids normally present only in low concentration. Pathways are indicated in Figure 8–5.

GLYCINEMIA WITHOUT KETOSIS. Besides the glycinemia which may occur secondary to the acidosis and ketosis in propionic or methylmalonic acidemia (see above), or rarely, in propionic acidemia, without acidosis or ketosis, there is another entity, *nonketotic glycinemia,* in which the primary defect is in glycine metabolism. Numerous patients with this entity have been studied during the past 10 years and numerous hypotheses developed concerning the nature of the biochemical defect(s). Recent studies in three different laboratories indicate that the basic defect is in the cleavage of glycine to form CO_2, ammonia and hydroxymethyltetrahydrofolate. Since the last normally reacts with another molecule of glycine to form serine, conversion of glycine to serine is also impaired. Some patients with nonketotic glycinemia have been reported to excrete less oxalic acid than normal, and defects have been postulated in the pathway from glycine to glyoxylic acid and thence to oxalic acid. Except for one case with a possible defect in the conversion of glyoxalate to oxalate, these patients have been shown to have a defect of the cleavage enzyme. Patients with nonketotic glycinemia are mentally retarded, are listless, fail to thrive and have seizures, but they do not have episodes of acidosis or ketosis and do not exhibit neutropenia or thrombocytopenia. A patient with nonketotic glycinemia and a proven defect of the cleavage enzyme, has been reported to have hyperammonemia. Normal values for carbamylphosphate synthetase, ornithine transcarbamylase and argininosuccinic acid synthetase were found. Thus, in both propionic acidemia and nonketotic glycinemia, occasional patients have an as yet unexplained elevation of blood ammonia.

SARCOSINEMIA. Increased concentrations of sarcosine (N-methylglycine) have been observed in both blood and urine in two siblings, one of whom was mentally retarded, had difficulty in swallowing, failed to thrive and died at 14 months of age. Loading tests in other family members suggest that this is a recessively inherited inborn error probably involving sarcosine dehydrogenase, the enzyme which converts sarcosine to glycine (Fig. 8–5). A third patient with hepatosplenomegaly and fatty metamorphosis of the liver has been described with this disorder, who at 8 months of age was apparently developing normally. A fourth patient was mentally retarded, whereas the fifth reported patient with sarcosinemia was a 10 year old boy with normal intelligence, short stature and contracture of the muscles of the lower limbs. In one of the original patients, who at 14 years of age seemed to be a healthy girl with an IQ of 77, hepatic tissue obtained at biopsy contained no sarcosine dehydrogenase.

TRIMETHYLAMINURIA. Choline is an important dietary source of methyl groups. It is normally converted to betaine, thence to dimethylglycine and to sarcosine and finally to glycine. Putrefaction, particularly in fish, yields trimethylamine. A 6 year old girl, smelling of stale fish, has been reported who excreted large amounts of trimethylamine. She had recurrent pulmonary infections, splenomegaly and a mild bleeding tendency. Both platelet and leukocyte adhesiveness to glass was reduced.

GLYCINURIA AND GLUCOGLYCINURIA. Glycinuria and glucoglycinuria have been identified as separate disorders of the renal tubules. Glycinuria is also observed in prolinemia and prolinuria, since there exists a common transport system for proline, hydroxyproline and glycine, in addition to the specific renal transport system for glycine alone.

PRIMARY OXALURIA AND OXALOSIS. Oxalic acid is a 2-carbon dicarboxylic acid which is derived mostly from the oxidation of the amino acid glycine via glyoxylic acid (Fig. 8–5). A storage disease, *oxalosis,* is characterized by the deposition of calcium oxalate crystals throughout the body tissues, excessive urinary excretion of oxalic acid, renal and vesical lithiasis, and nephrocalcinosis. Early in the course of the disease and in mild forms, only oxaluria may be present. Clinical manifestations appear in childhood, and death occurs in early adulthood. It is now known that primary oxaluria comprises two distinct disorders, each caused by a different enzymatic deficit, both presumably inherited as autosomal recessives.

In the first form, the more common and more severe, there is usually excess excretion of *glycolic acid* and glyoxylic acid as well as oxalic acid. The missing enzyme, α-ketoglutarate-glyoxylate carboligase, normally removes glyoxylic acid to form α-hydroxy-β-ketoadipic acid. In the absence of this enzyme the glyoxylic acid floods the pathways leading to glycolic and oxalic acids.

In the second type of hyperoxaluria, *L-glyceric acid is also excreted* in the urine in large amounts. This acid, which is not produced by normal persons, arises from the reduction of hydroxypyruvic acid (the keto-acid of serine) by lactic dehydrogenase. Ordinarily, hydroxypyruvic acid is reduced to D-glyceric acid by the specific enzyme D-glyceric acid dehydrogenase. This enzyme is also capable of reducing glyoxylic acid to glycolic acid. In its absence hydroxypyruvic acid is converted to and

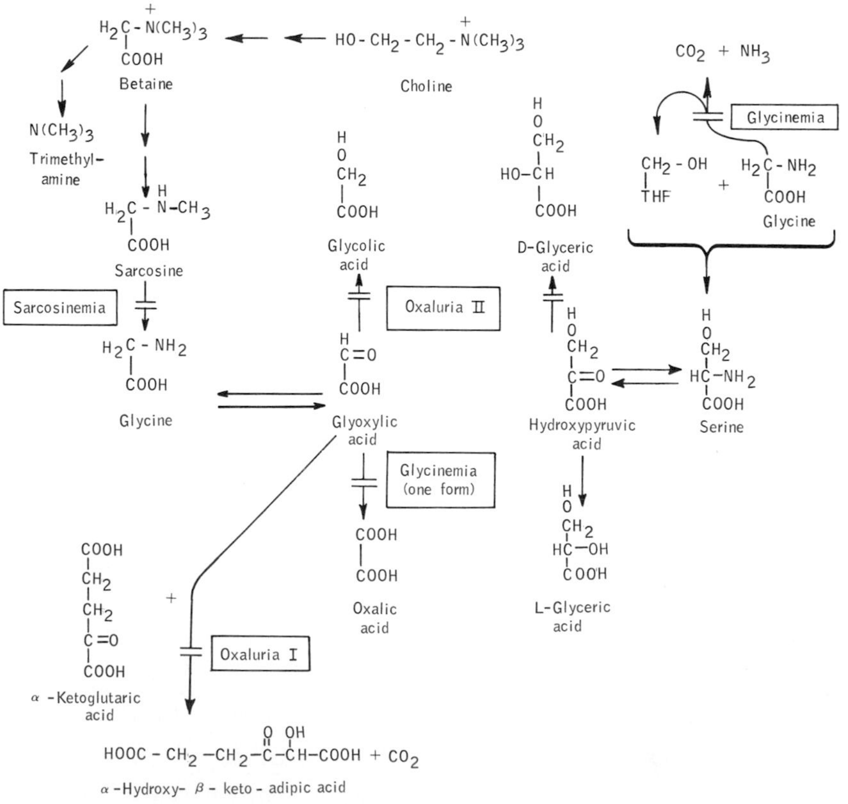

Figure 8–5 Pathways in the metabolism of glycine. See also legend for Figure 8–1.

excreted as L-glyceric acid, and glyoxylic acid is converted to and excreted as oxalic acid. Of about 30 fully studied cases with primary oxalosis, most have had glycolic aciduria and only four glyceric aciduria. Attempts at treatment, including renal transplantation, have not proved efficacious. In some patients, administration of large doses of pyridoxine has reduced the urinary excretion of oxalate, but values achieved remained well above normal limits.

PROLINE AND HYDROXYPROLINE

Proline and hydroxyproline are found in high concentration in collagen. Neither of these amino acids is normally found in urine in its free form except in early infancy. "Bound" hydroxyproline (dipeptides and tripeptides containing hydroxyproline) is excreted whenever there is rapid turnover of collagen such as may occur in such disorders as rickets and hyperparathyroidism.

PROLINURIA. A defect in renal tubular reabsorption of proline is inherited as an autosomal recessive. Since proline, hydroxyproline and glycine are all transported by a common mechanism, patients with familial prolinuria also excrete the other two amino acids in abnormal amounts; however, the concentrations of these amino acids in serum are normal. Many of the affected persons also have impaired intestinal transport of proline. An early impression of high coincidence of prolinuria and mental retardation may have arisen as an error of ascertainment. In a screening program in Australia involving 200,000 infants, persistent aminoglycinuria was found in 15, none of whom had any clinical abnormalities.

PROLINEMIA. Two distinct types of prolinemia are known in which excessive amounts of proline are present in both blood and urine. Hydroxyproline and glycine are also excreted in abnormal amounts in the urine, owing to the inhibition of the common tubular reabsorption mechanism. In the first type of prolinemia the enzymatic defect involves proline oxidase (Fig. 8–6). In the second type the defect is presumed to be in the enzyme of the next step, a dehydrogenase, since pyrrolidine carboxylic acid, as well as proline, accumulates abnormally. Type I prolinemia has been associated with mild mental retardation, renal abnormalities, nerve deafness and photogenic epilepsy. Whether there is a causal relation, however, is uncertain, since both types of prolinemia appear to be inherited on an autosomal recessive basis, and the other abnormalities were dominantly inherited. Prolinemia has also been an isolated finding in a large family. Type II prolinemia was originally observed in a young child who had only mild mental retardation. At least five other patients are now known, two of whom are not retarded.

HYDROXYPROLINEMIA. This disorder was first described in a severely retarded girl. Excessive hydroxyproline was found in serum and urine. In hydroxyprolinemia, in contrast to prolinemia, excessive urinary excretion of the other two amino acids (proline and glycine) which share the same transport mechanisms does not occur. The defect is in the enzyme hydroxyproline oxidase (Fig. 8–6). This enzyme is distinct from the corresponding enzyme which acts upon proline. The disorder is presumed to be inherited as an autosomal recessive.

Two new families have now been studied: in one, the child with hydroxyprolinemia was retarded; in the other, two adult siblings had hydroxyprolinemia and no other clinical abnormalities. The association with mental retardation may be fortuitous.

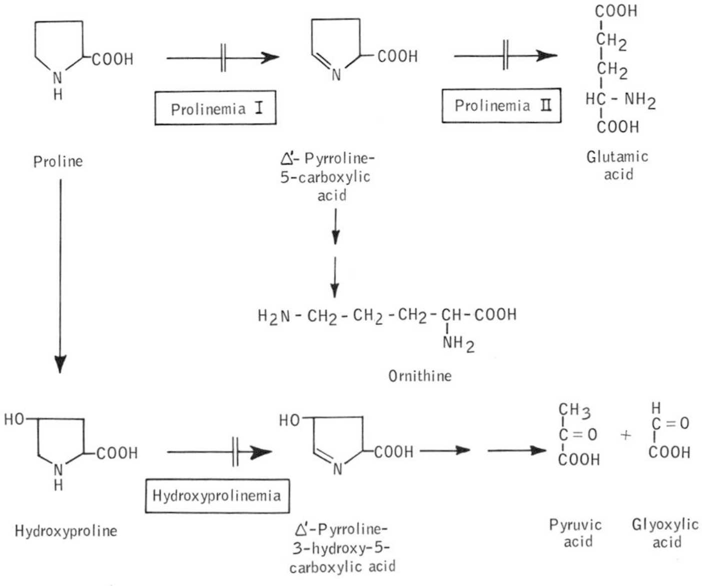

Figure 8–6 *Pathways in the metabolism of the imino acids. See also legend for Figure 8–1.*

GLYCYLPROLINURIA. Glycylproline has been found in the urine in two syndromes: In the first syndrome, though various other proline dipeptides were found in urine, only glycylproline was demonstrated in serum. The patient had hepatosplenomegaly and a peculiar face, but no bone disease. The electron microscopic appearance of collagen was similar to that seen in lathyrism. In the second syndrome, glycylproline could not be demonstrated in serum, but appeared in large amounts in urine. The patients, two sisters, had thickened bone cortices, macrocranium and frequent fractures.

GLUTAMIC ACID

Glutamic acid is a pivotal compound in amino acid metabolism. A number of inborn errors involving the metabolism of glutamic acid are known. Most involve one or more steps in the synthesis or breakdown of the tripeptide *glutathione* (γ-glutamylcysteinylglycine) in blood plasma or in the erythrocytes. Glutathione is also involved in a nonspecific amino acid transport system, particularly in the renal tubule and in the intestinal villus, where the cyclical synthesis and degradation of glutathione is involved in the formation of dipeptides with glutamic acid of the amino acids to be transported. An inborn error in one of the steps of this γ-glutamyl cycle has been described in a number of patients with pyroglutamic aciduria.

PYROGLUTAMIC ACIDURIA. Two patients, a 20 year old male with mental retardation, and a one year old girl without retardation but with metabolic acidosis, have been found to excrete massive amounts (6 to 20 gm/day) of pyroglutamic acid (also known as 5-hydroxyproline or pyrolidone-2-carboxylic acid). This compound is an intermediate in Meister's γ-glutamyl cycle for the transport of amino acids (Fig. 8–7). The genetic defect is in the enzyme 5-hydroxyproline hydrolase. It is presumably localized to the kidney and intestine, since the enzyme has been found in cultured skin fibroblast cells from one of the patients.

Although these patients have a defective cycle for generalized amino acid transport, this process remains intact since the defect is distal to the release of the transported amino acid. Instead, they excrete an amount of pyroglutamic acid equimolar with the amount of transported amino acid. Glutamic acid is present in the diet, is synthesized from other amino acids, and is produced through the citric acid cycle by transamination of α-ketoglutarate. Accordingly, the γ-glutamyl cycle can continue to operate despite defective hydrolysis of pyroglutamic acid, so long as there is a fresh supply of glutamic acid for the resynthesis of glutathione.

UREA CYCLE

Catabolism of amino acids results in the production of free ammonia, which is highly toxic to the brain. Ammonia is catabolized further to urea by a series of reactions known as the Krebs-Henseleit or urea cycle (Fig. 8–8). Defects are now known for each of the five enzymes of the urea cycle. In each instance the affected persons exhibit mental retardation, presumably resulting from intoxication with ammonia. In some instances a deficiency of an enzyme in the urea cycle has been directly demon-

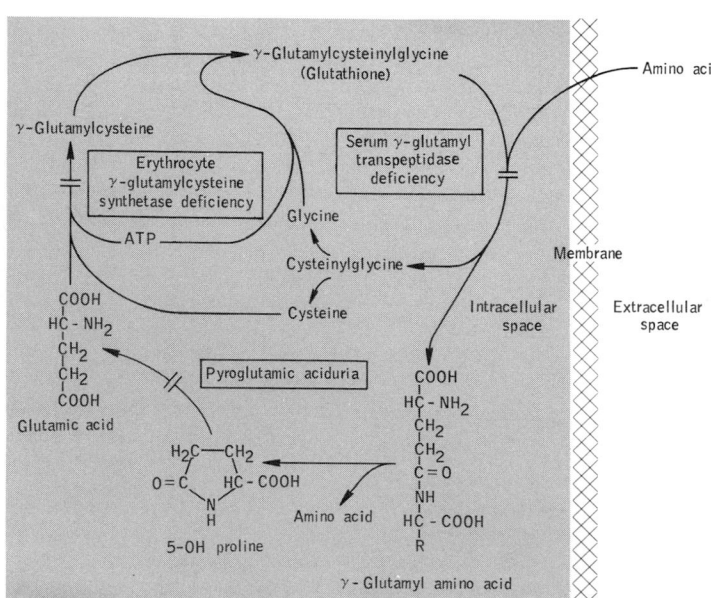

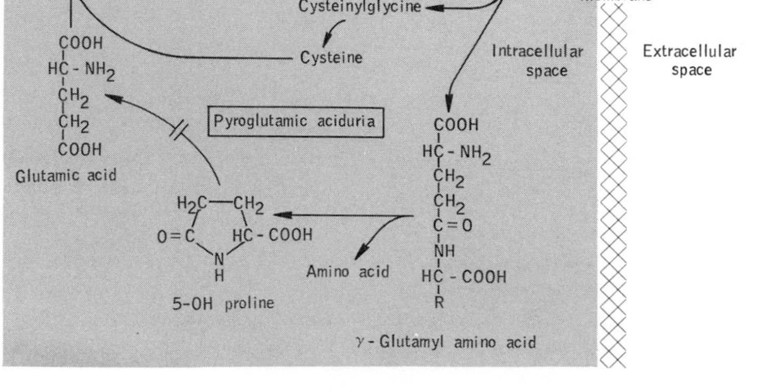

Figure 8–7 The γ-glutamyl cycle for nonspecific amino acid transport in kidney and intestine. Defects of glutathione synthesis and degradation found in plasma or erythrocytes are indicated.

strated in biopsy material; in other instances the defect in urea synthesis is only postulated. Since most patients with defects of the urea cycle excrete normal amounts of urea, it is presumed that the defect is either not present in all tissues or that other pathways exist for synthesis of urea. A new pathway for urea synthesis involving guanidosuccinic acid has been postulated recently, based upon the finding of this acid in the urine of patients with uremia.

Treatment consists of lowering the dietary protein intake. An infant with argininosuccinase deficiency with protein intake restricted to 1.5 gm/kg/day for two years has so far developed normally.

CARBAMYL PHOSPHATE SYNTHETASE DEFICIENCY. At least three children have demonstrated a defect in the initial step of urea synthesis. The patient described in the original investigation of hyperammonemia of this type died at 5 months of age after a stormy course that was aggravated by protein feeding. With restriction of dietary protein, the patient improved neurologically and blood ammonia levels became normal, but there were glycinemia, neutropenia and, terminally, acidosis. A second patient appeared normal at birth, but developed irritability, rigidity and hyperammonemia after protein feeding had begun, and died on the third day of life. Another died at 7½ months of age with a history of lethargy, convulsions and papilledema. Some patients with proven propionic acidemia and nonketotic glycinemia (see above) also have hyperammonemia.

ORNITHINE TRANSCARBAMYLASE DEFICIENCY. About a dozen patients have been described with this disorder of urea synthesis. All have had hyperammonemia. One died in the newborn period. Most of the others experienced severe vomiting, coma, and either retardation or seizures. Some excreted increased amounts of orotic acid (q.v.), presumably as a result of the accumulation of excess carbamyl phosphate and shunting of this compound into the pyrimidine biosynthesis pathway. In some instances the level of the enzyme ornithine transcarbamylase was reduced to less than 10 per cent of normal. In other cases the reduction in enzyme activity was much less severe. In one instance the total activity was not severely reduced, but it was shown that the K_m of the mutant enzyme for the substrate carbamyl phosphate was four times normal; accordingly, the affinity for this compound was much less than that of the normal enzyme. The affinity for the other substrate, ornithine, was normal. It is apparent, therefore, that ornithine transcarbamylase deficiencies are a heterogeneous genetic group. Despite the enzymatic heterogeneity, it would appear that this disorder follows X-linked inheritance and is lethal for males in the newborn period. Nearly all surviving the neonatal period have been female. No fa-

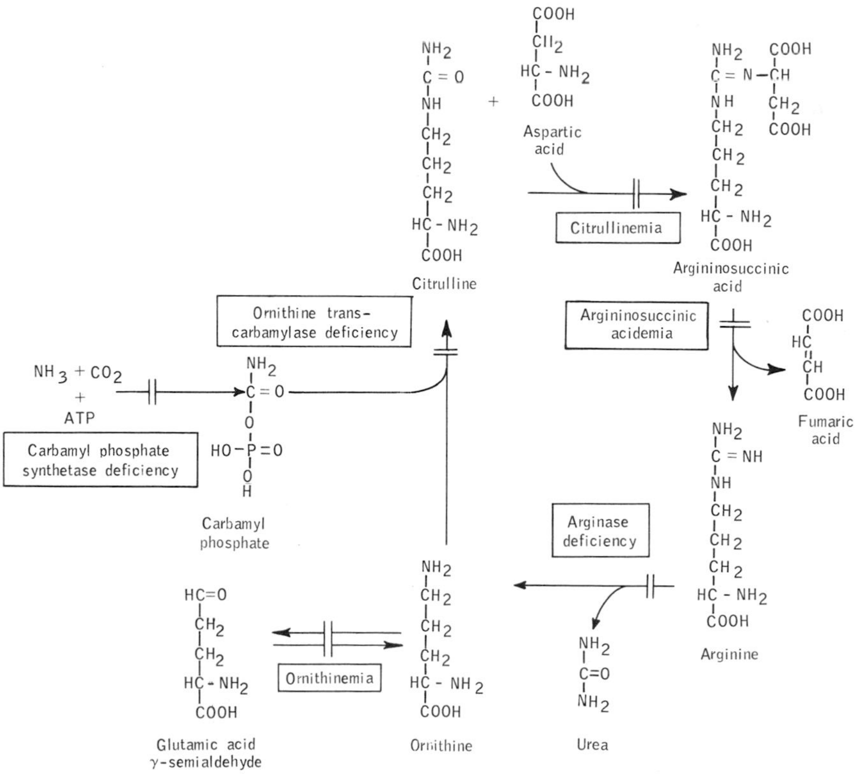

Figure 8–8 Pathways in the metabolism of ammonia and in the urea cycle. See also legend for Figure 8–1.

ther has transmitted the disorder, whereas some mothers of affected female patients have reduced enzyme activity and aversion to high protein foods.

CITRULLINEMIA (ARGININOSUCCINIC ACID SYNTHETASE DEFICIENCY). In the seven cases of this disorder which have been reported, there has been considerable biochemical and genetic heterogeneity. Mental retardation seems to be a constant feature. Some patients have hyperammonemia, others do not. The latter include an infant girl who died at 7 days of age and an adult male who is in apparently good health at 33 years of age. In most of the patients there is a virtual absence of argininosuccinic acid synthetase activity; in others the affinity of a mutant enzyme toward citrulline is reduced 25-fold. It has been suggested that in those cases without ammonia elevation citrulline is itself toxic to brain metabolism. Treatment with low protein diets seem efficacious in the mild form of the disorder.

ARGININOSUCCINASE DEFICIENCY (ARGININOSUCCINIC ACIDEMIA). About two dozen instances of this disorder have been reported, with hyperammonemia in some. Affected children have argininosuccinic acidemia and aciduria and have usually been mentally retarded; some have had abnormally friable hair (trichorrhexis nodosa). Not all patients with this type of hair abnormality, however, have argininosuccinic acidemia. The defect is in argininosuccinase, the enzyme which splits argininosuccinic acid to arginine and fumaric acid. The defect can be demonstrated in erythrocytes; heterozygotes have lower than normal activity. The disorder is transmitted as an autosomal recessive. Levels of argininosuccinic acid are higher in the cerebrospinal fluid than in the blood; concentrations of urea in the blood and urine are normal. The defect in the urea cycle in these patients may be limited to the brain. It has been postulated that there are two forms of the disorder: one with early onset, in which case failure to thrive and vomiting are noted in the first few months of life; and a second with the late onset, in which case developmental failure, seizures and ataxia are observed after a year of age.

ARGINASE DEFICIENCY (ARGININEMIA). Two sisters with hyperammonemia, spastic dysplegia, seizures and severe mental retardation have been found to have deficient arginase activity in erythrocytes. Their parents had lower than normal activity, and are probably heterozygous. Their hyperammonemia and increased urinary excretion of other dibasic amino acids such as lysine and cystine disappeared on a low protein diet (1.5 gm/kg/day). Argininemia, however, persisted.

ORNITHINEMIA. Three mentally retarded patients are known with this finding. One had hyperammonemia and homocitrullinuria and responded well to a low protein diet. The defect in this patient remains unknown. The other two patients did not exhibit hyperammonemia, but had liver disease; a defect was found in the liver enzyme ornithine transaminase, which equilibrates ornithine and glutamic acid semialdehyde.

HISTIDINE

HISTIDINEMIA. In histidinemia the activity of the enzyme histidase, which normally converts histidine to urocanic acid, is deficient in liver and skin. As a result, histidine is transaminated to imidazolepyruvic acid, which appears in the urine along with excessive amounts of histidine (Fig. 8–9). Imidazolepyruvic acid, like phenylpyruvic acid, reacts with ferric chloride to produce a blue-green color. Many patients with histidinemia have been detected in screening tests for phenylketonuria, and some cases have been misdiagnosed as such. Demonstration of elevation in plasma levels of histidine is necessary for the correct diagnosis of this disorder, and a definitive diagnosis depends on measuring histidase activity of cornified epithelium or of liver.

Some affected persons have had impaired speech, a few were retarded in growth, and some were mentally retarded. The relation of these defects to histidinemia is unknown inasmuch as routine amino acid screening has uncovered a significant number of asymptomatic persons with histidinemia. The metabolic defect is transmitted as an autosomal recessive character; in some families the heterozygous state can be identified by demonstration of decreased histidase activity in skin.

There is some evidence for genetic heterogeneity in histidinemia. In some but not in all affected children plasma levels of alanine as well as of histidine were elevated. The reason for this association is unknown. In some families with histidinemia the level of histidase in skin is normal, and perhaps the defect in enzymatic activity is limited to the liver.

Affected neonates do not excrete imidazole derivatives of histidine because there is a normal delay in the maturation of histidine transaminase.

HISTIDINE AND FOLIC ACID METABOLISM. After histidine has been converted to urocanic acid it is further metabolized to formiminoglutamic acid (FIGLU). The formimino group of this compound is normally transferred to folic acid, with the concomitant production of glutamic acid (Fig. 8–9). Measurement of the urinary excretion of FIGLU after loading with histidine has been used as a method for the detection of folic acid deficiency states. Both FIGLU and urocanic acid are excreted by patients with megaloblastic anemia. Urocanic acid is found in the urine of children with kwashiorkor.

A group of mentally retarded infants have been described in Japan who have defects in folic acid metabolism. Microcephaly and electroencephalographic abnormalities were frequent findings. Three distinct defects have been delineated, in

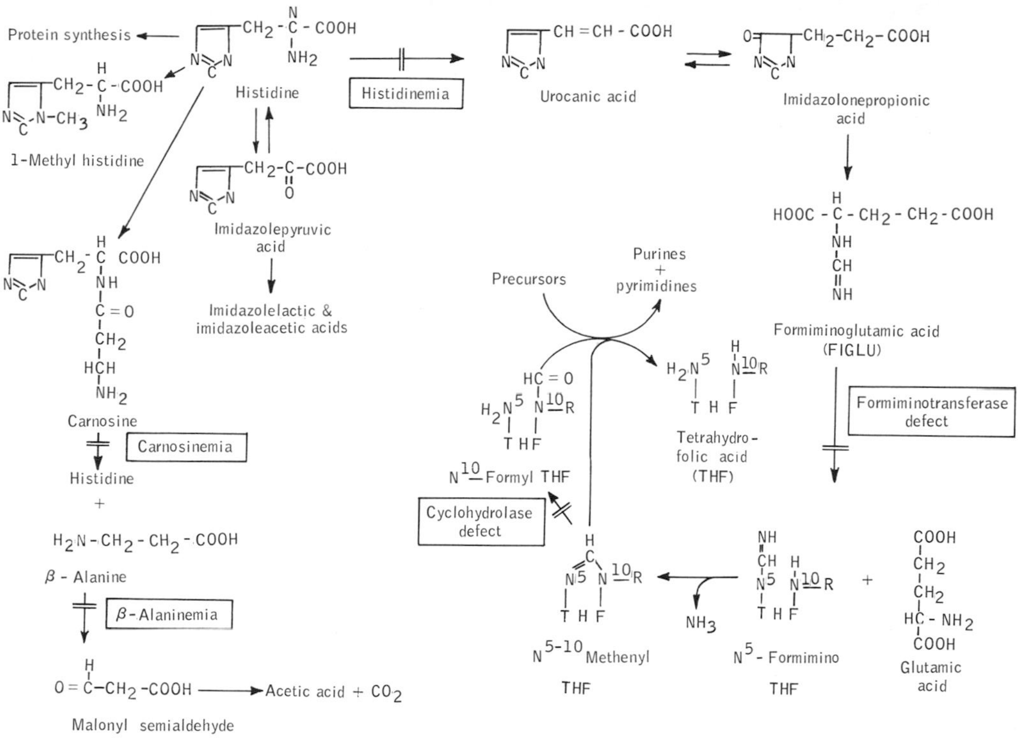

Figure 8–9 *Pathways in the metabolism of histidine, beta amino acids and folic acid. See also legend for Figure 8–1. (THF is an abbreviation for tetrahydrofolic acid.)*

each of which the blood values of folic acid are elevated. In the first, formiminoglutamic acid is increased after administration of histidine; the enzyme formiminotransferase is deficient. In the second disorder FIGLU is not excreted even after an oral load of histidine; the defect is in the enzyme cyclohydrolase. The third disorder is further down the metabolic pathway and involves a defect in the enzyme which normally transfers the methyl group of ^{5}N-methyltetrahydrofolate to homocysteine, forming methionine (Fig. 8–2 and text).

HISTIDINURIA. The urinary excretion of histidine normally increases in pregnant women. Histidinuria occurs as an overflow phenomenon in patients with histidinemia. Isolated histidinuria without histidinemia, owing to defective renal tubular reabsorption, has been found in a 15 year old boy whose parents and siblings were shown to be heterozygous for the defect.

DIPEPTIDES OF HISTIDINE. Carnosine (β-alanyl-histidine) and anserine (β-alanyl-1-methyl histidine) are dipeptides of histidine found in muscle, where their function is unknown. These peptides, as well as 1-methyl histidine derived from anserine, have been found in urine of normal persons, particularly after the ingestion of large amounts of turkey and chicken. In the disorders described below, the findings of the dipeptides of histidine in urine have been specific and independent of dietary intake.

IMIDAZOLE ACIDURIA. Excessive excretion of carnosine, anserine and occasionally of homocarnosine (γ-amino butyryl histidine), as well as of histidine and 1-methyl histidine, has been reported in a number of patients with a form of cerebromacular degeneration resembling juvenile Tay-Sachs disease. The use of labeled histidine provided some evidence for increased synthesis of the dipeptides. The genetic basis of the disorder is not clear; in the 3 families studied the cerebromacular degeneration was inherited on a recessive basis, whereas the histidine peptiduria appeared to be transmitted on a dominant one. Isolated increased excretion of 1-methyl histidine without 1-methyl histidinemia has been reported in three male siblings with precocious puberty who had no other clinical abnormality.

CARNOSINEMIA. Two unrelated children with severe mental retardation and myoclonic seizures have been found who excreted large amounts of carnosine. One child had persistent carnosinemia on a dietary regimen free of carnosine; both had a tenfold increase of homocarnosine in cerebrospinal fluid. The defect is in the enzyme carnosinase, which normally hydrolyzes carnosine to histidine and β-alanine and can be assayed in plasma. The disorder appears to be inherited as an autosomal recessive. A third patient has no detectable carnosine in plasma, low levels of carnosinase activity and similar clinical findings.

BETA AMINO ACIDS

BETA-ALANINEMIA. An infant with lethargy, somnolence and grand mal seizures who died at 5 months of age was found to have persistent β-alaninemia, at a concentration two to four times that of normal. Beta-alanine is derived from the hydrolysis of certain dipeptides and by the degradation of uracil. It is normally further metabolized by transamination to malonic acid, then to acetate and carbon dioxide. Preliminary evidence suggests a block in the transamination of this compound. Two interesting features of the disorder are the increased concentrations of β-aminoisobutyric acid and taurine as well as of β-alanine in urine. These findings have been used in support of the concept of a common renal transport mechanism for the β-amino acids. The affected child also had increased concentration of γ-aminobutyric acid in cerebral spinal fluid, plasma, and urine. The neurologic symptoms have been attributed to the increase in β-alanine and the decrease in γ-aminobutyric acid within the brain. Abnormal urinary excretion of β-alanine and β-aminoisobutyrate has been reported in a 3 year old girl with brittle hair. What appears to be an isolated transport defect for β-alanine has been reported in a 16 year old girl with physical and mental retardation.

BETA-AMINOISOBUTYRIC ACIDURIA. Excessive excretion of β-aminoisobutyric acid (BAIB) is a genetic variant in metabolism in a small percentage of the population; there are racial and geographic variations in incidence. In addition, β-aminoisobutyric aciduria occurs in a variety of illnesses in which there is tissue destruction and deoxyribonucleic acid is catabolized excessively. Beta-aminoisobutyric acid is a normal metabolite of both valine and thymine. Normal persons fed large amounts of β-aminoisobutyric acid have the ability to excrete it rapidly, which indicates that the renal tubular excretion of this compound is an adaptive process secondary to an increased plasma level. In any case, increased excretion of β-aminoisobutyric acid is not evidence of a renal tubular defect, since reabsorption in the tubules does not occur.

Affected persons with the congenital form are asymptomatic; they excrete 100 to 300 mg of β-aminoisobutyric acid daily in contrast to 10 to 40 mg in other persons. The condition is transmitted by a single recessive gene.

LYSINE

Lysine is an essential amino acid which shares a common renal transport mechanism with other dibasic amino acids. Lysinuria has been observed in some children with malnutrition. There are at least three enzymopathies in which elevations of plasma lysine occur.

LYSINEMIA. Persistent lysinemia and lysinuria have been observed in 6 children studied by three groups of investigators. One group studied 2 siblings who had severe mental retardation and muscle weakness. Another group studied 3 children (2 siblings and a third cousin) with even higher plasma lysine levels than in the first cases, but only one of the siblings was retarded. The third group reported a child in whom mental retardation may have been coincidental, since the mother and some unaffected siblings were also mentally retarded. There is an unexplained difference in the findings of two of the groups: in 1 patient almost no labeled carbon dioxide appeared in expired air after administration of carbon-labeled lysine, whereas in another one oxidation to carbon dioxide was unimpaired. These observations suggest at least two different biochemical defects.

Study of these patients has added to knowledge of the pathway of lysine degradation in man (see Fig. 8–10). One of the main routes of catabolism appears to be the condensation of lysine with alpha-ketoglutaric acid to form a compound known as saccharopine. In three patients with lysinemia, studies of cultured fibroblasts revealed marked reductions of activity of lysine ketoglutarate reductase, the enzyme which converts lysine to saccharopine. Minor pathways for lysine degradation have been shown; homocitrulline and homoarginine, ϵ-N-acetyl-L-lysine and alpha-N-acetyl-L-lysine are formed and excreted.

A seventh patient with this disorder was discovered in infancy as a result of routine screening. The diagnosis was confirmed by assay of lysine ketoglutarate reductase activity. He was treated with a low lysine diet, and at 15 months of age was clinically normal. It cannot be stated that dietary treatment prevented mental retardation, since it was mental retardation that brought the 6 other known cases to the attention of investigators, the lysinemia perhaps being coincidental. Moreover, the enzymatic defect has been found also in two nonretarded relatives of a mentally retarded propositus.

SACCHAROPINEMIA. A short, mentally retarded woman has been described who had lysinuria, citrullinuria, homocitrullinemia and saccharopinuria. These compounds were also elevated in the serum, and saccharopine was found in high concentrations in cerebrospinal fluid. A 3½ year old girl has also been described with saccharopinemia and saccharopinuria, who was slightly retarded and had spastic diplegia. At 4½ years of age this patient had 50 per cent of normal activity of the enzyme aminoadipic semialdehyde-glutamate reductase in fibroblasts and in muscle. This enzyme is responsible for the further catabolism of saccharopine (Fig. 8–10).

GLUTARIC ACIDEMIA. Glutaric acid is an intermediate in the degradation of lysine (Fig. 8–10), hydroxylysine and tryptophan (Fig. 8–3). Two siblings with chronic metabolic acidosis and glutaric acidemia and aciduria were neurologically normal in infancy, but later deteriorated, with

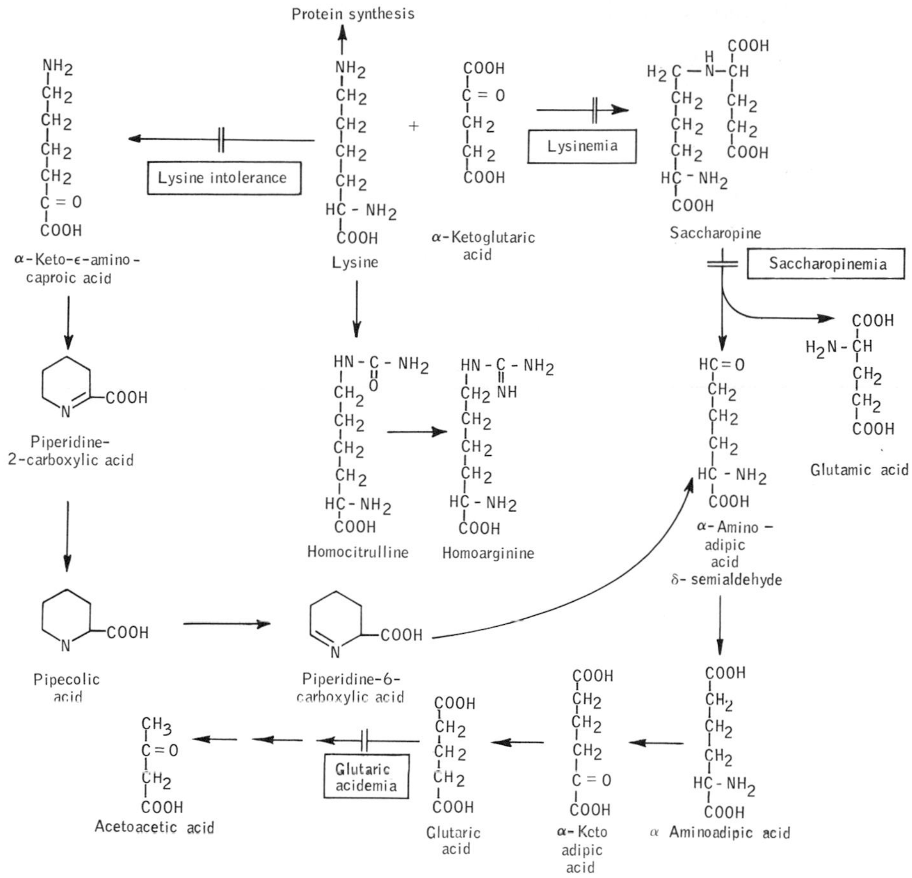

Figure 8–10 *Pathways in the metabolism of lysine. See also legend for Figure 8–1.*

opisthotonus and posturing. Administration of lysine increased and lowering the protein intake reduced glutaric acid excretion. An enzymatic defect could not be demonstrated in leukocytes.

CONGENITAL LYSINE INTOLERANCE. This disorder was first observed in a 3 month old infant who had episodes of ammonia intoxication. With normal intake of protein, blood levels of lysine and arginine were normal, but when the protein intake was raised to 2.5 to 3 gm/kg/day, plasma lysine, arginine and ammonia levels increased to at least double their control values. The increases in arginine and ammonia were thought to be due to inhibition of arginase by lysine, with consequent inability to detoxify ammonia by the formation of urea. The administration of lysine orally depressed erythrocyte arginase activity and led to an increase of blood ammonia to 680 μg/dl, and coma. There was a diminution in the activity of lysine dehydrogenase in liver; this enzyme converts lysine to alpha-keto-ε-aminocaproic acid (Fig. 8–10).

A second case has been reported. A 3 year old child, who was spastic at birth and had frequent seizures, was found to have slight hyperammonemia and lysine intolerance. During a lysine load, blood arginine also rose dramatically.

The experience with lysinemia, saccharopinemia and lysine intolerance serves to point out how the study of inborn errors of metabolism contributes to knowledge of normal biochemical pathways. It was the studies of patients with these rare disorders that led to our present knowledge of the enzymatic steps involved in lysine metabolism.

LYSINURIA (HYPERDIBASICAMINOACIDURIA). Lysine is a dibasic amino acid excreted in large amounts in cystinuria (q.v., this Section). Lysinuria also occurs without cystinuria in a number of other disorders. One set of patients with dibasicaciduria had severe mental and physical retardation with malabsorption of lysine, arginine and ornithine, both by intestinal villi and by renal tubules; all three amino acids were excreted in the urine in large amounts and the blood levels of all three were below normal. Another patient and 12 of his relatives had increased excretion of lysine, arginine and ornithine, but normal plasma levels. The propositus was short and had mild malabsorption, but these findings were thought to be incidental to the renal defect. In yet a third form of dibasicaciduria, only lysine and arginine were excreted in abnormal amounts, the serum levels of these amino acids being below normal; the patient was mentally and physically retarded and had severe hyperammonemia.

FAMILIAL PROTEIN INTOLERANCE. This disorder, which has been studied in 20 Finnish patients, has much in common with one or more types of lysinuria described above. The patients have an aversion to protein-rich foods, excrete large amounts of lysine and arginine, have physical but not mental retardation and low circulating levels of arginine, lysine, ornithine and glutamine, with high values of glutamate, alanine and citrulline. Most of the patients exhibited hyperammonemia at one time or another, particularly after high protein intake. Hepatomegaly and periods of diarrhea and vomiting have been noted in infancy. The hyperammonemia, which has been treated by the administration of arginine or ornithine, was not due to any demonstrable deficiency of enzymes of the urea cycle. It has been suggested that the defect may lie in the ability of the liver to transport urea cycle substances to the site of urea synthesis.

HYDROXYLYSINEMIA. At least 8 patients with a variety of symptoms (two had trisomy-21) have been reported with hydroxylysinuria. As hydroxylysine is usually not detectable in plasma, the small amount found in the plasma of these patients indicates that the defect is not one of renal absorption. The nature of the defect, presumably in the degradation of free hydroxylysine, is not yet known.

HYDROXYLYSINE DEFICIENT COLLAGEN. Three patients with the clinical appearance of Ehlers-Danlos syndrome (q.v.) have been shown to have collagen with an abnormally low hydroxylysine content. Two patients exhibited severe scoliosis, joint laxity, hyperextensible skin and thin scars. The third patient had, in addition, clubbed feet, retinal detachments, peptic ulcer and hiatal hernia. The latter patient had a brother with the same clinical disorder. Measurements of the activity of the enzyme lysyl-protocollagen hydroxylase in cultured fibroblasts from the first two patients revealed approximately one eighth of the normal value. There was a partial defect in the activity in one of the parents, indicating that the defect is inherited as an autosomal recessive character.

In another form of Ehlers-Danlos syndrome, the defect is of the enzyme procollagen peptidase.

DEFECTS IN METABOLISM OF CARBOHYDRATES

DEFECTS IN ABSORPTION OF CARBOHYDRATES

A variety of syndromes in infants and children are characterized by defective intestinal absorption and hydrolysis of monosaccharides and disaccharides. Affected patients have diarrhea as a presenting symptom. Absorption of monosaccharides and disaccharides takes place in the small intestine, and digestion of disaccharides involves at least two steps: absorption into the mucosal cells and splitting within the cells. Glucose, galactose and perhaps lactose are absorbed against a concentration gradient (active transport), apparently sharing the same mechanism. Fructose and probably sucrose are absorbed by passive diffusion.

Hydrolysis of the disaccharides occurs within the mucosal cells, and the resultant monosaccharides are released into the circulation. Lactase (beta-galactosidase) is responsible for the hydrolysis of lactose to glucose and galactose. Sucrase (invertase) hydrolyzes sucrose to glucose and fructose and also splits maltose into two glucose molecules, but at a slower rate. Isomaltase splits isomaltose and other 1–6 linked glucose residues; isomaltase also has some activity against maltose. In addition to these enzymes, the intestinal mucosa contains maltases which are specific for the disaccharide maltose.

Lactase is usually present in the intestine during infancy. Lactase deficiency occurs as a genetic defect, leading to lactose malabsorption (Section 11). Persons not genetically lactose intolerant who do not regularly ingest lactose will become physiologically lactose intolerant until they adapt to new regular feedings of lactose by producing the enzyme in their intestinal mucosa. Persistence of lactase activity after weaning or into adult life depends also upon the genetic and racial background of the child. Among Caucasians the enzyme tends to persist, so long as the individual continues to ingest lactose. On the other hand, most Orientals and Africans do not have an adult form of the enzyme. They are, therefore, lactose intolerant as adults even if persistently challenged with lactose. With lactose intolerance, the bacterial oxidation of lactose in the lower intestine produces acid, flatulence and diarrhea. *Lactosuria* may follow heavy ingestion of the disaccharide.

Sucrosuria is also a common finding in normal adults and children after a sucrose load. Severe diarrhea in children may lead to inability to hydrolyze disaccharides, which in turn prolongs the diarrhea if disaccharides are ingested.

A number of conditions are described (Section 11) in which inability to absorb or hydrolyze monosaccharides or disaccharides is due to abnormal genes. In lactose intolerance due to an inborn error of metabolism, the pathogenesis and symptomatology are the same as in lactose intolerant adults who had the enzyme during infancy but do not have any enzyme activity as adults. The consequences for the infant, however, are much more severe. Treatment for this and the other conditions always consists in removal of the offending carbohydrate from the diet.

DEFECTS IN MONOSACCHARIDE METABOLISM

The most common clinical disorder involving monosaccharides is diabetes mellitus. (See Section 16.)

DEFECTIVE PENTOSE METABOLISM. The pentose D-ribose is a constituent of many coenzymes and of ribonucleic acid; deoxyribose is a constituent of deoxyribonucleic acid. These pentoses are not derived directly from dietary sources, but are synthesized as needed from glucose via the pentose-phosphate pathway. Pentoses are absorbed slowly from the intestine, and renal tubular reabsorption of filtered pentose is also poor. Normal persons excrete up to 100 mg of pentose per day in the urine, and twice this amount when the intake of pentose-containing fruits is excessive. In such instances the urinary pentoses are xylose and arabinose.

Scurvy. The formation of ascorbic acid from gulonic acid requires a highly specific enzymatic transformation. Most species have this ability and are able to synthesize ascorbic acid (vitamin C). On the other hand, man, some monkeys, the guinea pig, the Indian fruit bat and the red-vented bulbul have a defect in this enzyme system and require exogenous vitamin C to prevent death from scurvy. It is appropriate to think of scurvy as an inborn error of monosaccharide metabolism which is limited to certain species. The administration of vitamin C to prevent this disorder exemplifies the ease with which certain enzymatic defects can be circumvented.

Essential Benign Pentosuria (L-Xylulosuria). This rare anomaly, transmitted as an autosomal recessive trait, is characterized by excessive excretion of L-xylulose (1 to 4 gm/day), regardless of diet. Found almost exclusively in Jewish families, it has an incidence of about one in 50,000. Most cases are not detected until adult life, but it has been found in a 19 month old infant. The heterozygous carrier can be detected by measurements of L-xylulose in serum or urine after the oral administration of D-glucuronolactone. Homozygous persons with pentosuria, unlike normal persons, cannot convert L-xylulose to xylitol, and thence back to glucose, owing to a defect of the enzyme NADP-linked xylitol dehydrogenase. Erythrocytes from pentosuric individuals have two xylitol dehydrogenases (NAD- and NADP-linked), the latter so altered genetically that its affinity for the cofactor NADP is one tenth to one twentieth of normal. The defect is in the same metabolic pathway as the one leading to scurvy.

L-Xylulosuria is usually harmless and symptomless. It is ordinarily discovered by urinalysis. Because L-xylulose reduces Benedict's and Fehling's solutions, it may be confused with glucose in urine. It does not react with glucose oxidase.

ESSENTIAL (BENIGN) FRUCTOSURIA. This rare and benign defect results from an inability to metabolize fructose (levulose). Fructose occurs as a monosaccharide in many fruits and vegetables and in honey. It is also derived from the intestinal hydrolysis of sucrose and of complex polysaccharides in certain vegetables.

Patients with the defect excrete from 10 to 20 per cent of ingested fructose in urine. Inherited as a recessive trait, essential fructosuria occurs in less than one in 100,000 persons. The defect resides in fructokinase, which normally converts fructose to fructose-1-phosphate (see Fig. 8–11, *B*).

Fructose reduces Benedict's and Fehling's solutions, but does not react with glucose oxidase. Other causes of fructosuria must be eliminated before it can be designated as genetic in origin. In acquired hepatic disorders with severe cellular damage such as infectious hepatitis, cirrhosis and syphilitic hepatitis, fructose is occasionally found in the urine. Since the loss of dietary fructose in the urine is apparently harmless, dietary restriction is not indicated.

FRUCTOSEMIA (FRUCTOSE INTOLERANCE). Absence of the activity of the hepatic enzyme fructose-1-phosphate aldolase occurs in patients with hereditary fructose intolerance. Effects include fructosemia and hypoglucosemia (Section 16). High doses of folic acid have recently shown promise as therapy. The disorder has variants. A patient with typical clinical fructosemia has no demonstrable defect of hepatic activity of either fructose-1-phosphate or fructose-1, 6-diphosphate aldolase. It may be that this patient's defect involves fructose-1, 6-diphosphatase (see below).

FRUCTOSE-GALACTOSE INTOLERANCE. An adult with a neurologic disorder has been reported who had hypoglycemia after oral challenge by either fructose or galactose. The precise defect is not known.

FRUCTOSE-1,6-DIPHOSPHATASE DEFICIENCY. Six patients with symptoms of severe fasting hypoglycemia, hepatomegaly and lactic acidosis have a defect in the liver enzyme fructose-1,6-diphosphatase, which hydrolyzes fructose-1,6-diphosphate to fructose-6-phosphate and phosphate. This step is one of the reactions unique to the process of gluconeogenesis. No activity for the phosphatase was found in hepatic tissue or in leukocytes. Most but not all the patients became hypoglycemic after the administration of fructose. Dietary restriction of fructose and fructose-containing sugars seems to be efficacious. Two patients have been successfully treated with large doses of folate, presumably owing to induction of the phosphatase by folate. It is important that this cause of hypoglycemia and acidosis be recognized

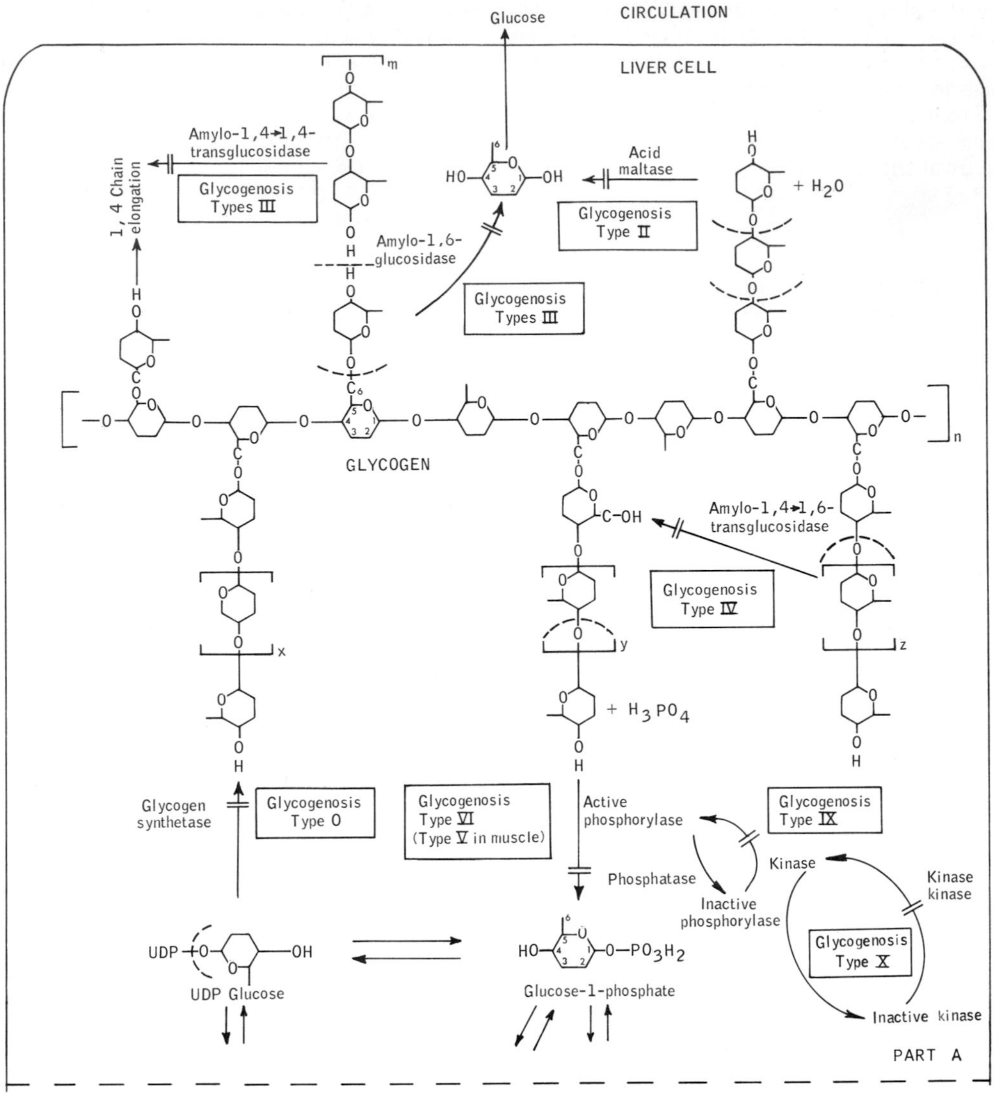

A

Figure 8–11 A *Pathways in the metabolism of glycogen. Stereospecificity of bonds and correct lengths of chains are not shown.*

Illustration continued on opposite page.

early; some untreated children with proven fructose-1,6-diphosphatase deficiency have died in the first year of life.

GALACTOSE

Abnormal elevations of the concentration of galactose in blood result from defects in its metabolism. Two different enzymatic defects are known to produce galactosemia, each with distinct clinical manifestations. In the more common form there is almost complete deficiency of galactose-1-phosphate uridyl transferase activity, the untreated disorder leading to death in infancy or to mental retardation in those who survive. The other disorder, in which there is a deficiency of galactokinase, is rare and, in contrast, relatively benign, being characterized clinically only by the presence of cataracts. Patients with the transferase defect have been further classified into several subtypes, depending largely upon the degree of enzymatic deficiency and the tissues involved. Each of the defects and variants represents a distinct genotype, and each is inherited in an autosomal recessive manner.

GALACTOSEMIA: TRANSFERASE DEFECT. When galactose is absorbed, it is phosphorylated in the tissues to galactose-1-phosphate. This compound reacts with uridine diphosphoglucose (UDPGlu) in the presence of the enzyme galactose-1-phosphate uridyl transferase to form uridine diphosphogalactose (UDPGal); glucose-1-phosphate is liberated. The UDPGal is then converted directly to UDPGlu by an epimerase; the new UDPGlu may again liberate glucose-1-phosphate on reaction with another molecule of galactose-1-phosphate (see Fig. 8–11, *B*). The transferase is normally found in liver,

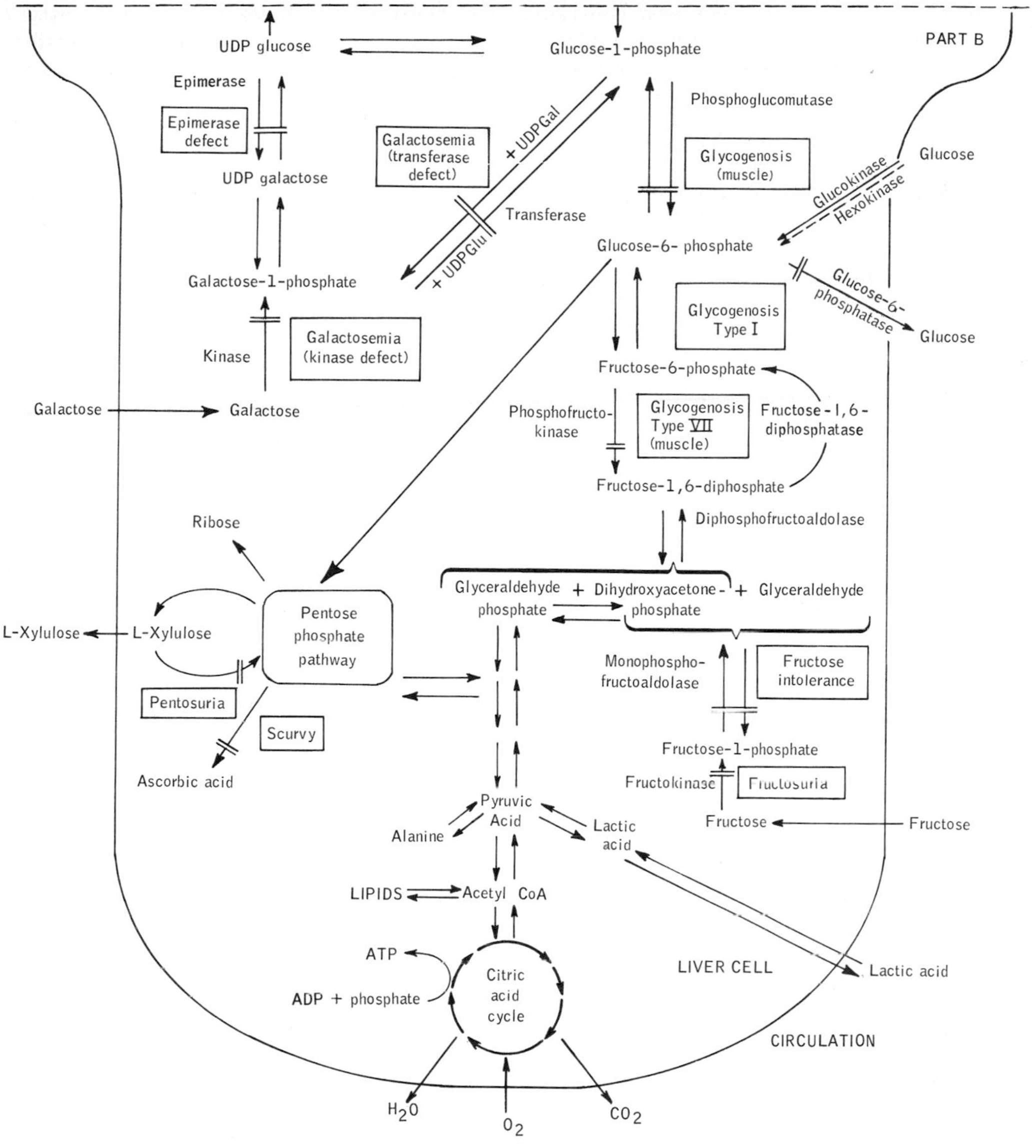

B

Figure 8–11 B *Pathways in the metabolism of hexoses and pentoses. See also legend for Figure 8–1.*

leukocytes and erythrocytes. If the enzyme activity is absent, galactosemia results. Sufficiently sensitive enzyme assays have been devised to allow not only for diagnosis of the homozygote, but also for the accurate detection of the heterozygote. The clinically normal heterozygote has approximately half of normal transferase activity.

Clinical Manifestations. Infants appear normal at birth, but in most instances symptoms appear soon after milk feedings have been instituted. Listlessness, feeding difficulties, vomiting and weight loss are the earliest manifestations. Jaundice is common and may seem to be a prolongation of the neonatal physiologic jaundice; this symptom is caused by early hepatic damage or interference with glucuronidation of bilirubin. Hepatomegaly and occasionally splenomegaly appear early in the untreated patient and may be accompanied by signs of portal obstruction; lenticular cataracts may appear about the same time. With the onset of hepatic failure, hemorrhages, due to prothrombin deficiency, occur in skin and mucous membranes, and generalized edema and ascites may develop. Hypoglycemic symptoms may result from the low blood glucose levels even in the presence of normal or elevated *total* blood sugar concentrations. The symptoms progress rapidly to emaciation, hypotonia and death from infection or severe hepatic failure.

Occasionally the manifestations of galactosemia evolve more slowly and are milder, and the diagnosis may not be suspected until later infancy or even early childhood. The presence of hepatomegaly and retarded physical and mental development, particularly in association with cataracts, should suggest the diagnosis. A significant degree of mental retardation occurs in most infants when diagnosis is delayed beyond the first month of life.

Laboratory Data. Galactosuria is a constant finding when milk is fed; it rapidly disappears, however, when milk feedings are replaced by oral or parenteral administration of glucose solution. Galactose will reduce copper (Fehling's or Benedict's solution), but will not be detected by Testape or Clinistix, each of which is impregnated with glucose oxidase and reacts specifically with glucose.

There is generalized aminoaciduria resulting from damaged tubular reabsorption. Cystathioninuria may occur secondarily to the hepatic disease. Proteinuria is present in all untreated infants and may amount to 1 gm per day. These findings are the result of the toxic effects of galactose-1-phosphate upon the kidney and disappear when galactose is removed from the diet.

Hepatic involvement is manifest by elevated levels of bilirubin and alkaline phosphatase, prolonged prothrombin time and positive cephalin flocculation test results. Blood levels of galactose are elevated, and galactose tolerance test results are abnormal. Galactose loading may result in sudden depression of glucose concentration and produce clinical manifestations of hypoglycemia. For this reason and because more specific diagnostic tests are available, galactose tolerance tests should not be performed.

The definitive diagnosis of galactosemia can be made by measurements of the specific enzyme in erythrocytes.

Treatment. Withdrawal of milk from the diet and substitution of a galactose-free diet result in cessation of galactosemia and galactosuria and, when done early in the clinical course, in disappearance of the abnormal clinical findings. Cataracts which persist require surgical treatment. The small quantities of galactose (less than 0.1 per cent) present in milk substitutes made with casein hydrolysates do not raise the blood galactose level high enough to cause galactosuria and are well tolerated by affected infants. Strict avoidance of milk, milk products containing galactose and such unsuspected sources as lactose-containing tablets and prepared dessert foods is essential. Galactose is an essential component of many brain lipids. Biosynthesis of these galactolipids uses UDPGal, which the body can make as needed from UDPGlu through the action of epimerase, even when the diet contains no galactose. Absence of transferase is irrelevant to this synthesis.

Dietary lapse should be suspected as a cause of an illness in a treated infant, especially if hepatomegaly or jaundice develops. In the absence of galactosuria, aminoaciduria is a sensitive indicator of the presence of galactose in the diet.

Two galactosemic women, one under dietary control, the other not, have delivered healthy infants. Both were black (see below).

TRANSFERASE VARIANTS. Most patients with the classic form of galactosemia cannot metabolize galactose to carbon dioxide, as demonstrated by administration of labeled galactose. A few patients, however, can metabolize galactose to a limited degree; they have clinical manifestations of galactosemia and proved absence of transferase activity in erythrocytes. All such patients thus far studied have been black, and they have an anomalous distribution of enzyme activity, the liver containing about 10 per cent of the normal transferase activity, though there is none in the red blood cells. This situation is in contrast to the usual one, in which the enzyme is inactive in all tissues. Some untreated black infants with absent erythrocyte transferase activity have mild clinical manifestations or none at all.

In another variant of the transferase defect the affected person is usually asymptomatic. In such persons the defect is in the same enzyme, but at a different locus. The defect was discovered during a population survey designed to determine the gene frequency of the classic form of galactosemia. The *Duarte variant,* as it is known, is characterized by a reduction of erythrocyte transferase activity to 75 per cent of normal in heterozygous persons, and consequently to 50 per cent of normal activity in persons who are homozygous for this variant gene. Persons who are heterozygous for both the classic and Duarte variants have also been detected.

Another transferase variant involves an unstable enzyme with different electrophoretic properties from the normal or Duarte enzymes. The patient presented clinically with a classic galactosemia of the transferase type.

GALACTOSEMIA: GALACTOKINASE DEFECT. A patient was described in the 1930's as having "galactose diabetes." Recent reinvestigation of this patient and observations on several new patients have revealed a deficiency of galactokinase, the enzyme responsible for the initial phosphorylation of galactose. The disease is characterized by galactosemia, galactosuria and cataracts, without mental retardation or aminoaciduria. One patient with galactokinase deficiency developed severe neurologic signs and symptoms at 17 years of age; the relationship to the enzymatic defect is unclear. In contrast to the transferase-deficient type of galactosemia in which both galactose-1-phosphate and dulcitol (galactitol) accumulate, in the kinase type of galactosemia only dulcitol accumulates. These observations and animal experiments suggest that the cataracts in both forms of galactosemia are caused by the abnormal accumulation of dulcitol, whereas damage to the developing brain and the renal tubules in the transferase-defect variety results from the accumulation of galactose-1-phosphate.

Galactokinase is also involved in racial polymorphism. The galactokinase activity of pregnant black women is lower than that of pregnant Caucasians, though there is significant overlap of values. Transferase activities in the two groups are virtually identical. A variant of galactokinase found in a clinically normal adult black woman had three times normal activity.

EPIMERASE DEFECT. One method for neonatal screening for galactosemia (transferase defect) depends on finding elevated blood levels of galactose-

1-phosphate. During such screening, a healthy infant was found with elevated galactose-1-phosphate levels who had no deficiency of transferase but less than 1 per cent of normal activity of UDP glucose–UDP galactose epimerase in erythrocytes. This genetic disorder seems to be without clinical consequences.

MISCELLANEOUS ASPECTS OF CARBOHYDRATE METABOLISM

BLOOD GROUP SUBSTANCES. The immunologic differences in blood groups are complicated. The distinguishing features of the ABO system depend on the structures of *glycoproteins,* which form the blood group substances within the red cell membrane and within body fluids. The differences in the glycoproteins are referable to the presence or absence of an N-acetylgalactosamine residue or a galactose residue. For example, in persons who have the A gene, N-acetylgalactosamine is combined with the basic "O" substance through the action of the specific enzyme N-acetyl-D-galactosaminyl-transferase. Persons who lack the A gene do not have this enzyme and have blood group B or O. Persons who carry the B gene (types AB or B) have the enzyme galactosyl transferase, which adds a galactose residue to the basic blood group glycoprotein to form B substance.

Persons who have blood type substance in soluble form in various body fluids, and particularly in saliva, are called "secretors." The quality of being a secretor resides in an enzyme, fucosyltransferase, which adds the monosaccharide fucose (6-deoxy-L-galactose) to the basic blood group glycoproteins of the ABO system. Those homozygous or heterozygous for this enzyme activity are "secretors." "Nonsecretors" cannot form fucosyltransferase. They have blood group substances only on the surface of their erythrocytes. The incidence of nonsecretors varies from about 40 per cent in American blacks to 25 per cent in Caucasians and to near zero in American Indians.

FUCOSIDOSIS (DEFICIENCY OF α-FUCOSIDASE). Absence or marked reduction in activity of the lysosomal enzyme α-fucosidase leads to storage of fucose-containing glycoproteins and glycolipids, and has been reported in 10 patients, in whom death usually occurred by 6 years of age. Their course has been characterized by frequent respiratory infections, hyperhidrosis, cardiomegaly, and hypotonia, followed by spastic quadriplegia and decerebrate rigidity. Some patients have presented a marked resemblance to Hurler syndrome. In the more severe cases, with early death, no α-fucosidase activity was found in liver, brain, lung, kidney, leukocytes or serum. The disorder is transmitted as an autosomal recessive. Leukocyte α-fucosidase activity currently appears to be the best index of the presence of the altered gene. Two variants of fucosidosis are known. In both, enzyme activity in cultured fibroblasts or leukocytes was 10 per cent of normal. One patient was a 20 year old mentally and physically retarded male with the cardinal sign of Fabry's disease, angiokeratoma corporis diffusum (q.v.), but his lysosomal α-galactosidase activity was normal. The other patient was a 9 year old boy with spondyloepiphyseal metaphyseal dysplasia and normal intelligence, who seemed to have a defect of α-fucosidase limited to bone. He had no other clinical manifestations of the disease.

MANNOSIDOSIS (DEFICIENT α-MANNOSIDASE ACTIVITY). In a boy who died at 4 years of age with signs and symptoms similar to those seen in Hurler syndrome, it was shown that the mannose content of tissue was abnormally high. The patient had had frequent infections, hepatosplenomegaly, hypotonia, abnormally structured bones, lenticular opacities and vacuolized lymphocytes. The lysosomal enzymes which hydrolyze sugars were all present; α-mannosidase activity was markedly deficient, whereas the other activities, including α-fucosidase, β-galactosidase and β-glucuronidase, were abnormally elevated. A similar genetic disorder with marked deficiency of α-mannosidase activity is known to occur in Angus cattle.

BETA-XYLOSIDASE DEFICIENCY. A nine month old girl with severe neurologic involvement, seizures, vomiting, and frequent upper respiratory infections has been found to have less than 10 per cent of the normal activity in lymphocytes of the lysosomal enzyme β-xylosidase.

ASPARTYLGLYCOSAMINURIA. The compound 2-acetamido-1 (β-L-aspartamido)-1,2 dideoxyglucose (AADG) is a substituted hexose which forms one of the linkage points between the carbohydrate moiety and the amino acid groups of many glycoproteins. Large quantities of AADG have been found in the urine of two mentally retarded siblings; one had petit mal seizures; the other, a manic-depressive psychosis. Other patients have had vacuolated lymphocytes, mental retardation, facial and osseous features similar to those of the mucopolysaccharidoses, hepatomegaly and lenticular opacities. The defect of glycoprotein metabolism is in the lack of the enzyme, normally demonstrable in seminal fluid, which hydrolyzes AADG to glucosamine and aspartic acid. In this disorder the lysosomal enzyme is deficient in liver, brain and spleen.

SIALIC ACIDEMIA. Neuraminic acid is a condensation product of pyruvic acid and mannosamine. The N-acetyl derivative is known as sialic acid and is widely distributed in the body mucopolysaccharides, mucoproteins and brain lipids such as gangliosides. Massive excretion in urine (5 to 7 gm/day) and elevated blood levels of sialic acid have been reported in a 4 year old boy who was retarded, and had a peculiar facial appearance and hepatomegaly. The nature of the defect is unknown.

GLYCOPROTEIN STORAGE DISEASE. An apparently dominantly inherited disorder of glycoprotein storage in the reticuloendothelial system has been reported. The propositus, a 52 year old man, had splenomegaly and a long history of vague abdominal pain.

LEIGH'S ENCEPHALOMYELOPATHY (PYRUVIC ACID CARBOXYLASE DEFECT). This disorder, also known as infantile subacute necrotizing encephalomyelopathy, is a progressive encephalopathy. Onset may be in the first weeks of life or be delayed for a year or so. Clinical manifestations are variable; most patients have failure to thrive and progressive mental retardation; some have seizures, vomiting and respiratory difficulty. Most patients have bulbar symptoms and die by 4 years of age; a few have survived into adolescence. Postmortem examination reveals symmetrical necrosis of the basal ganglia and brain stem. The disorder appears to be inherited as an autosomal recessive.

Children with Leigh's encephalomyelopathy have acidosis and hyperlacticacidemia, pyruvicacidemia, and alaninemia. In three patients assay of liver tissue did not reveal any activity for pyruvic carboxylase. This enzyme converts pyruvic acid to oxaloacetic acid, which can then either be oxidized in the citric acid cycle or participate in gluconeogenesis. In another patient hepatic pyruvate carboxylase activity early in the course of the disease tested normal, but was vanishingly low at post mortem. It was postulated that the fall in pyruvate carboxylase activity may have been a result of the disease and not its cause. The high blood levels of lactic acid have fallen temporarily in response to administration of lipoic acid, the cofactor required for the conversion of pyruvic acid to CoA. Lipoic acid is effective in reducing the lacticacidemia by aiding in the removal of excess pyruvate via the acetyl CoA pathway (See Fig. 16–1).

A substance found in the urine of many patients with Leigh's encephalomyelopathy inhibits the phosphorylation in brain of thiamine pyrophosphate to thiamine triphosphate. This inhibitor is not present in the urine of patients with a variety of other neurologic disorders. In the brains of 6 children with Leigh's disease the total thiamine content was higher than in control brains, but thiamine triphosphate was virtually absent. This inhibitor has also been demonstrated in urine and in blood of parents and siblings of patients with Leigh's disease. These findings may help to explain why thiamine has been of limited value in some patients with this disorder.

The definitive diagnosis of Leigh's encephalomyelopathy depends on postmortem examination of the brain. Other genetic and biochemical entities of unknown cause have been called Leigh's disease. Among these are: a boy with hereditary ataxia (Behr syndrome), who had thiamine pyrophosphate kinase inhibitor in his urine; and 8 year old and 3 year old girls with hypokalemia, hypomagnesemia and aldosteronism (Bartter syndrome). The urine and serum of the younger girl contained the inhibitor, which disappeared temporarily upon treatment with thiamine. Brains of both girls were diagnostic for Leigh's disease.

A patient who appears clinically and biochemically to have Leigh's disease has recently been described whose alaninemia and lactic acidosis responded dramatically to thiamine therapy, and whose hepatic pyruvate carboxylase activity had abnormal kinetic parameters. The patient lacked the component of pyruvate carboxylase activity that has a high affinity for the substrate, pyruvic acid, but the low affinity component was present. Since thiamine is not a cofactor for this enzyme system, it was postulated that the therapeutic effect of the vitamin was achieved through increasing the flow of pyruvate through the alternate pathway of pyruvate dehydrogenase, a thiamine-dependent step.

LACTIC ACIDOSIS. Lactic acidosis is a biochemical component of many different genetic disorders. Owing to the facile equilibrium between lactic acid and pyruvic acid and between pyruvic acid and alanine, the latter two compounds are usually also present in increased amounts. Lactic acidosis is a prominent finding in fructose-1, 6-diphosphatase deficiency, type I glycogenosis and diabetic coma, and in the entities collectively known as Leigh's encephalomyelopathy (above). In many other syndromes with lactic acidosis, the biochemical defects are not known. Many involved children have been mentally or physically retarded; others have had various neurologic signs. A set of siblings had enamel hypoplasia and diabetes mellitus. In some reported cases the patients developed lactic acidosis immediately after birth and died in the neonatal period. In some families the lactic acidosis has been intermittent, and death was delayed for a few years. Three patients with lactic acidosis and myopathy have been reported; two of these were sisters who also had growth failure and nerve deafness, and one sister died in acidosis, examination of muscle mitochondria indicating a probable defect of the respiratory chain; the third child with a myopathy and lactic acidosis had frequent vomiting and growth retardation, with muscle fibers described as "ragged-red" with the Gomori trichrome stain, again suggesting a defect of mitochondrial oxidation. Another patient, a 3 year old girl with severe mental and motor retardation, optic atrophy, hypotonia and lactic acidosis, had a 75 per cent decrease in ability to oxidize labeled citric acid in cultured fibroblasts; oxidation of isocitrate was unimpaired.

PYRUVATE DECARBOXYLASE DEFICIENCY. In a 9 year old boy with numerous episodes of ataxia and choreo-athetosis, levels of pyruvate and alanine were markedly elevated in both urine and blood, whereas lactic acid levels were usually not elevated. A defect of the enzyme pyruvate decarboxylase was demonstrated in fibroblasts and leukocytes; his parents had intermediate values, indicating autosomal recessive inheritance. Other patients with similar clinical features have been described who presumably have the same defect; and a patient with cerebellar ataxia in whom this enzyme defect was earlier postulated responded to massive doses of thiamine, the vitamin form of the cofactor for the reaction. Of three children with intermittent lactic acidosis and generalized neurologic disease and retardation, two of whom (sisters) died during acidotic episodes, the surviving brother had less than 10 per cent of normal activity of the pyruvic dehydrogenase complex in fibroblasts; his urine did not contain the inhibitor for thiamine triphosphate production (see above). Three patients with Friedreich's ataxia have shown defective oxidation of pyruvate in fibroblasts.

DEFECTS IN MUCOPOLYSACCHARIDE METABOLISM. The mucopolysaccharidoses are discussed elsewhere (Section 22). Other diseases also involve metabolism of mucopolysaccharides. In cystic fibrosis, in which yet undefined changes take place in mucus-secreting tissue, fibroblasts from both homozygous and heterozygous persons, grown in tissue culture, stain metachromatically, indicating an underlying abnormality of mucopolysaccharide metabolism.

Some increase in urinary excretion of normal mucopolysaccharides occurs in systemic lupus erythematosus, rheumatoid arthritis, leukemia, lymphoma and multiple myeloma.

There is some overlapping in classification between the mucopolysaccharidoses and the lipidoses. Farber's disease (Section 23) and generalized gangliosidosis (q.v.) involve deposition of both classes of compounds. This is also the case in fucosidosis (above). The defects have recently been defined in a number of disorders involving lysosomal enzymes, the function of which is to degrade or otherwise alter cellular macromolecules, including mucopolysaccharides, glycolipids, gangliosides, cerebrosides and the like.

GLYCOGENOSES: DISORDERS OF GLYCOGEN METABOLISM

(Glycogen Storage Diseases)

A variety of disorders result from derangements of synthesis or degradation of glycogen or of its subsequent utilization. This group of disorders has been known as the glycogen storage diseases, but this name is not sufficiently inclusive to encompass those disorders in which accumulation of glycogen is deficient or in which there is synthesis of glycogen with an abnormal structure. For this reason the collective term "glycogenoses" has been adopted.

In Table 8–2 the recognized entities are grouped for clinical purposes on the basis of the principal organ or systems involved. In the first group the liver is the principal organ affected, and the symptomatology can include hypoglycemia, ketosis, acidosis, hepatomegaly and failure to thrive. In the second group, cardiomegaly is the most prominent manifestation and patients usually die from cardiac failure in infancy, but there is also massive accumulation of glycogen in most other tissues. In the third group skeletal muscle is principally involved, and the main complaints are easy fatigability and muscular cramps. The glycogenoses have been assigned numbers (see under Type in Table 8–2) in the order in which the enzymatic defects were delineated, irrespective of clinical distinctions. When, for example, the Coris found diminished activity of the enzyme glucose-6-phosphatase in a patient with what was then known as von Gierke's disease, the disorder became known as type I glycogen storage disease.

Chemical and physiologic understanding of each of the known glycogenoses is far from complete. Uncritical acceptance of an arbitrary classification may unwittingly convert hypotheses to truths. These, in turn, may be perpetuated, and an apparently suitable working classification may actually hinder rather than help comprehension of this group of diseases. It is essential for the physician or student to know that he will encounter clinical patterns which do not fit in all details into any of the present categories and that ultimately some apparent variants may be found to be entities in their own right. Furthermore, one cannot always predict the enzymatic defect from the clinical pattern. Though it is assumed that all these disorders are genetically determined, some patients have been observed with more than one type of defect, and several different types have been noted within a single kindred. To add further uncertainty, some patients have a clinical pattern with metabolic derangements simulating one or the other of the glycogenoses without having any demonstrable enzymatic defect. All these features make it essential that any categorical scheme be recognized for what it is – an arbitrary arrangement of currently available data.

Glycogen is a branched polysaccharide of high molecular weight (range three to ten million) which is present in most animal tissues. It is composed entirely of glucose units linked together by alpha 1–4 and alpha 1–6 bonds; in this respect it resembles the starches of plants. Both muscle and liver store glucose in the form of glycogen, and both can degrade glycogen to glucose-1-phosphate and then to pyruvic and lactic acids via the Embden-Meyerhof pathway.

Certain features distinguish the carbohydrate metabolism of liver from that of muscle. Liver can and usually does synthesize glycogen from dietary glucose or by reversal of the Embden-Meyerhof pathway, using much of the lactic acid derived from muscle. Free glucose derived from stored glycogen or by synthesis from other compounds can be released into the circulation by liver after hydrolysis of glucose-6-phosphate by the enzyme glucose-6-phosphatase. Muscle, however, which does not have the enzyme glucose-6-phosphatase, cannot release glucose into the circulation; after glucose has been absorbed from the circulation, it can only be stored as glycogen, utilized with the concomitant production of lactic acid or, in the presence of sufficient oxygen, burned to carbon dioxide and water. Under anaerobic conditions, as during vigorous exercise, lactic acid accumulates and diffuses into the circulation. Part or all of the lactic acid

TABLE 8–2

PRINCIPAL ORGAN INVOLVED	EPONYM AND SYNONYM	TYPE	OTHER ORGANS INVOLVED	CLINICAL MANIFESTATIONS
Liver	von Gierke (hepatorenal)	Ia	Kidney, intestinal mucosa	Hepatomegaly, growth retardation, hypoglycemia, hyperlipemia, hyperlactic acidemia; may have bleeding diathesis
		Ib	?	Same
	Forbes, Cori (limit dextrinosis)	IIIa	Muscle, heart not severely	Hepatomegaly, ketosis, hypoglycemia with fasting, resembles type I; may have muscle weakness
		IIIb	None	Hepatomegaly, ketosis, hypoglycemia with fasting, resembles type I
		IIId	Muscle	Hepatomegaly, hypoglycemia with fasting, resembles type I; may have muscle weakness
	Andersen (amylopectinosis)	IV	Kidney, heart, muscle, reticuloendothelial system, nervous system	Hepatosplenomegaly, portal cirrhosis of liver, no ketosis or acidosis; may be icteric; esophageal varices in 2 patients
	Hers (liver phosphorylase)	VI	None	Hepatomegaly
	Hug	IXa	None	Same
	Huijing	IXb	Muscle	Same
	Hug (inactive liver phosphorylase)	VIII	Brain	Hepatomegaly, progressive brain degeneration
	Hug (phosphorylase kinase) kinase	X	Muscle	Hepatomegaly
	Lewis (aglycogenosis)	0	None	Severe hypoglycemia only after overnight fast. Mental retardation
	Edstrom		All tissue	Cirrhosis of the liver
Heart	Pompe (cardiac)	IIa	Muscle, liver, nervous system	Cardiomegaly hypotonia, death in first year of life
Muscle	Pompe	IIb	Liver, nervous system	Hypotonia; often survive more than 1 year
	Forbes, Cori (limit dextrinosis)	IIIc	None	Hypotonia, ketosis
	McArdle (muscle phosphorylase)	V	None	Manifest as a rule in adulthood. Muscular fatigability and pain with exercise, especially after ischemic activity; myoglobinuria
	Tarui	VII	None	Same as V
	Thomson		None	Variable generalized muscular dysfunction; shortening of the gastrocnemius muscle
	Rosenberg (intramitochondrial storage)		Nervous system	Muscle weakness and atrophy, hyperreflexia
	Satoyoski		None	Muscle pain after exercise

This table is an oversimplification of the categorization of the glycogenoses, many patients with disorders of glycogen metabolism do not fit within listed categories; however, patients have been observed and studied who qualify for each classification. Some patients have combined defects of the types noted.

TESTS	GLYCOGEN STRUCTURE	GLYCOGEN CONTENT*	ENZYME DEFECTS
Poor hyperglycemic response to glucagon or epinephrine. Galactose or DHA increase blood lactic acid. Prediabetic type glucose tolerance curve	Normal	5-15 (L)	Glucose-6-phosphatase absent or very low
Same	As above	Same	Unknown
Hyperglycemia after glucagon only after feeding. Enzyme defect may be detected in WBC	Abnormal Excessive branching, short outer chains	10-20 (L) 2-6 (M)	Amylo-1,6-glucosidase (debrancher) and amylo-1,4→1,4-transglucosidase absent or very low
Same	As above	10-20 (L)	Same
Same	As above	10-20 (L) 2-6 (M)	Amylo-1,4→1,4-transglucosidase absent or verylow
Poor hyperglycemic response to glucagon; some response to epinephrine; abnormal glycogen can be measured in RBC. Enzyme defect may be detected in WBC	Abnormal. Very little branching, long outer chain	1-10 (L)	Absence of amylo-1,4→1,6-transglucosidase (brancher enzyme)
Normal hyperglycemic response to glucagon or epinephrine, good response to galactose. Enzyme defect may be detected in WBC	Normal	5-20 (L)	Liver posphorylase levels below 50% of normal
Same	Normal	Same	Phosphorylase kinase (autosomal recessive)
Normal response to glucagon & epinephrine	Normal	Same	Phosphorylase kinase (sex-linked)
None	Normal	9-18 (L)	Unknown
No response to glucagon			3′5′ cyclic AMP dependent kinase
Poor hypoglycemic response to glucagon with fasting; normal response after feeding; no increase in urinary catecholamines after insulin	Normal	<0.5 (L)	UDPG-glycogen transglucosidase (glycogen synthetase) absent or very low
No response to glucagon	Abnormal low molecular weight	Normal	Unknown
Normal tolerance tests (glucagon, epinephrine, glucose, galactose, etc.). Enzyme defect may be detected in WBC	Normal	5-15 (L) 5-10 (H) 5-15 (M) >Normal (N)	Lysosomal alpha-1,4-glucosidase (acid and neutral maltase) absent or very low
Normal tolerance tests (glucagon, epinephrine, glucose, galactose, etc.)	Normal	5-15 (L) 5-15 (M) >Normal (N)	Lysosomal alpha-1,4-glucosidase (acid, and in some instances neutral, maltase) absent or very low
Normal liver function, but no increase in lactic acid after epinephrine in fasting	Abnormal. Excessive branching, short outer chains	2-6 (M)	Amylo-1,6-glucosidase (debrancher enzyme) absent or very low
No outpouring of lactic acid after epinephrine or ischemic muscular activity. Work capacity increased by glucose or fructose infusion	Normal	2-5 (M)	Muscle phosphorylase absent or very low
Same as V	Normal	2-5 (M)	Phosphofructokinase absent or very low
Very low outpouring of lactic acid after ischemic work, normal hyperglycemic response after epinephrine	Normal	3-13 (M)	Low activity of muscle phosphoglucomutase; also partial defects of other enzymes of glycolysis
None	Unknown	Normal (intramitochondrial storage of glycogen)	Unknown
No lactate after ischemic work	Normal	1.6-1.7	Low activity of phosphohexose isomerase

*Contents in grams per 100 gm of fresh tissue. Normal values and the symbols used are: Liver (L), 1–5 gm 100 gm fresh tissue. Heart (H), 0.2–1.5 gm 100 gm fresh tissue. Muscle (M), 0.2–1.5 gm 100 gm fresh tissue. Nerve (N) by histochemical techniques only.

can return to the liver and be utilized in the formation of glycogen, or it can be oxidized to carbon dioxide and water.

A large number of enzyme systems are involved in the synthesis and degradation of glycogen (Fig. 8–11, *A*). Deficiencies of activity of some of these have been implicated as causative factors for many of the clinical syndromes categorized as glycogenoses.

Glucose enters into the synthesis of glycogen as uridine diphosphoglucose (UDPG). The enzyme uridine diphosphoglucose-glycogen-transglucosylase (UDPG-glycogen synthetase) adds glucose units derived from UDPG, one at a time, to the growing outer chains of glycogen. The attachment of these glucose units as 1-4 bonded groups is always such that it extends the chain linearly. For practical purposes the action of glycogen synthetase is not reversible. After a particular outer chain has grown to about 15 glucose units in length, another enzyme called amylo-1,4→1,6-transglucosidase (branching enzyme) dislodges a portion of this chain and transfers it intact onto a glucose residue of another chain, where it is attached at the 6 position, thus creating a branched structure. The glycogen molecule continues to grow by the combined action of these two enzymes. Yet another enzyme (amylo-1,4→1,4-transglucosidase) breaks off and transfers short linear chains from one part of the glycogen molecule to another point. These, however, are added onto existing chains in 1-4 linkages. In this phase the arrangement is entirely in a straight line, and there is no branching. This mechanism leads to elongation of the chain without branching.

The degradation of glycogen involves phosphorylase, an enzyme which exists in active and inactive forms; these differ by two molecules of phosphate. The active form is produced from the inactive form in the presence of another enzyme, phosphorylase kinase, and ATP; a phosphatase converts the active form back to the inactive one. Phosphorylase kinase is itself activated by another kinase which is dependent on the presence of adenosine-3′, 5′-monophosphate (cyclic AMP). Cyclic AMP, known as the second messenger, is a compound whose formation is dependent upon the action of hormones such as epinephrine or glucagon. Phosphorylase removes glucose units, one at a time, from straight chains found at the outside of the glycogen molecule. From glycogen and inorganic phosphate this enzyme produces glucose-1-phosphate (G-1-P). The action of phosphorylase cannot proceed beyond a branch point in the glycogen formed by a glucose attached by a 1-6 bond and probably does not even reach to within two glucose residues from such branch points. Although phosphorylase can act in reverse to synthesize glycogen from glucose-1-phosphate in vitro, this is not its physiologic function, nor is it thought that much glycogen is synthesized by reversal of phosphorylase action in vivo. The few remaining glucose residues, other than the branch point itself, are removed by the action of amylo-1,4→1,4-transglucosidase. The enzyme which debranches glycogen at the 1-6 position, giving rise to free glucose, is called amylo-1,6-glucosidase. When the branch point is removed, phosphorylase may again proceed down the 1-4 linked chain, removing glucose units until it encounters the next branch point of this highly ramified molecule.

Another mechanism, entirely independent of the action of phosphorylase and amylo-1,6-glucosidase, exists within normal cells, capable of degrading glycogen to free glucose. Intracellular structures called lysosomes contain hydrolytic enzymes which act at acid pH to destroy virtually all the macromolecules normally found within the cytoplasm (glycogen, protein, nucleic acid). Among these enzymes is alpha-1,4-glucosidase (acid maltase), whose function is to hydrolyze glycogen. These lysosomal enzymes may hydrolyze the entire protoplasm of a cell and contribute to its destruction, but within viable functioning cells these enzymes destroy only selected portions of the protoplasm. It is the combined actions of the various enzyme systems that are responsible for the degradation and resynthesis which maintain the protoplasm in a viable state.

Available evidence, based on pedigrees with affected siblings and in some instances consanguinity, indicates that most of the glycogenoses are probably inherited in an autosomal recessive manner. It has been suggested that one form of phosphorylase kinase defect (type IX) may be transmitted as a sex-linked characteristic, since virtually all examples occur in males. (See also comments below in respect to multiple disorders of glycogen metabolism in an individual and to different disorders in a kindred.)

GLYCOGENOSES IN WHICH THE LIVER IS PRINCIPALLY INVOLVED

HEPATORENAL GLYCOGENOSIS (TYPE I). In this disorder of glycogen metabolism, also known as von Gierke's disease, glucose-6-phosphatase activity is deficient in hepatic, renal and intestinal mucosal cells; an accumulation of glycogen in these organs results. The inability to release glucose from glucose-6-phosphate leads to hypoglycemia. This is accentuated after overnight fasting and during intercurrent illness. The excessive accumulation of lactic acid in the blood is evidence of impaired hepatic oxidation of carbohydrates and glucogenic amino acids by the enzymes of the citric acid cycle. In the need for energy, fats (free fatty acids) are mobilized at an excessive rate and are metabolized in the liver to the 2-carbon level. As a consequence, glycogenolysis in liver proceeds only as far as pyruvic acid, which in turn is converted to lactic acid. These coeval events account for the acidosis, hyperlipemia and fatty infiltration of the liver. The hyperlactic acidemia and increased levels of free fatty acids in blood all disappear or ameliorate after administration of glucose. Since hypoglycemia is the normal state in these patients, increased mobilization of fat is almost constant and explains the hypertriglyceridemia. Whereas the response to intramuscular injection of glucagon in the normal subject is hyperglycemia, in these patients it causes further elevation of lactic acid in the blood. The presence of normal or relatively increased fat depots and the deficient development of skeletal muscle may account for the doll-like appearance of many of these patients.

The enlarged, smooth liver may contain 5 to 15 per cent of glycogen in fresh tissue; the average normal content is 3 per cent (range 1 to 5 per cent). The hepatic cells are large, with small, centrally placed nuclei; the cytoplasm is filled with glycogen and in stained preparations appears as an empty space if the tissue is not properly fixed in 90 per cent ethanol. Intracellular fat is increased. The kidneys are enlarged, owing to accumulation of glycogen in the renal convoluted tubules. Histologic demonstration of an apparent excess of glycogen in liver cells is not sufficient evidence of hepatic glycogenosis; quantitative and qualitative chemical determinations of liver tissue obtained by biopsy are essential and should reveal more than 5 per cent of glycogen having a normal molecular structure.

The presence of excess glycogen in hepatic or renal cells is not necessarily evidence of a deficiency in glucose-6-phosphatase. In a few patients who have otherwise conformed to the generally accepted criteria of this form of glycogenosis, no deficiency of glucose-6-phosphatase is demonstrable, the defect in these instances being unknown; the result of the administration of glycerol to such patients suggests that the phosphatase demonstrated in vitro is not functional in vivo. For the sake of categorization the disorder in these patients has been termed type Ib, type Ia indicating the form in which the enzyme deficiency is demonstrable.

Clinical Manifestations. Both the severity and the prognosis of the illness vary. In the majority of instances the onset is insidious. Hepatomegaly is present at birth, but the abdominal enlargement may go unnoticed, since there are often no other symptoms during the first year of life. Gradually symptoms of hypoglycemia appear. Vomiting, more common at night, is frequent. Drowsiness, twitching and occasionally coma or convulsions may occur. Clinical manifestations resulting from acidosis are common complications of inanition accompanying intercurrent infections. Retardation of growth commonly results in dwarfism.

Occasionally the disorder is manifest within the neonatal period by dehydration and acidosis. Such severely affected infants have fatty infiltration of the liver. Many die in early infancy.

The elevated levels of lactic acid in the blood reduce the plasma carbon dioxide content. The fasting level of blood glucose is low, though it is remarkable that hypoglycemic manifestations are often not evident even with blood glucose levels below 30 mg/dl. There are isolated reports of neurologic sequelae following hypoglycemic episodes. Hyperlipemia is common, and the serum inorganic phosphate levels may be low. A serious bleeding diathesis with thrombocytosis has been observed in a number of patients.

It has long been assumed that patients lacking glucose-6-phosphatase also have a fasting ketosis, but this is not the case. The first patient described as having von Gierke's disease with ketosis was proved, upon re-examination 36 years later, to have a defect of debranching (type III); such patients can exhibit ketosis.

Reports of adults with this disease suggest that the prognosis may not be so serious as was once felt. In a few adults a defect in glucose-6-phosphatase activity has been associated with tophaceous gout. This was undoubtedly related to the high levels of circulating uric acid found in most examples of the type I defect, even in childhood; these appear to be secondary to hyperlacticacidemia, lactate competing with urate for renal excretion. Hepatic carcinomas have been observed in 3 adolescent patients with this diagnosis.

Diagnosis. Clinical studies are essential to determine whether a liver biopsy is indicated. Fasting hypoglycemia, hepatomegaly without evidence of parenchymal liver disease, and an abnormal response to intramuscular injection of glucagon (100 micrograms per kg) suggest the diagnosis of hepatic glycogen disease. In the normal subject there is an increase in blood glucose of at least 70 mg/dl within 30 minutes after injection of glucagon, whereas in patients with this disorder the increase will not be greater than 30 mg/dl. The glucose tolerance curve is characterized by a low fasting blood level of glucose, a high elevation following ingestion of glucose, which decreases slowly over several hours. A further increase in the usually elevated level of lactic acid follows ingestion of a test load of galactose, glucagon or dihydroxyacetone (DHA), a change not observed in normal persons.

Treatment. There is no corrective therapy for the biochemical defect in the liver, but symptomatic measures can provide some relief through maintaining blood glucose at close to physiologic levels. Four or more meals daily are advisable, the last being given at midnight. There is some rationale for limiting intake of lactose (milk), since galactose will augment the hyperlacticacidemia. A diet high in protein, though without effect upon levels of glucose in blood, may produce less postprandial hyperglycemia and thereby lessen release of insulin, this reducing, in turn, the degree of hypoglycemia. The administration of zinc glucagon twice a day immediately postprandially has been of value in some children.

Prolonged withholding of food for diagnostic procedures should be avoided. The ease with which acidosis and hypoglycemia develop in the course of an infection should be anticipated and prevented by provision of adequate amounts of fluid containing glucose and sodium lactate or bicarbonate.

GLYCOGENOSIS OF LIVER AND MUSCLE (TYPE III; LIMIT DEXTRINOSIS; FORBES'S DISEASE). Debranching of glycogen involves two enzymes, amylo-1,6-glucosidase and amylo-1,4→1,4-transglucosidase. These enzymes are normally present in both liver and muscle. Deficiency of one or the other or of both enzymes can occur in liver or in muscle, or in both tissues in varying combinations. Of the 15 possible combinations of defects, four have been described (see Table 8–2); two involve both liver and muscle, one involves only liver, and one involves only muscle. In all instances, the glycogen which accumulates is abnormal not only in amount but also in its molecular structure. Analysis reveals an excessive number of branch points, owing to deficiency of the debranching system.

The clinical manifestations are dependent on the tissues involved. The hepatic disturbances in types IIIa, IIIb and IIId are similar to those of type I glycogenosis, but are often milder, although these patients may also manifest ketosis and acetonuria. Muscular involvement is manifested by variable degrees of weakness.

Diagnosis. The responses to the various tolerance tests (except that to glucagon) are similar to those in patients with type I glycogenosis (see above). The response of the blood glucose to administration of glucagon is negligible in fasting patients, but after a meal high in carbohydrate there is a significant increase in the level of glucose. The administration of epinephrine in the fasting state will not result in an increase in blood lactic acid when there is involvement of muscle. The amylo-1,6-glucosidase can normally be demonstrated in leukocytes and in fibroblasts; it is absent in some patients. Markedly increased amounts of abnormal glycogen have been demonstrated in erythrocytes in some patients and not in others. The significance of this discrepancy is not known; it is possible that it may be a distinguishing feature between subtypes, but in many of the earlier reported cases only one of the two enzymes was assayed.

Biopsy should include muscle as well as liver. Glycogen from affected tissue has an excess of short outer branches. In some instances of type III glycogenosis the activity of hepatic glucose-6-phosphatase has also been low. This activity was brought to normal levels in at least one case by treatment with triamcinolone.

GLYCOGENOSIS ASSOCIATED WITH HEPATIC CIRRHOSIS (TYPE IV; AMYLOPECTINOSIS; ANDERSEN'S DISEASE). In this rare type of glycogenosis (6 patients have been reported) an abnormally structured glycogen accumulates in liver, kidney, spleen, muscle and nervous system. Clinically there are growth retardation, hepatosplenomegaly, cirrhosis, and ascites, and in some instances icterus and esophageal varices. A child presenting primarily muscular symptoms was described as a "severely floppy infant." Hypoglycemic crises, ketosis and acidosis are absent, and the fasting blood sugar levels and the glucose tolerance curves are within normal ranges. The responses to epinephrine and glucagon are poor. Impaired hepatic function is manifest by abnormal results in thymol turbidity and cephalin flocculation tests, by low serum albumin and elevated serum globulin levels, by Bromsulphalein retention, by increased serum bilirubin concentration, and increased levels of such serum enzymes as transaminases and aldolase.

The glycogen is characterized by an abnormal molecule with decreased branching resembling amylopectin. A deficiency of the enzyme amylo-1,4→1,6-transglucosidase has been demonstrated in hepatic tissue and in leukocytes of affected patients. That any branching of glycogen occurs at all in the absence of branching enzyme is remarkable; it has been suggested that such branching results from reversible activity of the debrancher system. The abnormal glycogen can be demonstrated in erythrocytes. The fibrosis which occurs in liver and at times in other tissues containing abnormal glycogen has been attributed to a foreign body reaction. Patients have all died in infancy or childhood. Treatment is entirely symptomatic. In one patient intravenous administration for 4 days of α-glucosidase of fungal origin resulted in a decrease of hepatic glycogen content from 11 to 1 per cent without altering the clinical course of the disease.

GLYCOGENOSES DUE TO DEFECTS OF THE LIVER PHOSPHORYLASE SYSTEM (TYPES VI, VII, IX AND X). The conversion of glycogen to glucose-6-phosphate in the liver requires the activity of the enzyme phosphorylase. For phosphorylase to be in its active form, the activity of the enzyme phosphorylase kinase must be normal. Phosphorylase kinase activity is, in turn, dependent on the activity of phosphorylase kinase kinase (3′5′-cyclic AMP-dependent kinase). Glycogenoses involving all three enzymes have been reported. Historically the disorders are referred to as *Hers disease* (phosphorylase defect). Most of the patients reported as having deficient phosphorylase activity have, in fact, had a deficiency of phosphorylase kinase, early assays not differentiating the various entities.

In at least one patient, advanced methods have shown a defect of phosphorylase itself. This patient, with what may now be known as true type VI glycogenosis, was a 10 month old male with hepatomegaly, who was neither hypoglycemic nor ketotic; responses to glucagon and to epinephrine were normal.

A patient with hepatomegaly (and increased glycogen content) and progressive neural involvement has been reported in whom it seemed the enzyme phosphorylase was present but inhibited or somehow inactivated. The administration of glucagon led to normal levels of phosphorylase in a subsequent biopsy. This form of glycogenosis has been called type VIII. A second patient without neural involvement who may fit this category has been described.

Most of the patients with deficient phosphorylation have a defect of the enzyme phosphorylase kinase (type IX). They have hepatomegaly with increased glycogen content. Fasting hypoglycemia is sometimes observed. The response to glucagon is normal and this hormone has been administered therapeutically in order to reduce the size of the liver. There would appear to be two forms of type IX disorder: one appears to be inherited as an autosomal recessive and involves only the liver; the other is sex-linked, manifest almost exclusively in males, and besides hepatomegaly displays retarded growth and muscle weakness.

Deficiency of phosphorylase kinase kinase activity (type X) has been reported in a single patient, a 5 year old girl with hepatomegaly and no other clinical signs or symptoms. There was no response to glucagon, but she did not exhibit hypoglycemia. Although phosphorylase kinase kinase activity was deficient in both liver and muscle, there were no muscular symptoms.

AGLYCOGENOSIS (DEFECT IN SYNTHESIS OF GLYCOGEN). A form of glycogenosis in which the basic defect is inability to synthesize glycogen in adequate amounts has been described. Biopsy of the liver from one patient and autopsy material from another have revealed fatty metamorphosis, an abnormally low glycogen content (less than 0.5 gm per 100 gm of fresh tissue) and absence of activity of the enzyme UDPG-glycogen transglucosylase (glycogen synthetase). This enzyme is responsible for the glycogen synthesized in normal persons; a small amount of glycogen may possibly be produced by reversal of the phosphorylase action. Clinically the outstanding manifestation is severe hypoglycemia after overnight fasting. Hypoglycemic convulsions, lethargy, vomiting and mental retardation have been observed. Response to the glucose tolerance test is characterized by a sharp rise in blood glucose from a low fasting level and a delayed return to hypoglycemic levels. There is essentially no response to the epinephrine test in the fasting state while the patient is hypoglycemic; a normal response occurs after feeding.

LOW MOLECULAR WEIGHT GLYCOGEN. A male infant with hepatomegaly, failure to thrive, and cirrhosis of the liver died at 14 months of age with deposition in all tissues of a glycogen of extremely low molecular weight (8000 to 15,000 vs. over 1,000,000 for normal glycogen). The total content of this polysaccharide was within normal limits, but its relatively low solubility led to precipitation in the tissues. Low levels were found for numerous enzymes, but no specific defect identified. Brancher enzyme was present, differentiating this disorder from Type IV, in which cirrhosis has also been observed.

GLYCOGENOSES INVOLVING PRINCIPALLY CARDIAC MUSCLE

TYPE II; GENERALIZED GLYCOGENOSIS (POMPE'S DISEASE). In only one of the recognized glycogenoses (type IIa) is cardiac muscle sufficiently involved to be responsible for severe cardiac dysfunction. In types III and IV there is some deposition of abnormally structured glycogen in cardiac muscle, but no significant handicaps appear to be related to it. By contrast, in the classic form of Pompe's disease (type IIa), the significant clinical disorder is the cardiac involvement, though skeletal muscle and liver also have abnormal accumulations of glycogen (Table 8–2).

Massive glycogen deposition in the cardiac muscle produces a "lacework" appearance of the fibers in microscopic sections and is responsible for massive enlargement of the heart. Accumulation of glycogen also increases the diameters of voluntary muscle fibers. In fact, the storage of glycogen in skeletal muscle in this illness is greater than that usually observed in other glycogenoses. The enzymatic defect in liver and in cardiac and skeletal muscle is absence or deficient activity of the lysosomal enzymes, acid and neutral α-1, 4-glucosidase (acid and neutral maltase) (see below). These enzymes can be measured in cells cultured from amniotic fluid; accordingly, antenatal diagnosis of the severe infantile form of the disease is possible. There are no detectable derangements of the Embden-Meyerhof pathway; the results of tolerance tests with glucagon, epinephrine, glucose or galactose are within the normal ranges. Serum lipid concentrations are also within normal ranges.

Symptoms related to impaired cardiac function may be manifest at birth and in most instances become evident within the neonatal period. Cyanosis, dyspnea, tachypnea and restlessness are common. With advancing cardiac embarrassment, anorexia, listlessness and cough may appear. The heavy infiltration of glycogen in other tissues may produce clinical manifestations which are confusing. Mistaken diagnoses of Down syndrome, cretinism and amyotonia congenita have been made on the basis of thickening of the tongue and extreme muscular hypotonicity. Neurologic abnormalities may be prominent when there is massive infiltration of the central nervous system with glycogen. The heart is greatly enlarged and has a circular appearance in roentgenograms. Murmurs are usually absent. Electrocardiographic tracings may show pronounced left axis deviation, inverted T waves and widened QRS complexes.

Though this disorder is rarely diagnosed before death, it should be considered a possibility in all infants under a year of age with cardiac enlargement and failure not otherwise readily explained. Demonstration of increased glycogen content in muscle and liver obtained at biopsy supports the diagnosis, but demonstration of lack of activity of alpha-1,4-glucosidase is necessary for definitive diagnosis. Leukocytes from patients with the disorder have very low acid maltase activity, but some clinically normal persons also have deficiency of this enzyme.

Aberrant origin of a coronary artery from the pulmonary artery, acute interstitial myocarditis, and endocardial fibroelastosis, in particular, must be considered in the differential diagnosis.

Other than symptomatic therapy, no treatment is available. Alpha-glucosidase prepared from a mold has been used experimentally with only transient improvement. Death usually occurs within the first year of life.

GLYCOGENOSES WITH MUSCULAR MANIFESTATIONS

Muscle weakness is the predominant clinical manifestation of glycogenosis when the defect involves muscle enzymes. This symptom occurs occasionally in glycogenoses primarily involving liver (types IV and IX).

PHOSPHORYLASE DEFICIENCY (McARDLE SYNDROME). The disorder in glycogen metabolism in type V glycogenosis, or McArdle's disease, is limited to the skeletal muscle. There is an abnormal accumulation of glycogen, owing to an absence or deficiency of phosphorylase in striated but not smooth muscle. Although the disease is usually manifest in childhood, most patients have not been detected until adulthood. The disorder is characterized by muscular weakness and by pain following exercise which is out of proportion to the exertions; these symptoms may abate if exercise is continued. Exercise under ischemic conditions, with a cuff applied at greater than arterial pressure, can be carried out for only a short time. Under these conditions the usual increase in the lactic acid concentration of the venous blood returning from the ischemic muscle does not occur. Hyperlacticacidemia is not observed after the administration of epinephrine. Muscle biopsy reveals abnormal amounts of normally structured glycogen, and enzyme assays reveal absent or extremely low activity of muscle phosphorylase. Other enzymes involved in glycogenolysis are not altered. The heart is not involved, and patients tolerate the disorder well, provided they do not overexert. Myoglobinuria has been observed to follow prolonged exercise.

PHOSPHOFRUCTOKINASE DEFICIENCY. Four patients of both sexes, three of them siblings, have presented all the clinical manifestations of McArdle's disease, including easy fatigability, cramps, myoglobinuria and inability to produce lactic acid after ischemic muscular exercise, but have differed biochemically in that they had a deficiency in muscle of phosphofructokinase (Type VII) rather than of phosphorylase. In addition to elevated levels of glycogen, their muscles also accumulated abnormal amounts of glucose-6-phosphate and fructose-6-phosphate. Measurement of phosphofructokinase activity of blood cells revealed normal activity in leukocytes and about one-half normal activity in erythrocytes. In one of the studies both parents also had lower than normal levels in erythrocytes. The disorder appears to be inherited in an autosomal recessive manner.

PHOSPHOGLUCOMUTASE DEFICIENCY. Another form of glycogenosis with abnormal accumulation of normally structured glycogen in skeletal musculature has been described in one patient. The symptomatology was similar to that seen in McArdle's disease, but muscle phophorylase activity was normal. In this patient a deficiency in the activity of muscle phosphoglucomutase and partial defects of other aspects of glycolysis were demonstrated (Thomson). The patient was in good general health. His gastrocnemius muscles were bulky and were shortened to such an extent that he walked on the foreparts of his feet.

PHOSPHOHEXOSISOMERASE DEFICIENCY. Two adult brothers have presented symptoms and signs similar to those of McArdle's disease. There was no lactate elevation after ischemic work. Assays of muscle showed a 60 per cent reduction in activity of the enzyme phosphohexose isomerase. Oral administration of fructose bypassed this defect and ameliorated the symptoms of easy fatigability and muscle pain after work.

INTRAMITOCHONDRIAL GLYCOGEN STORAGE. Four children in one family have presented a myeloneuromyopathy characterized by distal weakness and atrophy, with a family history indicating dominant transmission. Muscle glycogen content was normal, as were many enzyme levels; electron microscopy revealed giant mitochondria with intramitochondrial glycogen.

AMYLO-1,4-GLUCOSIDASE DEFICIENCY (POMPE'S DISEASE). In type IIb of Pompe's disease there is little or no cardiac involvement, and the significant disturbance results from abnormal accumulations of glycogen in skeletal muscle and nervous tissue. The enzyme α-1, 4-glucosidase (acid maltase) is absent from liver, skeletal muscle, and presumably from the heart as well. The disorder presents childhood and the adult forms: the childhood form is clinically characterized by hypotonia, muscular weakness, moderate hepatomegaly and normal mental function; the adult form involves muscle weakness, particularly of the respiratory muscles, and mimics other chronic myopathies. The biochemical differences between type IIa (infantile form) and type IIb (childhood and adult forms) depend on the pattern of lysosomal acid and neutral maltase activities in muscle, liver and heart. Acid maltase activity is deficient in all three forms in liver and muscle. It is also deficient in the heart in the infantile and childhood forms; no measurements have been made in heart in the adult form. In the infantile form, neutral maltase activity is low in all three tissues. In the childhood form, it is deficient only in liver, and in the adult form the activity is normal in all tissues. Since no family has been observed with more than one form of the disease, they appear to be distinct genetic entities.

An adult with myopathy is known who presented symptoms of McArdle's disease, with one half of the normal amount of acid maltase activity in muscle. It was discovered that this patient had hypothyroidism, whereupon treatment with thyroxine for six months relieved the symptoms and returned the muscle acid maltase level to normal.

AMYLO-1,6-GLUCOSIDASE DEFICIENCY (LIMIT DEXTRINOSIS). In type III glycogenosis (limit dextrinosis, or Forbes's disease) there is muscular involvement in three of the four subtypes. In one type the disordered metabolism is limited to skeletal muscle and is manifest by hypotonia and weakness. The metabolic diagnosis is discussed above and outlined in Table 8–2.

DOUBLE ENZYMATIC DEFECTS

The simultaneous occurrence of two different enzymatic abnormalities such as those of phenylketonuria and cystathioninemia in the same person is very rare and is expected to happen by chance with a frequency which is the product of likelihoods of having each defect by itself. Among the glycogenoses, however, the occurrence of two enzymatic errors in the same person is not infrequent. This is particularly evident in type III, and in sorting out the subgroups of type II with respect to the presence or absence of different enzyme activities (acid and neutral maltase) in various tissues. Other combinations of two enzymatic defects have been reported, and a number of sibships have been studied in which 2 children have different types of glycogenosis. The genetic mechanisms underlying these associations are poorly understood. One consequence of such observations is that biopsy material should in every instance be assayed for as many enzymes involved in carbohydrate metabolism as is technically feasible.

DEFECTS IN METABOLISM OF PYRIMIDINES AND PURINES

Purines and pyrimidines are heterocyclic nitrogen-containing compounds which, in conjunction with ribose or deoxyribose and phosphate, form the nucleotides. Ribonucleotides containing adenine and uracil are important energy-producing compounds or cofactors (ATP, UDPG, NAD, NADP, and so on) involved in many metabolic reactions. The ribonucleotides make up ribonucleic acid, and the deoxyribonucleotides form deoxyribonucleic acid. Purines and pyrimidines are constantly being synthesized and degraded; genetic defects are recognized in each phase. The important purines are adenine and guanine; the important pyrimidines are thymine, cytosine and uracil.

OROTIC ACIDURIA. Orotic acid is an intermediate metabolite in the synthesis of pyrimidines. A block in the further metabolism of orotic acid, resulting in its excretion up to 1.5 gm/day, has been observed in 5 persons. All had a megaloblastic anemia which did not respond to therapy with vitamin C, folic acid or vitamin B_{12}, and all formed orotic acid crystals in urine. In two of the patients therapy with a corticosteroid resulted in general improvement, but disappearance of abnormalities in the marrow and of excretion of orotic acid were noted only after administration of the pyrimidine nucleotides or nucleosides.

Two enzymes in the pathway distal to orotic acid, orotidylic acid pyrophosphorylase and orotidylic acid decarboxylase (see Fig. 8–12), were absent in liver, erythrocytes, leukocytes and fibroblasts grown in tissue culture. Heterozygotes have approximately half of both enzyme activities.

The effect of pyrimidine derivatives in lowering the excretion of orotic acid indicates that the enzymes in the pathway leading to orotic acid synthesis are under feedback inhibition control. The hematologic response is directly due to the provision for DNA and RNA synthesis of essential material which cannot be made de novo. The fact that two enzymes in a sequence are missing indicates that the mutation probably involves a controller gene rather than a structural alteration of enzyme proteins. This view is further supported by the observation that fibroblasts from affected persons, grown in the usual tissue culture media, lack these enzyme activities, but exhibit near normal activities when grown in the presence of 6-azauridine, a compound which raises the activity of both enzymes in normal cells in tissue culture.

The administration of allopurinol or oxypurinol can result in increased excretion of orotidine and orotic acid. Orotic acid crystals appeared in the urine of a 3 month old infant later shown to have a partial deficiency of ornithine transcarbamylase activity. As a result of this defect in the urea cycle (q.v.), extra carbamyl phosphate was shunted into the pyrimidine synthesis pathway and led to the overproduction and excretion of orotic acid.

In all patients with orotic aciduria in whom orotidylic acid pyrophosphorylase (also known as orotidylic acid phosphoribosyltransferase) and orotidylic acid decarboxylase have been measured, they were deficient. A patient has now been described who lacks only the decarboxylase function and is phenotypically indistinguishable from the more usual genotype with orotic aciduria. The biochemical explanation of this observation must await further investigation. The possibility exists that there is multiple genetic control over shared or unshared subunits of the proteins involved.

XANTHINURIA. The catabolism of purines in man is completed at uric acid, which is then excreted in the urine. Xanthine is the immediate precursor of uric acid and is formed directly from certain purines, whereas hypoxanthine is formed

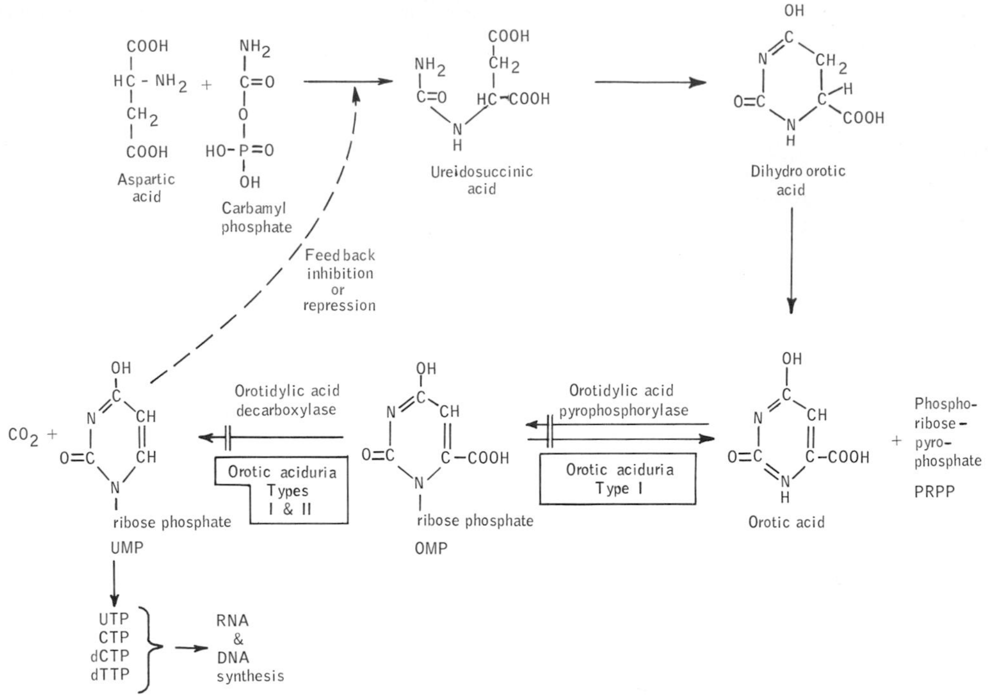

Figure 8–12 Pathways in pyrimidine biosynthesis. See also legend for Figure 8–1.

from others. The oxidation of hypoxanthine to xanthine and of xanthine to uric acid is mediated by the enzyme xanthine oxidase, found in liver and intestinal mucosa (Fig. 8–13).

Ten patients with xanthinuria have been reported. They have low levels of hypoxanthine and uric acid in the urine and plasma, and their excretion of uric acid decreases to zero on a purine-free diet. Some patients had xanthine stones and two, who complained of muscular pain after exertion, were shown to have deposits of xanthine and hypoxanthine in muscle. How many other persons with xanthine stones may have this defect is unknown. Xanthine stones have also been reported as a rare consequence of allopurinol administration. Jejunal biopsy of one of the affected adults revealed no activity of xanthine oxidase toward xanthine and only about 5 per cent of normal activity toward hypoxanthine. Increased renal clearances of xanthine and hypoxanthine are a natural consequence of their elevated blood levels.

HYPERURICEMIA (GOUT). Hyperuricemia is transmitted by a dominant autosomal gene with different degrees of penetrance in the two sexes; it has been estimated to occur six to seven times more frequently in males than in females. Primarily a disorder of adults, gout rarely occurs in children. A notable exception is the child with type I glycogenosis in whom hyperuricemia is common and gouty tophi may develop.

Among adults with gout there are at least two genetic forms of the disease. In one, available evidence suggests that hyperuricemia is due to overproduction of uric acid; the disordered mechanisms are not understood. In the other group there is diminution to about 5 per cent of normal of the enzyme hypoxanthine guanine phosphoribosyltransferase (Fig. 8–13). The enzyme has been measured in erythrocytes, leukocytes and fibroblasts; its connection with purine metabolism is discussed below. Otherwise healthy children with only 5 per cent of the normal activity of this enzyme have been reported, who have hyperuricemia and uric acid crystalluria, but no gouty arthritis. This latter disorder seems to be inherited in an X-linked manner.

Another biochemical cause of gout has been observed in two families in which the overproduction of purines was traced to abnormally high activity of the enzyme phosphoribosylpyrophosphate synthetase (Fig. 8–13), rather than to an enzyme defect involving loss of activity. The increase in enzyme activity seemed intrinsic rather than due to overproduction. This alteration pushed the regulatory mechanism of purine metabolism toward increased uric acid production. The error seems to be inherited in an X-linked manner.

The occurrence of hyperuricemia in conjunction with ataxia, deafness and gout has been described as a new syndrome in a large kindred. No biochemical lesion has been defined.

A 3 year old boy with hyperuricacidemia due to overproduction of purines has been studied who represents yet another syndrome. He was mentally retarded, with autistic behavior, produced no tears, and had dysplastic teeth. Hypoxanthine guanine phosphoribosyltransferase activity was normal, adenine phosphoribosyltransferase activity elevated. The latter finding occurs also in

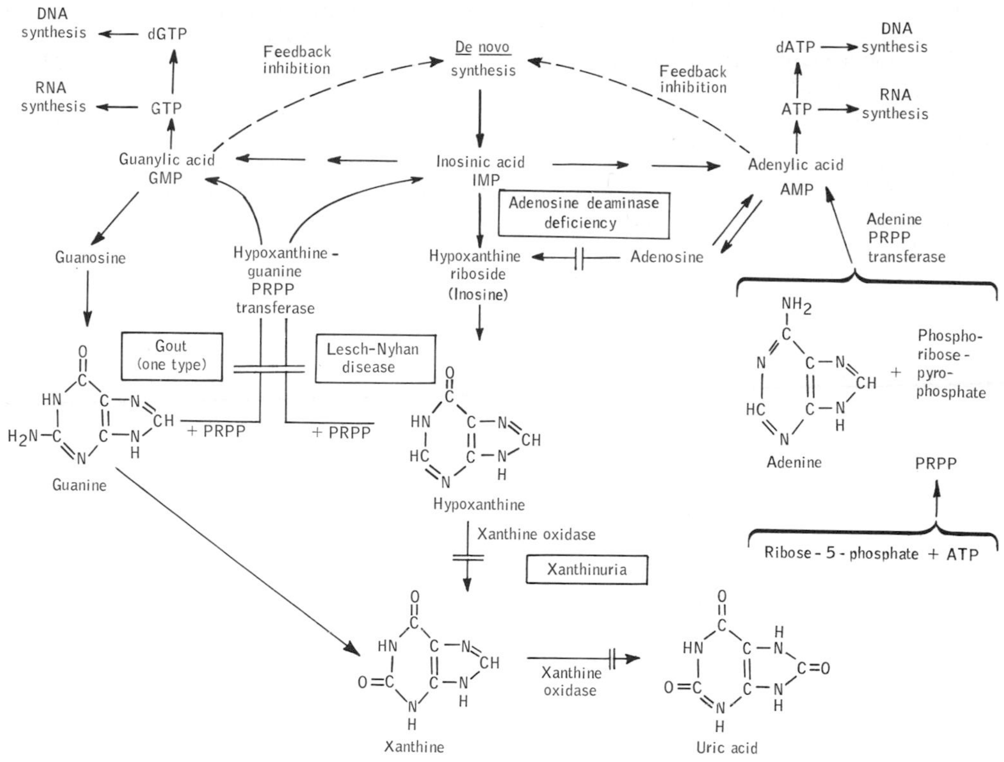

Figure 8–13 Pathways in purine metabolism and salvage. See also legend for Figure 8–1.

Lesch-Nyhan disease (see below), and implies deficiency of an unknown purine metabolizing enzyme.

An association has also been described between gout and a variant erythrocyte glutathione reductase. This particular form of the polymorphic enzyme has higher activity than the usual form; both heterozygotes and homozygotes for increased glutathione reductase activity have a greater incidence of primary gout than the normal population.

LESCH-NYHAN DISEASE. This disorder is characterized by mental retardation, choreoathetoid movements, scissoring position of the legs, self-mutilation and overproduction of uric acid. It is inherited by an X-linked gene; female carriers have been shown to have two populations of cells (Lyon hypothesis). The self-mutilation is not the result of an inability to feel pain, but of uncontrollable aggressive impulses which can be directed against others as well as self. Serum uric acid levels are in the same range (approximately 10 mg/dl) as in patients with gout, and daily urinary excretion of uric acid approaches 1 gm. Gouty tophi appear in older patients and can be controlled with allopurinol; although it is effective in adults with gout, azathioprine does not lower serum uric acid levels in Lesch-Nyhan disease.

The enzymatic defect consists in absence of hypoxanthine guanine phosphoribosyltransferase activity and has been demonstrated in erythrocytes and fibroblasts. The disorder can be diagnosed prenatally; after birth a single hair root provides sufficient material for enzyme determination. The role of this enzyme is of interest. Purines such as guanine and adenine, which are required for RNA, DNA and coenzyme synthesis, can be obtained from the diet or synthesized de novo from available metabolites. These same purine bases are normally catabolized via hypoxanthine and xanthine and excreted as uric acid. A reutilization mechanism conserves some of the hypoxanthine, which, with the addition of a ribose phosphate group, converts the base hypoxanthine to its nucleotide, inosinic acid. This is accomplished through the enzyme hypoxanthine guanine phosphoribosyltransferase. The same enzyme converts the base guanine to its nucleotide, guanylic acid (see Fig. 8–13). The concentrations of these two nucleotides and of adenylic acid (which is formed from the base adenine by a different enzyme) control by feedback inhibition the rate of de novo synthesis of inosinic acid. In the absence of these salvage mechanisms for reutilization of hypoxanthine and guanine there is an inability to maintain the nucleotide levels required for feedback inhibition of purine synthesis; excessive purines are synthesized and excess uric acid is excreted.

In Lesch-Nyhan disease the crucial enzyme for purine salvage is absent and the clinical manifestations of the disorder appear to be referable to this occurrence. Only a few patients with gout have a significant deficiency (5 to 10 per cent of normal) of hypoxanthine guanine phosphoribosyltransferase activity. It is surprising that complete absence of activity produces the severe neurologic manifestation of Lesch-Nyhan disease, whereas 90 to 95 per cent loss of enzyme activity leads only to gout.

Two variants of Lesch-Nyhan disease have been reported. In the first, a 3 year old girl presented the complete clinical picture but normal levels of uric acid. It was suggested that she had an autosomal recessive form of the disease; hypoxanthine guanine phosphoribosyltransferase activity was not measured. The second variant involved a 10 year old boy in whom enzyme assay in erythrocytes found approximately one fourth of normal activity. Further analysis showed alteration of the kinetic parameters with marked decrease in affinity of the enzyme for its substrates.

ADENOSINE-DEAMINASE DEFICIENCY. An absence of adenosine deaminase activity in erythrocytes, inherited as an autosomal recessive, has been observed in 13 infants and young children with severe combined immunodeficiency syndrome (see Section 9) and in an apparently healthy 10 year old boy. Although adenosine deaminase deficiency accounts for only a small portion of infants with such immunodeficiency, it is of special importance because it is the first specific enzymatic defect identified among the numerous inherited immunodeficiency syndromes. About half the infants with deficiency of the enzyme have also had cupping of the anterior ends of the ribs and other radiographic findings suggestive of defective development of cartilage. Both red cell and "tissue" isoenzymes of adenosine deaminase have been found to be absent from lymphocytes, liver, kidney and fibroblasts. These observations and the fact that conversion of normal erythrocyte enzyme to "tissue" enzymes has been accomplished indicate that both the tissue isoenzymes and the red cell enzyme are controlled by alleles at the same locus (on chromosome number 20). Prenatal diagnosis by assays on amniotic fluid fibroblasts will probably be possible; heterozygotes usually show a quantitative deficiency in red cell enzyme levels. The precise role of adenosine deaminase deficiency in defective lymphocyte proliferation, immunodeficiency and skeletal abnormalities remains to be elucidated.

MISCELLANEOUS DISORDERS INVOLVING PURINES. Pseudouridine is a nucleoside found in transfer RNA and microsomes and differs from uridine in that the ribose is attached to the uracil base at a carbon atom instead of a nitrogen atom. Some pseudouridine is normally excreted in urine, and increased amounts in persons with gout. Excretions of pseudouridine of two to three times the normal amount have been observed in two mentally retarded brothers. The cause is unknown.

Urinary stones consisting of uric acid have been found in 4 members in three generations of a family with normal serum uric acid levels and average daily excretion of uric acid. Uric acid crystals were found nevertheless in the distal urinary tract, leading to irritation. Studies suggested a specific disorder of tubular glutaminase as the causative factor responsible for a highly acid urine, precipitation of uric acid and formation of stones.

Hypouricemia has been demonstrated in one patient to result from a defect of renal tubular reabsorption of uric acid. This genetic defect is without clinical sequelae; the same defect is found in Dalmatian dogs.

The enzyme adenine phosphoribosyltransferase plays a role in purine reutilization. The activity of this enzyme, which is elevated in Lesch-Nyhan disease and in another disorder with hyperuricemia and mental retardation (see above), has been found defective in clinically normal heterozygotes. The homozygous condition, which might have clinical sequelae, is as yet unknown.

OTHER DEFECTS OF ENZYMES AND PROTEINS

We have thus far considered those inborn errors of metabolism which can be assigned naturally to certain biochemical systems, such as those involved in amino acid, carbohydrate, purine, or pyrimidine metabolism. Other natural assignments can be made to the areas lipid, porphryrin, mucopolysaccharide, immunoglobulin, clotting factor, hemoglobin and red cell metabolisms. Other inborn defects involving mineral metabolism (phosphate, iodine, copper, iron, and so on) are dispersed throughout this book. Aspects of vitamin metabolism other than the purely nutritional are treated in this chapter and elsewhere. Some disorders discussed elsewhere are mentioned here because of their nosologic significance as inborn errors. Other defects involve the soluble proteins and formed elements of blood and certain proteins and enzymes of other organs or tissues.

Defects in Plasma Proteins

ANALBUMINEMIA. Plasma albumin has two main functions: to maintain the oncotic pressure of blood, and to serve as a vehicle for the transport of many normal blood constituents, such as free fatty acids. A few persons have been observed in whom no circulating albumin could be demonstrated. Some were asymptomatic; others exhibited only slight edema. The first cases reported were siblings whose parents were double second cousins, suggesting that the disorder is genetic in nature. Periodic administrations of albumin result in disappearance of edema, but usually no treatment is necessary.

It may be speculated that lack of symptoms in analbuminemia depends on lifelong compensations in fluid dynamics which patients with such disorders as nephrosis or protein-losing enteropathy are unable to make in the face of acutely lowered oncotic pressure.

HAPTOGLOBIN DEFICIENCY. Haptoglobin is an alpha-2-globulin which binds free hemoglobin. There are numerous phenotypic variations (polymorphism) in the types of haptoglobins among normal persons. These are demonstrable by starch gel electrophoresis and are under genetic control. In the presence of severe hemolytic anemia, haptoglobin levels may be greatly decreased or absent. Healthy persons also have been found who have no demonstrable circulating haptoglobin, on a genetic basis, without apparent ill effect.

ABETA-LIPOPROTEINEMIA. Abeta-lipoproteinemia (see Sections 11 and 20), a defect in synthesis of beta-lipoprotein, is characterized by bizarrely shaped erythrocytes with thornlike projections (acanthocytes) and steatorrhea in infancy, followed by the development of ataxic neuropathy in childhood and retinitis pigmentosa in early adulthood. Characteristic pathologic changes have been observed in the intestinal mucosa; the columnar epithelium is filled with globules containing lipids. Plasma cholesterol, phospholipid and triglyceride levels are sharply reduced. Beta-lipoprotein and chylomicra are absent. There appear to be two forms of abeta-lipoproteinemia, each associated with a deficiency of an antigenically different beta-lipoprotein. In one form triglycerides are assimilated from jejunal epithelial cells; in the other the lipid cannot exit from the villous core. The disorder is transmitted in an autosomal recessive manner.

ANALPHA-LIPOPROTEINEMIA (TANGIER DISEASE). Tangier disease is a rare congenital metabolic defect first described in siblings residing on Tangier Island in Chesapeake Bay. This disorder is characterized by enlarged tonsils which have a distinctive orange color. Other clinical manifestations may include enlargement of the liver, spleen and lymph nodes.

Plasma levels of cholesterol and phospholipids are moderately reduced; there is storage of large amounts of cholesterol esters in reticuloendothelial tissues, including the tonsils.

The basic defect is absence in serum of alpha-lipoprotein (high-density lipoprotein). Inheritance is autosomal recessive. Heterozygotes have about half the normal concentrations of high-density lipoprotein, but are asymptomatic.

ABSENCE OF TRANSFERRIN. Transferrin, or siderophilin, is a plasma protein of molecular weight 90,000, with the electrophoretic mobility of a beta-2 globulin. It is assumed that it has a prominent role in the transport of iron. The only recorded instance of a congenital absence of transferrin at birth involved a physically retarded girl with hepatomegaly and splenomegaly, and anemia sufficiently severe to require multiple transfusions. The anemia did not respond to any of the antianemic agents used. Iron was absorbed from the intestinal tract and transported to the tissues. Erythrocytes were hypochromic, and the marrow contained many immature erythroblasts. Liver biopsy revealed cirrhosis and siderosis. Immunochemical studies revealed complete absence of transferrin. Antibodies to transferrin developed after multiple transfusions. Sudden death at 7 years of age was attributed to hemosiderosis. Both parents had lower than normal amounts of transferrin; this suggests autosomal recessive transmission.

C′-1 ESTERASE INHIBITOR. Reduced levels of C′-1 esterase inhibitor, an alpha$_2$-neuraminoglycoprotein, are associated with hereditary angioneurotic edema (giant urticaria). The protein is an inhibitor of the esterase activity of the complement component designated C′-1. The esterase rises to high concentrations during an attack and is thought to be responsible for increased capillary permeability. Prednisolone has been used successfully to treat the condition; during its administration the inhibitor becomes demonstrable and the enzyme activity decreases. The disorder can be caused by a number of different genetic defects: in some, the concentration of C′-1 esterase inhibitor is low; in others, an abnormally structured protein is produced. Transfusion of fresh frozen plasma has been reported to be of benefit if given during the acute phase of edema and/or abdominal pain.

Affected persons are apparently heterozygous for the condition and manifest their fluctuating levels of the inhibitor as episodic edema. No homozygous persons with the condition are known.

ALPHA$_1$-ANTITRYPSIN PROTEIN DEFICIENCY. Normal persons produce a circulating protein which in in-vitro assays inhibits trypsin activity. This inhibitor is not made by persons who are homozygous for a mutant gene. Many persons without alpha$_1$-antitrypsin protein suffer pulmonary emphysema as they grow older, and significant numbers of patients with emphysema can be shown to lack this protein. In families in which a patient with emphysema has been shown to be homozygous for deficient antitrypsin activity, there is an increased incidence of pulmonary disease in relatives heterozygous for the deficiency. It has been speculated that the protein inhibits bacterial proteinase which would otherwise destroy alveolar architecture.

Deficiency of circulating α_1-antitrypsin has also been described in children with cirrhosis who have had neonatal hepatitis and in adults with either hepatic cirrhosis or fibrosis. It would appear that both emphysema and cirrhosis may be consequences of the same primary defect involving the synthesis in the liver of an aberrant α_1-antitrypsin molecule, which if not released into the circulation accumulates in the liver. Low blood levels of α_1-antitrypsin have risen to normal in one patient who underwent liver transplantation.

TRANSCOBALAMINE II DEFICIENCY. Two different serum proteins bind vitamin B_{12}. One of these, transcobalamine I (an α-globulin), has been reported deficient in 2 siblings; there were no discernible clinical or hematologic sequelae. The other protein, transcobalamine II (a β-globulin), has been reported deficient in several infants with severe megaloblastic anemia, some of whom have also had neurologic changes. No abnormalities were found in reactions involving the coenzyme forms of vitamin B_{12}, homocysteine methyltransferase and methylmalonyl CoA mutase (q.v., this Section). Treatment consists of parenteral administration of large doses of vitamin B_{12}.

Defects in Plasma Enzymes

PSEUDOCHOLINESTERASE. Pseudocholinesterase is found in plasma, liver and neural tissue; its physiologic function is poorly understood.

Numerous presumably allelic forms of the altered enzyme are known. Some with reduced enzyme activity are characterized by the extent of inhibition by dibucaine or fluoride, whereas a "silent" form has no activity. Homozygotes for each form and mixed heterozygotes are known. About one in 25 persons is heterozygous for one or another of these defects.

The one person in 3000 who is homozygous for one of these genes is ordinarily asymptomatic. The defect was discovered because the enzyme participates in the destruction of a commonly used muscle relaxant, succinylcholine. In the normal person this drug is rapidly destroyed by pseudocholinesterase and therefore has a transient effect. Persons homozygous for mutant pseudocholinesterase split the drug abnormally slowly or not at all, and apnea results, lasting for hours. Artificial respiration is required, preferably through an endotracheal tube; the period of apnea can be shortened by transfusion with normal plasma.

Another genetic alteration of pseudocholinesterase has been described which leads to *increased* enzyme activity and hence to resistance to the pharmacologic effects of succinylcholine. These observations demonstrate how unusual sensitivity or resistance to the pharmacologic effects of drugs may be predetermined by the genetic constitution of the person. The study of such interactions is known as pharmacogenetics. Other well studied examples are primaquine sensitivity and variation in response to isoniazid.

LECITHIN-CHOLESTEROL ACYLTRANSFERASE DEFICIENCY. Three sisters with corneal opacity, normochromic anemia and proteinuria were shown to have the following abnormal blood chemical findings: decreased alpha-lipoprotein and prebeta-lipoprotein, increased concentration of free cholesterol, almost absent esterified cholesterol and, in two cases, hyperlipidemia. There were none of the changes of the tonsils seen in analpha-lipoproteinemia. The defect was demonstrated to be an almost complete absence of lecithin-cholesterol acyltransferase, a plasma enzyme which normally esterifies cholesterol; lecithin is the source of the fatty acid.

CARNOSINASE DEFICIENCY. Excessive carnosine (β-alanylhistidine) has been found in the urine and low levels of carnosinase in the serum of children with a progressive neurologic disorder beginning in infancy and leading to severe deterioration by childhood. The diet is the major source of carnosine, which carnosinase (q.v.) splits to β-alanine and histidine. Two electrophoretic forms of the enzyme occur; tissue studies in one patient revealed absence of one form but not of the other. The disorder is transmitted as an autosomal recessive. Infusion of fresh normal plasma has been shown to reduce the urinary excretion of carnosine.

GAMMA-GLUTAMYL TRANSPEPTIDASE DEFICIENCY. A moderately retarded adult with increased levels of glutathione in blood and urine has been shown to have a deficiency in serum of γ-glutamyl transpeptidase, which catalyzes the first step in the degradation of glutathione. There was no other abnormality in amino acid excretion. These observations must be seen in the perspective of the involvement of this enzyme in amino acid transport (Fig. 8–7). Apparently, the serum enzyme produced in the liver is under different genetic control from that synthesized in the renal tubule and intestine.

HYPOPHOSPHATASIA. There are several isoenzymes in plasma which have alkaline phosphatase activity. The one presumably derived from bone is markedly low in homozygous individuals who excrete large amounts of phosphoethanolamine and have a defect of ossification leading to severe bone disease. (See Section 22.)

Defects of Proteins of Other Tissues

CERULOPLASMIN DEFICIENCY (WILSON'S DISEASE) (see Section 11). Ceruloplasmin, a blue-colored alpha-2-globulin containing 8 copper atoms per molecule, constitutes 0.5 per cent of the total plasma proteins. The average normal serum concentration is 25 mg/dl (range, 16 to 33). Low levels are found in newborn infants and in patients with active nephrosis, in whom ceruloplasmin is lost in the urine. Wilson's disease, or hepatolenticular degeneration, is a hereditary disorder transmitted by an autosomal recessive gene, in which low serum levels of ceruloplasmin are characteristic; they average 5 mg/dl (range, 0 to 14). Several unequivocal cases, however, have been observed with normal levels of ceruloplasmin. Furthermore, the ceruloplasmin found in the blood of patients with Wilson's disease has been shown to be of normal structure. It appeared likely that the primary genetic defect in Wilson's disease was in the synthesis of ceruloplasmin, but recent evidence indicates that in this disorder an abnormal structure of the intracellular storage protein, *copperthionein*, results in a fourfold increase in affinity for copper, and all the clinical and biochemical manifestations can be explained on this basis.

Increased amounts of copper are absorbed from the intestinal tract and are present in tissue and urine, though levels in blood are typically decreased. Injury to parenchymatous organs (kidney, liver and brain), whether anatomic or functional, seems related to elevated concentrations of copper. The presence of the pathognomonic eye sign, Kayser-Fleischer rings, is also secondary to copper deposition.

Renal copper intoxication is presumably the cause of increased excretion of amino acids, uric acid, polypeptides, glucose and phosphate in urine. The disorder can be detected while it is still latent by ascertainment of the ceruloplasmin level, and therapy can be initiated with drugs, such as penicillamine, that lower the body content of copper.

MENKES KINKY HAIR SYNDROME. This sex-linked disorder is characterized by abnormal hair, growth retardation, progressive neurologic degeneration, and death in the first few years of life. There are defective absorption of copper and decreased levels of ceruloplasmin and copper in plasma. If copper is administered intravenously to these patients, the synthesis of ceruloplasmin occurs rapidly. Analysis of mitochondria from brain and muscle has revealed a diminished content of the copper-containing enzyme, cytochrome oxidase (cytochrome a + a_3). This finding may be secondary to the defect in copper absorption.

MYOGLOBIN. Myoglobin, a heme protein found in muscle, is responsible for the intracellular transport of oxygen. Two different variants of myoglobin have been identified by starch gel electrophoresis. Changes in amino acid sequence producing myoglobinopathies are analogous to the changes responsible for the hemoglobinopathies. In each of two families observed, mother and son were heterozygous for the normal and for the aberrant molecules. Each family had a distinctive aberrant molecule. Neuromuscular diseases were not found in these families.

Spectrophotometric analyses of myoglobin from a number of patients with various neuromuscular diseases have revealed consistent changes in those with the sex-linked form of pseudohypertrophic muscular dystrophy (Duchenne), and the persistence of fetal myoglobin in one patient with facioscapulohumeral dystrophy. Fetal myoglobin has also been found in a patient with recurrent myoglobinuria. The myoglobin isolated from patients with progressive spinal muscular atrophy and the limb-girdle type of muscular atrophy appears to be normal spectrometrically. Females who carry the defect for the Duchenne type of muscular dystrophy have moderately elevated serum levels of creatine phosphokinase, and biopsy discloses small areas of dystrophic muscle fibers intermingled with the normal muscle fibers. The genetic form of muscular dystrophy of mice responds therapeutically to the vitamin-like substance coenzyme Q, suggesting that perhaps one of the human forms of the disease may involve a derangement of the synthesis of coenzyme Q.

XERODERMA PIGMENTOSUM. Extreme dermal sensitivity to sunlight or ultraviolet light and the development of skin cancers which metastasize and lead to death are characteristic of this rare recessive disease (Section 23). Skin fibroblasts grown in tissue culture have a defect of the enzymatic mechanism for repair of DNA. In normal persons the rupture of one strand of DNA in the double helical form by a mutagenic agent such as ultraviolet light is rapidly repaired by a set of specific enzymes which ensure integrity of the genetic material. Persons with xeroderma pigmentosum lack one of these enzymes and are therefore subject not only to skin damage by what would normally be small doses of radiation, but also to the immediate potentially carcinogenic effects of other unrepaired breaks in DNA.

There seem to be at least three genetic forms of the disease, each with a different biochemical defect; in one patient with clinical xeroderma pigmentosum no defect in DNA repair can be demonstrated.

PANCREATIC ENZYME DEFICIENCIES. Malabsorption due to pancreatic dysfunction is a cardinal feature of the genetic disease cystic fibrosis (Section 11), but it is fairly certain that the *basic* genetic defect is not an inability to synthesize one or another of the pancreatic enzymes.

A number of patients have been described in whom malabsorption appears to result from a specific enzymopathy involving a pancreatic enzyme or proenzyme. They have none of the pulmonary or electrolyte abnormalities of cystic fibrosis.

A syndrome with inability to produce trypsin,

lipase and amylase in conjunction with hematologic evidence of bone marrow dysfunction has also been described, but in this case, as in cystic fibrosis, pancreatic dysfunction is presumed to be secondary to an underlying defect (Section 11).

Lipase Deficiency. Four children have been described with congenital inability to form active pancreatic lipase (two formed none, and two synthesized small amounts). They had malabsorption of lipids and fatty (and sometimes malodorous) stools. Treatment with pancreatin was effective.

Trypsinogen Deficiency. A number of children with severe malnutrition, growth failure and hypoproteinemic edema resembling kwashiorkor have been shown to lack the ability to synthesize pancreatic trypsinogen. As a result, chymotrypsin and carboxypeptidase activities are also low, since these enzymes need to be formed from the corresponding proenzymes by trypsin activity. Treatment with a protein hydrolysate diet and exogenous pancreatic enzymes is recommended.

Amylase Deficiency. Less defined deficiencies of pancreatic amylase activity have been described in at least 2 children with malabsorption who were shown not to have cystic fibrosis. One of the children also had reduced trypsin activity.

These observations indicate the need to investigate pancreatic function in children with malabsorption in whom the causative factors are unknown; these disorders may be more common than is indicated by the relatively few cases reported.

INTESTINAL ENTEROKINASE DEFICIENCY. Enterokinase, an enzyme secreted by the small intestine, initiates the reactions for the conversion of the pancreatic proenzymes to their active forms. A number of children with a proven deficiency of enterokinase activity have been studied. The clinical findings and recommended treatment are identical with those described above for trypsinogen deficiency. Many if not all of the cases originally described as trypsinogen deficiency may be instances of enterokinase deficiency, with the lack of trypsin activity secondary to inability to form trypsin from trypsinogen.

LYSOSOMAL ACID PHOSPHATASE DEFICIENCY. Lysosomal acid phosphatase was shown to be markedly reduced in many tissues and in cultured fibroblasts of an infant who died at 3 months of age following intermittent vomiting, and terminal hypotonia, opisthotonus and bleeding. Fibroblasts cultured from the parents had about one half the normal activity of lysosomal acid phosphatase. Cells obtained by amniocentesis from a subsequent pregnancy had low activity; the abortus was shown to be deficient in acid phosphatase.

COLLAGEN METABOLISM. A deficiency of the enzyme procollagen peptidase, which converts the protein procollagen to collagen, has been demonstrated in 3 patients with one of the variant forms of Ehlers-Danlos syndrome. Another form of this disorder has been shown to result from defective hydroxylation of lysine (above, this Section).

CARNITINE DEFICIENCY. The metabolism of long chain fatty acids requires carnitine (γ-trimethylamino-β-hydroxybutyrate). A patient with longstanding muscle weakness was found to have muscle fibers filled with lipid vacuoles. Oxidation of long chain fatty acids was depressed and the concentration of carnitine in muscle was shown to be one sixth of normal.

SUCCINYL-CoA, 3-KETO-ACID CoA-TRANSFERASE DEFICIENCY. Acetoacetate and β-hydroxybutyrate cannot be further metabolized unless the acetoacetate is activated by the addition of a molecule of coenzyme A, which is donated by succinyl CoA via a specific transferase. A boy with severe ketoacidosis who died at 6 months of age was shown to lack this transferase in all tissues studied. In another family, in which a 2 year old boy died during his third severe ketotic episode, the same enzymatic defect was found. Two siblings (one male, one female) had died in infancy under similar circumstances. Consanguinity of the parents indicates the probability of autosomal recessive inheritance.

ACATALASIA. Catalase is found in most tissues, including the erythrocytes. Persons with decrease of catalase activity in all tissues, to less than 1 per cent of normal, can be detected through the demonstration that blood placed in contact with hydrogen peroxide turns brown and does not produce the oxygen bubbles usually seen. The disorder is heterogeneous; some instances appear to be mutations of the controller gene, whereas others are alterations of the structural gene. In all instances the mode of inheritance is autosomal recessive; the heterozygote can be detected by quantitative catalase assays. Of the two main types, the Japanese variants have oral gangrene *(Takahara's disease),* whereas the Swiss variants are asymptomatic. A genetic strain of mice with acatalasia is known; catalase encapsulated in semipermeable membranes has been used successfully in their treatment.

TRUE CHOLINESTERASE. True cholinesterase, an enzyme essential for neural and muscular function, is also found in erythrocytes, where its function is unknown. A brother and a sister have been observed whose erythrocyte cholinesterase activities were decreased to about one third of normal. They appeared to be homozygous for the condition and their parents and 2 siblings to be heterozygous. There were no associated clinical manifestations. It has been suggested that a deficiency of true cholinesterase at the neuromuscular endplate may account for the defect in myotonia congenita (Thomsen's disease, Section 21).

SYNDROMES WITH IMPAIRED LEUKOCYTE FUNCTION. The ability of leukocytes to phagocytose foreign particles such as bacteria and to destroy the ingested material depends on a number of factors, both extrinsic and intrinsic to the cell. The role of various opsonizing factors which act upon the particle undergoing phagocytosis, and the effect of deficiencies of these factors is considered in Section 9. A tetrapeptide, L-threonyl-L-lysyl-L-prolyl-L-arginine, *tuftsin,* has been isolated from a leukophilic fraction of γ-globulin. Tuftsin is formed in the spleen, and splenectomized patients lack it. It has been shown to stimulate phagocytosis by acting directly upon leukocytes. Two children with recurrent severe infections have been reported to have *tuftsin deficiency.* The mode of inheritance is not clear since each child had at least one parent with the same tuftsin deficiency but no clinical manifestations.

Diminished bactericidal activity of leukocytes is observed in *chronic granulomatous disease,* in association with deficiency of the leukocytic enzyme, reduced nicotinamide-adenine dinucleotide oxidase. This enzyme normally converts the reduced form of the coenzyme NAD, produced when glucose is converted to pyruvate via the Embden-Meyerhof pathway, to the oxidized form; concomitantly, hydrogen peroxide is formed. The failure to form hydrogen peroxide may be responsible for the diminished ability to kill phagocytosed bacteria.

Myeloperoxidase is an enzyme in leukocytes which, in the presence of hydrogen peroxide, oxidizes many compounds. Its activity seems to be important in the killing of phagocytosed microorganisms. A patient with *disseminated candidiasis* has been shown to have a *myeloperoxidase deficiency* in his polymorphonuclear leukocytes and monocytes. Phagocytosis was normal, but ingested *Candida albicans* were not killed, and the ability to kill other microorganisms was diminished. No other abnormalities of immune response were observed in this patient.

EPILOGUE

The number of *recognized* inborn errors of metabolism is constantly increasing. This is due in part to the clinical identification of new syndromes and to description of the biochemical nature of the metabolic block responsible for the condition. In addition, as new biochemical techniques have become available, many disorders, such as phenylalaninemia and the glycogenoses, once thought to result from single enzymatic defects and manifesting a broad spectrum of clinical manifestations, are now being subdivided into several distinct clinical entities, each with a different enzymatic error.

The detection of many inborn errors of metabolism can now be made early in life; large-scale detection programs utilizing screening tests for blood or urine are currently carried out. Analyses of enzymes in readily available cells such as erythrocytes, leukocytes, and cultured fibroblasts for confirmation of clinical diagnoses are becoming increasingly available. For many conditions, particularly those associated with mental retardation, the earlier detection takes place and effective therapy is instituted, the better is the prognosis. A vigorous effort at early detection and subsequent treatment by dietary regulation has improved the mental development of children with phenylketonuria. Other inborn errors amenable to diet therapy include galactosemia, maple syrup urine disease, propionicacidemia and homocystinemia. The administration of massive amounts of certain vitamins can effectively overcome an enzymatic error when the mutant enzyme can no longer effectively bind the cofactor derived from the vitamin. This is exemplified by the beneficial effects of pyridoxine in one form of cystathioninemia and in hydroxykynureninuria (pyridoxine dependency) and by the beneficial effects of cobamide in some patients with methylmalonic acidemia.

Replacement of a missing enzyme has always seemed a logical and desirable goal of therapy, but has not been possible except in a very limited way. In cystic fibrosis the extracellular enzyme required for proper digestion can be administered conveniently, though the underlying defect is not ameliorated. When one is dealing with an intracellular enzyme, the problem is more complex. Nevertheless, the experimental administration of hydrolytic enzymes such as α-glucosidase in the treatment of some forms of the glycogenoses is a step in this direction. It has been shown in tissue culture of cells derived from deficient patients that the direct addition of purified enzymes is efficacious in correcting the metabolic defect in some disorders, but this has not been the case in others. The feasibility of injection of microencapsulated purified enzymes, avoiding the immunologic difficulties encountered by the repeated introduction of foreign proteins, has been demonstrated in animal studies. One form of microencapsulation is the loading of intact red cell ghosts with purified enzymes.

Detection of some inborn errors of metabolism can now be made in utero through culture of cells obtained by amniocentesis. These techniques permit prenatal diagnosis with the possibility of interruption of pregnancy.

Finally, there is reason to anticipate that with increasing knowledge of genetic mechanisms it will be possible in the future to alter the genetic constitution of an individual and to overcome some of nature's more undesirable errors. For example, the Gunn rat, which lacks the hepatic enzyme bilirubin uridine diphosphate glucuronyltransferase, has been "cured" by the implantation into its liver of small pieces of normal rat liver. Whether this "cure," which spread throughout the recipient's liver, represented genetic alteration or was due to some other effect is not known. In any case, the results are promising, as are those involving the injection of protein-coated pseudovirus particles containing new genetic information. In both cases, however, we must remember that until it is possible to employ specific purified genes in this manner, other alterations may be produced which might prove even less tolerable than the disorder whose correction is attempted.

VICTOR H. AUERBACH
ANGELO M. DIGEORGE

GENERAL

Bergsma, D. (ed.): Birth Defects, Atlas and Compendium. The National Foundation. Baltimore, The Williams & Wilkins Company, 1973.

Bickel, H., Hudson, F. P., and Woolf, L. I. (eds.): Phenylketonuria and Some Other Inborn Errors of Amino Acid Metabolism. Stuttgart, Georg Thieme, 1971.

Bondy, P. K., and Rosenberg, L. E. (eds.): Duncan's Diseases of Metabolism. 7th Ed. Philadelphia, W. B. Saunders Company, 1974.

Brock, D. J. H., and Mayo, O. R. (eds.): The Biochemical Genetics of Man. London, Academic Press, 1972.

Dickens, F., Randle, P. J., and Whelan, W. J. (eds.): Carbohydrate Metabolism and Its Disorders. New York, Academic Press, 1968.

Goodman, R. M. (ed.): Genetic Disorders of Man. Boston, Little, Brown and Company, 1970.

Harris, H.: The Principles of Human Biochemical Genetics. New York, American Elsevier Publishing Company, 1970.

Harris, H.: Garrod's Inborn Errors of Metabolism. London, Oxford University Press, 1963.

Hommes, F. A., and Van Den Berg, C. J. (eds.): Inborn Errors of Metabolism. London, Academic Press, 1973.

McKusick, V. A.: Mendelian Inheritance in Man, Catalogs of Autosomal Dominant, Autosomal Recessive and X-Linked Phenotypes. 3rd ed. Baltimore, Johns Hopkins Press, 1971.

Nyhan, W. L. (ed.): Amino Acid Metabolism and Genetic Variation. New York, McGraw-Hill Book Co., Inc., 1967.

Scriver, C. R., and Rosenberg, L. E.: Amino Acid Metabolism and Its Disorders. Philadelphia, W. B. Saunders Company, 1973.

Stanbury, J. B., Wyngaarden, J. B., and Fredrickson, D. S., (eds.): The Metabolic Basis of Inherited Disease. New York, McGraw-Hill Book Co., Inc., 1972. 3rd Ed.

THE LIPIDOSES

A "lipidosis" is a genetically determined syndrome in which expression of an inborn error of metabolism results in a specific alteration (usually an increase) in the lipid content of tissues or serum. The anatomic hallmark of the lipidosis process is the formation of the "foam cell"—a large histiocyte in which there is intracytoplasmic accumulation of lipid materials, generally in discrete organelles (distended lysosomes) (Fig. 8–14). Etiologic considerations are complicated by the observation that less specific foam cells may also develop in a wide variety of acquired disease conditions (e.g., granulomas, tumors, infections, toxic states) which may mimic the true lipidosis picture. Foam cell formation in an organ characteristically results in an increase in its size and weight, a paler color and a firmer texture, producing clinical "visceromegaly." Such an occurrence may also lead to a variety of functional problems, depending on the locus of the process (e.g., liver, spleen, lungs, marrow cavity). Frequent coordinate handicaps, of more critical clinical importance, are diffuse alterations in neurones, producing cellular changes in gray matter and difficulty in formation and maintenance of myelin.

For pedagogic purposes it is customary to make principal reference to the "type" lipid, accumulation of which is specific for any given syndrome (Fig. 8–15). This may be an unjustified oversimplification which obscures a wider consideration of the underlying pathogenesis. It is possible that the presently demonstrated lipid defects in the lipidoses are actually late or partial effects, and identification of each of these disorders may ultimately

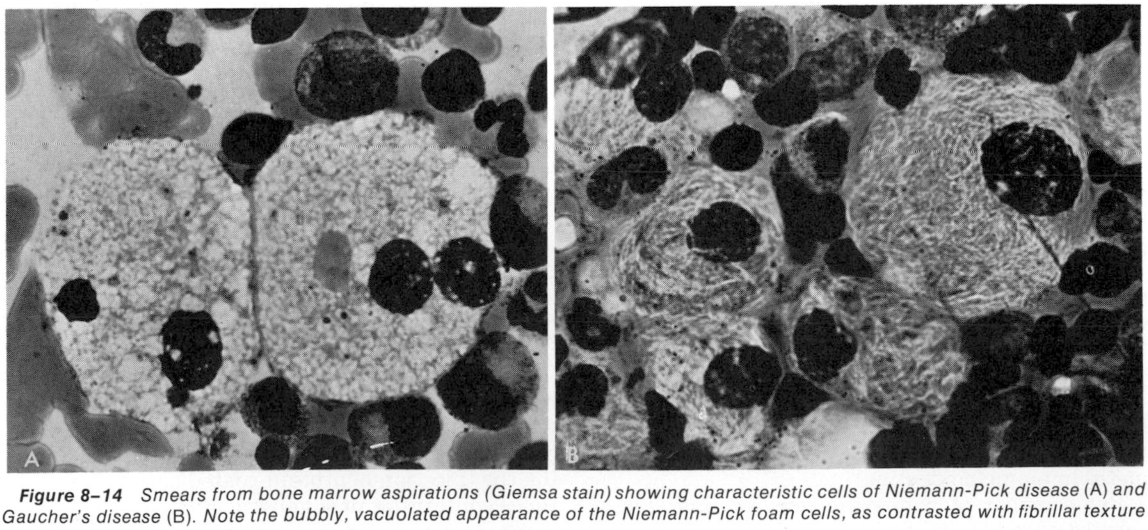

Figure 8–14 Smears from bone marrow aspirations (Giemsa stain) showing characteristic cells of Niemann-Pick disease (A) *and Gaucher's disease* (B). *Note the bubbly, vacuolated appearance of the Niemann-Pick foam cells, as contrasted with fibrillar texture of the Gaucher cell cytoplasm.*

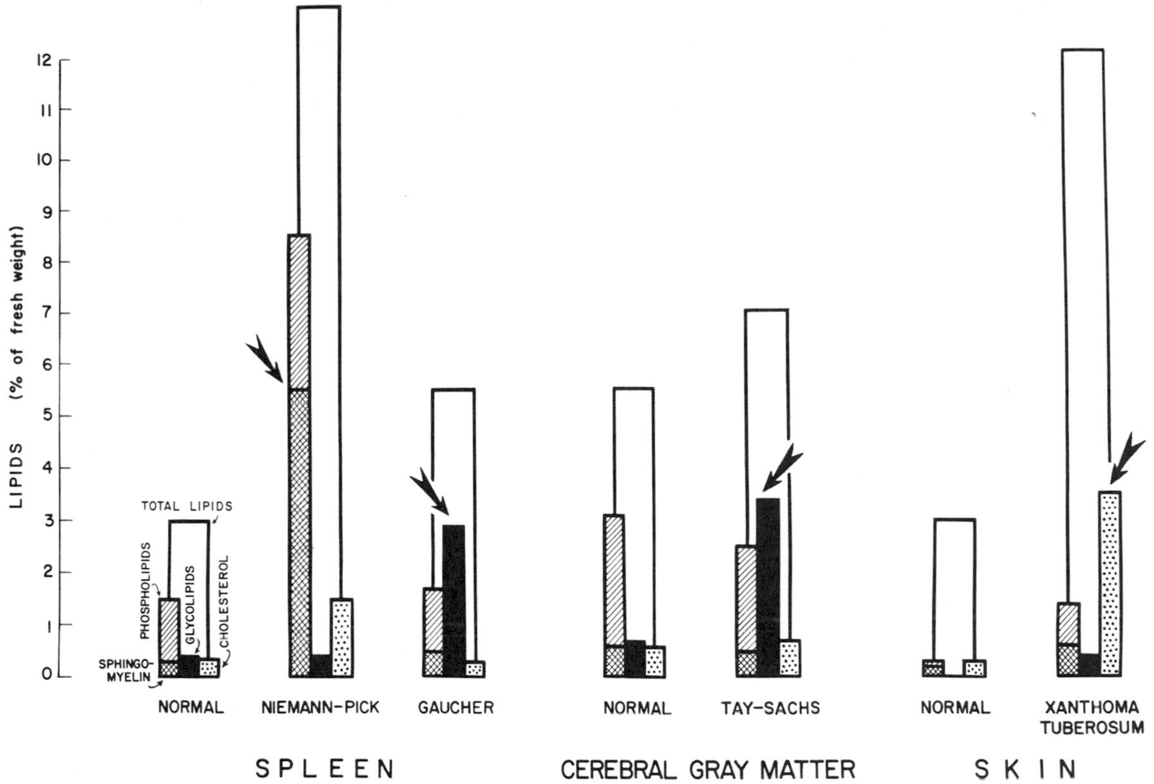

Figure 8–15 *Typical results of analyses of tissue specimens from various lipidosis syndromes. Arrows indicate the most characteristic element of the lipid increase in each disease. (Note key to lipid components, on left.)*

include the listing of other types of biochemical handicaps as well. For most of the syndromes under discussion, however, there are enzyme assay systems which demonstrate for each a deficient function of a lysosomal hydrolase of pertinence to the known lipid alteration, implying a specific defect in lipid turnover. Significant unknown components remain in the schemata for the actual mechanisms of the diseases. For the central nervous system changes, specifically, it is often difficult to understand the ultimate lesions.

The genetic pattern is that of autosomal recessive transmission in the majority of instances, both parents demonstrating a "carrier" (heterozygously involved) status, and the child with the disease (a one in four risk for each pregnancy) being homozygous. Identification of the carrier through study of enzyme levels in serum, white blood cells or cultured skin fibroblasts is often possible; in most instances prenatal diagnosis can be accurately established by assays on tissue cultures of fetal cells obtained through amniocentesis. Enzyme replacement therapy has not proved feasible in trials to date. To date, no morphologic alterations have been found in the chromosomes of patients with lipidoses. No genetic interrelations are known among the various syndromes. All affected members of any one pedigree will have a reasonably uniform clinical picture (e.g., early or late onset, neurologic defect).

GAUCHER'S DISEASE

Gaucher's disease is an uncommon disorder, encompassing a group of syndromes in which "Gaucher cells" can be demonstrated in the viscera. This cell has a characteristic morphology, with intracytoplasmic accumulation of cerebroside-type glycolipids (Fig. 8–15). The most common form of the disease is a relatively benign disorder, with clinical manifestations usually first evident within the pediatric age period. An unusual type, with fatal outcome, is seen in infancy.

ETIOLOGY. In Gaucher's disease the majority of the glycolipid in the viscera is a glucocerebroside, instead of the usual form with galactose; there is a deficiency in glucocerebrosidase activity in these tissues and in the white blood cells and an elevation of acid phosphatase activity in the same tissues and in the serum. The majority of pedigrees demonstrate recessive transmission of the disease, with no clinical abnormalities in the "carrier" heterozygotes; rare instances of undoubted dominant transmission for the chronic form have been described. About two thirds of all cases occur in Ashkenazi Jewish pedigrees.

PATHOLOGY. The Gaucher cell is sufficiently unique in its appearance to allow tentative identification by common tissue techniques. It is a large, often multinucleated, cell with a fibrillar or wrinkled-appearing cytoplasm which is nonvacuolated and pale-staining with most dyes. It is periodic acid–Schiff positive and gives a strong acid phosphatase reaction. In chronic forms of the syndrome it is found in the bone marrow, the red and white pulp of the spleen, between liver cells and in lymphoid tissue. Splenomegaly is common; splenic weights are five to eighteen times the normal for age.

In the *infantile form,* Gaucher cells are prominent in the lung, but are found in all areas of the body, even within the central nervous system. There are also some decrease in brain size, mild neuronal distention in the gray matter, neuronophagia, loss of nerve cells, gliosis and signs of poor myelination.

CLINICAL MANIFESTATIONS. There is a wide spectrum of clinical expression in Gaucher's disease. Two principal disease pictures exist, each of which is genetically distinct.

In the *acute* or *infantile* form there is an early onset of symptoms, which include slowed development, moderate enlargement of the liver and spleen, normal fundi, strabismus, retroflexion of the head, dysphagia and other signs of bulbar palsy, and increasing respiratory problems. Most of these infants do not survive beyond the first year of life, but occasional patients have lived until 2 to 6 years of age.

The *chronic* or *adult* form of the disease, about twenty times more common than the infantile type, has a great variation in time of onset of symptoms. Abdominal enlargement is the most frequent first complaint, with splenic increase more notable than hepatomegaly. Owing to the sustained splenomegaly, the clinical signs of "hypersplenism," with suppression of the blood cell counts and even hemorrhagic manifestations, will appear. Symptoms related to the bones and joints, such as bone pain, rheumatic-like joint swelling and discomfort (often episodic and not dependent on trauma) and pathologic fractures, may also be early manifestations. The bone and joint symptoms occur only where disease activity in the medullary cavity has already produced radiologically identifiable changes. Less frequently one finds a child who temporarily escapes the bone difficulties, but has poor growth and maturation and major enlargement of the liver. Even rarer are patients who develop hepatic fibrosis and portal hypertension, or who have chronic pulmonary difficulties.

The usual time for onset of symptoms in the chronic form is middle childhood, but some patients go on to adult life before presenting medical problems. The development of scleral *pingueculae* and dermal pigmentation does not occur until after adolescence. For patients without neurologic involvement there should be no mortality from the disease itself, although the course may prove distressing because of the orthopedic difficulties. Bone pain episodes decrease in intensity after puberty.

LABORATORY DATA. Examination of bone marrow is the critical diagnostic procedure; the characteristic Gaucher cell is demonstrable in all forms of the disease. In addition, by the time the child has clinical manifestations it is usually possible to show bone changes by radiologic examination. These include signs of chronic marrow cavity overactivity with bone texture changes, extension of the usual limits of the medullary space, failure of tubulation, and occasional rarefactions in bone, seen best in the femora, but also found elsewhere as in the tibiae and humeri. As the disease progresses, pathologic fractures of the femoral neck may develop, with local disintegration of bone and serious aseptic necrosis of the femoral head. Thrombocytopenia, anemia and leukopenia may reflect the effects of sustained splenomegaly. A mild myelophthisic anemia may also be present, which will be of a chronic but nonprogressive nature. The serum acid phosphatase level is elevated, best demonstrated by measurement with the Gutman procedure (phenyl phosphate substrate).

TREATMENT. Clinical management of the patient with *chronic Gaucher's disease* involves (1) surveillance for signs of hypersplenism, for which splenectomy may be indicated, and (2) orthopedic supervision for the care of bone complications. The disturbing periods of rheumatic-like bone pain should be conservatively managed (rest and analgesics). Collapse of vertebral bodies usually does not result in notable morbidity. Fractures of the femoral neck require careful support, with continuing attention to preservation of the structure of the femoral head. Permanent hip joint handicaps are frequent and usually represent the most significant effects carried into adult life. The psychologic effects of chronic and recurrent osseous problems may be severe and require much support. At present there is no effective chemotherapy or replacement therapy. For the *infantile patient* the care program is similar to that for any baby with serious central nervous system disease.

NIEMANN-PICK DISEASE

Niemann-Pick disease includes a small, heterogeneous collection of conditions which have in common the occurrence in the tissues of vacuolated foam cells whose most striking chemical feature is the cytoplasmic accumulation of sphingomyelin (a phospholipid). Originally Niemann-Pick disease was viewed as a syndrome with major neurologic handicaps, certain ethnic predilections and a uniformly fatal outcome in early life, but observations in recent years require a broader definition of the clinical picture.

ETIOLOGY. It is probable that the tissue changes in Niemann-Pick disease represent yet another example of specific lysosomal hydrolase deficiency, but current investigations have identified inadequate activity of a "sphingomyelinase" in only two of the four clinical phenotypes mentioned below (Groups A and B). Sphingomyelin accumulation is prominent in the viscera of the other types as well. Cholesterol and the monoaminophosphatides are also present in increased amounts (Fig. 8–15). The inconstant occurrence of simultaneous neurologic handicaps, and the otherwise wide variation in severity of the syndrome, require the postulation of several separate mutations, whose relationship may be rather superficial. To date, all pedigrees studied have demonstrated inheritance consistent with autosomal recessive transmission, and experience indicates that about one fourth of the patients in this country are of Jewish ancestry.

PATHOLOGY. The Niemann-Pick cell has obviously vacuolated cytoplasm, a strongly positive reaction with fat stains (most specifically the Smith-Dietrich procedure), and is pale-appearing with other routine tissue stains (Fig. 8–14). Such cells are most prominent in the bone marrow, spleen and lymphoid tissue of all types; they are commonly found in liver and lung, and may appear in the connective tissue or parenchyma of virtually any organ. Splenomegaly is important (the organ varies from two to ten times normal weight for age); there is often a proportionate enlargement of the liver. When there is neurologic involvement, the brain is underweight, the gray matter is soft, with widespread neuronal distention, and there are mild deficiencies of white matter. The sphingomyelinase deficiency, when present, can be demonstrated in white blood cells, in biopsies of the liver or brain, and in cultures of skin fibroblasts or fetal amnion.

CLINICAL MANIFESTATIONS. The clinical picture in Niemann-Pick disease has such broad variations, albeit relatively constant for any one pedigree, that generalizations do not pertain. At least four common clinical patterns are repeated, but even this list may need further extension or subdivision.

Group A. The originally described "classic" form of the syndrome has major hepatosplenomegaly, early and severe handicaps, frequent occurrence of macular degeneration and blindness. Death occurs usually by 2 years of age.

Group B. A number of patients have been identified who have pathologic and biochemical abnormalities in most viscera, but no evidence (up to early adult life) of nervous system involvement. It is possible that survival potential may be normal in this interesting group.

Group C. In the most common form, motor and intellectual handicaps appear in late infancy; the visceral abnormalities are quantitatively milder, and the fundi normal. The child survives to 3 to 6 years of age.

Group D. In this group affected persons (most often of Nova Scotian French Canadian ancestry) have normal early development, but manifest neurologic disease in middle childhood which progresses to full dementia and paresis. Death occurs by 12 to 20 years of age.

The basic pathology for each of these groups is qualitatively similar (except for the normal brain in group B), and all must, by present definitions, be described as having Niemann-Pick disease. Skin lesions are infrequent; occasional xanthomas are seen, but pigmentation of the skin is rarely observed.

LABORATORY DATA. Examination of the bone marrow is the most useful diagnostic procedure. Sometimes, however, aspirations fail to yield an adequate number of abnormal cells, and in a few instances odd histiocytes with granular cytoplasm are seen. Similar foam cells may also be found in the bone marrow in other conditions, such as during cortisone therapy, in some liver tumors and in chronic hyperlipemia. Vacuolated lymphocytes and monocytes in the peripheral blood smear are a characteristic, but not invariable, sign of Niemann-Pick disease. These odd vacuoles, of uncertain origin, which occur in 1 to 10 per cent of otherwise normal agranulocytes, are seen elsewhere in comparable form only in the Swedish type of juvenile amaurotic idiocy, Wolman's disease, G_{M1}-gangliosidosis, I-cell disease and fucosidosis (Table 8–3). In Niemann-Pick disease there is suppression of white cells and platelets in the peripheral blood, as occurs in any sustained splenomegalic syndrome; there is usually a moderate anemia. Roentgenographically there may be diffuse pulmonary parenchymal abnormalities, especially in the first two clinical groups described, and the bones may show undermineralization or signs of marrow cavity overactivity. Increase of serum lipids, with moderate hypercholesteremia and even a turbid serum, is also characteristic of the patients in these two groups. When marrow examinations are unconvincing, or the clinical course is atypical, lipid analysis of tissues obtained by biopsy from the liver, spleen or lymph nodes may be required to establish the diagnosis.

TREATMENT. In contrast to Gaucher's disease, orthopedic problems are not a major issue in Niemann-Pick disease. Splenectomy may be indicated when there are significant evidences of hypersplenism. Special support for the patient with neurologic handicaps is of great importance in respect to feeding problems, mucus difficulties, seizures, and the like. To date, no chemotherapeutic agent has been convincingly effective. Judicious trials of new drugs, however, are justified when adequate control can be maintained.

TAY-SACHS DISEASE

In this lipidosis one finds in the gray matter a large increase in the concentration of ganglioside, a water-soluble, neuraminic-acid-containing glycolipid (Fig. 8–15). It occurs in unique cytoplasmic organelles, masses of which distend the neuronal cell body. Many of the inborn-error syndromes have a slight increase in the content of brain ganglioside, but none to the magnitude of Tay-Sachs disease. Further, it has been shown that the increase is particularly in one special class of ganglioside, so-called G_{M2} or "Tay-Sachs" ganglioside. There are also minor electron microscopic

TABLE 8–3 PRINCIPAL FEATURES OF RECENTLY DESCRIBED LIPIDOSES

DESCRIPTIVE NAMES AND EPONYMS	AGE AT ONSET OF CLINICAL MANIFESTATIONS	PATHOLOGY	LIPID ACCUMULATED INTRACELLULARLY	INVOLVEMENT OF C.N.S.	COURSE
Primary familial xanthomatosis with involvement and calcification of the adrenals (*Wolman's disease*)	Early weeks of life	Diffuse foam cell formation in viscera, including small intestine Malnutrition	Cholesterol and triglycerides	Yes	Diarrhea, vomiting, nutritional failure Prominent calcification of the adrenals Familial involvement Death by 2-4 months of age
Angiokeratoma corporis diffusum universale (*Fabry's disease*)	Midchildhood to early adult life	Vacuolization of renal epithelial cells Changes in blood vessel walls and myocardium Neuronal distention	Ceramide trihexoside	Yes	X-linked transmission Cutaneous lesions Corneal dystrophy Renal failure
Generalized gangliosidosis; G_{M1}-gangliosidosis, Type 1	Early months of life	Foam cells in viscera Glomerular epithelial cells swollen Distention of neurons	Ganglioside (G_{M1}), especially in brain Mucopolysaccharides in viscera	Yes	Odd facies, varying visceromegaly, neurologic handicap, skeletal changes Death in 1-3 years
Tangier disease; familial high-density lipoprotein deficiency (*Frederickson's disease*)	Childhood	Foam cells in tonsils and other reticuloendothelial tissues	Cholesterol esters (Low blood levels of cholesterol and phospholipid)	No	Large tonsils, with orange or gray color Occasional enlargement of spleen, lymph nodes or liver
Phytanic acid storage disease (*Refsum's disease*)	Early childhood to fifth decade	Retinal pigmentation Peripheral neuropathy Cerebellar ataxia	Phytanic acid	Yes	Progressive motor weakness, muscular atrophy Deafness, cataracts, osteochondritis Cardiac and respiratory deaths
I-cell disease (*Leroy's disease*)	Early months of life	Foam cells in spleen, liver, endocardium Swollen clear cells in glomeruli Vacuoles and granules in white blood cells	Uncertain ? increased glycolipid	Yes	Delayed development Odd facies, gingival hyperplasia Skeletal dysplasia, growth failure Death by 3-8 years
Disseminated lipogranulomatosis (*Farber's disease*)	Usually early months of life Occasionally later in childhood	Granulomatous lesions of skin, synovia, viscera (some with foam cell formation); distention of neurons	Ceramide	Usual	Typically produces hoarse cry, subcutaneous nodules, arthropathy, irritability and nutritional failure Milder form also known
Fucosidosis	Early months of life	Thick skin, increased sweat Na and Cl Full forehead, beaked L_2 and L_3 vertebrae Hepatosplenomegaly Vacuolated lymphocytes	Fucose-containing polysaccharides and glycolipids	Yes	Progressive cerebral deterioration Spastic quadriplegia, weakness Recurrent respiratory infections Myocarditis Death around 5 years

and chemical changes in viscera other than the nervous system (e.g., liver). Analysis of serum for a deficiency of "hexosaminidase A" allows accurate identification of homozygotes (involved children) and of adults and others who are genetic carriers for Tay-Sachs disease. The procedure permits the screening of young adults at high risk (those of Ashkenazi Jewish background, among whom the carrier rate for the defect is approximately 1 in 30); definitive information may be secured thereby in advance about a couple's potential for having an involved infant.

See Section 20 for the clinical description of the syndrome.

RECENTLY DESCRIBED SYNDROMES

In the past decade a large number of newly identified syndromes have been described as belonging in the lipidosis category. The principal features of eight such diseases are given in Table 8–3. Most of these syndromes are rare, but it is likely that many more affected children will be found as familiarity is gained with the clinical and pathologic patterns. When tissue specimens are available from patients of this sort, it is advisable to retain portions in a frozen, unfixed state for study in one of the laboratories now doing investigative work with lipids and mucopolysaccharides.

SYNDROMES WITH INCREASED BLOOD FAT

SECONDARY HYPERLIPIDEMIA. The content of fat in the blood of children may be increased in a variety of circumstances. The most common situations are *secondary,* dependent for degree upon the evolution of medical diseases in which lipid metabolism is altered as a byproduct of disturbances in the metabolism of carbohydrate or protein, as, for example, in diabetic acidosis, the von Gierke type of glycogenosis and the nephrotic syndrome. During compensated phases of these illnesses the serum lipids return to normal or near-normal values. The hyperlipidemia provides an index of the progress of the disease, but it does not in itself require any special considerations in treatment beyond that directed at the primary metabolic disorder. The milky or lipemic appearance of the serum in the foregoing diseases is due principally to excess of triglycerides (neutral fat). One can expect a frank turbidity to appear whenever the triglyceride concentration exceeds 1000 mg/dl (normal level, 0 to 200 mg/dl). Characteristically, such patients also have moderate increases in the phospholipid and cholesterol values of the serum.

Significant increases in the blood lipids also occur, with a clear-appearing serum, in children with intrahepatic biliary atresia. In this instance the concentration of the triglycerides is not elevated, but there is a great increase in the phospholipid and cholesterol levels (up to 3000 to 5000 mg/dl). The use of vegetable oil supplements in the diet lessens this hyperlipidemia considerably, as does also the use of bile-acid-absorbing resins. Other less frequent causes of increased blood lipid levels in children include hepatic tumors, hypothyroidism, severe anemia and Niemann-Pick disease.

PRIMARY HYPERLIPOPROTEINEMIAS. More critical elevations of blood fat occur in the syndromes identified collectively as the *familial hyperlipoproteinemias.* In these hereditary biochemical disturbances the basic defect appears to be in lipid metabolism. Frederickson has provided a working classification of five major phenotypes, based on clinical features, enzymatic abnormalities and the serum lipoprotein electrophoretic patterns.

"Type I" Hyperlipoproteinemia. ("idiopathic familial hyperlipemia," Buerger-Grutz syndrome). This is characterized by the presence of extremely lactescent serum (triglyceride levels of 2000 to 4000 mg/dl or higher) in an otherwise well-appearing child who may have minor enlargement of the liver and spleen. On occasion there are bouts of abdominal pain and vomiting which may mimic an acute surgical crisis. Serum cholesterol levels are only mildly elevated; a deficiency of lipoprotein lipase ("clearing factor") can be demonstrated. The lipemia is responsive to a reduction in dietary intake of fat, but this is difficult to administer for long periods in children, and there seems little urgency to do so, since the prognosis for cardiovascular disease is not disturbing.

"Type II" Familial Hypercholesterolemia. In this most common of the constitutional hyperlipoproteinemias, the serum is clear, with the triglyceride levels usually measuring near zero. The condition is inherited as a simple mendelian character.

In *heterozygously involved* persons the serum cholesterol concentration characteristically is stable at about 300 to 450 mg/dl. Children with this disorder are asymptomatic and are identified only through family surveys. Adults, especially males, have a high incidence of coronary disease in the age range of 30 to 40 years.

When both parents have the trait, the child may be *homozygous.* Such a child will have a serum cholesterol concentration in the range of 700 to 1000 mg/dl, and will have skin and tendon xanthomas in the early years (see below). The homozygous state is incompatible with survival beyond early adult life, and deaths at 12 to 14 years of age are not infrequent from the complications of valvular and coronary atheromatosis. Lowering the hypercholesterolemia by dietary therapy should be the first effort made; for the heterozygously involved child the results may be of critical value. Diet should include a significant reduction in intake of dairy fats and fatty meats (especially pork and pork products), utilization of vegetable oils for food preparation, and emphasis on poultry and fish. Extreme restrictions, however, are not justified. Various chemotherapeutic agents are irregularly effective, but worthy of trial: *d*-thyroxine, clofibrate, cholestyramine, beta-sitosterol, nicotinic acid, and neomycin have each seemed helpful in some patients.

"Types III, IV and V" Familial Hyperlipoproteinemia. These are infrequently identified in childhood. Characteristically there is a family history of diabetes mellitus and often also of heart disease. Affected persons may have a mildly abnormal glucose tolerance test result. The serum is often turbid (increase in triglycerides), sometimes markedly but inconstantly so; the cholesterol value is moderately elevated, and electrophoresis shows an important "pre-beta" factor in the lipoproteins. Xanthomas appear in adult life, and the cardiovascular prognosis is poor. The hyperlipoproteinemia often seems to be potentiated by a high intake of carbohydrates rather than of fat. Within the pediatric age range it is significant to realize that there are kinds of constitutional hyperlipemia which do not qualify for the more common types I and II and which will require more detailed study for full understanding. The child should be followed with blood lipid measurements for an extended period, the glucose tolerance examined, and information sought about the cardiac and carbohydrate and lipid metabolism of other family members.

SKIN XANTHOMAS

Xanthomas of the skin have little direct importance in themselves, but serve as useful indicators of lipid disturbances, or of certain benign tumorlike syndromes. These "yellow tumors" (also orange, brown or red) represent nodular collections of lipidized histiocytes and other related elements; their color is probably due to deposition of carotenoid material. The most pertinent cytoplasmic abnormality is the local accumulation of cholesterol. Only rarely is it necessary to substantiate the clinical impression of xanthoma by biopsy. The evaluation requires a general pediatric examination and careful measurement of the serum cholesterol level.

XANTHOMAS IN PATIENTS WITH NORMAL SERUM CHOLESTEROL LEVELS. These lesions are typically distributed in an axial fashion on the scalp, face, trunk and, occasionally, in the mouth. Such lesions are relatively common and are called "juvenile xanthogranulomas" (previously referred to as nevoxanthoendotheliomas). The lesions, which may range from one to a hundred or more, usually appear in the first months of life, increase for the next year or so, and then fade spontaneously by the time the child is 3 to 5 years of age (Fig. 8–16, *A*). The lesions are apparently benign new growths and require no specific therapy. The resulting scars are innocuous. In the characteristic situation there is no familial aspect, but many involved children or their relatives will also have *café-au-lait* spots or other evidence of neurofibromatosis.

Other related disease pictures, with more extensive involvement, are also seen; these include minor degrees of hepatomegaly, light pulmonary infiltration, leukocytosis (monocytes and lymphocytes) and anemia. One of the rare forms is the so-called *leukemic xanthomatosis,* with a monocytic or monomyeloid leukemoid picture, in conjunction with manifestations of neurofibromatosis (Fig. 8–16, *B*). Such syndromes appear to be expressions of the overall histiocytosis reaction pattern, with an unknown type of provoking mechanism. There is similarity of the visceral lesions to those in true Letterer-Siwe disease. There may also be skin xanthomas and accumulation of cholesterol in foam cells in internal granulomatous lesions, especially in the dura, bone marrow and thymus in Letterer-Siwe disease. The differential diagnostic study of the child with normocholesteremic skin xanthomas requires consideration of the presence of leukocytic abnormalities and of Letterer-Siwe disease.

Another rare syndrome, termed "xanthoma disseminatum," also appears to be related. Clusters of brown xanthomas are found in the skin folds and on the oral mucosa, and at times in the larynx, on the meninges and on the cornea or sclera.

XANTHOMAS ASSOCIATED WITH AN INCREASE IN THE SERUM CHOLESTEROL LEVEL. *Eruptive xanthomas* may appear on the skin in any syndrome in which there is a sustained elevation of blood lipids (see Syndromes with Increased Blood Fat). Diseases with which they are associated include von Gierke's disease, poorly controlled diabetes mellitus, chronic obstructive liver disease (Fig. 8–16, *C*) and "familial hyperlipemia" (Frederickson type I hyperlipoproteinemia). Typically, the lesions occur in crops on the extensor surfaces of the extremities, where minor trauma is common, but occasionally they appear on the face, on the palate and on the sides of the toes. On the eyelids they are referred to as "xanthelasmata." When they first appear, there may be mild itching. Eruptive xanthomas tend to be transient and are dependent upon the course of the hyperlipidemia.

In instances of familial hypercholesterolemia (type II hyperlipoproteinemia) the xanthomatous lesions are more extensive. Heterozygously involved young adults may initially have xanthomas only on the eyelids and within the Achilles tendons, but with the passage of years more widespread lesions form, particularly in other tendons. Children are free of xanthomas in this syndrome unless they are homozygously involved (both parents have hypercholesteremia). In this circumstance, xanthomas begin to appear at 1 to 2 years of age and progress steadily. Lumpy cutaneous lesions, referred to as "xanthoma tuberosum" (Fig. 8–16, *D*), form on the elbows and knees. Tendon lesions become large (heels, toes, knees, elbows, knuckles) and interfere with local comfort and function. On occasion their surgical removal may

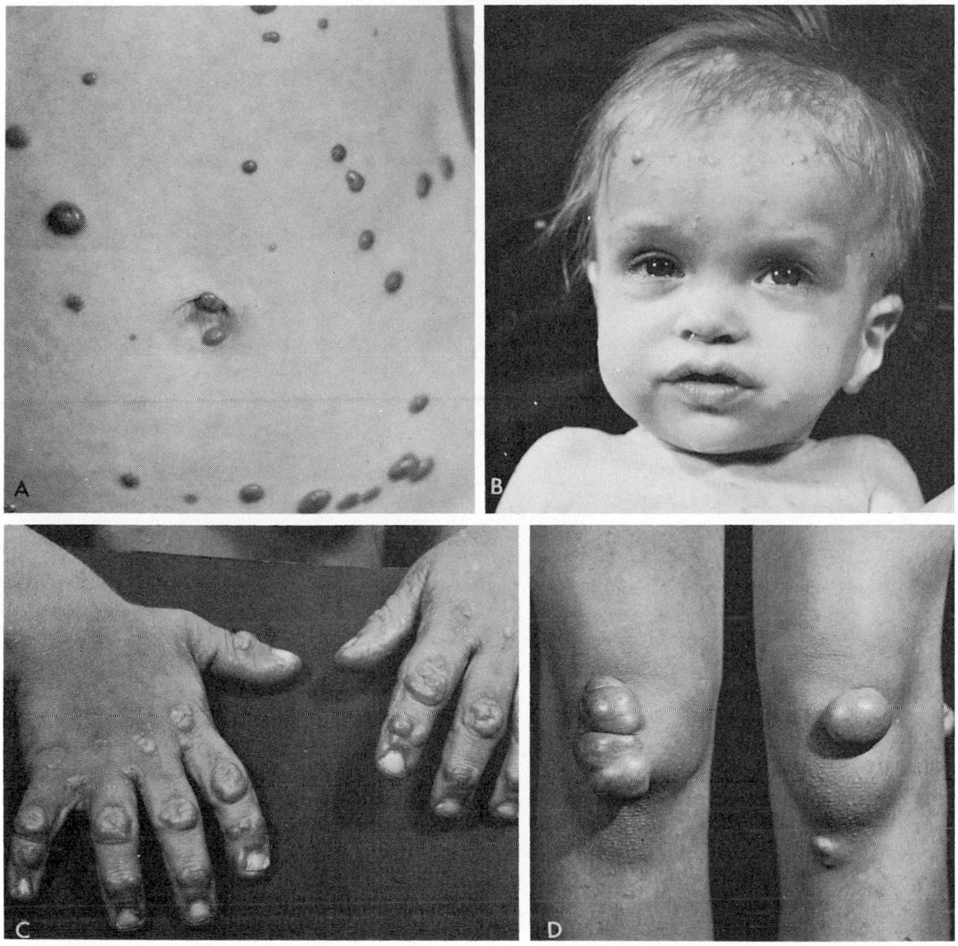

Figure 8–16 Skin xanthomas. A, *Juvenile xanthogranuloma lesions on the abdomen of a 17 month old girl.* B, *Xanthomas on the forehead and scalp of a 15 month old boy with a histiocytic syndrome which included leukocytosis, hepatomegaly and café-au-lait spots.* C, *Eruptive xanthomas on the hands of a 4 year old boy with intrahepatic biliary atresia.* D, *Xanthoma tuberosum lesions on the knees of a 12 year old girl with homozygous involvement in type II hyperlipoproteinemia.*

be justified as a temporary aid. In late childhood a corneal "arcus" may develop and, rarely, xanthomatous lesions within the medullary cavity of bone. Cardiovascular lesions (atheromas) are of critical importance.

ALLEN C. CROCKER

Lipidoses, General

Bernsohn, J., and Grossman, H. J. (eds): Lipid Storage Diseases; Enzymatic Defects and Clinical Implications. New York, Academic Press, Inc., 1971.

Crocker, A. C.: The cerebral defect in Tay-Sachs disease and Niemann-Pick disease. J. Neurochem. *7*:69, 1961.

Crocker, A. C., and Farber, S.: Niemann-Pick disease; A review of 18 patients. Medicine *37*:1, 1958.

Crocker, A. C., and Landing, B. H.: Phosphatase studies in Gaucher's disease. Metabolism, *9*:341, 1960.

Thannhauser, S. J.: Lipidoses; Diseases of the Intracellular Lipid Metabolism. 3rd ed. New York, Grune & Stratton, Inc., 1958.

Volk, B. W., and Aronson, S. M. (eds): Sphingolipids, Sphingolipidoses, and Allied Disorders. New York, Plenum Press, 1972.

Recently Described Syndromes

Bergsma, D. (ed): Birth Defects; Atlas and Compendium. Baltimore, The Williams & Wilkins Company, 1973.

Crocker, A. C., Cohen, J., and Farber, S.: The "lipogranulomatosis" syndrome—Review, with report of patient showing milder involvement. *In* Aronson, S. M., and Volk, B. W. (eds.): Inborn Disorders of Sphingolipid Metabolism. Oxford, Pergamon Press, 1966, p. 485.

Crocker, A. C., Vawter, G. F., Neuhauser, E. B. D., and Rosowsky, A.: Wolman's disease: Three new patients with a recently described lipidosis. Pediatrics *35*:627, 1965.

Frederickson, D. S., Gotto, A. M., Jr., and Levy, R. I.: Familial lipoprotein deficiency (Tangier disease). *In* Stanbury, J. B., Wyngaarden, J. B., and Frederickson, D. S. (eds): The Metabolic Basis of Inherited Disease. 3rd ed. New York, McGraw-Hill Book Company, 1972, p. 493.

Leroy, J. G., Spranger, J. W., Feingold, M., Opitz, J. M., and Crocker, A. C.: "I-Cell" disease; A clinical picture. J. Pediatr. *79*:360, 1971.

O'Brien, J. S.: Generalized gangliosidosis. J. Pediatr. *75*:167, 1969.

Philippart, M.: Fucosidosis: A novel neurovisceral sphingolipidosis. Neurology *19*:304, 1969.

Steinberg, D.: Phytanic acid storage disease (Refsum's syndrome): *In* Stanbury, J. B., Wyngaarden, J. B., and Frederickson, D. S. (eds): The Metabolic Basis of Inherited Disease. 3rd ed. New York, McGraw-Hill Book Company, 1972, p. 833.

Sweeley, C. C., Klionsky, B., Krivit, W., and Desnick, R. J.: Fabry's disease: Glycosphingolipid lipidosis. *In* Stanbury, J. B., Wyngaarden, J. B., and Frederickson, D. S. (eds): The Metabolic Basis of Inherited Disease. 3rd ed. New York, McGraw-Hill Book Company, 1972, p. 663.

Syndromes with Increased Blood Fat and Skin Xanthomas

Crocker, A. C.: Skin xanthomas in childhood. Pediatrics *3*:573, 1951.

Crocker, A. C.: The histiocytosis syndromes: *In* Fitzpatrick, T. B., Arndt, K. A., Clark, W. H., Jr., Eisen, A. Z., Van Scott, E. J., and Vaughan, J. H. (eds): Dermatology in General Medicine. New York, McGraw-Hill Book Company, 1971, p. 1328.

Crocker, A. C.: Inborn errors of lipid metabolism: *In* Gellis, S. S., and Kagan, B. M. (eds): Current Pediatric Therapy 5. Philadelphia, W. B. Saunders Company, 1973, p. 366.

Frederickson, D. S., and Levy, R. I.: Familial hyperlipoproteinemia: *In* Stanbury, J. B., Wyngaarden, J. B., and Frederickson, D. S. (eds): The Metabolic Basis of Inherited Disease. 3rd ed. New York, McGraw-Hill Book Company, 1972, p. 545.

Liebman, S. D., Crocker, A. C., and Geiser, C. F.: Corneal xanthomas in childhood. Arch. Ophthal., *76*:221, 1966.

Rausen, A. R., and Adlersberg, D.: Idiopathic hyperlipemia and hypercholesterolemia in children. Pediatrics, *28*:276, 1961.

DEFECTS IN PIGMENT METABOLISM

THE PORPHYRIAS

The porphyrias are a group of syndromes characterized biochemically by errors in pyrrole metabolism and clinically by photodermatitis and visceral and neuropsychiatric complaints. Incidence is estimated at 1:30,000 in the general population. Table 8–4 classifies them according to the organ system in which the error in pyrrole metabolism is localized: *erythropoietic* and *hepatic* forms are recognized. Most of the porphyrias have a dominant mode of inheritance. Family studies and close surveillance through adolescence are essential in order to identify cases in the latent stage; this is vital since most deaths occur during the late adolescent and early adult years and are attributable to delays in diagnosis which may lead to inappropriate and harmful therapy. Family studies entail determination of porphyrins in both urine and stool in all members; in cases of photosensitivity, measurements of erythrocyte protoporphyrin are also necessary. With early diagnosis, proper fluid and dietary therapy and avoidance of contraindicated drugs, the prognosis for survival and symptomatic relief during acute visceral attacks is good.

TABLE 8–4 A CLASSIFICATION OF THE PORPHYRIAS

Hepatic Porphyrias

A. Acute intermittent porphyria (AIP, Swedish genetic porphyria)
B. Porphyria variegata (PV, South African genetic porphyria)
C. Hereditary coproporphyria
D. The cutaneous porphyrias (PCT, porphyria cutanea tarda)
   1. Hereditary types
   2. Acquired (but possible genetic predisposition associated with alcoholism, etc.)
   3. Toxic (hexachlorobenzene-induced)

Erythropoietic Porphyrias

A. Erythropoietic protoporphyria
B. Congenital erythropoietic porphyria

RELATION OF ABNORMAL HEME BIOSYNTHESIS TO DISEASE STATES. Heme is the prosthetic group of hemoglobin, myoglobin, catalase, peroxidase and the cytochromes. It is formed via the metabolic pathway shown in Figure 8–17. This pathway is common to all mammalian cells, each cell synthesizing its own heme for the formation of its own particular hemoproteins. The initial step, formation of δ-aminolevulinic acid (ALA),* is mediated by ALA synthetase (Fig. 8–17). This mitochondrial enzyme is inductible, and its availability is rate-limiting for the entire process.

Four basic porphyrin isomers are known and are designated as types I, II, III and IV. Types I and III are the only naturally occurring isomers. Mammalian hemoproteins contain type III porphyrin isomers only. Protoporphyrin (PROTO) 9 is a type III isomer. Infinitesimal quantities of type I isomers are formed as byproducts of heme synthesis.

In *acute intermittent porphyria* excessive formation of ALA synthetase occurs in liver and is responsible for the increased amounts of ALA and porphobilinogen (PBG) which characterize this disease. It seems likely that excessive ALA synthetase is common to all the hepatic porphyrias; this enzymatic abnormality has also been observed in red cells of patients with erythropoietic protoporphyria. Factors not yet elucidated account for differences in pattern of excretion of pyrroles in the various porphyrias.

The fundamental metabolic defect in *congenital erythropoietic porphyria* resides in the inability of approximately half of the developing erythroblasts to convert PBG to uroporphyrinogen (UROGEN) III (Fig. 8–17). Instead, URO I accumulates within the nuclei of these defective erythroblasts, diffuses into the circulation, is deposited in various tissues, including teeth and bone, and is excreted in the urine as a mixture of URO I and coproporphyrin (COPRO) I, with URO I predominant. In

*See Table 8–6 for key to abbreviations used in this chapter.

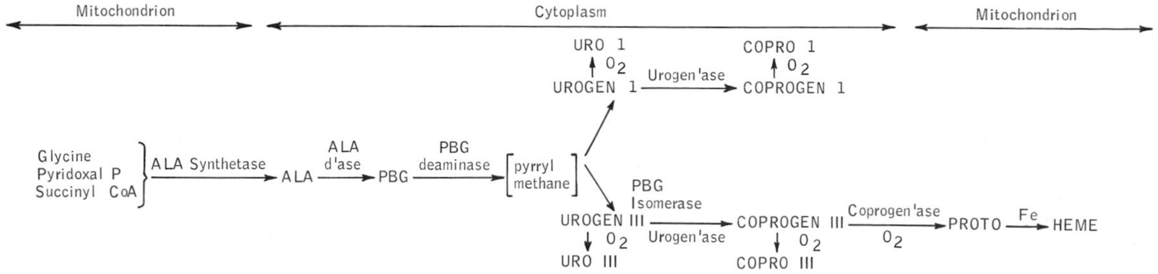

Figure 8–17 *Intracellular organization of biosynthesis of heme. The initial and final steps in heme synthesis occur within the mitochondria. ALA is released in the cytoplasm. The metabolites formed in the cytoplasm are the ones found in the plasma and urine. ALA synthetase is the rate-limiting enzyme. Only the fully reduced porphyrin intermediates UROGEN III and coproporphyrinogen (COPROGEN) III are utilized for heme formation. These substances are colorless and unstable and do not exhibit fluorescence. Oxidation stabilizes porphyrin molecules and renders them fluorescent. Those portions of UROGEN and COPROGEN not utilized for heme synthesis are oxidized to UROs I and III and COPROs I and III, and it is in this form that these porphyrins are usually detected in the tissues and excreta. PBG and ALA are also colorless and do not fluoresce; they are measured by chemical methods.*

erythropoietic protoporphyria excessive amounts of PROTO 9 are produced in the cytoplasm of erythrocytes, both in marrow and in the circulation. The accumulated PROTO 9 is excreted in feces, but not in urine.

Normally the urinary excretion of PBG and ALA does not exceed 3 mg a day. The qualitative Schwartz-Watson reaction for PBG (see below) is positive only with a pathologic excess of PBG. Porphyrins normally appear in the excreta in very small amounts: fecal COPRO and PROTO should not exceed 100 μg per gram of dry feces per day; COPRO appears in urine at a rate of 2.2 μg/kg (1 μg/lb) of body weight per day. Infections and accelerated erythropoiesis cause a two- to threefold increase in urinary COPRO; hepatitis (infectious and toxic) a ten- to fortyfold increase in urinary COPRO; and lead intoxication a ten- to fortyfold increase in both ALA and COPRO in urine. Porphyria may cause up to one thousandfold increases in pyrrole excretion. In acquired porphyria COPRO always exceeds URO in urine, but in the heritable forms the quantity of URO in urine always exceeds COPRO, if both are present. Increased fecal porphyrins virtually always indicate a heritable form of porphyria.

RELATION OF METABOLIC ERRORS TO CLINICAL MANIFESTATIONS

Photosensitizing Effects of Porphyrins. Some but not all the skin lesions of both erythropoietic and certain hepatic porphyrias are due to the photosensitizing effect of URO. Erythema, edema and vesiculation of the exposed skin result when persons with increased uroporphyrinemia are irradiated with a combination of near ultraviolet (4000 Å) and infrared (26,000 Å) monochromatic lights. Urticaria and eczematoid lesions may follow exposure to near ultraviolet light of subjects with greatly increased amounts of PROTO in their red blood cells and plasma. All the heme precursors (Fig. 8–17) have at one time or another been injected into both healthy and porphyric human subjects without demonstrable adverse effect other than photosensitization.

Toxic and Experimental Hepatic Porphyria. In patients with the hepatic forms of porphyria it is clear that the overproduction of ALA by the liver is responsible for the great accumulation of pyrroles in this organ and the excreta. What is not clear is how or whether this metabolic error is related to the visceral and neuropsychiatric disorders encountered in many such patients.

Acute intermittent porphyria is the first inborn error of metabolism in which the genetic defect causes an excess rather than a deficit of a specific enzyme (hepatic ALA synthetase). Table 8–5 lists the drugs, chemical agents and endogenous metabolites which may induce hepatic porphyria in experimental animals. Granick has demonstrated that formation of ALA synthetase can be induced in vitro by hexachlorobenzene, griseofulvin, barbiturates, dihydrocollidines and steroids. The cur-

TABLE 8–5 AGENTS USED TO INDUCE CHEMICAL HEPATIC PORPHYRIA IN ANIMALS

Chemicals	
Allylisopropylacetamide	
Allylisopropylacetylurea (Sedormid)	
Hexachlorobenzene	
3,5-dicarbethoxy-1,4-dihydrocollidine	
Drugs	
Sulfonal	
Barbiturates	
Sulfonamides	
Griseofulvin	
Chloroquine	
Endogenous Sex Steroids	
1. Potent porphyrin-inducing activity	
C-19 Steroids	C-21 Steroids
(Etiocholanolone)	(Pregnanediol)
(Etiocholandiol)	(Pregnanolone)
(Etiocholandione)	(11-Ketopregnanolone)
(Etiocholanolone-17)	(17-OH Pregnanolone)
2. Weak porphyrin-inducing activity	
Testosterone	
Progesterone	
Estradiol	
Estrone	
Estriol	

rent hypothesis is that the level of ALA synthetase is controlled by operator and repressor genes. Granick proposes that hepatic porphyria is caused by a mutation in the operator gene which renders it poorly responsive to the repressor substance, which may consist of a protein aporepressor and heme as a corepressor. The inducing chemicals (Table 8–5) compete with heme, with the result that more ALA synthetase is formed in their presence. Certain C-19 and C-21 sex steroids, such as etiocholanolone, pregnanediol and pregnanolone, are potent inducers of porphyrin synthesis. They are produced in significant quantities daily and in the past were considered inert metabolites of hormone metabolism; in Granick's in-vitro system for studying induction of porphyrin formation, the glucuronide conjugates of even the most potent steroid inducers are inert. The fact that sex steroid metabolites are potent endogenous inducers may explain the delay in appearance of symptoms in hepatic porphyria until after puberty. The inactivation of potent inducers of ALA synthetase by conjugation and the presence of other evidences of liver dysfunction in some acquired forms of porphyria (i.e., Bantu, alcoholic) suggest that optimal hepatic function may play a significant role in ameliorating the clinical course in hepatic porphyrias.

Balance studies in patients with hepatic porphyria show that both severe caloric restriction and negative nitrogen balance are accompanied by a sharp increase in the excretion of pyrroles. This increase in pyrrole excretion can be suppressed if adequate caloric intake is restored by the administration of carbohydrates. Return to positive nitrogen balance is also accompanied by diminution in pyrrole excretion. The maintenance of a diet high in carbohydrate and adequate in protein is of considerable clinical importance.

DIAGNOSIS AND MANAGEMENT OF THE PORPHYRIAS

Clinical Manifestations. Although the porphyrias are generally genetically determined and associated with some metabolic error present from birth, clinical symptoms are rare before puberty in the hepatic forms. Three groups of clinical manifestations are recognized: cutaneous, visceral and neuropsychiatric. Their onset is insidious, but once they occur, the complaints tend to run an undulating course throughout the remainder of the patient's life. The principal clinical syndromes and patterns of pyrrole excretion encountered in the porphyrias are summarized in Table 8–6.

Acute exacerbations of dermal lesions occur with exposure to sunlight. Visceral and neurologic complaints, which almost invariably occur together, may be precipitated by infection, menstruation, pregnancy, alcohol, barbiturates and other agents listed in Table 8–5. Although the skin lesions are bothersome and may be disfiguring, it is the acute visceral and neurologic problems that threaten life. The relative frequency of various abnormal clinical findings encountered during an acute attack are shown in Figures 8–18 and 8–19; none are pathognomonic. Early diagnosis depends upon recognition of the sequence in which the clinical manifestations appear, intensify and abate, and upon demonstration of excess pyrroles in the excreta. Colicky abdominal pain and varied neuropsychiatric symptoms are the usual presenting complaints.

Colicky abdominal pain is the initial symptom of an acute attack in most patients. The pain is most frequently in the epigastrium or right iliac fossa, but may be located anywhere in the abdomen or pelvis. There is considerable variation in its intensity; the pain tends to worsen in an undulating manner over a period of days. Severe colic may persist for hours and often causes the patient to writhe about or assume bizarre positions in bed. Vomiting and constipation shortly develop in all but the mildest attacks. Examination of the abdomen and pelvis reveals minimal signs which seem insignificant in comparison with the patient's pain. Diffuse tenderness of the abdomen is usually present, but does not localize; rigidity and muscle spasm are rare. Leukocytosis and fever are often present. The acute visceral pain of porphyria has been confused with virtually every acute surgical condition of the abdomen, various painful gynecologic disorders and "hysteria." In the absence of other features and objective findings characteristic of these other conditions, the presence of tachycardia and hypertension makes porphyria a likely diagnosis.

Uncommonly, pain, weakness and paresthesia in back and limb muscles occur as presenting complaints in the absence of abdominal pain. *Personality changes,* probably attributable to patchy cerebral demyelination, are observed in most patients suffering from visceral attacks, but they are rarely the predominating features. These patients are variously described as depressed, nervous, hysterical, lachrymose or "peculiar." These traits wax and wane with the severity of the pain. In severe colic, mental confusion, hallucinations and disorientation are often present.

After the patient with acute intermittent porphyria or porphyria variegata (Table 8–6) has had an exacerbation characterized by abdominal pain, vomiting, constipation, tachycardia and, in more severe cases, hypertension, the end of the attack may often be heralded by the return of blood pressure, pulse and weight to normal.

The urine is apt to be colorless at first, although PBG is always present in high concentration and is diagnostic. If the attack progresses, and especially if barbiturates are given, the urine usually becomes red, increasing motor restlessness is noted, and neurologic manifestations, rarely present initially, soon appear. These take the form of unpredictable, spotty weakness or paralysis, with diminished or absent tendon reflexes, and pain and tenderness in the involved muscle groups. These signs are attributable to patchy demyelination of peripheral nerves. Muscle paralysis is an ominous sign. Ill advised abdominal or pelvic surgery may

TABLE 8–6 CLINICAL SYNDROMES AND PYRROLE[1] EXCRETION PATTERNS IN HERITABLE FORMS OF PORPHYRIA

		HEPATIC PORPHYRIAS				ERYTHROPOIETIC PORPHYRIAS	
		Acute Intermittent Porphyria	*Porphyria Variegata*	*"Porphyria Cutanea Tarda"*	*Hereditary Coproporphyria*	*Erythropoietic Protoporphyria*[2]	*Congenital Erythropoietic Porphyria*
Transmission			Autosomal dominant				Recessive
Onset of clinical manifestations			Puberty or later[3]		Early childhood		Infancy
Acute visceral and neurologic attacks		Present	Present	Present	Present	Absent	Absent
Cutaneous lesions		Absent	Present	Present	?Absent	Present	Present
Pyrrole excretion[4] during acute visceral and neurologic attacks	*Urine*						
	ALA, PBG[5]	++++	++++	±	+ to ++		
	URO, COPRO	± to +++	± to +++	±	+ to ++		
	Feces						
	COPRO,	0	++++	++++	++++		
	PROTO	0	++++	+++	±		
Pyrrole excretion[4] during remission of visceral and neurologic symptoms	*Urine*						
	ALA, PBG	±	0	±	0	0	0
	URO, COPRO	±	0	0	±	0	++++
	Feces						
	COPRO,	0	++++	++++	++++	±	+++
	PROTO	0	++++	++++	0	++++	±

1. Strictly speaking, ALA is a heme precursor, but not a pyrrole. PBG is a monopyrrole. URO, COPRO and PROTO are tetrapyrroles.
2. Erythrocyte PROTO grossly increased in erythropoietic protoporphyria.
3. In each group rare cases have been observed before puberty.
4. Increased URO in feces found in some cases of each group.
5. ALA – δ-aminolevulinic acid.
PBG – porphobilinogen.
UROGEN – uroporphyrinogen.
URO – uroporphyrin.
COPROGEN – coproporphyrinogen.
COPRO – coproporphyrin.
PROTO – protoporphyrin.

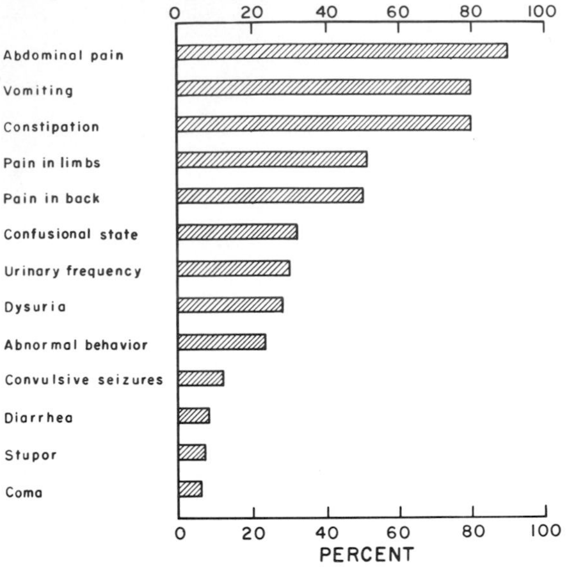

Figure 8–18 *The acute attack of porphyria—relative frequency of symptoms. Based on an analysis of 107 acute attacks in 80 patients. (Adapted from Eales, L.:* S. Afr. J. Lab. Clin Med., *9:151, 1963.)*

be quickly followed by catastrophic paralysis and coma. Weakness and paralysis may persist for months after the other features of an acute attack have subsided. Death, when it occurs, usually results from quadriparesis or respiratory failure.

There is a profound disturbance in water and electrolyte homeostasis in severe attacks of porphyria. The serum is hypotonic, with reduced concentrations of sodium and chloride (Fig. 8–19). The urine is hypertonic, owing in part to excessive loss of sodium, which is attributed to inappropriate secretion of antidiuretic hormone. The severity of neurologic injury may be related to the degree of hyponatremia. Hypocalcemia and hypomagnesemia may occur, with and without tetany.

Burgundy red urine in the porphyric patient is due to the presence of URO. It is a constant finding in congenital erythropoietic porphyria and a frequent finding in patients with cutaneous manifestations of hepatic porphyria.

A variety of *dermal lesions* may be observed in porphyria. Exposure to sunlight, particularly during the summer months, produces vesicles, bullae and edema on the exposed skin. These photosensitive lesions are prone to secondary infection and heal slowly, with chronic scars which become hyperpigmented. In some patients such lesions may also follow minor mechanical trauma and exposure to indoor sources of ultraviolet light. Macules, papules, eczematous plaques and urticaria are also seen. Nearly all patients with cutaneous forms of porphyria eventually have hypertrichosis and a violaceous hue to their skin. These changes develop insidiously over the years and are most prominent on the exposed parts of the body.

Differential Diagnosis. Examination of Figures 8–18 and 8–19 makes it clear that porphyria must be included in the differential diagnosis of essential hypertension, hyperthyroidism, painful gynecologic disorders, "hysteria," psychosis and all surgical conditions of the abdomen. Whenever diagnosis of such surgical conditions as ulcer, gallbladder disease or appendicitis cannot be made with confidence, a Schwartz-Watson test for PBG should be done prior to surgical exploration. A surprising number of porphyric patients are treated in error for hyperthyroidism. Serum protein-bound iodine may be elevated in hepatic porphyria without other laboratory evidence of hyperthyroidism. Cutaneous forms of porphyria should be included in the differential diagnosis of photosensitive dermatitides.

Laboratory Diagnosis. Accurate diagnosis of porphyria requires examination of both urine and feces, and, in the case of erythropoietic protoporphyria, of blood (Table 8–6). The excreta of the patient and of his relatives must be examined to establish the type of pedigree and to identify latent cases. In the hepatic porphyrias, pyrrole excretion patterns may vary according to the presence or absence of visceral symptoms. Porphyrin excretion may be increased a thousandfold or more over the normal values. The red color imparted to urine by URO must be distinguished from that due to urates, bile, anthocyanin (from beets), melanin, eosin, hemoglobin or myoglobin.

The *Schwartz-Watson reaction for PBG* is almost always positive in acute visceral attacks. In *freshly voided* urine the test is simple, and diagnostic when performed as follows:

Five ml of freshly voided urine (cooled to room temperature) is thoroughly shaken in a small separatory funnel for 30 seconds with 5 ml of Ehrlich's aldehyde reagent (0.7 gm of p-dimethylaminobenzaldehyde [ACS reagent grade], 150 ml of concentrated hydrochloric acid, and 100

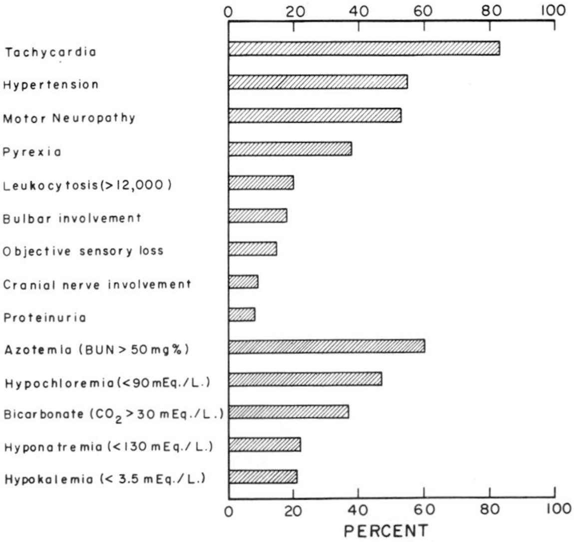

Figure 8–19 *The acute attack of porphyria—relative frequency of signs and pertinent laboratory findings. Based on analysis of 107 acute attacks in 80 patients. (Adapted from Eales, L.:* S. Afr. J. Lab. Clin. Med., *9:151, 1963.)*

ml of distilled water). The solution is then adjusted to pH 4 to 5 by mixing thoroughly with a saturated aqueous solution of sodium acetate (10 ml usually required). The formation of a cherry-red or red-violet color at this point indicates the presence of porphobilinogen, urobilinogen or certain indolic compounds. The red pigments formed with Ehrlich's reagent by each of these substances can then be separated on the basis of differential solubility.

If red pigment is present, the solution is next extracted with 10 ml of chloroform. Red color due to urobilinogen passes into the chloroform phase, which is discarded. Extraction with chloroform is repeated, until a clear chloroform phase is observed, indicating complete removal of urobilinogen pigment from the aqueous phase. If the remaining aqueous solution still contains red pigment, this aqueous solution is next extracted with 5 ml of n-butanol. Red pigment due to indoles and other Ehrlich reactors passes into the n-butanol phase, while only red pigment formed from porphobilinogen remains in the aqueous phase. Butanol-extractable red pigment, as well as porphobilinogen, has been found in the urine of some patients with acute intermittent porphyria; so both the butanol and aqueous phases may contain red pigment after the final extraction.

If this test gives equivocal results, the urine should be treated with heat and acetic acid to convert all precursors to URO, which is then readily identified. New simplified methods for measuring porphyrins in blood (primarily PROTO) should facilitate the clinical diagnosis of erythropoietic protoporphyria and possibly other porphyrias associated with photosensitive dermatitis. The bibliography contains further references to analytical methods.

Treatment. Disturbances in water and electrolyte homeostasis are not usually seen in mild attacks; nevertheless, they should be anticipated and the patient treated expectantly. When profound disturbances in water and electrolyte homeostasis are present, restriction of water and careful replacement of the sodium deficit may result in dramatic clinical improvement. Poor ventilation in depressed patients and respiratory paralysis may occur and require cardiopulmonary assistance.

Because many chemical agents are capable of inducing porphyria, drug therapy must be approached with extreme caution. Pain and restlessness can be controlled with morphine and chloral hydrate. Cortisone and chlorpromazine have been beneficial in some cases, without obvious effect in others, and deleterious in a few. Adequate caloric and nitrogen intakes should be restored as rapidly as possible.

Successful long-term management requires careful control of infections, and absolute avoidance of alcohol and of the drugs listed in Table 8–5. A diet adequate in nitrogen and high in carbohydrates is beneficial. Many patients are fearful of precipitating colicky episodes and indulge in food fads. In some women, attacks are clearly related to the menstrual cycle; some have been treated with ovulatory suppressants, androgens and even oophorectomy, with apparent beneficial results. Oral contraceptives in the lowest effective dosage have been beneficial in some but not all cases of acute intermittent porphyria; they are apparently contraindicated in pedigrees with dermal symptoms. Persons with latent or manifest hepatic porphyria should wear "Medic Alert" bracelets.

The cutaneous lesions are usually satisfactorily managed by avoidance of excessive exposure to sunlight. When this is inadequate, the application of *red veterinary petrolatum* to the skin may be beneficial. This petrolatum protects the skin from radiation in the near ultraviolet zone; the usual commercial sunscreens do not.

Infants of mothers with hepatic porphyria may have increased pyrrole excretion during the neonatal period; this *passive porphyria* is not associated with any symptoms. The infant's excretion of pyrroles soon returns to normal.

ACQUIRED HEPATIC PORPHYRIA

Most cases of hepatic porphyria are clearly of genetic origin. When it is not possible to demonstrate this in family studies, such cases are usually designated as "acquired," but the possibility of genetic predisposition cannot be entirely excluded. This is illustrated by an outbreak of toxic porphyria which occurred in Turkey following the introduction of a new fungicide to which the population may not have been exposed previously. Between 1956 and 1960, some 5000 cases of porphyria in southeastern Turkey were traced to the eating of seed wheat which had been treated with a fungicide, hexachlorobenzene. The resultant syndrome, seen predominantly in children, was characterized by cachexia, hepatomegaly, bullous skin lesions, photosensitivity, hyperpigmentation, hypertrichosis and increased porphyrin content of the excreta. "Rheumatoid" arthritic changes were noted ultimately in more than 50 per cent of the patients. A chronic porphyric state with all the features just enumerated persisted in most patients for at least 2 years after the cessation of hexachlorobenzene ingestion. Even 5 years later most still had hepatomegaly, arthritis, hypertrichosis and hyperpigmentation. Genetic factors were at first thought to be excluded but later work by Dogramaci suggests that those affected may have been genetically predisposed. For example, within a family unit, only one parent was usually affected and only a portion of the children.

The acquired forms of hepatic porphyria are clinically indistinguishable from the hereditary cutaneous syndromes (Table 8–6). Visceral manifestations are minimal or absent, and dermal features are usually less severe in the acquired disease, often being limited to hyperpigmentation and hypertrichosis. Acquired porphyria may occur as a rare complication of chronic alcoholism, cirrhosis, tumors involving the liver and such systemic diseases as Hodgkin's disease, disseminated lupus and leukemia. Red urine due to the presence of URO is usually the clue that leads to the diagnosis.

VARIANTS OF GENETIC PORPHYRIA

Congenital erythropoietic porphyria is one of the rarest inborn errors of metabolism. Vastly increased amounts of URO I are found in bone marrow, circulating erythrocytes, plasma, urine and feces. Lesser amounts of COPRO I are also found in the excreta. The excretion of other pyrroles is normal. The accumulation of URO I in the tissues (including the teeth) and the associated hemolytic anemia account for all the clinical manifestations of this disease. The photodermatitis of this disease is devastating, often causing severe permanent disfigurement. Splenomegaly results from the hemolytic anemia; splenectomy is beneficial in some cases. The excretion of urine which is burgundy red as passed, or becomes so upon exposure to light, begins at birth or shortly thereafter and continues for life.

Erythropoietic protoporphyria begins during childhood and continues through adult life. Two types of skin lesions follow exposure to sunlight: (1) a urticarial response which resolves without chronic dermal changes; and (2) erythema and edema followed by an eczematous eruption on the exposed parts. This eczematous eruption is chronic rather than recurrent and leaves considerable scarring. These patients also have dull, opaque fingernails without lunulae. Clinical manifestations are otherwise limited to the skin. Increased amounts of PROTO 9 are always found in erythrocytes, and usually in feces. Rigorous avoidance of sunlight is indicated.

Among the hepatic porphyrias the visceral, neurologic and dermal manifestations and the pattern of pyrrole excretion are usually constant within a given pedigree. There is, however, considerable variation from one pedigree to another. The features of four typical variants are shown in Table 8–6. Of these, *acute intermittent porphyria* and *porphyria variegata* are perhaps the most common. In kindreds with **acute intermittent ("Swedish") porphyria**, visceral and neurologic attacks are both most frequent and most severe in females of child-bearing age. The disorder probably has an autosomal dominant mode of transmission, but the fact that the excreta may not contain excess pyrroles during the asymptomatic phase has impeded genetic studies. In such kindreds acute attacks often occur without obvious precipitating factors. The occurrence of visceral attacks before puberty is rare, but has been reported.

In kindreds with **porphyria variegata, "South African porphyria,"** symptoms are most common between puberty and the fifth decade of life. Skin lesions are relatively more common in males, whereas acute visceral attacks are more frequent in females. A striking feature is the importance of barbiturates in the precipitation of severe acute visceral attacks. There is an autosomal dominant mode of transmission; 50 per cent of adult members of affected families have a constant increase in excretion of porphyrins in the feces whether symptoms are present or not.

Porphyria cutanea tarda presents with visceral as well as dermal manifestations, but the visceral complaints tend to be mild in comparison with those seen in acute intermittent porphyria. The existence of a purely cutaneous, hereditary form of hepatic porphyria has been disputed; it can be argued that these patients have never encountered an environmental agent which would precipitate a visceral attack.

Hereditary coproporphyria appears to be transmitted as an autosomal dominant, and it is not a symptomless trait, as previously thought. Clinically it resembles acute intermittent porphyria, except as symptoms may begin during childhood. There may be chronic "nervousness" and other psychiatric complaints, with or without recurrent abdominal pain. The unique biochemical feature of this disease is increased excretion of COPRO III in the feces; urinary COPRO III may or may not be increased. In the majority of cases severe visceral attacks are provoked by barbiturates and possibly by other anticonvulsant and tranquilizing drugs; during such attacks urinary excretion of ALA, PBG and COPRO III is increased. Photosensitivity has been described in only 1 of 30 cases.

HEREDITARY METHEMOGLOBINEMIAS

Normally the iron of both oxygenated and deoxygenated hemoglobin is in the ferrous state (ferrohemoglobin); this is essential for its oxygen-transporting function. Oxidation of hemoglobin iron to the ferric state yields methemoglobin (ferrihemoglobin), which is nonfunctional and imparts a chocolate hue to the blood; in sufficient concentration it causes cyanosis. The blood of healthy persons contains methemoglobin, but the intraerythrocytic methemoglobin-reducing system maintains its concentration at less than 2 per cent of the total hemoglobin. "Normal" methemoglobin has a characteristic spectral absorption band at 632 millimicrons, which is abolished by treatment of the blood sample with cyanide (technique of Evelyn and Malloy). This technique is specific for assaying methemoglobin produced by exposure to certain chemicals such as aniline dyes, but yields erroneous results when hemoglobin M type pigments are present. In familial cases both recessive and dominant patterns of inheritance are recognized; each has a distinct metabolic error.

HEREDITARY METHEMOGLOBINEMIA ASSOCIATED WITH DEFECTIVE METHEMOGLOBIN-REDUCING SYSTEM. Reduction of methemoglobin in normal erythrocytes can be effected by four known systems; ascorbic acid, glutathione, triphosphopyridine nucleotide (TPNH) diaphorase and diphosphopyridine nucleotide (DPNH) diaphorase. Among these, DPNH diaphorase (or DPNH methemoglobin reductase) is by far the most active.

In hereditary methemoglobinemia with a recessive pattern of inheritance there is complete absence of the DPNH-dependent methemoglobin reductase. In these patients the methemoglobin formed has the spectral and chemical properties of "normal" methemoglobin. Methylene blue is therapeutically effective because it is reduced to leucomethylene blue by both glutathione and TPNH diaphorase; leucomethylene blue, in turn, can reduce "normal" methemoglobin to hemoglobin.

Clinically the disorder is characterized by cyanosis, the intensity of which varies with season and diet. The time at onset of the cyanosis also varies; in some patients it appears at birth, in others as late as adolescence. No associated abnormalities which might explain the cyanosis are found. Despite the fact that up to 50 per cent of the total circulating hemoglobin may be in the form of nonfunctional methemoglobin, there is little or no cardiorespiratory distress except on exertion.

The daily oral administration of ascorbic acid (200 to 500 mg in divided doses) will gradually reduce the quantity of methemoglobin to about 10 per cent of the total pigment and will alleviate the cyanosis as long as therapy is continued. Methylene blue given intravenously (1 to 2 mg/kg) promptly eliminates both methemoglobin and cyanosis. and this effect can be maintained by the daily oral administration of methylene blue (3 to 5 mg/kg). Mental deficiency has been associated in a few cases, but not in most, and there is insufficient evidence to indicate that it is causally related to the methemoglobinemia.

HEREDITARY METHEMOGLOBINEMIA ASSOCIATED WITH ABNORMAL METHEMOGLOBINS (HEMOGLOBIN M DISEASES). The dominantly transmitted forms of methemoglobinemia are collectively known as the hemoglobin M diseases. When all the hemoglobin pigment in a blood sample is first oxidized to methemoglobin by treatment with potassium ferricyanide, the abnormal methemoglobin M type pigments can be separated from normal methemoglobin by means of starch gel electrophoresis. Amino acid "fingerprinting" of several hemoglobin M pigments reveals the substitution of an abnormal amino acid residue in the globin chain. Dissimilar substitutions have been found in different pedigrees. This situation is analogous to that of other hemoglobinopathies (hemoglobin S, hemoglobin C, and others). Theoretic considerations strongly suggest that the abnormal amino acid residue in each of the hemoglobin M pigments lies in a portion of the globin chain in close proximity to the prosthetic heme group where it can alter the properties of the heme moiety. Thus, cyanosis is probably due to the unusual stability of the methemoglobin form of the M hemoglobins. Such a hypothesis would also explain the variable response of patients to ascorbic acid and methylene blue as well as the abnormal spectral properties and differing response to cyanide treatment of various hemoglobin M pigments. Among the several hemoglobin M pedigrees examined, five different hemoglobin M pigments have been identified. Some of their properties are summarized in Table 8–7. It is possible that the entity previously described as "congenital sulfhemoglobinemia" may fall within the hemoglobin M disease group.

Clinically methemoglobinemia of the hemoglobin M type should be suspected when family studies suggest an autosomal dominant pattern of inheritance and when the blood of the cyanotic patient fails to show the absorption band at 632 millimicrons, characteristic of normal methemoglobin. The patient's methemoglobin may or may not react with cyanide (technique of Evelyn and Malloy) to yield a normal cyanomethemoglobin absorption curve. This varies with the pedigree (Table 8–7). In the hemoglobin M diseases the quantity of methemoglobin does not exceed 25 per cent of the total hemoglobin; the cyanosis, although persistent from early infancy, is not associated with any disability. There may be a compensatory polycythemia. Affected members of some pedigrees do not respond to ascorbic acid or methylene blue (hemoglobin M_B and hemoglobin $M_{M\text{-}1}$). Fortunately alleviation of cyanosis is not essential in the hemoglobin M diseases.

HEMOCHROMATOSIS

Hemochromatosis is one of several forms of iron storage disease. It is characterized by excessive

TABLE 8–7 SOME SPECTRAL AND CHEMICAL PROPERTIES OF THE HEMOGLOBINS M

Hb M TYPE*	ABNORMAL HEMOGLOBIN CHAIN	METHEMOGLOBIN SPECTRAL ABSORPTION MAXIMA IN VISIBLE RANGE† (mμ)	CYANOMETHEMOGLOBIN DERIVATIVE ABSORPTION SPECTRUM
Hb M_{Boston}	α	495 and 602	Abnormal
Hb $M_{Saskatoon}$	β	492 and 602	Normal
Hb $M_{Milwaukee-1}$	β	500 and 622	Normal
Hb $M_{Milwaukee-2}$	?β	490 and 588	Normal
Hb M_{Iwate}	α	485 and 590	Abnormal
Normal Hb A	–	502 and 632	Normal

*Geographic designation refers to residence of first pedigree studied; types are often abbreviated as follows: Hb M_B, Hb M_S, Hb $M_{M\text{-}1}$, Hb $M_{M\text{-}2}$, Hb M_I.

†In M/15 sodium phosphate buffer, pH 6.5.

Adapted from P. S. Gerald: *Pediatrics,* 31:780, 1963.

deposition in many organs of hemosiderin, an iron hydroxide-protein complex which in liver, pancreas or heart eventually causes impaired structure and function. The familial form of the disease is called **primary hemochromatosis**, and is associated with increased gastrointestinal absorption of iron. The nature of the metabolic defect is unknown. It is not associated with any known cause of excessive iron absorption, such as increased erythroid activity or excessive dietary iron intake, which can cause **secondary hemochromatosis**. Untreated cases of primary hemochromatosis eventually exhibit the classic triad of hepatic cirrhosis, slate or bronze pigmentation of the skin and diabetes mellitus. These symptoms and signs do not appear before adulthood. Serum iron levels are increased in both latent and symptomatic adult members of affected families, but not in the children. The pattern of inheritance has not been established. Depletion of iron stores is the aim of treatment and will improve both symptoms and the function of affected organs. This is most conveniently achieved by repeated phlebotomy; in anemic patients with secondary hemochromatosis or hemosiderosis, chelation therapy with deferoxamine is preferred.

J. JULIAN CHISOLM, JR.

Dean, G., and Barnes, H. D.: The inheritance of porphyria. Brit. M. J. *2*:89, 1955.

Debré, R., and others: Genetics of haemochromatosis. Ann. Human. Genet. *23*:16, 1958.

Dogramaci, I.: *In* Levine, S. Z. (ed.): Advances in Pediatrics. Chicago, Year Book Medical Publishers, Inc., 1964, Vol. 13, pp. 11–64.

Goldberg, A.: Acute intermittent porphyria. Quart. J. Med. *28*:183, 1959.

Goldberg, A., Rimington, C., and Lochhead, A. C.: Hereditary coproporphyria. Lancet *1*:632, 1967.

Granick, S.: The induction *in vitro* of the synthesis of δ-aminolevulinic acid synthetase in chemical porphyria: A response to certain drugs, sex hormones and foreign chemicals. J. Biol. Chem. *241*:1359, 1966.

Granick, S., and Kappas, A.: Steroid control of porphyrin and heme biosynthesis: A new biological function of steroid hormone metabolites. Proc. Nat. Acad. Sci. *57*:1463, 1967.

Heller, S. R., Labbe, R. F., and Nutter, J.: A simplified assay for porphyrin in whole blood. Clin. Chem. *17*:525, 1971.

Hellman, E. S., Tschudy, D. P., and Bartter, F. C.: Abnormal electrolyte and water metabolism in acute intermittent porphyria. Am. J. Med. *32*:734, 1962.

Hellman, E. S., et al.: Elevation of the serum protein-bound iodine in acute intermittent porphyria. J. Clin. Endocrinol. Metab. *23*:1185, 1963.

Keitt, A. S.: Hereditary methemoglobinemia with deficiency of NADH-methemoglobin reductase. *In* Stanbury, J. B., Wyngaarden, J. B., and Frederickson, D. S. (eds.): The Metabolic Basis of Inherited Disease. 3rd ed. New York, McGraw-Hill Book Company, Inc., 1972, pp. 1389–1397.

Lamont, N. McE., Hathorn, M., and Joubert, S. M.: Porphyria in the African. Quart. J. Med. *30*:373, 1961.

Marver, H. S., and Schmid, R.: The porphyrias. *In* Stanbury, J. B., Wyngaarden, J. B., and Frederickson, D. S. (eds.): The Metabolic Basis of Inherited Disease. 3rd ed. New York, McGraw-Hill Book Company, Inc., 1972, pp. 1087–1140.

Neuberger, A., Goldberg, A., and Magnus, I. A.: The porphyrias. Proc. R. Soc. Med. *61*:191, 1968.

Pollycove, M.: Hemochromatosis: *In* Stanbury, J. B., Wyngaarden, J. B., and Frederickson, D. S. (eds.): The Metabolic Basis of Inherited Disease. 3rd ed. New York, McGraw-Hill Book Company, Inc. 1972, pp. 1051–1084.

Ridley, A., Hierons, R., and Cavanagh, J. B.: Tachycardia and the neuropathy of porphyria, Lancet *2*:708, 1968.

Runge, W., and Watson, C. J.: Experimental production of skin lesions in human cutaneous porphyria. Proc. Soc. Exp. Biol. Med. *119*:809, 1962.

Schmid, R., Schwartz, S., and Sundberg, D.: Erythropoietic (congenital) porphyria: A rare abnormality of the normoblasts. Blood *10*:416, 1955.

Schwartz, S., Johnson, J. A., Stephenson, B. D., Anderson, A. S., Edmondson, P. R., and Fusaro, R. M.: Erythropoietic defects in protoporphyria: A study of factors involved in labelling of porphyrins and bile pigments from ALA-^{3}H and glycine-^{14}C. J. Lab. Clin. Med. *78*:411, 1971.

Tschudy, D. P., and others: Acute intermittent porphyria: The first "overproduction disease" localized to a specific enzyme. Proc. Nat. Acad. Sci. *53*:841, 1965.

Watson, C. J., Taddeini, L., and Bossenmaier, I.: Present status of the Ehrlich aldehyde reaction for urinary porphobilinogen. J.A.M.A. *190*:501, 1964.

Welland, F. H., and others: Factors affecting the excretion of porphyrin precursors by patients with acute intermittent porphyria. I. The effect of diet. Metabolism *13*:232, 1964.

Welland, F. H., and others: Factors affecting the excretion of porphyrin precursors by patients with acute intermittent porphyria. II. The effect of ethinyl estradiol. Metabolism *13*:251, 1964.

Zimmerman, T. S., McMillin, M., and Watson, C. J.: Onset of manifestations of hepatic porphyria in relation to the influence of female sex hormones. Arch. Intern. Med. *118*:229, 1966.

9

THE IMMUNOLOGIC SYSTEM, ALLERGY AND RELATED DISEASES

IMMUNITY AND ALLERGY

The prevention, diagnosis and treatment of infectious diseases and their complications occupy a large portion of the time of the pediatric physician. These functions require not only familiarity with available vaccines and the clinical pharmacology of antimicrobial drugs, but also knowledge of the epidemiology of the common viral, bacterial, fungal and parasitic infections and an appreciation of the variation of their clinical manifestations in children of different ages as a reflection of the anatomic, physiologic and immunologic development of the host. An attempt will be made in the following sections to summarize the present state of knowledge of the host factors which affect response to infection and allergens.

The immunologic system has two main functional divisions: the phagocytes, and the lymphoid system. *Phagocytic cells*, comprising polymorphonuclear leukocytes, monocytes, histiocytes and tissue macrophages, are responsible for the capture, killing and intracellular digestion of invading microorganisms. Lymphoid cells, which are responsible for the specificity of immunologic responses, differentiate from stem cells into two distinct lines, known as T (thymus-derived) and B (bursa or bone marrow-derived) cells (Fig. 9–1). **T lymphocytes** require the *thymus* to establish their immunologic competence and are concentrated in the paracortical zones of the lymph nodes and periarterial sheaths of the splenic white pulp. They mediate specific *cellular immunity*; i.e., the capacity (1) to develop specific resistance to infection with many viruses, fungi and mycobacteria, (2) to acquire specific delayed hypersensitivity, which influences the pathology and symptomatology of a wide variety of infections, and (3) to recognize cells in tumors or allografts as foreign and to mobilize lymphoid cells for their rejection.

B lymphocytes vary in morphology, depending upon their functional state, and are responsible for the synthesis of specific antibodies and, thus, for *humoral immunity*. B cells are found in the lymphoid follicles of the lymph nodes, spleen and bowel. When stimulated, they develop into plasma cells that secrete the specific immunoglobulin antibodies that protect against subsequent exposure to certain viruses, bacterial exotoxins and pyogenic bacteria. Immunologic "memory," upon which the accelerated cellular and antibody responses of the immune state depend, is a property of "instructed" lymphoid cells; it seems likely that both groups of lymphocytes have this functional capacity. Although the lymphoid system has two distinct functional subdivisions, recent work clearly indicates that cooperation between the different lymphoid cells is a feature of normal im-

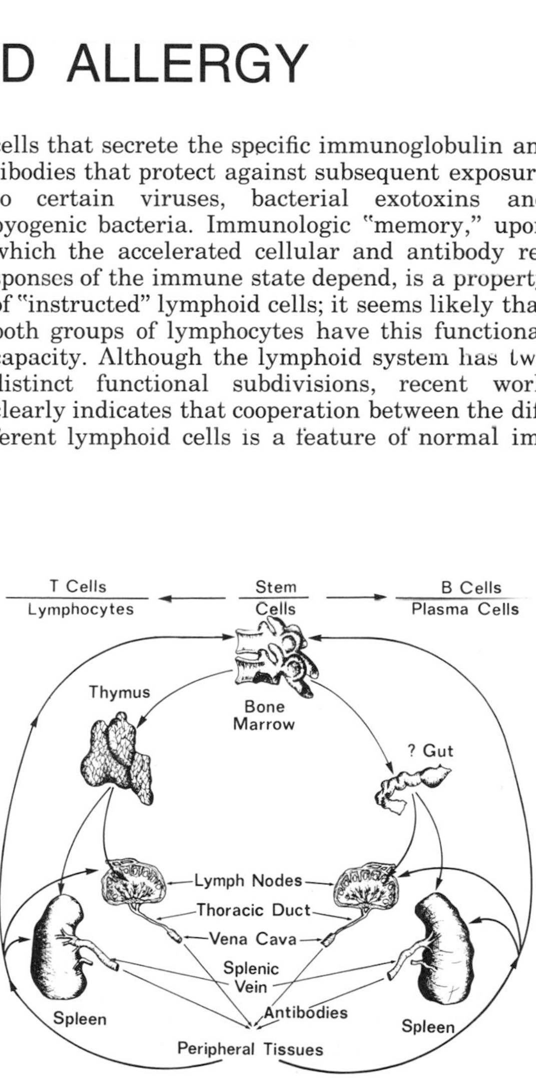

Figure 9–1 *Diagrammatic representation of the circulation and localization of the two types of lymphoid cells arising from stem cells. T cells, on the left, must either arise in or pass through the thymus to become competent, then localize in the spleen and paracortical areas of the lymph nodes, whence they recirculate constantly. B cells, on the right, are possibly activated in the gut wall, but localize in the follicles of spleen and lymph nodes. Some B cells circulate; antibodies are secreted into the lymph and blood by plasma cells formed from B cells in response to antigenic stimuli.*

munologic responses and that their activities have an important influence upon the function of phagocytic cells.

The term **allergy**, originally introduced by von Pirquet to describe the specifically altered state brought about by the immunologic response of the organism to an initial contact with a foreign substance or an infectious agent, has come to be used to describe the inherited tendency of certain individuals to overrespond to a variety of foreign chemicals upon their contact with the skin, mucous surfaces or vascular endothelium. Its cellular and humoral basis, giving rise to "immediate" reactions of the anaphylactic type, characterized by local exudation and smooth muscle contraction, will be described later.

THE IMMUNOLOGIC SYSTEM

COMPONENTS OF THE IMMUNOLOGIC SYSTEM

Although a great deal of new knowledge has been acquired in recent years about the various organs, cells and proteins comprising the immunologic system, the exact manner in which their functions are linked together in response to infection is still not entirely clear.

ORGANS

THYMUS. The thymus plays a dominant role in the development of immunologic competence by the fetus and young infant, and in the process, which occurs in early fetal life, whereby the ability of the immunologic system to distinguish between self and nonself is established. The epithelial portions of the thymus, destined to form its medulla, develop as paired structures arising from endoderm of the third and fourth pharyngeal pouches of the embryo; these fuse and descend into the upper mediastinum. Hassall's corpuscles begin to appear by about 8 weeks of gestational age. *Lymphoid cell* precursors appear first in the yolk sac, then in succession in the liver, bone marrow, thymus, gut mucosa, lymph nodes and spleen. Immunologic responsiveness appears to develop by about 13 weeks, when T cells, as shown by their response to phytohemagglutinin, can first be identified in the cortex of the thymus. By 18 weeks both T cells and B cells can be found in the spleen.

In the absence of intrauterine infection the development of the clear-cut follicular architecture of the mature lymphoid tissues and the appearance of plasma cells do not take place until 4 to 6 weeks after birth. Although the *relative* size of the thymus is greatest in the first few years of life, it continues to grow until puberty, when involution normally begins.

The thymus plays a key role in the development of immunologic competence by T lymphocytes as manifested by the capacity to reject allografts and to develop the delayed type of hypersensitivity. These functions are markedly depressed in certain animal species if the thymus is removed at birth. The fact that they can be restored, not only by reimplantation of the thymus, but also by its insertion in a millipore chamber, which prevents the ingress and egress of cells, suggests that the thymus may act in two ways: (1) possibly, by supplying competent lymphocytes to the peripheral lymphoid tissues; and (2) by secreting a hormone that affects the function of these cells. In animals thymectomized neonatally there is a paucity of lymphocytes in the paracortical areas of the lymph nodes and in the periarterial sheaths of the white pulp of the spleen; lymphocytes of these "thymus-dependent" areas are thought to be derived from or controlled by the thymus.

In chickens a second central lymphoepithelial organ, the bursa of Fabricius, arises from the cloaca. It controls the development of B lymphocytes. Antibody synthesis is markedly depressed by early bursectomy and is restored by the injection of bursal lymphocytes. These cells, in contrast to the thymus-derived lymphocytes, localize around the germinal centers to form the cortical lymphoid follicles of the lymph nodes. Efforts to identify, in man or other mammals, a second lymphoepithelial organ analogous to the bursa of Fabricius and essential for development of the capacity to synthesize antibodies have failed thus far; tonsils, appendix and Peyer's patches have all been suggested. Nevertheless, studies of patients with immunologi deficiency have revealed conditions in which the functional deficits and morphologic changes are those which would be predicted if there were two such lymphoid systems and if one were deficient while the other remained intact.

LYMPH NODES. These, the most important immunologically active organs, are located at strategic sites along the peripheral lymphatic vessels and serve to collect macromolecules and particulate matter. Their structure, consisting of sinusoids lined by macrophages, provides for phagocytosis of foreign and particulate material; the sinusoids are closely related to a cortex consisting of lymphoid follicles, the number and size of which reflect the activity of the node. The paracortical, thymus-dependent area with its accumulation of lymphocytes lies below the cortex; the medullary cords, which lead toward the efferent lymphatic channel, have the greatest concentration of plasma cells in a stimulated node (Fig. 9–2).

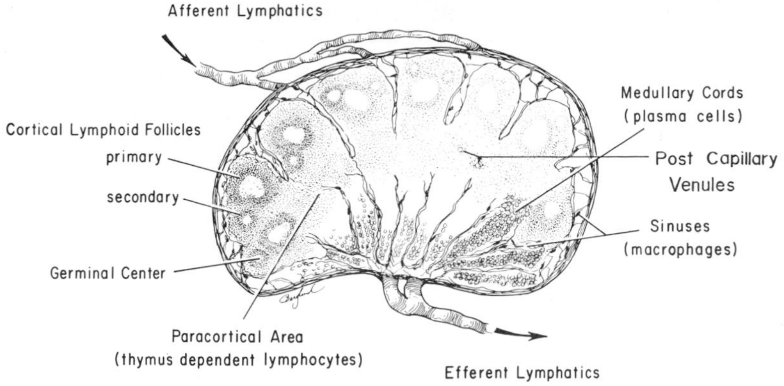

Figure 9–2 *Diagram of a normal lymph node after antigenic stimulation.*

SPLEEN. This organ bears a similar anatomic and functional relationship to the blood stream as do lymph nodes to the lymphatic vessels. It contains abundant sinusoids lined with macrophages, sheaths of lymphocytes around the arteries, lymphoid follicles in the white pulp, and plasma cells in the red pulp. Thus, both lymph nodes and spleen have (1) phagocytic elements which clear the lymph or blood during passage through the respective organ, and (2) lymphoid follicles, lymphocytes and plasma cells, which mediate the specific immunologic responses to foreign antigens.

CELLS

Three main groups of cells are involved in immunologic responses: phagocytes, T lymphocytes and B cells. The *phagocytes* include the "fixed" macrophages of the reticuloendothelial system in lungs, liver, spleen, lymph nodes and bone marrow, as well as the "wandering" phagocytes—polymorphonuclear leukocytes and monocytes of the blood and histiocytes of the connective tissues. Eosinophils seem to be involved in the phagocytosis of antigen-antibody complexes, basophils and tissue mast cells in the release of mediators of immediate allergic reactions.

T LYMPHOCYTES. These cells play a key role in specific immunologic responses to histoincompatible cells, to many viruses and to foreign chemicals or antigenic configurations of microorganisms which evoke delayed hypersensitivity. The lymphocytes in the blood are almost certainly a heterogeneous population. Cells with similar morphology may be derived from thymus, bone marrow and peripheral lymphoid tissues (lymph nodes, spleen and Peyer's patches); some may have a life span of only a few days, whereas others have been reported to survive in the body for as long as 10 years.

T lymphocytes are carried in the blood from the thymus to their localization in the peripheral lymph nodes and spleen, whence they undergo constant recirculation which permits them to perform their surveillance function. Passing into the great veins by way of the efferent lymphatic vessels and thoracic duct, T lymphocytes travel throughout the body in the circulation, returning to the paracortical areas of the lymph nodes through the specialized walls of the postcapillary venules (Fig. 9–2). T cells make up 70 to 80 per cent of the circulating lymphocytes. They are characterized by a size of 7 to 9μ, by responsiveness to stimulation by phytohemagglutinin, antigens and allogeneous cells, by moderate antigen uptake and by the release of macrophage *migration inhibitory factor* (MIF) upon contact with specific antigen. In mice they may be distinguished by a specific (θ) surface antigen, but such an antigen has not been identified in man. T cells appear to be the source of a considerable number of soluble substances, known as *lymphokines,* many of them released upon contact with the specific antigen to which the cells have been sensitized, such as MIF and a recently discovered mitogen that stimulates the proliferation and transformation of other lymphocytes. One important lymphokine is the *transfer factor,* described by Lawrence, which permits a lymphocyte to transfer its specific immunologic reactivity to other lymphocytes.

B CELLS. About 10 to 15 per cent of the peripheral blood lymphocytes are B cells, small (7μ), with very scant cytoplasm, characterized by surface immunoglobulins with a high affinity for antigens to which the donor has been immunized and by receptors for C3, as shown by the formation of rosettes with sensitized sheep red blood cells reacted with the first four components of complement (EAC1423). **Plasma cells,** which are derived from B cells after antigenic stimulation, are characterized by staining with methyl green pyronine of their more abundant cytoplasm, which contains an extensive endoplasmic reticulum upon electron microscopic examination, a feature associated with a high rate of protein synthesis and secretion.

In addition, the blood normally contains a small population of medium and large lymphoid cells, which are unresponsive to stimulation by mitogens, but which exhibit a high rate of spontaneous DNA synthesis and are capable of forming colonies when cultured in semisolid medium, and which are presumably progenitor cells.

IMMUNOLOGICALLY ACTIVE PROTEINS. The *immunoglobulins* are synthesized by B cells and their plasma cell derivatives and are molecules specifically reactive with the antigens which stimulated their formation. Three main classes of immunoglo-

TABLE 9–1 HUMAN PLASMA IMMUNOGLOBULINS

CLASS OF IMMUNO-GLOBULINS	MOLECULAR FORMULA	MOLECULAR WEIGHT	CARBO-HYDRATE CONTENT	TURNOVER HALF-TIME (DAYS)	CONCENTRATION IN NORMAL ADULT SERUM (MG. %)	MATERNO-FETAL TRANSFER	FUNCTIONAL COMPONENTS
IgM	$(\mu_2\kappa_2)_5$ or $(\mu_2\lambda_2)_5$	(19S) 900,000	10%	3–4	60–70	0	Antibodies formed in initial response; Anti-O (bactericidal to gram-neg. orgs.) isohemagglutinins, Forssmann
IgA	$\alpha_2\kappa_2$ or $\alpha_2\lambda_2$	(7–12S) 160,000–500,000	7%	4–7	150–250	0	Serum IgA probably derived from locally formed "secretory IgA"
IgG	$\gamma_2\kappa_2$ or $\gamma_2\lambda_2$	(6.7S) 150,000	2%	20–30	700–1400	+	Antibodies formed in later response; Antiviral; Antitoxic; Antibacterial; Anti-H
IgD	$\delta_2\kappa_2$ $\delta_2\lambda_2$	160,000	–	–	3	0	–
IgE	$\epsilon_2\kappa_2$ $\epsilon_2\lambda_2$	180,000	–	–	0.03	0	Atopic reagins

bulins (IgM, IgA, IgG) are recognized when the plasma of normal adults is analyzed by immunoelectrophoresis; two additional classes, which are present in trace amounts in normal serum (IgD, IgE) have been identified in recent years. The immunoglobulin molecules have a basic structure of two heavy (H) and two light (L) polypeptide chains joined by disulfide bonds. The L chains (κ or kappa and λ or lambda) are the same in all classes of immunoglobulins. Usually about two thirds of the molecules contains a pair of κ chains; one third of them, a pair of λ chains. On the other hand, the heavy or H chains of each class are different and account for the immunologic, structural and functional differences between the classes. Data concerning these differences are given in Table 9–1.

In addition, there are genetic differences between immunoglobulins from different persons. Four different γ H chains have been identified from studies in myeloma patients (γ_1, γ_2, γ_3, γ_4,). Therefore, one might write the formula for IgG globulins not just as $\gamma_2\,\kappa_2$ or $\gamma_2\,\lambda_2$, but as $\gamma 1_2\,\kappa_2$ or $\gamma 1_2\,\lambda_2$, $\gamma 2_2\,\kappa_2$ or $\gamma 2_2\,\lambda_2$, $\gamma 3_2\,\kappa_2$ or $\gamma 3_2\,\lambda_2$, and $\gamma 4_2\,\kappa_2$ or $\gamma 4_2\,\lambda_2$. Genetic variation in these γH chains is controlled by the GM locus, and more than 20 variants have thus far been identified. The Inv locus controls the structure of the κL chains, with 3 alleles thus far identified. Because κ chains are present in all classes of immunoglobulins, this form of genetic variation affects them all and not just the IgG globulins, as in the case of the GM locus.

Not to be confused with these subclasses are *chromatographically* distinguishable fractions of IgG. These represent mixtures which may be functionally distinct but which have not been completely characterized. One such fraction, separable on phosphocellulose, is of interest because of its tendency to bind to leukocytes and to carry the phagocytosis-stimulator, "tuftsin" (see p. 454).

Enzymatic and reductive cleavage of the immunoglobulin molecules has been used to investigate their structure and to alter them for therapeutic use. Three proteolytic enzymes—papain, pepsin and human plasmin—produce differing effects. Papain splits **IgG globulin** into three fragments, each with a sedimentation constant of approximately 3.5S, equivalent to a molecular weight of approximately 50,000; these fragments are known as the Fc fragment, which is without antibody activity, and two identical Fab fragments, each containing a single binding site for antigen. Pepsin digestion yields a single major 5S fragment ($F(ab')_2$) with a molecular weight of approximately 100,000, composed more or less of two Fab fragments, and with bivalent antibody activity. Properly controlled digestion of IgG globulin by human plasmin yields a major component with bivalent antibody activity and only slightly reduced molecular weight (6.5S), as well as smaller fragments. Purified and isotopically labeled fragments derived from pepsin and plasmin digestion of human IgG globulin have been shown to behave very differently after intravenous injection. The 5S $F(ab')_2$-like fragment of pepsin digestion has a very short half-life, while the 6.5S fragment obtained by plasmin digestion has a half-life close to that of normal IgG globulin (approximately 20 days). Both are much better tolerated on intravenous injection than are standard preparations of normal human serum gamma globulin, which contain small amounts of globulin complexes of higher molecular weight which produce severe reactions on intravenous injection, thus necessitating intramuscular administration. Gamma globulin fragments, some with molecular weights as low as 10,000, but still retaining bivalent antibody activity, are found in normal urine in very small amounts (5 to 10 mg per liter).

IgM globulins are macroglobulins with a sedimentation constant of 19S and with a much higher valence and lower affinity for antigens than the IgG globulins, from which they may be distinguished by their susceptibility to reductive cleavage by mercaptoethanol, which destroys their activity as antibody. IgM globulins are polymers composed of five 7S IgM subunits arranged around a core composed of a J chain, providing 10 antibody combining sites per molecule. This type of antibody is the first to be detected after immunization or infection and is the "natural" bactericidal antibody in adult serum against the endotoxins of the gram-negative enteric bacilli. **IgA globulins** appear to be the antibody contained in body secretions, in which they appear as polymers composed of two or, occasionally, three 7S IgA molecules joined by a J chain. Synthesis occurs locally in plasma cells. Secretory IgA also contains an immunologically distinct secretory or transport piece, which is contributed by the epithelial cells through which secretion occurs.

Complement, originally described by Ehrlich as the heat-labile factor in serum essential for immunologically determined hemolysis, is a very complex system. For many years it was considered to have four components, but nine separate proteins have now been identified. The complement system consists of a series of proteins (C1 through C9) that successively react with antigen-antibody complexes, with other macromolecular aggregates or with cells sensitized by antibody. In the course of this series of reactions, some of which require Ca^{++} or Mg^{++} ions, enzymes are activated which damage the bacterial or cell wall. Certain of the complement components themselves may be destroyed or altered by their participation in the reactions. In addition to the nine known components of complement in serum, there are inhibitors which help to maintain an equilibrium in this system of interacting proteins, some of which are extremely labile. Thus C1, the first component of complement, exists as a proesterase in serum, but is activated to an esterase (C1 esterase) in the first step of the complement fixation reaction. Normal serum contains a C1 inhibitor, which can neutralize its activity; deficiency of this inhibitor in patients with hereditary angioneurotic edema results in recurrent attacks of localized swelling.

Research upon complement was handicapped in the past by the lability of many of its components and by the necessity for using immune hemolysis as the indicator system for measuring its activity. Recent advances in the purification of a number of the components of complement have made possible their measurement by immunochemical methods. C3, or β_{1c} globulin, a relatively stable protein present in considerable amounts in normal serum, has turned out to be the limiting factor in immune hemolysis; its concentration is proportional to the hemolytic activity of fresh serum upon sensitized red cells. Thus immunochemical measurement of β_{1c} globulin concentration has been introduced as an easy method for measuring complement in clinical laboratories.

The components of complement appear to have a short half-life and rapid turnover in the body. Thus, the level of C2 or C3 (β_{1c} globulin) is lowered only when there is a fairly massive fixation of C by antigen-antibody complexes (e.g., in acute glomerulonephritis, serum sickness or lupus erythematosus) or when synthesis is depressed.

Complement, or at least some of its components, probably plays an essential role in certain responses to infectious agents mediated by specific antibody—immune adherence, immune bacteriolysis, enhancement of phagocytosis and intracellular killing of virulent bacteria. In addition, as the components of complement are successively activated after initiation of complement fixation by the attachment of C1 to antigen-antibody complexes, a series of factors are released that mediate the chemotaxis of phagocytic cells and the changes in vascular tone and permeability characteristic of inflammation, which are due to the action of a group of vasoactive peptides known as "kinins."

The **properdin system**, discovered by Pillemer, now appears to provide an alternate pathway through which, perhaps in the presence of very small amounts of antibody, C3 is directly activated without the previous activation of C1, 4 and 2, as occurs in the usual complement fixation reaction. Since C3 is central to the enhancement of phagocytosis, this may be quite important in the early response to infection.

Interferon is a substance produced by cells infected with a virus. It inhibits viral multiplication in such cells. It is rapidly produced, nonspecific toward many viruses, but relatively species-specific in its action on cells. It probably plays an important role in recovery from certain viral infections. Interferon production may be stimulated by the injection of certain macromolecular substances such as double-stranded RNA, as well as by viral infection.

IMMUNOLOGIC RESPONSES

INFLAMMATION. Most infections lead to inflammation, a nonspecific local response to injury characterized by migration, first of polymorphonuclear leukocytes and later of mononuclear cells from dilated capillaries and venules, and by exudation of plasma proteins into the tissues at the site of infection. Small thrombi in blood vessels and lymphatics tend to localize the infection. The nature and intensity of the inflammatory response vary with the microbial agent as well as with the physiologic and immunologic status of the host. In general, the inflammatory reaction tends to be less intense in infants than in older persons. Study of the inflammatory response with a Rebuck chamber on the skin in newborn infants shows a greater than usual outpouring of eosinophils and a slower appearance of mononuclear cells. While inflammation characterizes acute infections, granulomatous responses occur in more chronic ones, particularly when delayed hypersensitivity plays an important role.

Fever usually occurs in an infectious process, presumably as a result of the action upon hypothalamic nuclei of endogenous pyrogen released from leukocytes injured by bacterial endotoxins. Likewise, the *acute phase reaction,* which develops rapidly, is characterized by a series of changes in the plasma proteins which tend to parallel the intensity of the inflammation and to disappear when that subsides. These changes are (1) an increase in fibrinogen, producing a rapid sedimentation rate, (2) increases in α_1 antitrypsin, α_2 globulin and serum glycoprotein—principally haptoglobulins, (3) a rise in C3, and (4) the appearance of a new β-globulin, the C-reactive protein.

SPECIFIC IMMUNOLOGIC RESPONSES. While the local and systemic responses to infection are taking place, the immunologic response has already begun, with phagocytosis of the infecting organisms by the leukocytes at the site of infection. This process requires *recognition* of the foreign nature of the infecting agent and the presence of "opsonins" in the plasma, and is greatly enhanced in the case of most virulent organisms by specific antibody and complement. If organisms invade the blood stream, they are cleared through phagocytosis by the macrophages of the sinusoids of the liver and the spleen. The process of phagocytosis stimulates an increase in hexose monophosphate shunt activity and lipid turnover in the phagocytic cells, presumably to replenish the cell membrane pinched off to form the lining of the phagocytic vacuoles. Killing of the ingested bacteria is a complex process characterized by degranulation of the leukocytes and release of the lytic enzymes and bactericidal substances of the granules into the phagocytic vacuoles containing the ingested bacteria. The leukocytes may themselves be damaged or killed by the bacteria which they ingest, and release of their lytic enzymes, as well as toxic products derived from the bacteria, contributes to the intensity of the local inflammatory reaction.

Damaged cells, bacteria and the breakdown products derived from the action of the cellular enzymes on bacteria, tissues and plasma proteins are swept along in the lymph to the regional lymph nodes, where the macrophages ingest and digest these materials and somehow pass specific antigens along to the immunologically competent cells. Thus, the process of phagocytosis results in the capture of infecting bacteria and their chemical processing to the actual antigens which initiate specific immunologic responses.

These responses may be divided into two groups: (1) those dependent upon specific instruction of T lymphocytes; and (2) those dependent upon the specific instruction of the B cells. It is generally agreed that T lymphocytes are responsible for recognition of incompatible cells and, hence, for the rejection of allografts. They also are responsible for the delayed hypersensitivity which develops in varying degree in most infections. An intact thymus, at least in fetal and early neonatal life, seems essential for T lymphocytes to develop their functional capacity to respond. B cells, when stimulated by an antigen, undergo mitosis, proliferation and differentiation, first into plasmacytoid cells synthesizing specific IgM, and ultimately into plasma cells synthesizing specific IgG. Once "instructed" by an antigen, lymphocytes appear to carry "immunologic memory," so that subsequent encounter with the antigen evokes a rapid response. This memory may be due to gamma globulins, which have recently been separated from lymphocytes by chemical treatment and shown to be specifically reactive with antigens to which the donor had been immunized.

The cellular responses, which are the morphologic accompaniments to recognition of an antigen and to the antibody response, have been well described, but the biochemical events responsible for them are not clear. In vitro, when an antigen to which the host has been immunized is added to a culture of human peripheral blood lymphocytes, there is transformation of the cells to larger cells, and mitoses are induced in many of them. In vivo, the injected antigen is soon demonstrable in the lymph node draining the site of injection. The germinal centers of the primary follicles of the cortex enlarge, then secondary follicles develop at the periphery of the primary follicles, and, in a few days, plasma cells containing specific antibody appear in the margins of the follicles and, ultimately, in the medullary cords.

Von Pirquet, in his studies of vaccinia, and von Pirquet and Schick, in their classic work on serum sickness, recognized that the difference between the initial response to an infectious agent or antigen and the response to a subsequent contact lay in a shortening of the interval between contact with the antigen and the manifestations of the immune response. These fundamental observations have been elaborated and applied in a practical way in recent years. A summary of the differences between the primary and secondary responses to an antigen or to an infectious agent is given in Table 9–2.

Another observation with important practical consequences, which has not been completely explained, is the action of adjuvants, originally described by Freund. By precipitation of protein antigens, such as toxoids, on aluminum salts, or by adding oily substances or killed tubercle bacilli, the capacity of antigens to sensitize and to elicit antibody formation is greatly enhanced.

TABLE 9-2 CONTRAST BETWEEN PRIMARY AND SECONDARY RESPONSES TO ANTIGENIC STIMULATION

Basic process	PRIMARY RESPONSE	SECONDARY RESPONSE
Basic process	(1) *Recognition* (2) *Instruction* of immunologically competent cells	*Immunologic memory* permits stimulation of previously instructed cells
Effect upon T cells	Induction of state of delayed hypersensitivity (1–4 weeks)	Delayed hypersensitivity response (1–2 days)
Effect upon B cells	(1) Transformation to plasmacytoid cells (2) Synthesis of IgM globulin antibodies	(1) Proliferation of plasma cells (2) Synthesis of IgG globulin antibodies
Antibody response	(1) Low titer (2) Shorter duration of antibody	(1) High titer (2) Longer duration of antibody

MATURATION OF IMMUNOLOGIC FUNCTION

By analogy with animal studies, immunologic competence is probably lacking during most of the first trimester of fetal life, so that *tolerance* to foreign cells and possibly to certain infectious agents may be established. This time corresponds to the period preceding population of the fetal lymphoid system with immunologically competent cells. During the subsequent 6 months of intrauterine life the fetus has the capacity to develop delayed hypersensitivity and to form plasma cells capable of synthesizing specific immunoglobulins. These are usually of the IgM and IgA classes; more than 20 mg/dl of IgM globulin in cord blood provides suggestive evidence for prenatal infection. Although the human fetus is capable of synthesizing IgG, the evidence strongly suggests that IgG in the cord blood, which usually is at a slightly higher level than in the maternal blood and possesses the maternal spectrum of antibodies, is derived from transfer of maternal IgG to the fetus through the placenta. This transfer is dependent upon a property of γH chains in the Fc portion of the molecule.

Postnatal development of the immunologic system is conditioned by the experience of the growing child. Animals raised in a germ-free environment, like human newborn infants, continue to have small lymph nodes, few plasma cells and very low rates of immunoglobulin synthesis. Normally, soon after birth, the infant begins to respond to multiple antigenic stimuli from the bacterial flora which rapidly populate his skin, upper respiratory tract, and bowel, as well as from the vaccines he receives and the microbial and parasitic infections (estimated roughly at one every 6 weeks until age 12) acquired from the environment. If the immunologic system is normal, this immunologic experience is reflected in progressive hyperplasia of the follicles and gradual appearance of plasma cells in lymphoid tissues throughout the body, including enlargement of tonsils and lymph nodes from their relatively small size at birth. As the child's immunologic experience expands, there is an increase in immunoglobulin synthesis (Fig. 9-3).

An important aspect of immunologic development is that the maternally derived IgG antibodies are catabolized with a usual half-life of approximately 30 days, so that passive immunity is gradually lost; the duration of immunity to a particular infection depends upon the level of the particular antibody in the mother's plasma during pregnancy and upon the amount of antibody required to protect the infant from that type of infection. Protection against pyogenic bacterial infections seldom lasts more than 1 or 2 months, whereas protection against measles or infectious hepatitis may last from 6 to 10 months. This passive protection from maternally derived antibody may interfere with the response to active immunization. Thus, measles vaccine should not ordinarily be given before 12 months of age. Likewise, maternal diph-

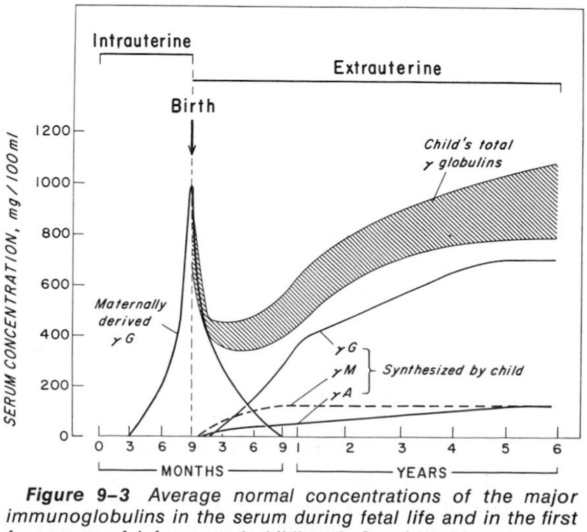

Figure 9-3 *Average normal concentrations of the major immunoglobulins in the serum during fetal life and in the first few years of infancy and childhood. Considerable variations may occur as a result of infection or delay in the initiation of immunoglobulin synthesis after birth.*

theria antitoxin may suppress the infant's response to diphtheria toxoid, but this is overcome by the practice of giving multiple injections of DPT. The striking frequency in newborn infants of sepsis or meningitis due to gram-negative enteric bacilli such as *Escherichia coli,* probably depends, in part at least, upon the fact that bactericidal antibodies to this group of organisms are IgM globulins which are not transferred from mother to fetus.

The increasing immunologic experience of the child, derived from his contacts with various viruses, bacteria and fungi, is inscribed upon the memory of his specifically instructed lymphocytes, which continue to circulate for several years and have the additional property of being able to transfer immunologic information to other lymphocytes through the "transfer factor" described by Lawrence. The induction of delayed hypersensitivity appears to have rather broad specificity for a whole species or group of organisms, whereas protective immunity is apt to be more strain- or type-specific. Thus, the child who has already experienced a type XIV pneumococcal infection, for example, will react to infection with a type I pneumococcus with an accelerated and intensified inflammatory response, because his T lymphoid cells produce a delayed hypersensitivity reaction to antigens common to all pneumococci. The residual protective antibodies to the type XIV polysaccharide, however, will not protect against the type I infection. One concludes, therefore, that the formation of protective antibody to type I polysaccharide is in the nature of a primary response. It would appear that many of the relatively unique clinical pictures of infectious diseases during the first 3 years of life are due to the fact that these are primary infections occurring in the unsensitized host. By contrast, in later childhood, delayed hypersensitivity to many of the common groups of organisms has already been established, thus altering the rate and intensity of the tissue response, even though protective immunity to the infecting strain may be absent.

Alper, C. A.: Complement. *In* Allison, A. C. (ed.): Plasma Proteins in Health and Disease. London, Plenum Press, 1974.

Bellanti, J.: Biologic significance of the secretory γA globulins. Pediatr. *48*:715, 1971.

Cooper, M., Peterson, R. D., South, M. A., and Good, R. A.: The functions of the thymus system and the bursa system in the chicken. J. Exp. Med. *123*:75, 1966.

David, J. R.: Lymphocyte mediators and cellular hypersensitivity. New Engl. J. Med., *288*:143, 1973.

Frommel, D., and Good, R. A.: Immunological mechanisms: *In* Gairdner, D., and Hull, D. (eds.): Recent Advances in Paediatrics. 4th ed. London, J. A. Churchill, Ltd., 1971. Chapter 12, p. 401.

Katz, D. H., and Benacerraf, B.: The regulatory influence of activated T cells in B cell responses to antigen: *In* Dixon, F. J., and Kunkel, H. G. (eds.), Advances in Immunology. Volume 15. New York, Academic Press, 1972.

Lawrence, H. S.: Transfer factor: *In* Dixon, F. T., and Kunkel, H. G. (eds.): Advances in Immunology. Volume 11. New York, Academic Press, 1969.

Pirquet, C. F. H. von, and Schick, B.: Serum Sickness. Baltimore, The Williams & Wilkins Co., 1951.

Ruddy, S., Gigli, I., and Austen, K. F.: The complement system of man: Activation, control and products of the reaction sequence. New Engl. J. Med. *287*:489, 1972.

Smith, R. T., and Robbins, J. B.: General physiology; The specific immune reponse; Developmental aspects of immunity: *In* Cooke, R. E. (ed.): The Biologic Basis of Pediatric Practice. New York, McGraw-Hill Book Co., Inc., 1968, Section 6, pp. 495, 507, 521.

Tomasi, T. B., Jr.: Secretory immunoglobulins. New Engl. J. Med. *287*:500, 1972.

IMMUNOLOGIC DEFICIENCY DISEASES

The frequent complaint that a child has "poor resistance to infection" requires careful analysis. It may be due to unreasonable parental expectations for the health of the child, or to environmental factors such as an overcrowded household into which older siblings bring multiple infections from their contacts at school or at play. If the child truly does have unusually frequent or severe infections, *host factors* must be considered. In so doing, the physician must distinguish between persistent or recurrent infections in one site, which suggest a local anatomic or physiologic defect, and exceptionally severe, persistent or frequent infections in different sites compatible with a generalized immunologic deficiency. The latter group of disorders will be described in this section on the basis of selective deficiencies of particular organs or cells, since this determines the type of functional impairment that expresses itself in the clinical picture of the disease.

DEFICIENCIES OF THE PHAGOCYTES

THE WANDERING PHAGOCYTES

The polymorphonuclear leukocytes are the body's first line of defense against bacterial infections; wandering macrophages (activated monocytes) play an important supporting role. The polymorphonuclear leukocytes may be quantitatively or qualitatively deficient.

NEUTROPENIA. (See also Section 14.) Quantitative deficiency of the neutrophils may arise from a variety of causes. Failure to form them adequately in the bone marrow may occur as a rare congenital defect, either *reticular dysgenesis,* in which all white cells are absent and the infant survives only a few days, or *familial neutropenia,* a genetic defect (there may be more than one) which may result in death from infection within the first 1 or 2 years of life. *Acquired neutropenia* or *agranulocytosis* may develop at any age, either from direct suppression of the bone marrow or by the destructive action of autoantibodies. Thus, it may be an expression of the toxic or sensitizing effects of various drugs, of invasion of the bone marrow by tumors, of the action of the therapeutic agents used to suppress them, of damage by ionizing radiation, or of bone marrow injury from certain infections. It also may occur in recurrent cycles *(cyclic neutropenia)* of unknown cause.

The most common infection in patients with severe neutropenia is staphylococcal, usually arising from a local skin lesion, but other pyogenic infections, or invasion by gram-negative bacilli or anaerobic organisms from ulcerations in the oropharynx or gastrointestinal tract, may also occur. With the use of antimicrobial agents and the resultant distortion of the body's bacterial flora, invasive infections with drug-resistant gram-negative bacilli or fungi have become the principal causes of death.

Treatment of severe neutropenia consists in supportive therapy, the rational use of antimicrobial drugs, and protection of the hospitalized patient from infections by "reverse" precautions. Elimination of any drug thought to be responsible for the neutropenia, intensive antitumor therapy in cases of leukemia, good nutrition, transfusion of fresh blood or concentrated white cells and bone marrow transplants are all part of the relatively unsatisfactory treatment of neutropenia. The condition is best avoided by great care in the use of potentially toxic drugs and of those to which the patient is known to be sensitive.

DEFICIENCY OF LEUKOCYTE FUNCTION. Two major disorders of leukocyte function have been identified thus far: chronic (fatal) granulomatous disease of children and the Chediak-Higashi syndrome. (See also Section 8.)

Chronic Granulomatous Disease. (See also Section 14). This is usually an X-linked recessive disease characterized by persistent and frequently fatal infections, often caused by organisms of low virulence, which may be suppressed but are not usually cured by antimicrobial therapy, and which result in lymphadenopathy, hepatosplenomegaly and hypergammaglobulinemia. The basic defect is an inability of both polymorphonuclear leukocytes and monocytes to kill ingested bacteria. There is a pronounced deficiency in the stimulation of oxidative metabolism which normally accompanies phagocytosis, although the granules themselves contain a normal complement of enzymes and bactericidal substances. The metabolic abnormality of the leukocytes is the basis of the nitroblue tetrazolium (NBT) test, which is diagnostic for this disease and can be used to recognize heterozygous carriers (Fig. 9–4). Occasional heterozygous females may have trouble with persistent infections, and several females with the full-blown disease have been described, suggesting an autosomal recessive inheritance in some cases. The exact enzymatic defect has not been identified, but is thought to be a DPNH oxidase deficiency; there may well be more than one form of the disease. Specific immunologic responses (delayed hypersensitivity and antibody formation) are normal.

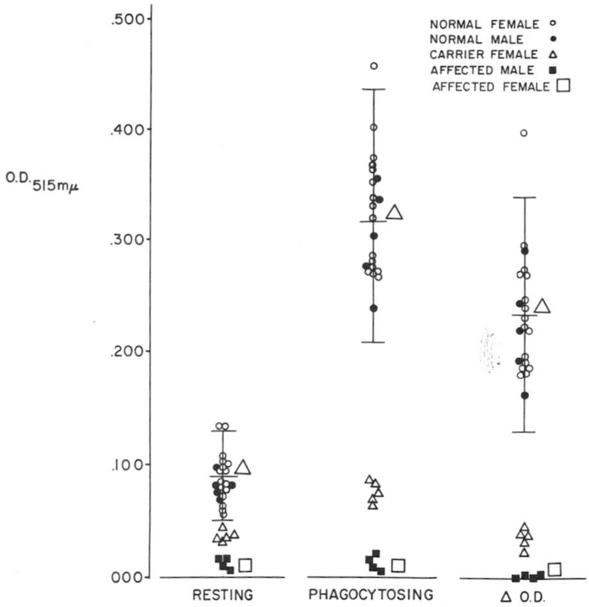

Figure 9–4 *Chronic granulomatous disease. Quantitative NBT dye test on normal controls, mothers of affected males, affected males and one affected female and her parents (large symbols). Note that increased dye reduction during phagocytosis (as shown by change in optical density, △ O.D.) is nil for affected persons, marked in normals and slight but definite in carrier females. (Reproduced from New Engl. J. Med., 278:973, 1968, with permission of authors and publishers.)*

The *clinical picture* of the disease usually begins with infection of the skin, cervical lymph nodes or parenchyma of the lung; the middle ear or gut may be involved early. Lymphadenopathy, hepatosplenomegaly, and pulmonary consolidation with enlargement of the hilar nodes and hypergammaglobulinemia usually develop within weeks or months as infection recurs soon after antimicrobial therapy has been discontinued. Staphylococcal infection is most common, but gram-negative bacilli are often implicated as well. Locally the pathologic reaction is a granulomatous one, with the formation of microabscesses, which may give rise to draining sinuses. The peripheral blood picture varies; generally there is moderate anemia and a moderate increase in eosinophils and monocytes.

Antimicrobial *treatment* is often successful in suppressing the signs of invasive infection, but it is difficult to eradicate the persistent low-grade infections or the immunologic responses which trouble these patients. The disease varies considerably in severity, but is generally fatal within the first 5 years in full-blown cases.

Chediak-Higashi Syndrome. (See also Section 14.) This is a rare autosomal recessive disease characterized by the presence of giant granules in the leukocytes, undue susceptibility to bacterial infection, and diminution in the pigment of skin, hair and eyes. There are pyoderma, pneumonia, ulceration of the oral mucosa and recurrent fever. Death usually occurs before adolescence with a terminal febrile illness characterized by enlargement of the reticuloendothelial organs, anemia, neutropenia and thrombocytopenia. Although the immunologic responses of these patients are normal, the giant granules found in the leukocytes represent a general phenomenon affecting many cells, apparently as a result of failure of integrity of the membrane limiting subcellular particles; thus, it appears to be a lysosomal disease, the connection of which with the abnormal susceptibility to infection remains unclear.

Since chemotaxis and a number of other aspects of the inflammatory reaction depend upon the activation of the complement sequence, there are instances of poor phagocyte function in which the defect is not cellular but humoral, resulting in recurrent or persistent bacterial infections.

DEFICIENCY OF THE FIXED PHAGOCYTES OF THE SPLEEN

Bacteria that enter the blood stream are usually rapidly cleared by the phagocytic action of the macrophages of the liver and the spleen. Smith demonstrated that when virulent pneumococci were injected intravenously into rabbits, the liver was responsible for removal of the majority of organisms in the immune animal, but that the spleen was principally responsible for this activity in the nonimmune animal. This experimental demonstration of the importance of the spleen has its counterpart in human disease, for clinical observation has shown that fulminating bacteremia and meningitis caused by the principal pyogenic invasive organisms—pneumococci, meningococci and *H. influenzae*—pose a very real threat to any child without a spleen. This has now been observed in four clinical situations: (1) *congenital absence of the spleen* (Section 14), which occurs in association with certain cardiac malformations; (2) *familial splenic hypoplasia,* observed in two families in which siblings with fulminating bacteremia were shown to have structurally normal but minute spleens, whereas parents and siblings with no such infectious history had normal spleens (Fig. 9–5); (3) *postsplenectomy syndrome* (Section 14), in which it has been statistically demonstrated that the younger the child in whom splenectomy is performed and the more serious the underlying disease, the greater the risk of subsequent fulminating bacteremia or meningitis; and (4) *functional asplenia of sickle cell disease,* which is reversible if the patient's normal red cells can be increased by transfusion to compose over 50 per cent of his total red cells. At present there is little one can do to prevent such infection except to be as conservative as possible in recommending splenectomy in young children, to warn the parents of a splenectomized child to be alert, and to provide them with an effective broad spectrum antimicrobial drug to be administered immediately at the onset of any febrile illness.

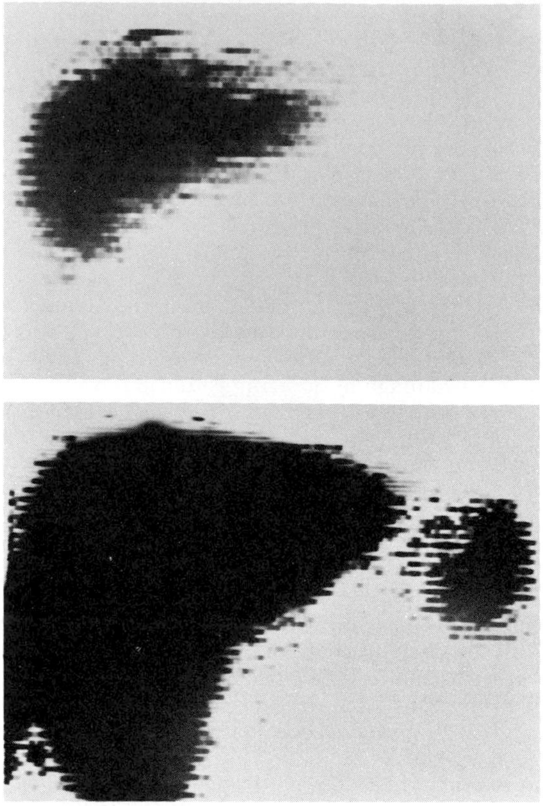

Figure 9–5 *Hereditary splenic hypoplasia. Scintillation scan of the upper portion of the abdomen after injection of colloidal* ^{198}*Au.* Lower, *Normal scan of liver and spleen of unaffected sibling.* Upper, *Normal scan of liver, but no demonstrable spleen, in affected sibling. (Reproduced from Pediatrics 42:755, 1968, with permission of the authors and publishers.)*

IMMUNODEFICIENCY STATES

Since the initial recognition of agammaglobulinemia by Bruton in 1953, and the description of lymphocytophthisis by Glanzmann in 1950, there has been an explosion of reports of various types of immunodeficiency, so that the clinician has become increasingly confused as terminology and interpretation have changed in this field. Since much basic knowledge concerning the biochemical and molecular events involved in the complex response of the cells of the immunologic system to the stimulus of infection or immunization is still lacking, any attempt at detailed classification of immunodeficiency diseases on the basis of their pathogenesis is difficult. Certain general statements can be made, however, on the basis of accumulated clinical experience and laboratory investigations; these can be of help in analyzing the problem of immunodeficiency in an individual patient.

PRIMARY VS. SECONDARY IMMUNODEFICIENCY

A number of *primary* disorders of the lymphoid system, many of them with a genetic basis, others due to multifactorial or unknown causes, will be described below and may be recognized as definite disease entities (Table 9–3). In addition, probably the most frequent type of immunodeficiency today is *secondary* to some other disease or therapeutic maneuver that results in injury to the hematopoietic tissues (e.g., use of immunosuppressive or antineoplastic agents), anatomic or functional impairment of the lymphoid system (e.g., leukemia or lymphoma), or blunting of the inflammatory response (e.g., corticosteroids).

By and large, the clinical manifestations of immunodeficiency fall into one of three general patterns, depending upon whether the functional deficit predominantly involves T cells or B cells, or a combination of the two.

PRIMARY T CELL DEFICIENCIES

The characteristic clinical manifestations of defective T cell function are frequent infections with a wide variety of microorganisms, particularly viruses, mycobacteria and fungi. Of the latter, the most ubiquitous is *Candida albicans;* thrush lasting longer than the usual week to 10 days or recurring after effective local treatment should make one suspicious of a T cell defect. These patients do not give the usual skin reactions of delayed hypersensitivity and do not reject skin grafts normally. Living attenuated virus vaccines or BCG vaccine may give rise to disseminated fatal infections in patients with impaired cellular immunity. The following definite clinical syndromes may be associated with defective T cell function.

THYMIC HYPOPLASIA (DIGEORGE SYNDROME). This disease is characterized by congenital hypoparathyroidism with neonatal tetany, increased susceptibility to infections, particularly those due to viruses and fungi, failure to thrive, and anomalies of the mouth, neck and great vessels.

The grouping of anomalies suggests a developmental defect of structures arising from the pharyngeal pouches and branchial arches. Since the parathyroids and thymus are formed from the third and fourth pharyngeal pouches, combined aplasia of them is readily understood. The difficulty of inducing mitoses in cultured lymphocytes has hampered the search for chromosomal aberrations in this syndrome, and no genetic basis has been found for it.

Clinically there are usually neonatal tetany and the low serum calcium and high serum phosphorus values seen in hypoparathyroidism. These manifestations respond to appropriate therapy, but within a few weeks or months a tendency to recurrent infections of the respiratory tract, diarrhea, moniliasis and failure to thrive becomes apparent. There are poor nutrition and growth, anomalies such as a fishmouth deformity of the lips and mal-

TABLE 9–3 PRIMARY IMMUNODEFICIENCIES

	SUGGESTED CELLULAR DEFECT			INHERITANCE		
	B Cells Circulating Ig bearing Lymphocytes					
PRIMARY IMMUNODEFICIENCIES	*Quantitatively deficient*	*Qualitatively deficient*	*T Cells*	*X-linked Recessive*	*Autosomal Recessive*	OTHER CAUSES
A. Deficiencies of T Cells						
1. Thymic hypoplasia			+			+
2. MIF (migration inhibitory factor) deficiency			+		?	
3. Mucocutaneous candidiasis			(+)			+
B. Deficiencies of B Cells						
1. Transient hypogammaglobulinemia of infancy		+				+
2. X-linked agammaglobulinemia	+	(+)		+		
3. X-linked immunodeficiency with increased IgM		+		+		
4. Selective Ig deficiency		+				+
5. Immunodeficiency with normal or hypergammaglobulinemia		+	(+)			+
6. Variable immunodeficiencies	+	+	(+)		(+)	+
C. Combined T and B Cell Deficiencies						
1. Severe combined immunodeficiency	+	(+)	+	+	+	
a. with dysostosis	+	(?)	+		+	
b. with adenosine deaminase deficiency	+		+		+	
c. with generalized hematopoietic hypoplasia	+		+		+	
2. Immunodeficiency with ataxia-telangiectasia		+	+		+	
3. Immunodeficiency with thrombocytopenia and eczema		(+)	+	+		
4. Immunodeficiency with thymoma	+		+			+

formations of the ears, esophagus or great vessels (especially double aortic arch), and upper or lower respiratory tract infections.

The number of circulating lymphocytes is usually normal, but they respond poorly to stimulation with phytohemagglutinin. Efforts to elicit delayed skin reactions to antigens normally provoking them, such as *candida* antigen, or attempts to induce delayed skin hypersensitivity with potent sensitizers like dinitrochlorobenzene (DNCB), are unsuccessful. Usually the levels of immunoglobulins and of isohemagglutinins are normal for age, but specific antibody responses to injected antigens may be poor.

Pathologically the stimulated lymph nodes display abundant follicles and plasma cells, but a depletion of lymphocytes in the paracortical ("thymus-dependent") areas (Fig. 9–6) and in the white pulp of the spleen. Thymic tissue usually cannot be found, and parathyroids are either absent or rudimentary.

Early diagnosis of these cases is essential and begins with suspicion of thymic deficiency in any young infant with a history of neonatal tetany or laboratory findings consistent with hypoparathyroidism. The degree of thymic deficiency in this syndrome is variable. The infants who manifest recurrent infections generally succumb before the age of 6 years to a viral infection such as varicella or measles. *Transplantation of fetal thymic tissue,* resulting in establishment of immunologic competence and clinical improvement in the wasting and susceptibility to infection, has been carried out successfully in several infants and would appear to be the treatment of choice.

DEFICIENCY OF MIF (MACROPHAGE MIGRATION INHIBITORY FACTOR). At least one family has been observed in which unusual susceptibility to bacterial infection, recurrent bouts of fever and a tendency to thrush were associated with marked to moderate hypergammaglobulinemia and subsequent development of autoantibodies, vitamin B_{12} deficiency, hypothyroidism and hypoadrenalism in different siblings. The only immunologic disturbance found in a study of the youngest affected child in this kindred was a deficiency of MIF

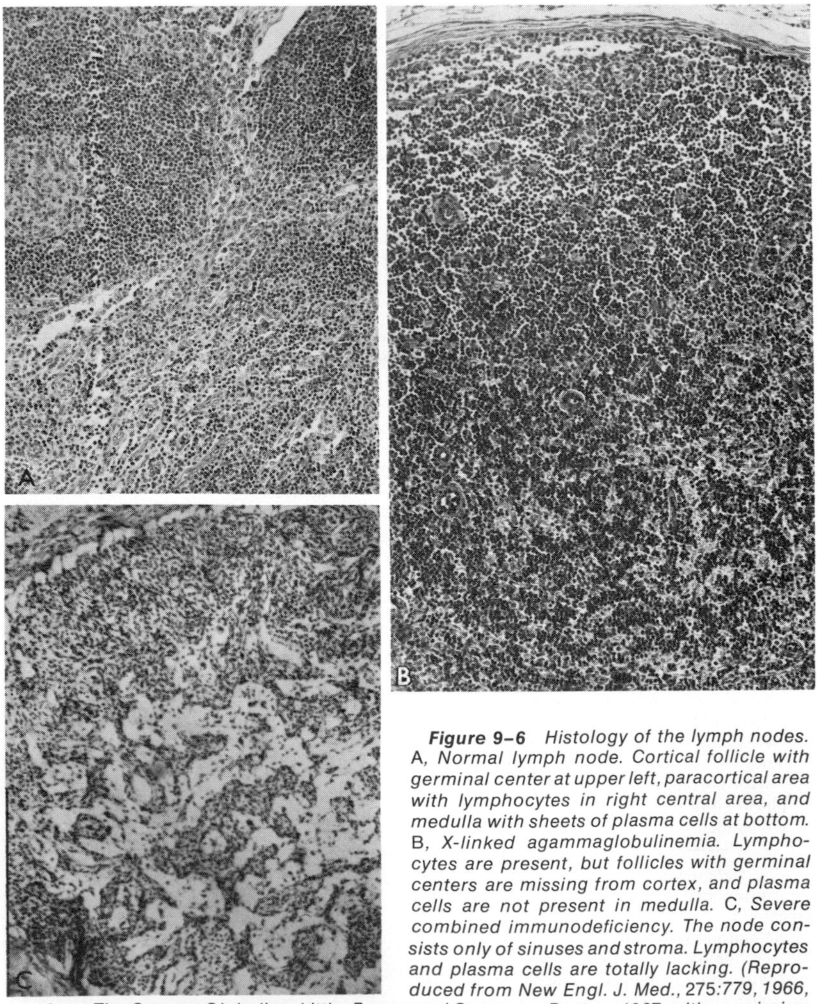

Figure 9–6 *Histology of the lymph nodes. A, Normal lymph node. Cortical follicle with germinal center at upper left, paracortical area with lymphocytes in right central area, and medulla with sheets of plasma cells at bottom. B, X-linked agammaglobulinemia. Lymphocytes are present, but follicles with germinal centers are missing from cortex, and plasma cells are not present in medulla. C, Severe combined immunodeficiency. The node consists only of sinuses and stroma. Lymphocytes and plasma cells are totally lacking. (Reproduced from New Engl. J. Med., 275:779, 1966, and from The Gamma Globulins, Little, Brown and Company, Boston, 1967, with permission of the authors and publishers.)*

production by his lymphocytes. Whether this defect had been present earlier in his older siblings, who survived and who appear to have outgrown their tendency to infections, is not known; their present MIF production is normal.

MUCOCUTANEOUS CANDIDIASIS. Persistent infection of the skin with *Candida albicans,* usually in large circular patches with centrifugal extension, infection of the nails and oral mucosa, but without systemic symptoms, is a stubborn and troublesome disease. These patients are not unduly susceptible to other types of infection, but seem unable to rid themselves of local infection with monilia. This syndrome has been shown to be associated with several different immunologic defects: (1) a specific inability of the T lymphocytes to respond to skin tests with, or in vitro exposure to, candida antigens; (2) a transient inability to respond to candida antigen—responsiveness can be restored by reducing the antigenic burden through appropriate therapy of the candida infection (mycostatin and amphotericin B); and (3) a few cases in which the immunologic responses appear to be normal. Once the local infection was reduced by appropriate fungistatic therapy, some patients in the first of the aforementioned groups have been cured by the administration of *transfer factor* prepared from the lymphocytes of individuals normally responsive to sensitization with candida. Transfer factor may have to be readministered periodically.

PRIMARY B CELL DEFICIENCIES

ANTIBODY DEFICIENCY SYNDROME. The outstanding clinical manifestation of patients with quantitative or qualitative defects of B cell function is recurrent, invasive infections with pyogenic bacteria. The infections (pyoderma, pharyngitis, sinusitis, otitis media, pneumonia, sepsis and meningitis) are notable for their frequency and/or severity, but are otherwise no different from those observed in normal individuals of the same age and respond normally to antimicrobial therapy. There is diminished or absent antibody response to injected antigens or to infection, which has given rise to the term *antibody deficiency syndrome,* introduced by Swiss workers. Since this basic pathogenetic defect results in failure of phagocytosis, an essential step in the control of invasion by pyogenic bacteria, it is not surprising that an indistinguishable clinical picture has been observed in patients with deficiency of the third component of complement (C3). Cellular immune responses of the T cells being preserved, these patients respond to most viral, fungal or mycobacterial infections normally. A number of different primary disorders can give rise to the antibody deficiency syndrome.

TRANSIENT HYPOGAMMAGLOBULINEMIA OF INFANCY. Normally the synthesis of immunoglobulins in response to infection and other antigenic stimuli begins after birth, with the result that the level of gamma globulins, which falls rapidly during the first month of life, levels off during the second month and soon begins to rise. Rarely, there is delay in the development of this important immunologic function; the level of IgG globulins received by passive transfer from the mother continues to fall and is not adequately replaced by immunoglobulins synthetized by the infant, so that within a few months the total gamma globulin level is much lower than usual for age. The infants have overt infections, unexplained episodes of fever and often bronchitis with wheezing. Regular injections of gamma globulin in full doses (see below) will protect them from severe, invasive infections. The injections may be discontinued when IgM appears in the serum and the IgG globulins begin to rise toward normal levels, usually before the age of 3 years. The cause of this transient hypogammaglobulinemia is not known.

X-LINKED AGAMMAGLOBULINEMIA (CONGENITAL AGAMMAGLOBULINEMIA; BRUTON'S DISEASE). This X-linked recessive disorder gives the classic picture of the antibody deficiency syndrome. Though abnormalities of one or more of the immunoglobulins may occur among relatives of patients with this disease, no method for detecting a carrier female has been found.

Pathology. The thymus is normal (Fig. 9–7), but lymph nodes and spleen lack the usual follicular architecture. Germinal centers are absent, and there are few, if any, plasma cells in the medullary cords or red pulp (Fig. 9–6). Although the number of lymphocytes in the tissues appears diminished, they are present in the thymus-dependent areas, and normal numbers are found in the blood. Study of the circulating lymphocytes has, in most cases, revealed normal numbers of T cells, but complete absence of B cells.

Clinical Manifestations. The disease usually manifests itself in the second year of life, although the onset of the characteristically severe, recurrent infections may begin at any age from 8 months to 3 years. The infections are those caused by the common pyogenic organisms—*Staphylococcus aureus,* pneumococci, meningococci, *H. influenzae,* and less often beta-hemolytic streptococci or salmonellae. They differ from infections in normal children only in their frequency, severity and the tendency for infection with the same organism to occur more than once. Pyoderma, purulent conjunctivitis, pharyngitis, otitis media, sinusitis, bronchitis, pneumonia, empyema, purulent arthritis, meningitis and sepsis occur with surprising frequency and may be associated with unusually high fever and unexpected elevation or depression of the leukocyte count. A rather indolent rheumatoid-like arthritis with sterile effusion into one of the large joints develops in about one third of patients and may be the presenting complaint. The children usually, but not always, handle most viral infections normally.

Diagnosis. There should be a high index of suspicion on the basis of the history of repeated severe bacterial infections. A careful family history may uncover instances of death from overwhelming infection or multiple severe infections in other male siblings, maternal uncles or male off-

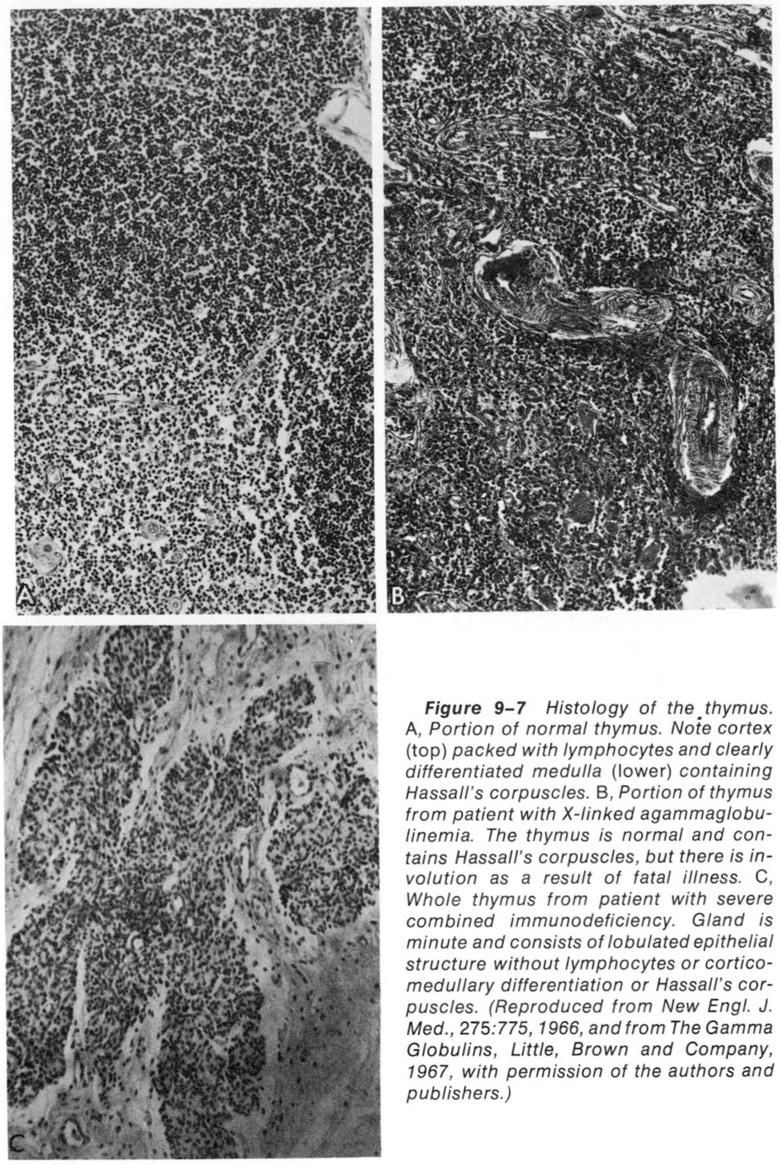

Figure 9–7 *Histology of the thymus.* A, *Portion of normal thymus. Note cortex* (top) *packed with lymphocytes and clearly differentiated medulla* (lower) *containing Hassall's corpuscles.* B, *Portion of thymus from patient with X-linked agammaglobulinemia. The thymus is normal and contains Hassall's corpuscles, but there is involution as a result of fatal illness.* C, *Whole thymus from patient with severe combined immunodeficiency. Gland is minute and consists of lobulated epithelial structure without lymphocytes or corticomedullary differentiation or Hassall's corpuscles. (Reproduced from New Engl. J. Med., 275:775, 1966, and from The Gamma Globulins, Little, Brown and Company, 1967, with permission of the authors and publishers.)*

spring of maternal aunts. Examination reveals little except the signs of infection, evidence of joint involvement if present, and unusually small, smooth tonsils. Lateral films of the pharynx fail to reveal an adenoid shadow. Lymph nodes are small but palpable; regional nodes may be swollen and tender during episodes of infection. Proof of the diagnosis can be obtained by immunoglobulin assay, which reveals a marked diminution of IgM, IgA and IgG globulins in the serum (Fig. 9–8). It is important to remember that, because of individual variations and the low levels of immunoglobulins normally found in the early months of life, the diagnosis cannot be firmly established by immunoelectrophoresis until 6 to 8 months of age. However, failure of IgM or IgA to appear in significant concentration and a steady fall in IgG during the first 3 or 4 months of life is highly suspicious. Isohemagglutinins are usually absent or in very low titer. Injection of vaccines is not followed by an adequate antibody rise, and removal of a stimulated regional lymph node discloses absence of the expected germinal centers, secondary follicles and plasma cells (Fig. 9–6).

Prognosis. Provided the diagnosis is made before repeated infections have produced serious anatomic damage (e.g., bronchiectasis, pulmonary insufficiency, middle ear deafness), the immediate prognosis for these children is excellent, and they gain and grow normally. However, in later childhood, adolescence or early adult life, a few of these patients may develop hepatitis, slowly progressive neurologic disease suggesting "slow virus" infection, or a dermatomyositis-like syndrome with brawny edema, perivascular mononuclear infiltrates and, terminally, severe systemic symptoms and death (Fig. 9–9). No consistent cause for these complications has been found, but an enterovirus

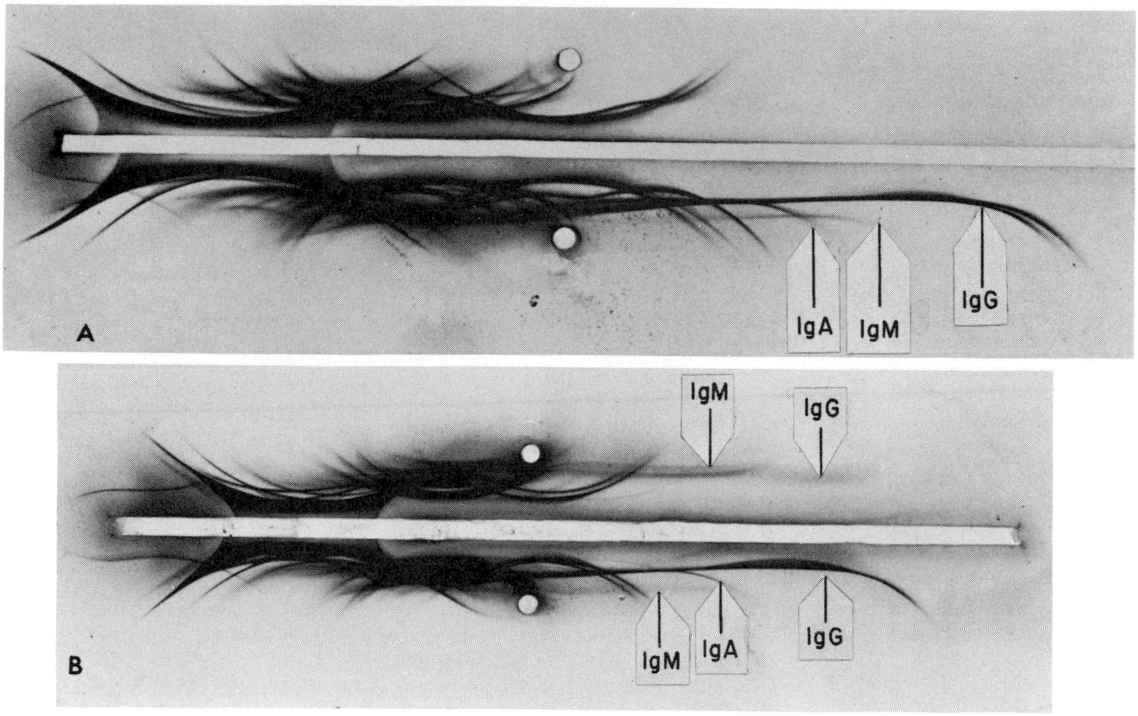

Figure 9–8 *Immunoelectrophoresis of serum.* A, Top, *X-linked agammaglobulinemia. Complete absence of IgM, IgA and IgG bands.* Bottom, *Hypergammaglobulinemia, showing increased amounts of IgM, IgA and IgG.* B, Top, *X-linked immunodeficiency with increased IgM. Marked increase in IgM, faint trace of IgG, absent IgA.* Bottom, *Normal serum.*

was repeatedly isolated from blood, stool and spinal fluid in the last patient to succumb with the dermatomyositis-like picture.

Treatment. Vigorous antimicrobial therapy is indicated for individual infections, which respond to treatment as in normal individuals. Regular injections of gamma globulin in doses adequate to maintain a plasma concentration of IgG globulin above 200 mg/dl are essential. Maintenance therapy is initiated with a loading dose of 0.3 gm (1.8 ml) per kg of IgG globulin. This may be given in divided doses over a period of a week in order to minimize discomfort. Thereafter an average dose of 0.1 gm (0.6 ml) per kg per month (the volume of the injection may be scaled down if injections are given every 2 or 3 weeks) is required to maintain a protective level of antibody. Intramuscular administration is necessary to avoid reactions with the standard preparation. A preparation satisfactory for intravenous administration has been shown to be effective in preventing infections in these patients and is being developed for clinical trials. Prophylaxis with gamma globulin is usually effective in preventing invasive bacterial infection and communicable disease, and its institution generally cures hydrarthrosis. It does not control localized superficial infection of skin or respiratory tract; in a few instances antimicrobial drugs may have to be given in addition to control chronic sinusitis, most frequently due to *H. influenzae.* Infections may be prevented for considerable periods by the administration of broad spectrum antibiotics without gamma globulin, but this does not protect against all types of infection.

Once a case of congenital agammaglobulinemia has been identified in a family, each subsequent male sibling or male offspring of a maternal aunt should be followed up carefully, with clinical examination and serial immunoelectrophoretic analyses of the serum at intervals of every 2 months from birth through the first year. Affected infants so detected, and given prophylactic gamma globulin before severe infections have occurred, seem to thrive particularly well, but the physician must be absolutely certain of the diagnosis before initiating such a program.

OTHER PATTERNS OF DEFICIENCY OF IMMUNOGLOBULINS. X-linked Immunodeficiency with Increased IgM. A few patients with clinical manifestations similar to those of X-linked agammaglobulinemia, but with higher immunoglobulin levels, turn out to have a marked deficiency of serum IgA and IgG but an elevation of IgM. The congenital form of this disease seems to occur almost entirely in males, suggesting an X-linked pattern of inheritance. Except for a greater frequency of hematologic disorders (cyclic neutropenia, autoimmune hemolytic anemia, thrombocytopenia), the clinical course is indistinguishable from that of X-linked agammaglobulinemia. Histologically there is disorganization of the follicular architecture of the lymphoid tissues, but PAS-positive plasmacytoid cells containg IgM are present, and tonsillar hypertrophy owing to these cells has been observed. Similar disturbances of the immunoglobulin picture associated with the antibody deficiency syndrome have been seen in occasional adults with frequent respiratory tract infections

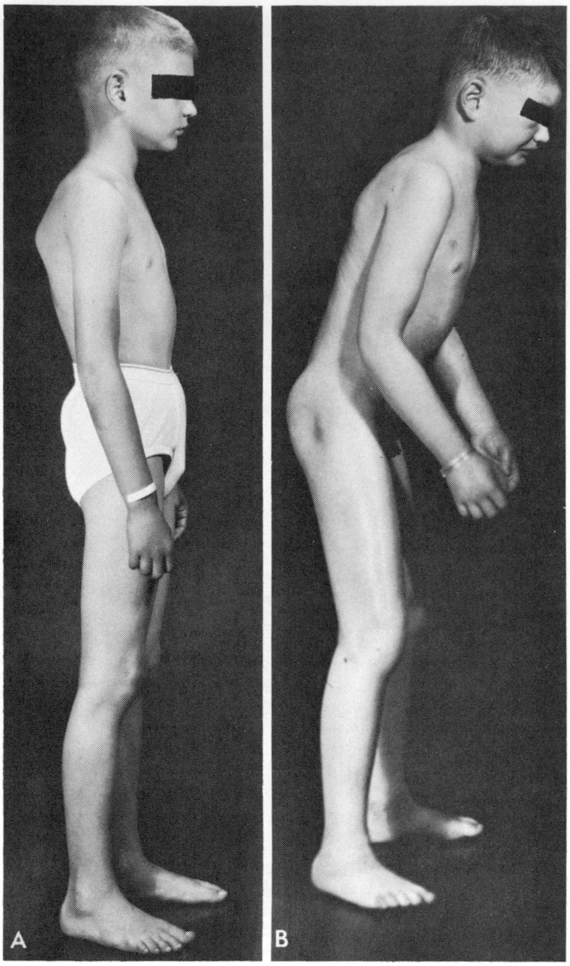

Figure 9–9 *X-linked agammaglobulinemia. A, Age 11 years, in normal health. B, Age 12. Same patient 7 months after onset of dermatomyositis-like syndrome. Note brawny edema and contractures. Patient died 1 month later.*

and bronchiectasis and in some infants with congenital rubella.

Selective Immunoglobulin Deficiencies (Dysgammaglobulinemia). This term is used to describe patients in whom there are consistent deficiencies of one or more of the recognizable plasma immunoglobulins. Although often associated with clinical manifestations of the antibody deficiency syndrome, some instances appear to be chance laboratory findings in otherwise normal individuals.

Selective Deficiency of IgG Subclasses. The patient may be unable to synthesize one or more of the IgG subclasses and fail to produce antibodies in one or more of the four presently identified γG subclasses. This results in failure to respond to particular types of antigens, to increased susceptibility to a limited spectrum of bacterial infections, and to a reduction in total serum IgG proportional to the percentage of the total IgG pool accounted for by the deficient IgG subclass.

Selective IgA Deficiency. This is observed with considerable frequency. In a few patients this may portend the development of ataxia telangiectasia (see later). An appreciable number of individuals with selective IgA deficiency remain healthy throughout life, but a high incidence of rheumatoid arthritis, systemic lupus erythematosus and malabsorption syndrome has been observed among them.

Deficiency of Secretory IgA. The form of antibody synthesized in plasma cells closely related to the mucous membranes and secreted into colostrum, saliva, respiratory and intestinal secretions as two subunits of IgA in combination with a "transport piece" synthesized by the epithelial cells, may well play a role in undue susceptibility to certain infections, particularly viral, of the respiratory and gastrointestinal tracts. Deficiency of this type of local immunity may contribute to the clinical picture of agammaglobulinemia and ataxia telangiectasia as well as to the tendency to recurrent otitis media or to chronic diarrhea in some patients with selective IgA deficiency. Likewise the greater efficacy of intranasally administered respiratory viral vaccines or of oral poliomyelitis vaccine may depend more upon the establishment of local immunity than upon the stimulation of systemic antibody formation.

Immunodeficiency with Normal or Increased Immunoglobulins. Rare cases have been observed in which the classic picture of the antibody deficiency syndrome was accompanied by the presence of plasma cells in the tissues and normal or even increased levels of immunoglobulins. Deficiency of circulating C3, with recurrent pyogenic infections since early childhood, and normal antibody responses and immunoglobulin levels, has been observed twice. The mechanism for the C3 deficiency differed in the two cases, in one being due to lack of an inhibitor for stabilization of the alternate (properdin) pathway to C3 activation, in the other to homozygous deficiency in the biosynthesis of C3.

Variable Unclassified Immunodeficiency (Acquired Hypogammaglobulinemia). This most common form of immunodeficiency probably includes a number of entities. It occurs in either sex at any age without any known genetic or acquired causative factor. A predisposition may be inherited, since it has been reported in siblings, but it has also been reported in only one of a pair of monozygotic twins.

The clinical picture is that of the antibody deficiency syndrome, but the immunoglobulin deficiency may be somewhat less severe than in the X-linked form of agammaglobulinemia. Pathologically there is necrobiotic change in the follicular architecture of the lymph nodes and spleen, or lymphadenopathy and splenomegaly as a result of reticulum cell hyperplasia. The predominant infections are sinusitis and pneumonia, often leading to bronchiectasis unless intensively treated. Although rheumatoid arthritis-like complications are occasionally seen, a sprue-like syndrome and pernicious anemia are more common. Recent work has demonstrated that this malabsorption syndrome is often due to giardia, demonstrated either in aspirates of duodenal fluid or in biopsy specimens of duodenal mucosa.

Management is the same as for X-linked agammaglobulinemia: substitution therapy with regular injections of large doses of immune serum globulin for prophylaxis and intensive antimicrobial therapy for acute infections. The chronic diarrhea and malabsorption due to giardiasis, which may give a picture of protein-losing enteropathy, usually responds promptly to metronidazole (Flagyl) in doses of 0.25 gm t.i.d. for 5 days.

COMBINED IMMUNODEFICIENCY

In combined immunodeficiency, there are defects in both T cell and B cell functions, with consequent susceptibility to a wide variety of infections due to viruses, fungi and bacteria.

SEVERE COMBINED IMMUNODEFICIENCY (SWISS TYPE AGAMMAGLOBULINEMIA, ALYMPHOCYTOSIS). This disease, originally described as *lymphocytophthisis* by Glanzmann in Switzerland, as *alymphocytosis* by Donahue in Canada, and as *thymic alymphoplasia* in this country, gives rise to a severe form of immunologic deficiency characterized by persistent infections in early infancy, failure to thrive and death within the first 2 years. It is a genetic disease with both sex-linked recessive and autosomal recessive inheritance; no defect is demonstrable in the carrier of the trait.

Pathologically the thymus is tiny, consisting only of a small, lobulated epithelial structure lacking corticomedullary differentiation, lymphocytes or Hassall's corpuscles (Fig. 9–7). The lymph nodes are tiny structures consisting mainly of stroma and sinusoids (Fig. 9–6), and the white pulp of the spleen and the lamina propria of the gut are devoid of lymphocytes and plasma cells; Peyer's patches are missing. The absence of lymphocytes in the tissues, except for a few in the bone marrow and blood, is striking.

The onset of persistent infection of the lungs, monilial infection of the oropharynx, esophagus and skin, chronic diarrhea and wasting, and runting begins in the early months of life and progresses with monotonous regularity to a fatal termination despite all attempts at therapy. Examination usually reveals absence of tonsils, very small lymph nodes despite chronic infection, chronic pneumonitis evidenced by a pertussis-like cough, inspiratory retractions of the chest and rales, a somewhat distended abdomen with much wasting, and oral thrush.

Roentgenographic signs include pulmonary infiltration and absence of a thymic shadow and of an adenoid shadow on lateral examination of the nasopharynx. There is usually an absolute decrease in the number of circulating lymphocytes, and occasionally neutropenia. In classic cases the immunoglobulins are markedly decreased, but variants have been described in which circulating immunoglobulins are normal or there is selective immunoglobulin deficiency. Plasma cells have been found in the tissues of such patients, but antibody formation is almost always somewhat impaired. Tests of delayed hypersensitivity give negative results: sensitization cannot be induced with dinitrochlorobenzene, cultured lymphocytes do not respond to phytohemagglutinin, and skin allografts are not rejected.

Treatment of the infections in these patients must be specific. Pulmonary infection is frequently due to *Pneumocystis carinii,* requiring pentamidine or pyramethamine and sulfadiazine. Routine antimicrobial therapy, fungistatic drugs and human gamma globulin are only temporarily effective and do not prevent the inexorable termination of the disease, if the immunologic deficiency is not overcome. The use of attenuated viral or BCG vaccines must be avoided, since the attenuated viruses or mycobacteria can produce fatal generalized disease, and natural infection with herpes, varicella or measles virus is uniformly fatal.

The induction of immunologic competence in these infants is still experimental and should be carried out only in centers with adequate manpower, clinical and laboratory experience, and physical facilities for what is an exacting ordeal for patient, family, nurses and physicians. Success depends upon attention to a number of factors:

1. *Early recognition.* For an index case in a family the diagnosis is seldom made until infection is already established. Every subsequent sibling should be carefully watched for early signs of the disease—absence of clinically demonstrable thymic tissue, low peripheral lymphocyte count, absence of serum IgM and IgA, and failure of cultured lymphocytes to respond to phytohemagglutinin.
2. *Treatment of established infection and reduction of microbial flora of skin, bowel and respiratory mucosa* with properly directed local and systemic chemotherapy.
3. *Protection against infection* by care in an environment from which microorganisms are excluded as far as possible, with injections of gamma globulin for passive protection.
4. *Identification of a donor* whose cells are HL-A identical and can be shown to be histocompatible in vitro; in practice this almost always means a sibling.
5. *Administration of* a suitable *dose of bone marrow cells* from this donor when the infant is as free of infection as possible.
6. *Careful observation* over a period of 3 to 8 weeks for signs of *graft versus host disease,* evidence that the graft has become established and that immunologic constitution (T cell function as shown by phytohemagglutinin responses, B cell function by immunoglobulin synthesis) has occurred.

In skilled hands, patients with this hitherto fatal disease have been cured and appear normal. Nevertheless, success is not universal, and the treatment is heroic. Intrauterine diagnosis of this disorder has not been accomplished, but might ultimately lead to its prevention in affected families.

Variant forms of severe combined immune deficiency have been described. These include patients with *dysostosis* (short-limbed dwarfism, cartilage-hair syndrome), with *adenosine deaminase defi-*

ciency, and with *generalized hematopoietic hypoplasia*. The latter has been called *reticular dysgenesis;* infants with this type of immunodeficiency lack white cells in the bone marrow and peripheral blood and survive for only a short time after birth.

IMMUNODEFICIENCY WITH ATAXIA-TELANGIECTASIA. This is an autosomal recessive disease in which abnormalities of the thymus have been found at postmortem examination. Gradually progressive cerebellar ataxia begins in early childhood. This is associated with increasing telangiectasia, which first becomes apparent as a rather inconspicuous dilatation of small blood vessels in the bulbar conjunctivae and ultimately is visible in the skin. Gonadal dysgenesis and failure of sexual maturation may be present in those who survive into the second decade. In late childhood recurrent sinobronchial infections begin in many patients, often leading to bronchiectasis. There is also a tendency toward development of malignant tumors, particularly of the lymphoid system. These reflect an immunologic disturbance affecting T cell function, as shown by blunting of delayed hypersensitivity reactions, failure to reject allografts normally, and reduced response of the lymphocytes to phytohemagglutinin. At postmortem examination late in the disease the thymus is abnormally small and has a decreased number of lymphocytes; there is a poor differentiation between cortex and medulla and decided diminution in Hassall's corpuscles. The number of circulating lymphocytes and the architecture of the lymph nodes vary considerably and do not always correlate well with the patient's history. The most consistent B cell defect is a low level or absence of IgA globulin in the serum, which occurs in about 70 per cent of affected persons and may precede clinical evidence of immunologic deficiency by a number of years.

IMMUNODEFICIENCY WITH THROMBOCYTOPENIA AND ECZEMA (WISKOTT-ALDRICH SYNDROME). (See also Section 14.) The Wiskott-Aldrich syndrome is an X-linked recessive disorder which is usually manifested by eczema, thrombocytopenia, and a wide variety of infections beginning late in the first year, although it may present rarely as thrombocytopenia alone. Death may occur from hemorrhage, infection, or the development of a malignant process similar to the Letterer-Siwe type of reticuloendotheliosis. The infections may be caused by a wide variety of microorganisms, including viruses, bacteria, fungi and *Pneumocystis carinii* Transient episodes of arthritis have been observed.

Results of studies of the pathogenesis of the Wiskott-Aldrich syndrome are confusing. The lymphoid tissues appear normal early in the course of the disease, but as it progresses there may be a loss of lymphocytes from the thymus and paracortical areas of the lymph nodes. The peripheral lymphocyte count may decrease, and there is a variable loss of cellular immunity resulting in increased susceptibility to viral or fungal disease. Studies of immunoglobulin production in these patients suggest normal responses to a variety of antigens. IgM values are often low, and isohemagglutinins and Forssmann antibodies, normally present as "natural" antibodies, are usually lacking. The failure of these patients to respond to pneumococcal polysaccharides has led to the postulation that they have a general inability to respond to polysaccharide antigens, as opposed to normal responses to protein antigens. Whether this failure resides in the recognition system of the lymphocytes, in a deficit of the macrophages in processing such antigens or in a qualitative deficiency of plasma cell function is not clear. Since polysaccharides are widely distributed and important constituents of bacteria and fungi, it is reasonable that such a selective immunologic deficiency might have a serious impact upon resistance. Transfer factor has been tried and found to induce cellular immunity and clinical improvement in some patients with this disease.

IMMUNODEFICIENCY WITH THYMOMA. In adults, tumors of the thymus, made up of spindle-shaped epithelial cells, have been associated with disturbances of both T and B cell function.

SECONDARY IMMUNODEFICIENCY

In the primary immunodeficiency states, there is a genetic or other inherent cause for defective function of one or more of the cells, organs or proteins involved in immunologic responses. However, immunodeficiency is a frequent secondary phenomenon, not only in certain diseases, but as a consequence of modern advances in therapy.

IMMUNODEFICIENCY IN NEOPLASTIC DISEASES OF THE LYMPHOID OR HEMATOPOIETIC TISSUES. In the leukemias and lymphomas, in which normal lymphoid tissues and bone marrow are replaced by malignant cells, immunologic function may be compromised by neutropenia, impaired cellular immunity, and deficient synthesis of secretory or plasma immunoglobulins, all consequences of the disease process, and all of which may be potentiated by treatment. The result is marked susceptibility to infection due to bacteria, fungi and viruses; varicella and measles are particularly dangerous for children with acute leukemia. Hypogammaglobulinemia may develop in some patients, giving rise to the antibody deficiency syndrome in approximately one third of adult cases of chronic lymphatic leukemia. In multiple myeloma there is marked increase in immunoglobulins, but this is monoclonal in type from the neoplastic cells and is often accompanied by a severe antibody deficiency syndrome, giving rise to recurrent sepsis, frequently due to pneumococci.

IMMUNODEFICIENCY FROM IMMUNOSUPPRESSIVE AND ANTINEOPLASTIC THERAPY. Since the rates of DNA and RNA synthesis are highest in the bone marrow, the stimulated lymphoid system and the gastrointestinal epithelium of normal individuals, it is not surprising that these groups of cells are most susceptible to the injurious effects of the chemical and physical agents used to destroy neoplastic cells. Consequently neutropenia and impaired T and B cell function are a constant threat in the patient undergoing radiation or antimetabolite therapy for diffuse neoplasia.

The same groups of agents have been shown experimentally to impair certain specific immune responses, particularly if given prior to the antigenic stimulus, so that they are now being used more and more extensively for "immunosuppression' to prevent rejection of allografts and as a means of treatment for diseases felt to have an "autoimmune' basis. These types of agents have been used: (1) *corticosteroids,* which blunt the inflammatory response, but principally affect T cells and thus impair cellular immunity; (2) *antimetabolites,* which probably affect both T cells and B cells; (3) *antilymphocyte globulin,* which probably affects a number of fundamental lymphocyte functions, such as recognition and memory, but particularly those of the T cells. Successful use of these agents depends upon very careful regulation of dosage, but infection due to viruses, mycobacteria, fungi and unusual organisms like *Pneumocystis carinii* poses a constant threat to the patient.

IMMUNODEFICIENCY IN MALNUTRITION. Severe malnutrition, particularly of the kwashiorkor type with protein deficiency, enhances susceptibility to infection. At the same time, infection often precipitates frank nutritional failure. In Africa in those areas where chronic protein deficiency is widespread in older infants and preschool children, measles is a major cause of death. In general, investigation has shown that B cell function (immunoglobulin antibody synthesis) is better preserved than T cell function, which is clearly impaired in patients with malnutrition.

IMMUNODEFICIENCY WITH GASTROINTESTINAL DISEASE. **Protein-losing enteropathy** is a common accompaniment of inflammatory bowel disease, with exudation of smaller plasma proteins into the bowel lumen and their loss in the feces or through digestion by the intestinal juices. The resulting shortened half-life and lowering of the plasma concentration of the affected proteins, principally albumin and gamma globulins, is seldom severe enough to produce the antibody deficiency syndrome. However, the picture of the malabsorption syndrome as part of a primary B cell deficiency, in which protein-losing enteropathy may occur, especially with giardiasis, may create considerable diagnostic confusion.

Lymphangiectasia of the bowel, with or without malformations of other lymphatic vessels, occurs as a rare congenital malformation in occasional infants. It may sometimes result not only in loss of plasma proteins, but of lymphocytes into the bowel lumen, with impairment of cellular immunity, as in animals experimentally subjected to chronic drainage of the thoracic duct to prevent allograft rejection. Thus, edema and recurrent infections may remain a problem in such an infant unless the diseased bowel can be removed.

IMMUNODEFICIENCY WITH HYPERCATABOLIC HYPOGAMMAGLOBULINEMIA. The level of circulating immunoglobulins may be markedly reduced if there is extensive loss or rapid catabolism of plasma proteins, which results in a distinct shortening of their half-lives in the circulation. There may be loss of proteins through the skin in pemphigus, severe eczema or burns, into the lumen of the bowel in exudative enteropathy, or lymphangiectasia of the bowel, or into the urine in the nephrotic syndrome. There is usually a reduction of circulating albumin as well as of gamma globulin, but rarely, except in the nephrotic syndrome, is the deficiency of gamma globulin sufficient to produce undue susceptibility to invasive infection; plasma cells develop and immunoglobulin synthesis and antibody formation are normal even though the half-life of the immunoglobulin is greatly shortened. In the nephrotic syndrome several factors seem to be responsible for the increased susceptibility to septic bacterial infection: (1) age, since most of the patients are young children in whom recurrent infections are normally prevalent; (2) the nature of the edema fluid in the tissues and body cavities, with its low protein content, which makes it a good culture medium for certain organisms, notably pneumococci; and (3) the extremely low concentrations of gamma globulin in the edema fluid. The administration of prophylactic gamma globulin is of little use in instances of hypercatabolic hypogammaglobulinemia, since it is rapidly lost from the bloodstream.

IMMUNODEFICIENCY WITH OTHER CONDITIONS. Functional failure of the lymphocytes and even quantitative lymphocyte deficiency may develop late in the course of *ataxia-telangiectasia,* the *Wiskott-Aldrich syndrome* and in a few instances of *agammaglobulinemia.* A few cases of *"immunologic amnesia"* have been observed, in which recurrent infections have been associated with a reduction in circulating lymphocytes apparently due to the presence of a cytotoxic substance in the serum, resulting in a loss of immunologic memory. Though delayed hypersensitivity could be induced, it could not be retained. There was no "second-set" accelerated rejection of an allograft, and the antibody response to reinjection of an antigen was of the primary rather than of the secondary type. This state is somewhat analogous to that induced by the injection of antilymphocyte serum in order to prevent graft rejection.

In *Hodgkin's disease* and also in *sarcoidosis,* both acquired diseases affecting the lymphoid system in a diffuse manner, many patients become "anergic." In Hodgkin's disease, antibody formation is usually not impaired, but the response to antigens normally eliciting delayed skin reactions is markedly reduced, allografts are tolerated by certain patients, and delayed hypersensitivity cannot be induced even by passive transfer of cells from sensitive donors. Thus there is a serious defect in cellular immunity to which the susceptibility of these patients to tuberculosis and fungal infections is probably related. Lepromatous *leprosy,* the progressive, ultimately fatal form of the disease, is also characterized by anergy with a negative skin reaction and hypergammaglobulinemia, whereas in the benign form of the disease (the tuberculoid type), the lepromin skin test is positive and the immunoglobulin level is normal. Improvement in the prognosis of the lepromatous form of the disease has been achieved by using transfer factor to induce hypersensitivity to lepromin, thus converting the process to the more benign tuberculoid form.

CHARLES A. JANEWAY

Ament, M. E., Ochs, H. D., and Davis, S. K.: Structure and function of the gastrointestinal tract in primary immunodeficiency syndromes. Medicine *52*:227, 1973.
Burke, B. A., and Good, R. A.: *Pneumocystis carinii* infection. Medicine *52*:23, 1973.
Chandra, R. K.: Immunocompetence in undernutrition. J. Pediatr. *81*:1194, 1972.
Claman, H. N.: Corticosteroids and lymphoid cells. New Engl. J. Med., *287*:388, 1972.
Cooper, M. D., Faulk, W. P., Fudenberg, H. H., Good, R. A., Hitzig, W., Kunkel, H., Rosen, F. S., Seligmann, M., Soothill, J., and Wedgwood, R. J.: Classification of primary immunodeficiencies. New Engl. J. Med. *288*:966, 1973.
Eraklis, A. J., Kevy, S. V., Diamond, L. K., and Gross, R. E.: Hazard of overwhelming infection after splenectomy in childhood. New Engl. J. Med. *276*:1225, 1967.
Frommel, D., and Good, R. A.: Immunological disorders: *In* Gairdner, D., and Hull, D. (eds.): Recent Advances in Paediatrics. 4th ed. London, J. A. Churchill, Ltd., 1971, Chapter 13, p. 420.
Hitzig, W. H., Barandun, S., and Cottier, H.: Die Schweizerische Form des Agammaglobulinämie. Ergeb. Inn. Med. Kinderheilkd. *27*:79, 1968.
Hughes, W. T., Price, R. A., Kim, Ho-K., Coburn, T. P., Grigsby, D., and Feldman, S.: *Pneumocystis carinii* pneumonitis in children with malignancies. J. Pediatr. *82*:404, 1973.
Johnston, R. B., Jr., and Baehner, R. L.: Chronic granulomatous disease: Correlation between pathogenesis and clinical findings. Pediatrics *48*:730, 1971.
Johnston, R. B., Jr., Newman, S. L., and Struth, A. G.: An abnormality of the alternate pathway of complement activation in sickle cell disease. New Engl. J. Med. *288*:803, 1973.
Kevy, S. V., Tefft, M., Vawter, G. F., and Rosen, F. S.: Hereditary splenic hypoplasia. Pediatrics *42*:752, 1968.
Kretschmer, R., Janeway, C. A., and Rosen, F. S.: Immunologic amnesia. Pediatr. Res. *2*:7, 1968.
Lawrence, H. S.: Immunotherapy with transfer factor. New Engl. J. Med. *287*:1092, 1972.
Lischner, H. W.: DiGeorge syndrome(s). J. Pediatr. *81*:1042, 1972.
Miller, J. F. A. P.: Thymus tissue as a therapeutic measure. New Engl. J. Med. *287*:818, 1972.
Nell, P. A., Amman, A. J., Hong, R., and Stiehm, E. R.: Familial selective IgA deficiency. Pediatrics *49*:71, 1972.
Pearson, H. A., Cornelius, E. A., Schwartz, A. D., et al.: Transfusion-reversible functional asplenia in young children with sickle cell anemia. New Engl. J. Med. *283*:334, 1970.
Rosen, F. S.: The thymus gland and the immune deficiency syndromes: *In* Samter, M. (ed.): Immunological Diseases. 2nd Ed. Boston, Little Brown and Company, 1971, Vol. 1, p. 497.
Ruddy, S., Gigli, I., and Austen, K. F.: The complement system of man: Inherited anomalies; acquired abnormalities. New Engl. J. Med. *287*:592, 642, 1972.
Schulkind, M. L., Ellis, E. F., and Smith, R. T.: Effect of antibody upon clearance of I^{125}-labelled pneumococci by the spleen and liver. Pediatr. Res. *1*:178, 1967.
Silverstein, A. M.: Fetal immune responses in congenital infection. New Engl. J. Med., *286*:1413, 1972.
Spitter, L. E., Levin, A. S., Stilco, D. P., Fudenberg, H. H., Pirofsky, B., August, C. S., Stiehm, E. R., Hitzig, W. H., and Gatti, R. A.: The Wiskott-Aldrich syndrome; results of transfer factor therapy. J. Clin. Invest. *51*:3216, 1972.
Stossel, T. P., Alper, C. A., and Rosen, F. S.: Opsonic activity in newborn. Role of properdin. Pediatrics *52*:134, 1973.
Walzer, P. D., Schultz, M. G., Western, K. A., and Robbins, J. B.: *Pneumocystis carinii* and primary immune deficiency diseases of infancy and childhood. J. Pediatr. *82*:416, 1973.

ALLERGIC DISORDERS

The terms allergy and allergic, as used here, describe adverse physiologic reactions resulting from the interaction of antigen with humoral antibody and/or lymphoid cells. This definition does not necessarily include a variety of as yet poorly characterized disorders, particularly those thought by some to result from ingestion of foods, in which no immunologic mechanisms have been demonstrated. For example, adverse reactions which clinically resemble typical allergic reactions are known to occur following ingestion of certain foods, particularly cow's milk. Some of these reactions appear to have a biochemical basis, such as disaccharidase insufficiency in some instances of diarrhea following ingestion of cow's milk, or reaction to nitrites in headache after eating of certain other foods ("hot dog headache"); however, the underlying cause in many of the syndromes following food ingestion is unknown.

Use of the term "allergy" to designate only those reactions involving humoral antibody or cellular immune responses, and occurring in a host sensitized by prior exposure to the antigen, imposes a restriction on the term not intended by von Pirquet when he originated the word. As originally defined, allergy referred to a "state of changed reactivity" in a host occurring as a result of contact with antigen. This altered reactivity could be either beneficial to the host, as in the case of immunity, or detrimental, as in anaphylaxis. In modern usage, allergy refers only to the adverse consequences of exposure to antigen or "allergen."

The terms antigen and allergen are generally used interchangeably, but not all antigens are good allergens, or vice versa. For example, tetanus and diphtheria toxoids are excellent antigens but are only rarely responsible for adverse reactions. On the other hand, ragweed pollen protein, one of the most potent allergens known, is not a particularly potent antigen by immunologic criteria. The immunochemical characteristics that determine why various antigens are potent or feeble allergens have not been identified.

"Atopy" and "atopic" are terms also used in reference to allergic diseases. The words originated 50 years ago in recognition of the fact that hay fever, asthma and eczema had a particular tendency to cluster in certain families. Atopy is not easy to define, an individual commonly being identified as atopic if he has a disease considered "atopic." Atopy implies a constitutional abnormality with the following characteristics: (1) a *hereditary factor* expressed in a high frequency of hay fever, asthma and atopic eczema in the immediate relatives of affected individuals; (2) *eosinophilia* of the blood and tissue secretions (an almost universal finding at some stage of asthma, hay fever or eczema); (3) a predisposition to *selective synthesis of IgE antibody* on exposure to environmental substances; (4) a *hyperactivity of the airways in asthmatics* upon exposure to various physical factors (cold air, irritant odors) and to certain endogenous body chemicals (acetylcholine, histamine), and/or *hyperreactivity of the skin in eczema* to certain physical and chemical factors (stroking, acetylcholine); and (5) a presumptive *disturbance in metabolism of cyclic 3′,5′-adenosine monophosphate (cAMP)* in asthmatics, manifest in abnormal responses to catecholamines (epinephrine, isoproterenol) and in abnormal synthesis of cAMP by leukocytes. (See Chemical Mediators of Allergic Injury, later in this Section.)

The tendency to form IgE antibodies is expressed clinically in atopic persons by "wheal and flare" skin test reactions to common inhalants and food substances. The nature of the defect resulting in increased production of reaginic IgE has not been identified, but evidence has been presented suggesting that atopic and normal persons differ in the disposition of antigens coming in contact with mucosal surfaces.

Not all the above characteristics of atopy are present in every individual with asthma, hay fever or eczema; those that do occur appear in varying degrees. But these criteria are rarely fully met by persons not afflicted with atopic disorders.

IMMUNOLOGIC BASIS OF ATOPIC DISEASE

The lymphoid system, through its cellular components (the lymphocytes) and their synthetic products (the immunoglobulins and lymphokines), has a primary role in immunity to bacteria, viral agents and fungi and in the elimination of mutant malignant cells. The same system, however, is also responsible paradoxically for a broad spectrum of diseases and much chronic illness of mankind, ranging from relatively mild conditions such as ragweed hay fever to such serious disorders as disseminated lupus erythematosus. Attempts to modulate the deleterious effects resulting from antigen-antibody or antigen-lymphocyte interaction by immunosuppression of the lymphoid system may result in serious infections or in the development of malignancy. Such complications have been particularly observed in patients receiving potent immunosuppressive agents in support of organ transplantation.

Allergic reactions in man are complex, resulting from a concatenation of factors. Allergic injury to tissues varies from the completely reversible to permanent pathologic change. Determinants of the extent of the tissue damage include both the character of the antigen and the target organs involved; but perhaps most important are the nature and degree of involvement of various components of the immune system, which include circulating antibodies, lymphoid and other hematopoietic cells, the complement system of proteins and a wide variety of physiologically active molecules that are either generated or released as a result of the interaction of antigen with antibodies and lymphoid cells. Because immunologic reactions leading to allergic tissue damage are so complex, it is useful to attempt to characterize them in terms of the reactants involved, in order to appreciate the mechanisms by which injury occurs. It is possible to dissect allergic reactions into several distinctive types, but it must be recognized that most clinical reactions are not pure. In a disorder in which one mechanism of tissue injury may predominate, there are frequently a number of interacting mechanisms.

Immunologically mediated tissue injury may occur as a result of the interaction of humoral antibody with antigen or of the interaction of antigen with lymphocytes (cell-mediated or delayed hypersensitivity). Humoral antibody-antigen reactions are recognizable in three forms, two of which occur on the surface of cells and the third in the extracellular fluids. Of the two reactions occurring on the surface of the cells, the type mediated by IgE (immediate, or anaphylactic) is of greatest interest to the allergist. In this circumstance, circulating basophils and their tissue counterparts, the mast cells which are strategically located around blood vessels, become "sensitized" by antibodies of the reaginic type belonging to the IgE class.

The terms *reaginic IgE* or *IgE reagins* or *homocytotropic antibodies* refer to specific IgE molecules formed against allergens, such as ragweed pollen, in contradistinction to "nonspecific" IgE molecules, which are found in the serum and tissues of all normal individuals. In species other than man, reaginic activity is not confined to antibodies of the IgE class; the bulk of the evidence indicates that in man IgE antibodies are the principal carriers of reaginic activity.

IgE antibodies, like IgA antibodies, are synthesized by plasma cells located predominantly under mucosal surfaces, and particularly in the respiratory and gastrointestinal tracts. Once formed, IgE antibody has the unique property of becoming "fixed" to the surfaces of mast cells and basophils for long periods of time. The precise nature of the fixation process is not known, but the Fc portion of the IgE molecule is known to be involved. Once this attachment is made, the basophils and mast cells may be considered as "sensitized," and upon subsequent contact with the antigen specific for the attached IgE, a sequence of energy-dependent reactions occurs which results in release of pharmacologically active substances (such as histamine), which are known as the chemical mediators of allergic reactions. The released mediators act on tissue receptors to cause the physiologic reaction expressed in the patient as symptoms. The reaction is largely reversible, both in terms of the cellular source of the mediators and in the effects of the mediator on the affected tissues. Although aggregated IgE can fix late components of the complement system through an alternate pathway, participation of the complement system in IgE-mediated hypersensitivity disorders has not been shown.

The prototypic *anaphylactic or IgE-mediated reaction* is ragweed hay fever. The allergist makes use of the IgE antibody-antigen reaction in mast cells when he tests for inhalant or food sensitivity. Small amounts of extracts of pollens, molds, danders and foods are introduced into the patient's skin by scratch, puncture or intradermal techniques. If IgE antibody specific for the test antigen is present on the subject's mast cells, the interaction of injected antigen with bound IgE will release histamine, a potent vasoactive material which causes increased capillary permeability and dilatation, leading to the familiar "wheal and flare" reaction characteristic of IgE sensitivity.

In the *second type of interaction* between antigen and antibody taking place at cell surfaces, immunoglobulins of the IgG or IgM class react with antigenic determinants* that either are an integral part of the cell membrane or have become adsorbed to or incorporated in the membrane. In contrast to the IgE or anaphylactic type of reaction, the complement system is activated in most reactions of this second kind and the target cell is destroyed.

A familiar example of immunologic injury of the second type occurs when incompatible red blood cells are transfused. The recipient's isohemagglutinins (antibodies directed against determinants on the surface of the red cells) react with the incompatible cells, the complement system is activated, and sequential action of complement proteins results in lysis of the cell. Immune injury to platelets, leukocytes and erythrocytes may involve this type of mechanism, and is sometimes induced by drugs.

The *third immunopathologic mechanism* of tissue injury involving humoral antibody and antigen does not occur on the surface of cells but in the extracellular spaces. In certain ratios of antigen to antibody, antigen-antibody complexes are formed which are "toxic" to tissues in which they are deposited. For example, complexes formed in moderate antigen excess have the capacity to activate the complement sequence and release histamine. Complexes so formed lodge in the filtering organs of the body such as the kidney and lung, and infiltrate the walls of small blood vessels. Complement components C5, C6 and C7 are chemotactic for polymorphonuclear (PMN) leukocytes, which are attracted to the site of the toxic complex deposition. With phagocytosis of the complexes, the polymorphonuclear leukocytes are lysed, and basic proteins and proteolytic enzymes are released which produce tissue damage. The glomerulonephritis of systemic lupus erythematosus is the prototype of human immune complex disease; immune complex injury is responsible for up to 90 per cent of immunologic glomerulonephritis in man.

Toxic complex injury is an excellent example of the cooperation that may take place between different antibodies in the production of tissue injury. It has been known for years that the deposition of complexes containing IgG and IgM in small blood vessels in the kidney in experimental serum sickness in animals could be prevented by prior treatment with antihistamines, and it has been recently shown that deposition depends on an increase in the permeability of these vessels. The increase in permeability to IgG and IgM complexes is brought about by histamine liberated in the course of a simultaneous interaction of IgE antibody and antigen which leads to "leakiness" of the capillaries and prepares them to receive the toxic complexes.

In the three foregoing types of immune injury humoral antibody interacts with antigen, either on the surfaces of cells or in tissue spaces. In cell-mediated or delayed hypersensitivity pathologic changes occur following interaction of antigen with specifically sensitized mononuclear cells, morphologically represented by the small lymphocyte. As a result of this interaction a host of biologically active molecules are either synthesized or released. These factors include what has been termed an "initiator molecule" (transfer factor) as well as a group of "effector" molecules (migration inhibitory factor, chemotactic factor, lymphotoxin, lymphocyte transforming factor and interferon).

The cell-mediated immune reaction is the immunologic basis for contact dermatitis and for most cases of rejection of organ transplants. In certain infectious diseases, exemplified by tuberculosis, much of the tissue damage observed is due to the cell-mediated hypersensitivity response of the host to antigenic components of the organism rather than to inherent toxicity of the organism.

CHEMICAL MEDIATORS OF ALLERGIC INJURY

Histamine is formed from the amino acid histidine by the action of histidine decarboxylase. Its pharmacologic effects include: (1) dilatation of small blood vessels; (2) increase in capillary permeability; (3) stimulation of mucous secretion; and (4) contraction of bronchial smooth muscle. His-

*An antigenic determinant is a restricted portion of an antigen molecule that determines the specificity of an antigen-antibody reaction. Antigenic determinants may be composed of only four or five amino acid residues. In complex antigens found in nature, such as pollens, there may be several hundred determinants on the surface of an antigen molecule, each capable of initiating an immune response and subsequently reacting with specific antibody.

tamine is also a potent stimulus of itching. Histamine liberation in ragweed hay fever produces the rhinorrhea, sneezing, nasal obstruction and itching characteristic of the ragweed-sensitive patient.

Slow reacting substance of anaphylaxis (SRS-A) is probably a group of several acidic lipids of unknown chemical composition which have potent contractile effects on human bronchial muscle. The bronchoconstrictor effects are typically slower in onset and more prolonged than those produced by histamine. Unlike histamine, SRS-A does not exist preformed in cells but appears to be synthesized following IgE antibody-antigen interaction. The source of SRS-A has not been established unequivocally in man but is probably the mast cell.

Plasma kinins are a group of peptides with capacities to stimulate capillary permeability and vasodilatation exceeding even those of histamine. Kinins cause contraction of nonvascular smooth muscle and stimulate pain receptors but not itching. Generation of kinin activity from precursors in plasma is initiated through a complex series of enzymatic reactions. The initial event in the generation of bradykinin (a nonapeptide) in human plasma is the activation of Hageman factor; the latter may be activated by immune complexes and appears to be in the chain of events leading to liberation of *bradykinin* by immune complexes.

Anaphylatoxins are vasoactive peptides derived from plasma protein precursors. Anaphylatoxins liberate histamine from mast cells and also have potent chemotactic activity for polymorphonuclear leukocytes. The human anaphylatoxins designated $C3_a$ and $C5_a$ are called "split products" of the complement system, because they are derived from interaction of immune complexes with C3 and C5. Intracutaneous injection of $C3_a$ causes itching, wheal formation and an axon reflex type of erythema. In addition to their formation from complement interaction with immune complexes, $C3_a$ and $C5_a$ fragments can be formed by the action on plasma protein precursors of various enzymes, including some of bacterial origin. As in the case of nonimmunologic release of histamine, these vasoactive molecules can be released by nonimmunologic mechanisms, with the potential of causing typical signs and symptoms of an allergic reaction. A typical "allergic" reaction may in reality, therefore, not represent antigen-antibody interaction at all.

The *eosinophil chemotactic factor of anaphylaxis (ECF-A)* is chemotactic for eosinophilic leukocytes. Its release by the interaction of IgE antibody and antigen has been proposed as the explanation for the eosinophilic infiltration of tissues undergoing allergic tissue injury.

Serotonin (5-hydroxytryptamine) is an important mediator of anaphylaxis in rodents. In man, however, only minute amounts are found in the lung, and the bronchiole does not constrict on exposure to serotonin in vitro. There is little evidence that serotonin plays a role in human allergic reactions.

Prostaglandins are 20-carbon fatty acids. The F and the E series are of special relevance in human allergic disease. Prostaglandin $F2_a$ is known to contract human bronchiolar smooth muscle; the E series act as bronchodilators. Both E2 and $F2_a$ are released in vitro following antigenic challenge of the sensitized lungs of experimental animals. Administration of prostaglandin E by aerosol has been reported to relieve airway obstruction in asthmatic patients.

Study of the IgE-mediated release of mediators has established that the intracellular nucleotide cyclic adenylate (cyclic adenosine monophosphate or AMP), which has a central role in numerous biologic processes as a regulator of cellular function, also plays an important role in regulation of allergic responses. The role of cyclic AMP in regulation of these allergic responses is an extension of its normal function as a control molecule. According to the "second messenger" hypothesis, when a circulating hormone (the first messenger) finds its receptor in a target cell, it alters the activity of adenyl cyclase, a membrane-bound enzyme. The resulting change in adenyl cyclase activity alters the intracellular level of cyclic AMP, generally (but not always) in the direction of increased intracellular cyclic AMP concentration. The change in concentration of cyclic AMP affects the metabolic behavior of the cell and evokes physiologic responses which vary with the type of cell involved. In the case of a smooth muscle cell, for example, the result of an increase in cyclic AMP is relaxation; an adrenal cortical cell secretes cortisol with increased intracellular cyclic AMP, and so on. Cyclic AMP has been called the second messenger in this system, and in the case of cells that secrete other hormones, these hormones are called third messengers.

The intracellular cyclic AMP concentration is determined not only by adenyl cyclase activity but also by a specific phosphodiesterase which rapidly catabolizes cyclic AMP as it is formed. Methylxanthines, and particularly theophylline, have been found to be potent inhibitors of this phosphodiesterase, thus tending to increase intracellular cyclic AMP concentrations.

The relevance of this system to allergic responses derives from studies on human lung tissue sensitized with reaginic IgE and then challenged with specific antigen. In this preparation β-adrenergic receptor agonists (epinephrine, isoproterenol) and theophylline inhibit antigen-induced release of histamine, SRS-A and ECF-A. On the other hand, α-adrenergic stimulation enhances release of histamine and SRS-A, in association with a decrease in cyclic AMP. In the same experimental system using sensitized human lung tissue, cholinergic stimulation enhances antigen-induced release of histamine and SRS-A, but the mechanism is apparently independent of any influence on cyclic AMP concentration; it involves another cyclic nucleotide, cyclic guanine monophosphate (cyclic GMP). The events described above are illustrated in Figure 9–10. The essence of the β-adrenergic receptor theory of Szentivanyi is that

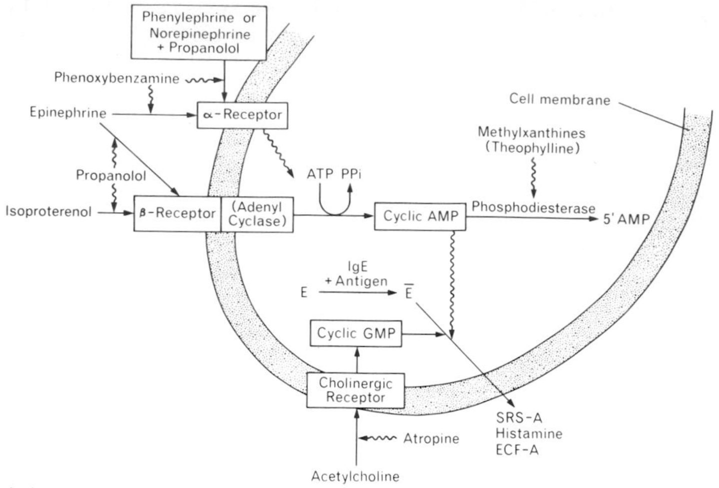

Figure 9–10 *The stippled structure represents the cell membrane of a mast cell. Three of many receptors are diagrammatically depicted: two adrenergic receptors, designated α and β, and a recently described cholinergic receptor. β-adrenergic stimulation with epinephrine or isoproterenol acts upon the β-receptor–adenyl cyclase complex to catalyze the formation of cyclic 3′,5′-AMP (cAMP) from ATP, which leads to a rise in intracellular cAMP. An increase in intracellular cAMP modulates (decreases) the release of mediators (SRS-A, histamine, ECF-A) from the cell, otherwise induced by activation of a hypothetical enzyme (E) when antigen interacts with IgE antibody.*

Cyclic AMP is hydrolyzed to 5-AMP by a specific phosphodiesterase, the activity of which is inhibited by methylxanthines, particularly by theophylline. The inhibition of hydrolysis of cAMP acts to maintain the level of intracellular cAMP. Accordingly, β-adrenergic agonists and theophylline may be looked upon as acting synergistically to elevate the level of intracellular cAMP.

Alpha-adrenergic stimulation by phenylephrine or by norepinephrine plus propranolol (the latter blocks the minimal β-adrenergic activity of norepinephrine, permitting relatively isolated α stimulant activity) acts to decrease intracellular cAMP, enhancing mediator release. The mechanism is unknown. Acetylcholine interacts with cholinergic receptors to increase intracellular cyclic guanosine monophosphate (cGMP) through an effect on guanyl cyclase. Cyclic GMP enhances mediator release.

The opposing actions on mediator release of β-adrenergic stimulation through cAMP and of cholinergic stimulation through cGMP are reminiscent of the opposing actions of the adrenergic and cholinergic divisions of the autonomic nervous system.

Certain prostaglandins, particularly among those of the E series, also act to increase intracellular cAMP; this effect is not depicted.

many of the abnormalities seen in asthmatic individuals can be explained on the basis of an abnormality in the structure or function of the β-adrenergic–adenyl cyclase complex.

GENERAL AND SPECIFIC METHODS OF DIAGNOSIS

Etiologic diagnosis of allergic disorders depends, as does all medical diagnosis, upon a carefully taken history supplemented by the judicious use of tests appropriate to the organ system involved in the disease.

ALLERGIC HISTORY. A carefully taken history is the single most important tool in arriving at a correct diagnosis in allergic diseases. After the elements of the general medical history have been obtained, information of particular interest to the allergist is sought. For example, inquiry is made as to whether the patient's symptoms are perennial or seasonal. Seasonal symptoms suggest the etiologic role of seasonal allergens, such as pollens, whereas perennial symptoms suggest exposure either to multiple seasonal allergens or to factors not influenced by season. Are the symptoms continuous or intermittent? Are they subject to diurnal variation? Has a change of location had any effect? All these questions help to focus on particular etiologic agents. For example, impressive amelioration of symptoms when the child spends time in a relative s home, or perhaps on a vacation in a different part of the country, suggests that there may be something in the patient's immediate environment responsible for his illness. In assessing the role of foods as etiologic agents, it is important to distinguish between what the parents have actually observed following ingestion of a food and what they may have been told by a physician, possibly on the basis of skin tests to foods, which are subject to frequent misinterpretation. (See Adverse Reactions to Foods, below.) One must be particularly critical in interpreting cause and effect relationships where foods are concerned, as it is very easy for parents to arrive at erroneous conclusions based on inconsistent relationships between ingestion of a particular food and the appearance of symptoms. The effect of drug therapy is sometimes of value in establishing the allergic etiology of the problem. Significant improvement in symptoms following the use of antiallergic drugs such as antihistamines, sympathomimetics, xanthines or corticosteroids supports the notion that an allergic reaction is the basis of the symptoms; on the other hand, symptoms occurring on a nonimmunologic basis might also respond to such therapy.

IN VITRO STUDIES. A white blood cell count and a differential count are useful in establishing the presence or absence of *eosinophilia.* A total eosinophil count gives a more accurate estimate of blood eosinophilia. Eosinophilia may be intermittent, and at least two or three normal determinations should be made before it is concluded that eosinophilia is not present. Eosinophilia in excess of 5 per cent on peripheral smear or of 250 cells/mm^3 is considered elevated. Eosinophilia of respiratory tract secretions, in a patient with rhinorrhea or cough, is a useful diagnostic sign. A smear of nasal secretions or bronchial mucus is easily prepared and stained on a microscope slide, preferably with an eosin-methylene blue stain (Hansel's stain).* Giemsa or Wright's stain is an acceptable, less effective alternative. The presence of more than 5 to 10 per cent eosinophils in nasal secretions supports the diagnosis of allergic rhinitis, and eosinophils in bronchial mucus are highly suggestive of asthma. The degree of blood eosinophilia in allergic conditions does not generally exceed 15 to 20 per cent, but one occasionally observes eosinophilia of as high as 35 per cent in allergic children in the absence of other disorders known to cause eosinophilia. Stool specimens should always be examined for the presence of ova or parasites before final judgment is reached regarding the cause of eosinophilia. Corticosteroids cause eosinopenia for up to 6 hours following a dose; the timing of a blood specimen collection should be appropriately adjusted.

A number of immunologic tests are of value in allergy diagnosis. These involve examining the total and specific IgE content of serum and determining the sensitivity of the patient's leukocytes for antigen-induced histamine release. Quantification of total IgE can be accomplished by the radioimmunoabsorbent test (RIST) or by a double antibody radioimmunoassay procedure. Mean concentrations of IgE are higher in individuals with such allergic disorders as hay fever, asthma, and atopic dermatitis than in normal persons. There are a significant number of allergic individuals, however, who have normal or low IgE concentrations, so that determination of total IgE for diagnostic purposes may be of limited value except in unusual circumstances. Occasionally in atypical forms of atopic dermatitis in which diagnosis is uncertain, the finding of grossly elevated IgE, an almost universal finding in active atopic dermatitis, will support the latter diagnosis.

The determination of IgE antibody levels against specific allergens is possible for such allergens as ragweed, grass, house dust or other inhalants, and various foods. Determination of specific IgE antibodies is accomplished by the radioallergosorbent test (RAST). The sensitivity of the RAST appears to be excellent and a technician can do 100 to 200 tests per day. The RAST technique may prove to be an acceptable alternative to direct skin testing of the patient under many circumstances, as an in vitro diagnostic tool in IgE-mediated allergic disorders.

In the *histamine release test,* the patient's leukocytes are tested for their sensitivity for antigen-induced histamine release. For example, leukocytes from individuals with ragweed hay fever, on exposure to various concentrations of ragweed antigen "E" (the major allergen of ragweed pollen) under appropriate in vitro conditions, will release histamine into solution, which can then be measured. The cells of individuals with high degrees of leukocyte sensitivity release histamine on exposure to very small quantities of specific antigen, whereas cells with lesser degrees of sensitivity require exposure to higher concentrations of antigen for release of comparable amounts of histamine. In the ragweed system, there is a rough correlation between sensitivity of leukocytes to histamine release on exposure to an antigen, the titer of specific IgE antibody and the titer of passive transfer (P-K) activity, and clinical sensitivity to the antigen on environmental exposure.

IN VIVO TESTS. Determination of allergic reactivity through direct **skin testing** of the patient has been in use for over 50 years; and owing to its simplicity and sensitivity it will remain for the foreseeable future an important diagnostic tool in the diagnosis of IgE-mediated sensitivity. A small quantity of potential allergen is introduced into the skin by the scratch, puncture or intracutaneous technique; if the allergen interacts with specific IgE antibody on the surface of mast cells in skin, a sequence of energy-dependent enzyme reactions culminates in release of histamine from the mast cell, which acts upon histamine receptors in capillaries to cause the increased permeability and dilatation observed clinically as the wheal and flare reaction. One infers from the positive skin test that specific IgE antibody is present also on the mast cells in the tissues of the clinically affected organ, the nasal or bronchial mucosa, for example. This inference is not completely trustworthy. *The positive wheal and flare reaction on skin testing establishes only the presence of specific IgE antibody on the surface of the mast cell; it does not indicate that the patient will necessarily have clinical symptoms on exposure to the allergen.* A significant number of atopic individuals have no symptoms whatsoever on natural exposure to allergens which give positive wheal and flare reactions on skin testing. Histamine release from tissue mast cells can be modified by various drugs (codeine, polymyxin, antihistamines), and by improper technique, including the use of unduly concentrated antigen solutions. In the latter instances, histamine release may be nonspecific or nonimmunologic; the resulting wheal and flare is identical, however, to that produced immunologically. All too often, owing to lack of appreciation of this possibility, patients are erroneously diagnosed as having reagin-mediated disease.

In the **passive transfer test** (Prausnitz-Küstner [P-K] test) serum from the allergic individual is injected intracutaneously into a nonallergic recipient. The specific IgE antibodies in the donor serum passively sensitize the recipient's mast cells in the injected sites. The passively sensitized sites are

*Lide Laboratories, Inc., 6828 Oakland Avenue, St. Louis, MO 63139.

challenged 24 to 48 hours later with various allergens and the effects of histamine release are read in the same way as with direct skin tests. Because the passive transfer technique is time-consuming, somewhat less sensitive than direct skin testing and carries the danger of transmission of serum hepatitis, it is not very often employed in clinical practice.

Because the appearance of symptoms on natural exposure is not infrequently poorly correlated with results of skin testing, **provocation testing** by direct exposure of the mucous membrane of the affected organ to the suspected allergen (usually in the form of an extract of the material) has received considerable attention, particularly in Scandinavian countries. Provocation testing using mucous membranes has been used mostly in asthma, and to a lesser extent in allergic rhinitis, in the latter instance primarily as a research tool. The method for bronchial provocation testing is fully described in the references. In our laboratory, increasing concentrations of extracts of various allergens are inhaled by the patient after nebulization with a Maxi-Myst vacuum pump. A positive response will be manifest by an increase in airway obstruction, as monitored carefully with an instrument that measures expiratory flow rate. The patient's degree of sensitivity should be determined by skin tests prior to provocation testing, in order to permit appropriate initial concentrations of allergic extract to be used. With appropriate precautions, the method is safe and the results of provocation testing correlate well with history. It is time-consuming, however, and not suitable for general use as an outpatient procedure. Bronchial challenge testing has its greatest utility in patients who have multiple positive skin tests, and allows the rational selection of those allergens which may be most clinically significant for inclusion in a hyposensitization mixture. Selection in this way permits a greater concentration of the more clinically significant allergens in the mixture than would be possible if all the allergens possibly implicated by skin testing were to be included.

Provocation testing with foods has been explored by both the subcutaneous injection and the sublingual administration of food extracts. As introduced by Rinkel and expanded upon by Randolph and Lee, the results have been the subject of controversy. In the hands of the proponents of the methods, symptoms referable to various organ systems are provoked by positive tests. These symptoms may then be "neutralized" by the injection of a weaker concentration (higher dilution) of extract of the same food that provoked the reaction, a response difficult to understand on immunologic or other grounds. In individuals who have IgE-mediated sensitivity to a food, there is little doubt that symptoms can be provoked when that foood is ingested or injected. The relationship of this reaction to the provocative food testing described by Rinkel and Randolph is unclear, however, and though there is great enthusiasm on the part of some proponents, the technique has not yet been validated by adequately critical evaluation.

The **Rebuck skin window test** has been used primarily as an investigational tool. In this procedure, the skin is abraded with a sharp edge just to the point of producing minute pinpoint areas of bleeding. Test allergens are then applied to the abraded area and covered with a clear plastic coverslip. The coverslip is maintained in place for periods of 4 to 24 hours and then examined for increased numbers of eosinophils when compared to a control site to which allergen has not been applied. When the test is positive, eosinophils are the predominating cell in the stained coverslip smears removed at 24 hours. In individuals with grass or ragweed pollenosis (hay fever) there has been a good correlation between positive skin window responses and clinical symptoms. In the diagnosis of food and drug allergy, the results with the skin window test have been inconsistent.

PRINCIPLES OF TREATMENT OF ALLERGIC DISORDERS

Successful treatment of allergic disorders requires consideration of four principles in management: avoidance of allergens, pharmacologic therapy, immunotherapy (hyposensitization or desensitization), and prophylaxis.

Avoidance of the substance or substances known to be responsible for the allergic symptoms is the treatment of choice, and in cases of inhalant, food or drug allergy, simple avoidance of the exposure to the allergen frequently manages the problem. For individuals with inhalant allergies, instructions for preparation of an "allergen-free" indoor environment, emphasizing the bedroom, may be found in Table 9–4.

Pharmacologic therapy is the mainstay of the symptomatic treatment of allergic disorders, inasmuch as pharmacologic agents can modulate antigen-induced mediator release or reverse its physiologic consequences. In significant numbers of patients, a great deal can be accomplished by the proper application of environmental control measures and the appropriate use of pharmacologic agents in the management of allergic disorders without resort to hyposensitization.

Immunotherapy or hyposensitization is used for allergic disorders mediated by IgE antibody-antigen interaction which involves allergens that can either not be or only partially be avoided. The techniques of hyposensitization and the results that may be anticipated are discussed below.

AVOIDANCE OF SUSPECTED ALLERGENS. Identification of allergens by a carefully taken history, supplemented by judicious use of allergy skin tests and followed by elimination of the allergens implicated, will be all the treatment needed in many cases of IgE-mediated disease. For example, if it is established by history and skin testing that reac-

TABLE 9–4 INSTRUCTIONS FOR MAINTENANCE OF A DUST-FREE ROOM

PREPARATION AND MAINTENANCE OF AN ALLERGEN-FREE (DUST-FREE) ROOM. The most important dust is ordinary house dust, which is a mixture of many things, such as the wool fiber of rugs, feather dust from pillows, molds, insect scales, and the wool and cotton dust from upholstery, draperies, clothing, and the like. Practically anything which can wear out can produce dust. Though it is impossible to make a whole house or even a single room safe for a child who is allergic to dust by ordinary cleaning methods, special cleaning measures in the bedroom can be helpful.

Cleaning the room. Everything possible should be taken from the room, including pictures, rugs and curtains. If there is a closet, it should be emptied, or if it is used only for storage, it should be sealed off by wide Scotch tape. The room should be made as dust-tight as possible by closing all holes or cracks in the walls, ceiling or floor. If there is a hot-air outlet, it should be turned off in the basement and covered airtight in the room by plastic material or oilcloth. It is not necessary to supply heat for this room, since it is intended mainly for a bedroom and since any source of heat tends to collect dust and circulate it.

Once the room is tightly closed to the entry of dust, it should be cleaned thoroughly with soap and water. Remove every speck of dust from floors, walls and ceiling, including the dust on molding strips above doors and windows, in cracks in floors, on light fixtures, around pipes, and so on. A vacuum cleaner can be used to clean the room of large dust particles, but final cleaning should always be done with a damp cloth.

Furnishing the room. Furniture can be returned after it has been completely freed of dust by cleaning with soap and water. The bed should be taken apart to be cleaned carefully in every niche. Springs should be carefully wiped with a damp cloth. Only the following furniture is permitted: a bed, a small table, a simple wooden chair or two, and a chest of drawers (if the child's clothes cannot be kept in some other place). These things should all be carefully cleaned inside and out and should be of a material that is easily kept clean.

The mattress of the bed should be covered by plastic material specially made for allergic protection. Heavy plastic is necessary, such as is used in shower curtains. If there is a box spring, it should also be covered with plastic material. Foam rubber pillows should be used and should have plastic covers unless they are brand new. Foam rubber mattresses are desirable, and even they should be covered with plastic material.

Cotton blankets are preferable to wool. If wool must be used, it should be kept from the child by 1 or 2 sheets, so that the wool does not touch the child or have a chance to add dust to the room. Blankets should be washed frequently. Wool clothes are preferably not worn by the allergic child and in any event should be kept out of the bedroom.

The following should not be permitted in the room: rugs, upholstered furniture, curtains or draperies, bookcases, venetian blinds, or anything likely to make dust or to give it a resting place. Stuffed toys, such as animals, are not permitted. Toys should be as few as possible and be made of wood, metal or plastic.

If a floor covering is desired, linoleum should be used. If there are cracks in the floor which collect dust and cannot be filled, the floor should be covered with linoleum from wall to wall.

Pets are preferably excluded from the house and in any case should not enter the allergen free room.

Maintenance. 1. Keep windows and doors closed except at night, when a window may be open. A screen door spring on the door will help to keep it closed.

2. Go over the room each day with a damp cloth, removing dust from all exposed surfaces.
3. Once a week clean room and furniture thoroughly with a damp cloth.
4. It is best if the child dresses and undresses in another room, using the bedroom only for sleeping.
5. The rest of the house should be kept as dust-free as possible by the measures outlined above and by frequent, careful damp cloth cleaning.

tivity to household inhalants such as house dust or molds or dog or cat dander is contributing to the patient's symptoms, elimination of these allergens as a first step is mandatory. The recommendation that a family pet be removed from a home is frequently difficult to implement, and occasionally one encounters families in which pets seem to be as deeply embedded in the social fabric of the family as the child or children. However, when the allergic disorder is a serious one, such as asthma, and when the child has a positive skin test to the dander of the pet, parents can generally be persuaded to remove the animal. When skin tests to danders are negative, the problem may be more difficult; most allergists feel that elimination of potentially sensitizing pets from the household of the allergic child is desirable on prophylactic grounds.

PHARMACOLOGIC THERAPY. Much relief can be provided children suffering from allergic diseases through the appropriate use of pharmacologic agents. Drugs useful in treatment fall into four general classes: sympathomimetics, methylxanthines, antihistamines and corticosteroids.

Sympathomimetics. The sympathomimetic drugs exert their activity by combining with adrenergic receptors on cell surfaces. According to the dual receptor theory, adrenergic receptors fall into two general types, α and β. In general, drugs which affect α receptors cause physiologic responses that are excitatory, whereas drugs that influence β receptors produce inhibitory responses. (There are several exceptions to this generality.) In a given tissue the response to a drug depends upon the relative proportion of α and β receptors and upon the intrinsic properties of the drug, i.e., whether it stimulates primarily α receptors, β receptors, or both. The identification of receptors has been made possible largely through the development of drugs which specifically block various classes of adrenergic receptors. These drugs, in turn, have assumed important roles in therapy of diseases in which it becomes advisable to block the physiologic response resulting from stimulation of a given receptor. Variations in sensitivity of β receptors in different organs to β agonists (stimulants) and differences in response to β blocking drugs of diverse chemical structure have led to separation of β receptors into two subclasses, β_1 and

TABLE 9–5 EFFECTS OF STIMULATION OF ADRENERGIC RECEPTORS IN VARIOUS TISSUES

TISSUE, ORGAN, OR FUNCTION AFFECTED	EFFECT OF STIMULATION OF ALPHA RECEPTORS	EFFECT OF STIMULATION OF BETA RECEPTORS
Blood vessels	Constriction	Dilatation
Heart	–	Increase in rate Increase in contractility
Lung	Bronchial muscle constriction	Bronchial muscle relaxation
Glycogenolysis	Hepatic glycogenolysis increased	Muscular glycogenolysis increased (lactic acid)
FFA mobilization	–	Lipase activation

β_2. Table 9–5 shows the physiologic effects resulting from stimulation of adrenergic receptors in different tissues.

Sympathomimetics are used in allergic disorders principally because their activity on smooth muscle in blood vessels can reverse physiologic responses resulting from allergen-induced mediator release. Stimulation of α adrenergic receptors reduces edema of nasal mucous membranes through vasoconstriction and decrease of capillary permeability, for example, whereas β adrenergic stimulation causes smooth muscle relaxation which relieves at least one component of obstruction of the airway in asthma. Sympathomimetic drugs include the catecholamines (epinephrine and isoproterenol) and the noncatecholamines (ephedrine, isoetharine, salbutamol, orciprenaline, and terbutaline). The importance of distinguishing between catecholamine sympathomimetics and noncatecholamine sympathomimetics is that the former group of drugs should not be administered orally, since they are rapidly inactivated by the enzyme catechol-o-methyl transferase found in the gastrointestinal tract and liver. Accordingly, the use of epinephrine and isoproterenol is limited largely to injection and to topical application to mucous membranes. Ephedrine, the oldest and most widely used of the noncatecholamine sympathomimetics, is a drug of relatively weak β-stimulant activity, and its use is associated with a significant incidence of adverse side effects, principally involving the central nervous system. A number of promising noncatecholamine sympathomimetics available in Europe are now undergoing clinical investigation in this country. The advantages of this latter group of drugs is that they may be given orally, have a somewhat longer duration of action (at least 6 hours) than ephedrine (4 hours), and have relatively selective activity on the β_2 receptors in the airways, with less of the cardiovascular effects of isoproterenol and epinephrine.

Methylxanthines. The methylxanthines include theophylline, theobromine and caffeine. Theophylline is the only member of this class of drugs used in treatment of allergic disorders; caffeine and theobromine, found principally in coffee and tea, respectively, have similar pharmacologic properties but produce significantly less smooth muscle relaxation than theophylline. Theophylline exerts its activity principally by virtue of its potent inhibition of the phosphodiesterase responsible for the degradation of cyclic AMP. Theophylline thus acts to maintain the intracellular concentration of this important cyclic nucleotide, with the result that tension decreases in smooth muscle and IgE-mediated histamine and SRS-A release are inhibited. As with other potent drugs, overuse of theophylline can result in serious adverse effects, chiefly in the gastrointestinal and central nervous systems. Analysis of the case reports of adverse effects of theophylline in children shows that toxicity has generally resulted from overdosage of the drug.

Antihistamines. Antihistamines include a group of drugs of diverse chemical structure which compete for tissue receptor sites with histamine released in an allergic reaction. Their optimal effects are exerted when antihistamine concentration at the receptor sites is maintained continuously. Antihistamines belong to four chemical families; in occasional patients drugs from one group will give better results or have fewer undesirable side effects than drugs of another group; the most bothersome side effect is excessive sedation. The aminoalkylether derivatives (e.g., diphenhydramine [Benadryl]) are particularly potent soporifics, and may be used for this effect alone, particularly in elderly persons. Antihistamines have anticholinergic activity which makes them particularly useful in allergic rhinitis in decreasing rhinorrhea. This drying effect is undesirable in severe asthma when there is marked airway obstruction due to mucous secretions; when used in the usual dosage necessary to control allergic rhinitis, however, there is generally no adverse effect on the day-to-day course of asthma.

Corticosteroids. Corticosteroids have potent anti-inflammatory activity and they have recently been reported to restore in vitro the adenyl cyclase sensitivity of leukocytes of asthmatic patients. They are of great value in treatment of allergic disorders. Their use is associated, however, with significant adverse effects, the most troublesome of which in children is the suppression of linear growth. This latter effect is related to dose and is almost always a result of the daily use of steroids. With alternate-day steroid regimens (a single dose of prednisone or methylprednisolone given early in the morning every 48 hours) suppression of linear growth is seen much less frequently, as are all other adverse effects. The short-term use of corticosteroids in self-limited allergic disorders such as severe contact dermatitis is benign, but the decision to initiate long-term corticosteroid therapy in a child with allergic disease must be carefully weighed. Long-term corticosteroid administration is used most often in and should be limited to children with asthma who have failed to respond to adequate tests of other allergic management, including avoidance, hyposensitization and the use of conventional drugs. With the appropriate use of corticosteroids, children who are otherwise home-bound invalids, unable to function normally in terms of school, play activity, and the like, can live relatively normal lives with minimal adverse effects, particularly if alternate-day regimens are used. Prednisone is the corticosteroid of choice; both cost and incidence of certain side effects are lower than with newer steroid preparations, some of which, such as dexamethasone and triamcinolone, are not suitable for alternate-day regimens because of their relatively long duration of action.

IMMUNOTHERAPY, OR HYPOSENSITIZATION. Hyposensitization was introduced in the early 1900's by Leonard Noon, who believed that hay fever plants contained a toxin that was responsible for the symptoms observed in sensitive patients. He injected patients with extracts of the offending plant in order to induce immunity, as had been

Patient's Name ____________________

Extract contains: Mixed grass, Ragweed, Alternaria, Hormodendrum

Vial #1 contains each antigen in a 1:10,000 dilution
Vial #2 contains each antigen in a 1:1000 dilution
Vial #3 contains each antigen in a 1:100 dilution

Desensitizing injections should be given once or twice a week, according to the following program:

	AMOUNT	DILUTION	DATE GIVEN	REACTION
1st dose	0.05 ml	1:10,000 (vial #1)		
2nd dose	0.075	"		
3rd dose	0.10	"		
4th dose	0.15	"		
5th dose	0.20	"		
6th dose	0.30	"		
7th dose	0.50	"		
8th dose	0.05	1:1000 (vial #2)		
9th dose	0.075	"		
10th dose	0.10	"		
11th dose	0.15	"		
12th dose	0.20	"		
13th dose	0.30	"		
14th dose	0.40	"		
15th dose	0.50	"		
16th dose	0.05	1:100 (vial #3)		
17th dose	0.075	"		
18th dose	0.10	"		
19th dose	0.15	"		
20th dose	0.20	"		
21st dose	0.30	"		
22nd dose	0.40	"		
23rd dose	0.50	"		
Maintenance dose	0.50	1:100		

INJECTIONS are given in the area of the triceps, subcutaneously, with precautions to prevent accidental intravenous administration. Serious reactions to these dosages are rare, but patients should remain under observation for 20 to 30 minutes after each injection, so that any immediate reactions can be promptly managed with a tourniquet, epinephrine, and so forth.

REACTIONS: A systemic reaction that appears within a few minutes of the extract injection may be quite serious and needs prompt treatment. A *local* reaction of erythema and edema occurring within 20 to 30 minutes is generally benign and gone within 6 to 12 hours. Delayed reactions include: (1) worsening of respiratory symptoms within 6 to 12 hours (usually more sneezing or coughing); (2) worsening of itching and redness of *eczema,* as late as 24 to 48 hours after injection; or (3) chronic worsening of an allergic condition during a course of treatment. If reactions continue, it is necessary to separate the allergens in the mixture to determine the role of each in causing the reaction.

Any of the above mentioned reactions indicates that *the optimum dose has been exceeded.* Delayed reactions are difficult to evaluate and may need to be confirmed by another dose given at the same level. In any event, if a reaction is suspected, the dose of extract *must not be increased.* Furthermore, *the dose should not be increased beyond any level at which a satisfactory clinical response has occurred.*

When satisfactory clinical improvement occurs, the interval between injections can be increased, first to every 2 weeks, then to every 3, but injections *should generally not be given at intervals more widely spaced than every 4 weeks,* since reactions may occur to previously well-tolerated doses if this interval is exceeded. Injections should be continued usually until the patient has been considerably improved for a year. This generally requires 2 to 3 years of injection therapy.

Figure 9–11 *Record and suggested regimen for desensitization program.*

done with other toxic agents, such as diphtheria toxin. Noon's technique has been modified remarkably little in the 60 years since it was introduced. Only recently have the immunologic changes that occur following hyposensitization begun to be extensively investigated. Patients undergoing immunotherapy for ragweed hay fever show the appearance in serum of IgG-blocking antibody, a reduction in the in vitro sensitivity of basophils from peripheral blood to release of histamine by antigen, and a prevention of the anamnestic rise in specific ragweed IgE antibody that occurs during the ragweed season. In view of the uncertainties of results following hyposensitization, there still exists doubt in the minds of some investigators concerning the value of its widespread application to persons with inhalant allergy. In spite of these uncertainties, hyposensitization is widely used by practicing allergists as a specific mode of therapy, and the evidence is good that some patients benefit from it.

Hyposensitization involves the repeated administration of extracts of inhalants such as house dust, pollens and molds in increasing doses, in an attempt to increase the patient's tolerance to natural exposure to these allergens. Many physicians believe a trial of hyposensitization is indicated, in addition to avoidance of allergens and appropriate drug therapy, when symptoms persist and when there is a reasonably good correlation between the clinical history and allergy skin tests. A typical hyposensitization regimen is seen in Figure 9–11. Doses are increased by 25 to 50 per cent of the previous dose, until a maintenance concentration is achieved. The amount of extract that an individual patient can tolerate is determined to a great extent by his sensitivity. Children who appear to be very sensitive by clinical history or by skin testing are frequently unable to tolerate high doses of extract without the appearance of severe local reactions at the site of the injection or the actual induction of symptoms in the form of a systemic reaction. Children with eczema may be able to tolerate only very small doses without flare-ups of activity of the skin lesions. The maintenance dose will therefore vary from patient to patient and the regimen suggested would be appropriate only for a patient with average sensitivity.

Injections may be given at first once or twice weekly, and then the intervals between injections lengthened to once every two weeks, three weeks, and then four weeks. Most allergists do not repeat the same dosage at greater than a four-week interval. If a delay of more than four weeks between hyposensitization injections occurs, a reduction in the dosage is made and the dose increased to the previous maintenance level upon subsequent injections. A reasonable course of therapy is considered to be from two to three years. If the patient is doing well at the end of this time, the hyposensitization regimen is discontinued and the patient observed for reappearance of symptoms. If a child fails to improve after 1 or 2 years of injection therapy, it is unlikely that improvement will be realized after this interval.

Physicians who undertake the administration of hyposensitization programs should be prepared to deal with adverse reactions, including systemic anaphylaxis, which may occur during the course of therapy and especially immediately following injections.

PROPHYLACTIC MEASURES. The tendency of allergic children to react with allergic symptoms to various stimuli will likely continue for an extended time. During this time the child should be protected as completely as possible from contact with those substances to which he is demonstrably reactive, but contacts should also be avoided with other substances of high sensitizing potential. Accordingly, it is appropriate to postpone the introduction into the diet of an allergic infant of substances such as wheat, egg, chocolate and the like, and perhaps to discourage exposure of the allergic child to other sensitizers such as feathers, animal danders, and the like, when this can be easily done.

RESPIRATORY ALLERGY

The respiratory tract is the organ system most frequently affected by allergic disorders during childhood.

ALLERGIC RHINITIS

Seasonal allergic rhinitis, seasonal pollinosis, and hay fever are terms used interchangeably to describe a symptom complex seen in children who have become sensitized to wind-borne pollens of trees, grasses and weeds. Symptoms vary in severity with the season.

In *perennial allergic rhinitis* the patient is symptomatic the year round, and the causative agents, when they can be identified, are generally found to be allergens to which the patient is exposed more or less continually, though exposure may be greater at one time of the year. Indoor inhalant allergens may be implicated most often, such as house dust, feathers and danders of household pets; in certain climates, particularly where the humidity is high, mold spores are frequent offenders. In an occasional patient foods appear to cause symptoms of allergic rhinitis, but their role must be critically evaluated. Anecdotally, one learns of patients who can apparently ingest certain foods with impunity except during a pollen season, when ingestion causes an aggravation of nasal symptoms.

DIAGNOSIS. The symptoms of allergic rhinitis include sneezing, which is frequently paroxysmal; rhinorrhea, which is often watery and profuse; nasal obstruction; and itching of the nose, palate, pharynx and ears. Itching, redness and tearing of the eyes may also be present and may cause severe discomfort.

Physical examination in the typical case of allergic rhinitis reveals bilateral nasal obstruction resulting from edema of the mucous membranes. There is frequently redundant mucosa on the floor of the nose. The mucous membranes are bluish in hue and rather pale, and a clear mucoid nasal discharge is seen. The child often has mannerisms involving the nose, which stem from itching or from attempts to increase the airway. The child wrinkles the nose (rabbit nose), and may rub it in characteristic ways ("allergic salute"). Rubbing in an upward direction may lead to a characteristic crease on the dorsum of the nose near the tip. The dark circles under the eyes which may be seen in some patients have been attributed to venous stasis resulting from interference with blood flow through the edematous nasal mucous membranes. Mouth breathing is common. The diagnosis of allergic rhinitis is substantiated by the finding of a predominance of eosinophils in a smear made of the nasal secretions.

TREATMENT. Successful treatment of either seasonal or perennial allergic rhinitis includes avoidance of exposure to suspected allergens, hyposensitization to those that cannot be avoided or can only partially be avoided, and the institution of drug therapy.

Avoidance. Although it is difficult or impractical to avoid exposure to seasonal pollens, a great deal can be done to eliminate exposure to such indoor inhalant factors as house dust, danders and molds. Environmental control of house dust, with special attention to the child's bedroom as outlined in Table 9–4, frequently leads to amelioration of symptoms in the dust-allergic child. As indicated in the section on general treatment principles, elimination of exposure to danders and feathers is mandatory in a child with perennial allergic rhinitis when these factors appear to contribute to the patient's symptoms. For the child sensitive to indoor molds, avoidance of damp basements and the application of measures designed to discourage mold growth in the house frequently lead to good results. These measures include dehumidifiers, air conditioners with efficient filters, and air cleaning devices, either of the electronic precipitator type or containing a HEPA filter. A 1:750 solution of Zephiran chloride is an effective agent in controlling mold growth. In areas that can be closed off, such as damp cellars, volatilization of paraformaldehyde (25 to 50 gm, depending upon the size of the area to be treated) from several open jars is also frequently effective in discouraging growth of mold.

Hyposensitization. Desensitization in allergic rhinitis is generally limited to house dust, pollens and molds, but occasionally includes other antigens. Vaccines against wind-borne pollens are the ones most frequently used.

Drug Therapy. Relief can usually be obtained in allergic rhinitis by the appropriate use of drug therapy. *Antihistamines* have been extremely useful, especially in the treatment of the seasonal variety of allergic rhinitis. For unknown reasons, some patients appear to respond better to an antihistamine of one chemical group than to drugs from another group. To achieve the desired effects it is frequently necessary to increase the dosage beyond that routinely recommended. Nasal itching, sneezing and rhinorrhea are usually well controlled by antihistamine therapy, whereas nasal obstruction is relieved to a lesser degree. The major adverse side effect of antihistamine therapy is somnolence. This is most noticeable during the early treatment period and lessens with continued therapy. Sometimes it necessitates a change to another class of antihistamine.

If nasal obstruction is particularly troublesome, the addition of *sympathomimetics* such as ephedrine, pseudoephedrine or phenylpropanolamine to the antihistamine is useful. Nose drops should be avoided except for short-term use, inasmuch as continued use may lead to progressively severe nasal obstruction due to rebound vasodilatation (*rhinitis medicamentosa*). The treatment of rhinitis medicamentosa requires complete cessation of use of medicated nose drops and the substitution of nose drops of physiologic saline solution.

Corticosteroids are rarely indicated in the treatment of allergic rhinitis. Occasionally, in the instance of a child who in the middle of the ragweed pollen season has severe ophthalmic and nasal symptoms unresponsive to antihistaminic and sympathomimetic therapy, the use of systemic corticosteroid therapy may be indicated. The need for control of symptoms will be limited by the length of the pollen season, and steroid withdrawal will be easily accomplished. In perennial allergic rhinitis, when severe symptoms are resistant to usual therapy, the topical use of a corticosteroid aerosol frequently brings dramatic results. Dexamethasone in a Freon propellant (Turbinaire) is used, initially with two puffs in each nostril three times a day. As symptoms improve, the dose and frequency of use are abated until a minimal effective dosage is reached. About one third to one half of the total dose administered is absorbed with systemic effect; this must be considered when long-term use is contemplated. Occasionally, temporary use of corticosteroid eye drops is necessary in a child with hay fever and particularly severe eye symptoms.

OTHER CONSIDERATIONS. *Nasal polyps* are only rarely seen in children with allergic rhinitis. They occur more often in patients with chronic infectious sinusitis and rhinitis, such as may be found in cystic fibrosis, Kartagener's syndrome and immunologic deficiency diseases. Consultation with an otolaryngologist is indicated when nasal polyps are observed in a child with allergic rhinitis. When nasal polyps occur in association with asthma, they suggest so-called *triad asthma,* in which ingestion of aspirin may produce an attack of asthma of life-threatening severity. Surgical procedures in the nose designed to relieve nasal obstruction (submucous resection) and destructive procedures including cautery of the inferior turbinates are rarely, if ever, indicated in children with allergic rhinitis. The improvement that follows these procedures is usually temporary and may be followed by a condition even more troublesome than that for which the surgery was done.

Vasomotor rhinitis designates a disorder with symptoms similar to those of allergic rhinitis but in which an allergic etiology cannot be identified. Characteristically the patients do not have eosinophils in their nasal secretions, and symptoms are particularly affected by environmental changes, including humidity and temperature. Although the underlying nature of the disorder is not clear, there appears to be some peculiar hyperreactivity of the vessels in the nasal mucous membranes in affected persons. Drug treatment is essentially that of allergic rhinitis.

Swelling of the mucous membranes of the sinuses frequently occurs in association with allergic rhinitis in childhood. Edema of the lining of the mucous membranes is seen as cloudiness in roentgenograms of the involved sinuses. Occasionally a fluid level is seen. Sinus infection is rare in these cases, and the symptoms generally are those of fullness and discomfort. Drug therapy aimed at reducing edema and relieving obstruction to the ostia opening into the nasal cavity usually results in amelioration of symptoms.

ASTHMA
(Bronchial Asthma)

Asthma is one of the leading causes of chronic illness in childhood and is responsible for a very significant proportion of school days lost due to chronic illnesses. Prior to puberty asthma is twice as common in boys as in girls; the disease affects males and females equally during adolescence and thereafter. Asthma may be defined as a diffuse obstructive disease of the airways characterized by a high degree of reversibility with appropriate therapy. Emphysema, which is an irreversible diffuse obstructive disease of the airways, rarely occurs in childhood. Both small airways (those less than 2 mm in diameter) and large airways are involved in asthma, with the extent of involvement varying from patient to patient.

PATHOGENESIS. The elements causing airway obstruction are edema of the mucous membranes, increased mucous secretions and spasm of smooth muscle. The relative contribution of each of these factors to the obstructive process varies from patient to patient and during the course of the disease. Early in an attack, particularly if the onset is sudden, it is likely that smooth muscle spasm plays a major role. As the attack progresses, however, mucous membrane edema and increased mucous secretions appear to play predominant roles in the obstruction. Patients dying during status asthmaticus essentially asphyxiate, owing to almost complete occlusion of airways by mucous plugs. All individuals with asthma have a characteristic hyperreactivity of the airways to a variety of environmental factors, including irritants of various kinds (sulfur dioxide, tobacco smoke and other pollutants), strong odors (wet paint), cold air and rapid changes in temperature and humidity. Appreciation of the irritability or increased reactivity of the airways of children with asthma is important in their management.

ETIOLOGY. Asthma is a complex disorder in which biochemical, immunologic, infectious, endocrine and psychologic factors play roles of varying degrees of importance in different individuals.

Biochemical Abnormalities. Both adults and children with asthma have been shown to have an abnormal biochemical response to injection of epinephrine. Normally epinephrine administration results in hyperglycemia and lactacidemia as a result of activation of β_2 receptors in muscle and liver. Asthmatics have a blunted hyperglycemic response to epinephrine and develop little if any increase in plasma lactic acid. This finding, with other observations and experiments, led Szentivanyi to postulate that there exists in individuals with asthma a generalized abnormality in structure or function of the β-adrenergic receptor–adenyl cyclase complex. Additional support for the concept derives from studies in vitro which show that leukocytes from asthmatics have deficient synthesis of cyclic AMP after stimulation by catecholamines when compared with leukocytes from normal individuals. The possibility that the abnormalities observed are due to treatment with adrenergic agents has not been excluded.

Immunologic Factors. In certain individuals with so-called extrinsic or allergic asthma, it is clear that attacks follow exposure to environmental factors such as dust, pollens, danders and foods. Increased concentrations both of total IgE and of specific IgE against the allergen implicated are generally but not invariably found in these individuals. In other asthmatics with clinically similar asthma, no evidence of IgE involvement can be found. In this group of patients, skin tests are negative and IgE concentrations low. This form of asthma, which is seen most often in the first two years of life and in women about the time of menopause, has been called intrinsic or nonimmunologic asthma. No differences in general immunologic reactivity have been found between the intrinsic and extrinsic groups.

Infectious Factors. Respiratory infection commonly provokes asthmatic attacks, particularly in patients with the intrinsic form. Bacterial respiratory tract infection has not been shown to play an etiologic role in exacerbation of asthma, nor has hyposensitization with bacterial vaccines been proved to be of value in therapy. On the other hand, certain viral agents have been shown to cause exacerbations of wheezing in a group of young children with asthma; these are respiratory syncytial and parainfluenza viruses. A specificity of these agents in terms of asthmagenic potential is suggested by the fact that infection with adenovirus and A_2/Hong Kong influenza virus did not result in exacerbations of asthmatic symptoms in the same group of children.

Endocrine Factors. Asthma may have exacerbations in relation to menses, particularly premenstrually, or may have its onset in women around the menopause. It improves in some children at puberty. Little else is known about the role of endocrine factors in the etiology and pathogenesis of asthma. It is said there is an increased incidence in Addison's disease, and that asthmatics with thyrotoxicosis do not respond to treatment until the endocrine problem is brought under control.

Psychologic Factors. Asthma has long been thought to be a disorder influenced to a great extent by emotional factors. Current thinking would not assign a primary etiologic role to psychologic factors but would recognize that emotional incidents play an important role as precipitants of symptoms in many children and adults. The effects of a severe chronic illness such as asthma on a child's view of himself, his parents' view of him, or his life in general can be devastating.

CLINICAL MANIFESTATIONS. The onset of asthma may be insidious or abrupt. Sudden onsets are often ushered in by a spell of coughing, which may be associated with itching of the chin, anterior part of the neck or chest. The onset is apt to be gradual and resolution to be slower when the asthmatic attack complicates a respiratory infection; wheezing may appear a day or more after rhinorrhea and may resolve over a period of hours or days.

The asthmatic paroxysm is characterized by increasing dyspnea, with prolongation of the expiratory phase of respiration, by wheezing, and coarse and fine musical rales. A severe asthmatic paroxysm greatly limits pulmonary ventilation; the resulting air hunger is manifest by such signs as flaring of the alae nasi, the use of accessory muscles of respiration, cyanosis and, at times, hypercapnia. The heart and respiratory rates are increased, and the child is restless and fatigued. Sweating may be prominent. There may be abdominal pain, particularly when coughing is severe, and the child may vomit. Vomiting may be followed by some relief of the dyspnea, but this is usually only temporary. The sputum of the child with acute asthma is tenacious and scanty until a response to treatment is seen, when it may become more abundant and loose. Then spirals of mucus which contain eosinophils are coughed up.

The chest is generally hyperresonant, with wheezing and musical and sibilant rales most prominent in the expiratory phase. Breath sounds may be suppressed, and occasionally the restriction of tidal air flow is so great that the breath sounds are barely audible. This is an ominous sign. The physical findings are those of generalized obstructive emphysema. (See Section 12.) If atelectasis, pneumothorax or pneumomediastinum occurs, the chest findings will be altered, with a shift of the mediastinum to the side of atelectasis or to the side opposite the pneumothorax. When emphysema is severe, the liver and spleen may be felt below the costal margins.

Many attacks of asthma over a long period may lead to chronic emphysema. These changes may be largely or completely reversible with adequate therapy during childhood. Children with moderate to severe chronic asthma are likely to have fine lanugo hair over the shoulders and arms. Pulmonary osteoarthropathy is rare; allergic rhinitis and sinusitis are common.

DIAGNOSIS. The history of recurrent episodes of coughing and wheezing, particularly accentuated by exercise, is so characteristic of asthma that the diagnosis is easily made in the majority of cases. However, there are a significant number of young children with asthma who have a persistent chronic nonproductive cough, particularly at night after going to bed, who cough and become short of breath on exercise, but in whom wheezing has not been conspicuous or obvious, and in whom, accordingly, a diagnosis of chronic bronchitis is often erroneously made. If these patients are old enough to undergo pulmonary function testing, the majority will be shown to have findings characteristic of asthma. Furthermore, when treated by measures that are specific for asthma, they show remarkable improvement.

Asthma in Early Life. In a significant number of children who are subsequently shown to have asthma, careful inquiry will indicate that symptoms of obstructive airway disease began early in life and frequently during the first year. Some physicians are reluctant to consider a diagnosis of asthma during the first two years of life, but recurrent episodes of coughing and wheezing are highly suggestive of this diagnosis regardless of age. A plethora of terms are used to describe such patients, including asthmatic bronchitis, wheezy cold, wheezy bronchitis and bronchiolitis, and many more. These terms serve no useful purpose, especially when they represent an evasion of the need to undertake adequate allergic study and management.

It is important to recognize that many other conditions besides asthma can cause partial airway obstruction resulting in wheezing (Table 9–6). Congenital anatomic malformations may lead to intrinsic or extrinsic obstruction; these include anomalies of the gastrointestinal, respiratory and cardiovascular systems. Aspiration of a foreign body can usually be suspected on the basis of a careful history of onset of the first attack, and in addition a foreign body almost always produces

TABLE 9–6 SOME CAUSES OF WHEEZING IN EARLY LIFE

1. Anatomic obstructions
   a. Congenital anomalies
      1. Bronchial—lobar emphysema
      2. Vascular—aberrant vessels
   b. Foreign bodies
2. Infections
   a. Bacterial
   b. Viral
3. Allergy
   a. Inhalants
   b. Food

TABLE 9–7 HISTORICAL, CLINICAL AND LABORATORY DIAGNOSTIC CLUES IN ETIOLOGY OF RECURRENT WHEEZING

1. Concurrent illness in family members or in the community
2. Past history of atopic disease
3. Family history of atopic disease
4. Eosinophilia of blood or of nasal or bronchial secretions
5. Skin tests to relevant allergens
6. Response to epinephrine
7. Response to corticosteroids

pneumonitis on a roentgenogram. Nonopaque materials such as plastics are, of course, not visualized, but fluoroscopy may be useful in diagnosing a unilateral obstructive process due to a foreign body.

During the early years of life, respiratory tract infections commonly cause symptoms of airway obstruction. Certain viral agents, such as respiratory syncytial virus and parainfluenza virus, are particularly prone to cause symptoms of airway obstruction in infants and young children. Bacterial infections of the lower airway are rare, and the concept that bacterial allergy causes asthma is unproved. A child with recurrent episodes of coughing and wheezing associated with bacterial infections should be investigated for cystic fibrosis of the pancreas or immunologic deficiency disease.

The role of food allergy as a major cause of obstructive airway symptoms during early life is a subject of controversy. Positive skin tests for IgE-mediated sensitivity to foods of clinical significance are unusual in early life, and elimination diets and provocative food tests rarely give consistent results. The temporary elimination of milk, wheat, eggs and chocolate from the diet of the asthmatic patient is recommended by some practitioners.

Table 9–7 lists some of the clues which may be helpful in raising or lowering the index of suspicion that the respiratory symptoms of an infant or child may be allergic. Each area should be examined in assessment of the patient.

Pulmonary Function Testing. The physiologic abnormalities seen on pulmonary function testing in patients with asthma reflect the obstructive process in the small airways. Tests that measure expiratory flow rate (EFR), forced expiratory volume in 1 second (FEV_1), maximal mid-expiratory flow (MMEF) and peak expiratory flow (PEFR) show evidence of obstructed airways. Testing the child before and after administration of a bronchodilator is frequently useful in establishing the reversibility of the obstructive process characteristic of asthma. Administration of aerosolized bronchodilators, such as isoproterenol, generally results in a significant increase in expiratory flow rate over baseline values. More sophisticated testing of lung function with the body plethysmograph shows increased total lung capacity and increased airway resistance, while helium or nitrogen washout techniques show evidence of uneven distribution of gas and, when combined with body plethysmography, of air trapping. Involvement of small airways (less then 2 mm in diameter) is determined by measurement of closing volume and MMEF. Reversibility is the outstanding characteristic of the asthma of childhood, and the patient can vary widely physiologically in accordance with his clinical state at the time of any examination. Serial measurements of pulmonary functions are much more valuable than an isolated test.

Blood gases and pH during an asymptomatic period are characteristically normal. During a symptomatic period, particularly if the symptoms are severe enough to warrant the attention of a physician, hypoxemia of some degree is almost always present. Measurement of blood gases and pH are most important in following the progress of the child hospitalized for status asthmaticus.

TREATMENT. The principles of avoidance of allergens outlined under treatment of allergic rhinitis also serve the child with asthma. The hyperreactivity of the asthmatic airway is an additional factor and is dealt with by minimizing exposure to nonspecific irritants such as tobacco smoke, and strong odors, such as wet paint and disinfectants, and by the avoidance of ice cold drinks and of rapid changes in temperature and humidity. Proper maintenance of humidified air is especially important in dry cold climates in the winter. If the clinical history suggests IgE-mediated sensitivity to inhalant factors that cannot be avoided or can be only partially avoided, institution of hyposensitization therapy should be considered. The principles of hyposensitization are the same as those outlined for allergic rhinitis.

Pharmacologic therapy is the mainstay of treatment of asthma. An acute episode of asthma of sufficient severity to cause obvious distress is effectively treated by the subcutaneous injection of 0.1 or 0.2 ml of a 1:1000 concentration of aqueous epinephrine hydrochloride (Adrenalin). In infants and small children a dose of 0.05 ml is often effective in relieving the symptoms. It may be necessary to repeat the same dose once or twice at 20-minute intervals to obtain optimal relief. The undesirable side effects of epinephrine, such as pallor, tremor and headache, can frequently be minimized by the administration of no more than 0.2 ml per dose. There are several repository forms of epinephrine available which provide more sustained bronchodilatation than aqueous epinephrine and are particularly useful for administration prior to sending a patient home from an emergency room late at night. Sus-Phrine is a 1:200 thioglycolate suspension of epinephrine. The dose of Sus-Phrine is 0.05 to 0.1 ml for children. Isoproterenol for inhalation, in 1:200 solution, generally gives rapid relief of symptoms. The drug is best given as an aerosol, using a plastic nebulizer to which 5 drops of isoproterenol 1:200 and 1 ml of saline have been added. The solution is nebulized over a few minutes with an air source from a vacuum pump, for example, a MaxiMyst compressor, or simply by using a bicycle pump. Isoproterenol is also available in Freon-propelled units which deliver, depending upon the apparatus used, measured doses of from 0.075 to 0.125 mg of isoproterenol per inhalation. Although these compact units are very convenient, their use should be reserved for *acute* episodes, particularly those occurring in the middle of the night or following exercise.

If the response to epinephrine and to isoproterenol is not satisfactory, some form of theophylline should be administered. Aminophylline (85 per cent theophylline and 15 per cent ethylenediamine) may be given intravenously in a dose of 4 mg/kg over 5 to 15 minutes at a rate no greater than 25 mg/min. The drug is quite safe in the patient who has had no theophylline in the past 8 hours, and is generally effective in relieving symptoms when so administered. Theophylline therapy may then be continued with oral preparations. Liquid formulations of theophylline are well absorbed, give prompt plasma concentrations and good therapeutic responses, and are particularly suited for small children. Theophylline in the form of aminophylline tablets is generally well absorbed from the gastrointestinal tract. A safe and effective oral dose of theophylline is 5 mg/kg given every 6 hours. Because theophylline has a relatively short half-life, administration at greater than 8-hour intervals results in wide fluctuations in plasma levels of theophylline and inadequate therapeutic responses. Theophylline is eliminated from the body by biotransformation in the liver; liver disease and the concomitant administration of other drugs which interfere with the metabolism of theophylline may significantly alter its biologic half-life and thus its plasma concentration. Moreover, there appear to be significant differences between patients in the rapidity of metabolism of theophylline. A child receiving theophylline should always, therefore, be observed for signs of theophylline toxicity; early signs include vomiting, especially of blood (hemorrhagic gastritis), along with such central nervous system signs and symptoms as restlessness, irritability, agitation and, later, seizures.

Status Asthmaticus

If the patient continues to have a significant amount of respiratory distress despite administration of sympathomimetic drugs and theophylline, the diagnosis of status asthmaticus should be considered. There is no precise definition of status asthmaticus. It is essentially a clinical diagnosis based upon the observation of increasingly severe asthma not responsive to drugs that are generally effective in treating an attack. A patient in whom the diagnosis of status asthmaticus is made should be admitted to a hospital, and preferably to an intensive care unit where he can receive careful monitoring of his condition. Analysis of arterial blood for determination of pO_2, pCO_2, and pH is indicated. For these determinations, well arterialized capillary blood is adequate but less desirable than arterial blood, particularly if the patient has had injections of epinephrine, which has a vasoconstrictive effect on the peripheral vascular bed.

Patients in status asthmaticus are invariably hypoxemic and oxygen in carefully controlled concentrations is therefore always indicated, even when the pCO_2 is elevated. In the face of hypercarbia, particular care should be taken to administer oxygen continuously and not intermittently. It may be administered very effectively by nasal prongs at a flow rate of 2 to 3 liters/min. Use of a mist tent should be avoided because it has been shown that the water does not reach the lower airway to any significant extent, and particularly because mist has an irritant effect on the airways of many asthmatics, leading to coughing and worsening of the wheezing. Furthermore, it is not possible adequately to observe a patient who is enveloped in a dense fog.

Dehydration is frequently present in the child with status asthmaticus, owing to inadequate fluid intake, greatly increased insensible water loss due to tachypnea and the diuretic effect of theophylline. Adequate fluid intake must be provided for correction and maintenance. Sodium bicarbonate, 1 to 3 mEq/kg, should be administered every 4 to 6 hours, or more often if signs of metabolic acidosis appear.

Corticosteroids in the form of hydrocortisone (Solu-Cortef) or methylprednisolone (Solu-Medrol) should be administered in large doses (2 mg/kg of prednisone, or its equivalent, every 4 to 6 hours). These soluble steroids may be conveniently injected directly into the intravenous tubing. Corticosteroid therapy can usually be maintained orally; prednisone is given in doses of 1–2 mg/kg/day in one or two doses until status asthmaticus subsides, following which the administration of steroids can be rapidly terminated, unless the decision is made to move to an alternate-day regimen.

If both gas and pH analysis indicate that respiratory failure is present (when pO_2 is less than 50 mm of mercury and pCO_2 greater than 50 mm of mercury), an anesthesiologist should be alerted and facilities and equipment for nasotracheal intubation and respiratory support with a volume-cycled respirator should be made ready.

Sedation of patients with status asthmaticus is hazardous unless careful monitoring of blood gases is done. If sedation is necessary, chloral hydrate is the safest drug to use. A chest roentgenogram should be obtained in all cases and repeated as indicated in order to detect complications such as mediastinal emphysema or pneumothorax. Antibiotics need not be administered routinely, but each case should be evaluated on its own merits.

DAY-TO-DAY MANAGEMENT OF THE ASTHMATIC CHILD

The day-to-day management of the asthmatic child builds on the measures previously described and includes a continuing effort to identify causative agents, avoidance of them when possible, and institution and maintenance of hyposensitization when indicated by history and appropriate testing. In the majority of children who have only intermittent episodes of asthma, oral theophylline therapy given every 6 hours during symptomatic periods will usually suffice. It may be desirable to add ephedrine in a dose of 0.5–1.0 mg/kg to the regimen for additional bronchodilator activity. Ephedrine is best given every 4 hours. Prescription of theophylline and ephedrine separately is preferred to the administration of a combination formulation because the dose of either drug can be adjusted without commitment to a fixed ratio.

Children with acute exacerbations of coughing and wheezing who also have such continuing symptoms of airway obstruction as night cough or coughing and wheezing on exercise will benefit from regular around-the-clock administration of bronchodilators. Theophylline given orally every 6 hours, with or without additional ephedrine, frequently results in significant improvement in cough, exercise tolerance and general well-being. Moreover, the number of acute exacerbations of asthma is lessened. The use of nebulized isoproterenol as previously described for treatment of the acute attack will enable parents to manage many acute episodes at home.

The decision to use corticosteroids in ambulatory outpatient children with asthma generally follows their need for the control of status asthmaticus and anticipates its possible recurrence. Steroids should be given in adequate doses (1–2 mg/kg/day of prednisone in one or two doses), and an attempt should be made to discontinue them as quickly as possible. A long "weaning" period following their use in the treatment of an acute attack of asthma is unnecessary and return of normal hypothalamic-pituitary-adrenal function is hastened by the *prompt* discontinuation of the drug when the acute episode is over.

In a small percentage of children with asthma, despite the best available allergic management, including the continuing use of bronchodilators in doses increased to maximum tolerance, unacceptable degrees of coughing and wheezing persist, which severely limit the child's play activities, school attendance, and the like. In such children the judicious administration of corticosteroids on an alternate-day basis frequently results in significant amelioration of symptoms and allows the child to lead a normal life without suffering the adverse effects of corticosteroids. If it is determined that alternate-day therapy is indicated either because of the chronicity of disability or the severity or frequency of attacks of status asthmaticus, the patient is given a few days of intensive daily therapy and then promptly switched to an alternate-day regimen using prednisone or methylprednisolone. A 12 year old child might be given 60 mg, 40 mg, 20 mg and 10 mg per day over a 4-day period for an exacerbation of asthma, to be followed by alternate-day therapy at a dose of 20 mg/day given as a single dose at 8 A.M. every 48 hours. (Administration early in the morning mimics the circadian rhythm of endogenous cortisol secretion.) If the patient responds well to this regimen, the prednisone given on alternate days may be reduced by 5 mg per dose at 10- to 14-day intervals until the lowest dose compatible with acceptable control of symptoms is reached. Conventional bronchodilator therapy (theophylline and perhaps ephedrine) should be maintained, inasmuch as addition of bronchodilator agents to the regimen almost always results in a need for less steroid than would be needed if the bronchodilator drugs were not given. Low-dose alternate-day therapy is associated with minimal adverse effects, so far as can be determined by current clinical or laboratory measurements. In a disease that can be so life-threatening or so capable of causing chronic invalidism, prudent use of chronic alternate-day therapy in selected cases should override the physician's reluctance to use corticosteroids in children. It is reprehensible, on the other hand, to let steroid therapy substitute for or delay a commitment to comprehensive allergic management.

A new group of corticosteroids have been synthesized for inhalational use. The idea of applying steroids topically to the airway in asthma is not new, but preparations available in the past have been absorbed systemically to a significant degree. Agents now becoming available have limited solubility and apparently act locally in the airway with little or no systemic absorption. Evidence for the latter comes not only from tests of the hypothalamic-pituitary-adrenal function, but also from the observation that well controlled eczema in asthmatics receiving oral steroids may relapse when they are changed to the inhalational preparation. The use of these agents in children has been studied in Great Britain with favorable results.

Disodium cromoglycate (Intal, Aarane) is a new anti-asthmatic drug now marketed in the United States after extensive testing and use abroad. The drug is a synthetic "cromone" derivative used *prophylactically, and not for treatment of acute attacks.* The drug is not an antagonist of chemical mediators, does not interfere with antibody synthesis nor prevent fixation of IgE to mast cells, and has no anti-inflammatory activity. It does prevent antigen-induced release of chemical mediators, but it is likely that other properties are responsible for its efficacy in certain respects (e.g., in preventing exercise-induced asthma). The drug is available as a white powder which is aerosolized with a special device. It was originally introduced for treatment of extrinsic or allergic asthma, but it is now evident that some individuals with intrinsic asthma also respond favorably. Disodium cromoglycate is not a drug of first choice in treatment of asthma in childhood. For a number of reasons, including its high cost, it should be reserved for cases resistant to the usual modalities of therapy.

Emotional tensions surrounding asthma are best handled by unhurried discussion of the child's difficulty with the parents, by avoidance of overdramatization of the child's illness, and by careful examination with the parents of those areas in which parent and child seem to be in conflict. The use of tranquilizers or sedatives as a substitute for more direct attempts to solve emotional problems should be avoided. As the allergic aspects of the child's disorder are brought under control, the emotional climate is often improved.

PROGNOSIS. With adequate treatment asthma can be brought under satisfactory control in the majority of affected children. Some will continue to have periodic attacks over months or years, but most will be able to lead active normal lives, within modest limitations imposed by their allergic condition. Rackemann and Edwards found that 20 years after the onset of asthma, 30 per cent of patients were entirely relieved of their symptoms; 19 per cent had no symptoms so long as they successfully avoided offending allergens; 21 per cent no longer had asthma, but did have some other allergic manifestation, usually hay fever; 26 per cent still had asthma of some degree, but in only 11 per cent was it considered a serious health problem; 1 per cent had died of asthma. It deserves emphasis that this generally favorable result was achieved for the most part with continuous and comprehensive allergic management. Although there is a tendency for asthma in some children to abate spontaneously with puberty, no purely expectant program of management is justified. Even with the best management some asthmatic children have chronic and disabling pulmonary and cardiopulmonary disability.

ATOPIC DERMATITIS

Atopic dermatitis is an inflammatory skin disorder characterized by erythema, edema, intense pruritus, exudation, crusting and scaling. Histologically, in the acute stages, intraepidermal vesiculation (spongiosis) is present. The disease tends to appear in individuals who have a genetically determined allergic predilection. The close association of atopic dermatitis with allergic rhinitis and asthma is well established, infants with atopic dermatitis having a high incidence of subsequent respiratory allergy, especially asthma. Individuals with atopic dermatitis have as a group extraordinarily high serum IgE concentrations, but there is no correlation between severity of eruption and elevation of IgE. However, the level of IgE does appear to fluctuate with the *stage* of the disease, serial studies indicating that levels return to normal when the disease has been quiescent for several years. The elevation of total IgE in atopic dermatitis has not been satisfactorily explained. It is not clear that atopic dermatitis is primarily caused by IgE-mediated allergy; and it is difficult to demonstrate an etiologic role for allergens, either of food or inhalant type, in the pathogenesis of the condition. Moreover, the typical dermal manifestation of the interaction of IgE antibody with antigen is the hive (wheal and flare) rather than the erythematous papule of atopic dermatitis; and, while patients with atopic dermatitis frequently possess IgE antibody specific for inhalants or food allergens, it is not generally possible to induce skin lesions of atopic dermatitis by intradermal injection of the suspected allergen. Typical lesions of atopic dermatitis may occur in individuals with immunologic deficiency disease who lack IgE reagins.

Individuals with atopic dermatitis have hyperreactive skin which differs from normal skin in its response to a variety of physical and pharmacologic stimuli. For example, a light mechanical stroke of the skin results within a minute in a white line, with a surrounding blanched area. This phenomenon, not seen in normal skin, has been called white dermographism. Involved skin presents abnormalities in the rates of cooling and warming in response to temperature changes, particularly in the flexural areas. A number of paradoxical responses to injections of various pharmacologic agents, such as histamine, acetylcholine ("delayed blanch phenomenon") and nicotinic acid ester have been described. The abnormal reactivity of the skin in individuals with atopic dermatitis is reminiscent of the airway hyperreactivity characteristic of asthma; in both disorders the hyperreactivity seems to be an intrinsic part of the disease and is independent of immunologic factors.

CLINICAL MANIFESTATIONS AND NATURAL HISTORY. Atopic dermatitis typically occurs in three stages with fairly distinctive features. The disease most often begins in infancy, usually during the first two to three months of life. The onset is sometimes delayed until the second or third year. The earliest lesions of infantile atopic dermatitis are erythematous weepy patches on the cheeks, with subsequent extension to the remainder of the face, neck, wrists, hands and extensor aspects of the extremities. Typical involvement of flexural areas characteristically appears later, but there may be popliteal and antecubital dermatitis in early life.

The markedly pruritic nature of the disease is evident in the affected infant's incessant efforts to scratch the skin by rubbing his face on bedclothes and against the sides of the crib. This trauma to the skin rapidly leads to weeping and crusting, and at this stage of the disease secondary infection is common and may be extensive.

The onset of dermatitis frequently coincides with the introduction of certain foods, particularly cow's milk, wheat or eggs, into the infant's diet. In most of these instances, however, a direct role of reaginic sensitivity in the pathogenesis of skin eruption is hard to prove, and wide divergences of opinion exist among allergists and dermatologists concerning the importance of food allergy in initiating or maintaining atopic dermatitis. In certain infants, on the other hand, there is unequivocal evidence of reaginic sensitivity, manifest by the appearance of urticaria, colic and a diffuse erythematous flush following ingestion of the offending food. The erythematous flush appears to be accompanied by intense itching, which results in scratching and then in the appearance of the skin lesions characteristic of eczema. The major role of scratching in the production of skin lesions has been demonstrated when an extremity has been occluded by surgical dressings; the lesions of atopic dermatitis occur only in the uncovered extremity. Scratching is thus necessary for the development of the dermatitis.

Studies of the natural history of atopic dermatitis show a tendency for remission between 3 and 5 years of age. In the majority of children the disease will be quiescent by the age of 5 years; in some, a mild to moderate degree of eczema may persist in the antecubital and popliteal fossae, the wrists, behind the ears and on the face and neck. During childhood, antecubital and popliteal involvement become common; extensor surfaces of the extremities may still be actively affected. With increasing age there is a tendency toward drying and thickening of the skin in the involved areas, particularly in the antecubital and popliteal fossae, and on the neck, forehead, eyelids, wrists and the dorsa of the hands and feet. The face takes on a whitish hue, presumably due to vasoconstriction, sometimes called the "mask of atopic dermatitis." Hyperpigmentation of the skin, scaling and lichenification (a particular kind of papular thickening of the skin, with accentuation of the normal surface lines) become prominent. There is a marked tendency toward healing of the disease in the 4th and 5th decades of life.

DIAGNOSIS. When pruritus is intense and the lesions characteristic, the diagnosis of atopic dermatitis may be easy. A family history of asthma, hay fever or atopic dermatitis, the finding of elevated serum IgE concentrations and of reaginic antibodies to a variety of foods and inhalants, the presence of eosinophilia and the demonstration of white dermographism support the diagnosis. Certain physical findings, such as the presence of a wrinkle or a fold of skin just below the eyelid (Morgan's fold) and an increased number of creases of the skin of the palm, are seen in affected individuals. The skin of individuals with atopic dermatitis has a tendency to lichenify in response to chronic irritation or rubbing, a phenomenon that is not seen in normal persons. Generalized dryness of the skin, even in uninvolved areas, and sparsity of the hair of the lateral portion of the eyebrows, thought to be secondary to chronic rubbing, are also characteristic of the disease.

DIFFERENTIAL DIAGNOSIS. The eczematoid skin reaction characterized by erythema, edema, exudation, crusting and scaling is not specific for atopic dermatitis. In infants and children the differential diagnosis includes: seborrheic dermatitis, primary irritant dermatitis, allergic contact dermatitis, infectious eczematoid dermatitis, ichthyosis, phenylketonuria, acrodermatitis enteropathica, histiocytosis-X, and four primary immunologic deficiency disorders, the Wiskott-Aldrich syndrome, sex-linked agammaglobulinemia, ataxia-telangiectasia and a deficiency of the C5 component of complement (Miller).

Seborrheic dermatitis typically begins on the scalp, often as "cradle cap," and involves the ear and contiguous skin, the sides of the nose and eyebrows and eyelids, with greasy, brownish scales that are usually easily distinguishable from the erythematous weeping, crusted lesions of infantile atopic dermatitis. On the other hand, it is sometimes difficult during the first few months of life to distinguish clearly between seborrhea and atopic dermatitis, particularly when the face is primarily involved. The course of seborrhea in infancy is shorter than that of atopic eczema and it responds much more rapidly to treatment. The difficulty in differentiating the two conditions is recognized in the use of the term seborrheic eczema by some dermatologists.

Primary irritant dermatitis is a nonallergic reaction due to exposure of the skin to irritants of various kinds and is most commonly seen in infancy in the diaper area. The localization of the lesions and rapid response to therapy permit the correct diagnosis to be made.

The skin lesions of *allergic contact dermatitis* (the prototype is poison ivy) are usually limited to the sites of exposure to the offending allergen. The lesions do not typically involve the flexural areas, as is the case in atopic dermatitis. Occasionally contact dermatitis is superimposed upon atopic dermatitis when sensitization occurs to chemicals used in treating the latter, such as neomycin, the parabens (used as preservatives in many ointments) or iodochlorohydroxyquin (Vioform).

Infectious eczematoid dermatitis is most often seen as a result of discharge of purulent material from a draining ear or other site of infection. The typical location of the lesions and rapid response to therapy support the diagnosis.

In *ichthyosis* dryness of the skin may lead to confusion with atopic dermatitis, but the scales in ichthyosis are usually larger than those in atopic dermatitis and the pruritus of ichthyosis, if any, is generally mild.

Histiocytosis-X (Letterer-Siwe Disease) and *acrodermatitis enteropathica* are serious systemic diseases occurring early in life in which failure to thrive is a prominent part of the clinical picture. Hemorrhagic manifestations in the skin are common in histiocytosis-X. The skin around the oral, nasal, genitourinary and rectal orifices is typically involved in acrodermatitis.

COMPLICATIONS. During early infancy and childhood, secondary infection of the lesions of atopic dermatitis with bacterial or viral agents is common. Staphylococci and β-hemolytic streptococci are the bacterial agents most often recovered from infected lesions. Herpes simplex (Kaposi's varicelliform eruption) and vaccinia are the viral agents that are of particular concern to individuals with atopic dermatitis. The greatest threat to a child with eczema does not occur as a result of vaccination of the child himself but arises from vaccination of siblings or playmates. In the latter circumstance, multiple inoculations of eczematoid lesions occur with greater frequency than is the case when the child himself is vaccinated. Infants and children with eczema should, therefore, neither be vaccinated nor exposed to siblings or playmates who have been vaccinated, nor exposed to adults with herpes simplex infections ("cold sores"). With smallpox vaccination no longer routine, eczema vaccinatum should virtually disappear in this country. An attenuated vaccinia virus developed by Kempe has been shown to be safe for primary vaccination of infants and children with atopic dermatitis in those rare instances when this is required. Keratoconus is occasionally seen in children with atopic dermatitis and is thought to occur as a consequence of chronic rubbing of the eyelids. Cataracts occur in 5 to 10 per cent of adults with severe atopic dermatitis, but are rarely seen during childhood.

TREATMENT. Effective treatment of atopic dermatitis requires control of the environmental precipitants of the itch-scratch-itch cycle that perpetuates the disease, beginning with avoidance of ingestant, injectant, contactant and atmospheric factors that are known or can be shown to trigger itching or scratching. Extremes of temperature and relative humidity should be avoided. A warm climate of moderate humidity appears to be optimal for the majority of patients. Sweating leads to itching and to aggravation of the disease. Exposure to sunlight and salt water has a beneficial effect on the skin of many patients.

Special attention should be paid to clothing, especially in infants and small children. Garments should be made of a smooth-textured cotton; wool should be avoided. Infants should not be allowed to crawl on wool carpeting.

Individuals with atopic dermatitis have generally dry skin, even in the noninvolved areas. Soaps and detergents which defat the skin should be avoided as much as possible. Bathing should be kept to a minimum. Bath oils are often misused. Since the purpose of the bath oil or other creams applied to the skin is to seal the water into the skin, the correct use of bath oil is to have the patient soak in the tub for 20 minutes while the skin becomes hydrated; then the bath oil is added, which acts now to seal the moisture into the skin rather than to exclude it as would occur if the oil were added before the patient enters the bath. The same principle applies to application of creams and lotions to the skin. They should be applied to the damp skin following a bath. Should bathing appear to make the patient worse, Cetaphil, a commercially available nonlipid lotion, can be applied to the skin when a nondrying cleansing agent is desired.

The role of dietary factors in exacerbation of the dermatitis must be critically evaluated. If it appears that a food or other ingestant leads to exacerbation of itching, then that food must be excluded from the diet. On the other hand, the arbitrary exclusion of numerous foods from the diets of infants with atopic dermatitis without clear-cut evidence that they are involved in the disease is irrational and can lead to malnutrition. The possibility that inhalant factors are causally related to the disease must be evaluated with the same concern for rules of evidence.

Local therapy is the mainstay of management of atopic dermatitis. During acute flare-ups of the disease, wet dressings (e.g., Burow's solution, 1:20) have an antipruritic and anti-inflammatory effect. The continuous application of wet dressings also has the advantage of immobilizing and protecting the affected parts and preventing scratching. Unless scratching can be controlled, it will be almost impossible to manage the disease successfully, particularly during infancy and early childhood. Fingernails must be kept cut as short as possible; restraints for the elbows which keep the hands from the face are sometimes necessary to control scratching during infancy and early childhood, especially at night. Itching is difficult to control with drugs. Drugs with both sedative and antihistaminic activity, such as diphenhydramine (Benadryl) or promethazine (Phenergan), appear to be of greatest value. In some patients, aspirin has a marked antipruritic effect.

When infection is present, antibiotics should be given systemically. Antibiotics incorporated in topical medicaments are not only of little therapeutic value, but can lead to sensitization to the agents applied, particularly in the case of neomycin. The possibility that contact sensitization is superimposed upon atopic dermatitis must be considered when there is a sudden exacerbation of eczema to which a topical medicament has been applied. Parabens, mercurial compounds and lanolin can all cause contact sensitization.

After the acute phase has subsided, topical application of corticosteroid creams and ointments is of great value in management of the disease. Unfortunately their cost may be a serious problem. Cost can be reduced by purchasing relatively concentrated creams in bulk, which the pharmacist can dilute to half strength with Aquaphor. A considerable saving is possible over the purchase of equivalent material in 15- or 30-gm amounts. Small amounts of steroid rubbed in well at frequent intervals appear to give better results than large amounts applied only infrequently. Percutaneous absorption of corticosteroid occurs, but it is not generally clinically significant. Long-continued use of topical steroids leads to an increase in growth of hair in some patients and eventually to some atrophy of the skin.

Systemic administration of corticosteroids should be avoided in treatment of atopic dermatitis in infancy and childhood at all costs. Systemic steroids are effective in clearing the skin, but their withdrawal almost invariably results in a severe exacerbation of the disease. The possible place of alternate-day steroid treatment in management of atopic dermatitis has not been adequately investigated.

Topical treatment with corticosteroids has

largely superseded the use of coal tar preparations. A 1.5 per cent tar preparation may occasionally be of value, particularly in areas of thickened skin. Coal tar is photosensitizing, and occasionally its use results in a sterile, pustular folliculitis.

With adequate control of factors known to trigger itching, with appropriate local treatment, and with understanding support for the parents of a child for whom no immediate cure is to be expected, reasonable control of the disease can generally be accomplished, with an ultimately satisfactory resolution.

URTICARIA
(Hives)

DEFINITION. Urticaria, or hives, is a common skin disorder characterized by the appearance of usually well circumscribed but sometimes coalescent, localized or generalized erythematous raised skin lesions (wheals or welts) of various sizes. The lesions may be intensely pruritic or itch little, if at all. The individual hive usually resolves within 48 hours, but new ones may continue to appear singly or in crops. When urticaria persists for longer than 6 to 8 weeks, the condition is arbitrarily called chronic urticaria. Physiologically urticaria has been attributed to edema of the upper corium due to dilatation and increased permeability of the capillaries.

In angio-edema (angioneurotic edema or giant urticaria) the involvement is in the deeper skin layers or submucosa and in subcutaneous or other tissues; the upper respiratory tract and the gastrointestinal tract are common target organs. The distinction between urticaria and angioedema is frequently not clear; the lesions appear to differ only in the depth of the tissue involvement.

INCIDENCE. As many as 20 per cent of persons experience hives at some time during life. Urticaria appears to occur somewhat more frequently in females than in males.

PATHOGENESIS. The hive is the dermal manifestation of interaction between antigen and IgE antibody fixed to mast cells. Histamine is the vasoactive agent most often implicated in production of urticarial lesions; other vasoactive peptides, particularly the kinins, also have potent action on capillary vasodilation and permeability. Anaphylatoxins C3a and C5a, generated either as a result of involvement of the complement system in an immunologic reaction or through the alternate complement pathway by mechanisms not involving antigen-antibody interaction, can liberate histamine and cause urticaria. It is unlikely that serotonin plays an important role in human urticarial reactions, despite the fact that hives occur in patients with the carcinoid syndrome.

ETIOLOGY. A clinical classification of urticaria is given in Table 9–8. Urticaria may be due to IgE-mediated allergy to *ingestants* (particularly fish, eggs, shellfish, nuts and peanuts, and drugs), *contactants* (plant substances and drugs applied to the skin surface; dog and cat saliva), *injectants* (drugs [particularly penicillin], therapeutic antisera, transfused blood, insect stings and bites, and allergenic extracts), *infection* (particularly parasitic infestation), and rarely *inhalants* (pollens, molds or danders). In some instances urticaria may reflect the direct action of vasoactive materials on vessels in the skin (particularly in the case of insect bites and certain ingestants).

TABLE 9–8 CLASSIFICATION OF URTICARIA

1. *Due to immunologic mechanisms*
   a. Ingestants (foods, drugs)
   b. Contactants (drugs, plants, other substances)
   c. Injectants (drugs, stinging insects)
   d. Infection (parasites)
2. *Due to unknown mechanisms*
   a. Papular urticaria
   b. Cholinergic urticaria
   c. Physical urticaria
      (1) Cold (immunologic mechanism, some cases)
      (2) Solar
   d. Urticaria pigmentosa and mastocytosis
   e. Erythema multiforme
   f. Dermatographism
   g. Malignant neoplasms
   h. Connective tissue disorders
   i. Psychogenic
3. *Due to biochemical mechanisms*
   a. Hereditary angioedema

DIFFERENTIAL DIAGNOSIS. *Papular urticaria* is usually seen in small children, generally on the extremities and other exposed parts at the site of insect bites. *Cholinergic urticaria* is characterized by the appearance of wheals 1 to 2 mm in diameter surrounded by large flares, and frequently involves the skin in the neck area. It is brought on by exercise or by heat, and particularly by emotional factors. There appears to be an increased sensitivity to acetylcholine in affected persons. *Cold urticaria* is a disease of unknown etiology which occasionally appears during childhood. Affected individuals respond to cold by the development of hives in exposed parts of the body. This form of urticaria may not be accompanied by pruritus. Occasionally the disease may be life-threatening, and deaths have been reported following immersion in cold water. Cold urticaria occurs in both sporadic and familial forms, and in adults is occasionally secondary to an underlying systemic illness. In some instances of acquired cold urticaria, a factor inducing urticaria has been passively transferred, with both IgE and IgM immunoglobulin fractions of serum.

Solar urticaria occurs in susceptible individuals upon exposure to light, particularly at 2850 to 3200 angstroms. *Urticaria pigmentosa* typically occurs in childhood and presents a distinctive clinical picture. (See Section 23.) Typically, urtication occurs following stroking of the skin (Darier's sign). *Systemic mastocytosis* is a serious form of urticaria pigmentosa, in which there is mast cell infiltration of the skeletal system, liver, spleen and lymph nodes. *Erythema multiforme* is a form of the urticaria-angioedema symptom complex in which typical iris or target lesions are seen. Mucosal involvement is particularly common in erythema multiforme. During the course of the eruption, some patients show typical hives, which spontaneously change into lesions of erythema multiforme. Erythema multiforme is particularly seen in young children in association with a viral illness and as a manifestation of drug hypersensitivity.

Dermatographism refers to the appearance of a wheal following application of pressure to the skin in the form of scratching or stroking. The physiologic basis in affected individuals is unknown. Urticaria has been described in adults with *malignant* and *connective tissue disorders. Psychogenic urticaria* is frequently suspected, but it is unlikely that emotions are of prime importance, except perhaps in certain cases of cholinergic urticaria.

Hereditary angioedema (HAE) is a serious form of angioedema transmitted as a mendelian dominant. The condition is characterized by recurrent, acute episodes of subepithelial edema of the skin or of the mucosa of the gastrointestinal and upper respiratory tracts. Typical hives do not occur. The edema is nonpitting, does not itch, is generally localized to the face or extremity, and is frequently precipitated by trauma. Gastrointestinal symptoms are commonly present, especially vomiting. Involvement of the glottis is life-threatening. The disease is due to the functional absence of an alpha-2 globulin inhibitor of the activated first component of complement (C1 esterase inhibitor deficiency). In the absence of inhibition, episodic activation of C1 leads to attacks of angioedema, presumably as a result of generation of a vasoactive substance causing increased capillary dilatation and permeability.

TREATMENT. In most instances urticaria is a self-limited illness requiring little treatment other than that aimed at relieving the associated pruritus. Antihistamines are the drugs of first choice for treatment of acute urticaria. Diphenhydramine (Benadryl) 1.25 mg/kg or chlorpheniramine (Chlortrimeton) 0.1 mg/kg may be given every 4 to 6 hours as required. Occasionally epinephrine 0.1 to 0.2 ml gives rapid relief of itching; Sus-Phrine 0.05 to 0.2 ml may give more sustained relief. When the urticaria persists for more than a few days, a careful search should be made for the causes listed in Table 9–8. Hydroxyzine (0.5 mg/kg) every 4 to 6 hours has been reported to be particularly useful in chronic urticaria, and cyproheptadine (Periactin) has been shown to be of value in treatment of cold urticaria. Corticosteroids are rarely required; in any case, their efficacy leaves much to be desired.

ANAPHYLAXIS

DEFINITION. Anaphylaxis is a word first used in 1902 by Portier and Richet following their observation of a heightened reactivity to venom in dogs they were attempting to immunize by repeated injections of foreign material. The term was meant to indicate the opposite of "phylaxis" or protection, and described immediate life-threatening reactions which are most often, but not necessarily, immunologic. Many anaphylactic reactions are the result of IgE-mediated sensitivity to foreign substances, most commonly drugs. As a typical example, a patient develops IgE antibodies to penicillin following its administration; upon its subsequent administration, particularly by injection, the patient may experience an immediate systemic reaction, with generalized urticaria, upper airway obstruction due to laryngeal edema or lower respiratory obstruction due to asthma, peripheral vascular collapse, or unconsciousness, or any combination thereof. Sometimes an immunologic mechanism cannot be identified for a reaction having these clinical features. Anaphylaxis is rare in children.

ETIOLOGY. Virtually any foreign substance is capable of producing anaphylaxis under appropriate circumstances. Drugs, sera, pollen extracts, venom of stinging insects, foods, injectable agents for roentgenographic contrast studies and hormone preparations have all produced anaphylactic reactions.

PATHOGENESIS. In the individual who has developed IgE-mediated anaphylactic sensitivity to a given antigen, subsequent administration of the antigen may result in an explosive antigen-antibody reaction, with massive release of chemical mediators such as histamine and slow-reacting substance of anaphylaxis (SRS-A). The action of the mediators on various tissue receptors throughout the body is responsible for the symptoms observed. Since there are certain dissimilarities between the effects of intravenously administered histamine and the symptoms of systemic anaphylaxis, there is reason to believe that other vasoactive substances besides histamine may be released in the course of human anaphylaxis. In those instances of anaphylaxis in which an immunologic mechanism cannot be identified, it is presumed that mediator release occurs as a direct effect of the causative agent on basophils and mast cells or perhaps by activation of the alternate complement pathway, with generation of anaphylatoxins.

CLINICAL MANIFESTATIONS. Anaphylactic reactions are characteristically explosive, particularly when the antigen is injected. Surviving patients describe a "feeling of impending doom." The more rapidly the symptoms appear after administration of the foreign material, the more serious is the reaction. In carefully studied fatal cases of anaphylaxis in man the shock organ has most often been the glottis, death resulting from acute upper airway obstruction. In other instances, profound circulatory collapse without upper airway obstruction has been reported, with essentially negative findings on autopsy. Besides upper airway obstruction and shock, wheezing, generalized urticaria, abdominal cramps, diarrhea and contractions of the uterus and other smooth muscle organs may occur. Hypotension is present in varying degree.

TREATMENT. Important aspects of treatment of anaphylaxis are the anticipation that the event may occur and being prepared for it. In particular, physicians who administer allergen extracts must be ready to treat this life-threatening complication of hyposensitization. If, for example, a generalized reaction were to follow an injection of pollen extract into an upper extremity, aqueous epinephrine 1:1000, 0.3 to 0.5 ml, should be administered immediately subcutaneously into the other arm and a tourniquet placed above the site of extract injection. In case the allergenic material has been given subcutaneously an additional injection of epinephrine may be administered subcutaneously at the site of injection to slow absorption; but if the extract has been given intramuscularly, aqueous epinephrine should *not* be injected into the site, owing to the fact that epinephrine has a vasodilatory effect on the smooth muscle of blood vessels of skeletal muscle, whereas its effect is vasoconstrictive in the case of subcutaneous blood vessels. An intravenous infusion must be started immediately for administration of aminophylline should wheezing occur and to facilitate administration of drugs such as metaraminol (Aramine) and/or levarterenol (Levophed) for hypotension. Oxygen should be administered by mask, and if there is evidence of upper airway obstruction (stridor, hoarseness), the patient should be intubated or a tracheostomy performed. Diphenhydramine in a dose of 25 to 50 mg should be administered intravenously. Corticosteroids are not administered as emergency drugs, but some physicians feel they are useful in prevention of the late complications of an anaphylactic reaction.

The incidence of drug-induced anaphylaxis would drop substantially if drugs were given only when indicated and then by the oral route unless some compelling reason for injection exists. Not only is anaphylactic sensitivity more easily induced by injection of drugs than by oral administration, but in the sensitized individual, anaphylaxis occurs more commonly following parenteral than oral administration. The incidence of anaphylaxis following Hymenoptera stings can be reduced significantly by the appropriate use of hyposensitization therapy. (See below.)

SERUM SICKNESS

DEFINITION. Serum sickness, or serum disease, is a rather characteristic systemic immunologic disorder which follows the administration of foreign antigenic material.

ETIOLOGY. The disorder was first described in 1905 by von Pirquet and Schick, as a consequence of antitoxin therapy for such diseases as diphtheria and tetanus. The illness was shown to be due to an adverse reaction to the serum proteins of the animal in which the antitoxin was prepared. Therapeutic antisera of animal origin, especially equine, are still occasionally used, but today the major cause of the serum sickness syndrome is drug allergy, particularly that due to penicillin. Cases also have been described following other therapeutic agents, including human gamma globulin, and following Hymenoptera stings. Preparations of immune globulin of human origin are presently available for treatment of diphtheria and tetanus in man, but antitoxins for treatment of rabies, crotalid envenomation, and clostridial intoxication (botulism, gas gangrene), and the antilymphocyte serum used for immunosuppression in transplantation procedures are still prepared in the horse. Fractionation of these antitoxins to eliminate the nonantibody equine plasma proteins has reduced the incidence of serum sickness to far below that which followed the administration of whole serum.

PATHOGENESIS. Serum sickness is the classic example of "immune complex" disease, at least in the experimental animal. In the "one shot" model for serum sickness in the rabbit, a single large dose of isotopically labeled antigen is injected. The symptoms of serum sickness occur coincidentally with the appearance of antibody formed against the injected antigen, at a time when the latter is still present in the circulation. Antigen-antibody complexes formed under conditions of moderate antigen excess have a number of properties which render them injurious to tissue: they lodge in small vessels and in filtering organs throughout the body; they fix complement; and they attract polymorphonuclear leukocytes to the site of deposition. Tissue injury results from the liberation of toxic molecules from the polymorphonuclear leukocytes. In this animal model, healing of the lesions occurs following elimination of the complexes from the circulation.

There are certain similarities between the rabbit serum sickness model and serum disease in man, but there are also outstanding differences. For example, glomerulonephritis is a major lesion of serum sickness in the rabbit, but rarely develops in man; and a fall in serum complement concentration characteristic of the animal disease is also, as a general rule, not seen in man.

Serum sickness demonstrates well how different molecular species of antibodies formed against the same antigen are responsible, by virtue of their differing biologic activities, for diverse parts of the clinical picture. For example, the urticaria of serum sickness is thought to be due to IgE antibody molecules reacting with horse serum proteins, whereas the joint symptoms are thought to occur as a result of deposition of antigen-antibody complexes of the IgG and IgM class. Prospective studies in man indicate that of those who received 1500 units of horse tetanus antitoxin, only those who developed hemagglutination titers against horse serum above 200 developed the disease. There was no correlation between the titer of hemagglutinating antibody and severity of illness.

CLINICAL MANIFESTATIONS. Typically the symptoms of serum sickness begin 7 to 12 days following injection of the foreign material. Urticaria, usually generalized, is the most common finding; fever, myalgia, lymphadenopathy, arthralgia and/or arthritis also occur. Intense pruritus accompanying the urticaria is the most distressing symptom in many patients. The site at which the foreign material was administered generally becomes red and swollen, commonly 1 to 3 days before the appearance of the systemic symptoms. In individuals who have had earlier exposure or previous allergic reactions to the same foreign antigen, symptoms may appear in an accelerated fashion, within 1 to 3 days following injection, or as anaphylaxis. The disease generally runs a self-limited course, and the patient recovers in a week to 10 days. Carditis and glomerulonephritis may rarely occur; the most serious complications of serum sickness are Guillain-Barré syndrome and peripheral neuritis.

LABORATORY FINDINGS. The peripheral leukocyte count may be either increased or decreased, and the sedimentation rate either normal or elevated. A sheep cell agglutinin of the Forssman type is usually found in elevated titer. Serum complement levels are generally normal to only slightly reduced. In the case of serum sickness due to horse serum proteins, antibodies of the IgG, IgA, IgM and IgE classes may be found directed against various horse serum proteins. Occasionally antibody titers against horse serum proteins will be of sufficient magnitude to permit their detection in gel diffusion.

TREATMENT. As noted, uncomplicated serum sickness is a self-limiting disease. Patients generally respond well to aspirin and antihistamines; when the symptoms are particularly severe, corticosteroids have been used with great efficacy. High doses are given, 1 mg/kg every 12 hours, the dose being rapidly reduced as the patient improves.

PREVENTION. The use of horse serum or other animal serum for therapeutic purposes should be limited to cases for which no alternative therapy is available. In particular, the availability of tetanus antitoxin of human origin makes the use of equine tetanus antitoxin unwarranted. Skin tests may be employed prior to administration of serum, beginning with 0.02 ml of a 1:100 dilution, to be followed, if negative, by 0.02 ml of 1:10 dilution. A negative reaction to the stronger solution of horse serum will indicate that anaphylactic sensitivity to horse serum is very unlikely in an individual requiring serum therapy, but skin tests do not predict the likelihood of development of serum sickness.

Occasionally, an individual will require horse serum therapy who has evidence of anaphylactic sensitivity to horse serum by virtue either of a previous reaction or a positive immediate wheal and flare skin test. In such a case the antitoxin can be successfully administered by a process of rapid desensitization. An intravenous infusion is started, the patient premedicated with epinephrine and antihistamines (some immunologists prefer not to premedicate the patient for fear of masking a reaction), and minute amounts of the diluted antitoxin are injected subcutaneously at 20-minute intervals. If the patient tolerates the previous injection well, the amount administered is doubled every 20 minutes. Generally the entire amount of antitoxin can be administered safely over a 4- to 6-hour period.

ADVERSE REACTIONS TO DRUGS

DEFINITION. An adverse reaction to a drug may be defined as any unwanted consequence of administration of the agent, during or following the course of therapy. Reactions may be classified into two broad categories, those dependent upon pharmacologic mechanisms and those dependent upon immunologic mechanisms; the majority of drug reactions are pharmacologic. Both kinds of reactions may be manifest in virtually any organ system, and vary from generalized anaphylaxis, serum sickness or drug fever to involvement of single organ systems such as the skin, bone marrow, gut, respiratory tract or central nervous system. Therapy of any adverse drug reaction depends upon understanding of its underlying nature.

CLASSIFICATION. Adverse reactions occurring on a pharmacologic basis include the following:

Overdosage. The toxic effects of the drug may be directly related to its concentration in the body. Overdosage may result from excessive intake of the drug, as in intentional poisoning; because of abnormalities of the absorption, metabolism or excretion of the drug; or owing to genetic factors, disease, or other interactions of the patient and the drug which allow toxic concentrations to accumulate in the body.

Intolerance. Some patients have an excessive pharmacologic response to an average dose of the drug; the reasons are unclear but may be related to drug receptor sensitivity. In this form of adverse reaction, the effects of the drug are qualitatively normal but quantitatively increased.

Side Effects. Undesirable but unavoidable pharmacologic effects of a drug can be defined as a side effect; for example, epinephrine given for its bronchodilator effect in asthma may also cause tachycardia, pallor and headache, which in this instance are undesirable side effects.

Secondary Effects. Effects of the drug that are not related to its primary pharmacologic action are known as secondary effects. A perianal eruption due to the disturbance of the bacterial flora of the gut by antibiotic therapy is an example of a secondary effect.

Idiosyncrasy. An idiosyncratic reaction to a drug is qualitatively abnormal. Many such reactions can be shown to be due to metabolic abnormalities. The hemolytic anemia occurring in patients with glucose-6-phosphate dehydrogenase (G-6-PD) deficiency following ingestion of primaquine is an example.

Drug Interaction. Drugs administered simultaneously interact with each other in a number of ways that are occasionally favorable for the patient, but are more often detrimental. Interactions may occur at the site of absorption, in the gastrointestinal tract, during excretion by the kidney, during transport of the drug in the blood, or at the receptor site in the tissue. For example, drugs may interact with each other through enzyme induction or inhibition in the liver, which may either accelerate or decelerate drug metabolism. In diseases in which multiple drug therapy is employed, the physician must know the drug interaction potential of the agents used.

Allergy. The above reactions occur on a pharmacologic basis; allergic reactions result from immunologic sensitization to a drug through previous exposure either to the same drug or to a chemically related substance. Allergic reactions are mediated by antigen-antibody interaction or by interaction of antigens with lymphocytes. It is frequently difficult in reactions designated as allergic to demonstrate antibody to the drug using current laboratory methods, and in most allergic reactions serologic evidence of an immunologic mechanism is lacking. On the other hand, allergic reactions have certain features that are useful in distinguishing them: first the clinical expression of an allergic reaction does not generally resemble a known pharmacologic property of the drug, and like an idiosyncratic reaction, is a qualitatively abnormal response; second, allergic reactions generally do not occur on initial exposure to the drug, but between initial exposure and the appearance of symptoms there is almost always a latent period during which allergic sensitization presumably develops. In the sensitized individual reactions may be immediate and explosive or delayed, with no relationship between severity of the reaction and the dose. Systemic anaphylactic reactions can be precipitated by exposure to exquisitely small amounts of drug, such as the amount of benzylpenicillin used in skin testing. Patients allergic to a drug frequently show similar adverse reactions to other drugs that are chemically related, the cross-reactivity being due to the sharing of antigenic determinants between the two drugs. In the case of chemically related but not identical drugs, sensitization may occur to an antigenic determinant which occurs in one drug but not in the other; for example, in a patient sensitive to penicillin G, the likelihood of a reaction to ampicillin depends upon whether the sensitivity involves antigenic determinants common to both drugs or found only on the penicillin G molecule. In the latter instance, a patient sensitive to penicillin G should tolerate ampicillin.

TREATMENT OF DRUG REACTIONS. Treatment of a drug reaction depends upon its mechanism and the clinical manifestations produced. Discontinuation of the drug is indicated in most cases. Under certain circumstances, and especially in infants and small children who develop rashes while receiving antibiotics, the circumstances may support a decision to continue administration of the drug until the etiology of the rash becomes clear. If, for example, an infant or small child with a febrile illness, receiving his first exposure to penicillin or ampicillin or another antibiotic, develops an exanthematous and nonurticarial rash, the rash is much more likely that of a viral illness than a cutaneous manifestation of allergy to the drug. Rather than on tenuous grounds labeling the child allergic to the drug and depriving him of its future use, it appears reasonable to continue therapy for any necessary further period while the course of the rash is observed. If the history suggests that the adverse reaction has a pharmacologic basis, the drug may be introduced again at a later date, at a lower dosage or a longer interval between doses while the plasma concentration of the drug is measured if possible. This may now, for example, be done during digoxin therapy. On the other hand, *if an allergic etiology is likely, the drug should not be reintroduced into the patient,* and an alternative drug should be sought.

Treatment of systemic anaphylaxis was discussed earlier.

Drug allergy in children most commonly manifests itself in the skin. The eruption is generally self-limited and disappears when the drug is discontinued. Treatment is therefore symptomatic. Antihistamines are most useful for urticarial rashes. Diphenhydramine (Benadryl) has both antihistaminic and sedative properties, which may be useful. It may be necessary to give from one and one half to two times the ordinarily recommended dose to achieve satisfactory control of the symptoms. Epinephrine 1:1000 in doses of 0.1 to 0.3 ml provides short-term relief of symptoms. For a more sustained effect, a suspension of epinephrine (Sus-Phrine) in doses of 0.1 to 0.2 ml subcutaneously every 6 hours may be prescribed. Ephedrine sulfate in a dose of 0.5 mg/kg by mouth every 4 to 6 hours can be given orally when prolonged therapy is indicated. Corticosteroids are reserved for those severe cases in which relief is not obtained from the foregoing measures. Prednisone in a dose of 2 mg/kg/24 hr given by mouth in a single dose or two divided doses is the corticosteroid of choice.

PREVENTION. In order to minimize adverse drug reactions, physicians should use drugs only when indicated, be wary of new drugs, and know the relationship between drugs. Concurrent use of two or more drugs should be avoided unless genuinely indicated. The oral route of administration is less sensitizing than the parenteral and is to be preferred whenever possible. Topical application of drugs should be avoided when possible owing to increased risk of sensitization by this route of administration. Drug interactions should be anticipated, and patients should be warned against self-medication.

INSECT ALLERGY

DEFINITION. Allergic reactions to insects are commonly seen in three clinical forms: (1) respiratory allergy secondary to inhalation of particulate matter of insect origin; (2) local cutaneous reactions to insect bites; and (3) anaphylactic reactions to stinging insects.

ETIOLOGY. Sensitization to antigenic material found in the debris and disintegrated bodies of dead insects may produce conjunctivitis, rhinitis or asthma. Inhalation of scales from the wings of insects such as the May fly, Caddis fly and moths is a particularly common cause of respiratory symptoms in the Great Lakes area, where large numbers of these insects appear each summer. Local cutaneous reactions are commonly observed following bites by mosquitoes, flies and various bugs. Anaphylactic reactions due to insect allergy are almost entirely due to the Hymenoptera order of insects (bees, wasps, hornets, yellow jackets and ants).

PATHOGENESIS. Inhalant allergy to insects is in many cases due to IgE-mediated sensitivity to antigenic materials found in the insects' bodies. The antigenic components responsible for the inhalant symptoms have not been thoroughly studied, but the allergenic material appears to reside usually in the cuticle or integument of the insect's body.

In the case of biting insects, the local reaction is frequently a wheal and flare lesion; it appears to be due to vasoactive or irritant materials deposited in the skin while the insect is feeding, but may, particularly with recurrent bites, be mediated by IgE. Some late or persisting cutaneous reactions represent delayed hypersensitivity.

The biochemical and immunologic properties of the venom of stinging insects have been well studied. Venom contains such vasoactive materials as histamine, acetylcholine and kinins, a number of enzymes and formic acid. Hymenoptera venom and whole body extracts have some antigens that are common to the Hymenoptera order and others that are species specific. Other antigens are specific for venom sac material. The majority of patients who experience systemic reactions following Hymenoptera stings are thought to have IgE-mediated sensitivity to antigenic material in the venom, but in a significant number of patients no evidence of IgE-mediated allergy can be demonstrated by skin testing with commercial whole-body extracts. In these individuals, it is suspected, but not proved, that components of the venom may produce symptoms directly or through release of chemical mediators of anaphylaxis. Alternatively, the whole-body extract may not contain a sufficient amount of the actual sensitizing antigen of the venom to give a positive skin test.

CLINICAL FINDINGS. The clinical findings in inhalant allergy due to insects are quite similar to those seen with the usual inhalant allergens such as pollens. Rhinitis, conjunctivitis and asthma have all been described.

The cutaneous reactions to biting insects are most often urticarial but may be papular, vesicular and erythematous, particularly as the lesion progresses. Typical delayed hypersensitivity reactions are also seen.

Clinical reactions to stinging insects range in severity from minimal pain and local erythema to life-threatening anaphylactic episodes. Local reactions vary from a papule or wheal at the site of the sting to edema of an entire extremity. The clinical manifestations of anaphylaxis due to sensitivity to stinging insects are identical to those observed in anaphylactic reactions due to other causes. The patient may develop generalized urticaria, symptoms of upper and lower airway obstruction and circulatory collapse. Death may occur within a few minutes if appropriate measures are not taken. Typical serum sickness or nephrotic syndrome may be seen as a late sequela of the reaction to a stinging insect.

DIAGNOSIS. The diagnosis is usually easily made on the basis of history and, in the case of biting insects, by examination of skin lesions. Papular urticaria, which is common in children, occurs almost always as a result of insect bites, particularly of fleas and bedbugs.

Skin testing with whole body extracts is useful in establishing the IgE-mediation of a systemic reaction to a stinging insect, but because the degree of sensitivity to the stinging insect antigens may be exquisite, caution is indicated. It is safest to begin testing with a whole body extract of mixed insects at a 1:10,000 dilution by the *puncture or scratch method,* progressing to a 1:1000 concentration of the extract if the former is negative. If the patient is skin test negative to 1:1000 by scratch or puncture, *intracutaneous testing* may be begun with a 1:1,000,000 or 1:100,000 concentration, progressing in tenfold increments up to a concentration of 1:100 or until a positive wheal and flare reaction results. Generally, concentrations greater than 1:100 are not employed in skin testing. Skin testing is useful not only to verify IgE-mediated sensitivity but also as a guide to the appropriate starting point for hyposensitization therapy.

TREATMENT. Hyposensitization is occasionally undertaken when it can be established that inhalant allergy is due to a specific insect such as the May fly or Caddis fly. Results of hyposensitization treatment have not been very satisfactory, and avoidance of the insect appears to be the preferred management.

For cutaneous reactions due to biting insects, treatment with topical medicaments to relieve itching and local discomfort, and occasionally the systemic use of an antihistamine, is all that is generally required.

In case of an anaphylactic reaction following a Hymenoptera sting, the acute treatment is essentially that of anaphylaxis. Epinephrine 1:1000 in a dose of 0.2 to 0.3 ml subcutaneously, or administration of a 1:100 solution of epinephrine by aerosol (available as Medihaler-Epi), will be effective in combatting both local respiratory symptoms and symptoms of peripheral vascular collapse. The sublingual administration of isoproterenol has been recommended, but its use may actually be contraindicated in anaphylaxis, since, though it may relieve asthma, it will be ineffective in relieving glottic edema, and because its vasodilator action on peripheral vasculature may aggravate hypotension. An antihistamine (for example, Benadryl 25 to 50 mg) should be given. Corticosteroids are of little use in treatment of the acute systemic reaction.

Kits are available commercially for emergency use in case of anaphylaxis following insect sting. They contain a syringe filled with epinephrine and an antihistamine tablet, and should be in possession of all individuals who have had a previous severe or anaphylactic reaction. An acceptable alternative to having epinephrine in the kit is possession of a 1:100 solution of epinephrine in an aerosol unit (Medihaler-Epi).

It is generally agreed that a course of hyposensitization should be given to those who have had a systemic reaction following a sting. Since the individual who has been stung is generally unable to identify precisely whether he was stung by a wasp, bee, yellow jacket or hornet, hyposensitization with a mixed extract of all four insects is usually administered. It is safe to start with a dilution of extract tenfold less than that to which the patient reacted on intracutaneous testing. The dose of extract is increased weekly in a manner similar to that used in pollen hyposensitization therapy for hay fever. The final and maintenance dose is usually 0.25 ml of a 1:10 dilution of aqueous whole body extract. Once this dose is reached, injections are then given at monthly intervals, and later at bimonthly intervals for three years. Some allergists prefer to continue the injections indefinitely. Whether hyposensitization should be initiated in a patient with a large *local* reaction, such as swelling of an entire extremity, has not been resolved. Extracts prepared from venom sac material are currently under investigation for both skin testing and hyposensitization.

OCULAR ALLERGIES

Allergic reactions involving the eye occur much less commonly in children than in adults. The eye may be involved as part of a generalized allergic reaction, in urticaria and angioedema, for example, or the eye alone may be affected. Allergic reactions in the eye are known to occur on the basis of IgE-mediated allergy, as conjunctivitis in a child with ragweed hay fever, for example, or on the basis of a cell-mediated (delayed hypersensitivity) immune reaction, as is seen in contact dermatitis of the eyelids.

EYELIDS. Eyelids are particularly prone to swelling because of their loose areolar connective tissue. Swelling may result from contact dermatitis to a variety of environmental substances. The lids are particularly involved because of the frequency with which offending contact sensitizers are carried to the eyelids with the hands. Occasionally contact dermatitis appears as a result of sensitization to medication applied to the eyes.

ALLERGIC CONJUNCTIVITIS. Allergic conjunctivitis is a frequent concomitant of allergic rhinitis in individuals with hay fever, particularly when it is due to pollens. In affected children, the eyes itch, the conjunctiva is reddened and edematous and there may be profuse tearing. Rubbing of the eyes aggravates the condition. The nature of the discharge is frequently watery, but if persistent, may become purulent in appearance. On examination, however, even the discharges which appear purulent consist predominantly of eosinophils; these permit differentiation from infectious conjunctivitis, in which the discharge is composed of polymorphonuclear leukocytes and bacteria.

Vernal Conjunctivitis. Vernal conjunctivitis is more common in children than in adults and appears most often during the spring and summer. The disease occurs in palpebral and limbal forms. In the **palpebral** form, the tarsal plate of the upper lid presents a characteristic "cobblestone" appearance as a result of hyperplasia and thickening of the conjunctiva. In the **limbal** form of the disease, there is involvement at the junction of the cornea and sclera, with thickening and opacity of the tissue in the area. Progression of the limbal form may scar the cornea ultimately and lead to blindness in the most severe cases. Symptoms of vernal conjunctivitis include lacrimation, itching, burning, and a particularly distressing photophobia. The seasonal occurrence, the finding of eosinophils and the frequent coexistence with other atopic diseases such as asthma, hay fever and eczema have suggested that IgE-mediated sensitivity is responsible for the condition; but a detailed study of patients with the condition usually fails to prove any specific etiologic agent, and hyposensitization is of little if any value. In essence, the etiology of vernal conjunctivitis is unknown.

TREATMENT. Contact dermatitis of the lids is best managed by identification of suspected sensitizers and their elimination. Topical corticosteroids are of value in managing the acute reaction. Allergic conjunctivitis in the patient with hay fever generally responds well to topical application of sympathomimetics in the form of eye drops, or, failing that, to eye drops or ointments containing corticosteroids. Hyposensitization for allergic conjunctivitis without concomitant allergic rhinitis has given unimpressive results. Vernal conjunctivitis may be treated with sparing use of corticosteroid eye drops or ointments. Ophthalmic preparations of disodium cromoglycate have recently been shown to be helpful.

ADVERSE REACTIONS TO FOODS

The incidence of adverse reactions to foods is not known, and unquestionably varies in different parts of the world. The average United States diet contains many food antigens, chemical food additives, antibiotics and other substances; accordingly, a significant frequency of reactions to foods

TABLE 9–9 ADVERSE REACTIONS ATTRIBUTED TO FOODS

Systemic	*Genitourinary*
Shock	Cystitis
Malaise	Enuresis
Fever	
Growth failure	*Musculoskeletal*
	Leg pains
Gastrointestinal	Arthritis
Cheilitis	Hydroarthrosis
Stomatitis	
Canker sores	*Respiratory*
Colic	Rhinitis
Abdominal pain	Asthma
Flatulence	
Diarrhea	*Cutaneous*
Malabsorption	Urticaria
Colitis	Eczema
Pruritus ani	"Rashes"
Central nervous system	*Auditory*
Headache	Serous otitis
Irritability	Meniere syndrome
Hyperactivity	
"Tension fatigue"	*Hematologic*
Seizures	Anemia
Psychosis	Heiner syndrome

should not be surprising. Reactions due to allergic mechanisms are estimated to occur in from 0.3 to 0.7 per cent of the population. Adverse reactions to foods have been reported to give rise to symptoms in many organ systems, with frequencies which vary markedly as reported by various investigators. Table 9–9 is a partial listing of allergenic symptoms which have been attributed to food ingestion.

ETIOLOGY. Possible mechanisms for adverse reactions to foods are summarized in Table 9–10. The most easily identified reactions occur on an immunologic (allergic) basis. IgE-mediated reactions are characteristically rapid in onset and may present as angioedema of the lips, mouth, uvula of glottis, as generalized urticaria, as asthma, or occasionally as shock. In such cases it is often not necessary for the physician to make the diagnosis; the patient usually recognizes the symptoms have followed ingestion of a certain food. Individuals with such IgE-mediated food allergy are at constant risk of exposure to the offending food hidden in a food mixture. For example, a nut-sensitive individual may have a serious reaction to ingestion of a cookie coated with almond extract.

TABLE 9–10 MECHANISMS OF ADVERSE REACTIONS TO FOODS

1. *Immunologic*
   a. IgE mediated
   b. ? Toxic complex
   c. ? Delayed hypersensitivity
   d. Immune deficiency
2. *Biochemical*
   a. Enzyme deficiency (e.g., disaccharidase)
   b. "Hot dog" headache – nitrite sensitivity
   c. Tyramine headache
   d. Malabsorption (α-gliadin)
3. *Unknown*
   a. Reactions to food additives (e.g., FD&C dyes)

Individuals with IgE-mediated food reactions consistently show positive skin tests to the suspected food. In fact, skin testing itself, particularly if done by the intracutaneous technique, can precipitate the clinical reaction in individuals with anaphylactic allergy. They should be tested with caution.

More difficult to diagnose are reactions which begin a few hours to 24 hours after ingestion of the offending food. Such reactions have been attributed without much convincing evidence to allergy to a digestive product of the food such as a proteose or polypeptide. The role of antigen-antibody complexes and cell-mediated (delayed hypersensitivity) immunity in the pathogenesis of these late-occurring reactions has been the subject of speculation. Individuals with certain forms of immune deficiency disorders, particularly those diagnosed as variable immunodeficiency (WHO classification) have diarrhea and malabsorption. Patients with isolated IgA deficiency may have malabsorption problems due to wheat.

Adverse food reactions having a biochemical basis are well known. Perhaps the best studied are those in individuals with disaccharidase deficiency, who have a variety of gastrointestinal complaints following milk ingestion, including abdominal pain, flatulence and diarrhea. Their inability to hydrolyze lactose, owing to absence of intestinal lactase, produces a disturbance of osmotic relationships in the gut lumen. An acid and gassy diarrhea results.

Sensitivity to cow's milk protein is probably overdiagnosed in infants and children. In the best documented cases symptoms appear during the first 6 months of life. Vomiting, watery or blood-streaked mucoid diarrhea and steatorrhea are observed in affected infants. Heiner has described in older infants the association of iron deficiency anemia, occult blood in the stools, recurrent pulmonary infiltrations and multiple precipitating antibodies to cow's milk proteins; and occult loss of blood in the stools leading to iron deficiency anemia in infants with a high intake of whole cow's milk seems to be a well established entity. Beta lactoglobulin and bovine serum albumin have been incriminated most often as the cause of adverse reactions to cow's milk. The precise mechanisms for these reactions are unknown; except in the case of anaphylactic reactions only rarely can an immunologic basis for symptoms and signs be clearly established.

Soy bean protein sensitivity with fever, vomiting and diarrhea has been reported. Wheat-sensitive individuals react adversely to alpha gliadin present in the gluten fraction of wheat; whether the symptoms result from a toxic reaction to the alpha gliadin or are due to immunologic factors involving IgA immune complexes has not been settled.

Certain individuals, particularly those who develop headaches after food ingestion, have been shown in clinical studies to be hyperreactive to tyramine present in the food or, in one well investigated case, to nitrate. It seems clear that some individuals react adversely to food additives, particularly to dyes used in foods, drugs and cosmetics. For example, tartrazine (yellow No. 5) will induce asthma in some aspirin-intolerant asthmatics. The mechanisms of the tartrazine reaction and other symptoms thought to be due to ingestion of food additives are not known.

DIAGNOSIS. An etiologic diagnosis in a child suspected of an adverse food reaction requires careful objective study. Elimination from the diet for a period of 7 to 10 days of a food causing difficulty should generally result in improvement in the patient's symptoms. Reintroduction of the food, preferably in large amounts for several meals, should result in the return of symptoms in a reasonable period of time, within 7 days at most. For example, when cow's milk allergy is suspected in an infant with vomiting, colic, diarrhea, eczema or chronic rhinitis, elimination of milk from the diet should result in amelioration of the symptoms. If this occurs, the infant should be maintained on a milk substitute, such as soy bean formula, for several weeks; the cow's milk is then reintroduced. The previously observed symptoms should promptly reappear and then disappear when the milk is again withdrawn. Unfortunately, when the child does well on the milk substitute, cow's milk rechallenge is often not done, and an erroneous diagnosis of milk allergy may be perpetuated. An equally critical diagnostic approach should be undertaken in children felt possibly to have "allergic tension-fatigue," a syndrome whose frequency varies among the patients of physicians according to their belief in the importance of foods as a cause of adverse clinical reactions.

The critical testing of foods by the elimination and provocation method is difficult, if patient or parent believes that he is food sensitive, owing to the emotional reaction incident to the ingestion of a food to which one believes he reacts adversely. Though not easy to accomplish, food challenges are best done in a blind manner whereby the food is given in a disguised form, for example, in capsules or mixed with another food. Diagnosis by the elimination and provocation method is most easily interpreted when the patient's symptoms are present on a more or less continuous basis. Under these circumstances, the results of elimination of a given food are readily appreciated. On the other hand, when symptoms such as headache are only intermittent, results of elimination and provocation testing are frequently equivocal.

Skin testing utilizing properly prepared food antigens will reveal the presence of any IgE antibody to the test antigen. A positive skin test does not necessarily indicate, however, that the particular food causes symptoms. In anaphylactic food allergy skin tests almost invariably show a positive reaction to the offending food, but in this instance the history alone usually establishes the diagnosis and skin testing is superfluous. Occasionally a positive skin test to a food not previously suspected of causing trouble will be clinically corroborated when the history is re-examined in light of the positive test. All too often, undue attention paid to clinically insignificant skin reactions to food extracts has eventuated in very restricted diets, with no attempt made to confirm the clinical importance of suspected foods through elimination and provocative testing. Overdiagnosis of food allergy has sometimes produced malnutrition in infants and children, as well as anxiety and depression in mothers who have found it impossible to adhere to severely restrictive diets.

In the provocative neutralizing method of diagnosis of food allergy, dilutions of food extracts are injected intracutaneously in an attempt to reproduce the patient's symptoms, which are then said to be relieved by successive intracutaneous injections of other dilutions of the same extract. Much attention is given by proponents of the method to the morphology of the wheal produced by the injection. "Whealing responses" are reported to be "neutralized" by injections of more dilute solutions of the extract used to produce the original wheal; and symptoms, if produced, may also be "neutralized," usually by higher dilutions of the original extract. The method has been enthusiastically presented, with no explanations as yet of its rationale, and the techniques used vary among the users of the method. For example, some users both "provoke" and "neutralize" by *sublingual* administration of the antigen solutions. There is little doubt that injections of appropriate extracts may produce skin wheals and clinical symptoms in individuals who have food allergies mediated by IgE, but it is difficult to understand how the symptoms thus provoked can be neutralized by a *higher* dilution of the same antigen extract used to elicit them. Following study, the Committee on Provocative Food Testing of the American College of Allergists concluded that the method could not be recommended as a valid procedure in the investigation of food sensitivity.

TREATMENT. The treatment of an adverse food reaction is directed at the clinical manifestations which may be anaphylaxis, urticaria, diarrhea, rhinitis, asthma, and so on. Offending foods should be eliminated from the diet. For reasons that are unclear, some persons shown to be highly reactive to foods will become "tolerant" as they grow older; this is particularly likely in infants and small children. With the passage of time, therefore, cautious reintroduction of offending foods into the diet may be tried, particularly in the case of those common foods which are difficult to avoid in the average diet. Hyposensitization by injection, sublingual or oral administration of extracts of offending foods has not gained acceptance among most allergists.

ELLIOT F. ELLIS

Immunologic Basis of Allergic Disease

Austen, K. F., and Becker, E. L. (eds.): Biochemistry of the Acute Allergic Reactions. 2nd International Symposium. Oxford, Blackwell Scientific Publications, 1971.

Becker, E. L.: Nature and classification of immediate-type allergic reactions. Adv. Immunol. *13*:267, 1971.

Ellis, E. F.: Immunologic basis of atopic disease. Adv. Pediatr. *16*:65, 1969.

Ellis, E. F.: Immunologic mechanisms in allergic disease. Pediatr. Clin. N. Am. *19*:373, 1972.

Ishizaka, K., and Ishizaka, T.: Mechanisms of reaginic hypersensitivity: A review. Clin. Allergy. *1*:9, 1971.

Johansson, S. G. O., Bennich, H. H., and Berg, T.: The clinical significance of IgE. Prog. Clin. Immunobiol., *1*:157, 1972.

Leskowitz, S., Salvaggio, J. E., and Schwartz, H. J.: An hypothesis for the development of atopic allergy in man. Clin. Allergy *2*:237, 1972.

Levy, D. A.: Immediate hypersensitivity. *In* Tice's Practice of Medicine. Hagerstown, Md., Harper and Row, 1973, Vol. 1, Chap. 31.

Lichtenstein, L. M.: Allergy. Clin. Immunobiol. *1*:243, 1972.

Middleton, E., Jr.: Autonomic imbalance in asthma with special reference to beta adrenergic blockade. Adv. Intern. Med. *18*:177, 1972.

Reed, C. E.: Beta adrenergic blockade, bronchial asthma, and atopy. (Editorial.) J. Allergy *42*:238, 1968.

Szentivanyi, A.: The beta adrenergic theory of the atopic abnormality in bronchial asthma. J. Allergy *42*:203, 1968.

Pharmacologic Therapy

Middleton, E., Jr., and Coffy, R. G.: Immediate hypersensitivity. II. Drugs in clinical use. Ann. Rep. Med. Chem. *8*:273, 1973.

Hyposensitization

Lichtenstein, L. M., Ishizaka, K., Norman, P. S., Sobotka, A. K., and Hill, B. M.: IgE antibody measurements in ragweed hay fever. Relationship to clinical severity and the results of immunotherapy. J. Clin. Invest. *52*:472, 1973.

Lichtenstein, L. M., Norman, P. S., and Winkenwerder, W. L.: A single year of immunotherapy for ragweed hay fever. Immunologic and clinical studies. Ann. Intern. Med. *75*:663, 1971.

Treatment of allergic rhinitis with injections of allergic extracts. Med. Lett. Drug Ther. *15*:55, 1973.

Allergic Rhinitis

Ellis, E. F.: Allergic rhinitis. *In* Gellis, S. S., and Kagan, B. M. (eds.): Current Pediatric Therapy-5. Philadelphia, W. B. Saunders Company, 1971, p. 654.

Seebohm, P. M.: Allergic rhinitis. *In* Tice's Practice of Medicine. Hagerstown, Md., Harper and Row, 1972, Vol. 1, Chap. 39.

Asthma

Austen, K. F., and Lichtenstein, L. M. (eds.): Asthma. Physiology, Immunopharmacology and Treatment. New York, Academic Press, Inc. 1974.

Chai, H., and Newcomb, R.: Pharmacologic management of childhood asthma. Am. J. Dis. Child. *125*:757, 1973.

Ellis, E. F.: Asthma in childhood. *In* Conn, H. F. (ed.) Current Therapy. Philadephia, W. B. Saunders Company, 1973, p. 538.

Porter, R., and Birch, J. (eds.): Identification of Asthma. Ciba Foundation Study Group No. 38. Edinburgh, Churchill-Livingstone, Ltd., 1971.

Rackemann, F. M., and Edwards, M. D.: Asthma in children (a follow-up study). New Engl. J. Med. *246*:815; 858, 1952.

Townley, R.: Mechanisms and management of bronchial asthma. *In* Tice's Practice of Medicine. Hagerstown, Md., Harper and Row, 1972, Vol. 1, Chap. 40.

Adverse Reactions to Drugs

Ellis, E. F.: Adverse reactions to drugs. *In* Conn, H. F. (ed.) Current Therapy. Philadelphia, W. B. Saunders Company, 1974.

Richards, D. J., and Rondell, R. K.: Adverse Drug Reactions. Their Prediction, Detection and Assessment. Edinburgh, Churchill-Livingstone, Ltd., 1972.

Wade, O. L.: Adverse Reactions to Drugs. London, William Heinemann Medical Books, 1970.

Atopic Dermatitis

Ellis, E. F., and Goltz, R. W.: Atopic dermatitis. *In* Tice's Practice of Medicine. Hagerstown, Md., Harper and Row, 1972, Vol. 1, Chap. 44.

Holt, L. E., Jr. (ed.): Conference on Infantile Eczema. J. Pediatr. *66*:153, 1965.

Jacobs, A. H.: Local management of atopic dermatitis in infants and children. Clin. Pediatr. *8*:201, 1969.

Norins, A. L.: Atopic dermatitis. Pediatr. Clin. N. Am. *18*:801, 1971.

Rostenberg, A., Jr., and Solomon, L. M.: Atopic dermatitis and infantile eczema. *In* Samter, M. (ed.): Immunological diseases. 2nd ed. Boston, Little, Brown and Company, 1971 p. 920.

Urticaria

Beall, G. N.: Urticaria. A review of laboratory and clinical observations. Medicine *43*:131, 1964.

Sheffer, A. L., and Austen, K. F.: Vascular responses: Urticaria and angioedema. *In* Fitzpatrick, T. B., Arndt, K. A., Clark, W. H., Jr., Eisen, A. Z., Van Scott, E. J., and Vaughan, J. H., (eds.): Dermatology in General Medicine. New York, McGraw-Hill Book Company, 1971, p. 1261.

Anaphylaxis

James, L. P., Jr., and Austen, K. F.: Fatal systemic anaphylaxis in man. New Engl J. Med. *270*:597, 1964.

Sheffer, A. L.: Current concepts. Therapy of anaphylaxis. New Engl. J. Med. *275*:1059, 1966.

Weiszer, I.: Allergic emergencies. *In* Patterson, R. (ed.): Allergic Diseases. Diagnosis and Management. Philadelphia, J. B. Lippincott Company, 1972, p. 327.

Serum Sickness

Chodirker, W. B., and Vaughan, J. H.: Serum sickness. *In* Fitzpatrick, T. B., Arndt, K. A., Clark, W. H., Jr., Eisen, A. Z., Van Scott, E. J., and Vaughan, J. H. (eds.): Dermatology in General Medicine. New York, McGraw-Hill Book Company, 1971, p. 1274.

Reisman, R. E.: Serum sickness. *In* Tice's Practice of Medicine. Vol. 1, Chap. 34. Hagerstown, Md., Harper and Row, 1971.

Smith, J. M., and Gell, P. G. H.: Serum sickness and acute anaphylaxis in man. *In* Gell, P. G. H., and Coombs, R. R. A. (eds.): Clinical Aspects of Immunology. Oxford, Blackwell Scientific Publications, 1968, p. 660.

Insect Allergy

Barnard, J. H.: Allergic reaction to insect stings and bites. N. Y. J. Med. *57*:1787, 1967.

Brown, H., and Bernton, H. S.: Allergy to hymenoptera. Arch. Intern. Med. *125*:665, 1970.

Feingold, B. F., Benjamini, E., and Michaeli, D.: The allergic responses to insect bites. Ann. Rev. Entomol. *13*:137, 1968.

Frazier, C. A.: Insect Allergy. St. Louis, Warren H. Green, Inc., 1969.

Schulman, S.: Insect allergy. Biochemical and immunological analyses of the allergens. Prog. Allergy *12*:246, 1968.

Ocular Allergy

Allansmith, M., and Frick, O. L.: Antibodies to grass in vernal conjunctivitis. J. Allergy *34*:535, 1963.

Sherman, W. B.: Hypersensitivity Mechanisms and Management. Philadelphia, W. B. Saunders Company, 1968, p. 386.

Theodore, F. H., and Schlossman, A.: Ocular Allergy. Baltimore, The Williams & Wilkins Company, 1958.

Adverse Reactions to Foods

Ament, M. E.: Malabsorption syndromes in infancy and childhood. Parts I and II. J. Pediatr. *81*:685; 867, 1972.

Bleumink, E.: Food allergy. The chemical nature of the substances eliciting symptoms. World Rev. Nutr. Diet. *12*:505, 1970.

Goldstein, G. B., and Heiner, D. C.: Clinical and immunological perspectives in food sensitivity. J. Allergy *46*:270, 1970.

Walker, W. A., and Hong, R.: Immunology of the gastrointestinal tract. I and II. J. Pediatr. *83*:517; 711, 1973.

RHEUMATIC DISEASES

(Inflammatory Diseases of Connective Tissue, Collagen Diseases)

The disorders described in this section are grouped because of similarities in symptomatology and pathology; in general, they are associated with inflammatory changes in various connective tissues throughout the body. Included are:

I. Juvenile rheumatoid arthritis (JRA)
II. Ankylosing spondylitis
III. Systemic lupus erythematosus (SLE)
IV. The vasculitis syndromes
  A. Schönlein-Henoch vasculitis
  B. Polyarteritis nodosa
    1. Infantile polyarteritis
    2. Wegener's granulomatosis
  C. Takayasu's arteritis
V. Dermatomyositis
VI. Scleroderma
  A. Morphea
  B. Progressive systemic sclerosis
VII. Miscellaneous
  A. Erythema multiforme exudativum (Stevens-Johnson syndrome)
  B. Erythema nodosum
  C. Goodpasture syndrome
  D. Relapsing nodular nonsuppurative panniculitis
  E. "Rheumatoid" nodules without rheumatic disease

Certain diseases, discussed elsewhere, have points of similarity to these disorders, i.e., acute rheumatic fever, serum sickness, glomerulonephritis, the idiopathic nephrotic syndrome, ulcerative colitis, regional enteritis and thrombotic thrombocytopenic purpura.

The causes and pathogenesis of these disorders are unknown, and precise diagnostic criteria are lacking. They usually appear as clinically distinct entities, each generally presenting a characteristic picture. For example, rheumatoid arthritis is associated with chronic arthritis, dermatomyositis with inflammation of muscle, scleroderma with induration of skin, and the like. But each of these diseases can affect many organs, and overlapping symptoms and signs sometimes make precise diagnosis difficult.

JUVENILE RHEUMATOID ARTHRITIS

Juvenile rheumatoid arthritis (JRA) is a disease or group of diseases characterized by chronic synovitis and associated with a number of extra-articular manifestations. The disease was first well described in 1897 by Still, who noted that chronic arthritis in children differs from rheumatoid arthritis of adult onset in both articular and extra-articular manifestations. JRA is an extremely variable disease which encompasses several broad clinical subgroups (Table 9–11): polyarticular disease (multiple joints involved), pauciarticular disease (only a few joints involved), and systemic disease (high fever and rheumatoid rash as well as polyarthritis). Polyarticular disease most closely resembles adult onset rheumatoid arthritis; pauciarticular and systemic types of disease occur rarely in adults. Recognition of these disease patterns is useful in diagnosis and care of children with JRA.

ETIOLOGY AND EPIDEMIOLOGY. The etiology of rheumatoid arthritis and the mechanisms for perpetuation of chronic synovial inflammation in the disease are unknown. Two frequently mentioned hypotheses are that the disease results from an infection with as yet unidentified microorganisms or that it represents a hypersensitivity or "autoimmune" reaction to unknown stimuli. There is as yet no convincing evidence for either hypothesis. Various microorganisms have been isolated from rheumatoid synovium, but none consistently. Organisms such as mycoplasma can cause chronic synovitis resembling rheumatoid arthritis in experimental animals. The possible roles of viruses or slow virus infections remain under investigation. Evidence that immune mechanisms are involved in pathogenesis is supplied by the association of rheumatoid factors (antibodies reactive with IgG) with adult onset rheumatoid arthritis. Although these antibodies do not cause the disease, recent work has suggested that immune complexes of rheumatoid factor and immunoglobulin

TABLE 9–11 FORMS OF JUVENILE RHEUMATOID ARTHRITIS

	POLYARTICULAR	PAUCIARTICULAR	SYSTEMIC
Sex	80% girls	70% girls	50–60% boys
Joints	Any	Large joints: knee/ankle	Any
Severe disability from arthritis	15%	Rare	20%
Iridocyclitis	Rare	25%	None
Rheumatoid factors	10–15%	Rare	None
Antinuclear antibodies	25%	25%	None

may perpetuate synovial inflammation and are responsible for the rheumatoid vasculitis seen in seropositive rheumatoid arthritis. Low synovial fluid complement levels in some rheumatoid patients and low serum complement levels in patients with rheumatoid vasculitis are consistent with such a mechanism. However, this mechanism fails to explain all rheumatoid inflammation, since chronic synovitis can occur in the absence of rheumatoid factors and with normal joint fluid complement levels. The occurrence of chronic arthritis in patients with IgA deficiency and hypogammaglobulinemia suggests that immunodeficiency may somehow predispose to rheumatoid arthritis; however, no blatant immunodeficiency has been identified in rheumatoid patients. There is no evidence that JRA is a hereditary disease; it rarely occurs in siblings. Clinical onset may follow an acute systemic infection or physical trauma to a joint, but no direct relation to such events has been shown. Exacerbations may follow intercurrent illness or psychic stress.

JRA is not a rare disease; it is estimated that there are one quarter of a million affected children in the United States. About 5 per cent of all cases of rheumatoid arthritis begin in childhood. The disease may start at any age, though rarely before the second birthday.

PATHOLOGY. Rheumatoid arthritis is characterized by chronic nonsuppurative inflammation of synovium. Microscopically, affected synovial tissues are edematous, hyperemic and infiltrated with lymphocytes and plasma cells. Secretion of increased amounts of joint fluid results in joint effusions. Projections of thickened synovial membrane form villi which protrude into joint spaces; hyperplastic rheumatoid synovium may spread over and become adherent to articular cartilage (pannus formation). With continuing synovitis, articular cartilage may become eroded and progressively destroyed. The mechanism of destruction of articular cartilage and other joint structures by chronic proliferating synovium remains unknown. The period of time before synovitis causes permanent joint damage varies from patient to patient; in general, lasting damage to articular cartilage occurs later in the course of JRA than in adult onset disease, and many children with JRA never incur permanent joint damage despite prolonged synovitis. Once joint destruction has commenced, erosions of subchondral bone, narrowing of the "joint space" (loss of articular cartilage), destruction or fusion of bones, and deformity, subluxation or ankylosis of joints may result. Tenosynovitis and myositis may be present. Osteoporosis, periostitis, accelerated epiphyseal growth and premature epiphyseal closure can occur adjacent to affected joints.

Rheumatoid nodules, less frequent in children than adults, are characterized by fibrinoid material surrounded by chronic inflammatory cells; palisading of cells and necrosis are less prominent than in rheumatoid nodules of adults. Pleura, pericardium and peritoneum may show nonspecific fibrinous serositis; progression to severe thickening, as in chronic constrictive pericarditis, occurs rarely if ever. The rheumatoid rash appears histologically as a mild vasculitis, with a few inflammatory cells surrounding small vessels in subepithelial tissues.

CLINICAL MANIFESTATIONS

Polyarticular Disease. Polyarticular disease is characterized by involvement of multiple joints, typically including the small joints of the hands (Figs. 9–12 and 9–13). Polyarticular disease unassociated with prominent systemic manifestations occurs in 40 per cent of children with JRA. Girls are predominantly affected. The polyarticular pattern is generally established early in the course of disease.

Onset of arthritis may be insidious, with gradual development of joint stiffness, swelling and loss of motion; or fulminant, with sudden appearance of symptomatic arthritis. Affected joints are swollen and warm but rarely red. Swelling results from periarticular edema, joint effusion and synovial thickening. Some children have joint stiffness and discomfort before objective changes appear. Affected joints may be tender to touch and painful on motion; however, severe tenderness and pain are unusual, and many children do not complain of any pain in obviously inflamed joints. Early in the disease limited joint motion is related to muscle spasm, joint effusion and synovial proliferation; later, limited motion may result from joint destruction and ankylosis or from contractures of soft tissues. Pronounced synovial proliferation may produce cystic swellings about affected joints; occasionally herniations of synovium and synovial fluid occur into neighboring structures, particularly in the popliteal area (popliteal cyst). Morning stiffness and "gelling" following inactivity are characteristic of rheumatoid arthritis in children, as in adults. Young children, particularly those with multiple joint involvement, are often irritable

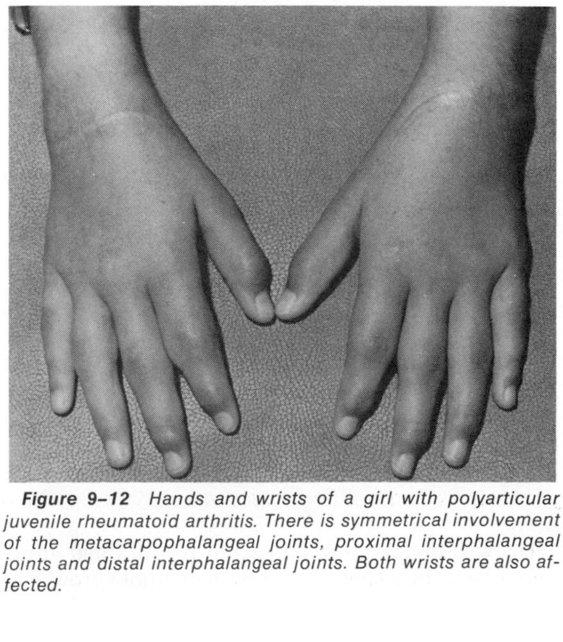

Figure 9–12 Hands and wrists of a girl with polyarticular juvenile rheumatoid arthritis. There is symmetrical involvement of the metacarpophalangeal joints, proximal interphalangeal joints and distal interphalangeal joints. Both wrists are also affected.

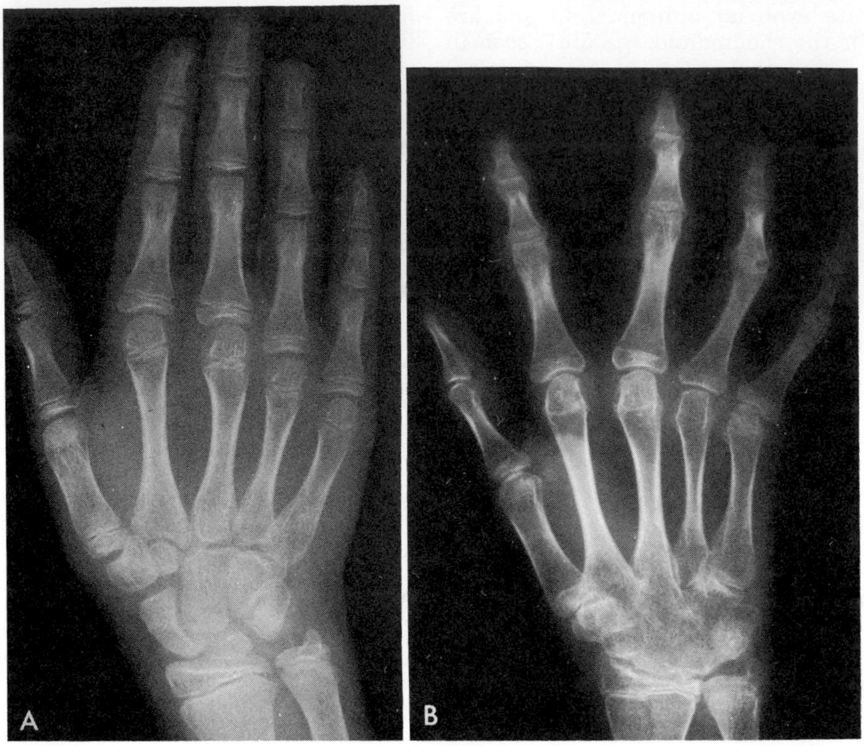

Figure 9–13 *Progression of joint destruction in a girl with juvenile rheumatoid arthritis despite doses of corticosteroids sufficient to suppress symptoms in the interval between* A *and* B. A, *Roentgenogram of hand at onset;* B, *roentgenogram four years later, showing loss of articular cartilage and destructive changes in the distal and proximal interphalangeal and metacarpophalangeal joints, and destruction and fusion of wrist bones.*

and assume a typical posture of anxious guarding of their joints against movement (Fig. 9–14).

Arthritis, which may affect any synovial joint, often begins in large joints such as knees, ankles, wrists and elbows. The involvement is often symmetrical. Inflammation of proximal interphalangeal joints produces spindling or fusiform changes of the fingers; metacarpophalangeal joint involvement is equally common, and distal interphalangeal joints may also be affected (Figs. 9–12 and 9–13). Arthritis of the cervical spine, characterized by neck stiffness and pain, occurs in about half the patients. Temporomandibular involvement with limited ability to open the mouth is common; the pain may be referred to as earache by young children. Hip involvement occurs in at least half the children with polyarthritis, usually beginning later in the disease process. Destruction of the femoral heads may ensue; severe hip disease is a major cause of disability in late JRA (Fig. 9–15). Radiographic changes in the sacroiliac joints occur in 25 per cent of patients, usually in association with hip disease; these changes differ from those of ankylosing spondylitis and are not associated with involvement of the lumbodorsal spine. Rarely, cricoarytenoid arthritis causes hoarseness and laryngeal stridor. Involvement of sternoclavicular joints and costochondral junctions may cause chest pain.

Growth disturbances adjacent to inflamed joints may result in either overgrowth or undergrowth of the affected part. For example, increased leg length may follow chronic arthritis of the knee, and micrognathia after temporomandibular arthritis is one of the late hallmarks of juvenile rheumatoid arthritis. Small, deformed feet may result from foot involvement in early childhood.

Extra-articular manifestations are not so dramatic as in systemic rheumatoid arthritis. However, the majority of patients with active polyarticular disease have malaise, anorexia, irritability and mild anemia. Low-grade fever, slight hepatosplenomegaly and lymphadenopathy may be present. Pericarditis is infrequent and iridocyclitis rare. Rheumatoid nodules sometimes occur over pressure points, usually in patients with positive agglutination tests for rheumatoid factor. Growth may be retarded during periods of active disease; growth spurts often occur with remission.

Pauciarticular Disease. Pauciarticular (Latin, *pauci* = few) disease is characterized by arthritis that remains limited to only a few joints, typically large joints such as the knees, ankles and elbows (Fig. 9–16). Occasionally the temporomandibular joints, single toes or fingers, the wrist or the neck are affected. The hips are generally spared. About 35 per cent of children with JRA have pauciarticular disease. Girls are predominantly affected. The clinical appearance of affected joints and the synovial histology are indistinguishable from those of polyarticular JRA. If arthritis remains limited to a few joints for the initial

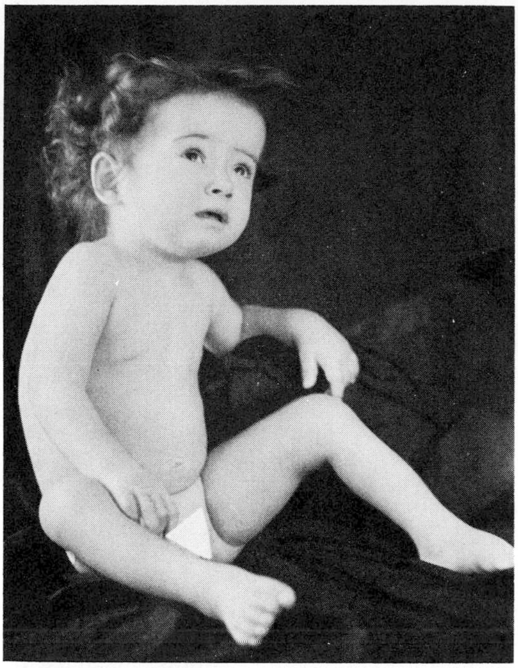

Figure 9-14 Characteristic posture of a child with rheumatoid arthritis, showing the anxious appearance and guarding of joints.

six months of disease, the disease generally remains pauciarticular throughout its course; additional large joints may be affected over the years, but widespread polyarticular disease does not usually occur. Although the arthritis may be chronic or recurrent, serious disability is uncommon. However, patients with pauciarticular disease are at risk for iridocyclitis; chronic iridocyclitis occurs in one of four children with pauciarticular arthritis sometime during the course of disease.

The **iridocyclitis** of JRA is characteristically chronic and unassociated with early symptoms or signs, activity of arthritis, or elevated sedimentation rate. Occasionally children note redness, pain, photophobia or decreased visual acuity early in the course of iridocyclitis. One or both eyes may be affected. If initial involvement is unilateral, the second eye usually remains uninvolved. Iridocyclitis is sometimes the presenting manifestation of JRA, but generally begins at or after the onset of joint complaints. Patients with iridocyclitis frequently have positive tests for antinuclear antibodies. The earliest signs of inflammation of the iris and ciliary body are increased numbers of cells and amounts of protein in the anterior chamber of the eye—changes detectable only by slit lamp examination. Sequelae of the ocular inflammation (Fig. 9-17) include posterior synechiae (adherence of the iris to the lens, causing an irregular or poorly reactive pupil), band keratopathy (deposition of calcium salts in the cornea and sclera), complicated cataracts, secondary glaucoma and phthisis bulbi (degeneration of the globe). Loss of vision may result; in severe cases permanent blindness occurs. Early detection and therapy before scarring are important for preservation of vision. For this reason, all children with pauciarticular disease should have slit lamp examinations three or four times yearly for the first five or more years of disease regardless of the activity of the joint disease.

Other extra-articular manifestations are usually mild in pauciarticular JRA; low-grade fever, malaise, modest hepatosplenomegaly and lymphadenopathy, and mild anemia may occur in association with active joint disease.

Systemic Disease. Systemic JRA is character-

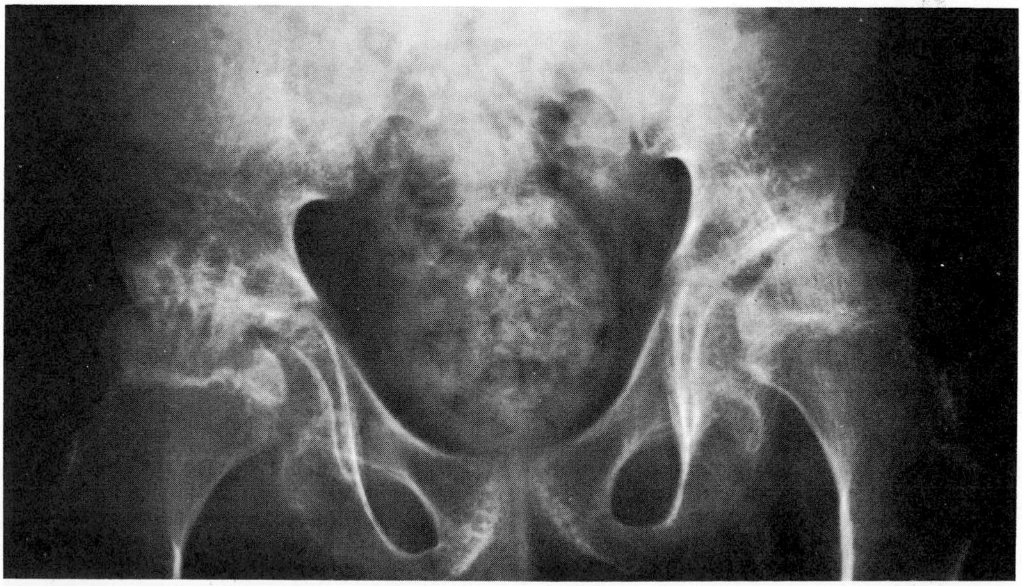

Figure 9-15 Severe hip disease in a 13 year old boy with long-active juvenile rheumatoid arthritis, showing destruction of femoral heads and acetabula, joint space narrowing, and subluxation of the left hip. The patient had received corticosteroids systemically for nine years.

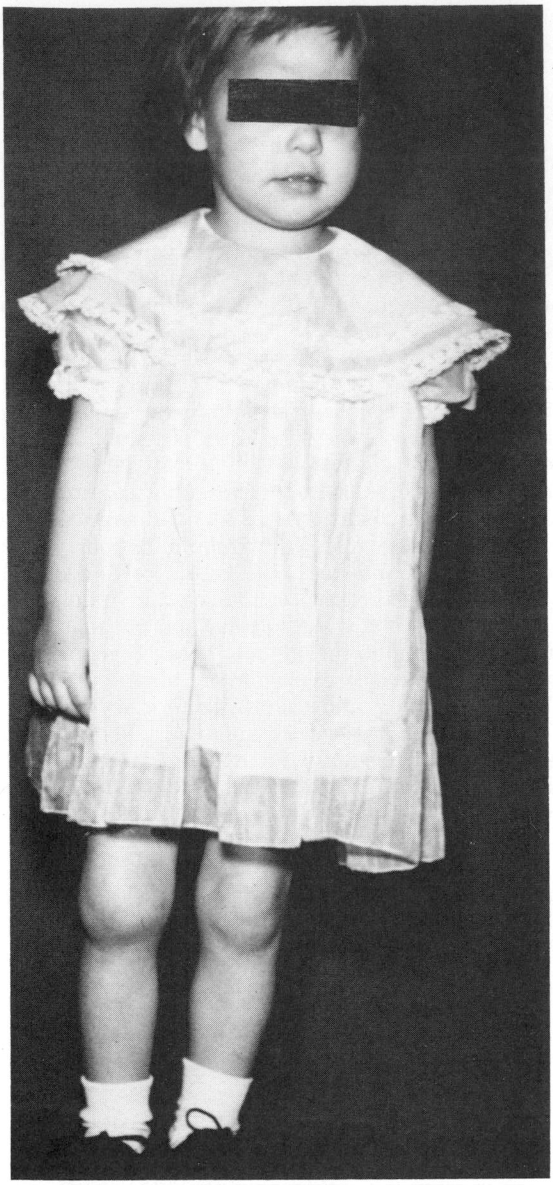

Figure 9–16 Characteristic appearance of a child with pauciarticular arthritis; there is obvious swelling of the right knee.

ized by prominent extra-articular manifestations (Table 9–12), particularly high fevers and rheumatoid rash. This type of disease occurs in 25 per cent of JRA patients. In contrast to other types of JRA, as many boys as girls are affected. Systemic symptoms are generally the presenting manifestations of disease.

The fever is intermittent, with daily or twice-daily elevations to 103° F or higher and rapid return to normal or subnormal levels (Fig. 9–18). Temperature elevations usually occur in the evening, but sometimes in the morning as well. Shaking chills are frequently associated. Patients may seem alarmingly ill during the period of fever and surprisingly well during its remission. Rheumatoid rash (Figs. 9–19 and 9–20) is characterized not

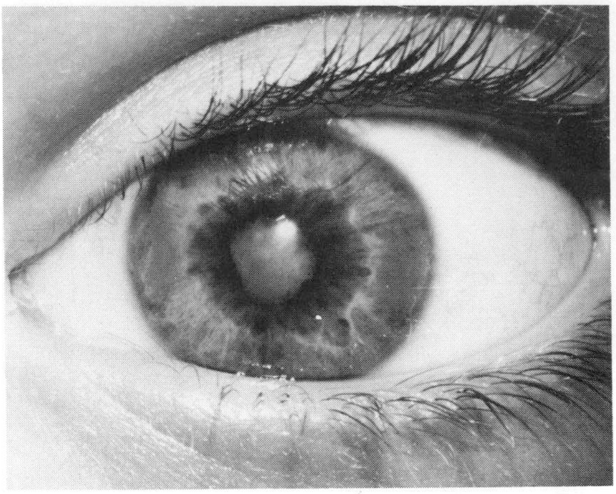

Figure 9–17 Chronic iridocyclitis of juvenile rheumatoid arthritis; extensive posterior synechiae have resulted in a small irregular pupil. There is a well developed cataract, and early band keratopathy can be seen at 3 and 9 o'clock positions in the cornea.

only by its appearance, but also by its evanescent, recurrent nature. Individual lesions are small (several millimeters), pale, red-pink macules, often with central pallor; extensive lesions may coalesce. The rash is most frequently found on the trunk and proximal extremities, but may occur anywhere on the body including the palms and soles. It usually appears during febrile periods but may also be induced by skin trauma (isomorphic response), heat and embarrassment. Hepatosplenomegaly and generalized lymphadenopathy occur in most children with active systemic disease. The degree of organomegaly may be great. Mild hepatic dysfunction may be present, and lymph node histology may simulate lymphoma. About one third of affected children have detectable pleuritis or pericarditis, often subclinical. Chest radiographs may show pleural thickening or small pleural effusions; pericardial effusion may be large and electrocardiographic changes present. The pericarditis of JRA is generally benign. Rarely, severe chest pain, dyspnea or cardiac failure, with or without evidence of myocarditis, demands vigorous therapy. Occasionally interstitial lung infiltrates occur during periods of active systemic disease, but chronic

TABLE 9–12 MANIFESTATIONS OF SYSTEMIC JUVENILE RHEUMATOID ARTHRITIS

	PER CENT
High intermittent fever	100
Rheumatoid rash	90
Hepatosplenomegaly and/or lymphadenopathy	85
Pleuritis and/or pericarditis	35
Abdominal pain	10
Marked leukocytosis	85
Polyarthritis	100
Iridocyclitis	0

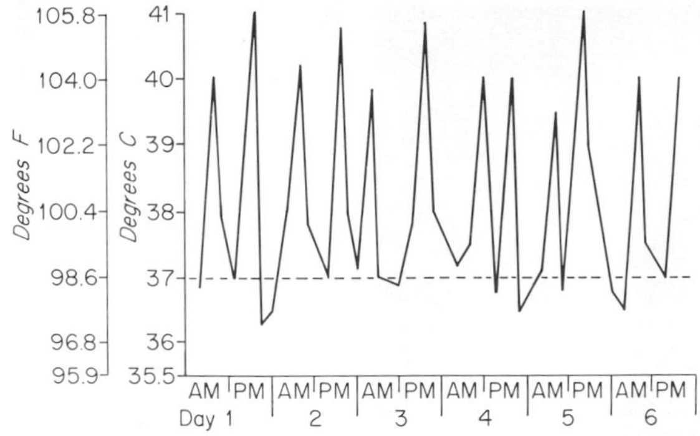

Figure 9–18 *Characteristic fever of systemic juvenile rheumatoid arthritis; there are one or two daily temperature elevations to 39°C or greater, with rapid return of temperature to normal or subnormal levels.*

rheumatoid lung disease rarely if ever occurs in children. A few children have episodes of severe abdominal pain during active disease. Leukocytosis and even leukemoid reactions are common. Anemia is also common during active disease and may occasionally be profound.

Most children with systemic JRA have joint manifestations at or within a few months of onset, although arthritis may initially be overlooked because of the overwhelming systemic symptoms. Some patients initially have only severe myalgia, arthralgia or transient arthritis. A few patients do not develop arthritis until months or years later. The pattern of joint involvement is ultimately polyarticular and resembles that described in polyarticular disease. The systemic manifestations generally run a self-limited course for several months but may recur. The real morbidity of systemic JRA, as in polyarticular JRA, lies in arthritis, which becomes chronic in some patients and persists after systemic symptoms have remitted. Systemic manifestations rarely recur after patients reach adulthood, even though chronic arthritis may persist.

COURSE AND PROGNOSIS. The major cause of morbidity in polyarticular and systemic JRA is chronic joint disease; in pauciarticular disease, the major morbidity is chronic iridocyclitis. The outcome is unpredictable in any individual patient. Even with severe systemic involvement, the disease is rarely life-threatening. There may be exacerbations and remissions, or symptoms may continue for years with mild arthritis causing little disability or, less commonly, with severe arthritis which progresses to joint destruction and permanent deformity. The disease does not always remit at puberty; some patients continue to have active arthritis into adulthood, and some have exacerbations after many years of apparently complete remission. Exacerbations may be associated with intercurrent illnesses, but hepatitis and other forms of liver disease may be followed by transient remission.

There appear to be no features which permit accurate prediction of outcome. The overall prognosis is good, however. At least 75 per cent of patients eventually enter long remissions without significant residual deformity or loss of function. A few patients are left with crippling joint deformities. Severe hip disease is particularly debilitating, as is loss of vision from iridocyclitis. Secondary amyloidosis, generally heralded by proteinuria and diagnosed by demonstration of amyloid in tissues, may cause morbidity in rare patients.

LABORATORY DATA. There are no specific laboratory tests. The sedimentation rate is usually, but not invariably, elevated during active disease. Anemia is common, usually with low reticulocyte counts and negative Coombs test results; iron deficiency may also be present. The white blood cell count is often elevated; leukemoid reactions sometimes occur, particularly in systemic JRA, in which counts of 10,000 to 30,000 per mm^3 are the rule, and counts as high as 75,000 per mm^3 may be detected. Urinalyses are normal; during salicylate therapy a few erythrocytes and renal tubular cells may be seen. Serum proteins may be altered, with increase in the alpha-2 and gamma globulin fractions and decrease in albumin. Any or all of the serum immunoglobulins may be elevated. Antinuclear antibodies are found in 25 per cent of children with polyarticular and pauciarticular disease, but are rarely present in systemic disease. Presence of antinuclear antibodies does not correlate with severity of arthritis, but 80 per cent of children with chronic iridocyclitis of JRA have them. Lupus erythematosus (LE) cells can at times be demonstrated.

Rheumatoid factors are antibodies which react with gamma globulin. They are generally detected by agglutination of gamma globulin-coated erythrocytes or latex or bentonite particles; rheumatoid factors detected by such agglutination techniques are usually IgM immunoglobulins. Such

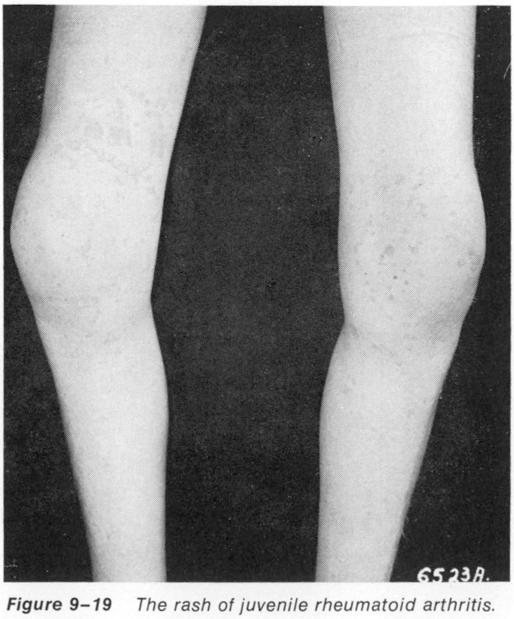

Figure 9–19 *The rash of juvenile rheumatoid arthritis.*

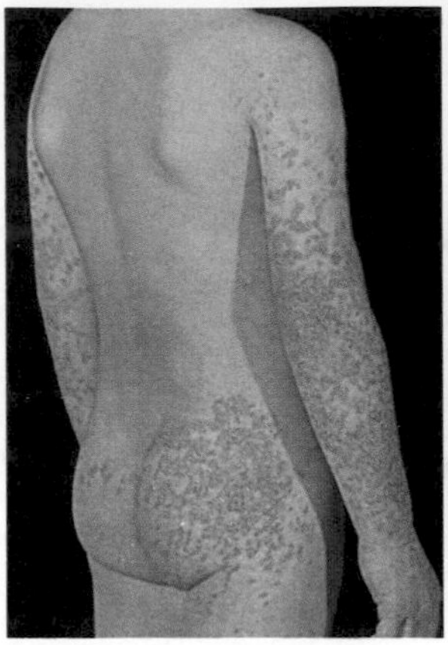

Figure 9–20 *Henoch-Schönlein purpura (anaphylactoid purpura). (From G. W. Korting:* Hautkrankheiten bei Kindern und Jugendlichen. *Stuttgart, Germany, F. K. Schattauer Verlag, 1969.)*

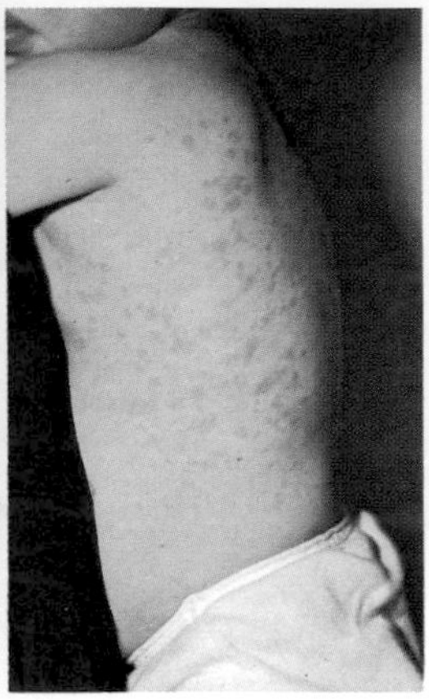

Figure 9–26 *Rash of rheumatoid arthritis.*

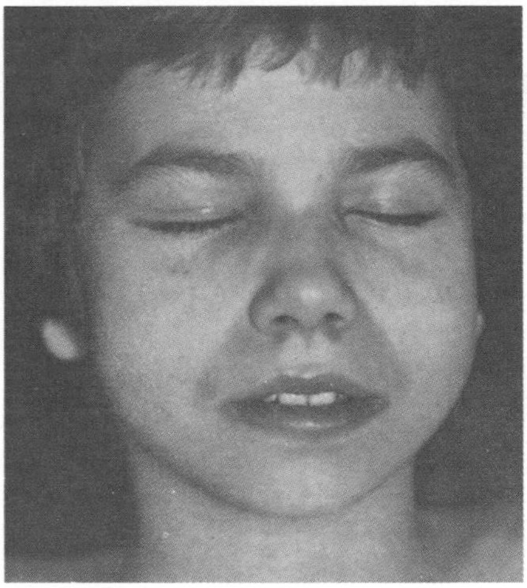

Figure 9–27 *The facial rash of dermatomyositis. Note the faint erythema over the bridge of the nose and malar areas, and the heliotrope discoloration of the upper eyelids.*

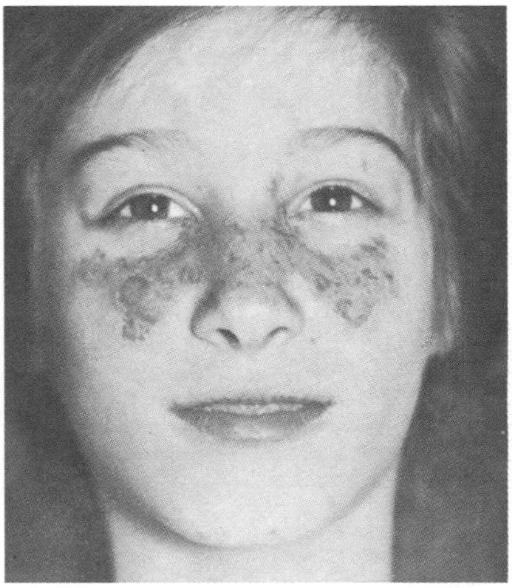

Figure 9–25 *The butterfly rash of systemic lupus erythematosus.*

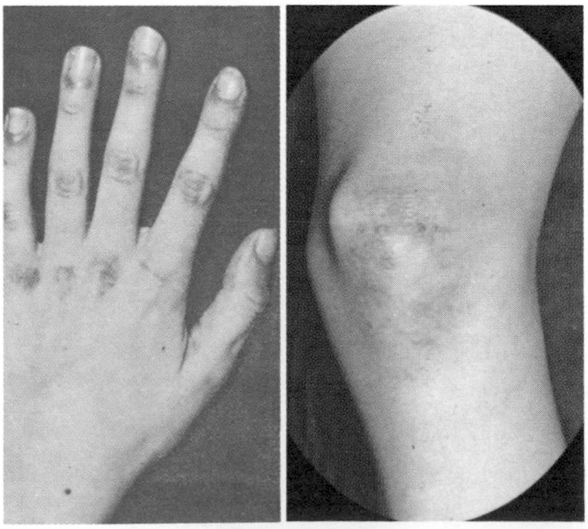

Figure 9–28 *Rash of dermatomyositis. Skin changes over the knuckles (left) and over the knee (right).*

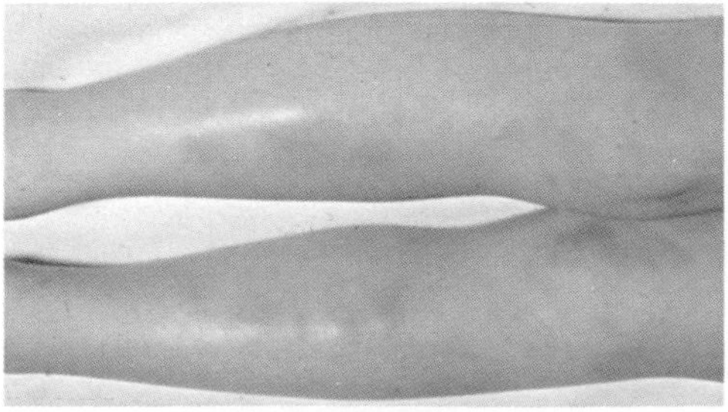

Figure 9–31 *Erythema nodosum.*

rheumatoid factors are demonstrable in 80 per cent of adults with rheumatoid arthritis, but are much less frequently found in children. Rheumatoid factors are not specific for rheumatoid arthritis, but are found also in other rheumatic diseases (for example, lupus erythematosus, scleroderma) and in association with certain infections and malignancies. It has recently been shown that IgG antibodies reactive with gamma globulin, demonstrable by techniques other than agglutination, are present in some seemingly seronegative children with JRA. The significance of this observation remains to be determined, but there is little reason to believe that such antibodies are specific for JRA.

Positive agglutination tests for rheumatoid factors correlate with age at onset of rheumatoid arthritis; positive test results are rarely found in children whose disease begins before the age of 8 years, but become progressively frequent with increasing age at onset. Tests do not convert from negative to positive despite long active JRA. Positive tests are most commonly associated with polyarticular disease, occur frequently in patients with rheumatoid nodules, but are rare with systemic or pauciarticular disease. A few patients with onset of disease in late childhood and positive tests for rheumatoid factors develop progressive erosive rheumatoid arthritis similar to severe disease of adult onset.

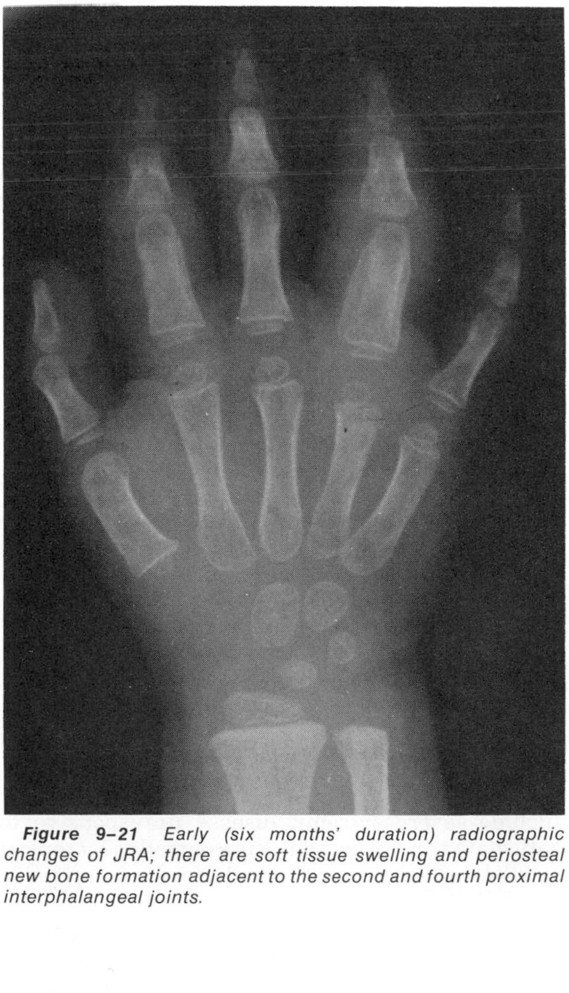

Figure 9–21 *Early (six months' duration) radiographic changes of JRA; there are soft tissue swelling and periosteal new bone formation adjacent to the second and fourth proximal interphalangeal joints.*

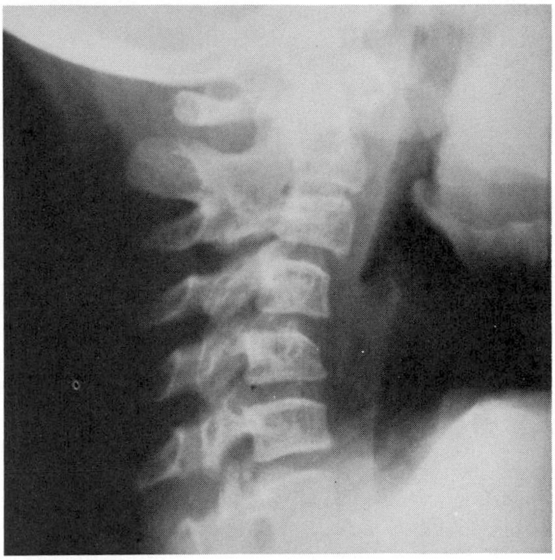

Figure 9–22 *Cervical spine in long-active juvenile rheumatoid arthritis, showing fusion of neural arch joints between C2 and C3, narrowing and erosions of the remaining neural arch joints, and resulting abnormal curvature.*

Synovial fluid in JRA is cloudy, may clot spontaneously and usually contains increased amounts of protein. The cell count varies from 5000 to 50,000 cells per mm^3; the cells are predominantly neutrophils. Levels of glucose may be low in the joint fluid; levels of complement may be normal or decreased. None of these findings is diagnostic.

Early radiographic changes consist of soft tissue swelling, osteoporosis and periostitis about affected joints (Fig. 9–21). Regional epiphyseal closure may be accelerated and local bone growth increased or decreased. In long-active joint disease, subchondral erosions and narrowing of cartilage spaces may occur, as may varying degrees of bony destruction and fusion. Late radiographic changes, as in the wrist and hand (Fig. 9–13), are characteristic. Characteristic changes may occur in the neck, with narrowing and eventual fusion of neural arch joints (most frequently seen at C2 and C3, Fig. 9–22), erosions of the odontoid process, atlantoaxial subluxation and underdevelopment of vertebral bodies.

DIAGNOSIS AND DIFFERENTIAL DIAGNOSIS. The diagnosis is clinical and depends on the presence of persistent arthritis or typical systemic manifestations for three or more months, as well as on the exclusion of other diseases.

Early in the disease *pyogenic or tuberculous joint infection, osteomyelitis, sepsis* or *arthritis associated with other acute infectious illnesses* must be considered. Culture of joint fluid, tuberculin test and radiographs of affected joints are helpful. Arthritis of limited duration may occur in association with a number of viral infections and after rubella immunization. Gonococcal infection may also result in arthritis. *Acute leukemia* and other malignancies occasionally present with pain and swelling of one or more joints and should be considered when onset is recent, particularly if severe anemia, thrombocytopenia or abnormalities of peripheral white blood cells are present.

In *acute rheumatic fever* the transient, migratory nature of the arthritis and the presence of valvular carditis help in differentiation. *Systemic lupus erythematosus* (SLE) can cause arthritis indistinguishable from rheumatoid arthritis, but the joint changes are usually milder and other clinical manifestations of lupus are usually present; it should be noted that antinuclear antibodies and occasionally LE cells occur in JRA as well as SLE. *Ankylosing spondylitis* may present with arthritis of a few peripheral joints which is indistinguishable from JRA before characteristic involvement of the spine becomes manifest; the presence of early radiographic sacroiliac joint changes associated with pain in the low back and hip girdles is suggestive. The *vasculitis syndromes, dermatomyositis, ulcerative colitis, regional enteritis, psoriasis* and *sarcoidosis* may be associated with arthritis similar to that of JRA, but are generally distinguishable on clinical grounds. *Reiter syndrome* (arthritis, urethritis and conjunctivitis) is uncommon in children. *Immunodeficiency diseases* may rarely be associated with chronic arthritis resembling JRA.

Various conditions such as joint trauma, Legg-Perthes disease (aseptic necrosis of the femoral head), Osgood-Schlatter disease (aseptic necrosis of the tibial tubercle), and slipped capital femoral epiphysis may initially mimic JRA. Acute toxic synovitis of the hip is a self-limited condition of uncertain origin; JRA rarely begins in or affects solely the hip. Pigmented villonodular synovitis, an uncommon synovial overgrowth, usually affects only one joint.

Synovial biopsy may be useful, especially to exclude infection in monarticular disease; however, synovial histology may not differentiate the synovitis of rheumatoid arthritis, various other rheumatic disorders, or even so-called postinfectious states.

TREATMENT. In planning therapy it is important to realize that although JRA may be of long duration and there is no specific cure, the ultimate prognosis is good for most patients and life is rarely threatened. Management of these children and their families constitutes a real test of the physician's ability to treat the whole child and requires sympathy, patience and understanding. Unpredictable exacerbations are discouraging and make evaluation of therapy difficult. There is an understandable tendency to shop for medical help and partake of fad or quack cures. The chronic nature of the disease may cause the family to give up, allowing unnecessary crippling to occur.

The aims of immediate and long-term treatment are twofold: (1) to preserve joint function and to provide adequate care of extra-articular manifestations without therapeutic harm; and (2) to support the outlook of the child and his family. Such care ideally requires the devoted attention of a primary physician, in consultation with specialists including a physiatrist or physical therapist, an orthopedist, an ophthalmologist, and sometimes a rheumatologist, an orthodontist and a psychiatrist or social worker.

A number of drugs are effective in suppressing the inflammatory process; these include salicylates, corticosteroids and gold salts. Acetylsalicylic acid (aspirin) is the safest and most satisfactory; in doses sufficient to maintain blood levels of 20 to 30 mg per dl it usually aleviates both arthritis and systemic manifestations. About 100 mg of aspirin per kg daily, divided into 4 or 6 doses, is needed to maintain such blood levels. There is considerable individual variation in required dosage; blood levels should be followed initially and the patient watched carefully for toxicity. Full therapeutic response may require weeks to months. When dosage and response are determined and stabilized, the medication can be continued for years. Chronic therapeutic salicylate administration is relatively safe even in small children if physician, patients and parents are aware of the potential toxic effects. Intoxication from overdosage can be avoided if the dose is calculated with care and parents are made aware that rapid or heavy breathing and drowsiness or other central nervous system changes are often the earliest signs of salicylism in children. Tinnitus, a common complaint of adults with salicylism is rarely noted by children. Salicylates should be given with food because of the possibility of gastric irritation. If patients complain of stomach ache, antacids can be added, or buffered salicylate preparations or choline salicylate substituted for ordinary aspirin. Children with persistent gastrointestinal complaints should be investigated for peptic ulcer. Hemorrhagic phenomena and hypersensitivity reactions are extremely uncommon with therapeutic doses of aspirin; if such reactions occur, they may be circumvented by substitution of choline salicylate or sodium salicylate. Elevated levels of hepatic enzymes have recently been described in the sera of patients with rheumatic diseases who were receiving large doses of salicylates; association of clinically significant liver disease appears to be rare.

There are few indications for systemic corticosteroids in JRA. Although they dramatically suppress symptoms, they do not induce permanent remission or prevent the occurrence of joint damage (Fig. 9–13). It is suspected that destruction of cartilage and aseptic necrosis of bone, particularly in the femoral heads, may be related to long-term steroid therapy (Fig. 9–15). Therapeutic doses of corticosteroids cause adrenal suppression, may suppress growth, and may produce a host of other potentially dangerous side effects. The dose required for suppression of symptoms is unpredictable and may actually increase with prolonged therapy.

Indications for use of corticosteroids in JRA include severe systemic disease unresponsive to salicylates and iridocyclitis uncontrolled by topical steroids. In severe systemic disease unresponsive to an adequate trial of salicylates, or in rare instances of cardiac decompensation from pericarditis or myocarditis, prednisone in initial doses of 1 to 2 mg/kg/day is indicated. As soon as symptoms are suppressed, the dose should be decreased and the drug gradually discontinued under a cover of salicylates. With decreasing doses there are often transient rebounds of symptoms which should be waited out. Since the systemic manifestations of JRA generally run a self-limited course, prednisone can usually be successfully discontinued within weeks or months. In iridocyclitis unresponsive to topical steroid therapy, systemic corticosteroids in doses sufficient to suppress ocular inflammation as monitored by the slit lamp are indicated; single doses given daily or on alternate days may be sufficient. Therapy should be managed in conjunction with an ophthalmologist.

Corticosteroids should rarely be used for relief of joint manifestations alone, since they do not cure arthritis or prevent joint damage, and since their chronic side effects may be even less tolerable than the joint disease. Other reasonable therapeutic possibilities should always be exhausted first. If corticosteroids are used, every effort should be made to employ the lowest effective dose, to use alternate day or single daily dosage, and to minimize the period of treatment.

Gold salts have not been widely used in JRA but appear to be no more toxic in children and as effective as in adults. They are useful if arthritis does not respond to an adequate trial of salicylates. Gold therapy requires weekly injections, each preceded by careful weekly follow-up for possible toxicity (skin rash, mucosal ulcers, leukopenia, thrombocytopenia and proteinuria). Initially 2.5 to 5.0 mg of gold sodium thiomalate (Myochrysine) should be given intramuscularly and repeated 1 week later, followed by a maintenance dose of 1 mg/kg/week intramuscularly; a total weekly dose of 25 mg is appropriate for children weighing 25 to 60 kgs; 50 mg can be given to larger teenagers. Several months are required for therapeutic response, but if none has resulted after 20 weekly injections the drug should be discontinued. If response occurs, injections should be gradually spaced out to three- or four-week intervals and continued indefinitely. Continuous surveillance for side effects must be maintained throughout the period of therapy; their appearance is almost always an indication for discontinuing the drug.

Chloroquine and hydroxychloroquine may benefit some children with JRA but must be used with extreme care because of possible retinal toxicity; ophthalmologic examinations should be made every three months. Indomethacin and phenylbutazone may also afford symptomatic relief in some patients. In the United States indomethacin is currently authorized only for experimental use in children; toxicity includes gastric irritation, headache and other central nervous system effects. Phenylbutazone may cause gastric irritation and hematopoietic toxicity. Although agents such as azathioprine and cyclophosphamide have recently been advocated as therapeutic agents in rheumatoid arthritis, their use in children for symptomatic relief of a disease which rarely threatens life does not seem warranted until more is known of their long-term side effects.

Physical therapy is important to maintain and to improve motion and muscular strength about affected joints. Patients and parents should be instructed in an appropriate exercise program to be carried out at home on a regular daily basis. Activities such as tricycle riding and swimming are beneficial and should be encouraged. Night splints for knees and wrists may aid in preventing and correcting deformity. Cylindrical casts or prolonged immobilization of joints should be avoided. Bed rest has little role in treatment of JRA. Children can usually determine their own activity; in general, they should avoid only those activities that cause overtiring and joint pain. Orthopedic surgery is sometimes required to correct joint deformities. Synovectomy of selected joints is occasionally helpful but does not appear to be curative. Injection of corticosteroids into selected joints may be helpful at times, but repeated injections should not be used. Children with micrognathia may require orthodontic management.

Iridocyclitis requires prompt diagnosis and therapy to preserve vision. The eyes should be examined at each medical visit. Ophthalmologic slit lamp examinations should be made at least once a year in children with systemic and polyarticular disease and three or four times yearly in children with pauciarticular disease. Parents should be cautioned to report any eye symptoms or decreased visual acuity at once. Therapy of iridocyclitis should be supervised by an ophthalmologist. Initially it consists of topical steroids and dilating agents. Systemic steroids or subconjunctival injections should be used if prompt resolution of ocular inflammation is not achieved with topical agents. Frequent long-term follow-up of eyes is essential. Ophthalmologic surgery may be required for chronic sequelae.

Children with JRA should be encouraged to lead as normal lives as possible. They and their parents need to know what to expect and to be treated optimistically. Affected children should not be led to believe that they are invalids, but should be taught to be as self-sufficient as possible. With encouragement most can lead active lives, attend school and participate in usual activities except strenuous sports. Long hospitalizations should be avoided. Children with residual handicaps need help in vocational planning for the future.

ANKYLOSING SPONDYLITIS

Ankylosing spondylitis is characterized by stiffness and pain in the back, with involvement of sacroiliac joints and variable progression to joints and periarticular tissues of the lumbodorsal and cervical spine. About half of patients also have arthritis of peripheral joints. It is usually a disease of young and middle-aged adults, but may begin in childhood, usually in males over 6 years of age. A striking association of ankylosing spondylitis with HLA antigen W27 has recently been demonstrated. The pathology of synovial tissue from affected synovial joints is similar to that of rheumatoid arthritis.

Clinically ankylosing spondylitis differs from rheumatoid arthritis in several respects: (1) characteristic involvement of sacroiliac joints and lumbodorsal spine, (2) predilection for males, (3) rarity of rheumatoid factor in affected adults, (4) extreme rarity of rheumatoid nodules, (5) high frequency of acute iridocyclitis, (6) occurrence of aortitis with resulting aortic insufficiency, and (7) significant familial incidence.

CLINICAL MANIFESTATIONS. Peripheral arthritis may be the first manifestation; large joints, particularly those of the lower extremities, are affected most frequently. Heel pain is common. Shoulders, feet and temporomandibular joints are also involved in a significant number of patients. Affected joints may be warm, swollen and painful. Peripheral arthritis is often transient.

Characteristic involvement of sacroiliac joints and lumbodorsal spine may be present at the onset of disease or appear months to years later. Pain in the low back, hip girdles and thighs is characteristic. The pain is often transient, more severe at night and relieved by moving about. Stiffness in the low back, with loss of normal spinal mobility, follows (Fig. 9–23). Spinal involvement characteristically begins in the sacroiliac joints and proceeds in an ascending fashion, involving the lumbar, the dorsal and, finally, the cervical spine. In contrast,

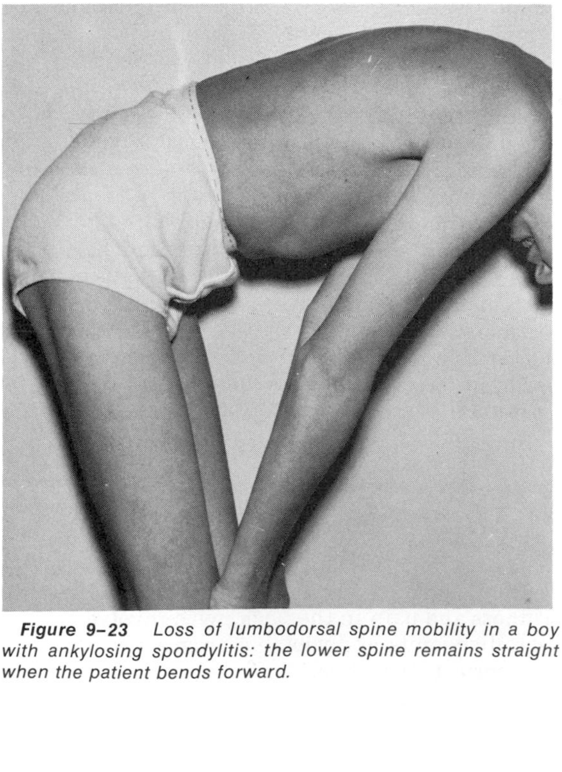

Figure 9–23 *Loss of lumbodorsal spine mobility in a boy with ankylosing spondylitis: the lower spine remains straight when the patient bends forward.*

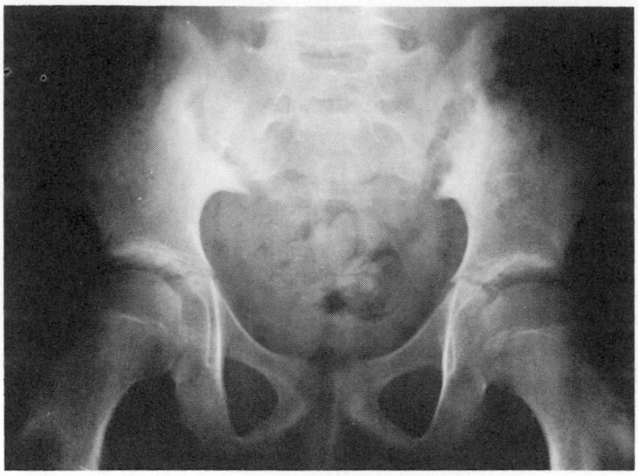

Figure 9–24 *Well developed sacroiliitis in a boy with ankylosing spondylitis; both sacroiliac joints show extensive sclerosis, erosions of joint margins and apparent widening of the joint space.*

in JRA the neck is involved but the lumbodorsal spine spared. Decreased expansion of the chest, related to involvement of costovertebral joints, may occur early in disease. Low-grade fever, anemia, anorexia, fatigability and growth retardation may occur.

Ankylosing spondylitis may arrest at any stage, or the entire spine may become involved over a number of years, with loss of virtually all vertebral mobility. Prognosis for functional outcome is usually good if good posture is maintained. Deformity of peripheral joints is uncommon, although some patients develop destructive hip disease. Acute iridocyclitis occurs in about 25 per cent of patients at some time; aortitis has not been described in children but occurs in a significant number of adults with ankylosing spondylitis.

LABORATORY DATA. There are no specific laboratory tests. Sedimentation rates may be elevated. Anemia similar to that of rheumatoid arthritis occurs. However, rheumatoid factors are rarely found. Involvement of the sacroiliac joints is demonstrable radiographically (Fig. 9–24), usually within the first 3 or 4 years; destruction is progressive, with eventual obliteration of the joints. Characteristic radiographic changes in the lumbodorsal spine occur some years later in the disease.

DIFFERENTIAL DIAGNOSIS. Ankylosing spondylitis should be suspected in any child with persistent pain in hips, thighs or low back, with or without peripheral arthritis. Radiographic changes in the sacroiliac joints are necessary for diagnosis, but several years may elapse before they appear. In addition to ankylosing spondylitis, spinal cord tumors, anatomic defects or infections of vertebrae or intervertebral discs and Scheuermann's disease must be considered in any child with persistent back pain. Legg-Perthes disease and slipped capital femoral epiphysis may cause persistent hip and thigh pain. Ulcerative colitis, regional enteritis, psoriasis and Reiter syndrome may have an associated spondylitis resembling ankylosing spondylitis.

TREATMENT. The aims of therapy are to relieve pain and to maintain good posture and function. For relief of pain, salicylates may suffice. Indomethacin and phenylbutazone may be helpful, but must be used with caution in children. (Indomethacin is still considered an experimental drug in children.) Gold is not usually effective, and corticosteroid therapy is rarely, if ever, indicated. Radiation therapy is contraindicated because of possible induction of leukemia. Maintenance of good posture is essential for preservation of good function; exercises designed to promote good posture and strengthen paraspinal muscles may be employed. A firm mattress or bed board should be used for sleeping and thick pillows should be avoided.

SYSTEMIC LUPUS ERYTHEMATOSUS

Systemic lupus erythematosus (SLE), recognized clinically during the 1800's, is a systemic disease characteristically affecting many organ systems. Its natural history is unpredictable; it is often progressive, terminating in death if untreated, but may remit spontaneously or smolder for many years. Lupus in children is generally more acute and severe than in adults.

ETIOLOGY AND EPIDEMIOLOGY. The cause remains unknown. Many observations are consistent with the hypothesis that SLE is a disease of altered immune reactivity, perhaps genetically determined. Hargraves' description of the LE cell in 1948 led to the discovery of the antinuclear antibodies and to extensive studies of immunologic mechanisms in this disease. Recent studies, including the finding of virus-like particles in tissues, suggest that viruses may play a role in pathogenesis. A variety of immune phenomena occur. Serum levels of immunoglobulins are increased. Antibodies are found which react with various nuclear constituents (the antinuclear antibodies), ribonucleic acid, gamma globulin (rheumatoid factors), red blood cells (positive Coombs test), platelets, white blood cells, antigens used in serologic tests for syphilis (false positive serology) and coagulation factors. Recent studies have shown an association between inflammation and circulating immune complexes, particularly complexes of deoxyribonucleic acid (DNA) and antibodies reactive with DNA. Such immune complexes are deposited in tissues, fix complement and initiate in inflammatory response that results in tissue injury. In SLE nephritis, for example, immunoglobulins and complement can be demonstrated in renal tissues by immunofluorescent techniques, and DNA and anti-DNA antibodies eluted from affected glomeruli; active SLE with nephritis is associated with circulating antibodies reactive with DNA and decreased levels of serum complement.

The onset of SLE or exacerbations of disease may appear related to intercurrent infections; it is suspected that there is increased susceptibility to infections, perhaps on the basis of faulty immune mechanisms. Available evidence, including recent studies showing decreased numbers of thymus-dependent cells in patients with SLE, suggests that an immunodeficiency state may underlie the disease. SLE is sometimes familial and has occurred in identical twins; hypergammaglobulinemia, antinuclear antibodies and other immune abnormalities have been found in relatives of lupus patients.

Lupus-like disease has been reported following exposure to a number of drugs, notably hydralazine, sulfonamides, procainamide and anticonvulsants. Drug-induced disease is generally mild and reversible when the inciting drug is withdrawn. Cutaneous manifestations of SLE, and sometimes systemic manifestations, may be exacerbated by sunlight.

The incidence is not known but the disease is not rare. SLE begins in childhood in 20 per cent of cases, usually in children over 8 years of age. Females are predominantly affected (8:1) in all age groups. All races may be affected.

PATHOLOGY. Changes occur at multiple sites and involve many organ systems. The presence of masses of amorphous, purple-staining extracellular material in hematoxylin-stained affected tissues is characteristic. These "hematoxylin bodies" probably represent degenerated cell nuclei and are considered similar to the inclusions of LE cells. Fibrinoid, an acellular, deeply eosinophilic material, is found in loose connective tissue or in walls of blood vessels of affected tissues. This substance, of uncertain composition, is not specific for SLE. Fibrinoid deposition is usually accompanied by an inflammatory cell reaction, predominantly with mononuclear cells. In the spleen, perivascular fibrosis about affected vessels results in characteristic "onion ring" lesions. Granulomas are sometimes found in affected tissues.

The renal pathology is described under Nephritis in Systemic Lupus Erythematosus in Section 15.

CLINICAL MANIFESTATIONS. The disease may begin insidiously or acutely. Sometimes symptoms antedate the diagnosis of SLE by years. The most frequent early symptoms in children are fever, malaise, arthritis or arthralgia, and rash. Fever occurs at some time in most affected children; it may be intermittent or sustained. Malaise, anorexia, weight loss and debility are common.

Cutaneous manifestations occur in most affected children at some time. The "butterfly" rash (Fig. 9–25), an erythematous blush or scaly erythematous patches, involves the malar areas and usually extends over the bridge of the nose. The rash may be photosensitive, may spread to the face, scalp, neck, chest and extremities, and may become bullous and secondarily infected. *Discoid lupus* (cutaneous manifestations only) is unusual in children. There are also other skin eruptions. Erythematous macules and punctate lesions on the palms, soles and fingertips are distinctive; such lesions are secondary to vascular changes, and local infarction of tissue may occur. Raynaud's phenomenon may be present. Vascular changes are seen at times in the nail beds. Macular and ulcerative lesions also occur on the palate and mucous membranes of the mouth and nose. Purpura, sometimes associated with thrombocytopenia, may appear on dependent or traumatized areas. Erythema nodosum or erythema multiforme are occasionally associated. Alopecia, from inflammation about hair follicles, may be patchy or generalized, and the hair coarse, dry and brittle.

Arthralgia and joint stiffness are common and often occur without objective changes. Sometimes affected joints are warm and swollen, but persistent deforming arthritis is rare. Aseptic necrosis of bone, particularly in the femoral heads, has been described, presumably secondary to vasculitis. Tenosynovitis and myositis may occur.

Polyserositis with pleurisy, pericarditis and peritonitis is characteristic. Hepatosplenomegaly and generalized lymphadenopathy are common. Cardiac involvement may be manifested by variable murmurs, friction rubs, cardiomegaly, electrocardiographic changes or congestive heart failure, with myocarditis, pericarditis or verrucous endocarditis (Libman-Sacks endocarditis) found at postmortem examination. Parenchymal lung infiltrates may occur; infection must be excluded, however, before pneumonia can be ascribed to SLE. Involvement of the nervous system may cause personality changes, seizures, cerebral vascular accidents and peripheral neuritis. Gastrointestinal manifestations include abdominal pain, vomiting, diarrhea, melena and even bowel infarction secondary to vasculitis. Ocular changes may include episcleritis, iritis or retinal vascular changes with hemorrhages or exudates (cytoid bodies).

Most children have clinical renal involvement. (See Nephritis in Systemic Lupus Erythematosus, Section 15.)

LABORATORY DATA. Antinuclear antibodies are demonstrable in all patients with active SLE and provide the best screening test for the disease. The antinuclear antibodies are a group of antibodies reacting with various nuclear constituents, including deoxyribonucleic acid (DNA) and deoxyribonucleoprotein (DNP), and are generally detected by immunofluorescent techniques. Antibodies to DNP are present in virtually all patients with SLE, but may be found also in rheumatoid arthritis and other diseases; these antibodies reactive with DNP cause the LE cell phenomenon. LE cells result when damaged cell nuclei coated with antibody to DNP are phagocytosed by neutrophils. Since relatively high titers of IgG antibody are necessary for the formation of LE cells, they are not invariably demonstrable in SLE patients, and are thus not a reliable screening test for the disease. Antibodies to DNA are relatively specific for SLE and are associated with active disease, and particularly with nephritis; DNA antibodies thus provide a useful index of severity and activity. Serum hemolytic complement and some of its components (C3 is most frequently measured) are decreased in patients with severe active SLE, particularly in those with nephritis; measurement of serum complement therefore provides another useful guide. Other antibodies may be demonstrated by a biologic false-positive test for syphilis or a positive Coombs test. Serum gamma globulin levels are usually elevated; alpha-2 globulin levels may be increased and albumin decreased. One or more of the individual immunoglobulins may be elevated.

Anemia, related to chronic inflammatory disease or hemolysis, is common. Difficulties in typing and crossmatching blood may arise from the presence of erythrocyte antibodies. Thrombocytopenia and leukopenia occur frequently. Platelet antibodies may be demonstrable; idiopathic thrombocytopenia purpura may be the first manifestation of SLE. The urine may contain red cells, white cells, protein and casts. Renal insufficiency is manifest by elevation of the blood urea nitrogen or creatinine and abnormal renal function studies.

PROGNOSIS. SLE has generally been considered a potentially or even uniformly fatal disease, particularly in children. Now, however, some children with milder disease are being recognized, and it is apparent that not all children with SLE have severe nephritis. Although spontaneous exacerbations and remissions of SLE occur, prolonged spontaneous remission appears unusual in children. Antibiotic and corticosteroid therapy prolong survival and improve the overall prognosis. The major cause of death in SLE is nephritis (Section 15); CNS complications and infections are also significant causes of morbidity. Whether the ultimate prognosis of severe lupus can be modified by vigorous drug therapy remains to be determined.

DIAGNOSIS AND DIFFERENTIAL DIAGNOSIS. SLE may mimic any rheumatic disease and many other diseases as well. Diagnosis is clinical and is confirmed by laboratory tests. Antinuclear antibodies are always present in patients with active SLE; even though they are not diagnostic, their absence makes the diagnosis unlikely. Antibodies to DNA are virtually diagnostic of SLE, but are present only in severe or widespread disease. LE cells are not always demonstrable. Hypergammaglobulinemia, elevated serum immunoglobulins, positive Coombs test, biologic false-positive test for syphilis, anemia, leukopenia or thrombocytopenia, and signs of nephritis may also be diagnostically helpful. Serum hemolytic complement and some of its components are lowered in some patients with active disease, particularly in those with nephritis. Renal biopsy may confirm the diagnosis, but histologic changes are not entirely specific. Thrombocytopenic purpura and hemolytic anemia may be presenting features; the differential diagnosis of these manifestations should include SLE.

THERAPY. Therapy of SLE should be based on the extent and severity of disease in the individual patient. Patients must be thoroughly evaluated, particularly for renal involvement. The type and severity of the renal lesion should be determined by renal biopsy on patients with clinical evidence of nephritis. Since decreased serum complement levels and circulating antibodies to DNA are associated with severe SLE, and particularly with active lupus nephritis, their determination is important in evaluation and follow-up of patients. There is no specific therapy; drugs used to treat the disease suppress inflammation and perhaps suppress the formation of immune complexes (although the latter mechanism remains unproved). In general, patients should be treated to maintain clinical well-being and normal serum complement levels.

In patients with mild SLE without nephritis, salicylates should be used to provide symptomatic relief of arthritis and other discomforts. Careful follow-up for possible development of nephritis is important. Chloroquine and hydroxychloroquine have long been used in discoid and systemic lupus, but extreme care must be taken because of retinal toxicity. Topical steroid preparations may suppress the facial rash. Corticosteroids in doses sufficient to suppress symptoms may be required. In patients with SLE and mild renal disease (viz., lupus glomerulitis), therapy is also symptomatic, with careful follow-up. Doses of corticosteroids sufficient to suppress symptoms should be given initially (1–2 mg/kg/day may be required) and then tapered to the lowest suppressive dose. Chloroquine may be a useful adjunctive drug. In patients with SLE and severe nephritis (lupus glomerulonephritis or membranous glomerulonephritis with the nephrotic syndrome) therapy must be geared to maintain not only clinical well-being of the patient but also suppression of the renal disease, as reflected by return of serum complement levels to normal and reduction of circulating antibodies to DNA. Large doses of corticosteroids for prolonged periods may be required; initial doses of 1–2 mg prednisone/kg/day are usual. All the undesirable side effects of steroid therapy may be expected if large doses are required for any significant period of time. Recent studies suggest possible effectiveness of agents such as azathioprine and cyclophosphamide in suppressing severe SLE; such therapy remains experimental and must be used with extreme care. Little is known of the long-term effects of such drugs, particularly in children; side effects include increased susceptibility to severe viral and other infections, gonadal suppression and possible induction of malignancies. Such agents should never be used in mild SLE, or in patients whose disease can be satisfactorily controlled with corticosteroids alone.

Seizures and other central nervous system manifestations of SLE should be treated with large doses of prednisone; they are generally associated with severe active disease. CNS disease occurs episodically in SLE and may never recur if the patient is tided over the acute episode and the disease can be subsequently controlled.

Because of the possibility of drug-induced disease, inquiry should be made about possible offending agents; drugs known to be associated with SLE should not be used in patients with the disease.

Meticulous follow-up is of paramount importance in the treatment of all patients with SLE; this requires monitoring of clinical, renal and serologic status. Any signs of worsening disease should be promptly recognized and appropriately managed. Since there is no cure, the disease is potentially life-long, and patients must be followed for years.

LUPUS PHENOMENA IN THE NEWBORN PERIOD

Infants of mothers with SLE may have transient manifestations of lupus in the newborn period, presumably mediated by transplacental factors. Transiently positive antinuclear antibody tests or LE cells are the most frequent abnormalities; there are generally no associated clinical manifestations, and the serologic abnormalities regress after several weeks. The most frequent clinical abnormality of infants born to mothers with SLE is a skin rash that is clinically and histologically typical of lupus and fades over a period of several months. Transient thrombocytopenia related to transplacental platelet antibodies has been noted, as have transient hemolytic anemia and leukopenia. Endocardial fibroelastosis has been recorded in infants of mothers with SLE. Few if any cases of true SLE in infants have been reported.

VASCULITIS SYNDROMES

In these syndromes of inflammation of blood vessels the various patterns of disease depend on the size and location of affected vessels. When small nonmuscular vessels are involved, the disease takes the form of Schönlein-Henoch vasculitis (anaphylactoid purpura). With involvement of larger muscular arteries the disease is called polyarteritis nodosa; many variants have been described, including infantile polyarteritis and Wegener's granulomatosis. Some overlap of these syndromes occurs; it is reasonable to expect that vessels of various sizes may sometimes be involved in the same patients. In Takayasu's arteritis the aorta and other great vessels are sites of inflammation.

Inflammation of blood vessels occurs also in other rheumatic disease in children, notably lupus erythematosus, dermatomyositis and scleroderma; in hypertension; and in vessels exposed to local infection, trauma or thromboemboli.

The causes of these disorders are unknown. Both Schönlein-Henoch vasculitis and polyarteritis may follow exposure to drugs or allergens. In serum sickness, a usually self-limited type of vasculitis occurring after exposure to foreign substances, vasculitis is caused by deposition of immune complexes. Recently several cases of polyarteritis nodosa have been associated with Australia antigen, vascular damage presumably being caused by immune complexes of Australia antigen and its antibody. In contrast to most other rheumatic diseases, Schönlein-Henoch vasculitis and polyarteritis nodosa predominantly affect males. In childhood Schönlein-Henoch vasculitis is the most commonly encountered type; polyarteritis and its variants are extremely rare in children.

SCHÖNLEIN-HENOCH VASCULITIS

(Anaphylactoid, Allergic or Rheumatoid Purpura)

This distinctive syndrome was described by William Heberden before 1800; Schönlein in the 1830's described the typical rash in association with joint manifestations, and Henoch in the 1870's recognized the association of gastrointestinal and renal manifestations. Osler pointed out the similarity between this disease and the hypersensitivity reactions, erythema multiforme and serum sickness. The skin lesion, which is not always purpuric, is the most obvious sign; the visceral lesions are less easily recognized, but are far more serious. The primary manifestations are due to vasculitis of small blood vessels.

The cause is unknown. Allergy or drug sensitivity seem to play a role in some cases. The disease may follow an upper respiratory tract infection, sometimes streptococcal, but this is of uncertain significance. The syndrome is not rare and may occur at any age; it is more common in children than in adults, most cases occurring in the age range from 2 to 8 years. Boys are affected twice as often as girls.

PATHOLOGY. In the skin small vessels of the corium are surrounded with an acute inflammatory exudate of polymorphonuclear and round cells; eosinophils and varying numbers of red blood cells may be present. Capillaries are most frequently involved, but small arterioles and venules may be affected. Scattered nuclear debris, edema and swelling of collagen fibrils are found adjacent to affected vessels.

For the pathology of the renal lesion, see the Nephritis of Anaphylactoid Purpura in Section 15.

There is a paucity of data on histologic changes in other organs, but inflammation or hemorrhage may occur at other sites, notably in synovium, the gastrointestinal tract and the central nervous system.

CLINICAL MANIFESTATIONS. Onset may be acute, with simultaneous appearance of several manifestations, or gradual, with sequential appearance of different manifestations over a period of weeks. Various combinations of symptoms and signs may occur. Malaise and low-grade fever are present in half the patients.

Skin lesions are present in all identified patients; it is not known whether visceral manifestations occur in the absence of rash. The lesions usually appear on the lower extremities, but may involve buttocks, upper extremities, trunk and face as well (Fig. 9–26). Dermatologic manifestations are extremely variable. The classic lesion begins as a small wheal or an erythematous maculopapule. Lesions initially blanch on pressure, but later lose this ability and generally become petechial or purpuric. Purpuric areas progress in the usual manner of ecchymoses, changing from red to purple, becoming rusty and eventually fading. Skin lesions appear in crops, and at any time a variety may be present. In addition to these characteristic lesions, the various patterns of erythema multiforme and erythema nodosum may occur. Such rashes are rarely pruritic. Angioneurotic edema involving the scalp, eyelids, lips, dorsa of the hands and feet, back and perineum is common and may be striking, especially in young children. Rarely an entire limb segment, such as the forearm, may be transiently swollen and tender.

Arthritis occurs in two thirds of affected children. Large joints, particularly knees and ankles, are most commonly involved. Affected joints may be swollen, tender and painful on motion. Effusions may be present; joint fluid is serous, with leukocytosis, not hemorrhagic. Joint symptoms usually resolve after a few days without residual deformity or articular damage, but may recur during the period of active disease.

Gastrointestinal symptoms appear in two thirds of affected children. The most common complaint is colicky abdominal pain, which may be severe and is often associated with vomiting. Stools show gross or occult blood in over half of patients, and hematemesis may occur. Failure to recognize this syndrome in children with sudden onset of acute abdominal pain may lead to unnecessary laparotomy. In such cases peritoneal exudate and enlarged mesenteric lymph nodes are usually found; segmental edema and hemorrhage into bowel wall may be present. Gastrointestinal radiographs may show decreased motility and segmental narrowing, presumably related to submucosal edema and hemorrhage. Rarely intussusception, obstruction or infarction and perforation of bowel may occur.

Renal involvement is potentially the most serious manifestation, since it can result in chronic renal disease. It occurs in 25 to 50 per cent of children during the acute phase, the frequency depending in part on the adequacy of examination. It is usually manifest during the first few weeks of illness, but sometimes appears after other manifestations have become quiescent. Moderate azotemia and hypertension, and even oliguria and hypertensive encephalopathy, can occur. Most children with renal involvement recover, although some continue to have abnormal urinary sediment, with or without abnormal renal function; a few suffer chronic renal disease within a few years of the acute phase. See also Section 15.

A rare but potentially serious manifestation is central nervous system involvement, with seizures, pareses and coma. Hepatosplenomegaly and lymphadenopathy may occur during acute phases of the disease. Rarely intramuscular hemorrhage, rheumatoid-like nodules, cardiac involvement, eye involvement or testicular swelling and hemorrhage have been reported.

Prognosis is excellent in the absence of significant renal disease. The course is variable. Often the disease is mild, lasting a few days and manifest only by transient arthritis and a few purpuric spots. In more seriously affected children the average duration is 4 to 6 weeks, but subsequent exacerbations and remissions may occur. Sometimes the illness may smolder for one or more years.

LABORATORY DATA. Laboratory tests are not diagnostic. The sedimentation rate may be elevated. The white blood cell count is often increased, and eosinophilia may be present. Coagulation studies are normal. With renal involvement red cells, white cells, casts and albumin are present in the urine. There may be gross or occult blood in the stools. Lupus erythematosus cells, rheumatoid factor and antinuclear antibodies are not associated. Serum complement titers are normal or elevated. Serum levels of IgA immunoglobulin may be elevated.

DIAGNOSIS AND DIFFERENTIAL DIAGNOSIS. The full-blown picture of Schönlein-Henoch vasculitis with rash, arthritis and gastrointestinal and renal manifestations is characteristic. However, diagnostic confusion may result when one symptom predominates or multiple system involvement is not recognized. The rash may suggest a hemorrhagic diathesis or septicemia; platelet counts, blood clotting tests and cultures will exclude these possibilities. In addition, the patient with septicemia usually appears more acutely ill. When gastrointestinal manifestations predominate, the syndrome may suggest a number of intra-abdominal emergencies. The possibility of Schönlein-Henoch vasculitis should be considered in any child with acute abdominal pain, and inquiry made for associated rash, nephritis or arthritis. With prominent renal findings, acute glomerulonephritis may be suggested; the presence of other manifestations of Schönlein-Henoch vasculitis should allow differentiation. In children with chronic renal disease a history of acute Schönlein-Henoch vasculitis in the past should be sought. Differentiation from other rheumatic diseases is rarely difficult. In polyarteritis nodosa, peripheral neurologic changes and cardiac manifestations are more common, but clinical distinction from Schönlein-Henoch vasculitis may occasionally be difficult.

PROGNOSIS. During the acute phase, death may rarely occur from gastrointestinal complications (massive hemorrhage, intussusception, bowel infarction), acute renal failure or central nervous system involvement. Chronic renal disease may cause later morbidity in a few patients. About 25 per cent of children with initial renal involvement have persistence of abnormal urine sediment for years; the eventual outcome for these patients is not known.

TREATMENT. There is no specific therapy. In the rare instance in which a specific allergen can be proved, the patient should be kept from contact with it. When the disease seems to follow a bacterial infection, particularly streptcococcal, the organism should be eliminated and, if the disease recurs, prophylaxis considered. Symptomatic treatment only is indicated for arthritis, rash, edema, fever and malaise. Salicylates will often alleviate these self-limited discomforts.

In the acute phase intestinal hemorrhage, obstruction or perforation may be life-threatening; these complications may perhaps be prevented by the early use of corticosteroids. Therapy with prednisone in dosage of 1 to 2 mg/kg/day is often associated with dramatic improvement. Corticosteroid therapy is also indicated in the rare instances of central nervous system manifestations. Steroids do not, however, seem to affect renal involvement in the acute phase, nor prevent chronic renal disease. Acute renal failure should be managed as in acute glomerulonephritis. Therapy of severe nephritis with drugs such as azathioprine and cyclophosphamide remains experimental. (See Section 15.)

POLYARTERITIS NODOSA

Medium-sized and small arteries are the sites of inflammation in polyarteritis nodosa. The disease can affect all age groups but is rare in childhood. Males are affected more frequently than females. As with Schönlein-Henoch vasculitis, the cause is not known, but the disease has been reported to follow drug exposures, and Australia antigen has been associated with a few cases. Pathologically lesions are characteristically located in medium-sized vessels; smaller vessels may be involved as well. Inflammation, with polymorphonuclear leukocytes, eosinophils and round cells, may involve the entire vessel wall. Necrosis, thrombosis or aneurysm formation may occur in affected vessels and result in infarction. Healed vessels become scarred or recanalized.

Clinical manifestations are diverse and depend on sites of vascular involvement. Signs of systemic illness, such as fever, anorexia, lethargy, weakness and loss of weight, are usually present. Arthralgia and arthritis are frequent; myalgia and myositis may be present. Various cutaneous manifestations are common and include erythematous rashes, nodular lesions, petechiae and purpuric spots, cutaneous ulcers and edema. Rarely, gangrene of extremities occurs. Peripheral neuropathy with pain, numbness, paresthesias and muscle weakness results from involvement of peripheral nerves adjacent to affected vessels. Abdominal pain, bleeding, ulcerations and infarction can follow involvement of gastrointestinal vessels. Renal involvement is a potentially serious manifestation which may result in kidney failure and death. Involvement of large renal vessels results in flank pain and gross hematuria, that of small vessels and glomeruli causes microscopic hematuria, proteinuria and cylindruria. Associated hypertension is usual. Inflammation of pulmonary vessels may cause cough, wheezing, pulmonary infiltrates and pleuritis. Central nervous system manifestations include seizures, encephalitic symptoms and stroke. Cranial nerve palsies may occur. Hepatosplenomegaly is common. Involvement of coronary vessels may produce tachycardia, congestive heart failure and myocardial infarction; pericarditis may also be present. Orchitis and epididymitis are common. Iridocyclitis may occur.

There are no specific laboratory tests. The sedimentation rate may be elevated and acute phase reactants present. Anemia is common; eosinophilia is sometimes found. There may be gross or microscopic hematuria, and renal function studies may be deranged.

Polyarteritis nodosa is readily confused with many other diseases. Differentiation from other rheumatic diseases may be particularly difficult. The diagnosis is based primarily on clinical suspicion and on histologic changes in involved tissues on biopsy. Muscle biopsies may fail to identify vasculitis. Testicular biopsies are said to be helpful, but are seldom done. Arteriograms of liver or kidney may be diagnostically helpful. The diagnosis in children is probably most frequently made at autopsy.

The prognosis is poor; death can occur from renal failure, heart failure or severe gastrointestinal or central nervous system disease. Corticosteroids may suppress acute manifestations of the disease and effectively lengthen survival. Certainly a trial of steroid therapy in doses sufficient to suppress symptoms is indicated with severe disease. Long-term therapy may be required.

Infantile Polyarteritis

Polyarteritis in infants less than 1 year of age, though rare, presents a rather characteristic clinical pattern. Both sexes are affected. The cause is not known, but as in other forms of vasculitis, this disease has been reported in association with drug exposure (sulfonamides, penicillin). There is also a suggestive relation to immunization and to viral and bacterial illnesses. Pathologic changes are similar to those of polyarteritis in older patients; fibrinoid necrosis of vessels is said to be less prominent.

The disease usually begins with a combination of fever, rhinitis, conjunctivitis and macular erythematous rash, suggesting an acute viral infection, but the illness persists. Involvement of the coronary arteries has been the predominant manifestation in most reported cases, resulting in tachycardia, cardiomegaly, congestive heart failure or pericarditis. The electrocardiogram may show right, left or combined ventricular hypertrophy, as well as evidence of myocardial ischemia or infarction. At autopsy, aneurysms of coronary arteries are frequently found, as well as myocardial infarcts and pericarditis. Aneurysms may perforate, causing hemopericardium.

Other reported manifestations include renal involvement (abnormal urinary sediment), hypertension, decreased blood pressure in or ischemia of an extremity, central nervous system manifestations (nuchal rigidity, pareses, cranial nerve palsies, seizures), hepatosplenomegaly, lymphadenopathy, gastrointestinal symptoms and cough. Involvement of vessels in skeletal muscle is apparently uncommon, and muscle biopsy is of little diagnostic usefulness. At autopsy widespread arteritis involving many organs has been found.

There are no specific laboratory tests. The white blood cell count is often elevated, with eosinophilia; sedimentation rates may be high. Diagnosis is usually made at autopsy, although awareness of this syndrome should permit presumptive clinical diagnosis.

The prognosis is very poor, all reported cases having terminated in death within an average of 1 month after onset. Death is usually sudden or related to progressive cardiac decompensation.

No satisfactory treatment has been found, but corticosteroid therapy appears worthy of trial.

WEGENER'S GRANULOMATOSIS
(Lethal Midline Granuloma)

Wegener's granulomatosis is a rare syndrome in which destructive granulomatous lesions of the upper respiratory tract and lungs are associated with a systemic necrotizing vasculitis, most prominent in lungs and kidneys. The upper respiratory and pulmonary granulomas may predominate in some cases, antedating recognition of systemic vasculitis by years. Limited forms of this syndrome, with only upper respiratory or pulmonary involvement, may occur. Males are predominantly affected (2 to 1). The cause is not known; as in other vasculitis syndromes, an association with drug sensitivity and allergy has been noted.

Respiratory symptoms are prominent. Persistent nasal discharge may be an early symptom, with crusted or pustular lesions in the nares. Lesions are progressively destructive and may result in perforation of the nasal septum, obliteration of nasal sinuses and ulcerations of the palate, pharynx, larynx and trachea. Pulmonary symptoms of cough or hemoptysis occur, and fever and prostration are common. Associated in most instances are other manifestations such as arthritis, neuropathy, rash, splenomegaly and severe progressive glomerulitis often terminating in renal failure. In cases with clinically inapparent systemic involvement, diffuse vasculitis may yet be found on postmortem examination.

There are no specific laboratory findings; eosinophilia may be present. Roentgenograms may reveal bone destruction in the nose and sinuses and pulmonary infiltrates suggestive of tuberculosis or neoplasm. Urinalyses usually show evidence of nephritis, and renal function studies may be abnormal.

Diagnosis is based on the clinical picture and confirmed by histologic demonstration of granulomatous lesions of the respiratory tract and systemic vasculitis, particularly nephritis. The prognosis is poor. Patients with more limited forms of the disease may survive for long periods of time, but the destructive lesions of the upper respiratory tract may be extremely disfiguring.

No curative treatment is known, but corticosteroids may suppress systemic vasculitis and prevent progression of destructive lesions in the upper respiratory tract. Recent evidence suggests that therapy with drugs such as azathioprine and cyclophosphamide may arrest the disease in some patients.

TAKAYASU'S ARTERITIS
("Pulseless Disease")

This uncommon condition, an inflammatory process involving the aorta and its major branches, occurs primarily in young women. Some cases have been reported in late childhood, a few in infants. Most reported cases have been from Asia or Africa. The cause is unknown; associated congenital defects of great vessels have been recorded.

The underlying pathology is a segmental panarteritis of the aorta and its major branches. Smaller vessels are spared. Aneurysmal dilatation and rupture may occur. Involvement of the great vessels can cause weak or absent pulses in the upper extremities—hence, "pulseless disease." Blood pressure in the legs may exceed that in the arms, the opposite of coarctation of the aorta. Renal arterial involvement may cause renal ischemia, resulting in hypertension. Decreased brain blood flow can result in neurologic disturbances. Visual disturbances are common in older patients.

Various rheumatic complaints including arthritis, myalgia, pleuritis, pericarditis, fever and rashes have been associated, sometimes antedating the symptomatic aortitis by years. There are no specific laboratory data. Sedimentation rates and gamma globulin levels may be elevated; positive LE preparations have been reported. Angiography may demonstrate changes in affected vessels.

The condition should be considered in any child with obscure hypertension, particularly when fever and an elevated sedimentation rate are associated. The prognosis is variable. Some adults have survived; most children have died. No specific therapy is known. Corticosteroids have been used. Endarterectomy or nephrectomy may be warranted.

DERMATOMYOSITIS

Dermatomyositis is a multisystem disease characterized principally by nonsuppurative inflammation of striated muscle. Affected children usually have characteristic associated cutaneous lesions. Adults may have polymyositis without skin manifestations.

ETIOLOGY AND EPIDEMIOLOGY. The cause of dermatomyositis is unknown. Recent studies suggest that cellular immune mechanisms play a basic role in pathogenesis. Lymphocytes from patients with dermatomyositis release lymphotoxins and kill muscle cells in tissue culture. Immunoglobulin and complement deposition have also been described in vessels in affected muscle. In adults, but not children, there is a frequent (20 per cent of cases) association with malignancies, chiefly carcinomas.

Dermatomyositis is less common than rheumatoid arthritis, systemic lupus erythematosus or Schönlein-Henoch vasculitis. It rarely begins before the second year of life. Girls are affected more frequently than boys (3:2). There seems to be no familial or racial predilection.

PATHOLOGY. Biopsy is not generally necessary for diagnosis but may provide supportive evidence. Lesions in skin, subcutaneous tissues and muscles are irregularly distributed; care must be taken to choose an involved site for biopsy. The most prominent lesion in children appears to be a vasculitis involving arterioles, venules and capillaries in connective tissues of skin, subcutaneous tissue and muscle. In muscle there is patchy degeneration, atrophy and regeneration of muscle fibers, interstitial edema and proliferation of connective tissue. In affected skin there is thinning of the epidermis, and edema and vasculitis in the dermis. In the chronic phase, calcium deposits with surrounding inflammation may occur in skin, subcutaneous tissue and muscle. In the gastrointestinal tract, vasculitis may result in mucosal ulcerations and tissue infarction. Mild renal glomerular changes have been described.

CLINICAL MANIFESTATIONS. Onset is usually insidious, with slowly developing muscle weakness, generally first apparent in proximal muscles of the extremities and trunk. The child may develop an awkward gait and slowly lose capacity for functions such as climbing stairs, riding a bicycle and dressing. Affected muscles tend to be stiff and sore and sometimes brawny, indurated and tender. Nonpitting edema and thickening of skin and subcutaneous tissues may be present. Although myositis is generally most pronounced in proximal muscles, any muscles can be affected, with varying sites and degrees of atrophy. Severe involvement of palatorespiratory muscles may lead to respiratory difficulty, aspiration and death. Arthralgia and arthritis sometimes occur.

The skin lesions are characteristic and often have a distinctive violaceous hue. The upper eyelids assume a pathognomonic violaceous discoloration (heliotrope eyelids) (Fig. 9–27). Periorbital and facial edema may be associated. A butterfly rash similar to SLE may be present. Lesions of palatal and nasal mucous membranes may occur in association with the malar rash. The skin over extensor surfaces of joints, particularly the knuckles, knees and elbows, becomes erythematous, atrophic and scaly (Fig. 9–28). These areas later develop pigmentary changes, resulting in hyperpigmentation or vitiligo. A dusky erythema may cover the upper trunk and proximal extremities. Other nonspecific skin changes may also occur. The skin over involved extremities may appear tight and glossy; in longstanding disease there may be cutaneous atrophy with binding of skin to underlying structures. Calcium may be deposited in affected subcutaneous tissues, muscles and fascia; these deposits sometimes break down and extrude in semisolid or solid form.

Low-grade fever is often present, and other evidence of systemic involvement such as lymphadenopathy, hepatosplenomegaly and gastrointestinal manifestations may occur.

In untreated cases the fatality rate is about 40 per cent. Most deaths are related to palatorespiratory involvement or such gastrointestinal complications as hemorrhage and perforation, and occur within 2 years of onset. Otherwise the disease slowly becomes inactive over a period of several years and subsequent exacerbations are unusual. Infrequently the disease may smolder for years. Most surviving patients are able to lead active lives, although they may have residual abnormalities. A few have severe contractures and crippling deformities. It is now apparent that the course of dermatomyositis can be favorably modified by early, vigorous treatment with corticosteroids and that the prognosis in adequately treated children is good.

LABORATORY DATA. Muscle inflammation is responsible for elevated serum levels of such enzymes as transaminases, creatine kinase and aldolase. The electromyogram of affected muscles is abnormal. The sedimentation rate may be elevated or normal. Tests for rheumatoid factors and antinuclear antibodies are generally negative. Urinalyses are usually normal. In patients with gastrointestinal involvement, there may be gross or occult blood in the stool. Roentgenograms may reveal calcium deposits in soft tissues.

DIAGNOSIS AND DIFFERENTIAL DIAGNOSIS. In its typical form dermatomyositis should present little diagnostic difficulty. The combination of muscle weakness and characteristic rash, elevated serum levels of enzymes, and abnormal electromyogram is diagnostic; muscle biopsy is not usually necessary. In the differential diagnosis various neuromuscular disorders such as poliomyelitis, Guillain-Barré syndrome, muscular dystrophy and myasthenia gravis should be considered, as should illnesses having predominantly muscular lesions, such as trichinosis. Transient myositis has been reported in association with influenza and may occur with other viral infections as well. Systemic lupus erythematosus, juvenile rheumatoid arthritis and scleroderma are distinguishable clinically and by laboratory tests. In the chronic phase, features of dermatomyositis and generalized scleroderma may overlap, making precise categorization difficult. When the onset is insidious, a period of observation may be needed to establish the diagnosis.

A rheumatic disease syndrome combining features of dermatomyositis, scleroderma, and SLE has recently been described and termed **mixed connective tissue disease.** Affected patients may have myositis and a dermatomyositis-like rash, as well as other manifestations including arthritis, swollen hands, Raynaud's phenomenon and abnormal esophageal motility. High titers of antinuclear antibodies (speckled pattern of nuclear immunofluorescence) and an antibody reactive with an extractable nuclear antigen are invariably present. This syndrome is probably distinct from dermatomyositis. The therapy is similar.

TREATMENT. During the acute phase, care in evaluating palatorespiratory function may be lifesaving. If swallowing mechanisms are impaired, soft or liquid diets should be provided under close observation. The patient should be closely watched for possible deterioration in respiratory function. Constant nursing care is mandatory for any child with palatorespiratory involvement, and equipment for nasopharyngeal suction, endotracheal intubation and tracheotomy should be available. A respirator may be required. The possibility of serious gastrointestinal manifestations during the acute phase of disease must also be considered.

Functional recovery depends on preservation of adequate muscle strength and prevention of crippling contractures. Corticosteroids effectively suppress the inflammatory process in most patients. Serial serum levels of transaminase, creatine kinase or aldolase provide a helpful gauge of activity and therapeutic response. Prednisone in initial dosage of 1–2 mg/kg/day (or 60 mg per square meter of body surface area per day) usually reduces enzyme levels toward normal values within 1 to 2 weeks; clinical improvement with decreased pain and swelling in muscles and increasing muscle strength usually follows. When enzyme levels have declined to normal, the steroid dosage should be slowly decreased, with continued monitoring of the clinical course and serum enzyme levels. If the dose of steroids is reduced too rapidly, rebound in enzyme levels may occur; such rebounds are followed by deterioration in the clinical condition within a few weeks unless corticosteroid dosage is promptly increased. A low dose of steroids sufficient to suppress clinical symptoms and serum enzyme levels should be found and maintained for months. Steroid therapy can generally be discontinued in 1 to 2 years. Steroid preparations such as triamcinolone and dexamethasone, which are associated with "steroid myopathy," should be avoided. Salicylates may occasionally be helpful as adjunctive drugs in relieving symptoms. Immunosuppressive agents such as methotrexate and cyclophosphamide are rarely warranted in childhood dermatomyositis.

Physical therapy is essential to avoid contractures and to rebuild muscle strength. During the acute phase when muscle weakness is pronounced, passive exercises can be used to maintain range of motion. With clinical improvement active exercises to strengthen muscles should be added. Appropriate splints to maintain good position of the limbs may be needed. Bed rest is not necessary, and immobilization without exercise is to be avoided at all times. Skin hygiene, especially around the neck, skin creases and axillae, is important.

SCLERODERMA

Scleroderma ("hard skin") is a chronic inflammatory disturbance of connective tissue which classically involves skin, but may also affect the gastrointestinal tract, heart, lung, kidney and synovium. Cutaneous involvement, the hallmark of the disease, may occur either in focal patches (morphea) or in a generalized, symmetric distribution. The latter is usually associated with systemic involvement (progressive systemic sclerosis) and is the usual form seen in adults. Scleroderma in children usually has a patchy, focal distribution (morphea); systemic involvement is uncommon.

The disease is rare and of obscure origin. It affects girls more frequently than boys and may begin at any time during childhood. There is no familial predisposition.

Histology of affected cutaneous tissues shows increased thickness and density of dermal collagen with perivascular infiltrates of mononuclear cells.

CLINICAL MANIFESTATIONS

Morphea. The first signs are patchy lesions of skin and subcutaneous tissues. These often have a linear pattern similar to the distribution of peripheral nerves and may occur primarily on one side of the body. During the early phases, involved areas are slightly erythematous and edematous or have an atrophic, shiny appearance. The child may complain of pain or a prickly sensation. As the disease progresses, the skin lesions become indurated with violaceous, sometimes elevated borders and pale waxy-appearing centers. Lesions enlarge peripherally and may coalesce to involve an entire extremity or a large portion of the body. Extensive scarring and fibrosis of the involved area can occur, with firm binding of cutaneous tissues to underlying structures ("hide-binding"). This may be severe enough to limit growth of the affected part and produce crippling contractures (Fig. 9–29). Chronically involved areas may be hyperpigmented or depigmented. Active disease may arrest over a period of months to years, or may smolder for years. Prognosis for life is good in the absence of systemic involvement.

Progressive Systemic Sclerosis. Cutaneous involvement is symmetrical, involving hands, feet and distal extremities, and sometimes the trunk and face as well. Induration, pigmentary changes and hide-binding of involved cutaneous tissues occur as with focal forms of the disease. Raynaud's phenomenon may be associated, and cutaneous ulcers occur. The disease may involve the gastrointestinal tract, heart, lungs, kidneys and joints. Systemic manifestations, particularly renal, cardiac and pulmonary, may be fatal. Esophageal dysfunction may result in chronic aspiration penumonia.

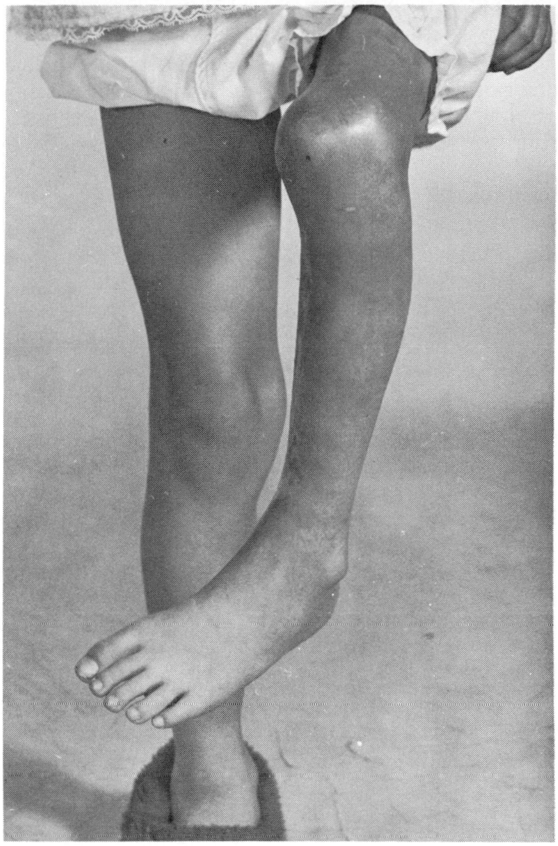

Figure 9–29 *Extensive morphea involving the entire left leg, causing scarring, shortening and flexion contractures. Note the shiny appearance and patches of hyperpigmentation and vitiligo of affected skin.*

LABORATORY DATA. There are no specific laboratory tests. The sedimentation rate is frequently normal. Rheumatoid factor and antinuclear antibodies may be found in both focal and disseminated forms of the disease. Radiographs may show dysfunction of esophageal and small bowel motility. Pulmonary function studies, electrocardiograms and chest radiographs may disclose cardiopulmonary involvement. Urinalyses and renal function studies are abnormal in the presence of renal involvement.

DIAGNOSIS. The clinical picture is characteristic in both morphea and progressive systemic sclerosis. The disease may bear some superficial resemblance to dermatomyositis, but absence of myositis and the characteristic rash of dermatomyositis should allow differentiation. Subcutaneous fat necrosis and Weber-Christian nonsuppurative panniculitis may be suggested in morphea, but the course and histology are distinctive. **Scleredema adultorum**, a self-limited benign induration of subcutaneous tissues, occurs acutely, sometimes following streptococcal infection; subcutaneous tissues of the neck, upper trunk and arms become indurated, but skin is spared.

TREATMENT. No specific therapy is known. Many therapeutic agents, including corticosteroids, salicylates, chelating agents, chloroquine, radiation, dimethyl sulfoxide, para-aminobenzoic acid and penicillamine, have been tried without clear-cut benefit. Surgical excision of local patches of morphea does not arrest the process. Systemic therapy with corticosteroids may be tried for severe systemic disease. Topical corticosteroids have been used for morphea. Vigorous physical therapy is important early in the course of morphea to prevent or minimize crippling contractures.

ERYTHEMA MULTIFORME EXUDATIVUM

(Stevens-Johnson Syndrome)

Erythema multiforme exudativum (bullosum), characterized by lesions of skin and mucous membranes, with fever and systemic prostration, was described by Hebra and Bazin over 100 years ago.

The disease occurs in children and young adults and affects males more frequently than females. Onset often follows an upper respiratory tract infection. Evidence for a viral etiologic agent, especially herpes virus, has been inconclusive. The association of Stevens-Johnson syndrome with patchy pneumonia, increased titers of cold agglutinins and the isolation of *Mycoplasma pneumoniae* have suggested a relation to mycoplasma infection. Association of the syndrome with ingestion of drugs, including sulfonamides, anticonvulsants, penicillin and barbiturates, has also been observed. The LE phenomenon has been demonstrated in a few patients.

The hallmark of the syndrome is an erythematous papular skin lesion that enlarges by peripheral expansion and usually develops a central vesicle. This eruption may involve most cutaneous surfaces, including the palms and soles, but spares the scalp. Lesions may be scattered or confluent. New lesions appear for 1 to 2 weeks after onset. Vesiculobullous lesions also occur on mucous membranes of the conjunctivae, nares, mouth, anorectal junction, vulvovaginal region and urethral meatus. Lesions have even been described in the larynx, trachea, bronchi, bladder and gastrointestinal tract.

The rash is often preceded by fever and general malaise. Severe prostration may occur at the height of the syndrome. About one third of the affected patients have pulmonary involvement, with a harsh, hacking cough and patchy changes on the chest radiograph. Periarticular swelling has been described. Involvement of cardiovascular, and renal systems does not usually occur. As the disease process reaches its peak, the patient presents a striking picture (Fig. 9–30). Stomatitis is particularly distressing; lesions erode, ulcerate, bleed and crust. Meatal involvement may make urination painful. Conjunctivitis results in photophobia, and purulent conjunctival discharge may be profuse. Corneal ulcerations can occur with resulting scarring and even blindness.

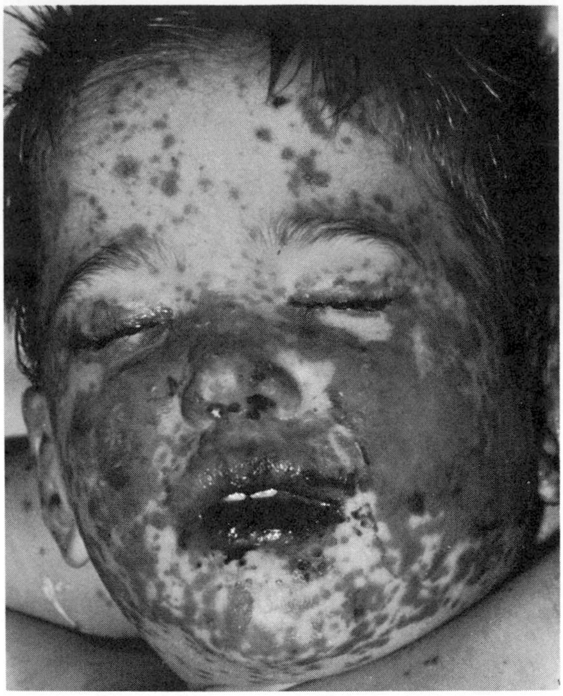

Figure 9–30 *Cutaneous, oral, nasal and conjunctival involvement in severe Stevens-Johnson syndrome.*

The mortality may be as high as 10 per cent during the acute phase, particularly in patients with pulmonary involvement. Subsequently the disease is self-limiting: skin lesions gradually subside without scarring in 1 to 4 weeks; mucous membrane lesions may persist for months. In about 20 per cent of patients the disease recurs, often in association with re-exposure to an offending drug.

During the acute phase, symptomatic treatment is of great importance. Fluid requirements are high, and intravenous administration is often required. Cutaneous hygiene should be maintained to prevent secondary infection. Ophthalmologic consultation should be sought if serious conjunctivitis is present. Prednisone, 1 to 2 mg/kg, is often used in children with serious disease. The efficacy of such therapy is not proved; it should be carefully supervised and is contraindicated whenever there is a possibility of herpetic infection of the eye. Appropriate antibiotic therapy is indicated if there is reasonable suspicion of infection with *Mycoplasma pneumoniae.*

ERYTHEMA NODOSUM

Erythema nodosum is characterized by the development of painful, indurated, shiny, red, hot, elevated, ovoid nodules 1 to 3 cm in diameter. They are most frequently distributed symmetrically over the shins (Fig. 9–31), but may also occur on the calves, thighs, buttocks and upper extremities. Fever, malaise and arthralgia may precede or accompany the rash, and hilar adenopathy may be present on chest roentgenograms. The skin lesions have a characteristic progression: Over a period of several days they become protuberant and present a brilliant display of violaceous colors. After 1 or 2 weeks, as induration decreases, a dull purple discoloration predominates, and then fades in the manner of a large bruise, leaving a brown residuum. The lesions come in crops, usually over a period of 3 to 6 weeks. The disease then becomes quiescent and rarely recurs. Erythema nodosum is uncommon in children under the age of 6 years, becoming progressively more frequent up to the third decade of life. Females are affected more frequently than males.

It is generally accepted that the skin lesions represent a reaction to a variety of provocative stimuli. The eruption has been induced experimentally in patients with the disease by local injection of a single specific bacterial antigen. Epidemiologically the disease was previously closely linked to tuberculosis, especially in Europe. In both the United States and Europe streptococcal infections are now more frequently implicated as provocative stimuli. The eruption may also appear as a concomitant of sarcoidosis, histoplasmosis, coccidioidomycosis and Yersinia infections; or in association with the administration of some drugs. It may also occur with diseases such as systemic lupus erythematosus, vasculitis, regional enteritis and ulcerative colitis.

Careful search for a precipitating infection, drug or underlying disease should be instituted. The sedimentation rate is usually elevated, and other nonspecific evidences of inflammatory disease, such as acute phase reactants, are found. Suggestive etiologic evidence may include the demonstration of beta-hemolytic streptococci in throat cultures or a rising antistreptolysin O titer; conversion of a previously negative tuberculin, histoplasmin or coccidioidin skin reaction; radiographic evidence of pulmonary tuberculosis or fungus disease; or evidence of an underlying disease such as systemic lupus erythematosus, inflammatory bowel disease or sarcoidosis.

Salicylates are usually adequate for symptomatic relief of erythema nodosum. The skin lesions and their constitutional manifestations may respond to corticosteroids, but such therapy is usually not warranted in a self-limited disease and may be contraindicated because of the presence of underlying active infection.

THE GOODPASTURE SYNDROME

The combination of pulmonary alveolar hemorrhage and glomerulonephritis, called the Goodpasture syndrome, appears to be a distinctive clinical entity, although there is some overlap with polyarteritis nodosa and with idiopathic pulmonary hemosiderosis. Young adult males are predominantly affected, but the disease has been reported in children. The cause is unknown. The disease often appears to begin after an acute illness and has been associated with influenza. Recent evidence suggests that antibodies reactive with glomerular and alveolar basement membranes are involved in pathogenesis.

The syndrome is characterized clinically by hemoptysis, anemia and nephritis. Dyspnea, cough, malaise and fever are often present; and rales and rhonchi may be heard on auscultation of the chest. Chest roentgenograms characteristically show bilateral flocculent infiltrates spreading from hilus to periphery of the lung fields. Hemosiderin-laden macrophages can be demonstrated in the sputum. Anemia, presumably related to pulmonary hemorrhage, is prominent. Urinalyses reveal varying degrees of proteinuria, hematuria, pyuria and cylindruria. Azotemia is frequent; progressive renal failure often ensues. Histologically, focal glomerulitis or widespread glomerulonephritis may be demonstrated. Intra-alveolar hemorrhages, hemosiderin-laden macrophages and thickening of alveolar septa are present in the lungs. Generalized vasculitis is not found; patients with concomitant vasculitis are usually considered to have polyarteritis nodosa.

The disease is usually rapidly fatal. Corticosteroid therapy has been considered helpful in a few cases, and recently alkylating agents and antimetabolites have been used on an experimental basis.

RELAPSING NODULAR NONSUPPURATIVE PANNICULITIS

(Weber-Christian Syndrome)

Recurrent nodular nonsuppurative panniculitis is a rare disorder. Its cause is not known; infection, drug reaction (especially to bromides and iodides), abnormal fat metabolism and hypersensitivity have all been suggested. It is probable that panniculitis does not represent a single disease. It has been reported in association with several rheumatic tissue diseases and with corticosteroid withdrawal. Adults are predominantly affected, although the syndrome has been reported in all age groups. Females are affected more frequently than males.

Histologically there are foci of degeneration and inflammation in subcutaneous fat. Mesenteric, perivisceral and periarticular adipose tissues may be affected; fatty metamorphosis of the liver and reticuloendothelial hyperplasia have been recorded. Laboratory findings are not specific. Leukopenia and elevated sedimentation rates may be present; rheumatoid factor, LE cells and cryoglobulins have been observed.

Clinically the disease is characterized by the appearance of crops of subcutaneous nodules on any part of the body; thighs, abdomen, breasts and arms are most frequently involved. Nodules vary in size from millimeters to several centimeters and may be painful, with redness and warmth of the overlying skin. Nodules regress in days to weeks, usually leaving a pigmented depression. Fever is common and a variety of rheumatic complaints may occur, including arthritis, arthralgia and myalgia. Hepatosplenomegaly, abdominal pain and episcleritis have been reported. Crops of nodules and systemic symptoms generally recur over long periods of time.

Diagnosis of Weber-Christian syndrome is made by the clinical picture and histologic changes. Differential diagnosis includes erythema induratum, sarcoidosis and postinjection subcutaneous fat necrosis. Fat necrosis with subcutaneous nodules, arthritis and visceral involvement can occur as a manifestation of pancreatic disease, presumably from enzymatic action on fat cells.

No specific therapy is known. Symptomatic relief has been reported after therapy with corticosteroids, chloroquine and phenylbutazone. Patients with underlying pancreatic involvement are benefited by appropriate therapy of the pancreatic disease.

"RHEUMATOID" NODULES WITHOUT RHEUMATIC DISEASE

Rheumatoid nodule-like lesions unassociated with rheumatic disease occur occasionally in children. Single or multiple lesions may be present. Nodules occur over various sites, including the pretibial areas, dorsa of the feet, scalp, hands and elbows, and may appear over pressure points or after trauma, as do true rheumatoid nodules. Clinically the nodules are subcutaneous or fixed to deeper tissues and resemble rheumatoid nodules. Histologically these lesions show central areas of fibrinoid necrosis with surrounding histiocytes and mononuclear cells; they may resemble well organized adult-type rheumatoid nodules. Histologically these subcutaneous lesions resemble the intracutaneous lesions of granuloma annulare and may occur in association with typical granuloma annulare.

The etiology of these nodules is unknown. Affected children are well; there are no associated rheumatic complaints. Laboratory tests are normal; tests for rheumatoid factor and antinuclear antibodies are negative. The nodular lesions wax, wane and may recur, but recurrences generally cease after months or years. It is important to realize that this is a benign condition, that affected children are not at risk for rheumatic disease, and that no therapy other than reassurance is required.

Nodules that occur in association with rheumatic disease (rheumatoid arthritis, acute rheumatic fever, scleroderma, systemic lupus) rarely if ever occur as sole manifestations, but rather appear in association with other signs of active rheumatic disease. Rheumatoid nodules in rheumatoid arthritis are generally associated with positive tests for rheumatoid factor.

JANE GREEN SCHALLER
RALPH J. WEDGWOOD

PATIENT EDUCATION

Arthritis in Children. Arthritis Foundation, 1212 Avenue of the Americas, New York, N.Y. 10036. (Obtainable from the Arthritis Foundation or from its local chapter offices.)

GENERAL

Mikkelsen, W. M. et al.: Twentieth Rheumatism Review. New York, Arthritis Foundation, 1973.

Rodnan, G. P. (ed.): Primer on the rheumatic diseases (7th ed.), J.A.M.A. *224*:662, 1973.

Hanson, V., and Kornreich, H.: Systemic rheumatic disorders ("collagen disease") in childhood: Lupus erythematosus, anaphylactoid purpura, dermatomyositis, and scleroderma. Bull. Rheum. Dis. *17*:435, 1967.

Hollander, J. L., and McCarty, D. J., Jr.: Arthritis and Allied Conditions. 8th ed. Philadelphia, Lea & Febiger, 1972.

Juvenile Rheumatoid Arthritis

Ansell, B. M., and Bywaters, E. G. L.: Prognosis in Still's disease. Bull. Rheum. Dis. *9*:189, 1959.

Ansell, B. M., and Bywaters, E. G. L.: Diagnosis of "probable" Still's disease and its outcome. Ann. Rheum. Dis. *21*:253, 1962.

Bianco, N. E., Panush, R. S., Stillman, J. S., and Schur, P. H.: Immunologic studies of juvenile rheumatoid arthritis. Arthritis & Rheum. *14*:685, 1971.

Bywaters, E. G. L.: Heberden Oration, 1966. Categorization in medicine: A survey of Still's disease. Ann. Rheum. Dis. *26*:185, 1967.

Calabro, J. J., and Marchesano, J. M.: The early natural history of juvenile rheumatoid arthritis. Med. Clin. N. Amer. *52*:567, 1968.

Calabro, J. J., and Marchesano, J. M.: Fever associated with juvenile rheumatoid arthritis. New Engl. J. Med. *276*:11, 1967.

Hanson, V., Drexler, E., and Kornreich, H.: The relationship of rheumatoid factor to age of onset in juvenile rheumatoid arthritis. Arthritis Rheum. *12*:82, 1969.

Isdale, I. C., and Bywaters, E. G. L.: The rash of rheumatoid arthritis and Still's disease. Quart. J. Med. *25*:377, 1956.

Jeremy, R., Schaller, J., Arkless, R., Wedgwood, R. J., and Healey, L. A.: Juvenile rheumatoid arthritis persisting into adulthood. Amer. J. Med. *45*:419, 1968.

Laaksonen, A. L.: A prognostic study of juvenile rheumatoid arthritis. Analysis of 544 cases. Acta Paediat. Scand. (Suppl.) *166*:1, 1966.

McMinn, F. J., and Bywaters, E. G. L.: Differences between the fever of Still's disease and that of rheumatic fever. Ann. Rheum. Dis. *18*:293, 1959.

Schaller, J., Kupfer, C., and Wedgwood, R. J.: Iridocyclitis in juvenile rheumatoid arthritis. Pediatrics *44*:92, 1969.

Schaller, J., and Wedgwood, R. J.: Is juvenile rheumatoid arthritis a single disease? A review. Pediatrics *50*:940, 1972.

Smiley, W. K., May, E., and Bywaters, E. G. L.: Ocular presentations of Still's disease and their treatment: Iridocyclitis in Still's disease: Its complication and treatment. Ann. Rheum. Dis. *16*:371, 1957.

Still, G. F.: On a form of chronic joint disease in children. Med. Chir. *80*:47, 1897. (Reprinted in Arch. Dis. Child. *16*:156, 1941.)

Ankylosing Spondylitis

Ladd, J. R., Cassidy, J. T., and Martel, W.: Juvenile ankylosing spondylitis. Arthritis Rheum. *14*:579, 1971.

Schaller, J., Bitnun, S., and Wedgwood, R. J.: Ankylosing spondylitis with childhood onset. J. Pediatr. *74*:505, 1969.

Wilkinson, M., and Bywaters, E. G. L.: Clinical features and course of ankylosing spondylitis; as seen in a follow-up of 222 hospital referred cases. Ann. Rheum. Dis. *17*:209, 1958.

Systemic Lupus Erythematosus

Baldwin, D. S., Lowenstein, J., Rothfield, N. F., Gallo, G., and McCluskey, R. T.: The clinical course of proliferative and membranous forms of lupus nephritis. Ann. Intern. Med. *73*:929, 1970.

Cook, C. D., Wedgwood, R. J., Craig, J. M., Hartmann, J. R., and Janeway, C. A.: Systemic lupus erythematosus. Description of 37 cases in children and a discussion of endocrine therapy in 32 of the cases. Pediatrics *26*:570, 1960.

DuBois, E. L. (ed.): Systemic Lupus Erythematosus. New York, McGraw-Hill Book Company, Inc., 1966.

Estes, D., and Christian, C. L.: The natural history of systemic lupus erythematosus by prospective analysis. Medicine *50*:85, 1971.

Hayslett, J. P., Kashgarian, M., Cook, C. D., and Spargo, B. H.: The effect of azathioprine on lupus nephritis. Medicine *51*:393, 1972.

Jacobs, J. C.: Systemic lupus erythematosus in childhood: Report of 35 cases, with discussion of seven apparently induced by anticonvulsant medication, and of prognosis and treatment. Pediatrics *32*:257, 1963.

Koffler, D., Agnello, V., Thoburn, R., and Kunkel, H. G.: Systemic lupus erythematosus: Prototype of immune complex nephritis in man, J. Exp. Med. *134*:169s, 1971.

Meislin, A. G., and Rothfield, N.: Systemic lupus erythematosus in childhood. Pediatrics *42*:37, 1968.

Peterson, R. D., Vernier, R. L., and Good, R. A.: Lupus erythematosus. Pediat. Clin. N. Amer. *10*:941, 1963.

Pincus, T., Hughes, G. R. V., Pincus, D., Tina, L. U., and Bellanti, J. A.: Antibodies to DNA in childhood systemic lupus erythematosus, J. Pediatr. *78*:981, 1971.

Pollak, V. E., Pirani, C. L., and Schwartz, F. D.: The natural history of the renal manifestations of systemic lupus erythematosus. J. Lab. Clin. Med. *63*:537, 1964.

Ropes, M. W.: Observations on the natural course of disseminated lupus erythematosus. Medicine *43*:387, 1964.

Schur, P. H., and Sandson, J.: Immunologic factors and clinical activity in systemic lupus erythematosus. New Engl. J. Med. *278*:533, 1968.

Winkelmann, R. K.: Chronic discoid lupus erythematosus in children. J.A.M.A. *205*:675, 1968.

Lupus Phenomena in the Newborn Period

Beck, J. S., and Rowell, N. R.: Transplacental passage of antinuclear antibody. Lancet *1*:134, 1963.

Jackson, R.: Discoid lupus in a newborn infant of a mother with lupus erythematosus. Pediatrics *33*:425, 1964.

Schönlein-Henoch Vasculitis

Ackroyd, J. F.: Allergic purpura, including purpura due to foods, drugs and infections. Am. J. Med. *14*:605, 1953.

Allen, D. M., Diamond, L. K., and Howell, D. A.: Anaphylactoid purpura in children (Schönlein-Henoch syndrome): Review with a follow-up of the renal complications. Am. J. Dis. Child. *99*:833, 1960.

Ayoub, E. M., and Hoyer, J.: Anaphylactoid purpura: Streptococcal antibody titers and β 1C globulin levels. J. Pediatr. *75*:193, 1970.

Bywaters, E. G. L., Isdale, I., and Kempton, J. J.: Schönlein-Henoch purpura; Evidence for a group A β-haemolytic streptococcal aetiology. Quart. J. Med. *26*:161, 1957.

Hurley, R. M., and Drummond, K. N.: Anaphylactoid purpura nephritis: Clinicopathological correlations. J. Pediatr. *81*:904, 1972.

Osler, W.: The visceral lesions of purpura and allied conditions. Brit. Med. J. *1*:517, 1914.

Vernier, R. L., Worthen, H. G., Peterson, R. D., Colle, E., and Good, R. A.: Anaphylactoid purpura. Pathology of the skin and kidney and frequency of streptococcal infection. Pediatrics *27*:181, 1961.

Wedgwood, R. J., and Klaus, M. H.: Anaphylactoid purpura (Schönlein-Henoch syndrome); Long term follow-up study with special reference to renal involvement. Pediatrics *16*:196, 1955.

Polyarteritis Nodosa

Fager, D. B., Bigler, J. A., and Simonds, J. P.: Polyarteritis nodsa in infancy and childhood. J. Pediatr. *39*:65, 1951.

Frohnert, P. P., and Sheps, S. G.: Long term follow-up study of periarteritis nodosa. Am. J. Med. *43*:8, 1967.

Gocke, D. J., Hsu, K., Morgan, C., Bombardieri, S., Lockshin, M., and Christian, C. L.: Vasculitis in association with Australia antigen. J. Exp. Med. *134*:330s, 1971.

Owano, L. R., and Sueper, R. H.: Polyarteritis nodosa—A syndrome. Am. J. Clin. Path. *40*:527, 1963.

Rose, G. A., and Spencer, H.: Polyarteritis nodosa. Quart. J. Med. *26*:43, 1957.

Infantile Polyarteritis Nodosa

Munro-Faure, H.: Necrotizing arteritis of the coronary vessels in infancy. Case report and review of the literature. Pediatrics *23*:914, 1959.

Roberts, F. B., and Fetterman, G. H.: Polyarteritis nodosa in infancy. J. Pediatr. *63*:519, 1963.

Wegener's Granulomatosis

Blatt, I. M., and others: Fatal granulomatosis of the respiratory tract (lethal midline granuloma—Wegener's granulomatosis). Arch. Otolaryng. *70*:707, 1959.

Carrington, C. B., and Liebow, A. A.: Limited forms of angiitis and granulomatosis of Wegener's type. Am. J. Med. *41*:497, 1966.

Novack, S. N., and Pearson, C. M.: Cyclophosphamide therapy in Wegener's granulomatosis. New Engl. J. Med. *284*:938, 1971.

Takayasu's Arteritis

Danaraj, T. J., Wong, H. O., and Thomas, M. A.: Primary arteritis of the aorta causing renal artery stenosis and hypertension. Brit. Heart J. *25*:153, 1963.

Lee, K., and others: Primary arteritis (pulseless disease) in Korean children. Acta Paediat. Scand. *56*:526, 1967.

Nakao, K., and others: Takayasu's arteritis. Clinical report of 84 cases and immunological studies of 7 cases. Circulation *35*:1141, 1967.

Strachan, R. W., Wigzell, F. W., and Anderson, J. R.: Locomotor manifestations and serum studies in Takayasu's arteriopathy. Am. J. Med. *40*:560, 1966.

Dermatomyositis

Banker, B. Q., and Victor, M.: Dermatomyositis (systemic angiopathy) of childhood. Medicine *45*:261, 1966.

Middleton, P. J., Alexander, R. M., and Szymanski, M. T.: Severe myositis during recovery from influenza. Lancet *2*:533, 1970.

Pearson, C. M.: Patterns of polymyositis and their response to treatment. Ann. Intern. Med. *59*:827, 1963.

Schaller, J.: Dermatomyositis. J. Pediatr. *83*:699, 1973.

Sharp, G. C., Irvin, W. S., Tan, E. M., Gould, R. G., and Holman, H. R.: Mixed connective tissue disease: An apparently distinct rheumatic disease syndrome associated with a specific antibody to an extractable nuclear antigen (ENA). Am. J. Med. *52*:148, 1972.

Sullivan, D. B., Cassidy, J. T., Petty, R. E., and Burt, M. T.: Prognosis in childhood dermatomyositis. J. Pediatr. *80*:555, 1972.

Wedgwood, R. J., Cook, C. D., and Cohen, J.: Dermatomyositis: Report of 26 cases in children with a discussion of endocrine therapy in 13. Pediatrics *12*:447, 1953.

Ziff, M., and Johnson, R. L.: Polymyositis and cell-mediated immunity. New Engl. J. Med. *288*:465, 1973.

Scleroderma: Morphea and Progressive Systemic Sclerosis

Bradford, W. D., Cook, C. D., Vawter, G. F., and Berenberg, W.: Scleredema of childhood. J. Pediatr. *68*:391, 1966.

Chazen, E. M., Cook, C. D., and Cohen, J.: Focal scleroderma. J. Pediat. *60*:385, 1962.

Christianson, H. B., Dorsey, C. S., O'Leary, P. A., and Kierland, R. R.: Localized scleroderma: Clinical study of 235 cases. Arch. Dermat. *74*:629, 1956.

Jaffe, M. O., and Winkelmann, R. K.: Generalized scleroderma in children. Arch. Derm. *83*:402, 1961.

Kass, H., Hanson, V., and Patrick, J.: Scleroderma in childhood. J. Pediatr. *68*:243, 1966.

Winkelmann, R. K., and others: Symposium on scleroderma. Mayo Clin. Proc. *46*:77, 1971.

Erythema Multiforme Exudativum (Stevens-Johnson Syndrome)

Ashby, D. W., and Lazar, T.: Erythema multiforme exudativum major. Lancet *1*:1091, 1951.

Bukantz, S. C.: The Stevens-Johnson syndrome. *Disease-A-Month,* p. 1. Chicago, Year Book Medical Publishers, Inc., Oct., 1968.

Foy, H. M., Kenny, G. E., and Koler, J.: *Mycoplasma pneumoniae* in Stevens-Johnson syndrome. Lancet *2*:550, 1966.

Stevens, A. M., and Johnson, F. C.: A new eruptive fever associated with stomatitis and ophthalmia. Am. J. Dis. Child. *24*:526, 1922.

Erythema Nodosum

A Group of Pediatricians: Aetiology of erythema nodosum in children. Lancet *2*:14, 1961.

Doxiadis, S. A.: Erythema nodosum in children. Medicine *30*:283, 1951.

James, D. G.: Erythema nodosum. Brit. Med. J. *1*:853, 1961.
Kirby, J. F., and Kraft, G. H.: Oral contraceptives and erythema nodosum. Obstet. Gynec. *40*:409, 1972.
Weinstein, L.: Erythema nodosum. *Disease-A-Month,* p. 1. Chicago, Year Book Medical Publishers, Inc., June, 1969.

The Goodpasture Syndrome

Benoit, F. L., Rulon, D. B., Theil, G. B., Doolan, P. D., and Watten, R. H.: Goodpasture's syndrome. Am. J. Med. *37*:424, 1964.
McCombs, R. P.: Diseases due to immunologic reactions in the lungs. New Engl. J. Med. *286*:1186; 1245, 1972.

Relapsing Nodular Nonsuppurative Panniculitis

Perry, H. O., and Winkelmann, R. K.: Subacute nodular migratory panniculitis. Arch. Derm. *89*:170, 1964.
Hallahan, J. D., and Klein, T.: Relapsing febrile nodular nonsuppurative panniculitis. Review of the literature and report of a case. Ann. Intern. Med. *34*:1179, 1951.
Sanford, H. N., Eubank, D. F., and Stenn, F.: Chronic panniculitis with leukopenia (Weber-Christian syndrome). Am. J. Dis. Child. *83*:156, 1952.

"Rheumatoid" Nodules Without Rheumatic Disease

Altman, R. S., and Caffrey, P. R.: Isolated subcutaneous rheumatic nodules. Pediatrics *34*:869, 1964.
Beatty, E. C.: Rheumatic-like nodules occurring in nonrheumatic children. Arch. Path. *68*:154, 1959.
Burrington, J. D.: "Pseudorheumatoid" nodules in children; Report of 10 cases. Pediatrics *45*:473, 1970.
Mesara, B. W., Brody, G. L., and Oberman, H. A.: "Pseudorheumatoid" subcutaneous nodules. Am. J. Clin. Path. *45*:684, 1966.

RHEUMATIC FEVER

Rheumatic fever is a multisystem disease, the acute manifestations of which may include arthritis and fever, carditis, emotional instability and choreiform movements and, less frequently, a characteristic rash (erythema marginatum) and subcutaneous nodules. It is by nature recurrent and derives its importance from the fact that it can result in chronic heart disease. Despite a decline in severity and prevalence of acute rheumatic fever in recent years, rheumatic carditis is still the leading form of acquired heart disease in children. Worldwide it is a common cause of heart disease among the poor and medically deprived.

Both acute and recurrent attacks are triggered by group A beta-hemolytic streptococcal infections of the upper respiratory tract. Knowledge of this has led to practical approaches to control through the prevention and treatment of streptococcal pharyngitis, tonsillitis and otitis.

HISTORICAL ASPECTS. Though acute rheumatic fever was apparently known to the ancient Greeks, it was many centuries before it became clearly separated from other forms of rheumatism. Sydenham, whose name is associated with chorea, also described the migratory arthritis pattern, but the association of the two manifestations was first recognized by Stoll a century later in 1780. Shortly thereafter Pitcairn, Jenner and Wells emphasized that rheumatic fever can damage the heart. Another century passed before the French pediatrician Roger recognized the relation of the various manifestations of the disease and before Cheadle pointed out the variations in the clinical patterns at different ages as well as the tendency of the disease to occur in families. Although earlier observers had described submiliary nodular reactions in the myocardium, Aschoff in 1904 is generally credited with stressing their specificity. The "criteria" introduced by Jones in 1944 brought order into the clinical classification.

The association of acute rheumatic fever with sore throat and the concept of a latent period were recognized during the nineteenth century, particularly by Haygarth, Fowler and Haig-Brown. The relation of scarlet fever and streptococcal tonsillitis to acute rheumatic fever was described by Schlesinger, Collis and Coburn in 1930 and 1931. The development of techniques for classifying streptococci by Lancefield and Griffith has led to firm documentation of the relation of group A streptococci to acute rheumatic fever. The description of the antistreptolysin O test by Todd in 1932 has permitted correlation of serologic with clinical, epidemiologic and bacteriologic findings.

MacLagon advocated salicylates for the treatment of acute rheumatism in 1876, and the era of steroid therapy was introduced in 1949 by Hench and coworkers. Control of recurrences by sulfonamide prophylaxis was demonstrated independently by Thomas and France and by Coburn and Moore in 1939. Treatment of acute streptococcal infections with penicillin was first shown to reduce recurrent attacks of rheumatic fever by Massell and colleagues and to prevent initial attacks by Rammelkamp and coworkers.

PATHOGENESIS. Rheumatic fever may properly be considered a *complication of streptococcal infection of the upper respiratory tract.* Although not all patients with acute rheumatic fever give a history of sore throat, evidence consistent with recent streptococcal infection can usually be obtained by careful laboratory examinations. Throat cultures taken at the time of the acute infection preceding an attack of rheumatic fever regularly yield beta-hemolytic streptococci serologically identifiable as group A, but by the time of onset of rheumatic fever the numbers of group A streptococci may have diminished naturally or may have been suppressed by penicillin therapy to the point at which they are difficult to identify in throat cultures. Serologic evidence of a recent streptococcal infection (elevation of antistreptolysin O or other streptococcal antibodies) can usually be obtained. The demonstrated association of acute rheumatic fever with outbreaks of streptococcal sore throat or scarlet fever provides epidemiologic evidence of a relation between rheumatic fever and these streptococcal diseases. The striking reduction of first attacks of rheumatic fever when streptococcal infections are treated with penicillin and of secondary attacks in patients who are receiving continuous antimicrobial prophylaxis provides additional support for the role of streptococcal infections in the pathogenesis of both initial and recurrent attacks.

Despite the large number of *antigens and biologically toxic or active factors* associated with group A streptococci, none has been definitely identified as causing rheumatic fever. The streptococcal factor(s) responsible for rheumatic fever must be common to most strains, since clinical and epidemiologic evidence suggests that many *serologic types* of group A streptococci infecting the throat can be associated with acute rheumatic fever. This is in contrast to acute nephritis, which is related to a limited number of serologic types. Further, again in contrast to acute nephritis, rheumatic fever tends not to follow streptococcal infections of the skin, indicating important pathogenetic differences with regard to the *location of infection,* and reflecting either differences (1) in host response (e.g., poor antibody response to skin infections, which has been demonstrated for at least one streptococcal antigen), or (2) in the capacity of strains with different biologic capacities to infect different sites.

The importance of *host factors* is suggested by the fact that group A streptococcal infections are common during childhood, yet relatively few children acquire acute rheumatic fever. The tendency for rheumatic fever to occur in families points to a possible genetic factor, but a clear-cut pattern has not been found; in a study of monozygotic twins, less than one fifth were concordant for rheumatic fever.

The resemblance of the clinical manifestations of acute rheumatic fever to those of serum sickness, including the presence of a latent period, has suggested *hypersensitivity* or *immunologic factors* in the pathogenesis of acute rheumatic fever. Although the delayed type of hypersensitivity of the skin to a variety of streptococcal products can be demonstrated in rheumatic patients, these reactions are also demonstrable in many healthy persons. A role for exaggerated antibody responses in the pathogenesis of acute rheumatic fever has been postulated on the basis that levels of antistreptolysin O and other streptococcal antibodies in patients with acute rheumatic fever are usually higher than those in patients after uncomplicated streptococcal infections. The view that rheumatic fever may be an *autoimmune disease* is supported by the demonstration of antigenic cross-reactions between components of the streptococcus and human heart muscle and valves, but circulating cross-reacting antibodies are found in persons who fail to acquire rheumatic fever as well as among those who do, and it is not known whether the cross-reactions are a cause or an effect of injury.

The possible significance of *living streptococci* in the pathogenesis of rheumatic fever is suggested by the demonstration that successful prevention of rheumatic fever by treatment of the preceding streptococcal infection depends upon eradication of the infecting organisms. Direct infection of heart valves is not supported by recent observations, and massive penicillin therapy during the course of acute rheumatic fever does not alter the course or prognosis of the disease. The possibility that penicillin-resistant, wall-less forms of streptococci *(protoplasts or L-forms)* may survive or propagate in tissues has been entertained, but successful attempts to produce these aberrant streptococcal forms in the test tube and in experimental animals have not been matched by convincing success of efforts to recover them from the pharynx, blood or hearts of patients.

No completely satisfactory *pathologic model* for acute rheumatic fever has been developed in experimental animals. This has hindered further exploration of the pathogenesis of this disease.

EPIDEMIOLOGY. The epidemiology of acute rheumatic fever is closely related to the epidemiology of streptococcal infections of the upper respiratory tract (pharyngitis, tonsillitis, scarlet fever and otitis media).

Rheumatic fever, like streptococcal infections, occurs most commonly in children between 5 and 15 years of age, with a peak incidence of first attacks at 6 to 8 years of age. The rarity of rheumatic fever in infants under 3 years of age and in older adults is probably attributable to the rarity of streptococcal infections at these extremes. Adults who have intimate and frequent exposures to streptococcal infections, as in military service or through close contact with school-age children, incur an increased risk of rheumatic fever.

The distinct *seasonal fluctuation* in onset of acute rheumatic fever coincides with the seasonal variation in streptococcal infections; the incidence is highest in the winter and spring months. This may be related to the increased opportunity for spread of streptococcal infection by close contact during the colder and damper months.

Traditionally considered to be a disease of temperate *climates,* rheumatic fever also occurs in the warmer ones. The high prevalence of rheumatic heart disease which may be found in some tropical or desert climates, as in India and Egypt, suggests that the pathologic process is common there but may be clinically modified. This is in keeping with the observation in the United States that acute rheumatic fever appears to be more frequent in the North than in the South, but rheumatic heart disease is found at autopsy as often in Southern as in Northern clinics.

Crowding due to socioeconomic factors or to military exigencies seems to play an important role in the spread of streptococcal infections and in the incidence of acute rheumatic fever. When allowance is made for the effect of crowding, due to differences in housing, no significant *racial differences* have been established.

The *attack rate* of acute rheumatic fever after documented streptococcal infections in epidemic situations is fairly constant at about 3 per cent; among children in nonepidemic situations it has been reported to be about 3 per thousand. The lower rate in nonepidemic situations may be more apparent than real, resulting from the misidentification of streptococcal carriers with viral respiratory infections as cases of streptococcal disease. Although rheumatic fever appears to be more common in certain *families,* it is not known whether this is due to an increased group exposure to streptococcal infections or to differences in host or genetic factors.

There is no striking *sex difference* in the overall incidence of rheumatic fever, but chorea and mitral disease are more common in females; aortic valvular disease is more common in males.

MORBIDITY AND MORTALITY. Over the past several decades there has been a decline in severity and mortality of attacks of acute rheumatic fever, and in prevalence of rheumatic heart disease; the incidence of recurrent attacks has been gradually declining, but a decline in the frequency of first attacks is less well established. Antibiotics have been generally held responsible for the *decline in the incidence of rheumatic fever,* but more credit is probably due to socioeconomic improvements leading to less crowded living conditions; wherever poverty and crowding persist, in developing countries or in the United States, rheumatic fever still flourishes. Changes in the infecting organism or in the infected host may also be factors, but have not been documented.

Annually in the United States about 100,000 new cases of rheumatic fever and rheumatic heart disease are identified. The *yearly incidence of first attacks* is estimated at about 5 per 10,000 children. In recent years *prevalence rates for rheumatic heart disease* among schoolchildren have been of the order of 7 to 16 per 10,000, as opposed to 60 to 90 per 10,000 among college students and servicemen. Congenital heart disease is more prevalent among schoolchildren, but rejection rates among military selectees are appreciably greater for rheumatic heart disease.

In the United States in 1972 about 14,000 *deaths* (or almost 1 per cent of all deaths) were attributed to rheumatic fever or chronic rheumatic heart disease, an overall mortality rate of 7 per 100,000 population. Most of the deaths occur in adults, although the initial attack usually dates back to childhood.

PATHOLOGY. The pathologic response to acute rheumatic fever includes both exudative and proliferative reactions. The *exudative reactions* when manifest as arthritis subside spontaneously, but more rapidly with anti-inflammatory drugs, and leave no evidence of permanent damage; when manifest as pancarditis, they may be life-threatening. *Proliferative reactions* accompanied by permanent damage appear to be confined to the myocardium and endocardium.

The unique pathologic lesion of rheumatic fever, the **Aschoff body**, does not develop in brain tissue, and its occurrence in joints is doubtful. Although generally considered to be a granuloma, developing from injury to collagen fibers, some pathologists contend that the Aschoff body results from primary injury to the myocardium; others believe that it may result from blockage of lymphatic channels in the heart. Biopsies of auricular appendages in patients with rheumatic heart disease may show Aschoff bodies many years after the last clinical evidence of rheumatic activity. Whether the *deposits of gamma globulin* which have been demonstrated in rheumatic heart tissue are a cause or a result of heart damage is not known. *Valvular damage* most frequently involves the mitral, less commonly the aortic, and rarely the tricuspid and pulmonary valves. Scarring sufficient to result in stenotic heart valves requires months or years to develop. There is little knowledge or understanding of the *pathology of Sydenham's chorea,* since patients do not often die with this form of rheumatic fever, and the histopathologic changes cannot be related to the clinical manifestations. Lesions similar to those of hyaline membrane disease of newborn infants have been reported in patients dying with rheumatic pneumonitis.

CLINICAL MANIFESTATIONS. The first symptoms of rheumatic fever usually do not develop until some time after the manifestations of the preceding streptococcal infection have disappeared. This *latent period* may last from 1 to 5 weeks, and in chorea may be 2 to 6 months.

The *presenting manifestation* of acute rheumatic fever is commonly arthritis or choreiform movements in school-age children and carditis in very young children. Abdominal pain, which may be suggestive of appendicitis, is occasionally the presenting complaint. The onset is usually abrupt when arthritis and fever are the initial manifestations, and may be with carditis when chest pain or shortness of breath appears suddenly. The onset with carditis, however, is more apt to be insidious and unsuspected until an enlarged liver or a significant murmur is detected. A subtle onset is especially common in chorea, and a diagnosis of emotional disturbance is often made initially.

A *history of a recent sore throat* is obtained in about 50 per cent of instances. A *family history* of rheumatic fever or rheumatic heart disease can sometimes be elicited, but must be carefully differentiated from other arthritic and cardiac diseases. Patients presenting with well established rheumatic heart disease should be meticulously questioned about possible earlier attacks.

Fever is almost invariably present in the early stage, except in patients whose only manifestation is chorea or in those receiving salicylates or a corticosteroid. Prolonged fever without development of other manifestations is unusual. Without suppressive drugs the fever will often become low grade after the first week and may persist at this level for 2 to 4 weeks.

The **arthritis** of acute rheumatic fever characteristically involves the large joints and migrates from one joint to another for a few days to several weeks. Involvement of the most distal joints, such as the small joints of the fingers and toes, and the central ones, such as the hips and the spine, is unusual. Infrequently such joints as the temporomandibular joint may be involved. Pain on pressure or movement is characteristically intense and aggravated rather than alleviated by massage. Exquisite tenderness is likely to be diffusely present over the entire joint. Swelling, heat and redness of the joint are commonly present. Pain without objective changes (*arthralgia*) may occur in some joints and frank arthritis in others. Myalgia is rare.

Carditis occurs in approximately 40 per cent of patients during the first attack of rheumatic fever and may be the only major manifestation, especially in infants and young children. It usually appears within the first week of illness. *Tachycardia* disproportionate to fever, present during sleep, and persisting after fever is under control, is highly suggestive of carditis. The first heart sound may be muffled, consistent with first-degree heart block, or both sounds may be distant in patients with pericardial effusion. Significant **murmurs** are almost always present with rheumatic carditis. Mitral valvulitis is manifested as an apical systolic murmur sometimes accompanied by an apical mid-diastolic murmur. The apical systolic murmur should be carefully differentiated from functional murmurs by its length (filling all of systole), by its blowing, high-pitched quality and by its persistence irrespective of position or phase of respiration. The low-pitched mid-diastolic murmur is more difficult to detect and must be differentiated from the third heart sound and the late-appearing murmur of mitral stenosis, with which there is presystolic accentuation. Involvement of the aortic valve, uncommon in children but relatively frequent in adult males, is manifest by the basal diastolic murmur of aortic regurgitation. Mitral stenosis and aortic stenosis are late manifestations of cardiac damage, which do not develop until months or years after the initial or repeated attacks. **Cardiomegaly, pericarditis,** with or without friction rub, and **congestive failure** may be present during the acute phase. In children with chronic rheumatic heart disease, changing murmurs or increasing heart size may be evidence of progressive or reactivated carditis.

Rheumatic pneumonia does occur, but is difficult to distinguish clinically from pneumonitis of other cause and from pulmonary congestion. It occurs especially in association with extensive heart damage. **Subcutaneous nodules** (Fig. 9–32) are also most often found in patients with well established rheumatic disease, often after multiple attacks of carditis. The nodules are firm and nontender, and range in size from 0.1 to 1.0 cm in diameter. They are usually found over the extensor surfaces of both large and small joints, over the scalp, or near the superficial bony prominences of the spine and scapulae. The skin overlying the nodules is freely movable and is not inflamed. **Epistaxis,** occasionally an early sign, occurs in less than 10 per cent of patients with acute rheumatic fever; by itself it is not sufficient grounds for a rheumatic work-up. Patients with severe active

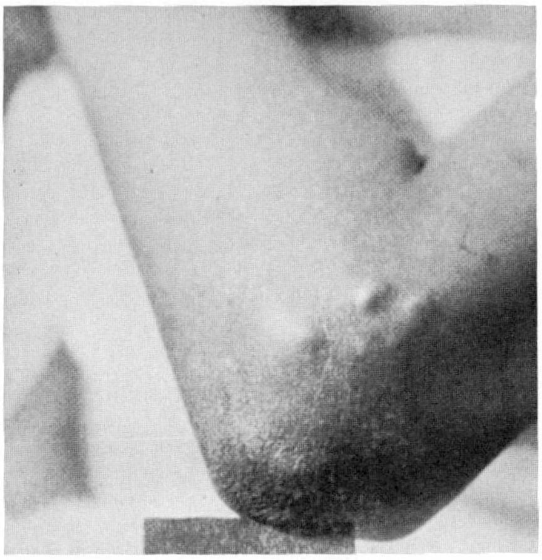

Figure 9–32 *Rheumatic nodules at the elbow in a black girl 10 years of age. She had polyarthritis, endocarditis and pericarditis. She died 3 weeks after the picture was taken.*

heart disease may also have striking *pallor,* often accompanied by anemia.

The distinctive skin rash associated with rheumatic fever is **erythema marginatum** (Fig. 9–33). It occurs in about 10 per cent of patients with acute rheumatic fever and is rarely found in other diseases. The pink, often slightly raised, macules of the early stages fade centrally and coalesce to form a serpiginous pattern. The lesions are most common over the protected parts of the body and may be elicited or accentuated by the local application of heat. They may disappear after a few hours or days and may occur intermittently over a period of weeks or months. Although commonly occurring in association with other manifestations of rheumatic fever, erythema marginatum sometimes appears as an isolated physical finding.

Chorea, known also as **Sydenham's chorea, St. Vitus' dance** or **chorea minor**, may appear as the only clinical sign, and without laboratory manifestations of inflammation (pure chorea). It may also precede, follow or exist concomitantly with other manifestations, including chronic rheumatic heart disease; the interval between chorea and other preceding or following manifestations may be short or a matter of years. It occurs most often in prepubertal girls and is rare among adults of either sex. Its most striking feature is involuntary purposeless movements. These are usually bilateral, but sometimes unilateral. They develop gradually over a period of weeks and vary in intensity from those that can be brought out only by excitement or conscious efforts to be still, to those that are so violent that they may result in self-injury. Deterioration in speech and in handwriting as well as general clumsiness may be noted. Serial samples of handwriting may be a useful manner of documenting the course of the affliction. The child may have difficulty in counting rapidly and in holding his protruded tongue still. He tends to hyperextend his fingers and wrists when holding his fingers outstretched and to turn his palms

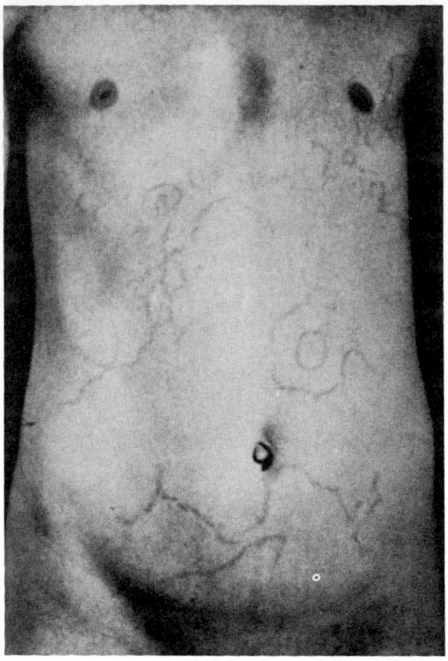

Figure 9–33 *Erythema marginatum. Annular erythema on the chest and abdomen of a boy 8 years of age who also had rheumatic carditis.*

outward when he holds his arms above his head. He has a weak hand grip, and the examiner may detect intermittent muscular contractions or twitchings. Other evidence of muscular weakness is usually present. The patellar reflex is often manifest by a "hung-up" type of response. Emotional lability is characteristic and may be expressed by inappropriate outbursts of crying or laughter.

LABORATORY DATA. Inflammatory activity can be confirmed by demonstration of a rapid *erythrocyte sedimentation rate* (ESR) or of circulating *C-reactive protein* (CRP). These and other so-called acute phase reactants are not specific for rheumatic fever, but they are almost always demonstrable in the early stages of the untreated disease (except with pure chorea or with isolated erythema marginatum) and are useful in objectively documenting the presence or persistence of activity. The ESR is increased in anemia and usually decreased in congestive heart failure. The CRP test is not influenced by anemia, but it may be positive in any type of heart failure.

Leukocytosis may occur in patients with acute rheumatic fever, but is not regularly present. A mild to moderate *anemia* is common during the active phase. Blood loss by epistaxis is usually not sufficient to account for the anemia, and the cause is ill defined.

Laboratory evidence of a preceding streptococcal infection can be obtained in most patients with acute rheumatic fever, but often not in those with chorea. The frequency with which *group A streptococci* can be isolated from the throat at the time rheumatic symptoms appear is related to the number of cultures taken and the care with which they are performed. The streptococci may be difficult to detect, owing to natural decline in numbers during the latent period or to suppression by antibiotics. *Streptococcal antibody tests* more regularly provide corroboration of recent streptococcal infection; each test in general use measures the neutralization of the hemolytic or enzymatic activity of one of the specific extracellular products of group A streptococci. Elevated values may be present even in the absence of clinical or bacteriologic evidence of streptococcal illness.

The antistreptolysin O (ASO) titer is the most widely used streptococcal antibody test. It measures the inhibition of hemolysis of rabbit red blood cells by specific antibody to streptolysin O, an extracellular product of beta-hemolytic streptococci, which in its reduced form is actively hemolytic for these cells. Normal levels of this and other streptococcal antibodies vary with the age of the population, the geographic location and the season of the year. Antistreptolysin O titers of 500 Todd units or greater are rarely found in normal school-age children and can be considered clear evidence of recent streptococcal infection (Fig. 9–34). About 20 per cent of normal school-age children have titers of 250 or greater, and 10 per cent have titers of 320 or greater. Therefore titers below 250 should be considered normal, and titers of 250 to 320 should be considered borderline elevated. About 80 per cent of patients with acute rheumatic fever have ASO titers of 250 or greater; about 60 per cent have titers of 500 or greater. In infants and older adults, who normally have lower levels of streptococcal antibodies, titers in the range of 200 to 250 may be significant. A demonstrated rise of two tubes or more on serially collected serums tested simultaneously is evidence of recent streptococcal infection regardless of the absolute level of the titers or the age of the patient.

In patients suspected of acute rheumatic fever who have normal or borderline elevated antistreptolysin O titers, the determination of antibody levels to another streptococcal antigen is often helpful. *Antistreptokinase* and *antihyaluronidase* titers have been used for this purpose but have been somewhat difficult to standardize. More recently antibody tests for streptococcal deoxyribonuclease B (DNase B) and streptococcal diphosphopyridine-nucleotidase (DPNase) or nicotinamide-adenine-dinucleotidase (NADase) have been developed (Fig. 9–34). The *anti-DNase B* and the *anti-DPNase (anti-NADase)* tests are dependent upon antibody neutralization of the activity of these specific enzymes produced by the streptococcus. Multiple antibody tests may be especially helpful in patients with pure chorea, who are less likely than other rheumatic patients to have distinct elevation of antistreptolysin O.

Patients whose disease is of several months' duration may have declining or normal titers of streptococcal antibodies. In patients receiving antistreptococcal prophylactic medication, serial

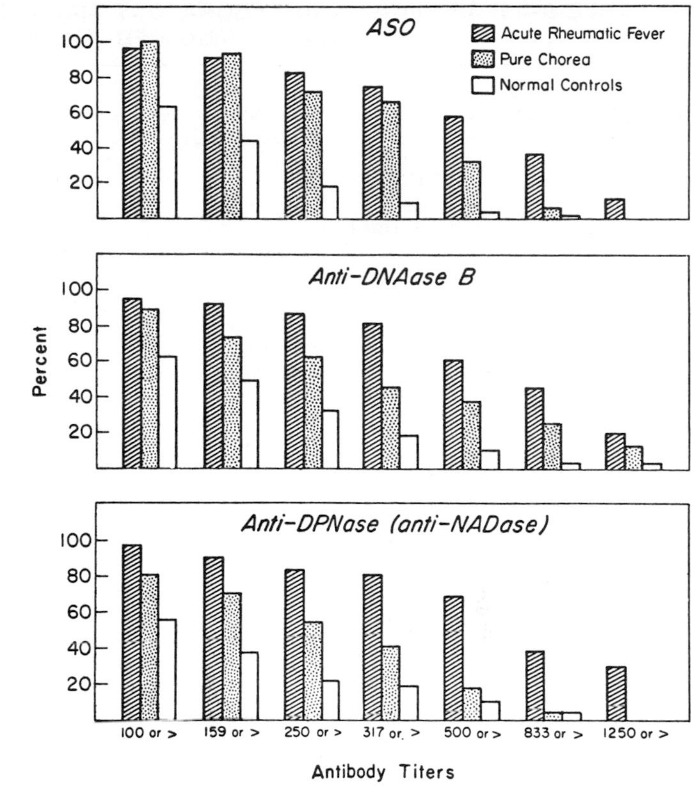

Figure 9–34 *Distribution of various streptococcal antibody titers at certain levels or greater in patients with acute rheumatic fever, patients with pure chorea, and normal controls. (Adapted from data of Ayoub and Wannamaker:* Pediatrics *29:527, 1962; 38:946, 1966.)*

streptococcal antibody titers may be useful in identifying new clinical or subclinical streptococcal infections which may result in recurrent attacks.

Measurement of *antibodies to some of the specific cellular constituents of group A streptococci* may be valuable in certain instances. The presence of type-specific antibody indicates immunity for that specific M type. Antibody to group A carbohydrate tends to persist in patients who develop chronic valvular disease. Heart-reactive antibody, absorbable by streptococcal membrane, is often present in higher titer in patients with acute rheumatic fever than in those with uncomplicated streptococcal infection, and its persistence may indicate susceptibility to recurrence.

Roentgen examinations are useful in documenting cardiac enlargement and pericardial effusion. The presence of pericarditis may be suggested or supported by elevation of the ST segment on the *electrocardiogram.* Carditis should not be diagnosed on the basis of prolongation of the P-R interval alone, since this finding may occur in many infectious diseases. Although careful auscultation is usually sufficient for the differentiation of innocent from organic murmurs by physicians experienced with cardiac examinations in children, *phonocardiographic studies* may be helpful in substantiating or documenting the clinical impression.

DIAGNOSIS AND DIFFERENTIAL DIAGNOSIS. Since no single clinical or laboratory finding is pathognomonic for acute rheumatic fever, the diagnosis is based on a combination of manifestations characteristic for the disease and on the absence of evidence of other diseases which may mimic it. For this purpose the *Jones criteria,* as modified over the years, have proved useful (Table 9–13). The major manifestations are much more likely to be indicative of acute rheumatic fever than the minor ones; for this reason a diagnosis based on two major manifestations is stronger than one based on one major and two minor manifestations. The possibility of other diseases should always be considered and, if possible, ruled out by appropriate tests, especially in patients with only one major manifestation, atypical findings or no serologic evidence of recent streptococcal disease.

The combination of *fever, arthritis and positive acute phase reactants* is found in many diseases, including rheumatoid and bacterial arthritis, serum sickness, penicillin hypersensitivity, systemic lupus erythematosus, subacute bacterial endocarditis, sickle cell anemia, Henoch-Schönlein purpura and acute leukemia. Some of these diseases, notably the latter three, may also present with *abdominal pain;* rheumatoid arthritis, serum sickness and penicillin hypersensitivity may also be accompanied by skin lesions, which must be differentiated from erythema marginatum. *Skin reactions,* such as hives, erythema multiforme and erythema nodosum, should not be confused with the lesions of erythema marginatum, which do not itch and are not markedly elevated or painful.

The diagnosis of acute rheumatic fever in patients with nonmigrating or monoarticular arthritis unaccompanied by other major manifestations is particularly hazardous. *Osteomyelitis* and *local*

TABLE 9–13 CLINICAL AND LABORATORY MANIFESTATIONS OF ACUTE RHEUMATIC FEVER* (MODIFIED JONES CRITERIA)

MAJOR MANIFESTATIONS	MINOR MANIFESTATIONS	SUPPORTING EVIDENCE OF STREPTOCOCCAL INFECTION	OTHER FINDINGS
Carditis	Fever	Recent scarlet fever	History of recent sore throat
Polyarthritis	Arthralgia†	Throat culture positive for group A streptococci	Family history of rheumatic fever
Chorea	Previous rheumatic fever or rheumatic heart disease	Increased ASO or other streptococcal antibodies	Abdominal pain Epistaxis
Erythema marginatum	Positive acute phase reactants: Increased erythrocyte sedimentation rate C-reactive protein		Tachycardia Rheumatic pneumonia
Subcutaneous nodules	Leukocytosis Prolonged P-R interval‡		Pallor and anemia Precordial pain Weight loss Malaise

Adapted from the recommendations of the Committee of the American Heart Association (Circulation, 32:664, 1965).

*The presence of 2 major or of 1 major and 2 minor manifestations supported by evidence of recent streptococcal infection indicates a high probability of acute rheumatic fever.

†Should not be counted as a minor manifestation in patients in whom polyarthritis is counted as a major manifestation.

‡Should not be counted as a minor manifestation in patients in whom carditis is counted as a major manifestation.

injuries to the bones and joints may be confused with the early stages of acute rheumatic fever. *Arthralgias,* such as *growing pains,* vaguely localized and confined to the lower extremities, most often presenting at night and disappearing in the morning, are a common complaint in children. There is no pain on motion, nor are there objective findings. In contrast to rheumatic joints, there is often relief from massage.

Pericarditis or myocarditis is often of viral origin, which should be considered in the absence of other clinical and laboratory manifestations typical of acute rheumatic fever. *Atrial myxomas* may also produce findings suggestive of rheumatic fever and rheumatic heart disease.

The movements of chorea must be carefully differentiated from simple fidgeting, tics and athetosis. Healthy children in close association with patients with chorea may mimic the disease sufficiently well to cause problems in differential diagnosis.

Subcutaneous nodules occur in rheumatoid arthritis, particularly in older persons without evidence of heart involvement. Because they usually occur as a late manifestation in children with well established rheumatic heart disease, they are rarely helpful in differential diagnosis.

Except in patients with pure chorea, the *absence of serologic evidence of streptococcal infection* in two or more antibody tests should stimulate a search for other possible diseases. On the other hand, elevated streptococcal antibody tests should *never* be the basis for diagnosis of rheumatic fever in the absence of definitive clinical criteria.

Every effort should be made to establish or disprove the diagnosis during the acute stage of the illness, as it is often difficult or impossible to make a diagnosis or to de-label patients years later. *Overdiagnosis of acute rheumatic fever on the basis of either clinical or laboratory findings should be assiduously avoided, since it may result in psychologic damage, a long-term commitment to unnecessary antimicrobial prophylaxis, and difficulties with regard to future insurability.*

TREATMENT. Therapy with salicylates or corticosteroids should *not* be initiated until a firm diagnosis has been established, since it may leave the physician in unresolvable doubt as to the nature of the disease process (see above). Ordinarily the disease is full-blown by the end of the first or second week, but some patients may have low-grade symptoms for a longer time, leaving the diagnosis in question. Although a therapeutic trial of aspirin or a corticosteroid has sometimes been used in such patients, the response is not sufficiently specific to make a certain diagnosis.

Bed rest is recommended during the acute stage of the disease. Strict bed rest, including feeding by an attendant, should be insisted upon in patients with congestive failure or cardiac enlargement without evidence of stabilization. *Sedatives* may be required in such patients. **Digitalis,** perhaps in conjunction with diuretics, should be used when heart failure is present. (See Section 13.) Although some patients may have unusual sensitivity to digitalis, requiring special caution in digitalization, there is consensus that rheumatic patients in congestive heart failure should be digitalized regardless of the presence or absence of active carditis.

The acute signs of rheumatic inflammation are quickly suppressed by **anti-inflammatory drugs**. Fever and joint manifestations disappear within a few days. The acute phase reactants, especially the sedimentation rate, may require several weeks to return to normal. *Corticosteroids* are more powerful suppressive agents than aspirin and may be somewhat more prompt in bringing the acute manifestations under control. They are the drug of choice for fulminating pancarditis. *Aspirin* may be the drug of choice for joint disease without evidence of carditis. Many physicians prescribe a corticosteroid when a firm diagnosis of carditis has been made in the acute stage. Opinions differ, however, and available evidence is conflicting as to the possible effect on residual heart disease.

The dosages of both aspirin and corticosteroids may have to be adjusted for individual patients to achieve suppression. For aspirin, a total daily dose of 60 mg per pound, not to exceed 10 gm per day, is usually adequate. Blood levels, occasionally helpful in patients who do not appear to respond to therapy or who show evidence of toxicity, should be maintained at about 25 to 35 mg/dl. Some patients tolerate aspirin poorly, responding with nausea and vomiting. Postprandial administration of enteric-coated pills may be helpful; sodium bicarbonate may reduce the effectiveness of salicylates. Tinnitus, decreased hearing acuity and hyperpnea may occur and require temporary discontinuance or adjustment of the dose. Prednisone is usually favored over other steroids because it may reduce the requirements for a low salt diet and added potassium. A dose of about 2 mg/kg/24 hr administered in divided doses is generally considered to be sufficient. High-dose (2.5–4 mg/kg/24 hr), short-term (7-day) therapy has been used in some clinics. Moonface, abdominal fullness and other mild manifestations of Cushing's disease occur in patients after several weeks of steroid therapy; severe reactions such as toxic psychoses, hypertension, overwhelming infection, growth retardation, gastric ulcers and compression fractures of the spine may occur with prolonged administration. In patients with mild or moderate disease who respond promptly, especially those without evidence of carditis, aspirin can often be discontinued in about 10 days or the dose of the steroid can be tapered and then discontinued after a similar time. Steroid treatment for periods up to 4 to 6 weeks or longer may be required for patients with severe carditis.

Rebounds occur after discontinuance of aspirin therapy and are even more common after steroid therapy. Arthralgia and fever are the usual manifestations; at times there is frank arthritis and, rarely, severe carditis. Subclinical rebounds may be detectable only by laboratory tests (acute phase reactants). The most reasonable explanation for rebounds is that anti-inflammatory drugs have been discontinued before the disease has run its natural course, which may be 1 to 5 weeks in patients with arthritis and 2 to 6 months or longer in patients with severe carditis. The clinical manifestations of rebound usually resolve spontaneously or respond to salicylate therapy.

There is no evidence that anti-inflammatory agents have any effect on erythema marginatum or Sydenham's chorea. It is questionable that they influence the disappearance of subcutaneous nodules.

The *management of chorea* is supportive. The disease subsides spontaneously after a few weeks or months; in unusual cases it may persist a year or more. Symptomatic care includes an environment free from noise and bright lights, patient and understanding attendants, and protection against tongue-biting and other self-injuries due to violent, uncontrollable movements. Phenobarbital or chlorpromazine may be helpful. Some patients manifest increased agitation during therapy with sedatives.

Antimicrobial agents are important in the prevention of further streptococcal insults, which may result in new or additional cardiac damage. They should be prescribed for all patients with acute rheumatic fever, including those with chorea. As soon as the diagnosis is established and cultures have been taken, therapeutic doses of penicillin should be prescribed to eradicate residual group A streptococci and then should be followed by continuous prophylaxis (see below).

Gradual *ambulation* should be started when the clinical and laboratory signs of acute disease have subsided, as soon as 7 to 10 days in children with no evidence of heart disease. Bed rest for periods of 3 weeks to 3 months may be required for patients with carditis, depending on the severity and evidence of progression or stabilization. Prolonged bed rest should be avoided, if possible, and due attention should be given to the psychologic needs and school activities of the child. *After recovery no restriction of physical activity* is ordinarily required, except in patients with persistent cardiac enlargement, who will usually tolerate moderate exercise, but may not tolerate the vigorous exercise of active competitive sports. Patients with rheumatic heart disease are susceptible to *subacute bacterial endocarditis*. They should be encouraged to maintain good oral and dental hygiene and should be protected against the possibility of this complication during dental and other surgical procedures that may result in bacteremia (Table 9–14).

PREVENTION. *Continuous antimicrobial prophylaxis* (Table 9–14) for patients with a well documented history of acute rheumatic fever or clear evidence of rheumatic heart disease has proved highly effective in preventing streptococcal infections and recurrences of acute rheumatic fever. Intramuscular benzathine penicillin is preferable to oral drugs, which depend heavily on patient cooperation and adequate absorption from the gastrointestinal tract. Ingestion histories have been shown to be a poor indication of compliance when com-

TABLE 9–14 PREVENTION OF RHEUMATIC FEVER AND BACTERIAL ENDOCARDITIS

PREVENTIVE AIM	RISK	APPROACH	RECOMMENDED REGIMENS*	EFFECTIVENESS	LIMITATIONS AND PRECAUTIONS
First attacks of rheumatic fever in general population	0 to 5 cases per 100 cases of streptococcal respiratory infection	*Eradication* of streptococcus by *prolonged* treatment of acute infection	*Single intramuscular injection of benzathine penicillin:* < 10 yrs., 600,000 units; > 10 yrs., 900,000 units; adults, 1,200,000 units *Oral penicillin for 10 days:* 200,000 to 250,000 units 3 or 4 times daily *Erythromycin* in penicillin-sensitive patients (20 mg/lb/day, up to 1 gm per day in older children and adults, for 10 days) Sulfadiazine and tetracyclines should not be used	90% effective with intramuscular benzathine penicillin; oral regimens generally less effective, usually due to failure to take drug regularly for 10 days	Dependent upon *recognition* of streptococcal infection and *differentiation* from viral infections *Subclinical infections* (comprising about 50% of total) usually escape detection except in cultured family or school epidemic contacts Reculture at 2 weeks to confirm effectiveness of oral therapy
Recurrent attacks of rheumatic fever in patients with well documented histor, rheumatic fever or definite evidence of rheumatic heart disease	10 to 50 cases per 100 cases of streptococcal respiratory infections	Prevention of streptococcal parasitism by *continuous administration* of antimicrobial agents (Acute streptococcal infections should receive vigorous and prolonged treatment, but complete reliance should not be placed on this approach)	*Intramuscular benzathine penicillin G*: 1,200,000 units at monthly intervals. *Oral sulfadiazine:*† < 60 lb, 0.5 gm once daily > 60 lb, 1.0 gm once daily *Oral penicillin:*† 200,000 to 250,000 units once or twice daily Erythromycin (250 mg twice daily) in patients sensitive to both sulfonamides and penicillin†	Intramuscular benzathine penicillin G is considerably more reliable than oral prophylaxis with either penicillin or sulfadiazine; oral sulfadiazine is at lease as effective, perhaps more effective than oral penicillin	Faithful patient cooperation is essential in oral prophylaxis; a simple urine test for penicillin is available for monitoring compliance‡ Monitor for possible reactions for first few months in patients receiving sulfadiazine. After this time reactions are extremely rare with either drug
Bacterial endocarditis in patients with rheu-	Transitory bacteremia from *dental and other*	Maintain high level of oral health. When	*For dental procedures likely to cause bleeding, tonsillectomy, adenoidectomy, and bronchos-*	Reduction in bacteremia has been demonstrated,	In patients with history of *sensitivity* to penicillin

matic or congenital heart disease	*operative and diagnostic procedures* is frequent; risk level of endocarditis not certain, but probably low	dental or other surgical procedures are required, *prevent* or minimize *bacteremia; eradicate implanted bacteria* before vegetation forms	*copy* (most likely organism: viridans streptococci): *Intramuscular penicillin.* Mixture of 600,000 units of *procaine penicillin G* and 200,000 units of *crystalline penicillin G,* 1 hour before procedure and once daily for 2 days after procedure *Oral penicillin V or phenethicillin.* 500 mg 1 hour before procedure and then 250 mg every 6 hours for at least 72 hours *Oral penicillin G.* 1,200,000 units 1 hour before procedure and then 600,000 units every 6 hours for at least 72 hours *For genitourinary or gastrointestinal tract surgery or instrumentation* (most likely organism: enterococci): *Penicillin (or ampicillin) + streptomycin.* Mixture of *procaine* and *crystalline penicillin* intramuscularly as outlined above or *ampicillin* 25–50 mg/kg orally or intravenously 1 hour before procedure and then 25 mg/kg every 6 hours for 72 hours plus *streptomycin* intramuscularly 40 mg/kg (up to 2 grams) 1 hour before procedure and once daily for 2 days after procedure, or *Vancomycin + streptomycin. Vancomycin* 20 mg/kg (up to 1 gm) intravenously 1 hour before procedure and then 10 mg/kg (up to 0.5 gm) every 6 hours for 72 hours plus *streptomycin* intramuscularly as indicated above. *For cardiac surgery* (most likely organism: staphylococci): *Penicillinase-resistant (semisynthetic) penicillin* or *cephalosporins* are drugs of choice.	but prevention of endocarditis is not documented	or ampicillin and in patients on *oral penicillin prophylaxis* undergoing dental or oropharyngeal procedures, substitute erythromycin 20 mg/kg (up to 500 mg) orally 1½ to 2 hours before procedure and then 10 mg/kg (up to 250 mg) every 6 hours for at least 72 hours. (Parenteral preparations also available.)

*Adapted from American Heart Association recommendations (Circulation, *43*:983, 1971).

†Before initiation of continuous prophylaxis, a full therapeutic course of penicillin or erythromycin should be given as outlined under treatment of acute infection (see above). This is to eradicate any possible residual streptococci which may or may not be demonstrable.

‡Markowitz, M., and Gordis, L.: Pediatrics *41*:151, 1968.

pared with urine tests for penicillin. Oral prophylaxis should be considered only in patients who are reliable, who have minimal or no heart disease, and who have not had repeated attacks of rheumatic fever. Prophylaxis should not be discontinued during childhood unless the original diagnosis is in doubt. Young adults should be urged to continue their prophylaxis, particularly while subjected to the hazard of exposure to streptococcal infections in the military service or by close contact with children as parents, baby-sitters, schoolteachers or in other occupations. Older adults, whose initial attack was many years previously, especially those without heart disease and with minimal exposure to streptococcal infection, may be in relatively little danger, but available information is insufficient to define their risk in discontinuing prophylaxis.

Prevention of first attacks of acute rheumatic fever (Table 9–14) is more difficult than prevention of recurrences because of problems in recognition and definition of streptococcal infection and assurance of adequate therapy. A throat culture, carefully taken and processed, will help to determine those who are harboring beta-hemolytic streptococci, but will not distinguish patients with streptococcal disease from streptococcal carriers with nonstreptococcal disease. This is a serious problem, since carrier rates among school-age children are often of the order of 20 to 25 per cent in the winter and spring and may on occasion be much higher. However, the risk of rheumatic fever may be small in such children, unless they have clear physical signs of pharyngeal or tonsillar inflammation, such as exudate, or association with an epidemic in their family or school.

Eradication of the infecting streptococcus is essential for successful prevention of rheumatic fever. Patients who harbor group A streptococci after oral therapy should be retreated with injectable benzathine penicillin. Examination of *family contacts* will reveal evidence of streptococcal infection in about 1 out of 4 persons. Treatment may be beneficial in those who have clinical evidence of infection or large numbers of beta-hemolytic streptococci in their throat culture. When there is a sequential pattern of infection within a family, treatment of all members should be considered.

Mass penicillin prophylaxis is rarely required in civilian populations and should be considered only when there is good evidence of epidemic streptococcal disease or multiple cases of acute rheumatic fever or acute nephritis. *Tonsillectomy* is ineffective in preventing initial or recurrent attacks of rheumatic fever and may increase the likelihood that streptococcal infections will go unrecognized clinically and therefore not be treated. Some *streptococcal vaccines* are currently being subjected to clinical trial, but the problem is a complex one because of the large number of serologic types, the question of whether primary immunization can be regularly achieved and the possible risks involved.

PROGNOSIS. Prognosis is related chiefly to the development and persistence of *heart disease.* Fulminating carditis progressing to death during or after a single attack occurs in only a few patients. In approximately one fourth to one third of patients with carditis, the heart disease will regress during the acute episode or over a 10-year follow-up period. Arthritis is never permanently crippling. The neurologic manifestations of chorea subside completely with time, but a high percentage of *psychiatric disturbances* has been reported in long-term follow-up studies. Since psychologic disturbances may commonly exist prior to the onset of chorea, it is not clear whether this finding is a cause or a result of the disease. Patients with pure chorea may be somewhat less likely to develop carditis than patients with other rheumatic manifestations, but some reports indicate that a considerable proportion will develop rheumatic heart disease if not protected by prophylaxis.

Most chronic disability and deaths are related to *recurrent attacks,* which occur with high frequency in rheumatic children not protected by antistreptococcal prophylaxis. In one study more than two thirds of patients had one or more recurrences during a follow-up period averaging 8 years. The risk of rheumatic fever following streptococcal infection is about 10 times greater in persons who have had one attack than it is in the general population. Recurrences are most likely to occur in younger children, in the years immediately after an attack, in patients with heart disease, and in those who have had multiple attacks.

LEWIS W. WANNAMAKER

PATIENT EDUCATION

You, Your Child and Rheumatic Fever. Available at no cost through your local Heart Association or from The American Heart Association, 44 East 23rd St., New York, N. Y., 10010.

GENERAL

Albam, B., and others: Rheumatic fever in children and adolescents: A long-term epidemiologic study of subsequent prophylaxis, streptococcal infections, and clinical sequelae. Ann. Intern. Med. *60*:(Supp. 5, No. 2, part II), 1964.

Ayoub, E. M., and Dudding, B. A.: Streptococcal group A carbohydrate antibody in rheumatic and nonrheumatic bacterial endocarditis. J. Lab. Clin. Med., *76*:322, 1970.

Aron, A. M., Freeman, J. M., and Carter, S.: The natural history of Sydenham's chorea. Am. J. Med. *38*:83, 1965.

Catanzaro, F. J., Rammelkamp, C. H., Jr., and Chamovitz, R.: Prevention of rheumatic fever by treatment of streptococcal infections. II. Factors responsible for failures. New Engl. J. Med. *259*:51, 1958.

Dorfman, A., Gross, J. I., and Lorincz, A. E.: The treatment of acute rhuematic fever. Pediatrics *27*:692, 1961.

Feinstein, A. R.: Standards, stethoscopes, steroids and statistics. The problem of evaluating treatment in acute rheumatic fever. Pediatrics *27*:819, 1961.

Goldring, D., Behrer, M. R., Brown, G., and Elliot, G.: Rheumatic pneumonitis. II. Report on the clinical and laboratory findings in twenty-three patients. J. Pediatr. *53*:547, 1958.

Gordis, L., Markowitz, M., and Lilienfeld, A. M.: The inaccuracy in using interviews to estimate patient reliability in taking medications at home. Med. Care, 7:49, 1969.

Inter-Society Commission for Heart Disease Resources: Prevention of rheumatic fever and rheumatic heart disease, Circulation *61*:A-1, 1970.

Kuttner, A. G., and Mayer, F. E.: Carditis during second attacks of rheumatic fever. Its incidence in patients without clinical evidence of cardiac involvement in their initial rheumatic episode. New Engl. J. Med. *268*:1259, 1963.

Lendrum, B. L., Simon, A. J., and Mack, I.: Relation of duration of bed rest in acute rheumatic fever to heart disease present 2 to 14 years later. Pediatrics *24*:389, 1959.

Marienfeld, C. J., Robins, M., Sandidge, R. P., and Findlan, C.: Rheumatic fever and rheumatic heart disease among U.S. college freshmen, 1956–60. Pub. Health Rep. *79*:789, 1964.

Markowitz, M., and Gordis, L.: Rheumatic Fever – Diagnosis, Management and Prevention, 2nd ed. Philadelphia, W. B. Saunders Company, 1972.

McCarty, M.: Missing links in the streptococcal chain leading to rheumatic fever. The T. Duckett Jones Memorial Lecture. Circulation *24*:488, 1964.

Stollerman, G. H.: Factors determining the attack rate of rheumatic fever. J.A.M.A. *177*:823, 1961.

Taranta, A.: Relation of isolated recurrences of Sydenham's chorea to preceding streptococcal infections. New Engl. J. Med. *260*:1204, 1959.

United Kingdom and United States Joint Report: The natural history of rheumatic fever and rheumatic heart disease: Ten-year report of a cooperative clinical trial of ACTH, cortisone and aspirin. Circulation *32*:457, 1965.

Wannamaker, L. W.: Medical progress: Differences between streptococcal infections of the throat and of the skin. New Engl. J. Med. *282*:23; 78, 1970.

Wannamaker, L. W., and Matsen, J. M.: Streptococci and Streptococcal Diseases. New York, Academic Press, Inc., 1972.

Wood, H. F., and McCarty, M.: Laboratory aids in the diagnosis of rheumatic fever and in evaluation of disease activity. Am. J. Med. *17*:768, 1954.

Zabriskie, J. B., Hsu, K. C., and Seegal, B. C.: Heart-reactive antibody associated with rheumatic fever: Characterization and diagnostic significance. Clin. Exp. Immunol. *7*:147, 1970.

10
INFECTIOUS DISEASES

CLINICAL USE OF THE MICROBIOLOGY LABORATORY

Much of the responsibility for attaining satisfactory laboratory diagnosis of infectious diseases rests with the clinician. It is he, not the laboratory worker, who decides what specimens to collect, when to collect them, how to obtain them and which laboratory procedures to request. He must also see that the specimens are preserved properly until they can be delivered to the laboratory. Finally, he should be competent to make the correct interpretation of the results.

The choice of specimens to be examined often makes the difference between diagnostic success and failure. The clinician will in many instances be guided by the patient's signs and symptoms as to the type of causative agent he should suspect. In other instances, however, the signs and symptoms may be so nonspecific that he must ask the laboratory s help in ruling out a variety of agents. Material from the system of the body chiefly involved should be collected; e.g., cerebrospinal fluid from a patient with meningeal symptoms or blood from a patient with fever of undetermined origin. Consideration should also be given to possible portals of entry, such as the upper respiratory tract in patients with meningeal involvement.

In the choice of specimens the clinician must decide whether an attempt should be made to isolate the causative agent or to demonstrate the antibody response, or both. More than one culture is advisable when seeking a pathogen.

BACTERIAL INFECTIONS

In bacterial infections the preferred diagnostic method is the demonstration of the responsible organism by smear and culture.

NASOPHARYNGEAL, THROAT AND SKIN SWABS. A dry cotton or alginate swab is most efficient for the collection of specimens from the skin and mucous membranes. The proper preservation of swab specimens is important. Since drying is rapidly destructive to some pathogenic bacteria, swab specimens should be placed promptly in about 0.3 ml of nutrient broth (Fig. 10–1).

Interpretation of results of cultures from skin and mucous membranes must take into account the fact that microbial flora are normally recovered from these areas. Some organisms will be considered pathogenic whenever found, such as *Corynebacterium diphtheriae* and beta-hemolytic streptococcus; others such as *Klebsiella pneumoniae* or staphylococci may or may not be pathogenic, depending on the circumstances; and still others, such as *Neisseria catarrhalis,* will rarely be considered pathogenic. It cannot be emphasized too strongly that there is poor correlation between flora of the upper airway and of the lower airway in cases of lower respiratory tract disease. Sputum specimens have value in determining lower respiratory tract flora; tracheal aspirates and lung punctures are even more useful.

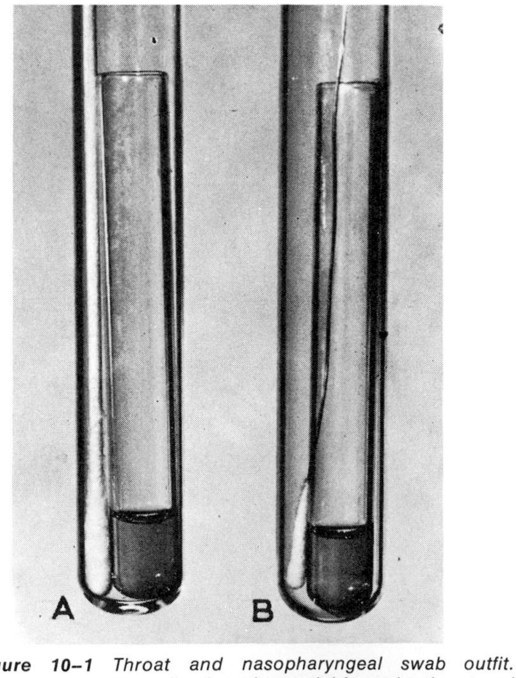

Figure 10–1 Throat and nasopharyngeal swab outfit. A, Wooden swab for collection of material from the throat and tonsils or for general use. B, Wire swab for collection of nasopharyngeal specimens. Both are contained in sterile cotton-plugged test tubes. After the test material has been obtained the swabs are immersed in the broth in the inner tube.

CULTURE OF FECES. Rectal swabs are cultured for two reasons: to identify common bacterial pathogens such as salmonella, shigella and enteropathogenic *Escherichia coli;* or to determine the predominant flora of the intestine in a patient with weakened host defenses whose endogenous flora may become pathogenic. It should be remembered that feces contain mostly anaerobic bacteria and that routine cultures identify only the predominant aerobic organisms among the billions of bacteria contained in each gram. Fortunately salmonella, shigella and enteropathogenic *E. coli* usually replace the normal aerobic flora when they cause acute infection, thus rendering their isolation easier. Even so, selective media are needed to suppress other organisms.

In patients on immunosuppressive therapy culture of the intestinal flora may have value in predicting the organism that will invade the blood stream through intestinal ulcerations. In certain epidemiologic situations vibrios *(Vibrio cholera, V. parahemolyticus)* may need to be sought by culture on alkaline peptone broth.

BLOOD CULTURE. Culture of the blood is one of the most fruitful procedures in the diagnosis of bacterial disease. It should be done carefully before administration of antibiotics, using iodine-alcohol for skin cleansing. After the venipuncture a fresh needle should be used for inoculating the blood into at least two flasks of medium prewarmed to room temperature. If only one sampling of blood is possible before antibiotic therapy begins, then a generous sample should be obtained: e.g., 10 ml from a newborn, 60 ml from an adult, and proportional amounts between these ages. Not more than 5 ml should be inoculated into each flask. If therapy with penicillins or cephalosporins has been started prior to culture, the bacteriologist may want to add penicillinase to help to destroy the antibiotics. Polyanethanol sulfate is included in modern blood culture media to inactivate leukocytes. If a positive isolate is reported, blood cultures should be repeated immediately to determine: (1) whether treatment has been successful when the patient is already on antibiotics; (2) whether the isolate is a contaminant when the organism reported is usually nonpathogenic; or (3) whether the organism is still present if the patient had not been given antibiotics in the interim.

CULTURE OF CSF. In addition to routine culture in appropriate media, cerebrospinal fluid from a patient with suspected bacterial meningitis should be incubated at 37° C for 12 to 18 hours for subsequent reculture. Turbid fluids may coagulate, thus rendering the detection of organisms difficult and accurate cell counts impossible. When turbid fluids are encountered, a portion of each specimen should be collected in an oxalate tube for smear and cell count. Gram stains of CSF are very helpful when the presence of organisms distinguishes bacterial from viral disease, but impressions gained from smears should not be relied on to limit treatment to that for a single bacterial organism. Errors are possible, even in experienced hands, and it is better to use broad-spectrum initial therapy in life-threatening disease than to wait for the culture report before ordering specific treatment. Fluorescent antibody identification of pathogens in the CSF is more accurate, but so long as ampicillin can be used for initial therapy it is probably preferable to await the results of culture before changing to antibiotics of narrower spectrum. If there are enough organisms in the CSF, a quellung reaction can be performed with antisera to *Hemophilus influenzae* type b, or to various types of meningococci and pneumococci.

URINE CULTURE. Urine for culture and colony count can be obtained in three ways: clean catch, catheterization or suprapubic puncture. The latter method is the most accurate, since urine so obtained should normally be sterile. Urine collected by catheter may have up to 100 organisms per ml in boys and up to 300 per ml in girls without signifying infection. Clean catch urine, if obtained after adequate cleansing, can be considered abnormal if more than 10^5 organisms/ml are present, and possibly abnormal if between 10^4 and 10^5 organisms are counted per ml. In practice it often happens that urine specimens from girls are obtained by the clean catch technique after inadequate washing and allowed to sit at room temperature for some time before being transported to the laboratories. This accounts for the high frequency in girls of putatively positive urine cultures which are not confirmed when repeated. Urine cultures should be done carefully or not at all, since false positives may condemn a patient to long courses of antimicrobials.

EXUDATES AND TRANSUDATES. Abscesses, pleural fluids, joint fluids and other miscellaneous exudates and transudates can be cultured directly on agar, but inoculation of some material into blood culture medium is desirable, since polyanethanol sulfate will stop leukocytic action on bacteria. One cannot overemphasize the necessity for prompt delivery of these specimens to the laboratory. In addition to cultures and stains, sugar and cell count determinations should be done on all transudates, for the same reasons they are done on CSF.

GRAM STAIN. The examination of a Gram stain should be carried out on all cultured fluids, including urine.

SPECIAL CULTURES. Most bacteria can be cultivated on blood agar, chocolate agar and eosin-methylene blue or MacConkey agar. In some cases, clinical circumstances may call for the use of additional media, such as those listed in Table 10–1. When an organism on this list is suspected, the microbiology laboratory should be informed in advance of sending the specimen. If the hospital's laboratory is not proficient in a particular culture technique, prior arrangements should be made with a reference laboratory that can do the necessary culture. The frequency of recovery of anaerobic organisms has increased in recent years, as media with low redox potentials have gained wide use.

TABLE 10–1 SOME PATHOGENS REQUIRING SPECIAL MEDIA FOR CULTIVATION

SUSPECTED ORGANISM	APPROPRIATE SPECIAL MEDIUM
Anaerobic organisms	Prereduced media, incubated under inert gas
Bordetella pertussis	Bordet-Gengou medium
Brucella sp.	Serum-glucose broth, under CO_2
Corynebacterium diphtheriae	Loeffler's and tellurite media
Francisella tularensis	Blood-dextrose-cystine agar
L-Forms of bacteria	Sucrose-containing hyperosmotic medium
Leptospira sp.	Tryptose phosphate–rabbit serum broth
Mycobacterium sp.	Löwenstein-Jensen or Middlebrook media
Mycoplasma pneumoniae	Horse serum agar
Neisseria gonorrhoeae	Thayer-Martin medium

FLUORESCENT ANTIBODY STAINS. Fluorescent antibody (FA) technique has widened the diagnostic scope of direct microscopy. Specific antisera are now available commercially for several common pathogens. In these sera the antibody molecules have been conjugated with a fluorescein dye. The specific dye-labeled serum is added to the smear containing the suspected organism and the slide examined microscopically under ultraviolet light. If the organism is present, the antibody molecules are concentrated about it and the observer sees a bright fluorescence. The presence of even a small number of organisms in the smear can be detected in this manner. This *direct method* can be used if specific fluorescein-labeled antisera are readily available. In the absence of such sera, the *indirect method* is useful, though more complex. In the indirect method there are two steps: (1) the slide is covered with the unlabeled specific antiserum, time is allowed for antibodies to fix, and then the excess of unfixed antibody is washed off; and (2) the slide is then overlaid with a fluorescein-labeled gamma globulin specific for the species in which the antiserum was made. The antigamma globulin antibodies are concentrated and fluoresce at the sites of specific microorganism-antibody complexes. The potential of fluorescence in bacteriology is great, but at this time its principal use has been in the identification of *Mycobacterium tuberculosis, Bordetella pertussis* and *Corynebacterium diphtheriae*. and in the grouping of streptococci. The case of *M. tuberculosis* is a special one, in that no antibody is used; rather, the smears are stained with auramine-rhodamine, which is taken up by the organisms, and which fluoresces under ordinary light. This fluorescent stain is more sensitive and specific than the acid-fast stain.

SKIN TESTS. The Schick test and the Dick test (for susceptibility to diphtheria and to scarlet fever, respectively) are no longer in general use. The principal indication for skin testing is suspicion of mycobacterial infection. Purified protein derivatives of *M. tuberculosis* (PPD-S) and other mycobacteria (PPD-B, PPD-Y, etc.) are not sensitizing in themselves, but dermal hypersensitivity to them often provides the quickest means of diagnosis. If skin tests are negative, but clinical suspicion remains high, skin testing for anergy should be conducted with one of the potent sensitizers like keyhole limpet hemocyanin (KLH).

SEROLOGIC TESTS. Bacteria are often typed through agglutination by specific sera, but determination of serum antibodies is useful in only a few bacterial infections, among which are those caused by streptococci, salmonella and brucella. In the case of streptococci, antibodies against exotoxins are assayed to determine whether there has been recent significant invasion. Salmonella antibodies must be measured for each group (A, B, C, D, etc.) and for both flagellar and somatic antigens. Unless positive and negative control sera are tested also, the results may be misleading.

ANTIBIOTIC SENSITIVITIES. Most laboratories now routinely test bacterial isolates for sensitivity to various antibiotics. Clinicians have come to depend on this information for selection of therapy, but are not always aware of how to obtain the best information from the laboratory and how to interpret it. The most prevalent technique of antibiotic testing is by the Kirby-Bauer method, in which a standardized inoculum of the organism is seeded onto a plate. Paper discs, each impregnated with an antibiotic, are placed on the plate, and the zone around each disc is measured. The concentration of antibiotic in the disc is supposed to reflect the achievable blood level, and for most antibiotics the zone size is generally correlated with the actual clinical sensitivity of the organism. However, there are many pitfalls in disc sensitivity testing. The geometry of the test indicates that the difference in area between a zone of 13-mm diameter and one of 12-mm diameter is 17 per cent, presumably equivalent to a 17 per cent difference in antibiotic activity. Small differences, therefore, have large effects, and the control of inoculum size, the rate of diffusion of antibiotics and the accurate measurement of zones are critical.

Apart from the technical artifacts in antibiotic testing, clinicians may misapply valid results. Antibiotic sensitivities cannot be interpreted correctly except in the pharmacologic context. Certain clinical situations, such as endocarditis or osteomyelitis, call for the use of bactericidal rather than bacteriostatic drugs. Although a staphylococcus might be sensitive to both semisynthetic penicillins and erythromycin, only the use of the former would be acceptable in a blood stream infection. Toxicity of drugs must also be taken into account: chloramphenicol is very active in vitro and in vivo, but the use of other agents is preferable when possible. Finally, attainable blood and tissue levels are the true touchstone of clinical efficacy: polymyxin B gives good zones of inhibition in vitro, but the highest blood levels that can be tolerated are often insufficient to achieve sterilization; on the other hand, carbenicillin may appear ineffective in vitro, but the high blood levels that are possible with this drug, and its synergism with certain other antibiotics like gentamicin, may make it useful even when in vitro results do not appear promising.

For more accurate measurement of antibiotic sensitivity, tube dilution procedures are used. An antibiotic is diluted in steps through the range of the attainable blood level and then each tube is inoculated with the test organism (about 10^4 organisms). After 24 hours the tubes are examined for turbidity; the first clear tube is the bacteriostatic concentration (minimal inhibitory concentration, or MIC). The tubes are then subcultured to agar plates; the concentrations of antibiotic in tubes that yield no organism on subculture are bactericidal (minimal bactericidal concentration, or MBC).

The bacteriostatic and bactericidal activity in the serum of a patient receiving antibiotics can be similarly measured by inoculation of the organism originally isolated from the patient into dilutions of serum obtained at known times after injection or infusion of antibiotics. The actual concentrations of certain antibiotics in the blood can be measured by chemical assays or by microbiologic assays using susceptible stock strains of bacteria. These measurements are mandatory when patients with renal disease are treated with potentially toxic antibiotics.

A good example of the utility of the above procedures is in the management of streptococcal endocarditis. First, the organism is tested by tube dilution against penicillin G. If sensitive, the bacteriostatic and bactericidal activities of serum are measured ½ hour and 6 hours after infusion of penicillin. Killing at ½ hour and at 6 hours should occur at dilutions at least as high as at one eighth and at one half, respectively. If the organism is relatively resistant to penicillin G and an aminoglycoside needs to be added to the regimen, actual measurement of the aminoglycoside will help to monitor the optimal blood level.

SPIROCHETES

Serologic procedures are heavily relied on for the diagnosis of treponemal infection. Many serologic tests have been developed for syphilis, including complement fixation, precipitin, and fluorescent antibody methods. Darkfield examination of lesions of skin and mucous membranes may strongly suggest the diagnosis, but serologic confirmation is necessary. Leptospira can be cultivated directly in special media, but serologic tests are more generally available. Other spirochetes can be visualized directly.

MYCOPLASMA AND L-FORMS

These organisms are discussed together because they both lack cell walls. *Mycoplasma pneumoniae* is an important cause of pneumonia and can be isolated on agar medium. Serologic tests on paired sera (by complement fixation, for example) are more often positive than cultures. If cold agglutinins are found in the blood, a presumptive diagnosis of mycoplasmal infection can be made, but both false negatives and false positives are common.

FUNGI

The diagnosis of fungal disease is often difficult, and all possible procedures should be employed. Direct visualization in pus or exudates using various stains is particularly helpful in candidiasis, cryptococcosis and actinomycosis. Culture on Sabouraud's medium is desirable for all fungi except candida, which grows well on ordinary bacterial media. Urine culture helps to identify candidal pyelonephritis. Blood and bone marrow cultures are frequently positive in disseminated histoplasmosis.

Fungal serology is just coming into wide use, including precipitin, hemagglutinating, complement fixing and agglutinating antibody systems. Currently, serologic tests are most valuable in candidiasis, coccidioidomycosis, cryptococcosis and histoplasmosis. In addition, cryptococcal antigen can be sought in serum or CSF by latex slide agglutination.

Reliance on skin tests for the diagnosis of acute fungal infection is to be condemned; many patients do not manifest hypersensitivity and many normal people have been sensitized by previous exposure. Furthermore, skin test antigens may produce confusing rises in serum antibody.

RICKETTSIAE

Ordinarily no attempt is made to culture rickettsiae. Instead, diagnosis relies on nonspecific and specific serologic tests. The latter are accomplished with complement-fixing antigens prepared from yolk sacs infected with each species of rickettsia. The nonspecific test is the familiar Weil-Felix reaction, which depends on a heterologous antibody response to Proteus OX organisms. It should be remembered that all serologic tests can be negative early in rickettsial infection.

PROTOZOA

Protozoan infection is identified mainly by direct visualization; for example, of amebae in feces, of

TABLE 10–2 MICROBIOLOGIC APPROACHES TO THE DIFFERENTIAL DIAGNOSIS OF FOUR SYNDROMES*†

SYNDROME	TESTS TO BE DONE
Exanthem of uncertain origin (See also specific conditions mentioned)	Blood culture for bacteria (e.g., meningococci, *Salmonella typhosa*)
	Throat culture for streptococcus
	Serologic test for streptococcal antibodies
	Serologic test for syphilis
	Serologic test for toxoplasmosis
	Serologic test for rickettsiae (Proteus OX and specific CF antibodies)
	Nose and throat swabs for viruses (measles, rubella, enteroviruses)
	Rectal swab for viruses (e.g., enteroviruses)
	Serologic tests for heterophile antibodies and EB virus antibodies (infectious mononucleosis)
	Serologic tests for viruses (e.g., measles, rubella)
Meningitis, suspected (See also specific conditions mentioned)	CSF stain and culture for bacteria
	Blood culture for bacteria
	CSF fluorochrome stain for mycobacteria
Meningitis, suspected (*continued*)	CSF culture for mycobacteria
	PPD–S skin test for mycobacterial hypersensitivity
	CSF culture for leptospira
	Serologic test for leptospirosis
	CSF culture for fungi
	India ink stain for cryptococci
	CSF and serum for cryptococcal antigen
	Serologic tests for cryptococcal and other fungal antibodies
	CSF culture on HeLa cells for amebae
	CSF culture for viruses
	Nasopharyngeal and rectal swabs for viruses (e.g., mumps, enteroviruses)
	Serologic tests for viruses (e.g., mumps, arboviruses)
Pulmonary infiltrates of uncertain nature (See also Section 12, and specific conditions)	Blood culture for bacteria
	Tracheal aspirate or sputum culture for bacteria
	Gram stain of tracheal aspirate or sputum

*Not all tests will necessarily need to be done in any given situation, but when the diagnosis is obscure most of these will be indicated.

†Where serologic tests are suggested, paired sera are required except in "Neonatal infection, suspected."

Pneumocystis carinii in lung aspirates, or of sporozoans in blood. Serologic tests, however, are extremely valuable in the diagnosis of toxoplasmosis and malaria. Screening for toxoplasma antibodies is widely practiced in newborns with possible congenital infection, and the absence of malarial antibodies is the most accurate means of excluding malaria.

HELMINTHS

Traditionally, direct examination of stool or of other materials has been the method of diagnosis of helminthic infection. When tissue invasion occurs, as in trichinosis, echinococcosis, toxocariasis, and so forth, serologic procedures become crucial in efforts to identify the parasite. These tests are done at the Center for Disease Control, Atlanta, Georgia.

VIRUSES

If viral disease is a diagnostic possibility when the patient is first seen, immediate steps should be taken to confirm the diagnosis, since delay usually nullifies attempts at isolation and makes serologic results more difficult to interpret.

MICROSCOPIC OBSERVATION. Electron microscopy and fluorescent antibody techniques provide opportunities for quick identification of viruses. Vesicle fluid can be examined by electron microscopy to distinguish smallpox (a poxvirus) from

TABLE 10-2 MICROBIOLOGIC APPROACHES TO THE DIFFERENTIAL DIAGNOSIS OF FOUR SYNDROMES (*Continued*)

SYNDROME	TESTS TO BE DONE	SYNDROME	TESTS TO BE DONE
Pulmonary infiltrates of uncertain nature (*Continued*)	Fluorescent stain of nasopharyngeal swabs for pertussis	**Pulmonary infiltrates of uncertain nature** (*continued*)	Serologic tests for viral antibodies (e.g., adenoviruses, respiratory syncytial viruses)
	Fluorescent stain of sputum or gastric washings for mycobacteria	**Neonatal infection suspected** (See also Neonatal Septicemia, Section 7, and specific conditions)	Blood culture for bacteria
	Sputum or gastric washings for mycobacterial culture		Throat cultures for bacteria
	PPD-S skin test for mycobacterial hypersensitivity		Rectal cultures for bacteria
	Sputum stain and culture for fungi		Urine cultures for bacteria
	Serologic tests for fungal antibodies		Gastric aspirate for bacterial stain and culture
	Lung biopsy (preferred) or aspiration for *Pneumocystis carinii* (patient on immunosuppressive therapy)		Serologic test for syphilis
	Throat culture for *Mycoplasma pneumoniae*		Serologic test for toxoplasma antibodies
	Serologic test for cold agglutinins (*Mycoplasma pneumoniae*)		Nasal swab for rubella virus
	Serologic test for antibodies to *M. pneumoniae*		Throat swab for viruses (e.g., herpes, coxsackie B)
	Serologic test for psittacosis		Rectal swab for viruses (e.g., coxsackie B, ECHO)
	Serologic test for Q fever antibodies		Urine culture for viruses (cytomegalovirus, herpes)
	Nasopharyngeal and rectal swabs for viruses		Serologic tests for cytomegalovirus, herpesvirus, rubella, equine encephalitis
			Serologic test for hepatitis B antigen

varicella (a herpesvirus). Smears of mucosal cells or urinary sediment can be stained by fluorescent antibody to identify the antigens of any virus for which one has a good animal antiserum. Rubella and respiratory syncytial viruses, among others, have been rapidly detected in this way.

Cytologic examination is an aid in diagnosis when inclusion bodies or syncytia are found, as in the urine of patients infected with cytomegalovirus, for example, and in the noses of patients with measles; but such demonstration should be buttressed with actual isolation of the virus.

ISOLATION. Viruses and rickettsiae require living cells for propagation; the cells used may be in the form of intact laboratory animals, embryonated hen's eggs or tissue cultures of human or animal cells. Some viruses are difficult to isolate, and since many different tissue culture systems must be employed to isolate a wide range of viruses, the unspecified request from the clinician for "virus isolation" is impractical. Virus laboratories can screen for the most common agents and are materially assisted if the clinician can name the virus he is looking for, or at least state the type of illness.

Prompt delivery of specimens to the laboratory is essential. In some cases bedside inoculation of cultures may increase the chance of virus recovery. Routinely, throat and stool or rectal swab specimens should be submitted. Throat specimens are best taken by means of vigorous throat swabbing, which results in removing some superficial cells. For certain viruses, e.g., rubella, swabs should be taken from the nasal turbinates. The swab should be rinsed thoroughly in a fluid medium (nutrient broth or 0.5 per cent gelatin in Hanks' solution), squeezed against the glass and discarded. Discarding of the swab is important because the chlorine used for bleaching the stick is toxic for tissue culture cells in which virus isolation will be attempted. If the laboratory is reasonably close, storage of specimens at 4° C for a few hours is permissible. If to be mailed, the specimen should be frozen and packed in sufficient dry ice for the journey.

Rectal swabs should not be heavily charged with feces, as the antibiotics present in viral transport media may be insufficient to kill a large inoculum of bacteria. Rectal swabs should be collected in respiratory and central nervous system syndromes, since many viruses replicate in the intestinal cells.

Cerebrospinal fluid is often positive during the acute stages of CNS inflammation. It is good practice to take a small extra amount of spinal fluid for viral diagnostic studies at the initial lumbar puncture. This can always be discarded if a positive diagnosis of bacterial meningitis is made.

Urine culture for viruses is most useful for the isolation of cytomegalovirus, but urine is also a good source of mumps and adenoviruses.

Vesicular fluid can be cultured to distinguish among vaccinia, variola, varicella, herpes and enteroviruses.

Blood is not routinely cultured for viruses, though viremia is part of many if not most viral infections.

The principal difficulties with virus isolation are: the fragility of some viruses such as the respiratory syncytial virus on removal from the patient; the need for living cell cultures or organisms as substrates for virus growth; and the uncertainty with which pathogenicity can be attributed to many isolates from the respiratory or gastrointestinal tracts.

SEROLOGIC TESTS. To establish a firm etiologic relationship between a viral isolate and a disease, serologic tests are required, unless the isolation was directly from tissues rather than from mucosal surfaces. To establish the etiologic diagnosis, it is necessary to demonstrate a fourfold rise in titer of specific antibody against the isolated agent in the convalescent serum over the titer in the acute serum.

Correct diagnosis from serologic tests requires at least two blood specimens: The first should be taken at the time of the first examination during the early acute phase of the disease ("acute serum"); the second ("convalescent"), 14 to 21 days later. If the second is taken earlier than 14 days, it is advisable to take a third blood specimen 4 to 6 weeks after the onset, since the rise of antibodies may be delayed, especially in infants. Great care must be taken to avoid contamination and hemolysis. An aseptic venous puncture, avoidance of air bubbles and early separation of serum are all important in obtaining the best results. Serum should be frozen for preservation; whole blood should never be.

Although the finding of a substantial titer against a suspected agent in a single late acute or convalescent specimen of serum will not differentiate between a recent and a past infection (two serum specimens usually being necessary for a definitive diagnosis), under the following circumstances the study of a single serum specimen can strongly support a clinical diagnosis: (1) a high antibody level in comparison with that of the population in general; (2) particularly in neonates, antibody in the IgM fraction; (3) antibody in the young infant not present in the mother; (4) antibody in both infant and mother which persists at the neonatal level in the infant; (5) in suspected mumps, the presence of antibody to the soluble ("S") fraction of the mumps virus in the acute serum (this antibody may be found as early as the second or third day of the disease, when that to the viral ("V") antigen may be absent or very low); and (6) in infectious mononucleosis, the presence of antibody to the early antigen in cells infected by EB virus.

Antibody can be detected by a variety of specific serologic methods, some methods being more appropriate than others for specific viruses. Complement-fixation (CF) antigens are available for a great range of viruses, and CF antibodies have the advantage of being generally correlated with recent infection. In poliomyelitis, for example, CF antibodies appear during acute infection and often disappear within a year. Neutralizing antibodies, on the other hand, remain for life, and unless one has obtained serum early in the disease, a rise in antibodies may be difficult to show. Furthermore, neutralization tests have the technical disadvantage of needing to be done in tissue cultures or in whole animals. Hemagglutination-inhibition (HI) antibodies correlate fairly well with neutralizing antibodies. Fortunately, many viruses such as the myxoviruses, rubella and some enteroviruses have the capacity to agglutinate erythrocytes. The presence of antibodies can be detected by the extent to which a particular serum specifically inhibits hemagglutination. Many of the viruses that agglutinate red cells will also cause adsorption of red cells to the membranes of infected cell monolayers. Inhibition of adsorption is a particularly useful test for parainfluenza virus antibodies. Fluorescent antibodies (FA) can be detected by the technique of indirect fluorescence (see above). FA antibodies are slightly less sensitive than HI antibodies, and for their demonstration require slides bearing cells infected with the specific virus against which antibodies are being sought. On the other hand, FA tests can be performed very quickly. Indirect hemagglutination tests are now in greater use in virology than heretofore; these depend on the attachment of viral antigens to glutaraldehyde or tannic acid-treated sheep erythrocytes.

APPLICATION OF MICROBIOLOGY TO DIAGNOSTIC PROBLEMS

When the diagnosis is uncertain but infection is a possibility, a systematic approach to the patient is necessary, involving multiple cultures and serologic procedures. Diagnostic strategies will, of course, depend on the severity of the illness, the epidemiology and the clinical likelihood of certain infections. Table 10–2 presents examples of complete microbiologic approaches to certain diagnostic problems, indicating the tests that *might* be considered for patients presenting: (1) an exanthem; (2) the possibility of meningitis; (3) pulmonary infiltrates of uncertain nature; or (4) possible infection in the neonatal period.

STANLEY A. PLOTKIN

Bodily, H. L., Updyke, E. L., and Mason, J. O.: Diagnostic Procedures for Bacterial, Mycotic and Parasitic Infections. Washington, D.C., American Public Health Association, Inc., 1970.
Lennette, E. H., and Schmidt, N. J.: Diagnostic Procedures for Viral and Rickettsial Infections. Washington, D.C., American Public Health Association, Inc., 1969.

GENERAL CONSIDERATIONS IN BACTERIAL INFECTIONS

There are principles in diagnosis and treatment of bacterial infections which are common to most, if not all, of the infections considered in this section. A grasp of these principles will help to indicate appropriate answers to specific questions.

DIAGNOSIS. Bacteriologic diagnosis by isolation of the offending agent is essential to selection of effective therapy and, in some instances, to outcome. Bacteriologic diagnosis requires collection of appropriate specimens from appropriate sites and use of effective transport media and culture techniques. Knowledge of the pathogenesis of the disease, of the expected spectrum of pathogens and of the best sites for recovery of the organism are all requisite to the proper collection of specimens.

In the initial phases of many infections, specific bacteriologic information is lacking; therapy must then proceed on empiric or presumptive bases. If certain agents can be logically anticipated, a wise selection of antibiotics can be made and "shot-gun" therapy or inappropriate choices avoided. For example, bacterial meningitis after 2 months of age is almost always due to *Hemophilus influenzae* type b, pneumococci or meningococci; accordingly, ampicillin will likely be the most appropriate and effective therapy.

Reliance on nonbacteriologic means of diagnosis is fraught with peril, but occasionally rewarding. For example, reliance on the total white count or the proportion of neutrophils to decide whether a particular instance of pharyngitis is due to group A β-hemolytic streptococci will be as often wrong as right. Therapy based solely on this criterion will treat many children needlessly; others who deserve therapy will remain untreated. On the other hand, a purulent spinal fluid with a low glucose content is characteristic of bacterial meningitis, even if a gram stain is negative; in such a case, therapy should not wait for isolation of an organism.

The urgency for etiologic identification is directly dependent upon the risk to the patient of imprecise diagnosis. A pulmonary infection in a patient who is immunodeficient may demand early lung aspiration or biopsy to obtain bacteriologic information, whereas in the infant with normal defenses these procedures may be unwarranted.

PRINCIPLES OF MANAGEMENT. The cornerstone of therapy in most bacterial infections is the employment of effective antimicrobials, but lack of attention to other modalities of therapy may be detrimental and even lethal.

Isolation must be considered whenever there is risk to patient or hospital personnel (see below). Staphylococcal infections, meningococcal infections and bacillary dysentery require attempts to prevent transmission to personnel and other patients. Patients with diminished capacity to respond to infections must not be exposed to additional infectious agents. A major defect of isolation is that its inconvenience may lead to fewer visits to the patient; personnel must be stimulated to submit to the inconvenience. Limitations should be removed promptly as the need for isolation diminishes (e.g., as bacteriologic cure of meningitis is achieved) in order not to hamper care during convalescence.

Malnutrition, metabolic derangements and disturbances in fluid balance may all contribute to the failure of recovery from infection. Optimal therapy requires timely correction to the extent possible.

For the poorly nourished patient, energy for metabolism must be provided. Ordinarily this can be accomplished in acute infections by intravenous administration of hypertonic (10 per cent) glucose solutions. For more chronic infections one may wish to use oral alimentation as soon as is feasible; when applicable, intravenous alimentation should be undertaken.

Disturbances in fluid balance and electrolytes should be corrected as rapidly as appropriate. When fluid loss through vomiting or diarrhea has occurred over a 24- to 48-hour period, replacement therapy may generally proceed rapidly; chronic losses must be replaced more slowly. Circumstances of the specific infection may also modify replacement or maintenance regimens in severe infection. In bacterial meningitis, for example, it is desirable to avoid excessive fluid administration to minimize cerebral edema or the effects of inappropriate ADH secretion.

Administration of blood or blood components has been a traditional practice in severe infections, but except for acute correction of significant anemia or for replacement of acute blood loss, there is no firm rationale for their use. On the contrary, administration of blood may worsen the patient's immediate condition (through febrile reactions, cardiac failure, fluid and oncotic overload, etc.) or result in long-term problems (sensitization to red or white blood cells, development of anti-IgA antibody in IgA deficient individuals, and the like).

Bed rest is generally advisable for patients with severe infections, and limitation of activity for those with milder disease, but this is also a time-honored but unproved prescription. In general, the child should be allowed to set his own level of activity within broad limits. Once he or she "feels better," it is fruitless and exasperating to attempt to enforce immobility in bed.

Other forms of therapy should be employed appropriately: oxygen for cyanosis; surgical procedures (drainage, biopsy, excision, etc.) when indicated; postural drainage of the respiratory tract; and so on. Shock, including "gram-negative" (endotoxic) shock, should be anticipated, recognized when it occurs, not overlooked because attention is concentrated upon the infection, and treated promptly and appropriately. Disseminated intravascular coagulation (DIC) frequently receives too little attention as a part of pediatric infections. It is particularly common in meningococcemia. Pathogenesis and treatment are discussed in Section 14.

Antimicrobial therapy must be appropriate to the individual infection, and given by an appropriate route in proper dose; possible toxic effects must be monitored.

The choice of route for administration is based upon: (1) pharmacology of the antibiotic; (2) desired tissue levels; and (3) toxicity. Intramuscular chloramphenicol is therapeutically useless and oral administration often associated with poor absorption; intravenous use may be safest and most reliable. Absorption of the penicillins is generally reduced in the presence of food; if predictable effect is urgently needed, then oral administration upon an empty stomach must be arranged or parenteral therapy substituted.

Intravenous therapy should be employed whenever it is desirable to penetrate tissue reached only with high blood levels. In osteomyelitis and meningitis only intravenous therapy will provide sufficient tissue levels for initial therapy. Only after almost total eradication of the organism can a change to oral therapy be made in osteomyelitis; in meningitis the period of therapy may be so brief that all can be accomplished by the intravenous route.

The choice of an antimicrobial agent for a given patient with a given disease should represent a considered balance between anticipated effectiveness, the risk of toxicity and the risk of the disease. In a patient with streptococcal pharyngitis who is allergic to penicillin, one employs an agent of second choice. On the other hand, if the same patient had staphylococcal septicemia and pneumonia or bacterial endocarditis, one might elect and risk a rapid desensitization procedure in order to employ penicillin or an appropriate derivative.

VINCENT A. FULGINITI

ISOLATION MEASURES FOR INFECTIOUS DISEASES

The care of a patient with a communicable disease should include measures to prevent others from contracting it. Certain quarantine practices, which vary with the specific infection (Table 10–3) and in different localities, have been set up for the protection of the community (Table 10–4). Quarantine regulations have at best a limited value in control of the spread of contagious diseases. In many places "placarding" is no longer practiced. Until effective vaccines for active immunization are widely available there are substantial arguments in favor of permitting children to contract certain viral infections in the preadolescent years, provided they are in good health at the time. For the control of poliomyelitis, diphtheria, smallpox, pertussis, measles and rubella, artificially induced immunity is of great importance.

Patients with contagious diseases should be isolated, not only to limit distribution of the disease, but also to protect them from secondary infection.

Isolation technique necessitates cooperation of physician, nurse and family, and, in hospitals, of all personnel, including those from laboratories, housekeeping or maintenance, who may come in contact with the patient or his environment. An error in technique by any of these persons may defeat the efforts of the others.

The patient and the area in which he

TABLE 10–3 PERIODS OF INFECTIVITY OF SELECTED INFECTIONS*

DISEASE	INFECTIVE	RECOMMENDED ISOLATION
Diphtheria	Two to 4 weeks; 1 to 2 days after start of therapy	Until 2 or 3 consecutive cultures are negative
Scarlet fever (scarlatina)	Variable; a day or two after start of therapy	One day after start of therapy
Measles (rubeola)	Five days of incubation through several days of rash	From onset of catarrhal stage through third day of rash
Rubella (German measles)	Seven days before rash to 5 days after; up to 10 to 12 months for congenital	None, except that women in the first trimester of pregnancy should not be exposed
Smallpox (variola)	Onset of rash until all crusts are shed	Until all crusts are shed
Chickenpox (varicella)	One day before rash until 5 to 6 days after onset, when all lesions crusted; longer in patients with immune deficiency	Until all lesions crusted; usually 5 to 6 days
Pertussis	From catarrhal stage through fourth week	Four weeks or until cough has ceased; protect infants from exposure
Poliomyelitis (enterovirus)	Variable respiratory excretion at onset; in feces later to several weeks	Enteric precautions
Mumps	Up to 7 days before and 9 days after onset of parotitis or other manifestation	Until swelling subsides
Infectious hepatitis	Variable; in feces up to 3 weeks after jaundice	Enteric precautions

*Adapted from Report of the Committee on Infectious Diseases. (Red Book, 17th Ed.) American Academy of Pediatrics, 1974.

is—whether a room in the home or the hospital, a cubicle or space in a ward—constitute a contaminated unit. The space between beds in an open ward should be at least 6 feet. Anything which comes into contact with the unit area must be considered contaminated. Isolation precautions for persons entering and leaving the unit area are based on "hand and gown technique"; all physicians and nurses should be familiar with an approved method. When the child is to be cared for by a nonprofessional attendant at home, e.g., the mother, adequate instruction should be given by the physician.

The adequate washing of hands before and after every contact with an infected patient is the essential element in isolation technique. Those caring for the patient should not touch anything in the contaminated area except with the commitment to adequate handwashing. The clothing of attendants should be protected by their donning clean or sterile gowns for each contact with the patient. These must be donned, worn, removed and disposed of in accordance with acceptable technique.

Infectious agents may also be transferred by air conduction. The control of airborne infection is still not adequately solved. The control of dust through use of oils on floors and blankets may be useful; air sterilization with ultraviolet irradiation or an aerosol has limited effectiveness in reducing the spread of infection in institutions. Antibiotic treatment of bacterial infections is the most effective means for limiting their spread.

The unit area must be properly equipped to care for the patient, and nothing should be taken into it that is not necessary or cannot later be destroyed or decontaminated. The trays and dishes—or the bottles for infants—should be sterilized after each use by boiling or autoclaving.

A bedpan should be provided for each patient. In the home a special bathroom reserved for the isolated area is a great convenience.

Bed linen and clothing, including diapers, should be adequately disinfected by washing in very hot water with an appropriate soap, detergent or bactericidal chemical; in the home they should be boiled before being sent to the laundry. The *hot* cycle of many home laundry machines is often adequate, so long as the water is hot enough (70° C or higher).

Secretions from the eyes, nose, mouth and throat should be received on soft paper squares which are placed in a paper bag and burned.

All attendants should be in good health and free of infection of the respiratory or intestinal tracts.

TABLE 10–4 SUGGESTIONS FOR QUARANTINE REGULATIONS*

DISEASE	PATIENT IS RELEASED FROM ISOLATION AND MAY RETURN TO SCHOOL	SUSCEPTIBLE CONTACTS MAY RE-ENTER SCHOOL	IMMUNE CONTACTS MAY RE-ENTER SCHOOL
Diphtheria	On recovery, and after 2 or 3 successive negative cultures; each from nose and throat; taken after cessation of antimicrobial therapy and at intervals of not less than 24 hours.	When two or more successive cultures of nose and throat are negative, or not for at least 7 days after last exposure	If bacteriologically negative
Scarlet fever	Upon clinical recovery, but not less than 7 days from onset	No restriction	No restriction
Measles (rubeola)	On recovery; at least 8 or 9 days (5 days after appearance of rash)	Exclusion from school of no practical value; when practiced, at least 14 days must elapse after last exposure	No restriction
Rubella (German measles)	Quarantine is usually not imposed. Period of infectivity estimated from 7 days before and 4 to 5 days after appearance of rash	No restriction; should avoid contact with women in first trimester of pregnancy until past incubation period	No restriction
Smallpox (variola)	On recovery and after disappearance of scabs and crusts; usually 3 to 6 weeks	16 days after successful vaccination	If there is not continued exposure and if successfully vaccinated within 5 years; the person should be vaccinated whenever exposure occurs even if there has been a previous successful "take"
Chickenpox (varicella)	On recovery and when crusts have formed; not sooner than 7 days after onset	Exclusion from school of no practical value; when practiced, at least 21 days must elapse after exposure	No restriction
Pertussis	Not before 3 weeks after onset of typical paroxysms	14 days after exposure, if clinically well	No restriction
Poliomyelitis (enterovirus)	One week after onset of symptoms or after defervescence, whichever is longer	No restriction	No restriction
Mumps	When swelling has disappeared	No restriction	No restriction
Infectious hepatitis	After first week of illness	No restriction	No restriction

*Adapted from several sources, principally from The Control of Communicable Diseases, The American Public Health Association, New York, 1960, and Report of the Committee on the Control of Infectious Diseases, American Academy of Pediatrics, 1974.

Patients should be discharged from their units only after thorough bathing with soap and warm water, including a shampoo. They should not, of course, return to the contaminated area.

Other materials, as well as the floor and furniture of the room, should be thoroughly washed with a disinfectant and water, and the room aired for at least 24 hours before again being occupied.

Material in the unit area which cannot be burned is cleansed as follows: all clothing and linen, as already described; mattresses and pillows are aired for 6 to 8 hours, preferably on two successive days; all glass, rubber, china, enamelware and any instruments which permit it are boiled for 5 to 10 minutes, or autoclaved or wiped down with an antiseptic solution.

When a patient is to be taken to an operating or x-ray room, or is transferred to another unit area, the accompanying attendant must wear a clean gown, and the patient should be wrapped in a clean sheet. Equipment in the operating or x-ray room which has been contaminated should be cleaned in the manner described for the unit area.

VICTOR C. VAUGHAN

BACTERIAL INFECTIONS

STREPTOCOCCAL INFECTIONS

Streptococci are among the commonest causes of bacterial infections encountered in pediatric practice. Group A β-hemolytic streptococci account for most cases of *bacterial* tonsillopharyngitis, though most upper respiratory infections are due to viruses. Apart from the discomfort of the acute illnesses caused by this organism, the potential risk of serious nonsuppurative sequelae of streptococcal infections makes it mandatory that all physicians who care for children should be knowledgeable in regard to the diagnosis and treatment of these infections.

ETIOLOGY. Streptococci belong to the Eubacteriales order and the *Lactobacillaceae* family. They occur as spherical cocci possessing rigid cell walls which contain specific antigens. Within the cell wall is a C-carbohydrate component which forms the basis for Lancefield grouping (groups A to O). Among the protein antigens is one identified as M-protein, which is closely related to the virulence of the organism. Different M-proteins determine type specificity within the Lancefield groups, there being more than 50 M-protein types. Streptococci elaborate a number of biologic products, including enzymes, toxins and hemolysins. Among the more important ones are streptokinase, streptodornase, diphosphopyridine nucleotidase, and a variety of hemolysins, including streptolysins O and S. The characteristics of hemolysis divide streptococci into those with hemolysins producing complete hemolysis of red blood cells (beta-hemolytic), those producing partial hemolysis (alpha-hemolytic) and those producing no hemolysis (gamma-hemolytic).

The classification of streptococci is confused. Four clinically relevant groups are usually recognized, but their separation is not based upon any single criterion: the *hemolytic streptococci* (beta-hemolytic, belonging to C-carbohydrate groups A to O) include important clinical pathogens, especially in groups A, B, C and G; *Streptococcus viridans* (variable hemolysis of alpha or gamma type, with no C-carbohydrate in the cell wall) is included among the normal flora and only occasionally produces disease; *Streptococcus faecalis* or *enterococcus* (variable, or no hemolysis with C-carbohydrate of the D group) is normally found in the gastrointestinal tract and rarely produces disease in children; *Streptococcus lactis* (variable hemolysis, C-carbohydrate of N type) is unimportant in human disease.

Streptococci are distributed in nature as part of the normal flora of many species, including man. Their capacity to produce disease is determined by their structure, the chemical products they elaborate and the response of host tissues to their presence. Pathogenic characteristics of streptococci include: (1) the M protein, which is responsible for immunologic reactions which may attack normal host tissue (cardiac muscle and other mesenchymal cells); (2) hemolytic toxins; (3) the erythrogenic toxin, the elaboration of which probably depends upon bacteriophage infection of the bacterium, and which is toxic to mucosal and dermal cells (scarlet fever) and may damage other tissues; and (4) a number of enzymes which contribute to penetration of tissues, to destruction of phagocytes and red blood cells, and to a favorable environment for microbial growth.

EPIDEMIOLOGY. Streptococcal infections may be sporadic, endemic or epidemic. The organisms are frequently encountered in healthy individuals who may subsequently become infected or who may infect others. Group A beta-hemolytic streptococci are spread from person to person and, some suspect, from animals to people. Infections due to group A β-hemolytic streptococci are usually spread by droplets expelled by infected individuals; they are more common in cold weather. Since these organisms are ubiquitous, the gathering of people into groups (schools, camps, military installations), personal contacts with infected individuals, and such stresses as fatigue or predisposing nonbacterial infection all contribute to the likelihood of infection. In confined populations the rate of infection may approach epidemic proportions.

Acquisition of streptococci is inhibited in early infancy, presumably owing to maternal immunity transmitted to the fetus through IgG type-specific antistreptococcal antibodies. Along with the loss of maternal IgG comes exposure to an increasingly widening circle of individuals potentially infected with various serotypes of group A β-hemolytic streptococci. Either overt infection or a transient carrier state may ensue, during which type-specific immunity usually develops. By adult life sufficient contacts have occurred to provide a broad spectrum of immunity to the common serotypes. Rates of clinical infection are highest among school-age children and young adults.

Streptococcal skin infection may also occur in epidemic fashion but is more often observed in warm seasons, unlike respiratory disease. Pharyngitis may accompany skin infections in summer; it appears to represent spread from skin to throat.

The epidemiologies of rheumatic fever and glomerulonephritis are discussed elsewhere. (See Index.)

PATHOLOGY. Changes in infected tissues are those of an acute inflammatory response. Edema, dilatation of capillaries, migration and accumulation of polymorphonuclear phagocytic cells and a lymphatic reaction are all observed. Regional nodes may demonstrate reactive and proliferative changes which can progress to frank suppuration.

In scarlet fever acute dilatation of vessels occurs,

with a superficial inflammatory infiltrate; death and desquamation of the epithelium follow. Injection of antitoxin into as yet unaffected skin prevents the appearance of the rash of scarlet fever.

In streptococcal pneumonia extensive tissue necrosis is added to the acute inflammatory changes. Streptococcal meningitis is not unlike other forms of pyogenic meningitis.

CLINICAL MANIFESTATIONS. The commonest infections due to group A β-hemolytic streptococci involve the respiratory tract, skin, soft tissues and blood. Nonsuppurative sequelae include acute rheumatic fever and glomerulonephritis, which are discussed elsewhere.

Respiratory Tract Infection. A marked difference in clinical expressions of upper respiratory tract infections with group A β-hemolytic streptococci is observed between early infancy and later childhood. The infant develops an insidious nasopharyngitis. A thin, clear or slightly cloudy nasal discharge is associated with the development of anorexia, irritability, lack of weight gain and other nonspecific symptoms. These signs and symptoms may develop over a period of several weeks without conspicuous nasopharyngitis. Cervical lymphadenopathy, rhinitis and signs of weight loss are apparent on physical examination, but the pharynx does not appear acutely inflamed nor is exudate present. This syndrome is referred to as **streptococcosis.**

In older children the more classic picture of **streptococcal pharyngitis** is likely. Acute onset of sore throat is accompanied by fever and vomiting. Listlessness, some dysphagia and anorexia occur. The tonsils and pharynx are intensely reddened and covered with a purulent, yellowish, patchy exudate. Marked edema is usually present; both edema and erythema may spread to the palate. In instances of severe disease tonsillar and pharyngeal edema may impose upon the airway and lead to respiratory obstruction. Palatal petechiae may be noted. Cervical lymphadenitis is usually present, and the pain associated with sore throat and tender nodes may result in meningismus. Whereas the above description represents severe forms of infection, many patients have more limited findings; as many as 20 per cent with acute infection may have few or no signs or symptoms.

If the infecting streptococcus elaborates an erythrogenic toxin to which specific antibody (antitoxin) has not previously been made by the host, then **scarlet fever** may occur. Erythrogenic toxin produces a bright red punctate or finely papular skin rash, which is often better felt than seen. The rash first appears in skin creases (axillae, groin, neck) and rapidly spreads to involve the trunk, extremities and face, save for the perioral area (circumoral pallor). The deep creases may contain linear streaks of rash that will not blanch on pressure (Pastia's lines, in the antecubital flexure). The rash usually appears on the first or second day of illness, reaches peak intensity by 3 to 7 days and slowly fades, frequently leaving a very fine desquamation which flakes spontaneously and upon friction of the surface. Given a history of sore throat and rash, the observation of this "branny" fine desquamation, particularly at the margins of the fingernails, on the fingertips and in the deep skin creases, will often suggest scarlet fever.

During the development of the toxic skin eruption, the mucous membranes may also be involved. The tongue is most notably affected, with a characteristic appearance: projecting above a diffusely coated white surface are prominent red papillae (white strawberry tongue). As desquamation occurs (3 to 7 days), a residual appearance supervenes, a denuded, deeply reddened surface with edematous, red papillae (red strawberry tongue).

Toxic manifestations of scarlet fever include severe headache, abdominal pain, vomiting, delirium and fever. Systemic effects of erythrogenic toxin may involve kidney (hematuria), joints (arthritis) or heart (myocarditis). The child may be profoundly ill, with severe apprehension or prostration.

Any of the secondary bacterial effects (as contrasted to the toxic) of group A β-hemolytic streptococcal infection may be seen in scarlet fever, as well as in pharyngitis without scarlet fever. If the host has antitoxic immunity to erythrogenic toxin, none of the manifestations of scarlet fever are seen despite production of erythrogenic toxin.

Streptococcal pharyngitis in adults is similar in appearance to that described for children, but the systemic symptoms are less severe and may be totally absent.

Streptococcal pharyngitis may be accompanied by infection of contiguous tissues (sinusitis, otitis media) or may be the precursor, if untreated, of more distant spread (bacteriuria, pneumonia, meningitis).

Pneumonia. Pneumonia due to group A β-hemolytic streptococcal infections produces a severe necrotizing pneumonitis, particularly in the neonate, in immunologically compromised individuals, and following severe viral pulmonary infections. There are no characteristic symptoms or signs which distinguish pneumonia due to group A β-hemolytic streptococci from that due to other pyogenic organisms such as pneumococci. The disease tends to be diffuse rather than lobar or lobular, to be rapidly progressive, to be associated frequently with pleuritis and/or empyema and to be resistant to antimicrobial therapy once the process is well established.

Skin Infections. The commonest form of skin infection due to group A β-hemolytic streptococci is pyoderma. Less frequently one may see cellulitis, lymphadenitis or lymphangitis.

Pyoderma takes several forms; the usual superficial infection **(impetigo)** is very common in young children, particularly of toddler and preschool age. Deeper infections also occur and may be associated with concurrent staphylococcal infection.

Typically, and frequently at the site of previous injury, a small blister develops; it is thin walled and easily ruptured. The lesions rapidly crust with thin, honey-colored scales. Multiple sites of involvement commonly appear, owing to spread of the organism by scratching. The individual lesions are very superficial, involving the outermost layers of the epidermis.

Deeper infections may occur secondary to impetigo or upon deeper implantation of streptococci. **Streptococcal cellulitis** presents a painful, diffuse induration in involved areas. Considerable overlying erythema and edema are observed. Lymphangitis ("streaking") is frequently seen cephalad to a lesion on the extremities, and regional nodes are commonly involved. **Erysipelas** (St. Anthony's fire) is a superficial, local cellulitis of skin characterized by a raised, irregular, advancing border. The border is frequently blanched in comparison with the main mass of the lesion, which is usually hot, red and very tender. Systemic symptoms are usually prominent, with fever, vomiting and irritability.

In the neonate a rapidly progressive cellulitis may follow group A β-hemolytic streptococcal infection; it is often associated with bacteremia and death. The progression may be so rapid that there is no response to usually effective therapy.

Bacteremia and Septicemia. Invasion of the blood stream most commonly occurs as a sequel to infection of the skin or respiratory tract in children. It may, however, be seen as a primary event without obvious antecedent disease. Streptococcal bacteremia is associated with fever and such "toxic" manifestations as chills, malaise, prostration, delirium and vomiting. Signs and symptoms of the localized infection may be present, and if seeding of other organs occurs, manifestations referable to those sites may develop (meningitis, pyelonephritis, arthritis, etc.).

Uncommonly, group A β-hemolytic streptococci may be the agents involved in acute or subacute bacterial endocarditis.

DIAGNOSIS. The certain diagnosis of infections due to group A β-hemolytic streptococci can be accomplished only by isolation of the organism in appropriate clinical syndromes. Identification of group A β-hemolytic streptococci is relatively precise and sensitive by common laboratory procedures. First, typical colonies with β-hemolysis are identified on primary isolation and subcultured to obtain pure cultures; then one of several methods may be employed to identify group A organisms (bacitracin disc sensitivity or fluorescent antibody staining). This series of procedures will give a reasonably reliable result within 48 hours of obtaining the material for culture. Some group A β-hemolytic streptococci (2 to 4 per cent) will fail to be identified by these techniques; less commonly a false identification will be made. Ultimate precision in bacteriologic diagnosis requires those serologic techniques for Lancefield grouping usually available only in reference laboratories.

Clinical criteria alone do not suffice in the identification of various streptococcal syndromes, since they may be mimicked by other disease processes (see differential diagnosis); the manifestations of pharyngitis are too variable to permit precise etiologic identification. Nonspecific laboratory tests such as total white blood cell count, differential count, erythrocyte sedimentation rate, C-reactive protein and other similar tests do not help to establish a specific diagnosis.

Specific host responses to streptococcal antigens can be identified. The only commonly employed technique is the measurement of antistreptolysin-O (ASO) titers in individuals suspected of having been infected by group A β-hemolytic streptococci. In 80 per cent of untreated children ASO titers increase within the first 3 weeks following infection. Prompt chemotherapy may modify the height of the response or completely forestall it. In patients in whom rheumatic fever develops, very high titers of ASO antibody are found. The response in glomerulonephritis is irregular and more variable.

Differential Diagnosis. In children with *acute pharyngitis,* viral pharyngitis and infectious mononucleosis are the most common diseases requiring differentiation. The only certain differentiation is by culture of specimens obtained by pharyngeal swab. Group A β-hemolytic streptococci may occasionally be isolated in infectious mononucleosis; the typical clinical manifestations, presence of atypical lymphocytes in the peripheral blood and rise in heterophil antibody titer should serve to identify this condition. Failure to isolate streptococci suggests viral pharyngitis, which can be specifically identified by viral studies or presumed by exclusion.

Less often, acute leukemia (with agranulocytosis), staphylococcal pharyngitis, tonsillar tuberculosis (unilateral, less erythema and edema), diphtheria (character of membrane, toxicity, low-grade fever, specific culture) or other infections (tularemia, toxoplasmosis) must be differentiated.

Scarlet fever must be differentiated from a variety of viral exanthems, including: rubeola (Koplik's spots, characteristic rash, respiratory and conjunctival involvement); rubella (postauricular adenopathy, mildness of disease, epidemic pattern in community, negative throat culture); enteroviruses (season of year, associated symptoms, epidemic nature, negative throat culture); fifth disease (reticulated rash, flushed, "slapped-cheek" appearance, lack of pharyngeal signs, negative cultures); roseola (three-day fever, transient nature of rash); and infectious mononucleosis (splenomegaly, adenopathy, hematologic and serologic changes).

Occasionally sunburn, scalded skin syndrome (toxic epidermolysis) and Stevens-Johnson syndrome require differentiation.

Skin infections are seldom confused with other conditions save for pyoderma and cellulitis due to staphylococci. Frequently only culture can establish the correct bacteriologic diagnosis.

In most instances of pneumonic, septicemic and meningitic forms of streptococcal disease, only isolation of the offending organism establishes the definitive cause.

COMPLICATIONS. Pyogenic complications usually involve contiguous spread and/or invasion of the blood stream. Local abscesses (peritonsillar, retropharyngeal), lymphangitis and regional lymphadenitis, bacteremia and distant dissemination (meningitis, osteomyelitis) have all been observed. Direct extension of nasopharyngeal infection into the middle ears, mastoids and sinuses may occur. Extension of upper respiratory tract infection into the lower airways produces pneumonia, frequently with empyema and occasionally with mediastinitis.

Nonsuppurative complications include acute rheumatic fever and acute glomerulonephritis. These entities and their relationship to prior streptococcal infection are discussed elsewhere.

PROGNOSIS. Untreated streptococcal infections may heal, but pyogenic or nonsuppurative complications are common. With early therapy, complete recovery from the infection is the rule except in such fulminant, progressive infections (pneumonia, sepsis) as may progress despite seemingly adequate therapy.

THERAPY AND PREVENTION. Antimicrobial therapy is the mainstay of treatment of streptococcal infections. Penicillin remains the preferred agent, since it is routinely effective and no streptococci have been isolated which are resistant to it. The goals of therapy are twofold: first, to control primary disease and prevent or treat pyogenic complications; and second, to prevent nonsuppurative sequelae through total elimination of the organisms. The essential principles of therapy are: (1) that the patient must be exposed to penicillin for at least 10 days continuously; (2) that the tissue level of penicillin must be sufficient to eradicate streptococci; and (3) that only conversion of positive cultures to negative will be adequate to achieve the goal of prevention of nonsuppurative sequelae. Many regimens achieve these goals, ranging from oral to parenteral therapy, and with a variety of forms of penicillin. Such factors as acceptability to the patient, cost, compliance, inconvenience and pain have all been considered in recommending one or another regimen. An effective therapeutic program can generally be found among the choices.

Oral Regimens. Breese and others have indicated that at least 800,000 units of penicillin G or its equivalent must be administered orally daily for 10 days to achieve eradication of streptococci. Most commonly, 300,000 to 400,000 units of penicillin are given four times daily. Most studies do not demonstrate a clear therapeutic superiority of other penicillins over penicillin G. Phenoxymethyl penicillin (penicillin V) has a theoretical advantage, however, in its capacity to be absorbed even in the presence of food. Compliance may be enhanced with the simpler instructions required. Therapy must be continued for a full 10 days.

Parenteral Regimens. Bass and others have demonstrated an advantage for regimens employing adequate doses of benzathine penicillin. The question of compliance of the patient is circumvented, the level of penicillin is adequate, and the lowest relapse rates are obtained with regimens employing benzathine penicillin. Bass claims a shorter clinical course for combinations of shorter acting penicillins with benzathine penicillin. Recommendations for dosage vary; we prefer a combination of 600,000 units of procaine penicillin with 600,000 units of benzathine penicillin. If the data of Bass are correct, it may be necessary to employ as much as 1.2 million units of benzathine penicillin, in which case the volume of the combination becomes too large and it would be preferable to administer the benzathine penicillin alone.

Patients *allergic to penicillin* should receive erythromycin (40 mg/kg/day) or lincomycin (at the same dose). Regimens using antibiotics other than penicillin are associated with higher relapse rates; reculturing after therapy is essential for evaluation of the effectiveness of the treatment. Sulfonamides and tetracyclines have *no* place in therapy of acute streptococcal illness. Sulfonamides may be used in *rheumatic fever prophylaxis.* (See Table 9–14.)

Periodically it has been suggested that newer antibiotics are equivalent to penicillins. Such claims have frequently been based upon studies with inadequate follow-up and little or no assessment of effect on the ASO response. Penicillin *does* reduce the incidence of rheumatic fever and, some believe, of glomerulonephritis. Another antimicrobial agent for streptococcal illness must match this record *and* have some superiority over penicillin in pharmacologic or safety characteristics.

For systemic infections or for severe infections outside the skin or upper respiratory tract, parenteral administration of soluble penicillin G is the treatment of choice. The intravenous route is often the best; doses are empiric. We usually assay the serum killing power (SKP) to assess the effectiveness of dosage in these instances.

Management of carriers of β-hemolytic streptococci is controversial. Some experts believe that therapy of the carrier may abort type-specific immunity, rendering the individual susceptible to reinfection and potentially only deferring illness to a later age. We have employed a family contact approach: "family" is defined as those living, eating and sleeping in, or otherwise closely associated with a household; cultures are made of family members, and, if positive, the members are treated as above. More casual contacts (in schools, on playgrounds, etc.) are excluded from such surveillance. Institutional epidemics may modify the definition of "family" to include contacts within the institution.

Children who have had rheumatic fever require continuous prophylactic therapy against streptococcal infection (Table 9–14). Such children should be examined promptly when respiratory infections occur; cultures are obtained, and if β-hemolytic streptococci are recovered, penicillin is administered.

Attempts to develop streptococcal vaccines have been frustrating. Imperfect understanding of streptococcal immunology has made selection of antigens difficult; at least one trial has resulted in an adverse immunologic effect.

Breese, B. B.: Beta-hemolytic streptococcal infections in children. Pediat. Clin. N. Amer. 7:843, 1960.
Dillon, H. C., Jr., and Derrick, C. W., Jr.: Streptococcal complications; The outlook for prevention. Hosp. Prac. 7:93, 1972.
Kaplan, E. L., Top, F. H., Jr., Dudding, B. A., and Wannamaker, L. W.: Diagnosis of streptococcal pharyngitis: Differentiation of active infection from the carrier state in the symptomatic child. J. Infect. Dis. *123*:490, 1971.
Lancefield, R. C.: Current knowledge of type-specific M antigens of group A streptococci. J. Immunol. *89*:307, 1962.
Stillerman, M., and Bernstein, S. H.: Streptococcal pharyngitis: Evaluation of clinical syndromes in diagnosis. Am. J. Dis. Child. *101*:976, 1961.
Wannamaker, L. W.: Differences between streptococcal infections of the throat and of the skin. New Engl. J. Med. *282*:23, 78, 1970.

PNEUMOCOCCAL INFECTIONS

The pneumococcus is one of the three major coccal pathogens; the others are the streptococcus and the staphylococcus. The early use of antibiotics for respiratory tract infections has reduced the incidence of severe disease due to the pneumococcus, except in areas of the world where access to medical care is limited and treatment delayed. In addition to classic lobar pneumonia, pneumococcal infection may be manifest as bronchopneumonia or otitis media and, less frequently, as meningitis, peritonitis, pericarditis or bacteremia. The pneumococcus is a normal inhabitant of the upper respiratory tract. Its role in pharyngitis and nasopharyngitis is generally believed to be that of a secondary invader.

ETIOLOGIC AGENT. The pneumococcus is a gram-positive, often "lancet"-shaped diplococcus, with a type-specific polysaccharide capsule with which one can identify 82 different strains. The presence of the capsule is variable; it is the most significant property of the organism relative to virulence, since it protects against phagocytosis. The capsule also permits rapid differentiation from *Streptococcus viridans*. Pneumococci can be recognized readily on blood agar plates through their flat umbilicated colonies and alpha hemolysis. Typing is accomplished by adding specific antisera to suspensions of the organism and observing for capsular swelling (quellung reaction), which is dependent upon the interaction between antibody and a capsular specific soluble substance (SSS). The pneumococcus produces no toxins.

EPIDEMIOLOGY. The peak incidence of pneumococcal disease occurs in the respiratory disease season, December to April. The neonate and very young infant are usually spared major pneumococcal disease, owing to transplacentally acquired type-specific immunoglobulin G antibody. The later absence of type-specific serum antibody is correlated with an increased incidence of nasal colonization and is associated with a peak incidence of disease from 1 to 4 years of age. The incidence of pneumococcal disease is therefore greatest in young children and in old age, falling with the acquisition of type specific antibodies in childhood and increasing as these are lost with diminishing exposure in old age.

Most clinical disease in infants and children is caused by types I, V, VI, XIV, XIX, XXIII. The presence of these or other strains in the nasopharynx does not reliably indicate their relationship to concurrent disease, since pneumococci are found in the nasopharyngeal flora of 20 to 50 per cent of asymptomatic individuals. On the other hand, the highly pathogenic strains are much less frequently found in asymptomatic carriers than are the nonpathogenic strains.

Pneumococcal disease is generally sporadic, but epidemics have occurred in closed communities (nurseries, orphanages). Pneumococcic infection is more frequent and more severe in children with immunoglobulin deficiencies, asplenia and sickle cell disease. The frequency and severity of pneumococcic meningitis is greater among children of disadvantaged socioeconomic status, probably owing to poor nutrition.

PATHOLOGY AND PATHOGENESIS. Changes in tissues in pneumococcal infection depend upon whether the infection is a first or a subsequent encounter for the host. To cause disease the pneumococcus must breach the body's nonspecific defenses against infection, especially those of the respiratory mucosa. Mucosal damage from a viral infection both favors the rapid and abundant implantation of pneumococci and impedes phagocytosis through accumulations of respiratory secretions. Once established in tissues, pneumococci multiply rapidly and may spread, either through bacteremia or by direct extension from a local site (such as from the ear or mastoid to the meninges); as many as 30 per cent of patients with pneumococcal pneumonia have bacteremia.

The pathologic sequence in pneumococcal infections of the lung is described in Section 12. Early in the course of infection capsular specific soluble substance (SSS) fosters spread of infection through its antiphagocytic action. An edema-producing factor also enhances rapid early spread of infection. As specific antibody is developed, fixed tissue macrophages become more numerous and SSS less protective against improved and more specific phagocytic mechanisms of the host. This sequence usually takes place during the first 7 days of the infection; it may be accelerated by administration of type-specific serum. The progression of intra-alveolar pulmonary exudation through consolidation to ultimate clearing of the tissue reaction by mononuclear cells completes the pathologic process in the lung. Antibiotic therapy modifies the spreading (edema) phase of pulmonary infection, with lysis of clinical signs and symptoms, and shortens the period of consolidation.

Pneumococcal meningitis is accompanied by an outpouring of protein into the cerebrospinal fluid; the resulting adhesions may be a factor in the incidence of sequelae, which is higher than in meningococcic meningitis.

CLINICAL MANIFESTATIONS. These are related to the site of localization. In most instances, the pneumococcus first produces a respiratory infection (pneumonia, otitis media, sinusitis). Subsequent spread may broaden the clinical spectrum to include mastoiditis, meningitis, brain abscess, osteomyelitis, arthritis, peritonitis, pericarditis or endocarditis.

The onset of the respiratory phase of pneumococcal disease usually follows an incubation period of 1 to 7 days. The symptoms vary with age and prior experience with pneumococcal antigens. Though fever and chills may have a sudden onset in a previously well child, in the absence of antibody due to prior exposure pulmonary involvement may be slow to develop. In the older child, as in the adult, rapidly progressive pulmonary disease may reflect a hypersensitivity reaction to pneumococcal protein. Respiratory symptoms and findings will vary with the severity of disease. (See Pneumococcal Pneumonia, Section 12.)

Convulsions or meningismus may occur in infants whose infection is basically respiratory in nature; but they suggest pneumococcal meningitis if there is otitis media or mastoiditis, and the spinal fluid must be examined. With pneumococcal bacteremia, gangrenous areas of the skin may appear on extremities and face, but are uncommon; disseminated intravascular clotting may occur concomitantly. Pneumococcal osteomyelitis and arthritis are common in patients with such predisposing factors as immunologic deficiency syndromes, congenital or traumatic asplenia, or sickle cell disease (autosplenectomy). Primary peritonitis, now rare, is usually pneumococcal in origin; children with untreated nephrotic syndrome appear to be particularly susceptible.

DIAGNOSIS. A definitive etiologic diagnosis is possible only with isolation of pneumococci from material obtained from a site of infection or from blood; isolation from the nasopharynx does not establish a causal relationship with clinical disease. Serologic testing is available, but not clinically useful at the present time. Blood cultures should be obtained in all cases of lobar or lobular pneumonia, meningitis, cutaneous gangrene, osteoarthritis, peritonitis or pericarditis.

Leukocytosis is usual and tends to be pronounced, with a marked predominance of neutrophils (more than 75 per cent) and an outpouring of immature cells (more than 20 per cent). Marked polymorphonuclear leukocytosis is characteristic enough of pneumococcal infections to suggest a pneumococcal etiology for childhood infections associated with peripheral blood leukocyte counts over 30,000/mm^3 and a predominance of neutrophils. The sedimentation rate is elevated.

In pneumococcal meningitis, as opposed to that due to *H. influenzae* or the meningococcus, the organism is almost always easily identifiable on gram stain of the cerebrospinal fluid. Rarely, many bacteria may be present in the cerebrospinal fluid early in the disease with little or no cellular reaction; accordingly, a stained smear must be examined even if the fluid appears clear. (See Meningitis.)

Differential Diagnosis. During the prodromal period prior to development of localizing disease it is often difficult to differentiate pneumococcal from other bacterial or from viral infections. The characteristic, marked polymorphonuclear leukocytosis is often helpful in differentiating pneumococcal disease; children with an unexplained febrile illness and marked polymorphonuclear leukocytosis should have a roentgenogram of the chest and a blood culture even if there are no auscultatory signs suggestive of pneumonia. A history of exposure is important in differentiating granulomatous and fungal diseases of the lung.

Signs of upper and lower airway infection, including stridor, hoarseness, bronchiolar spasm or wheezing, are frequently associated with respiratory syndromes of viral etiology. Roentgenograms of the chest are useful to delineate classic lobar pneumonia from lobular and other forms of infiltrative patterning less characteristic of pneumococcal infection. On the other hand, lobar pneumonia may also be caused by other pyogens, and pneumococcal pneumonia in small infants often does not assume the characteristic lobar form seen in older children and adults. Bacterial, fungal and granulomatous respiratory syndromes must be differentiated by microbiologic cultures as well as by skin and serologic tests. Pneumococcal meningitis can be differentiated from other causes of meningitis by examination and culture of the spinal fluid.

Pain may be referred to the right lower quadrant from the right hemidiaphragm in patients with right lower lobe pneumonia, and may suggest appendicitis, mesenteric adenitis or infection of the right kidney. A roentgenogram of the chest assists in differential diagnosis. Similarly, upper lobe pneumonia not infrequently causes **meningismus,** a term applied to resistance of the neck to anterior flexion in patients without meningitis. Meningismus is also sometimes seen in children with acute cervical adenitis, other respiratory infections with fever, brain abscess or brain tumors in the posterior fossa. With pneumococcal pericarditis or septicemia, elevation of the serum glutamic oxaloacetic transaminase (SGOT) is not uncommon.

COMPLICATIONS. Complications of pneumococcal infection usually occur as direct extensions of localized areas of infection (e.g., empyema from pneumonia, mastoiditis from otitis media, or meningitis from mastoiditis), are secondary to bacteremia (e.g., peritonitis, osteomyelitis, pericarditis, disseminated intravascular coagulation and cutaneous gangrene) or are secondary to obstructive processes which develop as a result of the inflammatory response initiated by the pneumococcus (e.g., bronchiectasis following pneumonia or hydrocephalus following meningitis). Response of pneumoccoccal infections to specific antibacterial therapy is usually dramatic, but it may be delayed, with 3 to 4 weeks required for resolution of fever in pneumococcal pneumonia with empyema.

PROGNOSIS. Prognosis is dependent on host factors such as race, sex, age, nutritional status and ability to localize infection to the lung, as well as on the type of infecting pneumococcus and on how early in the course of the disease adequate, specific antibacterial therapy is initiated. Mortality remains highest with meningitis, but may be as low as 5 per cent overall with adequate therapy for infections in other sites. When an impaired host response is evidenced by low white blood cell counts in peripheral blood or in spinal fluid, the prognosis becomes poor, as in any bacterial infection.

PREVENTION AND TREATMENT. There is no adequate means of immunization against pneumococcal infections; experimental vaccines are in development. Administration of gamma globulin to patients with hypogammaglobulinemic syndromes results in a reduced incidence of bacteremia, meningitis and other serious infections due to the pneumococcus, but the incidence and severity of upper respiratory infections and of pneumonia are not significantly affected.

All strains of pneumococcus are sensitive to penicillin G, which is the antibacterial agent of choice. The dose varies with the location of the infection and the presence or absence of complications. For uncomplicated pneumonia, 25,000–50,000 units/kg/day divided into 4 doses for 7 days is adequate. With pulmonary complications, septicemia, meningitis or osteomyelitis, 300,000–400,000 units/kg/day is indicated, and therapy should be continued until the patient has been afebrile for 5 days or the sedimentation rate has returned to normal.

For a patient with penicillin hypersensitivity, erythromycin or cephalosporin should be utilized. Sulfadiazine and sulfisoxazole (Gantrisin) are also effective in pneumococcal pneumonia. Since strains of pneumococci resistant to tetracyclines have now been described, these agents are not recommended.

STAPHYLOCOCCAL INFECTIONS

The staphylococci are a group of round gram-positive bacteria belonging to the family Micrococcaceae; they are frequent causes of pyogenic infection in infants and children.

Micrococci may grow aerobically or as facultative or obligate anaerobes. The staphylococcus is both an aerobe and a facultative anaerobe. It usually appears in clusters in smears made from pus or cultures. Staphylococci produce pigments which vary from white to deep yellow. These assist in differentiating potentially pathogenic strains from less pathogenic ones, but pathogenicity correlates better with the ability to coagulate plasma; the ability to produce hemolysis in culture on blood agar is of somewhat less pathologic significance. These features permit differentiation of the hemolytic *Staphylococcus aureus* from *S. epidermidis* and *S. albus.*

INFECTIONS DUE TO STAPHYLOCOCCUS AUREUS

Staphylococcus aureus is a sporadic and epidemic pathogen of infancy and childhood. It is the most common cause of pyogenic infections of the skin, and often involves the respiratory tract.

ETIOLOGIC AGENT. The pathogenicity of *S. aureus* is dependent upon a number of factors, some of which are intrinsic to or produced by the organism and some of which reflect the environment in which infection occurs.

Some diseases produced by *S. aureus* manifest specific properties of an invading strain. Staphylococcal gastroenteritis occurs primarily as a result of ingestion of food contaminated by an enterotoxin-producing strain. (See Section 28.) Diarrhea may also occur from secondary staphylococcal infection (superinfection) following suppression of normal or other enteric flora by antibiotic therapy. Certain strains of *S. aureus* produce a leukocyte-damaging factor (leukocidin) which inhibits phagocytosis, and an exotoxin (alpha hemolysin) which produces necrosis in tissue. Production of coagulase correlates best with staphylococcal pathogenicity.

Certain strains of *S. aureus* (phage types 3A, 3B, 3C, 55 and 71) have been reported to be responsible for cutaneous lesions in children in which there is a generalized separation within the skin at the level of the epidermis. (See toxic epidermolysis, below.) The factor responsible for this effect has not been identified.

Certain strains of staphylococci produce a penicillinase (β-lactamase) which inactivates penicillin. Such strains tend to cluster and be perpetuated in the hospital environment.

Strains of *S. aureus* are identified and classified in accordance with the numbers designating the bacteriophage or phages which lyse them. Routine typing is carried out with five sets of pooled phages: Group I (phages number 29, 52, 52A, 79 and 80); Group II (phages 3A, 3B, 3C, 55 and 71); Group III (phages 6, 7, 42E, 47, 53, 54, 75, 77 and 83A); Group IV (phage 42D); and Miscellaneous (phages 81 and 87); the organism is then classified as belonging to phage Group I, II, III, IV or Miscellaneous. More exact identification requires use of a large panel of individual phages. That in most common use is the WHO panel. Strains resistant to penicillin and prevalent in hospital settings generally fall into Groups I and II. Enterotoxin-producing strains are usually of phage types 42D or 6/47, but most staphylococci of these types do not produce enterotoxin. In the past, phage type 80/81 has been that most frequently identified in hospital epidemics of staphylococcal disease; it appears to have decreased in prevalence.

EPIDEMIOLOGY. Approximately one third of healthy persons carry *S. aureus* in their nasal passages; the organism is also frequently recovered as part of the normal flora of the rest of the respiratory and gastrointestinal tracts and of the skin.

In nurseries and hospitals penicillin-resistant strains tend to replace penicillin-sensitive organisms in the usual flora of patients and staff. Institutional transmission of disease-producing bacteria is chiefly by hand-to-patient contact; handwashing between attendance on successive patients is therefore of paramount importance in prevention. The umbilicus is an important reservoir in the newborn nursery, as may be circumcision wounds. Ventriculoatrial shunts, myelomeningoceles or skin disturbances (e.g., eczema) may predispose to the development of staphylococcal infection. Infants with immunologic deficiencies are at great risk. Viral infections of the lung (e.g., influenza) predispose to secondary bacterial infection with staphylococci.

Family epidemics of staphylococcal infection are common. Usually they are manifested by recurrent furunculosis (boils) or other skin infections passed back and forth from one family member to another; but any type of staphylococcal infection may be seen. Often such epidemics begin with the introduction to the home of a highly pathogenic strain acquired in the hospital or newborn nursery. The individual who introduces the infection into the home may have no clinical disease initially or later. (See also Staphylococcal Infections in Section 7.)

PATHOLOGY, PATHOGENESIS AND IMMUNOLOGY. Staphylococcal disease represents the concurrence of pathogenic factors in the organism and predisposing factors in the host. A normal host is able to withstand exposure to a large number of organisms; nonspecific protective factors of skin and mucous membranes are of great significance, along with immunologic defenses. Type-specific antibody transferred to the newborn transplacentally may provide some protection against staphylococcal strains for the first few months of life. As passive immunity decreases, infants colonized with pathogenic strains in the newborn nursery may later develop disease.

Staphylococcal strains which produce an exotoxin (enterotoxin) may cause disease in the absence of living bacteria; gastroenteritis, for example, may occur when infected food has been heated sufficiently to kill the bacteria but not to destroy the enterotoxin. Staphylococcal infection with other strains leads to abscess formation, with varying degrees of tissue necrosis. Localization of the infection is marked by an intense leukocytic response, with ingestion and killing of organisms. For some strains, effective phagocytosis requires the presence of strain-specific opsonins against polysaccharide surface antigens. Antibodies to various other staphylococcal antigens may also develop; their value in limiting disease is not known. If the immune response is successful, the staphylococcal abscess will be found to have a core consisting of leukocytes containing dead bacteria and cells of necrotic tissue, and a peripheral layer of viable cells of fibroblastic, phagocytic and bacterial origin. Dissemination of bacteria may occur from such lesions via blood or lymph, through interaction of the spreading factors of the staphylococcus and a less than optimal host response. The role of delayed hypersensitivity in the elimination or spread of staphylococcal disease is not yet clearly defined.

CLINICAL MANIFESTATIONS. The incubation period for staphylococcal infections may be hours (in gastroenteritis due to enterotoxin) or up to 7 days.

A pyogenic skin lesion is often considered to be the primary lesion of staphylococcal infections, but primary lesions may also localize in the paranasal sinuses, in the middle or external ear, in the parotid glands, in the lungs or in the gastrointestinal tract. Secondary localization follows blood stream invasion; bacteremic spread may occur to bones and joints, endocardium and pericardium, kidneys, brain and venous sinuses, and the lung and muscles (tropical pyomyositis).

Infection of the skin may be primary (furuncle, pyoderma, impetigo) or secondary (infected wounds or eczema). Another kind of staphylococcal cutaneous lesion is associated with intraepidermal separation and reflects a toxic effect of certain phage group II organisms. The lesions have been called bullous impetigo (or pemphigus neonatorum), Ritter's disease and "scalded skin syndrome" (toxic epidermal necrolysis, Lyell's disease). The various names reflect variations in clinical appearance and age of occurrence. In most instances, skin involvement follows a sequence of generalized erythema with marked tenderness of skin and subsequent formation of bullae, with exfoliation of the skin and a positive Nikolsky sign (dermal separation which follows the stroking of skin which appears normal). Staphylococcal *scarlet fever* also occurs as generalized erythema or scarlatiniform rash without exfoliation.

The umbilicus in the newborn and the periungual tissues are other frequent sites of colonization and localization of staphylococcal infection. Chronic or recurrent skin infection (furunculosis) is often indicative of reinfection within a family setting. (See also Section 23.)

Sinusitis due to staphylococcal infection is not common in childhood. Staphylococcal *tonsillopharyngitis* is rare but may be observed if there are predisposing immune defects, particularly of white blood cell function. *Neonatal parotitis* may follow nasal colonization. *Pneumonia* is usually primary but may complicate a preceding viral infection. Abdominal pain and distention are frequent presenting symptoms in staphylococcal pneumonia, the diagnosis being established only by roentgenographic examination of the chest. Staphylococcal pneumonia is a necrotizing process, with high likelihood of pneumatoceles, empyema, pyopneumothorax or bronchopleural fistula. (See Staphylococcal Pneumonia, Section 12.)

Food poisoning (Section 28) occurs within a few hours of ingestion of improperly handled food contaminated by a staphylococcus producing an enterotoxic exotoxin. *Staphylococcal enterocolitis* results when staphylococci overgrow normal bowel flora in patients in whom the latter has been eliminated or modified by prior antibiotic therapy (usually a tetracycline or other broad spectrum antibiotic).

Bacteremia disseminates staphylococcal infection and may follow any local infection; the onset is marked by chills and high fever. Metastatic foci occur most commonly in the lungs, brain, heart, kidney, bones, joints and skin. *Staphylococcus aureus* is the commonest cause of *osteomyelitis* and septic arthritis in children (Section 22). *Endocarditis* is a rare but serious accompaniment of staphylococcal bacteremia. Acute staphylococcal endocarditis often results in perforation of a cardiac valve and sudden death. Purulent *pericarditis* is caused most commonly by the staphylococcus and may develop either from direct extension from the lung or from bacteremia. *Renal or perinephric abscesses* may also follow staphylococcal bacteremia. Central nervous system involvement may follow bacteremia or neurosurgical procedures or occur from direct extension of otitis media, from infection of a disrupted myelomeningocele or from trauma. Following neurosurgical procedures the offending organism is likely to be *S. albus.* The staphylococcus is the second most common cause of *brain abscess,* and may also infect the cavernous and sagittal sinuses, either as a result of bacteremia or by direct extension from an area of venous drainage.

DIAGNOSIS. Diagnosis of staphylococcal infection is dependent upon isolation of the organism from pus, blood, cerebrospinal fluid or other appropriate clinical specimens. Determinations of coagulase reactivity, antibiotic sensitivity patterns and phage type are useful in establishing the organism as pathogenic or epidemic. There are no serologic tests of practical clinical value.

Differential Diagnosis. Staphylococcal skin lesions are usually clinically characteristic and easily diagnosed, but impetiginous lesions due to β-hemolytic streptococcus may be indistinguishable from those caused by staphylococci. In staphylococcal pneumonia the chest roentgenogram is often specifically suggestive, but other causes of necrotizing pneumonia must be differentiated. Characteristic features of staphylococcal pneumonia include dense lobar or lobular consolidation, a depressed fissure below a consolidated lobe, the presence of air-fluid levels (abscess or pyopneumothorax), and the development of pneumatocoeles. These changes are occasionally noted in other pyogenic pneumonias and are therefore not pathognomonic. Localized abscesses and infection sites other than the skin can be established as staphylococcal only by culture. The lesions of *cat-scratch disease* may simulate staphylococcal infection.

COMPLICATIONS. Pulmonary infection may be associated with residual fibrosis from loss of pulmonary parenchyma, though permanent sequelae are rare. With joint infection, destruction of articular cartilage may lead to permanent joint deformity. Chronic osteomyelitis may result from delayed or inadequate therapy.

PROGNOSIS. Untreated staphylococcal sepsis once carried a mortality rate of 80 per cent; with antibiotic treatment it is now approximately 25 per cent.

Absent or sluggish host response (white cell count less than 5000 or polymorphonuclear cells less than 70 per cent) and abdominal distention are grave prognostic signs. The prognosis of any staphylococcal infection varies with the invasiveness, general pathogenicity and antibiotic sensitivity of the strain involved, and with such host factors as immunologic adequacy, hypersensitivity to antibiotics and nutritional status.

PREVENTION AND TREATMENT. Prevention of staphylococcal infection is fostered in potentially epidemic situations such as an infection in a nursery by rigid attention to handwashing techniques and appropriately directed antibiotic therapy. (See Staphylococcal Infections, Section 7.) Careful monitoring of nosocomial infections in potential problem areas usually requires an active infections control committee and a full-time surveillance officer. Pre-emptive colonization of newborn infants with a nonvirulent strain of *S. aureus* (502A strain) has been carried out with variable success as a method of curtailing epidemics due to virulent strains.

Drainage of abscesses and removal of any foreign bodies (such as sutures, or artificial valves in the cardiovascular or central nervous systems, and the like) must be accomplished for permanent cure. For undrained abscesses or with persistent foreign bodies antibiotic therapy alone is almost always ineffective.

Appropriate antibiotic therapy requires in vitro sensitivity testing of the organism isolated. Every effort must be made to isolate the infecting staphylococcus early in the course of infection and before treatment is initiated. For example, in osteomyelitis aspiration of the suspected metaphysis and cultures of blood should be obtained immediately prior to institution of therapy and during the first hours of treatment.

Initial therapy for severe infections should always proceed on the assumption that the infecting staphylococcus is resistant to penicillin G, and a semisynthetic, penicillinase-resistant antibiotic should be chosen. We prefer methicillin, but other agents (nafcillin, oxacillin, etc.) are also effective. Some prefer the use of a cephalothin initially, particularly if the infecting organism may be other than a staphylococcus or if a mixed infection is suspected. In all severe infections therapy should be initiated by the intravenous route, employing at least 100/mg/kg/day of methicillin, divided into 6 doses. Daily doses as high as 400 mg/kg may rarely be utilized in life-threatening situations.

Continuing therapy is shaped by antibiotic sensitivity of the organism in vitro and by the specific type of infection, and is tempered by the patient's response to treatment. If the organism is found sensitive to penicillin G, therapy can be altered and this agent employed. In such diseases as pneumonia and bacteremia intravenous therapy is continued until fever is absent for at least 48 hours and other signs of infection have subsided. For osteomyelitis it is our practice to maintain intravenous therapy for 3 to 4 weeks. In meningitis intravenous therapy continues until the patient is afebrile for at least 5 days, the spinal fluid cultures are negative, and pleocytosis and protein are reduced to near normal, with a normal glucose level. In all serious infections oral therapy follows intravenous therapy until one is confident of eradication of the infecting organisms. It is difficult to establish absolute guidelines, but the following durations of therapy are usual: pneumonia, 2 to 3 weeks; meningitis, 3 to 4 weeks; osteomyelitis, 6 to 12 weeks.

Milder infections (skin, upper respiratory tract) may be managed with brief intravenous therapy or with initial oral therapy, depending on severity and extent of disease. We prefer dicloxacillin in a dose of 12.5 mg/kg/day. Others prefer nafcillin or an oral cephalothin.

In individuals who are hypersensitive to penicillin and its derivatives, other agents must be employed. The cephalothins demonstrate a 5 per cent cross-reactivity in penicillin-sensitive children (higher in adults) and can frequently be employed. Erythromycin, kanamycin, gentamicin and chloramphenicol can be used but are inferior to the penicillins. Vancomycin and ristocetin are effective but quite irritating and toxic. In life-threatening infections, however, they may offer the next best therapy to the penicillins. Another alternative in the patient allergic to penicillin is to attempt cautious "desensitization." To a continuous intravenous infusion 1 unit is added of the penicillin to which the patient is sensitive; every 20 minutes the dose is increased by a factor of 10, if tolerated, until a full dose is reached. Thereafter, therapy at that level is maintained without interruption. During this procedure the physician should remain at the bedside and a syringe containing epinephrine (1:1000, aqueous) should be at hand. Should an immediate systemic allergic reaction occur, intravenous administration of epinephrine will abort the episode and penicillin should be discontinued.

Occasionally it is desirable to enhance serum levels of penicillin(s) by oral administration of probenecid (25 mg/kg initially and 40 mg/kg/day thereafter). This is seldom necessary; upward adjustment of penicillin dosage is usually safe and effective when indicated.

The effectiveness of antibiotics should not result in other appropriate forms of therapy being overlooked or postponed when indicated. Incision and drainage of abscesses, drainage of osteomyelitis by aspiration or marsupialization, and drainage of empyema by chest tube or repeated transthoracic aspirations all contribute to resolution of typical staphylococcal infections. Instillation of proteolytic enzymes into abscesses or body cavities, once fashionable, is now condemned as useless; it may contribute to morbidity through irritation or sensitization, with fever and systemic symptoms.

In superficial skin infections, cleansing with soap and water or a mild antiseptic may suffice. Occasionally application of topical antibiotics (bacitracin) may be beneficial. Penicillin should not be applied topically.

INFECTIONS DUE TO STAPHYLOCOCCUS EPIDERMIDIS

This organism may produce bacteremia in infants and children with hydrocephalus who have had ventriculocardiac or ventriculojugular shunts using plastic tubing and valves. Recovery of the organism from blood or from the shunt in place or at time of removal is diagnostic. Appropriate antibiotics must be utilized, but recurrence is common. Bacteriologic cure can almost never be accomplished unless the foreign body (shunt) is removed.

Breckinridge, J. C., and Bergdoll, M. S.: Outbreak of food-borne gastroenteritis due to a coagulase-negative enterotoxin-producing staphylococcus. New Engl. J. Med. *284*:541, 1971.

Melish, M. E., and Glasgow, L. A.: Staphylococcal scalded skin syndrome: The expanded clinical syndrome. J. Pediatr. *78*:958, 1971.

Shinefield, H. R., Ribble, J. C., and Boris, M.: Bacterial interference between strains of staphylococcus aureus, 1960 to 1970. Am. J. Dis. Child. *121*:148, 1971.

Shurtleff, D. B., Foltz, E. L., Weeks, R. D., and Loeser, J. L.: Therapy of *Staphylococcus epidermidis*: Infections associated with cerebrospinal fluid shunt. Pediatrics *53*:551, 1971.

INFECTIONS DUE TO NEISSERIAE

Neisseriae are gram-negative kidney-bean or biscuit-shaped diplococci. Most Neisseriae are found normally in the nasopharynx. *Neisseria meningitidis* (or *intracellularis*) and *N. gonorrhoeae* are most commonly associated with human infection. *Neisseria catarrhalis, N. flava, N. subflava* and *N. flavescens* have been associated only sporadically with disease in man.

Neisseriae are aerobic and readily isolated on blood agar. However, because they do not withstand drying or other insults in transit, their accurate isolation is dependent upon rapid inoculation on appropriate media.

INFECTIONS DUE TO NEISSERIA MENINGITIDIS (N. INTRACELLULARIS)

(Meningococcemia; Cerebrospinal Fever; Epidemic Cerebrospinal Fever; Spotted Fever)

Neisseria meningitidis may be carried in the nasopharynges of asymptomatic persons or may cause acute infections characterized by septicemia and/or meningitis, often following an upper respiratory illness.

ETIOLOGIC AGENT. *Neisseria meningitidis* is a gram-negative, nonmotile coccus which is usually arranged in pairs, the opposing edges of which are flattened. In smears of infected blood or cerebrospinal fluid they are commonly, but not necessarily, seen in an intracellular location. Four main groups of *N. meningitidis* are distinguished (A, B, C, D) on the basis of type-specific capsular polysaccharides as determined by agglutination. The cell walls of all meningococci produce a potent lipopolysaccharide endotoxin.

EPIDEMIOLOGY. *Neisseria meningitidis* is the

cause of classic epidemic meningitis. Group A organisms formerly caused the majority of epidemics, whereas group B related primarily to sporadic infections. Group B subsequently became the predominant epidemic organism, only to be displaced recently by group C. Group D organisms are currently rarely associated with disease in man.

About 2 to 4 per cent of healthy persons normally carry meningococci in the nasopharynx; during epidemics this number may increase to 20 to 80 per cent. Meningococcal disease usually appears in winter and spring and affects previously healthy infants and children. It does not strikingly prefer children with underlying immunologic defects. About 75 per cent of infections occur in children under 10 years of age. Because maternal antibody protects the very young infant, meningococcal meningitis is rare under 2 months of age. Institutional or family crowding creates a situation favorable to an increase in both carriers and cases of meningitis and/or septicemia; infection occurs with significant frequency among family contacts.

PATHOLOGY AND PATHOGENESIS. Meningococci gain entry to the nasopharynx in respiratory droplets. After an incubation period of 2 to 7 days, there is lymphatic spread to the blood stream (meningococcemia) and then to the lungs, ears, eyes, meninges, skin, joints, adrenal glands and heart. Clinical manifestations may range from a simple upper respiratory infection to fulminant meningococcemia, with or without subsequent localization in one or more other areas.

The characteristic inflammatory response consists of necrosis, hemorrhage and pus formation. Primary targets in tissues include phagocytic cells and the endothelial lining of blood vessels. Small veins are frequently filled by leukocyte-platelet-fibrin thrombi, characteristic of the local Shwartzman reaction. Bleeding into the adrenals produces the Waterhouse-Friderichsen syndrome (adrenal hemorrhages in patients with septicemia and shock).

CLINICAL MANIFESTATIONS. Several clinical types of disease may be recognized: upper respiratory, septicemic and localizing (in the meninges and elsewhere).

An *upper respiratory infection* presumably due to meningococci may be observed during epidemic periods; it can be etiologically identified only by culture.

Meningococcemia may be mild or severe, acute or chronic. In the mild form, a petechial rash of the skin and mucous membranes may follow a 1- to 2-day prodromal period of upper respiratory symptoms, with headache, fever and gastrointestinal symptoms. Chronic meningococcemia is generally mild, recurrent or intermittent, producing a petechial or purpuric rash, with associated fever and, sometimes, joint symptoms. It may present as a fever of unknown origin. Chronic meningococcemia may be accompanied by bacterial endocarditis, as well as by other localizing manifestations, including splenomegaly.

Fulminant septicemia is the most severe form of meningococcemia and is rapidly progressive, with the development of endotoxic shock, disseminated intravascular coagulation and cutaneous and mucosal hemorrhages. The spinal fluid is in most instances normal.

The *rash* of meningococcemia may be erythematous, maculopapular, papular, petechial or hemorrhagic (purpuric and ecchymotic). (See Figure 10–2, p. 656.)

The meninges are the most common points of localization following meningococcemia, with the production of meningitis. Skin manifestations and shock are not so prominent a part of meningitis as they may be with meningococcemia alone.

DIAGNOSIS. The diagnosis of meningococcal infection can be confirmed by culture of blood, spinal fluid, nasopharynx or skin lesions. In some instances, blood obtained from papular or purpuric skin lesions by puncture may reveal organisms on gram stain which are not recoverable on blood culture. The organism may occasionally be demonstrated in the white blood cells of the buffy coat of the peripheral blood.

Leukocytosis with neutrophilia and an increase in immature forms is usually present. An elevated blood urea nitrogen, proteinuria and microscopic hematuria are not uncommon. When the infection localizes in the central nervous system, spinal fluid findings are usually consistent with a diagnosis of bacterial meningitis, but may be normal for 6 to 8 hours after the onset of symptoms. A second lumbar puncture is essential, therefore, if the initial specimen of spinal fluid is normal in a patient who continues to show symptoms pointing to infection of the central nervous system. It is not uncommon for meningococci to be recovered on culture of apparently normal spinal fluid obtained early in the course of the disease. Prior antibiotic therapy may obscure the etiologic diagnosis of meningitis.

Differential Diagnosis. The petechial skin lesions of meningococcemia must be differentiated from those of bacterial endocarditis and of rickettsial and enteroviral infections. Rocky Mountain spotted fever, echovirus types 6, 9 and 16, and coxsackievirus types A-2, A-4, A-9 and A-16 must particularly be considered.

The purpuric, ecchymotic, necrotic rash of overwhelming or fulminant meningococcemia must be differentiated from that seen with other forms of overwhelming sepsis, such as those due to *H. influenzae, E. coli, D. pneumoniae* and *S. aureus.* Meningococcal meningitis must be differentiated by specific isolation of the causative organism.

COMPLICATIONS. Herpes labialis frequently accompanies meningococcemia, appearing between the third and sixth days of illness. Complications of meningitis include deafness, blindness, paralysis of the 3rd, 4th, 6th and 7th cranial nerves, hemiplegia or localized muscle paralysis, brain abscess, obstructive hydrocephalus or herniation of the brain stem. Pericarditis or interstitial myocarditis may produce a fatal outcome in meningococcal septicemia. Arthritis may be toxic or purulent, but usually heals without sequelae. Rarely, pneumonia or otitis media may occur. Disseminated intravascular coagulation may occur (see Section 14).

PROGNOSIS. Few patients survive meningococcemia or meningococcal meningitis without treatment. Mortality may be as high as 15 per cent even with adequate therapy; most fatal cases are associated with the Waterhouse-Friderichsen syndrome. Poor prognostic signs include leukopenia, a low sedimentation rate or a total eosinophil count below 25/mm^3 in the peripheral blood. Encephalitis, shock and early appearance of a purpuric rash are also bad prognostic signs. A good prognosis is generally correlated with survival for 48 hours after the initiation of therapy, leukocytosis in the peripheral blood, presence of meningitis with meningococcemia, and an elevated sedimentation rate.

PREVENTION. A type-specific vaccine against meningococci of groups A and C, prepared from the capsular polysaccharide, has been shown to be protective for military recruits in potentially epidemic situations. Epidemiologic and clinical surveillance is managed through nasopharyngeal cultures.

Sulfonamides have been successful in prophylactic use against meningococcal disease until the mid-1960's. By 1969 three fourths of all meningococcal isolates had become resistant to sulfonamides. The change may be related to the new predominance of type C organisms, and has resulted in substitution of other antibiotics for prophylaxis. No completely satisfactory alternative exists, though rifampin has been effective in preliminary trials and is still under evaluation.

TREATMENT. Specific treatment consists of aqueous penicillin G, 400,000 units/kg/day in 4 doses given intravenously (See Meningitis, below, this Section.)

The treatment of disseminated intravascular coagulation is discussed in Section 14.

Abildgaard, C. F., Corrigan, J. J., Seeler, R. A., Simone, J. V., and Schulman, I.: Meningococcemia associated with intravascular coagulation. Pediatrics *40*:78, 1967.

Artenstein, M. S., Gold, R., Zimmerly, J. G., Wyle, F. A., Schneider, H., and Harkins, C.: Prevention of meningococcal disease by group C polysaccharide vaccine. New Engl. J. Med. *282*:417, 1970.

Ater, O. H., and Plunket, D. C.: Prolonged mild meningococcemia in an infant. Clin. Pediatr. *6*:125, 1967.

Bell, W. E., and Silber, D. L.: Meningococcal meningitis: Past and present concepts. Military Med. *136*:601, 1971.

INFECTION DUE TO NEISSERIA GONORRHOEAE

Gonorrhea is an acute infectious disease being reported with increasing frequency in children of all ages, from newborns to adolescents. In most instances the infection is limited to a local mucosal site. Rarely, hematogenous dissemination may involve bones, joints, skin, meninges or heart.

ETIOLOGIC AGENT. *Neisseria gonorrhoeae* resembles *N. meningitidis* in its fastidious requirements for growth as an aerobic and facultatively anaerobic organism. It is a gram-negative oval or spherical coccus usually found in pairs with flattened opposing edges. The organisms are usually found within polymorphonuclear leukocytes in acute infections but may also be extracellular, especially in chronic infections. Isolation is best accomplished on selective media such as chocolate agar or Thayer-Martin medium containing VCN (vancomycin, colistimethate, and nystatin) to inhibit organisms which could be mistaken for the gonococcus.

EPIDEMIOLOGY. Gonorrheal infection in infants and children may be acquired during birth, by venereal contact or from fomites. The general incidence of the disease has doubled in the United States since 1965, and now has its greatest incidence in adolescents. Newborn infants become infected while traversing the birth canal of an infected mother. Small children may be infected through contact with an infected caretaker. Most cases in older children and adolescents are the result of venereal contact. Communal living contributes heavily to the spread of gonorrhea among teen-agers.

PATHOLOGY AND PATHOGENESIS. Primary gonococcal invasion may take place on any mucosal surface which is not covered by squamous epithelium: the eye in the newborn; the vulva and vagina in the prepubertal girl; the anterior urethra in the pre- or postpubertal boy; the urethra and cervix in the postpubertal girl; the pharynx and the anus in case of orogenital or anogenital contacts. Gonococcemia may give rise to metastatic involvement of the joints, bones, skin, heart and meninges. Pathologically the gonococcus produces an acute pyogenic reaction.

CLINICAL MANIFESTATIONS. The clinical manifestations of primary gonorrheal infection vary with the site and the duration of infection. The usual incubation period is 3 to 5 days.

Between 15 and 30 per cent of infected postpubertal women may be asymptomatic. Symptoms of genital infection usually include vaginitis, with mucoid discharge, pruritus and dysuria. Adolescent males usually develop a purulent urethral discharge with burning on urination, but studies among military personnel indicate that gonorrhea may be asymptomatic in up to 60 per cent of infected male contacts of women with symptomatic gonorrhea. *Gonorrheal vulvovaginitis* may occur in preadolescent girls from sexual contact, or rarely from fomites. This type of infection seems to be related to the columnar epithelium in the vulva and vagina of young girls, which is more susceptible to gonococcal infection than the squamous epithelium of the vulva and vagina of postpubertal girls.

Gonococcal *ophthalmia neonatorum* may involve one or both eyes and is manifested by reddened and edematous lids and purulent conjunctivitis. (See Section 24.) Gonococcal meningitis must be considered when meningeal signs coexist with gonococcal urethritis. Skin lesions reflect gonococcemia, are more common in females and are frequently accompanied by arthritis. They may be purpuric or vesiculopustular on a broad erythematous base, or may form hemorrhagic bullae. Gonococcal arthritis is the most common cause of arthritis in the adolescent age group and occurs more frequently in females. It is rare in children under 10 years of age. Polyarthritis may occur with or without joint effusion and may be associated with skin lesions, chills and fever. An infected effusion is characteristic of the arthritis, and other clinical manifestations tend to be less prominent. Large joints are selectively affected. Tenosynovitis of the wrist and ankle may also occur.

DIAGNOSIS. The diagnosis of gonococcal infection is dependent upon continuing awareness of its epidemiology and clinical manifestations. A definitive diagnosis can be made with 99 per cent accuracy in the symptomatic male with urethritis, on identification of gram-negative intracellular diplococci in the urethral drainage. In the infected female, the cervical smear may be positive only early in the acute phase of infection; the only reliable method of diagnosis is by culture of vaginal or cervical specimens. To increase opportunity for positive isolation, non-cotton swabs should be used to obtain specimens; specimens should not be allowed to dry in the air but should be placed immediately in a transport medium (e.g., a modified Thayer-Martin medium); cultures should be incubated anaerobically in a candle jar. These same precautions are applicable to specimens obtained for culture from other sites. There are no reliable and clinically useful serologic tests for diagnosis of gonorrheal infections.

Differential Diagnosis. Gonococcal urethritis in the male and vulvovaginitis in the female must be differentiated from other infections (mycoplasma, trichomonas, fungi) and from trauma or nonspecific causes by specific culture for the offending organisms. In prepubertal girls vulvovaginitis due to beta-hemolytic streptococci and vaginal discharge secondary to foreign body are to be differentiated; the latter is often blood-tinged or malodorous. Vaginal moniliasis, oxyuriasis, infections with herpesvirus type 2, other pyogenic bacterial infections and adolescent leukorrhea must also be differentiated by appropriate culture techniques.

Gonococcal arthritis must be differentiated from acute rheumatoid arthritis, acute rheumatic fever, other bacterial causes of infectious arthritis, and arthritis due to rubella or to rubella immunization.

COMPLICATIONS. In the male, gonorrhea may produce epididymitis, prostatitis and urethral strictures; in the female, salpingitis, tubo-ovarian abscess and sterility; pelvic peritonitis and hepatitis may complicate primary gonorrhea. Gonorrheal conjunctivitis may lead to corneal opacity and blindness or to corneal ulceration with loss of aqueous humor and subsequent need for enucleation of the eye. In gonorrheal arthritis the articular cartilage may be rapidly destroyed, leading to ankylosis of the joint.

PROGNOSIS. With appropriate and adequate antibiotic therapy, the prognosis of primary gonorrhea is excellent. Permanent sequelae are common when complications of the disease occur.

PREVENTION AND TREATMENT. Neonatal gonorrheal conjunctivitis is effectively prevented by instillation of 1 per cent silver nitrate solution into the conjunctival sac shortly after birth. (See Section 7.) The use of a condom during and urethral prophylaxis after intercourse helps to prevent the acquisition of gonorrhea by the sexually active male, and may also offer protection to his partners. All patients with gonorrhea should have a serologic test for syphilis performed prior to treatment and again 3 months later because of the frequent concomitant occurrence of infection with *T. pallidum.*

Penicillin and ampicillin are the preferred drugs for treatment of gonorrhea. If the involved strain of *N. gonorrhoeae* is sensitive to penicillin, an adolescent or a contact should receive 2.4 to 4.8 million units of aqueous procaine penicillin G intramuscularly and 1 gm of probenecid orally; 1.2 million units of aqueous procaine penicillin is usually sufficient for infants and small children. For penicillin-resistant strains, ampicillin (3.4 gm intramuscularly) should be used.

Handsfield, H. H., Lipman, T. O., Harnisch, J. P., Tronica, E., and Holmes, K. K.: Asymptomatic gonorrhea in men. New Engl. J. Med. *290*:117, 1974.

Nazarin, L. F.: The current prevalence of gonococcal infections in children. Pediatrics *39*:372, 1967.

Recommended Treatment Schedules for Gonorrhea. Morbidity and Mortality Reports *21*:82, 1972.

Rudolph, A. A.: Control of gonorrhea: Guidelines for antibiotic treatment. J.A.M.A. *220*:1587, 1972.

Thatcher, R. W., and Pettit, T. H.: Gonorrheal conjunctivitis. J.A.M.A. *215*:1494, 1971.

OTTO F. SIEBER, JR.,
VINCENT A. FULGINITI

INFECTIONS DUE TO HEMOPHILUS INFLUENZAE

Hemophilus influenzae was first described in 1892 by Richard Pfeiffer, who mistakenly considered it to be the primary etiologic agent in influenza. This important bacterial species is primary in the etiology of certain acute life-threatening infections, of which meningitis and epiglottitis are the most common; others are pneumonia, empyema, septic arthritis, osteomyelitis, cellulitis and carditis. All are associated with septicemia and occur mainly between the ages of 1 month and 4 years, with the exception of epiglottitis, which occurs principally between 2 and 7 years of age. *Hemophilus influenzae* is also important in some less serious situations in which surface infections seem to follow the breakdown of local host resistance, as in bronchiectasis, cystic fibrosis, chronic sinusitis and otitis media. From clinical observations, it has been concluded that the infections begin in the nasopharynx and spread, either locally or via the blood stream. The great majority of nasopharyngeal infections with this species are probably mild and eventually lead to immunity in late childhood, thus limiting the age incidence of serious infections.

THE ORGANISM. *Hemophilus influenzae* is a fastidious, tiny, gram-negative, pleomorphic coccobacillus which requires factors X (hematin, heat stable) and V (phosphopyridine nucleotide, heat labile) for growth. For successful identification, culture media enriched by the heat labile components must not be subjected to sterilization by heat. Encapsulated strains are classified by the polysaccharides of the soluble capsular substance and designated as types a through f. Types a, b, c and f contain phosphates, while d and e contain neither phosphorus nor sulfur. Almost all the serious, invasive infections in children are due to encapsulated strains, usually type b, rarely types a, e or f. Nonencapsulated strains (nontypable) have been indicted as etiologic factors in chronic lung disease and in otitis media. Alexander and her colleagues demonstrated transformation into typable strains by interaction with DNA from capsular substance, thus magnifying the possible importance of the nonencapsulated strains, which are common in nasopharyngeal flora.

IMMUNITY. The exact role of serum antibodies in immunity is not fully understood. There is clear evidence, however, to indicate that the capsular polyribophosphate (PRP) of type b is antigenic, stimulating specific antibodies which promote bacterial killing and phagocytosis. Bactericidal activity, however, may be due to antibodies directed against multiple antigens, noncapsular as well as capsular. Somatic antigens of various strains of type b may be dissimilar, but capsular PRP seems to be identical in all.

In a longitudinal study of infants followed from birth, natural serum antibodies in cord blood, presumably of maternal origin, usually were lost by age 5 months. Transient peaks of bactericidal and opsonic activity were common in infancy and early childhood and became persistent in about one third of the subjects before age 5 years, apparently owing to repeated experiences with infections due to *H. influenzae* or to bacteria producing cross-reacting antigens.

MENINGITIS

See also Acute Bacterial Meningitis, below. *Hemophilus influenzae* type b is the leading cause of bacterial meningitis in the United States in children between the ages of 1 month and 3 years, occurring almost exclusively before school age. It is regularly accompanied by septicemia. The annual incidence in the United States is about 40 per 100,000 children under 4 years of age, similar to that of poliomyelitis in the preimmunization era. The peak incidence occurs in infants 6 to 9 months of age, with one half of the cases occurring during the first year of life. The highest attack and mortality rates are found in November, December and January, but cases occur the year around. Clinically, meningitis due to *H. influenzae* cannot be distinguished from that due to *N. meningitidis* or *D. pneumoniae.* The case fatality rates vary from 2 to 18 per cent, depending upon the facilities for rapid diagnosis and adequate treatment. It has been shown in two studies that nearly half of the survivors have long-term neurologic sequelae of varying degrees, ranging from the severe and obvious (e.g., retardation, paralyses and convulsions) to the more subtle (e.g., lowered intelligence quotient relative to siblings, language and learning problems, and hyperactivity).

For reasons not clear at present, the majority of infants recovering from influenzal meningitis develop only low levels of detectable serum antibodies against *H. influenzae* type b during convalescence; nevertheless, recurrences are rare. Meningitis may occur in family contacts.

ACUTE EPIGLOTTITIS

Acute epiglottitis is a dramatic, potentially lethal condition which occurs usually in children between the ages of 2 and 7 years. (See also Acute Infections of the Larynx and Trachea in Section 12.) It is characterized by a fulminating course of fever, sore throat, rapidly progressive respiratory obstruction (croup) and prostration. Within a matter of hours, epiglottitis may progress to complete obstruction of the airway and death unless adequate treatment is administered. The physical signs include absence of hoarseness and a large, shiny, cherry-red epiglottis brought into view when the posterior portion of the tongue is properly depressed. The large, sticky epiglottis tends to produce a ball-valve obstruction, being drawn down with inspiration and eventually completely blocking the intake of air. Establishment of an airway, either by nasotracheal tube or tracheostomy, is mandatory in the face of clear evidence of epiglottitis, even though the degree of apparent respiratory distress may not seem to indicate it. Since septicemia is also present, parenteral antibiotic therapy should be instituted promptly. Pneumonia or meningitis due to *H. influenzae* may be present simultaneously.

There is evidence to indicate that patients with acute epiglottitis have cellular antigens which are genetically different from those of siblings who contract meningitis. After epiglottitis, subjects develop high serum antibody titers against type b, whereas postmeningitic children do not. This may be a function of their older age, but further study is needed to explain these differences in response.

OTHER HEMATOGENOUS LESIONS

Hemophilus influenzae may also produce: (1) *pneumonia* and *empyema,* which occur most frequently in infants and young children, especially under 1 year of age, with clinical features which fail to differentiate pneumonia or empyema due to *H. influenzae* from that due to other bacteria, especially *D. pneumoniae* (failure of clinical response to the usual dosages of penicillin may alert the clinician to the nonpneumococcal etiology); (2) *osteomyelitis* and *pyarthrosis,* with the knees, elbows, wrists and hips as the most common sites (aspirated pus is characteristically yellowish green); (3) *cellulitis,* a hot, tender, purplish-red swelling, usually without a sharply defined edge, but occasionally with a border sharp enough to lead to confusion with streptococcal erysipelas; the face or cheek, neck and periorbital areas are most commonly reported as sites, but the extremities may be involved; and (4) *pericarditis* and *bacterial endocarditis,* which have no clinically distinguishing features as compared to those due to other bacteria.

All require bacteriologic studies for positive diagnosis. More than one of these clinical situations may occur concomitantly as consequences of bacteremia.

OTITIS MEDIA

Hemophilus influenzae has been identified in cultures of middle ear fluid removed by tympanocentesis from 20 to 35 per cent of children with acute otitis media. This proportion was found in school-age children as well as younger ones. Eighty-five to 90 per cent of the strains were nonencapsulated and seemed to be acting as primary pathogens. This finding was in contrast to the strains of *D. pneumoniae* identified in middle ear fluid, nearly all of which were encapsulated. Of the typable strains of *H. influenzae,* type b was the most common; a significant proportion of the patients also had systemic infection with the same organism.

TREATMENT. For invasive infections, ampicillin and chloramphenicol are in general favor at present. For otitis media and chronic lung disease, ampicillin, erythromycin plus a sulfonamide, and the tetracyclines have proved useful.

PREVENTION. An antigen prepared from purified polyribophosphate of *H. influenzae* type b is in early clinical trial as an immunoprophylactic agent. Preliminary results indicate immunogenicity with few untoward reactions. On the other hand, the antibody levels produced in young infants, the group for whom protection is most needed, are often low or undetectable by present methods. The exact levels of antibody which correlate with protection are not yet known. Hopefully the vaccine will prove to be effective in prevention of serious invasive infections, but further studies are required for definite conclusions.

Alexander, H. E.: Hemophilus influenzae infection. *In* Cooke, R. E. (ed.): The Biologic Basis of Pediatric Practice. New York, Blakiston Division, McGraw-Hill Book Co., 1968.

Fraser, D. W., Darby, C. P., Koehler, R. E., Jacobs, C. F., and Feldman, R. A.: Risk factors in bacterial meningitis: Charleston County, South Carolina, J. Infect. Dis. *127*:271, 1973.

Howie, V. M., Ploussard, J. H., and Lester, R. L.: Otitis media: A clinical and bacteriological correlation. Pediatrics *45*:29, 1970.

Pfeiffer, R.: Vorläufige Mittheilungen über die Erreger der Influenza. Deutsch. Med. Wschr. *18*:28, 1892.

Pittman, M.: Variation and type specificity in bacterial species of *H. influenzae.* J. Exp. Med. *53*:471, 1931.

Robbins, J. B., Parke, J. C., Jr., Schneerson, R., and Whisnant, J. K.: Quantitative measurement of "natural" and immunization-induced *Haemophilus influenzae,* type b, capsular polysaccharide antibodies. Pediatr. Res. *7*:103, 1973.

Sell, S. H. W.: The clinical importance of *Hemophilus influenzae* infections in children. Pediat. Clin. N. Amer. *17*:415, 1970.

Sell, S. H. W., and Karzon, D. (eds.): Hemophilus Influenzae. Nashville, The Vanderbilt University Press, 1973.

Sell, S. H. W., Merrill, R. E., Doyne, E. O., and Zimsky, E. P., Jr.: Long term sequelae of Hemophilus influenzae meningitis. Pediatrics *49*:206, 1972.

Sell, S. H. W., Webb, W. W., Pate, J. E., and Doyne, E. O.: Psychological sequelae to bacterial meningitis: Two controlled studies. Pediatrics *49*:212, 1972.

Smith, D. H., Peter, G., Ingram, D. L., Harding, A. L., and Anderson, P.: Children immunized against *Hemophilus influenzae,* type b. Pediatrics *52*:637, 1973.

HEMOPHILUS APHROPHILUS

This tiny, gram-negative, nonmotile, pleomorphic coccobacillus deserves special mention since it may be confused with *H. influenzae* on stained smears. It is infrequently identified and has been reported most often in cases of endocarditis and brain abscess. It must be distinguished, also, from other microaerophilic or fastidious gram-negative bacilli. *Hemophilus aphrophilus* requires X, but not V, factor for growth; grows best in moist air containing 10 per cent CO_2; reduces nitrates; ferments lactose and trehalose; and fails to produce indole or catalase or to split urea.

The natural habitat of the organism and the source of infections due to it are not definitely established, but brain abscesses and endocarditis have been reported to follow respiratory infection or dental disease, with an increased incidence among children with congenital heart disease. The possibility of transfer from canine pets with pharyngeal infections due to *H. aphrophilus* has been raised.

Clinically the symptoms are those of the illness caused by localization of the organism, most frequently endocarditis, less commonly brain abscess, sinusitis, miscellaneous abscesses and wounds, pneumonia and/or empyema, septicemia, otitis media, septic arthritis, osteomyelitis or meningitis.

For therapy, the drug of choice is penicillin G, with chloramphenicol, ampicillin, kanamycin, gentamicin, or rifampin as alternatives, to be indicated by sensitivity studies of the organism causing a particular infection.

SARAH H. W. SELL

Fischbein, C. A., Beckett, K. M., and Rosenthal, A.: Hemophilus aphrophilus brain abscess associated with congenital heart disease. J. Pediatr. *83*:631, 1973.

Khairat, O.: Endocarditis due to a new species of *Haemophilus.* J. Path. Bact. *50*:497, 1940.

Sutter, V. L., and Finegold, S. M.: *Haemophilus aphrophilus* infections: Clinical and bacteriologic studies. Ann. N.Y. Acad. Sci. *17*:468, 1970.

ACUTE BACTERIAL MENINGITIS

Bacterial meningitis is given separate consideration because of its clinical importance, its diverse etiology and the principles involved in diagnosis and therapy. The etiology, morbidity and mortality of meningitis vary with age. Few other kinds of infection so well illustrate how host response may relate to level of development; bacterial meningitis remains a challenge to physicians caring for children. At some stages in life this disease retains virtually the same morbidity and mortality as before the advent of the first effective antimicrobial agents, and the problems in management have remained in major degree unchanged.

ETIOLOGY. Consideration of how the etiology of bacterial meningitis relates to the age of the patient is of great clinical utility, having impact upon considerations of pathogenesis, diagnosis, complications and therapy.

Neonatal Period to Two Months of Age. From fetal life until an uncertain period after birth arbitrarily set at 2 months, the organisms responsible for bacterial meningitis predominantly reflect the maternal flora and immunologic experience. For example, vaginal flora related to maternal fecal flora may contaminate the intrauterine environment or be transferred to a susceptible infant during the birth process. Enteric bacilli lead the list of organisms responsible for meningitis and are followed by enteric cocci. Until recently it was rare to encounter the usual pathogens of later infancy (*H. influenzae, D. pneumoniae* and *N. meningitidis*); recently, however, *H. influenzae* has been more conspicuous in neonates with meningitis, possibly owing to decreased immunity in women of childbearing age. Infrequent but important causes of bacterial meningitis in this age period are *Listeria monocytogenes,* and *Mima* and *Brucella* species.

Two Months to Adolescence. Most bacterial meningitis in this age period is due to *H. influenzae,* pneumococci and meningococci. In special circumstances other organisms may be encountered such as staphylococci, listeria, salmonellae and coliform organisms.

Adult. *Hemophilus influenzae* rarely causes meningitis in adults; *N. meningitidis* assumes a more prominent role. Pneumococci infect all age groups except the neonate.

Special Circumstances. In the immunologically deficient or suppressed child, particularly those treated for some other infection with broad spectrum antimicrobial therapy, opportunistic organisms may cause meningitis. Pseudomonas, *Alcaligenes fecalis, Serratia* sp. and others may be isolated in such instances. In addition, recurrent infection with pyogenic organisms may occur.

Structural abnormalities of the neural apparatus may result in direct contamination of the meninges with organisms of skin or feces. The association of pseudomonas with meningomyelocele is an example. Therapeutic intervention resulting in abnormal communication between the cerebrospinal space and other body compartments is associated with introduction of staphylococci or enteric organisms. Trauma to the bony structures encasing the central nervous system may lead to minute fractures which permit entry of unusual organisms. Of course, direct penetration into the central nervous system by trauma may implant a wide variety of organisms.

Certain disease states may selectively permit susceptibility to specific pathogens which can result in meningitis of unusual etiology. The association of susceptibility to Salmonella with sicklemia is an example.

EPIDEMIOLOGY. The epidemiologic characteristics of each infecting agent will be discussed in connection with that agent (q.v.).

Neonatal meningitis reflects the environment of the fetus and newly born infant. In the case of purulent amnionitis due to infection ascending from the maternal vagina he will be exposed to a predominantly enteric flora; on the other hand, although rare, if he is exposed to maternal bacteremia, any of the pyogenic organisms can be transferred.

The acquisition of meningitis by older infants and children varies with the prevalence of the organism in the community. For example, the incidence of respiratory infections with Hemophilus or pneumococci tends to peak in the autumn, winter and early spring, following the pattern of viral respiratory disease. The high concurrence of prior respiratory infection with subsequent meningitis simply reflects this pattern. More subtle environmental influences may participate in the selection of children who develop meningitis, but our understanding is incomplete in this regard. Any condition that leads to an increased incidence of respiratory disease will enhance the incidence of meningitis; the crowding, ill health and poor nutrition associated with poverty result in higher rates of both respiratory disease and meningitis.

Males have a higher incidence than females of many bacterial infections. Neonatal meningitis follows this pattern, but a less distinct separation is seen thereafter. The reasons for this association are obscure.

Meningococcal infections may occur sporadically or as epidemics. (See above, this Section.) Conditions of crowding, fatigue and associated respiratory infections all contribute to a high potential for meningococcal spread in the young adult population (such as military recruits). Whether such factors are operative within groups of children in a civilian setting is not known.

PATHOGENESIS AND PATHOLOGY. Organisms can gain entry into the meninges in a variety of ways: by direct implantation (trauma, surgical procedures); by contiguous spread (upper respiratory infections, facial infections); by lymphatic drainage (mastoids and possibly sinuses); and by bacteremia with focal implantation. Once implanted the organisms multiply and spread into the cerebrospinal fluid and probably seed other areas of the meninges. Extension into the brain parenchyma is more common than has been realized; perivascular channels and deep meningeal folds provide access for the organism into surrounding brain substance. Such penetration may account, in part, for the profound sequelae frequently observed following meningeal infection.

The inflammatory response to most pyogens is pronounced, and fibrinous exudates form which may lead to obstruction of the flow of cerebrospinal fluid. Occasionally organisms become entrapped in these adhesions and resist antimicrobial therapy.

Subdural effusions occur frequently during the course of meningitis but their exact origin is not known. Brain abscess may follow extension of the infection into the parenchyma or may simultaneously result from the original bacteremia.

Occasionally an inappropriate secretion of antidiuretic hormone occurs. The cause of this phenomenon is unknown; it may, however, potentiate the cerebral edema of the acute inflammatory process to a life-threatening degree.

Extension of infection into the peripheral cranial nerves or compression necrosis of these nerves by increased intracranial pressure can produce blindness, deafness or paralysis of facial and other muscles of the head and neck.

CLINICAL MANIFESTATIONS

Neonatal Period. In marked contrast to later life, bacterial meningitis in neonates is an insidious process seldom displaying the classic findings associated with this disease. Generally the infant is born in circumstances which make infection possible, but not all such infants are infected. Rarely, the infant may be profoundly affected in utero, with manifestations at birth which may vary from an unresuscitable collapse to transient failure to breathe. More commonly, the infant appears well at birth, but within the first few days of life displays a pattern of behavior characterized by some or all of the following: poor tone, poor cry, lack of movement, poor sucking ability, vomiting, diarrhea and other nonspecific symptoms. If the diagnosis is not established, the infant may subsequently demonstrate cardiovascular collapse, convulsions, apnea and weight loss. Depending on maturity, fever or hypothermia may be noted. The common physical findings (bulging fontanel, nuchal rigidity) are frequently lacking or appear very late in the course of disease. In many instances the diagnosis is made only at post mortem.

Older Infants and Children. The onset is variable and frequently preceded by several days of respiratory or gastrointestinal symptoms. With a slow onset the infant becomes increasingly irritable and difficult to comfort. Frequently, it is a convulsion that first causes the parent to seek medical advice. On the other hand, with fulminant disease there may be virtually no symptom prior to the sudden onset of convulsions or excessive irritability with fever or shock. All variations between these extremes are encountered. Occasionally, a preceding or initiating respiratory infection has prompted antibacterial therapy and the signs of meningitis are masked and delayed.

Untreated, meningitis generally progresses steadily and inexorably through increasing irritability and convulsions to coma, shock and death.

Physical findings are characteristic at some point in the course of meningitis. The child is agitated, irritable when handled, resists flexion of the neck and, in infancy, the fontanelles become prominent and pulseless. Older children whose cranial sutures have fused develop papilledema. Ultimately meningeal irritation results in a constantly overextended neck (opisthotonus). Neurologic findings vary with the stage of illness; paralysis of cranial nerves (6th and 3rd most commonly), reflex changes (variable) and alterations in muscle tone may be noted.

Other manifestations include evidence of purulent respiratory infection (pneumococcus and *H. influenzae*), otitis media with or without mastoiditis (usually pneumococcal, but also with *H. influenzae*), septic arthritis (*H. influenzae,* meningococcus, gonococcus), and a papular or petechial skin rash (meningococcus and, rarely, other pyogens).

Special Circumstances. With any of the conditions listed above which dispose to meningitis, the onset may be atypical. Low-grade pathogens may produce a sluggishly invasive infection, in which symptoms and signs evolve slowly or, occasionally, there is abrupt onset of fever, irritability and focal signs.

DIAGNOSIS. The only certain diagnosis is achieved by examination of the cerebrospinal fluid. Lumbar puncture should always be considered in any newborn infant who is not doing well and displays signs detailed above. Many older infants are irritable, vomit and are febrile with relatively minor infections. If meningitis is suggested, however, good judgment requires that too many rather than too few lumbar punctures be done. There is a sound clinical basis for the principle that "if one obtains no normal cerebrospinal fluid examinations among diagnostic lumbar punctures, too few are being done." Of special note is the clinical judgment required in the child who presents with a febrile seizure. In many instances the child will have no other clinical signs suggesting meningitis, and continuing observation may be all that is required by an experienced physician. On the other hand, some children with febrile seizures will have either aseptic meningitis or early bacterial meningitis; lumbar puncture for spinal fluid examination is justified in many instances and probably in the majority of children with fever and convulsions.

Cerebrospinal fluid pressure should always be measured and sufficient fluid collected to determine glucose and protein content, and to permit a gram stain and culture. Caution should be exercised if increased intracranial pressure is indicated by a full fontanelle or papilledema. In doubtful situations it is advisable to seek neurologic or neurosurgical consultation. The puncture should be performed with a small bore needle and with caution in such circumstances.

The findings in spinal fluid are usually diagnostic in untreated and in some previously treated patients. There are an increase in white cells, predominantly polymorphonuclear, and decreased glucose and elevated protein levels. A gram stain of sediment may disclose the classic appearance of specific bacteria, but mistaken identity has often enough followed gram stain identification to suggest that therapy should not be guided by this finding. The most frequent mistake is that *H. influenzae* are identified as gram positive cocci or bacilli. Rarely, the initial specimen of spinal fluid may be normal except that organisms are isolated on culture; and occasionally, if lumbar puncture is performed early in the course of bacterial meningitis, lymphocytes may predominate.

Other laboratory procedures of little specific value in diagnosis of meningitis may be useful in managing the patient. Depression of the white blood count may reflect life-threatening disease and indicate more urgent and vigorous therapy. Depressed hemoglobin levels may necessitate blood transfusion, and disturbances of electrolyte levels guide fluid replacement. With infectious foci elsewhere, appropriate diagnostic cultures should be obtained. In immunosuppressed or immunodeficient patients, specific tests should guide replacement therapy. Blood cultures should always be obtained in patients suspected of having meningitis.

In meningococcal meningitis scrapings from the petechiae or purpuric skin lesions frequently permit identification of the organism. On occasion, a drop of peripheral blood or buffy coat may be similarly diagnostic.

Differential Diagnosis. Bacterial meningitis is most frequently confused with aseptic meningitis due to a variety of viruses. Usually the spinal fluid findings differentiate patients with similar clinical presentations. Rarely, aseptic meningitis and treated bacterial meningitis are confused, and in such instances it is necessary to treat the patient as if he had bacterial meningitis, pending cultures and evolution of the disease. On occasion therapy must be completed without definitive diagnosis. It is not known how frequently antibiotic therapy not designed for meningitis can alter spinal fluid findings sufficiently to cloud the diagnosis permanently. We feel that when treated patients presenting clinical findings compatible with meningitis have ambiguous spinal fluid findings, such patients must be treated as if they had bacterial meningitis modified by suboptimal antibiotic therapy.

Other causes of nonpurulent meningitis may need consideration: *tuberculous meningitis* (differentiated by history of exposure, positive skin test, negative culture for pyogens, usual predominance of lymphocytes in spinal fluid, evidence of pulmonary or other focal tuberculosis, ultimate identification of mycobacteria); *fungal meningitis* (differentiated by specific cultures, appropriate clinical associations, spinal fluid changes); *mass lesions of the brain* (differentiated by focal nature of findings, demonstration of abscess or tumor by abnormalities in brain scan, sonogram, arteriogram, etc.); and other encephalopathies.

Meningismus may be due to pneumonia or upper respiratory tract infection. Usually evidence of the primary infection and absence of specific central nervous system symptoms permit correct differentiation; lumbar puncture must sometimes be employed.

COMPLICATIONS. Complications of bacterial meningitis are related to the locations of the inflammatory process, to systemic infection, or to secondary pathophysiologic effects.

Adhesive arachnoiditis may result in obstruction to cerebrospinal fluid flow at the foramina. Internal hydrocephalus follows ventricular obstruction; communicating hydrocephalus is associated with basilar arachnoiditis.

Widespread inflammation may lead to acute cerebral edema, with compression and destruction of cranial nerves, compression of the medulla and pons into the base of the skull, and convulsions. Local compression necrosis or actual inflammation of the cranial nerves may produce blindness, deafness or other cranial nerve palsies.

Subdural effusions and empyemas are related to local infection. Their exact pathogenesis is unknown. Small fluid collections are common and most frequently asymptomatic. More extensive subdural effusions are common in Hemophilus meningitis, rare in meningococcal infection, and frequent in pneumococcal disease. Subdural collections which occur early in the course of meningitis may be detected because acute symptomatology does not resolve appropriately; more commonly, an initial favorable response to therapy is noted but a "second illness" develops, with recurrence of fever which may be associated with increased intracranial pressure, focal neurologic signs or frank seizure activity. Subdural collections can be suggested by abnormal sonograms (lateral displacement of the midline echo) or lateralizing electroencephalograms (diminished electrical amplitude), but definitive diagnosis rests with subdural puncture. In young infants this procedure can be accomplished through unclosed sutures; in children with sealed sutures trephine may be necessary. One can usually distinguish subdural fluid from subarachnoid fluid through comparison of its protein level with that of lumbar cerebrospinal fluid obtained at the same time. Subdural fluid protein is greatly elevated and may be as high as 2000 mg/dl or more. Occasionally subdural collections contain viable organisms and inflammatory exudate.

The effects of systemic infection may be manifested in sites distant from the meninges, and include joint infections, skin rashes, and other focal infections.

Disseminated intravascular coagulation may occur in any form of meningitis with bacteremia, but is most common in meningococcal meningitis.

Shock and respiratory failure may be noted initially or develop during the course of meningitis. Emphasis has been placed in the past on adrenal hemorrhage and adrenal failure (Waterhouse-Friderichsen syndrome), but steroid levels are frequently normal or elevated despite extensive adrenal damage. Shock in meningitis and other severe infections is a complex process and may be unrelated to adrenal failure.

Inappropriate secretion of antidiuretic hormone may complicate bacterial meningitis and lead to water retention and cerebral edema. This syndrome often develops acutely and may be heralded by convulsions. Edema may be noted, with increased intracranial pressure associated with hyponatremia and hypo-osmolality. The precise mechanism is unknown.

The therapy of bacterial meningitis may produce complications unrelated to the meningeal process, which may be confused with it. Chemical thrombophlebitis secondary to intravenous therapy can produce a rise in temperature at a point in the course of meningitis when subdural effusions occur. Drug fever may also be a source of confusion. Superinfection of other organs can result from antibiotic therapy and must also be taken into account in the differential diagnosis of persistent or recurrent fever.

PROGNOSIS. The prognosis of meningitis is related to age, specific bacterial etiology, prior therapy, the existence of predisposing or contributory structural factors, the severity and course of infection, the occurrence of complications, the allergic or other tolerance of the host for antibiotic therapy, and the pharmacology of the antibiotics employed.

Meningitis has the worst prognosis in the neonate. Despite increasing sophistication in diagnosis and therapy, mortality of bacterial meningitis has remained almost constant in this age period. As many as 65 to 75 per cent of infants succumb, particularly if the infection is acquired in utero and is due to enteric organisms. A significant percentage of the survivors will suffer such sequelae as brain damage, blindness, deafness or other focal neurologic deficits. Structural changes can result in hydrocephalus.

Enteric organisms carry the worst prognosis, owing to delays in diagnosis, to the fact they occur in fetal and neonatal situations, to their resistance to antibiotics which penetrate easily into the central nervous system, and to poor host response. Among the pyogenic organisms the pneumococcus carries the highest mortality. As many as 15 to 25 per cent of infants will die, and as many will suffer crippling sequelae. *Hemophilus influenzae,* partially because it affects very young infants, ranks next, with a 10 to 15 per cent mortality and similar, or slightly higher, morbidity. Most innocuous is meningococcal meningitis unassociated with fulminant meningococcemia; fewer than 5 per cent will die, and very little residual morbidity is observed.

The oral administration of antibiotics in suboptimal doses during the early stages of meningitis can delay diagnosis and permit the process to become well established prior to the initiation of effective therapy.

Structural disturbances, natural or iatrogenic, worsen the prognosis unless they can be corrected.

Fulminant infections of rapid onset produce greater mortality than do those with slow progression. If severe leukopenia accompanies a fulminant infection, mortality will approach 100 per cent. The observation of spinal fluid saturated with organisms but displaying a paucity or absence of leukocytes is ominous.

Complications of therapy may hamper its application and effectiveness, resulting in morbidity, mortality and sequelae in addition to those of the basic disease; prognosis is adversely affected in proportion to the degree that complications such as drug sensitivity interfere with optimal treatment.

If effective therapy depends on antibiotics which are difficult to administer or penetrate poorly to the central nervous system and cerebrospinal fluid, the prognosis is worsened. This is a major factor in neonatal meningitis due to enteric organisms.

TREATMENT. Antimicrobial therapy is second only to early diagnosis in effect on outcome. The choice of antibiotics is conditioned by the patient's age and the sensitivity spectrum of possible or identified infecting agents, by the pharmacology of the drugs and their interactions with the host.

In neonatal meningitis an agent effective against enteric bacilli must be employed, in combination with another antibiotic effective against the less commonly observed pyogens. This initial therapy is modified by the results of specific sensitivity testing in vitro. Various combinations have been recommended. Most clinics use a penicillin in combination with an aminoglycoside. The choice of penicillin is conditioned by prior experience in the nursery. If streptococci are anticipated, penicillin G or ampicillin is employed, but if resistant staphylococci occur, methicillin or an equivalent is selected. For all penicillins, dosage is reduced according to the degree of renal maturation.

One of the aminoglycosides (kanamycin or gentamicin) is selected as the major antibiotic. This choice is based upon prior knowledge of the prevalent sensitivity pattern of *E. coli* and the coliforms in the local neonatal environment. Unfortunately these drugs do not penetrate into the central nervous system as well or regularly as is wished, and some prefer the addition of intrathecal therapy. Our practice is to employ intrathecal therapy with polymyxin or kanamycin or gentamicin upon the diagnosis of bacillary meningitis. Others prefer to employ this route only if bacteriologic cure is not achieved within the first few days of therapy. Still others, concerned with the potential hazards of intrathecal therapy, do not use this route. A collaborative study of this form of therapy is under way. Pending the results of this study, our choice responds to the continuing high mortality of neonatal meningitis with conventional intravenous therapy alone.

In older infants and children therapy has been simplified by the nearly universal initial use of ampicillin. Ampicillin is employed in an initial dose of 150 mg/kg and followed by 150 mg/kg/day, divided into 6 intravenous doses given every 4 hours. Until recently, ampicillin has been uniformly effective against all three major pathogens; results with it have been equal or superior to those with other antibiotics. It has also been associated with very low toxicity.

Strains of *Hemophilus influenzae* have recently been identified which require higher levels of ampicillin than those attained with the above regimen. This finding has led to recommendations either that higher doses be given (200 to 400 mg/kg/day) or that chloramphenicol be substituted. Since the vast majority of strains are very sensitive and clinical experience has shown that few instances of clinically significant resistance to therapy occur, we prefer to modify the above regimen only if a clinical response has not occurred *and* viable organisms are still present in the cerebrospinal fluid. In these circumstances we change to chloramphenicol, 100 mg/kg/day, divided into 6 doses, with lower doses for the neonate in the first month of life. (See Section 7.)

Some physicians prefer to choose an antibiotic to fit the etiology, employing penicillin G if pneumococci or meningococci are identified, and giving ampicillin only in infections due to *H. influenzae.* Others will continue with ampicillin irrespective of specific etiology. It should be noted that sulfonamides have no place today in the routine therapy of bacterial meningitis, especially that due to the meningococcus. Sulfonamide-resistant meningococci became prevalent in the 1960's; a sufficiently large number of such strains now exist in civilian populations to contraindicate routine use of sulfonamides.

In certain special circumstances the selection of antimicrobial therapy may respond to knowledge that certain infecting agents are commonest under those circumstances. For example, methicillin or another semisynthetic penicillin is indicated in meningitis associated with shunts between the cerebral ventricles and other parts of the body. Gentamicin would be selected for treatment of meningitis accompanying meningomyelocele, because of the high incidence of Pseudomonas infections.

Successful therapy will lead to reduction in symptoms, to clearing of bacteria from the spinal fluid, and to other improvement in the abnormal elements of the spinal fluid. In many instances, rapid clinical clearing is associated sequentially with increase in spinal fluid glucose content, disappearance of viable bacteria, and more gradual reduction in cell count and protein levels. Matthies and Wehrle have suggested the following criteria for cessation of therapy: (1) five days with no fever; (2) a cell count of less than $30/mm^3$ with no polymorphonuclear cells; and (3) normal glucose and protein levels.

This formula is generally useful but exceptions will be made. The commonest is to have all criteria fulfilled except that the cell count persists higher than $30/mm^3$. We evaluate this criterion in the context of the clinical status of the patient and most often opt to discontinue therapy if only a few hundred or less cells persist and the other criteria are met. In general, fulfillment of these criteria requires a minimum of 8 to 10 days of therapy, with a maximum of 4 weeks, the average duration being 2 to 3 weeks.

Therapy should be by the intravenous route exclusively. It is a common error to switch from intravenous to intramuscular or oral therapy as the patient responds. Such changes are frequently associated with relapses and should be avoided.

Not all instances of bacteriologic response are accompanied by swift clinical improvement. In fact, a prolonged slow improvement is frequently observed in meningitis due to *H. influenzae.* It is easy to become anxious during this period, but if bacteriologic cure is evident, and if no complications are detected, then further interference may only be harmful, or at best of no use. So long as the patient shows steady improvement, however slight, the therapeutic regimen should not be altered.

Supportive therapy for meningitis must take into account the anticipated pathophysiologic changes and the occurrence of complications. Patients should be isolated initially, but with bacteriologic cure this constraint can be removed. Fluid therapy should be adjusted so that the patient receives minimal requirements for maintenance, in order to minimize the risk of cerebral edema. (See Fluid and Electrolytes, Section 5.) If inappropriate secretion of antidiuretic hormone occurs, severe fluid restriction may be necessary. Cerebral edema calls for one of a variety of regimens to reduce increased intracranial pressure; administration of urea or mannitol has been recommended, many neurologists preferring judicious use of mannitol during the acute phase, with water restriction. Urea is generally ineffective; dexamethasone has not been proved efficacious in this form of cerebral edema, and is associated with rebound increases in intracranial pressure.

Administration of whole blood or packed red blood cells may be useful in alleviating profound anemia. If slow administration is necessary, a second intravenous route may have to be established in order not to interfere with antibiotic therapy.

Subdural effusions should be evacuated daily until no further fluid is obtained. If fluid persists, neurosurgical intervention may be necessary.

Neuromuscular rehabilitation may be required during convalescence.

PREVENTION. Prevention of neonatal meningitis requires attention to good obstetric care, adequate therapy of maternal infections, and so on, with the possibility of using antimicrobial agents in those situations in which the fetus is at high risk.

Effective vaccines are being sought for *H. influenzae* type b, for meningococci, and for certain types of pneumococci. If the considerable problems in their development and application can be overcome, widespread use may be associated with a decline in the incidence of meningitis.

Benson, P., Nyhan, W. L., and Shimizu, H.: The prognosis of subdural effusions complicating pyogenic meningitis. J. Pediatr. *57*:670, 1960.

Converse, G. M., Gwaltney, J. M., Strassburg, D. A., and Hend-

ley, J. O.: Alteration of cerebrospinal fluid findings by partial treatment of bacterial meningitis. J. Pediatr. *83*:220, 1973.
Murray, J. D., Fleming, P. C., Anglin, C. S., Steele, J. C., and Fujiwara, M. W.: Acute bacterial meningitis in childhood. Clin. Pediatr. *11*:455, 1972.
Smith, D. H., Ingram, D. L., Smith, A. L., Gilles, F., and Bresnan, M. J.: Bacterial meningitis: A symposium. Pediatrics *52*:586, 1973.
Wehrle, P. F., Mathies, A. W., and Leedom, J. M. The critically ill child: Management of acute bacterial meningitis. Pediatrics *44*:991, 1969.

PERTUSSIS

Pertussis is an acute respiratory infection caused by *Bordetella pertussis.* It usually occurs in unimmunized children under 4 years of age, producing an illness characterized by a prolonged period of respiratory symptoms, the most striking of which are paroxysms of coughing which terminate in a spasmodic whoop or crow. A similar but milder clinical syndrome may be produced by *B. parapertussis* or *B. bronchiseptica.*

ETIOLOGY. *Bordetella pertussis* is a small, nonmotile gram-negative rod with rather fastidious growth requirements. Since it is easily overgrown, penicillin is usually added to freshly prepared Bordet-Gengou agar (glycerin-potato-blood agar) to inhibit other organisms. *Bordetella parapertussis* and *B. bronchiseptica* have similar growth requirements and morphology and must be differentiated by serologic reactions (agglutination). *Bordetella pertussis* organisms have variable characteristics; phase I organisms (freshly isolated without subculturing on artificial media) are required for transmission of infection or for production of pertussis vaccine.

EPIDEMIOLOGY. *Bordetella pertussis* is highly contagious for unimmunized individuals, comparable to the varicella and rubella viruses. Immunization does not produce lifetime immunity; adults are frequently susceptible. Infants born of mothers with low levels of immunity are particularly susceptible and are at high risk of serious disease. The avoidance of pertussis immunization in persons over the age of 5 years because of possibly serious side effects from the vaccine has resulted in mild pertussis in adolescents and adults. Recent reports of pertussis in medical personnel underscore this risk.

Pertussis has less seasonal variation than other respiratory diseases, maintaining a high incidence during spring and summer. The disease has a very high incidence in developing countries, and for unknown reasons occurs more frequently in females than males.

Infection follows direct contact with a patient; intimate family exposure gives an attack rate as high as 70 to 80 per cent among susceptibles.

PATHOGENESIS AND PATHOLOGY. Infection follows inhalation of infectious particles. After an incubation period of 7 to 14 days, respiratory symptoms appear, the organism growing diffusely throughout the respiratory mucosa, but primarily in the bronchi and bronchioles. Focal necrosis of the basilar epithelium is accompanied by a predominantly neutrophilic infiltration. Beyond these foci, lymphocytes are associated with areas of peribronchial interstitial pneumonitis. Chronic pulmonary changes have been attributed to pertussis and may be secondary to atelectasis following obstruction by mucopurulent exudate or to bronchiectasis. Bronchopneumonia is observed with secondary bacterial infection. Following severe disease, small foci of hemorrhage have been found in the brain, but whether an encephalitis exists is unclear. A prominent lymphocytosis is characteristic and has been attributed to a factor produced by *B. pertussis.*

CLINICAL MANIFESTATIONS. The clinical presentation varies with the specific etiology *(B. pertussis, B. parapertussis* or *B. bronchiseptica)*, the immunization status of the host, and the age of the host (children under 4 years are particularly susceptible).

The classic syndrome produced by *B. pertussis* lasts 6 to 8 weeks, with three stages of about equal duration being recognizable: catarrhal, spasmodic and convalescent. During the catarrhal phase symptoms are similar to those of a common cold, with rhinorrhea, cough and low-grade fever. Pertussis is seldom suspected during this period, but suspicion increases when there is worsening cough instead of expected improvement. As the spasmodic or paroxysmal phase develops, a strangling cough is present on expiration, associated with marked facial redness or cyanosis, bulging eyes and a protruding tongue, evident anxiety, and a characteristic inspiratory whoop. Tenacious mucus may bubble from the mouth and nose; the coughing may be associated with sweating and exhaustion; and vomiting frequently follows the paroxysms. The spectrum of disease is variable during this phase, paroxysms occurring from as few as two to three times to dozens of times daily. Younger infants (under 6 months of age) may have paroxysmal coughing without whooping, or may develop apneic spells. There may be no specific clues to pertussis in this age group. During the convalescent phase, whooping and vomiting diminish and the cough becomes less severe and less frequent.

Bordetella parapertussis is associated with a milder disease (parapertussis); the cough is less severe, with similar characteristics, but parapertussis lasts only 1 to 3 weeks.

In previously immunized individuals, or those with second attacks of pertussis, the illness may be modified and difficult to recognize.

DIAGNOSIS. Pertussis is recognized by the characteristic whoop of the paroxysmal phase. Milder symptoms or atypical disease may fail to suggest pertussis to parents or physicians and may delay or prevent diagnosis. Leukocytosis with an absolute lymphocytosis may appear near the end of the catarrhal stage, counts ranging from 20,000 to 45,000 cells per mm^3 of blood, with 70 to 80 per cent lymphocytes. In infants less than 6 months of age the white blood cell count and differential are not characteristic. In mild cases, the roentgenogram of the chest may show perihilar infiltration;

in severe cases there may be atelectasis or mediastinal emphysema and, with secondary bacterial infection, lobar infiltration. Pertussis organisms may be recovered best during the early phases of illness by nasopharyngeal swabs obtained during a paroxysm of coughing and cultured on fresh medium at the bedside (cough plates are no longer recommended). Fluorescent antibody staining of pharyngeal specimens permits rapid diagnosis. Culture is mandatory for specific diagnosis; isolation or identification of the organism is not always possible in atypical cases.

A rise in neutrophil count may indicate a secondary bacterial infection.

Differential Diagnosis. Most common infectious conditions of the respiratory tract must be differentiated from pertussis. This may be readily done in typical cases on the basis of history, bacteriologic data and roentgenograms of the chest. Such conditions as other bacterial pneumonias, cystic fibrosis, tuberculosis, bronchiolitis, bronchopneumonia and interstitial pneumonia must be considered. A foreign body may produce intermittent coughing. *Adenovirus infections* have recently been implicated in the production of a syndrome impossible to differentiate from pertussis.

COMPLICATIONS. Complications of pertussis may occur in the respiratory, nervous and digestive systems. Pulmonary infection is most commonly due to secondary bacterial invasion. Otitis media is also common and frequently due to the pneumococcus. Atelectasis and bronchiolitis may result in chronic disease. Rarely, pulmonary and subcutaneous emphysema may result from paroxysms. Convulsions are not uncommon in infants, but are not believed to be due to intracranial hemorrhage; it is rather thought that anoxia secondary to paroxysms may produce both. Cerebral edema may also occur. Subconjunctival hemorrhage is common, as are cutaneous petechiae. Nutritional disturbances may follow excessive vomiting.

PROGNOSIS. The prognosis for recovery is excellent except for infants under 5 months of age; mortality may reach 40 per cent in this age group. Most deaths in infancy result from bacterial infections of the respiratory tract (interstitial pneumonia). The risk of chronic disease is unknown and its link with pertussis disputed by some.

PREVENTION AND TREATMENT. Active immunization with DPT vaccine is an effective means of prevention of pertussis due to *B. pertussis. If a convulsion or other neurologic symptom occurs after a DPT or other injection of pertussis vaccine, no further pertussis vaccine should be given alone or in combination. Rare instances of encephalopathy with mental retardation and other neurologic sequelae have been reported when this precaution has not been observed.* There is no cross-immunity with parapertussis, the latter occurring in infants and children fully immunized for pertussis. The value of passive immunization with pertussis immune globulin is unproved in either prophylactic or therapeutic use. The Committee on Infectious Disease of the American Academy of Pediatrics does not encourage its use.

Antibiotic therapy does not shorten the paroxysmal phase but does eliminate the organism. Both ampicillin (150 mg/kg/day) and erythromycin (40 mg/kg/day) have been used. The efficacy of these regimens is controversial. Erythromycin has been useful in chemoprophylaxis of pertussis infection if given before the catarrhal phase begins.

Appropriate supportive care is essential. Complications may require specific forms of intervention.

VINCENT A. FULGINITI
OTTO F. SIEBER, JR.

Bass, J. W., Klenk, E. L., Kotheimer, J. B., Linnemann, C. C., and Smith, M. H. D.: Antimicrobial treatment of pertussis. J. Pediatr. *75*:768, 1969.

Bradford, W. L., and Slavin, B.: An organism resembling Hemophilus pertussis, with special reference to color changes produced by its growth upon certain media. Am. J. Pub. Hlth. *27*:1277, 1937.

Klenk, E. L., Gaultney, J. V., and Bass, J. W.: Bacteriologically proved pertussis and adenovirus infection. Am. J. Dis. Child. *124*:203, 1972.

Kurt, T. L., Yeager, A. S., Guenette, S., and Dunlop, S.: Spread of pertussis by hospital staff. J.A.M.A. *221*:264, 1972.

Nelson, J. D., Antibiotic treatment of pertussis. Pediatrics *44*:474, 1969.

Pittman, M.: Bordetella pertussis. Bacterial and host factors in the pathogenesis and prevention of whooping cough. *In* Mudd, S. (ed): Infectious Agents and Host Reactions. Philadelphia, W. B. Saunders Company, 1970, p. 239.

Preston, N. W.: Effectiveness of pertussis vaccine. Brit. Med. J. *2*:11, 1965.

Scherp, H. W., Bradford, W. L., Day, E., and Allen, R. M.: Humoral antibodies and intradermal reactions to chemical fractions of hemophilus parapertussis. Am. J. Dis. Child. *87*:724, 1954.

ENTEROPATHOGENIC ESCHERICHIA COLI

Enteropathogenic *Escherichia coli* (EEC) are those strains of this widely prevalent bacterial genus that have a selective capacity to cause enteritis. Disease caused by these organisms is one of the most common of the acute, infectious diarrheas of known etiology; it is endemic, but institutional outbreaks are well known. Infants are primarily affected. The two most common clinical manifestations, gastroenteritis or dysentery, reflect the defined pathogenic bacterial properties.

HISTORY. *Escherichia coli* are ubiquitous, being one of the major constituents of the intestinal tract of man and most animals. It was therefore widely held that these bacteria produce no gastrointestinal disease. However, epidemiologic studies in Germany about four decades ago suggested a role for certain *E. coli* in institutional epidemics of enteritis in infants. This thesis could not be adequately documented because methods for identification of individual isolates were unsatisfactory until the currently employed classification system was introduced by Kauffman in 1944. Within a decade thereafter, several serotypes were convincingly associated with outbreaks of diarrheal disease and were designated "enteropathogenic" *E.*

coli (EEC). The pathogenicity of certain of these types was confirmed by the induction of diarrhea in orally challenged individuals. Pooled antisera to known enteropathogenic *E. coli* have since been used for diagnosis. Recent studies have defined two mechanisms by which they produce diarrhea, have extended the list of disease-associated serotypes and have emphasized the deficiencies in available methods for diagnosis.

ETIOLOGY. *Escherichia coli* are facultative anaerobic, gram-negative rods which do not form spores and are generally motile. They are distinguished from other enteric bacilli by metabolic activities. Individual isolates can be classified by agglutination reactions with immune sera, the antibodies of which are directed to O (cell wall or endotoxin), K or B (capsular) and H (flagellar) antigens. There are more than 145 serogroups; approximately 50 K and 80 H antigens yield almost innumerable serotypes. Of these, only a small per cent have been implicated as causes of diarrhea. Single serotypes of the following O groups were the earliest associated with intestinal disease: 26, 44, 55, 86, 119, 125, 126, 127 and 128. The clinical disease produced by members of these groups is primarily a gastroenteritis. Subsequently, single types of O groups 28 a, c, 112 a, c, 115, 124, 136, 143, 144, 147 and 152 have been found to produce a shigella-like dysentery; many of these enteropathogenic *E. coli* also share antigens and certain metabolic characteristics (e.g., slow lactose fermentation) with shigella species.

The availability of assays for enteropathogenicity and renewed interest in the epidemiology of infectious diarrhea have provided evidence that the list of defined serotypes of enteropathogenic *E. coli* is incomplete and, in some instances, inaccurate. For example, serotypes of O114 and O142 have recently been associated with outbreaks of severe disease in Great Britain. Isolates of O serogroups 6, 12, 15, 23, 25, 75, 78 and 148 and nontypable groups have been implicated as causes of childhood diarrhea and found to produce enterotoxin(s). Finally, it is now evident that not all members of an "enteropathogenic" serotype are pathogenic.

EPIDEMIOLOGY. The epidemiology of the earliest defined serotypes of enteropathogenic *E. coli* has been well defined, but that of EEC with defined pathogenic mechanisms is still incomplete. Disease owing to enteropathogenic *E. coli* occurs worldwide; it is endemic, but outbreaks in institutions can be explosive in onset and difficult to eradicate. Although wide regional differences in prevalence are observed, enteropathogenic serotypes are isolated from up to 40 per cent of children hospitalized with diarrhea and 20 per cent of those with diarrhea seen as outpatients. That the incidence of disease caused by these organisms may be even higher is suggested by the recent observation that only 37 per cent of toxigenic *E. coli* producing diarrhea in young children had serotypes previously identified as enteropathogenic.

Disease caused by enteropathogenic *E. coli* is most prevalent in July through October, is more common in boys than in girls and occurs predominantly in infants less than 18 months of age. Approximately half of the children are under 3 months of age, and up to 80 per cent are under 6 months. Breast-fed infants appear to be more resistant to infection than those fed by bottle. The annual attack rate caused by enteropathogenic *E. coli* of "classic" serotypes in one community in this country was 60 per 1000 infants aged 0 to 12 months. Although gastroenteritis induced by *E. coli* has been thought to be rare in adults, enterotoxigenic strains have been found to be the cause of outbreaks of "traveler's" diarrhea, and dysentery of this origin among adults is being described with increasing frequency.

Most reports implicate direct interpersonal transmission, but infection via contaminated food, drink and inanimate objects is well described. Hospital epidemics have been associated with contaminated equipment (incubators, thermometers, instruments) but most transmission is due to breaks in handwashing techniques. During an outbreak, up to 20 per cent of asymptomatic infants and 7 per cent of professional staff may be asymptomatic intestinal carriers. The possibility that *E. coli* with human pathogenicity might have an animal reservoir which could produce human disease via contamination of foodstuffs is suggested by the observations that (1) the *E. coli* in man's stool flora is derived primarily from his diet, (2) a high proportion of those *E. coli* originate in farm animals, and (3) the enterotoxin(s) of *E. coli* of human and animal origin are probably identical and are mediated by transferable genetic units. A recent national outbreak of dysentery due to enteropathogenic *E. coli* spread by contaminated soft cheese illustrates the potential transmissibility via foods.

Fecal-oral transmission has been presumed to be the predominant route of interpersonal transmission. Ingestion of 10^8 to 10^9 enteropathogenic *E. coli* is required to produce disease in healthy adults; concomitant ingestion of alkali to neutralize gastric acidity, which is a nonspecific barrier, reduces the infectivity dose by a hundredfold. Acutely ill individuals excrete more than 10^8 enteropathogenic *E. coli* per gram of stool; stomach contents may contain up to 10^3 per ml and small intestine fluid 10^3 to 10^7 per ml. The role of respiratory transmission remains undefined, but nasopharyngeal cultures are more commonly positive than stool cultures among contacts of infected children, and transmission from children with positive throat but negative stool cultures does occur.

PATHOGENESIS. The earlier proposal that enteropathogenic *E. coli* cause disease only in conjunction with certain viruses has been discounted. Two mechanisms for the enteropathogenicity have been elucidated: production of an enterotoxin that promotes fluid and electrolyte loss from the small intestine, and the capacity to invade and multiply in the intestinal epithelium, primarily of the colon. The bacterial endotoxin and capsule play no apparent role in enteropathogenicity.

Colonization of the upper intestinal tract appears to be critical to the pathogenesis of toxigenic *E. coli,* being promoted by the attachment of the bacteria to the intestinal epithelium via specialized K antigens. Such attachment promotes local bacterial multiplication and facilitates interaction of released enterotoxin and epithelium. A heat-labile and heat-stable enterotoxin have been identified. The former resembles cholera toxin in that it binds specifically to ganglioside Gm_1 of the epithelial cells of the small intestine, activates cellular adenyl cyclase to increase intracellular cyclic AMP and promotes net secretion of water and chloride. This heat-labile toxin also has immunologic cross-reactivity, but not identity, with cholera toxin. Toxin production can be identified at present only by the induction of disease in man or certain animals, by production of fluid secretion in isolated ileal loops of animals or by the activation of adenyl cyclase in certain tissues treated in vitro.

Infant lambs, calves and pigs are susceptible to diarrhea caused by enteropathogenic *E. coli*; mortality rates are often high, resulting in a problem of major economic importance. The causative bacteria have serotypes different from those causing human disease, but they produce enterotoxins that appear to be identical to those produced by enteropathogenic *E. coli* of human origin.

The genetic basis for toxin production resides on nonchromosomal elements or plasmids which are potentially transferable between *E. coli* by bacterial conjugation or by virus mediation (transduction). Such transfer of plasmids (horizontal genetic inheritance) undoubtedly explains the variable association of toxigenicity with serologic type.

Although the molecular basis has not been defined, the enteropathogenicity of some *E. coli,* like that of shigella, correlates with their capacity to invade and multiply in epithelial cells, primarily of the large bowel. This property is determined by demonstration of invasiveness in rabbit intestine, production of keratoconjunctivitis in guinea pigs (the Serény test), and multiplication in tissue cultures of epithelial (HeLa) cells.

PATHOLOGY. Toxigenic *E. coli* are not invasive, and the enterotoxin produces no morphologic pathology. Local intestinal inflammation, metastatic abscesses, fatty hepatic necrosis and lymphoid depletion have been associated with serotypes of *E. coli* which produce "gastroenteritis." These observations preceded the availability of assays for enteropathogenicity; thus, pathogenic mechanisms and these histologic findings cannot be correlated. Moreover, involved children have generally been hospitalized with chronic, debilitating diseases or systemic infections of other etiologies, so that the direct role of enteropathogenic *E. coli* in the extraintestinal pathology remains undefined. Enteropathogenic *E. coli* with invasive capacity produce the characteristic findings of (shigella) dysentery: local inflammation with hyperemia, edema, erosion of blood vessels, ulceration of epithelium and intraluminal exudate composed of cellular debris, fibrin and acute inflammatory cells. Extension to the lymphatic system or serosa occurs only infrequently; peritonitis and invasion of lymphatics and the blood stream with resultant metastatic disease are uncommon.

CLINICAL MANIFESTATIONS. There is considerable variation in the clinical manifestations of individuals affected in an outbreak of disease caused by a single serotype of enteropathogenic *E. coli* and in separate outbreaks caused by different ones. Most children with gastroenteritis develop watery diarrhea without significant fever or other systemic symptoms or signs after an incubation period of about two days. The stools are watery, with mucus but not pus or blood, and generally number five to ten per day. Symptoms generally subside spontaneously in three to seven days, but protracted courses are observed. Relapse rates of up to 20 per cent are observed, even in children treated with antibiotics. Although respiratory colonization is common, respiratory symptoms are rare. Infants have more severe and prolonged manifestations, with significant dehydration, fever and electrolyte disturbances, particularly acidosis and often hypernatremia. Vomiting, probably as a result of metabolic disturbances, is common in infants. There may be peritonitis or metastatic infection in debilitated infants. Jaundice, hepatocellular dysfunction and hypoproteinemia with resultant peripheral edema have been observed in infants with other underlying illnesses involved in outbreaks characterized by severe clinical courses; the direct role of enteropathogenic *E. coli* in these manifestations remains undefined.

Dysentery produced by certain strains produces similar symptoms in children and adults. After an incubation period of 18 to 24 hours, there is a rather abrupt onset of fever up to 103° F, severe diarrhea (often bloody), nausea, crampy abdominal pain, tenesmus, myalgia, chills, malaise, vomiting and headache. Some individuals have severe systemic toxemia and even transient hypotension.

DIAGNOSIS. Blood cultures are only rarely positive. Cultures of the nasopharynx, throat, upper intestinal contents and stool are positive in children with gastroenteritis; stool, but not small bowel contents, is positive in those with dysentery. Immunofluorescence of bacteria from specimens or cultures or agglutination of cultured organisms is employed to confirm the presence of enteropathogenic serotypes. The correlation between immunofluorescence of stool specimens and culture results is about 70 per cent, the fluorescent antibody system yielding significantly more positive results. Some specimens with positive immunofluorescent smears but negative cultures come from children who previously or subsequently have positive cultures or who are receiving antibiotics; more than half, however, are false positives produced by cross-reacting antigens. Enteropathogenic *E. coli* may be cultured on most routine media, but selective media which identify lactose fermentation are most commonly used. Although healthy individuals excrete multiple serotypes of *E. coli,* in those with disease the etiologic serotype predominates.

Thus, slide agglutinations of (mixtures of) 5 to 10 colonies suffice to screen most specimens. Some problems encountered in interpreting the agglutination reactions are that antiserum to many pathogenic serotypes is not included in commercially available reagents, that some isolates of "pathogenic" serotypes do not cause disease, and that some enteropathogenic *E. coli* have nontypable antigens. Assessment of enterotoxin production or epithelial invasiveness can be performed in only a few research laboratories.

Some enteropathogenic *E. coli* ferment sorbitol, but this is not diagnostic. Strains which produce dysentery may ferment lactose slowly and often react with serum prepared against shigella species; careful evaluation of metabolic and serologic reactions is therefore often required to make this differentiation. Systemic antibody responses are observed in less than half of diseased individuals and are not commonly assayed.

Serum electrolytes are often abnormal, but are not diagnostic. There are no characteristic hematologic findings. Sigmoidoscopy of children with gastroenteritis may reveal hyperemia; in those with dysentery, hyperemia with bleeding points and superficial ulcers are often evident.

Differential Diagnosis. Clinical distinction between gastroenteritis produced by enteropathogenic *E. coli* and that caused by salmonellae or viruses is difficult. In endemic areas, enteropathogenic *E. coli* often cause vibrio-negative cholera. The relative lack of fever and vomiting and the age of the child affected by gastroenteritis due to enteropathogenic *E. coli* may be helpful in the differential diagnosis. Respiratory symptoms are rare in disease caused by enteropathogenic *E. coli* but relatively common with viral gastroenteritis. Dysentery due to enteropathogenic *E. coli* cannot be differentiated clinically from shigellosis. Ulcerative and granulomatous colitis, dysentery caused by anaerobic organisms, and acute surgical disorders must be distinguished (see Shigellosis). The stool in gastroenteritis due to enteropathogenic *E. coli* usually has a foul odor, is often green in color and may contain mucus, but no leukocytes or erythrocytes. On the other hand, as in shigellosis, the stool of patients with dysentery contains polymorphonuclear leukocytes and, often, erythrocytes. The presence of acute inflammatory cells, observed best in flecks of mucus in freshly passed stool, distinguishes this as one of the invasive bacterial causes of diarrhea.

PREVENTION. The interpersonal transmission of enteropathogenic *E. coli* is often difficult to prevent. Special precautions in the handling of the urine and feces of hospitalized children should be instituted, and consideration given to the use of masks if nasopharyngeal cultures are positive. Strict handwashing practices by (professional) contacts are the most important facet of prevention. During an institutional epidemic, all exposed patients and personnel should have cultures made and appropriate antibiotic therapy instituted. Outbreaks in nurseries often require a "cohort" system of admissions. Community outbreaks usually occur in the presence of inadequate housing, sanitation and personal hygiene.

Little is known of immunity to enteropathogenic *E. coli*. Resistance of nursing infants to infection by these organisms is thought to be consequent to the inhibitory effects of the intestinal flora associated with a breast milk diet. Experience with disease caused by other bacterial enteric pathogens suggests that circulating and copro-antibodies play a role in protection; antibody to cholera toxin reduces clinical symptoms but not infection rates, and it seems logical that similar observations will be found for toxigenic *E. coli*. The prevalence and importance of disease due to enteropathogenic *E. coli*, particularly in developing countries, suggest the need for active immunization. The potential of developing an enterotoxoid is under evaluation; the feasibility of oral vaccines of attenuated bacteria seems obviated by the number of strains involved.

PROGNOSIS. The prognosis depends on the type of disease, the properties of the etiologic bacterium, and the age and underlying state of health of the patient. Mortality rates of 30 to 50 per cent have been reported in certain dramatic outbreaks affecting infants, but generally this figure is 5 per cent or less.

TREATMENT. Older children and adults rarely require hospitalization, but infants often have significant morbidity, mortality and need for intravenous fluids. Therefore, the patient's age and the extent of symptoms, particularly hydration and vomiting, dictate the need for hospitalization. Correction of fluid and electrolyte imbalance is the major therapeutic consideration. The usual diet is restricted or stopped until fluid and electrolyte imbalances are corrected. Intravenous fluid therapy has been used commonly for dehydrated infants, but many will take sufficient oral fluids to correct their dehydration. The solution introduced for therapy of cholera and used successfully for other infectious diarrheas can be made as follows: glucose 20 gm (8 teaspoonfuls), sodium chloride 4 gm (1 teaspoonful), sodium bicarbonate 3.5 gm (3/4 teaspoonful), potassium citrate 1.6 gm (1/4 teaspoonful) dissolved in 1 liter of drinking water.

Drugs such as kaolin with pectin and tincture of opium that increase stool bulk or decrease bowel motility do not affect the loss of fluids and electrolytes into the intestinal tract. Their therapeutic effects may therefore promote a false assessment of the clinical state; accordingly, such agents are not recommended. Some experienced clinicians prescribe low doses of sedatives to control abdominal pain and cramps; antispasmodic drugs are usually not necessary.

Specific antibiotic therapy is indicated for patients ill enough to be hospitalized and outpatients with significant or prolonged symptoms. Spontaneous clinical recovery and eradication of intestinal colonization generally occur within 3 to 7 days. Thus, by the time the child is ill enough to seek medical attention and the disease is diagnosed clinically and in the laboratory, the need for specific antibiotic therapy may have passed.

No controlled studies of antibiotic therapy in disease caused by *E. coli* with defined pathogenic mechanisms have been published. Clinical experience indicates that antibiotics appropriate to the susceptibility of the etiologic organisms reduce the duration of symptoms and of intestinal excretion. Wide regional differences exist in the antibiotic sensitivities. When studied, the antibiotic resistances of enteropathogenic *E. coli,* like those of other gram-negative bacilli, are mediated by bacterial plasmids, the R factors. These mediate resistance to one or several antibiotics commonly used and are potentially transferable between all gram-negative, but not gram-positive, bacilli.

Most experience with antibiotic treatment of disease caused by enteropathogenic *E. coli* has been in the therapy of *gastroenteritis,* not dysentery. Neomycin, 100 mg/kg/day given in 3 to 6 divided doses, has been the most popular regimen; stool cultures become negative within 24 hours in about 75 per cent of children, and within 48 hours in 90 per cent. Relapse rates following cessation of therapy may be as high as 20 per cent and apparently are not affected by duration of treatment. Clinical response correlates with elimination of the pathogen from the stool. A therapeutic course of 3 to 5 days has all the advantages of one of 7 to 10 days, no disadvantages and is recommended. In areas where resistance of enteropathogenic *E. coli* to neomycin is prevalent, oral colistin at 10 mg/kg/day is recommended. Oral ampicillin at 50 to 100 mg/kg/day has also been used successfully, but the relative prevalence in many areas of ampicillin-resistant organisms precludes the general recommendation of this antibiotic.

Therapy of *dysentery* due to enteropathogenic *E. coli* has not been critically evaluated, but the clinical and pathologic similarities to shigellosis permit extrapolation from the considerable experience with that disease. Treatment of shigellosis with nonabsorbable antibiotics has been disappointing, but excellent responses have been obtained with absorbable ones which produce inhibitory concentrations in tissues. Ampicillin has been the most widely recommended agent for susceptible strains of both shigella and enteropathogenic *E. coli.*

Boris, M., Thomason, B., Hines, V., Montague, T., and Sellers, T.: A community epidemic of enteropathogenic *Escherichia coli* O126:B16:NM gastroenteritis associated with asymptomatic respiratory infection. Pediatrics *33*:18, 1964.

Danielsson, D., and Laurell, G.: The fluorescent antibody technique in the diagnosis of enteropathogenic *Escherichia coli,* with special reference to sensitivity and specificity. Acta Path. Microbiol. Scand. *76*:601, 1969.

DuPont, H. I., Formal, S. B., Hornick, R. B., Snyder, M. J., Libonati, J. P., Sheahan, D. G., LaBrec, E. H., and Kalas, J. P.: Pathogenesis of *Escherichia coli* diarrhea. New Engl. J. Med. *285*:1, 1971.

Gorbach, S. L., and Khurana, C. M.: Toxigenic *Escherichia coli;* A cause of infantile diarrhea in Chicago. New Engl. J. Med. *287*:791, 1972.

Marier, R., Wells, J. G., Swanson, R. C., Callahan, W., and Mehlman, I. J.: An outbreak of enteropathogenic *Escherichia coli* foodborne disease traced to imported French cheese. Lancet *2*:1376, 1973.

Nelson, J. D., and Haltalin, K. C.: Accuracy of diagnosis of bacterial diarrheal disease by clinical features. J. Pediatr. *78*:519, 1971.

Neter, E.: Enteritis due to enteropathogenic *Escherichia coli;* Present-day status and unsolved problems. J. Pediatr. *55*:223, 1959.

Riley, H. D.: Antibiotic therapy in neonatal enteric disease. Ann. N. Y. Acad. Sci. *176*:360, 1971.

Sakazaki, R., Tamura, K., and Saito, M.: Enteropathogenic *Escherichia coli* associated with diarrhea in children and adults. Japan J. Med. Sci. Biol. *20*:387, 1967.

South, M. A.: Enteropathogenic *Escherichia coli* disease: New developments and perspectives. J. Pediatr. *79*:1, 1971.

SALMONELLA INFECTIONS

Salmonellae are parasites of the intestinal tract of man and animals. Humans are affected by indirect or direct transmission from animals or man. Most human infections are asymptomatic, but some produce acute gastroenteritis, bacteremia, often with metastatic localization, or enteric (typhoid) fever. Currently, salmonella gastroenteritis is one of the most common infectious diseases in the United States, whereas typhoid fever is rare. In many developing areas of the world, however, typhoid fever is still endemic and occurs in epidemics.

ETIOLOGY. Salmonellae are gram-negative, nonencapsulated, nonsporulating rods. They are facultative anaerobes and utilize simple carbon and nitrogen compounds for biosynthesis and energy; they therefore grow readily on ordinary media. Both biochemical activities and serologic reactions are used to distinguish salmonellae from other bacteria.

Surface antigenic composition is used to distinguish individual types of salmonellae. The carbohydrate moieties of the lipopolysaccharide cell wall are the basis for identification of the more than 60 O antigens, which, in turn, are used to classify salmonellae into groups, designated A to I. Members of each O group can be further typed by their protein, flagellar (H) antigens, designated with arabic numerals and small letters. A few salmonellae, particularly *Salmonella typhosa,* produce a carbohydrate envelope (Vi) antigen. Certain of these antigens react with sera prepared against antigens of other enteric bacilli. This system of classification has been successfully employed in reference laboratories to identify more than 1400 distinct types of salmonellae, over 90 per cent of which are in groups A to E.

The nomenclature of this complex system is further complicated by the designation of certain strains by names. (Table 10–5 lists some of the common types.) Further classification of certain serotypes, e.g., *S. typhosa,* by susceptibility to a panel of bacteriophages has been useful in epidemiologic studies.

Salmonellae are only moderately resistant to physical agents. They are killed by heating to 130° F for 1 hour or 140° F for 15 minutes, but

TABLE 10–5 CERTAIN COMMONLY ISOLATED SALMONELLAE

Group A:	*S. paratyphi*
Group B:	*S. schottmuelleri* *S. typhimurium*
Group C_1:	*S. hirschfeldii* *S. cholerasuis* *S. oranienburg* *S. montevideo*
Group C_2:	*S. newport*
Group D:	*S. typhosa* *S. enteritidis* *S. gallinarum* *S. pullorum*
Group E:	*S. anatis*

remain viable for days at ambient or reduced temperatures, particularly in materials that are buffered by organic material or dried. Thus, contaminating organisms may survive for days or weeks in fecal material, sewage, dried foodstuffs and pharmaceuticals. Salmonellae in stool specimens, collected in the field and transported in appropriate carrier media, will be viable when cultured days later in the laboratory. Prolonged survival has also been observed in contaminated fresh and sea water. Resistance to certain chemicals and dyes, e.g., selenium salts, sodium tetrathionate, sodium deoxycholate and brilliant green, has been exploited for the development of media that selectively inhibit growth of other bacteria, particularly enterobacteria, present in fecal specimens.

The properties of salmonellae responsible for pathogenicity are incompletely defined. The basis for invasiveness and stimulation of fluid exsorption is not known, but there is no evidence that salmonellae produce an enterotoxin. The O antigen (an endotoxin) enhances resistance to phagocytosis, and strains deficient in it are avirulent. The pharmacologic effects of the endotoxin may produce certain of the clinical manifestations of systemic disease, but there is no evidence that they are important in gastroenteritis. Although the responsible mechanisms are not known, certain serotypes of salmonellae have marked host preferences and produce characteristic patterns of disease. *Salmonella typhosa* infects only man; *S. paratyphi A* and *C* are generally isolated from human sources, while *S. pullorum* is primarily a fowl pathogen, and *S. abortus equi* infects only horses. However, six or seven of the 10 types of salmonellae most commonly isolated from animal sources each year in the United States are among the 10 types most commonly isolated from man. Most salmonellae can cause human gastroenteritis and some are invasive; indeed, *S. paratyphi A* and *B* and, less often, *S. schottmuelleri, S. hirschfeldii* and *S. cholerasuis* may cause a syndrome of enteric fever that cannot be readily distinguished clinically from typhoid fever, the sole disease produced by *S. typhosa.* Since certain aspects of nontyphoidal salmonella infections (salmonellosis) differ significantly from those of typhoid fever, these will be considered separately.

NONTYPHOIDAL SALMONELLOSIS

EPIDEMIOLOGY. Approximately 25,000 culture-proved cases of salmonellosis are reported in the United States annually. Based on experiences with the inefficiency of case reporting in several large epidemics, epidemiologists estimate that the actual number of cases may be as great as 100 times that reported. Thus, 1 per cent of persons in the United States is thought to have a salmonella infection each year. Of reported individuals with salmonellosis, approximately two thirds are less than 20 years of age. The attack rates in this age group are highest for those under 9 years of age, particularly infants (Fig. 10–3), and for males. The largest number of isolates are reported from July through

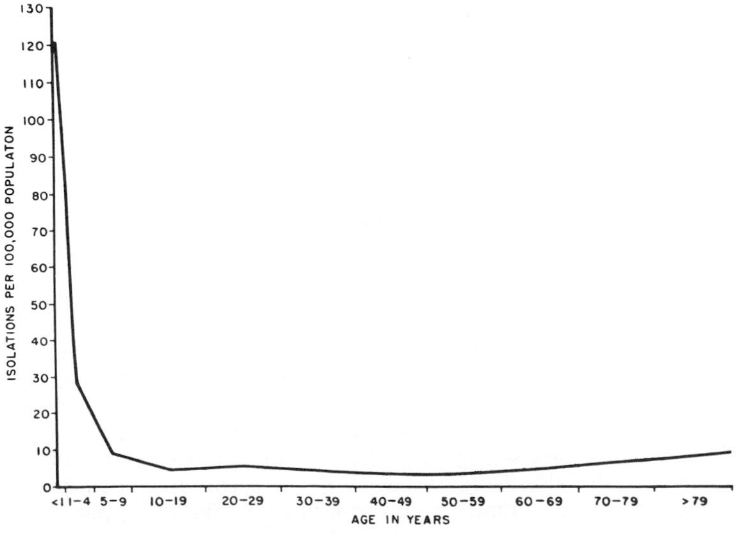

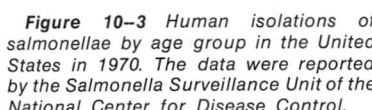

Figure 10–3 *Human isolations of salmonellae by age group in the United States in 1970. The data were reported by the Salmonella Surveillance Unit of the National Center for Disease Control.*

October, the lowest from January through April. Seventy per cent of isolates reported in 1970 involved the following 10 serotypes: *S. typhimurium* (25 to 30 per cent of the total), *enteriditis, newport, heidelberg, infantis, saintpaul, thompson, blockley, derby, typhi.*

Humans are infected primarily via contaminated food and drink. Abundant evidence indicates that the salmonellae that cause most human infections originate from animal sources. Salmonellae infect most animals, including fowl, e.g., chickens, turkeys, ducks and wild birds; mammals, e.g., swine, cattle, sheep, dogs, cats and rodents; reptiles, e.g., turtles, lizards and snakes; and insects. Essentially all surveys of domestic livestock have revealed infected animals, with up to 70 per cent of poultry, 33 per cent of cattle and 50 per cent of swine studied having positive fecal cultures. Most, but not all animal infections are asymptomatic.

The animal reservoir of salmonellae is self-generating. Animal feeds are frequently contaminated because constituents, e.g., animal by-products or fish used for protein supplementation, are infected. Feed may also be contaminated by unclean production machinery or personnel, or indirectly, during storage, by rodents and insects. Animals are also infected by other domestic and wild animals and birds, which, in turn, have been infected by human or domestic animal products which they have ingested. Water supplies contaminated by human or animal sources are often the source of new cycles of infection. Contemporary mass methods of food production and distribution amplify the animal reservoir of salmonellae and provide the link between it and man. Crowding of animals during transportation and in slaughterhouses, mechanized processing of carcasses and large scale handling of retail meat products all facilitate contamination. The prevalence of salmonellosis in chickens creates a high risk of contamination of eggs; salmonellae may contaminate the shell surface, from which they can penetrate into the egg, or be transmitted from an ovarian infection directly to the egg yolk. Pooling of large numbers of eggs prior to freezing, drying or use in the preparation of foodstuffs increases the risk of human infection.

Up to 50 per cent of poultry, 5 per cent of beef, 16 per cent of pork and 40 per cent of frozen eggs purchased in retail markets contain salmonellae. These foods pass inspection because the contamination cannot be visibly appreciated. Salmonellae introduced into kitchens on contaminated meat and poultry may be transferred to other foods from contaminated utensils, table surfaces or personnel. Salmonellae inside foods (e.g., large turkeys, soft-boiled eggs) may not be exposed to sterilizing temperatures during cooking. It is not surprising, therefore, that poultry, eggs and their products, such as eggnog, and meats are the most common food source of salmonellosis. Contamination of equipment in processing plants has been responsible for outbreaks associated with dried coconut, baker's yeast, dried milk, cottonseed protein and a remarkable list of pharmaceuticals. Presumably because of increased exposure, individuals working in slaughterhouses, food processing plants and commercial kitchens have an increased incidence of salmonellosis, and they are often the source of contamination of production equipment and utensils.

Certain dramatic examples of direct transmission of salmonellae from animals to man, e.g., an outbreak traced to sea gulls, produce a small percentage of human disease. Recently, pet chickens, mammals and turtles have been appreciated as sources of human disease, particularly among children. Indeed, the results from retrospective analysis of case surveys suggest that pet turtles may cause as much as 15 per cent of human salmonellosis!

The frequency with which humans transmit salmonellae to their contacts has not been defined, but the risk is real. During the acute stages of infection, 10^6 to 10^9 salmonellae are excreted per gram of stool, while concentrations of 10^2 to 10^5 per gram of stool are excreted for variable intervals thereafter. Seventy to 90 per cent of infected individuals still have positive stool cultures 2 weeks after infection, about 50 per cent at 4 weeks, and 10 to 25 per cent at 10 weeks. The duration of excretion is similar whether the infection has been symptomatic or asymptomatic, but is longer for infants under 1 year of age than for older children. Excretion is significantly prolonged by antibiotic therapy, regardless of the agent. Up to 60 per cent of family contacts of reported cases are infected at the time of surveillance by public health authorities, but it is rarely possible to determine whether salmonella infections have resulted from human transmission or from the common ingestion of contaminated foods. The high incidence of salmonellosis among people in closed communities who have contact with individuals infected by a common food source illustrates the potential for interpersonal transmission of salmonellae. Outbreaks in institutions and hospitals, particularly obstetrical suites and nurseries, are usually caused by direct transmission, but transmission by aerosol or on articles such as incubators, clothing and thermometers has been implicated.

PATHOGENESIS AND PATHOLOGY. Salmonellae produce gastroenteritis by stimulating excretion of intestinal fluid and by local inflammation. Bacterial penetration of intestinal epithelium and multiplication in the lamina propria produces the inflammation, but may not be required for fluid exsorption. The small intestine is predominantly involved, but disease of the large bowel is not unusual. Following local multiplication, organisms may penetrate to local lymphatic tissue, from which they invade lymphatic or vascular circulations. Disseminating organisms are usually cleared by the reticuloendothelial system, but focal invasion of distant organs can occur.

Invaded intestinal epithelial cells become shortened and villi irregular. The mucosa becomes hyperemic and edematous and is invaded by acute inflammatory cells, but necrosis, ulceration and intraluminal hemorrhage are unusual. Local lymphatic tissues hypertrophy and, when invaded, show evidence of acute inflammation.

The risk and type of infection are determined by the number and properties of the salmonellae ingested, and by host factors. Studies with healthy adult volunteers indicate that 10^5 to 10^6 bacteria generally produce disease, but this dose may vary by a hundredfold, depending on the type, or even subtype, of the salmonellae. Asymptomatic infection can be produced by much smaller numbers. Local factors, such as gastric acidity, to which salmonellae are sensitive, intestinal motility and bacterial flora, play major roles in resistance to colonization. Individuals with achlorhydria and gastric or intestinal bypasses are unusually susceptible to salmonellae. Studies with animals indicate that alteration of the intestinal flora by antibiotics may reduce the disease-producing dose of salmonellae by 100,000. Systemic invasion is much more common in individuals at the extremes of age and in those with diseases that impair reticuloendothelial or cellular immune functions. Thus, a high percentage of patients with salmonella septicemia have lupus erythematosus, hepatic cirrhosis, leukemia, lymphoma, Hodgkin's disease or disorders accompanied by hemolysis, such as malaria, bartonellosis and hemoglobinopathies. Individuals with ulcerative colitis may also have abnormally high attack rates of salmonellosis. The invasiveness of certain salmonellae is evidenced by the observation that up to one half of the infections caused by *S. cholerasuis* and *S. paratyphi A* and *B*, but less than 5 per cent caused by many other types, produce a septicemia. That *S. typhimurium* is the type most commonly isolated from blood cultures reflects the prevalence of this type rather than special invasive characteristics.

Salmonellae appear to localize preferentially in necrotic tissue, such as those associated with vascular aneurysm or infarction, neoplasia, hematomas and surgical sutures. Staphylococci cause at least 80 per cent of hematogenous osteomyelitis in the general population of children, but salmonellae cause more than 50 per cent of this disease in children with sickle cell disease.

CLINICAL MANIFESTATIONS. In the usual case of salmonella gastroenteritis, an incubation period of 8 to 24 hours (range 6 to 48 hours) is followed by nausea, vomiting, and colicky abdominal pain. Shortly thereafter, diarrhea starts, occasionally with blood and mucus. Initially, chills may occur and temperatures to 102° F are common. Hyperactive peristalsis and mild abdominal tenderness are found on physical examination. The symptoms are self-limited and usually subside within 5 days. This clinical picture is highly variable, however. Some patients remain afebrile and have only mild intestinal symptoms. Others develop higher fevers, with associated headache, drowsiness, confusion, seizures and meningismus. Some children, even afebrile ones, may pass multiple watery stools daily and become dehydrated. There may be moderate abdominal distention and severe, localized pain with associated rebound tenderness.

Septicemic spread of salmonellae is accompanied by chills and high temperatures. The symptoms of *enteric fever* are those described for typhoid fever, but the course is shorter and the mortality lower. Salmonellae may localize in any tissue, causing abscesses, meningitis, bronchopneumonia, empyema, osteomyelitis, endocarditis, septic arthritis and pyelonephritis; the clinical manifestations reflect inflammation of the organ involved.

DIAGNOSIS. The stool in salmonella gastroenteritis characteristically contains polymorphonuclear leukocytes, which can be demonstrated by staining a freshly passed specimen with methylene blue; erythrocytes and mucus may also be present. Salmonellae can be isolated from stool for variable periods after infection. Culture of stool itself is more often positive than a specimen from a rectal swab. Two swabs taken during the same examination increase the yield by 10 per cent over that obtained with one, but the results are still inferior to those obtained with a single specimen of stool. Optimal bacteriologic results are obtained by incubation of the specimen in an enrichment broth, e.g., tetrathionate broth, prior to plating on selective medium, e.g., brilliant green agar. Attempts have been made to adapt the direct fluorescent antibody technique to the rapid identification of salmonellae, since such a technique would have application in the food processing industry as well as in diagnostic laboratories. The large number of salmonella surface antigens, some of which are shared with other common enteric bacilli, and the natural fluorescence of many products pose serious problems, but promising results have been obtained with specimens incubated in enrichment broth prior to examination. Three consecutive negative stool cultures usually are evidence that infection has ceased, but excretion may be intermittent. Salmonellae can be isolated from blood, spinal fluid, urine and local tissues when they are infected.

A fourfold rise in serum agglutinins is considered diagnostic of infection, but cross-reactions and the large number of antigens make serologic tests difficult to perform accurately in routine laboratories. Individuals with chronic hepatic and gastrointestinal diseases may have unusually high titers of salmonella agglutinins in the absence of documented infection. It is presumed that the primary diseases facilitate excessive exposure of these individuals to cross-reacting antigens of other enteric bacilli. Patients with salmonella gastroenteritis have no outstanding hematologic findings, but those with metastatic infection have a marked leukocytosis.

Differential Diagnosis. Salmonella gastroenteritis must be distinguished from other causes of *food poisoning, viral gastroenteritis* and *dysentery* caused by *Shigella* or *E. coli. Meningitis,* acute *appendicitis* or *intussusception* are suggested in certain cases. Rarely a clinical course and even radiologic findings suggestive of *ulcerative colitis* are observed.

PROGNOSIS. Salmonella gastroenteritis has an excellent prognosis except in infants, debilitated children or those with underlying disease. The pronosis of salmonella meningitis and endocarditis is very poor; that of other systemic infections generally depends on the basic state of health of the infected individual.

TREATMENT. Correction of dehydration and electrolyte disturbances and symptomatic management are the most important aspects of the therapy of salmonella gastroenteritis. Antibiotics rarely alter the clinical course, and for reasons that are not clear, they usually do not eliminate susceptible salmonellae from the intestinal tract. Moreover, antibiotics prolong the duration of intestinal excretion. Antibiotics are indicated in gastroenteritis, therefore, only for individuals at highest risk, e.g., infants, children with immunologic deficiencies or those suffering a severe, protracted course.

Children with bacteremia, enteric fever or metastatic infection should be treated with systemically administered ampicillin (100–300 mg/kg daily, given at 6-hour intervals) or chloramphenicol (50-100 mg/kg daily for older children and 25 mg/kg daily for infants, given at 6-hour intervals). In vitro susceptibility to these agents should always be determined. Resistance to chloramphenicol is rare among salmonellae isolated in the United States but is not uncommon among those recovered in many other areas of the world. Up to 20 per cent of salmonellae isolated from humans in this country are resistant to ampicillin. Many clinicians prefer chloramphenicol for salmonella infections, but there is little evidence documenting its superiority over ampicillin, and its potential hematologic toxicity must be considered prior to use, particularly for diseases which are not life-threatening.

TYPHOID FEVER

EPIDEMIOLOGY. The prevalence of typhoid fever in the United States has declined steadily since 1900. About 500 new cases are now reported annually. It is estimated that more than half are newly recognized carriers, while the rest have acute disease. The majority with disease are less than 20 years of age. Several thousand chronic carriers are known to health departments.

Historically the highest attack rates of typhoid fever have occurred in crowded populations with impure water and inadequate housing and sanitation. Populations involved in major social upheaval, such as war or natural disaster, are particularly likely to be affected.

Since the typhoid bacillus infects only man, all cases ultimately have a human origin. Acutely infected patients excrete *S. typhi* in respiratory secretions, urine and feces for variable periods, but chronic carriers are responsible for most of the disease in this country. Characteristically the implicated carrier is an adult woman who has had contact with an acutely infected individual, who may have had an enteric illness herself or who prepares food consumed by the index case. Because foods may be contaminated in processing plants and in kitchens, many kinds of food have been sources of disease. The prolonged survival of *S. typhi* in nature facilitates transmission in water supplies or via inanimate objects. Water transmission generally involves inadequate plumbing or sanitation and is responsible for individual episodes in the rural United States and for endemic disease in developing countries. Because oysters and shellfish are often cultivated in waters polluted by sewage that has not been properly disinfected, and are generally consumed without cooking to sterilizing temperatures, they are not uncommon sources.

PATHOGENESIS. Studies with adult volunteers infected with laboratory strains of *S. typhi* indicate that 10^5 organisms cause disease in 25 per cent of individuals, 10^7 in 50 per cent and 10^9 in 95 per cent. The observation that naturally acquired disease may be produced by as few as a thousand organisms suggests that differences exist in the resistance of individual hosts and in the pathogenicity of individual strains, particularly between those transmitted in nature and in laboratories.

Infection with *S. typhi* always results in clinical disease. The pathogenesis involves several discrete but overlapping events. Organisms rapidly invade the blood stream from sites of minimal inflammation. Some early investigators argued that this initial septicemia arises from the oropharynx, but the upper small bowel is generally accepted as the predominant site of invasion. The septicemia is cleared by the reticuloendothelial organs, where the bacteria multiply to large numbers, primarily inside cells. Local inflammation is thus produced in lymph nodes, liver and spleen, from which sites the bacteria re-enter the blood stream. This secondary septicemia is usually prolonged and seeds many organs. The gallbladder appears to be particularly susceptible and is infected from the liver via the biliary system or from the blood. Local multiplication in the wall of the gallbladder produces large numbers of organisms which are discharged into the small intestine, which is then extensively reinfected.

PATHOLOGY. The morphologic changes are less striking in younger children but increase with age. The mesenteric lymph nodes, liver and spleen are hyperemic and usually have areas of focal necrosis, but hyperplasia of reticuloendothelial tissue with proliferation of mononuclear cells is the predominant finding. The hepatic cells may show cloudy swelling. The mucosa and lymphatic tissue of the intestinal tract show marked inflammation and necrosis. Ulceration, which heals without scarring, is common. Blood vessels may be interrupted, resulting in hemorrhage. Uncommonly the inflammatory lesion penetrates the muscularis and serosa to produce intestinal perforation. The bone marrow reflects the mononuclear response and may contain areas of focal necrosis. Inflammation of the gallbladder is inconstant, focal and markedly out of proportion to the extent of local bacterial multiplication. Bronchitis is common. Microscopically the so-called *rose spot* consists of focal congestion and infiltration with mononuclear cells and bacteria. Acute inflammation is observed in the uncommon local abscesses, pneumonia, pyelonephritis, osteomyelitis, arthritis and meningitis. Bacteria may be observed in all involved organs.

CLINICAL MANIFESTATIONS. Typhoid fever in infants has a much more variable presentation than it does in adults. The clinical picture may be that of mild gastroenteritis or of severe, undefined bacterial sepsis. Vomiting, abdominal distention and diarrhea are common. The temperature is irregular but high and may provoke seizures. Hepatosplenomegaly, jaundice, anorexia and weight loss may be marked.

In older children, an incubation period of 10 to 20 days (range 5 to 40 days) is followed by an irregular fever, headache, malaise, lethargy, myalgia and abdominal pain and tenderness. Diarrhea occurs in one half of infected children at this stage; constipation is less common. Cough is a common symptom, but the chest is clear to examination. Epistaxis may occur. In less than a week the fever rises and becomes less variable; fatigue, cough, abdominal pain, diarrhea, anorexia and weight loss increase and may be marked. The patient may become severely obtunded. Mental depression is common, and delirium and stupor may be observed. The child now appears acutely ill, depressed and often disoriented. There is usually an enlarged spleen, abdominal tenderness—often right-sided with associated rebound tenderness—abdominal distention, and rhonchi and scattered rales on auscultation of the lungs. The maculopapular rash, observed in up to 80 per cent of patients, is erythematous and occurs in the skin of the lower chest and abdomen in successive crops of 10 to 20 lesions that are 2 to 5 mm in diameter and that last 2 to 3 days. The disproportion between temperature (high) and pulse rate (low) is not so common as in adults. For those without complications the symptoms and physical findings resolve simultaneously within 2 to 4 weeks, but convalescence may require an equal interval.

COMPLICATIONS. Severe *intestinal hemorrhage* and/or *perforation* are the most common complications and occur in up to half of 1 per cent of children with typhoid fever. Both complications occur during the second stage of the disease; they are generally preceded by a drop in temperature and blood pressure and an increase in pulse rate. Perforation rarely occurs without preceding hemorrhage; it usually occurs in the lower ileum and is attended by markedly increased abdominal pain, tenderness, vomiting and signs of peritonitis. *Cerebral thrombi* and *toxic encephalopathy* may occur, but neurologic sequelae are rare; chorea and peripheral and optic neuritis have been reported. Gallbladder infection is usually asymptomatic, but acute typhoid cholecystitis is observed. Thrombosis and phlebitis occur occasionally. *Pneumonia* is common during the second stage of the illness, but it is often a superinfection produced by other bacteria. Metastatic abscesses may involve any organ. Endocarditis, pyelonephritis, meningitis and infection of bones and joints occur rarely.

LABORATORY FINDINGS. Patients with typhoid fever develop a normochromic, normocytic anemia as a result of intestinal blood loss and toxic inhibition of the bone marrow. The classic leukopenia is only relative; peripheral leucokyte counts are unexpectedly low for the patient's fever and toxicity but seldom lower than $3000/mm^3$. Thrombocytopenia may be striking and last several days. Disturbances of coagulation have not been critically evaluated. Proteinuria, caused by the fever, and melena are common.

DIAGNOSIS. Microscopic examination of the stool shows abundant leukocytes, more than 90 per cent of which are mononuclear. Bacteriologic cultures provide the diagnosis, but identification of *S. typhi* in most laboratories requires 3 to 5 days. Culture specimens planted on enriched media and examined with fluorescein-labeled antibody to Vi antigen may provide specific, rapid identification. The frequency with which *S. typhi* is found in the blood, stool and urine correlates well with the pathogenesis of the disease. Thus, blood cultures are most often positive early in the disease, whereas urine and stool cultures become positive following the secondary septicemia (Fig. 10–4). Up to 40 per cent of throat cultures are positive during the initial stage of the disease. Cultures of bone marrow and involved lymph nodes or other phagocytic tissues often remain positive after the blood has been sterilized. Aspirates of the skin rash are

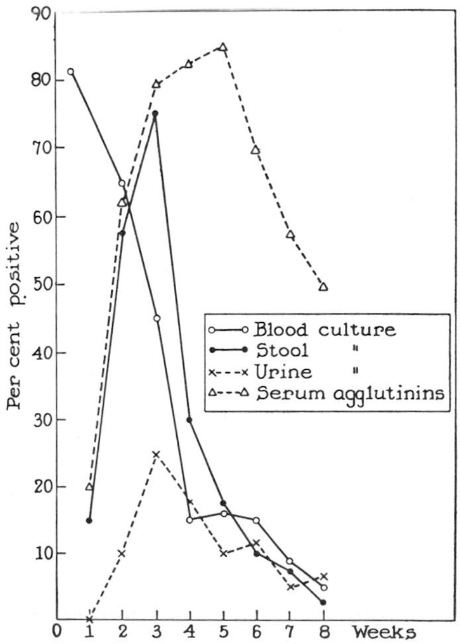

Figure 10–4 *Results of bacteriologic cultures and serum agglutinin titers during the course of typhoid fever. (From Morgan, H. R.: In Dubos, R. J., and Hirsch, J. G. (eds.): Bacterial and Mycotic Infections of Man. Philadelphia, J. B. Lippincott Company, 1965.*

positive in up to 50 per cent of patients. Stool and urine of suspected chronic carriers should be cultured; blood and bone marrow cultures are not positive. Enteric carriers usually excrete 10^6 to 10^9 *S. typhi* per gram of stool; in suspected cases with negative stool cultures, culture of aspirated duodenal fluid to evaluate biliary infection may be useful.

The interpretation of serologic results can be complicated; the agglutination test, as performed in most diagnostic laboratories, is not standardized; the O and H antigens of *S. typhi* are not unique to that serotype or even to salmonellae; chloramphenicol therapy may depress an antibody response, while titers, particularly H agglutinins, may be high as a result of prior typhoid immunization. Nonspecific agglutination is often observed in the serum of patients with underlying disease accompanied by macroglobulinemia. A fourfold rise in agglutinins of a nonimmunized individual usually is diagnostic when performed in the same laboratory. A rise in O agglutinins in an individual immunized more than 6 months earlier is suggestive of infection; H agglutinin titers are valueless in a previously immunized individual. In a nonimmunized child who has lived in nonendemic areas, single titers of 1:50 for H and 1:100 for O agglutinins during the first week of symptoms provide suggestive evidence of typhoid fever. Titers of Vi agglutinins of 1:5 or greater usually identify a chronic carrier in nonendemic populations.

Differential Diagnosis. During the initial stage, the patient with typhoid fever may be diagnosed as having influenza, bronchitis, bronchopneumonia or gastroenteritis. Later, tuberculosis, brucellosis, rickettsial diseases (including Rocky Mountain spotted fever), shigellosis and, when epidemiologically applicable, malaria and typhus must be differentiated. Sepsis of unknown etiology, particularly that caused by enteric bacilli, leukemia, lymphoma and Hodgkin's disease, may be suspected. Concern about acute surgical diseases of the abdomen may lead to unnecessary operative procedures. Herpes labialis is so rare in typhoid fever that its presence suggests another diagnosis.

PROGNOSIS AND TREATMENT. The prognosis in typhoid fever depends on the age of the patient, the previous state of health and the severity of complications. Of those not treated with antibiotics, at least 10 per cent of infants and a smaller percentage of older children succumb. Chloramphenicol therapy has reduced the mortality rate to less than 1 per cent in most institutions. Debilitation and underlying disease, as well as perforation and severe hemorrhage, increase the chance of death. Meningitis is nearly always fatal; the prognosis of endocarditis is grave.

Relapses occur in up to 10 per cent of those not treated with antibiotics, but in twice that percentage of those who receive chloramphenicol. The clinical manifestations generally become apparent about two weeks after defervescence or the cessation of antibiotic therapy; they resemble those of the acute illness but are generally milder and more abbreviated. Multiple relapses may occur.

Individuals excreting *S. typhi* 3 months after infection usually are excretors at one year and often for life. The risk of chronic carriage (longer than 1 year) involves few children but increases with age; up to 5 per cent of acutely infected adults become chronic carriers, who generally have chronic gallbladder infections and excrete the organisms in their stool. Chronic urinary carriage occurs but is rare except in individuals with schistosomiasis.

Maintenance of proper nutrition and of fluid and electrolyte balance are important, particularly for infants. Shock often accompanies intestinal perforation and severe hemorrhage, and requires expansion of intravascular volume. Transfusions may be required to correct anemia.

Chloramphenicol remains the preferred antibiotic for the therapy of typhoid fever. It can be given orally, but intravenous administration is preferable, especially when the patient is acutely ill, has significant diarrhea or has a complication. Daily doses of 50–100 mg/kg/day are given to children and 25 mg/kg/day to infants, divided at 6-hour intervals. Although the patient may feel improved after 1 or 2 days of therapy, objective evidence of that improvement may not be realized for 3 to 5 days. Most children will be afebrile within 7 days of beginning therapy, but treatment of uncomplicated cases should be continued at least 10 to 14 days, or for 5 to 7 days following defervescence. Complications, including hemorrhage and perforation, have been observed during therapy. Treatment with chloramphenicol increases the chance of relapse and does not prevent the development of chronic carriage.

Ampicillin therapy results in a slower clinical response and more treatment failures than treatment with chloramphenicol. However, patients who have a favorable response to ampicillin are less likely to have relapses or to become chronic carriers than those treated with chloramphenicol. Ampicillin should be given at 100–200 mg/kg/day divided at 6-hour intervals. Systemic administration is often preferable, as with chloramphenicol. *Salmonella typhi* have rarely been resistant to chloramphenicol or ampicillin in the past. Chloramphenicol-resistant strains have recently caused local outbreaks outside the United States and epidemics in Southeast Asia and Mexico. Such strains have been isolated from individuals returning to the United States from these areas, and from their local contacts. Most chloramphenicol-resistant strains are susceptible to ampicillin, and patients infected with them have responded to ampicillin therapy. Although *S. typhi* is often susceptible to other antibiotics in vitro e.g., penicillin, cephalosporins, aminoglycosides, furazolidone and nalidixic acid, none of these are effective in treatment of the disease.

Corticosteroid therapy is indicated for individuals with severe toxemia or prolonged symptoms despite appropriate antibiotic therapy. Corticosteroids do not increase the incidence of complications, provided antibiotic therapy is adequate. Thrombocytopenia may be severe enough to play a role in intestinal hemorrhage and to require platelet transfusions, particularly if surgery is required. Since most patients with intestinal hemorrhage or perforation respond to antibiotics and medical management, surgery is rarely required. Furthermore, the mortality rate associated with the surgery of these complications is very high.

Up to 80 per cent of carriers with chronic gallbladder infection can be cured by cholecystectomy, even without antibiotic therapy. High-dose ampicillin therapy for 4 to 6 weeks has cured the majority of carriers, including some with cholelithiasis.

IMMUNITY. Immunity to typhoid fever is only relative; reinfection may occur in 20 to 25 per cent of adults infected naturally or experimentally. Typhoid infection stimulates host resistance by inducing in the reticuloendothelial system a temporary nonspecific increase in phagocytic activity, as well as a longer lasting enhancement of specific bactericidal activity in the form of type-specific antibodies. Antibodies to O antigens are primarily of the IgM class, whereas those to H antigens are primarily of the IgG class. In the presence of complement, antibodies directed to O and Vi antigens are bactericidal for homologous strains in vitro, but not in vivo; such immune globulins do enhance the host's immunity, however, by slowing extracellular bacterial multiplication and by promoting opsonization. That antibody is only one factor in the host's resistance to typhoid is evidenced by the observation that susceptibility to initial or subsequent attacks does not correlate with titers of antibodies to O, H or Vi antigens. Little is known of the role in typhoid fever of specific local antibody or of cellular factors in the intestinal tract. Promising preliminary studies with attenuated oral typhoid vaccines suggest that local antibody activity may have importance in the host response to salmonellae.

Vaccines for typhoid fever have been available since 1898, but their use has not been enthusiastically recommended in the past, primarily because efficacy had not been adequately proved. Recent controlled studies conducted under the auspices of the World Health Organization have documented a reduction of up to 94 per cent in symptomatic, culture-proved disease for 2 to 3 years following single inoculations. Efficacy of up to 73 per cent was observed during the third to seventh years after immunization. These studies were conducted in endemic areas and, therefore, the vaccine's effectiveness may have been due, at least in part, to an enhancement of resistance acquired from subclinical infection(s). Immunization reduced significantly the attack rate among susceptible adult volunteers who were challenged with an oral dose of typhoid bacilli that caused disease in 25 per cent of nonimmunized individuals (ID_{25}); it did not affect attack rates among individuals challenged with ID_{50} doses. Thus, if comparison of the field and volunteer studies is valid, immunization probably reduces disease among individuals exposed to a dose of bacteria that produces disease in only a minority of susceptible individuals.

The indications for use of typhoid vaccine in the United States are: (1) intimate exposure to a known household carrier, (2) outbreak of typhoid fever in the community or an institution, and (3) travel to an endemic area. Attendance at summer camp and flood conditions are not accepted as specific indications. A dose of 0.5 ml administered subcutaneously is recommended for both primary and booster immunization of individuals over 10 years old, and 0.25 ml for those under that age. Febrile and local reactions are common, and prophylactic antipyretics in young children may be indicated. An intradermal dose of 0.1 ml may produce equal immunogenicity and fewer side reactions than the larger subcutaneous dose and therefore may be used as a booster injection. Unacceptable reactions occur with the intradermal administration of acetone-extracted vaccine.

CONTROL OF SALMONELLA INFECTIONS

The urine and feces of hospitalized patients should be handled with extreme precaution until three consecutive stool cultures are negative. Strict handwashing, personal hygiene and sanitary practices must be maintained by personnel involved in food preparation and patient care to minimize person-to-person and person-to-food transmission.

Every effort should be made to eradicate *S. typhi* from excreting individuals. When these efforts are unsuccessful, such individuals must be kept under strict surveillance by health departments and kept from working in food- and water-processing plants, kitchens and patient care. The prevalence of asymptomatic human infection, contaminated foodstuffs and other potential sources of infection makes quarantine of nonhospitalized individuals excreting other types of salmonellae impractical and of little meaning. Such individuals, if known, should be instructed regarding their potential contagiousness and the importance of handwashing and personal hygiene. Particular attention should be given food handlers. As mentioned previously, antibiotic therapy of exposed individuals is contraindicated; prophylactic ingestion of nonspecific antimicrobial agents, e.g., oxyquinolines, does not prevent infection.

Proper attention to potential cross-contamination of foodstuffs and proper cooking temperatures and the avoidance of holding potentially infected foods at warming temperatures are important control measures that should be practiced in kitchens. A requirement that pets be proved salmonella-free before sale would eliminate a real but unnecessary problem.

Control of typhoid fever in endemic areas can be accomplished only with improved housing and sanitation, and the availability of pure water. Large scale immunization programs will reduce, but not eliminate, the disease. International travel to endemic areas and the inability to prevent all transmission by chronic carriers rule out the eradication of typhoid fever from developed countries. The problem of human nontyphoidal salmonellosis in the United States would be markedly reduced by the eradication of the animal reservoir and improvement in the technology of food production. While feasible, these goals do not seem attainable in the immediate future.

Aserkoff, B., and Bennett, J. V.: Effect of therapy in acute salmonellosis on salmonellae in feces. New Engl. J. Med. *281*:636, 1969.

Aserkoff, B., Shroeder, S. A., and Brachman, D. S.: Salmonellosis in the United States—A five year review. Am. J. Epidem. *92*:13, 1970.

Cherry, W. B., and Thomason, B. M.: Fluorescent antibody techniques for salmonella and other enteric pathogens. Pub. Hlth. Rep. *84*:887, 1969.

Cherubin, C. E., Fodor, T., Denmark, L. I., Master, C. S., Fuerst, H. T., and Winter, J. W.: Symptoms, septicemia and death in salmonellosis. Am. J. Epidem. *90*:285, 1969.

Cvjetanovic, B., and Uemura, K.: The present status of field and laboratory studies of typhoid and paratyphoid vaccines. Bull. WHO *32*:29, 1965.

Giannella, R. A., Formal, S. B., Dammin, G. J., and Collins, H.: Pathogenesis of salmonellosis. J. Clin. Invest. *52*:441, 1973.

Harris, J. C., DuPont, H. L., and Hornick, R. B.: Fecal leucocytes in diarrheal illness. Ann. Intern. Med. *76*:697, 1972.

Hook, E. W.: Salmonellosis: Certain factors influencing interaction of salmonella and human host. Bull. N.Y. Acad. Med. *37*:499, 1961.

Hornick, R. B., Greisman, S. E., Woodward, T. E., Dupont, H. L., Dawkins, A. T., and Snyder, M. J.: Typhoid fever: Pathogenesis and immunologic control. New Engl. J. Med. *283*:686; 739, 1970.

Overtuf, G., Marton, K. I., and Mathies, A. W.: Antibiotic resistance in typhoid fever. New Engl. J. Med. *289*:463, 1973.

Robertson, R. P., Wahab, M. F. A., and Raasch, F. O.: Evaluation of chloramphenicol and ampicillin in salmonella enteric fever. New Engl. J. Med. *278*:171, 1968.

Rosenstein, B. J.: Salmonellosis in infants and children. Epidemiologic and therapeutic considerations. J. Pediatr. *70*:1, 1967.

Saphra, I., and Winter, J. W.: Clinical manifestations of salmonellosis in man; Evaluation of 7779 human infections identified at the New York Salmonella Center. New. Engl. J. Med. *256*:1128, 1957.

Wilder, A. N., and MacCready, R. A.: Isolation of salmonella from poultry. New Engl. J. Med. *274*:1453, 1966.

Woodward, T. E., and Smadel, J. E.: Management of typhoid fever and its complications. Ann. Intern. Med. *60*:144, 1964.

SHIGELLOSIS
(Bacillary Dysentery)

Shigellosis is an acute inflammatory disease of the colon that is produced by bacteria of the genus *Shigella* and is characterized by fever, general toxicity, crampy abdominal pain and frequent loose stools which generally contain mucus, pus and blood. The term shigellosis is preferable to that of bacillary dysentery, since bacteria of other genera may produce the same pathology and symptoms.

HISTORY. During his investigation of an epidemic of dysentery in Japan in 1896, Shiga isolated several distinguishable bacilli from the stools and intestinal wall of involved patients. One of these bacteria was agglutinated by the sera of convalescent, but not of healthy, individuals. The concentration of this organism in their feces correlated with the patients' symptoms, and it was not found in the feces of healthy individuals. Although this bacterium did not produce dysentery in animals, Shiga concluded that the organism caused the human disease. Similar observations were made in the Philippines by Flexner (1900) and in Germany by Kruze (1900).

ETIOLOGY. Shigella organisms are gram-negative, nonmotile, facultative anaerobic bacilli which ferment lactose very slowly, if at all. They are distinguished from other enterobacteria primarily by biochemical properties; most of the antigenic determinants of *Shigella* are unique, but some are shared with other enteric bacilli. *Shigella* are divided into four groups, in part by biochemical reactions, but more specifically by antigenic composition; the serotypes are designated by Arabic numerals. The *dysenteriae* species contains 10 subtypes, of which Shiga's bacillus is type 1; *flexneri* contains six types, some of which are further divided into an "a" and a "b" series; *boydii* contains 15 types, while *sonnei* is homogeneous. Susceptibility to bacteriophages or the capacity to produce a given colicin, an extrabacterial product lethal for certain other bacteria, can distinguish individual members of a group or serotype. Typing by these methods has been particularly useful in epidemiologic studies of disease caused by the serologically homogeneous *S. sonnei. Shigella* are not remarkably hardy bacteria, but under optimal conditions they may persist in nature for some time. At 65 to 70° F shigellae may survive up to 46 days when dried on linen and up to 12 days in soil. They may survive for days and even multiply in milk and certain foods, and they have been recovered from fresh and salt water naturally infected a few days earlier. Shigellae are killed by heating at 55° C for one hour, and by commonly used disinfectants. They are quite sensitive to a combination of low pH, volatile acids and anaerobiosis. Thus, they lose viability in a few hours in feces in which the bacteria are metabolically active, but if the feces are buffered, shigellae may remain viable for days.

PATHOGENESIS. Shigellae naturally produce dysentery in primates, but not other animals. Alterations of intestinal flora, motility or nutrition affect susceptibility. Thus, experimental disease can be produced in germ-free or starved animals, or those treated with agents such as carbon tetrachloride or oral antibiotics. The virulence of many bacteria correlates with the presence of a capsule; increased reactivity with antiserum to O antigens (cell wall) following heating of suspensions of shigellae is cited as evidence that they may have a heat sensitive capsule exterior to the cell wall; this thesis remains unproved. The cell wall of shigellae, like that of other gram-negative bacilli, is a lipopolysaccharide (endotoxin), but the role of this substance in the pathogenicity of shigellae remains undefined. *Shigella dysenteriae,* type 1 (Shiga's bacillus), produces an exotoxin whose neurotoxic properties were described by early investigators. Recent studies have indicated that this toxin is a protein with a molecular weight of 50,000 and that it is also a potent enterotoxin, producing dramatic loss of fluid in isolated ileal loops of rabbits. It also kills epithelial cells grown in tissue culture. The role of this toxin in humans is still being studied, but clinical observations indicate that among all shigellae, *S. dysenteriae,* type 1, produces the most severe disease, and that patients recovering from disease produced by such strains have antitoxin in their serum. The ability to penetrate intestinal epithelium correlates best with the pathogenicity of shigellae. This property, in turn, correlates with the ability of the organisms to multiply in tissue cultures of the epithelial HeLa cells, and to penetrate the conjunctival epithelium of guinea pigs, producing keratoconjunctivitis (the *Serény test*). The chemical composition of certain cell wall antigens appears to correlate with the capacity of shigellae to penetrate epithelial cells.

EPIDEMIOLOGY. Shigellae have a world-wide distribution; their prevalence is affected most by climate, living conditions and the predominant serotypes. Although reported cases constitute only a fraction of the actual total, the prevalence of shigellosis in the United States appears to have remained relatively constant over the past decade. More than 99 per cent of the isolates come from humans, most of whom reside in urban areas. Children under 9 years of age account for about 60 per cent of clinical cases, with more than one third occurring in those between 1 and 4 years of age. The peak incidence is in the late summer. Until 1966, in the United States, disease caused by *S. flexneri* was most prevalent, but at present *S. sonnei* causes about 60 per cent of cases and *S. flexneri* the bulk of the remainder; *S. boydii* and *S. dysenteriae* cause less than 2 per cent of the total, and most of these cases are acquired outside the United States, where the six serotypes most commonly isolated cause more than 90 per cent of the cases. For unexplained reasons, *S. sonnei* predominates in the northern United States, whereas *S. flexneri* is most prevalent in the southern states.

Since there is essentially no animal reservoir, shigellae are acquired directly or indirectly from infected individuals. The potential for interpersonal infection is considerable: ingestion of as few as 200 *S. flexneri,* type 2a, produces shigellosis in healthy adult volunteers, and concentrations of at least 10^8 shigellae per gram of feces are excreted during the period of acute symptoms. Lower concentrations are excreted during convalescence and by the uncommon chronic carrier. Direct contamination of hands with feces of infected individuals is a common route by which children are infected. Shigellae can be isolated from the seats and bases of toilets used by infected individuals; considerable contamination by air and droplets may occur during the flushing of infected feces. Spread via toys, inanimate objects and food contaminated by an infected individual also occurs. Despite the potential major common source, food- or water-borne outbreaks are relatively uncommon in the United States. Shigellae can be passively transferred by flies, but active multiplication in the insect does not occur. The role of this vector obviously relates to local practices of hygiene and sanitation. Most epidemiologic studies indicate, however, that flies are less important than the lack of water for washing in the transmission of shigellosis in areas with primitive sanitation.

In hospitals, the most important factor in spread of shigellosis is inadequate handwashing following contact with contaminated patients or bedclothes, combined with failure to give meticulous attention to isolation precautions in general.

Although most of the disease is endemic, considerable epidemics of shigellosis occur. High attack rates are characteristic of institutions with poor hygiene. Indeed, "asylum dysentery" has been well known for generations, and the role of dysentery in military campaigns is legendary. Currently the incidence of shigellosis among residents of mental institutions and American Indians on reservations is estimated to be 200 and 10 to 15 times greater, respectively, than that of the general population in the United States. A pandemic caused by a single strain of *S. dysenteriae,* type 1, has ravaged Central America since December 1968, involving several thousand individuals.

HOST RESISTANCE. Shigellae must traverse the barriers imposed by gastric acidity, proteolytic enzymes, certain antibacterial substances and intestinal motility before their potential for infection of the colon can be realized. Evidence from studies of clinical cases and experimental models indicates that the bacteria normally resident in the intestine adversely affect colonization by shigellae. Replication of shigellae in vitro is inhibited by the decreased pH, volatile acids and anaerobiosis produced by enteric bacilli found in the intestine, but further studies are needed to define the role of these factors in vivo. Although susceptibility to shigellosis is markedly increased among animals deprived of folic acid or starved, and the incidence of disease is greatest among populations with poor diets, the effect of nutrition on human resistance to shigellae has attracted little study. Reinfection with homologous strains occurs not uncommonly, and host resistance does not correlate with serum antibody concentrations. Despite these observations, individuals resident in endemic areas appear to have a lower incidence of shigellosis than travelers to the area but, even so, shigellosis is a rare cause of "traveler's diarrhea." The role of local (copro-) antibody and circulating antitoxin in host resistance is currently being evaluated. The factors involved in the rather remarkable capacity of the host to eliminate shigellae spontaneously also remain to be defined.

PATHOLOGY. The colon, and occasionally the terminal ileum, is involved. The organisms multiply in and penetrate the epithelium; further multiplication occurs in the submucosa and lamina propria, but spread to regional lymph nodes is uncommon and invasion of the blood stream occurs very rarely. The bacterial multiplication produces local inflammation, with edema, hyperemia and disruption of epithelial cell function, such as secretion of mucus. The cellular infiltrate is predominantly polymorphonuclear. Small abscesses form, coalesce and ulcerate into the intestinal lumen, discharging pus, pooled mucus and blood from disrupted vessels. Because of their superficial location, the ulcers do not perforate into the peritoneal cavity. A shaggy, fibrinosuppurative exudate containing polymorphonuclear leukocytes usually covers the mucosa. The local and mesenteric lymphoid tissue hypertrophies. Lesions generally begin to heal spontaneously and without scarring within 4 to 7 days.

CLINICAL MANIFESTATIONS. The onset of symptoms is variable but usually occurs between 24 and 72 hours after ingestion of shigella organisms. Initially, fever and crampy abdominal pain predominate; vomiting is rare. The body temperature may be as high as 105° F, and the patient may be toxic and appear septic. Convulsions occur in approximately 10 per cent of reported cases and are often associated with temperatures greater than 103° F, but they may occur in children with slight or no elevation of temperature. Only a minority of children who convulse with shigellosis have a preceding history of seizures. Headache is common, and nuchal rigidity and delirium are not rare. Subsequent symptoms are consistent with the intestinal pathology. Diarrhea generally starts 12 to 48 hours after onset and is usually watery, with mucus, pus and, occasionally, erythrocytes. A child may have 10 to 20 stools per day and develop significant dehydration, acidosis and electrolyte imbalance. Characteristically, abdominal cramps precede and tenesmus and straining follow each diarrheal stool. Rectal prolapse may occur in severely afflicted children, particularly among those who are malnourished at onset of the dysentery. Some individuals do not manifest constitutional symptoms or those of classic dysentery, but have only mild diarrhea without mucus or pus; a significant per cent of those infected remain asymptomatic. Culture-proved conjunctivitis may occur, probably resulting from local inoculation with contaminated fingers; corneal ulceration and iritis are rare complications.

Coryza, cough and radiologically proved pneumonia may occur in as many as one quarter of hospitalized children. Shigellae are not isolated from the respiratory tract of such patients, leaving the etiology of such symptoms undefined. Arthritis associated with shigellosis is uncommon in children. It usually consists of sterile effusions in weight-bearing joints, which characteristically are neither hot nor red. Since the joint manifestations often develop two to four weeks after the intestinal symptoms and may require months to resolve, their pathophysiology remains obscure. A few patients with shigellosis have manifested the symptom complex of *Reiter syndrome* during convalescence. Mild, localized and transient peripheral neuropathy may be associated with *S. dysenteriae* infections. Skin manifestations are rare. Metastatic suppurative lesions are very rare.

Symptoms generally subside spontaneously within 5 to 10 days, and the feces are usually clear of detectable shigellae by seven to 14 days. Less than 10 per cent of persons infected have positive cultures 3 months after the onset of symptoms, and no more than 3 per cent excrete shigellae for longer intervals. Intermittency of excretion by convalescents and carriers may be observed; *S. dysenteriae* predominates as the cause of such persistent infections. The chronic carrier may be asymptomatic or have episodes of diarrhea and abdominal pain; the latter pattern is more common with *S. dysenteriae* infections. Chronic disease, particularly in previously debilitated individuals, may be associated with weight loss, feeding disturbances, secondary anemia and nutritional deficiencies. There is no evidence that shigellosis plays a role in the etiology of ulcerative colitis.

DIAGNOSIS. The stool in shigellosis characteristically contains mucus and polymorphonuclear leukocytes; erythrocytes may also be present. The finding of acute inflammatory cells distinguishes bacillary dysentery, including shigellosis, from bowel disorders other than ulcerative colitis. Examination of a fleck of mucus obtained from a freshly passed stool and stained with methylene blue gives optimal results; specimens collected by rectal swab are less satisfactory. There are no characteristic hematologic findings. Many children, particularly those with convulsions, have a modest leukocytosis; leukopenia is seen in approximately 20 per cent of children. Thrombocytopenia, anemia and disturbances in coagulation are rare. The spinal fluid is sterile; it may contain a few cells, but a total count of greater than 100 cells per mm^3 and any significant number of leukocytes are unusual.

Less than 0.5 per cent of blood cultures of hospitalized children are positive; positive urine cultures are even more uncommon. Prompt inoculation of stool onto bacteriologic media and the selection for culture of a specimen containing blood-tinged mucus (which contains the highest concentration of shigellae) significantly increase the recovery of shigellae. Exact bacteriologic diagnosis rests on patterns of biochemical activities and of agglutination with standard sera of lactose-negative isolates identified on selective media. Xylose-lysine deoxycholate appears to be the best single selective medium for shigellae; SS medium may give slightly higher yields with *S. flexneri* strains but significantly poorer yields with *S. sonnei* strains. Most enriched broths have been formulated primarily to increase the recovery of salmonellae and are used by default for shigellae. Shigellae may remain viable for days in buffered glycerol saline, but the yield from this and other transport or enriched media is significantly lower than from inoculation of fresh specimens onto selective media. Shigellae can be identified in smears of stool by fluorescein-labeled, type-specific antisera, but such sera are not readily available and the technique is not commonly employed. Circulating type-specific antibodies often develop in individuals with severe disease but not in those with milder symptoms; serologic methods are therefore rarely used in the confirmation of shigellosis.

Differential Diagnosis. Shigellosis may not be

considered prior to the onset of diarrhea. However, it should be included in the differential diagnosis of any child who has an acute, febrile illness with toxicity and a seizure. Prior to the onset of diarrhea, appropriate laboratory tests may be needed to distinguish *meningitis, encephalitis, bacterial sepsis, pneumonia* and *urinary tract infection.* The absence of vomiting and of the characteristic findings on abdominal and rectal examination differentiates shigellosis from *appendicitis.* Children with a *Meckel's diverticulum* or *anaphylactoid purpura* may have abdominal pain and blood in their stools, but the former are not toxic and the latter generally have other manifestations, such as rash, arthralgia, arthritis or hematuria. The lack of a local abdominal mass, vomiting and the character of the stool rule against an *intussusception.* Children with toxin-induced gastroenteritis have less general toxicity and fever. The child with *salmonellosis* or *viral gastroenteritis* usually has more vomiting and less constitutional and large bowel symptoms than one with shigellosis. The acuteness of the symptoms and the clinical course usually distinguish shigellosis from *ulcerative colitis* and *granulomatous bowel* disorders. The epidemiology, the undetermined nature of the colonic ulcers and the clinical course help to distinguish *amebic dysentery;* identification of amebae in fecal specimens provides the diagnosis. Shigellosis cannot be distinguished clinically from dysentery produced by other bacteria such as certain *E. coli* and salmonellae.

PREVENTION. Prevention of shigellosis requires interruption of the "fingers, food and flies" transmission of the organisms. On a community basis water that is safe and readily available, appropriate sewage disposal and insect control are required. Rigid handwashing practices are the most important aspect of the prevention of individual cases. Children should be managed with special precautions when hospitalized. The frequency of asymptomatic infections makes it necessary to culture all patients and personnel associated with an institutional outbreak. In such situations, a program of mass antibacterial therapy may also be indicated.

Since susceptibility does not correlate with serum antibody concentrations, the failure of early attempts at immunization, using homogenates of virulent bacteria as a systemically administered vaccine, is not surprising. Orally administered, attenuated strains are currently being evaluated as vaccines. The most promising are streptomycin-dependent bacteria which cannot multiply in the absence of the drug, and a hybrid organism prepared from a genetic cross of *E. coli* and a strain of shigella that cannot multiply in epithelial cells. Titers of coproantibody are stimulated, and protection rates of up to 90 per cent have been observed in studies of military recruits and children. Reversion of the mutant bacteria to virulence may be a problem, and optimal results require several ingestions of high concentrations of bacteria, preceded by an antacid preparation. Since immunity develops only to homologous strains, a multivalent vaccine will be required to provide protection against even the limited number of strains causing disease in the United States. The possibility of antigenic drift of endemic strains following use of such vaccines remains a potential but unrealized problem. Future studies should indicate the value of such vaccines in high-risk environments.

PROGNOSIS. Dehydration and convulsions are the most common cause of hospitalization. Mortality is greater in infants, but is usually less than 1 per cent in developed countries. Infection of malnourished children or that caused by *S. dysenteriae* carries a poorer prognosis.

TREATMENT. Unlike the situation with salmonella gastroenteritis, antibiotic therapy eradicates shigellae and significantly reduces the duration of symptoms. The studies of Nelson and his collaborators clearly indicate that successful therapy can be obtained only with antibiotics which produce significant tissue concentrations. Nonabsorbed agents such as nitrofurantoin (Furadantin), kanamycin and neomycin are no more effective than a placebo, even though the causative isolate may be sensitive to these drugs by in vitro tests. Sulfonamides were formerly the preferred therapy, but these agents cannot now be generally recommended because of the high prevalence of resistance to them. The situation is generally similar for the tetracyclines. Ampicillin produces excellent results with strains of shigellae sensitive to it and has been the recent choice for therapy. A daily dose of 50 mg/kg, given in divided doses at 6-hour intervals, produces the same bacteriologic cure rates and clinical responses as 100 mg/kg; the response is less prompt with the lower dose, but overgrowth of Candida species occurs more commonly with the higher dose. Parenteral administration is preferable when the child is very ill or unable to take oral medication. Unfortunately, resistance to ampicillin has increased in the United States since 1972 to a point where it is moderately prevalent; in some areas, 50 to 90 per cent of isolates are resistant. Ampicillin is therefore recommended with reservations. Chloramphenicol remains a successful alternative, but its use for outpatient therapy of shigellosis (or other infections) can rarely be recommended because of its potential lethal toxicity. Thus, the need for, and the choice of, antibiotic therapy for shigellosis must be more selective than previously considered. The duration of symptoms and intestinal excretion are usually short enough that many outpatients are well before they are seen by physicians and their disease confirmed in the laboratory. The decision to treat hospitalized children and outpatients with more prolonged symptoms must be made on the basis of the clinical situation, laboratory evaluation of antibiotic sensitivities and regional experience.

The strain of *S. dysenteriae,* type 1, which is pandemic in Central America, is resistant to all sulfonamides and tetracyclines, streptomycin and chloramphenicol. Thus, an epidemiologic history may provide early insight into the optimal therapy for shigellosis acquired outside the United States.

The basis for the antibiotic resistance of shigellae is the extrachromosomal genetic elements, the *R (resistance) factors*. These elements were first appreciated in multiply resistant shigellae isolated in Japan in 1958. R factors are autonomous units of double standard DNA that are potentially transferable to all gram-negative bacilli by conjugation or transduction. They may mediate resistance to one or more antibiotics, but multiple resistance is more common. R factor-mediated resistances include those to ampicillin, cephalosporins, chloramphenicol, gentamicin, kanamycin, neomycin, paromomycin, spectinomycin, sulfonamides, streptomycin and tetracyclines. Many of the resistances are mediated by drug-inactivating enzymes. Recent studies indicate that R factors are the most common basis for clinically important antibiotic resistances in these bacteria.

DAVID H. SMITH

Barrett-Connor, E., and Connor, J. D.: Extraintestinal manifestations of shigellosis. Am. J. Gastroent. *53*:234, 1970.
Grady, G. F., and Keusch, G. T.: Pathogenesis of bacterial diarrheas. New Engl. J. Med. *285*:831, 891, 1971.
Haltalin, K. C., Nelson, J. D., Hinton, L. V., Kusmiesz, H. T., and Sladjoe, M.: Comparison of orally absorbable and nonabsorbable antibiotics in shigellosis: A double-blind study with ampicillin and neomycin. J. Pediatr. *72*:708, 1968.
Haltalin, K. C., Nelson, J. D., Kusmiesz, H. T., and Hinton, L. V.: Optimal dosage of ampicillin for shigellosis. J. Pediatr. *74*:626, 1969.
Mel, D., Gangarosa, E. J., Radovanovic, M. L., Arsic, B. L., and Litvinjenko, S.: Studies on vaccination against bacillary dysentery. 6. Protection of children by oral immunization with streptomycin-dependent Shigella strains.Bull. WHO *45*:457, 1971.
Morris, G. K., Koehler, J. A., Gangarosa, E. J., and Sharrar, R. G.: Comparison of media for direct isolation and transport of shigellae from fecal specimens. Appl. Microbiol. *19*:434, 1970.
Reller, L. B., Gangarosa, E. J., and Brachman, P. S.: Shigellosis in the United States: 5 year review of nationwide surveillance, 1964–1968. Am. J. Epidem. *91*:161, 1970.
Weissman, J. B., Gangarosa, E. J., and DuPont, H. L.: Changing needs in the antimicrobial therapy of shigellosis. J. Infect. Dis. *127*:611, 1972.

CHOLERA

Cholera is a severe diarrheal disease which usually occurs in epidemics among crowded and poorly nourished populations; the case fatality rate is high among untreated patients.

ETIOLOGY. *Vibrio cholerae* is a small, highly motile, comma-shaped, polymorphic gram-negative organism. It occurs in three serotypes which share a common group antigen (A). The serotypes are Inaba (AC), Ogawa (AB) and Hikojima (ABC). The validity of the Hikojima serotype is questioned by some authorities. *Vibrio El Tor* is also widely accepted as a cause of cholera, but there is disagreement as to whether it is actually a vibrio separate from *V. cholerae;* the two strains are identical in many respects, including the serotypes. Other "noncholera vibrios" with different serotypes have been identified in association with diarrheal disease when searched for; their possible relation to common epidemic diarrheal disease of unknown origin is currently under investigation.

EPIDEMIOLOGY. The human bowel is the chief reservoir for *V. cholerae.* The organism is known to have been shed for as long as 4 years by an asymptomatic carrier, although the vibrio usually disappears from stools of patients about the third to fifth day of the disease. During epidemics the carrier rate may approach 10 per cent in the community and 20 per cent among family contacts. Contaminated food and water supplies have been responsible for household and community outbreaks; cholera tends to disappear in endemic areas as modern sewage disposal and water systems are installed. The vibrio may survive up to 2 weeks in food or water stored at room temperature, and longer in refrigerated or frozen foods. It is sensitive to drying and to an acid environment.

Bengal (India and Bangladesh) is the chief endemic center from which cholera is spread to cause recurrent epidemics, which have occurred as far away as Afghanistan, Egypt, Iran, Thailand, the Philippines, New Guinea, Hong Kong and Korea. In recent years cholera has spread westward through the Middle East and across northern Africa to invade southern Europe.

Cholera is rare among infants under 1 year of age. In previously unaffected areas the incidence is equal among children and adults, but in endemic areas the incidence in young children may be as much as ten times that in adults, presumably because of previously developed immunity in the adults. Secondary cases of cholera are rare among medical personnel who have close contact with patients and fomites, but are common among family contacts.

IMMUNITY. It is rare for a person to have more than one attack of clinical cholera. Coproantibody appears early in the disease, but recovery takes place before there is a demonstrable rise in serum antibody. Both serum and coproantibody appear in response to parenteral immunization, but immunized persons who contract the disease do not get a "booster type" response.

PATHOLOGY AND PATHOPHYSIOLOGY. The intestines contain an almost clear, whitish, watery fluid with a notable absence of bile. The intestinal mucosa is congested and studded with enlarged solitary lymph follicles, and Peyer's patches are enlarged and hypertrophied, but the mucosal surface remains intact. The liver and the spleen are congested, and the gallbladder is distended with bile. Tubular necrosis and other renal changes may be present in patients dying of postcholeric uremia.

In vitro studies indicate that cholera toxin acts by increasing both adenyl cyclase activity and cyclic AMP (cyclic 3′,5′ adenosine monophosphate) in the intestinal mucosa. The mechanism of increase in adenyl cyclase activity is unknown, but the result appears to be an increase in synthesis of cyclic AMP, which, in turn, triggers the small intestine to secrete chloride actively. In vivo, cholera toxin also appears to increase bicarbonate secretion in the ileum.

CLINICAL MANIFESTATIONS. Typically, after an incubation period of 6 hours to 3 days (rarely it may be as long as 7 days) there is sudden onset of profuse, watery diarrhea without griping, tenesmus or irritation of the skin around the anus. The stools are intermittent at first, then almost continuous; they resemble whitish, almost clear water, and contain flecks of mucus. The term "rice-water stool" is derived from the resemblance to water in which rice is being boiled. They have only a slight, inoffensive fishlike odor. Many children complain of crampy abdominal pains just before, during or after the onset of the diarrhea, at which times vomiting is also common. When the child is first seen, the rectal temperature is usually slightly elevated (about 38° C), but may fall to levels below normal as shock deepens and death nears. Within a few hours the skin assumes a dusky hue, the eyes become sunken, with dark circles, the skin cold and clammy, and the facial expression anxious. The tips of the fingers may become shriveled ("washer-woman's hands") as dehydration becomes severe. As the disease progresses, there are intense thirst, restlessness and cramps in the legs and abdomen. The blood pressure falls, the radial pulse becomes imperceptible, and urine volume decreases. Although lethargy, thick speech and a somnolent state occur usually within a few hours of onset, the patient rarely loses consciousness. Migration of ascaris out of the intestinal tract may be a striking feature; a Bengali word for cholera is translatable as "madness of the worms."

The usual duration of the acute symptoms is about 3 days, with a range of 1 to 10 days. The first sign of recovery is usually the reappearance of pigment in the stools; the cessation of diarrhea is usually rapid.

COMPLICATIONS. *Anuria* of 24 to 36 hours' duration or longer is not uncommon. If it is prolonged, it may be evidence of irreversible renal damage, which results in death from renal failure. Dehydration, hypovolemic shock and circulatory failure in that sequence are the mechanisms to which anuria and renal damage were attributed in the past and are no doubt valid explanations among patients who are untreated or who first receive treatment late in the course of the disease. On the other hand, among children treated with the usual adult fluid regimens, anuria may be secondary to hypernatremia. Such patients, though their blood volume and plasma specific gravity have been restored to normal, remain extremely thirsty; relief of thirst and anuria follows the administration of "free water" by mouth or by vein. Fever, tachycardia, tachypnea, vomiting, twitching, delirium, coma, and convulsions occurring in children whose therapy included fluids with a high sodium content are likewise probably of hypernatremic origin.

Hypokalemia may be avoided by using solutions containing 15 to 20 mEq of potassium per liter and by avoiding the unnecessarily heavy sodium loads contained in most solutions widely used in the treatment of adults with cholera. *Hypoglycemia* may be avoided by making sure that all intravenous solutions contain 3 per cent dextrose. *Pulmonary edema* is rarely, if ever, seen if fluid and electrolyte therapy is appropriate for the age, size and condition of the patient. Fever and shock may result from pyrogens contained in bacterially contaminated undistilled water used in the manufacture of homemade solutions for intravenous use, as well as from hypernatremia.

PROGNOSIS. The case fatality rate is less than 0.5 per cent among adult patients who are treated early and adequately. With less than optimum treatment the mortality rate rises and is about 40 per cent in untreated cases. Reliable statistics are lacking for infants and small children, but the mortality rate among them is high for both treated and untreated patients.

PREVENTION. The avoidance of contact with patients and carriers and good personal and environmental hygiene, combined with good nutrition, are probably the best preventive measures against cholera. Patients with cholera should not be released from isolation until their stool cultures have been negative for 2 days; their contacts should be kept under surveillance. The effectiveness of immunization is variously estimated at 20 to 80 per cent. There is general agreement that single injections of cholera vaccine are not very effective and that protection lasts only a few months. Mass treatment with orally administered vibriocidal agents, particularly tetracycline, offers promise in epidemic situations and is currently under investigation.

TREATMENT. The treatment of cholera is fraught with problems related to the circumstances under which it must be carried out. Laboratory facilities tend to be inadequate or lacking, those responsible for management are rarely acquainted with the principles of intravenous therapy of children, and appropriate intravenous fluids and equipment are often not available. The children themselves often present the added complications of anemia and malnutrition.

Fluid therapy to combat dehydration, hypovolemia and circulatory failure is the essential element in the treatment of cholera. The results have been disappointing in children as compared to adults. This is probably related to differences between children and adults with respect to the electrolyte composition of choleric stools (Table 10–6), to the use of intravenous solutions with electrolyte contents appropriate for adults, but not for children, and to the difficulty in getting children to drink adequate amounts of "free" water along with the intravenous administration of electrolyte solutions.

The few studies which have been done in children with cholera indicate that the sodium, chloride and bicarbonate contents of their stools are lower and the potassium content higher than in adults (Table 10–6). The concentrations of sodium, chloride and potassium in the serum are usually

TABLE 10–6 ELECTROLYTE CONTENT OF CHOLERIC STOOL AND OF SOLUTIONS RECOMMENDED FOR INTRAVENOUS TREATMENT OF CHILDREN

	APPROXIMATE ELECTROLYTE CONCENTRATION (mEq/LITER)					
	Na	Cl	K	HCO_3	Ca	Mg
Adult's choleric stool	132	96	19	44	2	2
Child's choleric stool	97	74	23	32	2	2
Ringer's lactate solution	130	109	4	28	–	–
SEATO 5:4:1/2 solution*	133	92	7	48	–	–
Dacca solution†	133	99	14	48	–	–
Recommended solution (N.A.M.R.U.-2 Pediatric Cholera Solution)‡	90	64	15	45	2	2

*5 gm NaCl, 4 gm $NaHCO_3$, 0.5 gm KCl per liter.
†5 gm NaCl, 4 gm $NaHCO_3$, 1 gm KCl per liter.
‡2.6 gm NaCl, 3.8 gm $NaHCO_3$, 1.1 gm KCl, 0.1 gm $CaCl_2$, and 0.1 gm $MgCl_2$ per liter.
All solutions should contain 30 gm of dextrose (glucose) per liter.

Composition of N.A.M.R.U.-2 Pediatric Cholera Solution courtesy of Dr. Lawrence S. C. Griffith.

normal or slightly elevated at the time treatment is begun. Average fluid deficits at the start of treatment are approximately 100 ml/kg, and continuing losses in the stools may be as high as 200 to 350 ml/kg/24 hours.

Since peripheral vascular collapse with diminished or absent radial pulse is usually present when the patient is first seen, it is frequently necessary to expose a vein surgically for the initial rehydration. Ideally the initial treatment of hypovolemic shock should probably be with Ringer's lactate or Dacca solution (see Table 10–6), with a change to a more hypotonic solution after the radial pulse has returned to normal volume and the patient is out of clinical hypovolemic shock. But the practicalities of treatment of cholera under epidemic circumstances dictate the use of a single solution, if possible. The N.A.M.R.U.-2 solution (Table 10–6) is recommended as a single solution which may be used. Even it may be too hypertonic if insensible fluid loss is high and the loss is not replaced through intake of additional "free" water.

The *rate of infusion* is usually limited by the size of the intravenous needle which can be introduced, but probably should not exceed 1 ml/kg/min until a normal radial pulse volume has been restored; then the infusion should be slowed to a rate adequate to replace continuing gastrointestinal fluid losses milliliter for milliliter and to provide for the gradual recovery of normal skin turgor. Measurement of stool losses is accomplished by use of a "cholera cot," a canvas cot with a hole cut to accommodate the buttocks, under which a calibrated bucket is placed. Measurements of plasma specific gravity are helpful as a guide to treatment; a rule of thumb is rapid infusion of 5 ml of fluid per kg for each 0.001 over 1.025. Oral intake of water should be encouraged to replace insensible water loss, which is 500 to 1000 ml/M^2 of body surface per day in hot climates. If oral intake is impractical, this necessary "free" water should be supplied by vein.

A solution for oral use containing 120 mM of sodium, 25 mM of potassium, 97 mM of chloride, 48 mM of bicarbonate and 110 gm glucose per liter has been used with success in at least one epidemic, either as the sole treatment or after initial intravenous hydration. The solution is administered warmed to body temperature at a rate equivalent to that of the measured continuing loss of diarrheal fluid. A nasogastric tube may be used to avoid disturbing the patient.

Antibiotic Therapy. The oral administration of tetracycline, 10 mg/kg every 6 hours for the first 72 hours of treatment, reduces the duration of diarrhea from a mean of about 72 hours to a mean of about 24 hours, reduces the duration of need for intravenous therapy (an important practical consideration during an epidemic), and reduces the incidence of convalescent carriers. Furazolidone has been used with similar results but is probably less safe.

R. James McKay

Bushnell, O. A., and Brookhyser, C. S. (eds.): Proceedings of the Cholera Research Symposium, January 24–29, 1965, Honolulu. Washington, D.C., Superintendent of Documents, U.S. Government Printing Office.
Carpenter, C. J., Jr., and Hirschhorn, N.: Pediatric cholera: Current concepts of therapy. J. Pediatr. *80*:874, 1972.
Field, M.: Intestinal secretion: Effect of cyclic AMP and its role in cholera. New Engl. J. Med. *284*:1137, 1971.

PSEUDOMONAS INFECTIONS

Pseudomonas aeruginosa is representative of a large group of gram-negative bacilli whose natural habitat is soil and water. They are ubiquitous organisms only rarely pathogenic for man. Under appropriate circumstances, however, they can and do cause serious and even fatal disease. They are opportunists which exhibit their full pathogenic potentiality in debilitated persons whose resistance to infection is compromised by disease, malnutrition, trauma or foreign body, or by immunosuppressive drugs. Pseudomonads are not fastidious in their growth requirements and are somewhat more resistant to germicides than the gram-positive cocci. Pseudomonas strains can be differentiated one from another for epidemiologic purposes by serologic typing (O types), phage typing and pyocin typing. In contrast to the staphylococci, there is little evidence that "hot strains" of unusual epidemicity or pathogenicity exist. All strains are endowed with a highly sophisticated system for energy conversion which probably accounts for their resistance to most antibiotics.

DISTRIBUTION. Since Pseudomonads are widely encountered in nature, it is to be expected that even small children will have frequent contact with them. They can be recovered occasionally from the skin of most people. Between 5 and 10 per cent of older children and adults carry these organisms in their stools, but they rarely become the predominating organism. It is not unusual to recover them from the throats of sick infants. Perhaps 20 per cent of children develop low titers of agglutinating antibodies to Pseudomonas in their serums by the first year, and practically 100 per cent do so by later childhood. The defenses of the body against Pseudomonas seem to reside mainly in intact body surfaces and in such nonspecific forces as phagocytosis and the natural bactericidal action of human serum against "nonpathogens." Because these defenses are not so well developed in the newborn infant as later on, serious and fatal infections are apt to occur during the first month of life. (See Section 7.)

CLINICAL PATTERNS. Pseudomonas produces two kinds of lesions: (1) in healthy persons introduction of these organisms into minor wounds may be followed by transient self-limited cellulitis or by frank pus formation, with the pus traditionally green or blue in the case of contamination of large surface wounds; (2) in debilitated persons Pseudomonas may overpower impaired local defenses and multiply in interstitial tissues so as to elaborate sufficient toxin (protease) to prevent a local neutrophilic reaction and pus formation. In this latter case unrestrained bacterial multiplication occurs, prodigious numbers of organisms propagating along paths of least resistance in and around blood vessel walls. Hemorrhagic necrosis results, producing lesions pathognomonic of Pseudomonas infections. In the skin these lesions may start as pink macules which progress to small subcutaneous hemorrhagic nodules, with or without vesiculation, and eventuate in coin-sized areas of necrosis with eschar formation surrounded by a bright red areola (ecthyma gangrenosum).

In hospitalized children, Pseudomonas causes serious systemic infections in several well recognized classes of patients. These are (1) newborn infants in the period following surgery of the gastrointestinal tract or repairs of meningoceles, (2) burned patients, (3) children under treatment for leukemia or aplastic anemia, (4) children with chronic obstruction of the urinary tract, and (5) children with cystic fibrosis. When several instances of Pseudomonas infection occur in a hospital in rapid sequence, they can often be traced to contamination of inhalation apparatus, suction devices, antiseptic solutions or other items of hospital usage.

Secondary Infections of Wounds. Although the natural defenses of the body can eliminate a few bacilli of low virulence inoculated under the skin, such bacteria may easily colonize body surfaces compromised by trauma, obstruction or disease. The weeping proteinaceous surfaces of burns and the viscid bronchial mucus of children with cystic fibrosis are commonly populated by Pseudomonas and other gram-negative bacilli, which in such situations set up a low-grade inflammatory reaction. Since drainage is possible, however, deep and spreading invasion of the tissues usually does not occur. The mere presence of these bacteria in injured surfaces does not, therefore, necessarily require vigorous treatment with antibacterial agents.

Colonization, however, is the necessary forerunner of invasion. Should circulation be impaired, a foreign body be present or the leukocytic response of the patient deteriorate, or should protein synthesis be compromised by drug or disease, colonization is likely to be followed by spread of the infection. Although often difficult to achieve, the most satisfactory management of these wound infections lies in adequate removal of bacterially contaminated secretions, débridement of devitalized tissue and foreign material, protection from colonization by additional bacteria and maintenance of a positive nitrogen balance in the patient. Frequent changes of moist bacteriostatic dressings, or alternating applications of bacteriostatic salves and their removal by washing, as in the *Sulfamylon* treatment of burns, is usually effective in keeping the concentration of surface bacteria sufficiently low to prevent tissue invasion and spreading infection. Systemic administration of toxic antibiotics should be reserved for treatment of spreading infection.

Leukemia. Leukemic patients in relapse are especially susceptible to invasion by Pseudomonas as a terminal event. Invasion is commonly by way of the intestine; it is insidious in onset, usually heralded by anxiety, anorexia, fever and diarrhea. Vasculitis of the intestinal and mesenteric vessels and hemorrhagic necrosis lead to septicemia. Metastatic lesions occur in many organs; in the skin they take the form of purplish nodules or ecchymotic areas which become gangrenous. Since leukemic patients often have a tendency to purpura, the infectious nature of these lesions is often not appreciated. Another frequent characteristic lesion in these patients is perirectal cellulitis, which also becomes hemorrhagic and gangrenous. Septicemia may lead to ileus, hypotension and shock. The severely burned patient has abundant neutrophils and may weather several attacks of septicemia, but few leukemic patients survive more than their first episode, despite antibiotic treatment and transfusions.

Cystic Fibrosis. (See also Section 11.) The majority of patients with cystic fibrosis who are maintained on antibiotic therapy acquire Pseudomonas in their sputum. Colonization of the bronchial secretions is not equivalent to tissue involvement. There seems little doubt that bacteria growing in profusion in mucus encourage the migration of pus cells into the sputum and promote an increase in its volume and viscosity. Frequently strains of Pseudomonas may be isolated which produce huge, watery mucoid colonies (slime producers). Slime production appears to be induced by infection of ordinary Pseudomonas organisms by lysogenic bacteriophage. Such strains may produce less pigment than rough strains and may appear in vitro to be more sensitive to antibiotics, even though they are isolated from patients receiving such antibiotics. They seem to produce a greater antibody response in the patient, indicating that they may be more pathogenic.

Pseudomonas may occasionally be suspected to be the cause of pneumonia in cystic fibrosis when appropriate antistaphylococcal therapy fails and sputum freshly obtained by "postural drainage" shows massive overgrowth of Pseudomonas. Such sputa, digested with N-acetyl cysteine and diluted 1:100,000 before culture, will reveal 10^6 or 10^7 organisms per mm^3. Treatment of Pseudomonas pneumonia with systemic antibiotics is not very successful unless effective thinning and removal of bronchial secretions are possible through postural drainage and aerosol therapy.

TREATMENT. Systemic infections with Pseudomonas are always serious and usually yield only to systemic treatment with antibiotics which are bactericidal to Pseudomonas. Polymixin B and colistin have had limited usefulness and have been replaced by gentamicin and carbenicillin. Gentamicin is preferred as the initial drug. It is given intramuscularly, 2.5 mg/kg, every 12 hours in the first week of life (5 mg/kg/day), and every 8 hours after the first week (7.5 mg/kg/day). It can be used intravenously in the same dose, infused over a 1½- to 2-hour period. Gentamicin is ototoxic and one hesitates to use it longer than 10 days, or in the presence of impaired renal function. Carbenicillin is also effective and is given intravenously, 100 mg/kg, every 8 hours under a week of age (300 mg/kg/day), and every 6 hours after the first week (400 mg/kg/day). The daily dose may be increased to 600 mg/kg/day if necessary. Carbenicillin may be combined with gentamicin in desperation, in which case the drugs should be added to the infusion alternately.

In treating meningitis, if the cerebrospinal fluid is not rendered sterile promptly with the treatment above, intrathecal or intraventricular polymixin B may be given for two to three days in a total dose of 3 to 5 mg, given once daily. Gentamicin can also be used in this manner in a total daily dose of 1 to 2 mg. Note that the total dose is independent of the weight of the patient.

Mere colonization of infected body surfaces does not ordinarily demand antibiotic treatment. Abscesses demand drainage, and surface wounds demand cleansing and débridement.

OTHER GRAM-NEGATIVE BACILLI. With the exception of the characteristic lesion of hemorrhagic necrosis with vasculitis caused by Pseudomonas, most of the considerations in the foregoing discussion apply also to infections with other gram-negative environmental bacteria. These organisms frequently include *E. coli,* Klebsiella-Enterobacter and Proteus, and less commonly Alkaligenes, Paracolon bacilli, Serratia, Mima, Flavobacteria and Achromobacter. Infection by these organisms is fostered by debility, the postoperative state, the leukemic state, obstructive uropathy and the administration of steroids or immunosuppressive drugs. Prompt treatment even of septicemia is frequently successful if bactericidal drugs are used. Gentamicin is more frequently the drug of choice than any other, but antibiotic sensitivity to the individual strain involved should be determined, since some of these agents may have strange patterns of antibiotic resistance. Septicemia with any of them may lead to infectious shock due to gram-negative endotoxin. When shock occurs, antibacterial treatment is important, but the major part of management involves maintenance of blood volume, blood pressure, cardiac output and tissue perfusion, and the avoidance of intravascular clotting.

WARREN E. WHEELER

Cooper, R. G.: Systemic pseudomonas infection in childhood. Med. J. Aust., *1*:527, 1967.

Finland, M., and Hewitt, W. L. (eds.): Second International Symposium on Gentamicin. J. Infect. Dis. *124* (Suppl.):S1, 1971.

Kirby, W. (ed.): Symposium on Carbenicillin: A clinical profile. J. Infect. Dis. *122* (Suppl.):S1, 1970.

Teplitz, C.: Pathogenesis of pseudomonas vasculitis and septic lesions. Arch. Path., *80*:297, 1965.

YERSINIA INFECTIONS

Species of Yersinia have long been appreciated as a cause of human disease in Europe; only recently have physicians elsewhere become aware of their role in clinical medicine. Ahvonen and others in Finland have described syndromes of acute appendicitis (related to mesenteric adenitis and terminal ileitis), erythema nodosum, and nonsuppurative arthritis due to Yersinia infection.

There are two organisms responsible for human disease: *Yersinia enterocolitica* and *Y. pseudotuberculosis.* Formerly classified as Pasteurella, these organisms are gram-negative polymorphic, motile cocci. With experience they can easily be recognized in routine culture; if they are suspected, special methods may enhance recovery. The two types are differentiated serologically. Serotypes 3 and 9 of *Y. enterocolitica* and 1 of *Y. pseudotuberculosis* are found most commonly in human infections. Infected patients develop specific agglutinins, but there are cross-reactions with a variety of bacteria and the serologic methodology is relatively primitive.

The organisms are found in many animal species in nature. Transmission to humans probably occurs through contaminated food, direct contact with animals, and hand to mouth contact with infected humans. Preliminary data suggest a prevalence in cool months, with young infants and children most susceptible.

Yersinia pseudotuberculosis produces mesenteric adenitis and terminal ileitis which may mimic acute appendicitis. Rarely there may be accompanying septicemia, which may be lethal. Usually the gastrointestinal disease is benign and self-limited, with fever and abdominal pain similar to those of acute appendicitis. Leukocytosis with polymorphonuclear predominance is frequent.

Yersinia enterocolitica is associated with a gastroenteritis which may likewise simulate acute appendicitis. Severe, persistent abdominal pain is frequently observed, with vomiting and fever. Diarrhea is persistent, with watery or mucoid stools which contain abundant polymorphonuclear white blood cells.

Arthritis and erythema nodosum have been reported in Europe, but not as yet in the United States.

Diagnosis may be accomplished during the acute phase of illness by isolation of the organism. Serologic diagnosis may be possible in convalescence, but cross-reacting antibodies must be taken into account.

Yersinia sp. are sensitive in vitro to streptomycin, tetracycline, chloramphenicol and sulfonamides. The efficacy of therapy is uncertain since the disease usually subsides spontaneously. Most workers advocate streptomycin or tetracycline; some suggest that ampicillin may also be effective.

Ahvonen, P.: Human yersiniosis in Finland, I. Bacteriology and serology. Ann. Clin. Res. *4*:30, 1972.

Ahvonen, P.: Human yersiniosis in Finland, II. Clinical features. Ann. Clin. Res. *4*:39, 1972.

Gutman, L. T., Ottesen, E. A., Quan, T. J., Noce, P. S., and Katl, S. L.: An inter-familial outbreak of Yersinia enterocolitica enteritis. New Engl. J. Med. *288*:1372, 1973.

Weber, J., Finlayson, N. B., and Mark, J. B. D.: Mesenteric lymphadenitis and terminal ileitis due to Yersinia pseudotuberculosis. New Engl. J. Med. *283*:172, 1970.

Winblad, S.: Erythema nodosum associated with infection with Yersinia enterocolitica. Scand. J. Infect. Dis. *1*:11, 1969.

BRUCELLOSIS

Brucellosis is an acute or chronic disease of man caused by any of four species of *Brucella.* The source of infection may be any of four domestic animals (cow, dog, hog, goat), but strains of the organisms have also been isolated from wild rats, wild guinea pigs, ground squirrels, field mice, camels, fowl, gazelles, water buffalo, chamois, deer, elk, moose, bison and jack rabbits.

ETIOLOGIC AGENT. Four species of Brucella have been described in infections of man: *B. abortus* (cattle); *B. suis* (hogs); *B. melitensis* (goats) and *B. canis* (beagles). The organisms are small gram-negative nonmotile aerobic coccobacilli.

EPIDEMIOLOGY. Human infection occurs by transmission of the agent from the infected animal to humans. The organism may enter the body through breaks in the skin on direct contact with infected milk, flesh or products of conception (the fetus or placenta), or indirectly through consumption of unpasteurized milk or milk products from infected animals. Congenital infection in man is unknown.

PATHOLOGY AND PATHOGENESIS. Brucella organisms are obligate intracellular parasites. Once entry into the body occurs, they are phagocytized by leukocytes and monocytes, in which they multiply. They are then disseminated to the reticuloendothelial system, where they may persist in macrophages for several months and are not susceptible to attack by serum antibody or by antibiotics.

All brucella species produce granulomas, some (*B. melitensis* and *B. suis*) with a greater degree of suppuration than others (*B. abortus*). These lesions involve the bone marrow as well as the liver, spleen and lymph nodes. Plasma cell infiltration is not uncommon. Chronic brucellosis may also involve the skin, brain, kidneys and genitourinary organs. Tissue localization may be enhanced by erythrophagocytosis in certain organs.

CLINICAL MANIFESTATIONS. After an incubation period of 5 to 30 days, the disease begins insidiously with vague symptoms of sweating, chills, weakness, exhaustion, backache and arthralgia. Physical findings at this time may be limited to cervical and axillary lymphadenopathy and splenomegaly. The classic undulating fever is uncommon in children.

In the chronic form of the disease localizing findings may develop in the long bones and spine, liver, spleen or genitalia.

DIAGNOSIS. A history of exposure may suggest brucellosis. The diagnosis must be made in the laboratory. The white blood count is normal, but there is a relative lymphocytosis. Specimens for culture should be obtained from blood and urine, and also from tissues where localization may have occurred.

A brucella agglutination titer of 1:160 or more is diagnostic of infection. Cross-reactions occur with agglutinins against *Francisella tularensis* and tests against both should be performed. Usually the titer is high to the infecting agent and several dilutions lower to the other. Unless both tests are performed on the same specimen, however, a mistaken diagnosis may be made. A complement fixation titer is useful in differentiation and is diagnostic at a titer of 1:10. With central nervous system involvement, antibody determination may be made on spinal fluid; any positive titer is diagnostic. Skin tests should not be performed if serologic studies are available because the skin test antigen may stimulate production of antibody, rendering subsequent serology confusing.

Differential Diagnosis. Diseases which are associated with lymphocytosis, lymphadenopathy and hepatosplenomegaly or granuloma formation must be differentiated.

Infectious mononucleosis can be differentiated by serial heterophil antibody determinations. Tuberculosis, coccidioidomycosis, typhoid fever and tularemia must be differentiated by appropriate tests. Lymphoma and neoplastic disease must be differentiated from chronic brucellosis by bone marrow examination, appropriate biopsy and roentgenologic studies.

COMPLICATIONS. Localization in tissues such as the brain, lung, liver, kidneys, heart and bones accounts for the majority of complications. Hepatic necrosis may occur with extensive multiplication of the organism. Neurologic complications may occur at any time, and are usually due to adhesive arachnoiditis. Death is usually from cardiac involvement (endocarditis). A Herxheimer reaction may occur at the onset of therapy as massive bacterial death occurs.

PROGNOSIS. The prognosis is excellent with specific antibiotic therapy. If the infection does not localize, spontaneous recovery may take place within several weeks to 6 months after onset. About half of patients with brucellosis experience relapse, even with treatment. Immunity is related to improved phagocytosis and a decrease in intracellular survival of the organisms.

PREVENTION. Prevention rests on the avoidance of exposure, eliminating the infected animal reservoir by immunization of cattle, and slaughter of infected animals identified through testing programs. Avoidance of ingestion of raw milk and of unpasteurized products made from raw milk is important.

TREATMENT. Administration of one of the tetracyclines in standard oral doses (see Drug Table in Section 30) for 3 to 4 weeks is recommended. If relapse occurs, the dose is doubled *or* streptomycin is added to the tetracycline and treatment continued for another 21-day period. Streptomycin should be given for 2 to 3 weeks intramuscularly at a dose of 15–30 mg/kg/day divided into two equal doses given every 12 hours. Half the initial dose may be given during the second week.

Localized lesions should be drained surgically. Antibiotic therapy suffices for spondylitis, however, and surgical drainage should be avoided. Steroids may be useful in reducing the risk of a Herxheimer reaction at the onset of therapy.

Boycott, J. A.: Diagnosing brucellosis. Lancet *1*:255, 1969.

Bradstreet, C. M. P., Tannahil, A. J., Pollock, T. M., and Mogford, H. E.: Intradermal test and serological tests in suspected brucella infection in man. Lancet *2*:653, 1970.

Hall, W. H., and Khan, M. Y.: Brucellosis. *In* Hoeprich, P. D. (ed.) Infectious Disease—A Guide to the Understanding and Management of Infectious Processes. New York, Harper & Row, 1972. Chapter 123.

Hall, W. H., and Manion, R. E.: In vitro susceptibility of brucella to various antibiotics. Appl. Microb. *20*:600, 1970.

TULAREMIA

Tularemia is a disease of small mammals which can be transmitted to man. The syndrome produced reflects both the route of inoculation and the virulence of the organism. Classic syndromes include ulceroglandular, oculoglandular, oropharyngeal, glandular, pulmonic and gastrointestinal manifestations.

ETIOLOGIC AGENT. *Francisella tularensis (Pasteurella tularensis)* is a gram-negative, nonmotile, pleomorphic organism with both coccal and rod forms. It requires selective media such as glucose-cystine-blood agar for differentiation from other similar gram-negative bacteria. There is no antigenic variation in strains, but virulence does vary; tick-borne strains from rabbits are associated with increased virulence in humans. Water-borne strains of rodent origin are virulent for rabbits but cause only mild disease in man. An endotoxin has been described.

EPIDEMIOLOGY. The organism is harbored by cottontail rabbits, hares, muskrats, rats and mice and transmitted to humans from animal tissues or secretions, by insect vectors (ticks, lice, mosquitoes, fleas, deerflies), by contaminated water or by inhalation. Indirect transmission may occur from contamination of teeth or claws of household pets or snakes which have preyed on animals in the primary reservoir. The incidence of disease is greatest in summer. Human-to-human contact has been suggested but not proved.

PATHOGENESIS, PATHOLOGY AND IMMUNOLOGY. Inoculation of the host occurs through intact or broken skin, mucous membranes or the respiratory and gastrointestinal tracts. The organisms spread to and multiply in regional lymph nodes where they produce granulomas. Bacteremia may occur and lead to involvement of the liver and spleen.

Since *F. tularensis* is an intracellular parasite, cell-mediated immunity may be more important than circulating antibody. Recovery is usually associated with lifelong immunity, though mild second infections may occur.

CLINICAL MANIFESTATIONS. Though tularemia may produce a severe generalized disease, diagnostically the most significant reaction occurs at the portal of entry. This phenomenon serves to classify the various clinical syndromes. Localizing forms of infections are the ulceroglandular, oculoglandular, oropharyngeal and glandular types.

Ulceroglandular disease is the most common form. It begins as an ulcerating papule with regional lymphadenopathy. In *oculoglandular* disease, yellow conjunctival nodules form and ulcerate, with development of periorbital edema and purulent conjunctivitis. Regional lymph nodes are also increased in size. *Oropharyngeal* tularemia is characterized by purulent tonsillitis and severe ulcerative stomatitis unresponsive to penicillin therapy. The *glandular* form occurs without a local cutaneous lesion but with prominent lymphadenopathy.

Pulmonary and *gastrointestinal* (or typhoidal) forms occur much more rarely. Pneumonia may be primary from inhalation of organisms or secondary from bacteremia associated with other forms of the disease. A typhoidal syndrome may result from primary tularemic pneumonia; organisms invade the blood stream with production of high fever, headache and myalgia. This form rarely occurs from enteric inoculation of organisms.

Dissemination may occur in any form of tularemia and result in meningitis, osteomyelitis, endocarditis or pericarditis. Splenomegaly and a maculopapular rash are not uncommon in any of the forms of the disease.

DIAGNOSIS. A history of contact is helpful but generally absent. It should be sought in any illness compatible with tularemia. The protean nature of the manifestations in tularemia requires the clinician to be alert to the possibility of this disease. Nonspecific signs of infection (such as the sedimentation rate) may be normal. The white blood cell count is usually within normal limits.

A preparation of phenolized organisms for *skin-testing* has been employed in diagnosis; positive reactions by the third to seventh day of a tularemic infection may be diagnostic.

Serologic testing examines titers of agglutinins in paired sera. By the second week of illness the titer may be 1:160; by 4 to 8 weeks it may reach 1:1280. Such titers are diagnostic of tularemia in single specimens, but a demonstrated rise in titer provides a firmer diagnosis.

Confirmation of the diagnosis by *culture* is feasible but requires appropriate media and is potentially hazardous to laboratory personnel. The drainage from wounds, blood and gastric washings provides suitable material for isolating the organisms.

Differential Diagnosis. Each of the tularemic syndromes must be differentiated from numerous other clinical entities. Ulceroglandular tularemia may resemble cat scratch fever, infectious mononucleosis, bacterial lymphangitis (*Spirillum minus*, streptococcal or staphylococcal infections), sporotrichosis, plague and anthrax. Oropharyngeal tularemia must be differentiated from the same conditions, but also from herpes simplex gingivostomatitis, herpangina and blood dyscrasias. Nonbacterial pneumonias such as those due to mycoplasma, psittacosis, fungi or mycobacteria can be differentiated on the basis of either skin test responses (coccidioidomycosis and histoplasmosis), isolation of the organism, serologic response or response to tetracycline therapy.

PROGNOSIS. The prognosis with specific treatment is excellent. Untreated, localized forms of tularemia have a 4 to 5 per cent mortality; with dissemination, it is five to six times greater.

PREVENTION. Tularemia may be prevented by avoidance of exposure to small mammals or vectors and by utilizing appropriate clothing and repellents. Rubber gloves should be worn when handling the raw flesh of wild game. Cutaneous administration of an attenuated Russian strain of *F. tularensis* has received preliminary testing as a vaccine, but its usefulness has yet to be determined.

TREATMENT. Streptomycin is the drug of choice and may be given intramuscularly in a dose of 30–40 mg/kg/day, divided into two doses. Response may be noted in 48 hours; treatment should be continued for 7 to 8 days. The acute symptoms of tularemia respond to treatment with chloramphenicol or tetracycline, but relapses usually ensue and require the use of streptomycin in any event. Kanamycin and gentamicin may be effective, but have not received sufficient clinical trial.

Buchanan, T. M., Brooks, G. F., and Brachman, P. S.: The tularemia skin test. Serologic correlation and review of the literature. Ann. Intern. Med. *74*:336, 1971.

Foshay, L.: Tularemia. Ann. Rev. Microbiol. *4*:313, 1950.

Fulginiti, V. A., and Hoyle, C.: Oropharyngeal tularemia. Rocky Mtn. Med. J. *63*:41, 1966.

Hughes, W. T.: Tularemia in children. J. Pediatr. *62*:495, 1963.

Young, L. S., and Sherman, I. L.: Tularemia in the United States: Recent trends and a major epidemic in 1968. J. Infect. Dis. *119*:109, 1969.

DIPHTHERIA

Diphtheria is an acute infectious disease caused by *Corynebacterium diphtheriae;* it is characterized by local growth of the organism, usually in the respiratory tract, and by local and systemic manifestations related to production and transport of an exotoxin.

ETIOLOGIC AGENT. *Corynebacterium diphtheriae* (Klebs-Loeffler bacillus) is a gram-positive pleomorphic rod which is nonmotile and nonsporeforming. Isolation of the organism from clinical specimens is best accomplished on a medium containing selective inhibitors of other gram-positive organisms (such as the pneumococcus and streptococcus); media may include either serum or tellurite to accomplish this goal. With media containing tellurite, three strains of *C. diphtheriae* may be identified by variations in colonial forms and chemical reactions: gravis, mitis and intermedius. Each produces a toxin, varying in amount and virulence, which is related to the severity of the systemic manifestations; virulence seems to be commonly present with strains of the intermedius and gravis varieties, less so with mitis. This variation in virulence also seems to be associated with the presence of a specific phage, which can be transferred from virulent to avirulent strains, enhancing the virulence of the latter. Variability in toxin production is evaluated in the laboratory to enable one to determine the virulence of a given isolate. This is necessary, since *C. diphtheriae* may also be a member of the normal flora, unassociated with an exotoxin. Toxin production may be evaluated with either of two tests: (1) tissue necrosis in the guinea pig; or (2) gel diffusion in agar, this test being based on demonstration of a precipitin band between toxin and antitoxin.

EPIDEMIOLOGY. Diphtheria was once most common in children from 1 to 5 years of age; it seems now to be affecting older children and adults with increasing frequency as humoral immunity from childhood immunization diminishes. Newborn infants born of mothers with diminished immunity are susceptible, as are children unimmunized owing to lack of access to medical care for socioeconomic reasons. Though the occurrence of diphtheria is world-wide, it is more common in temperate climates. Crowding enhances spread. The overtly ill patient is least likely to account for spread of diphtheria; the more significant source is the individual incubating the disease or the asymptomatic carrier. Communicability occurs primarily by direct contact, but also by indirect contact with articles of clothing; communicability may persist for more than 2 weeks in untreated cases, but is diminished to 2 to 3 days with antibiotic therapy.

PATHOGENESIS AND PATHOLOGY. The infection associated with diphtheria is initiated by entry of *C. diphtheriae* into the nose, pharynx, larynx, tracheobronchial tree, eyes, genitalia or skin. After a 2- to 4-day incubation period, local bacterial growth occurs, with elaboration of a small amount of toxin. This toxin is adsorbed to adjacent mucous membranes, where it produces disruption of cellular protein synthesis and then tissue necrosis, enhancing further growth of the organism. This leads to increased toxin production and, as this cycle continues, the original patchy loci of infection deepen and widen. As the epithelium degenerates, a serous and fibrinous exudate develops, incorporating inflammatory and red blood cells, producing a membrane-like cover of the involved area (pseudomembrane). Because mucosal cells form an integral part of the developing membrane, removal of the adherent membrane disrupts blood vessels, producing a bleeding surface (a differential characteristic of the diphtheritic membrane). The color of the membrane depends upon the number of red cells present (white if few cells are present, or gray to black if bleeding has occurred into the membrane). The characteristics which permit local growth of the diphtheria bacilli also permit growth to occur across the usual anatomic boundaries of the respiratory tract, so that the membrane may extend beyond tonsillar tissue onto the oropharynx and into the nasopharynx and tracheobronchial tree (Fig. 10–5, p. 657). Once sufficient local spread has taken place, toxin overflows into the blood stream, with systemic dissemination. The amount of toxin taken up is greater with infections of the oropharynx and the tonsils than with infection of the lower respiratory tract and reflects the vascularity of the structures involved. On the other hand, lower respiratory tract involvement can produce serious respiratory embarrassment in the young child from the obstruction associated with proliferation of the membrane.

The distant systemic effects of diphtheria toxin are also related to cellular destruction and to changes in physiologic function. Heart, kidneys and adrenal glands, liver and the cranial and peripheral nerves are most often affected. Toxin adsorbs preferentially to cells in these organs and, following penetration, interferes with synthesis of cellular proteins. Diphtheria antitoxin may neutralize circulating toxin or toxin adsorbed to cells but is ineffectual once cell penetration has taken place. Because a latent period usually occurs between the penetration of the cell and clinical manifestations (10 to 14 days for degenerative myocarditis and 3 to 7 weeks for toxic peripheral neuritis), no prognostic implications can be drawn until these periods have passed. Liver necrosis may occur, with hypoglycemia, and adrenal hemorrhage may be noted. The kidneys may undergo tubular necrosis.

CLINICAL MANIFESTATIONS. Signs and symptoms of diphtheria will vary with the site of localization of the disease, the duration of illness, whether there has been sufficient time for systemic distribution of toxin to occur and the immunization status of the host. Following the incubation period, low-grade fever, malaise, headache and vague aches and pains are common early general symptoms. If sore throat is present, it is usually less painful than streptococcal infection of the throat. Subsequent development of local disease will depend upon the sites at which primary bacterial growth is occurring; nasal, tonsillar or faucial, laryngotracheal, cutaneous and genital diphtheria can be delineated. The respiratory syndromes tend to be mixed.

Nasal diphtheria begins usually with mild unilateral or bilateral rhinorrhea, which may persist for many days without change, occasionally becoming serosanguineous, often excoriating the upper lip, and having a foul odor. Though toxin absorption is usually low and systemic symptoms mild, a membrane may be present on the nasal septum. This form of disease accounts for significant spread of diphtheria organisms because the patient lacks severe symptoms and is not isolated. It occurs in approximately 2 per cent of all patients, most often infants (Fig. 10–6, p. 657).

Pharyngeal diphtheria is a more severe disease, accompanied by sudden onset of sore throat and headache and malaise, with a pulse rate out of proportion to the low-grade fever. Development of a membrane can be readily followed, with characteristics described above; in partially immune patients, a membrane may not develop. The membrane may extend superiorly into the nose, to present several of the findings of nasal diphtheria, or may extend inferiorly into the larynx. In severe cases, circulatory collapse occurs early. Palatal paralysis may be associated with difficulty in swallowing and regurgitation. With marked toxemia the sensorium becomes clouded. Evidence of bleeding appears, with hemorrhages from the nose and mouth and cutaneous petechiae. Edema of the neck and marked cervical lymphadenopathy may occur (bull neck). If secondary infection with group A beta-hemolytic streptococci is present, the pharyngitis and neck edema may be more marked.

Laryngotracheal diphtheria occurs in approximately one fourth of instances, more commonly as a downward extension from a pharyngeal diphtherial focus. When illness occurs from a primary focus in the larynx, there is less associated toxicity. This form is more common in infants; symptoms begin with noisy breathing, harsh cough and hoarseness and progressive stridor. Retractions and anxiety usually reflect increasing respiratory obstruction, which may be lethal unless alleviated.

Other forms of diphtheritic infection include eye, ear, vaginal and cutaneous disease. Ulcerative lesions occur on the skin, which may be an important source of person-to-person transmission of diphtheria organisms. Membrane formation takes place in the base of the ulcer or with palpebral conjunctivitis.

DIAGNOSIS. The diagnosis of diphtheria is and must be a clinical diagnosis because of the profoundly deleterious effects delay in therapy may have on the course and outcome of the infection. Undue reliance on bacteriologic confirmation prior to use of specific antitoxin is partly due to clinical inexperience in determining and acting upon a diagnosis based on signs and symptoms. It is imperative, however, that clinical diagnoses guide initiation of therapy. Delay of 48 to 72 hours may result in complications which could be avoided. Only in mild cases, where the greatest clinical indecision may occur, may regular, frequent evaluations of the throat detect increases in membrane which lead to the correct diagnosis.

For bacteriologic confirmation of infection due to *C. diphtheriae*, material to be cultured should be obtained from beneath the membrane, or a portion of the membrane itself should be obtained and placed on appropriate media (Loeffler's, tellurite). *Corynebacterium diphtheriae* may have characteristic mid-polar bars on methylene blue smear or may be identified by fluorescent antibody staining. In all instances laboratory proof of toxigenicity is necessary for definitive diagnosis.

Other laboratory findings are not diagnostic. The white blood count may be normal or slightly elevated. The hemoglobin may drop rapidly from hemolysis. If neuritis is present, the spinal fluid may show minimal changes, with elevation of protein and, less often, a mild pleocytosis. Glucosuria may indicate toxic changes in the liver. Elevation of the BUN reflects renal toxicity. The high incidence of myocarditis and conduction abnormalities is an indication for electrocardiography.

Schick testing to determine immune status has been utilized in the diagnosis of diphtheria infection. It does not contribute to rapid diagnosis since a delay of 24 hours or more is necessary for interpretation. The **Schick test** reflects circulating diphtheria antitoxin. The test employs a measured amount of diphtheria toxin injected intracutaneously, any reaction being compared with a control injection of heat-killed diphtheria bacteria, which are nontoxic. False positive reactions are ruled out if the control reaction is negative. False positive reactions indicate dermal sensitivity to bacterial proteins other than the toxin and occur within 48 hours. If serum antitoxin is present, there is no skin reaction at the toxin-injected site since the toxin is neutralized, indicative of sufficient immunity to prevent or, at least, modify diphtheria. A positive reaction consists of more than 10 mm of induration, followed by brownish discoloration in 4 to 7 days, and indicates un-neutralized effect of toxin, and susceptibility to diphtheria. Hypersensitivity (false positive) reactions appear in a shorter time (48 hours) than the Schick-positive reaction.

The current major use of Schick-testing is in immunodeficiency states to determine whether antibody production is occurring.

Differential Diagnosis. With the reduction in incidence and severity of diphtheria, it is seldom considered as a primary diagnosis today; rather, diphtheria is considered secondarily, as some other diagnosis loses its credibility. This is particularly true when milder forms of diphtheria are seen in the partially immunized host. The persistent bloody nasal discharge of nasal or nasopharyngeal diphtheria must be differentiated from that of congenital syphilis, of nasal foreign body or of trauma by careful physical examination of the nose for the presence of a septal membrane, foreign body or bleeding source. Viral rhinorrhea does not usually contain blood.

Membranous tonsillar or pharyngeal diphtheria must be differentiated from other causes of localized membranous disease: streptococcal (more throat pain on swallowing, higher temperature, beefy red pharynx, membrane limited to tonsils, response to penicillin); infectious mononucleosis (splenomegaly, atypical lymphocytes, lymphadenopathy, positive test for heterophil antibody); Vincent's angina (may be indistinguishable); blood dyscrasias (leukemia, agranulocytosis); post-tonsillectomy appearance of tonsils; adenoviral, toxoplasmal and tularemic oropharyngeal involvement; and monilia (linear anterior oral lesions).

Laryngeal diphtheria with stridor must be differentiated from croup, spasmodic or nonspasmodic (intermittent stridor); epiglottitis (sudden onset, air hunger, primary involvement of epiglottis); laryngotracheobronchitis; aspirated foreign body (direct and roentgenographic or bronchoscopic examination); peripharyngeal abscesses and laryngeal papillomata.

COMPLICATIONS. Complications remain the greatest cause of morbidity and mortality and reflect the specific diphtheria strain associated with the clinical infection. Local bacterial infection, respiratory obstruction and systemic effects of toxin also are factors which contribute to complications. Streptococcal infection is common (30 per cent of diphtheria cases), adding to cervical adenopathy and production of edema, with a greater tendency toward development of the "bull neck" appearance. Respiratory obstruction is mechanical and related to the relatively small size of the trachea and larynx of infants under 4 years of age, which are easily occluded by the proliferating diphtheritic membrane. A bacterial pneumonia or atelectasis may occur.

The toxic complications of diphtheria more often cause death than the infectious ones. When the local diphtheritic lesion is prominent and recognized, these toxic effects can be anticipated. In some situations the local diphtheritic process may have been mild and have healed or been missed as a specific etiologic diagnosis. Accordingly, toxic peripheral neuritis may be difficult to associate with *C. diphtheriae* infection. The most common toxic effects are circulatory, but neurologic, gastrointestinal, hepatic and genitourinary complications also occur. The earliest complications are primarily circulatory, as tachycardia, murmurs and delayed conduction time reflect acute toxic myocarditis on the second to seventh days of infection. Neurologic complications may involve local paralyses of cranial nerves VI and X, which occur at the earliest on the fifth day and may be associated with blurred vision, difficulties in swallowing, and nasal speech. Mild cases tend to have mild neurologic complications. Local unilateral diphtheria may show paralysis of the palate on the same side. Two to three weeks following onset, cardiac failure and a drop in blood pressure from degenerative involvement of the vasomotor centers and arterial musculature can be seen. The most common late neurologic complication is peripheral nonsensory neuritis, occurring as late as 12 weeks after the local lesion. An ascending generalized paralysis may also occur, with phrenic nerve paralysis and with gastritis and toxic hepatitis. Proteinuria and nephritis secondary to streptococcal disease have also been described.

PROGNOSIS. Many factors bear on the prognosis of diphtheria, but each therapeutic advance in the last century (e.g., diphtheria antitoxin; immunization; antibiotics) has led to a lowering of mortality. At present, overall mortality is less than 4 per cent and related to several predictive factors: virulence of the organism, severity of the disease as noted by extent and location of the membrane, immunization status, specific therapy (and the timeliness, dosage and route of administration of antitoxin), general nursing care and the development of complications. If death does not intervene, most complications are reversible, except for an occasional instance of myocarditis. The most serious prognostic associations are with myocarditis and atrioventricular dissociation, amegakaryocytic thrombocytopenia and isolation of the gravis strain of *C. diphtheriae.* Mortality may be decreased to approximately 0.5 per cent if specific treatment begins on the first day of disease, but a delay in instituting treatment may increase the mortality twentyfold by the fourth day.

A significant carrier state for *C. diphtheriae* is defined as the presence of virulent organisms in the nose or throat of individuals who have insufficient immunity (negative Schick test) and are without symptoms. The carrier state may develop in contacts of patients with diphtheria, or in those few found on routine survey to have virulent organisms. The latter situation may occur as bacteriophage converts nonvirulent to virulent strains in situ. Persistence of diphtheria occurs in as many as 5 to 10 per cent of convalescing patients more than 3 months after treatment, but may be lower when antitoxin and antibiotic are used simultaneously in the early treatment.

PREVENTION. Preventive measures for *C. diphtheriae* infection include immunization and management of contacts of known cases of diphtheria. In addition, isolation of the patient with diphtheria minimizes spread.

Active immunization for diphtheria has effectively reduced the incidence of diphtheria and is the basic tool in prevention. Immunization in infancy with an alum-precipitated toxoid combined with pertussis and tetanus (DPT) has the potential of eliminating *C. diphtheriae* as a cause of fulminating disseminated disease because of its effectiveness. (See Immunization, Section 4.) Diphtheria immunization provides protection for a limited period, the exact duration being uncertain. Hence, repeated boosters are recommended; currently a 10-year interval between "booster" doses after primary immunization is felt to be adequate. Beyond 6 years of age the pediatric combinations of diphtheria toxoid with other antigens (DPT, DT) are not employed, owing to the high incidence of reactions associated with their use. Instead, an adult form (Td) is used containing one twentieth to one tenth the dose of diphtheria toxoid in the pediatric preparations. Diphtheria vaccine is not available as a single preparation; it is always combined with tetanus or pertussis. Ideally, a separate diphtheria fluid toxoid would permit more accurate adjustment of diphtheria immunization to the older individual.

Diphtheria immunization does not always afford complete protection. Infection and the carrier state occur in a few who are fully immunized, but the disease is less severe, with fewer complications and very low mortality.

The major problem today is inadequate immunization of the population. Some groups of children are totally unprotected, particularly in the poor areas of our inner cities. Recent epidemics in Phoenix, Arizona, and San Antonio, Texas, occurred in just such areas with low rates of immunization.

Levels of immunity in adults are poorer than those in infants and children because of failure to maintain antitoxin levels by repeated "booster" doses. Such states of lapsed immunization have resulted in epidemics of diphtheria among adults, particularly in adverse social circumstances.

Contacts of cases of diphtheria may contract the disease if they are not immune. Many recommend that carriers of *C. diphtheriae* should be identified among these contacts by nasal and pharyngeal cultures, whether or not they have been immunized. Those carriers with prior immunization should be given a "booster" injection of diphtheria toxoid. On the other hand, the management of carriers who have not been immunized is controversial. Some recommend that each contact receive a Schick test and that Schick test-positive carriers be considered infected and be treated with both antitoxin and antibiotics; others forgo the Schick test and treat carriers with antibiotics alone.

Contacts with negative cultures should receive "booster" immunization or have immunization initiated, depending on their history of prior immunization.

To minimize spread of *C. diphtheriae* from patients with cultures positive for the organism, isolation is recommended until two to three consecutive cultures are negative.

TREATMENT. Treatment of uncomplicated diphtheria is based upon neutralization of free toxin and the elimination of organisms which might produce further toxin. The only specific treatment is antitoxin, and horse serum is the only source at present. Antitoxin must be administered as early in the disease as possible by the intravenous route to achieve a high level of antitoxin in a short time and to minimize late toxic complications, in sufficient dosage to neutralize all accessible toxin (by assessment of duration of illness, location and extent of membrane), and in a single dose to avoid the increased risk of sensitization from repeated injections of horse serum. Antibiotics cannot be used as a substitute to avoid the risk of sensitization to horse serum.

Tests for sensitivity to horse serum must be done prior to administration of antitoxin, by intracutaneous injection of 0.1 ml of a 1:100 saline dilution of the material to be used or by conjunctival instillation of 1 drop of 1:10 saline dilution. A positive reaction (1 cm cutaneous erythema in 20 minutes or conjunctivitis and tearing) will require desensitization before antitoxin may be administered intravenously. Suggested schedules all use progressively larger amounts of more concentrated dilutions of antitoxin, administered at first subcutaneously, then intramuscularly and, finally, intravenously at undiluted strength. One such regimen employs an initial subcutaneous injection of 0.05 ml of a 1:20 dilution of antitoxin. The dose is doubled at 20-minute intervals until 0.5 ml of undiluted antitoxin is tolerated intramuscularly; then 0.1 ml of the same material is given intravenously, followed by slow intravenous administration of the remainder. Reactions may be treated with intravenous aqueous epinephrine (1:1000), which should be ready in a syringe by the bedside. If tolerated, antitoxin dosage should approximate 40,000 units for mild nasal or pharyngeal diphtheria; 80,000 units for moderately severe pharyngeal diphtheria; and up to 120,000 units for severe pharyngeal or laryngeal diphtheria, for mixed types, for cases of over 48 hours' duration or for those with brawny edema. Some recommend the use of intramuscular antitoxin for asymptomatic, unimmunized carriers.

Both penicillin and erythromycin have been recommended in the treatment of diphtheria and of carriers. Penicillin may be used intravenously or by the intramuscular route in doses of 300,000 to 600,000 units daily for 7 days. Erythromycin is administered orally at 40 mg/kg/day for a similar period. The end point of therapy is three consecutive negative cultures. Each of these antibiotics is also effective in eliminating the group A beta-hemolytic streptococcus, which may complicate as many as 30 per cent of cases of acute diphtheria. Cephalexin is adequate for antistreptococcal therapy, but does not, with the usual oral dosage, reach sufficient blood levels to eliminate *C. diphtheriae.* If early diphtheria is a consideration in the differential diagnosis of pharyngitis, cephalexin should not be used in treatment. With complicating pneumonia, antibiotic coverage for anaerobes should be included. (See Other Anaerobic Infections.)

In treatment of the carrier state, procaine penicillin G, benzathine penicillin (for use in epidemics) or erythromycin may be utilized. With full compliance in courses of oral erythromycin, failure rates in treatment of carriers can be reduced virtually to zero, but this may require hospitalization.

Corticosteroids have been used in acute laryngeal diphtheria in an effort to reduce the incidence of myocarditis. If electrocardiographic changes occur, voluntary activity should be minimized and bed rest required until the EKG returns to normal. If respiratory obstruction develops in severe laryngeal diphtheria, tracheostomy may be required or bronchoscopy for removal of the membrane.

No specific therapy is available for treatment of the more common complications, myocarditis and neuritis. Activity has been associated with sudden death; accordingly, bed rest is mandatory. Digitalis may be contraindicated owing to arrhythmias, but it should be used for treatment of congestive cardiac failure. (See Diseases of the Myocardium, Section 13.) Generalized paralysis or phrenic nerve paralysis may produce respiratory failure, requiring assisted ventilation.

About half of patients recovering from diphtheria will not develop adequate immunity and will be susceptible to mild reinfection. Immunization is therefore indicated, once recovery is complete.

Brooks, G. F.: Recent trends of diphtheria in the United States. J. Infect. Dis. *120*:500, 1969.

Freeman, V. J.: Studies on the virulence of bacteriophage-infected strains of Corynebacterium diphtheriae. J. Bact. *61*:675, 1951.

McCloskey, R. V., Eller, J. J., Green, M., Mauney, C. U., and Richards, S.E.M.: The 1970 epidemic of diphtheria in San Antonio. Ann. Intern. Med. *75*:495, 1971.

Miller, L. W., Older, J. J., Drake, J., and Zimmerman, S.: Diphtheria immunization: Effect upon carriers and the control of outbreaks. Am. J. Dis. Child. *123*:197, 1972.

Report of Committee on the Control of Infectious Diseases. Evanston, Illinois, American Academy of Pediatrics, 1974, p. 45.

Tasman, A., Minkenhof, J. E., Vink, H. H., Brandwijk, A. C., and Smith, L.: Importance of intravenous injection of diphtheria antiserum. Lancet *1*:1299, 1958.

Wiester, M. J., Bonventre, D. F., and Grupp, G.: Estimate of myocardial damage induced by diphtheria toxin. J. Lab. Clin. Med. *81*:354, 1973.

LISTERIOSIS

Listeria monocytogenes is becoming more commonly recognized as a cause of both meningoencephalitis and septicemia (listeriosis) in newborn infants and in individuals with modified immunoresponsiveness (malignancy, diabetes mellitus, renal transplantation). The healthy host may also become infected.

ETIOLOGIC AGENT. *Listeria monocytogenes* is the only species of the genus Listeria known to be associated with human disease; of seven known serotypes of *L. monocytogenes* only two (types 1 and 4) are commonly isolated from man. Other types of listeria not yet fully defined may also be pathogenic for man. The organism is a short gram-positive and pleomorphic rod with tumbling motility, noncapsulated, and nonacid-fast. It may be mistaken for diphtheroids, streptococci or diplococci on gram stain, or discarded as a contaminant. It is both a facultative anaerobe and an aerobe, is catalase positive and produces beta hemolysis when grown on blood agar. The isolation rate can be increased by storage of tissue specimens at 4° C for several days prior to inoculation of media.

EPIDEMIOLOGY. Approximately 100 new cases of listeriosis are now being reported annually in the United States, though few infections were being reported prior to the early 1960's. One third of these new cases occur in infants less than 4 weeks of age. Wild and domestic animals and birds may serve as reservoirs, but infection is as common without as with a history of animal exposure. Man may therefore be as significant a reservoir in the urban setting as the animal in the wild. Rarely, spread from one infant to another has been noted. The organism has been found in soil, water, sewage and raw milk; inhalation of infected dust and ingestion of contaminated milk or other contact with fluids of infected animals have been sources of sporadic human diseases. The incidence of human disease seems lowest in the spring. Risk of infection is highest in the newborn period and in the adult over 40 years of age. A human carrier state may exist.

PATHOGENESIS AND PATHOLOGY. Infection with *L. monocytogenes* is intracellular. The mechanism of infection is unknown; neonatal infection is most likely related to transplacental infection of the fetus but may occur during delivery. The outcome of intrauterine exposure is dependent upon the time during pregnancy when the infection occurs; infection in the first and second trimester tends to be associated with fetal loss, and third trimester infection with neonatal meningitis. With blood stream invasion, all organs of the body are involved. When meconium is infected, respiratory infection is common from aspiration.

On pathologic examination, widely disseminated granulomas or micro-abscesses are found, with multiple small foci of necrosis, most commonly in the liver, lungs, spleen, adrenals and brain. The foci characteristically have a minimal amount of peripheral cellular infiltrate. *Listeria monocytogenes* produces a pyogenic meningitis.

CLINICAL MANIFESTATIONS. The clinical expression and the severity of *L. monocytogenes* infection are dependent upon the age of the host and the primary site of localization of the organism. The most severe form of the disease occurs in utero. Pregnancy is invariably shortened, with infection early in pregnancy resulting in abortion; infection later in pregnancy leads to premature delivery, with infection and death of the fetus within the first weeks of life. Maternal illness in the third trimester is usually mild, and listeriosis acquired by a newborn infant from contaminated meconium or by passage through the birth canal is also usually a relatively milder illness. The clinical pattern may be that of isolated meningitis or of severe overwhelming septicemia (*granulomatosis infantiseptica*). Neonatal infection is frequently accompanied by a transitory macular rash over the trunk and legs. Meningoencephalitis is the most common form of listeriosis in most age groups outside the newborn period. It resembles mycobacterial or fungal meningitis. An oculoglandular syndrome may also occur, with keratoconjunctivitis, corneal ulceration and regional adenitis. Meningitis may follow this form of disease. More rarely, skin infection, septicemia and endocarditis may occur. Rarely an asymptomatic carrier state has been found. In certain infants onset of disease occurs late (over 9 days after birth) and cannot be related to a specific exposure. The symptoms are comparable to those above, but the disease may be milder.

DIAGNOSIS. The absence of a history of animal exposure for the mother does not exclude *L. monocytogenes* as a potential cause of neonatal infection. Listeriosis must be considered whenever neonatal sepsis or meningitis is a possibility, and particularly when macular cutaneous lesions are present. A specific diagnosis is made through isolation and identification of this organism from the maternal lochia, or from the infant's meconium, skin lesions, blood or spinal fluid. This requires careful communication with the microbiology laboratory to avoid confusion and loss of isolates; the laboratory should be made aware that *L. monocytogenes* is a possible isolate. A characteristic finding in the peripheral blood is an increase in large mononuclear cells (or atypical lymphocytes), without a rise in titer of heterophil antibody.

Differential Diagnosis. Listerial meningitis is indistinguishable from that due to other bacteria. The atypical lymphocytosis observed in the peripheral blood may also be present in the spinal fluid.

In the newborn period, all conditions presenting as a meningoencephalitis or bacteremia must be differentiated. Except for a maternal history of recurrent fetal loss, there is little to help to identify this specific infection; the diagnosis depends upon isolation of the organism. Toxoplasmosis and infectious mononucleosis produce comparable changes in the peripheral blood but can be differentiated by rises in titer of related antibodies.

COMPLICATIONS. Without specific treatment, recovery is accompanied by marked residua, including mental retardation and hydrocephalus. A chronic form of listerial meningitis has been described.

PROGNOSIS. Antepartum fetal infection is usually associated with a fetal or neonatal mortality greater than 50 per cent. When infection develops later, the mortality is diminished. Early use of appropriate antibiotic therapy may decrease the mortality and minimize the complication rate.

PREVENTION AND TREATMENT. Intrauterine infections can be minimized by avoiding unpasteurized milk during pregnancy. The antibiotic sensitivity of *L. monocytogenes* should be specifically determined for each isolate. Prior to such determination, ampicillin should be used. Though penicillin G, chloramphenicol and tetracycline have been used successfully, ampicillin has the specific advantages of proved greater efficacy than penicillin (more strains are sensitive) and of being less toxic and having greater effectiveness and a lower mortality than either chloramphenicol or tetracycline. The hazard of tetracycline to the teeth contraindicates its use in pregnant women and in children under 8 years of age. If ampicillin is unavailable or if sensitivity testing cannot be performed, penicillin G in a dosage of 300,000 units/kg/day can be given.

Buchner, L. H., and Schneierson, S. S.: Clinical and laboratory aspects of listeria monocytogenes infections. Am. J. Med. *45*:904, 1968.

Lavetter, A., Leedom, M., Mathies, A. W., Jr., Ivler, D., and Wehrle, P.: Meningitis due to Listeria monocytogenes. A review of 25 cases. New Engl. J. Med. *285*:598, 1971.

Medoff, G., Kunz, L. J., and Weinberg, A. N.: Listeriosis in humans: An evaluation. J. Infect. Dis. *123*:247, 1971.

Ray, C. J., and Wedgwood, R. J.: Neonatal listeriosis: Six case reports and a review of the literature. Pediatrics *34*:378, 1964.

Zoonoses Surveillance, Listeriosis, Annual Summary 1971. Atlanta, Georgia, Center for Disease Control, 1972.

TETANUS

(Lockjaw)

Tetanus is a central nervous system disease produced by infection with the anaerobic spore-forming bacterium *Clostridium tetani.* It results from an exotoxin (tetanospasmin) produced by the organism at the point of entry into the body, with the subsequent transport and fixation of the neurotoxin in the nervous system.

ETIOLOGIC AGENT. *Clostridium tetani* is an obligate anaerobe which occurs in both vegetative and spore forms. It is a motile, nonencapsulated gram-positive bacillus found in soil, dust, water and the intestinal tracts of men and animals. In its sporulating form it is moderately resistant to disinfectants and to boiling, but is killed by ethylene oxide and autoclaving.

EPIDEMIOLOGY. *Clostridium tetani* and tetanus occur world-wide. The local incidences and expressions of the disease vary with several factors, such as regional differences in immunization practices and/or application of contaminated poultices to umbilical stumps or to vaccination sites. Tetanus most frequently occurs in unimmunized individuals, such as newborn infants delivered in contaminated environments, or among deprived populations. Wound contamination by soil is a frequent source of infection; the incidence of disease is greatest in the months of outdoor activity. In the United States, the incidence in children is highest in the southeast, and in boys.

PATHOGENESIS. Several conditions must be met for disease to be produced by *C. tetani.* These include a susceptible host, contact with the organism and an appropriate anaerobic environment. The newborn infant of an unimmunized mother, and the unimmunized child, are particularly susceptible to infection. Contamination of the umbilical cord is the usual source of infection in newborn infants. In the older child the introduction of the organism usually occurs at the time of a traumatic wound, perhaps trivial or even inapparent. Insect bites, wounds produced by contaminated surgical catgut and mucosal points (eyes, tonsils, intestinal tract) have also been described as portals of entry. The risk of tetanus infection is greatest in those wounds with tissue necrosis, those caused by puncture and those in which foreign bodies have been retained. Infections produced by aerobic bacteria may occasionally produce sufficient tissue destruction so that favorable conditions occur for growth of *C. tetani.* A history of contamination may not be obtained; survival and persistence in normal tissue of *C. tetani* spores introduced at time of injury may account for infection under such circumstances.

With local growth of *C. tetani,* production of the neurotoxin, tetanospasmin, occurs. Other toxins are also produced but are of no apparent significance in human disease. Tetanospasmin gains access to the central nervous system by either vascular or neural routes; toxin may be transferred by the lymphatics to the blood and then transported to the central nervous system, or it may be absorbed locally at the myoneural junctions, migrating via nerve trunks and their lymphatics to the brain and spinal cord. In the central nervous system the neurotoxin attaches to a ganglioside, producing hypertonicity and spasm similar to that seen with strychnine poisoning. Once bound to central nervous tissue, tetanospasmin is unaffected by antitoxin. Antitoxin does not prevent germination of *C. tetani* spores nor multiplication of the organisms in tissue. If binding has occurred only peripherally, antitoxin may still prevent binding in the central nervous system.

Additional neurovascular effects of tetanospasmin are suspected, but are as yet poorly defined in the pathogenesis of tetanus.

PATHOLOGY. There is a minimal cellular response to infections with *C. tetani.* Infection tends to remain localized, as the organism is not invasive. Pathologic changes result only from the effects of the primary injury and from toxic changes in the anterior horn cells of the spinal cord.

CLINICAL MANIFESTATIONS. The incubation period for *C. tetani* is generally 5 to 12 days, but depends upon the severity of the infection or the previous use of antitoxin. Mild or modified infections may have an incubation period as long as 50 days.

If the infection has been modified but there has been neural binding of toxin at the motor end-plates of muscles in the vicinity of a wound, the clinical manifestations will be restricted to the involved area; local pain and regional increase in muscle tone and spasm will be present without systemic findings.

More frequently, generalized involvement occurs in tetanus. The onset is usually insidious, heralded by stiffness of muscles in the jaw or neck. Spasm of the masseter muscle produces difficulty in opening the mouth (*trismus* or *lockjaw*) and difficulty in swallowing. Headache, increasing irritability and restlessness occur as nonspecific early symptoms. With progression of the disease, spasm of other muscle groups develops. Spasms of the muscles of the cheeks draw the perioral tissues up to produce a peculiar fixed sardonic grin (*risus sardonicus*). Opisthotonos develops, with spasm of the neck, back and extremity muscles. The abdominal wall becomes rigid. Apprehension is a prominent feature, as the sensorium remains clear. Spasms, which initially are of short duration with effective relaxation between episodes, become more frequent, prolonged and painful. The forcefulness of the contractions may produce intramuscular hemorrhage or compression fractures of the spine. Spasm of the respiratory and laryngeal muscles may produce respiratory obstruction and laryngospasm, with cyanosis and asphyxia. Urinary retention occurs with bladder sphincter spasm; on the other hand, relaxation of spasms of bladder and intestinal sphincters may produce involuntary urination and defecation. A generalized convulsive spasm of several minutes' duration may be precipitated by very minor auditory, tactile and visual stimuli such as turning of the patient, offering the patient a drink, or the switching on of lights.

The temperature is usually only mildly elevated in tetanus. Circulatory disturbances have recently been described as occurring early in the course of the disease, and consist of tachycardia, dysrhythmia, an elevated blood pressure and a shift in body fluids from the vascular to the interstitial spaces. There may be a mild polymorphonuclear leukocytosis. The cerebrospinal fluid is normal except for a slight increase in pressure owing to muscle contractions.

Neonatal tetanus is of the generalized type, presenting most often with progressive difficulty in sucking, which may begin as early as the third day of life.

DIAGNOSIS. The diagnosis of tetanus is made on clinical grounds and is not difficult except in infancy. Development of the various degrees and patterns of muscle spasm in an unimmunized person with clear sensorium following a wound, or in a newborn infant after a contaminated delivery, is highly suggestive of tetanus. Isolation of the organism in anaerobic culture of appropriately collected material is confirmatory, but is found in only one third of instances. In the absence of the clinical syndrome, isolation of *C. tetani* is not diagnostic of tetanus.

Differential Diagnosis. Both local conditions and other systemic illnesses must be differentiated. Local infection in the jaw or throat may produce a local muscular stiffness which can be confused with trismus but can be differentiated by physical examination and roentgenograms. The stiffness or spasm of early *poliomyelitis* can be differentiated by asymmetrical flaccid paralysis and the absence of trismus. In addition, in the child with poliomyelitis pleocytosis and an increase in protein in spinal fluid and/or isolation of poliovirus are usually found. Other forms of *viral meningitis* and *encephalitis* are not associated with trismus. The sensorium is clouded in encephalitis. Both *rabies* and tetanus may follow an animal bite, and they may be difficult to differentiate because trismus may be present in both conditions. Rabies tends to have intermittent clonic seizures and may have spinal fluid pleocytosis. Bacterial *meningitis* is seldom confused because there are obvious changes in the spinal fluid. In *strychnine poisoning*, trismus is less common and occurs after the rapid development of generalized tonic activity. A history of ingestion of poisons containing strychnine may be helpful. *Tetany* may be confirmed by a low level of calcium in serum. Intestinal obstruction, perforation and peritonitis may all be the sources of tetanus infections; abdominal rigidity in these conditions must be differentiated from the board-like abdomen of tetanus. The absence of a more diffuse pattern of muscle spasm should differentiate these conditions.

COMPLICATIONS. The frequency and type of complications of tetanus are determined by the age of the patient, the quality of supportive nursing care and the effectiveness of specific therapeutic efforts. Pulmonary complications follow aspiration or tracheostomy and include aspiration pneumonia, atelectasis, pneumothorax and mediastinal emphysema. Respiratory obstruction may result in asphyxia. Severe seizures may produce oral lacerations, intramuscular hematomas, and thoracic vertebral fractures. Fluid and electrolyte complications and malnutrition may develop. The use of heterologous serum antitoxin may be associated with serum sickness or anaphylaxis.

PROGNOSIS. Survival in tetanus after the newborn period has been improved by the application of newer supportive techniques. Neonatal mortality is still above 60 per cent; mortality is lowest for the 10 to 19 year age group (less than 20 per cent). Since recovery in patients surviving tetanus is complete, certain determinants for survival can be delineated. In addition to the age of the patient, the number of days required for the clinical manifestations to appear, the extent of muscle involvement and the height of fever correlate with survival. Regional tetanus and slow progression (over 3 days) of generalized muscle spasm to the onset of generalized convulsions are associated with a better prognosis. The prognosis is poorer if the temperature rises above 38.9° C. Fatalities usually occur during the first week in severe cases.

PREVENTION. The prevention of tetanus can best be accomplished by aseptic delivery of infants and by the administration of tetanus toxoid as part of programs of routine health maintenance. The efficacy of active immunization before exposure has been well demonstrated, and is best accomplished with a basic series of three intramuscular injections of a combined vaccine of tetanus toxoid, diphtheria toxoid and pertussis vaccine. The injections are given at 4- to 6-week intervals between 1 and 6 months of age, with booster doses at 1 and 4 years of age. This approach may be modified to meet local needs. In areas where the incidence of neonatal tetanus is high, immunization of nonimmune pregnant mothers will provide the fetus with adequate protection after delivery. Tetanus toxoid which has been alum-precipitated or aluminum hydroxide-adsorbed should be used for immunization prior to exposure, where the need is for suitable duration of antigenic effect. The duration of protection with active immunization is unknown but suspected to be as long as 30 years; adequate recall occurs if a routine booster dose is given every 10 years. Levels of tetanus antitoxin in serum of 0.01 IU/ml by the toxin neutralization assay are protective; hemagglutination titers also measure antibody, but in certain sera these titers do not correlate with the neutralization assay and should not, therefore, be used to set criteria for immunization, either active or passive.

Preventive measures following injury should be tailored to the specific situation and based on immunization status and the circumstances and characteristics of the injury. Specific prophylactic modalities available for use following trauma include fluid tetanus toxoid and human tetanus immune globulin (TIG); equine and bovine antitoxin preparations are also available, but TIG is to be preferred. Fluid toxoid produces a much more rapid secondary immune response than precipitated or adsorbed tetanus toxoids and is the agent of choice for booster injections after serious injury in children who have completed a series of at least four DPT injections. Since protective levels of antibody are maintained for at least 5 years, booster injection (for injury) need not be given more frequently. If the immunization status is incomplete, it may be completed. Frequently repeated injections of tetanus toxoid for minor injuries during childhood and early adulthood have led to hyperimmunization; immediate and delayed types of allergic reactions occur, including severe urticarial, anaphylactic and Arthus reactions.

The choice between fluid toxoid and TIG to protect against tetanus is dependent on the circumstances and the characteristics of the injury. In "tetanus prone" injuries (compound fractures, burns, crush injuries, wounds with retained foreign bodies, puncture wounds, wounds contaminated by barnyard or garden soil, or wounds unattended for over 24 hours), surgical treatment is carried out; 250 to 500 mg of TIG is given intramuscularly to the unimmunized or the inadequately immunized patient (less than two prior injections of tetanus toxoid). The half-life of TIG is two to three times greater than that of horse serum antitoxin and the dose is correspondingly reduced. TIG does not produce serum sickness; skin testing prior to injection is unnecessary. The objective is to prevent tetanus or to modify inevitable disease. If TIG is not available, 3000 to 5000 units of horse or bovine tetanus antitoxin (TAT) may be used, with appropriate precautions. Tetanus toxoid should be given to initiate active immunity; it may be given simultaneously in another site in a separate syringe to avoid interference with TIG or TAT. Prophylactic TIG or TAT is never indicated for wounds in fully immunized children.

TREATMENT. Therapy of tetanus must include administration of specific antitoxin, antibiotics and nonspecific measures including surgery, the control of muscular spasms and the use of tracheostomy and other supportive care.

The most specific agent is antitoxin. Intramuscular administration of 3000 to 6000 units of tetanus immune globulin (TIG) is presently recommended, with part of the dose to be infiltrated locally at the site of injury. TIG, like other gamma globulin, should not be given intravenously. If TIG is unavailable, TAT can be administered (after skin testing shows no hypersensitivity) in a single dose of 50,000 to 100,000 units, divided equally into intramuscular and intravenous injections. If sensitization to the animal serum exists, rapid desensitization may be undertaken. (See Diphtheria.) Antitoxin does not reverse the effects of bound toxin but is given to neutralize any circulating neurotoxin which is not yet fixed to tissue. Antitoxin does not penetrate the blood-brain barrier.

Antibiotic therapy terminates the production of neurotoxin only indirectly, as it controls the proliferation of the vegetative form of the organism at the site of infection. Aqueous penicillin G (600,000 units) may be used intravenously every 4 hours for 10 days. In patients sensitive to penicillin, tetracycline is effective.

Surgery reduces the number of proliferating organisms by eliminating conditions favorable to growth of clostridia, but surgery should not be undertaken until efforts have been made to control muscle spasms. An absolutely quiet environment is ideal for care of the patient with tetanus. Effort should be made to control or eliminate all stimulation from light or sound. Sedation and muscle relaxation should be attempted. Administration of *d*-tubocurarine to the point of respiratory paralysis, with artificial ventilation, has produced the best survival rates. This technique requires a skilled team. Diazepam is more readily available to less specialized centers for control of hypertonicity and spasms in less severe disease; it may be used intramuscularly or intravenously in a dose of 0.2 mg/kg every 3 to 5 hours as needed. Chlorpromazine and mephenesin have also been utilized but do not have the advantage of diazepam. Two to 6 weeks of muscle relaxant therapy may be required. Tracheostomy is often indicated and is best done prior to the development of severe involvement of respiratory muscles or of laryngospasm, before it becomes an emergency procedure. A gastrostomy may be indicated for feeding.

Once convalescence begins, active tetanus immunization should be undertaken with toxoid, since no permanent immunity results from *C. tetani* infection.

Brooks, V. B., Curtis, D. R., and Eccles, J. C.: Mode of action of tetanus toxin. Nature (London) *175*:120, 1955.

Burnett, J. V.: Tetanus. *In* Hoeprich, P. D. (ed.): Infectious Disease—A Guide to the Understanding and Management of Infectious Processes. New York, Harper & Row, 1972, Chapter 114.

Edsall, G., Elliott, M. W., Peebles, T. C., Levine, L., and Eldred, M. C.: Excessive use of tetanus toxoid boosters. J.A.M.A. *202*:111, 1967.

Klingler, H.: Tetanus of the newborn. J.A.M.A. *218*:1437, 1971.

Stanfield, J. P., Gall, D., and Bracken, P. M.: Single dose antenatal tetanus immunization. Lancet *1*:215, 1973.

Young, L. S., LaForce, F. M., and Bennett, J. V.: An evaluation of serologic and antimicrobial therapy in the treatment of tetanus in the United States. J. Infect. Dis. *120*:153, 1969.

INFECTION DUE TO CLOSTRIDIAL SPECIES

(Gas Gangrene, Food Poisoning and Necrotizing Enteritis)

Gas gangrene is caused by several species of Clostridia, usually as a complication of trauma or surgery which results in a necrotizing infection.

ETIOLOGIC AGENT. Gas gangrene is caused by certain members of the genus *Clostridium.* These bacteria are all anaerobic gram-positive bacilli. *Clostridium perfringens* is capsulated and nonmotile, whereas the remaining members of this group *(C. novyi, C. septicum, C. welchii)* are noncapsulated and motile. They exist in vegetative and spore forms. Vegetative forms produce powerful necrotizing exotoxins. The spores are extremely resistant to physical and chemical agents.

EPIDEMIOLOGY. Spores occur normally in soil, in the gastrointestinal tract and in the female genital tract. Infection has followed injections through improperly prepared skin.

PATHOGENESIS AND PATHOLOGY. Anaerobic conditions are required for growth of these bacteria; anaerobiosis is enhanced by toxic destruction of tissue after initial infection has been established. Affected tissues characteristically contain gas and are crepitant, owing to the production of CO_2 by the metabolizing organisms.

CLINICAL MANIFESTATIONS. Three syndromes are associated with *C. perfringens* infection: gas gangrene (or clostridial myositis), food poisoning and necrotic enteritis. Most common is *gas gangrene,* which may occur as anaerobic cellulitis, myositis or puerperal sepsis. Myositis is the most severe and follows infection in a heavily contaminated wound which has been inadequately debrided. Severe edema and pain occur, with discoloration and crepitation. Septicemia or toxemia may occur, with hemolytic anemia due to the toxin. Uterine infections may follow prolonged labor or instrumentation. Gas gangrene may progress to shock, renal failure and death.

Food poisoning may also be associated with *C. perfringens* infection. Sudden onset of illness occurs after an 8- to 22-hour incubation period, with nausea, vomiting and acute abdominal pain. Recovery is prompt.

Necrotic enteritis is marked by acute gangrene in the region of the jejunum and adjacent small bowel and has a high mortality.

Clostridium septicum has produced gas gangrene in patients with malignancies.

DIAGNOSIS. A rapid clinical diagnosis must be made in lieu of bacteriologic findings, owing to the gravity of this infection. Diagnosis is suggested by a contaminated injury or operation, rapidly spreading discoloration of a crepitant edematous wound, intense pain and changing affect of the patient. Roentgenographic evidence of gas in soft tissues or in the abdomen is confirmatory. Cultures may subsequently be positive for *Clostridium* sp.

Differential Diagnosis. Massive bullae may be observed with streptococcal gangrene, but crepitation or other evidence of gas formation is absent. Bacteroides infections may also form gas, but are not associated with gangrene.

PROGNOSIS. Untreated clostridial infections are fatal. With treatment, the mortality is 20 per cent.

PREVENTION AND TREATMENT. Early and adequate surgical debridement will eliminate suitable growth conditions for these organisms. High dose antibiotic therapy (penicillin G 150,000 units/kg/day intravenously in 4 doses) should be administered until there is clinical improvement. A polyvalent gas gangrene antitoxin is available as horse serum; the usual precautions are required against anaphylaxis. Its use is not necessary with adequate surgical and antimicrobial therapy and many experts question its value. Hyperbaric oxygen therapy may be helpful in conjunction with standard management.

Alpern, R. J., and Dowell, V. R., Jr.: Clostridium septicum infections and malignancy. J.A.M.A. *209*:385, 1969.

Altemeier, W. A., and Fullen, W. D.: Prevention and treatment of gas gangrene. J.A.M.A. *217*:806, 1971.

Lambertsen, C. J.: Oxygen in the therapy of gas gangrene. J. Trauma *12*:825, 1972.

Mackay, N. S., Grüneberg, R. N., Harries, B. J., and Thomas, P. K.: Primary Clostridium welchii meningitis. Brit. Med. J. *1*:591, 1971.

Morgan, T. H., and Chiu, S. H.: Gas gangrene of the extremities. Maryland Med. J. *22*:52, 1973.

Rifkind, D.: The diagnosis and treatment of gas gangrene. Surg. Clin. N. Amer. *43*:511, 1963.

OTHER ANAEROBIC INFECTIONS

Nonclostridial anaerobic bacteria are frequently overlooked as causes of infectious syndromes in infants and children, partially because of the relative ease with which aerobic bacteria can be identified and in spite of the overwhelming prevalence of

TABLE 10–7 MORPHOLOGIC CHARACTERISTICS OF ANAEROBIC ORGANISMS

	GRAM-POSITIVE	GRAM-NEGATIVE
Cocci	Microaerophilic streptococci	Veillonella
	Peptococcus	
	Peptostreptococcus	
Bacilli	Actinomyces	Bacteroides sp.
	Bifidobacterium	Fusobacterium
	Clostridium sp.	Sphaerophorus
	Eubacterium	Vibrio
	Propionibacterium	

anaerobic bacteria in normal flora. The association of anaerobic organisms with infectious states of significant mortality and morbidity emphasizes the need for increased clinical awareness of these bacteria as potential causes of serious pediatric disease.

ETIOLOGIC AGENTS. Anaerobes are microorganisms that grow only in the absence of molecular oxygen. In clinical terminology, however, "anaerobe" also refers to facultative anaerobes which can grow both with and without molecular oxygen.

The obligate anaerobes of clinical importance belong to the family Bacteroidaceae and include a variety of morphologic forms: gram-positive nonspore-forming bacilli (e.g., *Propionibacterium acnes*); gram-negative nonspore-forming bacilli (e.g., *Bacteroides fragilis*); gram-positive spore-forming bacilli (e.g., *Clostridium perfringens*); gram-positive cocci (e.g., *Peptostreptococcus* sp.); and gram-negative cocci (e.g., Veillonella) (Table 10–7).

Anaerobes are among the most primitive of microbial species and are found in the normal microflora of the skin and the respiratory, gastrointestinal and genitourinary tracts. They are opportunistic organisms whose capacity to produce infection is limited by their own characteristics (low virulence) and by the presence of nonanaerobic members of the microflora. Their numbers greatly exceed those of the aerobic bacteria in the normal flora (e.g., 10:1 in the skin, mouth and vagina and 1000:1 in the colon).

PATHOGENESIS. Anaerobic bacteria are of low pathogenicity unless extrinsic conditions are favorable for their growth, multiplication and invasion or dissemination. Local anoxia, absence of inhibitory nonanaerobic flora and abnormal communications between the respiratory or gastrointestinal tracts and other body compartments all contribute to the conversion of these normally innocuous bacteria from a saprophytic existence to a pathogenic one. Local extension with the production of focal lesions may occur in the brain following trauma, chronic otitis media or sinusitis; beneath the diaphragm as a subphrenic abscess; or as a complication of a preceding infection with another agent (trench mouth). Pulmonary lesions occur most commonly after aspiration of stomach or oral contents, or distal to inhaled foreign bodies which remain undiagnosed for extended periods of time. Neonatal infection occurs most commonly after prolonged rupture of maternal membranes, with pulmonary or blood stream invasion. Bacteremia is one of the most common forms of anaerobic infection and leads to infection in many organs.

PATHOLOGY. Anaerobic infection results in marked and widespread tissue destruction and abscess formation, modified in accordance with the route of infection and the organ system involved. Unifocal infection results most commonly by direct extension from local lesions, whereas septic emboli produce more diffuse disease. Generally, infection is followed rapidly by congestion, edema and a marked neutrophilic infiltration and progresses to liquefaction necrosis; in the lung this process may be surrounded by a wall of granulation tissue and a wide zone of consolidation. Both alveolar and bronchial tissues are destroyed, and extension may proceed in an interlobar manner. Lung parenchyma becomes friable and abscesses are produced.

CLINICAL MANIFESTATIONS. Factors predisposing to infection can be identified in most instances of anaerobic infection. Trauma productive of extensive tissue destruction, human or animal bites, surgery accompanied by leakage of bowel contents, malnutrition and retained pulmonary or genitourinary foreign bodies may be associated with the introduction of appropriate circumstances for propagation of these bacteria.

Infections produced by anaerobic organisms may occur in any part of the body; ears, nose, throat, bones and joints, and the respiratory, cardiovascular, genitourinary and central nervous systems are among the common sites.

Oral infections usually involve the periodontium or mucous membranes. Poor dental hygiene and malocclusion contribute to a favorable anaerobic environment deep in the periodontal tissues. Fetid oral odor is noted, along with edematous gum tissue, a purulent, foul-smelling periodontal exudate and pain on chewing. Ultimately periapical abscesses may develop, with severe pain and with intensely edematous tissue at the base of the teeth in the gingival sulcus.

Anaerobic infections of the ears, nose and throat are less commonly seen owing to early use of antibiotics in these conditions. These infections are a potential source of extension to the nervous system. In the nervous system a focal lesion or abscess may occur adjacent to the site of entry. If septic emboli or bacteremia has occurred, more diffuse disease is common, with multiple abscesses or meningitis. Symptoms depend upon the extent and the type of the central nervous system involvement. (See Brain Abscess and Meningitis.)

Infectious arthritis or chronic osteomyelitis, primarily of the long bones, may result from bacteremic spread or be secondary to compound, contaminated fractures.

Blood stream invasion by anaerobic organisms accounts for a significant and increasing percentage of gram-negative bacteremias. Bacteremia may occur following alteration of the normal flora of the intestinal or genitourinary tracts by use of antibiotics not effective against the anaerobe, or during adrenal corticosteroid therapy. Less commonly, anaerobic bacteremia may be associated with pulmonary, oropharyngeal and sinus infections.

Abdominal anaerobic infection occurs most frequently with appendicitis, with or without peritonitis. Abscesses of the liver or subphrenic abscesses may occur.

Since *pregnancy* may predispose to infection of the genital tract with anaerobic organisms, the fetus is at risk following premature rupture of the membranes and prolonged labor. Anaerobic infections in the mother may occur after a postpartum hemorrhage or abortion. A small percentage of urinary tract infections are caused by anaerobes and follow either bacteremia or the introduction of indigenous urethral flora by urologic instrumentation.

DIAGNOSIS. The diagnosis of anaerobic infection is predicated upon awareness of the possibility of its existence. This awareness should be heightened by consideration of an infectious illness with a subacute or chronic course. Predisposing circumstances may exist, such as: seizures, with potential aspiration of vomitus or foreign body; bronchiectasis; severe dental caries or periodontal disease; retained foreign bodies; especially following trauma, puncture wounds, surgery or insertion of foreign bodies into the nose, ears or vagina; human or animal bites; or gastrointestinal surgery or trauma. With tissue necrosis there is often a foul odor.

Anaerobic flora are normally present in many specimens. Accordingly, the significance of anaerobes isolated from expectorated sputum, tracheal intubation or bronchoscopically collected specimens is difficult to evaluate, whereas isolates from blood or from pleural or empyema fluid can be appropriately interpreted. Needle aspiration of wounds, abscesses or bladder is the most acceptable means by which adequate specimens for anaerobic culture can be collected. Material for anaerobic culture should remain in a container unexposed to air (e.g., a syringe) or should be placed in thioglycollate medium immediately after collection. A clue to the presence of anaerobic bacteria is the identification of bacterial organisms on gram-stained smears, with failure of growth to occur from the same specimen upon routine aerobic culturing. Many clinical laboratories are not adequately equipped to search for anaerobic bacteria. Since blood cultures are routinely planted in anaerobic as well as aerobic media in most laboratories, they are one of the most effective means of culturing for anaerobes. Blood cultures are most useful in diagnosing anaerobic bacteremia, liver abscesses or abdominal abscesses, but may also be positive in anaerobic pulmonary infections.

Differential Diagnosis. A possibly anaerobic etiology should be considered whenever any of the following clinical entities are being evaluated: abscesses of the brain, lung, liver or breast; intra-abdominal (subphrenic) abscess; chronic otitis media or otogenic meningitis; empyema of the spaces surrounding the brain (extradural or subdural) or lung; pneumonia associated with aspiration or obstruction by a foreign body; sepsis at or following delivery, or endocarditis; dental and soft tissue infections; appendicitis or peritonitis.

PROGNOSIS. If undiagnosed and untreated, anaerobic infections are associated with a high mortality, which varies with the type and cause of the infection. Even with adequate treatment, mortality may approximate 15 per cent. *Bacteroides* bacteremia has the highest mortality. When there is extensive tissue necrosis, infection may persist for several months and ultimately end fatally. The duration of illness seems related to the nature of any underlying disease as well as to the number of anaerobic foci, a shorter illness generally being associated with a single focus or with few foci.

TREATMENT. In anaerobic infections, treatment must be specific and prolonged if morbidity, complications, relapses and mortality are to be minimized. Identification of the organism and of its antibiotic sensitivity pattern are often delayed, however, because of the slow growth and the special techniques required for anaerobic bacteria. In such instances, empiric selection of antibiotics is appropriate, in accordance with knowledge of which strains of anaerobic organisms are likely associated with infections in various sites.

In general, respiratory tract anaerobes are susceptible to penicillin G, whereas anaerobes from the gastrointestinal tract are resistant. On the other hand, most anaerobes, regardless of source, are resistant to several of the more commonly employed antimicrobials such as the aminoglycosides (e.g., kanamycin or gentamicin). Effective agents include one or more of the following: ampicillin, cephalothin, chloramphenicol, erythromycin, clindamycin and carbenicillin. Because increasing numbers of strains are resistant to tetracycline, its use is no longer indicated without laboratory evidence that it may be effective.

In most situations a combination of penicillin and chloramphenicol would be the most appropriate initial regimen. Clindamycin has recently proved very effective and may supplant penicillin G as the drug of choice in infections with anaerobic bacteria. Clindamycin should not, however, replace chloramphenicol for treatment of anaerobic brain abscess since it does not penetrate the blood-brain barrier.

Penicillin G is effective against all anaerobes except *Bacteroides fragilis* and certain fusobacteria. Ampicillin and cephalothin are comparable to penicillin G in efficacy. Chloramphenicol is best suited for *B. fragilis* but may be replaced by clindamycin except in infections of the central nervous system. Erythromycin is very effective against the anaerobic coccal agents. The dosage of these antibiotics is comparable to that used for the treatment of aerobic infections.

For mixed aerobic/anaerobic infections, a combination of clindamycin or chloramphenicol with gentamicin or kanamycin would appear appropriate.

VINCENT A. FULGINITI
OTTO F. SIEBER, JR.

Braude, A. K.: Anaerobic infection: Diagnosis and therapy. Hosp. Pract. *3*:42, 1968.
Gelb, A. F., and Seligman, S. J.: Bacteroidaceae bacteremia: Effect of age and focus of infection upon clinical course. J.A.M.A. *212*:1038, 1970.
Sanders, D. Y., and Stevenson, J.: Bacteroides infections in children. J. Pediatr. *72*:673, 1968.

TUBERCULOSIS

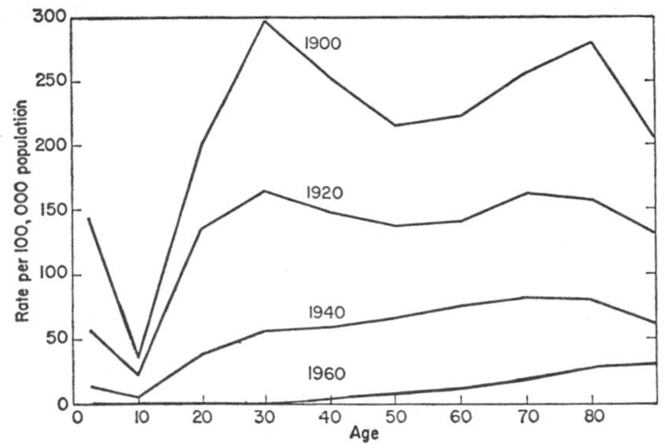

Figure 10–7 *Tuberculosis death rates by age, United States, 1900–1960 (Expanding Death Registration States). (Department of Health, Education, and Welfare, Public Health Service, Center for Disease Control, Tuberculosis Program, Atlanta, Georgia.)*

Tuberculosis has a uniquely important place in medical history. It has at all times been a main cause of illness and of death in all climates. It was one of the first diseases to elicit widespread organized public health efforts, and the degree of control attained has proved the value of detection and isolation of infected persons. It stands as the prototype of infections which exist in man most often without causing significant disease and yet capable of producing both acute and chronic disease patterns of sufficient seriousness to be one of the leading causes of death.

The steady decrease in death rates at all ages for many years (Figs. 10–7, 10–8) is evidence of gain in the battle with the tubercle bacillus. Only in recent years can credit be given to specific antimicrobial agents. It is essential to know by what means these gains have been made and to recognize that in our improving health situation, tuberculosis still remains a serious problem, demanding the common efforts of public health measures and medical therapy.

ETIOLOGY. Koch demonstrated in 1882 that tuberculosis is caused by the acid-fast bacillus *Mycobacterium tuberculosis.* Subsequently Smith showed that disease could be produced in man by bovine and human tubercle bacilli. (See also Other Mycobacterial Infections, below).

The tubercle bacillus does not contain or produce any chemical constituent which has measurable

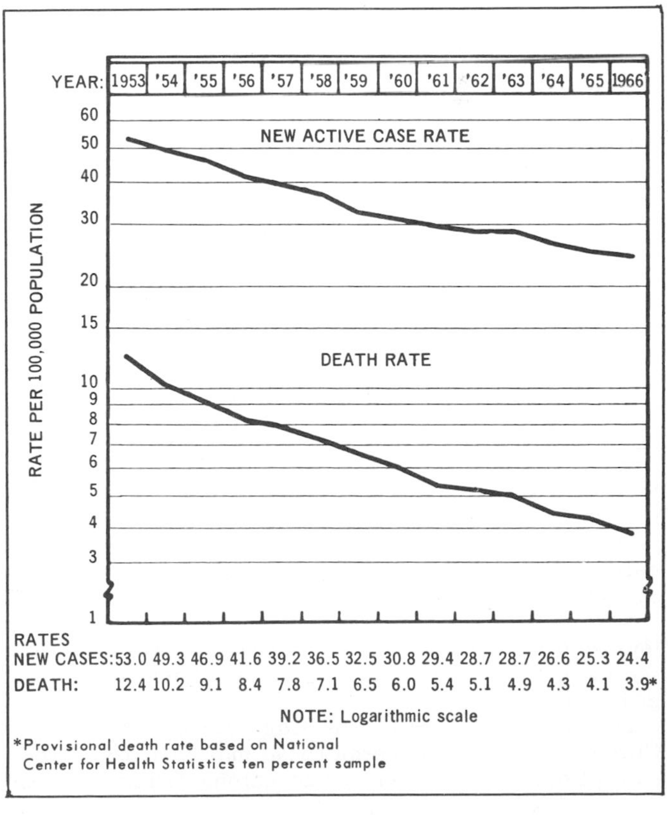

Figure 10–8 *New active tuberculosis case rate and death rate, United States, 1953–1966. (United States Department of Health, Education, and Welfare, Public Health Service, Bureau of Disease Prevention and Environmental Control, Center for Disease Control, Tuberculosis Program, Atlanta, Georgia.)*

toxicity for tissues not sensitized to tuberculin; its tissue-necrotizing capacity exists in the protein fraction. The lipids of the tubercle bacillus give it the property of acid-fastness and appear to be a factor in the production of fibrosis as well as in the formation of epithelioid cells and tubercles.

EPIDEMIOLOGY. The exact incidence of tuberculosis is not known. Evidence of its frequency is limited to surveys using the tuberculin test, roentgenographic films, clinical recognition of the disease and examination of autopsy material. Data indicate that the incidence of infection is declining throughout the world and in general is lowest in populations with high living standards. In all areas the incidence of tuberculous infection increases with age and is generally higher in urban than in rural areas.

PREDISPOSING FACTORS. The introduction of tubercle bacilli into the human body is not invariably followed by the development of significant disease. Certain persons have greater resistance to infection than others, and the resistance of a given person may vary from time to time.

Factors related to the tubercle bacillus which may affect the establishment of disease are principally of two orders: the relative virulence of the invading organisms and the number of organisms in the inoculum. There are distinct differences in the virulence of various strains of tubercle bacilli; strains of low virulence are rarely encountered in human infections.

Heredity. There is no evidence of an inherited tendency to tuberculous infection. Differences in constitutional patterns do, however, appear to influence resistance to disease. Animals of the same species vary in degree of resistance, and by selective breeding increased capacity for resistance can be transferred to offspring. The question in man is not so simply answered.

Differences in immunity among ethnic groups are not well defined. There is a higher mortality rate from tuberculosis in the United States among the nonwhite population, and especially among American Indians, than among the white, but much of this difference can be attributed to hygienic and environmental factors, such as poor housing conditions and opportunities for frequent reinfection from ambulatory patients.

Congenital or intrauterine infection occurs infrequently and is probably secondary to infection of the placenta.

Age. Age is a factor in resistance to tuberculous infection, the fatality rate being higher during infancy and adolescence than in the intervening years of childhood. There are also differences in the nature of the lesion which is initiated at various age levels. These are described under Pathology.

Sex. Sex appears to be a factor only in the latter part of childhood and during adolescence, when the morbidity and mortality rates are higher in girls than in boys.

Temporary Factors Affecting Resistance. Chronic illness and undernutrition may increase susceptibility to infection, as may chronic fatigue. Acute nontuberculous infections may activate a quiescent tuberculous lesion.

ALLERGY AND IMMUNITY. Two to 10 weeks after infection of a previously tuberculin-negative person with tubercle bacilli an allergic reaction can be demonstrated on intracutaneous injection of tuberculin. With the development of allergy there is an alteration in the host response to tubercle bacilli, evidenced by exudation and a tendency to localize the infection. Certain other immune reactions also develop which are neither complete nor as adequately measured as in some other infections. Immunity is not complete; it may be sufficient to protect against moderate infections, but not against large numbers of invading bacilli nor against those of exceptionally high virulence.

The relationship between allergy and immunity in tuberculosis is controversial. It is variously held (1) that they are related and perhaps identical, (2) that they are entirely separate phenomena, or (3) that they are opposing forces. The degree of hypersensitivity may be important; moderate degrees of hypersensitivity appear to be effective in localizing the lesion and in bringing the phagocytic cells in contact with the bacteria more quickly, whereas greater hypersensitivity is responsible for such extensive destruction of tissue that spread of the infection may be increased by it.

PATHOGENESIS. Inhalation and, to a lesser extent, ingestion are the principal routes by which tubercle bacilli gain entrance to the body. Infection through the intact skin probably does not occur, but infections may be acquired in open wounds and through inapparent abrasions, and have been transmitted by a human bite. Direct blood stream infection is a practical possibility only in placental transmission.

PATHOLOGY. The responses of infants and small children to tuberculous infection differ in certain respects from those of older children and adults. There is, however, a good deal of overlapping; lesions which have the characteristics of the "childhood type" are seen on occasion in adults, and the "adult" type of infection may occur in children, especially in the latter part of childhood.

In general, the age differences are as follows: (1) Though the pulmonary lesion in infants and children may be in any part of the lung, it has a tendency to be peripheral. The site is more likely to be in the lower than in the upper part of the lungs. By contrast, in adolescents and adults there is a predilection for localization of the lesion either in the apical region or just below it in the infraclavicular area. (2) The regional lymph nodes are more often involved in infants and children than in adolescents and adults. Initial infections in adults usually show little or no evidence of extensive involvement of the lymph nodes. (3) Both the parenchymal and nodal lesions in children exhibit a strong tendency to heal by calcification, whereas in adults the tendency is to heal by fibrosis. (4) Hematogenous dissemination is much more likely to occur in infants than in older children. Miliary tuberculosis and tuberculous meningitis occur with much greater frequency in the first few years of life than later.

At the site of the initial focus, e.g., in the parenchyma of the lung, there is at first an accumulation of polymorphonuclear leukocytes. This reaction is temporary and is followed by proliferation of epithelioid cells which surround the tubercle bacilli, forming the typical tubercle. Tubercles are usually surrounded by an accumulation of lymphocytes, and giant cells are usually present. The tubercles may remain discrete or may become confluent; central caseous necrosis is commonly present. Foci of the primary infection vary considerably in size, but the majority apparently remain small (1 cm or so in diameter). There is often only a single primary focus.

Lymph node involvement is an almost constant accompaniment of the initial parenchymal lesion in children. Lymph node involvement has generally been considered characteristic of the initial lesion of tuberculosis and not to occur with the lesion of reinfection. This concept does not appear to be wholly correct. Evidence suggests that the extent of involvement of regional lymph nodes is determined in part by age-related factors, being less with increasing age. The nodes become enlarged, often matted together, and tend to adhere to adjacent structures. In the mediastinum they may exert pressure on the trachea, bronchi or blood vessels, and at times rupture into them (Fig. 10–9).

The tendency of the primary lesions both in the parenchyma and in the lymph nodes is toward healing in the majority of instances. There are, however, three mechanisms by which the primary infection may be responsible for serious damage during its active phase: (1) progressive destruction at its initial site; (2) erosion of a bronchus with intrabronchial dissemination and the formation of other pulmonary lesions; and (3) hematogenous distribution resulting in one or more isolated foci in such parts of the body as the lungs, bones, kidneys, liver or brain, or in widespread miliary lesions involving some or all of the viscera.

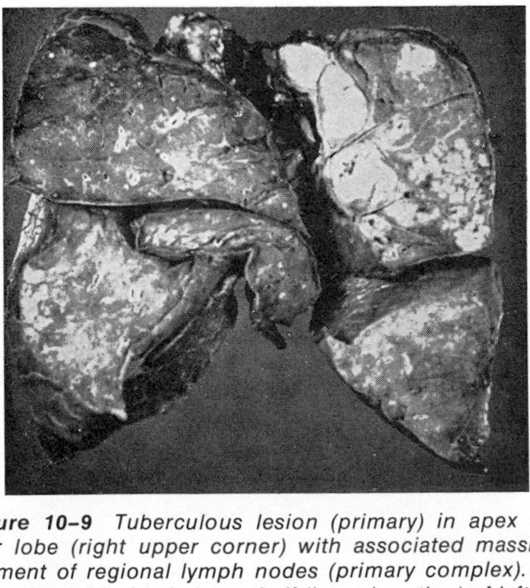

Figure 10–9 *Tuberculous lesion (primary) in apex of left upper lobe (right upper corner) with associated massive involvement of regional lymph nodes (primary complex). Large wedge-shaped lesion in lower half (lateral portion) of left upper lobe. This last lesion (tuberculous pneumonitis) is secondary to bronchial erosion from a tuberculous node. (Courtesy of Drs. Charles Dunlap and James B. Arey.)*

The progressive primary tuberculous focus is a large, irregularly demarcated area of caseation with no definite capsule. The tissue surrounding this area tends to be pneumonic and the overlying pleura to be thickened. Softening and liquefaction may be generalized in the nodular mass or localized in one or more small areas. If the liquefied material is evacuated, there remains an irregular, shaggy excavation with a poorly defined capsule. Hematogenous distribution is more likely to occur during the stage of softening before the stage of liquefaction, whereas bronchogenic spread tends to result from the breakdown of an area of liquefaction.

Consolidated lesions associated with primary infections are usually atelectasis or tuberculous pneumonia, or a combination of the two. Bronchi may be occluded by external pressure from caseous lymph nodes, or there may be erosion of the bronchus and occlusion of the lumen by the resultant intrabronchial lesion. When the obstruction is incomplete, there may be greater hindrance to the exit of respired air than to its entrance, so that obstructive emphysema may occur distal to the lesion; when obstruction is complete, resorption atelectasis occurs.

Massive hematogenous dissemination of tubercle bacilli from a tuberculous focus results in widespread formation of tubercles. The heaviest distribution is likely to be in the lungs, but any or all of the viscera may be involved, especially the liver, spleen and kidneys. Isolated hematogenous lesions may be located in the brain, kidneys and bones and occasionally in other structures. Rich and McCordock have shown that tuberculous meningitis is more likely to result from breakdown of a tuberculoma in contiguity with the meninges.

CLINICAL FORMS. Tuberculosis may involve practically any organ or tissue of the body. Exogenous foci are naturally limited to structures which have an epithelial covering or lining, whereas tuberculosis of structures of the body which have no outside contact are of necessity blood- or lymph-borne from a pre-existing focus. Symptoms of any tuberculous lesion may be varied and may simulate many other disease entities. In the differential diagnosis of the majority of chronic infections and of many acute ones, the possibility of tuberculosis must be considered.

Intrathoracic tuberculous infection accounts for at least 90 per cent of recognized tuberculous disease in children. Parenchymal and lymph node involvement always occurs, but the foci are not always apparent on clinical or roentgenographic examination. The extent of the infection in the pulmonary parenchyma or in the lymph nodes is largely responsible for the various clinical patterns. Table 10–8 classifies intrathoracic lesions according to clinical patterns rather than in the more traditional respect to primary tuberculosis or reinfection. Extrathoracic tuberculous lesions are tabulated in Table 10–10.

TABLE 10–8 CLASSIFICATION OF INTRATHORACIC TUBERCULOSIS

Hypersensitivity to tuberculin without clinically demonstrable disease
Apparently healed (calcified or fibrotic) pulmonary or tracheobronchial lymph node foci with hypersensitivity to tuberculin
Noncalcified pulmonary focus
Extensive pulmonary infiltration
Tuberculosis of the tracheobronchial lymph nodes
Intraluminal and extraluminal bronchial lesions
  Localized ulcerative or granulomatous endobronchial lesions
  Extraluminal bronchial compression
    Lesions distal to bronchial obstruction
      Emphysema
      Atelectasis
      Tuberculous pneumonitis
      Or any combination of above three lesions
Caseous bronchopneumonia
  Bronchogenic or hematogenous
Hematogenous tuberculosis
  Single or multiple pulmonary infiltrations (clinically indistinguishable from nonhematogenous lesions)
  Miliary tuberculosis
Apical and infraclavicular lesions
Pleurisy
(See Table 10–10 for Classification of Extrathoracic Tuberculosis)

INTRATHORACIC TUBERCULOSIS

CLINICAL MANIFESTATIONS. The initial lesion found in the lung is usually a localized one of 2 or 3 cm, from which tubercle bacilli colonize the regional lymph nodes. *The two lesions constitute the so-called primary complex.* Possible outcomes include: (1) healing; (2) persistence of indolent lesions; (3) extension at the local site with progressive destruction of tissue; (4) erosion of bronchial walls with partial or complete occlusion of the bronchial lumen (or such occlusions by external pressure of enlarged lymph nodes), with establishment of localized obstructive emphysema or atelectasis and at times with distribution of tubercle bacilli to other parts of the lung and establishment of a number of new lesions; (5) erosion of blood vessels with widespread distribution of tubercle bacilli (miliary tuberculosis) or with establishment of localized lesions at distant sites; (6) subsequent reactivity of the lesion; or (7) reinfection, endogenous or exogenous.

Detection of tuberculin sensitivity in any person requires careful study (1) to locate, if possible, any and all lesions; (2) to determine whether infection is active, quiescent or healed; and (3) to detect any tuberculous contacts.

When no lesion can be demonstrated in the child on physical examination or a roentgenogram of the chest, and there is no evidence of active infection such as fever, increased sedimentation rate or blood cell counts, the child may be diagnosed as *hypersensitive to tuberculin without clinically demonstrable disease.* Specific treatment is recommended for such children and for those of any age who are known to have become tuberculin-positive within recent months (see below).

When there are one or more *calcified foci in the pulmonary parenchyma or calcified lesions in the tracheobronchial lymph nodes* (Fig. 10–10) in a child with a positive reaction to tuberculin and no reaction to histoplasmin or coccidioidin and no evidence of active disease, he may be considered to be in an inactive state of tuberculosis. Calcified foci, especially those close to the hilus, can usually be distinguished roentgenographically from blood vessels, which tend to have a smooth circular or elliptical homogeneous density, whereas calcified foci are usually irregular in outline and density. Such a situation suggests a healed state, but the child must be watched for the possibility of an exacerbation, especially at adolescence.

Demonstrable Noncalcified Lesions. The **noncalcified small pulmonary focus** appears on the roentgenogram as a more or less circumscribed area, usually not more than 1 or 2 cm in diameter. There may or may not be evidence of associated hilar node involvement; in infants and children there is likely to be. As a rule, the child is not ill with this type of lesion. In the adolescent years such lesions are often located in the apex of the lung or the infraclavicular area, and in such circumstances initial tuberculous lesions may simulate the so-called reinfection lesions of adults.

On occasion the initial lesion in the lung is not confined to a small focal area, but extends into the surrounding lung tissue. Such an *extensive pulmonary infiltration* is often termed **"progressive primary tuberculosis"** (Fig. 10–11). Clinically there are no certain methods for determining whether such a lesion is the initial one or is an exogenous reinfection or one resulting from hematogenous or bronchogenic dissemination. Such lesions may involve several lobules or most of a lobe.

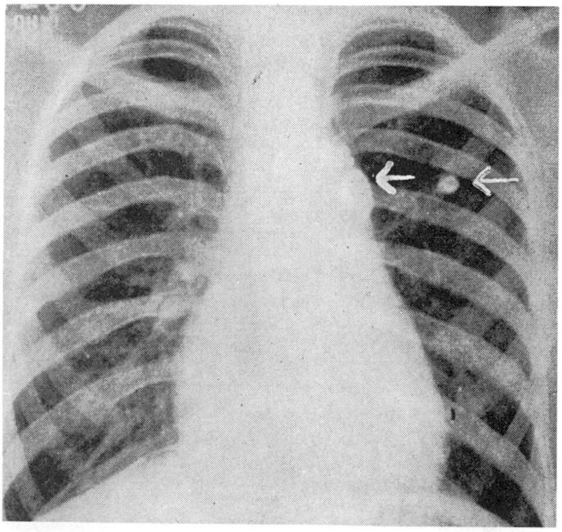

Figure 10–10 Calcified tuberculous focus (right arrow) and calcified tracheobronchial lymph node (left arrow) in a girl 10 years of age.

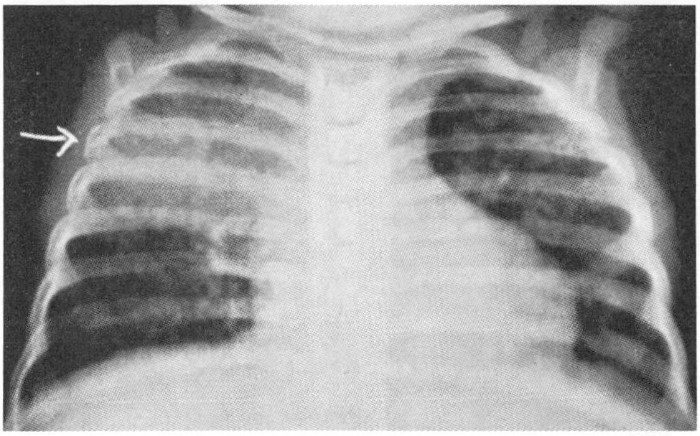

Figure 10–11 Extensive infiltrative lesion in the middle portion of the right lung in a boy 20 months of age.

Though there may be symptoms, not infrequently extensive pulmonary lesions are detected roentgenographically in children who have no complaints and whose parents have not observed any abnormalities.

Physical findings vary considerably. There may or may not be impairment to percussion. Rales may or may not be present. Cavitation occasionally occurs, but, because it is likely to be farther away from the chest wall than in apical lesions, it may be missed on physical examination and even on roentgenograms. Bullous emphysematous lesions have also been infrequently observed; these appear after initiation of therapy and may persist for months, apparently without inhibiting recovery. Tubercle bacilli can frequently be found in the sputum or in lavaged gastric contents.

Infection of the hilar lymph nodes is an almost constant accompaniment of pulmonary tuberculosis in infants and children. The nodes on the side of the parenchymal lesion are the ones usually involved, but the contralateral ones may also be infected. Frequently the only manifestation of the primary infection is the involvement of the tracheobronchial nodes, the parenchymal lesion being so small that it is not demonstrable on the roentgenogram. The infection in the lymph nodes goes through the same stages as that of the parenchymal lesion and, until calcification is complete, is attended by the same danger of local extension and hematogenous dissemination.

There are frequently no symptoms. Though a brassy, paroxysmal cough is often attributed to enlarged nodes, it occurs so infrequently that it can scarcely be considered characteristic. Enlargement of the nodes is rarely demonstrable by physical signs. Cyanosis, edema of the face and dilatation of the superficial veins have been observed in association with extremely enlarged nodes, owing to compression of the larger blood vessels. Paravertebral dullness is rarely demonstrable. Roentgenographic demonstration of enlarged nodes in conjunction with a positive tuberculin reaction constitutes the best evidence for diagnosis.

Intraluminal and **extraluminal bronchial lesions** are of considerable importance in tuberculosis in children. Involvement of the bronchus is almost invariably from a contiguous lesion, rarely by direct infection from an outside source.

Intraluminal lesions are produced by extension from an adjacent tuberculous process, usually in a lymph node, through the bronchial wall with establishment of an ulcerative or granulomatous lesion. The lesion may partially or completely obstruct the lumen of the bronchus and may also result in dissemination of infected material to

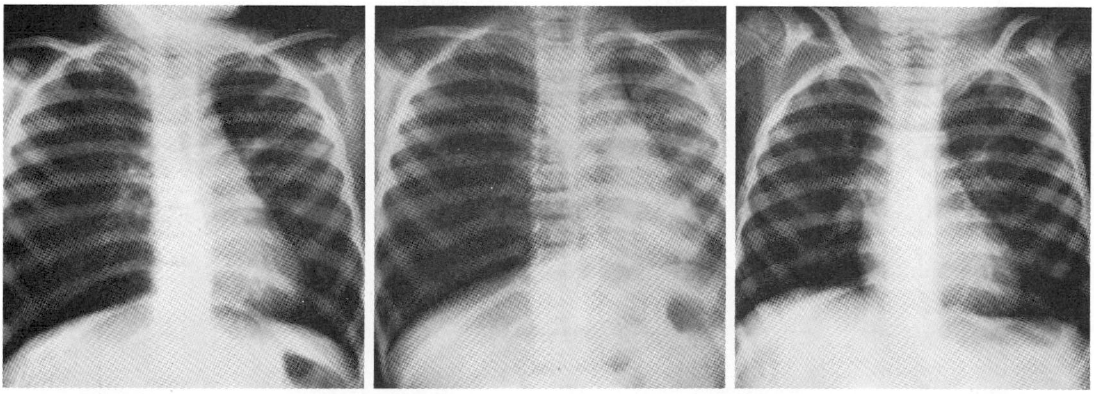

A B C

Figure 10–12 Obstructive emphysema of the right lung secondary to a granulomatous intrabronchial lesion. A, Inspiratory phase; B, expiratory phase, showing failure of right lung to contract, and shift of heart and mediastinal structures to left; C, film taken 24 hours after bronchoscopic removal of tuberculous tissue from right main stem bronchus, showing normal aeration of right lung.

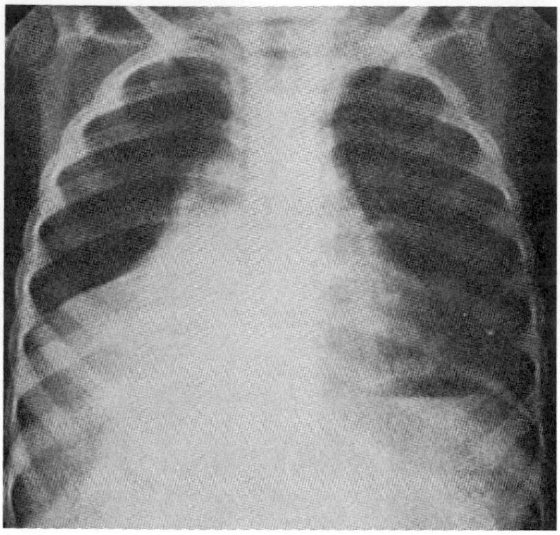

Figure 10–13 Atelectasis of right middle and lower lobes secondary to tracheobronchial tuberculous lymphadenitis and an endobronchial granulomatous lesion in a child 4 years of age. Gastric washings were positive for tubercle bacilli. Two months before the exposure of this film the child suffered a partial bronchial occlusion which resulted in obstructive emphysema. Subsequently complete bronchial occlusion resulted in absorption atelectasis illustrated here. At this time a portion of the endobronchial granuloma was removed endoscopically. There was no immediate effect, but re-expansion occurred over the next 2 months.

other portions of the tracheobronchial tree with establishment of tuberculous bronchopneumonia.

An *extraluminal lesion* is a partial or complete occlusion of a bronchus by enlarged adjacent and usually adherent tuberculous lymph nodes without erosion through the bronchial wall.

When a bronchus is partially obstructed by compression from without or by an intraluminal granulomatous lesion to a degree sufficient to interfere with the flow of air, the portion of the lung supplied by the bronchus becomes emphysematous (Fig. 10–12). When the obstruction is complete, absorption atelectasis occurs (Fig. 10–13). In each instance there may also be a tuberculous pneumonitis in all or part of the involved pulmonary area (Fig. 10–14).

Intrabronchial lesions may be responsible for cough, which may be brassy and may also be productive of variable amounts of sputum. Lesions in the major bronchi may be seen bronchoscopically. Biopsy material can often be obtained for histologic and cultural diagnostic purposes, and on occasion sufficient material can be removed to restore the bronchial airway.

Caseous bronchopneumonia may be localized in one area of the lung or widely disseminated. Material from a tuberculous focus in the parenchyma or in a lymph node discharged into a bronchus in a state of liquefaction is likely to be more widely distributed than when it is in a less fluid, caseous state. The lesions are particularly likely to be distal to the portion of the lung supplied by the eroded bronchus where conditions for localization are good, owing to interference with respiratory mechanics. In some instances all lobes are involved.

Children with caseous bronchopneumonia tend to be quite sick. There are usually fever, malaise and, not infrequently, a loose, productive cough. The physical findings vary considerably. There may or may not be impairment to percussion, bronchial breathing or rales. If there is cavity formation, there may be pectoriloquy unless the lesion is too deeply situated. The extent of the involvement can be determined only from the roentgenogram. Tubercle bacilli can usually be discovered in the sputum or lavaged gastric contents.

Acute miliary tuberculosis is a blood-borne infection characterized by multiple tubercle formations. It is more frequent in infants than in older children. Practically all organs of the body may be

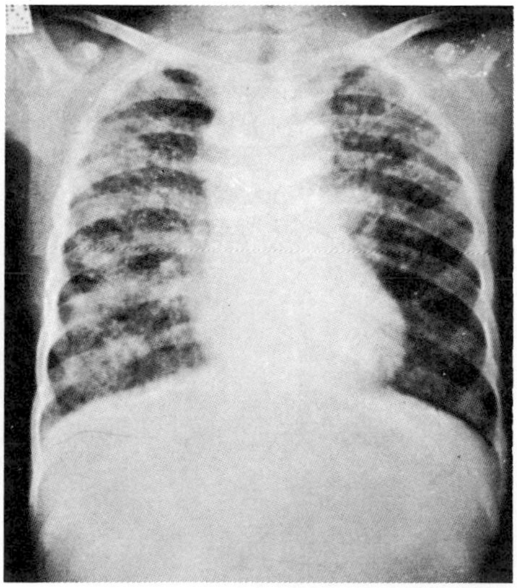

A

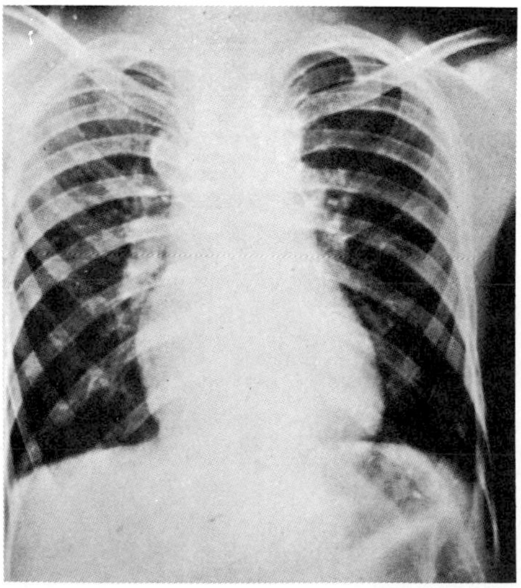

B

Figure 10–14 A, *Extensive tuberculous bronchopneumonia in a child 5 years of age, more prominent on the right side.* B, *Appearance of lungs at 9 years of age, after recovery (prior to availability of specific antimicrobial therapy).*

involved, as may any serous membrane. Tubercle bacilli become lodged in the small capillaries; a lesion develops at each site, and necrosis tends to develop rapidly in each of the small foci. If the life of the child is sufficiently prolonged, there is an epithelioid response, and the lesions in the lungs become visible on the roentgenogram.

The symptoms are usually those of a general infection. The onset may be abrupt, although at times it is insidious. Fever soon develops and tends to run an irregular course, frequently with peaks as high as 40° C (104° F), and the patient appears extremely ill. Initially there may be no physical signs to indicate the extent of the involvement. Choroidal tubercles may be an early manifestation and may be detected by funduscopic examination. The spleen is often enlarged and the abdomen distended; these findings with the high fever and absence of other physical findings may suggest the possibility of typhoid fever. At times the early pulmonary manifestations may be those of generalized obstructive emphysema, and acute bronchiolitis may be suspected. Localized signs which disclose the true identity of the infection frequently do not appear until the last week or so of the illness in the untreated patient. Fine crepitant rales may be heard at this time over all portions of the chest, and the roentgenogram which previously failed to reveal pulmonary changes will show the characteristic, widely distributed miliary lesions, which create a mottled appearance and are frequently described as resembling snowflakes (Fig. 10–15). The white blood cell count is not distinctive; it may be increased, but leukopenia is the more frequent response.

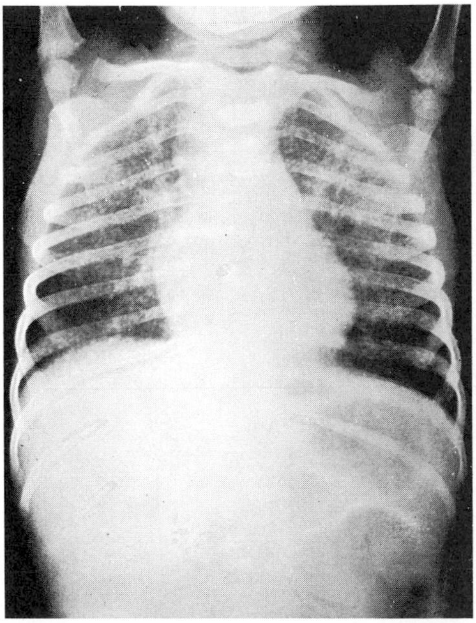

Figure 10–15 *Miliary tuberculosis of the lungs in a boy 3 years of age. His mother had pulmonary tuberculosis. The physical findings were fine, crackling rales throughout both lungs. Death occurred shortly after this roentgenogram was taken. The tuberculin reaction was positive.*

Death usually occurs within four to six weeks in untreated cases, but recovery is possible in the majority of instances if treatment is instituted sufficiently early.

Apical and infraclavicular lesions are most commonly seen in adult life and are often termed **"adult tuberculosis," "apical tuberculosis"** or **"reinfection tuberculosis."** They are relatively uncommon before the adolescent period, when they become the most frequent type of tuberculous involvement, being more common in females than in males. These lesions have generally been considered to be the result of endogenous or exogenous reinfection; their tendency to remain localized and the absence of any extensive involvement of the regional lymph nodes are attributed to an altered response of the host because of a previous infection with the tubercle bacillus. Lesions which are clinically indistinguishable will develop, however, in the upper portions of the lungs in previously tuberculin-negative as well as in tuberculin-positive adolescents and young adults. For this reason these lesions are described simply on the basis of their location and roentgenographic appearance.

The clinical courses of these lesions can in general be grouped into three categories. In some there is retrogression toward healing almost from the time of recognition; in others the lesion is indolent and resists healing. In this latter type, activation of the lesion may be associated with any factor which lowers the host's general resistance. In the third type the lesion is persistently progressive, and there is destruction of lung tissue with cavitation.

The symptoms and physical findings are also variable. In some instances no symptoms are elicited. In others there may be the general symptoms of a chronic infection. Physical examination may or may not reveal fine rales; they are likely to be most consistently detected at the beginning of an inspiration which follows a slight cough after forced expiration. Cavity formation of any extent can usually be suspected on the basis of bronchophony and pectoriloquy. The diagnosis is established by roentgenographic examination, the detection of tubercle bacilli in the sputum or lavaged gastric contents, and upon the response to the tuberculin test. Similar lesions can be produced by coccidioidomycosis and histoplasmosis.

Tuberculous pleuritis may occur as a dry fibrinous pleurisy, as a serous effusion and, rarely, as a necrotic involvement of the pleura stemming from a contiguous caseous focus in the lung. Most often the reaction is a serous one, and the process is nearly always unilateral.

Children rarely have complaints suggestive of pleural involvement. Occasionally during the dry stage there may be pleural pain with limitation of respirations on the affected side. Rarely an effusion may become so extensive that there is bulging of the intercostal spaces and respiratory embarrassment. The presence of pleural effusion is usually suspected from physical findings, and the diagnosis is confirmed roentgenographically and by pleural aspiration.

The prognosis is generally governed by the pulmonary lesion. Treatment is that of tuberculous infection; aspiration, other than for diagnostic purposes, is indicated only when there are severe symptoms of compression. Absorption of fluid is followed by pleural thickening and adhesions. There is no evidence that drainage will lessen such residuals or prevent reaccumulation of fluid.

DIAGNOSIS OF PULMONARY TUBERCULOSIS. The diagnosis of pulmonary tuberculosis is established with certainty by the demonstration of tubercle bacilli in the sputum, aspirated bronchial secretions or gastric contents. In the absence of such information the diagnosis is based on the history of symptoms and of contact with tuberculous infection, on the physical examination, on the reaction to tuberculin and on roentgenographic examination of the lungs.

The evaluation of the child suspected or proved to have tuberculosis should assess whether the tuberculous lesion is in an active, quiescent or healed stage. In the absence of fever and other clinical evidences of disease, such assessment is rarely clear-cut.

The appraisal is not complete without a careful search for the source of contact. Open tuberculosis will frequently be found in some member of the family or other close associate who is not aware of it (Figs. 10–16 and 10–17). For this reason tuberculin tests should be performed on all siblings; if the reaction is positive, roentgenograms of the chest should be obtained. All adult members should have a careful physical examination, tuberculin test and a roentgenogram of the chest. Grandparents and other older persons with whom there is contact should be included in this examination, since chronic, open tuberculosis is common among older people. It is a good policy to repeat after an interval of about six months the examination of the contacts who have no evidence of disease.

History. History of possible contact with open tuberculosis should be included in the appraisal of all children with or without symptoms of the disease (see above).

Symptoms of pulmonary tuberculosis vary considerably and to some extent are proportionate to the seriousness of the lesion. There are variations in this regard, however, and it is essential to know that pulmonary infections, even extensive ones, may not be productive of any recognizable symptoms. As a rule, symptoms in children are merely the general ones of chronic infection, such as fatigue, irritability and possibly some degree of undernutrition, and are usually not directly related to the respiratory system. When most of such symptoms as cough with expectoration, hemoptysis, fever, fatigue, malaise, loss of weight, and night sweats are present, one may be certain that the lesion is extensive.

Physical Examination. The examination should be complete, since tuberculous lesions may be present in other parts of the body and nontuberculous conditions of the lungs or other parts of the body may be coexistent.

The physical findings of the lungs vary with the nature and extent of the lesion and have been described above. Not infrequently, extensive lesions are found by roentgenogram when no or only slightly abnormal physical signs have been elicited. In general, physical signs of tuberculosis in children tend to be disproportionately few in relation to the extent of the pulmonary involvement.

Roentgenographic Examination. The common roentgenographic abnormalities have been described and illustrated in the descriptions of the various clinical types of intrathoracic tuberculosis. Chronic intrathoracic disease, such as histoplasmosis or coccidioidomycosis, cystic fibrosis, persistent bronchopneumonia, pulmonary changes following measles or pertussis, lymphoblastomas of

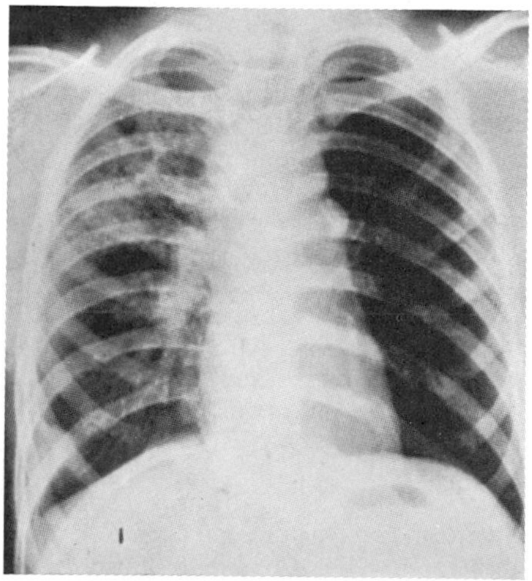

Figure 10–16

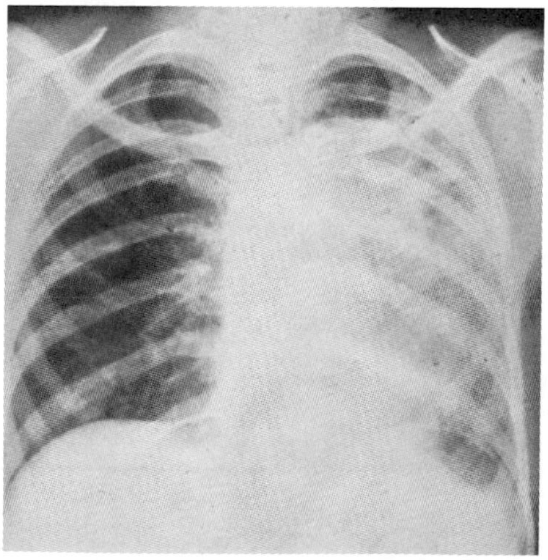

Figure 10–17

Figure 10–16 *Calcified node in left hilar area and tuberculous lesions in upper part of right lung in a child 12 years of age.*

Figure 10–17 *Extensive tuberculous lesion in the chest of the mother, who disclaimed any knowledge of illness or history of tuberculosis in any member of the family. Sputum was positive for tubercle bacilli. Roentgenogram of the mother was taken as part of a survey of the family because of detection of tuberculosis in the child.*

the mediastinum, lung abscess, aspiration of foreign material, pulmonary infiltrations due to ascariasis, toxocariasis or *Pneumocystis carinii*, Löffler's pneumonia, Letterer-Siwe disease and others, are likely to simulate the lesions produced by pulmonary tuberculosis. Interpretation of roentgenograms without adequate knowledge of the history, physical findings and laboratory data will lead to many erroneous diagnoses.

The Tuberculin Test

Significance of a Positive Reaction. A positive tuberculin reaction is evidence that the person has been infected with the tubercle bacillus or an unclassified acid-fast bacillus and is allergic or hypersensitive to its protein. The presence or absence of activity of a current lesion cannot be deduced from the extent of the reaction. Properly used, the test is the most reliable method for the detection of children who have had infection with the tubercle bacillus or with one of the unclassified mycobacteria and who need further examination to determine whether the lesion is active or quiescent. Certain of the unclassified mycobacteria pathogenic for man have an antigenic relation with the tubercle bacillus, and their respective "tuberculins" will elicit cross-reactions. The infecting bacterium can be determined with reasonable accuracy by comparative testing (see below).

With certain exceptions, failure to elicit a positive reaction to tuberculin eliminates the possibility of the presence of tuberculous infection. For several weeks after the entrance of tubercle bacilli into the body there is no cutaneous reaction to tuberculin. During advanced or terminal stages of tuberculosis, allergy to tuberculin may occasionally disappear; at times it is temporarily inhibited by such nonspecific factors as severe inanition, dehydration, acute febrile illness and administration of corticosteroids or immunosuppressive agents. Tuberculin hypersensitivity may also be temporarily suppressed after immunization with live measles vaccine and possibly with smallpox vaccine. Duration of allergy to tuberculin after healing of the lesion, and the factors that govern it are not completely understood. In most instances cutaneous allergy persists for years in association with apparently healed lesions. Injection of lymphocyte transfer factor from a tuberculin-positive donor into a tuberculin-negative recipient can render some recipients tuberculin-positive.

Choice and Dose of Tuberculin. Since human and bovine types of tubercle bacilli have a common allergen, the use of tuberculin from human tubercle bacilli is considered adequate to detect infection with either bacillus. (See below for use of "tuberculins" of unclassified mycobacteria.)

At present two tuberculins of the human tubercle bacillus are available: old tuberculin (OT) and purified protein derivative (PPD). The principal objection to OT has been the variation in potency of different batches of it. Purified protein derivative, now the most widely used tuberculin, contains no protein other than that of tubercle bacilli. Its antigenicity is reduced by heating. It is usually dispensed in the dried state in tablet form and is dissolved in a measured amount of diluent before use. PPD solutions should be stabilized with a substance such as Tween.

The recommendations for dosages of tuberculin by the American Lung Association are as follows:*

TECHNIQUE OF ADMINISTRATION

Intradermal (Mantoux) Test. This is performed by the intradermal injection of 0.1 ml of the desired concentration of PPD or OT into the cleansed skin of either the flexor or extensor surface of the forearm. Other skin areas may be used, but the forearm is preferred. The injection is made with a short (one fourth- to one half-inch), sharply beveled, platinum (26-gauge) or steel (27-gauge) needle with a tuberculin syringe. The injection should be made just beneath the surface of the skin, with the needle bevel upward. A discrete, pale elevation of the skin, 6 to 10 mm in diameter and resembling a mosquito bite, should be produced when the fluid is properly injected intradermally. If the wheal is smaller than 6 mm, the injection should be repeated at another site.

The standard dose for differential diagnosis and for surveys is 5 TU (TU = *tuberculin unit*, the activity contained in a specified weight of International Standard Mammalian PPD Tuberculin in a specified buffer). Only persons suspected of having active tuberculosis who fail to react to a repeat test with 5 TU need to be retested with 250 TU. However, a reaction to this larger dose is usually due to sensitivity caused by infection with atypical mycobacteria. A negative reaction to the larger dose is, therefore, of more value to the clinician in excluding a diagnosis of tuberculosis than is a positive reaction in supporting it.

Jet Injection. This method uses a jet gun to deliver 5 TU of PPD intradermally under high pressure. The wheal produced should be 6 to 10 mm, or the injection should be repeated at another site.

Tuberculins and other antigens, such as coccidioidin, histoplasmin and blastomycin, are difficult to remove from glassware and other materials. For this reason, syringes, bottles and jet guns used for one antigen should not be used subsequently for another.

Multiple-Puncture Tests. These tests use a skin puncture technique either by an applicator with points on which tuberculin is dried or by puncturing through a film of liquid tuberculin. Because all these tests use concentrated tuberculin, they may introduce more than 5 TU. There are several types of applicators for multiple-puncture tests available and others will undoubtedly be introduced.

READING AND RECORDING OF THE TESTS. The Mantoux and jet injection tests should be read 48 to 72 hours after injection. With multiple-puncture tests, the interval between injection and reading varies with the type of test given, and the manufacturer's instructions should be followed. Readings should be made in a good light, with the forearm slightly flexed. The basis of reading is the presence or absence of induration, which may be determined by inspection (from a side view against the light as well as by direct light) and by palpation with a gentle finger stroking.

For the Mantoux and jet injection tests, the diameter of induration should be measured transversely to the long axis of the forearm and recorded in millimeters. For multiple-puncture tests, coalescent reactions should be read and recorded as above; if the reaction is in the form of

---

*From Diagnostic Standards and Classification of Tuberculosis. New York, American Lung Association, 1969. Used by permission.

discrete papules, the diameter of the largest single papule should be recorded. Erythema without induration is without significance.

A record should always be made of the type of test used, including the type and dose of tuberculin, and the size of reaction in millimeters of induration.

INTERPRETATION OF SKIN TEST REACTIONS

Intradermal (Mantoux) and Jet Injection Tests with Standard Test Dose. The following interpretations are recommended:

10 mm or more of induration = POSITIVE REACTION

This is a positive tuberculin test and almost always reflects sensitivity resulting from infection with *M. tuberculosis.* The test does not need to be repeated for confirmation.

5 mm through 9 mm of induration = DOUBTFUL REACTION

This doubtful reaction reflects sensitivity which can result from infection with either atypical mycobacteria or *M. tuberculosis.* If PPD antigens for atypical mycobacteria are available, intradermal tests with such antigens should be applied at the same time as the repeat test with the standard test dose of PPD. If atypical antigens are not available, the standard test should be repeated at a different site. If the second reaction is 10 mm or more of induration, the person should be regarded as a positive reactor. If the second reaction is again in the 5 to 9 mm range, it is still a doubtful reaction. If the person with a reaction in this 5 to 9 mm range is known to have been in close contact with a case of proven active tuberculosis or has x-ray or clinical evidence of disease compatible with tuberculosis, he should be managed in the same fashion as a reactor with 10 mm or more of induration.

0 mm through 4 mm of induration = NEGATIVE REACTION

This reflects either a lack of tuberculin sensitivity, or a low-grade sensitivity which most likely is not due to *M. tuberculosis* infection. No repeat test is necessary unless there are other suggestive clinical evidences of tuberculosis. If the person is the contact of a case of tuberculosis, he should be followed according to the established routine for contacts, including repeated skin testing.

Multiple-Puncture (Tine and Mono-Vacc) Tests. In determining the size of induration, measure the diameter of the largest single reaction. If the reaction consists of discrete papules, the diameters of separate areas of induration should not be added. For screening tests done with presently available lots of OT and PPD, the following interpretation is suggested:

5 mm or more of induration = POSITIVE REACTION

The significance of the test and the management of the individual is the same as that for one who reacts with 10 mm or more of induration to the standard Mantoux test.

2 mm through 4 mm of induration = DOUBTFUL REACTION

Even though such reactions may be due to *M. tuberculosis,* a significant proportion of them may not be confirmed by a positive standard Mantoux test. Therefore, a Mantoux test should be done on all individuals in this group, and management should be based on Mantoux reactions.

Less than 2 mm of induration = NEGATIVE REACTION

There is no need for retesting unless the individual is a contact to a case of tuberculosis or there is suggestive clinical evidence of the disease.

Multiple-Puncture (Heaf and Sterneedle) Tests. It is suggested that all reactions to these two tests should be checked by retesting with the standard intradermal test. In screening programs, nonreactors can be considered negative.

In view of the similarity of certain fungus infections to tuberculosis, it may be wise to perform tests with their antigens simultaneously with the performance of the tuberculin test. This procedure is particularly applicable to histoplasmin in the central part of the United States and to coccidioidin in the Southwestern and Western states.

In extremely severe reactions to the intracutaneous test the inflammation may be decreased and sloughing of the necrotic center at times avoided by prompt application of an ice compress and a corticosteroid ointment.

Bacteriologic Examination. Tubercle bacilli can usually be isolated in children with active lesions if a diligent search is made. It is the only basis for definitive diagnosis of tuberculosis; *M. tuberculosis* must be distinguished from other acid-fast bacilli, including the unclassified strains of mycobacteria variously designated as anonymous or atypical strains. There are three principal means for detection of the tubercle bacillus: (1) by direct smear and staining of sputum, cerebrospinal fluid or discharges from such lesions as draining lymph nodes and sinuses of osseous lesions; (2) by guinea pig inoculation of any of these materials; and (3) by cultural methods in artificial media. The last is the most effective. In infants and children, who are apt to swallow sputum, the lavaged contents of the fasting stomach provide the best source of material for examination. The lavage should be performed early in the morning before the usual breakfast time.

Evaluation of Clinical Activity. The diagnosis of tuberculous infection is not complete without determining whether the lesion is active or quiescent. When there are such obvious signs of clinical activity as fever and malaise, no further evidence is required. When there are no apparent manifestations of active infection, however, other measures must be used. These include sedimentation rates, blood cell counts, serial roentgenograms, response to exercise and particularly continued observation of the child's apparent well-being and his growth pattern. Rectal temperature should not be taken for at least a half hour after active exercise, since it is normally elevated for a short time after physical activity. Failure to recognize this fact has often been responsible for unnecessarily confining a child to bed or reduced activity.

PROGNOSIS. Most children recover from primary tuberculous infection, and the majority are unaware of its presence even during its active phase. Although recovery is frequent, primary infection is not a benign lesion. There is a relatively high fatality rate during the first two years of life, owing to the fact that hematogenous and bronchogenic lesions may originate from the primary focus and, in such instances, are in reality a part of the primary infection.

Mortality rates have been relatively high in the first few years of life and during adolescence. The prognosis of pulmonary as well as of other forms of tuberculosis has been tremendously improved by the use of antimicrobial agents. Death, except in tuberculous meningitis, almost never occurs except in patients who are not treated or in whom the diagnosis is made in the terminal phase of the disease. Antimicrobial treatment of pulmonary tuberculosis has resulted in a striking decrease in hematogenous lesions. This observation has led to an extensive clinical trial of prophylactic administration of isoniazid to young children with positive tuberculin reactions with or without roentgenographically demonstrable lesions and to older children who are known to have become tuberculin-positive within recent months. This study demonstrated that progression of the localized lesion is usually prevented, and the incidence of hematogenous dissemination is decreased.

PREVENTION. The only certain means for the prevention of tuberculosis is avoidance of contact with tubercle bacilli. Maintenance of an adequate nutritional status and avoidance of fatigue and of debilitating infections are factors in natural resistance, but none of them is sufficient to prevent infection.

As yet no method exists for artificial induction of solid, specific immunity (see BCG, below).

Identification of Tuberculous Contacts. Perhaps the most important measure for the prevention of tuberculosis in children would be periodic tuberculin testing of all adults, with positive reactors examined roentgenographically at regular intervals. Unfortunately this method of case-finding has not yet become practical on a broad basis. It is desirable, however, that all children receive tuberculin tests at intervals of one to three years.

There is a high incidence of tuberculosis in urban and other areas where crowding and poor housing conditions prevail; correction of these conditions is an important public health measure.

Milk. If at all possible, only pasteurized milk from tuberculosis-free cattle should be used for the feeding of infants and children. Unpasteurized milk should not be used without boiling.

Vaccination with BCG. There have been numerous attempts to develop satisfactory methods for the stimulation of artificial immunity against tuberculosis. Of these, only vaccination with BCG (Bacillus of Calmette and Guérin) merits continued use. The vaccine is composed of bovine tubercle bacilli whose virulence has been reduced by special cultural procedures. Administration of the vaccine to animals or man produces a limited immunity to reinfection with virulent tubercle bacilli. Intradermal injections seem to be somewhat more effective than subcutaneous ones and less likely to result in indolent ulcers. An occasional infant vaccinated during the first few months of life may acquire suppurative adenopathy, but such a complication almost never occurs in older infants or children. The usual intradermal dose is in the range of 0.1 to 0.15 mg of freshly prepared vaccine. Positive tuberculin reactions develop in most instances after inoculation.

Controlled studies, chiefly in the Scandinavian countries and in the United States, have shown that BCG vaccination produces definite though incomplete protection against tuberculosis. The practice of administering BCG vaccine to children who live in areas with high tuberculosis mortality rates or to those who are intimately exposed to adults with inactive or "arrested" tuberculosis is less frequently recommended than previously, since equal or greater protection is afforded by the daily administration of isoniazid (see below).

At present BCG vaccine is prepared in only a few laboratories. Its distribution from these laboratories is usually controlled by local or state health departments.

Chemoprophylaxis. Extensive trials have demonstrated that the daily administration of isoniazid to children who have a high probability of exposure to tuberculosis significantly reduces the incidence of new tuberculous infections. The disadvantage of this form of prophylaxis is the need for continuous therapy. A significant advantage is the absence of any effect on the child's reaction to tuberculin, so that the test can continue to be useful in detecting an acquired infection.

TREATMENT. It is generally agreed that all children with demonstrable active lesions of whatever order and in whatever location in the body should receive antimicrobial therapy. In addition, it is recommended that all tuberculin-positive children up to 4 years of age, all older children who are known to have become tuberculin-positive within recent months, and all positive reactors who are or have been in recent contact with open tuberculosis, irrespective of the time of acquisition of their tuberculin sensitivity, should receive isoniazid in doses of 10 to 20 mg/kg/day for about a year whether or not they have demonstrable lesions. The reasons for this policy are the effectiveness of isoniazid in the control of progressive lesions, its apparently low degree of toxicity and, in particular, its effectiveness in the prevention of hematogenous dissemination.

The most useful drugs in the treatment of tuberculosis are isoniazid, streptomycin and aminosalicylic acid. Other agents include rifampicin, cycloserine and possibly pyrazinamide, ethionamide and ethambutol. Clinical experience with these drugs is limited in children. At the moment their usefulness is largely limited to patients infected with tubercle bacilli resistant to isoniazid and streptomycin.

Isoniazid is the most useful of the available agents. It can be administered orally or parenterally. Its toxicity is low, provided the daily dose does not exceed 10 to 20 mg/kg/day. The emergence of drug-resistant organisms is not rapid, and it can be used as a single agent in many patients with the less serious forms of tuberculosis. Patients with progressive, localized lesions, miliary tuberculosis and meningitis should receive an additional agent during the early part of their treatment (Table 10-9). Some adults receiving isoniazid for a long time have had convulsive disorders or hepatitis. So far as is known, such complications have not been observed in infants and small children. Such reactions have been minimized or averted by the continuous administration of pyridoxine.

TABLE 10–9 SUGGESTED SCHEDULES FOR ANTIMICROBIAL THERAPY OF PULMONARY TUBERCULOSIS IN INFANTS AND CHILDREN

TYPE OF DISEASE*	DRUG†	TOTAL DAILY DOSE PER KILOGRAM	DURATION
Positive tuberculin reaction in a child or a positive tuberculin reaction recently acquired by a person of any age	Isoniazid	10 to 20 mg (total daily dose should rarely exceed 500 mg)‡	One year
Asymptomatic pulmonary tuberculosis	Isoniazid	10 to 20 mg‡	One year or for a minimum of 6 months after lesion appears to be inactive
Progressive pulmonary lesions; progressive apical and infraclavicular lesions; pleurisy; miliary tuberculosis	Isoniazid and	10 to 20 mg (total daily dose should rarely exceed 500 mg)‡	12 to 18 months or for a minimum of 6 months after lesion appears to be inactive
	Streptomycin or	20 to 40 mg in 1 dose per day (dose not to exceed 1 gm/day)	Daily for 1 to 2 months, then 2 to 4 times weekly for 3 to 6 months (concurrently with isoniazid)
	Aminosalicylic acid (PASA) or	200 to 300 mg (dose not to exceed 12 gm/day)	For duration of isoniazid therapy; if streptomycin is given initially, then substitute PASA for it after its discontinuance.
	Rifampicin	15–20 mg/kg/day (not to exceed 300 mg/day)	Some prescribe it only for an arbitrarily determined shorter time

*See text for treatment of tuberculous adenitis and other forms of extrathoracic tuberculosis.
†See text for use of corticosteroids.
‡The smaller doses are used for large and overweight children. Pyridoxine is prescribed with isoniazid for adolescent children by some clinicians to lessen the likelihood of a convulsive disorder.

Streptomycin is an active agent against *M. tuberculosis,* and its use is probably indicated in addition to isoniazid in all serious tuberculous infections. The drug must be administered by intramuscular injection. Long-term treatment is occasionally complicated by labyrinthine disorders and less often by deafness, but these are uncommon if the drug is administered only once a day or less frequently. Streptomycin should not be used as the only antituberculous agent, owing to the rapid emergence of streptomycin-resistant organisms. This process can be retarded if another agent is administered concurrently. Dihydrostreptomycin is not recommended, since deafness is a common sequel.

Aminosalicylic acid (para-aminosalicylic acid or PAS) is tuberculostatic, but is not so effective as streptomycin or isoniazid. It rarely produces toxic reactions other than gastric irritation, which is occasionally sufficiently severe to prevent its administration. Drug-resistant tubercle bacilli have been infrequently observed. PAS inhibits the development of resistance by tubercle bacilli to both streptomycin and isoniazid and tends to increase serum levels of isoniazid by competing with it for acetylation.

Corticosteroid therapy in conjunction with antimicrobial drugs has not been clearly beneficial except in the treatment of endobronchial granulomas, in which improvement may be noted within a week or so, and possibly in the prevention of hydrocephalus in patients with tuberculous meningitis. Pleural effusions may also resolve more rapidly with such treatment. In such circumstances corticosteroid treatment is continued for about two months.

Bronchial obstruction owing to enlarged mediastinal lymph nodes is apparently not markedly benefited by the administration of corticosteroids.

Suggested plans for antimicrobial treatment of the various clinical forms of tuberculosis are detailed in Table 10–9.

When patients with progressive pulmonary tuberculosis are treated by the suggested plan, symptomatic improvement is usually noted in two to four weeks. Improvement, as measured by changes in the roentgenograms of the chest, is slow, but extension of the lesion rarely occurs.

Patients with miliary tuberculosis tend to show somewhat more rapid improvement in response to treatment. There is apt to be regression or even disappearance of the miliary densities observed in the roentgenograms within 6 to 10 weeks from the start of treatment. Coexisting extensive pulmonary lesions follow the same pattern of slow improvement noted with other progressive pulmonary lesions. If meningitis develops, the patient should be treated as outlined elsewhere below.

The use of antibacterial agents in the treatment of pulmonary tuberculosis does not eliminate the need for symptomatic and other general therapy.

Children with nonprogressive primary tuberculous lesions receiving isoniazid require no special care beyond that of assurance of adequate nutrition, avoidance of fatigue, prevention of exposure to open tuberculous infection and regular physical examinations, including roentgenograms of the chest. Active immunization against pertussis, measles and influenza is desirable for children with tuberculous lesions, as is the early treatment of all intercurrent infections in order to lessen the possibilities of activation of the tuberculous process.

Children who are sick with tuberculosis as evidenced by fever, malaise, loss of weight, anemia, abnormal white blood cell count, increased erythrocyte sedimentation rate or roentgenographic evidence of progression of the tuberculous lesion require general medical care.

Bed rest is indicated until there are substantial evidences of improvement. Other than maintenance of the necessary isolation procedures, the management is that of any child with a chronic illness, whether in an institution or at home. Most children with tuberculosis can be treated as ambulatory patients.

The *psychologic attitudes* of the child and his family are important. An atmosphere of cheerful optimism should prevail, in which the child is provided some regularity of schedule and even some purposeful duties. Except in severe illness, there is no reason why the child should not be permitted to continue with his schoolwork.

Fresh air and *sunshine* are not important in treatment except as they add to the child's sense of well-being. Heliotherapy is not contraindicated except in excessive amounts in patients with pulmonary lesions. Burning of the skin should be scrupulously avoided. Tanning is permissible if the tan is acquired gradually.

The *nutritional intake* should be adequate, but forced feeding should be avoided. Special attention should be given to the protein, mineral and vitamin content of the diet. There is need for additional amounts of vitamin C (100 to 200 mg of ascorbic acid will meet the daily requirement in the average patient); there is no reason why this cannot be supplied by natural foodstuffs. Vitamins of the B complex should also be supplied in amounts somewhat in excess of average requirements. There is no need for extra amounts of vitamin D or for more than a quart of milk a day. Fresh fruits and vegetables should be given freely. Feeding of tuberculous infants is, with the exception of those with gastrointestinal disturbances, not different from that of other infants. Low-residue diets should be prescribed when there is chronic intestinal involvement.

Surgical procedures, other than bronchoscopy, are rarely indicated in the treatment of pulmonary tuberculosis in infants and children. Lobectomy is occasionally required for those with persistent atelectasis or bronchiectasis following endobronchial lesions.

EXTRATHORACIC TUBERCULOSIS

Tuberculous Infection of Tonsils and Cervical Lymph Nodes

Infection of the cervical lymph nodes is, in most instances, secondary to tuberculous infection of the tonsils, which may constitute the primary lesion or may be secondary to a pulmonary lesion. When the tonsillar infection is primary, it constitutes, in conjunction with the cervical lymph node involvement, a primary tuberculous complex. Such infections have become much less frequent with the decrease in incidence of bovine tuberculosis.

CLINICAL MANIFESTATIONS. The local manifestations of tuberculosis of the cervical lymph nodes vary from slight enlargement of a single node to involvement of a number of them. The nodes of both sides are frequently affected, usually more on one side than on the other. The initial inflammatory changes are responsible for the enlargement, and at this stage the node or nodes are discrete, firm and usually freely movable. When the lesions of the individual nodes become caseous, however, there is a tendency to erosion of the capsule, and the nodes in the immediate vicinity become matted together in a single, irregular nodular mass, often with variable degrees of firmness in different portions. The mass becomes attached to other adjacent structures and to the overlying skin and is no longer freely movable. The skin is often discolored and may be irregularly retracted by the underlying adhesions, having an uneven contour.

If liquefaction of the caseous mass occurs, rupture into the adjacent tissues is likely. If the overlying skin is perforated, as it often is, one or more draining sinuses may be formed. When the nodes

TABLE 10–10 CLASSIFICATION OF EXTRATHORACIC TUBERCULOSIS

Tuberculosis of tonsils and cervical lymph nodes
Intra-abdominal tuberculosis
Enteritis
Mesenteric and retroperitoneal lymphadenopathy
Peritonitis
Liver
Fistula in ano
Tuberculosis of central nervous system
Tuberculoma
Tuberculous meningitis
Tuberculosis of skin
Tuberculosis of bones and joints
Tuberculous pericarditis
Tuberculosis of genitourinary tract
Kidney
Bladder
Female genital organs
Male genital organs
Tuberculosis of eye
Phlyctenular keratitis
Chorioretinitis
Tuberculosis of middle ear

of the retropharyngeal area are involved or when the discharge from other nodes or from an osseous lesion in the cervical vertebrae finds its way into the retropharyngeal area, a chronic, burrowing retroesophageal abscess results. The draining sinuses on the surface of the neck persist until the involved lymphatic tissue is broken down and evacuated, the course without antimicrobial therapy being measured in months or, at times, in years. Indolent skin lesions frequently result, and healing leaves permanent scarring, discoloration and contractural deformities.

Not all tuberculous lymph nodes undergo such a course, and resolution may take place before extensive caseation occurs, or the caseous mass may become calcified and a number of nodes remain matted together and indurated without suppurating. Calcification may be seen roentgenographically. During the period of active inflammation there may be a low-grade fever and other evidences of chronic infection.

DIAGNOSIS. The tonsillar lesion can be identified only by microscopic examination of the removed tonsil.

The differential diagnosis is from other conditions which may cause chronic lymphadenitis, and should include the lymphoblastomas, Hodgkin's disease, carcinoma of the thyroid, actinomycosis, cat-scratch disease and toxoplasmosis. Particular difficulty is experienced in residual or low-grade cervical lymphadenitis associated with chronic upper respiratory tract infections. The likelihood of a tuberculous origin is increased in the presence of a positive tuberculin reaction, but the diagnosis is established only by isolation of tubercle bacilli from the excretions of a draining sinus or by microscopic examination of an excised lymph node.

PROGNOSIS. This depends upon the stage at which diagnosis is established and treatment instituted. Most lesions eventually heal even when untreated. In such instances contractural deformities may be expected.

TREATMENT. Treatment varies with the stage of the lesion at the time of diagnosis. If the lymph nodes are still discrete, excision of the involved ones by careful surgical dissection is recommended. Streptomycin, 10 to 20 mg/kg/dose, should be administered two or three times at intervals of 12 hours before operation. After excision, streptomycin is continued for approximately two weeks, or longer if the operative site shows any drainage. Isoniazid is also administered postoperatively for 12 months in doses of 10 to 20 mg/kg/day.

If the lymph nodes have ruptured spontaneously, antibacterial therapy as recommended for progressive pulmonary tuberculosis in Table 10–9 should be instituted. If drainage persists after two weeks of treatment, secondary bacterial infection is probably present, and other antibiotic therapy should be given in addition to the antituberculous therapy. In most instances the sinus tracts will close within several weeks. Surgical excision can then be performed; antimicrobial therapy should be carried out postoperatively as recommended above.

If the mass of lymph nodes is so extensive that surgical excision is not feasible, antimicrobial therapy as recommended for progressive pulmonary lesions is suggested.

Whether tonsillectomy should be performed several weeks after excision of the lymph nodes is not established.

Infection of Other Superficial Lymph Nodes

Tuberculosis of other superficial lymph nodes, such as those of the axilla, groin or occipital region, may occur but is less frequent than infection of the cervical lymph nodes. Such infections are usually secondary to tuberculosis of the skin. The course of the infection is that described for cervical lymphadenitis.

Intra-abdominal Tuberculosis

Tuberculous enteritis may occur as a primary infection or may be secondary to a pulmonary lesion, the bacilli being transported in swallowed sputum. The stomach is rarely infected. Progressive ulcerative enteritis is more likely to be a secondary than a primary infection and is usually associated with advanced pulmonary disease. In both primary and secondary lesions the mesenteric and, at times, the retroperitoneal lymph nodes are involved. In primary infections the intestinal lesion is usually relatively unimportant and is overshadowed by the lymph node involvement, whereas the situation is essentially reversed in secondary infections. *Tuberculous peritonitis* may be part of a generalized hematogenous infection, but more frequently results from rupture of a caseous mesenteric lymph node or by extension from an ulcerative intestinal lesion. *Tuberculosis of the liver and spleen* is usually a part of generalized miliary tuberculosis. The incidence of intestinal tuberculosis in this country has decreased tremendously in recent years, owing in part to the almost complete eradication of bovine tuberculosis.

Fistula in ano may be secondary to tuberculosis, but is more frequently secondary to other gastrointestinal diseases such as granulomatous ileocolitis.

Tuberculous Enteritis

Small tuberculous ulcers frequently produce no symptoms and are discovered only at autopsy. With more extensive lesions the symptoms are those of ileocolitis with tenesmus and chronic diarrhea. There may be gross hemorrhage, but more often there is only slight bleeding. That the lesions are tuberculous may be suspected from the chronicity and also from the presence of tuberculous infection elsewhere in the body, especially in the lungs. Abdominal distention and tenderness may be present; there is irregular fever, wasting is often great, and anemia and debility are severe.

TREATMENT. The diet should be low in residue, but should have adequate caloric value and be high in vitamin content. In the more severe cases parenteral administration of vitamins may be indicated, as well as amino acids, blood and plasma. Antispasmodics such as paregoric and belladonna preparations may be given for the relief of tenesmus. Antimicrobial therapy for progressive pulmonary tuberculosis should be given (Table 10–9).

Tuberculous Peritonitis

The incidence of tuberculous peritonitis has decreased markedly, and the lesion is now rare in the United States. Scattered miliary tubercles may be found upon the peritoneum in acute, generalized miliary tuberculosis. Tuberculous peritonitis usually originates from erosion of a caseous or liquefied lesion in a mesenteric lymph node, less often from an intestinal lesion which has penetrated through the outer coat, usually without perforation.

CLINICAL MANIFESTATIONS. The onset is, as a rule, insidious and is characterized by gradually increasing abdominal distention, debilitation, vague abdominal pain or tenderness and low-grade fever. The onset may, however, be more abrupt and severe and may be suggestive of appendicitis when the pain and tenderness are in the right lower quadrant. Vomiting may occur, but usually is not severe, and there are no characteristic changes in the stools except in the presence of an associated enteritis.

Clinically, tuberculous peritonitis has been divided into three general types: the ascitic form, the fibrinous or plastic form and the caseous or ulcerative form. All these processes are frequently present in a single case, and there may be no sharp distinction into a particular clinical pattern.

PROGNOSIS. The natural course of tuberculous peritonitis is generally chronic. The outcome is determined not only by the type and extent of the local involvement, but also by the nature of the tuberculous lesions of other parts of the body. In general, the ascitic form has the most favorable prognosis, the caseous form the worst.

TREATMENT. The management of tuberculous peritonitis is essentially that of tuberculosis in general. If there is an associated enteritis, the diet should be low in residue; otherwise it may be adjusted to the patient's appetite. There should be adequate calories as well as a high vitamin and mineral content in the diet. Antimicrobial therapy as recommended for progressive pulmonary tuberculosis is indicated (Table 10–9).

Tuberculosis of the Central Nervous System

Tuberculoma

Tuberculomas of the brain or spinal cord may be single or multiple, and may or may not produce neurologic symptoms. They are often recognized only at autopsy, but may be responsible for symptoms of increased intracranial pressure or localized peripheral manifestations, and in such instances are indistinguishable clinically from intracranial neoplasms. Intracerebral calcification may be tuberculous in origin, but more often represents toxoplasmosis, cytomegalic inclusion disease, astrocytoma, Sturge-Weber syndrome or organized hemorrhage. Tuberculomas at the surface of the brain are the principal origins of infections of the meninges.

Tuberculous Meningitis

Tuberculous meningitis is the principal cause of death from tuberculosis and is most frequent in the first few years of life. It is always associated with primary tuberculous infection, usually in the lung, and is most likely to occur within a few months after the initial manifestation of the primary lesion. The incidence is especially high among black children. It is frequently the initial and only clinical manifestation of tuberculous infection, though always a secondary lesion. Generalized miliary tuberculosis is observed in about 25 per cent of cases.

PATHOGENESIS AND PATHOLOGY. The observations of Rich indicate that the meninges are rarely directly infected by the hematogenous route, but generally secondarily involved by the discharge of tubercle bacilli into the cerebrospinal fluid from contiguous older caseous foci such as a tuberculoma in the brain or spinal cord or osseous lesions of the vertebrae.

Tubercles are scattered over the pia and the surface of the brain. The dura is tense, the convolutions are flattened, and the subarachnoid space and ventricles contain serofibrinous exudate.

CLINICAL MANIFESTATIONS. The clinical manifestations may vary, and at times meningeal symptoms are not present until the terminal stage. In general, however, there is a more or less typical pattern which in the untreated child may be divided into three stages: (1) a prodromal stage of irritation, (2) a transitional stage of increased intracranial pressure and meningeal symptoms, and (3) a terminal stage of paralysis and coma. These stages are not sharply demarcated and not all may be present in a given case.

Prodromal Stage. The onset is usually slow, with little or no fever, rarely acute with high fever. The initial manifestations are often vague. Changes in disposition are frequent; a good-natured child becomes irritable. Periods of drowsiness are common, but sleep is frequently restless. Older children complain of headache. Anorexia, vomiting and constipation are common.

Transitional Stage. Convulsions may occur during this stage, and the drowsiness becomes much deeper. Most frequent, however, are the evidences of meningeal irritation. There is nuchal rigidity, and stiffness of the back and extremities, at times sufficient to produce opisthotonos. The deep reflexes tend to be exaggerated. There may be bulging of the fontanel. Ocular paralyses are common, or there may be nystagmus or strabismus;

the pupils are normal or contracted, and hippus may be present. Occasionally there is choking of the disk, and tubercles may be present along the vessels of the choroid. There is usually a well marked tache cérébrale and at times, because of vasomotor disturbances, irregular flushing of the trunk and face. The temperature is usually elevated, but is rarely high. The course is progressive, and the drowsiness tends to be replaced by stupor.

Terminal Stage. The evidences of meningeal irritation are replaced by those of paralysis in the final phase. The child lapses into a comatose state with dilated and unresponsive pupils, insensitivity of the cornea, widespread paralyses, irregular pulse which may be slow or accelerated, and irregular respirations which are at times of the Cheyne-Stokes type. The temperature rises abruptly at the terminal stage, at times to as high as 41.7° C (107° F), and there may be hyperglycemia and glycosuria. Death occurs without recovery of consciousness.

Variations. The duration of untreated tuberculous meningitis is generally not more than three weeks after definite symptoms appear. In general, each of the three stages described averages about a week, although the initial one may be somewhat longer and the last stage shorter. In unusual instances, however, the terminal stage may be prolonged for several weeks. The course is also subject to other variations. The prodromal stage may be absent, with the onset sudden and the total course brief. Temporary improvement and even remissions have been recorded. As a rule, the onset in infancy is more abrupt than in childhood; generalized convulsions are more frequent, the symptoms are less characteristic, and the course is shorter. A clinical course unmodified by treatment is now rarely seen.

DIAGNOSIS. A positive tuberculin reaction is only supportive evidence. As the illness advances, cutaneous sensitivity to tuberculin may be lost. The white blood cell count is not characteristic; in the early stages it may be decreased. In the late stage there is often a leukocytosis.

The *cerebrospinal fluid* provides the most important data, but an absolute diagnosis only when tubercle bacilli can be isolated from it. The fluid may be clear or only slightly turbid (the so-called ground-glass appearance). It is practically always increased in pressure. The cell count ranges from 20 to about 500 per mm^3. The cells are principally lymphocytes, though there is occasionally a predominance of polymorphonuclear cells in the early stage. The protein content of the cerebrospinal fluid is increased and is often more than 100 mg/dl; the sugar content is usually decreased, and the chloride concentration is usually significantly reduced in the latter phase of the disease.

On standing, the cerebrospinal fluid usually forms a fibrinous web or pellicle in which tubercle bacilli may be enmeshed and in which they can be demonstrated on staining. The fluid should also be centrifuged and the sediment examined. When the organisms cannot be demonstrated by direct examination, they usually can be by culture.

The *differential diagnosis* is chiefly from other conditions responsible for an increase in lymphocytic cells in the cerebrospinal fluid. (See Aseptic Meningitis Syndrome.) There is rarely any difficulty in the differential diagnosis of the various purulent meningitides, except as their course has been modified by suppressive but inadequate antimicrobial therapy. The demonstration of a tuberculous lesion in some other region of the body gives strong supportive evidence to the diagnosis of tuberculous meningitis.

PROGNOSIS. Complete recovery from tuberculous meningitis is now possible. The mortality rate is still high, ranging from 10 to 50 per cent in different series of treated cases; and the incidence of permanent physical and mental residuals among the survivors is also high. The promptness with which specific therapy is instituted would seem to be a determining factor, though recovery has occurred in patients considered to be hopeless.

TREATMENT. The treatment of choice is a combination of streptomycin and isoniazid and adequate supportive measures.

The plan currently used in our clinic is as follows: streptomycin, 50 mg/kg intramuscularly every 12 hours (but not over 2 gm/day) until there are signs of improvement, then 20 to 40 mg/kg every other day (but not over 1 gm/dose) for a total of three to six months; and isoniazid in total daily oral doses of 20 to 40 mg/kg until there is improvement. Thereafter the dose is reduced to 10 to 20 mg/kg and is continued for at least 18 months. Intrathecal therapy with antimicrobial drugs is not used. In some clinics aminosalicylic acid is administered in conjunction with isoniazid after the streptomycin has been discontinued (see Table 10–9). Administration of rifampicin has been recommended until the antibiotic sensitivity of the infecting strain is known.

One of the main obstacles in the management of tuberculous meningitis is the development of obstruction to the flow of cerebrospinal fluid. Obstruction may apparently be prevented or at times relieved by systemic administration of a corticosteroid during the first months of therapy.

Supportive measures include adequate nutrition, which often necessitates gavage feeding, vitamin supplements, attention to fluid and electrolyte balance (including sometimes a salt-losing syndrome), sedation, prophylaxis against bedsores, and early detection and treatment of intercurrent infections.

GENERAL

Diagnostic Standards and Classification of Tuberculosis. New York, American Lung Association, 1969.

Johnston, R. F., and Wildrick, K. H.: "State of the art" review. Impact of chemotherapy on the care of patients with tuberculosis. Amer. Rev. Resp. Dis. *109*:636, 1974.

Kendig, E. L.: Disorders of the Respiratory Tract in Children. Vol. I. 2nd ed. Philadelphia, W. B. Saunders Company, 1972.

Lincoln, E. M., and Sewell, E. M.: Tuberculosis in Children. New York, McGraw-Hill Book Co., Inc., 1962.

Epidemiology

Trauger, D. A.: Editorial. A note on tuberculosis epidemiology. Am. Rev. Resp. Dis. *87*:582, 1963.

Tuberculosis Programs 1971, DHEW Publication No. (HSM) 73-8189.

Pathology

Auerbach, O.: Tuberculosis in children. Am. J. Dis. Child. *75*:555, 1948.

Terplan, K.: Anatomical studies of human tuberculosis. Am. Rev. Tuberc. (Supp.) *42*:1, 1940.

Terplan, K.: Morphologic analysis of fatal tuberculosis in children. Am. Rev. Tuberc. *74*:7, 1956.

Factors Influencing Development of Infection

Johnston, J. A.: Nutritional Studies in Adolescent Girls, and Their Relation to Tuberculosis. Springfield, Ill., Charles C Thomas, 1953.

Lurie, M. B.: Heredity, Constitution and Tuberculosis; Experimental Study. Am. Rev. Tuberc. (Suppl.) *44*:1, 1941.

Pinner, M.: Pathogenesis of tuberculosis. J.A.M.A. *107*:475, 1936.

Rich, A. R.: The Pathogenesis of Tuberculosis. Springfield, Ill., Charles C Thomas, 1944.

Age Factors in Tuberculous Infection

High, R. H., and Zwerling, H. B.: Variation with age in the frequency of tuberculous pulmonary calcification. Pub. Health Rep. *61*:1769, 1946.

Israel, H. L., and Long, E. R.: Primary tuberculosis in adolescents and young adults. Am. Rev. Tuberc. *43*:42, 1941.

Lesions Simulating Tuberculosis

Christie, A., and Peterson, J. C.: Histoplasmin sensitivity. J. Pediatr. *29*:417, 1946.

Palmer, C. E.: Nontuberculous pulmonary calcification and sensitivity to histoplasmin. Pub. Health Rep. *60*:513, 1945.

Smith, C. E.: Coccidioidomycosis. Med. Clin. N. Amer. *27*:790, 1943.

Tuberculin

Furcolow, M. L., Hewell, B., Nelson, W. E., and Palmer, C. E.: Quantitative studies of tuberculin reaction. I. Titration of tuberculin sensitivity and its relation to tuberculous infection. Pub. Health Rep. *56*:1082, 1941.

Furcolow, M. L., Watson, K. A., Charron, T., and Lowe, J.: A comparison of the tine and Mono-vacc tests with the intradermal tuberculin test. Am. Rev. Resp. Dis. *96*:1009, 1968.

Nelson, W. E., Mitchell, A. G., and Brown, E. W.: Possibility of sensitization to tuberculin. Am. Rev. Tuberc. *37*:286, 1938.

Nelson, W. E., Seibert, F. B., and Long, E. R.: Technical factors affecting tuberculin test. J.A.M.A. *108*:2179, 1937.

Rosenthal, S. R.: The disc-tine tuberculin test (dried tuberculin—disposable unit). J.A.M.A. *177*:452, 1961.

Seibert, F. B., and Dufour, E.: A study of certain problems in the use of standard tuberculin. Am. Rev. Tuberc. *58*:363, 1948.

Statement of the Committee on Diagnostic Skin Testing: Tuberculin skin-testing techniques: Current status. Am. Rev. Resp. Dis. *87*:607, 1963.

Prophylaxis

A United States Public Health Service tuberculosis prophylaxis trial: Prophylactic effects of isoniazid on primary tuberculosis in children. Am. Rev. Tuberc. *76*:6, 1957.

Palmer, C. E., Shaw, L. W., and Comstock, G. W.: Community trials of BCG vaccination. Am. Rev. Tuberc. *77*:6, 1958.

Report of Ad Hoc Advisory Committee on BCG to the Surgeon General of the United States Public Health Service. Am. Rev. Tuberc. *76*:5, 1957.

Treatment

A Statement by the Committee on Tuberculosis and Respiratory Disease in Children: Treatment of tuberculosis in children. J. Pediatr. *57*:290, 1960.

Filler, J., and Porter, M.: Physiologic studies of the sequelae of tuberculous pleural effusion in children treated with antimicrobial drugs and prednisone. Am. Rev. Resp. Dis. *88*:181, 1963.

Matsaniotis, N., Kattamis, C., Economou-Mavrou, C., and Kyriazakou, M.: Bullous emphysema in childhood tuberculosis. J. Pediatr. *71*:703, 1967.

Nemir, R. L., Cardona, J., Lacoius, A., and David, M.: Prednisone therapy as an adjunct in the treatment of lymph node-bronchial tuberculosis in childhood. Am. Rev. Resp. Dis. *88*:189, 1963.

Smith, M. H. D.: Practical management of tuberculosis. Pediatr. Clin. N. Amer. *3*:427, 1956.

Steiner, P., and Portugaleza, C.: Tuberculous meningitis in children. Am. Rev. Resp. Dis. *107*:22, 1973.

INFECTIONS WITH UNCLASSIFIED MYCOBACTERIA (ATYPICAL OR ANONYMOUS MYCOBACTERIA)

The existence of acid-fast mycobacteria other than *M. tuberculosis* has been known for many years, but until recently these organisms were regarded as only occasionally pathogenic for man. In the past few years increasing evidence has shown that infections with these organisms can produce lesions which closely simulate tuberculosis in human beings and can also induce cutaneous sensitivity to tuberculin derived from human strains of *M. tuberculosis* as well as to their own specific antigens.

Currently the term "unclassified mycobacteria" is used to designate species obtained from human sources. According to the 1961 Diagnostic Standards and Classification of Tuberculosis they are grouped as follows:

Photochromogens (*M. kansasii, M. luciflavum,* the yellow bacillus, Runyon group I): these strains become yellow-pigmented only after exposure to light.

Scotochromogens (Runyon group II): the yellow-orange pigment of these strains is not completely light-conditioned.

Nonchromogenic strains (the "Battey" type, Runyon group III): characteristics include variable pigmentation, late in appearance, not light-conditioned.

Rapid growers (Runyon group IV): rapidly growing photochromogens.

EPIDEMIOLOGY. Human infections with unclassified mycobacteria have been reported from many areas of the world. In the United States the majority of the cases have been noted in the southeastern and southwestern or central states, where the most commonly isolated species are the "Battey" type and *M. kansasii,* respectively.

The unclassified mycobacteria have been isolated from a variety of sources, including soil, water, various animals and man. In man these organisms have most frequently been recovered from sputum, bronchial secretions, purulent discharges from infected lymph nodes, saliva and skin. In the rare instances of hematogenous dissemination they have been recovered from virtually every organ of the body.

Although the routes by which man acquires these infections are under intensive investigation, the epidemiologic pattern is not well understood. Outbreaks of cutaneous infections with *M. balnei* have been traced to infected water in swimming pools. Available data suggest that human contacts are relatively unimportant in the spread of these organisms.

PATHOLOGY. The macroscopic and microscopic lesions produced by infections with the unclassified mycobacteria simulate those produced by *M.*

tuberculosis. Differentiation must be made by appropriate bacteriologic studies.

CLINICAL MANIFESTATIONS. Human infections with the unclassified mycobacteria produce clinical manifestations which simulate those caused by *M. tuberculosis* and are therefore not described in detail. In adults the lungs are the most common site of infection, whereas in children most infections occur in lymph nodes, especially in the anterior cervical and submandibular areas. Isolated hematogenous foci of infection, such as osteomyelitis, have been noted. A few cases of fatal generalized infections have simulated miliary tuberculosis and the Letterer-Siwe variety of reticuloendotheliosis.

Cutaneous ulcers and chronic granulomas have been noted with infections caused by *M. ulcerans* and *M. balnei*.

DIAGNOSIS. Infections with the unclassified mycobacteria can be diagnosed only by appropriate bacteriologic studies. Pathologic studies, including the demonstration of acid-fast bacilli in tissues, purulent discharges, sputum, and the like, do not permit differentiation from disease produced by *M. tuberculosis*.

Tuberculin Tests. A number of antigens have been prepared from cultures of the unclassified mycobacteria by the method used for the production of PPD. These antigens are not commercially available, but may sometimes be obtained from state health departments or the United States Public Health Service. Intradermal tests with these antigens are applied and interpreted as described for the Mantoux test.

The results of intradermal tests with PPD-like material from the unclassified mycobacteria have shown that many persons react to one or more of the antigens and that such reactors commonly also react to the standard PPD of *M. tuberculosis*. In general, persons who have a strong reaction to the standard PPD are likely to show a lesser reaction to PPD preparations of one or more of the unclassified mycobacteria. The reverse is also observed.

Available evidence suggests that in instances when there are dermal reactions to PPD of the human tubercle bacillus and to one or more PPD preparations from the unclassified mycobacteria, the largest reaction is apt to be produced by the antigen of the infecting organism.

Differential Diagnosis. This is essentially the same as for tuberculosis.

PROGNOSIS. The outlook for spontaneous recovery from infections with the unclassified mycobacteria is generally good, probably more favorable than with infections caused by *M. tuberculosis*. Nevertheless, fatalities from these infections occasionally occur.

TREATMENT. Treatment of infections caused by the unclassified mycobacteria is largely symptomatic and supportive. Most species are moderately to strongly resistant to therapy with isoniazid and para-aminosalicylic acid. Some strains are moderately susceptible to streptomycin, cycloserine, or rifampicin. The choice of antimicrobial therapy should be controlled by in vitro sensitivity tests.

Infections of the lymph nodes or localized abscesses may be treated by excision or drainage.

ROBERT H. HIGH

Bialkin, G., Pollak, A., and Weil, A. J.: Pulmonary infection with Mycobacterium kansasii. Am. J. Dis. Child. *101*:739, 1961.

Diagnostic Standards and Classifications of Tuberculosis. New York, American Lung Association, 1961.

Edwards, L. B., and Palmer, C. E.: Epidemiologic studies of tuberculin sensitivity. Am. J. Hyg. *68*:312, 1958.

Hsu, K. H. K.: Nontuberculosis mycobacterial infections in children. J. Pediatr. *60*:705, 1962.

Kendig, E. L.: Disorders of the Respiratory Tract in Children. Vol. I. 2nd ed. Philadelphia, W. B. Saunders Company, 1972, Chap. 47.

Mellman, W. J., and Barness, L.: Unclassified mycobacteria. Am. J. Dis. Child. *104*:21, 1962.

Runyon, E. H.: Anonymous mycobacterium in pulmonary disease. Med. Clin. N. Amer. *43*:273, 1959.

Yakovac, W. C., Baker, R., Sweigert, C., and Hope, J. W.: Fatal disseminated osteomyelitis due to an anonymous mycobacterium. J. Pediatr. *59*:909, 1961.

LEPROSY

(Hansen's Disease)

Leprosy is a chronic infection caused by *Mycobacterium leprae*, which chiefly affects superficial neural and epithelial tissues.

The World Health Organization estimates that there are approximately 10.7 million infected persons, of whom about 3.8 million have some disability (including anesthesia). The Western hemisphere is estimated to have 385,000 cases, chiefly in Central and South America. In the United States patients are found now in states bordering on the Gulf of Mexico and in Hawaii; patterns of immigration and the deployment of military and civilian personnel in Asia may lead to more cases, especially in ethnic groups believed to be innately susceptible. The interval between first exposure and appearance of disease may be many years, especially in Caucasians.

There are no intermediate hosts in leprosy, transmission being dependent upon rather prolonged, intimate association with infected persons. Children are more easily infected than adults, but congenital infection does not occur. The basis for the variations in susceptibility among persons and races is probably genetic.

CLINICAL MANIFESTATIONS. Children may acquire either of the two main types of disease: *lepromatous* (nodular) or *tuberculoid* (cutaneous, neural) (Table 10–11). The two forms may coexist in the same child. Disfigurement and deformity result from destruction by the disease process itself and from burns and other traumatic injuries in areas with diminished sensation. Trophic and motor changes occur in portions of the body supplied by involved nerves.

There are numerous types of skin lesions; slightly raised erythematous plaques, elevated

TABLE 10–11 DISTINGUISHING FEATURES IN TUBERCULOID AND LEPROMATOUS LEPROSY

	TUBERCULOID	LEPROMATOUS
Usual lesions	Macules, plaques	Nodules
Distribution	Asymmetric, localized	Symmetric, general
Involvement	Skin, nerves	Skin, nerves, eyes, mucosa, viscera
Anesthesia; nerve damage	Early; in skin lesions	Late, not confined to skin
Fever	Rare	Common
Host resistance	Good	Poor
Lepromin test	Positive	Negative
Bacilli	Very sparse	Abundant
Cellular immune capacity	Usually normal	Markedly impaired

thick plaques, flat, pale anesthetic areas, and nodular lesions are among the more common. Associated anesthesia is common. Involvement of the nasal, ocular, pharyngeal and laryngeal mucosal surfaces is less frequent in children than in adults.

The *lepromatous* (nodular) lesions are the most infectious; they yield many organisms when scraped for diagnosis. These lesions tend to be symmetrical especially on the exposed parts such as face and hands. Bacteremia with *M. leprae* is common, subsiding after several months of specific therapy. Patients with lepromatous leprosy regularly have a negative lepromin skin reaction, poor resistance and progression of disease. Moreover, the incidences of active tuberculosis and of falsely positive serologic test results for syphilis are much higher in such patients than in those with tuberculoid leprosy. These patients have impaired cellular immune response.

In *tuberculoid* leprosy, skin lesions consist chiefly of asymmetrical localized macules or of plaques associated with rapid neural changes. Lesions may appear anywhere, including the clothed trunk of the body. Such lesions yield few organisms, and the patients have good resistance, often with spontaneous arrest of the disease within a few years. They usually have a positive lepromin test, seem to be less susceptible to tuberculosis than patients with lepromatous lesions, and seldom have a falsely positive serologic test for syphilis.

DIAGNOSIS. The diagnosis of leprosy is largely

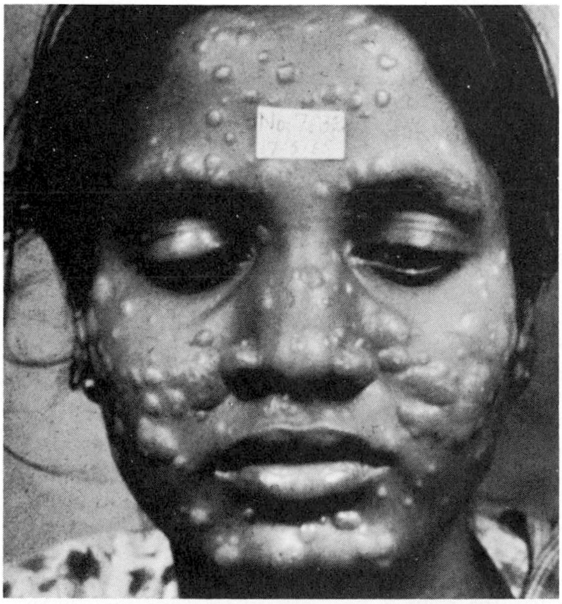

Figure 10–18 Lepromatous leprosy in an adolescent girl. Nodules are extensive, especially on exposed parts. The lepromin skin test result was negative.

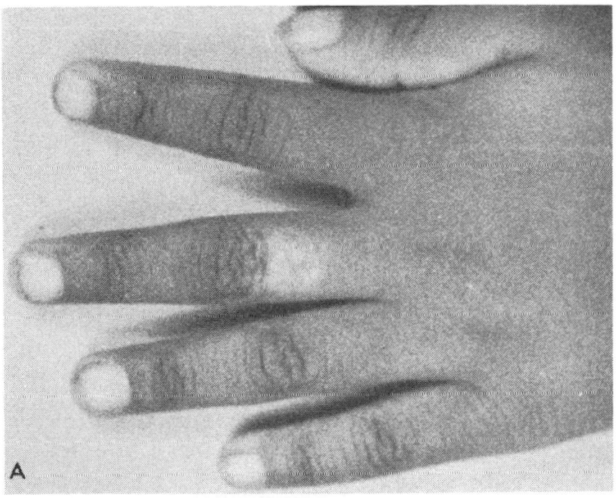

A

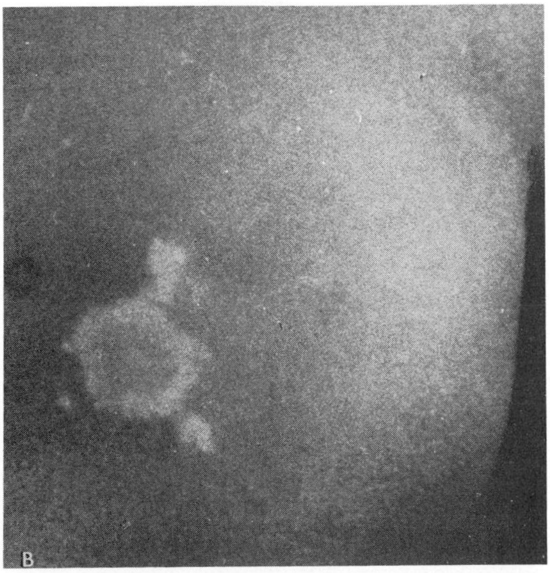

B

Figure 10–19 Tuberculoid leprosy. A, Early tuberculoid leprosy of finger: a hypopigmented anesthetic macule which had been present for 6 months. B, Tuberculoid leprosy on buttock. The well defined, anesthetic hypopigmented macule had been present for a year; the satellite lesions were of shorter duration. (Courtesy of Dr. A. B. A. Karat, India.)

clinical and may be difficult, especially in the early stages of the disease and in nonendemic areas.

In children who may have been exposed to leprosy the key to early diagnosis is to suspect any nonitching skin lesion which is hypopigmented, with reduced sweating, and which does not respond to simple treatments and displays diminished sensation progressively to light touch, temperature and pain. Similarly, any obscure peripheral nerve disorder arouses suspicion.

The **lepromin skin test** consists in the intradermal injection of autoclaved filtered human tissue containing *M. leprae.* A positive reaction in a leprous patient is more often seen in tuberculoid than in lepromatous leprosy. A positive test has limited value, however, in establishing a diagnosis; numerous persons living in areas where leprosy does not occur have positive reactions owing to cross-reaction with other animal and human strains of mycobacteria, including wild and BCG strains of *M. tuberculosis.*

Diagnosis is confirmed through demonstration of the typical acid-fast rods in scrapings and smears of affected tissues. In the past decade the technique of inoculation of murine foot pads with *M. leprae* has made it possible to study pathogenesis, response and resistance to drugs.

CONTROL AND TREATMENT. Isolation in leprosaria remains in vogue and is important for the *lepromatous* form until infectivity has been reduced by treatment. Bacteriologically negative patients need not be isolated. Unaffected children should, however, be removed from contact with infectious cases if possible. Recent trials have created hope that BCG vaccine may reduce the incidence of childhood leprosy.

Administration of diaminodiphenylsulfone (Dapsone) over a period of several years is effective in arresting progression of the disease. Prolonged maintenance therapy is important except in patients whose natural resistance is indicated by a strongly positive lepromin reaction. Except for residual nerve destruction and tissue mutilation, recovery often ensues.

Children with tuberculoid leprosy who have little disfigurement or neurologic involvement should be able to lead fairly normal lives. Surgical procedures are now available to restore usefulness of hands and feet affected by ulnar and peroneal nerve damage. Unfortunately most patients reside in parts of the world where optimal surgical and occupational and social rehabilitation are not easily achieved.

Alex. J. Steigman

Hart, D'A. P.: Biology of the mycobacterioses. Statement of the questions. Ann. N.Y. Acad. Sci. *154*:3, 1968.

Long, E. R.: Biology of the mycobacterioses. A retrospective review of mycobacteria and the diseases they cause. Ann. N.Y. Acad. Sci. *154*:8, 1968.

Sloan, N. R., Worth, R. M., Jano, B., et al.: Repository acedapsone in leprosy chemoprophylaxis and treatment. Lancet *2*:525, 1971.

WHO Expert Committee on Leprosy: Fourth Report. Geneva, WHO Tech. Rep. Ser. No. 459, 1970.

SPIROCHETAL INFECTIONS

CLASSIFICATION AND NOMENCLATURE. Spirochaetales is an order consisting of two families of motile spiral organisms: (1) Spirochaetaceae with its three genera (Spirochaeta, Saprospira, Cristispira) which do not cause human disease, and (2) Treponemataceae with its three genera (Treponema, Leptospira, Borrelia) which can cause human disease. These last three genera include species which are saprophytes, others which cause only animal disease, and still others, like certain leptospira, which may afflict man or animals.

The recognized spirochetal infections of man are listed in Table 10–12; they are major causes of human disease. There are numerous other species of Spirochaetales which are saprophytic in man; for example, *T. microdentium* resides in the mouth and gums.

SYPHILIS

Syphilis is a systemic communicable infection characterized by periods of clinical activity and prolonged latency. The requirement of a premarital serologic test for syphilis (STS) and the widespread use of penicillin (not necessarily given for syphilis) have dramatically reduced the occurrence of infectious syphilis in the United States until lately, when a rising incidence has been noted, particularly in adolescents. In 1957, 6251 cases of primary and secondary syphilis were reported; in 1971 the figure was 23,336.

The organism responsible for syphilis, *Treponema pallidum,* is a fine, pale, spiral motile thread 5 to 15 μ long and about 0.15 μ thick, which cannot be cultured in vitro and which survives poorly outside the body. It stains poorly even in tissue sections; its detection in fresh scrapings of lesions requires darkfield illumination and a competent observer. Lifelong persistence of the organism despite successful treatment has been documented, especially in the eye.

Fetal syphilis is contracted from the mother, whose infection is usually latent. Acquired syphilis requires close contact between an infective lesion and a break in the skin or mucosa of the genitalia, anus, lips, mouth, face, fingers or other parts of the recipient child or adult. Fomites, vectors, and the

TABLE 10-12 MEMBERS OF TREPONEMATACEAE WHICH CAUSE HUMAN DISEASE

Treponema		
*pallidum**	Human contact (venereal)	Syphilis
*pallidum**	Human contact (nonvenereal)	Endemic childhood syphilis
*pertenue**	Human contact (nonvenereal)	Yaws
*carateum**	Human contact (nonvenereal)	Pinta
Leptospira		
± 15 species	Direct or indirect contact with animals	Leptospiroses
Borrelia		
recurrentis	Lice, ticks	Relapsing fever
vincenti	Human (usually with B. fusiformis)	Vincent's angina, gingivitis, genital and topical ulcers, etc.

*These treponemata cannot be distinguished morphologically nor by the serologic reactions they engender. The clinical pictures produced are distinctive. Their relation is such that in places where yaws, pinta and endemic nonvenereal childhood syphilis flourish, the incidence of venereal syphilis is markedly curtailed.

like, appear to have no role in transmission. Transmission by blood transfusion is now extremely rare.

CONGENITAL (FETAL) SYPHILIS

EPIDEMIOLOGY. The incidence of fetal syphilis is determined by the incidence of syphilis in pregnant women and by whether or not the disease is detected and treated early enough in pregnancy to protect the infant. The effectiveness of preventive measures would be increased if the STS required before marriage in many places were to be repeated early in pregnancy, again in the third trimester, and in subsequent pregnancies, since fetal syphilis may be contracted from a mother whose syphilitic infection occurred during the current pregnancy or many years earlier and whose intervening pregnancies may have yielded infants without syphilis.

Congenital syphilis is often not recognized in early infancy when treatment is highly successful. A resurgence of concern with congenital syphilis is taking place. In 1965 less than 15 per cent of cases reported in the United States were diagnosed under 10 years of age; in 1971 this had risen to almost 25 per cent. Cases of congenital syphilis diagnosed after 10 years of age generally have serious sequelae. Prevention and control of congenital syphilis depends on a high level of clinical suspicion, supported by routine and diagnostic use of laboratory and radiologic aids.

PATHOLOGY. Fetuses of less than 5 months' gestation have not been observed to have syphilitic pathology. It was once believed that for some reason *T. pallidum* could not pass across the placenta until there was full development of the deciduate hemochorial placenta; but it is more likely that *T. pallidum* may cross the placenta at an early stage before the fetus has developed those sufficiently mature delayed-sensitivity (cellular) responses which are necessary for pathologic lesions to be detectable.

Syphilis only rarely causes abortion, but if the mother is untreated, stillbirths result in one fourth of cases. The other 75 per cent of untreated mothers deliver offspring who may manifest no *clinical* abnormality for weeks or even months. The severity of disease depends upon the time in pregnancy when the fetus is infected, upon the dose of *T. pallidum* and its capacity to multiply in a given fetus, upon the state of maternal immunity, and upon whether the pregnant mother received sufficient penicillin to cure or modify the infection. Penicillin might have been given to the mother inadvertently for some intercurrent infection or specifically for syphilis.

The fetal tissues most often extensively involved in stillborn infants or in those severely ill at or soon after birth are bone, bone marrow, lungs, liver and spleen. There may be considerable extramedullary hematopoiesis. Any organ system may be involved. Lesions of the skin and mucous membranes in early congenital syphilis, generally manifest a few weeks or months after birth, may occasionally be present at delivery.

When congenital syphilis is not treated in infancy, additional changes involving such tissues as cornea, teeth, bone, palate and nervous system become evident in later years.

CLINICAL MANIFESTATIONS OF EARLY CONGENITAL SYPHILIS. The infant may seem normal for the first few weeks or months of life. General symptoms such as fever, anemia, failure to gain weight or restlessness may first appear without any of the characteristic lesions of the skin or mucous membranes. On the other hand, local findings may erupt in an infant who appears quite well otherwise. This stage of congenital syphilis is roughly analogous to the systemic eruptive secondary stage of acquired syphilis. There is no lesion in congenital or in transfusion-acquired syphilis which corresponds to the primary or chancre stage of acquired syphilis.

The characteristic clinical changes of florid congenital syphilis include a variety of rashes, severe rhinitis ("snuffles"), moist lesions at the mucocutaneous junctions of the mouth, anus and genitalia, painful pseudoparalysis of limbs, and enlargement of liver, spleen and lymph nodes. Scrapings of the cutaneous and mucosal lesions reveal motile *T. pallidum* on darkfield examination.

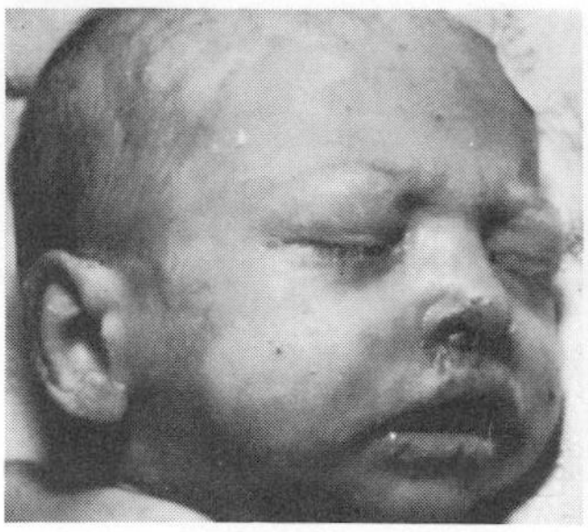
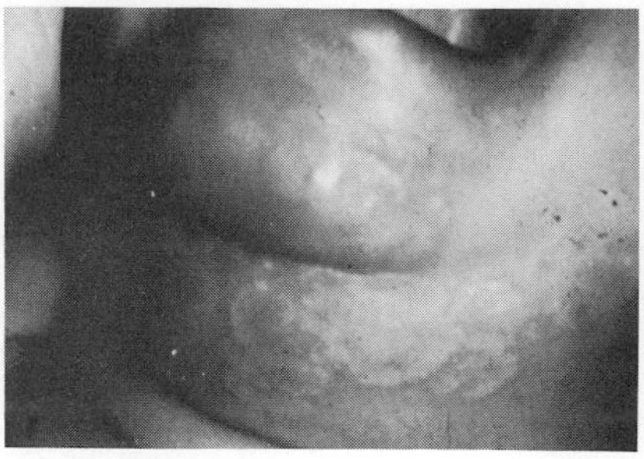
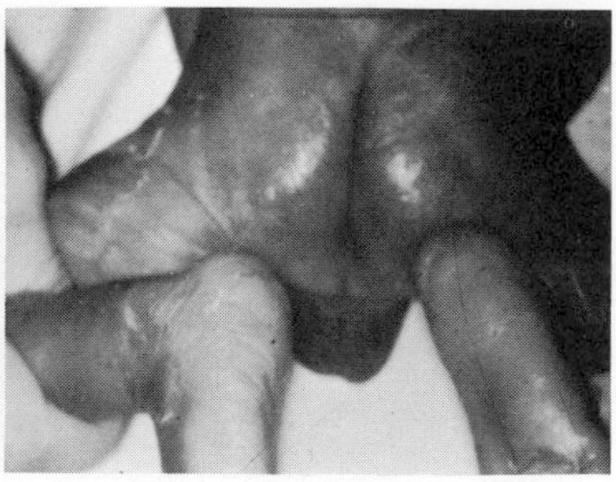

Figure 10–20 Figure 10–21 Figure 10–22

Figure 10–20 Nasal snuffles, labial excoriation, macular eruption of forehead.
Figure 10–21 Circinate syphilide.
Figure 10–22 Desquamation with shiny, parchment-like appearance following bullous eruption.

The eruption in skin may be scant or diffuse. It is reddish and maculopapular, sometimes bullous or circinate, and involves palms and soles. The nails may be ridged, and syphilitic paronychia may occur from finger sucking. The rash may disappear spontaneously, only to recur a few weeks or months later. No permanent stigma remains from such eruptions in skin, whether or not specific therapy is given. But the nasal discharge of syphilitic rhinitis ("snuffles") commonly excoriates the upper lip, leaving fine scars, and the nasal structures may ulcerate, leaving a flat nasal bridge. Mucocutaneous lesions about the mouth, anus and genitalia are also moist and irritating, and produce fissures which heal with permanent scars ("rhagades"), especially around the corners of the mouth and on the chin. During the florid eruptive stage of early congenital syphilis, raised plaques may be present in the perianal area, and even condylomata, which are more characteristic of later stages. The eruptions of early congenital syphilis do not itch.

A characteristic pseudoparalysis (Parrot's paralysis) may occur in one or more limbs, owing to the bone changes of syphilitic osteochondritis and periostitis. Lymph node enlargement is common, and involvement of the epitrochlear node is especially characteristic. Edema may be seen in severe cases, owing to hypoproteinemia and sometimes to renal involvement (syphilitic nephrosis). Anemia may stem from the syphilitic infection and from complicating secondary bacterial infection, especially of the respiratory tract.

Although the central nervous system is seldom clinically involved in early congenital syphilis, the spinal fluid should always be examined for cells, for abnormalities of protein content and for STS. Acute meningovascular syphilis in early infancy frequently has severe sequelae, which include mental retardation, low-grade hydrocephalus and convulsions. Other damage to the nervous system and organs of special sense may not become evident for years.

Radiologic changes in the skeleton are often diagnostic in early congenital syphilis and may be especially helpful when the serologic and clinical findings are ambiguous. Characteristic changes include multiple sites of osteochondritis at the elbows, wrists, ankles and knees, periostitis of several long bones and occasionally of the skull bones, widened and serrated epiphyseal lines and sometimes actual separation of epiphyses. Despite adequate therapy prenatally to the mother or to the infant after birth the periostitis may persist for many months.

Untreated, early congenital syphilis frequently subsides, but *T. pallidum* persists in the tissues. Recent evidence indicates that *T. pallidum* may persist in ocular tissues for five or six decades. The infant soon becomes noncontagious, however, and

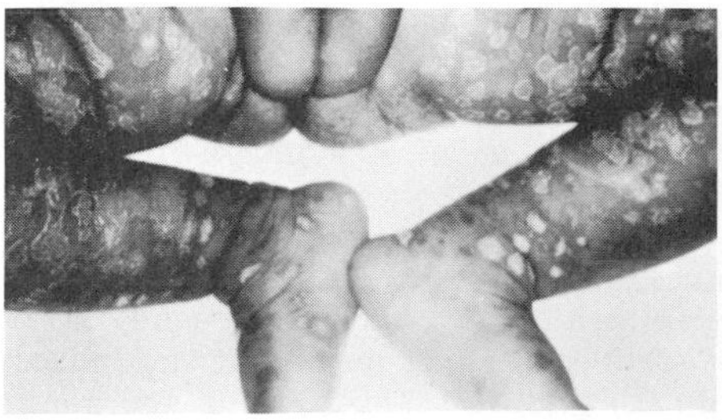
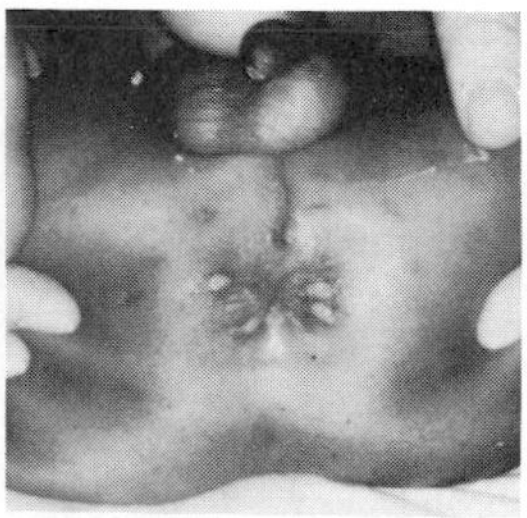
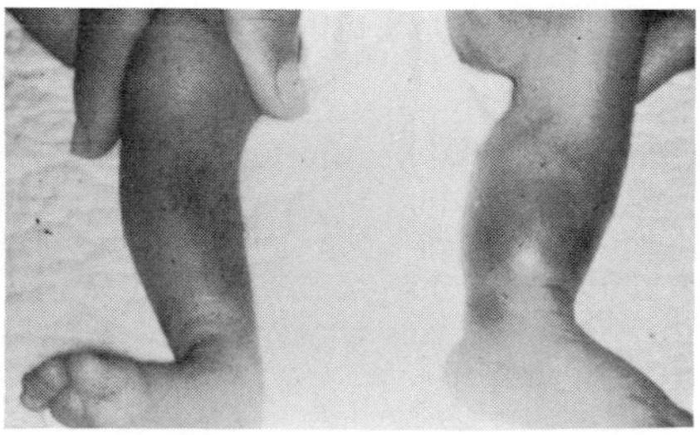

Figure 10–23 Figure 10–24 Figure 10–25

Figure 10–23 Generalized maculopapular syphilide.
Figure 10–24 Perianal condylomata.
Figure 10–25 Severe bilateral syphilitic periostitis.

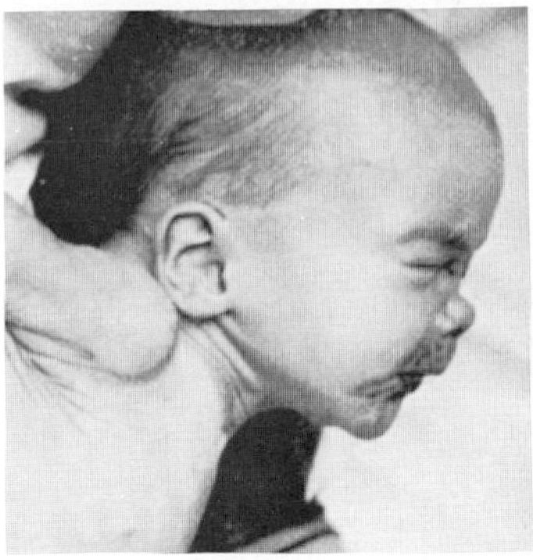
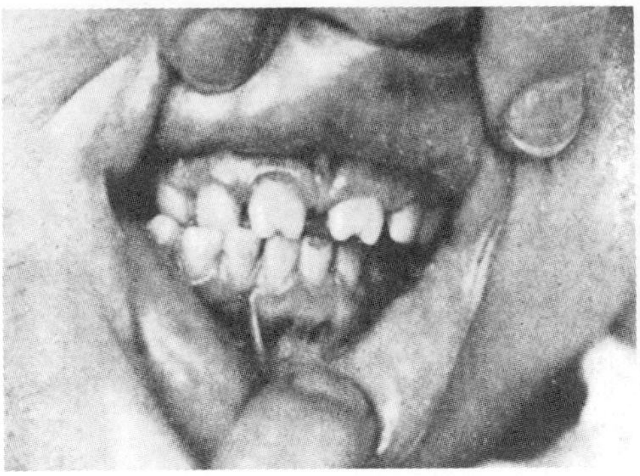
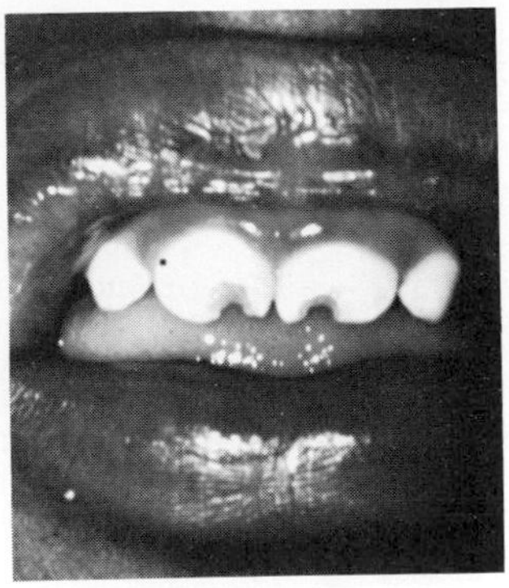

Figure 10–26 *Figure 10–27* *Figure 10–28*

Figure 10–26 *Saddle nose in early syphilis.*
Figure 10–27 *Hutchinson's teeth in congenital syphilis in a boy 10 years of age.*
Figure 10–28 *Dental dysplasia of deciduous incisors, nonsyphilitic, not to be confused with hutchinsonian incisors.*

probably cannot be reinfected with acquired syphilis. Nor will the female child be able to give congenital syphilis to her offspring ("third-generation syphilis"). The child may bear *stigma of the early manifestations* such as a flat bridge of the nose, a square high forehead (cranial bossing), and fine scars around the puckered mouth and chin (rhagades). Other changes which were initiated early take time to appear. For example, the buds of the permanent incisors and first permanent molars are being formed in the first weeks of extrauterine life, when the impact of early congenital syphilis may be great. Each permanent incisor may become notched **(Hutchinson's incisor),** and the cusps of the molar surfaces may appear squeezed together **(mulberry molar).** The deciduous teeth do not appear deformed.

CLINICAL MANIFESTATIONS OF LATE CONGENITAL SYPHILIS. The term "late congenital syphilis" refers to those clinical manifestations which appear only after infancy. The most frequent and important of these involve the skeleton, the eye and the central nervous system. Much rarer are subcutaneous gummas, paroxysmal hemoglobinuria and cardiovascular or other visceral changes more characteristic of late syphilis in adults.

The most frequent late ophthalmic change is *interstitial keratitis,* which may be unilateral or bilateral and appear at any age. Intense photophobia and lacrimation occur, and progressive corneal opacity may lead to blindness in a period of weeks, or months. Less common late ocular manifestations include choroiditis, retinitis, vascular occlusions and optic atrophy.

The nervous system may harbor latent *meningovascular syphilitic infection,* which may be abruptly manifest in prepubertal children by hemiplegia or convulsions. More often, however, the child with central nervous system syphilis is dull, retarded or irritable or exhibits antisocial behavior. *Juvenile paresis* is the counterpart of general paresis in the adult. *Juvenile tabes* with spinal cord involvement is rare. Involvement of the eighth cranial nerves may occur without other detectable central nervous system changes and may produce rapidly progressive *deafness.* The classic **Hutchinson's triad** of late congenital syphilis consists of nerve deafness, interstitial keratitis and hutchinsonian incisors.

The skeletal changes include persistent or recurrent periostitis which causes chronic thickening of bone, best exemplified in the tibia, where anterior curving produces the "saber shin." Dactylitis may occur as a late manifestation, and swollen joints

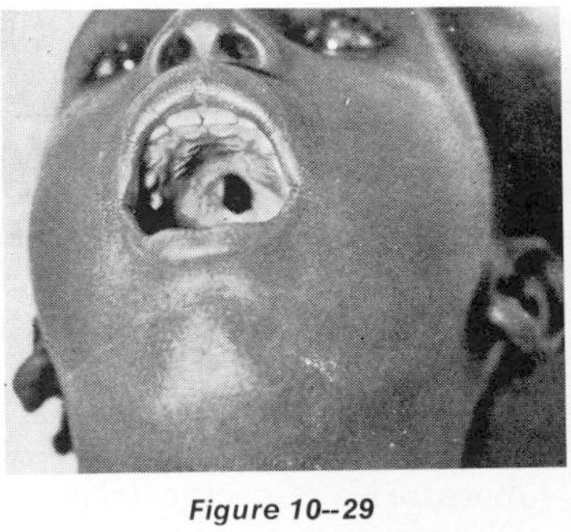
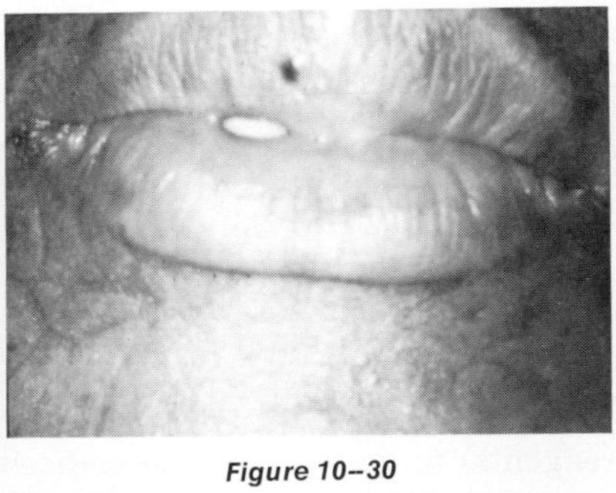
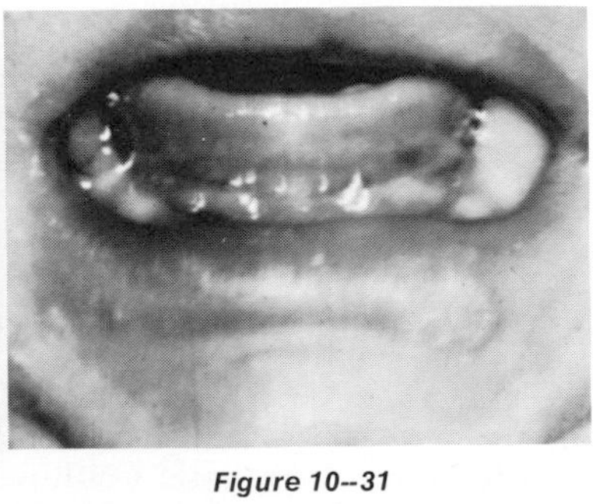

Figure 10–29 *Figure 10–30* *Figure 10–31*

Figure 10–29 *Syphilitic perforation of the palate in a girl 10 years of age.*
Figure 10–30 *Rhagades as long-term residua from infantile snuffles and eruption.*
Figure 10–31 *Chancre of lower lip, darkfield-positive.*

TABLE 10–13 CLINICAL MANIFESTATIONS OF CONGENITAL SYPHILIS

AREA AFFECTED	EARLY MANIFESTATIONS	STIGMAS	LATE MANIFESTATIONS
Skin	Maculopapular rash Diffuse inflammation of palms and soles Mucocutaneous lesions about nose, mouth and anus Condylomas Café-au-lait appearance Pemphigus Paronychia Deformities of nails Alopecia	Rhagades	Condylomas Syphilides Gummas
Mucous membrane	Rhinitis Mucous patches	Saddle nose	
Bones	Periostitis Osteochondritis (epiphysitis) Pseudoparalysis (Parrot's) Dactylitis	Bossing of head Hutchinson's teeth Mulberry molars	Osteoperiostitis Saber shin Gummas Hydrarthrosis Arthritis
Eye	Chorioretinitis Iritis	Keratotic scar Chorioretinitis Pupillary change Optic atrophy	Interstitial keratitis Chorioretinitis Optic atrophy
Nervous system	Meningitis Hydrocephalus	Deafness	Deafness Neurosyphilis
Other	Pneumonia alba Hepatitis Jaundice Splenomegaly Nephritis Lymphatic hyperplasia Orchitis Malnutrition Anemia Gastrointestinal disturbances Fever Hemorrhage	Syphilitic facies	Paroxysmal hemoglobinuria

may occur without evident cause from time to time, especially in adolescent boys and at the knee (**Clutton's joints**). Gummatous involvement of the bones of the nose or palate may lead to destruction of the nasal bridge or to perforation of the palate.

Table 10–13 lists most of the manifestations of late congenital syphilis.

DIAGNOSIS. The diagnosis of congenital syphilis depends on clinical judgment and appropriate use and evaluation of microscopic, serologic, radiologic and sometimes epidemiologic data.

Darkfield examination of scrapings from moist cutaneous and mucocutaneous lesions in early congenital syphilis may reveal the *T. pallidum* to the experienced observer. The organism cannot be cultured in vitro.

Serologic tests for syphilis fall into two main groups: (1) those using *nontreponemal* antigens (cardiolipin or synthetic lecithin reagents) to detect nonspecific *reagin* antibodies in complement-fixation tests (Wassermann, Kolmer), flocculation tests (VDRL, Kahn, Kline, Eagle, Hinton and others), or agglutination tests (RPR—Rapid Plasma Reagin); and (2) specific serologic tests with antigens harvested from *T. pallidum* inoculated into rabbit testis.

Within both groups of tests there are numerous variations in procedures; the physician should familiarize himself with those used in his region. The reagin tests are highly satisfactory for screening, especially in *early* congenital syphilis, when the tests using treponemal antigen are not often needed to clarify an ambiguous situation. The latter tests are most helpful in dealing with questionable cases of *late* congenital syphilis and in adults who have been treated.

The original treponemal serologic test described in 1949 is the TPI (*T. pallidum* immobilization) procedure. This test is highly specific and sensitive, but its complexities restrict its use to a few highly specialized laboratories. Specific treponemal antibody, unlike the nonspecific reagin, is detectable for many years, often for life; it is little influenced by therapy unless this is given early in the course of infection. Other treponema-specific serologic tests have been developed since 1949, of which the FTA-ABS (fluorescent treponemal antibody-absorbed) is most favored at present. Commercially prepared slides containing dried *T. pallidum* (nonviable) are overlaid with the serum being tested. Syphilitic antibody globulin will attach to the *T. pallidum,* and can be revealed when fluorescein-tagged antibody to human gamma globulin is added and the treponemata viewed for fluorescence under ultraviolet light microscopy. Human serums may contain nonspecific treponemal antibodies; these can be absorbed out with a sonicate of Reiter treponemes prior to the FTA-ABS test. When in case of an asymptomatic newborn infant there is doubt about the interpretation of a positive STS, whether reagin or treponemal, repeated *quantitative* serial tests should be performed. The half-life of gamma globulin is such that a falling titer in the first three to four months of life is the usual finding associated with the passive transfer of maternal antisyphilitic antibody. The passively transferred reagin antibody usually declines in titer before the passively acquired FTA antibody disappears. The maternal history of intrapartum illnesses and antibiotic therapy, the maternal serology and the roentgenographic examination of the infant's skeleton must all be taken into consideration in deciding whether a positive STS reflects active disease requiring therapy in an asymptomatic infant. When there remains reasonable doubt about the status of a newborn infant with a positive STS who does not have any clinical manifestations of syphilis, it would seem appropriate to treat him as if he had an active infection.

In response to various infections, including congenital syphilis, newborn and young infants have elevated serum levels of immunoglobulin M (IgM). IgM is not passively transferred via the placenta. The IgM fraction of umbilical cord or infant's serum can be tested by the indirect immunofluorescent technique (IgM-FTA-ABS.). A positive reaction gives highly specific evidence of *active* syphilis.

Biologic falsely positive reagin reactions (BFP) occasionally create problems in the diagnosis of congenital syphilis. Tests using crude lipoidal antigen may give more BFP's than tests using purified cardiolipin. A positive STS which does not fit the clinical picture should be repeated by several techniques. BFP reactions may be found if the infant or his mother has a current or recent infection or recent immunization. BFP reactions are common in some families, especially in those in which there have been so-called autoimmune diseases such as thyroiditis or lupus erythematosus. Apparently healthy pregnant women may occasionally have a BFP which appears in the newborn infant's cord blood. Such infants do not have elevated IgM levels, nor are specific treponemal test results positive.

Differential Diagnosis. The chief pitfall in diagnosis is not to think of syphilis. In *early congenital syphilis* the following diagnoses may be considered: diaper rash, scabies, epidermolysis bullosa, drug rashes, cutaneous moniliasis, pemphigus, Letterer-Siwe disease, the fetal rubella syndrome, cytomegalovirus infection, toxoplasmosis, acute poliomyelitis, scurvy, pyogenic osteomyelitis, Caffey syndrome, the "battered-child syndrome," and others. The sometimes bloody nasal discharge, excoriating the upper lip, may suggest nasal diphtheria.

Late congenital syphilis may suggest phlyctenular conjunctivitis, undifferentiated mental retardation, osteomyelitis, epilepsy, idiopathic hemiplegia, acquired toxoplasmic chorioretinitis and other conditions.

TREATMENT AND PROGNOSIS. In *early congenital syphilis* penicillin is the therapeutic drug of choice. *Only in the most severe forms of penicillin allergy* should erythromycin (15 mg/kg/day for 12 to 15 days) be substituted for penicillin. Injectable preparations are preferred to oral administration. Experience with semisynthetic penicillins and with cephalothin is too limited for any reliable recommendations to be made at this time. See Table 10–14 for treatment schedules.

When a full course of penicillin is given in early congenital syphilis, there is swift disappearance of lesions. Reversion to negative of the STS and of the reactivity of spinal fluid requires some months. Skeletal changes are more stubborn, especially those of the periosteum; these may not disappear radiographically for a long time, even when the mother received an adequate course of therapy during pregnancy.

Brief, febrile Herxheimer reactions occur in 15 to 20 per cent of patients, especially if excessive penicillin is given. These reactions are of little consequence and do not constitute an indication to change from penicillin to other drugs.

The general and social management of these infants must not be neglected. Secondary bacterial infections, anemia, malnutrition and parental negligence or dysfunction in extreme degree sometimes coexist with syphilis in such infants.

In *late congenital syphilis* the antibiotic therapy is generally similar to that for early congenital syphilis. Interstitial keratitis requires additional

TABLE 10–14 DOSE AND DURATION OF PENICILLIN THERAPY FOR CONGENITAL SYPHILIS

AGE	CHOICE OF	DURATION
Under 2 years	15,000 units APP*/kg /day	10 days
	or	
	50,000 units benzathine penicillin/kg	Weekly for 3 doses
Over 2 years	20,000 units APP*/kg /day	10 days
	or	
	100,000 units benzathine penicillin/kg	Weekly for 3 doses

*APP = aqueous procaine penicillin.

treatment, and will include topical corticosteroids and topical cycloplegics. In interstitial keratitis, optic atrophy, chorioretinitis and iritis the cooperation of an ophthalmologic consultant in planning treatment is highly desirable. These lesions are generally considered to be manifestations of hypersensitivity to endogenous spirochetes and may result in painful and deep corneal scars and iritis.

ACQUIRED SYPHILIS

Infants, children or adolescents may acquire syphilis from an infected adult. The older the patient, the more likely is the source of transmission through sexual play or exploration or participation in usual or unusual forms of intercourse. Transmission to a youngster by kissing or other innocent contact is not common, even from a parent or other adult in the rather highly infectious stage of secondary syphilis.

The primary sites of introduction of *T. pallidum* are chiefly on the genitalia, anus, face, neck, lips and mouth, but a detectable chancre is not common in children. It is often not until such manifestations of the secondary stage as rash, condylomata and mucous patches appear that the condition comes to medical attention.

When acquired syphilis is recognized and treated promptly, the infection is suppressed and seroconversion leads to negative reagin tests. Whether every *T. pallidum* is then entirely eradicated is doubtful. Recent evidence suggests long-term survival of *T. pallidum* even after seroconversion. The organism has been demonstrated in ocular fluids, spinal fluid, lymph nodes and liver by means of fluorescent antibody techniques. These organisms are relatively dormant, but may still be pathogenic, especially for ocular lesions. Penicillin acts most effectively on actively multiplying organisms; in these cases of dormancy the *T. pallida* are not reproducing regularly.

ENDEMIC NONVENEREAL CHILDHOOD SYPHILIS

This condition is not known in the Western Hemisphere. Children in the Balkans, Asia Minor, the Middle East and parts of Africa may be infected in early childhood by personal nonvenereal contact. Lesions in moist areas (mouth, axilla, inguinal region, rectum) abound with *T. pallidum*. There is no detectable chancre-like primary lesion. Congenital (fetal) infection is not known in this condition. Late changes may occur in the bones and elsewhere, but the majority of changes are confined to the skin.

YAWS

Yaws is an acute and chronically relapsing nonvenereal treponematosis, primarily of children, caused by the introduction of *T. pertenue* into a break in the skin. *Treponema pertenue* cannot be distinguished microscopically from *T. pallidum;* patients with yaws have serologic reagin and treponemal antibody reactions identical to those of patients with syphilis. Because the biologic relation between the two treponemes results in considerable cross-immunity, syphilis, including congenital syphilis, has a lowered incidence in regions where yaws is endemic. Congenital yaws is unknown.

Yaws occurs chiefly in the wet tropical climate of Africa, Southeast Asia and some South Pacific Islands. It is also found in Central and South America, and was probably brought to the New World by West African slaves. Instances are reported of children infected in these endemic areas in whom lesions erupt after they emigrate to areas where yaws is unknown.

One to two months after exposure to yaws a primary granuloma or papule appears at the inoculation site. An indolent papilloma usually persists some weeks to months, until the manifestations of the secondary stage appear.

The secondary stage is characterized by mild constitutional symptoms and by the eruption in crops of macules, papules and characteristic granulomas (*yaws* or *frambesiomas),* which are crusted granular lesions resembling raspberries. These lesions are infectious and may persist for months or years, after which they undergo spontaneous involution. Yaws may then become latent until the lesions of the tertiary stage appear.

The lesions of tertiary yaws may resemble cutaneous gummata, with some destruction of skin and subcutaneous tissues, and with painful thickening of the soles ("crab yaws") and sometimes of the palms. In a small percentage of patients, osteitis and periostitis of the extremities, and more rarely of skull, pelvis and spine, may occur, either in association with the infectious skin lesions or in later years after the skin lesions have regressed. In contrast to syphilis, yaws rarely if ever involves the nervous system, organs of special sense or viscera.

Diagnosis requires alertness to the possibility of yaws and use of the same laboratory tests for confirmation as syphilis.

Penicillin therapy in the doses used for syphilis is remarkably effective. Eradication of yaws may be obtained with mass use of penicillin in endemic areas, together with improved conditions of general health.

PINTA

Thought before 1938 to be a fungus infection, pinta is caused by *T. carateum,* which is morphologically indistinguishable from *T. pallidum.* This nonvenereal treponematosis is essentially confined to the skin. Visceral and osseous lesions do not occur. Congenital pinta is unknown. Patients with pinta have the same serologic reactions as do patients with syphilis or yaws.

Pinta is endemic in wide areas of Central and South America and, to a lesser extent, in the West Indies, tropical Africa and some South Pacific islands. Children and young persons are the chief victims, but marks of untreated pinta remain visible throughout life.

Treponema carateum enters a break in the skin. In several weeks the primary papular lesion occurs, which often looks like a patch of psoriasis or scaly eczema. The regional lymph nodes are slightly enlarged, and treponemata can be seen on darkfield microscopy of skin scrapings or in an aspirate of a lymph node. The primary lesion may spread slightly or seem to regress. After 6 to 8 months the secondary eruption occurs, which consists of small macules and papules, especially likely to appear on the face, scalp and other exposed parts. These are bluish to pink, nonpruritic, slightly scaly and darkfield-positive. Many lesions involute spontaneously; others coalesce, forming scaly pigmented patches resembling psoriasis. Their color ultimately changes to a violet-bluish tint. In time the skin becomes atrophic and depigmented, leaving areas of disfiguring vitiligo and mottled skin on the hands, wrists, ankles, feet, face and scalp. The chronic lesions of pinta may remain darkfield-positive for years.

Treatment with penicillin is as effective as for yaws.

LEPTOSPIROSIS

Many species of animals are carriers or victims of the 15 or more serotypes of Leptospira. The principal carriers throughout the world are wild rodents whose excreta—especially urine—may infect many species of domesticated and wild animals or contaminate water supplies. Cats, dogs, cattle, swine, deer, foxes, raccoons, skunks and opossums become infected with Leptospira through exposure to the excreta of rodents, and may become ill and die; but more often they become persistent urinary carriers. Human infection results from direct or indirect exposure to infected animals, their products or excreta. The diagnosis in man is considered frequently only in adults with occupational exposures, such as miners, veterinarians, herdsmen and farmers. The actual frequency of human infection is doubtless greater than reported.

Most human infections in the United States seem to be due to *L. icterohemorrhagica*, *L. canicola* and *L. pomona,* but all serotypes are potentially pathogenic for man. Unlike the treponemata causing human disease, Leptospira are fairly hardy and can be cultured in vitro and on chick embryo membranes. Direct contact with animals is not necessary for transmission; indirect contact, such as bathing in contaminated waters, is sufficient. The incubation period is one to two weeks. Leptospirosis produces a wide range of clinical illnesses, from inapparent to fatal.

Because of its severity, *Weil's disease (icterohemorrhagic fever)* is the best known manifestation of leptospirosis, but it is relatively uncommon. The liver, kidneys, muscles and blood vessels are especially involved. Jaundice, proteinuria, azotemia, hematuria, anemia and thrombocytopenia occur, with hemorrhages into the skin and many viscera, including the nervous system. Macular and maculopapular rashes with no particularly distinctive features may appear. Although *L. icterohemorrhagica* is classically associated with Weil's disease, this organism may cause a very mild general illness not involving the liver, and Weil's disease may be caused by other Leptospira species.

Leptospirosis may run a biphasic febrile course, with the initial period ushered in abruptly with fever, headache, conjunctivitis, photophobia with scleral pain and hemorrhage, myalgia and chills. The clinical picture of aseptic meningitis is probably the most common expression of leptospirosis. Even in patients without nuchal or spinal rigidity, pleocytosis is frequently found on spinal fluid examination, especially four to five days after onset of symptoms.

A mild febrile illness with a macular or maculopapular eruption over the pretibial area *(pretibial fever, Fort Bragg fever)* has been ascribed to *L. autumnalis,* and has been reported in children, who may develop recurring febrile episodes.

The diagnosis of leptospirosis begins with suspicion of the disease. Children taken abruptly ill with a grippe-like illness should be suspect, especially in summer or fall and if they have been swimming in questionably safe streams or otherwise exposed to animals. It is more usually epidemiologic data rather than clinical judgment that point toward the diagnosis of leptospirosis. Laboratory confirmation of the diagnosis is essential, and identification of the specific serotype of Leptospira involved is desirable as an aid in surveillance of disease in herds of domestic animals.

Blood, urine and spinal fluid may reveal Leptospira on culture. Serologic tests include agglutination, fluorescent antibody and other techniques. Direct darkfield examination of blood, urine or spinal fluid is *not* recommended, owing to the frequency of confusing artifacts. A polymorphonuclear leukocytosis occurs, but is too variable to be useful in diagnosis.

Leptospirosis must be differentiated from aseptic meningitis, acute brucellosis, hemolytic-uremic syndrome, dengue fever, typhoid fever, nephritis, hepatitis, and the like.

Patients severely ill with leptospirosis require skillful management of fluids, electrolytes and nutrition, and the use of blood components as indicated. Penicillin does not have the same dramatic effect as in treponemal diseases; it does, however, reduce fever and somewhat shorten the period of illness. Penicillin should be given in preference to the tetracyclines.

Treponematoses Research. Geneva, World Health Organization Technical Report Series No. 455, 1970.

VD Fact Sheet. 28th ed. Atlanta, Center for Disease Control, 1971.

RAT-BITE FEVER

Two forms of rat-bite fever may be distinguished clinically and bacteriologically. Despite the frequency of exposure to rats in depressed urban areas and in certain occupations, rat-bite fever is not common. Both forms have recently been observed following bites by laboratory rats.

In both types of rat-bite fever it appears that the nature of the illness is determined both by infection and by a cellular and humoral immune response to the organism on the part of the host.

SPIRILLARY RAT-BITE FEVER
(Sodoku)

The spirillary form of rat-bite fever is caused by *Spirillum minus* and produces a clinical picture known as Sodoku, first described in Japan.

The initial bite heals promptly, to be followed within 10 to 30 days by a painful indurated ulcer at the site of the original bite, and by regional lymphadenopathy. In a few days the temperature may rise and a rash will appear, which consists of violaceous macules, more or less ovoid in shape and up to several centimeters in diameter. There is no pruritus. The eruption is in some ways analogous to that of secondary syphilis. Within a few days to a week the temperature will subside, but cycles of fever recur at irregular intervals.

Laboratory confirmation of the diagnosis may be difficult. Darkfield examination of scrapings from the lesion may show the relatively thick spirillary forms with three curls. The organism cannot be cultivated in vitro. Animal inoculation in expert hands may be confirmatory, but animals used must be free of morphologically related organisms. Falsely positive reagin serologic reactions for syphilis are common.

There is a prompt therapeutic response to either penicillin or streptomycin.

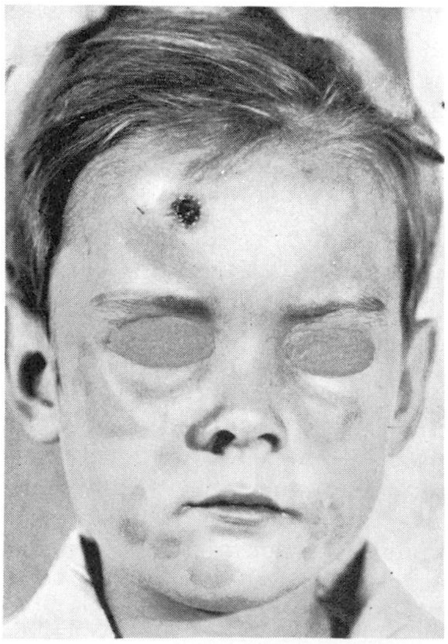

Figure 10–32 *Sodoku: chancre-like indurated ulcer at bite site on forehead; secondary macular eruption of face.*

STREPTOBACILLARY RAT-BITE FEVER AND HAVERHILL FEVER

Streptobacillus moniliformis is carried by many rats, presumably as a saprophyte. The organism is an aerobic gram-negative bacillus; it may assume a minute L form which is filtrable and resistant to penicillin. In old cultures, especially in solid media, it forms chains, with swellings resembling yeast buds; hence, the designation moniliformis.

The incubation period following an infectious rat bite ranges from two to seven days. The local lesion is not distinctive and may be overlooked even when fever erupts. In contrast to spirillary rat-bite fever, the streptobacillary form has a greater tendency to produce a maculopapular rash, arthralgia, arthritis, subcutaneous abscesses, endocarditis and erythema nodosum.

When *S. moniliformis* infects man by the respiratory or alimentary tract instead of by rat bite, the resulting condition is referred to as *Haverhill fever* The incubation period is short, often less than five days, with abrupt onset of fever, chills, vomiting, headache, muscle and joint pains and a maculopapular rash. Recurrent cycles of fever are characteristic, and at times large metastatic subcutaneous abscesses may appear. Arthritis is a prominent feature. Organisms may be recovered from any of the affected parts.

Laboratory tests are more readily confirmatory in streptobacillary rat-bite fever than in the spirillary form. The organism can be cultured in vitro or recovered by animal inoculation with patient's blood or material from an abscess or an affected joint. A rising titer of specific agglutinins is also helpful in diagnosis. The incidence of falsely positive reactions for syphilis is lower than in Sodoku.

Haverhill fever is more readily detectable in its epidemic form, such as may occur from ingestion of infected milk, than in individual sporadic cases, which are easily misdiagnosed. In epidemic form the fever, rash and intense muscle and joint pain may suggest dengue fever.

Penicillin therapy for seven to 10 days is the treatment of choice.

RELAPSING FEVER

Various species of *Borrelia* cause relapsing fever in many parts of the world. The disease has been observed in at least 12 of the western United States, where it is tick-borne. Relapsing fever spread by human body lice may be accompanied by typhus fever but has not occurred in the United States.

Clinically an unexplained fever of 103 to 104° F for 3 to 4 days occurs, resolves spontaneously, only to recur as many as 3 to 8 times, each attack being of lesser severity and generally without known residual effects. A mortality rate of less than 5 per cent has been reported.

The *Ornithodoros* ticks inhabit rodent burrows

and may lodge on persons who have been out camping, generally overnight. Old tree stumps, deserted shacks and cabins in the woods have been the source of ticks responsible for isolated cases and for cases in groups of Boy Scouts and others. A history of this type of exposure some days prior to the onset of recurrent bouts of unexplained fever is the most important clue. Laboratory confirmation comes from direct examination of peripheral blood smears; large, loosely coiled spirochetes are seen. Laboratory animals inoculated with the patient's blood develop recurring fever and spirochetes can be seen in their peripheral blood. Penicillin therapy is not always effective; tetracycline or chloramphenicol is often more efficacious.

ALEX. J. STEIGMAN

Center for Disease Control Morbidity and Mortality Weekly Report July 21, 1973, Atlanta, Georgia.

Southern, P. M., Jr., and Sanford, J. P.: Relapsing fever. Medicine *48*:129, 1969.

VIRAL INFECTIONS AND THOSE PRESUMED TO BE CAUSED BY VIRUSES

MEASLES
(Rubeola)

DEFINITION. Measles is an acute communicable disease characterized by three stages: (1) an incubation stage of approximately 10 to 12 days with few, if any, signs or symptoms; (2) a prodromal stage with enanthem (Koplik's spots) on the buccal and pharyngeal mucosa, mild to moderate fever, slight conjunctivitis, coryza and an increasingly severe cough; and (3) a final stage with a maculopapular rash erupting successively over the neck and face, body, arms and legs and accompanied by high fever.

ETIOLOGY. The virus is classified as an RNA-containing paramyxovirus with only one antigenic type known; it is similar in structure to the viruses of mumps and parainfluenza. It is present in the nasopharyngeal secretions, blood and urine, at least during the prodromal period and for a short time after the rash appears. It can remain active for at least 34 hours at room temperature.

The production of typical giant cells in successive passages in cultures of human renal cells and in human amnion cells by Enders et al. has made possible the development of neutralization, complement fixation and hemagglutination tests.

INFECTIVITY. Maximal virus dissemination by droplet spray from the respiratory tract occurs during the prodromal period (catarrhal stage). Transmission to susceptible contacts often occurs before the diagnosis of the original case has been established. An infected person becomes infective for others by the ninth or tenth day after exposure (beginning of the prodromal phase), in some instances as early as the seventh day. Isolation precautions to prevent spread, especially in hospitals or other institutions for children, should be maintained from the seventh day after exposure until about five days after the rash has appeared.

EPIDEMIOLOGY. The endemicity of measles is essentially world-wide. In the past, epidemics tended to occur irregularly, appearing in large cities at 2- to 4-year intervals as new groups of susceptible children were exposed. Before the use of measles vaccine approximately 90 per cent of susceptible children under 6 years of age with family exposure during an epidemic contracted the disease. Most of the remaining 10 per cent contracted it subsequently. There is no evidence that a carrier state exists, nor has any other mode of interepidemic transmission been established. During an epidemic the airborne route appears to be the commonest mode of spread, although direct contact and spread by droplet spray are important means of cross infection.

Infants acquire immunity transplacentally from mothers who have had measles. This immunity is usually complete for the first four to six months of life and disappears rapidly thereafter. Infants of susceptible mothers have no such immunity and may contract the disease with the mother before or after delivery.

PATHOLOGY. The essential lesion of measles is found in the skin, in the mucous membranes of the nasopharynx and bronchi, and in the conjunctiva. It is a reaction of the capillary bed to the invading virus. Serous exudate and proliferation of mononuclear cells and a few polymorphonuclear cells occur around the capillaries. There is usually hyperplasia of the lymphoid tissue, where multinucleated giant cells up to 100μ in diameter (Warthin-Finkeldey reticuloendothelial giant cells) may be found. In the skin the reaction is particularly notable about the sebaceous glands and hair follicles. Koplik's spots* consist of serous exudate and prolifer-

*So-called Koplik's spots were apparently first described by Dr. John Quier in his Fifth Letter written from the West Indies to London in 1774.

ation of endothelial cells similar to those in the skin rash. There is a general inflammatory reaction of the buccal and pharyngeal mucosa which extends into the lymphoid tissue and the tracheobronchial mucous membrane. Interstitial pneumonitis is occasionally associated with measles; in some instances it may be due to the measles virus. Hecht's giant cell pneumonia is an infrequent accompaniment. Bronchopneumonia due to secondary bacterial invasion is perhaps the most frequent pulmonary infection. Peripheral blood leukocyte cultures show a temporarily increased incidence of metaphase cells containing chromosomal breaks, a phenomenon also noted in some other viral diseases and in leukemia.

CLINICAL MANIFESTATIONS. The incubation period is approximately 10 to 12 days if the first symptoms are selected as the time of onset, or approximately 14 days if the appearance of the rash is selected; rarely it may be as short as 6 to 10 days. A slight rise in temperature may occur 9 or 10 days from the date of infection and then subside for 24 hours or so.

The prodromal phase, which usually lasts 4 to 5 days, is characterized by low-grade to moderate fever, a slight hacking cough, coryza and conjunctivitis. These practically always precede Koplik's spots, the pathognomonic sign of measles, by 2 or 3 days. An enanthem or red mottling is usually present on the hard and soft palates. Koplik's spots are grayish white dots, usually as small as grains of sand, with a slight reddish areola; occasionally they are hemorrhagic. They tend to occur opposite the lower molars but may spread irregularly over the rest of the buccal mucosa. Rarely they are found within the midportion of the lower lip, on the palate and on the lacrimal caruncle. They appear and disappear rapidly, usually within 12 to 18 hours. As they fade there may remain red, spotty discolorations of the mucosa. The conjunctival inflammation and photophobia lead one to suspect measles before Koplik's spots appear. In addition, a transverse line of conjunctival inflammation, sharply demarcated along the eyelid margin, may be of diagnostic assistance in the prodromal stage. As the entire conjunctiva becomes involved, the line disappears.

Occasionally the prodromal phase may be unusually severe, being ushered in by sudden high fever, at times with convulsions and even pneumonia. Usually the coryza, fever and cough are increasingly severe up to the time the rash has covered the body.

The temperature rises abruptly as the rash appears and often reaches 104 to 105° F. When the rash appears on the legs and feet, within about 2 days, the symptoms subside rapidly in uncomplicated cases. The patient up to this point may appear desperately ill, and yet within 24 hours after the drop in temperature, which is usually abrupt, he will appear to be essentially well.

The rash usually starts as faint macules on the upper lateral parts of the neck, along the hairline and on the posterior parts of the cheeks. The individual lesions become increasingly maculopapular as the rash spreads rapidly over the entire face, neck, upper arms and upper part of the chest within approximately the first 24 hours (Figs. 10–33, 10–34). During the succeeding 24 hours it spreads over the back, abdomen, entire arms and thighs. As it finally reaches the feet on the second or third day it is beginning to fade on the face. The fading of the rash proceeds downward in the same sequence as that of its appearance. The severity of the disease is directly related to the extent and confluence of the rash. In mild measles the rash tends not to be confluent, and in very mild cases there are few, if any, lesions on the legs. In severe measles the rash is confluent, the skin being completely covered, including the palms and soles, and the face is swollen and disfigured.

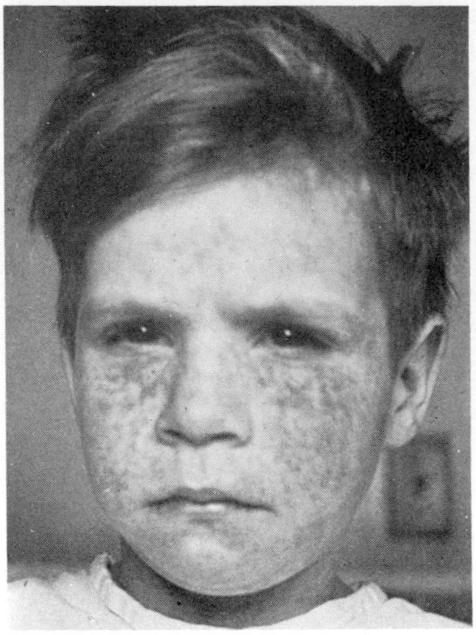

Figure 10–34 *Purpuric rash of measles.*

The rash is often slightly hemorrhagic; in severe cases with a confluent rash, petechiae may be present in large numbers, and there may be extensive ecchymoses. Itching is generally slight. As the rash fades, there is a branny type of desquamation and a brownish discoloration, which disappear within seven to 10 days.

Variations in types of rash may occur. Infrequently a slight urticarial, a faint macular or a scarlatiniform rash may appear during the early prodromal stage and disappear in advance of the typical rash. Complete absence of rash is rare except in patients who have received human antibodies during the incubation period, and possibly in infants under 8 months of age who have appreciable levels of maternal antibody. Occasionally death may occur before the rash has appeared. In the hemorrhagic type of measles (**black measles**) bleeding may occur from the mouth, nose or bowel. In mild cases the rash may be less macular and more nearly pinpoint, somewhat resembling that of scarlet fever.

Lymph nodes at the angle of the jaw and in the posterior cervical region are usually enlarged, and slight splenomegaly may be noted. Mesenteric lymphadenopathy may cause abdominal pain. Characteristic pathologic changes of measles in the mucosa of the appendix may cause obliteration of the lumen and symptoms of appendicitis. Changes of this type tend to subside with the disappearance of Koplik's spots. Gastrointestinal symptoms, such as diarrhea and vomiting, otitis media and bronchopneumonia are more common in infants and small children than in older children.

The white blood cell count tends to be low, with a relative lymphocytosis.

DIFFERENTIAL DIAGNOSIS. Diseases from which rubeola must be differentiated include exanthem subitum, rubella, infections due to echo-, coxsackie- and adenoviruses, infectious mononucleosis, toxoplasmosis, meningococcemia, scarlet fever, rickettsial diseases, serum sickness and drug rashes.

Koplik's spots are pathognomonic for rubeola, and the diagnosis of unmodified measles should not be made in the absence of cough.

Roseola infantum (exanthem subitum) is distinguished from measles because the rash appears as the fever disappears. The rashes of rubella and of enteroviral infections tend to be less striking than that of measles, as do the degree of fever and severity of illness. Although cough is present in many rickettsial infections, the rash usually spares the face, which characteristically is involved in measles. Headache is a more prominent feature of rickettsial infections. The absence of cough and the history of injection or ingestion of drug usually serve to identify serum sickness or drug rashes. Meningococcemia may be accompanied by a rash somewhat similar to that of measles; however, cough and conjunctivitis are usually absent. The diffuse, finely papular rash of scarlet fever, a confluent erythema with a "gooseflesh" texture most marked on the abdomen, is relatively easy to differentiate from that of measles.

The milder rash and the clinical picture of measles modified by gamma globulin, through partial immunity induced by measles vaccine, or in infants with maternal antibody, may be difficult to differentiate. Diagnostic tests for verification are of increasing importance and include neutralization, complement fixation, and hemagglutination inhibition, demonstrating rising antibody titers. Virus isolation and immunofluorescent studies are helpful.

COMPLICATIONS. The chief complications of measles are otitis media, pneumonia and encephalitis. Noma of the cheeks may occur in rare instances if the disease is severe. Gangrene elsewhere appears to be secondary to purpura fulminans or disseminated intravascular coagulation following measles.

Pneumonia (see also Giant Cell Pneumonia, Section 12) may be caused by the measles virus itself; when this is the case, the lesion is interstitial. Bronchopneumonia is more frequent, however; it is due to secondarily invading bacteria, particularly the pneumococcus, streptococcus, staphylococcus and *Hemophilus influenzae.* Laryngitis, tracheitis and bronchitis are common and may be due to the virus alone.

One of the potential dangers of measles is exacerbation of an existing *tuberculous process.* There may also be a temporary loss of hypersensitivity to tuberculin.

Myocarditis is an infrequent serious complication; transient electrocardiographic changes are said to be relatively common.

Neurologic complications are more common in measles than in any of the other exanthems. The incidence of *encephalomyelitis* is estimated to be 1 to 2 per 1000 reported cases of measles. There appears to be no correlation between the severity of the measles and that of the neurologic involvement, nor between the severity of the initial encephalitic process and the prognosis. Rarely, encephalitis has been reported in association with measles modified by gamma globulin and with the use of live attenuated measles virus vaccine. However, the measles virus has been implicated in slow virus infections such as subacute sclerosing panencephalitis (SSPE, *Dawson's encephalitis*), and the possibility of establishment of such slowly progressive infections must be kept in mind. In a few instances encephalitic involvement is manifest in the pre-eruptive period, but more often the onset is 2 to 5 days after the appearance of the rash. The cause of measles encephalitis remains controversial. It is suggested that when encephalitis occurs early in the course of the disease, viral invasion plays a large role, whereas that which occurs later is predominantly demyelinating in nature and may reflect an immunologic reaction. In this demyelinating type of reaction the symptoms and course do not differ from those of other parainfectious encephalitides. Other central nervous system complications, such as Guillain-Barré syndrome, hemiplegia, cerebral thrombophlebitis and retrobulbar neuritis, occur rarely.

PROGNOSIS. Case fatality rates in the United States have decreased in recent years to low levels for all age groups, in large part because of improved socioeconomic conditions, but also because of effective antibacterial therapy for the treatment of secondary infections.

When measles is introduced into a highly susceptible population, the results may be disastrous. Such an occurrence in the Faroe Islands in 1846 resulted in the deaths of about one quarter, nearly 2000, of the total population regardless of age. At Ungava Bay, Canada, where 99 per cent of 900 persons had measles, the mortality rate was 7 per cent.

PROPHYLAXIS. Quarantine is of little value, owing to the high communicability of the disease during its prodromal stage, when its presence is usually not suspected. Susceptibles known to have been exposed to the first case or group of cases may be permitted freedom for a week and then kept under strict isolation for 8 days. Under ordinary school or home conditions such attempts at isolation are ineffectual. The isolation of children with measles will decrease the opportunities for them to

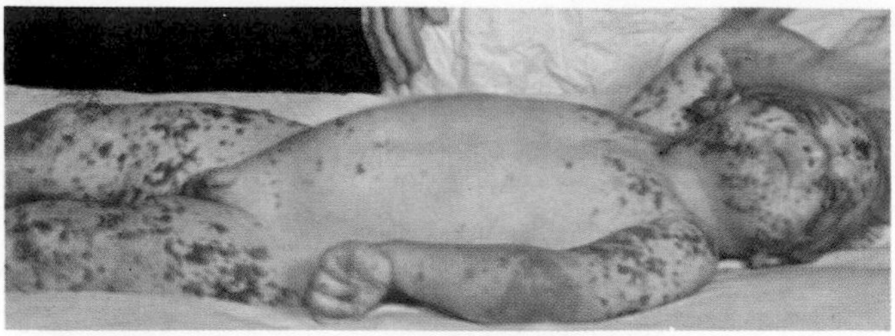

Figure 10–2 *Fulminating meningococcemia in a child 2½ years of age. Onset 36 hours before admission, with vomiting and fever; 18 hours before admission, extensive purpuric eruption began; death 8 hours after admission. Blood culture positive, Meningococcus type II. Nasal and cerebrospinal fluid cultures negative. One sibling had meningitis; another was found to be a carrier.*

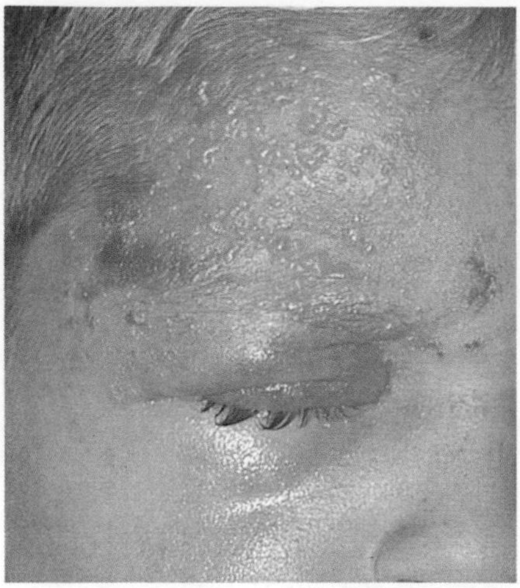

Figure 10–44 *Herpes zoster ophthalmicus. (From G. W. Korting: Hautkrankheiten bei Kindern und Jugendlichen. Stuttgart, Germany, F. K. Schattauer Verlag, 1969.)*

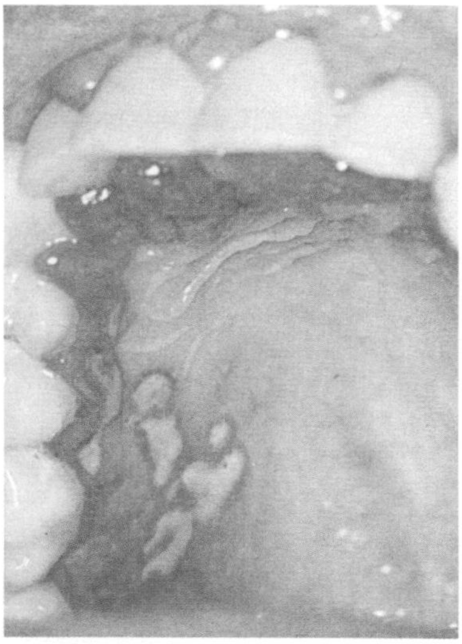

Figure 10–51 *Herpangina. (From G. W. Korting: Hautkrankheiten bei Kindern und Jugendlichen. Stuttgart, Germany, F. K. Schattauer Verlag, 1969.)*

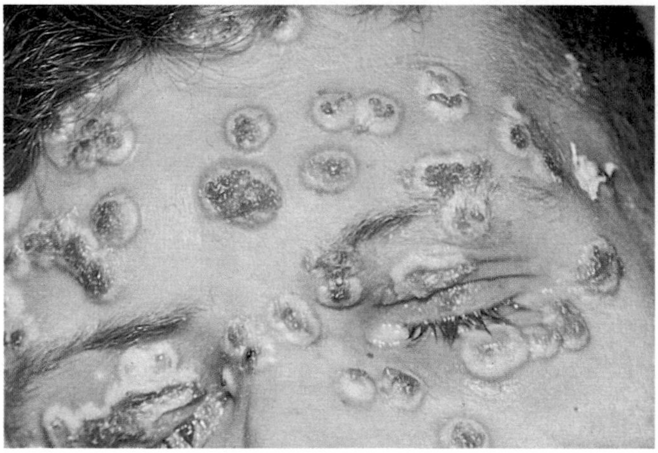

Figure 10–47 *Eczema vaccinatum. (From G. W. Korting: Hautkrankheiten bei Kindern und Jugendlichen. Stuttgart, Germany, F. K. Schattauer Verlag, 1969.)*

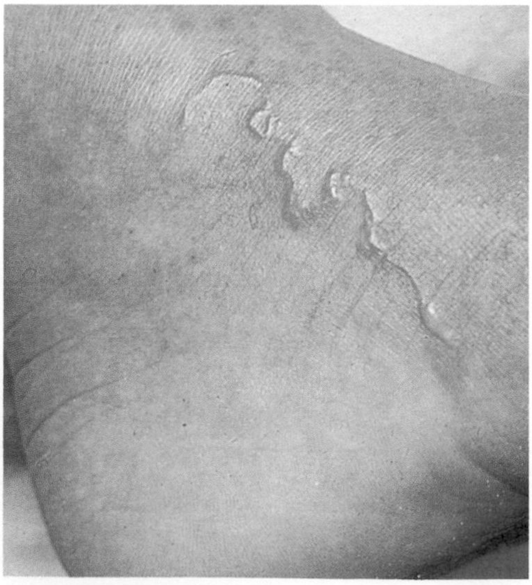

Figure 10–69 *Creeping eruption of cutaneous larva migrans. (From G. W. Korting: Hautkrankheiten bei Kindern und Jugendlichen. Stuttgart, Germany, F. K. Schattauer Verlag, 1969.)*

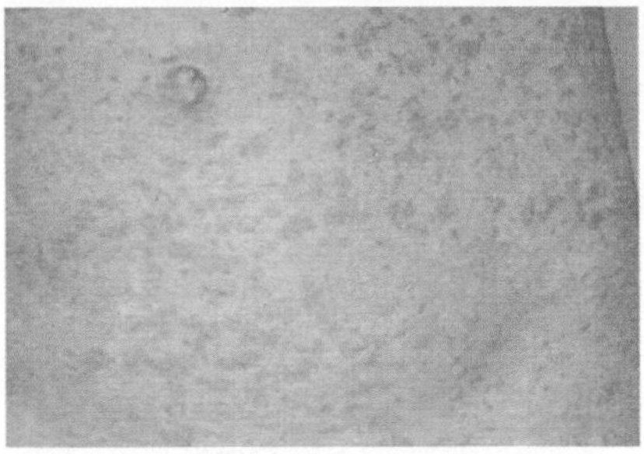

Figure 10–33 Maculopapular rash of measles. (From G. W. Korting: Hautkrankheiten bei Kindern und Jugendlichen. Stuttgart, Germany, F. K. Schattauer Verlag, 1969.)

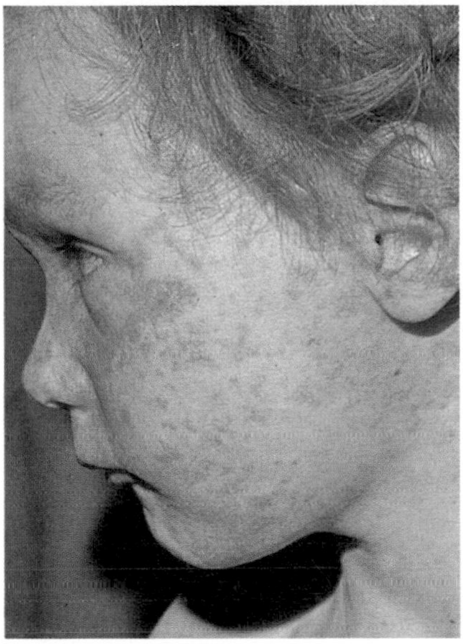

Figure 10–35 Rash of rubella (German measles). (From G. W. Korting: Hautkrankheiten bei Kindern und Jugendlichen, Stuttgart, Germany, F. K. Schattauer Verlag, 1969.)

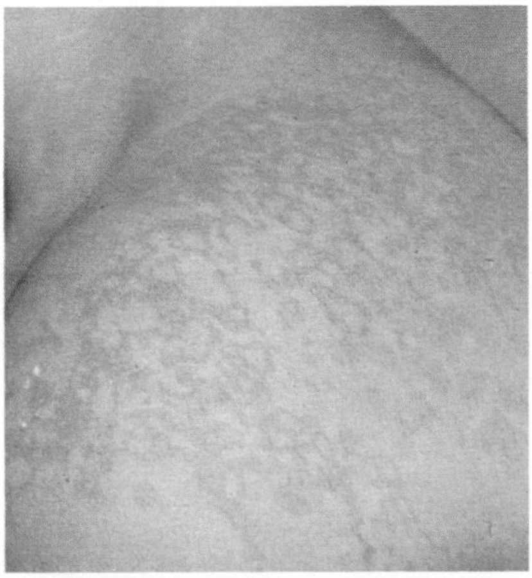

Figure 10–36 Erythema infectiosum. (From G. W. Korting: Hautkrankheiten bei Kindern und Jugendlichen. Stuttgart, Germany, F. K. Schattauer Verlag, 1969.)

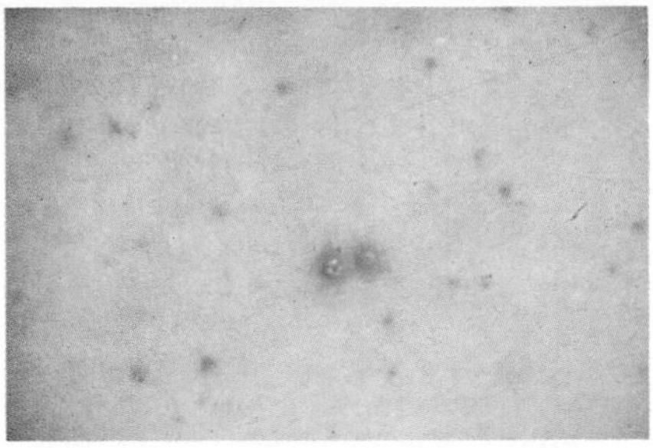

Figure 10–42 Skin lesions of chicken-pox. Note the varying stages of development (macules, papules and vesicles) present at the same time. (Courtesy of Dr. P. F. Lucchesi.)

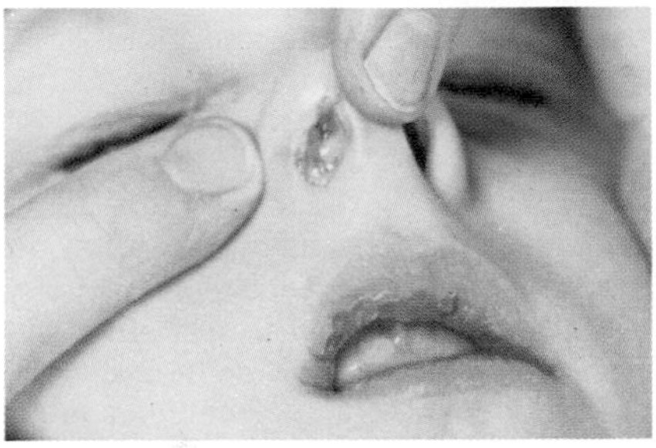

Figure 10–6 Nasal diphtheria. (Courtesy of Dr. Robert A. Lyon.)

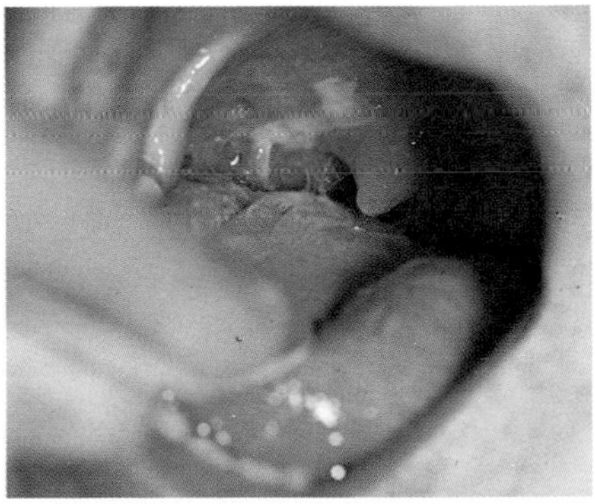

Figure 10–5 Pharyngotonsillar membrane of diphtheria. (Courtesy of Dr. Robert A. Lyon.)

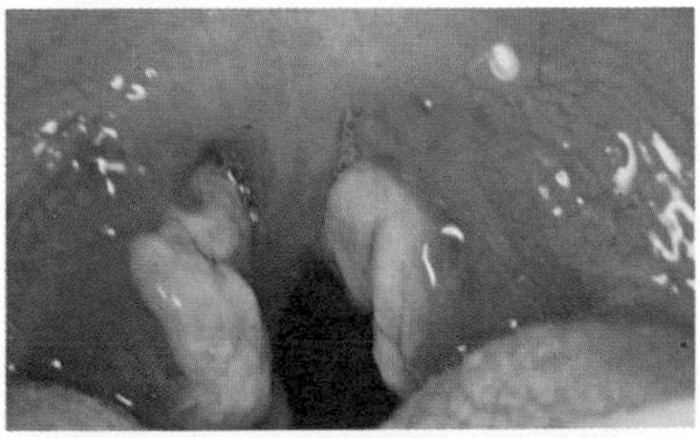

Figure 10–49 Pharyngitis with membrane formation in infectious mononucleosis. (Courtesy of Dr. Alex J. Steigman.)

acquire secondary bacterial infections. Quarantine of the patient may be lifted 1 to 2 days after return of the temperature to normal.

Active Immunization. Active immunization against measles has been achieved by vaccines. Currently in use are the Edmonston B vaccines prepared in chick embryo cells or canine renal cells, and the further attenuated virus vaccines derived from chick embryo culture (Schwarz and Moraten*). Vaccines are being prepared chiefly from the Edmonston strain of Enders. The live attenuated virus vaccine is administered as a single subcutaneous injection of 0.2 to 0.25 ml. There is often a short febrile (101 to 104° F rectally) illness of 2 to 3 days about a week after inoculation. Koplik's spots and mild skin eruptions may be seen. The use of immune globulin, 0.02 to 0.04 ml/kg given intramuscularly from a separate syringe at a different site immediately after the inoculation of the vaccine, lessens the reaction to the vaccine. The more highly attenuated live virus vaccines (Schwarz and Moraten) produce less reaction and are now used almost exclusively.

Antibody responses are satisfactory and lasting. Human immune serum globulin (ISG) may be used with Edmonston B chick cell vaccine at the discretion of the physician, but must be used with the canine renal cell preparation. Antibody level increases rapidly on subsequent exposure or challenge. During their febrile response vaccinated children do not appear to be an infection hazard for susceptible contacts.

As a rule, young infants who have received measles antibody from their immune mothers do not show a response to measles vaccine until about the eighth month of life, when the passively transferred maternal antibody has fallen to a low level. Effective immunization may not be achieved if the vaccine is given before 1 year of age.

Severe reactions, including neurologic involvement, following vaccination with live virus vaccine are rare. Regional lymphadenopathy, thrombocytopenic purpura and pneumonia have been recorded, as have febrile convulsions.

Allergic reactions have followed the use of chick embryo-cultured vaccine in persons sensitive to egg and the use of dog kidney-cultured vaccine in persons sensitive to canine antigens. When egg sensitivity is known, the use of dog kidney cell vaccine is recommended; when sensitivity to canine antigens is present, chick cell vaccine should be used. The response to live measles vaccine is unpredictable if immune globulin has been administered in the 3 months preceding immunization. Anergy to tuberculin may develop and persist for a month or longer after administration of live attenuated measles vaccine. A child with active tuberculous infection should be receiving antituberculosis treatment when live measles vaccine is administered. A tuberculin test prior to active immunization against measles is desirable.

*Coined from "more attenuated Enders."

Use of live measles vaccine is not recommended during pregnancy, nor for children with untreated tuberculosis. Live vaccine is contraindicated in children with leukemia and in those receiving immunosuppressive drugs because of the risk of persistent, progressive infection such as giant cell pneumonia. After exposure of susceptible children to measles, measles immune globulin (human) should be given intramuscularly in a dose of 0.25 ml/kg as soon as possible. A larger dose may be advisable in children with acute leukemia.

The use of inactivated (killed) virus measles vaccine is not recommended. Antibody response may be poor and short-lived and does not include secretory IgA against measles; secretory antibody is present in respiratory tract secretions after the natural disease or use of live virus vaccine. Unusual local or systemic reactions have occurred in recipients of killed virus measles vaccine who were later exposed to natural measles or were vaccinated with live attenuated measles virus. Such reactions to live virus vaccine have included severe local tenderness, swelling, erythema, heat and hemorrhagic or vesicular lesions, accompanied by malaise, fever and regional lymphadenopathy. Exposure to natural measles has resulted in a severe, atypical form of measles, with high fever, pneumonia and toxicity. The rash, which may be petechial, vesicular or urticarial, begins on the feet and extends upward, but is concentrated largely on the extremities. Such reactions do not seem to follow repeated inoculations of the attenuated live virus vaccine in children. Combined vaccines are being evaluated. The trivalent measles-mumps-rubella preparation, measles-rubella and measles-smallpox are available and appear to be effective.

Passive Immunization. Passive immunization with pooled adult serum, pooled convalescent serum, placental globulin and gamma globulin of pooled plasma is effective for prevention and attenuation of measles. Measles can be prevented by the use of immune serum globulin (gamma globulin) in a dose of 0.25 ml/kg given intramuscularly within 5 days after exposure, but preferably as soon as possible. Complete protection is indicated for infants, for children with chronic illness and for contacts in hospital wards and children's institutions. Attenuation may be accomplished by the use of gamma globulin in a dosage of 0.05 ml/kg. Gamma globulin, including that now prepared in the United States from placental blood, is approximately 25 times as potent in antibody titer as pooled adult serum, and it avoids the risk of hepatitis. Attenuation is variable, and the modified clinical patterns may vary from those with few or no symptoms to those with little or no modification.

After the seventh or eighth day of incubation the amounts of immune bodies must be increased greatly for any degree of protection. If the injection is delayed until the ninth, tenth or eleventh day, slight fever may already have started, and only slight modification of the disease may be expected.

TREATMENT. Sedatives, antipyretics for high fever, skin lotions for itching or irritation, complete bed rest and an adequate fluid intake are the usual requirements. Humidification of the room may be necessary for laryngitis or an excessively irritating cough, and it is best to keep the room comfortably warm rather than cool. Because of conjunctival irritation, the patient should be protected from exposure to strong light. The complications of otitis media and pneumonia require appropriate antimicrobial therapy.

In complications such as encephalitis, subacute sclerosing panencephalitis, giant cell pneumonia, and disseminated intravascular coagulation, each case must be assessed individually. Good supportive care is essential. Gamma globulin, hyperimmune gamma globulin and steroids are of limited value. The effectiveness of antiviral substances, such as IUDR (5-iodo-2-deoxyuridine), BUDR (5-bromo-2-deoxyuridine), pyran copolymer, and amantadine hydrochloride, has not been evaluated fully as yet. In some cases of subacute sclerosing panencephalitis antiviral substances have appeared to slow the progressive disease process.

American Academy of Pediatrics: Report of the Committee on Infectious Diseases. 17th ed. Evanston, Ill., 1974, p. 79.

Blattner, R. J. Live measles vaccine and the tuberculin reaction. Comments on current literature. J. Pediatr. *63*:174, 1963.

Blattner, R. J.: Myocarditis in prodromal measles. Comments on current literature. J. Pediatr. *64*:144, 1964.

Blattner, R. J.: Subacute sclerosing encephalitis. Comments on current literature. J. Pediatr. *71*:910, 1967.

Brem, J.: Koplik spots for the record: An illustrated historical note. Clin. Pediatr. *11*:161, 1972.

Enders, J. F., and others: Studies on an attenuated measles virus vaccine (series of papers). New Engl. J. Med. *263*:159, 1960.

Goldberger, J., and Anderson, J. F. An experimental demonstration of the virus of measles in mixed buccal and nasal secretions. J.A.M.A. *57*:476, 1911.

Goldfield, M. Boyer, N. H., and Weinstein, L.: Electrocardiographic changes during the course of measles. J. Pediatr. *46*:30, 1955.

Katz, S. L., and Enders, J. F.: Measles virus: *In* Horsfall, F. L., and Tamm, I. (eds): Viral and Rickettsial Infections of Man. 4th ed. Philadelphia, J. B. Lippincott Company, 1965, p. 784.

Katz, S. L., and Griffith, J. F.: Slow virus infections. Hosp. Prac. *6*:64, 1971.

Krugman, S.: Present status of measles and rubella immunization in the United States: A medical progress report. J. Pediatr. *78*:1, 1971.

Landrigan, P. J., and Witte, J. J.: Neurologic disorders following measles vaccination. J.A.M.A. *223*:1459, 1973.

Panum, P. L.: Observations Made During the Epidemic of Measles on the Faroe Islands in the Year 1846. Translated by A. S. Hatcher. New York, Delta Omega Society, American Public Health Association, 1940.

Payne, F. E., Baublis, J. V., and Itabashi, H. H.: Isolation of measles virus from cell cultures of brain from a patient with subacute sclerosing panencephalitis. New Engl. J. Med. *281*:11, 1969.

Scott, T. F., and Bonanno, D. F.: Reactions to live measles-virus vaccine in children previously inoculated with killed-virus vaccine. New Engl. J. Med. *277*:248, 1967.

Sever, J. L., and Zeman, W. (eds.): Conference on Measles Virus and Subacute Sclerosing Panencephalitis. U.S. Dept. HEW, P.H.S., N.I.N.D.B., held in Bethesda, Md., Sept. 13, 1967. Neurology *18*:192, 1968.

Starr, S., and Berkovich, S.: The effect of measles, gamma globulin modified measles and attenuated measles vaccine on the course of treated tuberculosis in children. Pediatrics *35*:97, 1965.

Stokes, J., Jr., Weibel, R. E., Villarejos, V. M., Arguedas, J. A., Buynak, E. B., and Hilleman, M. R.: Trivalent combined measles-mumps-rubella vaccine. Findings in clinical-laboratory studies. J.A.M.A. *218*:57, 1971.

GERMAN MEASLES

(Rubella, Three-day Measles)

DEFINITION. Rubella is a common communicable disease of childhood characterized ordinarily by mild constitutional symptoms, a rash similar to that of mild rubeola or scarlet fever, and enlargement and tenderness of the postoccipital, retroauricular and posterior cervical lymph nodes. In older children and adults the infection may occasionally be severe, with such manifestations as joint involvement and purpura.

Rubella in early pregnancy as a cause of severe congenital anomalies in the newborn infant was first recognized in 1941. Since the 1964 pandemic, attention has been given to other aspects of maternal rubella which have serious import for the newborn infant and significant epidemiologic implications. The congenital rubella syndrome is now recognized as an active contagious disease with multisystem involvement, a wide spectrum of clinical expression and, as a rule, a long postnatal period of active infection with shedding of virus.

HISTORY. Designated as *Röteln* by German physicians in the eighteenth century, German measles was regarded as a variant of measles or scarlet fever. Maton described it as a separate entity in 1815; Wagner emphasized its distinction from rubeola and scarlet fever in 1829; and in 1866 Veale in Edinburgh called the disease rubella. Gregg (Australia) in 1941 observed severe congenital malformations in newborn infants whose mothers had rubella early in pregnancy. The pandemic of 1964 brought to light a new concept of congenital rubella as mentioned above.

ETIOLOGY. Rubella is caused by a viral agent, probably a myxovirus. Krugman in 1953 showed that the infectious agent was present in the blood 2 days before and on the first day of the rash.

Early attempts at tissue culture isolation were not successful because of the absence of cytopathic effect. Two methods are now available for virus assay and antibody study: use of cell lines in which rubella virus shows a visible effect, e.g., human amnion cells, and rabbit kidney cells, and by interference phenomena, i.e., the presence of rubella virus interfering with the cytopathic effect of echovirus 11 and coxsackievirus A-9 subsequently introduced into the culture. During clinical illness the virus is present in nasopharyngeal secretions, blood, feces and urine. Virus has been recovered from the nasopharynx 7 days before the exanthem, and from 7 to 8 days after its disappearance. It has also been recovered in some cases of relatively common inapparent infection.

EPIDEMIOLOGY. Transplacental immunity is effective for the first 5 or 6 months of life. Epidemics occur approximately every 3 to 4 years. A single attack is thought to confer permanent immunity, and verified second attacks occur rarely.

When an adult population living in continental United States is screened for the presence of rubella hemagglutination-inhibition (HI) or neutralizing antibody, 80 per cent will show serologic evidence of previous rubella infection. If the population of islands such as Hawaii is screened, only 20 per cent of adults will have protective antibody. This curious epidemiologic finding has not yet been fully explained.

Epidemiologic studies have confirmed the spread of rubella in families. Up to 60 per cent of family members may be affected, with a 2:1 ratio of inapparent to overt infection.

In maternal rubella, the primary infection is in the mother and is transferred during the period of viremia to her offspring by way of the placenta. In a considerable number of instances in which therapeutic abortion was performed because of clinical rubella in the first trimester, the rubella virus was recovered from the products of conception, including chorionic villi. In one case the mother was thought to be in the first week of pregnancy at the time of clinical rubella. Therapeutic abortion was performed at 18 weeks; the fetus had cataracts, and its development was impaired. Rubella virus was recovered from various fetal tissues. Virus has also been recovered from a fetus aborted after active immunization of a nonimmune woman who did not know that she was pregnant, but malformations of the fetus were not identified.

In the congenital rubella syndrome, virus can be isolated from nasopharyngeal washings, stool, blood, urine and spinal fluid of the newborn infant. Virus shedding continues for periods as long as 12 to 18 months, making the infant a source of infection for contacts, such as older children who are not immune and nonimmune adults, including pregnant women and nursery personnel. The risk of malformations among the infants of women who contract rubella in the first weeks of pregnancy approaches 100 per cent; 40 per cent during the second month; 10 per cent in the third month; and 4 per cent in the second and third trimesters.

CLINICAL MANIFESTATIONS. The incubation period for rubella is generally 14 to 21 days. The prodromal phase of mild catarrhal symptoms is shorter than that of measles and may be so mild as to go entirely unnoticed. The most characteristic sign is retroauricular, posterior cervical and postoccipital adenopathy. No other disease causes the tender enlargement of all these nodes to the same extent as rubella. An enanthem may appear just before the onset of the skin rash. It consists of discrete rose spots on the soft palate which may coalesce into a red blush and may extend over the fauces.

Lymphadenopathy is evident at least 24 hours before the *rash* appears and may be present for a week or more. The exanthem is more variable than that of rubeola. It begins on the face (Fig. 10–35) and spreads quickly. Its evolution is so rapid that the rash on the face may be fading by the time it appears on the trunk. Discrete maculopapules are present in large numbers, but there are also large areas of flushing which spread rapidly over the entire body, usually within 24 hours. The rash may be confluent, particularly on the face. During the second day the rash may assume a pinpoint appearance, especially over the trunk, resembling that of scarlet fever. Mild itching may occur. The eruption usually clears by the third day. Any residual pigmentation disappears in a few days; desquamation is minimal. Rubella without a rash has been described.

The pharyngeal mucosa and the conjunctivas are inflamed slightly. In contrast to rubeola, there is no photophobia. Fever is slight or absent. When present, it occurs at the height of the rash, and persists for 1, 2 or occasionally for 3 days. The temperature seldom exceeds 101° F. Anorexia, headache and malaise are not common in rubella. The spleen is often slightly enlarged. The white blood cell count is normal or slightly reduced; thrombocytopenia is relatively rare, with or without purpura. Especially in older girls and women, polyarthritis may occur with arthralgia, swelling, tenderness and effusion, but usually without any residuum. Its duration is usually several days to 2 weeks; rarely it persists for months. Paresthesia also has been reported.

In the **congenital rubella syndrome** the most common permanent defects are cataracts, cardiovascular anomalies (especially patent ductus arteriosus and pulmonary artery branch stenosis), deafness and secondary mutism, microcephaly and mental deficiency. Less frequent conditions are microphthalmus, buphthalmus, glaucoma, retinal lesions, talipes equinovarus, syndactyly, hypospadias, generalized muscular weakness, cerebral diplegia, cleft palate and dental anomalies.

The degree of involvement of the infant at birth varies widely. In severe cases, growth retardation, particularly in weight, is the most common finding at birth. Within the first few days of life other evidences of widespread infection may appear, and the infant may experience a stormy course for the first 6 months or so with such manifestations as thrombocytopenia, anemia, hepatitis, pancreatitis, pneumonitis, encephalitis, rhinitis, otitis media, congestive heart failure and diarrhea. Radiographically demonstrable abnormalities of the skeleton are common in infants with the rubella syndrome. In the skull, mineralization of the calvaria is poor, and sutures are prominent. The anterior fontanel is often large and may extend well into the frontal bone, involving the metopic suture. The long bones have an altered trabecular pattern characterized by longitudinal streaks of poor mineralization. Bone manifestations are most pronounced at the knees and bear resemblance to syphilis. These skeletal abnormalities are self-correcting in about 3 months if the infant thrives.

Central nervous system involvement is striking; the degree may be masked in the very ill infant, the only clues in the first few months of life being a tense fontanel and hypotonia. Overt neurologic disease may not be apparent until later in infancy. Persistence of virus infection is reflected by virus recovery from the cerebrospinal fluid. Virus can be isolated from inner layers of the lens of the eye for as long as 3 years.

DIFFERENTIAL DIAGNOSIS. Since similar symptoms and rashes can occur with many other viral infections (see Infections by Enteroviruses), rubella is a difficult disease to diagnose clinically unless the patient is seen during an epidemic. A history of having had rubella is unreliable; immunity should be determined by testing for antibodies. Particularly in its more severe forms, rubella may be confused with the mild types of scarlet fever and rubeola. *Roseola infantum* (exanthem subitum) is distinguished from rubella by the appearance of the rash at the end of the febrile episode rather than at the height of the signs and symptoms. *Drug rashes* may be extremely difficult to differentiate from rubella. The characteristic enlargement of the lymph nodes would support the diagnosis of rubella. In *infectious mononucleosis* a rash may occur which resembles that of rubella, and enlargement of the lymph nodes in both diseases may lead to confusion. The hematologic findings in infectious mononucleosis should be sufficient to distinguish the two diseases. Enterovirus infections, which may be accompanied by a rash, can be differentiated by their shorter incubation period and the absence of suboccipital adenopathy.

Diagnostic tests include virus isolation from the pharynx by tissue culture, and serologic tests such as neutralization, complement fixation, hemagglutination inhibition and fluorescent antibody studies. In congenital rubella, virus can be isolated from throat, blood, urine, cerebrospinal fluid, lens and other involved organs.

COMPLICATIONS AND PROGNOSIS. Complications are relatively uncommon in childhood rubella. Neuritis and arthritis occur occasionally. Resistance to secondary bacterial infection is not altered significantly. Encephalitis similar to that seen with rubeola occurs rarely. The prognosis of childhood rubella is good; that of congenital rubella varies with the severity of the infection. The mortality of infants with neonatal thrombocytopenic purpura is about 35 per cent in the first 18 months of life, but tends to result from general debility, sepsis and heart failure rather than from bleeding. Only about 30 per cent of infants with encephalitis appear to escape residual neuromotor deficits, including an autistic syndrome. Spontaneous abortion occurs in about one third of women who acquire rubella in the first trimester of pregnancy.

PREVENTION. Preventive measures are of the greatest importance for the protection of the fetus. It is especially important that girls have immunity to rubella before the child-bearing age, either by contracting the natural disease or by active immunization. The immune status can be evaluated by appropriate serologic tests.

Pregnant women, especially early in pregnancy, but also during the entire gestational period, should avoid exposure to rubella, regardless of history of the disease during childhood, or of history of active immunization. Exposure of pregnant women to infants with congenital rubella syndrome should be especially guarded against; such infants may shed virus for 12 to 18 months. Risk of damage to the fetus is considered to be reduced after the fourteenth week of gestation (See Epidemiology.)

In an exposed susceptible, protection from or attenuation of the disease may or may not be afforded by intramuscular injection of immune serum globulin (ISG), given in large dosage (0.12 to 0.20 ml per pound) within the first 7 to 8 days after exposure. The effectiveness of immune globulin is not predictable, depending apparently upon the antibody content of the blood product used, or upon factors as yet undetermined. The value of ISG has been questioned also because in some instances rash was prevented, and clinical manifestations were absent or minimal, though viable virus was demonstrable in the blood. Nevertheless, the risk to the fetus appears to be reduced if the mother receives immune substance early and in adequate amount. Studies of a concentrated ISG with high globulin level, which is prepared from serum of patients with naturally occurring rubella, are in progress.

Management of Pregnant Women Exposed to or Acquiring Rubella. Since approximately 80 per cent of women in the child-bearing age are immune to rubella as a result of the natural infection, women who are at risk to become pregnant should have their immune status to rubella determined by the hemagglutination-inhibition (HI) technique. If shown to be susceptible and if they can be relied upon not to get pregnant for 2 months after immunization, they should be actively immunized.

If a pregnant woman of unknown immune status is exposed to rubella, an HI test should be performed *immediately and as an emergency measure* If determined to be immune, she can be reassured that the pregnancy can be continued without added risk. If found to be susceptible and therapeutic abortion is unacceptable or unavailable to her, passive immunization with immune serum globulin (ISG), 20 to 30 ml intramuscularly, should be attempted immediately.

If exposure to rubella occurs in a susceptible pregnant woman to whom abortion is available and desirable in case of significant potential hazard to the fetus, and in view of the uncertainty of protection and possibility of masking the infection in women receiving ISG, it is probably advisable to withhold ISG and observe her carefully. If rubella then develops at a stage of pregnancy at which she feels the risk (see Epidemiology) is greater than she wants to take, therapeutic abortion may be performed.

For **active immunization** against rubella the vaccines in current use are live virus vaccines prepared in tissue cell cultures of various origins. The vaccines are in chick or duck embryo, or mammalian tissue culture of canine or rabbit HPV-77-DE-5 (duck embryo), HPV-77-DK-12 (dog kidney), Cendehill (rabbit kidney), and RA 27/3 human embryonic lung fibroblasts of the WI-38 line. Vaccine is administered as a single subcutaneous injection. With few exceptions antibody response is good (about 95 per cent develop antibodies) with minimal clinical manifestations. Antibody levels are lower than those resulting from natural infection, and the duration of effective immunity is not as yet known. Following vaccination, viremia occurs but is transient and of low level. While virus may persist, especially in the nasopharynx, and shedding occurs between 18 and 25 days after immunization and may persist for up to 50 days after vaccination, communicability does not appear to be a problem. The serious risk is the possible spread to pregnant women. Antibody detection studies are often useful in this situation.

Live rubella virus vaccine is recommended for boys and girls between the age of 1 year and puberty, and for nonpregnant postpubertal females who have been demonstrated to have a negative hemagglutination-inhibition test and who can reasonably be relied upon not to become pregnant within 2 to 3 months of immunization. Vaccination in infants under 1 year is not recommended since persisting maternal antibody may interfere. Attention should be given particularly to kindergarten and elementary school children since these groups are a major source of community spread; nonimmunized adolescents have also been identified as an important source. Criteria for possible reimmunization remain to be determined.

Pregnant women should not be given live rubella virus vaccine. Other contraindications include immune deficiency states, severe febrile illness, hypersensitivity to vaccine components, therapy with antimetabolites, steroids, steroid-like substances, and so forth.

Clinical manifestations which may follow vaccination include fever, typical lymphadenopathy, rash and transient arthritis and arthralgia. The latter occur more frequently in older girls and adult women. In rare instances neurologic manifestations such as myeloradiculoneuritis have been reported.

Measles-mumps-rubella, measles-rubella and mumps-rubella combined vaccines are also available and apparently effective.

REINFECTION. The incidence of reinfection on exposure of serologically immune individuals to wild virus is 3 to 10 per cent among those demonstrating serologic immunity without a history of immunization, 14 to 18 per cent among those immunized with RA 27/3 vaccine, and 40 to 100 per cent among those immunized with HPV-77 or Cendehill vaccine. A significant incidence of infection has been demonstrated among the fetuses of reinfected pregnant women, as well as among pregnant women receiving rubella vaccine. The importance of reinfection of serologically immune pregnant women in the production of congenital malformations remains to be determined but is of obvious significance in the planning of large-scale immunization programs against rubella. The effectiveness of "herd immunity" in preventing rubella-induced malformations remains controversial. Until these questions are answered, *all* pregnant women should make every effort to avoid exposure to rubella.

TREATMENT. Unless bacterial complications occur, treatment is symptomatic.

Alford, C. A., Jr., Neva, F. A., and Weller, T. H.: Virologic and serologic studies on human products of conception after maternal rubella. New Engl. J. Med. *271*:1275, 1964.

American Academy of Pediatrics: Report of the Committee on Infectious Diseases. 17th ed. Evanston, Ill., 1974, p. 150.

Baylor College of Medicine, Rubella Study Group: Rubella: Epidemic in retrospect. Hosp. Prac. *2*:27, 1967.

Bunnell, C. E., and Monif, G. R. G.: Interstitial pancreatitis in congenital rubella. J. Pediatr. *80*:465, 1972.

Chang, T. W.: Rubella reinfection and intrauterine involvement. (Editorial.) J. Pediatr. *84*:617, 1974.

Desmond, M. M., and others: Congenital rubella encephalitis: Course and early sequelae. J. Pediatr. *71*:311, 1967.

Desmond, M. M., and others: The early growth and development of infants with congenital rubella. *In* Advances in Teratology. Vol. 4. New York, Academic Press, 1970, p. 39.

Gilmartin, R. C., Jabbour, J. T., and Duenas, D. A.: Rubella vaccine in myeloradiculoneuritis. J. Pediatr. *80*:406, 1972.

Gregg, N. M.: Congenital cataract following German measles in the mother. Trans. Ophthal. Soc. Austr. *3*:35, 1941.

Gregg, N. M., and others: The occurrence of congenital defects in children following maternal rubella during pregnancy. Med. J. Aust. *2*:122, 1945.

Hanissian, A. S., and Hashimoto, K.: Paramyxovirus inclusions in rubella syndrome. J. Pediatr. *81*:231, 1972.

Katz, M.: Rubella vaccine. (Editorial.) J. Pediatr. *84*:615, 1974.

Krugman, S.: Present status of measles and rubella immunization in the United States: A medical progress report. J. Pediatr. *78*:1, 1971.

Krugman, S. (Guest Editor), and others: International Conference on Rubella Immunization. Bethesda, Md., National Institutes of Health, February 18–20, 1969. Amer. J. Dis. Child. *118* (Nos. 1 and 2):1; 155, 1969.

Meyer, H. M., Jr., and Parkman, P. D.: Rubella vaccination: A review of practical experience. J.A.M.A. *215*:613, 1971.

Monif, G. R. G., Sever, J. L., Schiff, G. H., and Traub, R. G.: Isolation of rubella virus from products of conception. Am. J. Obstet. Gynec. *91*:1143, 1965.

Rawls, W. E., and others: Persistent virus infection in congenital rubella. Arch. Ophthal. *77*:430, 1967.

Rawls, W. E., Desmyter, J., and Melnick, J. L.: Serologic diagnosis and fetal involvement in maternal rubella. J.A.M.A. *203*:627, 1968.

Rudolph, A. J., and others: Transplacental rubella infection in newly born infants. J.A.M.A. *191*:843, 1965.

Weiss, D. I., Cooper, L. Z., and Green, R. H.: Infantile glaucoma: A manifestation of congenital rubella. J.A.M.A. *195*:105, 1966.

EXANTHEM SUBITUM

(Roseola Infantum)

DEFINITION. Exanthem subitum is an acute viral disease of infants and young children, usually occurring sporadically, but occasionally in epidemics. It is unique in that the diagnostic rash and clinical improvement occur almost simultaneously. The disease is characterized by a period of high fever lasting 3 to 4 days, during which time there are insufficient clinical findings to explain the hyperpyrexia, and by an abrupt termination with a precipitous drop of the temperature to normal and the appearance of a generalized eruption, which fades quickly.

ETIOLOGY. Available evidence supports viral origin. Blood serum, heparinized blood and throat washings obtained from patients on the third day of fever and also on the first day of the rash have been shown to be infective for susceptible infants, and for monkeys. Typical disease resulted after an incubation period of 9 to 10 days in infants and 4 to 5 days in monkeys.

Nothing is known of the pathologic changes of the disease.

EPIDEMIOLOGY. The degree of contagiousness is not known. There is a tendency for the disease to occur in the spring and fall. It attacks both sexes equally. In the rare epidemics described the incubation period was estimated to be from 7 to 17 days, usually about 10 days. The epidemiologic pattern is not clear. The occurrence of exanthem subitum sporadically in early life, with rare epidemics in older age groups, suggests the possibility of an endemic spread through most of the population in early infancy and childhood, with production of permanent immunity. Most of the cases occur between the ages of 6 months and 3 years, although the disease does occur infrequently in older children and even in adults. The peak incidence appears to be during the second year of life.

CLINICAL MANIFESTATIONS. The onset is sudden, with fever which rises abruptly as high as 103 to 105° F; convulsions may occur at this time. Although the pharyngeal mucosa is slightly inflamed at times and there may be slight coryza, there are no typical signs. The outstanding feature is the absence of physical findings sufficient to explain the height of the fever. The diagnosis is suspected chiefly by exclusion of other possible infections, particularly those which at this age are the most common causes of high fever and in which the diagnosis may not be evident, such as otitis media, acute pyelonephritis, pneumonia and meningitis.

During the first 24 to 36 hours of fever the blood cell count may be elevated, as high as 16,000 to 20,000 per mm^3 with an increase in neutrophils. By the second day leukopenia becomes evident, with counts from 3000 to 5000 on the third to fourth day of fever. There is an absolute neutropenia with a relative lymphocytosis, which may be as high as 90 per cent. Occasionally a large number of monocytes are present.

The fever falls by crisis on the third or fourth day, and just before or shortly after the return of the temperature to normal a macular or maculopapular eruption appears over the body, starting on the trunk and spreading to the arms and neck, with slight involvement of the face and legs. The rash soon fades, rarely remaining as long as 24 hours. Desquamation is rare, and no pigmentation remains. In the rare epidemic outbreaks, cases without a rash may be suspected, but a definite diagnosis cannot be made. Clemens described an enanthem on the soft palate consisting of small erythematous spots and streaks. Slight periorbital edema has also been described. Occasionally the lymph nodes, especially in the cervical area, may be enlarged, but not to the extent that they are in rubella. When present, postoccipital lymphadenopathy can be a helpful diagnostic sign.

DIFFERENTIAL DIAGNOSIS. The principal difficulty in differential diagnosis is with *rubella*, from which exanthem subitum is distinguished chiefly by the prodromal period of high fever. *Rubeola* and *dengue* can be distinguished primarily by the time of appearance of their rash in relation to fever and other clinical findings. In measles, though there is usually a fever of variable degree for 3 or 4 days just before the rash, the temperature becomes abruptly elevated to 103 to 104° F at the time of appearance of the rash and remains elevated for the next 2 days or so. The lack of Koplik's spots, severe coryza, conjunctivitis and cough also helps to distinguish exanthem subitum from rubeola. As a rule, distinction from viral diseases of the enterovirus and adenovirus groups does not present a problem. Certain allergic rashes, e.g., those resulting from sensitivity to drugs, may be difficult to distinguish from exanthem subitum, but the characteristic clinical pattern of the latter is usually sufficiently definite to establish the diagnosis.

PROGNOSIS. This is good except in the rare patient who has encephalopathy or extreme hyperpyrexia.

PROPHYLAXIS AND TREATMENT. There are no known methods for shortening the course of the disease or for prophylaxis. In infants and young children who are prone to convulsions the administration of a sedative at the appearance of the sharp febrile onset of exanthem subitum may be effective as prophylaxis against such seizures. An antipyretic may be of help in partially reducing the fever and in allaying restlessness.

RUSSELL J. BLATTNER

Berenberg, W., Wright, S., and Janeway, C. A.: Roseola infantum (exanthem subitum). New Engl. J. Med. *241*:253, 1949.
Burnstine, R. C., and Paine, R. S.: Residual encephalopathy following roseola infantum. Am. J. Dis. Child. *98*:144, 1959.
Clemens, H. H.: Exanthem subitum (roseola infantum): A report of eighty cases. J. Pediatr. *26*:66, 1945.
Hellström, B., and Vahlquist, B.: Experimental inoculation of roseola infantum. Acta Paediatr. *40*:189, 1951.
Kempe, C. H.: Exanthem subitum. *In* Horsfall, F. L., Jr., and Tamm, I. (eds.): Viral and Rickettsial Infections of Man. 4th ed. Philadelphia, J. B. Lippincott Company, 1965, p. 810.
Kempe, C. H., Shaw, E. B., Jackson, J. R., and Silver, H. K.: Studies on the etiology of exanthem subitum (roseola infantum). J. Pediatr. *37*:561, 1950.
Letchner, A.: Roseola infantum: A review of fifty cases. Lancet, *2*:1163, 1955.
McEnery, J. T.: Postoccipital lymphadenopathy as a diagnostic sign in roseola infantum (exanthem subitum). Clin. Pediatr. *9*:512, 1970.
Veeder, B. S., and Hempelmann, T. C.: A febrile exanthem occurring in childhood (exanthem subitum). J.A.M.A. *77*:1787, 1921.
Zahorsky, J.: Roseola infantum. J.A.M.A. *61*:1446, 1913.

ERYTHEMA INFECTIOSUM

(Fifth Disease)

ETIOLOGY. A viral etiology has been postulated. In one epidemic approximately 10 per cent of the patients studied had evidence of rubella infection. A strain of rubella virus isolated from one of these patients produced an exanthem resembling erythema infectiosum in adult volunteers. However, in most patients studied no laboratory evidence for a viral disease could be detected.

PATHOLOGY. Biopsy of the skin lesion shows edema and a nonspecific inflammatory infiltrate of lymphocytes.

EPIDEMIOLOGY. Erythema infectiosum is a moderately contagious disease affecting mainly children. Infants and adults are affected infrequently. There is no sex predilection. The incubation period has been estimated from family studies to range from 7 to 28 days (average, 16 days). Community epidemics involving mainly school-age children have been described. Distribution is world-wide.

CLINICAL MANIFESTATIONS. There are usually no prodromal symptoms. Fever is absent or low grade. The characteristic rash appears in three stages. The illness usually begins with the sudden appearance of livid erythema of the cheeks which gives the child a "slapped cheek" appearance. An erythematous maculopapular rash then appears on the trunk and extremities. The palms and soles may be involved. The rash fades with central clearing, giving a lacy or reticulated appearance (Fig. 10–36, p. 657), which is the most distinctive part of the disease. The duration of the rash is from 2 to 39 days (mean, 11 days). It is frequently pruritic. The rash resolves without desquamation, but periodic recrudescences may occur with exercise, warm baths, rubbing of the skin or emotional upset. Constitutional symptoms such as headache, pharyngitis, coryza and gastrointestinal disturbance are more frequent and more severe in adults.

LABORATORY DATA. There are no confirmatory laboratory tests.

DIAGNOSIS. Erythema infectiosum must be differentiated from rubella, enteroviral diseases, systemic lupus erythematosus, atypical measles and drug rashes.

COMPLICATIONS. Complications are rare. Arthritis, hemolytic anemia, pneumonitis and encephalitis have been reported.

TREATMENT. No treatment is indicated. Isolation is not required.

Balfour, H., et al.: Encephalitis associated with erythema infectiosum. J. Pediatr. 77:133, 1970.

Balfour, Henry H.: Erythema infectiosum. Clin. Pediatr. *8*:721, 1969.

Balfour, H., et al.: Erythema infectiosum: Recovery of rubella virus and echovirus 12. Pediatrics *50*:285, 1972.

HERPES SIMPLEX

Herpesvirus hominis (HVH) is a common parasite of man that can produce a variety of clinical manifestations. These can be classified under diseases of the skin, the mucous membranes, the eye, the central nervous system, the genital tract and generalized systemic disease.

Two types of infection are recognized: (1) Primary: This is the susceptible host's first experience with the virus, which results in a subclinical infection in most instances. In the remainder, local superficial lesions usually occur (see below) accompanied by a varying degree of systemic reaction. In newborn infants and severely malnourished infants a fatal systemic infection, often without superficial lesions, may occur. Circulating antibodies develop in nonfatal cases. (2) Recurrent: These lesions are the result of reactivation of a latent infection in an immune host with circulating antibodies. Reactivation follows such nonspecific stimuli as changes in the external milieu (e.g., cold, ultraviolet light) or the internal milieu (e.g., menstruation, fever or emotional stress). The lesions are localized and, as a rule, unassociated with systemic reaction.

CLINICAL PATTERNS

Systemic Infection

IN THE NEWBORN INFANT. Most neonatal herpes is caused by type 2 virus acquired by passage through an infected birth canal. Occasionally type 1 infection is seen, possibly due to transplacentally or postnatally acquired infection. The true incidence of neonatal herpetic disease is not known. Since most of the early reports were based on autopsy material, it was originally believed that the disease had a very high mortality rate. With improved techniques for viral isolation, a number of mild cases have been diagnosed with localized involvement of the skin, eye or mouth. Some infants have shown no clinical illness. The prognosis of disseminated disease or central nervous system involvement is poor. Severe sequelae are present in about 50 per cent of surviving infants.

The infant with typical generalized infection appears well until the fifth to ninth day, when appetite fails and evidence of a widespread infection rapidly follows. The fully developed illness may simulate septicemia; the infant may have fever or hypothermia, dyspnea, increasing jaundice, vomiting, lethargy or convulsions. Myocarditis has been described, and circulatory collapse is often the terminal event. Hepatosplenomegaly is common. Purpura or other bleeding results from liver failure or thrombocytopenia. Vesicular lesions on the skin or mucous membranes or conjunctivitis may or may not be present; when the esophagus is affected, thick, yellow mucus accumulates. A terminal septicemia with *Pseudomonas aeruginosa* is not unusual. Some infants recover after a mild infection characterized only by a vesicular eruption and low-grade fever.

HVH has been implicated as a cause of congenital malformations resembling those caused by rubella and cytomegalovirus. More studies are necessary to confirm this observation.

IN SEVERELY MALNOURISHED INFANTS. The primary infection in infants who have severe protein malnutrition, often in their second year, may be generalized and fatal. The clinical and pathologic findings are similar to those in the newborn.

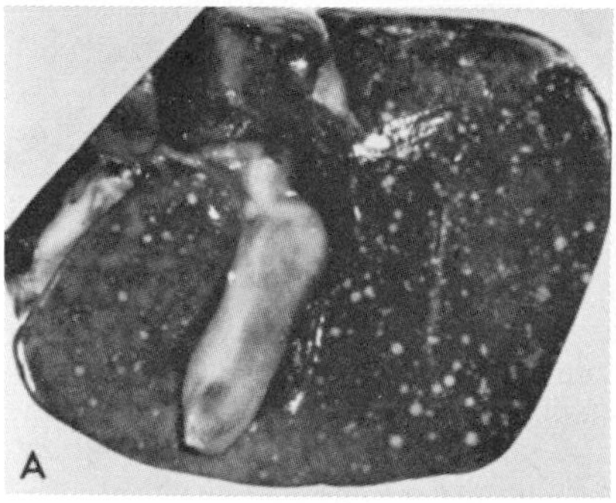

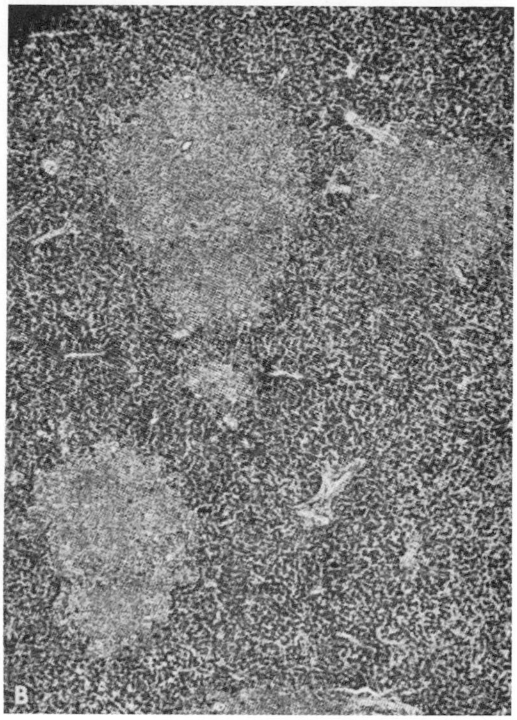

Figure 10–37 A, *Right lobe of liver of an infant with generalized herpes simplex, who died at 10 days of age. The mother had vesicles on both labia; there were no lesions on the skin of the infant. Note the multiple discrete areas of necrosis.* B, *Photomicrograph of liver from an infant with generalized herpes simplex. There are multiple sharply demarcated areas of necrosis scattered throughout the parenchyma (×38).*

Lesions of the Skin and Mucous Membranes

Lesions of the Skin
(Herpes Labialis, Facialis, Febrilis)

Primary infection may, uncommonly, result in a generalized vesicular eruption in which the lesions are small and may continue to appear over a period of 2 to 3 weeks. If the systemic manifestations are mild, the infection must be differentiated from varicella; if severe, from variola.

Clinical lesions of recurrent herpes infection occur on the skin or mucous membranes. On the skin the lesion consists of aggregates of thin-walled vesicles on an erythematous base. These rupture, scab and heal within 7 to 10 days without leaving a scar except after repeated attacks or secondary bacterial infections; temporary depigmentation occurs in blacks. The local lesions may be preceded by mild irritation or burning at the local site or by severe neuralgic pain in the region. In children the vesicles often become secondarily infected, introducing *impetigo contagiosa* into the differential diagnosis. The lesions tend to occur at mucocutaneous junctions, but may occur anywhere. They tend to recur at the same site. The sites most commonly affected are also those where lip cancer occurs most commonly.

Traumatic lesions of the skin can be readily infected by the ubiquitous herpesvirus. Primary lesions can also occur on apparently unbroken skin, as, for example, on the chin of a drooling infant with herpetic stomatitis, in whom scattered isolated vesicles appear (contrast the grouped vesicles of recurrent attacks). When the skin of a limb is infected, vesicles appear in 2 to 3 days at the site of the trauma. There is often centripetal spread along lymph channels, causing enlargement of regional lymph nodes and scattered vesicles on the intervening undamaged skin. The final clinical picture may be mistaken for that of *herpes zoster,* especially if accompanied by neuralgic pain, unless the lesions are recognized as not being confined to a dermatome. The lesions heal slowly, often taking 3 weeks; recurrences at the site of the local trauma are common and may assume a bullous nature. Wrestlers and medical personnel are liable to herpetic infections of superficial abrasions (herpes gladiatorum and herpetic Whitlow). In the latter, infection of minor trauma about the nails leads to extremely painful, deep-seated spreading lesions with vesicles which resolve spontaneously in 2 to 3 weeks. Similar lesions occur on the fingers of thumb suckers who are suffering from herpetic gingivostomatitis. Treatment is symptomatic only; the lesions should not be incised.

Eczema Herpeticum
(Kaposi's Varicelliform Eruption; Juliusberg's Pustulosis Vacciniformis Acuta)

This, the most serious manifestation of "traumatic herpes," results from a widespread and usually primary infection of the eczematous skin with herpesvirus. The severity of the complication varies; the attacks may be so mild as to be overlooked without a high index of suspicion and adequate laboratory facilities, or they may be fatal. In a typical severe primary attack, vesicles develop abruptly in large numbers over the area of eczematous skin. They continue to appear in crops for as long as 7 to 9 days. Isolated at first, they later become grouped and may occur on adjoining areas of normal skin. Wide denudation of the epidermis may occur. Scabs eventually form, and epithelization occurs. The systemic reaction varies, but temperatures of 103 to 105° F. for 7 to 10 days are not uncommon. Recurrent attacks develop on chronic atopic skin lesions. The systemic, presumably hypersensitivity, reaction is usually less than in primary infection. Death may occur as the result of profound physiologic disturbances from loss of fluid, electrolytes and protein through the skin, from dissemination of the virus to the brain and other organs, or from secondary bacterial invasion. A differentiation from *eczema vaccinatum* can usually be made clinically by determining with reasonable certainty that the child has not been exposed to vaccinia and by the occurrence of crops of vesicles in herpes. The diagnosis can be established quickly and accurately by examination of vesicular fluid with the electron microscope. Herpes simplex virus cannot be differentiated from varicella-zoster by this method but can easily be distinguished from vaccinia and variola.

Acute Herpetic Gingivostomatitis

(Acute Infectious Gingivostomatitis; Aphthous Stomatitis; Catarrhal Stomatitis; Ulcerative Stomatitis; Vincent's Stomatitis)

This primary infection is probably the commonest cause of stomatitis in children between 1 and 3 years of age. It can occur in adults. The symptoms may appear abruptly, with pain in the mouth, salivation, fetor oris, refusal to eat and fever, often as high as 104 to 105° F. The onset may be insidious, fever and irritability preceding the oral lesions by a day or two. The initial lesion is a vesicle, seldom seen because of its early rupture. The residual lesion is 2 to 10 mm in diameter and is covered with a yellow-gray membrane. When this membrane sloughs, a true ulcer remains. Although the tongue and cheeks are most commonly involved, no part of the oral lining is exempt. Except in edentulous infants, acute gingivitis is characteristic of the disease and may precede the appearance of mucosal vesicles. Submaxillary lymphadenitis is common. The acute phase lasts 4 to 9 days and is self-limited. Pain tends to disappear 2 to 4 days before healing of the ulcers is complete. In some instances the tonsillar regions are involved early, and acute tonsillitis of bacterial origin or herpangina may be suspected. Failure of the lesion to respond to antibiotic therapy differentiates a bacterial infection, and the spread of the vesiculation to the buccal mucosa rules out herpangina.

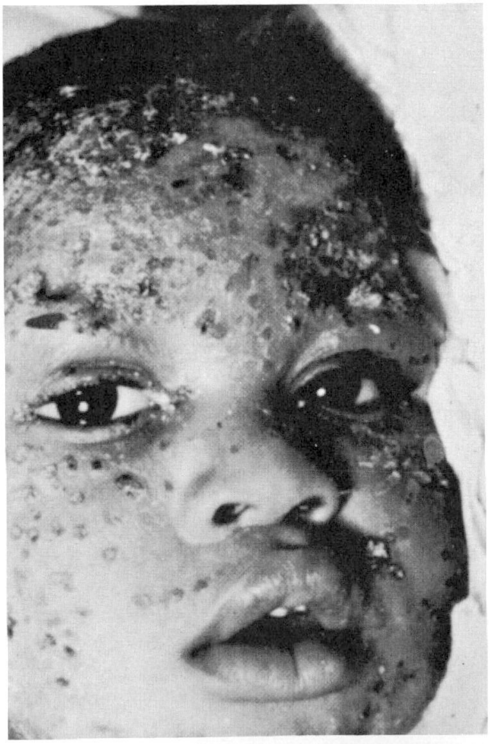

Figure 10–38 *Eczema herpeticum. Note similarity of umbilicated vesicular lesions on face to those of eczema vaccinatum.*

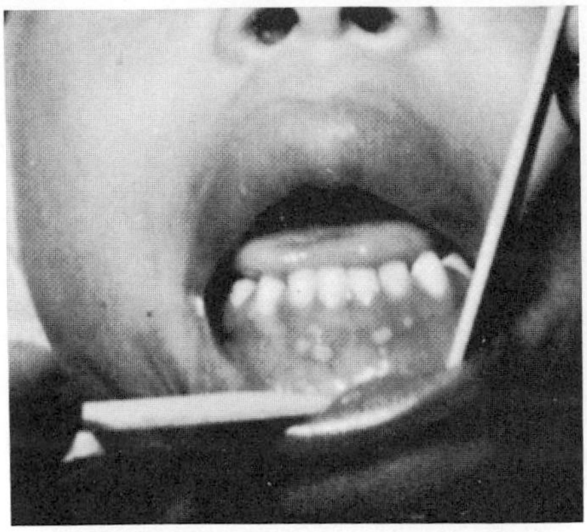

Figure 10–39 *Herpetic stomatitis.*

Recurrent Stomatitis

Localized lesions may occur on the palate in association with a febrile illness or on the mucosa ad-

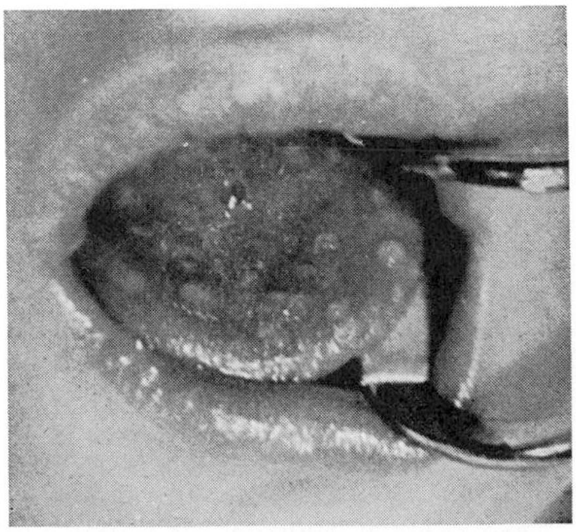

Figure 10–40 *Lesions of herpetic stomatitis on the tongue.*

jacent to a lesion on the lip; recurrent aphthous ulcers, however, are not caused by herpesvirus. In some persons a generalized stomatitis recurs consistently 7 to 10 days after a recurrent herpetic lesion of the lip or elsewhere, and is often accompanied by skin lesions of erythema multiforme; this lesion is a hypersensitivity reaction to virus protein.

Genital Herpes

Genital infections with herpesvirus occur most commonly in adolescents and young adults, are usually due to type 2 virus and are spread venereally. Five to 10 per cent of cases are caused by HVH-1. When the patient has no antibody to either type of herpes (approximately 30 per cent of cases), systemic symptoms such as fever, regional adenopathy and dysuria are more likely to occur. In adult women the vulva and vagina may be involved, but the cervix is the primary site of infection. Recurrence is common. Recurrent disease involving only the cervix is frequently subclinical, an important point since active disease in the cervix can easily infect an infant during passage through the birth canal.

In males, herpetic vesicles or ulcers are usually seen on the glans penis, prepuce or shaft of the penis. The scrotum is less frequently involved.

Epidemiologic studies as well as studies which report the in vitro transformation of cells inoculated with herpesvirus, type 2, suggest this agent as a possible factor in the etiology of carcinoma of the cervix.

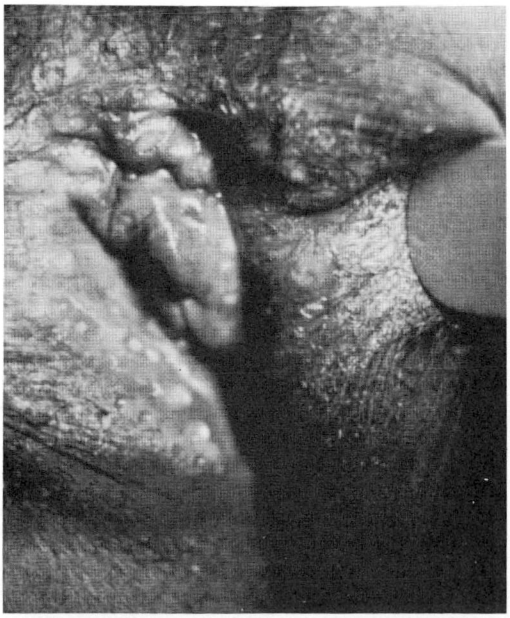

Figure 10–41 *Primary herpetic vulvovaginitis. Note the similarity of the lesions to those of herpetic gingivostomatitis. (From Scott, Coriell, Blank and Burgoon: J. Pediat., Vol. 41.)*

Lesions of the Eye

Conjunctivitis and keratoconjunctivitis may occur as manifestations of either a primary or a recurrent infection. The conjunctiva appears congested and swollen with little, if any, purulent discharge. In the primary infection the preauricular node is enlarged and tender. Cataracts, uveitis and chorioretinitis have been described in newborn infants.

Corneal lesions may be superficial in the form of a dendritic ulcer, or deep, as a disciform keratitis. The diagnosis is suggested by the presence of herpetic vesicles of the lids and established by the isolation of the virus. The highly contagious *epidemic keratoconjunctivitis* (shipyard conjunctivitis) due to one of several serotypes of adenovirus must be considered in the differential diagnosis.

Meningoencephalitis

(See also Encephalitis of Viral Origin in section on Encephalitis.) Herpes encephalitis is seen in all age groups. HVH-2 is the usual cause in newborns, HVH-1 in older patients. The pathogenesis is unknown, but it can occur in patients who already possess antibody against herpes simplex. It is the most common type of nonepidemic encephalitis in the United States, has a high mortality rate and frequently produces severe sequelae in survivors.

GENERAL FEATURES OF HERPETIC INFECTIONS

ETIOLOGY. *Herpesvirus hominis* (HVH) is a DNA-containing virus. Each particle (virion) is 150 to 200 mμ in diameter and is made up of 162 capsomeres surrounded by an envelope derived from the host. The virus readily infects rabbits, guinea pigs, hamsters and mice; suckling mice are especially susceptible. It produces pocks on the chorio-allantoic membrane of the embryonated hen's egg and characteristic cytopathic changes in a variety of cells growing in monolayer tissue cultures. Two strains are recognized from biologic and antigenic characteristics: type 1, which commonly infects skin and mucous membranes, and type 2, which infects primarily the genitalia.

EPIDEMIOLOGY. This virus is a parasite of man which has developed an extremely compatible relationship with its host. In the majority of instances (approximately 85 per cent) the infection is subclinical; even when clinical manifestations are present, the host is only rarely disabled or killed. Under exceptional circumstances the primary infection may lead to institutional or family outbreaks of stomatitis. The incubation period is 2 to 12 days (average, 6 days). *The spread of infection appears to be determined in large measure by two factors: trauma and close bodily contact.* Prior to the onset of symptoms there is often a history or implication of trauma to the site such as teething, or a break in the skin. Since trauma decreases production of interferon in infected guinea pigs, the clinical manifestations may be the result of the combination of incidental seeding of the virus and depressed body defenses.

The higher incidence of HVH antibody in lower socioeconomic groups correlates well with crowded living conditions. The epidemiology differs for the two types of HVH. Detailed serologic studies have been done only in low income groups. In these groups most infants show transplacental antibody for about the first 6 months of life. From 1 to 4 years there is a sharp rise in antibodies to type 1; a much slower rate of acquisition is seen from 5 to 14 years. After 14 there is again a sharp rise in antibodies to HVH—mostly to type 2. By adult life HVH antibodies are seen in 80 to 100 per cent of the population of lower socioeconomic groups. Antibodies to type 2 are seen in up to 60 per cent of adults in these groups. The incidence of type 2 antibody in higher socioeconomic groups is about 10 per cent and in nuns about 3 per cent.

Once infected, the majority of people continue to carry the virus in an occult state and maintain an almost constant level of circulating antibodies. It has been shown that the level of antibodies may fall after a primary infection, and that several subclinical reinfections may occur before a stable antibody level is established. Carriers may distribute virus without the presence of a manifest lesion. Herpes simplex virus can be isolated from the pharynx in about 5 per cent of asymptomatic adults.

PATHOLOGY. The pathologic changes vary with the tissue infected. In general, a specific lesion is characterized by the presence of intranuclear inclusion bodies. These are homogeneous masses lying in the midst of a severely disorganized nucleus in which the basichromatin has marginated to the nuclear membrane. In the area of the specific lesion there is always evidence of an acute inflammatory reaction. In the skin and mucous membranes the typical lesion is a unilocular vesicle. This is formed by breakdown of epidermal cells which have undergone ballooning degeneration. In the skin the vesicle is tense; the roof is formed by the outer cells of the prickle layer and the keratinized cells beyond. Ballooned epithelial cells containing intranuclear inclusions can best be seen at the margins of the vesicle. The vesicular fluid contains infected epithelial cells, including multinucleated "virus" giant cells and leukocytes. In the corium there is no necrosis, but capillaries are dilated and there is infiltration with mononuclear and polymorphonuclear cells. In the mucous membrane, owing to maceration, there is early leakage of the vesicular fluid, resulting in a collapsed vesicle, mainly filled with fibrin. The edematous roof cells form a gray membrane over the lesion.

In normal persons, the lesions are confined to the skin and mucous membranes; viremia has been described only rarely. Blood stream spread of the virus with resultant widely disseminated disease is seen mainly in the newborn, in severely malnourished children, in persons with skin diseases such as eczema and in those with defects in cell-mediated immunity. In these patients the virus spreads from the portal of entry by a primary viremia, and infection of most susceptible organs occurs. Virus increases within these organs and a secondary viremia occurs with evidence of extensive cell destruction. Healing begins with clearing of the viremia and decrease in the production of virus within the cells.

There is evidence that the method of spread to the central nervous system is different for type 1 and type 2 herpesvirus. It is probable that most cases of HVH-1 encephalitis in patients other than newborns are caused by neurogenic spread of the virus to the brain; HVH-2 is usually bloodborne.

LABORATORY DATA. Microscopic examination of properly fixed and stained scrapings from lesions reveals multinuclear giant cells and intranuclear inclusions. Immunofluorescent techniques applied to these specimens can be useful in diagnosing herpes infection and in differentiating the two types of herpes. Virus can be isolated from the lesions using tissue culture techniques. Such cultures are usually positive in 1 to 4 days. Serologic tests are less helpful except for tests to determine herpes-specific IgM in the newborn infant.

There is a moderate polymorphonuclear leukocytosis in acute herpetic gingivostomatitis, eczema herpeticum and meningoencephalitis. In meningoencephalitis there is a cellular increase in the cerebrospinal fluid up to about 1000 cells per mm^3, most of which are lymphocytes; the protein level is elevated, and the sugar is within the normal range.

DIAGNOSIS. The diagnosis is based on any two of the following: (1) a typical clinical pattern; (2) isolation of the virus; (3) development of specific neutralizing antibodies; (4) demonstration of characteristic cells or histologic changes in scrapings or biopsy material.

COURSE AND PROGNOSIS. Primary infection with the herpesvirus is a self-limited disease, usually lasting 1 to 2 weeks. Fatalities may occur in the newborn infant, in older infants with severe malnutrition and in patients with meningoencephalitis or severe eczema herpeticum; otherwise, the prognosis is usually good. There may be frequent recurrent attacks, but they seldom cause more than a temporary inconvenience except in the eye, where they may eventually cause scarring of the cornea and blindness.

TREATMENT. Since it is believed that most infants with neonatal herpes acquired the infection during passage through an infected birth canal, cesarean sections have been advocated in women with genital herpes close to term. If the membranes have been ruptured for longer than 6 hours, there is an increased risk for ascending infection, and cesarean section is unlikely to protect the infant.

Topical treatment of genital herpes with 5-iodo-2′-deoxyuridine (IDU) has been advocated, but its efficacy has not been proved. Application of a vital dye such as proflavine or neutral red, followed by exposure to light, has been reported to decrease severity of disease and incidence of recurrences of labial and genital herpes.

Topical IDU is usually effective in treatment of

herpetic keratitis but does not reduce the rate of recurrence. Topical corticosteroids may cause increased ocular involvement and should not be used.

Systemic IDU and other antiviral drugs such as cytosine arabinoside (Ara-C) and adenine arabinoside (Ara-A) have been used in treatment of neonatal herpes and herpes encephalitis. These drugs interfere with the synthesis of viral DNA but also affect the DNA of normal cells (particularly those which are actively dividing), producing toxicity such as bone marrow depression. Controlled studies are necessary to determine the efficacy of these drugs in antiviral therapy.

Many types of immunizing agents have been tried. Repeated smallpox vaccination has been advocated, but controlled studies have shown little benefit. BCG vaccination has also been suggested. Several inactivated herpes simplex vaccines have been developed and some of the studies have shown that they are useful in preventing recurrent infections. They appear to be more effective in prevention of type 1 infections. The possibility that herpesvirus may be oncogenic even when inactivated limits the usefulness of these vaccines.

The effectiveness of high doses of gamma globulin in the affected newborn infant needs further study.

Apart from this specific therapy, symptomatic and supportive therapy is of great importance. In infants especially, eczema herpeticum and stomatitis may lead to severe dehydration, shock and hypoproteinemia, requiring replacement of fluids, electrolytes and proteins.

Care of the mouth demands cleanliness by oral lavage; Ceepryn 1:4000 or Zephiran 1:1000 may be useful. Local analgesics, such as viscous lidocaine or benzocaine lozenges may allay pain and enable the older child to eat. Labial lesions may be helped by application of drying agents such as calamine lotion or glycerine with carbamine peroxide. Analgesics should be used systemically as required. Antibiotics are useful only in the treatment of secondary bacterial infections.

The intake of food and fluid will be facilitated by acquiescing to the child's whims. Ice-cold fluids or semisolids are often accepted when other food is refused. Recurrences are often due to emotional stress, which must be recognized and treated.

Nahmias, A. J., and Roizman, B.: Infection with herpes-simplex viruses 1 and 2. New Engl. J. Med. *289*:667, 719, 781, 1973.

Melnick, J., and Rawls, W.: Herpesvirus type 2 and cervical carcinoma. Ann. N.Y. Acad. Sci. *174*:993, 1973.

VARICELLA AND HERPES ZOSTER

Since the observations of Bokay (1888) there have been frequent reports that exposure of susceptible persons to a patient with herpes zoster could result in the acquisition of chickenpox. The work of Weller and his co-workers confirmed the belief that these two diseases are different clinical manifestations of the same causative agent.

ETIOLOGY. The common causative agent is now designated as *Herpesvirus varicellae.* The structure of viral particles as seen under the electron microscope is indistinguishable from that of *Herpesvirus hominis.* The agent can be grown in a variety of primary cultures of human and simian tissues. It cannot be transmitted to lower animals or grown in the embryonated hen's egg. Serum antibodies in patients recovering from varicella react equally with the agents derived from varicella and herpes zoster vesicles.

The reasons for different clinical manifestations of the two diseases are not understood. It seems probable that varicella is the primary response of a susceptible host, whereas herpes zoster may be the response of partial immunity when a latent infection is activated by some exogenous factor, e.g., stress, trauma, malignancy or x-radiation.

PATHOLOGY. The *skin lesions* of both diseases are identical and characteristic of the herpesvirus group and cannot be distinguished from those of *Herpesvirus hominis* (herpes simplex.) Although not usual in cases of average severity, necrosis with hemorrhage can be found in the mucous membranes of the mouth, trachea, esophagus and intestine.

Internally the lesions vary somewhat in the two diseases. In fatal cases of *varicella* intranuclear inclusions can be found in the endothelium of the blood vessels; the vessel walls may undergo necrosis. Intranuclear inclusions have also been found in most organs of the body, including the salivary glands and the nervous system, and in the cells of the myenteric plexus of the stomach and intestine. In the brain perivenous demyclination is similar to that of other postinfectious encephalitides; necrosis of nerve cells and leptomeningitis have been described.

In *herpes zoster* the characteristic lesions are in the nervous system, particularly in the dorsal root ganglia. Early in the disease the cells of the dorsal ganglia of the affected dermatome contain intranuclear inclusions. Shortly thereafter the ganglia show only necrosis of cells, sometimes associated with hemorrhage. As the disease progresses evidence of inflammation and degeneration is found in the posterior roots and in the peripheral portions of the nerves. Unilateral and segmental necrosis of the nerve cells in the posterior horn may be found (cf. poliomyelitis, which involves the nerve cells of the anterior horn). Leptomeningitis occurs in the region of the involved nerves. Intranuclear inclusions have been found in the sympathetic ganglia, the neurilemma cells of the nerve twigs in the corium and in the myenteric plexus, and, in visceral herpes, in the walls of the bladder and other viscera.

VARICELLA
(Chickenpox)

Varicella is characterized by the appearance on the skin and mucous membranes of successive crops of typical vesicles, generally accompanied by a mild constitutional reaction. Chickenpox, the term derived from *cicer* (chick-pea), was clearly distinguished from smallpox in 1767 by William Heberden.

EPIDEMIOLOGY. Varicella is a highly contagious disease. Ninety per cent of reported patients are less than 10 years of age. The peak age of incidence is 5 to 9 years, but the disease may occur at any age, including the neonatal period. Secondary attack rates among susceptible household contacts is about 90 per cent. The disease is seen mainly from January to May. It is spread by direct contact or by droplet. Infectious virus is present in the vesicles but, unlike smallpox, is not contained in the crusts. Patients are infectious from about 24 hours before the appearance of the rash until all lesions are crusted (usually 6 to 7 days after the eruption). Epidemics of chickenpox have been initiated by exposure to herpes zoster. Second attacks are rare.

CLINICAL MANIFESTATIONS. The incubation period varies from 11 to 21 days, and is between 13 and 17 days in the majority of instances. At the end of the incubation period prodromal symptoms, except in the mildest cases, precede the characteristic rash by 24 hours. There may be slight fever, malaise or anorexia, accompanied at times by a scarlatiniform or morbilliform rash. It is characteristic of the specific rash to appear rapidly. Typically, it begins as crops of small, red papules which almost immediately develop into clear, often oval, "teardrop" vesicles on an erythematous base. These vesicles are usually not umbilicated. The contents become cloudy within about 24 hours. The vesicles are easily broken and become scabbed. Occasionally they dry before becoming cloudy. Except for the mildest cases in which few lesions occur, crops of widely scattered vesicles continue to erupt for 3 or 4 days, starting on the trunk and later spreading to the face and scalp, with minimal, if any, involvement of distal parts of the extremities. There is some tendency for the lesions to be concentrated in areas of skin pressure or irritation, but not to the same extent as in smallpox. Characteristically, at the height of the disease the eruption consists of papules, early and late vesicles, and crusts present at the same time (Fig. 10–42, p. 657). Rarely, in severe disease, the lesions appear as hard, pearly lumps (mostly at the same stage of development) and resemble those of smallpox. Pruritus is a constant and annoying characteristic of the rash. Vesicles on the mucous membranes, particularly those of the mouth, rapidly become macerated. The top of the lesion sloughs to form a shallow ulcer. Less commonly, lesions are found on the genital mucous membranes and on the conjunctiva and the cornea, where they are potentially dangerous to sight. Laryngeal involvement is rare. There may be generalized lymphadenopathy.

The severity of the disease varies from a few lesions with little evidence of systemic illness to many hundreds of lesions, and extreme toxicity with temperatures ranging from 103 to 105° F. Systemic manifestations occur only during the first 3 to 4 days when the rash is erupting.

Infrequently the rash becomes hemorrhagic in association with a mild to severe thrombocytopenia. The more severe forms usually occur with other complications such as pneumonia or in patients receiving immunosuppressive therapy. Purpura fulminans, which occurs about the end of the first week, and is associated with gangrene, probably represents a Shwartzman-like reaction.

Varicella bullosa is an uncommon variant seen mainly in children under 2 years of age, in which many of the lesions appear as bullae instead of vesicles. The course of the disease is not changed.

Congenital varicella may be manifest at birth or appear within a few days in infants whose mothers have an active infection. Such infections have a mortality rate of about 20 per cent; in contrast, infections acquired postnatally by young infants are usually mild.

LABORATORY DATA. There may be a mild leukocytosis. Virus giant cells (see Herpes Simplex) can be demonstrated in scrapings from the floors of fresh vesicles. The virus can be isolated in a variety of human tissue culture cell lines.

DIAGNOSIS. This is not difficult in the average case. Most important is the distinction between chickenpox and smallpox, which may be exceedingly difficult in patients with mild smallpox or severe chickenpox. The following clinical points should be borne in mind: (1) The rash of chickenpox begins on the trunk and spreads toward the periphery, whereas that of smallpox tends to spread from the periphery toward the trunk. (2) The lesions of smallpox tend to be most frequent in areas of pressure or tightness of the skin, as over the bridge of the nose and the wrist or at the belt line, whereas those of chickenpox do not have this tendency to the same extent. (3) The lesions of chickenpox are more superficial and are not umbilicated, whereas the lesions of smallpox tend to be deeper and more "shotty" to the touch and are usually umbilicated. (4) The lesions of chickenpox are present in all stages of development at a given time, whereas those of smallpox are more or less in the same stage at each phase of the disease. (5) The prodromal symptoms of chickenpox are short (1 to 2 days) and usually mild; those of smallpox are longer (3 to 4 days) and may be severe, with high fever which drops with the appearance of the rash.

Material from vesicles can be examined by electron microscopy; varicella-zoster virus can be easily distinguished from variola virus by its morphologic appearance.

COMPLICATIONS. Secondary bacterial infection of the skin lesions is the most common complication. Thrombocytopenia with hemorrhage into the skin and mucous membranes may occur; internal hemorrhage from ulcerations or into an adrenal may be fatal.

Varicella pneumonia is uncommon in children, but 20 to 30 per cent of adults with chickenpox have clinical or radiologic signs of lung involvement. Recovery is usually prompt, but x-ray changes may persist for 6 to 12 weeks in the more seriously ill. Fatalities have been reported. Purpura fulminans (see Consumption Coagulopathies in Section 14) is most frequently seen following chickenpox. Lesions on the larynx may cause severe enough edema to produce respiratory distress. Myocarditis, pericarditis, endocarditis, hepatitis, glomerulonephritis and acute myositis of the limb muscles have been described. Keratitis and vesicular conjunctivitis are rare and usually benign. About 10 per cent of cases of Reye syndrome are associated with chickenpox. Congenital malformations have been described in infants whose mothers had varicella during the first trimester of pregnancy. The babies have been small for age, with scarring of the skin, muscular atrophy, chorioretinitis, seizures, mental retardation and an unusual susceptibility to infection.

The most common central nervous system complication is postinfectious encephalitis. Cerebellar signs such as ataxia, nystagmus and tremors are common. Encephalitis presenting mainly with cerebellar signs has a much better prognosis than cerebral symptoms of convulsions and coma. Overall mortality rates vary from 5 to 25 per cent. About 15 per cent of survivors have permanent sequelae of seizures, mental retardation or behavior disturbances. Other central nervous system complications include the Guillain-Barré syndrome, transverse myelitis, facial nerve palsy, optic neuritis with transient loss of vision, and the hypothalamic syndrome with obesity and recurrent fever. In contrast to herpes zoster, in which virus has been isolated from the cerebrospinal fluid, no virus has been isolated from the central nervous system of patients dying with chickenpox.

Children on steroids or antimetabolites are at risk for developing severe, often fatal, chickenpox. The greatest risk appears to be in children with leukemia, but deaths have been reported in children receiving steroids for acute rheumatic fever or nephrosis.

PROGNOSIS. The prognosis is usually good; fatalities occur from the complications.

TREATMENT. Symptomatic treatment should be directed to alleviating itching by the use of systemic antipruritic agents and sedation as required. Scratching should be minimized by use of mittens and keeping the nails short. Daily changes of clothes and linen and antiseptic baths will reduce the incidence of secondary bacterial infection. If secondary infection occurs, systemic antibiotic therapy is indicated.

Treatment of varicella pneumonia is supportive. Antibiotics are indicated only if secondary bacterial infection occurs. Steroids have not been shown to be useful.

Cytosine arabinoside, a pyrimidine nucleoside, has been shown to have some activity in vitro against DNA viruses, particularly of the herpes group. It has been used in a limited number of leukemic patients with varicella with some reported success. No control studies have been done. Cytosine arabinoside has marked toxicity, particularly for bone marrow. More studies are necessary to determine its usefulness in the therapy of varicella in immunocompromised patients.

PROPHYLAXIS. No vaccine is available for active prophylaxis. Passive immunity can be induced by use of zoster immune globulin (ZIG). ZIG is a gamma globulin fraction of plasma with high titer of antibody, obtained from patients recovering from herpes zoster infection. It is effective in preventing chickenpox when given within 72 hours of exposure. The recommended dose of ZIG is 5 ml given intramuscularly. Most of the studies of ZIG have been done in normal susceptible children, and doses as small as 2 ml have been effective in preventing infection. However, prophylaxis is indicated only in susceptible patients at high risk for developing severe varicella: those with immunodeficiency diseases, leukemia or other malignancies or those on immunosuppressive drugs. These children are not protected by ZIG as completely as normal children, and larger quantities of high titer ZIG seem indicated. Serum obtained from patients convalescing from herpes zoster has also been used. It appears to be less effective than ZIG and carries the added risk of transmitting hepatitis.

HERPES ZOSTER
(Shingles)

Herpes zoster is an acute infection characterized by crops of vesicles, usually confined to a dermatome and by neuralgic pain in the area of the affected dermatome.

EPIDEMIOLOGY. Herpes zoster is relatively uncommon under 10 years of age, after which its incidence increases steadily with each succeeding decade. Second attacks are rare, less than 1 per cent in one study of 206 patients. The patient with herpes zoster usually has a history of having had varicella. When this is not the case, the possibility must be considered that a mild case of varicella may have been misdiagnosed or that there had been exposure in the neonatal period which resulted in clinically unrecognized disease. There is an increased incidence of the disease in patients with malignancies and in those receiving immunosuppressive drugs. The severity of the disease increases with age. There is no sex, race or seasonal predilection. The factors which initiate an attack of herpes zoster are not understood.

CLINICAL MANIFESTATIONS. Herpes zoster has a pre-eruptive and a posteruptive phase. The patient usually has pain and tenderness along the involved dermatome. There is often generalized malaise and fever. Within a few days groups of red papules appear, distributed along one or two adjacent dermatomes; the individual lesions quickly vesiculate (Fig. 10–43), become pustular, dry up and scab in the course of 5 to 10 days. The lesions tend to appear first at a point nearest the central nervous system. Successive crops of lesions appear for 1 to 4 days. Occasionally they continue to appear for 7 days, extending along the course of the

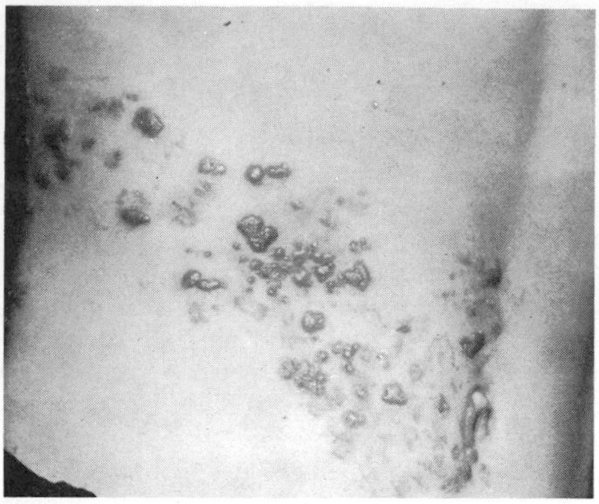

Figure 10–43 Herpes zoster. (Courtesy of Dr. Carroll S. Wright.)

nerve. The eruption clears in 7 to 14 days in most patients under 20 years of age, but when vesicles continue to appear for 7 days, healing may be delayed up to 5 weeks. The lesions, except in rare instances, are unilateral. Fever, pain and tenderness usually continue throughout the period of progression. The regional lymph nodes are invariably enlarged. Although the dermatomes of the second dorsal to the second lumbar nerves are the commonest sites under the age of 20 years, cephalic zoster and infection of the sacral nerves, producing lesions of the leg and genitalia, do occur in children. Transient paralysis of the affected part is a rare complication.

When there is infection of the fifth nerve, any or several of its branches may be affected; with involvement of the ophthalmic branch, lesions may appear over the forehead with local loss of hair, on the tip of the nose and on the cornea (herpes ophthalmicus, Fig. 10–44, p. 656), over the cheek and the homolateral palate, with infection of the maxillary branch, and over the homolateral mandible and tongue when the mandibular branch is affected. Infection of the seventh nerve or the geniculate ganglion results in the *Ramsay Hunt syndrome* of paralysis of the facial nerve and vesicles in the external ear canal.

A generalized rash may accompany herpes zoster; this tends to occur in elderly patients, but may occur in children who have had a mild attack of varicella in early infancy. Occasionally in children the first vesicles of varicella may be distributed along a dermatome.

LABORATORY DATA. Examination of the cerebrospinal fluid often reveals a mild lymphocytosis. Scrapings of the floors of vesicles in their initial stage contain virus giant cells. (See Herpes Simplex.)

DIAGNOSIS. Diagnosis may be difficult before development of the rash; the pain may resemble that of pleural, cardiac or peritoneal origin, depending on the site of the lesion. Once the rash has appeared, its distribution and characteristics along with the pain make the diagnosis relatively simple. Occasionally herpes simplex may simulate the distribution of herpes zoster.

COURSE AND PROGNOSIS. In children the course is usually mild, and the ultimate prognosis is good.

COMPLICATIONS. Postherpetic pain does not occur in children, and ocular complications are rare. Keratitis and uveitis may follow fifth nerve involvement in adults. Secondary bacterial infection is possible in any of the lesions.

TREATMENT. Treatment is symptomatic. Soaks and calamine or other drying lotions may be helpful. Pain is seldom a problem in children and can usually be controlled with aspirin. Steroids have been shown to be useful in adults in diminishing the amount and duration of postherpetic neuralgia, without affecting the rate of healing of the skin lesions or increasing the number of complications.

Cytosine arabinoside, a drug with antiviral properties, has been used for therapy. One study showed that patients receiving this drug had an increase in duration of dissemination of the lesions and a reduction in antibody titer and local interferon production. More controlled studies are needed. Treatment or prophylaxis with zoster immune globulin is not effective.

PROPHYLAXIS. The possibility that herpes zoster may follow exposure to chickenpox should be kept in mind. Conversely, since chickenpox can follow exposure to herpes zoster, it is unwise to admit to an open ward a child suffering from the latter disease.

Brunell, P., and Gershon, A.: Passive immunization against varicella-zoster infections and other modes of therapy. J. Infect. Dis. *127*:415, 1973.

Griffith, J., et al.: The nervous system diseases associated with varicella. Acta. Neurol. Scand. *46*:279, 1970.

McKendry, J.D.J., and Bailey, J. D.: Congenital varicella associated with multiple defects. Can. Med. Ass. J. *108*:66, 1973.

Meyers, J. D.: Congenital varicella in term infants: Risk reconsidered. J. Infect. Dis. *129*:215, 1974.

Stevens, D., et al.: Adverse effect of cytosine arabinoside on disseminated zoster. New Engl. J. Med. *289*:873, 1973.

Stevens, D. A., and Merigan, T. C.: Uncertain role of cytosine arabinoside in varicella infection of compromised hosts. J. Pediatr. *81*:562, 1972.

Triebwasser, J., et al.: Varicella pneumonia in adults. Medicine *46*:409, 1967.

SMALLPOX
(Variola)

Smallpox is an acute communicable viral disease characterized by a papulovesicular, pustular rash and usually by severe systemic symptoms.

ETIOLOGY. There appear to be two stable types of virus, variola major and variola minor, which can usually be distinguished by the severity of the disease they cause. They can be dried under relatively unfavorable conditions and remain viable for months, e.g., in house dust. The virus particles, studied in the form of the identical-appearing vaccinia virus, are the prototypes of the poxvirus group. Under the electron microscope the particles are roughly rectangular, measuring 300 by 250 mμ. There is a dense central region 100 to 150 mμ across. On or near the surface is a complex network of filamentous structures, 6 to 8 mμ in diameter, resembling a loose ball of yarn; some particles have an envelope. The nucleic acid is DNA. The virus grows on a variety of mammalian cells in tissue culture; it grows readily on the chorioallantoic membrane, where it produces small pocks similar to those of herpes simplex. In the rabbit it produces a keratoconjunctivitis after corneal inoculation (Paul's test).

EPIDEMIOLOGY. Man is the only natural host for smallpox. Although monkeys can be infected experimentally and develop a mild illness (usually without rash), natural outbreaks of pox in monkeys are caused by monkey pox (a virus that does not produce smallpox in man). There are no subclinical carriers. Infection is acquired by inhalation of droplets of aerosolized virus from sick patients, from handling of skin lesions even after scabbing or from fomites such as infected bedclothes. Close contact appears to be necessary, in most cases, for spread of the disease. Smallpox is not so contagious a disease as measles or influenza. The patient is infectious from the onset of symptoms until all the lesions have healed completely and no scabs remain. After recovery, the patient is immune for life. Most outbreaks of smallpox occur in family groups or in hospitals. Over 50 per cent of cases of smallpox seen in nonendemic countries are among hospital personnel. Smallpox during pregnancy usually results in abortion or premature birth of an infant with active disease.

The World Health Organization has been conducting an extensive program of smallpox surveillance and vaccination. Mainly because of this program, the disease is no longer endemic in large parts of the world. Only four countries (India, Bangladesh, Pakistan and Ethiopa) now report extensive disease.

The great danger of dissemination is from mild sporadic cases which may go unrecognized or be misdiagnosed as chickenpox, or from patients with severe hemorrhagic disease who die before they exhibit the characteristic rash. Laboratory assistance should be sought whenever there is suspicion of smallpox.

PATHOLOGY. The virus first infects the bronchiolar and upper respiratory tract epithelium and multiplies locally. A primary viremia then occurs, with dissemination to the reticuloendothelial system. A second and more intense viremia results, with spread to the skin and other organs producing a rash and systemic signs of illness. Specific changes are found in the skin, mucous membranes and many of the organs. The typical skin lesion starts with changes in the capillaries of the corium and is characterized by dilatation, endothelial proliferation and perivascular mononuclear infiltration. In the adjacent epidermis the cells of the middle and upper stratum spinosum swell, and the characteristic Guarnieri bodies make their appearance. These are spherical bodies lying close to the nucleus, consisting of collections of virus elementary bodies, and range in size from 2 to 8 μ; in rare instances intranuclear inclusions may be found. The swollen cells rupture, forming a vesicle divided into lobulations by thin septums of partially ruptured cellular membranes and thicker septums formed of the resistant ducts of sweat glands. The lower layer of the stratum spinosum and the basal layer beneath the growing vesicle also degenerate, and the vesicle eventually reaches the corium. The basal cells at the margin of the vesicle proliferate, leading to an increase in the thickness of the epidermis over that of the vesiculating portion. This gives rise to the early umbilication, which is accentuated when the vesiculation surrounds a hair follicle. Umbilication disappears as the fluid increases, but reappears as desiccation and crusting begin. Healing occurs without scarring except on the face, where necrosis of sebaceous glands characteristically occurs, and in other areas where there has been secondary bacterial infection.

In the squamous epithelium of the upper digestive tract, changes occur coincidentally with those of the skin and consist initially in localized and then diffuse necrosis of the superficial cells and congestion and hemorrhage in the tunica propria. Grossly, these lead to the appearance of a diffuse pseudomembrane in the pharynx by the third or fourth day, which disappears without scarring by the third week. The kidneys reveal the changes of interstitial nephritis. Orchitis occurs during the papulovesicular stage and consists in hyperplasia of the vascular endothelium followed in order by necrosis of the interstitial cells and of those of the seminiferous tubules; in boys the lesions resemble ischemic infarctions. There are hemorrhages in bone marrow in all types of smallpox; the megakaryocytes are profuse except in hemorrhagic smallpox, in which they are decreased. Small hemorrhages and mononuclear infiltrates may be found in other organs.

CLINICAL MANIFESTATIONS. The incubation period is usually 12 to 14 days, but may be as long as 21 days in previously vaccinated persons and in variola minor.

Variola Major. In a typical case the prodromal symptoms are severe and usually start abruptly. The initial clinical manifestations include headache, chills or chilliness, aching of the back and limbs, and fever, which mounts rapidly to 106 or 107° F. In children there may also be vomiting, drowsiness, convulsions and coma. Often delirium occurs, and the patient is prostrated.

During the first 2 days transient rashes are common and may resemble scarlet fever or measles or may be petechial. They tend to be most prominent over the upper thighs and buttocks and disappear rapidly by the third or fourth day, when the raised macules of the typical cutaneous lesion begin to appear over the face. Widespread prodromal rashes and the early appearance of macules presage a severe attack.

There is usually diminution in severity of symptoms as the rash becomes papular, and the temperature may even become normal and remain so until the pustular stage. The individual lesions ap-

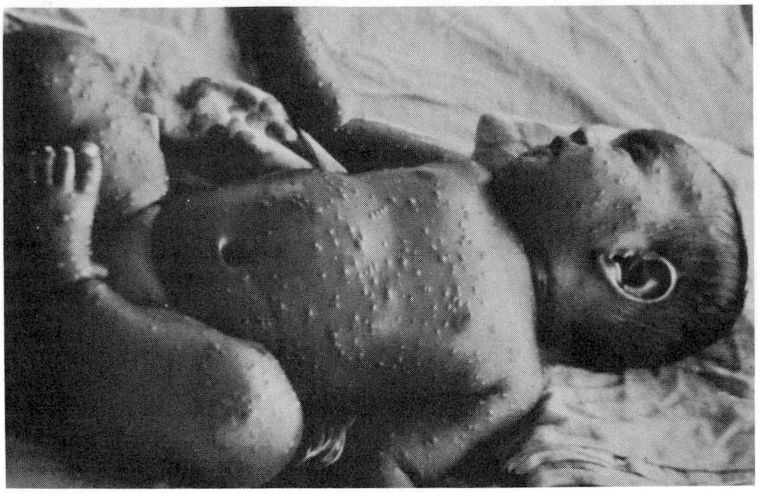

Figure 10–45 *Variola in an unvaccinated infant. (Courtesy of Dr. Roger Feldman.)*

pear in a single crop and progress at the same rate, unlike the multiple crops in chickenpox. Initially the papules are 2 to 4 mm in diameter and are firm and "shotty." Within about 24 hours the size of the papules increases and vesicles appear. They tend to be umbilicated in the early and again in the late stages. Some of the vesicles are superficial, and others deeper and less readily recognized. A small red areola encircles each vesicle.

About the fifth or sixth day of the disease the vesicles become cloudy and the pustular stage begins. The individual lesion is greenish or grayish yellow and has an elevation slightly greater than its diameter. About the ninth day of the disease the lesions begin to dry and the areolas disappear. They are usually crusted over by the end of the second week, and the scabs drop off about the end of the third or fourth week, leaving scars which are permanent in about 50 per cent of survivors. The scabs persist longest on the palms and soles, where they are known as "seeds," and may have to be enucleated with a needle.

The cutaneous areas chiefly involved in the early stages are those where the skin is tight, such as the wrists and the prominences of the face; the more exposed extensor surfaces of the forearms and upper arms are then involved, leaving the more protected flexor surfaces and the axillae relatively free. The rash then spreads to the chest. In severe cases the abdomen and the legs are heavily covered; in milder cases they may be only slightly involved. Concurrently with the skin lesions, the mucous membranes of the mouth, eyes and often the larynx become affected.

A striking feature of the disease, in contrast to chickenpox, is the profusion of lesions on the face, including the lips, and the presence of a relatively large number of lesions on the palms and soles. When the lesions become confluent, there is considerable edema of the face, so that there is difficulty in closing the eyes and mouth. The lesions on the mucous membranes also tend to be confluent. Scarring, greatest on the face, results from necrosis of sebaceous glands and is not greatly influenced by secondary infection. Intense pigmentation of the skin persists for a variable time after the scabs have fallen. In the fatal cases death usually occurs during the second week of the disease.

Hemorrhagic smallpox may occur in two forms: *vesicular hemorrhagic smallpox,* in which hemorrhages occur in the corium after the development of vesicles, and *true hemorrhagic* or *black smallpox,* in which a diffuse hemorrhagic rash begins on the second or third day of prodromal symptoms, followed by ecchymoses and hemorrhages into the mucous membranes. In the latter form the temperature may be subnormal, although the symptoms are severe. Death may occur before the characteristic rash of smallpox develops.

Variola Minor (Alastrim). Variola minor is a much milder disease, with a mortality rate of about 1 per cent. The virus of alastrim can be distinguished from that of variola major by growth on the chorioallantoic membrane at 38° C or in mouse brain, although they appear identical when examined with the electron microscope.

Modified Smallpox (Varioloid). Previously vaccinated persons with partial immunity may develop a modified illness. The prodrome is usually unchanged, but the rash evolves more rapidly and the lesions are fewer and more superficial. Fatalities are rare. Such patients are capable of transmitting severe smallpox to susceptible contacts. Since the disease may be quite atypical, diagnosis and isolation are frequently delayed. Such patients have been the source of extensive outbreaks of smallpox.

Abortive Type. In persons who have been vaccinated shortly before exposure to smallpox a condition known as "variola sine eruptione" may occur. Macules or papules may involute with great rapidity, or there may be no eruption at all, and the patient has only a mild, febrile illness. In this form, variola is not contagious.

LABORATORY DATA. A neutropenia is characteristic of the early stages of the disease. In hemorrhagic smallpox this may be associated with a reduction of platelets. Large lymphocytes are characteristically present in small numbers. During the pustular stage a polymorphonuclear leukocytosis occurs. There is prolongation of the prothrombin time and a decrease in fibrinogen associated with the hemorrhagic type, probably dependent on extensive liver damage.

DIAGNOSIS. The typical case of smallpox is readily diagnosed, but mild cases may be misdiagnosed as chickenpox, or missed altogether. In a doubtful case the patient should be isolated and viral studies obtained. (See Diagnosis of Varicella.)

COMPLICATIONS. Pyogenic infections of the skin and bacteremia, particularly with the streptococcus, were common before the availability of antibacterial agents. An enanthem of the larynx may lead to edema of the glottis and perichondritis of the laryngeal cartilages. Bronchopneumonia is relatively common. Viral osteomyelitis occurs occasionally in children and usually appears between the tenth and twentieth days of the disease. Multiple joints as well as bones are commonly infected, but severe systemic symptoms are not related to this involvement. Roentgenographic changes of bone destruction may be seen as early as the fourth day after onset of swelling and slight tenderness. Serious deformities such as flail joints, ankylosis, malformed bones and cessation of bone growth are common sequels. Central nervous system involvement is rare; symptoms usually begin 5 to 13 days after the appearance of the rash and resemble those of other postinfectious encephalomyelitides.

PROGNOSIS. The case fatality rate varies with the type of the disease and the age of the patient. The rate during epidemics of variola minor is less than 1 per cent, whereas an overall rate of about 10 per cent may be expected in epidemics of variola major. The case fatality rate is considered to be about 5 to 6 per cent in discrete smallpox, 60 per cent in confluent smallpox and 80 per cent or over in hemorrhagic smallpox. The mortality rate is greatest in children under 5 and in persons over 45 years of age.

TREATMENT. No effective specific therapy is available once the disease has developed. Marboran is effective as a prophylaxis (see below) but does not appear to be useful in treatment of established disease. Symptomatic treatment and nursing care are of extreme importance. The patient's room should be light and well ventilated; some odor-killing device is desirable. Severe cases of confluent and hemorrhagic smallpox should be treated for shock and dehydration by proper use of intravenous fluids, blood and plasma. Appropriate antibiotics in therapeutic doses should be used in severe disease when secondary bacterial infection is identified or suspected. Nutrition must be maintained, by tube feeding if necessary. Lesions of the eyes require frequent irrigation; this therapy should be supervised by an ophthalmologist. Crusts in the nose may be loosened with swabs moistened with oil. Sedation should be given as indicated. In the milder cases the general methods of treatment as outlined under Chickenpox are adequate.

PROPHYLAXIS. Vaccination (see below) is almost totally protective against acquiring variola major for 3 years and variola minor for 7 years; it reduces the severity of the disease for up to 20 years. A primary vaccination given within 3 to 4 days of exposure to smallpox gives some protection. Revaccination of a previously immunized person is effective in preventing the disease if given within 7 to 8 days of exposure. Hyperimmune vaccinia gamma globulin given at the time of vaccination raises the protection rate fourfold; Marboran (N-methylisatin beta-thiosemicarbazone) raises the protection rate sixteenfold. The drug is given orally as a 10 or 20 per cent suspension in syrup in doses of 200 mg/kg initially, followed by 50 mg/kg every 6 hours for 8 doses. There may be nausea and vomiting if the drug is not given after meals.

Patients should be strictly isolated until all the crusts have dropped off. Fomites, books, letters, and the like, must be sterilized, preferably by heat.

In the public health management of a smallpox epidemic the following steps, scrupulously enforced, can usually be relied on to control the spread of the disease without mass vaccination: (1) listing of contacts; (2) surveillance of contacts for 3 weeks for any evidence of illness; (3) vaccination of contacts, preferably within 24 hours of exposure. Vaccination must produce reliable evidence of a take, and must be repeated if negative or doubtful.

Bauer, D. J., St. Vincent, L., Kempe, C. H., and Downie, A. W.: Prophylactic treatment of smallpox contacts with N-methylisatin β-thiosemicarbazone. Lancet *2*:494, 1963.

Bras, G.: The Morbid Anatomy of Smallpox. Docum. Med. Geog. et Trop. *4*:303, 1952.

Cockshott, P., and MacGregor, M.: The natural history of osteomyelitis variolosa. J. Fac. Radiol. *10*:57, 1959.

Dixon, C. W.: Smallpox, London, J. & A. Churchill, 1962.

Downie, A. W.: Poxvirus group. *In* F. L. Horsfall, Jr., and I. Tamm (eds.): Viral and Rickettsial Infections in Man. 4th ed. Philadelphia, J. B. Lippincott Company, 1965, Chap. 44, p. 932.

Horne, R. W., and Wildy, P.: Virus structures revealed by negative staining. Adv. Virus Res. *10*:101, 1963.

Kempe, C. H., and others: The use of vaccinia hyperimmune gamma globulin in the prophylaxis of smallpox. Bull. WHO *25*:41, 1961.

VACCINATION AGAINST SMALLPOX

The use of cowpox virus for vaccination against smallpox was the first successful development of a method for the protection of human beings against a serious epidemic disease. Although used by Benjamin Jesty, a Dorsetshire farmer, in 1774 to protect his own family, it was Dr. Edward Jenner in 1798 who conclusively proved that the inoculation of human beings with material from cowpox led to immunity to smallpox. Cowpox and variola belong to the "pox" group of viruses which affect many species of animals, each animal having its own specific pox infection which, as a rule, is not transmissible to another host. Cowpox, however, is sufficiently related to the human "pox" virus, variola, that it can and does affect man with a specific disease of the skin of the hands on close contact. The stable pox virus of vaccinia may have been derived from hybridization between variola and cowpox viruses. In the laboratory such hybrids resemble the virus of vaccinia and could have occurred from documented early accidental contamination of vaccine virus batches with variola virus. The great diversity of vaccine strains that exist at present may also be the result of the past practice of mixing different strains of vaccinia virus in order to produce an effective vaccine.

Until recently vaccination against smallpox was considered a routine procedure for healthy children in the United States and most states required evidence of vaccination before entrance into school. In 1971 that policy was changed because (1) the risk of acquiring smallpox in the United States was very small, no cases having been reported since 1949; (2) the risks of primary vaccination were considerable, with a mortality rate of 1 to 2 per million primary vaccinations; (3) there was no evidence that the complication rate for primary vaccination was higher in adults than in children; and (4) the World Health Organization campaign to eradicate smallpox from the world had decreased the incidence of the disease to the point where it was considered endemic in only five countries.

The success of this new policy is dependent on continued efforts to eliminate smallpox in the remaining endemic countries, close surveillance for possible imported cases and prompt identification of all patient contacts.

Vaccination is still recommended for health care workers, military personnel and travelers into areas where the disease is endemic.

TYPE OF VACCINE. The usual type of vaccine is obtained from the pulp of vesicles of vaccinated calves, which is diluted 1:5 in 50 per cent glycerin-saline solution containing 1 per cent phenol. It is distributed in capillary glass tubes. The marketed vaccine is not completely free of bacteria; by law, it must contain less than 50 bacteria per dose and no pathogens. It is considered potent for 3 months if kept below 5° C; it deteriorates rapidly at room temperature. Avianized vaccine prepared from vaccinia-infected chorioallantoic membranes of embryonated hens' eggs is equally effective. Lyophilized dried vaccine which is stable at room temperature is advisable in the tropics or where refrigeration facilities are inadequate. A vaccine for subcutaneous administration, derived from a strain of virus attenuated by passage in chick embryo tissue culture, is under study.

SITE OF VACCINATION. Vaccination should be performed on the skin over the insertion of the deltoid muscle or on the posterior axillary fold. The latter site is exposed to a minimum of trauma, and the scars are inconspicuous. Vaccination on the thigh is more exposed to contamination in the infant and proves more incapacitating during the height of the reaction in older persons.

METHOD OF VACCINATION. Although there is good evidence that there is direct correlation between protection against the disease and the number and extent of the vaccination scars, the present policy, in nonendemic areas, is to make only one inoculation. Where smallpox is endemic or after exposure, two to four sites of inoculation are advocated. The technique is as follows:

The skin should be cleansed with a volatile antiseptic, e.g., ether or acetone, care being taken to avoid making abrasions in which the virus could "take." The tube of lymph should be removed from the freezing section of the refrigerator only at the moment of use, the ends broken off after filing, and the contents expressed on the skin by means of a small rubber bulb. Introduction of the virus can be accomplished by one of two methods.

1. The *multiple pressure method* is most generally recommended in the United States. The needle is held almost parallel with the skin and the point pressed up and down against the skin through a drop of lymph in such a way that the surface cells are picked off, thus exposing the deeper-growing cells of the epidermis to the virus. Two or three pressures over an area of about 1/8 to 1/4 inch in diameter are usually sufficient for primary vaccination after the age of 6 months. In very young infants and for revaccination, 30 pressures are recommended. The area should become erythematous, but should not bleed.

2. The *scratch method* is generally recommended in the British Isles and consists in making a scratch with a sterile needle through a drop of vaccine lymph. The scratch should be about 1/4 inch long and deep enough to get through the skin without drawing blood.

In each method the lymph is rubbed into the site with the shaft of the needle, the excess wiped off, and the remainder allowed to dry.

TYPE OF REACTION. The reaction to smallpox vaccination is considered to be due to hypersensitivity as well as to the necrotic action of vaccinia virus on the infected cells. The usual reactions vary according to the degree of host sensitivity and are classified as primary, accelerated or vaccinoid, "early" reaction or no visible reaction.

Primary Reaction. This is the reaction of the nonimmune unsensitized person. There is little reaction at the site except a fading erythema until the third to fifth day, when a red, slightly itching papule appears. This rapidly vesiculates within about 24 hours and becomes surrounded by a red areola. The vesicle grows in size, becomes umbilicated and pearly gray and is surrounded by an increasing area of erythema and induration. The reaction reaches its height about the ninth or tenth day, when the area is hot and tender, the regional lymph nodes are enlarged and painful, and the spleen may be enlarged. There is usually some systemic reaction, which may be mild, with low-grade fever, malaise and headache, or severe, with temperatures of 104° F or higher for 3 to 4 days. There is little change in the leukocyte count. After the peak of the reaction the vesicle undergoes desiccation, and becomes covered with a dark scab which is shed about the twenty-first day. The pink, pitted scar, which slowly fades to white, remains as the only evidence that successful vaccination has been performed.

Vaccinoid or Accelerated Reaction. This is the reaction of the partially sensitized person. The lesion goes through the same general stages as does the primary take, but more rapidly. The greater the sensitization, the more rapid is the evolution. A papule may become vesiculated within 2 days and reach the peak of its reaction in less than a week. The size of the reaction is smaller than with the primary take, and there are few, if any, general signs or symptoms.

"Early" Reaction. This reaction consists of a small area of redness and induration maximal at 8 to 72 hours; a vesicle may or may not be present. It occurs in highly sensitized persons and usually, but not always, indicates immunity. Nevertheless, a similar lesion can be produced by inactivated vaccine in such persons, so that they should be revaccinated with a known potent vaccine if exposed to smallpox.

No Reaction. In some persons repeated vaccinations do not result in a local lesion. Poor technique or the use of inactivated virus may explain some of these failures. Obviously such persons should be vaccinated several times with potent vaccine and by an approved technique before it is assumed that they have been immunized. Laboratory tests for neutralizing antibodies will provide definite proof of immunization.

REVACCINATION. Revaccination of health personnel is ordinarily indicated every 4 years, but must be performed whenever there is contact with a case of smallpox. In endemic areas revaccination is required at 6- to 12-month intervals. Under these circumstances a positive "take" is of such importance that at least two "insertions" should be made. Local skin immunity to vaccination can exist without systemic immunity; hence, the site of revaccination should be at a location other than the original one; the forearm appears to be particularly sensitive.

WHO suggests "major" for any reaction present on the seventh day and "minor" or "equivoid" for the earlier reactions.

CARE OF SITE OF VACCINATION. Maintenance of dryness and free flow of air about the vesicle is essential. Shields should never be used. A relatively sterile surface may be maintained on the entire area surrounding the reaction by sponging gently with alcohol at least twice daily, being careful to leave the surface of the vesicle intact. If the vesicle ruptures because of excessive tension or trauma, the area should be sponged with alcohol three or four times daily and loosely covered with a piece of gauze attached to the skin above and below by adhesive tape placed well outside the indurated area. When the dressing is changed, it should be cut off and the fresh one taped over the original adhesive tapes. These should not be removed until the inflammation has subsided to avoid secondary lesions in the adhesive abraded areas.

COMPLICATIONS

PYOGENIC INFECTIONS. As a result of scratching or neglect, the vaccination site can become contaminated with various bacterial pathogens, such as staphylococci and streptococci, giving rise to cellulitis, scarlet fever or septicemia. The size of the scar is always increased by such contamination. Vaccine lymph can be contaminated with tetanus spores; however, tetanus has occurred only in the presence of a tight shield or other occlusive dressing.

ABNORMAL DISTRIBUTION OF VIRUS

Local. Transfer of infection to other parts of the body can result from scratching the primary lesion. Such infections may occur at any site, especially when the skin is traumatized, and they have occurred on the eye, tongue, lip, penis, vulva and anus. In those autoinoculated, the secondary lesions heal, usually without scarring, at the same time as the primary lesion. When the lesion is at a potentially harmful site, as on the eye, specific treatment should be given (see below). Osteomyelitis from the viremia of a primary vaccination is a rare complication. A susceptible person can be infected by contact with the primary lesion of another person.

General. *Eczema vaccinatum* (Figs. 10–46 and 10–47, p. 656), or vaccinia superimposed upon eczematous skin, can result from autoinoculation, from infection of eczematous skin or from contact with a vaccinated person. There is probably spread of virus via blood stream and lymphatics in addition to local inoculation. The eczematous skin is covered with umbilicated vesicles which involute like the primary ones. Infants are seriously ill; the mortality rate is in the range of 30 to 40 per cent. The condition must be distinguished from eczema herpeticum, chiefly by history of exposure.

ABNORMAL HOST RESPONSE

Antibody Formation. In patients with defective cellular immunity (i.e., decreased globulins, thymic dysplasia, those receiving steroids, immunosuppressive drugs or x-ray therapy) progressive vaccinia may develop. This includes (1) *satellite or widespread vaccinal lesions,* which usually persist, along with the original lesion, for days or weeks beyond the normal time of healing until antibodies are eventually formed and all lesions heal together. Generalized vaccinia is sometimes mistakenly diagnosed when a coincidental skin eruption, e.g., varicella or impetigo, occurs in a child who has been vaccinated. Generalized vaccinia can be excluded if the original vaccination site is progressing normally without satellite lesions.

(2) *Prolonged progressive vaccinia or vaccinia*

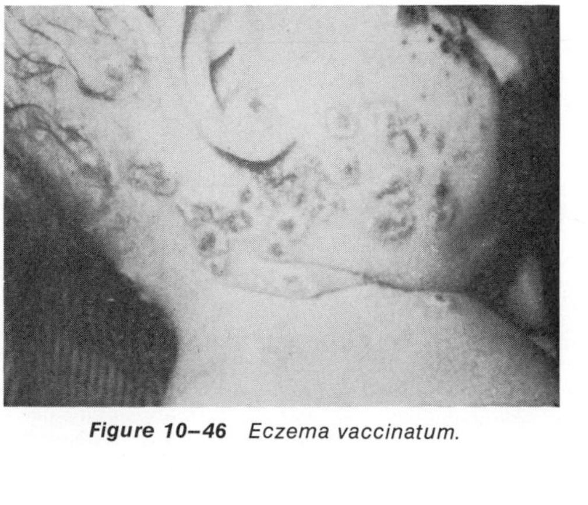

Figure 10–46 Eczema vaccinatum.

gangrenosa. There is spreading necrosis at the site of the primary inoculation which eventually destroys the area, and metastatic necrotic lesions occur throughout the body, including the bones. The mortality rate is high.

Hypersensitivity Reactions. A variety of rashes, which can be included under the general term "erythema multiforme," occur at 7 to 11 days in about 1 of 5000 vaccinations. They are commonly mild and maculopapular ("roseola vaccinosa") (Fig. 10–48), papulovesicular or urticarial. Less frequently, there is a severe, generalized bullous rash which may also involve the mucous membranes of the mouth, anus and genitalia (erythema multiforme pluriorificialis).

Central Nervous System. Postvaccinal encephalomyelitis is one of the allergic encephalitides. It usually appears 11 to 14 days after vaccination, but often earlier in infants. The clinical signs and symptoms include fever, meningismus, seizures, coma, paralysis, polyneuritis, myasthenia, transverse myelitis and signs of increased intracranial pressure. The cerebrospinal fluid may show pleocytosis and increased protein. Examination of the brain shows cerebral edema, perivascular mononuclear infiltration around cerebral vessels and some demyelinization. It occurs in approximately 1 of 100,000 vaccinations in the United States; in parts of Europe the incidence has been as high as 1 per 4000. The case fatality rate is approximately 50 per cent. There is no evidence that a particular batch of vaccine is involved, and there appears to be no correlation with the size or severity of the local reaction or the number of inoculations. Encephalitis appears to be less common and less severe after revaccination than after primary vaccination.

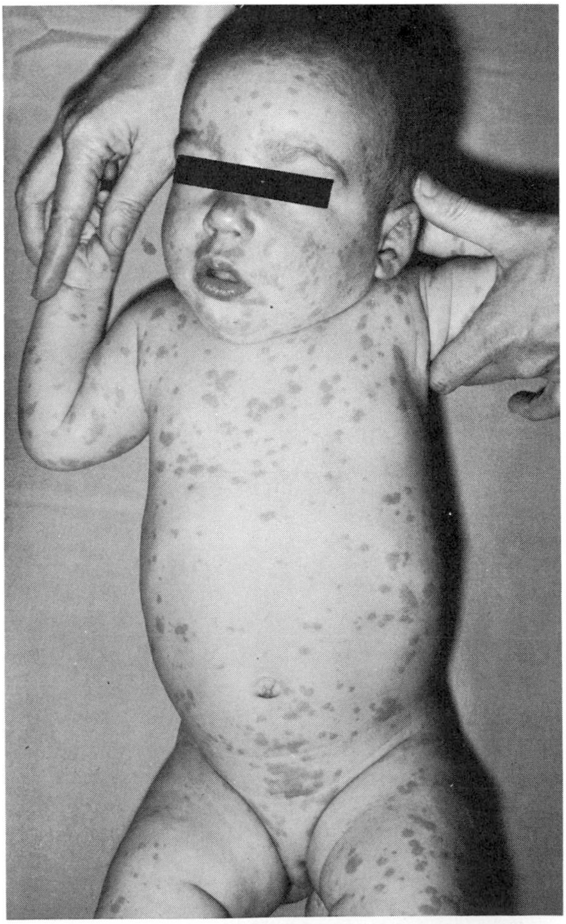

Figure 10–48 *Erythema multiforme (roseola vaccinosa) complicating smallpox vaccination. Rash appeared 8 days after primary vaccination. Vaccination site is just visible in upper lateral aspect of left thigh.*

TREATMENT OF COMPLICATIONS. Bacterial complications should be treated with appropriate antibiotic agents. Delay of antibody production leading to generalized vaccinia can be overcome by administration of hyperimmune vaccinal gamma globulin in a dose of 0.6 ml/kg, which can be repeated as required. A single injection of the same amount of gamma globulin can be given prophylactically to contacts with eczema or to eczematous subjects at the time of a mandatory vaccination. Lesions due to autoinoculation or heteroinoculation in potentially dangerous sites should be treated with a similar dose of hyperimmune globulin, except when the cornea is affected. Serotherapy aggravates this, and IUD drops should be used locally (see herpes). For *eczema vaccinatum,* two administrations may be required. For *progressive vaccinia* the administration must be repeated every week or two until healing is proceeding favorably and until vaccinia virus can no longer be demonstrated in the lesions. N-methylisatin β-thiosemicarbazone, given orally as a 10 per cent suspension, has appeared to be effective in some patients in whom serotherapy has failed. The therapy for encephalitis is supportive, and there is no reason to give hyperimmune gamma globulin, because the normal development of antibodies is indicated by normal healing of the vaccinal lesion. Hyperimmune gamma globulin, given at the time of the primary vaccination, has been useful prophylactically in areas where the incidence of encephalitis is high.

Kempe, H.: The end of routine smallpox vaccination in the United States. Pediatrics *49*:489, 1972.

Lane, J. M., et al.: Smallpox and smallpox vaccination policy. Ann. Rev. Med. *22*:251, 1971.

MUMPS

(Epidemic Parotitis)

Mumps is an acute contagious generalized viral disease in which painful enlargement of the salivary glands, chiefly the parotids, is the usual presenting sign.

HISTORY. The disease was recognized as early as the fifth century B.C. by Hippocrates, who mentioned the complication of orchitis. In 1790 Hamilton also noted orchitis and the involvement of the central nervous system in certain patients. The frequency of the latter complication has been recognized increasingly during the present century, as has the fact that other organs, e.g., the pancreas, can also be infected.

ETIOLOGY. The viral origin was firmly established by Johnson and Goodpasture in 1934. The virus is a member of the paramyxovirus group. In addition to mumps this group includes the parainfluenza and Newcastle disease viruses. The virus particle contains single-stranded RNA enclosed in an envelope of protein and lipid. The envelope is roughly spherical and is studded with numerous spike-like projections. The diameter of the virus particle ranges from 150 to 250 mμ. The envelope contains a hemagglutinin, a neuraminidase and a hemolysin. There is only one known serotype. The virus can be grown in cultures of human and monkey tissue, in embryonated eggs and in cell cultures of chick embryos. Primary cultures of human or monkey kidney cells are used for viral isolation. Sometimes cytopathic effect is observed, but hemadsorption is the most sensitive indicator of infection. Fixation and staining of cells shows syncytia formation with cytoplasmic inclusions. Virus has been isolated from saliva, cerebrospinal fluid, blood, urine, brain and other infected tissues of patients with mumps.

EPIDEMIOLOGY. Mumps is endemic in most urban populations; the virus is spread from a human reservoir by direct contact, airborne droplet nuclei, fomites contaminated by infectious saliva and possibly by urine. It has a world-wide distribution and affects both sexes equally; 85 per cent of the infections occur in children under the age of 15 years. Epidemics occur at all seasons of the year, although they are slightly more frequent in the late winter and spring. The source of infection may be difficult to trace, because 30 to 40 per cent of infections are subclinical.

It is uncertain how long a patient may be infectious, but virus has been isolated from saliva as long as 6 days before and up to 9 days after the appearance of salivary gland swelling. Under usual conditions, however, transmission does not seem to occur longer than 24 hours before the appearance of the swelling or later than 3 days after it has subsided. Virus has been isolated from the urine from the first to the fourteenth day after the onset of salivary gland swelling.

A lifelong immunity is produced by any type of clinical or subclinical infection; transplacental antibodies seem to be effective in protecting infants during the first 6 to 8 months of life. The serum neutralization test is the most reliable method for determination of immunity but is cumbersome and expensive. A complement-fixing antibody test is available. (See Diagnosis.) The presence of V antibodies alone suggests previous mumps infection.

A mumps skin test is available which uses killed mumps virus injected intradermally. A positive test is considered to be erythema and induration greater than 15 mm 24 to 48 hours after injection. Skin test material itself may stimulate the rise of serum antibody titers and confuse serologic diagnosis. Recent studies have seriously questioned the value of the skin test in predicting immune status, since both false positives and false negatives occur with considerable frequency.

PATHOGENESIS. The probable evolution of the disease is as follows: after entry and initial multiplication in the cells of the respiratory tract, the virus is blood-borne to many tissues, of which salivary and other glands seem to be the most susceptible. The swelling of the infected structures is probably the result of a hypersensitivity reaction to the locally multiplying virus, since the virus can be detected in the infected monkey parotid 4 to 5 days before clinical swelling occurs.

PATHOLOGY. Little information is available about the lesions caused by mumps in the human patient. In a parotid from which the virus was isolated 70 hours after onset of the disease the acini were well preserved, but there was periductal edema and lymphocytic infiltration extending slightly into the connective tissue. The main damage was to the ducts; the extent varied from slight epithelial swelling with a few polymorphonuclear cells in the lumen to complete desquamation of the epithelium and dilated lumens choked with debris. Some epithelial cells were observed with swelling of cytoplasm, but only rarely did one contain a large basophilic inclusion body. Other studies of parotid glands from patients with clinical mumps, without viral isolation, confirmed these general findings, although in some instances damage to the acini was observed. Changes in testes, when biopsies were taken within a day or two after onset of pain, have varied from mild interstitial edema and no disturbance of spermatogenesis in the majority of instances, to focal destruction of epithelium with extensive perivascular lymphocytic cuffing. The basic injury appeared to be vascular; irregular hemorrhages occurred in the more severe infections. Even in these, however, areas of normal germinal epithelium could be seen.

CLINICAL MANIFESTATIONS. The incubation period ranges from 14 to 24 days, with a peak incidence at 17 to 18 days. In children prodromal symptoms and signs are rare, but may be manifest by fever, muscular pain, especially in the neck, headache and malaise. The onset of illness is usually characterized by pain and swelling in one or both parotid glands. The parotid swells in a characteristic way; it begins by filling the space between the posterior border of the mandible and the mastoid and then extends in a series of crescents downward and forward, being limited above by the zygoma. Edema of the skin and soft tissues usually extends further and obscures the limit of the glandular swelling, with the result that the swelling is more readily appreciated by sight than by palpation. The swelling may proceed extremely rapidly, reaching a maximum size within a few hours, although the peak is usually reached in 1 to 3 days. The swollen tissues push the ear lobe upward and outward. The swelling slowly subsides within 3 to 7 days; occasionally it lasts longer. Usually swelling of one parotid gland precedes that of the other by a day or two, but swelling limited to one gland is common. The swollen area is tender and painful, pain being especially elicited by tasting sour liquids such as lemon juice or vinegar, a useful diagnostic sign. Redness and swelling are commonly noted about the opening of Stensen's duct. Accompanying the parotid swelling there may be edema of the homolateral pharynx and soft palate displacing the tonsil medially; acute edema of the larynx has been described. Edema over the manubrium and upper chest wall may be found, probably owing to lymphatic obstruction. The parotid swelling is usually accompanied by moderate fever, but normal temperatures are common (20 per cent) and temperatures of 104° F or over are rare; no correlation exists between extent of swelling and degree of fever.

Although the parotid glands alone are affected in the majority of patients, swelling of the submandibular glands occurs frequently and usually accompanies or closely follows that of the parotid glands. In 10 to 15 per cent of patients, however, only the submandibular gland(s) may be swollen. The swelling of the submandibular gland follows two patterns: the commoner is an ovoid enlargement extending forward and downward from the angle of the mandible; in the other, the enlargement extends more directly downward in a half-egg shape. The deep portion of the gland is only rarely affected. Little pain is associated with the submandibular infection, but the swelling subsides more slowly than that of the parotids. Redness and swelling at the orifice of Wharton's duct frequently accompany swelling of the gland.

Least commonly the sublingual glands are infected, usually bilaterally; the swelling is evident in the submental region and in the floor of the mouth.

COMPLICATIONS. Viremia early in the infection probably accounts for the widespread complications which are mainly manifestations of mumps infection in organs other than the salivary glands.

Meningoencephalomyelitis. This is the most frequent complication in childhood. The true incidence is hard to estimate because subclinical infection of the central nervous system, as evidenced by a pleocytosis in the cerebrospinal fluid, has been reported in over 65 per cent of patients with parotitis. Clinical manifestations have been reported in over 10 per cent of patients. The reported incidence of mumps meningoencephalitis is approximately 250 per 100,000 cases. Ten per cent of these cases occurred in patients over 20 years old. The mortality rate is about 2 per cent. Males are affected three to five times as frequently as females. Mumps is one of the most common causes of aseptic meningitis.

The pathogenesis of mumps meningoencephalitis has been described as both a primary infection of neurones by virus and a postinfectious encephalitis with demyelination. In the first type, parotitis frequently appears at the same time or following the onset of encephalitis. In the latter type, encephalitis follows parotitis by an average of 10 days. Parotitis may, in some cases, be absent. Mumps has been implicated as a possible etiologic agent in the production of aqueductal stenosis and hydrocephalus in children. Injection of mumps virus into suckling hamsters has produced similar lesions.

Meningoencephalitis begins typically with a rise in temperature, headache, vomiting, irritability and, occasionally, a convulsion. This clinical picture is indistinguishable from meningoencephalitis of other origins. Moderate stiffness of the neck is seen, but the remainder of the neurologic examination is usually normal. Occasionally neck, shoulder and leg weakness, resembling paralytic poliomyelitis, occurs. The CSF usually contains less than 500 cells, although occasionally the count may exceed 2000. The cells are almost exclusively lymphocytes, in contrast to enteroviral aseptic meningitis, in which polymorphonuclear leukocytes often predominate early in the disease. The CSF glucose is normal. Protein is slightly elevated. Mumps virus can be isolated from the CSF early in the illness.

Orchitis, Epididymitis. These lesions rarely occur in prepubescent boys, but are common (14 to 35 per cent) in adolescents and adults. The testis is most often infected with or without epididymitis, or epididymitis may occur alone. Rarely there is a hydrocele. The orchitis usually follows parotitis within 8 days, but sometimes is delayed, and it may occur without evidence of salivary gland infection. In about 30 per cent of patients with orchitis, both testes are affected. The onset is usually abrupt, with a rise in temperature, chills, headache, nausea and lower abdominal pain; when the right testis is implicated, appendicitis may appear to be a diagnostic possibility. The affected testis becomes tender and swollen and the adjacent skin edematous and red. The average duration is 4 days. As the swelling subsides, the testis loses its normal turgor; approximately 30 to 40 per cent of affected testes atrophy. Impairment of fertility is estimated to be about 13 per cent, but absolute infertility is probably rare.

Oophoritis. Pelvic pain and tenderness are noted in about 7 per cent of postpubertal female patients. There is no evidence of impairment of fertility.

Pancreatitis. Severe involvement of the pancreas is rare, but mild or subclinical infection may be more common than is recognized. It may be unassociated with salivary gland manifestations and be misdiagnosed as gastroenteritis. Epigastric pain and tenderness are suggestive; these may be accompanied by fever, chills, vomiting and prostration. An elevated serum amylase value is characteristically present in any patient with mumps, with or without clinical manifestation of pancreatitis. Serum lipase determination may be helpful. The possibility that diabetes mellitus may be an infrequent sequel should be investigated.

Nephritis. Viruria has been reported frequently. In one study of adults, abnormal renal function was observed at some time in every patient and viruria was present in 75 per cent. The frequency of renal involvement in children is unknown. Fatal nephritis, occurring 10 to 14 days after parotitis, has been reported.

Thyroiditis. Although uncommon in children, a diffuse, tender swelling of the thyroid may occur about a week after the onset of parotitis and has been followed by the development of antithyroid antibodies.

Myocarditis. Serious clinical manifestations are extremely rare, but mild infection of the myocardium is probably more common and overlooked. In one series of adults electrocardiographic tracings revealed changes, mostly depression of the S-T segment, in 13 per cent. Such involvement could explain the precordial pain, bradycardia and fatigue sometimes noted among adolescents and adults with mumps.

Mastitis. This is an uncommon occurrence in either male or female patients.

Deafness. Unilateral, or rarely bilateral, nerve deafness may occur after mumps; although the incidence is low (1:15,000), mumps is considered a leading cause of unilateral nerve deafness. The onset may be sudden or gradual. Hearing loss is complete and permanent.

Ocular Complications. These include *dacryoadenitis,* painful swelling of the lacrimal glands which is usually bilateral; *optic neuritis (papillitis)* with symptoms varying from loss of vision to mild blurring and with recovery in 10 to 20 days; *uveokeratitis,* usually unilateral, with photophobia, tearing, rapid loss of vision and recovery within 20 days; *scleritis; tenonitis* with resultant exophthalmos; and *central vein thrombosis.*

Arthritis. Arthralgia associated with swelling and redness of the joints is an infrequent complication which appears 12 to 14 days after the onset of parotitis; complete recovery is the rule.

Thrombocytopenic Purpura follows mumps on occasion, as it does other infections.

Mumps Embryopathy. There is no firm evidence that maternal infection with mumps leads to any damage to the developing fetus; a possible relation to endocardial fibroelastosis has been postulated but not established.

DIAGNOSIS. The diagnosis of mumps parotitis is usually readily apparent from the symptoms and physical examination. When the clinical manifestations are limited to those of one of the less common lesions, the diagnosis is not so clear but may be suspected, especially during an epidemic. The routine laboratory tests are nonspecific; there is usually a leukopenia with a relative lymphocytosis, but complications often result in a polymorphonuclear leukocytosis of a moderate degree. An elevation of serum amylase is found in most patients with mumps; the rise, paralleling the parotid swelling, reaches its peak in a week and generally returns to normal over the course of the next 2 weeks. The etiologic diagnosis depends on the isolation of the virus from the saliva, urine, spinal fluid or blood or the demonstration of a significant rise in circulating CF antibodies during convalescence. Serum antibodies to the S antigen reach their peak early in about 75 per cent of patients and are detectable at the time of the presenting symptoms. They gradually disappear within 6 to 12 months; antibodies against the V or viral antigen usually reach a peak titer in about a month, remain stationary for about 6 months and then slowly decline over the ensuing 2 years to a low level, at which they persist. The presence of a high anti-S titer and a low anti-V titer during the acute stage of an otherwise undiagnosed meningoencephalitis, for example, would be strongly suggestive of a mumps infection, which would be confirmed if a convalescent serum (taken 14 to 21 days later) revealed a fourfold rise of anti-V antibodies with little change in the titer of anti-S antibodies.

Differential Diagnosis. This includes *parotitis* of other origin, as in the rare instances of coxsackie A and lymphocytic choriomeningitis infections, which can be distinguished only by specific laboratory tests; *suppurative parotitis,* in which pus can often be expressed from the duct; *recurrent parotitis,* a condition of unknown origin, but possibly allergic in nature, which has frequent recurrences and a characteristic sialogram; *salivary calculus,* obstructing either a parotid or, more commonly, a submandibular duct, in which the swelling is intermittent; *preauricular* or *anterior cervical lymphadenitis* from any cause; *lymphosarcoma* or other rare *tumors* of the parotid; *orchitis due to infections other than mumps,* e.g., the rare infections by coxsackie A or lymphocytic choriomeningitis viruses; and *parotitis due to cytomegalovirus* in immune-compromised children.

TREATMENT. This is entirely symptomatic. Bed rest should be guided by the patient's needs; there is no statistical evidence that it prevents complications. The diet should be adjusted to the ability of the patient to chew. The headache of meningoencephalitis may be relieved by a lumbar puncture. Orchitis should be treated with local support and bed rest. Corticosteroids, preferably hydrocortisone in pharmacologic doses (10 mg/kg/day) for 2 to 4 days, relieve the pain, although evidence of any effect on length of illness or protection against atrophy is lacking.

PROPHYLAXIS

Passive. Present evidence suggests that the use of hyperimmune mumps gamma globulin not only does not significantly reduce complications, but also in some instances actually increases their incidence.

Active. A live, attenuated mumps virus vaccine has been developed (Mumpsvax [Merck, Sharp & Dohme]). It is given subcutaneously to children over the age of 12 months. Vaccinated children do not develop fever or other detectable clinical reactions. They do not excrete virus and are not contagious to susceptible contacts. The vaccine induces antibody in about 96 per cent of seronegative recipients. The antibody level produced is about one fifth of that achieved after natural infection, but a protective efficacy of about 97 per cent against natural mumps infection has been demonstrated. The protection afforded by the vaccine appears to be long-lasting. Mumps vaccine can be combined with measles and rubella in one immunization. There is no evidence that vaccination will protect any susceptible person after exposure to mumps, but there is no contraindication to its use in exposed adolescents or adults who presumably have not had mumps.

CAROL F. PHILLIPS

Bistrian, B., et al.: Fatal mumps meningoencephalitis. J.A.M.A. *222*:478, 1972.

Brunell, P. A., et al.: Ineffectiveness of isolation of patients as a method of preventing the spread of mumps. Failure of the mumps skin-test antigen to predict immune status. New Engl. J. Med. *279*:1357, 1968.

EPIDEMIC INFLUENZA

DEFINITION. Influenza is an acute communicable viral disease primarily affecting the respiratory tract. It occurs in pandemic waves usually separated by several decades, during which epidemics of less severity occur at 2- to 4-year intervals.

ETIOLOGY. Two viral agents of the myxovirus group appear to have been responsible for most of the outbreaks of respiratory infection resembling influenza since 1933: influenza A virus, identified by Smith, Andrewes and Laidlaw (1933); and influenza B virus, identified independently by Francis and by Magill in 1940. Subsequently two additional types of influenza virus have been isolated and identified. In 1949 Taylor isolated a virus which was designated as influenza C. Thus far it has been responsible for only mild epidemic disease. A viral agent isolated in 1953 in Japan (Sendai virus) was first identified as a possible influenza type D, but was later classified with the parainfluenza group of agents. It has been responsible for a severe form of pneumonitis in newborn infants in many parts of the world.

Of the parainfluenza viruses, types 1, 2 and 3 are associated with human disease; type 4, rarely associated, and mild. Clinical manifestations of infection with parainfluenza viruses include pharyngitis, rhinitis, bronchitis, bronchopneumonia, pneumonitis and croup. Types 1 and 2 appear to have affinity for the tissues of the trachea, larynx and bronchi; type 3 has been the agent commonly isolated in bronchitis and pneumonia.

Pandemic influenza, similar in worldwide prevalence but not in severity to that of 1918–19, occurred in 1957. The causative virus was a mutant strain – Asian strain – of type A influenza virus, to which immunity could not be produced by vaccines containing known strains of type A virus. Persons born before 1890 were usually found to have antibodies to the Asian strain, thus suggesting an antigenic relation of the new mutant to the virus responsible for the pandemic of 1889–90. In general, the type A strains have been associated with large epidemics, both animal and human; the type B, with lesser human outbreaks; and the type C, with small local outbreaks. Antigenic relationships among influenza types of human and animal origin are currently under study on a world-wide basis.

Influenza viruses A and B are distinct serologically with no cross immunity, and each type has a number of antigenic strains. In spite of antigenic differences the A and B viruses have common features. Both have an affinity for respiratory epithelium and produce the same type of lesion. A and B viruses multiply rapidly in embryonated eggs in contrast to type C, which multiplies slowly and requires amniotic transfer. They can be cultivated in tissue culture, and both are capable of producing hemagglutination.

After either experimental or natural infection with influenza virus, neutralizing and complement-fixing antibodies increase rapidly, reaching their peak within approximately 2 to 3 weeks, and then slowly diminish to their previous levels in approximately a year. A fourfold increase of antibodies in comparative tests of acute and convalescent serums is diagnostic.

The agglutination of red cells by strains of influenza virus and the inhibition of this phenomenon by previous addition to the viruses of an immune serum were developed independently by Hirst and Hare as a means of determining the presence and amounts of antibodies in unknown serums. This method of measuring antibody formation is more exact than the virus neutralization test, but not so accurate as the complement fixation test.

In both pandemic and epidemic influenza the mortality is, to an extent, dependent on secondarily invading bacteria, of which *Hemophilus influenzae,* hemolytic streptococcus, pneumococcus and *Staphylococcus aureus* are the most frequent. In the 1957 epidemic, however, it became evident that rapidly fatal cases were not always due to superimposed bacterial infection, but could be caused by the virus itself.

EPIDEMIOLOGY. Influenza is probably the only remaining pandemic disease over which no effective control has been established. The pandemic of 1918 is estimated to have caused approximately 22,000,000 deaths throughout the world in about 3 months.

Serologic data relating to the pandemics of 1889, 1918 and 1957, together with identification of different strains of influenza A virus from various epidemics since 1930, suggest a pattern of recurrent outbreaks of influenza A infections which depends primarily upon mutant strains of virus and secondarily upon the accumulation of susceptible hosts, especially among the young and the middle-aged. Epidemics from the same strain may recur every 3 to 4 years, but a subsequent pandemic does not occur until a new mutant strain of virus again becomes widespread. Epidemics from strains of A virus tend to occur every year or two, those of influenza B less frequently. Epidemics usually occur in the late winter and early spring. Antigenic strains vary from year to year; in recent years the occurrence of mutant strains appears to have been increasing, a situation which complicates strain identification, as well as the problem of protection by vaccination.

The viruses, which spread by the airborne route

and by direct contact, are present in the upper respiratory tract of patients from the first to the fifth day of disease. Viremia has not been demonstrated.

Both sexes and all races appear equally susceptible. Young adults and children over 5 years of age appear to be more susceptible than infants and older persons. Experimental human infection has indicated a direct relation between the titer of serum antibodies and resistance to infection. A large number of inapparent infections occurs in any epidemic, as indicated by the rise of antibody titers in asymptomatic persons. No reservoir of the viruses for interepidemic survival has been found, nor have carriers been discovered.

PATHOLOGY. Uncomplicated influenza in man may be considered analogous to the disease in ferrets, in which there is severe inflammatory reaction in the mucous membrane of the upper respiratory tract with a loss of ciliated epithelium. Regeneration occurs by development of epithelium of a more squamous type over a period of several weeks, with slower regeneration of the columnar epithelium. During this transitional period the epithelium is resistant to further influenzal virus infections.

In severe cases hemorrhages with serosanguineous exudate often occur in the pharynx, larynx, and tracheobronchial tree, with edema of the entire respiratory tract. The alveolar ducts and bronchioles may be dilated and their walls frequently covered with hyaline material. There is necrosis of the mucous membrane, and emphysema is usually present in localized areas.

The pathologic picture may be altered by bacterial pathogens. When several different organisms are present, the pathologic changes are less uniform than when there is a single pathogen. With pneumococcus there is typically a lobular pneumonia tending to become confluent; with the influenzal bacillus, severe destructive changes in the bronchioles and interstitial pneumonia, often leading to bronchiectasis; with *Staphylococcus aureus,* an overwhelming infection characterized by hemorrhagic edema and multiple pulmonary abscesses; and with hemolytic streptococcus, an interstitial reaction with hemorrhagic edema and frequently with pleurisy and empyema.

CLINICAL MANIFESTATIONS. The symptoms of pandemic and epidemic influenza are similar except for severity and extent of complications. Experimental infections of human susceptibles have simulated the milder cases of epidemics.

The incubation period is usually 36 to 48 hours. The onset is sudden, with a chill or a chilly sensation, frequently with a convulsion in children; a sharp rise in temperature to a range of 102 to 106° F.; flushing of the face, neck and chest; headache; vertigo; a dry sore throat; and pains in the back and extremities. A short, dry, hacking cough is usually present soon after the onset and rapidly increases in frequency and severity. It often becomes paroxysmal and resembles the cough of pertussis. In young children vomiting and diarrhea may be the principal manifestations at the onset. Severe croup, frequently requiring tracheotomy, has been reported. The accompanying prostration may be extreme and is related not only to the severity of the disease, but also to the lack of complete bed rest from the onset of symptoms. The fever is often diphasic, with the two peaks separated by a period of 24 to 48 hours.

The mucous membranes of the throat appear dry and red with no exudate; those of the nose are red, but usually there is little or no discharge except when purulent sinusitis is a late complication. Tingling of the back of the tongue may be experienced, followed by a loss of the sense of taste, which gradually returns over a period of several days up to several months. The conjunctivas are injected. Epistaxis is common. The pulse is usually rapid and often weak, as are the heart sounds when the cardiac muscle is seriously affected. Often the skeletal muscles are painful on pressure, and movements of the eyeballs cause considerable discomfort.

The usual increase in leukocytes during the early stages of the disease is soon replaced by a leukopenia with a relative lymphocytosis.

The milder uncomplicated cases rarely last more than 3 to 4 days.

In severe infections which extend into the lower respiratory tract fine moist rales may soon be detected bilaterally, and these may spread rapidly over the entire lung area, with diminution of breath sounds or a tendency to bronchial breathing if consolidation occurs. As the cough increases in frequency it becomes productive, often sanguineous at first and later mucopurulent. Diminution of breath sounds resulting from edema of the bronchial tree and alveoli is far more common than the localized consolidation of lobular pneumonia, and frequently the breath sounds almost disappear as patchy edematous and atelectatic areas are interspersed with areas of emphysema. In extremely severe infections the patient shows evidence of anoxia. Myocardial involvement results in distention of the right side of the heart, passive congestion of the liver and, finally, extensive pulmonary edema and cardiac failure.

When secondary bacterial infections are present, the symptoms depend to a considerable extent upon the type of organism involved.

DIAGNOSIS. During epidemics or pandemics the diagnosis is not difficult. The simplest diagnostic test is that of Hirst and Hare (see Etiology); the complement fixation test, however, appears to be more reliable. The isolation of virus by intra-amniotic inoculation of throat washings is diagnostic. Virus isolation can be accomplished also in primary tissue culture systems, minced chick embryo, and especially in monolayers of monkey or chick kidney cells.

COMPLICATIONS. In few other diseases are the complications such an integral part of the severe forms of the infection. Many of these have been mentioned under Clinical Manifestations and actually may be considered clinical variations.

Otitis media, mastoiditis, purulent sinusitis, pneumonia, bronchiectasis, pulmonary abscess and empyema are the more common respiratory variants of severe infections. Less common ones are pneumothorax and mediastinitis. Rare nonrespiratory complications include hematoma from rupture of the rectus muscles of the abdomen, epistaxis, intestinal hemorrhage, polyneuritis, postinfluenzal psychoses, nephritis, subcutaneous or intramuscular abscess, endocarditis, myocarditis, pericarditis, thrombophlebitis, meningitis and hemorrhagic encephalitis. Acute encephalopathy with fatty degeneration of the viscera (Reye syndrome) has been reported in association with various viral infections, including influenza.

PROPHYLAXIS. During epidemics, avoidance of fatigue and chilling and of crowds is important. Specific resistance can be increased by the use of vaccines. Vaccination is preventive and not therapeutic. Febrile and local reactions to the vaccines are proportional to the amount of contaminant (i.e., egg protein, etc.) they contain. Newer vaccines are purer, contain much more viral protein than previously, and produce fewer and milder side effects. In rare instances persons sensitive to chick embryo proteins may have allergic reactions, including vascular purpura.

As a rule, persons who have some circulating antibodies respond promptly to this antigenic stimulus, and antibodies can be increased within 7 to 10 days. Serum antibody levels of 1:128 measured by the hemagglutination inhibition test appear to be associated with a high degree of immunity. Antibody levels tend to fall to half the attained level in 6 months to a year.

At present, routine immunization is not recommended for normal children. The available influenza vaccines have been variable in effectiveness, and febrile reactions unaccountably high. However, children, especially those of school age and those residing in institutions, represent a major factor in the spread of the disease in the community. The new improved vaccines appear to be associated with less reaction, and in the future more widespread immunization of normal infants and children may prove to be important in the control of influenza. If an epidemic is anticipated, vaccination is recommended for high-risk individuals: those suffering from rheumatic heart disease, cardiovascular disorders, congenital heart disease, cystic fibrosis or other chronic bronchopulmonary disease, chronic metabolic or neurologic disorders, glomerulonephritis, nephrosis, and so forth.

Antigenic types in a given preparation are varied from time to time according to the strains seasonally prevalent. For example, a bivalent vaccine may be recommended which contains greater amounts of two current strains in preference to a polyvalent vaccine containing several strains. Under certain circumstances, when a new variant appears, a single strain vaccine may be recommended. Choice of vaccine must be individualized at the discretion of the physician. Vaccination during pregnancy, likewise, is at the discretion of the physician.

Primary immunization consists of an initial subcutaneous or intramuscular dose repeated 2 months later. Antibody response is good; an early second injection, when indicated, enhances the first response. Recent data suggest that a single dose of one of the newer, improved vaccines may be sufficient, with continuing protection afforded by an annual booster. A recommended basic bivalent vaccine contains antigenic type A_2, strain Aichi/2/68, which is a Hong Kong variant, and type B, the Massachusetts 3/66. In the event of epidemics, prior vaccination against influenza appears to reduce complications.

TREATMENT. No specific treatment is available. Complete bed rest from the earliest evidence of disease is essential and should be continued long into convalescence. Antimicrobial therapy is indicated for bacterial complications. The fluid intake should be ample. Aspirin and codeine may be used for discomfort and cough.

The status of chemotherapy in influenza is uncertain. In some instances, the synthetic antiviral substance amantadine hydrochloride (Symmetrel) has been considered useful in influenza A chemoprophylaxis, but is not therapeutically effective. During epidemic periods amantadine must be administered regularly, since the substance has no lasting antiviral effect within the body.

American Academy of Pediatrics: Report of the Committee on Infectious Diseases. 17th ed. Evanston, Ill., 1974, p. 138.

Blattner, R. J.: Neurologic complications of Asian influenza. Comments on current literature. J. Pediatr. *53*:751, 1958.

Blattner, R. J.: Virus isolation in fatal human cases of Asian influenza. Comments on current literature. J. Pediatr. *55*:113, 1959.

Center For Disease Control, U.S. Public Health Service: Recommendation of the Public Health Service Advisory Committee on Immunization Practices: Influenza vaccine. Morbidity and Mortality Weekly Report *23*:215, 1974.

Communicable diseases in 1971: Some aspects of the WHO programme: Virus and rickettsial diseases: Influenza. WHO Chronicle *26*:253, 1972. (See also Geneva Conference, Bull. WHO *45*:119, 1971.)

Francis, T., Jr.: Influenza viruses: *In* Horsfall, F. L., and Tamm, I. (eds.): Viral and Rickettsial Infections of Man. 4th ed. Philadelphia, J. B. Lippincott Company, 1965, p. 689.

Glick, T. H., Likosky, W. H., Levitt, L. P., Mellin, H., and Reynolds, D. W.: Reye's syndrome: An epidemiologic approach. Pediatrics *46*:371, 1970.

Hirst, G. K.: The agglutination of red cells by allantoic fluid of chick embryos infected with influenza virus. Science *94*:22, 1941.

Jackson, G. G.: Influenza: The present status of chemotherapy. Hosp. Prac. *6* (No. 11): 75, 1971.

Kilbourne, E. D.: Influenza: The vaccines. Hosp. Prac. *6* (No. 10): 103, 1971.

Langmuir, A. D.: Influenza: Its epidemiology. Hosp. Prac. *6* (No. 9): 103, 1971.

McClelland, L., and Hare, R.: The absorption of influenza virus by red cells and a new in vitro method of measuring antibodies for influenza virus. Canad. Pub. Hlth J. *32*:530, 1941.

Reynolds, D. W., and others: An outbreak of Reye's syndrome associated with influenza B. J. Pediatr. *80*:429, 1972.

Smith, W., Andrewes, C. H., and Laidlaw, P. P.: A virus obtained from influenza patients. Lancet *2*:66, 1933.

RABIES

(Hydrophobia)

DEFINITION. Rabies is an acute viral disease of the central nervous system which is transmitted by dogs, cats, bats and wild animals. In general, it is characterized by extreme excitation, severe and painful spasm of the muscles of the pharynx and larynx at the sight of food or liquids, which accounts for the name "hydrophobia," and finally by generalized paralysis and death within a few days.

HISTORY. Rabies is one of the oldest recorded diseases in Europe and Asia. Democritus in 500 B.C. and Aristotle in 322 B.C. described rabies; Celsus in A.D. 100 advised cauterization of bites by rabid dogs, and Galen in A.D. 200 advised surgical excision of the bite. Apparently rabies had not occurred in North and South America before colonization.

In 1804 Zinke infected a normal dog with saliva from a rabid dog. Pasteur in 1881 to 1884 demonstrated the infective agent in the central nervous system of rabbits and named it a virus, from the Latin word for poison. There followed the development in his laboratories of the fixed virus and the study of vaccination with attenuated virus. Fermi in 1908 treated infected nervous tissue with phenol for use as a vaccine. In 1903 Negri demonstrated the inclusion bodies now known by his name. In 1921 Haupt found the vampire bat to be a symptomless carrier of the virus, a finding of great epidemiologic importance.

ETIOLOGY. The rabies virus is neurotropic and travels by the peripheral nerves to the central nervous system. This natural virus is termed "street virus" and has a variable incubation period related to the distance of the injury from the head, the severity of the bite and the amount of virus in the wound. The "street virus" invades the salivary glands and is usually transmitted in saliva. The "fixed virus" is the natural virus modified by repeated intracerebral passages in laboratory animals. This virus has a 4- to 6-day incubation period and does not invade the salivary glands. The "street virus" through multiple passage in the chick embryo loses its pathogenic properties and may be used without inactivation for vaccination.

EPIDEMIOLOGY. Two categories of rabies have been suggested by Johnson: the sylvatic, existing in wild animals; and the urban, prevalent in domestic dogs. Rabies is significantly on the increase among wild animals (skunks, foxes, coyotes, bats, raccoons and bears) and in domestic animals (dogs, cats and cattle). Small wild rodents such as squirrels, chipmunks, rats and mice are less commonly infected. Recently the Rabies Committee of the National Research Council has made available a compendium of animal rabies vaccines with recommendations for their use. Pets such as mice, hamsters, gerbils, rabbits, and so forth, are susceptible to rabies virus and can be potential hazards to children, especially when brought to the schoolroom.

Symptom complexes in animals which in the past were not associated with rabies, such as "running fits" of dogs and paralytic syndromes in dogs and other animals, may be of rabid origin. In the United States and Canada deaths from rabies in human subjects have been estimated at less than 100 annually, although rabies appears to be increasing among dogs. In certain areas outside the United States the paralytic form of rabies has been more frequent. In Trinidad both man and cattle have been infected by vampire bats, which apparently are carriers and not victims of the disease.

The common insectivorous bat, widespread in the United States and Canada, is susceptible to infection and may transmit the disease. Sleeping, injured or obviously sick bats are particularly hazardous when disturbed. A few instances of unprovoked attack have occurred.

PATHOLOGY. Fresh virus from a rabid animal will cause widespread degeneration and necrosis of neurons. Demyelination and degeneration of the axis cylinders are present in the white matter. The areas chiefly involved are the red nucleus, substantia nigra, pons and particularly the nuclei of the cranial nerves in the medulla. Here neuronophagia and infiltration with mononuclear cells are extensive. The pathognomonic sign in the neuronal cytoplasm and dendritic processes is the Negri body, which apparently is an inclusion body. It has eosinophilic cytoplasm with a basophilic granular corpuscle in the center. Since the neurons of the salivary glands at times show similar changes with Negri bodies, it is conceivable that the rabies virus enters the saliva by this route. Examination of tissues (brain, salivary gland) by the fluorescent antibody test is a rapid, reliable means of diagnosis.

CLINICAL MANIFESTATIONS. Since prophylaxis against the disease in man depends to a great extent upon an understanding of the early manifestations in the dog, they are described first.

In the dog symptoms may be considered under two general types, although it is not possible to separate them completely.

1. The "furious" type results from increased excitation of the central nervous system, with fever, hyperesthesia and lack of appetite. The evidences of disease depend to a great extent upon the nature and training of the dog. The more aggressive dog will begin to snap and become excited and dangerous early in the course of the disease. The gentle dog in the early stages will more frequently seek seclusion and refuse food or will become excessively affectionate, after which it becomes agitated and restless. This is usually followed by irritability and snapping at strangers and a little later by snarling or snapping at imaginary objects and chasing and biting other animals. Finally, if free, it will run for miles, snapping at or biting all living things in its path until it falls paralyzed to the ground.

2. The "dumb" or paralytic type, despite its frequency (approximately 20 per cent), is rarely recognized by the dog's owners, primarily because no agitation or excitement is seen. The course is far more rapid, paralysis occurring in any group of muscles, but particularly in the lower jaw and in the muscles of deglutition. In such cases the tongue hangs out of the mouth, continuously dripping saliva; sympathetic persons, suspecting a foreign body in the dog's throat, may expose their hands to the infective saliva in an effort to relieve the dog. Rapidly extending

paralysis soon results in death; occasionally dogs die suddenly without signs of illness, and encephalitis with Negri bodies is found at autopsy.

In man the incubation period is approximately 4 to 8 weeks, but may be months and, rarely, as long as a year. It may be shorter than 4 weeks when the lacerations are about the head or neck.

Clinical cases are usually characterized by three stages. In the *prodromal* phase, numbness, formication, tingling, burning or a sensation of cold may be felt about the wound and along the involved nerve trunks, followed by mild excitation, with irritability, restlessness, dilatation of pupils, salivation, lacrimation, perspiration and insomnia or, at times, drowsiness and depression.

In the *second* phase, excitation increases rapidly, and there is apprehension and even terror. The neck is stiff, and there are delirium and twitching or mild convulsive movements. At this stage the sign appears which has characterized the disease, i.e., the strangulating and painful spasm of the throat at any attempt to swallow food or liquids and even at the sight of them (hydrophobia). Slight noises may initiate these spasms, as may tactile stimuli. At such times the patient is unable to breathe, and the body remains in a tonic convulsion during which death may occur. The temperature is usually elevated to 103 to 105° F, but may be lower. Blood-tinged vomitus or excessive saliva may give the impression of "frothing."

Within 1 to 3 days the patient passes rapidly into the *terminal* phase with increasing paralysis, cessation of spasms, coma and death within another day or two.

The paralytic form of the disease, which is far less common, begins with numbness or severe pains in the nerve trunks supplying the involved area, followed shortly by flaccid paralysis of the part, which extends first to the opposite side of the body, and then slowly ascends in a manner similar to Landry's paralysis, terminating with involvement of the respiratory and circulatory centers.

In each form there may be a polymorphonuclear leukocytosis, as great as 20,000 to 30,000 cells per mm^3. The cerebrospinal fluid usually has a slight increase of protein and occasionally of mononuclear cells, up to 30 to 100 per mm^3.

DIAGNOSIS. With classic symptoms and history of bite, the diagnosis is not difficult. History of bite may be lacking, however, and symptoms may be atypical. The paralytic form may be confused with poliomyelitis. In a few instances differentiation from tetanus has been a problem, since tetanus also may be transferred by animal bite. In rabies the incubation period is usually longer. In tetanus the cerebrospinal fluid shows no cellular response and no increase in protein level. Persistent muscle spasm, particularly trismus, is characteristic in tetanus, whereas the strangulating spasms of the muscles of deglutition characteristic of rabies are lacking. Also to be considered in the differential diagnosis are encephalitis, ascending myelitis, lead encephalopathy, tick paralysis and various forms of acute meningitis.

Occasionally a person who has been bitten becomes hysterical and may present signs and symptoms which simulate rabies; however, differential diagnosis in this instance should not be difficult.

PROGNOSIS. Except for a single case in a child, recovery from human rabies has not been recorded.

PREVENTION. The most important prophylactic measure is control of dogs. In England, the Scandinavian countries and Canada, rabies has been nearly eliminated by precautions in the general handling of dogs. In some countries these include strict quarantine practices on entry of dogs into the country. Stray dogs should be eliminated, and all other dogs should be muzzled, confined or on leash. A dog bitten by a rabid animal should be either killed or isolated for at least 6 to 8 months. Vaccination of such a dog to be successful must include a sufficient number of injections; the customary single prophylactic injection is totally inadequate. The disappearance of a dog after biting an animal or man should be regarded with suspicion, since a dog frequently seeks seclusion before death from rabies. Suspicion should also be attached to a previously gentle dog whose behavior suddenly changes. Any dog which has bitten a person, but which has no sign of rabies, should be kept under surveillance.

In the case of bat bite it has been recommended that treatment be initiated regardless of the clinical condition of the bat.

Suggestions for prophylactic therapy are detailed in Table 10–15. Although no form of prophylaxis is 100 per cent effective, the regimens now recommended can be expected to prevent rabies from minor exposures and in at least 90 per cent of the more severe exposures. Modifications of these basic recommendations have been suggested. Cases must be individualized, as in the suspected exposure of young children who cannot give a reliable history. Very minor exposures may be covered by hyperimmune serum while the animal is being observed. In such instances longer observation of the dog in question is recommended: 12 to 14 days instead of a minimum of 5 days.

Rabies Vaccine. Pasteur's method of active immunization consisted of daily injections of increasing quantities of attenuated ("fixed") virus in spinal cord suspensions from infected rabbits.

The Semple vaccine consists of infected rabbit brain sterilized by phenol. The multiple passage chick embryo vaccine (HEP Flury) is used widely in the vaccination of dogs, but in human subjects gives variable results. Duck embryo vaccine appears to be the preparation of choice for ordinary exposures.

Two vaccines have been approved for use: duck embryo vaccine (DEV) and rabbit nervous tissue vaccine (NTV). Treatment failures for the two vaccines do not differ significantly, but the lower frequency of central nervous system reaction with DEV makes it preferable to NTV. The dose recommended is that given by the manufacturer. In mild exposure, e.g., a single bite (except on the head and neck), a minimum of 14 daily injections of vaccine

TABLE 10–15 RABIES: INDICATIONS FOR SPECIFIC POSTEXPOSURE TREATMENT

NATURE OF EXPOSURE	CONDITION OF ANIMAL		RECOMMENDED TREATMENT
	At Time of Exposure	*During Observation Period of 10 Days*	
I. No lesions Indirect contact only	Rabid		None†
II. Licks			
1. Unabraded skin	Rabid	–	None†
2. Abraded skin and abraded or unabraded mucosa	(a) Healthy	Healthy	None
	(b) Healthy	Clinical signs of rabies or proved rabid	Start vaccine at first signs of rabies in animal
	(c) Signs suggestive of rabies	Healthy	Start vaccine immediately. Stop treatment if animal is normal on fifth day after exposure‡
	(d) Rabid, escaped, killed* or unknown	–	Start vaccine immediately
III. Bites			
1. Simple exposure	(a) Healthy	Healthy	None
	(b) Healthy	Clinical signs of rabies or proved rabid	Start vaccine at first signs of rabies in animal
	(c) Signs suggestive of rabies	Healthy	Start vaccine immediately. Stop treatment if animal is normal on fifth day after exposure‡
	(d) Rabid, escaped, killed* or unknown; or any bite by wolf, jackal, fox or other wild animal	–	Start vaccine immediately
2. Severe exposure (multiple; or face, head or neck bites)	(a) Healthy	Healthy	Hyperimmune serum immediately no vaccine as long as animal remains normal
	(b) Healthy	Clinical signs of rabies or proved rabid	As in III, 2, (a), but start vaccine at first sign of rabies
	(c) Signs suggestive of rabies	Healthy	Hyperimmune serum immediately, followed by vaccine. Vaccine may be stopped if animal is normal on fifth day after exposure
	(d) Rabid, escaped, killed* or unknown. Any bite by wild animal	–	Hyperimmune serum immediately, followed by vaccine

Hyperimmune serum to be effective must be given within 72 hours of exposure.
These indications apply equally well whether or not the biting animal has been previously vaccinated.
†Start vaccine immediately when a reliable history cannot be obtained.
‡Alternative treatment would be to give hyperimmune serum and not start vaccine as long as animal remains normal.
*The fluorescent antibody technique of examination of brain tissue may be used, if available, as a guide for vaccination.
Prepared by Expert Committee on Rabies of World Health Organization.

is given subcutaneously in the abdomen, lower back and lateral aspects of the thighs, with site rotation recommended. In more severe exposure such as multiple bites or bites about the face, head or neck, this treatment is continued for 21 days. In some instances of severe exposure, 14 doses have been administered during the first 7 days, in the form of either a double dose, or two separate daily injections, with the remaining 7 doses given singly each day for 7 days. A booster injection is recommended at 10 and again at 20 days after completion of the primary course. Two booster doses are considered more important if antirabies serum has also been given.

When an immunized person with previously demonstrable antibody is exposed, one booster dose is recommended for mild exposure, and for severe exposure, five daily doses, followed by a booster dose in 20 days.

Hyperimmune antirabies serum in combination with vaccine is considered the best postexposure prophylaxis. Hyperimmune antirabies serm is prepared by the immunization of horses; it is standardized by mouse tests. Hyperimmune serum is most effective when given within 24 hours after exposure, and is especially valuable in severe exposures. Sensitivity status of the patient to horse serum must be initially determined by skin or eye test. The recommended dose is one vial (1000 units) intramuscularly per 55 lb (25 kg) of body weight. A portion of the antiserum is used to infiltrate the wound. If 72 hours have elapsed since the bite, double the intramuscular dose is recommended.

Because sensitivity to horse serum may be a problem in a significant percentage of those requiring prophylaxis, a human preparation, rabies immune globulin human (RIGH), is being developed. It is not available as yet for general distribution.

The *wound* should be washed thoroughly with soap or detergent and water. Suturing should not be carried out immediately, since immediate closure is thought to contribute to virus spread. Cauterization of the wound with concentrated nitric acid has been a traditional procedure; this acid does destroy the virus. The procedure is painful, however, and disfiguring. The use of a freshly prepared 1 per cent solution of Zephiran chloride (benzalkonium chloride) has been recommended for final wound cleansing. The activity of such quaternary ammonium compounds is neutralized by soap, and the washed wound should be rinsed well with water before the application of Zephiran. Since tetanus spores as well as rabies virus may be introduced into the wound, tetanus toxoid or antitoxin is recommended if the patient has not been immunized within the past year.

Repeated exposure to rabies is not common; if it occurs within 3 months after vaccination, no retreatment is necessary beyond proper wound cleansing and prophylaxis for tetanus (see above). If re-exposure occurs within 3 to 6 months, two booster vaccine doses may be given a week apart. If the interval is longer than 6 months, antiserum and 7 daily injections of vaccine are recommended.

Reactions to Antirabies Vaccine. Minor reactions are those common in allergic conditions such as urticarial or erythematous rashes and edema, with occasional syncope. Of greater significance are such infrequent neurologic complications as polyneuritis of the Guillain-Barré type, ascending paralysis and meningoencephalitis. They are thought to be due to an antigen-antibody reaction in the perivascular tissues. Treatment of neurologic manifestations is chiefly symptomatic. In some cases antihistaminics or corticosteroids have been beneficial. When meningeal or neuropathologic reactions are manifest, the vaccine treatment should be discontinued.

TREATMENT. Active treatment, once the disease has developed, consists of supportive measures. Sedatives should be used in large doses, and the patient's room kept darkened and quiet. Anesthesia may be required as the disease progresses. Control of convulsions is to be emphasized. Attendants should be instructed carefully in the handling of the patient; human bite is possible, and contact with saliva from an infected person is hazardous.

American Academy of Pediatrics: Report of the Committee on Infectious Diseases. 17th ed. Evanston, Ill., 1974, p. 127.

Blattner, R. J.: Rabies infection transmitted by insectivorous bats: Human case with virus isolation from spinal fluid during life. Comments on current literature. J. Pediatr. *58*:433, 1961.

Briggs, G. W., and Brown, W. M.: Neurological complications of antirabies vaccine treated with corticosteroids. J.A.M.A. *173*:802, 1960.

Burns, K. F., Skelton, D. F., Lukeman, J. M., and Grogan, E. W.: Cortisone and ACTH impairment of response to rabies vaccine. Pub. Hlth. Rep. *75*:441, 1960.

Cox, H. R.: Rabies: Laboratory diagnosis and postexposure treatment. Am. J. Clin. Path. *57*:794, 1972.

Garfield, H. I., Kimbrell, R. A., and Kahn, B.: The problem of rabies prophylactic therapy: Case report and review of literature. South. Med. J. *64*:157, 1971.

Johnson, H. N.: Rabies virus: *In* Lennette, E. H., and Schmidt, N. J. (eds.): Diagnostic Procedures for Viral and Rickettsial Diseases. 3rd ed. New York, American Public Health Association, Inc., 1964, p. 356.

Johnson, H. N.: Rabies virus: *In* Horsfall, F. L., and Tamm, I. (eds.): Viral and Rickettsial Infections of Man. 4th ed. Philadelphia, J. B. Lippincott Company, 1965, p. 814.

Kent, J. R., and Finegold, S. M.: Human rabies transmitted by the bite of a bat. With comments on the duck embryo vaccine. New Engl. J. Med. *263*:1058, 1960.

Loofbourow, J. C., Cabasso, V. J., Roby, R. E., and Anuskiewicz, W.: Rabies immune globulin (human): Clinical trials and dose determination. J.A.M.A. *217*:1825, 1971.

McQueen, J. L., Lewis, A. L., and Schneider, N. J.: Rabies diagnosis by fluorescent antibody: I. Its evaluation in a Public Health laboratory. Am. J. Pub. Hlth. *50*:1743, 1960.

Veeraraghavan, N., and Subrahmanyan, T. P.: Value of antirabies vaccine with and without serum against severe challenge. Bull. WHO *22*:381, 1960.

Weis, Th., Stechschulte, J., and Hattwick, M.: Recovery from rabies. Morbidity and Mortality Weekly Report *19*(Nos. 50, 52) 479; 496; 1970–1971. Follow-up on probable human rabies, Ibid. *20*(No. 7): 1971.

World Health Organization, Expert Committee on Rabies. Fifth Report, Geneva, 1966, Technical Report Series 321. See also Morbidity and Mortality Weekly Report *16*:152, 1967, and United States Department of Health, Education, and Welfare, Public Health Service: New national recommendations for animal rabies vaccination, Ibid. *21*:317, 1972.

YELLOW FEVER

DEFINITION. Yellow fever is an acute viral disease with severe constitutional symptoms accompanied by jaundice, hematemesis, and renal and cardiac involvement. Distribution is essentially tropical.

HISTORY. Carlos Finlay in 1881 first suggested the mosquito *Aedes aegypti* as the vector. The classic experiments of Reed, Carroll, Agramonte and Lazear in 1900 and 1901 verified its essential role and the need for mosquito control, and established the viral origin.

ETIOLOGY. The virus of yellow fever is small, averaging 20 to 23 mμ. Affinity of the virus for host cells is of two main types: neurotropism, an affinity for nervous tissue, and viscerotropism, an affinity for liver, kidney and heart. Under natural field conditions the virus is pantropic. Both viscerotropism and neurotropism of the virus can be greatly reduced by repeated passage in tissue cultures, whereas neurotropism is increased and viscerotropism practically disappears after repeated intracerebral passage of the virus in mice.

In the laboratory the neurotropic strain developed from intracerebral mouse passage produces, when injected intracerebrally in the *Macaca mulatta,* fatal encephalitis with absence of hepatitis and other visceral lesions.

Immunologically the strains of yellow fever virus may not differ, but clinically a differentiation appears necessary between *jungle yellow fever* and *urban yellow fever.* Jungle yellow fever occurs occasionally in man in close contact with the jungle in the absence of *Aedes aegypti*, its usual vector. In South America the virus has been found in mosquitoes of the genus *Haemagogus* and in *Aedes leucocelaenus,* while in Africa it has been found in *Aedes simpsoni* and *A. africanus.*

EPIDEMIOLOGY. In transmission of the more common form of the disease the aegypti mosquito bites an infected person during the first 3 days of the disease when the virus is circulating in the blood. After 9 to 12 days the mosquito becomes infective, and a susceptible host acquires the disease by bite, with clinical manifestations beginning within 3 to 6 days. All ages are susceptible.

A possible mode of transmission in the laboratory without insect vector has been suggested. While the virus is circulating in the blood of monkeys it can apparently be transferred from one animal to another through minute cutaneous abrasions, or even through the intact skin. The passaged neurotropic virus may also be transmitted to mice and monkeys by intranasal instillation.

Outbreaks of urban yellow fever have occurred in areas adjacent to endemic areas of jungle yellow fever. In Central America jungle yellow fever has been spreading slowly northward from Panama since 1948. Urban yellow fever has not been present in the Western Hemisphere since 1934 and has not been reported in the Orient. Southeastern United States is considered a receptive area for yellow fever; constant vigilance against mosquitoes is essential. Epidemics of the urban type still occur in Africa, Central and South America, and in Trinidad, areas in which the World Health Organization is constantly on the alert.

PATHOLOGY. There is severe jaundice, combined with petechial hemorrhages or ecchymotic areas of the skin. Black bloody material may be present in the mouth, nasal passages and stomach. The liver is normal in size or slightly enlarged and is stained a deep yellow. Hepatic cells undergo fatty degeneration, with a distinctive type of necrosis, which is typically midzonal, although in severe cases the entire lobule may be involved. The architecture of the liver is preserved, and in healing no cirrhosis occurs. Coalescent acidophilic areas of hyaline necrosis, widely scattered in the parenchymatous cells, are termed "Councilman bodies." Superficial hemorrhages are often seen in the mucous membranes of the stomach, particularly in the pyloric region, and in the intestines. Although the spleen is fairly normal in size, there is usually degeneration of the malpighian corpuscles. The cardiac muscle and the tubular epithelium of the kidneys show involvement similar to that in the liver. The brain at times shows perivascular hemorrhages.

CLINICAL MANIFESTATIONS. The majority of infections are so mild that the diagnosis may not be suspected.

The onset is acute with severe headache, chills, backache, pain in the limbs, and flushing of the face. Photophobia and conjunctival injection are prominent features. At the onset, jaundice is absent or slight. Cough and evidence of upper respiratory tract infection are usually lacking. As a rule, during the first 2 or 3 days the temperature rises rapidly to 103 to 104°F with an increasing pulse rate, and then diminishes relatively more slowly than the pulse rate in what is often termed a temporary remission. During this period, albuminuria develops, and there are epigastric pain and tenderness, and vomiting.

Subsequently the temperature is again elevated and prostration and depression are prominent features. The face is pale with a cyanotic appearance. Jaundice increases slowly. Hemorrhages into the skin and often into the gums appear at this time with epistaxis, a dry, brown tongue and a decreasing pulse rate to less than 50 per minute in spite of high fever (Faget's sign). Degenerative changes in the heart result in cardiac dilatation and low blood pressure. The urine contains large amounts of albumin and casts. There is usually vomiting of dark brown material. The leukocyte count is often as low as 3000 cells per $mm.^3$ In severe and fatal cases bile appears in the urine; at times there is anuria followed by convulsions or coma.

In nonfatal cases improvement starts about the sixth day, and the temperature often is normal by the eighth day. When convalescence begins, progress is continuous without complications. There is permanent immunity to the disease.

DIAGNOSIS. Differential diagnosis may present a problem, especially in the milder cases. Early differentiation from leptospirosis is particularly difficult. In infectious and serum hepatitis the illness usually develops and subsides much more slowly. Cases of yellow fever with acute onset may be confused initially with influenza, malaria, typhoid and dengue fever.

Diagnostic aids include animal inoculations and neutralization and complement fixation tests of acute phase and convalescent serums. Increasing titer of type-specific antibody during clinical recovery constitutes good presumptive evidence of the disease. Isolation of the virus from blood obtained during the first 3 to 4 days of illness has been accomplished with regularity by intracerebral inoculation of mice, and is the most rapid and satisfactory diagnostic method.

PROGNOSIS. The overall case fatality rate is probably not over 5 per cent, but in any outbreak the fatality rate of recognized cases may be 50 per cent or more.

PROPHYLAXIS. Yellow fever vaccine is a live attenuated virus preparation made from one of two strains, 17-D and Dakar (French neurotropic). The Dakar vaccine, which is prepared by mouse brain passage, has been associated with a significant (0.5 per cent) incidence of meningoencephalitic reaction and is not recommended. The 17-D strain vaccine is attenuated virus grown in chick embryo tissue culture inoculated with a fixed-passage-level seed virus. The vaccine is a freeze-dried supernate of centrifuged embryo homogenate. Vaccine should be stored at the temperature recommended by the manufacturer until it is reconstituted for use by the addition of sterile physiologic saline: dilution 1:10. Unused vaccine should be discarded within one hour after reconstitution. A single subcutaneous injection of 0.5 ml of 1:10 dilution of vaccine is recommended. Immunity is afforded within about 8 days after inoculation and lasts for 8 years or longer.

Vaccination is recommended for all persons living in areas where the virus is known to occur or recur, and for those planning to visit such areas. A recall injection of the same dose is required every 10 years in high-risk areas. Pregnant women and children under 1 year should not be vaccinated unless under high risk of exposure.

About 5 per cent of all persons vaccinated have a mild reaction on the sixth to eighth day, principally headache, myalgia and low-grade fever. Untoward reactions appear to be more prevalent in infants, and all recorded cases of encephalitis have been in this age group and have occurred within 1 to 2 weeks after administration of the vaccine. In most recorded cases recovery was spontaneous within 4 to 5 days, with no apparent residual damage. In one instance, however, a 3 year old child died of encephalitis following subcutaneous inoculation. Virus (17-D strain yellow fever virus) was recovered from the brain.

In the event of suspected cases the patients should be protected from mosquitoes. Spraying of premises, house, room or ward with a satisfactory insecticide is recommended.

TREATMENT. Specific therapy is lacking; complete bed rest is essential to lessen the danger of cardiac failure and hepatic damage. Supportive treatment and good nursing care are important, with special attention to oral hygiene and control of fever. Vomiting should be kept under control; solid food should be limited. Maintenance of nutritional status and of fluid and electrolyte balance, and control of intercurrent infection are essential. Because of diminution in prothrombin and fibrinogen, vitamin K should be given, and, if possible, plasma concentrates which contain coagulation factors.

American Academy of Pediatrics: Report of the Committee on Infectious Diseases. 17th ed. Evanston, Ill., 1974, p. 30.

Clarke, D. H., and Casals, J.: Yellow fever: *In* Horsfall, F. L., and Tamm, I. (eds.): Viral and Rickettsial Infections of Man. 4th ed. Philadelphia, J. B. Lippincott Company, 1965, p. 608.

Feitel, M., Watson, E. H., and Cochran, K. W.: Encephalitis after yellow fever vaccination. Pediatrics *25*:956, 1960.

Langmuir, A. D., and others: Fatal viral encephalitis following 17-D yellow fever vaccine inoculation: Report of a case in a 3-year-old child. A joint statement. J.A.M.A. *198*:671, 1966.

Mortality and Morbidity Weekly Report: Yellow fever vaccine. *18*:189, 1969; Yellow fever vaccination centers. Ibid. (Summary supplement) *20*:9, 1971.

Reed, W., Carroll, J., Agramonte, A., and Lazear, J. W.: Yellow fever: A compilation of various publications. Washington, D.C., United States 61st Congr., Third Session, Senate Doc. No. 822, 1911.

WHO Chronicle: Prevention of Aedes aegypti-borne diseases in the Americas: Yellow fever. *25*:275, 1971; *26*:60, 254, 1972.

LYMPHOGRANULOMA VENEREUM

(Lymphogranuloma Inguinale)

The majority of children with lymphogranuloma venereum acquire the disease by direct transmission from an infected adult. The infectious agent is considered to be a virus closely related to those of the psittacosis-ornithosis group (Rickettsiales). The agent usually enters through a minor abrasion on the penis or vulva, or it may penetrate the urethra, resulting in a mild urethritis. Rarely, the primary lesion is at other sites, as the mouth or hand.

CLINICAL MANIFESTATIONS. Enlargement of the inguinal lymph nodes is the most prominent manifestation of the disease and may be the first and only sign. In children the primary lesion may not be recognized as such, or may not be discovered. Rectal and anal strictures are not common in children; when they do occur, obstruction from residual scarring may be the first indication. The site of the primary lesion determines the extent and location of the lymphadenitis. Cervical and axillary lymphadenopathy has been described following mouth and hand lesions, respectively.

The lymphadenopathy is chronic, and the involved nodes are tender and often painful. They suppurate frequently, draining sinuses form, and the nodes become matted together and to adjacent tissues. In some instances the nodes change little in consistency, remain firm and gradually become less tender. On biopsy, there is evidence of chronic inflammatory reaction in the involved nodes and surrounding tissues. Infiltration of mononuclear elements is widespread, especially by plasma cells, with fewer neutrophils and eosinophils. There is proliferation of macrophages with giant-cell configuration. Proliferation of fibrous tissue is marked.

Although early stages of the condition may be characterized by fever and malaise, in general the systemic symptoms are mild. Joint involvement has been observed roentgenographically in children, with the joint space slightly increased. There may be diffuse, mild rarefaction of the bones. Scarlatiniform eruptions and erythema nodosum have been described, and in some instances splenic enlargement and generalized lymphadenopathy have occurred.

Parinaud's oculoglandular syndrome, a unilateral conjunctivitis followed by a chronic enlargement of the parotid gland and the anterior cervical nodes, may be caused by the virus of lymphogranuloma venereum, as well as by other infectious agents.

Central nervous system involvement has been reported in only a few instances, some of which, however, progressed to fatal outcome. Headache, nuchal rigidity and mental confusion were the presenting symptoms. The cerebrospinal fluid is under increased pressure, with increased protein content and pleocytosis. The spinal fluid sugar content may be reduced moderately, and the colloidal gold curve may show a strong first-zone reaction. Encephalitis may develop in the absence of obvious lesions or enlarged nodes. The agent has been recovered from spinal fluid by chorioallantoic or yolk-sac inoculation of embryonated eggs.

DIAGNOSIS. Viremia may be demonstrated during most of the course. A fourfold or more increase in the titer of complement-fixing antibody during clinical recovery provides good presumptive evidence. A titer of 1:32 obtained on repeated tests is highly suggestive even without a further rise. The antigen commonly used is derived from virus grown in chick embryo tissue culture.

The skin test (Frei) with heat-inactivated virus, usually material from a bubo, is performed by injecting 0.1 ml of the antigen (Lygranum) intradermally into the flexor surface of the forearm, with a similar amount of control material injected into the other arm. A positive reaction consists of a firm papule 5 mm or more in diameter which appears within 48 to 72 hours, with a negative or only a slight reaction at the site of the control inoculation. The reaction usually becomes positive within 3 to 8 weeks from the time infection has occurred and may remain positive for years. Recently tissue-culture antigen has been used in the same manner. Transient positive skin reactions have been reported in patients with psittacosis, atypical pneumonias and syphilis. If the patient is receiving corticosteroids the diagnostic value of the skin test may be reduced.

Differential Diagnosis. This includes distinction from other types of lymphadenopathy such as in chronic pyogenic bacterial infection, tuberculosis, tularemia, cat-scratch disease, and lymphoma or other neoplasm.

TREATMENT. Sulfonamide drugs, penicillin and the tetracyclines have been given, singly or in combination. The tetracyclines are generally considered the drug of choice, penicillin and chloramphenicol being less effective. Treatment must be continued for 10 to 14 days. Surgical excision of lymph nodes is rarely necessary. Unless severe, rectal stricture may respond to carefully graduated dilation.

Banov, L., Jr.: Rectal lesions of lymphogranuloma venereum in childhood. Am. J. Dis. Child. *83*:660, 1952.

Beeson, P. B., Wall, M. J., and Heyman, A.: Isolation of virus of lymphogranuloma venereum from blood and spinal fluid of human being. Proc. Soc. Exp. Biol. Med. *62*:306, 1946.

Greaves, A. B., Hilleman, M. R., Taggart, S. R., Bankhead, A. B., and Feld, M.: Chemotherapy in bubonic lymphogranuloma venereum: A clinical and serological evaluation. Bull. WHO *16*:277, 1957.

Greaves, A. B., and Taggart, S. R.: Serology, Frei reaction and epidemiology of lymphogranuloma venereum. Am. J. Syph. *37*:273, 1953.

Levy, H.: Lymphogranuloma venereum in childhood. J. Pediatr. *11*:812, 1937.

Meyer, K. F.: Psittacosis–Lymphogranuloma venereum agents: *In* Horsfall, F. L., and Tamm, I. (eds.): Viral and Rickettsial Infections of Man. 4th ed. Philadelphia, J. B. Lippincott Company, 1965, p. 1006.

Roth, D., and Schulick, R.: Isolated cervical lymphogranuloma in a Child. Pediatrics *8*:480, 1951.

Sabin, A. B., and Aring, C. D.: Meningoencephalitis in man caused by the virus of lymphogranuloma venereum. J.A.M.A. *120*:1376, 1942.

INFECTIOUS MONONUCLEOSIS

Infectious mononucleosis, which seems to occur most frequently in older children and young adults, is not uncommon in children between the ages of 2 and 10 years, and during epidemic periods it has been observed in infants. The variable manifestations and common occurrence of this disease make it a diagnostic possibility in throat infections, colds, influenza-like disease and generalized rashes. The essential feature of the disease is an increase in the mononuclear elements of the blood at some time during its course. The infectious agent is considered to be viral; blood from patients in the acute phase has produced similar disease when injected into monkeys and rabbits.

Recently the EB virus (Epstein and Barr), similar in structure to viruses of the herpes group, has been implicated in the causation of infectious mononucleosis. This virus (EBV), originally observed by electron microscopy in cultures of Burkitt lymphoma cells, apparently replicates only in cells of the lymphoreticular system. Extensive seroepidemiologic studies by complement fixation, virus neutralization and indirect immunofluorescence techniques strongly suggest a causative relation between EB virus and infectious mononucleosis.

Evidence for this relationship has been strengthened by recent epidemiologic studies among college students which at the same time have delineated the nature of the antibodies involved in the disease. Specific antibody to EB virus appears regularly in the serum of patients with clinical infectious mononucleosis and seems to persist for life. Recurrence of clinical disease is rare. It is apparent that the EB virus is widespread, and that the presence of EBV antibody is protective against the development of infectious mononucleosis.

In tissue culture there is a marked tendency for infectious mononucleosis cells to undergo spontaneous lymphoblastoid transformation. However, the association of the EB virus with Burkitt lymphoma cells and its exact relationship with infectious mononucleosis and with the malignant lymphoproliferative diseases remains to be established. Extensive studies are in progress at present.

CLINICAL MANIFESTATIONS. The incubation period is variable; it averages about 11 days, but has been as long as 6 weeks. The onset may be insidious or acute. Common clinical manifestations are malaise, sore throat with pharyngitis, and prolonged fever characterized by morning remission. In children periorbital edema may be the initial sign. Enlargement of the lymph nodes may occur early or relatively late in the clinical course, with the anterior and posterior cervical nodes commonly involved. The enlarged nodes may be tender but seldom suppurate. The salivary glands are rarely inolved. The throat may be mildly or severely inflamed, at times with a membranous exudate which may simulate severe streptococcal disease or diphtheria (Fig. 10–49, p. 657). Splenomegaly is common and may persist for months. The spleen, not always tender, is palpable by about

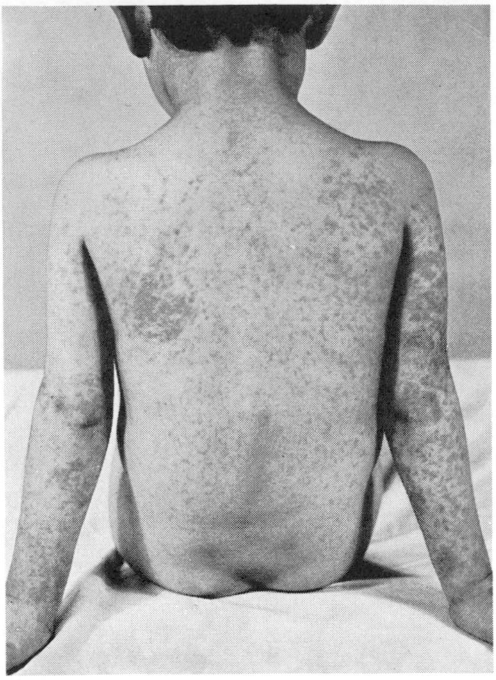

Figure 10–50 *Morbilliform rash in mononucleosis.*

the seventh day of illness. A skin rash is present in 10 to 20 per cent of the patients, appearing between the fourth and tenth days of the disease, usually in the form of a discrete macular eruption (Fig. 10–50). Most prominent over the trunk, it is rarely seen on the hands, thighs, legs and feet. The rash may also assume a petechial, vesicular, morbilliform or scarlatiniform appearance.

Hepatic involvement is nearly always present to some degree, and in many instances is associated with jaundice. Hepatic coma has been reported. Acute pancreatitis with glycosuria and enzyme changes has been noted as part of the disease process. Confusion of infectious mononucleosis with infectious hepatitis is possible in view of the lymphocytosis which may occur in hepatitis.

Neurologic manifestations occur occasionally and may precede, follow or occur simultaneously with the acute phase of the disease. The pattern may be that of an aseptic meningitis or a polyneuritis. Severe headache, nuchal rigidity, blurring of vision, mental confusion and, occasionally, convulsions have been noted. The cerebrospinal fluid may show an increase in mononuclear cells and in protein content. Concentration of sugar is normal.

Pericarditis and myocarditis have been reported, with clinical manifestations and electrocardiographic changes during the acute phase, prolonging the convalescence. Pneumonitis, thrombocytopenia and hemolytic anemia occur rarely.

DIAGNOSIS. Essential laboratory data are lymphocytosis with characteristic changes in the lymphocytes of the peripheral blood and a positive heterophil antibody test. Rising titer of antibody to EB virus is considered confirmatory.

The characteristic hematologic alteration is in the lymphocytes, which vary markedly in size and shape. Typically they are larger than mature lymphocytes and have basophilic cytoplasm which is excessively vacuolated, giving a foamy appearance. The nucleus in these larger cells is frequently placed eccentrically and is irregular or indented. Electron microscopic studies of the leukocytes in infectious mononucleosis have confirmed these characteristic features. Such atypical lymphocytes are also seen in smaller numbers (not more than 5 per cent) in other diseases such as infectious hepatitis, rubella and primary atypical pneumonia. In infectious mononucleosis, however, the increase in these atypical lymphocytes is characteristically greater, being 10 to 25 per cent of the leukocytes.

The leukocyte count is usually elevated, but may be normal or low. Although initially the polymorphonuclear cells are often increased in number, in a fully developed case the relative reduction in granulocytes is typical. The rise in lymphocytes usually begins on the fourth or fifth day, and by the seventh to the tenth day these cells constitute 60 to 90 per cent of the total leukocytes. In rare instances thrombocytopenia with purpura and prolonged bleeding time, agranulocytosis and anemia may occur.

The sheep cell or heterophil agglutination test (Paul-Bunnell-Davidsohn) for the diagnosis of infectious mononucleosis is a nonspecific serologic reaction, the exact nature of which is not known.

In 1932 Paul and Bunnell demonstrated a high titer of sheep red cell agglutinins in the serum of patients with infectious mononucleosis. These agglutinins proved to be different from other antibodies in human sera which agglutinate sheep red cells, such as the antibodies found in low titer in normal human serum, or those which occur in relatively high titer after the administration of horse serum (serum sickness). Titration of these heterophil antibodies has been a useful tool in the diagnosis of infectious mononucleosis, particularly after certain refinements were made in the test, i.e., differential absorption of the antibodies from the serum by beef red cells or guinea pig kidney cells. In infectious mononucleosis, the sheep cell agglutinins (antibodies) can be absorbed from the serum completely by beef red cells, but not by guinea pig kidney cells. The agglutinating antibodies present in serum sickness can be absorbed from the serum completely either by beef erythrocytes or by guinea pig kidney cells. The sheep cell agglutinins present in normal human serum are not absorbed by beef erythrocytes, but are almost completely absorbed by guinea pig kidney cells.

In each part of the test, the antibody level can be titrated. In the case of infectious mononucleosis, titers of 1:10 to 1:40 are considered negative or borderline; titers of 1:80 to 1:160 are presumptive; and titers above 1:160 are considered diagnostic. The best criterion in the early stages of the disease is a rising titer. In 60 per cent of cases of infectious mononucleosis the heterophil antibody reaction becomes positive during the first week of the disease and remains so for varying periods of time; the titer may reach a peak quickly and subside rapidly, or may persist at relatively high levels for several months. Falsely positive results may be obtained in patients who have received horse serum recently, as indicated above, and in rare instances in other infections. Although in very young children all the diagnostic criteria of infectious mononucleosis seem to be met, it appears that the full expression of the disease may not be seen, and the infection may not be accompanied by rise in heterophil antibody titer. In infants both the heterophil and anti-EBV antibody tests convert more slowly to positive.

Patients with infectious mononucleosis may have a falsely positive complement fixation (Wassermann or Kahn) reaction for syphilis, which usually appears during the second week of the disease and becomes negative within 2 or 3 weeks. Patients in whom a rash develops appear more likely to have this falsely positive reaction than those who do not have an eruption.

PROGNOSIS. In general the prognosis is good, even in prolonged and the more serious cases. The convalescent period, however, is usually long, especially in older children; weakness and easy fatigability may persist.

COMPLICATIONS. Liver involvement is usually mild, but chronic hepatitis may follow; hepatic coma has been reported. Other complications include pneumonitis, thrombocytopenia, hemolytic anemia, pericarditis and myocarditis. Neurologic complications have been common in certain outbreaks and vary widely in severity; they include Guillain-Barré syndrome, peripheral neuritis, cranial nerve involvement and psychoses. Reye syndrome (acute encephalopathy with fatty degeneration of the viscera) has been reported in association with infectious mononucleosis. Fatalities have occurred as the result of rupture of the spleen, severe neurologic complications, myocarditis, pulmonary edema, pneumothorax and hepatic necrosis.

TREATMENT. Therapy is supportive and nonspecific. Bacterial complications are not common and may be treated as indicated. An initial period of bed rest is usually indicated. Increase in activity should be gradual, based on the patient's temperature and evidence of fatigue. In patients with severe dysphagia, dyspnea, myocarditis, pericarditis, hepatitis or hemolytic anemia, a short course of corticosteroids usually affords prompt relief.

PROPHYLAXIS. Recent investigations concerned with the nature and structure of the surface antigens of sheep red cells have suggested the possibility that a vaccine might be developed on this basis.

Bender, C. E.: The value of corticosteroids in treatment of infectious mononucleosis. J.A.M.A. *199*:529, 1967.

Davidson, I., and Lee, C. L.: Serologic diagnosis of infectious mononucleosis: A comparative study of five tests. Am. J. Clin. Path. *41*:115, 1964.

Diehl, V., Henle, G., Henle, W., and Kohn, G.: Demonstration of herpes group virus in cultures of peripheral leukocytes from patients with infectious mononucleosis. J. Virol. *2*:663, 1968.

Epstein, M. A., Barr, Y. M., and Achong, B. G.: Studies with Burkitt's lymphomas. Wistar Institute Symp. Monograph *4*:69, 1965.

Evans, A. S., Niederman, J. C., and McCollum, R. W.: Seroepidemiologic studies of infectious mononucleosis with EB virus. New Engl. J. Med. *279*:1121, 1968.

Fernbach, D. J., and Starling, K. A.: Infectious mononucleosis. Pediat. Clin. N. Amer. *19*:957, 1972.

Henle, G., and Henle, W.: EB virus in the etiology of infectious mononucleosis. Hosp. Prac. *5*:33, 1970.

McMahon, J., Elliott, C., and Green, R.: Infectious mononucleosis complicated by hepatic coma. Am. J. Gastroent. *51*:200, 1969.

Paul, J. R., and Bunnell, W. W.: The presence of heterophile antibodies in infectious mononucleosis. Am. J. Med. Sci. *183*:90, 1932.

Rahal, J., Jr., and Henle, G.: Infectious mononucleosis and Reye's syndrome: A fatal case with studies for Epstein-Barr virus. Pediatrics *46*:776, 1970.

Rawsthorne, G., Cole, T., and Kyle, J.: Spontaneous rupture of the spleen in infectious mononucleosis. Brit. J. Surg. *57*:396, 1970.

Schnell, R. G., Dyck, P. J., Bowie, E. J. W., Klass, D. W., and Taswell, H. F.: Infectious mononucleosis: Neurologic and EEG findings. Medicine *45*:51, 1966.

Stevens, D. A.: Infectious mononucleosis and malignant lymphoproliferative diseases. J.A.M.A. *219*:897, 1972.

Wislocki, L. C.: Acute pancreatitis in infectious mononucleosis. New Engl. J. Med. *275*:322, 1966.

ACUTE INFECTIOUS LYMPHOCYTOSIS

This infection, originally thought to be a variant of infectious mononucleosis, was described and named by Carl Smith in 1941. The outstanding characteristic is the increase in the total number of lymphocytes in the peripheral blood and in the bone marrow, which persists over a relatively long time. Although the clinical course is usually mild, a variety of symptoms and signs has been recorded, such as fever, nasopharyngitis, abdominal complaints, skin rash and mild meningoencephalomyelitic manifestations.

ETIOLOGY AND EPIDEMIOLOGY. No bacterial or viral agent has been isolated as the cause of this condition. Multiple cases have been reported in institutional epidemics and in families. The incubation period is estimated to be 12 to 21 days. Most of the cases described have been in children under the age of 10 years. The disease has been observed in the Western Hemisphere and in Europe. Nothing is known about the development of immunity.

PATHOLOGY. Microscopic examination of excised lymph nodes reveals degeneration of the lymph follicles and proliferation of the reticuloendothelium of the sinuses.

CLINICAL MANIFESTATIONS. Many patients are asymptomatic, and there may be no abnormal physical findings. In some instances there may be fever at the onset and transient complaints. The manifestations may be those of an upper respiratory tract infection, sore throat predominating, or there may be gastrointestinal symptoms such as vomiting, diarrhea or abdominal pain. In a few instances symptoms simulating those of acute appendicitis have been present, suggesting a surgical emergency. The clinical pattern in a small number of recorded cases has been that of a meningoencephalitis with slight increase in the cerebrospinal fluid cell count. In one of these there was paralysis. A mild, generalized morbilliform rash similar to that in infectious mononucleosis may appear early in the course and last for several days. Slight enlargement of lymph nodes or the spleen has been observed, but is not common.

LABORATORY DATA. The only characteristic finding is the high white blood cell count, which ranges from 20,000 to 120,000 per mm^3, the proportion of lymphocytes varying from 62 to 97 per cent. The lymphocytes are normal in appearance and chiefly of the small variety. A slight eosinophilia may be present. There is no abnormality in the erythrocytes or platelets.

The heterophil agglutination reaction is negative. The bone marrow contains an increased number of normal or postmature lymphocytes; otherwise, it is not abnormal. These changes persist longer in the bone marrow than in the peripheral blood.

DIAGNOSIS. From the hematologic point of view the condition must be differentiated from infectious mononucleosis, acute leukemia and infections associated with a lymphocytosis, principally pertussis. Less frequently the disease must be distinguished from acute abdominal conditions such as acute appendicitis, and from meningoencephalitis of other causes.

Infectious mononucleosis can be identified by positive heterophil agglutination, complement fixation and immunofluorescent antibody tests, and by demonstration in the peripheral blood of the abnormal lymphocytes typical of this disease. In addition, the clinical manifestations in infectious mononucleosis are more severe, including fever, malaise, sore throat, rash, jaundice and enlargement of lymph nodes and often of the spleen.

Differentiation from *acute leukemia* may on occasion be impossible without examination of the bone marrow.

Though in some of the more severe cases of *pertussis* extremely high lymphocyte counts are observed, the characteristic clinical manifestations in pertussis are usually sufficient for differential diagnosis.

When abdominal manifestations suggest a surgical condition, the high lymphocyte count supports a period of watchful waiting, during which the diagnosis will usually become apparent, partly because in infectious lymphocytosis the abdominal complaints are of short duration.

COURSE AND PROGNOSIS. Clinical manifestations, as a rule, are of short duration, and the prognosis is excellent. The lymphocytosis persists for weeks, however, and in one case was observed for 7 months. No sequelae have been recognized and no deaths recorded.

TREATMENT. Therapy is symptomatic.

Barnes, G. R., Jr., Yannet, H., and Lieberman, R.: A clinical study of an institutional outbreak of acute infectious lymphocytosis. Am. J. Med. Sci., *218*:646, 1949.

Clement, D. H.: Reassurance regarding infectious lymphocytosis. Pediatrics *41*:547, 1968.

Horwitz, M. S., and Moore, G. T.: Acute infectious lymphocytosis: An etiologic and epidemiologic study of an outbreak. New Engl. J. Med., *279*:399, 1968. Editorial: Lymphocytopoietic viruses. *Ibid.*, p. 432.

Lemon, B. K., and Kaump. D. H.: Infectious lymphocytosis: A report of an epidemic in children. J. Pediatr. *36*:61, 1950.

Putnam, S. M., Moore, G. T., and Mitchell, D. W.: Infectious lymphocytosis: Long-term follow-up of an epidemic. Pediatrics *41*:588, 1968.

Ryder, R. J.: Acute infectious lymphocytosis. Am. J. Dis. Child. *110*:299, 1965.

Smith, C. H.: Acute infectious lymphocytosis. *In* Advances in Pediatrics. New York, Interscience Publishers, Inc., 1947, Vol. II, p. 64.

CAT-SCRATCH DISEASE

(Benign Inoculation Lymphoreticulosis; Cat-claw Disease; Cat-bite Fever)

The relation of cat-scratch disease in man to contact with the domestic cat seems to have been established.

ETIOLOGY. The causative agent, though not identified, has been thought to be a virus of the psittacosis-lymphogranuloma venereum group (Rickettsiales). Attempts to isolate the agent from suppurative lymph nodes have been unsuccessful, but transfer of the disease to monkeys and human volunteers has been accomplished. Stained sections of primary skin lesions and involved lymph nodes from both man and monkeys show large numbers of intracellular and extracellular granule-like bodies similar to those of psittacosis. On the basis of similarity in the type of elementary body, a possible relation between the causative agent of cat-scratch disease and that of feline pneumonitis has been suggested. This agent, which is related antigenically to the psittacosis-lymphogranuloma viruses, can be isolated readily and established in mice by intranasal passage. A similar transfer of material from infected nodes in cat-scratch disease has not produced disease in mice. Both complement fixation and hemagglutination studies support the concept of viral origin, and recent work has suggested relation of the agent to viruses of the herpes group.

EPIDEMIOLOGY. Initially recognized about 1930 in France and the United States, the disease occurs world-wide.

Cats which transfer the agent to human subjects show no evidence of illness and have no reaction to the intradermal injection of the antigen. Attempts to isolate the agent from cat saliva and cat claws have been without success.

PATHOLOGY. Examination of involved lymph nodes has revealed only nonspecific morphologic changes which can be classified into distinct phases: (1) an "elementary" phase of simple hyperplasia; (2) an "accentuated" phase in which, in addition to hyperplasia, areas of early cellular necrosis stain as acidophilic masses; and (3) the "ultimate" stage in which the lymph node architecture is displaced by multiple areas with central necrosis and by circumscribed foci of epithelioid cells and scattered giant cells of the Langhans type (pseudotubercles). The final phase corresponds to the clinical stage when the enlarged node becomes fluctuant.

CLINICAL MANIFESTATIONS. Cat-scratch disease is a nonfatal systemic illness characterized by malaise, headache, low-grade fever and lymphadenitis. Although as a rule the patient does not appear acutely or chronically ill, the size of the involved lymph node, or nodes, is often striking. The nodes may be tender, especially early in the course. In most instances the history will reveal association with cats, with or without the recollection of a specific abrasion. The incubation period varies from 10 to 30 days. In a volunteer subject regional adenopathy began in 8 days and progressed to fluctuation in about 20 days. At the height of the lymph node response a skin papule appeared at the site of the primary intradermal inoculation and persisted for several days.

The foregoing sequence appears to be characteristic of the natural infection. At the time medical advice is sought there is usually an exacerbation of redness and swelling at the site where a primary lesion is in the process of healing. This lesion tends to heal slowly and may resemble an insect bite, a small furuncle or a scab following simple trauma. The nodes involved are those which drain the area where the initial lesion occurred, commonly the epitrochlear, axillary, submandibular, cervical or inguinal nodes. The skin overlying enlarged nodes may show some redness, but more often is normal in appearance. Involved lymph nodes may be hard or soft and vary in diameter from 1 to 5 cm; on aspiration purulent fluid may be obtained.

Unusual clinical manifestations have included cervical adenitis, transient pulmonary infiltration and an oculoglandular form of the disease, with conjunctivitis and enlargement of preauricular and cervical nodes. Purpura and skin rashes of the erythema multiforme and nodosum types have been observed. In one instance an osteolytic lesion which healed spontaneously was reported.

Central nervous system involvement, classified as encephalitis, encephalomyelitis, myelitis, radiculitis and optic neuritis, may accompany or follow the acute phase. Onset of neurologic symptoms is usually abrupt, with high fever. The spinal fluid shows a moderate increase in lymphocytes and in protein level.

LABORATORY DATA. There may be a moderate leukocytosis with a slight shift to the left. Sedimentation rate may be elevated during the first few weeks of lymphadenitis; otherwise, there are no conclusive laboratory findings.

SKIN TEST. Patients with cat-scratch disease usually exhibit a skin reaction after the intradermal injection of an antigen prepared by the Frei procedure from an involved node of a known case. The skin test is performed by injecting intradermally 0.1 ml of the antigen; the site should be observed at intervals of 48 and 72 hours. A typically positive reaction consists of an indurated, raised erythematous wheal 5 mm or more in diameter, surrounded by a zone of erythema 30 to 40 mm in diameter. The erythema may disappear in 1 to 2 days, but as a rule the wheal can be recognized for 4 or 5 days longer. A positive skin reaction may be obtained for years after cat-scratch infection. No regional adenopathy is associated with a positive reaction to the intradermal injection. Although the skin test is considered to have diagnostic significance, it must be recognized that the material used for preparation of antigen varies considerably from case to case. The antigen is not available commercially.

DIFFERENTIAL DIAGNOSIS. Cat-scratch disease may be confused with simple pyogenic adenitis, but must be differentiated also from tuberculous adenitis, tularemia, bubonic plague, rat-bite fever, Hodgkin's disease, lymphoma, infectious mononucleosis, sarcoidosis, fungus infections and lymphogranuloma venereum.

PROGNOSIS. The prognosis is uniformly good; the enlarged nodes regress spontaneously in 1 to 3 months. In some instances fibrosis may result in persistent enlargement.

PREVENTION. At present, detection of cats carrying the infective agent is not possible, since they are asymptomatic and do not have a positive skin reaction to the antigen. There are no control measures other than avoidance of contact with cats. Other possible means of transfer include abrasions by thorns and wood splinters, and by fragments of bone. The obvious question in such instances is whether the persons involved had subsequent contact with cats.

TREATMENT. No therapeutic measures are known to be of benefit. Occasionally drainage by aspiration will hasten resolution of fluctuant nodes; this procedure carries the risk of a draining sinus, which, however, usually heals with minimal scarring.

Adams, W. C., and Hindman, S. N.: Cat-scratch disease associated with an osteolytic lesion. J. Pediatr. *44*:665, 1954.

Carithers, H. A., Carithers, C. M., and Edwards, R. O., Jr.: Cat-scratch disease: Its natural history. J.A.M.A. *207*:312, 1969.

Debré, R., and Job, J.-C.: La maladie des griffes du chat. Acta Paediatr. *43* (Suppl. 96):1; 386, 1954.

Kalter, S. S., Kim, C. S., and Heberling, R. L.: Herpes-like particles associated with cat-scratch disease. Nature (London) *224*:190, 1969.

Margileth, A. M.: Cat scratch disease: Non-bacterial regional lymphadenitis. Pediatrics *42*:803, 1968.

Mollaret, P., Reilly, J., Bastin, R., and Tournier, P.: Le virus de la lymphoréticulose bénigne d'inoculation. Présse méd. *64*:1177, 1956.

Naji, A. F., Carbonell, F., and Barker, H. J.: Cat scratch disease: A report of three new cases: Review of the literature, and classification of the pathologic changes in the lymph nodes during various stages of the disease. Am. J. Clin. Path. *38*:513, 1962.

Paxson, E. M., and McKay, R. J., Jr.: Neurologic symptoms associated with cat scratch disease. Pediatrics *20*:13, 1957.

Pollen, R. H.: Cat-scratch encephalitis. Neurology *18*:1031, 1968.

Rice, J. E., and Hyde, R. M.: Rapid diagnostic method for cat scratch disease. J. Lab. Clin. Med. *71*:166, 1968.

Small, W. T., and Sniffen, R. C.: Nonbacterial regional lymphadenitis (cat scratch fever): Evaluation of surgical treatment. New Engl. J. Med. *255*:1029, 1956.

Sweeney, V. P., and Drance, S. M.: Optic neuritis and compressive neuropathy associated with cat scratch disease. Canad. Med. Ass. J. *103*:1380, 1970.

CYTOMEGALIC INCLUSION DISEASE

Cytomegalic inclusion disease is seen predominantly in young infants as a congenitally acquired infection, but it is encountered also in older children and adults. It is a systemic disease characterized by the presence of intranuclear and intracytoplasmic inclusion bodies in enlarged cells of many viscera. Affected cells may be epithelial or mesenchymal. At necropsy inclusion-bearing cells have been demonstrated in almost all the organs of the body, including the respiratory system, kidneys, adrenals, liver, gastrointestinal system, hematopoietic tissues and brain. Involvement of the central nervous system may be extensive. Although the tissue adjoining the involved cells may show no significant inflammatory response, in some instances there is an associated infiltration of lymphocytes and, on occasion, focal areas of necrosis or fibrosis. Advanced periventricular cerebral necrosis has been observed in premature infants. Excessive extramedullary hematopoiesis may be present, especially in the spleen and liver of infants dying during the neonatal period. In premature and newborn infants who have acquired the infection in utero the inclusion bodies are prominent in the kidney. The intranuclear inclusion body occupies most of the enlarged nucleus of the infected cell and characteristically is separated from the nuclear membrane by a clear halo. Small, multiple intracytoplasmic inclusion bodies occur less frequently.

Strains of cytomegalovirus (DNA), which structurally resembles herpes simplex virus, are species-specific, affecting man, monkeys and other animals, especially rodents.

Serologic studies indicate that the virus is widespread. Antibodies have been demonstrated in a high proportion of human serums. After infection in the human subject the virus may be shed in the saliva for as long as 4 weeks, and in the urine for as long as 24 months. Infants may shed the virus in the saliva for as long as 4 months, and in the urine for several years. Human cytomegalovirus has been isolated from breast milk and from the placenta. Virus isolation can be accomplished readily in tissue culture, especially in human fibroblast preparations. At necropsy it has been recovered from a variety of tissues, including salivary gland, kidney, brain and liver. It has also been recovered from adenoid and tonsillar tissue undergoing spontaneous degeneration in tissue culture, and from the urine of infants and children with no overt evidence of cytomegalic inclusion disease or other signs of clinical illness. Characteristic inclusion bodies have been observed as an incidental finding in the salivary glands of 8 to 32 per cent of fetuses and infants dying from a variety of causes. Inclusion bodies of this type have been observed in the tissue of infants, children and adults dying from pertussis and from debilitating diseases such as cystic fibrosis, leukemia and lymphoma. The significance of these findings is under evaluation at present. It has been suggested that a latent viral infection may have been activated because of lowered host resistance. Cytomegaloviruses have been isolated from the peripheral blood and from lymph node tissue.

CLINICAL MANIFESTATIONS. Manifestations of the congenitally acquired infection are apparent most often in the neonatal period or early infancy. The congenital disease is acquired by passage across the placenta; viral placentitis has been reported, with description of the placental changes. Well defined inclusion bodies were observed in the cells of some areas. In the case of dizygotic twins, one infant only may be affected. Affected infants are often premature or below average birth weight for gestational age. Although any organ system may be involved, the manifestations are usually referable to the hematopoietic system, liver and central nervous system. Hepatomegaly, splenomegaly, icterus, anemia, thrombocytopenia, purpura, deafness and cerebral calcifications are common findings. The cerebral calcifications are classically paraventricular, occurring mainly in the subependymal regions of the lateral ventricles; there may be poor development of the convolutions and dilatation of the ventricles with resultant microcephaly or hydrocephalus. Chorioretinitis, similar to that of congenital toxoplasmosis, may be a manifestation. Virus has been isolated from aqueous humor obtained from the anterior chamber.

Acquired Infection. If a mother is excreting cytomegalovirus in her cervical secretions, her baby may become infected during passage through the birth canal. This occurs in spite of high titers of maternal antibody. Virus can be isolated from the throat and urine of these babies beginning in the third to twelfth week of life. Shedding of virus continues for at least 12 to 18 months, and infants do not develop clinical illness.

Young infants can acquire the infection in the nursery from infected babies who are shedding virus. Infants known to be excreting virus should be placed in strict isolation. Women working in such areas should be checked frequently for antibody titer, or preferably should be beyond child-bearing age. Pregnant women should not care for infants shedding virus.

In older children and infants whose first evidence of the disease is apparent some time after birth, the clinical manifestations are more varied. Hepatosplenomegaly may be a prominent sign, with or without evidence of hepatitis. Cytomegalovirus infection is a diagnostic possibility in any case of clinical hepatitis. However, in older infants and children, the more common signs and symptoms are those associated with interstitial pneumonitis and enterocolitis. Complications resulting from intestinal malabsorption have been reported: hypocalcemia and osteomalacia with spontaneous fractures. Subclinical infection with active shedding of virus is possible.

Acquired infection may follow transfusion with

large quantities of fresh (but not stored citrated) blood, a situation which may be a problem in open heart surgery and in patients on immunosuppressive therapy. An incubation period of 3 to 5 weeks following transfusion has been recorded. The virus appears to be carried in the leukocytes and to become less active with their deterioration.

DIFFERENTIAL DIAGNOSIS. The differential diagnosis in the neonatal period includes erythroblastosis fetalis, sepsis, toxoplasmosis, congenital syphilis, generalized herpes simplex, congenital hemolytic anemia and congenital leukemia. In older children infectious mononucleosis and hepatitis must be considered. The diagnosis is based on the demonstration of inclusion-bearing cells which may be seen in the urine, gastric washings, cerebrospinal fluid, fluid aspirated from the subdural space, and in liver biopsy cells. In older children and adults inclusion bodies have been seen in macrophages and in cells of the vascular endothelium; in infants, largely in epithelial cells.

PROGNOSIS. The prognosis is grave in *congenital cytomegalic inclusion disease.* The fatality rate in recognized cases of the congenitally acquired infection is extremely high; accumulating evidence suggests, however, that there may be a relatively high incidence of clinically inapparent infections. Permanent cerebral damage, often present in infants who survive the clinically apparent disease, varies widely in severity.

In general, the prognosis for future pregnancies is good in women who have borne a child with congenital cytomegalovirus disease. However, recent reports indicate that a mother may give birth to a second affected infant in a consecutive pregnancy, especially if it follows the first at short interval. In one such instance the first child, severely affected, died at 30 days of age; the second child demonstrated viruria but no obvious clinical manifestations.

TREATMENT. No satisfactory therapy is known; antibiotics, gamma globulin, corticosteroids and blood transfusions have been used without demonstrable benefit. Several antiviral substances have been under consideration. They are not available commercially, and their efficacy and toxicity are not assessed as yet. Transfusions of sedimented red blood cells have been recommended for anemia, and platelet-rich plasma or platelet concentrates for thrombocytopenia. Anticonvulsants have been employed for seizures.

Elliott, G. B., and Elliott, K. A.: Observations on cerebral cytomegalic inclusion disease of the foetus and the newborn. Arch. Dis. Child. *37*:34, 1962.

Embil, J. A., Ozere, R. L., and Haldane, E. V.: Congenital cytomegalovirus infection in two siblings from consecutive pregnancies. J. Pediatr. *77*:417, 1970.

Hanshaw, J. B.: Cytomegalovirus infection and cerebral dysfunction. Hosp. Prac. *5*:111, 1970.

Hanshaw, J. B.: Congenital cytomegalovirus infection: A fifteen year perspective. J. Infect. Dis. *123*:555, 1971.

Harnden, D. G., Elsdale, T. R., Young, D. E., and Ross, A.: The isolation of cytomegalovirus from peripheral blood. Blood *30*:120, 1967.

Hayes, K., Danks, D. M., Gibbs, H., and Jack, I.: Cytomegalovirus in human milk. New Engl. J. Med. *287*:177, 1972.

Kopelman, A. E., Halsted, C. C., and Minnefor, A. B.: Osteomalacia and spontaneous fractures in twins with congenital cytomegalic inclusion disease. J. Pediatr. *81*:101, 1972.

Lang, D. J., and Noren, B.: Cytomegaloviremia following congenital infection. J. Pediatr. *73*:812, 1968.

Medearis, D. N.: Observations concerning human cytomegalovirus infection and disease. Bull. Johns Hopkins Hosp. *114*:181, 1964.

Monif, G.R.G., and Dische, R. M.: Viral placentitis in congenital cytomegalovirus infection. Am. J. Clin. Path. *58*:445, 1972.

Reynolds, D. W., Stagno, S., Hosty, T., Tiller, M., and Alford, C. A.: Maternal cytomegalovirus excretion and perinatal infection. New Engl. J. Med. *289*:1, 1973.

Shearer, W. T., Schreiner, R. L., Marshall, R. E., and Barton, L. I.: Cytomegalovirus infection in a newborn dizygous twin. J. Pediatr. *81*:1161, 1972.

Starr, J. G., and Gold, E.: Screening of newborn infants for cytomegalovirus infection. J. Pediatr. *73*:820, 1968.

Stulberg, C. S., Zuelzer, W. W., Page, R. H., Taylor, P. E., and Brough, A. J.: Cytomegalovirus infections with reference to isolations from lymph nodes and blood. Proc. Soc. Exp. Biol. Med. *123*:976, 1966.

Weller, T. H.: The cytomegaloviruses: Ubiquitous agents with protean clinical manifestations. New Engl. J. Med. *285*: 203; 285; 267; 1971.

INFECTIOUS NEURONITIS

(Infectious Polyneuritis; Guillain-Barré Syndrome)

Infectious neuronitis is a disease of unknown origin involving the nervous system and manifested by varying degrees of motor and sensory disturbances. Characteristically there is bilateral ascending paralysis. The existence of this disorder as a distinct entity has been questioned on the basis that it may represent a hypersensitivity phenomenon, and because it has been reported in association with diseases of divergent causes. The condition frequently follows an acute infection and is thought by many to be a toxic effect of the original infection. Others have suggested that the nervous system involvement may be due to an activated latent virus or to a concurrent viral infection. Experimental studies on animals have failed to demonstrate a specific causative agent. Diseases with which infectious neuronitis has been associated include diphtheria, scarlet fever, typhoid fever, mumps, varicella, influenza, respiratory infections, rubeola, rubella, infectious mononucleosis, tuberculous meningitis and infections with mycoplasma and with some of the enteric viruses. It has also been observed as a complication following the administration of tetanus antitoxin and various vaccines, including those for smallpox and poliomyelitis.

The incidence of the disease in children appears to be increasing. Although recorded cases suggest a higher susceptibility between the ages of 4 and 10 years, the condition can occur in infants under 1 year of age. The sexes appear to be equally susceptible.

The clinical picture is variable and may consist of acute ascending motor paralysis, of motor and sensory disturbances, or of a combination of signs and symptoms referable to the peripheral and cranial nerves. In most instances signs of peripheral neuritis develop symmetrically in the legs several days after an upper respiratory tract infection. The muscles become tender, and the deep tendon reflexes are abolished or greatly diminished; cutaneous reflexes are maintained, as a rule. Sensory loss is variable, but in children it is not often prominent. Cramping pains and paresthesias may occur. The paralysis tends to be symmetrical and ascending in its pattern of development, often involving the abdominal and thoracic muscles. Involvement of the cranial nerves is not common, except for the facial nerves, in which it may be bilateral. As a rule, muscular atrophy is not a feature of this disease, and recovery is usually complete, especially in children. The course tends to be prolonged, with a gradual return of function to the paralyzed muscles. Fatalities are uncommon but may occur as a result of respiratory paralysis. Fever is an inconspicuous feature and may be absent.

When a cytoalbuminous dissociation coexists with polyneuritis, the condition has been designated as the Guillain-Barré syndrome. The characteristic increase in the protein level of the spinal fluid with little or no increase in cell count is an important diagnostic feature. The symmetry of the paralysis and the cerebrospinal fluid findings tend to distinguish the condition from acute anterior poliomyelitis.

PATHOLOGY. Pathologic changes are found in the peripheral nerves and nerve roots; these consist chiefly in degeneration in the myelin and in the axis cylinders. There may or may not be evidence of inflammatory reaction. Marked involvement of the roots of the cranial nerves and of the ventral roots along the spinal axis has been reported frequently. No characteristic central nervous system changes are found. Visceral lesions have been reported which consist in focal necroses with round cell infiltration in the liver, kidneys and adrenals.

PROGNOSIS. The prognosis in children is usually good, except in the most fulminating cases. Pneumonia is a common complication. The greatest danger is respiratory paralysis, in which early tracheotomy and mechanical respiratory aids may be lifesaving. Recovery is extremely slow and may require many months, but it is usually complete with no permanent residuals.

TREATMENT. Treatment is symptomatic; no specific therapy is available. Acceleration of recovery has been reported when therapy with a corticosteroid was initiated early in the course of the disease.

Russell J. Blattner

Berlacher, F. J., and Abington, R. B.: ACTH and cortisone in Guillain-Barré syndrome: Review of the literature and report of a treated case following primary atypical pneumonia. Ann. Intern. Med. *48*:1106, 1958.

Eden, A. N.: Guillain-Barré syndrome in a six-month old infant. Am. J. Dis. Child. *102*:224, 1961.

King, E. G., and Jacobs, H.: "Complications" of the Landry-Guillain-Barré-Strohl syndrome. Canad. Med. Ass. J. *104*:393, 1971.

Liebman, W. M., and St. Geme, J. W., Jr.: Management of migratory atelectasis and pneumonitis in Guillain-Barré syndrome. Clin. Pediatr. *9*:403, 1970.

Low, N. L., Schneider, J., and Carter, S.: Polyneuritis in children. Pediatrics *22*:972, 1958.

McFarland, H. R., and Heller, G. L.: Guillain-Barré complex: A statement of diagnostic criteria and analysis of 100 cases. Arch. Neurol. *14*:196, 1966.

Osler, L. D., and Sidell, A. D.: The Guillain-Barré syndrome: The need for exact diagnostic criteria. New Engl. J. Med. *262*:964, 1960.

Steele, J. C., Gladstone, R. M., Thanasophon, S., and Fleming, P. C.: *Mycoplasma pneumoniae* as a determinant of the Guillain-Barré syndrome. Lancet *2*:710, 1969.

DENGUE FEVER AND DENGUE-LIKE DISEASE

DEFINITION. Dengue fever is a benign syndrome caused by several arthropod-borne viruses and characterized by biphasic fever, myalgia or arthralgia, rash, leukopenia and lymphadenopathy.

HISTORY. Epidemic dengue-like disease was described by David Bylon in Java in 1779, and a year later in Philadelphia by Benjamin Rush. Large epidemics occurred frequently in temperate areas of the Americas, Europe, Australia and Asia until early in the twentieth century. Dengue fever and dengue-like disease are now endemic in tropical Asia, Africa and America. An extensive epidemic of dengue occurred in Oceania in 1971–72.

ETIOLOGY. Dengue fever is caused by dengue viruses, of which there are at least four distinct antigenic types. In addition, three other arthropod-borne (arbo) viruses are frequently the cause of a similar or identical febrile disease with rash (Table 10–16).

EPIDEMIOLOGY. Dengue viruses are transmitted by mosquitoes of the Stegomyia family.

TABLE 10–16 VECTORS AND GEOGRAPHIC DISTRIBUTION OF DENGUE-LIKE DISEASES

ARBOVIRUS GROUP	VIRUS AND DISEASE	VECTOR	GEOGRAPHIC DISTRIBUTION
A	Chikungunya	*Aedes aegypti* *Aedes africanus*	Africa, India, Southeast Asia
A	O'nyong-nyong	*Anopheles funestus*	East Africa
B	West Nile fever	*Culex molestus* *Culex univittatus*	Middle East, Africa, Southeast India

Aedes aegypti, a daytime biting mosquito, is the principal vector. All four virus types have been recovered from naturally infected *Aedes aegypti.* In most tropical areas *Aedes aegypti* is highly urbanized, breeding in water stored for drinking or bathing, or, alternatively in any container collecting rain water. Dengue viruses have also been recovered from naturally infected *Aedes albopictus,* and outbreaks in the Pacific area have been attributed to *Aedes scutellaris.* These species breed in water trapped in vegetation; *Aedes albopictus* frequently breeds in bamboo stumps. In Southeast Asia dengue may be maintained in a jungle cycle involving primates, since neutralizing antibody to dengue viruses is common in several species of Malaysian monkeys.

Dengue outbreaks in urban areas infested with *Aedes aegypti* may be explosive; as many as 70 to 80 per cent of the population may be involved. Because *Aedes aegypti* has a limited flying range, spread of an epidemic is mainly through movement of viremic human beings. For this reason such outbreaks follow main lines of transportation. Sentinel cases may infect household mosquitoes and result in a large number of nearly simultaneous secondary infections, giving the appearance of a contagious disease. Where dengue viruses are endemic, children and susceptible foreigners may be the only persons to acquire overt disease, adults having become immune.

Dengue-like diseases may occur in epidemic outbreaks. Important epidemiologic features are determined by the vectors and their geographic distribution (Table 10–16). Chikungunya virus is widespread in the most populous areas of the world. In Asia, *Aedes aegypti* is the principal vector of infection to man; in Africa other Stegomyia may be important vectors. In Southeast Asia, dengue and chikungunya outbreaks occur concurrently. Outbreaks of O'nyong-nyong and West Nile fever usually involve people living in villages or small towns, as opposed to the many urban outbreaks of dengue and chikungunya.

PATHOLOGY. Insufficient pathologic material has been obtained from virologically confirmed cases of dengue fever to present a comprehensive description. Fatalities are rare with chikungunya and West Nile infections; those recorded have been ascribed to viral encephalitis, hemorrhage or febrile convulsions. (See description of Dengue Hemorrhagic Fever.)

CLINICAL MANIFESTATIONS. Biphasic fever and rashes are the most characteristic features of dengue. Manifestations vary with age and from patient to patient. In infants and young children the disease may be undifferentiated or characterized by a 1- to 5-day fever, pharyngeal inflammation, rhinitis and mild cough. In outbreaks a majority of patients have most of the findings described below.

After an incubation period of 2 to 7 days there is a sudden onset of fever which rapidly rises to 103 to 106° F, usually accompanied by frontal or retroorbital headache. Occasionally back pain precedes the fever. A *transient,* macular, generalized rash which blanches under pressure may be seen during the first 24 to 48 hours of fever. The pulse rate may be slow in proportion to the degree of fever. Myalgia or arthralgia occurs soon after onset and increases in severity. Involvement of the knee may be particularly severe in patients with chikungunya or O'nyong-nyong infection. During the second to the sixth day of fever, nausea and vomiting are apt to occur, and during this phase generalized lymphadenopathy, cutaneous hyperesthesia or hyperalgesia, taste aberrations and pronounced anorexia may develop.

One or two days after defervescence a generalized, morbilliform, maculopapular rash appears, which spares the palms and soles. It disappears in 1 to 5 days; desquamation may occur. Rarely there is edema of the palms and soles. About the time of appearance of this second rash the body temperature, which has previously fallen to normal, may become slightly elevated and establish the biphasic temperature curve.

Epistaxis, petechiae and purpuric lesions, though uncommon, may occur at any stage of the disease. Swallowed blood from epistaxis passed by rectum or vomited may be interpreted by the unwary as bleeding of gastrointestinal origin. Convulsions may occur during extreme temperature elevations and are fairly common with chikungunya fever.

After the febrile stage prolonged asthenia, mental depression, bradycardia and ventricular extrasystoles, common in adults, occur infrequently in children.

LABORATORY DATA. Pancytopenia may be manifest on the third or fourth day of illness, and neutropenia may persist or reappear during the latter stage of the disease and may continue into convalescence. White blood cell counts as low as 2000 per mm^3 have been recorded. Platelets rarely fall below 100,000 cells per mm^3. Venous clotting, bleeding and prothrombin times and plasma fibrinogen values are within normal ranges. The tourniquet test infrequently is positive. Mild acidosis, hemoconcentration, increased transaminase values and hypoproteinemia have been described during primary dengue virus infections, particularly in infants. Sinus bradycardia, ectopic ventricular foci and prolongation of the P-R interval may be observed electrocardiographically.

DIAGNOSIS AND DIFFERENTIAL DIAGNOSIS. *Clinical diagnosis* derives from a high index of suspicion and a knowledge of the geographic distribution and environmental cycle of causal viruses. Activities of the patient during the period preceding the onset of illness may give important clues to the possibility of infection.

Differential diagnosis includes a number of viral respiratory and influenza-like diseases and the early stages of malaria, scrub typhus, hepatitis and leptospirosis. Abortive forms of these latter diseases modified by therapy or vaccine may never evolve beyond a dengue-like stage.

Three arbovirus diseases have dengue-like courses, but without rash: Colorado tick fever, sandfly fever and Rift Valley fever. Colorado tick fever occurs sporadically among campers and hunters in the western United States; sandfly fever in the Mediterranean region, the Middle East, southern Russia and parts of the Indian subcontinent; and Rift Valley fever in East, Central and South Africa.

Because of the variations in clinical findings and the multiplicity of possible causative agents, the descriptive term "dengue-like disease" should be used until a specific etiologic diagnosis is provided by the laboratory. *Etiologic diagnosis* can be made by serologic study or isolation of the virus. Blood for comparative and viral studies should be obtained during the febrile period, preferably before the fourth day of illness and during the convalescent phase, 14 to 21 days after the onset. The acute phase serum or plasma may be frozen, optimally at −65° C or colder, to preserve the specimen for later virus isolation. *Serologic diagnosis* is dependent on a fourfold or greater increase in antibody titer in the paired serums by hemagglutination inhibition, complement fixation or neutralization test. It may not be possible to distinguish the infecting virus by serologic methods alone, particularly when there has been prior infection with another member of the same arbovirus group, e.g., yellow fever immunization followed by dengue infection. For this reason, isolation of the virus should be attempted.

PROGNOSIS. Primary infections with the viruses of dengue fever and dengue-like diseases are usually self-limited and benign. Fluid and electrolyte losses, hyperpyrexia and febrile convulsions are the most frequent complications in infants and young children, particularly in tropical countries. There is evidence that the prognosis may be adversely affected by previous infection with a closely related virus. (See Dengue Hemorrhagic Fever.)

PROPHYLAXIS. An attenuated vaccine for dengue type 1 and a killed vaccine for chikungunya are efficacious but not available for general use. Prophylaxis consists in avoiding mosquito bite by use of insecticides, repellents, body-covering with clothing, and screening of houses. Destruction of *Aedes aegypti* breeding sites is also effective. If water storage is mandatory, a tight-fitting lid or a thin layer of oil may prevent egg-laying or hatching. A larvicide, such as Abate [O,O′-(thiodi-p-phenylene)O,O,O′,O′-tetramethyl phosphorothioate], available as a 1 per cent sand granule formulation and effective at a concentration of 1 part per million, may be added safely to drinking water. Ultra-low volume spray equipment mounted on truck or airplane effectively dispenses the adulticide malathion for rapid intervention during an epidemic. Only personal antimosquito measures are effective against mosquitoes in the field, forest or jungle.

TREATMENT. Treatment is supportive. Bed rest is advised during the febrile period. Salicylates or cold sponging should be used to keep body temperature below 104° F. Salicylates or mild sedation may be required to control pain. Fluid and electrolyte replacement therapy is required when there are deficits due to sweating, fasting, thirsting, vomiting or diarrhea.

Casals, J., and Clarke, D. H.: Arboviruses. *In* F. L. Horsfall and I. Tamm (eds.): Viral and Rickettsial Infections of Man. 4th ed. Philadelphia, J. B. Lippincott Company, 1965, pp. 583–684.

Sabin, A. B.: Research on dengue during World War II. Am. J. Trop. Med. Hyg. *1*:30, 1952.

Wisseman, C. L., and Sweet, B. H.: The ecology of dengue. *In* May, J. M. (ed.): Studies in Disease Ecology. New York, Hafner Publishing Co., Inc., 1961, pp. 15–40.

DENGUE HEMORRHAGIC FEVER

(Philippine, Thai or Singapore Hemorrhagic Fever; Hemorrhagic Dengue; Acute Infectious Thrombocytopenic Purpura)

DEFINITION. Dengue hemorrhagic fever is a severe, often fatal, febrile disease caused by dengue viruses. It is characterized by shock, hemoconcentration, hypoproteinemia and abnormalities of hemostasis, and is currently thought to represent a hypersensitivity to a second infection with dengue virus.

HISTORY. Hammon in 1956 established the causative relation of dengue infection to dengue hemorrhagic fever, which may have occurred in Australian children as early as 1897. Recent epidemics have involved most of Southeast Asia.

ETIOLOGY. At least four distinct types of dengue virus (types 1 through 4) have been isolated from patients with hemorrhagic fever.

EPIDEMIOLOGY. Dengue hemorrhagic fever occurs in areas where multiple types of dengue virus are simultaneously or sequentially transmitted. It is almost exclusively a disease of children. It is endemic in tropical Asia where warm temperatures and the practice of water storage in homes result in large, permanent populations of *Aedes aegypti.* Under these conditions, infections with dengue viruses of all types are frequent, and second infections with heterologous types are common. Nearly all patients with typical severe hemorrhagic fever have a secondary rise of antibody against dengue virus, indicative of a previous infection with a closely related virus.

Nonimmune foreigners, adults as well as children, exposed to dengue virus during an outbreak of hemorrhagic fever have classic dengue fever or even a milder disease. Since hemorrhagic fever has been described in a Caucasian child born in Thailand, the differences in clinical manifestations of dengue infections between natives and foreigners are probably related more to immunologic status than to racial susceptibility.

PATHOLOGY. Usually no gross or microscopic lesions are found which might account for death. In rare instances, death may be due to gastrointestinal or intracranial hemorrhages. Minimal to moderate hemorrhages are seen in the upper gastrointestinal tract, and petechial hemorrhages are frequent in the interventricular septum of the heart, on the pericardium and on the subserosal surfaces of major viscera. Focal hemorrhages are occasionally seen in the lungs, liver, adrenals and subarachnoid space. The liver is usually enlarged, often with fatty changes. Yellow, watery, at times blood-tinged, effusions are present in serous cavities in about three fourths of patients. Retroperitoneal tissues are markedly edematous.

Microscopically there is perivascular edema in the soft tissues and widespread diapedesis of red blood cells. There may be maturational arrest of megakaryocytes in the bone marrow, and increased numbers of them are seen in the capillaries of the lungs, in renal glomeruli and in sinusoids of the liver and spleen. Proliferation of lymphocytoid and plasmacytoid cells, lymphocytolysis and lymphophagocytosis occur in the spleen and lymph nodes. Granulomatous-appearing germinal centers are present in the spleen, and there is depletion of lymphocytes in the thymus. In the liver there are varying degrees of fatty metamorphosis, focal midzonal necrosis, hyperplasia of the Kupffer cells, and non-nucleated cells with vacuolated acidophilic cytoplasm, resembling Councilman bodies, in the sinusoids. Skin biopsies reveal minimal necrosis of endothelial cells during the acute stage of illness. Platelet or fibrin thrombosis or necrosis of vessel walls has not been described.

Dengue virus is almost invariably absent from tissues at the time of death; fluorescein-labeled antidengue gamma globulin has failed to reveal dengue antigen in tissues obtained either before or after death. These tissue suspensions, however, contain large quantities of dengue-neutralizing substances.

PATHOLOGIC PHYSIOLOGY. Dengue hemorrhagic fever is characterized by two stages. Two to 5 days after the onset of a usual dengue illness the second phase, that of shock or hemorrhage, or both, occurs. At this time the patient has begun to produce large quantities of antidengue immunoglobulin (IgG), which presumably forms a complex with viral antigens and complement, resulting in consumption of complement. Increased vascular permeability may be mediated by a C′3 anaphylatoxin or other substances of immunologic nature. A mild degree of disseminated intravascular coagulation, plus liver damage and thrombocytopenia, may contribute additively to produce hemorrhage. Capillary damage allows fluid, electrolytes, protein and, in some instances, red blood cells to leak into extravascular spaces. This internal redistribution of fluid, together with deficits due to fasting, thirsting and vomiting, results in hemoconcentration, hypovolemia, increased cardiac work, tissue hypoxia, metabolic acidosis and hyponatremia. The timing and sequence of dengue infections required to produce the aberrant host response are unknown.

CLINICAL MANIFESTATIONS. The incubation period of dengue hemorrhagic fever is unknown but is presumed to be that of dengue fever. The progression of the illness is characteristic in the severely ill child. A relatively mild first phase with abrupt onset of fever, malaise, vomiting, headache, anorexia and cough is followed after 2 to 5 days by rapid clinical deterioration and physical collapse. In this second phase the patient usually manifests cold, clammy extremities, a warm trunk, flushed face and diaphoresis. He is restless and irritable, and complains of mid-epigastric pain. Frequently there are scattered petechiae on the forehead and extremities; spontaneous ecchymoses may appear, and easy bruisability and bleeding at sites of venipuncture are common. A macular or maculopapular rash may be present, and there may be circumoral and peripheral cyanosis. Respirations are rapid and often labored. The pulse is weak, rapid and thready, and the heart sounds are faint. The pulse pressure is frequently narrow (20 mm Hg or less); the systolic and diastolic pressures may be low or unobtainable. The liver may become palpable two to three fingerbreadths below the costal margin and is usually firm and nontender. Less than 10 per cent of patients manifest gross ecchymosis or gastrointestinal bleeding.

After a 24- to 36-hour period of crisis, convalescence is fairly rapid in the children who recover. The temperature may return to normal before or during the stage of shock. Bradycardia and ventricular extrasystoles are common during convalescence. Infrequently there is residual brain damage due either to prolonged shock or occasionally to intracranial hemorrhage. Death occurs in 10 to 40 per cent of patients with shock.

In contrast to the fairly characteristic pattern in the severely ill child, secondary dengue infections are relatively mild in the majority of instances, ranging from an inapparent infection through an undifferentiated, upper respiratory or dengue-like disease to an illness similar to that described above, but without apparent shock.

LABORATORY DATA. The most common hematologic abnormalities during clinical shock are a 20 per cent or greater increase in hematocrit over the recovery value, thrombocytopenia, mild leukocytosis (seldom exceeding 10,000 per mm^3) with 1 to 5 per cent of Türk's cells, prolonged bleeding time, and moderately prolonged prothrombin time (seldom less than 40 per cent of control). Particularly after prolonged periods of shock and metabolic acidosis, fibrinogen levels may be subnormal and fibrinogen split-products elevated. The tourniquet test gives a positive result early in the illness, except in the moribund child.

Other abnormalities include moderate elevations of the serum transaminases, mild metabolic acidosis with hyponatremia and, at times, hypochloremia, slight elevation of serum urea nitrogen and hypoalbuminemia. Roentgenograms of the chest reveal bronchopneumonia and pleural effusions in somewhat less than 50 per cent of patients.

DIAGNOSIS AND DIFFERENTIAL DIAGNOSIS. In areas endemic for dengue, hemorrhagic fever should be suspected in children with a febrile illness who exhibit shock, hemoconcentration, hypoproteinemia and hemorrhagic manifestations with or without hepatic enlargement. Since many rickettsial diseases, meningococcemia and other severe illnesses caused by a variety of agents may produce a similar clinical picture, the diagnosis should be made only when epidemiologic or serologic evidence suggests the possibility of dengue fever. Hemorrhagic manifestations have been described in other diseases of viral or presumed viral origin; these include the hemorrhagic fevers observed in Argentina, Bolivia, Korea and the Soviet Union. These diseases differ clinically from dengue hemorrhagic fever. The bases for diagnosis of dengue fever are described on preceding pages.

Antibody response is of the secondary type, with rapid and pronounced rise of both hemagglutination-inhibiting (HI) and complement-fixing (CF) antibodies to dengue antigen. There are usually high and apparently fixed titers of HI antibody (1:640 or greater) and CF antibody (1:32 or greater) in both acute and convalescent serums. Such titers are regarded as presumptive evidence of recent dengue infection.

PREVENTION. Preventive measures are described earlier under Dengue Fever. The possibility exists that dengue vaccination may sensitize a recipient, so that ensuing dengue infection may result in hemorrhagic fever. Vaccination with yellow fever 17D strain has no effect on dengue illness.

TREATMENT. Management requires immediate evaluation of vital signs and degrees of hemoconcentration, dehydration and electrolyte imbalance. Close monitoring is essential for at least 48 hours, since shock may occur or recur precipitously early in the disease. Patients who are cyanotic or have labored breathing should be given oxygen. Intravenous replacement of fluids and electrolytes is frequently sufficient to sustain patients until spontaneous recovery occurs. When elevation of the hematocrit value persists after replacement of fluids, plasma or plasma protein preparations are indicated. Care must be taken to avoid overhydration, which may contribute to cardiac failure. Transfusion of fresh blood or of platelets suspended in plasma may be required to control bleeding, but should not be given during hemoconcentration, and then only after evaluation of hemoglobin or hematocrit value.

Paraldehyde or chloral hydrate may be required for children who are markedly agitated. Pressor amines, alpha-adrenergic blocking agents, aldosterone, hydrocortisone and heparin have been widely utilized; their use has not resulted in a significant reduction of mortality over that observed with simple supportive therapy.

Cohen, S. N., and Halstead, S. B.: Shock associated with dengue infection. I. The clinical and physiological manifestations of dengue hemorrhagic fever in Thailand, 1964. J. Pediatr. *68*:448, 1966.

Ehrenkranz, N. J., Ventura, A. R., Cuadrado, R. R., Pond, W. L., and Porter, J. E.: Pandemic dengue in Caribbean countries and the southern United States—past, present and potential problems. New Engl. J. Med. *285*:1460, 1971.

Halstead, S. B., Nimmannitya, S., and Cohen, S. N.: Observations related to pathogenesis of dengue hemorrhagic fever: IV. Relation of disease severity to antibody response and virus recovered. Yale J. Biol. Med. *42*:311, 1970.

Halstead, S. B.: Observations related to pathogenesis of dengue hemorrhagic fever: VI. Hypotheses and discussion. Yale J. Biol. Med. *42*:350, 1970.

Russell, P. K., Intavivat, A., and Kanchanapilant, S.: Anti-dengue immunoglobulins and serum β1c/a globulin levels in dengue shock syndrome. J. Immunol. *102*:412, 1969.

OTHER VIRAL HEMORRHAGIC FEVERS

Viral hemorrhagic fevers are a loosely defined group of clinical syndromes in which hemorrhagic manifestations are either common or especially notable in the severe illness. Since overt hemorrhagic manifestation or abnormal hemostasis is relatively common in many viral diseases, the designation "viral hemorrhagic fever" should be regarded as noninclusive and largely of historical interest. For most hemorrhagic fevers, both the etiologic agents and the clinical syndromes differ. A list of the more important viral hemorrhagic fevers is given in Table 10–17.

ETIOLOGY. As shown in Table 10–17, six of the "viral hemorrhagic fevers" are caused by arthropod-borne (arbo) viruses. Four are members of arbovirus group B: (OHF, KFD, YF and DHF); one, a group A arbovirus (chikungunya); and one, ungrouped (Congo virus). Junin (AHF) and Machupo (BHF) are arenaviruses, a newly established morphologic and ecologic viral group. Although it is commonly thought that all viral hemorrhagic fevers are arthropod-borne, three are contracted from an environmental contamination caused by animals or animal cells (AHF, BHF, Marburg disease); this mode of transmission is also suspected for HF with renal syndrome.

EPIDEMIOLOGY. With rare exception, the viruses causing viral hemorrhagic fever are transmitted through a nonhuman agency. Since a specific ecosystem is required for viral survival, these are diseases of place. To initially consider a diagnosis, the physician must first establish that the patient has had an appropriate geographic or ecologic exposure. Laboratory infections with these agents have occurred, and this occupational hazard should be considered in a diagnostic evaluation. The geographic distribution, relative prevalence and ecologic aspects of the more common viral hemorrhagic fevers are summarized below. Yellow fever and dengue hemorrhagic fever are discussed in preceding sections.

Tick-borne Hemorrhagic Fevers

Omsk Hemorrhagic Fever (OHF). The disease occurs throughout the south central Soviet Union into northern Rumania. Vectors of OHF virus may include *Dermicentor pictus* and *D. marginatus,* but direct transmission from moles and muskrats to man seems well established. Human disease occurs in a spring-summer-autumn pattern, paralleling the activity of vectors. OHF occurs most frequently in persons with outdoor occupational exposure.

Kyasanur Forest Disease (KFD). Human cases, chiefly in adults, occur in one area of Mysore State,

TABLE 10–17 VIRAL HEMORRHAGIC FEVERS

MODE OF TRANSMISSION	DISEASE	VIRUS
Tick-borne	Omsk HF (OHF)	Omsk
	Crimean HF (CHF)	Congo
	Kyasanur Forest disease (KFD)	Kyasanur Forest disease
Mosquito-borne	Yellow fever (YF)	Yellow fever
	Dengue hemorrhagic fever (DHF)	Dengue (4 types)
	Chikungunya* (CHIK)	Chikungunya
Infected animals or materials to human	Argentine HF (AHF)	Junin
	Bolivian HF (BHF)	Machupo
	Marburg disease†	Marburg agent
Unknown	Hemorrhagic fever with renal syndrome	Not identified

*Associated at low frequency with petechiae, petechial hemorrhages and epistaxis. More severe hemorrhagic manifestations have been alleged in some studies.

†Marburg disease is caused by an agent tentatively classified as a rhabdovirus. The disease is characterized by sudden onset, myalgia, gastrointestinal distress, prostration and a second phase febrile period accompanied by hemorrhagic and encephalitic manifestations. A total of 31 human cases, all laboratory workers, are described. The agent was present in a shipment of African green monkeys shipped to various European countries in 1967. Infection was acquired by handling monkey tissues. Some human-to-human transmission occurred. Little is known of the epidemiology of this virus.

India. The principal vectors are two Ixodidae ticks, *Haemaphysalis turturis* and *H. spinigera.* Monkeys and forest rodents may be amplifying hosts.

Crimean Hemorrhagic Fever (CHF). Recognized in western Crimea, on the Kersch peninsula and in the Rostov-Don and Astrakhan regions, a somewhat similar disease occurs in Kazakstan and Uzbekistan. The vectors are *Hyalomma marginatum* and *H. anatolicum* which, along with hares and birds, may serve as a viral reservoir since transovarial transmission is likely. Disease occurs from June to September, largely among farmers and dairy workers.

HF Transmitted Through Environmental Contamination

Arenavirus Hemorrhagic Fever (AHF and BHF). The first described arenavirus, lymphocytic choriomeningitis virus (non-HF) establishes a persistent tolerant infection in the young of the common house mouse, *Mus musculus.* These rodents excrete virus continuously throughout life, contaminating food and fluids and creating an airborne infection hazard. There is experimental evidence that Machupo and Junin viruses have similar host-parasite relationships with several South American rodents. A highly fatal member of the group, *Lassa fever* (non-HF), is occasionally transmitted between humans and is the cause of sporadic outbreaks in West Africa.

Argentine Hemorrhagic Fever (AHF). First recognized in 1955, hundreds to several thousand cases occur annually from April through July in the maize-producing area northwest of Buenos Aires which reaches to the eastern margin of the Province of Córdoba. Junin virus has been isolated from the rodents *Mus musculus, Akodon arenicola* and *Calomys laucha laucha.* It is transmitted to migrant laborers who harvest the maize and who inhabit rodent-contaminated shelters.

Bolivian Hemorrhagic Fever (BHF). The recognized endemic area consists of the sparsely populated province of Beni in Amazonian Bolivia. Sporadic cases occur in farm families who raise maize, rice, yucca and beans. In the town of San Joaquin a disturbance in the domestic rodent ecosystem may have led to an outbreak of household infection caused by *Callomys callosus,* ordinarily a field rodent. Mortality rates are high in young children.

Hemorrhagic Fever with Renal Syndrome. The endemic area includes far eastern Siberia, parts of eastern Manchuria, Korea north of Seoul, an area west of the Ural mountains, Scandinavia, Czechoslovakia, Rumania and Bulgaria. Although the incidence and severity of hemorrhagic manifestations and mortality are lower in European Asia than in northeast Asia, the renal lesion is the same. Cases occur predominantly in the spring and summer. There appears to be no age factor in susceptibility, but because of occupational hazards, young adult men are most frequently attacked. Rodent plagues or evidence of rodent infestation have accompanied endemic and epidemic occurrences.

CLINICAL, PATHOLOGIC AND LABORATORY FEATURES

Omsk HF and Kyasanur Forest Disease. After an incubation period of 3 to 8 days, both diseases begin with sudden onset of fever and headache. In OHF there is moderate epistaxis, hematemesis and a hemorrhagic enanthem, but no profuse hemorrhage; bronchopneumonia is common. KFD is characterized by severe myalgia, prostration, bronchiolar involvement, often without hemorrhage, but occasionally with severe gastrointestinal bleeding. Severe epistaxis is regarded by some observers as a good prognostic sign. Severe leukopenia and thrombocytopenia occur in both diseases. In many patients recurrent febrile illness may follow an afebrile period of 7 to 15 days. This second phase takes the form of a meningoencephalitis.

Pathology and detailed pathophysiologic studies are scant. In KFD acute degeneration of renal tubules may correlate with the urinary changes noted. There also may be focal liver damage. In both diseases there is evidence of vascular dilatation, increased vascular permeability, gastrointestinal hemorrhages and numerous subserosal and interstitial petechial hemorrhages.

Crimean HF. The incubation period of 7 to 12 days is followed by a febrile period of 5 to 12 days and a prolonged convalescence. Disease begins with sudden onset of fever, malaise, severe myalgia, weakness, irritability and anorexia. The patient may develop an erythematous facial and truncal flush and injected conjunctivae. This is followed by a hemorrhagic enanthem on the soft palate and a fine petechial rash on the chest and abdomen. Less frequently there are large areas of purpura and bleeding from gums, nose, lungs, uterus and intestine. Hematuria and proteinuria are rare. Leukopenia with relative lymphocytosis and marked thrombocytopenia are common. Case fatality ranges from 2 to 50 per cent.

Argentine and Bolivian HF. The incubation period is commonly 10 to 14 days. Recognized clinical illnesses range from undifferentiated fever to the characteristic severe illness. Onset is usually gradual, with increasing fever, headache, diffuse myalgia and anorexia. A petechial enanthem appears on the soft palate 3 to 5 days after onset; about the same time a petechial exanthem is seen on the trunk. The tourniquet test may be positive. This may be followed by microscopic hematuria and frank hemorrhages from the stomach, intestines, nose, gums and uterus. Hypotension frequently occurs 6 to 8 days after onset, usually with defervescence. Twenty per cent of patients develop late neurologic involvement characterized by intention tremor of the tongue and associated speech abnormalities. In the severe case there may be intention tremors of the extremities, seizures and delirium. The cerebrospinal fluid is normal. The prolonged convalescence is accompanied by signs of autonomic nervous system lability such as postural hypotension, spontaneous flushing or blanching of the skin and intermittent diaphoresis. Marked leukopenia and mild to moderate thrombocytopenia are common. Pathologic studies are scant and without pathognomonic features. Usually focal hemorrhage, bleeding by diapedesis and little inflammatory reaction are seen.

HF with Renal Syndrome. In most cases the disease is characterized by fever, petechiae, mild hemorrhagic phenomenon and mild proteinuria followed by relatively uneventful recovery. In 20 per cent of recognized cases, the disease may progress through four rather distinct phases: The *febrile phase,* which lasts 3 to 8 days, is ushered in with fever, malaise and facial and truncal flushing, and is terminated by thrombocytopenia, petechiae and low-grade proteinuria. The *hypotensive phase* of 1 to 3 days follows defervescence. Loss of fluid from the intravascular compartment may result in marked hemoconcentration. Proteinuria and ecchymoses increase. The *oliguric phase,* usually 3 to 5 days in duration, is characterized by a low output of protein-rich urine, with increasing nitrogen retention, nausea, vomiting and dehydration. Confusion, extreme restlessness and hypertension are common. The *diuretic phase,* which may last for days or weeks, usually initiates clinical improvement. The kidneys show little concentrating ability, and the rapid loss of fluid may result in severe dehydration and shock. Potassium and sodium depletion may be a serious problem.

The fatal case manifests abundant protein-rich retroperitoneal edema. There is a marked hemorrhagic necrosis of the renal medulla.

DIAGNOSIS. Diagnosis rests upon a high index of suspicion in endemic areas. In nonendemic areas a history of recent travel, a recent laboratory exposure or, in rare instances, history of exposure to a previous human case might evoke suspicion of viral hemorrhagic fever.

In all viral hemorrhagic fevers except HF with renal syndrome, the viral agent circulates in the blood at least transiently during the early febrile stage. The diagnostic specimens and virus isolation systems required for group A and B arboviruses are as described previously under Dengue Fever. The principles for establishing an etiologic diagnosis of Argentine and Bolivian HF are similar. Acute phase blood or throat washings from patients can be inoculated intracerebrally into guinea pigs, infant hamsters or infant mice. Group reactive complement-fixing antibodies and specific neutralizing antibodies appear in convalescent serum 3 to 4 weeks after onset of illness. HF with renal syndrome is a clinical diagnosis only.

Differential Diagnosis. The mild case of hemorrhagic fever might be confused with almost any self-limited systemic bacterial or viral infection. In the more severe cases it is important to consider typhoid fever, epidemic, murine or scrub typhus, leptospirosis or a rickettsial spotted fever. With the exception of leptospirosis, effective chemotherapeutic agents are available for these diseases. Many of them may be acquired in geographic or ecologic locations similar to those which may provide exposure to a viral hemorrhagic fever.

PREVENTION. A form of inactivated mouse brain vaccine is said to be effective in preventing OHF. A similar vaccine for KFD was produced experimentally but is no longer available. Prevention of tick bite includes careful examination of the skin after outdoor exposure. Tight-fitting clothing which fully covers the extremities is helpful, as is the use of tick repellents. Disease transmitted from a rodent-infected environment can be prevented by any of several methods of rodent control. Elimination of refuse and rodent breeding sites is particularly successful in urban or suburban environments.

TREATMENT. The principle involved in all these diseases, especially HF with renal syndrome, is the careful reversal of any specific physiologic derangement such as dehydration, hemoconcentration, renal failure and protein, electrolyte or blood losses. Although some have claimed that disseminated intravascular coagulation (DIC) occurs in all viral hemorrhagic fevers, the contribution of this phenomenon to the hemorrhagic manifestations has not been well established; heparin should be used only if severe DIC is documented. The therapeutic efficacy of steroids, pressor amines or alpha-adrenergic blocking agents has not been established. Sedatives should be selected with regard to the possibility of kidney or liver damage. The successful management of HF with renal syndrome may require renal dialysis.

SCOTT B. HALSTEAD

Benenson, A. S. (ed.): Control of Communicable Diseases in Man. 11th ed. Washington, D.C. American Public Health Association, 1970.
Casals, J., Henderson, B. E., Hoogstraal, H., Johnson, K. M., and Shelokov, A.: A review of Soviet viral hemorrhagic fevers, 1969. J. Infect. Dis. *122*:437, 1970.
Clarke, D. H., and Casals, J.: Arboviruses: Group B. *In* Horsfall, F. L., Jr., and Tamm, I. (eds.): Viral and Rickettsial Infections of Man. 4th ed. Philadelphia, J. B. Lippincott Company, 1965.
Johnson, K. M., Halstead, S. B., and Cohen, S. N.: Hemorrhagic fevers of Southeast Asia and South America, a comparative appraisal. Progr. Med. Virol. *9*:106, 1967.
Kissling, R. E., Murphy, F. A., and Henderson, B. E.: Marburg virus. Ann. N.Y. Acad. Sci. *174*:932, 1970.

INFECTIONS BY ENTEROVIRUSES

The enteroviruses are members of a large family of picornaviruses, so called for their small size (pico) and ribonucleic acid (RNA) core. The picornaviruses are also represented by the rhinoviruses, as well as by a number of viruses of animals.

Enteroviruses primarily inhabit the alimentary tract of man and include polioviruses, coxsackieviruses and echoviruses. Additional types discovered since 1969 have been designated and numbered only as enteroviruses. These agents have many properties in common. They are small (20 to 30 nm in diameter) and have a single-stranded ribonucleic acid core surrounded by 32 protein subunits; they lack a lipid component, as reflected by their resistance to inactivation by ether. Infection has been induced by RNA extracted from representative enteroviruses. Viral activity is relatively stable at room temperature and well preserved at −20 to −70° C. Thermostability varies under different conditions, but inactivation is probably complete at 60 to 65° C for 30 minutes. Viral activity persists at pH 3. Interference has been noted between different enteroviruses as well as between members of this group and other viruses. Enteroviruses have maximal incidence in warm weather (summer season in temperate zones) and other similarities of epidemiologic pattern. Serologic surveys for detection of antibody in various populations have shown that human experience with these agents is ubiquitous and cumulative. Many of these viruses produce disease in man, and all induce recognizable infection in one or more experimental hosts, including primates, rodents and cells in tissue culture. The principal associations of enteroviruses with human diseases, as currently recognized, are indicated in Tables 10–18 and 10–19.

COXSACKIEVIRUS INFECTIONS

ETIOLOGY. Coxsackieviruses, named for the town in New York state where they were first encountered, have in common the capacity to induce fatal infection, frequently with paralysis, in newborn mice and hamsters. The manifestations of infection depend upon route of inoculation, strain of virus and size of dose, as well as age of the host. Dalldorf classified these agents into two groups, differentiated by the features of the diseases induced in newborn mice. Group A viruses characteristically cause flaccid paralysis attributable to extensive necrosis of skeletal muscle; there are no lesions elsewhere, except that massive excretion of myoglobin may result in renal damage. Group B viruses cause tremors, spasticity and paralysis, with focal myositis and encephalomyelitis, myocarditis, hepatitis, pancreatitis, necrosis of brown fat and, less regularly, lesions in other organs. Some group B viruses also induce carditis and hepatitis, and a form of pancreatitis in mature mice in which the islets of Langerhans are spared and the acinar tissue first becomes necrotic and then is replaced by fat. A strain of B-4 virus has been shown to damage islet as well as exocrine cells. The greater susceptibility of newborn as compared to older mice may be attributable to the fact that only the latter produce interferon after infection by coxsackieviruses. Corticosteroids, which increase susceptibility of mature mice, inhibit formation of interferon. Lymphocyte-mediated defenses may contribute to recovery from coxsackievirus infections.

Twenty-four coxsackieviruses of group A (designated A-1 to A-24) and six of group B (designated B-1 to B-6) have been recognized to date (A-23 is identical with echovirus type 9). Each of these agents is antigenically distinct and can be identified and differentiated by neutralization and complement fixation tests, and some strains (B-1, B-3, B-5, A-7, A-20, A-21, A-24) are identifiable by hemagglutination reactions with specific immune animal serums. A-9 and all the group B viruses share a common antigen which is detected by agar gel diffusion. In patients infected with group B viruses, homologous viral antigen has been detected by immunofluorescent techniques in exfoliated cells in urine and in affected organs examined post mortem. Circulating antibodies can usually be found in the animal or human host within 2 weeks of infection or of the onset of symptoms and reach maximum titer in about 3 weeks. Neutralizing antibodies persist for years, apparently associated with resistance to homologous reinfection. Antibody is transferred passively from mother to offspring.

Animals other than mice have been infected experimentally with some strains of coxsackieviruses, but in general are less susceptible and have not been extensively used. A-7, A-14, A-16 and B-2 viruses induce poliomyelitis-like lesions in monkeys. Acute carditis and mitral stenosis have also been induced in monkeys. All six group B and all but six Group A viruses (types A-1, A-4, A-5, A-6, A-19 and A-22) produce characteristic cellular

TABLE 10–18 ASSOCIATION OF ENTEROVIRUSES WITH HUMAN DISEASE

Enteroviruses	
Poliovirus Types 1, 2, 3	Paralytic poliomyelitis (mild to severe) Polioencephalitis Ataxia (type 1) Nonparalytic poliomyelitis Abortive poliomyelitis, pharyngitis or undifferentiated febrile disorder
Coxsackievirus, group A Types 1-24 (type 23 same as Echovirus type 9)	Aseptic meningitis (epidemic, types 7, 9–16; sporadic, many types) Paralysis (types 4, 7, 9) Encephalitis (types 2, 5, 6, 7, 9, 16) Ataxia (types 4, 7, 9) Guillain-Barre syndrome (types 2, 5, 6, 9) Exanthem (see Table 10–19) Herpangina and other enanthems (see Table 10–19) Lymphonodular pharyngitis (type 10) Lymphadenitis (types 5, 6) Acute respiratory illness (types 9, 21, 24 in addition to herpanginal strains), pharyngitis or undifferentiated febrile disorder (many types) Hepatitis (types 4, 9, 10) Myocarditis or pericarditis (types 1, 4, 9, 16, 23)
Coxsackievirus, group B Types 1-6	Aseptic meningitis (types 1-6) Paralysis (types 1-5) Encephalitis (types 1, 2, 3, 5) Epidemic myalgia (types 1-6) Encephalomyocarditis in early infancy (types 1-5) Myocarditis or pericarditis (types 1-5) Exanthem (see Table 10–19) Enanthem (see Table 10–19) Orchitis (types 1-5) Hepatitis (type 5) Acute respiratory illness, pharyngitis or undifferentiated febrile disorder (types 1-5)
Echovirus Types 1-33 (types 10 and 28 deleted, type 8 same as type 1, type 9 same as coxsackievirus A type 23)	Aseptic meningitis (types 1-7, 9, 11-23, 25, 30, 31) Paralysis (types 1, 2, 3, 4, 6, 7, 9, 11, 16, 18, 30) Encephalitis (types 2, 3, 4, 6, 7, 9, 11, 14, 18, 19) Guillain-Barré syndrome (types 6, 7, 22) Ataxia (types 9, 19) Acute glomerulonephritis (type 9) Acute pleurodynia (types 1, 6, 9, 19) Acute pericarditis (types 1, 9, 19) Acute myocarditis (types 3, 6, 9) Exanthem (see Table 10–19) Enanthem (see Table 10–19) Diarrhea (types 11, 14, 18) Acute respiratory illnesses, pharyngitis or undifferentiated febrile disorder (types 1, 3, 6, 9, 11, 19, 20 and others)

Modified from Committee on the Enteroviruses, National Foundation: the Enteroviruses. Am. J. Pub. Hlth. *47*:1556, 1957.

damage or cytopathic effect (CPE) in cultured normal or malignant primate cells. Cultivation in cells of other animals has been less successful. Plaques produced by coxsackieviruses, when grown in susceptible cells under agar, are round and resemble those of polioviruses but develop more slowly. Coxsackievirus B-3 has been observed to have an oncolytic effect after serial passage through HeLa tumors in rats.

Coxsackieviruses are small, approximately 28 nm in diameter, and have a ribonucleic acid core which carries the hereditary determinants of infectivity and virulence. An A-10 strain has been purified and crystallized. By means of electron microscopy, crystalline arrays of B-5 virus have been observed within the cytoplasm of infected cells.

Coxsackieviruses are unusually stable. Viral activity is maintained at room temperature for many days and can be preserved for a long time if in-

TABLE 10–19 ENTEROVIRAL EXANTHEMS AND ENANTHEMS

Exanthems	
Occurrence	
Epidemic	Echovirus 16 (Boston exanthem) Echovirus 9 Coxsackievirus A-9 Coxsackievirus A-5, A-16 (hand, foot and mouth disease)
Smaller outbreaks	Coxsackievirus A-4, 9, 10, B-5 Echovirus 2, 4, 11
Sporadic	Coxsackievirus A-2, 4, 5, 9, 16 Coxsackievirus B, types 1-5 Echovirus 1-7, 9, 11, 14, 16, 18, 19, 25, 32
Type of rash	
Maculopapular ("rubelliform")	Coxsackieviruses A and B and Echoviruses—all types associated with rash
Vesicular	Coxsackievirus A, types 5, 16 (hand, foot and mouth disease); Coxsackievirus A, types 4, 9; Coxsackievirus B, types 1, 4
Petechial	Echovirus 3, 4, 6, 9, 11, 14, 19, 25 Coxsackievirus A-9, B-3
Urticarial	Coxsackievirus A-9, A-16, B-5 Echovirus 11
Telangiectatic	Echovirus 25, 32
Enanthems	
Herpangina	Coxsackievirus A, types 1-10, 16, 17, 22 Coxsackievirus B, types 1-5; Echovirus 9, 17
Lymphonodular pharyngitis	Coxsackievirus A-10, Echovirus 30
Gingivostomatitis	Coxsackievirus A-3, A-5
Miscellaneous	Coxsackievirus A-5, A-9, A-16 Coxsackievirus B-2, B-3, B-5 Echovirus 6, 9, 16

Modified from Horstmann, D. M.: Pediatrics *41*:867, 1968.

fected tissues are stored in glycerin or in a frozen state. In aqueous suspensions activity disappears after exposure to a temperature of 60° C for 30 minutes. When these viruses are suspended in milk or ice cream, higher temperatures are required for their inactivation. Like polioviruses, these agents retain their activity through a wide range of pH (2.3 to 9.4 for a day and 4.0 to 8.0 for a week). They are not inactivated by ether, 70 per cent ethyl alcohol, 5 per cent Lysol, 1 per cent Roccal or antibiotics, but are inactivated rapidly by tenth-normal (0.1N) hydrochloric acid, 2 per cent tincture of iodine and 0.3 per cent formaldehyde.

EPIDEMIOLOGY. Coxsackieviruses have been encountered throughout the world in epidemic and sporadic distribution. Like other enteroviruses, they have been recovered most commonly from human feces and pharyngeal swabbings, and also from sewage and flies. Recently coxsackieviruses B-1, B-3 and B-5, as well as echovirus 6, have been isolated repeatedly from nasal, pharyngeal and rectal swabbings of beagle dogs which had presumably acquired infection from human sources. Neutralizing antibodies to polioviruses, coxsackieviruses and echoviruses have been found in serum of dogs and other domestic animals. Strains of all the group B types and many different group A viruses have been recovered from the cerebrospinal fluid of patients with viral meningitis. Recovery of a coxsackievirus during life from blood, urine or other human sources has been less common. Virus in relatively high titer has been detected in the heart, brain and other organs of infants, but rarely of older persons, after death. No natural reservoir of infection other than man has been found, though flies, dogs and possibly cockroaches are able to transport these agents.

In temperate zones coxsackieviruses have been recovered mainly during the summer and fall; in tropical areas and to a lesser extent elsewhere they may be encountered throughout the year. Infection is more common in children. Atypically, infection by coxsackievirus A-21 and associated acute respiratory illnesses have been observed more frequently in young adults during the winter. The types of virus prevalent in a community vary from year to year. Enteroviruses may pass from mother to fetus in utero, and studies of enterovirus infections during pregnancy have revealed a relation between maternal infection with some of these viruses and malformations in the offspring: coxsackievirus B-2 and B-4 infections with urogenital, A-9 with digestive, and B-3 and B-4 with cardiovascular anomalies. Transmission (fecal-oral vs respiratory) and strain differences may influence clinical manifestations. Spread is rapid through susceptible members of a household. Rates of infection may be higher under poor living conditions. Some of these viruses cause epidemics of human disease, but at unpredictable intervals and locations. Successive infections with different enteroviruses are common; with strains of the same type, extremely rare. Immunity appears to be type-specific and relatively lasting. Communicability of infection by coxsackieviruses is similar to that in poliomyelitis.

PATHOLOGY. Maculopapular, petechial, vesicular and telangiectatic lesions of skin, and papules, vesicles, ulcers and lymphonodular lesions of mucous membranes have been noted. Myocarditis, encephalitis, hepatitis, pancreatitis, pneumonia, pulmonary hemorrhage and inflammatory changes in the spinal cord have been observed in newborn infants with fatal disease attributed to a group B virus. Fatal myocarditis, pericarditis and endocarditis have occurred in older persons. For example, coxsackievirus B-3 was recovered post mortem from the pericardial fluid of a 15 year old girl with fever, aches, exanthem, lymphadenopathy, diarrhea and cardiomegaly who at autopsy had meningoencephalitis, hepatitis, myopericarditis and terminal bronchopneumonia. In a few instances myositis and degenerative changes have been observed in biopsies of skeletal muscle. In cases of sudden death among infants from whom group A and other enteroviruses have been isolated, the principal pathologic lesions were laryngitis, epiglottitis, pneumonia, bronchitis, myocarditis and erythroblastosis. Calcific pancarditis has been observed in a stillborn infant with immunofluorescent evidence of coxsackievirus B-3 infection. Myocarditis associated with group B viruses is not uncommon in the fetus and newborn. Immunofluorescent techniques provide a ready way to detect viral antigen.

CLINICAL MANIFESTATIONS. Probably the commonest clinical expression of infection by an enterovirus is an acute, self-limited, febrile illness without distinctive features, occurring during the summer months and mainly affecting children. In some cases attention may be attracted to particular manifestations or lesions such as meningitis, myalgia, carditis, rash or exanthem. Two or more of these features may be encountered among different patients in a household, in a community outbreak or even in the same patient; in other persons infection is clinically inapparent, recognized only by recovery of virus or demonstration of an antibody response. Usually, as shown in Tables 10–18 and 10–19, more than one but not every enterovirus can induce each of the various clinical syndromes which have been etiologically associated with these agents.

Aseptic Meningitis. This syndrome (see below, this Section) can be caused by any of a large number of viruses. Coxsackieviruses have frequently been found in association with sporadic cases and in epidemics during summer and fall. All the group B viruses and 16 different group A viruses have been recovered from patients with this disorder, with the group B, A-7, A-9 and A-16 viruses appearing in epidemic distribution. All the group B types and at least 12 of group A have been recovered from spinal fluid. Some patients have experienced successive episodes of enteroviral meningitis, each usually attributable to a different virus. In two infants the same virus, coxsackievirus B-5, has been isolated during two attacks approximately a year apart.

The clinical picture of aseptic meningitis caused by a coxsackievirus is not distinctive. The onset may be sudden or gradual; in approximately half the instances it is initiated by a prodromal phase. In one patient viremia with a B-2 strain was demonstrated 5 days before the appearance of meningeal signs. Anorexia, malaise, fever, nausea and abdominal pain are frequent early complaints. The temperature may be elevated to 40° C (104° F). Ultimately headache, drowsiness, vomiting and discomfort or stiffness of the neck or back may appear, occasionally with focal or generalized myalgia. Physical examination may reveal hyperemia of the pharynx, occasionally with discrete vesicles or ulcers, and some degree of resistance to flexion of the neck and back. Persistent muscular stiffness or weakness is usually equivocal or absent. The tendon reflexes remain normal.

The white blood cell count is normal or only slightly elevated. The cells of the cerebrospinal fluid are increased, usually not in excess of 500 per mm^3 but occasionally as high as 2000 or more. Initially 10 to 50 per cent are polymorphonuclear cells; later, lymphocytes predominate. Glucose levels are usually normal; protein may be slightly elevated.

The course is characteristically uncomplicated and terminates in complete recovery; in older patients fatigue and irritability may persist for several months.

Other Neurologic Disorders. Paralysis, encephalitis, ataxia and infectious neuronitis have infrequently been associated with coxsackieviruses. Paralysis, in most instances mild and transitory, has been observed in patients infected with group A viruses types 4, 7 and 9 and with B viruses types 1 to 5. Exclusive of newborn infants, encephalitis has been found in association with A types 2, 5, 6, 7, 9 and 16 and B types 1, 2, 3 and 5. Group A viruses types 4 and 9 have been recovered from fecal specimens of patients with ataxia, and types 2, 5, 6 and 9 have been encountered in patients with the Guillain-Barré syndrome.

Pleurodynia (Epidemic Myalgia; Devil's Grip; Bornholm Disease). Pleurodynia, recognized in 1856 by Finsen in Iceland, has occurred in epidemics throughout the world, usually in summer or fall. The monograph by Sylvest in 1934 presents a classic description of an outbreak on the Danish island of Bornholm. Since 1949 coxsackieviruses of group B have been shown to cause this disorder. Association with other enteroviruses has also been reported.

The incubation period is usually 2 to 4 days. The illness begins suddenly with fever, headache and pain in the muscles of the chest or abdomen on one or both sides. Characteristically sharp or stabbing, the pain may be extreme and is accentuated by respirations. Sometimes pain is localized in the lower part of the abdomen and may simulate an acute surgical condition. Superficial tenderness and palpable swelling of muscles in affected areas may be detected. The extremities are rarely involved. Although pleurisy may be suggested, auscultation and roentgenographic examination of the chest seldom reveal abnormalities. Splenomegaly is infrequent. The white blood cell count is not unusual.

Fever and pain subside within 2 or 3 days, but in about a fourth of the cases recur on one or more occasions after asymptomatic intervals of 2 or 3 days. Often several members of a family are affected, usually with somewhat different manifestations and degrees of severity. Signs of cardiac disease may be associated. Involvement of the central nervous system may be evidenced by convulsions, encephalitic manifestations or pleocytosis of the cerebrospinal fluid. Except for occasional cardiac or meningeal involvement and orchitis in mature males, complications are unusual and recovery is spontaneous.

Encephalomyocarditis in the Newborn Infant. Gear and his associates in South Africa first showed that group B coxsackieviruses may cause generalized and sometimes fatal intrauterine or neonatal infection in human infants. Cases have occurred in relation to pleurodynia, meningitis or other acute febrile illnesses in the mother about the time of delivery.

The infant usually becomes ill suddenly, most often within the first 10 days of life and sometimes shortly after a brief episode of diarrhea and anorexia. Tachycardia, dyspnea and cyanosis may appear early, and lethargy, grayish pallor and mild jaundice are typical manifestations. The temperature may be depressed or elevated. The heart, liver and sometimes spleen are enlarged. Electrocardiographic changes are characteristic of myocarditis. The cerebrospinal fluid may be xanthochromic and the leukocytes and protein may be increased.

The clinical course may be rapidly fatal or progress to complete recovery. In fatal cases viruses have been recovered from the blood, brain and spinal cord as well as from the myocardium and other organs. Postmortem examinations have revealed lesions in the brain, heart, liver and other organs resembling those seen in experimentally infected newborn mice. Not all neonatal infections are severe or fatal; some are mild or even inapparent, as found in a nursery outbreak associated with coxsackievirus B-5.

Acute Myocarditis or Pericarditis. Myocarditis, pericarditis or endocarditis may occur in older children or adults infected with a coxsackievirus of group B or, less frequently, group A. The virus has been recovered from pericardial fluid, or in fatal cases from the myocardium. The etiologic role of enteroviruses recovered only from the oropharynx or stools of surviving patients with acute cardiac disorders has been difficult to establish. Nonetheless, enteroviruses, especially those capable of inducing muscle lesions in mice, are prominent among known causes of acute inflammatory cardiac disease.

Herpangina. Herpangina, an acute, self-limited febrile disorder, is characterized by distinctive papular, vesicular and ulcerative lesions on the anterior tonsillar pillars, soft palate, tonsils, pharynx and posterior buccal mucosa. First described by Zahorsky in 1924, it was shown by Heubner and his associates in 1951 to be etiologically associated with six different group A coxsackieviruses (types 2, 4, 5, 6, 8, 10). Since then additional group A viruses (types 1, 3, 7, 9, 16, 17, 22) have been found in typical cases, and the characteristic enanthem has also been observed in patients infected with group B types 1 through 5 and echovirus types 9 and 17, including some patients with such additional manifestations of enteroviral infection as meningitis, pleurodynia or rash.

After an incubation period of 2 to 4 days the illness is usually initiated by an abrupt elevation of temperature to as high as 40.5° C (105° F). Anorexia and dysphagia are common, and patients over 2 years of age complain of sore throat. Headache and abdominal pain are encountered less often. Infrequently convulsions occur with the fever. The pharynx is usually hyperemic. Characteristic discrete lesions appear initially as white or grayish papules or later as shallow ulcers 1 to 5 mm in diameter, each surrounded by a red areola. They range from one to about 15 in number and are commonly located on the anterior pillars of the fauces, less frequently on the palate, tonsils, uvula or tongue (Fig. 10–51, p. 656). These lesions are not invariably present, however. Genital ulceration attributed to infection by A-10 virus has been described in a 7 year old girl with herpangina. Acute parotitis complicating herpangina has also been reported. Rhinitis, cough, otitis media, sinusitis, diarrhea, generalized myalgia and meningeal irritation are not typical features of herpangina. The illness generally follows an uncomplicated course to recovery. Fever may last 1 to 4 days and the ulcers heal within a week. The white blood cell count is usually normal or only slightly elevated.

Acute Lymphonodular Pharyngitis. Coxsackievirus A-10 was encountered in an outbreak of illness resembling herpangina. Patients complained of fever, headache and sore throat. Examination revealed small white or yellowish nodular lesions of the uvula, anterior pillars and posterior pharynx which subsided without vesiculation or ulceration. Histologic examination showed the papules to be heavily infiltrated with lymphocytes.

Fever with Lymphadenitis. Coxsackieviruses A-5 and A-6 were associated in Africa with a febrile disorder resembling glandular fever which lasted 4 to 10 days. The illness was characterized by an abrupt onset and tender, swollen lymph nodes; stiffness of the neck and splenomegaly were noted in a few instances.

Hand, Foot and Mouth Disease. Coxsackieviruses A-16 and A-5 especially, but also A-4, 9 and 10, have been recovered from infants and children with a syndrome called "hand, foot and mouth disease" characterized by vesicular and ulcerative lesions in the mouth, a maculopapular rash, and vesicles on the hands and feet. In some cases a transient erythematous rash has been seen on the buttocks as well as the extremities. The course is acute and usually self-limited, but fatal cases in infants infected with A-16 have been reported.

Exanthems. Rashes have also been reported in association with other types of coxsackieviruses. These are generally maculopapular, though vesicles and urticaria or petechiae have been seen in some cases. (See Table 10–19.)

Hepatitis. Hepatic lesions occur in newborn infants with generalized infection by coxsackieviruses of group B. Other coxsackieviruses may affect the liver in infants or older subjects. A-10 and B-5 viruses have been encountered in outbreaks of mild hepatic disorder; and A-4 and A-9 viruses have been recovered post mortem from the blood and from the liver, respectively, of patients with signs of hepatitis.

Acute Respiratory Illness and Other Undifferentiated Disorders. In addition to herpangina and other illnesses characterized by pharyngitis, coxsackieviruses have been found in association with acute respiratory illnesses, including both undifferentiated and typical forms. In an outbreak of illness among infants and children attributed to A-9 virus, three had pneumonia and the virus was recovered from the liver and lung of one who died. A-21 virus (Coe) has been encountered repeatedly in outbreaks of acute respiratory infection, mainly among military recruits, and has been shown to cause "common colds" or mild febrile upper respiratory tract illness in human volunteers. A-24 virus (Pett) was recovered from the feces of children during an institutional outbreak of respiratory disease.

Infection with each of the group B viruses has produced a varied spectrum of clinical manifestations within a community and often within a single family. Sore throat or other respiratory symptoms may occur during the prodromal stage in patients with aseptic meningitis or pleurodynia and may be the only features of illness in other members of the household. Coxsackieviruses of several serotypes have been encountered in outbreaks of febrile respiratory illness in families, camps and institutions. B-3 and B-5 viruses were found in association with respiratory disease among infants and children during serial long-term studies in an orphanage. B viruses have also been recovered occasionally from patients with croup, bronchiolitis, vesicular pharyngitis, pneumonia and pleurisy, but are not considered to be principal causes of these clinical entities. On the other hand, mild respiratory illnesses are probably frequently attributable to coxsackieviruses, especially during the summer and fall.

DIAGNOSIS AND DIFFERENTIAL DIAGNOSIS. Diagnosis of infection by a coxsackievirus is suggested by clinical and epidemiologic findings and confirmed by the recovery of virus and the demonstration of a related increase in titer of homologous neutralizing antibodies in paired sera obtained during the acute and convalescent phases of illness. Primary recovery of virus may be achieved by inoculation of newborn mice, or preferably in the case of group B types 1 to 6, A-9 and A-23 viruses, by propagation in tissue cultures. Coxsackieviruses which agglutinate human group 0 erythrocytes at 37° C (in maximum titer with red blood cells from newborn infants) can be identified by hemagglutination inhibition tests. Since infection by any one of these viruses may stimulate complement-fixing antibodies to heterologous strains, determinations by this technique are of limited diagnostic value. Tests for presence of viral antigen or antibody using immunofluorescence techniques may provide early presumptive evidence of infection. It should be emphasized that the establishment of a causative relation between a coxsackievirus and associated disease requires careful correlation of pertinent clinical, epidemiologic and laboratory evidence.

Differentiation of *aseptic meningitis* caused by a coxsackievirus from bacterial meningitis, leptospirosis or space-occupying lesions, or from infections of the central nervous system caused by other viruses such as poliovirus, echovirus, mumps, lymphocytic choriomeningitis, equine encephalitis or herpes simplex virus, is often indicated by clinical and epidemiologic evidence and can usually be verified in the laboratory. Recovery of a coxsackievirus from cerebrospinal fluid collected during the acute stage of illness is positive diagnostic evidence. When both a coxsackievirus and another viral agent, especially a poliovirus or echovirus, are isolated simultaneously from a patient, it may be difficult to determine the etiologic significance of each virus to the associated disease.

Paralysis caused by an enterovirus other than a poliovirus has been encountered occasionally in individual patients, but not in epidemic distribution except with coxsackievirus A-7.

Pleurodynia attributable to a coxsackievirus must be differentiated from other causes of thoracic pain, particularly pneumonia and pleurisy, and from other causes of abdominal pain, including acute gastroenteritis, appendicitis, volvulus, intussusception, peptic ulcer and disease of the gallbladder. Whether a group B coxsackievirus can cause pancreatitis in man as in mice has not been determined, but epidemiologic evidence has suggested an association between coxsackievirus B-4 infection and diabetes. The superficial quality of the pain, the absence of deep abdominal or rectal tenderness, the relatively normal leukocyte count and the absence of abnormal roentgenologic findings should aid in the recognition of pleurodynia. Consideration of pleurodynia, particularly during the season of prevalence or in the presence of a local outbreak, may avert unnecessary surgery. *Orchitis* complicating pleurodynia or aseptic meningitis must be differentiated from that of mumps.

Generalized infection with myocarditis caused by a group B coxsackievirus is suggested in the newborn infant by tachycardia, signs of myocarditis and circulatory collapse, particularly when epidemic myalgia is prevalent in the vicinity, or following an acute illness of the mother possibly attributable to infection by the same virus. This disorder must be differentiated from congenital heart disease and other neonatal infections.

In older patients *carditis* attributable to a coxsackievirus may be difficult to distinguish from acute cardiac disease of different or undetermined origin.

Herpangina is suggested by its occurrence in seasonal outbreaks in the community, and in individual patients by the presence of discrete vesicular or ulcerative lesions in characteristic distribution on the anterior pillars of the tonsils, the soft palate or uvula. In this last respect the lesions differ from those attributable to herpes simplex virus; the latter may occur in the faucial areas, but are commonly distributed more diffusely in the gingival and buccal mucosa, on mucocutaneous borders and on skin. Occasionally lesions typical of herpangina are seen in patients infected with coxsackievirus of group B or echovirus. Coxsackieviruses of group A and herpesviruses are readily isolated from human sources by tests in suckling mice, but differ in their capacity to grow in various tissue cultures; each can be identified by appropriate procedures in the laboratory. The oral lesions of other bacterial and viral diseases, moniliasis, infectious mononucleosis, blood dyscrasias, deficiency diseases and heavy metal poisoning are unlikely to be confused.

Exanthems or *enanthems* occurring during the warm seasons, especially in epidemic distribution, should suggest enteroviral infection. The vesicular stomatitis and rash of the syndrome designated hand, foot and mouth disease should suggest infection with coxsackievirus A-16 or A-5, also A-4, A-9 or A-10. The rash associated with A-23 (Echo 9) infection often appears with violaceous lesions on the cheeks, spreading to the trunk and extremities and even to the palms and soles. The rashes associated with enteroviral infections are frequently described as maculopapular or rubelliform, but may be vesicular, petechial or urticarial; they must be distinguished from those encountered in other exanthematous diseases of childhood and from those resulting from administration of drugs.

Enteroviruses are not generally regarded as important in the causation of *respiratory diseases,* and their role in these disorders may be overlooked or difficult to prove. The forms of enterovirus-related respiratory illnesses are multiple, not distinctive and, in most instances, relatively mild. Enteroviral infection should be suspected in patients with respiratory disorders occurring during the seasonal prevalence of these viruses and especially in affected members of a household in which other members are experiencing enterovirus-related disease.

PROGNOSIS. Complete recovery from disease caused by coxsackieviruses can usually be expected except in newborn infants, in whom infection with a group B virus may prove fatal, and in some older patients with severe neurologic or cardiac disorders.

TREATMENT AND CONTROL MEASURES. No definitive therapy is known. Treatment is supportive and symptomatic. Specific measures to control infection by coxsackievirus are not available.

ECHOVIRUS INFECTIONS

The introduction of tissue culture techniques for recovery of virus from the alimentary tract led to the accidental discovery of a hitherto unrecognized group of enteroviruses, referred to initially as enteric human cytopathogenic "orphan" or ECHO viruses and now called echoviruses. Many of these agents have since been shown to cause human disease.

Echoviruses, though less extensively studied, appear to have in common many of the biologic, chemical and physical properties of other enteroviruses, including comparable size and structure, RNA core, relative thermal stability and resistance to inactivation by ether, common antiseptics and antimicrobial agents. They are all cytopathogenic in variable degree for human or monkey cells in tissue culture and, when grown in appropriate cells under agar, produce distinctive plaques.

The echoviruses can be separated into two groups based on capacity for growth and kind of plaques found in cultures of cells from rhesus and patas monkeys. In general, echoviruses do not cause disease in suckling mice with the exception of type 9, which in this and other respects appears indistinguishable from coxsackievirus A-23. Type 6 has been adapted to mice, causing lesions in muscle resembling coxsackievirus B infections. Some of the echoviruses (types 1, 4, 6, 13) produce neuronal lesions in monkeys after experimental injection into the central nervous system or muscle; paralysis has been induced in these animals with virus types 7 and 14, and meningitis with types 6 and 16. Clinically inapparent infection associated with excretion of virus and with homologous antibody response has been demonstrated in chimpanzees after oral administration of virus types 4 or 6. Interference has been observed between echoviruses and other enteroviruses, including active poliovirus vaccine strains, the latter in man as well as in the laboratory. Interference by rubella virus with the propagation in tissue culture of echovirus type 11 has been widely used as an indirect technique for detecting the presence of the former.

Currently, echoviruses are identified by types, numbered 1 to 33, utilizing neutralization and complement fixation techniques and, when possible, tests for hemagglutination of human group 0 erythrocytes (types 3, 6, 7, 11–13, 19–21, 24, 29). Types 1 and 8 are now both regarded as type 1; type 9 is also recognized as coxsackievirus A-23. Types 10 and 28 have been reclassified as type 1 rheovirus and rhinovirus, respectively. Considerable variation has been observed between individual strains of certain types, especially of types 4 and 6. Although weak antigenic relations with other enteroviruses have been suggested, the echoviruses appear to be distinct entities, clearly distinguishable from other viruses which affect man. Similar viruses, however, have been encountered as natural parasites of other mammals.

EPIDEMIOLOGY. In general, echoviruses have exhibited the same epidemiologic characteristics as other enteroviruses. They have been detected in many parts of the world both by recovery of virus and by demonstration of specific antibody in individual sera or gamma globulins. Infection has been more common among children in warm seasons and among those living under poor socioeconomic conditions; virus has been recovered from the oropharynx, feces, urine and other sources. At different times in widely separated localities, epidemics of meningitis have occurred which were caused by echoviruses of types 3, 4, 6, 9, 11, 14, 16 and 30. In sporadic distribution, meningitis has been attributed to 24 different types; strains of at least 17 types have been recovered from cerebrospinal fluid of patients with meningitis.

Exanthems have been associated with infection by 15 types of echoviruses, often in epidemics. Some patients infected with type 3, 4 or 9 had exanthems and meningitis. Patients infected with type 16 have shown either rash or meningitis. Whenever meningitis or rash attributable to an echovirus has been epidemic, instances of less distinctive and inapparent infections have also been prevalent in the same vicinity. The attack rate and rapid dissemination of infection by these viruses within families have indicated a high degree of communicability and a relatively short incubation period.

PATHOLOGY. A virus identified as echovirus type 2 was recovered from the spinal cord of a child who died of a disease which clinically and pathologically resembled bulbospinal poliomyelitis. Type 9 virus was found in the medulla of another patient and type 6 virus in the blood of other fatal cases with paralysis. Types 3, 6, 14 and 19 have been recovered from body fluids and organs of newborn infants, some with petechiae and ecchymosis, who died of overwhelming infection and on postmortem examination showed hemorrhagic lesions and hepatic necrosis.

CLINICAL MANIFESTATIONS. Clinical disorders associated with echoviruses are indicated in Tables 10–18 and 10–19. The manifestations of illness resemble those seen with other enteroviruses, but, with the exception of meningitis and rash, they tend to occur in sporadic rather than epidemic distribution.

Neonatal Infections. Neonatal infections may be epidemic but clinically inapparent (types 22, 31), or result in individual cases in mild to abruptly lethal disease (types 3, 6, 9, 14, 17, 19, 31). They have been associated with respiratory symptoms, diarrhea, aseptic meningitis or exanthems and, in fatal cases, with disseminated intravascular coagulation and hepatoadrenal necrosis.

Aseptic Meningitis. The clinical features and laboratory findings in meningitis caused by echoviruses generally correspond to those observed in patients infected with coxsackieviruses. The illness is usually initiated abruptly with headache, often retrobulbar, and ensuing stiffness of the neck or back. Sore throat, nausea, vomiting and myalgia of the extremities may be present. In many patients with meningitis attributable to type 9 and, less frequently, in patients infected with type 4 virus, a fine or blotchy, sometimes morbilliform, maculopapular, erythematous rash may appear on the face and spread to the trunk and extremities. Occasionally small ulcerations of the oral mucosa resembling the lesions of herpangina are also seen during infection with some echoviruses, particularly types 9 and 16. Cervical or generalized lymphadenopathy is not unusual. The illness in most patients is self-limited and relatively mild, although the duration and intensity of symptoms are extremely variable.

In most patients with echovirus meningitis the blood leukocyte count is normal. In the cerebrospinal fluid the leukocyte counts usually range up to 500 per mm^3 and in cases of type 9 infection may exceed 1000. Virus has been recovered from cerebrospinal fluid both with and without pleocytosis. Polymorphonuclear leukocytes may be numerous (up to 90 per cent) early; lymphocytic cells predominate eventually, and with type 4 infections may do so throughout the course of illness. The protein content is normal or slightly elevated; the glucose level is normal.

Other Neurologic Disorders. Individual cases of muscular weakness or paralysis with associated alterations of reflexes similar to poliomyelitis have been seen in association with at least 11 types of echovirus (types 1, 2, 3, 4, 6, 7, 9, 11, 16, 18, 30), and fatal cases of infection with types 2, 3, 6, 7, 9 and 11 are recorded. Thus, clinical as well as experimental evidence indicates that some echoviruses induce poliomyelitis-like neuropathy.

Sporadic cases of encephalitis have been reported in association with 10 types of echovirus (types 2, 3, 4, 6, 7, 9, 11, 14, 18, 19), but the clinical pattern has been diverse and the evidence for a causative relationship inconsistent. Similarly, the role of echovirus types 6, 7 and 22 recovered from patients with the Guillain-Barré syndrome remains uncertain. Cerebellar ataxia has been seen in patients infected with types 9 and 19.

Pleurodynia. Myalgia of the extremities is a common feature of echovirus infections, but typical pleurodynia has been reported infrequently in patients infected with types 1, 6, 9 or 19.

Myocarditis and Pericarditis. Echoviruses types 1, 9 and 19 have been detected in cases of pericarditis; myocardial involvement has been suggested by electrocardiographic changes observed in patients during infection with types 3, 6 and 9, and type 9 virus has been isolated from the myocardium.

Nephritis. Acute glomerulonephritis associated with echovirus type 9 infection has been observed in 2½ year old twins.

Exanthem. Maculopapular exanthems have been recognized as a characteristic feature of infection with types 4, 9 and 16 echoviruses. Rashes have been especially common in association with epidemics of type 9 infection in patients both with and without meningeal involvement. A rash (Boston exanthem) has also been a conspicuous feature in outbreaks of a mild febrile illness caused by strains of echovirus type 16. Rashes have also been observed in association with other echoviruses. The exanthems have most frequently been maculopapular, but vesicles, urticaria and petechiae have also been described. Transitory telangiectatic lesions have been associated with acute infections attributed to echoviruses types 25 and 32. These manifestations of infection appear to be more common in infants and children than in adults.

Diarrhea. The association of certain echoviruses, particularly types 11, 14 and 18, with diarrheal disease in infants and children has been observed and a causative relationship suggested.

Acute Respiratory Illness. A number of echoviruses have been associated with acute respiratory illnesses. Echovirus type 11 (U or Uppsala) virus was recovered in Sweden from children with nondiphtheritic croup. It was also found in children and adults with acute respiratory infections and with brief febrile illnesses in experimentally infected human subjects. Echovirus type 6 has been recovered from patients with mild illnesses during epidemics of meningitis attributable to this agent and from cases of pharyngitis and conjunctivitis among children and adults in Japan. Echovirus type 1 was reported among infants in a Japanese institution and was associated with upper respiratory tract infection, diarrhea and a rubella-like rash. A diagnosis of pneumonia was made in some cases during an epidemic of infection with echovirus type 9. Echovirus type 19 has been encountered in infants and children with mild respiratory disease and was recovered from a fatal case during an outbreak of severe respiratory disease in premature infants. Echovirus type 20 was found in infants with minor respiratory disorders and diarrhea. Volunteers experimentally infected with this agent had fever, pharyngitis and, in two instances, coryza. Echoviruses, however, do not appear to be of great importance in the causation of respiratory disease.

DIAGNOSIS. As with other enteroviruses, diagnosis of infection by an echovirus can be confirmed in the laboratory, but diagnosis of disease can be established only by careful correlation of associated clinical, epidemiologic and laboratory evidence. All the echoviruses are cytopathogenic and can be identified by neutralization tests with specific immune serum in cultures of renal cells from rhesus monkeys. The presence of infection may be demonstrated by the detection of virus in the feces, oropharyngeal swabbings, urine, blood, cerebrospinal fluid or other specimens from the patient and by the demonstration of a related antibody response in the patient's serum. In the newborn, echoviruses can cause life-threatening illness clinically indistinguishable from bacterial sepsis, coxsackievirus or herpes simplex virus infection. Vesicles are more characteristic of herpes and should be cultured for this agent. Leukocytosis or leukopenia may be associated.

For further discussion of differential diagnosis see Coxsackievirus Infections, above.

PROGNOSIS. Disease caused by an echovirus is usually self-limited and uncomplicated and progresses rapidly to complete recovery. In patients with involvement of the central nervous system, muscular paralysis is an occasional complication. Fatal infection is rare except in the newborn.

TREATMENT AND CONTROL MEASURES. No definitive therapy is known. Treatment is supportive and symptomatic. Specific measures to control infection by echovirus are not available.

E. C. CURNEN

Andrewes, C. H.: Viruses and Noah's ark. Bacterial Rev. *29*:1, March 1965.

Brown, G. C., and Karunas R. S.: Relationship of congenital anomalies and maternal infection with selected enteroviruses. Am. J. Epidemiol. *95*:207, 1972.

Curnen, E. C.: Immunology, epidemiology and clinical aspects of coxsackie virus infections. *In* Poliomyelitis, compiled and edited for the International Poliomyelitis Congress. Philadelphia, J. B. Lippincott Company, 1952.

Dalldorf, G., and Melnick, J. L.: Coxsackie viruses. *In* Horsfall, F. L., Jr., and Tamm, I. (eds.): Viral and Rickettsial Infections of Man. 4th ed. Philadelphia, J. B. Lippincott Company, 1965.

Dalldorf, G., and Sickles, G. M.: An unidentified filtrable agent isolated from the feces of children with paralysis. Science *108*:61, 1948.

Gear, J.: Coxsackie Virus infections in southern Africa. Yale J. Biol. Med. *34*:289, 1961–62.

Huebner, R. J., and others: Herpangina; Etiological studies of a specific infectious disease. J.A.M.A. *145*:628, 1951.

International Enterovirus Study Group: Picornavirus group. Virology *19*:114, 1963.

Kibrick, S.: Current status of Coxsackie and ECHO viruses in human disease. *In* Melnick, J. L. (ed.): Progress in Medical Virology. Houston, Hafner Publishing Company, 1964, Vol. 6.

Kibrick, S., and Benirschke, K.: Severe generalized disease (encephalohepatomyocarditis) occurring in the newborn period and due to infection with coxsackie virus group B: Evidence of intrauterine infection with this agent. Pediatrics *22*:857, 1958.

Lerner, A. M., Klein, J. O., Cherry, J. D., and Finland, M.: New viral exanthems. New Engl. J. Med. *269*:678, 736, 1963.

Melnick, J. L.: Echoviruses. *In* Horsfall, F. L., and Tamm, I. (eds.): Viral and Rickettsial Infections of Man. 4th ed. Philadelphia, J. B. Lippincott Company, 1965.

Sylvest, E.: Epidemic Myalgia: Bornholm Disease. London, Oxford University Press, 1934.

Wenner, H. A.: The ECHO viruses. Ann. New York Acad. Sci. *101*:398, 1962.

POLIOMYELITIS

Poliomyelitis is an acute viral infection of man, without any established extrahuman reservoir, producing a wide range of clinical illness from none to rapidly progressive paralysis and death. Both sporadic cases and the characteristic summertime epidemics of yesteryear are uncommon in countries whose people are properly immunized with attenuated oral poliovaccine.

ETIOLOGY. Much more is known about poliovirus than about the predisposing factors which influence the clinical outcome.

The Virus. Poliovirus is an RNA virus whose diameter is only 28 mμ. The lack of lipid in the virus' coat is responsible for resistance to ether, chloroform, bile in the gut and various detergents. The virus is inactivated by strong oxidants, chlorine, formalin and ultraviolet radiation. Unfortunately poliovirus deteriorates on desiccation; hence, freeze-dried oral vaccine which would not require refrigeration is not feasible. There are three serotypes (I, II, III). The occurrence of two separate paralytic illnesses, each due to a different serotype, is rare but documented.

Other viruses on rare occasion cause nonparalytic and paralytic disease distinguishable from poliomyelitis only by special virologic study; these are the enteroviruses (echo and coxsackie) and mumps virus.

Predisposing Factors

Immune Status. Previous adequate exposure to a natural wild or a vaccine strain will protect against disease due to that serotype of virus.

Neurovirulence or Invasiveness of Strain. This characteristic affects the severity of epidemics as well as the neural response of infected persons.

Host Factors. Host factors are poorly understood; they operate at the cellular level, affecting the rate and perhaps the sites of virus multiplication. The influences of hormonal factors and of stress are evidenced by such observations as the following: (1) prepubertal boys have twice the paralytic rate of girls; (2) the incidence and severity of paralytic disease are higher in pregnant women than in the nonpregnant of similar age; (3) clinical severity of the disease increases with the age of the patient; (4) such stresses as muscular exhaustion, chilling and surgical procedures have deleterious effects once the virus has entered the body (concurrent or very recent tonsillectomy predisposes to bulbar poliomyelitis, and even remote tonsillectomy has a similar but less marked effect; excessive exertion and trauma may localize what might have been a nonclinical infection into a paralytic form, as may the injection of an arm with an irritating substance, such as alum-precipitated vaccine); and (5) cortisone increases the severity of certain forms of *experimental* poliomyelitis.

EPIDEMIOLOGY. Man is the sole natural reservoir for poliovirus and transmits infection by the oropharyngeal-fecal circuit. Casual unrecognized contact with alimentary tract content is probably the main source of virus transmission.

Most large outbreaks of poliomyelitis occur in the summer and early autumn months. Nevertheless poliovirus may be recovered from urban sewage in varying amounts through the entire year, and some outbreaks have occurred during periods of freezing weather.

The greatest communicability from known cases occurs during the latter part of the incubation period and the first week of illness. During outbreaks it is wise to postpone elective surgery on susceptible persons, especially nasal, throat and dental operations.

Community outbreaks of poliomyelitis can now be brought under control by widespread oral immunization with attenuated monovalent oral poliomyelitis vaccine (Sabin) of the same wild virus serotype causing the outbreak.

Acutely ill paralytic patients should be managed in general or children's hospitals equipped to care for emergencies and to provide intensive aftercare. Isolation precautions to be observed are the same as those for typhoid fever.

PATHOGENESIS. In man the virus generally enters the body by the oropharyngeal route and multiplies in the alimentary tract and in its related lymph nodes and other reticuloendothelial structures. Viremia of short duration is followed by the appearance of type-specific humoral antibody. Antibody also appears in the alimentary tract. If the responses are of sufficient speed and magnitude, the virus particles are neutralized, no clinical disease occurs, and immunity to that type of poliovirus ensues. In this infectivity-antibody contest the virus may proliferate and become invasive before sufficient antibody is formed.

If virus gains *direct access* to nerve structures or to the blood-lymphatic system, direct infection of the central nervous system may occur. Thus, bulbar poliomyelitis occurring soon after tonsillectomy may be due to virus gaining direct access to the medulla through severed cranial nerve filaments. Subcutaneously injected virus may follow nerve pathways and cause paralytic consequences, initially in the injected limb, as it did in 1935 with the trial of incompletely inactivated vaccines and again in 1954. The virus then made its way centrifugally *from* the nervous system and appeared in the pharynx and feces, causing secondary cases in noninjected persons. There is no evidence that biting insects "inject" poliovirus into man.

PATHOLOGY

Neuropathology. The neuropathology of poliomyelitis is usually pathognomonic; only certain cells and areas of the neuraxis are susceptible to the virus. There is little histologic evidence of meningeal reaction. There are perivascular cuffing and some interstitial glial infiltration.

Neuronal damage is due directly to virus multiplication. The clinical picture is dependent upon the number and location of involved neurons. Not all affected neurons are killed. The injury may be reversible, and restoration of function may occur within 3 to 4 weeks after onset.

Histologic sections generally reveal more widespread lesions than would be estimated from the clinical findings. Considerable destruction of scattered neurons may occur without clinical disability.

The regions in which neuronal lesions occur are (1) spinal cord (anterior horn cells chiefly and to a lesser degree the intermediate and dorsal horn and dorsal root ganglia); (2) medulla (vestibular nuclei, cranial nerve nuclei and the reticular formation which contains the vital centers); (3) cerebellum (nuclei in the roof and vermis only); (4) midbrain (chiefly the gray matter, but also the substantia nigra and occasionally the red nucleus); (5) thalamus and hypothalamus; (6) the pallidum; and (7) cerebral cortex (motor cortex). The virus *spares* the following areas, although they are invaded by the viruses of the arthropod-borne encephalitides: (1) the entire cerebral cortex *except* the motor area, (2) the cerebellum *except* the vermis and deep midline nuclei, and (3) the white matter of the spinal cord. It is the *distribution* of lesions which permits a histologic diagnosis of poliomyelitis.

Flaccid paralysis is the most obvious clinical expression of the neuronal changes. The ensuing muscular atrophy is due to denervation plus the atrophy of disuse. The pain, spasticity, nuchal and spinal rigidity and hypertonia of early illness are probably due to lesions of the brain stem, spinal ganglia and posterior columns. Respiratory arrhythmias, blood pressure and vasomotor fluctuations, cardiac arrhythmias, and the like, are reflections of damage to vital centers in the medulla.

Extraneural Pathology. Although the virus seldom causes lesions outside the central nervous system, secondary lesions do occur elsewhere. When nervous control of ventilation is disturbed, secondary bronchopulmonary changes occur, viz., aspiration pneumonia, atelectasis and purulent bronchitis, owing to the inability to cough and to interference with thoracic movements. The cardiovascular changes may result in hypertension, cardiac failure and pulmonary edema. Long immobilization leads to negative nitrogen and calcium balances, with urinary lithiasis, renal failure, hypertension with encephalopathy and convulsions; thrombophlebitis and pulmonary embolism are less common than might be expected. Treatment itself may cause untoward complications, such as urinary tract infection from improper catheterization, decubitus ulcers and psychotic disturbances. The virus does not affect the intellectual structures of the cerebral cortex. Ulcerations in the alimentary tract may result in serious bleeding and occasional perforation. Respiratory failure results in anoxic changes and respiratory acidosis.

CLINICAL MANIFESTATIONS. The diagnosis of acute poliomyelitis rests upon clinical grounds; there is no generally available diagnostic laboratory test. Careful history, close examination of the unclothed patient, and recollection of conditions which may mimic poliomyelitis will obviate most diagnostic pitfalls.

When a susceptible person has had effective contact with poliovirus, one of the following responses may occur in this order of frequency: (1) *asymptomatic infection,* (2) *abortive poliomyelitis,* (3) *nonparalytic poliomyelitis,* (4) *paralytic poliomyelitis.* Any of these results in durable resistance to reinfection. One response may blend into a more severe form. This feature may result in a biphasic course ushered in by a minor febrile illness, a symptom-free interlude of a few days succeeded by symptoms and signs referable to the nervous system.

Abortive Poliomyelitis. This presumptive clinical diagnosis is applicable only during obvious poliomyelitis outbreaks, especially in patients known to have been exposed to a clearly recognizable form of the disease. A brief febrile illness occurs, with one or more of the following symptoms: malaise, anorexia, nausea, vomiting, headache, sore throat, constipation and unlocalized abdominal pain. The following are *uncommon* in abortive poliomyelitis: coryza, cough, pharyngeal exudate, diarrhea, localized abdominal tenderness and rigidity. A definitive diagnosis is impossible without viral identification. The fever seldom exceeds 103° F, and the pharynx shows little despite the frequent complaint of sore throat.

During poliomyelitis outbreaks patients presumed to have the abortive clinical form should have complete rest for about a week after defervescence and should be examined carefully about 2 months later to exclude muscular involvement previously undetected.

Nonparalytic Poliomyelitis. The subjective symptoms are those enumerated for abortive poliomyelitis, except that headache, nausea and vomiting are more intense, and there is soreness and stiffness of the posterior muscles of the neck, trunk and limbs. Fleeting paralysis of the bladder is not uncommon, and constipation is frequent. Approximately two thirds of the children have a short symptom-free interlude between the first phase (minor illness) and the second phase (central nervous system or major illness). This two-phase course is less common in adults, in whom the evolution of symptoms is more insidious. Nuchal and spinal rigidity is a necessity for the diagnosis of nonparalytic poliomyelitis during the second phase.

Detection of Nuchal-spinal Signs. With cooperative patients the signs are first sought by *active tests.* The child is asked to sit up unassisted. If this causes undue effort, if the knees flex upward and he writhes a bit from side to side in sitting up and then places his hands on the bed behind him in the *tripod* supporting position, there is unmistakable spinal rigidity (Fig. 10–52). While he is still sitting, ask him to flex his chin to his chest and observe whether nuchal rigidity is apparent. Then from the supine position, holding the knees down gently, ask him to sit up and *kiss his knees* (Fig. 10–53). If the knees draw up sharply or if the maneuver cannot be adequately completed, there is stiffness of the spine due to muscle spasm.

If still uncertain, the *passive tests* should be applied; these include the maneuvers which elicit Kernig's and Brudzinski's signs. Gentle forward flexion of the occiput and neck will elicit nuchal rigidity, which may antedate spinal rigidity.

Next one looks for *head drop* by placing the hands under the patient's shoulders and raising the trunk (Fig. 10–54). Normally the head follows the plane of the trunk, but in poliomyelitis it often falls backward limply. The frequency of the head-drop sign even in nonparalytic poliomyelitis with no subsequent residuals indicates that it is not due to true paresis of the neck flexors.

In struggling infants it may be difficult to distinguish voluntary resistance from clinically impor-

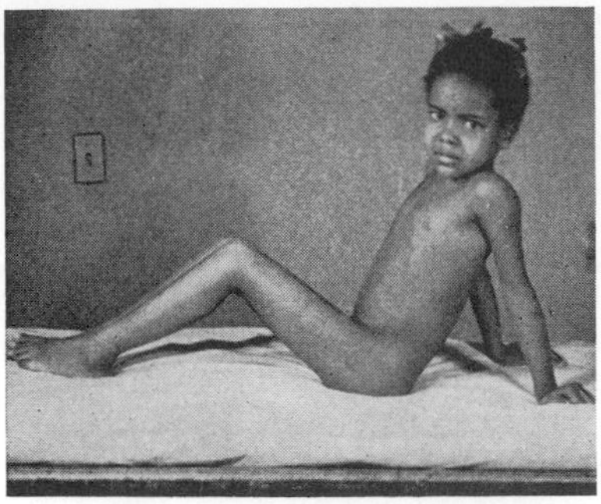

Fig. 10–52

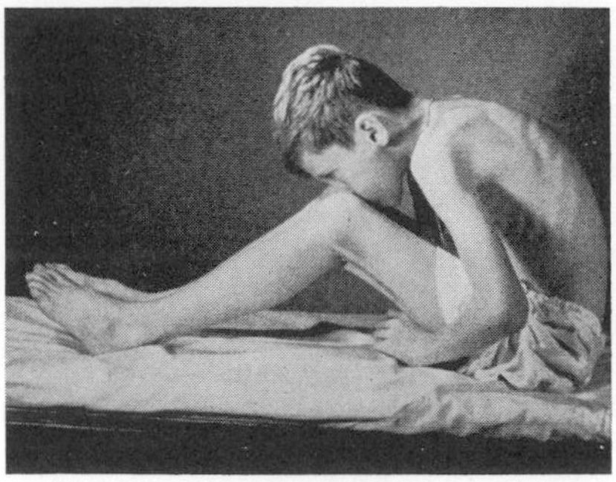

Fig. 10–53

Figure 10–52 Tripod sign: characteristic position associated with stiffness of the spine. (From A. J. Steigman: Diagnosis and General Care of Acute Poliomyelitis. Pediat. Clin. N. Amer., Vol. 1, No. 1A.)

Figure 10–53 Kiss-the-knee test: ability to complete the maneuver only by flexing the knee. Note tense appearance of the hamstrings. (From A. J. Steigman: Diagnosis and General Care of Acute Poliomyelitis. Pediat. Clin. N. Amer., Vol. 1, No. 1A.)

tant involuntary nuchal rigidity. One may place the infant's shoulders flush with the edge of the table, support the weight of the occiput in the hand, and then flex the head anteriorly (Fig. 10–55). Nuchal rigidity that persists during this maneuver may be interpreted as involuntary. When not closed, the anterior fontanel may be tense or bulging as in meningitis.

In poliomyelitis the nuchal rigidity detected in the supine position (Fig. 10–56, *A*) often disappears when the patient is turned over (Fig. 10–56, *B*). The nuchal rigidity associated with purulent meningitis generally persists in either position. This paradoxical sign, though helpful, is not pathognomonic.

Superficial and Deep Reflexes. In the early stages the reflexes are normally active and remain so unless paralysis supervenes. Changes in reflexes, either increased or depressed, may *precede weakness* by 12 to 24 hours; hence, it is important to detect them, especially in nonparalytic patients managed at home.

The *superficial* reflexes, i.e., cremasteric, abdominal, and the reflexes of the spinal and gluteal muscles, are usually the first to be diminished. The spinal and gluteal reflexes are elicited by tapping segmentally downward on each side of the spine and buttocks. These reflexes may disappear before the abdominal and cremasteric ones.

Changes in the *deep* tendon reflexes, whether exaggerated or depressed, generally occur 8 to 24 hours after depression of superficial reflexes and indicate impending paresis of the extremities. There is absence of tendon reflexes with paralysis. Objective evidence of sensory defects does not occur in poliomyelitis.

Differential Diagnosis of Nonparalytic Poliomyelitis. A wide variety of diseases must be considered in an alert, febrile patient with meningeal signs whose muscular power and reflexes are still intact. In such a patient, when the cerebrospinal fluid reveals pleocytosis, no organisms and a normal sugar level, the differential diagnosis must include all causes of the acute *aseptic meningitis syndrome*. Serologic procedures may be helpful in excluding many of these diseases. The clinical diagnosis of nonparalytic poliomyelitis is made by exclusion of other conditions and the epidemiologic

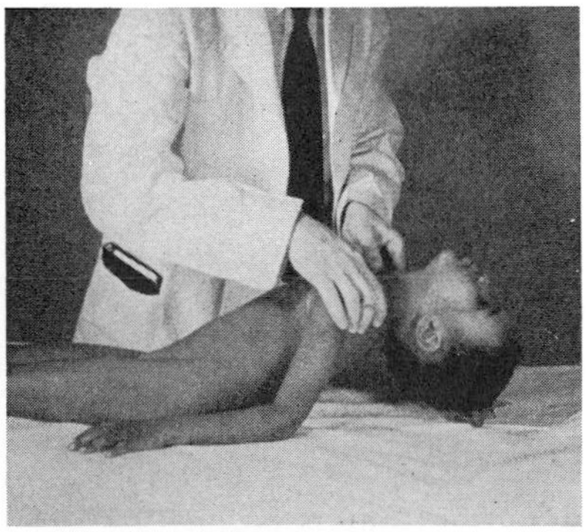

Fig. 10–54

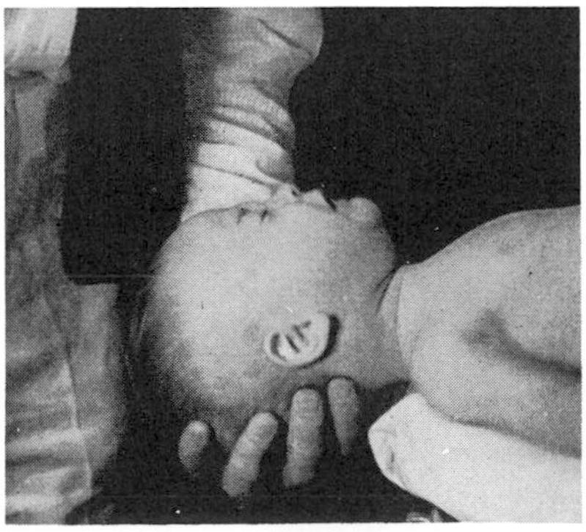

Fig. 10–55

Figure 10–54 Head-drop sign: the head fails to continue in the plane of the body when the shoulders are elevated. This child had nonparalytic poliomyelitis. Tripod and head-drop signs appear in nonparalytic and paralytic poliomyelitis. (From A. J. Steigman: Diagnosis and General Care of Acute Poliomyelitis. Pediat. Clin. N. Amer., Vol. 1, No. 1A.)

Figure 10–55 Testing nuchal rigidity in uncooperative, struggling infant: Place the shoulders at the edge of the table, supporting the occiput manually. Flex anteriorly. Only true involuntary rigidity persists. (From A. J. Steigman: Diagnosis and General Care of Acute Poliomyelitis. Pediat. Clin. N. Amer., Vol. 1, No. 1A.)

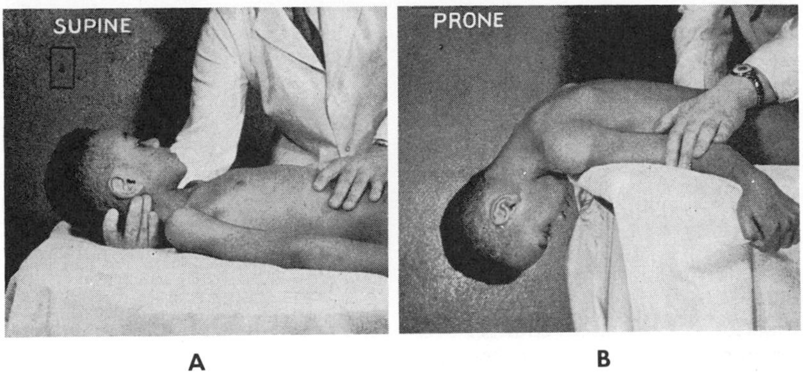

Figure 10–56 Supine versus prone postural test for nuchal rigidity in poliomyelitis. A, Nuchal rigidity elicited in conventional supine position. B, In prone position nuchal rigidity disappears in poliomyelitis, but generally persists in pyogenic meningitis. (From Steigman, A. J.: Pediat. Clin. N. Amer., Vol. 1, No. 1A.)

probability. Specific virus studies are now more feasible.

In their early stages *tuberculous* and *purulent meningitis* may simulate nonparalytic poliomyelitis. A lumbar puncture should be done; in addition to bacterial smears and cultures and a cell count, particular attention should be paid to the sugar content, since it is not depressed in the viral infections. Headache, fever and stiffness of the neck and back with tender extremities may occur in *acute rheumatic fever, rheumatoid arthritis* and *serum sickness;* the cerebrospinal fluid is normal, however, as it also is in the *meningismus* which may accompany the early stages of pneumonia, dysentery, typhoid, pyelitis and other infections. *Acute tonsillitis* and other conditions associated with cervical adenitis may cause a child to hold his head and neck immobile; this should not be confused with true nuchal rigidity.

Paralytic Poliomyelitis. The manifestations are those enumerated for nonparalytic poliomyelitis plus weakness of one or more muscle groups, either skeletal or cranial. These symptoms may be followed by a symptom-free interlude of several days and then a recurrence of symptoms, culminating in paralysis. Bladder paralysis of 1 to 3 days' duration occurs in approximately 20 per cent of patients, and bowel atony is common, occasionally to the point of paralytic ileus. In infants muscular paralysis may be the first evidence noted.

Clinical Classification. The distribution of clinical paralysis is characteristically spotty and haphazard. To detect mild muscular weakness it is often necessary to apply gentle resistance in opposition to the muscle group being tested.

SPINAL FORM. There is weakness of some of the muscles of the neck, abdomen, trunk, diaphragm, thorax or extremities.

BULBAR FORM. There is weakness in the motor distribution of one or more *cranial nerves* with or without dysfunction of the *vital centers of respiration and circulation.*

BULBOSPINAL FORM. Components of the preceding forms occur together.

ENCEPHALITIC FORM. There are irritability, disorientation, drowsiness and coarse tremors not explained by inadequate ventilation. Even during poliomyelitis epidemics this group can be recognized *only* if some peripheral or cranial nerve *paralysis* coexists or ensues. Hypoxia and hypercapnia due to inadequate ventilation from respiratory insufficiency may produce disorientation without true encephalitis.

Differential Diagnosis of Paralytic Poliomyelitis.

CONDITIONS CAUSING MUSCULAR WEAKNESS. (1) *Infectious neuronitis* (Guillain-Barré syndrome) is the most common and difficult differential problem in this group. Generally the fever, headache and meningeal signs are less notable; characteristically there are few cells but elevated globulin content in the cerebrospinal fluid. Paralysis is characteristically symmetrical in distribution. Sensory changes and pyramidal tract signs are common, but are absent in poliomyelitis. (2) *Peripheral neuritis*—postinjectional, toxic (lead, avitaminosis, and so forth), paralytic cranial herpes zoster, postdiphtheritic neuropathies—is excluded by history, sensory examination and related findings. (3) Arthropod-borne viral *encephalitis, rabies* and *tetanus* have been confused with bulbar poliomyelitis. (4) *Botulism* may closely simulate bulbar poliomyelitis; nuchal-spinal rigidity and pleocytosis are absent. (5) *Demyelinizing types of encephalomyelitis* are associated with or follow the exanthems and other infections or occur as an untoward sequel of antirabies vaccination. (6) *Tick-bite* paralysis is uncommon; meningeal signs are absent, and removal of the tick is followed by swift recovery. (7) *Neoplasms* originating in and around the spinal cord may rarely have a fairly abrupt onset. (8) *Familial periodic paralysis, myasthenia gravis* and *acute porphyria* are uncommon causes of weakness. (9) *Hysteria* and *malingering* are rare in children.

CONDITIONS CAUSING PSEUDOPARALYSIS. In these, nuchal-spinal rigidity and pleocytosis are absent. (1) *Unrecognized trauma* as from contusions, sprains, fractures and epiphyseal separation is a common cause of diagnostic confusion. (2) *Nonspecific (toxic) synovitis* produces a limp, usually unilaterally; the hip and the knee are the most common sites. There may be low-grade fever for several days. (3) *Acute osteomyelitis* has a more septic course; there is polymorphonuclear leukocytosis, with localized signs, positive blood culture and later roentgenographic changes. (4) In *acute rheumatic fever* the clinical pattern is usually diagnostic. (5) *Scurvy* is revealed by history of inadequate intake of vitamin C and by roentgenographic changes in the bones. (6) *Congenital syphilitic osteomyelitis* of the acute painful type is found only in early infancy; serologic tests are indicated.

Bulbar and Respiratory Forms of Poliomyelitis. A number of components acting together may produce insufficiency of ventilation (see Table 10–20). The most serious biochemical changes are hypoxia and hypercapnia. These states produce effects on many other systems, such as the cardiovascular-renal one.

Respiratory insufficiency should be detected early in order to diminish its widespread effects. Since the situation may shift rapidly, continued clinical analysis is essential.

Despite weakness of the respiratory muscles, the patient may respond with so much respiratory effort that normal alveolar ventilation is maintained. In fact, the increased effort (associated with anxiety and fear) may actually produce overventilation at the outset, resulting in respiratory alkalosis. Such effort is fatiguing and soon leads to respiratory failure.

For clarity, certain terms will be defined: (1) *Pure spinal poliomyelitis with respiratory insufficiency* refers to tightness, weakness or paralysis of respiratory muscles (chiefly the diaphragm and intercostals) without discernible clinical involvement of cranial nerves or vital centers. The cervical and thoracic spinal cord segments are chiefly involved. (2) *Pure bulbar poliomyelitis* refers to paralysis of motor cranial nerve nuclei with or without involvement of the vital centers which control respiration, circulation and body temperature. Involvement of the ninth, tenth and twelfth cranial nerves is most important, since there is paralysis of the pharynx, tongue and larynx with resultant obstruction of the airway. (3) *Bulbospinal poliomyelitis with respiratory insufficiency* refers to involvement of the respiratory muscles with coexisting bulbar paralysis.

TABLE 10–20 COMMON SOURCES OF HYPOXIA AND HYPERCAPNIA IN POLIOMYELITIS

1. Cranial nerves IX to XII involved, with
   a. Pharyngeal paralysis and pooling of secretions
   b. Laryngeal involvement—either spasm of laryngeal muscles or paralysis of vocal cords
   c. Lingual paralysis
   d. Tracheal accumulation of secretions due to inability to cough
   e. Aspiration of vomitus
2. Vital center involvement with
   a. Inefficient, irregular respiration
   b. Cardiovascular disturbance
   c. Hyperpyrexia causing increased oxygen consumption
3. Cervical and spinal cord involvement causing paresis of the primary and accessory muscles of respiration
4. Pulmonary complications, viz., pneumonia, atelectasis, edema
5. Contributory factors
   a. Panic
   b. Gastric dilatation
   c. Sedation
   d. Inadequate equipment, viz., small-bore tracheostomy tubes, unsuitable respirator settings, and the like

The clinical findings resulting from involvement of the *respiratory muscles* are (1) anxious expression; (2) inability to speak without frequent pauses, resulting in short, jerky, "breathless" sentences, which can be demonstrated by asking the child to count numbers serially; (3) increased respiratory rate; (4) movement of the alae nasi and of the accessory muscles of respiration; (5) inability to cough or sniff with full depth; (6) paradoxical abdominal movements due to diaphragmatic immobility from spasm or weakness of one or both leaves; (7) relative immobility of the intercostal spaces, which may be segmental, unilateral or bilateral. When the arms are weak, and especially when deltoid paralysis occurs, it is well to beware of impending respiratory paralysis, since the phrenic nerve nuclei are in adjacent areas of the spinal cord. In order to bring out minor degrees of paresis, splint the abdominal muscles manually and observe the patient's capacity for thoracic breathing. By lightly splinting the thoracic cage manually, the effectiveness of diaphragmatic movement may be assessed.

The clinical findings of *bulbar poliomyelitis* with respiratory difficulty (other than paralysis of extraocular, facial and masticatory muscles) include (1) nasal twang to the voice or cry, due to palatal and pharyngeal weakness—hard-consonant words such as "cookie" or "candy" bring this out best; (2) inability to swallow smoothly, resulting in accumulation of saliva in the pharynx and in partial immobility on holding the larynx lightly and asking the patient to swallow; (3) accumulated pharyngeal secretions which may cause irregular respiration, since each inspiration must be "planned" and cannot be "subconscious" in view of the risk of aspirating; the respirations may thus appear interrupted and abnormal even to the point of falsely simulating intercostal or diaphragmatic weakness; (4) the impossibility of effective coughing with resultant constant fatiguing efforts to clear the throat; (5) nasal regurgitation of saliva and fluids due to palatal paralysis with inability to separate the oropharynx from the nasopharynx during swallowing; (6) deviation of the palate, uvula or the tongue; (7) involvement of vital centers as reflected by irregularity in rate, depth and rhythm of respiration; by cardiovascular alterations which include blood pressure changes, especially upward, alternate flushing and mottling of the skin, and cardiac arrhythmias; and by rapid changes in body temperature; (8) paralysis of one or both vocal cords causing hoarseness, aphonia and ultimately asphyxia unless recognized by laryngoscopy and managed by tracheotomy immediately; (9) the "rope sign," an acute angulation between the chin and larynx, due to weakness of the hyoid muscles. The hyoid bone is pulled posteriorly, narrowing the hypopharyngeal inlet.

Lumbar Puncture in Poliomyelitis. This procedure has diagnostic but not prognostic value. Although there are generally fewer than 500 leukocytes per mm^3, the count may be higher, and rarely there may be no cellular increase. Early the cells are predominantly polymorphonuclear, but they soon become predominantly lymphocytic and decrease to normal numbers as early as 10 to 14 days after the onset. Absence of organisms on smear and culture and normal to elevated sugar content support the diagnosis of poliomyelitis. The protein content in the early stages is normal (up to 40 mg/dl) or slightly elevated. Within 2 to 3 weeks after onset the pleocytosis diminishes, but the protein content frequently rises to as high as 300 mg/dl.

COMPLICATIONS

Gastrointestinal Tract. Striking complications arise occasionally, including melena, which may be severe enough to require transfusion and is due to single or multiple superficial erosions. Gastrointestinal perforation is rare. Acute gastric dilatation may occur abruptly during the acute or convalescent stage, causing further embarrassment of respiration; immediate gastric aspiration and external application of ice bags are indicated.

Cardiovascular System. Mild hypertension of a few days' or weeks' duration is common in the acute stage, probably related to lesions of the vasoregulatory centers in the medulla, and especially to underventilation. In the later stages, owing to the protracted immobilization, hypertension may occur along with hypercalcemia, nephrocalcinosis and vascular lesions. Dimness of vision, headache and a lightheaded feeling in association with hypertension should be regarded as premonitory of a frank convulsion. Anticonvulsive therapy is then indicated, and a program favoring increased mobilization should be instituted. Cardiac irregularities are uncommon; they vary from unexplained tachycardias (which may yield to digitalization) to cardiac arrest, for which measures to restore cardiac action are indicated. Electrocardiographic abnormalities indicative of myocarditis are not rare.

Acute pulmonary edema occurs occasionally, particularly in patients with arterial hypertension. Immediate management may be lifesaving. Pulmonary embolism is uncommon despite the immobilization.

Urinary Tract. Transitory paralysis of the bladder in the acute stage has been mentioned. Skeletal decalcification begins soon after immobilization and results in hypercalciuria, which in turn predisposes to calculi, especially when urinary stasis and infection are present. A high fluid intake is the only effective prophylactic measure. The patient should be mobilized as much and as early as possible.

PROGNOSIS. Recorded case fatality rates in large urban epidemics in the United States have approximated 5 to 7 per cent. Most deaths occur within the first 2 weeks after onset. Fatality rates and the degree of disability appear to be greater after the age of puberty.

In general, the more extensive the paralysis in the first 10 days of illness, the more severe will be the ultimate disability. Unexpected improvement may appear soon after defervescence and again about 6 weeks after the onset, a time which corresponds to functional restoration of temporarily inactive neurons. The degree of functional recovery depends also upon the adequacy and promptness of therapy as related to proper body positioning, active motion, use of assistive devices and, of great importance, the psychologic motivation to return to as full and normal a life as possible.

TREATMENT. The broad principles of management are to allay fear, to minimize ensuing skeletal deformities, to anticipate and meet complications in addition to the neuromusculoskeletal ones, and to prepare the child and family for the prolonged treatment which may be required and for permanent disability, when this seems likely. A highly individualized approach with optimism blended with candor is essential.

Patients with the *nonparalytic* and mildly *paralytic* forms may be treated at home. No antibiotics are effective against poliovirus, and human immune globulin is ineffective after the onset of illness.

For the *abortive* form simple analgesics, sedatives, an attractive diet and bed rest until the child's temperature is normal for several days suffice. Avoidance of exertion for the ensuing 2 weeks is desirable, and there should be a careful neuromusculoskeletal examination 2 months later for any minor involvement.

Treatment for the *nonparalytic* form is similar to that for the abortive one, relief being indicated in particular for the discomfort of muscle tightness and spasm of the neck, trunk and extremities. Analgesics alone are not so effective as when combined with the application of hot packs for 15 to 30 minutes every 2 to 4 hours. Hot tub baths are sometimes useful. A firm bed is desirable and is improvised at home by placing table-leaves or a sheet of plywood beneath the mattress. A footboard should be used to keep the feet at a right angle with the legs. Muscular discomfort and spasm may continue for some weeks even in the nonparalytic form, necessitating hot packs and gentle physical therapy. Such patients should also be *carefully* examined 2 months after apparent recovery to detect minor residuals which might cause postural problems in later years.

Most patients with the *paralytic* form require hospitalization. A calm atmosphere is desired. Suitable body alignment is necessary to avoid excessive skeletal deformity. A neutral position with the feet at a right angle, knees slightly flexed, hips and spine straight, is achieved by use of boards, sandbags and occasionally light splint shells. Active and passive motions are indicated as soon as the pain has disappeared. Opiates and sedatives are permissible only if no impairment of ventilation is present or impending. Constipation is common, and fecal impaction should be prevented.

When bladder paralysis occurs, a parasympathetic stimulant such as bethanechol (Urecholine), 5 to 10 mg orally, 2.5 to 5.0 mg subcutaneously, may induce voiding in 15 to 30 minutes; some patients do not respond, and others have nausea, vomiting and palpitation. Bladder paresis rarely lasts more than a few days. If Urecholine fails, manual compression of the bladder and the psychologic effect of running water should be tried. If catheterization must be performed, the strictest asepsis is essential.

An interesting diet and a relatively high fluid intake should be started at once unless there is vomiting. Additional salt should be provided if the environmental temperature is high or if the application of hot packs induces sweating. Anorexia is common initially. An indwelling polyethylene gastric tube may be necessary to ensure adequate dietary and fluid intake.

The orthopedist and the physiatrist should see these patients as early in the illness as possible, and assume responsibility before fixed deformities develop.

The management of *pure bulbar poliomyelitis* consists essentially in maintaining the airway and avoiding all risks of inhalation of saliva, food or vomitus. Gravity drainage of accumulated secretions is favored by the head-low (foot of bed elevated 20 to 25 degrees) *prone* position with the face to one side. Aspirators with rigid or semirigid tips are preferred for direct oral and pharyngeal use, and soft flexible catheters may be used for nasopharyngeal aspiration.

Fluid and electrolyte equilibrium is best maintained by intravenous infusion, since tube or oral feeding in the first few days might incite vomiting. After the first few days an indwelling polyethylene gastric tube may be used and sips of sterile water given from a spoon, with increments as indicated by ability to swallow. In addition to close observation for respiratory insufficiency, the blood pressure should be taken at least twice daily. Hypertension is not uncommon and occasionally leads to hypertensive encephalopathy. Patients with pure bulbar poliomyelitis may require tracheotomy because of vocal cord paralysis or because of a "rope sign" with constriction of the hypopharynx.

The majority of patients with pure bulbar poliomyelitis who recover have little residual impairment; some patients exhibit mild dysphagia and occasional vocal fatigue with slurring of speech.

Management of Respiratory Failure Due to Inadequacy of Respiratory Muscles. This consists essentially in providing artificial mechanical respiration; familiarity in the use of the equipment selected is essential. Indications for use of assisted ventilation will include mounting anxiety, restlessness, fatigue and hypoxia or hypercapnia in a patient with evidence of respiratory paralysis.

When placing a child in a respirator, it is essential to conceal any sense of haste or anxiety. The child and the parents should be told what is to take place; often the presence of the parents at the time of transfer reduces the child's terror and permits smoother synchronization to the machine. Clinical evidence of improvement is detected by disappearance of restlessness, pallor or cyanosis, by adjustment to the machine's rhythm with cessation of extra efforts with the accessory muscles, and by an ability to doze.

Fever increases the oxygen requirement and should be controlled; in desperate instances the author has used induced therapeutic hypothermia. During the early febrile days it is better to err on the side of hyperventilation. If patients are hyperventilated too long, they may become "addicted," making the process of weaning from the respirator more difficult.

The amount of ventilation needed to maintain normal levels of oxygen and carbon dioxide in the arterial blood may vary widely within a short time. When blood gas determinations are not readily obtained, close clinical supervision is required. Respiratory acidosis from accumulation of carbon dioxide may occur despite normal oxygenation achieved by oxygen therapy. The only effective way to remove excess carbon dioxide is by augmented ventilation.

A combination of positive and negative pressures may be used with a cumulative net effect. A patient on occasion may require minus (−) 25 cm of water pressure or more; this makes nursing care difficult because of the need to maintain a tight seal at the portholes. A combination of negative and positive pressures is then preferred, as for patients with hypotension and poor cardiac filling in whom "atmospheric" pressures, e.g., of minus (−) and plus (+) 10 cm, yield a net pressure of 20 cm. The amount of ventilation prescribed must be "enough"; individualized judgment is required at *frequent* examinations. The thoracic cage of recumbent poliomyelitic patients acquires a lack of compliance or resistance to distensibility, so that pressures required to yield "enough" ventilation may be high.

Measurement of ventilation provides an index of the patient's requirement for artificial respiration and is especially useful in establishing the degrees of progress during the recovery stage.

Tracheotomy. Tracheotomy is required for some patients with pure bulbar poliomyelitis, for some with pure spinal respiratory paralysis and for most patients with bulbospinal respiratory involvement. During epidemics it is generally possible for a busy nurse to maintain the airway more readily in respirator patients with a tracheostomy than by oropharyngeal aspiration alone. The operation is best done with a bronchoscope in situ to maintain ventilation, if necessary by attachment of the anesthetist's manual bag. An opening of the second tracheal ring is preferred, and the *largest* size tube admissible is inserted in order to reduce resistance to airflow. Respirator collar depressors are available for tracheotomized respirator patients. Standard tracheostomy tubes are often too long for these recumbent, head-low patients and may impinge upon the anterior tracheal wall, so that it may be advisable to cut 1 to 2 cm from the distal end. The aftercare requires extremely close attention to details. Strict asepsis is mandatory. Since the "prophylactic" administration of antibiotics may permit colonization of resistant bacteria, routine use of them is not advised. Nasopharyngeal wire swabs can be inserted down the tracheostomy tube to obtain material for bacterial culture. Frequent but swift endotracheal aspiration is required and is facilitated by instillation of a broncholavaging solution such as saline. Humidification of air or oxygen is important in preventing inspissation.

The tracheotomized patient with bulbospinal poliomyelitis differs from patients with tracheostomy for other acute airway problems in being unable to cough, frequently for many months. Tubes should not be removed too early, but may be corked and left in place until some tussive strength is restored.

Electronically activated mechanical devices ("exsufflators") are designed to produce sudden periodic high pressures on the chest wall of respirator patients during exhalation, thus forcing the bronchial secretions toward the glottis. Convalescent respirator patients whose cough is ordinarily feeble can also be trained to clear their bronchi several times daily by coughing while the chest is squeezed together by the attendant.

Weaning a Patient from Dependency on a Respirator. In this part of the necessary rehabilitation, much depends upon the initial psychologic and physical handling of the patient. The respirator should be opened periodically even if only for a few seconds, beginning on the first day of acute illness. *Strong verbal reassurance is given to the patient.* Gradually the pressure settings are lowered and the periods out of the respirator increased in duration and frequency. Cuirass respirators and the rocking bed are valuable devices in the weaning process, during which fatigue must be avoided. Speech therapists may be helpful in training these patients in glossopharyngeal ("frog") breathing. The weaning from respirators and the total rehabilitation of the severely involved ex-respirator patient may require several years of active work plus a supervised program for life. With adequate artificial devices and maintained motivation, patients with apparently overwhelming disabilities have been returned to productive lives.

PREVENTION

Immunity and Vaccines. Newborn infants whose mothers' serum contains antibodies to all three serotypes of poliovirus are *passively immune* only for the duration of protective levels of transplacentally derived IgG. Pooled Human Immune Globulin contains poliomyelitis antibody, but this biologic preparation has no place in therapy and, in practical terms, no role in prophylaxis.

Prior to the advent of effective vaccines, lifelong natural active immunity without illness came from adequate contacts with wild natural poliovirus strains. The increasing use of poliomyelitis vaccines will reduce the quantity of natural poliovirus in the general population. This situation underscores the importance of maintaining a high level of artificially acquired active immunity in the population by appropriate vaccination procedures.

Poliovirus Vaccines. In the United States and in other countries in which large segments of the population have been vaccinated, reported cases of poliomyelitis are now infrequent. From 1950 through 1954 the number of cases reported in the United States totaled 190,000, i.e., approximately 25 per 100,000 population per year, mostly in children. The average of almost 40,000 cases reported per year has now dropped to approximately 100; these occur mostly in nests of unvaccinated children. The oral poliovaccine (OPV) developed by Sabin consists of attenuated strains of the three serotypes of virus. (See p. 212.)

ALEX J. STEIGMAN

International Conference on the Application of Vaccines Against Viral, Rickettsial and Bacterial Diseases of Man. Washington, D.C., Pan American Health Organization, Scientific Publication No. 226, 1971.

Sabin, A. B.: Oral Poliovirus vaccine. History of its development and prospects for eradication of poliomyelitis. J.A.M.A. *194*:872, 1965.

Steigman, A. J.: The control of poliomyelitis. J. Pediatr. *59*:163, 1961.

Steigman, A. J.: Clinical paralytic poliomyelitis due to enteroviruses other than poliovirus. Arch. Gest. Virusforsch. *13*:169, 1963.

ACUTE ASEPTIC MENINGITIS SYNDROME

The term "acute aseptic meningitis syndrome" includes a number of disorders which have in common an acute onset, usually a self-limited course with meningeal manifestations of varying degree, an increase in the cells of the spinal fluid and an absence of organisms on direct smear. (Also see Encephalitis.) The clinical significance is considerable in view of the frequency of this syndrome.

The majority of these disorders are caused by viruses, especially enteroviruses with or without rashes, and by mumps virus with or without accompanying parotitis. There are numerous other causes, infectious and otherwise, as noted in Table 10–21, which may present this clinical picture.

The term "acute aseptic meningitis syndrome" is discarded in favor of a specific diagnostic one when clinical and laboratory data make this possible.

The epidemiology and the clinical patterns vary with the causative agent. The incidence tends to be higher in males with mumps and in certain enterovirus outbreaks. The Sections relevant for the individual agents should be consulted for details.

Immunity to a specific virus is long lasting. More than one attack of this syndrome may occur, how-

TABLE 10–21 CLINICAL CONDITIONS WHICH MAY INDUCE THE ACUTE ASEPTIC MENINGITIS SYNDROME

DISEASE	AGENT
I. Infectious	
A. Viral	
Man to man	
Enteric, upper respiratory, neurologic infections	Enteroviruses (coxsackieviruses A and B, echoviruses, polioviruses); mumps virus
Common exanthems	Viruses of measles, rubella, herpesviruses (simplex, varicella-zoster)
Infectious mononucleosis	Epstein-Barr (EB) virus
Infectious hepatitis; influenza	Viruses of hepatitis, influenza
Rodent to man	
Lymphocytic choriomeningitis (LCM)	Lymphocytic choriomeningitis virus
Febrile meningeal reaction	Encephalomyocarditis viruses
Arthropod to man ("arbo" or arthropod-borne)	
Meningeal and systemic illness	Arboviruses A, B and nongroup; e.g., Eastern, Western, Venezuelan equine (group A); St. Louis, Japanese, Murray Valley, tickborne encephalitis viruses (group B); California group of viruses
B. Presumed viral	
Infectious lymphocytosis	Agent unknown
Cat-scratch disease	Agent unknown
C. Rickettsial	
Rocky Mountain spotted fever	*Rickettsia rickettsii*
D. "Allergic" or "Reactive"	
Postinfectious	E.g., viruses of measles, rubella, mumps, varicella, variola
Postvaccinal	E.g., vaccines against smallpox, rabies, influenza, pertussis
E. Bacterial	
Incipient or partially treated meningitis	*M. tuberculosis;* common pathogens, especially *H. influenzae*
F. Spirochetal	
Leptospirosis	*Leptospira icterohemorrhagica, L. canicola, L. pomona*
Syphilis	*Treponema pallidum*
G. Fungal	
Disseminated coccidioidomycosis, moniliasis, cryptococcosis, histoplasmosis	*Coccidioides immitis, Candida albicans, Cryptococcus neoformans, Histoplasma capsulatum*
Nocardiosis	Nocardia (several species)
H. Protozoal	
Toxoplasmosis	*Toxoplasma gondii*
Acanthamoebiasis	Acanthamoebae (Hartmanella)
II. Noninfectious	
A. Meningeal irritation from contiguous lesion	E.g., abscesses, granulomas, hematomas, tumors, thromboses adjacent to or within central nervous system
B. Tumor	
Meningoencephalitis with increased intracranial pressure	Medulloblastoma
C. Allergy	
Meningeal reaction	
After vaccinations or infections	See I, D above
After other causes, e.g., serum sickness	Horse serum, antibiotics
D. Miscellaneous	
Leukemic meningitis	Leukemic infiltration
Meningeal reactions to systemic poisoning	E.g., lead, toxins of gram-negative bacilli
Intrathecal injections	E.g., serum, antibiotic, contrast media
Implanted valves for treatment of hydrocephalus	Immediate postoperative or later bacterial infection

ever, owing to the variety of etiologic agents, including, for example, the numerous serotypes of enteroviruses.

CLINICAL MANIFESTATIONS. Although the onset may be insidious over a week or so, or even be preceded by a nonspecific acute febrile illness for a few days, it is generally fairly acute. The presenting manifestations in older children are headache and hyperesthesia; in infants, irritability and resentment at being handled. Fever, nausea and vomiting are frequent, but convulsions are rare. Preceding or accompanying exanthems may occur, especially with the echoviruses (q.v.).

Examination reveals nuchal-spinal rigidity (see Poliomyelitis for technique of the examination) without significant localizing neurologic changes.

LABORATORY DATA. The cerebrospinal fluid contains from 20 to several thousand cells per mm^3; early in the disease these are often polymorphonuclear; later they are chiefly mononuclear. No organisms are seen on direct smears (bacteria, mycobacteria, protozoans, yeasts), and there are normal or slightly elevated levels of protein and of glucose. A decrease in glucose level can occur with medulloblastoma, leukemic infiltration and, rarely, in certain viral infections. In all instances the spinal fluid should be cultured for bacteria and mycobacteria, and in some instances special examinations are indicated for fungi, protozoa and other pathogens. Careful examination of the spinal fluid is most important, especially to assure that stains used for smears do not introduce artifacts and that the standard solutions used for glucose levels are accurate. A simultaneous blood glucose level is taken at the time of spinal puncture.

For special laboratory procedures to be used in the identification of viruses and other agents, refer to the various agents.

DIFFERENTIAL DIAGNOSIS. Careful analysis of the history and epidemiologic circumstances may point toward one of the specific causes listed in Table 10–21. Especially during the summer and autumn, the presence of pleurodynia or of unexplained febrile eruptions in the community suggests the possibility of coxsackie- or echovirus infections; the coexistence of acute paralytic disorders in other patients suggests poliomyelitis; encephalitic infections in horses point to the possibilities of an arbovirus infection; a history of swimming in waters contaminated by dead animals may suggest leptospiral infection. Knowledge of clear-cut exposure to or concurrent evidence of mumps or one of the common exanthems can be helpful in the differential diagnosis.

Most difficult from the diagnostic, therapeutic and prognostic points of view are instances of incipient or partially treated bacterial (especially when due to *H. influenzae*) or mycobacterial meningitis. The clinical findings, the dosage of antibiotic previously used and the spinal fluid smear, culture and glucose level may be helpful in the former. When tuberculous meningitis is suspected, a careful evaluation of contacts, a positive Levinson test and a positive tuberculin reaction may suggest the correct diagnosis. Medulloblastoma must be considered in the differential diagnosis, particularly if there are hypoglycorrhachia and prominent signs of increased intracranial pressure.

Finally, the possibility that the observed meningeal reaction is of neither viral nor bacterial origin must be recognized.

TREATMENT. Symptomatic measures, including aspirin, sponging and a cool room for relief of headache, hyperesthesia and fever, are useful. The withdrawal of spinal fluid for diagnosis often relieves headache. Codeine, morphine and the phenothiazine derivatives are best avoided, since they may induce misleading signs and symptoms. Assurance that recovery is likely may be considered part of therapy.

Several weeks after apparent recovery, careful neuromuscular assessment should be conducted to assure that muscular weakness has not been missed. Bilateral audiometry is recommended, especially when mumps virus was involved.

When the specific cause has been identified, the parents should be so informed. This is especially useful in the case of mumps in order to avoid anxiety following exposure to mumps in later life.

ENCEPHALITIS

(Meningoencephalomyeloradiculitis)

The term "encephalitis" often conjures up a picture of a severe acute viral infection of the brain. In the actual clinical situation, however, this is too simplistic. Infectious and noninfectious causes, inflammatory and noninflammatory reactions, and signs and symptoms arising from all portions of the complex central nervous system may be considered "encephalitic" from a general clinical standpoint. For the individual sick child opinions may differ as to definitions: must there be fever, or pleocytosis, or convulsions, or drowsiness or coma, or focal neurologic signs, or other specific signs before a child's condition is called "encephalitic"? The term "encephalopathy" adds further confusion except when definite causal factors can be ascertained, such as uremia, hypernatremia, plumbism, water intoxication or botulism.

Various terms are applied for clinical convenience, but conceptually the following are regarded as related to encephalitis: the *aseptic meningitis syndrome*—in which there is little or no external evidence of neuronal involvement; the *Guillain-Barré syndrome,* with or without detectable involvement of cranial nerve nuclei and roots; and *Landry syndrome,* in which the initial findings occur in the spinal cord but ascending changes reach the brain. When there is a marked disturbance in cerebral functions and there is no discernible metabolic or toxic cause, the term is simply "encephalitis."

It is difficult in many instances to classify, to prognosticate or to assess various modes of preven-

TABLE 10–22 CLASSIFICATION OF ENCEPHALITIS BY ETIOLOGY AND SOURCE

I. Infections–Viral
  A. Spread man to man only
    1. RNA viruses
      Mumps: frequent; often mild
      Measles:not rare; may have serious sequelae
      Enterovirus group: frequent all ages; more serious in newborns
      Rubella: uncommon; sequelae rare except in congenital rubella
    2. DNA viruses
      Herpesvirus group
        a. Herpesvirus hominis (types 1 and 2: relatively common; sequelae frequent; devastating in newborns
        b. Varicella-zoster virus: uncommon; serious sequelae not rare
        c. Cytomegaloviruses–congenital or acquired: may have delayed sequelae in congenital CMV
        d. EB virus (infectious mononucleosis): not common
      Pox group
        a. Vaccinia and variola: uncommon, but serious CNS damage occurs
  B. Arthropod-borne agents
    Arboviruses (RNA viruses): spread to man by mosquitoes (Powassan from tick bites); seasonal epidemics depend upon ecology of the insect vector; the following occur in the U.S.A.:

Eastern equine	St. Louis
Western equine	California
Venezuela equine	Powassan

  C. Spread by warm-blooded mammals:
    Rabies: saliva of many domestic and wild mammalian species
    Herpesvirus simiae ("B" virus): monkeys' saliva
    Lymphocytic choriomeningitis: rodents' excreta

II. Infections–Not Viral
  A. Rickettsial: encephalitic component from cerebral vasculitis
  B. *Mycoplasma pneumoniae*: interval of some days between respiratory and CNS symptoms
  C. Bacterial: tuberculous and other bacterial meningitis; often has encephalitic component
  D. Spirochetal: syphilis, congenital or acquired; leptospiroses
  E. Fungal: immunologically compromised patients at special risk; cryptococcosis; histoplasmosis; aspergillosis; mucormycosis; moniliasis; coccidioidomycosis
  F. Protozoal: Hartmanella amebae; *Toxoplasma gondii*
  G. Metazoal: trichinosis; echinococcosis; cysticercosis; schistosomiasis

III. Para-infectious–Post-infectious, Allergic
  Patients in whom an infectious agent or one of its components plays a contributory role in etiology, but the intact infectious agent is not isolated in vitro from the nervous system. It is postulated that in this group the influence of cell-mediated antigen-antibody complexes plus complement is especially important in producing the observed tissue damage
  A. Associated with specific diseases (These agents may also cause direct CNS damage–see I above)

Measles	Rickettsial infections
Rubella	Pertussis
Mumps	Influenza
Varicella-zoster	Hepatitis
Mycoplasma pneumonia	

  B. Associated with vaccines:

Rabies	Pertussis
Measles	Yellow fever
Influenza	Typhoid
Vaccinia	

IV. Human Slow-Virus Diseases.
  Accumulating evidence that viruses acquired earlier in life, not necessarily with detectable acute illness, participate somehow in later chronic neurologic disease (similar events also known to occur in animals) (see Section 20)
  A. Subacute sclerosing panencephalitis (SSPE)
  B. Jakob-Creutzfeldt disease (spongiform encephalopathy)
  C. Progressive multifocal leukoencephalopathy
  D. Kuru (Fore tribe in New Guinea only)

V. Unknown–Complex Group
  This group comprises more than half the cases of encephalitis reported to the Center for Disease Control, Atlanta, Georgia.

There is also a miscellaneous group with eponyms which are based on clinical criteria: Reye syndrome is one current example. Others include the extinct von Economo encephalitis (epidemic from 1918 to 1928); myoclonic encephalopathy of infancy; retinomeningoencephalitis with papilledema and retinal hemorrhage; recurrent encephalomyelitis (? allergic or autoimmune); pseudotumour cerebri; and epidemic neuromyasthenia–Iceland disease.

An encephalitic clinical picture may be presented by a patient who has ingested unknown toxic substances, as well as recognized instances of lead or methyl mercury ingestion or excessive absorption of hexachlorophene.

---

tion and treatment of the encephalitides. Consequently in two thirds of patients in the United States officially reported as having encephalitis the disease is classified as being of "unknown complex etiology." Knowledge is increasing, however, especially with regard to those patients with encephalitis due wholly or in part to infectious agents, especially viruses.

Table 10–22 presents an abbreviated catalog of encephalitic categories. Many of the specific agents listed produce other syndromes and are discussed more fully elsewhere. (See the index.)

GENERAL CLINICAL PATTERNS. The conditions called encephalitis are more correctly thought of as meningoencephalomyeloradiculitis. The clinical findings are determined by: (1) the severity of involvement and anatomic localization of the affected portions of the nervous system; (2) the inherent pathogenicity of the offending agent; and (3) the immune and other reactive mechanisms of the patient ("host factors"). There is, accordingly, a wide range of severity of clinical manifestations even with the same etiologic agent. Some children may appear to be mildly affected initially, only to lapse into coma and sudden death. Others may have their illness ushered in by high fever, violent convulsions interspersed with bizarre movements, and hallucinations alternating with brief periods of clarity, ending nevertheless with relatively few sequelae.

Most commonly the initial manifestation resembles an undifferentiated acute systemic illness with fever, with headache or, in infants, with screaming spells, and with abdominal distress, nausea and vomiting. Signs of an associated mild nasopharyngitis may suggest a mere respiratory infection. As the temperature rises, new findings direct attention to the nervous system: mental dullness eventuating in stupor; bizarre movements; convulsions; nuchal rigidity, often not so pronounced as in a purely meningitic illness; and focal neurologic signs which may be stationary, progress or fluctuate. Loss of bowel and bladder control and unprovoked emotional bursts may be noted.

With some exceptions, the neurologic findings observed at the bedside hour by hour and day after day seldom give clues as to the etiologic diagnosis, but serve as baselines for prognosis. Careful serial descriptions of patients may help to establish specific clinical patterns such as emerged in the 1918 to 1928 epidemic of (presumed viral) von Economo's encephalitis.

A meticulous history is essential and must evaluate exposure in the past 2 or 3 weeks to illness in contacts; exposure to mosquitoes, ticks and animals during recent vacations, picnics, and so forth; recent travel from the home area; recent injections of any kind; and the possibility of accidental exposure to heavy metals, pesticides or other questionable substances.

The *cerebrospinal fluid* must be examined carefully in order to exclude disorders which require and respond to urgent specific therapy, which is unfortunately not the case in most instances of encephalitis. Smears for bacteria and cultures of the cerebrospinal fluid are mandatory; the history and clinical findings may indicate the need for acid-fast stain and culture of the sediment for Mycobacteria. Other circumstances may indicate the need for excluding fungal or protozoal infection; atypical cells may require cytopathologic study to exclude neural neoplasms which may present acutely.

In viral encephalitis the fluid is generally clear; the leukocyte count ranges from none to several thousand, often with a significant percentage of polymorphonuclear cells initially, moderate or no elevation of protein, and an initially normal level of glucose in ratio to the simultaneously determined blood glucose level. More sophisticated tests for the presence or absence of endotoxin, specific enzymes, globulin fractions, antigen detection by immunoprecipitation and fluorescent staining of cells are not generally available. Expert advice should be sought early for any patient suspected of having an encephalitic illness. At the very least, in any patient suspected of having viral meningoencephalitis, spinal fluid, blood, feces and throat swabs should be collected and sent via the hospital laboratory to an institutional or governmental laboratory offering viral diagnostic services. An additional serum specimen should be collected 10 to 14 days later. They give no immediate diagnostic assistance, but such studies are useful for the following reasons: etiologic diagnosis may give early warning of a specific epidemic; the cautious experimental use of specific antiviral chemotherapy may be indicated by the preliminary results; if evidence is produced for a specific virus the patient can generally be assured of subsequent lasting immunity to that virus, which in the case of mumps is useful since subsequent exposures are likely.

DIFFERENTIAL DIAGNOSIS. A patient with concurrent or recent mumps, measles, and so forth (see Table 10–22, I, A) is a likely candidate for that infection, but neurologic involvement at times precedes the classic general disease, and mumps meningoencephalitis commonly occurs without parotitis. When mumps parotitis occurs without clinical evidence of involvement of the central nervous system, cerebrospinal fluid pleocytosis often indicates that such involvement is present. In measles, moreover, some 40 per cent of patients without clinical evidence of encephalitis have electroencephalograms suggestive of an active disturbance. The relation of acute non-neural diseases in early life to neural syndromes appearing in later life is an important enigma. (See Table 10–22, IV.)

Inquiry regarding recent illnesses, recent injections and especially recent exposures away from the home environment are sometimes helpful. The incubation periods of some arboviruses are such that mosquito bites acquired a week or more earlier or insect bites now healed may give a clue. Occasionally, patients who have traveled in Africa or Asia in recent weeks will present with encephalitis due to viruses, trypanosomiasis or falciparum malaria.

Children whose immunologic status is compromised (e.g., lymphoma, cytotoxic drugs, immunogenetic defects) are at increased risk, especially with respect to infections in which protective cell-mediated immunity is important (e.g., chickenpox, cytomegalovirus, fungal infections). Children with leukemia who have had prophylactic radiation to the central nervous system and intrathecal drugs may develop an acute meningoencephalitis after cessation of such prophylaxis.

ENVIRONMENTAL FACTORS. Sporadic cases of encephalitis occur in any season. The summer months bring an increased incidence of encephalitis, in large measure due to enteroviruses (coxsackie and echo groups, and poliomyelitis when the latter has not been controlled by vaccination) and the arboviruses. The incidence of presumably viral encephalitis rises in the summer months, however, even when there is little or no evidence of the prevalence of arboviruses or enteroviruses. Continued research may disclose additional viruses whose activity is amplified by summer weather or activities.

Geographic considerations are alluded to above. Consultation with health departments may provide clues to etiology. Terms used for arboviruses, such as Eastern, Western, Venezuelan, California, indicate only where those viruses were first discovered and not where they are now observed.

SOME VIROLOGIC FEATURES

Arboviruses. (See Table 10–22, I,B.) These single-stranded RNA viruses are really zoonoses in which man is infected accidentally by an arthropod vector, man not being essential in the life cycle of arboviruses. Most commonly mosquitos or other insects are infected through biting birds, which often have prolonged viremia without illness. The insect vectors, though preferring birds, bite other vertebrates, including man and horses. Encephalitis in horses and mules ("blind staggers") may be the first indication of incipient trouble in an area; veterinarians are often the first to detect an impending epidemic.

Eastern Equine Encephalitis. This appears to have a predilection for young infants; it is devastating, with high mortality and severe sequelae.

St. Louis Virus Encephalitis. This produces inapparent infection (demonstrated only by seroconversion) as well as disease, and has a lower incidence in young children than in adolescents and adults.

Western Equine Encephalitis. Many infections are mild or clinically inapparent, demonstrated only by seroconversion. The case fatality is much less than with Eastern equine encephalitis, but sequelae may be severe in young children and adolescents.

California Virus Encephalitis. Outbreaks occur mostly in the midwestern United States. Some cases are mild, but a significant number are severe, with important sequelae.

Powassan Virus Encephalitis. Transmitted by the bite of infected wood ticks, more cases occur in Canada than in the United States; few cases have been found in children so far.

Venezuelan Equine Encephalitis. Infection with this has begun to appear in the United States. Thus far the incidence of human disease has been low and the illness mild, though devastating equine outbreaks have occurred.

The Human Herpesvirus Group. Man is the sole source of the following four DNA viruses: (1) herpesvirus hominis, types 1 and 2; (2) chickenpox-zoster virus; (3) cytomegalovirus; and (4) the Epstein-Barr (EB) virus of infectious mononucleosis. In addition to the more usual general clinical syndromes known to be caused by these agents, acute encephalitis may occur. Members of this group may become latent and induce late neurologic damage as a result of a variety of circumstances which compromise host resistance, especially conditions associated with depression of cellular immunocompetence (e.g., malignancy, immunodepressant drugs, organ transplants).

Herpesvirus hominis, types 1 and 2, are relatively frequent causes of sporadic acute encephalitis, which may occur during primary contact with the virus or in persons who had an earlier primary infection, either subclinical or long forgotten. Herpesvirus encephalitis in newborn infants is part of a generalized viremia; the infection is usually due to type 2 virus harbored in the maternal genital tract, but type 1 neonatal encephalitis also occurs. In older patients infections may produce diffuse encephalitis, simulate brain abscess, or simulate fatal bulbospinal poliomyelitis, even when the patient's serologic status indicates nonprimary infection. The cerebrospinal fluid may contain erythrocytes in a nontraumatic spinal tap.

Chickenpox-zoster virus (VZV) may cause acute encephalitis in close temporal relationship to chickenpox. The VZV appears capable of secluding itself in spinal and cranial nerve roots and ganglia as a latent or suppressed infection, to express itself later as herpes zoster.

Cytomegaloviruses (CMV) may produce intrauterine infection with involvement of the central nervous system. Severe cases may be recognized at birth, but more often subtle evidence of brain damage is not apparent for months or several years after birth. As with other herpesviruses, CMV has a talent for latency in various tissues, including latency within leukocytes. Blood transfusions may be responsible for transmission of disease. Under situations compromising host immunity, recrudescence may occur.

Epstein-Barr virus (EBV) encephalitis may occur during infectious mononucleosis, but there is no evidence at present for its becoming latent in any portion of the nervous system.

The Enterovirus Group. There are 66 members of this group, all small RNA-containing viruses. The three serotypes of poliovirus have become less important as agents of disease among well vaccinated populations. Not all the 63 coxsackie and echo serotypes have as yet been definitely associated with neurologic disease, either as the chief clinical feature or as a complication, for example, of pleurodynia or myocarditis. The severity of disease ranges from mild meningoencephalitis (aseptic meningitis) to severe encephalitis with significant sequelae or fatality.

Epidemics have been observed in newborn nurseries in many parts of the world, sometimes with devastating effects.

PATHOGENESIS. The sequence of events varies with the agent of disease and with the host. In general, the viruses of encephalitis get into the lymphatic system, whether from ingestion of an enterovirus, or from a mosquito or other insect bite. There multiplication begins, and seeding of the blood stream leads to infection of several organs. At this stage (the extraneural phase) a non-neural systemic illness is present, but if further viral multiplication takes place in the seeded organs, a secondary propagation of large amounts of virus may occur. Invasion of the central nervous system may then be followed by clinical evidence of neurologic disease.

A formerly held, simplistic view of viral encephalitis was that the disease was caused either: (1) by direct invasion and destruction of neural tissues by actively multiplying viruses; or (2) by a reaction

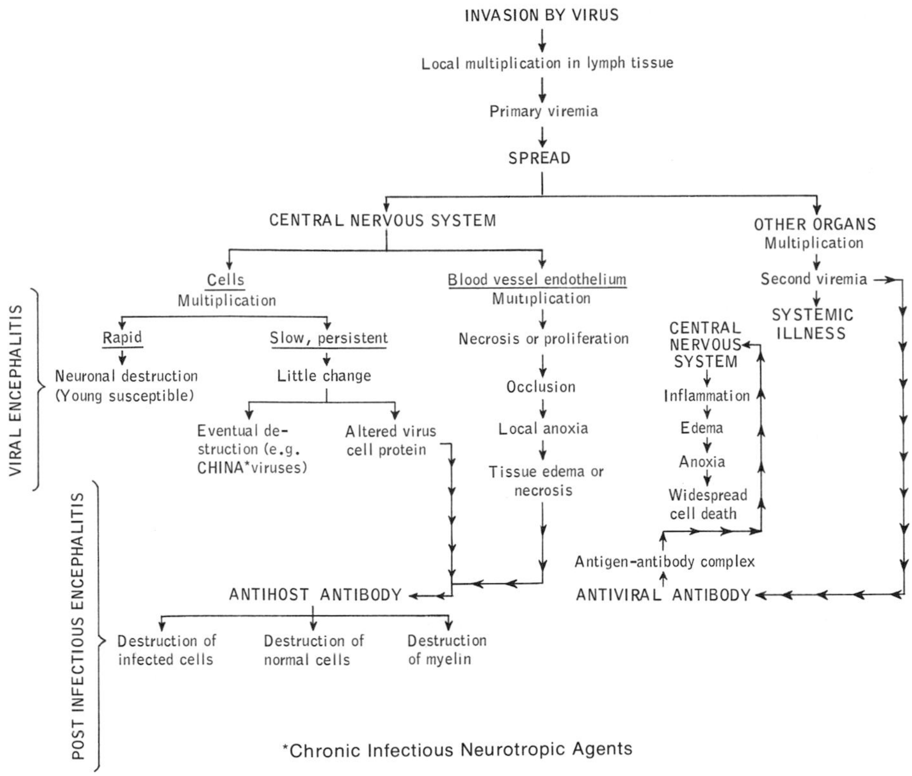

Figure 10–57 *Pathogenetic mechanisms of encephalitis.*

of the patient's nervous tissue to antigens of the virus (the so-called postinfectious or allergic encephalitis). It is more likely that elements of both occur in many instances. Direct viral damage is likely associated with neuronal destruction, and the host's vigorous tissue response associated with demyelinization, vascular and perivascular destruction. The latter process leads to impaired circulation and to corresponding signs and symptoms. Figure 10–57 portrays diagrammatically some of the numerous events which may occur in acute encephalitis, along with early and remote tissue responses.

The etiology and pathogenesis of cases of inflammatory encephalitis in which there is no evidence of the direct or indirect involvement of any infectious agent remains shrouded in mystery. There is a distinctly elevated ratio of male to female patients with encephalitis due to mumps or the enteroviruses. Neither this nor the disparity between the large numbers infected and the relatively few who become ill is explained. Every case of encephalitis deserves intensive investigation, clinically, epidemiologically and in the virus and microbiologic laboratories.

PATHOLOGY. The etiologic diagnosis of encephalitis is difficult to make even post mortem. Exceptions involve such nonviral causes as falciparum malaria, trypanosomiasis and fungal encephalitis, in which morphologic identification is possible. (See Table 10–22, II, A to E.) In viral encephalitides, the histopathologist may recognize rabies (cytoplasmic Negri bodies) or an agent of the herpesvirus group (intranuclear inclusion bodies), but generally special viral studies are needed. This requires that tissues be collected *without fixation in preservatives*, so that viral isolation and identification can be attempted; immunofluorescent studies and electron microscopic study may provide critical diagnostic information.

Tissue sections of the brain generally reveal meningeal congestion and mononuclear infiltration, perivascular cuffs of lymphocytes and plasma cells, some perivascular tissue necrosis with myelin breakdown, neuronal disruption in various stages including ultimately neuronophagia, and endothelial proliferation or necrosis. When there is a marked degree of demyelination with preservation of neurons and their axons, one tends to consider this as predominantly "postinfectious" or "allergic" encephalitis. With the above exceptions, specific viral etiology is not generally determined by histopathology. The severity and the extent of observed lesions does vary somewhat with the viral agent, as well as with the degree of exuberance in the reaction of the host. The cerebral cortex, especially the temporal lobe, is often severely affected by herpesvirus; the arboviruses tend to affect the entire brain; rabies has a predilection for the basal structures. The degree of involvement of the spinal cord, nerve roots and peripheral nerves is quite variable.

Extraneural pathology varies with the responsible cause, the duration of the illness and the complications stemming from the urgencies of intensive treatment. Seen are pneumonia with and without tracheostomy, congestive heart failure, urinary tract infection associated with catheterization, thrombophlebitis at the sites of infusions, hemolytic-uremic syndrome and, in cases of fatal neonatal encephalitis and chickenpox encephalitis, the syndrome of disseminated intravascular coagulation.

MANAGEMENT. A guarded prognosis is in order with respect to both immediate outcome and sequelae. Sequelae involving the central nervous system may be intellectual, motor, psychiatric, epileptic, visual or auditory. Cardiovascular, intraocular, pulmonary, hepatic and other systems are sometimes permanently affected. The short-term and long-term prognoses depend to some extent on etiology. Age is a factor; young infants generally have severe disease and sequelae. In general, herpesvirus types 1 and 2 carry a worse prognosis for survival and residual disability than do the enteroviruses. Fetal rubella encephalitis is very ominous, as is acute generalized cytomegalovirus infection accompanied by encephalitis. The latter may be insidious, with evidence of disability deferred for some months.

Acute Stage. Treatment is nonspecific and empirical, aimed at maintaining life and the support of each involved organ system. It has been impossible to evaluate objectively the effectiveness of various recommended regimens.

Until a bacterial etiology is substantially excluded, parenteral antibiotic therapy should be administered.

It is crucial to anticipate and be prepared for *convulsions, cerebral edema, hyperpyrexia, inadequate respiratory exchange, disturbed fluid and electrolyte balance, aspiration and asphyxia, abrupt cardiac and respiratory cessation of central origin* and *cardiac decompensation.* The syndrome of *disseminated intravascular coagulation* may be an additional complication. For these reasons all patients with severe encephalitis should be cared for in hospitals equipped for full-time intensive care. A cardiac monitor should be attached for continuous surveillance and for periodic recording. All fluids, electrolytes and medications are given parenterally initially. The syndrome of *inappropriate secretion of antidiuretic hormone* is fairly common in acute central nervous system disorders, infectious or not; its possible occurrence adds to the importance of frequent clinical and laboratory evaluation of the fluid and electrolyte equilibrium. Normal blood levels of glucose, magnesium and calcium must be maintained in order to minimize the threat of convulsions.

Phenobarbital, 5 to 8 mg/kg/24 hr, is given in an effort to prevent convulsions. The use of phenobarbital may make clinical assessment of progress difficult, but the importance of preventing convulsions is paramount. If frequent or sustained convulsions appear, it may then be necessary to give diazepam (Valium) intravenously (0.1 to 0.2 mg/kg).

A number of methods are proposed to minimize cerebral edema and to diminish the consequences of cerebral anoxia; these measures are difficult to evaluate and are generally reserved for patients with very severe illness, whose condition appears desperate:

1. *Dexamethasone,* 0.25 to 0.5 mg/kg/24 hr is given intramuscularly. This large dose should be reduced gradually after a few days if recovery or improvement is evident.

2. Substances employed in an effort to reduce elevated intracranial pressure include:
   a. *Mannitol,* given intravenously as a 20 per cent solution in a dose of 1.5 to 2.0 gm/kg over a 2-hour period. This may be repeated every 8 to 12 hours.
   b. *Glycerol,* by nasogastric tube, using 1.5 ml/kg diluted with twice that volume of orange juice. This is nontoxic and may be repeated every 8 hours for an extended period of time.
   c. *Urea,* given intravenously as a 30 per cent solution in 10 per cent invert sugar (Urevert), in a dose of 1.0 to 1.5 gm slowly over a 30- to 60-minute period. Repeated doses of Urevert may yield a rebound effect, resulting in increased intracranial pressure.

3. Artificial *hypothermia* may be tried, and should maintain a body temperature of approximately 31.5°C (89°F). The use of an autoregulated coolant blanket is required. If shivering retards the desired decrease in temperature, chlorpromazine (Thorazine), 1 mg/kg, may be injected. After 3 to 4 days of hypothermia the patient is restored to normothermia; if neurologic signs and convulsions reappear, a new trial of induced hypothermia may be made.

Equipment and personnel for handling emergencies such as cardiac and respiratory arrest must be constantly at hand. Early consultation with an anesthesiologist is useful in anticipation of the need for artificial assisted respiration. (See Section 5.) For the management of associated cardiac arrhythmias and congestive failure, see Section 13.

Only when the specific etiology is recognized or surmised are there therapeutic agents which may be considered at all specific. These occasions are few (Table 10–22, II). In conditions listed in table under III, the empiric use of dexamethasone or immunosuppressive agents may be tried.

At the present time there are no generally available safe and effective chemical or biologic agents of proved value in the management of viral encephalitis. Current study of the DNA viruses of the herpesvirus group indicates that three pyrimidine nucleosides (iododeoxyuridine, cytosine arabinoside and adenine arabinoside) may soon be shown to be helpful, but limited observations at this time are inconclusive for any beneficial effect on acute encephalitis.

Interferon, a biologic product of infected host cells, produces antiviral effects through inducing a state of resistance to virus infections of host cells. It may be responsible in part for the natural arrest of certain viral infections. Interferon production can be stimulated by the administration of inducing substances such as polyionosinic and polycytidylic acid complex (poly I:C). Experimental results have been interesting, but there is at present no evidence that poly I:C is useful in management of acute encephalitis.

Certain difficult phases of management begin only after the patient recovers. Supportive and rehabilitative efforts are very important during the follow-up period. Motor incoordination, convulsive disorders, squint, total or partial deafness, or behavioral disturbances may appear only after an interval of time. Visual disturbances due to chorioretinopathy and perceptual amblyopia may also make a delayed appearance. Special facilities and at times institutional placement may become necessary.

ALEX. J. STEIGMAN

Balfour, H. H., Jr., et al.: California arbovirus (La Crosse) infections I: Clinical and laboratory findings in 66 children with meningoencephalitis. Pediatrics *52*:680, 1973.
Brody, J. A., Henle, W., and Koprowski, H.: Chronic Infectious Neuropathic Agents (CHINA) and other slow virus infections. Curr. Top. Microbiol. Immunol. *40*:1, 1967.
Byington, D. P., Castro, A. E., and Burnstein, T.: Adaptation to hamsters of neurotropic measles virus from subacute sclerosing panencephalitis. Nature (London) *225*:554, 1970.
Carter, R. F.: Primary amoebic meningo-encephalitis. Trans. Roy. Soc. Trop. Med. Hyg. *66*:193, 1972.
Casals, J.: Arboviruses. Amer. J. Clin. Path. *57*:762, 1972.
Gibbs, C. J., and Gadjusek, D. C.: Infection as the etiology of spongiform encephalopathy (Creutzfeldt-Jakob disease). Science *165*:1023, 1969.
Holzel, A., Smith, P. S., and Tobin, J. O'H.: A new type of meningo-encephalitis associated with a rhinovirus (retino-meningoencephalitis). Acta Paediat. Scand. *54*:168, 1965.
Johnson, R. T., and Mims, C. A.: Pathogenesis of viral infections of the nervous system. N. Engl. J. Med. *278*:23; 84; 1968.
Kennedy, C., and Scott, T. F. McN.: The management of acute febrile encephalopathies. *In* Eichenwald, H. (ed.): The Prevention of Mental Retardation Through Control of Infectious Disease. Bethesda, Md., Department of Health, Education, and Welfare, NIH, 1966, p. 309.
Lerer, R. J., and Kalavsky, S. M.: Central nervous system disease associated with mycoplasma pneumoniae. Pediatrics *52*:658, 1973.
Link, H., Panelius, M., and Salmi, A. A.: Immunoglobulins and measles antibodies in subacute sclerosing panencephalitis: Demonstration of synthesis of oligoclonal IgG with measles antibody activity within the central nervous system. Arch. Neurol. *28*:23, 1973.
Liu, C., and Llanes-Rodas, R.: Application of the immunofluorescent technique to the study of pathogenesis and rapid diagnosis of viral infections. Amer. J. Clin. Path. *57*:829, 1972.
McIntosh, S., and Aspnes, G. T.: Encephalopathy following CNS prophylaxis in childhood lymphoblastic leukemia. Pediatrics *52*:612, 1973.
Melnick, J. L.: Classification and nomenclature of viruses. Prog. Med. Virol. *14*:32, 1972.

RICKETTSIAL DISEASES

The rickettsiae are microorganisms which commonly inhabit the alimentary canal of certain insects and may be associated with disease in man. Stained preparations appear under the ordinary microscope as pleomorphic coccobacilli 0.3 to 0.5 μ in diameter. Most species are retained by bacterial filters, and all require the presence of living cells for multiplication. Biologically the rickettsiae have some of the characteristics of bacteria and some of viruses and are classified in an intermediate position.

The rickettsial diseases of man, with the exception of Q fever, are febrile illnesses with rashes. They may be separated into four groups on the basis of clinical characteristics, insect vectors, etiologic agent and epidemiology (Table 10–23).

Epidemic typhus and endemic typhus are almost identical clinically and pathologically. The causative agents are so similar antigenically that cross-reactions occur in Proteus or rickettsial agglutination tests. The two forms of the disease may be distinguished by specific complement fixation tests and by the inability of epidemic typhus to produce a scrotal reaction in guinea pigs. Brill's disease is a recrudescence of epidemic typhus.

There are many related strains of rickettsiae which cause spotted fever of variable severity in different parts of the world. The list includes boutonneuse fever of the Mediterranean regions; São Paulo, Tobia and pinta fevers of South America; Kenya or Nigeria fever of Africa; and many others. Rickettsialpox is included in the spotted fever group because of antigenic relations of *Rickettsia akari* to the causative agent of Rocky Mountain spotted fever.

Tsutsugamushi fever, or scrub typhus, was known in certain areas of Japan for many years, but not until the beginning of World War II was it learned that the disease was present also among the populations of India, Australia, Indonesia (Dutch East Indies) and Malaya. Effective vaccines are not available, and scrub typhus continues to be a hazard to those who enter endemic areas.

Q fever differs clinically, histologically and epidemiologically from the other diseases listed and is classified with them only because it is caused by a rickettsia.

The immunity, pathology, methods for making a laboratory diagnosis, and manner of treatment of each of the rickettsial diseases in man are so similar that it seems appropriate to discuss these topics as a whole before describing the individual diseases.

IMMUNITY. Prolonged immunity to specific rickettsial agents following recovery from disease has been shown by clinical and epidemiologic observations. In laboratory animals experimentally infected, immunity has been proved by unsuccessful attempts to reinfect. A significant degree of cross-immunity to related organisms may result from infection with one member of a group, i.e., the individual who has had Rocky Mountain spotted fever

TABLE 10–23 RICKETTSIAL DISEASES OF MAN: SUMMARY OF PERTINENT INFORMATION

GROUP	DISEASE	CAUSATIVE AGENT	ARTHROPOD VECTOR	ANIMAL HOST	PROTEUS AGGLUTINATION*	GEOGRAPHIC DISTRIBUTION
Typhus	Epidemic typhus	*R. prowazeki*	Body louse	None	OX19	World-wide; rarely U.S.A.
	Brill's disease	*R. prowazeki*	None		OX19	Eastern coastal cities of U.S.A.; Israel
	Murine typhus	*R. mooseri*	Rat flea, louse	Rat	OX19	World-wide; southern states of U.S.A.
Spotted fever	Rocky Mountain spotted fever	*R. rickettsii*	Tick	Rodents, mammals	Variable OX2 or OX19	North and South America; related diseases world-wide
	Rickettsial-pox	*R. akari*	Mite	House mice	None	Reported from eastern U.S.A.
Tsutsugamushi fever	Scrub typhus	*R. orientalis* (tsutsugamushi)	Mite	Rodents	OXK	Far East
Q fever	Q fever	*R. burnetii (Coxiella burnetii)*	Rarely ticks ?	Ticks, cattle, sheep, goats	None	World-wide; western U.S.A.

*Specific serologic procedures using rickettsial antigens in complement fixation, agglutination or neutralization tests are more reliable.

is protected against other tickborne spotted fevers; immunity to epidemic and murine typhus are linked, but an attack of scrub typhus which confers good homologous immunity protects only transiently against heterologous strains of *R. orientalis.* Protection produced by vaccines is generally less effective and of shorter duration than that produced by natural infection. Chronic or recurrent infections with rickettsiae may occur. Brill's disease is the well known example, but exacerbations of scrub typhus with repeated isolation of the same strain of *R. orientalis* have been observed. Cell-mediated immune mechanisms may play an important role in limiting the intracellular persistence of rickettsiae, but investigations in this area are rudimentary.

PATHOLOGY. The lesion of the arthropodborne rickettsial diseases is sufficiently distinctive to be diagnostic in patients with a history of an exanthem. The main changes involve the small blood vessels, chiefly of the skin, subcutaneous tissue and central nervous system. The endothelial cells swell and occlude the small blood vessels, and thrombosis results. The occluded vessels are surrounded by cuffs of mononuclear cells, plasma cells and macrophages. Rickettsiae localize in the endothelium of capillaries and extend via the intima into larger vessels. Rocky Mountain spotted fever may be distinguished histologically from other rickettsial diseases by the presence of rickettsiae in the smooth muscle cells of the media. This results in severe destruction of blood vessels and may explain the occurrence of necrosis of skin in sites such as the ear lobes, fingers, toes and scrotum.

The symptomatology of vector-transmitted rickettsial diseases correlates with the degree of involvement and the location of affected vessels. For example, the fall in blood pressure, an outstanding clinical feature of rickettsial disease, is generally conceded to be the result of changes in the peripheral vessels. Perivascular reactions in the lung may result in atelectasis and pneumonia. Vascular changes in the brain may produce central nervous system symptoms.

Q fever, which is not accompanied by a rash and does not require an insect vector, differs pathologically from the other rickettsial diseases. The principal, and usually the only, lesions occur in the lungs, where there is a patchy interstitial pneumonitis with copious exudate composed of fibrin and mononuclear cells. Alveolar walls, alveolar ducts and terminal bronchioles are infiltrated by large mononuclear cells.

DIAGNOSIS. The diagnosis of a rickettsial infection in man usually requires laboratory confirmation, which is most readily established by demonstration of acquired specific antibodies. In unusual cases when serologic tests are unobtainable or equivocal, it may be necessary to identify the causative agent.

Serologic Diagnosis. During etiologic studies of typhus fever, Felix isolated a strain of *Proteus vulgaris* from the urine of a patient. This strain (OX19) was not the causative agent of typhus, but had sufficient antigenic similarity to *Rickettsia* *prowazeki* so that serum from patients convalescent from typhus fever contained high titers of OX19 agglutinin. Additional strains of Proteus related to the causative agents of tsutsugamushi (OXK) and Rocky Mountain spotted fever (OX2) were also discovered. These easily prepared antigens are used for agglutination tests in patients' serums (the Weil-Felix reaction).

In epidemic typhus fever the agglutination to OX19 usually reaches a titer greater than 1:160 during the second week of illness; the OX2 and OXK titers remain low. The agglutinin pattern observed with murine typhus is similar to that of epidemic typhus, and the two infections cannot be distinguished by this method. The Proteus agglutination test is of little value in the diagnosis of Rocky Mountain spotted fever, owing to the variations in the degree and types of response; classically, the patient should have a high titer of OX2 agglutinins and little, if any, antibody against OX19 and OXK. Proteus OXK agglutinin titers are high after tsutsugamushi disease. Convalescent serum from patients with Q fever or rickettsialpox does not agglutinate to significant titer the Proteus strains used in the Weil-Felix reaction. Proteus titers do not persist and are usually below a significant level within 3 months after the illness.

Specific serologic procedures using rickettsial antigens in complement fixation, agglutination or neutralization tests are much more reliable than the Weil-Felix reaction and should be used to confirm the diagnosis of rickettsial infections. Two samples of serum, one obtained during the first week of illness, and the other, 2 or 3 weeks later, should be available to determine whether a significant increase in titer has occurred during the illness.

Culturing of Rickettsiae. Rickettsiae may be propagated by inoculating susceptible experimental animals or developing chick embryos. These techniques are seldom required to diagnose rickettsial infections, but may be used to study the effectiveness of various antibiotics or to detect the presence of rickettsiae in milk, dust or insects.

The culturing of rickettsiae in the laboratory is extremely hazardous and has been the source of infection for many investigators. This is a task for a special laboratory with proper facilities and immunized personnel. Serologic procedures, using killed antigen and heat-inactivated serums, involve little risk to the laboratory worker.

PROGNOSIS. In general, there is a rather striking relationship between age and mortality from rickettsial disease; children do better than adults or the aged. Epidemics of typhus in the 19th century had an average mortality rate of 20 per cent, ranging from less than 3 per cent in the pediatric age group to 50 per cent in those in their fifth decade of life. The range was similar in severe outbreaks of scrub typhus or Rocky Mountain spotted fever. Mortality rates are markedly diminished by prompt use of antibiotics. Murine typhus, Q fever and rickettsialpox are relatively mild diseases with low mortality rates even when untreated.

TREATMENT. Treatment of rickettsial infections is much more effective since the discovery of the broad spectrum antibiotics. Mortality rates have fallen greatly, the morbidity rate has decreased and complications have become infrequent. These drugs, however, are not immediately or invariably effective in influencing the course of the disease, and clinical relapses are not uncommon. Rickettsiae have been isolated from the blood of patients who received presumably adequate doses of an antibiotic. These difficulties are related to the fact that chloramphenicol and the tetracyclines suppress, but do not destroy, the rickettsiae. Final eradication of the microorganism depends upon the immune processes of the host.

The recommended dose of the tetracyclines or chloramphenicol for children is 50 to 100 mg/kg/day orally in 4 divided doses. The maximum or adult daily dose is 4 gm. When the intravenous route is used, 30 to 40 mg/kg/day of either drug should be administered in 3 equal doses. Drug therapy should be continued until the patient is afebrile for 48 hours; this is usually 5 to 9 days after initiation of treatment.

Early diagnosis and the proper use of antimicrobial agents are all that is necessary in the management of most rickettsial infections. Vigorous supportive therapy, parenteral fluids, transfusions, sedation and oxygen are necessary for the severely ill patient.

Good results with added corticosteroids have been reported in cases apparently refractory to antibiotics alone, but this therapy remains to be critically evaluated. Corticosteroids are not recommended for the average case.

TYPHUS FEVER

(Epidemic Typhus; Louse-borne Typhus)

HISTORY. Typhus fever has been associated with misery since man donned clothing. Typhus was probably responsible for the plague of Athens, 430 B.C.; it existed during the Middle Ages and was associated with each of the serious famines in England. Typhus was spread through Europe by louse-infected soldiers and was often the most important factor in determining the outcome of battles or the survival of nations.

In more recent years typhus has been an Old World disease with large outbreaks during time of war. In October, 1943, the disease broke out in Naples as the Allied occupation troops arrived. Typhus was encountered in Nazi concentration camps and was spread through Europe by escaping inmates. Epidemics have occurred among immigrants in coastal cities in America, but typhus has not been common in the United States during recent years. The existence of endemic areas within a few hours of travel distance, however, makes epidemics of typhus in any country a possibility.

ETIOLOGY AND TRANSMISSION. Man is the sole reservoir of *Rickettsia prowazeki,* the causative agent of epidemic typhus. The body or head louse may become infected by feeding upon the blood of a person with rickettsemia. The ingested organisms multiply within the cells lining the alimentary tract of the insect and are eliminated in the feces.

Contaminated feces may be introduced into a susceptible human host through abrasions or perforations in the skin, or by way of the conjunctival sac or upper respiratory tract. Inhalation of dried, infected louse excreta present in the clothing, bedding or furniture of a typhus patient is probably an important source of infection.

The infected louse dies soon after contracting typhus and seldom has more than a week to spread disease. The louse cannot fly or jump, but may crawl short distances to another human being, especially if his original host becomes uncomfortably hot or cold.

PATHOLOGY. See preceding pages.

CLINICAL MANIFESTATIONS. Typhus fever was a much milder disease in children than in adults even before the availability of chemotherapeutic agents.

The clinical manifestations of typhus in children may include fever, transient rash and only a few constitutional symptoms, which often make recognition of the disease difficult.

The incubation period is usually less than 14 days and is followed by an abrupt onset with severe frontal headache, weakness, malaise, generalized aches and pains, chills, and fever of 104° F or more. Four to 7 days later the rash appears.

Faint, rose-colored spots of irregular outline 2 to 4 mm in size which fade with pressure appear first over the chest and spread gradually over the abdomen, back and extremities. In 24 to 48 hours the lesions become dark red and no longer fade with pressure. The lesions may spread to include the palms and soles, but the face and scalp usually remain free. Petechial lesions occur in severe cases. The rash may be present for only a few hours or persist after the temperature has returned to normal. In general, the more profuse the rash, the more severe is the disease.

The appearance of the rash marks the beginning of the critical period. The fever remains high and unremitting, and periods of stupor are interrupted by bouts of violent delirium. The blood pressure is low, and renal output decreased. Oral intake is low and requires parenteral supplementation. In the absence of complications such as pneumonia, severe central nervous system involvement or renal insufficiency, which are frequently fatal, the patient begins to improve during the third week. The temperature gradually falls, the central nervous system symptoms disappear, and the headache ceases. Recovery from typhus is complete, and even in patients with evidence of diffuse involvement sequelae are rare.

LABORATORY DATA. (See also prior pages.) Leukopenia with a relative lymphocytosis early in the disease is usually followed by a leukocytosis during the second and third weeks; a normocytic anemia is common. Urinary findings vary with the degree of renal involvement; albuminuria and microscopic hematuria are frequent.

DIFFERENTIAL DIAGNOSIS. Meningococcemia, typhoid, measles or smallpox may be confused with typhus, but the history, clinical course and laboratory data usually permit a proper diagnosis.

CONTROL MEASURES. The immediate destruction of vectors with an insecticide with persisting effect such as DDT is an important measure in the control of an epidemic. Dust containing excreta from infected lice is also capable of transmitting typhus, and care must be taken to prevent its inhalation. This usually requires washing the patient's clothing, bedding and other possessions with hot water and a disinfectant after they have been dusted with DDT. Vaccination of persons likely to come in contact with typhus is recommended. The preferred vaccine is a killed preparation of a rickettsia grown in the yolk sac of the chick embryo. Insufficient data are available as to differences in sensitivity to broad spectrum antibiotics by strains of rickettsiae, but if resistant forms do not occur, the administration of an antibiotic may be adequate prophylaxis for brief exposures to typhus.

TREATMENT. See prior pages.

MURINE TYPHUS

(Endemic Typhus)

ETIOLOGY AND TRANSMISSION. Unlike epidemic typhus, which is not seen among children in the United States, endemic typhus is fairly common, particularly in Texas and the southeastern states, and has been seen in most regions of this country. It usually occurs in the summer and fall, in contrast to typhus, which is characteristically a disease of winter and spring.

Murine typhus is a disease of rats caused by *Rickettsia mooseri.* It is usually transmitted from rat to rat by the rat louse or flea. In both the rat and the insect vectors murine typhus is a mild disease with no apparent effect on their life span. The eggs laid by infected fleas or lice do not transmit *R. mooseri* to the next generation. Man usually acquires murine typhus when bitten by an infected rat flea, but can also be infected by inhaling or possibly ingesting infected excreta of fleas.

PATHOLOGY. See prior pages.

CLINICAL MANIFESTATIONS. Murine typhus is a mild, seldom fatal illness that can be distinguished from epidemic typhus only by special laboratory procedures.

The incubation period is usually about 8 days. Prodromal symptoms such as headache, arthralgia and backache are followed by a gradually increasing temperature which may reach 106°F in children and last 9 to 14 days. Anytime from the first to the eighth day of fever, most often by the fifth day, the rash appears. The eruption begins on the trunk and spreads to the periphery, rarely involving the face, palms or soles. Initially the skin lesion is a dull red macule with ill defined margins which becomes slightly papular as it matures. It persists for a much shorter period than the rash of epidemic typhus, and rarely, if ever, becomes purpuric. Twenty per cent or more of children may have no rash, or such a transient one that it is not noted. Central nervous system symptoms are uncommon, as is peripheral vascular collapse or other complications.

DIAGNOSIS. See prior pages.

CONTROL MEASURES. Control of murine typhus requires elimination of the rat reservoir or the insect vector, or both. Immunization of personnel in contact with possibly infected rats is recommended. The vaccine is different from that used for epidemic typhus, although most persons who have recovered from one form of typhus are also immune to the other.

TREATMENT. See prior pages.

BRILL'S DISEASE

Brill's disease is an unusual phenomenon in which a patient with a history of typhus suffers a recrudescence of his illness. It has been observed among immigrants from eastern Europe in the coastal cities of the United States and more recently in Israel. The strains of rickettsiae isolated from such patients are indistinguishable from those of epidemic typhus. It is presumed that organisms have persisted in the tissues of the host for years, and then, for reasons not understood, they increase in number and produce clinical symptoms. A patient with Brill's disease can infect lice and is a potential point of origin for a typhus epidemic when the vector is present. Brill's disease is not a problem in children.

SCRUB TYPHUS

(Tsutsugamushi Fever; Mite Typhus)

Scrub typhus has been recognized in Japan and Formosa for centuries, but not until World War II was it realized that this disease could be found in localities stretching from India to the Philippines, including Burma, Malaysia, New Guinea, the Solomon Islands and Queensland. The incidence of scrub typhus among United States Army personnel in bases north of Australia during 1942 and 1943 was about 10 per 1000 troops per year, with a case fatality rate of 3 to 10 per cent.

ETIOLOGY AND TRANSMISSION. *Rickettsia tsutsugamushi,* also known as *R. orientalis,* is the causal agent of scrub typhus. The vectors which carry the agent are the larval forms of the chigger or trombiculid mites. The larvae feed on rats or other rodents and when not feeding are present on low-lying vegetation, whence they can attack man. *Rickettsia tsutsugamushi* has been isolated from many species of rodents, and it seems likely that both mites and rodents serve as reservoirs of rickettsiae.

Scrub typhus is mainly a disease of persons whose occupations bring them into contact with infected mites.

PATHOLOGY. See prior pages.

CLINICAL MANIFESTATIONS. The symptomatology of scrub typhus, although showing some distinctive features, is similar to that of other rickettsial infections. The disease may vary in severity but characteristically has an abrupt onset 12 to 18 days after the bite by the infected mite. The initial symptoms are fever and headache, sometimes accompanied by anorexia and vomiting.

The mite bite usually results in a local skin lesion, which begins as an asymptomatic, pink papule, increases in size and becomes either an eschar, consisting of a central, black scab 4 to 8 mm in diameter surrounded by a red areola, or, in moist areas (axilla, perineum), a pinched-out shallow ulcer. By the end of the first week of illness a maculopapular rash develops on the chest and abdomen and gradually spreads to involve the entire body, but rarely the hands and face. Diffuse, tender adenopathy, greater in the region of the primary lesion, is common.

Laboratory confirmation may be obtained by isolation of the causative agent in mice. The Weil-Felix reaction for Proteus OXK may become positive by the third week of the illness, but this is not invariable, especially in patients treated with antibiotics.

In severe cases signs of pulmonary or cardiac involvement may develop during the second week of illness, and death results. In mild or treated cases improvement begins by the end of the second week, fever decreases, the rash fades, and the eschar heals. The mortality rate when antibiotics are used is less than 5 per cent.

CONTROL MEASURES. The difficulties encountered in attempting to eliminate the widely prevalent mite vector of scrub typhus have led to investigations of control by vaccines. Unfortunately the vaccines tested have not proved entirely satisfactory, owing to the many antigenically different strains of *R. tsutsugamushi* which are pathogenic for man. It is hoped that an effective polyvalent vaccine can be prepared. Until such time, protective clothing and early treatment with broad spectrum antibiotics are the most useful aids to prevention of death from scrub typhus.

TREATMENT. See prior pages.

ROCKY MOUNTAIN SPOTTED FEVER

HISTORY. Rocky Mountain spotted fever is an exanthem of man first recognized in the Rocky Mountain region of the United States by Maxey in 1899. Ricketts inoculated monkeys and guinea pigs with infected human blood and was able to transmit the infection and demonstrate the causative agent. He later showed that the disease is spread by the wood tick and discovered infected ticks in the Bitterroot Valley of Montana. The name "Rocky Mountain spotted fever" gives a false impression of geographic limitation to a disease that has been observed throughout the United States. The attack rate in Virginia, Delaware and Maryland, for example, is as high as or higher than that in Nevada, Idaho and Montana.

ETIOLOGY AND TRANSMISSION. The causative agent of Rocky Mountain spotted fever, *Rickettsia rickettsii*. is maintained in nature by many hosts, including the ground squirrel, jack rabbit, chipmunk, wood rat, meadow mouse and weasel; the animal hosts do not become ill. Transmission among animals and from animal to man is most commonly via the wood tick, *Dermacentor andersoni* or the dog tick, *Dermacentor variabilis*.

Sheepherders, hunters, woodsmen or others whose occupation or recreation brings them into the isolated tick-infested woods of Montana or Idaho are most likely to be bitten by an infected wood tick. In the eastern United States, however, more infections occur in children and women, who are probably bitten by infected dog ticks encountered during outings in the woods or while handling the family dog. More cases occur in summer than in other seasons.

Infected female ticks may pass rickettsiae through eggs to the progeny and thus maintain a reservoir without infecting man.

PATHOLOGY. See prior pages.

CLINICAL MANIFESTATIONS. The incubation period in children varies from 1 to 8 days. The disease usually begins with such nonspecific symptoms as headache, fever, anorexia and restlessness. There is a history of tick bite in approximately half the cases; many others report exposure to tick-infected dogs or woods. Local reaction at the site of the bite is uncommon. Discrete, pale, rose-red macules or maculopapules appear 1 to 5 days after the onset of illness; rarely there may be little or no rash. The rash characteristically begins peripherally on the ankles, wrists or lower legs and then spreads, often rapidly, to involve the entire body, including the scalp, palms and soles. Early, the rash fades with pressure, but after 1 or 2 days it becomes more purple, papular and frequently petechial. Fever and headache persist; intense myalgia and malaise are frequent complaints. Splenomegaly is present in approximately 33 per cent of patients and shock

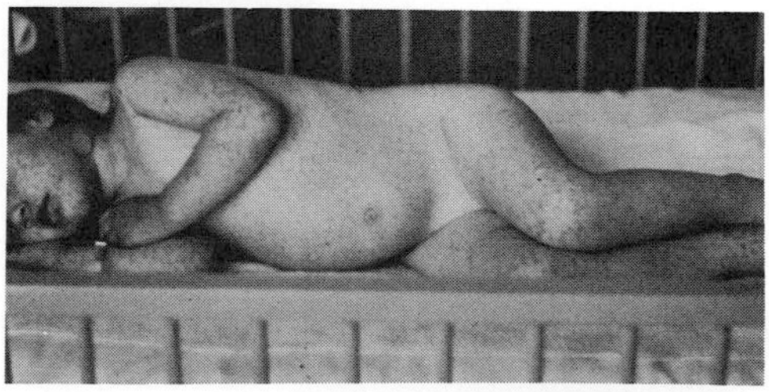

Figure 10–58 Patient with Rocky Mountain spotted fever. Note the greater concentration of skin lesions on the ankles, wrists and lower legs. (Courtesy of William H. Wood, M.D., Cleveland.)

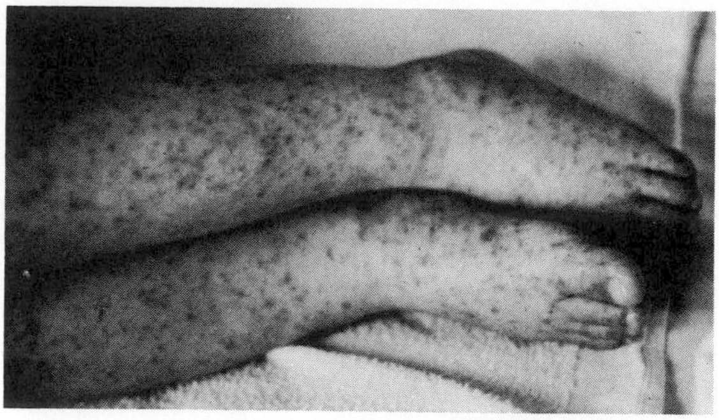

Figure 10–59 Ninth day of rash in Rocky Mountain spotted fever, showing hemorrhagic nature of rash and puffy edema of feet. (Courtesy of William H. Wood, M.D., Cleveland.)

in 7 to 10 per cent. Bizarre central nervous system symptoms, edema of the face, electrocardiographic evidence of myocarditis, renal involvement, peripheral collapse and pneumonitis are the more severe manifestations. Thrombocytopenia is present in nearly half the patients. Patients with multiple coagulation disturbances (disseminated intravascular coagulation) are being reported with increasing frequency and may constitute the group with highest risk of death. Fatality rates among unvaccinated children before the availability of antibiotics varied from 10 to 40 per cent; in 1970–1971 the case fatality ratio was 5.1 per cent. It is generally accepted that rickettsial strains of high and low virulence exist throughout the United States. Recovery in uncomplicated cases occurs in the third week, initiated by a fall in temperature and gradual subsidence of symptoms.

LABORATORY DATA. The clinical laboratory findings are not specific. See prior pages re serologic tests.

DIFFERENTIAL DIAGNOSIS. Infectious mononucleosis, rubella, measles, echovirus exanthems, and meningococcemia are diseases frequently considered in patients with Rocky Mountain spotted fever. The spread of rash from distal portions of the extremities to the trunk and face, with involvement of palms and soles, is often the clue that leads to the diagnosis. Season of the year, negative blood cultures and normal spinal fluid are additional aids in reaching a correct diagnosis.

CONTROL MEASURES. The reservoirs and vectors of spotted fever are so numerous and widespread that removal of the source of infection is not feasible. Protection from tick bite is best accomplished by the use of proper wearing apparel plus tick repellents or, optimally, the avoidance during the tick season of areas known to be infested.

Ticks rarely transmit infection until they have fed on the person for several hours; thus careful examination of children who have been playing in the woods and prompt removal of ticks may prevent disease. This is best accomplished by the use of gloves or forceps which will protect the operator from becoming infected by the crushed insect. The use of a hot match head or a coating of petrolatum to provoke the tick to remove his mouth parts is often recommended.

Vaccines are available and should be used by those whose pursuits require unusual exposure to virulent strains of rickettsiae.

TREATMENT. See prior pages.

FIÈVRE BOUTONNEUSE

Fièvre boutonneuse is a relatively benign rickettsial disease, limited almost exclusively to Europeans in the countries surrounding the Mediterranean. The natives in this area are apparently infected early in life and develop long-lasting immunity. *Rickettsia conorii,* the causal agent, is transmitted by the dog tick, *Rhipicephalus sanguineus.* As in rickettsialpox or scrub typhus, a local lesion known as *tâche noire,* or primary eschar, develops, followed by a diffuse, maculopapular rash which later becomes petechial. Severe systemic manifestations are uncommon. The diagnosis is usually made on the basis of the clinical symptoms in an exposed person with a primary skin lesion. Agglutinins to both OX19 and OX2 occur during the second week of the disease and may be used to confirm the diagnosis if the more specific complement fixation test is not available. Treatment with broad spectrum antibiotics is followed by rapid clinical improvement.

RICKETTSIALPOX

HISTORY. In 1946 an epidemic of an unusual febrile disease with varicelliform rash occurred in a New York housing development. The disease was recognized as a new entity caused by a previously unknown rickettsia, *Rickettsia akari,* and transmitted by the mouse mite, *Allodermanyssus sanguineus.* The illness, named rickettsialpox, has continued endemic in New York, and isolated cases have been reported from Boston, Philadelphia and Cleveland. The mite vector has been found in many cities of the United States.

CLINICAL MANIFESTATIONS. Rickettsialpox is a mild illness characterized by an initial skin lesion followed by fever, chills, headache and a papulovesicular rash.

The initial lesion, presumed to be the site of the mite bite, has been observed in more than 90 per cent of cases. It may be located anywhere on the body, beginning as a nontender, nonitching, firm, red papule, 0.5 to 2.0 cm in diameter. A deeply entrenched vesicle develops in the center of the papule and ruptures after several days, leaving a crusted, pigmented lesion or eschar which may persist 3 weeks or longer. Adjacent lymph nodes become enlarged and tender, but do not suppurate.

The initial lesion is followed in 2 to 7 days by fever, headache, chills and sweats. Temperature varies between 102 and 105°F, but the patient remains oriented and does not appear severely ill.

Within 24 to 72 hours after the onset of fever, scattered erythematous maculopapules appear over the body, showing no preference for trunk, head or extremity. The lesions enlarge, become more papular and develop vesicles on the summit of each papule. The secondary lesions (rash) resemble the initial lesion except that they are smaller in size and heal, without leaving scars, in 4 to 7 days.

The duration seldom exceeds 7 to 10 days. Complications, sequelae and fatalities are rare.

Except for leukopenia with relative lymphocytosis early in the disease, studies of blood, urine or stool show no characteristic changes.

DIFFERENTIAL DIAGNOSIS. The rash of rickettsialpox may be confused with that of chickenpox. In the latter the vesicles are superficial, thin, dewdrop lesions which appear in successive crops beginning on the chest. These differ from the deeply seated, randomly distributed firm vesicles of the rickettsial disease. The initial lesion and the presence of chills and fever before the rash may also help in differentiation. Other diseases to be considered include infectious mononucleosis, meningococcemia, Rocky Mountain spotted fever and typhus.

CONTROL MEASURES. Preventive measures should include the eradication of rodent reservoirs as well as the mite vector. *Rickettsia akari* grows well in the yolk sac of the developing chick embryo, and a vaccine could be prepared if there were substantial need.

TREATMENT. See prior pages.

Q FEVER

HISTORY. Q fever, a febrile disease without rash and often associated with an interstitial pneumonia, was originally observed among Australian abattoir workers in 1935. Initially the disease was infrequently diagnosed in this country except among laboratory workers. During World War II, epidemics of "pneumonia of unknown etiology" and "Balkan grippe" among military personnel in the Mediterranean theater were shown to be Q fever. Since that time the disease has been reported from all parts of the world.

ETIOLOGY AND TRANSMISSION. Q fever occurs naturally in cattle, sheep, goats and many wild animals. The causative agent of Q fever, *Coxiella burnetii* has been found in many species of ticks, in which it may pass from the adult through ova to progeny.

Experimentally, Q fever has been transmitted by insect vectors through the skin and by inhalation. Careful studies of outbreaks of the disease in human beings have failed to incriminate insect vectors, although this mode of transmission may be important among animals. Person-to-person spread, if it occurs, is rare. Q fever epidemics in Italy during the war remained localized and involved only the inhabitants of specific quarters, a fact which led to the idea that Q fever was a "place infection." Later studies suggest that excreta from infected animals or insects may be a source of infection. In the endemic areas of California, human infections are related to contact with animals which show evidence of *Coxiella burnetii* infection. In northern California, sheep are the probable source of infection; in southern California, the dairy cow. The main route of infection appears to be inhalation of contaminated material from domestic animals or by direct exposure to or contact with wool, hides, hay or other contaminated materials.

Milk may be another source of infection for man. In a study of sporadic cases of Q fever in England, Marmion isolated *Coxiella burnetii* from 10 of the 20 (raw) milk sources used by the patients; *Coxiella burnetii* may survive pasteurization temperatures.

PATHOLOGY. See prior pages.

CLINICAL MANIFESTATIONS. Q fever may be a mild disease diagnosed only in retrospect by serologic survey, but, as commonly recognized, it is a disease of moderate severity with a duration in children of 2 to 3 weeks. The onset is characteristically sudden, but in some instances symptoms may increase slowly in intensity. Malaise, fever, chilliness and generalized weakness appear early, but the most prominent symptom is severe frontal headache, often associated with pain upon movement of the eyes. There is no rash. Complaints referable to the respiratory tract are mild and infrequent. Cough may occur late in the first week of illness, with production of small amounts of blood-streaked sputum, and chest pain may be associated with pneumonitis or infrequently with pleural effusion.

Pneumonitis is common; rales may be audible, but the pulmonary involvement is usually established roentgenographically. Pulmonary consolidation is usually patchy and in the peripheries of the lower lobes; hilar involvement is rare. Resolution is slow and may require 3 to 6 weeks.

During the acute phase the temperature may reach 104 to 105°F, but may be remitting with wide daily swings. After 5 to 15 days the temperature gradually returns to normal and most symptoms disappear. Convalescence may be prolonged for several weeks, but complications are rare. The mortality rate is less than 1 per cent.

Routine hematologic data are not significant. Serologic tests for syphilis may give falsely positive results during the illness.

CONTROL MEASURES. Complete control of Q fever is not possible because of ignorance of the exact mode of spread. Recognition of the disease in livestock should alert communities to the risk of infection. Stockyard workers and others exposed to infected material might receive the formalinized vaccine, which at present is not generally available. Milk from infected herds must be pasteurized at temperatures sufficient to destroy the rickettsiae. Person-to-person spread of Q fever is not a problem, and special isolation measures are not necessary.

TREATMENT. See prior pages.

ELI GOLD
FREDERICK C. ROBBINS

Atkin, M. D., Strauss, H. S., and Fisher, G. U.: A case report of "Cape Cod" Rocky Mountain spotted fever with multiple coagulation disturbances. Pediatrics *36*:627, 1965.

Commission on Acute Respiratory Diseases: Epidemics of Q fever among troops returning from Italy in the spring of 1945. Am. J. Hyg. *44*:88, 1946.

Cooke, J. V.: Rocky Mountain spotted fever in children. Yale J. Biol. Med. *16*:495, 1944.

Greenberg, M., Pellitteri, O., Klein, I. F., and Huebner, R. J.: Rickettsialpox–Newly recognized rickettsial disease; Clinical observations. J.A.M.A. *133*:901, 1947.

Ley, H. L., Jr., and Smadel, J. E.: Antibiotic therapy of rickettsial diseases. Antibiotics Chemother. *4*:792, 1954.

Luoto, L., Casey, M. L., and Pickens, E. G.: Q fever studies in Montana. Detection of asymptomatic infection among residents of infected dairy premises. Am. J. Epidemiol. *81*:356, 1965.

Marmion, B. P.: Q fever; Natural history and epidemiology of Q fever in man. Tr. Roy. Soc. Trop. Med. Hyg. *48*:197, 1954.

Murray, E. S., et al.: Brill's disease; Clinical and laboratory diagnosis. J.A.M.A. *142*:1059, 1950.

Ormsbee, R. A., Parker, H., and Pickens, E. G.: The comparative effectiveness of Aureomycin, Terramycin, chloramphenicol, erythromycin and Thiocymetin in suppressing experimental rickettsial infections in chick embryos. J. Infect. Dis. *96*:162, 1955.

Pan American Health Organization: Vaccine against viral and rickettsial diseases of man. WHO Bulletin No. 147, 1967.

Robbins, F. C., Ragan, C., and Rustigian, R.: Q fever in Mediterranean area; Report of its occurrence in Allied troops; Laboratory outbreak. Am. J. Hyg. *44*:64, 1946.

Smadel, J. E., Intracellular infections. Bull. N.Y. Acad. Med. *39*:158, 1963.

MYCOTIC INFECTIONS

ACTINOMYCOSIS

DEFINITION AND ETIOLOGY. Actinomycosis is a chronic infection, more suppurative than granulomatous, characterized by the formation of abscesses with multiple draining sinuses. The disease is more frequent in adults than in children, but must be considered in chronic infections of the lung and draining sinuses in the jaw, neck or thoracic or abdominal region.

The causative agent, the anaerobic gram-positive *Actinomyces israeli,* appears in the lesion as small, hyaline-like to yellow "sulfur granules." On microscopic examination the crushed granule is a mass of branched mycelial filaments of approximately the same width as bacteria. The filaments in the periphery of the granule may be clubbed. The organisms must be cultured anaerobically, preferably in thioglycolate broth or brain-heart infusion agar. They can often be recovered from the mouth, tonsils and pyorrheal pus of patients without actinomycosis, suggesting an endogenous source of infection. The disease is not contagious.

PATHOLOGY. The lesion are those of a chronic granulomatous infection with a great tendency to suppuration with abscess formation, fibrosis, the formation of scars and multiple draining sinuses. Direct extension occurs without regard to anatomic structures or boundaries. The presence of typical "sulfur granules" is characteristic but not pathognomonic.

CLINICAL FORMS

Cervicofacial Actinomycosis (57 per cent of cases). The fungus enters through a carious tooth or the mucous membrane of the mouth or pharynx and produces a gradually enlarging hard or "woody" swelling in the jaw or neck. The tense overlying skin is often reddish or purple. The swelling later softens and drains to the outside through multiple sinuses, but can penetrate deeper to involve the bone and meninges. "Sulfur granules" may be found in the pus. Pain is minimal, and the general health is not greatly affected.

Abdominal Actinomycosis (22 per cent of cases). Infection may appear several months after an appendectomy or a penetrating lesion of the gut as a hard, irregular mass in the ileocecal region. This mass tends to soften and drain to the outside. Frequently, however, the infection extends through the diaphragm, after involving the liver and other abdominal organs, to produce thoracic lesions. With a severe infection there are chills, fever, night sweats and loss of weight.

Thoracic Actinomycosis (15 per cent of cases). The clinical pattern (occurring frequently following aspiration of a foreign body) is that of a chronic pulmonary infection with cough, sputum, fever, dyspnea, hemoptysis and loss of weight. Roentgenograms generally reveal bilateral involvement, usually in the lower lobes. Extension to the pleura causes accumulation of pleural fluid and involvement of the ribs and subcutaneous tissues with multiple sinus formation.

DIAGNOSIS. The diagnosis requires finding the organisms in the pus or biopsy material from the sinus walls. A drop of pus is crushed under a coverglass and examined under the low power of the microscope for the typical "sulfur granules." The disease closely simulates tuberculosis, but other chronic bacterial and fungus diseases and amebic hepatic abscess must be considered.

PROGNOSIS. This varies; widespread infection may be fatal.

PREVENTION AND TREATMENT. Removal of chronically infected tonsils and treatment of pyorrhea may eliminate possible sources of infection. Penicillin is the drug of choice. Massive doses (250,000 to 400,000 units/kg/day intravenously for 6 to 8 weeks) may be necessary in severe infections. Penicillin can be used alone or preferably in combination with a sulfonamide. The broad spectrum antibiotics (tetracyclines, chloramphenicol and erythromycin) may be used if the patient is sensitive to penicillin. Hyperbaric oxygenation may help in resistant cases, since the organism is anaerobic. Potassium iodide (see Sporotrichosis for dose and administration) may be useful in chronic actinomycosis and may be given with the more specific drugs for several months after the patient is apparently well. Surgical excision and drainage may be necessary.

NORTH AMERICAN BLASTOMYCOSIS

DEFINITION AND ETIOLOGY. North American blastomycosis (Gilchrist's disease) is an infection with *Blastomyces dermatitidis* characterized by chronic granulomatous lesions and microabscess formation in any part of the body, but with a predilection for lungs, skin and bone. This disease is confined almost solely to the North American continent and especially to the southeastern and Mississippi Valley states. Evidence suggests that the usual portal of entry is the lungs and that both skin and bone lesions are metastatic.

The source of the infection is unknown. Blastomyces have been found in domestic animals (dog and horse), but only rarely living free in nature (soil and wood). In tissues and in pus the fungus appears as a thick-walled, double-contoured, single-budding organism averaging 8 to 12 μ in diameter. On Sabouraud's medium at room temperature it grows slowly as a mold composed of branching filaments and small spores. Budding yeast-like forms are obtained on blood agar at 37° C. Small forms of the organism must be distinguished by cultural means from histoplasma and monilia. The disease is not spread from man to man.

PATHOLOGY. The acute phase and the advancing portions of the lesion are characterized by the formation of minute (micro-) abscesses. In the older portions of the lesion the reaction is essentially chronic and granulomatous, resembling tuberculosis. Necrosis and fibrosis are present.

CLINICAL FORMS. The disease, like coccidioidomycosis and histoplasmosis, may exist more frequently as a mild primary infection than as the more severe form usually recognized. In a well documented epidemic 7 of 10 patients were children, and the majority of these had only mild pulmonary lesions and few systemic manifestations; 1 patient cleared spontaneously without therapy.

Pulmonary Blastomycosis. The usual history is of an acute respiratory tract infection which persists despite therapy. Cough, chest pain, weakness and loss of weight may occur. Erythema nodosum may be present. The roentgenogram may reveal lymph node enlargement, infiltrations resembling virus pneumonia, diffuse miliary lesions, nodular or homogeneous areas of consolidation or abscesses of various size. With progression, the symptoms increase in severity and the patient has irregular bouts of fever and bloody, purulent sputum, and loses weight. Spread may be either local or hematogenous.

Cutaneous Blastomycosis. Cutaneous blastomycosis may result from direct inoculation of the organism into the skin or from dissemination to the subcutaneous tissue from a pulmonary lesion which may be unrecognized. The initial lesion is a small papule, usually on an exposed area of the body. It undergoes ulceration and crusting, and spreads by peripheral extension, with a tendency to heal in the center. The periphery of the lesion tends to be serpiginous, with a raised, ulcerated granulomatous border in which there are many microabscesses. The pus expressed from them usually contains the budding organisms. Systemic symptoms are rare unless there is involvement of other organs.

Disseminated Blastomycosis. The usual sequence is extension from a primary lesion in the lungs to many organs, in particular to bones, skin, subcutaneous tissues and internal organs. Skeletal involvement results in localized or diffuse osteomyelitis, with destruction of bone and formation of cutaneous sinuses. Subcutaneous nodules and abscesses, which may be painful, have a tendency to break through the skin and then assume the characteristics of the cutaneous lesions. Systemic symptoms may be relatively mild in the predominantly osteomyelitic form, but severe in the widely disseminated disease.

DIAGNOSIS. Diagnosis is established by demonstration (smear and culture) of the organisms in sputum or, in children, in gastric washings. Pus from draining sinuses should be mixed with a drop of 10 per cent potassium hydroxide and examined for the characteristic refractile, thick, double-contoured, walled organisms.

The pulmonary lesions may resemble those of tuberculosis, neoplasms, pneumonia, abscess, sarcoidosis and other fungus diseases. The cutaneous lesions can be mistaken for syphilis, tuberculosis, pyoderma, cat-scratch disease, carcinoma, bromide rashes, granulomas and other fungus infections.

Infection results in a positive delayed skin reaction to blastomycin or blastomyces vaccine. A negative skin reaction does not exclude the diagnosis, and a positive reaction may be obtained in persons without clinical manifestations. Severe and disseminate lesions tend to produce complement-fixing antibodies in the blood.

PROGNOSIS. The localized, mild pulmonary lesions have a good prognosis, as do the localized cutaneous lesions. Widespread pulmonary and disseminate lesions are usually fatal without extensive treatment. A negative skin reaction with a positive complement fixation reaction indicates a poor prognosis and the probability of relapse after therapy. A positive skin reaction with a negative complement fixation reaction is a good prognostic sign.

TREATMENT. Amphotericin B (see end of section) is the treatment of choice. If it is not effective or cannot be tolerated, hydroxystilbamidine diisethionate should be tried. The initial dose of the latter for adults is 50 to 100 mg given intravenously in 100 ml of 5 per cent glucose. It is followed by daily intravenous doses of 225 mg in 300 ml of 5 per cent glucose for 30 days, or in several series of 10 to 14 days each with a rest period between series. Proportionately smaller amounts are given to children, with a total dose of 100 mg/kg. Weakness, nausea and circulatory collapse may result from too rapid administration. Hydroxystilbamidine is stored in the tissues and exerts its effect for months after the course has been completed. In addition, iodides may be used, but the patient should first be desensitized to blastomyces vaccine if the skin reaction is strongly positive. Operation, performed under a mistaken diagnosis of neoplasm, has occasionally been curative in localized pulmonary lesions, but may precipitate dissemination. Appropriate antimicrobial agents should be used for secondary bacterial infections.

CRYPTOCOCCOSIS

(Torulosis)

DEFINITION AND ETIOLOGY. Cryptococcosis is a subacute or chronic infection caused by *Cryptococcus neoformans (Torula histolytica),* a fungus which can invade the lungs, skin, joints and subcutaneous tissues, but has a predilection for the central nervous system. The disease is world-wide in distribution and occurs at all ages. The organism has been found on various fruits, in soil, pigeon excreta and cow's milk. It probably enters the body through the respiratory tract, but may also enter through the skin.

PATHOLOGY. The early lesion is a cyst-like cavity containing gelatinous material with little cellular reaction. Older lesions may become granulomatous, but cryptococcosis usually remains a nonsuppurative disease. The earliest pulmonary lesion is probably a subpleural nodule which may go on to spontaneous healing. In the brain and meninges there is a chronic inflammatory reaction, with giant cells, macrophages and lymphocytes but relatively few neutrophils.

CLINICAL MANIFESTATIONS. Symptoms of central nervous system cryptococcosis are those of meningitis or brain abscess, with headache, dizziness and stiffness of the neck. Signs of increased intracranial pressure appear after weeks or months. Coma ensues, and death results from respiratory failure.

The clinical picture of pulmonary cryptococcosis is not diagnostic. There are low-grade fever, mild cough, and infiltrative lesions in the lungs which are of variable size and are frequently bilateral. Although pulmonary involvement may cause death, the chief danger is dissemination to the central nervous system.

Infection of the skin usually occurs on the face, beginning as an acneiform, firm, nodular, painless eruption which may enlarge, become necrotic and ulcerate. The lesions resemble carcinoma, sarcoidosis, tuberculosis and other fungus infections.

Infection with cryptococcosis and dissemination

of the disease probably depend largely on host factors. For example, there is a great susceptibility in patients with malignant lymphoma, Hodgkin's disease, leukemia, sarcoidosis and diabetes mellitus, and during corticosteroid therapy.

DIAGNOSIS. Diagnosis is established by finding encapsulated budding yeast cells in the cerebrospinal fluid or sputum, or in biopsies of lesions by direct examination and culture. The fungus appears as a thin-walled budding yeast surrounded by a large gelatinous capsule. Growth on Sabouraud's medium is creamy white, mucoid and glistening. The cerebrospinal fluid shows slight to marked lymphocytic pleocytosis and usually elevated protein and reduced glucose; fungus cells may easily be mistaken for lymphocytes unless an India ink preparation is used to demonstrate the capsule. Cryptococcal antigens may be present in serum or spinal fluid.

In differential diagnosis, tuberculosis and infections by other fungi must be considered.

PROGNOSIS AND PREVENTION. The prognosis is serious in all forms of the disease, especially in meningitis. Early treatment of pulmonary, cutaneous and subcutaneous infections is advisable to obviate the danger of central nervous system involvement. The disease is not communicable from man to man.

TREATMENT. Treatment of localized lesions consists in surgical excision and drainage. The drug of choice is amphotericin B, given intravenously and occasionally intrathecally. (See later.) Iodides may be helpful. Sulfonamides have but slight effect, and other antibiotics are valueless. Recently 5-Fluorocytosine (flucytosine—Ancobon [Roche]) has been shown to be of value in cryptococcus and candida infections. The dose is 100 to 150 mg/kg/day, divided into 4 doses, given for weeks to months. Kidney function, liver enzyme concentrations and bone marrow activity should be monitored before and during therapy. The addition of 5-fluorocytosine may permit a decrease in the dose of amphotericin B to one half or one third the usual amounts, with a resulting marked reduction in toxicity.

PHYCOMYCOSIS

(Mucormycosis)

DEFINITION AND ETIOLOGY. The fungus class *Phycomycetes* causes a spectrum of diseases ranging from benign epidermal infections to bizarre, acute, usually fatal, invasive diseases characterized by a necrotizing and inflammatory process in which broad, nonseptate hyphal strands can be seen in histologic section. The causative organisms include the genera *Mucor, Rhizopus, Absidia* and *Basidiobolus.* These organisms are generally saprophytes of widespread distribution (bread molds) and achieve pathogenic invasiveness when resistance has been lowered by debilitating illness. The organisms grow well on Sabouraud's medium at room temperature.

PATHOLOGY. The organism causes an intense inflammatory reaction with a polymorphonuclear response and extensive necrosis. The hyphae penetrate and grow in the walls of arteries and veins, breaking out in some sections through the adventitia and in other parts rupturing the intima. Thrombosis occurs, and the organisms can be seen in the clot. The resulting infarction accounts for much of the necrosis. In addition, there may be a striking invasion of nerves and perineural lymphatics. Involvement of the cranial cavity ("cerebral mucormycosis") may cause leptomeningitis, infarctions due to vascular thromboses, direct nerve involvement by invasion and acute necrotizing encephalitis.

CLINICAL FORMS. The disease usually develops in association with a severe and prolonged metabolic disturbance as in uncontrolled diabetes, uremia, chronic diarrhea, burns, corticosteroid therapy, prolonged chemotherapy and malignancies but has been reported in normal children.

Pulmonary. Infection occurs by direct or hematogenous invasion of the lungs, resulting in the pathologic processes described above. The clinical picture is that of an extremely acute, severe lobular pneumonia or infarction. The patient complains of chest pain and has bloody sputum, friction rub, fever and leukocytosis.

Craniofacial. In this type the organism probably enters the nasal cavity or the sinuses. Ulceration of the palate and nasal septum may occur. Necrosis and acute inflammation extend to the orbit, palate, meninges and brain. Symptoms and signs of orbital cellulitis, sinusitis, cavernous sinus thrombosis, nerve involvement or meningoencephalitis result.

Other Systemic Forms. The organism may invade the digestive tract, the heart and other organs. Symptoms are those of inflammation and infarction of the involved organs.

Subcutaneous. An unusual form of phycomycosis, occurring in children otherwise in good health, has been reported from Indonesia and Africa. The disease begins as a painless subcutaneous nodule which gradually increases, sometimes to massive proportions. After several months to years of growth, spontaneous healing may occur. Histologically the lesion resembles an eosinophilic granuloma containing the nonseptate hyphae of Basidiobolus species.

DIAGNOSIS. The appearance of acute inflammation, infarction or necrosis in the lungs, gastrointestinal tract, nasopharynx, orbits or intracranial cavity in a patient debilitated by a chronic disease should suggest this serious complication. Bloody nasal discharge and a gray-black, ischemic necrotic lesion resembling dried blood are characteristic. The diagnosis depends upon recognition of the fungus in specimens of tissue or body fluid.

PREVENTION AND TREATMENT. Prevention and treatment require scrupulous care of the underlying, predisposing debilitating illness. Amphotericin B is the drug of choice. (See later). Additional therapy includes surgical debridement or excision where possible, administration of large doses of iodides, desensitization with vaccine made from the fungus and antimicrobial treatment of any intercurrent bacterial infection.

NOCARDIOSIS

DEFINITION AND ETIOLOGY. Nocardiosis is a noncontagious, subacute or chronic suppurative disease primarily of the lungs, but with a tendency to hematogenous dissemination. The causative organisms belong to the same family as does Actinomyces. They are gram-positive with branching filaments, but, in contrast to Actinomyces, may be partially or strongly acid-fast, can be grown aerobically on simple media at room temperature and are found living free in nature (soil). Of the nine recognized species, *N. asteroides* is the commonest cause of systemic infection.

PATHOLOGY. The basic histologic lesion is a focal area of necrosis surrounded by a variable cellular infiltrate. These abscesses are characteristically not encapsulated but may show secondary fibrosis, or they may caseate and cavitate. Pulmonary infection (probably produced by inhalation of contaminated dust) begins as an acute pneumonitis which may become chronic. The lesions may extend locally and spread hematogenously to the subcutaneous tissues and to other organs, especially the brain. Differentiation from tuberculosis may be extremely difficult because of the histology, the acid-fastness of the organisms and their ready fragmentation into bacillary forms.

CLINICAL MANIFESTATIONS. Aside from the localized primary cutaneous and subcutaneous infections which are uncommon in the United States, the clinical picture of nocardiosis is that of a chronic suppurative pulmonary disease, usually in persons with lowered resistance. Local and metastatic spread may occur. Twelve per cent of these cases have occurred in children—as early as 4 weeks of age. Because of a reported association, the physician should be alert to the possibility of chronic granulomatous disease in children with nocardiosis. Common manifestations are cough, fever, anorexia, weight loss, malaise, night sweats, fatigue, dyspnea, chest pain and leukocytosis up to 50,000 cells per mm^3. Local extension may result in empyema. A characteristic sequence is pulmonary disease followed by pustular eruption of the skin. There is a pronounced tendency to chronicity, with remissions and exacerbations over many years. Secondary intracranial involvement results in cerebral abscess or meningitis. When the organisms, particularly *Nocardia madurae,* gain entrance through abrasions in the feet, they produce a burrowing infection of the subcutaneous tissues and bone, *mycetoma pedis.*

DIAGNOSIS. Roentgenograms of the lungs are not diagnostic but usually show small infiltrative lesions or large lobular areas of consolidation, with the lower lobes of the lungs involved most often. Suppuration and cavitation may occur. The important features are chronicity, with gradual progression, multiple lesions, refractoriness to antibiotic therapy and inability to establish the diagnosis by routine methods.

Differentiation must be made from tuberculosis and actinomycosis by cultural means and by examination of the pus ("sulfur granules" are seldom present in *N. asteroides* infections). This is important, since therapy is different in the three conditions. When the lesion metastasizes to other organs, the resemblance to staphylococcal pyemia is striking. The chronic pulmonary disease has also been mistaken for cystic fibrosis. Cutaneous involvement may mimic tuberculosis, infections with atypical mycobacteria or cat-scratch disease.

PROGNOSIS AND TREATMENT. The overall mortality rate is probably over 50 per cent in untreated cases. Lesions respond well to symptomatic care and sulfonamide therapy in their early stage. Surgical excision may be necessary. The organisms are partially susceptible to the broad spectrum antibiotics and streptomycin but resistant to penicillin. Several recent reports indicate that the addition of trimethroprim or cycloserine to sulfonamide therapy may be advantageous. Trimethoprim and sulfamethoxazole may be given in a one to five combination (cotrimoxazole) in doses of 250 mg trimethoprim per M^2 daily divided into 2 doses. The adult dose of cycloserine is 250 mg 2 to 4 times daily. Proportionately smaller amounts are given to children.

SPOROTRICHOSIS

ETIOLOGY. Sporotrichosis is caused by *Sporotrichum schenckii,* a fungus which most frequently infects skin and subcutaneous tissues, producing a series of nodules and ulcerations. The fungus also may infect mucous membranes, lungs and other organs. It has been isolated from soil, plants and timber. Man is probably inoculated through abrasions in the skin.

PATHOLOGY. Section of a nodule usually shows granulation tissue, with epitheloid cells and giant cells surrounding a necrotic area, a lesion similar to that produced by other fungus infections or tuberculosis.

CLINICAL MANIFESTATIONS. The lesion begins usually in the skin or in the subcutaneous tissue as a small, hard nodule not attached to the skin. This nodule later adheres to the overlying skin, which becomes darker and finally ulcerates, discharging a small amount of purulent material. This primary "chancre" may persist for months and is usually followed by a chain of nodules along the course of the lymphatic drainage. These nodules may subsequently become attached to the skin and ulcerate. The patient is afebrile, and the general health is not affected. Sporotrichotic infections of the mucous membranes, lungs, bones, joints and other organs occur.

DIAGNOSIS. The disease may resemble tuberculosis, syphilis or infections by other fungi. The local lesions suggest tularemia, but the general symptoms are not those of an acute bacterial infection. Diagnosis depends upon culturing the fungus from the chancre or subcutaneous nodule.

The fungi occur in the lesions as intracellular, small "cigar-shaped" bodies, 3 to 4 μ in length, and are demonstrated with difficulty. Direct smears cannot be depended upon as a diagnostic procedure. On Sabouraud's medium the fungus grows as a white or black mold identified as clusters of small, delicate, pear-shaped spores borne on short branches of narrow mycelial filaments.

PROGNOSIS. Though the disease may persist for many months, the prognosis is good under adequate therapy.

TREATMENT. Oral administration of potassium iodide in increasing amounts up to tolerance is almost specific for the lymphocutaneous forms. It is given orally as the saturated solution (1 gm/ml), beginning with 1 to 10 drops 3 times a day, depending on the size of the patient, and increased by 1 drop per dose per day until a final dose of 10 to 40 drops 3 times a day is reached or until symptoms of iodism appear (skin eruptions, lacrimation, parotid swelling, nausea, vomiting). The medication should be continued for at least a month after healing has occurred. Abscesses may be aspirated, but incision and curettage should be avoided. For patients who are sensitive to iodides or have systemic lesions, amphotericin B may be helpful.

ASPERGILLOSIS

ETIOLOGY. Aspergillosis is caused by various species (especially *Aspergillus fumigatus*) of the widely distributed, usually nonpathogenic genus *Aspergillus*. The organism most frequently causes granulomatous inflammatory lesions of the skin (external ear) and vagina, and may invade the nasal sinuses, orbit, bones, meninges and lungs. In the lungs the organism may grow in large masses ("fungus balls") in pulmonary cavities without eliciting much reaction or may invade the pulmonary parenchyma, causing necrosis and cavitation. Rarely dissemination occurs by the hematogenous route.

PATHOLOGY. Little reaction is seen to the fungus ball. Invasion of the pulmonary parenchyma or blood vessels results in obstruction, thrombosis and extensive necrosis.

CLINICAL MANIFESTATIONS. Disease caused by Aspergillus may be classified as follows:

Superficial. They are granulomatous inflammatory lesions of the skin (particularly external ear) and genitalia.

Saprophytic. The fungus grows as masses of matted mycelia in bronchiectatic, tuberculous or histoplasmotic cavities. They form fungus balls (aspergilloma) without invasion and the main symptoms relate to the underlying disease rather than to the fungus.

Invasive. In patients debilitated by neoplasm, tuberculosis or systemic mycosis or in whom immunity has been depressed by long corticosteroid, intensive antibiotic, antineoplastic or immunosuppressive therapy, a rapidly invasive infection may spread from the bronchus to cause a necrotizing parenchymatous pneumonitis. Symptoms are cough, fever, severe malaise, episodic pleuritic pain and dyspnea (? due to emboli), hemoptysis and purulent sputum in which hyphae may be seen. Further and usually fatal dissemination may occur to the brain, heart, liver, kidneys, bone and skin.

A rapidly fatal invasive pulmonary aspergillosis has been reported in infants and young children, presumably because of massive inhalation of spores, but possibly because of an unrecognized immunologic defect.

Aspergillus, like Candida, has been reported as an infective agent in endocarditis following intracardiac surgery with or without the insertion of prosthetic devices.

Allergic Bronchopulmonary Aspergillosis. In this condition the patient presumably is sensitized by and is sensitive to endogenous saprophytic aspergillus in his own respiratory tract. Essential features are usually occupational exposure, episodes of wheezing with low-grade fever, expectoration of characteristic brown plugs, transient pulmonary infiltrates and eosinophilia of blood and sputum. Reaginic (immediate positive) skin reactions and precipitins to aspergillus extracts are present. Treatment consists of corticosteroid therapy to depress the production of antibodies. Antifungal agents in the form of aerosol therapy with amphotericin B or nystatin may be used as adjuncts to steroid therapy.

DIFFERENTIAL DIAGNOSIS. Aspergillosis, as well as other "opportunistic" fungus diseases, should be suspected in severely debilitated patients or in those whose immune responses have been suppressed. The roentgenogram of the fungus ball in a pulmonary cavity is characteristic. Cultures may be misleading, since the organisms are widespread in nature and may be present as contaminants in routine cultures.

TREATMENT. Treatment must be directed against the underlying disease. For pulmonary aspergillosis, inhalation or direct intrabronchial instillation of amphotericin B or nystatin may be helpful. Surgical therapy is indicated for localized lesions. For patients with the invasive type of disease, systemic amphotericin B, sulfonamides and potassium iodide may be tried; none is particularly effective.

THERAPY WITH AMPHOTERICIN B

Amphotericin B (Fungizone [Squibb]) is a polyene antifungal antibiotic produced by a strain of streptomyces. It is insoluble in water, but may be dispersed in a colloidal suspension for intravenous use with deoxycholate and phosphate buffers. The colloidal suspension may be diluted with 5 per cent glucose, but not with salt solutions or any other diluents which may cause precipitation of the drug. The drug is poorly absorbed from the gastrointestinal tract, and subcutaneous or intramuscular injections are inefficient. The drug must be given intravenously. Little of it penetrates the cerebrospinal fluid. Because of a high renal threshold and slow excretion the drug is administered once daily or every other day. Solutions must be protected against prolonged exposure to light and should be discarded after 24 hours.

METHOD OF ADMINISTRATION. The drug is used intravenously in sufficient 5 per cent dextrose solution to permit giving the fusion over a 4- to 6-hour period (250 to 500 ml). The maximum concentration should not exceed 0.1 mg/ml. Rapid administration or the use of high concentrations may lead to convulsions, ventricular fibrillation and cardiac arrest. Therapy starts with a test dose (0.1 mg/kg with a maximum of 1.0 mg) to exclude hypersensitivity and is increased gradually by approximately 0.1 mg/kg each day, if tolerated, to a maximum of 0.75 to 1.0 mg/kg/day or 1.5 mg/kg given on alternate days. The total dose should be tailored to the needs of the patient. Relapses are significantly less with a total dose of 40 mg/kg than with doses of 20 mg/kg, but recent reports indicate good results with the smaller total dose, provided peak serum levels are twice those necessary for inhibition of the infecting fungus. The duration of therapy depends upon the nature, severity and type of infection. Relapses may occur and require additional courses of therapy.

In fungal meningitis, amphotericin may be administered intrathecally on alternate days or twice weekly beginning with 0.025 mg dissolved in 2 to 3 ml of spinal fluid or distilled water and increasing to a maximum of 0.5 mg (total single dose) if tolerated. The dosage must be kept small and given in dilute solution in order to avoid adhesive arachnoiditis, transverse myelitis and visual disturbances. An Ommaya reservoir connected to the ventricular system may be helpful. See also Coccidioidomycosis.

The drug is also given topically (into cutaneous lesions), intra-articularly, intrathoracically, by direct intrabronchial infusion (as a solution containing 0.5 mg/ml) and as an aerosol inhalant spray (1 mg/kg/day as a solution containing 5 mg/ml).

TOXICITY. The reactions to intravenous administration of amphotericin are legion. Fortunately they seem to be less serious in children and tend to decrease during a prolonged course of therapy. Anxiety, anorexia, chills, fever and malaise are common and may be partly controlled by the prior (30 minutes) administration of aspirin, antihistaminics or chlorpromazine. Headaches, nausea, vomiting, abdominal pain and chest pains require a diminution in the total daily dose, particularly if these symptoms increase in severity or duration. With increasing doses, renal function is affected and the blood urea nitrogen level tends to rise. If the BUN is increased (over 20 to 40 mg/dl) the drug should be discontinued until the level returns toward normal. The drug may then be given either in diminished doses or preferably every other day. Fortunately the effect on the kidneys seems to be temporary in most instances and disappears on discontinuation of the drug. Rarer toxic effects include proteinuria and other renal difficulties, anemia, thrombocytopenia, hypokalemia causing muscular weakness, renal tubular acidosis, renal calcinosis, duodenal ulcerations and hemorrhagic gastroenteritis. Observation should be made to detect these complications at an early stage, when they usually are reversible. Thrombophlebitis may occur, unfortunately probably more commonly in children, owing to their small veins, and cause technical difficulties in prolonged courses of therapy. The addition of heparin (500 USP units per 100 ml) may be helpful. Simultaneous administration of 20 to 100 mg of soluble hydrocortisone in the intravenous infusion has been advocated to prevent toxicity, particularly from intrathecal injections.

ACTION AND USES. Amphotericin B is probably fungistatic rather than fungicidal, but has a broad spectrum of action, including *Coccidioides immitis. Histoplasma capsulatum, Cryptococcus neoformans,* Phycomyces species, Blastomyces species, Candida, Nocardia and Sporotrichum among others. There is no effect on bacteria or actinomyces.

In view of the many toxic effects of the drug and the difficulty of administration, amphotericin B should be reserved for the more serious infections and particularly for those which do not respond to other forms of therapy. It is the drug of choice in blastomycosis, cryptococcosis, disseminated coccidioidomycosis, chronic histoplasmosis and systemic moniliasis.

Treatment failures may be due to premature discontinuation of the drug, far advanced disease, insufficient amount of drug, death from associated diseases (e.g., leukemia), relapses (with steroid treatment, and metabolic disturbances), and disease due to resistant organisms.

JEROME S. HARRIS

GENERAL

Baker, R. D., and others: The pathologic anatomy of mycoses. *In* Handbuch der Speciellen Pathologischen Anatomie und Histologie. Vol. 3, part 5, pp. 1–1191, 1971. (Written in English.)

Conant, N. F., Smith, D. T., Baker, R. D., and Callaway, J. L.: Manual of Clinical Mycology. 3rd ed. Philadelphia, W. B. Saunders Company, 1971.

Emmons, C. W., Binford, C. H., and Utz, J. P.: Medical Mycology. 2nd ed. Philadelphia, Lea & Febiger, 1970.

Fetter, B. F., Klintworth, G. K., and Hendry, W. S.: Mycoses of the Central Nervous System. Baltimore, The Williams & Wilkins Company, 1967.

Moss, E. S., and McQuown, A. L.: Atlas of Medical Mycology. Baltimore, The Williams & Wilkins Company, 1969.

Actinomycosis

Bronner, M., and Bronner, M.: Actinomycosis. 2nd ed. Bristol, John Wright & Sons, Ltd., 1971.

Halldorsson, T. S.: Actinomycosis in childhood. Clin. Pediatr. *6*:221, 1967.

Peabody, J. W., Jr., and Seabury, J. H.: Actinomycosis and nocardiosis—A review of basic differences in therapy. Am. J. Med. *28*:99, 1960.

Blastomycosis

Duttera, M. J., and Osterhout, S.: North American blastomycosis: A survey of 63 cases. South. Med. J. *62*:295, 1969.

Harrell, E. R., and Curtis, A. C.: North American blastomycosis. Am. J. Med. *27*:750, 1959.

Smith, J. G., Jr., Harris, J. S., Conant, N. F., and Smith, D. T.: An epidemic of North American blastomycosis. J.A.M.A. *158*:641, 1955.

Turner, D. J., and Wadlington, W. B.: Blastomycosis in childhood: Treatment with amphotericin B and a review of the literature. J. Pediatr. *75*:708, 1969.

Cryptococcosis

Goodman, J. S., Kaufman, L., and Koenig, M. G.: Diagnosis of cryptococcal meningitis: Value of immunological detection of cryptococcus antigen. New Engl. J. Med. *285*:434, 1971.

Littman, M. L., and Walter, J. E.: Cryptococcosis: Current status. Am. J. Med. *45*:922, 1968.

McDonald, R., Greenberg, E. N., and Kramer, R.: Cryptococcal meningitis. Arch. Dis. Child., *45*:417, 1970.

Phycomycosis (Mucormycosis)

Harris, J. S.: Mucormycosis. Report of case. Pediatrics *16*:857, 1955.

Landau, J. W., and Newcomer, V. D.: Acute cerebral phycomycosis (mucormycosis). J. Pediatr. *61*:363, 1962.

Nocardiosis

Ballenger, C. N., Jr., and Goldring, D.: Nocardiosis in childhood. J. Pediatr. *50*:145, 1957.

Bates, R. R., and Rifkind, D.: Nocardia brasiliensis lymphocutaneous syndrome. Am. J. Dis. Child. *121*:246, 1971.

Gundersen, G. A., and Nice, C. M., Jr.: Nocardiosis. A case report and brief review of the literature. Radiology *68*:31, 1957.

Sporotrichosis

Lynch, P. J., and Botero, F.: Sporotrichosis in children. Am. J. Dis. Child. *122*:325, 1971.

Orr, E. R., and Riley, H. D., Jr.: Sporotrichosis in childhood: Report of 10 cases. J. Pediatr. *78*:951, 1971.

Aspergillosis

Blattner, R. J.: Pulmonary aspergillosis in children. J. Pediatr. *70*:139, 1967.

Slavin, R. G., Laird, T. S., and Cherry, J. D.: Allergic bronchopulmonary aspergillosis in a child. J. Pediatr. *76*:416, 1970.

Young, R. C., Bennett, J. E., Vogel, C. L., Carbone, P. P., and DeVita, V. T.: Aspergillosis—The spectrum of the disease in 98 patients. Medicine *49*:147, 1970.

Therapy

Buechner, H. A. (ed.): Management of Fungus Diseases of the Lung. Springfield, Ill., Charles C Thomas, 1971.

Cherry, J. D., Lloyd, C. A., Quilty, J. F., and Laskowski, L. F.: Amphotericin B therapy in children. J. Pediatr. *75*:1063, 1969.

Hildick-Smith, G., Blank, H., and Sarkany, I.: Fungus Diseases and Their Treatment. Boston, Little, Brown and Company, 1964.

Utz, J. P. (ed.): Treatment of the systemic mycoses. Mod. Treat. 7:509, 1970.

Treatment of Fungal Diseases. A statement by the Committee on Therapy. Am. Rev. Resp. Dis. *100*:908, 1969.

HISTOPLASMOSIS

Histoplasmosis is an acute, subacute or chronic infectious disease caused by the fungus *Histoplasma capsulatum.* Once thought invariably fatal, it is now recognized as a relatively common benign (often clinically inapparent) or only moderately severe disease. At least 30 per cent of cases have occurred in children.

ETIOLOGY. *Histoplasma capsulatum* has two distinct growth phases. When cultivated on artificial media at room temperature, it produces a white, cottony, aerial, mycelial growth and a brownish-yellow subsurface growth. In tissues and when first cultivated on enriched media at 37° C, it grows in a yeast cell phase, having a relatively thick, translucent capsule. It can be identified in the mycelial culture by the tuberculate chlamydospores.

EPIDEMIOLOGY. Histoplasmosis was first described by Darling as a rare tropical disease occurring in Panama, but between 1930 and 1940 a large number of persons living in the central and southern United States, especially in the Mississippi Valley and along the western Appalachian slope, were found to have calcified lesions in the lungs and tracheobronchial lymph nodes, with negative reactions to tuberculin and positive skin test reactions to histoplasmin. It is now apparent that they had been infected with *H. capsulatum,* in most instances without having been aware of any illness, and that histoplasmosis, like tuberculosis and coccidioidomycosis, is geographically widespread in this country and abroad.

The fungus has been isolated from dogs, cats, mice, rats, horses, brown (Kodiak) bears, shrews, woodchucks, skunks, opossums, ground squirrels, foxes and raccoons; from soil adjacent to chicken houses and pigeon lofts, or under the roosting places of starlings, grackles, blackbirds, oil birds and bats; from damp places along streams or in caves or cellars; and even from air samples. Human epidemics have been most frequently identified among individuals involved in disturbing apparently contaminated chicken, pigeon, bird or bat manure, especially while engaged in dusty cleaning of places inhabited by these creatures. It is not clear whether the various birds and bats from whose feces *H. capsulatum* has been isolated are infected carriers or merely serve as a means of transporting the organism; available evidence favors the latter. The disturbance of contaminated dirt while spelunking and while digging worms for fishing has also been implicated. There is no evidence of direct man-to-man or animal-to-man transmission.

PATHOGENESIS AND PATHOLOGY. The fungus apparently enters the body through the skin or through the mucous membrane of the mouth, nasopharynx, respiratory tract or intestinal mucosa, producing an ulcerative lesion.

The granulomatous lesions of histoplasmosis may simulate those of tuberculosis. For example, the initial lesion in the pulmonary parenchyma, with subsequent involvement of the regional lymph nodes, simulates the primary complex of tuberculosis. The yeast form of the fungus proliferates in the macrophages, initiating new cycles. Unlike that of tuberculosis, this reaction produces relatively little inflammation in adjacent tissues. Foci tend to become surrounded with giant cells and macrophages and to progress to central caseous necrosis. Calcium is often deposited in the healing lesion.

In infants and debilitated older persons there is a tendency toward hematogenous dissemination, and the disease may manifest itself as a generalized process involving bone marrow, lung, liver, spleen, and lymph nodes.

As in tuberculosis, the spread of the organism

TABLE 10–24 CLINICAL FORMS OF HISTOPLASMOSIS

1. Primary, usually pulmonary—may be intestinal with mesenteric adenitis
2. Postprimary complications
   a. Intrathoracic
      (1) Miliary "atypical" pneumonia
      (2) Mediastinal adenopathy
      (3) Chronic progression with cavity formation (adults)
   b. Extrathoracic
      (1) May affect any tissue of the body; e.g., regional adenopathy; meningitis; lytic bone lesions; Addison's disease; eye, skin and mucous membrane ulcerations; myocarditis and endocarditis; ulcerative colitis
   c. Disseminated progressive varieties

varies with the tissue resistance of the host, the size of the inoculum and the virulence of the strain. Hypersensitivity similar to that in tuberculosis occurs. Histoplasmin reactivity is established about 3 to 6 weeks after the primary inoculation.

CLINICAL MANIFESTATIONS. Histoplasmosis has a wide spectrum of clinical manifestations strikingly analogous to those of tuberculosis. Benign and subclinical forms of the disease are common in endemic areas; severe or progressive forms are relatively rare. Histoplasmosis is probably best thought of as a primary infection, usually mild, which may be followed by postprimary complications of varying clinical form and severity. (Table 10–24).

The lesions of the primary forms heal by calcification (Fig. 10–60 *A*), but noncalcified single and multiple focal lesions have been demonstrated. When children with calcified pulmonary lesions have positive skin test reactions to histoplasmin and negative ones to tuberculin, it can be assumed that they have healed calcified histoplasmosis.

There may be a single primary lesion, completely asymptomatic, or multiple miliary calcifications (Fig. 10–60*B*) may be found on roentgenographic examination with no history of clinical manifestations. Occasionally a mediastinal node is of such size and location as to cause obstruction to venous return. Such instances may require bronchoscopy or thoracotomy for diagnosis and relief. On the other hand, infection in children may commonly produce such symptoms as fever (38 to 39°C), malaise and fatigue, with a desire to rest rather than to play after school, nonproductive cough, weight loss or failure to gain weight, vomiting, or diarrhea which is occasionally blood-streaked. Depending on the resistance of the host, virulence of the organism or frequency of reinfection, such as might occur in young infants or debilitated older persons, there may be hematogenous dissemination, with progressive and usually fatal varieties of this disease (Table 10–24, Fig. 10–61).

The physical examination, particularly of the chest, may be normal. If efforts to explain the fever include skin tests, a positive reaction to histoplasmin may be found. Pneumonitis with pulmonary infiltration is common. In most cases there is enlargement of the spleen and liver. Roentgenograms of the chest may reveal scattered parenchymal le-

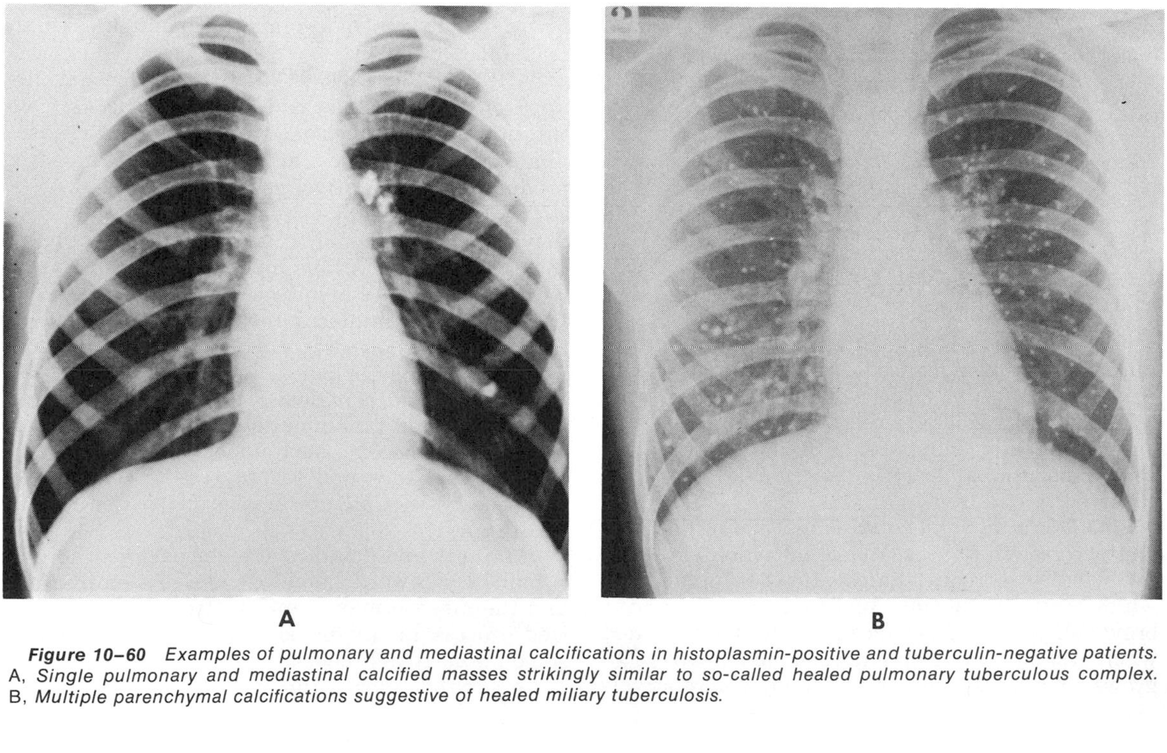

A B

Figure 10–60 *Examples of pulmonary and mediastinal calcifications in histoplasmin-positive and tuberculin-negative patients.* A, *Single pulmonary and mediastinal calcified masses strikingly similar to so-called healed pulmonary tuberculous complex.* B, *Multiple parenchymal calcifications suggestive of healed miliary tuberculosis.*

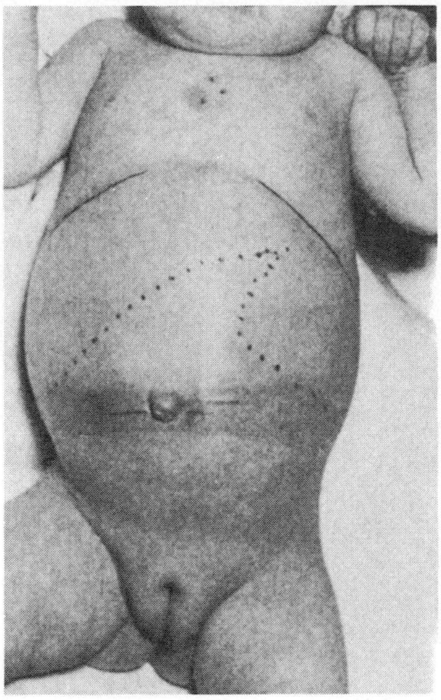

A

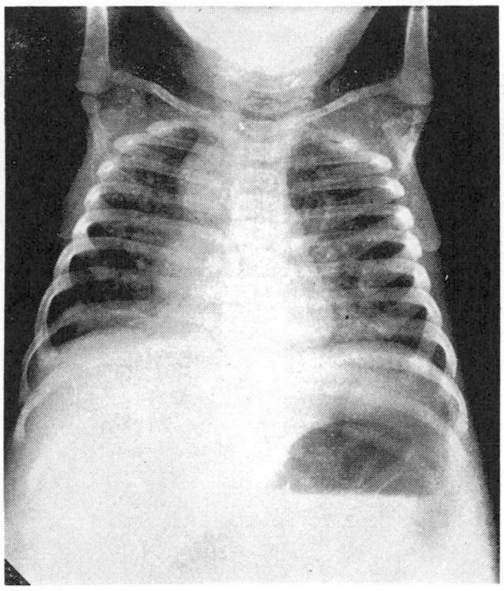

B

Figure 10–61 *Histoplasmosis in an infant aged 5½ months, with pyrexia, anemia, hepatosplenomegaly and leukopenia.* A, *Note site of sternal puncture; yeast cells of* H. capsulatum *were found in smears and cultures of the sternal marrow.* B, *Chest roentgenogram shows diffuse pneumonitis and a mediastinal mass. Diagnosis confirmed by autopsy. (Hild: Am. J. Dis. Child., Vol. 63.)*

sions or enlarged mediastinal nodes, or occasionally localized obstructive emphysema. Purpura, ecchymoses and melena may be present in terminal stages. Peripheral or generalized lymphadenopathy of a severe degree is uncommon in children, an important difference from the adenopathy of leukemia. Meningitis and cerebrospinal fluid changes similar to those of tuberculous meningitis have been observed. Until recently the prognosis has been grave for a child with these postprimary complications.

In addition, a wide variety of other manifestations occur with considerable frequency, depending on the localization of infection. These include ulcerative lesions of eyes, skin and mucous membranes, ulcerative colitis, adrenal insufficiency, pericarditis, myocarditis, endocarditis and lytic lesions of the long bones (Table 10–24).

Between the asymptomatic, benign forms of histoplasmosis and the severe disseminated and fatal forms are the illnesses of children with splenomegaly, ulcerations of the skin or mucous membranes, and pulmonary infiltrations, who have spontaneously recovered. These children also have complement-fixing antibodies and skin sensitivity to histoplasmin.

LABORATORY DIAGNOSIS. Changes in the blood usually include a progressive hypochromic anemia and a leukopenia with a relative lymphocytosis. There may be pancytopenia, suggestive of an aleukemic phase of leukemia; the platelets, however, are usually not reduced until late in the course of the disease.

On occasion the parasites can be demonstrated in the white blood cells in the peripheral blood or in bone marrow. The yeast phase of the fungus as it occurs in the cells of the body appears as a small (1 to 5 μ), encapsulated oval body in large mononuclear cells. Thick-drop preparations or smears of the peripheral blood and bone marrow should be stained with Wright's or Giemsa's stain. Biopsy material from lymph nodes or from the liver or spleen, as well as bone marrow, sputum or material swabbed from an ulcerative lesion, can also be smeared and stained by one of these methods and cultured. It is possible to identify *H. capsulatum* morphologically with routine stains, but silver stains are advantageous in identifying the yeast cells in tissue.

Technique of Culture. The technique to be followed varies somewhat with the material. Biopsy specimens are ground to a thin paste, using a minimal amount of sterile saline solution. Swabs from infected areas are placed in test tubes containing 1 to 2 ml of sterile saline solution. Blood is mixed with heparin, rather than citrate, as an anticoagulant and is centrifuged at sufficiently high speed to allow separation of the white cells, which are pipetted off and placed in a test tube containing 1 to 2 ml of sterile saline solution. After 1 hour, and again after 24 to 48 hours of incubation, the material is streaked heavily in each of two screw-cap bottles (25 by 50 mm) containing slants of peptone or meat extract agar to which has been added 50 units/ml of penicillin and 0.4 mg/ml of streptomycin and plasma or blood serum to a concentration of 5 per cent. The use of bottles instead of Petri dishes or plates decreases the chances of air contamination by fungi and permits small amounts of material to be studied. The bottles must be sealed; one bottle is incubated at 37° C, the other at room temperature. The cultures should be examined at intervals of 3 to 4 days and should not be considered negative until after an observation period of 4 weeks. Positive cultures which have

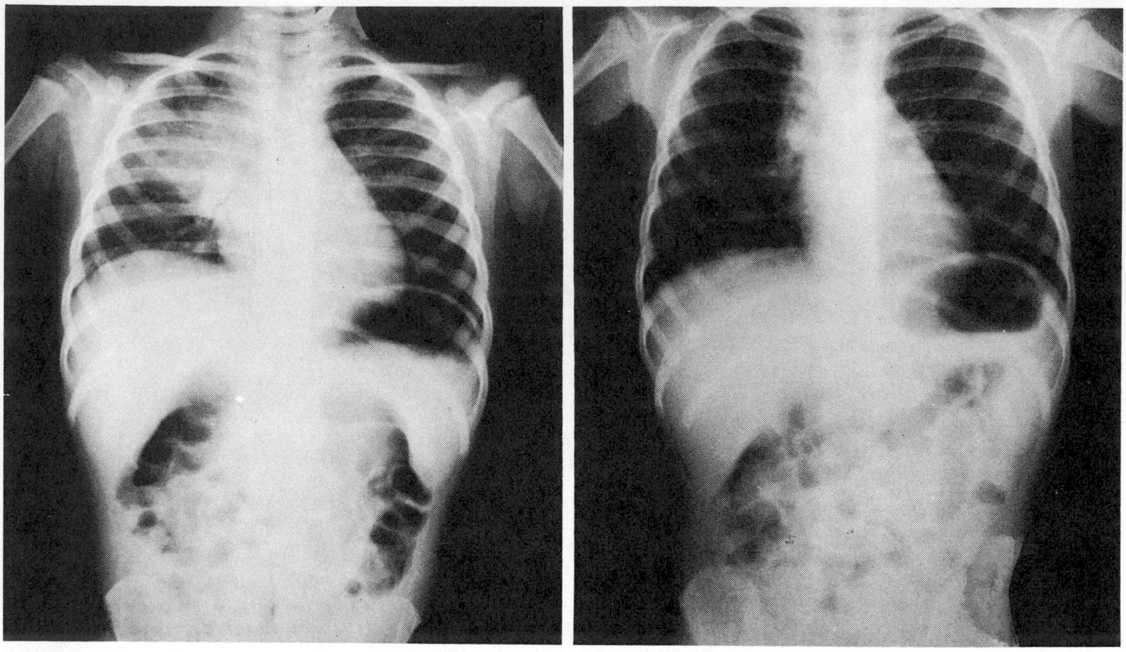

Figure 10–62 Primary histoplasmosis with resolution during sulfonamide therapy over a period of 7 months.

been kept at 37° C will frequently have colonies of yeast cells rather than of mycelium. At room temperature *H. capsulatum* grows only in the mycelial phase, producing the characteristic tuberculate chlamydospores. The older the mycelial culture, the more likely are chlamydospores to be present.

Histoplasmin Test. The histoplasmin skin test resembles the tuberculin test. The testing material, a filtrate of a broth culture of *H. capsulatum,* is injected intracutaneously. The reaction is read at 48 hours; a positive reaction consists of an area of erythema with induration of at least 0.5 cm in diameter. A positive reaction is evidence of sensitization to *H. capsulatum,* but does not indicate whether the infection is active. Conversion from a negative to a positive reaction within a few weeks or a positive reaction in infants is suggestive of an active infection. Persons with progressive disseminated histoplasmosis frequently fail to react to histoplasmin.

It has been recently shown that healthy adults with positive histoplasmin skin tests, who are initially serologically negative, will develop complement-fixing antibodies after the reapplication of a single histoplasmin skin test. This serologic response is limited to the mycelial antigen only; it has not been studied in children. This stimulation of mycelial complement-fixing antibodies does not seem to be an adequate reason to discard the skin test (which is the most practical diagnostic and epidemiologic aid for histoplasmosis), since there is no interference with the complement fixation test for yeast cell antibody, and it is the yeast cell which is involved in clinical infections. A two-tube response to yeast cell antigen by standard complement fixation antibody techniques therefore supplies an adequate index for diagnosis and leaves the road open for continued use of the skin test. In any case, a positive skin test indicates current or active infection only if conversion from negative to positive has been shown.

Serologic tests are useful to establish the presence of progressive infection.

DIFFERENTIAL DIAGNOSIS. Histoplasmosis may simulate a number of clinical conditions besides tuberculosis and coccidioidomycosis. Progressive anemia, leukopenia and hepatosplenomegaly require differentiation from leukemia, the lipid storage diseases, Banti syndrome, malaria and brucellosis. Ulceration of the skin or mucous membranes must be differentiated from actinomycosis, leishmaniasis and toxoplasmosis; irrespective of lymph node enlargement, Hodgkin's disease and other malignant lymphomas must be ruled out, as must other systemic mycotic diseases.

TREATMENT. No chemotherapeutic or antibiotic agent has been found which satisfactorily inhibits the growth of *H. capsulatum* without injuring the tissue of the host. The commonly used antibiotics are completely without effect, and some may facilitate growth of the fungus. In the author's experience sulfonamides (triple sulfonamides) in doses sufficient to obtain blood levels of 10–12 mg/dl have seemed to offer the most benefit, especially in the more benign primary form of the disease. Amphotericin B may be used for the severe progressive disseminated infections. The drug is toxic, however, and should be used only by an experienced person. (See Therapy with Amphotericin B on a prior page.)

AMOS CHRISTIE

Schwarz, J., and Baum, G. L.: The history of histoplasmosis, 1906 to 1956. New Engl. J. Med. *256*:253, 1957.

COCCIDIOIDOMYCOSIS

(San Joaquin Fever; Valley Fever; Desert Rheumatism; Coccidioidal Granuloma)

ETIOLOGY. Coccidioidomycosis is an infection caused by the fungus *Coccidioides immitis.* The minute spores of its mycelial saprophytic phase are inhaled or, rarely, enter through an abrasion. They round up into spherules which develop endospores within doubly refractile walls, the characteristic sporangium of the so-called parasitic phase. These spherules do not spread from person to person or from animal to man. Viable *C. immitis* does occur in pulmonary cavities, often in the mycelial as well as spherule form, but no cases of man-to-man infection have been discovered. As they occur naturally, however, and on surface cultures, the arthrospores (chlamydospores) of the "saprophytic phase" are highly infectious. Although isolation is unnecessary, precautions should be taken with dressings and casts over open lesions lest the mycelial arthrospores develop as they do on surface cultures. Within the arid endemic areas of California's San Joaquin Valley, in scattered regions in central and southern California, in central and southern Arizona and even in western and southern Texas, from three quarters to nine tenths of long-time residents have been infected, along with cattle, sheep, dogs and wild rodents. Infection apparently confers permanent immunity; therefore, where the population is stable, it is a childhood infection.

CLINICAL FORMS. The human infection must be considered under three broad headings: (1) a benign, self-limited primary infection; (2) residual pulmonary lesions; and (3) a rare, disseminating, generally fatal disease. The disease tends to be milder in children; however, in those requiring medical attention, dissemination to bones and meninges is fairly common.

Primary Coccidioidomycosis. The incubation period varies from 1 to 3 weeks, with an average of 10 to 16 days. Sixty per cent of infected persons show no clinical manifestations. Symptoms are influenzal in type; the onset may be insidious, or abrupt with malaise, chills and fever. Night sweats and anorexia are common. On occasion there is a persistent dry cough with which there may be a painful throat. There may be headache, backache and chest pain, which may vary from a mere sense of constriction to excruciating pleurisy.

A generalized, fine, macular erythema or urticarial eruption may appear within the first day or two. It may be evanescent and present only in the groin. The most frequent dermatologic manifestation is erythema nodosum with or without erythema multiforme. These lesions develop at the time sensitivity to coccidioidin is maximal, 3 to 21 days after onset of symptoms. Skin lesions may occur, however, in persons otherwise asymptomatic. Other allergic manifestations, arthritis and phlyctenular conjunctivitis may occur concomitantly.

Physical examination of the chest rarely dicloses positive findings, even though roentgenography reveals extensive consolidation. Infrequently dullness, a friction rub or fine rales may be detected. Pleural effusions occur at times and may be so massive as to embarrass respiration. Like tuberculous pleural effusions, they may develop without preceding respiratory symptoms.

Residual Pulmonary Coccidioidomycosis. Infrequently a cavity may develop in an area of pulmonary consolidation during the primary infection and close shortly. More often, however, after a variably prolonged period a persistent cavity may form. There are usually no symptoms related to it, and the diagnosis is made roentgenologically. Occasionally there is hemoptysis which, although it may recur and be alarming, is seldom so severe as to impair health. Rarely, fatal hemorrhage has occurred. Dissemination of the fungus from cavities to cause lesions in other areas is rare. Pulmonary residual "granulomas" sometimes persist. They are not harmful, but do pose problems of differentiation from tuberculosis or neoplasms.

Disseminated or Progressive Coccidioidomycosis (Coccidioidal Granuloma). Certain persons seem to lack ability to localize coccidioidal infection. Dissemination, which is rare and occurs mainly in males, especially in Filipinos and blacks, usually follows the initial illness within 6 months, often without any interlude. The closest analogy is to progressive primary tuberculosis. Meningitis is the most serious of the disseminated lesions, being clinically similar to tuberculous meningitis. In white persons it is not unusual for meningitis to be the only extrapulmonary lesion. Papillomatous skin lesions and cold abscesses, both subcutaneous and osseous, occur most frequently in the dark-skinned races. Miliary dissemination and peritonitis are clinically and pathologically indistinguishable from tuberculosis, except by demonstration of the causative agent. The case fatality rate of the untreated disseminated infection is at least 50 per cent, and of meningitis practically 100 per cent.

DIAGNOSIS. Diagnosis of the disseminated infection may be established by biopsy or at autopsy. If histologic examination demonstrates the characteristic double-contoured spherules with endospores and without budding, the diagnosis is certain. In both primary and disseminated infections demonstration of the fungus by culture and animal inoculation is also diagnostic. Coverglass identification is not sufficient, since the diphasic nature of the fungus should be demonstrated. Sputum is generally scanty in the primary infection, so that gastric lavage may be advisable, especially in children. The fungus will not withstand the concentration procedures usually used for tubercle bacilli. The material should be cultured or, after treatment with penicillin and streptomycin, chloramphenicol or 0.05 per cent copper sulfate, injected intraperitoneally into a mouse or intratesticularly into a guinea pig. Any suspicious, white fluffy fungus should be injected into a mouse or guinea pig to demonstrate diagnostic spherules. Only especially qualified laboratories should undertake such hazardous procedures.

Coccidioidin Test. The test is specific except for occasional cross-reactions in histoplasmosis and blastomycosis. Like the tuberculin test, a positive reaction does not distinguish between a recent or old infection unless preceded within a reasonably short time by a negative test result. *A negative skin test does not rule out coccidioidal infection.* Coccidioidin is administered intradermally as 0.1 ml of a 1:1000, 1:100 or even 1:10 dilution. The reaction generally reaches its peak at 36 hours and should be read at 24 and 48 hours. The criterion for a positive result is an area of induration more than 5 mm in diameter. Patients with suspected coccidioidal erythema nodosum are likely to be hypersensitive and should receive the 1:1000 dilution. Patients with disseminated infections are much less sensitive; on occasion even a 1:10 dilution may not elicit a reaction. Dermal sensitivity to coccidioidin is less durable than to tuberculin. There is no danger of disseminating or activating a coccidioidal infection by a strong coccidioidin reaction, although there may be a systemic reaction as well as a local one. Coccidioidin does not evoke humoral coccidioidal antibodies in the human, so that the skin test may precede serologic tests and provides information useful in their interpretation.

Blood and Cerebrospinal Fluid Tests. Serum precipitins and complement fixation appear after coccidioidin sensitivity has become demonstrable and persist during periods of anergy associated with disseminated coccidioidomycosis. In general, the more severe the infection, the higher the complement fixation titer. Humoral antibodies are generally not demonstrable in asymptomatic infections. The sedimentation rate is rapid in both primary and disseminated infections and is helpful in evaluating clinical status. Eosinophilia is common. The cerebrospinal fluid findings, other than a frequently encountered paretic type of colloidal gold curve, are similar to those of tuberculous meningitis. Fixation of complement by cerebrospinal fluid occurs in three fourths of patients with coccidioidal meningitis and is usually diagnostic. Occasionally epidural coccidioidal lesions may also lead to complement fixation by the cerebrospinal fluid. Complement-fixing antibody may be detected in cisternal and lumbar fluid but may be deceptively absent from the ventricular fluid. Complement-fixing antibodies do not pass the blood-brain barrier, but are found in cord blood at the same titer as in the mother's blood. Passively transferred antibody in the infant disappears within 6 months. Congenital coccidioidal dissemination has been reported, but is rare.

Roentgenography. During the primary infection, roentgenograms of the chest may reveal no pulmonary changes, and those that occur are not diagnostic. Hilar adenopathy is frequent, and there may be single or multiple, sharply circumscribed or soft, feathery, small pulmonary densities or larger consolidated areas. Pulmonary cavities, when present, tend to be thin-walled. There may be pleural effusions of variable extent. The osseous lesions of the disseminated infection are usually multiple, with a predilection for cancellous bone; the lesions often show considerable proliferation and are generally indistinguishable from those of tuberculosis.

TREATMENT. The treatment of primary coccidioidal infection consists in restriction of activity and in symptomatic measures. Treatment should be continued until the sedimentation rate is returning to normal, precipitins have vanished, the complement-fixing titer of serum is regressing, and radiographic improvement is noted. Pulmonary cavities frequently close spontaneously. When a cavity persists or is located peripherally, or if there is recurrent bleeding or secondary infection, excision should be considered. Infrequently, bronchopleural fistulas or recurrent cavitation may occur as surgical complications; rarely dissemination may result. When extensive thoracic surgery is required, therapy with amphotericin B may be desirable.

Amphotericin B is the only available agent effective in the treatment of disseminated coccidioidomycosis. It is ineffective by mouth and is given intravenously. See Therapy with Amphotericin B on a prior page for details of dosage. Immediate febrile reactions are frequent, but may be reduced by pretreatment with thorazine or a similar drug. Its nephrotoxicity is reflected best by diminished creatinine clearance, but also by an elevation of the blood urea nitrogen level and at times by depletion of potassium. Once the full dose is achieved, administration of the amphotericin can be on every other day or 2 or 3 times a week in the face of reduced renal function. Thrombophlebitis is common even with scrupulous care in the intravenous administration. Anemia is constant during adequate administration of the drug, but is effectively controlled by transfusions and terminates when treatment is stopped. Agranulocytosis is rare, but hepatic insufficiency develops occasionally, mainly in those with pre-existing liver damage. The drug should not be used in primary infections except when dissemination seems imminent. Although the response is occasionally dramatic in the disseminated form of the disease, generally treatment must be continued for months and, if possible, until improvement is demonstrated by a significant reduction in complement-fixing antibodies. An increase in sensitivity to coccidioidin is evidence of a favorable immunologic response. Immunologic reconstitution with leukocyte transfer factor may be helpful in patients anergic to coccidioidin. Cold abscesses should be drained, and if osseous lesions are accessible, excision should be considered. Amphotericin may be used locally in selected cases.

Amphotericin B does not pass the blood-brain barrier in therapeutic amounts, but it may mask meningitis during intravenous treatment. Early treatment of coccidioidal meningitis is important. Intrathecal administration of the drug in doses of 0.5 mg 2 or 3 times a week is usually necessary.

Arachnoiditis is a hazard of intraspinal administration, and at least one instance of transverse myelitis has been reported.

Treatment of coccidioidal meningitis should begin with both intravenous and intrathecal or intraventricular administration of amphotericin B. The intrathecal administration of amphotericin B is preferably in the cisterna magna. Recent limited experience indicates that amphotericin in 10 per cent glucose solution may be administered via the lumbar route with the patient's head tilted down at −30 degrees from the horizontal. This has not been accompanied by the serious arachnoiditis which usually results from the administration of amphotericin by this route. Intravenous therapy may be discontinued when the physician feels confident that the meningitis is the only extrapulmonary site of involvement, and when the patient appears clinically well and laboratory findings (complement fixation titer, erythrocyte sedimentation rate, total and differential leukocyte counts) support the clinical impression of improvement. Treatment of coccidioidal meningitis should continue for at least 3 months after the cerebrospinal fluid has normal cells, glucose and protein, and has become negative by complement fixation test. Follow-up should include examination of the cerebrospinal fluid at intervals of 1 to 3 months (and immediately if there is headache or any change in behavior or personality) for a period of at least 2 years (Winn). Clinical surveillance should be continued for some years longer.

In patients with subcutaneous or osseous lesions, surgical intervention may be necessary. In these cases intravenous and local therapy with amphotericin B may be used, depending on the extent of involvement. Again, therapy should be guided by clinical status and the laboratory parameters mentioned above.

Demosthenes Pappagianis

PATIENT EDUCATION

Coccy (Coccidioidomycosis), The Facts. Published by the American Lung (Christmas Seal) Association and available through its local Chapter offices.

GENERAL

Ajello, L. (ed.): Symposium on Coccidioidomycosis. Tucson, Ariz., University of Arizona Press, 1967.

Birsner, J. W.: The roentgen aspects of five hundred cases of pulmonary coccidioidomycosis. Am. J. Roentgenol. *72*:556, 1954.

Einstein, H.: Coccidioidomycosis. *In* Buechner, H. A. (ed.): Management of Fungus Diseases of the Lungs. Springfield, Ill., Charles C Thomas, 1971, Chap. 4, pp. 86–144.

Fiese, M. J.: Coccidioidomycosis. Springfield, Ill., Charles C Thomas, 1958.

Pappagianis, D.: Epidemiology of Coccidioidomycosis. Proceedings of International Symposium on Mycoses. Scientific Publication Pan Amer. Hlth. Org. No. 205, 1970.

Richardson, H. B., Anderson, J. A., and McKay, B. M.: Acute pulmonary coccidioidomycosis in children. J. Pediatr. *70*:376, 1967.

Seabury, J. Coccidioidomycosis. *In* Kendig, E. L. (ed.): Pulmonary Disorders of Infancy and Childhood, 2nd ed. Philadelphia, W. B. Saunders Company, 1972.

Smith, C. E.: Coccidioidomycosis. Pediat. Clin. N. Amer. *2*:109, 1955.

Winn, W. A.: The treatment of coccidioidal meningitis. The use of amphotericin B in a group of 25 patients. Calif. Med. *101*:78, 1964.

PARASITIC INFECTIONS

Helminthic Diseases

The parasitic helminths of man fall into three major groups: the Nematoda or roundworms, the Cestoda or tapeworms, and the Trematoda or flukes. A fourth group, the Acanthocephala or thorny-headed worms, are mentioned only to point out that records of Acanthocephala infections in children are extremely rare.

As a rule, parasitic worms do not multiply in the host. Therefore, the number of worms in the body depends on the intensity and frequency of exposure, and especially on the intensity or amount of the *first* exposure. Prior and existing infections, more particularly the latter, tend to bar entirely or to limit to some extent any additional or subsequent infection. In general, whereas light and very light helminthic infections in children tend to be asymptomatic, worms of all kinds are pathogenic when present in large numbers.

The helminths commonly found in children and the usual modes of transmission are listed in Table 10–25.

INFECTIONS PRODUCED BY ROUNDWORMS (NEMATODA)

All important roundworm infections are produced by species belonging to the phylum Nematoda, which includes the true roundworms. These are elongated, cylindroid, unsegmented animals covered with a tough, relatively impermeable cuticula secreted by the underlying tissue layer, the hypodermis. They have a complete digestive tract, consisting of a mouth which is frequently provided with lips, teeth or other organs designed for penetration and attachment, a muscular esophagus, a midgut, and a rectum. The nervous system is prim-

TABLE 10–25 MODES OF TRANSMISSION OF SOME HELMINTHIC INFECTIONS

MEDIUM	TRANSMISSION SOURCE	HELMINTH AND STAGE INVOLVED	COMMON NAME OF WORM OR INFECTION
		Peroral Exposure	
1. Raw foods	Fruits, vegetables (night-soil fertilized)	Ascaris, Trichuris (embryonated eggs)	Roundworm Whipworm
	Watercress	Fasciola (encysted metacercaria)	Sheep liver fluke
	Water nuts	Fasciolopsis (encysted metacercaria)	Intestinal fluke
	Meat Pork	Trichinella (encapsulated larva) *Taenia solium* (cysticercus)	Trichinosis Pork tapeworm
	Beef	*Taenia saginata* (cysticercus)	Beef tapeworm
	Bear	Trichinella (encapsulated larva)	Trichinosis
	Fish (fresh-water)	*Diphyllobothrium latum* (sparganum) Clonorchis, Opisthorchis (encapsulated metacercaria)	Fish tapeworm Liver fluke
	Crabs, crayfish	Paragonimus (encapsulated metacercaria)	Lung fluke
2. Drinking water	Cyclops, Diaptomus	Dracunculus (infective larva) Sparganum (procercoid larva)	Guinea worm Sparganosis
3. Immediate environment Person-to-person	Anus to fingers and fomites to mouth	Enterobius *Hymenolepis nana* (embryonated egg)	Pinworm Dwarf tapeworm
Dog-to-person	Dog coat to hands; fomites, food, to mouth	Echinococcus (egg)	Hydatid
4. Soil contaminated with feces of: Man	Dirt (food contamination, geophagy)	Ascaris (embryonated egg) Trichuris (embryonated egg)	Roundworm Whipworm
Dog	Dirt (contamination, geophagy)	Echinococcus (egg) *Toxocara canis* (embryonated egg)	Hydatid Visceral larva migrans
Cat	Dirt (contamination, geophagy)	*Toxocara cati* (embryonated egg)	Visceral larva migrans
5. Feces-eating insects	Fleas of dog or cat	*Dipylidium caninum* (larva in flea)	Dog and cat tapeworm
	Rodent fleas, grain beetle	*Hymenolepis diminuta* (larva in vector)	Rat tapeworm
		Percutaneous Exposure	
1. Soil contaminated with feces of: Man	Damp ground (skin contact)	Necator, Ancylostoma (filariform larva) Strongyloides (filariform larva)	Hookworm Threadworm
Dog, cat	Damp ground (skin contact)	Ancylostoma species (filariform larva)	Creeping eruption (cutaneous larva migrans)
2. Infested water	Mollusca—intermediate hosts in water	Schistosoma species (cercarial larva)	Schistosomiasis, schistosome dermatitis
3. Blood-sucking insects	Mosquitoes, black flies, etc.	Filarial worms (filariform larva)	Filariasis

itive and is elaborated only at the oral end. A conspicuous body cavity contains the organs of excretion and reproduction. With few exceptions the sexes are separate. The female reproductive opening (vulva) is midventral in position, near the equatorial plane or anterior to this level. The male reproductive system joins the rectum to form a cloaca, which opens externally at or near the posterior end of the body.

The most important roundworm infections (nematodiases) are ascariasis, toxocariasis (visceral larva migrans), enterobiasis, trichuriasis, the hookworm infections, strongyloidiasis, trichinosis, the filariases and dracontiasis, or dracunculosis.

ASCARIASIS

ETIOLOGY. Ascariasis is produced by the giant roundworm, *Ascaris lumbricoides,* which normally lives in the lumen of the host's small intestine. The mature female worm measures 20 to 35 cm in length by 3 to 6 mm in greatest diameter, and the male is about one fifth smaller. Both sexes have three fleshy lips surrounding the triangular mouth, and both taper to a sharp posterior end, with the male curved ventrally at the posterior extremity. The female lays approximately 200,000 eggs each day. These are infertile if males are lacking, and some may be infertile if the female is just

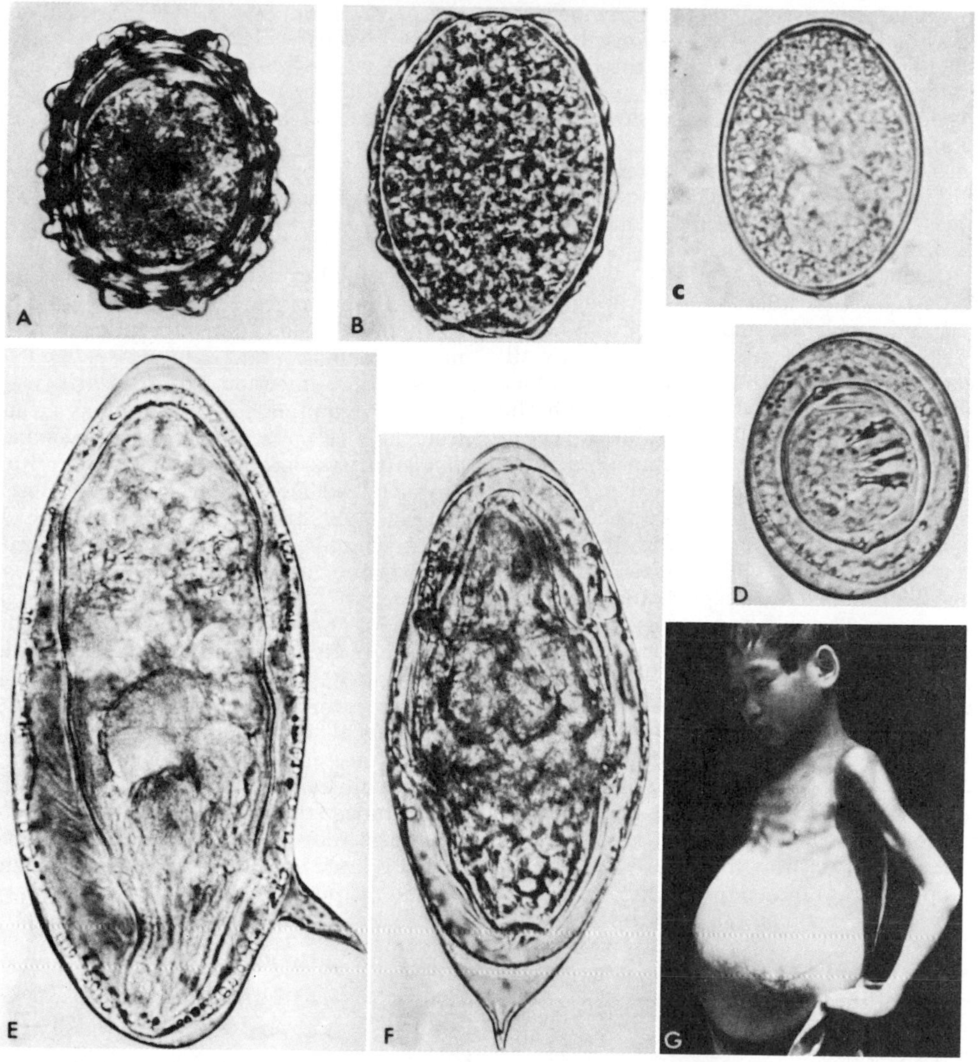

Figure 10–63 A, *Fertilized egg of* Ascaris lumbricoides. × *550.* B, *Unfertilized egg of* Ascaris lumbricoides. × *550.* C, *Egg of* Diphyllobothrium latum. × *550.* D, *Egg of* Hymenolepis nana. × *550.* E, *Egg of* Schistosoma mansoni *from feces.* F, *Egg of* Schistosoma haematobium *from urine.* × *550.* G, *Advanced stage of schistosomiasis japonica in a 13-year-old Chinese boy, with ascites resulting from hepatic cirrhosis, splenomegaly, fever, anemia and dysentery. (After E. G. Nauck. Lehrbuch der Tropenkrankheiten. Courtesy of Georg Thieme Verlag, Stuttgart.)*

beginning to oviposit. The fertile eggs are passed in the patient's feces in the one-celled stage. They are broadly ovoidal, measure 35 to 50 μ in cross section by 65 to 75 μ in greatest diameter and are provided with a thin, resistant inner shell, a thick hyaline middle shell and a mammillated outer covering which is usually bile-stained. Within the shell covering is a densely granular, more or less spherical egg cell (Fig. 10–63).

EPIDEMIOLOGY. Ascariasis is widely distributed throughout the tropics and extends into the temperate zones as far north and south as latitude 40 degrees. The fertile eggs are able to survive practically all external conditions except heat and extreme desiccation. When the egg is deposited on the soil or any suitably moist medium it proceeds to embryonate and in warm weather within 9 days or more contains a motile first-stage larva. A week later, during which the larva molts once, the egg is infective. It does not hatch on the soil, but only after being swallowed. In favorable environments, as in the Gulf Coast area of the United States, the embryonated eggs may remain viable and infective for months or even for several years. The worms are harbored principally by young children. The infective eggs develop in the soil, and children take some of them into the mouth on contaminated fingers or play objects, or as a result of eating dirt. Where these unsanitary conditions prevail, 60 to 100 per cent of children from 1 to 10 years of age are infected with Ascaris. Older children and adults are parasitized to a lesser degree and can usually trace their infections to sources provided by the younger groups.

Ascariasis is encountered occasionally among children in the northern United States, but the southern Appalachians and their extension into the Ozarks and the Gulf Coast states constitute the regions of high endemicity in the United States. Clay soils are most favorable for the development of Ascaris eggs, in contrast to moist, sandy humus for those of hookworms.

Hogs are infected with an Ascaris morphologically indistinguishable from that in man, but the hog Ascaris, though infective for human beings under natural conditions, usually does not develop to full maturity in man.

PATHOLOGY. When infective Ascaris eggs are swallowed and reach the duodenum, they hatch, and the escaping larvae enter the intestinal wall. The larvae penetrate into the mesenteric lymphatics or venules, commonly migrating through the liver, and are carried to the lungs. An acute cellular infiltration typically occurs in the immediate vicinity of the larvae. Large numbers of larvae migrating through the lungs produce Loeffler syndrome or an atypical pneumonia (Fig. 10–64).

After growth and one molt in the lungs, the third-stage larvae reach the epiglottis, are swallowed and become established in the small intestine, where they grow into adult worms. Between the sixtieth and seventy-fifth days after the eggs have been swallowed, mature worms mate, and the females begin their egg-laying. If the worms become irritated by their environment, as, for example, owing to digestive disturbances or fever, they may pass down the bowel and be spontaneously evacuated; or they may enter the stomach to be vomited, or escape through the nares. They may block the appendiceal lumen, perforate the intestinal wall, block the common bile duct, migrate into the parenchyma of the liver or reach the pleural cavity. Extensive destruction of the hepatic parenchyma and abscess formation may occur as a result of their movements, death and disintegration.

CLINICAL MANIFESTATIONS. During their development in the lungs the larvae may cause an atypical pneumonia. The sensitization produced by them is responsible for the manifestations of ascaris allergy frequently observed, including asthma, urticaria and eosinophilia. In some regions **Loeffler syndrome**, which is characterized by transient, migratory infiltration and peripheral eosinophilia, is a common manifestation of pulmonary ascariasis.

Intestinal infection with Ascaris may be apparently symptomless, or there may be such manifestations as nausea and vomiting, anorexia, loss of weight, insomnia, slight fever, irritability, or physical and mental languor. The most common complaint of children is intestinal colic. As a rule, acute symptoms accompany ectopic excursions of the worms. A mass of writhing worms knotted together frequently produces acute intestinal obstruction, at times resulting in perforation of the wall, in intussusception or in paralytic ileus.

DIAGNOSIS. The diagnosis is commonly made by the recovery of fertile or infertile eggs in microscopic fecal films. Direct unconcentrated films usually provide this evidence after the mature females have begun to oviposit. If only male worms occur (in less than 5 per cent of infections), clinical diagnosis may be confirmed by the therapeutic test. From time to time adult or immature worms passed in the stool or vomited or discharged from the nostril require diagnosis. Occasionally, during

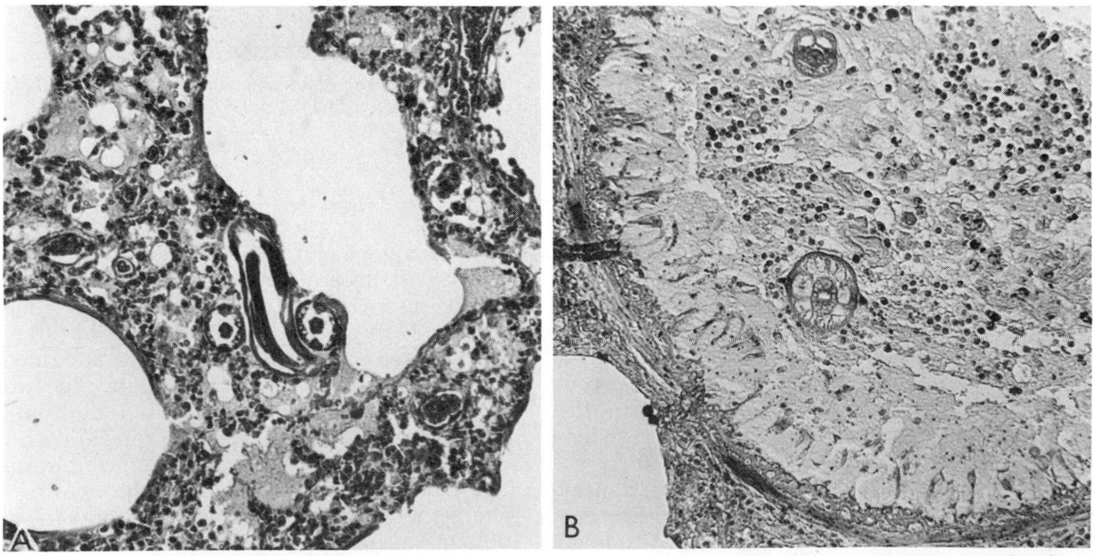

Figure 10–64 *Larva of Ascaris in human lung. (× 170.)* A, *Longitudinal and transverse sections of developing larva in parenchyma with minimal inflammation;* B, *transverse sections through esophageal and midintestinal regions of mature pulmonary-stage larva in migration to the intestine via bronchiole filled with mucopurulent material. Both larvae are presumed to be* A. lumbricoides *though morphologically indistinguishable from pig Ascaris,* A. suum, *which also causes pneumonitis. In both* A *and* B *numerous other larvae were found in the lungs, and in both cases death was attributed to pulmonary ascariasis. The patient in* A, *1 year old, was reported by Piggott et al. in 1970; photomicrograph made from slide received courtesy of R. C. Neafie. The other case* (B) *was reported by Beaver and Danaraj in 1958.*

barium studies of the gastrointestinal tract for other purposes, the worms are demonstrated.

PROGNOSIS. Except when large numbers of Ascaris larvae in the lungs initiate lobular pneumonia or when adult worms produce intestinal obstruction or migrate into abnormal foci, the prognosis is good to excellent, provided a specific anthelmintic is administered.

PREVENTION. In highly endemic areas re-exposure is the rule, and reinfection takes place about every 3 months. Thus, both the physician and the public health officer are concerned with problems of control. Community sanitation combined with periodic treatment is an effective measure for control.

TREATMENT. There is no specific treatment that is effective against the larval stages in the lungs. For removal of both young and old worms from the intestine, *piperazine citrate* is almost ideal. No pretreatment or post-treatment purgation or fasting is required, and the recommended dosage produces no side effects. The syrup of piperazine citrate is given orally in a single dose of 3 or 4 gm (see Drug Table 30–1) and may be repeated in 2 days. It may be introduced by tube to children suspected of having intestinal or biliary obstruction resulting from ascariasis. Also effective and relatively nontoxic are Pyrantel, given in a single dose of 10 mg/kg, and thiabendazole in a dosage of 25 mg/kg twice a day for 2 days.

VISCERAL LARVA MIGRANS
(Toxocariasis)

ETIOLOGY. Intestinal infections with adult-stage *Toxocara canis* and *T. cati* have been reported in children, but all such records are questionable. By contrast, infections with the larval stage of *T. canis* are very common in children, and similar infections with *T. cati,* though less common, have also been reported. The larvae invade the tissues and, though they remain alive for many months or years, they neither grow nor develop beyond the infective stage. The larvae of *T. canis* are less than 0.5 mm long and 18 to 20 μ wide; those of *T. cati* are slightly smaller. They are readily distinguishable from other types of larvae found in human tissues. *Visceral larva migrans* was first described in 1952 as a disease of toddler-age children, caused by the prolonged migration of nematode larvae such as Toxocara in the deep tissues, producing trails of focal eosinophilic infiltration followed by a granulomatous reaction.

EPIDEMIOLOGY. *Toxocara canis* is among the most common species of intestinal worms found in dogs; *T. cati* is similarly common in cats. Both are cosmopolitan in distribution, though there are areas where *T. canis* is less common than is a morphologically similar species *(Toxascaris leonina),* which is not known to cause disease in man. *Toxocara canis* infection in dogs is acquired in four different ways: (1) by ingesting infective eggs in soil; (2) by eating small mammals earlier infected by ingesting eggs from soil (paratenic hosts); (3) by migration of larvae from the tissues of the mother to the fetal pup (prenatal infection); and (4) by ingesting larvae passed in the feces of hyperinfected suckling pups. Children acquire infections primarily through "dirt eating." Since even lightly infected dogs pass enormous numbers of eggs in the feces daily for many months, and though the fecal matter is variously and quickly dissipated, the eggs accumulate in the soil, so that in any area where dogs habitually defecate the soil becomes highly infectious. Further, through the sorting action of rain the eggs tend to be both widely disseminated and, in certain places, highly concentrated, so much so that a few milligrams of soil may contain hundreds of viable, infective eggs, making it possible for a dirt-eating child to ingest at one "sitting" enormous numbers of infective eggs. Though reported from essentially all parts of the world, the majority of cases have occurred in the United States and Europe.

PATHOLOGY. On reaching the intestine, the eggs hatch and the mobile larvae migrate to the liver and eventually to all major organs of the body including the brain and eye (Figure 10–65). Following the early period of migration the larvae are relatively immobile, and eventually they become encapsulated in dense fibrous tissue. In the migratory phase, which may last several months, there are eosinophilic inflammation and granuloma formation in the wake of the moving larva.

CLINICAL MANIFESTATIONS. The most striking feature of visceral larva migrans caused by Toxocara is hypereosinophilia of the blood. Even in asymptomatic cases the levels of eosinophilia often exceed 50 per cent. Levels above 90 per cent of 90,000 leukocytes have been reported, and absolute levels of 25,000 per mm^3 are not uncommon. Other typical manifestations are hepatomegaly, pulmonary infiltration, neurologic disturbances and endophthalmitis, each condition resulting from the presence of larvae in the affected organs. Low-grade fever usually is noted, along with recurrent upper respiratory complaints, cough and, occasionally, asthmatic breathing. The disease is seen mostly in children 1 to 4 years of age, usually with a history of pica. As *Ascaris lumbricoides* and *Trichuris trichiura* infections are acquired in the same manner as is Toxocara infection, they often are acquired simultaneously, and together they produce signs and symptoms that are not readily interpreted.

DIAGNOSIS. Toxocara infection can be diagnosed with certainty only by identifying the larvae in tissues removed by biopsy or at autopsy, usually from the liver or in the enucleated eye. Serodiagnostic tests and skin tests are of little value and often may be misleading.

PROGNOSIS. Deaths attributed to exceptionally heavy infections with larval toxocariasis have been recorded. However, the prospect of complete recovery within a period of 6 to 12 months is good if exposure to further infection can be barred. Of continuing concern, even after all evidences of infection have disappeared, is the prospect of invasion

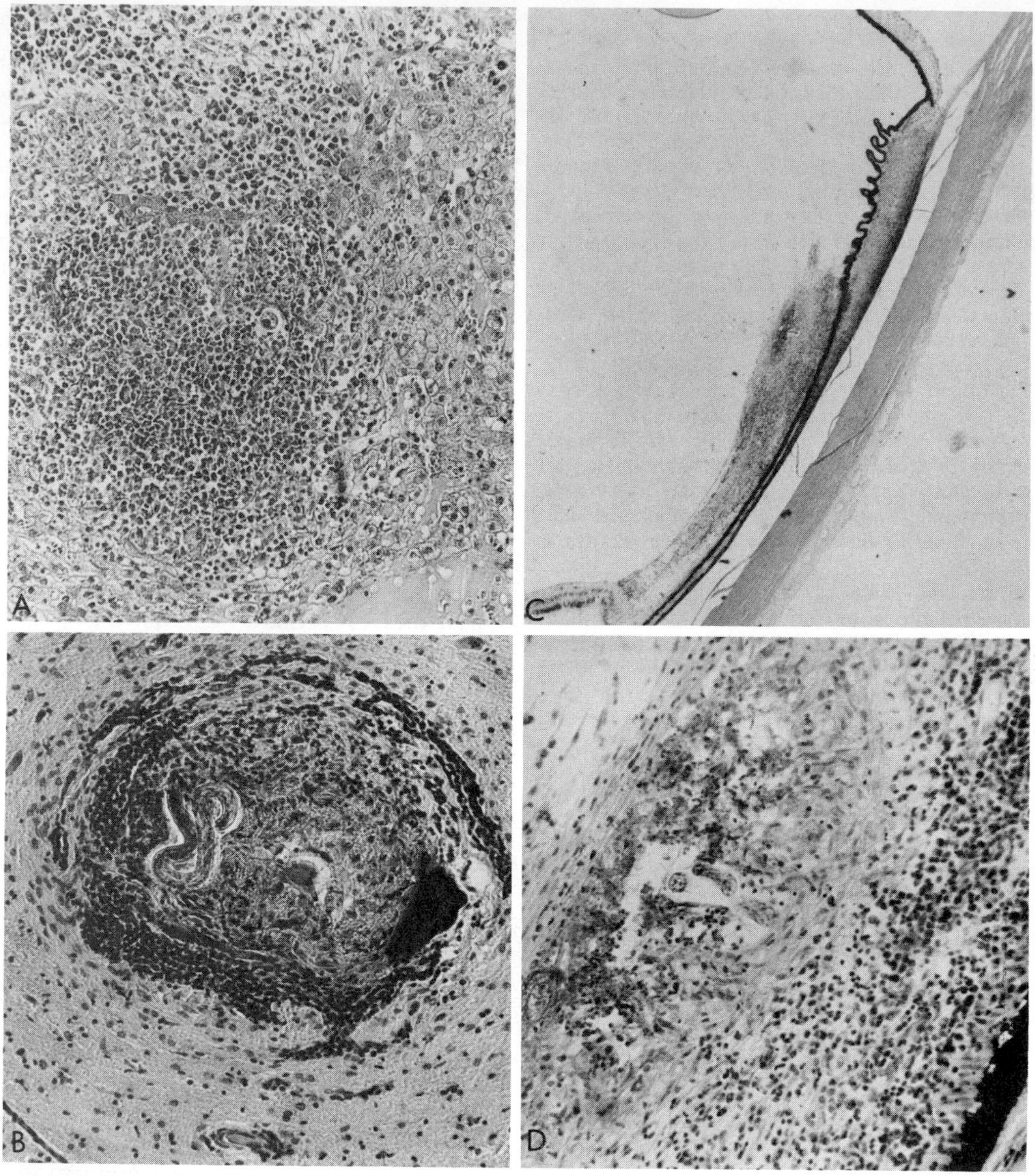

Figure 10–65 *Visceral larva migrans produced by larvae of the dog ascarid,* Toxocara canis. A, *Larva in area of intense eosinophilic inflammation in liver; biopsy from a 4 year old girl in South Africa.* B, *Larva in granuloma in thalamus discovered at autopsy of 6 year old girl who died with poliomyelitis in England.* C *and* D, *Larva in eosinophilic granuloma in enucleated eye of 4 year old boy in California.* (A, B, D, × *ca. 150;* C, × *17.) Photomicrographs courtesy of Dr. Leonard Sagorin* (A), *Dr. A. L. Woolf* (B), *and Dr. A. R. Irvine, Jr.* (C *and* D).

of the eye and the consequent loss of vision. Endophthalmitis caused by Toxocara has generally occurred in older children with no other signs or symptoms of toxocariasis and often without a clinical history suggestive of the infection.

PREVENTION. Protection of toddler-age children from contact with soil known or presumed to be contaminated with feces of dogs, and the periodic (monthly) deworming of household dogs are reasonable preventive measures.

TREATMENT. Though not definitely known to be effective, thiabendazole has in two instances been thought to be beneficial. For relief of severe symptoms, corticosteroids may be used.

ENTEROBIASIS
(Pinworm Infection)

ETIOLOGY. Enterobiasis is caused by the pinworm, *Enterobius vermicularis* (seatworm, oxyuriasis of older textbooks). The adult worms are small (males, 2 to 5 mm in length, and curved ven-

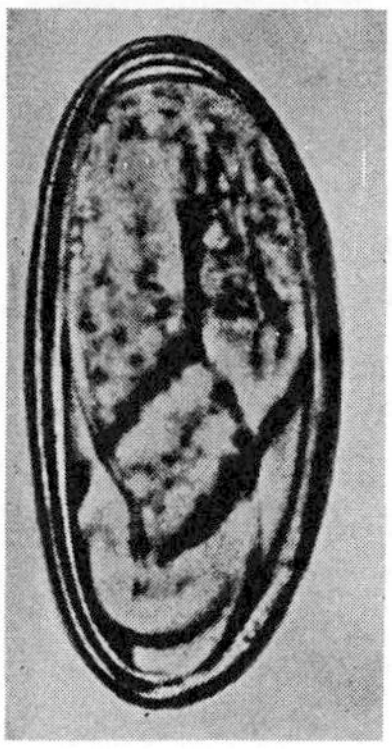

Figure 10–66 *Fully embryonated egg of* Enterobius vermicularis *obtained by perianal swabbing.* × *800. (From Cram: Introduction to Nematology. Bureau of Plant Industry, Washington, D.C.)*

trally at the posterior end; females, 8 to 13 mm in length, robust in the middle and drawn out into a long sharp point posteriorly). The worms live in the cecum and appendix. When worms become gravid they migrate down the bowel and characteristically crawl out the anus onto the perianal and perineal skin, where each female deposits several thousand eggs. Eggs are seldom laid within the bowel, and if so, are usually infertile or immature. The eggs laid outside the anus are elongated, ovoidal, somewhat flattened on one side, with a thick, slightly opalescent shell, and measure 50 to 60 by 20 to 30 μ. They contain a coiled larva at the time of oviposition (Fig. 10–66). They require only a few hours after deposition to become infective.

EPIDEMIOLOGY. This infection is world-wide in distribution. Children are particularly susceptible, and those in large families, schools in slum areas, and dormitory groups are more heavily parasitized than the population at large. They are exposed to infection by scratching the itching skin around the anus, where the eggs are lodged, or from soiled night garments or undergarments, bed linen or contaminated objects in the room; they get the infective eggs onto their fingers and then into their mouths, or may breathe in and ingest airborne eggs. Eggs remain viable in humid environments for several days.

PATHOLOGY. When viable eggs are swallowed and pass down the digestive tract, they hatch at the duodenal level, and the escaping larvae migrate to the cecum, become attached and develop into adults in the upper colon in 15 to 28 days. They usually produce no appreciable damage inside the body, but gravid worms, crawling out the anus, usually at night, frequently cause a severe pruritus, and the inevitable scratching results in scarification and secondary infection of the skin. In the female patient the gravid worms may enter the genital tract, cause a salpingitis, become encapsulated in the tubes or enter the peritoneal cavity and provoke encapsulation.

CLINICAL MANIFESTATIONS. The appendiceal lesions occasionally produce symptoms of acute or subacute appendicitis, with indications for excision of the organ. Pruritus ani is frequently complicated by bacterial invasion of the skin and the production of weeping, eczematous areas. Children, especially young girls, may exhibit irritability, loss of appetite and weight, and insomnia, resulting in chronic emotional disturbances. Vaginitis has been ascribed to direct invasion by the worms. Eosinophilia does not necessarily occur.

DIAGNOSIS. Fecal examination is not effective in the diagnosis of enterobiasis. The eggs (Fig. 10–65) can usually be recovered in one to several swabbings of the perianal and perineal skin, preferably in the morning before dressing, bathing or defecation.

A simple and probably the most efficient anal swabbing technique consists in the use of adhesive cellulose tape, with the sticky surface pressed firmly against the perianal folds. After swabbing, the tape is placed flat, sticky side down, on a slide. It may be examined microscopically at any convenient time after lifting the tape and allowing a drop of toluene to enter between tape and slide.

PROGNOSIS. As treatment usually is effective, at least temporarily, prognosis usually is good.

PREVENTION. Scrupulous personal and group hygiene is advised, but in itself will not eradicate infection. Accurate diagnosis and treatment of all infected persons in a household, repeated several times if necessary, will delay reinfection, though in normal circumstances complete prevention is not feasible.

TREATMENT. Pyrvinium pamoate, a cyanine dye, is used for single-dose treatment (5 mg/kg). Piperazine, administered as piperazine citrate syrup, is highly efficient and well tolerated. It is administered by mouth, 65 mg/kg/day (maximum 2.5 gm/day) for 8 days. Pyrantel is effective in a single dose of 10 mg/kg given as a suspension.

It is sometimes recommended that all persons, or at least all infected persons, in a household or dormitory receive treatment simultaneously. However, even if the infection is completely eradicated from a household, its return through outside contacts can be expected.

TRICHURIASIS

(Whipworm Infection)

ETIOLOGY. Whipworm infection in man is produced by *Trichuris trichiura,* whose body is composed of a capillary anterior three fifths and a fleshy posterior two fifths. The males measure 30 to 45 mm in length and are coiled ventrally at the posterior end. The females measure 35 to 50 mm in length and have a club-shaped posterior end. These worms live with their anterior ends threaded into the mucosal epithelium of the cecum and appendix and, in heavy infections, the ascending colon, and even the sigmoid colon and rectum. The females daily lay a few thousand barrel-shaped eggs, which have mucus-like polar plugs and are commonly bile-stained (Fig. 10–67).

EPIDEMIOLOGY. Whipworm infection is widely

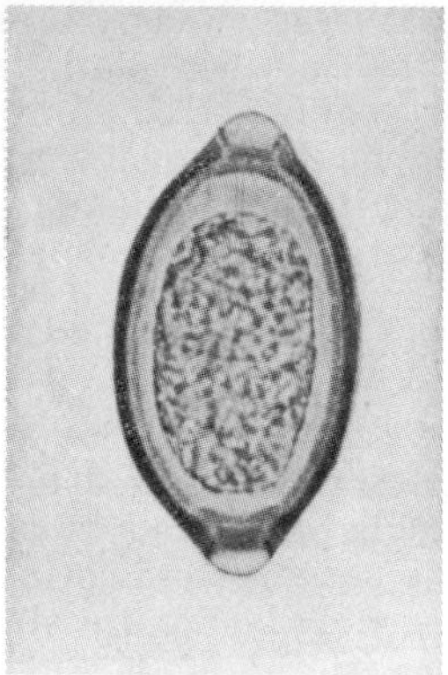

Figure 10–67 *Egg of* Trichuris trichiura, *as seen in freshly passed feces.* × *666. (After Faust, in Brennemann's Practice of Pediatrics. Courtesy of W. F. Prior Co.)*

distributed in warm, moist climates. It is most common in children over 5 years of age, but may be prevalent in younger patients. The eggs passed in feces and deposited on moist, shaded soil require 10 to 14 days to develop to the infective stage, at which time each contains a motile larva. When ripe eggs are swallowed and hatch, the escaping larvae migrate to the cecum or appendix, penetrate or become attached to the mucosal epithelium, and in about 3 months develop into adult worms.

PATHOLOGY. Usually the infection is well tolerated unless the worm burden is heavy (i.e., several hundred), as it frequently is in the tropics or the moist subtropics. In heavy infections the worms colonize the intestinal mucosa from the lower level of the ileum almost to the anal sphincter.

CLINICAL MANIFESTATIONS. Many persons, especially in the southern United States, harbor a few worms without apparent symptoms, but in heavy infections there is chronic irritation of the bowel wall, resulting in a bloody, mucous diarrhea, at times with an associated prolapse of the rectum.

DIAGNOSIS. Diagnosis is made on the recovery of the characteristic eggs (Fig. 10–67) in direct or concentrated fecal films. Worms in the lower colon are readily seen by sigmoidoscopy, even when immature and not yet laying eggs.

PROGNOSIS. Prognosis is good in most patients. With the removal of the worms, recovery is immediate and complete.

PREVENTION. Sanitary toilet facilities and disposal of sewage, along with the protection of children against dirt eating, are sound preventive measures. Children must be trained not to take contaminated objects and dirt into their mouths.

TREATMENT. For rapid treatment in hospitalized or clinic patients, high enemas of 0.2 per cent hexylresorcinol retained for 20 to 30 minutes are effective in removing a large proportion of the worms, and thus produce clinical cure. Before instilling the solution it is necessary to coat the buttocks, thighs and perineum with petroleum jelly to prevent burning of the skin from returned or spilled solution. Colon-filling amounts should be used; the procedure can be repeated after 1 week. Cleansing enemas given 1 to 2 hours before the treatment are beneficial, except in patients with dysentery. None of the standard orally administered anthelmintics is effective for trichuriasis, though thiabendazole, 25 mg/kg twice a day for 2 days, is sometimes recommended. Mebendazole has given satisfactory results in recent trials.

HOOKWORM INFECTIONS

(Uncinariasis; Ancylostomiasis)

ETIOLOGY. The hookworms which parasitize man are *Necator americanus*, the so-called American hookworm; *Ancylostoma duodenale*, the so-called Old World hookworm; *A. ceylanicum* and *A. braziliense*. The first two are exclusively parasites of man; *A. ceylanicum* and *A. braziliense* are typically parasites of dogs and cats. Hookworms are 7.5 to 13 mm long and 0.3 to 0.4 mm in greatest breadth. The males are slightly smaller than the females. The mouth of Necator is provided with a pair of upper and a pair of lower cutting plates; that of Ancylostoma, with two or three pairs of incurved upper teeth. The females have a bluntly pointed caudal extremity and a vulvar opening midventral in position near the equatorial plane. The caudal extremity of the male is drawn out into an umbrella-like expansion, the copulatory bursa, used to grasp the female during copulation. These worms are attached by their mouth capsule to the mucosa of the small bowel, typically at the level of the duodenum, jejunum and adjacent portion of the ileum.

After insemination each female hookworm lays several thousand eggs a day. These eggs (Fig. 10–68) are broadly ovoidal, thin-shelled and hyaline; they measure 60 to 76 by 36 to 40 μ. They are in an early stage of development when evacuated in the feces, but in stools passed several hours before examination they may be more advanced in development (Fig. 10–68 B).

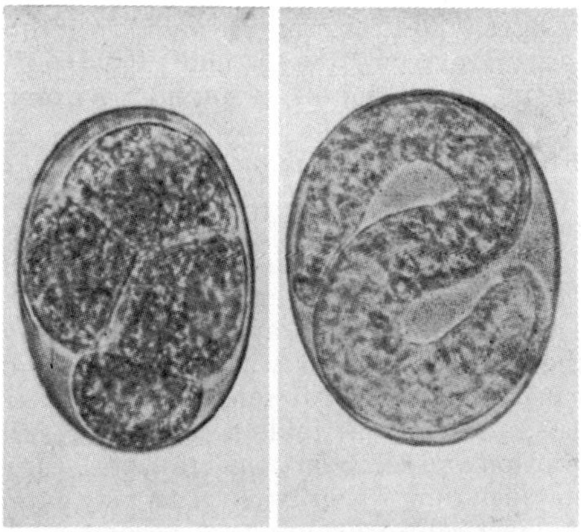

A B

Figure 10–68 *Eggs of hookworm,* Necator americanus. *(× 666.)* A, *Four-cell stage as seen in freshly passed feces;* B, *maturing embryo, as seen in feces passed several hours earlier. (After Faust, E. C.:* In *Brennemann's Practice of Pediatrics. Courtesy of W. F. Prior Co., Hyattsville, Md.)*

EPIDEMIOLOGY. *Necator americanus* is the tropical hookworm of the Western Hemisphere; it is the only widely distributed hookworm in the Americas, including the southern United States. *Ancylostoma duodenale* is the hookworm of the Mediterranean basin and similar latitudes in Asia and is the more common species on the Pacific coast of South America. *Ancylostoma ceylanicum* is found in Southeast Asia and Brazil. In all essential clinical respects it so closely resembles *A. duodenale* that a specific diagnosis is not required.

Eggs of Necator and *A. duodenale* evacuated from the human bowel and deposited on a moist, sandy humus soil in a shaded site in warm climates embryonate rapidly and hatch in 24 to 48 hours. The escaping larvae feed on fecal and soil bacteria and organic debris, grow, molt, feed again and, between the fifth and tenth days, transform into infective-stage filariform larvae. Exposure occurs when these larvae come in contact with the skin. Infants and small children are seldom exposed to infection except in hyperendemic areas. Older children and adults, especially males, in highly endemic areas are subject to repeated infection; thus, man initiates the extrinsic phase of the life cycle by discharging hookworm eggs on the soil and, in turn, picks up the infection by direct contact with the soil. The larva of *A. duodenale* is infective by mouth as well as by skin; that of Necator by skin only. Man occasionally acquires intestinal infection with *A. ceylanicum* and incurs cutaneous larva migrans (creeping eruption) after exposure to *A. braziliense*.

PATHOLOGY. The infective-stage larvae of the hookworm can invade the human skin through hair follicles or under particles of desquamating epidermis. They migrate to the cutaneous blood vessels, enter the venules, are carried to the lungs through the right side of the heart and lodge in the pulmonary capillaries, where, in Necator, a molt occurs. From the capillaries they penetrate the alveoli, migrate up the respiratory tract, pass over the epiglottis and are swallowed. In the small intestine they become sexually mature and copulate, and in 7 or 8 weeks after invasion of the skin the females begin to lay eggs.

Temporary trauma and tissue reaction develop at the sites where the larvae invade the skin and where they pass from the pulmonary capillaries into the air sacs, but these manifestations are not serious unless the cutaneous lesions become secondarily infected or the number of invading larvae is large. After attachment to the mucosa of the intestine the worms move from place to place, especially when crowded, leaving lacerations through which relatively large amounts of blood are lost.

CLINICAL MANIFESTATIONS. The effects of the migrating larvae of hookworms differ somewhat according to the species. The two common species, *N. americanus* and *A. duodenale*, differ as regards the normal mode of infection and the site of early development in the tissues. In Necator the larvae normally enter the body through the skin, whereas in *A. duodenale* the larvae may enter either by mouth or by skin. Also, in the migration from skin to intestine through the lungs, the larvae of Necator undergo essential development in the lungs, whereas the larvae of *A. duodenale* pass through the lungs unchanged and undergo growth and early development in the intestinal mucosa. It can be expected, therefore, that the migrating larvae of Necator affect the lungs more severely than do those of *A. duodenale*, whereas in the intestine *A. duodenale* may be more disturbing than Necator.

The skin reactions to both species are more or less severe, depending on the number of larvae penetrating and the degree of prior sensitization. After repeated exposure, migration of Necator larvae in the skin may cause transient but otherwise typical creeping eruption.

In the lungs, Necator larvae may cause cough, fever and sensations of bronchial and tracheal irritation that in timing and character resemble those of pulmonary ascariasis. In *A. duodenale* infection, the most notable pulmonary reactions are those seen in Japan one or two days following ingestion of larvae on green vegetables. In this condition, referred to as *Wakana disease*, there are nausea, vomiting, severe cough and sputum, and high eosinophilia of the blood. These reactions apparently develop whether or not any of the larvae reach the lungs.

Eggs appear in the feces during the sixth week of infection with *A. duodenale*, one or two weeks later with Necator. About one week before eggs can be found in the stools, symptoms of enteritis may appear and may be severe and sudden in onset. At the same time, abundant Charcot-Leyden crystals are found in the feces and there is eosinophilia of the blood. In light or moderate infections symptoms subside a week or so after eggs appear in the feces, but the Charcot-Leyden crystals and eosinophilia persist for several weeks. In infants with very heavy infections, intestinal bleeding and symptoms of enteritis may occur much earlier.

The anemia resulting from chronic, heavy hookworm infection is well known. Blood loss from mucosal laceration and perhaps from feeding activities of the worms, when greater in amount than can be replaced, results eventually in a hypochromic microcytic anemia. The manifestations of chronic hookworm disease are essentially the same as those caused by blood loss from other causes.

Creeping eruption, or **cutaneous larva migrans**, results mainly from infection with the dog and cat hookworm *A. braziliense;* less commonly, the cosmopolitan dog hookworm *A. caninum*; and rarely, the human hookworms *N. americanus* and *A. duodenale*. The larvae penetrate to the deeper layers of the epidermis, but instead of entering the dermal tissues and blood vessels, continue to migrate for several days, even several months (larva migrans) through serpiginous tunnels in the skin (Fig. 10–69, page 656). This produces an inflamed appearance of the somewhat elevated channels, which often become infected as a result of scratching the pruritic lesions.

DIAGNOSIS. Diagnosis of an intestinal infection is based on identification of eggs (Fig. 10–68) in the feces. Species identification can be made by examination of infective-stage larvae obtained from cultures.

PROGNOSIS. Prognosis is usually good with specific treatment, provided reinfection is prevented, the hemoglobin content is returned to normal and an adequate, balanced diet is provided.

PREVENTION. At the community or national level, prevention is accomplished through the periodic detection and treatment of infected persons and the provision of sanitary facilities to reduce soil contamination. The individual can prevent infection by avoiding contact with contaminated soil at times when the surface is wet or damp.

TREATMENT. The iron-deficiency anemia of hookworm disease is treated as such. For removal of the worms, tetrachloroethylene is used for Necator, bephenium hydroxynaphthoate for Ancylostoma. As the eggs of these worms are indistinguishable, species diagnosis can be made most readily by examination of infective larvae obtained from fecal cultures. This is always time-consuming (7 to 10 days of incubation required) and often unreliable (technicians are rarely trained for the task). It therefore is better to assume that the worms present are Necator, and if after two or three attempts at removal with tetrachloroethylene, significant numbers of eggs are still being passed in the stools (more than 5 per mg of feces), to turn to the other drug. The dosage of tetrachloroethylene is 0.12 ml/kg (up to 4 ml total) in a single dose, after overnight fasting, without pre- or post-treatment purgation; food may be taken after 2 or 3 hours. The treatment can be repeated after 1 week. Bephenium is given in a single 5-gm dose after overnight fast. For children under 5 years the dose can be reduced to half, and for adults the 5-gm dose can be repeated later the same day.

Creeping eruption of hookworm origin can be effectively treated with thiabendazole ointment or suspension applied locally, or with tablets or suspension given orally, 25 mg/kg twice daily for 2 days, repeated after 2 days if needed.

STRONGYLOIDIASIS

ETIOLOGY. The parasitic stage of the threadworm, *Strongyloides stercoralis,* is a delicate, threadlike female, barely more than 2 mm in length, living primarily in the mucosal epithelium of the duodenum and jejunum, but at times extending forward into the pyloric stomach and downward as far as the upper colon. Eggs are laid in the mucosal epithelium; on hatching, the larvae move into the intestinal stream and are evacuated in the feces. In the evacuated feces or in warm, moist soil the larvae grow and develop rapidly, becoming infective-stage filariform larvae in one or two days. Alternatively, they may undergo one or more free-living cycles before the infective stage is produced. Reproduction in the free-living cycle is bisexual, both males and females being of a "rhabditoid" morphology, i.e., relatively short and stout and with a complex type of esophagus, whereas in the parasitic females the body is filariform and the esophagus is simple.

Infection ordinarily is acquired when the larvae reach infectivity outside the body, penetrate the skin, migrate to and through the lungs and, on reaching the intestine, enter the mucosal epithelium, mature, and produce eggs parthenogenetically. Under conditions and at frequencies not yet determined the larvae after hatching may develop to the infective stage in the intestine, penetrate the mucosa of the large intestine and migrate via the blood stream to the lungs, then return to the intestine by the trachea and esophagus, completing the cycle without leaving the body. This is referred to as internal autoinfection.

EPIDEMIOLOGY. Strongyloidiasis is relatively common in warm, moist climates, but in the Western Hemisphere it is occasionally seen as far north as Canada. Exposure results from direct contact of the skin with long-voided feces from an infected person or with contaminated soil, especially where there is a high ground-water level, as in the bayou regions of the Gulf coast of the United States. There are no known reservoir hosts of significance.

PATHOLOGY. The sites and methods of entry of Strongyloides into the skin and its migration to the intestine by way of the lungs are essentially the same as in hookworm infection. Occasionally, as these worms escape from the pulmonary capillaries, there is considerable cellular infiltration into the alveoli and bronchioles. After a brief period of essential development, the young migrate to the bronchi and trachea and move on to the intestine where they enter the mucosa and, in about 2 weeks after exposure, begin to deposit eggs. The continued burrowing of the worms, together with the infiltration of their eggs, and the hatching and escape of the larvae contribute to the trauma and frequently to the sloughing of portions of the mucosa. There is a general irritation of the involved mucosa, with secretion of excess mucus and impaired absorption.

CLINICAL MANIFESTATIONS. Reactions to the invading larvae in the skin and lungs are generally mild and are not specific. Attributable to the intestinal stages are malabsorption, abdominal pain suggestive of peptic ulcer, general abdominal discomfort and diarrhea. Eosinophilia when present usually is not remarkable. When there is internal autoinfection there may be reinvasion at the anus and a characteristic type of creeping eruption in which there are rapidly developing and rapidly disappearing progressive linear lesions radiating from the anus to the buttocks, trunk and more distant sites.

DIAGNOSIS. The infection is diagnosed by finding and identifying the larvae in the feces or in material aspirated from the duodenum (Fig. 10–70).

PROGNOSIS. The prognosis is fair to good in the recently acquired infection, provided specific treatment is adequately carried out. Patients with undiagnosed strongyloidiasis and receiving cortico-

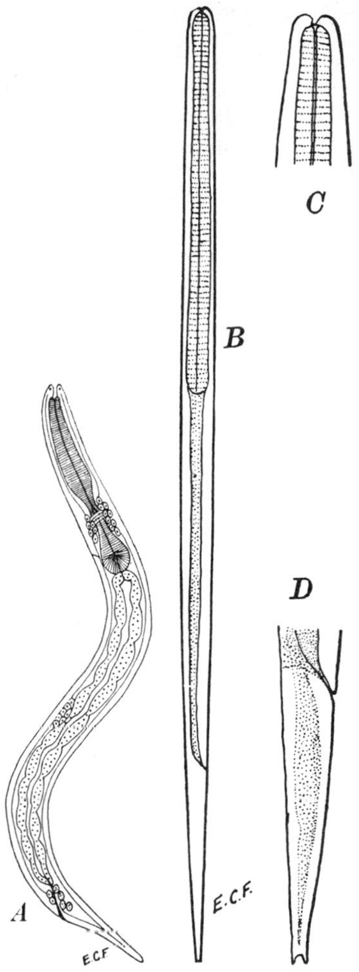

Figure 10–70 Strongyloides stercoralis. A, *Rhabditoid larva, × 310;* B, *filariform larva, × 120;* C, D, *anterior and posterior ends of filariform larva, × 640. (Faust, E. C., et al.: Clinical Parasitology. 8th ed. Philadelphia, Lea & Febiger, 1970.)*

steroid treatment for other conditions may develop an overwhelming internal autoinfection.

PREVENTION. Preventive measures consist in the sanitary disposal of human feces, treatment of infected persons and protection against contact with wet polluted soil.

TREATMENT. Thiabendazole is generally effective in doses of 25 mg/kg twice daily for 2 days. Also satisfactory is pyrvinium pamoate in a single dose of 5 mg/kg (to a maximum of 250 mg), repeated after 2 weeks.

TRICHINOSIS

ETIOLOGY. Infection with *Trichinella spiralis* involves two stages: the lodging of adult males and females in the mucosa of the upper small intestine, and liberation of their larvae into the tissues. The larvae find their way into the skeletal muscles where they grow and differentiate to an advanced stage (subadult) that becomes encapsulated during the fifth week of infection. The encapsulated larval stage in the human muscles is the same stage as that which was ingested, usually in rare pork, when the infection was acquired.

EPIDEMIOLOGY. The encapsulated larva is a long-persisting infective stage. In nature it is found primarily in rats and pigs, and in carnivorous-omnivorous mammals which feed on either. Though human infection has become increasingly uncommon in this country, it still occurs in the United States and elsewhere among people who eat rare or poorly cooked pork or, occasionally, the meat from wild boar, bear, walrus and other such animals. Outbreaks of trichinosis usually result from the sharing of the meat from a single, heavily infected, home-butchered hog.

PATHOLOGY. During the first 2 days in the intestine the young worms mature and mate. Production of the new generation of larvae begins at 5 days of infection, reaches a peak during the second week, and continues at a rapidly diminishing rate to about the fifth week. Reactions to the intestinal stages are variable and usually relatively mild. On reaching the muscles, the minute invasive larvae enter the muscle fibers, and as they grow and differentiate they destroy the occupied portion of the fiber. This and the encapsulation induced by them cause acute inflammatory reactions which collectively, when numerous, produce severe changes in the muscles. In extremely heavy infections larvae may accumulate and perish in the brain, causing many minute inflammatory lesions.

CLINICAL MANIFESTATIONS. The clinical picture which most firmly suggests infection with *T. spiralis* is seen in the second and third weeks of infection when hordes of larvae produced by worms in the intestine invade the striated muscles. Typically there are fever, muscle pain, periorbital edema and eosinophilia of the blood. Other conditions such as conjunctivitis, dyspnea and dysphagia also occur frequently, but in the absence of muscle soreness, facial edema and hypereosinophilia, they would not suggest trichinosis. Serious complications, not often seen in children, are encephalitis from larval invasion of the brain, usually during the third week, and myocarditis, which characteristically comes later. Deaths attributable to this complication usually occur after the fourth week of infection. Retrospectively, gastrointestinal signs and symptoms such as nausea, vomiting, abdominal pain and diarrhea are often associated with the earliest phase of the infection, during the first few days when the infective larvae are invading the intestinal mucosa and developing to maturity.

DIAGNOSIS. The most reliable diagnosis is that based on identification of the larvae in a muscle biopsy. As the larvae are small and lie parallel to the muscle fibers until late in the third week of infection, it is advisable to do the biopsy 3 weeks after the presumed infective meal was eaten, or later, when the larvae coil and become encapsulated and are then more readily detected. At times a remaining portion of the suspected infective meat can be found and examined for the presence of larvae. The biopsy specimen should be generous in amount and submitted to the laboratory in fresh condition, unfixed and unfrozen.

An intradermal test with Trichinella antigen can be regarded as highly reliable if it gives an immediate positive reaction after the third or fourth week of infection, especially if a test in the second week was negative. Serodiagnostic tests may be useful, especially if done in the period of increasing eosinophilia and repeated later for titer comparison. Usually the choice of test(s) (fluorescent antibody, hemagglutination, precipitin, flocculation, complement-fixation) and their interpretations will be governed by the laboratory services available. None will be entirely conclusive without substantial support from a muscle biopsy.

PROGNOSIS. Except in very heavy infections the chances of recovery are good. The fatality rate for reported cases in the United States for the 20-year period to 1968 was approximately 21 per 1000.

PREVENTION. Avoiding rare and poorly cooked pork or pork products will prevent infection. Larvae in pork are killed by deep-freezing.

TREATMENT. There is no specific therapy and, except in severe cases, treatment is merely supportive. When there is involvement of the central nervous system or heart, steroid treatment is indicated. Thiabendazole in doses of 25 mg/kg twice daily for 5 to 7 days has appeared to be beneficial in some cases.

FILARIASIS

ETIOLOGY. Filariasis is produced by any of several filarial worms, the most important being *Wuchereria bancrofti, Brugia malayi, Onchocerca volvulus* and *Loa loa*. The adult worms are threadlike objects characteristically living in certain body tissues. *Wuchereria bancrofti* and *B. malayi* inhabit lymphatic vessels and lymphoid tissues; Onchocerca adults are immured in fibrous subcutaneous nodules; *Loa loa* migrate through subcutaneous tissues. These worms all produce microscopic embryos called microfilariae, which eventually migrate through the superficial blood vessels or skin.

EPIDEMIOLOGY. *Wuchereria bancrofti* is widely distributed through the tropics in both hemispheres; *B. malayi* occurs in India, the Far East and the Southwest Pacific. Onchocerca is found in tropical Africa, in areas where Guatemala and Mexico are contiguous, in Venezuela and in one limited focus of Colombia, South America. The loa worm is found exclusively in tropical Africa.

Microfilariae are picked up by bloodsucking insects and develop to the infective-stage larvae in their thoracic muscles. *Wuchereria bancrofti* and *B. malayi* utilize mosquitoes; Onchocerca, species of black gnats (Simulium); *Loa loa*, the mango fly (Chrysops). After incubation in the appropriate insect host, the larvae migrate to the tip of the fly's proboscis and enter the victim's skin in or near the puncture wound made by the fly. In endemic areas children as well as older persons are infected.

PATHOLOGY. The developmental period in Bancroft's filariasis may be as long as a year, but is not definitely known. Indirect evidence indicates that the larvae, on entering the skin, invade lymphatic vessels and may make long migrations through the lymphatic system before they reach the sites where they mature and mate, and the females begin to produce microfilariae. During this period, if they block lymph flow, they may produce an acute lymphangitis and associated lymphadenitis. At the end of the incubation period the microfilariae discharged by the female appear in the tissues around the parent worms, and within a short time those of Wuchereria, Brugia and *Loa loa* may be found in the blood. Tissue reaction may be temporary during the migration of larvae or adults, but in Bancroft's and Malayan filariasis there is usually a series of acute episodes of lymphangitis, often with fever, and subsequently there is fibrosis of the dead or dying parent worms, resulting at times in permanent blockage of lymphatic vessels. In onchocerciasis, fibrosis around the adult worms develops without acute local reaction, but almost invariably with systemic sensitization. In Loa infection there is only temporary swelling in the subcutaneous tissues through which the worm is migrating.

CLINICAL MANIFESTATIONS. In infection with Bancroft's and Malayan filariasis the incubation period may be marked by acute lymphangitis or allergic states. A second period, usually symptomless, begins when microfilariae are first recoverable, a year or more after exposure. Most patients have repeated attacks of lymphangitis, usually with fever. With fibrotic obstruction of lymph flow, elephantiasis gradually develops and the skin becomes thickened.

Onchocerca adults produce a painless swelling on any site of the body, but particularly at the junction of the long bones and on the temporal and occipital areas of the head. Their microfilariae, especially from parent nodules in the upper part of the trunk, neck and scalp, tend to migrate to the eyeball and optic nerve, causing diminished vision and, eventually, blindness. Loa usually produces only pruritus, but at times there is generalized edema or giant urticaria.

DIAGNOSIS. Infection is suggested by the clinical manifestations, is confirmed by recovery of microfilariae in blood at night *(W. bancrofti, B. malayi)*, in the daytime *(Loa loa)* or in biopsies of skin (Onchocerca). When parent worms have died and during biologic incubation, microfilariae will be absent.

PROGNOSIS. The prognosis, usually good following treatment, depends on the degree of involvement and on the location of the lesions.

PREVENTION. This is difficult and requires control of breeding of the vector insects. DDT and other insect toxicants have provided a moderately effective means of control.

TREATMENT. For *W. bancrofti* and *B. malayi* infections diethylcarbamazine usually is satisfactory and can be used without special precautions. It is given orally, about 2 mg/kg three times daily for 2 weeks. The same treatment, but with special caution in the form of small starting dosage, is used for *Loa loa*. Even greater caution is required when treating Onchocerca infection with diethylcarbamazine. Also necessary for successful treatment of onchocerciasis is suramin, which is available in the United States only from the Parasitic Disease Drug Service, National Center for Disease Control, Atlanta, Georgia 30333. Information on its use is provided with the drug. Onchocerca nodules if present should be excised as soon as they are discovered. The adult *Loa loa* occasionally can be removed when it appears under the conjunctiva.

ERNEST CARROLL FAUST
PAUL C. BEAVER

TROPICAL EOSINOPHILIA

Eosinophilia in the absence of an evident cause suggests occult helminthic infection. Trichinosis and larval toxocariasis (visceral larva migrans) are common forms of helminthic infection in which eosinophilia may be conspicuous while the causative worms are difficult to detect. Certain helminths, such as ascaris and hookworms, whose presence in the adult stage is easily detected by finding eggs in the feces, characteristically produce transient pulmonary infiltration and eosinophilia (Löffler syndrome) during the period of larval migration through the lungs.

In tropical countries, particularly in India and some countries of southeastern Asia, there occurs, more frequently in adults than in children, a syndrome known as *tropical eosinophilia*. In addition to hypereosinophilia, the outstanding features are chronic or recurrent bronchial asthma and pulmonary infiltration (eosinophilic lung), both of which are relieved by diethylcarbamazine given orally in daily doses of 12 mg/kg in 3 divided doses for 4 days.

Tropical eosinophilia is an aberrant form of filariasis in which the mature worms produce microfilariae that are filtered out of the blood stream and destroyed in the lungs, causing small granulomas. The species involved may be *W. bancrofti, B. malayi, B. pahangi,* and probably others. The symptoms are those of bronchial asthma, and the lesions are demonstrable on roentgenograms of the lung. In visceral larva migrans caused by larval Toxocara infection, the lungs are not usually affected, and in Löffler syndrome caused by larval ascariasis, the pulmonary phase and peripheral eosinophilia are notably transient, rarely persisting at remarkable levels for more than 3 weeks.

PAUL C. BEAVER

Beaver, P. C.: Toxocariasis (visceral larva migrans) in relation to tropical eosinophilia. Bull. Soc. Pathol. Exot. *55*:555, 1962.
Beaver, P. C.: Filariasis without microfilaremia. Am. J. Trop. Med. Hyg. *19*:181, 1970.
Danaraj, T. J., Pacheco, G., Shanmugaratnam, K., and Beaver, P. C.: The etiology and pathology of eosinophilic lung (tropical eosinophilia). Am. J. Trop. Med. Hyg. *15*:183, 1966.
Gelpi, A. P., and Mustafa, A.: Seasonal pneumonitis with eosinophilia. A study of larval ascariasis in Saudi Arabia. Am. J. Trop. Med. Hyg. *16*:646, 1967.

DRACUNCULOSIS
(Guinea Worm Infection)

Dracunculosis, caused by the Guinea worm *(Dracunculus medinensis),* is prevalent in the arid and semiarid areas of India and westward through the Middle East into tropical Africa. The infection is acquired by ingesting infected copepods (small crustacea) in drinking water from pools, step-wells or ponds used also for bathing and washing. The adult worms develop slowly, the meter-long female reaching maturity in the deep layers of the skin in about 1 year. In the skin over the anterior end of the gravid worm a blister 15 to 20 mm in diameter is formed which, on sloughing, allows thousands of motile microscopic larvae to be expelled from the worm into the water during bathing or washing of the affected parts, usually the feet or legs, less commonly the genitalia or upper extremities. On reaching the water, larvae are immediately infective for copepods, and within a few days after ingestion by these microcrustacea the larvae are infective for man. Lesions produced by worms at the ankle or knee often cause crippling ankylosis.

TREATMENT. Extraction of the worm by slowly and intermittently winding it on a stick or cord and removal by surgical means, still widely practiced, were once the only forms of treatment. Drugs are now available which act directly against the developing or adult worm, or reduce inflammation and facilitate extraction of the gravid female. Diethylcarbamazine (Hetrazan), given as for filariasis, was the first such oral medication to be used against the adult worm. It was thought to be effective also as a prophylactic. More recently niridazole (Ambilhar), as given for schistosomiasis, was found to be effective against the guinea worm, as was also thiabendazole, a drug commonly used for ascariasis, strongyloidiasis and creeping eruption. Probably the most effective is metronidazole (also used for trichomoniasis and amebiasis), given orally in a dosage of 250 mg three times daily for 7 days.

The most effective preventive measure is the provision of piped clean water.

INFECTIONS PRODUCED BY TAPEWORMS (CESTODA)

Tapeworms are flatworms (Platyhelminthes); they are invertebrate animals which have either a simplified digestive tract or none at all, a protonephridial excretory system, male and female genitalia usually in the same organism (hermaphroditism), no body cavity and, primitively, a ciliated ectodermal covering. Each tapeworm consists of a group of coordinated units: (1) a scolex or "head," provided with suckers and frequently with rostellar hooklets for attachment; (2) a "neck" or region of growth; (3) a series of proglottids or segments, beginning with immature ones arising from the distal part of the neck and becoming increasingly developed and finally gravid in the distal portion of the worm. The entire worm is called a strobila. Each mature proglottid contains a full set of male and female genitalia. The gravid proglottids are filled with eggs. Tapeworms have the following stages in their life cycle: egg, embryo, larva, adult.

The important tapeworm infections of man are teniasis (including the larval-stage infection cysticercosis), hymenolepiasis, diphyllobothriasis and hydatid disease. Dog tapeworm *(Dipylidium caninum)* infection occasionally occurs in children who fondle infected dogs or cats. The epidemiologic aspects of these infections are summarized in Table 10–25.

TENIASIS

ETIOLOGY. Teniasis is produced by the beef tapeworm, *Taenia saginata,* and the pork tapeworm, *Taenia solium.* The former has a length of 15 feet or more, contains about 1000 to 2000 proglottids or "segments" and has a head with four suckers, but no rostellar hooklets. *Taenia solium* generally attains a length of between 5 and 8 feet, has less than 1000 proglottids and has an apical ring of rostellar hooklets, as well as four head suckers. The most distal proglottids are gravid and contain fully embryonated eggs which may be passed in feces, but are more commonly excreted in proglottids (Fig. 10–71) which are detached from the parent worm.

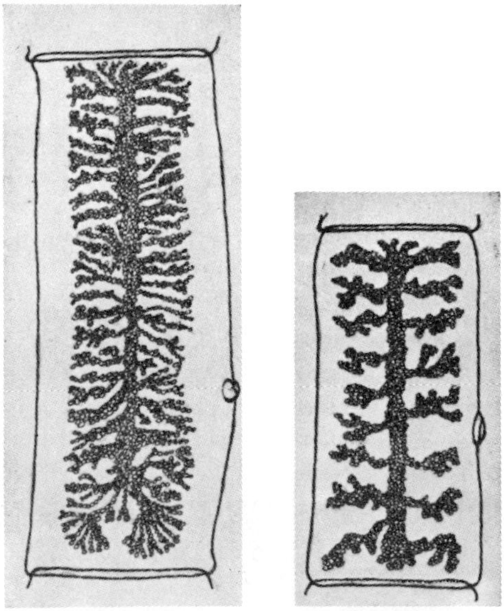

A B

Figure 10–71 Gravid proglottids of Taenia saginata *and* T. solium, *as passed in the feces or as they migrate from the anus, showing differential patterns of uteri.* A, T. saginata; B, T. solium. *(After Faust, E. C.:* In *Brennemann's Practice of Pediatrics. Courtesy of W. F. Prior Co., Hyattsville, Md.)*

EPIDEMIOLOGY. *Taenia saginata* infection is common in beef-eating peoples such as the Mohammedans and also occurs in the United States. *Taenia solium* infection occurs most often in eastern and southeastern Europe, is no longer indigenous in the United States, but is as common as *T. saginata* in Mexico and certain other Latin American countries. Gravid proglottids, discharged in human feces, disintegrate, and the contaminated soil is infective for cattle *(T. saginata)* or hogs *(T. solium).* The larval stage (cysticercus) develops in striated muscle of these animals, and the flesh becomes infective in about 3 months. Human beings who consume raw or rare beef or pork containing the cysticercus larvae are liable to infection.

PATHOLOGY. The larvae are digested out of the meat in the human stomach, become attached in the mucosa of the upper small intestine and, in about 3 months, develop into mature worms. Although there is slight inflammatory reaction at the site of attachment, the important pathogenic action is toxic and allergenic, with systemic reactions. Occasionally obstruction of the bowel may result from a tangled mass of the worm or from a free proglottid which becomes lodged in the lumen of the appendix.

CLINICAL MANIFESTATIONS. Toward the end of the incubation period there is considerable digestive disturbance, including mucous diarrhea due to the irritative action of the worm's by-products on the intestinal mucosa. There may be false hunger pains, especially at night. When the worm is mature, there may be no intestinal disturbance, but there may be other evidences, including (1) inconvenience from gravid proglottids which, having migrated from the anus, crawl down the leg; (2) nutritional drain on the patient; (3) appendiceal inflammation from detached proglottids; and possibly (4) neurotoxic symptoms.

Man is also subject to infection with the cysticercus stage of *T. solium* by swallowing eggs in contaminations from his own or another person's intestinal infection. These cysticerci lodge in any soft tissue, including the brain, the meninges and the eyeball. Involvement of the brain usually results in a jacksonian type of epilepsy.

DIAGNOSIS. Teniasis can be diagnosed by recovery of Taenia eggs in the stool or from anal swabs, but most patients do not pass eggs in appreciable numbers. Specific diagnosis can be made from a gross examination of gravid proglottids passed in the stool or migrating from the anus. When these are freed of debris and flattened in the fresh condition (not hardened in alcohol or formalin) between glass slides, it is easy to count the number of main lateral arms of the uterus. In *Taenia saginata* the number is 15 to 21; in *T. solium,* 7 to 13 (Fig. 10–71).

PROGNOSIS. This is good in intestinal teniasis if the worms are removed. Rarely, acute intestinal or appendiceal obstruction is a hazard. In cysticercosis the cerebral lesions may have serious consequences.

PREVENTION. Teniasis may be prevented by eating only previously frozen or well cooked beef and pork. More fundamental is the sanitary disposal of human feces.

TREATMENT. A drug that is generally effective in expelling all kinds of tapeworms of man is quinacrine hydrochloride (Atabrine). Failures with quinacrine usually can be attributed either to intolerance of the patient or ineffectiveness of the post-treatment purge. In emotionally unstable patients and those with a history of psychosis the drug may cause an acute psychotic reaction. In some cases quinacrine causes nausea and vomiting despite countermeasures. A newer drug, niclosamide, is now preferred for the removal of *T. saginata* and all other types of tapeworms except *T. solium.* The drug causes *T. solium* to disintegrate in the intestine, and it is considered possible that the mature eggs thus freed may be stimulated to hatch and allow the larvae to invade the intestinal wall, become disseminated in the body, and produce cysticercosis.

Quinacrine is given on an empty stomach after overnight fasting, in a single dose or in divided doses at 5- to 10-minute intervals in total amounts of 500 mg for children under 6 years to 800 mg for older children and adults, preceded 30 minutes earlier by an antiemetic. One hour later a strong castor oil or (for adults) saline purgative is given to expel the worm. Food may be taken as desired any time after the purge has been effective. At times the quinacrine itself acts as a purge and the worm, deeply stained and alive, will be evacuated within 1 or 2 hours.

Niclosamide is given in a single oral dose of 4 tablets of 500 mg each (2 gm total) chewed well and taken with a light meal. Children under 6 years take two tablets (1 gm). Purgation is not required. In the United States, niclosamide is available from the Parasitic Disease Drug Service, Center for Disease Control, Atlanta, GA 30333.

HYMENOLEPIASIS

ETIOLOGY. Hymenolepiasis is produced by the dwarf tapeworm, *Hymenolepis nana,* and the rat tapeworm, *H. diminuta.* The former is a small worm, only 1 to 2 cm in length. Its head is provided with four suckers and a crown of rostellar hooklets. *Hymenolepis diminuta* is considerably larger (20 to 60 cm in length) and has suckers but no hooklets on the head. The most distal gravid proglottids disintegrate as they become fully ripe, setting the characteristic eggs (Figs. 10–63, *D*; 10–72) free in the small bowel to be evacuated in the feces.

EPIDEMIOLOGY. The dwarf tapeworm, *H. nana,* is cosmopolitan in distribution, except in cold climates. It is most commonly a parasite of children. Although this species is found in rats and mice, the strains are thought to be distinct and not infective for man. Human infection with *H. diminuta* results from accidental ingestion of an insect that had earlier eaten the feces of an infected rat. *Hymenolepis nana* infections are common in children in the southern United States, in many countries of Latin America, India and in the Mediterranean area. *Hymenolepis diminuta* infections have been recorded from several countries, including the United States.

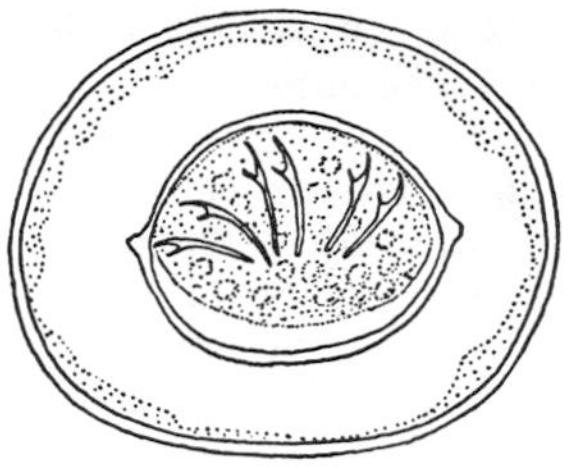

Figure 10–72 Egg of Hymenolepis diminuta. *(× 500.) (Faust, E. C., et al.: Clinical Parasitology. 8th ed. Philadelphia, Lea & Febiger, 1970.)*

Eggs of *H. nana* passed in human feces are directly infective for man. They hatch soon after ingestion. On reaching the duodenum the escaping embryos bore into the villi, transform into larvae, return to the intestinal lumen, become attached, and grow into adults within a few weeks. Eggs of *H. diminuta* must undergo larval development in certain insects, usually rat fleas. Ingestion of these intermediate hosts is the source of infection for human beings.

PATHOLOGY. Except in heavy infections, the damage produced is largely local. There is suggestive evidence that in continued heavy infections with *H. nana,* internal autoinfection occurs repeatedly, causing extensive damage to the intestinal mucosa.

CLINICAL MANIFESTATIONS. There may or may not be clinical evidence of infection. Light to moderate infections usually are asymptomatic. In heavy infections with internal autoinfection there are gastrointestinal and allergic manifestations.

DIAGNOSIS. This is made by demonstration of eggs in the feces (Figs. 10–63, *D*; 10–72).

PROGNOSIS. This is almost always good, provided specific medication is instituted.

PREVENTION. Dwarf tapeworm infection can be controlled by personal and group hygiene and by treatment of infected persons. Rat tapeworm infection may be eliminated as a human infection by campaigns against rats.

TREATMENT. For the removal of either *H. nana* or *H. diminuta,* niclosamide is given as for other tapeworms, except that treatment is repeated daily for 5 days. The daily dose is 500 mg for children under 2 years, 1 gm for ages 2 to 8, and 2 gm for older children and adults.

DIPHYLLOBOTHRIASIS

ETIOLOGY. Diphyllobothriasis is produced by the fish tapeworm, *Diphyllobothrium latum,* which measures up to 30 feet in length and has possibly as many as 3000 proglottids. The head is spatulate and is provided with a pair of longitudinal sucking grooves, one dorsal and one ventral in position.

The proglottids never become strictly gravid, but discharge immature eggs.

EPIDEMIOLOGY. Fish tapeworm infection is prevalent in the lake districts of Minnesota and northern Michigan, adjacent territory in Canada and in the lake districts of Chile and Argentina, northern, eastern and southeastern Europe, U.S.S.R. including Siberia, Palestine, Syria, Japan and Australia. Elsewhere it is rarely endemic. Gefüllte fish may be a source of infection if it is eaten before it has been cooked. The immature eggs passed in feces are broadly ovoidal and operculate (Fig. 10–63, *C*). When discharged into cold fresh water, they must incubate for about 2 weeks, whereupon the shell opens to release a ciliated embryo. This swimming organism is eaten by little "water fleas" of the genera Diaptomus and Cyclops, in the bodies of which the embryos transform into procercoid (first-stage) larvae. Small fresh-water fish consume the infected water fleas and acquire infection in their flesh, the plerocercoid or sparganum (second-stage) larvae. Larger fish, in turn, consume the smaller ones and acquire the infection in their muscular tissues. Man, dogs or bears eat the fish in a raw or inadequately processed condition and become infected.

PATHOLOGY. Fish tapeworm infection frequently produces a toxic state, possibly due to absorption of unsaturated fatty acids, particularly if the worms are attached to the duodenal mucosa, where they prevent absorption of vitamin B_{12}.

CLINICAL MANIFESTATIONS. In addition to the usual symptoms, fish tapeworm may be associated with a primary anemia. It is believed that the tapeworm, when attached to the duodenal or jejunal mucosa, precipitates an anemic state in persons having an unstable equilibrium with respect to the antianemic intrinsic factor.

DIAGNOSIS. This is made on recovery of the eggs (Fig. 10–63, *C*) in the patient's feces.

PROGNOSIS. This is good with specific treatment.

PREVENTION. Thorough cooking of all fresh-water fish prevents infection.

TREATMENT. See Teniasis, above.

HYDATID DISEASE
(Echinococcosis)

ETIOLOGY. Hydatid disease is produced by the larval stage (hydatid cyst) of *Echinococcus granulosus* and *E. multilocularis,* minute worms which live as adults in the small intestine of the dog and its wild relatives. A third species of Echinococcus, *E. oligarthrus,* has recently been reported to cause human infection in Panama and Colombia; wild cats are the usual definitive hosts.

EPIDEMIOLOGY. *Echinococcus granulosus* is widely distributed wherever sheep, cattle and hogs are associated with dogs. It is particularly common in man in Australia, New Zealand, Palestine, Syria, Argentina, Uruguay, southern Brazil and Chile. Occasionally autochthonous cases occur in the United States. *Echinococcus multilocularis* is common in the highlands of Central Europe, where foxes replace dogs and wood mice replace sheep, cattle and hogs in the natural evolution of the infection (see below). This cycle also occurs in northern Alaska, Siberia and on a small adjacent island of Japan.

The eggs of *E. granulosus* passed in an infected dog's feces initiate the infection in practically any mammal (except a rodent) which ingests the eggs. These hatch in the duodenum; the escaping embryos bore into the intestinal wall, gain access to mesenteric venules or lymphatics and are carried to various parts of the body where they are filtered out. Dogs become infected from eating the carcasses of animals which have died of the disease. Man's association with infected sheep and cattle dogs and parasitized pet dogs provides the means for exposure to the disease.

PATHOLOGY. Unless the young larvae lodge in some vital location in the human body, they will usually develop to a considerable size before their presence is discovered. Thus, infection acquired in childhood may not be detected until middle life. The little hydatid cyst provokes an acute inflammatory reaction at the site of implantation; nonetheless, it proceeds to vacuolate, to develop its germinative layer with many viable heads (scolices) and to accumulate fluid within the cavity. The cysts grow slowly, but in several years may reach the size of a grapefruit or larger. The outer layer is essentially a noncellular laminated structure which is friable; the entire cyst is surrounded by adventitia. The fluid of the *E. granulosus* cyst contains considerable foreign protein and is extremely toxic for the host if there is appreciable leakage. Rupture of a cyst may cause anaphylactic shock or may only set free a large number of viable scolices which become implanted elsewhere and develop secondary cysts. If the cyst reaches the shafts of long bones, it may proceed to grow as a syncytium (osseous hydatid). The most common sites of hydatid cysts in man are, in descending order, the liver, lungs, brain, peritoneal cavity and bone, but no tissues are exempt. The hydatid of *E. multilocularis* is alveolar and has no circumscribing membrane or adventitia. It almost invariably develops in the liver and is essentially malignant in its growth.

CLINICAL MANIFESTATIONS. If the larvae of *E. granulosus* lodge on a heart valve or in the brain or eye, the lesion causes grave symptoms relatively early in the infection. If it develops in the lungs, the first evidence may be a violent paroxysm of coughing with discharge of the contents of a ruptured cyst. If a unilocular cyst is hepatic in location, 20 or more years may pass before the weight of the mass causes sufficient discomfort to bring the patient to a physician. However, a blow on the abdomen may rupture the cyst and cause death from anaphylactic shock. The hydatid of *E. multilocularis* produces symptoms of hepatic disease.

DIAGNOSIS. This is difficult before operation. Eosinophilia is suggestive, but depends on leakage from the cyst. Hydatid thrill is suggestive, but difficult to elicit. Serologic tests are the most reliable. These include complement fixation, bentonite flocculation, indirect hemagglutination and intradermal tests with antigen prepared from sterile hydatid fluid, which is usually obtained from infected sheep.

PROGNOSIS. The prognosis of a unilocular cyst is fair if it is in an operable site. Recurrence resulting from the spilling of scolices from the parent cyst at the time of operation is difficult to avoid. Osseous hydatid disease is serious, and surgical intervention is rarely helpful. In alveolar hydatid disease the prognosis is always grave because the lesion is uncircumscribed.

PREVENTION. Control in endemic areas involves the deep burying of dead sheep, hogs and cattle. Periodic deworming of dogs greatly reduces the amount of exposure to eggs. Man must be careful to keep dog feces from contaminating his food, drink or cooking utensils. Children should not be allowed to play with dogs which have access to sheep in endemic areas.

TREATMENT. No chemotherapy is available for treating the larval stage of the hydatid infections which occur in man. If the cyst is unilocular and in a favorable location for operation, an incision is made down to the outer cyst wall and the hydatid fluid is aspirated, with precaution against spillage in the operative area. Then the cyst wall is incised and enough 10 per cent formaldehyde is introduced into the cavity to sterilize the germinative layer. If possible, the entire cyst should be enucleated; if this is not feasible, the cyst should be collapsed and closed with sutures separately from closure of the operative wound.

INFECTIONS PRODUCED BY FLUKES (TREMATODES)

Flukes belong to a group of flatworms (Platyhelminthes) that have an incomplete digestive tract and are either unisexual or hermaphroditic. The flukes which parasitize man have a complicated life cycle, with required stages of multiplication in certain species of snails. Some flukes require a second intermediate host in which encystation occurs. The most important fluke infections are the schistosomiases, due to blood flukes. Other types of flukes live in the intestine, liver and lungs. (See Table 10–25).

SCHISTOSOMIASIS
(Blood Fluke Infections)

Schistosomiasis in man is produced by three species of blood flukes, two of which *(Schistosoma mansoni* and *S. japonicum)* inhabit the veins draining the intestines and one of which *(S. haematobium)* lives in the veins of the urinary bladder. A slender female worm embraced by a larger and much stouter male lives in the small vessels in or on the wall of the organ, and eggs deposited in the submucosal vessels lodge there; as develop-

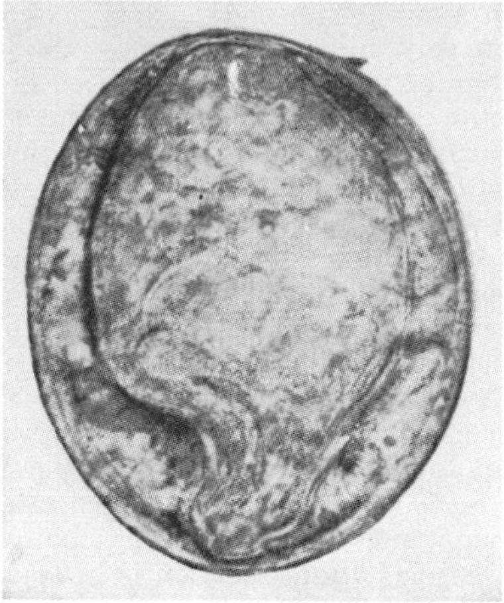

Figure 10–73 Egg of Schistosoma japonicum *as seen in freshly passed feces. (×660.) (After Faust, E. C.:* In *Brennemann's Practice of Pediatrics. Courtesy of W. F. Prior Co., Hyattsville, Md.)*

ment of the contained embryo progresses toward a ciliated larva, the miracidium, the egg gradually moves through the tissues to the mucosal surface and into the lumen. On reaching fresh water in the feces or urine, the miracidium hatches and enters the tissues of an appropriate snail which serves as an intermediate host for development and reproduction of two generations of asexual stages. Finally emerging from the snail are hordes of minute, free-swimming, fork-tailed larvae (cercariae) which on contact with the skin of man or certain other mammals grasp the surface and within moments penetrate to the deeper tissues; then via the blood and lymph vessels they move on to the lungs. After essential growth and development in the pulmonary tissues the young flukes move on to the liver (apparently via the pulmonary arterial and the hepatic vessels), where they reach maturity, mate and move to the intestinal or vesicular vessels to deposit eggs and repeat the cycle. The eggs are relatively large, and for each species the size and shape are distinctive (Figs. 10–63 *E, F* and 10–73).

EPIDEMIOLOGY. Blood fluke infections have an extensive distribution and involve millions of people in endemic territory. *Schistosoma japonicum* occurs in the Orient, especially in central, west and south China, in the Philippines and in certain foci of Japan, Thailand, Laos and Celebes; *S. mansoni,* in Africa, Arabia, Puerto Rico, some of the Lesser Antilles, extensive areas of Brazil, coastal Surinam and foci in central north Venezuela; *S. haematobium,* in Africa, the Near East, Iran, Iraq, western India and the southern tip of Portugal. Children are frequently exposed to infection at an early age.

PATHOLOGY. The approximate prepatent period, during which the larval worms develop to maturity, mate and produce eggs which appear in the feces or urine, is 4 to 5 weeks for *S. japonicum,* 6 to 7 weeks for *S. mansoni* and 10 to 12 weeks for *S. haematobium.* Until eggs begin to pass through and accumulate in the tissues, the infection causes only relatively minor, nonspecific tissue changes. In heavy infections eggs are produced in massive numbers and the walls of the intestine or bladder become heavily infiltrated with and thickened by inflammatory reactions which form granulomas around the eggs individually or in clumps. As the wall becomes progressively more reactive to the eggs and increasing numbers of the mucosal vessels become involved, there is a proportionate increase in the numbers of eggs that are deposited in the larger vessels and carried in the blood stream to the liver. Here, as elsewhere, the eggs cause a granulomatous reaction; since all persist until they die and are resorbed, the destruction of liver parenchyma and the inflammatory changes in the hepatic vessels, when infection is heavy, are proportionately great and lead eventually to extensive cirrhosis of the liver and obstructive circulatory changes, with hepatosplenomegaly and ascites (Fig. 10–63, *G*).

As in helminthic infections in general, light infections with the schistosomes are well tolerated and the pathologic changes and associated symptoms range from the imperceptible and trivial to the conspicuous and fatal.

CLINICAL MANIFESTATIONS. At each site of invasion of the skin by the cercariae there is a minute lesion, with sharp needling pain which lasts only a few hours. As the larval worms pass through the lungs and later lodge elsewhere, there is considerable local and generalized reaction, particularly in the liver, which becomes greatly enlarged and tender, and hypereosinophilia and giant urticaria may develop. Toward the end of the incubation period there are late afternoon fever and night sweats. In the intestinal types there is a prodromal toxic diarrhea. Then, with the discharge of eggs, there is dysentery *(S. japonicum, S. mansoni)* or hematuria *(S. haematobium)*. The patient may become very ill and, in the intestinal types, bedridden. After a few weeks of rest the dysentery is arrested, but on physical exertion is reactivated. Digestive disturbances are increased as fibrosis of the intestinal wall develops and papillomas and cicatricial tissue prevent the normal passage of food or feces. There is periportal hepatic cirrhosis, the spleen becomes greatly enlarged, and the thoracic cavity is reduced in capacity by the increase in size of the abdominal viscera. In the vesical type the urinary bladder gradually becomes thickened and fibrosed; as masses of eggs become calcified in the wall, the inner surface assumes a granular appearance and stones may form in the bladder lumen. In the intestinal types, ascites develops in the chronic stage, which occurs relatively early in the Oriental type. In the vesical type there is incontinence of urine. In both intestinal varieties of schistosomiasis, sepsis may be anticipated in the chronic stage, and carcinoma of the liver, intestinal wall or urinary bladder may develop as a result of constant irritation.

During the acute stage there is pronounced eosinophilia. Later there is a neutropenia, with a moderate eosinophilia and monocytosis.

DIAGNOSIS. This is made by recovery of the typical eggs in the stool (*S. japonicum,* Fig. 10–73; *S. mansoni,* Fig. 10–63, *E*) or in the urine (*S. haematobium,* Fig. 10–63, *F*).

PROGNOSIS. This is fair to excellent in the acute or early chronic stage with specific therapy, but is poor in longstanding or inadequately treated chronic infections. In highly endemic areas of China and the Philippines, children who are subjected to heavy exposure may die of the disease before reaching maturity.

PREVENTION. The use of the molluscicide sodium pentachlorophenate (Santobrite) to kill the snails which are intermediate hosts and prohibition of wading or bathing in suspected water are temporary and relatively inadequate measures. Permanent control can be effected by health education, along with the curbing of ditches and sanitary disposal of excreta. In endemic areas of *S. japonicum* infection the control problem is complicated by many mammalian reservoir hosts which can perpetuate the disease in the absence of human infection.

TREATMENT. Sodium antimony tartrate and potassium antimony tartrate (tartar emetic) are the drugs most likely to be effective in a single course of treatment. Tartar emetic, most effective against *S. japonicum,* is given intravenously in a 0.5 per cent solution slowly, on alternate days, in increasing amounts; 8 ml is the first dose, followed by 12, 16, 20, and 24 ml, respectively, in the next four doses, and then 28 ml each in 10 additional doses, the total dosage for adults being 360 ml (containing 0.648 gm antimony), with proportional reductions for children. The drug is toxic, causing cough, nausea, vomiting and hypotensive reactions, and may produce hepatic and cardiac damage. It can be used with relative safety only in patients with early infection, without marked signs of hepatic or cardiac disease.

Among the drugs that are effective against *S. mansoni*, the one commercially available in the United States is stibophen (Fuadin), a trivalent antimonial. Stibophen is given intramuscularly in a solution containing 8.5 mg/ml; the dosage for adults and children 9 years of age or older is 4 ml daily five times per week to a total of 80 to 100 ml. Antimony sodium dimercaptosuccinate (Astiban), somewhat less toxic and easier to administer, is used against *S. mansoni* where available, the adult dose being 40 mg/kg total, in five divided doses given intramuscularly once or twice per week. A promising new drug, considered to be less toxic and more effective than the antimonials, is niridazole (Ambilhar); it has the added advantage of being given orally. The dosage is 25 mg/kg daily for 7 days.

For *S. haematobium* infection any of the above drugs is effective, but, where available, niridazole currently is the drug of choice, especially for children. The dosage for children is 25 mg/kg daily for

7 days (as for adults), or 12.5 mg/kg twice daily for 7 days. As children tolerate the drug better than do most adults, daily dosages up to 40 mg/kg are sometimes recommended.

Cercarial (Schistosome) Dermatitis

Cercarial dermatitis, or swimmer's itch, is caused by penetration of cercariae of blood flukes which are not able to complete their development in the human body. These are usually blood flukes of aquatic birds, occasionally of passerine birds or of domestic mammals. "Cercarial dermatitis" is widely distributed throughout the world, including the lake districts of northern United States and both fresh- and salt-water areas along the east and west coasts. These cercariae on entry into the epidermis do not move immediately into the deeper tissues, and their presence causes a pruritic dermatitis (Fig. 10–74). Children are highly susceptible.

INTESTINAL FLUKE INFECTIONS
(Intestinal Trematodiasis)

Intestinal flukes are uncommon in children except in China and Southeast Asia, where a large species, *Fasciolopsis buski,* may be acquired by eating aquatic plants, and in the Far East, parts of India, Egypt and the Balkans, where several minute species of heterophyids are acquired by eating fresh- or brackish-water fish. The infections rarely cause serious disturbances except in isolated localities where extremely heavy infections are acquired. Diagnosis is made by detecting and identifying the characteristic eggs in the feces. Tetrachloroethylene, as administered for hookworm infection, can be used for the removal of intestinal flukes.

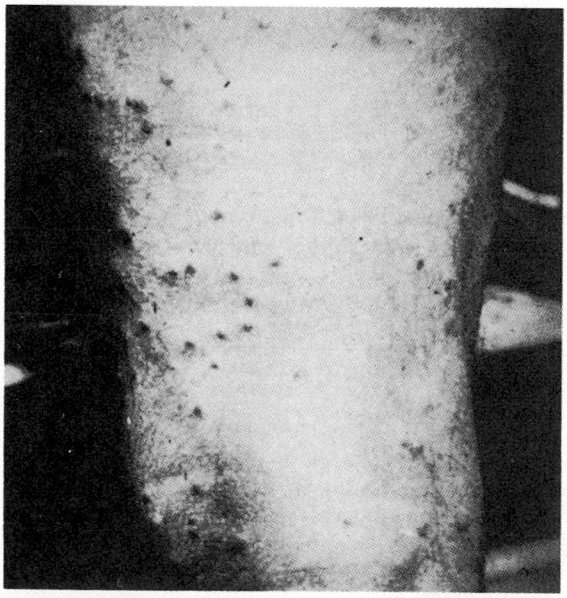

Figure 10–74 Papular eruption of leg in cercarial dermatitis (swimmer's itch) acquired in a Michigan lake. (After D. B. McMullen, Army Medical Graduate School. In Hunter, G. W., III, Frye, W. F., and Swartzwelder, J. C.: Manual of Tropical Medicine. 4th ed. 1966.)

LIVER FLUKE INFECTIONS
(Hepatic Trematodiasis)

Two kinds of flukes may be found in the human liver: (1) a large form, *Fasciola hepatica,* which is the common liver fluke of sheep and is acquired by eating aquatic plants such as watercress; and (2) smaller forms represented by the Chinese liver fluke, *Clonorchis sinensis,* and two closely related species, *Opisthorchis felineus* and *O. viverrini,* both of which are common in cats. All three of the small forms are acquired by eating raw fish. *Fasciola* lives mainly in the large proximal bile ducts, whereas the smaller species inhabit the smaller bile passages. The eggs of *Fasciola* are large (140 by 75 μ) with regular contours; those of the smaller species are relatively minute (approximately 30 by 15 μ) and with a seated operculum at one end and a small knob at the other.

Fasciola is widely distributed in sheep-raising areas. The eggs require development in water before hatching and the intermediate snail hosts are pulmonate species which are adapted to living in small lakes and ponds or slow-flowing streams and ditches. Cercariae emerging from infected snails encyst on vegetation, and when eaten by man, sheep or other herbivorous mammals they migrate through the intestinal wall to the liver, penetrate the capsule, and after development in the parenchymal tissue move into the bile ducts and begin to lay eggs 3 to 4 months after exposure.

Clonorchis and Opisthorchis eggs are infective when shed in host feces, and the snail intermediate hosts are infected by ingesting the egg along with food elements in the ooze of the stream bottom. Cercariae emerging from the snail penetrate and encyst in the tissues of fish. Infection is acquired when the infected fish is eaten uncooked, and eggs appear in the feces in about 1 month and continue to be passed for many years.

Liver flukes cause dilatation and hypertrophy of the bile ducts. In heavy infections there are biliary and circulatory obstruction and associated symptoms. In the early acute phase of symptomatic cases, hypereosinophilia is often marked. Diagnosis is made by finding characteristic eggs in the feces or bile. For removing *Fasciola* emetine hydrochloride is effective in a dosage of 1.0 mg/kg/day intramuscularly for 10 days. For Clonorchis and Opisthorchis there is no readily available satisfactory drug. Bithionol, and information about its use, is available through the USPHS, Center for Disease Control, Atlanta, Georgia 30333.

LUNG FLUKE INFECTION
(Pulmonary Trematodiasis; Paragonimiasis)

The list of worms which may be found in the lungs of children includes a number of zoonotic and ectopic nematodes such as the true lung worms of rats and pigs (*Angiostrongylus* and *Metastron-*

gylus), the heartworm of dogs (*Dirofilaria immitis*) and the large intestinal roundworm (*Ascaris*), which occasionally finds its way into the lungs. The larval form of the tapeworm *Echinococcus* (hydatid) also occurs in the lung, as well as in the liver and elsewhere. The only natural worm-parasite of man whose normal habitat is the lung is the lung fluke, *Paragonimus westermani* which also occurs in cats, dogs and some other animals. This worm is widely distributed in Japan, the Philippines, Korea, China and elsewhere in the Orient. When *P. westermani* has been occasionally reported from other regions, the diagnosis has been erroneous. In West Africa, Central and South America and throughout much of Asia there are zoonotic species of *Paragonimus* which may infect man. Infection is acquired by eating raw crab or crayfish, and eggs appear in the sputum and feces 1½ to 3 months after exposure. Infection may persist up to 20 years.

The worms, up to 13 mm long by 8 mm wide, are encapsulated singly or in pairs in the lung tissue, with a communicating channel between the capsule and a bronchiole or bronchus for the flow of eggs. The eggs are broadly ovoidal, approximately 90 by 55 μ, and have a relatively flat operculum and a distinctly amber color. When numerous in the sputum, the eggs are visible grossly as brownish streaks and flecks which may be mistaken for blood. Light infection is well tolerated.

The drug of choice for paragonimiasis is bithionol administered as for clonorchiasis and other small liver fluke infections.

ERNEST CARROLL FAUST
PAUL C. BEAVER

GENERAL

Anonymous: The Medical Letter on Drugs and Therapeutics: Handbook of Antimicrobial Therapy. Revised ed. 1974.

Faust, E. C., Beaver, P. C., and Jung, R. C.: Animal Agents and Vectors of Human Disease. 4th ed. Philadelphia, Lea & Febiger, 1974.

Faust, E. C., Russell, P. F., and Jung, R. C.: Craig and Faust's Clinical Parasitology. 8th ed. Philadelphia, Lea & Febiger, 1970.

Markell, E. K., and Voge, M.: Medical Parasitology. 3rd ed. Philadelphia, W. B. Saunders Company, 1971.

Marsden, P. D., and Schultz, M. G.: Intestinal parasites. Gastroenterology *57*:724, 1969.

Most, H.: Treatment of common parasitic infections of man encountered in the United States. *New Engl. J. Med. 287*:495; 698, 1972.

Neva, F. A.: Parasitic diseases of the GI tract in the United States. Disease-a-Month, June, 1972.

Nematodes

Antani, J. A., Srinivas, H. V., Krishnamurthy, K. R., and Borgaonkar, A. N.: Metronidazole in dracunculiasis. Report of further trials. Am. J. Trop. Med. Hyg. *21*:919, 1972.

Beaver, P. C.: The Detection and identification of some of the common nematode parasites of man. Am. J. Clin. Path. *22*:481, 1952.

Beaver, P. C.: The nature of visceral larva migrans. J. Parasit. *55*:3, 1970.

Beaver, P. C., and Danaraj, T. J.: Pulmonary ascariasis resembling eosinophilic lung. Am. J. Trop. Med. Hyg. *8*:100, 1958.

Beaver, P. C., and Orihel, T. C.: Human infection with filariae of animals in the United States. Am. J. Trop. Med. Hyg. *14*:1010, 1965.

Bird, A. C., Smith, J. L., and Curtin, V. T.: Nematode optic neuritis. Am. J. Ophthal. *69*:72, 1970.

Botero, D., and Castano, A.: Comparative study of pyrantel pamoate, bephenium hydroxynaphthoate, and tetrachloroethylene in the treatment of *Necator americanus* infections. Am. J. Trop. Med. Hyg. *22*:45, 1973.

Brown, D. H.: Ocular *Toxocara canis*. Part II. Clinical review. J. Pediatr. Ophthalmol. *7*:182, 1970.

Clark, P. S., Brownsberger, K. M., Saslow, A. R., Kagan, I. G., Noble, G. R., and Maynard, J. E.: Bear meat trichinosis. Epidemiologic, serologic, and clinical observations from two Alaskan outbreaks. Ann. Intern. Med. *76*:951, 1972.

Duke, B. O. L.: Onchocerciasis. Brit. Med. Bull. *28*:66, 1972.

Edeson, J. F. B.: Filariasis. Brit. Med. Bull. *28*:60, 1972.

Gelpi, A. P., and Mustafa, A.: Seasonal pneumonitis with eosinophilia. A study of larval ascariasis in Saudi Arabia. Am. J. Trop. Med. Hyg. *16*:646, 1967.

Gelpi, A. P., and Mustafa, A.: Ascaris pneumonia. Am. J. Med. *44*:377, 1968.

Hall, W. J., and McCabe, W. R.: Trichinosis. Report of a small outbreak with observations of thiabendazole therapy. Arch. Intern. Med. *119*:65, 1967.

Jones, C. A.: Clinical studies in human strongyloidiasis. I. Semeiology. Gastroenterology *16*:743, 1950.

Jung, R. C., and Beaver, P. C.: Clinical observations on *Trichocephalus trichiurus* (whipworm) infestation in children. Pediatrics *8*:548, 1952.

Lampkin, B. C., and Mauer, A. M.: Clinical manifestations of visceral larva migrans. Variability as related to duration of ingestion. Clin. Pediatr. *9*:683, 1970.

Marshall, C. L., and Yasukawa, K.: Control of bancroftian filariasis in the Ryukyu Islands: Preliminary results of mass administration of diethylcarbamazine. Am. J. Trop. Med. Hyg. *15*:934, 1966.

Martin, L. K.: Hookworm in Georgia. I. Survey of intestinal helminth infections and anemia in rural school children. Am. J. Trop. Med. Hyg. *21*:919, 1972.

Martin, L. K.: Hookworm in Georgia. II. Survey of intestinal helminth infections in members of rural households of southeastern Georgia. Am. J. Trop. Med. Hyg. *21*:930, 1972.

Most, H.: Trichinellosis in the United States. J.A.M.A. *193*:871, 1965.

Nelson, J. D., McConnell, T. H., and Moore, D. V.: Thiabendazole therapy of visceral larva migrans: A case report. Am. J. Trop. Med. Hyg. *15*:930, 1966.

Padonu, K. O.: A controlled trial of metronidazole in the treatment of dracontiasis in Nigeria. Am. J. Trop. Med. Hyg. *22*:42, 1973.

Pena Chavarria, A., Swartzwelder, J. C., Villarejos, V. M., and Zeledon, R.: Mebendazole, an effective broad-spectrum anthelmintic. Am. J. Trop. Med. Hyg. *22*:592, 1973.

Piggott, J., Hansbarger, E. A., Jr., and Neafie, R. C.: Human ascariasis. Am. J. Clin. Path. *53*:223, 1970.

Schmitt, N., Bowmer, E. J., Simon, P. C., Arneil, A. S., and Clark, D. A.: Trichinosis from bear meat and adulterated pork products: A major outbreak in British Columbia, 1972. Canad. Med. Ass. J. *107*:1087, 1972.

Smith, P. H., and Greer, C. H.: Unusual presentation of ocular toxocara infestation. Brit. J. Ophthalmol. *55*:317, 1971.

Stone, O. J., and Mullins, J. F.: First use of thiabendazole in creeping eruption. Texas Rep. Biol. Med. *21*:422, 1963.

Swartzwelder, J. C., Miller, J. H., and Sappenfield, R. W.: The treatment of cases of ascariasis with piperazine citrate. With observations of the effect of the drug on other helminthiases. Am. J. Trop. Med. Hyg. *20*:842, 1971.

Villarejos, V. M., Arguedas-Gamboa, J. A., Eduarte, E., and Swartzwelder, J. C.: Experiences with the anthelmintic pyrantel pamoate. Am. J. Trop. Med. Hyg. *20*:842, 1971.

Waller, C. E., and Othersen, H. B., Jr.: Ascariasis: Surgical complications in children. Am. J. Surg. *120*:50, 1970.

Wilkinson, C. P., and Welch, R. B.: Intraocular toxocara. Am. J. Ophthalmol. *71*:921, 1971.

Cestodes

Anderson, O. W.: *Dipylidium caninum* infestation. Am. J. Dis. Child. *116*:328, 1968.

von Bonsdorff, B.: *Diphyllobothrium latum* as a cause of pernicious anemia. Exp. Parasitol. *5*:207, 1956.

Botero, R. D.: Paromomycin as effective treatment of *Taenia* infections. Am. J. Trop. Med. Hyg. *19*:234, 1970.

Edelman, M. H., Spingarn, C. L., Nauenberg, W. G., and Gregory, C.: *Hymenolepis diminuta* (rat tapeworm) infection in man. Am. J. Med. *38*:951, 1965.
Moore, D. V., and Connell, F. H.: Additional records of *Dipylidium caninum* infections in children in the United States with observations on treatment. Am. J. Trop. Med. Hyg. *9*:604, 1960.
Most, H., Yoeli, M., Hammond, J., and Scheinesson, G. P.: Yomesan (niclosamide) therapy of *Hymenolepis nana* infections. Am. J. Trop. Med. Hyg. *20*:206, 1971.
Rausch, R. L., and Bernstein, J. J.: *Echinococcus vogeli* sp. n. (Cestoda: taeniidae) from the bush dog, *Speothos venaticus* (Lund). Z. Tropenmed. Parasitol. *23*:25, 1972.
Rausch, R. L., and Wilson, J. F.: Rearing of the adult *Echinococcus multilocularis* Leuckart, 1863, from sterile larvae from man. Am. J. Trop. Med. Hyg. *22*: 1973.
Schultz, M. G., Hermos, J. A., and Steele, J. H.: Epidemiology of beef tapeworm infection in the United States. Pub. Hlth. Rep. *85*:169, 1970.
Swartzwelder, J. C., Beaver, P. C., and Hood, M. W.: Sparganosis in southern United States. Am. J. Trop. Med. Hyg. *13*:43, 1964.
Verster, A.: Redescription of *Taenia solium* Linnaeus, 1758 and *Taenia saginata* Goeze, 1782. Z. Parasitenk. *29*:313, 1967.
Williams, J. F., Lopez Adaros, H., and Trejos, A.: Current prevalence and distribution of hydatidosis with special reference to the Americas. Am. J. Trop. Med. Hyg. *20*:224, 1971.
Wittner, M., and Tanowitz, H.: Paromomycin therapy of human cestodiasis with special reference to hymenolepiasis. Am. J. Trop. Med. Hyg. *20*:433, 1971.

Trematodes

Doby, J. M., and Beaucournu, J. C.: A propos des formes erratiques et abortives de deux parasitoses non exceptionelles chez l'homme (distomatose par *Fasciola* et hypodermose). Difficultés du diagnostic clinique différentiel. Bull. Soc. Pathol. Exot. *63*:227, 1970.
Hardman, E. W., Jones, R.L.H., and Davies, A. H.: Fascioliasis—A large outbreak. Brit. Med. J. *3*:502, 1970.
Jordan, P.: Epidemiology and control of schistosomiasis. Brit. Med. Bull. *28*:55, 1972.
Most, H., and others: Schistosomiasis japonica in American military personnel: Clinical studies of 600 cases during the first year after infection. Am. J. Trop. Med. *30*:239, 1950.
Sadun, E. H.: Studies on *Opisthorchis viverrini* in Thailand. Am. J. Hyg. *62*:81, 1955.
Sadun, E. H., and Maiphoon, C.: Studies on the epidemiology of the human intestinal fluke, *Fasciolopsis buski* (Lankester) in central Thailand. Am. J. Trop. Med. Hyg. *2*:1070, 1953.
World Health Organization: WHO Expert Committee on Bilharziasis. Third Report. WHO Tech. Rep. Ser. No. 299, 1965.
World Health Organization: Chemotherapy of Bilharziasis. Report of a WHO Scientific Group. WHO Tech. Rep. Ser. No. 317, 1966.
Wykoff, D. E., Chittayasothorn, K., and Winn, M. M.: Clinical manifestations of *Opisthorchis viverrini* infections in Thailand. Am. J. Trop. Med. Hyg. *15*:914–918, 1966.
Yokogawa, M., and others: Chemotherapy of paragonimiasis with bithionol: V. Studies on the minimum effective dose and changes in abnormal x-ray shadows in the chest after treatment. Am. J. Trop. Med. Hyg. *12*:859, 1963.
Yokogawa, S., Cort, W. W., and Yokogawa, M.: *Paragonimus* and paragonimiasis. Exp. Parasitol. *10*:81; 139, 1960.

Arthropods

The role of arthropods (i.e., insects and their allies) in the production of disease is fourfold: (1) certain arthropods elaborate venoms which they introduce into the human body; (2) some are bloodsucking ectoparasites; (3) others are tissue invaders; and (4) many arthropods are mechanical transmitters of pathogenic microorganisms, and others are obligate incubators and transmitters of disease-producing microorganisms.

VENENATING ARTHROPODS

This group of arthropods includes centipedes, scorpions, spiders, ticks, mites and several species of insects.

CENTIPEDES. These animals have a pair of hollow jaws which serve as fangs to introduce into the skin toxic substances elaborated in their heads. The venom is relatively weak, and at most, even in an infant, will produce an inflammatory reaction at the puncture site and mild lymphangitis. It may be treated with local compresses and an antiseptic.

SCORPIONS. Many species of scorpions, including the dangerous ones in the southwestern United States, Latin America, many areas in Africa, southern Europe, Israel and India, have potent venom. This is elaborated in the swollen caudal segment and is introduced through the sharp, caudal sting into the skin of a person who accidentally steps on the animal or brushes it unaware with an arm.

The venom of some species produces only local tissue reaction (swelling at puncture site is distinctive), while that of other species is primarily neurotoxic in its action. The latter type of venom contains several fractions, including hemolysins, endotheliolysins, and neurotoxins. In addition to an intense aching pain and numbness radiating from the site of the injury, and lymphadenitis, there is typically an ascending motor paralysis, with convulsions resembling those observed in strychnine poisoning, a rapid weak pulse, excessive salivation, extreme thirst and dysuria; at times there is evidence of an acute pancreatitis. Deaths from scorpion stings occur particularly in children under 4 years of age.

Initially, spread of venom from the site of the sting may be retarded by prompt application of a temporary tourniquet and (without incision) prolonged, but not excessive, cooling with ice packs. In most countries where the more dangerous species are common, standardized species-specific or group-specific antivenin is available for intramuscular administration.* Supportive treatment consists initially in infiltrating into the puncture wound a 2 per cent solution of procaine containing 1:1000 epinephrine to relieve pain, then parenteral administration of glucose and amino acid solutions. Shock should be treated with parenteral solutions, including blood plasma. Morphine is not indicated. Such patients can be controlled effectively by phenobarbital. Relatively large doses of sodium phenobarbital are necessary for irrational patients and those with convulsions. For example, 6 mg/kg of sodium phenobarbital may be injected subcutaneously initially in infants and children; subsequent doses of similar amounts are given at intervals of 20 or 30 minutes, up to 4 or 5 administrations.

*Specific scorpion antivenin is available from the Poisonous Animals Research Laboratory, Arizona State University, Tempe, Arizona 85281.

The application of creosote and oil as repellents or of residual sprays of available insecticides such as DDT, BHC, lindane or malathion to hiding places around homes and outbuildings will reduce the number of scorpions and the risk of stings.

SPIDERS. All spiders produce venoms to stun or kill their prey, but relatively few species have powerful enough fangs or potent enough venom to endanger human beings as does the black widow spider of the United States, *Latrodectus mactans.* This is a black spider with a red ventral spot and variable red dorsal spots, attaining a body length of 13 mm and a leg spread of 40 mm. The spider may bite on chance contact or attack when her web is touched, striking with a pair of anterior fangs. There is an immediate sharp pain at the site, with a burning, swollen, inflamed area around the puncture wound. The venom enters the blood stream and, in about 30 minutes, produces dizziness, weakness, tremors, abdominal cramps and typically a spastic contraction of the muscles, particularly those of the abdomen, simulating acute abdominal conditions and sickle-cell crisis.There is rapid shallow respiration, tachycardia and high arterial blood pressure. Acute nephritis may develop as a result of the intoxication. Hemoglobinuria has been reported in small children. The double fang markings at the site of inoculation may provide a diagnostic clue, but diagnosis is usually from the clinical history.

Treatment consists in intramuscular injection of standardized species- or group-specific antivenin.* Pain can be reduced by slow intravenous or intramuscular injection of a 10 per cent solution of calcium gluconate, 0.05-0.1 ml/kg repeated as necessary, or by subcutaneous morphine sulphate, alone or with intramuscular phenobarbital. Prolonged hot baths are also effective. Barbiturates may be needed to allay muscle spasm and pain. Neostigmine bromide, USP, may also be used to reduce spasms of smooth muscle. Acute symptoms usually abate after 24 hours, but there may be a long convalescence. Most of the reported deaths, within 36 hours, have occurred because the patients were brought to the hospital too late for supportive or antivenin treatment.

Species of the genus *Loxosceles,* which are domestic in their habitats, produce necrotic arachnidism. *Loxosceles laeta* and *L. rufipes* in South America cause topical necrosis and, at times, systemic hemolysis. In the central and southern United States *L. reclusa,* the brown recluse spider and related species (body 7 to 12 mm long, leg spread 30 to 40 mm; yellowish to reddish brown with dark violin-shaped mark dorsally between legs, and with 6 eyes), inhabit dry cellars, closets and outbuildings. They are not aggressive, but when crushed or entangled in clothing both the male and the female bite, causing severe local pain, with rapid development of an indurated wheal which transforms into a large violaceous sloughing ulcer, leaving a deep granulating base. Healing occurs very slowly over a period of weeks if the lesion is not excised. Systemic reactions vary but may include restlessness, fever and sometimes a scarlatiniform rash; rarely, deaths have been reported. Experimentally the venom has been found to contain a powerful necrotoxin. Parenteral administration of corticotropin to victims of Loxosceles bites will hasten healing of the wound.

Contact insecticides, such as lindane in kerosene sprayed on the spider's web, are lethal to *Latrodectus* and to *Loxosceles.*

TICKS AND MITES. Ticks are macroscopic and mites microscopic arthropods with unsegmented flat or swollen bodies and 6 or 8 legs. Ticks are brown or gray, whereas mites may be colorless, reddish or dark. Many species of ticks and several species of mites cause serious local irritation at the sites on the skin which they pierce to feed on blood or (chiggers) tissue fluid. The most notorious mites are the chigger (red bug) and the rat mite. These are particularly irritating for small children. The local lesion at the site of attachment can be effectively treated by application of phenolated camphor solution in pure mineral oil, or of Quotane ointment (containing dimethisoquin hydrochloride), or by coating chigger bites with collodion or nail polish. Dusting sulfur into socks and pants or rubbing dimethyl phthalate on the ankles and legs will usually prevent infestation with chiggers. Nonparasitic mites may be involved in house-dust allergy (Dermatophagoides sp. and others) and, infrequently, in contact dermatitis (grain-itch and produce mites).

Tick Paralysis. Certain ticks, including the Rocky Mountain wood tick, introduce saliva which sometimes produces a flaccid ascending motor paralysis which usually begins in the legs. Recovery is usually rapid and complete if the tick is removed quickly, but if it is allowed to remain, death may result from respiratory paralysis. The application of petrolatum or heat to induce the tick to detach will avoid the risk of leaving the imbedded mouth parts in the skin by forceful removal.

INSECTS. These include bees, wasps, ants, blister beetles, moth caterpillars and many bloodsucking insects. The honeybee worker, unlike bumblebees and wasps, may leave the stinger imbedded in the skin; it should be scraped off carefully to avoid pressure on the attached poison sac. The venoms of bees, wasps and ants are complex mixtures of peptides, proteins and amines, including histamine and hyaluronidase. Hypersensitive people who go into shock require prompt use of epinephrine, and then should be gradually desensitized with whole bee extract to minimize subsequent reactions.

Blister beetles produce a painful blister when their juices are brought into contact with the skin. Ammonia will partly neutralize the blister fluid, and a corticosteroid ointment will ease the pain. Certain caterpillars elaborate venom in nettling hairs which, on contact with the skin or mucous membranes, produce an intense stinging sensation and a painful burn which heals slowly. Prompt

---

*Antivenin *Latrodectus mactans* (Merck Sharp and Dohme) is specific.

washing with soap and water or alcohol is advisable, and a palliative such as calamine lotion may be applied. The pain is partially eased by a corticosteroid ointment, but systemic effects (e.g., from the puss caterpillar), which may be severe during the first day or longer, sometimes require sedation and bed rest.

Blood-sucking Insects. Insects such as mosquitoes, gnats, deerflies, stable flies, fleas, lice and assassin bugs introduce saliva into the skin while taking a blood meal. This foreign protein produces allergic manifestations in many persons. Specific desensitization may alleviate hypersensitivity. *Papular urticaria* in children may result from sensitivity to insect bites, particularly by fleas or bedbugs in the home, and requires appropriate control or protective measures. Repellents applied to exposed skin provide temporary protection out of doors, while indoors flying insects can be killed by household fly sprays or dichlorvos (DDVP)-impregnated plastic strips.

TISSUE-INVADING ARTHROPODS

Among the arthropods which invade tissues the following are important: the itch mite *(Sarcoptes scabiei),* which produces scabies; the chigoe *(Tunga penetrans)*; and the maggots or larval stage of many species of filth flies and their relatives, which cause myiasis.

SCABIES. This disease, produced by *Sarcoptes scabiei,* is world-wide in distribution and is most frequent in lower economic groups where personal hygiene is neglected. The adult mite is a minute 8-legged organism which burrows into the stratum corneum of the skin and forms a tunnel nearly parallel to the surface. At the blind end of the tunnel the female lays about 10 eggs a week for 4 or 5 weeks. In 3 to 5 days the eggs hatch, and 6-legged larvae emerge. These young mites either make lateral tunnels or come out of the tunnel and re-enter the skin. Since an entire life cycle may be completed in 11 to 15 days, an infestation, once established, develops rapidly. The mites are usually transferred from person to person by direct contact but can survive as long as a week on fomites. A severe and chronic form of infestation, "Norwegian scabies," characterized by crusts teeming with mites, occasionally occurs, especially in mongoloid or debilitated children. (See also Section 23.)

CHIGOE INFESTATION. *Tunga penetrans,* a flea, is a common skin parasite of dogs, pigs and barefooted persons in the American tropics and tropical Africa. The most common sites of infestation are the spaces between the toes, into which the fleas burrow. The females swell to the size of a pea and produce painful, festering lesions. The gravid fleas should be removed with a sterile needle and the wounds painted with tincture of iodine to kill the remaining fleas and eggs. Since infestation is usually acquired from direct contact of the bare foot with dust or dirt harboring fleas from dogs or pigs, well shod feet practically guarantee safety from attack.

MYIASIS. This results from invasion of tissues and organs by the larvae (maggots or grubs) of various species of flies, which may be specific obligate parasites or semispecific or accidental facultative parasites. Myiasis may affect the skin, connective tissue, eye, nasopharynx, ear, intestines or urethra, and the clinical effects range from benign intestinal infestations or localized lesions to severe mutilation and even death from deep penetration into vital organs. Children are particularly vulnerable to myiasis through either outdoor exposure or the ingestion of fly-contaminated food. The larvae are active, whitish, headless, segmented and wormlike, found imbedded in tissues or in freshly passed stools that have been protected from contamination by flies.

In specific myiasis, the gravid fly deposits eggs or larvae on skin, hair, mucous membranes or (tropical warble fly) on carrier arthropods. The natural hosts are animals, and infestation of man is incidental. Individual larvae of the tropical warble fly (*Dermatobia hominis*) and fox, mink and rodent parasites (*Wohlfahrtia* and *Cuterebra* species) produce furuncular lesions, horse bots (*Gasterophilus* species) (a cutaneous creeping eruption), sheep bots (*Oestrus ovis*) (conjunctival invasion), and cattle bots (*Hypoderma* species) (deep migratory invasion), while multiple larvae of the primary screwworm (*Cochliomyia hominivorax*) burrow deeply and destructively into the skin or head.

Semispecific and accidental myiasis may result from attraction of saprophagous flies to open lesions or soiled skin, or by ingestion of food containing eggs or larvae of flies. Blowflies (species of *Calliphora, Lucilia, Phaenicia,* and others, and *Cochliomyia macellaria)* and flesh flies *(Sarcophaga* species*)* are semispecific and most frequently involved, while other species, including the house fly *(Musca domestica),* are rare accidental intestinal parasites.

Maggots burrowing into tissues or breeding in wounds should be removed as soon as possible. The lesions should be irrigated, treated with a bactericidal ointment and covered with a sterile dressing. In intestinal myiasis frequent saline purgation and enemas may be helpful. Young children, particularly those around stock farms, should be protected from flies by screening or mosquito netting, and any discharges from the eyes, nares, or skin lesions should not be allowed to accumulate, since these attract myiasis-producing flies. Fly control measures should be applied, especially around domestic animals and fur-breeding farms.

ARTHROPODS AS TRANSMITTING AGENTS OF DISEASE

Arthropods serve in two ways to transmit disease-producing microorganisms to man: mechanically, and as essential biologic hosts or incubators of pathogens.

MECHANICAL TRANSMITTERS. The most important group of mechanical transmitters is that of the filth flies, including the common housefly, the lesser houseflies, stable flies, greenbottles, bluebottles, blowflies, flesh flies and fruit flies. During epidemics or when food and water are grossly polluted with human excreta, they are often responsible for the transmission of typhoid and other salmonella infections, shigellosis, cholera and amebiasis. Evidence is less conclusive that they play a conspicuous role in the spread of poliomyelitis and epidemic conjunctivitis. Cockroaches may also transmit enteric disease organisms to food.

ESSENTIAL TRANSMITTERS. Arthropods which are biologic vectors of pathogens include: (1) the ticks, which transmit spotted fever, Q fever, Colorado tick fever, hemorrhagic fever, relapsing fever and tularemia; (2) red mites, which transmit scrub typhus, rat and mouse mites, which transmit murine typhus and rickettsialpox; (3) lice, which transmit epidemic typhus fever, trench fever and relapsing fever; (4) fleas, which transmit plague, murine typhus and several other infections; (5) mosquitoes, which transmit malaria, yellow fever, dengue, a large number of other arboviruses causing viral encephalitis, filariasis and tularemia; (6) sandflies, which transmit kala-azar, cutaneous and mucocutaneous leishmaniasis, Oroya fever and pappataci fever; (7) *Glossina* (tsetse) flies, which transmit African trypanosomiasis; (8) black gnats, which transmit onchocerciasis; and (9) assassin bugs, which transmit Chagas' disease.

Children are particularly susceptible to all these diseases. In some instances protection can be afforded by vaccine, as in yellow fever, Rocky Mountain spotted fever and typhus fever. In some, individual prophylaxis consists in avoiding endemic territory. In certain diseases the only practical safeguard consists in dusting the exposed person's clothing with DDT, as in louse-borne typhus fever, or using this or other insecticides as a residual spray, as in areas of rodent plague. Another method of attack is the destruction of the reservoir host (rats in the case of plague and murine typhus). Vector arthropods are man's greatest enemy and today constitute one of his most serious challenges.

ERNEST CARROLL FAUST
ALBERT MILLER

Baker, E. W., and others: A Manual of Parasitic Mites. New York, National Pest Control Assoc., Inc., 1956.

Blattner, R. J.: Necrotic arachnidism. J. Pediatr. *53*:377, 1958.

DeBusk, F. L., and O'Connor, S.: Tick toxicosis. Pediatrics *50*:328, 1972.

Frazier, C. A.: Diagnosis and treatment of insect bites. Clin. Symp. (Ciba) *20*:75, 1968.

Frazier, C. A.: Insect Allergy: Allergic and Toxic Reactions to Insects and Other Arthropods. St. Louis, W. H. Green, Inc., 1969.

Goldman, L., and others: Investigative studies of skin irritation from caterpillars. J. Invest. Dermatol. *34*:67, 1960.

Haller, J. S., and Fabara, J. A.: Tick paralysis. Case report with emphasis on neurological toxicity. Am. J. Dis. Child. *124*:915, 1972.

Horen, W. P.: Insect and scorpion stings. J.A.M.A., *221*:894, 1972.

Horsfall, W. R.: Medical Entomology. Arthropods and Human Disease. New York, The Ronald Press Co., 1962.

James, J. A., and others: Reactions following suspected spider bite. Am. J. Dis. Child. *102*:395, 1961.

James, M. T.: The Flies That Cause Myiasis in Man. Washington, D. C., U.S. Department of Agriculture, Misc. Publ. No. 631, 1947.

James, M. T., and Harwood, R. F.: Herm's Medical Entomology. 6th ed. London, The MacMillan Co., 1969.

Mallis, A.: Handbook of Pest Control. 5th ed. New York, MacNair-Doland Co., Inc., 1969.

Maretic, Z., and Stanic, M.: The health problem of arachnidism. Bull. WHO *11*:1007, 1954.

O'Rourke, F. J.: The toxicity of black widow spider venom. *In* Venoms. Washington, D.C., American Association for the Advancement of Science, Publ. 44, 1956.

Reed, H. B., Jr., and others: Variation in severity of loxoscelism. J. Tenn. Med. Ass. *61*:1097, 1968.

Stahnke, H. L.: Scorpions. Tempe, Arizona, Arizona State College Bookstore, 1956.

Vorse, H., and others: Disseminated intravascular coagulopathy following fatal brown spider bite (necrotic arachnidism). J. Pediatr. *80*:1035, 1972.

Wand, M.: Necrotic arachnidism: A new entity in the Northwest. Northwest Med. *71*:292, 1972.

SYSTEMIC PROTOZOAN INFECTIONS

MALARIA

Malaria results from the invasion of erythrocytes by one of four species of protozoan parasites of the genus *Plasmodium.* It is characterized by high fever, which is often intermittent, and by anemia and splenic enlargement. Despite world-wide campaigns aimed at eradication of malaria through interruption of its life cycle in the intermediate host (female mosquitoes of the genus *Anopheles*), the disease continues to be the principal health problem of warm climates; it is frequently imported to countries in the temperate zones where, in the summer months, it may be spread locally by mosquitoes.

For clinical and diagnostic purposes, malaria may be regarded as two disease entities: the more dangerous one, caused by *Plasmodium falciparum* and formerly termed "subtertian" or "malignant tertian malaria," can produce a great variety of acute clinical manifestations and may, if untreated, be fatal within a few days of its onset; the other, caused by *P. vivax* (benign tertian malaria), *P. ovale* (a rarity resembling *P. vivax*) or *P. ma-*

lariae (quartan malaria), is more typically paroxysmal and is almost never fatal. The latter may recur weeks after a primary attack has apparently been cured, in contrast to falciparum infections, which, except in the case of drug-resistant strains, rarely recrudesce after standard treatment.

ETIOLOGY. Malaria is usually acquired from the bites of previously infected female anopheline mosquitoes. In other instances, malaria, particularly of the quartan type, has developed after the transfusion of infected blood, in which circumstances the pre-erythrocytic phase of the parasite's development in the liver is avoided. The usual evolution of the disease is as follows:

Pre-erythrocytic Phase. The *sporozoites* injected by the biting mosquito reach the sinusoids of the liver through the blood stream and enter the cytoplasm of hepatic cells. Growth and nuclear division are rapid, and microscopic cysts (*schizonts*) are formed which contain *merozoites.*

At the end of approximately 6 days of development of falciparum cysts in the liver the cysts rupture, liberating some 40,000 merozoites from each cyst, which penetrate red blood cells. In vivax infections as many as 10,000 merozoites develop in each cyst in 8 days, in ovale 15,000 in 9 days, and in quartan 15,000 in 15 days. Not all merozoites enter erythrocytes; some are believed to return to hepatic cells, paving the way for a relapse at a later date.

The prepatent or incubation period (the period between the infecting mosquito bite and the presence of parasites in the blood) varies with the species; *P. falciparum* is 10 to 13 days; *P. vivax* and *ovale,* 12 to 16; and *P. malariae,* 27 to 37, depending on the size of the inoculum. Malaria transmitted by the transfusion of infected blood becomes apparent in a much shorter time. Clinical manifestations of infection induced by any means may be suppressed for many months by subcurative doses of medications; this is particularly so in the cases of vivax and quartan malaria.

Erythrocytic Phase. The merozoites which invade red blood cells appear first in stained smears as bluish rings or (*P. malariae*) bands of cytoplasm, with one or occasionally two red dots of nuclear chromatin. The growing parasites are named *trophozoites,* and appearing with them in the red cells are granules of yellow-brown pigment which consist of hematin derived from the hemoglobin consumed by the parasite to meet its protein requirements. The shape of the organism varies during growth until it becomes round and, with the scattered or clumped pigment, almost fills the red blood cell, which in the case of *P. vivax* is enlarged and stippled.

The nucleus of the parasite now divides asexually several times, its cytoplasm is arranged around the new nuclei, and the pigment aggregates into large clumps; this segmenter, or mature *schizont,* contains a varying number of merozoites, depending on the species: 8 to 28 in *P. falciparum,* 12 to 24 in *P. vivax,* and 6 to 12 in *P. ovale* and *malariae.* The erythrocytes containing these merozoites rupture, and naked merozoites, pigment and erythrocytic debris are freed in the plasma. Those merozoites that escape phagocytosis enter fresh red blood cells. Thus, an asexual cycle is begun each time a new crop of merozoites invades red cells, and this cycle, whose duration is of considerable clinical importance, lasts 48 hours in falciparum, vivax and ovale malaria and 72 hours in quartan malaria. The malarial paroxysm does not take place until enough cycles have occurred to produce the amount of parasitic material, pigment and red cell debris required to induce febrile or other reactions.

Certain of the growing parasites fail to divide, the nucleus remaining intact during the period of maturation. They are differentiated into male or female forms called *gametocytes,* which are of no clinical importance but are capable of infecting mosquitoes feeding on the patient.

Mixed Infections and Broods. Although mixed infections with two species may occur, almost invariably one species is responsible for the clinical pattern. Falciparum strains usually dominate vivax, and vivax dominate quartan; only when sufficient immunity is developed to the dominant strain does the other one begin to produce clinical manifestations.

In an infection with a single species distinct broods may develop. Since the merozoites in the liver are not released simultaneously and the erythrocytic schizonts do not all rupture at the same time, some groups of parasites begin their existence in red blood cells before or after the majority, often maturing in sufficient numbers to produce an independent clinical reaction. In vivax infections single broods will produce a febrile reaction every other day, whereas if two broods develop, there will be daily paroxysms; though this may also be the case initially in falciparum malaria, the classic picture of intermittent fever is soon disrupted. Two broods of *P. malariae* can be responsible for fever 2 days out of 3; and three broods, for daily temperature rises.

EPIDEMIOLOGY. Only in regions where the people have gametocytes in their blood can anopheline mosquitoes become infected. Children may be especially important vectors. Transmission of malaria occurs in most tropical and some temperate zones; although North America is now free of indigenous malaria, focal outbreaks have occurred through infection of local mosquitoes by travelers and returning students and servicemen.

Congenital malaria, due to the transfer of the causative agent across the placental barrier, is believed to occur, but is extremely rare, particularly in endemic areas where mothers have acquired some immunity to the disease. Neonatal malaria, on the other hand, is less uncommon and may result from mingling of infected maternal blood with that of the infant during the birth process.

PATHOLOGY. The extent of destruction of red blood cells characteristic of malaria depends upon the duration and severity of the infection. Hemolysis often leads to an increase in the serum bilirubin, and in falciparum malaria it may be sufficiently intense to result in hemoglobinuria (blackwater fever). In any malarial infection the degree of anemia is greater than that attributable solely to the destruction of cells by parasites. Hemolysis is probably contributed to by autoantigenic changes produced in the red cell by the parasite. Autoantigenic changes and increased osmotic fragility occur in all erythrocytes whether infected or not. Hemolysis may also be induced by quinine or primaquine in persons with hereditary glucose-6-phosphate dehydrogenase deficiency.

The pigment extruded into the circulation upon red cell disintegration accumulates in the reticuloendothelial cells of the spleen, the follicles of which become hyperplastic and sometimes necrotic, in the Kupffer cells of the liver, and in the bone marrow, brain and other organs. Deposition of sufficient pigment and of hemosiderin results in a slate-gray color of the organs.

The malignancy of falciparum malaria is peculiar to that species. The merozoites emerging from the liver are considerably more numerous than those of other species; there are as many in young children as in adults, so that children have a proportionately greater initial wave of infection. Young children are particularly prone to severe, often lethal, parasitemia.

Eight to 18 hours after the parasite has entered the red blood cells, these cells become increasingly sticky and tend to adhere to the endothelial lining of blood sinuses and vessels, especially when the circulation is slow. A cross section of a small venule from a fatal case will usually reveal the remains of parasites or pigment in most of the red cells adjacent to the endothelium, and not in those lying in the lumen. The sticky cell is thus fixed and unable to return to the general circulation, although the parasite within it matures in the normal manner. As more cells adhere, flow within the vessel is progressively impeded, and occlusion or even rupture may occur.

The site and extent of this interference with vascular function, coupled with a selective localization of parasitized cells in various organs or systems, are responsible for the variety of symptoms from falciparum infections. Thus, pneumonitis, encephalitis or enteritis may be manifest when the bulk of the infection is in the lungs, brain or intestinal tract, respectively. In the pregnant woman damage to the placenta may result in death of the fetus or in premature birth; infants born at full term to infected women have birth weights averaging one sixteenth less than those of infants born to uninfected mothers living under similar conditions.

The release of merozoites where the circulation is slowed facilitates the invasion of nearby red blood cells, so that falciparum parasitemia may be heavier than that of other species in which the rupture of schizonts takes place in the active circulation. Whereas *P. falciparum* invades all erythrocytes irrespective of age, *P. vivax* attacks primarily reticulocytes, and *P. malariae* invades mature red cells, features which tend to limit parasitemia of the latter two forms to less than 20,000 red cells per mm^3. Falciparum infections in the nonimmune child may develop densities of as much as 500,000 parasites per mm^3; the prognosis is correspondingly grave.

Successful treatment stops the growth of parasites. Homologous immunity is vested in specific antibodies which may be associated with increased levels of 7S (IgG) gamma globulin in the serum of people repeatedly infected with a particular species. Antibody facilitates the phagocytosis of naked merozoites and of parasite-containing erythrocytes, which are ingested by reticuloendothelial cells and by large lymphocytes and neutrophils and particularly by monocytes. These antibodies do not, however, interfere with development of the parasite in the liver. A passive immunity, effective in restraining the severity of attacks of malaria for several weeks after birth, is conferred on infants born to mothers who have the disease. The beneficial effect of this transplacental acquisition of humoral immunity may be enhanced by persistence of fetal hemoglobin and by a diet limited to milk (low in PABA, hence inimical to growth of parasites). Certain hemoglobinopathies are also protective and tend to be genetically selective in endemic malarious regions. *Plasmodium falciparum* may fail to mature in children with the sickle-cell trait; *P. vivax,* in those with thalassemia and enzyme deficiencies; and *P. falciparum* is unable to attain high densities in children deficient in glucose-6-phosphate dehydrogenase.

CLINICAL MANIFESTATIONS. Children who acquire malaria fall into two groups: those who have not had previous contact with the disease have little or no immunity and become severely ill unless treated; those who have been exposed to repeated infection since birth may survive early childhood to acquire a high degree of tolerance by about 10 years of age, though growth and development may be impaired. In the partially immune child heavy parasitemia may occur with a few symptoms, or an intercurrent infection may initiate renewed activity of a quiescent malarial infection. Tolerance to malaria is most apparent among Africans and persons of African descent; it appears to be based on inherited factors that modify the severity of the disease.

In a nonimmune child clinical signs usually appear 8 to 15 days after infection and may not be distinctive. Behavioral changes such as fretfulness, anorexia, unusual crying, drowsiness or disturbances of sleep may have been observed. Fever may be absent or increase gradually for 1 or 2 days, or the onset may be sudden with temperature up to 40.6° C (105° F) or higher, with or without prodromal chill. After varying periods of time, the temperature falls to normal or below, and sweating occurs.

The febrile paroxysm may be extremely short or may last for 2 to 12 hours; its characteristic pattern is usually obscured in children less than 5 years of age. Complaints may be made of headache, nausea, generalized aching, particularly of the back, and occasionally of pain in the abdomen, when the spleen has swollen quickly and is tender. In vivax and quartan infections dominated by a single brood the fever is the characteristic manifestation, occurring at intervals of 48 hours in the former and 72 in the latter. If convulsions occur, they abate when the fever falls. Herpetic lesions of the mouth are not uncommon. The red blood cell count and hemoglobin level may decrease rapidly; leukopenia is variable, but monocytosis is common.

In falciparum infections the fever is less characteristic and may even be continuous; it may be overshadowed by severe manifestations related to the cerebral, pulmonary, intestinal or urinary systems. Cerebral complications are evidenced by convulsions or coma, with few localizing neurologic signs and (unless bacterial or viral infections of the central nervous system are superimposed) a normal cerebrospinal fluid. In cases of algid malaria, coma is preceded in the child by medical shock. Persistent nausea and vomiting, an enlarged and tender liver and progressive jaundice may evolve into hepatic failure; severe diarrhea may occur; or occasionally the signs of acute appendicitis may be imitated.

The spleen is more commonly enlarged in vivax than in falciparum infections; perisplenitis, infarction, even rupture may occur, and after repeated attacks the spleen may become very large and hard. "Idiopathic splenomegaly" (so-called big spleen disease of Africa) may constitute an abnormal immune response to *P. malariae* in malnourished children in underdeveloped countries. Enlargement of the spleen is accompanied by lymphocytic infiltration of liver sinusoids and an elevated fluorescent antibody titer for malaria, with or without scanty parasitemia.

Disturbances of renal function are shown by oliguria, and anuria may supervene. The *nephrotic syndrome* is associated with *P. malariae* in children inhabiting endemic malarious areas and is characterized by gross edema, massive proteinuria and severe hyproteinemia; the prognosis is poor. *Blackwater fever*, now rarely seen, is associated with *P. falciparum*. Hemoglobinuria results from severe and sudden intravascular hemolysis, which may lead to anuria and to death from uremia.

DIAGNOSIS. The diagnosis of malaria depends upon identification of parasites in the blood. In falciparum malaria, only ring forms are likely to be seen initially, crescents (gametocytes) joining them after 10 days; up to 20 per cent of the erythrocytes may be infected. All stages of the other species of parasites appear in the blood, but less than 2 per cent of red cells will contain them.

In the properly stained blood smear the parasites within the red cells have a red chromatin and bluish cytoplasm. In some leukocytes, particularly monocytes, remnants of phagocytized parasites and pigment may be seen. The parasites should first be looked for in thick blood films, since in light infections it may not be possible to find plasmodia in the thin film; the latter is best used for species differentiation. As parasites may not be seen at the height of the fever, examinations should be repeated preferably at intervals of 12 hours. Of the various stains available, the most suitable is Giemsa diluted 1:25 with distilled water preferably buffered to pH 7.0 to 7.2. Wright's stain may be used, 0.75 gm of the powder being repeatedly shaken for 2 days with 65 ml of pure methyl alcohol and 35 ml of pure glycerin.

A falsely positive Wassermann reaction will be found in many cases.

PREVENTION. Natural infection of man does not occur where breeding of anopheline mosquitoes is prevented, where the adult mosquitoes are kept from contact with man by screens or bed nets, or where they are killed by natural enemies or insecticides before sporozoites have had time to mature. Children visiting endemic malarious areas should be protected by screens during the hours of mosquito activity, but as this is rarely entirely effective, they should also be given one of the chemoprophylactic drugs *regularly* throughout their stay and for 4 weeks thereafter. At least during this period, malaria should be suspected if febrile illness or chronic debility affects the child.

Chemoprophylactic drugs in common use are the following: the slightly bitter but extremely safe chloroguanide (Proguanil), taken daily in amounts of 25 mg (to 2 years), 50 mg (2 to 6 years) or 100 mg (older than 6); the tasteless but more toxic pyrimethamine (supplies of which should be particularly well guarded from inquisitive children), taken weekly in amounts of 6.25 mg (to 2 years), 12.5 mg (2 to 6 years) or 25 mg; and chloroquine or amodiaquine taken weekly in amounts of 37.5 mg of the base (to 1 year), 75 mg (1 to 2 years), 112.5 mg (2 to 6 years), 150 mg (6 to 12 years) or 300 mg. The bitterness of chloroquine diphosphate and sulfate has been partially concealed in syrups which are available commercially, and tasteless products are the silicate salt of chloroquine and the base preparation of amodiaquine.

Proguanil and pyrimethamine not only suppress the development of parasites in the red blood cells, as do chloroquine and amodiaquine, but also interfere with the pre-erythrocytic stage in the liver. Unfortunately cross-resistance of the organism to the first two drugs is widely distributed, for which reason chloroquine and amodiaquine are generally preferred in prophylaxis. When resistance to the latter compounds also occurs, as in northern South America and southeast Asia, potentiating combinations of pyrimethamine with long-acting sulfonamides or sulfones may be taken by mouth, or an injectable repository preparation containing cycloguanil pamoate and diacetylaminodiphenylsulfone may prove effective.

TREATMENT. *Clinical treatment* falls into four categories: (1) specific chemotherapy of the attack, whether fresh infection, recrudescence or relapse; (2) supportive treatment and treatment of complications; (3) specific chemotherapy to prevent late relapse of vivax, ovale or quartan infections; (4) specific chemotherapy to destroy or sterilize gametocytes, and thus to protect the community should vector mosquitoes be present.

1. Any one of the drugs listed in Table 10–26 will effect a clinical cure of all types of malaria and provide a radical cure of falciparum malaria, unless drug-resistant parasites are present. Children who have inhabited malarious regions and acquired some immunity may be cured by one half of the quantities listed. Treatment must be repeated if vomiting occurs within an hour of ingestion of the drug; persistent vomiting is an indication for parenteral therapy.

Although specific treatment should not usually be undertaken until the diagnosis has been established, many experienced physicians, when con-

TABLE 10–26 TREATMENT OF UNCOMPLICATED MALARIA ATTACK

DRUG (USP)	SCHEDULE	DOSAGE IN MG BASE (CHLOROQUINE AND AMODIAQUINE)* OR MG SALT (QUININE)				
		Age Under 1 Year	*Age 1-3 Years*	*Age 3-6 Years*	*Age 6-12 Years*	*Older Children*
Chloroquine or Amodiaquine	Day 1 – first dose	75	75	150	150	300
	6 hours later	75	75	150	150	300
	6 hours later	37.5	75	75	150	300
	Day 2 – first dose	37.5	75	75	150	150
	6 hours later	–	–	–	–	150
	Day 3 – first dose	37.5	75	75	150	150
	6 hours later	–	–	–	–	150
Quinine	Daily†	249	416	666	1000	2000

*Commercial tablets usually contain 250 mg of chloroquine diphosphate or sulfate, of which 150 mg is base: the quantity of base is stated on the label of the container, and should be prescribed as such.

†Given for 10 days in divided doses every 4 or 8 hours, as tolerated.

fronted with a critically ill or comatose child whose history is suggestive of malaria or exposure thereto, would consider it advisable to administer quinine or chloroquine parenterally while awaiting the result of blood film examination.

Parenteral administration of chloroquine or quinine, although hazardous in children bordering on shock, is often essential for those who are vomiting persistently, who are in coma or who cannot be induced to swallow the drugs even if the bitterness is concealed. Parenteral therapy with antimalarial drugs should be replaced by oral administration as soon as possible. Chloroquine may be given intravenously by slow drip in a glucose-saline solution, but it is preferable to inject it intramuscularly; the dose by either route should not exceed 5 mg base per kg and should be repeated once, 6 hours later, if treatment still cannot be given by mouth. Quinine dihydrochloride is administered intravenously in a dose of 10 mg/kg and may be repeated 12 hours later; it should be given well diluted (1 mg/ml) and slowly (no faster than 1 ml/minute) by drip.

2. Supportive treatment includes that for hyperpyrexia; tepid sponging may add to the comfort when the temperature exceeds 40° C (104° F). Particular attention should be paid to fluid and electrolyte needs, as indicated in the discussion of deficit fluid therapy in Section 5.

Metabolic requirements of the parasite rapidly deplete the reserves of glucose, vitamins and coenzymes, as well as of hemoglobin. Vitamin B_1 may be given, and when the acute phase is passed, ferrous sulfate should be prescribed for a considerable time. Transfusion of packed red cells may be beneficial to children who have had longstanding infections and consequently severe anemia (hemoglobin 5 gm/dl or less).

It is essential that children with severe falciparum infections receive fluids intravenously if dehydrated or in shock. Rapid expansion of the circulating blood volume with whole blood is more satisfactory than with dextran, plasma or glucose-saline solution. Renal failure, which may have to be dealt with by peritoneal dialysis, is a rare development. The full course of antimalarial therapy should not be instituted until the child is hydrated, out of shock and urinating, and quinine and primaquine are contraindicated in the presence of hemoglobinuria; nevertheless, high parasitemia must be combated by the judicious use of chloroquine or amodiaquine.

In the comatose stage of cerebral malaria, in addition to specific parenteral antimalarial treatment, use has recently been made in adults of dexamethasone sodium phosphate (3 mg every 8 hours) to reduce cerebral edema, but this has not proved particularly beneficial in children. Dextran-75 is useful for the prevention of intravascular sludging. Convulsions may be controlled with paraldehyde or barbiturates.

The nephrotic syndrome associated with quartan malaria is managed by the regimen described in Section 15, together with a course of chloroquine and primaquine.

3. Late relapse of vivax or ovale malaria rarely occurs more than 5 years after the primary attack, but much longer intervals have been recorded in the case of quartan malaria. Such relapses may be prevented by treatment of the child with primaquine (commencing on the second day of a concomitant clinical curative course of chloroquine, amodiaquine or quinine). The primaquine is given for 14 days in a daily dose of 2.5 mg (base) for children aged 1 to 3 years, 5 mg for those aged 4 to 6 years, and proportionately more up to the adult dose of 15 mg daily.

Children receiving primaquine should be watched for toxic manifestations such as methemoglobinemia, hemolytic anemia (sometimes accompanied by hemoglobinuria in children with G-6-PD deficiency), neutropenia and renal dysfunction. Quinacrine (mepacrine) should not be used simultaneously with primaquine, but since the former is obsolete as an antimalarial drug, the problem need not arise. Other synthetic antimalarial drugs are relatively nontoxic in therapeutic doses.

4. Gametocytes do not give rise to symptoms and disappear from the circulation soon after destruction of their asexual precursors by chloroquine, amodiaquine or quinine. Gametocytes may be destroyed by a single dose of primaquine, or their further development in the mosquito inhibited by single doses of chlorguanide or pyrimethamine, provided the parasite is not resistant to these drugs.

Drug resistance is of growing concern. Many strains of plasmodia are now resistant to chlorguanide and pyrimethamine, but a greater problem is posed by the spread in northern South America and in southeast Asia of *P. falciparum* resistant to chloroquine and amodiaquine; some strains are also tolerant to quinine. These strains are being introduced into countries such as the United States, where focal outbreaks may occur in the summer months, and children may become infected. Should the malarial attack not respond to chloroquine or amodiaquine, quinine should be used immediately. If this has only a temporary effect, the course should be repeated with the addition, on the first day, of a long-acting sulfonamide (age or weight equivalent of 1 gm adult dose). There is evidence that the same amount of sulfonamide given with the single dose of pyrimethamine specified under "Prevention" has a potentiating effect in the cure of multidrug-resistant falciparum malaria.

David F. Clyde

Gilles, H. M.: Malaria in children. Brit. Med. J. *2*:1375, 1966.
Reid, H. A.: The treatment of malaria in children. Med. Today *2*:10, 1968.
Reid, H. A., and Nkrumah, F. K.: Fibrin-degradation products in cerebral malaria. Lancet *1*:218, 1972.
Trowell, H. C., and Jelliffe, D. B.: Diseases of Children in the Subtropics and Tropics. London, E. Arnold, 1958.
Young, M. D.: Malaria. *In* Hunter, G. W., III, Frye, W. W., and Swartzwelder, J. C.: A Manual of Tropical Medicine. 4th ed. Philadelphia, W. B. Saunders Company, 1966.

KALA-AZAR IN CHILDREN

(Leishmaniasis)

Leishmaniasis in children includes three different clinical entities: (1) kala-azar, or visceral leishmaniasis; (2) cutaneous leishmaniasis, or Oriental sore; and (3) naso-oral leishmaniasis, or espundia. Though clinically these are three different entities and each one has a definite geographical distribution, they are caused by morphologically identical and possibly the same protozoal parasites, *Leishmania donovani.*

KALA-AZAR (VISCERAL LEISHMANIASIS)

Kala-azar means black sickness in the Indian language; it is also known in India as tropical splenomegaly, sirkari disease or Dumdum fever, as ponos in Greece, and as mard el bicha in Malta. The condition is the result of infection of cells of the reticuloendothelial system by *Leishmania donovani.* The usual characteristics of the disease are: long incubation period, insidious onset and prolonged course, during which the child has irregular fever, loss of weight, progressive enlargement of spleen and liver, leukopenia and anemia. If untreated, mortality is high and death may occur within 2 to 24 months.

EPIDEMIOLOGY AND GEOGRAPHIC DISTRIBUTION. Kala-azar is endemic in India, particularly in the eastern states of Assam, Bengal and some areas of Madras; small foci have been detected in Bombay. It also occurs in Ceylon and throughout Africa, particularly in the eastern region, especially the Sudan. It has been reported from China, U.S.S.R., many countries of Central and South America (Paraguay, Argentina, Brazil, Colombia, Venezuela, Guatemala, a few cases from Mexico) and recently 3 cases in the U.S.A. In certain areas of the Mediterranean (Malta) it occurs mainly in infants and is termed "infantile kala-azar." The outstanding features of the disease in India and China are that it is confined to rural areas, especially alluvial plains, and that it does not usually occur at elevations above 730 meters (2000 feet). Favorable climatic conditions include a temperature between 20 and 45° C and a humidity of not less than 70 per cent. Usually the disease is transmitted by the bites of sandflies; dogs, foxes and jackals are important reservoirs of infection. Two stages in the life history of *L. donovani* are known: the aflagellate leishmania stage in man and reservoir mammals, and a flagellated leptomonad stage in the sandfly and in culture media.

ETIOPATHOLOGY. When a person is bitten by a sandfly the leptomonad form of the parasite is introduced into the skin and is engulfed by macrophages where the parasite changes into the leishmania form, which multiplies in the spleen, bone marrow and lymph glands. The parasite is 2 to 4 μ in diameter and is ovoid or roundish in shape. With Leishman's stain it shows lilac-colored chromatin masses of different sizes enclosed in cytoplasm having a faint blue tint about the periphery. The presence of Leishmania in the cells of the reticuloendothelial system leads to great proliferation of macrophages. This results in progressive enlargement of the spleen and liver and expansion of the red bone marrow. At times the reticuloendothelial cells are heavily infected, even in the lymph nodes, lungs, intestines and skin. Histologically the main feature of the tissue involved is an enormous proliferation of cells of macrophage type which distorts the normal structure of the organ. The spleen becomes very large and may fill the whole abdomen. There is very little fibrous tissue formation. In the liver, parasites proliferate in Kupffer cells. There is little fibrous tissue formation in the liver; the so-called leishmanial fibrosis of the liver is probably due to associated malnutrition. Peripheral blood shows marked leukopenia, usually below 4000 per mm^3. Neutrophils are mainly affected and there is an associated mononucleosis. Neutropenia may progress to agranulocytosis, and this may lead to severe septic complications. With the involvement of the bone marrow by the parasites and at times with the complication of hypersplenism, there is progressive anemia and the platelet count may be reduced. Red cell fragility is increased and the sedimentation rate is high. The indirect serum bilirubin level may be increased. Serum protein levels are low, with reduction of albumin, increase in globulins and reversal of albumin:globulin ratio.

CLINICAL MANIFESTATIONS

Incubation Period. Following a bite by an infected sandfly the symptoms may develop during a period of 2 weeks to 2 years or more.

Infantile Kala-azar. The onset is acute and there are high fever, vomiting and toxemia. The fever rises gradually to a peak in 1 or 2 weeks, becomes remittent or continuous, and comes down by lysis. There is enlargement of lymph nodes, mild generalized edema, enlargement of spleen and liver, leukopenia and anemia. If untreated, the patient develops agranulocytosis; this may lead to cancrum oris, septicemia, pneumonia and gastroenteritis, which may prove fatal. Infantile kala-azar occurs in the Mediterranean region, particularly in Malta. The youngest baby involved was 4 months old, though the majority are between 1 and 2 years. Sudden death may occur from hyperpyrexia, vomiting, intense dyspnea or hemorrhage.

Congenital Kala-azar. That kala-azar may rarely be a congenital infection was proved by Low and Cook (in 1926), when they diagnosed this disease in a child of 7 months born in England. The mother of this child had suffered from kala-azar during pregnancy. Similar cases have been reported by Hindel and Banerjee.

Chronic Form. The chronic form of the disease occurs in older children. The onset is insidious and patients often present late. In the early stages there are lassitude, ill health, weakness and pallor. There is low-grade fever, rarely above 38.5° C (102° F), and often there are two remissions in a 24-hour period. The fever may be continuous or remittent in the first 2 to 6 weeks of the disease, and later there may be periods of low-grade or no fever. The child develops abdominal distention and progressive enlargement of the spleen. Initially the spleen is soft; it later becomes firm. It may enlarge as rapidly as 2.5 cm every month and may ultimately extend into the pelvis. Enlargement of the liver occurs a little later in the disease, and in advanced cases there may also be gross enlargement of the liver. Liver and spleen are not tender. Moderate enlargement of lymph nodes may be observed in patients who live in the Mediterranean areas and China, but not those in India. The skin becomes dry and rough and there is an earthy gray pigmentation of the skin, of the malar bones, temples, hands, feet and abdomen; hence, the name kala-azar. The child may develop edema of the feet and puffiness of the face. The hair becomes sparse and brittle. In spite of the chronicity of this disease, the appetite is often good and the tongue is clean but pale. In advanced stages secondary bacterial infections may supervene. Gastroenteritis, dysentery and pneumonia may cause death. Septic infection of the mouth may lead to cancrum oris and loss of the teeth. Purpura, gingivitis and stomatitis are common. Though patients with comparatively mild cases of kala-azar may recover without treatment, the mortality of the untreated disease is very high; death usually occurs within 2 years of the onset.

Postkala-azar Dermal Leishmaniasis. This is an important and not uncommon sequel of kala-azar in India, but less so in China and Sudan. It is due to the peculiar localization of the parasite in the skin, which occurs a year or so after kala-azar has been cured by specific treatment. The skin lesions may be erythematous patches on the face, particularly nose and cheeks, and may take the form of hypopigmented macules or nodules on the face and trunk. The nodules may resemble leprosy. They rarely ulcerate. The diagnosis of postkala-azar dermal leishmaniasis can be made from the history of kala-azar in the past and recovery of donovan bodies from skin lesions.

DIAGNOSIS AND DIFFERENTIAL DIAGNOSIS. In the early stage kala-azar may be confused with malaria, typhoid fever and disseminated tuberculosis. Prolonged recurring fever may simulate protracted hematogenous tuberculosis, particularly abdominal tuberculosis with enlargement of liver and spleen (Udani), amebic abscess of the liver (Parekh et al.), brucellosis, leukemia, Hodgkin's disease, and at times rheumatoid disease and disseminated lupus erythematosus. The chronic stage may be confused with Indian childhood cirrhosis, myeloid leukemia, the tropical splenomegaly syndrome described in Uganda and New Guinea (usually due to malaria or other antigenic complexes in a genetically determined abnormal response of IgM antibody), and rarely with splenomegaly of extrahepatic portal hypertension. Diagnosis depends fundamentally on the recovery and recognition of Leishman-Donovan bodies in material aspirated from bone marrow, spleen, liver or peripheral blood. The smears or cultures of the bone marrow are stained by the Leishman or Giemsa method. Splenic puncture provides the highest percentage of positive results (about 95 per cent); there is a risk of hemorrhage, however, when there is anemia with bleeding tendency. In smears of peripheral blood and of material obtained from lymph nodes the organisms are less likely to be detected, but a blood culture on NNN medium may increase the percentage of identifications.

The characteristic blood changes indicating visceral leishmaniasis are gross neutropenia with relative mononucleosis. Various serum tests helpful in the diagnosis are not specific. They depend on marked increase in the globulin content of the serum. The formol-gel (aldehyde) test is performed by adding two drops of commercial formalin to 2 ml of the patient's serum in a test tube. The mixture is shaken and left to stand at room temperature. A positive reaction is indicated by opacity of the serum; it becomes solid in 20 minutes and resembles boiled white of egg. This test becomes positive within a month or two of the development of the disease and becomes negative within 6 months of successful treatment. The test is positive in other infections in which there is hypergammaglobulinemia. Chopra's antimony test is also useful in the diagnosis of chronic kala-azar. The complement fixation test (using an antigen from Kedrowsky's acid-fast bacillus) is useful for diagnosis during the early stage of the disease. Fluorescent tests are being used for the identification of visceral and other forms of leishmania infection.

Leishmanin Skin Test (Montenegro Test). This test depends upon the delayed hypersensitivity reaction following intracutaneous injection of 0.5 ml of suspension of leptomonads in formolized saline. The test is read 48 to 72 hours after the injection. A local induration of more than 5 mm suggests a positive reaction and signifies immunity against reinfection with a homologous strain of leishmania. The test is not meant for the diagnosis of active kala-azar, in which it is negative; it becomes positive within 2 months of successful treatment and remains positive for many years thereafter. It is of value in surveying for prevalence of the disease in an area. A positive leishmanin rate above 5 per cent is suggestive of endemic kala-azar.

TREATMENT. The susceptibility of kala-azar to specific drug therapy appears to vary considerably in different parts of the world. Three drugs are useful in its treatment: (1) pentavalent antimonial drugs; (2) aromatic diamidines such as pentamidine and stilbamidine; and (3) amphotericin-B.

Pentavalent antimonial drugs include sodium antimony gluconate (sodium stibogluconate, Solustibosan, Stibatin, Pentostam) made up in solution ready for injection (100 mg/ml). Children tolerate this drug well. For patients between 5 and 15 years of age the dose is 400 mg (4 ml) daily intramuscularly. The dose for those below the age of 5 years is 200 mg (2 ml) daily. For Indian kala-azar the total dose is 2.4 gm for children between 5 and 15 years and 1.2 gm for those below 5. For kala-azar occurring in other parts of the world the dose is 12 gm above 5 years and 6 gm below 5 years. The tests for cure are absence of fever, regression of enlargement of spleen and liver, improvement in bone marrow, and so forth. The serum protein level returns to normal, and various serum tests become negative. If the patient fails to respond satisfactorily, a second course should be tried. Urea stibamine is another pentavalent antimony compound successfully used in the treatment of kala-azar. It is given in solution in water on alternate days intravenously for 6 to 10 doses. Intramuscular injection is painful. The dose is 125 mg intravenously for children above 5 years and 65 mg for children below 5. Six doses are given for Indian kala-azar. During treatment with these compounds anaphylactic shock may rarely occur. Epinephrine should be kept ready for injection.

Aromatic diamidine drugs such as hydroxystilbamidine isethionate should be used when pentavalent antimony therapy has failed. Children under 15 years should receive 150 mg daily, and under 5, 65 mg daily intravenously for 10 days. A second and a third course should be given at 10-day intervals for complete cure. Since this compound produces a fall in blood pressure by release of histamine, antihistaminic drugs should be given.

Amphotericin B is necessary when there is failure to improve with repeated courses of pentavalent antimony and diamidine drugs. The initial dose is 0.25 mg/kg; it should be gradually increased to 1 mg/kg. This should be given in a 5 per cent solution of dextrose, and the concentration of the drug should not exceed 0.1 mg per ml of solution. This is to be given intravenously slowly over a period of 3 to 6 hours on alternate days for 3 to 8 weeks. Toxic reactions such as fever, headache, and so forth, should be treated with antipyretics, antihistaminics and steroids.

The intercurrent infections should be treated with appropriate antibiotics. Nutrition should be improved through a diet adequate in calories and proteins. In children with severe neutropenia, anemia and thrombocytopenia, repeated blood transfusions may be required. Apart from combating malnutrition, oral hygiene is necessary to prevent stomatitis and cancrum oris.

PREVENTION. Sandfly control is not difficult to achieve with insecticides and other measures, as has been done for malaria. Early diagnosis and specific treatment of the human host have also helped to reduce the incidence of the disease. The adequate treatment of postkala-azar dermal leishmaniasis is important, since these patients are highly infectious. Destruction of infected dogs in Crete was followed by a decrease in the incidence of kala-azar. A strain of leptomonad cultures of this protozoan obtained from ground squirrels has been used for mass inoculation of those exposed to infection in North Kenya. Animal strains of leishmania are dermatotropic and capable of producing skin immunity without causing kala-azar. Some populations in East Africa have a high incidence of immunity to experimental infections with human strains of leishmania, possibly owing to previous exposure to nonhuman strains. The use of repellent cream, insecticidal sprays and protective nets may help in personal prophylaxis against sandflies.

P. M. Udani

Adams, A. R. D., and Maegrith, B. G.: Clinical Tropical Diseases. London, English Language Society and Blackwell Scientific Publications, 1971.

Manson-Bahr, P. E. G.: Manson's Tropical Diseases, London, English Language Book Society and Baillière, Tindall and Cox, Ltd., 1968.

Manson-Bahr, P. E. G.: Leishmaniasis. *In* Gellis, S. S., and Kagan, B. M. (eds.): Current Pediatric Therapy. Philadelphia, W. B. Saunders Company, 1973.

Parekh, U. C., Udani, P. M., and Mukerjee, S.: Amoebic Abscess of Liver in Children. Proc. XIIIth International Pediatric Congress, Vienna, 1971.

Udani, P. M. Tuberculous hepatic and splenic lesions and hepatosplenomegaly. Ind. J. Child Health *11*:372, 1962.

Udani, P. M.: Tuberculosis in childhood. Pediatr. Clin. India *3*:163, 1968.

Zavoral, J. M., Paloucek, J. T., and Yaeger, R. G.: Kala-azar imported into U.S.A. Pediatrics *50*:471, 1972.

TOXOPLASMOSIS

This disease results from infection with *Toxoplasma gondii,* an intracellular protozoan parasite first described in 1908 in animals in both North Africa and Brazil. In 1939 Wolf, Cowen and Paige demonstrated that toxoplasma caused human illness by isolating the organism from infants with congenital encephalomyelitis. It soon became apparent that there are two forms of infection: congenital, transmitted in utero, and acquired, usually asymptomatic. Sabin described congenital toxoplasmosis as being manifested typically by a syndrome consisting of chorioretinitis, cerebral calcification, psychomotor retardation, hydrocephalus or microcephaly, and convulsions. With the description of the dye and complement fixation tests in 1948, serologic studies of toxoplasmosis became feasible, and intensive investigation of the disease began. More recently, indirect fluorescent antibody and hemagglutination tests have been described and their usefulness demonstrated.

ETIOLOGY. *Toxoplasma gondii* is a protozoon which recently was determined to be a coccidian of cats. Trophozoites are oval or crescent-like, measuring 2 to 4 by 4 to 7 μ and best stained with Giemsa or Wright's stain. These multiply by endodyogeny, only in the presence of living cells. Tissue cysts containing hundreds of parasites, which appear to remain alive indefinitely, are produced early in infection. Toxoplasma is unique in that it can multiply in all tissues of mammals and birds except for non-nucleated erythrocytes. Its disease spectrum is expressed with remarkable similarity in different hosts, perhaps because the parasite adapts to such an unparalleled variety of cells. Only one species is known, and all known strains are serologically similar.

Recently, Hutchison, Frenkel and others demonstrated that newly infected cats (and other *Felidae*) excrete toxoplasma oocysts in their feces. The oocysts are infectious for all animals studied, including the chimpanzee and, by inference, man. Toxoplasma acquired by susceptible cats, presumably by eating infected meat, behave as coccidia, multiplying through schizogonic and gametogonic cycles in the intestinal epithelium. Oocysts containing two sporocysts are formed and excreted. Under proper conditions of temperature and moisture, each matures into four sporozoites resembling trophozoites in appearance. The cat excretes oocysts for about 1 to 2 weeks. Under proper conditions the oocysts can retain viability for a year or more. Given suitable circumstances, these sporulate in 1 to 5 days and become infectious. Although very resistant, oocysts are killed by drying, boiling and some strong chemicals. Several isolations have been reported from soil and sand frequented by cats, but the role of this stage in the causation of human disease is as yet obscure. Oocysts have not been identified in the excreta of animals other than *Felidae.* There is ample evidence for incriminating tissue cysts as a significant source of animal and human infections.

EPIDEMIOLOGY. Based upon serologic evidence, the prevalence of toxoplasma infections varies considerably among people and animals in different parts of the world. Significant titers of dye test and other antibodies have been detected in 50 per cent or more of residents of some localities, but in less than 5 per cent in other areas. The higher frequencies are more often, but not always, noted in the warmer and more humid climates. Similar variations have been observed in wild and domesticated animals and birds. The interpretation of positive serologic findings in older children and adults may be difficult unless changing titers in serial samples suggest recent infection.

Except for transmission from mother to fetus and, rarely, by organ transplant or transfusion, toxoplasma is not communicated from person to person. The high prevalence of subclinical infections in animals and man make it difficult to relate a human case to a specific animal. Desmonts found in an institution in Paris, France, that young children acquired antibodies for toxoplasma without exhibiting significant clinical symptoms at the rate of 4.8 per cent per month, but this almost doubled when their diets were supplemented with additional undercooked beef and mutton. Jacobs has shown that freezing and thawing usually renders meat noninfectious. While contaminated meat may explain some instances of infection in man, the sources of parasites for vegetarians and herbivorous animals remain undefined.

Two longitudinal studies among families residing in Cleveland and Syracuse demonstrated very few acquisitions of toxoplasma infections and no clinical illness that could be related to them. In the first study, only four serologic conversions were detected in a 10-year period, whereas in the second the comparable rate was 1 per 2392 person months. On the other hand, acquisition rates are very high among young adult Parisian women, leading apparently to significant numbers of congenital cases.

PATHOLOGY. In both the congenital and acquired forms of toxoplasmosis histologic changes may be found in almost all tissues. In the congenital form these are especially frequent in the central nervous system, the retina and the choroid; similar lesions occasionally have been noted in acquired toxoplasmosis. Toxoplasma usually will be seen as cysts, especially in muscle, often with surprisingly little associated tissue reaction. In severe acute infections, free trophozoites may be noted. Gross or microscopic areas of necrosis may be present in many tissues, especially in heart, lungs, skeletal muscle, liver and spleen. Areas of calcification occur in the brain in the congenital form, but not in acquired cases. The lesions of toxoplasmosis are not sufficiently characteristic to permit a specific diagnosis unless the parasite can be identified or other information supports the impression. Parasites have been found in lymph nodes and tonsils, and their identity confirmed by animal inoculation. In congenital infection, tissue damage stabilizes early and tends not to progress, but live parasites may remain in tissue cysts for years.

CLINICAL MANIFESTATIONS

Congenital Toxoplasmosis. Fetal infections can result only when the initial maternal acquisition of toxoplasma occurs during pregnancy. Maternal antibody acquired at any time prior to pregnancy is fully protective. While clinical severity may vary, all fetuses in the same pregnancy usually are infected. Desmonts and Couvreur recently provided the first prospective data on the products of pregnancies in which susceptible women acquire toxoplasmosis. The maternal infections are usually asymptomatic and their offspring, contrary to previous impressions, usually are not infected at all. Thus, in 118 such pregnancies, there were 109 live births with 70 uninfected babies and 28 with subclinical infections. There were two perinatal deaths and only four with both cerebral and ocular lesions. But the significant finding is that 98 (90 per cent) of the 109 completed pregnancies ended with normal offspring.

The fetus infected with toxoplasma may be stillborn, born prematurely or at full term. Illness may be apparent at birth or may not become evident for some days. Manifestations include poor feeding, fever, maculopapular rash, lymphadenopathy, hepatomegaly, splenomegaly, icterus, hydrocephalus, microcephaly, microphthalmia and convulsions, singly or in combination. Cerebral calcifications (often a single, semilunar line in the area of the striate body) and chorioretinitis (usually bilateral) may be present at birth or appear subsequently.

Active congenital infection may terminate fatally in days or weeks, or become inactive with residuals of varying degrees and combinations of hydrocephalus or microcephaly, chorioretinitis, psychomotor retardation, ocular palsies and convulsive disorders. The full impact of the infection upon development may not become evident until some weeks or months after its apparent cessation.

In a large series of cases of symptomatic congenital toxoplasmosis (Feldman), premature birth was common (31 per cent), with an expected higher mortality rate (27 per cent) than among infants born at term (12 per cent). Chorioretinitis was noted in 99 per cent, cerebral calcification in 63 per cent, psychomotor retardation in 56 per cent and hydrocephalus or microcephaly in about half of these infants. Chorioretinitis was bilateral in 85 per cent of instances, but residual damage in some cases was as slight as a minute peripheral patch of chorioretinitis or a single oculomotor palsy.

The Desmonts-Couvreur data suggest that the later in pregnancy the fetal infection occurs, the lower the infection rate and the less severe the involvement. Though toxoplasma may be responsible for premature birth, cerebral palsy, blindness and mental retardation, it does not appear to be a prominent cause of any of them. The disease can occur only in the offspring of one pregnancy of a given mother, so that subsequent pregnancies may be undertaken without fear of its repetition.

Acquired Toxoplasmosis. Although postnatally acquired toxoplasmosis is a relatively common inapparent infection, clinically expressed disease is rare. Parasitemia probably occurs in all cases and is the presumed route by which the fetus acquires infection from its mother. Except for occasional instances of lymphadenopathy, clinical evidence of maternal infection is usually not detectable.

When clinical manifestations are apparent in acquired toxoplasmosis, they may include almost any combination of malaise, fever, myalgia, maculopapular rash, generalized lymphadenopathy, hepatomegaly, encephalitis, pneumonia and myocarditis. Chorioretinitis (usually unilateral) occurs in less than 1 per cent of cases. The rash, if it occurs, persists for about 3 days. Symptoms may be evident for a few days or for some weeks; most patients recover spontaneously. The incubation period and mortality rate are unknown.

Siim has reported generalized lymphadenopathy to be frequent in acquired toxoplasmosis in Denmark. Such cases may resemble infectious mononucleosis, Hodgkin's disease or other lymphadenopathies. The Paul-Bunnell test is negative, and splenomegaly is rare. The involved lymph nodes are generally firm, nontender and nonsuppurative. Owing to the vagueness of this syndrome, the correct diagnosis usually is not considered until too late in its course to obtain serologic confirmation. Persistently negative serologic tests exclude the diagnosis.

LABORATORY DATA. Congenital toxoplasmosis may be diagnosed in its active stage shortly after birth by demonstration of parasites in smears of sediments from cerebrospinal and ventricular fluids. These may be xanthochromic and contain cells (sometimes eosinophils) and increased protein. Otherwise, identification depends upon isolation of the parasites in laboratory-reared mice. The inoculum should consist of suspensions of fresh tissue or of sediment from body fluids. Organisms, especially cysts, may be found in sections of tissue.

The dye test is the most sensitive and reliable indicator of toxoplasma antibody in human and animal sera, but requires employment of live parasites, heat-labile serum factors and meticulous detail. Toxoplasma antibodies identified by the dye test appear early in the course of infection and remain in high titer for months or years. Antibody diminishes gradually, but some may persist for life. In the sera of infants or young children with congenital disease and of their mothers, titers of 1:1000 to 1:16,000 are usual for at least some months. If the infant's antibodies have been acquired only by passive transfer, there will be a sharp decline in titer by 3 months of age and almost total disappearance by 6 months.

The complement fixation test, not too commonly

performed, may offer additional aid. It becomes positive more slowly, so that early in the course there may be a strongly positive dye, but a negative complement fixation reaction. The latter tends to decrease relatively quickly so that within months or a year or two after the initial illness, there again may be a negative complement fixation and a positive dye reaction. An infant born with active disease and a positive dye titer may have a negative complement fixation reaction, even though the mother has high titers by both procedures.

The skin test, which is of the delayed type, has little clinical diagnostic usefulness since negative reactors may have high titers of serum antibodies and antigen cannot be standardized. The time required for the development of skin sensitivity is unknown, but may be as long as a year. The indirect hemagglutination test is enticing because of its relative simplicity. Its results may parallel the dye test, but there are sufficient differences so that they cannot be substituted for each other.

More recently, indirect fluorescent antibody (IFA) systems have been adapted to measuring toxoplasma antibodies of both the IgM and IgG classes. The former has been used to identify early acquired infections. Screening cord bloods for elevated IgM levels may disclose cases of toxoplasmosis as well as other congenital infections. Persisting antibodies of the IgG class also can be detected by IFA. Given proper reagents and controls, this method most closely approaches the dye test in sensitivity and specificity.

DIFFERENTIAL DIAGNOSIS. Any manifestation of congenital toxoplasmosis may occur in other diseases, especially that caused by cytomegalovirus. Neither the cerebral calcification nor the chorioretinitis is pathognomonic. In our experience fewer than 50 per cent of children less than 5 years of age with chorioretinitis satisfy the serologic criteria for congenital toxoplasmosis. Most of the others are due to unknown causes. The clinical picture in the newborn infant also may be compatible with sepsis, syphilis or hemolytic disease.

TREATMENT. A combination of pyrimethamine (Daraprim) and sulfadiazine is superior to either drug alone in the treatment of experimental toxoplasma infections. The combination has also been used in human patients. Experience suggests it has been effective during acute, acquired disease, but owing to the variable natural course of toxoplasmosis, satisfactory evaluation of any therapeutic regimen is difficult. Sulfadiazine should be administered in usual therapeutic dosage, and pyrimethamine, 1 mg/kg/day, in divided doses. The total daily dose of pyrimethamine should not exceed 25 mg, except that twice the calculated daily dose is usually prescribed for the initial 24 to 48 hours. Treament should be continued for about 4 weeks, but this is arbitrary. Both pyrimethamine, an antifolic agent, and the sulfonamide may produce severe leukopenia and—the former especially—thrombocytopenia. Thus, frequent leukocyte counts should be obtained. The hematologic complications induced by pyrimethamine may be alleviated by the simultaneous administration of leucovorin and fresh yeast cakes. Frenkel suggests that infants receive 1 mg of leucovorin and 100 mg of fresh baker's yeast daily. This will not interfere with the antiparasitic activity of the drug, but will counteract its hematologic effects. Unfortunately there is no evidence that this treatment affects intracellular or encysted organisms. In newborn infants with active disease the most that can be hoped for is that further damage will be prevented, but its regression cannot be expected.

PREVENTION. The identification of the cat as a producer of infective oocysts has led to much interest in potential sources of infection for humans, especially the pregnant female. Because unjustifiable conclusions as to the risk of acquiring toxoplasmosis often have been drawn both by physicians and lay persons, a few simple guidelines may be in order: Those women who have antibodies prior to pregnancy are safe from further difficulty. Those who do not have antibodies or who have not been tested should be guided as follows: eat only thoroughly cooked meat during pregnancy and avoid handling cat litter. A cat known to have antibodies presents no problem. Cats kept indoors, maintained on prepared diets and not fed fresh, uncooked meat also should present no problem. At its worst, the overall risk is small, both for mother and fetus.

HARRY A. FELDMAN

Desmonts, G. and Couvreur, J.: Congenital toxoplasmosis: A prospective study of 378 pregnancies. New Engl. J. Med. *290*:110, 1974.

Feldman, H. A.: Toxoplasmosis (Medical Progress). New Engl. J. Med. *279*:1370; 1431, 1968.

Hentsch, D. (ed.): Toxoplasmosis. Bern, Hans Huber Publishers, 1971.

Hutchison, W. M., and Dunachie, J. F.: The life cycle of the coccidian parasite, *Toxoplasma gondii,* in the domestic cat. Trans. Roy. Soc. Trop. Med. Hyg. *65*:380, 1971.

PRIMARY AMEBIC MENINGOENCEPHALITIS

ETIOLOGY. Acute meningoencephalitis in children or young adults with a history of recent swimming in stagnant fresh water lakes or pools, or warm mineral springs, may be caused by a type of amebic organism which, though free-living in nature, is capable of invasion of the central nervous system, apparently via the olfactory mucosa. The amebae that have been firmly identified with this type of infection belong to the genus *Naegleria,* characterized as medium in size and elongate in shape when moving (average dimensions, 22 by 7 μ), and as having a nucleus with a large central karyosome, a clear ectoplasm and a more granular endoplasm containing vacuoles. The amebae are capable of forming spherical, smooth-walled, resistant cysts or of transforming into actively free-swimming biflagellate forms, ameboflagellates, which may again become trophic amebae.

EPIDEMIOLOGY. Human infections were first reported in Australia and the United States in 1965. By early 1972 more than 60 cases had been reported from various parts of the world, including Australia, the United States, Czechoslovakia, New Zealand, Great Britain, Belgium and East Africa. With few exceptions, the disease has been reported in young people 7 to 20 years of age who apparently acquired the infection while swimming. In one locality of South Australia, strains of *Naegleria* pathogenic for mice were isolated from domestic water supplies as well as from surface water.

PATHOLOGY. The amebae invade the meninges, olfactory bulbs and brain substance, particularly the gray matter of the frontal, temporal and cerebellar regions. Invasion may extend to the spinal cord. Massive amebic reproduction and extension along the vessels and channels results in disorganization and necrosis of the invaded tissues. Clusters and space-filling masses of amebae can be readily demonstrated in histopathologic sections of the affected areas.

CLINICAL MANIFESTATIONS. Following a brief incubation period of 3 to 7 days, usually 3 or 4 days, there is in most cases sudden appearance of frontal or occipital headache and fever, which rapidly increase and are followed by vomiting, neck rigidity and coma; death from increased intracranial pressure and cardiorespiratory failure may occur as early as the fourth day of illness. The disease closely resembles acute bacterial meningitis, and failure to find pathogenic bacteria in purulent cerebrospinal fluid during specific examination of the fluid for amebae may offer an early clue to diagnosis.

DIAGNOSIS. Motile trophozoites can be demonstrated in temporary wet mounts of uncentrifuged and unrefrigerated cerebrospinal fluid, examined microscopically at a magnification and with lighting that is optimal for viewing leukocytes. The amebae are readily distinguishable from other cells by the relatively rapid directional movement and greater size. Although the direct wet mount examination is the most rapid and reliable means of diagnosis, the organisms can occasionally be recognized in stained smears and can be isolated in culture (plain agar seeded with *Escherichia coli*).

PROGNOSIS. Of the 60 or more patients reported with a firm diagnosis of primary amebic meningoencephalitis, few have survived. In one case with a confirmed diagnosis of *Naegleria fowleri* infection, treatment with amphotericin B was started on the fourth day of illness and the patient recovered. One other patient survived when similarly treated. In three other cases the patients recovered, but the diagnosis was uncertain and different forms of treatment were used.

PREVENTION. Swimming in warm, stagnant, fresh water lakes, ponds or pools should be avoided. No other preventive measure is known.

TREATMENT. The scant experience to date indicates that the drug of choice is amphotericin B. In the one clear-cut record of success (a 14 year old boy reported by Carter in 1972), the drug was given in a dose of 1 mg/kg/day intravenously beginning on the fourth day of illness, and three other drugs that had been given during the 3 previous days (penicillin, ampicillin, sulfadiazine) were continued. Marked improvement was noted in 2 days, but amebae were still present in the cerebrospinal fluid even after 5 days. Amphotericin B was then given intrathecally and later intraventricularly in doses of 0.1 mg on alternate days. Survival was attributed to the amphotericin B, but it was felt that sulfadiazine should always be used as well because the involved organism might possibly prove to be a different type of soil ameba which in experimental studies appeared to be affected by sulfadiazine. It was noted also that use of corticosteroids should be avoided, since they may combine with amphotericin B.

PAUL C. BEAVER

Anderson, K., and Jamieson, A.: Primary amoebic meningoencephalitis. Lancet *2*:379, 1972.

Butt, C. G.: Primary amebic meningoencephalitis. New Engl. J. Med. *274*:1473, 1966.

Callicott, J. H., Jr.: Amebic meningoencephalitis due to free-living amebas of the Hartmannella (Acanthamoeba)-Naegleria group. Am. J. Clin. Path. *49*:84, 1968.

Carter, R. F.: Primary amoebic meningoencephalitis. An appraisal of present knowledge. Trans. Roy. Soc. Trop. Med. Hyg. *66*:193, 1972.

Cerva, L., Novak, K., and Culbertson, C. G.: An outbreak of acute, fatal amebic meningoencephalitis. Am. J. Epidemiol. *88*:436, 1968.

Culbertson, C. G.: The pathogenicity of soil amebas. Ann. Rev. Microbiol. *25*:231, 1971.

Duma, R. J., Ferrell, H. W., Nelson, C., and Jones, M. M.: Primary amebic meningoencephalitis. New Engl. J. Med. *281*:1315, 1969.

Duma, R. J., Rosenblum, W. I., McGehee, R. F., Jones, M. M., and Nelson, E. C.: Primary amoebic meningoencephalitis caused by *Naegleria.* Two new cases, response to amphotericin B, and a review. Ann. Intern. Med. *74*:923, 1971.

Hecht, R. H., Cohen, A. H., Stoner, J., and Irwin, C.: Primary amebic meningoencephalitis in California. Calif. Med. *117*(1):69, 1972.

INTESTINAL PROTOZOA

The severity of disease produced by protozoa is not necessarily proportional to the size of the inoculum. Though protozoa are capable of developing colonies of limitless size, the ultimate population is limited by the area of suitable habitat and other factors. Once the colony is established, its reproductive potential is in part used for production of transfer stages which infect other hosts.

The life cycle of an intestinal protozoan colony typically begins with a single cell, a *trophozoite* (vegetative stage), which has one or more nuclei and specialized structures for locomotion. The trophozoite grows and reproduces by binary fission (*Isospora* excepted). In some of the trophozoites the vegetative functions are interrupted, an enveloping membrane is secreted by the organism, and, thus immobilized, it is eliminated in the feces. In this stage it is infective and is referred to as a *cyst*, not to be confused with the eggs of higher animals or spores of other organisms. The protozoan cyst is fairly resistant to external conditions, but it rarely reaches a new host in a viable state except in relatively cool, moist media. When the cyst is ingested and reaches its normal habitat in the intestine, it ruptures its membrane, and the organism resumes its vegetative functions. Then by a succession of generations a new colony is formed, and the cycle is repeated.

Of the several species of protozoa found in the human intestine, six are amebae (*Entamoeba histolytica, E. hartmanni, E. coli, Endolimax nana, Iodamoeba buetschlii, Dientamoeba fragilis*), three are flagellates (*Giardia lamblia, Chilomastix mesnili, Trichomonas hominis*), one is a ciliate (*Balantidium coli*) and two are sporozoa (*Isospora* species). Only two, *E. histolytica* and *B. coli*, produce serious disease in man, though *D. fragilis*, *E. hartmanni* and *G. lamblia* are frequently classified as pathogens. Isospora infection rarely occurs in man; it usually produces only mild symptoms and tends to be self-terminating.

AMEBIASIS

ETIOLOGY. Amebiasis is usually regarded as synonymous with *Entamoeba histolytica* infection. If one of the other species is suspected of producing symptoms, treatment for the illness can be the same as for infection with *E. histolytica*.

Entamoeba histolytica inhabits the colon. It is frequently found in symptomless carriers and is thought by some to be a harmless commensal in the majority of instances. It is capable of deep invasion of the bowel wall, however, and of being transported to other organs, especially the liver, where it may cause serious damage.

EPIDEMIOLOGY. Amebiasis is found in all parts of the world, especially in the tropics, but, like other filth-borne diseases, its distribution and prevalence correlate more closely with standards of personal hygiene and sanitation than with climate. Infection rates may exceed 50 per cent in densely populated unsanitary areas and may be extremely low in well sanitated groups. In the United States amebiasis is probably most prevalent in the South Central States. In the Charity Hospital at New Orleans routine examinations reveal *E. histolytica* in approximately 2 per cent of stools. Possibly because amebiasis is more difficult to diagnose in children than in adults, surveys usually show a higher incidence in adults. Infrequently the disease appears in epidemic form. The mortality rate in the United States is less than 0.1 per 100,000 population.

Infection is passed from person to person by means of relatively nonresistant but extremely abundant cysts in feces which, in diverse but mostly unproved ways, contaminate food and water.

Infective cysts passed in stools vary from too few to be detected by ordinary means to many millions a day. Stools from 10 consecutive patients averaged 241 cysts per mg of feces. A housefly or cockroach may ingest much more than a milligram of feces, the amebic cysts passing through its intestine unharmed.

Cysts are killed immediately by desiccation and by temperatures above 55° C, but may survive for months in water at temperatures below 20° C. They are killed by all commonly used disinfectants, but not by ordinary chlorination of water. There are no important animal reservoirs of amebic infection, though monkeys, apes and dogs may harbor natural infections, and other animals are readily infected in the laboratory. Amebic infection in dogs is relatively common, but as they rarely pass cysts they are not an important source of human infection.

PATHOLOGY. Some strains of *E. histolytica* are more pathogenic than others, and some which fail to produce symptoms in one person may readily produce disease in another. Infection may exist without evidence of disease, other than an abundance of cysts in the stools, and later develop into frank dysentery. Conversely, dysentery may be followed by a carrier state without evidence of disease.

Although massive colonization over its unbroken surface may deleteriously affect the mucosa, the only known means by which amebae produce disease is by tissue destruction in the colon or in other organs secondarily colonized by way of the bloodstream. The colon is most frequently invaded at the cecal and sigmoidorectal levels, but involvement varies greatly in area and in depth, the extreme being the full length of the organ and all layers, even to or through the serosa. The older lesions are complicated by secondary bacterial invasion, and there are various degrees of inflammation and suppuration. Microscopically the presence of amebae is diagnostic.

The hepatic lesion, the amebic liver abscess, is more characteristic. It usually contains a pasty, liver-colored material. Occasionally this material is mixed with purulent exudate, and the demonstration of amebae, essential for positive diagnosis, is more difficult.

CLINICAL MANIFESTATIONS. The signs and symptoms of intestinal amebiasis are largely those of nonspecific regional ulcerative colitis. Varying from mild irritation to extensive destruction of the bowel wall, from involvement of one or more local areas to that of the entire organ and from transient minor clinical disturbances to severe chronic disease, the manifestations of amebic infection are so diverse that presence or absence of intestinal amebiasis can be established only with the aid of a microscope. Any abnormal bowel activity, unusual stools, abdominal complaints or physical findings suggestive of colonic disease should be an indication for microscopic examination of stools for amebae.

In severe amebic colitis, in contrast to bacillary dysentery, the onset is not likely to be sudden. Fever and leukocytosis are slight or absent, and the stools lack the odor and appearance of containing pus; i.e., the mucus is clear instead of being whitish or yellowish, and the odor is reminiscent of autolytic rather than suppurative processes. In this latter respect the diarrheas caused by *E. histolytica* and by whipworm *(Trichuris trichiura)* infections are identical.

The presence of an *amebic abscess of the liver* is suggested by chills, fever, leukocytosis and right upper quadrant tenderness or pain, especially if accompanied by physical signs or roentgenographic evidence of a bulging mass. The demonstration of colonic amebiasis would be supportive evidence, but other causes should be considered. In regions where *Ascaris lumbricoides* is endemic, abscess formation around adult worms in the liver, or enlargement and tenderness of the liver resulting from migrating larvae, is much more frequent in children than is hepatic amebiasis.

DIAGNOSIS. The diagnosis of parasitic infections by stool examination presents two distinct problems: the detection of some stage of the organism and its identification.

Since all stages of amebae in feces or other material retain their normal appearance longer at room temperature than at body temperature and even longer under refrigeration (but not frozen), stools should be refrigerated promptly if examination is to be delayed more than 1 hour.

Abnormal elements in stools, such as mineral oil, fats, bismuth, kaolin, barium, certain foods such as bananas and milk and excessive amounts of undigestible pulpy fruits and vegetables, diminish the chances of finding amebae in the stools.

The specimen obtained by purgation, saline enema or proctoscopy has only the advantage of being delivered fresh and at a convenient time. A large specimen permits selection of favorable samples, but overemphasis of this factor may delay diagnosis, especially of waning dysentery. An ideal microscopic preparation contains only 1 to 2 mg of feces, and most concentration methods require less than 1 gm. A fleck of feces obtained from the rectum on the gloved finger or from a saline enema may be sufficient.

If reliable diagnostic service is not locally available, fecal specimens and material aspirated from the colon or from liver abscesses may be satisfactorily preserved and mailed to distant laboratories by using one of the procedures described below. The material *must* be freshly collected and well mixed with the fixative-preservative.

Methods for Preservation of Stools. Full-strength commercial formaldehyde diluted 1 part with 9 parts of water is a good general fixative-preservative. An adequate specimen is 1 ml of feces in 10 ml of fixative. On reaching the laboratory the material is examined directly or after concentration by centrifugal sedimentation. This is not satisfactory for dysenteric stools.

Preferred for dysenteric stools, and satisfactory for other types, is a fixative-preservative consisting of two solutions, stored separately and mixed immediately before use. Solution I is 40 parts of tincture of Merthiolate (Lilly), 5 parts of formaldehyde (USP) and 1 part of glycerin. Solution II is freshly prepared Lugol's solution (5 per cent iodine in 10 per cent aqueous potassium iodide solution). For use, combine 15 parts of solution I with 1 part of solution II. An adequate specimen is 1 ml of feces in 8 to 10 ml of preservative. Wet smears of the mixed specimen or the sediment are examined microscopically without further staining.

Cultures of fecal or aspirated material are generally not practical. Serologic tests are not used routinely.

PROGNOSIS. Once a diagnosis of colonic amebiasis has been made, prompt eradication of the parasite is possible. Chronic refractory infections requiring long, varied treatments are exceptional. With proper corrective and supportive measures even severe dysentery can usually be controlled within a few days and cured within 2 or 3 weeks. Except for amebic abscess of the brain, which is rare even in adults, the prognosis is also good in extraintestinal infections diagnosed early.

PREVENTION. Contaminated water and food are probably the only important sources of amebic infection. In children the transfer of infection occasionally may be more direct. Water may be made safe by boiling. When this is impractical, hyperchlorination or halogenation with iodine by means of commercially available preparations is possible. Thoroughly dried foods may be regarded as safe. Rooty vegetables and fruits can be washed and peeled, and leafy vegetables can be safely eaten after immersion in aqueous iodine disinfectant or in full-strength vinegar (5 per cent acetic acid) for 15 to 20 minutes at room temperature.

TREATMENT. For children with mild or asymptomatic intestinal amebiasis the choice between a number of relatively safe and effective drugs can be somewhat arbitrary. Diiodohydroxyquin (Diodoquin), glycobiarsol (Milibis), iodohydroxyquinoline (Chiniofon, Anayodin, Yatrin), iodochlorhydroxyquin (Entero-Vioform) and others are often satisfactory. Recently it was found that metronidazole (Flagyl) is effective for acute amebic dysentery or severe diarrhea caused by *E. histolytica,* as well as for mild infections. Tetracycline or emetine may be given for more rapid control of symptoms, but because of cost, toxicity and cure rates they usually are not recommended as curative. Metronidazole is administered orally in a dosage of 50 mg/kg/day in two or three divided doses for 10 days for children 4 to 8 years of age, 750 mg three times daily for 5 to 10 days for older children and adults.

Two or more fecal examinations should be made at weekly intervals after completion of treatment. Because amebae may appear in the stools within a few days after reinfection, positive findings on treated outpatients should not be interpreted as necessarily indicating failure of treatment.

Hepatic amebiasis, in the presence of demonstrated or suspected infection of the colon, was until recently usually treated with chloroquine diphosphate. The current drug of choice is metronidazole, given for 10 days in the same daily dosage as for intestinal amebiasis. If treatment with metronidazole is unsuccessful, emetine or dehydroemetine may be used. Emetine is obtainable in 1-ml ampules containing 65 mg of emetine hydrochloride and is injected intramuscularly in a dosage of 1 mg/kg body weight daily for not more than 10 days, and never in excess of 65 mg per day. As emetine may produce neuritis or severe myocarditis, its use should not be repeated in less than a month. Dehydroemetine, possibly less toxic than emetine and comparable in action, is administered in the same manner and dosage. To obtain higher cure rates, treatment with emetine or dehydroemetine can be supplemented with a course of chloroquine diphosphate: for children less than 6 years of age, 250 mg twice daily for 2 days followed by 125 mg twice daily for 12 additional days; for older children and adults, the dose is doubled.

GIARDIASIS

Giardia lamblia is most frequently found in the tropics and subtropics, its distribution seeming to vary with economic, hygienic and sanitary conditions. Prevalence rates, generally highest in children 5 to 10 years of age, exceed 10 per cent in some communities. The parasite may be transmitted by food and water and by houseflies, or directly from person to person.

The flagellate usually lives in the duodenum and upper jejunum, where it may persist for years, or disappear spontaneously, especially in older children and adults. Trophozoites die within a few hours outside the body, but cysts may remain viable for several days.

As in the case of *E. histolytica* and some other organisms, the pathogenicity of *G. lamblia* is unpredictable and the virulence factors are poorly understood. The organism frequently occurs in stools of children with a variety of complaints referable to the intestinal tract, and conditions resembling sprue or celiac disease have been attributed to it.

Fortunately the infection is easily eradicated by drugs that are neither expensive nor very toxic. Quinacrine dihydrochloride (Atabrine) administered orally in 0.1-gm tablets for 5 days in the following dosage rarely if ever fails to result in complete removal of Giardia: for adults and children over 8 years of age, 1 tablet three times daily; for children 4 to 8 years, 1/2 tablet on the same schedule; and for younger children, 1/2 tablet twice daily. Metronidazole (Flagyl) is also effective; it is given in doses of 250 mg twice daily for children 4 to 8 years of age, or three times daily for older children and adults, for 5 days.

BALANTIDIASIS

Balantidium coli is a parasite which, like *E. histolytica*, colonizes the colon. More often than in man it is found in monkeys and pigs, both of which tolerate the infection without apparent damage. Although *Balantidium coli* is the only ciliate protozoon known to parasitize the human colon, numerous morphologically similar organisms are frequent in stools as contaminants and may lead to errors in diagnosis. Diagnosis is established by the presence of either the more or less uniformly ciliated, large, rapidly motile trophozoites or the large spherical cysts.

Balantidiasis is rare in the United States, but is relatively common in Puerto Rico, Mexico and various parts of South America. In 1971 an epidemic involving 110 persons occurred on Truk in the Caroline Islands following a typhoon. Most of the human infections apparently are derived from pigs. Under crowded or unsanitary conditions, person-to-person transfer of infective cysts can occur. As a rule, however, cysts are formed only sparingly or not at all in the human intestine.

Typically the infection is of short duration, producing in children a disease similar to amebic dysentery. The pathologic changes are similar in distribution and nature. The chief difference is the greater tendency of balantidiasis toward spontaneous cure. This factor has led to variable interpretations of the curative value of tested drugs. Satisfactory results appear to be obtained with tetracycline given orally in doses of 8 to 10 mg per pound three times daily for 10 days, the total dose not to exceed 2 gm.

PAUL C. BEAVER

GENERAL

Faust, E. C., Beaver, P. C., and Jung, R. C.: Animal Agents and Vectors of Human Disease. 3rd ed. Philadelphia, Lea & Febiger, 1968.

Jelliffe, D. B. (ed.): Diseases of Children in the Subtropics and Tropics. 2nd ed. London, Edward Arnold, Ltd., 1970.

Most, H.: Treatment of common parasitic infections of man encountered in the United States. New Engl. J. Med. *287*:495; 698, 1972.

Neva, F. A.: Parasitic diseases of the GI tract in the United States. Disease-a-Month, June, 1972.

Amebiasis

Beaver, P. C.: The exudates in amebic colitis. Proc. VI Int. Congr. Trop. Med. & Malaria, Lisbon, 1958, *3*:419.

Brooke, M. M.: Epidemiology of amebiasis in the U.S. J.A.M.A. *188*:519, 1964.

Gilman, R. H., and Prathap, K.: Acute intestinal amoebiasis—Proctoscopic appearances with histopathological correlation. Ann. Trop. Med. Parasitol. *65*:359, 1972.

Neal, R. A.: Pathogenesis of amebiasis. Bull. N.Y. Acad. Med. *47*:462, 1971.

Powell, S. J.: Therapy of amebiasis. Bull. N.Y. Acad. Med. *47*:469, 1971.

Scragg, J. N., and Powell, S. J.: Metronidazole and niridazole combined with dehydroemetine in treatment of children with amoebic liver abscess. Arch. Dis. Child. *45*:193, 1970.

Giardiasis

Cortner, J. A.: Giardiasis, a cause of celiac syndrome. Am. J. Dis. Child. *98*:311, 1959.

Moore, G. T., and others.: Epidemic giardiasis at a ski resort. New Engl. J. Med. *281*:402, 1969.

Balantidiasis

Arean, V. M., and Koppisch, E.: Balantidiasis: A review and report of cases. Am. J. Path. *32*:1089, 1956.

Shookhoff, H.: *Balantidium coli* infection, with special reference to treatment. Am. J. Trop. Med. *31*:442, 1951.

Walzer, P. D., Judson, F. N., and others.: Balantidiasis outbreak in Truk. Am. J. Trop. Med. Hyg. *22*:33, 1973.

11

THE DIGESTIVE SYSTEM

THE ORAL CAVITY

The condition of the oral cavity is important to physical and psychologic health and the sense of well-being. The recognition and treatment of oral abnormalities and diseases, particularly in infancy and early childhood, require cooperative effort between physicians and dentists. Initially the physician's role is predominant; later it is the dentist who has the most opportunity for periodic observation of the child as well as of his mouth. Many oral abnormalities are associated with systemic conditions and are best handled through coordinated efforts; the physician should identify and utilize the services of those dentists in his community, usually pedodontists or orthodontists, who share his concern for the psychologic and physical health of children.

The principal consideration in the oral health of children is the establishment of an intact, balanced, self-maintaining permanent dentition. Dental examination at 2½ to 3 years of age permits a careful evaluation of oral health, including the pattern of eruption and completeness of the dentition, tooth-to-tooth and arch-to-arch relations, facial growth, and condition of the enamel and dentin. Needed restorations may be made at this time, as well as plans for the treatment of other abnormalities. Regular, periodic surveillance is necessary throughout childhood to ensure that teeth are not lost through caries and that malocclusions receive timely correction; periodontal disease of adults is often traceable to caries or malocclusion not treated during childhood.

ABNORMALITIES IN GROWTH AND DEVELOPMENT OF THE JAWS AND TEETH

DEVELOPMENT OF THE JAWS

The lower portions of the head mature much later than the cranium. The jaws and teeth continue to undergo change until late adolescence.

MAXILLA. The maxillary bone is formed in utero from a fusion of the maxilla and premaxilla; the latter contains the upper incisors and anterior portion of the palate. Sutures are formed with the adjoining maxillary, zygomatic, frontal and palatine bones. The inclination of the sutures determines the direction of enlargement of the maxillary bone. Growth at these sutures results in forward and downward movement of the maxilla in relation to the base of the cranium. Remodeling and appositional bone growth result in the maxillary sinuses, alveolar ridges and mature facial contours. Transverse growth is by proliferation of bone at the median palatal suture and at the outer surface of the maxilla. As with other sutures, bony union occurs and growth terminates during adolescence.

MANDIBLE. The mandible arises both from centers of ossification and from bony replacement of portions of Meckel's cartilage. Longitudinal growth is accomplished by interstitial bone growth at the condyles. The ramus maintains its configuration through resorption on the anterior border and deposition of bone on the posterior border. The body of the mandible also undergoes appositional growth at the alveolar ridges and inferior border. Condylar growth normally stops with adolescence, but the potential for further growth remains.

ABNORMALITIES OF JAW GROWTH. The upper and lower jaws have dissimilar patterns of longitudinal growth. The maxillary bone moves forward and downward through appositional and sutural growth, whereas the mandible enlarges in a similar direction through interstitial bone growth. Consequently, disturbances which affect connective tissue alter maxillary growth; abnormalities in cartilaginous growth alter mandibular growth. For example, in cleidocranial dysostosis and craniofacial dysostosis sutural growth is retarded, and the maxillary complex is relatively smaller than the mandible. On the other hand, in acromegaly cartilage grows more rapidly than connective tissue, and the mandible becomes much larger than the maxilla, resulting in class III malocclusion.

FACIAL ASYMMETRY. Molding of the head during birth is possible because the bones of the cranium are not fused and can override. No such mechanism of adjustment to the narrow birth canal is present in the face. The mandible is the only movable bone in the face and is attached to the cranium only at its condylar head by the muscles of mastication. Facial asymmetries resulting from excessive molding of the cranium or from displacement of the mandible during breech or face presentations are fairly common and are usually self-correcting. Facial asymmetry resulting from injury to the growing cartilage or fracture of the condylar head during birth, infancy or early childhood is also common, but the effects may be permanent. Traumatic injuries may occur during birth from the placing of obstetric forceps over the area or may result from blows on the chin during infancy and childhood.

Injuries, acute infections or arthritis of the growing condylar cartilage may result in partial (fibrous) or complete (bony) *ankylosis of the temporomandibular joint* and failure of that side of the mandible to grow. The normal side, meanwhile, continues to grow and pushes the midline toward the affected side. The midline deviation is exaggerated during mouth opening. Roentgenograms of the affected side reveal an increased preangular notch or displaced condylar head. Bilateral injuries to the growing cartilage result in failure of the mandible and chin to grow downward and forward, causing the entire mandible to be considerably smaller than normal and much retruded.

HYPOPLASIA OF THE MANDIBLE

Pierre Robin Syndrome. The Pierre Robin syndrome consists of micrognathia with associated pseudomacroglossia, glossoptosis and high-arched or cleft palate. Posterior displacement of the attachment of the genioglossus muscle to the hypoplastic mandible prevents the normal anchorage of the tongue. Under the influence of gravity the tongue assumes a retruded position, obstructing the pharynx. A postalveolar cleft of the hard and soft palates is a common but not constant feature. In some instances the palate is high-arched.

Although the tongue is usually of normal size, the floor of the mouth is foreshortened and the buccal cavity reduced in size. The lack of space further contributes to the glossoptosis. The obstruction of the air passages, particularly on inspiration, usually requires treatment in order to avoid suffocation. The infant should be placed in the prone or partially prone position so that the tongue falls forward to relieve respiratory obstruction. In a number of instances further treatment, such as temporarily suturing the ventral surface of the tongue to the lower lip, or tracheotomy, is not necessary, since sufficient mandibular growth usually takes place within a few months to relieve the glossoptosis. A variety of splints and traction devices designed to pull the mandible forward have been unsuccessful. The feeding of infants with mandibular hypoplasia requires great care and patience, but can usually be accomplished without resort to gavage. Often the growth of the mandible will progress so that an essentially normal profile is achieved within 4 to 6 years. A variety of dental anomalies usually require individual treatment.

Mandibulofacial Dysostosis. In mandibulofacial dysostosis (Treacher Collins syndrome, Franceschetti-Klein syndrome) there is less severe micrognathia than in the Pierre Robin syndrome. The facial appearance is characterized by palpebral fissures sloping downward toward the outer canthi, coloboma of the lower eyelids, sunken cheekbones, blind fistulas opening between the angles of the mouth and the ears, deformed pinna, atypical hair growth extending toward the cheeks, receding chin and large mouth. Facial clefts, diseases of the ears and deafness are common. The disorder is transmitted as a dominant trait, but expression is often incomplete. The mandible is almost always hypoplastic; the undersurface is often pronouncedly concave, the ramus may be deficient, and the coronoid and condyloid processes are flat or even aplastic. The palatal vault may be either high or cleft (about 40 per cent). Infrequently, unilateral or bilateral macrostomia, or failure of embryonic fusion of the maxillary and mandibular processes, may occur. Owing to poor maxillary development and palatal deformity, dental malocclusions are frequent. The teeth may be widely separated, hypoplastic, displaced or have an open bite. Orthodontic and routine dental treatments are indicated.

Unilateral Hypoplasia of the Mandible is sometimes part of an anomaly that includes partial paralysis of the facial nerve, macrostomia, blind fistulas between the angles of the mouth and the ears, and deformed ear lobes. Owing to the absence or hypoplasia of the mandibular condyle on the affected side, severe facial asymmetry and malocclusion develop. When there is early roentgenographic evidence of congenital condylar deformity, the deformity tends to increase with age. Plastic surgical procedures may be indicated early to minimize the deformity.

DISEASES OF THE JAWS

CAFFEY'S DISEASE (INFANTILE CORTICAL HYPEROSTOSIS). See Section 22.

OSTEOMYELITIS. (See Section 22.) In the newborn infant, osteomyelitis tends to occur in the area of the premaxillary suture, but during childhood the mandible is the more common location. The infection is marked by swelling and redness of the oral mucosa or skin, associated with pain, fever and lymphadenopathy. Drainage should be established and the exudate cultured so that an appropriate antibiotic may be administered. Large sequestra may require surgical removal.

RETICULOENDOTHELIOSIS (HISTIOCYTOSIS X). (See Section 26). Oral lesions may occur in any of the syndromes and may be an early manifestation. Lesions of the jaws may produce pain, swelling, loosening of teeth and fetid breath. Healing is often delayed after dental extraction. Dental roentgenograms may reveal spongelike patterns in bones with distinct "punched-out" areas.

NEOPLASMS. (See Section 25.) **Benign Tumors.** ***Ossifying Fibroma.*** This is perhaps the most common tumor of the jaws. Prior to puberty its growth is rapid, after which it may slow or even cease. Cell-rich connective tissue invades bone and undergoes gradual ossification. Since the lesion is painless, a unilateral soft tissue swelling is usually the first sign. The radiologic features vary with the degree of mineralization; there is a transition from radiolucency to a mottled, "ground-glass" appearance. The tumor is benign; most patients do not require treatment. If the lesion is extensive, curettage or further surgical correction may be required.

Cysts of Jaw. *Multiple basal cell nevoid syndrome.* See Section 23.

Malignant Tumors. The malignant tumors of the jaws which occur in children include Burkitt's sarcoma, osteogenic sarcoma, lymphosarcoma and, more rarely, fibrosarcoma.

DEVELOPMENT OF THE TEETH AND ASSOCIATED ABNORMALITIES

INITIATION. The teeth form in dental crypts which arise from a band of epithelial cells incorporated into each developing jaw. Prior to the calcification of the maxilla and mandible a ribbon of epithelial cells grows inward from the oral epithelium into the underlying mesenchyme. By the twelfth week of fetal life these epithelial bands, the *dental lamina,* each have five areas of rapid growth, which result in rounded, budlike enlargements. An accompanying organization of the mesenchyme adjacent to each area of epithelial growth takes place, and the two elements together constitute the beginning stages of a tooth. Five such areas on each side of the maxilla and of the mandible initiate the primary dentition.

The *permanent teeth* form in two groups. After the formation of the primary crypts a bandlike extension of the dental lamina proliferates lingually from each side to form another generation of tooth buds for the permanent incisors, cuspids and premolars, which erupt into sites previously occupied by primary teeth. This takes place from about the fifth gestational month for the central incisors to about 10 months of age for the second bicuspids. The permanent molars, on the other hand, arise from a backward extension of the dental lamina beyond the site of initiation of the second primary molars. Three budlike enlargements form sequentially at approximately 4 months of gestation, and 1 year and 4 to 5 years, respectively, for each of the three permanent molars.

Both failures and excesses of tooth initiation are observed. *Anodontia,* or absence of teeth, occurs when no tooth buds form. *Total anodontia* often occurs with ectodermal dysplasia. *Partial anodontia* results when a normal site of initiation is disturbed, as in the area of a palatal cleft, or from genetic failure, frequently familial, to code the formation of specific teeth. The third molars, maxillary lateral incisors and mandibular second premolars are the teeth which most commonly fail to form.

If the dental lamina produces more than the normal number of buds, *supernumerary teeth* occur. These are most often seen in the area of the maxillary central incisors. Since they tend to disrupt the position and eruption of the adjacent normal teeth, their identification as supernumerary teeth by radiologic examination is important. *Natal teeth,* present at birth or erupting shortly thereafter, may be members of the normal primary dentition, but this should be verified radiologically, since they are often supernumerary teeth, which should be removed (see Natal Teeth, below).

HISTODIFFERENTIATION-MORPHODIFFERENTIATION. As the epithelial bud proliferates, the deeper surface invaginates and a mass of mesenchyme becomes partially enclosed. Beginning with the crown, the epithelial cells assume the shape of the tooth they represent, lay down the organic matrix for calcification of the enamel, and induce the underlying mesenchymal cells to become columnar. These cells, in turn, lay down the organic matrix for calcification of dentin. The vascular, nerve and lymph structures (the *dental pulp* of the mature tooth) are confined in the mesenchyme of the hollow central portion of the tooth bud. Disturbances during histodifferentiation-morphodifferentiation may result in gross alterations in dental morphology. *Macrodontia* and *microdontia,* large and small teeth, respectively, are caused at this formative point. The maxillary lateral incisors not only may be absent owing to failure of initiation, but also may assume a slender, tapering shape *("peg-shaped laterals").*

Twinning, in which two teeth are joined together, is most often observed in the mandibular incisors of the primary dentition. It may result from three separate causative possibilities: germination, fusion or concrescence. *Germination* is the result of division of a single tooth germ to form a bifid or cloven crown on a single root with a common pulp canal. An extra tooth is then present in the dental arch. *Fusion* is the joining of incompletely developed teeth that under pressure of trauma or crowding continue to develop as a single tooth. Fused teeth are sometimes joined through their entire length; in other instances a single wide crown is supported on two roots. *Concrescence* is the attachment of the roots of closely approximated adjacent teeth by an excessive deposition of cementum. This type of twinning, unlike the others, is found most often in the maxillary molar region. *Dens in dente,* a "tooth in a tooth," is a radiologic finding in a tooth of normal appearance. It results from an invagination in the lingual surface, usually of a maxillary incisor, at the site of fusion between separate sites of calcification in the same tooth. Enamel continues to be formed, and an enamel-lined hollow space results. The dental radiogram shows the outline of a second dental structure within a tooth.

Congenital syphilis affects differentiation of permanent teeth, resulting in screwdriver-shaped incisors, often with central notches in their incisive edges *(Hutchinson's incisors),* and *mulberry molars,* with lobular occlusal surfaces and narrow, pinched crowns.

CALCIFICATION. Calcification, the deposition of

the inorganic mineral crystals of mature enamel and dentin, takes place after the organic matrix has been laid down. Disturbances at this time affect the color, texture and thickness of the tooth surface. All teeth form from several sites of calcification which later coalesce. The characteristics of the inorganic portions of a tooth can be altered by (1) disturbances in formation of the matrix, (2) decreased availability of one or more of the minerals involved, and (3) the incorporation of foreign materials.

Amelogenesis imperfecta, a dominant genetic trait, results in faulty production of matrix. The teeth are covered by only a thin layer of abnormally formed enamel through which the yellow coloration of the underlying dentin is seen, giving a darkened appearance to the dentition. Usually all the teeth, both primary and permanent, are affected. Although susceptibility to caries is low, the enamel is subject to destruction from abrasion. Restorations offering complete coverage of the crowns are often placed for protection and improved appearance.

Dentinogenesis imperfecta, or hereditary opalescent dentin, is an analogous condition in which the odontoblasts fail to differentiate normally, and brown, poorly calcified dentin results. The junction between the enamel and dentin is altered, the enamel has a tendency to flake away, and the exposed dentin is then susceptible to abrasion. The teeth are opaque and pearly, and the pulp chambers are obliterated by calcification. Both primary and permanent teeth are usually involved. Unless the crowns of these teeth are covered early and completely, the abrasion of chewing often reduces them to the level and contour of the supporting alveolar bone.

Localized disturbances of calcification which correlate with periods of illness or malnutrition are frequent; they are analogous to the "growth disturbance lines" often seen in the long bones. An example is the *neonatal line* commonly observed on all the primary teeth and on the permanent central incisors and tips of cuspids at coronal levels consistent with the stage of calcification present at birth. Two general disturbances of the surface of the enamel are seen: Discoloration of the smooth surface, usually a more opaque white patch, is referred to as *hypocalcification.* A more severe disturbance, *hypoplasia,* may be manifest as pitting, or areas devoid of covering enamel. Hypoplasia is uncommon in the primary dentition because of the relative infrequency of intrauterine stress, as opposed to the frequent occurrence of illness or malnutrition during early infancy when the enamel of the outer third of the permanent incisors, cuspids and first molars is forming. Dental restoration of such areas is desirable to eliminate the sensitivity of exposed dentin, to prevent caries and to improve the appearance.

Mottled enamel is found in persons whose early life is spent in areas where the fluoride content of the drinking water is greater than two parts per million; it is probably due to ameloblastic dysfunction. It varies from small, inconspicuous white patches to severe, brownish discoloration and hypoplasia; the latter changes are usually seen with fluoride concentrations over 5 parts per million.

Disturbances due to mineral deficiency are rare, but irregular dentin and enlarged pulp chambers have been observed with vitamin D-resistant rickets, and hypoplasia with vitamin D-deficient rickets.

Discolored teeth may result from incorporation of foreign substances into developing enamel. The hemolysis accompanying *erythroblastosis fetalis* may produce blue to black discoloration of the primary teeth, beginning at the neonatal line; the tips of the permanent first molars may also be affected. *Tetracyclines,* extensively incorporated into bones and teeth, may result in ugly, brownish yellow discoloration and even hypoplasia of the enamel, if administered during the period of formation of enamel. This period extends from about the fourth month of gestation to the tenth month of life for the primary teeth and from about the fourth month to the sixteenth year of life for the permanent teeth. The enamel is completely formed on all but the third molars by about 8 years of age. Therefore, if possible, tetracyclines should not be prescribed for pregnant women or for children under 8 years of age. Discoloration of the teeth has been observed with *all* the tetracycline antibiotics. Fluorescence of the teeth under ultraviolet light is diagnostic.

ERUPTION. At the time of tooth bud formation each tooth begins a movement outward in relation to the bone; this movement is continuous. The full chronology of human dentition is given in Table 2–4; the relative times of eruption and shedding of the primary teeth and the times of eruption of the permanent teeth are listed in Tables 11–1 and 11–2.

The mandibular teeth usually erupt before their maxillary counterparts, as do those of girls before boys. As the teeth penetrate the gums, inflammation and sensitivity sometimes occur, a condition

TABLE 11–1 TIME OF ERUPTION AND SHEDDING OF THE PRIMARY TEETH*

	ERUPTION		SHEDDING	
	Lower Age (Months)	Upper	Lower Age (Years)	Upper
Central incisor	6	7½	6	7½
Lateral incisor	7	9	7	8
Cuspid	16	18	9½	11½
First molar	12	14	10	10½
Second molar	20	24	11	10½
Incisors	Range ± 2 mos.		Range ± 6 mos.	
Molars	Range ± 4 mos.			

*From Massler and Schour: Atlas of the Mouth. Chicago, American Dental Association.

TABLE 11–2 TIME OF ERUPTION OF THE PERMANENT TEETH*

	LOWER AGE (YEARS)	UPPER AGE (YEARS)
Central incisors	6– 7	7– 8
Lateral incisors	7– 8	8– 9
Cuspids	9–10	11–12
First bicuspids	10–12	10–11
Second bicuspids	11–12	10–12
First molars	6– 7	6– 7
Second molars	11–13	12–13
Third molars	17–21	17–21

*From Massler and Schour: Atlas of the Mouth. Chicago, American Dental Association.

termed *difficult eruption.* The child may become irritable, and salivation may increase markedly. Bacterial invasion through a break in the tissue or under a gingival flap covering the teeth may be responsible. A blunt, firm object for the infant to bite on is useful; incision of the gums is seldom indicated. There is no definite evidence to support claims of accompanying temporary systemic disturbances. Such disturbances, the most common of which are low-grade fever, facial rashes and mild diarrhea, are not attributable to eruption of teeth.

Delayed eruption of all teeth may indicate systemic or nutritional disturbances such as hypopituitarism, hypothyroidism, cleidocranial dysostosis and rickets. Local causes such as malpositioning of teeth, supernumerary teeth, cysts or retained primary teeth may be responsible for failure of eruption of single or small groups of teeth.

Early loss of primary predecessors is the most common cause of *premature eruption* of teeth. If the entire dentition is advanced for age and sex, an endocrine disorder such as hyperpituitarism must be considered.

Natal Teeth. Erupted teeth are observed in approximately one of 2000 newborn infants. Usually there are two in the position of the mandibular central incisors. Their attachment is generally limited to the gingival margin, with little root formation or bony support; such teeth should not be considered supernumerary until a radiologic examination has proved them to be; a natal tooth may be a prematurely erupted primary tooth, an indication that generally early dental eruption may be expected.

The presence of teeth at birth may result in complications. Pain secondary to looseness and movement may interfere with nursing, as may maternal discomfort due to abrasion or biting of the nipple during feeding. There is danger of detachment with subsequent aspiration of the tooth. Since the tongue lies between the alveolar processes during birth, it may become lacerated, and occasionally the tip is amputated (Riga Fide's disease).

Supernumerary teeth should be extracted; the decision to extract prematurely erupted primary teeth must be made on an individual basis. Should extraction seem indicated, it should be performed by carefully dissecting away the gingival attachment to prevent tearing of the tissue and excessive hemorrhage.

Exfoliation Failure. This occurs when a primary tooth fails to exfoliate prior to the eruption of its permanent successor. The primary tooth should be extracted if the erupting permanent tooth becomes visible. The mandibular incisor region is the most common location for this occurrence.

DISORDERS OF THE TEETH ASSOCIATED WITH OTHER CONDITIONS

Osteogenesis imperfecta is usually accompanied by *hereditary opalescent dentin,* also termed *dentinogenesis imperfecta.* Treatment is usually not indicated.

In *cleidocranial dysostosis* there are a number of oral-facial variations. Frontal bossing, mandibular prognathism and a broadened base of the nose may be seen. Eruption of teeth is characteristically delayed. The primary teeth are abnormally retained, and the permanent teeth may remain unerupted. The presence of supernumerary teeth is common, especially in the premolar area. Erupted teeth are free of hypoplasia, but variations in size and shape are frequent. The primary dentition and those permanent teeth which do erupt should be restored if they become carious. Extraction of a primary tooth rarely results in the eruption of its permanent successor. The removal of the unerupted permanent teeth is also contraindicated. Their roots are usually crooked and curved, often leading to fracture during attempted removal.

In *ectodermal dysplasia* the teeth are totally or partially absent. Since alveolar bone does not develop in the absence of teeth, the alveolar processes are usually either totally or partially absent, and the resulting overclosure of the mandible causes the lips to protrude. Cephalometric growth studies have shown, however, that facial development is otherwise not disturbed. Teeth, when present, are small and conical in form. Aplasia of the buccal and labial mucous glands, leading to dryness and irritation of the oral mucosa, has also been observed. Persons with ectodermal dysplasia need either partial or full dentures. The vertical height between the jaws is thus restored, improving the position of the lips and facial contours. Masticatory function is restored, and eating habits are thereby improved.

DISEASES OF THE TEETH

Dental Caries

Dental caries, or decay of the teeth, is a progressive, destructive lesion of the calcified dental tissues. Untreated, it eventually results in total destruction of involved teeth. Dental caries is the

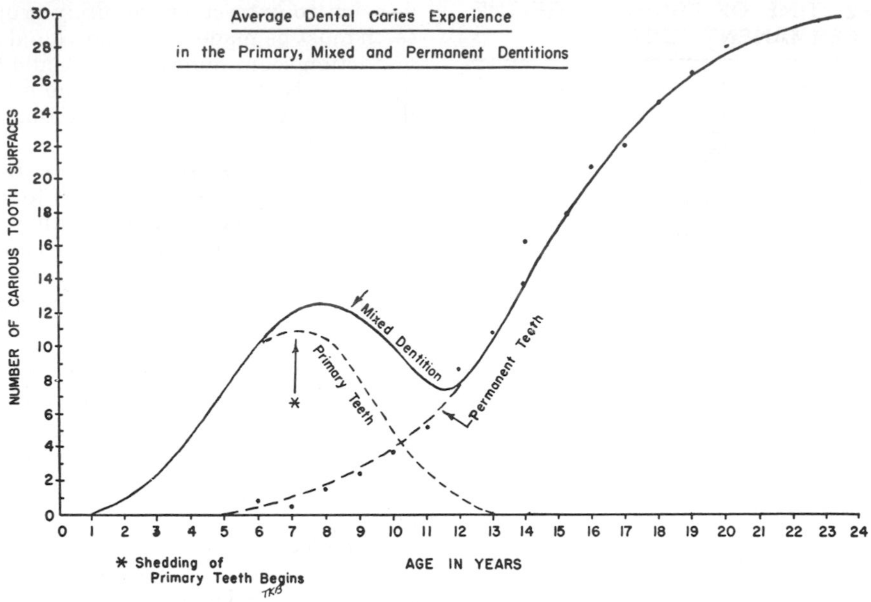

Figure 11–1 *Average number of carious surfaces at different age periods. (Brauer, J. C. et al.: Dentistry for Children. 4th ed. New York, The Blakiston Division, McGraw-Hill Book Company, Inc., 1959.)*

principal oral problem of children; by 2 years of age the average child has two carious lesions (Fig. 11–1).

ETIOLOGY. Dental caries is a bacterial disease, but many factors influence susceptibility. The causative organisms are principally streptococci; they produce extracellular polysaccharides that form a gelatinous plaque over the tooth to which the organisms adhere. Fermentable carbohydrates, and especially sucrose, are the main substrate for the production of metabolic acids by the adherent bacteria (Fig. 11–2). The acids first decalcify the enamel, and then cause lysis of the protein of the organic matrix and destruction of the tooth structure.

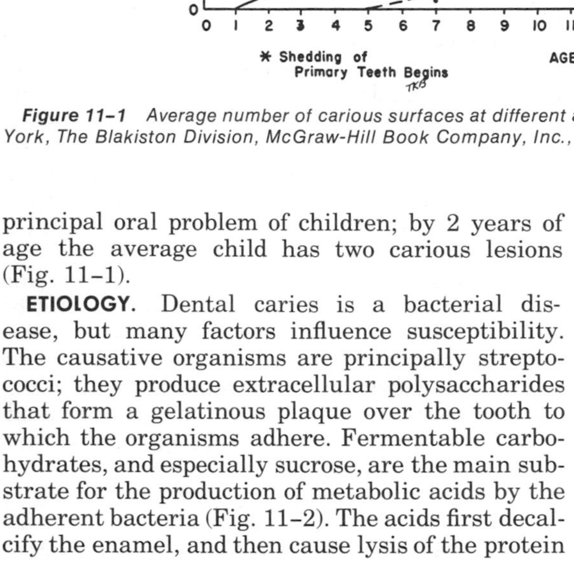

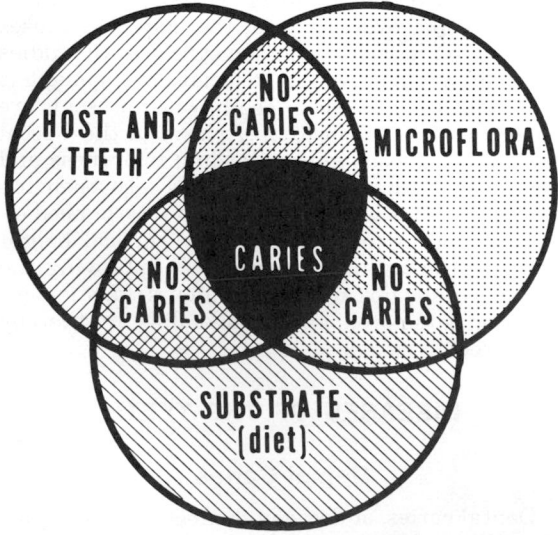

Figure 11–2 *Factors involved in causation of dental caries. All factors must be operative before caries will develop. (Keyes: Etiologic Factors of Dental Caries. Med. Ann. D.C. 34:463–7, 1968.)*

Factors Influencing Caries

Age. Caries is primarily a disease of childhood and adolescence. The periods of greatest carious activity are 4 to 8 years in the primary dentition and 12 to 18 years in the permanent dentition (Fig. 11–1). Ninety per cent of rampant caries occurs during the latter period.

Fluoride. The incorporation of fluoride into mineral apatite crystals appears to increase their resistance to acid dissolution. Children living in communities where the drinking water contains 1.0 part per million (p.p.m.) or more of fluoride have 40 to 60 per cent less caries than those in areas where the fluoride content is under 0.5 p.p.m. The maximal reduction in dental caries appears to occur when the drinking water contains 1.0 to 1.5 p.p.m. of fluoride. If the fluoride content is 2.0 to 2.5 p.p.m. or more, mottling of the enamel becomes evident.

Diet. An important factor contributing to caries is the ingestion between meals of foods or fluids containing sucrose, particularly in forms which cling, such as taffy, or promote prolonged contact with the teeth, such as lollipops and lozenges. Such ingestion provides the substrate for production of tooth-destroying acid by the bacteria adherent to the teeth. Sugars ingested at mealtime are less injurious, since the buffering capacity of other foods and saliva tends to neutralize the acid.

The practice of putting small children to sleep with a bottle of milk or other sweetened fluids results in pooling in the oral cavity. The acids produced by bacterial action on the substrate may also result in early, rampant caries. A prominent diagnostic feature of the condition is the progression of the destruction from the maxillary anteriors to the posterior teeth, with the lower anteriors relatively protected by the nipple and tongue. This practice is probably the most common cause of severe caries in children under 3 years of age.

Oral Hygiene. Lack of oral hygiene (rinsing and brushing, particularly after meals) permits the accumulation of food debris upon which the bacteria feed. The primary purpose of brushing and the use of dental floss is the removal of the bacteria-laden plaque, thereby reducing the quantity of oral microorganisms. The prevention of caries and of the early stages of periodontal disease depends upon the assistance of parents in the performing and supervising of oral hygiene procedures.

State of Health. In chronic debilitating diseases both the quantity and the bacteriostatic quality of saliva may be reduced. Oral hygiene after each meal is even more important than for the healthy person.

CLINICAL MANIFESTATIONS. Caries originates most often in areas where food may become impacted, as in the pits and fissures on the occlusal surfaces of the posterior teeth, between the teeth, or along the gum line at the neck of the tooth. The lesions may penetrate rapidly through the substance of the tooth, or their progress may be intermittent and slow. Rapidly burrowing caries is characteristic in children; the slow, intermittent type predominates in middle age.

PREVENTION. The most effective preventive measure against dental caries is *natural or artificial fluoridation of the water supply.*

If an adequate amount of fluoride (1.0 p.p.m.) is not present in the water supply either naturally or by municipal fluoridation, 0.5 mg of fluoride daily can be mixed with a quart of the water used for the formula, or added directly to cow's milk. Although fluoride absorption from milk is delayed in comparison to that from water, it is essentially complete. Children over 1 year of age should receive 0.5 to 1.0 mg of fluoride (1.1 to 2.2 mg of sodium fluoride) per day. Recent studies have shown that a beneficial effect is obtained with oral fluoride preparations even after teeth have erupted. This is probably due to topical incorporation of fluoride into the surface dental enamel. Therefore, when liquid preparations containing fluoride are given, the dose should be deposited into the buccal area with the head turned slightly sideways, or the *chewable* tablet should be prescribed in order to encourage oral retention and give time for surface contact. Such fluoride preparations are not recommended in areas where the water supply contains fluoride in excess of 0.7 part per million.

The prescription of *fluoride supplements* is not a substitute for fluoridation of community water supplies, since the latter ensures availability of adequate fluoride to *all* children in the area at a safe level and at a considerably lower cost. There is no definitive evidence that administration of fluoride to the pregnant woman reduces the incidence of caries in the child.

After dental eruption, biannual *topical application of fluoride* to the teeth increases the concentration of fluoride in the surface enamel where decay begins. Such applications are effective in areas with an adequate content of fluoride in the water supply, as well as in areas where the fluoride content of the water is inadequate.

Reduction of frequency of eating and *avoidance of sucrose-containing snacks, candies or drinks between meals* can markedly reduce the incidence of new carious lesions. The small child's "bedtime bottle" of milk should be avoided. If the habit has become established, replacement of the bottle with a cup of milk before brushing the teeth at bedtime is more effective than attempts at gradual withdrawal.

The *elimination of active lesions* by restoration of primary as well as permanent teeth reduces the bacterial population in the oral cavity and thereby the hazard to uninvolved teeth. When a child exhibits the rapid appearance and progression of new carious lesions, the usual 6-month interval between dental examinations may be inadequate; examination, particularly of the teenage child, may be repeated at 3-month intervals.

Proper *oral hygiene* also is most helpful in preventing caries. The mechanical removal of plaque and debris from tooth surfaces by brushing is important. Small children can be held in the lap. One hand can retract the lips while brushing is accomplished with the other. Brushing should be initiated on eruption of the first primary teeth. The child perceives the pattern and will eventually accomplish the procedure routinely without assistance. Parental assistance has usually been found to be necessary until at least 9 years of age. Visual inspection with or without staining can be substituted for parental brushing with more responsible children.

Malocclusion

The oral cavity can be viewed as a masticatory machine. The cusps of the opposing posterior teeth interdigitate and slide around each other to reduce foodstuffs to a soft, moist bolus. The cheeks and tongue force the food into the areas of tooth contact. The incisal edges of the anterior teeth are apposed by mandibular manipulation for the purpose of biting off increments of larger food items.

The masseter and temporal muscles are the main forces of mandibular closure. Acting in conjunction with the internal pterygoid muscles, they produce very high pressures on contact of opposing teeth. If a number of teeth meet simultaneously, the force is distributed over a large area of bone to tooth attachment. In malocclusion, when only a few teeth touch, the same force is exerted over a much smaller area. In adulthood occlusal deformi-

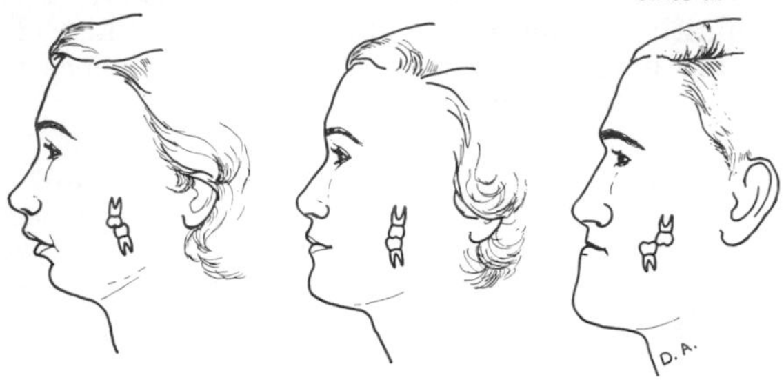

Figure 11–3 *Angle classification of occlusion. The typical correspondence between the profile and molar relationship is shown. (Moyers, R. E.: Handbook of Orthodontics. 2nd ed. Chicago, Year Book Medical Publishers, Inc., 1963.)*

ties are a leading cause of loss of teeth. For this reason preventive measures in childhood should be directed at establishing proper relations between upper and lower dental arches for physiologic as well as cosmetic reasons. The Angle classification categorizes the variations in growth patterns into three main types of occlusion (Fig. 11–3).

Class I (Normal). The cusps of the posterior mandibular teeth interdigitate ahead of and inside the corresponding cusps of the opposing maxillary teeth.

Class II. The cusps of the posterior mandibular teeth are behind and inside the corresponding cusps of the maxillary teeth. This is the most common occlusal discrepancy; about 45 per cent of the population exhibits some form of it. There is an increased space between upper and lower anterior teeth which results in a receding chin and encourages sucking and tongue-thrust habits.

Class III. The cusps of the posterior mandibular teeth oppose cusps which are a tooth or more ahead of their maxillary counterpart. The anterior teeth are directly opposed, or the mandibular incisors are protruded beyond the maxillary incisors; the chin is prognathic.

Cross Bite. Normally the mandibular teeth are in a position just inside the maxillary teeth, so that the outside mandibular cusps or incisal edges meet the central portion of the opposing maxillary teeth. A reversal of this relation is referred to as a *cross bite.*

OPEN AND CLOSED BITES. If the posterior mandibular and maxillary teeth contact each other, but the anterior ones do not, the situation is termed an open bite. If the mandibular anterior teeth fit inside the maxillary anterior teeth in an overclosed position, the situation is referred to as a closed bite. If the overclosure is extreme, the mandibular incisors may strike the gingiva behind the maxillary incisors. The occlusal relation is determined by observing the positions of the teeth when the jaws are closed and the heads of the condyles are in the most posterior position within the glenoid fossa of the temporal bone.

Genetic factors are by far the most common cause of malocclusion. Nevertheless, malocclusion may also result from abnormal growth; the mandibular protrusion seen with acromegaly is an example of abnormal growth leading to class III malocclusion. Habits such as thumb-sucking and tongue-thrusting are also important causative factors.

The severity of the malocclusion is the principal factor which determines the timing of treatment. Many cross bites, open bites and closed bites, and a few mild class II malocclusions can be corrected as early as they are diagnosed. Most class II and class III malocclusions are more easily correctable after the eruption of all the permanent dentition except the third molars.

The congenital absence of teeth also may cause occlusal discrepancies. These may be corrected either by prosthetic replacement of the missing tooth or teeth or by moving other teeth to close the vacant space. Early roentgenographic appraisal is important in establishing a plan for treatment.

Periodontal Disease

The roots of teeth are usually essentially conical in shape. Their retention and stability depend on the integrity of the surrounding alveolus and on a healthy periodontal membrane, with its fibers running from cementum to bone. In otherwise healthy adults, prolonged local insults may disturb one or both of these elements. This type of breakdown is relatively rare in childhood; apart from the normal sequence of eruption, either trauma or an underlying systemic condition is likely to be responsible for looseness or exfoliation. The differential diagnosis of noneruptive loss of teeth in children includes scurvy, osteomyelitis of the jaw, juvenile periodontitis, dysplasia of dentin, leukemia, acrodynia, vitamin D deficiency, vitamin D-refractory rickets, hypophosphatasia, Papillon-LeFevre syndrome (hyperkeratosis of palms and soles and disintegration of alveolar bone) and reticuloendotheliosis.

Poor oral hygiene may set the stage for more severe periodontal breakdown. Inflammation of the gingival margins may lead to irreversible changes in the capillary vessels. The resistance to further insult can be reduced. The inflammatory response results from plaque accumulations in the gingival sulci and the toxic products of bacterial growth.

PERIAPICAL INFECTION (ALVEOLAR ABSCESS). Teeth may become devitalized as a result of deep caries or trauma without accompanying pain. Grayish discoloration, looseness and sensitivity on mastication are frequent symptoms. Localized alveolar swelling and redness are most commonly due to infection around the roots of nonvital teeth, which may also lead to chronic draining fistulas visible in the alveolus at the level of the apex of the root. Periapical infections of primary teeth may cause defects in the underlying permanent teeth. The roots of nonvital primary teeth may not follow the normal pattern of resorption, thus inducing abnormalities in eruption and decalcification of the enamel of the underlying teeth.

Periapical infections and nonvital teeth, which are potential foci for infection if not treated, should be referred promptly for dental treatment; surveillance for these conditions should be routine during pediatric physical examinations. After the reduction of acute symptoms the involved tooth may be extracted. Root canal therapy can be carried out on primary teeth, and is especially valuable in the retention of permanent teeth.

IMPACTED TEETH. Though not actually a disease, impaction of teeth is a common dental problem in children. Previously erupted permanent teeth may prevent the subsequent eruption of another tooth which must occupy the same area of the alveolar ridge. The teeth most frequently involved are the maxillary canines and the mandibular third molars. The impacted tooth becomes lodged against the one impeding its eruption. Ectopic eruption, or resorption of the offending tooth, may result. Pain is common. Formation of a dentigerous cyst is the most serious consequence. Treatment consists in surgical removal of the impacted tooth. Unless otherwise contraindicated, impacted teeth should be extracted. If they are retained, periodic roentgenographic examinations should be made to be certain that complications do not arise.

DENTIGEROUS CYSTS. Impacted teeth retained in alveolar bone for long periods of time are the source of dentigerous cysts or of cystic degeneration of the enamel epithelium around the crown. The teeth most frequently involved are the mandibular third molars and the maxillary canines. Roentgenographically the crown of the unerupted tooth is surrounded by a well demarcated radiolucent zone. A dentigerous cyst may dislodge the tooth with which it is associated, e.g., to the inferior border of the mandible or to the floor of the nasal cavity. The lesion requires complete enucleation or curettage; cysts arising from enamel epithelium have the potential of becoming ameloblastomas.

DENTAL INJURIES

The risk of accidental damage to the teeth is exaggerated with the protruding anterior teeth of class II malocclusions or protrusions of maxillary incisors due to finger-sucking or tongue-thrusting; protruding teeth should be brought into a less vulnerable position as soon as possible after the eruption of the permanent incisors. Sports are responsible for many dental injuries. Individually fitted protective mouthpieces are available and should be used. When injury does occur, prompt treatment of a fracture or displacement improves the prognosis for subsequent alignment. Dental therapy usually should precede soft tissue treatment.

FRACTURED INCISORS. Blows on the mouth usually strike the maxillary incisors, since they are the most anteriorly located hard structures. Fractures of the crowns and roots of these teeth are therefore frequent. If the cleavage of the crown does not include a portion of the pulpal cavity, treatment is limited to covering any exposed dentin, followed by placement of an esthetic restoration. If a small area of exposed pulp is covered very quickly, recovery may take place. With more extensive injury, the pulpal tissue must be removed. Treatment of the root canal, necessary to prevent possible periapical abscess, varies according to whether or not the root is fully developed.

DISLOCATED TEETH. When the force of a blow is not dissipated by fracture of a tooth, dislocation is common, usually accompanied by fracture of the cortical plate of the alveolar bone. The blood supply to the fractured portion of alveolar bone almost always remains intact, and healing is complete in 3 or 4 weeks. On the other hand, because the alveolar ridge acts as a fulcrum, the apex of a tooth may be forced out of position, frequently severing the blood vessels and nerve which enter through the small apical foramen.

Dislocated teeth should be promptly repositioned and splinted. After a week, if the sensitivity of the tooth has not returned, root canal therapy will probably be required to prevent abscess formation.

AVULSED TEETH. Completely avulsed teeth should be placed in saline and taken immediately to a dentist for reimplanting. The devitalized tooth usually becomes firmly attached once again, but retention is limited, varying from 6 months to 12 years. Even so, reimplantation increases the success of ultimate prosthetic replacement, because it allows adjacent dental structures to mature normally.

HABITS INJURIOUS TO THE TEETH. The positions of the teeth significantly determine the contour of the alveolar bone and the shape of the face. The positions of the teeth, in turn, are dependent on a balance of forces. Normal pressure from the tongue is opposed by buccal and labial pressures; the force of eruption offsets the depression of mastication. Alteration in equilibrium between these forces can change the positions of teeth, disturb the interarch relations and, with time, change facial appearance.

Tongue Thrust. Since swallowing occurs about once every 2 minutes during the waking hours, the common oral habit of thrusting the tongue forward during swallowing produces almost continuous lingual pressure on the teeth. Anterior inclination of the incisors, with frequent anterior open bite and a tight, protruding upper lip results. Pursing of the lips during swallowing identifies the habit. The placement on the palate of an appliance with a guard-reminder section is useful. Tongue exercises directed by a speech therapist may also be effective in treatment.

Finger-sucking. Sucking thumb, fingers or a pacifier between feedings is common in infants. Many children continue this habit well beyond infancy, frequently in response to stress. Weaning from a pacifier is usually less difficult than from a thumb or fingers. The outward pull, particularly of thumb-sucking, may produce a forward movement of the primary maxillary incisors and, in turn, may induce the associated alveolar bone to shift anteriorly. The permanent incisors then erupt in a more forward position. If the habit persists during eruption of these permanent teeth, they are frequently directed into a protruding inclination. Finger-sucking should be terminated by 5 years of age in order to prevent the displacement of permanent teeth when they erupt the following year.

After the age of 4 years finger-sucking is usually self-correcting in response to social pressures. Persuasion by the pediatrician or dentist may help furnish the motivation to stop. If the habit is very strong, an appliance with a guard in the region of the anterior palate may be successful. With the guard a palatal vacuum is unattainable, and interest in sucking is lost. An emotional problem usually underlies protracted cases.

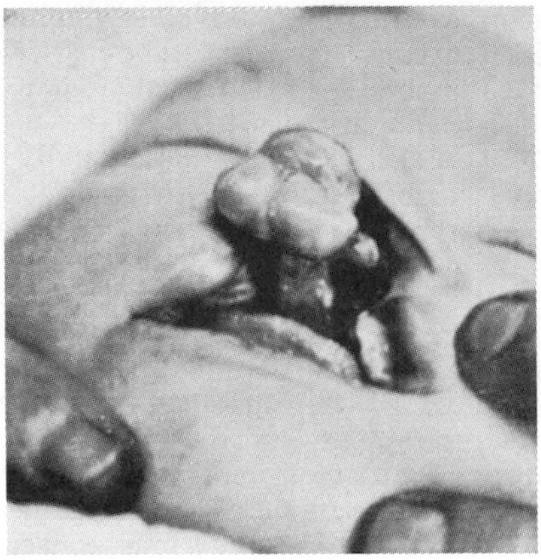

Figure 11–4 Double cleft lip and cleft palate in an infant 2 months of age. Note the intermaxillary process between the clefts.

ABNORMALITIES OF DEVELOPMENT OF THE PALATE AND SOFT TISSUES OF THE MOUTH

CLEFT LIP AND CLEFT PALATE

The incidence of cleft lip or cleft palate is from one in 600 to one in 1250 births according to various studies. Twin studies indicate that genetic factors are of more importance in cleft lip with or without cleft palate than in cleft palate alone. The incidence of cleft lip with or without cleft palate is about one in 1000 births; the incidence of the cleft palate alone is about one in 2500 births. Cleft lip (harelip) with or without cleft palate is more frequent in males; cleft palate alone is more frequent in females. There appears to be an increased incidence of associated congenital malformations and of intellectual impairment among children with cleft defects; both are more common with cleft palate alone. These findings are partially explained by an increased incidence of impairment of hearing in children with cleft palate and by the frequency of cleft defects among children with chromosomal abnormalities; many of the latter are stillborn or die in early infancy or childhood. The risks of recurrence of cleft defects within families are enumerated in Section 6 and in Table 11–3.

Animal studies suggest that nongenetic influences may also be responsible for clefts if applied to a susceptible host at a critical period of organogenesis. Associated malformations are especially frequent in structures derived from the first branchial arch.

TABLE 11–3 APPROXIMATE RISK OF RECURRENCE OF CLEFT LIP AND CLEFT PALATE*

AFFECTED	RISK FOR SUBSEQUENT OFFSPRING	
	Cleft Lip with or Without Cleft Palate (%)	*Cleft Palate Alone* (%)
Propositus	4–7	2–5
One parent	2	7
Propositus and one parent	11	17
Propositus and one sibling	10	No data

*From Fraser, F. C.: Pediat. Clin. N. Amer. *5*:475, 1958.

CLEFT LIP. Cleft lip may vary from a small notch in the vermilion border to a complete separation extending into the floor of the nose. Clefts may be unilateral (more often on the left side) or bilateral, and usually involve the alveolar ridge. Deformed, supernumerary or absent teeth are additional anomalies. The nasal alar cartilage may also be displaced or deformed. Bilateral clefts of the lip are frequently associated with a deficiency of the columella and an elongation of the vomer producing a protrusion of the anterior aspect of the cleft premaxillary process (Fig. 11–4).

CLEFT PALATE. Clefts of the palate may occur alone or in association with cleft lip. Isolated cleft palate occurs in the midline and may involve only the uvula or extend into or through the soft and hard palates to the incisive foramen. When associated with cleft lip, the palatal defect may involve the midline of the soft palate and extend into the hard palate on one or both sides, exposing one or both of the nasal cavities as a unilateral or bilateral cleft palate.

MANAGEMENT. The immediate problems of the infant with a cleft lip or palate are concerned with feeding and prevention of aspiration and infection. Most infants can be adequately managed by feeding in an upright position, using softened nipples with slightly enlarged openings. In some instances a medicine dropper or gavage feedings may be used to advantage. Special cleft palate nipples and plastic palatal coverings are usually not necessary.

Surgical Correction. Operation should be performed by a qualified plastic surgeon. Operation for *cleft lip* is usually at a month or two of age after the infant is gaining weight satisfactorily and is free of any oral, respiratory or systemic infection. The most common technique utilizes a staggered suture line to minimize notching of the lip from retraction of scar tissue. A Logan clamp (a wire bow attached by adhesive to the cheeks) is applied immediately after the operation to take tension off the suture line. The initial repair may be revised at 4 to 5 years of age. In most instances corrective surgery on the nose is better delayed until adolescence. Cosmetic results are dependent on the extent of the original deformity, absence of infection and the skill of the surgeon.

Since *clefts of the palate* vary considerably in size, shape and degree of deformity, the timing for operation should be individualized. Criteria such as width of the cleft, adequacy of the palatal parts, the morphology of the surrounding areas (such as the width of the oropharnyx) and the neuromuscular function of the soft palate and pharyngeal walls affect the decision. The goals of operation are union of the cleft parts, intelligible and pleasant speech and avoidance of injury to the growing maxilla. The optimal time for palatal surgery varies from 6 months to 5 years of age, depending on the need to take advantage of the palatal changes which occur with growth. When operation is best delayed beyond the third year, a contoured speech bulb can be attached to the posterior of a denture so that contraction of the pharyngeal and velopharyngeal muscles can accomplish occlusion of the nasopharynx and help the child to develop intelligible speech. Almost always the cleft crosses the alveolar ridge and interferes with the formation of teeth in the area. The missing elements of the dentition must be replaced by prosthetic devices; alterations in the positions of teeth may also be necessary.

Pre- and Postoperative Management. Even the suspicion of infection is a contraindication to operation. If the child is in good nutritional state and in fluid and electrolyte balance, feeding may be permitted to within 6 hours of the operation. Fluid management is discussed in Section 5.

During the immediate postoperative period *special nursing care is essential.* Gentle aspiration of the nasopharynx minimizes the chances of the common complications of atelectasis or pneumonitis. The primary considerations in postoperative care are maintenance of a clean suture line and avoidance of strain on the sutures. For these reasons the infant is fed with a medicine dropper, and the arms are restrained with elbow cuffs. A fluid or semifluid diet is maintained for 3 weeks, and feeding is with a dropper or spoon. The patient's hands as well as toys and other foreign bodies must be kept away from the palate.

Complications. Recurrent otitis media and hearing loss are frequent complications. Excessive dental decay is not unusual and requires special care. Displacement of the maxillary arches and malpositions of the teeth usually require orthodontic correction.

Speech. Speech defects may be present even after good anatomic closure of the palate. Such speech is characterized by emission of air from the nose and by a hypernasal quality when certain sounds are made. The speech defect before and, at times, after palatal surgery is due to inadequacies in function of the palatal and pharyngeal muscles. The muscles of the soft palate and the lateral and posterior walls of the nasopharynx constitute a valve which functions to separate the nasopharynx from the oropharynx during swallowing and in the production of certain sounds. If the valve does not function adequately, it is difficult to build up enough pressure in the mouth to make such explosive sounds as p, b, d, t, h, g or the sibilants s, sh and ch, and such words as "cat," "boats" and "sisters" are not intelligible. After operation or the insertion of a speech appliance it may be necessary to institute speech therapy to lessen the persisting speech defect.

A *complete program of habilitation* for the child with a cleft lip or palate may require years of special medical, surgical, dental and speech treatment. Representatives of the specialties involved function more effectively on a team basis than individually. One of these, however, must be responsible for parental counseling and guidance. Ideally, this is the child's physician. Pediatrician, plastic surgeon, orolaryngologist, children's dentist, prosthetic dentist, orthodontist, speech therapist, medical social worker, psychologist, child psychiatrist and public health nurse may make up such a *cleft palate team.* The child's physician may need to avail himself of such a group, usually located in the larger medical centers. Most states have programs for financial assistance for the medical care when the economic status of the family warrants.

PALATOPHARYNGEAL INCOMPETENCE

The speech disturbance characteristic of the child with a cleft palate can also be produced by other osseous or neuromuscular abnormalities in the oral and pharyngeal areas. The common denominator is the inability to form an effective muscular seal between oropharynx and nasopharynx during swallowing or phonation. The anomaly may be in the bony structures of the palate or pharynx or in the muscles attached to these structures. An adenoidectomy may precipitate the speech defect in a child who previously spoke normally, and the defect may be attributed to a previously unrecognized submucous cleft palate. In such instances it is assumed that the adenoid had a static function as a mass protruding into the epipharynx, allowing the soft palate to make contact with it when elevated. This became impossible after removal of the adenoid. If there is sufficient reserve neuromuscular function, compensation in palatopharyngeal movement may take place, and the speech defect disappears, although often some symptoms of palatopharyngeal incompetence may persist. In other instances slow involution of the adenoids may allow for gradual compensation in palatal and pharyngeal muscular function. This may explain why a speech defect does not become apparent in some children who have a submucous cleft palate or similar anomaly predisposing to palatopharyngeal incompetence.

Manifestations of Palatopharyngeal Incompetence

1. Hypernasal speech defect especially noted in the articulation of pressure consonants, such as p, b, d, t, h, v, f, s
2. Conspicuous constricting movement of the nares during speech
3. Inability to whistle, gargle, blow out a candle or inflate a balloon
4. Loss of liquid through the nose when drinking with the head down
5. Otitis media and hearing loss

Signs on Oral Inspection

1. Cleft palate or a relatively short palate with a large oropharynx
2. Absent, grossly asymmetric or minimal muscular activity of the soft palate and pharynx during phonation or gagging
3. A submucous cleft, as evidenced by the following pathognomonic signs:
   (a) Bifid uvula
   (b) Translucent membrane in midline of soft palate revealing lack of continuity of muscles
   (c) Palpable notching in posterior border of hard palate instead of a posterior nasal spinous process
   (d) Forward or V-shaped displacement of grooving on the soft palate during phonation or gagging

The symptoms of palatopharyngeal disturbances are similar, although clinical signs will vary. The diagnosis can usually be made without difficulty if there is sufficient awareness of the entity.

Palatopharyngeal incompetence can be demonstrated roentgenographically. The head should be carefully positioned to obtain a true lateral view; one film is obtained with the patient at rest and another during continuous phonation of the vowel "u" as in "boom." The soft palate contacts the posterior pharyngeal wall in normal function, while in palatopharyngeal incompetence such contact is absent.

Treatment of palatopharyngeal incompetence is either surgical or prosthetic. In selected cases the palate may be retropositioned or a pharyngoplasty performed, utilizing a flap of tissue from the posterior pharyngeal wall. Dental speech appliances have also been used successfully. *Adenoidectomy should be avoided when there is a submucous cleft palate or a potential palatopharyngeal incompetence.*

DISEASES OF THE ORAL MUCOSA AND GUMS

BEDNAR'S APHTHAE (PTERYGOID ULCER). Abrasions of the palatal mucous membrane of the newborn infant, resulting from efforts to clear the mouth of debris, are termed Bednar's aphthae. Superficial trauma denudes a region of the posterior hard palate, over which a grayish necrotic membrane forms typically on either side of the midline just anterior to the junction with the soft palate. The lesions heal spontaneously within 7 to 10 days.

EPSTEIN'S PEARLS (BOHN'S PEARLS). Epithelial retention cysts may appear on either side of the median raphe of the palate of the newborn infant. They disappear within a few weeks.

MUCOCELE (MUCOUS CYSTS). At any age from infancy to adulthood small mucus-containing cysts may occur in salivary gland-bearing areas of the oral cavity. They have a circumscribed, translucent, bluish appearance. Though usually elevated, they may be deep-seated and mobile on palpation. The cysts form after traumatic rupture of the excretory ducts of minor salivary glands. They are usually lined by granulation tissue, rarely by epithelium. Since recurrence is frequent if only drainage is accomplished, surgical removal of the cyst and the superficially located gland is recommended.

FORDYCE GRANULES. Almost 80 per cent of adults have multiple, yellowish white granules in clusters or plaque-like areas on the oral mucosa, most commonly on the buccal mucosa or lips. Histologically, normal sebaceous glands are seen in the lamina propria and submucosa. The glands are present at birth, but they hypertrophy and first appear as discrete yellowish papules during the preadolescent period in approximately 50 per cent of children. No treatment is necessary.

EPULIS. See Section 25.

ORAL MONILIASIS (THRUSH). Oral infection with the fungus *Candida albicans* is fairly common in the newborn infant. The organisms are regular inhabitants of skin, and of oral, vaginal and intestinal mucosa and are spread to the infant during birth. The oral lesions in children are white, flaky plaques covering all or part of the tongue, lips, gingiva and buccal mucous membranes. They are removable, leaving a brightly inflamed base. Discomfort may interfere with food ingestion. The condition is likely to be acute in newborn infants and chronic in infants and young children with nutritional deficiencies and other debilitating conditions. Alterations in the oral flora due to antibiotic therapy also may be responsible. The diagnosis can usually be confirmed by direct microscopic examination and culture of scrapings from mucous membranes.

Though the infection in the newborn infant is usually self-limited, treatment is advisable to limit spread within the nursery and to avoid the occasional protracted infection. The simplest plan at the moment, and as effective as any, is the oral instillation of 1 ml of a solution of nystatin (100,000 units/ml) 4 times a day at intervals of 6 hours. The solution should be slowly and gently instilled so that there is an opportunity for it to be widely distributed throughout the oral cavity before it is swallowed.

Topical application of 1 per cent aqueous gentian violet is also effective, but it is temporarily disfiguring and stains clothing and bed linen (stains can be removed with a paste of sodium bicarbonate). Applications should be made on individual lesions, and care should be taken to avoid an excess of the solution, which may be irritating when swallowed. This can also be lessened if the infant is placed face downward after the application, so that saliva containing the drug will drain outward.

Of primary importance in the chronically ill or malnourished infant or child is the correction of the underlying disturbance. Topical treatment as described above is of course indicated.

HERPANGINA. See Coxsackievirus infections, Section 10.

HERPETIC STOMATITIS. See Herpes simplex, Section 10.

APHTHOUS ULCERS (CANKER SORES). Aphthous ulcers are commonly painful lesions found on the oral mucosa, including the tongue and palate. An initial erythematous macule ruptures to form a highly sensitive crater surrounded by an indurated zone of inflammation. The lesions, which resemble somewhat those of herpetic stomatitis but are more localized, occur singly and multiply, usually following situations of stress. It has been suggested that an L-form of streptococcus may be the pathogen responsible when in the transitional state. Topical applications of tincture of benzoin are of value in the control of pain. The ulcer usually heals in one to two weeks without scar formation.

NECROTIZING ULCERATIVE GINGIVITIS (VINCENT'S INFECTION; VINCENT'S ANGINA). Necrotizing ulcerative gingivitis is characterized by the formation of a gray necrotic membrane and small ulcers which are localized upon painful hyperemic gingivae. Fever, malaise and a prominent fetid odor are common. The infection is not a communicable disease as was once thought, but most often represents a decrease in resistance of gingival tissue to infection with the usual oral flora and with an especially heavy overgrowth of fusiform bacilli and spirochetes. Such infections are largely limited to chronically ill, malnourished children. The acute stage of the infection responds dramatically usually within 48 hours to thorough cleansing of the mouth with oxidizing sprays or mouth rinses; hourly rinses with half-strength (3 per cent) hydrogen peroxide while the child is awake are a useful regimen.

Since necrotizing ulcerative gingivitis is extremely rare in childhood, except in areas of extreme poverty, the diagnosis should be made with caution. Herpetic stomatitis and the oral manifestations of acute leukemia and the reticuloendothelioses may be similar and should be excluded.

NOMA (GANGRENOUS STOMATITIS; CANCRUM ORIS; INFECTIVE GANGRENE OF THE MOUTH). Noma is a rare progressive gangrene of the buccal mucosa which results in a perforating ulcer of the cheek (Fig. 11-5). It is caused by invasion of the buccal tissues by fusospirochetal organisms and other bacteria in children whose resistance has been lowered by concurrent disease or nutritional deficiency. The lesion usually begins as a small ulcer with few constitutional symptoms, but soon results in a gangrenous, greenish-black area on the gums, buccal mucosa or mucocutaneous borders. The gangrenous area spreads slowly but inexorably until the cheeks are perforated and the jaws denuded.

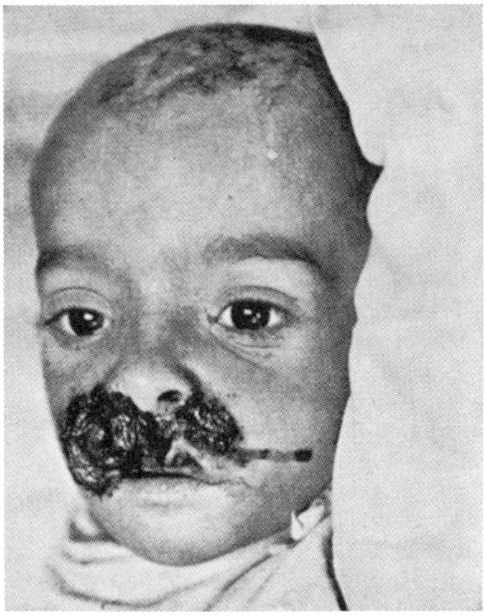

Figure 11-5 *Gangrenous stomatitis, beginning in the lip.*

Intensive antibacterial therapy, based on susceptibility tests in vitro, should be instituted as soon as the diagnosis is made and continued until all necrotic tissue, whether soft tissue or bone, has sloughed. Since malnutrition is frequent in these patients, an adequate diet should be introduced gradually, with special emphasis on adequate amounts of protein and vitamins. Plastic surgical procedures may be indicated when healing is complete.

CHEMICAL BURNS. In addition to accidental ingestion of acids, alkalis or other caustic substances, incorrect self-medication may cause burns of the oral mucosa, which usually appear as white lesions. The most common example is the holding of an aspirin tablet locally against a painful tooth or gingival area so that the tablet dissolves slowly. The result is a white, irregular patch of coagulated tissue. Camphor held in the mouth is another frequent cause of oral burns. The only treatment required is elimination of the practice; healing is spontaneous.

DILANTIN HYPERPLASIA. A generalized enlargement of the gingiva occurs in about 10 to 30 per cent of patients who receive diphenylhydantoin sodium (Dilantin) for control of seizures. The gingiva is pale, firm and granular and may hypertrophy to the point of covering the crowns of the teeth. Superimposed trauma or infection may cause inflammation and discomfort. Careful oral hygiene helps to avoid discomfort.

FIBROMATOSIS GINGIVAE. Fibromatosis gingivae is a rare familial idiopathic gingival hyperplasia which resembles Dilantin hyperplasia. It may be associated with other developmental defects such as mental deficiency and hypertrichosis. The firm, smooth-surfaced, generalized enlargement of the gingiva consists of collagen covered by stratified squamous epithelium. The swelling may produce protrusion of the lips and migration of the teeth. The only effective treatment is surgical removal of the excess gingiva, but recurrence is common. Particular attention must be devoted to oral hygiene to prevent irritation and stimulation of further gingival overgrowth.

THE LIPS

PROMINENT LABIAL FRENUM. In some instances the labial frenum appears prominent and thick. The fibers may pass between the maxillary central incisors, rather than attaching to the labial mucosa, and may appear to cause spacing, or diastema, of deciduous or permanent incisors.

A space between the primary maxillary incisors is common. If a wide band of the frenum with an attachment to the lingual side of the alveolar ridge persists after eruption of the permanent canines, the frenum may be suspected as being the cause of a diastema. In most cases the downward growth of the alveolar bone raises the attachment, and the lateral force of the erupting canines closes any existing space. When necessary, the attachment can be raised surgically, and a simple appliance can be used to bring the incisors together.

CHEILITIS. Dryness of the lips followed by scaling and cracking and accompanied by a characteristic burning sensation is common in children. It is usually caused by sensitivity to contact substances (from toys and foods) plus photosensitivity to the sun's rays. It is aggravated by the habit of alternate wetting with the tongue and drying by the wind, especially in cold weather. Cheilitis also often occurs in association with fever. Frequent application of a bland ointment permits healing and is also preventive.

ANGULAR FISSURES. Maceration and fissuring at the angles of the mouth may be caused by an infection with *Candida albicans.* It usually causes no constitutional symptoms or pain. The infection usually extends inside the mouth. Treatment with a mild antiseptic is successful.

When fissuring is caused by a nutritional deficiency, it is termed *cheilosis.* Cheilosis is an early sign in riboflavin deficiency and is often accompanied by moniliasis. Fissuring also occurs in mentally deficient children who drool (rhagades in the Down syndrome).

HERPES SIMPLEX (HERPES LABIALIS; COLD SORE; FEVER BLISTER). Herpes simplex (see Section 10) is an aggregate of small transparent vesicles on an inflammatory base and is accompanied by itching or burning. It usually affects the mucocutaneous junction, but may affect the skin of the face or the mucous membrane of the mouth. It is self-limited, disappearing in 8 to 14 days.

ALLERGIC ERUPTIONS. Certain substances such as lipsticks and toothpastes may produce eruptions where they come in contact with the lips. The lesions may be vesicular or elevated reddish wheals *(urticaria),* and there may be a glossitis. There is usually a history of other allergic manifestations.

Angioneurotic edema (see also Section 9) is a variety of urticaria which may be responsible for a sudden diffuse swelling of short duration (1 to 2 days) in children with allergic tendencies. It often itches but is seldom painful. There is no erythema, and the tissues appear to be normal in color and firm and do not pit.

MUCOUS RETENTION CYSTS. These are single teatlike projections covered by a thinned-out mucous membrane and filled with a clear fluid. They are caused by occlusion of the orifice of a labial or buccal mucous gland, resulting in retention of the secreted fluid.

POSTANESTHETIC TRAUMA. Local anesthetic blockage for dental procedures or minor surgery may leave a portion of the lips temporarily senseless. Young children will occasionally traumatize the area with their teeth. Swelling results, accompanied frequently by ulceration. Spontaneous remission usually occurs in 2 to 3 days. Antibiotic therapy is occasionally necessary to control secondary infection.

THE TONGUE

The tongue in certain instances may assume an unusual appearance without undue clinical significance. The patient is often not aware of the unusual appearance.

ANKYLOGLOSSIA (TONGUE-TIE). Occasionally the lingual frenum extends to near the tip of the tongue and interferes with its free protrusion; if the attachment reaches the anterior border, a notch may be visible. Owing to the possibility of bleeding or infection, and because it usually stretches with time, it is no longer thought advisable to clip the lingual frenum at birth. Should surgical correction be necessary (which it rarely is), the procedure can be carried out at any time after 8 to 10 months of age.

FISSURED TONGUE. The pattern may be foliaceous (leaflike) or cerebriform. The tongue may be somewhat enlarged and show imprints of the teeth at the sides. Fissured (scrotal) tongue is usually congenital, but may be acquired, especially in the Down syndrome. Occasionally fissuring may follow certain diseases such as scarlet fever, syphilis or typhoid fever.

BLACK HAIRY TONGUE (LINGUA NIGRA). This condition is characterized by an elongation of the filiform papillae into hairlike projections as long as ½ to 1 inch. It is generally concentrated in a triangular area in front of the V-shaped line of circumvallate papillae. The patch may vary from brown to black. The condition is usually chronic, but often disappears spontaneously.

A similar condition also occurs in association with chronic intra-oral hemorrhage, as in purpura and hemophilia. The filiform papillae become hypertrophied and are colored dark brown by the blood pigments. There is always a characteristic *fetor ex ore,* owing to the presence of blood in the mouth.

Hairy tongue may occur during prolonged antibiotic therapy, especially with oral troches.

GEOGRAPHIC TONGUE (WANDERING RASH). This benign lesion is characterized by one or more smooth, bright red patches, often showing a yellowish, grayish or whitish membranous margin upon the dorsum of an otherwise normally roughened tongue. The patches are areas in which the filiform papillae have become completely desquamated, leaving a smooth, slick surface. The patches may be single or multiple, discrete or confluent (maplike). They travel by an extension of desquamation of the papillae at one edge and a regeneration of the normal papillae at the other. The condition is usually chronic, and a single cycle may last 2 to 7 days.

Temporary smooth red patches on the dorsum of the tongue simulating geographic tongue are frequent in children with low-grade fevers, particularly those accompanying the common cold and chronic systemic infections. Treatment is contraindicated.

MACROGLOSSIA. The tongue in infants occasionally appears proportionately larger than the other oral structures because it grows at a relatively faster rate and is not confined by the teeth. In stocky infants the tongue is frequently so large and unconfined that it protrudes from the mouth, and may be mistaken for a manifestation of hypothyroidism. As the infant grows, the other oral structures gradually catch up and confine the tongue, so that its relative size is decreased.

A true hypertrophy of the tongue is rare. It may exist congenitally, as a diffuse lymphangioma or as a muscular hypertrophy (rhabdomyoma). The tongue may reach such a size that it cannot be retained in the mouth, with the result that nursing and, later, speech are interfered with. In such cases the teeth are pushed into a malocclusion by the action of the tongue.

Treatment is surgical, although some relative adjustment usually occurs as the child grows older.

Hemangiomas and cysts may be responsible for diffuse or localized enlargement of the tongue. Enlargement is also present in cretinism, acromegaly, Beckwith syndrome and, occasionally, gargoylism.

WHITE-COATED TONGUE. The accumulation of food debris and bacteria among hypertrophied filiform papillae causes a *moist coated tongue.* The filiform papillae are present at birth, but are much shorter than even the fungiform papillae until about 5 years of age, so that the tongue appears smooth. Thus, in the young child the cause should be sought for any coating of the tongue.

The condition of *dry furry tongue* (hypertrophied filiform papillae) is seen early in states of mild dehydration and low-grade fever.

A transitional stage from the white-coated tongue to the raw red tongue is known as the *white strawberry tongue.* The appearance is that of an unripe strawberry. The engorged and enlarged fungiform papillae appear prominently above the level of the white, desquamating filiform papillae. It is seen early in scarlet fever and other acute febrile states.

RAW RED TONGUE (GLOSSITIS). When the filiform papillae of the white strawberry tongue or the coated tongue are shed, leaving the engorged fungiform papillae raised above the smooth, denuded surface of the tongue, the condition is known as red raspberry or red strawberry tongue. This is seen often in the later stages of febrile states and about the sixth or seventh day of scarlet fever.

When the papillae become flattened and edematous (mushroom-shaped), but not atrophied or shed, the *raw pebbly tongue* results. The color is a characteristic purplish red (magenta) instead of pink. Edema of the tongue is common, and the indentations of the teeth can easily be seen. The edges of the tongue often become denuded and raw, resulting in a burning, painful sensation. Fissuring is common. Such lesions occur in *ariboflavinosis* in association with cheilosis, photophobia and lacrimation.

Complete atrophy of both the filiform and fungiform papillae results in a *smooth atrophic tongue.* The desquamated surface is usually dry and extremely sensitive (glazed tongue). *Atrophic glossitis* with a fiery red (scarlet) coloration of the tongue is characteristic of *niacin deficiency (pellagrous glossitis),* especially when accompanied by infection. Atrophic glossitis with a pale salmon coloration of the tongue *(Hunter's glossitis)* occurs in *pernicious anemia,* and also in *sprue, achlorhydria* and *hypochromic anemia.*

Taste buds may be reduced or absent in the tongue in familial dysautonomia (Riley-Day syndrome).

TRAUMA. Accidental biting of the tongue, irritation by carious teeth, injuries by sharp objects placed in the mouth, and burns by hot foods occur frequently in children. Such injuries may result in a simple blister or ulcer which disappears in a few days, but even superficial ulcers are painful. In extreme cases the tongue may become swollen and edematous. Ice may be used to reduce the swelling. The food should be cool and in liquid form; it may be necessary to feed young infants through a nasal tube. A mild antiseptic mouthwash such as 1 per cent tincture of iodine in physiologic saline solution may be used.

Accidental injuries and burns resulting from ingestion of poisons are not uncommon in young children. Immediate care is determined by the poison ingested and the extent of the injury. In severe cases particular attention should be given to adequacy of the airway; occasionally tracheotomy is essential as a lifesaving measure.

Ulcerations of the frenum and the margins of the tongue are usually the result of herpetic infection; those limited to the frenum may be secondary to biting the tongue during paroxysms of coughing in pertussis. Such ulcers have also been observed in association with familial dysautonomia (q.v.).

SALIVARY GLANDS

Salivary secretions originate from three pairs of glands: the parotid, submaxillary and sublingual. The parotid fluid is serous and contains amylase and secretory immunoglobulin (IgA); that of the submaxillary glands is a mixed seromucoid fluid, and that of the sublinguals is a mucoid viscous fluid. The volume and composition of the mixed saliva are a function of the degree of secretory stimulation to each of the three pairs of glands and are subject to many local and systemic influences.

With the exception of epidemic parotitis (mumps, see Section 10), disease of the salivary gland is rare in children. Bilateral enlargement of the submaxillary glands may occur in cystic fibrosis, malnutrition and, transiently, during acute asthmatic attacks. Chronic vomiting and aspiration, as in achalasia, may also be accompanied by enlargement of the parotids.

Infants exhibit salivary discharge or drooling until muscular reflexes which initiate swallowing and lip closure are developed. Later, the irritation of teething in conjunction with the accompanying increase in oral activity may also lead to drooling. In some children with mental retardation, drooling is never overcome.

If salivary flow rates are decreased by medications, disease or irradiation, an increase in dental decay usually follows. In addition to the obvious washing action, saliva also appears to furnish the materials from which the cell-free film which covers dental enamel is formed. This film influences the surface equilibria between enamel and bathing fluids; its absence is accompanied by a pronounced increase in caries.

Excessive secretion of saliva occurs during teething, as a reflex to anticipated feeding or pain, from irritative lesions in the mouth, in conjunction with nausea, after administration of mercurial compounds, and in certain nervous affections such as encephalitis and chorea.

XEROSTOMIA (DRY MOUTH). Temporary dryness of the mouth occurs with fever, dehydration and the ingestion of drugs such as the phenothiazine derivatives, atropine and other anticholinergic substances. In *congenital xerostomia* the mouth becomes glazed, dry and filled with debris. The condition responds to the administration of pilocarpine.

RECURRENT PAROTITIS. Recurrent idiopathic swelling of the parotid gland may occur in otherwise healthy children. The swelling is usually unilateral, but parotid glands may be involved simultaneously or alternately. Up to ten or more recurrences may be observed in an individual child. There is little pain associated with the swelling, which is limited to the gland and usually lasts 2 to 3 weeks. Subsidence is spontaneous and may be complete or partial. The incidence appears to be higher in the spring.

Suppurative parotitis, most often due to *Staphylococcus aureus,* may occur as a primary disease or as a complication of parotitis due to another cause. It is usually unilateral and may be accompanied by fever, and the gland becomes swollen, tender and painful.

Recurrent parotitis requires no treatment, but it may be confused with suppurative parotitis, which responds to appropriate antibacterial therapy based on culture of purulent discharge from Stensen's duct, or of pus obtained by infrequently required surgical drainage. Radiotherapy appears to shorten the attacks of recurrent parotitis and to decrease the number of recurrences. Owing to the potential hazards of radiation to the growing child, it should be considered only in severe or prolonged cases.

MIKULICZ'S DISEASE. This is a term applied to idiopathic bilateral, painless enlargements of the parotid and lacrimal glands, usually associated with dryness of the mouth and an absence of tears. The manifestations may also occur in diseases such as tuberculosis, leukemia and lymphosarcoma.

RANULA. Because of resemblance to the appearance of a frog's belly, a cyst associated with one of the major salivary glands in the sublingual area is termed a ranula. The large, soft, mucus-containing swelling occurs in the floor of the mouth and may be seen at any age, including infancy. The cyst should be excised and the severed duct exteriorized.

FREDERICK M. PARKINS
GIULIO J. BARBERO

Blayney, J. R., and Hill, I. N.: Fluorine and Dental Caries. J. Am. Dent. A., *74*:225, 1967.

Brauer, J. C., and Lindahl, R. L.: Dentistry for Children. 5th ed. New York, McGraw-Hill Book Company, Inc., 1964.

Finn, S. B.: Clinical Pedodontics. 4th ed. Philadelphia, W. B. Saunders Company, 1973.

Gorlin, R. J., and Pindborg, J. J.: Syndromes of the Head and Neck. New York, McGraw-Hill Book Company, Inc., 1964.

Keyes, P. H.: Research in Dental Caries. J. Am. Dent. A., *76*:1357, 1968.

Kraus, B. S., and Jordan, R. E.: The Human Dentition Before Birth. Philadelphia, Lea & Febiger, 1965.

Moyers, R. E.: Handbook of Orthodontics. 3rd ed. Chicago, Year Book Medical Publishers, 1972.

Richmond, J. B. (Ed.): Symposium on the Child's Mouth. Pediat. Clin. N. Amer., *3*:845–1137, 1956.

THE ESOPHAGUS

Symptoms suggestive of esophageal disease in infants and children are cough or choking on ingestion of fluids, dysphagia, complete inability to swallow, pain on swallowing, regurgitation of undigested food or fluids, and hematemesis. With any of these symptoms, swallowing function should be studied by cinefluoroscopy. Barium is the usual contrast medium used unless a tracheo-esophageal fistula or a complete esophageal obstruction is suspected, in which case an iodized oil should be used to avoid aspiration of barium into the trachea or bronchi. The esophagus may be examined directly with the esophagoscope, generally without anesthesia, in infants or children of any age. If a general anesthetic is preferred, airway patency must be maintained by an intratracheal tube to avoid compression of the soft tracheal walls by the esophagoscope.

CONGENITAL ANOMALIES

The esophagus is developed from the first part of the primitive gut, its upper part from the retropharyngeal segment, and the lower from the pregastric segment. As the neck differentiates and the heart, lungs and stomach move caudad, the esophagus elongates rapidly. Vacuoles appear in the epithelium to form a lumen by the eighth week. During the fourth week the laryngotracheal groove develops to become the larynx and trachea and the primordia of the lungs. Two furrows course longitudinally along the sides of this respiratory primordium and cut inward to separate it from the esophagus. This separation progresses in a cephalic direction. Congenital anomalies develop through a failure of one of these critical steps to be completed correctly, and vary from complete absence of the esophagus to duplication throughout its length.

ATRESIA AND FISTULA
(Tracheo-Esophageal Fistula)

ETIOLOGY. Atresia and fistula of the esophagus, the most common congenital anomalies, may be due to a deviation of the septum between trachea and esophagus or to altered cellular growth along the septum. Absence of growth along the septum results in a fistula to the trachea; deficient growth of entodermal cells of the dorsal wall results in atresia.

TABLE 11–4 AVERAGE MEASUREMENTS OF THE ESOPHAGUS AT VARIOUS AGES

AGE	TEETH TO CRICOID	TEETH TO BIFURCATION	TEETH TO CARDIA
Birth	7 cm	12 cm	18 cm
1 year	9 cm	14 cm	21 cm
3 years	10 cm	16 cm	23 cm
5 years	11 cm	17 cm	25 cm
10 years	12 cm	19 cm	27 cm
15 years	14 cm	23 cm	33 cm
Adult	16 cm	25 cm	40 cm

CLINICAL FORMS. Of the five types of atresia or fistula, the most common one (Fig. 11–6, *A*) consists of an upper segment which ends in a blind pouch at or slightly above the level of the bifurcation of the trachea, and a lower segment from the stomach which is connected to the trachea by a short fistulous tract. The *symptoms* are characteristic. The first swallow or two by the newborn infant is normal; then suddenly the fluids return through the nose and mouth; the child coughs, struggles, turns cyanotic and may stop breathing. The cycle is repeated with each attempt at nursing, and between feedings there is constant drooling from the dependent corner of the mouth. The stomach becomes distended with air, and bile and gastric secretion may be collected from the regurgitated material, owing to the fistula between the lower segment and the trachea. Pneumonia from aspiration of gastric secretions refluxed into the trachea is a serious problem prior to surgical correction.

In the second commonest type (Fig. 11–6, *B*) both segments are blind, neither being connected to the air passages. The *symptoms* are like those of the first type, but the roentgenogram shows an opaque abdomen devoid of gas in the stomach and intestines (Fig. 11–7). Since no gastric juice can enter the tracheobronchial tree, the pulmonary symptoms are produced entirely by overflow of milk and saliva from the esophagus, so that postural drainage and suction of the trachea are effective in clearing the obstruction. The lower segment is often rudimentary, and generally primary anastomosis is impossible.

Tracheo-esophageal fistula without atresia, the so-called H type (Figs. 11–6, *C*; 11–8), may be suspected in infants or children who show signs of respiratory embarrassment and choking and coughing associated with fluid, as opposed to solid, feedings. There are usually gastric distention, and excessive amounts of mucus in the oropharynx. Repeated episodes of pneumonitis are common and may lead to the diagnosis only after the child is several months to a year or so of age. The fistula may be found at any point from the level of the cricoid cartilage to the midesophagus. The opening, which may be no more than pinpoint in size, is usually at a higher level in the trachea than in the esophagus.

In the least common types (Fig. 11–6, *D, E*) the upper segment of the esophagus opens into the trachea, and the infant may "drown" with the first feeding; coughing and cyanosis with feeding are prominent.

DIAGNOSIS. Maternal polyhydramnios, com-

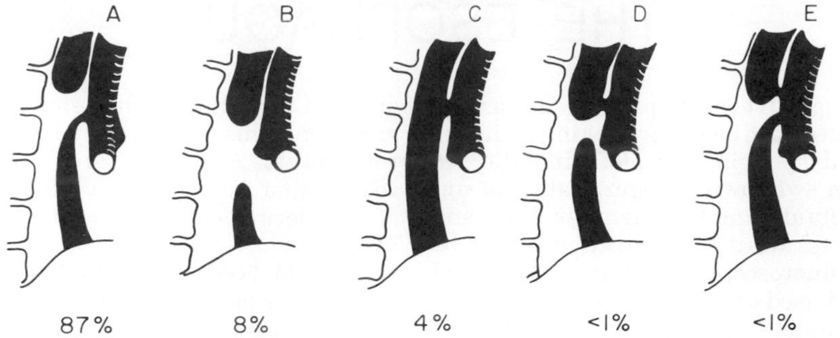

Figure 11–6 *Diagrams of the five most commonly encountered forms of esophageal atresia and tracheo-esophageal fistula, in order of frequency.*

monly associated with atresia of the upper digestive tract, and excessive salivation or drooling in the newborn infant should arouse suspicion of esophageal atresia before the diagnosis is evident from choking, cyanosis or regurgitation on feeding. Roentgenologic confirmation may be obtained by demonstration that a radiopaque catheter will not pass into the stomach, or by use of contrast media. Iodized oil rather than barium should be used as the contrast medium for roentgenologic studies to avoid the danger of aspiration of barium. One half milliliter of the contrast material given by mouth with a medicine dropper or instilled in the esophageal pouch with a catheter is adequate for diagnostic purposes. The roentgenogram of the chest and abdomen taken in the upright position shows the round blind end of the esophagus at the level of the tracheal bifurcation, or it may demonstrate the fistulous tract into the trachea or the absence of air below the diaphragm, depending on the type of malformation.

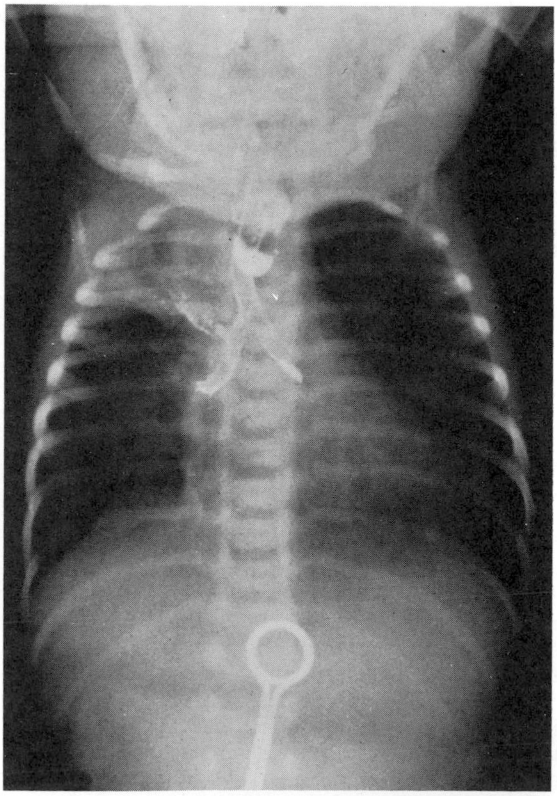

Figure 11–7 *Roentgenogram of a newborn infant with esophageal atresia without tracheo-esophageal fistula (Fig. 11–6, B). Note absence of air in the gastrointestinal tract. Lipiodol was given by mouth, thereby demonstrating the upper blind pouch; some of the contrast material spilled over into the trachea and bronchi. The atelectasis of the right upper lobe is a common associated finding.*

The demonstration of an H type of fistula usually requires lateral or oblique cinefluoroscopy (Fig. 11–8) with contrast medium. Cinefluoroscopy is also helpful in distinguishing between a small fistula high in the trachea and pharyngeal overflow into the larynx in pharyngeal paralysis due to neurogenic abnormalities in the newborn infant.

TREATMENT. Most of the malformations can be corrected surgically. The success of operation is dependent on early diagnosis, before bronchopneumonia, dehydration and inanition have progressed to an irreversible degree.

The condition of the infant, particularly when the weight is less than 5 pounds, occasionally does not permit end-to-end anastomosis. In such instances a gastrostomy may be performed, the tracheal fistula to the lower segment ligated, and the upper segment exteriorized to avoid the otherwise inevitable pneumonia from aspiration. Later, when the infant's condition permits, the two ends are anastomosed to establish oral-gastric continuity.

Adequate preoperative and postoperative management is essential for the successful outcome of esophageal surgery. The following preoperative factors are considered important: (1) broad-spectrum antibiotic therapy for the treatment of pneumonia; (2) intermittent suction drainage of the upper esophageal pouch through an indwelling catheter, the tip of which should be maintained just above the lower end of the pouch; (3) maintenance of the infant in an upright position to avoid reflux of gastric juice into the trachea and lungs; (4) parenteral administration by slow, continuous intravenous drip of 5 to 10 per cent glucose in 0.2 per cent saline solution containing potassium (1 to 2 mEq/dl, or 10 to 20 mEq/l) until the condition is deemed favorable for operation; (5) strict isolation technique, preferably in an enclosed incubator; (6)

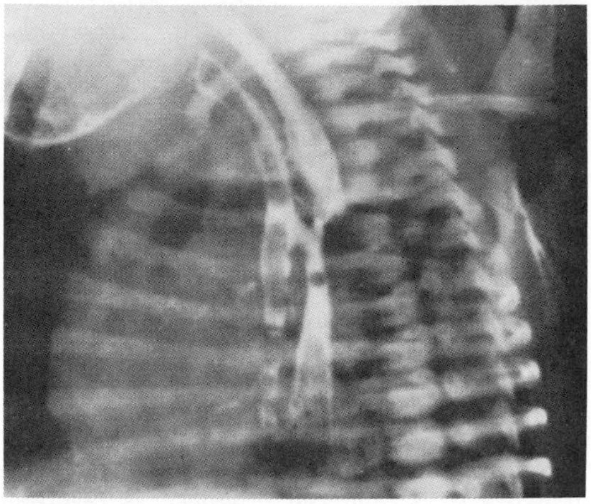

Figure 11–8 *Tracheo-esophageal fistula (H type) without esophageal atresia. The infant was born prematurely; birth weight was 3 pounds 14 ounces. Respiratory distress appeared soon after birth and was progressive; it was accentuated when liquids were swallowed. The large fistula was demonstrated after the tip of the catheter had been positioned in the upper end of the esophagus and contrast material introduced through it. There is narrowing of the esophagus just above the site of the fistula.*

constant nursing supervision and care. Immediately before operation a cannula should be placed in a vein for administration of blood during the operation. Bronchoscopic aspiration may be required preoperatively or postoperatively if atelectasis persists; atelectasis of the right upper lobe is common.

Postoperatively the infant should be placed in an oxygen tent or enclosed incubator. Feedings through the gastrostomy tube or through an esophageal-passed polyethylene tube may be started in 2 or 3 days. (Some surgeons are opposed to nasogastric intubation immediately postoperatively.) The first two or three feedings should consist of 0.5 per cent physiologic saline solution and then of 5 per cent glucose solution. If these are tolerated, a milk formula of gradually increasing strength may be given. Oral feedings are usually tolerated 8 to 10 days after the operation. There is a trend away from the use of prophylactic antibiotic therapy.

TABLE 11–5 SURVIVAL OF PATIENTS WITH TYPE A TRACHEO-ESOPHAGEAL FISTULA AS RELATED TO SOME ASSOCIATED ANOMALIES*

ASSOCIATED ANOMALY	PATIENTS AFFECTED	SURVIVORS
None	478 (52%)	373 (78%)
Congenital heart disease	171 (19%)	37 (22%)
Genitourinary	98 (11%)	22 (22%)
Imperforate anus	88 (10%)	38 (43%)
Intestinal atresia	30 (3%)	4 (13%)
Other	51 (5%)	– – – –

*Adapted from T. M. Holder, D. T. Cloud, J. E. Lewis, Jr., and G. P. Pilling, IV: Pediatrics *34*:542, 1964.

Stenosis at the operative site is not uncommon. A swallow of contrast material 10 days postoperatively observed fluoroscopically and recorded by spot films will determine the adequacy of the lumen. If there is stenosis, soft rubber mercury-filled bougies may be used to establish and maintain a satisfactory lumen. Too often the diagnosis of stenosis at the site of anastomosis is delayed because the diet is entirely liquid and the degree of obstruction is not apparent until semisolids are added at 2 or 3 months of age. It must be stressed that early esophageal dilatations of the soft stenosis at the point of anastomosis are more successful in maintaining a satisfactory lumen than later dilatations of fibrous scars.

The survival of patients with tracheo-esophageal fistula is influenced not only by prompt diagnosis and skilled surgical treatment, but also by the presence of other anomalies (Table 11–5).

SHORT ESOPHAGUS

The esophagus may be abnormally short, with a portion of the stomach displaced upward through the diaphragm into the thoracic cavity. Occasionally, temporary obstruction by a foreign body leads to a roentgenologic study which reveals a stricture in the midthorax at the esophagogastric junction, with the short esophagus above it and true gastric mucosa with rugae below. These rugae can be followed through the diaphragm as a continuation of the rugae of the subdiaphragmatic stomach. The fact that the cardia becomes stenotic accounts for the symptoms. It has been suggested that the stricture may be the result of reflux of gastric contents due to an incompetence of the gastroesophageal mechanism as described under chalasia. The clinical picture is characterized by dysphagia, regurgitation, malnutrition and frequent attacks of complete obstruction of the esophagus.

TREATMENT. When there is no evidence of stricture, treatment consists in propping the infant in an erect position during and after feeding, as described for chalasia. When there is stenosis, repeated dilatations are indicated; the lesion is peculiarly resistant to therapy, and occasionally one must resort to gastrostomy and retrograde dilatation or, more rarely, to surgical reconstruction. Ulcers in the supradiaphragmatic stomach should be treated in a manner similar to other gastric ulcers.

STENOSIS

Congenital stenosis of the esophagus without a fistula can be found at any point, but usually occurs in the distal third as either a web or a long segment of esophagus with only a threadlike lumen. The symptoms are those of esophageal obstruction, usually first apparent when the infant begins to eat semisolid or solid food. The diagnosis is made by roentgenographic and esophagoscopic examinations. The treatment is esophagoscopic dilatation; these strictures respond more readily than does that of a congenitally short esophagus.

EXTERNAL COMPRESSION

Partial obstruction of the esophagus may be caused by compression from congenital cardiac or vascular anomalies and by mediastinal tumors such as tracheogenic or bronchogenic cysts, cystic duplications of the esophagus, teratomas or neurogenic tumors. Fluoroscopic studies of the esophagus with contrast material and recognition of both esophageal and tracheal compression by esophagoscopy and bronchoscopy assist in establishing the diagnosis. Angiocardiography is of value in questionable cases in which symptoms are severe. Treatment consists in surgical relief of the obstruction.

NEUROGENIC SWALLOWING DYSFUNCTION

Congenital anomalies of the medulla or cerebral birth injuries occasionally result in a lack of nervous stimulation of the muscles of deglutition. The infant is unable to swallow, and food and mucus constantly fill the pharynx and the trachea. Esophagoscopy, gavage and roentgenograms show the esophageal lumen to be entirely patent. Similar symptoms may occur in amyotonia congenita and bulbar poliomyelitis. Death may result from pneumonia.

TREATMENT. Postural drainage and suction of mucus are necessary to prevent pulmonary aspiration and pneumonia. Feedings must be entirely by gavage or gastrostomy.

CARDIO-ESOPHAGEAL RELAXATION
(Chalasia)

This clinical syndrome is manifest by vomiting following feeding when the infant is in the horizontal position. The vomiting is the result of persistent relaxation of the lower end of the esophagus (chalasia). The cause in most instances is not demonstrable. The course tends to be self-limiting, and for this reason chalasia has often been assumed to be the result of temporary neuromuscular imbalance. Chalasia has been associated with cerebral defects, with obstruction at the pylorus or just below it, and in one reported instance with a hemangioma at the cardia.

Vomiting begins a few days after birth, is more or less effortless, and can usually be avoided if the infant is maintained in the erect position. It may occur during feeding, but usually begins after the infant has been returned to the crib. In untreated cases the infant loses weight and becomes dehydrated. It may be that an occasional instance of rumination is the result of chalasia.

The diagnosis is established by observing the swallowing of barium under the fluoroscope. Persistent relaxation of the esophageal hiatus is observed with retrograde filling of the esophagus during inspiration or with increase of intra-abdominal pressure.

Therapy consists in feeding a relatively thick milk formula and in maintenance of the infant in an erect (propped sitting) position for several hours after feedings. Permanent relief is usually obtained after a month or two of such management.

ACQUIRED DISEASES

ESOPHAGITIS

Acute esophagitis may complicate practically any acute infectious disease; it may be associated with inflammation of other parts of the digestive tract or may follow lacerations produced by swallowing of foreign bodies or injuries caused by ingestion of hot liquids. The lesions generally last but a few days, and the prognosis is favorable. Symptoms may be substernal pain on swallowing, dysphagia and hematemesis, or may be entirely absent. Some benign esophageal strictures seen in later life originate from acute esophageal ulcers associated with infectious diseases in childhood.

The so-called *Rokitansky-Cushing ulcer,* which is an occasional accompaniment of severe lesions of the central nervous system, may be located in the lower third of the esophagus, in the fundus of the stomach or in the duodenum. Most often these lesions are identified at necropsy; occasionally they perforate before death.

Chronic esophagitis is not rare in early life. It may follow an acute process or be the result of venous congestion in chronic pulmonary or cardiac disease. Most commonly it is associated with congenital strictures or with a short esophagus.

Infrequent causes of esophagitis include diphtheria, thrush, variola, varicella and perforation by a caseous lymph node.

Inflammatory strictures may follow any of the conditions mentioned as esophagitis. Symptoms and treatment are those of corrosive strictures. The diagnosis must be established from the history and from the roentgenographic and esophagoscopic appearances.

CORROSIVE STRICTURES

The most common cause of stricture of the esophagus (see also Section 28) is ingestion of caustic and corrosive agents such as lye, ammonia (readily available in the kitchen as cleansing agents and for flushing drains), acids—acetic, lactic, carbolic, nitric, sulfuric and hydrochloric—and bleaches (hypochlorite). Most accidents in children are due to the fact that these agents are carelessly kept in a soft drink bottle, cup or jar similar to one the child uses for food or drink. The lesions vary from superficial pharyngitis and esophagitis to ulceration and necrosis of the esophageal or gastric wall with a chemical mediastinitis or peritonitis which may result in death in a few hours.

CLINICAL MANIFESTATIONS. When a child swallows lye or an acid, the first mouthful causes intense burning and pain, and tends to inhibit further swallowing, but the damage has already been done. The lips, chin, tongue and pharynx become edematous and covered with exudate; similar changes occur in the esophagus and, infrequently, in the stomach. In many cases the edema subsides after the first week, and the swallowing function returns to normal in 2 to 4 weeks.

The ensuing period may be symptomless, but if treatment is not carried out, difficulty in swallowing usually recurs insidiously over weeks or months as strictures develop in the burned areas. At first the child has difficulty in swallowing solid food. Eating becomes slow, food is frequently regurgitated, and, later, difficulty in taking liquids becomes apparent. Often the child is considered a "feeding problem" because the accident has been forgotten and the dysphagia is so gradual in its progress. Roentgenograms then reveal strictures of the esophagus, most pronounced in the areas of anatomic narrowing: the cervical region, the cardia and the point at which the left bronchus crosses the esophagus. Children with longstanding esophageal strictures have numerous evidences of nutritional deficiencies.

TREATMENT. Emergency management for ingestion of alkalis consists in oral administration of large amounts of water, dilute vinegar or citrus fruit juices, and milk, egg whites, olive or mineral oil. For acid ingestion, milk, lime water, soap solution or aluminum hydroxide gel, followed by egg whites or olive or mineral oil, is appropriate. *Gastric lavage and emetics should not be used in either case.* For bleaches, gastric lavage with warm water, emetics and saline cathartics are recommended. Patients with severe reactions following ingestion of any of these agents must be fed intravenously or by gastrostomy and may require a tracheotomy because of pharyngeal or laryngeal edema.

After emergency treatment there is considerable variation in management, but it is imperative that an active regimen be initiated immediately. Hospitalization for observation is advisable. Ampicillin is usually prescribed for a week or so. Some use corticosteroids to lessen scar tissue formation, but the incidence of spontaneous hemorrhage or perforation of the esophagus or stomach associated with their use in acute esophageal burns is appreciable; furthermore, steroids alone do not prevent stricture formation. Their use may be of some advantage, but should be limited to 10 to 14 days.

Esophagoscopy should be performed within 48 hours by an experienced endoscopist; if no esophageal damage is seen, further treatment is unnecessary. With mild burns the initial medication (usually ampicillin and systemic corticosteroids) should be continued for a week or two, and the patient then followed with esophagrams at 6, 8 and 12 weeks after ingestion.

Early dilation of the esophagus after severe alkali and bleach burns is the sine qua non of their treatment. On the second or third day after ingestion, well lubricated, rubber, Hurst-type mercury-filled bougies are passed into the stomach. Beginning with bougies No. 14F and 16F, dilatations are done daily for the first week, every second day for the second week, then twice a week, weekly, twice monthly and then at monthly or bimonthly intervals. The size of the bougies is gradually increased to No. 24F for infants, 32F for children and 40F for adults. In mild acid burns this same routine may be followed. In severe acid burns early instrumentation is strictly avoided; a jejunostomy may be necessary for feeding purposes because of the severity of esophageal and gastric destruction.

With failure of early treatment, stricture formation or actual atresia may become apparent within 2 to 4 months; in some instances many years elapse before the stricture becomes severe enough to produce dysphagia. The generally accepted method of treatment of definitely formed strictures consists in esophageal dilatations, which may be guided by a swallowed string, or visually through an esophagoscope. If the stricture is extremely tight, retrograde dilatation is preferred, the bougie being guided by a string advanced through a gastrostomy. When complete atresia of the esophagus follows ingestion of a caustic substance, endoscopic efforts at recannulization are generally successful, but occasionally external surgical procedures must be considered. Replacement of the esophagus by a section of colon or small bowel is preferred to resection of the stricture and gastroesophageal anastomosis.

SPASM OF THE ESOPHAGUS

(Achalasia; Mega-esophagus)

Esophagospasm, including cardiospasm, may be present even in newborn infants. Esophagospasm is usually characterized by severe sudden obstruction to swallowing and reverse peristalsis and, in older children, may be initiated by emotional stress. *Cardiospasm* (achalasia, preventriculosis) is the syndrome of nonorganic obstruction of the cardia associated with dilatation and hypertrophy of the esophagus (mega-esophagus). It is generally considered to be a failure of coordination of the mechanism at the cardia, preventing normal passage of food from the esophagus to the stomach. In longstanding cases there is fibrosis and disorganization of musculature of the lower end of the esophagus.

CLINICAL MANIFESTATIONS. These are difficulty in swallowing, regurgitation of undigested food and fluid, cough from overflow of fluids into the larynx, especially at night, and failure to gain or loss of weight. The diagnosis is made by fluoroscopy or roentgenograms, which demonstrate the barium column in the dilated esophagus terminating in a fine point as it approaches the diaphragm. Pulmonary infections, including bronchiectasis, may result from the constant overflow of food from the esophagus into the larynx.

TREATMENT. In uncomplicated cases treatment includes dilatations of the cardia by a pneumatic bag accurately placed under fluoroscopic guidance, by a Hurst mercury bougie, by an esophagoscope or by string-guided, olive-tip bougies. Psychotherapy should be considered. In advanced cases retention of food and fluids produces esophagitis, periesophageal inflammation and fibrous strictures at the cardia. Surgical intervention may become necessary in extreme situations; such procedures as a Heller esophagocardial myotomy (similar to the Fredet-Ramstedt operation for pyloric stenosis) or an esophagogastrostomy may give permanent relief. Unfortunately, however, reflux esophagitis often leads to a recurrence of the symptoms and of the stricture itself, necessitating a return to dilatations or reoperation. Belladonna derivatives may be of some benefit if administered early, but are of no avail in advanced cases.

ESOPHAGEAL VARICES

Esophageal varices may occur in children with portal hypertension as one of the evidences of the attempt to return blood to the heart by circumventing the liver. The principal **symptoms** of the varices are recurrent, profuse hematemesis of bright red blood, tarry stools and systemic signs of severe hemorrhage. Careful roentgenographic studies with barium may outline the varices. Their presence may be confirmed by esophagoscopic examination.

TREATMENT. Treatment of portal hypertension is discussed elsewhere (p. 897). Acute hemorrhage may at times be controlled by some form of tamponade. The varices may be injected with sclerosing solutions, special long needles being used through the esophagoscope. These procedures are palliative in most instances, but prolong life, reducing the number and severity of the hemorrhages.

RETROESOPHAGEAL ABSCESS

The most frequent cause of retroesophageal abscess is extension of a retropharyngeal abscess downward to the retroesophageal component of this single, potential space; other causes are esophageal perforations, foreign bodies, spinal caries, pleuritis, pericarditis, ulceration from an intubation or tracheostomy tube, diphtheria of the pharynx or suppurating mediastinal lymph nodes. The abscess forms behind and around the esophagus and often displaces it to one side, while at the same time it compresses the more firmly seated trachea.

The **symptoms** are dyspnea, brassy cough, dysphagia and, as the trachea is pushed forward, swelling of the neck. Toxemia, pain, tenderness on palpation of the neck, and cervical emphysema may be present. The increased retrotracheal space can be demonstrated on lateral roentgenograms of the neck without the use of contrast medium; if the abscess is due to esophageal perforation, barium is contraindicated.

PROGNOSIS. The abscess may rupture into the pleura, trachea or lung. Death may result from pressure of the abscess upon the vagus nerve or on the trachea with consequent asphyxia, or by an erosion into the great vessels of the neck with exsanguinating hemorrhage.

TREATMENT. Prompt surgical drainage is indicated. If the abscess is high, the retroesophageal space may be opened in the neck along the anterior border of the sternocleidomastoid muscle. Drainage here is effective to the level of the fourth dorsal vertebra. For retroesophageal abscesses occurring below this point a posterior mediastinotomy is generally indicated. Appropriate antibiotic therapy is indicated, but it should be recognized that such therapy could mask an advancing mediastinal infection and that only repeated lateral roentgenograms of the neck and chest will indicate the situation in the post-tracheal area.

FOREIGN BODIES IN THE ESOPHAGUS

Infants and children swallow an unlimited variety and number of inedible objects which, in most instances, reach the stomach and pass through the gastrointestinal tract without complications. Occasionally they lodge in one of the three anatomically narrow points of the esophagus, from which they must be extracted.

The point of lodgment of most foreign bodies is the cervical esophagus, immediately below the cricopharyngeus muscle. Here the musculature is weak in comparison with the strong muscles immediately above. The narrowing at the hiatus of the diaphragm and the cardia constitutes the second most common site for the lodgment of foreign bodies, although few lodge there. The third and infrequent site for lodgment is the normal narrowing of the esophagus at the level of the arch of the aorta. Open safety pins are found most frequently in infants 7 to 15 months of age, and coins, small toys, buttons, marbles and jackstones in children from 3 to 6 years.

Strictures of the esophagus, congenital or acquired, are often responsible for the lodgment of foreign bodies which would pass through the normal esophagus. They are a constant problem in infants and children who have had a repair of a congenital esophageal atresia.

CLINICAL MANIFESTATIONS. Initial symptoms of coughing, gagging, choking and dyspnea usually occur with ingestion of an object, no matter where it lodges. If it remains in the esophagus, pain localized in the region of the thyroid cartilage, dysphagia and drooling may follow. Once a foreign body becomes fixed, there is frequently a symptomless interval until edema around it produces evidence of obstruction, or until signs of infection resulting from esophageal perforation become evident.

Laryngeal symptoms may be produced by foreign bodies in the cervical esophagus. Dyspnea resulting from compression of the trachea may be severe enough to require a tracheotomy before the foreign body can be removed. This is especially true of marbles or jackstones. Cough and hoarseness follow obstruction of the cervical esophagus because of the irritation from secretions overflowing into the larynx. Similar symptoms occur if the foreign body erodes into the trachea.

DIAGNOSIS. The diagnosis of a foreign body in the esophagus is most frequently made from the history. The child may state that he swallowed a button or coin, or the mother may state that the child placed some object in his mouth and choked on it. A history of difficulty in swallowing or the refusal of a child to take solid or liquid food suggests an esophageal foreign body.

A complete search of the gastrointestinal tract as well as of the respiratory system must be made to locate the object. Fluoroscopic examinations and roentgenograms of the cervical esophagus, with the introduction of radiopaque media if necessary, and of the chest and the abdomen in the anteroposterior and lateral projections are indicated. On anteroposterior projection of the chest, the face of a flat foreign body, such as a coin or safety pin, is usually visible if it lies in the esophagus; if it lies in the larynx, the edge is visible.

TREATMENT. *Foreign bodies in the esophagus should be removed under direct vision through the esophagoscope.* The use of blind instrumentation in an attempt to force the foreign body into the stomach or attempted extraction by means other than by direct vision is likely to lead to esophageal perforation, mediastinitis and death. Attempts to force the foreign body into the stomach with dry bread, cabbage, cotton or roughage diets not infrequently necessitate the removal of this material as well as the foreign body. Such procedures may also wedge the foreign body more firmly into the esophageal mucosa.

PAUL H. HOLINGER

Berenberg, W., and Neuhauser, E. B. D.: Cardioesophageal relaxation (chalasia). Pediatrics *5*:414, 1950.

Carré, I. J., Astley, R., and Smellie, J. M.: Minor degrees of partial thoracic stomach in childhood. Lancet *2*:1150, 1952.

Chunn, V. D., and Geppert, L. J.: Spontaneous rupture of the esophagus in the newborn. J. Pediatr. *60*:404, 1962.

Cleveland, W. W., Chandler, J. R., and Lawson, R. B.: Treatment of caustic burns of esophagus: Early esophagoscopy and adrenocortical steroids. J.A.M.A. *186*:262, 1963. (See comment in Year Book of Pediatrics, 1964–65 Series, S. Gellis ed., Chicago, Ill., Year Book Medical Publishers.)

Herweg, J. C., and Ogura, J. H.: Congenital tracheoesophageal fistula with esophageal atresia. J. Pediatr. *47*:293, 1955.

Holder, T. M., Cloud, T. C., Lewis, J. E., Jr., and Pilling, G. P., IV: Esophageal atresia and tracheoesophageal fistula (a survey). Pediatrics *34*:542, 1964.

Holinger, P. H., Johnston, K. C., and Potts, W. J.: Congenital anomalies of the esophagus. Acta Oto-Lar., Suppl. 100, 1952.

Holinger, P. H., Johnston, K. C., Potts, W. J., and da Cunha, F.: The conservative and surgical management of benign strictures of the esophagus. J. Thorac. Surg. *28*:(Oct.) 1954.

THE GASTROINTESTINAL TRACT

Gastrointestinal Symptomatology

Gastrointestinal symptoms may result from disturbances outside the gastrointestinal tract, from the central nervous and genitourinary systems, from systemic infections, and from psychogenic factors. The common symptomatic expressions of the gastrointestinal tract are lack of appetite, abdominal pain, vomiting, diarrhea, disturbance in fecal elimination and bleeding.

POOR APPETITE

Whenever a child is said to eat poorly, the first step is to evaluate the complaint in terms of the child's activity, appearance and growth. Records of height and weight should be plotted on a growth chart to find if they deviate from the expected growth pattern. Poor appetite in any acute or chronic illness warrants further examination in those instances where growth failure develops. In the absence of growth failure, the complaint frequently arises from a misconception about normal food intake, especially in the second or third year of life when diminished intake accompanies a decreased rate of growth. The dawdling of young children as they begin to explore self-feeding is sometimes viewed as poor appetite, and adults may fail to recognize or accept that normal children have day-to-day variations in food intake. Predilections for limited varieties of foods and refusals to explore others, particularly of different appearance and textures, occur in many children. In the social atmosphere of the family meal familial tensions commonly emerge and become focused upon both the type and amount of food eaten by the child. Pressures at such times can lead to strong aversions to certain foods or even to the whole eating process. A complaint of poor appetite most frequently involves an only child, a child born many years after the last previous child, a child of elderly parents, or children of families experiencing marital and other stresses. In certain instances of lack of appetite, parental anxiety is occasioned by remembered illness in an earlier offspring or from the parent's own childhood.

Neither the physician's blunt statement that the child is well nor the administration of a "tonic" (which may be requested by the parent) will alone resolve the problem of poor appetite. In the child with adequate growth, thorough physical examination and growth evaluation, followed by a search for the factors responsible for parental apprehension, may provide the atmosphere in which sympathetic explanation of the evidence of the health of the child will lead to reduction of parental anxiety.

Gastrointestinal surgery in the first year of life may lead to a wide range of subtle and gross derangements of feeding patterns with psychologic impact. Such disturbances often require detailed explanation and specific empiric individual approaches. Some of the children involved show chronic growth failure.

Later psychosomatic or emotional difficulties may be partly rooted in early parent-child conflict over eating. In chronically ill children efforts to allay parental anxiety and improve the poor appetite are rarely successful. On the other hand, the poor appetite of children with severe iron deficiency anemia or other treatable disease often responds dramatically to specific therapy.

ANOREXIA NERVOSA. Anorexia nervosa is an extreme form of poor appetite or self-starvation, most often observed in adolescent girls. It is accompanied by severe weight loss and, in girls, by amenorrhea or delayed puberty. Anorexia nervosa frequently starts as an attempt to lose weight by dieting. Normal physical activity may be maintained at a high level despite much loss of weight. Children with this disorder often appear to have broken down in their ability to compete adequately in school and play; they manifest many patterns of emotional restriction, such as flat facial expressions and diminished verbal responses.

Treatment. Treatment often initially includes separation from the family into a hospital environment and intensive psychiatric therapy; hyperalimentation may be necessary for survival. In general, it is sound to avoid punitive approaches such as nasogastric feeding unless a clear danger to survival is present and alternatives have proved ineffective. It will be useful if staff and parents attenuate pressure around food intake. The patient should know clearly at what weight level the physician will feel he must intervene. See also Anorexia Nervosa, Section 2.

The pattern of illness clearly suggests a self-inflicted "suicidal" starvation with many phobic elements. The ultimate prognosis for survival is good; only rarely do irreversible cachexia, heart failure and death occur.

FAILURE TO THRIVE. "Failure to thrive" has come to be used to describe the symptom of failure to gain or loss of weight without superficially evident cause. The symptom is discussed in Section 26. See also Neglect and Abuse of Children, Section 2.

ABDOMINAL PAIN

Almost all children experience abdominal pain at some time. Of the many causes, some can be serious; no symptom presents so much uncertainty and disquietude for the physician. It is particularly difficult to interpret in young children who cannot help significantly with the history and physical examination. A number of critical questions help to define the pattern of the pain for diagnosis and management. Its localization, manner of onset, character and severity are all important, along with its frequency, the duration of an episode, and the possible existence of prior episodes. A brief pang of pain at infrequent intervals is considerably different from acute, persistent distress of increasing intensity. Recurrent episodes are less suggestive of such serious causes as appendicitis. A periumbilical localization is one of the more common, and also less likely to mean major organic disease. Pain that changes its localization is less likely to result from some anatomic or intra-abdominal disease. The major exception to this is that the pain of acute appendicitis may start in the periumbilical or epigastric area and later settle in the right lower abdominal quadrant. The severity of pain does not necessarily indicate serious disease; many instances of severe pain in childhood are due to a spastic colon. It must be determined whether pain is getting better or worse; it is also of value to learn what brings on the pain, makes it worse or eases it. The character of the pain should be explored. Is it sharp, stabbing, burning, colicky, throbbing, or a steady ache? The more consistent the description, the more one searches for an underlying organic disease; the more erratic or inconsistent the pattern and character of the pain, the more likely that no major underlying organic disease is present. It is useful also to elicit associated symptoms. Diarrhea, constipation and the like will suggest an intestinal origin, and dysuria or other urinary symptoms an origin in the urinary tract, whereas headache, dizziness and other vague subjective complaints will suggest a functional disturbance.

The examination of the child must be complete, since many sources of abdominal pain are extra-abdominal. It is important to examine the child in the position which permits greatest ease and least anxiety, sometimes with the child standing up or in the parent's lap. It is important that the physician palpate the abdomen with a very light touch and warm hand, while he addresses soothing or reassuring words to the child and looks at his face, which will tell more by its expression than an answer to "Does it hurt?" In case of acute abdominal pain, rectal examination is necessary, but it may be delayed beyond a first visit if there have been recurrent episodes of abdominal pain. Auscultation of the abdomen will reveal increased intestinal motor activity, or absence as in ileus.

The causes of pain are many, an ever-present

question being "appendicitis?" During infancy, abdominal pain may be caused by obstructions associated with intestinal atresia, or by volvulus, duplication, visceral hernias, annular pancreas, incarcerated hernia, intussusception or appendicitis. Pain as a subjective complaint is difficult to evaluate in the infant. The paroxysmal fussiness of infantile colic is often interpreted as the result of abdominal pain. Pain may be produced by infection, inflammation, changes in bowel activity, anatomic obstruction, and visceral distention that can accompany many medical illnesses. The following incomplete list includes some conditions quite rare in childhood:

Urinary tract anomalies and infection
Gastroenteritis
Mesenteric adenitis
Duodenal ulcer
Asthmatic attacks
Lower lobe pneumonia
Rheumatic fever
Acute nephritis
Mumps and other viral infections
Infectious mononucleosis
Infectious hepatitis
Anaphylactoid purpura
Diabetic acidosis or hypoglycemia
Sickle cell crises
Lead poisoning
Cystic fibrosis
Meckel's diverticulum
Regional ileitis or enterocolitis
Ulcerative colitis
Abdominal tumors
Ovarian cyst or torsion of ovarian pedicle
Torsion of the testes
Drugs
Pancreatitis
Primary peritonitis
Periodic disease
Porphyria

Ascariasis can cause acute attacks of pain when active adult worms temporarily obstruct the intestinal lumen. The evidence that *pinworm infestation* causes abdominal pain is not firm. *Giardiasis* has been associated with recurrent attacks of abdominal pain.

RECURRENT ABDOMINAL PAIN. Recurrent abdominal pain without detectable disease of the urinary or gastrointestinal tract is a frequent complaint of children. It is often emotionally frustrating to the child and his parents, and diagnostically and therapeutically frustrating to the physician.

In many instances recurrent abdominal pain may represent a spastic form of the *irritable colon syndrome* (see later, this Section).

The frequent association of recurrent abdominal pain with signs of hyperactivity of the autonomic nervous system and with emotionally charged situations such as ambivalence about going to school gives support to the hypothesis that the syndrome of recurrent abdominal pain in children is often a psychosomatic illness. Further support for this hypothesis lies in the behavioral characteristics exhibited by children with the syndrome, such as generally strong sensitivity to other persons, varying degrees of fear for the health and happiness of parents and other persons close to them, and fears of being unacceptable to others in appearance or competence. Frequently, the life of the family has been punctuated by illness and acute situational crises, such as deaths, separations and accidents.

The physician must make a careful and unbiased exploration of possible organic causes for recurrent abdominal pain, as well as a search for areas which may be recognized as emotionally stressful. When organic illness has not been found and the evidence supports the hypothesis that emotional tensions may account for the pain, *treatment* consists in reassurance and helping the child and his parents to gain insight into the nature of the problem. Implication that the abdominal pain is "in the head," "made up," or "put on" must be carefully avoided; the pain is real. Glib statements that the pain is "psychologic" or "emotional" are also hard for the parents to accept; they tend to have an unusual sensitivity to and sense of responsibility for pain of the body or spirit of their child.

Since anxiety over pain originally initiated by anxiety may result in a vicious circle, breaking the cycle may be helpful; a few patients respond to mild sedation or to the symptomatic relief sometimes offered by antispasmodics. Such therapy should be intermittent and used only as seems necessary, in the early phase of psychosocial therapy. Dependence on drugs by family or child should be avoided. The ritual of administration of an appropriate number of drops of tincture of belladonna in water 30 minutes before each meal may be more effective than the swallowing of a pill.

If the abdominal pain is interfering with play or attendance at school, or if it has become an overwhelming focus of anxiety in the life of the family, hospitalization may be helpful in providing reassurance that every reasonable attempt has been made to rule out organic causes. The temporary removal from the home of the child who has become the focus of parental anxiety may break the cycle of anxiety and in itself be therapeutic. The usual diminution of the complaint during hospitalization offers additional reassurance to both physician and family that the diagnosis is correct, and there is opportunity for calm and unhurried exploration of possible precipitating factors.

The measures outlined above are usually successful in temporarily or permanently alleviating the complaint of recurrent abdominal pain, but relapses are frequent. Fortunately, most children with recurrent abdominal pain recover promptly or gradually or learn to accept the symptom as a part of life; a few continue to have recurring episodes disruptive to their own and their parents' lives. Even these latter children usually ultimately become free of pain. Psychiatric referral may be helpful for identified emotional problems with which the physician and parents are unable to cope on a more superficial basis.

ABDOMINAL EPILEPSY. Very rarely, recurrent

abdominal pain may occur as an epileptic aura or equivalent. The diagnosis is based on the electroencephalographic demonstration of clear-cut cerebral dysrhythmia. The presence of minor electroencephalographic abnormalities in patients with recurrent abdominal pain, even if apparently relieved by anticonvulsant therapy, does not suffice to justify a diagnosis of epilepsy with its lifelong implications.

GASTROINTESTINAL BLEEDING

Since many of the specific entities resulting in gastrointestinal bleeding are discussed elsewhere, only general comments will be made here. Gastrointestinal bleeding raises many questions of diagnosis and management, the resolution of which depends on the severity and duration of bleeding, associated symptoms, site of origin, and the age of the child. Of first importance are estimating the amount of bleeding and assessing its impact on the child. Pulse rate and blood pressure must be measured at frequent intervals, rising pulse rate and falling blood pressure being signs of major blood loss. If major bleeding is suspected or possible, hospitalization may be indicated. Blood of an appropriate donor should be typed and cross-matched, and hemoglobin level and hematocrit determined to establish baseline levels. It may take several days for the hematocrit to stabilize after an acute hemorrhage. Placement of a catheter for measurement of central venous pressure may be useful to follow the need for blood replacement in intensive bleeding. Some intravenous line should be readily available. Diagnostic maneuvers are then necessary to locate the site of bleeding and identify its source. Passage of a nasogastric tube may help to establish that bleeding is occurring in stomach or duodenum, but observations may be confusing, and the procedure is arduous for the child. Arteriography has been used to locate severe bleeding of unexplained origin. The passage by rectum of bright red blood does not rule out a lesion of the upper gastrointestinal tract, but the passage of altered blood is more frequent in such lesions.

The age of the child has considerable diagnostic significance in gastrointestinal bleeding. Below 1 year of age intussusception, Meckel's diverticulum, volvulus and gangrene of the small bowel, and hiatal hernia are important causes of intestinal hemorrhage (Fig. 11–9), but *anal fissure, also more common under 1 year of age, is the most frequent cause of rectal bleeding in both infancy and childhood.* In newborn infants hemorrhagic disease of the newborn and the "swallowed blood syndrome" may result in the passage of either bright red or altered blood. Polyps, esophageal varices and ulcerative colitis occur beyond 1 year of age. Localized lesions are responsible for about 50 per cent of cases of gastrointestinal bleeding, and systemic disturbances (sepsis, hemorrhagic

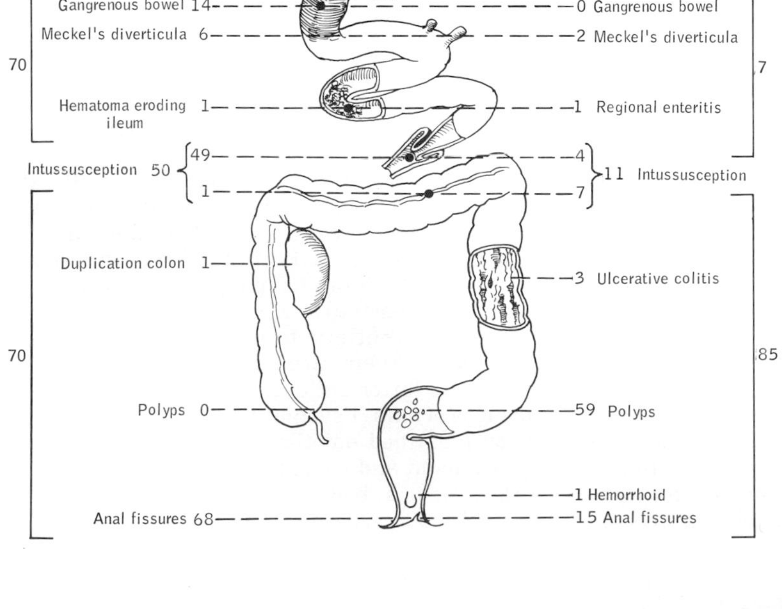

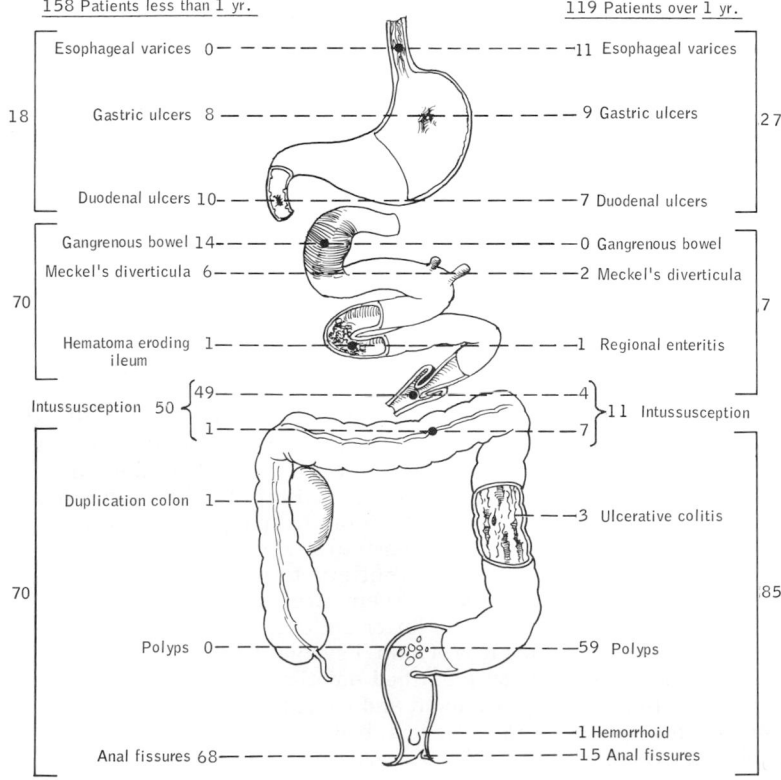

Figure 11–9 *Lesions producing gastrointestinal hemorrhage in children under and over 1 year of age. (After Spencer: Surgery, 1963.)*

diseases, allergy) are responsible for 10 to 20 per cent. About one third of cases of gastrointestinal bleeding are not etiologically identifiable, even after exhaustive investigation. About half of the localized lesions causing bleeding from the intestinal tract are in the anus, rectum or colon; about one third are in the small intestine, and only about 10 per cent are above the ligament of Treitz.

HEMATEMESIS. Hematemesis in childhood may result from blood swallowed during epistaxis or after a surgical or dental procedure. Such bleeding or accumulation of a large amount of blood in the gastrointestinal tract may be responsible for leukocytosis or fever. Blood-tinged vomitus and minor hematemesis are quite frequent after repeated vomiting of any origin. Otherwise, hematemesis suggests upper gastrointestinal lesions such as esophageal varices, erosive esophagitis secondary to gastroesophageal hiatal hernia, peptic ulcer, poisons and drugs such as aspirin, or, rarely, hemangioma or aberrant gastric mucosa in the esophagus.

RECTAL BLEEDING. Gross rectal bleeding may result from anal fissure, peptic ulcer, marginal ulcer associated with a Meckel's diverticulum or an intestinal duplication, gangrenous bowel secondary to volvulus, intussusception, gastrointestinal infection, ileitis, polyps, ulcerative colitis or amebiasis. Tarry stools may result from peptic ulcer, esophageal varices or bleeding diatheses. The association of vomiting, abdominal pain or shock with rectal bleeding suggests the possibility of a surgical emergency. Rectal bleeding with diarrhea suggests infectious enterocolitis, ulcerative colitis, amebiasis or intussusception. Minimal or microscopic bleeding with recurrent or chronic anemia suggests Meckel's diverticulum, amebiasis, ulcerative colitis, infectious enterocolitis, hiatal hernia, or polyps; in infants, *cow's milk allergy* is an occasional cause of such bleeding.

If the blood is bright red, diagnosis of the cause of rectal bleeding begins with careful examination of the anus for a fissure or "sentinel tag." If any one of these is found, and the bleeding is minor or consists chiefly of blood-streaked stools or blood spots on the paper used to wipe the anus after defecation, particularly if there is a history of hard, large or painful bowel movements, the blood may be presumed to be from an *anal fissure.* Treatment consists in meticulous cleansing of the anus with soap and water after each defecation and in use of mineral oil to lubricate passage of stool until the lesion heals.

If an anal lesion is not found, thrombocytopenia, hypoprothrombinemia and other bleeding disorders should be ruled out; the rash associated with anaphylactoid purpura usually serves to identify it as a cause of intestinal bleeding. Sigmoidoscopic examination is useful to identify ulcerative colitis or polyps in the distal colon. Barium studies can serve to diagnose duodenal ulcer (because of the relative shortness and motility of the child's intestine, blood from a bleeding ulcer may be passed in virtually unaltered form), ileitis, ulcerative colitis, polyps, intussusception and volvulus; they are rarely informative for Meckel's diverticulum or duplication. Occasionally air contrast study of the colon is useful in the diagnosis of polyps. Pigmented lesions on the lips suggest polyposis of the small bowel as part of the *Peutz-Jeghers syndrome.*

Exploratory laparotomy may be indicated in selected cases of severe bleeding without historical, physical, laboratory or roentgenographic findings to explain the bleeding.

VOMITING

Vomiting is one of the commonest symptoms of infancy and childhood; its causes tend to vary with age. There may be nonspecific association with almost any infection or emotional stress; otherwise, vomiting is most frequently related to abnormalities of the central nervous, urinary and gastrointestinal systems.

VOMITING IN THE NEONATAL PERIOD. See Section 7.

VOMITING IN INFANCY AFTER THE NEONATAL PERIOD. Certain infants regurgitate or spit up small amounts of feeding at frequent intervals. They are usually well nourished, very active and responsive, and tend to regurgitate more when excited or exposed to an emotionally charged environment. Neither overfeeding nor other aberration in care seems to be a common causative factor. Formula changes rarely help. The vomiting tends to subside spontaneously in the second year of life, suggesting a maturational process. Treatment consists in reassuring the parents that organic disease is absent. Barium studies may be useful as much for parental reassurance as for ruling out abnormalities of the esophagus, stomach and duodenum. In rare instances, hospitalization of the infant for observation and thorough study may be therapeutic and relieve a parent, exasperated from the continual cleaning up of vomitus, who has been unable to accept reassurances from the physician of the basic health of the infant. In such situations, it may be helpful to determine whether there may be basic fears about the baby rooted in events of pregnancy or birth which have produced anticipatory anxiety in the parent. The need for intensive study is signaled whenever vomiting is accompanied by failure to grow.

Infants may respond with vomiting to the frustration of inhibition of free movement by body or leg casts applied for orthopedic treatment. The disturbance usually clears spontaneously within a few days.

Infants with neurologic disease or damage may have pharyngeal and esophageal dysfunction which results in vomiting and aspiration. Tracheostomy or gastrostomy may be required temporarily; in spite of progressive or persisting neurologic abnormality, the pharyngeal dysfunction usually improves sufficiently to permit oral feeding without complications by 2 years of age.

The validity of the popular assumption that vomiting is associated with *teething* is open to question. In some instances it is a manifestation of allergy to cow's milk.

RUMINATION (MERYCISM). Rumination is a rare but serious form of chronic regurgitation, leading to severe growth failure in infancy. The onset is usually in the latter half of the first year of life. The condition appears to be of psychogenic origin and is often associated with the mother's difficulty in establishing a warm, maternal relationship with the baby. There may be a general inability of the mother to develop a mature marital or parental role, or she may be unable to mother her infant because of a deep-seated fear that the baby will die; occasionally conception or birth has taken place near the time of the tragic death of a sibling. It has been thought that the rumination is a repetitive self-stimulatory pattern of the infant as a substitute for the lack of appropriate external stimuli.

Chewing movements and mouthing of the regurgitated material and fingers often precede or accompany the regurgitation. Careful observation may disclose that the infant actively gags himself with his tongue or fingers. The large loss of nutrient may appear deceptively small; the infant lies continuously in a small pool of regurgitated liquid. In some cases such infants have been left for protracted intervals without soothing tactile, visual or auditory stimulation. A barium swallow and upper gastrointestinal series as well as urinalysis, blood urea nitrogen determination and a hemogram are valuable in ruling out chronic renal disease and upper gastrointestinal lesions such as hiatal hernia, esophageal stricture, chalasia, achalasia or duodenal ulcer.

Treatment involves an intensive relationship with a warm, interested caretaker; rumination tends to stop while eye contact and verbal contact are established and maintained until the stomach empties. This usually leads to decreased regurgitation and to a gain in weight. Concomitant exploration of mother-child relationships, together with warmth and support to combat the mother's feeling of inadequacy engendered by her malnourished infant, may allow her to regain her sense of adequacy, develop a warmer relation with the infant, and gradually take over the care of her child in the hospital. The prognosis is usually good for these infants if such a setting can be instituted. Otherwise death may result from malnutrition.

VOMITING IN CHILDHOOD. Beyond infancy acute episodes of vomiting are usually due to readily ascertainable infectious or psychologic causes. Community epidemics of nausea, vomiting and diarrhea are common and presumably of viral origin. Appendicitis should always be considered when vomiting is coupled with abdominal pain and fever. Ingestion of drugs or other toxic substances may lead to vomiting, which also may be an important symptom of chronic lead poisoning. Recurrent or prolonged vomiting should always arouse suspicion of an intracranial neoplasm.

CYCLIC, PERIODIC OR RECURRENT VOMITING. Some children experience periodic attacks of unexplained vomiting. These episodes may be mild and accepted as a matter of course after intense activity or emotional stress. Other children, particularly preadolescent girls, have recurrent attacks of severe vomiting. The bouts are characterized by violent retching, often of mildly bloodstained material, severe drooling and salivation, lethargy, withdrawn behavior and a striking facial flush. Intense thirst, headache and abdominal pain are frequent. The severity of the attacks often leads to suspicion of organic disease of the central nervous system or gastrointestinal tract, but physical, neurologic and roentgenographic examinations are normal. Occasionally electroencephalographic variations may arouse suspicion of an epileptic equivalent, but therapy with anticonvulsant drugs is usually disappointing. In some children, cyclic vomiting appears to be the childhood equivalent of migraine.

TREATMENT OF VOMITING. Vomiting should in all instances be viewed as a symptom, with principal attention directed toward determination and correction of its cause. Withholding oral intake for 4 to 6 hours, followed by frequent sips of clear fluids containing carbohydrate for the rest of the day, may be helpful. Phenothiazine derivatives are of limited value and may lead to disturbing central nervous system symptoms (Drug Table). Severe or prolonged vomiting may lead to dehydration and hypochloremic alkalosis requiring parenteral fluid and electrolyte therapy, which should include glucose, most importantly, and potassium. (See Section 5.) Nonobstructive vomiting may also commonly be associated with acidosis and ketosis. Attacks of *cyclic vomiting* may be aborted by hospitalization, administration of fluids intravenously, or both. In addition, a search should be made for sources of unrecognized or unadmitted frustration in the life of the child or the parents; environmental adjustment or the mere fact that the patient and parents gain insight into the existence of a problem may be sufficient to diminish recurrences. In any event, the attacks tend to subside as the child becomes older, though migraine may be a sequel during later life.

FECAL ELIMINATION

NORMAL STOOLS. The characteristics of the meconium stools of the first few days of life and of the transitional stools are described elsewhere. When breast feeding is well established and the infant's intake is composed entirely of milk, the stools are yellow to golden, of salvelike consistency, faintly acid in reaction (pH 4.7 to 5.1), and may contain seedlike particles *(birdseed stools)*.

With cow's milk feedings, the stools vary from pale yellow to light brown, are firmer in consistency, less acid in reaction and may be slightly alkaline (pH 6 to 8); there is a more fecal odor, owing to decomposition of protein. Oral administration of acids or alkalis has little effect on the pH of the stools.

The number of stools per day varies considerably; the comfort and well-being of the infant are more important than the number and type of stools. Breast-fed infants average from 2 to 4 stools a day with a range of 1 to 7 during the first 3 or 4 months of life, whereas artificially fed infants average 1 or 2 stools. Occasionally the breast-fed infant may comfortably and normally have a bowel movement only once in 4 to 7 days, with movements that remain of the usual consistency. By the end of the first year of life many infants have only 1 stool a day, but more or less than that need not be abnormal.

Normal stools contain approximately 80 per cent water; the residue consists preponderantly of cellular elements, mucus and bacteria. Fat is present in the form of neutral fat, fatty acids and soaps. The fat is largely a residue from unabsorbed foods; some comes from bile, bacteria and cellular detritus, and some from lipids excreted from the blood. The fat content of infants' stools varies widely. It is usually less than 20 per cent of ingested fat in the young infant, becoming less than 5 per cent of ingested fat by the end of the first year. The sugar of the infant's diet is well absorbed. Starch is not completely digested and may be demonstrated in the stool by the iodine test. Only about 8 per cent of the protein ingested is lost in normal stools. From 8 to 10 per cent of the dried stool consists of mineral matter, chiefly calcium.

Curds may be found in the stools of both breast-fed and artificially fed infants and are of no particular significance. They are whitish, with an outer coating of yellow or brown; they are composed of a casein coagulum; those of breast milk stools are smaller and less firm in consistency than those of cow's milk. The small white curds which appear in diarrheal stools represent undigested neutral fat.

Various enzymes are present in the stools, such as diastase, lactase, invertin, trypsin, rennin and a fat-splitting ferment.

Microscopically the stools of an infant exhibit fat globules of various sizes, needles of fatty acids, innumerable bacteria, cholesterin plates, epithelial cells, small round cells, calcium salts in crystalline form, granular detritus, and occasionally bilirubin crystals, yeast fungi and protein matter.

As the infant grows older and the proportion of the diet contributed by milk becomes less, the stools acquire more of the characteristics of those of adults in both color and odor. By 2 years of age, stools are expected to be formed, but even young infants may pass fully formed stools.

The odor of putrefaction may be present in the stools of infants who ingest large amounts of protein or whose digestion of protein is impaired. The color is brownish yellow or sometimes greenish black, and mucus may be present. Tough, yellowish, bean-like protein curds are often present after ingestion of unboiled milk. Stools from diets high in carbohydrate are of normal consistency, smooth, brown or yellowish brown, and have an acid reaction. When there is deficient digestion of carbohydrate and decomposition of it in the intestinal tract, the stools become thin, frothy, light yellow, or often green, with an acid reaction and an odor suggestive of acetic acid. It is difficult to distinguish a fatty stool by observation; however, such stools sometimes are yellow to gray, bulky and soft, with a greasy appearance. If protein is also present in large amount, the odor is cheesy and offensive; when there is also undigested carbohydrate, the stool is frothy. Such stools are seen in the malabsorption syndromes.

Mucus is often present in the stools of infants, and in small amounts may have no significance. During starvation the stools consist of thin mucoid secretions of the intestine which are stained a brownish tint *(starvation stool)*. Mucus is generally present in considerable quantity after administration of a purgative such as castor oil. In older children it may represent a functional disturbance and is present in inflammatory conditions. Stools composed almost entirely of bloodstained mucus occur in dysenteric conditions and intussusception. Undigested starch may resemble mucus in appearance, but can be distinguished by the iodine reaction.

GREEN STOOLS. A faint pea-green color when the stool is passed or developing shortly thereafter is not abnormal; it results from oxidation of bilirubin (responsible for the yellow color) to biliverdin. Green watery stools are common in diarrhea.

BLACK STOOLS. Black or reddish black stools may be seen after large amounts of blood have been swallowed or after extensive bleeding high in the gastrointestinal tract. Ingested iron causes the stools to become black.

DIFFICULTIES IN FECAL ELIMINATION

In many families the control and organization of the nature, timing and frequency of bowel movements are the focus of undue concern. Few people other than physicians know that the number of bowel evacuations may vary in normal persons from 3 or 4 a day to as few as one in 5 or 6 days; when the family's concept of the normal pattern differs, their reassurance may require not just an adequate explanation, but often repeated explanations and reinforcement.

When parents complain that their child has "diarrhea," they may mean any increased frequency or any degree of decreased firmness of bowel movements. The term "constipation" may be applied by parents to painful or infrequent passage of bowel movements of normal consistency and size, or to hard or large bowel movements of normal or decreased frequency. The significance of the soiling which frequently accompanies fecal withholding is less well recognized. Chronic fecal retention may present as a complaint of liquid stools *(paradoxical diarrhea)*.

Certain items of history should be explored in every child with a disorder of elimination. These are (1) whether the disorder has been continuous since birth or emerged subsequently, and, if so, when; (2) whether there is fecal retention; (3) whether the stools are bulky, scybalous or soft; (4) whether blood has ever stained or been passed with bowel movements; (5) whether there is fecal soiling; and (6) whether behavior suggestive of voluntary withholding of stool is evident.

ACUTE DIFFICULTIES IN ELIMINATION (CONSTIPATION). In infancy acute difficulty in elimination may be manifested by straining and irritability at scattered times of the day. Quiescence follows an episode of straining with stool passage. A blood-streaked stool indicates anal fissure. The stools may vary from hard pellets to soft, pasty or loose, unformed feces. Such episodes may occur during acute infantile colic, an upper respiratory tract illness, travel, or a period of intensive emotional stimulation. Anal irritation due to diaper rash or fissure may result in discomfort and difficulty in passing feces. On occasion, particularly in infants between 1 and 2 years of age, the difficulty may arise in association with family upset caused by death, parental separation or strife, major illness or a move to a new home.

Both infants and older children may withhold feces because of fear of pain on defecation. In such children there is often a history of an obviously painful, large, hard or blood-streaked bowel movement at the time of onset of the difficulty. Examination of the anus may reveal a small raw or bleeding fissure. Older children may withhold feces because of unavailability of a toilet at times of an urge to defecate. The unavailability may be actual or psychologic, owing to embarrassment in asking to use the toilet in school, or to aversion to using cold, unclean or malodorous facilities.

Most *acute disorders of elimination* are temporary, provided causative factors are eliminated and the condition not complicated by parental or medical manipulation. The physician should lend psychologic support in order to minimize parental inclination to intervene aggressively. The anal area is very sensitive and can easily be traumatized by manipulations. Most acute disorders of elimination, including anal fissures, will subside spontaneously with minimal hygienic measures. Gentle cleansing of the anus with soap and water after each bowel movement is more effective than the application of topical anesthetics. The gentle application of a protective zinc oxide ointment or petroleum jelly to the anal orifice will decrease the burning sensation. Warm baths may also be helpful prior to such applications. Stool softeners seem to have very limited utility, particularly since the stool is often already quite soft. The use of suppositories and anal dilators may lead to undesirable alterations in the child's bowel habits and result in sensory disruption which may perpetuate a disorganized bowel habit rather than permit the establishment of a normal pattern for the child. At times there may be justification for temporary use of a mild laxative or stool softener. Dietary changes such as increased intake of fruit or fluid, or a change of formula have little value in small children. The common notion that increased fluids will make softer stools has little basis in fact.

In instances of sudden inability to defecate, the possibility of acute mechanical obstruction, as by incarcerated hernia or volvulus, must be considered.

CHRONIC DIFFICULTIES IN ELIMINATION. Failure to pass bowel movements is a symptom rather than a primary illness. Constipation dating from the neonatal period suggests hypothyroidism or aganglionic megacolon. The latter may present as acute intestinal obstruction in the first few weeks of life or as insidious difficulty in passage of stools, with chronic abdominal distention. Table 11–6 summarizes some of the characteristics which distinguish aganglionic megacolon from functional constipation and to some extent from encopresis. Constipation is also not uncommon among mentally retarded children. If stool retention is protracted, there is a tendency for the colon to become dilated.

CHRONIC CONSTIPATION. An important disorder of elimination is infrequency of bowel movements and difficulty in passage of stools. During the second and third years of life, as bowel control is being established in most children, bowel difficulty is often manifest by voluntary retention of feces while the body is held taut, by episodes of florid-faced straining, by holding the buttocks compressed together, and by crossing the legs, walking on the tips of the toes, or by jumping around in a tight, restrained fashion. Fecal soiling may occur during some of these episodes. Some young children will be considerably distressed if placed on the toilet at this time. About two thirds of such children have a history, dating from the neonatal period, of straining at stool, of colic and of parental manipulations such as enemas, suppositories and formula changes. A few children have a history of chronic diarrhea during the second year, clinically misdiagnosed as a type of celiac disease. Boys are involved approximately four times as frequently as girls. The bowel movements are infrequent and, at times, very large. Approximately two thirds of the children have fecal soiling as retention of stool persists. Enuresis or occasional urinary retention is also reported in about two thirds of the cases. Such children usually have a primary behavioral disturbance which seems contributory to the fecal retention.

Secondary emotional problems are frequent as a result of interaction between parent and child over the stool difficulty. Many children shut out any reference to stools and give no outward sign of awareness of an urge to defecate, an urge that they may deny on questioning. They often prefer to be alone in a corner or lying on the floor during episodes of resistance to colonic peristalsis, and they may hide their soiled underclothing. Other children who withhold bowel movements are unable to tolerate even minor uncleanliness, such as dirty hands. Similarly, some parents of children who withhold bowel movements, particularly mothers,

TABLE 11-6 DIFFERENTIATING FEATURES OF AGANGLIONIC MEGACOLON AND THE COMMON PATTERN OF FUNCTIONAL CONSTIPATION

	AGANGLIONIC MEGACOLON	FUNCTIONAL CONSTIPATION
Onset	Birth or neonatal period Symptoms of intestinal obstruction	About 60% in first year of life; most of remainder from 1 to 4 years
Course	Failure to pass formed bowel movements except by enema	Huge bowel movements at long intervals
Withholding efforts	Not present	Present
Soiling	None	At least two thirds of cases
Growth	Impaired	Usually normal
Abdominal findings	Distended; large fecal mass remains in same site	Variable distention and masses
Rectal examination	Rectum not dilated and usually empty of stool	Cavernous rectum, often filled with soft feces
Roentgenographic findings	Colon dilated proximal to an area of normal caliber; post-evacuation film shows poor evacuation of barium	Colon dilated to anus; post-evacuation film shows effective evacuation
Rectal biopsy	Absence of ganglion cells, large nerve bundles	Normal

tend to have a fetishistic devotion to housework and cleanliness as a compensation for feelings of inadequacy which also make them unable to tolerate any level of discomfort in their offspring. Adverse experiences during their own childhood may make it difficult for them to comfort a child over minor distress without intervening in some physical, manipulative fashion. With respect to their child's bowel movements, many such parents go through stages of use of laxatives, cajoling, rewarding and punishing, all culminating in a feeling of desperation. They seem to interpret the whole process as a failure on their part and as defiance or "laziness" on the part of the child. They frequently describe the child as stubborn and "hard to understand." The children themselves tend to play poorly with peer groups and to be "loners," a problem contributed to by the malodor of their fecal soiling. Feeding problems, overall restraint in expression of feeling, reading disability and infantile speech may be present in some cases.

Abdominal palpation in cases of chronic constipation reveals masses of retained feces of variable size, consistency and movability. On rectal examination there is a markedly dilated rectal ampulla which is often filled with soft stool.

Chronic fecal retention may lead to urinary stasis, as evidenced in urograms, with distortion and displacement of the urinary bladder and some dilatation of the ureters and occasionally of the renal pelves. An increased frequency of urinary tract infection has also been observed in chronic constipation.

Treatment. Treatment involves (1) attenuating parental fear of danger from retention of stool, and of physical defect beyond dilatation of the colon, and (2) assisting the child in interrupting the patterned withholding response to colonic peristalsis and in re-establishing a normal, regular bowel habit. This may be accomplished in many children by the oral administration of 1 or 2 teaspoonfuls (5 or 10 ml) of mineral oil twice a day for a protracted period, usually 3 to 9 months. In cases of severe or longstanding retention of stool, particularly when accompanied by much parental anxiety, hospitalization may occasionally be justified for a more intensive period of observation and study and to interrupt the adverse interaction between parent and child. Roentgenographic studies may be necessary to provide convincing evidence of the absence of serious organic diseases such as aganglionic megacolon. Some physicians utilize this period to initiate emptying of the dilated colon through a series of warm saline enemas (a heaping teaspoonful of table salt per liter or quart of water) 2 or 3 times a day until the returns are clear. Subsequent administration of mineral oil will then usually suffice to maintain a regular pattern of bowel movements. The medication must be continued for at least 3 to 9 months in order to allow time for the colon to return to an undilated and more physiologically effective state, as well as for establishment of a regular bowel habit. In some instances a regular bowel habit may follow such a period of hospitalization. Dietary approaches have little value in most of these children, many of whom have concurrent feeding problems. Because manipulations such as enemas and suppositories place abnormal emphasis on bowel movements, they cause a strain on the parent-child relationship, so it is usually wise to use these procedures to the absolute minimum within the home.

In many instances of chronic constipation the precipitating factor has long since been removed, so that the condition itself has become a self-perpetuating automatic process in the child, resulting in conflict between parent and child. In such cases, relief of the symptoms of constipation and fecal soiling is sufficient to allow favorable psychologic readjustment, although exacerbations of the problem may recur under the stress of illness or emotional upset. In other cases, in which the underlying problem is a more deep-seated emotional one, psychiatric treatment is indicated. Psychiatric referral should be on the basis of the emotional disorder, however, rather than for the constipation itself, since the latter is usually refractory to purely psychiatric therapy.

As improvement in the bowel problem takes place, the child may become more self-reliant, aggressive and outspoken, a situation in which parents frequently need the sympathetic support of the physician, as they do with the relapses and exacerbations which may characterize the problem. Management must be focused upon the long-range outlook rather than immediate fluctuations.

CONSTIPATION WITH RECTAL SCYBALA. In this type of constipation there tend to be more abdominal pain, shorter periods of no stool passage, little abdominal distention, no bulky stools, some soiling with mucus or feces, less evidence of withholding and greater awareness of toilet and stool passage than in children with the previously described form of chronic constipation. There may be vague abdominal tenderness, fecal masses or balls palpable in the sigmoid, and minimal dilatation demonstrable by rectal examination or barium enema. These patients may be appropriately classified as having a variety of the irritable colon syndrome (see below) and can be similarly managed, with the addition, on occasion, of small doses of mineral oil. This form of stool retention tends to be milder and less refractory than the more intense disorder previously described.

ENCOPRESIS. This term, which connotes the involuntary passage of feces unrelated to organic defect or illness, is used commonly to designate fecal soiling without voluntary withholding of bowel movements or physical signs of retention. The pattern may be continuous from infancy, during which it is normal, or it may arise after establishment of normal bowel control. Abdominal distention and dilatation of the rectal ampulla are not present. The anal sphincter usually has adequate tone, but anal tonometry as a measure of the integrative reflexes of the rectum and anal sphincter has shown occasional failures of anal sphincter responses, which may explain passage of feces at unpredictable times. Children with encopresis may also be hyperactive and have dyslexia or other learning disabilities suggesting a degree of neural incoordination. Emotional instability is frequent, with a wide spectrum of manifestations ranging from intensive motor responses without facial expression to great sensitivity to criticism or a high level of basic anxiety, with easy crying. In most instances there is a disturbance in relations with both parents and peers. The condition is relatively rare in girls.

Consultation with a physician is usually sought under the social impact of beginning school without bowel control. Older children seem to be able to maintain some control of their bowel passage during school hours, only to drop their guard and to soil when they get home after school. They are usually exquisitely sensitive to the problem the soiling presents with respect to their relations with parents and peers and view themselves as failures because of it.

Since the natural history of encopresis is that it frequently, like enuresis, may become an organized habit if it is not resolved, careful neurologic examination, psychologic evaluation and psychiatric consultation are indicated. Since behavioral features predominate in this picture, pediatric and child psychiatric approaches are of importance in the management of encopresis. The outcome is frequently good with even minimal approaches to the emotional area in these children unless severe psychosocial disorders exist in the family setting.

DIARRHEA

Diarrhea, the passage of loose or watery stools, usually with increased frequency, is an important clinical manifestation of a large number of gastrointestinal disorders. The problem is more serious during infancy than in later childhood, mainly because of the infant's greater susceptibility to infection and to water and electrolyte imbalances. The decrease in mortality from diarrheal disorders in countries with high standards of living and improved hygienic conditions has been largely responsible for the large overall decrease in infant mortality in these areas. In countries with a high incidence of infectious diarrhea there is an increased number of cases during the warmer period of the year, whereas there is little seasonal variation in areas with a low incidence.

ETIOLOGY. The causes of the majority of acute diarrheal disturbances are unknown. The clinical disturbances of the recognized enteric infections in which diarrhea is a significant manifestation are described elsewhere (see Bacillary Dysentery, Amebiasis, Salmonella Infections, Typhoid Fever, Cholera and Food Poisoning).

Diarrhea in the newborn (see also Section 7) is more serious when it occurs in epidemic form in a hospital nursery. Most of the intestinal pathogens, including enteropathogenic *Escherichia coli,* have been incriminated in individual epidemics. In addition, various bacteria not ordinarily considered pathogens, such as those of the paracolon, proteus, pseudomonas, staphylococcal and streptococcal groups, have been suspected in some epidemics in the neonatal period.

The problem *in infancy after the neonatal period* varies greatly in different socioeconomic groups. In situations of poverty and poor sanitation, contamination of milk feedings and foods is probably an important source of infection. Most infections in infants from higher socioeconomic groups are probably transmitted by infected persons or "carriers." Perhaps the most frequent causes at present are enteropathogenic *E. coli,* dysentery bacilli, salmonella and various viral agents. In addition to enteric viruses, it appears that some respiratory viruses may be responsible for mild diarrheal disturbances in conjunction with respiratory infections; it is not uncommon to observe diarrhea in an infant of a family whose older members have an epidemic respiratory infection. Diarrhea may also arise by direct enteric infection by the staphylococcus in association with staphylococcal infections elsewhere in the body. Diarrhea associated with infections in the middle ear or in the urinary or respiratory tract is termed *parenteral diarrhea.* This form usually lasts only as long as the parenteral infection. Whether parenteral diarrhea represents a secondary intestinal infection with the agent causing the parenteral infection, or an intestinal reaction to the parenteral infection has not been determined.

In *childhood,* acute diarrheal disturbances become less frequent and relatively less severe. Erratic eating, fatigue, nervous excitement and infection may precipitate mild diarrheal disorders.

Diarrhea induced by therapy with antibacterial agents administered by mouth occurs, and may be related to changes in the normal balance among the flora of the intestinal tract. Ampicillin, chloramphenicol and the tetracyclines are the drugs frequently involved. Staphylococci, candida, proteus or pseudomonas are organisms which frequently become predominant in the stools. *Treatment* is cessation of oral administration of the offending drug so that the normal balance of intestinal flora can be re-established. Diarrhea usually ceases in 2 to 5 days. In some instances it may be necessary to stop *all* antibacterial therapy.

A number of *noninfectious conditions* may be responsible for diarrhea. These include allergy or intolerance to specific foods (see Adverse Reactions to Foods, Section 9); metabolic disorders such as hyperthyroidism, uremia and acidosis; emotional upset and fatigue; excessive ingestion of certain foods or unripe fruits; so-called starvation diarrhea, in which the stools contain an excessive amount of mucus and little fecal material; and malabsorption syndromes (see later, this Section). Diarrhea may be a symptom of aganglionic megacolon, as a form of exudative colitis in the dilated bowel proximal to the aganglionic segment.

Chronic or Persistent Diarrhea. This may be a manifestation of genetic disorders in which there is an absence of intestinal sugar-splitting enzymes (Section 8). Temporary absence of such enzymes may be the reason for persistence of diarrhea after an acute diarrheal disorder; the diarrhea ceases if the specific disaccharide is eliminated from the diet. In areas in which amebiasis is endemic it is responsible for chronic diarrhea. *Acrodermatitis enteropathica (Danbolt-Closs syndrome)* is characterized by severe chronic diarrhea accompanied by areas of denuded skin around the mucocutaneous junctions, especially of the mouth and anus. This ill defined condition was formerly considered fatal, but some cases have responded to diiodohydroxyquin. Cohlan has described a form of mild, chronic diarrhea in otherwise healthy infants and young children, usually from homes of good socioeconomic status and whose parents, especially the mother, are emotionally tense and insecure. Although amebic infection cannot be proved, some of these infants apparently respond to diiodohydroxyquin (Diodoquin), which usually must be continued for 6 to 12 months (potentially toxic).

Recurrent Mild Diarrhea (Irritable Colon Syndrome). (See also later.) Recurrent mild diarrhea is a common disturbance of childhood observed preponderantly between the ages of 1 and 3 years. It rarely leads to dehydration and almost never affects growth. It often begins or is exacerbated by a respiratory illness. There are usually 2 to 8 stools a day. The first stool of the day may be formed, the others progressively looser. Occasionally the diarrhea alternates with episodes of constipation. A bacterial or amebic basis for the diarrhea is rarely found, and clinical or laboratory signs of maldigestion or malabsorption are absent. The children are characteristically intense and hyperactive. First children are commonly involved. The fathers often work night and day; the young mothers are often lonely and find it hard to let their very active toddlers determine their own pattern of activity. If these children are hospitalized, they tend to improve promptly without medication. Diets and drugs are of little value; in some instances they seem deleterious. Diiodohydroxyquin has sometimes seemed to produce nonspecific improvement, but has limited value. Clarification of the various diagnostic possibilities through reasoning rather than therapeutic action, together with understanding and sympathetic discussion with the parents about their questions and personal problems, usually provides the reassurance and support necessary to relieve the child of his emotionally reactive symptoms.

CLINICAL MANIFESTATIONS. The descriptions here apply principally to infants and very young children; see also Diarrhea in the Newborn and the various specific infections responsible for diarrheal disturbances.

Mild Diarrheal Disturbances. Occasionally

there are such prodromal symptoms as slight fever, irritability and a disinclination to eat. Severe vomiting is not common. The frequency of stools varies; there may be only 2 or 3 a day or as many as 10 or 12. Temporary reduction in oral feeding usually results in abatement of the diarrhea, and there is little or no evidence of dehydration.

Severe Diarrheal Disturbances. These can be placed in two groups: (1) patients in whom the upset is only moderately severe and toxic manifestations are greatly accentuated when dehydration and electrolytic disturbances have become a factor; (2) patients in whom the onset is abrupt with higher fever and extreme toxicity.

In the first group there may or may not be fever. There is often vomiting at the onset, but it is usually not persistent. It may return in the later stages. Diarrhea appears within 24 hours of onset; the stools are at first chiefly fecal, often contain small white curds, and are usually strongly acid. They quickly become liquid and greenish or greenish yellow, contain increasing amounts of mucus, and at times are blood-tinged. Initially there are evidences of irritability and, at times, stupor and convulsions; these symptoms often disappear after the first day, but the irritability and lassitude return if dehydration and acidosis develop. The number of stools varies from a few to 20 or more a day. Evacuation is often preceded by pain, and the stools may be expelled with force.

The extent of dehydration and the rapidity of its development depend upon the amount of fluid lost in the stools, the presence or absence of vomiting, and the extent to which fluids are replaced parenterally. In untreated cases there is loss of subcutaneous tissues and elasticity of the skin. The pulse is rapid and weak, and there is increasing prostration. The output of urine is progressively decreased; the urine has a high specific gravity and often contains albumin and casts. Hemoconcentration varies with the severity of dehydration. Owing to the decrease in renal function and to the hemoconcentration, urea nitrogen levels of the blood are increased to as much as 50 mg/dl or more. Acidosis is usually a prominent manifestation; in untreated cases plasma carbon dioxide levels may be less than 3 mEq/l and the pH may approach 7. Hypertonic dehydration may be a problem, especially when skim milk feedings or concentrated oral electrolyte solutions are given. See also Section 5.

Cases which fall in the second category have been variously termed "acute toxic diarrhea" and food poisoning. They are characterized by an abrupt onset with high fever, often 40 to 40.5° C (104 to 106° F), and extreme prostration. Vomiting is frequently severe. An infant who has been otherwise well suddenly becomes very ill. In some instances there is evidence of irritability, restlessness and even convulsions, but symptoms of collapse are more frequent. The infant in this latter instance is flaccid, and pallor is present. Respirations are rapid and may be hyperpneic. Diarrhea may be an early and severe manifestation or may not appear for some hours or even a day. Rarely, shock and death may occur without a diarrheal movement; at autopsy the bowel is filled with fluid of high electrolyte content. The fatality rate is high, and death occurs within the first 24 hours. Though acidosis and hemoconcentration are likely to be extreme, such peripheral manifestations of dehydration as loss of subcutaneous tissue and inelasticity of the skin are not prominent in the infants who die in the first day or two of the disease.

DIAGNOSIS. Occasionally the history may indicate the source and nature of the infection or the possibility of food poisoning, but in most instances the cause can be determined, if at all, only by bacteriologic and virologic cultures of the stool. Samples of several stools in the first 24 hours of observation or, preferably, several rectal swabs at an interval of 8 to 12 hours should be cultured.

Since the metabolic disturbances of diarrhea in infants are an important part of the clinical situation, no severe case can be adequately appraised without the assistance of laboratory data. (See Section 5.)

PREVENTION. Diarrheal disturbances are more frequent in artificially fed infants than in breast-fed ones. With artificial feeding the mother should be instructed in the proper preparation, storage, use, and disposal of formulas, so that contamination is prevented. During periods of unusually high environmental temperature and humidity or during any febrile disturbance, infants should be supplied with adequate amounts of hypotonic fluid and the intake of food should be temporarily reduced. Excessive clothing should be avoided.

TREATMENT. Specific therapies are discussed under the various diarrheal entities. See the index for references to appropriate text.

Congenital Anomalies of the Gastrointestinal Tract and Intestinal Obstruction

A variety of congenital anomalies of the gastrointestinal tract may be responsible for partial or complete obstruction. The majority of obstructions involve the rectum and the anus; the remainder are preponderantly in the small intestine. The important congenital anomalies may be listed as follows:

- Pyloric stenosis
- Atresia and stenosis
- Anomalies of rotation (malrotation)

Duplications
Diverticula (Meckel's)
Anomalies of innervation (aganglionic megacolon)
Intra-abdominal hernias
Extra-abdominal hernias
Abnormalities of the pancreas

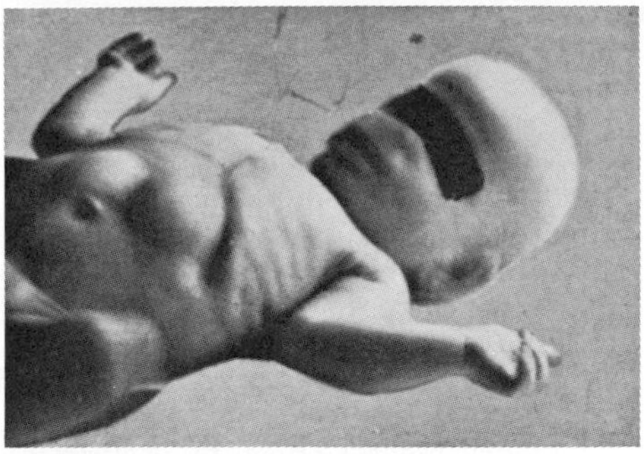

Figure 11–10 Gastric peristaltic waves of pyloric stenosis in an infant 3 weeks of age. (Courtesy of Dr. Carl Wagner, Cincinnati.)

CONGENITAL HYPERTROPHIC PYLORIC STENOSIS

Pyloric stenosis is characterized by vomiting starting usually in the second or third week of life and becoming increasingly projectile. It affects approximately one in every 150 male and one in every 750 female infants. It has been thought to occur more frequently in first-born male infants, but recent observations do not support this impression. Familial incidence has been observed, but genetic study has not disclosed a specific pattern of inheritance.

ETIOLOGY. The cause of pyloric stenosis is not known. In favor of a congenital origin is its high incidence in both of monovular twins, in contrast to relative infrequency in both of binovular twins. It appears probable there is an undetermined, acquired factor involved in the pathogenesis of the lesion.

PATHOLOGY. The pylorus is elongated, thickened to as much as twice its usual size and almost cartilaginous in consistency. There is severe narrowing of the lumen, due principally to the hypertrophy of the circular muscular layer. The stomach is usually dilated, and in longstanding cases there may be hypertrophy of its muscular coat.

CLINICAL MANIFESTATIONS. Initially there is only regurgitation or occasional nonprojectile *vomiting*. The onset rarely occurs before 1 week of age, is usually in the second or third week, and is seldom delayed until the second or third month. The vomiting becomes projectile, usually within a week after onset, and generally occurs during or shortly after feeding, but at times as much as several hours later. In some instances there is vomiting after each feeding; in others it is intermittent. The infant is hungry and will take another feeding immediately. The vomitus consists only of gastric contents, but may be blood-tinged; it is not bile-stained. The stools may become very small and infrequent, depending on the amount of food that reaches the intestinal tract.

Weight loss and *dehydration* may be extensive; weight may decrease to a level below that at birth. There is decreased elasticity of the skin and loss of subcutaneous tissue. The eyes may be sunken and the fat pads of the cheeks lost, so that the infant has a wrinkled, "old man" appearance.

Gastric peristaltic waves are visible as they progress from the left upper quadrant toward the pylorus in a manner suggesting the slow rolling of balls beneath the abdominal wall; they are most prominent immediately after feeding or just before vomiting (Fig. 11–10). At times the infant appears to be uncomfortable, but pain is not a prominent feature.

The pyloric tumor, which is usually the size and consistency of a medium-sized olive, can be palpated in the majority of instances midway between the umbilicus and the costal margin and just lateral to the right rectus muscle; its detection may require repeated examinations. Success in palpation depends on a relaxed, comfortable baby who is being fed by a relaxed, comfortable person while a relaxed, comfortable examiner sits with his hand gently lying across the upper portion of the infant's abdomen with the fingertips on the right upper quadrant. Kneading usually prevents the relaxation necessary to allow the fingers to sink and feel the tumor as it comes up during feeding. If the pyloric tumor cannot be felt, feeding should be continued until vomiting occurs, because this is followed by a momentary period of great relaxation during which the tumor can best be palpated.

Protracted jaundice, with hyperbilirubinemia of the indirect type, has been observed in some infants with pyloric stenosis. The relation to the pyloric stenosis is, thus far, unexplained.

METABOLIC ALTERATIONS. Extensive and protracted vomiting in pyloric stenosis, as in other forms of high intestinal obstruction, may lead to critical deficits of potassium and sodium which, owing to dehydration, may or may not be reflected by low values in the serum. Much more striking are the decrease in chloride concentration and increases in pH and in carbon dioxide content which constitute the characteristic serum chemical changes of *hypochloremic alkalosis.* (See Section 5.) These chemical changes of hypochloremia and alkalosis cannot be corrected through the intravenous administration of ammonium chloride solution, which is contraindicated. Rather, there is a need for sodium and especially for potassium replacement. Intravenous administration of 5 per cent glucose in isotonic sodium chloride solution, to which, after the infant has been observed to urinate, potassium chloride is added (to a concentration of 3 to 5 mEq/dl, or 30 to 50 mEq/l), will gradually and satisfactorily replace the calculated deficits (Table 5–16) of potassium, chloride and sodium and avoid the danger of hyponatremia which may ensue if hypotonic electrolyte solutions are used for replacement of fluid and electrolytes in dehydrated infants who have had protracted vomiting. The serum chloride level, which may vary from nearly normal to as low as 70 mEq/l, may be used as a rough index of potassium deficit; if the serum chloride is normal, the potassium deficit may be minimal, and care should be taken not to overload the infant with this ion. When maintenance fluids are given, following correction of dehydration, hypotonic solutions will be appropriate (Section 5).

DIAGNOSIS. The usual case can be diagnosed by the characteristic clinical pattern and the identification of a pyloric mass. Congenital obstructions of the duodenum, if complete, are responsible for symptoms within a few hours after birth; if incomplete, as with stenosis, malrotation or constricting bands, vomiting may not become evident for days or even weeks after birth; there is no pyloric tumor, however, and the vomitus contains bile if the constriction is below the ampulla of Vater. Gastric waves are occasionally visible in small, emaciated infants who do not have pyloric stenosis. Chalasia of the esophagus and hiatal hernia usually result in vomiting in the first week of life and can be differentiated from pyloric stenosis by roentgenographic studies. Adrenal insufficiency may simulate pyloric stenosis, but the absence of a palpable tumor and the metabolic acidosis and elevated serum potassium and urinary sodium concentrations of adrenal insufficiency aid in differentiation. Allergy to cow's milk may be accompanied by projectile vomiting, but this vomiting is rarely so forceful as with pyloric stenosis. A family history of allergy and the presence of other signs of milk allergy usually indicate the diagnosis. (See Section 9.)

The principal diagnostic difficulty is with hyperkinetic infants who are exceptionally reactive to external stimuli and vomit frequently in the earlier weeks of life. Such infants may bear a resemblance to infants with pyloric stenosis. The vomiting may be persistent and even projectile, but often diminishes or subsides completely when the feedings are given by a comfortable caretaker other than the mother. For this group of infants the term pylorospasm has been used, but it has limited functional or pathologic significance. A pyloric tumor is not palpable. Gastric waves are absent. Roentgenographic studies may show delayed emptying of the stomach, but the pyloric lumen is normal.

If the pyloric tumor can be palpated, roentgenographic studies are unnecessary, but they should be done if a pyloric tumor cannot be palpated and the picture is not otherwise classic. With pyloric stenosis there is not only delayed emptying and vigorous peristaltic activity of the stomach, but also delayed prepyloric opening time and, most importantly, a narrowed, elongated pyloric canal with a single streak of barium, the "string sign," or a double-track of barium outlining the canal, an antral "beak" at the beginning of the pylorus, and a curve of the pylorus upward and to the left.

PROGNOSIS. When the diagnosis is made early in the course of the disease and the infant is properly prepared for operation, the operative fatality rate is less than 1 per cent. Medical therapy has a higher mortality rate and, even when beneficial, must be continued for 2 to 8 months.

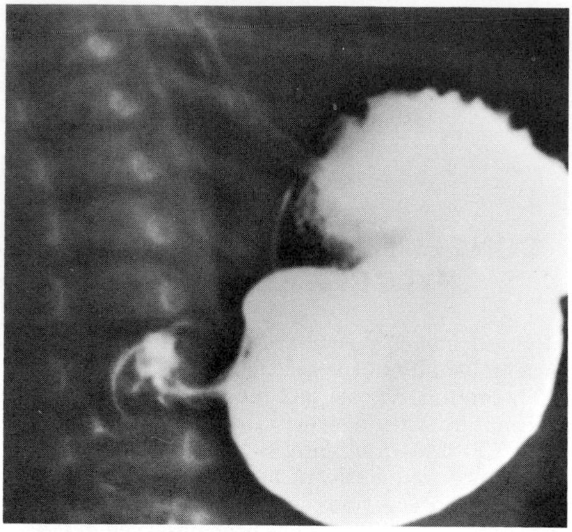

Figure 11–11 Hypertrophic pyloric stenosis. Note the elongated, narrow pyloric canal (string sign) as well as the blunt antrum. The base of the duodenal bulb is concave. Hyperperistalsis was noted fluoroscopically.

TREATMENT. Surgical relief of the pyloric obstruction as soon as the diagnosis is established and the metabolic imbalances have been corrected is the treatment of choice. The correction of dehydration and electrolyte deficits with parenteral fluids has been described under Metabolic Alterations and in Section 5. Well hydrated infants without evidence of electrolyte imbalance may be operated on without delay; delays of 24 to 36 hours for replacement therapy without oral intake are indicated in severely dehydrated infants. Gastric lavage with isotonic saline solution prior to operation is advised by some in the hope of diminishing gastric irritation which may cause postoperative vomiting; the tube is left in the stomach during the operation in order to remove secretions and swallowed air. At operation the pyloric musculature is incised and separated longitudinally down to the mucosa (Fredet-Ramstedt pyloromyotomy). Four to six hours postoperatively, oral feedings are begun in small amounts and increased gradually. An acceptable regimen is to give 4 ml of 5 per cent glucose in saline solution hourly for 4 feedings. If no vomiting develops, 8 ml are given hourly for the next 4 feedings, then 16 ml hourly for 4 feedings. If these feedings are retained, 1 ounce of formula is given an hour after the last feeding of clear fluid and repeated 2 hours later. By stepwise increment the amount of feedings and the interval between them are increased until a full feeding program is in effect, usually within 48 hours. If vomiting occurs before formula feedings are begun, oral feedings are withheld for 4 hours, and the regimen is reinstituted from the beginning. Persistence of vomiting suggests an incomplete pyloromyotomy or possibly concomitant hiatal hernia or chalasia;

occasional episodes of vomiting are not uncommon after operation, probably as the result of persisting gastritis. Feedings should ordinarily be maintained, but not increased, until a clear pattern of retention is sustained, at which time increases may be resumed. During the initial period of small feedings, intravenous administration of fluids is often required, depending on the fluid and electrolyte balance of the infant. If vomiting persists for 3 to 5 days after operation, it suggests an incomplete division of the hypertrophied pyloric muscle, and may indicate exploratory laparotomy. Complete cessation of vomiting is the rule after operation, even though postoperative roentgenographic studies have shown that the pyloric canal may remain narrow for many months in the asymptomatic infant.

Nonsurgical Treatment. The slowness of improvement (2 to 8 months), the higher case fatality rate, and the current high cost and probable adverse effect on emotional development of prolonged hospitalization have led to a virtual abandonment of nonsurgical treatment for pyloric stenosis. If, for some reason, medical rather than surgical management is necessary, slow improvement will usually take place on a regimen of small, frequent feedings thickened with cereal, maintenance of a semi-upright position for an hour or so after feedings, sedation, administration of a cholinergic blocking agent, and parenteral administration of fluids as required. Emptying of the stomach by lavage when there is epigastric distention before a feeding may likewise decrease the chance of vomiting.

The same measures may be used with equivocal or varying success in the treatment of infants with recurrent vomiting or regurgitation. Phenobarbital is used for sedation in doses of 8 to 15 mg half an hour before feeding 3 or 4 times a day; if drowsiness or apathy appears, the administration of the drug should be suspended until normal alertness is regained, at which time it may be resumed at a lower dose. Some babies treated with phenobarbital may become markedly agitated by this drug. The common anticholinergic drugs for infants are atropine as a 1:1000 solution, tincture of belladonna, and a 0.6 per cent alcoholic solution of atropine methylnitrate (Eumydrin). Each is given by placing 1 drop on the infant's tongue about 20 minutes before each of 3 feedings a day. The dose may be increased first by giving it before more feedings, later by increasing the number of drops, until vomiting is controlled or flushing of the face or dilatation of the pupils appears, when the dose should be decreased. Care should be exercised that fresh solutions of these drugs are used; there is easy danger of overdosage into toxic ranges.

CONGENITAL INTESTINAL OBSTRUCTION

GENERAL CONSIDERATIONS. Intestinal obstruction is observed in approximately one out of 1500 newborn infants. The cardinal signs of obstruction are (1) vomiting, (2) abdominal distention, and (3) failure to pass feces. Since a number of days may go by prior to full certainty that the infant has an obstructive lesion, early diagnosis depends on appreciation of the significance of vomiting and distention. *High intestinal obstruction* is characterized by vomiting, which tends to be persistent even when feedings have been stopped; distention may be absent. *Low obstruction* is characterized principally by distention, and vomiting may be only a later manifestation.

From an anatomic standpoint congenital obstructive lesions of the intestines can be viewed as *intrinsic*, e.g., atresia, stenosis, meconium ileus and aganglionic megacolon, or *extrinsic*, e.g., malrotation, constricting bands, intra-abdominal hernias, duplications. Clinically, whether an intestinal obstruction is intrinsic or extrinsic is often not definable and is of secondary importance, since operation is always indicated. An attempt should be made, however, to locate the lesion preoperatively in order to guide the surgical approach.

When the obstruction is *complete,* there should be little difficulty in clinical recognition, but when incomplete, there may be considerable difficulty. Polyhydramnios is frequently an accompaniment of high intestinal obstruction, as it is of esophageal atresia. When polyhydramnios has been noted, an attempt to aspirate the infant's stomach immediately after birth may provide an important diagnostic clue. Failure to pass the tube into the stomach may disclose an esophageal atresia. Aspiration of 10 to 15 or more ml of gastric fluid, especially if it is bile-stained, is suggestive of a high intestinal obstruction. When the obstruction is in the duodenum, symptoms may become manifest within a few hours; if it is in the large intestine, symptoms may be delayed for more than 24 hours.

Meconium stools may be passed initially if the obstruction is in the upper part of the small intestine. The absence, on microscopic examination of the stool, of lanugo hairs and cornified epithelial cells, which are swallowed in amniotic fluid, is suggestive of complete obstruction *(Farber test).* This test has limited value, since a partially obstructive lesion may on occasion constitute as much of a surgical emergency as a completely obstructive one. In any event, the specimen to be examined should be taken from the center of the stool, since epithelial cells from the rectum and perianal area may adhere to the outside of the stool and be misinterpreted as swallowed epithelial cells.

Obstruction in the duodenal area is responsible for epigastric distention and, at times, for gastric waves similar to those of pyloric stenosis. The distention may not be persistent, however, since it may be relieved by vomiting. The vomiting may be projectile, and the vomitus will contain bile if the obstruction is below the ampulla of Vater, as it usually is.

Obstructions in the lower ileum, colon or rectum cause more generalized distention, often with bulging of the flanks. When the liver dullness is obliterated, there is a strong possibility that intestinal perforation has occurred. Vomiting with lower bowel obstruction may be delayed a day but eventually may become fecal in type.

When the obstruction is *incomplete,* as, for example, with intestinal stenosis, constricting bands, duplications and incomplete volvulus, symptoms (vomiting, abdominal distention, obstipation) may appear shortly after birth or may be delayed an indeterminate time. They may approach in severity those of a completely obstructive lesion, or they may be sufficiently mild and infrequent as to be overlooked until either an acute episode or diagnostic studies disclose the lesion.

Meconium ileus, meconium plug, aganglionic megacolon, and anal and rectal obstructions are described later in this Section (see Index).

Valuable information on the location of congenital obstructive lesions in the intestine may often be obtained from flat and upright roentgenograms of the abdomen without ingestion of contrast media, since with completely obstructive lesions there will be distention of the bowel above the obstruction and there may be a series of fluid levels with superimposed gas in the distended loops. An air-contrast study of the colon following an enema containing radiopaque material may provide additional localizing information, especially in respect to the possibility of a displaced cecum with malrotation of the intestine. Under usual circumstances, air is demonstrable roentgenographically in the stomach of the normal infant immediately after birth. Within an hour the proximal portion of the small intestine and segments of the colon are demonstrable. The distal parts of the colon may be visible as early as the third hour.

PROGNOSIS. If a complete obstruction is not relieved promptly, the clinical course progresses rapidly. Vomiting is persistent; dehydration, loss of weight, and prostration become severe, and the infant dies within a few days. When the obstruction is not complete, the infant may survive for weeks; minor obstructions may be compatible with life even without treatment. Recovery from both complete and incomplete obstructions can be expected in many instances with early diagnosis and appropriate management.

TREATMENT. Not every obstructive lesion is amenable to surgery, but infants can withstand massive resection of the small intestine when the lesion necessitates it. Preoperative preparation, including constant gastric aspiration, and postoperative care are of the greatest importance, especially in relation to the correction of dehydration and electrolyte deficits and to the maintenance of fluid balance and nutrition by parenteral means (Section 5).

ATRESIA AND STENOSIS

Atresia (complete occlusion) and stenosis (partial occlusion) of the gastrointestinal tract account for about one third of cases of intestinal obstruction. *Atresia* is the more common. The obstructive lesion is most frequently in the ileum (50 per cent) and duodenum (25 per cent), less frequently in the jejunum, rare in the colon and almost never in the stomach. There is an increased incidence of duodenal atresia, as well as of imperforate anus, in babies with the Down syndrome. About 15 per cent of intestinal atresias are multiple. The types of atresia are (1) a diaphragm-like occlusion of the lumen, (2) a blind end not in continuity with a distal segment, and (3) segments of bowel with cord-like connections.

The *diagnosis* of intestinal atresia should be suspected in the presence of maternal hydramnios, of the Down syndrome, and of vomiting or abdominal distention in the newborn infant. Upright roentgenograms of the abdomen show that the air in the intestinal tract has failed to progress beyond the level of the atresia. Intestinal stenosis results in signs of intestinal obstruction, the severity of which depends on the degree of the stenosis.

Treatment is surgical. In duodenal atresia or stenosis the surgical procedures of choice are duodenoduodenostomy or duodenojejunostomy to bypass the obstruction. Jejunal or ileal atresias are often associated with errors in rotation of the intestine, are subject to gangrene of the blind end of the bowel proximal to the atresia, and have a greater incidence of complications and of death.

ANOMALIES OF ROTATION
(Malrotation)

Incomplete rotation, also incorrectly termed *malrotation of the intestine,* represents a failure of the bowel to rotate and become fixed normally. The normal embryologic sequence is as follows: the cecum rotates around the superior mesenteric artery, which acts as an axis, counterclockwise from a position in the middle of the abdomen just below the stomach. The colon, which lies on the left side of the abdomen, follows as the cecum rotates into the right upper quadrant and finally into the right lower quadrant. When rotation is completed, the ascending and descending mesocolon fuse to the back of the abdomen, anchoring the mesentery from the ligament of Treitz obliquely downward to the cecal area. In some instances rotation may be complete, but the mesentery is incomplete, so that there is abnormal mobility of the midgut and colon.

Most often in malrotation the cecum has failed to move into the right lower quadrant, and the bands fixing it to the posterior abdominal wall cross over and may obstruct the duodenum (Fig. 11–12). The narrow mesenteric stalk which suspends the small intestine in the area of the superior mesenteric vessels is liable to volvulus, resulting in intermittent or acute obstruction which may progress to strangulation. Obstruction occurs first at the upper portion of the duodenum, then at the lower end of the loop. Volvulus is present in more than half of the patients operated on for intestinal obstruction when the cecum is in the right upper portion of the

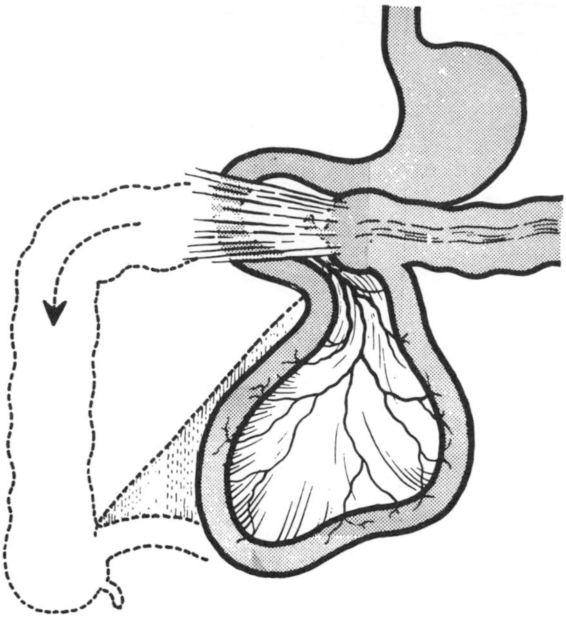

Figure 11–12 The mechanism of intestinal obstruction with incomplete rotation of the midgut ("malrotation"). The dotted lines show the course the cecum should have taken. Failure to rotate has left obstructing bands across the duodenum, and a narrow pedicle for the midgut loop, making it prone to volvulus. (Nixon and O'Donnell: The Essentials of Pediatric Surgery, 1961.)

abdomen. This problem usually presents with symptoms of acute or recurrent intestinal obstruction at birth or in the first year of life. An occasional child with malrotation presents the clinical picture of celiac disease, which is relieved by surgical repair. Nonrotation is associated with midgut volvulus, gastroschisis, omphaloceles, and hernia through the foramen of Bochdalek. Malrotation may be present with an annular pancreas and congenital atresia or stenosis of the duodenum.

Roentgenograms of the abdomen may show an abnormal colonic gas pattern, and barium enema confirms the abnormal position of the cecum. In acute obstruction, diagnosis is at laparotomy, and only an upright film of the abdomen is made in order to disclose the gas and fluid shadows.

Management includes fluid therapy to combat shock and disturbance of body fluids and electrolytes, followed by laparotomy, at which the volvulus is unwound, transduodenal bands are divided, and the large intestine is straightened and placed in the left side of the abdomen with all the small bowel on the right.

DUPLICATION OF THE GASTROINTESTINAL TRACT

Duplications are congenital tubular or oval structures which have a smooth muscle wall and a mucous membrane similar to some part of the gastrointestinal tract, and which are intimately connected to the gastrointestinal tract. They vary widely in size and shape. Clinical manifestations usually arise during infancy and early childhood. Symptoms and signs include: (1) obstruction of adjoining intestine by compression; (2) intestinal bleeding from peptic ulceration secondary to gastric mucosa in the lining of a duplication which communicates with the intestine; (3) pain from secretory distention of a noncommunicating duplication; (4) gangrene of the bowel from obstruction of segmental vasculature; and (5) a movable abdominal mass palpated on routine examination of the abdomen. Duplications are most frequent in the ileum, ileocecal region and esophagus, but may occur in any part of the gastrointestinal tract. In the abdomen a duplication may be the leading point of an intussusception. Duplications in the thorax are usually of the esophagus or the stomach, and only rarely communicate with either. They are evident through dysphagia and respiratory symptoms produced by esophageal and pulmonary compression and are demonstrable roentgenographically. Associated anomalies of vertebrae are not uncommon and often are at a higher level than the intrathoracic mass. Some intrathoracic duplications are of duodenal or jejunal origin.

Roentgenographic studies may show stenosis or compression of the intestinal lumen, but more frequently are normal. An intrathoracic duplication is usually visible as a mediastinal mass in roentgenograms of the chest. Very rarely barium studies may fill a communicating duplication.

Surgical removal is indicated, but is complex and usually involves removal of both duplication and adjoining intestine because of the common wall and blood supply, followed by primary anastomosis of the remaining ends of intestine.

DIVERTICULOSIS, DIVERTICULITIS AND ASSOCIATED DISORDERS

With the exception of Meckel's diverticulum, congenital and acquired single and multiple diverticula of the intestinal tract are extremely rare in children. *Diverticulosis,* the presence of multiple outpouchings of the intestinal tract, usually in the colon, and *diverticulitis,* or inflammation of diverticula, are essentially diseases of adult life.

The omphalomesenteric duct, which connects the ileum with the yolk sac and disappears by the fifth or sixth week of fetal life, may persist in all or part of its course and be responsible for a variety of anomalies (Fig. 11–13). Of these, the most frequent is Meckel's diverticulum, which is estimated to occur in 2 to 3 per cent of all persons and is more frequently symptomatic in males than in females.

PATHOLOGY. Meckel's diverticulum is located on the antimesenteric side of the ileum within 45 to 90 cm (18 to 36 in) of the ileocecal valve. Its mucosal lining may be gastric and ileal, or colonic and ileal, in that order of frequency. Sixty per cent of clinically significant Meckel's diverticula contain gastric mucosa. Pancreatic cells, including those of the islets of Langerhans, may also be present.

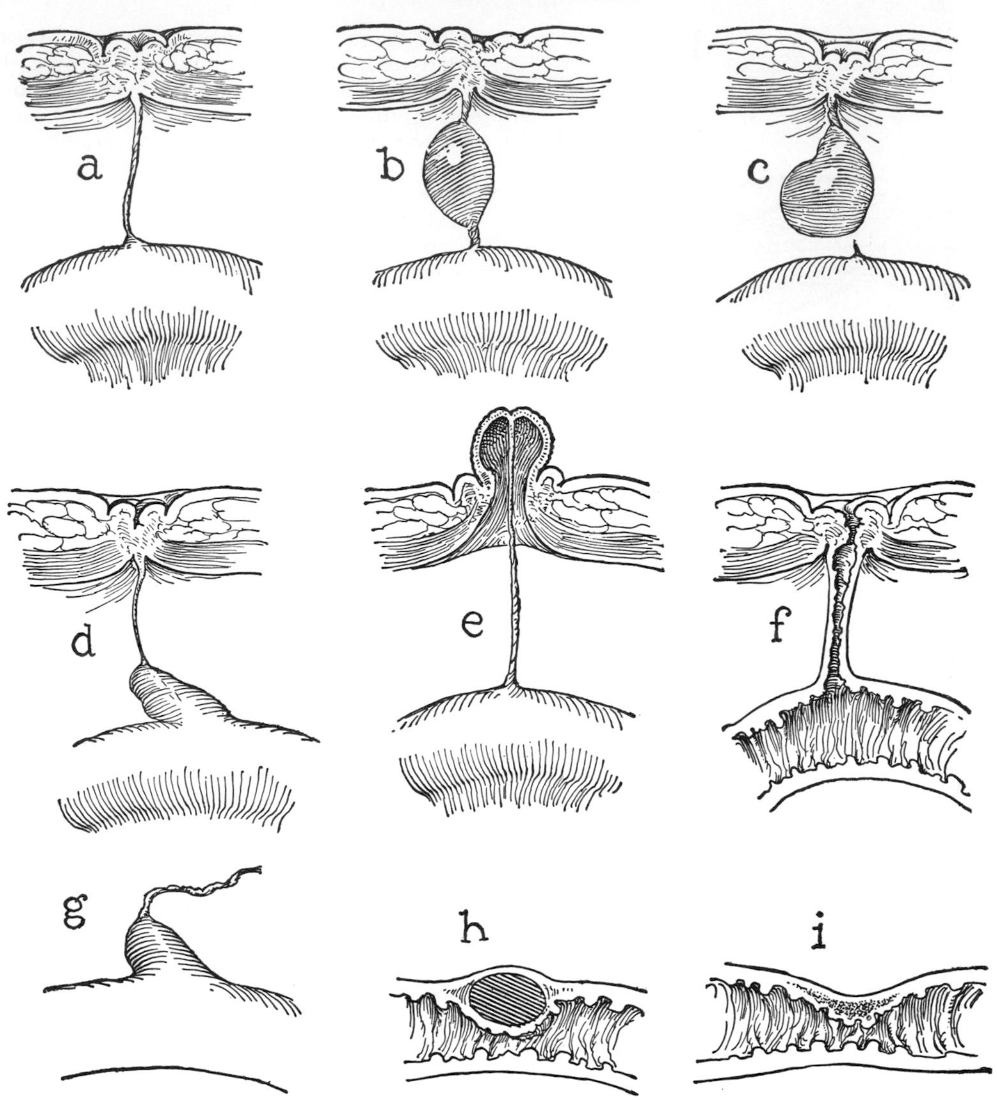

Figure 11–13 *Diagrammatic representation of structures derived from remnants of the omphalomesenteric duct.* a, *Cord extending between umbilicus and ileum;* b, *cyst suspended between umbilicus and ileum;* c, *cyst suspended from umbilicus;* d, *Meckel's diverticulum with cord extending to umbilicus;* e, *everted mucocele attached by cord to ileum;* f, *fecal fistula between ileum and umbilicus;* g, *Meckel's diverticulum with free intraperitoneal cord;* h, *enterocystoma;* i, *stenosis from excessive evolution. (Brennemann: Practice of Pediatrics. Hyattsville, Md., W. F. Prior Co., Vol. 3.)*

CLINICAL MANIFESTATIONS. Symptoms from Meckel's diverticulum can arise at any age, but occur more frequently in the first 2 years of life. *Hemorrhage* from a small peptic ulcer in or adjacent to aberrant gastric mucosa at the neck of the pouch is the most common symptom. The bleeding is unaccompanied by pain, a point which differentiates it from bleeding from an intussusception. Although the bleeding is usually acute, it may be intermittent and recurrent over an extended period of time. With mild recurrent bleeding, a chronic iron deficiency anemia may develop and be refractory to iron therapy. Repeatedly positive tests for occult blood in the stool in an anemic young child suggest Meckel's diverticulum. The blood may be dark red at first but with massive bleeding it is bright red. *Abdominal pain* is the next symptom in frequency. It may be acute and due to diverticulitis, with a clinical picture resembling that of acute appendicitis, or it may be vague and recurrent. Referral of the (ileal) pain to the umbilicus may suggest the true diagnosis. Perforation of an ulcer in the diverticulum may be responsible for peritoneal bleeding or inflammation. Meckel's diverticulum may invert and become the leading point of an intussusception, or intestinal obstruction can result from herniation of a loop of bowel through a "ring" formed by the atrophied cord of the diverticulum. Volvulus may result from twisting of the intestine around or in association with persistence of an omphalomesenteric duct or cord. *Littre's hernia* is a rare condition in which Meckel's diverticulum protrudes, along with the adjacent portion of the intestine, into the sac of an inguinal, femoral or umbilical hernia. The diverticulum is likely to become inflamed and adherent to the hernial sac with resultant incarceration.

Persistence of the omphalomesenteric duct may result in an umbilical sinus which discharges intestinal contents; if the ileal end is closed, there is only mucoid secretion. When both ends are closed, a cyst may form in the tract; the cyst may protrude through the umbilicus.

Roentgenographic studies are generally of little use in the diagnosis of Meckel's diverticulum. Very rarely abdominal films taken after the barium has cleared from the intestinal tract following gastrointestinal series or barium enema will show residual barium in the diverticulum. This is differentiated from barium in the appendix because it does not occupy a fixed position in the abdomen.

TREATMENT. If Meckel's diverticulum or other anomaly of the omphalomesenteric duct is responsible for signs or symptoms, surgical extirpation is indicated. A diverticulum discovered during an abdominal operation for other conditions should be removed, if the situation otherwise permits.

MEGACOLON

The term "megacolon" denotes gross enlargement of the colon irrespective of cause; the principal factors are chronic constipation from a variety of causes, chief of which are: (1) voluntary withholding of feces because of physical discomfort or emotional conflict (chronic constipation, above); (2) congenital aganglionic megacolon; (3) anorectal stenosis; or (4) the rare obstruction from a tumor in the pelvic area.

Congenital Aganglionic Megacolon
(Hirschsprung's Disease)

Congenital aganglionic megacolon is characterized clinically by fecal retention dating from birth, abdominal distention and, in severe cases, retardation of physical development. It is more common in males, and a familial pattern has been reported. Aganglionic megacolon accounts for about 20 per cent of neonatal intestinal obstruction.

PATHOLOGY. The colon is greatly dilated and filled with feces and gas proximal to a distal spastic area, usually in the rectum or rectosigmoid. The muscular coat of the dilated bowel is hypertrophied, but in longstanding cases the wall of the dilated intestine may be extremely thin. Perforation is rare, but ulceration of the mucosa is not uncommon, particularly in infants.

Histologically there is absence of the ganglion cells of the intramural and submucous plexuses of the spastic distal portion of the bowel. The *functional abnormality* is an increase in muscular tone and contractile activity of the aganglionic segment of bowel, without the reciprocal relaxation necessary to facilitate the onward movement of feces by the peristaltic activity of the colon proximal to the aganglionic segment.

In 90 per cent of instances the aganglionic segment of bowel extends for 4 to 25 cm proximally from the anus. Instances of involvement of the entire colon, of portions of the small bowel, and rarely of several aganglionic segments between normal areas have been reported.

CLINICAL MANIFESTATIONS. In newborn infants the symptoms may be present at birth, with failure to pass meconium, or may appear during the first week and be those of partial or even complete intestinal obstruction with vomiting, abdominal distention and failure to pass stools. Temporary relief of symptoms may occur after a rectal examination, which is characteristically followed by an explosive discharge of feces and gas. Bile-stained and even fecal vomiting may occur, and the infant may lose weight and become dehydrated. Diarrhea may be a prominent symptom in the neonatal period and occur in association with symptoms of intestinal obstruction. Hypoproteinemia and edema may develop in association with protein-losing enteropathy. Infants with aganglionic megacolon are prone to a severe, life-threatening enterocolitis.

When the symptoms are mild enough that the diagnosis is not made in early infancy, the clinical course is one of gradually increasing fecal retention and abdominal distention. Spontaneous bowel movements are rare, even in response to a laxative; enemas are usually necessary to produce evacuations. A large fecal mass is palpable in the left lower portion of the abdomen, but on rectal examination the rectum is not dilated and is usually empty of feces, in contrast to the dilated, full rectum of children with chronic constipation due to withholding of feces. The stools, when passed, may consist of small pellets, be ribbon-like or have a fluid consistency; the large stools and fecal soiling of patients with functional constipation are absent. In mild cases the nutrition may not be greatly disturbed; in severe cases there is likely to be loss of subcutaneous tissue and failure to grow. The wasted extremities and large, protruding abdomen of such patients create a typical appearance, but one which may be confused with some of the *malabsorption syndromes* (below), especially when diarrhea is present. Hypochromic anemia may be present. Intermittent attacks of intestinal obstruction from retained feces may be associated with pain and fever.

DIAGNOSIS. Anorexia, obstipation, abdominal distention and vomiting in the absence of readily demonstrable anatomic obstruction are suggestive of aganglionic megacolon in early infancy. When liquid stools are passed around the obstruction, they may confuse the picture. Later the diagnosis is suggested by a history of obstipation and abdominal distention from early infancy.

Roentgenographic studies in the young infant with intestinal obstruction due to aganglionic megacolon show dilated loops of bowel throughout the abdomen on anteroposterior films taken in the erect position. In lateral erect films rectal air, which is usually visible in the presacral area, is absent. The diagnostic findings on barium enema are

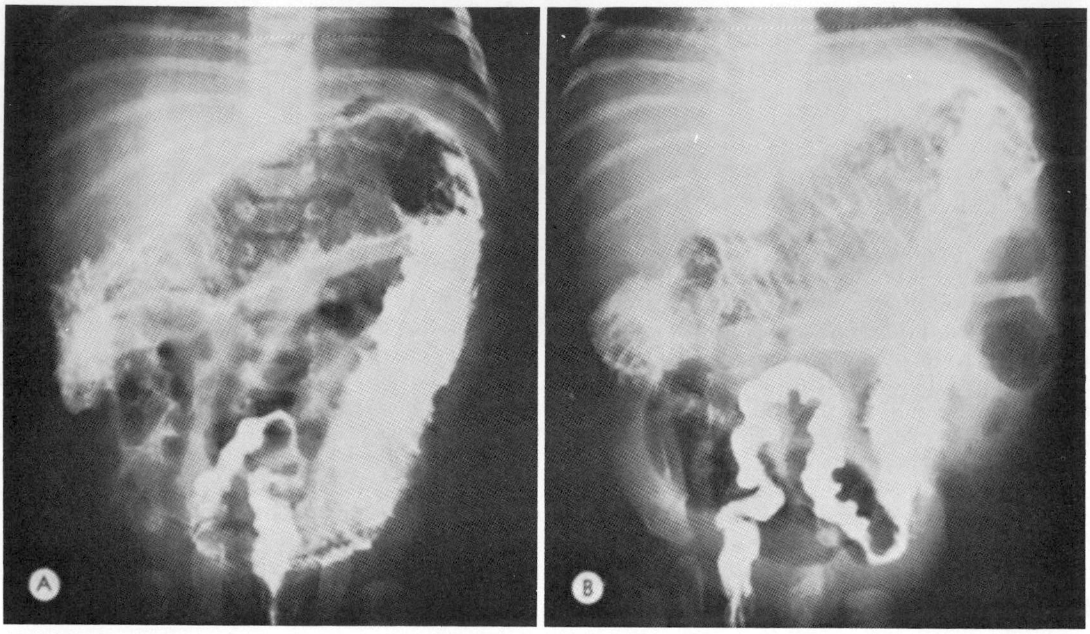

Figure 11–14 Roentgenographic findings in 8 week old identical male twins with congenital aganglionic megacolon. Diarrhea gradually changed to constipation during the first 3 weeks of life in each. Both developed generalized edema and hypoproteinemia at 6 weeks of age. Plain roentgenograms of the abdomen of each twin showed a distended bowel with a relatively narrow rectum. A, *Anteroposterior roentgenogram of the barium-filled colon of one of the twins shows irregular, bizarre, "sawtooth" contractions of the rectum and sigmoid. A zone of demarcation is noted at the junction of the sigmoid and descending colon, and parallel transverse folds are visible in the dilated proximal colon. Above this the colon is thick, nodular and edematous, producing a "shaggy" border suggestive of ulcerative colitis. This is the picture of exudative enteropathy. Histologic examination of the distal segment revealed the absence of ganglion cells.* B, *Anteroposterior roentgenogram of the barium-filled colon of the twin. (From Hope, J. W., Borns, P. F., and Berg, P. K.: Am. J. Roentgen. 95:217, 1965.)*

(1) an abrupt change in caliber between the ganglionic and aganglionic sections of bowel; (2) irregular, "sawtooth" contractions of the aganglionic segment; (3) parallel transverse folds in the dilated proximal colon; (4) a thickened, nodular edematous proximal colon characteristic of protein-losing enteropathy (Fig. 11–14); and (5) failure to evacuate the barium. In infants only a small amount of barium should be injected, slowly, through a small catheter whose tip is inserted barely beyond the anal sphincter, while the patient, in an oblique position, is being observed under the fluoroscope; the characteristic abrupt transition in caliber may be missed if the lower colon is flooded with too much barium. Roentgenographic studies may not show a spastic distal segment in the first weeks of life. In such infants, a postevacuation film in 12 to 48 hours may be helpful. The possible existence of mechanical obstructions such as stenosis or stricture of the anus and membranous valve-like lesions in the rectum or rectosigmoid may be determined by sigmoidoscopic examination.

When the clinical history is highly suggestive, but the roentgenographic studies are not diagnostic, *rectal biopsy* is useful. This is particularly true in early infancy and in cases in which the thrust of the stool mass produces dilatation of a short aganglionic segment. The first 2 cm of rectum are normally hypoganglionic so that biopsy should be taken above this level. Rectal suction biopsy can be done, but it is helpful only when demonstration of ganglion cells in the submucous plexus rules out aganglionic megacolon. Otherwise, full thickness surgical biopsy is much more definitive through revealing absence of ganglion cells from both plexuses, and frequently enlarged nerve bundles as well. *Anal tonometry* demonstrates absence of the normal reflex relaxation of the internal sphincter on rectal dilation with a balloon. This technique, carefully carried out, has been found to correlate well with evidence from biopsy.

Roentgenographic examination of the urinary tract should also be made, since megaloureters have occasionally been demonstrated in conjunction with aganglionic megacolon.

TREATMENT. Retention enemas of 3 to 4 ounces of mineral oil followed by repeated colonic irrigations with *isotonic saline solution* will usually remove most of the fecal accumulation. The rectal catheter should be inserted beyond the constricted segment. The use of solutions other than isotonic saline solution for rectal irrigation should be avoided. Attacks of syncope, shock and death have been attributed to water intoxication following the use of tap water or soapsuds enemas. Magnesium poisoning has been reported following retention of enemas of magnesium sulfate in patients with congenital megacolon.

Removal of the spastic segment of bowel by a variety of surgical techniques results in relief of symptoms and a return to normal bowel habits in the majority of instances. During operation it is essential to ascertain from biopsies of the bowel that ganglion cells are present in the proximal end of the resected bowel before the final anastomosis is made.

If an infant's condition prohibits the extensive surgery involved in an operation, a colostomy should be performed in the distal portion of the normal part of the colon. Preoperative correction of anemia and of water and electrolyte deficits and adequate maintenance postoperatively are important. Later, when the infant is in good nutritional state and has been gaining weight, the appropriate form of resection of the abnormal segment of bowel can be performed. Various modifications of current procedures are under evaluation.

INTRA-ABDOMINAL HERNIAS

An intra-abdominal hernia occurs when loops of intestine are trapped by an anomalous fold of peritoneum created by malrotation or malfixation of the duodenum or colon to the posterior abdominal wall. Loops of intestine also may herniate through congenital defects of the mesentery, particularly near the terminal ileum. The symptoms and signs are those of intermittent or acute intestinal obstruction. Gangrene of the intestine can occur if there is compression of the vasculature. Surgical reduction of the hernia and repair of the anomaly in order to prevent recurrence require great care and a knowledge of embryologic anatomy because of the danger of interference with intestinal blood supply.

EXTRA-ABDOMINAL HERNIAS

See Umbilical Hernia. (See Section 7 and Index.)

ABNORMALITIES OF THE PANCREAS

See Meconium Ileus, Pseudomeconium Ileus, and Annular Pancreas, later in this Section and in Index.

ACQUIRED INTESTINAL OBSTRUCTION

Paralytic ileus is an important cause of acquired intestine obstruction. It is likely to occur as a complication of acute infections, especially pneumonia and peritonitis, and of electrolyte imbalance or uremia. It is likely to present as distention, with absence of bowel sounds and minimal pain. Pneumonia is probably the most frequent cause of paralytic ileus in infants; peritonitis, the most frequent in older children.

Incarcerated inguinal hernias and intussusception are the most frequent mechanical causes of intestinal obstruction in infants. Intestinal obstruction may also result from postoperative adhesions or those produced by acute peritonitis from which recovery occurred, or by chronic peritonitis, e.g., tuberculous peritonitis. Other causes are foreign bodies in the intestine, including fecal concretions and inspissated meconium in the newborn infant, late obstruction by intraluminal contents in cystic fibrosis (pseudomeconium ileus), and by masses of roundworms; tumors of the bowel, including mesenteric cysts, may also be obstructive.

INTUSSUSCEPTION

Intussusception, an invagination of a portion of the intestine into a distal adjacent part, is a cause of intestinal obstruction in infants and young children from 3 to 24 months of age, but is rare both earlier and later. It is more common in males and in all infants from 3 to 11 months of age.

ETIOLOGY. In most instances intussusception develops in healthy infants without demonstrable cause. Correlations between intussusception and adenovirus infections have been equivocal. In about 5 per cent of the cases a specific lesion such as a Meckel's diverticulum, polyp, nodule of ectopic pancreas, duplication of the ileum, hypertrophied Peyer's patch, lymphoma of the bowel or intramural hemorrhage in anaphylactoid purpura serves as a lead point for the intussusception.

PATHOLOGY. Intussusceptions are most frequently ileocolic, ileo-ileocolic, and ileo-ileal in type, with the upper portion (intussusceptum) invaginating into the lower (intussuscipiens), pulling the mesentery with it. Swelling begins promptly from edema and hemorrhage secondary to venous engorgement, with resultant intestinal incarceration and obstruction. Most intussusceptions do not strangulate the bowel in the first 24 hours, but may lead subsequently to intestinal gangrene and systemic shock.

CLINICAL MANIFESTATIONS. In typical cases there is sudden onset of severe paroxysmal pain, which recurs at frequent intervals and is accompanied by straining efforts and loud outcries. Initially the infant may be comfortable and play normally between the paroxysms of pain, but if the intussusception is not reduced, he becomes progressively weaker and goes into a shock-like state, with an elevation of body temperature to as high as 41° C (106° F). The pulse becomes weak and thready, the respirations shallow and grunting, and the pain may be manifested only by moaning sounds. Vomiting occurs in most instances and is usually more frequent at the beginning. In the later phase the vomitus becomes bile-stained. Fecal matter of normal appearance may be evacuated during the first few hours of symptoms. After this time fecal excretions are small, or more often do not occur, and little or no flatus is passed. Blood generally appears in the first 12 hours, but at times not for 1 or 2 days and infrequently not at all. Stools consisting chiefly of blood and mucus are common and are termed *"currant jelly stools."*

Palpation of the abdomen usually reveals a sausage-shaped mass, sometimes ill defined, which may increase in size and firmness during a paroxysm of pain and is most often in the right upper portion of the abdomen. It is more readily located by bimanual rectal and abdominal palpation between paroxysms of pain. The presence of bloody mucus on the finger as it is withdrawn after rectal examination supports the diagnosis of intussusception. Abdominal distention and tenderness develop as intestinal obstruction becomes more acute. On rare occasions the advancing intestine prolapses through the anus. This can be distinguished from prolapse of the rectum by the separation between the protruding intestine and the rectal wall, which does not exist in prolapse of the rectum.

Ileo-ileal intussusception may have a less typical clinical picture, the symptoms and signs being chiefly those of small intestinal obstruction. *Recurrent intussusception* is rare, with an incidence of no more than 2 per cent. *Chronic intussusception*, in which the symptoms exist in milder form at recurrent intervals, is more likely to occur with or following acute enteritis and may arise in older children as well.

DIAGNOSIS. In intussusception the clinical history and physical findings are usually sufficiently typical for diagnosis. Roentgenographically, abdominal scout films may show a mass-like density in the area of the intussusception. The film after a barium enema will show cupping in the head of barium as its advance is obstructed by the intussusceptum (Fig. 11–15). A central linear column of barium may be visible in the compressed lumen of the intussusceptum, and a thin layer of barium may be seen trapped around the invaginating intestine (coil-spring sign), especially after evacuation. Retrogression of the intussusceptum under the pressure of the enema, and gaseous distention of the small intestine from obstruction are also useful roentgenographic signs. Ileo-ileal intussusception is usually not demonstrable by barium enema, but is suspected because of gaseous distention of the intestine above the intussusception.

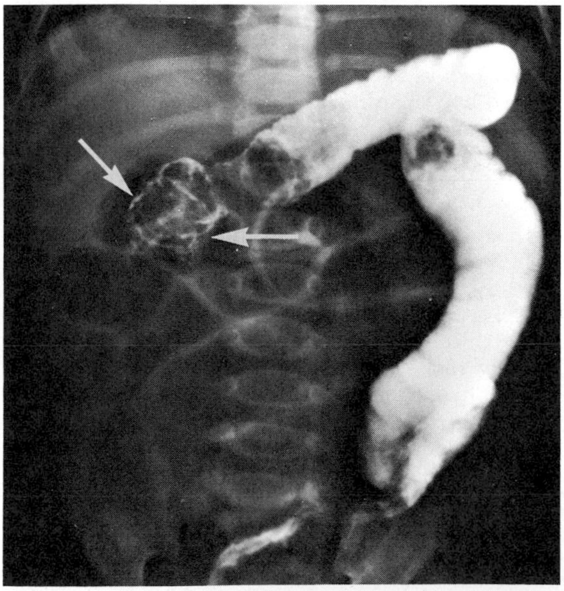

Figure 11–15 Intussusception in an infant. The obstruction is evident in the proximal transverse colon. Contrast material between the intussuseptum and the intussuscipiens is responsible for the coilspring appearance.

Differential Diagnosis. Bloody bowel movements and abdominal cramps accompanying *enterocolitis* may usually be differentiated from intussusception because the pain is less severe and less regular and because the infant is recognizably ill between pains from the time of onset. Bleeding from *Meckel's diverticulum* is usually painless. The intestinal hemorrhage of *anaphylactoid purpura* is usually accompanied by joint symptoms or purpura elsewhere. *It is important to keep in mind that intussusception may be a complication of any of the foregoing conditions,* none of which is accompanied by a palpable abdominal mass in the absence of intussusception. Since tenesmus and a discoverable tumor are usually absent in ileo-ileal intussusception, it may be confused with *ileal obstruction* from other causes. This is of little clinical importance, since surgical exploration is indicated in any case.

PROGNOSIS. Untreated intussusception in infants is nearly always fatal; the chances of recovery are directly related to the duration of intussusception before reduction. The majority of infants will recover if the intussusception is reduced within the first 24 hours, but the mortality rate rises rapidly after this time, and recoveries are unusual when reduction is deferred to the third day. Spontaneous reduction during transport or preparation for operation is not uncommon.

TREATMENT. Reduction of the intussusception is an emergency procedure to be carried out immediately after diagnosis and after rapid preparation for operation with fluids and blood for shock and water and electrolyte repair. In many cases of short duration, when there are no signs of prostration, shock or peritoneal irritation, it may be possible to reduce the intussusception by hydrostatic pressure under fluoroscopic guidance and with the consultation and close proximity of a surgeon. The technique is described by Ravitch as follows:

> The stomach is aspirated, intravenous administration of fluids is started, and a nonlubricated Foley bag catheter is placed in the rectum and inflated. The buttocks are compressed tightly and taped with adhesive plaster. A barium solution is then allowed to flow by gravity into the colon from a height of not more than 3 to 3½ feet above the fluoroscopic table. The abdomen is *not touched* during the procedure. Reduction of the intussusception is manifest by free filling of the small intestine, disappearance of the mass, passage of flatus or feces and improvement in the infant's condition. Charcoal is then administered by mouth, and its recovery in an enema 6 hours later is further evidence of intestinal patency. If there is any doubt about the completeness of the reduction, an exploratory operation is performed immediately.

Reduction by the hydrostatic technique is not effective in ileo-ileal intussusception and will resolve only the colonic component of ileo-ileocolic intussusception. With adequate surgical management, operative reduction carries a very low mortality rate in early cases, and has the advantage of more certainty of reduction and of demonstration of any lead points, some of which may be removable. The recurrence rates for operative and nonoperative methods are apparently about equal. When the intussusception is irreducible or the bowel gangrenous, the involved intestine must be resected promptly.

NEOPLASMS OF THE GASTROINTESTINAL TRACT

Neoplasms of the gastrointestinal tract occur less frequently in children than in adults; polyps, carcinoma, sarcoma, lymphosarcoma, lipomas, polypoid adenomas and teratomas are described elsewhere (Section 25).

FOREIGN BODIES IN THE STOMACH AND INTESTINES

An object which reaches the stomach will in most instances pass through the gastrointestinal tract. Certain types of foreign bodies, however, are potentially dangerous. Needles, hairpins or bobby pins pass easily through the esophagus on their long axis, but may be unable to round the turns of the duodenum, where they become fixed and eventually perforate the intestine. Such potentially dangerous foreign bodies can usually be removed gastroscopically. Special attention should be paid to safety pins in the stomach. If they are small, they will probably pass without difficulty, whether open or closed. If they are large, either closed or open, peroral removal is safe and is indicated.

If the foreign body has passed through the pylorus into the intestine, its progress should be observed by means of roentgenograms, and every stool should be examined for its presence. The stool can be placed in a fine-meshed sieve and disintegrated by allowing water to run through the sieve with some force. If serial roentgenograms show the foreign body to move progressively down the intestinal tract, perforation is not likely. If it remains stationary for a week, operation is indicated because of the dangers of ulceration and perforation of the bowel. If at any time such signs of perforation as tenderness, rigidity, pain, nausea or vomiting develop, surgery is indicated immediately. The diet should be normal, with no change from that to which the child has been accustomed. The bizarre roughage and wool or cotton diets sometimes recommended are valueless and may be dangerous. Laxatives are contraindicated, since the accelerated activity of the intestine increases the danger of perforation.

BEZOARS

Occasionally infants and children, particularly if emotionally disturbed or mentally retarded, acquire the habit of swallowing hair from their head or from dolls or brushes, or they may swallow fur, wool or cotton from wearing apparel or blankets. Some of this material is passed through the intestines, but when the habit is persistent, there is an accumulation in the stomach with formation of the so-called *hairball* or *trichobezoar*. The symptoms are indefinite, but indigestion and gastric distress may be present. The tumor mass is often palpable and may give a soft crackling sensation on palpation. A roentgenogram after administration of barium may disclose a mass outlined by barium. A portion of the bezoar may be dislodged and subsequently become impacted in the intestine and cause obstruction. The diagnosis may be suspected from observation of the child in the act of swallowing these materials, and hair may occasionally be observed in the mouth or stools. The tumor should be removed surgically. The child's mental and psychologic status should be evaluated, and treatment provided as indicated.

Phytobezoars are accumulations of fibrous or mucilaginous materials such as that in persimmons and various tar products. The accumulation is usually rapid in comparison with that of the hairball.

Diseases of the Gastrointestinal Tract

EPIDEMIC GASTROENTERITIS (INTESTINAL "FLU" OR GRIPPE). Community and family epidemics of highly contagious infections in which vomiting and diarrhea are prominent manifestations are common throughout the world. They are presumed to be due in large part to as yet unidentified pathogenic agent(s), probably viruses. Endemic gastroenteritis usually begins abruptly, with vomiting during the first 6 to 24 hours and then diarrhea for 3 to 10 days. Since the illness is likely to be much more severe in infants than in older children, every attempt should be made to protect infants from contact with affected persons.

The affected child, often with a fever, begins to vomit, and then has diarrhea. Abdominal pain, distention, and increased bowel sounds are often present. Some children show symptoms and signs of upper respiratory infection, such as a reddened pharynx. Children do not usually appear very sick in spite of the degree of vomiting.

Since this illness is self-limited, the key to management is to maintain hydration. During the vomiting phase, the child may be fasted for several hours, after which a teaspoonful or two of sugar syrup (Emetrol or Coca-Cola syrup) can be given. Then weak, sweetened tea, electrolyte solution

(Pedialyte, Lytren) or decarbonated soda preparations may be given at 15 to 30 minute intervals, beginning with a teaspoonful and doubling the amount with each interval. As vomiting subsides, larger amounts of these fluids can be given. In the later phase a soft diet of applesauce, bananas, custards, flavored gelatin desserts, soup and toast with jelly can be offered. In general, medication is not required. Antibiotics, sedatives, anticholinergic drugs and antidiarrhea preparations have not been demonstrated to shorten significantly the natural course of this illness.

If dehydration becomes apparent, the child should be hospitalized, serum electrolytes measured, and appropriate parenteral fluids administered.

SPECIFIC INFECTIONS. Infections of the gastrointestinal tract due to identified agents are discussed elsewhere. See Typhoid Fever, Escherichia Coli Infections, Bacillary Dysentery, Salmonella Infections, Tuberculous Enteritis, Enterovirus Infections, Intestinal Protozoa and Intestinal Parasites.

ACUTE GASTRITIS. Objective evidence of gastritis in children is not clinically apparent, and as an isolated lesion it must be rare. Gastric lesions are usually unsuspected during life since vomiting and anorexia are symptoms common to many infections. Bleeding may occur and be evident in the vomitus. Inflammatory lesions are occasionally observed at autopsy. Acute infections such as gastroenteritis, moniliasis, chickenpox, diphtheria, smallpox or scarlet fever may produce an inflammatory process in the stomach. *Drugs* such as acetylsalicylic acid, antibiotics and antileukemic agents may also cause acute or chronic gastritis in children, and an indwelling nasogastric tube may produce erosive lesions.

Corrosive gastritis is produced by strong acids or alkalis or by other irritants, such as calcium chloride, and may be accompanied by lesions of the mouth, pharynx and esophagus. Quantities of a swallowed irritant sufficient to produce an extensive gastritis frequently cause collapse and death. In most instances the esophageal lesion is the one of greatest importance.

Treatment. The general treatment of burns from acids and alkalis is discussed in Section 28, and of esophageal lesions earlier in this Section. Administration of irritant drugs should be discontinued or they should be administered after a meal; protective demulcents such as aluminum hydroxide gel may be helpful. The only practical immediate treatment of possible infectious gastritis is to diminish the oral intake until the primary infectious process subsides.

GASTRIC DILATATION. *Acute dilatation of the stomach,* and of the intestine as well (paralytic ileus), may occur during the acute stages of pneumonia and other severe infections, after abdominal and thoracic operations or trauma, during peritonitis, with diabetic acidosis, hypokalemia and intestinal obstruction, and occasionally without discoverable cause. Gastric dilatation denotes a serious condition, especially when it occurs with pneumonia and peritonitis. Temporary relief can be provided by deflation through a stomach tube or, when there are accumulated gastric contents, by lavage. The use of the suction drainage in postoperative conditions is helpful in avoiding and in treating paralytic ileus.

Chronic gastric dilatation may result from mechanical obstructions such as pyloric stenosis, external traction by adhesions, or pressure of a tumor in the pyloric area. During infancy a cause is atony of the muscular wall in such conditions as rickets and extreme malnutrition.

The treatment depends upon the cause. A mechanical obstruction should be relieved. Chronic nutritional disturbances should be corrected.

GASTRIC HEMORRHAGE. Bleeding from the stomach may occur in association with purpura, hemophilia, hypoplastic anemias, leukemia, scurvy, peptic ulcer, cirrhosis of the liver, varices associated with other obstructions of the portal or splenic vein, and polypoid adenoma of the stomach. Traumatic rupture of the stomach, injury from a swallowed foreign body, generalized infections, diabetic acidosis and persistent vomiting as in pyloric stenosis may also be responsible for gastric hemorrhage. Hemorrhagic disease of the newborn may result in gastric bleeding.

Blood which is vomited from the stomach may originate elsewhere, in the nose, mouth, esophagus or lungs, or from the fissured nipple of the nursing mother. Blood expectorated from the lungs without swallowing is frothy. When hemorrhage from the stomach is copious, the blood is usually bright red, but if bleeding has taken place slowly and the blood has remained for some time in the stomach, the color will be dark brown or black (coffee-ground vomitus).

The **prognosis** depends upon the cause; extensive gastric hemorrhage usually has serious implications.

Treatment. With extensive hemorrhage immediate steps should be directed toward its control, treatment of shock and replacement of lost blood. The child should be put at rest, and blood transfusions should be given as soon as possible to replace lost blood. When the bleeding is continuous, gentle but constant aspiration through a large-holed nasogastric tube may aid in putting the stomach at rest, removing irritation from gastric secretions, and providing an index of the extent of active bleeding. Irrigation with iced saline until the returns are clear may help.

GASTRIC PERFORATION. Perforation of the stomach or adjacent portions of the esophagus or duodenum is uncommon in infants and children; it is more often recognized at autopsy than during life. Rupture of the stomach in newborn infants may be recognized during life and repaired surgically, with recovery. In some cases, spontaneous gastric perforation in otherwise apparently healthy newborn infants has been explained at autopsy through presence of obstructive lesions, such as atresia of the pylorus or duodenum, or defects of the gastric musculature.

The perforation of ulcers is the most readily explained; though infrequent, ulcers may be caused by an indwelling nasogastric tube, be associated with systemic diseases, usually acute, and especially with intracranial lesions (Rokitansky-Cushing ulcers) or be a rare sequel to corticosteroid therapy. Rupture of chronic gastric and duodenal ulcers is uncommon.

Abdominal distention occurring suddenly in an infant should always suggest the possibility of perforation somewhere in the gastrointestinal tract, especially if there is obliteration of liver dullness. Vomiting, however, is usually the first symptom, and both the vomitus and the stool may contain blood. Cyanosis may appear if the distention is sufficient to interfere with respiration, and shock may be an early sign. The demonstration of air in the peritoneal cavity on a roentgenogram of the abdomen taken in the upright position is diagnostic.

Treatment consists in surgical repair as quickly as the infant can be prepared. Postoperatively, nasogastric suction is necessary and parenteral alimentation and hydration will be required.

PEPTIC ULCER

Gastric and duodenal ulcers are not common in childhood, but may occur at any age, including the neonatal. There is a high incidence of recurrent abdominal pain in children; the erroneous diagnosis of ulcer is too frequently made in children with this complaint. Gastric ulcers occur more frequently in early infancy; duodenal ulcers, more frequently in later infancy and childhood. Overall, the incidence of duodenal ulcer is at least five times that of gastric ulcer. Ulcerations of the upper gastrointestinal tract are more apt to be acute than chronic in the pediatric age range and are frequently secondary to conditions such as extensive burns (Curling's ulcer), neurologic lesions (Rokitansky-Cushing ulcer), intensive therapy with adrenocorticosteroids, severe infections (sepsis, gastroenteritis, meningitis, bronchiolitis) and marasmus.

SYMPTOMS. The symptoms related to the ulcer may dominate the clinical picture, but often they are obscured by the primary disorder. Vomiting is the most common manifestation in infancy, but the ulcer may present with bleeding (hematemesis and melena) or with abdominal distention associated with perforation. In older children, as in adults, the chief symptom may be epigastric pain during the night or before meals; it is often relieved by eating. Frequently, however, in younger children the pain is periumbilical, erratic in timing and aggravated by eating, or the chief symptom may be vomiting. Many children with ulcers are intense, competitive youngsters who do well in school and are faced with emotional conflicts in their families. Peptic ulcer also appears to be somewhat more frequent in children with other chronic functional disorders of the gastrointestinal tract such as constipation or the irritable colon syndrome.

DIAGNOSIS. The diagnosis of peptic ulcer should not be made without roentgenographic confirmation. In the very young infant free intraperitoneal air visible in abdominal films taken in the erect position should raise suspicion of a perforated gastric or duodenal ulcer. In such instances administration of contrast media is contraindicated; the nature of the perforation is determined at surgical exploration. The roentgenographic diagnosis of duodenal ulcer, most frequently located in the bulb, is based on a constant deformity of the bulb when it is well filled with barium: a persistent filling defect indicative of a crater, and a surrounding clear halo with convergent mucosal folds. Most duodenal ulcers are on the posterior wall; gastric ulcers are most frequently on the anterior wall and only rarely on the greater curvature. Postbulbar duodenal ulcers and ulcers of the pyloric canal (sometimes in conjunction with hypertrophic pyloric stenosis) are equally rare.

The roentgenographic identification of an ulcer in a child is difficult. A collection of barium caught between mucosal folds may resemble a crater, and it is difficult to obtain good compression films of the duodenum. Failure to fill the duodenal bulb with barium is not necessarily evidence of deformity or irritability, but may be solely the result of pyloric spasm and increased duodenal reactivity in a frightened child; subsequent study usually shows that suspected "craters" or deformities are not present.

Gastric analysis, utilizing the augmented maximum histamine stimulation test, is of limited value in children; correlation with peptic ulcer has not yet been shown in children.

PROGNOSIS. The case fatality rate is high among infants with perforated ulcers. Intractability and scarring of the duodenum is a rare sequel of peptic ulcer in childhood, and the necessity for gastric or duodenal resection is rare. An estimated 50 per cent of children with chronic ulcers have recurrent ulcers or ulcer-like pain as adults.

TREATMENT. Acute perforation requires immediate surgical closure. With acute hemorrhage the hematocrit should be followed closely and transfusions of blood given as indicated. (See Gastric Hemorrhage, above.) Infants with moderate hemorrhage but without perforation should be maintained on milk feedings; older children, on a bland diet. Hospitalization is usually warranted for initial therapy and a thorough investigation of the emotional interactions of the child and his family. After a few days on a bland diet a free diet is generally advocated. Gastric antacids or feedings between meals and at bedtime, as well as anticholinergic drugs shortly before meals, are therapeutically useful in children as in adults. It is almost impossible to maintain hourly antacid therapy in children, so that interval antacids are used between meals, and anticholinergic drugs at bedtime in double the usual recommended doses. Fortunately, most ulcers of childhood heal rapidly, so that treatment need not be maintained beyond 3 or 4 weeks in most instances. If the pain does not improve with therapy, another origin of the pain is more likely than intractability of the ulcer. Follow-up roentgenographic studies should be carried out 1 or 2 months after treatment has been initiated.

ZOLLINGER-ELLISON SYNDROME

The Zollinger-Ellison syndrome is rarely responsible for multiple duodenal or jejunal ulcers in childhood. The symptoms are severe, intermittent abdominal pain with little response to medical therapy, vomiting, hematemesis, melena and diarrhea. Radiographic study shows marked gastric rugal hypertrophy, marked duodenal dilatation and rapid transit time. Nocturnal gastric secretion is markedly increased in volume and in titratable acidity. Islet cell tumors or hyperplasia of the pancreas have been found, which produce a gastrin-like material responsible for the gastric hypersecretion and ulcer diathesis. Total gastrectomy has been found the treatment of choice.

MESENTERIC LYMPHADENITIS

ACUTE MESENTERIC LYMPHADENITIS. Acute mesenteric lymphadenitis is an ill defined and somewhat questionable entity frequently associated with an acute infection of the upper respiratory tract, especially of the pharynx. So much attention has been directed to this combination of inflammatory lesions, and the possibility that it may simulate acute appendicitis, that the physician may fail to recall that both acute and chronic involvement of the mesenteric lymph nodes may also be associated with infections of the appendix and the intestines.

Clinical Manifestations. There are fever, abdominal pain, vomiting and at times constipation or diarrhea. The pain may be spasmodic, is often in the right lower quadrant, but may be in any part of the abdomen.

Differential Diagnosis. When the pain is in the right lower quadrant and there is localized tenderness and muscular resistance, the possibility of appendicitis cannot be eliminated except by laparotomy. It has been suggested that in mesenteric adenitis there is a tendency for the area of tenderness to shift when the patient is rolled from side to side, whereas it remains fixed in appendicitis. Tenderness along the route of the mesentery on a line from McBurney's point upward to the left of the umbilicus is also said to favor a diagnosis of mesenteric adenitis. In the absence of physical signs of peritonitis or abscess, it is more common for the white blood cell count to be over 20,000 per mm^3 with mesenteric adenitis than with appendicitis.

Complications. Suppuration of the lymph nodes is rare, but it may be responsible for localized or generalized peritonitis.

Treatment. Whenever appendicitis is a reasonable possibility, operation is indicated, since the danger of operation in mesenteric adenitis is much less than the danger of rupture of an inflamed appendix. Otherwise, treatment is symptomatic, and the illness usually self-limited.

CHRONIC MESENTERIC LYMPHADENITIS. Chronic infection of the lymph nodes may be the sequel to an acute infection, or the involvement may be low-grade from the onset. In addition to conditions which may be responsible for acute adenitis, tuberculosis and histoplasmosis are causative possibilities. Involvement of lymph nodes is a nearly constant accompaniment of chronic intestinal infections, but is usually overshadowed by the manifestations of the primary disease. Noninfectious lymph node involvement occurs with Hodgkin's disease, lymphosarcoma, and neoplasms of the abdominal or pelvic organs.

NECROTIZING ENTEROCOLITIS

Necrotizing enterocolitis is a serious idiopathic disease of the newborn which occurs primarily in premature infants. It is characterized by gastric retention, abdominal distention, vomiting of bile, and blood-streaked and occasionally diarrheal stools. Earlier reports of "functional ileus," perforation of the ileum and colon, and colitis in the newborn infant probably represented forms of this condition.

The ileum and the colon are the most common sites of involvement; the duodenum is the least common. The condition is a complication of exchange transfusion or severe infections such as pneumonia, meningitis or omphalitis. *Pathologically* the intestine is dilated, necrotic and friable, with superficial ulcerations and submucosal hemorrhage. Perforation is common. Pneumatosis (intramural gas) of the intestinal wall may be present and often is a premonitory sign of perforation. The *roentgenographic findings* are (1) multiple dilated loops of small intestine with air-fluid levels in the erect position and separation of loops suggesting mural edema or peritoneal fluid, (2) intramural gas, (3) free air in the peritoneum, and (4) gas in the portal vein. Therapy is mainly supportive; intravenous alimentation and hydration are usually necessary. Gastric suction, blood transfusions and antibiotic therapy are always indicated. Surgical treatment is required for intestinal perforation.

IRRITABLE COLON SYNDROME

The irritable colon syndrome is a frequent cause of recurrent abdominal pain in childhood. Its tendency to occur in emotionally sensitive children of overconcerned parents, together with accompanying signs and symptoms of autonomic hyperreactivity, suggests that it has a strong psychosomatic component. See also Abdominal Pain and Chronic Diarrhea (earlier, this Section).

CLINICAL MANIFESTATIONS. Characteristically there is recurrent, intermittent, crampy abdominal pain which may be punctuated by acute, sharp episodes. It may occur at any time of day but usually not at night; there is no consistent relation to eating or to bowel movements. Headache, facial pallor, dizziness, nausea and vomiting are frequent concurrent symptoms and signs. The stools are commonly described as hard pellets, suggesting spastic contractile activity of the colon, but diarrhea is also a manifestation. There is abdominal tenderness over the colon, especially over the sigmoid and cecum. It is sometimes possible to palpate pellets of stool almost like a string of beads in the sigmoid colon of the left lower abdomen. Anorexia, weight loss and low-grade fever are sometimes present.

DIAGNOSIS. Transmural enterocolitis, ulcerative colitis, amebic and bacillary dysentery, and disorders of the urinary tract are ruled out by roentgenographic studies of the intestinal tract and colon using barium as the contrast medium, by intravenous urography and by microscopic examination and culture of the stools and urine. *Sigmoidoscopy* may show intense pallor of the rectal and colonic mucosa, prominence of the blood vessels, areas of erythematous flushing, increased mucus and prominent lymphoid follicles, which are nonspecific. The *family history* and relationships suggest the possibility of psychosomatic factors. The parents tend to be strikingly concerned about their children and to set high standards of performance for themselves as well as their children. Illness during pregnancy has often led to both prenatal and postnatal anxiety about the child, and a history of death or severe illness in the family is frequent. Parental concerns have often led to an atmosphere of hovering anxiety over normal processes of behavioral development. As a result, the child often appears to be looking constantly for direction, reassurance and safety; relations with peers become restricted, and there is interference with normal childhood activities. School phobia is common.

PROGNOSIS. Most children with the irritable colon syndrome gradually lose their symptoms with time, but a few retain them well into adulthood. As a group, their level of intellectual and material accomplishment is generally satisfactory.

TREATMENT. Parent and child must learn that the child can cope with new environmental situations much better than either had believed possible. Ascertainment that no serious organic disease is present may help to relieve parental anxiety. Care should be taken not to imply to parent or child that the pain is "in the head." The physician's recognition of the reality of the pain should be stressed at the same time that an understanding and sympathetic explanation of its psychosomatic nature is made. Exploration of sensitive stress factors with parents and patient separately may often develop understanding and relief for the child. Symptomatic therapy with an anticholinergic drug as needed is helpful in some instances. Older children with the irritable colon syndrome tolerate competitive sports poorly; prescribed relief from such compulsory school activities may on occasion be helpful.

On occasion hospitalization may be required, owing to the severity of symptoms and fears of parents and patient. At this time, laboratory and radiologic examinations will rule out serious disease and relieve family and patient of their fears. Various emotional areas of possible importance may be explored. Most frequently, symptoms improve during hospitalization, but a few children with this disorder have severe unabated pain during long periods of hospitalization.

INFLAMMATORY DISEASE OF THE INTESTINE

The inflammatory diseases of the bowel are divided into three categories: (1) infectious (amebic or bacterial, Section 10); (2) chronic ulcerative colitis; and (3) transmural enteritis and colitis.

ULCERATIVE COLITIS

Ulcerative colitis is a chronic inflammatory disease of the large intestine in which the mucous membrane becomes hyperemic and bleeds easily. The clinical course is marked by chronicity punctuated with acute exacerbations.

ETIOLOGY. Many theories based on infectious, immunologic, and psychogenic causes have been proposed for ulcerative colitis; none has been substantiated. The condition occurs more frequently among relatives of patients with the disease than would be expected from its incidence in the general population, and an inherited susceptibility to unidentified environmental factors has been suggested.

PATHOLOGY. The rectum and distal colon are principally involved, but all or any part of the colon may be affected. The disease extends into the ileum in less than one third of patients. The inflammatory process is generally limited to the mucosa, rarely involving the submucosa, and is generally continuous from distal to proximal colon. The mucosa of the rectum shows diffuse erythematous involvement, with easy friability and, rarely, ulcers. Histologically the mucosa is infiltrated by lymphocytes, mast cells and plasma cells. An early finding is the movement of polymorphonuclear leukocytes into the lamina propria below the tip of gland crypts, with decreased secretion of mucus and degenerative changes of the crypt epithelium. Crypt abscesses develop with necrosis of the crypt epithelial cells and underlying lamina propria. Pus moves from the abscess into the lumen of the crypt and to the surface of the mucosa. Fibrosis is not a characteristic response in the healing process. The colon decreases in length and caliber, owing to shortening of the muscle fibers. As the disease progresses, pseudopolyps may become prominent as the ulcerative process extends and excavates.

CLINICAL MANIFESTATIONS. Diarrhea and abdominal pain are the most frequent symptoms, along with rectal bleeding. The onset may be mild or very acute, and the course one of recurrent episodes of diarrhea and rectal bleeding, with periods of remission or long chronicity. Repeated urges to defecate during the night and on awakening in the morning are common. Abdominal cramps often precede the passage of stool, and tenesmus follows. Perianal disease is uncommon in ulcerative colitis, common in transmural colitis. Other symptoms such as anorexia, weight loss, malaise, nausea and vomiting may occur. Growth and sexual maturation may be retarded. There may be severe headaches and abdominal cramps, particularly early in the course of the disease or during remissions. Pallor and iron deficiency anemia may develop as the result of bleeding and diminished dietary intake. In severe cases hypoproteinemia and edema may accompany emaciation. There is frequently mild to moderate tenderness on abdominal palpation, particularly in the left lower quadrant over the sigmoid colon.

Children with ulcerative colitis tend to be anxious and dependent, anticipating the worst from any experience; they are often closely attached to the parents, and especially to the mother, with strong ambivalence of feeling. At least one parent has intense chronic anxiety, which is communicated to other family members. It is difficult to know how much the behavioral features in the child with ulcerative colitis are primary components or secondary developments; behavioral disturbances of some intensity are common.

Extra-intestinal manifestations are not uncommon in childhood. There may be erythema multiforme, erythema nodosum, and pyoderma gangrenosum. Other complications include arthritis, liver disease, and iritis.

DIAGNOSIS. The diagnosis is suspected on the basis of the clinical pattern and through failure to isolate a specific agent. It is confirmed by sigmoidoscopy: early in the disease the mucosa is hyperemic and bleeds easily, with a dull appearance and a loss of vascular markings; in later stages multiple ragged ulcers, a plum-colored granular mucosa and pseudopolyps are seen. The demonstration of polymorphonuclear infiltration in a mucosal biopsy specimen is diagnostically helpful early in the disease. *Rectal biopsy* should be taken at sigmoidoscopy because it may help differentiate ulcerative colitis from transmural colitis; moreover, it is often abnormal when sigmoidoscopic findings are normal or equivocal. A mucosal smear shows eosinophils and polymorphonuclear leukocytes. *Roentgenographic studies* with barium enema early in the disease may be normal, showing only increased irritability of the involved segment at fluoroscopy or distorted mucosal surface on films taken after evacuation of barium. Later, ulcers appear as shaggy, barium-filled niches extending beyond the lumen of the colon. As the disease progresses, there is shortening and rigidity of the colon with loss of haustral markings ("pipestem colon"), particularly in the transverse and descending colon.

The colon of a child with ulcerative colitis is very sensitive to diagnostic procedures such as sigmoidoscopy and barium enema during the very acute phases of the disease, and the child is often very frightened. It is usually sound to withhold diagnostic procedures until the patient has had a chance to settle down in the hospital; otherwise, exacerbations of symptoms may be provoked.

COURSE AND PROGNOSIS. The course is chronic and is usually marked by exacerbations and remissions over many years. Relapses may occur after remissions lasting up to 5 years. An acute situation called toxic megacolon (acute dilatation of the colon) with distention and vomiting is rarely seen in children, but appears to be induced in certain instances by ill timed procedures or manipulations during the acute phases of disease. Death may occur from cachexia (during a fulminating episode with toxic megacolon), thrombosis of major blood vessels or perforation of the colon. Some patients develop carcinoma of the colon years after the disease has appeared to be quiescent or nearly so. The risk of neoplastic degeneration increases with the duration of disease, particularly in those who have had their disease for 10 or more years. Overall, about 20 per cent of patients die of the disease, 30 to 40 per cent have prolonged remissions, and the remainder have symptoms persisting into adulthood.

TREATMENT. Hospitalization for initial evaluation and institution of therapy usually seems to produce better results than attempts at initial ambulatory management, perhaps because the child is removed from his usual psychologic stresses and the physician is able to develop a more effective relationship with patient and parents. Hospitalization is essential in children with severe attacks of ulcerative colitis to diminish the "toxic" anxiety of the family and for whatever therapy is required. Symptomatic treatment with tranquilizers, antidiarrheal and anticholinergic agents is of limited value. On rare occasions, opiates may be necessary for severe pain; they should be used with great caution.

It is common to restrict diets for adults with ulcerative colitis, but restrictions often interfere with an adequate intake of food in children. Children with ulcerative colitis are frequently anorexic or difficult to please with food, and will generally do better with an unrestricted diet. By the same token, activity should be as tolerated rather than limited. Supplements of vitamins and iron are indicated in children with severe diarrhea, malnutrition and anemia.

Some patients benefit from the oral administration of salicylazo-sulfapyridine (Azulfidine) in a dosage of 0.5 to 1.0 gm two to three times a day for children less than 10 years, and 1 to 2 gm two to three times a day for children over 10 years; this serves as maintenance therapy during the chronic or intermediate phases of disease. If the process is limited to the distal part of the colon, nightly retention enemas of 100 to 150 ml of saline solution containing a soluble corticosteroid (50 to 100 mg of hydrocortisone or 20 to 40 mg of methylprednisolone) may provide some relief of symptoms in a course of 10 to 14 days. If the disease is more widespread, severe or resistant to other modes of medical therapy, trial with a corticosteroid or corticotropin (ACTH) is usually justified. Initial high dose therapy with cortisone (8 mg/kg/24 hr) or prednisone (2 mg/kg/24 hr) may be necessary to achieve improvement. A maximum dose of 300 mg of hydrocortisone or 75 mg of prednisone is rarely exceeded. After one week the dose is reduced at weekly intervals by one fifth of the starting dose to the lowest maintenance dose which will keep the patient in remission, and is maintained at that level for at least 4 to 6 months.

The chronic administration of steroids in this disease is sometimes necessary if other measures fail, and it appears that some of these patients are benefited by small doses of prednisone (5 to 15 mg per day). Alternate day therapy is still of uncertain clinical value and not now recommended. On rare occasions an immunosuppressive drug, such as azathioprine (Imuran) has been used with some benefit, but the value and place of such drugs have not been adequately assessed. They are an alternative for the child refractory to steroid therapy who has not responded to other measures and is not an immediate candidate for colectomy.

Surgical treatment by colectomy and ileostomy is indicated for patients with unsatisfactory response to other medical treatment. The indications for colectomy are perforation, growth failure lasting 2 to 4 years or fulminating symptoms which do not respond to medical management. Whenever possible, surgery should be elective and planned so that proper preparation of the patient can be made for the procedure and for the management of the ileostomy. Response to surgery can be striking, with freedom from symptoms, considerable growth and abatement of extra-intestinal manifestations. Ileostomy is attended with problems in about 25 per cent of patients.

Psychotherapy by the physician should be directed towards minimizing the reactions to chronic illness and developing the child's strengths and aspirations toward health. The child should be seen regularly even when well, so that a positive relationship can be established which will support child and family in dealing with the stresses of family life and disease.

The proper care of children with ulcerative colitis requires a major, long-term commitment of interest on the part of the physician responsible for the patient. If this is not possible, he should consider referral to another physician who has a particular interest in the care of patients with the disease.

TRANSMURAL ENTEROCOLITIS

(Regional Enteritis; Granulomatous Colitis or Enterocolitis; Crohn's Disease)

Transmural enterocolitis is a chronic inflammatory disease of the intestinal wall of unknown etiology. Previously recognized in the ileum as regional ileitis, it has in the past decade been described in every part of the gastrointestinal tract. When it involves the colon, it must be differentiated from ulcerative colitis, from which in 10 per cent of cases it cannot be separated by the usual clinical and pathologic criteria. It is as common among children as ulcerative colitis.

PATHOLOGY. The ileum is the commonest site of this inflammatory process; the cecum is frequently involved along with the ileum. About 40 per cent of cases will involve the colon; in half, the illness is found only in the colon, where discontinuity is a characteristic feature of the disease. Less than 10 per cent of patients will have lesions set apart some distance in the small intestine. The wall of the involved intestine is thickened and indurated. The mesentery is edematous and thickened, with the fat encroaching on the wall of the involved intestine. The lumen is narrowed and the mucosa has a cobblestone appearance. Between the mounds there are deep ulcerated fissures. Internal fistulas develop when these ulcerations burrow into another viscus or to the skin. All layers of the intestinal wall are involved in the inflammatory process, but most strikingly the submucosa. The lymphoid tissue of the intestine is hyperplastic, as are the mesenteric lymph nodes. The common cells of the inflammatory infiltration are lymphocytes and plasma cells; polymorphonuclear leukocytes are scarce. Noncaseating granulomas containing giant cells and epithelial cells occur in about half the patients. Neoplastic degeneration is less common in transmural enterocolitis than in ulcerative colitis.

CLINICAL MANIFESTATIONS. In childhood, transmural enterocolitis usually begins in the preadolescent period. The onset may be acute, with a clinical pattern resembling that of acute appendicitis (acute regional enteritis). More often the onset is insidious, and the course is that of a low-grade chronic infection. There may be periodic bouts of fever without significant intestinal or abdominal symptoms or signs, or there may be recurrent abdominal pain, particularly after eating, mild diarrhea, intermittent constipation, low-grade fever, anorexia and a sensation of filling of the stomach at meals. The diarrhea may consist only of slightly loose stools which the patient considers to be unremarkable, or the stools may contain mucus, pus and, at times, blood. Loss of weight, delay of linear growth and delayed puberty in the absence of gastrointestinal symptoms other than anorexia may rarely lead to a mistaken diagnosis of anorexia nervosa. Iron deficiency anemia may occur. Pain is usually periumbilical or in the right lower quadrant; it is characteristically intermittent and cramping, but may be dull, aching or burning. Anal fissures or fistulas are important signs of transmural enterocolitis. Erythema nodosum, clubbing of the digits, aphthous stomatitis, arthritis, and oxalate renal stones have been noted in some patients. Complete or partial intestinal obstruction may be the presenting symptom.

Abdominal examination is uninformative unless there is a tender, fixed mass in the lower part of the abdomen, more often on the right than on the left or in the midline. Rarely, polypoid masses are palpable on rectal examination. With extensive disease abdominal fistulas can arise.

Children with transmural enterocolitis tend to be emotionally labile, to cry readily, to adapt poorly to new situations and to take a gloomy anticipatory view of any coming event. They often appear to be striving for high levels of performance in school and at home despite, or because of, lack of self-confidence or strong feelings of insecurity. Sometimes the onset of disease accompanies or follows a series of major family stresses, such as death or serious illness, a circumstance which minimizes the strength necessary to cope effectively with chronic illness. As in ulcerative colitis, it is not crucial how psychosocial factors may have contributed to causing the disease, but it is important to therapy that when psychosocial tensions exist, the pattern of illness and of the patient's coping are highly influenced by them.

DIAGNOSIS. *Laboratory data* are of little aid in diagnosis. The erythrocyte sedimentation rate is elevated in about half the patients, and the normal ratio of albumin to globulin in the serum is reversed in an equal number.

Roentgenographic studies early in the disease may show thickening of the bowel wall manifested by an increase in the distance between gas or barium shadows in adjacent loops; later there are visible mucosal irregularities or rigidity of a segment of bowel wall, followed in turn by ulcerations, fissures, fistulas, pseudodiverticula, the cobblestone pattern, or narrowing of a segment of bowel lumen. *Sigmoidoscopy* is useful in that patients with low colonic involvement show an irregular, inflamed surface with little friability or bleeding. Punched-out fissures or ulcers may be visualized, a finding not usually observed in ulcerative colitis. Rectal biopsy may confirm the diagnosis or add information when sigmoidoscopic and radiologic examination are equivocal.

DIFFERENTIAL DIAGNOSIS. When the onset has been abrupt, appendicitis may be suspected. Functional abdominal pain, ulcerative colitis, tuberculosis, abdominal actinomycosis, anorexia nervosa, Hodgkin's disease or lymphosarcoma may be confused with the chronic form of transmural colitis.

PROGNOSIS. The prognosis for life is usually good, but the course of the disease is persistent and chronic; spontaneous cures are infrequent, especially if fistulous tracts have developed. Rarely, an acute attack simulating appendicitis subsides spontaneously within a few weeks.

TREATMENT. No treatment is entirely satisfactory. Dietary restrictions have not been shown to be of benefit and may decrease food intake in a situation in which malnutrition is already a problem. Initially, corticosteroid therapy should be used, especially in patients with involvement of multiple or extensive segments of bowel and with disruption of a normal living pattern from weakness, loss of weight, anorexia and absence from school. Hydrocortisone (8-10 mg/kg/24 hr) or preferably prednisone (2 mg/kg/24 hr) is recommended. A maximum dose of 300 mg of hydrocortisone or 75 mg of prednisone is rarely exceeded. The dose should be reduced by one fifth at 1- to 2-week intervals, depending on response, to a dose not much above the physiologic one. This therapy may be maintained for 6 to 12 months. The dose should be sufficient to eliminate symptoms and perhaps to maintain a mildly "cushingoid" appearance of the patient; it has been suggested that those who do not have a "cushingoid" appearance often fail to benefit from such treatment.

Anticholinergic and antidiarrheal agents have some symptomatic value. Immunosuppressive therapy with azathioprine, along with chronic administration of antibiotics has shown sufficient promise in uncontrolled studies to merit consideration in cases of considerable illness.

Surgical resection of the involved area of bowel when it is an isolated segment may be accompanied by a long remission or apparent cure. Other indications for surgery are intestinal obstruction and management of abdominal fistulas. In acute cases resembling appendicitis, surgery is not indicated because of the possibility of spontaneous recovery.

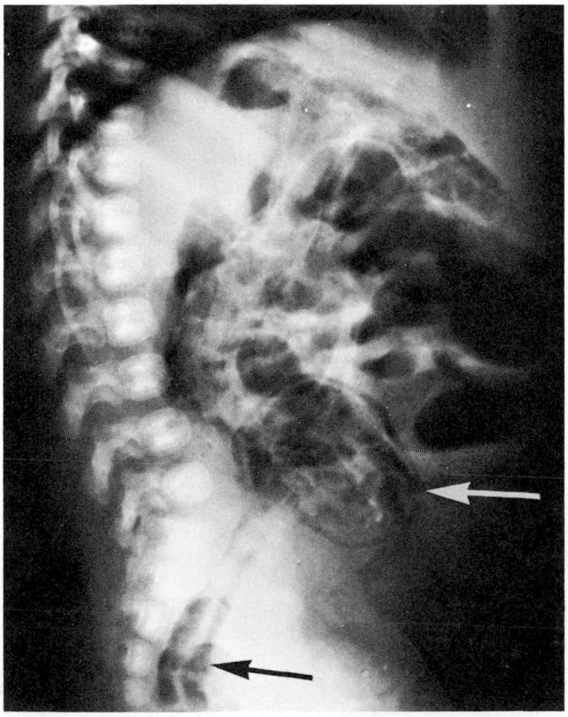

Figure 11–16 *Lateral roentgenogram of the abdomen of an infant with aganglionic megacolon involving the entire colon. Pneumatosis of the colon was demonstrated before and after death in the walls of the rectum and sigmoid; note the apparent double contour of the intestinal walls (arrows).*

Because of a high rate of recurrence after surgery, an initial trial of medical therapy is indicated, particularly if the disease is extensive and would require resection of large segments of intestine. Many patients eventually require resection.

On occasion such symptoms as abdominal pain and diarrhea may diminish or disappear during hospitalization or other change of environment. Since the disease is a distressing one which frequently results in emotional depression in the child or parents, a strong supportive role by the physician is of considerable assistance to them.

PNEUMATOSIS CYSTOIDES INTESTINALIS

This is a condition characterized by multiple gas-filled cysts in the wall of the bowel. The cysts may be located in the small intestine, the colon, or both; in infants they are predominantly submucosal. The condition may occur at any age. In infants it is often associated with intrinsic disease of the gastrointestinal tract, e.g., necrotizing enterocolitis or pyloric stenosis. No symptoms directly related to pneumatosis in infancy are recognized. The diagnosis has been established roentgenographically (Fig. 11–16) and at laparotomy, but more frequently at autopsy. The pathogenesis of the cysts is not known, but may be related to mucosal defects with escape of intestinal gases into the lymphatics and wall of the bowel. Pneumatosis intestinalis occurs in the course of other serious illnesses and is a serious prognostic sign. In some instances it will disappear if the primary disease improves. Death appears to result from some cause other than the pneumatosis.

GIULIO J. BARBERO

Feeding Difficulties

Apley, J., and MacKeith, R.: Infant feeding and its difficulties. *In* The Child and His Symptoms: A Psychosomatic Approach. Oxford, Blackwell Pub., 1962, Chaps. 12 and 13.

Barbero, G. J., and Shaheen, E.: Environmental failure to thrive: A clinical view. J. Pediatr. *71*:639, 1967.

Bliss, E. L., and Branch, C. H. H.: Anorexia Nervosa. New York, Paul B. Hoeber, 1960.

MacKeith, R., and Wood, C.: Infant Feeding and Feeding Difficulties. 4th ed. London, J. & A. Churchill, Ltd., 1971.

Patton, R. G., and Gardner, L. I.: Growth Failure in Maternal Deprivation. Springfield, Ill., Charles C Thomas, 1963.

Shaheen, E., Alexander, D., Truskowski, M., and Barbero, G. J.: Failure to thrive—A retrospective profile. Clin. Pediatr. *7*:255, 1968.

Abdominal Pain

Apley, J.: The Child with Abdominal Pain. Springfield, Ill., Charles C Thomas, 1959.

Kopel, E., Kim, I. C., and Barbero, G. J.: Comparison of rectosigmoid motility in normal children, children with recurrent abdominal pain and ulcerative colitis. Pediatrics *39*:539, 1967.

Stone, R. T., and Barbero, G. J.: Recurrent abdominal pain in childhood. Pediatrics *45*:732, 1970.

Wood, J. L., Hardy, M. L., and White, H.: Chronic Vague Abdominal Pain in Children. Pediat. Clin. N. Amer. *2*:465, 1955.

Gastrointestinal Bleeding

Abrams, B., and Lynn, H. B.: Rectal bleeding in children. Am. J. Surg. *104*:831, 1962.

Brayton, D.: Gastrointestinal bleeding of "unknown origin." A study of cases in infancy and childhood. Am. J. Dis. Child. *107*: 288, 1964.

Kiesewetter, W. B., Cancelmo, R., and Koop, C. E.: Rectal bleeding in infants and children with a hitherto unreported etiological factor. J. Pediatr. *47*:660, 1955.

Spencer, R.: Gastrointestinal hemorrhage in infancy and childhood: 476 cases. Surgery *55*:718, 1964.

Swenson, O.: Gastrointestinal bleeding in infants and children. *In* Pediatric Surgery. New York, Appleton-Century-Crofts, 1969, p. 709.

Vomiting

Craig, W. S.: Vomiting in the early days of life. Arch. Dis. Child. *36*:451, 1961.

Hoyt, C. S., and Stickley, G. B.: Study of 44 children with the syndrome of recurrent (cyclic) vomiting. Pediatrics *25*:775, 1960.

Hughes, J. G.: The etiology of vomiting in infancy and childhood. Pediat. Clin. N. Amer. *2*:483, 1955.

Menking, M., Wagnitz, J. G., Burton, J. J., Coddinton, R. D., and Sotos, J. F.: Rumination—A near-fatal psychiatric disease of infancy. New Engl. J. Med. *280*:802, 1969.

Richmond, J. B., Eddy, E. J., and Green, M.: Rumination—A psychosomatic syndrome of infancy. Pediatrics *29*:49, 1958.

Constipation

Anthony, E. J.: An experimental approach to the psychopathology of childhood; Encopresis. Brit. J. Med. Psychol. *30*:146, 1957.

Bellman, M.: Studies on encopresis. Acta Paediatr. Scand. Suppl. 170, 1966.

Davidson, M., Kugler, M. M., and Bauer, C. H.: Diagnosis and management in children with severe and protracted constipation. J. Pediatr. *62*:261, 1963.

Mercer, R. D.: Constipation. Pediat. Clin. N. Amer. *14*:175, 1967.

Neumann, P. Z., deDomenico, I. J., and Nogrady, M. B.: Constipation and urinary tract infection. Pediatrics *52*:241, 1973.

Pinkerton, P.: Psychogenic megacolon in children: The implications of bowel negativism. Arch. Dis. Child. *33*:371, 1958.

Shopfner, C. E.: Urinary tract pathology associated with constipation. Radiology *90*:865, 1968.

Diarrhea

Avery, G. B., Villaviccncio, O., Lilly, J. R., and Randolph, J. G.: Intractable diarrhea in early infancy. Pediatrics *41*:712, 1968.

Barness, L. A. (Ed.): Symposium on fluid and electrolyte problems. Pediat. Clin. N. Amer. *11*:789, 1964.

Davidson, M., and Wasserman, R.: The irritable colon of childhood (chronic non-specific diarrhea syndrome). J. Pediatr. *69*: 1027, 1966.

Karelitz, S.: Diarrhea in infants and children. Pediat. Clin. N. Amer. *3*:137, 1956.

Congenital Hypertrophic Pyloric Stenosis

Bell, M. J.: Infantile pyloric stenosis: Experience with 305 cases at Louisville Children's Hospital. Surgery *64*:983, 1968.

Bishop, H., and Hope, J. W.: Postoperative roentgen studies and their clinical significance. J. Pediatr. *60*:62, 1962.

Boggs, T. R., Jr., and Bishop, H.: Neonatal hyperbilirubinemia associated with high obstruction of the small bowel. J. Pediatr. *66*:349, 1965.

Schärli, A., Sieber, W. K., and Kiesewetter, W. B.: Hypertrophic pyloric stenosis at the Children's Hospital of Pittsburgh from 1912 to 1962: A critical review of current problems and complications. J. Pediatr. Surg. *4*:108, 1969.

Shuman, F. I., Darling, D. B., and Fisher, J. H.: The radiographic diagnosis of congenital hypertrophic pyloric stenosis. J. Pediatr. *71*:70, 1967.

Intestinal Obstruction

Estrada, R. L.: Anomalies of Intestinal Rotation and Fixation. Springfield, Ill., Charles C Thomas, 1958.

Fonkalsoud, E. W., de Lorimer, A. A., and Hays, D. M.: Congenital atresia and stenosis of the duodenum. Pediatrics *43*:79, 1969.

Hope, J. W., and O'Hara, A. E.: Use of air as a contrast medium in the diagnosis of intestinal obstruction of the newborn. Radiology *70*:349, 1958.

Nixon, H. H.: Intestinal obstruction in the newborn. Arch. Dis. Child. *30*:13, 1955.

Nixon, H. H., and Tawes, R.: Etiology and treatment of small intestinal atresia: Analysis of a series of 127 jejunoileal atresias and comparison with 62 duodenal atresias. Surgery *69*:41, 1971.

Singleton, E. B.: X-ray Diagnosis of the Alimentary Tract in Infants and Children. Chicago, Year Book Medical Publishers, Inc., 1959.

Swenson, O.: Pediatric Surgery. New York, Appleton-Century-Crofts, Inc., 1969.

Wasch, M. G., and Marck, A.: The radiographic appearance of the gastrointestinal tract during the first day of life. J. Pediatr. *32*: 479, 1948.

Intussusception

Bjarnason, G., and Pettersson, G.: The treatment of intussusception: Thirty years' experience at Gothenburg's Children's Hospital. J. Pediatr. Surg. *3*:19, 1968.

Gross, R. E., and Ware, P. F.: Intussusception in childhood: Experiences from 610 cases. New Engl. J. Med. *239*:645, 1948.

Ravitch, M. M.: Intussusception in Infants and Children. Springfield, Ill., Charles C Thomas, 1959.

Aganglionic Megacolon

Bodian, M., Carter, C. O., and Ward, B. C. H.: Hirschsprung's disease. Lancet *1*:302, 1951.

Campbell, P. E., and Noblett, H. R.: Experience with rectal suction biopsy in the diagnosis of Hirschsprung's disease. J. Pediatr. Surg. *4*:410, 1969.

Ehrenpreis, T.: Hirschsprung's Disease. Chicago, Year Book Medical Publishers, Inc., 1970.

Hope, J. W., Borns, P. F., and Berg, P. K.: Roentgenologic manifestations of Hirschsprung's disease in infancy. Am. J. Roentgenol. *95*:217, 1965.

Madsen, C. M.: Hirschsprung's Disease. Springfield, Ill., Charles C Thomas, 1964.

Tobon, F., Nigel, C. R. W., Talbert, J. L., and Schuster, M. D.: Nonsurgical test for the diagnosis of Hirschsprung's disease. New Engl. J. Med. *278*:188, 1968.

Peptic Ulcer

Abramson, D. J.: Curling's ulcer in childhood: Review of the literature and report of 5 cases. Surgery *55* 321, 1964.

Chenoweth, A. D., and Dimick, A. R.: Stress ulcers in infants and children. Ann. Surg. *161*:977, 1965.

Judd, D. R., Heimburger, I. L., Vellios, F., and Waldhausen, J. A.: Zollinger-Ellison syndrome in adolescents. Surgery *54*: 673, 1963.

Michener, W. M., Kennedy, R. L. J., and DuShane, J. W.: Duodenal ulcer in childhood. Am. J. Dis. Child. *100*:814, 1960.

Roselund, M. L., Crean, G. P., Johnson, D. G., Holzapple, P. G., and Brooks, F. P.: The Zollinger-Ellison syndrome in a 10-year old boy. J. Pediatr. *75*:443, 1969.

Schuster, S. R., and Gross, R. E.: Peptic ulcer in childhood. Am. J. Surg. *105*:324, 1963.

Singleton, E. B., and Faykus, M. H.: Incidence of peptic ulcer as determined by radiologic examinations in the pediatric age group. J. Pediatr. *65*:858, 1964.

Walker, E. E., and Grove, W. J.: Gastroduodenal ulcers in children with brain disease. Arch. Surg. *89*:559, 1964.

Gastric Perforation

Inouye, W. Y., and Evans, G.: Neonatal gastric perforation. Arch. Surg. *88*:741, 1964.

Pertsemlidis, D.: Neonatal gastric perforation. J. Mt. Sinai Hosp. *31*:97, 1964.

Transmural Enterocolitis

Kyle, J.: Crohn's disease. London, William Heinemann, Ltd., 1972.

Lindner, A. E., Marshak, R. H., Wolf, B. S., and Janowitz, H. D.: Granulomatous colitis. New Engl. J. Med. *269*:379, 1963.

Marshak, R. H., and Lindner, A. E.: Ulcerative and granulomatous colitis. J. Mt. Sinai Hosp. *33*:444, 1966.

McCaffrey, T. D., Khosrow, N., Lawrence, A. M., and Kirsner, J. B.: Severe growth retardation in children with inflammatory bowel disease. Pediatrics *45*:386, 1970.

Rudhe, U., and Keats, T. E.: Granulomatous colitis in children. Radiology *84*:24, 1965.

Necrotizing Enterocolitis

Mizrahi, A., Barlow, O., Berdon, W., Blanc, W. A., and Silverman, W. A.: Necrotizing enterocolitis in premature infants. J. Pediatr. *66*:697, 1965.

Stevenson, J. K., Oliver, T. K., Jr., Graham, C. B., Bell, R. S., and Gould, V. E.: Aggressive treatment of neonatal necrotizing enterocolitis: 38 patients with 25 survivors. J. Pediatr. Surg. *6*: 28, 1971.

Touloukian, R. J., Berdon, W. E., Amoury, R. A., and Santulli, T. V.: Surgical experience with necrotizing enterocolitis in the infant. J. Pediatr. Surg. *2*:389, 1967.

Ulcerative Colitis

Broberger, O., and Lagerkrantz, R.: Ulcerative colitis in childhood and adolescence. Adv. Pediatr. *14*:9, 1966.

Davidson, M., Bloom, A. A., and Kugler, M. M.: Chronic ulcerative colitis of childhood; An exhaustive review. J. Pediatr. *67*: 471, 1965.

Kirsner, J. B., Raskin, H. F., and Palmer, W. L.: Ulcerative colitis in children. A.M.A. J. Dis. Child. *90*:141, 1955.

Michener, W. M., Brown, C. H., and Turnbull, R. B. J.: Ulcerative colitis in children. I. Diagnosis. II. Medical and surgical treatment. Am. J. Dis. Child. *108*:230; 236, 1964.

Pneumatosis Cystoides Intestinalis

Coello-Ramirez, P., Guitierres-Topete, G., and Lifshitz, F.: Pneumatosis intestinalis. Am. J. Dis. Child. *120*:3, 1970.

Stone, H. H., Webb, H. W., and Kowalchik, M. T.: Pneumatosis intestinalis of infancy. Surg. Gynec. Obstet. *130*:806, 1970.

Intestinal Malabsorption

EVALUATION OF INFANT OR CHILD FOR MALABSORPTION

A carefully taken history and physical examination are basic to the correct diagnosis of malabsorption syndromes. The necessary data base should include: (1) a precise feeding history; (2) a plot of growth data on growth grids; (3) the type and time of onset of symptoms; and (4) the character of stools excreted.

A careful feeding history is necessary because certain diseases are related to the introduction of specific nutrients into the diet. The content of the foods physicians prescribe for their patients may give clues to the cause of malabsorption. The physician's knowledge of the content will enable him to plan rational therapy when dietary management is indicated.

Growth data indicate whether the infant or child is thriving, and may tell when a disease began to affect growth. Normal growth does not exclude malabsorption, but malabsorption is unlikely if normal growth is supported by normal caloric intake and stools.

Malabsorption syndromes occur with different frequencies during various periods of infancy and

TABLE 11–7 MALABSORPTION SYNDROMES WHICH MAY PRESENT AT DIFFERENT AGES

I. Neonatal Period
  A. Congenital lactase deficiency
  B. Secondary disaccharidase malabsorption
  C. Congenital glucose-galactose malabsorption
  D. Secondary monosaccharide malabsorption
  E. Cystic fibrosis
  F. Cow's milk protein intolerance
  G. Soy protein intolerance
  H. Short bowel syndrome
  I. Congenital chloridorrhea
  J. Primary hypomagnesemia
  K. Enterokinase deficiency
  L. Primary immune defects: Wiskott-Aldrich syndrome
  M. Transcobalamin II deficiency (vitamin B_{12} malabsorption)
  N. Acrodermatitis enteropathica
II. One Month to Two Years
  A. Sucrase-isomaltase deficiency
  B. Secondary disaccharidase deficiency
  C. Secondary monosaccharide malabsorption
  D. Cystic fibrosis
  E. Pancreatic insufficiency with bone marrow failure
  F. Celiac sprue
  G. Cow's milk protein sensitivity
  H. Soy protein sensitivity
  I. Intestinal lymphangiectasia
  J. Parasites
  K. Abetalipoproteinemia
  L. Enterokinase deficiency
  M. Biliary obstruction: neonatal hepatitis; biliary atresia; choledochal cyst
  N. Primary immune defects: Wiskott-Aldrich syndrome; thymic aplasia with agammaglobulinemia
  O. Whipple's disease
  P. Amino acid malabsorption
  Q. Wolman's disease
  R. Vitamin B_{12} malabsorption syndromes: juvenile pernicious anemia; Immerslund-Gräsbeck syndrome
  S. Congenital malabsorption of folic acid
  T. Stasis syndrome
  U. Acrodermatitis enteropathica
III. Two Years to Puberty
  A. Secondary disaccharidase deficiency
  B. Celiac sprue
  C. Tropical sprue
  D. Parasites
  E. Stasis syndrome
  F. Primary immune defects
  G. Biologically inert intrinsic factor

childhood. Some have their onset only during the early neonatal period (Table 11–7). These differences are important in choosing diagnostic tests.

The fecal consistency in malabsorption may be normal or watery or contain excessive fat. Knowledge of consistency may help to determine the most likely type of nutrient or mineral malabsorbed, and may aid in precise diagnosis. When there are both steatorrhea and excessive water loss, it is impossible to tell from the history if steatorrhea is present. Table 11–8 lists the types of malabsorption syndromes that characteristically have watery stools, steatorrhea or normal stools. In some of these, both normal and abnormal stools have been described. In the pages that follow are listed and discussed the tests used to diagnose malabsorption syndromes.

EVALUATION OF ABSORPTION OF CARBOHYDRATES

Dietary carbohydrates are almost entirely in the form of starch and the disaccharides, sucrose and lactose. In early infancy carbohydrate may be almost entirely lactose. Within the stomach little digestion of starch and disaccharides occurs despite the presence of salivary amylase. Pancreatic alpha-amylase hydrolyzes starch to maltose, a disaccharide, and maltotriose, a trisaccharide. This

TABLE 11–8 TYPES OF STOOLS IN MALABSORPTION SYNDROMES

I. Watery Stools
  A. Congenital, developmental and secondary lactase deficiency
  B. Sucrase-isomaltase deficiency
  C. Glucose-galactose malabsorption
  D. Primary immune defects
  E. Congenital chloridorrhea
  F. Enterokinase deficiency
  G. Cow's milk protein sensitivity
  H. Soy milk protein sensitivity
  I. Parasites
    1. *Giardia lamblia*
    2. *Strongyloides stercoralis*
    3. *Capillaria philippinensis*
    4. Coccidia
  J. Vitamin B_{12} malabsorption
  K. Transcobalamin II deficiency
II. Fatty Stools
  A. Cystic fibrosis
  B. Pancreatic insufficiency and bone marrow failure
  C. Celiac sprue
  D. Short bowel syndrome
  E. Abetalipoproteinemia
  F. Intestinal lymphangiectasia
  G. Whipple's disease
  H. Wolman's disease
  I. Tropical sprue
  J. Stasis syndrome
  K. Biliary tract obstruction
  L. Acrodermatitis enteropathica
III. Normal Stools
  A. Primary hypomagnesemia
  B. Amino acid malabsorption
  C. Vitamin B_{12} malabsorption
    1. Juvenile pernicious anemia
    2. Immerslund-Gräsbeck syndrome
    3. Adult-type pernicious anemia
    4. Biologically inert intrinsic factor
  D. Congenital malabsorption of folic acid

enzyme is an endo-enzyme and splits the interior 1–4 glucose-glucose linkages of the starch molecule but does not hydrolyze the outermost links of the polymer. Inasmuch as starches have 1–6 branching points along the 1–4 glucose-linked straight chain, branched saccharides of varying molecular size are also formed. Four disaccharidases (maltase, isomaltase, sucrase and lactase) hydrolyze the oligosaccharides and disaccharides; these enzymes are located within the microvillous membrane of the brush border of the intestinal absorptive cell throughout the entire length of the small bowel; their concentration is greatest in the jejunum. The quantity of lactase in each absorptive cell is the lowest among the intestinal disaccharidases; this is the limiting factor in lactose digestion. Other disaccharides and oligosaccharides are rapidly hydrolyzed; the rate-limiting step in their absorption is the monosaccharide transport system. Trace amounts of disaccharides may diffuse past the intestinal mucosal barrier and be excreted in the urine since there are no disaccharidases in other body organs. Glucose and galactose are both transported across the absorptive cells by an active sodium-dependent transport process. Fructose, which is released by hydrolysis of sucrose, is the only other important dietary monosaccharide; it is transported by a separate mechanism, and may be actively transported.

STOOL pH AND REDUCING SUBSTANCES

Patients with diarrhea who are suspected of carbohydrate malabsorption should have stools tested for both pH and reducing substances. Stool pH determinations measured by using pH paper (range 4.5 to 7.5) accurately indicate if significant amounts of organic acids are being produced from unabsorbed carbohydrates. Tests with Clinitest for reducing substances indicate if unabsorbed carbohydrate is present. Several factors must be considered in interpreting stool pH and reducing substance determinations: (1) the patient's age; (2) whether breast or formula feeding is being used; (3) the type of formula and its carbohydrate content; (4) whether antibiotics are being taken which can alter the intestinal flora and affect acid production; (5) the possibility of false positive reactions for reducing substances with Clinitest due to drugs; and (6) contamination of stools with urine.

Stool pH in the neonatal period ranges from 5.5 to 7.4. Neonates who are breast fed usually have a stool pH which is less than 6 and stools that contain more than 0.25 per cent reducing substances. Those neonates who are fed cow's milk formulas which contain 4.8 per cent lactose rarely have 0.25 per cent reducing substance in their stool and usually have stool pH of greater than 6. After the neonatal period stool pH is greater than 6.3 and only trace amounts of reducing substance are normally present. Stools are considered abnormal if pH is less than 6 and they contain greater than 0.25 per cent reducing substances. Tolerance tests for the specific disaccharide or monosaccharide should be done to define the type of carbohydrate malabsorbed, if screening tests are abnormal or equivocal.

Reducing substances may be tested for by the Clinitest method:

1. To 1 volume of stool in a test tube is added 2 volumes of water.
2. The mixture is shaken and 15 drops are transferred to a second test tube. (The mixture may be spun in a centrifuge after shaking, to remove excess sediment.)
3. A Clinitest tablet is added to the second tube.
4. The color determination for reducing substances is made when the chemical reaction stops.

DISACCHARIDE AND MONOSACCHARIDE TOLERANCE TESTS

Optimally the patient should be free of diarrhea for 24 hours before any of the tolerance tests are done, and the stool should have a pH greater than 6 and be free of reducing substances. In this way it can be determined if the stool changes its characteristics following challenge. Patients should be fasting for 6 hours before any of the tolerance tests. Accurate tolerance tests in infants may require gavage of the sugar solution through a gastric feeding tube. The dose of lactose or sucrose used for tolerance tests is 2 gm/kg up to a maximum of 100 gm. Lactose is given as a 10 per cent solution, sucrose as a 20 per cent solution.

Capillary blood specimens for glucose are taken fasting, at 30 minutes, and at one hour. The peak rise in blood glucose normally occurs between 30 and 60 minutes after feeding the solution. Stools should be tested for pH and reducing substances during the 24 hours following the test.

Lactose intolerance may be diagnosed if the capillary blood glucose level does not rise more than 20 mg/dl and if the patient develops diarrhea with greater than 0.25 per cent reducing substances in the stool and a decrease in stool pH to less than 6.

Sucrose intolerance may be diagnosed if the rise in blood glucose is less than 40 mg/dl and if the patient develops diarrhea. Stool pH may decrease to 6 or less, but significant amounts of reducing substances may not be found because sucrose is not a reducing sugar. If sufficient hydrolysis of sucrose by colonic bacteria occurs, however, significant amounts of reducing substances (>0.25 per cent) will be detected.

The *glucose-galactose tolerance* test is done in a manner similar to the lactose tolerance test, except that glucose, 1 gm/kg, and galactose, 1 gm/kg, are substituted for lactose. A normal response is a rise of 40 mg/dl or more in blood glucose.

The *fructose tolerance* test is done in a manner similar to the glucose-galactose tolerance test. The dose of fructose is 2 gm/kg, and a normal response is a rise of 40 mg/dl or more in blood glucose.

EVALUATION OF FAT ABSORPTION

Most dietary fat consists of long-chain triglycerides (fatty acid side-chain 16 to 18 carbon atoms) insoluble in water. They cannot be absorbed directly, but must first be hydrolyzed by pancreatic lipase to more polar monoglycerides and free fatty acids. In addition to lipase, the pancreas produces sodium bicarbonate to neutralize gastric hydrochloric acid and provide optimal pH near neutrality for the enzymatic hydrolysis. The efficiency of lipolysis is increased by bile salts, which aid in the dispersion of triglycerides in luminal water through their ability to lower surface tension.

Unsaturated free fatty acids have some solubility in water and can be absorbed readily without bile salts. Monoglycerides, cholesterol and fat-soluble vitamins are virtually insoluble in water, but in the presence of bile salts they can be solubilized as macromolecular aggregates called micelles. The solubilized lipids then passively diffuse into the intestinal absorptive cells. In the upper small intestine bile salts are not absorbed appreciably and are therefore available to shuttle more lipids to the absorptive cell surface. The long-chain fatty acids are resynthesized within the cell to triglycerides and, in the presence of cholesterol and lipoprotein, form chylomicrons which are transported via the lymphatics. Medium-chain triglycerides are lipids whose constituent fatty acids contain 6 to 8 carbon atoms. Some are absorbed directly without hydrolysis by pancreatic lipase. The medium-chain fatty acids released by hydrolysis are water soluble and do not need bile salts for solubilization. In the absorptive cell, medium-chain fatty acids are not re-esterified to triglycerides, but instead appear as free fatty acids unchanged in the portal venous blood.

In newborn infants fecal lipids include glycerides, which reflect a defect in lipolysis. Monoglycerides are also present and may indicate that micellization and/or mucosal transport of lipids may be insufficient for optimal lipid absorption.

MICROSCOPIC EXAMINATION OF THE STOOL FOR STEATORRHEA, USING SUDAN III OR IV DYE

The microscopic examination of random stools for the presence of steatorrhea is not a worthwhile screening test in infants and is of limited value in older children. Since infants normally excrete a greater percentage of their fat intake than older children and adults, examination of their stools usually shows an excessive number of large fat globules. Beyond infancy, if excessive fat is recognized microscopically, other studies should be done to confirm the presence of steatorrhea; examination of a stool suspension is not enough to exclude steatorrhea.

SERUM CAROTENE LEVELS

Vitamin A occurs only in animal tissues. Plants are devoid of vitamin A, but contain a group of substances called carotene, which act as a precursor of vitamin A in mammals. Carotene is neither manufactured nor stored long in the body. Consequently, a low level of serum carotene indicates that the patient either has not been eating carotene-containing foods or has not absorbed available carotene. The carotene level does not distinguish between pancreatic and mucosal origins of steatorrhea, but it is the simplest and best test to exclude steatorrhea. Serum carotene values less than 50 μg/dl indicate steatorrhea; values between 50 and 100 μg/dl may be found in normal individuals and some patients with mild steatorrhea; values greater than 100 μg/dl almost always indicate normal fat absorption. The test is 75 per cent accurate in predicting steatorrhea.

FAT BALANCE

The most reliable index of steatorrhea is a quantitative chemical determination of fat in complete collections of the feces over periods of 3 to 6 days. In clinical practice measurement of fecal fat may be used to detect steatorrhea in those individuals who have equivocal screening tests. The examination is unnecessary in those patients whose clinical histories, physical examinations and screening tests indicate steatorrhea. The purpose of the procedure is to measure the percentage of dietary fat absorbed. This percentage, called the coefficient of absorption (CA), is calculated from the formula:

$$CA = \frac{(\text{gm of fat ingested} - \text{gm of fat excreted}) \times 100}{\text{gm of ingested fat}}$$

It is difficult to prescribe a specific fat intake for infants because they spontaneously limit their intake by stopping feeding when full. In infants, therefore, it is best to keep an accurate record of the volume of formula or milk taken and the amounts of other foods eaten. After infancy it is easier to prescribe a specific fat intake appropriate for age and weight, since most children can be persuaded to complete their meals if they do not finish them spontaneously. It is easy to determine the number of grams of fat which should be included in the diet. Approximately 40 to 50 per cent of caloric intake is in the form of fat. First, determine the patient's caloric needs; then, determine the number of calories provided by fat; finally, divide by 9 to determine the number of grams of fat to be prescribed for the diet. Following an initial two-day period of dietary equilibration, feces are collected for three days. Individuals who do not excrete feces daily and who have equivocal evidence of malabsorption should have stool collections for six days. Many adults and children can be induced to have a daily bowel movement by the administration of a small amount of milk of magnesia each evening. The stools must be kept refrigerated to prevent bacterial utilization of fat. If the patient is hospitalized for the study of fat balance, it is wise not to do any interim studies which might alter the patient's appetite or pattern of defecation. This study can be done at home successfully with proper instruction. In this circumstance the child defecates into a paint can lined with plastic, which is easily sealed between periods of defecation. Contents of diapers may be emptied into the can. Diapers should be carefully scraped to remove as much stool as possible.

Normal excretion of fat by infants fed human milk or formulas with fat supplied as vegetable oils is less than 1 gm/kg/day. Excretion of fat by infants fed homogenized cow's milk is 2 gm/kg/day. From 180 days to 1 year, the coefficient of absorption is greater than 87 per cent; from 1 year to 2 years, 93 per cent; and from 2 years to adulthood, >95 per cent.

EVALUATION OF PROTEIN ABSORPTION

Pancreatic proteolytic enzymes hydrolyze proteins to amino acids, but the rate of hydrolysis of pancreatic origin is too slow to account for the rate of digestion in vivo. When pancreatic enzymes have reduced the proteins partially to oligopeptides, then peptidases in the brush borders of absorptive epithelial cells complete the hydrolysis to amino acids. Leucyl beta-naphthylamide hydrolase (amino-peptidase) is the only peptidase primarily associated with the microvilli of intestinal absorptive cells. Within the absorptive cells are cytoplasmic peptidases; it is not known whether they are under the same control as amino-peptidases. In patients with severe pancreatic insufficiency, up to 80 per cent of dietary protein can be absorbed. In patients with intact pancreatic function who have decreased epithelial cell peptide hydrolase activity due to damage to absorptive cells, the absorption of protein is delayed to a greater degree than is the absorption of free amino acids. The amino acids are transported across the epithelial cells of the intestine by three mechanisms: simple diffusion, facilitated diffusion and active transport. Since protein malabsorption usually correlates with steatorrhea, the finding of normal fecal fat excretion will exclude most instances of protein maldigestion.

TEST FOR PROTEIN-LOSING ENTEROPATHY

Exudation of protein from the blood into the intestinal lumen can be detected with reasonable convenience and reliability by means of intravenous injection of a suitable radio-labeled substance and determination of radioactivity of the stools. Suitable substances are ^{125}PVP, ^{131}I-albumin and ^{51}chromic chloride; the intravenous injection of ^{51}chromic chloride is the current method of choice. The test requires10 daily blood samples and collection of all stools for 8 of the 10 days. The procedure is difficult in infants and children because it requires keeping urine separate from stool. The disappearance curve of the isotope from the blood may be used alone as an indication of exudative enteropathy, but it will not give quantitative data showing the amount of plasma lost. Normal values for protein exudation in infants are not available. Adults excrete approximately 50 ml of plasma per day in feces.

TESTS OF PANCREATIC FUNCTION

Tests of pancreatic function are not useful in diagnosing early pancreatic disease because the pancreas is an organ with great reserve. Disordered function becomes apparent only when there is advanced involvement. Cystic fibrosis is the commonest cause of chronic malabsorption and pancreatic insufficiency in children, and a sweat chloride determination will establish that diagnosis; tests of pancreatic function are unnecessary. If a patient with steatorrhea does not have cystic fibrosis and mucosal disease is excluded, the possibility of pancreatogenous steatorrhea must be explored.

Pancreatic function tests such as the secretin test require skill at duodenal intubation and are time-consuming and expensive. The secretin test involves administering the hormone in a standard manner while pancreatic secretion is collected through a tube in the duodenum before and after administration of the hormone. The volume of fluid secreted and its pH, bicarbonate concentration, chloride concentration and levels of pancreatic enzyme activity are determined. An indirect diagnosis of pancreatic insufficiency may be made by adding pancreatic enzyme supplements to the diet and weighing the patient weekly for a month. If significant weight gain occurs, the supplement should be discontinued for a month and the patient reweighed at the end of that time to demonstrate lack of weight gain without replacement therapy.

Screening tests for pancreatic insufficiency such as determinations of stool trypsin and chymotrypsin activities have not been adequately compared with the secretin test. Chymotrypsin assay in the stool is a better screening test for pancreatic proteolytic enzyme insufficiency than trypsin assay because chymotrypsin is more stable than trypsin in intestinal fluid. Determination of stool chymotrypsin activity is a useful screening test for pancreatic proteolytic enzyme insufficiency, but it gives a false positive test in patients with enterokinase deficiency. Normal values for chymotrypsin in stool: birth to adulthood, 75 to 839 μg/gm of stool.

TESTS TO LOCATE ABNORMALITIES

D-XYLOSE EXCRETION TESTS

Examination of the excretion of D-xylose has been used to differentiate jejunal from ileal and mucosal from luminal abnormalities as causes of steatorrhea. Xylose is a 5-carbon sugar which is not normally found in the body. It is absorbed by facilitated diffusion in the upper small bowel. Approximately 60 per cent of the xylose absorbed is metabolized; the remainder is excreted in the urine. The absorption of xylose depends upon a structurally intact small bowel. It will be decreased in any condition that alters the absorptive area or the absorptive capacity of the small intestine. If gastric emptying is delayed, if the volume of the extravascular volume compartment is expanded (from liver, kidney or heart failure), if effective blood volume is decreased, or if renal excretion is impaired, then the urinary excretion may be low without implicating malabsorption. The results may be normal with a mucosal lesion that is not extensive. Bacterial overgrowth proximal to the absorptive site may consume enough sugar to produce falsely low values. In infants and in young children who cannot void on command, the test is of little value because urine collections are usually incomplete. The range of normal values cited for infants and toddlers makes it difficult to separate normal individuals from those with mucosal disease. In older children the D-xylose excretion test may be used to distinguish between mucosal and luminal causes of steatorrhea, but it is not diagnostic for any specific mucosal disease. Biopsy of the small intestine should be done in patients with mucosal disease or if such disease is suspected.

SERUM FOLATE LEVEL

A fasting serum folate level is a useful screening test to determine whether steatorrhea is of luminal or mucosal origin. Folic acid is a water-soluble vitamin which is absorbed in the proximal small bowel, in part by simple diffusion and possibly also by an active transport mechanism. Any disease which damages absorptive cells and decreases the absorptive surface area will affect the absorption of folic acid. In patients with limited areas of mucosal damage or mild degrees of injury, the serum folate level may be normal. Studies comparing fasting serum folate levels with D-xylose excretion tests and with fat balances have not been done. The normal fasting serum folate level is greater than 5 ng/ml.

SCHILLING TEST
(Vitamin B_{12} Absorption Test)

The Schilling or vitamin B_{12} absorption test determines if ileal absorptive function is normal. When the test dose of radioactive vitamin B_{12} is given orally after mixture with intrinsic factor, any possible inability of the stomach to make intrinsic factor is bypassed as a possible cause of impaired vitamin B_{12} absorption; under these circumstances the finding of impaired absorption leaves an ileal defect as the most likely cause. Two hours after the labeled oral dose is administered 1000 μg of nonradioactive vitamin B_{12} is given parenterally. This large amount of nonradioactive vitamin B_{12} spills into the urine over the next 24 hours, carrying with it a proportion of the radioactive mixture. In patients with defective renal function, bacterial overgrowth in the proximal small intestine, contracted vascular spaces or expanded extravascular spaces, falsely low urinary excretions may be found. Contamination of urine with feces containing unabsorbed radioactive vitamin B_{12} can give falsely elevated values.

With normal absorption, more than 7 per cent of the labeled vitamin B_{12} will appear in the urine within 24 hours; less than 2 per cent indicates severe malabsorption; 2 to 7 per cent, mild to moderate malabsorption.

ROENTGENOGRAPHIC STUDIES IN MALABSORPTION

Roentgenographic studies of the upper gastrointestinal tract which include the esophagus, stomach, duodenum and jejunum may give clues for diagnosis of malabsorption syndromes. Patients with congenital or surgically created defects of the small intestine may have specific radiographic findings. Examples of such defects are intestinal lymphangiectasia, diverticula, blind loops, webs and strictures. Diseases in which the mucosa of the small intestine is damaged are the most likely to show nonspecific abnormalities. During infancy and childhood, the disease most likely to show these nonspecific findings is celiac sprue (gluten-sensitive enteropathy). The abnormalities most frequently seen include prolonged transit time and jejunal dilatation. Patients with cystic fibrosis do not show abnormalities in upper gastrointestinal studies.

PERORAL BIOPSY OF THE MUCOSA OF THE INTESTINE

The most definitive method of diagnosing mucosal disease is by peroral biopsy of the small intestine. Several instruments are available, including the infant multipurpose biopsy tube and the pediatric Crosby capsule. Perforation and hemorrhage are the two possible complications of intestinal biopsy. Since the special models of the biopsy tube and capsule have been available, these complications have rarely been reported.

The most common indication for biopsy of the small intestine in infants and children is to establish the diagnosis of celiac sprue. This diagnosis cannot be made in any other way. The changes seen in the mucosa of patients with celiac sprue are characteristic, but they are not specific. The flat mucosa of celiac sprue is also seen in kwashiorkor, tropical sprue, unclassified sprue and soy protein intolerance. There are other diseases in which the mucosa may be flat, but other changes are present which are unique to the illness. The illnesses in which such specific flat lesions occur include hypogammaglobulinemic sprue, Whipple's disease, Zollinger-Ellison syndrome, eosinophilic gastroenteritis and primary intestinal lymphoma.

The diagnosis of intestinal lymphangiectasia is established by biopsy of the small intestine, because lymphangiograms are difficult to perform in an infant. Abetalipoproteinemia may be diagnosed by characteristic morphologic changes. The congenital disaccharidase deficiencies may be confirmed by the finding of normal small intestinal morphology and the determination of disaccharidase activities.

Four parasitic diseases which can cause diarrhea and malabsorption syndromes may be diagnosed by small intestinal biopsy; they are: giardiasis, strongyloidiasis, capillariasis and coccidiosis.

MALABSORPTION SYNDROMES

CONGENITAL, DEVELOPMENTAL AND SECONDARY LACTASE DEFICIENCY

CLINICAL MANIFESTATIONS. Congenital lactase deficiency is an exceedingly rare inborn error of metabolism. Its mode of inheritance has not been established. Some investigators question its existence, because long-term follow-up studies of some of the reported children have shown they developed normal lactase levels within months to a year or so after the deficiency was first diagnosed.

Watery diarrhea, abdominal distention, dehydration and vomiting are the characteristic symptoms of lactase deficiency; they develop within hours after feeding of human or cow's milk. The commonest type of lactase deficiency is that which develops in adolescents or young adults, who in early childhood have had no indications of lactose intolerance; as they grow older, they learn to avoid gastrointestinal symptoms by not drinking milk. Blacks and Orientals have high incidences of lactase deficiency as adults, though as infants they have no greater incidence of lactose intolerance than Caucasian infants. Lactase deficiency is also present in certain diseases, such as cystic fibrosis, at a greater than normal incidence.

Secondary lactase deficiency is common and may develop after any disease that damages the small intestinal epithelium. During infancy, gastroenteritis is the commonest cause of secondary lactase deficiency and lactose intolerance. Steatorrhea and azotorrhea may accompany lactose malabsorption in secondary lactase deficiency. Stools in these patients may not be characteristically watery. The duration of lactose intolerance in patients with secondary lactase deficiency may vary from a few days to several weeks and relates to the nutritional status of the patients; the worse the nutritional status, the more likely intolerance will be prolonged. When lactose intolerance persists for more than three weeks, intolerance usually exists to all other disaccharides, and possibly monosaccharides. After clinical recovery from the primary gastrointestinal illness, lactase is the last disaccharidase to return to normal. In older infants, children and adults, the symptoms are similar to those in congenital lactase deficiency, but these patients may also complain of bloating, crampy abdominal pain, nausea and borborygmi.

PATHOGENESIS OF DIARRHEA. Lactase deficiency has received more attention than any of the other disaccharidase deficiencies and can be considered as a prototype of carbohydrate malabsorption. In this condition dietary lactose is incompletely hydrolyzed and poorly absorbed. Presumably owing to osmotic effects generated by nonabsorbable disaccharide, fluid moves into the lumen of the gut, distending the small bowel, and intestinal transit time is reduced. In the colon disaccharide disappears from the luminal contents and the pH of the contents falls. The abnormal pH in the colon probably impairs water absorption. Bacterial hydrolysis of disaccharides to monosaccharides and subsequent hydrolysis of monosaccharides into even smaller molecules, such as organic acids of 2- to 4-carbon chains, may provide osmotically active compounds that retain water in the colon. Anions of short-chain organic acids are absorbed poorly by the colon and may act as osmotic cathartics.

DIAGNOSIS. Testing the stool for pH and reducing substances is an excellent way to screen for significant lactose malabsorption. If stool pH is 6 or less and reducing substances measure greater than 1+ with Clinitest, significant carbohydrate malabsorption is occurring. Diagnosis of lactose intolerance is established by performing lactose tolerance tests, using venous or capillary blood. The deficiency may be confirmed by disaccharidase determinations in tissue obtained by biopsy of the small intestine.

TREATMENT. If significant lactose malabsorption occurs, eliminating all sources of lactose from the diet will ameliorate symptoms. Labels of prepared foods should be read carefully, because many contain lactose.

SUCRASE-ISOMALTASE DEFICIENCY

Sucrase-isomaltase deficiency is the commonest congenital disaccharidase deficiency. This inborn error of metabolism is inherited as an autosomal recessive characteristic. Thus far, only the Eskimos have been shown to have an increased incidence of this combined enzymatic deficiency. The biochemical explanation for the combined defect rests on the fact that these two enzymatic activities appear to be located at independent sites on the same protein molecule.

CLINICAL MANIFESTATIONS AND COMPLICATIONS. Watery diarrhea is the presenting symptom in all cases and its pathogenesis is the same as in lactase deficiency. Abdominal distention and crampy abdominal pain are other frequent manifestations of the illness. Growth failure and dehydration are characteristic of those infants with sucrase-isomaltase deficiency who are fed sucrose-containing formulas beginning in the first weeks of life. Infants who are breast fed or given cow's milk formulas that do not contain sucrose or Dextrimaltose supplementation will not develop symptoms until juices or puréed fruits and vegetables are added to the diet. If sucrose and isomaltose are not introduced into the diet for several months, infants may grow and gain weight normally. Most cases go undiagnosed for long periods of time because physicians and parents fail to recognize the association between symptoms and eating of sucrose-containing foods or formulas. Physicians must know the carbohydrate content of the formulas they prescribe if they are going to recognize this condition. Many therapeutic formulas contain sucrose as the primary or secondary carbohydrate; these include all soy formulas, Nutramigen, Portagen, Probana, Bremil and MBF (meat base formula).

DIAGNOSIS. Diagnosis is established with a flat sucrose tolerance test and the development of acid diarrheal stools within 4 hours after the test dose of sucrose. Reducing substances may not be present in the stool. Disaccharidase determinations in small intestinal biopsies confirm the diagnosis. There is virtual absence of both sucrase and isomaltase activities.

TREATMENT AND PROGNOSIS. Treatment consists of providing a diet containing food with less than 2 per cent sucrose. Starches are usually not limited because their isomaltose content is low. Dextrose is substituted for sucrose in cooking and baking. Amelioration of symptoms occurs within 24 hours of beginning the diet. Most patients with this condition do not develop increasing tolerance for sucrose as they grow older.

SECONDARY SUCRASE-ISOMALTASE DEFICIENCY

This condition may develop in any intestinal disease in which the absorptive cells of the small intestine are severely damaged. It is almost always associated with lactase deficiency.

CONGENITAL GLUCOSE-GALACTOSE MALABSORPTION

Congenital glucose-galactose malabsorption is the rarest of the carbohydrate malabsorption syndromes and is inherited as an autosomal recessive trait. Because the transport of sodium ion is normal, the defect in this condition is believed to be at the step of entry of glucose and galactose into intestinal absorptive cells. The transport defect is not limited to the intestinal absorptive cells but is found also in the renal tubular epithelium, for nearly all these patients have renal glycosuria.

CLINICAL MANIFESTATIONS. The symptoms consist of watery diarrhea, which develops after the first glucose, breast milk or formula feeding. All prepared formulas will cause these symptoms. If the condition is unrecognized, dehydration and metabolic acidosis develop.

DIAGNOSIS. Stools in these patients contain significant amounts of reducing substances and usually have acid pH. Diagnosis is established by flat lactose and glucose-galactose tolerance tests, associated with diarrhea and a normal fructose tolerance test. It is confirmed by normal levels of disaccharidases in small intestinal biopsies, in association with normal morphology.

TREATMENT. Dietary management of these infants is difficult because of the severe carbohydrate restriction. A specially prepared formula base (Cho-free) to which fructose is added stops the diarrhea. As these patients grow older, they may tolerate limited amounts of sucrose. Long-term follow-up studies on these patients have not been reported.

SECONDARY GLUCOSE-GALACTOSE MALABSORPTION

Patients with this condition are intolerant of all monosaccharides and disaccharides. They have diarrhea with any type of feeding. This severe intolerance may develop secondary to infectious gastroenteritis or to intractable diarrhea of infancy caused by cow's milk protein sensitivity. Decreased and severely damaged numbers of absorptive cells are responsible for the condition.

DIAGNOSIS. All monosaccharide and disaccharide tolerance tests are flat and are accompanied by diarrhea. Stools may be acid and contain significant amounts of reducing substances.

TREATMENT AND PROGNOSIS. Intravenous fluids and electrolytes must be used to maintain these patients in positive fluid balance until the monosaccharide transport mechanism returns to normal. Severely malnourished infants may require parenteral hyperalimentation for two to three weeks before the monosaccharide transport mechanisms and disaccharidases return to normal. A carbohydrate-free formula base should not be fed, because hypoglycemia and seizures may develop.

PRIMARY IMMUNE DEFECTS

During infancy Wiskott-Aldrich syndrome and thymic dysplasia with agammaglobulinemia are the only primary immune defects with gastrointestinal symptoms as one of their major characteristics. Patients with Wiskott-Aldrich syndrome have thrombocytopenia, eczema, recurrent infections and diarrhea containing blood. The cause of diarrhea is unknown but may be an intolerance to specific dietary proteins. Patients with this syndrome who survive infancy have a gradual disappearance of gastrointestinal symptoms and are eventually able to eat a normal diet.

The cause of diarrhea in thymic dysplasia is unknown. Death usually occurs within the first year of life; malnutrition secondary to diarrhea and malabsorption is a contributing factor. Antibiotics, gluten-free and milk-free diets have not been successful in controlling the gastrointestinal symptoms.

After infancy, giardiasis is the commonest cause of chronic diarrhea in patients with primary immune defects. Giardia trophozoites can cause severe small intestinal damage that results in secondary disaccharidase deficiency, lactose intolerance, steatorrhea, vitamin B_{12} malabsorption and protein-losing enteropathy. Both the lesions and malabsorption are reversible if the parasite is eradicated. (See this Section, Giardiasis, below.)

Some patients with primary immune defects have severely damaged small intestinal mucosa and unexplained malabsorption. They do not respond either to gluten-free diets or to antibiotics. Intramuscular gamma globulin and fresh frozen plasma have been advocated as measures to control unexplained diarrhea in such patients. Neither form of treatment has been shown objectively to be useful.

Colonization of the proximal small bowel with colonic organisms occurs commonly in patients with primary immune defects, but their presence does not correlate with gastrointestinal symptoms or disease.

CONGENITAL CHLORIDORRHEA

Congenital chloridorrhea is a rare familial disease. In this condition chloride cannot be transported against electrochemical gradients in the ileum, nor probably in the colon; it can, however, be secreted, or absorbed down electrochemical gradients (diffusion). Affected individuals have normal sodium-hydrogen exchange but a chloride-bicarbonate exchange that is incapable of transporting chloride against an electrochemical gradient. Diarrhea occurs because the unabsorbed chloride in ileal and colonic luminal contents acts as an osmotic cathartic and causes a secondary loss of sodium and potassium in the diarrheal stools.

CLINICAL MANIFESTATIONS AND DIAGNOSIS. Affected infants are born before term and polyhydramnios is usually present as a prenatal sign of the disease. Symptoms begin in the first two weeks of life and consist of watery diarrhea, jaundice, abdominal distention and ileus. Diagnosis is established by the high chloride content of fecal fluid and hypoelectrolytemia. Metabolic alkalosis is not consistently found in the neonatal period but develops later in the course of the disease.

TREATMENT AND PROGNOSIS. Acid or alkaline salts of potassium are administered daily. With treatment, patients may live a normal life span.

ENTEROKINASE DEFICIENCY

Enterokinase is found in the microvilli of intestinal absorptive cells. It activates proteolytic enzymes secreted by the pancreas into the duodenum. Congenital deficiency of the enzyme is rare and is characterized by diarrhea, edema and hypoproteinemia. Diagnosis is established by pancreatic function tests which demonstrate normal levels of amylase and lipase but low proteolytic activity. The absence of enterokinase in duodenal juice and the appearance of normal proteolytic activity after incubation with exogenous enterokinase confirm the diagnosis. Pancreatic replacement treatment is used as therapy.

COW'S MILK PROTEIN SENSITIVITY AND INTRACTABLE DIARRHEA OF INFANCY

There are two clinically recognizable types of intestinal injury induced by cow's milk protein. The first type has its onset at any time from birth to 6 months of age.

CLINICAL MANIFESTATIONS. Affected infants have a spectrum of severity in symptoms and signs. The clinical picture may include several of the following: fever, vomiting, blood-tinged or watery diarrhea, steatorrhea, failure to gain weight or weight loss, anemia, eosinophilia, hypoproteinemia and anaphylaxis. Some infants develop an intractable diarrhea so severe that they are unable to absorb any nutrients; unless parenteral hyperalimentation is used, most of them die from complications of enterocolitis. The second type appears at any time from 6 months to 2 years of age and is typified by edema, diarrhea, intermittent vomiting, protein-losing enteropathy and eosinophilia.

PATHOGENESIS. Various cow's milk proteins have been shown to induce steatorrhea and lactose intolerance; betalactoglobulin is the protein most frequently injurious to the intestinal mucosa. The mechanism of injury is unknown.

DIAGNOSIS. Neither skin tests, milk antibody titers nor coproantibodies have been found useful in diagnosing the condition. Diagnosis requires withdrawal of cow's milk from the diet, observing amelioration of symptoms with a hypoallergenic formula, and reappearance of symptoms when the patient is challenged with the suspected protein or with whole cow's milk. Challenge with cow's milk should be done in the hospital under controlled conditions. If the patient has a history of severe gastrointestinal symptoms, then an intravenous infusion should be started before the challenge to provide a way of administering drugs and fluids if they become necessary for treatment. The dosage of whole milk or prepared cow's milk formula used for the initial challenge should be small; 5 to 15 ml is the usual starting dose. If overt symptoms do not develop within an hour, the dose is doubled. This procedure is repeated every hour until the dose reaches 4 ounces or the patient develops gastrointestinal symptoms. If symptoms develop, lactose intolerance and steatorrhea may occur. Failure to develop symptoms by the fifth day excludes the diagnosis.

A lactose tolerance test should be done before challenge to determine whether lactose intolerance is present. A normal test indicates absorptive cell function is normal. If lactose intolerance is present, challenge should be delayed until it is reversed; this may take 2 to 4 weeks.

TREATMENT. After diagnosis is established, hypoallergenic formula and diets free of milk protein should be fed to susceptible individuals for 1 year before rechallenge.

SOY MILK PROTEIN SENSITIVITY

Soy protein isolate, the primary protein in all soy milk formulas, can cause a violent gastrointestinal reaction in susceptible infants. The mechanism of intestinal injury is unknown, but it is not mediated by complement. Intestinal mucosa loses villous structure and becomes flat within 24 hours of challenge with soy protein isolate; recovery occurs within a few days.

CLINICAL MANIFESTATIONS, DIAGNOSIS AND PROGNOSIS. Symptoms are nonspecific and may consist of fever, leukocytosis, vomiting, blood-tinged mucoid diarrhea, lactose intolerance, dehydration and metabolic acidosis. These patients are frequently misdiagnosed as gastroenteritis. Reappearance of gastrointestinal symptoms may make the diagnosis apparent when the infants are refed soy milk. Sensitivity to the protein persists throughout infancy. Diagnosis may be established in the same manner as cow's milk protein sensitivity. Persistence of the sensitivity for two years has been reported.

MALABSORPTION DUE TO PARASITES

Four parasites have been documented to cause diarrhea and malabsorption in man: *Giardia lamblia, Strongyloides stercoralis, Capillaria philippinensis* and Coccidia. These parasites can invade the intestinal mucosa. Their mechanisms of injury are not understood.

GIARDIA LAMBLIA. *Giardia lamblia* is a protozoan that has man for its host. It may be transmitted from hand to mouth or in contaminated water. Giardiasis is the commonest cause of parasitic malabsorption in the United States. Infants, children, foreign travelers, campers and patients with hypogammaglobulinemia are especially susceptible to infection with *Giardia lamblia.*

Clinical Manifestations. Vomiting, diarrhea and steatorrhea may be preceded by a prodrome of anorexia, crampy abdominal pain and borborygmus which lasts for several days. Diarrhea may last for several weeks if the condition remains undiagnosed and untreated; this is one of its unique characteristics. Fever and eosinophilia are uncommon in this illness.

Diagnosis. The best way to establish the diagnosis is to examine fasting jejunal aspirates or small intestinal biopsies and smears of biopsy mucus for trophozoites. Stool examination for cysts is unsatisfactory because only 30 per cent of infected patients will demonstrate cysts.

Treatment. Metronidazole (Flagyl) is the drug of choice for treatment of giardiasis. It is taken orally for 7 days in divided doses (10–20 mg/kg/day). If the patient is asymptomatic at the conclusion of treatment, stools should be re-examined and, if necessary, duodenal aspirate or intestinal biopsies repeated to look for persistence of the parasite. Quinacrine (Atabrine) is recommended for patients who do not respond to metronidazole.

STRONGYLOIDES STERCORALIS. *Strongyloides stercoralis* is a nematode which has man for its host. Strongyloidiasis is primarily a disease of the tropics, but it may become endemic in vulnerable populations such as the institutionalized mentally retarded. It is found sporadically in areas of temperate climate. Malabsorption, pulmonary symptoms and pruritic rash typify the condition. Diagnosis is established by examination of jejunal aspirate for rhabditiform larvae. Thiabendazole (Metimazole) is the drug of choice for treatment.

CAPILLARIA PHILIPPINENSIS. Intestinal capillariasis is caused by a roundworm, *Capillaria philippinensis.* It is seen only in the Philippine Islands. Diagnosis is made by examination of stools for the characteristic eggs. Treatment consists of fluid and electrolyte replacement and antihelminthic therapy with thiabendazole.

COCCIDIA. The Coccidia are protozoa. Three species of Coccidia infect man. They are *Isospora belli, hominis* and *natalensis.* Fever, eosinophilia and diarrhea are the characteristic symptoms of coccidiosis. The disease is self-limited but may last for weeks to months. The best diagnostic technique has not been established. Schizonts may be detected in biopsies of the small intestine or in eggs in stool specimens. An accepted form of treatment has not been established.

CYSTIC FIBROSIS

In the United States cystic fibrosis is the commonest cause of chronic malabsorption in children. Pancreatic enzyme secretion is deficient in most patients with this illness from birth; decreased lipolysis and proteolysis result. Some patients secrete normal amounts of enzymes but have impaired pancreatic ductular function; they do not secrete pancreatic water or bicarbonate normally, but have no gastrointestinal symptoms.

Malabsorption of bile acids occurs in untreated cystic fibrosis, but not in celiac sprue. This suggests that unhydrolyzed fat or other products of maldigestion may interfere with bile acid absorption.

The discussion of cystic fibrosis here will be limited to those aspects pertinent to the consideration of malabsorption. For further discussion of these and other aspects, see Cystic Fibrosis, under Pancreas, this Section, below.

CLINICAL MANIFESTATIONS AND DIAGNOSIS. Infants with cystic fibrosis and malabsorption who have not had meconium ileus are usually recognized because of their chronic recurrent pulmonary infections. Diagnosis is established by an abnormally increased sweat chloride determination. Occasionally gastrointestinal symptoms are severe and pulmonary symptoms are mild or not present. Such infants overeat but do not gain weight normally. They have frequent diarrheal stools and steatorrhea.

Hypoproteinemia and anasarca develop in some infants because of their inability to hydrolyze and absorb peptides. This may occur with both breast and formula feeding, and is especially likely with feeding soy-protein milk substitutes. Decreased hepatic synthesis of proteins and protein-losing enteropathy rarely are responsible for hypoproteinemia. Vitamin K deficiency in undiagnosed infants may produce easy bruisability and seizures secondary to intracranial hemorrhage. The deficiency is due to malabsorption and to decreased synthesis of vitamin K by colonic bacteria, owing to antibiotic therapy. When unexplained bleeding in early infancy is associated with diarrheal stools or steatorrhea, the diagnosis of cystic fibrosis must be considered.

Vitamin A malabsorption may result in pseudotumor cerebri in infants and night blindness in older children. Clinically apparent vitamin D or E malabsorption in cystic fibrosis occurs rarely, if at all.

DIFFERENTIAL DIAGNOSIS. Patients with cystic fibrosis must be differentiated from those with *primary pancreatic insufficiency and bone marrow failure* (see Shwachman-Diamond syndrome), and from others with celiac sprue.

TREATMENT. Infants with cystic fibrosis may be fed formulas which contain either medium-chain triglycerides or long-chain triglycerides. With either type of formula, pancreatic enzyme supplements should be given in order to obtain optimum hydrolysis of fat and protein as well as micellization of fat-soluble vitamins. Formulas containing long-chain triglycerides are less expensive.

The goal of pancreatic replacement therapy is to improve luminal digestion of foods with doses of pancreatin that the patient can tolerate. Two preparations are available: triple strength pancreatin U.S.P., an alcoholic extract of hog pancreas which is standardized for amylase and trypsin but not for lipase activity; and pancrelipase U.S.P., a lipase-rich hog pancreatin marketed as Cotazym or Viokase and prepared from raw pancreas by azeotropic desiccation. The latter two are assayed for trypsin, amylase and lipase. The preparations come in the form of powders, tablets or capsules. In infants and children who have difficulty swallowing tablets and capsules, it is preferable to mix the powder with a portion of some food to disguise its taste. The preparation should be fed at the beginning of the meal to ensure that it is taken. In order to minimize decomposition of the powder it should be added to the food just prior to its administration, and by the same token, it should not be combined with warm food. The appropriate amount of pancreatic replacement therapy varies from patient to patient. Adequate replacement is judged in accordance with the decrease in the number and improved character of the stools, and decreased caloric intake. The dosage is increased until there is maximum improvement in growth and in weight gain. Infants may require from one quarter to one teaspoon of powder per feeding; 5 to 10 year old children, from 2 to 4 tablets per meal. Overdosage may produce constipation.

Pancreatic replacement therapy is less effective when pancreatic bicarbonate output is reduced and gastric acid production is normal. If pancreatic replacement therapy appears ineffective, then antacids should be administered at the same time as pancreatic enzymes.

Lactase deficiency occurs in some patients with cystic fibrosis. It does not ordinarily become apparent until late in the first decade of life and is usually not severe enough to require elimination of milk from the diet.

PANCREATIC INSUFFICIENCY AND BONE MARROW FAILURE

(Shwachman-Diamond Syndrome)

Pancreatic insufficiency and bone marrow failure is a rare illness characterized by normal sweat chloride values, pancreatic insufficiency and neutropenia. The pathogenesis of this syndrome is not understood and its mode of genetic transmission has not been defined. A variant of the syndrome has been described in which dwarfism and metaphyseal dysostosis of the hips are present.

Acinar pancreatic function is more impaired than ductular function because trypsin, lipase and amylase secretion (acinar function) are either totally absent or greatly reduced, whereas water and electrolyte production (ductular function) is intact. The defect results in growth failure in early infancy because of steatorrhea and azotorrhea. Neutropenia may be accompanied by anemia and/or thrombocytopenia. Ecchymoses and epistaxis are the primary hemorrhagic manifestations, but death from hemorrhage is rare. Infections occur with greater than expected frequency and may be related to neutropenia. Patients with this syndrome should receive pancreatic replacement therapy in adequate dosage to promote normal growth.

See also Pancreas, later, this Section.

CELIAC SPRUE

Celiac sprue is the second commonest chronic malabsorption syndrome in childhood. It has many synonyms: *childhood celiac disease, nontropical sprue* and *gluten-induced enteropathy.* Celiac sprue in childhood is the same disease as adult celiac disease. It is inherited, but the mode of genetic transmission is undetermined. Ten per cent of patients with celiac sprue have other family members with the disease. The true incidence of the disease is unknown; in England and Ireland it is estimated to be 1 in 300. The condition has not been reported in blacks or Orientals.

PATHOGENESIS. Celiac sprue is caused by a permanent intolerance for gluten, which is one of the protein fractions of wheat, barley, rye and oats. Only the glutens in wheat and rye have definitely been shown to be harmful to the small intestinal mucosa and to cause morphologic and functional damage. Gluten consists of two protein fractions, glutenin and gliadin; it is the gliadin fraction that does the damage. The mechanism for gluten-induced injury is unknown. Two theories have been proposed—toxic and immunologic; there is more evidence for impaired immunologic function than for some specific toxic factor in gluten.

CLINICAL CHARACTERISTICS. Symptoms of celiac sprue may begin at any time after introduction of gluten-containing foods into the diet. Onset is most commonly in the first 2 years of life, but may be delayed for years and, in rare cases, for decades. Chronic diarrhea, irritability, vomiting and failure to grow and to gain in weight are the most common symptoms. In some patients growth failure and delay in pubarche or menses are the only symptoms. At the time of diagnosis, two thirds of the patients are below the third percentile for weight and one third are below the third percentile for height. Growth retardation and anemia are more commonly seen in children diagnosed at an older age. Anorexia is far more common than overeating. Crampy abdominal pain, tetany, rectal prolapse, constipation and dermatitis herpetiformis are some of the less common symptoms. The majority of patients with celiac sprue have stools that are rancid in odor, bulky in volume and poorly formed.

Abdominal distention, decreased subcutaneous tissue, wasted proximal musculature, smooth tongue, dependent edema and long eyelashes are the commonest physical signs. Delayed dentition and clubbing of the fingers occur less frequently. Rarely, ecchymoses are observed, secondary to depletion of clotting factors dependent on vitamin K. Clinical signs of rickets have not been described, but typical radiologic changes in the bones have been observed on rare occasions.

DIAGNOSIS. Three criteria establish the diagnosis of celiac sprue: (1) demonstration of impaired intestinal absorption; (2) characteristic histologic changes in mucosa from the region of the duodenojejunal junction, as shown in peroral biopsy specimens; and (3) a beneficial clinical response to a strict gluten-free diet. Fat absorption is assessed in suspected cases by means of screening tests such as serum carotene levels or with quantitative determination of the fecal fat excreted in a 72-hour stool collection. Malabsorption of fat does not occur in all cases, since some patients are anorexic and eat decreased amounts of fat; they have sufficient effective absorptive area to absorb limited quantities. In other patients the mucosal lesion is limited to the proximal small intestine; such patients eat normally, with no malabsorption; they are almost invariably asymptomatic.

The D-xylose excretion test has limited value in screening patients for celiac sprue because one third of patients with the disease excrete between 15 and 25 per cent of the dose, which is within the normal range in children. Lactose intolerance may be present in some patients because of damage to the proximal mucosa that results in secondary lactase deficiency. Owing, however, to reserve lactase in distal small bowel, many patients are not intolerant of lactose. Celiac sprue should be considered as a possible diagnosis in any patient who has unexplained anemia associated with iron or folate deficiency or who has impaired calcium absorption. Small intestinal biopsy should be performed in any patient with poor growth or unexplained anemia, even in the absence of laboratory evidence of steatorrhea, and biopsy must be done *before* a gluten-free diet is instituted in patients suspected of celiac sprue.

The characteristic changes seen in biopsies taken from the proximal small intestine consist of a flat mucosa with elongated crypts containing increased numbers of mitotic figures, increased numbers of mononuclear cells in the lamina propria, and damaged surface epithelial cells (Fig. 11–17). This lesion is not specific for celiac sprue (see section on Intestinal Biopsy), but the diagnosis

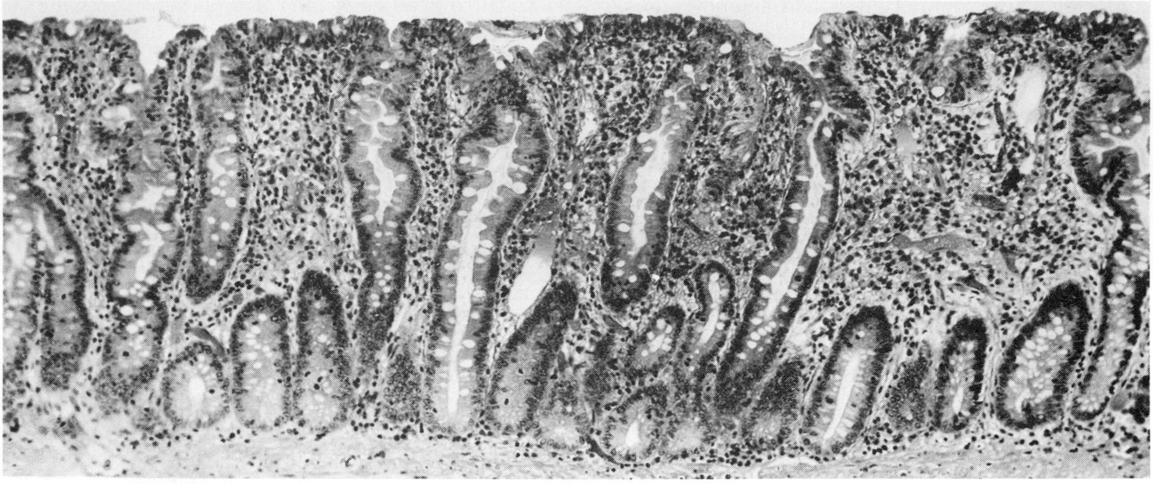

Figure 11–17 *Proximal jejunal biopsy from a patient with untreated celiac sprue. The biopsy is severely abnormal. Villous structure is absent and crypts extend the entire height of the biopsy. The lamina propria has an increased content of mononuclear cells and the surface epithelium is irregular and contains vacuoles. There is an increased transmigration of mononuclear cells across the surface epithelium.*

cannot be made without it. Mucosal changes in celiac sprue are most severe in the proximal small intestine, but the area of damaged mucosa may extend the entire length of the upper gastrointestinal tract. With a gluten-free diet, reversal of the lesion first becomes apparent in the least damaged areas and proceeds proximally. The intestinal lesion of celiac sprue may revert completely to normal within months (Fig. 11–18).

TREATMENT. After the intestinal biopsy is shown to have the characteristic changes, the patient is given a gluten-free diet. Foods that contain gluten from wheat, barley, rye and oats are totally excluded. Labels on prepared foods must be read carefully to determine if gluten has been added. Sometimes labels do not mention gluten or specific grains but indicate "HVP" (hydrolyzed vegetable protein) or "vegetable protein added." To use a gluten-free diet properly requires education and time, including extra time needed to shop for food; it is more expensive to prepare. The diet causes patient and family some inconvenience, but is worth the effort because of the improved health which results.* The patient should plan to be on a gluten-free diet for as long as he lives; it is for this reason that each patient must have the diagnosis established by biopsy before treatment is initiated. With

*Mrs. E. Hartsook, Clinical Research Center Dietitian at the University of Washington Hospital, Seattle, Washington, will provide to physicians and dietitians upon request the strict gluten-free diet used at the University of Washington. This includes recipes and food product lists of gluten-free foods.

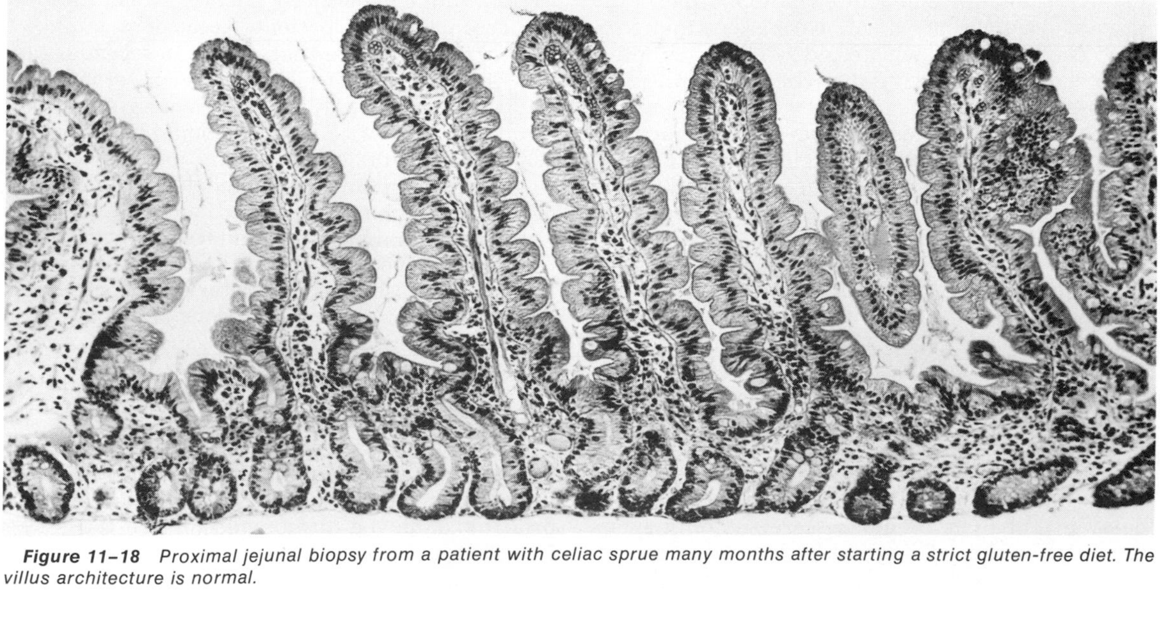

Figure 11–18 *Proximal jejunal biopsy from a patient with celiac sprue many months after starting a strict gluten-free diet. The villus architecture is normal.*

the diet begun, improvement in mood is usually the first change observed and appears within days. Improved appetite, weight gain and change in stools may take weeks. If significant improvement is not apparent within a month, either the diagnosis is incorrect or the patient is not being maintained on a strictly gluten-free diet. Failure to adhere to a gluten-free diet is the most common reason for lack of clinical response. Patients who fail to respond should have a second, confirmatory biopsy and must be re-educated in the use of the diet. If after another month improvement does not occur, the patient should be hospitalized and fed the diet under strict supervision. Within six months to one year of beginning a gluten-free diet, patients with celiac sprue should be within the normal range for weight. Height and bone age do not fully recover until after two years of treatment, but the measurements may no longer be significantly depressed after one year on the diet. Patients who remain on a gluten-free diet continue to gain weight and grow normally. Relapses occur in every child who returns to eating gluten. The younger children's symptoms become apparent sooner; in older children clinical relapse may be delayed for months or years. The symptoms may be insidious, consisting of suboptimal growth, chronic ill health, iron deficiency and megaloblastic anemia. An increasing number of adults with celiac sprue are being found who die of lymphoma of the small intestine; it is not known whether gluten in the diet contributes to this occurrence.

SHORT BOWEL SYNDROME

Massive resection of small bowel may be necessary to preserve life in infants with anomalies of the small intestine, most frequently in the neonatal period for volvulus and atresias. Survival following small bowel resection is related to the length of the remaining intestine, the presence or preservation of the ileocecal valve, birth weight, success of surgical management and problems of associated anomalies. Infants left with more than 38 cm of small intestine, not including the duodenum, have more than 90 per cent probability of survival; there is a 50 per cent chance with 15 to 38 cm of small bowel and an intact ileocecal valve.

Following massive resection patients may have gastric hypersecretion, which may be limited to the postoperative period or persist for months. The intraluminal pH postprandially is normally 5.4 to 6.0 at the duodenojejunal junction; when the intraluminal pH falls owing to gastric hypersecretion pancreatic enzymes may be inactivated, with resultant azotorrhea and steatorrhea. To combat excessive duodenal acidity, effective antacid therapy should be maintained. Vagotomy and pyloroplasty or gastroenterostomy should not be considered as primary therapy in such patients, since the hypersecretion may be self-limited and the decreased gastric emptying time following surgery may worsen steatorrhea.

Almost all the conjugated bile salts are actively reabsorbed in the terminal ileum. If it is resected, an insufficiency of bile salt results, and dietary fat and fat-soluble vitamins will not be made adequately soluble. Furthermore, if the resection includes the mid- and distal jejunum as well as the ileum, the patient may be unable to maintain positive fluid balance. For these reasons it is advisable to begin feeding with a glucose and electrolyte solution and to advance the formula from the simplest to the more complex. If the infant being fed only glucose and electrolytes has frequent, watery, acid bowel movements that contain significant reducing substances, oral feeding will not be successful. Parenteral hyperalimentation should then be used to provide essential nutritional support until compensatory growth of bowel occurs and intestinal absorption is sufficient to maintain the patient in positive fluid and nitrogen balance. When oral feeding is tolerated with dextrose and electrolytes, a special therapeutic formula, Pregestimil, should be considered first, because it contains all the basic nutrients in the most easily assimilable form. If this fails, an elemental diet such as unflavored Vivonex should be used, starting with a dilute concentration and with continuous infusion through a gastrostomy or nasogastric feeding tube. As the infant grows, a low fat diet or one in which medium-chain triglycerides are substituted for long-chain triglycerides should be used.

Malabsorption of water-soluble vitamins usually does not occur except for folic acid and vitamin B_{12}. When extensive resection occurs in the proximal half of the small bowel, absorption of folic acid may be impaired. Vitamin B_{12} is absorbed as a B_{12}-intrinsic factor complex by ileal receptor sites. Monthly injections of 100 μg of vitamin B_{12} need to be given for the duration of life to infants who have the ileum resected. In some cases cholestyramine will ameliorate the diarrhea induced by bile acids.

Vitamins A, D and E are available in water-miscible form and should be used to prevent or to correct deficiencies of absorption of the naturally occurring forms. The doses of vitamin D necessary to prevent rickets in such patients may be quite large. There is no good method to monitor this therapy. Determination of the prothrombin time every two weeks will indicate whether supplemental vitamin K is necessary.

After the first year of life, many surviving infants will have body weights within the normal range for their ages.

ABETALIPOPROTEINEMIA

This extremely rare condition is inherited in an autosomal recessive pattern. The biochemical basis of the disease is the inability of the endoplasmic reticulum of intestinal absorptive cells to syn-

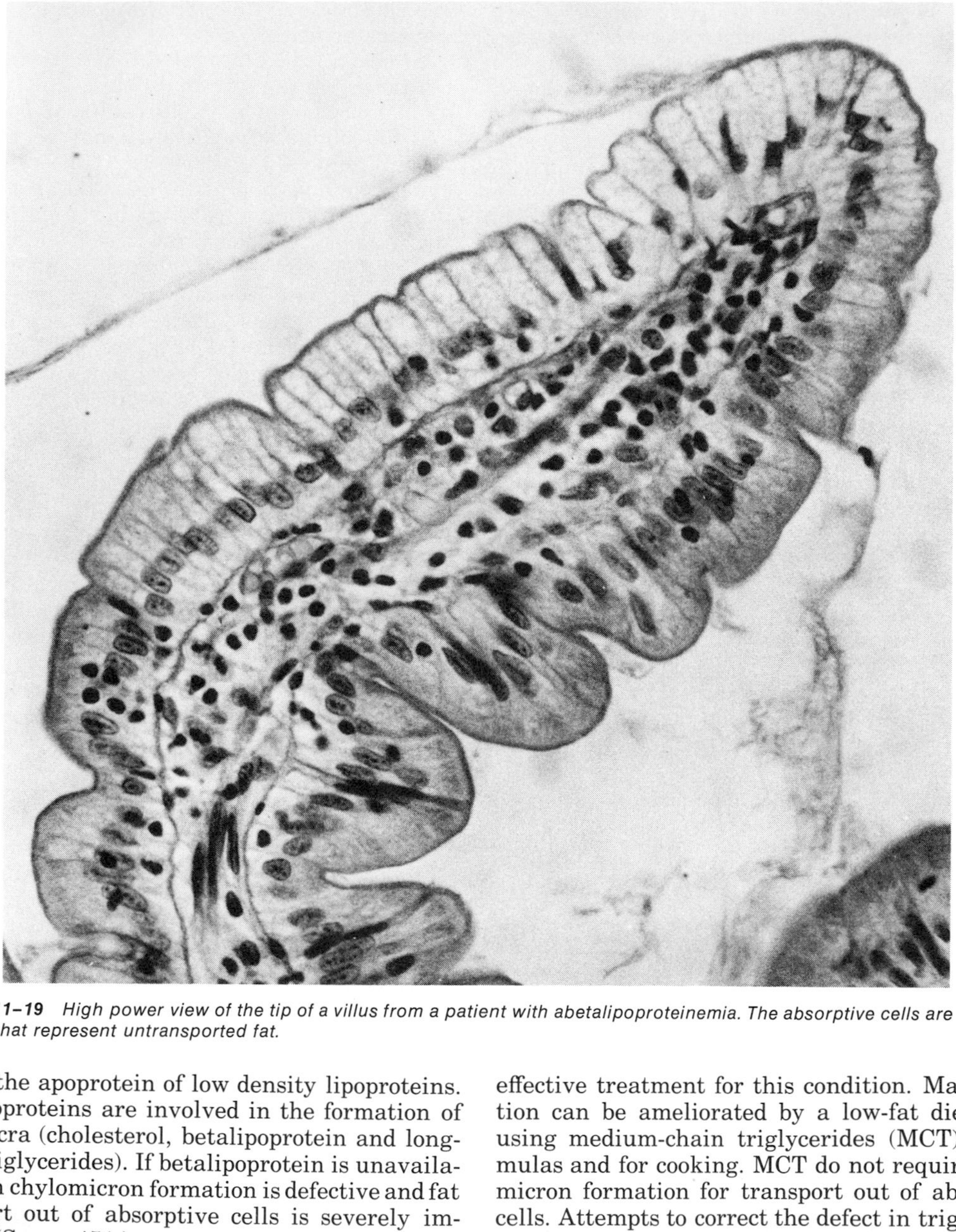

Figure 11–19 *High power view of the tip of a villus from a patient with abetalipoproteinemia. The absorptive cells are filled with vacuoles that represent untransported fat.*

thesize the apoprotein of low density lipoproteins. Betalipoproteins are involved in the formation of chylomicra (cholesterol, betalipoprotein and long-chain triglycerides). If betalipoprotein is unavailable, then chylomicron formation is defective and fat transport out of absorptive cells is severely impaired. (See p. 451.)

CLINICAL MANIFESTATIONS. Steatorrhea and acanthocytosis are the primary presenting features in early infancy. Prior to the availability of small intestinal biopsy these patients were often misdiagnosed as having celiac sprue because of the nonspecific symptoms of malabsorption. Diffuse degeneration of the central nervous system and retinitis pigmentosa may develop after many years.

DIAGNOSIS. Diagnosis is established by the absence of betalipoproteins on lipoprotein immunoelectrophoresis and by the characteristic morphologic changes in biopsy of the small intestine. These changes consist of vacuolated absorptive cells which represent untransported triglycerides (Fig. 11–19).

TREATMENT, COURSE, PROGNOSIS. There is no effective treatment for this condition. Malabsorption can be ameliorated by a low-fat diet or by using medium-chain triglycerides (MCT) in formulas and for cooking. MCT do not require chylomicron formation for transport out of absorptive cells. Attempts to correct the defect in triglyceride transport with betalipoprotein infusions have been unsuccessful, suggesting that the defect is not due simply to the lack of circulating betalipoprotein. These patients ultimately become blind and severely crippled neurologically.

INTESTINAL LYMPHANGIECTASIA

Intestinal lymphangiectasia is a rare congenital or acquired disorder of lymphatics associated with steatorrhea, protein-losing enteropathy, generalized hypoproteinemia and lymphopenia.

CLINICAL MANIFESTATIONS. The initial symptom may be conjunctival, scrotal or labial swelling and may occur in the neonatal period. Abdominal distention with chylous ascites may be the initial symptom, or may not be apparent for days or weeks. Because these patients usually have a generalized disorder of lymphatics, asymmetrical swellings of the upper or lower extremities may be the initial manifestations. The severity of diarrhea and steatorrhea is variable and depends on the extent of lymphatic obstruction.

DIAGNOSIS. Diagnosis is made by biopsy of the small intestine. The characteristic lesion shows dilated lymphatic channels in the mucosa and submucosa with distortion of villous architecture (Fig. 11–20). Lymphangiograms are rarely done to establish the diagnosis in childhood because they are difficult to perform in infants and children.

Radiographic examination of the small bowel may be normal or may show enlargement of the intestinal folds in both jejunum and ileum, dilution of the barium column distally and minimal dilatation of the bowel.

COMPLICATIONS. An immune deficiency state with abnormalities of both the humoral and cellular immune systems is associated with lymphangiectasia. Plasma immunoglobulin levels are reduced as a result of protein-losing enteropathy, whereas synthesis rates of immunoglobulin are normal. The cellular immune system is more severely impaired, as evaluated by intradermal delayed hypersensitivity skin tests or by skin allograft survival. These findings are associated with peripheral lymphocytopenia and with a particular loss of the recirculating long-lived lymphocytes which are responsible for in vitro blast transformation. Only a minority of these patients have more severe and frequent infections than usual.

TREATMENT, COURSE AND PROGNOSIS. Portagen, a therapeutic formula which contains medium-chain triglycerides (MCT), is fed to infants and children with intestinal lymphangiectasia, because the MCT are transported by the venules and not the lymphatics. A low-fat diet is used as the infants grow older. Most patients respond to treatment with a decrease in frequency of stools, a change to formed stools and diminution of ascites and edema. Serum proteins and lymphocyte counts increase with treatment but seldom reach normal levels. Normal growth and gain in weight may occur in response to dietary treatment in some patients. Despite good diet therapy, some patients with lymphangiectasia have frequent unexplained spontaneous exacerbations of symptoms. Intussusception and internal hernias causing intestinal obstruction are infrequent complications of this condition.

WHIPPLE'S DISEASE

Whipple's disease is a rare syndrome usually seen in Caucasian men, middle-aged or older. Except for one confirmed case in an infant, all others reported in childhood are questionable. It is likely

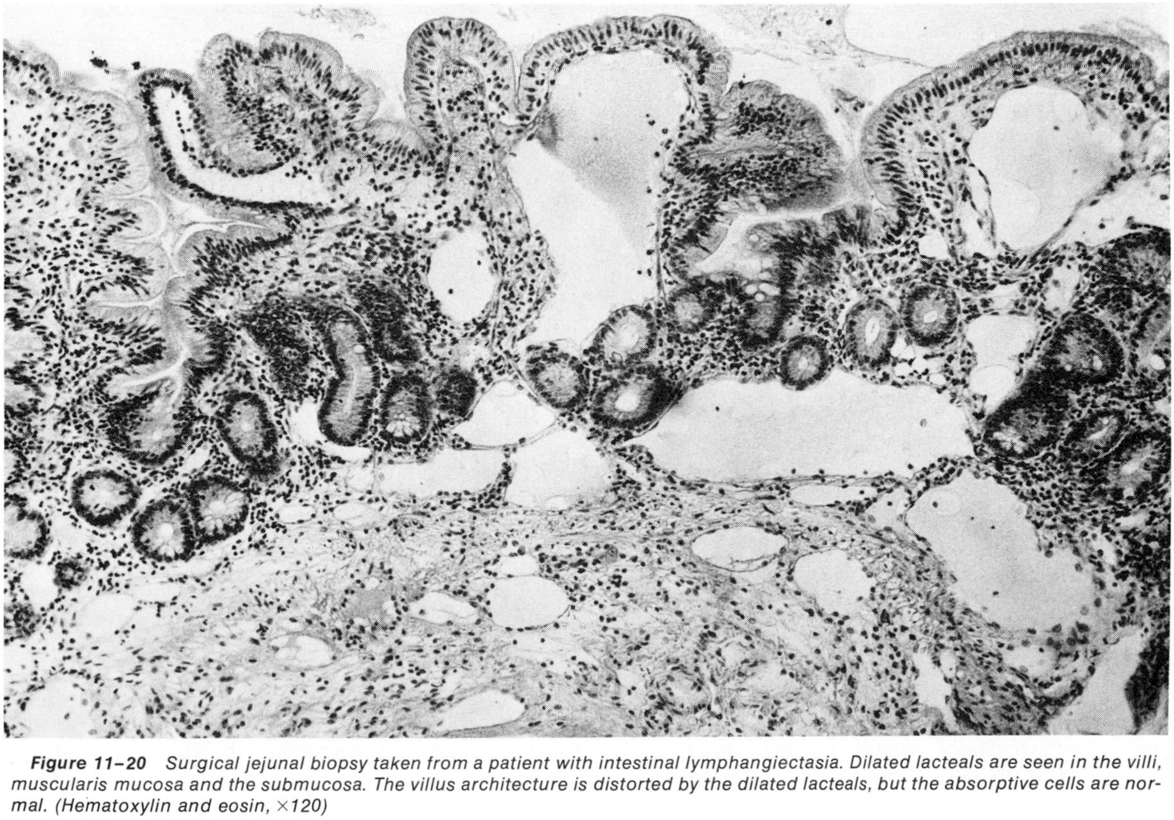

Figure 11–20 Surgical jejunal biopsy taken from a patient with intestinal lymphangiectasia. Dilated lacteals are seen in the villi, muscularis mucosa and the submucosa. The villus architecture is distorted by the dilated lacteals, but the absorptive cells are normal. (Hematoxylin and eosin, ×120)

the illness is caused by bacterial infection; electron micrographs show bacteria-like, rod-shaped bodies extracellularly and intracellularly in cells of small bowel biopsies from patients with this illness.

CLINICAL MANIFESTATIONS, DIAGNOSIS AND TREATMENT. The major signs and symptoms are diarrhea, fever, weight loss, arthralgia, abdominal pain and hyperpigmentation of skin. Steatorrhea in this illness is attributed to blockage of intestinal lymphatic channels by macrophages containing a glycoprotein derived from the bacillum-like bodies.

Diagnosis of Whipple's disease is established by finding the characteristic PAS-positive macrophages in biopsies of the small intestine and lymph nodes. Confirmation of the diagnosis is made by demonstration of the bacillary bodies in 1-micron-thick sections.

This illness is curable if it is recognized and treated with antibiotics.

WOLMAN'S DISEASE

Wolman's disease is a rare, usually lethal lipidosis resulting from deficiency of an intracellular lipase which acts on triglycerides and cholesterol esters in tissues such as the liver and spleen. Storage of these lipids in visceral organs results from the enzymatic deficiency.

CLINICAL MANIFESTATIONS, DIAGNOSIS AND TREATMENT. Most cases present early in infancy and are characterized by vomiting, diarrhea, steatorrhea, abdominal distention, hepatomegaly, splenomegaly, anemia and vacuolization of lymphocytes. In contrast to the other lipidoses, neurologic involvement does not occur. Steatorrhea may be due to obstruction of lymphatics by lipid-filled histiocytes in the lamina propria and submucosa.

A flat plate of the abdomen is usually diagnostic because the roentgenographic appearance of the adrenal glands is unmistakable; they are enlarged and show multiple punctate calcifications evenly distributed throughout both glands. Serum lipids are normal; but the cholesterol, triglyceride and neutral fat contents of the liver and spleen are abnormally high, while their phospholipid and glycolipid contents are normal.

No therapy is helpful in this illness. Death occurs from inanition.

TROPICAL SPRUE

The illness occurs in either epidemic or endemic form in individuals living in the tropics and where living conditions are unhygienic.

CLINICAL MANIFESTATIONS, DIAGNOSIS AND TREATMENT. Patients with tropical sprue have steatorrhea, malabsorption of vitamin B_{12} and bacterial overgrowth of colonic types of microorganisms in the proximal small intestine; biopsies of the small intestine vary in abnormality from flat lesions without villi to others in which there are only epithelial cell abnormalities. Abdominal distention, borborygmi, anorexia and vomiting are the most common symptoms. Fever occurs infrequently. The stools are semiformed or watery and may contain blood and mucus. Dehydration, metabolic acidosis and hypoelectrolytemia may cause death in a small proportion of patients. The mechanism of small intestinal injury by bacteria or their by-products of metabolism is unknown. This is a poorly understood clinical entity.

The most suitable therapy for patients with tropical sprue is undetermined. The first step in treatment is to control the diarrhea and make up deficiencies of fluids, electrolytes and vitamins. Some cases remit without further therapy. Antibiotics and folic acid are the other modes of treatment. The dosage of tetracycline is 50 mg/kg/day for 2 weeks. Folic acid is given orally, 5 mg 3 times a day for 2 weeks, and then 5 mg daily for 4 to 6 months. Absorptive function returns to normal within 2 weeks. Gluten-free diets have no place in treatment of this disease.

MALABSORPTION DUE TO SMALL INTESTINAL STASIS

Small intestinal stasis is characterized by stagnation of intestinal contents, secondary bacterial proliferation, and malabsorption of fat and sometimes of vitamin B_{12}. Congenital or surgically acquired partial small bowel obstruction is the commonest cause of the condition in children. Malrotations, with bands across the duodenum, and duodenal and jejunal diaphragms are the anomalies most frequently associated with stasis. The surgical procedures producing stasis with the highest frequencies are end-to-side and side-to-side anastomoses of small bowel following surgical resection for atresia and stenosis, because these types of anastomoses can eventuate in a blind loop. Other rare causes of the stasis syndrome are idiopathic intestinal pseudo-obstruction, with basal ganglia calcification, hypothroidism, scleroderma and jejunal diverticulosis.

CLINICAL MANIFESTATIONS AND TREATMENT. Diarrhea, vomiting and abdominal distention are the most frequent symptoms. The mechanism of steatorrhea in these patients is not definitely known but may be related to bacterial overgrowth.

Surgical correction of congenital or surgically acquired defects will eliminate stasis. If narrow areas of bowel are excised, end-to-end anastomoses should be performed to prevent recurrence. In those conditions not correctable by surgery, antibiotics can be used to reduce the number of bacteria in the proximal small bowel and to improve absorptive cell function. If the primary defect in motility cannot be corrected, the improvement in absorption may not last.

MALABSORPTION IN BILIARY TRACT OBSTRUCTION

Patients with biliary atresia of either intra- or extrahepatic types and choledochal cysts develop steatorrhea because insufficient bile salts are secreted into the lumen of the duodenum for micelle formation. Following surgical correction of the obstructed extrahepatic biliary ducts in cases amenable to surgery, steatorrhea is reversed. For further discussion of biliary obstruction, see The Liver, later, this Section.

ACRODERMATITIS ENTEROPATHICA (AE)

Acrodermatitis enteropathica is a poorly understood condition that is characterized by chronic diarrhea, alopecia and dermatitis of the extremities and mucocutaneous areas. Most cases present within the first weeks of life or when susceptible breast-fed infants are weaned; the condition has been reported, however, later in infancy. Diarrhea is usually the first symptom; it is followed by dermatitis weeks to months later. Abnormalities of absorptive function have been poorly documented, both normal absorption and generalized malabsorption having been described. Mucosal abnormalities may occur in both small intestine and colon. Several types of therapy have been recommended, but failures have occurred with each. Breast milk and diiodohydroxyquin (Diodoquin) have been most frequently used. (See p. 819.)

PRIMARY HYPOMAGNESEMIA

Primary hypomagnesemia is a rare congenital disorder of magnesium absorption in which magnesium depletion is associated with secondary hypocalcemia. Hypocalcemia occurs because magnesium deficiency results in impaired synthesis or release of parathyroid hormone. The mechanism of magnesium malabsorption has not been defined.

CLINICAL MANIFESTATIONS. Affected patients present tetanic convulsions in the first two months of life. Diarrhea may be present, along with edema, ascites and hypoalbuminemia.

TREATMENT, COURSE AND PROGNOSIS. Parenteral administration of 2.5 mEq of magnesium as 50 per cent magnesium sulfate stops the convulsions. Oral therapy with up to 24 mEq of magnesium salts per day is given, after parenteral repletion, to maintain positive magnesium balance. Infusions of calcium correct the hypocalcemia but do not affect hypomagnesemia or tetany. All clinical abnormalities are reversible, and these patients grow and develop normally as long as they receive magnesium therapy. (See also p. 393.)

AMINO ACID MALABSORPTION

There are four syndromes associated with intestinal malabsorption of amino acids in infants and children: cystinuria, Hartnup's disease, blue diaper syndrome and methionine malabsorption. The last syndrome has diarrhea as one of its major manifestations. The other amino acid malabsorption syndromes do not have gastrointestinal symptoms. See also Section 8.

VITAMIN B_{12} MALABSORPTION

There are five vitamin B_{12} malabsorption syndromes: juvenile pernicious anemia, adult-type pernicious anemia, Immerslund-Gräsbeck syndrome, biologically inert intrinsic factor, and hereditary transcobalamin II deficiency.

Juvenile pernicious anemia is a rare disorder in which the intrinsic factor activity necessary for vitamin B_{12} absorption is not produced by gastric parietal cells. Affected patients have histologically normal gastric mucosa and lack circulating antibodies to intrinsic factor or parietal cells. They have profound megaloblastic anemia and growth failure. Irreversible psychomotor retardation may develop if diagnosis is delayed.

Adult-type pernicious anemia is characterized by gastric atrophy, achlorhydria, deficient intrinsic factor production and circulating antibodies to intrinsic factor and parietal cells.

Immerslund-Gräsbeck syndrome is characterized by selective malabsorption of vitamin B_{12} in the terminal ileum despite normal intrinsic factor activity. The ileal mucosa is normal to light and electron microscopy. Proteinuria is usually present. Anemia and neurologic symptoms develop late in the first year of life and may be accompanied by diarrhea and steatorrhea. The mode of inheritance is autosomal recessive. Treatment with vitamin B_{12} reverses all signs of malabsorption and anemia.

An adolescent boy has been shown to have *biologically inert intrinsic factor.* He had acid gastric juice and normal quantities of immunologically identifiable intrinsic factor; gastric mucosa was normal. His gastric juice did not correct the vitamin B_{12} malabsorption of a totally gastrectomized volunteer, but he was able to absorb normal quantities of vitamin B_{12} when it was bound to normal human gastric juice. His clinical findings included anorexia, fatigue, a smooth tongue and enlarged liver and spleen.

Transcobalamin II deficiency is an autosomal recessive condition, in which there is a lack of a protein necessary for the absorption and transport of vitamin B_{12} into and through ileal absorptive cells. Patients with this inborn error of transport proteins typically develop diarrhea, vomiting and infections as neonates. Characteristic hematologic findings include leukopenia, granulocytopenia, thrombocytopenia, anemia and the bone marrow changes of megaloblastic anemia. Surprisingly, the serum folic acid and vitamin B_{12} levels are normal. Diagnosis is established by demonstrating absence of transcobalamin II in serum, either by diethylaminoethylcellulose chromatography or by polyacrylamide gel electrophoresis.

TREATMENT. Treatment of the first four conditions requires intramuscular injection of 100 μg of vitamin B_{12} once a month for life. Patients with transcobalamin II deficiency require 1000 μg/wk of vitamin B_{12} to maintain clinical remission.

CONGENITAL MALABSORPTION OF FOLIC ACID

This rare defect in absorption is characterized by relapsing megaloblastic anemia beginning early in infancy, and by ataxic or athetotic movements, mental retardation and central nervous system degeneration, with cerebral calcification and convulsions. The diagnosis is established by the findings of low serum folate levels and normal vitamin B_{12} absorption.

Intramuscular folic acid is used for therapy. There is some question whether the therapy can precipitate convulsions.

M. E. Ament

Carbohydrate Absorption

Ament, M. E.: Letters to the Editor. Screening tests for sugar malabsorption. J. Pediatr. *82*:893, 1973.

Davidson, A. G. F., and Mullinger, M.: Reducing substances in neonatal stools detected by Clinitest. Pediatrics *46*:632, 1970.

Gray, G. M.: Intestinal digestion and maldigestion of dietary carbohydrates. Ann. Rev. Med. *22*:391, 1971.

Kerry, K. R., and Anderson, C. M.: A ward test for sugar in faeces. Lancet *1*:981, 1964.

McGill, D. B., and Newcomer, A. D.: Comparison of venous and capillary blood samples in lactose tolerance testing. Gastroenterology *53*:371, 1967.

Soeparto, P., Stobo, E. A., and Walker-Smith, J. A.: Role of chemical examination of the stool in diagnosis of sugar malabsorption in children. Arch. Dis. Child, *47*:56, 1972.

Fat Absorption

Christiansen, P. A., Kirsner, J. B., and Ablaza, J.: D-Xylose and its use in the diagnosis of malabsorptive states. Am. J. Med. *27*:443, 1959.

Drummey, G. D., Benson, J. A., Jr., and Jones, C. M.: Microscopical examinations of the stool for steatorrhea. N. Engl. J. Med. *264*:85, 1961.

Fomon, S. J., Ziegler, E. E., Thomas, L. A., Jensen, R. L., and Filer, L. J.: Excretion of fat by normal full term infants fed various milks and formulas. Am. J. Clin. Nutr. *10*:1299, 1970.

Johnston, J. M.: Mechanism of fat absorption. In *Handbook of Physiology.* Vol. III, Section 6, "Alimentary Canal," Chap. 70. Washington, D.C., American Physiological Society, 1968.

Shmerling, D. H., Forrer, J. C. W., and Prader, A.: Fecal fat and nitrogen in healthy children and in children with maldigestion or malabsorption. Pediatrics *46*:690, 1970.

Watkins, J. B., Bliss, C. M., Donaldson, R. M., Jr., and Lester, R.: Characterization of newborn fecal lipid. Pediatrics *53*:511, 1974.

Weijers, H. A., and van de Kamer, J. H.: Coeliac disease. I. Criticism of the various methods of investigation. Acta Paediatr. Scand. *42*:24, 1953.

Protein Absorption

Fisher, R. B.: Absorption of proteins. Br. Med. Bull. *23*:241, 1967.

Protein-losing Enteropathy

Rootwelt, K.: Direct intravenous injection of ^{51}chromic chloride compared with ^{125}I-polyvinyl-pyrrolidone and ^{131}I-albumin in the detection of gastrointestinal protein loss. Scand. J. Clin. Lab. Invest. *18*:405, 1966.

Pancreative Function

Ammann, R. W., et al.: Diagnostic value of fecal chymotrypsin and trypsin assessment for detection of pancreatic disease. Am. J. Dig. Dis. *13*:123, 1968.

Barbero, G. J., et al.: Stool trypsin and chymotrypsin. Am. J. Dis. Child. *112*:536, 1966.

Hadorn, B., Zoppi, G., Shmerling, D. H., Prader, A., McIntyre, I., and Anderson, C. M.: Quantitative assessment of exocrine pancreatic function in infants and children. J. Pediatr. *73*:39, 1968.

D-Xylose Test

Hamilton, J. R., Lynch, M. J., and Reilly, B. J.: Active celiac disease in childhood. Q. J. Med. *38*:135, 1969.

Lanzkowsky, P., Madenlioglu, M., Wilson, J. F., and Lahey, M. E.: Oral D-xylose test in healthy infants and children. N. Engl. J. Med. *268*:1441, 1963.

Marin, G. A., Clark, M. L., and Senior, J. R.: Distribution of D-xylose in sequestered fluid resulting in false positive tests for malabsorption. Ann. Intern. Med. *69*:1155, 1968.

Sladen, G. E., and Kumar, P. J.: Is the xylose test still a worthwhile investigation? Brit. Med. J. *2*:223, 1973.

Serum Folate

Magnus, E. M.: Low serum and red cell folate activity in adult celiac disease. Am. J. Dig. Dis. *11*:314, 1966.

Schilling Test

McIntyre, P. A., Hahn, R., Conley, C. L., and Glass, B.: Genetic factors in predisposition to pernicious anemia. Bull. Hopkins Hosp. *104*:309, 1959.

Schilling, R. F.: Intrinsic factor studies. II. The effect of gastric juice on the urinary excretion of radioactivity after the oral administration of radioactive vitamin B_{12}. Lab. Clin. Med. *42*:860, 1953.

Peroral Biopsy

Ament, M. E., and Rubin, C. E.: An infant multipurpose biopsy tube. Gastroenterology. *65*:205, 1973.

Partin, J. C., and Schubert, W. K.: Precautionary note on the use of the intestinal biopsy capsule in infants and emaciated children. N. Engl. J. Med. *274*:94, 1967.

Lactose Malabsorption

Bayless, T. M., Paige, D. M., and Ferry, G. D.: Lactose intolerance and milk drinking habits. Gastroenterology *60*:605, 1971.

Christopher, M. L, and Bayless, T. M.: Role of the small bowel and colon in lactose induced diarrhea. Gastroenterology *60*:845, 1971.

Gray, G. M.: Intestinal digestion and maldigestion of dietary carbohydrates. Ann. Rev. Med. *22*:391, 1971.

Launiala, K.: The mechanism of diarrhea in congenital disaccharide malabsorption. Acta Paediatr. Scand. *57*:425, 1968.

Lifshitz, F., Coello-Ramirez, P., Gutierrez-Topete, G., et al.: Carbohydrate intolerance in infants with diarrhea. J. Pediatr. *79*:760, 1971.

Kretchmer, N.: Lactose and lactase. Sci. Am. *227*:70, 1972.

Welsh, J. D., Zschiesche, O. M., Anderson, J., et al.: Intestinal disaccharidase activity in celiac sprue (gluten sensitive enteropathy). Arch. Intern. Med. *123*:33, 1969.

Sucrase-Isomaltase Deficiency

Ament, M. E., Perera, D. R., and Esther, L.: Sucrase-isomaltase deficiency: A frequently misdiagnosed disease, J. Pediatr. *83*: 721, 1973.

Antonowicz, I., Lloyd-Still, J. D., Khaw, K. R., and Schwachman, H.: Congenital sucrase-isomaltase deficiency. Pediatrics *49*:847, 1972.

Eheart, J. F., and Mason, B. S.: Sugar and acid in the edible portion of fruit. J. Am. Diet. Assoc. *50*:130, 1967.

Gray, G. M.: Intestinal digestion and maldigestion of dietary carbohydrates. Ann. Rev. Med. *22*:391, 1971.

Glucose-Galactose Malabsorption

Hyman, C. J., Reiter, J., Rodnan, J., and Drash, A. L.: Parenteral and oral alimentation in the treatment of the nonspecific protracted diarrheal syndrome of infancy. J. Pediatr. *78*:17, 1971.

Lifshitz, F., Coello-Ramirez, P., and Gutierrez-Topete, G.: Monosaccharide intolerance and hypoglycemia in infants with diarrhea. II. Metabolic studies in 23 infants. J. Pediatr. *77*:604, 1970.

Lifshitz, F., Coello-Ramirez, P., Gutierrez-Topete, G., et al.: Carbohydrate intolerance in infants with diarrhea. J. Pediatr. *79*:760, 1971.

Schneider, A. J., Kinter, W. B., and Stirling, C. E.: Glucose-galactose malabsorption. N. Engl. J. Med. *274*:305, 1966.

Malabsorption with Immune Defects

Ament, M. E., Ochs, H. D., and Davis, S. D.: The structure and function of the gastrointestinal tract in 39 cases of primary immunodeficiency syndromes. Medicine *52*:227, 1973.

Schaller, J., David, S. D., and Wedgwood, R. J.: Failure of development of the thymus, lymphopenia and hypogammaglobulinemia. Am. J. Med. *41*:462, 1966.

Congenital Chloridorrhea

Bieberdorf, F. A., Gorden, P., and Fordtran, J. S.: Pathogenesis of congenital alkalosis with diarrhea. Implications for the physiology of normal ideal electrolyte absorption and secretion. J. Clin. Invest. *51*:1958, 1972.

Launiala, K., Perheentupa, J., Pasternack, N., and Hallman, N.: Familial chloride diarrhea—chloride malabsorption. Mod. Probl. Pediatr. *11*:137, 1968.

Enterokinase Deficiency

Hadorn, B., Tarlow, M. J., Lloyd, J. K., and Wolff, O. H.: Intestinal enterokinase deficiency. Lancet *1*:812, 1969.

Tarlow, M. J., Hadorn, B., Arthurton, M. W., and Lloyd, J. K.: Intestinal enterokinase deficiency. Arch. Dis. Child *45*:651, 1970.

Intolerance to Cow's Milk and Soy Protein

Ament, M. E., and Rubin, C. E.: Soy protein—Another cause of the flat intestinal lesion. Gastroenterology *62*:227, 1972.

Davidson, M., Burnstein, R. C., Kugler, M. M., et al.: Malabsorption defect induced by ingestion of beta lactoglobulin. J. Pediatr. *66*:545, 1965.

Davis, S. D., Bierman, C. W., Pierson, W. E., et al.: Clinical nonspecificity of milk coproantibodies in diarrheal stools. N. Engl. J. Med. *282*:612, 1970.

Freier, S., Kletter, B., Gery, I., Lebenthal, E., and Geifman, M.: Intolerance to milk protein. J. Pediatr. *75*:623, 1968.

Kranis, L., Donsky, G., and Leeks, I.: Upper and lower gastrointestinal tract bleeding induced by whole cow's milk in an atopic infant. Pediatrics *40*:661, 1967.

Liu, H.-Y., Tsao, M. U., and Moore, B.: Bovine milk protein-induced malabsorption of lactose and fat in infants. Gastroenterology *54*:27, 1967.

Waldmann, T. A., Wochner, R. D., Laster, L., and Gordon, R. S., Jr.: Allergic gastroenteropathy. N. Engl. J. Med. *276*:761, 1967.

Parasites and Malabsorption

Ament, M. E.: Diagnosis and treatment of giardiasis. J. Pediatr. *80*:633, 1972.

Ament, M. E., and Rubin, C. E.: The relation of giardiasis to abnormal intestinal structure and function in gastrointestinal immunodeficiency syndromes. Gastroenterology *62*:216, 1972.

Brandborg,, L. L., Goldberg, S. B., and Breidenbach, W. C.: Human coccidiosis—A possible cause of malabsorption. N. Engl. J. Med. *283*:1306, 1970.

Stemmerman, G. N.: Strongyloides in migrants. Gastroenterology *53*:59, 1967.

Whalen, G. E., Strickland, G. T., Cross, J. H., Rosenberg, E. B., Gutman, R. A., and Watten, R. H.: Intestinal capillariasis. Lancet *1*:13, 1969.

Malabsorption in Cystic Fibrosis

Hadorn, B., Johansen, G., and Anderson, C. M.: Pancreozymin-secretin test of exocrine pancreatic function in cystic fibrosis. Aust. Paediatr. J. *4*:8, 1968.

Keating, J. P., and Feigin, R. D.: Increased intracranial pressure associated with probable vitamin A deficiency in cystic fibrosis. Pediatrics *46*:41, 1970.

Littman, A., and Hansoom, P. H.: Pancreatic extracts. N. Engl. J. Med. *281*:201, 1969.

Petersen, R. A., Petersen, U. S., and Robb, R. M.: Vitamin A deficiency and night blindness in cystic fibrosis. Am. J. Dis. Child. *116*:662, 1968.

Strober, W., Peter, G., and Schwartz, R. H.: Albumin metabolism in cystic fibrosis. Pediatrics *43*:416, 1969.

Torstenson, O. L., Humphrey, G. B., Edson, J. R., and Warwick, W. J.: Cystic fibrosis presenting with severe hemorrhage due to vitamin K malabsorption: A report of three cases. Pediatrics *45*:857, 1970.

Weber, A. M., Roy, C. C., Morin, C. L., and La Salle, R.: Malabsorption of bile acids in children with cystic fibrosis. New Engl. J. Med. *289*:1001, 1973.

Pancreatic Insufficiency and Bone Marrow Failure

Shwachman, H., Diamond, L. K., Oski, F. A., and Khaw, K.: The syndrome of pancreatic insufficiency and bone marrow dysfunction. J. Pediatr. *65*:645, 1964.

Shmerling, D. H., Prader, A., Kitzig, W. H., Giedion, A., Hadorn, B., and Kuhni, M.: The syndrome of exocrine pancreatic insufficiency, neutropenia, metaphyseal dysostosis and dwarfism. Helv. Paediatr. Acta *24*:547, 1969.

Celiac Sprue

Anderson, C. M., Gracey, M., and Burke, V.: Celiac disease—Some still controversial aspects. Arch. Dis. Child. *47*:292, 1972.

Barr, D. G. D., Shmerling, D. H., and Prader, A.: Catch-up growth in malnutrition, studied in celiac disease after institution of a gluten-free diet. Pediatr. Res. *6*:521, 1972.

Egan-Mitchell, B., and McNichol, B.: Constipation in childhood celiac disease. Arch. Dis. Child. *47*:238, 1972.

Hamilton, J. R., Lynch, M. J., and Reilly, B. J.: Active celiac disease in childhood. Q. J. Med. *38*:135, 1969.

Hamilton, J. R., and McNeill, L. K.: Celiac disease—Duration of therapy. J. Pediatr. *81*:885, 1972.

MacDonald, W. C., Dobbins, W. O., and Rubin, C. E.: Studies of the familial nature of celiac sprue using small intestinal biopsy. New Engl. J. Med. *272*:448, 1965.

Rubin, C. E., Eidelman, F., and Weinstein, W. M.: Sprue by any other name. Gastroenterology *58*:409, 1970.

Young, W. F., and Pringle, E. M.: 110 children with celiac disease, 1950 to 1969. Arch. Dis. Child. *46*:421, 1971.

Short Bowel Syndrome

Heird, W. C., Driscoll, J. M., Schullinger, J. H., Grebin, B., and Winters, R. W.: Intravenous alimentation in pediatric patients. J. Pediatr. *80*:351, 1972.

Wilmore, D. W.: Factors correlating with a successful outcome following extensive intestinal resection in newborn infants. J. Pediatr. *80*:88, 1972.

Abetalipoproteinemia

Gotto, A. M., Levy, R. I., John, K., and Fredrickson, D. S.: On the protein defect in abetalipoproteinemia. N. Engl. J. Med. *284*:813, 1971.

Lees, R. S., and Ahrens, E., Jr.: Fat transport in abetalipoproteinemia. N. Engl. J. Med. *280*:1261, 1969.

Intestinal Lymphangiectasia

McGuigan, J. E., Purkerson, M. L., Trudeau, W. L., and Peterson, M. L.: Studies of the immunologic defects associated with intestinal lymphangiectasia with some observations on dietary control of chylous ascites. Ann. Intern. Med. *68*:398, 1968.

Pomerantz, M., and Waldmann, T. A.: Systemic lymphatic abnormalities associated with gastrointestinal protein loss secondary to intestinal lymphangiectasia. Gastroenterology *45*:703, 1963.

Strober, W., Wochner, R. D., Carbone, P. P., and Waldmann, T. A.: Intestinal lymphangiectasia: A protein-losing enteropathy with hypogammaglobulinemia, lymphocytopenia and impaired homograft rejection. J. Clin. Invest. *46*:1643, 1967.

Weiden, P. L., Blaese, R. M., Strober, W., Block, J. B., and Waldmann, T. A.: Impaired lymphocyte transformation in intestinal lymphangiectasia: Evidence for at least 2 functionally distinct lymphocyte populations in man. J. Clin. Invest. *51*:1319, 1972.

Wolman's Disease

Queloz, J. M., Capitanio, M. A., and Kirkpatrick, J. A.: Wolman's disease. Radiology *104*:357, 1972.

Young, E. P., and Patrick, A. D.: Deficiency of acid esterase activity in Wolman's disease. Arch. Dis. Child. *45*:664, 1970.

Whipple's Disease

Aust, C. H., and Smith, E. B.: Whipple's disease in a 3 month old infant. Am. J. Clin. Path. *37*:66, 1962.

Maizel, H., Ruffin, J. M., and Dobbins, W. O.: Whipple's disease: A review of 19 patients from one hospital and a review of the literature since 1950. Medicine *49*:175, 1970.

Tropical Sprue
Mathan, V. I., Joseph, S., and Baker, S. J.: Tropical sprue in children. Gastroenterology *56*:556, 1969.
Santiago-Borrero, P. J., Maldonado, N., and Horta, E.: Tropical sprue in children. J. Pediatr. *76*:470, 1970.

Malabsorption Due to Stasis
Ament, M. E., Shimoda, S. S., Saunders, D. R., and Rubin, C. E.: The pathogensis of steatorrhea in 3 cases of small intestinal stasis syndrome. Gastroenterology *63*:728, 1972.
Anderson, C. M., Townley, M. R. A. C. P., Freeman, M., and Johansen, P.: Unusual causes of steatorrhea in infancy and childhood. Med. J. Aust. *2*:617, 1961.
Bayes, B. J., and Hamilton, J. R.: Blind loop syndrome in children. Arch. Dis. Child. *44*:76, 1969.
Cockel, R., Anderson, C. M., Hill, E. E., et al.: Familial steatorrhea with calcification of the basal ganglia and mental retardation. Gut *11*:1064, 1970.
Soderlund, S.: Anomalies of midgut rotation and fixation: Clinical aspects based on sixty-two cases in childhood. Acta Paediatr. *51*:(Suppl.) 135, 1966.

Acrodermatitis Enteropathica
Ament, M. E., and Broviac, J.: Acrodermatitis enteropathies (AE)—Demonstration of small and large intestinal mucosal lesions; Failure of hyperalimentation, Intralipid and Diodoquin to reverse the intestinal lesions and generalized malabsorption syndrome. Gastroenterology *64*(A-8):691, 1973.
Cash, R., and Berger, C. J.: Acrodermatitis enteropathica: Defective metabolism of unsaturated fatty acids. J. Pediatr. *74*:717, 1969.
Frier, S., Faber, J., Goldstein, R., and Mayer, M.: Treatment of acrodermatitis enteropathica by intravenous amino acid hydrolysate. J. Pediatr. *82*:109, 1973.

Hypomagnesemia
Friedman, M., Hatcher, G., and Watson, L.: Primary hypomagnesemia with secondary hypocalcemia in an infant. Lancet *1*:703, 1967.
Palmer, L., Radde, I. C., Kook, S. W., Conen, P. E., and Fraser, D.: Primary hypomagnesemia with secondary hypocalcemia in an infant. Pediatrics *41*:385, 1968.
Woodward, J. C., Webster, P. D., and Carr, A. A.: Primary hypomagnesemia with secondary hypocalcemia, diarrhea and insensitivity to parathyroid hormone. Am. J. Dig. Dis. *17*:612, 1972.

Vitamin B_{12} Malabsorption
Gräsbeck, R.: Intrinsic factor and the other vitamin B_{12} transport proteins. Progr. Hematol. *6*:233, 1969.
Hakami, N., Neiman, P. E., Canellos, G. P., and Lazerson, J.: Neonatal transcobalamin II deficiency in two siblings. N. Engl. J. Med. *285*:1163, 1971.
Katz, M., Lee, S. K., and Cooper, B. A.: Vitamin B_{12} malabsorption due to biologically inert intrinsic factor. N. Engl. J. Med. *287*:425, 1972.
Lillibridge, C. B., Brandborg, L. L., and Rubin, C. E.: Childhood pernicious anemia: Gastrointestinal, secretory, histological and electron microscopic aspects. Gastroenterology *52*:792, 1967.
MacKenzie, I. L., Donaldson, R. M., Jr., Trier, J. S., et al.: Ileal mucosa in familial selective vitamin B_{12} malabsorption. N. Engl. J. Med. *286*:1021, 1972.

Folate Malabsorption
Lanzkowsky, P.: Congenital malabsorption of folate. Am. J. Med. *48*:580, 1970.

ANUS, RECTUM AND SIGMOID

Congenital anomalies of the anus and rectum are relatively common. The true incidence is not known, but it has been estimated that an anal or rectal anomaly of some extent can be expected in about one of each 400 births. Major anomalies which require surgical correction have been estimated to occur in about one of 1000 births.

MALFORMATIONS OF THE ANUS AND RECTUM

The term "imperforate anus" should be abandoned in favor of the more inclusive term "anorectal malformation." The most useful clinical classification separates "low" and "high" lesions, in accordance with whether the rectum does or does not pass through the puborectalis muscle, which is a major portion of the levator ani muscle of defecation. In the low type the bowel passes through the puborectalis sling; it may end abruptly at the skin, in a fistula to the median raphe of the perineum or, in girls, in a fistula to the vestibule. In the high type the muscle is not traversed; if there is a fistula, it leads most often to the urinary tract in males or to the upper part of the vagina in females.

EMBRYOLOGY AND PATHOGENESIS. In the normal embryology of the anus, after the cloacal stage there is a division of the cloacal cavity by a downgrowth of the mesoderm (the urorectal septum) into a ventral part, which will form the bladder and urethra, and a dorsal part, which forms the rectum. There is a small communication, the cloacal duct, between the two systems which is closed by the seventh week of gestation by a downgrowth of the urorectal septum. An ingrowth of mesoderm divides the cloacal membrane into the urogenital membrane ventrally and the anal membrane dorsally. During the seventh week the urogenital portion of the original cloaca has acquired an external opening, but the anal membrane does not open until later. The anus develops by an external invagination known as the proctodeum, which deepens toward the rectum, but is separated by the anal membrane. This membrane ruptures by the eighth week of gestation.

Interference with the development of anorectal structures at varying stages gives rise to a variety of anomalies which range from anal stenosis, incomplete rupture of the anal membrane or anal agenesis (the "low" types) to complete failure of descent of the upper portion of the cloaca and failure of invagination of the proctodeum (the "high" types). The persistence of the communication between the urinary and rectal portions of the cloaca is responsible for fistulas, which are more common in the male. In the female, fistulas connect the rectum more commonly with the vagina than with the urinary system.

Since the muscle of the anal sphincter is derived from exterior mesoderm, it is usually intact and not involved with the obstructive lesions of the anus and rectum.

DIAGNOSIS. Evaluation of the newborn infant with an anorectal malformation should be directed toward establishing whether a low or high lesion is present, since initial treatment, definitive treatment and prognosis differ for these two lesions.

Stenosis of the anorectal canal may occur at any point or extend its entire length. The constriction can be identified by digital and endoscopic examination. Imperforate anal membrane is readily identified as a thin translucent membrane which becomes progressively distended by the meconium just behind it.

More than 90 per cent of the other low anomalies are associated with an external fistula to the perineum or vestibule. These fistulas may not be apparent at birth, but peristalsis will gradually force meconium through the fistula. Repeated careful examinations during the first 24 hours of life will eventually in most cases reveal a tiny speck of meconium at the opening of the fistula. Roentgenograms employing contrast media injected through a tiny catheter inserted into the fistula will confirm the diagnosis.

A poorly developed anal dimple, a rounded perineum, or vertebral anomalies suggest a high lesion. Passage of meconium in the urine is diagnostic of a rectourinary fistula and a rectal pouch ending above the puborectalis muscle. In equivocal cases, a lateral roentgenogram in the upside down position (Wangensteen-Rice view, Fig. 11–21) may be obtained after clinical distention is evident. A distance of less than 1.5 cm from the bowel to the perineal marker is indicative of a low anomaly.

If none of these measures clearly identifies the level of the rectal pouch it is safest to assume the infant has a high lesion. Blind exploration of the perineum in hopes of finding a low lying rectal pouch should not be done.

Associated anomalies are common in these babies. Significant urinary tract and vertebral abnormalities occur in about half the patients with high anorectal malformation and one quarter of those with low types. Excretory urography should be done in all cases, and should precede definitive therapy in high lesions. The anatomy of the bony pelvis may reveal sacral anomalies, which may be important to later bowel or urinary functions.

TREATMENT. Anal stenosis can generally be treated by manual dilatations. All other forms of imperforate anus should be surgically corrected.

In the low types the bowel has the proper levator relationship, so that they can be repaired from below. A careful mucocutaneous reconstruction is essential.

The high types are best treated by a preliminary

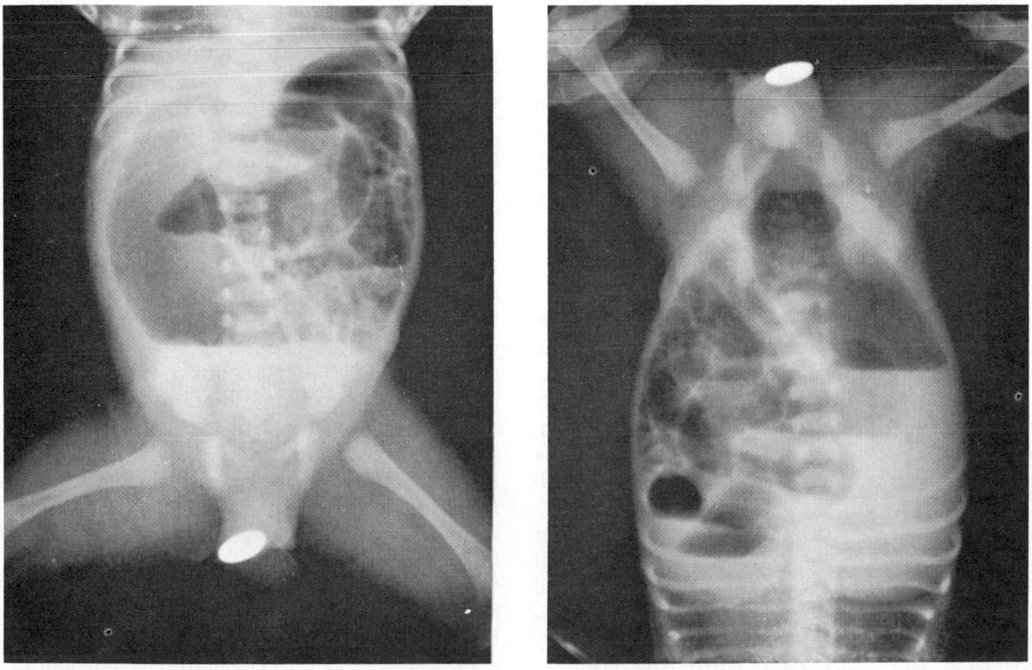

A B

Figure 11–21 Wangensteen-Rice roentgenographic technique for demonstration of the position of the blind colonic pouch in the case of an imperforate or absent rectum. The infant is held head downward, causing the intestinal gas to rise to the blind end of the gut. A, Roentgenogram of child in upright position, showing transverse level of gas. The level of the obstruction is not demonstrated. B, The level of the obstruction is apparent when the roentgenogram is taken with the child in the inverted position. The site of the anus is marked by a lead disk.

colostomy followed by a definitive repair in 6 to 12 months by an abdominoperineal, sacroperineal or sacroabdominoperineal approach, depending on the lesion and the preference of the surgeon. Careful positioning of the anus in the region of the external sphincter, and anatomic positioning of the bowel in the puborectalis sling are essential. Recognition of a fistula so that it can be eliminated is most likely when the reparative operation is delayed.

The surgical care of anorectal malformations is not complete until the child has adequate bowel control. The surgeon who knows the nature and degree of the disturbed anatomy and physiology must work closely with the child, the family and the pediatrician in order to achieve optimal results.

The higher the blind pouch and the more extensive the operation, the more difficulty one encounters in the postoperative period. Significant sacral anomalies are usually associated with deficient development of the pelvic parasympathetic plexus; this may interfere with neurologic control of defecation. With continuing care through the period of training a satisfactory functional solution can usually be expected. In a few instances there will be continuing problems due to stenosis, poor anal control or poor guidance. In the postoperative period constipation rather than, as one might expect, incontinence is the principal problem. The lack of sensation of fecal material in the rectum leads to fecal impactions with paradoxical or overflow diarrheal stools and gives rise to the acquired type of megacolon. Early attention to ensure regular evacuations will prevent massive fecal impactions. As a rule, the child should be taught to defecate at a given time of day rather than await the urge. In some instances a daily enema may be needed.

FISSURE IN ANO

Fissure in ano, a small slit or crack at the mucocutaneous line, is a common acquired lesion in infancy and childhood. The cause is often not evident, but the lesion may be caused by trauma secondary to overzealous cleaning or to constipation, by scratching induced by irritation from *Enterobius vermicularis,* and by eczema and other perianal conditions.

CLINICAL MANIFESTATIONS. Pain on defecation and often refusal to defecate are the principal manifestations. Bright red blood on the surface of the stool and sometimes bleeding following defecation may be observed. The diagnosis is made by inspection of the anal area while the child is straining.

TREATMENT. Most fissures will heal spontaneously if the local irritation is lessened or eliminated. This can usually be accomplished by the use of bland suppositories or instillations of mineral oil and by gentle dilatations of the anus. Oral medication to soften the stool may be indicated, and sitz baths may provide relief from the pain. A neglogic disturbances from fecal soiling. Surgery is serious constipation problems and eventually in acquired megacolon, with the associated psychologic disturbances from fecal soiling. Surgery is rarely necessary. (See Constipation, p. 816.)

PRURITUS ANI

Anal itching in childhood is generally secondary to enterobiasis, anal fissures and other local inflammatory lesions and to coarse or moist undergarments. Nocturnal itching is perhaps the most frequent evidence of pinworm infestation. Treatment consists in eradication of the underlying cause, and in cleansing the anal area with a mild soap and drying it with a soft cloth or tissue. Powders or solutions such as witch hazel may be used. In small infants exposure to sunlight or dry heat for as long as possible is helpful when the anal area is inflamed.

PROLAPSE AND PROCIDENTIA OF THE RECTUM AND SIGMOID

Prolapse is abnormal descent of the mucous membrane of the rectum with or without protrusion through the anal orifice; *procidentia* is abnormal descent of all the coats of the rectum or sigmoid with or without protrusion through the anus. These conditions are most common from 3 to 5 years of age. The infantile rectum lies on a lower plane than the other pelvic organs. This anatomic arrangement, combined with the effect of the nearly vertical infantile sacrum, predisposes to prolapse. Any factor causing suddenly increased intra-abdominal pressure may precipitate abnormal descent of the bowel wall. Malnutrition with absorption of ischiorectal fat is a contributory factor. Children with cystic fibrosis are particularly prone to develop prolapse. Protrusion at stool initially recedes spontaneously, but later requires manual replacement. Bleeding and the passage of mucus may occur. The protruding mass varies from bright to dark red; it may be as much as 6 inches in length. In prolapse the striations or furrows radiate from the center of the anal aperture, in contrast to the concentrically arranged rosette of procidentia.

Treatment should be directed to dietary correction of constipation, to proper toilet training and to the elimination of any underlying disturbance, such as parasitic infection, diarrhea or polyps. Oral administration of mineral oil, rectal instillations of olive oil and strapping the buttocks together with adhesive tape, having first placed a cotton ball over the anal area, may be helpful.

Reduction of protrusion is aided by pressure with hot compresses. Cold packs are contraindicated.

An easy method of reduction is to cover the finger with a piece of toilet paper, introduce it into the lumen of the mass and gently push it into the rectum. The finger is then immediately withdrawn. The toilet paper adheres to the mucous membrane, permitting release of the finger; the paper, when softened, is later expelled. For intractable cases perineal operation may be indicated. In procidentia of the rectum and sigmoid, abdominal sigmoidopexy is required.

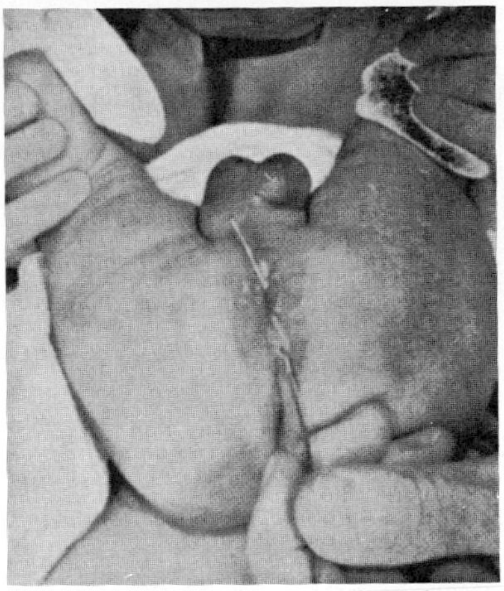

Figure 11–22 Complete anorectal fistula in a child 15 weeks of age; probe demonstrating external and internal openings. (Bacon, H.: Anus, Rectum and Sigmoid Colon. Philadelphia, J. B. Lippincott Company.)

ANORECTAL ABSCESS

An anorectal abscess is usually located in the ischiorectal fossa. Infection usually gains entrance through the anal crypts and the preformed spaces. The symptoms are pain and swelling. Defecation is painful, and the child is unable to sit comfortably. The temperature is not much elevated unless the perirectal space is invaded. A painful swelling overlies the ischiorectal fossa, with redness, heat, induration and fluctuation. Treatment consists in immediate incision and drainage under anesthesia. Hot sitz baths, 3 times daily, are helpful in the postoperative period.

FISTULA

Fistulas originating in the anus or rectum may be congenital or acquired and may extend to and communicate with the urinary bladder, urethra, vagina or perianal skin. Acquired fistulas are residuals of an abscess and usually open on the skin surface. There is frequently a history of one or more incisions into the abscess.

SYMPTOMS. The symptoms of an acquired fistula are those of a painful swelling which recurs intermittently, followed by a purulent discharge. Diagnosis is based on the presence of an opening into the skin beside the anal orifice into which a probe may be introduced (Fig. 11–22).

TREATMENT. Conservatism is indicated in the care of fistulas in infants. Many will close spontaneously without surgery. If surgical extirpation is necessary, care must be taken to incise rather than excise the sphincter in order to prevent incontinence. Simple incision and removal of the fistulous tract with packing of the resultant defect is usually effective.

HEMORRHOIDS

Hemorrhoids are uncommon in infants and children. When they are encountered, one must look for the underlying cause, such as a venacaval or mesenteric obstruction, cirrhosis, portal hypertension, or other reasons for venous obstruction. Occasionally, chronic constipation, fecal impaction and straining at stool result in hemorrhoids as they do in adults. Operation is rarely indicated except for an acute external thrombus. The condition generally subsides when the primary condition is corrected.

NEOPLASMS

See Section 25.

CONGENITAL DEFECTS OF THE SACROCOCCYGEAL REGION

PILONIDAL SINUS AND CYST. *Pilonidal sinus* is a congenital defect which probably results from faulty coalescence or invagination of the ectoderm in the midline over the sacrococcygeal region during early embryonic development. It is characterized by formation of a sinus tract in which are collected the products of dermal activity. Infection enters through the original site of invagination or through aberrant tracts which become manifest after puberty. A *pilonidal dimple* is commonly encountered, but is asymptomatic.

Pilonidal cysts and sinuses do not cause symptoms unless infection has occurred. The presence of swelling, heat, redness, tenderness, and fluctuation over the sacrococcygeal region is characteristic of an infected sinus. Purulent material may be discharged from one or more openings. If infection occurs, total excision should be performed. (See Section 20 for a discussion of complications occurring within the spinal canal.)

TUMORS OF THE SACROCOCCYGEAL REGION. See Section 25.

Kiesewetter, W. B., and Nixon, R. H.: Imperforate anus. I. Its surgical anatomy. J. Pediatr. Surg. *2*:60, 1967.
Rehbein, F.: Imperforate anus: Experiences with abdominoperineal and abdominosacro-perineal pull through procedures. J. Pediatr. Surg. *2*:99, 1967.
Santulli, T. V., et al.: Malformations of the anus and rectum. Surg. Clin. N. Amer. *45*:1253, 1965.
Santulli, T. V., et al.: Anorectal anomalies: A suggested international classification. J. Pediatr. Surg. *5*:281, 1970.
Santulli, T. V., et al.: Imperforate anus: A survey from the members of the surgical section of the American Academy of Pediatrics. J. Pediatr. Surg. *6*:484, 1971.

APPENDICITIS

Appendicitis, rare in the first year of life, has been noted in early infancy. The incidence increases after the first year of life; most cases occur in the first three decades. Males are slightly more prone to appendicitis than females. The mortality of this disease has progressively declined; on the other hand, the percentage of children hospitalized with a ruptured appendix and localized or generalized peritonitis has not changed significantly. Further reduction in the morbidity from appendicitis can be accomplished only by earlier recognition and treatment of the disease, before the inflamed appendix ruptures.

ETIOLOGY. Obstruction is the primary factor in the pathogenesis of appendicitis. The obstruction may be secondary to inflammatory changes from blood-borne or enteric infections or may be mechanical, as by pinworms, a fecalith, other foreign body, stenosis or kinking. Soft fecal material is commonly found in the lumen of the appendix, but has doubtful pathologic significance. In some instances appendicitis appears to be related to an infection of the upper respiratory tract, but a significant correlation is not established. Such systemic infections as rheumatic fever, measles, scarlet fever and other exanthems are infrequently responsible for appendicitis.

Peritonitis or appendiceal abscess eventually occurs from perforation of the inflamed appendix. Coliform organisms predominate in cultures, but a mixed flora is usually responsible for the infection. Recent improvements in microbiologic techniques have identified anaerobic organisms as major contributors to appendiceal infections.

PATHOLOGY. Inflammation begins in the mucosa, which may ulcerate; the wall is edematous and infiltrated with neutrophils; the lumen is distended, often enough to impair the blood supply and produce gangrene and perforation. In milder types there may be mucosal ulceration without obstruction. Bacteria may escape through a perforation or the intact gangrenous wall to produce diffuse peritonitis or an abscess confined by adherence of adjacent omentum and intestines.

CLINICAL MANIFESTATIONS. Epigastric pain shifting to the right lower quadrant and accompanied or followed by nausea, vomiting and low-grade fever is the classic pattern of acute appendicitis. It is the one observed commonly in older children, but relatively infrequently in infants and young children. About 70 per cent of children 5 years of age or younger who have acute appendicitis have a perforation of the appendix and peritonitis when first seen medically. The prodromal manifestations are usually not appreciated in the very young; perforation of the appendix takes place relatively quickly in the thin-walled appendix, and the omentum is not sufficiently developed to afford adequate protection against diffuse peritoneal spread.

Most children 4 years of age and under have difficulty in localizing pain; a finger pointed at the umbilicus or the mother's description of the positions of preference taken by the child, such as knees drawn up or reluctance to move the legs, is as much aid in localization as one may get. When perforation of the appendix has occurred in the very young child, he appears acutely ill with grunting respirations, a rigid abdomen, flaring of the alae nasi, an ashen color and an anxious expression. Extreme prostration may be preceded by an unaccustomed period of inactivity. Fever prior to rupture of the appendix may be absent or of low grade. After development of peritonitis the temperature is usually elevated to 39.5° C or more (103 to 105° F). Subnormal temperature in a prostrated child has serious implications. Active peristalsis may persist for some time with generalized peritonitis.

The initial symptom in the older child is pain, usually persistent rather than intermittent, which increases progressively in severity. With localized ileus, secondary to appendiceal inflammation, the pain may be intermittent or crampy. The amount of vomiting appears to be somewhat related to the position of the appendix; if the organ is retrocecal or deep in the pelvis, no vomiting may occur. Peritoneal irritation and pain may also be masked by the position of the appendix. Constipation is more common than diarrhea, though a pelvic appendix irritating the bowel in the cul-de-sac may produce mucus and diarrhea. Frequency of urination may be produced by an inflamed appendix adjacent to the bladder.

DIAGNOSIS. Persistent pain in the abdomen, insidious or abrupt in onset, accompanied by *persistent* localized tenderness in the right lower quadrant, involuntary muscular spasm and rigidity are evidence of localized intraperitoneal irritation. Nausea and vomiting are frequently present, and low-grade fever is more characteristic than chills and high fever at the onset of the disease. The distinction between voluntary and involuntary muscle spasm or guarding is important. When the frightened young child tenses his abdominal muscles at the sight of a white coat or the touch of a large, cold hand, the abdominal examination becomes unreliable. A gentle, unhurried approach gains the confidence of the child, and involves time well spent. In some cases, sedation with a short-acting barbiturate will allay apprehension and eliminate voluntary muscle guarding. Narcotic analgesics should not be given since they may mask signs of intraperitoneal inflammation.

Other signs of peritoneal irritation such as cough and rebound tenderness are helpful when elicited. An inflamed retrocecal appendix, however, may have deep tenderness as the only physical finding, and, when the appendix is in the pelvic area, there may be no abdominal findings. The rectal examination should be the final step in the physical examination, but must never be omitted, since it may provide valuable information.

Peristalsis is generally decreased or absent in the presence of intraperitoneal infection, but it may be hyperactive during the early stages. A positive psoas sign, or the tendency of the patient in bed to draw his legs up, is also suggestive of a right lower quadrant inflammatory lesion.

There is usually a mild leukocytosis of 14,000 to 16,000 cells per mm^3 with a preponderance of immature polymorphonuclear cells. Excessively high total leukocyte counts are suggestive of an abscess or peritonitis. Leukopenia associated with prostration and a shocklike state may indicate overwhelming sepsis.

Differential Diagnosis. A history of antecedent or concomitant respiratory or enteric disease, poorly localized pain, fever out of proportion to the abdominal findings or variations in the intensity of pain may suggest *mesenteric adenitis*, but an exact differential diagnosis can be made only by laparotomy.

Prolonged, severe *constipation* may also simulate an acute surgical condition of the abdomen. When feces are easily palpated, and one has reason to suspect fecal obstruction of the bowel, a saline enema of moderate amount may be given. In contrast to the valid objections to catharsis under such a situation, an enema judiciously given may be valuable diagnostically.

Infection of the urinary tract may mimic appendicitis. Urinalysis is indispensable in evaluation of abdominal pain. The urinalysis may be within normal limits, however, in the presence of completely obstructed hydronephrosis. On occasion an intravenous pyelogram may be required for differential diagnosis.

Pneumonia, especially of the right lower lobe, may simulate appendicitis. Abdominal tenderness and muscular tightness are apt to be somewhat higher with the pulmonary infection than with appendicitis. A roentgenogram of the chest will usually clarify the diagnostic situation.

The abdominal pain of *acute gastroenteritis* may on occasion suggest the possibility of appendicitis. Persistent *diarrhea* is rare as a symptom of appendicitis, though several loose stools may herald the onset of disease. If diarrhea persists after an acute abdominal episode, the possibility of a *pelvic abscess* should be considered. The differential diagnosis depends mainly on the physical findings. The two conditions may occur concomitantly.

Meckel's diverticulitis may simulate appendicitis. Blood, with or without mucus, in the stool favors diverticulitis. *Intussusception* must be considered, particularly in children under 5 years of age. Intermittent sharp pain, the presence of an abdominal mass and blood by rectum are the differential features. A barium enema, which is contraindicated in appendicitis, may be useful in confirming and localizing the intussusception.

Ovarian lesions, such as cysts, ruptured follicles or a twisted pedicle, must be considered in girls, especially in the older ones.

Acute rheumatic fever, diabetes mellitus, regional enteritis, abdominal epilepsy, sickle cell crisis, infectious mononucleosis and nonicteric infectious hepatitis must also be considered diagnostic possibilities; these are described in their respective sections.

When one is confronted with evident peritonitis, the possibility of a primary infection as well as one secondary to a ruptured appendix must be considered. The former lesion is now encountered so infrequently, however, even in patients with nephrosis, and the consequences of continued drainage from a ruptured appendix are so serious that the differential diagnosis should be established by laparotomy.

COMPLICATIONS. Whether localized abscess formation and diffuse secondary peritonitis (see below) are to be considered complications or part of the natural course of acute appendicitis may be debatable, but they are the only common sequels. Perforation occurs earlier and more frequently in children than in adults, and there is less tendency for the infection to become localized. This failure to localize has been attributed to the relatively small size of the omentum in young children. A pelvic abscess occasionally occurs, but subphrenic abscess is rare. Less common complications are paralytic ileus and thrombophlebitis.

Postoperative complications of acute appendicitis include abscess of the operative wound, multiple intra-abdominal abscesses, intra-abdominal adhesions and intestinal obstruction.

PROGNOSIS. There is great danger in postponing operation for appendicitis, since local or diffuse peritonitis consistently follows perforation, and almost negligible risk attends operation before perforation. Even when perforation has occurred, the mortality rate may be less than 1 per cent. This low rate is probably due to several factors, including improvements in preoperative preparation, operative technique, anesthesia, parenteral fluid therapy and antibacterial therapy.

TREATMENT. Appendectomy, with adequate external drainage in cases of abscess formation, is the only appropriate treatment of acute appendicitis. High fever, dehydration, overwhelming sepsis and a shocklike state are reasons for delay until appropriate preoperative correction can be attained. Convulsions during anesthesia are common in children with high fever. Induced hypothermia, hydration and antibiotic therapy are indicated. The temperature should be below 39° C

(102° F) and the pulse below 120 before anesthesia is initiated.

Managements of appendiceal abscess and of diffuse peritonitis are considered below, and that of preoperative and postoperative fluid therapy in Section 5. Reasonably early ambulation after removal of an unperforated appendix and dismissal from the hospital within a few days are usually possible.

Fields, I. A., and Cole, N. M.: Acute appendicitis in infants thirty-six months of age and younger. Am. J. Surg. *113*:269, 1967.
Holder, T. M., and Leape, L. L.: The acute surgical abdomen in children. New Engl. J. Med. *277*:921, 1967.

PERITONEUM AND ALLIED STRUCTURES

MALFORMATIONS OF THE PERITONEUM

Congenital peritoneal bands may be responsible for intestinal obstruction; numerous other anomalies may occur in the course of the development of the peritoneum, but are rarely of clinical importance. Intra-abdominal herniations infrequently occur through ringlike formations produced by anomalous peritoneal bands. Absence of the omentum or duplications of it are rare anomalies. Omental cysts and torsion of the omentum are unusual causes of acute abdominal crises leading to laparotomy.

ASCITES

ETIOLOGY. The term "ascites" indicates an accumulation of fluid in the peritoneal cavity, but it is usually applied to accumulations of serous fluid. Renal, especially nephrotic, and cardiac conditions are most often responsible for ascites. It may represent an accumulation of fluid secondary to chronic adhesive pericarditis, or it may be part of a polyserositis in so-called Pick syndrome. Other causes include obstruction of the portal circulation as in hepatic cirrhosis or by enlarged lymph nodes, tumors, thrombosis, chronic tuberculous peritonitis, rheumatic peritonitis or obstruction of the splenic vein.

CLINICAL MANIFESTATIONS. The abdomen is distended; when distention is great, there is flattening or pouting of the umbilicus. Fluctuation can be detected on palpation; a wavelike impulse is obtained by sharp tapping on one side of the abdominal wall while the other hand is placed on the opposite side of the abdomen and an assistant's hand compresses it in the midline; shifting percussion dullness can often be demonstrated.

Ascites must be differentiated from other conditions which cause distention of the abdomen. These include gaseous distention of the intestines, fecal distention as in megacolon, tumor masses, including cysts of the mesentery, acute or chronic peritonitis, peritoneal hemorrhage, extreme distention of the bladder and simple obesity.

PROGNOSIS AND TREATMENT. The course, prognosis and treatment depend entirely upon the cause.

CHYLOUS ASCITES

The accumulation of chyle is an uncommon form of ascites which may occur at any age of childhood and is occasionally congenital in origin. True chylous ascites is caused by some anomaly, injury or obstruction of the thoracic duct within its abdominal portion. In the case of anomalies the condition is present at birth or shortly thereafter. There may be an associated chylothorax. Obstructions may be produced by enlarged lymph nodes or neoplasms. The fluid has the appearance of milk, owing to its high fat content. In chronic peritonitis, peritoneal fluid may have a somewhat similar color from degeneration of inflammatory products.

The prognosis of chylous ascites is unfavorable, but recovery may occur. The accumulation of chyle can be reduced by providing a diet containing medium-chain triglycerides which are absorbed directly into the portal circulation. Since there is a loss of considerable protein in this fluid, high protein diets should be prescribed. Abdominal exploration is justified to search for the site of the leak, if a trial of dietary management is unsuccessful.

PERITONITIS

Acute infections of the peritoneum are arbitrarily designated as *primary* when the focus is outside the abdominal cavity and the infection is blood- or lymph-borne. The infection is termed *secondary* when it is disseminated by extension from or rupture of an intra-abdominal viscus or of an abscess of one of the solid organs.

Peritonitis in the neonatal period may arise from a transplacental infection in utero; more frequently it is the result of infection acquired during or shortly after birth. It may be a manifestation of septicemia, a direct extension from an umbilical infection, perforation of the intestine or, rarely, the sequel of a ruptured appendix. Meconium peritonitis is described in Section 7. After the neonatal period, peritonitis is uncommon until later childhood, when appendicitis becomes relatively frequent.

ACUTE PRIMARY PERITONITIS

ETIOLOGY. Primary peritonitis has become rare in children. In the past it was caused most often by the pneumococcus and the beta-hemolytic streptococcus, but now staphylococci and gram-negative organisms are being recovered more frequently. Ascites from nephrosis or cirrhosis is a major predisposing factor, but the disease may occur in otherwise healthy children. It is more common in girls than in boys and in some instances a nongonorrheal vaginitis appears to be the portal of entry. Gonococcal peritonitis is a rare complication of gonorrheal vaginitis.

CLINICAL MANIFESTATIONS. The onset may be insidious or rapid, with extreme prostration, some abdominal pain and vomiting. Intestinal peristalsis usually continues until late in the disease, and diarrhea is common. The facial expression is likely to be anxious; there is often cyanosis, and the child appears toxic and weak. The temperature usually rises and may be as high as 40° C or more (104 to 105° F); in very ill patients, and especially in young infants, it may be normal or subnormal. The pulse is rapid, small and compressible, and the respirations are rapid and shallow because of the pain which abdominal respiration produces. There is usually distention of the abdomen, moderate diffuse tenderness and a doughy resistance. Evidence of free fluid may be present. Rectal examination reveals tenderness. The white blood cell count is high, ranging from 20,000 to 35,000 cells per mm^3; 90 to 95 per cent are polymorphonuclear cells, with an increase in immature forms.

DIAGNOSIS AND TREATMENT. In most cases the clinical picture is indistinguishable from appendicitis with or without perforation, and the diagnosis should be established at laparotomy. If primary peritonitis is suspected preoperatively, paracentesis may be helpful. Gram-stain and culture showing only gram-positive organisms exclude an enteric source of infection and obviate the need for exploration. Supportive therapy and intravenous antibiotics chosen on the basis of the smear and culture are generally effective treatment.

ACUTE SECONDARY DIFFUSE PERITONITIS

ETIOLOGY. This type of peritonitis usually results from perforation of an abdominal viscus, most often an inflamed appendix. Peritonitis secondary to intussusception, volvulus, incarcerated hernia, perforation of the intestine by a foreign body or rupture of a Meckel's diverticulum is infrequent. Perforation of the intestine in meconium ileus and spontaneous rupture of the stomach or intestines are infrequent causes in the neonatal period, and perforation of a peptic ulcer, though infrequent, is more common in early infancy than in later childhood. The invading bacteria are most often coliform bacilli with varying numbers of other organisms belonging mainly to the streptococcal and staphylococcal groups.

CLINICAL MANIFESTATIONS. The manifestations of shock from a ruptured viscus or the early symptoms of acute appendicitis are followed by an increasing toxemia, as evidenced by greater restlessness and irritability, by a higher temperature, often 39.5° C or more (103 to 105° F), by an increase in the pulse rate and, at times, by chills or convulsions. In extreme situations, and especially in early infancy, the temperature may be normal or subnormal. Vomiting, if previously present, is usually increased. The pain tends to be more diffuse over the abdomen, but may not be too notable if the patient remains quiet. Constipation is marked.

The child has an anxious expression, and there is progressive evidence of prostration. Dehydration and loss of electrolytes through vomiting are contributory factors. There are rapid pulse, splinting of the diaphragm, and rectal tenderness. Peristalsis may persist until late in the course of disease.

The white blood cell count is usually 16,000 to 25,000 per mm^3, the polymorphonuclear elements usually being above 90 per cent.

TREATMENT. Adequate preoperative preparation is essential and may require 6 to 8 hours. These measures include rehydration, correction of electrolyte imbalance, gastric suction and antimicrobial therapy. Combinations of antibiotics will improve the spectrum of effectiveness against aerobic and anaerobic organisms. Relief of pain by meperidine (Demerol), morphine or codeine contributes to improvement. The pulse rate should be reduced below 120 and the temperature below 39° C (102° F) if possible prior to operation. Severely ill patients may require mild hypothermia. Operative therapy consists in drainage and repair of the perforated viscus.

ACUTE SECONDARY LOCALIZED PERITONITIS
(Peritoneal Abscess)

ETIOLOGY. A single, localized pyogenic abscess, most often secondary to perforation of an inflamed appendix, is somewhat less common in children than in adults. The poor ability of young children to localize a peritoneal infection of appendiceal origin has been attributed to lower general resistance and to a relatively smaller omentum. Though localized peritoneal abscesses occur most often in the appendiceal region, they may be at any site, originating from various sources; or appendiceal infections may gravitate to other areas, notably the pelvis. An abscess in the subdiaphragmatic area may originate from an appendiceal or other intra-abdominal infection or, rarely, from an empyema.

CLINICAL MANIFESTATIONS. The general symptoms of *peritoneal abscess* are continued fever or recurrences of it, poor appetite and vomiting following ingestion of food. The white blood cell count is increased, with a predominance of polymorphonuclear cells. With *appendiceal abscess*, tenderness in the right lower quadrant is extended, and there is often a palpable mass.

A *pelvic abscess* is suggested by abdominal distention, rectal tenesmus with or without the passage of small stools containing mucus, or bladder irritability. Rectal examination may reveal a tender mass anteriorly.

A *subphrenic abscess* is evidenced by physical signs at the base of the lung, usually on the right, owing to elevation of the diaphragm and frequently to the presence of pleural fluid. The diagnosis can often be established roentgenographically. The diaphragm is elevated and the liver depressed if the infection is on the right side, and there is frequently a pocket of air just below the diaphragm, owing to production of gas by bacteria.

TREATMENT. The abscess should be drained and appropriate antibiotic therapy provided. Initial broad-spectrum coverage should be modified, if indicated, by the results of sensitivity tests of the bacteria obtained from cultures. If the appendix cannot be removed at the initial operation, an appendectomy should be performed subsequently within 3 months.

TUBERCULOUS PERITONITIS

See Section 10.

HERNIA AND HYDROCELE

Hernias of various types may be present at birth or develop subsequently, often because of congenital defects. The uncommon femoral hernia and the rare internal hernias other than that of the diaphragm will not be discussed. Congenital omphalocele and umbilical hernia are discussed in Section 7.

INGUINAL HERNIA

ETIOLOGY AND PATHOLOGY. Most inguinal hernias are of the indirect rather than the direct type and occur much more frequently in boys than in girls. These hernias may be present at birth or may appear at any age thereafter; they are situated more often on the right side than on the left, but frequently are bilateral.

During embryonic life, as the testis descends retroperitoneally from the genital ridge, a sac of peritoneum (the processus vaginalis) precedes it into the scrotum. The lower portion of this sac envelops the testis to form the tunica vaginalis, and the remainder normally atrophies by the time of birth. The indirect inguinal hernia results from a persistence of the processus vaginalis and becomes manifest as a mass in the inguinal region when an abdominal structure or peritoneal fluid is forced into it. The persistent sac may vary from a short one not extending beyond the external inguinal ring to one which extends into the scrotum and maintains its continuity with the tunica vaginalis. The hernial sac is thus present at birth, but it usually remains empty for a variable period of time. Later, commonly by 2 or 3 months of age, when the infant becomes more active and is able to increase his intra-abdominal pressure sufficiently to open the sac, peritoneal fluid or an abdominal organ is forced into it. The hernial sac then appears as a bulge in the inguinal region, extending into the scrotum or toward the labia.

CLINICAL MANIFESTATIONS. There are no symptoms associated with an empty hernia sac. When abdominal contents are intermittently forced into it, symptoms of incomplete bowel obstruction with pain, fretfulness, difficult defecation, poor appetite and local pressure may result. On the other hand, there may be few or no symptoms associated with a filled hernial sac. If a loop of intestine becomes incarcerated in the sac, there may be all the manifestations of intestinal obstruction ultimately leading to strangulation of the bowel and death. In female infants the ovary may prolapse into the hernial sac and appear as a 1- to 2-cm movable, nontender, usually transient inguinal mass. Prompt surgical exploration and abdominal replacement of the ovary are indicated unless strangulation has destroyed the ovary, when excision is indicated. Occasionally the neck of the sac closes after peritoneal fluid has been forced into it and traps the fluid as an encysted, nontender irreducible hydrocele in the cord in the male or in the canal of Nuck in the female.

DIAGNOSIS. A history of the intermittent appearance of a mass in the inguinal region of an infant or child is characteristic. If the hernial sac is full at the time of examination and can be emptied by gentle compression, or if it can be made to fill when the infant cries or strains or the older child stands or coughs, the diagnosis is established. Often, however, the history is only suggestive. Inspection may reveal a fullness on the affected side, especially after recent incarceration. Palpation for an enlarged internal ring by invaginating the scrotum is fruitless during the early developmental stage of the hernia, since the ring is not enlarged, nor are the muscles weakened. Gentle palpation by rolling a finger over the spermatic cord at the level of the pubic tubercle will reveal thickening of the cord on the involved side, and often the "silk glove" sensation may be elicited by rubbing together the two sides of the empty hernial sac. This maneuver should be performed as part of routine physical examinations in infants in order to discover a hernial sac so that it can be removed before incarceration occurs.

The only difficulty in diagnosis is in distinguishing hernia from hydrocele. A hernial sac is often opaque to transmitted light, whereas the hydrocele is translucent. A hernia, however, may also be translucent if the sac contains only distended and empty bowel. The inguinal hernia is usually reducible with gentle manipulation and tends to slip suddenly into the peritoneal cavity. By contrast, the encysted hydrocele is not reducible; the communicating one is, but reduction is usually accomplished with great difficulty and without sudden emptying of the sac. Characteristically it is reduced most readily after the patient has been in the horizontal position for a prolonged time, as during a night's sleep. The coexistence of a communicating hydrocele and an inguinal hernia is relatively common.

TREATMENT. The treatment of inguinal hernias in healthy infants and children is by surgical repair as soon as the defect is diagnosed. The operation consists essentially in removing the hernial sac and transfixing the neck at the internal ring. It is well tolerated even by small infants and obviates the possibilities of incarceration, testicular atrophy, secondary enlargement of the internal ring and weakening of the floor of the canal from prolonged pressure. Treatment by injection of sclerosing agents is contraindicated in infants and children. Trusses are not recommended even for temporary use. They are difficult to apply correctly and impossible to keep clean. Every effort should be made to prepare the infant or child for early surgical repair.

The need for bilateral rather than unilateral inguinal exploration in the child with unilateral hernia is controversial. There is a high incidence of patent processus vaginalis contralateral to a hernia in infants under the age of 2 years. Some studies show that as many as 47 per cent of children in this age group who have unilateral herniorrhaphy will return later with a hernia on the opposite side. Arguments against routine bilateral exploration are that the additional surgery is unnecessary in 50 to 90 per cent of the children, that the duration of anesthesia is prolonged, and that there is a small but definite risk of injury to the testicle. We believe that with experienced pediatric anesthesiologists and surgeons these risks are minimal. Our own policy is routinely to perform bilateral exploration in children under 2 years of age.

Incarcerated Inguinal Hernia

Incarceration of inguinal hernias is common in children and occurs most often in the first 6 months of life. It is manifest by the appearance of a firm, tender, globular, irreducible swelling below the external inguinal ring. The infant is fretful and often vomits. Unless the condition is relieved, abdominal distention, cessation of bowel movements, persistent vomiting, fever and leukocytosis will develop as impairment of the blood supply progresses.

Manipulative reduction is the treatment of choice for an incarcerated hernia which has been present for less than 12 hours and has not been accompanied by a bloody stool. The infant is adequately sedated (with a barbiturate if under 6 months of age or with morphine in an older patient). He is then placed in the Trendelenburg position with a roll of cloth under the buttocks, and an ice bag is placed on the affected side to decrease the edema. A parent is kept at the bedside, if possible, to comfort and quiet the infant. After an hour or more, when the sedation has taken effect and the infant is asleep, the mass is gently grasped with all fingers of the physician's warmed hand and squeezed with gentle equal pressure by all digits toward the inguinal canal. This maneuver frequently leads to reduction. The patient should be admitted to the hospital and observed closely for several hours for signs of peritoneal irritation to make certain that nonviable bowel has not been reduced. Herniorrhaphy should be performed within a 24- to 48-hour period, following correction of any metabolic disturbance. Delay in operation increases the risk of recurrent incarceration.

If the incarcerated hernia cannot be reduced or if it is inadvisable to attempt reduction, owing to the duration of incarceration, emergency surgical correction must be undertaken.

HYDROCELE

A hydrocele is the presence of fluid anywhere within the course of the processus vaginalis.

Newborn male infants whose processus vaginalis has been obliterated often have residual peritoneal fluid in the tunica vaginalis of the testis. This common type of *noncommunicating hydrocele* forms an oval, fluctuant, tense, translucent sac, and the spermatic cord and ring can usually be felt above it. The fluid gradually absorbs during the first year of life, and surgical correction is rarely required.

If the processus vaginalis remains open, peritoneal fluid may be forced into it, forming a hydrocele of the spermatic cord or of the canal of Nuck in the female. An inguinal hernia is often associated. Frequently the parents note that the "testis seems larger" in the evening after an active day, and smaller the following morning. This history is highly suggestive of the *communicating hydrocele* (see Diagnosis under Inguinal Hernia). The length of the hydrocele is dependent upon the extent of the patency of the processus vaginalis. If it extends into the tunica vaginalis, then the elongated fluctuant mass extends to the lower part of the scrotum. When the occlusion is at a higher level, the hydrocele is a fluctuant swelling above the scrotum or extends only a short way into it. Occasionally the fluid becomes trapped in the sac and forms a firm globular mass which is irreducible and resembles an incarcerated inguinal hernia. If the fluid is at some distance below the external inguinal ring or has been present for several days and is neither tender nor symptomatic, the diagnosis of a hydrocele may safely be made.

Since the appearance of a hydrocele some time after birth is evidence of a persistent processus vaginalis, the hydrocele should be extirpated by the inguinal route and the hernial sac removed. Aspiration of the tunica vaginalis or injection of sclerosing solutions is not warranted; either may cause adhesions which make the ultimate operation more difficult, or may damage the testis.

EPIGASTRIC HERNIA

Epigastric hernias occur in the midline between the umbilicus and the lower end of the sternum. They are not common and, except for their location, are similar to umbilical hernias. They may become acutely painful and tender when a bit of preperitoneal fat becomes incarcerated. They should be repaired surgically.

INCISIONAL HERNIA

Postoperative hernias should be repaired as soon as the local condition of the wound and the general condition of the child warrant it. There is no justification for permitting children to continue with the discomfort attendant on this type of hernia. Incisional hernias tend to enlarge and may also become incarcerated.

DIAPHRAGMATIC HERNIA

Diaphragmatic hernias may be congenital (Fig. 11–23) or acquired. Acquired hernias are usually traumatic in origin and are not considered here. Congenital herniation of abdominal contents into the thoracic cavity may be responsible for serious embarrassment of respiration and usually constitutes a medical-surgical emergency in the immediate neonatal period. Infrequently there is little or no respiratory embarrassment, and the hernia may not be detected until later in infancy or childhood. In addition to herniation through a defect in the diaphragm (see below), there may be partial herniation of the stomach through the esophageal hiatus (Section 11), phrenic paralysis with displacement of abdominal contents upward, but not herniated (Section 7), and eventration of the diaphragm. *Eventration is not a herniation,* but is also an upward displacement of abdominal contents into an outpouching or saclike structure of the diaphragm resulting from a weakness or absence of diaphragmatic musculature without an abnormal opening. The clinical manifestations of an eventration may simulate those of a diaphragmatic hernia. Rarely there is complete absence of the diaphragm.

ETIOLOGY. Herniation occurs most often in the posterolateral segments of the diaphragm, and more often on the left than on the right side. The defect represents failure of the pleuroperitoneal canal to close completely during embryonic devel-

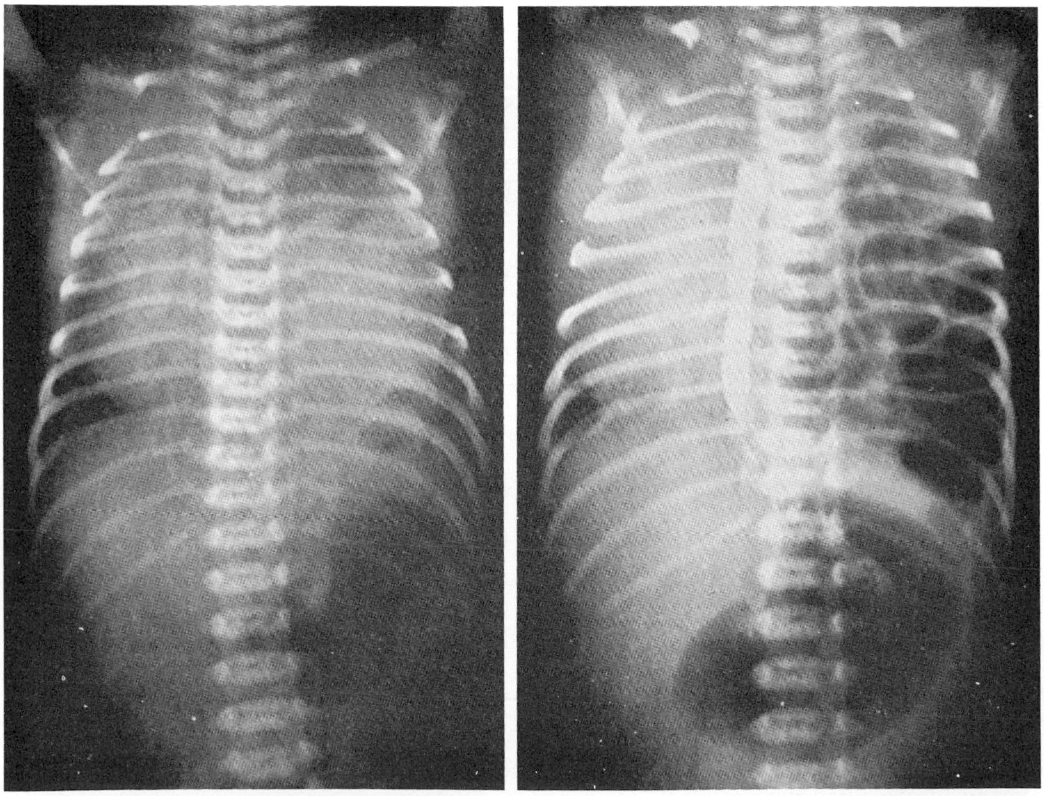

A B

Figure 11–23 Congenital diaphragmatic hernia. A, Film exposed shortly after birth: distortion of shadow of left leaf of diaphragm, with huge, masslike density in left hemithorax displacing heart to right. B, Film exposed about 20 minutes after A. As the result of swallowed air, coils of air-filled small bowel are now demonstrated in the left hemithorax. The esophagus is outlined by swallowed contrast material. Operative correction was attempted because of extreme dyspnea. Infant died 5½ hours after birth.

opment (foramen of Bochdalek). Much less frequently the herniation is in the anterior portion of the diaphragm in the retrosternal area; this defect represents failure of midline fusion of the two anlagen of the diaphragm with elements of the pericardium (foramen of Morgagni). With this defect there may be herniation of intestine into the pericardial sac or, conversely, ectopia cordis with displacement of the heart into the peritoneal cavity. Umbilical defects are commonly associated with herniation through the foramen of Morgagni.

PATHOLOGY. There are various degrees of protrusion of the abdominal viscera through a diaphragmatic hernia into the thoracic cavity. In severe cases the stomach and a large part of the intestines and even, in rare instances, the spleen, liver and kidneys displace the lungs and heart. There may be associated incomplete rotation of the cecum, umbilical defects and duodenal constricting bands. The lung on the affected side is compressed and often hypoplastic. Hypoplasia of the opposite lung has also been observed.

DIAGNOSIS. Severe respiratory distress, including dyspnea and cyanosis, is frequently present from birth. If symptoms are not present at birth, they may appear at any time during the neonatal period or later. These include vomiting, severe colicky pain, discomfort after eating and constipation as well as dyspnea. Symptoms and signs of acute intestinal obstruction may occur at any time. Infrequently there are no symptoms, and the condition may be discovered by chance roentgenographic examination.

The physical examination varies considerably, depending on the degree of displacement of abdominal contents into the thoracic cavity. When there is extensive displacement in the newborn infant, the abdomen is usually small and scaphoid in contour, and the infant is cyanotic and has obvious respiratory retractions. If the respiratory embarrassment is not relieved, shock and rapidly progressive hypoxia occur. In contrast, in mildly affected patients there may be no or only minimal respiratory distress and no digestive disturbance.

The percussion note over the part of the thorax containing the stomach and intestines may be more tympanic or duller than usual and the breath sounds absent, decreased or increased. Occasionally sounds of intestinal peristaltic movements can be heard over the chest.

The diagnosis can usually be established by roentgenographic examination, usually without the aid of contrast medium, or, if such is needed, air injected into the stomach may be sufficient. Characteristically, in the neonatal period there are fluid and air-filled loops of intestine in the chest which simulate cysts. The mediastinum is displaced toward the unaffected side, usually the right. Occasionally, in the case of cystic adenomatoid malformations of the lung or congenital lobar emphysema, it may be necessary to use contrast material to demonstrate that the stomach and intestines are in the abdominal cavity.

TREATMENT. Resuscitation of the newborn is mandatory prior to undertaking reduction of the hernia and closure of the diaphragmatic defect. As soon as the diagnosis is suspected, the newborn infant should be positioned with his head and thorax higher than the abdomen and feet to facilitate the downward displacement of the abdominal organs. Nasogastric intubation with intermittent suction will decrease entrapment of air and fluid within the herniated viscera and lessen the degree of ventilatory compromise. Positive pressure ventilation, if needed, should be administered cautiously through an endotracheal tube since pneumothorax may result, owing to the uneven distribution of intrapulmonary pressures in lungs affected by compression atelectasis or pulmonary hypoplasia. Arterial blood gas determinations, including pH, should be obtained preoperatively and metabolic and respiratory acidosis corrected with appropriate intravenous doses of sodium bicarbonate.

Emergency and definitive surgical correction is indicated. A subcostal incision provides excellent exposure of the diaphragm, and the herniated contents can be reduced into the peritoneal cavity after the pressures in the pleural and peritoneal cavities are equalized. Re-expansion of the hypoplastic ipsilateral lung may take several days. No attempt should be made to forcefully inflate the lung as this invariably causes a pneumothorax.

ROBERT J. TOULOUKIAN
JOHN H. SEASHORE
LAWRENCE K. PICKETT

Baran, E. M., and others: Foramen of Morgagni hernias in children. Surgery *62*:1076, 1967.

Golden, G. T., and Shaw, A.: Primary peritonitis. Surg. Gynec. Obstet. *135*:513, 1973.

Jackson, T. M.: Congenital diaphragmatic hernia. Arch. Surg. *95*:102, 1967.

McNamara, J. J., Eraklis, A. J., and Gross, R. E.: Congenital posterolateral diaphragmatic hernia in the newborn. J. Thorac. Cardiovasc. Surg. *55*:55, 1968.

Swenson, O.: Diagnosis and treatment of inguinal hernia. Pediatrics *34*:412, 1964.

THE LIVER

ANATOMY. The liver of the full-term infant weighs 120 to 160 gm at birth. The weight is doubled at 2 years and tripled at 3 years; at 9 years it has increased six times, and at puberty, ten times. The liver of the adult is twelve to thirteen times as large as that of the newborn infant. The relative sizes of the lobes of the liver change with age; at birth the right lobe is twice as large as the left lobe; in young children and adolescents it is about three times as large. The functional right and left lobes, drained by the right and left hepatic ducts and supplied with corresponding portal venous branches and hepatic veins, differ from the anatomic lobes. In the newborn infant the liver edge is usually less than 2 cm below the costal margin in the right midclavicular line. The upper border of hepatic dullness is at the level of the fifth or sixth rib in the mammary line and extends nearly horizontally. In the axillary line it is usually in the seventh intercostal space and posteriorly in the ninth space. The lower border of the liver may be normally palpable about 1 cm below the costal margin throughout childhood.

Extramedullary hematopoiesis, varying inversely in amount with the birth weight, may be found normally in the liver of infants for a few weeks after birth.

CONGENITAL ANOMALIES AND MALPOSITIONS. *Absence* of the liver has been reported in stillborn fetuses in association with other severe anomalies. The lobes of the liver may vary in size and shape; either one may be absent, or there may be more than two. Riedel's lobe is the tonguelike downward projection of the right lobe. A "floating liver" occurs when there is congenital elongation of the ligaments which support the organ. In situs inversus the liver is on the left side; rarely, with diaphragmatic hernia it may be located in the thorax.

Downward displacement of the liver is produced by contractural deformities of the thorax (rickets), relaxation of the abdominal musculature (severe malnutrition, amyotonia congenita and other paralyses) or increased intrathoracic pressure (empyema, pneumothorax or pulmonary hyperaeration). Subphrenic abscess or a collection of air (perforation of the gastrointestinal tract) will also push the liver downward. The less common upward displacement may be caused by ascites, abdominal tumors or paralysis of the diaphragm.

METABOLIC FUNCTIONS. Owing to its important role in the metabolism of foodstuffs, the liver has been aptly termed the commissariat of the body.

The liver plays the leading role in maintenance of the normal blood sugar level. It *forms and stores glycogen* from glucose, levulose, galactose and dextrolactate. It converts the glycogenic amino acids and the glycerol fraction of fats into dextrose, which is deposited as glycogen (glycogenesis). Glycogen can be reconverted into glucose by the liver (glycogenolysis). Thus, the liver serves as a storehouse of readily available glucose which can be delivered to the blood when required. The livers of infants contain proportionately less glycogen than those of children.

The liver is the site of both *synthesis and oxidation of fat.* Hepatic lipogenesis from acetate and pyruvate depends upon the normal functioning of both the anaerobic glycolytic (Embden-Meyerhof) and phosphogluconate pathways of carbohydrate metabolism. Most, if not all, of the fat mobilized in the liver is combined with lecithin and changed to *phospholipid,* a change which is apparently necessary for its transport and subsequent use. Dietary deficiency of lipotropic factors (e.g., choline, inositol or compounds which can contribute methyl groups for the formation of choline) prevents the formation of the more soluble phospholipid, so that fat accumulates in the liver. *Cholesterol* is formed in the liver from its esters or by synthesis from acetic acid. Cholesterol esters, i.e., compounds of cholesterol and fatty acids, which constitute 70 per cent of the plasma cholesterol, are also formed in the liver and are a means for the rapid transport of cholesterol. The plasma *lipoproteins* which transport triglycerides also appear to be, in part, formed in the liver.

The liver (and kidney) breaks down long-chain fatty acids into *ketone bodies,* which are burned by and supply energy to the muscles and other tissues which cannot form them. When fat is burned in excess (starvation and diabetes), large amounts of ketone bodies accumulate and are excreted in the urine.

Urea is formed exclusively in the liver by the deamination of amino acids. The liver is concerned with the formation of many fractions of the *serum proteins.* Fibrinogen, a globulin, is formed exclusively in the liver. Prothrombin and other coagulation factors and probably all the serum albumins are of hepatic origin. The liver also serves as a storage depot for protein. There is a large labile fraction of the hepatic proteins which increases with a high protein diet and decreases during starvation. In many disease states of the liver there is an increased concentration of serum globulins.

Vitamins A, C and D are stored in the liver, and considerable amounts of A and D remain for a long time after the administration of single large doses. The precursors of vitamin A are converted into vitamin A in the liver. The damaged liver has a reduced storage capacity for vitamin A and a lowered capacity for the conversion of its precursors. Riboflavin and vitamins E and K have important metabolic storage relations to the liver.

Influence of Diet upon the Liver. The vulnerability of the liver to toxic agents may be reduced or eliminated by various dietary constituents. A high carbohydrate diet has a protective action for the liver. This has been attributed to the resultant increased glycogen content of the liver, but may be due to other factors. An adequate protein intake also shields the liver from toxic injury; *methionine* and *cystine* are recognized as some of the protective elements in protein.

Dietary deficiencies lead to hepatic injury. A low protein diet results in massive hepatic necrosis, specifically as a result of cystine deficiency. Absence of tocopherol from the diet also predisposes to this type of liver damage. Protein deficiency of lesser degree or a high fat diet produces fatty infiltration of the liver which slowly progresses to diffuse hepatic fibrosis. This sequence of hepatic injury may be prevented by the inclusion of choline or methionine in the diet.

BLOOD FORMATION. The fetal liver is a site of active blood formation. Hematopoiesis is common in the livers of premature and occasionally of full-term infants as a remnant of this fetal function. In conditions such as hemolytic anemias in which excessive demands are placed on the blood-forming mechanisms, the liver undergoes myeloid metaplasia and resumes its hematopoietic activity. During the early months of infancy the liver also serves as a storehouse for iron which is used when the infant's diet is chiefly milk and is low in iron. With depletion of this store by about the fifth month, hypochromic anemia develops if the diet does not contain an adequate iron content.

DETOXIFYING FUNCTIONS. The liver can alter various exogenous toxic substances by conjugating them with sulfuric acid, glucuronic acid (an oxidation product of glucose) or amino acids. The conjugation mechanism is probably more concerned with increasing the solubility of the toxic substance so that it can be more easily transported through the body fluids and excreted than it is with a direct reduction in toxicity. Thus sulfanilamide is converted into the more soluble but more toxic compound, acetyl sulfanilamide. The liver also appears to be the principal site for removal of ammonia from the blood. The natural and synthetic estrogenic and androgenic substances are inactivated by the liver. Excesses of these hormones in the body, when the damaged liver fails to dispose of them, result in abnormal physiologic effects.

Biochemistry of Liver Disease and Liver Function Tests

Knowledge of the wide variety of functions performed by the normal liver has led to the development of biochemical methods for their evaluation. Among these are tests useful in defining the ability of the liver to conjugate and excrete bilirubin, to synthesize serum proteins and coagulation factors, to contribute to carbohydrate homeostasis, to dispose of ammonia as urea, and to conjugate various drugs and hormones. Other indices of hepatic disturbance which are generally less specific reflect the immunologic response of the organ to injury. In this category are the flocculation and turbidity tests and electrophoretically determined alteration in gamma globulin concentration.

The acutely injured liver cell may permit spillage of intracellular enzymes into the blood, where their increased levels are measurable. Most widely studied of this group are the serum transaminases, glutamic-oxaloacetic (SGOT) and glutamic-pyruvic (SGPT).

Clinical evaluation of liver function may include examination of excretory capacity for certain dyes such as Bromsulphalein as well as physiologic substances normally excreted by this organ: cholesterol, bile acids, alkaline phosphatase and bilirubin. The quantities of bilirubin metabolites in the stool and urine give valuable information relating to the adequacy of metabolic and anatomic excretory pathways.

Radiologic techniques are of great value in evaluating hepatic disorders. Cholangiography with introduction of contrast medium by oral, intravenous, transhepatic and direct injection into the gallbladder plays a part in the study of patients suspected of having disease of the gallbladder or of the extrahepatic biliary system. Contrast radiographic studies may disclose varices of the esophagus or, by distortion of the normal duodenal configuration, give suggestive evidence of the presence of obstructive dilatation of the common duct or mass lesions in the pancreas or its adnexa.

Transabdominal splenoportal venography with concomitant portal pressure measurements may confirm the presence of portal hypertension and document the presence of collateral circulation between portal and systemic venous systems. The same information may also be achieved by cannulation of the tiny lumen of the obliterated umbilical veins found in the falciform ligament as it passes extraperitoneally beneath the linea alba. The vessel is dilated to its entrance into the left portal vein, after which pressure measurements are made and venography is carried out. This procedure is more likely to show successfully the portal vein than is splenic venography, but it fails more often to show collaterals. It merits consideration also because it may be carried out under local rather than general anesthesia, avoids the occasional rupture of the spleen encountered in the usual venographic procedure, and also permits study of patients who have been subjected to splenectomy. Dye injected into the celiac axis through a catheter introduced into the femoral artery and threaded up the iliac to the aorta may give a good view of the intrahepatic arterial circulation, the portal vein and existent collaterals. Distortion of the intrahepatic circulation may disclose the presence of tumors or inflammatory masses. These lesions may also be seen by scintillation scanning techniques utilizing radioactive substances such as colloidal gold or ^{131}I-labeled rose bengal.

The hepatic circulation can also be evaluated by sampling hepatic venous and systemic arterial blood, utilizing dyes or radioactive substances extracted by the liver.

BILIRUBIN METABOLISM

Bilirubin is a linear tetrapyrrole formed by cleavage of the cyclic tetrapyrrole, protoporphyrin. Protoporphyrin and iron form a complex (heme), which is the prosthetic group of hemoglobin and other hemoproteins. Bilirubin is freely soluble in organic solvents, but only slightly soluble in aqueous solutions at physiologic pH. The levels of pigment can be measured accurately after it is coupled with diazotized sulfanilic acid (diazo or van den Bergh reaction). Unconjugated bilirubin reacts in aqueous solution only in the presence of accelerator substances, methanol or ethanol (indirect reaction), whereas conjugated bilirubin reacts in their absence (direct reaction). After the newborn period, the total bilirubin in plasma does not exceed 1.0 mg/dl, with 0.2 mg/dl reacting directly. The accuracy of measurement does not warrant attaching clinical significance to elevations in concentration of the direct reacting pigment up to 0.4 mg/dl.

The conversion of heme to bilirubin involves cleavage of the ferroprotoporphyrin ring by microsomal heme oxygenase to yield biliverdin. The latter compound is reduced to bilirubin by biliverdin reductase.

The serum bilirubin concentration reflects a dynamic process of production and excretion. Bilirubin is derived from several sources. Studies using labeled precursors of bilirubin have shown the label to appear first in the fecal bilirubin (urobilinogen) within 1 to 2 days. This "early labeled" fraction, representing 10 to 20 per cent of the daily bilirubin production, is derived from chromoproteins such as myoglobin, cytochromes, catalase and peroxidases, and also from maturing red blood cells in bone marrow. The remaining 80 per cent of bilirubin appears later, as senescent red blood cells, aged around 120 days, are removed from the blood. Each of these sources represents potential overproduction.

Unconjugated bilirubin is a potentially toxic, end-stage metabolite which must be eliminated from the body. The efficient process evolved for the accomplishment of this involves enzymatic degradation of heme compounds, binding of bilirubin by albumin in the circulation, uptake and conjugation in the hepatocyte, transport to the intestine, and reduction to compounds (urobilinogen) which are minimally reabsorbed and thus largely excreted in the stool.

Essentially all the bilirubin in blood is tightly bound to albumin. In addition to conferring solubility in water, the linkage of bilirubin with albumin restricts its transfer across cell membranes and protects cells from bilirubin toxicity. The total bilirubin-binding capacity of plasma is approximately 20 to 25 mg/dl. In competition with bilirubin for binding sites on albumin are sulfonamides, thyroxine and possibly acetylsalicylates. The displacement of bilirubin by these substances from its linkage to albumin is of particular importance to the icteric neonate in whom bilirubin concentrations may rise to levels which saturate the total binding capacity of albumin.

HEPATIC UPTAKE AND CONJUGATION. Within the liver cell, mechanisms exist which establish a gradient for the movement of unconjugated bilirubin from plasma to cell and facilitate its removal into bile. The lipid-soluble unconjugated bilirubin easily crosses the lipid-containing membrane of cells. A specific carrier system in the membrane of the hepatocyte has been postulated, but not demonstrated. Well characterized, however, are the Y and Z cytoplasmic acceptor proteins of the hepatocyte, which are capable of binding unconjugated bilirubin, preventing its back-diffusion from the hepatocyte, and fostering further transfer of the pigment from the plasma. This process may be competitively inhibited by other organic anions which are excreted in the bile, such as flavaspidic acid and certain cholecystographic agents.

The liver cell owes its unique capacity to remove bilirubin from the plasma to its ability to convert cytoplasmic pigment to water-soluble conjugates of glucuronic acid. Their ionic nature and increased molecular size limit their back-diffusion across the plasma membrane and at the same time foster their excretion into bile.

The conjugation of bilirubin with glucuronic acid requires uridine diphosphoglucuronic acid, which donates its glucuronic acid to the two propionic acid side chains of bilirubin. The reaction is catalyzed by the microsomal enzyme glucuronyl transferase. The enzyme may be induced by phenobarbital and other compounds.

The bacterial flora of the lower bowel reduces conjugated bilirubin to a group of chromogens designated urobilinogen. Urobilinogen is poorly reabsorbed from the bowel, and about 100 to 200 mg/day are excreted in the stool of adults. Of the small amount reabsorbed, most is excreted by the liver, with approximately 4 mg/day appearing in urine; this amount is not detectable by the usual semiquantitative tests for urobilinogen.

From the above considerations it will be clear that increased plasma levels of unconjugated bilirubin may derive from overproduction of bilirubin by hemolysis, from impaired hepatic uptake, or from impaired glucuronide conjugation. Increased plasma concentrations of conjugated bilirubin will stem from situations which permit bilirubin to gain access to the hepatocyte and undergo conjugation but interfere with its transport into the intestine (parenchymal cell injury, obstruction of the biliary tree, or functional disorders of secretion into the bile).

The color of feces yields important clues to the origin of jaundice. Acholic stools are commonly seen during the early stages of hepatitis and are usual in complete obstruction of the extrahepatic biliary tree. Under these circumstances small amounts of bile pigment measured as urobilinogen may be found. Bilirubin may reach the intestine with intestinal secretions, where it is reduced by bacteria to urobilinogen. Quantitative estimations of fecal urobilinogen are difficult, but have a place in obscure situations when increased hemolysis is suspected.

The Harrison spot and commercial tablet or strip tests for conjugated bilirubin are useful and easily performed. Bilirubin conjugates are not usually detected in urine unless the plasma concentration exceeds approximately 1 mg/dl. In acute viral hepatitis, bilirubin appears in the urine before urobilinogenuria and jaundice are noted. Its presence in urine is an early sign of hepatotoxic effects in patients receiving chlorpromazine or iproniazid, or who are exposed to carbon tetrachloride.

SERUM ENZYMES. For enzymes present in large quantities in liver tissue, the serum levels rise when they are lost to the circulation as a result of injury to the liver cell or when egress of a particular enzyme is blocked by obstructive processes. Liver cells are particularly rich in enzymes exhibiting transaminase, dehydrogenase, peptidase, nucleotidase and alkaline phosphatase activities. Since enzymes are rarely organ-specific, changes in serum concentrations may indicate possible injury of more than one organ. The enzymes responsible for serum activity have been shown to be heterogeneous (isoenzymes); with further delineation of these, organ specificity will no doubt be increased.

Phosphatases catalyze the hydrolysis of phosphoric acid esters. The International Unit for alkaline phosphatase is currently standard and applicable to results of the Bessey-Lowry procedure (Table 11–9). The enzyme is normally secreted in bile; with hepatocellular disease its production is decreased, and with obstruction of the biliary tract its excretion is impaired. In starch gel electrophoresis bone and hepatic alkaline phosphatases take similar positions. The serum of patients with intrahepatic or extrahepatic obstruction has three additional bands, in the beta lipoprotein, and alpha-2 and beta globulin regions. Since this picture is also exhibited by normal bile, it appears that the changes in the serum result from regurgitation of bile from the biliary passages.

TABLE 11–9 NORMAL VALUES OF SERUM ALKALINE PHOSPHATASE (INTERNATIONAL UNITS PER LITER)

AGE	RANGE
1 to 3 months	73–226
3 to 10 years	57–151
Puberty	57–258
16 years and older	13.8–38.4

TABLE 11–10 NORMAL VALUES OF TRANSAMINASES (IU PER LITER)

AGE	SGOT	SGPT
Infants	67 to 118	0 to 54
Older children	3 to 27	1 to 30

In obstructive jaundice, serum alkaline phosphatase concentrations usually markedly exceed normal limits. Concurrent elevation of serum 5-nucleotidase activity serves to confirm the phosphatase as of biliary origin. In jaundice due to hepatocellular injury, the elevation is of lesser degree. The levels in incomplete biliary obstruction, as found in common duct stenosis or primary biliary cirrhosis, are particularly high and out of proportion to the serum bilirubin concentration. It thus appears that the alkaline phosphatase level is a more sensitive indicator of bile stasis than is the serum concentration of bilirubin. Alkaline phosphatase levels are commonly elevated in the presence of hepatic tumors, even in the absence of jaundice. The level is also raised with other space-occupying hepatic lesions such as amyloidosis, leukemia, abscess, tuberculosis or sarcoidosis. Elevation of alkaline phosphatase also accompanies disease of the bone, particularly rickets and hyperparathyroidism.

The serum *transaminases* are of particular value in indicating the presence of active hepatocellular injury (Table 11–10). Glutamic oxaloacetic transaminase (GOT) is present in large amounts in heart, liver, skeletal muscle and kidney and appears in increased amounts in the circulation when cell destruction occurs in these tissues. Particularly high values accompany hepatocellular necrosis and myocardial infarction. There is more glutamic pyruvic transaminase (GPT) in liver cells than in cardiac or skeletal muscle cells; it is therefore a more specific index of hepatocellular injury. The differentiation of hepatic disease from myocardial infarction is not a significant clinical problem, and SGOT determinations alone are adequate.

Transaminase determinations are of particular value in the early diagnosis of viral hepatitis, especially in anicteric patients. Values above 800 units for SGOT are strongly suggestive of viral hepatitis and may also be seen in infectious mononucleosis. The elevation may be transient, with return to normal within a week of onset. Sustained elevations suggest continued activity of the disease. Transaminase determinations are also helpful in detecting toxic hepatitis. Levels in cirrhosis are variable, with relatively higher concentrations in active juvenile cirrhosis. Moderate elevations, usually below 100 units, are found in obstructive jaundice; in biliary atresia, however, levels as high as 800 units have been encountered.

The *dehydrogenases* are catalysts in oxidation-reduction reactions. Lactate dehydrogenase (LDH) is separable into five isoenzymes, each of which is comprised of combinations of two polypeptide chains. The highest serum LDH activity in hepatitis is found in the slowest moving electrophoretic band. Normal values in infants up to 10 days of age range from 308 to 1780 IU per liter (avg. 815), and in older subjects from 87 to 186. Values two to five times normal have been observed in acute and chronic hepatitis and in cirrhosis. The enzyme is not elevated in obstructive jaundice.

The *5-nucleotidase* of liver catalyzes the alkaline hydrolysis of phosphomonoesters only of the pentose 5′-phosphate nucleotides. It is therefore more specific than alkaline phosphatase. Its normal serum concentration is 0.3 to 3.2 Reis units. It is particularly elevated in obstructive jaundice, in contrast to hepatocellular disease.

DYE EXCRETION TESTS. The determination of the hepatic clearance of *Bromsulphalein (sulfobromophthalein, BSP)* is the most sensitive test of liver function. The injected dye is bound to albumin in the plasma and after clearance by the liver is excreted into the bile. BSP excretion by the liver involves selective uptake and concentration by the liver cell and the rate-limiting transport of both glutathione-conjugated and unconjugated dye into the bile canaliculi. In the standard test 5 mg/kg of the dye are injected intravenously. The normal person clears 90 and 96 per cent of the injected dye at 30 and 45 minutes, respectively. Additional information involving storage and excretory capacity for BSP may be obtained by measuring plasma clearance when the dye is infused intravenously. One or both of these values may be reduced when other usual tests of liver function give normal results. Changes in hepatic blood flow may reduce clearance of the dye in congestive heart failure or portal vein thrombosis. Clearance is also reduced with hepatocellular injury, metabolic abnormalities or obstructions to bile flow.

PROTEINS AND HEPATIC FUNCTION

Albumin. When albumin synthesis is depressed as a result of hepatocellular disease, the serum albumin concentration and total body pool decrease. These changes are not rapid, owing to the slow rate of albumin degradation (half-life 12 to 18 days).

Globulins. In clinical laboratory evaluations, electrophoretic analysis of the serum globulin fractions is becoming routine. Alpha and beta globulin concentrations increase in a variety of infectious processes and in obstructive jaundice. They decrease when liver cell failure reduces their synthesis. Immunoglobulins increase in response to antibody formation stimulated by exogenous or tissue antigens. Although production of gamma globulin is not a function of the liver, its determination may be helpful in hepatic diagnosis. Extreme elevation may be found in children with postnecrotic or biliary cirrhosis as well as in lupoid hepatitis.

Serum Haptoglobins. Haptoglobins are alpha-2 globulins which have the property of combining stoichiometrically with hemoglobin. It has been reported but not confirmed that their level falls in cirrhosis and rises with obstructive jaundice. A decreasing concentration with increasing jaundice is characteristic of infectious hepatitis.

Flocculation and Turbidity Tests. These are not specific for liver disease. Flocculation or precipitation of the plasma proteins depends upon changes in various serum factors which tend to maintain the serum proteins in solution.

Hepatitis Associated Antigen (Australia Antigen). This plasma protein is discussed below. (See Infectious Hepatitis.)

COAGULATION FACTORS. Many of the blood clotting factors are synthesized by the liver and may be reduced in hepatic parenchymal injury. Among these are fibrinogen (factor I), prothrombin (factor II) and factors V, VII, IX, X, XI and XIII. Reduction in any of these factors may cause prolongation of the one-stage prothrombin time. Vitamin K is a requirement for hepatic synthesis of prothrombin and factors VII, IX and X. Deficiency of vitamin K may result from decreased bacterial synthesis in the intestine following antibiotic treatment or from impaired absorption, with biliary tract obstruction and consequent reduction in bile salt concentration in the small bowel.

Specific alterations in coagulation factors are characteristic of particular types of liver disease. In cirrhosis, factor VII is decreased more than factors II, V and X. Factor V is more reduced in acute hepatitis. Factor XIII is low in acute hepatitis and normal in obstructive liver disease. Thrombocytopenia and intravascular coagulation can also contribute to the bleeding characteristic of liver disease.

Because of the rapid turnover (half-life 2 to 4 days) of a number of the coagulation factors, the one-stage prothrombin test serves as a sensitive indicator of changes in liver function in patients with acute liver disease. If abnormal values persist after vitamin K has been given parenterally to correct any deficiency secondary to malabsorption or impaired synthesis, severe liver damage is indicated.

FETAL ALPHA-1 GLOBULIN (α_1-FETOPROTEIN). The embryonic liver cell synthesizes an alpha-1 globulin which is present in fetal serum and cord blood. Shortly after birth the protein disappears and its presence late in life has been associated with hepatoma. In children this alpha-1 globulin is particularly characteristic of hepatoblastoma and teratoblastoma. Its determination is a valuable diagnostic test and assists in evaluating completeness of removal of a hepatoma.

BILE ACIDS. Recent advances in methodology,

including thin-layer and gas-liquid chromatography, have given new dimensions to the study of bile acid synthesis, excretion and metabolism, and are affording new understanding of liver disease, especially in pathologic processes of cholestatic nature, and in the pathophysiology of gastrointestinal disease in the adult. They will eventually aid in the evaluation of liver disease in the newborn, but current techniques for bile acid determination are complex and not available for routine clinical evaluation. Normal plasma values are less than 5 nanomoles/ml.

CHOLESTEROL. Variations in serum cholesterol concentrations reflect changes in serum lipoproteins. Cholestasis results in impaired excretion of cholesterol and bile acids, so that with normal synthesis of cholesterol, serum concentrations of lipoproteins and cholesterol are increased. Impaired synthesis of hepatic lipoprotein with hepatocellular disease leads to decreased serum cholesterol levels.

NEEDLE BIOPSY OF THE LIVER. Percutaneous needle biopsy of the liver by an intercostal approach under local anesthesia is a relatively safe procedure. The Menghini needle (size 1.0 to 1.8 mm), utilizing suction aspiration of the tissue, provides a more rapid and effective means of obtaining tissue than the Vim-Silverman needle. In young infants, in whom liver disease is almost invariably associated with hepatomegaly, a subcostal rather than a transthoracic approach is safer. Heavy sedation is necessary for all pediatric patients. The procedure is indicated in patients with otherwise unexplained jaundice, hepatomegaly and splenomegaly, as well as in evaluating progress in patients with subacute or chronic liver disease. It may also be useful in the diagnosis of unexplained fever, when biopsy may establish the presence of tuberculosis, sarcoidosis, brucellosis or neoplasia.

The procedure is contraindicated in patients with anemia, coagulation defects (prothrombin less than 60 per cent of control) and in infants in whom liver enlargement is not sufficient to permit a subcostal approach. The procedure should not be performed in patients suspected of having a vascular tumor of the liver. Hemorrhage from the biopsy site and leakage of bile from perforation of dilated intrahepatic ducts are unusual.

(See section on portal hypertension for discussion of venography and portal pressure measurements.)

Disorders Affecting Excretion of Bilirubin

Hyperbilirubinemia may be encountered with hepatic disease or with little or no evidence of it. The elevation in serum bilirubin which may be either of the conjugated or unconjugated type is the result of a failure of one or more steps involved in the normal pathway for excretion of bilirubin (Fig. 11–24): uptake by the liver cell, glucuronide conjugation, transport from the conjugation site in the smooth endoplasmic reticulum, and excretion via the bile canaliculi.

These disturbances may be temporary or permanent and appear at birth or in later infancy and childhood. For purposes of diagnosis it is convenient to group hyperbilirubinemias on the basis of whether the increase is predominantly of unconjugated or conjugated bilirubin (Table 11–11).

UNCONJUGATED HYPERBILIRUBINEMIAS

BILIRUBIN EXCRETION IN THE NEWBORN. Unconjugated lipid-soluble bilirubin formed by the fetus freely crosses the placenta and is excreted by the maternal liver. During the first week of extrauterine life, hepatic function is not adequate to prevent its accumulation in the plasma. This situation has been regarded as physiologic when it is limited to this age group and does not lead to a bilirubin concentration above 12 mg/dl in the absence of hemolytic disease. Several factors operative in the excretory process for bilirubin contribute to the deficiency observed in the newborn.

A transient deficiency of glucuronyl transferase is found in livers of the newborn of many animals, and in man (premature infants), and presumably accounts in part for impaired neonatal clearance of unconjugated bilirubin. Impaired hepatic uptake of unconjugated bilirubin is also characteristic of newborn animals and suggests that the cytoplasmic acceptor proteins have a role in physiologic jaundice. The Z protein appears to reach full development during fetal life, whereas the Y protein is almost absent at birth, reaching mature levels during the second week of life. Also important in the hyperbilirubinemia of the newborn is decreased effectiveness of the intestinal component of bilirubin elimination, which is dependent upon the intestinal flora for reduction of conjugated bilirubin to urobilinogen. The newborn infant has a relatively sterile bowel and is at a disadvantage. Furthermore, glucuronidases in the intestinal epithelium of the infant at birth are capable of splitting bilirubin glucuronide, re-forming unconjugated bilirubin. The latter pigment passes freely into the circulation and subjects the already disadvantaged infant to the additional burden of an enterohepatic recirculation of bilirubin. The above considerations contribute particularly to increased bilirubinemia in infants with intestinal obstruction. Early feeding of newborn infants serves to hasten

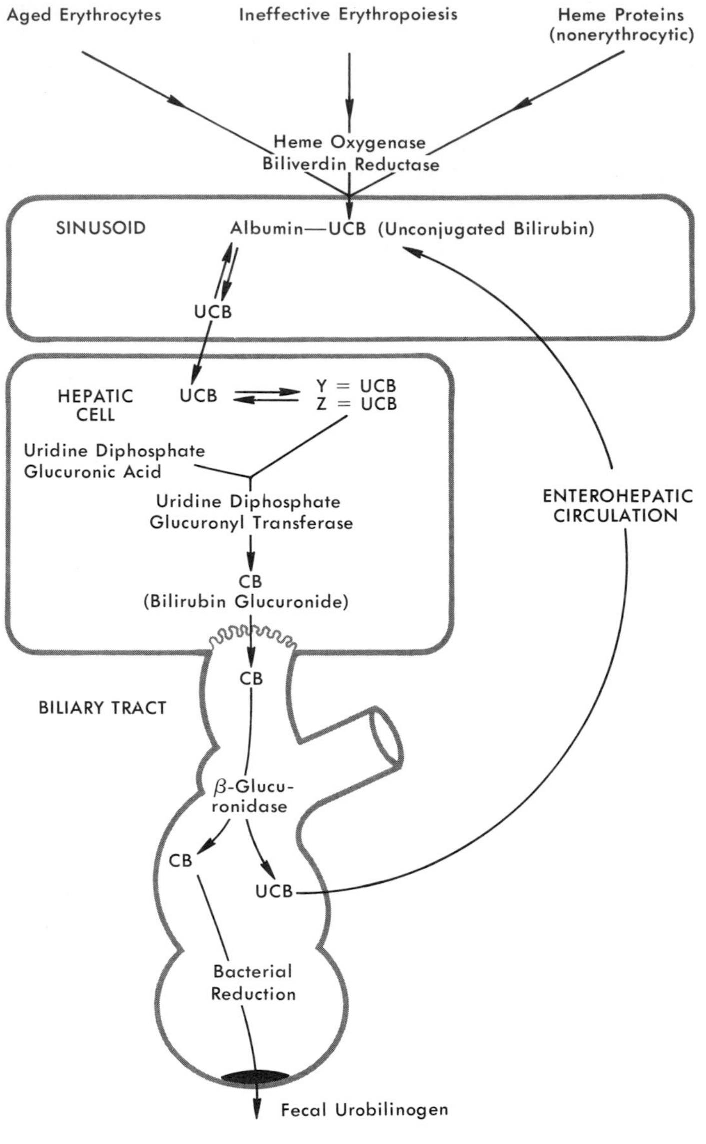

Figure 11–24 *Scheme of bilirubin metabolism in the neonate.*

the bacterial colonization of the intestinal tract and is effective in reducing the level of unconjugated hyperbilirubinemia.

An additional factor contributing to elevated levels of bilirubin in some newborns is continued patency of the ductus venosus, which permits a portion of the portal blood flow to bypass the liver. This occurs in babies with the respiratory distress syndrome.

Estrogens and progestins of maternal origin may contribute to physiologic jaundice through inhibiting bilirubin conjugation.

A variety of therapeutic approaches enhance the ability of the newborn infant to eliminate bile pigments. Phenobarbital is capable of inducing bilirubin glucuronyl transferase activity and increasing the concentration of the Y acceptor protein. Owing to the sedative properties of phenobarbital, its favorable effect on bilirubin excretion is of limited clinical application. Purgation and the feeding of agar gels decrease the enterohepatic recirculation by sequestering bilirubin and accelerating its passage through the intestinal tract. Phototherapy reduces the plasma bilirubin level in patients with unconjugated hyperbilirubinemia (see below).

TRANSIENT NEONATAL HYPERBILIRUBINEMIA (PHYSIOLOGIC JAUNDICE OF THE NEWBORN). See also Section 7.

Delayed Development of Bilirubin Conjugating System. Most full-term infants have mild unconjugated hyperbilirubinemia during the first 3 to 8 days of life. This is believed to be chiefly the result of delayed development of the bilirubin conjugating system, particularly involving glucuronyl transferase. Decreased activity of UDPG dehydrogenase has also been shown in guinea pig liver. Reabsorption of bilirubin which escapes conversion to stercobilinogen because of the relative sterility of the intestinal tract may be of greater importance. Production of increased quantities of bilíru-

TABLE 11-11 DISORDERS OF BILIRUBIN PRODUCTION, HEPATIC UPTAKE, CONJUGATION AND EXCRETION

I. Unconjugated hyperbilirubinemias
  A. Transient neonatal hyperbilirubinemia
    1. Delayed development of hepatic uptake and conjugating system
      a. Physiologic jaundice in full-term infant
      b. Physiologic jaundice in low-birth-weight infant
    2. Inhibitors of conjugation
      a. Lucey-Driscoll syndrome
      b. Breast-fed infant of certain mothers
    3. Increased enterohepatic recirculation of bilirubin
      a. Gastrointestinal obstruction
  B. Overproduction of bilirubin
    1. Hemolysis due to maternal-fetal blood group incompatibilities
      a. Rh system
      b. ABO system
    2. Deficiency of red cell enzymes
    3. Other hemolytic disorders
      a. Congenital
      b. Acquired
    4. Shunt hyperbilirubinemia
    5. Drugs
  C. Mixed or undefined
    1. Septicemia
    2. Hypothyroidism
    3. Drugs
  D. Persistent jaundice with defective conjugation
    1. Gilbert syndrome
    2. Crigler-Najjar syndrome
      a. Type I
      b. Type II
II. Conjugated hyperbilirubinemia due to impaired bilirubin excretion
  A. Transient neonatal hyperbilirubinemia
    1. Following Rh isoimmunization
  B. Chronic nonhemolytic jaundice
    1. Dubin-Johnson syndrome (pigment in hepatic cells)
    2. Rotor syndrome (without pigment in hepatic cells)
  C. Benign familial cholestasis
  D. Drugs
  E. Biliary obstruction

bin by "shunt" pathways and bypass of the liver through a patent ductus venosus as described above may also be contributing factors.

The serum unconjugated bilirubin usually does not exceed 10 mg/dl in the full-term infant or 15 mg/dl in the low-birth-weight infant (see Section 7). Increased hemolysis does not play a significant role in this process, since it is usually not associated with declining hemoglobin or rising reticulocyte values. The risk of kernicterus in physiologic jaundice has not been clarified. It is generally believed to be less than in hemolytic disorders.

Inhibitors of Conjugation. *The Lucey-Driscoll syndrome* is a form of intense, transient unconjugated hyperbilirubinemia which affects all newborn infants of certain mothers. The pathogenesis of this syndrome is not clear; the serums of the infants and their nonicteric mothers are several times more inhibitory to bilirubin conjugation by rat liver slices than the serums of unaffected infants and their mothers.

Certain breast-fed infants may exhibit a syndrome of severe and prolonged unconjugated hyperbilirubinemia. Rapid clearing of jaundice usually follows interruption of breast feeding. Pregnane-3 (alpha), 20 (beta)-diol isolated from inhibitory breast milk depresses glucuronyl transferase activity in vitro. Administration of this compound to infants is followed by unconjugated hyperbilirubinemia, which clears after administration is discontinued.

Deficiency of Red Cell Enzymes. (See Section 14.) Deficiency of red cell glucose-6-phosphate dehydrogenase is a common cause of neonatal hemolysis in the Mediterranean area. The incidence of especially severe cases in certain families suggests the presence of additional genetically determined hepatic factors. Deficiencies of other red cell enzymes such as fructokinase have been similarly implicated.

Septicemia. Unconjugated hyperbilirubinemia may accompany septicemia, which should be considered in patients with anemia and jaundice not resulting from blood group incompatibility. (See neonatal sepsis, Section 7.)

Drugs. Administration of certain drugs to pregnant women prior to delivery or to the newborn infant may accentuate unconjugated hyperbilirubinemia and increase the risk of kernicterus. Competition by the drug for bilirubin-binding sites on albumin may increase the quantity of bilirubin free to enter brain tissue. Sulfonamide drugs, especially sulfisoxazole (Gantrisin), have this effect and should not be administered to mothers before term or to newborn infants. Novobiocin appears to interfere with the excretory phase of bilirubin transport through the liver. Synthetic vitamin K in doses larger than 1 mg may act as an oxidizing agent, producing hemolysis. The presence of glucose-6-phosphate dehydrogenase deficiency increases susceptibility to the potential toxic effects of excess administration of vitamin K.

Gastrointestinal Obstruction in Newborn Infants. Unconjugated hyperbilirubinemia is relatively common in this situation, especially in pyloric stenosis. Increased shunting of blood through the ductus venosus and the consequent reduction in portal vein flow possibly related to increased intra-abdominal pressure may be an important factor in the increase in the unconjugated fraction of bilirubin. Reabsorption of bilirubin which escapes conversion to urobilinogen may also be a factor.

Hypothyroidism. Delayed development of the bilirubin conjugating system is thought to be the basis for the unconjugated hyperbilirubinemia which may accompany hypothyroidism in the young infant.

PHOTOTHERAPY

See also Section 7.

When the usual mechanisms for elimination of bilirubin from the body are impaired, as in the newborn infant or in the Crigler-Najjar syndrome, alternate routes of excretion may become significant. In such instances unconjugated bilirubin may undergo degradation to a series of water-soluble derivatives exhibiting progressively less yellow color and diazo reactivity. A similar decomposition of bilirubin occurs on exposure to white or blue light. This photolability has led to the use of phototherapy to reduce elevated levels of unconjugated bilirubin in infants with physiologic jaundice and hemolytic disease. Photo-oxidation of bilirubin in the skin produces derivatives which can be excreted in the bile and urine without prior conjugation. Light therapy reduces the need for exchange transfusions.

The sources of light most effective in the photo-oxidation of bilirubin have a high energy output near the maximum absorption peak of bilirubin (450 to 460 nm). The effective intensity of light is closely related to the particular spectral range emitted. A blue light at 68 foot-candles is more effective than daylight lamps at 350 foot-candles. Blue light has the advantage of requiring shorter periods of exposure, and may encounter less retinal sensitivity than daylight lamps. In most patients without hemolytic disease, however, use of daylight or white light will be adequate and its safety is better established.

Information is inadequate concerning the long-term effects of phototherapy; accordingly, prophylactic use in either premature or full-term infants is not indicated. Only 10 to 25 per cent of premature infants are exposed to bilirubin concentrations of 15 mg/dl or more; it is unwarranted to subject the rest to potential risks of phototherapy. Phototherapy may be justified when its benefits in preventing kernicterus outweigh the possible risks of its use and those associated with exchange transfusion. It should not be started until a significant rise in bilirubin (at least 10 mg/dl has occurred. In infants in whom exchange transfusion is indicated, there should be no delay for a trial of phototherapy. When there is an adequate response to phototherapy after 12 to 24 hours, the therapy should be discontinued for 6 to 12 hours, during which time the changes in bilirubin concentration should guide decisions about additional treatment. Serum bilirubin levels should be determined during and after the procedure. The infant's eyes must be shielded during exposure.

PERSISTENT JAUNDICE WITH DEFECTIVE CONJUGATION

(Chronic Nonhemolytic Unconjugated Hyperbilirubinemia with Glucuronyl Transferase Deficiency)

The severe form of this disorder was described by Crigler and Najjar and the syndrome bears their names. Arias has proposed the designation *chronic nonhemolytic unconjugated hyperbilirubinemia with glucuronyl transferase deficiency.* Clinical and laboratory data permit assignment of patients to Types I or II (Table 11–12). Type I presents autosomal recessive inheritance, onset at birth, higher levels of serum bilirubin, secretion of colorless bile lacking in bilirubin glucuronide, failure of administration of phenobarbital (5 mg/kg/day) to produce a fall in serum bilirubin concentration, and death in infancy with kernicterus. Type II is characterized by autosomal dominant inheritance, often a later onset of jaundice, lower concentrations of serum bilirubin following phenobarbital

TABLE 11–12 CRIGLER-NAJJAR SYNDROME (CHRONIC NONHEMOLYTIC UNCONJUGATED HYPERBILIRUBINEMIA WITH GLUCURONYL TRANSFERASE DEFICIENCY)

	TYPE I	TYPE II
Onset of jaundice	At birth	From birth to 10 years
Life expectancy	Death in infancy	Adult survival
Bilirubin (mg/dl) levels	17 to 43 (M = 27)	6 to 22 (M = 13)
Kernicterus	Usual	None
Bile		
Color	Colorless	Normal
Bilirubin glucuronide	Trace	Abundant
Urinary urobilinogen	Decreased	Decreased
Menthol glucuronide excretion	Decreased	Decreased
Hepatic glucuronyl transferase activity	Decreased	Decreased
Phenobarbital effect on:		
Bilirubin concentration	None	Marked reduction
Transferase activity	None	Increased
Fecal urobilinogen	None	Increased
Inheritance	Autosomal recessive	Autosomal dominant

treatment, and absence of kernicterus. The glucuronide conjugation of menthol in vivo and hepatic glucuronyl transferase activity in vitro are abnormally low in both types. Other liver function tests, as well as histologic appearance and cholangiography, are normal in both types. There is no hemolytic process in either.

The *Gilbert syndrome* may be included in the designation of chronic nonhemolytic unconjugated hyperbilirubinemia with glucuronyl transferase deficiency. Certain differences from the Crigler-Najjar syndrome warrant its retention as a separate diagnostic entity: unconjugated bilirubin concentrations have not exceeded 6.2 mg/dl; onset of jaundice is delayed to 10 years or older; there is a slight reduction in ^{51}Cr RBC survival; there is a predilection for males (4.2:1); and there are often significant associated symptoms of fatigue and malaise, as well as gastrointestinal complaints of nausea, abdominal pain, dyspepsia, constipation or diarrhea. As in the Crigler-Najjar syndrome, other tests of liver function and liver histology are normal. Inheritance is autosomal dominant. Treatment with phenobarbital is effective, and clearing of jaundice may be of considerable psychic benefit.

Berk has studied a group of subjects without structural liver disease in whom the hepatic clearance of unconjugated bilirubin was reduced to approximately one third of normal. Some of these patients exhibited obvious signs of increased hemolysis, but the bilirubin concentration was elevated to a level out of proportion to the increase in bilirubin production. It may be that the Gilbert syndrome should include these patients as well as those with little or no decrease in red cell survival.

There are additional causes of unconjugated hyperbilirubinemia to be differentiated from the above:

Compensated Hemolytic Disease Without Overt Signs of Hemolysis, Except During Crises. Affected persons have a decreased red cell survival time. They should be identified, since they are at risk of intermittent hemolytic crises. (See Hemolytic Anemias, Section 14.)

Mild Unconjugated Hyperbilirubinemia Following Viral Hepatitis. The serum bilirubin value is usually less than 5 mg/dl. Red cell survival and fecal urobilinogen excretion are normal. This syndrome may occur without evident antecedent viral hepatitis and with a variety of metabolic and infectious disorders. The cause is not known; reduced glucuronyl transferase activity and menthyl glucuronide excretion have been observed.

Chronic Unconjugated Hyperbilirubinemia in Cirrhotic Patients with Portocaval Shunts.

Chronic Hyperbilirubinemia at High Altitudes, Presumably Due to Anoxia.

Unconjugated Hyperbilirubinemia Due to Drugs. Impaired cytoplasmic binding of bilirubin has occurred following administration of flavaspidic acid for treatment of hookworm infestation and after administration of cholecystographic agents; both result in transient increases of unconjugated bilirubin.

Shunt Hyperbilirubinemia (Israel Syndrome). Jaundice in this disorder results both from hemolysis and from increased production of bile pigment from sources other than circulating red blood cells. Affected patients have exhibited splenomegaly, reticulocytosis and spherocytosis. Splenectomy corrects the shortened erythrocyte survival time, but jaundice persists. The principal source of bilirubin appears to be increased destruction of erythrocytes within the bone marrow.

Hemolysis Due to Maternal-Fetal Blood Group Incompatibilities. See Section. 7.

Other Hemolytic Disorders. See Section 14.

CONJUGATED HYPERBILIRUBINEMIAS

TRANSIENT NEONATAL HYPERBILIRUBINEMIA. Some infants with Rh hemolytic disease exhibit a sharp rise in serum conjugated bilirubin during the recovery phase when serum levels of unconjugated bilirubin are falling. Prolonged episodes of jaundice associated with evidence of hepatocellular obstruction have been called the *"inspissated bile syndrome"*; they apparently are less frequent since the widespread use of exchange transfusions for the primary disorder. The syndrome reflects diffuse hepatic cellular injury rather than mechanical plugging of ducts with bile as the name implies. These may be marked conjugated hyperbilirubinemia in the infant with hemolytic disease who has received intrauterine transfusions.

CHRONIC NONHEMOLYTIC JAUNDICE WITH CONJUGATED BILIRUBIN IN SERUM WITH AND WITHOUT PIGMENT IN LIVER CELLS. The Dubin-Johnson and Rotor syndromes were distinguished initially by liver biopsy. In Rotor syndrome the liver is histologically normal. The liver in the Dubin-Johnson syndrome is macroscopically black, and microscopically dark brown pigment granules are seen in parenchymal cells, particularly in the centrilobular areas. In some families with the Dubin-Johnson syndrome, jaundiced patients without abnormal pigmentation of liver cells have been observed. Differences in the two syndromes with respect to the excretion of Bromsulphalein and cholecystographic agents do not appear to be clear-cut, and Scheuer and Williams recommend abandoning the effort to distinguish between the disorders. The main defect in both is excretory: regurgitation of conjugated bilirubin occurs from the liver cell to the plasma. The excretory defect also involves cholecystographic agents, Bromsulphalein and other dyes. In 16 per cent of cases described by Dubin the onset was in the first 5 years of life. All patients exhibit jaundice, and approximately half have hepatomegaly and dark urine. The liver is frequently tender, and complaints of abdominal pain and weakness are common, along with nausea or vomiting, anorexia and diarrhea. Total bilirubin in the serum varies from 2 to 24 mg/dl. Bromsulphalein retention may be relatively normal or exceed 50 per cent of the injected dose. The gallbladder is usually not visible with cholecystographic agents, though visualization was achieved in the cases initially described by Rotor. Other tests of hepatocellular function give essentially normal results.

The pigment in the liver cells in the Dubin-Johnson syndrome differs from lipofuscin histochemically and structurally, and may be related to melanin and catecholamines. Mutant Corriedale sheep, which have a disorder apparently identical with the Dubin-Johnson syndrome, incorporate tritiated epinephrine or one of its metabolites into the pigment granules.

Recognition of these relatively benign syndromes permits their differentiation from other chronic liver diseases with jaundice.

BENIGN FAMILIAL RECURRENT CHOLESTASIS. This syndrome, initially described by Summerskill and Walshe, is characterized by recurrent episodes of jaundice accompanied by chemical and histologic evidence of cholestasis. Approximately half of the cases reported have been familial. The clinical pattern is characterized by recurrent attacks, usually beginning with pruritus, anorexia and weight loss followed within an interval of 1 to 3 weeks by obstructive jaundice with clay-colored stools and dark urine. Serum alkaline phosphatase levels are elevated, and the elevated serum bilirubin level is predominantly of the conjugated form. Biopsy during symptomatic periods reveals bile stasis and cellular infiltration of the portal areas. Despite repeated episodes starting as early as 1 year of age and encompassing intervals as long as 38 years in one instance, there has not been persistent impairment of liver function. Cholestyramine may be helpful in relieving distressing pruritus.

Infections of the Liver

NEONATAL HEPATITIS

The inflammatory processes which affect the liver in the early weeks or months of life have several features which distinguish them from those with onset in later childhood. Chief among these are greater tendencies to chronicity and to postnecrotic cirrhosis and death in hepatic failure. The formation of multinucleated giant cells is particularly prominent among the histologic changes with which the liver of the affected infant responds to injury. This response, though not unique to the infant, is exaggerated beyond that usually seen in older subjects and may be so extensive that it appears to involve the entire hepatic parenchyma in a giant cell or syncytial transformation. This response has led to the use of the term "giant cell hepatitis" as a synonym for neonatal hepatitis.

ETIOLOGY. No single agent has been shown to be the cause of neonatal hepatitis. Most infections are probably viral. Among the viruses incriminated by immunologic evidence or from isolation and transmission studies are those of serum hepatitis, cytomegalic inclusion disease, herpes simplex, rubella and Coxsackie infections. The virus of infectious hepatitis has not been proved to be a causative agent. Newborn infants of women who had infectious hepatitis during pregnancy have not had evidence of fetal infection.

Schweitzer and others have studied the relationship of illness in the neonate to positive tests during pregnancy for the hepatitis B antigen. (See Infectious Hepatitis, below.) They found that of 27 mothers with acute infection, especially in the third trimester of pregnancy or within two months post partum, 13 had babies who were chronically positive for HBAg, whereas only one infant of 21 asymptomatic maternal carriers was so affected.

A relatively high incidence of neonatal hepatitis and biliary atresia has been noted in infants with trisomy 18 and in infants with intrauterine rubella. These associations have led to the suggestion that a viral infection in utero may be the basis both for trisomy and for hepatic and biliary lesions.

The protozoan parasite toxoplasma has been found in newborn infants with hepatomegaly and jaundice, usually as a part of a generalized infection involving the central nervous system, the eye and the heart.

Hepatic involvement may also occur in such bacterial infections as septicemia, pneumonia, pyelonephritis and listeriosis. Syphilis may be responsible for neonatal hepatitis, but clinical evidence of significant hepatic dysfunction is not common. Hepatocellular damage with jaundice and giant cell alteration occurs occasionally with Rh or other acquired hemolytic disease and commonly with uncontrolled galactosemia.

PATHOLOGY. The characteristic lesion of neonatal hepatitis is giant cell transformation of the hepatic cells. In severe involvement essentially the entire parenchyma may be so transformed, but even in the most severe examples the hepatic parenchyma may undergo repair. Unknown factors related to host resistance and the virulence of the infecting organism apparently influence the course toward recovery or toward chronicity with postnecrotic cirrhosis. In infants with apparent recovery, the liver tissue may appear normal on histologic examination, and biochemical evidence of residual damage may be limited to decreased excretory capacity for sulfobromophthalein.

CLINICAL MANIFESTATIONS AND DIAGNOSIS. Affected infants commonly present with persistent jaundice, and the passage of acholic stools may suggest complete interruption of the flow of bile pigments from the liver to the intestinal tract. Approximately one third of infants presenting these signs prove to have hepatitis; most of the remainder have atresia of the extrahepatic biliary tree. The more or less characteristic clinical pattern of neonatal hepatitis consists of onset of jaundice in the second or third week of life, of initially normally colored stools which become acholic after several weeks, of persistent conjugated hyperbilirubinemia, and of positive qualitative tests for urobilinogen in urine and stool. Such a pattern suggests acquired disease with partial obstruction; similar clinical findings have been noted, however, in infants with proved extrahepatic biliary atresia.

The differentiation between obstructive jaundice on the basis of hepatocellular disease and that due to obstruction of the extrahepatic biliary tree is made difficult by a variety of factors. Among these are the frequency with which hepatitis leads to prolonged, essentially complete obstruction to the passage of bile into the intestinal tract, and the imperfect correlation of tests for hepatic parenchymal damage (flocculation, turbidity and transaminase) and the underlying disease process. Some clinicians have placed considerable reliance on serial determinations of serum bilirubin. Patients with hepatitis may exhibit initially high levels (often above 10 mg/dl), with a tendency toward an irregular decline with time. The infant with biliary atresia initially has lower values, followed by a gradual increase in concentration.

Esophageal varices, ascites and severe secondary biliary cirrhosis occasionally develop as early as the third month of life in the patient with biliary atresia. Accordingly, most workers feel urged to attempt a definite differential diagnosis of neonatal hepatitis from biliary atresia by about 2 months of age, so that the patient with operable biliary atresia may be spared the development of advanced biliary cirrhosis. Generally, operative liver biopsy and cholangiography have been relied on to accomplish the differentiation. The risks of these procedures may not be so great as originally thought when surgical exploration of the extrahepatic ducts was commonly practiced, but there are obvious reasons to avoid subjecting patients with neonatal hepatitis to them. Additional considerations are the significant number of infants with neonatal hepatitis who have spontaneous resolution of their disease and the relatively small number (about 10 per cent) of infants with biliary atresia whose lesions are potentially correctable by surgery.

Certain diagnostic procedures may support the clinical impression of hepatitis and afford additional time to determine whether there will be spontaneous clearing of the process, uncompromised by the hazards of anesthesia, open biopsy and cholangiography.

The radioactive rose bengal test may be helpful in this situation. Patients with obstructive jaundice who have patent bile ducts excrete 5 to 20 per cent of the injected dye in their stools, whereas patients with biliary atresia excrete 8 per cent or less. If equivocal results are obtained during the first month of life, the test should be repeated at monthly intervals until the situation is clarified.

Radioactive scanning techniques may demonstrate rapid passage of tagged rose bengal from the liver into the gastrointestinal tract, indicating patency of the extrahepatic biliary system.

Javitt has suggested that analysis of serum bile acids and their response to cholestyramine may be helpful in distinguishing biliary atresia from cholestatic syndromes such as neonatal hepatitis. The elevation of bile acid levels in serum in biliary atresia predominantly involved chenodeoxycholate. Cholestyramine treatment resulted in little change either in total serum bile acid level or in the ratio of cholate to chenodeoxycholate. In a small group of infants with intrahepatic cholestatic syndromes, elevations were largely due to cholic acid, and cholestyramine was effective in lowering the total level.

Administration of phenobarbital or cholestyramine increases the rose bengal fecal excretion, and lowers the serum levels of bilirubin and bile salts in those patients whose pathology indicates an intrahepatic process rather than extrahepatic biliary atresia.

The fat soluble vitamin E may be poorly absorbed when bile salts are excluded from the intestinal tract in biliary atresia; accordingly, the demonstration of vitamin E deficiency by the hydrogen peroxide hemolysis test is suggestive evidence of atresia.

Persistence of hepatitis B antigen supports the diagnosis of neonatal hepatitis; on the other hand, the antigen has been found in association with biliary atresia.

We rely heavily on information derived from needle biopsy of the liver in the differential diagnosis of prolonged obstructive jaundice in infants. The values for hemoglobin level and for bleeding, coagulation and prothrombin times must be adequate prior to the procedure. If the biopsy section is strongly suggestive of hepatitis, with giant cell transformation of the hepatic parenchyma and only minor evidence of portal fibrosis and bile duct proliferation, operation and cholangiography are delayed for 3 to 4 weeks to see whether the process will clear. If the histologic changes suggest biliary atresia, with relatively little alteration of the normal pattern of hepatic cell plates and definite evidence of portal fibrosis and proliferation of bile ducts, operative biopsy and cholangiography are undertaken. There is, however, considerable overlapping in the histologic changes observed in the two conditions. Some patients with biliary atresia have extensive giant cell transformation, and some patients with hepatitis have significant proliferation of bile ducts. Nor have cholangiographic studies proved to be infallible in distinguishing between neonatal hepatitis and biliary atresia.

Hays and colleagues have reviewed the variety of observations in a carefully studied series of patients with persistent jaundice.

MANAGEMENT. When the diagnosis of hepatitis is established and a few weeks of observation show no amelioration of jaundice, corticosteroid therapy should be tried. Prednisone in a dosage of 2 mg/kg/day is given in divided doses, initially for 2 to 3 months. If no significant clearing of jaundice occurs during this time, there appears to be little likelihood of benefit from continued therapy. When a favorable effect is achieved clinically as well as in the lowering of serum bilirubin and transaminase values, an attempt should be made to maintain the dose at the lowest possible amount adequate to avoid exacerbation of jaundice. Though there is no reason to believe that steroids exert a curative effect, the anti-inflammatory action may lessen the obstructive process and foster excretion of bilirubin. The improvement in appetite induced by the steroid may also be beneficial.

Not uncommonly patients are seen at 4 to 6 weeks of age with clinical and laboratory findings suggesting neonatal hepatitis, in whom the process rapidly subsides without sequelae. It appears that the likelihood of recovery falls with the longer duration of disease. In our experience, approximately one third of patients recover completely, and equal numbers die or progress to postnecrotic cirrhosis. Only one infant has achieved complete recovery after remaining jaundiced for more than 6 months.

HEPATITIS IN THE OLDER INFANT AND CHILD

A few families have more than one child affected by hepatitis presumed to be transmitted transplacentally. The apparent onset of hepatic injury may be delayed for 6 to 8 months after birth. In these infants the course may be unremittent and progress to postnecrotic cirrhosis and death.

INFECTIOUS HEPATITIS

Infectious hepatitis has its highest incidence, but lowest mortality, among children of school age. It is the leading viral disease in the United States for which no vaccine exists.

ETIOLOGY. The social impact of this illness is severe; between 50,000 and 70,000 cases are reported each year. This probably represents no more than 10 per cent of the actual number of cases.

The viral etiology of hepatitis has been suspected for years, but inability to isolate a viral agent or to identify a viral marker has frustrated the development of preventive measures and has retarded the delineation of two types of hepatitis: Type A, MS-1, short-incubation, "infectious" hepatitis; and Type B, MS-2 long-incubation, "serum" hepatitis.

Early in 1960 a group of investigators interested in protein polymorphism discovered precipitating antibodies against low density lipoproteins in persons exposed to multiple transfusions. Serologic surveys of different populations disclosed varying incidence of a serum marker ("Australia" antigen), which was found to be prevalent in the blood of patients with leukemia and Hodgkin's disease, in institutionalized patients with Down syndrome, in patients with lepromatous leprosy and in patients with viral hepatitis. Confirmation of the high incidence of Australia antigen was made by many other investigators, and it soon became apparent that this antigen was associated with the type of hepatitis formerly identified as serum hepatitis. The Australia antigen has also been called "SH antigen," "hepatitis associated antigen" (HAA), and "hepatitis-B antigen" (HBAg). We prefer the last.

The incidence of the hepatitis-B antigen (HBAg) in reported studies varies with the methods used for its detection. The incidence in the normal North American population is estimated at 0.1 per cent, so that detection of the antigen in a patient suspected of hepatitis carries the implication of clinical disease. As more and more sensitive techniques have been employed in testing for the antigen, including complement fixation, counterimmunoelectrophoresis, hemagglutination and hemagglutination-inhibition, and radioimmunoassay methods, the antigen has been reported more frequently in patients with the long-incubation type of hepatitis.

Serial observations of patients exposed to the long-incubation type of hepatitis have revealed that the antigen becomes detectable during the incubation or prodromal period of the illness. The absence of detectable antigen does not eliminate long-incubation hepatitis from consideration, since the antigen may disappear from the serum prior either to development of clinical symptoms or to the discovery of abnormal biochemical findings; additionally, the test employed may be insensitive to low serum concentrations of the antigen. The antigen may remain detectable in serum for periods of time ranging from days to years. In most patients the antigenemia is transient, especially in patients who develop icterus. Persistence of the antigenemia is of concern; it may indicate continuing infection or activity of the disease or may represent a carrier state. It is of importance to the public health, since transmission of the antigen may occur by other than parenteral contact.

The detection of this transmissible agent has had important preventive implications. Blood banks are now able to screen donor blood for the antigen, and already a reduction in the incidence of posttransfusion hepatitis has been recorded. The finding of an appropriate culture technique will eventually allow for the development of effective vaccines needed for the eradication of this type of hepatitis.

To date no specific virus has been identified as responsible for the initiation of the short-incubation type of ("epidemic") hepatitis. On the other hand, a number of different viral pathogens have been isolated from patients with hepatitis. These include strains of ECHO and coxsackieviruses, herpesvirus and adenoviruses. In most instances the presence of these viruses has been regarded as coincidental rather than etiologic; a number of "candidate viruses" are under study. Of interest in the search for a suitable experimental animal host is the recent occurrence of more than 20 cases of hepatitis in persons caring for primates, and especially for chimpanzees newly imported into the United States. In this animal there is a spontaneously occurring disease clinically resembling human viral hepatitis. In the South American marmoset histologic and biochemical evidence of hepatitis has been produced by serial passages of serum from a patient with typical viral hepatitis.

CLINICAL MANIFESTATIONS. The incubation period of infectious hepatitis prior to onset of jaundice is 14 to 40 days; if measured to the onset of initial symptoms, it may be 3 to 5 days less. The incubation period of serum hepatitis is 60 to 160 days. Clinical differentiation is more often suggestive than definitive. Infectious hepatitis is usually marked by an abrupt onset, with fever; by a peak of incidence in autumn and winter; and by a predilection for children and young adults. Serum hepatitis, on the other hand, usually exhibits an insidious onset, with little or no fever; and a year-round incidence without an age preference.

In the first phase (preicteric), symptoms usually begin 4 to 5 days before the appearance of jaundice. Fever, malaise, mild headache and chilliness are present at the onset. Signs of a mild upper respiratory tract infection are common. Anorexia is invariably an early symptom, frequently followed by nausea and vomiting. The breath is often foul, and older children may complain of a sour or bitter taste. Upper abdominal distress and pain are frequent complaints. Constipation is more common than diarrhea. Bile is usually present in the urine 1 to 3 days before the appearance of jaundice.

On occasion jaundice appears without any preceding symptoms. Jaundice may vary from a slight discoloration of the scleras, where it is first seen, to a deep pigmentation involving the entire body. Fever usually disappears with the onset of icterus, but anorexia continues, and severe prostration and vomiting secondary to pylorospasm may occur, especially in deeply jaundiced patients. The stools are light or clay-colored at this stage. Pruritus is infrequent.

The second phase (icteric) continues usually for 2 to 4 weeks, with gradually increasing clinical and laboratory measures of bilirubinemia during the first weeks; there is then a gradual diminution in the icterus. For 1 to 2 months following complete resolution of the jaundice the child may still complain of malaise and fatigue. Many children recover completely and resume full activity without this prolonged convalescent period.

The liver is commonly enlarged, and tenderness can be elicited either by direct palpation or by percussion with the fist over the right upper abdomen and lower thoracic cage. The spleen is palpable in as many as 15 per cent of patients and lymphadenopathy, including cervical adenopathy, may be present. Spider angiomata may develop during the acute illness, which will then disappear; they need not indicate chronic disease.

DIAGNOSIS. The increase in the serum concentration of bilirubin consists mainly of the conjugated (direct) form during the early days of jaundice. As recovery begins the unconjugated (indirect) form increases, and in the late phase it may account for the total increase. Serum bilirubin levels may be as high as 10 mg/dl or more. With the onset of jaundice there is an increase in the urinary excretion of urobilinogen, owing to the inability of the damaged liver to excrete reabsorbed urobilinogen formed from that decreased amount of bile which continues to enter the intestine. Subsequently, with complete failure of bile to reach the intestine and its complete regurgitation into the circulation, urobilinogen disappears from the urine. With resumption of excretion of bile into the intestine, urobilinogen is again formed and appears in the urine in large quantities, the liver still being incapable of removing it completely from the blood.

The Bromsulphalein retention test results tend to parallel the retention of bilirubin in the blood, but often remain abnormal for a longer time. The serum glutamic oxaloacetic or glutamic pyruvic transaminases are elevated early in the course of the disease; their return to normal heralds the end of active disease and the beginning of recovery. The sedimentation rate is increased in most cases. There are no significant changes in the total serum protein concentration, but an increase in gamma globulin can be demonstrated by electrophoretic analysis. The total white blood cell count remains normal in most cases of viral hepatitis. A fall in the granulocytes may appear early in the course of the illness, so that a relative lymphocytosis is apparent. Many of the lymphocytes appear large or atypical.

Differential Diagnosis. The diagnosis of infectious hepatitis is dependent on the elimination of other causes of jaundice or of hepatitis with or without jaundice. In *leptospirosis* labial herpes, a hemorrhagic exanthem, fever, leukocytosis, muscle pains and albuminuria occur, which should serve to distinguish it clinically. The specific agglutination test, the isolation of the spirochete from blood or serum, or the successful inoculation of a guinea pig confirms the diagnosis of leptospirosis. Involvement of the liver in *infectious mononucleosis* may mimic that of infectious hepatitis and is relatively common.

In the early preicteric phase of infectious hepatitis, symptoms may be suggestive of influenza or gastroenteritis. Abdominal pain may resemble that of pneumonia or acute appendicitis. Drug-induced or toxic hepatitis must also be considered. Consideration should also be given to other types of conjugated hyperbilirubinemia discussed elsewhere in this section and to the possibility of an exacerbation of chronic liver disease.

PATHOLOGY. Serial biopsy studies in adults reveal that similar pathologic changes occur in the liver in both types of hepatitis. The hepatic lobules show varying degrees of cellular necrosis and autolysis, beginning in the center of the lobules and spreading radially as the disease advances. There is thickening of the reticular fibers. Evidences of cellular regeneration (increased mitotic figures) are prominent in the early stages of the disease. Widespread infiltration with inflammatory cells, polymorphonuclear leukocytes, lymphocytes, macrophages and plasma cells accompanies the hepatocellular necrosis. In the later stages, lymphocytes predominate. There is a diffuse reticuloendothelial reaction; the reticulum becomes thickened and assumes the staining properties of collagen. The periportal areas are widened because of infiltration with large numbers of inflammatory cells. Proliferating bile ducts appear in the perilobular portal areas, and bile stasis is visible. The clinical manifestations of viral hepatitis are expressions of hepatocellular necrosis, intrahepatic biliary obstruction, portal obstruction and the diffuse inflammatory reaction in the liver. With recovery, complete regeneration of the liver cells occurs without scarring. In fulminating and fatal cases the hepatic changes are typical of yellow atrophy.

VARIANTS OF VIRAL HEPATITIS. Atypical hepatitis usually follows two courses: first, the illness may be very benign, and confusing to the clinician who is not familiar with its presentation; second, a variant may be so severe as to threaten the patient's survival.

Mild Anicteric Hepatitis. Mild anicteric hepatitis is more common among infants than the icteric form. (In an institutional epidemic of infectious hepatitis, which involved 36 infants, only one of them was jaundiced.) The symptoms are those of a mild gastroenteritis or systemic infection, and include anorexia, diarrhea and vomiting. The infants may excrete the virus in their stools for many months and constitute a potential source of infection to their attendants.

Hepatitis With Predominant Cholestasis. Hepatitis with predominant cholestasis is uncommon in children; it is also referred to as *cholestatic hepatitis* and *cholangiolitic hepatitis.* It is characterized principally by obstruction and dilatation of bile canaliculi, with little evidence of hepatocellular necrosis. The clinical manifestations include jaundice with pruritus, bilirubinuria, pale stools with decreased fecal urobilinogen, and an enlarged, nontender liver. Laboratory examinations show increases in alkaline phosphatase and 5-nucleotidase values in the serum, with only slight increases in the serum transaminases.

Chronic Hepatitis. Except in the very young infant, infectious hepatitis in childhood is usually a brief, self-limited illness. Occasionally a patient is seen in whom is found only an elevation of serum levels of indirect reacting bilirubin or serum transaminases, which may persist for months without either clinical disease or pathologic changes on liver biopsy. Only rarely do children with apparently typical bouts of hepatitis continue for months with hepatomegaly and biochemical evidence of continued hepatocellular injury. This occurrence has been designated "prolonged hepatitis." Perhaps even more uncommon in children is "recurrent" hepatitis, with exacerbation during the recovery phase. Patients with this course may be expected to recover ultimately unless subacute hepatic necrosis progresses to postnecrotic cirrhosis.

LIFE THREATENING COMPLICATIONS OF HEPATITIS. Fulminant Hepatitis. Fulminant hepatitis, or *acute massive necrosis,* is usually fatal within a few weeks after onset. Systemic manifestations during the preicteric phase are usually severe. Particularly prominent are high fever, abdominal pain and severe vomiting. Also indicative of an unfavorable outcome are rapid decrease in liver size, such mental changes as lethargy, drowsiness and confusion, electroencephalographic changes of encephalopathy, and an increase in prothrombin time not corrected by parenteral administration of vitamin K. Jaundice is usually intense, but death may precede its development. Serum levels of transaminases may not be very high, perhaps reflecting failure of their hepatic synthesis. Bleeding into skin and mucous membranes, ascites and deep coma are among the terminal manifestations.

Aplastic Anemia. This is an unusual complication of hepatitis in children. The mechanism of the bone marrow depression is unknown. Death is common, usually with massive hemorrhage.

Hepatic Failure. In viral hepatitis as well as in toxic reactions and chronic liver disease severe alteration in the function of or reduction in the mass of parenchymal cells may result in serious clinical liver failure. When this occurs, specific measures may have to be taken in order to control such consequences of failure as ascites, encephalopathy and hemorrhage.

Fluid Retention and Ascites. The formation of ascitic fluid in the abdomen is a result of many factors, among them that obstruction to blood leaving the liver sinusoids leads to increased filtration of protein-rich fluid into the hepatic lymphatics, from which it exudes from dilated lymphatic vessels on the surface and in the hilus of the liver; also, that increased portal venous pressure reduces the reabsorption of this protein-rich fluid by the splanchnic capillaries. Impaired hepatic synthesis of albumin is usually not the main cause of ascites. Once the fluid accumulates, renal and hormonal changes occur which result in increased tubular reabsorption of sodium.

Therapy is designed to reverse the positive sodium balance. Dietary treatment involves rigid restriction of sodium intake; the use of sodium-free milk may be necessary in order to maintain adequate intake of protein. Combined use of hydrochlorothiazide (2–4 mg/kg/day) and an aldosterone-blocking agent, spironolactone (10–20 mg/kg/day), is usually required to promote adequate diuresis. In severe cases, furosemide (1–2 mg/kg) may be given either intravenously or orally to replace the hydrochlorothiazide. Potassium deficiency may complicate therapy with these agents, and supplements may be necessary. Salt-poor albumin may be helpful in treating edema if the serum albumin concentration is below 2.5 gm/dl. Hyponatremia is usually dilutional and is best treated by restriction of water intake. Abdominal paracentesis for ascites should be avoided unless abdominal or respiratory distress is severe.

Hepatic Encephalopathy. Impaired liver function and shunting of portal blood to the systemic circulation are the chief factors responsible for the neurologic manifestations of severe hepatic disease. Most of the current theories of development of hepatic coma incriminate rising levels of ammonia in serum as the toxic factor producing alterations in cerebral metabolism. Ammonia is normally converted to urea in the liver; excesses arise from such nitrogen loads as are imposed by increased dietary intake of protein, by gastrointestinal hemorrhage, or by increased enterohepatic circulation of urea in azotemia. Infections, fluid or electrolyte imbalances induced by vigorous diuresis, or injudicial use of sedatives in patients with liver disease may at times precipitate hepatic coma.

To control the intestinal production of ammonia, protein should be eliminated from the diet, and adequate calories as carbohydrate should be provided to limit endogenous breakdown of protein. The gut lumen should be purged of its nitrogenous content by laxatives, and bacterial breakdown of protein reduced by the use orally of a nonabsorbable antibiotic such as neomycin (250 mg, four times daily) or by neomycin enemas.

The feeding of an unabsorbable disaccharide, lactulose, appears to induce an acidic diarrhea that traps ammonia in the colonic contents; its use in hepatic failure seems promising. Exchange transfusion is indicated in patients in whom biopsy indicates acute, toxic, potentially reversible disease, but should not be undertaken in patients with chronic disease or massive necrosis.

Hemorrhage. The massive bleeding accompanying liver failure is best managed by the infusion of fresh frozen plasma or fresh heparinized blood. Vitamin K should be administered to all patients with jaundice; an improvement in prothrombin time may be seen in patients whose disease is less than completely destructive of hepatic function.

TREATMENT. Treatment is symptomatic and aimed at supporting the patient during the interval required for his own immunologic defenses to control the invading virus. Maintenance of a reasonable state of nutrition during the illness appears to be beneficial; regeneration of damaged liver requires an adequate supply of protein and calories. An effort should be made to provide at least basal caloric requirements each day, utilizing the intravenous route if necessary.

After the initial anorexia has passed, a diet providing adequate calories and 1.5 to 2.5 gm/kg/day of protein should be provided. Restriction of fat intake is not necessary beyond the removal of gross fat from meats, and avoidance of fried foods and of oily dressings. Milk, eggs and butter are usually well tolerated. Frequent feedings are helpful in achieving an adequate dietary intake. When vomiting or anorexia is prominent, intravenous infusion of a solution of 10 to 15 per cent glucose with maintenance levels of electrolytes should be given. Unusual gastrointestinal losses due to vomiting may require additional amounts of sodium and potassium chlorides.

There has been controversy concerning the importance of restriction of physical activity during the acute phases of hepatitis. Recent evidence does not indicate that recovery is prolonged when the patient is allowed to be ambulatory while he is jaundiced. Bed rest does not appear to produce more rapid recovery than physical activity held within the limits of fatigue. Periodic rest periods for the child during the day seem more reasonable than a struggle to keep the child at rest continuously.

Adrenocortical steroids are capable of inducing a prompt clinical remission in acute viral hepatitis, but this is not accompanied by an increased rate of resolution of the hepatic injury. Among the beneficial effects of steroid treatment are improved appetite and sense of well-being, increased extrahepatic clearance of bilirubin, lessening of intrahepatic obstruction by decreasing inflammation, and increased renal excretion of water. More specific effects of these agents occur when hepatic disease is caused by allergy to drugs or by autoimmune processes.

Prednisone may be indicated in patients with acute viral hepatitis only for the following reasons: coma, persistent fever, severe bleeding and excessively abnormal blood chemical values, especially in respect to serum bilirubin and prothrombin time. A dose of 2 mg/kg/day is administered until the desired effects are noted; the drug is then discontinued gradually at a rate adequate to maintain clinical improvement.

PREVENTION. Isolation precautions appropriate for patients with intestinal infections are indicated during the period of hospitalization. Preparations of normal human gamma globulin offer effective prophylaxis in short-incubation (HAA-negative) hepatitis, but not against long-incubation (HAA-positive) hepatitis. Prevention of the short-incubation hepatitis is accomplished by administration of 0.04 ml/kg of pooled normal gamma globulin. The use of special gamma globulin preparations selected for their high-titer of anti-HAA appears to offer some potential for prevention of hepatitis in the contacts of patients with the HAA-positive type.

LIVER ABSCESS

Hepatic pyemia is uncommon in children. Consideration of this diagnosis should be made in prolonged fevers, especially after pyogenic infections, or in patients with impaired immunity. In patients with sepsis, multiple abscesses are the rule, whereas seeding from within the abdomen by way of the portal vein results in solitary abscesses in the right lobe of the liver. The more common organisms cultured from liver abscesses include *Staphylococcus aureus, Streptococcus fecalis,* and *Escherichia coli* and other gram-negative organisms. Amebic abscess, the commonest solitary abscess of adults, is relatively unknown in children.

CLINICAL MANIFESTATIONS. An abscess of the liver may occasionally be latent if it is well encapsulated, or it may be overshadowed by the symptoms of the disease from which it has its origin. Symptoms include fever, chills, sweating, prostration and nausea and vomiting. Pain is usually present over the liver and may be severe; at times it may be referred to the right shoulder or back. Encroachment upon the diaphragm may produce cough or dyspnea through irritation of the pleural surface. Mild icterus may be present in many cases and ascites in a few. There is moderate enlargement of the liver. The diagnosis can be established by a radioactive liver scan which demonstrates filling defects within the liver. Displacement of intrahepatic vessels by the enlarging abscess can be shown by selective hepatic arteriography.

TREATMENT. Solitary abscesses are best treated surgically with extraperitoneal drainage and irrigation. The selection of antibiotics is determined by the nature of the organism found at surgery and its antibiotic sensitivities. Multiple abscesses are best treated by aggressive antibiotic therapy; the mortality rate is high.

Acute Liver Disease

ACUTE ENCEPHALOPATHY AND HEPATOMEGALY WITH FATTY INFILTRATION

(Reye Syndrome)

The Reye syndrome is a poorly understood but acute and frequently fatal condition now reported in over 150 children. The diagnosis depends upon a constellation of clinical and pathologic findings. The acute illness frequently follows a mild "viral" illness from which recovery seems to be occurring. There is an abrupt onset of protracted vomiting, followed within hours by a change in the state of consciousness, leading to delirium and stupor.

Clinical examination discloses mild to moderate hepatomegaly and central nervous system depression, which may include signs of brain stem involvement, altered pupillary reflexes and increased intracranial pressure. Selected liver function tests are abnormal. There are marked increases in serum levels of transaminases and ammonia, with little or no increase in the serum bilirubin. Bleeding may be a problem, with reduction in the level of the liver-dependent components of coagulation. Hypoglycemia occurs commonly and may be resistant to therapy. Spinal fluid is normal, except that increased pressure may be found.

Liver tissue obtained by percutaneous biopsy is grossly abnormal, pale and at times white. Microscopically, diffuse fatty vacuolization of enlarged hepatocytes is seen. Ultrastructurally, mitochondrial swelling and pleomorphism are found. Lipid stains are positive, and chemical analysis of the liver tissue indicates large increases in content of triglycerides, and fatty acids. Fatty degeneration of the other organs, such as the heart, pancreas and kidney, has also been reported. The myocardial and renal tubular changes account for the occurrence of arrhythmias and aminoacidurias.

The cause of the Reye syndrome is unknown. A relationship to influenza B is suggested. Herpes simplex and varicella viruses have been found in a few patients, and in others, serologic evidence of recent infection with other viruses. Such exogenous agents as isopropyl alcohol, salicylates and aflatoxins have been found in gastrointestinal secretions, blood or autopsy material in other cases. The relationship between these infective or exogenous agents and the altered metabolism and pathology of the disease is unclear.

Since the pathophysiology of this disease is poorly understood, there is no specific therapy. Attention should be paid to correcting the hypoglycemia; infusions of 10 per cent glucose and insulin should be given to all patients in an attempt to correct central nervous system metabolism and reconstitute glycogen stores. If ketosis and acidosis are found, they should be corrected. Cerebral edema is managed by the infusion of mannitol and the administration of dexamethasone, and by the initiation of hypothermic measures. Exchange transfusion (using one and one half to two times the patient's blood volume every 12 hours) has been reported to improve mortality figures and reduce neurologic sequelae. This is not uniformly helpful, however, and is not established as a definite therapeutic measure. On the other hand, it appears that early exchange transfusion, before brain stem impairment or cerebral edema appears, results in a more favorable outcome than any of the above measures instituted after central nervous system signs are found.

TABLE 11–13 TOXIC AND DRUG-INDUCED HEPATITIS

Accidental and Industrial Poisoning:
Beryllium, carbon tetrachloride, chlorinated naphthalenes, copper, DDT, iron, manganese, phosphorus, Senecio alkaloids, toluene

Anesthetic Agents:
Chloroform, cyclopropane, halothane

Antiarthritic Agents:
Cinchophen, desacetylmethylcolchicine, indomethacin (Indocin), phenylbutazone (Butazolidin), probenecid (Benemid)

Antibiotics:
Erythromycin (Ilosone), griseofulvin, novobiocin, oxacillin, penicillin, intravenous chlortetracycline (Aureomycin), intravenous tetracycline (Achromycin), triacetyloleandomycin (Cyclamycin)

Anticonvulsants, Muscle Relaxants and Sedatives:
Diphenylhydantoin (Dilantin), mephenytoin (Mesantoin), phenobarbital, trimethadione (Tridione)

Chemotherapeutic Agents:
Antimony, arsenic, bismuth, isoniazid, nitrofurantoin, para-aminosalicylic acid, pyrazinamide, sulfonamides

Cytotoxic and Immunosuppressive Agents:
Azathioprine (Imuran), 6-mercaptopurine, methotrexate, chlorambucil, nitrogen mustard, urethane

Food Poisoning:
Aflatoxin, mushroom poisoning

Hormonal and Metabolic Agents:
Methyltestosterone, norethandrolone (Nilevar), methandrostenolone (Dianabol), fluoxymesterone (Halotestin), methimazole (Tapazole), propylthiouracil, cortisone

Estrogenic and Progestational Agents:
Stilbestrol, oral contraceptives (mixture of synthetic estrogens and progestins)

Hypoglycemic Agents:
Biguanides, chlorpropamide, tolbutamide

Psychopharmacologic Agents:
Chlorpromazine (Thorazine), prochlorperazine (Compazine), promazine (Sparine), thioridazine (Mellaril), trifluoperazine (Stelazine), chlordiazepoxide (Librium), Imipramine (Tofranil), Meprobamate

Miscellaneous:
Chlorothiazide, cholecystography dyes, male fern, methyldopa (Aldomet), radiation, transfusion reactions, trimethobenzamide (Tigan)

HEPATIC DRUG REACTIONS

The liver may be injured by a variety of chemical agents. Some of these are hepatotoxins and the liver injury may be considered "predictable." In the case of other compounds, hepatic damage is much less frequent and may be considered "nonpredictable" or of immunologic, allergic or idiosyncratic origin. Among the "predictable" agents are carbon tetrachloride, toluene and trichlorethylene solvents and mithramycin (used in cancer therapy). These agents are generally toxic in animals, injurious after short exposure and produce characteristic hepatic lesions. In contrast, the "nonpredictable" hepatotoxins may not produce lesions in experimental animals and usually exhibit evidence of hepatic toxicity after relatively prolonged use. Prominent among this group are chlorpromazine, isoniazid, antithyroid drugs, erythromycin estolate and oxyphenisatin (a component of some laxatives).

A variety of clinical presentations are seen which vary from mild elevation of serum transaminase with or without hepatomegaly to a picture simulating fulminant hepatitis. Withdrawal of the offending agent is usually associated with reduction of the hepatic injury. Children are relatively less susceptible than adults to these effects. Extensive treatment of this subject is given in recent reviews by Klatskin and by Perez, Schaffner and Popper. A list of agents with potential hepatic toxicity is given in Table 11–13.

Chronic Liver Disease

In children chronic liver disease may present as a manifestation of a wide variety of disorders (Table 11–14). In some it constitutes the principal clinical problem, e.g., the cirrhosis secondary to biliary atresia, whereas in others it is an associated disability of a systemic disturbance, e.g., cystic fibrosis.

The term "cirrhosis" indicates extensive destruction of hepatic parenchyma, with replacement by diffuse fibrosis. When hepatic cells are destroyed, new cells form from the cellular remnants. When death of cells is confined to individual lobules, orderly restoration of histologic and functional relations is possible. Destruction of many adjacent

TABLE 11–14 CLASSIFICATION OF CHRONIC LIVER DISEASE IN CHILDHOOD

I. Acquired
  A. Postnecrotic cirrhosis
  B. Chronic active liver disease
  C. Biliary cirrhosis
    1. Primary
    2. Secondary
      a. Bile duct obstruction (atresia, stenosis, choledochal cyst)
      b. Inspissated secretions, stones, tumors, pancreatitis
      c. Drugs
  D. Vascular obstruction
    1. Cardiac failure, constrictive pericarditis
    2. Hepatic vein obstruction (Budd-Chiari syndrome)
    3. Veno-occlusive disease
    4. Hemangioma
II. Hereditary
  A. Developmental
    1. Polycystic liver disease
    2. Congenital hepatic fibrosis
    3. Hereditary hemorrhagic telangiectasia
  B. Metabolic
    1. Hepatolenticular degeneration (Wilson's disease)
    2. Galactosemia
    3. Cystic fibrosis
    4. Fructose intolerance
    5. Sickle cell disease
    6. Glycogen storage disease
    7. Other storage diseases
      a. Mucopolysaccharidoses
      b. Gaucher's disease
      c. Niemann-Pick disease
      d. Gangliosidosis M_I
    8. Tyrosinosis
    9. Cystinosis
    10. Porphyria
    11. Hemochromatosis
    12. Amyloidosis
    13. Progressive familial hepatic cholestasis
    14. Alpha-1-antitrypsin deficiency
III. Miscellaneous disorders
  A. Idiopathic cirrhosis
  B. Indian childhood cirrhosis
  C. Sarcoidosis
  D. Inflammatory bowel disease

lobules with collapse of intervening stroma leads to regeneration of nodules which increase in size by growth at their periphery. New blood vessels surround the margins of the nodules and are compressed with continued growth. Compression impairs the flow of blood more in the low-pressure portal and hepatic veins than in the high-pressure arteries. This leads to dependence of the nodule on hepatic arterial blood for its nutrition, owing to shunting of portal blood past it and to impedance to outflow in the hepatic veins. Progress of the cirrhotic process occurs through further destruction of hepatic parenchyma, growth of regenerating nodules, and contraction of scar tissue.

Although fibrosis may be the most striking pathologic finding in cirrhosis, the amount of functional parenchyma may be of greater importance to the health and survival of the patient. Fibrosis may be largely reversible, for example, in hemochromatosis if excess iron is removed, or in secondary biliary cirrhosis if the obstruction is removed. In conditions characterized chiefly by hepatic fibrosis, portal hypertension rather than parenchymal insufficiency may become the major clinical problem, as, for example, in congenital hepatic fibrosis, multiple hemangiomas, scarring after abscess or hepatic schistosomiasis.

In children it is convenient to classify chronic liver disease as acquired or hereditary. In some instances a combination of hereditary and acquired factors may be operative, as in neonatal hepatitis, where both maternal viral infection and fetal genetic susceptibility may determine the manifestations of infection, or in such apparently acquired liver disease as lupoid hepatitis and primary biliary cirrhosis, where unidentified genetic factors may be important.

ACQUIRED HEPATIC DISEASE

POSTNECROTIC CIRRHOSIS

In children, in contrast to adults, most instances of postnecrotic cirrhosis are diagnosed because of a known preceding insult, e.g., hepatitis, or as a continuing active process, e.g., chronic hepatitis. Diffuse portal or Laennec's cirrhosis is rarely seen in children. Children have fewer opportunities than adults for contact with such hepatic toxic agents as chloroform, carbon tetrachloride and other chlorinated hydrocarbons. Diagnostic efforts should be directed toward those diseases of childhood with which cirrhosis is associated, e.g., cystic fibrosis, Wilson's disease or neonatal hepatitis.

Pathologically, postnecrotic cirrhosis differs from Laennec's cirrhosis in exhibiting larger nodules and wide bands of scar tissue. There is usually evidence of active inflammation, regeneration and irregular vacuolated or multinucleated cells. Uninvolved lobules are also usually observed. These features are not always sufficiently developed to permit a clear differentiation from portal cirrhosis.

CHRONIC ACTIVE LIVER DISEASE

The term "chronic active liver disease" (CALD) is herein used to describe a variety of conditions, previously including plasma cell hepatitis, lupoid hepatitis, Kunkel syndrome of hypergammaglobulinemia in young females, active juvenile cirrhosis and chronic active hepatitis. None of these terms accurately describes the etiology of this condition, which remains unknown.

CLINICAL MANIFESTATIONS. Chronic active liver disease may affect individuals at any age, from as early as 1 year up to 80 years. The peak incidence occurs in the 10 to 20 age group. In most series, females predominate, even in the prepubertal age group. In approximately one third of the patients, symptoms occur abruptly and the onset resembles that of acute infectious hepatitis. However, the clinical course is prolonged and jaundice does not resolve at the expected time as it does with infectious hepatitis. In the remainder of the patients, the onset is insidious, with symptoms of malaise, fatigue, weight loss, anorexia and fever developing over a period of weeks to months. These nonspecific symptoms may not alert the clinician to the possibility of liver disease. Portal hypertension with bleeding esophageal varices or ascites occurs late in the course of the illness, but may be the only specific sign implicating liver disease at the time of initial evaluation. About 20 per cent of patients have significant disease in other systems as the presenting complaint. Consequently these patients may appear with hematuria, bloody diarrhea, acne, malar flush or jaundice. Amenorrhea is common in females. Clinical evaluation will disclose the presence of nephritis, thyroiditis, myositis, arthralgias, colitis or hemolytic anemia. These multisystem symptoms may also develop during the course of the illness and suggest an "autoimmune" mechanism as either the etiologic factor or an important factor in the progression of the illness.

LABORATORY FINDINGS. Mild hyperbilirubinemia and mild elevation of the serum transaminases and gamma globulins are the more frequently found biochemical changes. The diagnosis of chronic active liver disease is supported if the serum glutamic-oxaloacetic transaminase is elevated more than ten times normal for longer than 8 weeks or if the serum gamma globulins are more than twice normal values. The hyperglobulinemia is a result of elevation of all the fractions (IgG, IgM, IgA). The findings of serologic abnormalities, including LE phenomena, antinuclear antibodies, smooth muscle antibodies, positive Coombs reaction and false-positive salmonella agglutination titers, indicate the presence of the dysproteinemia which frequently accompanies this clinical condition. Hypoalbuminemia indicates the possibility of cirrhosis, but may be present during the acute exacerbations of the illness.

PATHOLOGY. A liver biopsy is necessary to establish the diagnosis to assess the severity of the disease and to aid in evaluation of therapy. Characteristically the perilobular region shows degeneration and "piecemeal" necrosis of cells, with lymphocytic and plasma cell infiltration. The limiting plate separating the portal tract and lobule is eroded. Varying degrees of fibrosis, including features of multinodular cirrhosis, can be seen as well.

TREATMENT. If the disease is not treated, over 80 per cent of patients will die within five years. With treatment, improvement of early survival and quality of life is favorably influenced. The autoimmune mechanism apparently operative in this disease provides the rationale for corticosteroid therapy, which results in clinical, biochemical and histologic improvement in the majority of patients. If complications of corticosteroid therapy become too burdensome, reduction of steroid dosage and addition of azathioprine may alleviate the complications and continue to suppress the immunologic activity of the disease. It remains to be shown that survival longer than five years is favorably affected by early and persistent therapy, although complete resolution of the inflammatory process and even of the cirrhosis has been described in some patients. The multisystem symptomatology is usually brought under control with this regimen.

BILIARY CIRRHOSIS

In children, biliary cirrhosis develops after prolonged obstruction of the biliary system by inspissated bile, from extrahepatic atresia, or by choledochal cyst. Less frequent causes in childhood are stone or sludge in the common bile duct and tumor. It may also result from recurrent attacks of pancreatitis. In endemic areas the liver fluke, *Clonorchis sinensis,* may be responsible for a similar process.

Primary Biliary Cirrhosis

The syndrome of primary biliary cirrhosis simulates the clinical picture of extrahepatic biliary obstruction. This disorder primarily affects older women, in whom pruritus usually precedes the appearance of jaundice by months or years. Marked elevations of alkaline phosphatase and cholesterol, with mild to moderate increases in bilirubin levels, are characteristic and suggest extrahepatic biliary obstruction. More specific features are marked elevations of IgM, and in almost all cases positive tests for mitochondrial antibody. The histologic picture is pathognomonic in the early stages, showing damage to interlobular bile ducts and a dense cellular infiltrate composed of lymphocytes, histiocytes, plasma cells and a few eosinophils. In the latter stages, scarring and cirrhotic changes are seen.

VASCULAR OBSTRUCTION

Cardiac failure is the principal cause of passive congestion of the liver. Acute myocardial decompensation such as that associated with the crises of hemolytic anemias or with hypertensive acute glomerulonephritis will produce temporary passive hyperemia of the liver, but the more striking changes result from the prolonged passive congestion associated with chronic disease of the heart. *Longstanding pulmonary disease* with stasis in the right side of the heart will also engorge the liver. Occasionally a collection of pleural fluid or a thoracic tumor, through *compression of the inferior vena cava,* may retard the return of blood from the liver. *Constrictive pericarditis* will produce the same passive vascular congestion as either myocardial or valvular disease and is often unsuspected in the differential diagnosis of cirrhosis.

As the liver becomes congested, the central veins are distended, but the liver cords remain intact. With continuation of the hyperemia the liver cells surrounding the central vein undergo degenerative changes due to anoxemia and become atrophic, giving the liver the appearance described as the nutmeg liver. The large, firm liver of either of these two stages may produce some pain or tenderness in the hepatic region. Subclinical or mild jaundice may be present. With longstanding and particularly with recurrent episodes of congestive cardiac failure, cirrhosis may occur. Cirrhosis of this origin is rare in childhood.

Occlusion of the hepatic veins (Budd-Chiari syndrome) usually occurs suddenly as a thrombus or tumor obstructs the outflow from the liver. Congenital webs in the hepatic veins may be the structures upon which engraftment of the thrombus or tumor occurs. Clinically, abdominal enlargement, jaundice, splenomegaly and ascites occur in a period of a few days. Surgical treatment is difficult and not often successful, but should be attempted.

Veno-occlusive disease of Jamaican children is associated with cirrhosis. It is believed to be due to prolonged ingestion of toxic substances in "bush teas," which contain Senecio alkaloids.

HEREDITARY HEPATIC DISEASE

DEVELOPMENTAL DISORDERS

POLYCYSTIC LIVER DISEASE. This relatively uncommon disease, in which multiple cysts occur in the liver, is usually associated with polycystic renal disease. The renal component more often leads to symptoms and has therefore been more fully studied.

Polycystic disease in adults is inherited as an autosomal dominant, whereas autosomal recessive inheritance is typical for subjects who become symptomatic in infancy. The hepatic cysts are thought to represent dilated intralobular bile ducts which failed to undergo involution during embryonic development. They are invested with connective tissue, which may become extensive enough to obstruct hepatic venous circulation and lead to portal hypertension. When definitive determination of hepatic polycystic disease is warranted or indicated, a biopsy specimen should be obtained. Portal hypertension may require treatment.

CONGENITAL HEPATIC FIBROSIS. This developmental disorder is marked by irregular broad bands of fibrous tissue located chiefly in the portal areas. Hepatocellular function is usually well maintained, but portal hypertension often occurs and has been ascribed to defects in the terminal portions of the portal vein. Abdominal enlargement, hepatosplenomegaly and hematemesis usually lead to diagnosis by midadolescence. Portal pressure has been elevated in all instances in which it has been measured. Operative biopsy may be required to obtain sufficient tissue for diagnosis. Portacaval shunts have been successful in reducing portal pressure. A relationship to polycystic liver disease is suggested by the occurrence of polycystic kidneys in 1 of 3 siblings with hepatic fibrosis.

HEREDITARY HEMORRHAGIC TELANGIECTASIA (OSLER-RENDU-WEBER DISEASE). This condition, inherited as an autosomal dominant, is rarely associated with clinically significant liver disease. Hepatic involvement may be of several types: (1) telangiectases, (2) telangiectases with fibrosis, (3) postnecrotic cirrhosis, and (4) discrete massive hemangiomas. Postnecrotic cirrhosis without hepatic telangiectases may be related to chronic active hepatitis, inasmuch as these patients may also have immunologic defects.

METABOLIC DISORDERS

WILSON'S DISEASE

(Hepatolenticular Degeneration)

Wilson's disease is an autosomal recessive disease, occurring predominantly in young children. Symptoms become apparent as early as 5 years of age. By the beginning of the fourth decade of life, 95 per cent of patients will have developed symptoms, either of chronic liver disease or of a chronic neurologic disturbance. The symptoms are associated with an increase in the copper content of the liver and the central nervous system.

CLINICAL MANIFESTATIONS. There are varied modes of presentation of Wilson's disease. One of these modes reflects the hepatic dysfunction only. This form is usually seen in the younger patients and may resemble acute hepatitis. These patients have an acute onset of jaundice, have hepatomegaly, and may rapidly progress over a period of a few weeks into hepatic coma and death if treatment is not quickly instituted. In older patients, symptoms of involvement of the basal ganglia, such as rigidity, tremors, bradykinesia, dysarthria and abnormal posturing may mark the clinical onset. Psychic disturbances may accompany the neurologic form. Clinical jaundice may be absent, or hematemesis from esophageal varices be the only symptom; hepatosplenomegaly may, however, be evident, or the Kayser-Fleischer ring, a characteristic greenish orange discoloration at the superior and inferior borders of the cornea. Examination with slit lamp may be necessary to demonstrate early deposition of copper in Descemet's membrane; the absence of corneal changes does not exclude the diagnosis of Wilson's disease, especially in the younger patient during the first decade of life.

A more unusual method of presentation is as an acute hemolytic anemia. The anemia has been ascribed to a rapid shift of copper from storage sites into the blood, an abrupt increase in erythrocyte copper content resulting in hemolysis.

DIAGNOSIS. The diagnosis of Wilson's disease is

made by the demonstration of a decreased serum ceruloplasmin. The level of this specific alpha-2-globulin is low (less than 20 mg/dl) in 97 per cent of symptomatic patients. This protein can be measured either by virtue of its oxidase activity toward a number of polyphenols and polyamines or by a quantitative immunologic procedure. Low ceruloplasmin levels have been found in cord bloods of newborn infants, in diseases in which there is loss of protein, such as protein-losing gastroenteropathies, or in the nephrotic syndrome, kwashiorkor, and terminal liver failure.

Approximately 95 per cent of serum copper is incorporated into this protein. In spite of the general decrease in ceruloplasmin in Wilson's disease, the serum copper value may be normal; it is usually decreased. The fraction of serum copper bound to albumin apparently increases, so that the decrease in serum copper may not be so large as the reduction in serum ceruloplasmin.

Hypercupriuria (greater than 50 μg/day) also occurs in patients with Wilson's disease, who may excrete as much as 1.5 mg of copper per day. Since urinary excretion of copper may be increased in other forms of cirrhosis, especially biliary, examination of this alone does not establish the diagnosis of Wilson's disease. In Wilson's disease the copper content of the liver usually exceeds 100 μg per gm of dry weight.

When Wilson's disease has been found in one member of a family, the other family members must be screened with liver function tests, including levels of serum ceruloplasmin and urinary copper excretion, to exclude the presence of disease in otherwise asymptomatic siblings. Patients with asymptomatic disease may have higher hepatic copper levels than their symptomatic siblings. At any stage of presentation, however, mild to moderate changes in liver function are present. Even in the asymptomatic patient, elevations of serum transaminases are found, and pathologic changes can be seen on liver biopsy.

Renal tubular dysfunction occurs in patients with Wilson's disease. Deposition of copper in the tubular cell probably accounts for the incomplete acidification of the urine, the decreased tubular reabsorption of phosphate, and the glycosuria, aminoaciduria and uricosuria. The tubular defect accounts for the low serum urate levels which are typically seen in these patients.

PATHOLOGY. Early in the course of the illness, the changes in liver cells may be mild, including glycogen degeneration, vacuolization of nuclei and fatty cytoplasmic changes. In fulminant hepatic disease, diffuse pseudoglandular transformation of the lobule occurs, with diffuse mesenchymal reaction. In the older patient, portal fibrosis is more common. The basic defect of Wilson's disease is thought to be either insufficient biliary excretion of lysosomal copper or increased copper binding by a cytoplasmic protein, metallothionine, or copperthionein. (See also Section 8.)

TREATMENT. The goal of therapy is to deplete the body of excess stores of copper. To meet this goal, several approaches are necessary. The normal adult ingests about 2.5 to 5.0 mg of copper daily. To reduce the dietary intake, copper-rich foods such as liver, shellfish, nuts and chocolate must be avoided. Drinking water should be tested; if its copper content is high, distilled water should be substituted. Potassium sulfide (10 to 40 mg) is given with meals to decrease further the intestinal absorption of dietary copper. D-Penicillamine (β,-β-dimethylcysteine), an effective copper chelator, is given orally (0.02 gm/kg/day) on an empty stomach; an increase in urinary excretion of copper will result. Asymptomatic patients discovered by screening of siblings should also be treated with this regimen. Toxic reactions to penicillamine are common and include fever, a maculopapular rash, thrombocytopenia, leukopenia and nephrosis. Since these reactions may be transient, repeated therapeutic attempts are indicated. Early and prolonged treatment yields excellent results. The untreated disease is progressive and invariably fatal.

OTHER METABOLIC DISORDERS

GALACTOSEMIA. The liver is altered in nearly all patients with galactosemia, and frank cirrhosis is common. Fatty metamorphosis is present in the first weeks of life; later, liver plates are altered to pseudoglandular structures. The lesion progresses to cirrhosis with regenerative nodules. (See also Section 8.)

CYSTIC FIBROSIS. Focal cirrhosis has been found by Bodian in one fourth of 62 patients with cystic fibrosis examined at necropsy, and in almost all patients living beyond 1 year. Juvenile cirrhosis occurred in 16 per cent of patients in the study of di Sant'Agnese and Blanc, but it does not often produce hepatic symptoms. Cirrhosis may, however, antedate clinical evidence of pancreatic insufficiency in cystic fibrosis, and cystic fibrosis should be considered in the differential diagnosis of portal hypertension in childhood.

FRUCTOSE INTOLERANCE. Postnecrotic cirrhosis resembling that found in galactosemia may occur in patients with hereditary fructose intolerance. (See Section 8.)

SICKLE CELL DISEASE. Sickle cell disease is commonly associated with significant hepatic injury, which may be of several types: portal cirrhosis, ischemic necrosis and hemochromatosis. Hepatic damage appears to be secondary to ischemic infarcts produced by blockage of sinusoids with sickled erythrocytes, and by thromboses resulting from release of thromboplastin when sickle cells are impacted in the sinusoids. Gallstones occur in approximately one third of patients and are usually asymptomatic. Viral hepatitis secondary to transfusion and hemosiderosis consequent to hemolysis may also contribute to the hepatic damage.

GLYCOGENOSES (GLYCOGEN STORAGE DISEASE). Glycogen storage disease of several types produces hepatic enlargement. However, only one, type IV (brancher deficiency) storage disease, produces cirrhosis. (See Section 8.)

OTHER STORAGE DISEASES. Hepatomegaly, usually without cirrhosis or serious disturbance in liver function, is a common finding in several of the lysosomal storage diseases. Included in this category of chronic liver involvement are the generalized gangliosidoses, mucopolysaccharidoses, I-cell disease, Sandhoff's disease, Gaucher and Niemann-Pick diseases and cholesterol ester storage disease.

TYROSINOSIS. Tyrosinosis (Sakai) usually presents with multiple renal tubular defects and an enlarged cirrhotic liver and rickets. It may present as a fulminating neonatal disease with many of the characteristics of neonatal hepatitis. In some patients bouts of hypertension and symptoms suggesting acute intermittent porphyria have been seen. Autosomal recessive inheritance is likely. Biochemical findings include a high plasma level of tyrosine, generalized aminoaciduria with a marked excretion of tyrosine, and a large urinary excretion of phenolic acid derivatives of tyrosine, of δ-aminolevulinic acid and of catecholamines. Urinary excretions of protein, glucose and phosphate are increased, and hypophosphatemia results in rickets. The activity in the liver of p-hydroxyphenyl-pyruvate oxidase is reduced or absent. Reduction of the intake of phenylalanine and tyrosine is followed by a marked improvement in renal tubular function. The effect of dietary restriction on hepatic function is not clear.

A number of cases of neonatal cirrhosis described in the past are probably examples of this disorder. The lesion in the liver may resemble biliary cirrhosis, hepatic cholestasis, portal fibrosis or a focal nodular cirrhosis. The disease has certain features resembling cystinosis and Wilson's disease. (See also Section 8.)

CYSTINOSIS (FANCONI SYNDROME). Cirrhosis may accompany this condition, but the renal tubular dysfunction and hypophosphatemic rickets are its paramount clinical manifestations.

HEPATIC PORPHYRIA. Cirrhosis has been observed in all forms of hepatic porphyrias except the acquired form. Fibrous changes, increased storage of hepatic iron and hepatomas may also occur.

HEMOSIDEROSIS AND HEMOCHROMATOSIS. Excessive storage of iron without tissue damage may be defined as hemosiderosis and a generalized increase in body stores of iron in association with tissue damage as hemochromatosis. Idiopathic hemochromatosis (Section 8) may be mimicked by the late stages of other iron storage states such as those following repeated blood transfusions or excessive parenteral or oral administration of iron, hemolysis, or hepatocellular necrosis. The disease presents a classic tetrad of pigmentation, liver disease, diabetes mellitus and heart failure. Diagnosis involves demonstration of an increased plasma iron level (greater than 0.15 mg/dl), 75 to 100 per cent saturation of iron-binding protein and a positive liver biopsy. Treatment is by repeated phlebotomies. In anemic patients, intramuscular desferrioxamine may foster the removal of approximately 15 mg of iron per day.

PROGRESSIVE FAMILIAL CHOLESTASIS. This newly recognized progressive disorder presents with clinical and chemical evidence of obstructive jaundice. Early histologic changes consist of bile staining of hepatic cells and varying degrees of plugging of canaliculi with bile. The process progresses to fibrosis and biliary cirrhosis.

Clinical manifestations have included severe itching, which may antedate jaundice by months or years. On the other hand, jaundice has appeared as early as 6 to 7 weeks of life. Hepatosplenomegaly, growth retardation, abdominal pain and a facies marked by full cheeks and prominent eyes are common manifestations. Steatorrhea is common, and there is an increase in concentrations of bile acids in the plasma. The skin may be greatly thickened as the result of scratching. Mental retardation and a fatal course terminating in infancy or childhood have been observed in some but not all kindreds.

The syndrome was first reported by Clayton and associates in 1969 in seven members of four Amish families. Additional cases have been reported from Great Britain, Japan and the United States. Autosomal recessive inheritance is indicated.

Williams and associates studied the metabolism of ^{14}C-chenodeoxycholate in one of three siblings, all of whom died in childhood of liver failure. Plasma bile acids were increased to 325 nanomoles per ml (N<5). Lithocholate, a secondary bile acid derived from chenodeoxycholic acid and normally undetectable in plasma, constituted 16 per cent of the plasma bile acids. Its concentration was also elevated in bile and jejunal fluid. An increase in the per cent of the chenodeoxycholic acid pool which was present in the plasma (5 per cent) was also found (N<1 per cent). Since lithocholate produces cirrhosis, cholestasis and ductular hyperplasia in animals, an abnormality involving synthesis of bile acids or intestinal absorption may be the underlying basis for this disorder.

Additional biochemical features include impaired storage and clearance of Bromsulphalein, elevations of conjugated bilirubin, alkaline phosphatase and transaminases, and a decrease in prothrombin time with the development of cirrhosis.

ALPHA-1-ANTITRYPSIN DEFICIENCY. A deficiency of alpha-1-antitrypsin in association with neonatal hepatitis and cirrhosis has been reported in several families. Deficiency of this serum alpha globulin was earlier associated with the development of emphysema in young adults; recent reports indicate that changes in the liver tissues of these young adults resemble those found in these children with chronic liver disease. Clinically there are no specific features, except that the family history may indicate juvenile cirrhosis or emphysema. Serum levels of antitrypsin can be determined by a radioimmunodiffusion technique.

Histologically, periportal hepatocytes contain cytoplasmic globules which are amylase-fast and PAS-positive. These inclusions have been shown by immunofluorescence staining techniques to be related to alpha-1-antitrypsin. The relationship of the glycoprotein in the hepatocyte to the cirrhosis remains to be established.

THE LIVER IN INFLAMMATORY BOWEL DISEASE

Involvement of the liver may take various forms in inflammatory bowel disease (ulcerative colitis, and the like). *Fatty changes* are the most frequent and appear in the periphery of the lobule and progress centrally. This alteration results from undernutrition secondary to anorexia, anemia and intestinal loss of protein. *Postnecrotic cirrhosis* is common and probably results from serum hepatitis due to transfusion or other parenteral injections. *Pericholangitis* may result from portal toxemia and bacteremia arising from the inflamed colon. It may be benefited by prolonged treatment with a broad spectrum antibiotic. *Chronic intrahepatic cholestasis* has also been described; the clinical picture resembles that of primary biliary cirrhosis.

NUTRITIONAL LIVER DISEASES

Dietary protein deficiency produces two types of hepatic injury in experimental animals: One, acute massive hepatic necrosis with postnecrotic scarring, is caused by deficiency of sulfhydryl groups (cystine and methionine) and of alpha tocopherol. Its analogue in human disease is the necrosis seen in fulminating viral hepatitis and various kinds of poisoning. The second type, fatty liver with fibrosis, results from the dietary deficit of lipotropic labile methyl groups (lecithin, choline and methionine) (see below). A number of clinical syndromes of human nutritional liver disease, collectively designated as *protein malnutrition* or *kwashiorkor,* occur among native populations of tropical and subtropical regions.

Other identified syndromes include the following: *protein malnutrition complicated by Senecio (ragwort) poisoning* in South Africa. The Senecio alkaloids are hepatotoxic and are apparently ingested as a contaminant of wheat bread. Hepatomegaly and ascites are characteristic.

Protein malnutrition with siderotic cirrhosis of the liver in native South African children. The iron pigment in the cirrhotic liver appears to come from the iron cooking utensils in which carbohydrate foods are prepared.

Vomiting sickness of Jamaica is probably due to toxic substances in "bush teas" made from the bitter cassava or unripe ackee fruit. It produces severe hepatic damage in malnourished children, and is epidemic in the winter months. Severe vomiting after meals is characteristic, and associated with *hypoglycemic manifestations.* Death occurs in many instances in 2 to 3 days.

ROBERT KAYE
PHILIP G. HOLTZAPPLE

INDIAN CHILDHOOD CIRRHOSIS

A greater prevalence of cirrhosis of the liver in children in the tropics and subtropics than in the temperate zones is generally recognized, but in two widely separated regions, Jamaica and India, it is sufficiently common to constitute a public health problem. There seem to be certain differences, however, between the types encountered in these two areas. The Jamaican cases, known also as *veno-occlusive disease,* have an abrupt onset with acute hepatomegaly and ascites followed by a subacute phase with persistent hepatomegaly, with or without ascites, and finally by chronic cirrhosis.

By contrast, the onset of illness in Indian childhood cirrhosis is insidious or subacute in nearly three fourths of patients, and acute, resembling viral hepatitis, in the others; ascites is a late manifestation. Cirrhosis due to neonatal hepatitis, congenital atresia of bile ducts and certain vascular and metabolic disorders occurs in infants in India, as in Europe and America, but the frequent occurrence of cirrhosis of unknown origin in India among children between 1 and 5 years of age justifies the separate clinical designation "Indian childhood cirrhosis."

ETIOLOGY. An intriguing aspect of Indian childhood cirrhosis is that its maximum prevalence has been approached only in India, though a few such cases have been reported from Ceylon, Burma, Indonesia, West Africa, Costa Rica and Middle Eastern countries. The disease was once confined to coastal areas of India and predominantly to some communities, but is now seen in all areas. A preponderance of cases in certain communities still exist. The familial incidence of the disease is well established, but no consistent pattern of hereditary transmission has been observed, nor any chromosomal abnormality. The familial occurrence may indicate either a recessive gene or a dominant gene of low penetrance.

Gross malnutrition does not lead to Indian childhood cirrhosis. On the other hand, cirrhosis due to malnutrition associated with tuberculosis or aflatoxin is not uncommon in India and may in the later stages be difficult to differentiate from Indian childhood cirrhosis both clinically and histopathologically.

The similarity of histologic changes in the liver to those in the chronic phase of viral hepatitis, along with the frequency of an onset like viral hepatitis, has given rise to the speculation that Indian childhood cirrhosis may be a sequela of viral hepatitis, with or without jaundice. Clinical, epidemiologic and pathologic data collected over the past two decades lend support to this view. The recent findings of hepatitis-associated antigen in 10 to 20 per cent of cases of Indian childhood cirrhosis with insidious onset strengthens the view that a viral infection may be a major factor in the etiology of this disease.

PATHOLOGY. In the early stage the most constant change seen in liver biopsy specimens is damage of the liver cells. Fatty vacuolation of the liver cells is absent at all stages. Cellular infiltrates are often present. In the stage of cirrhosis there is postnecrotic scarring, with regenerating and degenerating nodules. Occlusion of hepatic vein radicles, a common feature in the Jamaican cases, is uncommon in the Indian ones.

CLINICAL MANIFESTATIONS. The onset is usually insidious, with vague symptoms of poor appetite and slight abdominal distention. The child lacks pep and is often peevish; nutrition is fair in early stages. Intermittent phosphaturia has been reported. Occasionally in some patients the onset is acute, comparable to that of viral hepatitis. Enlargement of the liver is invariably present from the beginning. Usually the liver extends to the umbilicus within a few months, contracting to some extent in the late stages, when it becomes increasingly firm. Jaundice is common in the late stages, and also often occurs for a short period in the early phase; occasionally there is a history of preceding jaundice.

Fever is inconstant, but never high. At times there is a discoverable cause such as an upper respiratory tract infection, but more often there is none, and the fever seems to be due to further hepatic parenchymal destruction. The child deteriorates during such febrile episodes. Portal hypertension with ascites, evidences of collateral circulation and hematemesis may be terminal manifestations. Splenomegaly and hypoproteinemic edema are also common in the late stages. The clinical manifestations can be attributed to hepatic dysfunction (peevishness, poor appetite, pale stools), to portal hypertension (ascites, tympanites, hematemesis) and in the late stages to hypersplenism (anemia, leukopenia and purpura due to thrombocytopenia).

The course is from a few months to a year or two; even in the more severe and prolonged cases, recovery may rarely occur and be complete as shown by clinical and by liver biopsy studies.

TREATMENT. Treatment is mainly symptomatic. Although a nutritious diet with moderate amounts of protein and vitamins, including vitamin B_{12}, can be expected to help these children, unusually large amounts of protein or lipotropic substances have not been beneficial and indeed may be harmful. Cortisone used over periods of months or years seems beneficial. Surgery may be indicated for esophageal varices. Hematemesis may necessitate transfusion, and extensive ascites may require drainage.

V. Balagopal Raju

Achar, S. T., Raju, V. B., and Sriramachari, S.: Indian childhood cirrhosis. J. Pediatr. *57*:744, 1960.

Balagopal Raju, V., Sundaravalli, N., Madhavan, T. V., and Sriramachari, S.: Proceedings of Indian Council of Medical Research Expert Committee on Liver, Chandigarh, India, February, 1972.

Chandra, R. K., Ramalingaswamy, V., et al.: Proceedings of Indian Council of Medical Research on Immunological Studies in Indian Childhood Cirrhosis, Chandigarh, India, February, 1972.

Jelliffe, D. B., Gerrit Bras, and Mukherjee, K. L.: Veno-occlusive disease of the liver and Indian childhood cirrhosis. Arch. Dis. Child. *32*:369, 1957.

Sriramachari, S., Sundaravalli, N., Madhavan, T. V., and Balagopal Raju, V.: Proceedings of Indian Council of Medical Research Expert Committee of Pathologists on Liver, Delhi, India, May, 1972.

FATTY INFILTRATION

Fatty infiltration of the liver results from deposition of dietary or mobilized tissue fat in the hepatic cells. Various lipotropic factors prevent the accumulation or accelerate the removal of excessive hepatic fat in the experimental animal. Choline and a large number of its chemical analogues inhibit the deposition of neutral fats and cholesterol esters and cause more rapid removal of these lipids from the livers of animals fed excessive fat. Methionine has also been shown to be lipotropic.

Fat is deposited in normal liver cells and, in larger amounts, in damaged liver cells in a variety of clinical conditions. Fatty infiltration of the liver occurs in many metabolic disorders such as obesity, starvation, galactosemia, diabetes mellitus and familial hyperlipemia. It is encountered frequently in chronic tuberculosis and osteomyelitis and occasionally after pneumonia. It may occur rapidly during corticosteroid therapy. Large fatty livers occur in poisoning with phosphorus, phlorhizin, chloroform, alcohol, arsenic and mushrooms, and in severe anemic states, presumably owing to anoxia. Fatty infiltration of the liver is also a common secondary condition in childhood.

Fatty infiltration of the liver should not be confused with *fatty degeneration* of hepatic cells, in which pre-existent cell lipids are altered chemically and become visible as fat droplets. In fatty infiltration the normal lipid content of the liver (3 to 5 per cent) may increase to 40 per cent. In fatty degeneration there is an alteration in the normal proportion between hepatic cholesterol and other hepatic lipids, but no absolute increase of liver fat. Occasionally, with hyperlipemia, the Kupffer cells of the liver will phagocytize fat droplets and become swollen.

CLINICAL MANIFESTATIONS. Infiltration of the liver by fat is usually not directly responsible for symptoms or abnormalities in hepatic function. When hypoglycemia and ketosis are present, the hepatomegaly may be confused with glycogen storage disease. The usual clinical finding is hepatic enlargement, which may be extreme in some instances.

TREATMENT. Reduction of fat intake with a liberal allowance of protein is indicated. Beneficial effects have been described after administration of choline and its analogues (betaine), but are difficult to evaluate. Reduction of corticosteroid dosage or improved control of the hyperglycemia in diabetes will result in decreased lipolysis and excretal clearing of the fat from the liver in appropriate instances.

PORTAL HYPERTENSION

See also Congestive Splenomegaly (Banti Syndrome).

ETIOLOGY. In children, in contrast to adults, obstruction of the portal vein exceeds cirrhosis as a cause of symptomatic portal hypertension. Thrombosis may be secondary to omphalitis in the neonatal period or to cannulation of the umbilical vein for exchange transfusion or other purposes. The development of collaterals in the connective tissue around the thrombosed portal vein is a response to obstruction rather than a malformation.

At the time of birth the ductus venosus branches off the left portal vein to enter the inferior vena cava. The umbilical vein is in continuity with both the ductus venosus and the left branch of the portal vein. Sepsis in the umbilical region may, therefore, spread along the umbilical vein to the left branch of the portal vein and then to the main portal vein. Umbilical infection may also spread to the hilus of the liver, producing portal vein obstruction there. Rarely, the normal obliterative process involving the umbilical vein and ductus venosus may extend to the portal vein. Anomalies of the portal venous system are rare: obstructive valves in the portal vein have been reported, as well as fistulas between the hepatic artery and portal vein and between the splenic artery and vein. Obstruction of the portal vein by neoplastic invasion is uncommon.

Portal hypertension is a common sequel to the cirrhosis which follows extrahepatic biliary obstruction or to postnecrotic hepatocellular disease. Because of the poor prognosis in these conditions, documentation of the presence of portal hypertension is often of only academic interest.

Acute thrombosis of the portal vein is usually followed by spread to the mesenteric veins, with diarrhea, peritonitis and intestinal gangrene.

CLINICAL MANIFESTATIONS. In portal vein thrombosis, hepatic function is usually normal and the presenting signs are those resulting from portal hypertension. Hematemesis is common and is often accompanied by the passage of bright red blood per rectum.

The opportunities for development of collateral communications between the portal and systemic circulations are many. They include: from vessels of the liver, esophagus and cardia of the stomach to diaphragmatic and intercostal veins; from vessels in the falciform ligament to umbilical veins; and from the surfaces of abdominal organs to vessels in the abdominal wall and in the retroperitoneal tissues; and from hemorrhoidal and portal veins to the azygos and bronchial ones. Because many of the collateral vessels enter the azygos vein, a widened mediastinum may be demonstrated by tomography.

Collateral circulation between portal and systemic vessels may produce dilated veins on the abdominal wall; such vessels radiating from the umbilical region are referred to as "caput Medusae." With development of extensive collateral circulation, venous hums may be audible over the xiphoid or umbilicus. The Cruveilhier-Baumgarten syndrome consists of cirrhosis and portal hypertension with a patent umbilical vein; this permits development of a particularly prominent caput Medusae. The varicosities arising in the *esophagus and stomach* are the most important, owing to their tendency to bleed massively (see below).

Pancytopenia commonly results from hypersplenism in the enlarged spleen (the Banti syndrome).

Ascites has generally not been considered to result from portal hypertension without cirrhosis, but it has been recognized in extrahepatic portal obstruction as a consequence of hypoproteinemia due to hemorrhage.

DIAGNOSIS. Radiographic examination of the esophagus for varices is the simplest and safest means of detecting collateral circulation secondary to portal hypertension. The mucosa of the normal esophagus appears on contrast study to exhibit long, narrow, evenly spaced lines; these may be displaced by varices, which appear as filling defects. Small, flexible fiberoptic esophagoscopes facilitate direct visualization; varices appear as blue, rounded projections beneath the mucosa.

Percutaneous measurement of intrasplenic pressure yields a good approximation of portal venous pressure. Portal venous pressure is normally about 7 mm Hg; presinusoidal pressure in the spleen is slightly above this value. Measurement of an elevated intrasplenic pressure provides a baseline for evaluating the effectiveness of shunting procedures.

Splenic venography should be carried out, but demonstration of collaterals alone does not establish the presence of portal hypertension, since the collaterals may effectively decompress the portal system. Demonstration of normal wedged hepatic vein pressure with elevated intrasplenic pressure establishes the site of the vascular obstruction as being in the extrahepatic portion of the portal vein. This procedure is not often necessary in children, since the distinction between intrahepatic and extrahepatic portal vein obstruction is readily made on clinical and biochemical grounds.

In a normal splenoportogram the opaque medium reaches the liver in 2 to 3 seconds, and the only vessels seen are the splenic and portal veins. The procedure is useful in investigating the cause of intestinal bleeding and essential before creating an anastomosis between portal and systemic circulations. It is also of value in the investigation of splenomegaly and in the delineation of liver masses. There is a 1 per cent risk of serious hemorrhage following splenoportography and this procedure should be undertaken only when definitive surgery is contemplated and scheduled.

Umbilical vein catheterization has been utilized as an alternate method of visualization of portal vein collaterals and determination of portal venous pressure. It can be carried out under local anesthesia and avoids the occasional splenic rupture which may follow percutaneous splenoportography.

Intrahepatic presinusoidal portal hypertension without elevation of wedged hepatic vein pressure has been encountered in schistosomiasis, in congenital hepatic fibrosis and in infiltrations of the portal tracts with primitive hematopoietic tissue, as in myeloproliferative disease, myeloid leukemia, Hodgkin's disease or sarcoid.

In cirrhosis with portal hypertension, wedged hepatic venous pressure is also elevated (*intrahepatic postsinusoidal portal hypertension*). Connective tissue proliferation in the portal tracts may lead to anastomoses between portal and hepatic vein radicles (internal Eck fistulas). In cirrhosis the main obstruction is to outflow from the hepatic vein, in which wedged pressures may remain elevated even after successful shunting procedures. In veno-occlusive disease, phlebitis of minute hepatic vein radicles also results in postsinusoidal intrahepatic portal hypertension.

Obstruction to outflow of the main hepatic veins by cardiac failure or constrictive pericarditis results in postsinusoidal extrahepatic portal hypertension.

Primary portal hypertension has been described; it may be the result of excessive blood flow through an enlarged spleen.

TREATMENT. In infants and children with portal hypertension secondary to cirrhosis, the prognosis of the underlying liver disease is often so poor as to contraindicate surgical treatment. On the other hand, in patients with Wilson's disease who have massive esophageal bleeding, amelioration of the portal hypertension by surgery may be indicated in view of expected improvement in the hepatic disease with penicillamine treatment.

Extrahepatic portal obstruction leading to symptomatic portal hypertension requires careful consideration of operative intervention. There are a number of reasons for conservatism in relation to a surgical approach. The surgical problems are more difficult in young children because of the small size of vessels available for portal to systemic vein anastomosis. If acute bleeding can be adequately controlled, the normal hepatic functions of these patients enable them to tolerate recurrent hemorrhages. A further basis for conservatism in respect to shunting procedures in children is the observation that variceal bleeding may cease spontaneously after repeated episodes. These considerations make the delay of surgical intervention until at least 4 to 6 years of age or older a reasonable course in most instances.

In most instances of portal hypertension secondary to portal vein thrombosis the vessel is unsuitable for anastomosis. In some patients patent proximal segments of the vessel seen on venography may be used for anastomosis to the inferior vena cava. The collateral branch most used for relief of portal hypertension in children is the splenic vein, which is anastomosed to the left renal vein, with removal of the spleen. Unfortunately the splenic vein may be unsuitable owing to small size, extension of thrombosis, perisplenitis involving the vessels at the splenic pedicle, previous splenectomy, or thrombosis of an earlier splenorenal shunt. It should be emphasized that splenectomy without a shunt procedure should not be done for obstruction of the portal vein, because it is ineffective in relieving portal hypertension and sacrifices the vessel most useful in definitive shunting procedures. Alternative approaches must be devised when the splenic vein is unsuitable for anastomosis.

ESOPHAGEAL AND GASTRIC VARICES

The clinical features are those of gastrointestinal bleeding, with the added manifestations of portal hypertension. The bleeding may be slow, and productive of melena, anemia and increased red cell production, or it may occur as massive hematemesis; it may continue for days until controlled by treatment. Patients with intact hepatic function whose portal hypertension is caused by thrombosis of the portal vein tolerate hemorrhage much better than those with cirrhosis.

When the source of bleeding is in doubt, a water-soluble barium solution may be used even in the presence of bleeding to establish its site. The Sengstaken tube, for compression of varices, may be used diagnostically as well as therapeutically. In obscure situations splenic venography may be used to detect varices.

In emergency treatment of bleeding varices, transfusion of whole blood is indicated, preferably guided by measurement of blood volume. Intensive care may be needed to prevent brain damage from hemorrhagic shock and anoxia. Esophageal tamponade employs the Sengstaken tube, a three-lumen tube connected to balloons placed in the esophagus and in the upper part of the stomach, and permitting aspiration of blood from the stomach; this will usually control bleeding. The gastric balloon is filled with radiopaque material in order to verify by radiography its proper placement. The balloons are distended to a pressure of approximately 30 mm Hg and traction is applied over a pulley. The technique has the disadvantages of being uncomfortable and giving rise at times to ulceration of the esophagus and pharynx.

CYSTS OF THE LIVER

Conditions which may simulate hepatic cyst include hydrops of the gallbladder, choledochal cyst, hydronephrosis, mesenteric cyst, duplication of the intestine and tuberculous peritonitis.

Hepatic cysts are relatively uncommon in children. They may be classified as follows:

A. Parasitic
   1. Echinococcal
B. Nonparasitic
   1. Solitary—retention
   2. Multiple—polycystic disease
   3. Cystadenoma—proliferative
   4. Pseudocyst—degenerative
   5. Teratomas
   6. Lymphatic-lymphangiomatous
   7. Endothelial—ciliated epithelial

Large cysts may be manifest by abdominal enlargement and vague gastrointestinal symptoms. Displacement of adjacent structures may be apparent on radiologic studies of the upper gastrointestinal tract. Echinococcal cysts are under relatively high tension, and the cyst wall characteristically exhibits calcification roentgenographically. Nonparasitic cysts have a predilection for the anteroinferior surface of the right lobe of the liver and may grow intrahepatically or extrahepatically. They are responsible for little or no impairment of liver function.

Treatment is by elective surgery, unless bleeding into or rupture of a cyst makes surgical intervention an urgent matter. A plane for excision can usually be established between the fibrous layers of the cyst wall and the liver substance. When resection is not feasible, simple drainage or marsupialization is usually effective in causing regression of the cyst.

The Gallbladder

The gallbladder of the newborn infant is elongated, deeply embedded in the liver, and usually does not reach the liver edge. It gradually assumes its pear shape in later infancy. The volume is approximately 3 ml in the young infant, 40 ml in the adult.

CONGENITAL ANOMALIES. Congenital anomalies of the gallbladder are rare. It may be bilobed or duplicated, or it may be absent with or without atresia of the hepatic ducts. Other anomalies include diverticulum, the so-called floating gallbladder, which is suspended from the liver by a mesentery and is freely movable, and various other malpositions, which may be left-sided, intrahepatic or retrodisplaced. These anomalies may be confusing radiologically but usually have little clinical significance.

CHOLECYSTITIS. Acute inflammation of the gallbladder is uncommon in childhood, but not so rare as generally thought. It may accompany a variety of acute infections, including bacterial pneumonia, meningitis, peritonitis and typhoid fever. The symptoms are nausea, vomiting, fever, abdominal distention and pain in the right upper quadrant. In some instances the gallbladder may be palpable as a tense, excruciatingly tender mass in the right upper quadrant. The diagnosis is not easily made, since most pain in the right upper quadrant in children is not of gallbladder origin. In many instances a preoperative diagnosis of intestinal obstruction is made. With advancing symptoms surgery is advisable, although with treatment of the associated infection symptoms and signs diminish rapidly.

CHOLELITHIASIS. Biliary calculi are uncommon in early life, but more common than cholecystitis. Calculi have been reported even in stillborn fetuses. In Ullen's series of 30 cases of cholecystitis in children, 43 per cent were jaundiced and 57 per cent exhibited stones. In 7 per cent of his cases the stone was in the common bile duct. Cholelithiasis in childhood occurs frequently as a complication of the congenital hemolytic anemias in white children and of sickle cell anemia in blacks. The stones are composed almost entirely of the excessive blood pigment liberated by hemolysis, but calcium is deposited in some, yielding a shadow visible roentgenographically. Pure pigment stones cast no shadow and are demonstrable only by the use of contrast medium. Even gallstones associated with idiopathic cholecystitis in children may fail to be visualized by such means. The treatment of symptomatic cholelithiasis is surgical. Dissolution of cholesterol gallstones by chenodeoxycholic acid appears efficacious in adults. Detection of those individuals susceptible to development of gallstones and their early use of chenodeoxycholic acid or other similar agents may ultimately diminish the importance of cholelithiasis as a gastrointestinal disease.

The Bile Ducts

CYSTIC DILATATION AND PERFORATION

(Choledochus Cyst)

Choledochus cyst, or cystic dilatation of the common bile duct, is generally considered to be an idiopathic congenital condition. Often there is no demonstrable mechanical obstruction. The dilatation is usually localized to the common duct, in contradistinction to the dilatation resulting from obstruction, which involves the entire biliary tract and usually the gallbladder. Occasionally the dilatation may involve the cystic and hepatic ducts. Lee and Mitchell have described bile peritonitis in infants secondary to perforation of the common bile duct and have related the latter to choledochal cysts. Exudate and fibrosis at the site of perforation may presumably result in formation of a bile-containing sac. A choledochus cyst may grow to large dimensions; cysts with a capacity of 2 liters are recorded.

The clinical manifestations of choledochus cyst are pain, jaundice and abdominal tumor. The liver may become enlarged and cirrhotic, and frequently there is cholangitis. Fever is indicative of infection. The pain is in the upper abdominal or umbilical region and is usually "dragging." Jaundice may be present.

Prolonged obstructive jaundice with serum alkaline phosphatase levels of 200 to 300 IU is suggestive of choledochal cyst or other incomplete obstruction to the common bile duct, as by stenosis or tumor. Radiographic visualization using oral or intravenous cholangiography may be diagnostic. Distortion of or impression on the duodenal loop on roentgenographic examination of the upper gastrointestinal tract suggests obstruction and dilatation of the common duct secondary either to intrinsic disease or to infiltrative disease of the pancreas.

Treatment is surgical, the operation of choice being a primary anastomosis between the biliary system and the intestinal tract. The results are usually good, if cirrhosis has not developed.

ATRESIA OF THE EXTRAHEPATIC BILE DUCTS

ETIOLOGY. Biliary atresia is generally thought to be a developmental anomaly. In early fetal life the liver and its ductal system develop as a diverticulum from the ventral floor of the endodermal foregut. The bile ducts and the gallbladder originate from the caudal portion; the liver arises from the cephalad portion. The ducts are initially patent, but become obliterated by epithelial proliferation to form solid cords, which with further development are recanalized. Failure of this last phase may involve all or part of the extrahepatic biliary tree, to give the clinical conditions of biliary atresia.

It has also been suggested that biliary atresia may represent an acquired lesion related to neonatal hepatitis. This relationship is suggested because biliary atresia has rarely been found in stillborn infants and occurs only rarely in premature infants, and also because some infants with obstruction of the extrahepatic bile ducts have histologic giant cell transformation.

PATHOLOGY. The tissues are deeply bile-stained, and the liver is enlarged and firm. During the first 4 to 6 months of life these changes are progressive. Histologically there is strikingly little distortion of the normal architecture of the hepatic plates. The outstanding feature is the extensive fibrosis within the portal triads, in which proliferating bile ducts are embedded. These changes have been noted in tissue obtained by needle biopsy during the first month of life. With further fibrosis and the development of cirrhosis there is interference with portal circulation and the development of portal hypertension. The spleen becomes enlarged, and during the second half of the first year of life esophageal varices, ascites and the hematologic changes of hypersplenism make their appearance. In cases of long duration the bones may show osteomalacia as a result of the associated severe malabsorption.

Effective surgical correction depends upon the presence of a patent portion of the extrahepatic ductal system in continuity with the intrahepatic biliary tree. This favorable circumstance has been reported to occur in 4 to 50 per cent of patients; its actual frequency is probably closer to the lower figure.

CLINICAL MANIFESTATIONS. Jaundice and hepatomegaly are the most striking signs, but may not be detected for several weeks after birth. The hyperbilirubinemia is predominantly of the conjugated variety. The concentration of bilirubin in the serum is usually below 10 mg/dl during the first 6 to 8 weeks of life, after which it steadily increases. Growth is impaired, especially in the latter part of the first year of life. The general appearance of well-being of these infants in the early phase is in striking contrast to their deep icterus. In the second half of the first year of life nutritional failure to the point of cachexia is common, and signs of portal hypertension and of liver cell failure may appear, with hypoproteinemic edema, bleeding secondary to prothrombin deficiency, and hyperammonemia. By this time the infant presents a pathetic, irritable appearance, with a skin color of greenish gray or bronze.

The stools are putty-like in consistency and white or clay-colored. Small amounts of bile pigments may be excreted on the surface of the stool. These are derived from intestinal secretions and epithelium and are responsible in a minority of patients for unexpectedly positive reactions for urobilinogen (stercobilinogen) in the face of complete obstruction of the extrahepatic biliary system.

The urine is always dark, resembling strong tea in color, and contains large amounts of direct-reacting bilirubin and bile salts. Urobilinogen is usually absent from the urine, except, as indicated above, when small amounts represent bilirubin which has entered the bowel with intestinal secretions and desquamated cells.

LABORATORY FINDINGS. There is moderate anemia and a steady increase in the conjugated hyperbilirubinemia. Transaminase values in the serum are elevated, but in most instances remain below 400 units; the serum leucine aminopeptidase is usually elevated above 250 units. Serum alkaline phosphatase is also moderately elevated. Early in the course of the disease prothrombin concentrations are maintained in the normal range. When low values occur, correction is usually possible by parenteral administration of vitamin K until the late stage when hepatic cellular failure has developed.

DIAGNOSIS. Congenital malformation of the bile ducts must be differentiated from other causes of obstructive jaundice in early infancy. The principal diagnostic problem is differentiation from neonatal hepatitis. (See earlier for suggested plan of study.) Occasionally an infant with the early manifestations of biliary atresia will, during operative cholangiography, expel a mucous plug from the common duct, with complete clearing of symptoms.

Prior to the general use of exchange transfusion in the treatment of erythroblastosis fetalis, some affected infants had a prolonged episode of obstructive jaundice which was inappropriately labeled "the inspissated bile syndrome" on the assumption that the obstruction was related to excessive excretion of bilirubin. This syndrome results from hepatocellular injury associated with hemolysis rather than mechanical obstruction; it has become quite rare.

TREATMENT. When a patent portion of the extrahepatic biliary tree is demonstrated on cholangiography, surgical correction of the obstruction is mandatory. Interposition of a segment of small intestine between the biliary tree and small intestine will usually prevent pyogenic bacterial cholangitis owing to ascending infection.

Occasionally at necropsy potentially operable lesions are found which were not detected at laparotomy, or impressive dilatation of portions of the intrahepatic biliary system. These observations suggest that in patients found to be inoperable initially, a second operative procedure should be considered after several months. Late dilatation of intrahepatic bile ducts may account for some reports of successful treatment of biliary atresia with implantation of tubes into the substance of the liver. Successful liver transplantation appears to be the ultimate therapy for extrahepatic biliary atresia, but complications of infection and rejection remain formidable problems.

The infant with an inoperable lesion requires symptomatic treatment. Vitamin K in an oral dose of 5 mg/day may delay bleeding due to hypoprothrombinemia. Vitamin D in a water-soluble medium in a dose of 1000 units/day will usually prevent clinical rickets. Antihistamines and starch baths should be given for itching, though they may be of little help. Paracentesis for relief of ascites should be withheld in favor of diuretics, as discussed above with the management of chronic liver disease.

PROGNOSIS. Patients with inoperable lesions usually succumb by the end of the second year of life. Correction of operable biliary atresia by 3 to 4 months of age should be followed in most instances by satisfactory regression of biliary cirrhosis. Good results are occasionally attained by surgery in older infants.

ATRESIA OF THE INTRAHEPATIC BILE DUCTS

Intrahepatic atresia of bile ducts has been observed most often in association with atresia of the extrahepatic biliary system and especially in infants with an unusually long survival time. It is likely that in such instances the intrahepatic atresia represents an atrophy of disuse of structures deprived of their normal function. It is possible that atresia of the intrahepatic biliary system might coexist with patent extrahepatic bile ducts, given the separate origins of the two portions of the biliary system from the cephalad and caudad portions of the foregut diverticulum. The outstanding clinical features of intrahepatic biliary atresia are prolonged survival, often to the end of the first decade, and hyperlipidemia with prominent cutaneous xanthomata. Treatment is symptomatic, including that for pruritus. Phenobarbital and cholestyramine increase the extrahepatic excretion of bilirubin and bile salts and decrease the serum lipids in these patients.

ROBERT KAYE
PHILIP G. HOLTZAPPLE

GENERAL

Popper, H., and Schaffner, F.: Progress in Liver Diseases. Vol. IV. New York, Grune & Stratton, 1972.

Schiff, L.: Diseases of the Liver. 3rd ed. Philadelphia, J. B. Lippincott Company, 1969.

Sherlock, S.: Diseases of the Liver and Biliary System. 4th ed. Oxford, Blackwell Scientific Publications, 1971.

Silverman, A., Roy, C. C., and Cozzetto, F. J.: Pediatric Clinical Gastroenterology. St. Louis, The C. V. Mosby Company, 1971.

Biochemistry and Function Tests

Combes, B., and Schenker, S.: Laboratory tests. *In* Schiff, L.: Diseases of the Liver. 3rd ed. Philadelphia, J. B. Lippincott Company, 1969.

Hong, R., and Schubert, W. K.: Menghini needle biopsy of liver. Am. J. Dis. Child. *100*:42, 1960.

Numerof, P.: Radioisotopes in liver and pancreatic disease. Radiol. Clin. N. Amer. *8*:115, 1970.

O'Brien, D., Ibbott, F. A., and Rodgerson, D. O.: Laboratory Manual of Pediatric Microchemical Techniques. 4th ed. New York, Harper and Row, 1968.

Sharp, H. L., Krivit, W., and Lowman, J. T.: The diagnosis of complete extrahepatic obstruction by rose bengal I-131. J. Pediatr. *70*:46, 1967.

Sherlock, S.: The immunology of liver disease. Am. J. Med. *49*:693, 1970.

Wheeler, H. O., Meltzer, J. I., and Bradley, S. E.: Biliary transport and hepatic storage of sulfobromophthalein sodium in the unanesthetized dog, in normal man, and in patients with hepatic disease. J. Clin. Invest. *39*:1131, 1960.

Disorders of Bilirubin Metabolism

Arias, I. M.: Inheritable and congenital hyperbilirubinemia; Models for the study of drug metabolism. New Engl. J. Med. *285*:1416, 1971.

Arias, I. M., Gartner, L. M., Cohen, M., Ezzer, J. B., and Levi, A. J.: Chronic nonhemolytic unconjugated hyperbilirubinemia with glucuronyl transferase deficiency. Am. J. Med. *47*:395, 1969.

Behrman, R. E., and Hsia, D. Y.-Y.: Summary of a symposium on phototherapy for hyperbilirubinemia. J. Pediatr. *75*:718, 1969.

Berk, P. D., Bloomer, J. R., Howe, R. B., and Berlin, N. I.: Constitutional hepatic dysfunction (Gilbert's syndrome). A new definition based on kinetic studies with unconjugated radiobilirubin. Am. J. Med. *49*:296, 1970.

Black, M., and Billing, B. H.: Hepatic bilirubin UDP–Glucuronyl transferase activity in liver disease and Gilbert's syndrome. New Engl. J. Med. *280*:1266, 1969.

Dubin, I. N.: Chronic idiopathic jaundice: A review of fifty cases. Am. J. Med. *24*:268, 1958.

Fleischner, G., and Arias, I. M.: Recent advances in bilirubin formation, transport metabolism and excretion. Am. J. Med. *49*:576, 1970.

Gartner, L. M., and Arias, I. M.: Formation, transport, metabolism and excretion of bilirubin. New Engl. J. Med. *280*:1339, 1969.

Levi, A. J., Gatmaitan, Z., and Arias, I. M.: Deficiency of hepatic organic anion-binding protein, impaired organic anion uptake by liver and "physiologic" jaundice in newborn monkeys. New Engl. J. Med. *283*:1136, 1970.

Maurer, H. M., Shumway, C. N., Draper, D. A., and Hossaini, A. A.: Controlled trial comparing agar, intermittent phototherapy and continuous phototherapy for reducing neonatal hyperbilirubinemia. J. Pediatr. *82*:73, 1973.

Odell, G. B.: "Physiologic" hyperbilirubinemia in the neonatal period. New Engl. J. Med. *277*:193, 1967.

Poland, R. L., and Odell, G. B.: Physiologic jaundice: The enterohepatic circulation of bilirubin. New Engl. J. Med. *284*:1, 1971.

Powell, L. W., Hemingway, E., Billing, B. H., and Sherlock, S.: Idiopathic unconjugated hyperbilirubinemia (Gilbert's syndrome). A study of 42 families. New Engl. J. Med. *277*:1108, 1967.

Schmid, R.: Bilirubin metabolism in man. New Engl. J. Med. *287*:703, 1972.

Sherlock, S.: Biliary secretory failure in man: Problem of cholestasis. Ann. Intern. Med. *65*:397, 1966.

Spiegel, E. L., Schubert, W., Perrin, E., and Schiff, L.: Benign recurrent intrahepatic cholestasis with response to cholestyramine. Am. J. Med. *39*:682, 1965.

Neonatal Hepatitis

Alpert, L. I., Strauss, L., and Hirschhorn, K.: Neonatal hepatitis and biliary atresia associated with trisomy 17–18 syndrome. New Engl. J. Med. *280*:16, 1969.

Brent, R. L.: Persistent jaundice in infancy. J. Pediatr. *61*:111, 1962.

Norman, A., Strandvik, B., and Zetterstrom, R.: Bile acid excretion and malabsorption in intrahepatic cholestasis of infancy ("neonatal hepatitis"). Acta Paediatr. Scand. *58*:59, 1969.

Poley, J. R., Smith, E. I., Boon, D. J., Bhatia, M., Smith, C. W., and Thompson, J. B.: Lipoprotein-X and the double 131-I rose bengal test in the diagnosis of prolonged infantile jaundice. J. Pediatr. Surg. *7*:660, 1972.

Schweitzer, I. L., Moseley, J. W., Ashcavai, M., Edwards, V. M., and Overby, L. B.: Factors influencing neonatal infection by hepatitis B virus. Gastroenterology *65*:277, 1973.

Sharp, H. L., and Mirkin, B. L.: Effect of phenobarbital on hyperbilirubinemia, bile acid metabolism and microsomal enzyme activity in chronic intrahepatitis cholestasis of childhood. J. Pediatr. *81*:116, 1972.

Strauss, L., and Bernstein, J.: Neonatal hepatitis in congenital rubella. Arch. Path. *86*:317, 1968.

Thaler, M. M., and Gellis, S. S.: Studies in neonatal hepatitis and biliary atresia. I. Long-term prognosis of neonatal hepatitis. II. The effect of diagnostic laparotomy on long-term prognosis of neonatal hepatitis. III. Progression and regression of cirrhosis in biliary atresia. IV. Diagnosis. Am. J. Dis. Child. *116*:257, 1968.

Acute Liver Disease

Breen, K. J., and Schenker, S.: Hepatic coma: Present concepts of pathogenesis and therapy. *In* Popper, H., and Schaffner, F.: Progress in Liver Diseases. Vol. IV. New York, Grune & Stratton, 1972.

Carver, D. H., and Seto, D. S. Y.: Current concepts concerning the hepatitis viruses. Pediatrics *51*:115, 1973.

Ginsberg, A. L., Conrad, M. E., Bancroft, W. H., Ling, C. M., and Overby, L. R.: Prevention of endemic HAA-positive hepatitis with gamma-globulin. New Engl. J. Med. *286*:562, 1972.

Huttenlocher, P. R.: Reye's syndrome: Relation of outcome to therapy. J. Pediatr. *80*:845, 1972.

Klatskin, G.: Toxic and drug-induced hepatitis. *In* Schiff, L.: Diseases of the Liver. 3rd ed. Philadelphia, J. B. Lippincott Company, 1969.

Krugman, S., Giles, J. P., and Hammond, J.: Viral hepatitis. Type B. (MS-2 strain). Studies on active immunization. J.A.M.A. *217*:41, 1971.

Perez, V., Schaffner, F., and Popper, H.: Hepatic drug reactions. *In* Popper, H., and Schaffner, F.: Progress in Liver Diseases. Vol. IV. New York, Grune & Stratton, 1972.

Saunders, S. J., Hickman, R., MacDonald, R., and Terblanche, J.: The treatment of acute liver failure. *In* Popper, H., and Schaffner, F.: Progress in Liver Diseases. Vol. IV. New York, Grune & Stratton, 1972.

Schubert, W. K., Partin, J. C., and Partin, J. S.: Encephalopathy and fatty liver (Reye's syndrome). *In* Popper, H., and Schaffner, F.: Progress in Liver Diseases. Vol. IV. New York, Grune & Stratton, 1972.

Schweitzer, I. L., Wing, A., McPeak, C., and Spears, R. L.: Hepatitis-associated antigen in 56 mother-infant pairs. J.A.M.A. *220*:1092, 1972.

Shulman, N. R.: Hepatitis-associated antigen. Am. J. Med. *49*:669, 1970.

Silverberg, M., Wherrett, B., Worden, E., and Neumann, P. Z.: An evaluation of rest and low-fat diets in the management of acute infectious hepatitis. J. Pediatr. *74*:260, 1969.

Chronic Liver Disease

Conn, H. O.: The rational management of ascites. *In* Popper, H., and Schaffner, R.: Progress in Liver Disease. Vol. IV. New York, Grune & Stratton, 1972.

Page, A. R., Good, R. A., and Pollara, B.: Long-term results of therapy in patients with chronic liver disease associated with hypergammaglobulinemia. Am. J. Med. *47*:765, 1970.

Sherlock, S., and Scheuer, P. J.: The presentation and diagnosis of 100 patients with primary biliary cirrhosis. New Engl. J. Med. *289*:674, 1973.

Soloway, R. D., Summerskill, W. H. J., Baggenstoss, A. H., Geall, M. G., Gitnick, G. L., Elveback. L. R., and Schoenfield, L. J.: Clinical biochemical, and histological remission of severe chronic active liver disease: A controlled study of treatments and early prognosis. Gastroenterology *63*:820, 1972.

Summerskill, W. H. J.: Ascites: The kidney in liver disease. *In* Schiff, L.: Diseases of the Liver. 3rd ed. Philadelphia, J. B. Lippincott Company, 1969.

Weber, A., and Roy, C. C.: The malabsorption associated with chronic liver disease in children. Pediatrics *50*:73, 1972.

Hereditary Liver Disease

Bearn, A. G.: Wilson's disease. *In* Stanbury, J. B., Wyngaarden, J.

B., and Frederickson, D. S. (eds.): The Metabolic Basis of Inherited Disease. 3rd ed. New York, McGraw-Hill Book Co., Inc., 1972.
Bensel, R. W., and Peters, E. R.: Congenital hepatic fibrosis presenting as hepatomegaly in early infancy. J. Pediatr. *72*:96, 1968.
Gray, O. P., and Saunders, R. A.: Familial intrahepatic cholestatic jaundice in infancy. Arch. Dis. Child. *41*:320, 1966.
Halvorsen, S., Pande, H., Loken, A. G., and Ghessing, L. R.: Tyrosinosis: A study of 6 cases. Arch. Dis. Child. *41*:238, 1966.
Jagenburg, R., Landblad, B., Magnus de Maré, J., and Rodjer, S.: Hereditary tyrosinemia: Metabolic studies in a patient with partial p-hydroxyphenylpyruvate hydrolase activity. J. Pediatr. *80*:994, 1972.
Linarelli, L. G., Williams, C. N., and Phillips, M. J.: Byler's disease: Fatal intrahepatic cholestasis. J. Pediatr. *80*:485, 1972.
Scriver, C. R., Partington, M., and Sass-Kortsak, A. (eds.): Conference on hereditary tyrosinemia. Canad. Med. Ass. J. *97*:1045, 1967.
Sharp, H. L., Desnick, R. J., and Krivit, W.: The liver in inherited metabolic diseases of childhood. *In* Popper, H., and Schaffner, F.: Progress in Liver Disease. Vol. IV. New York, Grune & Stratton, 1972.
Sharp, H. L., and Freier, E.: Alpha-1-antitrypsin and familial cirrhosis. Gastroenterology *60*:179, 1971.
Slovis, L., Dubois, R. S., Rodgerson, O., and Silverman, A.: The varied manifestations of Wilson's disease. J. Pediatr. *78*:578, 1971.
Sommerschild, H. C., Langmark, F., and Maurseth, K.: Congenital hepatic fibrosis: Report of two new cases and review of the literature. Surgery *73*:53, 1973.
Sternlieb, I., and Scheinberg, I. H.: Prevention of Wilson's disease in asymptomatic patients. New Engl. J. Med. *278*:352, 1968.
Tyson, R. T., Schuster, S. R., and Shwachman, H.: Portal hypertension in cystic fibrosis. J. Pediatr. Surg. *3*:271, 1968.
Williams, C. N., Kaye, R., Baker, L., Hurwitz, R., and Senior, J. R.: Progressive familial cholestatic cirrhosis and bile acid metabolism. J. Pediatr. *81*:493, 1972.

Portal Hypertension

Clatworthy, W. H., Jr., and de Lorimier, A. A.: Portal decompression procedures in children. Am. J. Surg. *107*:447, 1964.
Mikkelsen, W. P., Edmondson, H. A., Peters, R. L., Redeker, A. G., and Reynolds, T. B.: Extrahepatic portal hypertension in children. Am. J. Surg. *111*:333, 1966.
Voorhees, A. B., Harris, R. C., Britton, R. C., Crice, J. B., and Santulli, T. V.: Portal hypertension in children: 98 cases. Pediatr. Surg. *58*:540, 1965.

The Bile Ducts

Danks, D. M., and Campbell, P. E.: Extrahepatic biliary atresia: Comments on the frequency of potentially operable cases. J. Pediatr. *69*:21, 1966.
Hays, D. M., et al.: Diagnosis of biliary atresia: Relative accuracy of percutaneous liver biopsy, open liver biopsy, and operative cholangiography. J. Pediatr. *71*:598, 1967.
Javitt, N. B., Morrissey, K. P., Siegel, E., Goldberg, H., Gartner, L. M., Hollander, M., and Kok, E.: Cholestatic syndromes in infancy: Diagnostic value of bile acid pattern and cholestyramine administration. Pediatr. Res. *7*:119, 1973.
de Lorimier, A. A.: Surgical management of neonatal jaundice. New Engl. J. Med. *288*:1284, 1973.
Stiehl, A., Thaler, M. M., and Admirand, W. H.: The effects of phenobarbital on bile salts and bilirubin in patients with intrahepatic and extrahepatic cholestasis. New Engl. J. Med. *286*:858, 1972.
Warren, K. W., Kune, G. A., and Hardy, K. J.: Biliary duct cysts. Surg. Clin. N. Amer. *48*:567, 1968.

The Gallbladder

Morales, L., Taboada, E., Toledo, L., and Radrigan, W.: Cholecystitis and cholelithiasis in children. J. Pediatr. Surg. *2*:565, 1967.
Natar, G.: Gall bladder disease in childhood. Aust. Paediatr. J. *8*:147, 1972.
Strauss, R. G.: Cholelithiasis in childhood. Am. J. Dis. Child. *117*:689, 1969.

THE PANCREAS

The pancreas contains two types of secreting glands: the acinar tissue is responsible for the exocrine secretion, and the islands of Langerhans for the endocrine secretion.

This section is concerned only with the disorders of the exocrine pancreas. Disturbances of the endocrine function (diabetes mellitus and hypoglycemia) are discussed in Section 16.

PHYSIOLOGY OF THE EXOCRINE GLANDS OF THE PANCREAS

Pancreatic juice is collected by a branching system of ducts and conveyed through the ducts of Wirsung and Santorini into the second portion of the duodenum. The principal ferments in pancreatic juice are trypsin, chymotrypsin, carboxypeptidase, amylase and lipase. Trypsin is secreted as a precursor, trypsinogen, which must be activated by the action of enterokinase, an intestinal hormone. Chymotrypsin is secreted as chymotrypsinogen and is activated by trypsin. Pro-carboxypeptidase is also activated by trypsin. Trypsin and chymotrypsin, acting separately, digest proteins to peptides, which are then split to amino acids by pancreatic and intestinal carboxypeptidase (erepsin). Amylase is secreted in active form and digests starch to maltose, which later is hydrolyzed to glucose by intestinal maltase. Pancreatic lipase is activated by bile salts and splits the neutral fat molecule into its component fatty acid and glycerol. Trypsin and to some extent lipase and amylase are present at birth.

Pancreatic secretion is under both autonomic nervous (parasympathetic and sympathetic) control and hormonal regulation. Secretin, a hormone liberated by the mucosal cells of the upper intestinal tract in response to ingestion of food, is transported by the blood to the pancreas, where it stimulates the secretion of pancreatic juice, principally its water and inorganic constituents. Pancreozymin, a second pancreatic excitant, is also obtained from extracts of duodenal mucosa. Unlike secretin, it stimulates the secretion of enzymes, but exerts little or no effect on the volume of secretion.

TESTS OF PANCREATIC FUNCTION

Direct measurements of enzymatic activity of fluid obtained by duodenal drainage are the most reliable tests of pancreatic function. Good hydration and a reasonably good clinical condition of the patient are important prerequisites in order to ensure ample volume and enzyme content of the material obtained. An ordinary Levin tube can be used for the procedure, especially in infants and young children. It is important that no openings of the tube be in the stomach. A double-lumen tube can be used to advantage in older children.

Normally the duodenal fluid is clear, watery and of varying shades of yellow, depending on its bile content. Its pH is between 6.5 and 9; fluids of a lesser pH should not be accepted for testing. The volume obtained by drainage increases with advancing age: from an average of 3 to 5 ml per hour in infants to as much as 6 to 30 ml per hour in older children. The proteolytic enzymes, lipase and amylase, then can be measured by viscosimetric or enzymatic methods. A pancreozymin-secretin test to stimulate both bicarbonate and water secretion and enzymatic production also can be used: it has been studied in children by Hadorn et al.

ABSORPTION TESTS. Pancreatic function can be assessed indirectly by studies of fecal fat and nitrogen content or by fat absorption tests (*q.v.*). The rise of amino acid levels in blood after ingestion of a test meal of casein or gelatin has also been used as an indirect measure of pancreatic function.

The presence of tryptic activity in stools has been estimated by their capacity to digest the gelatinous coating of photographic film. The value of this test is limited, since proteolytic activity of bacterial origin may be present in stools. Ingestion of honeydew melon, pineapple or pancreatin may also give false positive results. Assessment of pancreatic enzymes from the tryptic and chymotryptic activity of fresh stool specimens on specific synthetic substrates as described by Barbero et al. may be more satisfactory.

DIFFERENCES BETWEEN STEATORRHEAS DUE TO PANCREATIC MALDIGESTION AND THOSE SECONDARY TO FAILURE OF ABSORPTION

Irrespective of etiology there are important differences between pancreatogenous maldigestion and other types of steatorrhea secondary to failure of absorption (e.g., gluten-induced enteropathy). In addition to steatorrhea, azotorrhea is always present in pancreatic deficiency, but fecal nitrogen excretion is normal in most other types of malabsorption.

In pancreatogenous steatorrhea there is a striking lack of correlation between level of fecal fat and nitrogen and clinical symptoms, and states of relatively good health and adequate nutrition and growth are compatible with great losses of both these nutrients through the feces. Conversely, most patients with steatorrheas secondary to impaired absorption states (e.g., gluten-induced enteropathy) are apt to be sick clinically, with relatively small increases in fecal fat excretion.

In patients with steatorrhea and maldigestion due to pancreatic deficiency (e.g., cystic fibrosis, inherited pancreatitis, and other conditions) hypocalcemia has never to our knowledge been reported and serum calcium and phosphorus levels are normal. In many other types of malabsorption hypocalcemia and its consequences are frequently seen in severe cases (e.g., gluten-induced enteropathy, agammaglobulinemia). Presumably this is due to the fact that in patients with pancreatic deficiency the fats are not split by pancreatic lipase; throughout most of the intestine, therefore, they are present as neutral fats, which do not form soaps with calcium as do fatty acids.

SWEAT TESTS FOR CYSTIC FIBROSIS

Determination of chloride and sodium levels in sweat is the principal diagnostic test for cystic fibrosis. The eccrine sweat glands number over 2 million in man. Their function is to help control body temperature through production of sweat. The sweat glands can be stimulated to secrete by environmental heat, by injection of cholinergic drugs or by iontophoresis.

QUALITATIVE SWEAT TESTS. These have been used for screening purposes. The reaction of chloride in palmar sweat with an appropriately treated agar plate or filter paper has been used for such testing. Conductivity of sweat, which is increased when the electrolyte concentration is increased, has also been measured, using modifications of the conventional Wheatstone conductivity bridge.

None of these procedures should be relied upon for a definitive diagnosis. If cystic fibrosis is suspected, a *quantitative sweat test* should be obtained. Quantitative tests of sweat induced by thermal stimulation are used primarily in research; the iontophoresis of pilocarpine is recommended for diagnostic purposes.

QUANTITATIVE SWEAT TEST BY IONTOPHORESIS OF PILOCARPINE. Iontophoresis of pilocarpine, which utilizes a small electric current to carry this cholinergic drug into the skin and stimulate sweat glands locally, is safe, painless and reliable for diagnostic purposes.

The electric current source should supply direct current at a voltage between 0 and 22 volts. The current passing between electrodes is measured by a milliamperemeter which records accurately variations between 0 and 5 milliamperes. A simple wiring diagram for a battery-operated machine has been given by Gibson and Cooke; various models are also commercially available.

The area to be iontophoresed is washed with distilled water and dried. The flexor surface of the forearm is used except in small infants, in whom the thigh may be substituted. Two milliliters of 0.2 per cent pilocarpine nitrate are pipetted onto a 2- by 2-inch gauze square placed on a positive copper electrode (1.8 by 1.8 inches in size), which is then applied to the washed area. A negative copper electrode of similar size (permanently covered with gauze) is placed elsewhere on the same extremity, its gauze covering wet with 0.9 per cent sodium chloride solution. Both electrodes are firmly attached with rubber straps of the kind used for electrocardiography. The lead wires are then connected, and the current is gradually raised to 4 milliamperes in 15 to 20 seconds. Iontophoresis is continued for 5 minutes.

A current of 4 milliamperes passing through 4 square inches of skin is barely detectable. But if the positive electrode is not completely covered with gauze or the contact with the skin is poor, the current passes through a much smaller area and gives rise to a burning sensation. In this case momentary pressure should be applied to the offending electrode, or the strap should be tightened.

After completion of iontophoresis, the electrodes are removed, the gauze with pilocarpine solution is discarded, and the area of skin under the positive electrode is washed with distilled water and dried.

A thin pad of dry gauze, 2 inches square (a brand with low sodium content), or a low-ash filter paper of similar size is removed from a bottle, in which it was previously weighed, and placed over the area of skin in which the pilocarpine was iontophoresed. The gauze or filter paper is then covered with a plastic square (2½ by 2½ inches) and sealed at the edges with waterproof adhesive tape to prevent evaporation.

The collecting gauze or filter paper is left in place for 30 to 45 minutes and then reweighed in the same flask. The difference between the second and the first weights represents the amount of sweat collected (usually 100 to 600 mg. NOTE: amounts less than 100 mg do not give reliable analytic results if a flame photometer is used.) In order to avoid contamination of the gauze or filter paper by fingers, a forceps should be used for all steps.

The sweat is then eluted from the gauze or filter paper with distilled water or other appropriate solution and analyzed for chloride by one of the titration methods and for sodium by flame photometry.

ANOMALIES OF THE PANCREAS

Annular pancreas is often associated with obstruction of the descending duodenum, which it partially or completely surrounds. The condition may cause symptoms in the neonatal period or early childhood or may cause no disturbance until adult life. Duodenoduodenostomy or duodenojejunostomy has proved effective and safer than divisions of the pancreatic ring.

Ectopic pancreatic tissue (pancreatic heterotopia) is occasionally found in the wall of the duodenum or in other sites in the alimentary tract. In rare instances ectopic pancreatic tissue has served as the lead point of an intussusception. If present in Meckel's diverticulum or in a duplication, it may lead to ulceration and hemorrhage.

CYSTIC FIBROSIS*

(Fibrocystic Disease of the Pancreas; Pancreatic Fibrosis; Mucoviscidosis)

Cystic fibrosis is a hereditary disease of children, adolescents and young adults due to a generalized dysfunction of exocrine glands. In fully manifested cases there is chronic pulmonary disease, pancreatic deficiency, abnormally high sweat electrolyte levels and at times cirrhosis of the liver. Absence or only partial involvement of organs or glandular systems usually affected in cystic fibrosis is characteristic of the disorder and leads to many variations in the clinical pattern.

In the United States cystic fibrosis accounts for the great majority of cases of progressive chronic (nontuberculous) pulmonary disease in children, adolescents, and young adults, for almost all cases of pancreatic deficiency, for most of the cases of chronic malabsorption in children, for some of the patients with hepatic cirrhosis, and for a substantial number of newborn infants with intestinal atresia or obstruction.

HISTORY. Before the recognition of cystic fibrosis as a clinical entity, most patients died in infancy of bronchopneumonia; a small number in whom symptoms of malabsorption predominated were thought to have "celiac disease."

Cystic fibrosis was first noted as a separate entity by Fanconi in 1936; Andersen in 1938 gave the first complete pathologic and clinical description of the disorder. In recent years, owing to greater awareness of the entity, improved diagnostic techniques and the use of effective antibiotic agents to increase the life span of patients, the condition is recognized with increasing frequency.

Several distinct phases evolved in the study of cystic fibrosis: (1) The pathologic changes in the pancreas and the clinical effects of pancreatic deficiency attracted the attention of the early investigators and accounted for the name of the disease (Fanconi, Andersen, Blackfan and May). (2) In 1944 Farber pointed out that a widespread defect in mucous secretions could explain many symptoms of this disorder, and the name "mucoviscidosis" was suggested (Shwachman, Bodian). (3) With the demonstration in 1953 (di Sant'Agnese) of consistent involvement of sweat and salivary glands in this disorder, it became evident that cystic fibrosis is in reality a generalized disease affecting many and perhaps all exocrine glands, mucus-producing and others. (4) Recent evidence further suggests that the abnormal gene is expressed in every cell of the body. There also is reason to believe that in reality cystic fibrosis is a symptom complex common to more than one genetic error; it may, therefore, be more than one disease.

*The description of this disorder is given in this book under The Pancreas only as a matter of convenience and to avoid unnecessary repetition. For some aspects, see also Malabsorption Syndromes, this Section.

Cystic fibrosis is not, therefore, limited to the pancreas; this organ is frequently but not necessarily involved. The name traditionally given this generalized disorder is a misnomer, to be used only with realization of its limitations.

ETIOLOGY AND INCIDENCE. The basic defect in cystic fibrosis is unknown, but there is general agreement that it is genetically transmitted as an autosomal recessive trait. Most authors believe that a single mutant allele causes the disease; but the presence of multiple alleles at different loci cannot be excluded. The overall incidence of the disorder among siblings is one in four, and both sexes are affected with approximately equal frequency, as would be expected from this hypothesis. Its occurrence in more than 25 per cent of siblings in small family groups is presumably due to chance distribution. The finding of the disease in first cousins, the rarity of affected offspring in remarriages of parents, and the recent observation that all 11 children of 10 mothers with cystic fibrosis were phenotypically normal, offer additional support for the thesis of a recessive transmission. Homozygotes for the gene of cystic fibrosis have all or almost all of the clinical manifestations of the disease, whereas heterozygotes have no clinically recognizable symptoms.

From 2 to 4 per cent of autopsies in various children's hospitals in this country and abroad are in patients with cystic fibrosis. Several surveys indicate that the incidence of the fully manifested disease (homozygotes) is about 1 in 2000 live births in countries with populations predominantly of Caucasian descent. It follows that about 5 per cent of the general population in the same areas are carriers of the cystic fibrosis gene (heterozygotes); this implies a very high mutation rate since heterozygote survival advantage has not as yet been demonstrated. Cystic fibrosis is, therefore, the most common substantially lethal hereditary disease among young Caucasians. Fibrocystic disease is less common in blacks than in Caucasians; homozygotes are born in one in ten to twelve thousand black live births in the U.S., which indicates that about 2 per cent of American blacks are carriers of the gene. Cystic fibrosis is rare in Oriental peoples and in native African blacks.

PATHOLOGY. In the *mucus-producing glands* throughout the body abnormal secretions may accumulate and dilate them (Fig. 11–25). In some organs (e.g., pancreas and intrahepatic bile ducts) the secretions precipitate or coagulate to form eosinophilic concretions in the glands and ducts and obstruct the outflow of their secretions. Most of the pathologic changes and consequent clinical symptoms (e.g., pancreatic fibrosis and achylia) are thought to be secondary to this obstruction and not due directly to an abnormality of the secretions.

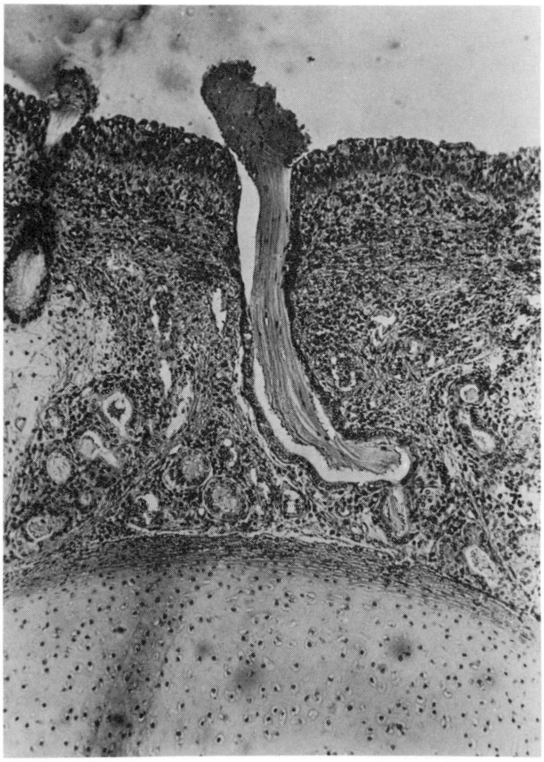

Fig. 11–25

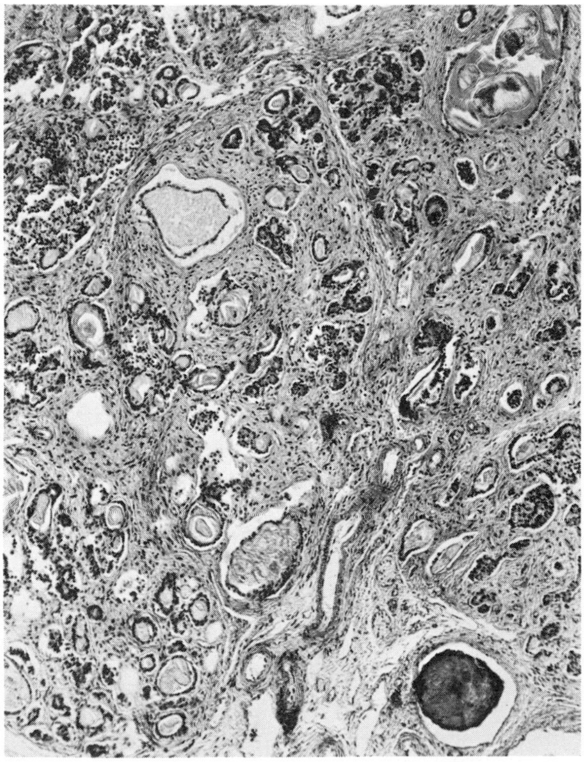

Fig. 11–26

Figure 11–25 *Microscopic section from trachea of patient who died at 6 months of age. Dense eosinophilic concretion obstructs a duct of the tracheal gland.*

Figure 11–26 *Microscopic section from pancreas of patient who died at 14 months of age. Note fibrosis, dilatation of ducts by eosinophilic inspissated secretion, calcified concretions and almost complete disappearance of acini.*

The most striking changes are characteristically observed in the *pancreas*, which grossly is smaller, thinner and firmer than normal. Microscopically the findings include obstruction of the pancreatic ducts by concretions, dilatation of the secretory acini and ducts and secondary degeneration of the exocrine parenchyma of this organ (Fig. 11–26). The pancreatic lesions are progressive. In the newborn infant most acinar cells appear normal, although the lumen contains concretions with initial fibrosis and inflammatory changes. After several years the picture is one of pancreatic atrophy with extensive fibrosis or replacement with fat. The entire process proceeds at variable speeds, and at a given age the pancreas of a patient may show different stages of evolution. The islands of Langerhans are usually normal, although they tend to decrease in number and exhibit increasing fibrosis with advancing age. Hyalinization or vascular changes in the islets are generally not present even when glucose intolerance and glycosuria are present.

Submaxillary, sublingual and labial *salivary glands* may be involved, with findings similar to those in the pancreas, although these changes are less widespread. In about one fifth of patients the *gallbladder* is small and contains a firm, gelatinous material which also fills the cystic duct.

Localized foci of biliary obstruction and fibrosis are common in the *liver* at necropsy, even in infants. These changes become progressively more extensive and may give rise to a distinctive type of multilobular biliary cirrhosis with large irregular nodules, at times with clefts. A trigger mechanism (e.g., nutritional injury or vital hepatitis) is postulated to account for the spreading of localized lesions. The onset of hepatic lesions before birth or in early infancy and the different growth rates of scar tissue and liver parenchyma may account for some of the bizarre morphologic findings. The fatty liver infiltration due to severe malnutrition described in earlier reports is uncommon nowadays, but is occasionally found even when nutrition has been adequate. Hepatic hemosiderosis may be seen in patients not treated with pancreatic replacement therapy. This is an expected finding, since pancreatic achylia of any cause is known to increase intestinal absorption of iron.

The *lungs* appear normal in most infants dying of complications other than chronic lung disease in the first few weeks of life. The initial lesion is a bronchiolar obstruction; later, the main bronchi also are blocked by mucopurulent material. Acute and chronic bronchitis, peribronchitis, patchy atelectasis, bronchiolectasis and bronchiectasis are commonly found at autopsy in cases of long standing. Destructive emphysema as such is not commonly seen in patients with cystic fibrosis; rather, a diffuse "obstructive overinflation" is usually prominent at necropsy.

Right ventricular hypertrophy is the dominant adaptive *cardiac change* and is probably directly related to the obstructive bronchial disease and pulmonary hypertension. Significant thickening of the arteriolar wall may be present in pulmonary vessels and has been considered a reversible change. It tends to increase with age and is probably secondary to contraction of the arteriolar muscle due to chronic hypoxia and acidosis. Occasional instances of perivascular myocardial fibrosis in scattered areas, predominantly of the left ventricle, have been reported.

Reproductive organs may be affected. Dilatation of cervical mucous glands is usually present in females. In males the mesonephric derivatives (epididymis, vas deferens and seminal vesicles) are generally abnormal, probably because of obstruction of the mesonephros by abnormal secretions early in fetal life, with consequent maldevelopment. The defects consist of anomalous or absent bodies and tails of the epididymides, with the globus major usually remaining intact; atretic or absent vasa deferentia; and dilated or absent seminal vesicles. In contrast, the prostate gland has usually been found to be normal, and examination of testes at biopsy and autopsy has revealed normal histology and active spermatogenesis, though abnormal forms of sperm often have been seen. Occasionally, especially when careful dissection is performed at autopsy, entirely normal male genital tracts are found.

Considerable deposition of *ceroid pigment* as a consequence of vitamin E deficiency is present in the smooth muscle of the gastrointestinal tract of patients dying after the age of 3 years. Lesions in the striate muscle due to deficiency of vitamin E, however, have never been substantiated.

Nonmucus-producing glands (e.g., sweat glands or parotid glands) show no pathologic histologic changes, although the chemical composition of their secretions may be abnormal.

PATHOGENESIS. The nature of the inborn error of metabolism which leads in the homozygotes to the generalized disease, cystic fibrosis, is as yet unknown. Present concepts as to pathogenesis are summarized in Figure 11–27. The unknown basic defect gives rise to two principal anomalies: (1) the "mucous secretion" abnormality; and (2) the electrolyte defect, most conspicuously expressed in the secretions of eccrine sweat glands but evident also in secretions of minor salivary glands.

"Mucous Secretion" Abnormality. Because of their abnormal physicochemical behavior mucous secretions precipitate in and obstruct passages of various organs, leading to virtually all the main clinical manifestations of cystic fibrosis: obstruction of bronchi and bronchioles, with chronic pulmonary disease; obstruction of pancreatic ducts, with pancreatic achylia; obstruction of biliary ductules, with cirrhosis of the liver; and various forms of intestinal obstructions.

Cystic fibrosis was at one time considered likely to be an inborn error of glycoprotein metabolism, but the evidence is far from conclusive. Dische et al. suggested that the primary alteration in glycoprotein fractions in cystic fibrosis might be in the carbohydrate moiety, with an increase in fucose (a methylpentose) changing the fucose:sialic acid

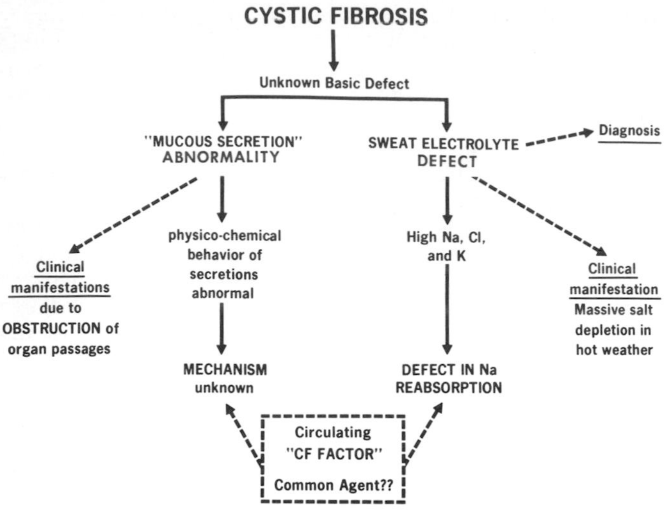

Figure 11–27 *Present concepts as to pathogenesis of cystic fibrosis.*

ratio. Some studies supported thse conjectures, but detailed chemical analyses of urinary macromolecules, Tamm-Horsfall urinary glycoprotein, salivary glycoprotein fractions, rectal mucus, and the like, disclosed no significant qualitative differences from normal, though at times the quantity or relative content of some components was increased or decreased.

In some tissue culture studies total acid mucopolysaccharides (AMPS) have been found increased, but there is no pathologic evidence of AMPS accumulation in the tissues of patients with cystic fibrosis. Moreover, in the majority of patients with cystic fibrosis there are no consistent or striking abnormalities in the amount and composition of urinary AMPS.

Electrolyte Defects. The sweat electrolyte abnormality is present from birth and throughout life and unrelated either to severity of the underlying disease or to whether other organs such as the pancreas or lungs are involved. It leads in patients with cystic fibrosis to concentrations in sweat of chloride, of sodium and, to a lesser extent, of potassium which are greatly in excess of the markedly hypotonic sweat levels found in normal individuals or in patients with almost any other type of disease (Fig. 11–28). The principal exceptions are renal diabetes insipidus and untreated adrenal insufficiency. In patients with cystic fibrosis, on the other hand, adrenal function is normal, and conservation of electrolytes by the kidney is normally preserved. From a practical standpoint, therefore, the abnormal increase in sweat electrolyte levels is extremely useful in diagnosis. The important clinical consequence is that massive salt depletion through sweating in hot weather may lead to serious and even fatal consequences through cardiovascular collapse.

In contrast to the elevated sweat concentrations of sodium, chloride and potassium, the levels of

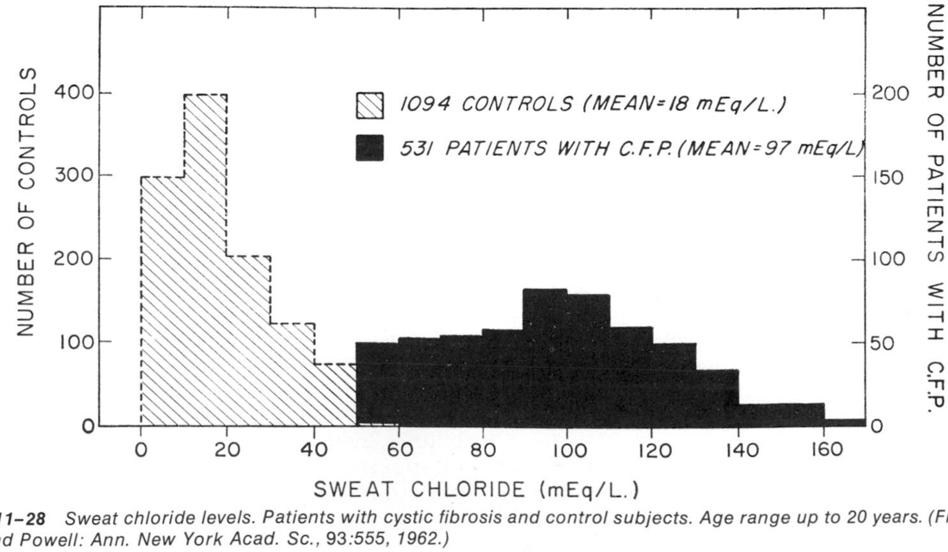

Figure 11–28 *Sweat chloride levels. Patients with cystic fibrosis and control subjects. Age range up to 20 years. (From di Sant'-Agnese and Powell: Ann. New York Acad. Sc., 93:555, 1962.)*

most other solutes, the rate of sweating, and other morphologic, physiologic and chemical factors of eccrine sweat gland function studied to date are either normal or close to normal. These include the calcium levels and the composition of the precursor solution in the sweat gland coil, as assayed by micropuncture methods. A defect in reabsorption of sodium and chloride in the sweat gland duct, therefore, has been postulated. Mangos and McSherry have found, in the sweat of patients with cystic fibrosis, a factor inhibiting sodium reabsorption. This gives a reasonable explanation of the increased sweat electrolyte levels. (See below.)

The only other exocrine gland system, in addition to the eccrine sweat glands, which constantly manifests the abnormality in sodium levels in cystic fibrosis consists of the small salivary glands found throughout the buccal mucosa. The sodium concentration in this type of saliva is markedly increased in patients with cystic fibrosis, but all other ions determined, including potassium and calcium, are found to be within normal limits. In contrast, sodium, chloride and potassium levels appear to be normal in submaxillary and parotid gland saliva, as well as in serum.

Studies of duodenal contents in patients who had cystic fibrosis but no pancreatic deficiency led Hadorn et al. in 1968 to suggest that failure in transport of electrolyte-containing fluid (bicarbonate as well as Cl and Na) and consequent concentration of macromolecules in organs throughout the body might result in many of the pathologic features of the disease. This hypothesis has not so far been proved.

Tissue Culture Abnormalities. In 1969 Danes and Bearn reported the occurrence of cytoplasmic metachromasia in tissue culture fibroblasts obtained from skin biopsies of patients with cystic fibrosis and of their parents (obligatory heterozygotes). This was soon followed by reports of a number of chemical anomalies in tissue culture fibroblasts for homozygotic patients with cystic fibrosis, though various laboratories have had different results, presumably owing to slight but important differences in the media and methods of tissue culture. The variety of abnormalities which have been identified in fibroblasts in tissue culture in patients with cystic fibrosis (metachromasia, increased total AMPS, glycogen increase, and others), as well as the varying results obtained by different investigators, presumably indicate that these findings are relatively nonspecific, though they may reflect a metabolic or catabolic defect.

"Cystic Fibrosis Factors." Spock et al. showed in 1967 that there is a factor in the serum of homozygotic patients and in the euglobin fraction of heterozygotes that induces "dyskinesia" in the ciliary epithelium of rabbit tracheal explants. Subsequently many investigators have tried with limited success to develop simple assay systems utilizing a variety of lower forms, on the theory that cilia behave in a similar manner regardless of whether the organism is a mammal, a clam, an oyster or another species. The factor appears to be heat labile, nondialyzable, has a molecular weight of 150,000 to 200,000, and on Sephadex or DEAE columns is eluted with IgG.

Also in 1967 Mangos and McSherry demonstrated that mixed saliva and sweat of cystic fibrosis patients (homozygotes) contains a factor which inhibits sodium reabsorption in an animal model (rat parotid). This was confirmed by Kaiser et al. in Switzerland for the human sweat gland in situ, by use of similar techniques. Experimental models give reason to believe that sodium transport in the gut of animals also may be affected. The factor was characterized by Mangos and McSherry as a strongly basic macromolecule, heat labile, destroyed by freezing and nondialyzable. They also showed that other basic polyelectrolytes have similar action, whereas the addition to the reactants of heparin, which is strongly negatively charged, eliminates the activity.

The demonstration of both of these factors depends at present on technically difficult biologic assay systems difficult to reproduce. Speculation is justified as to whether the factors described by Spock and Mangos and their associates are not in reality one and the same factor, perhaps in association with diverse fractions in various biologic fluids, and having different behavior and action in serum, sweat, and mixed saliva. There is some evidence this may be true.

Several investigators have shown that lymphoid cells and fibroblasts in culture produce a ciliotoxic factor. Interestingly, the tissue culture medium of fibroblasts does not become ciliotoxic until commercially available human IgG is added. The factor which becomes active after addition of this immunoglobulin is thought at present to be a small molecule of between 1000 and 10,000 molecular weight.

In addition, Rao and Nadler have recently shown that patients with cystic fibrosis have a deficiency in a trypsin-like enzyme (thought by them to be kallikrein-like). There is reason to believe that this deficient enzyme is not part of the kallikrein system, but perhaps another esterase of similar activity. In any case, this raises speculation as to whether the basic defect in cystic fibrosis may not be absence or deficiency of an enzyme which inactivates a small molecule produced even by normal people and which binds IgG. This molecule, perhaps a polypeptide, might be ciliotoxic when bound to IgG and not inactivated, and be inhibitory of reabsorption when unbound.

Calcium Abnormalities. Calcium abnormalities have been reported in cystic fibrosis, though calcium balance in this disease appears to be normal and serum levels of calcium and phosphorus are within normal limits.

Barbero et al. found some years ago a high calcium level in submaxillary (but not parotid) saliva of patients with cystic fibrosis. Later Gugler demonstrated that the gross appearance and the polyacrylamide-gel electrophoretic pattern of this secretion were quite distinctive in cystic fibrosis but could be normalized by chelating calcium with

EDTA. It was possible also by increasing calcium levels to transform both grossly and on electrophoresis the saliva of normal persons into saliva resembling that of patients with cystic fibrosis.

It was felt, therefore, that submaxillary saliva in both normal subjects and patients with cystic fibrosis contains some protein fractions which combine or interact with calcium present in high concentrations to form a reversible precipitate of high molecular weight that cannot travel in gel. There is evidence that even in submaxillary saliva calcium levels are normal at first, but that as time passes and as pathologic changes in this gland become increasingly severe (regardless of the degree of involvement in other organs of the body), calcium levels rise for unknown reasons. It is then that precipitation of calcium-protein complexes occurs, and presumably this is irreversible in vivo. The sequence in other organs may be similar.

Fortifying these observations, Bader found that the calcium transport ATPase in red blood cells of patients with cystic fibrosis was depressed, with a clear correlation between degree of depression and severity of the disease. He felt this might well account for the rising calcium levels in some of the secretions from cystic fibrosis patients and for the sequence of events.

Autonomic Nervous System. Abnormal function of the autonomic nervous system leading to overstimulation of cholinergic glands throughout the body has been proposed as a common denominator in cystic fibrosis. It would be an attractive explanation for many of the features of cystic fibrosis, especially since this system innervates all exocrine glands. Supportive evidence to date is not substantial.

Conclusions. It has been suggested that cystic fibrosis may be a syndrome or symptom complex common to two or more genetic errors. This unproved contention is supported by some tissue culture studies, by some clinical observations, and by the potential heterogeneity of genetic disease. The precipitation of calcium protein complexes (as exemplified in submaxillary saliva) may not be a primary defect, but suggests a possible mechanism for the kind of obstruction of glandular passages which gives rise to most of the clinical symptoms in this disease. There is some indication that an enzymatic deficiency may be responsible for failure of inactivation of a normally produced molecule, possibly having deleterious effects if unrestrained. When better, simpler and more reliable assay systems have been developed for "cystic fibrosis factors," these may lead not only to detection of heterozygotes and to antenatal diagnosis, but also to the elucidation of a basic defect responsible for the protean manifestations of cystic fibrosis.

PATHOLOGIC PHYSIOLOGY

Cardiopulmonary Involvement. Bronchial and bronchiolar obstruction by abnormally viscous and tenacious secretions is the primary and cardinal manifestation of the pulmonary involvement in cystic fibrosis. Ventilatory dysfunction is characteristic of obstructive pulmonary disease, and the increase in airway obstruction parallels the advance in clinical severity. The changes include an increase in residual lung volume and its ratio to total lung capacity, a decrease in ventilatory flow rates and vital capacity, an increase in airway resistance and uneven gas distribution throughout the lungs.

Compression of pulmonary blood vessels, variable degrees of atelectasis, acidosis, hypercapnia and hypoxia frequently lead to pulmonary hypertension and cor pulmonale. Catheterization studies show that intrapulmonary pressures are frequently increased and that they may decrease with administration of oxygen. The fact that the effects of bronchiolar and bronchial obstruction may be reversible is a strong argument for the use of all methods for evacuating mucopurulent secretions by physical and inhalational therapy, as well as combating infection by the judicious use of antibiotics.

Pancreatic Insufficiency. In more than 80 per cent of patients there is pancreatic achylia; trypsin, lipase and amylase are absent from duodenal contents. Steatorrhea and azotorrhea are excessive, reflecting the disturbances of alimentary absorption. In contrast to fats, proteins, though poorly absorbed, are well tolerated, making possible the attainment of positive nitrogen balance through increased dietary intake. Utilization of carbohydrates is less significantly impaired. Variable but large amounts of liposoluble vitamins are lost in the stools.

Owing to impaired intestinal absorption in patients with pancreatic deficiency, vitamin E levels are low in serum and in liver. It was found unexpectedly, however, by Underwood and Denning that while serum vitamin A levels were low even in patients receiving supplements, the content of vitamin A of liver tissue at post mortem was normal or increased in the same patients. This suggested to the investigators a defect in the transport of this vitamin. Smith et al. subsequently demonstrated that the serum retinol-binding protein (RBP) (needed for transport of unesterified vitamin A alcohol) is decreased in many patients with cystic fibrosis, perhaps as a consequence of impaired liver function.

Immunology. Except in the respiratory tract, fibrocystic patients do not have greater susceptibility to infections than normal subjects of comparable ages. This is exemplified by the almost complete absence of pleural complications or of blood stream infections in patients, the vast majority of whom have chronic pulmonary disease. Patients with cystic fibrosis are able to develop good levels of circulating antibodies to pathogenic bacteria and have excellent immunoglobulin responses in serum to infection. Immunofluorescent techniques indicate that IgA in bronchial cells is increased in patients with this disease who have pulmonary infection. Levels of IgA in saliva and in the gastrointestinal tract are normal or increased. The rate of synthesis of IgA in intestinal biopsy material has, by measurement of labeled leucine incorporation, been found to be increased in fibrocystic patients, presumably because of greater local antigenic stimuli.

The fact that the immune responses of fibrocystic patients are normal makes their unusual susceptibility to respiratory infection difficult to understand; although bronchial obstruction precedes the pulmonary infection, it does not appear to be the whole answer.

CLINICAL MANIFESTATIONS

Meconium Ileus. (See also Section 7.) In about 5 to 10 per cent of patients with cystic fibrosis intestinal obstruction occurs with consequent symptoms within hours after birth (so-called meconium ileus); the lumen of the small intestine is plugged by putty-like, grayish meconium, usually near the ileocecal valve. Proximal to it the loops are distended by accumulation of viscid meconium, and volvulus occurs in about one third of patients. Perforation may occur. Occasionally the obstruction is higher in the small intestine, usually from antenatal volvulus. Meconium peritonitis and congenital peritoneal adhesions are not uncommon as a result of perforation in utero.

Chronic Pulmonary Disease. Chronic pulmonary disease is present in almost all patients, frequently severe and progressive. The time of onset is variable; clinical manifestations may appear weeks, months or years after birth. For some time the patient has a dry, nonproductive cough. Later, usually after an acute respiratory infection, the signs of generalized bronchial or bronchiolar obstruction and secondary infection appear. At this stage some degree of respiratory distress is present. At times it is severe, and the patient is quite ill. The infection may be brought under temporary control with antibiotic therapy, but some degree of bronchial obstruction usually persists. The cycle is repeated with subsequent respiratory infections and may eventuate in a fatal episode.

According to Waring, so-called mucoid impaction of the bronchi occurs frequently. It consists of an accumulation of viscous mucus in one or more bronchi, resulting in their obstruction and dilatation. If the bronchi are irreversibly damaged, the pulmonary disease is progressive and eventually leads to pulmonary insufficiency, resulting in death through various complications within an average of 1 to 3 years. This sequence of events may be much shorter or endure for many years. If permanent damage has not been done to the bronchial wall, antibiotic and other therapy may be effective in keeping the disease in check.

As the pulmonary involvement progresses, compensatory emphysema or overaeration of the functioning alveoli tends to distend the chest, which becomes barrel-shaped. Except over large areas of atelectasis or other consolidations, the percussion note is tympanitic and rales are commonly heard. Typically there is roentgenographic evidence of generalized emphysema and bilateral parenchymal infiltrations (Fig. 11–29). Clubbing of fingers and toes is common in chronically ill patients.

In these patients the bacterial flora from the nasopharynx, sputum, and lungs consists primarily of *Staphylococcus aureus* and/or *Pseudomonas aeruginosa,* the latter probably secondary to antibiotic treatment. *Hemophilus influenzae, Escherichia coli, Proteus,* and other organisms are isolated less frequently. In the pre- and early antibiotic era usually only *S. aureus* was found in the respiratory tract of fibrocystic patients even at autopsy, a striking association of a specific microorganism with a disease. In recent years, since *Pseudomonas* has become so prevalent in such patients, the clinical course and pathologic findings have not changed significantly. When anti-*Pseudomonas* antibiotics are used, there is some clinical improvement, but the role of this organism and its importance in the pulmonary disease of cystic fibrosis is not clear.

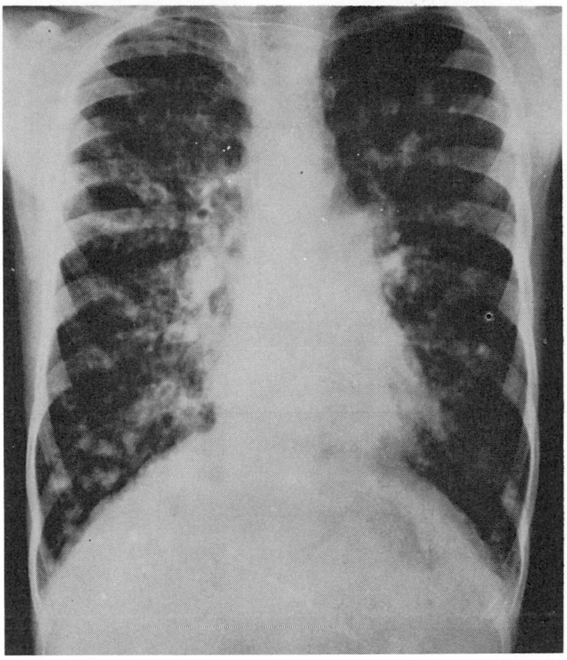

Figure 11–29 Advanced pulmonary disease in a 13 year old boy with cystic fibrosis. There is a diffuse infiltrate with thickening of the walls of the bronchi and dilatation of bronchi. Note the evidence of overaeration.

Numerous complications arise in the course of severe pulmonary disease. In 5 to 10 per cent of patients *lobar atelectasis* (Fig. 11–30) with collapse of one or more lobes, usually on the right side, occurs early in the course of the illness. Small and multiple *lung abscesses* are common. Sudden death may occur from *asphyxia* due to flooding of the trachea with copious amounts of thick, tenacious bronchial secretions in a debilitated infant or small child. Minor or massive (at times exsanguinating) *hemoptysis* and *recurrent pneumothorax* may be encountered, especially in older children. *Chronic cor pulmonale* with clinical and roentgenographic evidence of enlargement of the heart and cardiac failure may be seen with longstanding severe and progressive pulmonary disease. *Acute cor pulmonale* with dilatation of the heart may

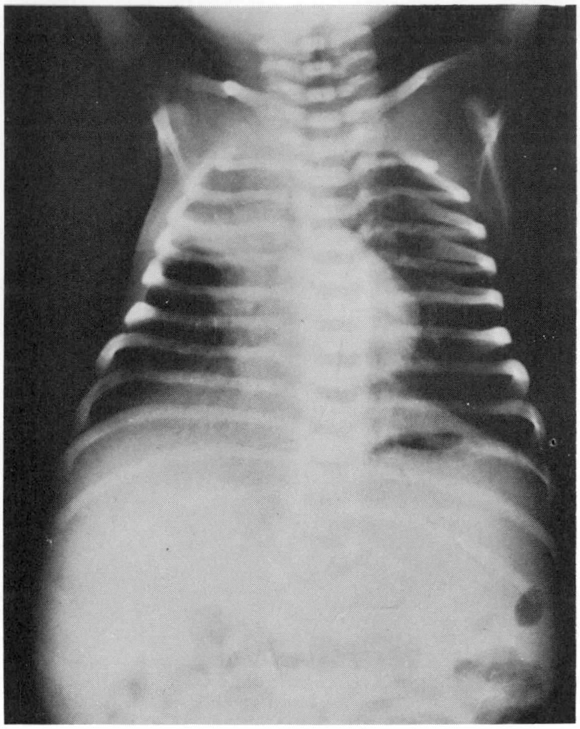

Figure 11–30 *Cystic fibrosis in a 2 month old infant. The lungs are overaerated, and there is evidence of generalized emphysema. The right upper lobe is atelectatic.*

occur during attacks of sudden and severe bronchial obstruction. If the patient survives and responds to antibiotic treatment, the heart may return to its normal size.

Involvement of the paranasal sinuses is usually demonstrable roentgenographically. A nasal voice, postnasal drip and polyps are common manifestations. Polyps often require surgical removal and tend to recur. Two cases of mucocele with complete nasal obstruction and extensive bony destruction have been reported.

Pancreatic Insufficiency. This is present in over 80 per cent of patients and gives rise to symptoms of intestinal malabsorption. Malnutrition may be striking despite excessive appetite and apparently adequate caloric intake. The abdomen is distended, and the stools are increased in number, bulky, greasy and foul. In most patients pancreatic achylia is present at birth, but in some children involvement of this gland may not be evident until later.

Because of the large amounts of preformed vitamin administered orally to most children, vitamin A deficiency is rarely a problem, though xerophthalmia was noted in the past. Vitamin D deficiency (rickets) has rarely been seen in patients with cystic fibrosis, a fact not clearly explained. Vitamin K deficiency leading to prolonged prothrombin time and subcutaneous bleeding is occasionally observed. Gordon and Nitowsky have shown that most children with cystic fibrosis have a deficiency of vitamin E; one manifestation is creatinuria, which ceases on administration of the vitamin.

Cirrhosis of the Liver. Focal biliary cirrhosis does not give rise to clinical manifestations, even if extensive. Only when there is progression to the diffuse type of multilobular biliary cirrhosis does the liver become hard and nodular. In about 2 per cent of patients there is portal hypertension with splenomegaly and at times hypersplenism, ascites and gastrointestinal bleeding. Owing to the focal nature of the process, the results of liver function tests may be within the normal range, and jaundice is usually absent or slight.

Other Complications. Cystic fibrosis is by far the commonest cause of *prolapse of the rectum* in infancy and childhood. It is more frequent in the younger age group but occurs at times in older children. The pathogenesis is not clear, but relief follows pancreatic replacement therapy.

Irrespective of age, all patients with cystic fibrosis are subject to intestinal obstruction due to inspissated or impacted feces, owing to the abnormality of their fecal content (so-called *meconium ileus equivalent*). *Adhesions* from previous surgery coupled with the abnormality of the intestinal content also increase the chance of obstructive complications. Small, hard *fecal masses* are frequently found in the large intestine, most often in the right lower quadrant. They are usually passed spontaneously, though fecal impaction has resulted from such masses. *Intussusception* is an occasional complication, even in older children and young adults. It appears to be precipitated by adherent intestinal content that cannot be propelled along the gut or through the ileocecal valve. As previously mentioned, *volvulus* is a frequent complication of neonatal meconium ileus; it may occur also in older patients.

Hypoalbuminemia is an occasional complication. There are three recognized causes: improper absorption and utilization of soybean protein in infancy; decreased synthesis of albumin with extensive hepatic cirrhosis; and hemodilution due to increased blood volume secondary to severe pulmonary disease and cor pulmonale. The last is the most common. In severely ill patients a combination of these factors may contribute to the hypoalbuminemia.

A progressively abnormal oral glucose tolerance curve and eventually *glycosuria* become manifest in some patients. Ketonuria, acidosis or vascular changes are not common, as they are in classic diabetes mellitus. Dietary measures are usually sufficient for adequate control, though insulin may occasionally be needed. This inability to metabolize glucose adequately seems to be associated with increasing age and duration of the disease. When such patients are examined at autopsy, the islets seem to be disorganized by pancreatic fibrosis, which presumably interferes with their function. This type of glucose intolerance is thus different from familial *diabetes mellitus,* which undoubtedly occurs coincidentally in some patients with cystic fibrosis.

Unexplained is the occurrence of *lactosuria* and *sucrosuria* in some patients with cystic fibrosis. Also unexplained is the *reduced lactase activity* in peroral intestinal specimens from some fibrocystic patients, in the absence of clinical symptoms or histologic changes. Occasionally, however, lactase deficiency may cause persistent diarrhea, even after adequate measures are taken to compensate for the effects of pancreatic deficiency.

Recurrent attacks of *acute pancreatitis* in patients with cystic fibrosis are uncommon, but have been observed. These patients may be the ones who have a late onset of pancreatic deficiency and spill enzymes into the surrounding tissues as a result of obstruction of the ducts. *Pancreatic lithiasis* also has been seen in rare instances.

Peptic ulcer has been mentioned as a complication, but we do not have the impression it occurs with greater frequency than in the general population.

A few cases of *neonatal obstructive jaundice* presumably due to the abnormal behavior of secretions in cystic fibrosis (see gallbladder in Pathology) have been reported. They are difficult to differentiate from cases of neonatal hepatitis and biliary atresia.

High atmospheric temperatures, especially sudden heat, cause profuse sweating. Since the concentration of sodium and chloride in sweat of patients with cystic fibrosis is close to that in the serum, *massive salt loss* and hypoelectrolytemia may occur. The accompanying dehydration is made worse by vomiting, which occurs regularly when the loss of electrolytes is sufficiently great; reduction in extracellular fluid volume results and may lead to cardiovascular collapse. Hyperthermia, coma and death may then follow in fairly rapid succession.

Two types of *ocular lesions* are encountered; they may coexist in children with severe pulmonary involvement. Exudative retinopathy is present at times with severe pulmonary disease; the arteries and veins of the fundus are dilated, and hemorrhages and papilledema may be present. These changes parallel the extent of pulmonary involvement and do not appear to affect vision. Optic neuritis with diminution of visual acuity has been observed in patients receiving prolonged therapy with chloramphenicol. Discontinuance of the drug has resulted in variable degrees of visual improvement.

As in other types of chronic pulmonary disease, *pulmonary hypertrophic osteoarthropathy* develops occasionally and may give rise to arthritis and chronic periostitis. At times no symptoms are present, but periosteal new bone formation can be seen roentgenographically in the lower extremities.

Infertility occurs in more than 95 per cent of adult males with cystic fibrosis, owing to aspermia. (See Pathology.)

DIAGNOSIS. The four criteria required for diagnosis of cystic fibrosis are (1) increase in electrolyte concentration of sweat, (2) absence of pancreatic enzymes, (3) chronic pulmonary involvement, and (4) family history of the disorder. Frequently not all four criteria are present, but in addition to high concentration of sweat electrolytes, either chronic pulmonary disease or pancreatic insufficiency should be present. In the majority of instances the correlation of symptoms of chronic pulmonary disease and of intestinal malabsorption suggests the diagnosis. Recognition of cystic fibrosis may present difficulties in patients in whom only malabsorption or only chronic pulmonary disease is present. Such ancillary manifestations as malnutrition despite ravenous appetite, history of rectal prolapse, nasal polyps, hepatic cirrhosis, heat prostration in summer, meconium ileus or recurrent abdominal obstructive complications should suggest the diagnostic possibility of cystic fibrosis. The sweat test will be "positive" in all instances. All children and adolescents with recurrent respiratory infections or malabsorption should have a sweat test as part of their diagnostic work-up.

Reliable sweat tests are difficult to obtain in the first three to four weeks of life, as the sweat glands do not yet appear to function adequately. Diagnosis of cystic fibrosis may be difficult also in patients seen for the first time as adolescents or young adults, since they are not apt to present the classic picture of the disease. The criteria for a definitive diagnosis should be more rigid than in children; this is especially so in view of the moderately higher normal concentrations of sweat electrolytes after the age of 18 or 20 years.

The *sweat test* (above) is the simplest and most reliable laboratory method for the diagnosis of cystic fibrosis. Up to the age of 20 years a level of more than 60 mEq/L of sweat chloride is diagnostic of cystic fibrosis, and values between 50 and 60 mEq/L are highly suggestive. Values for sweat sodium are about 10 mEq/L higher than those for chloride. Potassium concentration in sweat and sodium and chloride concentrations in saliva are not useful for diagnostic purposes. There are few conditions other than cystic fibrosis in which sweat electrolytes may be elevated. Untreated adrenal insufficiency is the most important one; occasionally elevations have been observed with glucose-6-phosphatase deficiency, glycogen storage disease, Pitressin-resistant diabetes insipidus, and, in one family group, with ectodermal dysplasia and sensorineural deafness.

Most children with pancreatic deficiency have cystic fibrosis; however, other causes of pancreatic achylia in this age group exist (see later, this Section). All such patients have been found to have normal sweat test results and usually do not have chronic pulmonary disease.

Demonstration of characteristic pathologic changes in specimens of rectal mucosa and of labial salivary glands obtained by biopsy has been advocated as a diagnostic aid. We have not so far found it necessary to use these methods.

Roentgenography. Persistent, generalized obstructive emphysema, though not pathognomonic, is highly suggestive of cystic fibrosis. Children with chronic lung disease, but without the signs of generalized emphysema, usually have other disease entities. In moderately advanced and severe pulmonary lesions, there are a variety of additional roentgenographic changes which include disseminated infiltrative lesions of bronchopneumonia (Fig. 11–29), lobular and lobar atelectasis (Fig. 11–30) and widely disseminated miliary infiltrations often indistinguishable from those of tuberculosis. At times mucoid impactions of the bronchi are demonstrated as grape-like nodular densities.

Changes in the roentgenographic patterns of the small intestine related to motility may be found in patients with pancreatic deficiency as in patients with other malabsorptive disorders. Similar intestinal patterns may be seen in healthy infants and young children. In most of the patients with cystic fibrosis abnormalities also are found in barium studies of the duodenum. These consist of markedly thickened folds, nodular filling defects, mucosal smudging and dilatation. The etiology of these duodenal changes is obscure, but they most likely represent contractions of the muscle layer secondary to irritation from unbuffered gastric acid. It is important to recognize these abnormalities so that faulty diagnoses, especially of peptic ulcer disease, are not made. A moderate degree of osteoporosis is occasionally demonstrated on roentgenograms of the skeleton.

Cor Pulmonale. Recognition of cor pulmonale may be difficult: cardiac signs are usually masked by the pulmonary manifestations; tachycardia may occur as the result of hypoxemia; the liver is frequently displaced downward by the emphysema; and overt edema occurs rarely and usually as a terminal feature. Roentgenograms, electrocardiograms and vectorcardiograms are unreliable. According to Moss, clinical evidence of severe disease with a poor clinical score, a vital capacity of less than 60 per cent of the predicted normal and inability to raise the oxygen tension above 300 mm Hg after breathing 100 per cent oxygen for 10 minutes should suggest cor pulmonale. As hemodilution is by far the commonest cause of hypoalbuminemia in cystic fibrosis, a level of serum albumin of less than 3 gm/dl in the presence of severe pulmonary disease is suggestive of increased plasma volume due to incipient heart failure and may appear months or years before demise. In the later stages of the chronic lung disease other evidences of hemodilution also frequently appear, such as low serum electrolyte levels and a drop in hemoglobin values.

Pancreatic Deficiency. Examination of duodenal contents for pancreatic enzyme activity as a confirmatory test and to evaluate pancreatic function may be performed when the diagnosis is uncertain (above). For practical purposes *only* tryptic activity need be measured; it is absent in over 80 per cent of patients. The fluid obtained from patients with cystic fibrosis and pancreatic achylia is diminished in volume; its viscosity, though variable, is frequently much increased.

Intestinal Malabsorption. Steatorrhea (*q.v.*) is present in more than 80 per cent of patients who have pancreatic achylia and can be demonstrated by tests described elsewhere. Intestinal mucosa obtained by peroral biopsy is generally normal. The decrease or absence of lactase activity in oral biopsy specimens from many patients with cystic fibrosis is unexplained. Tests using polyvinylpyrrolidone and chromium-tagged albumin reveal slightly increased loss of serum protein through the gastrointestinal tract in some patients, not enough, however, to account for any decrease in serum albumin levels which may be present.

Blood Chemical Studies. Serum electrolytes are within the normal ranges in patients with cystic fibrosis when they are reasonably well clinically. When there is severe pulmonary disease, the serum electrolyte pattern is apt to be that of uncompensated or more frequently of compensated respiratory acidosis. There is hypoelectrolytemia in patients with heat prostration and shock resulting from the massive outpouring of electrolytes in sweat. Serum potassium levels may remain within apparently normal limits under these circumstances if the process is rapid, but will decrease if the loss occurs over a longer time. Hypoelectrolytemia has also been observed in infants with cystic fibrosis during cold weather, owing to moderate losses of salt through sweat, combined with inadequate intake of salt. Such patients may erroneously be thought to have adrenal insufficiency.

Serum calcium and phosphorus levels are within normal limits. Serum protein values are usually normal in patients in reasonably good clinical condition. Hypoalbuminemia is discussed above. The globulin moiety may be increased by a rise in IgG and IgA related to the respiratory involvement. IgM is generally within normal limits.

The usual limited tests of liver function frequently give no evidence of hepatic impairment. On the other hand, a recent study of 49 patients with cystic fibrosis, aged 3 to 41 years, revealed that about one third had serologic evidence of hepatobiliary disease before clinical signs were evident. The transaminases, γ-glutamyl-transpeptidase, and the liver isoenzyme of alkaline phosphatase appeared to be the most reliable indicators of this complication.

Anemia is rarely a problem, and serum iron and iron-binding capacity are usually normal except as anemia due to chronic infection develops. Leukocytosis and elevation of the erythrocyte sedimentation rate reflect pulmonary or other infectious processes.

PROGNOSIS. The pulmonary involvement usually dominates the clinical picture and determines the fate of the patient. The effects of pancreatic deficiency are less important to the ultimate outcome, though proper attention should be paid to maintenance of good nutrition, including avoidance of vitamin deficiencies. Infants who survive the operation for meconium ileus have essentially the same outlook as do other patients with cystic fibrosis. Uncontrollable bleeding due to portal hypertension and massive loss of salt in hot weather are occasional hazards in this disease.

No precise figures on survival are available, but a reasonable estimate is a mean survival of 15 to 20 years. Some patients with cystic fibrosis will die in infancy or early childhood, while an increasingly large number now survive to the age of 20 or 30 years or longer. Prognosis will improve further as diagnostic and therapeutic methods become more effective. Reported instances of cystic fibrosis above the age of 30 years must be regarded with suspicion unless all or substantially all diagnostic criteria are met. The oldest patient we are following at the present time who meets all of these criteria is 42 years of age.

Though early diagnosis, early treatment and aggressive therapy during serious pulmonary complications are effective in prolonging the life of the patient, the natural variation in the severity of cystic fibrosis is an important factor in determining the outcome.

It is important for the physician and the patient's family to assess as accurately as possible the individual patient's current status and to estimate prognosis. The scoring system of Shwachman and Kulczycki has been used in the past. In the past few years, however, the average age of patients has increased; some of the pulmonary complications (e.g., recurring pneumothorax, massive hemoptysis) have become more prevalent, and the intestinal and other consequences of pancreatic insufficiency have become less important. Accordingly, Taussig et al. have developed a new, simple scoring system which permits assessment of a patient's past history, current status and prognosis, and reflects any current situation more precisely; it is especially accurate and helpful in patients older than 3 years.

Adolescents and Young Adults. As a group, patients over the age of 15 to 20 years are doing better than average, perhaps because their survival to this age depended on the relatively mild degree of respiratory involvement. Males have a slightly better outlook than females, a fact which is unexplained. Despite the handicap of chronic pulmonary disease, many of the older patients have been able to carry on a full-time occupation, and several are married.

The clinical picture, in general, is similar to that of children with the disease, and the chronic pulmonary involvement is still the major problem. On the other hand, sinusitis and polyps, abdominal obstructive complications, hemoptysis and spontaneous pneumothorax, often recurring and sometimes bilateral, are more common in this age group than in younger children. Despite the lack of pancreatic enzymes and the persistence of steatorrhea and azotorrhea, patients appear to need less dietary restrictions with advancing age. Retardation of growth has been traditionally considered an accompaniment of cystic fibrosis, but the eventual height achieved is generally within normal limits and there is little relation to the age at which the diagnosis was established.

Sexual maturation has been achieved in both males and females, though it is at times delayed in patients severely affected. The great majority of adult males with cystic fibrosis are infertile owing to aspermia (see Pathology), but the testicles are normally developed and all secondary sexual characteristics and sexual functions are normally preserved in patients not severely debilitated by their disease. Three cases of fertile males with cystic fibrosis have been reported, as well as other probable cases. It is imperative, therefore, to examine adequately all adult males with cystic fibrosis before counseling with regard to probable fertility. This should require, (at a minimum, a semen sperm count and assessment of the volume of the ejaculate.) There is reason to believe that females with cystic fibrosis are less fertile than average, but a number of pregnancies have been reported. These have resulted, in the patients known to us, in normal children; this might be expected as the overall risk of having an affected child in the random mating of a mother with cystic fibrosis with a male of unknown genetic status is only 2.5 per cent. If the affected mother, on the other hand, mates with a male carrier, 50 per cent of the offspring will have cystic fibrosis. At the time of writing there is as yet no practical method for positively identifying the heterozygote in the population or performing an antenatal diagnosis. The difficulties of the mother with cystic fibrosis during pregnancy and delivery have generally correlated with the degree of preceding pulmonary involvement. Pregnancy in cystic fibrosis is a potential hazard, therefore, to the patient who has severe lung disease.

TREATMENT. Until the basic defect in cystic fibrosis is uncovered, a rational, effective and truly lasting treatment cannot be devised. At present, therapy is mainly palliative and aimed at combating, slowing or preventing some of the secondary effects or complications of this disease.

General Care and Principles of Treatment. A normal life for the patient should be the ultimate goal, whenever possible. Activities (school, competitive sports, and so forth) should be restricted only as indicated by the patient's tolerance.

Routine immunizations against diphtheria, tetanus, pertussis and poliomyelitis should be performed at appropriate ages. Booster doses should be given when indicated. Live virus measles vaccine is mandatory in all susceptible patients if their condition permits, as complications following rubeola may be serious or even fatal. Influenza vaccine is recommended, especially in patients with pulmonary involvement, even if minimal; a bout of influenza may initiate serious pulmonary disease or cause a severe relapse.

A multidisciplinary approach is needed to the manifold problems presented by the patient with cystic fibrosis and his family. The role of the physician should be complemented by that of the social worker, the physical therapist and, at times, the psychiatrist. The parents must clearly understand all the therapeutic measures to be carried out at home so that they can cooperate to the fullest extent, and information regarding genetic aspects of the disease should be available to the family.

Social and Psychologic Considerations. Cystic fibrosis is not only a medical problem but a social one as well, owing to the devastating effects of the emotional and financial stresses on the family. There is need for a compassionate, helpful, understanding attitude on the part of the physician, and support and assistance when needed by psychologist or psychiatrist. Every effort must be made to prevent the patient from dominating the family emotionally and to allay the guilt feelings and consequent overconcern or hostility of the parents, which are apt to develop in relation to an inherited, severe and progressive disease. The support of a medical social worker familiar with the problems of this disorder is desirable to help deal with the family's emotional responses and practical problems, as well as to help them to utilize to the fullest extent the resources of the community.

Adolescents and young adults with cystic fibrosis grow up with an unusual number of stresses related to their physical appearance, conflicts in their upbringing and increased awareness of the future. Recent studies have shown that generally the father needs to be encouraged to become involved with the patient and that, conversely, the mother needs to be helped to allow the patient greater independence and let him take more responsibility. Both parents and patients need to be aware of the benefits of an environment in which there is free communication about cystic fibrosis.

The role of the physician is very important in helping the parents to allow the patient to develop normally emotionally, in listening professionally to the patient's concerns, in leading group discussions of parents (and at times of older patients themselves), in terms of offering practical and concrete ways to deal with daily concerns (e.g., handling separation, going to college, seeking employment, reorienting their goals more realistically). Patients (male and female) who marry need special counseling both before and after marriage to deal with common fears and frustrations. Specific concerns about sterility or adoption need to be discussed and then discussed again after the patient has had time to digest the facts. If the patient is a child, he should be encouraged to attend school; if an adolescent or a young adult, to continue his studies or to obtain a job and work within the limit of his capacities. Those who have had to stop, for whatever reason, have become lonely and depressed and have had low self-esteem.

Treatment of Pulmonary Involvement. Active therapy of the pulmonary involvement deserves the major emphasis. It is based on (1) evacuation of mucopurulent secretions by physical methods and, at times, by use of aerosol solutions; and (2) on the appropriate and timely use of antimicrobial agents to combat infections. Both these modes of therapy are essential to therapeutic success.

Physical Therapy. It is generally agreed that physical therapy is needed on a continued basis by patients with even minimal pulmonary involvement in order to relieve bronchial obstruction due to accumulated secretions. Frequency, duration of treatment and positions to be used should be individually prescribed on the basis of careful segmental auscultation of the chest and a review of the chest x-ray. After positioning the patient appropriately, clapping, cupping, deep breathing, assisted coughing, thoracic squeezing and vibration are used. Mechanical vibrators are less effective than hand vibration; in the case of the young adult living away from home, however, or where assistance with physical therapy is not available, mechanical devices may be useful.

Aerosol Therapy. One should distinguish between *interrupted inhalational treatments* usually done in conjunction with postural drainage and *mist tent therapy.* The object in both cases is to hydrate bronchial secretions and to assist in their evacuation by physical therapy methods. To penetrate to the smaller bronchial subdivisions aerosol particles must be 0.5 to 5.0 μ in size; hand-operated nebulizers do not deliver particles small enough. A small nebulizer such as those used in the treatment of asthma is sufficient for interrupted aerosol therapy, but for continuous nebulization in a "mist tent," a large capacity nebulizer is needed. Compressed air can be used as a propellant, with use of an appropriate pump. Frequently employed are ultrasonic nebulizers which produce a very thick mist with particles of small diameter and are quiet to operate. Solutions generally recommended contain 10 per cent propylene glycol in distilled water.

A recommended schedule for *interrupted nebulization* consists of three steps: *Step 1.* Postural drainage for 5 to 10 minutes to be done at least twice a day in the morning and evening and, if necessary, at midday. *Step 2.* Nebulization with the solution described for 10 to 15 minutes. (Following Step 1, this permits the moisture particles to penetrate farther along the bronchial tree.) *Step 3.* Following nebulization, repeat the postural drainage for 15 to 20 minutes.

In contrast to the universal acceptance of physical therapy methods *mist tent therapy* is quite controversial, following the demonstration that radioactive aerosolized solutions are almost entirely deposited in the esophagus and stomach and do not achieve satisfactory distribution in the lungs. Additional objections are that many physicians (notably in England) who do not use mist tent therapy have results equal to those of physicians who do. If it is to be employed, a large capacity nebulizer with a compressor or an ultrasonic nebulizer should be used, with the solution indicated above. According to the severity of the illness, the patient can be in a mist tent for 24 hours/day or just for the night and for naps. We tend to use mist tent therapy in patients hospitalized in acute relapses of pulmonary disease in conjunction with all the other physical therapy and antibiotic treatments, but are very selective in choosing patients to use the tent at home during the sleeping hours. It may become quite hot inside the tent; during the summer, air conditioning of the room is helpful. Mist tent therapy has also been advocated as a prophylactic treatment to prevent the onset of pulmonary involvement. This has not found general acceptance and we do not subscribe to this notion.

Whether interrupted nebulization or mist tent therapy is used, clean equipment in good working order is essential to successful treatment and to avoidance of complications. Daily or at least weekly thorough cleaning of inhalation therapy equipment decreases the chances of significant contamination.

Antibiotic Therapy. Therapeutic courses of intensive antibiotic therapy are indicated during acute exacerbation of the pulmonary disease and in an attempt to halt progressive deterioration.

The choice of the antibiotic agent should be based whenever possible upon in vitro susceptibility tests of the bacterial pathogens isolated by culture from the respiratory tract. If the situation is so acute, however, that it is not possible to wait for one to three days until the bacteriologic reports are received, patients may be started on one of the broad spectrum antibiotics, usually chloramphenicol, which is generally the most effective. And if a greenish color of the sputum suggests Pseudomonas, parenteral gentamicin or carbenicillin may be used.

The routes of administration selected (e.g., parenteral, oral, inhalation, or all three simultaneously) depend on the severity and acuteness of the disease and on the antibiotic agents to be used. As in all antibiotic therapy, drugs should be given for a long enough period and in sufficient doses to be effective. A therapeutic course of antibiotic therapy, therefore, is usually not less than 7 days and up to 15 days or even longer if necessary, and full therapeutic doses of the agent(s) of choice should be given. Because of the possible need for parenteral administration of antibiotic agents, the need for good physical therapy, and the need for other types of supportive treatment (e.g., oxygen therapy) hospitalization is recommended during most of the periods of intensive antibiotic therapy.

A fairly wide variety of antibiotic agents is available. In view of the bacterial flora most likely present in the respiratory tract, an antistaphylococcal agent is most commonly chosen, alone or in combination with a drug effective against Pseudomonas. If the Staphylococcus is resistant to penicillin G, penicillinase-resistant semisynthetic penicillins or cephalosporins usually have been selected, the dosage depending on the route of administration chosen as well as on the age of the patient. Gentamicin and carbenicillin have been effective against Pseudomonas. The combination of gentamicin and carbenicillin is usually considered synergistic; they can be used together when severe illness is life-threatening.

Among the broad spectrum antibiotics chloramphenicol has been the most effective agent, but because of the risks of suppression of the bone marrow and of optic neuritis (the latter especially after prolonged administration), its use should be avoided whenever equally efficacious antibiotics are available. If used, it should be given for only a short time (1 to 4 weeks), parents forewarned to seek immediate medical advice if diminution of visual acuity appears, and blood counts obtained at least once per week.

If possible, an antibiotic with fewer or milder side effects should be used. For the child below the age of 8 years, a penicillin should be used in conjunction with ampicillin, the latter of course being useful also against *Hemophilus influenzae* and *Proteus mirabilis.* If the patient is over the age of 8, a tetracycline drug is usually preferred.

Erythromycin, colistin, streptomycin and kanamycin have been widely used in the past with variable success; they have been generally supplanted, however, by newer antibiotic agents, especially in view of the potential toxicity of the latter two.

Aerosol antibiotic therapy is a form of topical treatment to be used only as an adjunct to systemic administration during periods of intensive antibiotic therapy. Penicillin G, nafcillin, ampicillin, gentamicin and other antibiotics have been used. We have found neomycin, polymyxin-B, or colistin not useful when administered in this manner.

In our experience and that of most others, some severely ill patients cannot be controlled effectively without *continued antibiotic therapy* for long periods of time (months or years). One of the oral antistaphylococcal agents or one of the tetracyclines (always provided the child is older than 8 years) is usually chosen, in the smallest dose sufficient to prevent reappearance of symptoms, as determined by experience. We do not favor rotation of antibiotics. The principal arguments against continuous therapy are the risks of development of increased resistance to antibiotics by strains of *Staphylococcus aureus* and of colonization with *Pseudomonas aeruginosa* and other resistant bacteria. This may occur, but if no treatment is given, there are at times such frequent and persistent recurrences of symptoms, with the menace of a rapidly progressive pulmonary disease, that continuous therapy seems essential.

Surgical and Other Treatment. *Pulmonary surgery* is rarely indicated, owing to the generalized nature of the lung involvement in most patients. Approximately 2 per cent of patients with cystic fibrosis have, however, a pulmonary disease sufficiently localized so that resection can be attempted. In the case of *massive hemoptysis,* especially if recurrent, lobectomy and even pneumonectomy have been attempted, with some success provided the localization was certain. Repeated episodes of *pneumothorax* pose a problem in treatment. If the pneumothorax is unilateral and not more than 15 per cent, hospitalization and observation alone are indicated; if more than 15 per cent or bilateral, closed thoracotomy is performed, with insertion of a tube. Intrapleural instillation of a sclerosing agent (e.g., atabrine, properly diluted) and open thoracotomy with resection of blebs and pleural scarification or pleural stripping have been performed with some success. *Tracheotomy* and *nasotracheal intubation* have been carried out in very ill patients in order to permit mechanical ventilation with a respirator, with results that have, in general, been unsuccessful; there is agreement that such procedures should be avoided, or reserved for carefully selected patients. The use of intermittent positive pressure machines (IPPB) should be limited to special circumstances and under close observation in the hospital. *Bronchoscopy for drainage* has been used with some success by skilled operators; in general, owing to the risks involved in the procedure, it should be done only in selected cases. A fiberoptic bronchoscope may facilitate this procedure; its use is being evaluated. *Pulmonary lavage* may be done, using a total volume of saline of many liters. This should be done only by an experienced person. It is mandatory in some other conditions (e.g., alveolar proteinosis), but of limited use in patients with cystic fibrosis, owing to technical difficulties (size of equipment needed, and so forth) and possible complications, and effectiveness is questionable. Its use should be restricted to selected older patients who have had previously good pulmonary function. Probably any possible benefit gained by *tracheobronchial lavage* without complete filling of the lavaged lung is outweighed by the risks of bronchoscopy. On the other hand, *deep tracheal aspiration* is often effective and should be used in severely ill patients; it must of necessity be limited to older patients who cooperate with the procedure. It is generally agreed that the use of isotonic saline solution is better for all types of lavage than solutions containing acetylcysteine (Mucomyst), which may cause severe irritation of tracheobronchial mucosa and bronchial spasm.

When *oxygen therapy* is necessary, the child should be observed carefully, preferably with frequent monitoring of blood gas levels, in order to avoid excessive accumulation of carbon dioxide in the blood and so-called carbon dioxide narcosis. As little oxygen concentration as needed to improve the oxygenation of blood should be used: 28 to 40 per cent. In general, concentrations of oxygen of more than 50 per cent for more than a few hours should be considered hazardous. Notwithstanding the dangers of oxygen therapy, it should be kept in mind that the degree of pulmonary hypertension is correlated with the severity of hypoxia. Digitalization for cor pulmonale and cardiac failure has been useful, but the dangers of administration of *digitalis* to anoxic patients should also be kept in mind. Many pediatric cardiologists feel that when digitalization has been initiated, it should be maintained for the lifetime of the patient. *Diuretics* are important adjuncts to the treatment of cor pulmonale; in general, only short courses of diuretic treatment are needed in patients with cystic fibrosis, usually lasting from one day to one week; there are times in very severely ill patients when continued diuretic therapy may be necessary. If cardiac failure is present, dietary salt restriction may be considered, but frequent determination of serum electrolyte levels is needed, because patients with cystic fibrosis lose excessive salt in sweat.

Expectorants are useful at times; caution is urged, however, in the use of iodides, which have produced hypothyroidism and goiters in patients with cystic fibrosis. *Antihistamines* are generally to be avoided because of their drying effect on secretions. *Bronchodilators* seem to be effective primarily when there is an associated allergic component. *Mucolytics* are usually not very effective and can be irritating if their use is prolonged. *Enzyme preparations* by inhalation (e.g., trypsin, hyaluronidase) are irritating and have not been beneficial. *Corticosteroid* therapy has not been helpful. Changing *climate* has not had strikingly beneficial effects on the course of the pulmonary involvement.

Dietary Therapy. (See also the discussion of malabsorption in cystic fibrosis, with Malabsorptive Syndromes, above.) The pancreatic achylia is readily compensated by a diet of high caloric, high protein and moderate fat content in conjunction with one of the pancreatic extracts. The patient's appetite should be a guide to the dietary intake. Commercially available powdered high-protein milk preparations can be used to advantage in the first few weeks of life; subsequently skim milk is advised until later childhood, when homogenized milk can be given if the patient tolerates it. Soybean milks do not provide adequate protein and should not be used for infants with cystic fibrosis; hypoproteinemic edema has been a consequence of such feeding. Supplements of vitamins A, D and E in water-miscible preparations should be provided every day in double the recommended dose. If hypoprothrombinemia is present, administration of vitamin K is indicated. Pancreatic extract, which improves intestinal absorption and the nature of the stools, is needed with each meal. Many commercial products are available, and there is little evidence that any one has therapeutic advantage over the others. Dosage depends on the preparation selected and, in particular, on the patient's clinical response. Constipation and anorexia may result if the dose of the pancreatic extract is excessive. Medium-chain triglycerides are absorbed better than other longer chain fats, and dietary supplements of them have been advocated. At times anabolic steroids have been useful in increasing appetite and promoting weight gain, but to avoid side effects only short repeated courses are recommended. Claims that they have been effective in improving the respiratory disease do not seem to have been substantiated. Recently oral arginine has been advocated to improve steatorrhea, but careful metabolic studies have shown it to be ineffective and, owing to side effects, probably contraindicated for this purpose. If symptoms of lactase deficiency are present, it may be necessary to limit the dietary lactose intake.

Dietary measures appear to become less necessary with advancing age, but individual variations are found in the need for dietary restrictions at all ages. The nutritional state is more closely correlated with the severity of the pulmonary infection than with pancreatic function.

Treatment of Abnormal Loss of Salt. Massive salt depletion through sweating in hot weather may present a real medical emergency. The administration of saline solution intravenously is urgently needed in such instances to reconstitute the extracellular fluid volume and to avoid cardiovascular collapse; as much as 10 ml of isotonic saline solution per kg within 15 minutes may have to be given, followed by appropriate replacement therapy. Additional sodium chloride (2 to 4 gm a day) should be taken orally by all patients in hot weather, regardless of their pancreatic status.

Other Therapy. For management of *meconium ileus,* see Section 7. As early as 2 to 3 days postoperatively, 10 ml of a 5 per cent solution of pancreatin powder should be administered every 6 hours through a nasogastric tube. When feeding by mouth is deemed advisable, a dilute formula of one of the protein milk preparations and glucose can be started and increased in caloric value as rapidly as tolerated. Most infants with fibrocystic disease eventually will need as much as 150 cal/kg/24 hr in order to gain weight. Pancreatin powder should be put in each bottle (e.g., 1/2 teaspoonful in each of 6 bottles, equivalent to 3 teaspoonfuls when given with each of 3 meals).

Alternatively, preparations containing predigested amino acids and monosaccharides in a high-protein, low-fat milk (e.g., Probana [Mead-Johnson]) have been used to advantage for the first few weeks.

Rectal prolapse responds well to medical and dietary treatment and surgical intervention is rarely, if ever, needed. In patients in whom *fecal masses* are occasionally present, constipation should be avoided; dioctyl sodium sulfosuccinate (Colace) may be given in a dose of 50 mg orally once or twice a day, along with a temporary moderate increase in dietary fat intake and a concomitant decrease in pancreatic enzyme therapy. *Meconium ileus equivalent* (intestinal obstruction in the older age group) and *intussusception* often result in incomplete obstruction and may respond to reduction by barium enema in the case of intussusception or to repeated high colonic enemas in the case of partial obstruction. Acetylcysteine (Mucomyst) has been used orally with satisfactory results. In such cases, time is of the essence in instituting treatment, because if adhesions have already formed, surgery will be inevitable. In the occasional case of *volvulus* in the older age group, surgery is needed. If hematemesis or melena occurs as a consequence of *multilobular biliary cirrhosis and portal hypertension,* it should be treated as in any other patient, with the performance of shunting operations if they are eventually needed. Surgeons usually prefer not to perform such procedures in a child who is still growing rapidly, owing to the small size of the vessels and the change in caliber due to age. There is no consensus as to the best treatment of the rare cases of *obstructive neonatal jaundice* in cystic fibrosis. Surgical intervention may be necessary in some cases, but a more conservative approach has generally been successful.

In severe *glucose intolerance with glycosuria,* dietary measures usually suffice, sometimes supplemented by oral antidiabetic agents; some patients require insulin. For the occasional case of coincidental *genetic diabetes mellitus* treatment should follow the same lines as in other patients with this condition, with attention to the additional problems and dietary limitations indicated by pancreatic achylia and consequent malabsorption. *Nasal polyps* may require repeated polypectomies for recurrent nasal obstruction. *Mucoceles* respond to surgical drainage. *Associated allergic conditions* should be treated as outlined in Section 9.

GENETIC PANCREATIC DEFICIENCIES NOT DUE TO CYSTIC FIBROSIS

Most infants and children with pancreatic achylia have cystic fibrosis, but several other rare entities have been recognized in which pancreatic insufficiency is part of the clinical picture.

Congenital hypoplasia of the exocrine pancreas associated with pancreatic achylia and malnutrition was described in infants by Bodian. At autopsy there was complete replacement of the parenchyma by fatty tissue, but notably there was neither fibrosis nor dilatation of pancreatic ducts. The islands of Langerhans appeared normal. In 1964 Shwachman et al. reported 6 children ranging in age from 2 months to 10 years, 3 in one family, with shortness in stature, *pancreatic achylia* and *hematologic abnormalities,* including anemia, thrombocytopenia and neutropenia (Shwachman-Diamond syndrome). All these children had normal sweat test results and were without pulmonary disease. By 1969 Shmerling found 40 cases reported, including the original ones of Shwachman. All had pancreatic deficiency, frequently with mild symptoms of malabsorption, normal sweat tests, and no pulmonary involvement; neutropenia was an almost constant feature. A hypercellular marrow and thrombocytopenia were usually present, but the hematologic abnormalities had their onset at times only after some years. Dwarfism was present in 21 out of 36 patients for whom data were available. Metaphyseal dysostosis, Hirschsprung's disease and hepatic cirrhosis were present in some. Many patients were unusually susceptible to upper and lower respiratory infections, otitis, sinusitis and even skin infections. Immunoglobulin levels were usually normal, but deficiencies were reported in a few instances. Nine of the 40 patients had died, but young adults are known who are doing fairly well. After cystic fibrosis, this syndrome appears to be the most common cause of exocrine pancreatic insufficiency. It seems probable that these cases represent more than a single genetic error and that there may be overlap between congenital hypoplasia of the pancreas, Shwachman-Diamond syndrome, Wiskott-Aldrich syndrome and perhaps other entities.

Trypsinogen deficiency has been identified in 2 unrelated infants with severe growth failure, hypoproteinemia and edema. The congenital absence of trypsinogen led to failure of activation of trypsin, chymotrypsin and carboxypeptidase and thus to impaired capacity to hydrolyze ingested protein. Pancreatic lipase and amylase activities were normal, as were sweat test results; there was no pulmonary involvement. Both patients were anemic, and one had neutropenia. The importance of recognizing this disorder is emphasized by the dramatic response to dietary management with protein hydrolysates.

Enterokinase deficiency has been reported in 3 infants, with consequent failure of activation of proteolytic enzymes. The clinical picture was similar to that in trypsinogen deficiency disease. There is some question as to whether the two conditions may coexist.

Pancreatic deficiency has been observed with the XXY Klinefelter syndrome, in a patient with pancreatic achylia, hypothyroidism, nerve deafness, chronic lung disease and dwarfism.

For pancreatic insufficiency secondary to *familial pancreatitis* see Pancreatitis, below.

PANCREATITIS

Primary inflammatory disease of the pancreas is not common in childhood; acute pancreatitis is more common than chronic relapsing pancreatitis. About one third of patients reported with acute pancreatitis have signs suggestive of an acute surgical condition of the abdomen. The cause of acute pancreatitis is varied and often not identified. Presumed or proved causative factors have included trauma, blocking of the pancreatic duct by *Ascaris lumbricoides,* obstruction of the common bile duct and administration of corticosteroids. Malnutrition, especially protein deficiency, may lead to inflammatory changes in the pancreas and to eventual functional deficiency.

Pancreatitis may occur as a complication of *mumps.* Symptoms of severe epigastric pain, nausea and vomiting make an abrupt appearance 4 to 5 days after the onset of the parotid lesion. In rare instances there may be only pancreatic involvement. There frequently are fever, diarrhea and leukocytosis. Transient hyperglycemia and glycosuria may occur occasionally during or after an acute attack. The prognosis is generally good, and complete recovery takes place in about a week. In mumps pancreatitis the finding of increased serum amylase concentration is not diagnostic, since it may be caused by inflammatory disease of the salivary glands.

Hereditary pancreatitis is a recently described autosomal dominant disease characterized by recurring episodes of severe abdominal pain. Though the onset of this illness is usually in early childhood, the diagnosis is generally obscure until pancreatic calcifications, pancreatic deficiency and intestinal malabsorption eventually occurs, as they do most frequently in early adult life. There are now 18 kindreds reported, with 231 proved or suspected patients. So far all have been of Caucasian ancestry, and all but two kindreds from the United States.

The disorder is marked by recurrent attacks of acute pancreatitis, with progressive impairment of exocrine pancreatic function. Episodes may occur as often as once or twice a month or with symptom-free intervals of several years. The single attacks last one to three days and are similar to those which occur in chronic relapsing pancreatitis of adults. In hereditary pancreatitis, however, in addition to the family history there are such definite differences as age of onset and absence of such etiologic factors as alcoholism or gallstones; there is an equal sex incidence. Pathology of the pancreas is similar in the two conditions and fibrosis is equally extensive in both, but there appears to be less destruction of the islands of Langerhans in the genetic type. Various complications (e.g., glucose intolerance, pseudocysts) may occur in the course of hereditary pancreatitis, but they are less common than in the classic relapsing pancreatitis of adults.

Two of the original families described by Gross had aminoaciduria involving cystine, arginine and lysine. This has not been found again, and it now appears that these two families probably had coincident hereditary pancreatitis and incompletely recessive cystinuria.

It is important to consider the possibility of hereditary pancreatitis in the differential diagnosis of recurrent abdominal pain in children so that unnecessary diagnostic and therapeutic procedures may be avoided. In pancreatitis, irrespective of etiology, serum amylase will be increased during acute attacks; in the absence of trauma or mumps, other causes of pancreatitis must be excluded, including the rare instances of pancreatitis associated with *hyperparathyroidism* and *hyperlipoproteinemia.* Differentiating hereditary pancreatitis from cystic fibrosis is a simple matter because patients with hereditary pancreatitis generally have negative sweat tests and carry none of the stigmata of cystic fibrosis such as chronic pulmonary disease. Pancreatic calcifications have been seen in hereditary pancreatitis as early as 13 years of age. Cystic fibrosis is the other main cause of pancreatic calcifications in childhood in the United States.

Treatment of an acute attack is largely symptomatic, as in other types of acute pancreatitis. The principle is one of restoring electrolyte balance and putting the pancreas at rest by discontinuing oral feedings. The acute attack nearly always subsides with conservative medical management; chronic pancreatic insufficiency and its complications eventually ensue. In such cases surgery has been tried with some success.

CYSTS AND PSEUDOCYSTS OF THE PANCREAS

Congenital cysts of the pancreas are usually multiple. They are asymptomatic and are frequently associated with polycystic involvement of other organs.

Pseudocysts of the pancreas may occur as a complication of mumps or other acute pancreatitis or may follow trauma. Falls from bicycles and tricycles have been one of the most frequent causes. Pseudocysts should be considered in the differential diagnosis of abdominal masses in children, especially after blunt abdominal trauma. Surgical drainage and *marsupialization* followed some time later by excision may be needed. Pancreatic enzyme activity can be demonstrated in the contents of the pseudocysts, though the addition of enterokinase as an activator may be needed.

INVOLVEMENT OF THE PANCREAS IN SYSTEMIC DISEASE

Acute and chronic changes in the pancreas are often associated with a variety of systemic diseases without producing symptoms that would lead to clinical recognition of pancreatic involvement. Infiltration of the pancreas by leukemia, Hodgkin's disease and other lymphogranulomatous conditions is common. Severe congenital syphilis involving the pancreas causes widespread fibrosis. Fibrotic changes with extensive atrophy of acinar tissue result from chronic passive congestion of the pancreas produced by longstanding cardiac decompensation. Miliary abscesses occur in association with septicemia; tubercles, with miliary tuberculosis.

NEOPLASMS OF THE PANCREAS

Neoplasms of the pancreas in childhood are rare; they are discussed in Section 25.

PAUL A. DI SANT'AGNESE

PATIENT EDUCATION

For the Family of the Child with Cystic Fibrosis

Your Child and Cystic Fibrosis. A pamphlet available from National Cystic Fibrosis Research Foundation, 3379 Peachtree Road, N.E., Atlanta, Georgia 30326.

For the Patient

Living with Cystic Fibrosis. A guide for the young adult. A pamphlet available from National Cystic Fibrosis Research Foundation, 3379 Peachtree Road, N.E., Atlanta, Georgia 30326.

GENERAL

Davenport, H. W.: Physiology of the Digestive Tract. 3rd ed. Chicago, Year Book Medical Publishers, Inc., 1971.

Beck, I. T., and Sinclair, D. G. (eds.): The Exocrine Pancreas. London, J. & A. Churchill, Ltd., 1971.

Tests

Andersen, D. H.: Pancreatic enzymes in the duodenal juice in the celiac syndrome. Am. J. Dis. Child. *63*:643, 1942.

Barbero, G. J., Sibinga, M. S., Marino, J. M., and Seibel, R.: Stool trypsin and chymotrypsin. Am. J. Dis. Child. *112*:536, 1966.

Gibson, L. E., and Cooke, R. E.: A test for the concentration of electrolytes in sweat in cystic fibrosis of the pancreas utilizing pilocarpine by iontophoresis. Pediatrics *23*:545, 1959.

Hadorn, B., et al.: Quantitative assessment of exocrine pancreatic function in infants and children. J. Pediatr. *73*:39, 1968.

Anomalies

Barbosa, J. J. de C., Dockerty, M. B., and Waugh, J. M.: Pancreatic heterotopia: Review of the literature and report of 41 authenticated cases of which 25 were clinically significant. Surg. Gynec. Obstet. *2*:527, 1946.

Hays, D. M., Greaney, E. M., Jr., and Hill, J. T.: Annular pancreas as a cause of acute neonatal duodenal obstruction. Ann. Surg. *153*:103, 1961.

Cystic Fibrosis

Andersen, D. H.: Cystic fibrosis of the pancreas and its relation to celiac diseases; A clinical and pathologic study. Am. J. Dis. Child. *56*:344, 1938.

Bodian, M.: Fibrocystic Disease of the Pancreas. London, William Heinemann, Ltd., 1952.

Bowman, B. H., McCombs, M. L., and Lockhart, L. H.: Cystic fibrosis: Characterization of the inhibitor to ciliary action in oyster gills. Science *167*:871, 1970.

Danes, B. S., and Bearn, A.: Cystic fibrosis of the pancreas: A study in cell culture. J. Exp. Med. *129*:775, 1969.

di Sant'Agnese, P. A., and Blanc, W. A.: A distinctive type of biliary cirrhosis of the liver associated with cystic fibrosis of pancreas. Pediatrics *18*:387, 1956.

di Sant'Agnese, P. A., Darling, R. C., Perera, G. A., and Shea, E.: Abnormal electrolyte composition of sweat in cystic fibrosis of the pancreas. Pediatrics *12*:549, 1953.

di Sant'Agnese, P. A., and Talamo, R. C.: Medical progress: Pathogenesis and physiopathology of cystic fibrosis of the pancreas. New Engl. J. Med. *277*:1287; 1344, 1399, 1967.

Doershuk, C. F., Matthews, L. W., Tucker, A. S., and Spector, S.: Evaluation of a prophylactic and therapeutic program for patients with cystic fibrosis. Pediatrics *36*:675, 1965.

Guide to Diagnosis and Treatment of Cystic Fibrosis of the Pancreas. National Cystic Fibrosis Research Foundation, 3379 Peachtree Road, N.E., Atlanta, Georgia 30326.

Handwerger, S., et al.: Glucose intolerance in cystic fibrosis. New Engl. J. Med. *281*:451, 1969.

Holsclaw, D. S., Grand, R. J., and Shwachman, H.: Massive hemoptysis in cystic fibrosis. J. Pediatr. *76*:829, 1970.

Huang, N. N. (ed.): Guide to Drug Therapy in Patients with Cystic Fibrosis. National Cystic Fibrosis Research Foundation, 3379 Peachtree Road, N.E., Atlanta, Georgia 30326.

Kaiser, D., Drack, E., and Rossi, E.: Inhibition of net sodium transport in single sweat glands by sweat of patients with cystic fibrosis of the pancreas. Pediatr. Res. *5*:167, 1971.

Kattwinkel, J., Taussig, L. M., Statland, B. E., and Verter, J. I.: The effects of age on alkaline phosphatase and other serologic liver function tests in normal subjects and patients with cystic fibrosis. J. Pediatr. *82*:234, 1973.

Lobeck, C. C.: Cystic fibrosis. *In* Stanbury, J. B., Wyngaarden, J. B., and Frederickson, D. S. (eds.): The Metabolic Basis of Inherited Disease. 3rd ed. New York, McGraw-Hill Book Co., 1972, p. 1605.

Mangos, J. A., and McSherry, N. R.: Studies on the mechanism of inhibition of sodium transport in cystic fibrosis of the pancreas. Pediatr. Res. *2*:378, 1968.

Matalon, R., and Dorfman, A.: Acid mucopolysaccharides in cultured fibroblasts of cystic fibrosis of the pancreas. Biochem. Biophys. Res. Commun. *33*:954, 1968.

Matthews, L. W., et al.: A therapeutic regimen for patients with cystic fibrosis. J. Pediatr. *65*:558, 1964.

Mullins, F., Talamo, R. C., and di Sant'Agnese, P. A.: Late intestinal complications of cystic fibrosis. J.A.M.A. *192*:741, 1965.

Schulz, I. J.: Micropuncture studies of the sweat formation in cystic fibrosis patients. J. Clin. Invest. *48*:1470, 1969.

Schuster, S. R., Shwachman, H., Harris, G. B. C., and Khaw, K-T.: Pulmonary surgery for cystic fibrosis. J. Thorac. Cardiovasc. Surg. *48*:750, 1964.

Shwachman, H., and Khaw, K-T.: Cystic fibrosis. *In* Shirkey, H. C. (ed.): Pediatric Therapy. 4th ed. St. Louis, The C. V. Mosby Company, 1972, p. 573.

Shwachman, H., and Kulczycki, L. L.: Long term study of 105 patients with cystic fibrosis. Am. J. Dis. Child. *96*:6, 1958.

Smith, F. R., Underwood, B. A., Denning, C. R., and Goodman, DeW.: Depressed plasma retinol binding protein levels in cystic fibrosis. J. Lab. Clin. Med. *80*:423, 1972.

Spock, A., Heick, H. M. C., Cress, H., and Logan, W. S.: Abnormal serum factor in patients with cystic fibrosis of the pancreas. Pediatr. Res. *1*:173, 1967.

Taussig, L. M., Lobeck, C. C., di Sant'Agnese, P. A., Ackerman, D. R., and Kattwinkel, J.: Fertility in males with cystic fibrosis. New Engl. J. Med. *287*:586, 1972.

Taussig, L. M., Kattwinkel, J., Friedewald, W. T., and di Sant'Agnese, P. A.: A new prognostic score and clinical evaluation system for cystic fibrosis. J. Pediatr. *82*:380, 1973.

Wiesmann, U. N., Boat, T. F., and di Sant'Agnese, P. A.: Flow rates and electrolytes in minor salivary gland saliva in normal subjects and patients with cystic fibrosis. Lancet *2*:510, 1972.

Genetic Pancreatic Deficiencies Not Due to Cystic Fibrosis

Grand, R. J., Rosen, S. W., di Sant'Agnese, P. A., and Kirkham, W. R.: Unusual case of XXY Klinefelter's syndrome with pancreatic insufficiency, hypothyroidism, deafness, chronic lung disease, dwarfism and microcephaly. Am. J. Med. *41*:478, 1966.

Shmerling, D. H., Prader, A., Hitzig, W. H., and Giedion, A.: The syndrome of exocrine pancreatic insufficiency, neutropenia, metaphysical dysostosis and dwarfism. Helvet. Paediatr. Acta *24*:547, 1969.

Shwachman, H., Diamond, L. K., Oski, F. A., and Khaw, K-T.: The syndrome of pancreatic insufficiency and bone marrow dysfunction. J. Pediatr. *65*:645, 1964.

Tarlow, M. J., Hadorn, B., Arthurton, M. W., and Lloyd, J. K.: Intestinal enterokinase deficiency. A newly-recognized disorder of protein digestion. Arch. Dis. Child. *45*:651, 1970.

Townes, P. L., Bryson, M. F., and Miller, G.: Further observations on trypsinogen deficiency disease: Report of a second case. J. Pediatr. *71*:220, 1967.

Pancreatitis

Frey, C., and Redo, S. F.: Inflammatory lesions of the pancreas in infancy and childhood. Pediatrics *32*:93, 1963.

Hendren, W. H., Greep, J. M., and Patton, A. S.: Pancreatitis in childhood: Experience with 15 cases. Arch. Dis. Child. *40*:132, 1965.

Kattwinkel, J., Lapey, L., di Sant'Agnese, P. A., and Edwards, W. A.: Hereditary pancreatitis: Three new kindreds and a critical review of the literature. Pediatrics. *51*:55, 1973.

Stein, D.: Pancreatitis—acute and relapsing—in infancy and childhood. S. African Med. J. *37*:1066, 1963.

Pseudocysts of the Pancreas

Kilman, J. W., Kaiser, G. C., King, R. D., and Shumacker, H. B.: Pancreatic pseudocysts in infancy and childhood. Surgery *55*:455, 1964.

12

THE RESPIRATORY SYSTEM

RESPIRATORY PHYSIOLOGY AND ITS APPLICATION TO PULMONARY DISEASE

Respiratory failure is the commonest cause of morbidity and death during the neonatal period, and respiratory disease is one of the most frequent reasons for hospitalization of infants and children. Basic knowledge of the development and functions of the respiratory system is essential for understanding many of these respiratory illnesses. The respiratory system, whose function is to maintain adequate oxygen and carbon dioxide exchange between the body and the environment, is made up of (1) a control system which consists of respiratory centers in the brain stem, chemoreceptors in the midbrain and in the carotid and aortic bodies, and peripheral nerves, both motor (efferent) and sensory (afferent); (2) the respiratory muscles and "thorax" (including diaphragm, rib cage, abdominal wall and abdominal contents); (3) the lungs and air passages; and (4) the pulmonary vasculature. Any one or a combination of these parts may be involved in disease processes which may contribute to respiratory disability.

DEVELOPMENT OF THE RESPIRATORY SYSTEM AND INITIATION OF RESPIRATION

The respiratory centers in the midbrain are sufficiently developed early in gestation (at least by 20 or 22 weeks) to respond to sensory stimuli and changes in pH, pCO_2 and pO_2 by initiating gasps and even sustaining rhythmic, although frequently periodic, respiration. In the immature infant these centers are particularly sensitive to the depressant effects of severe hypoxia, severe hypercapnia, acidosis or drugs. Even with a normally functioning respiratory center, extrauterine survival is usually not possible until after 27 or 28 weeks' gestation because of limiting factors within the lungs themselves. Capillarization of the alveoli is usually not far enough advanced until 28 weeks to permit adequate gas exchange. In addition, until approximately the same stage of development, pulmonary vascular resistance is probably so high, even after lung expansion, that pulmonary blood flow is significantly reduced.

The *ability of the lungs to resist collapse* is dependent upon the appearance (also at approximately 28 weeks' gestation) of certain surface active phospholipids (surfactant) in the alveolar lining membrane. The important role of these phospholipids can best be appreciated when one considers the Laplace Equation, $P=\frac{2T}{r}$ representing the relation between the tension *(T)* of the wall of a sphere, its radius *(r)*, and the pressure *(P)* within the sphere. If *T* were the same for all lung units (e.g., alveoli), then the smaller units would tend to collapse and the larger would expand. Actually, studies on extracts of lung lining layers suggest that, because of specific phospholipids, dipalmitoyl lecithin primarily and sphingomyelin in small part, the alveolar lining layer has a surface tension which varies with its degree of contraction (low surface tension) or expansion (high surface tension). This apparent adjustment of surface tension can explain the ability of air spaces of different sizes to coexist with equal pressures. Studies of experimental animals and of material obtained at autopsy from newborn infants indicate that the critical phospholipids are probably produced in type II (giant) alveolar cells in increasing amounts until enough is excreted into the alveolar spaces to allow formation of a continuous alveolar lining layer when the lungs are expanded for the first time with air. If only marginal amounts of the surface active compounds are present, production is apparently significantly decreased by various forms of cellular injury (e.g., hypoxia or acidosis) and by hypothermia. Thus, the atelectasis of the respiratory distress syndrome may be the result of immaturity of the phospholipid-producing cells of the alveoli alone or, in some cases, of immaturity combined with a variety of factors depressing the metabolism of the type II alveolar cell. On the other hand, it has now been shown that the appearance of surfactant can be accelerated by certain intrauterine stresses (e.g., infection) and by pharmacologic agents (e.g., heroin, corticosteroids, thyroxine). Clinical utilization of this information has been reported but such therapy must be considered experimental until there are more data concerning short- and long-term toxic side effects.

The *onset of respiration* is the most critical adjustment required of the infant. During fetal life there is some inhibitory mechanism which ordinarily prevents anything more than occasional respiratory movements. At birth, if the infant is to survive, a series of important events must occur in the respiratory system. Sensory (tactile and thermal) and chemical (pH, pO_2 and pCO_2) stimuli initiate respiration and, together with intrathoracic and intrapulmonary reflexes, sustain it. If the neuromuscular-thoracic structures are intact and adequately developed and the air passages are unobstructed, lung expansion will occur. For the initial inspiration, when air is introduced into the fluid-filled lung for the first time, large surface forces must be overcome. Transpulmonary pressures required for the first breath vary from 15 to 50 cm of water. Although these high pressures are normally produced by the infant himself, alveolar rupture may occur either spontaneously or as a result of artificial respiration. If the surface-active phospholipids are present in adequate quantities, air will tend to remain in the lung at the end of expiration, and subsequent respiration will require much smaller transpulmonary pressures, finally stabilizing at about 5 cm of water for the quiet respiration of normal infants.

Concomitant with lung expansion in the normal infant is a striking reduction in pulmonary vascular resistance, an increase in pulmonary blood flow, and a rapid decrease in the shunting of blood from the right to the left side of the heart. This pulmonary vasodilatation is apparently the result of changes in blood gases and pH as well as lung expansion itself.

As part of the process of lung expansion, the fluid which fills the potential air spaces during fetal life must be rapidly removed. Some is removed through the nose and mouth, while much is apparently picked up by the capillaries and lymphatics. After the initiation of respiration the stiffness of the lungs gradually decreases, presumably as a result of removal of the fluid.

The respiratory mechanism at birth is most likely to fail as the result of (1) central nervous system depression or (2) abnormalities within the lungs. Drugs, intrauterine hypoxia and trauma may all depress the respiratory center. Unless morphine antagonists are indicated, little can be done to improve the responsiveness of the center except to supply it with oxygen and to remove excess carbon dioxide. Good obstetric and anesthetic procedures should greatly reduce the occurrence of respiratory center failure.

Serious acidosis ($pH < 7.25$) is almost always present when significant intrauterine asphyxia has occurred. In order to improve the function of the respiratory center as well as cardiac output, the acidosis should be corrected; overcorrection ($pH > 7.45$) should be stringently avoided since cerebral blood flow is indirectly related to pH, being greater with acidosis and less with alkalosis.

Expansion of the lungs may be limited because of airway obstruction, which can be removed if it is in the pharynx, trachea or main bronchi. If the obstruction is in the smaller air passages, as may occur with aspiration of meconium-containing amniotic fluid or with plugging of alveolar ducts with hyaline membrane material, the lungs may be resistant to expansion. The latter type of respiratory obstruction is the greatest single cause of death in the neonatal period.

Congenital malformations such as diaphragmatic hernias, lung cysts, intrathoracic tumors and tracheo-esophageal fistulas may also be the cause of respiratory difficulty in the neonatal period and may at times simulate conditions which have less specific therapy.

After the adjustments of the neonatal period, further development of the respiratory system is primarily a matter of growth. The surface area of the lungs is calculated to be approximately 2 to 3 M^2 at birth and increases to approximately 70 M^2 in the adult male. The larger air passages increase in radius by a factor of 3 from birth to adulthood. Alveoli continue to increase in number until the age of 8 years; after 8 years the increase in lung size is accomplished by expansion of the alveoli. The various lung volumes in the normal person can best be related to body size, particularly height, and these relations are approximately constant from shortly after birth through young adulthood.

CONTROL OF RESPIRATION

Regulation of alveolar ventilation and maintenance of normal arterial pO_2, pCO_2 and pH are the principal functions of the medullary and peripheral chemoreceptors. The respiratory center in the brain stem is affected by reflexes from the lungs, the skeletal muscles and the carotid and aortic bodies, and also by its chemical environment. Proprioceptive impulses from the lungs are carried in the vagi and diminish inspiratory activity when the lungs are inflated and increase this activity when the lungs are deflated (Hering-Breuer reflex). Impulses transmitted by sensory nerves from the muscles and joints also stimulate activity of the respiratory center and are probably responsible for much of the hyperventilation of exercise.

In the newborn infant, ventilation is initially adjusted to achieve a relatively low pCO_2 (28 mm Hg versus 41 for the older child and the adult), presumably to compensate for metabolic acidosis. Periodic respiration occurs frequently in newborn and especially premature infants, and is usually diminished by the administration of oxygen.

Reduced arterial oxygen saturation stimulates chemoreceptors in the aortic and carotid bodies which, in turn, increase the activity of the respiratory center. Increases in arterial carbon dioxide stimulate the respiratory center directly without the mediation of a reflex arc. The actual stimulus to the center is probably due to the change in pH induced by the increase in pCO_2. Although both hypoxia and hypercapnia stimulate the respiratory center at first, when they are prolonged and severe, they act as depressants. For this reason the primary aim in the management of central depression of respiration should be to increase the oxygen supply to the respiratory center. Drugs are useful as respiratory stimulants only as they improve the general circulation, specifically counteract a respiratory depressant (e.g., naloxone), or correct severe acidosis (e.g., sodium bicarbonate).

Protective reflexes such as coughing and sneezing can alter the usual breathing patterns and act to eliminate foreign or obstructing matter from the respiratory tract. Respiration is also modified during swallowing and is altered reflexly by pain and variations of blood pressure.

Patients with weakened abdominal muscles cannot cough well. Manual pressure over the abdomen after a maximal inspiration can produce a fair cough when the glottis is opened suddenly, but this technique is limited to cooperative patients. When muscular function is diminished, as with poliomyelitis or other neuromuscular disease, the forces developed may be so limited that artificial respiration is required.

The weak respiratory muscles and the pliable thoracic cage of the premature infant may seriously limit his abilities to achieve normal ventilation, particularly when his lungs are abnormally stiff, as in the idiopathic respiratory distress syndrome. In addition, the premature infant's gag reflex is depressed and his ability to clear secretions markedly limited.

MUSCLES OF RESPIRATION

In quiet, normal breathing only the inspiratory muscles are used; expiration occurs as a result of the elastic recoil of the lung as the inspiratory muscles are relaxed. The diaphragm is the most important muscle of inspiration, but with increasing inspiratory effort the intercostal, spinal extensor and neck muscles become active in that order. They increase the thoracic diameter and thus its volume; the intercostal muscles also serve to stabilize the rib cage so that the diaphragm can function more effectively.

The abdominal muscles are the ones primarily used for a forced expiration; they are assisted by the "spinal flexors," which increase intrapulmonary pressure for coughing. The intercostal muscles also assist expiration, but here, too, they function largely to stabilize the rib cage.

LUNG VOLUMES

The static or semistatic subdivisions of lung volume are shown in Figure 12–1, which represents a series of tidal volumes and a vital capacity. The *vital capacity* is made up of the inspiratory capacity and the expiratory reserve volume, the proportion occupied by each varying with the position of the patient and with different respiratory conditions.

After each expiration a considerable volume of air, the *functional residual capacity,* remains in the lungs. This air serves as a buffer, minimizing changes in the partial pressure of carbon dioxide and oxygen in the alveoli and arterial blood during the respiratory cycle. Since most air spaces remain open at end-expiration, surface forces are also reduced.

The volume of the functional residual capacity (the resting end-expiratory volume) is determined

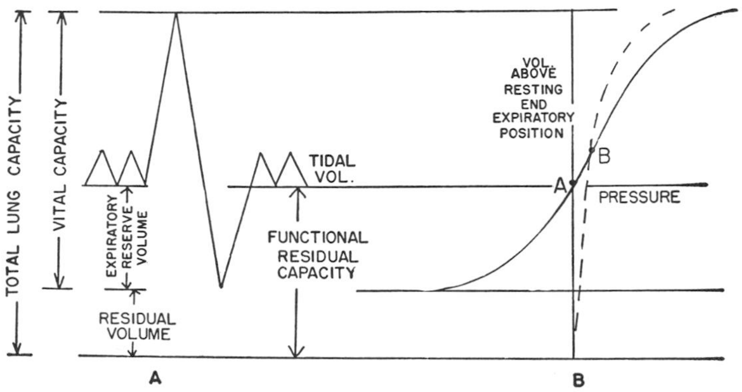

Figure 12–1 A, *Static or semistatic subdivisions of lung volume.* B, *Pressure-volume relationships of lungs (dashes) and thorax (solid curve). The resting end-expiratory volume has been continued as a horizontal line and also represents the pressure axis. Volume is represented by the vertical axis. Pressure changes to the right of the vertical axis are equivalent to positive airway or negative tank pressure, and pressures to the left represent negative airway or positive tank pressure. The volume-pressure characteristics of the lungs and "thorax" over the vital capacity range are represented by the solid curve. There is no scale because the values for subjects of different sizes are different; the shape of the curves, however, is similar. In the region of the tidal volume (between A and B on the curve) the relation of volume to pressure is essentially linear. With spontaneous respiration the effective strength of the respiratory muscles is an important factor in determining the magnitude of the maximum volume change. In addition, maximum inspiration is limited at large lung volumes by the decreased compliance of the lungs, the rib cage, and the abdominal wall and abdominal contents. Expiration, on the other hand, is limited by the compliance of the rib cage and the diaphragm.*

by the balance between the elastic recoil of the lungs and the tendency of the thorax to expand. The effective "thoracic" forces stem from the elastic characteristics of the rib cage, from the diaphragm and the abdominal wall, and from the hydrostatic force of the abdominal contents. The movement of the abdominal contents with shifts in position is largely responsible for the changes in the functional residual capacity; it is this movement on which the tilting method for artificial respiration is based. For example, in the supine position the diaphragm is pushed up and resting lung volume decreases, while in the upright position resting lung volume increases.

The *residual volume* is the amount of gas remaining in the lung at the end of a forced expiration; it is normally about 25 per cent of the total lung capacity. The functional residual capacity and especially the residual volume are increased when air is trapped beyond obstructed air passages, as in bronchiolitis, asthma or cystic fibrosis. These lung volumes may be calculated by measuring the amount of nitrogen washed out of the lungs during the breathing of pure oxygen or by the dilution of known amounts of an inert gas such as helium in the lungs. In addition, plethysmographic methods allow rapid measurements of lung volumes.

MECHANICS OF RESPIRATION

The mechanical properties of the respiratory system may be divided into 2 components—one concerned with static or elastic forces and the other with the dynamic or flow-resistance forces. The resting end-expiratory position or functional residual capacity results from two forces—the tendency of the lungs to collapse and the tendency of the "thorax" to expand. This can be likened to the balance between two springs; any deviation from the balance point requires work or an applied force; when the force is released, the springs return to their relaxation or balance point. In a comparable manner in normal breathing when the respiratory muscles contract, the thorax and lungs expand. When the muscles relax, the intrapleural pressure falls toward the resting end-expiratory pressure and expiration occurs.

The elastic or spring-like characteristic is called *compliance* and is expressed as milliliters or liters per cm of water pressure. In the case of the lungs it represents the change in pulmonary volume for a unit change of interpleural (i.e., transpulmonary) pressure and must be measured when there is no flow of air so that there is no flow-resistance component. The less the volume change produced by a given pressure change, the stiffer or less compliant are the lungs. Conversely, if the volume change for this same pressure difference is large, the lungs are highly distensible or compliant.

The lungs of infants are less compliant than those of older children and adults (Table 12–1), but when the difference in lung or body size is considered, they are found to be similar, and at all ages nearly the same transpulmonary pressure difference is required to produce the resting tidal volume. In order to measure the compliance of the lungs one must know the transpulmonary pressure changes. Pressure change in the thoracic esophagus may be used as an index of the transpulmonary pressure change; this measurement and direct interpleural pressure measurements, although useful in understanding pathophysiologic changes, have little application to clinical pediatrics.

Knowledge of the volume-pressure relation of the lungs and thorax (Fig. 12–1, *B*) is particularly useful during artificial respiration. In the older child and the adult, pressures required to produce

TABLE 12–1 NORMAL VALUES FOR PULMONARY STUDIES (RANGES INCLUDE APPROXIMATELY 95% OF NORMAL VALUES; VOLUMES IN LITERS, BTPS)

AGE (YEARS)	NEWBORN	6	10	14	♂ 18	18 ♀
LENGTH, HT. (CM.)	51	115	138	160	175	163
Vital capacity (L)	0.100	1.0–1.8	1.7–2.9	2.6–4.5	3.4–6.3	2.7–4.8
Total lung capacity (L)	0.140*	1.4–2.3	2.2–3.8	3.5–6.0	4.4–7.6	3.6–6.2
RV/TLC%	?	14–34	14–34	14–34	14–34	14–34
Vital capacity (2 sec) % total—average	?	>90%	>90%	>90%	>90%	>90%
$\dot{V}_{max}$ at 25% VC (L/sec)**	—	?	1.57	2.36	2.62	2.2
Peak expiratory flow rate (L/min.)	7.1–10.1	130–236	217–391	294–534	370–770	295–535
Lung compliance (ml/cm H_2O)	1–10	32–96	46–142	64–194	78–245	67–204
Flow resistance (cm H_2O/L/sec)	4–41†	3–14‡	2–9‡	2–6‡	1–5‡	2–6‡
Anatomic dead space (ml)	5.6–12.8	40–78	59–120	84–170	105–205	82–162

BTPS = 37° C saturated with water vapor at ambient pressure.
RV = residual volume; TLC = total lung capacity; VC = vital capacity
Newborn values in supine position, all others in sitting position.
*Values represent extrapolation and need further verification.
†Nose-breathing.
‡Mouth-breathing.
**Peak flow at 25% VC

TABLE 12–2 CHANGES IN PULMONARY FUNCTION IN 6 TYPES OF RESPIRATORY DIFFICULTY

	RESPIRATORY DISTRESS SYNDROME	CYSTIC FIBROSIS	ASTHMA	RESPIRATORY MUSCLE PARESIS	EMPHYSEMA	CONGESTIVE FAILURE
Total lung capacity	↓	↓	N or ↓	↓	↑	↓
Functional residual volume	↓	N or ↑	N or ↑	N	↑	N or ↑
Residual volume	?	↑	↑	↑	↑	↑
Vital capacity	↓	↓	N or ↓	↓	↓	↓
Timed vital capacity	?	↓	↓	N	↓	N or ↓
Lung compliance	↓	N or ↓	↓	↓	N or ↑	↓
Flow resistance	±	↑	↑	N	↑	N or ↑
Arterial blood pCO_2	↑	Late ↑	N or ↑	N or ↑	↑	±
Arterial blood pO_2	↓	Late ↓	N or ↓	N or ↓	↓	↓

suitable volume changes of the lungs plus thorax are approximately twice those required for the lungs alone. In the newborn infant, however, the thorax is so compliant that it requires little pressure for expansion.

A considerable part of the elastic characteristics of the lungs is the result of surface tension forces created by the fluid-air interface within the air spaces. Particularly important is the surface-active material lining the lung (cf. above).

Thus far the force required to maintain the lungs under static conditions has been considered. During inflation and deflation dynamic factors are also present. These are the resistance of the airway to the flow of gases and the viscous resistance of the pulmonary tissues. They are combined in the measurement of pulmonary flow resistance, which is the force or pressure difference required to produce a specific flow of air and is expressed as centimeters of water per liter per second (Table 12–1). In diseases such as asthma or cystic fibrosis the pulmonary resistance may be increased to 10 to 15 times the normal value (Table 12–2). Since resistance to the flow of air through a tube is inversely related to the fourth power (to the fifth power when turbulence is present) of the radius of the tube, inflammation or mucus (e.g., croup, bronchiolitis) is most likely to produce serious obstruction and increases in flow resistance in infants and small children.

The respiratory muscles must have sufficient work capacity to overcome the elastic and flow resistance of the respiratory system. During normal resting respiration the amount of work is small, approximately 1 per cent of the resting metabolism. As ventilation is increased, the expenditure of energy for breathing increases more rapidly than the effective ventilation, especially at high ventilatory rates.

VENTILATION

Ventilation involves the exchange of gas in the alveoli with gas in the external environment and normally serves to maintain the body in oxygen and carbon dioxide equilibrium. When ventilation is adequate, alveolar oxygen tension (P_AO_2) and, secondarily, arterial oxygen tension (PaO_2) are approximately 100 mm Hg, and carbon dioxide tension (P_ACO_2 and $PaCO_2$) is about 40 mm.

The partial pressures of gases at sea level in the normal person are presented in Figure 12–2. These are not valid at altitudes much above sea level, since the lower barometric pressure reduces the partial pressure for all gases except that of water vapor. The latter is related to the temperature of the air and remains fixed at 47 mm Hg at 37° C. If the patient is febrile, the vapor tension increases; an elevation of 2 to 3° C adds about 10 mm Hg to the partial pressure of water vapor, which then occupies more space and displaces other gases.

Owing to the differences in the pO_2 of alveolar gas and arterial blood, the sum of the partial pressures in the arterial blood does not equal the ambient barometric pressure. In normal persons vir-

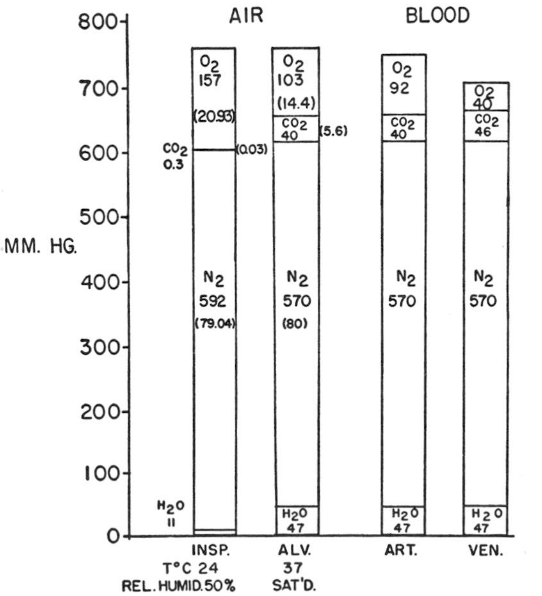

Figure 12–2 *Partial pressures of gases in various physiologic media at sea level (barometric pressure, 760 mm Hg).*

tually all this difference is due to a small venous admixture and ventilation-perfusion imbalance.

The volume of gas breathed into or out of the lungs with each breath is defined as the tidal volume (V_T). This volume multiplied by the respiratory rate (f) gives the minute volume ($\dot{V}_E$). Not all the tidal volume is effective in gas exchange; in the normal person about one third of each quiet respiration ventilates the nonfunctioning air passages or dead space (V_D), while the remaining portion (V_{Te}) enters the air sacs and alveoli and participates in gas exchange. Since alveolar ventilation ($\dot{V}_A$) is a function of carbon dioxide production ($\dot{V}_{CO_2}$) and the partial pressure of carbon dioxide in the arterial blood or alveoli, the following expressions are useful for defining the effective or alveolar ventilation:

$$V_T - V_D = V_{Te}$$

$$V_{Te} \times f = \dot{V}_A = k\frac{\dot{V}_{CO2}}{PaCO_2}$$

As metabolism and carbon dioxide production increase, the alveolar ventilation must increase if the blood carbon dioxide tension is to remain at the usual level. Conversely, if $\dot{V}_A$ were doubled for a given $\dot{V}_{CO_2}$, then $PaCO_2$ would be halved. It is also apparent that when the dead space increases secondary to disease or the use of anesthetic apparatus, V_T or f must increase to maintain a constant $PaCO_2$. The most effective way to increase alveolar ventilation is to increase the tidal volume. In this way alveolar ventilation is increased with a minimal increase in dead space ventilation.

In certain diseases, such as emphysema or cystic fibrosis, parts of the lung which should participate in gas exchange are essentially functionless because of obliteration of their blood supply or large reduction in their ventilation due to local obstruction. Even in normal subjects, owing to varying degrees of resistance of the different air passages to the alveoli, there is a small degree of uneven ventilation and an imbalance in the ventilation-perfusion ratios. When parts of the lung are involved in diseases associated with either varying amounts of obstruction or regional differences in lung compliance, there will be a greater degree of uneven ventilation. Regions which, as a result, are underventilated will not fully saturate the blood which perfuses them; the overventilated regions cannot compensate, since they cannot supersaturate blood with oxygen. Therefore, even when the total amount of ventilation is normal, uneven ventilation causes an impairment in the uptake of oxygen. When ventilation is uneven with respect to pulmonary capillary blood flow, a fall in PaO_2 occurs which is not accompanied by a rise in $PaCO_2$ until the ventilation-perfusion imbalance is severe.

Alveolar ventilation may be impaired not only by intrapulmonary disease, but also by conditions interfering with control of respiration, e.g., depression of the respiratory center, paralysis of nerves supplying respiratory muscles, primary weakness of the muscles, and mechanical disorders of the lungs, chest or abdomen (including obesity as in the Pickwickian syndrome). When hypoventilation results from such extrapulmonary causes, a rise in $PaCO_2$ is accompanied by a fall in PaO_2.

Normally there is a large reserve of ventilatory capacity. For example, a normal child may have a ventilation of 3 liters per minute at rest, but can increase this to 100 liters per minute for brief periods. When a disease is so severe that there is no longer any ventilatory reserve, the clearance of gas is impaired, and the composition of the alveolar gas is changed, the P_ACO_2 increasing and the P_AO_2 decreasing. This affects the arterial tension of oxygen and carbon dioxide, but, because of the shape of the oxygen-hemoglobin dissociation curve, the ventilation has to be seriously impaired before there is much change in arterial oxygen saturation. On the other hand, $PaCO_2$ and PaO_2 change proportionately with changes in alveolar ventilation. Since arterial blood is a mixture from all the alveoli, its pCO_2 may be regarded as equal to the mean of all the different pCO_2's in various parts of the lung. Indeed, $PaCO_2$ is particularly useful in measuring the level of alveolar ventilation because, unlike PaO_2, which may be affected by diffusion defects (cf. below) and the distribution of ventilation and blood flow in the lungs, carbon dioxide has a high solubility and the carbon dioxide-hemoglobin dissociation curve is almost linear. Its level, thus, is primarily a function of alveolar ventilation.

When the arterial pCO_2 rises, there is an accumulation of hydrogen ions, and pH decreases (uncompensated respiratory acidosis). In the course of a day or more the fall in pH is reversed by the retention of bicarbonate ions by the kidneys. When this occurs, the increased pCO_2 remains unchanged, but the pH will be near normal (compensated respiratory acidosis). In some respiratory disorders, when there is also an impairment in oxygen supply to the tissues, intermediate metabolites such as lactic acid accumulate in the blood, diminishing its buffering capacity (mixed respiratory and metabolic acidosis).

DIFFUSION

The uptake of oxygen by the lungs depends upon diffusion of the gas across the pulmonary membrane and chemical combination within the pulmonary capillary blood. Thus, the total diffusing capacity of the lungs for oxygen, or for a test gas such as carbon monoxide, is the result of the diffusing capacity of the pulmonary membrane and the ràte of uptake of the gas by the blood in the pulmonary capillaries. It is apparent that decreases in the diffusing capacity of the lungs may be the result of thickening of the alveolar membranes or a decrease in pulmonary capillary surface. Since carbon dioxide diffuses through living tissues approximately 20 times as rapidly as oxygen, its excretion is rarely limited by diffusion defects.

Although diffusion defects are rare in children, such conditions as pulmonary hemosiderosis, interstitial fibrosis, the Hamman-Rich syndrome, Niemann-Pick disease with pulmonary involvement and primary pulmonary artery hypertension with obliteration of many pulmonary capillaries are examples of pulmonary diseases associated with oxygen unsaturation secondary to abnormal diffusion. In adults, inhalation of a variety of toxic substances such as silica and beryllium leads to granulomatous lesions and fibrosis in the lungs and to diffusion defects.

PULMONARY VASCULATURE

The interdependence of the pulmonary vasculature and pulmonary function is obvious, but frequently overlooked. For maintenance of normal oxygen and carbon dioxide equilibration there must be a normal ventilation-perfusion relation throughout the greater part of the lung (cf. above).

In a number of pulmonary diseases, particularly those prolonged over months and years, pulmonary artery hypertension may develop. This may be due to actual compression of the pulmonary vascular system, as is apparently the case in scoliosis, or to vasoconstriction secondary to hypoxia and hypercapnia, as in scoliosis or cystic fibrosis. In either case the chronic pulmonary hypertension tends to be progressive, and cor pulmonale finally ensues, so that many of the children with the most severe pulmonary disease terminally exhibit a combination of cardiac *and* pulmonary failure. In some cases the pulmonary vasoconstriction may be temporarily reversed by the administration of oxygen and the reduction of hypercapnia accomplished by assisted ventilation, but the course of the disease is rarely more than temporarily slowed.

When pulmonary vascular congestion occurs in infants as a result of left-to-right shunts associated with congenital heart disease, respiratory acidosis occurs. Respiratory function is further altered, since these infants are particularly apt to have serious difficulty with respiratory tract infections.

VENTILATION-PERFUSION RELATIONS

Ventilation ($\dot{V}_A$) and perfusion ($\dot{Q}$) relations vary from one part of the lungs to another, but the average $\dot{V}_A/\dot{Q}$ ratio is 0.8. Although in the upright position both ventilation and perfusion are less at the apices than at the bases of the lungs, the difference is greater for blood flow and, hence, $\dot{V}_A/\dot{Q}$ is relatively higher at the top of the lungs and pO_2 is higher and pCO_2 lower than at the bases.

Congenital heart disease may affect ventilation-perfusion ratios. For example, the average value for $\dot{V}_A/\dot{Q}$ is decreased when there is a left-to-right shunt and increased when there is decreased perfusion of the lungs as in pulmonic stenosis.

Ventilation-perfusion relations may be measured in several ways. When ventilated areas are not well perfused, the difference between the physiologic and anatomic dead space (the alveolar dead space) will be increased. The alveolar-arterial (A-a) gas tension gradient increases when there are uneven $\dot{V}_A/\dot{Q}$ ratios in various parts of the lung, but an increased A-a pO_2 gradient may also be due to changes in diffusion or direct venous admixture. Yet if the A-a pO_2 gradient is measured at ambient *and* at high inspired oxygen tensions, uneven $\dot{V}_A/\dot{Q}$ ratios will be associated with little change. If, on the other hand, the A-a pO_2 gradient increases at low inspired oxygen tensions, a diffusion abnormality is likely, whereas a large A-a pO_2 gradient at high oxygen tensions suggests a direct venous admixture.

Nonuniform $\dot{V}_A/\dot{Q}$ ratios will also result in an increased A-a gradient for P_{N2}, and this has been the basis for another technique for indirectly estimating such changes. Since the P_{N2} of urine is a reflection of arterial P_{N2}, the A-a P_{N2} gradient can be measured in the steady state without drawing blood. In the newborn infant the normal value for A-a P_{N2} gradient is about 20 mm Hg or more, but within a few days of birth it approaches the adult value of 10 mm or less.

CILIARY ACTIVITY

No discussion of the ventilatory system is complete without some consideration of the cilia and their activity. Normally, cilia line the air passages down to the level of the terminal bronchioles. The continuous activity of the cilia has been described as the natural defense mechanism against extraneous agents. In animal studies, at least, the cilia have been shown to beat approximately 1300 times a minute and to move mucus toward the upper part of the respiratory tract at about 1.5 cm per minute.

Ciliary activity is directly related to the level of humidity in the inhaled gas, a fact which provides at least a partial scientific basis for the use of humidified air in infections of the upper respiratory tract. In addition, there is considerable evidence that any irritant, including inhaled cigarette smoke, may reduce the effectiveness of the cilia in keeping the air passages free of mucus and foreign material.

The ciliary activity of respiratory epithelial cells is adversely affected in vitro by perfusion with sera from patients with cystic fibrosis and their parents. The clinical significance of this finding remains to be determined.

Normally the lower respiratory tract is free of

bacteria, but bacteria may be introduced by techniques for inhalation therapy or respiratory assistance. In addition, various conditions, such as cystic fibrosis, bronchiectasis, malignancy and chronic bronchitis, and broad spectrum antibiotic therapy may predispose to lower respiratory tract infection. According to animal experiments, alveolar macrophages are effective in clearing these organisms from the lung, although the mucociliary "escalator" may also contribute.

METHODS OF ASSESSING VENTILATORY FUNCTION

Scrupulous history and physical examination combined with selected studies, including roentgenograms, bacterial and viral cultures and, on occasion, biopsy of the lung, are essential for the diagnosis of ventilatory abnormalities. *Pulmonary function tests are rarely helpful in establishing specific diagnoses; rather they are useful in assessing the severity of disease, following the course of pulmonary conditions, evaluating the effect of therapy, or providing a better understanding of the disordered physiology.*

Conditions affecting the function of the ventilatory system may be classified into five main groups: (1) restrictive disorders which limit the inflation and deflation of the lungs (e.g., respiratory muscle weakness), (2) obstructive diseases which lead to increased resistance to the flow of air within the lungs (e.g., asthma), (3) abnormalities in ventilatory control (e.g., central nervous system depression), (4) rarely, defects in the diffusion of gases, especially oxygen, across the alveolar membrane (e.g., idiopathic pulmonary hemosiderosis), and (5) abnormalities in the pulmonary circulation (e.g., primary pulmonary arterial hypertension). Fortunately the three most frequently encountered types of conditions, restrictive disorders, obstructive diseases and abnormalities in control, are the most readily studied with pulmonary function tests (see Table 12–2). To quantitate ventilatory function, the appropriate test should be applied. Although many complex techniques are available, those mentioned below are either easily applicable or, in some cases, necessary for the quantitation of the type of condition suspected by the clinical examination. *The fact that a high proportion of the tests require understanding and active participation on the part of the patient limits the use of many of the techniques.*

TESTS FOR RESTRICTIVE DISORDERS. In restrictive disorders the total excursion of the chest is limited and the vital capacity is thus reduced. Predicted values for vital capacity can be obtained from the following formulas:

	5–15 YEARS	16+ YEARS
Males	250 ml/yr age	25 ml/cm height
Females	200 ml/yr age	20 ml/cm height

These estimations are clinically useful, but not sufficiently accurate for research purposes. Normal values for children of various heights are given in Table 12–1.

Crying vital capacities have been measured in newborn infants by means of a face mask connected to a spirometer with low inertia. The average vital capacity for a full-term (3.0 kg) infant is approximately 140 ml.

If the restrictive disorder is thought to be secondary to muscle weakness, effective muscle strength can be measured directly with an anaeroid manometer. In order for the results to be comparable to predicted values, it is necessary to measure expiratory strength starting at full inspiration and inspiratory strength starting at full expiration.

TESTS FOR OBSTRUCTIVE DISEASES. Obstruction to the flow of air is the primary physiologic derangement in many of the acute (e.g., bronchiolitis and croup) and chronic (e.g., asthma and cystic fibrosis) diseases of childhood. The direct measurement of airway resistance involves complex research techniques. Resistance *(R)* is related to pressure *(P)* and flow *(F)* in the following fashion:

$$R = \frac{P}{F}$$

If pressure or muscle strength is normal, measurement of flow provides a good index of airway obstruction. Air passages are compressed during forced expiration, and obstruction is more readily detectable during such a maneuver.

A number of different techniques are available for measuring flow rates. Recording a forced expiratory vital capacity on a rapidly revolving drum allows the measurement of the peak flow rate. In predicting normal values the effect of body size on lung volume can be disregarded when the proportion of the total vital capacity forcibly expired in the first 1, 2 or 3 seconds is calculated from a recording spirometer. It should be emphasized that the absolute values should also be recorded and will be influenced by body size and starting lung volume. The peak flow meter of Wright is also useful and is available in two sizes, one for small children and one for older children and adults. Predicted values for the Wright peak flow meter can be obtained from equation 1 (below).

In children 3 to 5 years of age a sensitive flow meter (a pneumotachygraph) has proved useful. In this age group, peak expiratory flow rates for children of both sexes may be obtained from the formula below (equation 2).

1. For boys: Peak flow rate (l/min) $= 5.70 \times$ ht (cm) $- 480$ (S.D $= \pm 14.5\%$)
   For girls: Peak flow rate (l/min) $= 4.65 \times$ ht (cm) $- 344$ (S.D. $= \pm 14.3\%$)
2. Peak flow rate (l/min) $= 11.62 \times$ age (yr) $+ 2.862 \times$ ht (in) $- 60.12$ (S.D. $= \pm 24\%$)

Recently it has been demonstrated that measurement of maximal flow in relation to various lung volumes provides a more sensitive method of demonstrating obstruction in patients with such conditions as asthma and cystic fibrosis. This technique allows for comparison of maximal expiratory flow rates at various lung volumes (usually at 25 and 50 per cent of vital capacity) with normal values.

TESTS FOR REGULATION OF VENTILATION. Depression of the central nervous system secondary to asphyxia, trauma, infection, increased intracranial pressure or drugs is frequently associated with inadequate ventilation. There may be a decreased respiratory rate or disturbed rhythm (e.g., Cheyne-Stokes respiration). In addition, paralysis or muscle weakness may lead to hypoventilation.

The adequacy of ventilation can be estimated by measuring the minute volume ($\dot{V}_E$) by means of a recording spirometer or a ventilation meter. The measured tidal volumes are then compared with the predicted values obtained from a nomogram (Fig. 12–3) at the observed frequency of breathing. The use of the nomogram involves the assumption that the lungs themselves are relatively normal and that the body weight is a good index of the person's metabolism or carbon dioxide production. Knowing the weight and the frequency of breathing, one can then predict the required tidal volume. This calculation is most applicable when regulating artificial respiration in respiratory muscle weakness or during apnea or anesthesia. Use of the nomogram is demonstrated by the following example:

A 40-pound male child requires artificial ventilation. His temperature is 40° C, he is breathing through a tracheostomy tube, he is not in coma, and he is at an altitude of 3000 feet. Respiratory frequency is set at 30 per minute. Corrections to be applied to basal tidal volume are listed on the nomogram (Fig. 12–3) and demonstrated below:

Basal tidal	135 ml
Awake + 10%	14 ml
Fever + 3 × 9 = 27%	36 ml
Altitude + 1.5 × 5 = 7.5%	10 ml
	195 ml
Tracheostomy − 40/2	−20 ml
	175 ml predicted required V_T by tracheostomy tube

Predicted required minute volume ($\dot{V}_E$) is V_T times f; i.e., $\dot{V}_E$ is 175 × 20, or 3500 ml per minute.

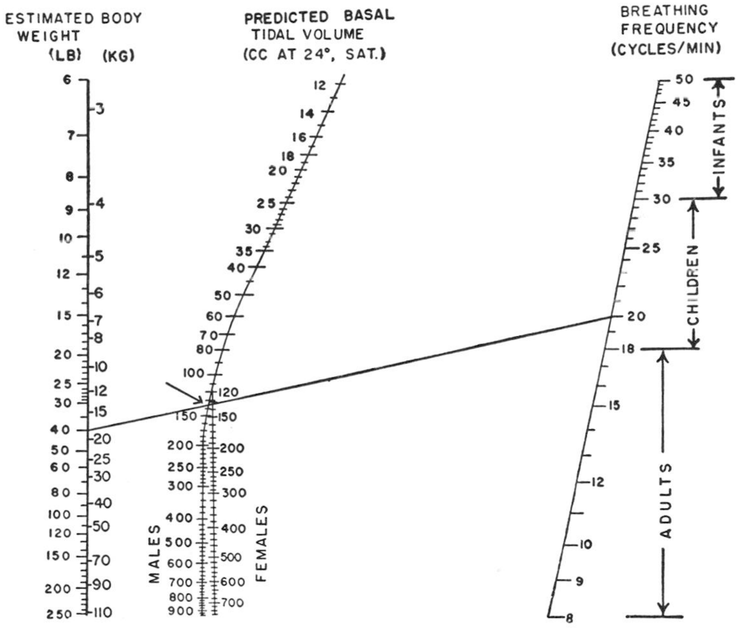

Figure 12–3 *Nomogram for regulation of artificial respiration.*

Corrections to be applied to basal tidal volume:

For metric system:

1. *Add 10 per cent for daily activity (i.e., patient not in coma).*
2. *Add 9 per cent for each 1° C above 37° C rectal temperature.*
3. *Add 8 per cent for each 1000 M altitude above sea level.*
4. *Subtract 1 cc/kg weight if patient is breathing through a tracheostomy or endotracheal tube.*

For English system:

1. *Add 10 per cent for daily activity (i.e., patient not in coma).*
2. *Add 5 per cent for each 1° F above 99° F rectal temperature.*
3. *Add 5 per cent for each 2000 ft above sea level.*
4. *Subtract volume (cc) equal to one half body weight expressed as pounds if patient is breathing through a tracheostomy or endotracheal tube.*

The adequacy of ventilation may be evaluated more accurately by measuring the alveolar or, more directly, arterial partial pressure of carbon dioxide. The determination of "alveolar" or end-tidal pCO_2, which can be continuously measured and recorded with an infrared carbon dioxide analyzer, is the most practical. End-tidal pCO_2, however, will not reflect the alveolar gas tension unless the physiologic dead space is completely cleared.

Cyanosis is, of course, an indication of respiratory insufficiency except in patients with shock, cardiovascular disease or methemoglobinemia. If cyanosis occurs in spite of adequate ventilation as judged either by minute volume or, better still, by arterial pCO_2 measurements, then the need is for higher concentrations of oxygen and not for an increase in ventilation. Increased ventilation produces relatively little change in arterial oxygen saturation, but removes significant amounts of carbon dioxide from the body, lowers the pCO_2 and increases pH. Alkalosis, in turn, decreases cerebral blood flow and should therefore be avoided. A decreased pCO_2 even in the presence of a compensated pH is not a normal state and may cause temporary personality changes.

TESTS FOR DIFFUSION DEFECTS. Although rare in children, pulmonary diffusion defects may be suspected from roentgen findings consistent with generalized interstitial fibrosis or a clinical history consistent with pulmonary hemosiderosis. Since the oxygen diffusing rate is approximately one twentieth that of carbon dioxide, the principal failure of gas exchange in the presence of diffusing difficulties involves oxygen. Thus, with partial compensation resulting from hyperventilation, the typical blood gas findings are a low PaO_2 and a normal or low $PaCO_2$. Further quantitation and definition (defective membrane diffusion or a decrease in pulmonary capillaries) of the diffusion defect require the actual measurement of lung diffusing capacity, most easily performed by using carbon monoxide as the indicator gas. This technique is difficult, however, especially in small children, and requires complex apparatus. Furthermore, when uneven ventilation is present, any interpretation of diffusion studies is of limited value.

TESTS FOR PULMONARY CIRCULATION. The pulmonary circulation, whether primarily involved in a disease process as in pulmonary artery hypertension or secondarily as in scoliosis, always requires for its investigation a fluoroscopic examination and usually necessitates cardiac catheterization (Section 13). Measurement of pulmonary diffusing capacity at 2 oxygen tensions allows calculation of the pulmonary capillary blood volume, which tends to increase with left-to-right shunts and to decrease with various forms of interstitial fibrosis.

DIFFERENTIAL BRONCHOSPIROMETRY. Localization of pulmonary dysfunction depends primarily on physical and roentgen examination. The insertion of a divided catheter is possible in children 12 years of age and older, and the ventilation, vital capacity and oxygen uptake of the right and left lungs may be compared. Another useful and less traumatic technique for the localization of pulmonary circulatory abnormalities and maldistribution of inspired gas involves scanning of the lungs for the presence of injected or inspired radioactive substances.

EXERCISE TOLERANCE TESTS. Provided the lungs alone are abnormal, their functional capacity may be measured indirectly by measuring exercise tolerance and comparing the results with standards established for children of comparable age and sex.

ARTIFICIAL RESPIRATION

Although obvious technical and quantitative differences exist, the basic principles of artificial respiration are the same for all ages and are as follows:

1. Maintenance of an adequate airway by
   a. Extension of neck with forward traction on mandible.
   b. Gentle suction.
   c. Intubation or tracheotomy.
2. Institution of adequate ventilation as quickly as possible.
3. Avoidance of injury to the patient.
4. Suppression of spontaneous respiratory efforts.

Severe hypoxia of only a few minutes may lead to irreversible damage, especially to the brain. Fortunately the newborn infant can tolerate hypoxia better than older persons, but, since the duration and severity of intrauterine hypoxia are impossible to gauge accurately, one should not delay resuscitative procedures even in the newborn. Oxygen administration is a useful adjunct, but is no substitute for adequate ventilation.

The methods of producing artificial respiration are (1) manual, (2) positive pressure applied to the airway, or negative pressure about the body, (3) rhythmic rocking of the patient, and (4) electrical stimulation of the phrenic nerve.

NEWBORN INFANT. See Resuscitation of the Newborn Infant, Section 7. Since hypoxia causes depression of the respiratory center itself, supplemental oxygen should be supplied in all instances until spontaneous respiration is established. The apneic infant is already hypercapneic and acidotic, and the administration of carbon dioxide may only lead to further depression. In the newborn infant particularly, but in anyone subjected to artificial respiration, the effectiveness of the procedure should be checked not only by observation of the excursion of chest and abdomen and auscultation of the lungs, but also by measurements of the ventilation and alveolar pCO_2 and blood gases.

For the infant whose lungs have never expanded, rocking will accomplish little; subsequently the effectiveness of rocking is in direct proportion to the size of the infant. Hence, rocking is of little direct use in small infants as a ventilating maneuver. Central nervous system stimulants (other than oxygen) are of little or no use and, in some instances, may be harmful. Tubbing, spanking, jackknifing and manual compression of the thorax are all dangerous and ineffective. Phrenic nerve stimulation produces a more natural type of breathing, but has limited practical use because of the need for special equipment and a trained operator.

INFANTS AND OLDER CHILDREN. Positive pressure (e.g., mouth-to-mouth) is useful once a free airway has been established. In addition, manual compression and expansion of the thorax as in the back pressure–arm lift method or back pressure–hip lift method can produce adequate ventilation, provided there is no respiratory obstruction. Electrical stimulation of the phrenic nerve is more practical than it is in the newborn infant. For more prolonged artificial ventilation the tank type of respirator, endotracheal positive pressure, the rocking bed and special chest-type or cuirass respirators can be used; the latter types have limited usefulness in infants and small children because the chest is compressed and ventilation may be insufficient. When mechanical artificial ventilation is required for a prolonged period (hours or days), the patient should be given deep breaths at regular intervals (two or three times an hour) in order to minimize the development of atelectasis.

When apnea has been present for more than a few minutes, the resulting acidosis should be treated as soon as ventilation has been restored.

The effectiveness of various types of ventilating devices is shown in Figure 12–4. The endotracheal positive-pressure technique produces the greatest tidal volume, owing to the compression of the gas within the lungs. The effectiveness of cuirass respirators varies with the amount of the body enclosed within them and the freedom of motion allowed. Rocking beds are not included, since there is great variation, depending on the size of the patient.

There is no special pressure that should be used

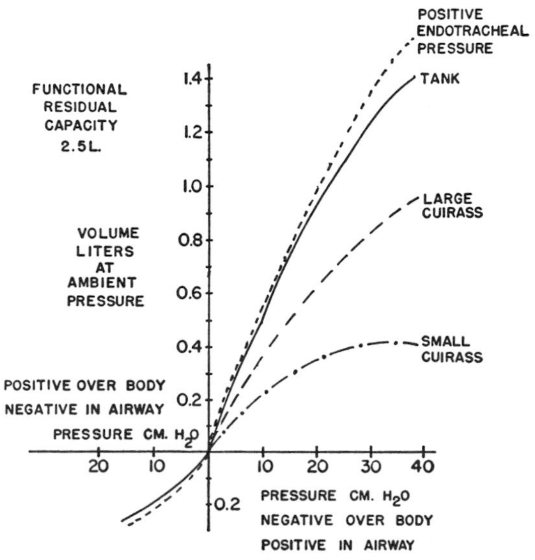

Figure 12–4 Effectiveness of breathing machines.

for different age groups. The pressure or degree of tilting should be set so that the required tidal volume or an end-tidal pCO_2 of 40 mm Hg is obtained. This requires measuring the tidal volume and comparing it with the predicted values from the nomogram (Fig. 12–3) or measuring the end-tidal pCO_2. If the device is unable to produce sufficient pressure at a given frequency, adequate ventilation may be obtained by increasing the frequency, which in turn usually increases the pressure developed. A new calculation from the nomogram will be necessary, since the predicted tidal volume will be different. Optimally, blood gas tensions should be checked in order to evaluate the adequacy of ventilation.

INHALATION THERAPY

Besides oxygen, the most frequently used agents for inhalation therapy are water, antibiotics and bronchodilators, which are administered in compressed air or oxygen.

OXYGEN. The therapeutic use of oxygen is not without danger. In premature infants, concentrations above that of room air increase the incidence of retrolental fibroplasia. When 40 or even 30 per cent oxygen is administered at sea level, alveolar oxygen tensions may reach approximately 240 and 185 mm Hg, respectively. If a mildly cyanotic infant is placed in such concentrations of oxygen, depending on the type of pathophysiologic change in the lungs, the possibility of raising the arterial oxygen tension above the safe (for retrolental fibroplasia) level is very real. In addition to administering oxygen to premature infants with primary pulmonary disease, it is sometimes necessary to give oxygen to those with episodes of apnea; under such circumstances, since the lungs are normal, arterial oxygen tensions will approach the alveolar oxygen tension as soon as regular respiration is reinstituted. Thus, if the risk of retrolental fibroplasia is to be minimized in the premature infant, it is imperative that the use of oxygen be limited to those infants who are cyanotic, to the minimum concentration necessary to prevent cyanosis, and should be discontinued as promptly as possible. There are, however, instances when oxygen therapy is necessary for the survival of a premature infant with severe hypoxemia; in such instances the potential benefit of the increased concentration of oxygen outweighs the potential risk of retrolental fibroplasia.

Oxygen therapy is also potentially dangerous in patients with chronic underventilation who are cyanotic. These patients may stop breathing and die, because the drive to breathe, which came from the low blood oxygen tension, is removed. Owing to chronic underventilation, blood carbon dioxide is high, and the respiratory center is no longer responsive to carbon dioxide. If the $PaCO_2$ is initially about 80 mm Hg, a further increase may reach narcotic levels, and the patient will become comatose. In such a situation artificial respiration may be necessary.

Environmental concentrations of oxygen greater than 60 per cent for a period of days are also toxic to the lungs themselves; hence, the prolonged use of such high concentrations should be avoided if possible.

WATER. The administration of air or oxygen supersaturated with water has long been used when there are increased or tenacious secretions and narrowing of the larger air passages (as with laryngitis or tracheobronchitis). Similarly, inhalation of water vapor is important in the management of patients breathing through a tracheostomy tube, when the normal humidifying action of the upper respiratory system is bypassed. In the premature infant, relatively high humidity (more than 60 per cent) helps to prevent heat loss and, hence, stabilizes the body temperature.

The use of vaporized water in peripheral pulmonary disease is less certainly effective. The air from the lower part of the trachea to the periphery of the lung is normally saturated with water at body temperature, whereas air saturated with water at room temperature (24° C) is only 50 per cent saturated when raised to body temperature. Thus, a saturated atmosphere does not necessarily supply saturated gas to the peripheral air passages.

ANTIBIOTICS. Inhalation of antibiotics in compressed air or oxygen (aerosols) is occasionally useful in the control of severe, diffuse pulmonary disease (e.g., cystic fibrosis). In most instances, however, the same agents may be as effective and more easily administered orally or parenterally. Furthermore, the distribution of ventilation, as well as the size of the droplets, the growth of the droplets, the polarization of the particles, and possibly other factors severely limit the penetration of an aerosol into the smaller pulmonary units and thus impose limitations on aerosol therapy.

BRONCHODILATORS. A number of bronchodilators can be effectively administered by inhalation. This route has the physical advantage that it is easy for the patient and the psychologic advantage that it is a means of treating directly the bronchoconstriction and, thus, the patient's symptoms. However, dosage is difficult to control, particularly when the frequency of administration is determined by the patient. Such uncontrolled inhalation of isoproterenol (Isuprel), and possibly of other sympathomimetic drugs, may exacerbate and perpetuate asthma by increasing mucosal edema and by drying respiratory secretions, may induce refractoriness to other forms of therapy, and is thought to be associated with an increased death rate among severe, chronic asthmatics.

CHARLES DAVENPORT COOK

Abramson, H. (Ed.): Resuscitation of the Newborn Infant. St. Louis, The C. V. Mosby Company, 1960.

Avery, M. E., and Fletcher, B. D.: The Lung and Its Disorders in the Newborn Infant. 3rd ed. Philadelphia, W. B. Saunders Company, 1974.

Barcroft, J.: Researches on Pre-Natal Life. Springfield, Ill., Charles C Thomas, 1947.

Bengtsson, E.: The working capacity in normal children, evaluated by submaximal exercise on the bicycle ergometer and compared with adults. Acta Med. Scand. *154*:91, 1956.

Bucci, G., Cook, C. D., and Barrie, H.: Studies of respiratory physiology in children. V. Total lung diffusion, diffusing capacity of pulmonary membrane and pulmonary capillary blood volume in normal subjects from 7 to 40 years of age. J. Pediatr. *58*:820, 1961.

Comroe, J. H., Jr.; Physiology of Respiration. Chicago, Year Book Medical Publishers, Inc., 1965.

Cook, C. D., and Hamann, J. F.: Relation of lung volumes to height in healthy persons between the ages of 5 and 38 years. J. Pediatr. *59*:710, 1961.

Cross, K. W., Klaus, M., Tooley, W. H., and Weisser, K.: The response of the newborn baby to inflation of the lungs. J. Physiol., *151*:551, 1960.

Daily, W. J. R., and Smith, P. C.: Mechanical ventilation of the newborn infant, Part I. Curr. Probl. Pediatr. *1* (No. 8) June, 1971.

Daily, W. J. R., and Smith, P. C.: Mechanical ventilation of the newborn infant, Part II. Curr. Probl. Pediatr. *1* (No. 9) July, 1971.

Dalhamn, T.: Mucous flow and ciliary activity in the trachea of healthy rats and rats exposed to respiratory irritant gases (SO_2, H_3N, HCHO). Acta Physiol. Scand., *36*(Suppl.), 123, 1956.

deLemos, R. A., Shermeta, D. W., and Avery, M. E.: Acceleration of appearance of pulmonary surfactant in the fetal lamb by administration of corticosteroids. Am. Rev. Resp. Dis. *102*:459, 1970.

Ferris, B. G., Jr., Mead J., Whittenberger, J. L., and Saxton, G. A.: Pulmonary function in convalescent poliomyelitis patients. III. Compliance of lungs and thorax. New Engl. J. Med. *240*: 390, 1952.

Gaensler, E. A.: Analysis of the ventilatory defect by timed vital capacity measurements. Am. Rev. Tuberc. *64*:256, 1951.

Gluck, L., Motoyama, E. K., Smits, H. L., and Kulovich, M. V.: The biochemical development of surface activity in mammalian lung. I. The surface active phospholipids; the separation and distribution of surface active lecithin in the lung of the developing rabbit fetus. Pediat. Res., *1*:237, 1967.

Harned, H. S., Jr., Rowshan, G., MacKinney, L. G., and Sugioka, K.: Relationships of P_{O_2}, P_{CO_2}, and pH to onset of breathing of the term lamb as studied by a flow-through cuvette electrode assembly. Pediatrics *33*:672, 1964.

Humphreys, P. W., Normand, I. C. S., Reynolds, E. O. R., and Strang, L. B.: Pulmonary lymph flow and the uptake of liquid from the lungs of the lamb at the start of breathing. *J. Physiol. 193*:1, 1967.

Liggins, G. C., and Howie, R. N.: A controlled trial of antepartum glucocorticoid treatment for prevention of the respiratory distress syndrome in premature infants. Pediatrics *50*:4, 1972.

Long, E. C., and Hull, W. E.: Respiratory volume-flow in the crying newborn infant. Pediatrics *27*:373, 1961.

Mead, J.: Mechanical properties of lungs. Physiol. Rev., *41*:281, 1961.

Murray, A. B., and Cook, C. D.: Measurement of peak expiratory flow rates in 220 normal children from 4½ to 18½ years of age. J. Pediatr. *62*:186, 1963.

Nelson, N. M.: Neonatal pulmonary function. Pediat. Clin. N. Amer. *13*:769, 1966.

Rivera, L. M., and Snider, G. L.: Ventilatory studies in preschool children. I. Peak expiratory flow rates in normal and abnormal preschool children. Pediatrics. *30*:117, 1962.

Sanchis, J., Dolovich, M., Rossman, C., Wilson, W., and Newhouse, M.: Pulmonary mucociliary clearance in cystic fibrosis. New Engl. J. Med., *288*:651, 1973.

Spock, A., Heick, H., Cress, H., and Logan, W.: In Vivo Study of Ciliary Motility: Asymmetrical Ciliary Beat Associated with Sera of Patients with Cystic Fibrosis. In 4th International Conference on Cystic Fibrosis, Berne, Switzerland, September, 1966.

Sutherland, J. M., and Ratcliff, J. W.: Crying vital capacity. Am. J. Dis. Child., *101*:67, 1961.

Zapletal, A., Motoyama, E. K., Woestijne, C. van de, Hunt, V. R., and Bouhuys, A.: Maximum expiratory flow volume curves and airway conductance in children and adolescents. J. Appl. Physiol. *26*:308, 1969.

Zapletal, A., Motoyama, E. K., Gibson, L. E., and Bouhuys, A.: Pulmonary mechanics in asthma and cystic fibrosis. Pediatrics *48*:64, 1971.

RESPIRATORY DISTURBANCES

GENERAL CONSIDERATIONS. Disturbances in respiration are not necessarily related to lesions in or disease of the respiratory tract, because the process of breathing is influenced by the function of many organs other than lungs, and because the amount of respiratory exchange required depends on many factors extrinsic to the lung. Accordingly, in the differential diagnosis of respiratory disturbances, one must consider genetic (anatomic and metabolic) anomalies, traumatic, chemical (poisoning) or infectious factors. From an anatomic standpoint, the primary lesions may be in the respiratory system, or in the central nervous, cardiovascular, endocrine, urinary or gastrointestinal systems. The disturbed respiratory patterns found with disorders of other systems are discussed in their respective sections; here we shall deal with primary diseases of the respiratory tract, excluding the conditions peculiar to the neonatal period.

AGE AS A FACTOR IN INFECTIOUS RESPIRATORY DISEASE. The clinical pattern of respiratory illness varies in considerable degree with the age of the patient. Differences in susceptibility to infection occur, the younger child being either more or less susceptible, according to the particular agent involved. Rates of infection among infants exposed to group A beta-hemolytic streptococci are lower than among their older siblings, and a similar pattern has been demonstrated for influenza. Moreover, streptococcal disease in the young may differ strikingly from that in older children and adults. In the child under 2 years streptococcal infection rarely produces exudative pharyngotonsillitis, but is usually manifested as an insidious, subacute, protracted illness whose common manifestation is rhinorrhea. On the other hand, the infant may suffer severe disease from certain agents which produce relatively trivial illness in the older child. Whooping cough, a relatively harmless tracheobronchitis of childhood, is a serious and often fatal disease in the infant under a year of age. Tuberculosis is strikingly more severe in the infant, with a decided tendency toward hematogenous dissemination. The respiratory syncytial virus, the parainfluenza viruses and the adenoviruses produce generally mild illnesses in older children, but are often associated in infants with severe lower respiratory tract disease such as bronchiolitis, pneumonia, and croup. Why these differences should exist is not completely understood. They are believed to be due in part to anatomic differences between the two age groups (distances between corresponding points of the respiratory tract are shorter, orifices are smaller, and connective tissue is less dense, so that swelling can occur more readily). It is also possible that prior experience with some viral agents serves to protect the older child from serious disease when reinfection occurs.

Aside from considerations of severity of illness in infants as compared to older children, the manifestations themselves may be different, and organ systems may be involved in one age group which are not affected in another. For example, adenovirus type 3 infection in an older child is often associated with the syndrome of pharyngoconjunctival fever; in infants this same agent may cause diarrhea without associated respiratory tract disease. The changes in susceptibility and the different manifestations of infection that occur with age are the products of interaction of three basic factors: immunologic, environmental and metabolic. These are influenced in turn by a number of others such as anatomy, heredity and nutrition. The complexity of the situation is great, and little is known of the mechanisms through which these factors operate.

THE UPPER RESPIRATORY TRACT

THE NOSE

In man the primary functions of the nose are to adjust the humidity and temperature of inspired air and to remove foreign particles and bacteria from the air stream. Passage through the nose raises air temperature nearly to that of the body, and adjusts the relative humidity to approximately 80 per cent.

Bacteria and other foreign matter are impinged on the "mucous blanket" covering the ciliated pseudocolumnar epithelium of the nasal passages. This blanket is continuously propelled toward the pharynx by ciliary action, the movement being sufficiently rapid to require the replacement of the mucous layer approximately every 10 minutes.

The principal defense mechanism of the nose appears to consist of the mechanical removal of bacteria and other noxious elements by means of this mucous blanket. Intranasal medication which affects adversely the production or integrity of mucus, or the behavior of the ciliary cells will reduce the efficiency of the protective barrier.

Nasal secretions contain specialized IgA antibodies, which offer an immunologic barrier to infection, and the enzyme lysozyme, whose action is capable of destroying bacteria, but whose exact protective function remains unknown.

MALFORMATIONS. Congenital structural nasal abnormalities are uncommon, in contrast to acquired malformations. Occasionally nasal bones are congenitally absent, so that the bridge of the nose fails to develop, resulting in nasal hypoplasia. Congenital absence of the nose, complete or partial duplication, or a single centrally placed nostril occasionally occurs, but usually as a part of malformation syndromes incompatible with life. Rarely, supernumerary teeth may be found in the nose, or teeth may grow into it from the maxilla and be absent from their usual site.

Hypertelorism is a common defect, resulting from overdevelopment of the lesser wings of the sphenoid. The most prominent physical manifestation is widening of the base of the nose, with the eyes widely separated.

On occasion, nasal bones are sufficiently malformed to produce severe narrowing of the nasal passages. Often such narrowing is associated with a high and narrow hard palate. Children with these defects may suffer from chronic or recurrent infections of the nasal and paranasal passages. Rarely, the alae nasi may be sufficiently thin and poorly supported to result in inspiratory obstruction.

Choanal atresia is the most common congenital abnormality of the nasal passages. If only one side is affected, it does not give rise to severe symptoms at birth. If both nares are blocked by a membranous, cartilaginous or bony septum, obvious symptoms occur in most but not all babies; some infants are unable to breathe through their mouths when both nares are blocked, while others can. Those unable to breathe through their mouths make increasingly vigorous efforts at inspiration, with a sucking in of their lips, become cyanotic quickly, and may soon die. Infants able to breathe through their mouths experience difficulty only in sucking and swallowing and become cyanotic as they attempt to nurse. Bilateral choanal occlusion should be suspected in a newborn infant who persistently breathes through his mouth, or is cyanotic when at rest with his mouth closed, but returns to normal color when he cries. Unilateral choanal obstruction is usually asymptomatic until the first respiratory infection, at which time the diagnosis may be suggested by unilateral nasal discharge or disproportionately severe nasal obstruction.

The obstruction can be demonstrated by the failure of a firm catheter or probe to pass into the nasopharynx. Other diagnostic possibilities can be eliminated with the instillation through a catheter of a radiopaque substance into each nostril while the infant is lying on his back. The anterior nasal cavity will be outlined and the block readily seen radiographically.

With bilateral choanal atresia, prompt establishment of an airway is urgent. In an emergency this is done most readily either by propping the jaws open with any suitable device or by inserting an airway from the lips into the nasopharynx. The infant can then be fed by gavage until such time (usually 2 or 3 weeks) as he learns to eat and breathe without the airway. Immediate surgery was formerly recommended, but can be delayed for weeks, months or even years in patients who adapt well to the obstruction. With unilateral obstruction it is usually desirable to postpone operation until infection has been controlled and the infant is in otherwise satisfactory physical condition.

Deviation of the nasal septum is generally an acquired rather than a congenital condition and is rarely seen in young children. Surgery is indicated only in the rare instances of obstruction and is best deferred until 14 or 15 years of age, since earlier operation often results in external deformities of the nose. **Perforation of the nasal septum** may rarely be congenital. It is more likely to be caused by syphilis, tuberculosis, or trauma. Other malformations of the septum, of the floor and of the external nose are frequently associated with harelip and cleft palate. An **encephalocele** protruding through a defect in the cribriform plate into the nasal cavity is a rare anomaly, but must be differentiated from polyps and tumors of extracranial origin.

FOREIGN BODIES IN THE NOSE. Foreign bodies such as vegetables, nuts, erasers, paper wads, beads and stones are frequently introduced into the nose by children. The object is usually situated anteriorly at first, but through the unskillful efforts of the patient or others it may be forced deeper into the nose.

Initial symptoms are local obstruction, sneezing, relatively mild discomfort and, rarely, pain. Irritation results in mucosal swelling, and, because some foreign bodies are hygroscopic and increase in size as water is absorbed, signs of local obstruction and discomfort may increase with time. Infection usually follows and gives rise to a purulent, malodorous or bloody discharge. Tetanus is a rare complication in nonimmunized children. *Unilateral nasal discharge and obstruction should suggest the presence of a foreign body,* which can usually be readily seen upon examination with a speculum or nasoscope. Removal should be carried out promptly in order to minimize the danger of aspiration of the object and to prevent local tissue necrosis. In most children, removal can be performed with topical anesthesia, using either forceps or nasal suction apparatus. Infection usually clears promptly upon removal of the object, and generally no further therapy is necessary.

The most frequent nasal growths are polyps, but rarely other tumors of the nose and nasopharynx occur. (See Section 25.) Polyps are most often associated with allergic rhinitis or cystic fibrosis; they usually produce obstructive symptoms as well as chronic nasal discharge. Treatment consists in removal of the growths and attention to the underlying cause.

EPISTAXIS

ETIOLOGY. Nosebleeds are rare in infancy, common in childhood, and decrease in incidence after puberty. They are more common in males. The source of the bleeding is usually the vascular plexus on the anterior septum or the mucosa of the anterior turbinates. By far the most common cause is trauma, including picking of the nose. There appears to be a familial predisposition, and susceptibility is increased during respiratory infections. Epistaxis is also encountered with adenoidal hypertrophy, with allergic rhinitis, sinusitis or polyps, and with a variety of acute infections such as rheumatic fever, scarlet fever, influenza, measles, varicella, typhoid fever, congenital syphilis, and diphtheria. In the last two conditions the discharge is generally both bloody and purulent. Especially severe bleeding may be encountered with such vascular abnormalities as telangiectasias or varicosities or if the child has thrombocytopenia, deficiency of clotting factors, hypertension or venous congestion. Adolescent girls occasionally have epistaxis at the time of menarche.

CLINICAL MANIFESTATIONS. Epistaxis usually occurs without warning, blood flowing slowly but freely from one nostril, occasionally from both. In children with nasal lesions, bleeding may follow physical exercise. When bleeding occurs at night, the blood is usually swallowed and may become apparent only when the child vomits or passes blood in his stools. Most nosebleeds stop spontaneously in a few minutes, but if bleeding continues, the child should be kept as quiet as possible in an erect position with the head tilted forward to eliminate blood trickling posteriorly into the pharynx. Local control of the hemorrhage can usually be achieved by compressing the nares. If these simple measures do not stop the bleeding, local application of a solution of epinephrine (1:1000) with or without topical thrombin may on occasion be useful. A tampon consisting of a suitably shaped wedge of "fat back" (salt pork) has been shown to be highly effective. If bleeding persists, an anterior nasal pack should be inserted; if bleeding originates in the posterior nares, combined anterior and postchoanal packing is necessary. After bleeding has been controlled, and if a bleeding site can be identified, its obliteration by cautery with silver nitrate may prevent further difficulties. In patients with severe or repeated nasal hemorrhages, blood transfusions may be necessary. Special blood products and derivatives may be required for patients who have an underlying hematologic disorder.

ELONGATED UVULA

Persistent enlargement of the uvula is rare; it may be congenital or may be associated with a chronic upper respiratory tract infection such as adenoiditis. The long uvula coming into contact with the base of the tongue produces an annoying cough and a constant desire to clear the throat. These symptoms tend to be exaggerated when the child is lying on his back. Enlargement associated with chronic infection may disappear with eradication of the infection. Otherwise, amputation of the tip of the uvula may be indicated.

Infections of the Upper Respiratory Tract

GENERAL CONSIDERATIONS. By a generally accepted definition, upper respiratory tract infections are those infectious processes primarily affecting the structures of the respiratory tract above the larynx. Most respiratory illnesses, however, affect the upper and lower portions of the tract simultaneously or sequentially; others predominantly involve specific portions of the respiratory tree. Diagnostic classification on an anatomic basis is arbitrary and depends largely upon which organ or area the physician or the patient concludes is most obviously involved.

Because large numbers of different microorganisms (chiefly viruses) are capable of causing primary upper respiratory tract disease, with few producing distinctive clinical syndromes, etiologic classification is of limited use. The same organism may cause clinical symptoms or syndromes of differing severity and extent in accordance with such host factors as age, sex, previous contact with the agent, allergy, nutritional status, and the like. For example, among different members of the same family a single virus may simultaneously produce typical colds in the parents, bronchiolitis in the infant, croup in a somewhat older child, pharyngitis in another, and a subclinical infection in another. Most of these agents, whether viral, bacterial or mycoplasmal, can affect the respiratory tract in much the same way. There is, in a clinical sense, no true "cold" virus or "pharyngitis" agent; rather, any clinical syndrome involving the upper tract may be caused by a number of different organisms, not identifiable except by suitable laboratory investigations.

ETIOLOGIC CONSIDERATIONS OF NONBACTERIAL INFECTIONS OF THE RESPIRATORY TRACT. It has become increasingly apparent that most acute respiratory tract infections are caused by viruses and mycoplasma. Exceptions are acute epiglottitis and the pneumonias of lobar distribution. Formerly it was widely held that various bacteria, and especially *Hemophilus influenzae,* were responsible for significant proportions of these illnesses. With the advent of modern methods of virology it has been clearly established that group A and B beta-hemolytic streptococci and the diphtheria organism are the only bacterial agents capable of causing primary nasal or pharyngeal disease; even in cases of acute tonsillopharyngitis, most illnesses are of nonbacterial origin.

VIRUSES AND MYCOPLASMAS WHICH MAY PRODUCE ACUTE RESPIRATORY DISEASE. The viruses and mycoplasmas which can cause acute respiratory disease are listed in Table 12–3. Each of these organisms produces a spectrum of effects ranging from inapparent infection to severe respiratory tract illness. Though considerable overlapping exists, some microorganisms are more likely to produce a given respiratory syndrome than others. Certain agents have a greater tendency than others to produce severe disease. Many other viruses (e.g., rubeola) may be associated with varying amounts of upper and/or lower respiratory tract symptomatology as part of their clinical picture.

The **respiratory syncytial virus** (RSV) is the most important respiratory tract pathogen of the first years of childhood. It is the principal single cause of bronchiolitis, accounting for about one third of all cases. It is a common cause also of pneumonia, croup and bronchitis, as well as of undifferentiated febrile disease of the upper respiratory tract. Because of the severity of illnesses produced by infection with this agent, it accounts for a disproportionately large number of infants hospitalized with respiratory disease.

The **parainfluenza viruses** account for the majority of cases of the croup syndrome, but may also produce bronchitis, bronchiolitis and febrile upper respiratory tract disease. Type 1 is the agent most commonly associated with croup; type 3 is associated with croup as well as with other varieties of respiratory infection. Type 4 virus does not appear to be as pathogenic as the other three.

Except during epidemics, **influenza viruses** do not play much part in the various respiratory syndromes. In infants and children, influenza viruses account for more disease of the upper than the lower respiratory tract. Croup severe enough to require tracheostomy is occasionally seen during influenza epidemics.

The **adenoviruses** account for less than 10 per cent of respiratory illnesses, many of which are mild. A large proportion may be asymptomatic.

The activity of the **rhinoviruses** is limited almost entirely to the upper tract, most commonly the nose. They account for a significant proportion of the "common cold" syndrome. Rarely do they produce lower tract disease.

The **Coxsackie A and B** viruses produce primarily disease of the nasopharynx. This may be expressed as an undifferentiated febrile respiratory illness or, in the case of the group A organisms, as herpangina or exudative pharyngotonsillitis. **Mycoplasma** can produce both upper and lower respiratory tract illness, including bronchiolitis, pneumonia, bronchitis, pharyngotonsillitis and otitis media. The frequency with which each of these organisms occurs in any age group varies from year to year, but in general mycoplasmas produce more disease in late childhood and early adult life than during infancy.

The ecology of infection, the seasonal pattern, the epidemiology, and the risk of reinfection are shown in Table 12–4. Several of these agents are encountered primarily during infancy, others at older ages, and some at all ages. They vary in contagiousness from very high to relatively low. With

TABLE 12–3 VIRUSES AND MYCOPLASMAS WHICH CAUSE RESPIRATORY DISEASE IN INFANTS AND CHILDREN

	SEROTYPES		RELATIVE IMPORTANCE IN INDICATED SYNDROME*				
GROUP	TOTAL NUMBER	NUMBER ASSOCIATED WITH RESPIRATORY ILLNESS	BRONCHIOLITIS	PNEUMONIA	CROUP	BRONCHITIS	URI
Myxovirus:							
Influenza	3	2 (A,B)	+	+	+	+	++
Parainfluenza	4	4 (1,2,3,4)	++	++	++++	+++	+++
Resp. syncytial	1	1	++++	++++	++	+++	+++
Adenovirus	30+	8 (1,2,3,4,5,7, 14,21)	++	+++	+	+++	+++
Picornavirus:							
Coxsackie A	24	8 (2,4,5,6,8, 10,21,22)					++
Coxsackie B	6	3 (2,3,5)					++
Rhinoviruses	60+	60+ (?)	?	?		++	++
Mycoplasmataceae	8	1 (M. pneumoniae)	+	++		++	+(?)

*Relative importance graded on a scale of 0 to ++++.
Table modified from R. M. Chanock and R. H. Parrott: *Pediatrics, 36*:21, 1965.

TABLE 12-4 ECOLOGY OF INFECTION WITH VARIOUS RESPIRATORY TRACT PATHOGENS

GROUP	SEROTYPE	USUAL TIME OF PRIMARY INFECTION	PERSON-TO-PERSON SPREAD	PATTERN OF INFECTION	RISK OF INDICATED ILLNESS DURING PRIMARY INFECTION	REINFECTION
Myxovirus: Influenza	A,B	Infancy and childhood; any age for minor antigenic variants	Highly effective	Epidemic – every 2-4 years, usually winter	Influenza – 75%	Common with new variants – less common with same variant
Parainfluenza	1,2,3,4	Infancy – type 3 Childhood – types 1,2,4	Highly effective – type 3; less effective – types 1,2,4	Endemic or sporadic – occasionally epidemic (types 1,3)	Febrile respiratory illness – 50-75% (types 1,2,3)	Common – can be associated with URI
Resp. syncytial	–	Infancy	Highly effective	Epidemic, every year – fall, winter or spring	Febrile lower respiratory tract illness – 45%	Common – often associated with URI
Adenovirus	1,2,3,5, 7	Infancy (1,2) Childhood (3,5,7)	Effective (1,2,5) or moderately effective (3,7)	Endemic (occasionally epidemic types 3,7)	Febrile respiratory disease – 55-90%	Uncommon
Picornavirus: Coxsackie B		Infancy and childhood	Moderately effective	Epidemic – summer	Not known	Not known
Rhinovirus	60 or more	All ages	?	Endemic sporadic flurries of different types	URI 50%*	Occurs
M. pneumoniae	–	2nd and 3rd decades	Ineffective	Endemic or occasionally epidemic	Pneumonia 3–10%*	Uncommon

*Data for adult infection.
Table modified from R. M. Chanock and R. H. Parrott: *Pediatrics, 36*:21, 1965.

some, although reinfection occurs readily, a previous encounter may protect against subsequent serious disease.

METHODS OF CONTROL. At present, vaccines exist only for influenza, and these are only moderately effective in preventing illness. See Section 10.

No vaccines are available to protect children against infection from the other agents, nor are there likely to be in the near future. The multiplicity of viruses and strains alone would make the development of a "broad spectrum" immunizing agent difficult; furthermore, potent vaccines even to the more important viruses are difficult to produce for a variety of technical reasons. The immunologic response is poor to vaccines against respiratory agents, and the protective effect of antibodies produced is relatively low. Even after the naturally acquired disease, reinfection occurs with many of these microorganisms. Some volunteers immunized against certain of these viruses and then challenged with the live agent have experienced severe illness.

It is not surprising that little protective effect can be expected from normal human gamma globulin. This substance is often administered to children with repeated respiratory infection, but its antibody content against the principal agents is low or undetectable, and even significant levels of antibody do not necessarily protect against disease.

Since bacteria do not play either a primary or secondary role in the undifferentiated upper respiratory tract diseases, the so-called bacterial cold vaccines can be expected to be ineffectual either in preventing illness or in changing the duration of disease.

ACUTE NASOPHARYNGITIS

("The Common Cold")

The term "acute nasopharyngitis" designates that disease of children which corresponds to the common cold in adults. This difference in nomenclature is desirable because the disease in children differs clinically from that encountered among older persons. In children the infection is more extensive and involves the accessory paranasal sinuses, and usually the middle ear as well as the nasopharynx. It is usually accompanied by fever in children, whereas in adults the illness is usually afebrile as well as more limited in extent. Acute nasopharyngitis is the most common infectious condition of children, but its importance in pediatric practice depends primarily on the relative frequency with which complications occur.

ETIOLOGY. The illness is caused by a large number of different viruses; the principal agents appear to be the rhinoviruses. The period of infectivity is short, lasting from a few hours prior to the appearance of symptoms to a day or two after the illness has appeared. Since the activity of a virus in the respiratory tract impairs local host defense mechanisms, invasion of tissue by potentially pathogenic bacteria may occur during the course of the infection and be responsible for complications in the sinuses, ears, mastoids, lymph nodes and lungs. Bacteria most frequently involved in these complicating conditions are group A streptococci, pneumococci, *H. influenzae* and staphylococci, the last two principally in the young child. These bacterial complications may respond to appropriate antimicrobial therapy, but bacteria play no role in the course of the uncomplicated infection or in the pathogenesis of symptoms.

CONTRIBUTORY FACTORS. For reasons poorly understood, susceptibility to acute nasopharyngitis appears to vary in the same person from time to time. It is widely believed that factors such as chilling, dampness, wet feet, and the like greatly increase susceptibility to the infection, but there is no direct evidence to support this view. The "predisposing" events produce vasomotor effects and reduce the temperature of the nasal mucous membranes through vasoconstriction; this is later followed by vasodilatation and, on occasion, by nasal irritation and discharge. These physiologic effects may exacerbate a chronic infection, but they do not cause a cold. The state of nutrition appears to have a moderate effect on susceptibility; frank malnutrition greatly increases the incidence of purulent complications.

Age does not appear to be a determining factor in susceptibility, but there is a higher incidence of purulent complications in the young child. Infants under 6 months of age are susceptible, but do not commonly acquire colds because of the relative infrequency of exposure. In general, the frequency with which acute nasopharyngitis occurs in a child is directly proportional to the number of exposures to it.

EPIDEMIOLOGY. Susceptibility to the agents causing acute nasopharyngitis is universal. Infection can occur throughout the year, but in the north temperate zone there are usually three peaks: (1) in September about the time school opens; (2) in late January; and (3) toward the end of April. It has been estimated that the incidence in children ranges from three to six infections a year, but some children have a greater number. The illness is most common during the second and third years of life, and is virtually endemic in nursery schools.

PATHOLOGY. The first changes are edema and vasodilatation in the submucosa. A mononuclear cellular infiltrate follows, which within a day or two becomes polymorphonuclear. The superficial epithelial cells separate and may slough, and there is profuse production of mucus, at first thin, later thicker and usually purulent.

CLINICAL MANIFESTATIONS. Colds are more severe in the young child than in the older child and the adult. In general, children between the ages of 3 months and 3 years have fever early in the course of the infection, occasionally a few hours before localizing signs have appeared. Younger infants are usually afebrile; older children may have low-grade fevers. Purulent complications occur with increased frequency and severity in inverse relation to age. Persistent sinusitis, however, is more common in the older child, occurring rarely in infants.

The initial manifestations in infants more than 3 months of age are the sudden onset of fever, often in the range of 39 to 40° C (102 to 104° F), and irritability, restlessness and sneezing. Nasal discharge begins within a few hours, quickly leading to nasal obstruction which interferes with nursing; in small infants with relatively great dependence on nose-breathing, signs of moderate respiratory distress may occur. During the first 2 to 3 days the eardrums are usually congested, and fluid may be noted behind the drum, whether or not purulent otitis media subsequently occurs. A few infants may vomit, and some have diarrhea. The febrile phase of the illness may last from a few hours to 3 days; the fever may recur with purulent complications.

In older children characteristically the initial symptoms are dryness and irritation in the nose and at times in the pharynx. This is followed within a few hours by sneezing, chilly sensations, muscular aches, a thin nasal discharge, and sometimes cough. Headache, malaise, anorexia and low-grade fever may be present. The secretions become thicker, usually within a day, and eventually purulent. The discharge is irritating, particularly during the purulent phase. Nasal obstruction leads to mouth-breathing, and this, through drying of the mucous membranes of the throat, increases the sensation of soreness. The acute phase lasts from 4 to 10 days.

DIFFERENTIAL DIAGNOSIS. Nasopharyngitis occurs early in the course of many contagious and acute infectious diseases of children. In the differential diagnosis one must also consider acute exacerbations of chronic upper respiratory tract infections such as adenoiditis, allergies, vasomotor responses to cold, diphtheria, and streptococcal infection.

The initial manifestations of measles and pertussis and, to a lesser extent, of poliomyelitis, hepatitis and mumps, are those of nasopharyngitis. A persistent nasal discharge, particularly if it is bloody, suggests nasal diphtheria or a foreign body and, in the first weeks of life, choanal atresia or congenital syphilis.

Allergic rhinitis differs from infectious rhinitis in that it is not accompanied by fever, the nasal discharge usually does not become purulent, and there is usually persistent sneezing, with itching of the eyes and the nose. The nasal mucous membranes in allergic rhinitis are usually pale rather than inflamed, and nasal smears will often contain many eosinophils rather than the polymorphonuclear leukocytes associated with infection. Antihistamines may produce rapid and relatively complete disappearance of signs and symptoms; in infectious rhinitis their effect is slight. The proof of allergic rhinitis rests on the demonstration that removal of a specific allergen results in distinct improvement.

COMPLICATIONS. Complications of acute nasopharyngitis are primarily due to the invasion of paranasal sinuses and other portions of the respiratory tract by bacteria. The cervical lymph nodes may also become involved and occasionally suppurate. The commonest complication is otitis media, seen most frequently in the infant. Ear involvement may occur early in the course of infection, but usually appears after the initial acute phase of the nasopharyngitis is past. It can therefore be suspected if fever recurs. Complications in the lower respiratory tract such as laryngitis, bronchitis and pneumonia occur much less frequently, but again are more common in the infant. Purulent sinusitis occurs more frequently in older children than in the infant; in the latter, however, acute ethmoiditis may occur.

PREVENTION. Effective vaccines to the viruses causing acute nasopharyngitis remain to be developed. Gamma globulin does not reduce the frequency of infection; its use is not recommended for frequent respiratory infections.

Because of the ubiquity of the common cold, it is not possible to isolate children from this condition. Since in the very young infant complications may be relatively serious, however, some attempt should be made to protect him from contact with potentially infected persons, particularly other children.

THERAPY. There is no specific therapy. Antimicrobial agents do not affect the course of the illness, and when given during the acute phase not only fail to reduce the incidence of bacterial complications, but may even increase it. When bacterial complications do occur, they are usually obvious and can then be suitably treated.

Though rest in bed is generally recommended, there is no evidence that this shortens the course of the illness or has any effect on the outcome. Aspirin is usually helpful in reducing irritability, aching and malaise for the first day or two of the infection. Excessive use should be avoided.

Most of the distress of the child is related to nasal obstruction, and attempts should be directed at relieving this condition. Relief usually will permit the child to sleep and to take fluids and food, which he may previously have been unable to do.

The most consistently effective method for the relief of nasal obstruction is nasal instillation of suitable medications. Effective and relatively harmless are ephedrine or epinephrine in isotonic salt solutions, in concentrations approximately one half to one third of those used in adults. Phenylephrine in a concentration of 0.25 to 0.50 per cent is widely used in North America. The more potent, longer acting nose drops useful in adults tend to be too irritating for use in infants and occasionally are associated with the development of hyperexcitability or sedation (naphazoline). Nose drops in oily vehicles must be avoided because these are readily aspirated. Addition of antibiotics, corticosteroids or antihistamines to nose drops increases their expense and adds nothing to their effectiveness.

Nose drops are best administered 15 to 20 minutes before feeding, and at bedtime. One to 2 drops are instilled in each nostril while the child is lying on his back with the neck extended. Since this will usually produce shrinkage only of the anterior mucous membranes, an additional 1 or 2 drops are instilled 5 to 10 minutes later. Introducing nasal decongestants by cotton-tipped applicators is not generally recommended in infants and small children, although this method is useful in the older child. Care must be taken that the cotton pledget extends beyond the anterior nares.

Bottles of nose drops should be used by only one person and for only one illness, since they usually become quickly contaminated with bacteria. Only older children should use a nasal spray, and then only under adult supervision, since such applicators tend to be overused. In general, no medicament instilled into the nose should be used for periods in excess of 4 to 5 days; after this time any drug may become irritating and produce a chemically induced nasal congestion mimicking acute nasopharyngitis.

Nasal obstruction is most difficult to treat in infants. Various types of apparatus for suction of secretions from the nose have been used, but are relatively ineffective and sometimes dangerous. However, they are occasionally essential to clear nasal mucus sufficiently to permit the young infant to nurse. Best drainage can usually be obtained by placing the infant in the prone position, if this does not further embarrass respiration. A highly humidified environment such as that provided by an efficient vaporizer usually provides substantial benefit.

Orally administered decongestants are now widely employed in the belief that they result in shrinkage of engorged nasal mucosa, thereby relieving stuffiness and preventing otitis media. Most available preparations combine antihistaminics and a phenylephrine-like agent. There is little doubt that, in many patients, the atropine-like action of the antihistaminic causes some drying of mucous membranes; little evidence exists that mucosal shrinkage is produced in a majority of children or that otitis media is prevented.

If the child is coughing, but has a profuse nasal discharge, potent antitussives should be avoided. Depressing the cough reflex may greatly increase the danger of aspiration of material from the nasopharynx.

Most children with acute nasopharyngitis experience decreased appetite. There is no advantage in compelling them to take nourishment. Fluids of the child's choice should be offered at frequent intervals. Transient constipation is common; this usually does not require treatment and will rapidly disappear when the child returns to his normal diet.

After the acute phase of the illness it is usually wise to limit the patient's contact with other children for a few days, because after such an infection the child appears to have increased susceptibility to the acquisition of potentially pathogenic bacteria and other viruses.

ACUTE PHARYNGITIS

The term "acute pharyngitis" refers to all acute infectious conditions of the pharynx, including tonsillitis and pharyngotonsillitis; the presence or absence of tonsils does not affect the frequency, the course or the complications of the illness or susceptibility to it. Pharyngeal involvement is part of most upper respiratory tract infections, and is also found with various acute generalized infections. When used in a strict sense, however, the term "acute pharyngitis" refers to conditions in which the principal involvement is in the throat. The disease is uncommon in children under 1 year of age. The incidence then increases to a peak between the fourth and seventh years, but the disease continues to occur throughout later childhood and adult life. In diphtheria, herpangina and infectious mononucleosis pharyngeal involvement may be prominent.

ETIOLOGY. Acute pharyngitis, whether febrile or not, is generally caused by viruses. The only common bacteria other than the diphtheria bacillus that cause this condition are group A beta-hemolytic streptococci; except during epidemics this organism accounts for less than 20 per cent and probably less than 15 per cent of cases. *Mycoplasma hominis* and group B streptococci may account for some cases. There are no epidemiologic data to suggest that pneumococci, *H. influenzae*, staphylococci or other bacteria are capable of producing acute pharyngitis; these organisms often proliferate during acute viral infections and may therefore be cultured in large numbers from the pharynx of an affected person.

CLINICAL MANIFESTATIONS. These differ somewhat, depending on whether streptococci or viruses are the cause. There is, however, much overlapping of signs and symptoms, and it is often impossible to distinguish clinically one form of pharyngitis from another.

Viral pharyngitis is generally a disease of relatively gradual onset, which usually has as early signs fever, malaise and anorexia with moderate throat pain. Sore throat may be present initially, but more commonly begins a day or so after onset of symptoms and reaches its peak by the second or third day. Hoarseness, cough and rhinitis are also common. Even at its peak, pharyngeal inflammation may be relatively slight; but on occasion it is severe, and small ulcers may form on the soft palate and the posterior pharyngeal wall. Exudates may appear on lymphoid follicles of the palate and of the tonsils and be indistinguishable from those encountered with streptococcal disease. The cervical lymph nodes are usually moderately enlarged and firm, and may or may not be tender. Laryngeal involvement is common, but the trachea, bronchi and lungs are rarely involved. White blood cell counts may range from 6000 to above 30,000, an elevated count (16,000 to 18,000) with predominance of polymorphonuclear cells being common in the early phase of illness. Leukocyte counts are therefore usually of little value in differentiating viral from bacterial disease. The entire illness may last less than 24 hours and usually does not persist more than 5 days. Significant complications are rare.

Streptococcal pharyngitis in the child over 2 years often begins with complaints of headache, abdominal pain and vomiting. These symptoms may be associated with fever as high as 104° F, although occasionally a temperature elevation is not noted for 12 hours or so. Hours after the initial complaints, the throat may become sore, and in approximately one third of patients tonsillar enlargement, exudation and pharyngeal erythema are found. The degree of pharyngeal pain is inconstant and may vary from slight to sufficiently severe to make swallowing difficult. Two thirds of patients with acute streptococcal pharyngitis may have only mild erythema, with no particular enlargement of the tonsils and with no exudate. Anterior cervical lymphadenopathy usually occurs early, and the nodes are often tender. Fever may continue for 1 to 4 days; in very severe cases the child may remain ill for as long as 2 weeks. The physical findings most likely to be associated with streptococcal disease are diffuse redness of the tonsils and of the tonsillar pillars, with a petechial mottling of the soft palate whether or not lymphadenitis or follicular exudation is found. These features, though common in streptococcal pharyngitis, are not diagnostic and occur with some frequency in nonstreptococcal infections.

Conjunctivitis, rhinitis, cough and hoarseness occur rarely with proved streptococcal pharyngitis, and the presence of two or more of these signs or symptoms suggests the diagnosis of viral infection.

The term **streptococcosis**, proposed in the 1940's, although not widely adopted as a diagnostic term, may be suitably applied to certain variations of streptococcal disease in early childhood. In general, it suggests that infection with the beta-hemolytic streptococcus has its pattern of clinical expression altered by an initial invasion of the host, in a manner somewhat analogous to tuberculous infection. Contact with the streptococcus is frequent, and it is postulated that the first infection is most likely to occur within the first few years of life. This first infection tends to be indolent and poorly localized, whereas subsequent infections tend to be localized, particularly in the throat, with acute manifestations of relatively short duration ("strep throat"). Scarlet fever, with its expression of the erythrogenic toxin, is included in this secondary infectional pattern, and glomerulonephritis and rheumatic fever are considered systemic manifestations of it. The presumption is that initial infection with one strain of group A beta-hemolytic streptococcus will alter the reaction to subsequent infections with all strains.

The following is the description of the clinical patterns by Powers and Boisvert:

> In the simplest form, the infant under 6 months shows irregular fever, under 102° F, a thin mucoserous nasal discharge causing some excoriation and crusting around the nostrils and some pharyngeal injection. There may be slight vomiting and diarrhea early in the course, and loss of appetite. The acute episode may last less than a week and except for persisting nasal discharge the patient may seem only somewhat peaked and slightly indisposed for . . . five or six weeks. Sometimes the disease . . . is almost asymptomatic with little or no complaint.
>
> In the form most frequently demanding medical attention . . . the patients are children between 6 months and 3 years of age; they are more severely ill than those just described. The early symptoms and signs are those of coryza with postnasal discharge, a diffusely reddened pharynx, fever, vomiting, and loss of appetite. For a few days the temperature curve shows elevations of from 100° to 103° F and continues, in typical cases, to be irregular for . . . four to eight weeks, gradually becoming normal. Within a few days of onset the cervical nodes begin to enlarge; they are usually modest in size and moderately resistant in consistency, there is some tenderness and pain when the mouth is opened. The course of the adenopathy follows roughly the fever with subsidence in about six weeks in the typical case. This is one of the several "glandular fevers" and "catarrhal fevers." Swelling, reddening, softening, and suppuration may occur at any time in the six weeks' course; this complication is usually unilateral. Catarrhal otitis media, like persisting cervical adenopathy, is so frequently an accompaniment of streptococcal upper respiratory infections in infants that the conditions in some form may be regarded . . . as integral parts of the disease rather than as complications.

A similar syndrome may be associated with pneumococcal infection in the child of 6 to 36 months.

DIFFERENTIAL DIAGNOSIS. It has been pointed out that it is difficult or impossible to differentiate viral from streptococcal disease on a clinical basis. The only reliable method is a throat culture. From 10 to 15 per cent of normal children carry group A streptococci in their throats, however, so that even a positive culture in a sick, febrile child is not necessarily conclusive evidence of streptococcal disease.

A syndrome of purulent nasal discharge, pharyngitis and fever (39 to 40° C) may be associated with positive pharyngeal cultures for pneumococci or *H. influenzae.* Some consider this a complication of viral pharyngitis; a few of these patients appear to respond to appropriate antimicrobial therapy.

When a membranous exudate is present on the tonsils or pharynx, specific culture for diphtheria must be performed even though the clinical course of the patient may not suggest this diagnosis. The membranous exudate of infectious mononucleosis closely resembles that found in the partially immunized child with a diphtheritic infection. Herpangina, a specific viral infection, is not usually associated with tonsillar exudates, but rather with many vesiculoulcerative lesions on the anterior pillars, fauces and soft palate.

Agranulocytosis often is first manifested by symptoms of acute pharyngitis. The tonsils and the posterior pharyngeal wall may be covered by a yellowish or dirty white exudate. The mucous membranes under this exudate will usually become necrotic, and ulceration will extend into the mouth and tongue. The lesions are very painful, and dysphagia is severe. Enlargement of cervical lymph nodes commonly occurs, as do mucosal hemorrhages.

Pharyngoconjunctival fever is a form of epidemic sore throat described in both military and civilian populations. Adenoviruses account for the majority of cases. The condition is characterized by fever, sore throat, which is often rather mild, and conjunctivitis. The most striking feature is follicular injection of bulbar and palpebral conjunctivae, often affecting only one eye. There usually is scanty serous exudate which produces slight matting of the eyelids and increased lacrimation. Submandibular lymphadenopathy is common, as is involvement of the preauricular node on the side of the conjunctivitis.

COMPLICATIONS. With viral infections the complication rate is very low, although purulent bacterial otitis media may occur. In debilitated children both viral and streptococcal infections may lead to large, chronic ulcers in the pharynx associated with the presence of a variety of normal mouth flora. With streptococcal disease, peritonsillar abscess occasionally occurs, as do sinusitis, otitis media and, rarely, meningitis. Since acute glomerulonephritis and rheumatic fever may follow streptococcal infections, it is desirable to re-examine children with proved streptococcal disease within 2 to 3 weeks after illness.

Mesenteric adenitis is occasionally associated with pharyngitis of either viral or bacterial origin. This may result in abdominal pain with or without vomiting which may closely simulate appendicitis.

MANAGEMENT OF THE CHILD WITH SORE THROAT. Optimally, following examination of the pharynx, mouth, nares, sinuses, cervical lymph nodes, ears and lungs, a nasopharyngeal culture should be obtained to screen for beta-hemolytic streptococcal infection; the value of identifying other bacterial pathogens is questioned by most experts in infectious disease. In areas where diphtheria is likely, culture for *Corynebacterium diphtheriae* should be done.

Since even exudative tonsillitis is usually of viral origin, for which there is no specific therapy, use of antimicrobial drugs should be deferred, pending the results of culture, unless there are strong clinical and epidemiologic grounds to suspect a streptococcal infection, which is best treated with penicillin, given orally if possible. This drug produces a prompt clinical response; if the patient is not afebrile within 24 hours after an appropriate dose of penicillin, the illness is not of streptococcal origin unless there is an existing complication. There is no reason, therefore, to continue administration of penicillin if the patient is not greatly improved within one day after start of therapy. In proved streptococcal disease it is generally recommended that the duration of therapy be 10 days. If penicillin cannot be used, owing to an allergy to the drug, erythromycin is a satisfactory alternative (Section 5).

Most children prefer to remain in bed during the acute phase of illness. When throat pain is severe, aspirin is often useful, as are hot or cold compresses to the neck, depending on the patient's preference. Gargles of warm saline solution offer some symptomatic relief for throat pain in children old enough to cooperate; in the younger patients the inhalation of steam occasionally produces similar effects. Because of pain on swallowing, cool bland liquids such as ginger ale are usually more acceptable to the child than solids or hot foods. No attempt should be made to force the child to eat.

The child with streptococcal infection is noninfectious to others within a few hours after penicillin therapy has begun. Children with viral disease remain infectious for several days. It is not possible to prevent viral pharyngitis. In children who require protection against streptococcal disease, such as those with a past history of rheumatic fever, penicillin or sulfonamide prophylaxis is usually satisfactory. (See Table 9–14.)

RETROPHARYNGEAL ABSCESS

During early childhood the potential space between the posterior pharyngeal wall and the prevertebral fascia contains several small lymph nodes, which usually disappear during the third or fourth year of life. The lymphatic channels which communicate with these nodes drain portions of the nasopharynx as well as the posterior nasal passages. With purulent infections of these areas, the nodes may become infected; this may, in turn, progress to breakdown of the nodes and to suppuration. The offending organism is usually a group A hemolytic streptococcus; staphylococci are occasionally involved. Occasionally a penetrating injury of the posterior pharyngeal wall, such as by a fishbone, can produce a retropharyngeal abscess.

CLINICAL MANIFESTATIONS. The patient usually has a history of an acute nasopharyngitis or pharyngitis, and the clinical features of the earlier illness may still be present. There is generally an abrupt onset of high fever, with difficulty in swallowing, refusal of feeding, hyperextension of the head, and noisy, often gurgling respirations. Respirations become increasingly labored, and secretions accumulate in the mouth, owing to the difficulty in swallowing.

A bulge in the posterior pharyngeal wall is usually readily apparent. Sometimes the abscess is located in an area of the nasopharynx where it may cause nasal obstruction and a bulging forward of the soft palate. A digital examination to determine whether the abscess is fluctuant or not must be performed with the patient in the Trendelenburg position and with provision for adequate suction in case the abscess ruptures. Retropharyngeal abscesses not detectable by simple inspection are uncommon, but roentgen examination of the neck may reveal abscesses too low to be visible or palpable through the mouth.

DIFFERENTIAL DIAGNOSIS. Nonfluctuant lymphadenitis may produce a tender bulge in the retropharyngeal space. Tuberculous caries of the cervical spine may on occasion produce a lateral retropharyngeal abscess; in this condition there are usually considerable rigidity of the neck and other signs of spinal involvement.

COURSE. If left untreated, the abscess may rupture into the pharynx spontaneously, resulting in aspiration of pus. The process may also dissect laterally and present externally on the side of the neck, or burrow into the esophagus, the mediastinum or auditory canal. Sudden death may occur if the abscess presses on the larynx, produces edema of the glottis, or erodes into major blood vessels.

If the abscess is incised as soon as it becomes fluctuant and proper antimicrobial therapy is given, the prognosis is good.

TREATMENT. If the condition is recognized in the prefluctuant stage, intensive treatment with parenteral penicillin G (100,000 to 250,000 units/kg/24 hr) may prevent suppuration and abscess formation. Analgesic drugs may be needed for pain, such as aspirin for the younger child or meperidine for the older one. As soon as fluctuance is present, the abscess should be incised; the operation is best performed under general anesthesia. Before incision is made, the mass should be aspirated to see whether retropharyngeal hemorrhage may not also be present from erosion of blood vessels. If no blood is obtained, an incision is made where the abscess is pointing, and the pus is carefully aspirated. If serious bleeding has occurred, ligation of the carotid artery is necessary.

LATERAL PHARYNGEAL ABSCESS

This condition occurs later in childhood than a retropharyngeal abscess. The process is usually so extensive that the entire pharyngeal wall is displaced medially, including the tonsil, the soft palate and the uvula.

CLINICAL MANIFESTATIONS. The patient usually has high fever, appears acutely ill, and complains of severe pain and difficulty on swallowing. The bulge in the lateral pharyngeal wall is obvious. Cervical adenitis is usually present, and nuchal rigidity is common, owing to muscular spasm.

TREATMENT. Antibiotic and analgesic therapy is identical to that of retropharyngeal abscess. As soon as the lesion is fluctuant, it should be incised.

PERITONSILLAR AND RETROTONSILLAR ABSCESSES

Both peritonsillar and retrotonsillar abscesses are uncommon in childhood. Since these diseases rarely appear in patients who have had a tonsillectomy, the tonsil apparently represents the initial focus from which the process develops. The abscesses are almost always caused by group A beta-hemolytic streptococci, rarely by *Staphylococcus aureus* or *H. influenzae*.

CLINICAL MANIFESTATIONS. The abscesses are usually preceded by an attack of acute pharyngotonsillitis. There may be an afebrile interval of several days, or the fever of the primary infection may not subside. The patient complains of severe throat pain, has progressive difficulty in opening his mouth because of spasm of the pterygoid muscles and often refuses to swallow or speak. Occasionally there is sufficient spasm of the homolateral muscles of the neck to produce torticollis. The fever may be septic and reach 40.5° C (105° F). The affected tonsillar area is markedly swollen and inflamed; the uvula is displaced to the opposite side. In untreated patients the abscess becomes fluctuant within a few days and usually points in the region of the anterior faucial pillar. If the abscess is not incised, spontaneous rupture will occur.

TREATMENT. Therapy is as for lateral pharyngeal abscess.

Subsequent attacks of peritonsillar abscess may be prevented by removal of the tonsils 3 to 4 weeks after inflammation has subsided.

SINUSITIS

The maxillary antrums and the anterior and posterior ethmoid cells are present at birth and are usually of sufficient size to harbor infection. Each of the frontal sinuses develops from an anterior ethmoid cell. Though invasion of the frontal bone and pneumatization of the sinuses are demonstrable some time during the first 2 to 4 years of life, the frontal sinus is rarely a site of significant infection until the sixth to the tenth year. When there is severe ethmoidal disease in the first few years of life, the development and pneumatization of the frontal sinuses may be curtailed or even completely prevented. The sphenoidal sinus is present at birth; though there are variations in its development, it usually does not assume clinical significance until the third to the fifth year of life.

It can be assumed that the paranasal sinuses are involved in an exudative process in practically all acute nasal infections, but, as a rule, the sinus involvement does not persist after the nasal infection has subsided unless there has been a pre-existing sinus infection. The incidence of both acute and chronic sinus infections increases in the latter part of childhood.

ACUTE PURULENT SINUSITIS

In addition to involvement of the sinuses during acute nasal infections, there may be acute empyema of one or more sinuses of sufficient severity to dominate the clinical picture.

CLINICAL MANIFESTATIONS. The symptoms of acute sinusitis, in addition to those of rhinitis, are fever, localized pain, or a sense of fullness, localized tenderness to pressure or direct percussion, headache and, at times, edema over the affected sinus. So-called sinus headaches, which tend to involve the region of the affected sinus, may assist in localization. In sphenoidal sinusitis the headache may be in the suboccipital region; in anterior ethmoidal sinusitis, in the region of the temples and over the eyes; and in posterior ethmoidal sinusitis, over the distribution of the trigeminal nerve, especially over the mastoid area. In maxillary sinusitis, there may be aching or tenderness on tapping of the underlying teeth. Unless the sinal ostia are obstructed, there is a purulent discharge which can be observed directly through a nasoscope. Pus in the middle meatus suggests involvement of the maxillary, frontal or anterior ethmoid sinuses; in the superior meatus, of the sphenoid or posterior ethmoid cells.

In acute ethmoiditis, especially in infants and small children, periorbital cellulitis with edema of the soft tissues and redness of the skin is a common manifestation.

DIAGNOSIS. A frontal or maxillary sinus filled with pus is roentgenographically opaque; a similar appearance may also be produced by thickening of the lining membrane. Transillumination may be helpful in older children, but not in young ones; it has greater limitations than the roentgenographic examination. It is rarely necessary in children to puncture a sinus simply to establish a diagnosis. Clouding of the ethmoid cells may be demonstrated on the roentgenogram in acute and chronic ethmoiditis. Serious complications are otitis media, meningitis, cavernous sinus thrombosis, optic neuritis, orbital cellulitis and abscess, and nephritis.

TREATMENT. Treatment is essentially that of the rhinitis. Shrinkage of the nasal mucous membranes will often facilitate drainage from the sinus. Gentle suction or aspiration may be used, but may be more of an annoyance than a help, especially in infants. Drainage of a sinus is rarely necessary, but if there is persistence of local and systemic manifestations, it may be justified. Appropriate antimicrobial therapy should be used in full dosage.

CHRONIC SINUSITIS

Even though it is a common ailment of persons living in harsh climates, chronic infection of the paranasal sinuses should suggest the possibility of a local or generalized disturbance which facilitates persistence of the infection. Search should be made for nasal deformities or infected and hypertrophied adenoids which might cause obstruction, for infected teeth as a source of maxillary sinusitis, and for such general disturbances as allergy and cystic fibrosis. Chronic or recurrent sinusitis is common in patients with absence of secretory antibodies and in other immunodeficiency states. The incidence of sinusitis is said to be greater in children who have had their tonsils and adenoids removed.

CLINICAL MANIFESTATIONS. Symptoms of chronic sinusitis vary considerably. Fever, when present, is low-grade. There is frequently malaise, easy fatigability, difficulty in mental concentration and anorexia. Nasal discharge, which may be bilateral or unilateral, varies from day to day and may be greater during a certain portion of the day. Frequently there is sufficient swelling of the middle turbinates to cause complete nasal obstruction. Postnasal discharge or drip is common and, in the absence of infected adenoids, is practically diagnostic. Headaches are frequent, and pain or tenderness to palpation or percussion is helpful in localization. There are frequent attacks of sneezing; when there is an associated watery, nasal discharge, the possibility of allergic rhinitis must be considered.

Constant pharyngeal irritation or inexplainably persistent mouth-breathing suggests sinusitis. Any of the complications of acute sinusitis may occur with chronic sinusitis, but probably the most frequent association is chronic bronchial infection. The term **"sinobronchitis"** is frequently used to designate the relationship. Actually, a considerable proportion of children with this condition have cystic fibrosis as the underlying disease. Children with a hereditary deficiency in α_1-antitrypsin may show among early manifestation of their condition repeated upper respiratory infections, including acute and chronic sinusitis associated with severe bronchopulmonary infections.

TREATMENT. Nasopharyngeal cultures are not useful as a diagnostic tool; the offending organism can be accurately identified only by culturing aspirates from the involved sinus. There is little agreement about the organisms most commonly involved in children; prominently mentioned usually are staphylococci, pneumococci, and *H. influenzae.*

Antibiotics are of no proven benefit. Locally obstructive nasal deformities should be corrected, if possible, and infected or hypertrophic adenoid tissue should be removed. Shrinkage of the mucous membranes by ephedrine or related compounds with the head in such a position as to facilitate entrance of the solution into the sinuses may be of some benefit, particularly if followed two or three times a day by exposure of the sinus areas to local heat. Either the so-called displacement method of Proetz or the lateral head-low posture of Parkinson may be used.

In the Parkinson method the child lies on his side with the shoulder elevated by a firm pad such as a folded blanket, and the head is bent down to a dependent position. The nasal solution which is then instilled can be expected to have contact with the various sinal ostia on both sides. The child should breathe through the mouth to prevent drawing the medication into the pharynx. The position is maintained for 5 to 6 minutes, and the face is then turned downward for a few moments to permit drainage of the nasal contents, or the child may sit up and place his head down between the knees.

Such therapy should be continued for about 2 weeks. Prolonged use of nasal solutions should be discouraged.

Every effort should be made to avoid operative procedures; but when there is persistence of chronic purulent sinusitis in spite of all nonoperative measures, surgery is indicated.

GENERAL CONSIDERATIONS OF CHRONIC INFECTIONS OF THE UPPER RESPIRATORY TRACT

THE PROBLEM OF CHRONIC COLDS

One of the disturbing problems of pediatric practice is that of the child with persistent or recurring upper respiratory tract infection with or without associated chronic bronchial involvement. Children with such chronic infections cannot be placed in any one category; each must be studied to determine, if possible, the underlying factor or factors.

The age of greatest incidence of respiratory infections is from the latter part of the first year of life to 6 or 7 years. During this time it can be expected that the average child will have 3 to 6 "colds" a year. Recovery should occur after each attack, and the child should appear healthy between episodes. In the so-called chronic cases the child seems to recover from one acute attack, only to enter another, or there are more or less persistent rhinitis, cough and a general failure to do well. Such patterns may reflect what appears to be a familial or individual susceptibility or repeated exposure to respiratory infection within the home. Rarely there is some underlying disturbance. Specifically included in the "chronic respiratory group" are chronic rhinitis, sinusitis, infected adenoids and tonsils, chronic otitis media, chronic bronchitis, bronchiectasis, tuberculosis, allergy, and respiratory tract infections associated with immune deficiency states.

CHRONIC RHINITIS

Chronic nasal discharge, with or without a tendency to acute exacerbations, is usually a reflection of an underlying disturbance such as infected adenoids, nasal polyps, chronic sinusitis, cystic fibrosis, allergy, foreign bodies, deviated septum, various congenital malformations, nasal diphtheria or syphilis. In addition, the possibility of a chronic debilitating infection or some nutritional, immunologic or metabolic (as of the thyroid) deficiency must be considered.

CLINICAL MANIFESTATIONS. Symptoms vary, but chronic nasal discharge is common to all cases. In the persistent cases the odor may be foul, and there may be excoriation of the anterior nares and upper lip. Bloody discharge is common in syphilitic and diphtheritic lesions and with foreign bodies, but may also occur in other conditions, especially if there is persistent picking of the nose. Disturbances of taste and smell are frequent. During exacerbations or superimposed infections, fever is common, but is otherwise usually absent. Chronic sinusitis, otitis media, pharyngitis and bronchitis are frequently associated.

Nasal polyps are commonly associated with allergy, sinusitis or cystic fibrosis; the symptoms are often predominantly unilateral. Their presence is determined by direct examination. They should be removed and the underlying disturbance treated. The possibility of an encephalocele or nasal tumor should always be considered prior to surgery.

Persistent **hypertrophic rhinitis** is also most often associated with chronic sinusitis or allergy. Especially in allergy, the mucous membrane tends to be pale; the soft tissues are swollen and resistant to pressure. Nasal obstruction may occur in a cyclic pattern.

Atrophic rhinitis is uncommon; it is usually associated with some general debilitating condition, or it may be a sequel to long-continued nasal infection. The sense of smell is impaired. There may be little or no discharge, but considerable crusting and a sense of dryness in the nose and throat. In some instances there is a profuse, excessively foul nasal discharge **(ozena).**

TREATMENT. The frequent application of a lanolin, silicone or petrolatum-base ointment protects against excoriation. Otherwise, treatment is directed toward the underlying disturbance. Particular emphasis must be placed upon eradicating foci of infection in sinuses, ears, adenoids or tonsils and upon the removal of or desensitization to known allergens. Attention should be given to such factors as nutritional status, rest and prevention of exposure to reinfection. In an attempt to provide symptomatic relief it is often difficult to avoid the use of such mucosal shrinking solutions as ephedrine and related compounds. It must be borne in mind, however, that their use is not without danger and that they may cause further damage. The use of antibiotics locally should be avoided, but systemic administration may be indicated in selected cases.

CHRONIC PHARYNGITIS

Chronic pharyngitis is rare. It is essentially a secondary condition resulting from chronic infections of the sinuses, adenoids or tonsils, although on occasion there is no evidence of infection other than hypertrophied lymphoid tissue on the posterior pharyngeal wall and on the base of the tongue. The latter type of involvement occurs with frequency only in children whose faucial tonsils have been removed; some of these children have infected tonsillar tags.

CLINICAL MANIFESTATIONS. There are likely to be repeated acute exacerbations; in the intervals there are complaints of discomfort in the throat such as dryness and raspy irritation. Frequent efforts to clear the throat and an irritative cough are common. The mucous membrane is usually inflamed, though on occasion it is pale, and the blood vessels are prominent. The pharyngeal wall is frequently covered with a mucopurulent secretion, and the lymphoid tissue is often hypertrophied and has a pebbled appearance.

TREATMENT. Treatment should be directed toward any disturbance in the sinuses, nose (deformities), adenoids or tonsils. Attention should also be given to the general nutrition and hygiene of the child.

TONSILS AND ADENOIDS

The term "tonsils" is used in its commonly accepted sense of indicating the two faucial tonsils; the term "adenoids," as synonymous with hypertrophy of the pharyngeal tonsil. The tonsils and adenoids are part of the lymphoid tissues which circle the pharynx and are known collectively as **Waldeyer's ring.** This consists of the lymphoid tissue on the base of the tongue (lingual tonsil), the two faucial tonsils, the adenoids (pharyngeal tonsil) and the lymphoid tissue on the posterior pharyngeal wall. This tissue serves naturally as a defense against infection; when its defense mechanism is overcome, it may become a site of acute or chronic infection.

The principal disturbances of the tonsils and adenoids are infection and hypertrophy. The latter is in most instances temporary and secondary to infection. The most important medical issue is the decision as to if and when they are to be removed. Though both tonsils and adenoids are usually removed at the same operation, there are good reasons for making the decisions for tonsillectomy and adenoidectomy separately, especially in children under 4 or 5 years of age. Tonsillar disturbances are uncommon in infancy.

NEOPLASMS OF THE TONSILS. Neoplasms of the tonsils are rare, although papilloma, lipoma, angioma, teratoma, fibroma, plasmocytoma and lymphosarcoma have been reported.

ACUTE TONSILLITIS. Acute infections of the tonsils are considered in the same category as acute pharyngitis and are discussed earlier in this Section, as is peritonsillar abscess.

CHRONIC TONSILLITIS

(Chronically Hypertrophic and Infected Tonsils)

The "tonsil problem" is of particular concern in pediatric practice, not only because of the frequency of chronic tonsillar involvement, but also because of its distortion by physicians and laity who have been too ready to attribute all sorts of complaints and ills to tonsillar involvement and have not been sufficiently critical in respect to their apparent improvement after tonsillectomy.

CLINICAL MANIFESTATIONS. These vary considerably; the more significant ones are recurrent or persistent sore throat, and obstruction to swallowing or breathing; the last is more often due to adenoids. There may be a sense of dryness and irritation in the throat, and the breath may be offensive, although neither of these is diagnostic. Constitutional symptoms are neither characteristic nor, as a rule, striking. Rarely, hypertrophied tonsils and adenoids obstructing the upper airway are associated with the development of pulmonary hypertension.

INDICATIONS FOR TONSILLECTOMY. The most frequent reason (*not* indication) for tonsillectomy and adenoidectomy is probably pressure from parents that SOMETHING be done about the child with frequent respiratory infections, allergic bronchitis, mouth-breathing, recurrent purulent or serous otitis, poor appetite, failure to gain weight, or recurrent or chronic fever. Improvement after "T & A" done for these reasons has been noted frequently enough to lead to wide acceptance among the laity and many physicians of the therapeutic benefits of the operation. Yet there is remarkably little, if any, evidence to indicate that the incidence of improvement is any greater than among comparable children not subjected to the procedure. Physicians may frequently interpret apparent parental despair over the failure of the medical profession to cure their child's complaints as irresistible pressure; many parents when queried preoperatively as to the reasons the operation is being done are either unclear about them or are actively wondering themselves why their child is undergoing the surgery. Until better means are available to identify those children who may truly benefit from tonsillectomy and adenoidectomy done for the above reasons, it would seem prudent to avoid it in most cases.

Decision for removal of tonsils should be based so far as possible on symptoms and signs directly related to the tonsils; tonsillectomy should not be recommended as a possible panacea for unrelated disturbances. In general, the conditions for which tonsillectomy should be considered are (1) factors directly related to the tonsils, and (2) disturbances in closely related structures.

Local indications for removal are symptomatic hypertrophy and chronic infection. True hypertrophy is often the result of infection, acute or chronic, but may occur independently. Benign hypertrophy unassociated with signs or symptoms of obstruction is not an indication for tonsillectomy. Furthermore, the frequency with which episodes of acute pharyngitis occur is not favorably altered by tonsillectomy, so "frequent sore throats" do not represent a valid indication. *Many or even most tonsils considered to be hypertrophic actually are normal in size; the misinterpretation results from failure to appreciate that tonsils are normally relatively larger during childhood than in later years.* Tonsils may, however, virtually meet in the midline in some children who are quite asymptomatic. Tonsils of average size are projected toward the midline when the child is gagged and may be interpreted as being hypertrophic. On the other hand, infection does not always produce hypertrophy, and chronically infected tonsils may be small and embedded behind the faucial pillars. There is no certain way to demonstrate by direct observation whether tonsils are harboring chronic infection. The consistency or size of the tonsil and the presence of cheesy material within the crypts are not reliable guides. Persistent hyperemia of the anterior pillars is a more reliable sign, and enlargement of the cervical lymph nodes is supporting evidence. Persistent enlargement of the node just below and slightly in front of the angle of the jaw is especially significant. In contrast to the difficulty in determining the presence of chronic infection, hypertrophy sufficient to obstruct swallowing or breathing is readily detectable. Such tonsils practically meet in the midline when the throat is examined without gagging the patient. Before tonsillectomy is recommended it should be ascertained that the hypertrophy is chronic and not the result of a recent acute infection. Tonsils can increase in size greatly during an acute infection and recede after its subsidence.

Removal of tonsils and adenoids may be recommended for persistent carriers of diphtheria bacilli (Section 10). Clinical diphtheria is rare among nonimmune individuals whose tonsils have been removed, as compared with those who have retained their tonsils.

Among the *disturbances in adjacent tonsillar structures,* peritonsillar (and retrotonsillar) abscess is the only definite indication for tonsillectomy. Other indications are less clear-cut. The removal of tonsils is of no value in the prevention or treatment of acute or chronic sinusitis. Perhaps in some instances of recurrent sinusitis removal of the adenoids is indicated, but even in this instance the benefits achieved are usually minor. This is also probably true in cases of chronic otitis media and of middle ear deafness. Suppurative cervical adenitis, when the focus of infection is not traceable to structures other than the tonsils, may also be considered an indication for tonsillectomy. There is no evidence to indicate that the removal of tonsils is justified for infections in the lower respiratory tract, although such conditions are not a contraindication if there are other reasons for tonsillectomy.

No *systemic disturbance* in itself is an indication

for tonsillectomy. The decision should be based on local indications. This applies to children with rheumatic fever or glomerulonephritis as well as to those with other infections in which the tonsils may be removed in a blind search for a focus of infection or as a remedy for undernutrition.

Tonsillectomy in Relation to Age of Child. Rarely it seems advisable to recommend tonsillectomy for children 2 or 3 years of age. Every attempt should be made, however, to postpone the operation. Frequently when the operation is postponed for reasons of age, the apparent need for it disappears within the next year or so. In the first few years of life the indications for adenoidectomy, though infrequent, are present more often than those for tonsillectomy. Neither procedure should be performed as a prophylaxis against the "common cold" at any age.

Tonsillectomy in Relation to Active Infection. Tonsillectomy should be postponed until 2 or 3 weeks after subsidence of an infection. This, however, is not always possible; an occasional child seems never to be free of infection in and about the tonsils. In such a case it is justifiable to perform the operation if an antibiotic is administered in therapeutic doses for a day or two before and 2 or 3 days after the operation.

TYPE OF OPERATION. Careful removal by dissection should be carried out to ensure that all the tonsillar tissue is removed without destruction of adjacent tissues. Too frequently small amounts of tonsillar tissue are allowed to remain which later become infected and hypertrophied, or there is removal of adjacent tissue from the lateral pharyngeal wall, from the soft palate and even at times from the uvula. Aspiration of the throat during the operation will lessen the chances of pulmonary abscess or pneumonia. Bleeding should be completely controlled, and the child should not leave the operating room until he has dry tonsillar fossae.

PREOPERATIVE PREPARATION. A careful preoperative work-up not infrequently uncovers unsuspected underlying conditions, recognition of which explains the apparent indication for the surgery and at the same time contraindicates it. The medical history should include questions related to recent infection, to exposure to contagious diseases and to bleeding tendencies in the patient and his family. A thorough physical examination should include observation for loose or carious teeth, which should be removed or repaired before tonsillectomy. Bleeding and clotting times are usually obtained but a careful history of bleeding tendencies is a more effective screening method than the commonly used poorly discriminating tests. The child should be told of the operation and the procedure explained, preferably by informed parents. Though food is withheld for several hours before the operation, feeding should be adequate up to this time. In children who are undernourished or readily susceptible to ketosis, preoperative intravenous administration of glucose is indicated.

POSTOPERATIVE CARE. The child should be kept in bed for the remainder of the day and at rest for several more; it is wise to encourage eating and drinking as soon as the nausea from the anesthetic has disappeared. Rinsing the mouth with an alkaline solution has certain esthetic advantages. Aspirin may be prescribed for discomfort. Avoidance of contact with infection is of the greatest importance. The membrane which forms at the operative site is at times interpreted as being diphtheritic. Fusiform bacilli (Vincent's organisms) may be cultured from it with considerable regularity, but this by itself is not an indication for treatment.

COMPLICATIONS. Complications are not particularly frequent, but postoperative hemorrhage, lung abscess, pneumonia and septicemia do occur. Hemorrhage is the most frequent problem and should be controlled by packing or, in the case of severe bleeding, by ligation. Transfusion may be necessary to prevent hemorrhagic shock and death if bleeding is extensive or prolonged.

RESULTS TO BE EXPECTED FROM TONSILLECTOMY. No reduction in the incidence of respiratory infections is to be expected. Obstructive symptoms due to hypertrophied tonsils can be relieved. Otitis media and sinusitis are not benefited by tonsillectomy; the incidence of sinusitis may even be increased. Nasal allergy is not affected, nor is the incidence of laryngitis or of pulmonary infections. Neither the incidence of initial attacks of rheumatic fever nor that of recurrences appears to be affected by the operation. Eradication of diphtheria bacilli from the throats of carriers after tonsillectomy is achieved sufficiently often to justify the operation in otherwise persistent carriers. The incidence of cervical lymphadenitis is decreased. In a few instances nutrition is improved after tonsillectomy. In part this may be due to psychologic factors, but it is reasonable that general benefit should accrue when a focus of infection is removed. Care should be taken, however, in making predictions in this respect.

ADENOIDS

(Hypertrophy of Pharyngeal Tonsil)

Disturbances of the lymphoid tissue of the nasopharynx (adenoids) tend to parallel those of the faucial tonsils. Hypertrophy and infection may occur separately, but often occur together, infection, as a rule, being primary. The soft adenoid structure, which is normally widespread in the nasopharynx, especially on the posterior wall and the roof, undergoes hypertrophy, and masses of varying size up to 2 or 3 cm are formed. These masses may almost fill the vault of the nasopharynx and interfere with the passage of air through the nose and obstruct the eustachian tubes.

CLINICAL MANIFESTATIONS. Mouth-breathing and more or less persistent rhinitis are the most characteristic symptoms. Mouth-breathing may be present only during sleep, especially when the child is on his back, and in this position snoring is also likely to occur. With severe adenoid hypertrophy the mouth is kept open during the day as well, and the mucous membranes of the mouth and lips are dry. Chronic nasopharyngitis may be constantly present or recur frequently. The voice is altered, developing a nasal, muffled quality. The breath is offensive, and taste and smell are impaired. A harassing cough may be present, especially at night, resulting from irritation of the larynx by inspired air which has not been warmed and moistened by passage through the nose. Impaired hearing is common. Chronic otitis media may be associated with infected, hypertrophied adenoids, but it is not clearly established that the otitis is directly or indirectly the result of adenoid disease.

DIAGNOSIS. The diagnosis can be confirmed by direct digital palpation, examination of the vault of the pharynx by pharyngeal mirror, or roentgenographic examination. Otherwise the presence of adenoid hypertrophy can be suspected from such symptoms as mouth-breathing, snoring and persistent rhinitis with or without chronic otitis media.

An abscess in the adenoid tissue is uncommon, but may be a cause of protracted fever. Identification and drainage of the abscess have been achieved by digital expression.

TREATMENT. Adenoidectomy is indicated when there are symptoms such as persistent mouth-breathing, "nasal" speech, repeated attacks of otitis media, deafness and persistent or recurring nasopharyngitis which seem to be related to infected hypertrophied adenoid tissue. Although it is customary to remove the adenoids when tonsillectomy is performed, there are occasions, particularly in young children, when only adenoidectomy should be recommended. Chronic serous otitis media may improve after adenoidectomy in some patients. The same precautions for complete removal and control of bleeding points as recommended for tonsillectomy should be observed; for this reason, removal under direct vision is preferable to the use of the adenotome.

HEINZ F. EICHENWALD
GEORGE H. MCCRACKEN, JR.

PATIENT EDUCATION

Alfaro, V. R.: Nasal sinus disease in children. Ped. Clin. N. Amer. *9*:1061, 1962.

Breese, B. B., and Disney, F. A.: The accuracy of diagnosis of beta streptococcal infections on clinical grounds. J. Pediatr. *44*:670, 1954.

Cain, W. A., Amman, A. J., Hong, R., Ishizaka, K., and Good, R. A.: IgE deficiency associated with chronic sinopulmonary infection. J. Clin. Invest. *48*:12A, 1969.

Cate, T. R., Couch, R. B., and Johnson, K. M.: Studies with rhinoviruses in volunteers: Production of illness, effect of naturally acquired antibody, and demonstration of a protective effect not associated with serum antibody. J. Clin. Invest. *43*:56, 1964.

Chanock, R. M., Mufson, M. A., and Johnson, K. M.: Comparative biology and ecology of human virus and mycoplasma respiratory pathogens. Progr. Med. Virol. *7*:208, 1965.

Chanock, R. M., and Parrot, R. H.: Acute respiratory disease in infancy and childhood: Present understanding and prospects for prevention. Pediatrics *36*:21, 1965.

Freeman, G. L., and Todd, R. H.: The role of allergy in viral respiratory tract infections. Am. J. Dis. Child. *104*:330, 1962.

Glazen, W. P., Loda, F. A., Clyde, W. A., Jr., Senior, R. J., Shaeffer, C. I., Conley, W. G., and Denny, F. W.: Epidemiologic patterns of acute lower respiratory disease in children in a pediatric group practice. J. Pediatr. *78*:397, 1971.

Greenwald, H. M., and Messeloff, C. R.: Retropharyngeal abscess in infants and children. Am. J. Med. Sci. *177*:767, 1929.

Gwaltney, J. M., Jr., and Jordan, W. S., Jr.: Rhinoviruses and respiratory disease. Bact. Rev. *28*:409, 1964.

Hartline, J. V., and Zelkowitz, P. S.: Kartagener's syndrome in childhood. Am. J. Dis. Child. *121*:349, 1971.

Haynes, R. E., and Cramblett, H. G.: Acute ethmoiditis: Its relationship to orbital cellulitis. Am. J. Dis. Child. *114*:261, 1967.

Hope-Simpson, R. E., and Higgins, P. G.: A respiratory virus study in Great Britain. Progr. Med. Virol. *11*:354, 1969.

Johnson, F.: Bleeding factors and tonsils and adenoid surgery. Arch. Otolaryng. *86*:584, 1967.

Maletzky, A. J., Cooney, M. K., Luce, R., Kenny, G. E., and Grayston, J. T.: Epidemiology of viral and mycoplasmal agents associated with childhood respiratory disease. J. Pediatr. *78*:407, 1971.

Mazodier, P.: Hereditary deficiency of α_1-antitrypsin. Pédiatre *6*:7, 1970.

Moresh, M. M.: Paranasal sinuses from birth to late adolescence. Am. J. Dis. Child. *60*:55, 1949.

Powers, G. F., and Boisvert, P. L.: Age as a factor in streptococcosis. J. Pediatr. *25*:481, 1944.

Stillerman, M., and Bernstein, S. H.: Streptococcal pharyngitis: Evaluation of clinical syndromes in diagnosis. Am. J. Dis. Child. *101*:476, 1961.

Stillerman, M., Bernstein, S. H., Smith, M. L., Gittelson, S. B., and Karelitz, S.: Antibiotics in the treatment of beta-hemolytic streptococcal pharyngitis: Factors influencing the results. Pediatrics *25*:27, 1960.

Tracey, V. V., De, N. C., and Harper, J. R.: Obesity and respiratory infection in infants and young children. Brit. M. J. *1*:16, 1971.

THE EAR

MALFORMATIONS. The complex embryology of the ear allows for the possibility of many developmental abnormalities. Minor malformations are common, but serious anomalies rare. There are no precise definitions of normal size, configuration or position of the external ear; anything esthetically acceptable is considered normal. Occasionally the auricle is grotesquely small (*microtia*), large (*macrotia*) or entirely absent (*anotia*). Malformed, low-set ears may be associated with serious renal anomalies, mandibulofacial dysostoses and other congenital anomalies. Absence of the antihelix and superior crus results in "lop ear," which can be cosmetically improved by plastic surgery.

Hereditary cutaneous dimples or sinus tracts anterior to and above the tragus are common. They do not require surgical correction unless recurrently infected. Accessory auricular skin tags can be ligated, but if there is cartilage or a broad base, they should be removed surgically.

Atresia of the external auditory canal is often associated with abnormalities of the external or middle ear. Roentgenographic examination is necessary to evaluate the bony canal, the ossicles and the middle ear cavity. If the conductive elements of hearing are present, reconstructive surgery can be attempted.

Chondromas and exostoses of the auditory canal are generally small and do not require removal. Rare congenital tumors of the ear in childhood include hemangiomata, lymphangiomata and dermoid tumors.

Sebaceous cysts located in or near the lobule of the ear are common. They are prone to periodic enlargement, with minimal tenderness, and to regress spontaneously.

Acquired malformation may result from trauma, frostbite or perichondritis. The treatment of frostbite, aside from prevention, is moderately rapid warming to body temperature. Hematomas of the auricle should be evacuated promptly or the clot may organize and produce the deformity known as cauliflower ear.

CAUSES OF PAINFUL EAR. Any acute inflammatory process in the external canal, middle ear or mastoids may cause pain. When suppurative material under pressure is allowed to drain, pain abates.

The sensory innervation of the ear involves branches of the fifth, ninth and tenth cranial nerves and the second and third cervical spinal nerves. Pain may be referred to the ear by disease in the parotid gland, temporomandibular joint, cervical spine, posterior ethmoid and sphenoid sinuses, third molars and the pharynx. *Herpesvirus zoster* affecting the fifth cranial nerve may cause pain interpreted as earache in the pre-eruptive phase.

EXTERNAL AUDITORY CANAL

The outer, cartilaginous portion of the canal contains sebaceous glands and the specialized apocrine glands that secrete cerumen. These are not present in the inner, osseous portion. The normal extrusion of wax cleanses the canal. Cerumen may be impacted against the tympanic membrane from attempts to clean the ears with swabs. Excessive cerumen is most easily removed by irrigation with water or isotonic saline, which should be at body temperature to avoid causing vertigo from labyrinthine stimulation. The syringe nozzle should be small enough that there is an adequate outflow space or damage may be done by pressure. Hard wax can be softened by twice daily instillation of mineral or lanolin oil for several days before irrigation, or a proprietary softener may be used. Cleaning the canal with a cerumen spoon or ear curette is often a painful, traumatic procedure and should be done only when there is urgency about examination of the ear and irrigation has been unsuccessful. Too often one exchanges cerumen for blood in the canal after probing with the cerumen spoon.

The auditory canal of the newborn infant is filled with detritus of vernix caseosa which disappears after a few days.

FOREIGN BODIES. A few children are prone to insert an astonishing variety of vegetable and mineral matter into the auditory canal. Insects which find their way into the canal are particularly distressing because of their movement. They can be immobilized by alcohol or mineral oil before removal. Vegetable matter, such as paper, may absorb moisture and become more tightly impacted during attempted irrigation and should instead be removed with small forceps. Most small objects can be removed by irrigation or with small forceps if the child can hold still during the procedure. General anesthesia is necessary if the child cannot cooperate and for removal of large objects or those deeply impacted.

OTITIS EXTERNA. Inflammatory conditions of the external auditory canal include furunculosis, acute bacterial and viral infections, and chronic disease related to bacteria, yeasts or dermatoses. The normal bacterial flora of the canal consists of nonpathogenic *Corynebacteria* ("diphtheroids") and *Staphylococcus epidermidis*. Acute external otitis is commonly caused by *Staphylococcus aureus* and streptococci. Subacute or chronic inflammations are likely to be associated with *Proteus, Pseudomonas, Klebsiella-Enterobacter* and fungi such as *Candida* and *Aspergillus*. Primary *Herpesvirus hominis* infection of the auricle and canal may be confused with impetigo.

With severe acute infections and furunculosis there are pain, fever and lymphadenitis. The pain is accentuated by movement of the tragus, a differential point from otitis media in which this manipulation does not increase pain. Pre-auricular, postauricular or cervical lymphadenitis also is helpful in differential diagnosis from otitis media because adenitis is not a feature of middle ear disease. The inflammatory process may obliterate the canal lumen, but if the tympanic membrane can be visualized, it may be normal or red.

Severe, acute external otitis is treated with parenteral penicillin, but milder infections respond satisfactorily to frequent instillation of antibiotic drops (not ointment) or insertion of a wick saturated with antibiotic solution or half-strength Burow's solution. Local steroids are commonly employed for anti-inflammatory effect but their efficacy is dubious. Analgesics and local heat assuage pain. As the inflammatory process subsides, mechanical cleansing to remove debris is useful.

Furunculosis due to *S. aureus* occurs in the outer cartilaginous portion of the canal. It is treated with incision and drainage and systemic penicillin or penicillinase-resistant penicillin, depending on the antibiotic susceptibility of the organism.

In subacute or chronic infections there is discomfort or itching rather than pain, and there may be decreased hearing and foul-smelling discharge. Because of the itching, cleaning of the canal may be pleasurable rather than painful. The canal and tympanic membrane become quite insensitive to pain in chronic external otitis. Systemic antibiotic therapy is not helpful. Therapy consists of thorough cleaning of the canal and instillation of antibiotic or antifungal ointments, depending upon the type of infection.

The condition known as "swimmer's ear" is due to loss of protective cerumen and chronic irritation and maceration from moisture in the canal. Pseudomonas organisms are commonly incriminated in the disease but are a secondary manifestation, not the basic cause. The distressing itching is temporarily alleviated by ointments, but the most effective therapy is cleansing and drying of the canal with alcohol after swimming and baths, and instillation of lanolin oil. Acute infection may supervene and necessitate antibiotic therapy.

THE TYMPANIC MEMBRANE

The tympanic membrane (myrinx, myringa) is situated obliquely, with the superior and posterior portion most lateral. The major portion, or pars tensa, has a fibrous layer between the outer epithelial surface and the inner mucosal lining. At the periphery the fibrous layer forms a thick annulus attached to a groove in the temporal bone. The annulus is incomplete superiorly and traverses the membrane to the short process of the malleus forming the malleolar folds or ridges. Above these, the fibrous layer is absent in the pars flaccida, or Shrapnell's membrane.

The handle of the malleus can be visualized through the normal tympanic membrane slanting downward and backward. From the umbo, or point of greatest concavity of the drum at the end of the handle of the malleus, a cone of light reflex fans out anteriorly and inferiorly.

EXAMINATION. The tortuous S-shaped course of the auditory canal is protective to the tympanic membrane but interferes with visualization. In the older child the canal can be straightened by pulling the auricle up, back and out; however, in young infants maximum exposure is obtained by pulling the auricle back and slightly downward. Visualization of the tympanic membrane can be accomplished with a speculum and head mirror for reflected light, but most pediatricians prefer the illuminated otoscope with magnifying lens. Optimum examination is with the binocular otoscope. The canal must be unobstructed and a bright light is necessary since even a normal tympanic membrane looks red and dull in dim light. Familiarity with normal variations in anatomy and the appearance of a normal membrane in a febrile, crying child is essential. Pneumatoscopy allows evaluation of the mobility of the tympanic membrane and is the best single aid for diagnosis of fluid in the middle ear.

The tympanic membrane of the newborn infant is difficult to evaluate. The canal is filled with debris and the drum appears dull. Lack of development of the osseous portion of the canal accentuates the normal obliquity of the tympanic membrane.

Spontaneous **perforation** may occur secondary to foreign bodies, pressure or infection. Before myringotomy or needle aspiration of the tympanum is performed, the canal and drum should be cleaned with an antiseptic. A semilunar incision is made with the knife, or the needle is introduced through the posterior inferior portion of the pars tensa. Perforations which fail to seal spontaneously predispose to chronic infection and require surgical correction.

Myringitis, or inflammation of the tympanic membrane, may accompany otitis externa or otitis media but also occurs independently. Myringitis without bacterial infection is commonly seen in rubeola and roseola and must be differentiated from secondary bacterial otitis media. In bullous myringitis there is pain, with or without fever and adenopathy, associated with serous blebs on the membrane; occasionally these are hemorrhagic. The disease has been produced experimentally by *Mycoplasma pneumoniae,* but it is not certain whether mycoplasmas account for all cases. Pain is relieved by rupture of the bullae. Secondary bacterial infection is rare, and antibiotic therapy is not indicated.

OTITIS MEDIA

PATHOGENESIS AND EPIDEMIOLOGY. Several factors contribute to the predisposition of infants to middle ear infection. The eustachian tube is short, the orifice patulous and easily compressed, and its horizontal position hinders drainage. Drainage is further impaired by the supine position in which the infant spends much of his time. The route of infection is presumed to be through the eustachian tube in most cases, although hematogenous infection is conceivable. Infection through the auditory canal probably occurs only with penetrating wounds. During the act of swallowing, fluid in the nasopharynx may be propelled up the eustachian tube to the middle ear. Thus, otitis media is a constant accompaniment of cleft palate and is also common in patients with submucous clefts. Bottle-fed babies have a higher incidence of otitis media than breast-fed infants. This is particularly true when bottle-propping is practiced, since the supine position during swallowing favors ingress of nasopharyngeal material to the eustachian tube.

Nasopharyngeal tumors, malocclusion, developmental defects such as cleft palate, connective tissue diseases, barotrauma and allergy are the primary factors underlying recurrent or chronic middle ear disease.

In infancy the commonest sequence of events is

viral upper respiratory infection, interference with tubal function, and bacterial invasion of the middle ear cleft. This has long been apparent with clinically obvious viral infections such as measles but more recently has been documented for other viral infections. The bacterial invaders of acute otitis media are those normally resident in the nasopharynx of infants: pneumococcus, *H. influenzae* and hemolytic streptococcus. Tuberculous and diphtheritic middle ear diseases are now exceedingly uncommon.

Otitis media is most common during the winter months. During infancy males are affected slightly more often than females. Eskimos, American Indians and other socioeconomically disadvantaged segments of our population have an inordinately high incidence of middle ear disease. Because reduced hearing from otitis media may have life-long impact on learning and occupational functioning, this condition is a major health challenge.

OTITIS MEDIA IN THE NEWBORN. Until recently little was known about otitis in the newborn, mostly because of technical difficulties in examination. Pneumatic otoscopy is essential for detection of middle ear fluid in this age group. Chronic otitis of infancy may have its onset in the first month of life but be unrecognized then because of the vagueness of symptomatology. The infant has low-grade fever, feeding problems, diarrhea, irritability and failure to thrive. The infecting bacteria are most commonly *Escherichia coli, Klebsiella pneumoniae* and *S. aureus* rather than the pyogenic bacteria found in older infants. Needle aspiration of middle ear fluid or myringotomy for culture and antibiotic susceptibility testing is a requisite for selecting specific chemotherapy.

SEROUS OTITIS MEDIA. Serous effusions of the middle ear are believed to originate as a physical phenomenon secondary to blockage of the eustachian tube and negative pressure in the middle ear cavity. The inciting cause of the obstructing edema or lymphoid hyperplasia may be nasopharyngeal inflammation, allergy or barotrauma, as from rapid descent in a nonpressurized aircraft cabin. The increasing recognition of serous otitis in the antibiotic era suggests that some cases represent incompletely resolved bacterial infections of the middle ear, but proof of this hypothesis is lacking. Attempts to isolate viruses from serous effusions have generally been unsuccessful, but viruses may play an indirect role by setting the stage for tubal dysfunction accompanying nasopharyngitis.

The serous fluid produces a sensation of fullness in the ear, decreased hearing and a popping or clicking sound with swallowing or jaw movement. The tympanic membrane is bulging and dull, with a few injected vessels or a diffuse, dusky hue, but there is much variation in the appearance, and pneumatoscopy may indicate fluid when the membrane looks almost normal. Later in the course when the fluid becomes viscous ("glue ear") there may be retraction, with prominence of the short process of the malleus, and the drum may acquire a blue-white coloration.

Initial **management** includes nasopharyngeal decongestants, and attention should be directed to treatable causes of tubal dysfunction such as allergy, neoplasms or adenoidal hypertrophy.

Many cases resolve after a few weeks, but if glue ear supervenes, most otologists recommend myringotomy and removal by suction of the viscid material because of the belief that the fluid eventually will undergo fibrinous changes with resulting permanent damage to the middle ear structures and decreased hearing. This opinion is not universally shared; others believe conclusive evidence is lacking that glue ear results in permanent deafness or that myringotomy affects long-term outcome.

For recurrent or chronic effusions the therapy of choice is disputable. In the past decade it has been common practice to implant plastic grommets in the tympanic membrane for ventilatory equalization of pressure. This produces an immediate improvement in hearing which may be of importance to the learning of the schoolchild and to the safety of the child exposed to motor traffic. The tubes are left in place for several months until they are spontaneously extruded. *Long-term benefits or disadvantages of this approach over older methods are unknown.* A more conservative approach is to perform adenoidectomy and myringotomy with suction. Controlled middle ear inflation is done postoperatively if fluid recurs. Adjunctive management of predisposing causes is important to either surgical method.

ACUTE SUPPURATIVE OTITIS MEDIA. Acute bacterial infection of the middle ear is due to *Diplococcus pneumoniae* in over half of cases. Streptococci are less common and staphylococci are found in fewer than 5 per cent of patients. *Hemophilus influenzae* accounts for approximately one third of cases in infancy but becomes progressively less frequent with increasing age. It should be kept in mind that the preceding are overall figures for etiologic incidence. At any one time in any one community there may be wide variation from them, depending on the locally prevalent pattern of bacteriologic infection.

Pain, fever and constitutional signs occur early. At this time the tympanic membrane may show only redness, but as purulence accumulates there is bulging of the drum with loss of landmarks. The young infant may indicate pain by head-shaking or tugging or batting at the ears, but there may be only constitutional signs of fever, irritability, vomiting and loose stools. If spontaneous perforation occurs, pain is relieved and fever decreases.

MANAGEMENT. Therapy includes antibacterials, analgesics and nasal decongestants. The use of decongestants is based more on tradition than on proof of efficacy. Past infancy, penicillin is the preferred agent. It can be given orally as penicillin V in a dosage of 40,000 units/kg/day in divided doses to a maximum of 800,000 to 1,200,000 units daily. Ampicillin (75–100 mg/kg/day in divided doses) is preferred for infants because of the likelihood of *H. influenzae* infection. Penicillin plus a sulfa drug is an acceptable alternative for infants. Erythromycin is a commonly used alternative drug, but there are doubts about its efficacy against *H. influenzae.* Lincomycin is ineffective against *Hemophilus.* Tetracyclines should not be used because some streptococci and pneumococci are resistant, because concentrations in middle ear exudate are low, and because their use prior to the age of 8 or 10 years frequently results in disfiguring discoloration of the teeth. Cephalosporins have not been adequately evaluated. Therapy is continued for approximately 10 days until signs of inflammation have cleared.

Myringotomy is not necessary routinely. For the patient with intense pain and imminent rupture of the membrane it provides dramatic relief. Myringotomy or needle aspiration should be performed to obtain pus for bacterial stains and culture if the patient fails to show any improvement after 48 to 72 hours of antibiotic therapy. This should also be done initially when otitis occurs in compromised hosts because of their propensity for infection with unusual or resistant bacteria. Discrepancy between the bacteriology of the middle ear and nasopharynx is so common that nasopharyngeal cultures are ordinarily of no value.

Recurrent Otitis Media. Recurrence of infection within a few days or weeks of cessation of therapy is common in infancy, accompanied by a change in spectrum of etiologic bacteria; pneumococci are much less common but *S. aureus, H. influenzae* and a variety of other bacteria may be involved. With recurrent infections, the tympanic membrane may become thickened and fail to show bulging or marked inflammation, so the physician does not appreciate the presence of pus in the middle ear.

To establish drainage and to identify the etiologic organism and its antibiotic sensitivity, myringotomy may be indicated in persistent or frequently recurrent otitis media. Investigation and treatment for predisposing causes should be undertaken.

Chronic Otitis Media. The chronically infected ear always has some degree of associated mastoid infection and a perforation of the membrane. Characteristically there is decreased hearing and a painless discharge from the ear through the permanent defect in the tympanic membrane. A **cholesteatoma** (a mass of desquamated epithelium with or without cholesterol crystals) may develop and lead to eventual destruction of middle ear structures.

Cultures of the discharge generally reveal enteric gram-negative organisms, staphylococci or a mixed growth. Acute exacerbation of infection may develop periodically and require antibiotic therapy, but, in general, systemic antibiotics are ineffective in chronic otitis media. Repeated, thorough cleansing of the ear, plus antibiotic ointments or drops may clear the infection and allow patching of the perforation, but if cholesteatoma is present surgery is necessary. Ultimately most patients with chronic ear infection require tympanoplasty, with or without mastoidectomy, and reconstruction of damaged ossicles.

COMPLICATIONS OF OTITIS MEDIA

Decreased hearing is the most serious long-term consequence of secretory or suppurative otitis media. Acute infectious complications may occur in the temporal bone, may extend to intracranial structures or may be metastatic to other organs.

MASTOIDITIS. Once the commonest complication of otitis media, mastoiditis has become quite rare in the antibiotic era. Inflammation of mastoid air cells occurs as part of acute otitis media but is usually aborted with antibiotic treatment. Untreated, the progressive inflammation leads to accumulated pus under pressure and coalescence of air cells into larger cavities. Osteitis may ensue. The pus follows the path of least resistance through the tympanomastoid fissure in infants, leading to redness and swelling behind the ear. The redness, swelling and tenderness over the mastoid process typical of acute mastoiditis in older children and adults is not seen in infants because this structure is undeveloped.

Normal variations in development may mimic the roentgenographic changes of mastoid infection. The mastoid antrum is present at birth and pneumatization of the temporal bone starts in infancy. This is not an orderly, predictable process from individual to individual or in the two temporal bones of one individual, making interpretation of roentgenographic changes before adolescence difficult.

Early infection of the mastoid cells sometimes responds adequately to massive antibiotic therapy alone. Penicillin is usually used because the pneumococcus and streptococcus are the most frequent etiologic organisms; 250,000–300,000 units/kg/day intravenously is recommended. In addition, simple mastoidectomy for drainage of pus is usually required.

Extension to the petrous portion may produce the constellation of pain, aural discharge and sixth nerve palsy known as **Gradenigo's syndrome.** Facial palsy can occur because of the vulnerable propinquity of the seventh nerve to the middle ear. Suppurative labyrinthitis with vertigo, pain and fever is rare.

INTRACRANIAL COMPLICATIONS. Extension to intracranial structures may proceed through vascular or nerve channels or by direct extension from osteitis. Otitis media is considered a major antecedent event in meningitis, but the precise mechanism by which this occurs and the factors responsible for selecting one infant for this complication from the vast number who go through an episode of otitis media without meningitis are unknown. Autopsy studies have revealed middle ear infection in virtually all cases of meningitis even when it was not diagnosed antemortem.

Thrombophlebitis of the lateral sinus may extend to involve other intracranial venous sinuses.

Brain abscess complicating chronic ear disease occurs in the temporal lobe or cerebellum. Cerebrospinal fluid otorrhea may be secondary to necrotizing middle ear infection of the sort that used to be seen with virulent scarlet fever, or may result from fractures. These patients are at great risk for developing meningitis. Epidural or subdural empyema may follow petrositis.

SYSTEMIC COMPLICATIONS. The clinical syndrome of septicemia rarely complicates otitis media, but hematogenously distributed bacteria may lodge in lung, bone, synovium or other structures to produce focal disease. The importance of middle ear disease as a primary focus for subsequent metastatic disease is impossible to assess.

JOHN D. NELSON

Beauregard, W. G.: Positional otitis media. J. Pediatr. *79*:294, 1971.
Berglund, B., Salmivalli, A., and Toivanen, P.: Isolation of respiratory syncytial virus from middle ear exudates of infants. Acta Otolaryng. *61*:475, 1966.
Bland, R. D.: Otitis media in the first six weeks of life: Diagnosis, bacteriology, and management. Pediatrics *49*:187, 1972.
Glorig, A., and Gerwin, K. S.: Otitis Media. Springfield, Ill., Charles C Thomas, 1972.
Gottschalk, G. H.: Serous otitis: A conservative approach to treatment. Arch. Otolaryng. *96*:110, 1972.
Howie, V. M., and Ploussard, J. H.: The "in vivo sensitivity test"—Bacteriology of middle ear exudate during antimicrobial therapy in otitis media. Pediatrics *44*:940, 1969.
Howie, V. M., Ploussard, J. H., and Lester, R. L., Jr.: Otitis media: A clinical and bacteriological correlation. Pediatrics *45*:29, 1970.
McGovern, J. P., Haywood, T. J., and Fernandez, A. A.: Allergy and secretory otitis media: An analysis of 512 cases. J.A.M.A. *200*:124, 1967.
Paradise, J. L., Bluestone, C. D., and Felder, H.: The universality of otitis media in 50 infants with cleft palate. Pediatrics *44*:35, 1969.
Rifkind, D., Chanock, R., Kravetz, H., Johnson, K., and Knight, V. Ear involvement (myringitis) and primary atypical pneumonia following inoculation of volunteers with Eaton agent. Amer. Rev. Resp. Dis. *85*:479, 1962.
Roddey, O. F., Jr., Earle, R., Jr., and Haggerty, R.: Myringotomy in acute otitis media: A controlled study. J.A.M.A. *197*:849, 1966.
Ronis, B. J., Ronis, M. L., and Liebman, E. P.: Acute mastoiditis as seen today. Eye, Ear, Nose, Throat Monthly *47*:502, 1968.
Silverstein, H., Bernstein, J. M., and Lerner, P. I.: Antibiotic concentrations in middle ear effusions. Pediatrics *38*:33, 1966.
Silverstein, H.: Surgery for chronic suppurative otitis media. New Engl. J. Med. *287*:287, 1972.
Tilles, J. G., et al.: Acute otitis media in children: Serologic studies and attempts to isolate viruses and mycoplasmas from aspirated middle-ear fluids. New Engl. J. Med. *277*:613, 1967.
van Dishoeck, H. A. E., Derks, A. C. W., and Voorhorst, R.: Bacteriology and treatment of acute otitis media in children. Acta Otolaryng. *50*:250, 1959.
Warren, W. S., and Stool, S. E.: Otitis media in low-birth-weight infants. J. Pediatr. *79*:740, 1971.

THE LARYNX

Symptoms referable to the larynx are dyspnea, stridor, wheezing, hoarseness and aphonia. The dyspnea of laryngeal obstruction is characteristically associated with deep inspiratory indrawing at the suprasternal notch and supraclavicular spaces, as well as with stridor. Not all inspiratory indrawing at the suprasternal notch is the result of high obstruction; it occurs whenever the accessory muscles of respiration are brought into play, as in generalized obstructive emphysema. In the latter situation the indrawing is more shallow. Stridor of laryngeal disease occurs in the inspiratory phase in contrast to the wheezing of asthma and other bronchiolitic disturbances, which is predominantly in the expiratory phase.

The only method of examining the larynx of a child under 6 or 7 years of age is by direct laryngoscopy. Direct laryngoscopic examination is indicated in the presence of the symptoms mentioned and may afford a means of treatment as well as diagnosis. Thorough physical examination, appropriate roentgenographic examination and bacteriologic studies may also be essential for the appraisal of laryngeal disease.

CONGENITAL MALFORMATIONS

CONGENITAL LARYNGEAL STRIDOR

Noisy, crowing respiratory sounds, usually associated with inspiration, are relatively common in the neonatal period and during the first year of life. Some infants merely have noisy breathing, whereas others have a laryngeal "crow," hoarseness or aphonia, dyspnea and inspiratory retractions in the supraclavicular, intercostal and subcostal spaces. If inspiratory retractions are severe, deformity of the thorax may result. Infants with severe dyspnea frequently have difficulty in nursing, so that undernutrition is common. Cyanosis is rarely observed. Respiratory infections tend to exaggerate all the symptoms.

In the first few days of life it may be difficult to distinguish between congenital disturbances of the larynx and transient disturbances such as laryngospasm of tetany of the newborn or laryngeal edema secondary to trauma or aspiration of irritant substances at birth. The history of aspiration at birth, hoarseness or aphonia and laryngoscopic examination establish the presence of postnatal laryngeal edema.

Stridor persisting or appearing after the first few days of life usually results from disturbances in or adjacent to the larynx. The most common of these is congenital deformity or flabbiness of the epiglottis and supraglottic aperture (laryngomalacia). Developmental malformations may be present, or there may be merely an exaggeration of the normal "omega" shape of the infantile epiglottis.

Anomalies of the larynx include malformations of the laryngeal cartilages, intraluminal webs and malformations or duplication of the vocal cords. At times generalized chondromalacia of the larynx and trachea may be observed. In such instances the larynx and the trachea tend to collapse with inspiration and to expand with expiration. Congenital tumors such as fibromas of the larynx are rare. Mucous retention cysts, branchial cleft cysts and thyroglossal duct remnants are other infrequent causes of stridor. Birth trauma must also be considered in the differential diagnosis (see below).

Stridor may also be produced by extralaryngeal causes. Hypoplasia of the mandible permits the base of the tongue to displace the epiglottis posteriorly and cause laryngeal obstruction. Macroglossia from hypertrophy of the muscles, hemangioma, lymphangioma or cysts may have the same effect. In the Pierre-Robin syndrome a combination of hypoplasia of the mandible, pseudomacroglossia and glossoptosis is responsible for laryngeal stridor and dyspnea. Compression of the larynx by congenital goiters has been reported. Congenital vascular anomalies may also cause stridor. Enlargement of the thymus is rarely, if ever, responsible for stridor.

DIAGNOSIS. Most cases of congenital laryngeal stridor can be diagnosed only by direct laryngoscopy. Abnormalities of the epiglottis, the vocal cords and other parts of the larynx can be seen.

Extralaryngeal causes of stridor can often be established without the aid of direct laryngoscopy. Vascular anomalies which partially occlude the trachea and esophagus can often be detected by fluoroscopic observation during a barium swallow.

TREATMENT. The most common cause of laryngeal stridor, laryngomalacia, rarely requires treatment. The condition is seldom serious, and symptoms gradually become less severe, generally disappearing by about 1 year of age. Cysts, webs, tumors and malformations of the larynx require various specialized procedures, such as excision, dilatation, laryngoplasty or tracheotomy. The stridor associated with macroglossia or hypoplasia of the mandible can be relieved by pulling the tongue and mandible forward.

Particular attention must be given to the feeding of infants with stridor. Aspiration is an ever-present danger. Moreover, the respiratory efforts preclude normal sucking and swallowing in some infants. Slow, careful feedings from a small nipple or by dropper or glass are usually adequate. Feeding by gavage or even gastrostomy is occasionally necessary.

Infants with stridor must be protected from respiratory infections.

CONGENITAL WEB

This condition is not common, but its immediate diagnosis is essential. If the web is complete or almost complete, the newborn infant will quickly be asphyxiated. Laryngeal atresia has been associated with anophthalmia. In a few instances a web has been perforated or removed with sufficient promptness to save the infant's life. Often the obstruction is not complete, and there are only stridor and mild dyspnea.

DIAGNOSIS AND TREATMENT. Direct laryngoscopy affords the means for both diagnosis and treatment. In some instances it may be necessary to insert a tracheostomy tube while a series of dilatations is carried out. Direct laryngoscopic incision or excision of a congenital web is nearly always followed by prompt re-formation and is, thus, rarely successful. An operative approach, usually consisting in anterior division of the web by an external approach and the use of a nonirritating metal or silicone "keel" until epithelialization is complete, may be helpful when the patient has reached 8 or 10 years of age.

TRAUMA OF THE LARYNX

BIRTH TRAUMA. Injury of the larynx during birth is not infrequent. It may result in dislocation of the cricothyroid or cricoarytenoid articulations. Such an injury will result in hoarseness and at times in wheezing or fluttering respiratory sounds. The diagnosis is made by direct laryngoscopic examination. Treatment by direct laryngoscopic manipulations, using a laryngeal dilator, may occasionally be effectual, but tracheotomy should be done when there is evidence that the infant is not getting enough air.

Unilateral or bilateral recurrent laryngeal paralysis may also be produced by birth trauma, especially during instrumental delivery. When only one cord is paralyzed, there may be only hoarseness and slight stridor. There is usually no dyspnea. In bilateral paralysis there is dyspnea with stridor. Direct laryngoscopic examination will establish the diagnosis. Tracheotomy is usually necessary for bilateral paralysis. The older child may wear a valvular cannula, or a laryngoplasty with lateral fixation of one vocal cord may be done to improve the airway and permit decannulation, unless breathing through the larynx has improved spontaneously.

POSTNATAL TRAUMA. Any trauma such as that brought about by a fall against a hard object may produce acute or chronic stenosis of the larynx, as may high tracheotomy and prolonged intubation. Immediate tracheotomy is required in the acute stage if there are signs of high obstruction.

LARYNGEAL STENOSIS

ACUTE LARYNGEAL STENOSIS

Acute stenosis may result from any acute infection, diphtheritic or nondiphtheritic, which is responsible for edema of the subglottic region or epiglottis and arytenoids; from inflammation secondary to the inspiration of a vegetal foreign body such as a peanut, and especially after instrumentation in the removal of such an object; from edema resulting from allergic factors or cardiorenal disease; or from a foreign body lodged in the larynx.

TREATMENT. This consists in immediate provision of an airway by intubation or tracheotomy, after which appropriate medical treatment can be instituted.

CHRONIC LARYNGEAL STENOSIS

Chronic laryngeal stenosis is a frequent sequel of high tracheostomy, that is, a tracheostomy in which the first tracheal ring or cricoid cartilage has been damaged, resulting in perichondritis and subsequent overgrowth of cartilage or fibrous tissue. It is rare when care is taken to keep these two structures intact. The laryngeal diseases which may be responsible for chronic stenosis include laryngeal diphtheria, syphilis, tuberculosis, burns by roentgen rays or radium, and external trauma.

PATHOLOGY. Scarring and stenosis most often develop in the subglottic region, and at times there is necrosis of cartilage.

CLINICAL MANIFESTATIONS. These are generally limited to inability to decannulate the tracheotomized patient or to extubate the intubated patient. When neither intubation nor tracheotomy has been done, there will be dyspnea with audible stridor and indrawing at the suprasternal notch and at the supraclavicular and intercostal spaces.

DIAGNOSIS. Diagnosis is by direct laryngoscopy, supplemented by palpation of the larynx and by roentgenographic examination.

The prognosis for eventual cure is good, though many patients require treatment for months or years.

TREATMENT. In the milder cases replacement of the tracheostomy cannula by a smaller one, and occlusion of this tube with a cork (at first a partial occlusion and then a complete one), will re-educate the patient to breathe through the mouth and permit removal of the cannula. If this is not successful, dilatation through a direct laryngoscope may accomplish the desired result. Such dilatation should not be done at too frequent intervals. When neither of these methods has sufficed to re-establish adequate breathing through the larynx, external surgery, with or without use of an indwelling mold, may be required.

NEOPLASMS OF THE LARYNX

Papilloma is the most common benign tumor of the larynx in children. The lesions may grow profusely from any portion of the larynx, though usually from the vocal cords. The tumor rarely, if ever, becomes malignant and often disappears after puberty. Initially the only symptom is hoarseness; but if the condition is allowed to persist, there is likely to be dyspnea; asphyxia has occurred in unrecognized cases (Fig. 12–5). The diagnosis may be made by direct laryngoscopy during

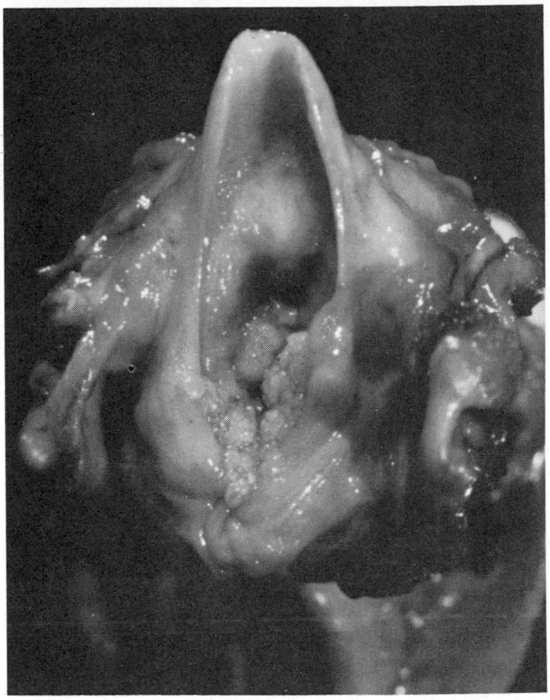

Figure 12–5 Obstructive glottic papilloma in a 5 year old girl with a history of progressive dyspnea and aphonia (postmortem specimen). Although examined by a physician on several occasions, she was referred for treatment only when dyspnea became extreme; she died of asphyxia en route to hospital.

the stage of hoarseness, even in an infant. The lesions are pinkish, warty tumors, which scalp off easily when grasped with the forceps. The diagnosis should be confirmed histologically.

The best treatment is superficial removal of the tumors by forceps through the direct laryngoscope. Care should be taken not to damage normal tissues. Cure will ultimately be obtained, even though at first there is usually rapid recurrence. If recurrence is too rapid to be kept under control by this method, and asphyxia threatens, a tracheotomy should be done; a cannula should be left in place while the tendency to recurrence persists. More extreme therapeutic measures such as radical excision or intensive irradiation are absolutely contraindicated. Recent evidence suggests that use of an autogenous vaccine prepared from freshly removed papilloma may retard growth of the tumor. Ultrasonic treatment, cryosurgery and laser surgery have recently been advocated as adjuvant forms of treatment, but are not yet widely used. There is some possibility that the use of ultrasonic therapy may inhibit normal growth of the larynx.

Vocal nodules are small tumors which occur in children at the junction of the anterior and middle thirds of the vocal cords; they are generally bilateral. They have been called "screamer's nodes" or "singer's nodes." The only symptom is slight hoarseness. Regression may occur if strenuous use of the voice is avoided. Otherwise the nodules may be removed by small cupped forceps under direct laryngoscopic view.

FOREIGN BODIES IN THE LARYNX, TRACHEA AND BRONCHI

The air passages of children are frequent sites for the lodgment of foreign bodies; the carelessness of adults is the most important contributory factor.

PATHOLOGY. The changes produced by foreign bodies depend upon their nature and upon the degree of obstruction of the air passage. A sharp or irritating object lodged in the larynx will produce severe edema and later suppurative perichondritis. In the bronchus a nonobstructive foreign body may produce little pathologic change, whereas an obstructive object will produce atelectasis and later bronchiectasis, pulmonary abscess or empyema. A vegetal object, such as a peanut, may immediately produce a generalized inflammatory condition involving not only the portion of the tracheobronchial tree obstructed, but also the entire respiratory tract.

CLINICAL MANIFESTATIONS. The initial symptoms of a foreign body in the air passages are choking, gagging, wheezing or cough. After the initial period there is often a symptomless interval which may last for hours, days or weeks. By the time symptoms reappear the initial ones may have been forgotten. The secondary symptoms usually give a clue to whether the foreign body is lodged in the air or food passage and may indicate the level of lodgment. On occasion, however, dysphagia may occur from the swelling that results from lodgment of a foreign body in the region of the larynx, and foreign bodies in the upper esophagus may cause symptoms referable to the air passages by compression or by the overflow of food or secretions into the larynx.

LARYNGEAL FOREIGN BODY

CLINICAL MANIFESTATIONS. A foreign body in the larynx causes hoarseness, a cough which soon becomes croupy, and aphonia. Hemoptysis, dyspnea with wheezing, and cyanosis may occur. Obstruction resulting from the foreign body or the combination of it and the inflammatory reaction may prove fatal if the signs of high respiratory tract obstruction are not promptly recognized and appropriate treatment given.

DIAGNOSIS. Roentgenographic and direct laryngoscopic examinations reveal the presence of a foreign body in the larynx (Fig. 12–6). An opaque foreign body in the neck will be clearly demonstrated on a lateral roentgenogram. When it is lodged anteriorly, it is obviously in the larynx; when it is behind the soft tissue shadows of the larynx, it is in the hypopharynx or the cervical esophagus. The plane in which the foreign body lies is another differential point in its localization. If it lies in the sagittal plane, it is in the larynx. If it is in the coronal plane, it is probably in the food passage. Even if the foreign body is not opaque, indirect evidence of its presence may be afforded by

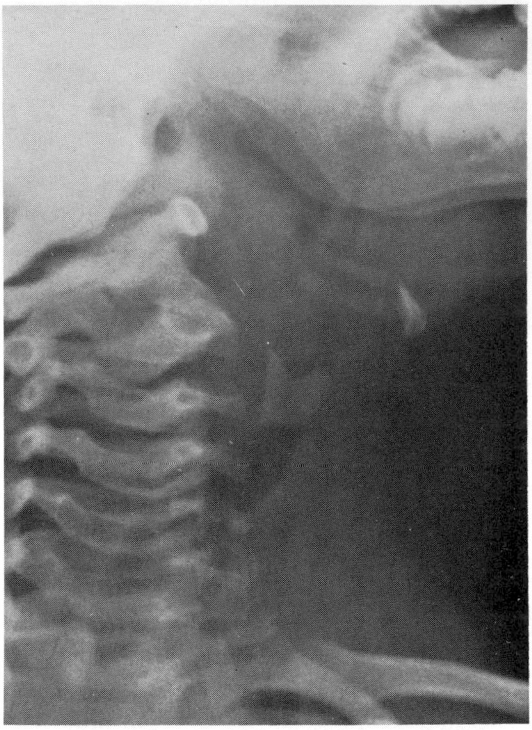

Figure 12–6 Foreign body (fragment of sea shell) in larynx of a 2 year old child treated for "croup" 6 days before foreign body was suspected. Fortunately tracheotomy was not required despite the presence of moderately severe laryngeal edema due to prolonged sojourn of the foreign body.

the roentgenographic examination. Films should always be taken from both the lateral and the anteroposterior projections. In some instances administration of a small amount of opaque material may be helpful. Direct laryngoscopy will confirm the diagnosis and provide access for instrumental removal of the foreign body. When there is a severe degree of dyspnea, it may be advisable to do a tracheotomy before the laryngoscopic examination.

TRACHEAL FOREIGN BODY

Though a foreign body in the trachea may be responsible for cough, hoarseness, dyspnea and cyanosis, the characteristic signs are the audible slap and palpable thud due to momentary expiratory impaction at the subglottic level, and the asthmatoid wheeze. The diagnosis of tracheal foreign body may occasionally be made from the symptoms, physical signs and roentgenogram of the chest, but in most instances a definite diagnosis can be made only by bronchoscopy.

BRONCHIAL FOREIGN BODY

CLINICAL MANIFESTATIONS. The initial symptoms are usually similar to those of foreign bodies in the larynx or trachea. Cough, blood-streaked sputum and metallic taste in the case of metallic foreign bodies are other symptoms that may be produced by bronchial foreign bodies. The degree of obstruction produced by a bronchial foreign body is a determining factor in the symptomatology as well as in the pathologic changes. A nonobstructive nonirritating foreign body may produce few symptoms even after prolonged sojourn. An obstructive foreign body quickly produces symptoms and signs and pathologic changes. When there is only a slight obstruction, a wheeze will be noted. When obstruction is of greater degree, obstructive emphysema or obstructive atelectasis will be produced; if either is allowed to persist, chronic bronchopulmonary disease may be a sequel. When both main bronchi are obstructed, there may be severe dyspnea and even asphyxia. If the foreign body is vegetal, e.g., a peanut, a severe condition known as vegetal or arachidic bronchitis will result. This is characterized by cough, a septic type of fever and dyspnea. Chronic pulmonary suppuration may be expected when a bronchial foreign body has been present for a long time.

DIAGNOSIS. The symptoms of a bronchial foreign body depend upon the stage in which the patient is seen. The possibility of a foreign body must be considered in acute or chronic pulmonary lesions regardless of whether there is a history of a foreign body accident. The physical signs of bronchial obstruction from foreign bodies include limited expansion, decreased vocal fremitus, impaired (atelectasis) or hyperresonant (emphysema) percussion note and diminished breath sounds distal to the foreign body. When there is complete obstruction, with a so-called drowned lung or with atelectasis, there is absence of vocal resonance and vocal fremitus, which may lead to an erroneous diagnosis of empyema. Varying degrees of tympany may be noted over areas of obstructive emphysema, which may persist for a time. Rales are more likely to be on the uninvaded side than on the invaded one.

Fluoroscopic examination is invaluable in detecting and localizing bronchial foreign bodies.

In order to understand the physical signs and the roentgenographic appearance of bronchial obstruction, it is helpful to recognize the analogies between the types of obstruction produced by foreign bodies and the different types of valves used to control the flow of fluids in pipes (Fig. 12–7).

A first-degree obstruction may be compared to a bypass valve, which allows passage of air or fluid in both directions, with only slight interference. In such cases a wheeze will be produced.

In a second-degree obstruction there is sufficient interference with the passage of air to permit it to go in one direction only. A "check-valve" action of this sort in the bronchial tree depends primarily upon the physiologic expansion of the bronchus on inspiration and its contraction on expiration. If the lumen is obstructed by an object which is of just the right size to cause complete obstruction in the expiratory phase, but to allow air to pass in the inspiratory phase, air will enter the distal portion of the lung on inspiration, but little or none will escape during expiration. This type of obstruction produces obstructive emphysema (Fig. 12–8).

If blockage of the bronchus is complete, either by corking of the bronchus by the object itself or by an obstruction produced by the foreign body in combination with the inflammatory swelling of the bronchial mucosa, a stop-valve obstruction results, and the air in the distal portion of the lung is soon absorbed, leaving an area of obstructive atelectasis (Fig. 12–9).

These phenomena are most readily appreciated by observation under the fluoroscopic screen. In a bypass valve obstruction there is little or no roentgenographic evidence produced by a nonopaque foreign body.

When there is a check-valve type of obstruction, the obstructive emphysema makes it possible to localize a bronchial foreign body. The obstructed lung will remain expanded during expiration, while the heart and the mediastinum will shift to the opposite side as the unobstructed lung empties. The diaphragm is low, flattened and fixed on the obstructed side; its excursion will be free and exaggerated on the unobstructed side. The differences between the lungs are much more evident on expiration than on inspiration. If a permanent record is desired, two films should be taken, one in full inspiration and one at the end of expiration.

When there is complete obstruction of the bronchus, producing obstructive atelectasis, the heart and the mediastinum are drawn toward the obstructed side and remain there during both phases of respiration. The diaphragm on the obstructed side remains high, while that on the unobstructed side moves normally. Films taken at

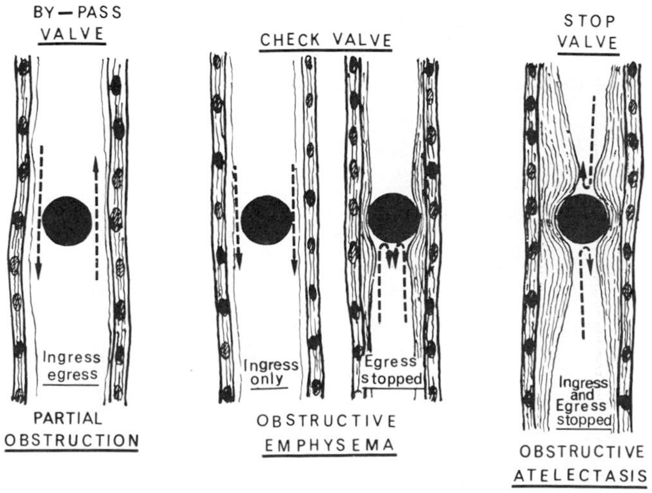

Figure 12–7 *Valvular mechanisms in bronchial obstruction (see text).*

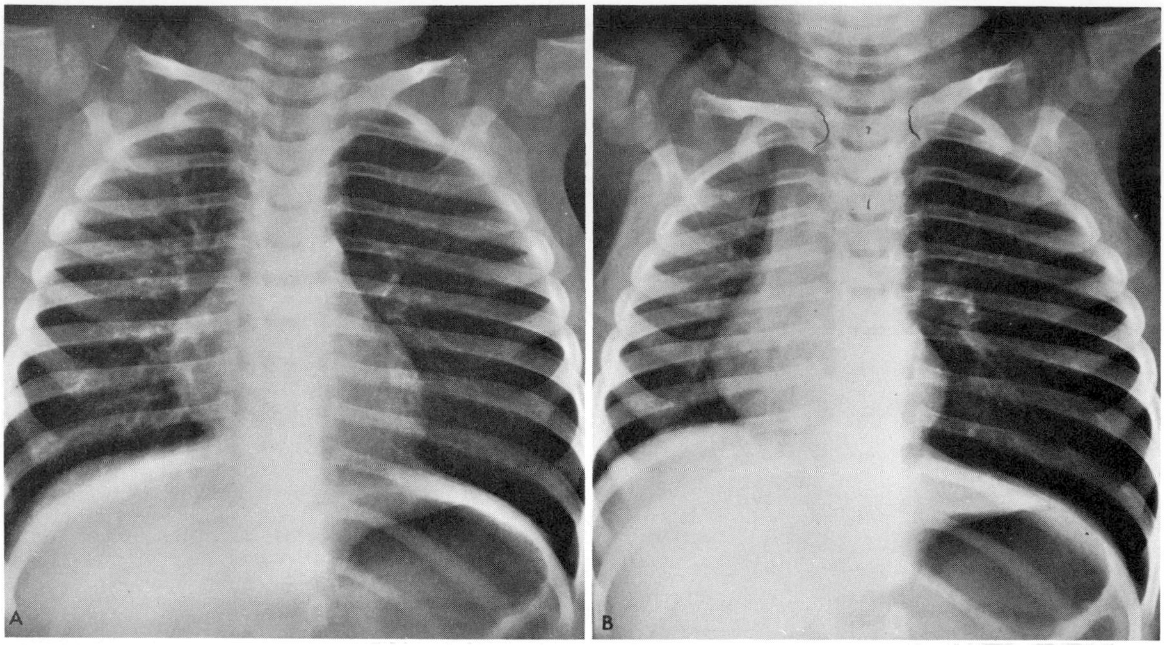

Figure 12–8 *Obstructive emphysema due to peanut fragment in left main bronchus. Inspiratory film* (A) *appears relatively normal except for slight mediastinal shift to the right. In expiration* (B) *the left lung remains overaerated (check-valve mechanism), and the mediastinum moves far to the right.*

the end of inspiration and of expiration will show only the slight difference resulting from the filling and emptying of the unobstructed lung. Observation of these phenomena under the fluoroscope and appreciation of the principles of the valvular mechanisms make it easier to understand the physical signs.

Opaque foreign bodies are clearly revealed on the roentgenogram. It is necessary to take films from both the anteroposterior and the lateral positions, with a sufficiently heavy exposure in the anteroposterior view to show a foreign body behind the heart.

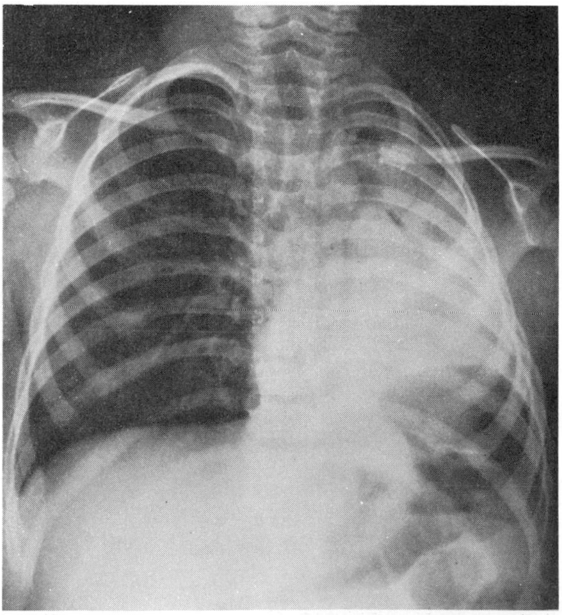

Figure 12–9 *Foreign body lodged in left main bronchus, producing atelectasis of left lung. Note that the heart is drawn completely into the left side of the chest.*

PROGNOSIS. Foreign bodies in the air passages that are not removed are sooner or later fatal in the majority of instances. Only 2 to 4 per cent of foreign bodies are coughed up spontaneously. About 99 per cent can be removed safely by the skilled bronchoscopist, and at least 98 per cent of patients so treated should recover completely.

PREVENTION. Much can be done to avoid foreign body accidents. If small objects are kept out of the reach of children, if children too young to masticate are not given candy containing nuts, and if toys that contain small parts loosely attached are not given to children, many serious cases of foreign body in the air passages will be prevented. Beads, the button box and coins should not be given to children as playthings. Safety pins should always be closed and not left near the baby. The closed safety pin is not a dangerous foreign body, but the open one is among the most dangerous and the most difficult to remove safely.

Adults should not set a bad example by holding pins or other objects in the mouth. The impulse to imitate is strong in a young child; frequently foreign body accidents occur because a baby or young child has imitated an adult by putting foreign objects in his mouth.

TREATMENT. The treatment of foreign body in the air passages consists in removal by direct laryngoscopy or bronchoscopy, with due consideration for the mechanical problem involved in the particular case. In some instances treatment of complicating conditions may be of equal importance. Removal of opaque foreign bodies lodged in the peripheral bronchi should be performed under the biplane fluoroscope. Any secondary infection should be treated with appropriate antimicrobial agents as indicated by laboratory sensitivity tests of the pathogenic organism. Attempts to dislodge foreign bodies from the respiratory tract by postural methods, the use of bronchodilators and pulmonary physiotherapy are inadvisable, not only because of the delay and the increased likelihood of complications, but because impaction of a dislodged foreign body at the subglottic level may result in asphyxia.

CHARLES M. NORRIS

Ferguson, C. F., and Kendig, E. L.: Pediatric Otolaryngology. Philadelphia, W. B. Saunders Company, 1972.
Holinger, P. H., Johnson, K. C., and Schiller, F.: Congenital anomalies of the larynx. Ann. Otol. *63*:581, 1954.
Jackson, C., and Jackson, C. L.: Bronchoesophagology. Philadelphia, W. B. Saunders Company, 1950.

Acute Infections of the Larynx and the Trachea

GENERAL CONSIDERATIONS. Acute infections of the larynx are of relatively greater importance in infants and small children than in older children. This is true in part because of a somewhat greater incidence in younger children, but principally because the younger child has a smaller airway which is thus predisposed to greater narrowing with the same degree of inflammation.

The term "croup" is commonly applied to a heterogeneous group of infectious conditions characterized by a peculiarly brassy ("croupy") cough, which may or may not be accompanied by inspiratory stridor, hoarseness and signs of respiratory distress due to varying degrees of laryngeal obstruction. The infection in infants and small children is rarely limited to a single area of the respiratory tract, usually affecting in varying degrees the larynx, the trachea, the bronchi and even the upper respiratory portion.

When there is sufficient involvement of the larynx to produce symptoms, the laryngeal part of the clinical picture is likely to overshadow other manifestations, owing to the severe effects upon vocalization and breathing.

Although an exact classification of acute laryngeal infection is not possible, there are several clinical varities which seem to justify the following classification:

Acute diphtheritic laryngitis (Section 10)
Acute nondiphtheritic infections
  Epiglottitis
  Laryngitis
  Laryngotracheobronchitis
  Spasmodic laryngitis

ACUTE NONDIPHTHERITIC INFECTIONS
(Infectious Croup)

ETIOLOGY. A large number of infectious agents, most often viruses, cause croup. Viral agents can now be identified for 60 to 75 per cent of patients studied, and it appears likely that they account for all or nearly all croup except that associated with diphtheria, pertussis and acute epiglottitis.

The agents most commonly isolated from patients with infectious croup are the parainfluenza viruses, which account for approximately two thirds of cases. The adenoviruses, respiratory syncytial, influenza and measles viruses cause most of the remaining cases for which an agent can be identified.

PREDISPOSING FACTORS. Regardless of cause, a number of factors predispose a child to this syndrome.

The majority of patients with viral croup are between the ages of 3 months and 3 years, whereas croup due to *H. influenzae* and *C. diphtheriae* is more common between 3 and 7 years of age. For unknown reasons, the incidence of croup is higher in males. The disease occurs most commonly during the cold season of the year.

In approximately 15 per cent of cases there is a strong family history of croup, and laryngitis does tend to recur in the same child.

CLINICAL FORMS. *In the hypoxic (cyanotic, pale or obtunded) child, any manipulation of the pharynx, including use of a tongue depressor, sometimes produces a vagal response which may result in sudden cardiorespiratory arrest.* Pharyngeal manipulation of the hypoxic child should therefore be deferred until after transfer to the hospital, administration of oxygen and, preferably, an anesthesiologist is on the scene to advise and to help to cope with any emergency.

Acute Epiglottitis. This form of croup is a severe, rapidly progressive infection of the epiglottis and surrounding areas. Although *H. influenzae* type b is the organism classically associated with this severe illness, pneumococci and group A streptococci may produce an identical disease. A milder and superficially similar clinical picture due to moderate inflammation of the supraglottic area is commonly caused by viruses. The onset is often abrupt, being preceded by a minor upper respiratory illness in about one fourth of the patients. The younger patient usually presents with sudden onset of high fever and difficulty in breathing. The older child often complains initially of severe sore throat and dysphagia. Severe respiratory distress may ensue within minutes or hours of the apparent onset, with inspiratory stridor, hoarseness, brassy cough, dysphagia, irritability and restlessness. Fever ranges between 38 and 40.5° C (100 to 105° F) with an average of 39.5° C (103° F). Drooling, due to dysphagia, is commonly present.

The young child may assume a position of hyperextension of the neck, although other signs of meningeal irritation are absent. The older child may prefer a sitting position, leaning forward, with mouth open and tongue somewhat protruding. Some children may progress rapidly to a shocklike state characterized by pallor, cyanosis and impaired consciousness.

On physical examination the patient presents severe respiratory distress, with inspiratory and sometimes expiratory stridor. There is flaring of the alae nasi and inspiratory retraction of the suprasternal notch, the supraclavicular and intercostal spaces and the subcostal area. The pharynx is usually inflamed, and excessive mucus is present in the faucial regions. The diagnosis may be missed unless the tongue is depressed with a blade to show the large, edematous, cherry-red epiglottis, which is pathognomonic. When the diagnosis is suspected in a seriously ill child, this procedure should be done only if tracheotomy can be performed at once. The maneuver may lead to sudden and complete obstruction. Mild to moderate cervical adenitis may be noted. The breath sounds are usually diminished bilaterally, indicating poor air exchange; there may be rhonchi due to mucus in the upper respiratory tract. When laryngoscopy is performed, intense inflammation is noted in the areas surrounding the epiglottis, as well as in the arytenoids and arytenoepiglottic folds, the vocal cords and subglottic regions. A pharyngeal or laryngeal membrane is rarely encountered.

The white blood cell count is usually between 15,000 and 25,000, with a striking polymorphonuclear leukocytosis. Bacteremia is common when *H. influenzae* or the pneumococcus is the causative agent.

Acute Infectious Laryngitis. Laryngitis is a common illness, and, except where diphtheria is common, all or nearly all cases are caused by viruses. The onset is usually characterized by an upper respiratory tract infection during which sore throat, cough and croup appear. The illness is generally mild, respiratory distress being unusual except in the young infant.

In severe cases, however, hoarseness is marked, and the patient may present with severe inspiratory stridor, retractions, dyspnea and restlessness. As the process progresses, air hunger and fatigue become evident, and the child alternates between periods of agitation and exhaustion.

Physical examination is usually not remarkable except for the evidences of pharyngeal inflammation and, when there is respiratory distress, the evidences of high respiratory obstruction: deep suprasternal and substernal retractions and diminished breath sounds on auscultation.

Inflammatory edema of the vocal cords and subglottic tissue may be demonstrated laryngoscopically. The principal site of obstruction is usually the subglottic area.

Acute Laryngotracheobronchitis. Laryngotracheobronchitis is the most common form of croup, and is believed to be caused only by viruses. Secondary bacterial infection is rare. Most patients have an upper respiratory tract infection for several days before the brassy cough, inspiratory stridor and respiratory distress become apparent. As the infection extends downward, to involve the bronchi and bronchioles, respiratory difficulty increases and the expiratory phase of respiration also becomes labored and prolonged. The child appears extremely restless and frightened. The temperature may be only slightly elevated or as high as 39 to 40°C (103 to 104°F). There are usually bilaterally diminished breath sounds, rhonchi and scattered rales.

This form of viral croup may usually be distinguished from bacterial epiglottitis by the more acute, explosive onset of the latter and its more rapid course. The duration of illness in viral croup ranges from several days to a week or more.

Acute Spasmodic Laryngitis. Acute spasmodic laryngitis, or spasmodic croup, is a distinctive clinical entity which occurs most often between the ages of 1 and 3 years. The cause is uncertain but is believed in most instances to be one of several viral agents. Allergy and psychologic factors are thought to be implicated in some cases. The anxious and excitable child is more prone to this syndrome; in some instances there is a familial predisposition.

Spasmodic croup occurs most frequently in the evening or at night and is usually preceded by mild to moderate coryza and hoarseness. The child awakens with a characteristic barking, metallic cough and noisy inspirations, and appears anxious and frightened. Respiratory distress is present. Retractions of the supraclavicular spaces, sternum, epigastrium and intercostal spaces are noted. Breathing is slow and labored; the pulse, accelerated; the skin, cool and moist; and the patient is usually afebrile. Dyspnea is aggravated by excitement, and intermittent episodes of cyanosis may occur. Usually within several hours the severity of the symptoms diminishes. The following day the patient often appears well except for slight hoarseness and cough; a similar but less severe attack may occur on the following night and occasionally on the third night; these are usually not accompanied by extreme respiratory distress. The distinguishing features of this syndrome are absence of fever and of signs of severe inflammation, sudden onset during the night with remission during the daytime, history of recurrent attacks and eventual complete recovery.

DIFFERENTIAL DIAGNOSIS. *Diphtheria* (Section 10) must be considered in the differential diagnosis of acute infectious croup. This illness may also be preceded by signs of an upper respiratory tract infection for 3 to 4 days. A clear, serous or serosanguineous nasal discharge is often present, and pharyngeal examination may reveal the typical gray-white membrane, or the membrane may be limited to the larynx and trachea. The symptoms of diphtheritic croup usually develop slowly, but signs of obstruction may occur relatively suddenly. The diagnosis is established by the identification of the organism in stained smears of scrapings of the membrane and its culture on Loeffler's medium.

Sudden onset of respiratory obstruction may be due to the inhalation of a *foreign body*. The child is usually between 6 months and 2 years of age, and the clinical picture is one of sudden onset of choking and coughing. There is absence of signs of inflammation, though the patient may look sick and be febrile; auscultation may reveal diminished to absent breath sounds on one or both sides of the chest. Fluoroscopic and roentgen examination of the chest will often suggest the diagnosis, which endoscopy will confirm.

A *retropharyngeal abscess* may present as respiratory obstruction. Palpation of the posterior pharyngeal wall usually reveals a fluctuant mass. Lateral x-ray films of the neck demonstrate an abnormal soft tissue density between the pharynx and cervical vertebrae.

A croupy cough may be the first symptom of *asthma* in some children. Development of the characteristic clinical and auscultatory wheezes and musical rales distinguish it from croup.

Angioneurotic edema may present as acute respiratory obstruction, but is rarely encountered in infancy or early childhood. The obstruction is due to edema of the supraglottic area. The swelling usually responds to epinephrine and antihistamines.

Croup is occasionally associated with *hypocalcemic tetany*, particularly in the young infant. Obstruction is secondary to spasm of the glottis, is of short duration and may recur many times during the day. Respiratory obstruction may also be associated with *trauma* to the laryngeal region or with *tumors* or *congenital malformations* of the larynx.

COMPLICATIONS. Complications occur in approximately 15 per cent of patients with viral croup. The most common one is extension of the infectious process to involve other regions of the respiratory tract such as the middle ear or the terminal bronchioles and pulmonary parenchyma. Otitis media characteristically presents several days to a week after recovery from croup. Interstitial pneumonia may occur, but is difficult to distinguish from patchy areas of atelectasis secondary to obstruction. Bronchopneumonia is unusual, unless aspiration of stomach contents has occurred during a period of severe respiratory distress. Secondary bacterial pneumonias are rarely found; suppurative tracheobronchitis is an occasional complication of laryngotracheobronchitis.

Mediastinal emphysema and pneumothorax occur, but are most commonly complications of tracheotomy.

PROGNOSIS. The outcome of infectious croup depends on the type and severity of infection, age of the patient, duration of illness prior to therapy, adequacy of therapy and the development of complications. In general, the length of hospitalization and the mortality increase as the infection extends to involve a greater portion of the respiratory tract, except in epiglottitis, in which the localized infection itself may prove fatal. Most deaths from croup are due to laryngeal obstruction or to the complications of tracheotomy.

MANAGEMENT. Therapy of infectious croup consists primarily in maintaining or providing for adequate respiratory exchange and is dependent in part on the primary location of the disease and its cause. In the bacterial forms antimicrobial therapy is also important.

The afebrile child with only a *croupy cough* complicating an upper respiratory infection should be kept indoors. Sleeping with a humidifier near but out of reach of the bedside is thought by some to reduce the likelihood of development of spasmodic croup in children known to be susceptible to it.

Most afebrile children with *acute spasmodic croup* can be safely and effectively managed at home. Placement in a closed bathroom filled with steam from a hot shower or bath often terminates acute laryngeal spasm and respiratory distress within minutes. The same effect has been noted by many parents as they take their child out into the cold night air on the way to the physician's office. Induction of vomiting either by coughing or by syrup of ipecac may also break the laryngeal spasm. Ipecac may also be effective in subemetic doses (2 to 4 ml). Once laryngeal spasm has been broken, it is believed by some that its return can be prevented on occasion by having the child sleep near a source of warm or cool (safer) humidification until the characteristic cough has subsided, usually after 2 or 3 days. If necessary, as simple a device as an ordinary teakettle can be used to provide the humidification. Antimicrobial agents are not indicated.

Children with croup and temperatures over 39° C (102.2° F) should be considered for hospitalization, but many can be safely managed at home. Indications for hospitalization are: presence or serious suspicion of epiglottitis, progressive stridor and respiratory distress, especially during the daylight hours; presence of hypoxia, restlessness, cyanosis, pallor, depressed sensorium; and high fever in a toxic-appearing child. In all instances the decision for hospitalization is made on the premises that reliable observation and relatively safe tracheotomy, should it become necessary, are more available in the hospital. Should these premises not be valid it may be safer to treat the child at home.

In the presence of *H. influenzae* epiglottitis with severe respiratory embarrassment, immediate tracheotomy must be considered.

At home or in the hospital, any patient with *croup* should be watched carefully for intensification of the symptoms of respiratory obstruction. The child is usually placed in an atmosphere of high humidity in order to lessen irritation and drying of secretions. Atomized water ("cold mist") is believed preferable to hot steam. In children with respiratory distress frequent, regular monitoring of the cardiac rate is essential; a rapid and rising rate may be the first sign of hypoxia and approaching total respiratory obstruction.

The patient should be disturbed as little as possible. With severe respiratory distress, fluids should be administered parenterally rather than orally to lessen physical exertion and vomiting with its potential for aspiration. The child should not be given a sedative, since restlessness is one of the clinical guidelines used to determine the severity of obstruction and the need for tracheotomy. In the rare instance when the patient is extremely agitated and frightened, chloral hydrate (5 to 10 mg/kg) or paraldehyde (0.1 ml/kg) may be administered; these agents do not depress the respiratory center or dry secretions.

Oxygen therapy may be used to alleviate anoxia and apprehension, but since cyanosis may be an indication for early tracheotomy, patients receiving oxygen must be observed particularly closely.

Children suspected of bacterial epiglottitis should receive parenteral ampicillin in dosage of 150 mg/kg/day. In viral croup, antimicrobial therapy is of no value, either in therapy or in the prevention of superinfections.

Expectorants, bronchodilating agents or antihistamines are not helpful. Opiates are contraindicated because they may depress necessary respiratory effort and have a drying effect on secretions.

Corticosteroids have been advocated as a means of diminishing the edema and spasm of croup and epiglottitis. Controlled studies have shown no benefit of these agents in this syndrome, and they are not indicated.

Dramatic results have been reported in the treatment of croup (not epiglottitis) with intermittent positive pressure breathing (IPPB) and nebulized racemic epinephrine (2.5 per cent, diluted 1:8 with water) for 15 minutes at intervals of 1 to 4 hours as necessary. The chief limiting factors have been malfunctioning equipment or a therapist unskilled at handling the equipment or the child.

Indications for Tracheotomy. The decision to perform a tracheotomy is based on the clinical examination, and experience is of the utmost importance. The aims of this procedure are to improve exchange of air and to facilitate the removal of secretions from the lower respiratory tract. The operation should be performed for patients who show increasing signs of respiratory obstruction with conservative therapy. Tracheotomy should not be delayed until cyanosis and extreme restlessness have developed; the patient then is often close to unconsciousness and death. A pulse rate over 150 and rising, especially in a tiring child, is an earlier sign that tracheotomy may be indicated. In acute epiglottitis, tracheotomy will be required in about half the patients and should not be delayed once the indications are present; indeed, it has been suggested by some that elective tracheotomy should be done on any patient with unequivocal (marked or severe) epiglottitis. In laryngotracheobronchitis, tracheotomy is rarely needed, but may be necessary occasionally to provide an airway and a means of clearing the trachea of sticky secretions. A severe form of laryngotracheobronchitis has been observed during several influenza A virus epidemics; tracheotomy was required in a fair portion of hospitalized patients.

The tracheostomy tube must remain in place until edema and spasm have subsided and the patient is able to handle secretions satisfactorily. The cannula should always be removed as soon as possible, usually within a few days.

The use of plastic nasotracheal tubes in place of a tracheotomy has recently been recommended. Although these devices can be used to secure an adequate airway under emergency conditions, their prolonged use may result in increased spasm and edema of the larynx. Furthermore, the incidence of complications (stenosis, granuloma formation, and permanent damage to the vocal cords) following the removal of the tube may be greater than with a tracheostomy, and adequate suctioning of the trachea is not possible.

George H. McCracken, Jr.
Heinz F. Eichenwald

Adair, J. C., Ring, W. H., Jordan, W. S., and Elwyn, R. A.: Ten-year experience with IPPB in the treatment of acute laryngotracheobronchitis. Anesth. Analg. *50*:649, 1971.

Berenberg, W., and Kevy, S.: Acute epiglottitis in childhood. A serious emergency, readily recognized at the bedside. New Engl. J. Med. *268*:870, 1958.

Cramblett, H. G.: Croup—Present day concept. Pediatrics *25*:1071, 1960.

Holinger, P. H., and Johnston, K. C.: The infant with respiratory stridor. Ped. Clin. N. Amer. *2*:403, 1955.

Rapkin, R. H.: Acute epiglottitis. Clin. Pediatr. *10*:312, 1971.

Rapkin, R. H.: Tracheostomy in epiglottitis. Pediatrics *52*:426, 1973.

Wolfsdorf, J., Swift, D., and Avery, M.: Mist therapy reconsidered: An evaluation of the respiratory deposition of labelled water aerosols produced by jet and ultrasonic nebulizers. Pediatrics *43*:799, 1969.

THE THORACIC CAVITY

For neoplasms of the lung, see Section 25.

MALFORMATIONS OF THE TRACHEA, BRONCHI AND LUNGS

Tracheo-esophageal fistula is the most important congenital anomaly of the trachea (Section 11). Rarely the trachea may be absent, or there may be tracheal stenosis of varying degrees. *Tracheal compression* may be produced by an anomalous aortic arch or other large vessel (Section 13). **Tracheal diverticula** are blindly ending bronchus-like projections, which infrequently terminate in normal-appearing lung tissue (tracheal lobe). Other tracheal abnormalities are mentioned on page 955 and with Fig. 22–13.

Bronchogenic cysts are usually located in the region of the bifurcation of the trachea. They rarely produce symptoms, and their clinical importance is based on the need to differentiate them from malignant tumors.

Anomalous fissures and lobes of the lungs are frequently observed roentgenographically and at autopsy but are usually of no clinical significance. The so-called **azygos lobe** is actually a part of the right upper lobe. During fetal development the azygos vein normally shifts medially into the mediastinum and onto the vertebral column. If such a migration fails to occur, the vein cuts into the growing right upper lobe, leaving a deep azygos fissure, which separates the more medially placed azygos lobe from the remainder of the right upper lobe; there is no abnormality of the bronchial tree.

Congenital absence *of both lungs* is extremely rare. **Bilateral hypoplasia** *of the lungs* may occur in anencephalic monsters or may be associated with congenital diaphragmatic hernia; in the latter instance the lung on the side of the defect in the diaphragm shows greater reduction in size.

Unilateral pulmonary agenesis *or hypoplasia* is compatible with life. The heart and other mediastinal structures are shifted to the affected side, and the other lung is hyperexpanded and partially fills the thoracic cavity on the involved side. The stem bronchus on the affected side may be absent, rudimentary or of normal length and covered by a small rudimentary lung. Associated extrapulmonary anomalies may be present, especially hemivertebrae. Ipsilateral facial anomalies may occur with unilateral agenesis.

A lower **accessory lung** is a rare congenital anomaly. The accessory lung does not communicate with the tracheobronchial tree, and its blood supply is usually systemic rather than pulmonary in origin. It is almost always situated at the base of the left lung, rarely below the left diaphragm. Its structure varies from normal-appearing lung to that of a cystic space containing bronchial elements, but few or no alveoli.

Anomalous (nonpulmonary) circulation in a portion of a lower lobe (**sequestered lobe**) has been observed; there is a bronchial communication, but some maldevelopment of it. The blood supply is from the systemic circulation by way of an anomalous artery from the aorta. The lung tissue is usually replaced by multiple bronchial cysts or bronchiectatic cavities. Surgical removal of the involved lung is indicated.

Cysts *of the lungs* are occasionally present in infants early in the neonatal period and may be single or multiple, restricted to one lobe or distributed in two or more lobes. There is lack of agreement about the origin of many of them. It has been considered that those with an epithelial lining were congenital anomalies and that those without such a lining were the result of postnatal destructive processes. There is doubt whether this distinction is valid or whether the presence of cartilage in the wall of a cyst is in itself evidence of a congenital origin.

Cysts of congenital origin have been described in association with **adenomatoid malformations** of the lungs. The lesion, which is usually limited to one lobe, may initially appear on the roentgenogram as a solid structure. The bronchi are malformed. As the lobe is irregularly aerated during the first few days of life, air accumulates in the potential cystic structures. These enlarge progressively and may cause severe respiratory distress. In the left lower lobe the condition may be confused with diaphragmatic hernia.

Most cystic structures in the neonatal period or later are acquired and result from destruction of the pulmonary architecture. This may occur during artificial respiration (see Pneumomediastinum, Section 7) and on occasion may be responsible for an accumulation of air (cyst) within one or more lobes (see Bullous Emphysema, Section 7). Partial blockage of a bronchus with creation of a ball-valve type of mechanism will permit retention of an increasing amount of air. Under such circumstances, whether the obstruction is inflammatory or purely mechanical and whether it is intra- or extrabronchial, a so-called tension cyst is created. In other circumstances connection with the tracheobronchial tree is broken, alveolar sacs are ruptured, and the accumulation of air (bullous emphysema) remains for a long time before it is finally absorbed and the architecture of the lungs is realigned. Many factors can be responsible for such obstructions of the bronchi, some of which may be congenital in origin, but the majority are probably the result of postnatal disturbances, usually inflammatory. An unusual association with cytomegalic inclusion disease has been recorded. The cysts may be filled entirely with air or fluid or with a combination of them.

Most cysts eventually disappear without interference, but when a tension cyst continues to ex-

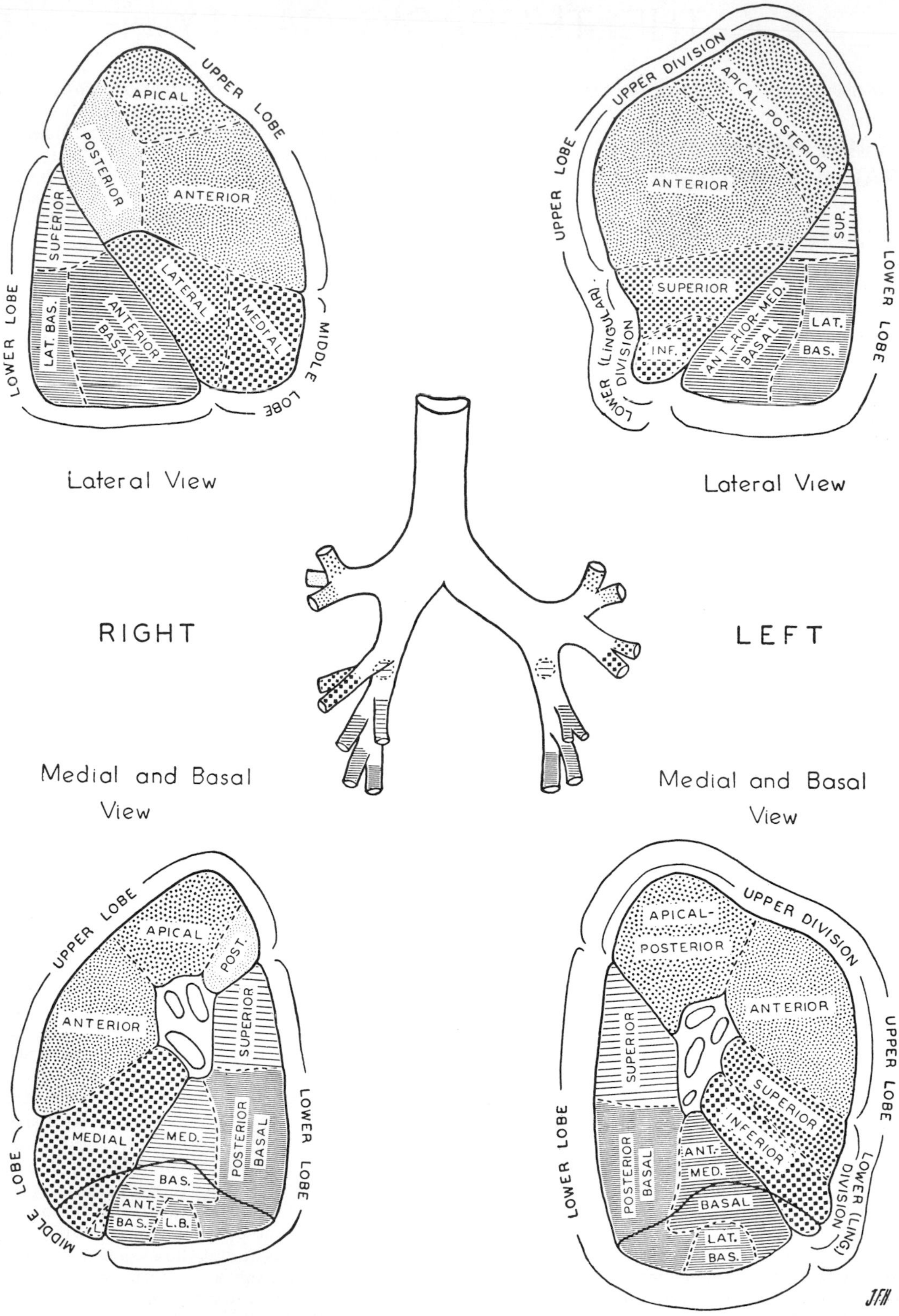

Figure 12–10 The lobar and segmental bronchi and the corresponding subdivisions of the lungs.

The subdivision of the lungs into parts smaller than the lobes aids in accurate localization of pathologic lesions and permits more economical resections in such diseases as bronchiectasis and tuberculosis. Although the lobes are classically identified by the interlobar fissures, the real basis of the division of the lungs into lobes is bronchial distribution. Each lobe is similarly subdivided by the branches coming from the lobar bronchus. For example, there are usually three branches of the right upper lobe bronchus, each of

Legend continued on opposite page.

pand and compress other lobes, it is usually necessary to remove the lobe containing it. Even such cysts, however, may establish an equilibrium with the uninvolved portions of the lung, become closed and eventually disappear. The decision for surgical removal must be based on the degree of respiratory embarrassment and whether it is progressive.

Lobar emphysema is discussed later.

Boyden, E. A.: Developmental anomalies of the lungs. Am. J. Surg. *89*:79, 1955.

Browder, J. A., and Billingsley, J. G.: Regional obstructive lung disease in childhood. Am. J. Dis. Child. *119*:322, 1970.

Caffey, J.: On the natural regression of pulmonary cysts during early infancy. Pediatrics *11*:48, 1953.

Campbell, P. E.: Congenital lobar emphysema. Aust. Paediatr. J. *5*:226, 1969.

Craig, J. M., Kirkpatrick, J., and Neuhauser, E. B. D.: Congenital cystic adenomatoid malformation of the lung in infants. Am. J. Roentgenol. *76*:516, 1956.

Ferencz, C.: Congenital abnormalities of pulmonary vessels and their relation to malformations of the lung. Pediatrics *28*:993, 1961.

Gallagher, H. S.: Cytomegalic inclusion disease of infancy: Report of case associated with cysts of lung with recovery following lobectomy. Am. J. Clin. Path. *22*:1147, 1952.

Gruenfeld, G. E., and Gray, S. H.: Malformations of the lung. Arch. Path. *31*:392, 1941.

Huber, J. F.: Practical correlative anatomy of the bronchial tree and lungs. J. Nat. Med. A. *41*:49, 1949.

Kergin, F. G.: Congenital cystic disease of lung tissue associated with anomalous arteries. J. Thorac. Surg. *23*:55, 1952.

Laipply, T. C.: Cysts and cystic tumors of the mediastinum. A.M.A. Arch. Path. *39*:153, 1945.

Potter, E. L., and Bohlender, G. P.: Intrauterine respiration in relation to development of the fetal lung, with report of two unusual anomalies of the respiratory system. Am. J. Obstet. Gynec. *42*:14, 1941.

Sperling, D. R., and Finck, E. J.: Intralobar bronchopulmonary sequestration. Am. J. Dis. Child. *115*:362, 1968.

BRONCHITIS

ACUTE BRONCHITIS

Though the diagnosis of "acute bronchitis" is frequently made, there is doubt that this condition exists in children as an isolated clinical entity. Rather, bronchitis occurs in association with a number of other conditions of the upper and lower respiratory tracts. The trachea is nearly always involved, and thus a more correct term would be "acute tracheobronchitis." The term "capillary bronchitis" (bronchiolitis) represents an entirely different illness, more closely related to the interstitial pneumonias.

Asthmatic bronchitis, a form of asthma with obscure pathogenesis, is often confused with acute bronchitis. Apparently, with a variety of upper respiratory tract infections, some children experience an exaggerated response of bronchi, with spasm and exudation similar to those encountered in older children with asthma.

Acute tracheobronchitis is most commonly found in association with an upper respiratory tract infection such as nasopharyngitis, but is also associated with such specific infections as influenza, pertussis, measles, typhoid fever (and other salmonelloses), diphtheria and scarlet fever. An acute, primary, undifferentiated tracheobronchitis also occurs, most commonly in older children and adolescents. It is likely that except for the bacterial diseases mentioned, acute tracheobronchitis is of viral origin. Pneumococci, staphylococci, *H. influenzae* and various hemolytic streptococci may be isolated from the sputum, but their presence does not imply a bacterial origin, and antimicrobial therapy does not appreciably alter the course of the illness.

Some children appear to be far more susceptible to acute tracheobronchitis than others. The reasons are unknown, but it is thought that allergy, poor health, climate, air pollution and chronic infections of the upper respiratory tract, particularly sinusitis, are contributory factors.

Evidence has recently been presented to indicate that the syndrome **bronchiolitis obliterans** may be caused by adenovirus type 21. This peculiar condition begins with an episode of acute bronchitis, bronchiolitis or bronchopneumonia and then progresses over several weeks to severe chronic pulmonary disease characterized by bronchiolar and bronchial obliteration and bronchiectasis.

CLINICAL MANIFESTATIONS. Generally the clinical manifestations of bronchitis are preceded by those of an upper respiratory tract infection. The illness is ushered in by a cough of relatively gradual onset, usually dry, hacking and unproductive. At this time the patient will often complain of low substernal discomfort, which is often aggravated by coughing. The child is frequently afebrile, but there may be fever to about 38.5° C (102° F). As the illness progresses, the patient will complain of soreness of the chest, occasionally of shortness of breath. Within 1 or 2 days the cough becomes productive, and the sputum, which may be clear initially, quickly becomes purulent. Vomiting is not uncommon and is generally related to gagging on secretions or to the violence of the cough. Usually within 5 to 10 days the mucus thins and

---

Figure 12–10 *Continued.*

which supplies or branches out to form a definitive part of the lobe. The term "bronchopulmonary segment" is applied to that portion of a lobe supplied by a branch of the lobar bronchus. The smaller subdivisions identified on the basis of the distribution of the branches of the segmental bronchus are referred to as "subsegments." Each segment is named according to its position in the lobe of which it is a portion. For example, the three segments of the right upper lobe are termed anterior, apical and posterior. The bronchi are correspondingly named anterior, apical and posterior segmental branches of the right upper lobe bronchus.

At an intersegmental plane the alveoli at the periphery of one segment are separated from the alveoli of the adjacent segment by a small amount of fibrous connective tissue containing the tributaries of the pulmonary veins. The branches of the pulmonary arteries follow the bronchial branchings. (Prepared by Dr. John Franklin Huber, Professor of Anatomy, Temple University School of Medicine.)

the cough gradually disappears. The considerable malaise often associated with the illness may continue for a week or more after acute symptoms have subsided.

Physical findings vary with the age of the patient and the stage of the disease. Early signs of nasopharyngitis and conjunctival injection are often noted. Later there may be some roughening of breath sounds, and rhonchi, coarse and fine moist rales and occasionally very fine bubbly rales may be heard over the entire chest.

In the otherwise healthy child, few if any complications occur. In undernourished children, or infants in poor health, such complications as otitis media, sinusitis or pneumonia are relatively common.

TREATMENT. There is no specific therapy. In small infants pulmonary drainage should be encouraged by frequent shifts in position. Older children are most comfortable in a highly humidified atmosphere, but there is no evidence that this shortens the duration of illness. Cough medicines are frequently given for symptomatic relief or for a supposed expectorant value, but none of the medications which can be safely given to children have been proved clearly beneficial. Potent cough remedies may suppress the cough reflex, but coughing is needed to clear the airway. If it is suppressed, obstruction of the bronchi by mucus may occur, which increases the possibility of suppuration. Antihistamines have an atropine-like action which tends to dry the secretions and should be avoided. Antimicrobial therapy does not shorten the duration of the viral illness or decrease the low incidence of bacterial complications.

Children with repeated attacks of bronchitis should be carefully evaluated for the possibility of anomalies of the respiratory tract, foreign bodies, bronchiectasis, hypogammaglobulinemia, tuberculosis, allergy, and such chronic upper respiratory tract infections as sinusitis, tonsillitis or adenoiditis.

CHRONIC BRONCHITIS

There is considerable doubt whether chronic bronchitis as an isolated clinical entity exists in children. This condition is frequently diagnosed, but generally the child with a chronic cough and the chest signs of bronchitis either has an underlying allergy, so that wheezing is a common finding, or has a chronic infection of the sinuses or nasopharynx (adenoiditis) with postnasal discharge. Rarely, bronchial irritation may be secondary to the chronic inhalation of dust or noxious fumes. The condition is frequently confused with mild cases of bronchiectasis and cystic fibrosis. In older children chronic bronchitis is occasionally a manifestation of hereditary α_1-antitrypsin deficiency but then usually is associated with progressive emphysema.

CLINICAL MANIFESTATIONS. The chief symptom is cough, with or without expectoration. The child will usually complain of soreness of the chest; characteristically these signs and symptoms are worse at night. Physical findings are similar to those of acute bronchitis. The condition is usually associated with other respiratory or systemic disease.

DIFFERENTIAL DIAGNOSIS. Every attempt should be made to find the underlying condition which may be associated with chronic bronchitis. Roentgenograms of the chest and of the sinuses should be obtained, and bronchograms are essential for elimination of bronchiectasis. A nasal smear should be examined for eosinophils and a search undertaken for inhalant allergens or other noxious factors in the child's environment.

COURSE AND PROGNOSIS. Both the course and the prognosis depend upon the possibility of appropriate management or eradication of any underlying illness. Complications will be those of the underlying illness.

TREATMENT. When an underlying cause for chronic bronchitis has been found, this should receive appropriate management. Allergic management may be helpful on occasion even when an underlying cause cannot be discovered. There is no evidence that autogenous vaccines or inhalation of antibiotics will serve a therapeutic purpose.

Feingold, B. F.: Infection in bronchial allergic disease: bronchial asthma, allergic bronchitis, asthmatic bronchitis. Pediat. Clin. N. Amer. *6*:709, 1959.

MacKeith, R.: Respiratory disorders in infants and young children, with special reference to recurrent stress bronchitis. Practitioner, *175*:692, 1955.

Williams, A.: Bronchitis, asthma and emphysema in childhood. Med. J. Aust. *1*:781, 1957.

PNEUMONIA

No clinical classification of pneumonia is entirely satisfactory. It has been common practice to separate the various clinical forms on the basis of their anatomic distribution, the principal designations being lobar pneumonia, lobular pneumonia or bronchopneumonia, and interstitial pneumonia or bronchiolitis. If separate categories are provided for the various aspiration pneumonias and for hypostatic pneumonia, most pneumonic infections can be grouped under these anatomic headings.

More or less characteristic lesions are produced by certain causative agents. For example, the pneumococcus produces an inflammatory lesion of the mucosa and an alveolar exudate, usually without destruction of the mucosal cells or extensive involvement of the interstitial tissues. The gross lesion is a consolidation of all or part of a lobe in the lobar variety, or of scattered lobules in the bronchopneumonic variety. In contrast, viral agents, *H. influenzae* and certain strains of the viridans group of streptococci invade or destroy the mucous membrane and produce principally bronchiolitis, peribronchiolitis and interstitial lesions. Secondary infections, especially in association with the primary viral infections, are often responsible for suppurative bronchiolitic, alveolar and interstitial lesions. Both the staphylococcus and

Friedländer's bacillus tend to destroy tissue and to produce multiple small abscesses.

Most bacteriologic infections can be identified not only as to the causative agent, but also as to the specific type or strain of a given species. Such identification or the failure of it has both therapeutic and prognostic significance. Since, however, it is not possible to identify the etiologic agent in all instances, it is necessary to supplement etiologic classification with grouping on a pathologic basis. Most etiologically unclassified infections occur in infancy and are probably of viral origin.

Within limits a clinical distinction can also be made on the basis of response to antimicrobial therapy; most bacterial infections are susceptible, whereas viral infections usually are not.

The following classification is presented as a working basis:

I. Bacterial Infections
- Pneumococcus
- Streptococcus
- Staphylococcus
- *H. influenzae*
- Friedländer's bacillus
- Tubercle bacillus
- *Treponema pallidum*

II. Viral or Probable Viral Infections
- Bronchiolitis and interstitial pneumonitis
- Giant cell pneumonia
- Influenza

III. Other Infections
- *Pneumocystis carinii* pneumonia
- *Q fever* (Section 10)
- *Mycoplasma pneumoniae* pneumonia

IV. Mycotic Infections
- Coccidioidomycosis
- Histoplasmosis
- Blastomycosis
- Cryptococcosis
- Mucormycosis
- Nocardiosis
- Sporotrichosis
- Thrush

V. Aspiration of
- Amniotic contents (fetal anoxia)
- Food
- Foreign bodies
- Zinc stearate
- Dust
- Kerosene
- Lipoid substances

VI. Löffler's Syndrome

VII. Hypostatic Pneumonia

BACTERIAL PNEUMONIA

GENERAL CONSIDERATIONS. In infants and young children with infection of the lower respiratory tract, signs and symptoms of pulmonary involvement are often nonspecific, and findings on physical examination may be sparse. Accordingly, roentgenographic evidence of pneumonia is frequently found in infants who clinically appear to have only upper respiratory tract infections, or only tachypnea and fever, without physical findings suggesting pulmonary involvement.

The defense mechanisms of the lower respiratory tract are extraordinarily efficient in preventing infection of the lungs. The defenses include: (1) the epiglottal reflex, which prevents aspiration of infected secretions; (2) ciliary action of the intact respiratory epithelium, which serves to carry microorganisms away from the lung; (3) the cough reflex, which propels foreign material out of the lower tract; (4) the viscous secretions of the respiratory tract, to which airborne organisms adhere; (5) the lymphatics which drain the terminal bronchi and bronchioles; and (6) phagocytic cells which line the normal alveoli. In addition, the normal flora of the upper respiratory passage inhibits growth of nonindigenous microorganisms. When one or more of these defense barriers is altered, inhibited or destroyed, pulmonary infection may result from aspiration of infected secretions or the inhalation of droplets or particles containing bacteria.

The most common event disturbing the defense mechanisms is a viral infection, which alters the properties of normal secretions, inhibits phagocytosis, modifies the bacterial flora, and may temporarily disrupt the normal epithelial layer of the respiratory passages. A viral respiratory disease often precedes the development of bacterial pneumonia by a few days. Once pneumonia has occurred, a series of intricate mechanisms brings about resolution of infection and recovery. These include such systemic phenomena as fever, the mobilization of leukocytes, the stimulation of antibody production, and changes in the circulation surrounding the involved area. Local activities include an increase in acidity of the pulmonary exudate, the phagocytosis and digestion of pathogens and cellular debris by macrophages, the cytolytic action of substances released by disintegration of leukocytes, the local release of antibacterial (neutralizing antibody) from immunologically competent cells, and the formation of antiviral substances (interferon).

Children with defects in defense mechanisms, or in the chain of events involved in recovery from infection, experience recurrent pneumonias or failure to resolve the disease completely. These defects occur with abnormalities of antibody production (agammaglobulinemia), cystic fibrosis, cleft palate, congenital bronchiectasis, tracheoesophageal fistula, abnormalities of the polymorphonuclear leukocytes, neutropenia, increased pulmonary blood flow, deficient gag reflex, and so forth. Among iatrogenic factors promoting pulmonary infection are trauma, anesthesia, aspiration and inappropriate antimicrobial therapy.

Pneumococcal Pneumonia

Though the incidence of pneumococcal pneumonia has declined over the last several decades, the disease remains the most common form of bacterial pneumonia encountered in childhood.

EPIDEMIOLOGY. Pneumococcal pneumonia most commonly occurs during the late winter and early spring when respiratory infections are at their peak. Serotypes 1 through 8 account for over 80 per cent of pneumonia in adults, but in children, types 14, 1, 6 and 19 are found most frequently.

Nontypable pneumococci and those with high type numbers are frequently encountered in the respiratory tracts of normal subjects. In contrast, the prevalence of carriers of the highly pathogenic serotypes is relatively low, except for type 3, which is a common inhabitant of the normal pharynx. Asymptomatic carriers of pneumococci play a more important role in the dissemination of infective types than do patients ill with pneumonia. Upon recovery from pneumococcal pneumonia, the possession of type-specific antibody not only protects the person from reinfection, but also renders him less likely to become a carrier of that specific serotype of organism.

When high carrier rates of pathogenic types are encountered in a relatively closed community (e.g., orphanages, nurseries, schools), the occurrence of widespread viral disease of the respiratory tract may be followed by an epidemic of pneumococcal pneumonia. Except for these unusual instances, the disease occurs as a sporadic illness.

In childhood the highest attack rates are found during the first 4 years of life and then decline with increasing age.

PATHOGENESIS AND PATHOLOGY. Pneumococci gain entrance to the lungs through the respiratory passages, usually by aspiration of infected secretions. Engorgement of interalveolar capillaries with outpouring of edema fluid supports proliferation of the organisms and aids in the spread of infection into adjacent portions of the lung. The involved lobe undergoes early consolidation, and polymorphonuclear leukocytes, fibrin, edema fluid, red blood cells and pneumococci fill the alveoli. This is the stage of *red hepatization,* which passes rapidly into that of *gray hepatization,* characterized by the deposition of fibrin over the pleural surfaces and the presence of fibrin and polymorphonuclear leukocytes in the alveolar spaces, where phagocytosis of pneumococci now rapidly takes place. The interalveolar capillaries are no longer engorged. The final stage involves the *resolution* of infection. Increasing numbers of macrophages appear in the alveolar spaces, the neutrophils undergo fatty degeneration and necrosis, and the fibrin threads are digested and disappear. The clinical crisis in the untreated case occurs about the seventh day of illness; resolution and re-expansion require an additional 1 to 3 weeks. When antimicrobial therapy is instituted in the first several days of illness, the course is interrupted and the characteristic stages are not seen.

In most infants and children pneumococcal pneumonia characteristically involves one or more lobes, or parts of lobes, leaving the remaining bronchopulmonary system uninvolved. In some infants the lesions may follow a bronchial distribution without the localization of lobar pneumonia.

CLINICAL MANIFESTATIONS. The classic history of a shaking chill followed by a high fever, cough and chest pain described for adults with pneumococcal pneumonia may be seen in older children, but is rarely observed in infants and young children, in whom the clinical pattern is considerably more variable. In addition, the widespread use of antimicrobial therapy for upper respiratory tract infections has altered the symptoms, physical findings and characteristic course.

In Infants. A mild upper respiratory tract infection characterized by stuffy nose, fretfulness and diminished appetite usually precedes the onset of pneumococcal pneumonia in infants. This mild illness of several days ends with the abrupt onset of fever of 39 to 40.5° C (103 to 105° F), restlessness, apprehension and respiratory distress. A generalized convulsion may accompany the high fever. Examination reveals an acutely ill infant with moderate to severe air hunger. Flushed cheeks and circumoral cyanosis are often noted. The respiratory distress is manifest by grunting respirations, flaring of the alae nasi, retractions of the supraclavicular, intercostal and subcostal areas, tachypnea and tachycardia. Cough is unusual at the onset of illness, but may be noted later.

Percussion of the chest is often unrevealing; dullness localized to one lobe is not a common finding. Auscultation may reveal diminished breath sounds and fine, crackling rales on the affected side, but these findings are not noted so consistently as in older children and adults. On the opposite side the breath sounds may be exaggerated and almost tubular in nature. If dullness is found on percussion in young infants, the presence of pleural effusion or empyema should be suspected. Abdominal distention usually reflects gastric distention due to swallowed air or paralytic ileus. The liver may seem enlarged, owing to downward displacement of the right diaphragm or to superimposed congestive heart failure. Nuchal rigidity without meningeal infection (meningismus) is not uncommon, especially with involvement of the right upper lobe. Occasionally the infant may be slightly jaundiced.

The physical findings change little during the course of illness, although moist rales may become audible during resolution.

In Children. The signs and symptoms of pneumococcal pneumonia in older children are similar to those of adults. After a brief upper respiratory tract infection the child usually experiences a shaking chill followed by high fever of 40 to 40.5° C (104 to 105° F). This is accompanied by drowsiness with intermittent periods of restlessness, rapid respirations, a hacking, unproductive cough, anxiety and occasionally delirium. Circumoral cyanosis may be present. The child is often noted to be splinting the affected side because of pleuritic chest pain and may lie on this side with the knees drawn up to the chest. Abnormal findings in the chest include dullness, diminished tactile and vocal fremitus, diminished breath sounds and fine and crackling rales on the affected side. On the first day of illness, dullness over the affected lobe is usually not evident, and the suppression of breath sounds on the affected side may lead to misinterpretation of the exaggerated breath sounds in the opposite lung as tubular breathing.

In older children, in contrast to young infants, the physical findings undergo greater change during the course of illness. Classic signs of consolidation are noted on the second or third day of illness and are characterized by dullness, increased fremitus, tubular breath sounds and the disappearance of rales. As resolution occurs, moist rales are heard and the signs of consolidation disappear. The initial dry, hacking cough loosens and becomes productive of large amounts of blood-tinged mucous material.

The development of a pleural effusion or empyema may cause a visible lag in respiration on the affected side, with exaggerated excursion on the opposite side. Examination usually reveals dullness over the area of the effusion, with diminished fremitus and breath sounds. Tubular breathing is often noted immediately above the fluid level and on the unaffected side.

LABORATORY FINDINGS. The white blood cell count is usually elevated to 15,000 to 40,000 cells per mm^3, with a preponderance of polymorphonuclear cells. White blood cell counts below 5000 per mm^3 are often associated with a grave prognosis. The hemoglobin value is usually normal or only slightly diminished.

In most patients with pneumococcal pneumonia, pneumococci can be isolated from the nasopharyngeal secretions, but this finding cannot be considered proof of a causative relation; the isolation of pneumococci should be attempted from secretions obtained upon deep coughing, from gentle tracheal aspiration or from pleural fluid obtained at thoracentesis. Bacteremia is found in about 30 per cent of cases of pneumococcal pneumonia.

ROENTGENOGRAPHIC FINDINGS. The roentgenographic changes in pneumococcal pneumonia do not always correspond to the clinical observations. Consolidation may be demonstrated on x-ray film before it is detectable by physical examination, and resolution of the infiltrate may not be complete until several weeks after the child is clinically well. Lobar consolidation is not so common in infants and young children as in the older child. Pleural reaction with the presence of fluid is not uncommon; it may be seen early in the course of illness and, even in the untreated patient, is not necessarily indicative of developing empyema.

DIFFERENTIAL DIAGNOSIS. Pneumococcal pneumonia cannot be differentiated from other bacterial and viral pneumonias without suitable microbiological studies. Conditions which may be confused with pneumonia are bronchiolitis, allergic bronchitis, congestive heart failure, acute exacerbations of bronchiectasis, aspiration of a foreign body, sequestered lobe, atelectasis, pulmonary abscess and endotracheal tuberculosis with secondary bacterial pneumonia.

An older child with right lower lobe pneumonia may have pain referred to the right lower quadrant of the abdomen. Since ileus may accompany pneumonia, right-lower quadrant pain and absent bowel sounds may be misinterpreted as indicative of acute appendicitis.

When meningismus is severe and presents with opisthotonos or positive Kernig and Brudzinski signs, it can be differentiated from meningitis only by examination of the spinal fluid.

COMPLICATIONS. With the use of antimicrobial therapy bacterial complications of pneumonia have become unusual. The most common complication is empyema, resulting from extension of infection to the pleural surfaces. This complication occurs most commonly in the young infant who has received medical attention late in the course of illness or has been inadequately treated. Purulent complications such as otitis media, meningitis, pericarditis, osteomyelitis and peritonitis are infrequent.

PROGNOSIS. In the preantibiotic era the mortality rate from pneumococcal pneumonia in infants and small children ranged from 20 to 50 per cent and in older children from 3 to 5 per cent. Furthermore, the incidence of chronic empyema with altered pulmonary function was relatively high. With appropriate antimicrobial therapy instituted early in the course of the illness, the mortality rate during infancy and childhood is now less than 1 per cent, and long-term morbidity correspondingly low.

TREATMENT. The drug of choice is penicillin G, since all pneumococci are highly susceptible to this agent. In infants and young children a dose of 25,000 to 50,000 units/kg/day is administered parenterally; a single daily intramuscular injection of the procaine form usually suffices. In older children the total dose of penicillin need not exceed 1,000,000 units per day unless empyema or another suppurative complication is being treated concurrently. If allergy prevents the use of penicillin, erythromycin, a cephalosporin or a sulfonamide may be substituted.

The majority of older children with pneumonia can be treated at home, the decision to hospitalize depending on the degree of certainty of diagnosis and the severity of illness, the physical adequacy of the home and the ability of the mother or other members of the family to supply good nursing care. Pneumonia in the young infant is best treated in the hospital, since fluids may have to be administered intravenously. Furthermore, the course of illness in young infants is more variable and complications more common. Pneumonia associated with pleural effusion or empyema is best treated in the hospital. Bed rest, liberal oral intake of fluids and the administration of aspirin for high fever are the principal adjuncts to therapy. The prompt administration of oxygen in patients with significant respiratory distress will greatly reduce the need for sedatives and analgesics, and it should be given long before the patient becomes cyanotic.

Streptococcal Pneumonia

Group A streptococci most commonly cause disease limited to the upper respiratory tract, but the organisms may spread to other areas of the body, including the lower respiratory tract. Streptococcal pneumonia and tracheobronchitis are uncommon, but certain viral infections, particularly the exanthems and epidemic influenza, predispose to these diseases, which are most frequently encountered in the child 3 to 5 years of age, and very rarely in the infant.

PATHOLOGY. Streptococcal infection of the lower respiratory tract may result in tracheitis, bronchitis or interstitial pneumonia. Lesions consist of necrosis of the tracheobronchial mucosa with formation of ragged ulcers and large amounts of exudate, edema and localized hemorrhage. The process may extend into the interalveolar septa and involve the lymphatic vessels. Infection may spread by way of the lymphatics to the mediastinal and hilar lymph nodes, or may proceed in a retrograde direction in occluded vessels and reach the pleural surfaces. Pleurisy is relatively common with streptococcal pneumonia; the effusion is often large and serous, occasionally serosanguineous, or thinly purulent, with a lower fibrin content than the exudate of pneumococcal pneumonia.

CLINICAL MANIFESTATIONS. The signs and symptoms of streptococcal pneumonia are similar to those of pneumococcal pneumonia. The onset may be sudden and characterized by high fever, chills, signs of respiratory distress and, at times, extreme prostration. On occasion the child appears only mildly ill, with cough and a low-grade fever. If an exanthem or influenza precedes the pneumonia, the onset may be seen only as an increasingly severe clinical course of the viral illness. Since streptococcal pneumonia is commonly an interstitial inflammatory process, the clinical findings on examination of the chest may be less impressive than the disseminated infiltration noted on x-ray examination. Serous or purulent pleurisy will be evidenced by the clinical findings characteristic of pleural fluid.

LABORATORY FINDINGS. The peripheral leukocyte count is elevated, with a predominance of polymorphonuclear cells. A rise in the serum antistreptolysin titer is supportive diagnostic evidence. Cultures should be taken from the nasopharynx and blood, and from pleural fluid when present. Isolation of group A streptococci from the nasopharynx alone does not establish the cause of the pneumonia; bacteremia occurs in approximately 10 per cent of cases.

DIFFERENTIAL DIAGNOSIS. The clinical course and radiographic findings of patients with streptococcal pneumonia with purulent pleurisy are often similar to those found with staphylococcal pneumonia. Pneumatoceles may be noted on x-ray examination in both conditions. The roentgenographic changes of uncomplicated streptococcal pneumonia may be indistinguishable from those of other interstitial pneumonitides, including those caused by *Mycoplasma pneumoniae* (primary atypical pneumonia). Chills and leukocytosis are more commonly observed in streptococcal pneumonia than in mycoplasma pneumonia.

COMPLICATIONS. Bacterial complications are common, as is long-term morbidity in the untreated patient. Empyema occurs in about 20 per cent of children. Occasionally septic foci develop in other areas such as the bones or joints, but otherwise, extension of the disease is uncommon. Acute glomerulonephritis occurs rarely.

THERAPY. Penicillin G is the drug of choice and should be given parenterally in a dose of 25,000 to 50,000 units/kg/day in infants and from 500,000 to a million units per day in children. If empyema develops, a thoracentesis should be performed for diagnostic purposes and to remove the fluid. On occasion, closed drainage with indwelling chest tubes may be required if the fluid reaccumulates. The intrathoracic administration of antimicrobial agents or enzymes to liquefy pus or dissolve fibrin does not contribute to the effectiveness of therapy.

Staphylococcal Pneumonia

(See also Section 7)

Pneumonia caused by *S. aureus* is a serious and rapidly progressive infection which, unless recognized early and treated appropriately, is associated with prolonged morbidity and high mortality. It occurs less frequently than pneumococcal or viral pneumonias and is more common in infants than in children.

EPIDEMIOLOGY. The incidence of staphylococcal pneumonia is highest during the winter months (October through May), corresponding to the season of greatest incidence of upper respiratory tract infections. As with other bacterial pneumonias, it is frequently preceded by a viral upper respiratory tract infection. Although staphylococcal pneumonia may occur at any age, 30 per cent of all cases occur under 3 months of age and 70 per cent before 1 year.

Although *S. aureus* is commonly found on normal human skin and mucous membranes, serious disease is comparatively rare. Colonization of these surfaces begins early; nearly 90 per cent of normal infants become nasal carriers in the neonatal period. The carrier rate gradually declines to approximately 20 per cent during the first 2 years of life, and then rises so that by age 4 to 6 years the adult rate of 30 to 50 per cent is achieved.

The occurrence of epidemics of staphylococcal disease in nurseries is usually associated with certain specific pathogenic strains, identifiable by phage or serologic typing; they are commonly resistant to many antibiotics. Even during these outbreaks most of the colonized infants and hospital personnel or family contacts remain free from staphylococcal disease, but these healthy contacts may serve to spread the infection to others. The infant may exhibit disease within a few days after colonization or not until weeks later; most staphylococcal pneumonias of infancy are caused by organisms acquired in the nursery. Viral respiratory infections play a significant role in promoting dissemination of the staphylococcus among infants, and in converting colonization to disease.

PATHOGENICITY AND PATHOLOGY. *Staphylococcus aureus* produces a variety of toxins and enzymes. Among the more important of these are the following: (1) hemolysin, which has been shown in certain animals to lyse red blood cells, to produce local necrosis after intradermal injection, and to be lethal if given intravenously; (2) leukocidin, which destroys human leukocytes by causing degranulation and membrane disruption; (3) staphylokinase, which causes clot dissolution by activation of plasma plasminogen; and (4) coagulase, which interacts with a plasma factor to produce an active principle which converts fibrinogen to fibrin and thereby causes clot formation. A good correlation exists between coagulase production and virulence. Coagulase-negative staphylococci rarely produce serious disease.

Staphylococci cause confluent bronchopneumonia characterized by the presence of extensive areas of hemorrhagic necrosis and irregular areas of cavitation. The pleural surface is usually covered by a thick layer of fibrinopurulent exudate. Multiple abscesses occur, containing clusters of staphylococci, leukocytes, erythrocytes and necrotic debris. Rupture of a small subpleural abscess may result in a pyopneumothorax, which in turn may erode into a bronchus, producing a bronchopleural fistula. Septic thrombi may form in pulmonary veins in regions of extensive destruction and inflammation.

CLINICAL MANIFESTATIONS. Most commonly the patient is an infant less than a year of age, often with a history of staphylococcal skin lesions and signs and symptoms of an upper or lower respiratory tract infection for several days to a week. Abruptly the infant's condition changes, with the onset of fever, cough and evidence of respiratory distress. Signs and symptoms include tachypnea, grunting respirations, sternal and subcostal retractions, cyanosis and anxiety. If left undisturbed, the infant appears lethargic, but upon arousal is irritable. Severe dyspnea and a shock-like state may be present. Some infants have associated gastrointestinal disturbances characterized by vomiting, anorexia, diarrhea and, occasionally, abdominal distention. The rapid progression of symptoms is characteristic of staphylococcal pneumonia.

Physical findings depend on the stage of pneumonia. Early in the course of illness diminished breath sounds, scattered rales, and rhonchi are commonly heard over the affected lung. With the development of effusion or pyopneumothorax, dullness on percussion is noted, and breath sounds and vocal fremitus are markedly diminished. A lag in respiratory excursion often occurs on the affected side. Physical examination may, however, be misleading, particularly in the young infant with meager findings disproportionate to the degree of tachypnea.

LABORATORY FINDINGS. In the older infant and child a leukocytosis of 20,000 or more cells per mm^3 usually occurs, with the increase primarily among the polymorphonuclear cells; in the young infant the white blood cell count may remain within the normal range. As in other forms of bacterial infection, a count below 5000 cells is a poor prognostic sign. Mild to moderate anemia is common.

Material for diagnostic cultures should be obtained by tracheal aspiration or from a pleural tap. The finding of staphylococci in the nasopharynx is of no diagnostic value. Bacteremia is demonstrable in 10 per cent or less of affected infants.

ROENTGENOGRAPHIC FINDINGS. Most patients with staphylococcal pneumonia will have radiographic evidence of bronchopneumonia early in the illness. The infiltrate may be patchy and limited in extent or be dense and homogeneous and involve an entire lobe or hemithorax. The right lung alone is involved in about 65 per cent of cases; bilateral involvement occurs in fewer than 20 per cent of patients. A pleural effusion or empyema will be noted during the course in most patients; pyopneumothorax occurs in about one fourth. Pneumatoceles of varying size are common

Though no roentgenographic change can be considered diagnostic, progression over a few hours from bronchopneumonia to effusion or pyopneumothorax with or without pneumatoceles is highly suggestive of staphylococcal pneumonia. Chest films should be obtained at frequent intervals if the diagnosis of early staphylococcal pneumonia is suspected. Clinical improvement usually precedes x-ray clearing by days or weeks, and pneumatoceles may persist asymptomatically for months.

DIFFERENTIAL DIAGNOSIS. The recognition of early staphylococcal pneumonia in the infant is often difficult. Abrupt onset and rapid progression of symptoms of pneumonia should be considered due to staphylococci until proved otherwise. A history of furunculosis, a preceding viral upper respiratory tract infection, a recent hospital admission or maternal breast abscess should also alert the physician to the possibility of this diagnosis in the infant.

Other bacterial pneumonias cause empyema or pneumatoceles and may thus be readily confused with staphylococcal disease. These include streptococcal, klebsiella, *H, influenzae* and pneumococcal pneumonias and primary tuberculous pneumonia with cavitation. Occasionally the aspiration of a nonradiopaque foreign body followed by pulmonary abscesses may lead to a similar clinical and radiologic picture.

COMPLICATIONS. Since empyema, pyopneumothorax and pneumatoceles are so commonly seen with staphylococcal pneumonia, they are considered part of the natural course of the illness and not complications. Septic lesions outside the respiratory tract occur rarely except in the young infant, in whom staphylococcal pericarditis, meningitis, osteomyelitis and multiple metastatic abscesses in soft tissue have been recorded.

PROGNOSIS. The case fatality rate ranges from 5 to 40 per cent and varies with the length of illness prior to hospitalization, the age of the patient, adequacy of therapy, and the presence of other illnesses and complications. Early recognition and immediate, adequate therapy are usually effective. The course is usually prolonged, the hospital stay often being 6 to 10 weeks. The long-term morbidity is very low. Five-year follow-up examinations of recovered patients with staphylococcal pneumonia generally have revealed normal growth and development, with no increase in susceptibility to pulmonary infections and with normal pulmonary function.

THERAPY. Treatment of staphylococcal pneumonia consists in control of microorganisms with antimicrobial therapy and surgical drainage of collections of pus. The infant should be placed in oxygen in a semireclining position to relieve cyanosis and allay anxiety. During the acute phase of illness, caloric intake and hydration should be maintained intravenously. If the patient is severely anemic, blood transfusion may be beneficial.

Upon completion of diagnostic procedures, antimicrobial therapy must be initiated immediately when staphylococcal pneumonia is suspected. Methicillin in a dosage of 250 to 300 mg/kg/day should be administered parenterally. Since methicillin is potentially nephrotoxic, urinalysis should be performed daily to detect hematuria and increasing proteinuria. If the culture demonstrates that the responsible staphylococcus is susceptible to penicillin G, then this agent should be given in a dosage of approximately 100,000 to 200,000 units/kg/day. There is no advantage to the concurrent use of several drugs; such use increases the frequency of adverse reactions. The duration of antimicrobial therapy should be in accordance with the clinical response of the patient; in the average patient 3 weeks is adequate.

When infection extends to the pleural surfaces, surgical intervention usually becomes necessary. With small effusions or empyema, repeated pleural taps may on occasion result in adequate removal of fluid, but generally pus reaccumulates so rapidly and is of such high viscosity that closed drainage is necessary, with a chest tube of the largest possible caliber. The appearance of pyopneumothorax is another indication for the immediate insertion of a catheter into the pleural space. It is often necessary to utilize several chest tubes when loculation occurs. Once the infant begins to improve and the lung has re-expanded, the tubes may be removed, even if they are still draining small amounts of pus. In general, tubes should not remain in the chest more than 5 to 7 days.

The instillation of antimicrobial agents or enzymes into the chest cavity does not help to control the infection or to promote drainage; in infants this procedure is associated with an increased incidence of pneumothorax and systemic toxic reactions.

Pneumonia Caused by Gram-negative Organisms

Gram-negative organisms have accounted for fewer than 1 per cent of pneumonias in infants and children beyond the immediate postnatal period. (See Section 7) The number, however, has increased in recent years, owing to the widespread use of antibiotics, to contamination of hospital equipment such as oxygen and humidification apparatus, and to the increasing use of immunosuppressive agents in the treatment of malignant disorders. The gram-negative organisms most commonly encountered are *H. influenzae* type b, *Klebsiella pneumoniae* and *Pseudomonas aeruginosa;* other organisms have occasionally been incriminated. The morbidity and mortality from these infections are rather high as a result of the pathogenicity of the bacteria and the altered host resistance in many of these patients.

HEMOPHILUS INFLUENZAE PNEUMONIA. *Hemophilus influenzae* type b is one of the more frequent causes of serious bacterial infections in infants and young children. Nontypable *H. influenzae* are routinely found in the nasopharynx of normal persons; initial encounter with a type-specific encapsulated strain, however, especially with type b, usually results in a mild, febrile upper respiratory tract infection followed by lasting immunity. Nasopharyngeal infection precedes virtually all the clinical varieties of localized *H. influenzae* disease, such as otitis media, epiglottitis, pneumonia and meningitis. The factors that determine whether a child will have a mild upper respiratory tract infection or serious disease are not understood. A synergistic action has been demonstrated between *H. influenzae* and certain respiratory viruses, such as the influenza virus, or certain bacteria, such as the staphylococcus. This synergism in some way alters the dynamics of the bacterial population on respiratory epithelium and promotes the growth of bacteria which may result in pyogenic disease. An example of this phenomenon occurred in the viral influenza pandemic of 1918, when a high incidence of serious lower respiratory tract disease due to *H. influenzae* was noted.

Hemophilus influenzae pneumonia is usually lobar in distribution. Disseminated pulmonary disease and bronchopneumonia have also been described. Microscopic examination of lung tissue usually reveals extensive destruction of the bronchial and bronchiolar epithelium, interstitial inflammation and hemorrhagic edema. As with *H. influenzae* infection of the larynx, edema is often striking.

Clinically *H. influenzae* pneumonia is difficult to differentiate from pneumococcal pneumonia; in contrast to pneumococcal infection, however, the onset of illness is often insidious, and the clinical course is usually subacute and prolonged over several weeks. In the young infant the disease is often associated with bacteremia and frequently with empyema.

The diagnosis may be difficult to establish. Predominant growth of *H. influenzae* type b in the nasopharynx is suggestive evidence of the cause, but only isolation of the organism from the blood, pleural fluid or lung aspirate confirms the diagnosis. The usual radiographic findings are those of a lobar pneumonia. There is a moderate leukocytosis, with a relative lymphopenia.

Complications are frequent, particularly in the young infant, and include bacteremia, pericarditis, cellulitis, empyema, meningitis and pyarthrosis.

Treatment consists of the same symptomatic and supportive measures utilized in pneumococcal and staphylococcal pneumonias. When *H. influenzae* is suspected as the causative agent, ampicillin is the antimicrobial agent of choice and is given parenterally in a dosage of 100 to 150 mg/kg/day. The development of empyema or pyarthrosis usually necessitates immediate surgical drainage.

FRIEDLÄNDER'S BACILLUS (KLEBSIELLA PNEUMONIAE) PNEUMONIA. *Klebsiella pneumoniae* is found in the respiratory and gastrointestinal tracts of approximately 5 per cent of normal persons. It is known to cause pneumonia in elderly patients and in those with diabetes mellitus, and frequently occurs as a secondary invader in the lungs of patients with chronic bronchiectasis, influenza or tuberculosis. Primary *Kl. pneumoniae* infection is unusual in infants and young children; it may occur, rarely, in nursery epidemics. During these epidemics many infants will carry the organism in their nasopharynges without signs of clinical illness; only an occasional baby will have severe disease. Contaminated fomites, including nursery equipment and humidification apparatus, are the primary source of nosocomial infection with the organism.

Pneumonia due to *Kl. pneumoniae* may be difficult to distinguish clinically from pneumonia due to other causes. In nursery epidemics, diarrhea and vomiting may be the presenting symptoms; the

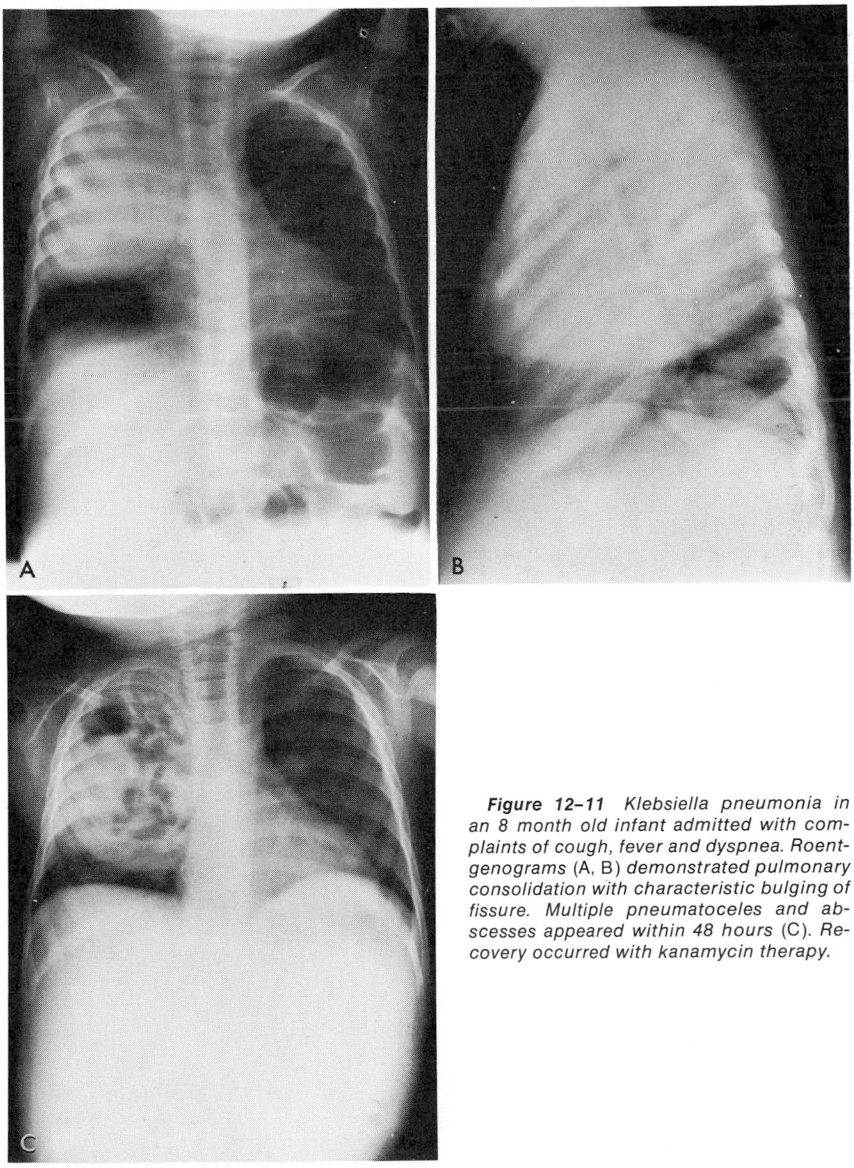

Figure 12–11 *Klebsiella pneumonia in an 8 month old infant admitted with complaints of cough, fever and dyspnea. Roentgenograms (A, B) demonstrated pulmonary consolidation with characteristic bulging of fissure. Multiple pneumatoceles and abscesses appeared within 48 hours (C). Recovery occurred with kanamycin therapy.*

onset of respiratory difficulty is often abrupt. The disease may have a fulminant course characterized by copious, thick, purulent secretions and the formation of pulmonary abscesses and cavitation. A lobar infiltrate with bulging fissures on radiographic examination is suggestive of klebsiella pneumonia (Fig. 12–11). Complications are common and include bacteremia, empyema and residual parenchymal damage. The case fatality rate in sporadic cases is about 50 per cent, but is lower during epidemics.

Isolation of the organism from purulent tracheal secretions, blood or lung aspirate establishes the diagnosis. Supportive treatment is similar to that given for other bacterial pneumonias; surgical intervention may be necessary to drain empyema or abscesses. The antimicrobial agent of choice is usually kanamycin, 15 mg/kg/day given intramuscularly every 8 hours for 10 to 14 days. If the organism is resistant to kanamycin, gentamicin may be employed with equally favorable results.

PSEUDOMONAS AERUGINOSA PNEUMONIA. (See also Section 10.) *Pseudomonas aeruginosa* produces a severe, progressive, usually fatal, necrotizing bronchopneumonia. It is rarely a primary infection of the lung, but occurs with chronic debilitating illnesses such as cystic fibrosis and malignant disorders, with altered immunologic function, during prolonged antimicrobial therapy and in premature infants exposed to contaminated hospital equipment. Carbenicillin administered alone or in combination with gentamicin represents the most effective therapy.

GEORGE H. MCCRACKEN, JR.
HEINZ F. EICHENWALD

GENERAL

Shuttleworth, D. B., and Charney, E.: Leukocyte count in childhood pneumonia. Am. J. Dis. Child. *122*:393, 1971.

Pneumococcal Pneumonia

Hodges, R. C., and MacLeod, C. M.: Epidemic pneumococcal pneumonia. V. Final considerations of factors underlying epidemic. Am. J. Hyg., *44*:237, 1946.

MacLeod, C. M.: The pneumococci: *In* Dubos, R., and Hirsch, J. (eds.): Bacterial and Mycotic Infections of Man. 4th ed. Philadelphia, J. B. Lippincott Company, 1965, Chap. 16.

Smith, M. H. C.: Pneumococcal pneumonia: *In* Kendig, E. L., Jr. (ed.): Disorders of the Respiratory Tract in Children. 2nd ed. Philadelphia, W. B. Saunders Company, 1972.

Wood, B. W.: Pneumococcal pneumonia: *In* Beeson, P., and McDermott, W. (eds.): Cecil-Loeb Textbook of Medicine. 13th ed. Philadelphia, W. B. Saunders Company, 1971.

Streptococcal Pneumonia

Keefer, C. S., Rantz, A., and Rammelkamp, C. H.: Hemolytic streptococcal pneumonia and empyema: A study of 55 cases with special reference to treatment. Ann. Intern. Med. *14*:1533, 1941.

Kevy, S. V., and Lowe, B. A.: Streptococcal pneumonia and empyema in childhood. New Engl. J. Med. *264*:738, 1961.

Staphylococcal Pneumonia

Ceruti, E., Contreras, J., and Neira, M.: Staphylococcal pneumonia in childhood; Long term follow-up. Am. J. Dis. Child. *122*:386, 1971.

Eichenwald, H. F., and Shinefield, H. R.: The problem of staphylococcal infection in newborn infants. J. Pediatr. *56*:665, 1960.

Forbes, G. B., and Emerson, G. L.: Staphylococcal pneumonia and empyema. Pediat. Clin. N. Amer. *4*:215, 1957.

Huxtable, K. A., Tucket, A. S., and Wedgwood, R. J.: Staphylococcal pneumonia in childhood; long-term follow-up. Am. J. Dis. Child., *108*:262, 1964.

Rebhan, A. W., and Edwards, H. E.: Staphylococcal pneumonia: A review of 329 cases. Canad. Med. Assoc. J. *82*:513, 1960.

Pneumonia Caused by Gram-negative Organisms

Nyhan, W. L., Rectanus, D. R., and Fousek, M. D.: Hemophilus influenzae type b pneumonia. Pediatrics *16*:31, 1955.

Riley, H. D., and Bracken, E. C.: Empyema due to Hemophilus influenzae in infants and children. Am. J. Dis. Child. *110*:24, 1965.

Friedländer's Bacillus (Klebsiella Pneumoniae) Pneumonia

Morgan, H. R.: The enteric bacteria. *In* Dubos, R., and Hirsch, J. (eds.): Bacterial and mycotic infections of man. 4th ed. Philadelphia, J. B. Lippincott Company, 1965.

Thaler, M. M.: Klebsiella-Aerobacter pneumonia in infants. Pediatrics *30*:206, 1962.

PNEUMONIAS OF VIRAL ORIGIN

Acute Bronchiolitis

Acute bronchiolitis, a syndrome of respiratory tract obstruction at the bronchiolar level, is a common disease of the lower respiratory tract of infants. It occurs during the first 2 years of life, with a peak incidence at approximately 6 months of age, and, in many localities, is the most frequent cause of hospitalization of infants. The incidence is highest during the winter and early spring months. The illness occurs both sporadically and epidemically.

ETIOLOGY. Acute bronchiolitis is a viral illness. The respiratory syncytial virus has been incriminated as the causative agent in over 50 per cent of cases; the parainfluenza 3 virus, the Eaton agent (mycoplasma), some adenoviruses and occasionally other viruses, some probably not yet identified, produce the remaining cases. There is no firm evidence to support the view that bacteria cause this condition. Occasionally, bacterial bronchopneumonia may produce generalized obstructive emphysema and thus be confused clinically with bronchiolitis.

PATHOPHYSIOLOGY. The most important pathologic lesion of acute bronchiolitis is bronchiolar obstruction due to edema and accumulation of mucus and cellular debris, and invasion of the smaller radicles of the bronchial tree by virus. Since resistance to airflow in a tube is inversely related to the cube of the radius, even minor thickening of the bronchiolar wall in infants may produce a profound effect on airflow. Resistance to airflow in the small air passages is increased during both the inspiratory and expiratory phases, but is relatively greater during expiration. Partial (ball-valve) respiratory obstruction leads to air trapping and emphysema. Atelectasis occurs when obstruction becomes complete and trapped air is absorbed.

The pathologic process impairs the normal exchange of gases in the lung. Diminished ventilation of the alveoli results in hypoxemia. Carbon dioxide retention (hypercapnia) usually does not occur in mild cases of bronchiolitis, since adjacent functioning alveoli can compensate for the poor ventilation of their neighbors. But if a critical proportion of the alveoli are obstructed, such compensation becomes inadequate, and hypercapnia and respiratory acidosis occur. Generally the higher the respiratory rate, the lower the arterial oxygen tension. Carbon dioxide retention is usually not found until respirations exceed 60 per minute; it then increases in proportion to the tachypnea.

CLINICAL MANIFESTATIONS. Most affected infants have a history of exposure to older children or adults with minor respiratory diseases within the week preceding onset of illness. The infant is first noted to have a serous nasal discharge and sneezing. These symptoms usually last several days and may be accompanied by fever of 101 to 102° F and diminished appetite. There is then the gradual development of respiratory distress, characterized by paroxysmal, wheezy cough, dyspnea and irritability. On occasion, in the more severely affected patients, these symptoms may develop more rapidly, within several hours. Other systemic manifestations such as vomiting and diarrhea are usually absent; the infant is commonly afebrile or has only a low-grade fever or may be hypothermic.

Examination reveals a tachypneic infant, often in extreme distress. Respirations range from 60 to 80 per minute; severe air hunger and cyanosis may be present. There is flaring of the alae nasi, and use of the accessory muscles of respiration results in intercostal and subcostal retractions, but these are shallow, owing to the persistent distention of the lungs by the trapped air. (See Respiratory Physiology in earlier pages.) The liver and the spleen may be palpable several centimeters below the costal margins as a result of depression of the diaphragm due to emphysema.

Widespread fine rales may be heard at the end of inspiration and in early expiration. The expiratory phase of breathing may be prolonged, and wheezes are audible, particularly in the later course of illness. In the most severe cases, breath sounds are barely audible when bronchiolitic obstruction is nearly complete.

Roentgenographic examination reveals hyperinflation of the lungs and an increased anteroposterior diameter on lateral view. Scattered areas of consolidation are found in about a third of patients and are due either to atelectasis secondary to obstruction or to inflammation of the alveoli. Early bacterial pneumonia cannot be excluded as a diagnostic possibility on radiographic grounds alone.

The white blood cell count is usually within normal limits. Lymphopenia, commonly associated with many viral illnesses, is usually not found. Nasopharyngeal cultures reveal normal flora except when the viral pathogen alters the ecology of the flora to allow growth of such microorganisms as *H. influenzae,* pneumococci or staphylococci. The presence of these bacteria does not imply that they are responsible for the illness.

DIFFERENTIAL DIAGNOSIS. The condition most commonly confused with acute bronchiolitis is bronchial asthma. Asthma occurs uncommonly in the first year of life, but frequently after this period. The presence of one or more of the following favors the diagnosis of asthma: a family history of asthma, repeated attacks in the same infant, sudden onset without preceding infection, markedly prolonged expiration, eosinophilia, and an immediate favorable response to the administration of a small dose of epinephrine. Repeated attacks represent an important differential point: fewer than 5 per cent of recurrent attacks of clinical bronchiolitis with obstructive emphysema have viral infections as a cause. Other entities which may be confused with acute bronchiolitis are congestive heart failure, foreign body in the trachea, pertussis, cystic fibrosis and bacterial bronchopneumonias associated with generalized obstructive emphysema.

COURSE AND PROGNOSIS. The most critical phase of illness occurs during the first 48 to 72 hours after the onset of cough and dyspnea. It is during this period that the infant appears desperately ill, when apneic spells occur in the very small infant and when respiratory acidosis is likely to be noted. After the critical period improvement occurs rapidly and often dramatically. Recovery is complete in a few days. The case fatality rate is below 1 per cent; death may result from prolonged apneic spells, severe uncompensated respiratory acidosis, or profound dehydration secondary to loss of water vapor from tachypnea and the inability to drink fluids. Infants with such complications as congenital heart disease or cystic fibrosis have a higher mortality. Bacterial complications, such as bronchopneumonia or otitis media, are uncommon. Cardiac failure during bronchiolitis is rare. It has been reported that a significant proportion of infants with bronchiolitis have asthma during later childhood, but the interrelation of these two entities, if any, is not understood.

TREATMENT. Treatment is symptomatic. It is common practice to place the patient in an atmosphere of high humidity, produced by cold vapor, but there is no evidence to indicate that this procedure is of benefit. Patients with dyspnea, whether cyanotic or not, should receive oxygen therapy. This serves not only to relieve the dyspnea and cyanosis, but also to allay anxiety and restlessness. Sedatives should be avoided whenever possible, owing to potential depression of respiration. When a sedative must be given, paraldehyde or chloral hydrate is preferred. The infant is usually more comfortable if head and chest are slightly elevated in such a way that the neck is slightly extended. Tachypnea has a dehydrating effect, and oral intake of fluids must often be supplemented by parenteral fluids. In the event of respiratory acidosis, electrolyte balance and pH should be adjusted by suitable intravenous solutions.

Since acute bronchiolitis is a viral illness, antimicrobial agents have no therapeutic value. Even in cases caused by the Eaton agent, no drug has been shown to have an effect on the course or outcome of the illness. The low incidence of bacterial complications is not made lower by antimicrobial therapy. Corticosteroids have not proved to be beneficial in bronchiolitis and may, under certain conditions, be harmful. Bronchodilating drugs are of no value; their use is, in fact, contraindicated, since they increase restlessness and oxygen requirement. Because the obstruction of bronchiolitis occurs at the bronchiolar level, tracheotomy cannot be expected to produce much benefit. The theoretical advantage which might be obtained by decreasing the dead air space of the respiratory passage is outweighed by the risk of performing this procedure in the acutely ill infant and the high rate of complications.

When bronchial asthma is considered a diagnostic possibility, a therapeutic trial of a single dose of hypodermically administered epinephrine may be tried. If there is no response to this therapy within a short time, no additional epinephrine or other bronchodilators should be administered.

Primary Atypical Pneumonia
(Eaton Agent Pneumonia)

In the late 1930's the term "primary atypical pneumonia" was coined to describe a group of nonbacterial pneumonias presenting with an acute onset, moderate to severe constitutional symptoms, cough, and pulmonary infiltrates on radiographic examination with minimal or absent physical signs. Cold agglutinins were often found.

ETIOLOGY. It has become evident that atypical pneumonia represents a syndrome with multiple causes. The respiratory syncytial virus, influenza viruses A and B, parainfluenza type 3 and adenoviruses as well as certain of the rickettsiae are proved causative agents. These agents, however, are not regularly associated with those cases of atypical pneumonia characterized by elevated levels of cold agglutinins. In adults atypical pneumonia with cold agglutinins is a distinct epidemiologic and etiologic entity caused generally by *M. pneumoniae* (Eaton agent), which is one of the Mycoplasmataceae, the smallest free-living organisms, similar in size to the myxoviruses).

EPIDEMIOLOGY. Unlike the influenza and respiratory syncytial viruses, *M. pneumoniae* does not produce sharply defined epidemics. Instead, infection occurs throughout the year, but most frequently during the early fall and winter months. The incidence and morbidity of mycoplasma pneumonia are higher in males than in females, particularly in the younger age groups. Though the organism causes lower respiratory tract illness in all ages, the majority of cases occur in childhood and through the third decade of life.

In an urban population the yearly incidence of mycoplasma pneumonia was found to be 1 to 1.5 cases per 1000 persons; in such closed populations as in military installations or institutions for the mentally retarded the annual incidence may be as high as 10 per 1000. These limited epidemics are caused by direct transmission by way of respiratory secretions, the degree of contact determining the contagiousness. The disease is not limited in its geographic distribution, and wide fluctuations in prevalence can occur in a given locality.

PATHOLOGY. The pathology of *M. pneumoniae* infection is not well known, since few patients die. The lungs usually have normal pleural surfaces, but occasionally there are patches of fibrinous pleural exudate. Areas of inflammation may be extensive or discrete, circumscribed and multiple. Nodular focal lesions resembling miliary granulomas may be present. Various stages of consolidation are seen, as well as areas of atelectasis and emphysema.

Microscopically the principal pathologic process consists of an interstitial pneumonia with areas of necrotizing bronchitis and bronchiolitis. There is necrosis of the epithelial lining cells of the respiratory passages, with desquamation and ulceration of the mucosa. The alveolar walls are hyperemic, and the septa are thickened, with round cell infiltration and edema.

CLINICAL MANIFESTATIONS. The effects of *M. pneumoniae* range from inapparent infection to pharyngitis, bullous myringitis, bronchitis, bronchiolitis and pneumonia. Most human infections do not become clinically apparent; it is estimated that only 3 to 10 per cent of infected persons develop pneumonia.

The incubation period ranges from 1 to 3 weeks, averaging 12 to 14 days. The course of illness is extremely variable, particularly in the younger age groups. The onset is usually insidious; the initial complaints are often constitutional and nonspecific, such as headache, malaise, fever, chilliness, fatigue and anorexia. The principal respiratory symptoms include sore throat and cough. The cough is the most frequent and characteristic feature; it is usually dry in the initial stages, but may become productive of moderate amounts of blood-streaked sputum later in the illness. Headache is often a complaint, particularly in the older child. The duration and degree of fever vary widely; it is usually remittent and terminates by lysis in 4 to 14 days.

Generally the older child and the adult do not appear to be as ill as the degree of fever might indicate. The pulse is slow in relation to the fever, and the respiratory rate is normal or slightly increased. Severe degrees of dyspnea are uncommon, and cyanosis is rare. The paucity of abnormal physical findings is striking; often there are none at all. The throat may be mildly injected, and there may be slight enlargement of the cervical lymph nodes. The most characteristic finding late in the course of illness is the presence of fine, crepitant rales over the chest, with no signs of consolidation. A few patients have a maculopapular or urticarial rash, which usually disappears within 48 hours.

Roentgenographic examination often shows evidence of pneumonia before physical signs are apparent. Characteristically the infiltrate appears to be most dense at the hilus and becomes progressively more feathery toward the periphery. The lesions may be confined to one lobe, more commonly a lower lobe, or may be present in several or all lobes. It is not uncommon for the infiltrate to spread, with resolution of early lesions as new infiltrates appear. Small pleural effusions are seen in approximately 20 per cent of patients. The roentgenographic changes are not distinctive or diagnostic.

LABORATORY FINDINGS. The white blood cell count usually remains within normal limits. *Mycoplasma pneumoniae* may be recovered from pharyngeal swabs or sputum for as long as 4 weeks after infection. A specific serologic response can be demonstrated by immunofluorescent techniques or by complement fixation and hemagglutination inhibition tests.

Some patients with atypical pneumonia have a variety of nonspecific immunologic reactions. Most adults with mycoplasma pneumonia develop cold hemagglutinins for group O human erythrocytes. Maximum titers are usually reached by the third or fourth week after onset of illness. Many of these patients also develop agglutinins for the MG strain of nonhemolytic streptococci. In children the development of cold agglutinins is erratic, and only a minority of patients have increases in titer. Cold agglutinins are also associated with lung infections due to other agents; the appearance of this antibody in children is related more to the degree of pulmonary involvement than to the specific cause.

DIAGNOSIS. The clinical picture of atypical pneumonia associated with *M. pneumoniae* is not sufficiently distinctive to allow differentiation from pneumonic processes caused by viral and rickettsial agents. In children a specific diagnosis can be made only if the causative agent is recovered or a rise in titer of specific antibody is demonstrated.

COURSE AND PROGNOSIS. The duration of the acute illness averages 8 to 10 days, with a convalescent period of an additional week. Complications are unusual, and the prognosis is excellent.

TREATMENT. Treatment is symptomatic, and hospitalization is rarely necessary. *Mycoplasma pneumoniae* is susceptible in vitro to the tetracyclines and to erythromycin. Although several studies have shown these agents to be useful in adults, the course of illness in children is not significantly altered by antibiotics.

Giant Cell Pneumonia
(Hecht's Pneumonia)

Giant cell pneumonia is an uncommon interstitial pneumonitis of infancy and childhood. A definitive diagnosis depends on histologic demonstration of characteristic multinuclear giant cells with intranuclear and intracytoplasmic inclusion bodies in the lung. There are also a mononuclear infiltrate, squamous metaplasia of the bronchial and bronchiolar epithelium, proliferation of the alveolar lining cells and the occasional occurrence of giant cells in organs other than the lungs. There are some clinical and histologic similarities to distemper (a measles-like illness of animals); moreover, patients often develop giant cell pneumonia after measles. Rubeola virus has been recovered from the lung tissue of patients with giant cell pneumonia who had no clinical evidence of measles or had leukemia complicated by measles infection. The giant cell formation seen in Hecht's pneumonia and in cystic fibrosis is not, on the other hand, a histologic feature of the pneumonia commonly encountered with clinical measles. In the former group the process of giant cell formation originates in or near terminal bronchioles or alveoli, whereas in the latter it is of bronchial origin. Hecht's pneumonia may also follow immunization with attenuated measles vaccine in children who have leukemia or lymphomas, and in patients with deficiency of cell-mediated immunity.

Clinically patients with giant cell pneumonia have moderate to severe respiratory distress manifest principally by tachypnea and dyspnea. Inspiratory and early expiratory rales and musical sounds are heard, but dullness is rarely present. Some patients continue to excrete rubeola virus from the upper respiratory tract for weeks after the onset of illness. Roentgenographically there are usually generalized, patchy infiltrates with areas of overinflation.

The course of illness may be prolonged over several weeks; clinical improvement may occur days to weeks prior to roentgenographic improvement. Occasionally bacterial superinfection may occur. The mortality rate is high, particularly in patients with debilitating diseases such as leukemia, cystic fibrosis and immunologic deficiency states. Treatment is symptomatic; gamma globulin is of no value.

PNEUMONIAS OF MISCELLANEOUS CAUSES

Pneumocystis Carinii Pneumonia
(Interstitial Plasma Cell Pneumonia)

Interstitial plasma cell pneumonia is an unusual infection of newborn infants and occasionally of children and adults with altered host resistance. The disease is caused by the protozoan *Pneumocystis carinii,* a ubiquitous organism whose exact affinities remain unknown, since it has not been grown in vitro.

PATHOGENESIS AND PATHOLOGY. The majority of cases of *P. carinii* pneumonia occur among three different groups of patients: (1) premature and full-term infants; (2) patients under treatment for chronic debilitating illnesses, particularly leukemia and lymphoma; and (3) patients with primary immunologic deficiency syndromes.

In newborn infants an incompletely developed immunologic responsiveness and exposure to a humidified atmosphere contaminated with the parasite may interact synergistically to produce sporadic or epidemic disease in the nursery. In some infants intensive treatment of a respiratory tract infection with antibiotics may produce activation of a latent pneumocystic infection. Infants with cytomegalic inclusion disease or children with lymphoreticular malignancies treated with cytotoxic agents, corticosteroids or prolonged antimicrobial therapy are particularly susceptible to *P. carinii* pneumonia, as are patients with congenital or acquired immunologic deficiency diseases such as agammaglobulinemia and primary lymphopenic immune deficiency.

Infection with *P. carinii* produces a characteristic intra-alveolar exudate of lace-like appearance which contains histiocytes, lymphocytes and plasma cells. The plasma cells are diminished or absent in agammaglobulinemia and hypogammaglobulinemia. Pneumocystic cysts are demonstrable in the exudate by a special silver staining technique. In the alveolar septa there are varying degrees of edema, inflammation and fibrosis.

CLINICAL MANIFESTATIONS. The usual age at onset in infants is from the third to fifth week of life; in children with immunologic deficiency syndromes, onset ranges from 3 months to mid-childhood. It may be seen at any age in patients with acquired temporary or permanent loss of host resistance. The disease usually begins insidiously with cough and proceeds over a period of 1 to 4 weeks to severe respiratory distress. There is low-grade or no fever, and the absence or paucity of pulmonary findings to percussion and auscultation in a patient with severe distress is remarkable.

Roentgenographic findings are fairly characteristic. The lung fields are hyperexpanded and have a generalized granular pattern; bilateral pulmonary infiltrates, which originate at the hilus, extend peripherally and eventually create a nearly solid appearance. The overaeration is most pronounced in the periphery. The white blood cell count is usually within normal limits or moderately elevated.

DIAGNOSIS. The diagnosis of *P. carinii* pneumonia should be suspected in newborn infants and patients with altered host resistance who have severe respiratory distress with minimal physical findings and suggestive radiologic changes. The definitive diagnosis rests on the demonstration of the organism. At present a lung biopsy is the most satisfactory means of demonstrating the presence of *P. carinii;* silver stains of tracheal aspirates or of tonsillar smears may occasionally be satisfactory. A complement fixation test has been developed but is not generally available.

COURSE AND PROGNOSIS. *Pneumocystis carinii* pneumonia usually lasts from 3 to 6 weeks, but may continue over many months. The death rate is variable; in infants with no complicating illness the most recent European case fatality rate is about 15 per cent.

THERAPY. Pentamidine isothionate (obtainable from the Center for Disease Control of the U.S. Department of Health, Education, and Welfare, Atlanta, Georgia) results in a cure rate of at least 60 per cent if used early. Recent reports suggest that pyrimethamine and sulfadiazine may be a reasonable alternative type of therapy. Gamma globulin is usually not helpful, even in children with immunologic deficiency diseases or lymphoreticular malignancies. If the disease develops in a patient on immunosuppressant or corticosteroid therapy, it is usually advisable to reduce dosage or discontinue these drugs.

Acute Bronchiolitis

Heycock, J. B., and Noble, T. C.: 1230 cases of acute bronchiolitis in infancy. Brit. Med. J. *2*:879, 1962.

Reynolds, E. O. R.: Bronchiolitis. *In* Kendig, E. L., Jr. (ed.): Disorders of the Respiratory Tract in Children, 2nd ed. Philadelphia, W. B. Saunders Company, 1972, Chap. 11.

Wright, F. H., and Beem, M. O.: Diagnosis and treatment: Management of acute viral bronchiolitis in infancy. Pediatrics, *35*:334, 1965.

Primary Atypical Pneumonia (Eaton Agent Pneumonia)

Sussman, S. J., and others: Cold agglutinins, Eaton agent and respiratory infections of children. Pediatrics, *38*:571, 1966.

Pneumocystis Carinii Pneumonia (Interstitial Plasma Cell Pneumonia)

Bazar, G. R., Manfredi, O. L., Howard, R. G., and Claps, A. A.: Pneumocystis carinii pneumonia in three full-term siblings. J. Pediatr. *76*:767, 1970.

Marshall, W. C., Weston, H. J., and Bodian, M.: Pneumocystis carinii pneumonia and congenital hypogammaglobulinemia. Arch. Dis. Child. *39*:18, 1964.

Patterson, J. H., Lindsey, I. L., Edwards, E. S., and Logan, W. D.: Pneumocystis carinii pneumonia and altered host resistance. Pediatrics, *38*:388, 1966.

Robbins, J. B.: Pneumocystis carinii pneumonitis. A review. Pediat. Res., *1*:131, 1967.

Walzer, P. D., Perl, D. P., Donald, J. K., Rawson, P. G., and Schultz, M. G.: Pneumocystis carinii pneumonia in the United States. Ann. Intern. Med. *80*:83, 1974.

MYCOTIC PULMONARY INFECTIONS

See also Coccidioidomycosis, Histoplasmosis, Blastomycosis, Cryptococcosis, Mucormycosis, Nocardiosis and Sporotrichosis in Section 10.

Thrush Pneumonia
(Pulmonary Candidiasis)

Pulmonary infections with *Candida albicans* are rare in the pediatric age group in spite of the relatively high incidence of oral thrush (Section 11) in early infancy. This fact has been attributed to a natural resistance of columnar epithelium to invasion by the fungus. Emanuel summarized data on 17 cases (15 from the literature) in infants; the oldest was 8 weeks. All had respiratory distress; about half had oral thrush, but there was no clinical or roentgen characteristic to suggest the cause of the pulmonary infection. Cystic fibrosis may dispose to pulmonary candidiasis in infancy.

Emanuel, B., Lieberman, A. D., Goldin, M., and Samson, J.: Pulmonary Candidiasis in the Neonatal Period. J. Pediatr. *61*:44, 1962.

BRONCHIAL AND PULMONARY LESIONS SECONDARY TO ASPIRATION OF FOREIGN MATERIALS

Aspiration Pneumonia

For Fetal Anoxia with Excessive Aspiration of Amniotic Debris, see Section 7.

ASPIRATION OF FOOD. Infants with obstructive lesions, such as tracheo-esophageal fistula and duodenal obstruction, and weak and debilitated infants who have no obstructive lesions may aspirate, or regurgitate and then aspirate, an amount of food sufficient to cause significant pulmonary damage. Aspiration may rarely be an immediate cause of death by asphyxiation. More frequently the irritated mucous membrane becomes a site for bacterial invasion. Prophylaxis is of the greatest importance. Care should be taken to avoid amounts of feedings that will overdistend the stomach; this is especially true for infants whose feeding is by gavage. After the infant has been fed he should be placed on his abdomen or on his right side. When he is in the supine position, his head should not be lower than the rest of his body. While the infant is lying on his abdomen, however, drainage from the lungs may be materially aided by lowering the head of the bed.

ASPIRATION OF ZINC STEARATE. Aspiration pneumonia resulting from inhalation of zinc stearate powder, once relatively common, has become rare because of efforts discouraging the use of this powder for infants. Containers have also been equipped with an automatic closing device, but this is not infallible. Severe respiratory distress follows inhalation almost immediately. There is a generalized obstructive emphysema with an expiratory type of dyspnea. The embarrassment to respiration appears to be the result of an inflammatory reaction caused by the irritation of the zinc stearate. Owing to the extreme lightness of the powder, it is almost immediately drawn into the finer bronchioles, and for this reason bronchoscopic aspiration is of little avail except to remove the secretions which subsequently accumulate.

Immediate treatment is by oxygen therapy in an atmosphere of high humidity. Bronchoscopic aspiration is indicated when there is an excessive accumulation of secretions in the larger air passages.

Kerosene Pneumonia

Pulmonary disturbances are frequently associated with the ingestion of kerosene. (See Hydrocarbons [Section 28] for other manifestations of kerosene poisoning.)

PATHOGENESIS. Although there are conflicting interpretations of the pathogenesis of the pulmonary lesions, the most plausible explanation is that kerosene reaches the lungs following aspiration during swallowing, vomiting, or gastric lavage. Because of this, gastric lavage after the ingestion of kerosene or other hydrocarbons is usually contraindicated. The pulmonary changes observed in animals are edema, inflammation and hemorrhage.

Coughing and vomiting follow ingestion almost immediately. There is an elevation of temperature (100 to 104° F), and the child may be drowsy or comatose. The pulmonary findings may be diminished resonance on percussion, suppressed or tubular breath sounds and rales. Pneumonic involvement is disclosed more frequently by roentgenographic examination than by physical findings. Occasionally radiologic findings may be minimal a few hours after ingestion, only to progress rapidly after that time.

COMPLICATIONS. Pneumothorax, subcutaneous emphysema of the chest wall and pleural effusion, including empyema, have occurred as complications. In spite of the stormy clinical course, which averages 2 to 5 days, recovery occurs in most instances.

TREATMENT. Vomiting must never be induced. When only small amounts of kerosene have been ingested, and especially if several hours have elapsed, gastric lavage should be omitted. When large quantities of kerosene or other hydrocarbons have been ingested, lavage should be performed with great care to avoid aspiration. The administration of an oil apparently decreases absorption from the gastrointestinal tract, but is not useful in practice. If there is dyspnea or cyanosis, the child should be placed in an oxygen tent. The routine use of antibiotics is not recommended; the occurrence of secondary infection of the affected lung can usually be readily detected by the reappearance of fever on the third to fifth day following ingestion, and can then be suitably treated with penicillin G and kanamycin. Corticosteroids have no beneficial effect on the course of the illness.

Lipoid Pneumonia

Lipoid pneumonia is a chronic, interstitial proliferative inflammation resulting from aspiration of lipoid material; it occurs principally in debilitated infants.

The factors which may be responsible for aspiration of oil include: (1) intranasal instillation of medicated oils; (2) any condition which interferes with the swallowing act, such as cleft palate, debilitation or a horizontal position during feeding; and (3) forced feeding and especially the administration of cod liver oil, castor oil or mineral oil to crying children.

The severity of the pulmonary reaction depends upon the kind of oil inhaled. Vegetable oils are generally the least irritating, such oils as olive, cottonseed and sesame producing no inflammation; chaulmoogra, a vegetable oil, on the other hand, produces extensive damage. Animal oils, owing to their high fatty acid content, are the most damaging. Cod liver oil belongs in this category. Liquid petroleum is chemically inert and not so irritative as some of the other oils, but does act as a foreign body.

The reaction within the lung begins as an interstitial proliferative inflammation with which there may be an exudative pneumonia. In the second stage there is diffuse, chronic, proliferative fibrosis. Acute bronchopneumonia is not infrequently superimposed in this stage. In the third stage there are multiple localized nodules, the so-called tumor-like paraffinomas. Microscopically there are numerous macrophages in the involved areas, with giant cell formation of the foreign body type. The lipoid substance is both intracellular and extracellular. The oil-laden cells may be carried through lymphatic channels to the hilar lymph nodes.

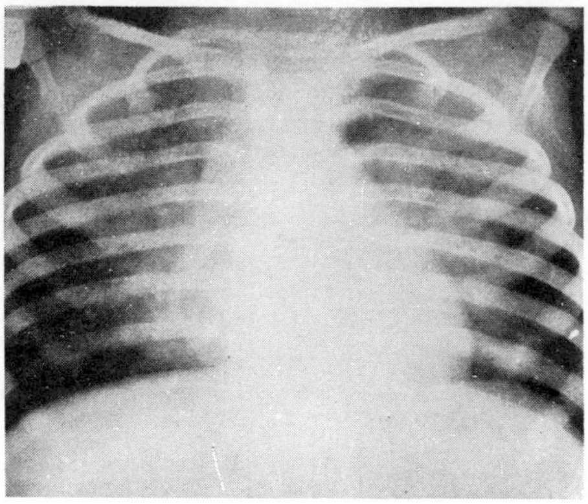

Figure 12–12 *Roentgenogram showing increased density radiating from the hilus of each lung in an infant 13 months of age after intranasal application of liquid petrolatum 3 times a day for 5 months.*

CLINICAL MANIFESTATIONS. There are no characteristic signs or symptoms. The most common symptom is cough, and in severe cases there may be dyspnea. Unless there is a superimposed infection, there is usually no fever or physical sign. With extensive involvement there may be some impairment to percussion and increased or decreased voice and breath sounds. Secondary bronchopneumonic infections are common.

The only characteristic finding is the roentgenographic appearance. With mild involvement, there is only an increase in the density and the extent of the hilar shadows. With increasing involvement there is greater density of the perihilar shadows with widening in all directions (Fig. 12–12). In a few instances the pulmonary changes have been limited to the right lung, and in the infant who is recumbent most of the time the changes may be mainly in the right upper lobe.

PROGNOSIS. The prognosis is guarded. It depends upon the extent of pulmonary damage, the discontinuance of oil inhalation, the general condition of the infant, and the avoidance of intercurrent infections.

PREVENTION. Intranasal medication in an oily vehicle should never be used. Concentrated preparations of vitamins A and D in water-miscible vehicles should be substituted for cod liver oil. Administration of mineral oil and castor oil should be avoided. Infants who regurgitate or vomit frequently should be placed on their abdomens to lessen the likelihood of aspiration.

TREATMENT. There is no specific treatment. The infant's position should be changed frequently to lessen the chances of hypostatic pneumonia.

Zinc Stearate

Heiman, H., and Aschner, P. W.: Aspirations of stearate of zinc in infancy. Am. J. Dis. Child., *23*:503, 1922.

Kerosene Pneumonia

Ashkenazi, A. E., and Berman, S. E.: Experimental kerosene poisoning in rats. Pediatrics, *28*:642, 1961.

Gerarde, H. W.: Toxicological studies on hydrocarbons. V. Kerosene. Toxicol. Appl. Pharmacol., *1*:462, 1959.

Marks, M. I., Chicoine, L., Legere, G., and Hillman, E.: Adrenocorticosteroid treatment of hydrocarbon pneumonia in children – A cooperative study. J. Pediatr. *81*:366, 1972.

Lipoid Pneumonia

Bromer, R. S., and Wolman, I. J.: Lipoid pneumonia in infants and children. Radiology, *32*:1, 1939.

Nathanson, L., Frenkel, D., and Jacobi, M.: Diagnosis of lipoid pneumonia by aspiration biopsy. Arch. Intern. Med. *72*:627, 1943.

Silo Filler's Disease

This condition is an acute interstitial pneumonia, seen rarely in farm children, which occurs following the inhalation of nitrogen dioxide, a gas generally encountered only in freshly filled silos. Cough and dyspnea occur immediately after exposure. An asymptomatic phase of several days follows, but then the patient suddenly experiences chills and fever associated with progressive cough, dyspnea and cyanosis. Auscultation of the chest reveals rales throughout both lungs; radiologic examination shows widespread pulmonary infiltration. The disease usually progresses rapidly to death. There is no known effective treatment.

Lowry, T., and Schuman, L. M.: Silo-filler's disease – A syndrome caused by nitrogen dioxide. J.A.M.A. *162*:153, 1956.

Olson, E. T.: Occurrence of silo-filler's disease in children. J. Pediatr., *64*:724, 1964.

Pearlman, M. E., Finklea, J. F., Creason, J. P., Shy, C. M., Young, M. M., and Horton, R. J. M.: Nitrogen dioxide and lower respiratory illnesses. Pediatrics *47*:391, 1971.

HYPERSENSITIVITY TO INHALED MATERIALS

Since 1932, when a condition due to the inhalation of moldy hay was described ("farmer's lung"), a series of pulmonary diseases has been reported which appear to be caused by hypersensitivity to various inhaled substances such as maple bark ("maple bark strippers' disease"), sugar cane bark (bagassosis), redwood tree bark, pigeon droppings and feathers ("pigeon breeders' disease") and the dusty output from air conditioners. In general, the responsible antigen is a fungus or mold associated with the specific material to which the patient is exposed. It is likely that other pulmonary parenchymal diseases of a similar nature exist and will be described in the future.

The clinical manifestations of all these diseases are more or less identical. Several hours following exposure there is acute onset of chest pain, fever and dyspnea associated with few physical findings, although on occasion wheezes and moist rales may be audible. Roentgenologic examination may show minimal emphysema, but is usually normal. If no further exposure occurs, the symptoms abate over a period of several days, but if contact with the responsible antigen continues, symptoms progress to severe dyspnea and cyanosis associated with a diffuse, usually rather fine, infiltrate on chest roentgenogram. Histologically this infiltrate consists of subacute granulomatous inflammation with accumulation of plasma cells, lymphocytes, epithelioid cells and giant cells of the Langhans type. With continued exposure the inflammatory lesions may be replaced by fibrosis. The immunologic basis of the disease is demonstrated by the development of hypergammaglobulinemia with elevation of the IgG, IgM and IgA fractions. Specific precipitins to the antigen occur in the serum of the affected patient, and the intradermal injection of this antigen causes a vigorous delayed hypersensitivity response.

Treatment consists of immediate removal of the patient from the environment in which the antigen occurs. The use of corticosteroids usually results in a prompt remission of symptoms, and the continued use of these drugs for a period of one to six months may prevent the subsequent development of pulmonary fibrosis in the more chronic cases.

Banaszak, E. F., Thiede, W. H., and Fink, J. N.: Hypersensitivity pneumonitis due to contamination of an air conditioner. New Engl. J. Med. *283*:271, 1970.

Hughes, W. F., Mattimore, J. M., and Arbesman, C. E.: Farmer's lung in an adolescent boy. Am. J. Dis. Child. *118*:777, 1969.

Stiehm, E. R., Reed, C. E., and Tooley, W. H.: Pigeon breeders' lung in children. Pediatrics *39*:904, 1967.

LÖFFLER'S SYNDROME
(Eosinophilic Pneumonia)

This syndrome is characterized by widespread, transitory pulmonary infiltrations which roentgenographically vary in size, but may resemble those of miliary tuberculosis, and by a blood eosinophilia which may be as high as 70 per cent. The clinical course is, as a rule, not particularly severe and varies from a few days to several months. Features more or less common to the reported cases are paroxysmal attacks of coughing, dyspnea, pleurisy and little or no fever. Zuelzer and others called attention to the association of hepatomegaly in this syndrome, especially in infants and young children. Biopsy sections of the liver reveal multiple focal areas of necrosis, granuloma formation and eosinophilic infiltration. These children have hyperglobulinemia, presumably as the result of hepatic dysfunction and in response to parasitic invasion of tissue. Autopsy studies have revealed evidences of eosinophilic infiltrations in the lungs and in other organs. Instances have been recorded of localized pneumonic consolidation with an associated eosinophilia.

Löffler's syndrome is not a clinical entity. It has been considered by some to be an unusual allergic manifestation to a variety of antigens. In children it would appear to be most often a manifestation of helminthic infections. The term *visceral larva migrans* is used for extraintestinal invasion by the larvae of a variety of roundworms. Perhaps the most common pathogen in this country is the larva of the dog ascarid, *Toxocara canis,* and less often of the cat ascarid, *Toxocara cati* (see Toxocariasis, Section 10). Other roundworms may also be responsible for the syndrome; these include *Ascaris lumbricoides* (usually responsible for transient pulmonary lesions), *Strongyloides stercoralis* and hookworms. So-called tropical eosinophilia (Section 10) may be manifest as Löffler's syndrome, and is probably caused by a number of different helminths. Paragonimiasis caused by a lung fluke (Section 10) may produce the syndrome, as well as extrapulmonary manifestations.

Beaver, P.: Wandering nematodes as a cause of disability and disease. Am. J. Trop. Med. Hyg. *6*:433, 1957.

Yun, D. J.: Paragonimiasis in children in Korea. J. Pediatr. *56*:736, 1960.

Zuelzer, W. W., and Apt, L.: Disseminated visceral lesions associated with extreme eosinophilia: Pathologic and clinical observations on a syndrome of young children. Am. J. Dis. Child., *78*:153, 1949.

HYPOSTATIC PNEUMONIA

Hypostatic pneumonia occurs after prolonged passive pulmonary congestion and may occur in any marantic state. Lying for a long time in one position favors its development. Pathologically there is dependent congestion, edema and pneumonia.

CLINICAL MANIFESTATIONS. The symptoms are not characteristic. There is neither dyspnea nor fever, unless these symptoms are dependent upon some other factor. The physical signs are principally slight dullness on percussion, feeble respiratory sounds and the presence of moist rales. Hypostatic congestion is usually a terminal event.

TREATMENT. Treatment is that of the primary affection. Prophylaxis is of the greatest importance; the position of any immobile patient should be changed frequently.

PULMONARY HEMOSIDEROSIS

The term "pulmonary hemosiderosis" is used to describe a number of rare conditions characterized by an abnormal accumulation of hemosiderin in the lungs. Hemosiderin deposits follow diffuse alveolar hemorrhage and may occur either as a primary disease of the lungs or secondary to cardiac or systemic vascular disease. In children primary hemosiderosis occurs more frequently than the secondary varieties. There appear to be three types of primary pulmonary hemosiderosis: an idiopathic form, a form occurring in association with myocarditis, and a form associated with progressive glomerulonephritis (Goodpasture's syndrome). Two types of secondary pulmonary hemosiderosis are recognized; one occurs with mitral stenosis and chronic left ventricular failure of any cause, and the other is associated with collagen diseases and anaphylactoid purpura.

IDIOPATHIC PRIMARY PULMONARY HEMOSIDEROSIS. The cause of this illness is unknown. Onset is usually in childhood, rarely later than early adult life. Symptoms are those of recurrent or chronic pulmonary disease and include cough, hemoptysis, dyspnea, wheezing and occasional cyanosis, associated with fatigue and pallor. The cough may be productive of bloody sputum or the infant or child may simply vomit large quantities of blood. During acute attacks, which usually last 2 to 4 days, the child may be febrile.

The usual clinical features of fever, tachycardia, tachypnea, leukocytosis, respiratory distress and abnormal radiologic findings may suggest a bacterial pneumonia, and only prolonged follow-up will reveal the correct diagnosis. In some children, however, the early manifestations of the illness are related to chronic iron deficiency anemia, often refractory to therapy, and the characteristic pulmonary symptoms do not appear until much later. Paradoxically the child may have severe pulmonary manifestations without roentgenographic abnormalities, or the roentgenographic picture may be abnormal before pulmonary symptoms have occurred.

The anemia is typically microcytic and hypochromic; serum iron concentrations are low. The stool usually contains occult blood, presumably swallowed. Hemosiderin can usually be demonstrated in macrophages of the sputum and in material obtained by gastric lavage. Roentgenographic changes range from minimal infiltrates to massive pulmonary involvement with secondary atelectasis, emphysema and hilar lymphadenopathy; significant changes may be seen from day to day. A biopsy may be necessary to establish the diagnosis. Histologic features are alveolar epithelial hyperplasia, large numbers of macrophages containing hemosiderin, varying amounts of interstitial fibrosis, and sclerosis of small blood vessels. Approximately 50 per cent of patients die within 1 to 5 years of the onset, usually from acute pulmonary hemorrhage and respiratory failure.

In some patients, corticosteroids may have produced remissions; in others these drugs have not been beneficial. Maintenance corticosteroid therapy has been used between attacks with variable results. Immunosuppressant drugs and deferoxamine have also been advocated, but there are inadequate data to evaluate them.

PRIMARY PULMONARY HEMOSIDEROSIS WITH MYOCARDITIS. Some patients with idiopathic pulmonary hemosiderosis have inflammation of the myocardium, varying from minimal lesions to extensive disease. If significant myocardial disease is present when pulmonary symptoms are first noted, it may be impossible to determine whether the pulmonary hemosiderosis is a primary or secondary phenomenon. The clinical picture does not differ from that of idiopathic disease except that the heart may be enlarged, owing to the myocarditis, and electrocardiographic signs compatible with this cardiac lesion may be present.

PRIMARY PULMONARY HEMOSIDEROSIS WITH GLOMERULONEPHRITIS (GOODPASTURE'S SYNDROME). (See also Sections 9 and 15.) This is a disease primarily of young adults and is rarely observed in children. The clinical picture is initiated by pulmonary involvement with hemoptysis and iron deficiency anemia. At this stage the disease may be virtually identical to idiopathic pulmonary hemosiderosis, but careful study will disclose a proliferative or membranous glomerulonephritis at the time of the first pulmonary attack. Patients with this syndrome usually have progressive renal disease which leads to renal failure and death.

PRIMARY PULMONARY HEMOSIDEROSIS WITH PRECIPITINS TO COW'S MILK. A small number of patients with signs and symptoms of primary pulmonary hemosiderosis have had unusually high titers in serum of precipitins to multiple constituents of cow's milk. These patients may also have chronic rhinitis, otitis media and growth retardation. On a cow's-milk-free diet some patients with these serologic findings of milk reactivity appear to improve, others do not. The causative relation of milk reactivity to pulmonary hemosiderosis remains unknown; in any event, the majority of children with this condition do not have unusual amounts of precipitins to milk proteins.

PULMONARY HEMOSIDEROSIS SECONDARY TO HEART DISEASE. Any form of heart disease producing chronic increase in pulmonary capillary pressure can lead to secondary pulmonary hemosiderosis. The most common primary lesion is mitral stenosis.

PULMONARY HEMOSIDEROSIS AS A MANIFESTATION OF DIFFUSE COLLAGEN DISEASE OR ANAPHYLACTOID PURPURA. The vascular changes of polyarteritis nodosa occasionally are initially limited to the lungs and may cause pulmonary hemosiderosis. In most instances polyarteritis progresses to involve other organs. Other collagen diseases such as rheumatic fever have occasionally produced pulmonary hemosiderosis as an effect of a generalized, diffuse vasculitis.

A few patients have had pulmonary hemosiderosis in association with anaphylactoid purpura or thrombocytopenic purpura.

Gilman, P. A., and Zinkham, W. H.: Severe idiopathic pulmonary hemosiderosis in the absence of clinical or radiologic evidence of pulmonary disease. J. Pediatr., *75*:118, 1969.

Heiner, D. C., Sears, J. W., Kniker, W. T.: Multiple precipitins to cow's milk in chronic respiratory disease. A syndrome including poor growth, gastrointestinal symptoms, evidence of allergy, iron deficiency anemia, and pulmonary hemosiderosis. Am. J. Dis. Child., *103*:634, 1962.

Irvin, J. M., and Snowden, P. W.: Idiopathic pulmonary hemosiderosis: Report of a case with apparent remission from cortisone. Am. J. Dis. Child., *93*:182, 1957.

Launay, C., Bach C., Thiriez, H., et al.: Idiopathic pulmonary hemosiderosis. Ann. Pediat. (Paris) *10*:379, 1963.

Soergel, K. H., and Sommers, S. C.: Idiopathic pulmonary hemosiderosis and related syndromes. Am. J. Med., *32*:499, 1962.

DESQUAMATIVE INTERSTITIAL PNEUMONITIS

This condition, sometimes classified as one of the collagen diseases, has been reported to occur in children, although most cases have been described in adults. The pathologic changes are characteristic, consisting of massive proliferation and desquamation of alveolar cells with thickening of the walls of the distal air spaces. The etiology remains unknown.

Initial symptoms consist of progressive dyspnea, followed by nonproductive cough and weight loss; there is no fever. Cyanosis and severe clubbing eventually occur. Radiologically a "ground glass" appearance of both lung bases is demonstrated, along with poorly defined densities in the hilar regions. Corticosteroid therapy arrests the progress of the disease in most patients and occasionally produces a remission of symptoms. Chloroquine has also been successfully employed in an occasional patient.

Buchta, R. M., Park, S., and Giammona, S. T.: Desquamative interstitial pneumonia in a 7-week old infant. Am. J. Dis. Child. *120*:341, 1970.
Liebow, A. A., Steer, A., and Billingsley, J. G., Desquamative interstitial pneumonia. Am. J. Med., *39*:369, 1965.
Rosenow, E. C., III, O'Connell, E. J., and Harrison, E. G., Jr.: Desquamative interstitial pneumonia in children. Am. J. Dis. Child. *120*:344, 1970.

PULMONARY ALVEOLAR PROTEINOSIS

In children, pulmonary alveolar proteinosis is a rare disease of unknown etiology. The first symptoms are usually cough and dyspnea or vomiting and diarrhea, most often presenting before the age of 1 year. Fever is present in about one third of the patients. Physical findings are relatively few, but radiologic changes generally are characteristic and consist of a fine, diffuse infiltrate radiating from the hilus to the periphery in a typical "butterfly" distribution. Some patients demonstrated bilateral lower lobe infiltrates, while others initially show nodular densities progressing to complete lobar consolidation.

The diagnosis of pulmonary alveolar proteinosis must usually be confirmed by biopsy. Tissue sections show alveoli distended by fine, granular, eosinophilic material which stains positively with PAS stain. Silver staining must be performed to rule out the possibility of *P. carinii* infection.

Immunologic examination of some children with this disease will indicate various types of immunologic deficiency states, including thymic alymphoplasia. Not surprisingly, therefore, various fungal and bacterial superinfections may be associated with the disease.

No effective treatment exists. There is no evidence that administration of corticosteroids or use of pulmonary lavage alters the relentless, progressive course of the illness. Maximum duration of survival from the time symptoms are first noticed is two years; most children die of respiratory failure less than 12 months after onset.

The adult form of pulmonary alveolar proteinosis, which occurs somewhat more commonly, has a much more favorable prognosis.

Colon, A. R., Jr., Lawrence, R. D., Mills, S. D., and O'Connell, E. J.: Childhood pulmonary alveolar proteinosis. Am. J. Dis. Child. *121*:481, 1971.
Sutherland, W. A., Campbell, R. A., and Edwards, M. J.: Pulmonary alveolar proteinosis and pulmonary cryptococcosis in an adolescent boy. *J. Pediatr. 80*:450, 1972.

IDIOPATHIC DIFFUSE INTERSTITIAL FIBROSIS OF THE LUNG
(Hamman-Rich Syndrome)

Idiopathic diffuse interstitial fibrosis of the lung is a rare chronic, usually progressive and fatal disorder of unknown origin, ordinarily observed in adults, but occasionally in infants and children. The clinical pattern is characterized by progressive pulmonary insufficiency resulting from interstitial fibrosis and alveolar-capillary block. Onset is usually insidious, with dyspnea generally the first symptom, initially occurring only with exercise, but later present even at rest. Cough is frequent and may be productive of blood. The patient is usually afebrile. As the disease progresses, anorexia, weight loss and fatigability occur, and finally cyanosis, clubbing of the fingers and evidences of right-sided cardiac failure. Serial roentgenograms show progressive, widespread granular or reticular mottling or small nodular densities. Intercurrent infections are frequent and often serious.

The pulmonary pathology is variable. During the early stage of the disease, fibrosis is usually not present, but there is cellular infiltration of the walls of the alveoli, alveolar ducts and peribronchial tissue by lymphocytes, plasma cells and occasionally eosinophils. This usually progresses to extensive and diffuse proliferation of fibrous tissue throughout all the lobes of the lung, associated with organization of intra-alveolar exudate.

The cause is unknown; some cases may be familial in origin.

Corticosteroids appear to give some symptomatic relief, but do not alter the progression of the disease or improve the degree of pulmonary function. Other therapy is also symptomatic.

Bradley, C. A.: Diffuse interstitial fibrosis of the lungs in children. J. Pediatr. *48*:442, 1956.
Ivemark, B. I., and Wallgren, C. G.: Diffuse interstitial pulmonary fibrosis (Hamman-Rich syndrome) in an infant. Report of a case with histologic and respiratory studies. Acta Paediat. *51* (Supp. 135):97, 1962.
Rubin, E. H., and Lubliner, R.: The Hamman-Rich syndrome: Review of the literature and analysis of 15 cases. Medicine *36*:397, 1957.
Sheridan, L. A., Harrison, E. G., Jr., and Divertie, M. B.: The current status of idiopathic pulmonary fibrosis (Hamman-Rich syndrome). Med. Clin. N. Amer. *48*:993, 1964.

PULMONARY ALVEOLAR MICROLITHIASIS

This rare disease appears often to have its onset during childhood, but the clinical manifestations tend to be delayed to later years. It is characterized by widely disseminated intra-alveolar calculi, which create a rather characteristic pattern on the roentgenogram (Fig. 12–13). The appearance has been likened to that of an overfilled normal bronchogram. If the disease is identified in childhood, it is apt to be by roentgenographic examination before symptoms have appeared or when they are still minimal. The disease usually progresses slowly and terminates in cardiopulmonary failure during the middle years of adulthood.

The cause is unknown; there are no known metabolic abnormalities, including those of calcium and phosphorus. Some cases have shown a familial pattern; there is no sex predilection.

There is no known effective treatment.

Clark, R. B., III, and Johnson, F. C.: Idiopathic pulmonary alveolar microlithiasis. Pediatrics, *28*:650, 1961.

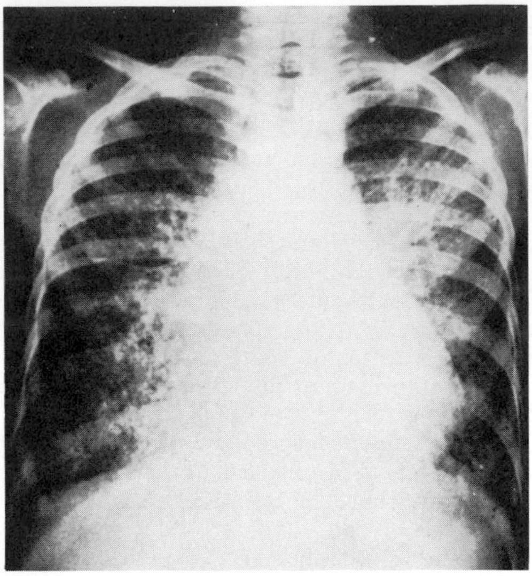

Figure 12–13 Roentgenogram of chest of a 7 year old boy with pulmonary alveolar microlithiasis. (From Clark, R. B., III, and Johnson, F. C.: Pediatrics, Vol. 28, 1961.)

EOSINOPHILIC GRANULOMA OF THE LUNG

See The Histiocytosis Syndromes, Section 26.

ATELECTASIS

Congenital atelectasis is discussed in Section 7.

ACQUIRED ATELECTASIS

ETIOLOGY. Atelectasis, the imperfect expansion or the collapse of air-bearing tissue of the lung, is relatively common in infants and children. Collapse may be produced by any factor which completely obstructs the intake of air into the alveolar sacs and persists sufficiently long to permit absorption of alveolar air into the blood stream. In general, the causes may be divided into two groups: (1) external pressure directly upon the pulmonary parenchyma or a bronchus or bronchiole, and (2) intrabronchial or intrabronchiolar obstruction. Any factor responsible for a continuously decreased amplitude of respiratory excursion or for respiratory paralysis may be contributory. Reflex stimuli have also been considered initiating factors. De Takats demonstrated that at least three distinct stimuli, namely, pulmonary embolism, intra-abdominal manipulation and trauma to the chest wall, are capable of initiating bronchoconstriction and increased bronchosecretion. Allergy may be responsible for atelectasis through spasm of the bronchial or bronchiolar musculature and production of an exudate which occludes the lumen. This latter may also be responsible for atelectasis in patients with cystic fibrosis.

Atelectasis from External Pressure. External factors may be operative in one of four ways: (1) interference with the movements of the thoracic cage (neuromuscular abnormalities as in cerebral palsy, poliomyelitis, spinal muscular atrophy, myasthenia gravis; osseous deformities as in rickets, scoliosis, kyphosis; scleroderma; splinting of the chest by casts and surgical dressings); (2) defective movement of the diaphragm (paralysis of phrenic nerve, increased abdominal pressure); (3) direct interference with expansion of lungs (pleural effusion, pneumothorax, intrathoracic tumors, diaphragmatic hernia); and (4) external compression of a bronchus completely obstructing ingress of air (enlarged lymph node, tumors, cardiac enlargement).

Atelectasis from Intrabronchial or Intrabronchiolar Obstruction. (See also Bronchial Foreign Body earlier in this Section.) Complete intraluminal obstruction of a bronchus may be produced by a foreign body, by a neoplasm, by granulomatous tissue as in tuberculosis or by secretions, as with cystic fibrosis, bronchiectasis, pulmonary abscess, allergy, chronic bronchitis or acute laryngotracheobronchitis.

Obstruction of one or more bronchioles in a given area may be produced by any of the conditions mentioned, but widespread bronchiolar obstruction is most often produced by bronchiolitis or interstitial pneumonitis and by asthma. Generalized obstructive emphysema is the initial result of such bronchiolar obstructions; but as the pathologic changes progress, some of the bronchioles may become completely obstructed, and there are then interspersed small areas of atelectasis and emphysema. Patchy atelectasis is relatively common in acute bronchiolitis or asthma, and is probably always present in advanced chronic diffuse infections such as the pulmonary infection associated with cystic fibrosis.

PATHOLOGY. The atelectatic areas are airless, congested, deep red, of a firm consistency, and depressed below the neighboring healthy or emphysematous lung. When there is extensive atelectasis of one or more lobes, there is usually compensatory emphysema of the air-bearing lung.

CLINICAL MANIFESTATIONS. Symptoms vary with the cause and extent of the atelectasis. A small area of atelectasis is likely to be asymptomatic. When a large area of the lung becomes atelectatic, and especially when it does so suddenly, there is dyspnea with rapid shallow respirations, tachycardia, and often cyanosis. If the obstruction is removed, the symptoms disappear rapidly. Even atelectasis of an entire lobe may not be responsible for changes in the percussion note, owing to the compensatory emphysema of the adjacent lung tissue. Breath and voice sounds are decreased or absent over extensive atelectatic areas.

DIAGNOSIS. The diagnosis can usually be established by roentgenographic examination (Fig. 12–14). Small areas may be indistinguishable from pneumonic consolidations, but those that involve as much as several lobules of a lobe can usually be identified by the contraction of the area. When one or more lobes are atelectatic, the roentgenographic

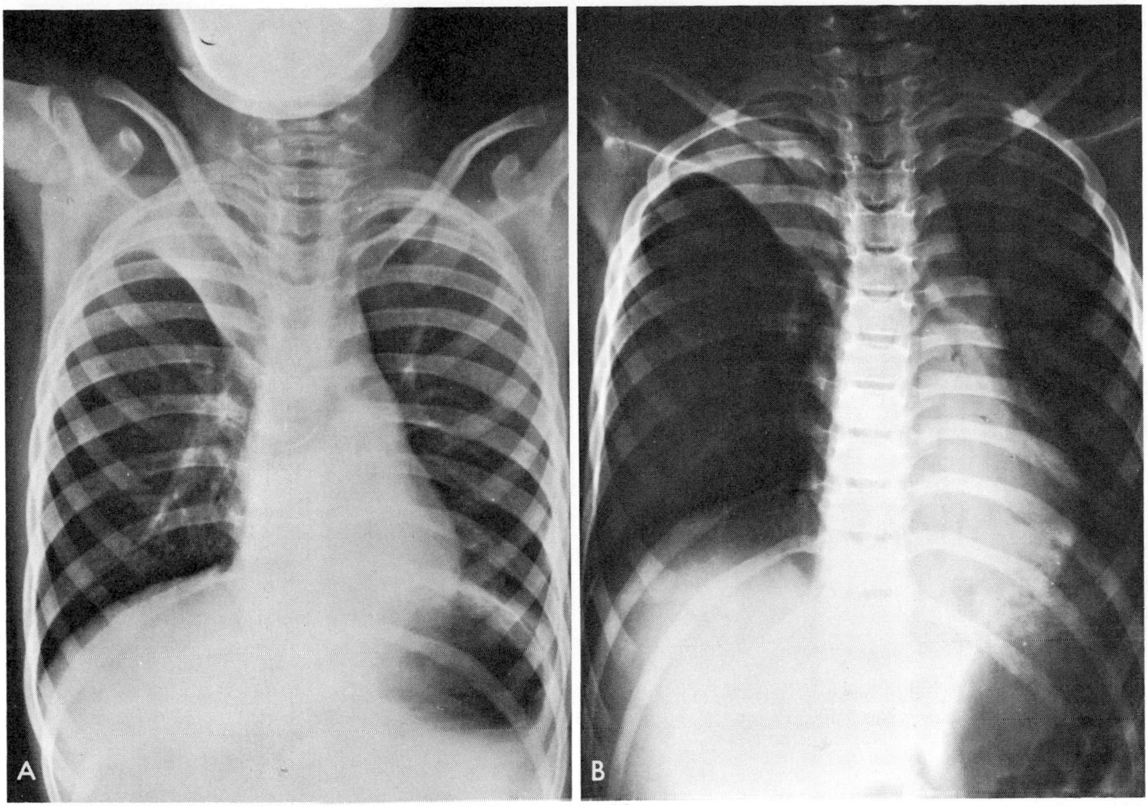

Figure 12–14 *Atelectasis. The right upper lobe and the left lower lobe are collapsed. The atelectasis of the left lower lobe is demonstrated on the overpenetrated film* (B). *The atelectasis occurred postoperatively and disappeared spontaneously.*

findings are those of massive collapse. Bronchoscopic examination will reveal a collapsed main bronchus when the obstruction is at the tracheobronchial junction and may also disclose the nature of the obstruction.

PROGNOSIS. If the obstruction disappears spontaneously or is removed, the atelectasis usually disappears unless there is secondary infection. In persistent cases bronchiectasis is a frequent complication and pulmonary abscess an occasional one.

TREATMENT. Bronchoscopic examination is indicated when an isolated area of atelectasis persists for several days, and immediately if it is the result of a foreign body or if there is reason to believe that it is due to any bronchial obstruction which may be relieved. Frequent changes in the child's position and deep breathing may be beneficial. Various types of positive pressure mechanical breathing devices may aid in re-expanding the involved pulmonary segment. Oxygen therapy is indicated when there is dyspnea. Morphine and atropine are contraindicated.

MASSIVE PULMONARY ATELECTASIS

Massive collapse of one or both lungs is most often a postoperative complication, but occasionally results from other causes such as trauma, asthma, pneumonia, tension pneumothorax, the aspiration of foreign material (either a solid object large enough to obstruct a main stem bronchus or liquids such as water or blood) or paralysis such as that in diphtheria or poliomyelitis. Massive atelectasis is usually produced by a combination of factors: immobilization or decreased use of the diaphragm and the respiratory muscles, obstruction of the bronchial tree and abolition of the cough reflex.

CLINICAL MANIFESTATIONS. The onset in postoperative cases is usually within 24 hours after operation, but may not occur for several days. There is dyspnea, cyanosis and tachycardia. The child is extremely anxious, there is likely to be prostration, and, if he is old enough, he usually complains of pain in the chest. The temperature may be as high as 103 or 104° F.

The physical signs are characteristic. The chest appears flat on the affected side, where there is also decreased respiratory excursion, dullness to percussion, and feeble or absent breath and voice sounds. Lower lobes are more frequently involved than upper ones. The heart and the mediastinum are displaced toward the affected side. Roentgenograms show the collapsed lung, elevation of the diaphragm, narrowing of the intercostal spaces and displacement of the mediastinal structures and heart toward the affected side (Fig. 12–15).

PROGNOSIS. Bilateral massive collapse is usually rapidly fatal, although prompt bronchoscopic aspiration and artificial respiration may be

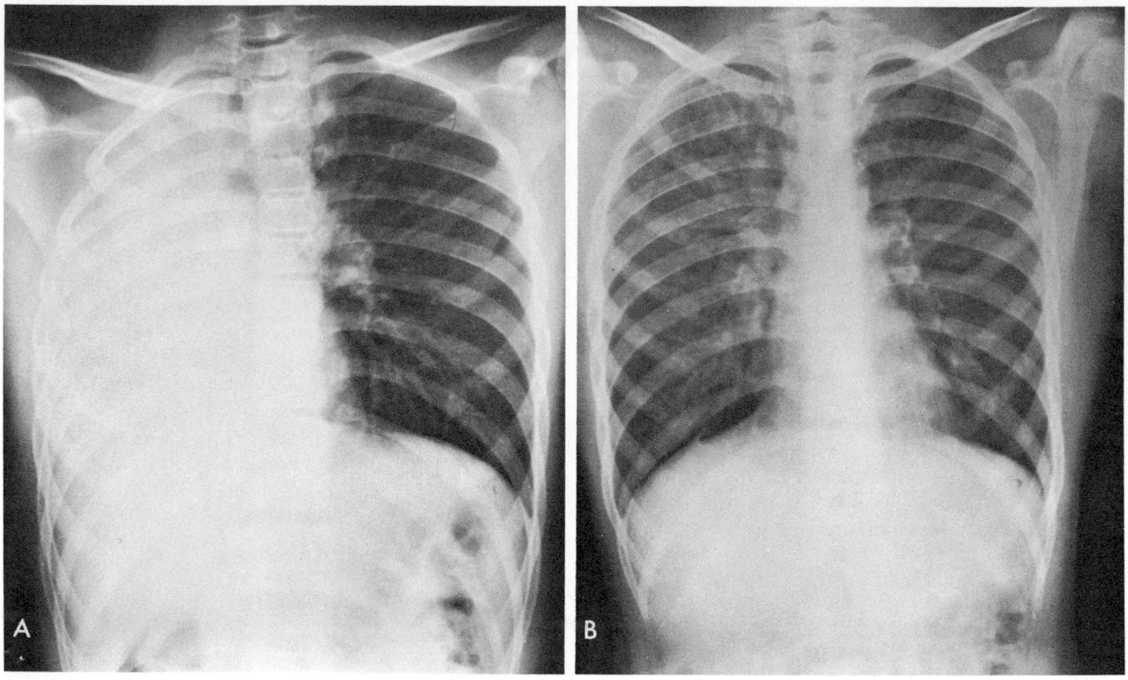

Figure 12–15 (A), *Massive atelectasis of the right lung, with* (B) *comparison study after reaeration following bronchoscopic removal of a mucous plug from the right stem bronchus. The patient is asthmatic. The heart and the other mediastinal structures are shifted to the right during the atelectatic phase.*

lifesaving. In the unilateral cases the prognosis is usually good.

PREVENTION. Prophylaxis is of the greatest importance. The incidence of postoperative atelectasis can be reduced by adequate ventilation during anesthesia. After operation the child's position in bed should be changed frequently, collections of secretions in the oropharynx should be aspirated, and when consciousness returns, the child should be encouraged to breathe deeply. Tight thoracic or abdominal binders should be avoided.

TREATMENT. When there is bilateral atelectasis, bronchoscopic aspiration should be performed immediately. When there is only unilateral atelectasis, the child should be placed on the unaffected side. Forced coughing or crying while the child is lying on the unaffected side may also be helpful, as is positive pressure ventilation. When these measures are not successful, bronchoscopic aspiration should be performed.

Relapses are not infrequent, and the child should be kept under constant observation.

EMPHYSEMA

Pulmonary emphysema is a distention or rupture of the alveoli. It may be generalized or localized and involve part or all of one lung. From a causative standpoint it may be compensatory or obstructive.

COMPENSATORY EMPHYSEMA. This may be either acute or chronic. It occurs in normally functioning pulmonary tissue when for any reason a sizable portion of the lung is partially or completely airless, as may occur with pneumonia, atelectasis, empyema and pneumothorax.

OBSTRUCTIVE EMPHYSEMA

Obstructive emphysema results from partial obstruction of a bronchus or bronchiole when the difficulty of getting air out of the alveoli becomes greater than getting it in, so that there is a gradually increasing accumulation of air distal to the obstruction. This is the so-called bypass or check-valve type of obstruction. Such obstructions may be intrabronchial or extrabronchial. (See Bronchial Foreign Body earlier in this Section.)

Localized Obstructive Emphysema

When a bypass type of obstruction partially occludes the main stem bronchus, the entire lobe is emphysematous; only individual lobules are affected when the obstruction is that of a secondary bronchus. Localized obstructions which may be responsible for emphysema include foreign bodies and the inflammatory reaction to them, intrabronchial tuberculosis or tuberculosis of the tracheobronchial lymph nodes and intrabronchial and mediastinal tumors. When most or all of a lobe is involved, the percussion note will be hyperresonant over the area and the breath sounds decreased in intensity. The distended lung may extend across the mediastinum into the opposite hemithorax. Fluoroscopically, during expiration the emphysematous area does not decrease in size, and the heart and the mediastinum shift to the opposite side.

Congenital obstructive lobar emphysema may account for severe respiratory distress in early infancy. Symptoms may become apparent in the neonatal period or may be delayed for as much as 5 or 6 months. A part or usually all of a lobe may be involved, the left upper lobe being most often affected. In some instances the obstruction is not demonstrable, but it is assumed to be produced by a check-valve type of mechanism. Such obstructions have been attributed to defective cartilage in the bronchi, mucosal folds which create a valvelike obstruction, bronchial stenosis and external compression by aberrant vessels, tumors, and the like. When the distention is considerable, the emphysematous lung compresses the unaffected lung below or above it and the opposite lung by extending across the mediastinum (Fig. 12–16). In most instances lobectomy is indicated.

Emphysema of all three lobes of the right lung has been produced by anomalous location of the left pulmonary artery, which partially constricts the right main bronchus.

Generalized Obstructive Emphysema

This depends upon widespread involvement of the bronchioles. It occurs more commonly in infants than in children and may be secondary to a number of clinical conditions, including respiratory infections associated with cystic fibrosis of the pancreas, acute bronchiolitis, interstitial pneumonitis, atypical forms of acute laryngotracheobronchitis, aspiration of zinc stearate powder, chronic passive congestion secondary to a congenital cardiac lesion, and miliary tuberculosis. Asthma is a relatively frequent cause in older children, but an uncommon one in infants.

The emphysematous portion of the lung is paler than usual, usually a light pink, and is distended and does not readily collapse. In chronic emphysema there is permanent loss of elasticity; many of the alveoli are ruptured and communicate with one another, producing distended saccules. As a result of the rupture of the alveoli, air may enter the interstitial tissue *(interstitial emphysema)* and result in pneumomediastinum and pneumothorax. (See Section 7.)

CLINICAL MANIFESTATIONS. Generalized obstructive emphysema is characterized by an expiratory type of dyspnea. Owing to the relatively greater difficulty in expiration than in inspiration, air is trapped in the alveoli, the lungs become increasingly overdistended, and the chest remains expanded during expiration. Just the reverse happens in laryngeal obstruction, in which interference with exchange of air is relatively greater during inspiration and the lungs do not become fully inflated. There are an increased respiratory rate and decreased respiratory excursions in emphysema, owing to the overdistention of the pulmonary alveoli and their inability to be normally emptied through the narrowed bronchioles. Air hunger is responsible for forced respiratory movements. Overaction of the accessory muscles of respiration results in indrawing at the suprasternal

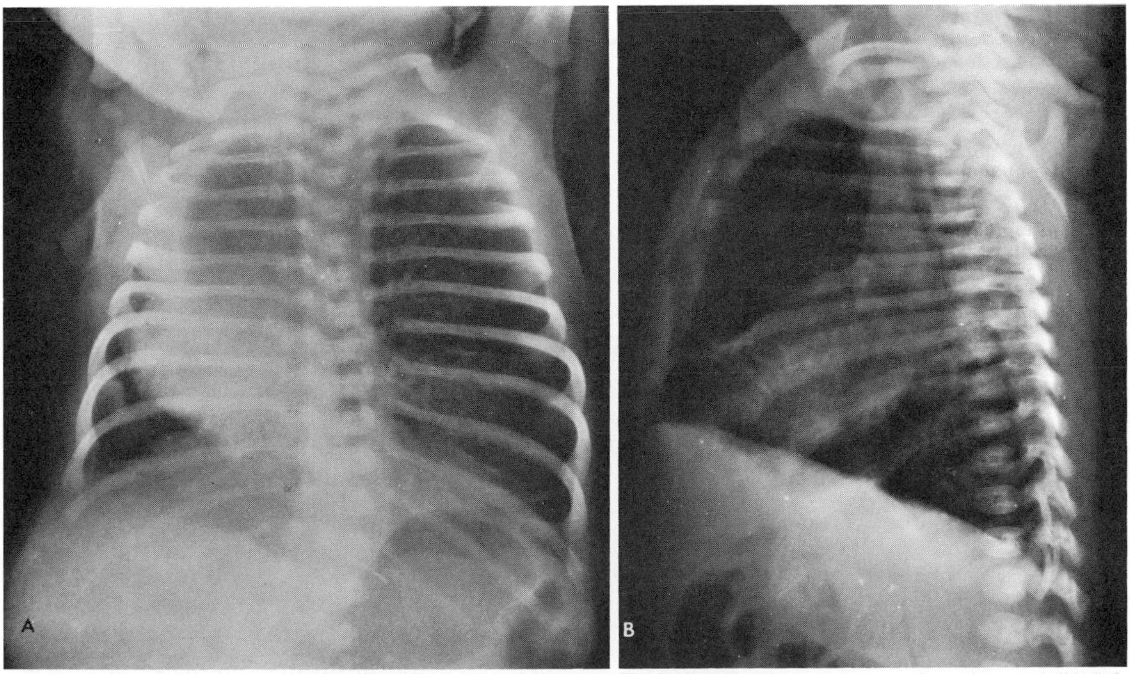

Figure 12–16 *Congenital lobar emphysema in an infant 4 weeks of age. Severe dyspnea and wheezing of 4 days' duration. The left upper lobe is emphysematous and protrudes across the midline anteriorly (note lateral projection). The mediastinal structures are displaced to the right. Relief of symptoms followed removal of the left upper lobe.*

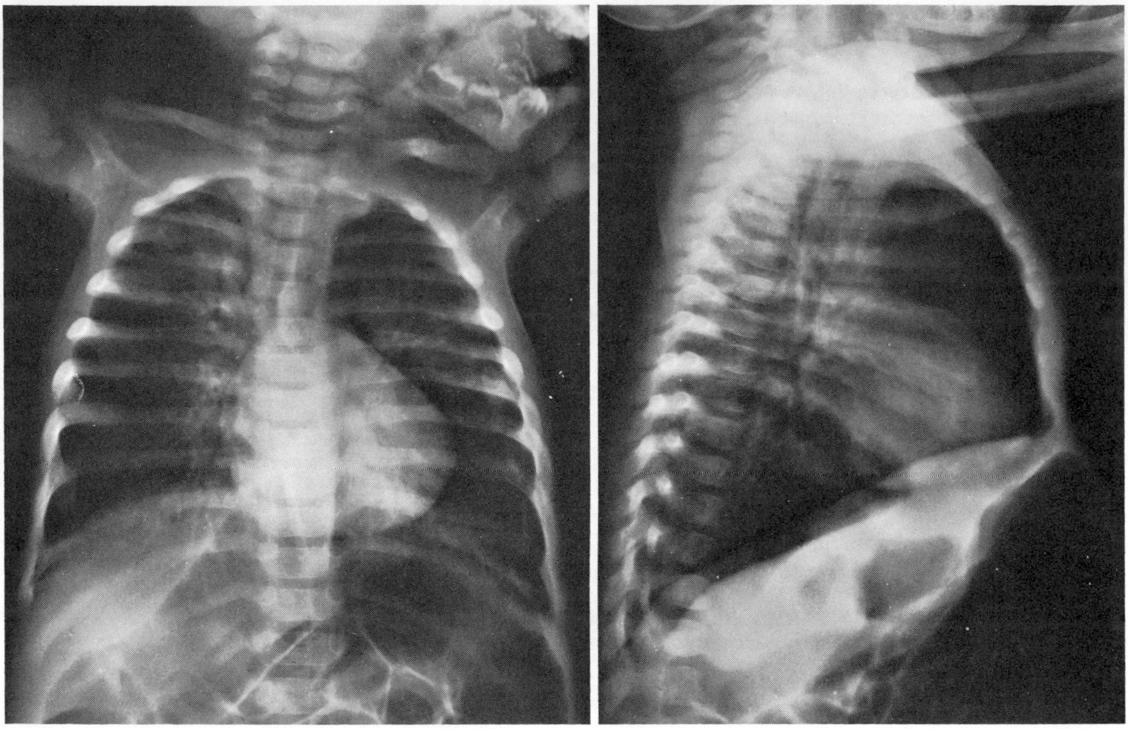

Figure 12–17 Generalized obstructive emphysema: dorsal projections of thorax in inspiratory and expiratory phases of respiration. Notice the relative failure of the lungs to empty in the expiratory phase. The left lung is less obstructed than the right (empties to a greater degree in the expiratory phase). This difference between the lungs is not apparent from a study of the diaphragm, which moves very little during respiration; it is evident, however, in the upper portions of the left lung space.

notch, the supraclavicular spaces, the lower margin of the thorax and the intercostal spaces. This indrawing is not nearly so great, however, as it is in laryngeal or tracheal obstruction, since the overinflated lungs will not permit it. There is scarcely any reduction in size of the overdistended emphysematous chest during expiration, in contrast to the flattened chest during both inspiration and expiration when there is laryngeal obstruction. There is no hoarseness or stridor as there is in laryngeal obstruction; there is usually audible wheezing in asthma. Cyanosis is common in the severe cases. The percussion note is hyperresonant, and on auscultation the inspiratory phase is usually less prominent than the expiratory phase, which is prolonged and roughened. Fine or medium rales may be present.

Roentgenographic and fluoroscopic examinations of the chest are of the greatest help in establishing the diagnosis. Both leaves of the diaphragm are low and flattened, the ribs are farther apart than usual, and the lung fields are less dense (Fig. 12–17). There is a decided restriction in the movement of the diaphragm, demonstrated best by fluoroscopic examination. The normal "doming" of the diaphragm during expiration is decreased, and the excursion of the low, flattened diaphragm in the severe cases is barely discernible. Another evidence of retention of air in the lungs during expiration is a paradoxical increase in the horizontal diameters of the chest during this phase, suggesting that the emphysematous lungs are merely being forced into a different position by the diaphragmatic activity (the abdominal respiratory effort is relatively stronger than that of the intercostals) rather than emptied of any significant amount of trapped air.

Bullous Emphysema

Bullous emphysematous blebs or cysts (**pneumatocele**) result from overdistention and rupture of alveoli during birth or shortly thereafter (Section 7), or they may be sequels of pneumonia and of other infections. They have been observed in tuberculous lesions while the patient was being treated with specific antibacterial therapy. These emphysematous areas presumably result from rupture of distended alveoli so that a single or multiloculated cavity is formed. At times the cysts may assume large proportions (Fig. 12–11). They may contain some fluid, and an air-fluid level may be demonstrated on the roentgenogram. The differential diagnosis must be made from pulmonary abscess. In most instances the cysts disappear spontaneously within a few months, although they may persist for a year or so.

There is almost never any indication for treatment; aspiration or surgery should be avoided unless there is severe respiratory and cardiac embarrassment.

Subcutaneous Emphysema

Subcutaneous emphysema occurs whenever free air finds its way into the subcutaneous tissue. It may be a complication of a fracture of the orbit permitting air to escape from the nasal sinuses. In the neck and over the thorax, emphysema may follow tracheotomy, deep ulcerations in the pharyngeal region, esophageal wounds or any perforating lesion of the larynx or trachea. It is an occasional complication of thoracentesis, of asthma, or following abdominal surgery. Air may also be formed in the subcutaneous tissues by gas-producing bacteria.

Caffey, J.: Pediatric X-ray Diagnosis. 4th ed. Chicago, Year Book Medical Publishers, Inc., 1961.
Currarino, G., and Silverman, F. N.: Roentgen diagnosis of pulmonary disease of the newborn infant. Pediat. Clin. N. Amer., *4*:27, 1957.
Kress, M. B., and Finklestein, A. H.: Giant bullous emphysema occurring in tuberculosis in childhood. Pediatrics, *30*:269, 1962.
Landing, B. H.: Anomalies of the respiratory tract. Pediat. Clin. N. Amer., *4*:73, 1957.
Nelson, W. E., and Smith, L. W.: Generalized obstructive emphysema in infants. J. Pediatr., *26*:36, 1945.

PULMONARY EDEMA

ETIOLOGY. Pulmonary edema results from the escape of serous fluid from the pulmonary capillaries into the alveolar spaces and the bronchioles. It is usually associated with circulatory or neurocirculatory collapse and consequently is often a terminal event in a variety of diseases. Though pulmonary edema may vary in severity, even in its mildest stages it is an ominous finding. It is a common manifestation of myocardial failure in acute or chronic rheumatic carditis and in congenital heart disease, or it may be due to hypervolemia from too rapid or too large an intravenous infusion. It may be a manifestation of acute or chronic nephritis or, rarely, of pneumonic and other infections with substantial degrees of toxicity. Poisoning by such substances as barbiturates, morphine, epinephrine and alcohol may be responsible for the development of pulmonary edema, as may the inhalation of toxic gases, such as illuminating gas, ammonia and nitrogen dioxide, or the ingestion and consequent aspiration of highly volatile hydrocarbons such as lighter fluid.

CLINICAL MANIFESTATIONS. The onset is variable, but rapid in most instances. The child often complains of a sense of oppression or pain in the chest. Cough is usually present and often produces a frothy, pink-tinged sputum. Pulse is rapid and feeble. The child is usually very pale and may be cyanotic. On physical examination, dullness to percussion and moist, bubbly rales are heard in the lower portions of the chest.

TREATMENT. Treatment is directed at the primary disease causing the pulmonary edema. Management of myocardial failure, nephritis and the various poisonings is discussed elsewhere. The administration of oxygen is often useful in relieving some of the chest pain, and when possible is best accomplished by intermittent positive pressure. Dyspnea can often be relieved by morphine sulfate in a dosage of 0.15 mg/kg. Antifoaming agents are not useful, and though atropine has been recommended, it is of doubtful value. If pulmonary edema is secondary to excessive parenteral administration of fluids or blood or to cardiac failure, the application of tourniquets or inflated blood pressure cuffs to the extremities or the withdrawal of blood may be lifesaving.

PULMONARY EMBOLISM AND INFARCTION

Pulmonary embolism as a recognized cause of disturbance in infants and children is rare. Emboli most often arise from thrombi in the femoral and pelvic veins and are usually postoperative complications. Fat emboli are most likely to be derived from fractured bones; on occasion they stem from necrotic tissue in the bone marrow of patients with sickle cell disease. Multiple pulmonary infarcts resulting from small emboli may be associated with severe dehydration in diarrheal disease, cyanotic heart disease, bacterial endocarditis and longstanding nutritional deficiencies. The clinical pattern is apt to be interpreted as a pneumonic process, and the diagnosis is usually made at autopsy. Emboli carrying bacteria may be responsible for multiple pulmonary abscesses.

Embolism of the pulmonary artery or its larger branches has a characteristic clinical picture. There is sudden pulmonary pain which is usually substernal, but may be pleural and radiate to the shoulder. There are dyspnea, tachycardia and signs of collapse. Though there are often no physical signs, if the infarct is sufficiently large (the base at the periphery and the apex toward the midline at the point of infarction), there may be impaired resonance and a pleural friction rub. Breath sounds may be distant or absent, and there may be moist rales. Expectorated material, which may be profuse, often contains blood. The case fatality rate is high, but recovery may occur even when the area of infarction is relatively large. Secondary infection may result in abscess formation.

PREVENTION. The prevention of pulmonary infarction depends essentially upon (1) prevention of vascular stasis, and (2) maintenance of a good nutritional status. The latter is especially important in bedridden children. Substances which decrease the coagulability of the blood such as heparin have a limited usefulness in pediatric practice.

TREATMENT. Embolism of the larger branches of the pulmonary artery is a medical emergency. The child should be given morphine sufficiently often to induce quietness and allay fears and should be placed in an oxygen tent for the relief of dyspnea and cyanosis.

Robbins, S. L.: Pathology. 3rd ed. Philadelphia, W. B. Saunders Company, 1967.

PULMONARY SUPPURATION

BRONCHIECTASIS

The term "bronchiectasis," as commonly used, is somewhat misleading. In the strict sense the connotation is simply dilatation of bronchi, whereas the process identified consists in inflammatory destruction of bronchial and peribronchial tissue, which permits accumulation of exudative material in dependent bronchi and hence distention of them in some instances. The classification of bronchiectasis based on such anatomic terms as cylindrical, fusiform, saccular or cystic has little clinical value.

Bronchiectasis is frequently misdiagnosed as chronic bronchitis, asthma or recurrent pneumonia; on the other hand, it may be present for some time without producing respiratory symptoms or may produce only minor ones. *The possibility that a nonopaque foreign body may be the cause of bronchiectasis is often overlooked.*

ETIOLOGY. Some cases probably represent **congenital bronchiectasis.** Though its pathogenesis is obscure, it has been postulated that an arrest in bronchial development has occurred which leads to formation of cysts; if these become infected, there is apt to be destruction of the bronchial wall. Another mechanism of congenital bronchiectasis is defective development of the bronchial cartilaginous supports. **Kartagener's syndrome** consists of dextrocardia, sinusitis and bronchiectasis, and has been reported to be manifest as early as infancy. Approximately 5 per cent of children with dextrocardia eventually have bronchiectasis; the bronchial defect is unknown but has been thought to include defective cartilage rings. Rarely, extreme forms of pectus excavatum or scoliosis may be associated with bronchiectasis, probably as a result of inadequate pulmonary drainage. There is evidence that some cases of bronchiectasis may be familial.

In the majority of instances bronchiectasis is probably acquired after birth without relation to congenital factors, but the mechanisms involved are poorly understood. Obstruction of the bronchial tree followed by infection is one possible inciting cause. For example, it is likely that atelectasis or aspiration followed by pulmonary infection during early infancy may be a contributing factor. Measles, pertussis and pneumonia in general, once regarded as frequent antecedent infections, are rare causes of bronchiectasis. At present cystic fibrosis is the single most common underlying factor in children. Here the bronchial involvement is generalized rather than localized. Other predisposing factors include aspiration of a foreign body, often a nonopaque one, enlarged bronchopulmonary nodes due to tuberculosis, recurrent and chronic lung infections, sarcoidosis, neoplasm, lung abscess, localized cysts and emphysema with compression of other lung parenchyma, allergy and asthma. Patients with agammaglobulinemia and dysgammaglobulinemia may have bronchiectasis, usually after repeated attacks of bacterial pneumonia and bronchitis. Bronchiectasis and sinusitis frequently coexist, but their interrelationship is not clear.

It has been postulated that the most common cause of bronchiectasis is gastroesophageal reflux leading to chronic aspiration of gastric contents; this view is not generally accepted.

The **"middle lobe syndrome"** consists of subacute or chronic pneumonitis, bronchial obstruction and atelectasis, and is generally caused by extrinsic compression of the middle lobe bronchus by hilar nodes, followed by peribronchitis and chronic infection. On occasion this syndrome is related to congenital anomalies of the bronchi.

Reversible bronchiectasis, or "pseudobronchiectasis," occurs relatively commonly after pertussis as well as with lobar and interstitial pneumonias. Shortly after or during these illnesses the bronchi will appear cylindrically dilated on bronchography, but if these studies are repeated some months later, the changes have disappeared.

Tracheobronchomegaly is a rare congenital condition in which the distal trachea and the main bronchi are grossly dilated. A similar condition may be associated with recurrent pneumonia.

PATHOLOGY. The exact mechanism producing dilatation of peripheral bronchi is unknown, but the first destructive change is a loss of ciliated epithelium, which is regenerated as cuboidal and squamous epithelium. Concurrently the elastic tissue within the bronchial walls disappears and thickening occurs, owing to interstitial edema, fibrosis and round cell infiltration, together with involvement of adjacent parenchymal and peribronchial tissue. In these peribronchial areas multiple abscesses may develop, and there usually is characteristic obstructive endarteritis of the small pulmonary vessels. Generally bronchiectasis follows a segmental distribution, except in cystic fibrosis. The areas most frequently involved depend somewhat on the basic cause; most frequently affected are the right middle lobe segments, the basal segments of the lower lobes, and the lingular segments of the left upper lobe. The right lower lobe is commonly involved by aspiration of a foreign body, whereas the right middle lobe is most frequently affected by hilar lymphadenopathy.

CLINICAL MANIFESTATIONS. In symptomatic cases cough is invariably present and produces copious mucopurulent sputum during acute respiratory infections. The sputum is generally swallowed by young children. Physical activity of the patient or change in position, particularly while reclining, will often initiate a bout of coughing.

Recurring infections of the lower respiratory tract are common; they tend to persist and are difficult to control. The patient may be afebrile, or fever may be the only symptom. Later in the course, particularly during acute exacerbations, hemoptysis may occur, varying in severity from streaking of the sputum to exsanguinating hemorrhage. Bronchiectasis characteristically follows a remitting and relapsing course; new pulmonary areas may or may not become involved.

Physical findings are often few, and may be absent. Moist or musical rales may be heard; during acute exacerbations physical signs of atelectasis or diffuse pneumonitis are often present. The usual roentgen examination is never pathognomonic, although such predisposing factors as mediastinal lymph nodes or radiopaque foreign bodies may be demonstrated, as well as suggestive increased bronchovascular markings near the hilus of the lung. Atelectasis is relatively common.

With extensive bronchiectasis there is persistent dyspnea, and physical development is retarded. Ventilatory and diffusion studies may reveal more widespread or severe pulmonary involvement than suspected otherwise. Pulmonary osteoarthropathy occurs relatively late, and probably represents a systemic reaction to arteriovenous shunting.

Bronchography is essential for diagnosis, as well as to delineate the extent of disease and the segments involved. To exclude the possibility of foreign bodies, strictures or tumors, bronchoscopy is essential. When the procedure is performed, secretions of the bronchi should be obtained for culture.

Every patient with suspected or proved bronchiectasis should be examined for the presence of such possible causative factors as sinusitis, agammaglobulinemia, tuberculosis, asthma or other respiratory allergy, and cystic fibrosis.

THERAPY. Therapy of bronchiectasis in children is primarily medical. Surgery should be contemplated only in patients with localized, severe disease who fail to respond to adequate medical management. Conservative treatment includes elimination of all foci of infection in the respiratory tract, effective postural drainage and, when indicated, antimicrobial therapy. Postural drainage must be carried out intensively as long as secretions are being formed and is one of the most important aspects of medical management. Its effectiveness may be enhanced by such measures as cupped-hand percussion.

Systemic antimicrobial therapy is usually administered only during acute exacerbations in short courses of 5 to 7 days or, rarely, up to 2 weeks. A few patients with bronchiectasis require more prolonged antimicrobial therapy for maximum benefit. Prolonged treatment, however, increases the risk of acquisition of resistant flora and reactions to the drugs employed. The appropriate drug is selected on the basis of the tested antimicrobial susceptibility of bacteria isolated from sputum, obtained preferably by bronchoscopy. If cultures contain only normal flora, antibiotic therapy should not be used. The administration of antimicrobial agents by aerosol inhalation immediately following appropriate postural drainage may also be helpful, but should not be continued for excessively long periods of time, since this will encourage the establishment of a drug-resistant bacterial flora, pseudomonas being particularly likely and troublesome.

In the infrequent instances when localized disease progresses despite adequate medical management, segmental or lobar resection should be considered, even though the long-term results are often discouraging. Surgery may also be indicated when an extrinsic anatomic obstruction of the bronchus is found or when suppurative lesions exist due to aspiration of fragmented foreign bodies, especially such vegetable objects as grass fibers or fragments of peanut which elude bronchoscopic removal.

PULMONARY ABSCESS

Abscesses of the lung occur when pulmonary parenchyma becomes obstructed, infected, and then suppurative and necrotic. Abscesses may be single or multiple, and be caused by a single organism, usually aerobic, or by anaerobic flora, usually mixed. Klebsiella and staphylococcal pneumonias often result in multiple abscesses, which occur infrequently in pneumococcal, streptococcal and *H. influenzae* pneumonias. Multiple abscesses may also be associated with tuberculous or mycotic infections. More often multiple abscesses occur in patients with such chronic pulmonary disease as cystic fibrosis or bronchiectasis, or with illnesses associated with diminished host resistance (agammaglobulinemia, agranulocytosis, chronic granulomatous disease of childhood, leukemia).

Solitary lung abscesses may be tuberculous, may follow pneumococcal or staphylococcal pneumonia, may stem from infected cysts or may be found in sequestered pulmonary tissue. Most commonly, however, a solitary lung abscess follows aspiration of a foreign body or other infected material or such surgical manipulations as tonsillectomy, adenoidectomy and tooth extractions. Abscesses associated with aspiration of tissue or foreign bodies are usually infected by bacteria normally found in the nasopharynx, such as anaerobic bacteroides, spirochetes, and various streptococci, generally not group A.

Whatever the cause, the pathologic evolution of abscess formation is similar. Initial inflammatory changes are followed by suppuration and thrombosis of the local blood vessels, which result in necrosis and liquefaction. Granulation tissue forms around the periphery of the abscess and may succeed in walling off the area, but more commonly the abscess will rupture into a bronchus and be evacuated. Contents of the abscess may be coughed up, or aspirated into other parts of the pulmonary tree, with additional abscess formation. Sputum is usually fetid, may separate into layers, and usually contains elastic fibers.

Peripheral abscesses may involve the adjacent pleura, with development of a plastic or occasionally a serofibrinous pleurisy. Abscesses may rupture into the pleural cavity and produce empyema.

On occasion, pulmonary abscesses may occur within interlobar fissures, where they are usually well encapsulated and respond poorly to antimicrobial therapy.

CLINICAL MANIFESTATIONS. The onset of lung

abscess is occasionally insidious, but more commonly there is the sudden appearance of fever, cough and chest pain, often associated with dyspnea and tachypnea. The fever curve is often septic in type, and leukocytosis is usually marked. Physical examination may or may not reveal an area of pulmonary consolidation, depending on the location of the abscess and its size. At an early stage roentgenographic examination will usually show a wedge-shaped area of consolidation.

In untreated patients the abscess will often rupture into a bronchus within a week to 10 days after onset, with production of purulent or putrid sputum; hemoptysis is common in older children. At this time roentgenographic examination will usually reveal a cavity, with or without a fluid level, surrounded by an area of consolidation. Spontaneous drainage of the abscess may result in disappearance of symptoms within about a month. During this interval, clubbing of the fingers may appear and recurrent hemoptysis may be seen.

TREATMENT. Adequate treatment of pneumococcal pneumonia with penicillin will usually prevent pulmonary cavitation. With staphylococcal and klebsiella pneumonias, cavitation often occurs despite treatment but rarely requires special therapy. It is generally enough if the underlying pneumonia is treated vigorously with suitable antimicrobial therapy. When a foreign body is suspected, bronchoscopic examination should be performed promptly for verification and removal, if possible. Bronchoscopy should be done also, as soon as an abscess ruptures into a bronchus, to aspirate the purulent material and to secure bacteriologic cultures by aerobic and anaerobic techniques. Repeated bronchoscopic aspirations may be needed for the patient who continues to cough up large quantities of purulent material. Intensive and appropriate antimicrobial therapy should be continued for at least 2 weeks. The instillation of proteolytic enzymes or antibiotics into the abscess cavity has not contributed significantly to therapy. As long as the patient continues to bring up sputum, he should receive postural drainage and physical therapy to the chest.

When patients do not respond to initial bronchoscopic aspiration and intensive antimicrobial therapy, repeated aspirations of the abscess may lead to eventual closure of the cavity. If conservative management has not given satisfactory results in 1 month, surgical removal of the affected segment or lobe is usually carried out.

PULMONARY GANGRENE

Gangrene of the lung is extremely rare in children. It occasionally follows measles, and is seen in persons with severe immunologic deficits. The onset is usually sudden and is associated with early pulmonary hemorrhage; there is rapid development of pneumothorax and putrid empyema, death occurring quickly. Treatment consists of adequate pleural drainage and intensive antimicrobial therapy.

PULMONARY SEQUESTRATION

Pulmonary sequestration is a congenital condition in which nonfunctioning embryonic and cystic lung tissue supplied by systemic arteries is contained within otherwise normal lung parenchyma, or, less commonly, is found at an extralobar location.

This condition apparently results from maldevelopment of the primitive vascular and respiratory tissue during the time when the lungs bud from the main tracheobronchial apparatus. Histologically the tissue is of fetal appearance and is cystic and disorganized. Most commonly, sequestered lung tissue is found in the region of the lower lobes.

Pulmonary sequestration becomes symptomatic if the tissue is infected; this may occur either by way of a fistula to normal lung tissue or through a similar connection to the digestive tract. Sequestered lung may also become infected by extension of pneumonia from neighboring lung. The primary manifestations of the condition become those of a recurrent, progressive, persistent pulmonary infection, often with suppuration and abscess formation. The patient is febrile and has cough, hemoptysis and weight loss; the signs and symptoms are indistinguishable from those found with other types of lung abscess. Roentgenographic findings do not differentiate the process from pneumonia and other lung abscesses, except that the process is generally limited to the basal segments of the lower lobes. The diagnosis of pulmonary sequestration is suggested by repeated episodes of infection involving the same basal area of the lung. Definitive diagnosis can be accomplished by bronchography or aortography. On bronchography the area of sequestration will not fill with dye, but its borders can be outlined by bronchi which are filled. Aortography will demonstrate anomalous arterial supply and give proof of the nature of the pulmonary density.

When the diagnosis has been established, resection of the sequestered area should be performed. Antimicrobial therapy is indicated prior to surgery.

Bronchiectasis

Becroft, D. M. O.: Bronchiolitis obliterans, bronchiectasis and other sequelae of adenovirus type 21 infection. J. Clin. Path., *24*:72, 1971.

Biering, A.: Childhood pneumonia, including pertussis pneumonia and bronchiectasis: A follow-up study of 151 patients. Acta Paediat., *45*:348, 1956.

Clark, N. S.: Bronchiectasis in childhood. Brit. Med. J., *1*:80, 1963.

Field, C. E.: Bronchiectasis in childhood. I. Clinical survey of 160 cases. II. Aetiology and pathogenesis, including a survey of 272 cases of doubtful irreversible bronchiectasis. Pediatrics, *4*:21, 231, 1949.

Field, C. E.: Bronchiectasis: Third report of a follow-up study of medical and surgical cases from childhood. Arch. Dis. Child., *44*:551, 1969.

Visconti, R. J.: Agammaglobulinemia with bronchopulmonary manifestations. Report of a case. Dis. Chest, *48*:530, 1965.

Williams, H., and O'Reilly, R. N.: Bronchiectasis in children: Its multiple clinical and pathological aspects. Arch. Dis. Child., *34*:192, 1959.

Williams, H. E., Landau, L. I., and Phelan, P. D.: Generalized bronchiectasis due to extensive deficiency of bronchial cartilage. Arch. Dis. Child., *47*:423, 1972.

Pulmonary Abscess
Bernhard, W. F., Malcolm, J. A., and Wylie, R. H.: Lung abscess: A study of 148 cases due to aspiration. Dis. Chest, *43*:620, 1963.
Collins, H. A., and Daniel, R. A., Jr.: Primary lung abscess. J. Thorac. Cardiov. Surg., *47*:383, 1964.
Pickar, D. N., and Ruoff, W. F.: Pulmonary abscess: A study of 70 cases. J. Thorac. Surg., *37*:452, 1959.

Pulmonary Gangrene
Lewis, J. M., and Barenberg, L. H.: Pulmonary gangrene due to spirochetes and fusiform bacilli. Am. J. Dis. Child., *37*:351, 1929.

Pulmonary Sequestration
Asp, K., Heikel, P. E., and Pasila, M.: Pulmonary sequestrations in children. Ann. Paediat. Fenn., *9*:270, 1963.
Simopoulos, A. P., Rosenblum, D. J., Mazumdar, H., and Kiely, B.: Intralobar bronchopulmonary sequestration in children: Diagnosis by intrathoracic aortography. Am. J. Dis. Child., *97*:796, 1959.
Talalak, P.: Pulmonary sequestration. Arch. Dis. Child., *35*:57, 1960.

Diseases of the Pleura

PLEURISY

Inflammatory processes in the pleura are usually divided into three general types: dry or plastic, serofibrinous or serosanguineous, and purulent pleurisy or empyema.

DRY OR PLASTIC PLEURISY

Dry or plastic pleurisy may be associated with pneumococcal pneumonia, or other acute bacterial pulmonary infections. Occasionally there is no obvious pulmonary involvement; in such instances the signs and symptoms usually develop during the course of an acute upper respiratory tract illness. The condition also is associated with tuberculosis and with mesenchymal diseases such as rheumatic fever.

The pathologic process is usually limited to the visceral pleura, which is roughened in appearance and covered with thick, yellowish green fibrin. There are usually small amounts of yellow serous fluid, which clots rapidly upon removal. Adhesions between the pleural surfaces develop rapidly, particularly in tuberculosis, in which thickening of the pleura often occurs. Occasionally fibrin deposition and adhesions may be sufficiently severe to produce a fibrothorax, which markedly inhibits the excursions of the lung.

CLINICAL MANIFESTATIONS. Signs and symptoms are often overshadowed by the primary disease. The principal symptom of dry pleurisy is pain, which is exaggerated by deep breathing, coughing and straining. Often the pain is not only localized over the chest wall, but also may be referred to the shoulder or the back. Pain with breathing is responsible for grunting and guarding of respirations, the child often lying on the affected side in an attempt to decrease respiratory excursions. Early in the illness a leathery, rough, to-and-fro friction rub may be audible, but this usually disappears rapidly. Occasionally increased dullness on percussion and suppressed breath sounds are heard when the layer of exudate is thick. On occasion, pleurisy is asymptomatic and is detected only on roentgenography. Two different radiologic pictures may be found; one consists of a diffuse haziness at the pleural surface, the other of a dense shadow which may be sharply demarcated. The latter finding may be indistinguishable from small amounts of pleural exudate. Chronic pleurisy is occasionally encountered with such conditions as atelectasis, pulmonary abscess, mesenchymal diseases and tuberculosis.

DIFFERENTIAL DIAGNOSIS. Plastic pleurisy must be distinguished from other diseases such as epidemic pleurodynia or trauma to the rib cage, particularly fracture of a rib, and from lesions of the dorsal root ganglia, tumors of the spinal cord, herpes zoster, gallbladder disease and trichinosis. Even if evidence of pleural fluid is not found on physical or x-ray examination, a pleural tap in suspected cases will often result in the recovery of small amounts of exudate, which, when cultured, will usually reveal the underlying bacterial cause in cases associated with an acute pneumonia. When pleurisy and pneumonia continue for more than a week, tuberculosis must be considered a causative possibility.

TREATMENT. Treatment should be aimed at the underlying disease. In the presence of pneumonia neither immobilization of the chest with adhesive plaster nor therapy with drugs capable of suppressing the cough reflex should be undertaken. If pneumonia is not present, or is under good therapeutic control, strapping of the chest to restrict expansion may afford relief from pain.

SEROFIBRINOUS PLEURISY

Serofibrinous pleurisy is most commonly associated with infections of the lung or with inflammatory conditions of the abdomen or mediastinum. Less commonly it is found with such mesenchymal diseases as lupus erythematosus, periarteritis or rheumatic fever. On occasion this type of effusion is seen with neoplasms of the lung, pleura or mediastinum, which may be primary or metastatic; tumors are, however, more commonly associated with a hemorrhagic pleurisy. Of infectious diseases, tuberculosis has been the most frequent cause of serofibrinous effusion, but in population groups where mycobacterial disease occurs infrequently, pneumococci have become the most common infectious agents.

CLINICAL MANIFESTATIONS. Since serofibrinous

pleurisy is often preceded by the plastic type, the early signs and symptoms may be those of the latter illness. As fluid accumulates, pleuritic pain may disappear and the patient become asymptomatic so long as the effusion remains small, or there may be only the signs and symptoms of the underlying disease. If a large amount of fluid collects, there may be cough, dyspnea, tachypnea, orthopnea or cyanosis. Physical findings depend to some degree on the amount of effusion. Dullness to flatness may be found on percussion. There is a decrease or absence of breath sounds, a diminution in tactile fremitus, a shift of the mediastinum away from the affected side, and, on occasion, fullness of the intercostal spaces. If the fluid is not loculated, these signs may shift with changes in position. In infants, physical signs are less definite; sometimes, instead of decreased or absent breath sounds, bronchial breathing will be heard. If extensive pneumonia is present, rales and rhonchi may also be audible. Friction rubs are usually present only during the early or late plastic stage. The process is usually unilateral.

Roentgenographic examination shows a more or less homogeneous density obliterating the normal markings of the underlying lung. Small effusions may cause only obliteration of the costophrenic or cardiophrenic angles or a widening of the interlobar septa. Examination should be performed both in the supine and in the upright positions to demonstrate a shift of the effusion with change in position. The decubitus position may also be helpful.

DIFFERENTIAL DIAGNOSIS. Thoracentesis should always be done when pleural fluid is known to be present or is suspected. Examination of the fluid is essential to identify acute bacterial infections and may disclose tubercle bacilli. Furthermore, thoracentesis can differentiate between serofibrinous pleurisy, empyema, hydrothorax, hemothorax and chylothorax. In hydrothorax the fluid has a low specific gravity, below 1.015, and only a few mesothelial cells rather than leukocytes. Chylothorax and hemothorax usually have fluid distinctive in appearance. It is not possible to differentiate serofibrinous from purulent pleurisy without bacterial examination of the fluid. The fluid of serofibrinous pleurisy is clear or slightly cloudy and contains relatively few white cells and, occasionally, some red cells. Serofibrinous fluid may rapidly become purulent; its nature may depend on the time during the course of illness when thoracentesis is performed.

COURSE. Unless the fluid becomes purulent, it usually disappears relatively rapidly, particularly with bacterial pneumonias. It persists somewhat longer with mesenchymal diseases and tuberculosis and may remain or recur for a long time with neoplasms. As the effusion is absorbed, adhesions usually develop between the two layers of the pleura, but no functional impairment results. Pleural thickening may develop and is occasionally mistaken for small quantities of fluid or for pulmonary infiltrates. Residual pleural thickening may persist for a long time. In general, however, the process disappears, leaving no residua.

TREATMENT. The treatment is that of the underlying disease. When a diagnostic thoracentesis is done, as much fluid as possible should be removed. If the underlying disease is adequately treated, there is usually no necessity for further drainage, but if sufficient fluid reaccumulates to embarrass the patient's respiration, repeated drainage should be performed.

PURULENT PLEURISY
(Empyema)

Purulent pleurisy, or empyema, is an accumulation of pus in the pleural spaces. At present the condition is most often associated with pneumonia due to staphylococci, less frequently with pneumococci and *H. influenzae.* In pediatric practice, empyema is most frequently encountered during infancy.

The disease may be produced also when a lung abscess ruptures into the pleural space, by contamination introduced from trauma or thoracic surgery, or rarely by mediastinitis or by the extension of intra-abdominal abscesses.

PATHOLOGY. Most commonly, purulent pleurisy is an extensive process, consisting of a series of loculated areas involving a large portion of one or both pleural cavities. Thickening of the parietal pleura occurs. If the pus is not drained, it may dissect through the chest wall *(empyema necessitatis),* into lung parenchyma, producing bronchopleural fistulas and pyopneumothorax, or into the abdominal cavity. Pockets of loculated pus may eventually develop into thick-walled abscess cavities, or, as the exudate organizes, the lung may collapse and be surrounded by a thick, inelastic envelope.

CLINICAL MANIFESTATIONS. Since most purulent pleurisy occurs early in the course of bacterial pneumonia, the initial signs and symptoms are primarily those of the underlying disease. Patients treated inadequately or with inappropriate antimicrobial agents may have an interval of a few days between the clinical phase of pneumonia and the evidence of empyema. In infants, manifestations of the disease may consist only of moderate exacerbation of respiratory distress. The older child is apt to appear more toxic and in greater respiratory difficulty. Physical and radiologic findings are identical to those described for serofibrinous pleurisy; the two conditions can be differentiated only by thoracentesis, which should always be performed when empyema is suspected. The maximum amount of pus obtainable should be withdrawn. The physical appearance of pus produced by different organisms is not particularly distinctive; cultures must always be obtained and Gram-stained smears examined for the presence of microorganisms. Staphylococci are usually numerous and thus easily identified; pneumococci and *H. influenzae* occasionally are present only in small numbers, particularly if antimicrobial therapy has been given previously,

COMPLICATIONS. With staphylococcal infections, bronchopleural fistulas and pyopneumothorax commonly develop. Other local complications encountered with any bacterial agent include purulent pericarditis, pulmonary abscesses, peritonitis secondary to rupture through the diaphragm, osteomyelitis of the ribs, and such septic complications as meningitis, arthritis and osteomyelitis. With staphylococcal empyema, septicemia occurs infrequently; it is often encountered in *H. influenzae* and pneumococcal infections.

TREATMENT. If pus is obtained by thoracentesis, closed drainage should be instituted immediately and controlled either by an underwater seal or by continuous suction. A catheter with the largest possible internal diameter should be inserted into the site where accumulation of pus is suspected; sometimes several tubes are required to drain loculated areas. Closed drainage is usually necessary only for a week or so, even though small amounts of material will continue to drain after this time; this material is usually formed in response to the presence of the tube in the pleural cavity. There is no need to withdraw the tube gradually; rather, it should be removed all at once.

The introduction of fibrinolytic agents or proteolytic enzymes commonly produces severe systemic reactions in small children, and they do not appear to promote drainage substantially. If the chest tube is of sufficient caliber and is kept clear, a free flow of pus is obtained. The instillation of antibiotics into the pleural cavity does not improve results obtained with systemic antimicrobial therapy alone and is associated with local reactions. No attempt should be made to control empyema by multiple aspirations of the pleural cavity rather than by closed continuous drainage.

Systemic antimicrobial therapy is required; the selection of the antibiotic should be based on the in vitro sensitivities of the responsible organism. Staphylococcal empyema in infancy is best treated by parenteral routes with methicillin or, when applicable, with penicillin G. Pneumococcal infection responds to penicillin, and *H. influenzae* to ampicillin. There is no advantage in the use of multiple antimicrobial agents. With staphylococcal infections, resolution of the process is slow, and systemic antimicrobial therapy is required for 3 or 4 weeks. In patients with inadequately treated empyema, extensive fibrinous changes may take place over the surface of the collapsed lungs; these may require decortication at a future date. If pneumatoceles form, no attempt should be made to treat them surgically, or by aspiration, unless they reach sufficient size to embarrass respiration or become secondarily infected.

Bechamps, G. J., Lynn, H. B., and Wenzl, J. E.: Empyema in children. Mayo Clin. Proc. *45*:43, 1970.

Middlekamp, J. N., Purterson, M. L., and Burford, T. H.: The changing pattern of empyema thoracis in pediatrics. J. Thorac. Cardiov. Surg. *47*:165, 1964.

Ravitch, M. M., and Fein, R.: The changing picture of pneumonia and empyema in infants and children. A review of the experience at the Harriet Lane Home from 1934 through 1958. J.A.M.A. *175*:1039, 1961.

Riley, H. D., Jr., and Bracken, E. C.: Empyema due to hemophilus influenzae in infants and children. Am. J. Dis. Child. *110*:24, 1965.

PNEUMOTHORAX

Pneumothorax in the neonatal period may be related to factors incident to birth and be associated with interstitial emphysema and pneumomediastinum (Section 7). In staphylococcal pneumonia in infancy the incidence of pneumothorax is relatively high. Aside from the accidental introduction of air into the pleural cavity during thoracentesis, pneumothorax is uncommon during childhood. Pneumothorax may occur in pneumonia, usually in connection with empyema; it may also be secondary to pulmonary abscess, gangrene, infarct, rupture of a cyst or an emphysematous bleb (as in asthma), foreign bodies in the lung and external thoracic trauma or surgical procedures. In association with mediastinal emphysema it is an occasional complication of tracheotomy.

Pneumothorax may be associated with a serous effusion *(hydropneumothorax)* or a purulent effusion *(pyopneumothorax)*. In pneumothorax the lung collapses toward the hilus, unless prevented by adhesions. Bilateral pneumothorax is rare.

CLINICAL MANIFESTATIONS. The onset is usually abrupt. When the pneumothorax is extensive, there may be pain, dyspnea and cyanosis. In infancy both symptoms and physical signs may be difficult to recognize. If the pneumothorax is only moderate in extent, there may be little displacement of intrathoracic organs and few or no symptoms.

The percussion note over the involved area is tympanitic; on auscultation respiratory sounds are feeble or absent. Larynx, trachea and heart may be shifted toward the unaffected side. The breath sounds may have an amphoric quality if there is an open fistula from air-bearing tissues into the pleural cavity. When fluid is present, there is usually a sharply delimited area of tympany above a level of flatness to percussion. It is important to determine whether the pneumothorax is an open *(tension pneumothorax)* or a closed one. The presence of amphoric breathing or of gurgling sounds synchronous with respirations when fluid is present in the pleural cavity is suggestive of an open fistula. Confirmatory evidence is provided when the pneumothorax fills rapidly after aspiration of it. Another means for determining whether a fistula is open is examination of the aspirated air for its oxygen content. If a fistula is present, the oxygen content of the air in pneumothorax remains constant. If there is no connection with the bronchial tree, the oxygen content is low, since it is rapidly absorbed. The diagnosis can usually be estab-

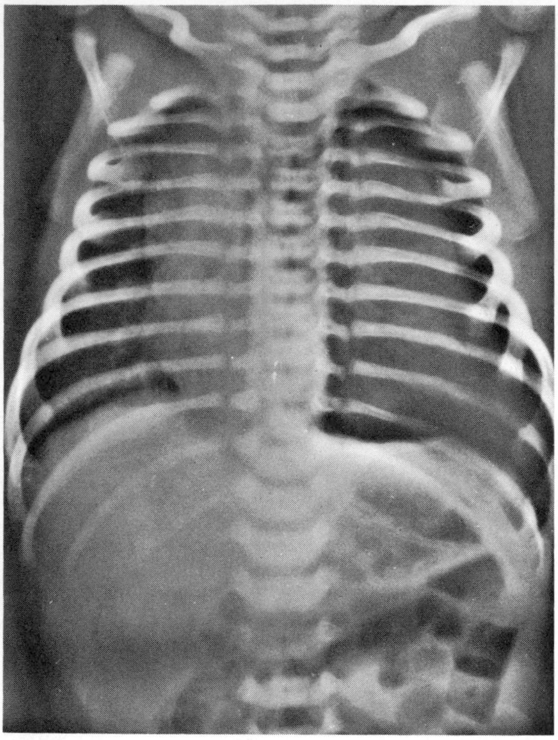

Figure 12-18 *Pneumothorax in a newborn infant. The air in the left pleural cavity has resulted in partial collapse of the left lung and shift of the heart and mediastinal structures to the right.*

lished by roentgenographic examination (Fig. 12-18).

DIFFERENTIAL DIAGNOSIS. Pneumothorax must be differentiated from localized or generalized emphysema, from an extensive emphysematous bleb, from large pulmonary cavities or other cystic formations, from diaphragmatic hernia and from gaseous distention of the stomach. In most instances a simple roentgenogram will be all that is necessary for the differentiation. In the case of diaphragmatic hernia, however, a small amount of barium may be necessary to demonstrate that a portion of the gastrointestinal tract is in the thoracic cavity.

PROGNOSIS AND TREATMENT. The prognosis depends upon the cause. When there is no fistula connecting the air-bearing tissue and the pneumothorax, the air is usually absorbed within a week or so, and no treatment is necessary unless there are symptoms of excessive pressure, in which case the air should be aspirated.

Tension pneumothorax with a communicating fistula is usually best managed with a closed thoracotomy and drainage of the trapped air through a catheter whose external opening is kept in a dependent position under water. If the bronchopleural fistula is large, negative pressure in the drainage tube may be necessary. If the tension pneumothorax is not relieved by this means, surgical closure of the fistula should be considered. Treatment of a coexisting empyema is of course essential.

HYDROTHORAX

In hydrothorax the fluid is noninflammatory in origin and has a lower specific gravity (less than 1.015) than that of a serofibrinous exudate. It contains less protein and fewer cells, which are mesothelial rather than leukocytic, and is usually associated with an accumulation of fluid in other parts of the body such as the peritoneal cavity and the subcutaneous tissues. Hydrothorax is most often associated with cardiac or renal disease, although on occasion it may be a manifestation of severe nutritional edema, and rarely it results from venous obstruction by neoplasms, enlarged lymph nodes or adhesions. Hydrothorax is usually bilateral in renal disease and in nutritional edema and may be in myocardial disease, although in this instance it may be limited to the right side or greater on the right than on the left side. The physical signs are those described under Serofibrinous Pleurisy, but there is more rapid shifting of the level of dullness with changes of position. The treatment is that of the primary disorder; aspiration may be necessary when pressure symptoms are notable.

HEMOTHORAX

Extensive bleeding into the pleural cavity may result from erosion of a blood vessel in association with such inflammatory processes as tuberculosis and empyema, but is not common. It is also an occasional manifestation of intrathoracic neoplasms and blood dyscrasias, and may be the result of thoracic trauma. Rupture of an aneurysm is not likely during childhood. When a pleural hemorrhage occurs in association with a pneumothorax, it is termed *hemopneumothorax.* The diagnosis of a hemothorax can be made only by thoracentesis. In every instance an effort must be made to determine the cause, the treatment obviously depending upon it. Surgical intervention may be required to control active bleeding, and transfusion is necessary when loss of blood is excessive.

CHYLOTHORAX

Chylothorax is a rare condition at any age, but especially in childhood, though it has been observed even during the neonatal period. It depends upon the escape of chyle from the thoracic duct into the thoracic cavity. In most instances thoracic trauma has produced rupture of the duct, but the escape of chyle apparently can occur without rupture as a result of the pressure of enlarged lymph nodes or neoplasms. Thrombosis of the duct or the subclavian vein and congenital anomalies of the duct system have also been reported as causes. Chylothorax is rarely bilateral, usually being on the left side.

The symptoms and physical signs are those related to the presence of fluid in the thoracic cavity. The diagnosis is established when thoracentesis demonstrates a chylous effusion, a milky fluid containing fat, protein and other constituents of chyle. In newborn infants who have not yet been fed the fluid may be clear. A pseudochylous milky fluid has been reported in cases of serous effusion in which the fatty material was assumed to be due to the degenerative changes within the fluid and not the presence of lymph. It has been suggested that this type of fluid can be distinguished from one containing chyle by shaking it with alkalis or ether; the fluid containing chyle tends to become clear.

Spontaneous recovery has occurred in over half of the reported cases in infants under a year of age. Repeated aspirations may be required to relieve the symptoms of pressure. The aspirated chyle has been reinjected intravenously without untoward reactions, although there is some doubt whether it has any particular benefit. The diet should be low in fat and high in protein. The lowered intake of fat is thought to be associated with a decreased production of chyle. The high protein intake is required because of loss of protein in the chyle. The total caloric intake must be above the average requirement, and several times the daily requirements of the various vitamins, especially the fat-soluble vitamins A and D, should be added. (See Section 7 for Chylothorax in the newborn infant.)

HEINZ F. EICHENWALD
GEORGE H. MCCRACKEN, JR.

Decancq, H. G., Jr.: Treatment of chylothorax in children. Surg. Gynec. Obstet. *121*:509, 1965.

Riker, W. L.: Lung cysts and pneumothorax in infants and children. Surg. Clin. N. Amer. *36*:1613, 1956.

Watson, E. H., and Foster, L. F.: Spontaneous chylothorax in infancy: Prognosis and management. Am. J. Dis. Child. *72*:89, 1946.

13
THE CARDIOVASCULAR SYSTEM

EVALUATION OF THE HEART AND CIRCULATION IN HEALTH AND DISEASE

INSPECTION AND PALPATION. In early life the heart is situated somewhat higher in the chest than in later years. The apex beat in the newborn infant may be palpated in the fourth left interspace in or just lateral to the left midclavicular line. After the age of 2 years the apical impulse is usually in the fifth intercostal space in or just medial to the midclavicular line. The flexibility of the mediastinum permits the heart to shift toward the side on which the patient lies. Although the relation of the apical thrust to the position of the midclavicular line is not an accurate index of cardiac size, it is helpful in making an estimate.

A hyperdynamic thrust, often extending over one or more interspaces, may accompany hypertrophy and dilatation of the ventricles. When the left ventricle is enlarged, the apex is likely to be one or two interspaces lower and farther to the left than normally. Enlargement of either ventricle, but especially of the right, tends to push the left side of the chest wall forward if the cardiac disease develops in early life. Displacement of the apex beat to the right or left without cardiac enlargement may be caused by pulmonary conditions such as empyema, atelectasis or the collapse of one lung, and sometimes by scoliosis of the spine or defects of the diaphragm.

A clinical evaluation of ventricular hypertrophy can be made by palpation of the apical impulse. In the presence of right ventricular hypertrophy the sensation of a *tap* is transmitted to the hand, whereas in left ventricular hypertrophy the apical impulse is *heaving.* Right ventricular hypertrophy is usually associated with clockwise rotation of the heart, so that the right ventricle accounts for nearly all the anterior surface of the heart. This can be appreciated by palpation of a sternal and a parasternal lift. Epigastric pulsations are commonly seen and felt in the presence of right ventricular hypertrophy, owing to the proximity of that chamber to the diaphragm. Biventricular hypertrophy can be suspected by a combination of the foregoing signs, namely, a sternal and parasternal lift associated with a left ventricular apical thrust.

Thrills may be detected during palpation; they should be timed in relation to the cardiac impulse. If the child is able to cooperate with the examiner, thrills should be felt during full expiratory apnea. Apical thrills are felt more easily in the left lateral position, and basal thrills with the patient sitting and leaning forward. Abnormal pulsations may also be detected, such as those produced by aneurysms or collateral vessels.

PERCUSSION. Percussion of the cardiac borders in infants is difficult, owing to the thick layers of subcutaneous fat on the chest wall and the barrel shape of the thorax. The value of percussion in the diagnosis of heart disease is frequently overstressed. This method can be helpful in the evaluation of pericardial effusion, dextrocardia and movement of the mediastinum secondary to pulmonary or pleural space disease. Accurate assessments of cardiac size, shape and position can usually be made only by radiography.

AUSCULTATION. The origin of the normal **first heart sound** is debatable. It is clearly related to events occurring in early systole and for many years was attributed solely to closure of the atrioventricular valves. Other factors contributing to this sound are the rapid rise of pressure during isometric contraction, the opening of the semilunar valves and the acceleration of blood in the great arteries. The first sound is louder when cardiac output is increased, as with fever, anemia, emotion and hyperthyroidism. It is also augmented in mitral stenosis and when the P-R interval is short.

The **second heart sound** is primarily due to closure of the semilunar valves. Normally the ventricles contract asynchronously, the left preceding the right. Therefore, at the end of systole, aortic valve closure precedes pulmonary valve closure. This results in physiologic splitting of the second sound, which is best heard at the upper left sternal edge and can be detected in most normal children

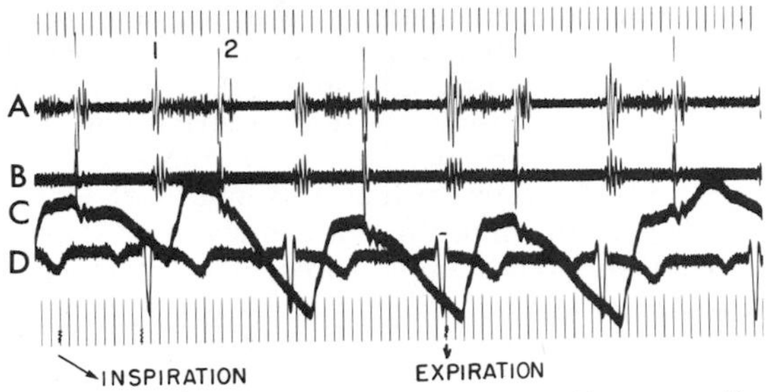

Figure 13–1 *Physiologic splitting of second heart sound in a 5 year old child with an innocent systolic murmur. Tracings from above are (A) phonocardiogram at pulmonary area, (B) phonocardiogram at apex, (C) carotid pulse, (D), electrocardiogram. Time lines 0.04 second. 1, First heart sound; 2, second heart sound.*

(Fig. 13–1). Furthermore, the split widens in inspiration and narrows in expiration, owing to the respiratory variation of pulmonary valve closure. The inspiratory delay of closure of the pulmonary valve is probably due to an increase in right ventricular stroke volume during this phase of respiration.

Recognition of the variations in the normal splitting of the second heart sound is of considerable diagnostic importance. Wide splitting of this sound is often associated with conditions causing left-to-right shunting of blood such as may occur in atrial septal defect. In the presence of severe pulmonary stenosis the intensity of the systolic murmur frequently obscures the aortic element of the second heart sound. This produces a single soft second sound which arises from late closure of the pulmonary valve. In tetralogy of Fallot the pulmonary element of the second sound may not be audible, resulting in a single second sound due to aortic valve closure.

A **third heart sound** is common in normal children. It occurs in early diastole (100 to 160 msec after the second sound), is best heard toward the cardiac apex and is of low intensity and frequency. This sound has been associated with rapid ventricular filling, as may occur in a normal heart. It is also audible when there is increased flow across the atrioventricular valves, as with large left-to-right shunts or incompetence of these valves. The pathologic counterpart of this sound produces the cadence of **protodiastolic gallop rhythm** and has been attributed to abrupt change in early ventricular filling because of abnormal compliance of the ventricle. Ventricular gallop rhythms are heard in myocarditis and in congestive heart failure. Generally they are associated with a poor prognosis.

The **fourth heart sound** occurs at the time of atrial systole and may be audible in normal children. Systolic overload of either ventricle may result in vigorous atrial contraction in order to fill the hypertrophied ventricle; therefore, the presence of a fourth sound is generally associated with significant obstruction to ventricular ejection.

Ejection Sounds. Aortic or pulmonic ejection sounds occurring early in systole are related to dilatation of or hypertension in the aorta and pulmonary artery. They are frequently heard in aortic or pulmonic stenosis and may be mistaken for a split first heart sound. The aortic variety is more widely transmitted and may be heard at the apex, whereas pulmonary ejection sounds are heard best along the left sternal border, especially during expiration.

Systolic Clicks. Early systolic clicks are synonymous with ejection sounds described above. The mechanism of midsystolic and late systolic clicks and multiple systolic clicks is unknown. They are heard best at the left sternal border and apex, and their intensity and timing are affected by respiration and position of the body. In the majority of instances the clicks are innocuous and are not indicative of heart disease. It is important to recognize their benign nature and to differentiate them from pathologic sounds such as a diastolic gallop rhythm, widely split second sound and an opening snap. A functional systolic murmur may be initiated by a click. Also, a systolic click may initiate a late systolic murmur of mitral incompetence.

Systolic Murmurs. A practical and clinically applicable classification of systolic murmurs based on abnormal hemodynamics has been described by Leatham. These murmurs have been divided into ejection and pansystolic types based on the timing of the murmur in relation to the first and second heart sounds.

Ejection Systolic Murmurs. These are produced by (1) stenosis of the pulmonary or aortic valves or infundibular stenosis, (2) dilatation of the aorta or pulmonary artery, (3) increased blood flow through a semilunar valve, and (4) combinations of these factors. These murmurs are found clinically in aortic and pulmonary stenosis and in conditions associated with a large left-to-right shunt. Their nature is related to the timing of valve closure on the side of the heart from which it originates. Ejection murmurs start after the first heart sound because blood flow, and consequently the murmur, only begins when the ventricle raises its pressure sufficiently to open its respective semilunar valve. The murmur increases in intensity in early, mid or late systole and ends before the normal or delayed semilunar valve closure of the affected side of the heart.

Pansystolic (Regurgitant) Murmurs. These are caused by the flow of blood from a ventricle or artery that retains a higher pressure throughout systole than the receiving chamber or vessel. They are heard most frequently in patients with mitral or tricuspid insufficiency and in ventricular septal defect. Blood flow, and consequently the murmur, begins soon after the first heart sound and continues up to the second heart sound.

Diastolic Murmurs. Diastolic murmurs may be divided into the following: (1) rumbling mid-diastolic mitral or tricuspid murmurs due to increased atrioventricular flow (as in left-to-right shunts) or atrioventricular valve disease with or without stenosis, (2) early, high-pitched diastolic murmurs due to incompetence of the aortic or pulmonary valves, and (3) atrial systolic murmurs (presystolic) due to active atrial contraction in the presence of stenosis of the atrioventricular valve or to increased atrial stroke volume.

Sounds and murmurs produced by valves are not always heard at the positions of the chest wall to which these sounds might be expected to be transmitted. For example, the ejection systolic murmur of aortic stenosis may be heard best at the apex. Therefore care should be taken to auscultate the whole precordium and not to localize the examination to certain predetermined points on the left side of the chest. Murmurs of congenital heart disease in children may be widely transmitted, so that it is necessary also to auscultate both sides of the neck and the back. On the other hand, the friction of a pericardial rub may be localized fairly accurately over the areas from which it emanates.

In older, cooperative children, sounds and murmurs may be more easily heard by varying the child's position, listening in various phases of respiration and noting the effects of exercise. Thus, mitral systolic and diastolic murmurs are more easily heard with the child in the left lateral position, especially after exercise, and basal murmurs may be more obvious in the forward sitting position with the patient in full expiratory apnea.

Innocent Murmurs. The terms "functional," "accidental" and "insignificant" have been used synonymously to designate murmurs unrelated to any demonstrable cardiac disturbance or anatomic abnormality. Though common usage has been responsible for their continuation, the term "innocent" is preferred because it stresses the innocuousness of the murmur. At a single, random auscultation, approximately 30 per cent of children may be found to have an innocent murmur; the number is higher with repeated auscultations of the same children over a period of years.

A common early or midsystolic innocent murmur, variously described as vibratory, musical, pure-pitched or squeaky, is heard especially at the lower left sternal edge (Fig. 13–2). In others, the systolic ejection murmur is short and of high frequency at the left second intercostal space. The intensity of innocent murmurs decreases, or they may disappear completely, when the patient changes position. These murmurs may also disappear with the Valsalva maneuver and reappear after release of the maneuver. The loudness and even the presence of the murmur may be variable from examination to examination. Occasionally they remain constant under all conditions and persist until adolescence. Soft murmurs often develop during an acute illness or severe anemia and disappear during convalescence. The intensity of innocent systolic murmurs is usually increased during an intercurrent acute infection. The quality, location and variability of these murmurs usually indicate their innocuousness, and these patients have normal electrocardiograms and x-ray films.

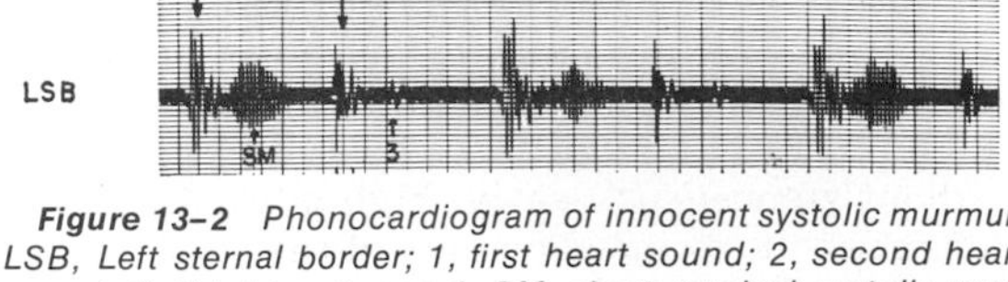

Figure 13–2 Phonocardiogram of innocent systolic murmur, LSB, Left sternal border; 1, first heart sound; 2, second heart sound; 3, third heart sound; SM, short musical systolic murmur. Time lines 0.04 second.

The mechanism of these murmurs is not understood clearly. They may represent an increase in intensity of normal vibrations in the pulmonary artery, or a series of systolic clicks may simulate a murmur.

It is important to reassure the parents of the innocence of the murmur and to avoid unnecessary limitations of the child's activities.

A **venous hum** is produced by turbulence of blood in the jugular venous system. The hum has no pathologic significance and may be heard in the neck or anterior portion of the upper chest. It consists of a soft humming sound heard in both systole and diastole, which can be exaggerated or made to disappear by varying the position of the head or by light compression over the jugular venous system in the neck. These simple maneuvers are sufficient to differentiate a venous hum from the murmurs produced by organic cardiovascular disease, particularly patent ductus arteriosus, from which the sound is frequently indistinguishable.

Innocent cardiac murmurs may also be produced by the **straight-back syndrome.** This consists of loss of the concavity of the upper thoracic spine with resultant decrease of the anteroposterior diameter of the chest. This syndrome results in innocent systolic ejection murmurs; at times the murmur is accentuated in late systole. Sometimes the murmur is associated with wide splitting of the second heart sound, electrocardiographic signs of incomplete right bundle branch block and radiographic prominence of the pulmonary arterial trunk. These signs simulate those produced by atrial septal defects or mild pulmonic stenosis. Lateral chest x-rays are diagnostic, since they demonstrate the straight dorsal spine and narrow anteroposterior diameter of the chest (Fig. 13–3). The straight back syndrome is benign and requires no therapy.

ARTERIAL PULSE. The **cardiac rate** of newborn infants is rapid and subject to wide fluctuations. The average rate, ranging from 120 to 140 beats per minute, may increase to 170 or more during crying and activity and drop to between 70 and 90 during sleep. As the child grows older the average pulse rate becomes slower. Table 13–1 lists rates compiled from several sources.

Throughout childhood the pulse rate is labile and increases rapidly in response to muscular activity or emotional stimuli. The average rate is generally higher in the afternoon than in the morning and more rapid after than before eating.

Tachycardia persisting for weeks or months has been observed in adolescents, especially girls, without any discernible cause. Persistent tachycardia (over 200 in newborns, 150 in infants or 120 in older children) should be investigated to exclude pathologic arrhythmias. The apprehension induced by a visit to the physician will often cause a fast rate at the time of examination. In order to determine the cardiac rate when it is not influenced by external stimuli, the pulse rate should be recorded several times throughout the day or night when the child is quiet or asleep.

Slow pulse rates are rare in children until the adolescent period, when rates as low as 40 per minute may be encountered, particularly in athletic boys.

The **rhythm** of the cardiac beat in the newborn infant is often irregular and seems to be closely related to respiration. When the infant is asleep, there may be periods of apnea and a slow cardiac rate, but when respiratory movements are resumed, the pulse rate speeds up again. This arrhythmia is exaggerated in premature infants and in those who have suffered from shock or intracranial hemorrhage.

Diagnostic information may also be obtained by analysis of the *quality* and *amplitude* of the peripheral pulse. A *water-hammer pulse* in the forearm or a *Corrigan pulsation* in the carotid arteries signifies a large pulse pressure commonly found in patent ductus arteriosus, aortic insufficiency or general vasodilatation. Capillary pulsation often accompanies such a finding. An anacrotic or plateau pulse of small volume signifies aortic stenosis, and pulsus bisferiens suggests combined aortic insufficiency and stenosis. Examination of the peripheral pulse should not be localized to the radial artery, but should include inspection and palpation of all major accessible arteries. Comparison of the amplitude of pulsation of the arteries on both sides of the body may help to localize a point of proximal compression. Routine examination of all infants and children should include palpation of the femoral vessels. Characteristically, the femoral pulsation is diminished or delayed in nearly all cases of coarctation of the aorta.

TABLE 13–1 AVERAGE PULSE RATES AT REST

AGE	LOWER LIMITS OF NORMAL		AVERAGE		UPPER LIMITS OF NORMAL	
Newborn	70		120		170	
1-11 months	80		120		160	
2 years	80		110		130	
4 years	80		100		120	
6 years	75		100		115	
8 years	70		90		110	
10 years	70		90		110	
	Girls	*Boys*	*Girls*	*Boys*	*Girls*	*Boys*
12 years	70	65	90	85	110	105
14 years	65	60	85	80	105	100
16 years	60	55	80	75	100	95
18 years	55	50	75	70	95	90

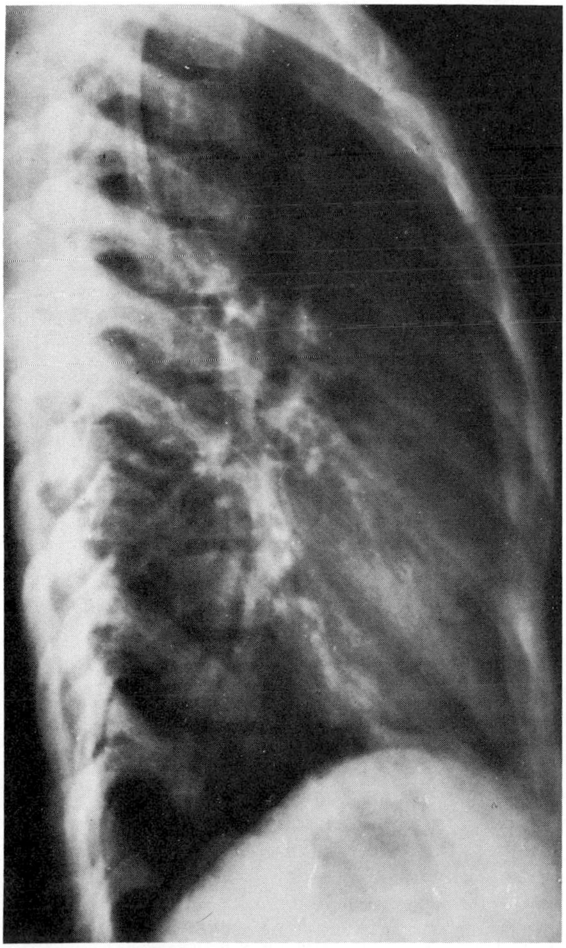

Figure 13–3 Straight-back syndrome which was associated with an innocent systolic murmur. Lateral teleroentgenogram shows absence of normal kyphosis of upper thoracic spine and narrow anteroposterior diameter of the chest.

ARTERIAL BLOOD PRESSURE. It is often difficult to determine arterial blood pressure with accuracy in infants and young children. The patient must be quiet, and the arm cuff should be wide enough to cover about two thirds of the upper arm. Erroneously high readings are obtained with narrower cuffs, and the converse with wider cuffs. When the thigh is used as the site for measuring blood pressure, the cuff should likewise cover two thirds of its surface area, especially when the pressure in this location is to be compared with that in the arm. Ordinarily the pressure in the legs with the cuff technique is about 20 mm Hg higher than in the arms.

The **flush method** for estimating blood pressure is frequently used in infants because of the difficulties of the auscultatory method in these small patients. The infant must be quiet and in the supine position. A blood pressure cuff is applied to the wrist or ankle. The part of the extremity distal to the cuff is compressed by firm wrapping. The cuff is inflated to about 200 mm Hg and the wrapping removed. The pressure in the cuff is released slowly until the blanched part of the extremity flushes. This point is an approximate index of mean arterial pressure. See Section 7 for the Doppler method.

The **oscillometric method** is also applicable to infants. As the pressure in the inflated cuff is lowered, an abrupt increase in oscillations indicates the systolic pressure; subsequent diminution indicates the diastolic pressure.

The blood pressure varies with the age of the child and is closely related to his height and weight. Significant increases occur during adolescence, with many temporary variations before the more stable levels of adult life are attained. Exercise, excitement, coughing and straining may raise the systolic pressure of children as much as 40 to 50 mm above their usual levels. Variability of blood pressure among children of approximately the same age and body build must be expected. (See Figure 13–70 for blood pressures of normal children.)

VENOUS PULSE. Inspection of the cervical veins may yield considerable diagnostic information. The patient should be propped in bed at an angle of about 45 degrees with his neck muscles relaxed. Distention of the external jugular veins, owing to constriction of their passage through the deep cervical fascia, occurs in many normal children. Distention and pulsation of veins situated above the sternal angle are otherwise abnormal. Increased venous pressure transmitted to the internal jugular vein may appear as venous pulsations without visible distention. Such pulsation does not occur in normal children reclining at an angle of 45 degrees. The height of venous pressure can be measured by observing the vertical height to which the distended and pulsating portion of the vein rises above the sternal angle. This clinical observation is of great help, since the difficulties of measuring the resting venous pressure by venipuncture in small patients often preclude the determination of exact pressure.

Venous pulsations may be distinguished from those of arteries in the following ways (Wood): (1) Venous pulsations undulate, yield readily to pressure, vary with the position of the patient, and usually have multiple components, whereas those of the carotid artery are single, abrupt, only compressible with moderate pressure and do not vary with the patient's position. (2) Abdominal pressure, especially over the right hypochondrium, increases the height of the venous pulse, but has no effect on the arterial pulsation. (3) Mild compression of the external jugular vein in the supraclavicular fossa will abolish venous pulsations and distend the vein, but will not affect the carotid pulsation. (4) The height of venous pulsation will increase with expiration and decrease with inspiration. Arterial pulsations are not affected by respiration.

The normal jugular phlebogram or direct tracings from the superior vena cava show three positive components, corresponding to each cardiac cycle; they are termed "a," "c" and "v," respectively (Fig. 13–4). The "a" wave is synchronous with atrial systole, the "c" wave with early ventricular systole, and the "v" wave with atrial diastole. Since the great veins are in direct communication with the right atrium, changes of pressure and volume of the chamber are transmitted to the veins.

For example: (1) In congestive cardiac failure the

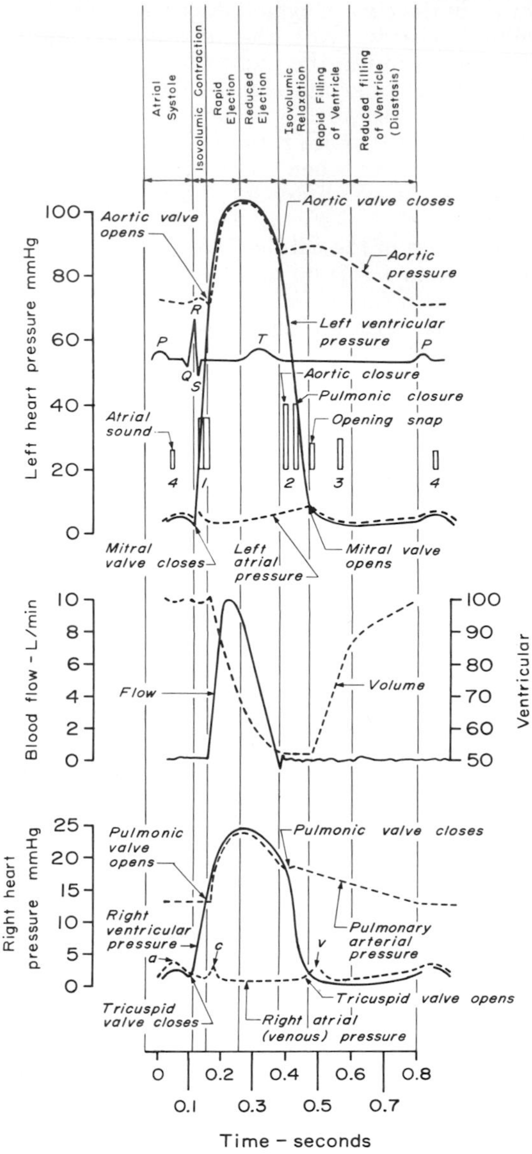

Figure 13–4 *Idealized diagram of temporal events of a cardiac cycle.*

increased right atrial pressure is transmitted to the cervical veins. The main pulsation at the upper part of distribution of these veins appears to be in late diastole. (2) Cardiac compression due to pericardial effusion or constriction increases the jugular pressure, but the amplitude of venous pulsation is small. (3) In relatively severe pulmonic stenosis the right ventricular diastolic pressure may be elevated. Emptying of the right atrium is dependent upon a systolic pressure in excess of the right ventricular diastolic pressure. A conspicuous presystolic "a" wave is present under these conditions. Similar "a" waves may be detected in patients with pulmonary stenosis and right ventricular hypertrophy with a normal right ventricular end-diastolic pressure. In these instances the mechanism of the "a" wave is due to a decreased distensibility of the right ventricle during diastole. (4) A presystolic "a" wave may be present in tricuspid stenosis or atresia, and the transmission of this wave to the inferior vena cava and hepatic veins produces presystolic hepatic pulsations. (5) In tricuspid insufficiency some of the right ventricular systolic pressure is transmitted to the right atrium, resulting in large, conspicuous venous pulsations, which correspond to ventricular systole and produce a fusion of the "c" and "v" waves. (6) In complete heart block the occurrence of cervical venous pulsations will depend on the position of the tricuspid valve at the time of atrial systole. If the right atrium contracts when the tricuspid valve is closed, a large venous pulsation will occur. (7) In superior vena caval obstruction the jugular venous pressure is increased, but the veins do not pulsate.

Direct determinations may be made by inserting a needle in a peripheral vein. The venous pressure may be read on a water manometer, using the sternal angle as the reference point. By this method the average venous pressure of children over the age of 3 years is about 50 mm of water.

ROENTGENOGRAPHIC EXAMINATIONS. Roentgenographic examinations furnish the most accurate information about cardiac size and shape. Many variations occur, owing to differences in body build, the phase of respiration or cardiac cycle, abnormalities of the thoracic cage, subdiaphragmatic pressure or pulmonary disease which may displace the heart to one side or the other.

Teleroentgenograms. Taken with the roentgen tube approximately 6 feet from the patient, teleroentgenograms represent fairly accurately the size of the heart and chest. For a complete assessment of cardiac configuration, posteroanterior, oblique and lateral views are essential. The positions of the various cardiac chambers and great vessels are shown in Figure 13–5.

The most frequently used measurement of cardiac size is the maximum width of the cardiac shadow in posteroanterior teleroentgenograms. When the cardiac width is more than half of the maximal chest width,* the heart is usually enlarged. The cardiothoracic ratio is a less accurate index of cardiac enlargement in infancy than in subsequent years, because the horizontal position of the heart may increase the ratio to more than half in the absence of true enlargement. In children with vertical hearts the cardiothoracic ratio will tend to give an erroneously low impression of the true heart size.

The width of the heart also bears a fairly definite relation to other body measurements. The transverse diameter is approximately 7 or 8 per cent of the body height and is more closely related to this factor than to age or weight.

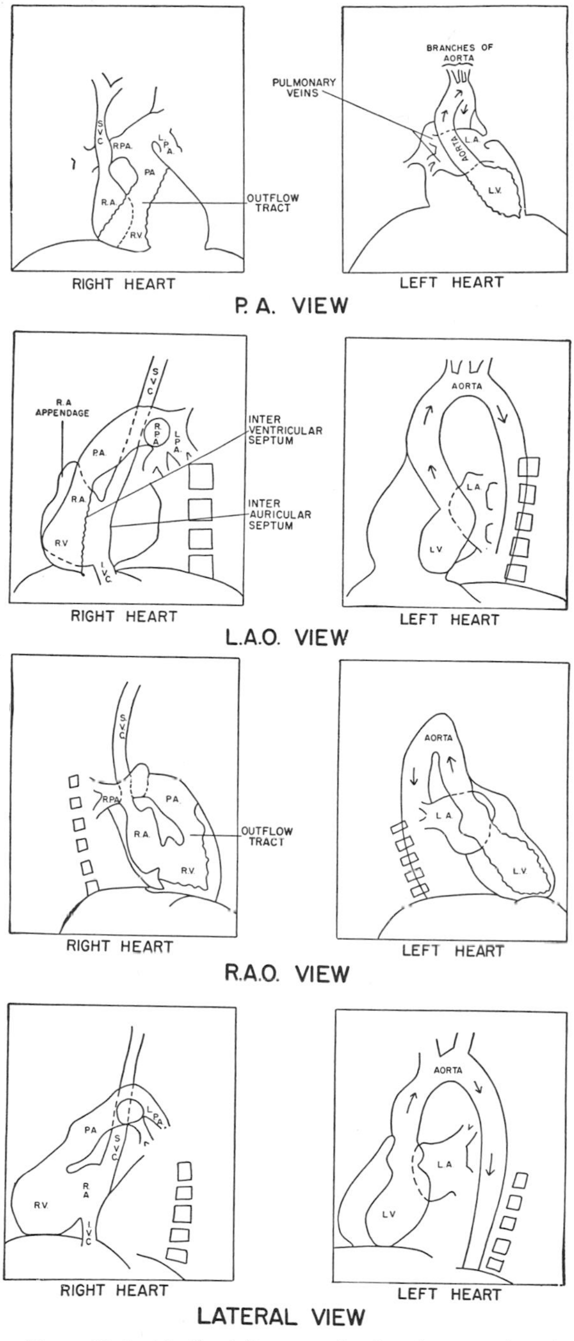

Figure 13–5 Idealized diagrams showing the normal position of the cardiac chambers and great blood vessels. Abbreviations are as follows: P.A., posteroanterior; L.A.O., left anterior oblique; R.A.O., right anterior oblique; S.V.C., superior vena cava; R.A., right atrium; R.V., right ventricle; P.A., pulmonary artery; R.P.A., right pulmonary artery; L.P.A., left pulmonary artery; L.A., left atrium; L.V., left ventricle; I.V.C., inferior vena cava. (Adapted and redrawn from Dotter and Steinberg: Angiocardiographic Interpretation. Radiology 53:513, 1949.)

In infants the thymic shadow may overlap the shadow cast by the base of the heart. In the posteroanterior view the left border of the cardiac shadow consists of three convex shadows produced from above downward by the aortic knob, the pulmonary arc and the left ventricle, respectively

*To obtain the maximal cardiac width in a posteroanterior midinspiration teleroentgenogram, a vertical line is drawn down the middle of the sternal shadow, and perpendicular lines are then drawn from the sternal line to the extreme right and left borders of the heart. The sum of the lengths of these lines is the maximal cardiac width. The maximal chest width is obtained by drawing a horizontal line between the right and left inner borders of the rib cage at the level of the top of the right diaphragm.

(Fig. 13–5). In cases of moderate to gross left atrial enlargement the atrium may project between the pulmonary artery and the left ventricle. Angiocardiographic and cardiac catheterization studies have conclusively proved that the outflow tract of the right ventricle or the pulmonary conus does not contribute to the shadows formed by the left border of the heart (Fig. 13–5). The aortic knob is not so easily seen in infants and children as in adults. Three structures also contribute to the right border of the cardiac silhouette; from above downward they are the superior vena cava, the ascending aorta and the right atrium. It is of fundamental importance also to assess the degree of pulmonary vascularity as represented by the intrapulmonary shadows. Angiocardiographic studies have shown that the hilar shadows are mainly vascular. Pulmonary overcirculation is usually associated with left-to-right shunts, and undercirculation with stenosis of the outflow tract of the right ventricle or of the pulmonary valve.

Roentgenographic examination is not complete until the cardiac shadows have been studied in both posteroanterior and lateral views (Fig. 13–5). Sometimes oblique views yield added information. The right anterior oblique view is optimal for the study of the left atrium and main pulmonary artery, whereas the left anterior oblique view is used for evaluation of the left and right ventricles, the aorta and the left atrium.

The esophagus is closely related to some of the cardiac chambers and great blood vessels, and its visualization with a barium emulsion helps further to delineate these structures, especially in the right anterior oblique view. The esophagus is indented in turn by the aorta, pulmonary artery and left atrium from above down.

Interpretation of atrial or ventricular enlargement in infants and children by radiographic means is difficult. A hypertrophied ventricle may displace a normal chamber, giving a false impression of ventricular enlargement. Thus, posterior displacement of a normal left ventricle by a hypertrophied right ventricle may cause the radiographic picture to resemble that of biventricular enlargement. The roentgenograms of patients with tetralogy of Fallot may not indicate the presence of right ventricular hypertrophy; conversely, the cardiac silhouette of patients with tricuspid atresia and an underdeveloped right ventricle may give the false impression of right ventricular hypertrophy. It is therefore apparent that the radiographic findings should be complemented by an electrocardiogram, which is a more sensitive and accurate index of ventricular enlargement.

FLUOROGRAPHY. *Routine* fluoroscopy, even with image intensification and video tape or cine recording, is not necessary for the diagnosis of heart disease in children. However, judicious use of this technique is of value in identifying impressions produced by cardiac chambers (e.g., left atrium) or by vascular rings on the barium-filled esophagus. Late postoperative complications such as ventricular aneurysms or calcifications in pericardial patches or homografts are also best evaluated by fluorography.

THE ELECTROCARDIOGRAM. The electrocardiogram in pediatric practice is not only of diagnostic aid in congenital and rheumatic heart diseases, but also is frequently helpful in the detection and management of disturbances of electrolyte metabolism, endocrine and metabolic diseases, and acute infections. Electrocardiographic examination is not complete unless the standard leads are supplemented by the unipolar limb leads and multiple chest leads. It is beyond the scope of this text to discuss the physiologic concepts of unipolar electrocardiography. A study of standard leads is valuable in the diagnosis of arrhythmias and for measurements of the duration of various parts of the cardiac cycle.

A wide electrocardiographic exploration of the chest is advised in children, and especially in infants. In addition to the conventional leads of V_1 through V_6, leads over the right chest (V_{4R} or V_{3R}) are essential for adequate assessment of right ventricular activity.

Normal Electrocardiogram.* The evolution of the electrocardiogram in the normal neonate is a dynamic process, with acute changes occurring in the first month of life, especially in the first week; these changes primarily involve the QRS voltage and T wave axis. Thereafter, changes are more gradual with growth of the infant and normally show slow regression of right ventricular dominance and progression of left ventricular forces (Fig. 13–6). In infants the right ventricular surface leads show an Rs pattern which usually persists for the first 2 years of life and may be found up to the age of 4 years (Fig. 13–7). The T waves are inverted in V_{4R}, V_{3R}, V_1, V_2 and V_3 in almost all infants and may remain inverted in V_{4R}, V_{3R} and V_1 up to the middle of the second decade of life.

*In this text capitalized letters refer to waves of high voltage (tall or deep waves), and small letters are used to designate waves of low voltage.

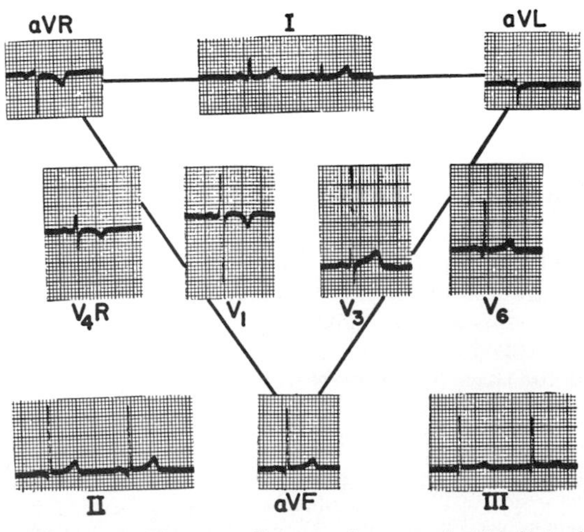

Figure 13–6 *Electrocardiogram of a normal child. Note the relatively tall R waves and inversion of the T waves in V_{4R} and V_1*

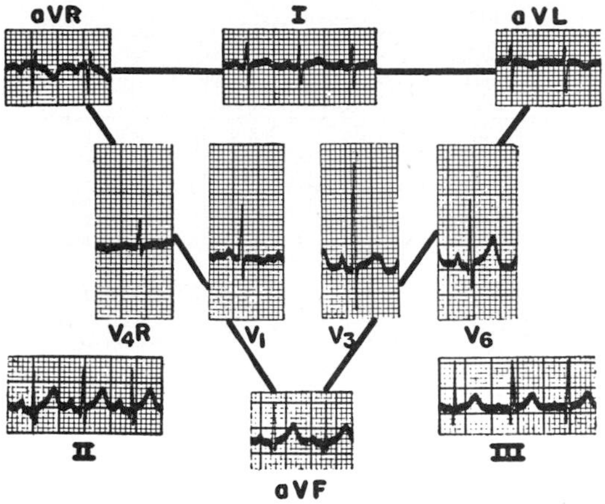

Figure 13–7 Normal infant's electrocardiogram. Note the tall R and small s waves in V_{4R} and V_1 and the inverted T wave in these leads.

In the normal *full-term newborn infant* the mean frontal QRS axis is 125 to 135°. The precordial leads show right ventricular dominance, with a tall R wave in V_4R and V_1, an R/S ratio greater than 1 in V_1 and an rS complex in V_6. The lack of precordial R wave progression is strikingly different from that in the older child or adolescent. *At birth* the direction of the T wave axis results in an upright T wave in leads I, aVL and the precordial leads. From *age 1 hour to 3 days* the T waves are normally inverted in leads I, aVL and V_6 and strikingly positive in V_4R and V_1. These signs occasionally persist for more than 3 days. Generally, however, after 3 days of age, the T wave axis changes so that these waves are upright in leads I, II, aVF and V_6, inverted in aVR, V_4R and V_1 and variable in leads III and aVL. The T wave changes have been attributed to the sudden increase in left ventricular volume and systemic vascular resistance that occur in the first few hours and days of life.

Because of these normal patterns of the QRS-T in infants and children, the changes produced by right ventricular hypertrophy are different from those in adults. The diagnosis of ventricular hypertrophy is sometimes based on the increased voltage of the R and S waves in the unipolar chest leads. Nevertheless, since the height of these waves is mainly governed by the proximity of the exploring electrode to the surface of the heart, and since the chest wall of infants and children is relatively thin, the diagnosis of ventricular hypertrophy should not be based on voltage changes alone. Normal *adolescents* may also show a large QRS voltage (tall RV_6 and deep SV_1) and early repolarization with elevation of the ST segment. These findings should not be confused with left ventricular hypertrophy.

The electrocardiogram of the *premature infant* may be indistinguishable from that of the full-term baby, but in some prematures generalized low voltage is present. In others there is a wide range of the frontal QRS axis, with left ventricular dominance; V_6 shows a well defined qR, and V_1 has an R/S ratio equal to or less than 1. Thus, the R wave progression across the precordium simulates the pattern seen in the older child.

Electrocardiographic Abnormalities. See Disturbances in Rate and Rhythm of the Heart later in this Section. Cardiac arrhythmias are uncommon in normal full-term babies. However, premature infants have a high incidence of intermittent sinus arrhythmia, sinus bradycardia and junctional rhythm.

The P Wave. Tall, narrow and spiked P waves are seen in congenital pulmonary stenosis (Fig. 13–8), Ebstein's anomaly of the tricuspid valve, tricuspid atresia and sometimes in cor pulmonale. These abnormal waves are probably due to right atrial hypertrophy, are usually taller than 2.5 mm and are most obvious in standard lead II and leads V_{4R}, V_{3R} and V_1. Similar waves are sometimes seen in thyrotoxicosis. Flat and widened P waves, commonly bifid, are seen in some patients with large ventricular septal defects, in communications between the aorta and the lesser circulation and in severe mitral stenosis. They are probably due to left atrial enlargement. Flat P waves may be found in hyperkalemia. Inverted P waves are seen in junctional rhythm and in atrial inversion, as occurs in dextrocardia with situs inversus.

Prolongation of the P-R Interval. This abnormality is a form of heart block. Permanent

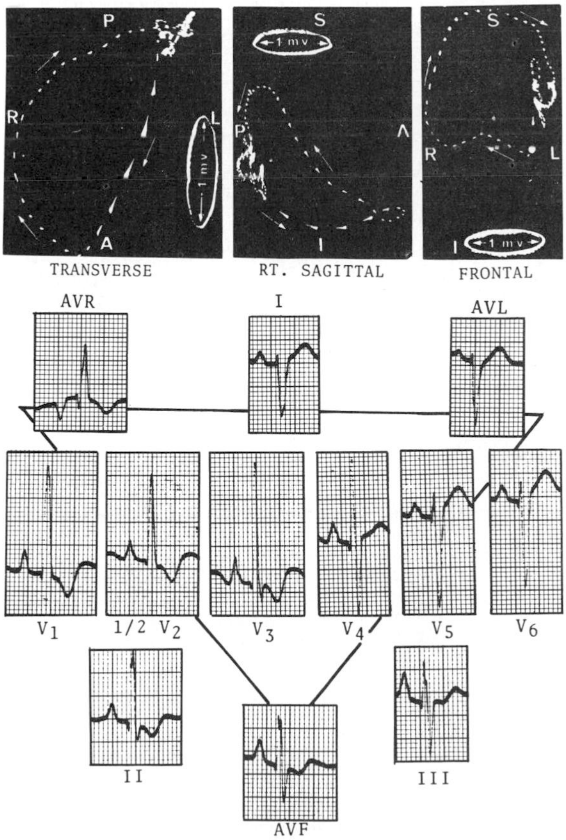

Figure 13–8 Electrocardiogram and vectorcardiogram of a 10 year old girl with severe pulmonary hypertension. Right atrial and ventricular hypertrophy is evident. Note prominent P waves and qR in right precordial leads. The QRS loop is of large voltage and is displaced anteriorly and to the right.

prolongation of the P-R interval may be congenital or due to scarring from rheumatic carditis. Any active carditis, including acute rheumatic fever, may produce transient prolongation of the P-R interval. Other causes of temporary prolongation include digitalis therapy and carotid sinus pressure. No specific treatment is required for this abnormality.

Right Ventricular Hypertrophy. *Right ventricular surface leads* of infants and children differ from those of adults, and tracings of the right side of the chest (V_{4R} or V_{3R}) are essential in young children. Review of electrocardiographic tracings in infants with known *right ventricular hypertrophy* has shown that the following changes may occur singly or in combination (Fig. 13–9): (1) a qR pattern in the right ventricular surface leads; (2) a positive T wave in leads V_{4R} through V_3 after the first 48 hours of life; (3) a monophasic R wave in V_{4R}, V_{3R} or V_1; (4) prolongation of the ventricular activation time in right ventricular surface leads to greater than 0.03 second; (5) the R wave in the right chest leads is usually taller than 7 mm, but this sign alone is not sufficient for the diagnosis; (6) aVR may show a QR pattern; and (7) in the presence of incomplete right bundle branch block, right ventricular hypertrophy is indicated by a tall secondary R wave.

Older children and adolescents who have right ventricular hypertrophy show the same changes, but in addition may have the following abnormalities of the R and S waves of the unipolar leads: (1) the sum of RV_1 or RV_{3R} and SV_5 or SV_6 totals 11 mm or more; (2) the depth of the S wave in V_1, V_{3R} or V_{4R} is less than 2 mm. It cannot be overstressed that the evaluation of ventricular hypertrophy should not be based on voltage changes alone.

Abnormal hemodynamics can be correlated with abnormal electrocardiographic patterns. Obstruction to right ventricular and pulmonary flow (e.g., pulmonary stenosis) is associated with a *systolic overload pattern.* This is characterized by an increasingly tall and late R wave in the right precordial leads. In these leads the T wave is initially

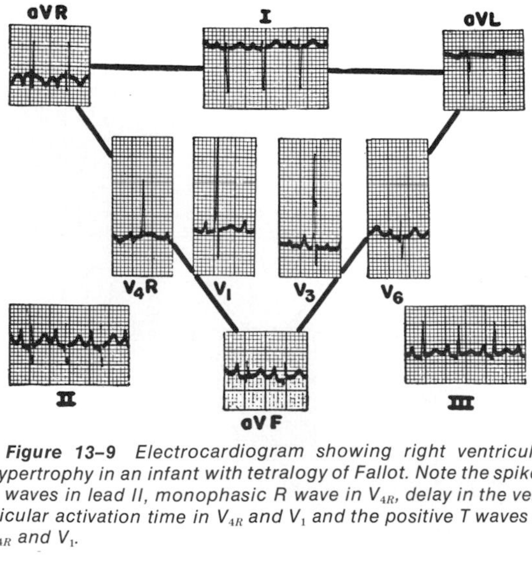

Figure 13–9 Electrocardiogram showing right ventricular hypertrophy in an infant with tetralogy of Fallot. Note the spiked P waves in lead II, monophasic R wave in V_{4R}, delay in the ventricular activation time in V_{4R} and V_1 and the positive T waves in V_{4R} and V_1.

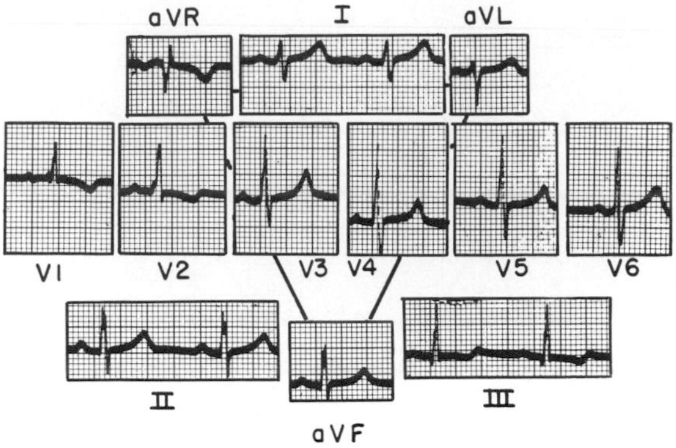

Figure 13–10 Electrocardiogram showing right ventricular outflow hypertrophy in a patient with an ostium secundum atrial septal defect. Note rsR′ in V_1 and deep, stumpy S in V_6.

upright and later becomes inverted (Figs. 13–8, 13–9). In contradistinction, *diastolic overload* of the right ventricle (e.g., with atrial septal defect) is characterized by the pattern of incomplete or occasionally complete right bundle branch block (Fig. 13–10). Although this concept appears to be true in extreme examples, there are many instances in which the dynamics of systolic overload may be associated with right ventricular hypertrophy, showing a pattern of incomplete right bundle branch block.

Left Ventricular Hypertrophy. The following features, alone or in combination, suggest dominance of the left ventricle (Fig. 13–11): (1) depression of the S-T segment and inversion of the T waves in left ventricular surface leads (i.e., V_5, V_6 or V_7; aVF if the heart is vertical and aVL if the heart is horizontal); (2) delayed onset of the ventricular activation time in V_5 or V_6 (greater than 0.04 second); (3) increased voltage of the QRS

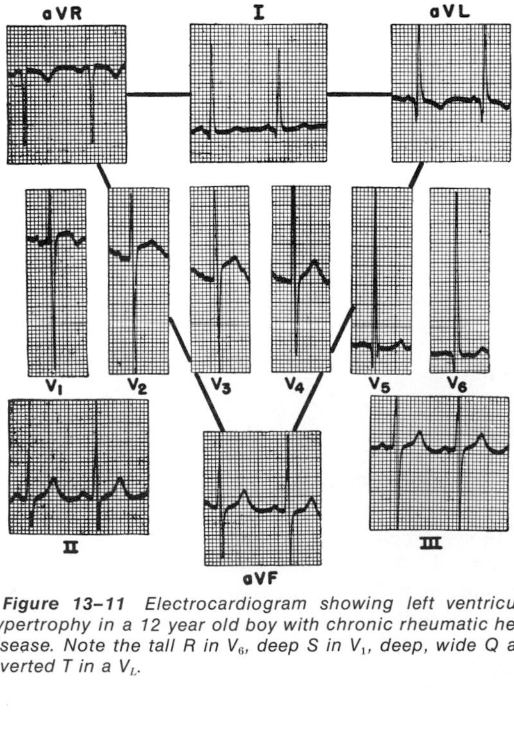

Figure 13–11 Electrocardiogram showing left ventricular hypertrophy in a 12 year old boy with chronic rheumatic heart disease. Note the tall R in V_6, deep S in V_1, deep, wide Q and inverted T in a V_L.

complex; and (4) a significant Q wave in left ventricular surface leads. In older children or adolescents the sum of the left ventricular potentials (i.e., RV_6 and SV_1) is greater than 35 mm. Also RV_5 or RV_6 exceeds 26 mm. If the heart is vertical the RaVF exceeds 20 mm, and in a horizontal heart RaVL exceeds 11 mm. It is again stressed that the evaluation of ventricular dominance should not be based on voltage changes alone.

Overload of the left ventricle is also reflected in an abnormal electrocardiogram. It is suggested that *systolic overload of the left ventricle* is characterized by depression of the S-T segment and inverted T waves in the left precordial leads. *Diastolic overload of the left ventricle* is suggested by tall R waves with a late activation time and tall, upright and symmetrically peaked T waves in the left precordial leads. The foregoing electrocardiographic diagnoses, especially diastolic overload of the left ventricle, are frequently difficult to establish.

Bundle Branch Block. *Complete right* or *left bundle branch block* is not frequently encountered in pediatric practice, except in patients who have undergone ventriculotomy during open-heart surgery. The electrocardiographic pattern does not differ from that in adults. *Incomplete right bundle branch block* with or without right ventricular hypertrophy is not uncommon. Incomplete right bundle branch block is suggested by an early r wave and a late R′ in the right precordial leads and a relatively broad SV_6. This can be a normal variant. Right ventricular hypertrophy, however, especially of the outflow, may produce the same pattern. In these patients the secondary R wave may be taller (Fig. 13–10). If there is associated right ventricular hypertrophy, the secondary R wave in the right precordial leads is tall and usually exceeds 10 mm. It is often difficult to differentiate incomplete right bundle branch block from right ventricular hypertrophy, and it has been suggested that the pattern of incomplete right bundle branch block may in fact be due to right ventricular outflow hypertrophy.

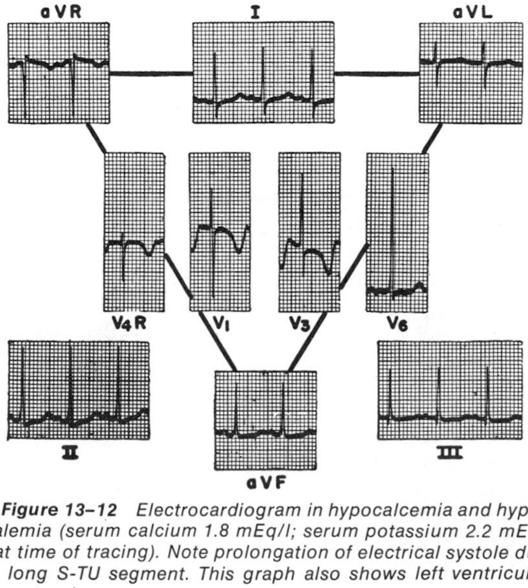

Figure 13–12 *Electrocardiogram in hypocalcemia and hypokalemia (serum calcium 1.8 mEq/l; serum potassium 2.2 mEq/l at time of tracing). Note prolongation of electrical systole due to long S-TU segment. This graph also shows left ventricular hypertrophy.*

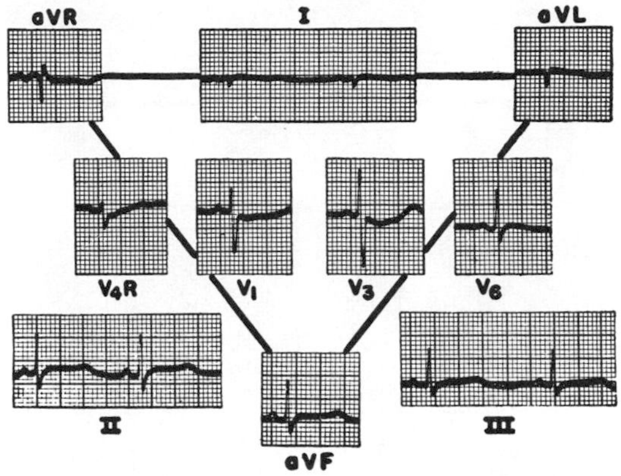

Figure 13–13 *Electrocardiogram in hypokalemia (serum potassium 2.7 mEq/l; serum calcium 4.8 mEq/l at time of tracing). Note the prolongation of electrical systole due to a widened TU wave, especially in leads II, III and aV_r; also depression of the S-T segment in V_{4R}, V_1 and V_3.*

Duration of Electrical Systole (Q-T Interval). The duration of the Q-T interval (electrical systole) varies with the cardiac rate, and many formulas have been devised in an attempt to adjust this differential. Taran and Szilagyi's modification of Bazett's formula states that the corrected Q-T interval (Q-TC) equals the measured Q-T interval divided by the square root of the cycle length (R-R interval). The normal Q-TC is variously given as 0.38 ± 0.04. It is often lengthened in children with hypokalemia, hypocalcemia and in some patients with myocarditis (Figs. 13–12 and 13–13). In hypokalemia and hypocalcemia prolonged electrical systole is due to a lengthened Q-U interval. A shortened Q-TC may be found after administration of digitalis and with pericarditis or hyperkalemia.

S-T Segment and T Wave Abnormalities. Elevation of the ST segment in normal teenagers has been attributed to early repolarization of the heart. In generalized pericarditis superficial epicardial involvement may cause elevation of the S-T segment, followed by abnormal T wave inversion as healing progresses. Administration of digitalis is associated with sagging of the S-T segment and abnormal inversion of the T wave. Depression of the S-T segment may also occur in conditions producing myocardial hypoxia, e.g., anemia, carbon monoxide poisoning, endocardial sclerosis, and aberrant origin of the left coronary artery from the pulmonary artery, as well as in glycogen storage disease of the heart, myocardial tumors and gargoylism. Aberrant origin of the left coronary artery from the pulmonary artery may lead to changes indistinguishable from those seen in acute myocardial infarction in adults. Similar changes may occur in progeria with degenerative coronary artery lesions and calcinosis of the coronary arteries.

In any form of carditis, especially diphtheritic, simple inversion of the T wave may occur. Hypothyroidism may produce flat or inverted T waves in

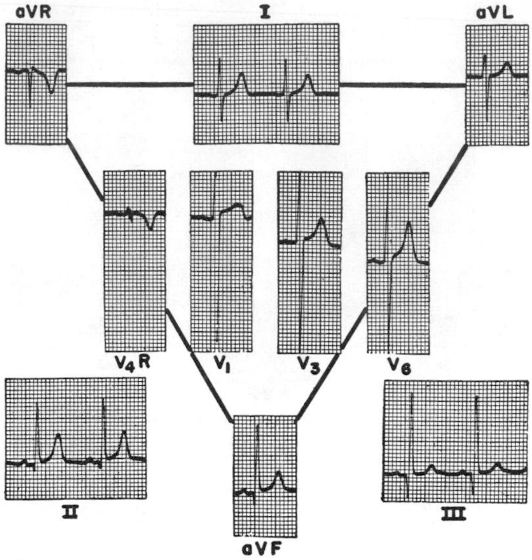

Figure 13–14 *Electrocardiogram in hyperkalemia (serum potassium 6.5 mEq/l; serum calcium 5.1 mEq/l). Note the tall, tent-shaped T waves, especially in leads, I, II and V_6.*

association with generalized low voltage. In hyperkalemia the T waves are commonly of high voltage and are tent-shaped (Fig. 13–14).

VECTORCARDIOGRAPHY. Vectorcardiography (VCG) is a study of the whole electrical activation of the heart. The spread of depolarization and repolarization through the heart muscle is a succession of innumerable instantaneous electrical forces or vectors. The recording of the direction, magnitude and orientation of these vectors in a single curve constitutes the vectorcardiographic loop (VCGsE). It is considered that these electrical forces arise from a common site, the so-called electromotive (E) point or zero (0) point. Three loops are recorded with each cardiac cycle: P loop (PsE), QRS loop (QRSsE) and T loop (TsE). Reference lead systems have been devised to record the vectorcardiogram in three planes: transverse or horizontal, sagittal and frontal. Analysis of vectorcardiographic loops includes evaluation of spatial position, magnitude, direction of rotation (clockwise or counterclockwise), speed of inscription and spatial relation of QRS and T loops. Normal loops end at their point of origin (E point), resulting in a closed loop.*

The normal P loop is small, is inscribed slowly, rotates counterclockwise in the horizontal or frontal plane and is usually oriented to the left, forward and downward. Beyond about 6 months of age the normal QRS loop has a great amplitude, is inscribed rapidly, rotates counterclockwise in the horizontal plane and clockwise in the sagittal plane. In the frontal plane the rotation is either clockwise or counterclockwise. QRSsE is oriented to the left downward and backward. The intermediate portion of the loop is inscribed most rapidly. The normal T loop is inscribed slowly, is small and is enclosed in QRSsE in at least two planes. In the child it is directed backward.

Right ventricular hypertrophy or overload is associated with QRSsE located to the right and forward. In the horizontal plane the loop is oriented clockwise and counterclockwise in the sagittal plane (i.e., opposite to normal). *Left ventricular hypertrophy or overload* is associated with an exaggeration of the normal physiologic dominance of the left ventricle. QRSsE shows a predominance of the electrical forces directed to the left and backward.

HEMATOLOGIC DATA. The normal variations of the blood picture in infancy should be borne in mind in evaluation of cardiovascular disease. These include the normal polycythemia of the neonatal period and the relative anemia and leukocytosis of infancy. Persistent polycythemia after the first month of life is frequently associated with right-to-left shunts and cyanosis. Polycythemia of any cause in the neonate results in plethora and cyanosis and may also result in cardiorespiratory symptoms even in infants with structurally normal hearts. In some instances, cardiomegaly and congestive cardiac failure are present. (See Disturbances of the Blood in Section 7 and Polycythemia in Section 14.)

Patients with right-to-left shunts and polycythemia have a delicate balance between intravascular thrombosis and a bleeding diathesis. It is important to recognize this *abnormal hemostasis* prior to any surgical procedure. The most frequent abnormalities are accelerated fibrinolysis, thrombocytopenia, abnormal clot retraction, hypofibrinogenemia, prolonged prothrombin time and prolonged partial thromboplastin time or thromboplastin generative time. These abnormalities occur singly or in combination and appear to be related to the severity of the polycythemia. The mechanism of the abnormal hemostasis is not clear. It has been suggested that low-grade chronic intravascular coagulation is present, but this has not been confirmed and heparin therapy is not used. Others have speculated that abnormal coagulation is related to the effects of hypoxia and polycythemia on platelet production and/or consumption, together with the effects of chronic liver dysfunction on procoagulants and fibrinolysis. The preparation of cyanotic polycythemic patients for elective surgery, e.g., dental extraction, includes evaluation for and treatment of abnormal coagulation. Accelerated fibrinolysis has been suppressed with epsilon-aminocaproic acid. Thrombocytopenia and hypofibrinogenemia have been improved by repeated small phlebotomies; this procedure is not without risk, especially in polycythemic patients with extreme elevation of pulmonary vascular resistance. These patients do not tolerate wide fluctuations in circulating blood volume, so the phle-

*All vectorcardiograms in this text were obtained with the Frank lead system. In all instances the loop is interrupted at 2.5 milliseconds so that every 4 teardrops represent 1/100 second. The stout part of the teardrop represents the front end. Sensitivity mark indicates 1 millivolt. Abbreviations in all vectorcardiograms are as follows: A, anterior; P, posterior; L, left; R, right; S, superior; I, inferior.

TABLE 13–2 ANALYSIS OF OXYGEN CONTENT IN BLOOD (CARDIAC CATHETERIZATION)

	VENAE CAVAE	RIGHT ATRIUM	RIGHT VENTRICLE	PULMONARY ARTERY	ARTERIAL OXYGEN SATURATION	REMARKS
Patent ductus arteriosus	←Comparable→			Higher than RV, RA and VC	Normal	(a) Rarely, with right-to-left shunt, arterial unsaturation present (b) If associated pulmonary valve insufficiency, high RV samples comparable to PA
Atrial septal defect	Lower than RA, RV and PA	←Comparable→			Normal	
Ventricular septal defect	←Comparable→		←Higher than RA and VC→		Normal	Rarely, direct shunt into PA without mixing in RV when PA higher than RV, RA and VC
Anomalous pulmonary veins	(a) If empty into SVC, IVC lower than SVC, RA, RV and PA (b) If empty into IVC, SVC lower than IVC, RA, RV and PA	If empty into RA, VC lower than RA, RV and PA	←Comparable→		Normal	Arterial saturation may be decreased with total anomalous pulmonary venous return
Isolated pulmonary stenosis	←Comparable→				Normal	If right-to-left shunt, e.g., through foramen ovale, arterial unsaturation
Aorticopulmonary septal defect	←Comparable→			Higher than RV, RA and VC	Normal	
Tetralogy of Fallot	←Comparable→				Usually gross unsaturation	In many instances RV and PA samples higher than RA and VC Venous blood grossly unsaturated
Tricuspid atresia	←Comparable→		—	—	Usually gross unsaturation	
Transposition of great vessels	Depends on presence of associated defects such as atrial defect, ventricular septal defect and patent ductus arteriosus				Gross unsaturation	Contents vary in same chamber because shunt is in both directions
Eisenmenger "physiology," i.e., pulmonary hypertension with bidirectional shunt	Depends on site of defect. Commonest is ventricular septal defect when RV and PA higher than RA and VC				Unsaturation	In atrial defect, VC lower than RA, RV and PA; in patent ductus PA higher than RV, and brachial artery higher than femoral artery

Normally the difference in oxygen content between the venae cavae and right atrium is less than 1.9 volumes per cent, between the right atrium and right ventricle less than 0.9 volume per cent, and between the right ventricle and pulmonary artery, less than 0.5 volume per cent.

PA = pulmonary artery; RV = right ventricle; RA = right atrium; VC = venae cavae; SVC = superior vena cava; IVC = inferior vena cava.

botomy is performed in the same way as an exchange transfusion, with blood being replaced with fresh frozen plasma or albumin. In some patients, screening tests prior to surgery do not predict an abnormal coagulation, and unexpected hemorrhage occurs during or after operation. The abnormal hemostasis is treated with fresh frozen plasma or corticosteroids.

Iron deficiency anemia is very poorly tolerated in cyanotic patients with right-to-left shunts, especially infants and toddlers. Such babies have an increase in frequency of hypercyanotic spells, in severity of attacks of dyspnea and in heart size. Iron therapy produces improvement, but surgical treatment of the cardiac anomaly is often required within months after alleviation of the iron deficiency.

Because of the high viscosity of polycythemic blood, infants with cyanotic congenital heart disease are at risk to develop vascular thrombosis, especially of cerebral veins. Polycythemic babies with iron deficiency are at even greater risk for cerebrovascular accidents, probably because thrombosis is enhanced by a decrease in velocity of blood flow as well as by altered deformability of the red cells.

CARDIAC CATHETERIZATION. All the chambers of the heart and the great vessels entering or leaving them are accessible for measurements of pressure, sampling of blood, injection of contrast and

TABLE 13–3 PRESSURES DURING CARDIAC CATHETERIZATION (mm Hg)

	VENAE CAVAE	RIGHT ATRIUM	RIGHT VENTRICLE	PULMONARY ARTERY	PULMONARY CAPILLARY	REMARKS
Normal	0–5	0–5	18–30/0–5	18–30/6–12 Mean 13–17	6–12	Normal left atrial pressure 4–8
Patent ductus arteriosus	Normal	Normal	Normal to increased	Normal to increased	Normal to increased	Right atrial and caval pressures increased in congestive failure
Atrial septal defect	Normal	Normal	Normal to increased	Normal to increased	Normal	
Ventricular septal defect	Normal	Normal	Normal to increased	Normal to increased	Normal to increased	Right atrial and caval pressures increased in congestive failure
Anomalous pulmonary veins (partial)	Normal	Normal	Normal to increased	Normal to increased	Normal	
Isolated pulmonary stenosis	Normal to increased	Normal to increased	Increased	Normal to decreased	Normal	Left atrial pressure normal, and right atrial pressure curve may show prominent "a" wave
Aorticopulmonary septal defect	Normal	Normal	Increased	Increased	Normal to increased	
Tetralogy of Fallot	Normal	Normal	Increased	Normal to decreased	Normal	Pressure differentials may be noted in continuous tracing as catheter passes from pulmonary artery to infundibular chamber and to right ventricle
Tricuspid stenosis	Increased	Increased	——	——	——	Left atrial pressure normal Right atrial pressure curve shows prominent "a" wave
Transposition of great vessels	Normal	Normal	Increased	Increased	Increased	Right atrial and caval pressures increased in congestive failure
Eisenmenger physiology	Normal to increased	Normal to increased	Increased	Increased	Normal	

TABLE 13–4 NORMALS AND FORMULAS FOR DETERMINATION OF HEMODYNAMICS IN CARDIAC CATHETERIZATION

1. Cardiac index 3.1 ± 0.4 liter/min /square meter
2. Arteriovenous oxygen difference 4.5 ± 0.7 ml/dl
3. Oxygen consumption 140-160 ml /square meter/min
4. Arterial oxygen saturation 94-100%
5. Difference in oxygen content between venae cavae and right atrium < 1.9 vol %
6. Difference in oxygen content between right atrium and right ventricle < 0.9 vol %
7. Difference in oxygen content between right ventricle and pulmonary artery < 0.5 vol %
8. Normal mean left atrial pressure 4 to 8 mm Hg
9. Pulmonary arteriolar resistance 50-150 dyne sec cm $^{-5}$(1 unit = 80 dynes)
10. Cardiac output ml /min =
$$\frac{O_2 \text{ intake (ml /min)}}{\left\{\begin{array}{l}O_2 \text{ content arterial blood (vols \%)} \\ \text{minus } O_2 \text{ content of mixed venous blood}\end{array}\right.} \times 100$$
11. Cardiac index = cardiac output (l/min) per square meter of body surface area
12. Pulmonary artery flow =
$$\frac{O_2 \text{ intake (ml /min)}}{\left\{\begin{array}{l}O_2 \text{ content of pulmonary venous blood (vols \%)} \\ \text{minus } O_2 \text{ content of pulmonary arterial blood (vols \%)}\end{array}\right.} \times 100$$
If a pulmonary venous sample is not obtained, it is assumed to be saturated to 95% of capacity
13. Systemic flow =
$$\frac{O_2 \text{ intake (ml /min)}}{\left\{\begin{array}{l}\text{systemic arterial } O_2 \text{ content (vols \%)} \\ \text{minus mixed venous } O_2 \text{ content (vols \%)}\end{array}\right.} \times 100$$
14. Effective pulmonary artery flow =
$$\frac{O_2 \text{ intake (ml /min)}}{\left\{\begin{array}{l}\text{pulmonary venous } O_2 \text{ content (vols \%)} \\ \text{minus mixed venous } O_2 \text{ content (vols \%)}\end{array}\right.} \times 100$$
15. Total left-to-right shunt = pulmonary artery flow minus effective pulmonary artery flow
16. Total right-to-left shunt = systemic flow minus effective pulmonary artery flow
17. Pulmonary arteriolar resistance $R = \frac{PA - PC}{PF} \times 1332$

Where R = pulmonary arteriolar resistance in dyne seconds cm^{-5}
PA = mean pulmonary artery pressure in mm Hg
PC = mean pulmonary "capillary" pressure in mm Hg
PF = pulmonary flow in ml /sec

indicator materials and introduction of intravascular transducers. The majority of congenital cardiac lesions can be diagnosed after a careful clinical history and examination, and cardiac catheterization should not be used indiscriminately in young patients, owing to the hazards of injury and even death. These sophisticated methods of study do not supersede careful clinical evaluation and routine laboratory techniques. They should be undertaken only with the specific objective of gaining information not available otherwise to help in management of the patient. Abnormal findings which may be encountered in patients with congenital heart disease are shown in Tables 13–2 and 13–3.

Cardiac catheterization in infants and children presents problems not encountered in adults. In many instances it is necessary to sedate or even anesthetize the patient. The calculations of cardiac output, shunts, resistances and valve areas should be interpreted cautiously if the study is made during anesthesia because their validity depends upon the patient's being in a "steady state," which is difficult to obtain during deep narcosis.

Routine evaluation of both the greater and lesser circulations during cardiac catheterization is now common practice. This is accomplished by the passage of radiopaque catheters with the aid of fluoroscopy via a peripheral vein into the right heart or via a peripheral artery in a retrograde manner into the left heart. The left atrium is entered by catheter passage across the interatrial septum (via a defect in the foramen ovale or by puncturing the septum) or in a retrograde manner from the left ventricle. In some congenital cardiovascular abnormalities the catheter may pass through intracardiac defects or into abnormally placed vessels. Oxygen consumption and carbon dioxide production may be calculated from samples of expired air. These studies are of value in determining the presence of intracardiac shunts, as well as for measurements of cardiac outputs and indices (Table 13–4). Calculations may also be made of the pulmonary and peripheral arteriolar resistances, the work of the heart, the volume of various shunts and the areas of intracardiac defects and valves.

INDICATOR DILUTION AND APPEARANCE TECHNIQUES. If a bolus of indicator material is injected intravenously or into the right side of the heart, it traverses the pulmonary circulation and enters the left side of the heart and then the arterial circulation. This indicator material may then be detected in the arterial blood. A continuous record of the circulation of indicator in normal subjects shows two peaks (Fig. 13–15). The time between the instant of injection and the detection of the indicator

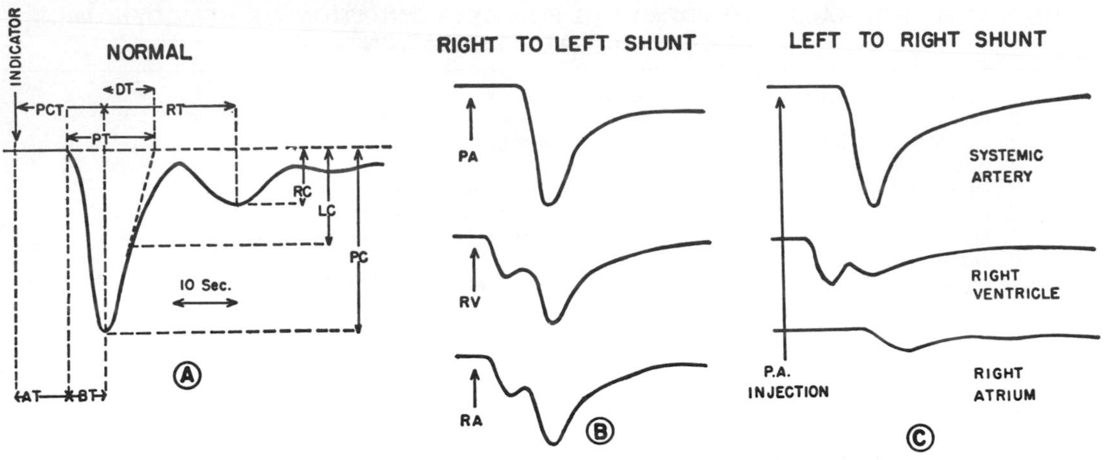

Figure 13–15 *Idealized diagrams of indicator dilution curves.* A, *Normal curve showing time and concentration components. Instant of indicator injection in right side of heart shown by arrow at top left. Curve obtained from indicator detector in a systemic artery. Abbreviations: AT, appearance time; BT, build-up time; PCT, peak concentration time; RT, recirculation time; PT, passage time; DT, disappearance time; PC, peak concentration; RC, maximal recirculation concentration; LC, least concentration. Extrapolation of declining slope of concentration is easier if the curve is plotted on a logarithmic scale. Cardiac output may be computed by the formula* $\frac{60I}{c\,(PT)}$, *where I = amount of indicator, c = mean concentration of indicator, PT = passage time.*

B, *Localization of* right-to-left shunt. *Instant of injection of indicator shown by arrows. Example illustrates shunt at ventricular level. Site of injection: PA, pulmonary artery; RV, right ventricle; RA, right atrium. Indicator detector in systemic artery in all instances. PA injection (i.e. downstream from shunt level) shows normal appearance time. RV and RA injections (i.e. at and upstream from shunt level) show early appearance times.*

C, *Localization of* left-to-right shunt. *Example illustrates shunt at ventricular level. Indicator injected into distal pulmonary artery (PA) in all instances. In upper tracing indicator detector is in a systemic artery, and curve shows prolonged disappearance time. Middle curve is from indicator detected in right ventricle and shows an early appearance time because of ventricular septal defect. Right atrial curve shows normal appearance time.*

in arterial blood is known as the appearance time and is a measure of circulation time. The first peak of the indicator curve is due to the passage of indicator past the arterial detector, and the second to recirculation through the systemic arterial and venous systems, pulmonary circulation and reappearance in the arterial tree. If the concentration of circulating indicator is known, cardiac output can be computed (Fig. 13–15).

Localization of intracardiac and extracardiac shunts may be facilitated by the use of these methods. *Right-to-left shunts* are characterized by an abnormally short transit time for some of the indicator from the site of injection to the point of intra-arterial detection. Curves obtained after the injection of indicator at or upstream from the site of a right-to-left shunt show a short appearance time because of the escape of indicator across the defect (Fig. 13–15). This initial curve is followed by a second peak produced by the indicator which has traversed the longer normal pathway through the lungs. In contradistinction, curves obtained from injection of indicator downstream from the site of a right-to-left shunt show a normal appearance time.

In the presence of *left-to-right shunts* some of the indicator has a normal transit time to the detection site, whereas the remaining indicator recirculates through the lungs, resulting in a prolonged transit time. Curves recorded from systemic arterial blood have normal appearance times, reduced peak concentration and prolonged disappearance times (Fig. 13–15). Similar curves may be obtained in the presence of valvular regurgitation. Left-to-right shunts may be *localized* by the following methods: (1) Indicator is injected upstream or downstream from the site of the shunt, and curves are recorded from a systemic arterial detector. Downstream injections result in normal curves. If indicator is injected at or upstream to the site of shunt, the curve is as described above (Fig. 13–15). (2) The second method requires the use of two cardiac catheters. The first is placed in the distal pulmonary artery or left side of the heart for injection of indicator. The second is placed in the lesser circulation for sampling of blood containing indicator from the vena cava, right atrium, right ventricle or pulmonary artery. After injection of indicator into the distal pulmonary artery, it traverses the pulmonary circulation and appears in the left side of the heart and systemic circulation. If a left-to-right shunt is present, detectable indicator re-enters the right side of the heart and pulmonary circulation (Fig. 13–15), and comparison of curves localizes the site of left-to-right shunt. (3) A third method uses the same principle as (2), but the indicator detector is incorporated in the cardiac catheter, avoiding the necessity of inserting a second catheter and the sampling of blood (see Ascorbic Acid Polarography).

Generally, indicator dilution methods are more sensitive than blood oxygen analyses for the detection of intravascular shunts. Available techniques for indicator curves include the following:

1. ***Dyes.*** The most frequently used material is indocyanine green. The detector is either an oximeter or densitometer. Accurate application of this method usually requires the continuous with-

drawal of blood for the inscription of the dye dilution curve.

2. *Ascorbic Acid Polarography.* Anodically polarized platinum electrodes are depolarized and hence allow current to flow by certain readily oxidizable substances such as ascorbic acid. This technique has a particular advantage in infants and children because the platinum detector is placed intravascularly, avoiding the necessity for withdrawal of blood for the inscription of the ascorbate dilution curve. The platinum electrode may be inserted intra-arterially for localization of right-to-left shunts and incorporated in the wall of the cardiac catheter for detection of left-to-right shunts.

3. *Physiologic Saline Solution.* This is used as the indicator and is detected by the continuous withdrawal of blood through a conductivity cell.

4. *Radioactive Materials. Radioactive gases* such as krypton-85 have also been used for the localization of left-to-right shunts by principles similar to those described under The Hydrogen Electrode.

The Hydrogen Electrode. A platinized platinum electrode capable of sensing hydrogen is incorporated in a cardiac catheter which is inserted intravascularly or in the cardiac chambers (usually right). The detection and localization of *left-to-right shunts* depend on the fact that the electrode develops a potential in the presence of blood which has been exposed to hydrogen in the lungs; this is accomplished by having the patient take a breath of hydrogen. The instant the hydrogen appears in the nasal passages may be timed with another hydrogen electrode mounted in a flexible tube which has been brought into contact with the mucosa of the nose (airway signal). Some prefer to use an arterial hydrogen electrode for timing. Thus, it is possible to time accurately the inhalation of hydrogen and its subsequent appearance in any part of the circulatory system. For example, in patients with ventricular septal defect and left-to-right shunt, the hydrogen appearance time will be normal in the venae cavae and right atrium (Fig. 13–16, *B*). Curves obtained from the right ventricle and pulmonary artery will show an early appearance time because left heart blood containing hydrogen has been shunted across the ventricular defect (Fig. 13–16, *B*).

The detection and localization of *right-to-left shunts* depend on the fact that saline solution saturated with hydrogen is completely cleared of hydrogen after passing through the normal lung. After the hydrogen electrode has been inserted into the aorta, hydrogenated saline is injected via a cardiac catheter into the various right heart chambers. If the injection is made upstream from the site of right-to-left shunt, the arterial electrode will instantly detect the dissolved hydrogen. For example, in a patient with tetralogy of Fallot and right-to-left shunt across the ventricular defect, hydrogenated saline solution injected into the right atrium or right ventricle will immediately be detected by the aortic electrode. But if the injection is made downstream (i.e., in the pulmonary artery), the hydrogen is cleared by the lung and is not detected by the electrode.

The hydrogen electrode technique is particularly useful in infants and children because of its simplicity, extreme sensitivity and elimination of repeated sampling of blood. The principal disadvantages are that the method is not quantifiable, and hydrogen gas is explosive.

ANGIOCARDIOGRAPHY. The great blood vessels and individual cardiac chambers may be seen by selective angiocardiography, i.e., injection of contrast material into specific cardiac chambers or great vessels. This method allows identification of specific abnormalities without the superimposition

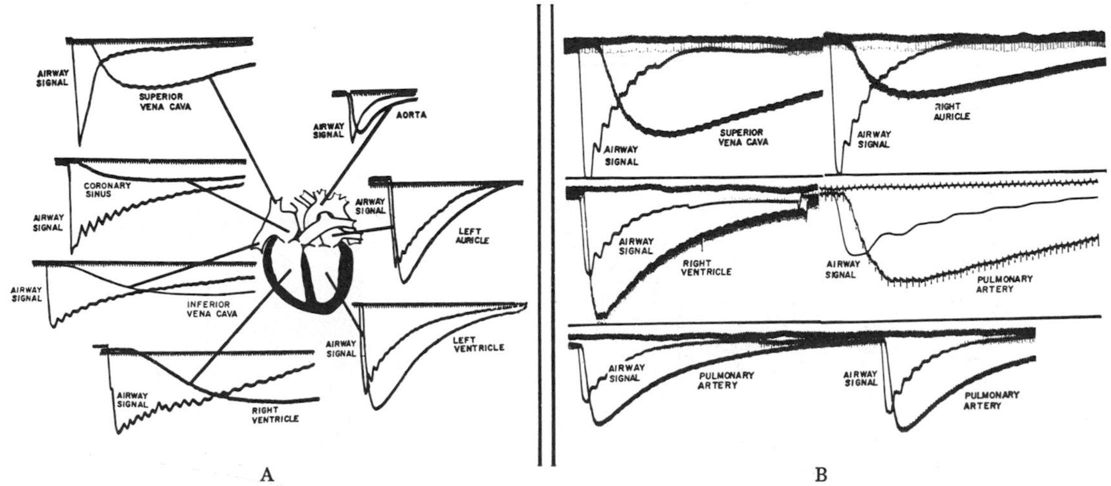

Figure 13–16 Hydrogen electrode curves. Airway signal curves from electrode in nasal passage, and these serve to time entrance of hydrogen into respiratory passages. A, Normal curves from various chambers of the heart. Note normal early appearance time in left as compared to right side of heart. B, Ventricular septal defect. Early appearance of hydrogen in right ventricle as compared to right atrium demonstrates left-to-right shunt at ventricular level. Right middle curve (pulmonary artery), at faster paper speed, demonstrates intracardiac electrocardiogram superimposed on hydrogen curve. (Courtesy of Dr. Leland C. Clark, Jr.)

of the shadows of normal chambers. Serial roentgenograms may be obtained in two planes at a rate of 6 to 14 per second.

Photofluorography with image intensification has made possible simultaneous cardiac catheterization and selective angiocardiography. The method has been combined with closed-circuit television to monitor the fluoroscopic screen and allow visualization of the cardiac silhouette and the cardiac catheter. After the cardiac catheter has been introduced into the specific chamber to be studied, a small amount of contrast medium is rapidly injected, and moving pictures are exposed at 30 to 60 frames per second. Biplane cine-angiocardiography allows detailed evaluation of specific cardiac chambers and blood vessels in two planes with the injection of a single bolus of contrast material.

The injection of contrast medium into the circulation is not without hazard and should be used with discrimination. Deaths have been reported from iodine sensitivity, cardiac arrhythmia, cerebrovascular complications and pulmonary edema. The risk has been reduced, however, by the introduction of better contrast agents.

"Idealized" diagrams of the normal angiocardiogram are shown in Figure 13–5. The indications for this study are outlined under the individual congenital lesions.

PHONOCARDIOGRAPHY. Graphic records of heart sounds and murmurs are recorded simultaneously with electrocardiograms and intravascular pressure pulses. The function of phonocardiography is not to replace, but to corroborate the findings of clinical auscultation. In many instances hemodynamic abnormalities may be evaluated fairly accurately. For example, the severity of isolated valvular pulmonary stenosis may be assessed by clinical auscultation supplemented with phonocardiography.

Sound pickups incorporated in cardiac catheters may be introduced intravascularly for recording sounds and murmurs (intracardiac phonocardiography). This method localizes the cardiac chamber or blood vessel from which murmurs or abnormal sounds originate.

NONINVASIVE TECHNIQUES. These are diagnostic maneuvers which can be applied without penetrating the skin or, in some instances, require only simple venipuncture. They have a particular attraction in the diagnosis and management of cardiovascular disease in infants and children, since the traditional invasive maneuvers such as cardiac catheterization are not without risk. The noninvasive methods of electrovectorcardiography, phonocardiography, evaluation of the arterial and venous pulses and chest roentgenography have been discussed earlier in this chapter.

Echocardiography. Echocardiography utilizes pulsed ultrasound with frequencies above the audible range. Ultrasound waves, harmless to body tissues, travel through fluid in a straight line but are reflected at the interface of substances of differing densities. When traversing living tissues, they are returned as echoes when they strike zones of differing acoustic impedance (Fig. 13–17). They also have a constant transit time, so that the distance can be measured between the transducer on the skin and the interface from which the echoes are returned. Echocardiography is now utilized to measure left and right ventricular dimensions and stroke volume; to record mitral, tricuspid, aortic and pulmonic valve motion; to define the left ventricular outflow tract and the left atrium; and to detect pericardial effusions. Since this method provides reliable information without risk or stress, it can be used repeatedly in seriously ill patients, and has proved to be particularly useful in the diagnosis of critical cardiovascular disease in the newborn infant; with further experience and technical improvements it may soon rival the more commonly used invasive techniques in diagnostic accuracy.

Systolic Time Intervals. These provide useful information concerning left ventricular function. The division of the various segments of electrome-

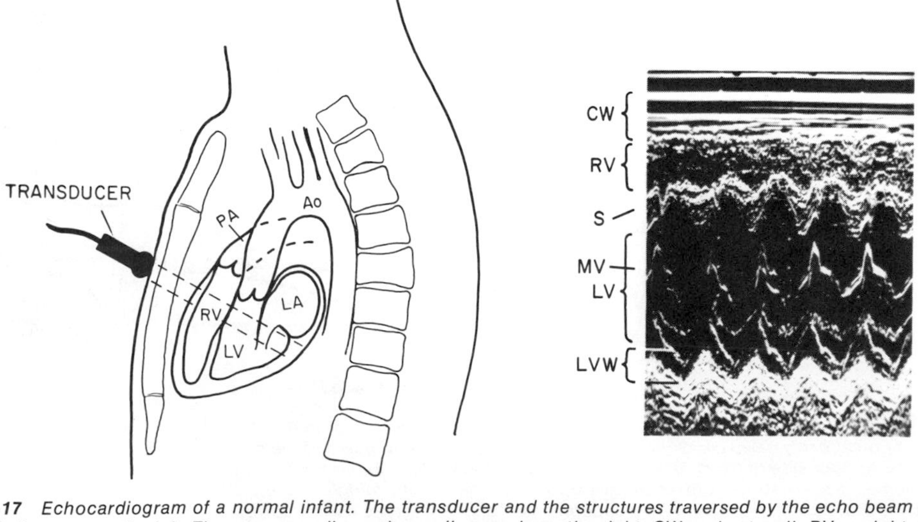

Figure 13–17 Echocardiogram of a normal infant. The transducer and the structures traversed by the echo beam are shown in the idealized diagram on the left. The corresponding echocardiogram is on the right. CW = chest wall; RV = right ventricle; S = interventricular septum; MV = mitral valve; LV = left ventricular cavity; LVW = posterior left ventricular wall. (From Meyer, R. A., and Kaplan, S.: Progr. Cardiovasc. Dis. 25:341, 1973. By permission of Grune & Stratton, Inc.)

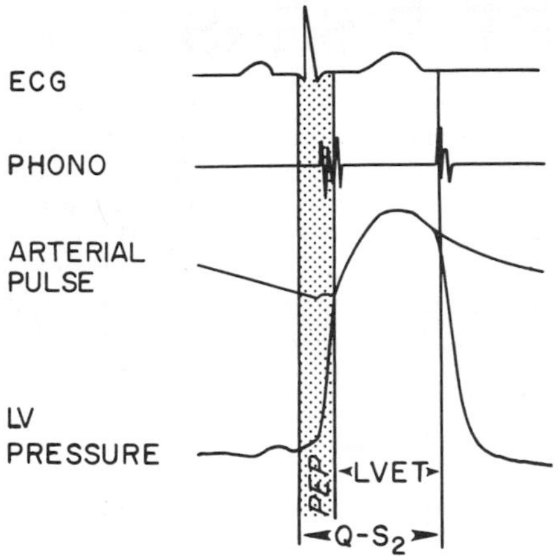

Figure 13–18 Temporal events of cardiac cycle to illustrate method of measurement of systolic time intervals. PEP, preejection period; LVET, left ventricular ejection time; Q-S2, total electromechanical systole; ECG, electrocardiogram; PHONO, phonocardiogram; LV, left ventricular (From Meyer, R. A., and Kaplan, S.: Progr. Cardiovasc. Dis. 25:341, 1973. By permission of Grune & Stratton, Inc.)

chanical systole is indicated in Figure 13–18. Much of the information concerning these measurements has been derived from adults; information from children is still meager. In adults with heart failure the pre-ejection period is prolonged and left ventricular ejection time abbreviated. Study of a small group of babies with left heart failure showed that they differed from adults in that the babies had normal pre-ejection periods and prolonged ejection times with respect to heart rate. Since significant alterations in systolic time intervals accompany changes in stroke volume and heart rate, repeated measurements of these intervals are useful in the follow-up evaluation of left ventricular function.

Graded Exercise. Major changes in cardiovascular dynamics accompany the increased oxygen demand of graded exercise up to a maximal capacity. The major response is increase in cardiac output, primarily because of increased heart rate, but stroke volume, systemic venous return and pulse pressure are also increased. Systemic vascular resistance is greatly decreased by immediate vasodilatation. This test is performed on a treadmill or bicycle ergometer. It provides objective and reliable data relevant to diagnosis and management. During submaximal exercise, S-T segment depression and a narrow pulse pressure occur in aortic stenosis with a resting systolic gradient exceeding 50 mm Hg. Even after adequate surgical resection of aortic coarctation, significant increases in pulse pressure and systolic hypertension may persist. In cyanotic congenital heart disease (e.g., tetralogy of Fallot), the resting arterial oxygen saturation is low; it is further reduced on exercise, and the time taken for recovery to the control level is prolonged. Postexercise unifocal and multifocal ventricular extrasystoles have also been recorded many years after total correction of Fallot's tetralogy.

Radioisotope Angiography. After intravenous infusion of a radioisotope, scintillation scanning over the chest will detect left-to-right shunts by use of pulmonary vascular isotope dilution curves. This method also delineates the orientation of the aorta and pulmonary artery and the position of the cardiac chambers. The objective information derived from this test is useful in detecting the presence of left-to-right shunts and helps in the differentiation of innocent from organic murmurs. The radioisotope used most frequently at this time is ^{99m}technetium.

GENERAL

Friedman, W. F., Lesch, M., and Sonnenblick, E. H.: Neonatal Heart Disease. New York, Grune & Stratton, Inc., 1972 and 1973.
Gasul, B. M., Arcilla, R. A., and Lev, M.: Heart Disease in Children. Philadelphia, J. B. Lippincott Company, 1966.
Kaplan, S.: Symposium on pediatric cardiology. Pediat. Clin. N. Amer. *18*:1009, 1971.
Keith, J. D., Rowe, R. D., and Vlad, P.: Heart Disease in Infancy and Childhood. 2nd ed. New York, The Macmillan Company, 1966.
Moss, A. J., and Adams, F. H.: Heart Disease in Infants, Children and Adolescents. Baltimore, The Williams & Wilkins Company, 1968.
Nadas, A. S., and Fyler, D. C.: Pediatric Cardiology. 3rd ed. Philadelphia, W. B. Saunders Company, 1972.
Oakley, C. M.: Advances in congenital heart disease. *In* Yu, P. N., and Goodwin, J. F. (eds.): Progress in Cardiology 2. Philadelphia, Lea & Febiger, 1973, pp. 75–134.
Rowe, R. D., and Mehrizi, A.: The Neonate with Congenital Heart Disease. Philadelphia, W. B. Saunders Company, 1968.
Taussig, H. B.: Congenital Malformations of the Heart. 2nd ed. Cambridge, Harvard University Press, 1960.
Watson, H.: Paediatric Cardiology. St. Louis, The C. V. Mosby Company, 1968.

Cardiac Sounds and Phonocardiography

Caceres, C. A., and Perry, L. W.: The Innocent Murmur: A Problem in Clinical Practice. Boston, Little, Brown and Company, 1966.
Leatham, A.: Systolic murmurs. Circulation *17*:601, 1958.
Rushmer, R. F., and Morgan, C.: Meaning of murmurs, Am. J. Cardiol. *2*:722, 1968.

Roentgen Examination

Caffey, J.: Pediatric X-Ray Diagnosis. 6th ed. Chicago, Year Book Medical Publishers, Inc., 1972.
Edwards, J. E., Carey, L. S., Neufeld, H. N., and Lester, R. G.: Congenital Heart Disease: Correlation of Pathologic Anatomy and Angiocardiography. Philadelphia, W. B. Saunders Company, 1965.

Electrocardiogram and Vectorcardiogram

Ellison, R. C., and Restieaux, N. J.: Vectorcardiography in Congenital Heart Disease. Philadelphia, W. B. Saunders Company, 1972.
Guntheroth, W. G.: Pediatric Electrocardiography. Philadelphia, W. B. Saunders Company, 1965.
Hoffman, I., Hamby, R. I., and Glassman, E.: Vectorcardiography 2. Philadelphia, J. B. Lippincott Company, 1971.

Cardiac Catheterization

Braunwald, E., and Swan, H. J. C.: Cooperative study on cardiac catheterization. Circulation *37*: Supplement 3, 1968.
Clark, L. C., and Bargeron, L. M.: Detection and direct recording of left to right shunts with the hydrogen electrode catheter. Surgery *46*:797, 1959.
Wood, E. H.: Diagnostic applications of indicator dilution technics in congenital heart disease. Circulation Res. *10*:531, 1962.
Zimmerman, H. A.: Intravascular Catheterization. 2nd ed. Springfield, Ill., Charles C Thomas, 1966.

Angiocardiography and Arteriography

Abrams, H. L.: Cinefluorographic equipment in cardiovascular studies. Prog. Cardiovasc. Dis. *5*:440, 1963.
Björk, L.: Cineangiocardiography or full-sized angiography? Experiences in diagnosis of congenital heart disease in early infancy. Radiol. Clin. (Basel) *39*:102, 1970.
Sones, F. M., Jr.: Cinecardioangiography. *In* American College of Chest Physicians: Clinical Cardiopulmonary Physiology. 2nd ed. New York, Grune & Stratton, Inc., 1960.

CONGENITAL HEART DISEASE

FETAL CIRCULATION. Oxygenated blood from the placenta flows to the fetus through the umbilical vein at an average rate of about 175 ml/kg and at a pressure of about 12 mm Hg. The oxygen saturation of this blood is almost 85 per cent, with a pO_2 of about 30 mm Hg. Approximately one half of the umbilical venous blood bypasses the liver and flows through the ductus venosus into the inferior vena cava, where it mixes with the remainder of the blood returning from the caudal part of the body. This stream of blood entering the right atrium from the inferior vena cava has the highest pO_2 for fetal perfusion, preferentially passes across the foramen ovale to the left atrium, flows into the left ventricle and is ejected into the ascending aorta. Therefore the coronary and cerebral arteries, and those of the upper extremities, are perfused with blood having a higher pO_2 than that perfusing other parts of the body, except for the liver. The superior vena caval blood is considerably less oxygenated and traverses the tricuspid valve to flow primarily to the right ventricle and pulmonary arterial trunk. The major portion of this blood (which has a pO_2 of 19 to 22 mm Hg) bypasses the lungs and flows through the ductus arteriosus into the descending aorta to perfuse the caudal part of the body and the placenta via the umbilical arteries. The effective fetal cardiac output, i.e., the sum of the left ventricular output and the ductal flow, amounts to about 220 ml/kg/min. Approximately 65 per cent of this blood returns to the placenta; the remaining 35 per cent perfuses the fetal organs and tissues (Fig. 13–19).

Since the fetal ventricles work in parallel rather than in series, the distribution of their ejected blood depends on resistance and flow and the fact that the large ductus arteriosus equalizes aortic and pulmonary arterial pressures. The high pulmonary vascular resistance diverts pulmonary arterial blood from the lungs to the ductus arteriosus and descending aorta. The mechanisms which result in pulmonary arteriolar constriction are not all understood. Fetal alveoli filled with fluid mechanically impede pulmonary flow. The resistance produced by the tortuous and kinked small blood vessels of the unexpanded lung also retard blood flow. However, it is generally agreed that the level of pO_2 of the blood perfusing the lung has the greatest influence on pulmonary vascular resistance; when pulmonary arterial pO_2 exceeds about 35 mm Hg, pulmonary vascular resistance falls and pulmonary flow increases.

NEONATAL CIRCULATION. Dramatic changes occur as the fetal circulation adapts to extrauterine life and gas exchange is transferred from the placenta to the lung of the newborn infant. These changes do not occur instantaneously but are effected over hours or days. After an initial and temporary fall, there is a progressive rise in systemic blood pressure and slowing of the heart rate as a result of an increase in systemic vascular resistance as the low-resistant placental circulation is eliminated. The average central aortic pressure in the neonate is 75/50 mm Hg. With the onset of ventilation a dramatic increase in pulmonary blood flow occurs because of the dilatative effect of oxygen on the constricted pulmonary blood vessels. This increases pulmonary venous return, with a resultant increase in left ventricular output. In the normal neonate, ductal closure and fall of pulmonary vascular resistance result in a fall of pulmonary arterial and right ventricular pressures. The major decline of pressure from the high fetal levels to the low "adult" levels in the human infant at sea level occurs within the first 2 to 3 days of life but may be prolonged for 7 days or more.

The significant differences between the neonatal circulation and that of older infants may be summarized as follows (Dawes): (1) right-to-left shunting may persist across the patent foramen ovale; (2) continued patency of the ductus arteriosus may allow bidirectional shunting, but the dominant shunt is from left to right because of the decreased pulmonary vascular resistance; (3) the neonatal pulmonary vasculature retains the ability to constrict vigorously in response to hypoxemia, hypercapnia and acidosis; (4) the muscular mass of the left and right ventricles is almost equal; (5) the neonate has a lower systemic arterial pressure and an unusual tolerance to hypoxemia; and (6) newborn infants at rest have a relatively high oxygen consumption, which is associated with their relatively high cardiac output.

After birth the foramen ovale, the ductus arteriosus and ductus venosus are no longer needed, but their closure proceeds gradually. The foramen ovale is functionally closed by the third month of life, though it is possible to pass a probe through the overlapping flaps in 25 per cent of adults. The ductus arteriosus has become functionally closed in 88 per cent of infants by the end of the eighth week, and the foramen ovale in 87 per cent by the end of the twelfth week. During this period of adjustment there are rarely physical signs of patency of these structures. Nevertheless, in some premature and occasional normal newborn infants an evanescent systolic murmur with late accentuation may be audible and is attributed to ductal flow. On rare occasions emboli to the abdominal aorta and its branches (especially mesenteric) may arise from thrombosis in the ductus arteriosus.

Oxygen is the most important factor controlling ductal closure. When the pO_2 of the blood passing through the ductus reaches about 50 mm Hg the ductal wall constricts; the mechanisms by which oxygen activates ductal constriction are still controversial. It has been suggested that oxygen releases bradykinin to trigger ductal closure. Others consider that the media of the ductal wall contains cells which act as oxygen receptors. The impor-

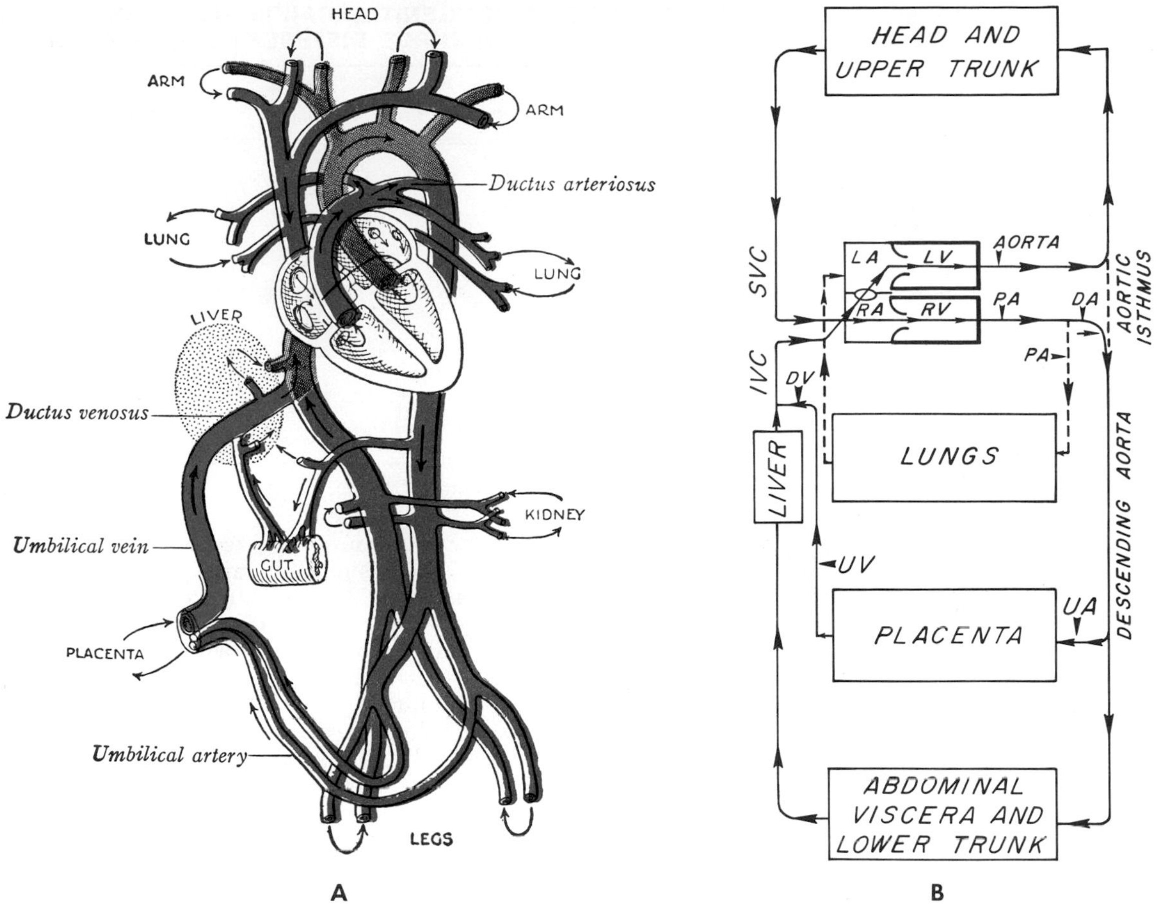

Figure 13–19 *A, Plan of the human circulation before birth (partly after Dodds). Colors show the quality of the blood, and arrows indicate its direction of flow (Arey).*

B, In the fetus a large fraction of the umbilical venous blood enters the ductus venosus (DV) and bypasses the liver. This relatively well oxygenated blood flows across the foramen ovale to the left heart, which preferentially perfuses the head and upper trunk. Superior vena caval blood (SVC) is ejected by the right heart into the pulmonary artery (PA) and ductus arteriosus (DA). This blood circulates to the placenta as well as to the abdominal viscera and lower trunk. Interrupted lines indicate a low pulmonary blood flow and the flow from the ascending aorta across the aortic isthmus is also diminished. DV = ductus venosus; IVC = inferior vena cava; SVC = superior vena cava; RA = right atrium; LA = left atrium; RV = right ventricle; LV = left ventricle; PA = pulmonary artery; DA = ductus arteriosus (From Kaplan, S., and Assali, N. S.: Pathophysiology of Gestation, 1972).

tance of genetic factors is unknown, but it is of interest that patent ductus arteriosus has been reproduced in a colony of dogs.

INCIDENCE OF CONGENITAL HEART DISEASE. The two important conditions which produce cardiovascular disease in children are congenital heart disease and rheumatic fever. The introduction of antimicrobial agents for the treatment and prophylaxis of streptococcal infections has resulted in a large decrease in the incidence of rheumatic fever in North America. Simultaneously, great advances have been made in the diagnosis and surgical treatment of congenital cardiovascular diseases. In centers where diagnostic and surgical facilities are available new patients with congenital heart disease are almost ten times more frequent than those with acute rheumatic fever.

The incidence of cardiovascular malformations at birth is about 8 per 1000, and they account for about 50 per cent of the deaths caused by congenital defects in the first year of life.

Table 13–5 provides a reasonable estimate of the incidence of selected malformations in different age groups; there is, however, considerable variation in different clinics. The development of palliative and corrective procedures has changed the frequency with which various malformations, especially transposition of the great vessels, are seen in older children. Patent ductus arteriosus is now seldom seen in adults, since surgical treatment is undertaken even in asymptomatic young children. Although small ventricular septal defects are common in children, they are uncommon in adults.

ETIOLOGY

Maternal Infection. This may result in congenital heart disease. Congenital rubella is associated particularly with patent ductus arteriosus and pulmonary arterial branch stenosis. Coxsackievirus B has been implicated in the causation of endocardial fibroelastosis and has been demonstrated as a cause of acute myocarditis in neonates. Although a positive skin reaction to mumps antigen may be present in patients with endocardial

TABLE 13–5 PERCENTAGE INCIDENCE OF CONGENITAL CARDIOVASCULAR MALFORMATIONS AMONG AFFECTED PERSONS IN THREE DIFFERENT AGE GROUPS

	INFANTS	CHILDREN	OLDER CHILDREN AND ADULTS
Ventricular septal defect	28.3	24	15
Patent ductus arteriosus	12.5	15	15.5
Atrial septal defect	9.7	12	16
Coarctation	8.8	4.5	8
Transposition	8	4.5	2
Fallot's tetralogy	7	11	15.5
Pulmonary stenosis	6	11	15
Aortic stenosis	3.5	6.5	5
Truncus	2.7	0.5	–
Tricuspid atresia	1	1.5	1
All others	12.5	9.5	7
Total	100.0	100.0	100.0

Adapted from Campbell, M.: *In* H. Watson (ed.): Paediatric Cardiology. London, Lloyd-Luke, Ltd., 1968, Chap. 5.

fibroelastosis, the role of mumps virus as a teratogen is not clear. The protozoa of toxoplasmosis may be found in the heart, but functional cardiac disturbance seldom occurs. Late manifestations of congenital syphilis only rarely include aortitis and aneurysm. Cytomegalovirus and adenovirus have been isolated from cultures of cells (especially from the kidney) obtained from infants who have succumbed with congenital heart disease, but the mechanism and time of infection are not clear.

The teratogenic effect of *drugs and radiation* is well recognized. To date the highest incidence (about 10 per cent) of congenital heart disease has been associated with the thalidomide syndrome. The offspring of mothers on anticonvulsant therapy also have a higher incidence of congenital cardiovascular disease and cleft lip and palate.

The incidence of patent ductus arteriosus appears to be higher among populations living at high altitudes, and cardiac malformations, especially arterial transposition and ventricular septal defect, appear to be more common among the offspring of prediabetic mothers.

Family Studies. These studies indicate that whereas the incidence of congenital heart disease in the population as a whole is about 8 per 1000, the incidence in liveborn siblings of probands is between 14 and 22 per 1000. The reported concordance of the lesions in siblings varies from 35 to 56 per cent. Information concerning the incidence of congenital heart disease in parents, other relatives and offspring of probands is scanty, but this incidence appears to be low. Generally only one of a pair of twins is affected by congenital heart disease.

The incidence of *atrial or ventricular septal defects* among siblings with these anomalies is about 1 per cent. Isolated instances of atrial septal defect have also been reported in several generations. *Patent ductus arteriosus* may aggregate in families and has been reported in three successive generations. *Truncus arteriosus* has been reported in siblings, as has *primary pulmonary hypertension.* Patients with *aortic stenosis* have occasionally had similarly afflicted siblings. The incidence of *coarctation of the aorta* in siblings is low, but that of *pulmonary stenosis* is probably highest of any form of congenital heart disease (almost 3 per cent). A relatively high incidence of consanguinity of the parents has been reported with *situs inversus.* Primary endocardial fibroelastosis has been reported in siblings.

Associated noncardiac malformations are common, especially with ventricular septal defects and double outlet right ventricle, whereas they are relatively uncommon with arterial transposition and aortic atresia; renal anomalies and cleft palate are the commoner ones. Scoliosis occurs more frequently with cyanotic congenital heart disease. The common cardiovascular diseases associated with specific syndromes are listed in Table 13–6.

Genetic counseling concerning recurrence risk is of great practical importance. Generally parents can be supported in a decision to have additional children when one child has congenital heart disease, since the recurrence rate is about 2 per cent. But if two siblings are affected, it is probable that the recurrence rate is higher. The incidence of cardiovascular malformation in the offspring of patients who have been treated for congenital heart disease is less than 3 per cent. Cyanotic women who become pregnant have an increased risk of spontaneous abortion, and, if they go to term, the infant is usually small.

DIAGNOSIS OF CONGENITAL HEART DISEASE. The development of surgical procedures effective for certain congenital cardiovascular defects has made accurate diagnosis essential. Most often the diagnosis can be established from the history, physical findings and customary roentgenographic and electrocardiographic examinations. When doubt exists, cardiac catheterization, selective angiocardiography and aortography often supply the necessary confirmatory information. Because early surgical intervention may save many of them from death, severely ill newborn and young infants with cardiovascular malformations should be subjected to any necessary diagnostic procedures.

CLASSIFICATION OF CONGENITAL HEART DISEASE. Abbott established the custom of dividing congeni-

TABLE 13-6 CARDIOVASCULAR INVOLVEMENT IN SYNDROMES

SYNDROME	COMMON CARDIOVASCULAR INVOLVEMENT
Heritable and Possible Heritable Syndromes and Disorders	
Ellis-van Creveld	Single atrium (other defects in 30%)
Holt-Oram	Atrial septal defect (other defects common)
Kartagener	Dextrocardia
Laurence-Moon-Biedl	Variable, including tetralogy of Fallot
Neurologic and muscular diseases:	
Friedreich's ataxia	Cardiomyopathy
Muscular dystrophy	Cardiomyopathy
Riley-Day	Episodic hypertension, postural hypotension
Refsum's	Arrhythmia, sudden death
Tuberous sclerosis	Rhabdomyoma, cardiomyopathy
Rendu-Osler-Weber	Arteriovenous fistula (lung, liver, mucous membranes)
Familial deafness	Occasionally arrhythmia, sudden death
Familial dwarfism and nevi	Cardiomyopathy
Congenital hypertrophic subaortic stenosis	Obstructive cardiomyopathy
Familial elfin facies, mental retardation, infantile hypercalcemia	Supravalvular aortic stenosis, pulmonary arterial branch stenosis
Scimitar syndrome	Hypoplasia of right lung, anomalous pulmonary venous return to inferior vena cava
Rubenstein-Taybi	Patent ductus arteriosus
Chromosomal Abnormalities	
Down	Endocardial cushion defect, atrial septal defect, ventricular septal defect, patent ductus arteriosus
Trisomy E	Ventricular septal defect, patent ductus arteriosus, pulmonic stenosis
Trisomy D	Ventricular septal defect, double outlet right ventricle, patent ductus arteriosus, atrial septal defect
Cri-du-chat	Ventricular septal defect in a minority
Turner syndrome:	
Phenotypic female	Coarctation of aorta, pulmonic stenosis, aortic stenosis
Phenotypic male	Pulmonic stenosis, aortic stenosis
Inborn Errors of Metabolism	
Pompe's disease	Glycogen storage disease of heart
Homocystinuria	Pulmonary arterial and aortic dilatation, intravascular thrombosis, flushing of skin
Connective Tissue Disorders	
Marfan	Aortic dilatation with aortic incompetence, mitral incompetence, dilatation of pulmonary artery
Hurler	Multivalvular and coronary artery disease
Morquio-Ulrich	Aortic incompetence
Scheie	Aortic incompetence
Pseudoxanthoma elasticum	Peripheral arterial disease
Ehlers-Danlos	Arterial dilatation
Osteogenesis imperfecta	Aortic incompetence
Arterial calcification of infancy	Calcinosis of coronary arteries

Adapted from Neill, C. A.: *In* Moss, A. J., and Adams, F. A. (eds.): Heart Disease in Infants, Children and Adolescents. Baltimore, The Williams & Wilkins Company, 1968, Chap. 3.

tal heart diseases into two groups: (1) those with cyanosis at rest, and (2) those without cyanosis or manifesting it only under certain adverse conditions, e.g., high pulmonary resistance. Taussig makes a similar division on the basis of malformations which do or do not permit an adequate supply of oxygen to the body. This classification has been criticized, and other, more complicated ones have been suggested; they depend on hemodynamic and anatomic factors, including the direction of shunt. In congenital heart disease persistent cyanosis is usually caused by the shunting of venous blood from the right to the left side of the heart, so that it passes into the systemic circulation without being oxygenated in the lungs. In this text the following classification of the more common anomalies will be used: (1) right-to-left shunts (i.e., with cyanosis), (2) left-to-right shunts (i.e., without cyanosis), and (3) no shunt at all. It is appreciated that there is overlappping in these groups.

Congenital Cardiac Disease with Cyanosis (Dominant Right-to-Left Shunt)

TETRALOGY OF FALLOT

The combination of (1) obstruction to right ventricular outflow (pulmonary stenosis), (2) ventricular septal defect, (3) dextroposition of the aorta and (4) right ventricular hypertrophy constitutes the tetralogy of Fallot. Obstruction to pulmonary arterial flow is usually at the right ventricular infundibulum and pulmonary valve, though the pulmonary arterial trunk is generally smaller than usual. The pulmonic valve may have a small ring, be bicuspid, and occasionally be the only site of stenosis. Hypertrophy of the crista supraventricularis contributes to the infundibular stenosis and results in the formation of an infundibular chamber of variable size and contour. The ventricular septal defect is generally large, just below the aortic valve, and related to the posterior and right aortic cusps. The normal continuity of the mitral and aortic valves is maintained. The aorta arches to the right in 20 per cent of these patients, is large, and straddles the ventricular septal defect. The aorta is dextroposed because a varying proportion of its origin is from the right ventricle.

HEMODYNAMICS. Systemic venous return to the right atrium and right ventricle is normal. When the right ventricle contracts, the outflow of blood is resisted by the pulmonary stenosis and blood is shunted across the ventricular septal defect into the aorta. This results in persistent arterial unsaturation and cyanosis. The pulmonary blood flow is restricted by the obstruction to right ventricular outflow, but may be supplemented by bronchial collateral circulation and occasionally by a patent ductus arteriosus. The systolic and diastolic pressures in each ventricle are usually similar, as are the mean pressures in the atria. A measurable gradient of pressure is always detected across the outflow of the right ventricle, owing to the pulmonary stenosis.

The major defects in the tetralogy of Fallot are the obstruction to right ventricular outflow and the ventricular septal defect. When these conditions exist without right-to-left shunt, the anomaly is termed *acyanotic Fallot* (see Pulmonary Stenosis and Ventricular Septal Defect).

CLINICAL MANIFESTATIONS. *Cyanosis,* one of the outstanding manifestations, may not be present at birth. Apparently, as long as the ductus arteriosus remains open, sufficient blood passes through the lungs to prevent cyanosis. As it closes during the first months of life, cyanosis may become apparent gradually or develop suddenly when the infant has an infection. The cyanosis is most prominent in the mucous membranes of the lips and mouth and in the fingernails and toenails, but the entire skin surface has a dusky, bluish color. The sclerae are gray, and the blood vessels at the periphery are likely to be engorged, giving the appearance of mild conjunctivitis. The blood vessels of the retina are large and dark. The mucous membranes of the pharynx are purple, and the tongue is deep blue and often large and fissured, with prominent papillae. The gums are frequently inflamed and bleed easily from light pressure. The eruption of the teeth may be delayed; histologic examination reveals dilatation and engorgement of the capillaries in the dental pulp and poor calcification of the dentin. *Clubbing* of the fingers and toes is a conspicuous sign, generally present by the age of 1 or 2 years. *Hemoptyses* may be recurrent, but are rare.

Dyspnea occurs on exertion. Infants and toddlers will play actively for a short time and then sit or lie down. Older children may be able to walk a block or so before stopping to rest. The capacity for exercise depends on the severity of the cardiac lesion, which is often reflected by the intensity of the cyanosis. Characteristically, children assume a *squatting* position for the relief of dyspnea due to physical effort. This results in an increase in arterial oxygen saturation, so that the child is able to resume physical activity within a few minutes. Assumption of the squatting position may result in decreased venous return and increased systemic arterial resistance, each of which would tend to decrease the right-to-left shunt and increase pulmonary blood flow.

Paroxysmal dyspneic attacks (anoxic "blue" spells) are a particular problem during the first two years of life. The infant becomes dyspneic and restless, cyanosis increases, and gasping respirations ensue. During the spell the cry is usually weak, but may be loud. Occasionally some infants clutch or scratch over the anterior portion of the chest as if they had precordial pain. Temporary disappearance or decrease in intensity of the systolic murmur is usual. The spells may last from a few minutes to a few hours and are occasionally fatal. Shorter episodes are followed by generalized weakness and sleep. Severe spells may progress to unconsciousness and occasionally convulsions or hemiparesis. Their onset is spontaneous and unpredictable, though they may follow feeding (especially breakfast), crying or a bowel movement, or may be precipitated by infection or iron deficiency anemia. The spells are associated with a reduction of an already compromised pulmonary blood flow, which results in hypoxia and metabolic acidosis. The disappearance or attenuation of the systolic murmur and reduction of arterial oxygen saturation and pulmonary arterial pressure suggest that blue spells are associated with spasm of the right ventricular outflow tract. Guntheroth et al. postulate that hyperpnea precipitates an attack by increasing systemic venous return. In the presence of fixed or decreased pulmonary blood flow, the right-

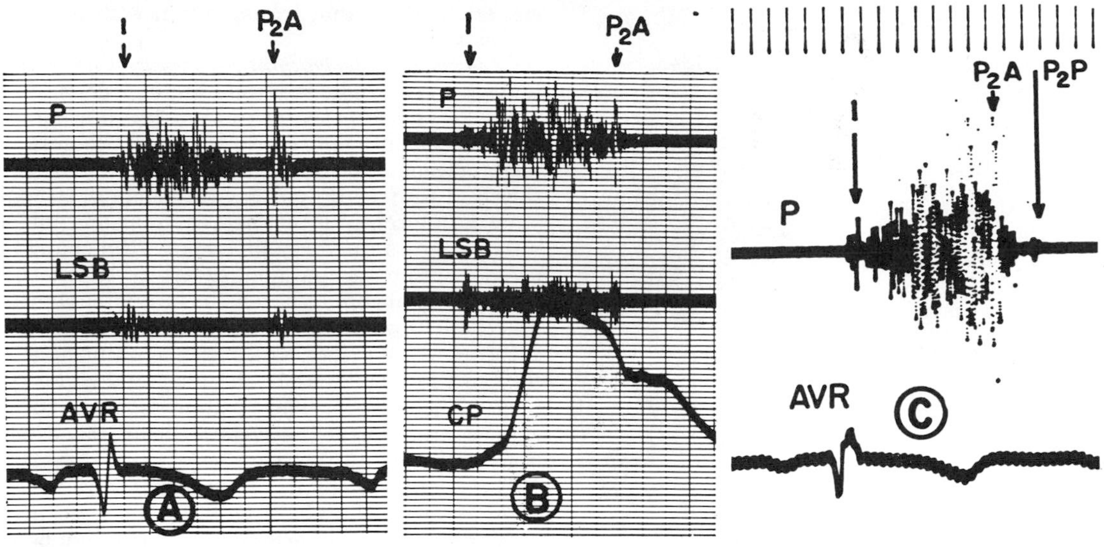

Figure 13–20 *Phonocardiograms illustrating the variability of auscultatory findings in cyanotic tetralogy of Fallot. Abbreviations: P, pulmonary area; LSB, left sternal border; AVR, electrocardiogram; CP, carotid pulse; 1, first heart sound;* P_2A*, aortic component of second heart sound,* P_2P*, pulmonic component of second heart sound. The systolic murmur may be early* (A)*, or when long* (B) *or accentuated in late systole* (C)*, it ends at* P_2A*. The second heart sound is single, owing to aortic valve closure* (A *and* B) *or split with a delayed soft pulmonic component* (C)*. Time lines 0.04 second.*

to-left shunt is increased. The resultant arterial hypoxia, metabolic acidosis and increased pCO_2 further stimulate the respiratory mechanism to maintain continuing hyperpnea. Depending on the frequency and severity of the attacks, one or all of the following procedures should be tried in sequence: (1) placement of the infant on his abdomen in the knee-chest position, making certain that there is no constricting clothing; (2) administration of oxygen; (3) injection of morphine subcutaneously with the dose not exceeding 0.5 mg per 10 pounds of body weight; this is especially effective. Since metabolic acidosis develops when the arterial pO_2 is below 40 mm Hg, rapid correction (within several minutes) is necessary if the spell is severe and there is lack of response to the foregoing therapy. This may be accomplished with intravenous administration of sodium bicarbonate or tri-hydroxyaminomethane (THAM). Recovery from the spell is rapid once the pH is returned to normal. Repeated blood pH measurements are necessary because rapid recurrence of acidosis is common. Beta-adrenergic inhibition by intravenous administration of propranolol (0.1 to a maximum of 0.2 mg/kg) has been used successfully in some patients with severe spells.

Growth and development may be delayed. The stature and nutritional status are usually below the average for the age, and the muscles and subcutaneous tissues are flabby and soft. Puberty is delayed.

The *pulse* is usually normal, as are the venous and arterial pressures. The left anterior hemithorax may bulge forward. The heart is usually normal in size, and the apical impulse is tapping. A *systolic thrill* is felt in 50 per cent of cases along the left sternal border in the third and fourth parasternal spaces.

The *systolic murmur* is frequently loud and harsh; it may be transmitted widely, but is most intense at the left sternal border. The murmur may be either ejection or pansystolic (Fig. 13–20), and it may be preceded by a click. In many instances the second heart sound is single and is produced by closure of the aortic valve. When closure of the pulmonary valve is audible, it is delayed and diminished. In a small number of instances the systolic murmur is followed by a diastolic murmur. This continuous murmur may be audible in any part of the chest, anteriorly or posteriorly; it is produced by enlarged bronchial collateral vessels or rarely by persistence of a patent ductus arteriosus and occurs frequently in pulmonary atresia.

ROENTGEN EXAMINATION. The typical configuration in the anteroposterior position shows a narrow base, concavity of the left border in the area usually occupied by the pulmonary artery and a normal heart size. The rounded apical shadow situated rather high above the diaphragm is produced chiefly by the hypertrophied right ventricle and has been likened to the shape of a sheep's nose; the entire cardiac silhouette, to that of a wooden shoe **(coeur en sabot)** (Fig. 13–21). In the lateral projection the anterior clear space may or may not be encroached upon by the hypertrophied right ventricle. In many patients the right ventricle displaces the normal left ventricle posteriorly so that the posterior border of the heart may overlap the spine in the left anterior oblique view. Although all these features suggest right ventricular enlargement, the electrocardiogram is a more sensitive index of right ventricular hypertrophy.

The aorta is usually large, and its position is important. In about 20 per cent of instances the aorta arches to the right instead of the left; this may be clearly visible in the anteroposterior view or may be confirmed by displacement of the barium-filled

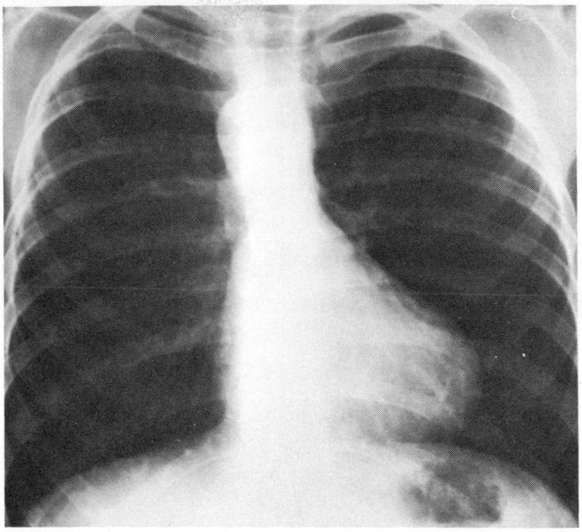

Figure 13–21 Teleroentgenogram of an 8 year old boy with tetralogy of Fallot. Note the normal heart size, some elevation of the cardiac apex, concavity in the region of the main pulmonary artery, diminished pulmonary vascularity and right aortic arch.

esophagus to the left. In the left oblique view a right aortic arch may indent the esophagus.

The hilar areas of the lungs are relatively clear and usually pulsate little or not at all, owing to the diminished pulmonary blood flow. The lung fields are remarkably clear for the same reason; this constitutes an important diagnostic sign.

Variations from the typical radiographic picture include poststenotic dilatation of the pulmonary artery, which is usually associated with valvular pulmonic stenosis. Occasionally pulmonary vascularity is made prominent by a reticular pattern of collateral bronchial circulation which radiates from the hilus of the lungs. Localized proximal infundibular stenosis with an infundibular chamber may produce a bulge at the upper left cardiac border in the frontal projection, which is distinguished from that of the pulmonary artery because it remains prominent in the right anterior oblique view.

ELECTROCARDIOGRAPHY. The electrocardiogram reveals evidence of right axis deviation and right ventricular hypertrophy. Evidence of right ventricular dominance, without which the diagnosis of tetralogy of Fallot is unlikely, is found in the right precordial chest leads where the configuration of the QRS complex is Rs, R, qR, qRs, rsR′ or RS. In these leads the T wave may be positive, which is further evidence of right ventricular hypertrophy. The P wave is tall and peaked or sometimes bifid in about one third of patients (Fig. 13–9).

OTHER TESTS. In the majority of instances the diagnosis of tetralogy of Fallot can be made with the aid of the foregoing studies. Preoperative cardiac catheterization and angiocardiography are essential, however, in order to elucidate the anatomic abnormalities and to exclude other defects which may mimic the tetralogy of Fallot, especially double outlet right ventricle with pulmonic stenosis and arterial transposition with pulmonic stenosis.

Cardiac catheterization reveals systolic hypertension in the right ventricle and a sudden fall of pressure as the catheter enters the infundibular chamber or pulmonary artery. Serial pressure determinations taken from the region of stenosis of the right ventricular outflow tract may in some instances differentiate between valvular and subvalvular stenosis. In valvular stenosis the change in pressure from the pulmonary artery to the right ventricle is abrupt, whereas in infundibular stenosis three pressure differentials are recorded as the catheter tip is withdrawn from the pulmonary artery to the infundibular chamber and right ventricle (Fig. 13–22). The systolic pressure in the right ventricle is at the systemic level, usually between 80 and 110 mm Hg.

The mean pulmonary arterial pressure is commonly between 5 and 10 mm Hg; the right atrial pressure is usually normal. The aorta may be entered from the right ventricle through the ventricular septal defect. The degree of arterial unsaturation depends on the magnitude of the right-to-left shunt and at rest is usually 75 to 85 per cent. Samples of blood from the venae cavae, right atrium, right ventricle and pulmonary artery are frequently similar in oxygen content, indicating absence of a left-to-right shunt. In many patients, however, a left-to-right shunt is demonstrated at the ventricular level (Table 13–3). Indicator dilution curves localize the site of right-to-left or bidirectional shunt at the ventricular level.

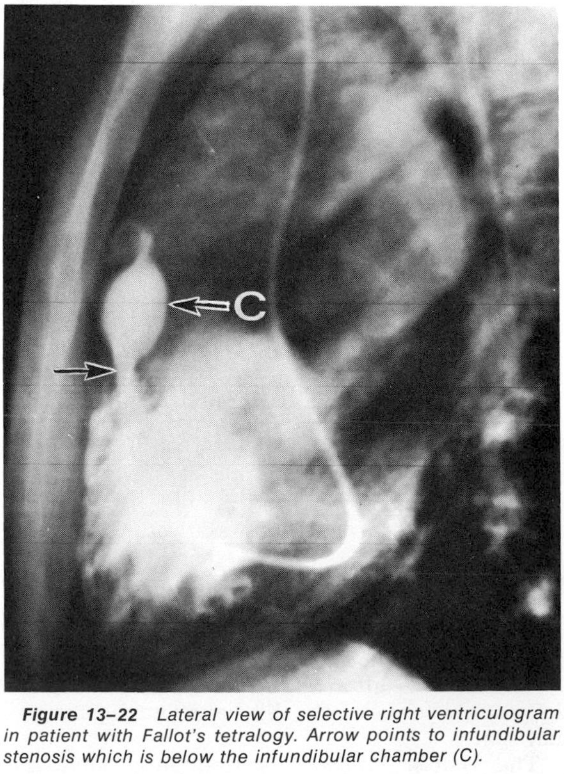

Figure 13–22 Lateral view of selective right ventriculogram in patient with Fallot's tetralogy. Arrow points to infundibular stenosis which is below the infundibular chamber (C).

Selective right ventriculography is of great diagnostic value. The contrast medium outlines the heavily trabeculated right ventricle. The infundibular stenosis varies in length, width, contour and distensibility. An infundibular chamber may also be demonstrated. The pulmonary valve may be normal, but frequently the leaflets are thickened and domed and the valve ring is small. Nearly simultaneous opacification of the aorta and pulmonary artery is usual. The size of the pulmonary trunk varies considerably. In severe cases it is small or hypoplastic. The ventricular septal defect is usually large and is situated below the hypertrophied crista supraventricularis. The large aorta is usually well opacified (Fig. 13–22).

PROGNOSIS. Without operation the prognosis varies with the severity of the pulmonary stenosis and the amount of collateral circulation. Deeply cyanotic children who have dyspnea on slight exertion rarely live until late childhood. Others may succumb during the adolescent period, and a few may live beyond the third decade.

COMPLICATIONS. The principal complications are as follows: (1) *Cerebral thromboses,* usually in the cerebral veins or dural sinuses and occasionally in the cerebral arteries are more common in the presence of extreme polycythemia and may be precipitated by dehydration. They occur more frequently in patients under the age of 2 years. Of great importance is the fact that one third of these patients with cerebral vascular accidents have iron deficiency anemia; these infants with microcytic hypochromic anemia may have hemoglobin and hematocrit levels in the normal range, so that microscopic examination of the blood smear and measurement of cell indices are essential. Therapy includes adequate hydration, especially in the comatose patient. Phlebotomy and volume replacement with fresh frozen plasma is indicated in the extremely polycythemic patient. Heparin is of little value since it does not influence blood viscosity and may not prevent extension of venous thrombosis; it is contraindicated in hemorrhagic cerebral infarction. Physical therapy to the affected extremities should be instituted as early as possible. (2) *Brain abscess* is rarer than cerebral thrombosis, but in some instances the differential diagnosis is difficult. Patients with brain abscess are usually over the the age of 2 years; the onset of the illness is often insidious; fever is usually of low grade; localized skull tenderness may be present; and the erythrocyte sedimentation rate and white cell count may be elevated. In others there is acute onset of symptoms, which may develop after a recent history of headache, nausea and vomiting. Epileptiform seizures may occur; localizing neurologic signs depend on the site and size of the abscess and the presence of increased intracranial pressure. Echograms, brain scans and cerebral angiography are helpful in identifying the site of abscess. Massive antibiotic therapy may help to localize the infection, but surgical drainage of the abscess is frequently necessary. (3) *Bacterial endocarditis* is rare in unoperated patients but is common in children who have had a palliative shunt procedure during infancy. Prophylaxis, preferably with penicillin, is essential in all surgical procedures during which the patient is at risk to develop bacteremia. These include especially dental surgery and procedures in the throat, nose and ear. (See Table 9–14.) (4) *Bleeding tendencies* (see p. 1158). (4) *Congestive heart failure* is rare, but in infancy may be precipitated by iron deficiency anemia.

ASSOCIATED CARDIOVASCULAR ANOMALIES. These are common and are difficult to recognize clinically. *Patent foramen ovale* and *patent ductus arteriosus* are frequent during infancy. Recognition of the drainage of a persistent left superior vena cava into the coronary sinus is important prior to surgical correction, since temporary occlusion of systemic venous return is essential prior to cardiotomy. *Atrial septal defects* of the secundum type are recognized during cardiac catheterization. Closure of defects in the atrial septum, including patent foramen ovale, is advised during radical surgery, since high venous pressure in the immediate postoperative period may result in cyanosis from a right-to-left shunt. *Absence of the pulmonic valve* produces a distinct syndrome; cyanosis is mild or absent, the heart is large and hyperdynamic, and loud to-and-fro murmurs are present. Aneurysmal dilatation of the pulmonary artery often produces wheezing respiration and recurrent pneumonitis from bronchial compression. The incidence of *stenosis of a branch of the pulmonary artery* has been estimated to be as high as 25 per cent. The diagnosis depends on visualization of the areas of obstruction by selective pulmonary arterial or right ventricular angiocardiography. Significant stenosis of major pulmonary arteries must be relieved during radical surgical correction. *Absence of a pulmonary artery* can be suspected if the roentgenographic appearance of the pulmonary vasculature differs on the two sides. Generally the left pulmonary artery is absent, so that the right lung appears more vascularized. This may be associated with hypoplasia of the left lung. Sometimes it is difficult to differentiate absence of the left pulmonary artery from severe stenosis with occlusion. It is of utmost importance to recognize absence of a pulmonary artery prior to the creation of an anastomosis between the systemic circulation and the single remaining pulmonary artery, since occlusion of the latter during operation seriously compromises the already reduced pulmonary blood flow. Other associated anomalies include *relative hypoplasia of the left heart, aortic or subaortic stenosis, bicuspid aortic valve, aberrant coronary artery* and *anomalies of the aortic arch.*

TREATMENT

General Management. Although the majority of patients require surgical treatment, astute management is necessary before operation. The prevention or prompt treatment of dehydration is important to avoid hemoconcentration and possible thrombotic episodes. The treatment of paroxysmal dyspneic attacks has been described. In infancy these attacks may be precipitated by a relative iron deficiency. Iron therapy may decrease their frequency and also improve exercise tolerance and general well-being. It appears that the safest level of the hematocrit is between 55 and 65 per cent. In some infants the frequency of dyspneic episodes may be decreased with mild sedation, as by promethazine (Phenergan). Oral propranolol (1 mg/kg every 6 hours) has also been used successfully to decrease the frequency and severity of dyspneic spells.

Surgical

Anastomotic Procedures. Taussig observed that the prognosis was better when the ductus arteriosus was patent. She and Blalock devised the operation whereby an artificial ductus is created by anastomosis of a branch of the aorta to the homolateral branch of the pulmonary artery. The most common procedure is anastomosis of the end of the left subclavian artery to the side of the pulmonary artery. Potts and his associates achieved the same objective by side-to-side anastomosis of the upper descending thoracic aorta to the pulmonary artery. Pulmonary blood flow may also be increased by side-to-side anastomosis of the ascending aorta to the right pulmonary artery (Waterston). Palliative therapy with shunt procedures carries an operative mortality of about 7 per cent and is advised in severely handicapped patients under 1 year of age; total correction is generally undertaken in older children.

The *postoperative course* of patients with a successful anastomosis is generally smooth. In addition to the usual postoperative complications following a thoracotomy, chylothorax, Horner's syndrome and postoperative cardiac failure may occur. Chylothorax is due to trauma to the thoracic duct or its tributaries and is treated with repeated thoracenteses. Suture of the duct is undertaken if chylothorax persists. Horner's syndrome is usually temporary and does not require treatment. Postoperative cardiac failure may be due to the large size of the anastomosis; its treatment is described later. Vascular problems in the upper extremity supplied by the subclavian artery which has been used for anastomosis are rare.

After a successful anastomosis there is a striking improvement in symptoms. Exercise tolerance is increased, and the habit of squatting is discontinued. The degree of cyanosis and clubbing diminishes. A machinery-type murmur, sometimes accompanied by a thrill, is detected after operation and is indicative of a functioning anastomosis.

The duration of symptomatic relief tends to be short-lived after the Blalock-Taussig operation, especially if it is done during infancy. Relief of symptoms of hypoxia is maintained well after the Potts operation, but late complications are frequent; they include cardiac failure, bacterial endocarditis and pulmonary hypertension. At present the Waterston operation is advised in infants because palliation is prolonged, and during later corrective surgery the shunt is closed with greater ease than after a Potts anastomosis. Late complications following the Waterston shunt are similar to those following the Potts anastomosis.

Brock Procedure. Brock suggested a direct surgical attack on the right ventricular outflow obstruction with infundibular resection or pulmonary valvotomy. With these procedures about two thirds of patients are greatly improved, and one sixth are benefited. It is possible that this approach steadily improves the size of the right ventricular outflow tract so that eventual surgical correction can be undertaken without the frequent need to use overlay patches.

Direct-vision Intracardiac Surgery (with a Pump Oxygenator). The preferred surgical therapy is relief of obstruction to right ventricular outflow, together with closure of the ventricular septal defect. The ideal therapy is a single corrective operation without previous palliation. This can be accomplished when there is dominant infundibular stenosis with pulmonary arteries and pulmonary valve ring of near normal size. In these patients surgery is advised after the age of 1 to 2 years but preferably delayed until after the age of 5. Symptomatic infants with grossly deformed right ventricular outflow tracts, and especially those with small pulmonary valve rings and arteries, are palliated with a shunt to await later corrective surgery, preferably after the age of 5.

While the patient's circulation is temporarily maintained by an artificial heart-lung machine, the right ventricle is opened extensively, the infundibular stenotic area resected, coexistent pulmonary stenosis relieved, and the ventricular septal defect closed. The outflow tract of the right ventricle is enlarged with a pericardial patch if a significant gradient of pressure persists between the right ventricle and the pulmonary artery. If the pulmonary valvular ring and pulmonary trunk are small, it may be necessary to enlarge this area with a pericardial patch, even though it produces pulmonary valvular incompetence. A previously established systemic-pulmonary shunt must be closed prior to cardiotomy. The Blalock-Taussig anastomosis is dissected and ligated immediately after establishing a cardiopulmonary bypass. The Potts anastomosis is closed from within the pulmonary artery after the induction of deep hypothermia and temporary total circulatory arrest. The Waterston shunt is closed from within the aorta after total cardiopulmonary bypass has been established, and after temporary occlusion of the ascending aorta just below the level of the innominate artery.

The surgical risk of total correction has currently fallen to less than 10 per cent. Factors that have contributed to this increasing success include optimal total body perfusion, adequate myocardial protection during bypass, relief of right ventricular outflow obstruction and prevention of air embolism. The presence of a previous anastomosis does not increase the operative risk significantly. Increased bleeding in the immediate postoperative period is common in markedly polycythemic pa-

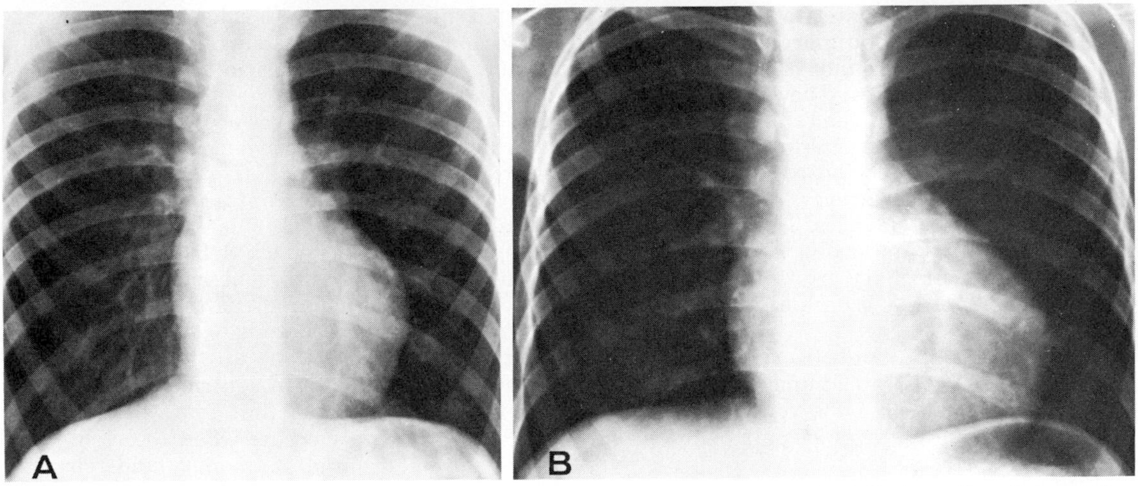

Figure 13–23 Teleroentgenogram of a 6 year old boy with tetralogy of Fallot. A, Preoperative. B, Postoperative, after resection of right ventricular outflow obstruction and closure of ventricular septal defect. Some increase in heart size is not infrequent after operation.

tients, but should not seriously affect the outcome. The operative risk is higher if there is marked deformity of the right ventricular outflow tract, and in older adolescents and adults.

After successful total correction (Fig. 13–23) the patients are asymptomatic and able to lead unrestricted lives. The shunt at the ventricular level is abolished and the resistance to right ventricular outflow is reduced greatly. The long-term effects of right ventricular outflow prostheses are unknown. They appear to be well tolerated if the ventricular septum is intact and the right ventricular pressure is near normal. The long-term effects of isolated pulmonary valvular incompetence are likewise unknown. Patients who have a significant left-to-right shunt postoperatively, or obstruction to right ventricular outflow, exhibit moderate to marked cardiac enlargement. A right ventricular outflow aneurysm may also be present at the site of ventriculotomy or outflow patch. Reoperation is generally necessary in such patients. The incidence of permanent complete heart block has decreased, but artificial pacing may be necessary for a few days or weeks because of temporary heart block.

Follow-up of patients 5 to 15 years after operation indicates that the spectacular improvement in symptomatology is maintained. However, in a small number (less than 5 per cent) sudden unexpected death has occurred and has been attributed to the late onset of complete heart block or other arrhythmias. The latter may be precipitated by graded exercise and consist of multifocal ventricular extrasystoles or ventricular tachycardia.

ORIGIN OF BOTH GREAT VESSELS FROM THE RIGHT VENTRICLE, WITH PULMONARY STENOSIS

The importance of this anomaly is that in many instances it cannot be distinguished from tetralogy of Fallot. In this condition both the aorta and pulmonary artery arise from the right ventricle, and the only outlet for the left ventricle is through the ventricular septal defect. The aortic and mitral valves lose their normal continuity, and the ventricular defect is inferior to the crista supraventricularis. The history, physical examination, electrocardiogram and roentgenograms are similar to those described under Tetralogy of Fallot. A clue to the diagnosis is the echocardiographic demonstration of lack of mitral-aortic continuity. Selective angiocardiography shows that the aortic and pulmonary valves lie in the same horizontal body plane. This study also demonstrates the abnormal anterior position of the aorta, which arises exclusively from the right ventricle. The angiocardiographic distinction between Fallot's tetralogy and the anomaly under discussion may be difficult because of the anterior position of the aorta in some patients with Fallot's tetralogy. Corrective surgical treatment is difficult, since a tunnel must be produced which allows an adequate outlet from the left ventricle to the aorta and at the same time closes the ventricular defect. The pulmonary obstruction also is removed. Palliative anastomotic procedures to increase pulmonary blood flow result in significant symptomatic improvement.

PULMONARY ATRESIA

WITH VENTRICULAR SEPTAL DEFECT. Sometimes called *pseudotruncus arteriosus,* this condition is an extreme form of Fallot's tetralogy. There is no direct communication between the right ventricle and pulmonary artery, since the pulmonary valve is atretic, rudimentary or absent. The pulmonary trunk is also atretic or hypoplastic. The entire ventricular output is ejected into the aorta. Pulmonary blood flow is dependent on bronchial collaterals or a patent ductus arteriosus.

The clinical manifestations are much the same as those of the tetralogy with the following exceptions: Cyanosis usually appears within a few days after birth in contrast to later in the first year in the tetralogy. The systolic murmur is absent or soft. The first heart sound is frequently followed by an ejection click. The second sound at the base is moderately loud and single. Continuous murmurs due to a patent ductus arteriosus or bronchial collateral flow may be heard anywhere in the chest, anteriorly or posteriorly, but are usually heard best under the clavicles. The heart may be enlarged roentgenographically, with a striking concavity of the pulmonary arterial segment. The reticular pattern of the bronchial collateral flow may be present.

The best diagnostic study is *right ventriculography,* which demonstrates immediate opacification of a large aorta from the ventricular septal defect and also the pathway of pulmonary blood flow from the aorta.

Since hypercyanotic spells and increasing hematocrit are frequent during infancy, a surgical systemic-pulmonary arterial anastomosis is indicated. The ideal patient has two reasonably sized pulmonary arteries available for anastomosis. In later years corrective surgery can be undertaken by closure of the ventricular septal defect and insertion of a conduit to act as the pulmonic valve and main pulmonary artery. Unfortunately, many patients have malformations of the primary divisions of the pulmonary arteries in the form of hypoplasia, multiple branch stenosis or absence of a pulmonary artery, with large bronchial collaterals. These are difficult to treat surgically even with anastomotic procedures.

Acquired total obstruction of right ventricular outflow may occur after a systemic-pulmonary anastomosis for Fallot's tetralogy. In these patients the right ventricular outflow tract is stenotic but patent before the anastomotic procedure. Some time after operation there may be a return of symptoms in association with total obstruction at the infundibulum or pulmonic valve. The systolic murmur due to pulmonic stenosis is attenuated or disappears, and the completeness of outflow obstruction is confirmed by right ventriculography. Corrective surgery is similar to that for Fallot's tetralogy.

WITH INTACT VENTRICULAR SEPTUM. In the majority of instances this anomaly is associated with a hypoplastic but thick-walled right ventricle lined by thick endocardium; the orifice of the tricuspid valve is small. In 15 to 20 per cent of patients the right ventricle is normal or large and the tricuspid valve functionally incompetent. Intermediate forms between the two extremes are common. Since there is no egress from the right ventricle, right atrial blood is shunted into the left atrium via the foramen ovale or an atrial septal defect, mixes with pulmonary venous blood, and is pumped by the left ventricle into the aorta. Pulmonary flow is via a patent ductus arteriosus and bronchial vessels.

Cyanosis occurs in early infancy, but may not be intense if the ductus is widely patent. Cardiac failure occurs early, especially in the presence of tricuspid incompetence. Cardiomegaly is usual. The second heart sound is single, and continuous murmurs are common, especially in older infants and children. In others only systolic murmurs are audible. Tall, spiked P waves are usual in the electrocardiogram. If the right ventricle is small, electrocardiographic signs of left ventricular hypertrophy are usual and the frontal QRS axis is either normal or to the right. This helps to exclude tricuspid atresia, in which left axis deviation is common. If the right ventricle is normal or large, right ventricular hypertrophy is noted. *Roentgenographically* there is extreme variability in size of the heart. Generally it is normal in neonates with a small right ventricle, but enlarges progressively during the first few weeks of life. Marked cardiomegaly occurs when the right ventricle is normal or large. Pulmonary undercirculation is usual.

Cardiac catheterization demonstrates right atrial and ventricular hypertension. Right ventriculography shows the size of the ventricular cavity, the atretic pulmonary valve, the tricuspid regurgitation and the successive filling of the right atrium, left atrium (via the interatrial septal defect), left ventricle, aorta, ductus arteriosus and pulmonary arteries. Large sinusoids may fill from a hypoplastic right ventricle; these drain in a retrograde manner into the coronary arterial system. Sometimes the angiographic findings simulate those found in tricuspid atresia.

Pulmonary valvotomy will relieve obstruction if the tricuspid valve, right ventricle, pulmonary valvular ring and pulmonary artery are nearly normal in size. If the right ventricle is hypoplastic, as in the majority of cases, the surgical treatment is a systemic-pulmonary arterial anastomosis and the creation of a large atrial septal defect, if this latter cannot be accomplished by balloon atrial septostomy. Later, pulmonary valvotomy may be undertaken with the hope that growth of the right ventricular cavity will follow. Surgical treatment is associated with a high risk, especially in neonates with a small right ventricular cavity.

TRICUSPID ATRESIA

In tricuspid atresia the tricuspid orifice is absent and the right ventricle hypoplastic. The presence and size of a ventricular septal defect determine the size of the pulmonary valve and trunk. Generally the ventricular defect is small and pulmonary arterial hypoplasia is present. Pulmonary atresia is usual if the ventricular septum is intact. In a minority of instances the pulmonary artery is nearly normal in size, especially if the ventricular septal defect is large. Tricuspid atresia with transposition of the great arteries is discussed elsewhere. When pulmonic stenosis is present with tricuspid atresia and arterial transposition, the hemodynamics and clinical picture simulate those of tricuspid atresia with normal relations of the great arteries.

Since there is no inflow into the right ventricle, right atrial blood escapes into the left atrium via the foramen ovale or an atrial septal defect. Here the blood mixes with pulmonary venous blood and enters the left ventricle. The larger portion of the mixed blood passes into the aorta, but some is shunted through the ventricular septal defect and passes from the hypoplastic right ventricle into the pulmonary artery. A patent ductus arteriosus provides pulmonary blood flow if the pulmonary trunk is hypoplastic.

CLINICAL MANIFESTATIONS. Cyanosis, polycythemia, easy fatigability, exertional dyspnea and anoxic hypercyanotic (paroxysmal dyspneic) attacks develop early, especially if pulmonary blood flow is seriously compromised. After infancy, clubbing is usual, but squatting is not so common as in tetralogy of Fallot. If the interatrial communication is small, right atrial hypertension results in a prominent jugular "a" wave and presystolic pulsations of an enlarged liver. These signs are easy to elicit but uncommon in infants. The heart may or may not be enlarged, with a heaving left ventricular apical impulse. In very ill small infants, murmurs may not be prominent, but in the majority a pansystolic or ejection systolic murmur is audible maximally down the left sternal border. The second heart sound is single, owing to absence of the pulmonary element.

Roentgenographic studies show pulmonary undercirculation and deficiency of shadows of the pulmonary artery (Fig. 13–24). The heart is normal in size or slightly enlarged. The cardiac contour is variable. In the postero-anterior view the right border may be straight or rounded by the large right atrium; the apex is high. In the left anterior oblique view the posterior border of the heart overlaps the spine because of the large left ventricle. The anterior border may be normal, recede from the sternum or be displaced forward by the large left ventricle. In many patients the cardiac silhouette is indistinguishable from that seen in Fallot's tetralogy, or is nonspecific in contour.

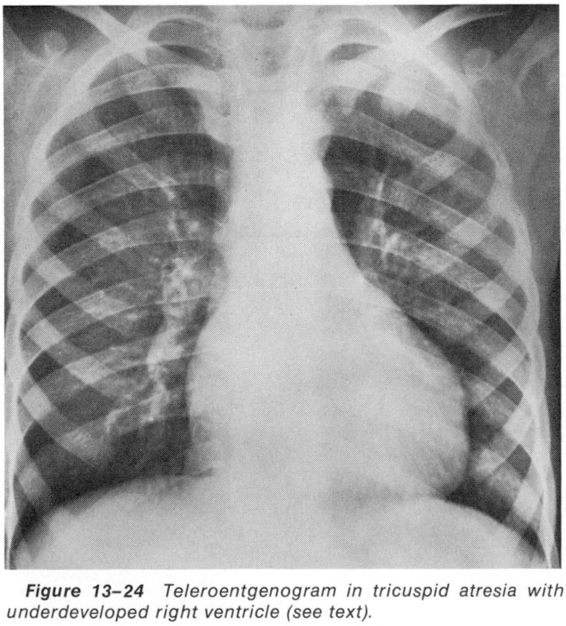

Figure 13–24 Teleroentgenogram in tricuspid atresia with underdeveloped right ventricle (see text).

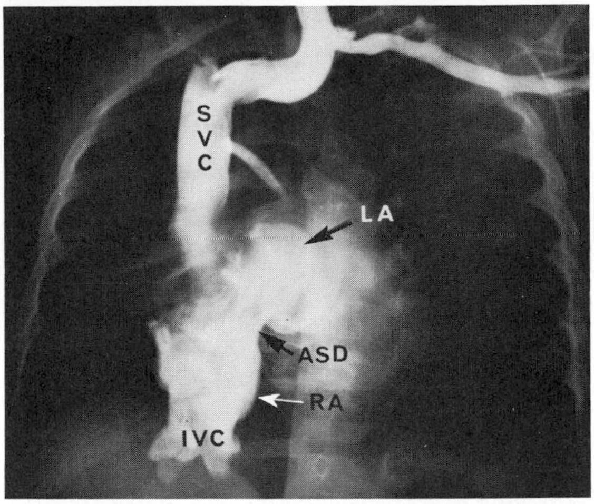

Figure 13–25 Angiocardiogram to demonstrate the course of the circulation in tricuspid atresia with underdeveloped right ventricle. Systemic venous blood flows from the right to the left atrium. Absence of right ventricular opacification due to tricuspid atresia. Abbreviations: SVC, superior vena cava; IVC, inferior vena cava; RA, right atrium; LA, left atrium; ASD, interatrial communication through atrial septal defect.

The *electrocardiogram* is a much more sensitive index of the state of the ventricles. Left axis deviation, left ventricular hypertrophy and abnormal P waves are the usual findings. In the right precordial leads the normally prominent R wave is replaced by an rS complex. The left precordial leads show a qR complex followed by a normal, flat, diphasic or inverted T wave. R_{V6} is normal or tall and S_{V1} generally deep. Although the P waves may be normal, they are usually tall and spiked, but sometimes diphasic or bifid.

Cardiac catheterization shows normal or elevated right atrial pressure with a prominent "a" wave. If the catheter is introduced from the saphenous vein into the inferior vena cava and right atrium, it usually passes with ease across the foramen ovale or atrial septal defect into the left side of the heart.

With *selective angiocardiography* there is immediate opacification of the left atrium from the right atrium followed by left ventricular filling and visibility of the aorta (Fig. 13–25). Absence of flow to the right ventricle results in a filling defect between the right atrium and left ventricle in early films in frontal projection. The tiny right ventricle is opacified if a ventricular septal defect is present. Otherwise, pulmonary arteries are filled via a patent ductus arteriosus. The presence of associated transposition of the great vessels and pulmonic stenosis may be demonstrated by selective left ventriculography.

PROGNOSIS AND TREATMENT. The prognosis is poor, and many infants fail to survive the first few months of life unless pulmonary flow is adequate and the interatrial communication large. Surgical treatment is designed to increase pulmonary blood flow. This may be accomplished by a systemic-pulmonary arterial anastomosis, preferably of the Waterston type. If the interatrial defect is small, it may be enlarged by a balloon septostomy or the Blalock-Hanlon operation. Although improvement after surgery may be striking, generally it is not so gratifying as with treatment of Fallot's tetralogy. Disappointing results are due to left ventricular failure or failure to recognize and enlarge a small interatrial communication. Good results may also be obtained from end-to-end anastomosis of the superior vena cava to the right pulmonary artery. Recently attempts have been made to increase pulmonary blood flow by the insertion of a valve-bearing conduit from the right atrium to the pulmonary artery. At the same operation a valve is also inserted at the junction of the inferior vena cava and right atrium to prevent regurgitation of blood down the inferior vena cava during atrial systole.

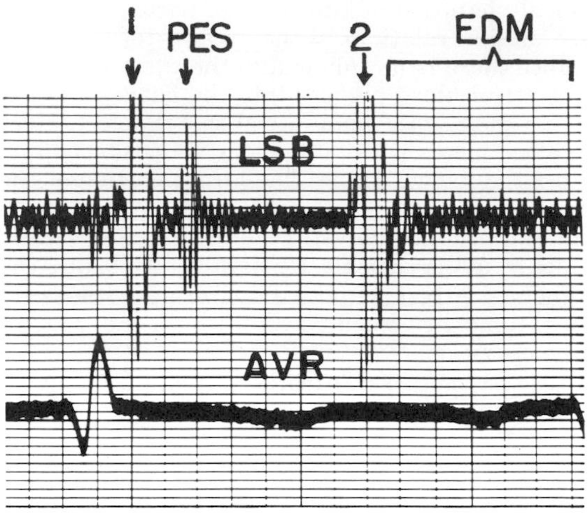

Figure 13–26 *Phonocardiogram which illustrates auscultatory findings of patient with Eisenmenger syndrome associated with a ventricular septal defect. Abbreviations: LSB, left sternal border; AVR, electrocardiogram; 1, first heart sound; 2, second heart sound; PES, pulmonic ejection sound; EDM, early diastolic murmur due to pulmonary valve incompetence. Time lines 0.04 second.*

EISENMENGER SYNDROME

The term "Eisenmenger syndrome" is used here for the combination of pulmonary hypertension with reversed or bidirectional shunt through either a ventricular septal defect, atrial septal defect or patent ductus arteriosus (or other communications between the aorta and lesser circulation). This concept implies that the principal physiologic abnormality is elevation of the pulmonary vascular resistance. In normal infants at, or soon after, birth the pulmonary vascular resistance is high. Within a few weeks the structure of the pulmonary arterioles changes to that of the adult with a thin wall and a large lumen, and the pulmonary vascular resistance falls to normal adult levels. In the Eisenmenger syndrome the pulmonary vascular resistance remains high. This abnormal resistance is probably present from birth, although in a minority of patients with large ventricular septal defects pulmonary resistance falls somewhat, only to rise again in later childhood or adult life.

CLINICAL MANIFESTATIONS. Symptoms are usually present in the first year of life, especially in patients with ventricular septal defect. These include dyspnea, feeding difficulties, fatigue, failure to gain weight and recurrent pneumonia. As the child gets older dyspnea on effort is obvious, especially when there are ventricular and atrial septal defects. Squatting, angina pectoris, hemoptysis and episodes of syncope occur occasionally. Cyanosis, which may be present early, increases in intensity as the child approaches puberty and is associated with clubbing and polycythemia. If there is a patent ductus arteriosus, venous blood from the pulmonary artery is shunted down the descending aorta and results in differential cyanosis (blue lower extremities and pink upper extremities).

Venous pressure is increased when congestive heart failure or functional tricuspid insufficiency is superimposed. Heart size is extremely variable, being normal in many cases with ventricular defect, but usually enlarged with atrial defect. A conspicuous left parasternal, right ventricular heave with palpable pulmonary arterial pulsations is frequent. A systolic murmur of varying intensity is usual and is frequently preceded by a pulmonic ejection click. The second heart sound is loud and booming. It is closely split or single in many cases of ventricular defect, but widely split with atrial defect. Functional incompetence of the pulmonary valve resulting in a blowing diastolic murmur down the left sternal border (Graham Steell mur-

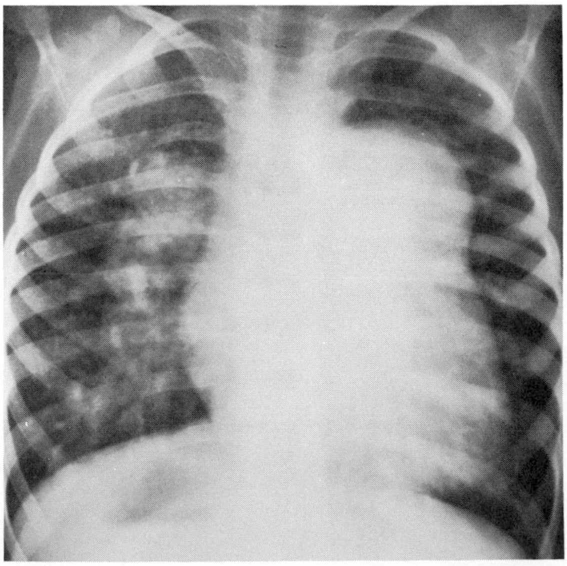

Figure 13–27 *Teleroentgenogram in Eisenmenger syndrome due to a ventricular septal defect. Note the dilatation of the pulmonary artery and gross pulmonary overvascularity.*

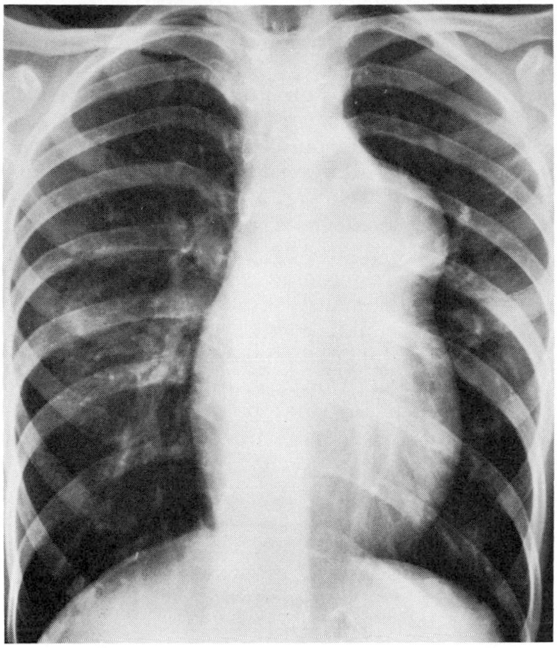

Figure 13–28 *Teleroentgenogram in Eisenmenger syndrome due to a patent ductus arteriosus. The heart size is normal, the pulmonary artery segment is dilated, and the pulmonary vascularity is normal or slightly increased.*

mur) (Fig. 13–26) is common and is associated with a normal peripheral arterial pulse.

Roentgenographically the heart varies in size from normal to greatly enlarged. The larger hearts are seen with atrial defects and the smaller ones with ventricular defects and patent ductus arteriosus (Figs. 13–27 and 13–28), but there is a large overlap. The pulmonary artery is usually enlarged. The pulmonary vessels are enlarged in the hilar areas and diminish in caliber in the peripheral branches. The right ventricle and atrium are prominent.

The *electrocardiogram* frequently shows right ventricular hypertrophy, occasionally associated with incomplete right bundle branch block. The P wave may be tall and spiked. Sometimes the electrocardiogram is balanced, with signs of biventricular hypertrophy.

Cardiac catheterization usually shows a bidirectional shunt at the site of the defect; e.g., in patients with a ventricular septal defect a left-to-right shunt is demonstrated at the ventricular level and is associated with a decrease in the arterial oxygen saturation due to the right-to-left shunt. There is, of course, a definite decrease in arterial oxygen saturation when there is only a right-to-left shunt. The catheter frequently traverses the defect, especially with a patent ductus arteriosus or atrial septal defect. The systolic pressures are usually equal in the systemic and pulmonary circulations. The pulmonary vascular resistance is elevated. *Indicator dilution curves* demonstrate the bidirectional shunts or the unidirectional right-to-left one. *Selective angiocardiography* is helpful in locating the site of the shunt. With patent ductus arteriosus contrast medium enters the descending aorta from the pulmonary artery.

TREATMENT. The presence of the Eisenmenger syndrome contraindicates surgical closure of the defect. But pulmonary hypertension with increased pulmonary blood flow, but without a right-to-left shunt, is not the Eisenmenger syndrome, and surgery may be lifesaving. Medical treatment of the Eisenmenger syndrome is entirely symptomatic. Older children and adolescents with significant polycythemia may be improved by cautious, repeated small venesections.

TRANSPOSITION OF THE GREAT VESSELS (ARTERIES)

In this condition the aorta arises from the right ventricle and the pulmonary artery from the left ventricle. The systemic veins return to the right atrium, and the pulmonary venous return is to the left atrium. Thus, the blood from the right side of the heart passes to the aorta; the pulmonary venous blood is returned to the lungs. The two independent circuits do not support life unless the foramen ovale or the ductus arteriosus remains open or unless there is a defect in the atrial or ventricular septum to permit some mixture of blood. This condition accounts for the majority of deaths in infants under the age of 1 year with cyanotic congenital heart disease. It is of interest that this condition occurs predominantly in males and that a significant number have a family history of diabetes mellitus.

Generally the aorta is anterior and to the right of the pulmonary trunk. Less commonly the aorta is directly in front of the pulmonary artery, or anterior and to the left of it, or the vessels are side by side. The pulmonary valve is continuous with the mitral valve (normally the mitral and aortic valves are continuous). Defects of the ventricular septum occur in about 50 per cent and are situated anywhere in the septum. Generally the right coronary artery arises above the posterior sinus of Valsalva and the left above the left sinus (in the normal the right coronary artery arises above the right sinus and the left above the left sinus).

The hemodynamics depend on the reaction of the pulmonary arterial and venous circulations and on the presence of associated defects. Neonates with a virtually intact ventricular septum show an increase in pulmonary arterial and venous pressure and gross arterial oxygen desaturation. Marked increase of pulmonary vascular resistance may be present early, but is generally found in older children, and usually with a large ventricular septal defect.

CLINICAL MANIFESTATIONS. Cyanosis, congestive cardiac failure, dyspnea, tachypnea and retardation of growth dominate the clinical picture, but the method of presentation depends on the associated defects. Cyanosis appears shortly after birth or in the first few weeks of life. It is present at rest and progressive in intensity. Polycythemia and arterial unsaturation are usual in older infants. Occasionally cyanosis of moderate intensity appears late in patients who have a torrential pulmonary flow. In some patients the legs are less cyanotic than the rest of the body because of the flow of arterialized blood across a patent ductus arteriosus from pulmonary artery to descending aorta. Differential cyanosis is usually seen only if there is associated preductal aortic coarctation. Hypercyanotic blue spells are rare. Congestive cardiac failure occurs early, frequently in the neonatal period, and generally before the age of 4 months. Cardiomegaly with a hyperactive precordium and a right ventricular lift is usual, especially after the first month of life, but the heart size may be normal in the neonate. The first heart sound is sharp, and the second sound is single or narrowly split.

With pulmonary vascular obstruction and reduced pulmonary blood flow, cyanosis is intense, but heart failure is minimal. Clubbing is marked in older children. Signs of pulmonary hypertension are obvious on auscultation and include a systolic ejection click, a booming second heart sound, a short systolic ejection murmur and sometimes an early diastolic murmur of pulmonary incompetence.

DIAGNOSIS. The typical *roentgenogram* (Fig. 13–29) reveals progressive cardiomegaly, increased pulmonary vasculature and a narrow cardiac base in frontal projection. During the first week of life these signs are not obvious. Progressive generalized cardiomegaly develops rapidly, however, and is much more striking if pulmonary blood flow is excessive. There is increased pulmonary vasculature bilaterally. The narrow cardiac base in frontal projection is due to superimposition of the shadows of the aorta and pulmonary trunk; it may be obscured by a large thymic shadow. When pulmonary vascular obstruction is present, cardiomegaly is only mild to moderate, and the pulmonary vessels are prominent in the hilar areas but appear narrow peripherally.

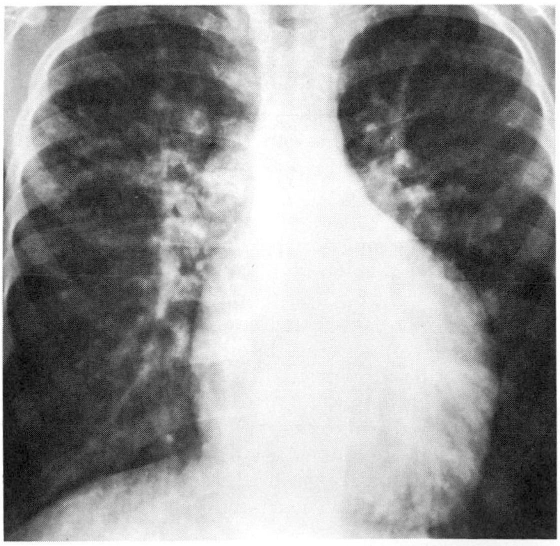

Figure 13–29 *Teleroentgenogram in complete transposition of the great vessels (arteries) with intact ventricular septum, showing cardiomegaly, gross pulmonary overcirculation and a narrow cardiac base.*

The *electrocardiogram* shows right axis deviation, right ventricular hypertrophy and frequently P pulmonale. In patients with a large pulmonary flow the axis is usually either to the right or normal, but occasionally it is to the left; there may be biventricular hypertrophy or occasionally dominance of the left ventricle. Right ventricular hypertrophy is usual when pulmonary vascular obstruction supervenes. In the newborn the electrocardiogram may be normal or show right ventricular hypertrophy.

Echocardiography is helpful in establishing the diagnosis, especially when it is possible to demonstrate that the anterior great vessel is in front of or to the right of the posterior vessel.

ISOLATED (SIMPLE) TRANSPOSITION OF THE GREAT ARTERIES

In these patients the ventricular septum is intact, and mixing of the circulation occurs from bidirectional shunting across the foramen ovale.

CLINICAL MANIFESTATIONS. Cyanosis and tachypnea appear within the first weeks of life and generally within the first days. If the foramen ovale is patulous, significant mixing may occur, so that the recognition of cyanosis is difficult and may be delayed for a few weeks. *However, the neonate of normal weight whose cyanosis and tachypnea are unexplained should be suspected of having the disease, which constitutes a medical emergency.* In the first days of life physical examination of these babies may be normal except for hepatomegaly. Significant cardiomegaly is unusual, and murmurs are absent in the majority.

DIAGNOSIS. The audibility of two distinct components of the second heart sound helps to exclude the diagnosis of hypoplastic left or right heart syndromes. *The electrocardiogram* shows the normal neonatal right-sided dominance. *Roentgenograms* of the chest may be entirely within normal limits or may show cardiomegaly, a narrow cardiac waist and increased pulmonary arterial and venous circulation. If cyanosis is in doubt, confirmation of desaturation may be obtained from pO_2 measurements of arterial blood; in these patients the arterial pO_2 is low and does not rise significantly after the patient breathes 80 to 100 per cent oxygen.

Cardiac catheterization shows right ventricular hypertension. The catheter enters the aorta directly from the right ventricle; it also may pass across the foramen ovale or an atrial septal defect into the left heart chambers and out the pulmonary artery. The blood in the pulmonary artery has a higher oxygen content than that in the aorta.

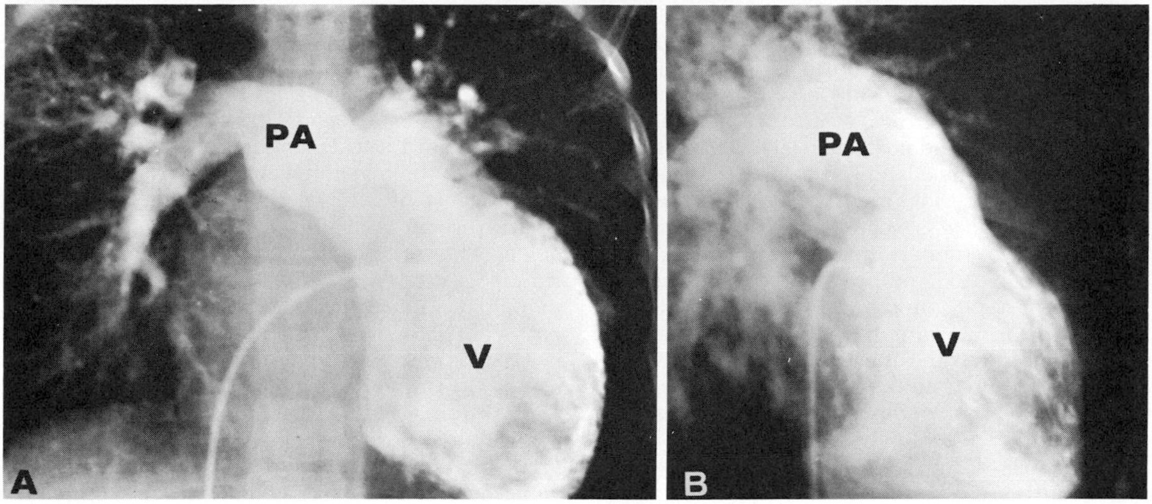

Figure 13–30 *Transposition of great vessels. Injection of contrast medium into a smooth-walled posterior (left) ventricle. Pulmonary artery arises exclusively from the posterior ventricle, and the interventricular septum is intact.* A, *Anteroposterior view;* B, *lateral view. Abbreviations: PA, pulmonary artery; V, posterior (left) ventricle.*

Marked systemic venous unsaturation is usual. The degree of arterial desaturation is variable and can be extreme. The left ventricular and pulmonary arterial pressures are variable; they are frequently at systemic levels but at other times are much lower. A pressure gradient across the atrial septum is usual, with the left atrial pressure exceeding that of the right. *Right ventriculography* is diagnostic. It demonstrates the origin of the anteriorly placed aorta from the right ventricle and the fact that the ventricular septum is intact, and excludes an associated patent ductus arteriosus. The aortic valve is cephalad to the pulmonic valve (reverse of normal). The origin of the coronary arteries is also shown. *Left ventriculography* demonstrates that the pulmonary artery arises exclusively from the posterior ventricle and that the ventricular septum is intact (Fig. 13–30).

Some patients with simple transposition of the great arteries have adequate mixing of blood across the interatrial septum and may only present at the age of 2 to 4 weeks or occasionally even at the age of a few months. These babies have the same clinical picture as described above. In addition to intense cyanosis and hypoxemia, the heart is obviously enlarged. The electrocardiogram shows signs of right ventricular or biventricular hypertrophy with or without prominent P waves. The chest x-ray is characteristic (Fig. 13–29), with progressive cardiomegaly and significant increase in pulmonary vascularity due to prominence of both arterial and venous shadows. The narrow cardiac base in the frontal projection is due to superimposition of the shadows of the aorta and pulmonary trunk. These patients also have a poor prognosis.

TREATMENT. The *prognosis* of the hypoxic neonate is extremely poor, and without treatment about one half die in the first week of life. Particular attention must be paid to maintaining a normal body temperature, since hypothermia intensifies the signs of metabolic acidosis, which occurs frequently from hypoxemia. The early recognition of the disease, the prevention of hypothermia and the rapid correction of acidosis and hypoglycemia, which may also occur in these infants, are essential. After the diagnosis has been confirmed in the catheterization laboratory on an emergency basis, a large interatrial communication is created by the **balloon atrial septostomy** technique of Rashkind. This method consists of advancing a catheter from a peripheral vein (usually the femoral) into the right atrium and across the interatrial septum into the left atrium. The balloon at the catheter tip is then inflated to a diameter of 1.0 to 1.5 cm and is abruptly withdrawn into the right atrium and inferior vena cava. The effect of this maneuver is to rupture the foramen ovale. It is repeated until there is no resistance to withdrawal of the balloon across the interatrial septum. After an adequate septostomy, mixing of the blood occurs at the atrial level, the high pressure in the left atrium and pulmonary veins is restored to normal, significant elevation of arterial oxygen saturation occurs, and tachypnea is relieved because of reduction of pulmonary venous pressure.

Surgical Treatment. Following atrial septostomy, adequate mixing is maintained at the atrial level, so that further treatment is unnecessary until surgical correction is undertaken. However, in some babies there is a recurrence of cyanosis due either to inadequate shunting at the atrial level or to the development of subvalvular pulmonic stenosis. These patients have polycythemia, effort intolerance, irritability, poor weight gain, and are at risk to develop cerebrovascular accidents. After significant pulmonic stenosis has been excluded, balloon atrial septostomy may be repeated or surgical atrial septectomy undertaken, especially if the patient is under 6 months of age. Intra-atrial surgical correction (Mustard operation) is advised in older babies.

Intra-atrial correction should not be postponed indefinitely in infants beyond the age of 1 year even if only moderate cyanosis is present. In this operation an atrial baffle of Dacron or pericardium is developed which directs systemic venous blood to the mitral valve and posterior (left) ventricle. Pulmonary venous blood flows through the tricuspid valve to the anterior (right) ventricle. Thus, systemic venous blood is ejected by the left ventricle to the lungs for oxygenation, and arterialized pulmonary venous blood is pumped by the right ventricle into the aorta. Symptomatic improvement after this operation is dramatic, with disappearance of cyanosis and marked increase in effort tolerance, but careful follow-up is necessary for many years because of the following complications: (1) *Arrhythmias* are common and are primarily atrial in origin. They consist of bradytachyarrhythmia owing to the "sick sinus syndrome," atrial tachycardia with block, atrial flutter and junctional rhythm. Occasionally complete heart block occurs. In some patients these arrhythmias occur after the Blalock-Hanlon operation (atrial septectomy) and precede the Mustard procedure. (2) *Recurrence of cyanosis* may occur as a result of rupture of the baffle and bidirectional atrial shunting. (3) *Superior or inferior caval syndrome* or *pulmonary venous obstruction* may result from obstruction by the baffle of the entry of these veins into the atria. (4) *Tricuspid valve incompetence* may result, with an increase in left atrial pressure, pulmonary edema and congestive cardiac failure.

TRANSPOSITION OF THE GREAT ARTERIES WITH VENTRICULAR SEPTAL DEFECT

If the defect is small the clinical picture, laboratory findings and treatment are similar to those described under Isolated (Simple) Transposition. However, a long systolic murmur is usually audible along the left sternal edge because of flow across the defect. A significant number of these small defects close spontaneously.

When the ventricular septal defect is large and nonrestrictive to ventricular ejection, significant mixing of blood occurs and the clinical picture is dominated by signs of congestive cardiac failure. The onset of cyanosis is subtle and frequently delayed and its intensity is variable. With careful observation, cyanosis can usually be recognized within the first month of life, but in some babies several months elapse before it is apparent. If the presence of cyanosis is dubious, a low arterial pO_2 and its failure to rise when the patient breathes 80 to 100 per cent oxygen resolves the problem. The hypoxemia is usually associated with polycythemia. The heart is significantly enlarged. The murmur is parasystolic and generally indistinguishable from that produced by a large simple ventricular septal defect with normally related arteries. The electrocardiogram shows prominent P waves, isolated right ventricular hypertrophy or biventricular hypertrophy. Usually the QRS axis is to the right, but sometimes it is normal or even to the left. Occasionally isolated dominance of the left ventricle is present. The chest x-ray shows marked cardiomegaly, a narrow cardiac waist and extreme pulmonary plethora. The diagnosis is confirmed by cardiac catheterization and angiocardiography. Right and left ventriculography indicate the presence of arterial transposition and demonstrate the site and size of the ventricular septal defect. The catheter may cross the ventricular septum from the right ventricle and enter the pulmonary artery. Peak systolic pressures are equal in both ventricles, the aorta and the pulmonary artery. The ventricular end-diastolic pressures are elevated in the presence of cardiac failure.

At the time of cardiac catheterization a balloon septostomy is also performed to decompress the left atrium even though adequate mixing occurs at the ventricular level. Elective but urgent pulmonary arterial banding with or without atrial septectomy is advised, since pulmonary vascular disease develops rapidly. These patients also require maintenance digitalis and diuretic therapy. Surgical therapy in later childhood is difficult and associated with a significant risk, especially if subpulmonic stenosis has developed. The operation consists of pulmonary artery debanding, closure of the ventricular septal defect and the Mustard procedure.

The *prognosis* in these patients is poor, the majority succumbing in the first year of life because of congestive cardiac failure, hypoxemia and pulmonary hypertension. Some patients survive infancy with medical and anticongestive therapy and without surgical treatment. The clinical picture and treatment in these patients is almost identical to that described under Eisenmenger Syndrome due to a large ventricular septal defect. Surgical palliation with a Mustard operation has been performed successfully if the patient is intensely cyanosed. This relieves the hypoxemia but does not affect the pulmonary vascular disease.

TRANSPOSITION OF THE GREAT ARTERIES WITH A LARGE PATENT DUCTUS ARTERIOSUS

In the neonate a large patent ductus arteriosus may be of benefit. However, persistent patency beyond the first few weeks of life aggravates the situation, since the dominant flow across the duct is from aorta to pulmonary artery, further increasing the pulmonary blood flow. This clinical picture is dominated by signs of congestive cardiac failure, and cyanosis may not be obvious. After effective palliation with balloon atrial septostomy, many of these babies remain in uncontrollable congestive cardiac failure and require surgical closure of the duct.

TRANSPOSITION OF THE GREAT ARTERIES WITH PULMONARY STENOSIS

This condition assumes importance because it may mimic tetralogy of Fallot. The site of obstruction is either valvular or subvalvular and may be associated with a hypoplastic pulmonary arterial trunk. A ventricular septal defect may or may not be present. It is important to recognize that subvalvular obstruction may be acquired after successful atrial septostomy or pulmonary arterial banding. The onset of symptoms varies from soon after birth to late infancy and is manifest by cyanosis, hypercyanotic (paroxysmal dyspneic) episodes, decreased exercise tolerance and poor physical development. Congestive heart failure is not common in infancy but may occur in later years. On examination the findings are similar to those described under tetralogy of Fallot. The cyanosis is usually more intense, however, and the heart may be enlarged. The pulmonary vasculature as seen on roentgenogram is somewhat diminished or normal and in some instances may be increased, especially if the pulmonic stenosis is not severe. The electrocardiogram usually shows right axis deviation, right ventricular hypertrophy and sometimes tall, spiked P waves.

Cardiac catheterization shows that the pulmonary arterial pressure is low, and its oxygen saturation exceeds that of the aorta. Selective right and left ventriculography demonstrates the origin of the aorta from the right ventricle, the origin of the pulmonary artery from the left ventricle, the ventricular defect and the pulmonary stenosis.

Treatment is difficult. Surgical correction by the Mustard operation with simultaneous closure of the ventricular septal defect and relief of left ventricular outflow obstruction has been done successfully but is associated with a high risk if the subvalvular obstruction is long and narrow and if the main pulmonary artery is hypoplastic. Another form of treatment consists of (1) repair of the ventricular septal defect with a patch to connect the left ventricle and aorta, (2) division of the pulmonary artery, and (3) reconstruction of the pulmonary artery with a valve-bearing conduit, which is anastomosed between the right ventricle and the distal stump of the pulmonary artery (Rastelli et al.). Systemic-pulmonary arterial anastomosis is undertaken in cyanotic infants who are not in congestive cardiac failure. At the same time an atrial septal defect may be created surgically (Blalock-Hanlon), especially if left atrial hypertension is present or if there is an insignificant rise in systemic arterial oxygen saturation from the shunt alone. Although anastomosis of the superior vena cava to the right pulmonary artery (Glenn) may result in palliation, later surgical correction may be compromised.

TRANSPOSITION OF THE GREAT ARTERIES WITH TRICUSPID ATRESIA

If arterial transposition is associated with tricuspid atresia and pulmonic stenosis, the syndrome is similar to that described under Tricuspid Atresia. If pulmonic stenosis is absent, however, and pulmonary flow excessive, cyanosis is mild and seldom conspicuous. Tachypnea, feeding difficulties, poor weight gain, recurrent respiratory infections and heart failure are usual. Increased venous pressure may result in presystolic pulsations of a large liver and a prominent "a" wave in the jugular venous pulse. Cardiac enlargement is moderate or marked. Systolic ejection murmurs of varying intensity are usual, and the second heart sound is loud and single. Although the electrocardiogram may show prominent P waves, left axis deviation and left ventricular hypertrophy, many patients have right axis deviation. Cardiac enlargement is confirmed roentgenographically; increased pulmonary vascularity is usual. The diagnosis is confirmed by selective left ventriculography, which delineates a large left ventricle, small right ventricle, arterial transposition and the relative size of the pulmonary artery and aorta. Generally the prognosis is poor, especially when the aorta is hypoplastic and pulmonary flow torrential. Surgical palliation is achieved with pulmonary arterial banding, which is most effective when the aortic root is near normal in size.

TRANSPOSITION OF AORTA AND OVERRIDING PULMONARY ARTERY
(Taussig-Bing Syndrome)

In this malformation the aorta arises from the right ventricle, and the pulmonary artery, which is large, overrides the ventricular septum. A ventricular septal defect is always present. The clinical picture is dominated by the presence of severe pulmonary hypertension. Cyanosis of varying intensity is usually present from birth. Tachypnea, frequent respiratory infections, decreased exercise tolerance and poor physical development are usual. Cardiac enlargement may be present during infancy, but in older children the heart is near normal in size because pulmonary vascular disease restricts pulmonary blood flow. Auscultatory findings are produced by pulmonary hypertension and include an early systolic ejection click, a midsystolic ejection murmur, a booming second heart sound and sometimes an early diastolic murmur of pulmonary valvular incompetence. The systolic murmur is longer and louder if pulmonary blood flow is torrential. Pulmonic stenosis is rarely present.

The *electrocardiogram* shows right ventricular hypertrophy with prominent P waves. Left ventricular hypertrophy is seen in infancy when a large pulmonary flow is present. The chest x-ray shows cardiomegaly and increased pulmonary vasculature during infancy. As pulmonary vascular obstruction develops, the heart size decreases, the major branches of the pulmonary artery become prominent, and there is attenuation of the vascular pattern in the outer lung fields. Cardiac catheterization reveals right ventricular and pulmonary hypertension, and the pulmonary arterial oxygen saturation exceeds that of the aorta. Selective right ventriculography demonstrates the abnormal anatomic positions of the aorta and pulmonary artery. The prognosis is variable, but many patients survive to adult life. Surgical correction now appears to be feasible by closure of the ventricular septal defect and interatrial venous transposition (Mustard operation). Pulmonary vascular obstruction contraindicates closure of the ventricular septal defect, but palliation of hypoxemia may be obtained by the Mustard operation. Extreme polycythemia is treated with repeated cautious venesection with volume replacement.

EBSTEIN'S DISEASE

This abnormality consists in downward displacement of an abnormal tricuspid valve into the right ventricle. The anterior cusp of the valve retains some attachment to the valve ring, but the other leaflets are attached to the wall of the right ventricle. The latter chamber is divided into two parts by the abnormal valve; the first is continuous with the cavity of the right atrium, and the second consists of a thin-walled ventricle. The right atrium is huge, and the tricuspid valve may or may not be competent. The effective output from the right side of the heart is decreased because of the small size of the functioning right ventricle and possible obstruction produced by the large, sail-like, anterior tricuspid leaflet. Similar hemodynamics are produced by thinning of the right ventricular wall due to hypoplasia of the myocardium (**Uhl's anomaly**).

The severity of symptoms appears to depend on the degree of displacement of the tricuspid valve. In many patients, symptoms are mild and the only complaint is fatigue. Cardiac dysrhythmias are frequent, the commonest being numerous extrasystoles or attacks of paroxysmal tachycardia, usually supraventricular. The presence of cyanosis depends on the integrity of the atrial septum. If the foramen ovale is open or an interatrial defect is present, a right-to-left shunt at this level produces cyanosis and polycythemia. This symptom can appear at any age and in some patients is intense. The venous pressure is normal or, if there is associated tricuspid insufficiency, increased. On palpation the precordium is quiet. A systolic murmur, sometimes accompanied by a thrill, is audible over most of the anterior left side of the chest. Gallop rhythm is common, as is a diastolic murmur at the left sternal border. This murmur is superficial and may mimic a pericardial friction rub. A series of systolic ejection clicks and an opening snap of the tricuspid valve may also be audible.

Although some patients may be asymptomatic until well into adult life, newborn infants with Ebstein's disease may present with cyanosis, cardiomegaly and long systolic murmurs. The mortality rate is high in these patients because of cardiac failure and hypoxemia. Rapid improvement does occur in some and has been attributed to a decrease in pulmonary vascular resistance.

The *electrocardiogram* shows incomplete or complete right bundle branch block, normal or tall and broad P waves and normal or prolonged P-R interval. Sometimes the pattern of the Wolff-Parkinson-White syndrome is present.

On *x-ray examination* the heart size varies greatly. In some instances it is normal, and in others there is cardiomegaly because of great enlargement of the right atrium and ventricle. In patients with large hearts the amplitude of cardiac pulsations is decreased; the intrapulmonary vasculature is normal or decreased, and the aorta is small.

Cardiac catheterization and selective angiocardiography confirm the presence of a large right atrium and demonstrate the right-to-left shunt at the atrial level, if this exists. The right atrial pressure may be normal, but it is frequently elevated, as is the right ventricular diastolic pressure. Simultaneous intracardiac electrocardiograms and pressures are of great value when they reveal the following 3 patterns: (1) right ventricular pressure with a right ventricular intracavity electrocardiogram, (2) from the atrialized portion of the right ventricle—atrial pressure curve with a right ventricular intracavity electrocardiogram, and (3) from the right atrium—atrial pressure curves and atrial intracavity electrocardiogram. These studies should not be undertaken lightly because of the hazard of precipitating cardiac arrhythmias or even rupture of the right atrium.

The *prognosis* is extremely variable, many patients living well into adult life. Medical treatment is directed toward control of cardiac failure and supraventricular dysrhythmias. Surgical treatment is seldom necessary in childhood. In deeply cyanotic patients, anastomosis of the superior vena cava to the right pulmonary artery (Glenn) has resulted in symptomatic improvement. Replacement of the abnormal tricuspid valve with a prosthesis has been performed successfully but is associated with a very high risk.

TRUNCUS ARTERIOSUS

This condition is characterized by a single arterial trunk leaving the ventricular portion of the heart and supplying the systemic, pulmonary and coronary circulations. A ventricular septal defect is always present, and the number of semilunar valve cusps varies from 2 to 6. In the majority of instances the pulmonary arteries arise from the ascending portion of the truncus proximal to the origin of the innominate artery. The pulmonary arteries may arise as a single vessel from the truncus or as two separate arteries. In some instances the pulmonary arteries and ductus are absent, so that the pulmonary blood flow is derived from collateral vessels, usually bronchial. If there is a remnant of a pulmonary artery leaving the right ventricle and pulmonary blood flow is supplied from the aorta via a ductus arteriosus, the condition is considered to be pulmonary atresia (see Pulmonary Atresia).

HEMODYNAMICS. Both ventricles empty their

blood at systemic pressure into the truncus. In the presence of a normal pulmonary vascular resistance, the blood flow to the lungs is greatly increased, the arteriovenous oxygen difference small, and cyanosis is minimal or absent. When the pulmonary resistance is high, the pulmonary circulation is inadequate, and cyanosis is intense. If pulmonary arteries are absent and collateral bronchial vessels supply the lungs, pulmonary blood flow is usually inadequate and cyanosis appears in early life.

CLINICAL MANIFESTATIONS. Owing to the extremely variable hemodynamics, the clinical picture varies. In the majority of infants pulmonary blood flow is torrential, and the clinical picture is dominated by dyspnea, fatigue, heart failure, recurrent respiratory infections and poor physical development. Cyanosis is minimal or absent. This situation closely simulates that produced by an isolated large ventricular septal defect. The runoff of blood from the truncus to the pulmonary circulation may result in a wide pulse pressure. The heart is usually enlarged, and the precordium is hyperdynamic. A systolic ejection murmur, sometimes accompanied by a thrill, is usual down the left sternal border. The murmur is frequently preceded by an ejection click. The second heart sound is loud and generally single, though it may be closely but clearly split. A mid-diastolic apical rumbling murmur is audible. In older children with restricted pulmonary blood flow, progressive cyanosis, polycythemia and clubbing develop. When pulmonary arteries are hypoplastic, cyanosis and dyspnea are present from infancy; cardiomegaly is moderate, and continuous murmurs may be produced by the bronchial collateral flow.

The *electrocardiogram* is variable and shows pure right, pure left or combined ventricular hypertrophy. There is considerable variation of the appearance of the chest on *roentgen examination*. Cardiac enlargement is due to prominence of both ventricles. The truncus may produce a prominent shadow which follows the normal course of the ascending aorta and aortic knob; it arches to the right in one third to one half of the patients. The shadow of the main pulmonary artery is not clearly discerned. Sometimes a high bulge, seen to the left of the aortic knob, is produced by the main or left pulmonary artery. The pulmonary vascularity is increased in the presence of normal pulmonary resistance; it decreases as the resistance rises. A diffuse reticular pattern in the lung fields with retroesophageal vessels demonstrated by barium esophagogram may be seen in patients with bronchial collateral blood flow to the lungs.

DIAGNOSIS. The diagnosis is confirmed by cardiac catheterization and by selective right ventriculography. The catheter may enter the pulmonary arteries from the truncus. A left-to-right shunt is demonstrated at the ventricular level, and the systolic pressures in both ventricles and the truncus are similar. Selective angiocardiography reveals the large truncus arteriosus and the origin of the pulmonary arteries.

PROGNOSIS. The prognosis is variable, but the majority of patients succumb during the first 2 years of life. Nevertheless, if pulmonary blood flow is via adequate collateral vessels, the patient may survive well into adult life with little incapacity.

TREATMENT. Treatment is not standardized. Infants with large pulmonary blood flow have been treated with banding of both pulmonary arteries. Corrective surgery is possible with closure of the ventricular septal defect and insertion of a conduit to act as a pulmonic valve and main pulmonary artery. Severe pulmonary vascular obstruction or hypoplastic pulmonary arteries preclude surgical treatment.

SINGLE VENTRICLE

With a single ventricle, both atria empty through two separate atrioventricular valves into a single ventricular chamber from which the aorta and pulmonary artery arise. Associated cardiac anomalies are usual and consist of one or any combination of the following: (1) a rudimentary outlet chamber in the region usually occupied by the right ventricular outflow and separated from the single ventricle by a muscular ridge, (2) transposition of the aorta and pulmonary artery, (3) pulmonic stenosis, (4) dextrocardia or other cardiac malposition, (5) aortic outflow obstruction with or without coarctation, (6) defects of the atrial septum, (7) common atrioventricular canal. The more frequent associations are (1) single ventricle, arterial transposition and rudimentary outlet chamber from which the aorta arises; and (2) single ventricle with pulmonic stenosis.

The hemodynamics and clinical picture are extremely variable because they depend on the associated intracardiac anomalies and the degree of pulmonary blood flow. If a single ventricle is associated with pulmonic stenosis, cyanosis is present in infancy and increases in intensity during childhood when clubbing and polycythemia also appear. Dyspnea and fatigue are frequent, and paroxysmal dyspneic spells may occur. Cardiomegaly is mild or moderate; a left parasternal lift is palpable, and a systolic thrill common. The systolic ejection murmur is usually loud; an ejection click may be audible, and the second heart sound is single and loud. When a single ventricle is associated with a rudimentary systemic outflow tract, pulmonary blood flow is torrential. These patients have tachypnea, dyspnea, poor physical development, recurrent pulmonary infections and congestive heart failure. Cyanosis is only mild or moderate. Cardiomegaly is generally marked, and a left parasternal lift is palpable. The systolic ejection murmur is generally not intense, and the second heart sound is loud and closely split. A third heart sound is frequent and may be followed by a short mid-diastolic murmur. The development of pulmonary vascular disease may restrict pulmonary blood flow so that cyanosis increases in intensity, heart size decreases, and signs of cardiac failure appear to improve.

The *electrocardiogram* is nonspecific. P waves are normal, spiked or bifid. Usually right axis deviation is present, but occasionally left axis deviation is observed. The precordial lead pattern suggests right ventricular hypertrophy, combined ventricular hypertrophy or sometimes left ventricular dominance. The initial QRS forces are usually to the left and anterior. *Roentgenographic examination* confirms the degree of cardiomegaly. The rudimentary systemic outflow chamber may produce a bulge on the upper left border of the cardiac silhouette in the postero-anterior projection. In the absence of pulmonic stenosis, pulmonary vasculature is increased, with prominence of the major branches of the pulmonary artery. Attenuation of the size of the peripheral pulmonary arteries occurs with the development of obstructive pulmonary hypertension. If pulmonic stenosis is present, pulmonary vasculature is decreased to varying degrees. *Echocardiography* is very useful. It demonstrates a large atrioventricular valve leaflet which moves far anteriorly; ventricular septal echos are absent.

Cardiac catheterization reveals a left-to-right shunt at the ventricular level. Varying degrees of arterial unsaturation are present. The arterial oxygen saturation is markedly decreased in the presence of severe pulmonic stenosis or obstructive pulmonary hypertension, but is near normal when pulmonary blood flow is increased. The pressure in the single ventricle is high, and a gradient may be demonstrated between it and the rudimentary outflow tract or the pulmonary artery in the presence of pulmonary stenosis. Severe pulmonary hypertension is present when pulmonary stenosis is absent. Selective ventriculography is diagnostic and demonstrates the single ventricle and the position and relation of the pulmonary artery and aorta. Also, the presence or absence of pulmonic stenosis or a rudimentary outflow chamber is identified.

A number of these patients succumb during infancy from congestive heart failure and superimposed pulmonary infection. Others may survive to adolescence and early adult life, but finally succumb to the effects of pulmonary hypertension. The prognosis appears to be better if there is associated pulmonary stenosis. If pulmonary stenosis is present, a systemic-pulmonary arterial anastomosis can result in improvement, but some patients suffer heart failure some months after operation. Anastomosis of the superior vena cava to the right pulmonary artery may be beneficial in patients with pulmonary stenosis. Pulmonary artery banding is advised for patients with a large pulmonary flow.

HYPOPLASTIC LEFT HEART SYNDROME
(Aortic Atresia)

The term "hypoplastic left heart syndrome" is used to describe varying degrees of underdevelopment of the left side of the heart. The anomalies include underdevelopment of the left atrium and ventricle, stenosis or atresia of the aortic or mitral orifices, and hypoplasia of the ascending aorta. Associated defects include endocardial fibroelastosis of the left ventricle, and atrial and ventricular septal defects. The left ventricular cavity is small, but the wall may be thick if obstruction to left ventricular outflow is associated with mitral stenosis. If aortic atresia and mitral atresia coexist, the left ventricular cavity is minute.

Since the left ventricle is virtually nonfunctional, the right ventricle maintains both pulmonary and systemic circulations. Pulmonary venous blood passes through an atrial or ventricular septal defect from the left to the right side of the heart, where it mixes with systemic venous blood. If the ventricular septum is intact, all the right ventricular blood is ejected to the pulmonary arteries; the systemic circulation is supplied via the ductus arteriosus. With a ventricular septal defect and a patent but small aortic orifice, right ventricular blood is ejected to the small left ventricle and ascending aorta as well as to the pulmonary artery. The major hemodynamic abnormalities are inadequate maintenance of the systemic circulation and pulmonary venous hypertension.

Signs of heart failure appear within the first few weeks of life and include dyspnea and hepatomegaly. All peripheral pulses are weak or impalpable. Although cyanosis may not be obvious in the first 48 hours of life, a grayish blue color of the skin is soon apparent. Differential cyanosis may be striking if the aortic valve has a small opening. In these patients oxygenated blood from the left ventricle enters the ascending aorta and innominate artery, resulting in a normal color in the right arm and right side of the head and neck with a contrasting cyanosis in the rest of the body. Cardiac enlargement is usual, with a palpable right ventricular parasternal lift. In many cases, murmurs are not audible and, if present, are short and midsystolic. *Roentgenographically* the heart is variable in size in the first few days of life, but moderate or gross cardiomegaly develops rapidly and is associated with increased pulmonary vascularity. In the first few days of life the *electrocardiogram* may show only the normal right ventricular dominance. If the patient survives, P waves become prominent and right ventricular hypertrophy is usual.

Echocardiograms are diagnostic (Fig. 13–31). They show absence or gross distortion of the normal mitral valve echo, absent or small aortic root, a small posterior ventricle, a large anterior ventricle and an easily identifiable tricuspid valve. These findings are so characteristic that the diagnosis of aortic atresia can be made without resorting to cardiac catheterization and angiocardiography. If the latter study is done, most of the contrast medium flows from the right ventricle to the pulmonary artery, through a patent ductus arteriosus and into the descending aorta. The hypoplastic ascending aorta is best demonstrated by aortography, which may also show the coronary arterial system.

Most patients succumb during the first month of

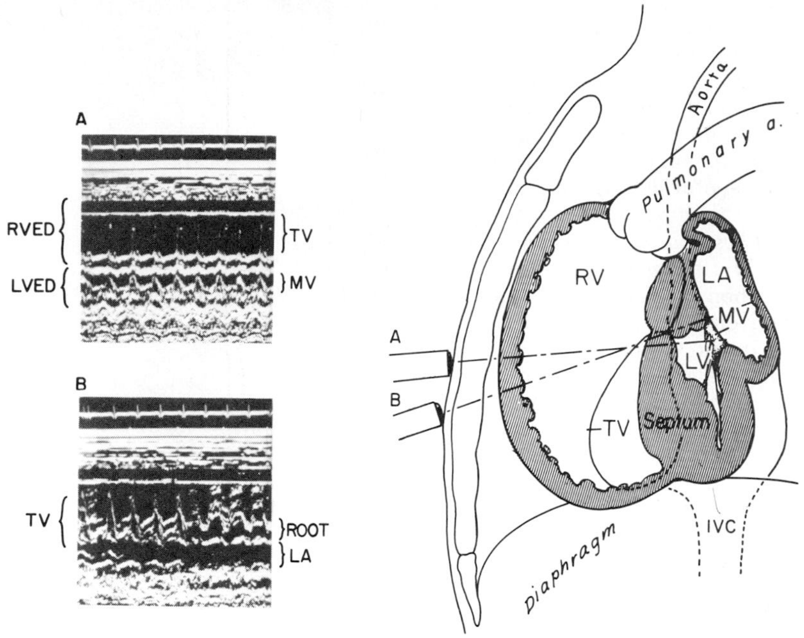

Figure 13–31 Idealized diagram in sagittal view of patient with aortic valvular atresia. Echogram A depicts the structures recorded from transducer position A. Echogram B depicts the structures recorded as the transducer is rotated from position A to position B. RVED, right ventricular end diastolic dimension; LVED, left ventricular end diastolic dimension; TV, tricuspid valve; MV, mitral valve: ROOT, aortic root; LA, left atrium; LV, left ventricle: IVC, inferior vena cava. (From Meyer, R. A., and Kaplan, S.: Progr. Cardiovasc. Dis. 25:341, 1973. By permission of Grune & Stratton, Inc.)

life, usually during the first week. Treatment is symptomatic.

ABNORMAL POSITIONS OF THE HEART: DEXTROCARDIA AND LEVOCARDIA

An approach to the classification and diagnosis of abnormal cardiac position has been suggested by Van Praagh et al. *Atrial localization* is facilitated by radiologic demonstration of the position of the abdominal organs and tracheal bifurcation for recognition of the situs of the right and left bronchi. Usually atrial situs is the same as visceral situs; if the viscera are in normal position, the atria have a normal position. Abdominal situs inversus is associated with the left atrium to the right and right atrium to the left. If the abdominal situs cannot be determined, as with a centrally located liver, atrial localization is difficult and asplenia or rudimentary spleen is common. *Localization of the ventricles and great arteries* depends on the direction of development of the embryonic cardiac loop. Initial protrusion to the right (d-loop) carries the future right ventricle to the right, and the left ventricle remains on the left. Protrusion to the left (l-loop) carries the future right ventricle to the left, and the left ventricle is on the right. In both types of loop the relations of the great arteries may be normal or transposed. Angiographic demonstration of the relations of the aorta and pulmonary artery indicates the type of cardiac loop and the relative location of the ventricle. The clinical picture of abnormal cardiac position is dominated by the associated cardiovascular anomalies.

DEXTROCARDIA WITH OR WITHOUT SITUS INVERSUS. This is frequently complicated by severe malformations, including combinations of single ventricle, arterial transposition, pulmonic stenosis, ventricular and atrial septal defects, complete atrioventricular canal, anomalous pulmonary venous return, tricuspid atresia, and pulmonary arterial hypoplasia or atresia. The patient with dextrocardia, cyanosis and signs of pulmonic stenosis generally has arterial transposition, pulmonic stenosis and ventricular septal defect. Surveys of older children and adults indicate that dextrocardia with situs inversus and with normally related great arteries (so-called mirror-image dextrocardia) is probably associated with a functionally normal heart. Some of the older patients have **Kartagener's syndrome** (complete situs inversus, paranasal sinusitis and bronchiectasis).

Abnormalities of the lung, diaphragm and thoracic cage may result in displacement of the heart to the right, mimicking dextrocardia. Hypoplasia of a lung may be accompanied by anomalous pulmonary venous return from that lung. The *electrocardiogram* is helpful in diagnosis, but frequently difficult to interpret. Inversion of the P wave in lead I is indicative of atrial inversion. Q waves produced by right ventricular hypertrophy may make interpretation of ventricular dominance difficult. Deep Q waves or QS in V_1, V_2 and aV_L are seen in patients with dextrocardia and normally related great arteries.

LEVOCARDIA WITH VARYING DEGREES OF VISCERAL HETEROTAXY (partial or complete situs inversus). This is usually associated with severe cardiovascular defects, frequently of the cyanotic type. These include combinations of abnormal systemic venous return (bilateral superior vena cava; absence of inferior vena cava with venous drainage of the lower part of the body into the azygous system), anomalous pulmonary venous return, arterial transposition, pulmonary stenosis or atresia, atrial or ventricular septal defect, common atrioventricular canal, single ventricle and patent ductus arteriosus. *These patients have a high incidence of asplenia or rudimentary spleen,* which may be suspected when Howell-Jolly bodies (nuclear remnants) or Heinz bodies (precipitated hemoglobin) are seen in the red cells.

Treatment of abnormal cardiac position is determined by the underlying defect. Cyanotic infants with pulmonic stenosis and ventricular septal defect as a part of the malformation improve after anastomosis of the systemic and pulmonary blood supplies. Lesions such as atrial or ventricular septal defect and Fallot's tetralogy have been repaired successfully.

PULMONARY ARTERIOVENOUS FISTULA

Fistulous vascular communications in the lungs may be large and localized or multiple, scattered and small. They may be a manifestation of the Rendu-Osler-Weber syndrome (hereditary hemorrhagic telangiectasia) with angiomas of the nasal and buccal mucous membranes, gastrointestinal tract or liver. A rare variant is a direct communication between the pulmonary artery and left atrium.

Venous blood in the pulmonary artery is shunted through the fistula into the pulmonary vein without exposure to alveolar air, enters the left heart and results in systemic arterial unsaturation. The shunt across the fistula is at low pressure and resistance, so that pulmonary arterial pressure is

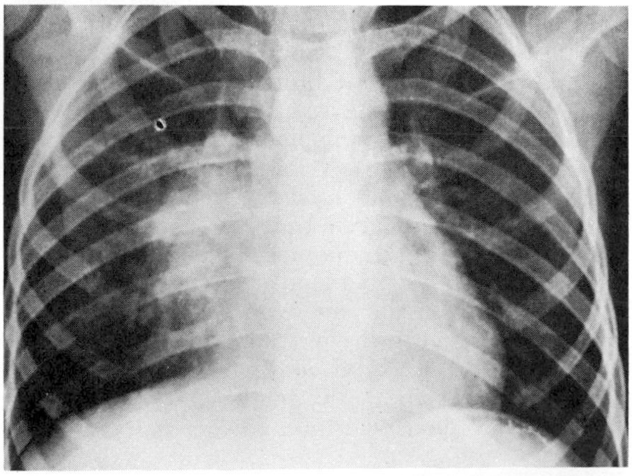

Figure 13–32 *Teleroentgenogram in pulmonary arteriovenous fistula, showing a localized increase in pulmonary vascularity in the right lung.*

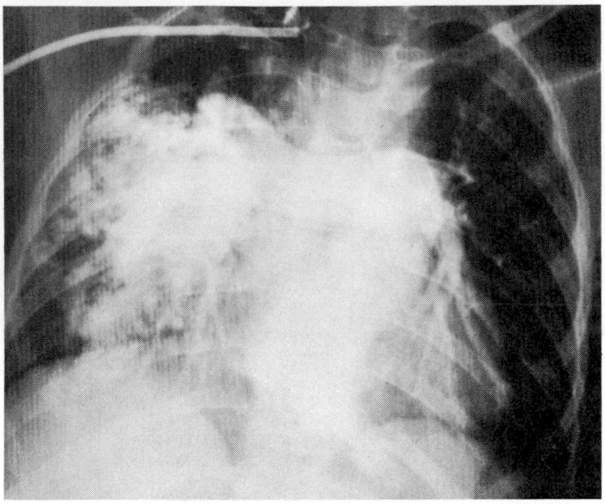

Figure 13–33 *Angiocardiogram in pulmonary arteriovenous fistula. (Same patient as Figure 13–32.) The contrast medium has delineated the extent of the fistula in the right lung.*

normal, cardiomegaly unusual, and heart failure rare.

The clinical picture depends on the magnitude of shunt. Dyspnea, cyanosis, clubbing and polycythemia occur with large fistulas. Hemoptysis is rare, but may be massive. Features of the Rendu-Osler-Weber syndrome occur in about half of the patients (or other members of their family) and include recurrent epistaxis and gastrointestinal bleeding. Transitory dizziness, diplopia, aphasia, motor weakness or convulsions may result from cerebral thrombosis, abscess or paradoxical emboli. The heart is normal on examination, but soft systolic or continuous murmurs may be audible over the site of the fistula.

The *electrocardiogram* is normal. *Roentgenographic examination* of the chest (Fig. 13–32) may show opacities produced by large fistulas; multiple small fistulas may be visualized by fluoroscopy (abnormal pulsations) or tomography. Selective *pulmonary arteriography* demonstrates the site, extent and distribution of the fistulas (Fig. 13–33).

Excision of solitary or localized lesions by lobectomy or wedge resection results in complete disappearance of symptoms. If the fistulas are widely distributed, extensive pulmonary resection may be followed by postoperative growth of smaller fistulas and recurrence of symptoms. Direct communications between the pulmonary artery and left atrium are obliterated by division and suture.

ECTOPIA CORDIS

This is a rare malformation in which the heart is in an abnormal location. In the commonest form, thoracic in type, the sternum is split, and the heart protrudes outside the chest. In others the heart protrudes through the diaphragm into the abdominal cavity, or may be situated in the neck. Associated intracardiac anomalies are common. Death occurs in the first few days of life in the majority of instances. Occasional patients with the abdominal type have survived to adulthood, but surgical attempts to replace the heart in the chest have failed.

DIVERTICULUM OF THE LEFT VENTRICLE

In this rare anomaly a diverticulum of the left ventricle protrudes into the epigastrium. The lesion may be isolated, or associated with complex cardiovascular anomalies. A pulsating mass is visible and palpable in the epigastrium. Systolic or systolic-diastolic murmurs produced by blood flow in and out of the diverticulum may be audible over the lower sternum and the mass. The *electrocardiogram* shows a pattern of complete or incomplete left bundle branch block. *Roentgenograms* of the chest may or may not show the mass. Associated abnormalities include defects of the sternum, abdominal wall, diaphragm and pericardium. Surgical treatment of the diverticulum and associated cardiac defects may be considered in the presence of uncontrollable heart failure or anoxemia.

Congenital Heart Disease with Little or No Cyanosis (Dominant Left-to-Right Shunt or No Shunt)

VENTRICULAR SEPTAL DEFECT

Isolated defects of the ventricular septum are among the commonest cardiac malformations. The majority lie inferior to the crista supraventricularis in close relation to the aortic valve and septal leaflet of the tricuspid valve; they may be between the crista supraventricularis and the papillary muscle of the conus or postero-inferior to this area to include the membranous portion of the septum. Defects superior to the crista supraventricularis are uncommon; they lie just below the pulmonic and aortic valves. Defects involving the inflow portion of the ventricular septum are muscular in type and may be isolated or multiple.

Effects on the cardiac chambers and pulmonary vascular tree depend to a large extent on the size of the defect and the response of the pulmonary vasculature. If the defect is small, the cardiac chambers and pulmonary vascular bed are normal. The significant left-to-right shunt and pulmonary hypertension produced by large defects result in varying degrees of right and left ventricular hypertrophy and dilatation, as well as in enlargement of the left atrium. The pulmonary arterial trunk is large. During infancy the media of the small muscular pulmonary arteries and arterioles are thick; this may represent retention of the normal fetal pulmonary vasculature, or a response to pulmonary hypertension. Intimal changes are variable; nonspecific intimal fibrosis may be the only lesion. In other instances there may be a plexiform lesion consisting of a papillary mass of endothelial cells in the lumen of the small vessel, with peripheral dilatation and thinning of the wall. Necrotizing arteritis may occur, but is uncommon.

HEMODYNAMICS. The fetal circulation (Fig. 13–19) is probably not jeopardized even with a large communication between the ventricles because the high pulmonary vascular resistance of the fetus limits the left-to-right shunt. It is possible that some right-to-left shunting occurs in utero, but this does not appear to be detrimental. After birth the magnitude of the left-to-right shunt is determined by the size of the defect and the ratio of systemic to pulmonary vascular resistance. Left-to-right shunting occurs as pulmonary vascular resistance falls, but this fall may be delayed for several weeks. Therefore, torrential pulmonary flows are unusual in the neonate, and death with overt congestive heart failure is unusual in isolated ventricular septal defects in the first month of life. In premature infants the fall of pulmonary vascular resistance may be more rapid, with an early onset of heart failure if the defect is large.

In older children defects ordinarily do not permit large left-to-right shunts, and right ventricular and pulmonary arterial pressures are normal. Larger defects allow enough communication between the left and right ventricles that the magnitude of the shunt is inversely related to the pulmonary vascular resistance; a marked increase in pulmonary vascular resistance may not only limit the magnitude of a left-to-right shunt, but also may result in a bidirectional shunt or a predominantly right-to-left shunt (see Eisenmenger Syndrome).

Levin and his co-workers have demonstrated that shunting of blood from left ventricle to right ventricle through a septal defect occurs throughout the cardiac cycle as long as right ventricular pressure is normal or moderately elevated. When ventricular pressures are nearly equal, right-to-left shunting occurs during isovolumic relaxation. In all patients a left-to-right shunt into the body of the right ventricle is present during diastole. Also, a left-to-right shunt is augmented during isovolumic contraction immediately preceding opening of the aortic valve.

In the presence of a left-to-right shunt the right ventricular output is supplemented by blood shunted across the defect; pulmonary arterial flow is increased, as is the return of pulmonary venous blood to the left atrium and ventricle. The resultant left ventricular diastolic overload produces a larger stroke volume and left ventricular hypertrophy with dilatation. The factors which determine pulmonary hypertension are not clear; although increased pulmonary flow contributes to increased pressure (hyperkinetic pulmonary hypertension), closure of the shunt is not always followed by immediate reduction of pulmonary arterial pressure.

CLINICAL MANIFESTATIONS. The manifestations of ventricular septal defects are determined by the hemodynamics; they vary according to the size of the defect and the reaction of the pulmonary circulation. **Small defects** with trivial left-to-right shunts and normal pulmonary arterial pressures are the most frequent. The patients are asymptomatic and the cardiac lesion is found accidentally during routine physical examination. Characteristically, there is a loud, harsh or blowing left parasternal pansystolic murmur, heard best over the lower left sternal border and frequently accompanied by a thrill. In a few instances the murmur ends well before the second sound, presumably because of closure of the defect during late systole; this atypical murmur becomes pansystolic after the administration of phenylephrine. It has already been indicated that pulmonary vascular resistance remains elevated in neonates with ventricular septal defects and that this limits the left-to-right shunt. Thus, the long systolic murmur which is the hallmark of ventricular septal defects may be inaudible in the first few days of life. This explains the common clinical experience of hearing this murmur for the first time when the baby returns for the "6-week checkup." In prematures the murmur is audible early, since the pulmonary vascular resistance falls early.

Roentgenograms are usually normal, although minimal cardiomegaly and a debatable increase in pulmonary vasculature may be observed. The electrocardiogram is usually normal, but may suggest isolated left or combined ventricular hypertrophy.

Ventricular defects of moderate size may result in large left-to-right shunts and mild to moderate increases in pulmonary arterial pressures and resistances. During infancy the symptoms are chiefly tachypnea, dyspnea, feeding difficulties, slow physical development and recurrent pulmonary infections with or without congestive cardiac failure. Improvement after the first year or two of life is usual, presumably due to relative or absolute decrease in size of the defect. Some prominence of the left precordium and sternum may be observed. A systolic thrill is usual. The characteristic pansystolic murmur is loud and harsh, has a wide distribution over the whole precordium, and is sometimes audible in the back, but is loudest at the lower left sternal border. The second heart sound at the apex is normal or moderately split and is

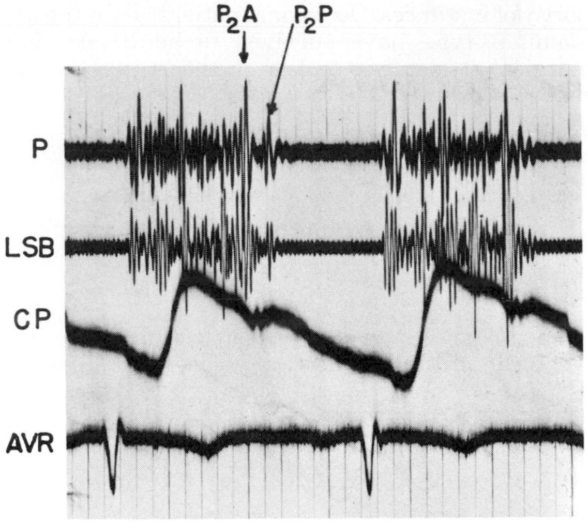

Figure 13–34 Phonocardiograms (P, pulmonary area; LSB, left sternal border) to illustrate auscultatory findings in moderate-sized ventricular septal defect with normal pulmonary arterial pressure. Long pansystolic murmur is evident. Abbreviations: CP, carotid pulse; AVR, electrocardiogram; P_2A, aortic components of second sound; P_2P, pulmonary component of second sound.

normal or somewhat accentuated at the upper left sternal border. The increased pulmonary blood flow produces a systolic ejection murmur heard best at the upper left sternal border (Fig. 13–34). The increased pulmonary venous return results in a large flow across the mitral valve, which, in turn, generates a rumbling mid-diastolic murmur best heard at the apex. This murmur may be preceded by a third heart sound.

Roentgenograms of the chest show mild to moderate cardiomegaly with some prominence of both ventricles and the left atrium. The shadow of the main pulmonary artery may be normal or prominent, and pulmonary overcirculation is usual. The *electrocardiogram* generally shows biventricular hypertrophy. Prominence of Q and R waves over the left precordium indicates left ventricular dominance; mild right ventricular overload is suggested by RS or rSr′ in the right precordial leads.

Large defects with excessive pulmonary blood flow and pulmonary hypertension produce symptoms in infancy. These babies are dyspneic, have feeding difficulties, grow poorly, perspire profusely and suffer from recurrent pulmonary infections and episodes of heart failure. Cyanosis is absent, but a dusky plethora is sometimes noted during infections or crying. In the absence of heart failure, arterial and venous pulses are normal. Protrusion of the anterior portion of the chest is common, especially of the left precordium and sternum. Cardiomegaly is usual, with a palpable parasternal lift and apical thrust. Systolic thrills are common. The characteristic systolic murmur is similar to that of moderate-sized defects, but the sound of pulmonary valvular closure is louder and the second sound is narrowly split. The presence of an apical diastolic murmur indicates an appreciable left-to-right shunt.

Roentgenographically gross cardiomegaly is usual, with prominence of both ventricles, the left atrium and pulmonary artery. The ascending aorta and aortic knob are relatively small. The *electrocardiogram* shows biventricular hypertrophy or dominance of either the left or right ventricle. P waves may be notched or peaked.

If the shunt across the defect is limited by a significant elevation of pulmonary arterial resistance, the symptoms may appear to be less severe. Nevertheless physical underdevelopment and easy fatigability are usual. Mild cyanosis due to concomitant right-to-left shunt may be observed during intercurrent pulmonary infections. A precordial bulge is usual. Cardiomegaly is moderate, with a prominent left parasternal lift. A pulmonic ejection click is frequent and initiates a systolic ejection murmur. The second sound is narrowly split, with a booming pulmonary component. An early diastolic murmur of pulmonary valvular incompetence is sometimes heard. *Roentgenographic examination* confirms the moderate cardiomegaly; there is some prominence of both right and left ventricular shadows. Minimal left atrial enlargement may also be present. Prominence and increased pulsation of the pulmonary arterial trunk and its primary divisions may contrast with the relatively narrow peripheral branches of the pulmonary arterial tree. The *electrocardiogram* shows dominance of the right ventricle, but associated signs of left ventricular hypertrophy may also be seen. The P waves are either peaked or notched.

SPECIAL STUDIES. The effects of a ventricular septal defect on the pulmonary and systemic circulations may be quantitated by cardiac catheterization, which also serves to determine if there are any clinically undetected anomalies. Since oxygenated blood passes across the defect from the left ventricle, blood from the right ventricle is significantly higher in oxygen than that from the right atrium. Occasionally mixing of blood in the right ventricle is inadequate, so that a definite rise in oxygen content is apparent only in the pulmonary arterial blood. If the right ventricular blood sample is obtained close to the defect, a falsely high oxygen content may be obtained. Conversely, small shunts may not result in a detectable increase in oxygen content of blood from the right ventricle, but may be demonstrated by indicator dilution tests (preferably hydrogen [Fig. 13–16] or indocyanine green [Fig. 13–15]), intracardiac phonocardiography or left ventriculography.

The nature of hemodynamic changes may be quantitated by pressure and flow measurements. Small defects are associated with normal right heart pressures and pulmonary vascular resistance. Pulmonary and systemic blood flow in patients with large defects with nearly equal pulmonary and systemic pressures is determined primarily by the resistance of the pulmonary and systemic circuits.

The location and number of ventricular defects may be demonstrated by left ventriculography. Contrast medium passes across the defect to opacify the right ventricle and pulmonary artery. Passage of the cardiac catheter across the defect into the left ventricle furnishes indisputable evidence for the presence of a ventricular septal defect. Intracardiac phonocardiography may show that the murmur is localized to the right ventricle and pulmonary artery and is inaudible in the right atrium.

PROGNOSIS AND COMPLICATIONS. The natural course of ventricular septal defects is a spectrum which includes the following: (1) A significant number (estimated by some to be 50 to 80 per cent) of small defects close spontaneously, most frequently during the first year of life but even in later years. It is unusual for moderate or large defects to close spontaneously, but this has been reported. (2) A large number of children remain asymptomatic without evidence of increase in heart size, pulmonary arterial pressure or resistance. (3) Subacute bacterial endocarditis occurs in less than 1 per cent. (4) A small but significant number of infants have repeated episodes of respiratory infection and congestive heart failure with a high case fatality. (5) Some have pulmonary hypertension. The majority of reports indicate lack of progression of pulmonary hypertension during childhood, but pulmonary resistance probably does increase in some children, and especially in adolescents and adults. (6) A small number acquire pulmonary stenosis, which serves as a protection to the pulmonary circulation. In these patients the clinical picture changes from that of ventricular septal defect with large left-to-right shunt to that of ventricular septal defect with pulmonic stenosis (see later).

TREATMENT. With open-heart surgery ventricular septal defects can be repaired. The left-to-right shunt is obliterated (Fig. 13–35), the hyperdynamic heart becomes quiet, thrills and murmurs are abolished, and the pressures in the lesser circulation return toward normal. In some instances after successful operation systolic ejection murmurs of low intensity persist for some months.

The most clear-cut candidate for surgical treatment is the symptomatic patient over the age of 2 years who has moderate pulmonary hypertension and a large left-to-right shunt. In these patients the surgical mortality rate is 3 per cent or less. Patients who have pulmonic systolic pressures at or approaching the systemic level, but without demonstrable right-to-left shunt and with large left-to-right shunts, are still good candidates for surgery, but the surgical mortality rate is higher. It appears that patients with significant right-to-left shunts and small left-to-right shunts are inoperable (see Eisenmenger Syndrome). Infants with large ventricular septal defects, torrential pulmonary flow, pulmonary hypertension and uncontrollable congestive cardiac failure present a difficult problem in management. Diligent and careful use of digitalis and diuretics and treatment of intermittent infections (especially pneumonitis) and anemia may improve the clinical course significantly. When this therapy fails surgical therapy is

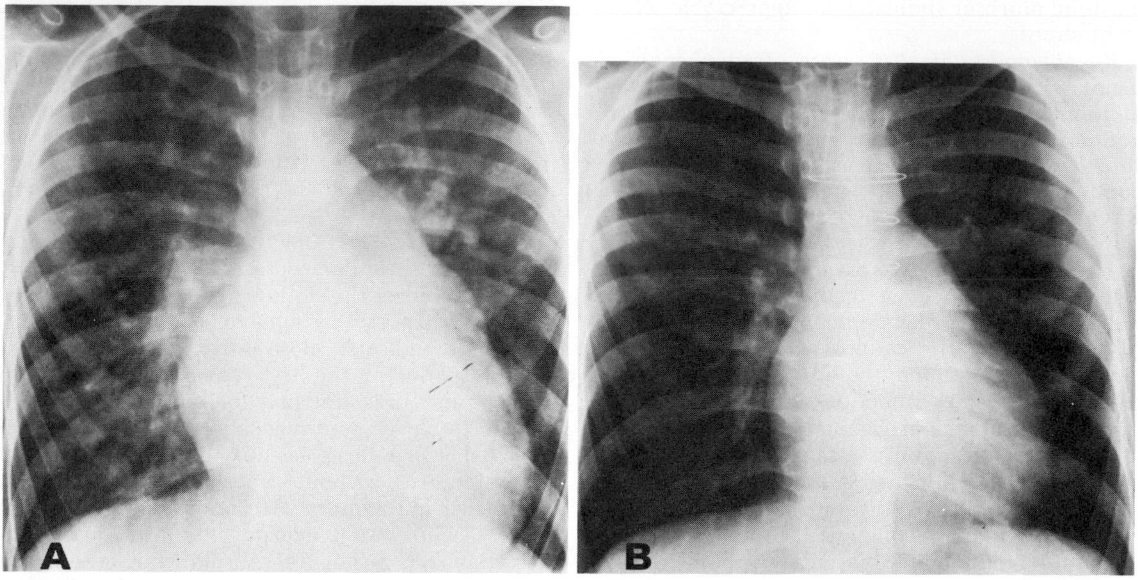

Figure 13–35 A, *Preoperative teleroentgenogram in ventricular septal defect with large left-to-right shunt and pulmonary hypertension. Significant cardiomegaly, prominence of the pulmonary arterial trunk and pulmonary overcirculation are evident.* B, *Three years after surgical closure of defect. There is marked decrease in heart size, and the pulmonary vasculature is normal.*

urgently indicated. At the present time this is not standardized. Pulmonary blood flow can be decreased by pulmonary arterial banding, which relieves congestive cardiac failure and decreases the frequency of intermittent pneumonitis. In later years the pulmonary artery is debanded and the ventricular septal defect closed. At present primary closure of the ventricular defect in infancy is being re-evaluated because of improvement of methods for total body perfusion as well as the experience gained by closure of the defect during deep hypothermia with circulatory arrest.

Surgical treatment is not recommended for patients who are asymptomatic, and have a normal-sized heart, normal electrocardiogram and normal pressures in the lesser circulation.

Medical management in the years before operation is important. Therapy for the symptomatic infant has been mentioned. As a protection against subacute bacterial endocarditis, the integrity of the primary as well as the permanent teeth should be carefully maintained, and the child should receive large doses of penicillin to cover dental extractions, tonsillectomy and adenoidectomy. Similarly, intercurrent infections should be treated diligently with suitable antibiotics. (See Table 9–14.)

VENTRICULAR SEPTAL DEFECT WITH AORTIC INSUFFICIENCY

This is a distinct syndrome in which the ventricular septal defect is complicated by prolapse of the aortic valve and aortic insufficiency. Frequently the septal defect, which is small or moderate in size, is anterior and subpulmonic; in other patients it is infracristal. The prolapsed cusp of the aortic valve is the right or sometimes the noncoronary one. The physical signs of aortic insufficiency (diastolic murmur and wide pulse pressure) are added to those of ventricular septal defect and may be confused with patent ductus arteriosus or other defects associated with aortic runoff.

The clinical spectrum varies widely from the asymptomatic child with trivial aortic regurgitation and small left-to-right shunt to the symptomatic adolescent with florid aortic incompetence, congestive cardiac failure, angina pectoris and massive cardiomegaly. The latter patients urgently require surgical closure of the defect and relief of aortic incompetence. Aortic valve repair may be possible only with a prosthesis. The *asymptomatic patient* presents a therapeutic dilemma. Some prefer to close the ventricular defect with the object of preventing progression of aortic incompetence. Others believe that the course of the aortic insufficiency is unaffected by septal defect closure and prefer to treat the patient conservatively.

VENTRICULAR SEPTAL DEFECT WITH LEFT VENTRICULAR, RIGHT ATRIAL SHUNT

Ventricular defects may be closely associated with an abnormal septal leaflet of the tricuspid valve. During left ventricular systole arterialized blood is ejected through the defect into the right atrium. The physical signs are those of ventricular septal defect or ostium primum defect. High right atrial pressure is manifest as a large systolic venous pulsation in the neck. Cardiac catheterization reveals a left-to-right shunt at the atrial level and may result in a misdiagnosis of atrial septal defect. The diagnosis may be confirmed by left ventriculography; the right atrium opacifies immediately after delivery of contrast medium to the left ventricle. Also, the pansystolic murmur is recorded in the right atrium with intracardiac phonocardiography. These patients are treated surgically by closure of the ventricular defect.

ORIGIN OF BOTH GREAT VESSELS FROM THE RIGHT VENTRICLE

In this anomaly both the aorta and the pulmonary artery arise from the right ventricle. The only outlet from the left ventricle is a ventricular septal defect. The clinical picture closely simulates that of an uncomplicated ventricular septal defect with a large left-to-right shunt. In the majority of instances pulmonary hypertension is present. The electrocardiogram simulates that seen in ostium primum defects. Echocardiography is diagnostic since it shows discontinuity of the mitral and aortic valves. The condition may be recognized by right ventriculography, which demonstrates the site of origin of the aorta and the fact that the aortic and pulmonary valves are at the same level. Although this anomaly has been treated successfully, surgical therapy is more complicated than for simple ventricular septal defect. Therefore it is important to differentiate these conditions before operation.

CORRECTED TRANSPOSITION OF THE GREAT VESSELS

(L-Transposition or Ventricular Inversion)

In this malformation the systemic venous blood returns normally through the venae cavae into a normal right atrium. Venous blood then passes through a bicuspid atrioventricular valve into a right-sided ventricle and is ejected to the pulmonary artery. Pulmonary venous blood returns to a normal left atrium, passes through a tricuspid atrioventricular valve into a left-sided ventricle and is then ejected into the aorta. The right-sided ventricle has the internal appearance of a normal left ventricle, and the internal structure of the left-sided ventricle is that of a normal right ventricle. The pulmonary artery and ascending aorta are parallel, and the former is medial. Thus, the course of the blood is normal in patients with uncomplicated corrected transposition. In the majority of instances, however, associated anomalies coexist, the common ones being ventricular septal defect, abnormalities of the left atrioventricular valve with or without incompetence, pulmonary valvular stenosis and atrioventricular conduction disturbances, frequently with complete atrioventricular dissociation.

Symptoms and signs are dominated by the associated lesions, since patients with uncomplicated corrected transposition have normal hemodynamics. Posteroanterior chest teleroentgenograms may suggest the abnormal position of the great arteries, since the ascending aorta occupies the upper left border of the cardiac silhouette. In addition to atrioventricular conduction disturbances, electrocardiograms may show abnormal P waves, absent QV_6, initial Q waves in leads III, aVR, aVF and V_1 and upright T waves across the precordium. The position of the great vessels is confirmed by cardiac catheterization or ventriculography.

Surgical treatment of the associated anomalies, especially of ventricular septal defects, has been difficult because of the unusual course of the coronary arteries, associated preoperative heart block and unrecognized disease of the left atrioventricular valve.

OTHER DEFECTS ASSOCIATED WITH VENTRICULAR SEPTAL DEFECT

The availability of surgical treatment for ventricular septal defects makes the diagnosis of associated cardiovascular malformations of paramount importance.

PATENT DUCTUS ARTERIOSUS. During cardiopulmonary bypass for the repair of ventricular defects arterialized blood from the heart-lung apparatus is returned to a branch of the aorta. If there is an associated patent ductus arteriosus, blood leaks into the pulmonary artery, flooding the surgical field with blood and contributing to postoperative pulmonary complications. In some instances the signs of the ventricular septal defect dominate, so that the murmur of the patent ductus is inaudible. In such cases the passage of the cardiac catheter from the pulmonary artery through the ductus and into the descending aorta is diagnostic.

In other instances the signs of patent ductus arteriosus predominate, although a systolic murmur and thrill are often present along the lower left sternal border. In these cases cardiac catheterization, hydrogen electrode and indicator dilution studies and angiocardiography reveal the left-to-right shunt at the ventricular level, as well as the patent ductus arteriosus.

The ventricular defect and the patent ductus are closed at the same operation. If the presence of the ductus is appreciated, the surgical risk is the same as that for the ventricular defect.

MULTIPLE VENTRICULAR SEPTAL DEFECTS. In rare instances there are multiple defects involving the ventricular septum. Generally these patients present in infancy with signs of a large left-to-right shunt and pulmonary hypertension. Usually, multiple defects cannot be appreciated clinically or by cardiac catheterization, but can be recognized by left ventriculography. Exploration of the entire ventricular septum is indicated during open cardiotomy to ensure that all defects have been treated. Nevertheless, even with careful exploration some defects may be missed. The postoperative period can be hazardous in these patients, especially if significant left-to-right shunts and pulmonary hypertension persist.

ATRIAL SEPTAL DEFECT. In patients with a ventricular defect and an ostium secundum the physical signs are usually dominated by the ventricular defect. The clinical picture is similar to that of moderate-sized or large ventricular septal defects. This combination of defects may be suspected during cardiac catheterization if left-to-right shunts are demonstrated at both the atrial and ventricular levels. During right ventriculotomy or atriotomy for closure of ventricular defects the atrial septum is easily explored; if both defects are present, they can be repaired during the same procedure.

COARCTATION OF THE AORTA. The signs of coarctation of the aorta are clear, but those of the ventricular defect may be confused with the signs produced by the collateral circulation secondary to the coarctation. It may be necessary to repair these lesions at separate surgical procedures.

PERSISTENT LEFT SUPERIOR VENA CAVA. This condition is not clinically diagnosable. It is proved by cardiac catheterization when the catheter enters the persistent left superior vena cava from the coronary sinus. Surgical treatment of ventricular defects with cardiopulmonary bypass requires occlusion of the venous inflow; if the left superior vena cava is not occluded, large volumes of venous blood enter the heart during cardiotomy. The persistent left superior vena cava in itself does not require treatment.

ENDOCARDIAL SCLEROSIS. Thickened white areas are frequently found in the endocardium of the right ventricle in patients with ventricular septal defect. These areas are presumably produced by the jet of blood shunting across the defect to the opposite right ventricular wall. Endocardial sclerosis involving the left atrium and ventricle is infrequent with ventricular defects.

COMPLETE HEART BLOCK. This arrhythmia is rare in patients with ventricular septal defect, although systolic murmurs of varying intensity are not unusual in patients with complete heart block. They are produced by the turbulence associated with the large stroke volume. Patients with ventricular septal defect and complete heart block should be suspected of having corrected transposition of the great vessels. These abnormalities do not contraindicate closure of the ventricular defect, but surgical treatment is more difficult.

ATRIAL SEPTAL DEFECT

PATENT FORAMEN OVALE

At or soon after birth the foramen ovale closes. In about 80 per cent of normal hearts the closure is permanent; in the remainder a small slitlike opening persists.

An isolated patent foramen ovale is of no clinical significance. If the right atrial pressure is increased (e.g., secondary to pulmonary stenosis or pulmonary hypertension), venous blood may be shunted across the patent foramen ovale into the left atrium and result in cyanosis. A cardiac catheter introduced from the saphenous vein into the inferior vena cava and right atrium may pass easily across a patent foramen ovale into the left atrium.

Because of the anatomic structure at the valve of a patent foramen ovale, blood cannot be shunted from the left atrium to the right atrium.

An isolated patent foramen ovale does not require treatment.

OSTIUM SECUNDUM DEFECT

This is a defect in the region of the fossa ovalis and is associated with normal atrioventricular valves. The defects may be multiple, and in symptomatic older children openings of 2 cm or more diameter are not unusual. Large defects may extend inferiorly toward the inferior vena cava and ostium of the coronary sinus, superiorly toward the superior vena cava, or posteriorly.

HEMODYNAMICS. A considerable shunt of oxygenated blood flows from the left to the right atrium. This blood is added to the normal venous return to the right atrium and is pumped by the right ventricle to the lungs. Pulmonary blood flow is usually two to four times systemic flow. Since the defect is closely related to the orifices of the right pulmonary veins, a greater volume of blood passes through it from the right lung than from the left. Although the left atrial pressure exceeds that of the right atrium by a few millimeters of mercury, the principal factor which determines the direction of shunt is the compliance of the chambers of the right side of the heart. The greater distensibility of the right atrium and ventricle and the low pulmonary vascular resistance allow a torrential left-to-right shunt. The paucity of symptoms in infants with atrial septal defects has been related to the structure of the right ventricle in early life when the ventricle is thick and less compliant, thus limiting the left-to-right shunt. As the infant gets older the right ventricular wall becomes thinner and the left-to-right shunt across the atrial defect increases. The large blood flow through the right side of the heart results in enlargement of the right atrium and ventricle and dilatation of the pulmonary artery. In spite of the large pulmonary blood flow, the pulmonary arterial pressure is usually normal or only moderately elevated. The left ventricle and aorta are smaller than usual, owing to the decreased amount of blood they carry. Progressive dilatation of the right ventricle may lead to heart failure. Cyanosis is extremely rare; it is seen occasionally with congestive heart failure or with the complicating features of the Eisenmenger syndrome.

CLINICAL MANIFESTATIONS. An ostium secundum defect may be asymptomatic in many instances; it is often discovered during routine physical examination. Ostium secundum defects rarely produce heart failure in infancy. The history in older children usually includes recurrent episodes of pneumonitis, frequently complicated by segmental pulmonary collapse, and varying degrees of exercise intolerance. Although physical development may be significantly retarded (*gracile habitus*), it is normal in the majority of patients.

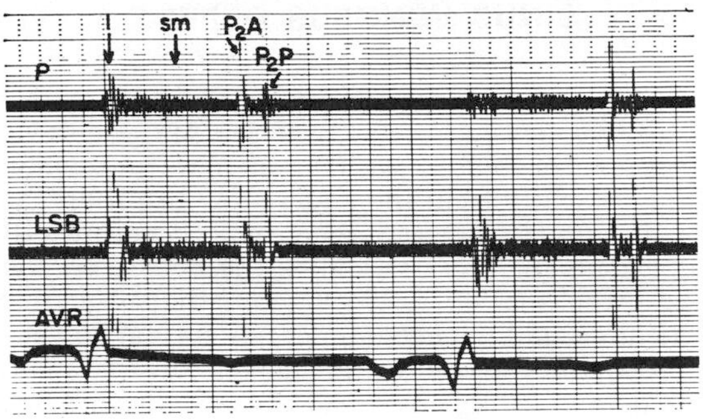

Figure 13–36 Phonocardiograms (P, pulmonary area; LSB, left sternal border) to illustrate auscultatory findings in ostium secundum atrial septal defect. Abbreviations: AV_R, Electrocardiogram; 1, first heart sound; sm, systolic murmur: P_2A, aortic component of second sound; P_2P, pulmonary component of second sound. Note wide splitting of second sound. This splitting persisted in all phases of respiration. Time lines 0.04 second.

The pulse is normal or small and the venous pressure normal unless there is associated tricuspid insufficiency or heart failure. The heart may be normal in size or moderately or greatly enlarged. A hyperdynamic right ventricular systolic lift is usually palpable and extends from the left sternal border to the midclavicular line. The systolic murmur is ejection in type, soft, and seldom accompanied by a thrill. It is best heard at the upper left sternal border and is produced by turbulence of the torrential flow in the dilated pulmonary artery. In some patients with thin chests the murmur may be loud and accompanied by a thrill. The murmur is preceded by a loud first heart sound and sometimes by a pulmonic ejection sound. In 95 per cent of patients the second heart sound at the upper left sternal edge is widely split and fixed in all phases of respiration. This auscultatory finding is so characteristic that the diagnosis of uncomplicated atrial septal defect is questionable in its absence (Fig. 13–36). The widely split second sound is probably due to prolongation of right ventricular systole because of large stroke volume which cannot be reduced (as in the normal) on expiration. A mid-diastolic murmur produced by the torrential flow across the tricuspid valve may be audible at the apex or at the lower left sternal edge. The diastolic murmur of pulmonary incompetence may be heard, but is rare.

Associated abnormalities which may be found on physical examination include pigeon chest, kyphoscoliosis and high-arched palate. Congenital or rheumatic mitral stenosis with atrial septal defect (**Lutembacher syndrome**) is rare.

Roentgenograms show varying degrees of cardiac enlargement owing to prominence of the right ventricle and atrium. The pulmonary artery is large, the pulmonary vascularity greatly increased, and the left ventricle and the aorta are small. These signs vary and may not be conspicuous in less advanced cases.

The *electrocardiogram* shows right axis deviation and right ventricular hypertrophy (the so-called incomplete right bundle branch block); the diagnosis of an uncomplicated secundum atrial septal defect is in doubt if they are absent. Infrequent electrocardiographic abnormalities include tall P waves, prolonged P-R intervals, dysrhythmias (e.g., atrial fibrillation and complete heart block), Wolff-Parkinson-White syndrome, complete right bundle branch block and left axis deviation. Occasionally the electrocardiogram is normal.

The *echocardiogram* shows findings which are characteristic of right ventricular volume overload: (1) increased right ventricular end-diastolic dimension, and (2) abnormal motion of the ventricular septum. The normal septum moves posteriorly during systole and anteriorly during diastole. In patients with right ventricular volume overload and normal pulmonary vascular resistance the septal motion is reversed (i.e., anterior movement in systole), or the motion is intermediate so that the echo remains straight.

The diagnosis may be confirmed by *cardiac catheterization,* which demonstrates a significantly higher oxygen content of the blood from the right atrium as compared to samples from the superior vena cava. This finding is not diagnostic, since it may be evident with anomalous pulmonary venous return to the right atrium, with ventricular septal defect with tricuspid insufficiency, with ventricular septal defects associated with left ventricular-right atrial shunts, and with aortic-right atrial communications (e.g., ruptured sinus of Valsalva). The physical signs produced by these anomalies generally differ greatly from those of atrial septal defects, and their presence can usually be confirmed by selective angiocardiography. In a minority of patients, mixing of blood is incomplete in the right atrium, so that the principal site of shunt appears to be at the ventricular level.

The catheter frequently enters the left atrium from the right atrium, especially if it is introduced into the heart from the inferior vena cava. Indicator dilution curves may be used to demonstrate the site of the left-to-right shunt and the presence of anomalous pulmonary veins. Streaming of inferior vena caval blood across the defect to the left atrium occurs in some patients with uncomplicated atrial septal defects. This minute right-to-left shunt may be demonstrated by indicator dilution curves, but does not result in arterial unsaturation or cyanosis. The pressures in the right side of the heart are frequently normal, but may show moderate right ventricular and pulmonary hypertension. Pressure gradients may be measured across the right ventricular outflow in the absence of organic pulmonic stenosis and are probably produced by functional pulmonic stenosis due to the large pulmonary flow. The pulmonary arteriolar resistance is usually normal, but occasionally may be increased. The shunt is also variable, but is usually considerable (as high as 20 liters per minute per square meter of body surface).

Intracardiac phonocardiography demonstrates

an ejection systolic murmur in the pulmonary artery, sometimes preceded by a click. A mid-diastolic murmur may be recorded in the inflow of the right ventricle, owing to the large flow across the tricuspid valve.

COMPLICATIONS AND PROGNOSIS. Secundum atrial septal defects are well tolerated during childhood, so that symptoms usually appear only in the third decade or later. Pulmonary hypertension, atrial dysrhythmias, tricuspid incompetence and heart failure are uncommon in childhood, although these complications are seen occasionally in infants. Bacterial endocarditis is rare; if it occurs, it suggests the presence of an associated cardiovascular anomaly. The principal guides to prognosis appear to be the presence or absence of symptoms and of continuing cardiac enlargement.

Secundum atrial septal defects are usually isolated, although they may be associated with partial anomalous pulmonary venous return, pulmonary valvular stenosis, ventricular septal defect, pulmonary arterial branch stenosis and persistent left superior vena cava.

TREATMENT. Direct-vision, open-heart surgery during cardiopulmonary bypass allows accurate closure. The mortality rate from surgery is less than 1 per cent and is advised even in asymptomatic patients prior to entry into school. Surgery is preferred during childhood because the surgical mortality is higher in adults, especially those with pulmonary hypertension, cardiac failure, tricuspid incompetence or atrial arrhythmias.

The results after operation are gratifying, especially in children with large shunts (Fig. 13–37). Symptoms disappear rapidly, and frequently physical development is enhanced. Although the heart size may decrease to normal, persistent cardiomegaly of moderate degree is not unusual. Many years after operation atrial arrhythmias may occur, including atrial tachycardia, flutter or fibrillation.

SINUS VENOSUS DEFECT

These defects are situated in the upper part of the atrial septum in close relation to the entry of the superior vena cava. One or more pulmonary veins (usually from the right lung) drain anomalously into the superior vena cava. Sometimes the superior vena cava straddles the defect, so that some systemic venous blood enters the left atrium. The abnormal hemodynamics are similar to those of secundum atrial septal defect, consisting primarily of a volume overload of the right ventricle. The clinical picture, electrocardiogram and chest x-ray are similar to those of secundum atrial defect. Generally the anomalous pulmonary veins are not recognized on routine chest x-ray, although a bulge of the superior vena caval shadow may suggest the diagnosis. During cardiac catheterization the catheter may enter the pulmonary veins from the superior vena cava. Anatomic correction usually requires the insertion of a patch to ensure the entry of anomalous veins into the left atrium; surgical results are good.

OSTIUM PRIMUM DEFECT AND COMMON ATRIOVENTRICULAR CANAL
(Endocardial Cushion Defects)

These abnormalities are grouped together because they have a common embryologic relation, and the clinical pattern may be similar.

An *ostium primum defect* is situated in the lower portion of the atrial septum and overlies the mitral and tricuspid valves. In the majority of instances there is a cleft in the anterior leaflet of the mitral valve. The tricuspid valve is usually normal, although some thickening of the septal leaflet may be present. The ventricular septum is usually intact functionally, but its proximal part is anatomically deficient.

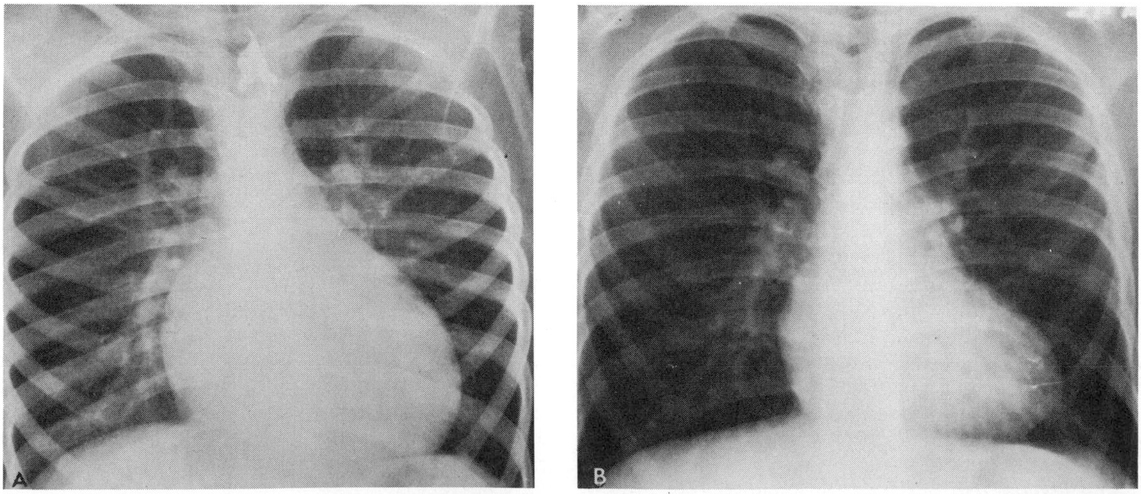

Figure 13–37 *Preoperative* (A) *and 1 year postoperative* (B) *teleroentgenograms in atrial septal defect (ostium secundum). Preoperative x-ray film shows cardiomegaly, prominent pulmonary artery segment and pulmonary overcirculation. Postoperative x-ray film shows decrease in heart size and normal pulmonary circulation.*

Common atrioventricular canal consists of an interatrial and interventricular defect with an atrioventricular valve which is common to both ventricles and consists of an anterior and a posterior leaflet related to the ventricular septum with a lateral leaflet in each ventricle. The lesion is more common among children with Down's syndrome than among other children; other congenital heart defects may also occur in association with Down's syndrome.

Transitional varieties of these defects also occur. These include ostium primum defects with clefts in the anterior mitral and septal tricuspid valve leaflets, and, less commonly, ostium primum defects with normal atrioventricular valves. In others the atrial septum is intact, but the ventricular septal defect simulates that found in common atrioventricular canal. These defects are also associated with deformities of the atrioventricular valves.

HEMODYNAMICS. In *ostium primum defects* the basic abnormality is a left-to-right shunt across the atrial defect, with associated mitral incompetence. The shunt is usually moderate or large. The degree of mitral incompetence is ordinarily mild or moderate. Pulmonary arterial pressures are usually normal or only moderately increased.

In *common atrioventricular canal* the left-to-right shunt is transatrial as well as transventricular. Pulmonary hypertension and increased pulmonary vascular resistance are common. Atrioventricular valvular incompetence results in regurgitation of blood from the ventricles to the atria. Some right-to-left shunting occurs at both atrial and ventricular levels, but is usually small in volume and seldom results in significant arterial unsaturation. Established or progressive pulmonary vascular disease increases the right-to-left shunt, however, so that clinical cyanosis may develop.

CLINICAL MANIFESTATIONS. Many children with *ostium primum defect* are asymptomatic, and the anomaly is discovered during routine physical examination. In these patients with moderate shunts and trivial mitral incompetence the physical signs are similar to those of atrial defect of the secundum type. Clues to the correct diagnosis include an apical systolic murmur and a classic electrocardiogram (see below).

A history of effort intolerance, easy fatigability and recurrent pneumonitis may be obtained, especially in patients with large left-to-right shunts and significant mitral incompetence. In these patients cardiac enlargement is moderate or marked, a precordial bulge is common, a hyperdynamic parasternal right ventricular lift is palpable, and a left ventricular apical heave suggests significant mitral incompetence. The auscultatory signs produced by the left-to-right shunt include a normal or accentuated first sound, wide, fixed splitting of the second sound, a pulmonary ejection systolic murmur sometimes preceded by a click, and a rumbling mid-diastolic murmur at the lower left sternal edge (Fig. 13-38). Signs of mitral incompetence are superimposed and usually consist of an apical pansystolic murmur which radiates to the left axilla; this murmur is variable in nature and may be short or musical.

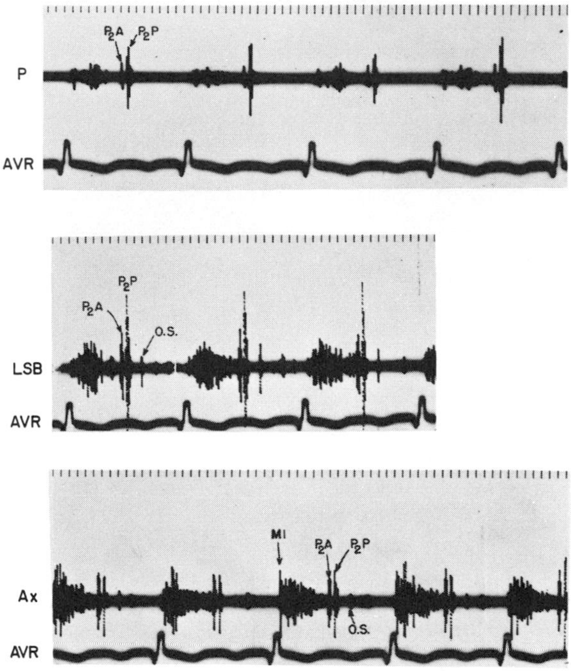

Figure 13-38 *Phonocardiograms to illustrate auscultatory findings in ostium primum atrial septal defect. Abbreviations: P, Pulmonary area; LSB, left sternal border; Ax, apex; AVR, electrocardiogram; P_2A, aortic component of the second sound; P_2P, pulmonary component of second sound; MI, mitral component of first sound; OS, opening snap. The systolic murmur is ejection in type at the pulmonary area and pansystolic at the left sternal border and apex. Splitting of the second sound is fixed. The opening snap is either tricuspid or mitral in origin. Time lines 0.04 second.*

In the majority of patients with common *atrioventricular canal,* congestive heart failure and intercurrent pulmonary infection appear in infancy. During these episodes minimal cyanosis may be evident. The jugular venous pressure may be increased because of pulmonary hypertension, congestive heart failure or incompetence of the atrioventricular valve. Cardiac enlargement is moderate or marked, and a systolic thrill is frequently palpable. The first heart sound is normal or accentuated and is followed by a widely distributed, harsh systolic murmur. The second heart sound is widely split if pulmonary flow is torrential; if severe pulmonary hypertension develops, the width of splitting may not be striking, but pulmonary valve closure is loud. A low-pitched mid-diastolic murmur is audible at the lower left sternal edge, and a pulmonic systolic ejection murmur is produced by the large pulmonary flow.

Roentgenograms in endocardial cushion defects confirm the cardiac enlargement, which is due to prominence of both ventricles. The pulmonary artery is large; pulmonary vascularity is increased, and hilar dance is not unusual. The aorta is small or normal in size (Fig. 13-39).

The *electrocardiogram* in endocardial cushion

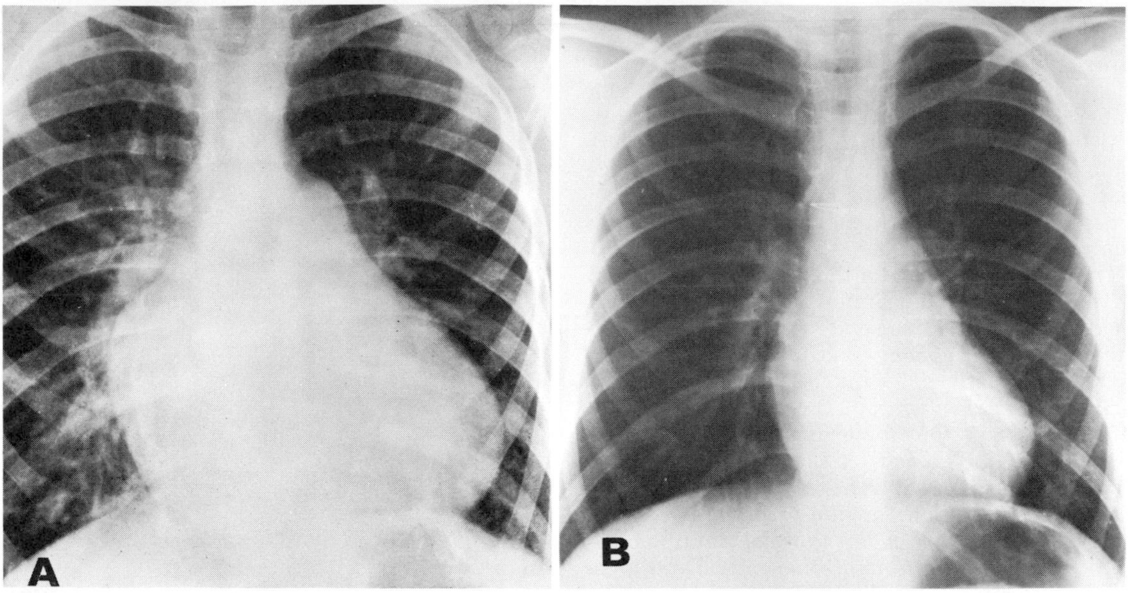

Figure 13–39 Ostium primum atrial septal defect with torrential pulmonary flow and normal pulmonary arterial pressure. A, Preoperative. Cardiomegaly is associated with prominence of the main pulmonary trunk, pulmonary overcirculation and an inconspicuous aorta. B, Postoperative. The cardiac silhouette and pulmonary circulation are within normal limits.

defects is unusual and diagnostic. The principal abnormalities are (1) superior orientation of the mean frontal QRS axis, with left axis deviation or occasionally extreme right axis deviation, (2) counterclockwise inscription of the superiorly oriented QRS vector loop, (3) signs of biventricular hypertrophy or sometimes isolated right or left ventricular hypertrophy, (4) normal or tall P waves, and (5) prolongation of the P-R interval.

Cardiac catheterization and *angiocardiography* confirm the diagnosis. These studies demonstrate the magnitude of the left-to-right shunt, the severity of pulmonary hypertension and increased pulmonary vascular resistance, and the degree of atrioventricular valve incompetence. The shunt is usually demonstrable at the atrial level; in some patients with inadequate mixing of blood it appears to be primarily at the ventricular level. The arterial oxygen saturation is normal except when severe pulmonary hypertension is present. In these patients a small right-to-left shunt may be demonstrable. Patients with ostium primum defects usually have normal or only moderate elevation of the pulmonary arterial pressure and resistance. Nevertheless common atrioventricular canal is usually associated with right ventricular and pulmonary hypertension as well as a moderate increase in pulmonary vascular resistance. The cardiac catheter enters the chambers of the left side of the heart with ease from the right side, especially if there is a common atrioventricular canal.

Selective left ventriculography is extremely helpful in the diagnosis of endocardial cushion defects. This study demonstrates the deformity of the mitral or common atrioventricular valve and the distortion of the outflow of the left ventricle. The latter has been described as a "gooseneck" deformity. The abnormal anterior leaflet of the mitral valve is serrated, and mitral incompetence may be demonstrable.

PROGNOSIS. The prognosis of endocardial cushion defects depends on the magnitude of the left-to-right shunt, the degree of pulmonary vascular resistance and the severity of mitral incompetence. Death from congestive cardiac failure during infancy is not uncommon with common atrioventricular canal, but many patients with ostium primum defects are asymptomatic or have only minor, nonprogressive symptoms until they reach the third or fourth decade of life.

TREATMENT. Direct-vision intracardiac surgery with an artificial heart-lung machine and cardiopulmonary bypass is now a feasible form of treatment for endocardial cushion defects. Ostium primum defects are approached from an incision in the right atrium. The cleft in the mitral valve is located through the atrial defect and is repaired by direct suture. A cleft in the tricuspid valve is also treated by direct suture. The defects in the atrial and ventricular septa are usually closed by insertion of a prosthesis. The surgical mortality rate for primum defects is low. Surgical treatment for complete atrioventricular canal is difficult, especially in infants with congestive cardiac failure and pulmonary hypertension. Pulmonary arterial banding has been successful in patients with dominant shunts at the ventricular level. Complete correction of these defects is difficult but has been accomplished successfully.

PATENT DUCTUS ARTERIOSUS

During fetal life a large percentage of pulmonary arterial blood is shunted through the ductus arteriosus into the aorta. Functional closure of the ductus normally occurs soon after birth, but if the ductus remains patent, aortic blood is shunted into the pulmonary artery. The aortic end of the ductus is opposite and usually distal to the origin of the left subclavian artery, and it enters the pulmonary artery at its bifurcation. Patent ductus arteriosus is peculiar among congenital cardiac defects in that it occurs frequently as an isolated anomaly. It occurs about twice as frequently in females as in males and is one of the commonest congenital cardiovascular anomalies associated with maternal rubella during early pregnancy.

HEMODYNAMICS. As a result of the higher aortic pressure the blood flow through the ductus is from the aorta to the pulmonary artery. The degree of shunt depends on the size of the ductus and the pressure gradient between the aorta and the pulmonary artery. In extreme cases one half to two thirds of the left ventricular output may be shunted through the ductus, and the oxygenated blood recirculates through the pulmonary circulation. In the majority of instances the pressures within the pulmonary artery, the right ventricle and right atrium are normal, but the pulmonary arterial and right ventricular systolic pressures may be elevated moderately or even to systemic levels (see Eisenmenger Syndrome). There is a wide pulse pressure. The total blood volume is increased; it returns to normal limits after surgical closure of the ductus.

CLINICAL MANIFESTATIONS. There are usually no symptoms, but symptoms may develop at any age and include slowly progressive exertional dyspnea, followed by left ventricular failure or frank congestive cardiac failure. Retardation of physical growth may be the main manifestation. Rarer symptoms include precordial pain, probably due to complicating neurocirculatory asthenia, and hoarseness from involvement of the adjacent recurrent laryngeal nerve.

The paucity of symptoms contrasts with the striking physical signs. Dynamically, a patent ductus arteriosus is an arteriovenous shunt of considerable extent; signs of a large pulse pressure are produced, including water-hammer radial pulsations and conspicuous arterial Corrigan pulsations in the neck. The low diastolic blood pressure may fall further after exertion. The heart is usually normal in size, but may be moderately or grossly enlarged. The apical impulse is normal or left ventricular and, with cardiac enlargement, is heaving. A thrill, maximal in the second left interspace, is present in many instances and may radiate toward the left clavicle, down the left sternal border, or toward the apex. The thrill is usually systolic in time, often extends into diastole and in some instances may be palpated throughout the cardiac cycle. The classic murmur has been variously described as machinery, humming top, millwheel or rolling thunder in quality. It begins soon after the onset of the first sound, reaches maximum intensity at the end of systole and wanes in late diastole. It may be localized to the second left intercostal space or radiate down the left sternal border or to the left clavicle. The murmur is harsh and does not have the blowing quality common in acquired lesions. A few patients have atypical murmurs, especially if there is pulmonary hypertension, when there is only a systolic murmur. Rarely the murmur is confined to diastole; this is probably due to pulmonary valvular insufficiency. In patients with a large left-to-right shunt a low-pitched mitral diastolic murmur may be audible and is probably due to the large blood flow across the mitral valve. The second heart sound may be split paradoxically.

The *electrocardiogram* is normal in the majority of instances. If the ductus is large, left ventricular hypertrophy may be present. The diagnosis of uncomplicated patent ductus arteriosus is untenable in the presence of electrocardiographic evidence of isolated right ventricular hypertrophy.

Roentgenographic studies commonly show a prominent pulmonary artery with increased intrapulmonary vascular markings. The cardiac size depends on the degree of left-to-right shunt; it may be normal, or moderately or grossly enlarged (Fig. 13-40). The chambers involved are the left atrium and ventricle. The aortic knob is normal or prominent and pulsates vigorously. Rarely, there may be calcification in the wall of the ductus.

The clinical pattern is sufficiently distinctive to allow an accurate diagnosis in the majority of patients. In patients with atypical murmurs further confirmatory studies are indicated.

Cardiac catheterization reveals a normal or increased pressure in the right ventricle and pulmonary artery. The presence of oxygenated blood in the pulmonary artery confirms a left-to-right shunt, as do hydrogen and indicator dilution curves. Samples of blood from the venae cavae, right atrium and right ventricle have a comparable oxygen content. With pulmonary valvular insufficiency some oxygenation of right ventricular blood may be present. The catheter may pass through the ductus into the descending aorta. Injection of contrast material into the outflow tract of the right ventricle may show a washing away of the dye in the pulmonary artery by the shunt of blood from the aorta. Aortography by injection of contrast medium into the ascending aorta shows opacification of the pulmonary artery from the aorta.

Patent Ductus Arteriosus in Infancy. Aside from the symptoms described above, an uncomplicated patent ductus arteriosus may on occasion produce symptoms of left-sided heart failure or severe congestive failure during the first 2 years of life. These symptoms are frequently precipitated by respiratory infections.

As in older children, the presence or absence of the diastolic component of the murmur depends on the pressure relations between the aorta and the pulmonary artery. If secondary pulmonary hypertension has developed, there is little or no flow of blood during diastole and only a systolic murmur is present. If the pulmonary arterial pressure is normal or only moderately elevated, the typical ma-

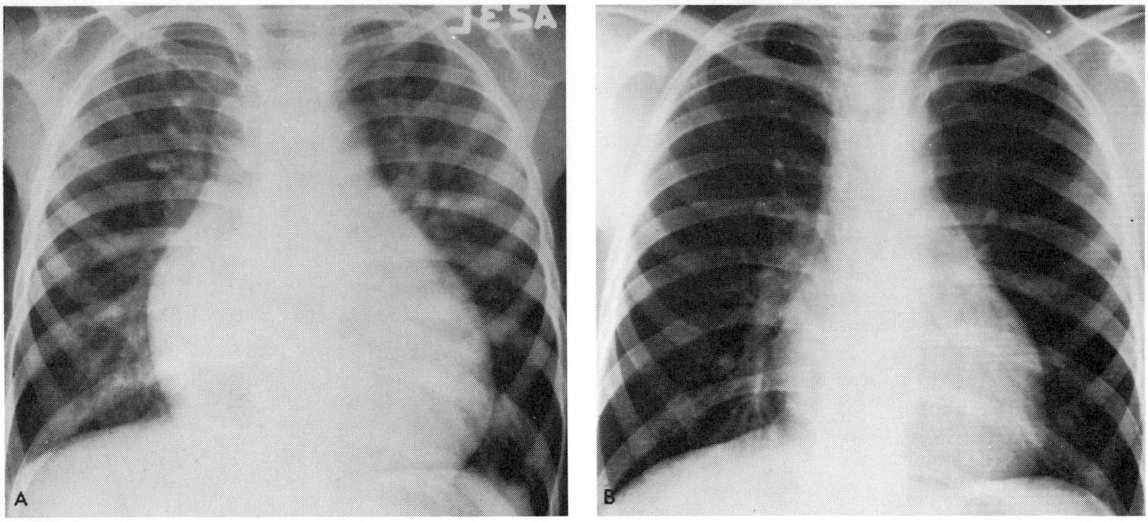

Figure 13–40 *Preoperative (A) and 3 years postoperative (B) teleroentgenograms in patent ductus arteriosus. Preoperative x-ray film shows cardiac enlargement, prominent aorta and pulmonary artery and increased pulmonary vascularity. The decrease in heart size and degree of pulmonary vasculature is evident in the postoperative x-ray film.*

chinery murmur may be present early, even in infants a few weeks of age. In addition, the pulse pressure is wide, and the heart is moderately to grossly enlarged, the main chambers involved being the left ventricle and atrium.

Roentgenographic studies confirm the enlargement of the chambers and also reveal prominent pulmonary arteries and increased aortic pulsations. The *electrocardiogram* may be normal or show evidence of left ventricular dominance or biventricular hypertrophy.

The diagnosis of symptomatic uncomplicated patent ductus arteriosus in infancy is important because surgical treatment of the lesion produces dramatic relief of symptoms. Surgical therapy is indicated in all symptomatic patients irrespective of age and has been successfully performed in very young infants.

Patent Ductus Arteriosus in Premature Infants. It has been estimated that the ductus remains patent in 10 to 15 per cent of premature babies, especially those weighing less than 1500 gm. This has been attributed to the precipitous fall in pulmonary vascular resistance at birth owing to a diminished amount of smooth muscle in the pulmonary arteries of premature infants. Many of these babies are asymptomatic and do not require specific therapy. The peripheral pulses are jerky and the majority have the typical continuous murmur. Sometimes the murmur is audible only in systole, with mid or late systolic accentuation. The ductus closes spontaneously, usually within 12 weeks.

In others the shunt across the duct is moderate or large and is complicated by cardiomegaly, pulmonary edema and heart failure. Many respond to digitalis and diuretics, with subsequent spontaneous closure, but in some the response to therapy is inadequate, and surgical obliteration of the duct is necessary to control cardiac failure.

The role of the ductus in premature infants with idiopathic respiratory distress is difficult to evaluate. Generally, adequate assisted ventilation and correction of anemia improves the signs produced by the patent ductus. Prolonged assisted ventilation with high oxygen concentrations may result in bronchopulmonary dysplasia. The clinical picture of this syndrome may be aggravated by a large flow across a patent ductus, and surgical obliteration may be necessary.

DIFFERENTIAL DIAGNOSIS. The diagnosis of uncomplicated patent ductus arteriosus is usually not difficult at any age. There are other conditions, however, which, in the absence of cyanosis, produce systolic and diastolic murmurs in the pulmonic area and may be misinterpreted.

The characteristics of a *venous hum* have been described elsewhere. Aorticopulmonary septal defect may be clinically indistinguishable from a patent ductus. Similarly, difficulty in diagnosis may occur in patients with a *ruptured sinus of Valsalva into the right side of the heart or pulmonary artery* and in patients with *coronary arteriovenous fistulas.* In these three conditions the dynamics are those of an arteriovenous fistula with a machinery murmur and a wide pulse pressure. Sometimes the murmur is not maximal in the pulmonic area, but is heard along the lower left sternal border. *Truncus arteriosus* with torrential pulmonary flow may be extremely difficult to differentiate from patent ductus, especially in infancy. *Pulmonary branch stenosis* is associated with systolic and diastolic murmurs, but the pulse pressure is normal. *Arteriovenous fistulas* of medium-sized intrathoracic vessels, e.g., the internal mammary, also produce signs which may be indistinguishable from those of patent ductus.

Ventricular septal defect with aortic insufficiency and *combined rheumatic aortic and mitral insufficiency* may be confused with patent ductus arteriosus because the combination of murmurs produced by these lesions superficially resembles those of patent ductus arteriosus. Careful auscultation and the absence of pulmonary overcirculation usually resolve the diagnostic problem.

Symptomatic infants with a large patent ductus arteriosus and pulmonary hypertension may have a clinical picture resembling a large ventricular septal defect. In others a widely patent ductus is associated with a ventricular septal defect; a wide pulse pressure may suggest the presence of the ductus, and confirmatory cardiac catheterization is indicated.

PROGNOSIS AND COMPLICATIONS. Because many patients with patent ductus arteriosus are asymptomatic, the impression may be gained that this lesion is benign. Keys and Shapiro estimated that a patent ductus was responsible for an average reduction of life expectancy of about 23 years in men and 28 in women. There are occasional instances of patients living a normal span with little or no cardiac embarrassment. Children and young adults who have this anomaly are subject to complications, however (see below), the frequency of which is great enough to make it clear that the lesion is not an innocuous one. Spontaneous closure of the ductus after infancy is extremely rare.

It has been mentioned that infants may succumb to congestive cardiac failure. This complication, which is not infrequently preceded by attacks of left ventricular failure, may occur at any age, but is most common in the third decade of life. Cardiac failure is treated along the usual medical lines, but it is an urgent indication for operation when the patient's condition permits.

Subacute bacterial endarteritis, the most frequent complication in late childhood, may occur at any age. Pulmonary emboli are common, and when the ductus is involved, systemic emboli may occur. This complication should be vigorously treated with suitable antibiotics and surgical closure of the ductus. The optimum time for surgical treatment is about 3 months after cure of the infective process.

Rarer complications include aneurysmal dilatation of the pulmonary artery or the ductus, calcification of the ductus, noninfective thrombosis of the ductus with embolization, paradoxical emboli and acquired rheumatic heart disease. Patent ductus arteriosus with pulmonary hypertension (Eisenmenger syndrome) has been described.

TREATMENT. Irrespective of age, patients with a patent ductus arteriosus or similar shunt will derive great benefit from surgical closure of the abnormality (see above). If congestive cardiac failure develops, surgical treatment should not be postponed too long after adequate digitalis, diuretic and low-salt diet therapy, even if some signs of failure persist.

Because the mortality rate with surgical treatment is less than 1 per cent, and the risk otherwise is greater, ligation or division of the ductus is indicated in the asymptomatic patient, preferably between the ages of 3 and 10 years. Operation in this age group is performed with relative facility, whereas in older persons the regional vessels are more rigid or associated with degenerative changes, and the cardiac reserve is reduced (Gross). The upper age limit for surgical repair in the asymptomatic patient is about 35 years. If serious symptoms develop at any age, there should be no hesitation to operate. Pulmonary hypertension is not a contraindication to operation if it can be demonstrated that the shunt is from aorta to pulmonary artery and not reversed.

Surgical closure is by ligation or by division and suture of the ductus; the latter is preferred if technically feasible.

After closure, symptoms of frank or incipient cardiac failure rapidly disappear. If the patient was physically stunted, there is usually an improvement in physical development within a year or two. The pulse and blood pressure return to normal, and the machinery murmur is replaced by two normal heart sounds. In a small number of patients a systolic murmur over the pulmonary area may persist; the murmur may be the result of turbulence in a persistently dilated pulmonary artery or rarely an unsuspected associated ventricular or atrial septal defect. The roentgenographic signs of cardiac enlargement and pulmonary overcirculation also disappear (Fig. 13–40), and the electrocardiogram becomes normal. Pulmonary hypertension, if present preoperatively, also recedes.

AORTICOPULMONARY SEPTAL DEFECT

This defect is a communication between the ascending aorta and main pulmonary artery. The presence of pulmonary and aortic valves and an intact ventricular septum distinguishes this anomaly from truncus arteriosus. Symptoms resembling those of a large ventricular septal defect may appear at any age and include recurrent pulmonary infections, congestive heart failure and occasionally minimal cyanosis. In the absence of severe pulmonary hypertension, physical signs are a wide pulse pressure, cardiac enlargement and a variety of cardiac murmurs. The murmurs may be only systolic, systolic and diastolic or continuous. The electrocardiogram shows either left, right or biventricular hypertrophy. Roentgenographic studies confirm the cardiac enlargement and demonstrate prominence of the pulmonary artery and intrapulmonary vasculature.

This condition may simulate a patent ductus arteriosus. Cardiac catheterization reveals a left-to-right shunt at the level of the pulmonary artery with varying degrees of pulmonary hypertension. The course of the catheter may be diagnostic. In patent ductus arteriosus the catheter enters the pulmonary artery and passes across the ductus into the descending aorta; in aorticopulmonary septal defect the catheter enters the ascending aorta from the pulmonary artery. Selective aortography with injection of contrast medium into the ascending aorta can demonstrate the lesion accurately.

Aorticopulmonary defects can be cured by surgical treatment. In the majority of instances the defect is in the intracardiac portion of the aorta, and cardiopulmonary bypass is necessary for the surgical repair.

FISTULA OF A CORONARY ARTERY

A congenital fistula may exist between a coronary artery and vein, or a coronary artery may empty directly into the heart, usually the right ventricle. In both instances the signs are similar to those of patent ductus arteriosus, but the machinery murmur may be more diffuse. In patients with *coronary arteriovenous fistula* arterialized blood enters the coronary veins, which in turn empty into the coronary sinus. In such cases the right atrial blood has a higher oxygen content than samples from the cavae. When a *coronary artery empties directly into the right ventricle*, there is a left-to-right shunt at the ventricular level. The anatomic abnormality is demonstrable by injection of contrast medium into the ascending aorta. Treatment consists in surgical abolition of the fistula.

RUPTURED SINUS OF VALSALVA

One of the sinuses of Valsalva of the aorta may be weakened by congenital or acquired disease and result in aneurysmal formation and rupture, usually into the right atrium or ventricle. The clinical manifestations are similar to those of patent ductus arteriosus, except that the machinery murmur may be in an unusual site. Cardiac catheterization demonstrates the left-to-right shunt at the atrial or ventricular level. Aortography with injection of contrast medium into the ascending aorta demonstrates the site of aneurysm and rupture. Surgical obliteration of the shunt during cardiopulmonary bypass is usually necessary.

PULMONIC STENOSIS (WITH NORMAL AORTIC ROOT)

Pulmonic stenosis may exist as an isolated abnormality or with defects in the atrial or ventricular septa. In all instances, however, the origin of the aorta is normal. This distinction aids in separating the malformation under discussion from tetralogy of Fallot, in which the aorta is dextroposed. Experience from direct-vision open-heart surgery indicates that in many instances dextroposition of the aorta (even in tetralogy of Fallot) may be more apparent than real.

The following is a modification of the classification of pulmonic stenosis with normal aortic root, as suggested by Abrahams and Wood:

1. Simple pulmonic stenosis
   a. Valvular
   b. Infundibular
   c. Combined valvular and infundibular
2. Pulmonic stenosis (valvular or infundibular or both) with arteriovenous shunt
   a. Pulmonic stenosis with atrial septal defect
   b. Pulmonic stenosis with ventricular septal defect (acyanotic Fallot)
   c. Pulmonic stenosis with patent ductus arteriosus
3. Pulmonic stenosis (valvular or infundibular or both) with veno-arterial shunt
   a. Pulmonic stenosis with ventricular septal defect (hemodynamically similar to tetralogy of Fallot)
   b. Pulmonic stenosis with reversed interatrial shunt (through patent foramen ovale or atrial septal defect)

SIMPLE VALVULAR PULMONIC STENOSIS

In this, the commonest type of isolated pulmonic stenosis, the valve cusps exist as a dome-shaped membrane of varying thickness with a small central or eccentric opening. The ventricular and atrial septa are intact.

HEMODYNAMICS. The obstruction to passage of blood from the right ventricle to the pulmonary artery results in increased systolic pressure and hypertrophy of the right ventricle. The degree of these changes depends on the degree of pulmonic stenosis. In severe cases right ventricular pressure may be much higher than systemic systolic pressure. Pulmonary artery pressure is low or normal. Arterial oxygen saturation is normal, and in severe cases the cardiac output is low and fixed.

CLINICAL MANIFESTATIONS. With mild or moderate pulmonic stenosis there are usually no symptoms. If the stenosis is severe, there is usually some degree of effort dyspnea, and exercise tolerance may be reduced to walking a few yards. Squatting may occur, but is not as common as with tetralogy of Fallot. Substernal pain and effort syncope are rare manifestations in severe cases.

The physique is frequently normal. The facies of patients with a severe type of pulmonic stenosis have been described as being round, bloated or moon-shaped. Pulmonary stenosis, frequently with a dysplastic valve, is the common abnormality in *Noonan syndrome.*

With *stenosis of a mild degree* the venous pressure and pulse are normal. The heart is not enlarged; the apical impulse is normal and the right ventricle is not palpable. A loud pulmonary systolic ejection murmur, frequently accompanied by a thrill, is audible maximally over the pulmonic area. The murmur is usually preceded by a pulmonic ejection sound. The second heart sound is

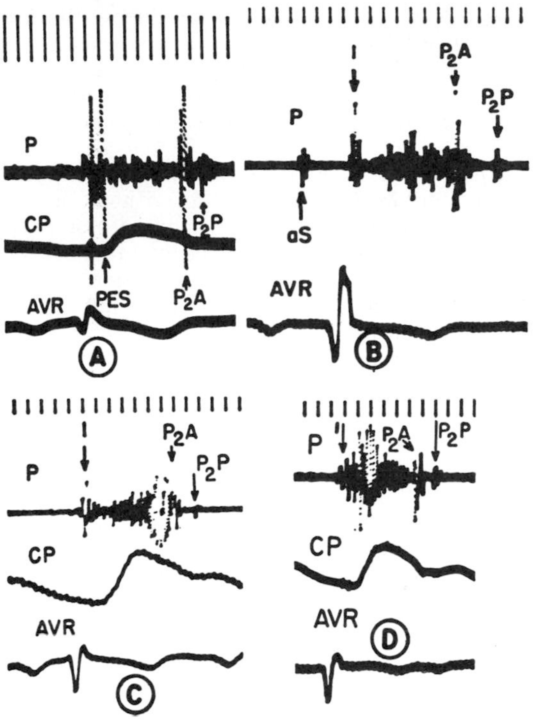

Figure 13–41 *Phonocardiograms to illustrate auscultatory findings in valvular pulmonic stenosis of varying severity. Abbreviations: P, Pulmonary area; CP, carotid pulse; AVR, electrocardiogram; PES, pulmonic ejection sound; P_2A, aortic component of second sound; P_2P, pulmonary component of second sound; aS, atrial sound. Time lines 0.04 second.*

A, Mild pulmonic stenosis. *Ejection sound followed by midsystolic murmur. Second sound split with delayed, diminished pulmonic component.* B, Severe pulmonic stenosis. *Systolic murmur accentuated in late systole and extends beyond P_2A. P_2P delayed and diminished.* C, Severe pulmonic stenosis (preoperative). *Compare with* B. D, *Same patient as in* C, *1 week postoperative. Murmur is now in early systole and midsystole. P_2P more accentuated and closer to P_2A. Compare with* A.

split, with a delayed pulmonary element of normal intensity (Fig. 13–41). The electrocardiogram is normal, or reveals minimal right ventricular hypertrophy. The only abnormality on roentgenographic examination is poststenotic dilatation of the pulmonary artery. The heart size, the right ventricle and the pulmonary vascularity are within normal limits.

In *stenosis of a moderate degree* the physical signs are those described above with variable exaggeration. The venous pressure may be slightly elevated, with an intrinsic "a" wave. A right ventricular sternal lift may be palpable. The systolic ejection murmur is accentuated in later systole, and a pulmonic ejection sound may or may not be present. The second heart sound is split, with a delayed and diminished pulmonary component. The electrocardiogram reveals varying degrees of right ventricular hypertrophy (systolic overload), sometimes with a prominent spiked P wave. Roentgenographic examination reveals the heart to be normal in size or mildly enlarged, owing to prominence of the right ventricle; intrapulmonary vascularity may be decreased.

In *stenosis of a severe degree* peripheral cyanosis is sometimes present, owing to a small cardiac output, to compensatory vasoconstriction and to sluggish blood flow through the skin. The arterial oxygen saturation is normal. The venous pressure is usually elevated, owing to a large presystolic jugular "a" wave, which is sometimes transmitted to the liver as a presystolic pulsation. Occasionally a large jugular "c" wave is evident and is due to functional tricuspid incompetence. The heart is moderately or greatly enlarged, with a conspicuous sternal and parasternal right ventricular lift which frequently extends to the midclavicular line. A loud systolic ejection murmur, frequently accompanied by a thrill, is audible maximally in the pulmonic area and may radiate widely over the whole precordium, into the neck and to the back. The murmur has late systolic accentuation, frequently encompasses the aortic component of the second sound, and is sometimes preceded by an ejection sound. The pulmonary element of the second sound is either inaudible or very late and soft. A right atrial presystolic gallop is usually heard in the presence of a large venous "a" wave. The electrocardiogram shows gross right ventricular hypertrophy frequently accompanied by a tall spiked P wave (**P pulmonale**). *Roentgenographic studies* confirm the moderate or gross cardiac enlargement with prominence of the right ventricle and atrium. The pulmonary artery segment is prominent, owing to poststenotic dilatation (Fig. 13–42). The intrapulmonary vascularity is decreased.

Cardiac catheterization demonstrates an abrupt gradient of pressure across the pulmonary valve, the magnitude of which depends on the severity of obstruction. The pulmonary arterial pressure is normal or low. The right ventricular systolic pressure is about 30 to 50 mm Hg in mild cases, about 50 to 100 mm in moderate cases, and in severe

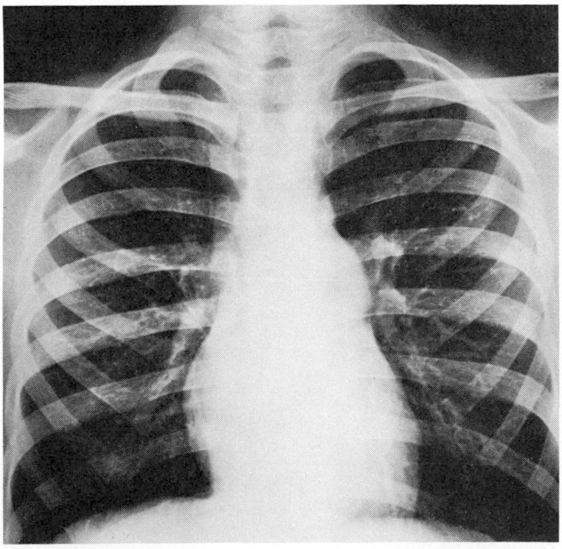

Figure 13–42 *Teleroentgenogram in valvular pulmonic stenosis with normal aortic root. The heart size is within normal limits, but there is poststenotic dilatation of pulmonary artery.*

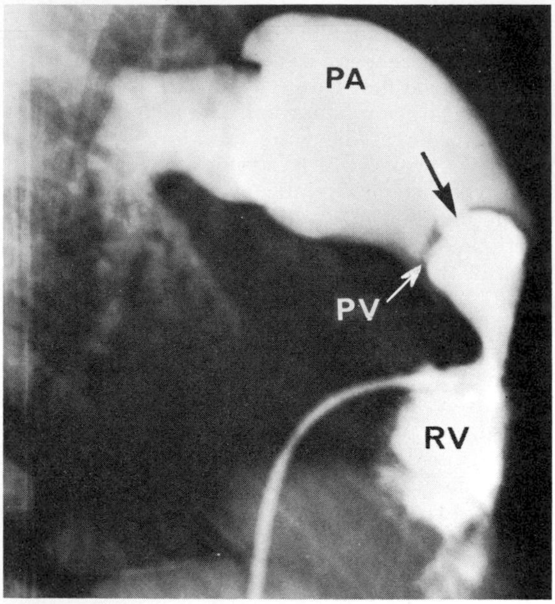

Figure 13-43 *Lateral projection of selective right ventriculogram in severe valvular pulmonic stenosis. Arrow points to jet of contrast medium through minute opening of pulmonary valve. Subvalvular infundibular hypertrophy is also present. Abbreviations: PV, thickened pulmonary valve; PA, poststenotic dilatation of pulmonary artery; RV, right ventricle.*

cases is frequently higher than the systemic systolic pressure. In severe and in some moderate cases the right atrial pressure shows a prominent, frequently giant, "a" wave (Fig. 13-45). *Selective right ventriculography* clearly demonstrates the obstruction. The flow of contrast medium through the stenotic valve in ventricular systole produces a jet of dye which fills the dilated pulmonary artery. The abnormal pulmonary valve is frequently visible. Subvalvular hypertrophy, which may intensify the obstruction, is also demonstrated (Fig. 13-43). This study also indicates that the ventricular septum is intact.

COMPLICATIONS. Congestive cardiac failure, the most common complication, occurs only in severe cases and at any age, even during the first month of life. The development of cyanosis from a right-to-left shunt across a foramen ovale is described below under Pulmonic Stenosis with Venoarterial Shunt. Subacute bacterial endocarditis is not common.

COURSE AND PROGNOSIS. Children with mild stenosis can lead a normal life without specific treatment, as may many with moderate stenosis, although their progress should be evaluated at regular intervals. Progression of obstruction to right ventricular outflow is indicated by change in the systolic murmur with the development of late systolic accentuation. Generally, there is good correlation between the width of splitting of the second heart sound and peak right ventricular pressure, so that the duration of split (in milliseconds) approximates the peak pressure (mm Hg); e.g., right ventricular systolic pressure is about 80 mm Hg when the duration of split of the second sound is 80 msec. Progressive electrocardiographic signs of right ventricular hypertrophy also indicate increasing obstruction to right ventricular outflow. With severe stenosis the course is rapidly downhill, with the development of congestive cardiac failure. Even newborn infants with severe stenosis require surgical treatment as promptly as possible.

TREATMENT. As indicated above, mild cases and many of moderate severity do not require specific treatment, and such patients should be encouraged to lead normal lives. Dental, ear, nose and throat surgery must be covered with prophylactic penicillin as described in Table 9-14.

All patients with severe isolated pulmonic stenosis require surgical therapy (*pulmonary valvotomy*). During cardiopulmonary bypass the valve is approached through an arteriotomy in the pulmonary artery. The valve leaflets are separated by incisions at the fused commissures.

Good results should be obtained in the majority of instances (Fig. 13-44). The gradient across the pulmonary valve is reduced or abolished. A pulmonary diastolic murmur due to surgically created pulmonary valvular incompetence is not unusual, but appears to have little clinical significance.

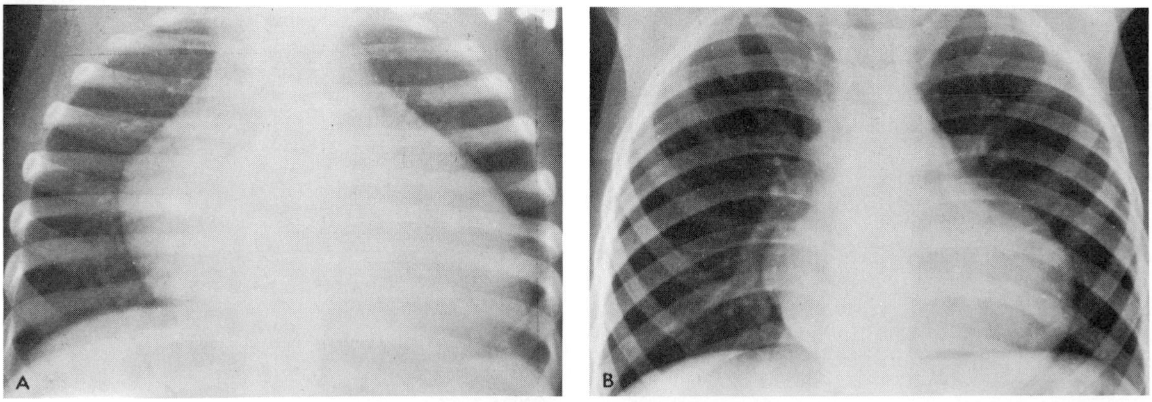

Figure 13-44 *Teleroentgenograms in an infant with valvular pulmonic stenosis.* A, *Preoperative, showing massive cardiomegaly;* B, *2 years after operation, showing decrease in heart size.*

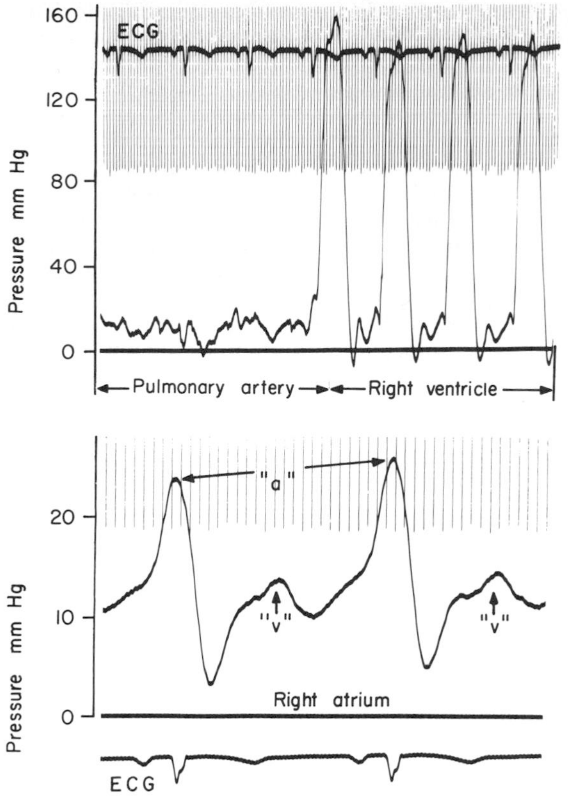

Figure 13–45 *Pressure curves in severe valvular pulmonic stenosis.* Top, *Pressure record as catheter is withdrawn from pulmonary artery to right ventricle demonstrates a high peak systolic pressure gradient.* Bottom, *Right atrial pressure curve shows prominence of "a" wave.*

INFUNDIBULAR STENOSIS

This condition is due to failure of involution of the bulbus cordis, resulting in a muscular or fibrous obstruction in the outflow tract of the right ventricle. The site of obstruction may be close to the pulmonary valve or well below it; an infundibular chamber is present between the right ventricular cavity and the pulmonary valve. When the pulmonary valve is abnormal (*combined valvular and infundibular stenosis*), the infundibular stenosis is frequently due to hypertrophy of the right ventricular outflow tract secondary to pulmonary valvular stenosis.

The *hemodynamics* and *clinical manifestations* are similar to those described under Simple Valvular Pulmonic Stenosis with the following exceptions: (1) The systolic thrill and murmur are frequently maximal in the third and fourth left parasternal spaces, but radiate widely. The murmur is long and seldom preceded by an ejection sound, and pulmonary valvular closure is soft and delayed. (2) Poststenotic dilatation of the pulmonary artery may be present, but is not usual. (3) With an infundibular chamber and valvular pulmonic stenosis, two pressure gradients may be noted during cardiac catheterization: between the right ventricle and the infundibular chamber and between it and the pulmonary artery. (4) Selective angiocardiography can be diagnostic in the majority of instances. When contrast material is injected into the right ventricle, the site of the infundibular stenosis is demonstrated, the presence of an infundibular chamber is evident, and associated abnormalities of the pulmonary valve are shown. It is important to prove that the ventricular septum is intact because the clinical picture of isolated infundibular stenosis closely mimics that of acyanotic tetralogy of Fallot.

The complications, course and prognosis are similar to those described under Simple Valvular Pulmonic Stenosis.

In severe cases surgical treatment is indicated. The infundibular stenosis is relieved under direct vision, and a pulmonary valvuloplasty performed if there is associated pulmonic stenosis. After operation the pressure gradients are reduced or abolished.

PULMONIC STENOSIS WITH ARTERIOVENOUS SHUNT

Valvular or infundibular pulmonic stenosis, or both, may be associated with a left-to-right shunt across an atrial septal defect, a ventricular septal defect or a patent ductus arteriosus. The clinical features depend on the degree of stenosis and the magnitude of the left-to-right shunt.

PULMONIC STENOSIS AND ATRIAL SEPTAL DEFECT. In patients with dominant valvular pulmonic stenosis and a small left-to-right shunt across an atrial septal defect, the clinical picture is indistinguishable from that described under Simple Valvular Pulmonic Stenosis. If the shunt across the atrial defect is large and the pulmonic stenosis slight, the clinical manifestations are similar to those described under Atrial Septal Defect, but the systolic murmur is harsh and frequently accompanied by a thrill. The diagnosis can be made during cardiac catheterization when a left-to-right shunt is demonstrated at the atrial level, and the pulmonic stenosis is shown by the presence of a pressure gradient across the valve. Selective angiocardiography also shows the presence of pulmonic stenosis, and indicator dilution curves confirm the left-to-right shunt across the atrial defect.

PULMONIC STENOSIS AND VENTRICULAR SEPTAL DEFECT. When the ventricular septal defect is dominant and the pulmonic stenosis is slight, the clinical picture is that of ventricular septal defect, and the presence of pulmonic stenosis is not recognizable. During cardiac catheterization, however, a gradient is demonstrated across the pulmonary valve, and the left-to-right shunt is demonstrated at the ventricular level. The recognition of a small ventricular septal defect with dominant valvular or infundibular pulmonic stenosis is also difficult. Rarely in patients with ventricular septal defects, progressive ventricular hypertrophy may result in the development of infundibular pulmonic stenosis, which obscures the presence of the septal defect. Even during cardiac catheterization the small shunt across the ventricular defect may not be demonstrated, and the diagnosis of isolated pulmonic stenosis may be made erroneously. Selective left ventriculography proves whether the ventricular septum is intact.

PULMONIC STENOSIS AND PATENT DUCTUS ARTERIOSUS. In addition to the signs of pulmonic stenosis, a machinery murmur is audible over the pulmonic area. This combination of anomalies is suspected in patients with the signs of patent ductus arteriosus and right ventricular hypertrophy. Pulmonary atresia is excluded by the absence of cyanosis and the presence of poststenotic dilatation of the pulmonary artery.

TREATMENT. These anomalies are treated by direct-vision surgery. Defects in the atrial or ventricular septa are closed and the pulmonic stenosis is relieved by infundibular resection or pulmonary valvuloplasty. If the ductus is patent, it is divided during the same procedure. Surgery is recommended only for severe or progressive cases. If operation is successful, the left-to-right shunt is obliterated, and the gradient across the valve is reduced or abolished.

PULMONIC STENOSIS WITH VENO-ARTERIAL SHUNT

WITH ATRIAL SEPTAL DEFECT OR PATENT FORAMEN OVALE (TRILOGY OF FALLOT). As indicated above, patients with moderate or severe valvular or infundibular stenosis have right ventricular systolic hypertension. If, in addition, the right atrium has difficulty in emptying during right ventricular diastole (which occurs during right atrial systole), the right atrial pressure rises. This results in reversal of the shunt to a right-to-left one across the atrial septal defect and in cyanosis. A similar sequence of events occurs if the foramen ovale is patent.

Cyanosis may be present at birth or appear later, frequently during adolescence, and is accompanied by clubbing of the digits and polycythemia. The jugular venous pressure is increased in many instances, with an intrinsic "a" wave. Other physical signs and technical data are similar to those described under severe valvular pulmonic stenosis. The right-to-left shunt produces arterial oxygen unsaturation.

Surgical therapy is required in all cases and consists in valvotomy and closure of the atrial septal defect.

WITH VENTRICULAR SEPTAL DEFECT. This condition is similar to tetralogy of Fallot (see earlier).

PULMONARY ARTERIAL BRANCH STENOSIS

Single or multiple constrictions may occur anywhere along the major branches of the pulmonary artery. The type and degree of stenosis vary from mild and localized to extensive and multiple. This condition may occur as an isolated anomaly, but frequently is associated with other types of congenital heart disease, especially pulmonary valvular stenosis, tetralogy of Fallot, patent ductus arteriosus, ventricular septal defect, atrial septal defect and supravalvular aortic stenosis. A familial tendency has been recognized in some patients with peripheral stenosis. A high incidence has been found in infants with the congenital rubella syndrome. Supravalvular aortic stenosis with pulmonary arterial branch stenosis has been observed with idiopathic hypercalcemia of infancy.

If the constriction is mild, there is little effect on the pulmonary circulation. In patients with multiple severe constrictions there is an increase in pressure in the right ventricle and pulmonary artery proximal to the site of obstruction. When the anomaly is isolated, the diagnosis is suspected by the presence of murmurs in unusual locations over the chest, anteriorly or posteriorly. These murmurs are usually midsystolic, but may be continuous or systolic and diastolic. Frequently the physical signs are dominated by the associated anomaly, e.g., tetralogy of Fallot. If the stenosis is severe, there is electrocardiographic evidence of right ventricular and right atrial hypertrophy.

Cardiomegaly and prominence of the main pulmonary artery are present in severe lesions. Generally, the pulmonary vasculature is normal; in some cases small intrapulmonary vascular shadows are seen which may be shown by pulmonary arteriography to be areas of poststenotic dilatation. Pressure gradients across the areas of obstruction are demonstrable by cardiac catheterization. These gradients may not be easily identified if right ventricular outflow obstruction coexists, since the pressure in the main pulmonary artery is normal or low in such patients. In severe bilateral pulmonary arterial branch stenosis without other malformations the pulse pressure curve from the pulmonary artery shows a deep dicrotic notch and a flattened diastolic descent. Severe obstructions of the main pulmonary artery and its primary branches should be resected. This is especially important during corrective surgery for Fallot's tetralogy or valvular pulmonic stenosis.

PULMONARY VALVULAR INSUFFICIENCY

Pulmonary valvular insufficiency usually accompanies other cardiovascular diseases, especially those which result in severe pulmonary hypertension. Incompetence of the valve is also frequent after surgery for right ventricular outflow obstruction, e.g., pulmonary valvotomy and infundibular resection. Isolated congenital incompetence of the pulmonary valve is rare and usually is asymptomatic, since the incompetence is mild. The prominent abnormal sign is a diastolic murmur at the upper left sternal border which simulates in quality the murmur of aortic incompetence. In pulmonary incompetence, however, the murmur may start later, has a lower pitch and may increase in intensity during inspiration. Roentgenograms of the chest show prominence of the main pulmonary artery. The electrocardiogram is normal or shows minimal right ventricular hypertrophy. The diagnosis is confirmed by cardiac catheterization, which demonstrates a low pulmonary arterial diastolic pressure. Selective pulmonary arteriography shows the incompetent valve, and intracardiac phonocardiography identifies systolic and diastolic murmurs in the region of the pulmonic valve and outflow tract of the right ventricle. Aortography excludes the presence of aortic incompetence. Generally, isolated pulmonary valvular incompetence is well tolerated and does not require treatment other than prophylactic measures against bacterial endocarditis (Table 9–14).

Absence of the pulmonic valve is usually associated with other defects, especially tetralogy of Fallot and ventricular septal defect. The pulmonary arteries become markedly dilated and compress the bronchi, resulting in recurrent episodes of wheezing, pulmonary collapse and pneumonitis. Florid pulmonary valvular incompetence is not well tolerated, and death may occur in infancy from bronchial compression and heart failure. Though a homograft valve may be inserted at the time of correction of the ventricular defect and infundibular stenosis, gross dilatation of the pulmonary arteries remains.

COARCTATION OF THE AORTA

Constrictions of varying length may occur at any point between the arch and the bifurcation of the aorta, but 98 per cent of them occur as a localized stricture just below the origin of the left subclavian artery. They are about twice as frequent in males as in females. Coarctation of the aorta occurs frequently in Turner (XO) syndrome.

HEMODYNAMICS. Owing to the obstruction of the aorta, extensive collateral circulation usually develops, chiefly from the branches of the subclavian artery, the superior intercostal artery and the internal mammary with its intercostal, superior epigastric and musculophrenic branches. The thoracic and subscapular branches of the axillary artery may also enlarge as collateral channels. These vessels unite with the intercostal branches of the descending aorta and inferior epigastric branches of the femoral artery to create a channel for arterial blood to bypass the area of coarctation. The vessels contributing to the collateral circulation become enormously enlarged and tortuous by early adulthood.

The blood pressure is elevated in the vessels arising proximal to the coarctation; below it the amplitude of pulsation is diminished, and the pressure below the constriction is lower than that above it. The basis for the hypertension is not clear. It does not appear to be due to the mechanical obstruction alone, nor does renal ischemia play a large role.

CLINICAL MANIFESTATIONS. Although incapacitating symptoms are not usual during the first decade of life, they may develop at any age and are the result of the hypertensive state, decreased myocardial performance or a deficient circulation in the legs. Hypertension may result in epistaxes and throbbing headaches, and the symptoms of left ventricular or frank congestive cardiac failure may occur secondary to the hypertensive state. Cerebral hemorrhages are not uncommon. Deficient circulation to the legs may be evidenced by cold feet and, occasionally, by intermittent claudication.

The classic sign of coarctation of the aorta is the disparity in pulsations and blood pressures between the arms and legs. The femoral, popliteal, posterior tibial and dorsalis pedis pulsations are weak and delayed or absent, in contrast with the bounding pulses of the arms and carotid vessels. In normal persons the systolic blood pressure in the legs as obtained by the cuff method is about 20 to 40 mm Hg higher than that in the arms. In coarctation of the aorta the blood pressure in the legs is much lower than that obtained in the arms; frequently it cannot be obtained. Elevation of blood pressure in the arms may appear at any age from infancy, but hypertension of some degree is the rule in older patients. There is also a rise of blood pressure in response to exercise. It is essential to determine the blood pressure in both arms; a difference of more than 30 mm between the right and left arms suggests involvement of the left subclavian artery in the area of coarctation.

The collateral arterial circulation may give rise to visible and palpable pulsations and to systolic murmurs, especially in the back between the scapulae and at their angles. These signs are usually more striking after the first decade of life, as is cardiac enlargement with a left ventricular apical impulse. Murmurs are variable in location, intensity and quality and are not diagnostic. The common murmur is systolic in time, ejection in nature and maximal over the base of the heart; it radiates down the sternum to the apex and to the interscapular area and frequently is loudest in the back. The murmur may be produced by the coarctation, by tortuous collateral vessels, by abnormalities of the aortic valve or by associated structural anomalies of the heart such as septal defects. Occasionally there is also a diastolic element, which may be due to associated congenital or rheumatic aortic insufficiency; it is heard best over the base of the heart and down the left sternal border. A continuous murmur over the pulmonic area radiating to the left clavicle suggests an associated patent ductus arteriosus. Rarely a diastolic murmur is heard in the back. A rumbling, apical diastolic murmur of uncertain origin may also be present.

The findings on *roentgenographic examination* depend on the age of the patient and on the effects of hypertension and collateral circulation. In infancy there are usually no changes except cardiac enlargement if congestive cardiac failure develops. During childhood the findings are not striking except when the left ventricle is prominent. After the first decade the heart tends to be mildly or moderately enlarged, owing to left ventricular prominence. The enlarged left subclavian artery commonly produces a prominent shadow in the left superior mediastinum. Notching of the inferior border of the ribs due to pressure erosion from enlarged collateral vessels is common by late childhood, except in the upper or lower two or three ribs. Rarely erosion is unilateral and is due to one of the subclavian arteries arising below the area of coarctation. In the majority of instances there is an area of poststenotic dilatation of the descending aorta. This may be manifest by displacement of the barium-filled esophagus and by discontinuity of the lateral margin of the aorta below the arch (Fig. 13–46). Prominent serrations on the posterior aspect of the barium-filled esophagus suggest the presence of large intercostal arteries entering the aorta below the coarctation. Occasionally scalloping in the soft tissues may be seen retrosternally; it is due to dilated internal mammary arteries.

The *electrocardiogram* is usually normal in children but may reveal evidences of left ventricular hypertrophy and occasionally of left bundle branch block. In scalar tracings, right ventricular hypertrophy may be erroneously diagnosed because of prominence of primary or secondary R waves in the right precordium. This finding is related to the rightward and posterior maximum QRS vector. This pattern is probably the result of hypertrophy of the posterobasal portion of the left ventricle or is a manifestation of left posterior hemiblock.

Most often the diagnosis can be made by physical examination. Routine examination of all hypertensive subjects and of all infants in whom cardiovascular defects are suspected should include palpation of all the major accessible peripheral arteries. This simple maneuver should make the correct diagnosis obvious. The segment of coarctation can be demonstrated by aortography (Fig. 13–47) or angiocardiography, but these are seldom indicated except when the site of coarctation is considered to be unusual, e.g., involvement of the abdominal aorta.

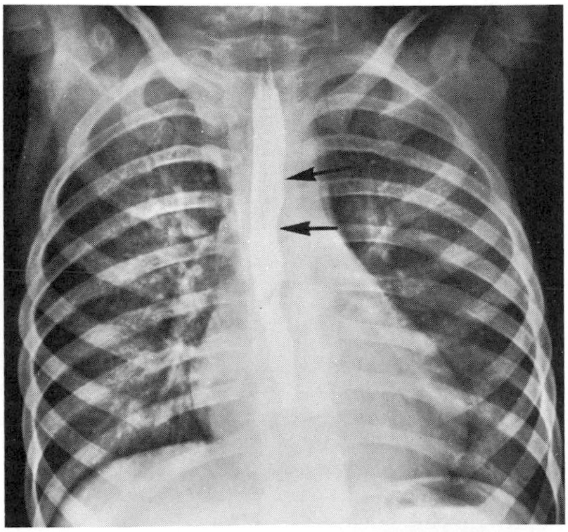

Figure 13–46 *Teleroentgenogram of a 6 year old boy with coarctation of the aorta. The barium-filled esophagus shows indentations produced by the aortic knob and left subclavian artery* (upper arrow) *and poststenotic dilatation* (lower arrow). *These two indentations produce the E sign. The left ventricle is prominent, but there is no evidence of rib notching.*

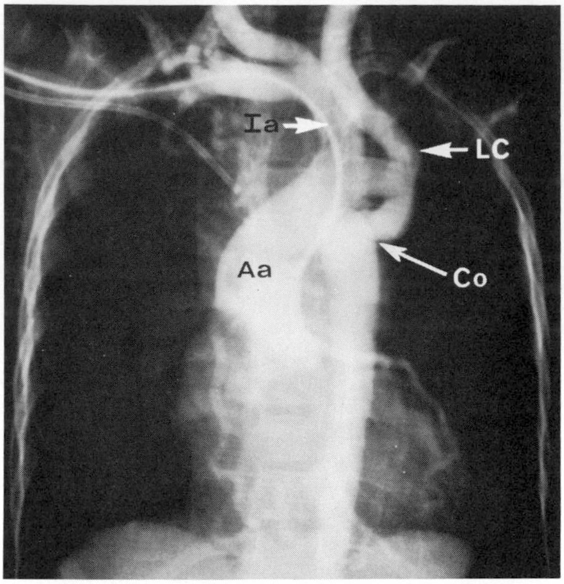

Figure 13–47 *Aortogram in coarctation of the aorta. The left subclavian artery was hypoplastic and at operation was found to arise at the site of coarctation. Abbreviations: Aa, ascending aorta; Ia, innominate artery; LC, left carotid artery; Co, site of coarctation.*

ASSOCIATED ABNORMALITIES. Associated defects may produce gross physical signs which allow a correct diagnosis. Aortic valve abnormalities are said to occur in 70 per cent of patients. Bicuspid aortic valves are common, but usually do not produce signs unless aortic incompetence or stenosis develops. Rheumatic mitral stenosis and aortic insufficiency are rare complications. The association of patent ductus arteriosus and coarctation of the aorta is discussed later. Ventricular and atrial septal defects may be suspected by the additional signs of left-to-right shunt.

Severe neurologic damage or even death may occur from associated cerebral vascular disease. Subarachnoid or intracerebral hemorrhage may result from rupture of congenital aneurysms in the circle of Willis, of other vessels with defective elastic and medial tissue or of normal vessels; these accidents are secondary to the hypertensive state. Abnormalities of the subclavian arteries may also occur and include involvement of the left subclavian artery in the area of coarctation, stenosis of the orifice of the left subclavian artery and anomalous origin of the right subclavian artery.

PROGNOSIS AND COMPLICATIONS. The majority of untreated patients with coarctation of the aorta succumb between the ages of 20 and 40 years, though some may live well into middle life without serious handicap. Symptoms may appear in infancy and are nearly always present by the age of 25 years. The common serious complications are related to the hypertensive state, which may result in congestive cardiac failure or intracranial hemorrhage. Heart failure is frequently related to complicating anomalies, e.g., bicuspid aortic valve with aortic stenosis or insufficiency. Subacute bacterial endocarditis or endarteritis is also a frequent complication and most commonly involves abnormal aortic valves. Rupture of the aorta may occur and is due to defective elastic and medial tissue. Aneurysms of the descending aorta or of the enlarged collateral vessels are not unusual. The natural course in the individual case is unpredictable.

TREATMENT. In view of the natural course of coarctation of the aorta, most patients should be treated surgically. The optimum age for operation is between 8 and 15 years, because at this time the aorta has good elasticity and few if any degenerative changes, the lumen after anastomosis is adequate to carry the patient through adult life, and the mortality rate at this age is less than 2 per cent. After the second decade the operation is more hazardous, owing to decreased cardiac reserve and degenerative changes or even aneurysms around the area of coarctation. Nevertheless, if the cardiac reserve is sufficient, the condition may be satisfactorily repaired well into midadult life. The mortality rate in this age group is about 5 per cent. Associated valvular lesions producing severe hemodynamic changes greatly increase the hazards of surgery.

The operation of choice is excision of the area of coarctation and primary anastomosis. If the length of aortic constriction does not allow primary anastomosis, Dacron grafts may be used.

After operation there is a striking improvement in the amplitude of pulsations in the femoral artery. Patients may note a definite increase in the temperature of their legs. Headaches and epistaxes disappear, and symptoms of cardiac failure are improved. The relief of hypertension may be delayed for 3 or 4 weeks. Murmurs may not disappear after operation; they are probably due to persistent enlargement of the collateral vessels or to aortic valvular disease.

THE POSTCOARCTECTOMY SYNDROME

Postoperative mesenteric arteritis may cause hypertension with abdominal pain in the immediate postoperative period. The pain varies in severity and may subside without treatment. In other instances it is associated with anorexia, nausea, vomiting, leukocytosis and even signs of small bowel obstruction. These patients usually respond to therapy with antihypertensive drugs and intestinal decompression; corticosteroids may help to alleviate the symptoms and thus avoid surgical exploration for bowel obstruction.

Although most patients are asymptomatic for many years after operation, they should continue to be observed because of the frequency of associated aortic valve abnormalities. Also, hypertension may persist or recur after many years, and the blood pressure response to exercise is abnormal (systolic hypertension and wide pulse pressure).

THE COARCTATION SYNDROME OF INFANCY

In infancy, especially under the age of 1 month, coarctation of the aorta is a common cause of heart failure. The lesion is frequently associated with other cardiovascular anomalies, including patent ductus arteriosus, ventricular and atrial septal defects, aortic valvular disease and transposition of the great vessels. Endocardial sclerosis may complicate the picture in older infants with isolated coarctation. The clinical picture is variable and depends on the effects of the associated malformations and on the pulmonary vascular resistance. In *isolated coarctation* the classic signs described earlier are present. Femoral pulses are delayed or absent and systemic hypertension may be significant. In the presence of a *large ventricular septal defect*, pulmonary blood flow is increased and pulmonary hypertension is usual. These infants are seriously ill, with signs of heart failure and pulmonary edema superimposed on those produced by both the coarctation and ventricular septal defect. However, this clinical picture is variable, since the reaction of the pulmonary vascular bed is labile, with hypoxemia resulting in pulmonary vasoconstriction. Critical left ventricular outflow obstruction produced by complicating stenosis of the *aortic valve* may be associated with endocardial sclerosis and a thick-walled left ventricle with a small cavity. These patients are critically ill, with severe congestive cardiac failure and pulmonary edema. *Coarctation of the aorta and transposition of the great arteries* may result in differential cyanosis, the lower body being less cyanotic than the upper in patients with an associated *patent ductus arteriosus*, which is frequent.

Many anatomic and physiologic classifications have been devised in an attempt to describe the nature of the coexisting abnormalities. The anatomic classifications depend on the site and length of coarctation, the site of the aortic opening of the ductus and the size of the aorta proximal to the coarctation. The direction of blood flow across the ductus depends primarily on the pulmonary vascular resistance. If the pulmonary vascular resistance is lower than the systemic resistance, the shunt is from aorta to pulmonary artery. This occurs irrespective of the site of aortic opening of the ductus in relation to the coarctation. In babies with a large ductus inserting distal to the coarctation and with greatly elevated pulmonary vascular resistance, right ventricular blood is ejected through the ductus to the descending aorta. Thus, the clinical picture in these babies is confusing, since femoral pulses are readily palpable (because the right ventricle is acting as a systemic ventricle) and one of the cardinal signs of coarctation is absent.

Symptoms occur early and include dyspnea, cyanosis, superimposed pulmonary infections and feeding difficulties. Congestive cardiac failure also occurs early. Because the descending aorta is supplied with venous blood, differential cyanosis may be expected below the pelvic brim and a normal color of the upper half of the body. Unfortunately this sign is not always conspicuous, even if carefully looked for. The heart is enlarged. The murmur is systolic, is heard over the whole precordium and is usually followed by a loud second sound. The electrocardiogram shows right ventricular hypertrophy. Roentgen examination confirms the cardiac enlargement and also reveals increased pulmonary vascularity.

The prognosis of the coarctation syndrome of infancy is poor and therapy difficult. Intensive medical therapy includes the judicious use of digitalis, diuretics and other anticongestive measures. Hypoglycemia is frequent and has been attributed to compromise of hepatic arterial perfusion as a result of intermittent or permanent closure of the ductus. If there is no response to therapy or if there is recurrence of symptoms with progression of heart failure, surgical therapy is undertaken even though the risk is high. It consists of resection of the coarctation, division of the ductus arteriosus, and pulmonary artery banding if severe hyperkinetic pulmonary hypertension is due to a large ventricular septal defect. Congestive cardiac failure due to isolated coarctation may respond to medical therapy alone, so that surgery can be postponed to late childhood, but significant hypertension during infancy may require treatment, usually with diuretics.

ANOMALOUS PULMONARY VENOUS RETURN

Abnormal development of the pulmonary veins may result in their anomalous drainage into the systemic venous circulation. The abnormal entry may be into the right atrium, into the superior or inferior vena cava or one of their major tributaries or into a persistent left superior vena cava which opens into the coronary sinus. The pulmonary veins may join a common trunk which enters the venous circulation infradiaphragmatically (portal vein, ductus venosus or inferior vena cava). An associated atrial septal defect is frequently present. All or only part of the pulmonary venous return may empty into the systemic venous circulation.

PARTIAL ANOMALOUS PULMONARY VENOUS RETURN. A varying number of pulmonary veins may enter the systemic venous circulation or right atrium. This results in a left-to-right shunt of oxygenated blood, which is increased if there is an associated atrial septal defect. Partial anomalous pulmonary venous return usually involves some or all of the veins of only one lung, more frequently the right (see Sinus Venosus Defect). The history, physical signs, electrocardiogram and roentgenographic findings are indistinguishable from those of atrial septal defect (ostium secundum). Occasionally an anomalous vein draining into the inferior vena cava is visible radiologically as a crescentic shadow of vascular density along the right border of the cardiac silhouette.

During *cardiac catheterization* the catheter may enter the anomalous pulmonary vein from the superior vena cava or right atrium or may traverse the associated atrial septal defect. The site of left-to-right shunt depends on the point of entry of the pulmonary veins and may be in the superior vena cava or right atrium. Frequently the oxygen content and saturation of the caval and right atrial blood are indistinguishable from those of atrial septal defect. Indicator dilution curves are valuable to demonstrate the presence of anomalous pulmonary veins. They may also be demonstrated by *selective pulmonary arteriography.*

The prognosis is similar to that for atrial septal defect (ostium secundum).

In symptomatic patients surgical therapy is indicated during cardiopulmonary bypass. An associated atrial septal defect should be closed in such a way as to direct the pulmonary venous return to the left atrium.

TOTAL ANOMALOUS PULMONARY VENOUS RETURN. There is no venous connection with the left atrium, and all the blood returning to the heart (the systemic and pulmonary venous blood) enters and mixes in the right atrium. Some of the blood passes into the right ventricle and pulmonary artery, and the remainder passes through an atrial septal defect or patent foramen ovale to the left atrium.

Usually the pulmonary veins form a single trunk before entering the systemic venous circulation at one of the following sites: left superior vena cava (43 per cent), coronary sinus (19 per cent), right atrium (14 per cent) and right superior vena cava (12 per cent) (Keith et al.). The remainder enter the portal vein or ductus venosus.

Most often symptoms occur during the first 2 years of life and include tachypnea, poor weight gain and congestive heart failure. Cyanosis may not be definite, especially in early life, but in some infants with undue elevation of pulmonary vascular resistance it may be striking. The left side of the chest is frequently protuberant and the heart enlarged. Gallop rhythm is usual. In early life, murmurs may not be audible, but in the majority of instances a systolic murmur is heard maximally down the left sternal border and may be followed by a diastolic murmur. A continuous murmur with the quality of a venous hum may be audible over the pulmonary area and sometimes under the right clavicle. Clinical signs of pulmonary edema may be present.

The *electrocardiogram* demonstrates right ventricular hypertrophy (usually a qR pattern in V_{4R} and V_1), and the P waves are frequently tall and spiked. *Roentgenograms* are pathognomonic if the pulmonary veins enter the innominate vein and

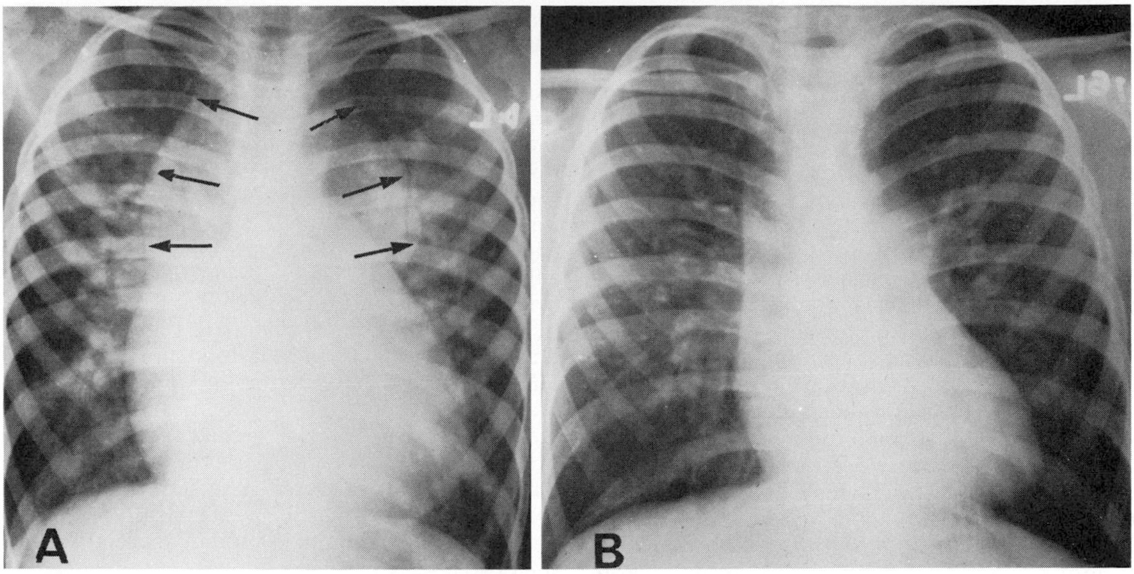

Figure 13–48 *Teleroentgenogram in total anomalous pulmonary venous return to the left superior vena cava.* A, *Preoperative. Arrows point to the supracardiac shadow, which produces the* snowman or figure-of-8 *configuration. Cardiomegaly and increased pulmonary vascularity are evident.* B, *Postoperative, showing decrease in size of the heart and supracardiac shadow.*

persistent left superior vena cava (Fig. 13–48). There is a large supracardiac shadow with a *figure-of-eight* or *snowman* appearance. The supracardiac shadow is produced by the dilated left superior vena cava, left innominate vein and right superior vena cava. If the pulmonary veins drain elsewhere, the heart is enlarged, the pulmonary artery and right ventricle are prominent, and the pulmonary vascularity is increased.

Cardiac catheterization shows that the oxygen saturation of blood in both atria, both ventricles and the aorta is more or less similar and higher than that of peripheral systemic venous blood. In older patients the pulmonary arterial and right ventricular pressures may be only moderately elevated, but in infancy pulmonary hypertension is usual. *Selective pulmonary arteriography* shows the anatomy of the pulmonary veins and their point of entry into the systemic venous circulation (Fig. 13–49).

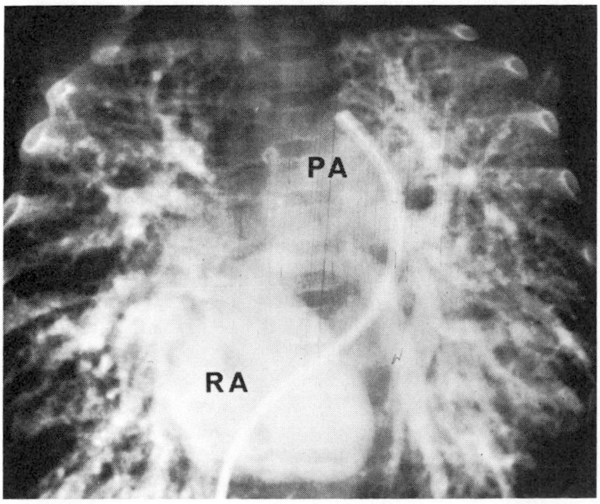

Figure 13–49 *Total anomalous pulmonary venous return to the coronary sinus. Injection of contrast medium into the pulmonary artery (PA) opacifies the pulmonary arterial tree. The contrast medium returns to the coronary sinus, which drains into the densely opacified right atrium (RA).*

The *prognosis* is usually poor, and survival beyond infancy is unusual; death is due to congestive heart failure. Patients who survive beyond 2 years of age may have surprisingly few symptoms. Surgical treatment is now possible and is undertaken preferably during cardiopulmonary bypass. The common pulmonary venous trunk is anastomosed to the left atrium, the atrial septal defect is closed, and the connection to the systemic venous circuit is obliterated. The surgical results are good in older children. The operative risk is high in symptomatic infants because of the hypoplastic left ventricle (which is unable to sustain cardiac output after correction) and poor lung compliance (due to pulmonary hypertension and edema). These babies present a therapeutic dilemma, since their prognosis is poor without operation and surgical risks are high.

INFRADIAPHRAGMATIC TOTAL ANOMALOUS PULMONARY VENOUS RETURN. The clinical picture of this anomaly differs somewhat from that described above. Symptoms are usually present within the first few months of life and are dominated by grayish cyanosis and signs of increased pulmonary venous pressure (pulmonary edema). Radiographically the heart may be normal in size, but the intrapulmonary vasculature is stippled because of prominent pulmonary veins and pulmonary edema; the chest films may superficially resemble those of newborn infants with hyaline membrane disease. The prognosis is extremely poor. This condition is potentially treatable by surgical anastomosis of the common pulmonary vein to the left atrium.

CONGENITAL AORTIC STENOSIS

Congenital aortic stenosis accounts for about 5 per cent of all cardiac malformations; it is more common in males (3:1). In the majority of instances the stenosis is valvular, the leaflets are thickened and the commissures fused in varying degrees. In others the stenosis is subvalvular (subaortic), with a discrete fibrous or muscular obstruction to the left ventricular outflow below the aortic valves. In rare instances the stenosis is supravalvular. Supravalvular aortic stenosis is sometimes associated with pulmonary arterial branch stenosis, and it may be sporadic, familial or associated with a syndrome of mental retardation and a typical facies (full face, broad forehead, flattened bridge of nose, long upper lip and rounded cheeks). Idiopathic hypercalcemia of infancy (see Section 22) has been associated with this syndrome (Fig. 13–50).

Most often the child with aortic stenosis is asymptomatic, the physical development is good, and the abnormality is discovered during routine physical examination. But with severe obstruction to left ventricular outflow, fatigue and effort intolerance may be present. In these patients, angina pectoris, dizziness, syncope or episodes of pulmonary edema as a result of left ventricular failure indicate the presence of critical aortic stenosis. The pulse is usually normal; it sometimes has a small volume and is anacrotic when obstruction is critical. The heart size and apical impulses are usually normal. In severe cases the heart may be enlarged, with a left ventricular apical thrust. A coarse, rasping systolic ejection murmur, usually accompanied by a thrill, is audible maximally in the aortic area and radiates to the neck and down the left sternal border and toward the apex. In some patients the systolic murmur may be maximal down the left sternal border or even at the apex, but retains its ejection nature. In valvular aortic stenosis the murmur is usually preceded by an aortic ejection click best heard at the apex and left sternal edge (Fig. 13–51). Clicks are unusual in discrete subaortic stenosis. Diastolic murmurs are not infrequent. Concomitant aortic insufficiency, which in some instances may dominate the picture, produces an aortic blowing diastolic murmur. Rarely an apical mid-diastolic rumbling murmur is audible in the presence of a normal mitral valve. The normal splitting of the second heart sound is present in mild cases. In patients with severe obstruction aortic valve closure is diminished, or the second sound may be split paradoxically. A prominent fourth heart sound is audible, especially when the obstruction is severe.

If the gradient of pressure across the aortic valve is small, the *electrocardiogram* is normal. It may also be normal in some children with severe obstruction, but evidence of left ventricular hypertrophy and strain is frequent in these patients. Children with severe obstruction and a normal electrocardiogram may have an abnormal vectorcardiogram. *Roentgenograms* (Fig. 13–52) may show signs of left ventricular enlargement. The ascending aorta is frequently prominent, but the aortic knob is normal. Valvular calcification has been noted even in children. *Left cardiac catheterization*

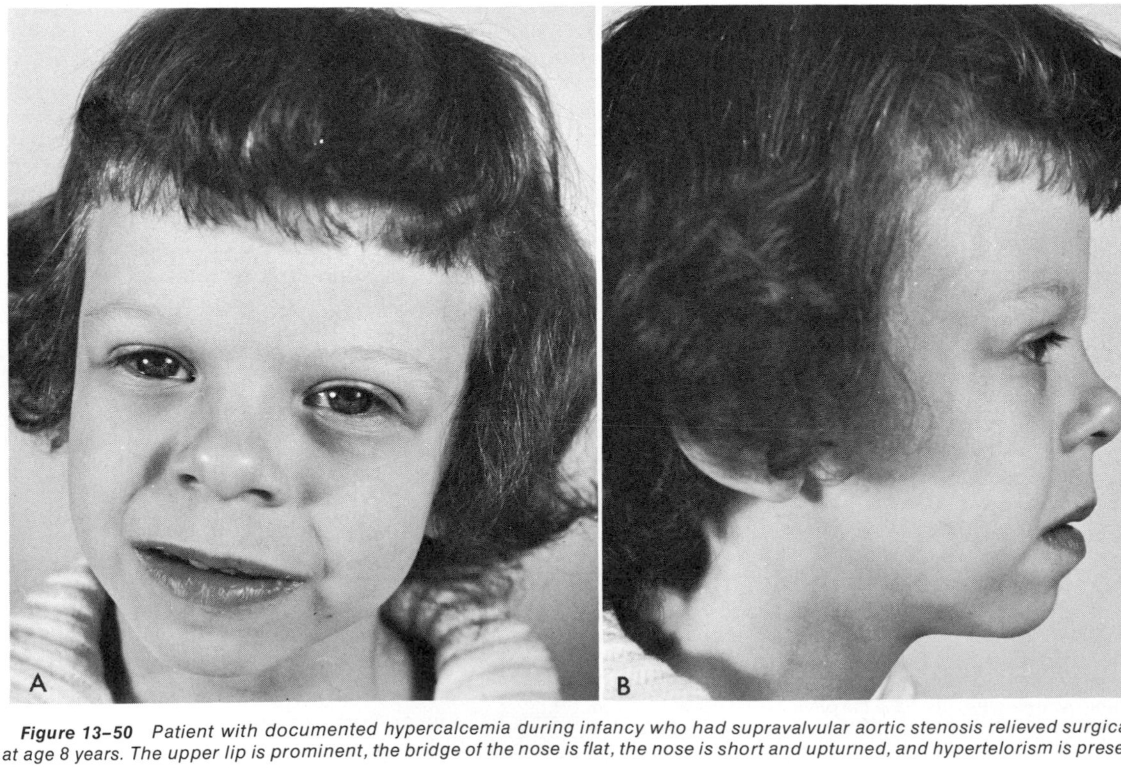

Figure 13–50 Patient with documented hypercalcemia during infancy who had supravalvular aortic stenosis relieved surgically at age 8 years. The upper lip is prominent, the bridge of the nose is flat, the nose is short and upturned, and hypertelorism is present.

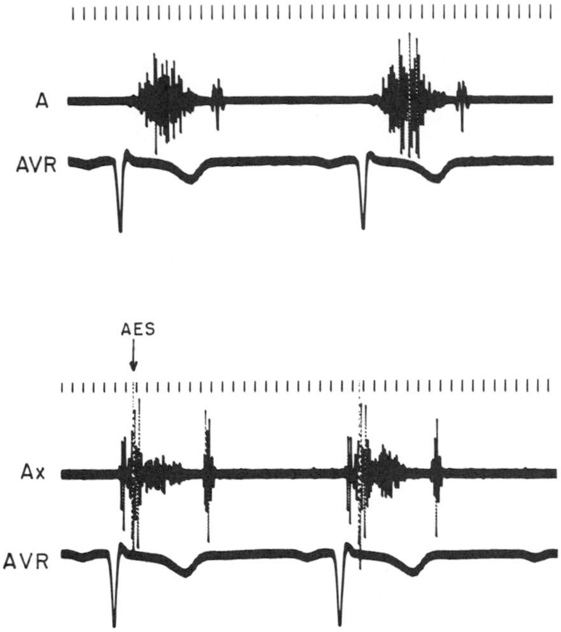

Figure 13–51 *Phonocardiogram to illustrate auscultatory findings in congenital aortic valvular stenosis. At the aortic area the systolic murmur is ejection in type. At the apex the systolic murmur is initiated by an aortic ejection sound. Abbreviations: A, aortic area; Ax, apex; AVR, electrocardiogram; AES, aortic ejection sound.*

demonstrates the magnitude and site of pressure gradient from the left ventricle to the aorta. The site of obstruction can also be identified by selective left ventriculography. The aortic pressure curve is abnormal if obstruction is severe; there are an early-appearing anacrotic notch, a slow, prolonged and delayed systolic upstroke, a narrow pulse pressure and a delayed dicrotic notch. In patients with severe obstruction the left atrial pressure is increased. Since a patient with severe aortic stenosis may be asymptomatic and have a normal electrocardiogram, vectorcardiogram and roentgenogram, whenever there is doubt otherwise about the severity of the lesion, left cardiac catheterization should be undertaken.

The *prognosis* is good in the majority of children; however, in a small number sudden death, frequently precipitated by severe physical exertion, has been reported. In these patients there is usually, but not always, evidence of gross left ventricular hypertrophy. The prognosis is also affected by associated malformations, including ventricular and atrial septal defects, coarctation of the aorta and pulmonary stenosis. Infants with aortic stenosis who die from congestive heart failure frequently have endocardial sclerosis of the left ventricle and atrium and of the mitral valve.

Surgical treatment is indicated in symptomatic patients and in those with electrocardiographic evidence of gross left ventricular hypertrophy. Obstructions to left ventricular outflow are treated during cardiopulmonary bypass. After the ascending aorta has been occluded just below the innominate artery, the aorta is incised and the site of obstruction identified.

Aortic valvular stenosis is usually treated by valvotomy, but a minority of patients may require valve replacement. Discrete subaortic stenosis can usually be resected without damage to the aortic valve, anterior leaflet of the mitral valve or the conduction system. Relief of supravalvular stenosis can be achieved if the area of obstruction is discrete and is not associated with a hypoplastic aorta. Postoperative evaluation is difficult, especially when aortic insufficiency is produced or aggravated by surgery. Nevertheless, the disappearance of angina pectoris, dizziness, syncope or effort intolerance and the electrocardiographic improvement with alleviation of signs of left ventricular hypertrophy indicate that the gradient across the

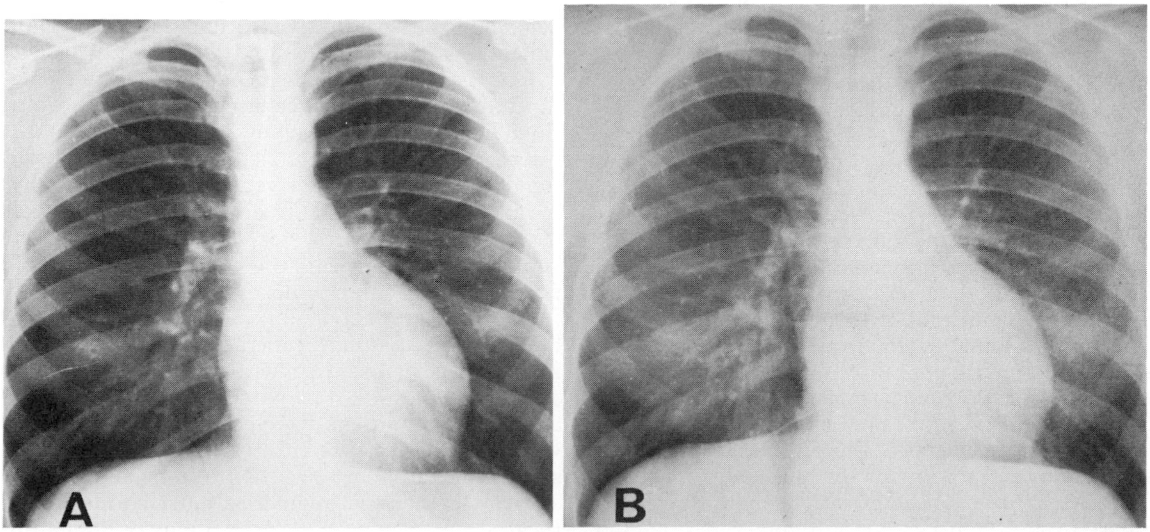

Figure 13–52 *Teleroentgenograms in congenital discrete subaortic stenosis with a resting systolic gradient of 120 mm Hg across the left ventricular outflow.* A, *Preoperative. Some prominence of the left ventricle is present, but in spite of the severity of the lesion, cardiomegaly is not prominent. The aorta is normal in size.* B, *Postoperative, after adequate resection of obstruction.*

aortic valve has been abolished or improved. Surgery is not indicated in the absence of definite evidence of left ventricular hypertrophy or of a significant gradient across the aortic valve. The definition of a "significant gradient" is difficult because the gradient depends on the degree of left ventricular obstruction as well as on cardiac output. The latter is difficult to measure in many small children, and a low cardiac output in the presence of severe aortic stenosis can result in the measurement of a relatively small gradient. It is generally agreed that surgery should be considered when the peak systolic gradient between the left ventricle and aorta exceeds 50 mm Hg at rest or when the calculated aortic valve orifice is less than 0.7 square centimeter per square meter of body surface. When these dynamics are present, significant ST segment depression is evident during and immediately after graded exercise. Even after successful surgery, careful follow-up is essential, since recurrence of obstruction 5 to 15 years after operation is frequent.

There is probably some danger in allowing patients with aortic stenosis to participate in active competitive sport, but otherwise they should lead normal lives. The status of each patient should be reviewed annually and surgery advised if progression of signs is definite. Since subacute bacterial endocarditis may develop in these patients, penicillin prophylaxis is indicated at the time of tonsillectomy, dental extractions or oral surgery (Table 9–14).

CONGENITAL MITRAL STENOSIS

This relatively rare anomaly can be isolated or associated with other defects, the commonest ones being patent ductus arteriosus, aortic stenosis and coarctation of the aorta. The role of endocardial sclerosis in its origin is not clear. The mitral valve is funnel-shaped, its leaflets are thickened, and the chordae tendineae are shortened and deformed.

Symptoms usually appear within the first 2 years of life. The infants are underdeveloped and usually have obvious dyspnea; cyanosis or pallor is not infrequent. Episodes of pulmonary edema and congestive heart failure are common. The heart is usually enlarged, owing to dilatation and hypertrophy of the right ventricle and left atrium. Although a variety of murmurs have been described (mainly systolic in time), our cases had rumbling diastolic murmurs followed by a loud first sound. The second sound is loud and split. An opening snap of the mitral valve may be present. The electrocardiogram reveals right ventricular hypertrophy, with normal, bifid or spiked P waves. Roentgenograms usually show left atrial and right ventricular enlargement and pulmonary congestion. At cardiac catheterization there is an increase in right ventricular, pulmonary arterial and wedge pressures, and associated anomalies such as patent ductus arteriosus may be demonstrated. Angiocardiography may show delayed emptying of the left atrium.

The prognosis is usually poor; the majority of children succumb during the first 2 years of life. The results of surgical treatment have been poor, but occasional patients have been salvaged.

CONGENITAL MITRAL INSUFFICIENCY

This anomaly can be isolated or associated with patent ductus arteriosus, coarctation of the aorta, ventricular septal defect, corrected transposition of the great vessels, anomalous origin of the left coronary artery from the pulmonary artery, endocardial fibroelastosis and Marfan's syndrome. It is frequently associated with congestive cardiomyopathy. Mitral incompetence is an integral part of many endocardial cushion defects.

The mitral valve annulus is usually dilated; the chordae tendineae are short and may insert anomalously; the valve leaflets are deformed; and endocardial sclerosis of varying degree is usual. In significant mitral incompetence the left atrium enlarges to accommodate the regurgitant flow. The left ventricle hypertrophies and dilates, further increasing the degree of mitral incompetence. Increased pulmonary venous pressure results, with ultimate right ventricular and atrial hypertrophy and dilatation. Mild lesions produce no symptoms; the only abnormal sign is the murmur of mitral incompetence. In the majority of patients, however, significant regurgitation results in symptoms which can appear at any age. These include poor physical development, frequent respiratory infections, fatigue on exertion and episodes of pulmonary edema or congestive heart failure. Some degree of cardiac enlargement is usual, as is the typical apical pansystolic murmur of mitral insufficiency. An associated apical mid-diastolic or late diastolic rumbling murmur is frequent. The pulmonary component of the second heart sound is accentuated in the presence of pulmonary hypertension. The electrocardiogram usually shows bifid P waves, signs of left ventricular hypertrophy and sometimes signs of right ventricular hypertrophy. X-ray examination shows enlargement of the left atrium, which at times is aneurysmal. The left ventricle is prominent, the aorta small, and the pulmonary vascularity normal or increased.

Selective left ventricular angiocardiography outlines the left atrium by contrast medium which has regurgitated across the mitral valve. Cardiac catheterization shows an elevated left atrial pressure and at times pulmonary hypertension. Mitral valvuloplasty has resulted in striking improvement in symptoms and heart size. Before consideration for surgery, associated anomalies must be identified. In children beyond 3 or 4 years it may be difficult to exclude rheumatic fever as the cause of the mitral insufficiency.

LATE SYSTOLIC MITRAL REGURGITATION

This is a distinctive syndrome resulting from an abnormal mechanism which allows billowing of the mitral leaflets (especially the posterior one) into the left atrium toward the end of systole. The abnormality may be congenital and associated with other anomalies, especially atrial septal defects of the ostium secundum type. In others the mitral regurgitation appears to be a complication of rheumatic or viral myocarditis which results in papillary muscle dysfunction. The syndrome is more common in girls and may affect siblings. Although generally asymptomatic, these patients may suffer from incapacitating chest pain. The pain is left precordial, stabbing, may last for several hours or days, and does not have the characteristics of classic angina pectoris. Its mechanism is unknown. The dominant abnormal signs are auscultatory. The apical murmur is late systolic in timing and may be preceded by a click, but these signs vary in the same patient, so that at times only the click is audible. In the standing position, the click appears earlier in systole and the murmur is longer. Arrhythmias may be present, primarily unifocal or multifocal premature ventricular contractions. The *electrocardiogram* may be normal, but characteristically shows diphasic T waves, especially in leads 2, 3, VF and V_6; the T waves may vary in the same patient, so that at times the electrocardiogram is normal. The chest *roentgenogram* is normal. The *echocardiogram* shows a characteristic posterior movement of the posterior mitral leaflet during mid or late systole. The condition does not progress in childhood; so that specific therapy is not indicated. However, these patients are at risk to develop bacterial endocarditis; prophylaxis (preferably with penicillin) is essential to cover dental and ear, nose and throat surgery (Table 9–14).

PULMONARY VENOUS HYPERTENSION

A variety of lesions may result in pulmonary venous hypertension followed by pulmonary arterial hypertension and congestive heart failure. These include congenital mitral stenosis, mitral insufficiency, some varieties of total anomalous pulmonary venous return and left atrial myxomas, as well as less frequent ones, such as *cor triatriatum* (stenosis of the common pulmonary vein), *individual pulmonary venous stenosis* and *supravalvular stenosing ring of the left atrium.* In these conditions the symptoms are irritability, episodes of pulmonary edema, recurrent pulmonary infections and congestive heart failure. Physical signs are dominated by the presence of pulmonary hypertension. The electrocardiogram shows right ventricular hypertrophy with spiked P waves. X-ray studies show cardiac enlargement, and prominence of pulmonary veins, the right ventricle and atrium and the main pulmonary artery; the left atrium is normal in size or only slightly enlarged. Cardiac catheterization excludes the presence of a shunt and demonstrates pulmonary hypertension with an elevated pulmonary arterial wedge pressure. The left atrial pressure is normal. Selective pulmonary arterial angiocardiography may delineate the anatomic lesion. It is important to recognize this clinical pattern, since cor triatriatum and some cases of supravalvular stenosing ring can be cured surgically.

ANOMALIES OF THE AORTIC ARCH

RIGHT AORTIC ARCH. In this abnormality the aorta curves to the right and descends on the right side of the vertebral column; it is usually asso-

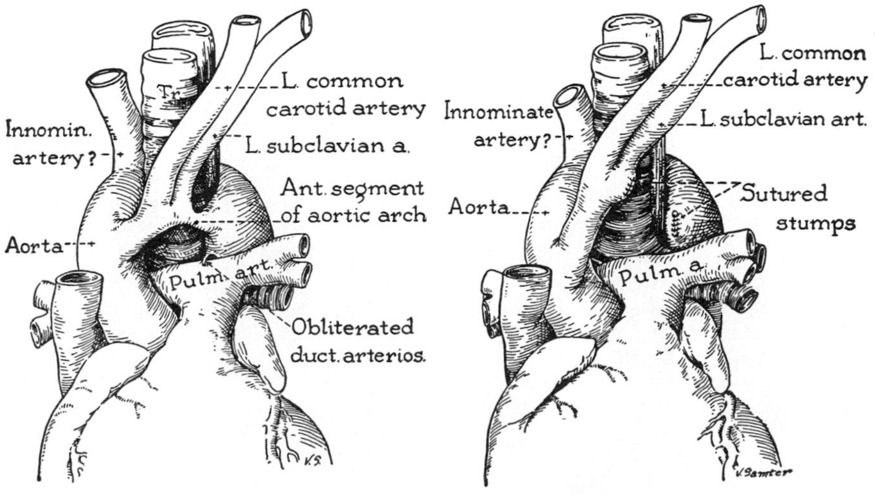

Figure 13–53 *Double aortic arch.* A, *Small anterior segment of double aortic arch (most common type).* B, *Operative procedure for release of vascular ring. (Courtesy of Dr. Willis J. Potts.)*

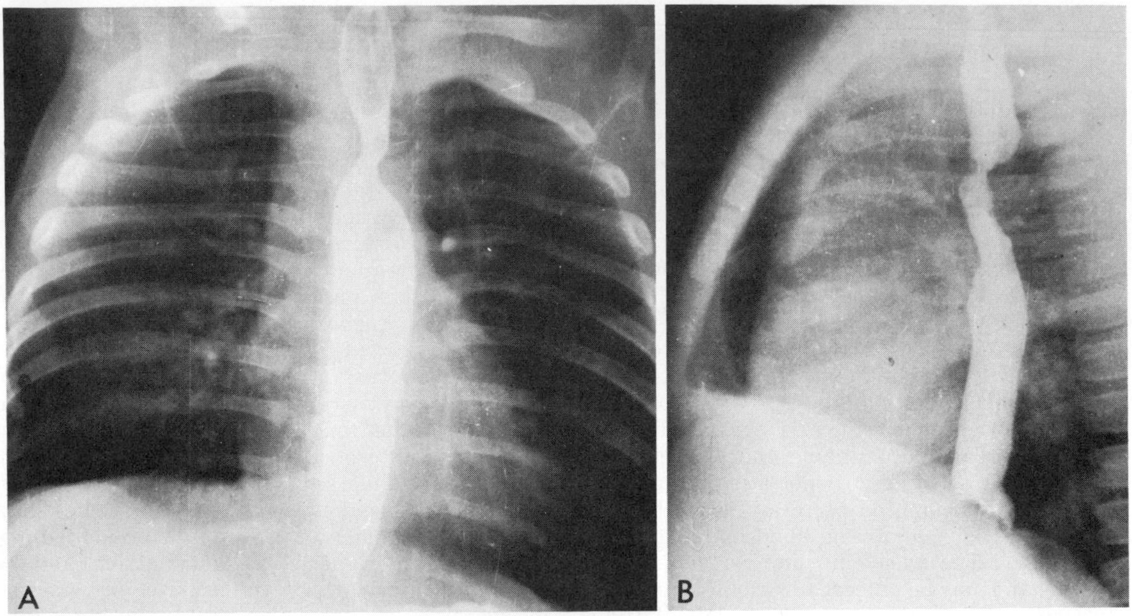

Figure 13–54 Double aortic arch in an infant aged 5 months. A, Anteroposterior view. The barium-filled esophagus is constricted on both sides. B, Lateral view. The esophagus is displaced forward. The anterior arch was the smaller and was divided at operation. (Courtesy of Drs. Eugene Saenger, Frederick Silverman and Edward McGrath.)

ciated with other cardiac malformations. It is found in 20 per cent of cases of tetralogy of Fallot and is common in truncus arteriosus. A right aortic arch without other anomaly is asymptomatic. It can be demonstrated roentgenographically, to the right of the sternum. The barium-filled esophagus is indented on its right border at the level of the aortic arch.

VASCULAR RINGS. Congenital abnormalities of the aortic arch and its major branches result in the formation of vascular rings around the trachea and esophagus with varying degrees of compression on them. The following are the more common anomalies: (1) double aortic arch (Figs. 13–53 and 13–54), (2) right aortic arch with left ligamentum arteriosum, (3) anomalous right subclavian artery arising as the last major thoracic branch of a normally placed aorta (Fig. 13–55), (4) anomalous innominate artery arising further to the left on the arch than usual, (5) anomalous left carotid artery arising further to the right than usual and passing anterior to the trachea, and (6) anomalous left pulmo-

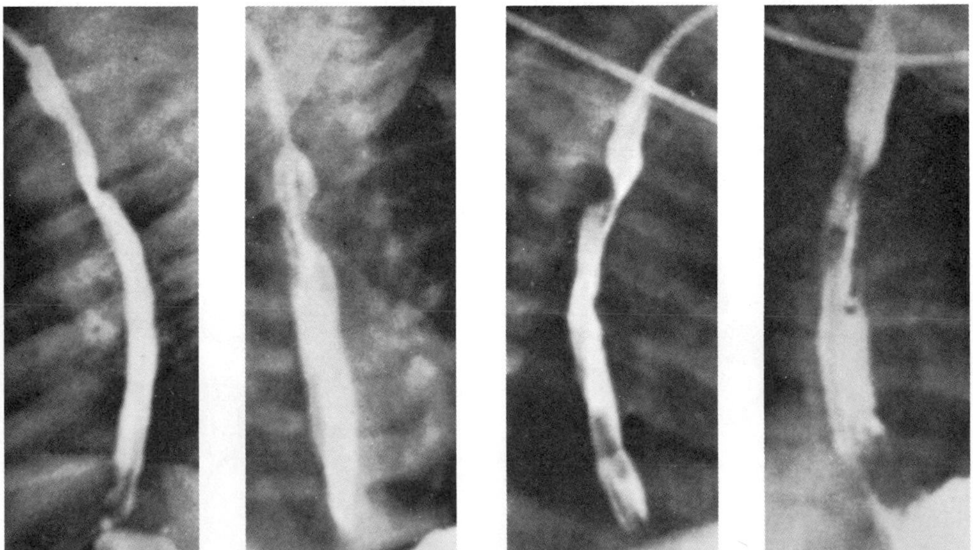

Figure 13–55 Esophagogram of a child with aberrant origin of the right subclavian artery as a last branch from the arch of the aorta. The positions from left to right are lateral, left anterior oblique, right anterior oblique, anteroposterior. A constant defect is visualized on the posterior aspect of the esophagus.

nary artery (vascular sling). This abnormal vessel arises from an elongated main pulmonary artery or from the right pulmonary artery. It courses between and compresses the trachea and esophagus.

The clinical patterns are extremely variable. In some instances, especially with anomalous right subclavian artery, the condition is asymptomatic. If the vascular ring produces compression of the trachea and esophagus, symptoms are frequently present during infancy. Respirations are wheezing and are aggravated by crying, feeding and flexion of the neck. Extension of the neck tends to relieve the noisy respiration. Vomiting is frequent. There may be a brassy cough, and pneumonia is common. Examination of the barium-filled esophagus and of the air- or Lipiodol-filled trachea, during fluoroscopy and on roentgenograms (Figs. 13–54 and 13–55), discloses the anomaly.

Surgery is advised in symptomatic patients with radiographic evidence of tracheal or esophageal compression. The appropriate vessel is divided in patients with double aortic arch (Fig. 13–53). Compression produced by a right aortic arch and left ligamentum arteriosum is relieved by division of the latter. An anomalous right subclavian artery is divided at its origin from the aorta. Anomalous innominate or carotid arteries cannot be divided; the tracheal compression is relieved by attaching the adventitia of these vessels to the sternum. Anomalous left pulmonary artery is treated by division at its origin and reanastomosis to the main pulmonary artery after the anomalous vessel has been brought in front of the trachea.

ANOMALOUS ORIGIN OF CORONARY ARTERIES

ANOMALOUS ORIGIN OF THE LEFT CORONARY ARTERY FROM THE PULMONARY ARTERY. In this condition there is a compromise of blood supply to the left ventricular myocardium. Soon after birth the pulmonary arterial pressure falls, so that the perfusion pressure to the left coronary artery is inadequate. Interarterial anastomoses may develop between the right and left coronary arteries. This results in reversal of flow, so that blood flows from the left coronary artery to the pulmonary artery. The left ventricle becomes dilated and somewhat hypertrophied, with patchy fibrosis and microscopic deposition of calcium. Complicating mitral incompetence is frequent and is due to papillary muscle infarction. Localized aneurysms may develop in the left ventricle.

In the majority of instances, symptoms occur during the first few months of life and are those of congestive heart failure, frequently associated with or precipitated by respiratory infections. Recurrent attacks of discomfort, restlessness, irritability, sweating, dyspnea and pallor with or without mild cyanosis could be interpreted as being produced by angina pectoris. Cardiac enlargement is moderate to marked. Gallop rhythm is common. Murmurs may be absent, nonspecific or ejective in quality, or regurgitant because of mitral incompetence. Older patients with abundant intercoronary anastomoses may have continuous murmurs. *Roentgen* examination confirms the cardiomegaly, but the contour and pulsations are not specific unless there is a complicating ventricular aneurysm. The *electrocardiogram* resembles the pattern described in anterior myocardial infarction in adults. A QR pattern followed by inverted T waves is seen in leads I and aVL. The left ventricular surface leads (V_5 and V_6) show deep wide Q waves and may also exhibit elevated S-T segments and inverted T waves (Fig. 13–56). *Aortography* is diagnostic; there is immediate opacification of only the right coronary artery. Generally this vessel is large and tortuous. After filling of the intercoronary anastomoses, the left coronary artery and the

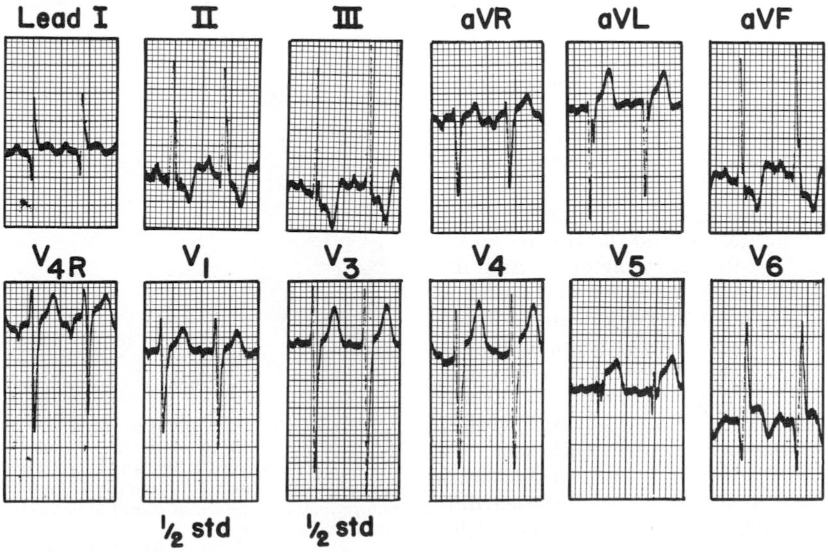

Figure 13–56 Electrocardiogram of a 3 month old child with anomalous origin of the left coronary artery from the pulmonary artery. Anterolateral myocardial infarction is present because of abnormally large and wide Q waves in leads I, V_5 and V_6, elevated S-T segment in V_5 and V_6 and inversion of TV_6.

pulmonary artery are in turn opacified. Selective pulmonary arteriography may opacify the anomalous left coronary artery. Selective left ventriculography reveals a dilated left ventricle which empties poorly.

In the majority of instances death from heart failure occurs within the first 6 months of life. The exceptional patients who survive have unusually abundant intercoronary anastomoses. The variable prognosis depends on the severity of the heart failure and the extent of myocardial infarction. Treatment is not standardized. Seriously ill infants with retrograde drainage of left coronary artery blood into the pulmonary artery have been treated by ligation of the left coronary artery to prevent run-off of blood from the coronary circuit and to increase myocardial perfusion via collaterals. Others have preferred vigorous medical management with digitalis and diuretics, so that surgery can be postponed beyond infancy. At that time the anomalous left coronary artery is detached from the pulmonary artery and reattached to the ascending aorta to establish normal arterial perfusion.

ANOMALOUS ORIGIN OF BOTH CORONARY ARTERIES FROM THE PULMONARY ARTERY. This is extremely rare and may be associated with other severe cardiac malformations. After birth, blood flow to the myocardium is severely compromised because the coronary arteries are perfused with venous blood at a low pressure. The prognosis is usually poor.

ANOMALOUS ORIGIN OF THE RIGHT CORONARY ARTERY FROM THE PULMONARY ARTERY. This is also rare; it does not produce signs or symptoms. The prognosis is good.

PRIMARY PULMONARY HYPERTENSION

Primary pulmonary hypertension is a disease of unknown origin characterized by hypertension of the lesser circulation and right-sided heart failure. The disease may occur at any age and may be clinically recognizable during childhood and adolescence. The pulmonary hypertension is associated with precapillary obstruction of the pulmonary vascular bed, owing to hyperplasia of the muscular and elastic tissues and the thickened intima of the small pulmonary arteries and arterioles. Atherosclerotic changes may be found in the larger pulmonary arteries. Other causes of pulmonary heart disease (chronic cor pulmonale) are absent, and there is no evidence of emphysema, pancreatic fibrosis or kyphoscoliosis. Recurrent pulmonary emboli may produce the same clinical picture, but this disease is rare in childhood. Severe pulmonary hypertension may result from myriads of minute microemboli from the cardiac end of a ventriculojugular shunt tube inserted for the treatment of hydrocephalus. Significant pulmonary hypertension may also result from persistent obstruction of the upper airway, e.g., by gross enlargement of the tonsils and adenoids; it may also be an accompaniment of extreme obesity, as in the Prader-Willi syndrome.

HEMODYNAMICS. The pulmonary hypertension places a mechanical burden on the right ventricle and pulmonary artery with resultant right ventricular hypertension and dilatation of the pulmonary artery. Frequently the cardiac output is decreased. Sooner or later right-sided heart failure develops, at times with tricuspid insufficiency.

CLINICAL MANIFESTATIONS. The predominant symptoms include effort intolerance and fatigability; occasional patients complain of precordial chest pain, dizziness or syncope. Peripheral cyanosis may be present and is associated with cold extremities and a nearly normal arterial oxygen saturation. If right-sided heart failure has supervened, the jugular venous pressure is elevated, and hepatomegaly and edema are present. Jugular venous "a" waves are present, and if functional tricuspid insufficiency has supervened, a conspicuous jugular "c" wave develops, with systolic hepatic pulsations. The heart is slightly to moderately enlarged, with a right ventricular apical tap. Thrills are absent, and murmurs may be insignificant. The first heart sound is frequently followed by a pulmonic ejection click. The systolic murmur is soft and short and is sometimes followed by a blowing diastolic murmur owing to pulmonary incompetence. The second heart sound is closely split, loud, sometimes booming, and

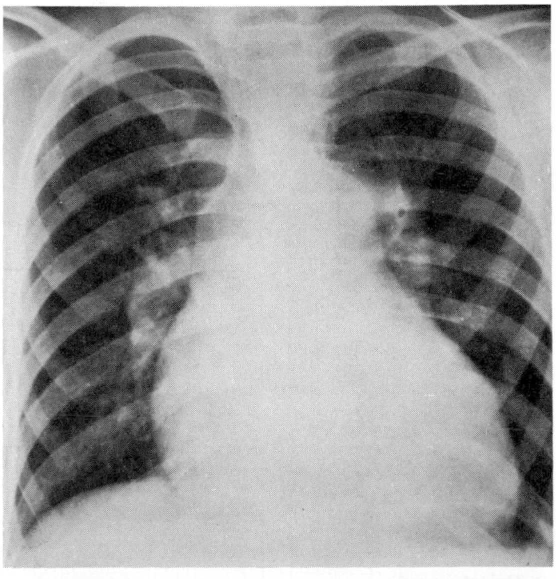

Figure 13–57 Teleroentgenogram in primary pulmonary hypertension, showing moderate cardiac enlargement, dilatation of the pulmonary artery and relative pulmonary undervascularity in the outer two thirds of the lung fields. This roentgen picture may simulate that found in valvular pulmonic stenosis with normal aortic root.

frequently palpable. A presystolic gallop rhythm may be audible down the left sternal border.

Roentgenograms reveal a prominent pulmonary artery and right ventricle (Fig. 13–57). The pulmonary vascularity in the hilar areas may be prominent and contrast with the peripheral lung fields, which are clear. The *electrocardiogram* shows right ventricular hypertrophy with spiked P waves.

DIAGNOSIS. The diagnosis is confirmed by *cardiac catheterization,* which reveals right ventricular and pulmonary hypertension with a normal pulmonary arterial wedge pressure. The cardiac output is usually low, and the arterial oxygen saturation is nearly normal.

Difficulty may arise in differentiating this condition from the Eisenmenger syndrome. Generally these may be differentiated by cardiac catheterization, which demonstrates the site, direction and magnitude of the shunt which has resulted in pulmonary hypertension. This study also excludes left-sided lesions which result in pulmonary venous hypertension; in these conditions the pulmonary arterial wedge pressure is elevated significantly. If primary pulmonary hypertension is associated with a reversed intra-atrial shunt through a foramen ovale, the clinical picture may simulate that of the Eisenmenger syndrome.

TREATMENT. Primary pulmonary hypertension is progressive, and the results of treatment are disappointing. Some relief may be obtained by the usual measures adopted for congestive cardiac failure.

MARFAN SYNDROME: CARDIOVASCULAR MANIFESTATIONS

The frequency of congenital malformations of the heart in Marfan syndrome (Section 22) has probably been overstressed. The common lesion is dilatation of the aorta, beginning at the aortic valve and usually confined to the ascending portion. The valve ring is stretched, and the resultant aortic insufficiency may be pronounced. Progressive left ventricular failure occurs with or without angina pectoris. Dissecting aneurysm of the aorta is a common terminal event or may result in the development of aortic valvular incompetence. Cardiac symptoms may occur as early as the fifth year of life, but frequently do not appear until adult life.

The pulmonary artery and valve may be involved in a similar way to that of the aorta, resulting in dilatation of the pulmonary artery. This syndrome may explain some cases of *idiopathic pulmonary arterial dilatation.* Mitral insufficiency may result from redundant cusps and chordae tendineae. Subacute bacterial endocarditis may be a complication. Congenital cardiac malformations have been reported in occasional patients. These include atrial and ventricular septal defects, Fallot's tetralogy, patent ductus arteriosus, coarctation of the aorta, pulmonary arterial stenosis and anomalous pulmonary venous return.

PRINCIPLES OF TREATMENT IN CONGENITAL HEART DISEASE

The following principles of treatment apply to all patients with congenital heart disease. Owing to rapid advances in diagnosis and surgical treatment, an attitude of guarded optimism should be adopted. A level of life as nearly normal as possible should be encouraged because untold psychologic trauma is imposed by unnecessary restriction. The parents' attitude toward the child can be more relaxed if it is pointed out that sudden death is rare in congenital heart anomalies in contradistinction to some degenerative diseases in adults. Rigorous restriction of physical activities in usually not indicated, since children soon learn their own capacity for exercise. If cardiac enlargement is present or if there is a history of congestive heart failure, competitive sports should be discouraged.

General management includes a well-balanced diet, a supplementation of iron and vitamins during the first few years of life and the usual immunization program.

The prevention or prompt treatment of dehydration in cyanotic patients is important, so that hemoconcentration and possible thrombotic episodes will be averted. Infections should be vigorously treated with suitable antibiotics to prevent the onset of bacterial endocarditis or congestive heart failure. Ear, nose and throat surgery and dental extractions must also be covered with antibiotics, preferably penicillin. Treatment with iron of a "relative hypochromic anemia" in cyanotic patients may improve their exercise tolerance and general well-being. The treatment of congestive heart failure is described later under that heading. For treatment of paroxysmal dyspneic attacks, see Tetralogy of Fallot.

SURGICAL TREATMENT. The standardized surgical therapy of patent ductus arteriosus, coarctation of the aorta and vascular rings has been described.

Open-heart Surgery. This technique is used when surgical treatment of intracardiac defects under direct vision is indicated. The systemic venous return to the heart is diverted to an artificial heart-lung machine, and arterialized blood is returned to the systemic arterial system *(cardiopul-*

monary bypass). Thus, the principal source of blood flow through the heart and lungs is diverted, and the chambers of the "bloodless" heart may be opened widely. The systemic venous return to the heart is picked up by cannulae in the superior and inferior venae cavae, usually inserted through the right atrium. The arterialized blood is returned from the heart-lung machine to the ascending aorta. With this system of cannulation coronary and bronchial flows are not disturbed, and the heart continues to beat. Mild or moderate hypothermia can be induced by controlling the temperature of the extracorporeal blood. Prolonged deep hypothermia without perfusion is used in severely ill neonates and in infants in whom prolonged cardiopulmonary bypass may be inadvisable; body temperature is reduced to about 20°C by a combination of surface cooling and decreasing extracorporeal blood temperature. During deep hypothermia cardiopulmonary bypass is discontinued because the brain appears to be protected at this temperature for periods up to 1 hour without perfusion. Normal temperature is restored by rewarming the blood extracorporeally. If it is desired to abolish coronary flow in a child with normal temperature or mild hypothermia, this is accomplished by intermittent occlusion of the ascending aorta.

The Postoperative Period. With successful total body perfusion and direct-vision open-heart surgery, the postoperative course is frequently benign. Nevertheless, many of these patients may be in a delicate or precarious state. The following complications are listed as a guide to management.

PLEURAL SPACE COMPLICATIONS. Pneumothorax and hemothorax are treated along usual lines.

PULMONARY COMPLICATIONS. Patchy areas of pulmonary atelectasis with or without edema and hemorrhage occur more frequently in patients with pulmonary hypertension and elevated pulmonary resistance. Decompression of the pulmonary vascular tree by cannulation of the left atrium or ventricle during cardiopulmonary bypass probably decreases the severity.

PULMONARY VENTILATION. Respiratory exchange may be improved by the use of respirators or continuous positive airway pressure. This can be accomplished via an endotracheal tube, but tracheostomy may be necessary if artificial ventilation is prolonged for more than a few days. Care must be exercised to avoid pulmonary damage from excessive concentrations of oxygen.

SHOCK. This complication is encountered within the first few hours or days after operation and may be seen after prolonged perfusion, in the presence of hypovolemia or cardiac tamponade, or when surgical correction is incomplete (e.g., inadequate relief of obstruction to right ventricular outflow). The clinical picture is dominated by hypotension, increased venous pressure (except in some patients with hypovolemia), peripheral vasoconstriction and cyanosis, oliguria and acidosis. In patients in whom hypovolemia and cardiac tamponade have been excluded artificial ventilation and correction of acidosis are usually required. The effects of small transfusions should be assessed by measurement of venous and arterial pressures, cardiac output and urinary volume. Although the use of corticosterioids with or without epinephrine or isoproterenol is debatable, these agents have had a salutary effect in some critically ill patients.

CARDIAC FAILURE. If heart failure was present before operation, many days or weeks may elapse before compensation is restored; anticongestive therapy is continued during this time. The appearance of heart failure for the first time after operation suggests volume overload of the ventricle (e.g. the development of aortic incompetence after aortic valvotomy) or inadequate relief of an obstructive lesion (e.g. persistent right ventricular outflow tract obstruction in pulmonic stenosis). Temporary increase of venous pressure is common after correction of Fallot's tetralogy and is probably related to the high pressure necessary to fill the recently incised right ventricle.

HEMORRHAGE. Although operation is conducted with the patient heparinized, postoperative bleeding should not be a problem. If it occurs, it may be an expression of inadequate perfusion. Deeply cyanotic patients may have an abnormal clotting mechanism preoperatively (see Hematologic Data in first pages of this Section).

COMPLETE HEART BLOCK. Trauma to the bundle of His during an intracardiac procedure may be produced by a suture or may result from local edema and myocardial anoxia. Fortunately, permanent heart block is becoming less frequent, but temporary episodes lasting from a few hours up to 3 or 4 weeks are seen. This complication is usually recognized at operation, but may develop during the first few postoperative days. If the slow heart rate results in inadequate cardiac output, treatment is required and consists of artificial pacing, with an external pacemaker delivering the stimulus to an internal electrode sutured into the wall of the ventricle at the time of operation. This myocardial wire electrode is removed when sinus rhythm is restored. If heart block is permanent, an implanted pacemaker with a transvenous catheter is indicated. Generally the pacing electrode is advanced from the jugular vein to the apex of the right ventricle and is attached to the permanent pacemaker, which is buried under the tissue below the right clavicle. Intravenous administration of isoproterenol (Isuprel) is useful in emergency situations. Although we have observed a number of children with surgically induced permanent heart block who have not required artificial pacing, the implantation of a pacemaker is advisable because of unpredictable Stokes-Adams attacks.

OTHER DYSRHYTHMIAS. The common causes of ventricular dysrhythmias after open-heart surgery are digitalis intoxication and hypokalemia; atrial dysrhythmias are common after extensive incision of the right atrium for correction of atrial septal defect or especially after interatrial correction of transposition of the great vessels. The dysrhythmia may take the form of ectopic atrial rhythms, atrial flutter or fibrillation, intra-atrial block, atrioventricular dissociation or sinus bradycardia. Generally these disturbances of rhythm are transient, but they may be recurrent or permanent, especially after treatment of arterial transposition.

Acidosis. Minor degrees of respiratory acidosis are common and do not require therapy. Severe metabolic acidosis may occur and is usually an indication of inadequate blood flow during cardiopulmonary bypass or inadequate cardiac output after operation. See Section 5 for treatment.

Postcardiotomy Syndrome. Toward the end of the first postoperative week, or sometimes weeks or months after operation, a febrile illness due to pericarditis and pleurisy with or without fluid may develop. In most patients the condition is benign. In others, fever, chest pain and pleurisy may be complicated by collections of pericardial fluid and the resulting danger of cardiac tamponade. Symptomatic patients usually respond to salicylates and bed rest. If there is no response, corticosteroids may be used. In some patients there is a tendency for the condition to recur.

Postperfusion Syndrome. Within 3 to 12 weeks after cardiopulmonary bypass, fever, malaise and splenomegaly may develop, with or without hepatomegaly and a maculopapular rash. The total leukocyte count varies from 3000 to 15,000 per mm^3, of which 40 to 80 per cent are atypical lymphocytes. The heterophil antibody test result may be positive. It is suspected that the disease is due to cytomegalovirus infection, possibly from donor blood. Its recognition and differentiation from bacterial endocarditis are important. The course is usually benign; salicylates may relieve the general discomfort.

Hemolytic Anemia. Hemolysis of probable mechanical origin may be seen after treatment of endocardial cushion defects or the insertion of an artificial prosthetic valve. It may be due to unusual turbulence associated with jets of blood at high pressure, since it tends to occur if there is residual mitral incompetence after treatment of an ostium primum defect when jets of blood impinge on the plastic prosthesis used to close the defect. Intravascular hemolysis may also be seen after insertion of an artificial valve, especially if the valve is incompetent. The anemia may be controlled with iron therapy, although reoperation may be necessary in patients with severe and progressive hemolysis who require frequent blood transfusions.

Infection. Sepsis with bacterial endocarditis is a serious complication, especially when prosthetic patches or valves are used. Common infecting organisms are *Staphylococcus aureus, Staphylococcus albus* and *Pseudomonas aeruginosa.* Less often, unusual bacteria and fungi, including some that are generally considered noninvasive, have also been the offending organisms. Treatment is difficult, but prolonged and diligent therapy with combinations of antimicrobial drugs have occasionally been successful. Infected prostheses may require replacement before the infection can be eliminated.

GENERAL

See under Evaluation at beginning of Section.

The Neonatal Circulation

Dawes, G. S.: Fetal and Neonatal Physiology. Chicago, Year Book Medical Publishers, Inc., 1968.

Heymann, M. A., and Rudolph, A. M.: Effects of congenital heart disease on fetal and neonatal circulations. Prog. Cardiovasc. Dis. *15*:115, 1972.

Kaplan, S., and Assali, N. S.: Disorders of circulation. *In* Assali, N. S. (ed.): Pathophysiology of Gestation. Vol. 3. New York, Academic Press, Inc., 1972, pp. 1–71.

Rudolph, A. M.: The changes in the circulation after birth: Their importance in congenital heart disease. Circulation *41*:343, 1970.

Incidence and Etiology

Campbell, M.: The incidence and later distribution of malformations of the heart. *In* Watson, H. (ed.): Paediatric Cardiology. St. Louis, The C. V. Mosby Company, 1968, pp. 71–83.

Neill, C. A.: Genetic aspects of congenital heart disease. *In* Moss, A. J., and Adams, F. H. (eds.): Heart Disease in Infants, Children and Adolescents. Baltimore, The Williams & Wilkins Company, 1968, pp. 36–46.

Nora, J. J.: Etiologic factors in congenital heart diseases. Ped. Clin. N. Amer. *18*:1059, 1971.

Warkany, J.: Congenital Malformations. Chicago, Year Book Medical Publishers, Inc., 1971, pp. 459–470.

Tetralogy of Fallot and Pulmonary Atresia

Guntheroth, W. G., and Morgan, B. C.: Physiologic studies of paroxysmal hyperpnea in cyanotic congenital heart disease. Circulation *31*:70, 1965.

Kaplan, S.: The treatment of tetralogy of Fallot. *In* Yu, P. N., and Goodwin, J. F. (eds.): Progress in Cardiology, 2. Philadelphia, Lea and Febiger, 1972, pp. 229–240.

Kirklin, J. W., and Karp, R. B.: The Tetralogy of Fallot: From a Surgical Viewpoint, Philadelphia, W. B. Saunders Company, 1970.

Ponce, F. E., et al.: Propranolol palliation of tetralogy of Fallot. Pediatrics *52*:100, 1973.

Eisenmenger Syndrome

Wood, P.: Pulmonary hypertension. Mod. Con. Cardiovas. Dis. *28*:513, 1959.

Transposition of the Great Vessels

Bonham-Carter, R. E.: Progress in the treatment of transposition of the great arteries. Brit. Heart J. *35*:573, 1973.

Mustard, W. T., Keith, J. D., Trusler, G. A., Fowler, R., and Kidd, L.: The surgical management of transposition of the great vessels. J. Thorac. Cardiovasc. Surg. *48*:953, 1965.

Noonan, J. A., Nadas, A. S., Rudolph, A. M., and Harris, G. B. C.: Transposition of the great arteries. New Engl. J. Med. *263*:592, 1960.

Rashkind, W. J.: Transposition of the great arteries. Pediat. Clin. N. Amer. *18*:1075, 1971.

Rashkind, W. J., and Miller, W. W.: Creation of an atrial septal defect without thoracotomy: A palliative approach to complete transposition of the great vessels. J.A.M.A. *196*:991, 1966.

Ebstein's Disease

Genton, E., and Blount, S. G.: The spectrum of Ebstein's anomaly. Am. Heart J. *73*:395, 1967.

Kumar, A. E., Fyler, D. C., Miettinen, O. S., and Nadas, A. S.: Ebstein's anomaly. Am. J. Cardiol. *28*:84, 1971.

Watson, H.: Electrode catheters in the diagnosis of Ebstein's anomaly of the tricuspid valve. Brit. Heart J. *28*:161, 1966.

Atrial Septal Defect

Evans, J. R., Rowe, R. D., and Keith, J. D.: Clinical diagnosis of atrial septal defect in children. Am. J. Med. *30*:345, 1961.

Kaplan, S.: Atrial septal defect. *In* Watson, H. (ed.): Paediatric Cardiology. St. Louis, The C. V. Mosby Company, 1968, p. 376.

Leatham, A., and Gray, L.: Auscultatory and phonocardiographic signs of atrial septal defect. Brit. Heart J. *18*:193, 1956.

Rastelli, G. C., Kirklin, J. W., and Titus, J. L.: Anatomic observations on complete form of persistent common atrioventricular canal, with special reference to atrioventricular valves. Proc. Mayo Clin. *41*:296, 1966.

Weyn, A. S., Bartle, S. H., Nolan, T. B., and Dammann, J. F., Jr.: Atrial septal defect, primum types. Circulation *32* (Supp. 3):13, 1965.

Zaver, A. G., and Nadas, A. S.: Atrial septal defect secundum type. Circulation *32* (Supp. 3):24, 1965.

Ventricular Septal Defect

Edwards, J. E.: The pathology of ventricular septal defect. Seminars Radiol. *1*:2, 1966.

Henry, J., Kaplan, S., Helmsworth, J. A., and Schreiber, J. T.: Management of infants with large ventricular septal defects. Ann. Thorac. Surg. *15*:109, 1973.

Hoffman, J. I. E.: Natural history of congenital heart disease: Problems in its assessment, with special reference to ventricular septal defects. Circulation *37*:97, 1968.

Hoffman, J. I. E.: Ventricular septal defect: Indications for therapy in infants. Pediat. Clin. N. Amer. *18*:1091, 1971.

Kaplan, S., et al.: Natural history of ventricular septal defect. Am. J. Dis. Child. *105*:581, 1963.

Levin, A. R., et al.: Intracardiac pressure-flow dynamics in isolated ventricular septal defects. Circulation *35*:430, 1967.

Ritter, D. G., Feldt, R. H., Weidman, W. H., and DuShane, J. W.: Ventricular septal defect. Circulation *32*(Supp. 3):42, 1965.

Pulmonary Stenosis with Normal Aortic Root

Abrahams, D. G., and Wood, P. H.: Pulmonary stenosis with normal aortic root. Brit. Heart J. *13*:519, 1951.

Brock, R. C.: The surgical treatment of pulmonary stenosis. Brit. Heart J. *23*:337, 1961.

Leatham, A., and Weitzman, D.: Auscultatory and phonocardiographic signs of pulmonary stenosis. Brit. Heart J. *19*:303, 1957.

Levine, O. R., and Blumenthal, S.: Pulmonic stenosis. Circulation *32* (Supp. 3):33, 1965.

Anomalous Pulmonary Venous Return

Burroughs, J. T., and Edwards, J. E.: Total anomalous pulmonary venous connection. Am. Heart J. *59*:913, 1960.

Cooley, D. A., Hallman, G. L., and Leachman, R. D.: Total anomalous pulmonary venous drainage. Correction with the use of cardiopulmonary bypass in 62 cases. J. Thorac. Cardiovasc. Surg. *51*:88, 1966.

Hastreiter, A. R., Paul, M. H., Molthan, M. E., and Miller, R. H.: Total anomalous pulmonary venous connection with severe pulmonary venous obstruction. Circulation *25*:916, 1962.

Snellen, H. A., and Dekker, A.: Anomalous pulmonary venous drainage in relation to left superior vena cava and coronary sinus. Am. Heart J. *66*:184, 1963.

Aortic Stenosis

Friedman, W. F., and Pappelbaum, S. J.: Indications for hemodynamic evaluation and surgery in congenital aortic stenosis. Pediat. Clin. N. Amer. *18*:1207, 1971.

Hohn, A. R., VanPraagh, S., Moore, A. D., Vlad, P., and Lambert, E. C.: Aortic stenosis. *Circulation 32*(Supp. 3):4, 1965.

Mitral Stenosis

Daoud, G., Kaplan, S., Perrin, E. V., Dorst, J. P., and Edwards, F. K.: Congenital mitral stenosis. *Circulation 27*:185, 1963.

Dextrocardia and Levocardia

Liberthson, R. R., et al.: Levocardia with visceral heterotaxy-isolated levocardia: Pathologic anatomy and its clinical implications. Am. Heart J. *85*:40, 1973.

VanPraagh, R.: Malposition of the heart. *In* Moss, A. J., and Adams, F. H. (eds.): Heart Disease in Infants, Children and Adolescents. Baltimore, The Williams & Wilkins Company, 1968, p. 602.

Principles of Treatment

Benzing, G., and Kaplan, S.: Late complications of cardiac surgery. Pediat. Clin. N. Amer. *18*:1225, 1971.

Caul, E. O., et al.: Cytomegalovirus infections after open heart surgery: A prospective study. Lancet. *1*:777, 1971.

Drusin, L. M., Engle, M. A., Hagstrom, J. W. C., and Schwartz, M. S.: The postpericardiotomy syndrome, A six year epidemiologic study. New Engl. J. Med. *272*:597, 1965.

Kaplan, M. H.: Symposium on immunity and the heart. Am. J. Cardiol. *24*:459, 1969.

Pirofsky, B., Sutherland, D. W., Starr, A., and Griswold, H. E.: Hemolytic anemia complicating aortic valve surgery. New Engl. J. Med. *272*:235, 1965.

Reyman, T. A.: Postperfusion syndrome: A review and report of 21 cases. Am. Heart J. *72*:116, 1966.

Williams, J. F., Morrow, A. G., and Braunwald, E.: The incidence and management of "medical" complications following cardiac operations. Circulation *32*:608, 1965.

DISTURBANCES OF RATE AND RHYTHM OF THE HEART

SINUS ARRHYTHMIA
(Respiratory Arrhythmia)

This rhythm, an acceleration of the heart rate during inspiration and a decrease during expiration, is physiologic in childhood. It is usually associated with cardiac rates under 90 to 100 per minute. It is exaggerated during convalescence from febrile illness and by drugs which increase vagal tone, such as digitalis, and is usually abolished by exercise or atropine. Some children have such great degrees of sinus arrhythmia that the presence of other arrhythmias such as extrasystoles is suspected, and an electrocardiogram is necessary for diagnosis.

EXTRASYSTOLES
(Premature Contractions)

Extrasystoles are produced by the discharge of an ectopic focus situated anywhere in atrial, junctional or ventricular tissue. They occur less frequently in children than in adults. In the majority of instances extrasystoles are of no clinical or prognostic significance. Under certain circumstances premature beats may be due to organic heart disease, e.g., in acute rheumatic or diphtheritic carditis. Drugs, especially digitalis and epinephrine, may also produce extrasystoles. Atrial premature contractions may precede atrial fibrillation in rheumatic mitral stenosis.

The clinical signs of extrasystoles include the prematurity of the beat followed by a compensatory pause, especially if the ectopic beat arises in the ventricles. In the majority of instances, extrasystoles disappear during the tachycardia of exercise. If they remain or become exaggerated during exercise, associated organic heart disease is suggested. Ectopic beats produce a smaller stroke and pulse volume than normal and, if very premature, may not be audible with a stethoscope or palpable at the radial pulse. Extrasystoles may assume a definite rhythm, e.g., alternating with normal beats (**pulsus bigeminus**) or occurring after two normal beats (**pulsus trigeminus**). This rhythmicity is frequent in digitalis intoxication. The site of origin of the extrasystoles is determined by the electrocardiogram.

Most patients are unaware of premature contractions. The basis of therapy is convincing reassurance that the arrhythmia is not the result of structural heart disease. If extrasystoles are produced by digitalis, the drug should be discontinued or its dose reduced. If relief is sought for palpitations, sedatives, quinidine sulfate or procainamide may be used.

PAROXYSMAL TACHYCARDIA

Paroxysmal tachycardia is produced by ectopic beats arising from the same focus in rapid succession. The ectopic focus may be anywhere in the atrial, junctional or ventricular tissue. Paroxysmal tachycardia may occur at any age and has been reported in the last month of fetal life. In the majority of instances the ectopic focus is situated in an atrium (paroxysmal atrial tachycardia or flutter). Paroxysmal ventricular tachycardia is rare in infants and children.

In older children, attacks of **paroxysmal atrial tachycardia** are characterized by abrupt onset and cessation. If an attack is not witnessed, its occurrence may be elicited by an accurate history. It may be precipitated by an acute infection. Attacks may last from a few seconds to several weeks, but usually persist for a few hours and seldom exceed 2 or 3 days. The cardiac rate usually exceeds 180 and occasionally may be as rapid as 300 per minute. The only complaint may be awareness of the rapid cardiac rate. If it is exceptionally rapid or if the attack is prolonged, precordial discomfort and congestive cardiac failure may supervene.

In young infants the diagnosis may be more obscure. Since the normal cardiac rate at this age is rapid and increases greatly with crying, a persistent tachycardia during quiet periods or sleep suggests the diagnosis. The cardiac rate during paroxysms is frequently in the range of 300 per minute, and signs of congestive cardiac failure rapidly supervene if the attack lasts a few hours or more. The infant is acutely ill, has an ashen and slightly cyanotic color and is restless and irritable. Tachypnea and hepatomegaly are the prominent signs of cardiac failure. Paroxysms may be associated with fever and leukocytosis. The diagnosis is confirmed by the electrocardiogram (Fig. 13–58), which also identifies the site of the ectopic focus.

TREATMENT. In supraventricular paroxysmal tachycardia (atrial or junctional) simple procedures of vagal stimulation such as pressure over the eyeballs or over the carotid sinus may abort the attack. Older children may have discovered some maneuver to abolish the paroxysm, such as self-induced vomiting, breath-holding, drinking ice water or the adoption of a particular posture. In infants and many older patients these measures fail, and digitalis should be given in full therapeutic doses. This drug abolishes the tachycardia in more than 95 per cent of patients. In infants, digitalis should be used even if the paroxysm was abolished by vagal stimulation, since the recurrence rate is high; therapy should be maintained for about one year after the paroxysm. In rare instances when paroxysms persist and congestive heart failure progresses, electrical cardioversion or beta-adrenergic antagonists (propranolol) are used. Other agents which have been used to abolish paroxysmal supraventricular tachycardia include infusions of phenylephrine (Neo-Synephrine), diphenylhydantoin (Dilantin) and oral quinidine sulfate. It is important to relieve the apprehension associated with a prolonged paroxysm by sedation, preferably with morphine.

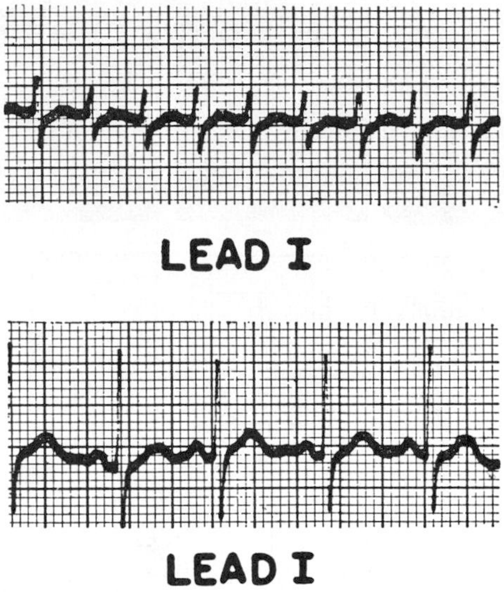

Figure 13–58 Electrocardiogram in paroxysmal atrial tachycardia. Upper tracing taken during paroxysm with heart rate of 240 per minute. Lower tracing, taken during recovery, is within normal limits.

In most instances of paroxysmal atrial tachycardia there is no underlying structural cardiac disease. If cardiac failure supervenes during the paroxysms, cardiac function rapidly returns to normal after cessation of the attack. Between attacks some children may exhibit the electrocardiographic signs of the **Wolff-Parkinson-White syndrome,** which is probably due to an anomalous connection by special conducting fibers between the right atrium and the ventricles. Electrocardiography shows a widened QRS complex at the expense of a shortened P-R interval, so that the P-S interval as measured from the beginning of the P to the end of the S is normal (Fig. 13–59). In the majority of instances there is no associated cardiac disease. Paroxysmal atrial tachycardia occurs in about 50 to 60 per cent of patients with the Wolff-Parkinson-White syndrome, and about 5 per cent of patients with paroxysmal tachycardia exhibit this syndrome between attacks of tachycardia.

Spontaneous **ventricular tachycardia** is rare in children. It may be seen in the immediate post-

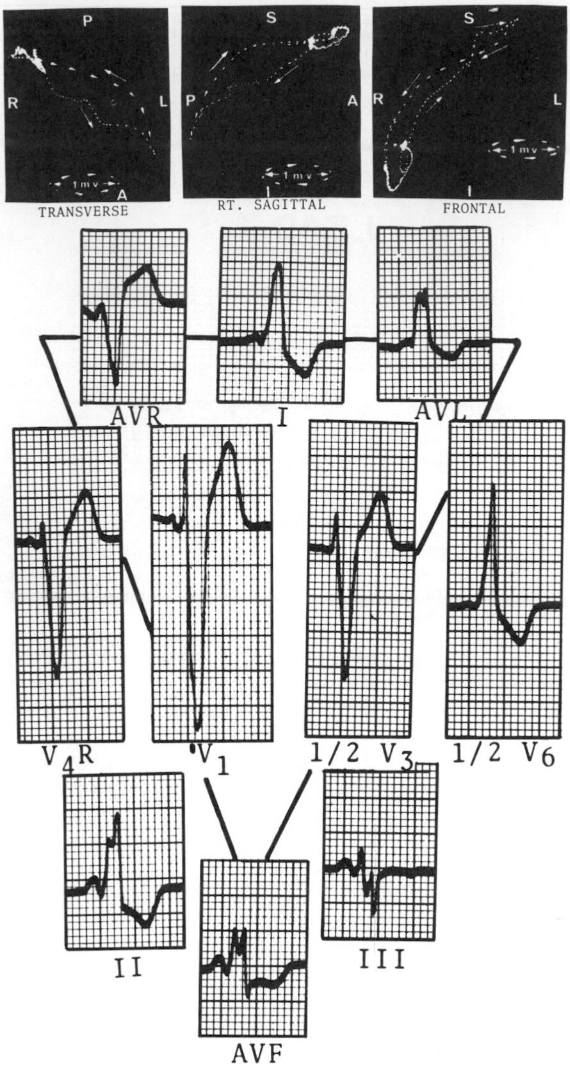

Figure 13–59 Electrocardiogram and vectorcardiogram in Wolff-Parkinson-White syndrome. Short P-R interval and wide QRS are present. The vectorcardiogram shows a slow inscription of the initial QRS.

operative period after cardiac surgery or occasionally during severe myocarditis. Patients with ventricular tachycardia usually appear critically ill, with restlessness, pallor and hypotension. The diagnosis is confirmed by electrocardiography. Abolition of the paroxysm is urgently indicated and is best accomplished by electrical cardioversion. Drugs of choice are lidocaine, procainamide and quinidine sulfate.

ATRIAL FLUTTER

This arrhythmia is due to rapid and regular but abnormal atrial contractions. Lewis attributed these contractions to a circus movement in the atria; Prinzmetal suggested that they are due to an irritable focus in the atrial muscle similar to that of paroxysmal atrial tachycardia and atrial extrasystoles. The rate of atrial beats ranges from 250 to 400 per minute. Because the atrioventricular node cannot transmit such rapid impulses, the ventricles respond to every second, or even to every third or fourth, atrial beat.

Atrial flutter is not frequent in children, but may sometimes complicate myocarditis of any cause and occasionally acute infectious diseases. It has also been recognized and has persisted after palliative or corrective intra-atrial surgery, e.g., for transposition of the great arteries, ostium secundum defect or total anomalous pulmonary venous return. It should be suspected in patients with a regular tachycardia which is not influenced by effort, emotion or posture. Atrial flutter may precipitate congestive cardiac failure. Carotid sinus pressure frequently produces a temporary slowing of the cardiac rate. The diagnosis is confirmed by electrocardiography, which demonstrates the rapid and regular atrial flutter or "f" waves (Fig. 13–60).

Treatment is by digitalization to convert the arrhythmia into atrial fibrillation. Normal sinus rhythm may then be restored when the digitalis is discontinued. If atrial fibrillation persists, quinidine sulfate is used. If atrial flutter still continues, the administration of digitalis is resumed. Uncontrollable atrial flutter may also be treated with electrical cardioversion.

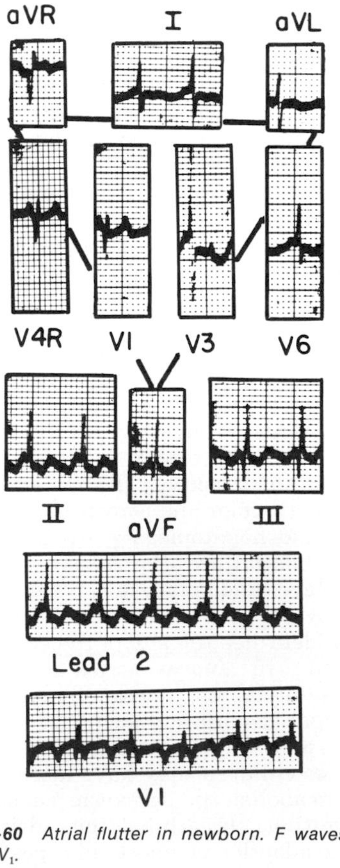

Figure 13–60 Atrial flutter in newborn. F waves present in leads II and V_1.

ATRIAL FIBRILLATION

The mechanism of this abnormality is similar to that of atrial flutter; the atrial excitation is irregular and more rapid (300 to 500 per minute). The arrhythmia occurs most frequently in older children with rheumatic mitral valve disease. It has been reported as a complication of atrial septal defect and patent ductus arteriosus.

The rhythm is grossly irregular (Fig. 13–61) and associated with a pulse deficit. Atrial fibrillation may complicate or precipitate congestive cardiac failure.

Treatment is by digitalization, which restores the ventricular rate to normal, although the rhythm remains irregular. Normal sinus rhythm may then be restored with quinidine sulfate. Electrical cardioversion also restores sinus rhythm. Maintenance of sinus rhythm is not usual in the patient whose atrial fibrillation was associated with florid mitral valve disease and cardiomegaly. Continuation of prophylactic therapy with digitalis and quinidine is usually required in these patients.

VENTRICULAR FIBRILLATION

This irregular ventricular action (Fig. 13–62) results in death unless an effective ventricular beat is restored. Occasionally this arrhythmia occurs during or shortly after cardiac surgery and explains some of the deaths that result from intravenous drug therapy. The only effective therapy is cardiac massage (preferably external) and electrical defibrillation.

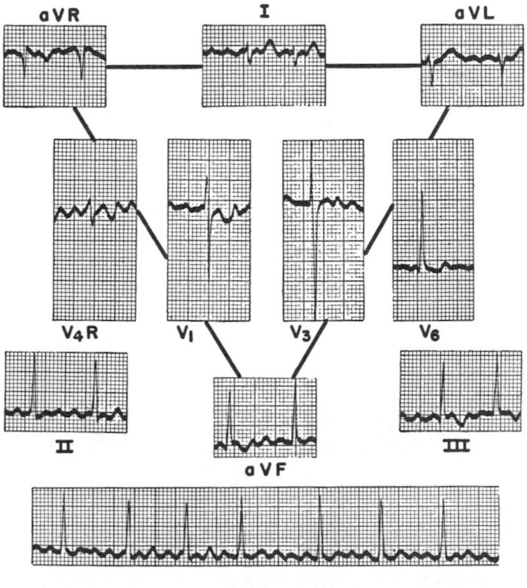

Figure 13–61 Electrocardiogram of an 11 year old girl with rheumatic heart disease and mitral stenosis. The tracing reveals the presence of atrial fibrillation, rarely seen in U.S. children in recent years.

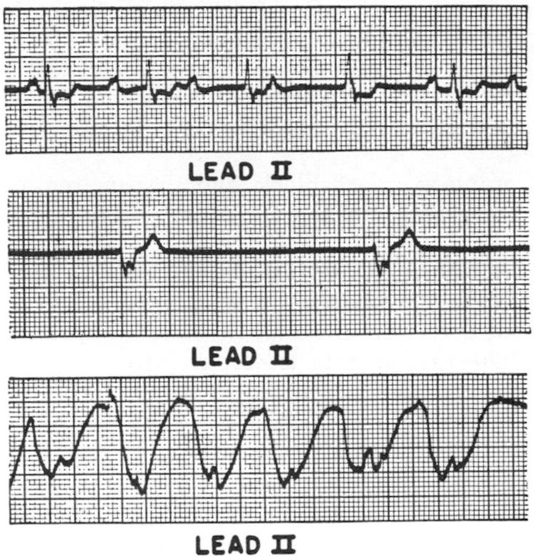

Figure 13–62 Electrocardiogram tracings showing various types of arrhythmias. Upper tracing shows the Wenckebach phenomenon. Note progressive prolongation of the P-R interval. Middle tracing shows idioventricular rhythm with a heart rate of 30 per minute. Lower tracing shows ventricular fibrillation.

BRADYCARDIA

A slow pulse rate may occur during convalescence from acute infections such as rheumatic fever, typhoid fever or infectious hepatitis and in association with lesions of the brain which cause increased intracranial pressure. Older children and young adults who lead active lives frequently have pulse rates of about 60 per minute at rest. Bradycardia of this degree may occur as a family trait. Rates of less than 80 per minute in the first 2 years of life and less than 50 in older children may be the result of heart block.

HEART BLOCK

The conductive system includes the sinoatrial node, the internodal pathways, the atrioventricular node, the bundle of His with its left and right branches, and the Purkinje network. The conductive system may be blocked at any site along this pathway. When the block occurs at the sinoatrial node, so that occasional beats are delayed or dropped, it is designated **sinoatrial block.** When the impulse is blocked in its pathway from the sinoatrial node through the atrioventricular node, it is termed **atrioventricular block.** *Partial atrioventricular block* may have only a prolonged P-R interval **(first-degree block)** or may be associated with dropped ventricular beats **(second-degree block).** Second-degree block may occur at regular intervals so that there are two or three atrial beats to one ventricular beat (2:1 or 3:1 partial atrioventricular block). Another type of partial atrioventricular block is a progressive lengthening of the P-R interval from cycle to cycle until a ventricular beat is dropped **(Wenckebach phenomenon,** Fig. 13–62). When no impulses pass through the atrioventricular node so that the atria and ventricles contract independently of each other, the condition is known as **complete atrioventricular block.** Finally, the impulse may be blocked in either the left or right branch of the bundle of His, and the condition is designated as **left** or **right bundle branch block.**

Complete heart block and first-degree partial block are the common types encountered in children.

CONGENITAL COMPLETE HEART BLOCK. In children complete block is probably the result of a congenital defect in the main stem of the bundle of His. The arrhythmia is occasionally suspected in the fetus. In an international study of almost 600 patients with congenital complete heart block, about 70 per cent had no other evidence of heart disease. At greatest risk were babies in the first few weeks of life who were in congestive cardiac failure with associated congenital heart disease and whose atrial rates exceeded 150 per minute while the ventricular rate was less than 55. The most frequently associated cardiac malformations were corrected transposition of the great vessels with ventricular septal defect, single ventricle, and patent ductus arteriosus. Isolated ventricular septal defect is seldom associated with complete heart block.

In older children with otherwise normal hearts the condition is commonly asymptomatic, although attacks of syncope may occur. The peripheral pulse is of the water-hammer type, owing to the large ventricular stroke volume and peripheral vasodilatation, and the systolic blood pressure is elevated. Jugular venous pulsations occur irregularly and may be large when the atrium contracts against a closed tricuspid valve. Inconspicuous venous pulsations may occur independently of ventricular contractions. The first cardiac sound has a changing intensity, and isolated atrial contractions may be audible down the left sternal border or at the apex. Taussig observed that exercise and atropine, which have no effect in increasing the cardiac rate of adults with complete heart block, may produce an acceleration of 10 to 20 beats per minute in the child. Heart block in itself produces cardiac enlargement. Systolic murmurs along the left sternal border are frequent and do not indicate the presence of a ventricular septal defect. Apical mid-diastolic murmurs are not unusual.

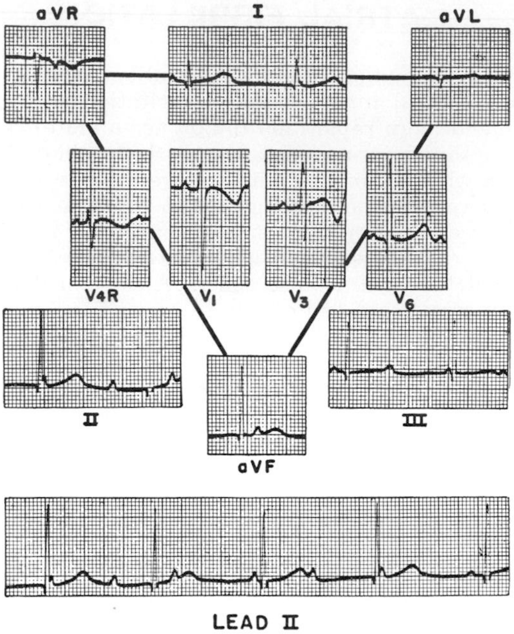

Figure 13–63 *Electrocardiogram of 5 year old boy showing complete heart block (see text).*

The diagnosis is confirmed by electrocardiograms; the P waves and QRS complexes have no constant relation (Fig. 13–63). The shape and amplitude of individual waves are generally normal.

The prognosis is usually favorable; patients who have been observed to the age of 30 to 40 years have lived normally active lives. In some patients, however, episodes of dizziness with or without syncope (Stokes-Adams attacks) may occur. This complication requires the implantation of a permanent pacemaker.

Engle, M. A., and Ehlers, K. H.: Cardiac dysrhythmias as a pediatric problem. *In* Yu, P. N., and Goodwin, J. F. (eds.): Progress in Cardiology, 2. Philadelphia, Lea & Febiger, 1973, pp. 135–179.

Michaëlson, M., and Engle, M. A.: International Cooperative Study of Congenital Complete Heart Block. *In* Engle, M. A. (ed.): Cardiovascular Clinics: Pediatric Cardiology. Philadelphia, F. A. Davis Company, 1972.

Nadas, A. S., Daeschner, C. W., Roth, A., and Blumenthal, S. L.: Paroxysmal tachycardia in infants and children: Study of 41 cases. Pediatrics *9*:167, 1952.

Paul, M. H.: Cardiac Arrhythmias in infants and children. Prog. Cardiovasc. Dis. *9*:136, 1966.

DISEASES OF THE ENDOCARDIUM

ACUTE OR MALIGNANT ENDOCARDITIS

Acute endocarditis has been observed at all ages, including the neonatal period; it may have been acquired during fetal life. The infection may occur suddenly in a previously well child or may complicate congenital or rheumatic heart disease. The commonest infecting agent is *Staphylococcus aureus.* Less frequently encountered organisms are gram-negative bacilli, enterococci, pneumococci and fungi. Vegetations develop on the endocardium of the valves and cardiac chambers, more frequently on the left side than on the right. They consist of bacteria in an exudate of fibrin and blood. Ulceration and the formation of friable granulation tissue occur early. Destruction of valvular tissue progresses rapidly, resulting in acute incompetence of valves, usually the mitral or aortic. Cardiac performance is further impaired by extension of the infection into the myocardium. Parts of the vegetations or necrotic tissue may embolize to any part of the body, obstructing blood flow and establishing secondary foci of infection.

CLINICAL MANIFESTATIONS. The onset of acute endocarditis is explosive, with high fever and prostration. Abdominal pain, hematuria, diarrhea or paralysis of parts of the body may be produced by septic emboli. Cardiomegaly may or may not be present. Cardiac murmurs are either absent or produced by previously underlying heart disease. Retinal hemorrhages, splenomegaly or the loss of pulsation of a major artery may be detected. In many patients the cause of the infection is not clear, but in some there is a history of recent furunculosis, osteomyelitis or infected pilonidal cyst. Polymorphonuclear leukocytosis is usual. Albuminuria, microscopic hematuria and pyuria are common. Blood cultures are usually positive.

PROGNOSIS. The prognosis is generally grave, and death usually occurs within a few days unless treatment is started early. The cause of death is either toxicity from infection or relentless progression of cardiac failure. The latter complication may occur weeks or months after the infection is cured, owing to rupture or development of defects in the valves (usually mitral or aortic).

TREATMENT. Since the prognosis is so poor if therapy is delayed, three blood cultures should be drawn within 1 to 2 hours and treatment started on the presumption that the causal organism is *Staphylococcus aureus*. Large intravenous doses of methicillin, oxacillin or nafcillin should be used until the results of the cultures and the antibiotic sensitivity of the organism are available. The duration of therapy should never be less than 4 weeks. Penicillin G (20 to 40 million units daily) may be used if the organism is sensitive to this antibiotic; the blood level may be increased with probenecid. Supportive therapy, including blood transfusions and intravenous fluids, is the same as for other acute infections. The complication of heart failure is treated with the usual anticongestive measures. Emboli to major vessels, especially in the lower extremities, should be removed surgically as an emergency.

SUBACUTE BACTERIAL ENDOCARDITIS

This disease resembles the acute form in many ways, but its course is more insidious and protracted. The infection usually develops at the site of congenital or acquired defects of the heart. It rarely occurs in infancy, but has been noted occasionally in children 3 or 4 years of age; the incidence increases with advancing age.

The commonest causative organism is *Streptococcus viridans*. Other infecting agents include enterococci (group D streptococci), *Staphylococcus albus* or *aureus* and fungi. Although predisposing factors are not clear in all patients, infection with *S. viridans* may follow oral or pharyngeal surgery, especially dental extractions. Enterococci may enter the bloodstream after instrumentation of the genitourinary or gastrointestinal tract. Organisms which are generally considered to be nonpathogenic may result in subacute (or acute) bacterial endocarditis after open-heart surgery.

The vegetations are usually smaller than those in the acute type. They may destroy the endocardial lining and underlying muscle and even perforate valves or septa. When superimposed upon acquired cardiac disease, the subacute form usually attacks the left rather than the right side of the heart. In congenitally malformed hearts the bacterial invasion begins at or near the site of the defect.

CLINICAL MANIFESTATIONS. Initially, symptoms are obscure and ill defined, including pyrexia, malaise, lassitude, pallor, anorexia, weight loss and arthralgia. Chills and night sweats may occur. Signs of pre-existing heart disease are present, and new murmurs may appear during the course of the disease, e.g., from mitral or aortic incompetence. Unexplained heart failure in a previously well compensated patient may be an early sign. Petechiae are common and are usually located in oral mucous membranes, conjunctivae and around the ankles and wrists. Splinter hemorrhages may be seen under the fingernails and toenails; occasionally retinal hemorrhages are present. The older literature stressed other classic signs of subacute bacterial endocarditis such as Osler's nodes (small, tender, palpable erythematous lesions in the pads of fingers or toes), Janeway's lesions (painless, hemorrhagic nodules in the palms and soles), Roth spots (hemorrhagic areas with a white center seen in the retina) and clubbing of the fingers. These signs are late manifestations of the disease and are now rarely seen. Splenomegaly may be present, but is not constant. Left upper quadrant pain may be produced by splenic infarction. A normochromic, normocytic anemia is usual. Proteinuria is common; microscopic hematuria may be present. The emphasis of the clinical picture may be altered by systemic embolization, which may result in infarction, hemorrhage, abscess formation or gangrene. When the underlying cardiac disease is associated with a left-to-right shunt, pulmonary infarction may occur. Occasionally bacterial endocarditis presents with meningitis, convulsions, hemiparesis or subarachnoid hemorrhage.

DIAGNOSIS. Anemia and leukocytosis are common and the sedimentation rate is increased. Identification of the causative organism by blood culture is the most important laboratory finding. Six blood cultures (aerobic and anaerobic) taken over a period of 2 to 4 days usually suffice; if these are negative, subsequent cultures are rarely positive.

PROGNOSIS. With early adequate treatment most children recover completely. The disease may run a mild course during its first weeks or even months so that the diagnosis may not be suspected until severe valvular disease has resulted. If therapy is inadequate, recurrences are usual.

TREATMENT. Identification of the infecting organisms is essential to successful therapy, but antibiotic treatment may be initiated, pending the results of in vitro sensitivity tests after the organism has been isolated. It is important that the blood level of antibiotics exceed the minimal inhibiting concentration of antibiotic in broth. Bactericidal agents should be used whenever possible, since bacteriostatic drugs are seldom successful in eradicating bacteria from cardiac vegetations.

Streptococcus viridans is almost always exquisitely sensitive to penicillin; i.e., growth is inhibited by 0.005 to 0.2 μg of penicillin per ml of serum. Infection with this organism is treated with a combination of penicillin and streptomycin, since the latter is synergistic with penicillin. The route of administration of penicillin and the duration of therapy are controversial. In many institutions penicillin G is given intravenously or intramuscularly in doses varying from 600,000 to 3,000,000 units every 4 hours for 2 to 6 weeks. We have had great success with oral phenoxymethyl penicillin (penicillin V) in a dose of 600 to 750 mg every 4 hours for 2 weeks. We have not encountered instances in which the antibiotic had to be abandoned because of inadequate absorption or gastrointestinal symptoms (nausea, vomiting, diarrhea). Streptomycin is given intramuscularly every 12 hours, and the dose should not exceed 1 gm per day even in adolescents. It is advisable to measure the antistreptococcal activity of the patient's serum against his own organism. Treatment is progressing satisfactorily if a serum dilution of 1:8, 1:16 or more inhibits growth of the organism.

Enterococci (group D streptococci) are usually more resistant to penicillin; patients infected with these organisms require intravenous therapy with penicillin G (15 to 25 million units daily) for 4 to 6 weeks. Streptomycin is used concomitantly; the dose should not exceed 1 gm daily.

Endocarditis due to *gram-negative bacteria* is difficult to manage and in children is generally seen as a complication of open-heart surgery. The choice of antibiotic depends on the in vitro sensitivity of the causal organism.

Penicillin sensitivity should be carefully confirmed by history. Barring a history of serious reaction, it is the drug of choice, and the following regimen may be used: (1) oral prednisone; (2) a gradual buildup in penicillin dosage (given at half hourly intervals) as follows: *(a)* 10 units intradermally, *(b)* 100 units subcutaneously, *(c)* 1000 units subcutaneously, *(d)* 10,000 units intramuscularly, *(e)* 100,000 units intramuscularly. If no reaction occurs, the usual schedule of penicillin therapy may be followed, even if urticaria is observed during the course of treatment.

Clinically acceptable but *bacteriologically unproved* endocarditis is a difficult therapeutic problem. Generally it is assumed that the organism is sensitive to penicillin, and so it is infused intravenously in a dose of at least 10 million units daily for not less than 4 weeks, frequently supplemented with intramuscular streptomycin. The adequacy of therapy is gauged by the clinical course. When there is lack of response to therapy, the dose of penicillin is increased or other bactericidal agents are added. Probenecid may be used to increase the blood level of penicillin.

A condition clinically indistinguishable from subacute bacterial endocarditis or endarteritis may be seen in children with *ventriculocardiovascular shunts* for the treatment of hydrocephalus. The colonization of bacteria is usually in the valve of the artificial shunt. Management is similar to that for subacute bacterial endocarditis, except that it is rarely successful without removal of the shunt and replacement with an uncontaminated substitute.

PROPHYLAXIS. All children with rheumatic heart disease and congenital cardiovascular anomalies are exposed to the hazard of subacute bacterial endocarditis. Therefore, these patients should be protected with large doses of penicillin before and after dental extractions and operations on the ears, nose or throat (Table 9–14). Acute bacterial infections should be vigorously treated with suitable antibiotics.

RHEUMATIC ENDOCARDITIS

Rheumatic infections (Section 10) are not limited to the endocardium, but involve other parts of the heart and other organs of the body; only the endocardial changes will be mentioned here.

Rheumatic involvement of the valves and endocardium is by far the most common type of endocarditis in children. The lesions begin as small verrucae composed of fibrin and blood cells along the borders of the valves. The mitral valve is affected most often, and aortic next most frequently, and the tricuspid and pulmonary valves less commonly. As the infection subsides, the verrucae tend to disappear and leave scar tissue. With each repeated infection more small lesions of this type form near the previous ones, and the mural endocardium and chordae tendineae also become involved.

CLINICAL PATTERNS OF VALVULAR DISEASE

Mitral Insufficiency. Mitral insufficiency that prevents normal closure of the mitral valve is most frequently rheumatic in origin. There is usually some loss of substance of the valve, and the chordae tendineae may be shortened and thickened. There is often associated mitral stenosis as a result of sclerosis of the base of the mitral ring and cusps.

During ventricular systole, blood regurgitates

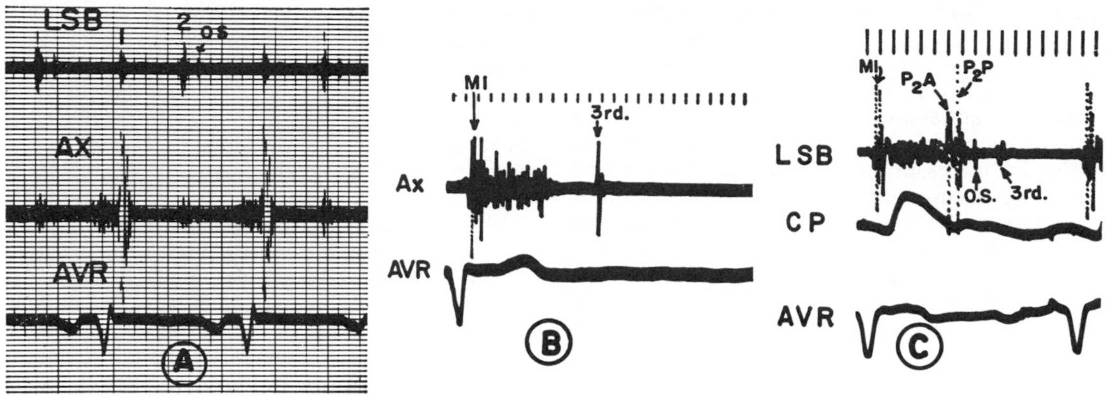

Figure 13–64 *Phonocardiograms to illustrate auscultatory findings in proved cases of mitral valve disease. Abbreviations: LSB, Left sternal border; AX, apex; AVR, electrocardiogram; CP, carotid pulse; 1, first heart sound; 2, second heart sound;* P_2A, *aortic component, second sound;* P_2P, *pulmonary component, second sound; OS, mitral opening snap; 3, third heart sound.* A, *Pure mitral stenosis. Note presystolic murmur, loud first sound, opening snap, prolonged Q-1 interval and 2-OS interval of 0.06 second.* B, *Pure mitral insufficiency. Note pansystolic murmur and loud third sound.* C, *Combined mitral insufficiency and stenosis. Note pansystolic murmur, opening snap and third heart sound.*

from the left ventricle to the left atrium. This may result in left atrial enlargement, which is sometimes aneurysmal. Owing to the greater work load and filling pressure of the left ventricle, this chamber may also enlarge. The increased left atrial pressure may be reflected through the pulmonary bed to the right side of the heart, producing enlargement of the right ventricle and atrium, with subsequent congestive cardiac failure. In the majority of children the lesion is of mild or moderate severity, is well tolerated, and is asymptomatic. The principal physical sign is the apical systolic murmur of mitral incompetence (see below). In moderately severe or florid lesions the dominant symptoms are fatigue, poor weight gain, weakness, dyspnea on effort, and palpitations. The heart is enlarged, and an apical systolic thrill may be palpable. The first heart sound is normal; the second sound may show wide expiratory splitting because of the shortened duration of left ventricular systole. Pulmonary valvular closure is loud in the presence of complicating pulmonary hypertension. A third heart sound is prominent and is due to the large early diastolic filling of the left ventricle. The usual murmur is pansystolic (Fig. 13–64) and radiates to the left axilla and to the left sternal edge; in a minority of instances it is short and on rare occasions may be absent. A diastolic murmur due to increased blood flow from the left atrium across the mitral valve may be audible even in the absence of mitral stenosis.

The electrocardiogram and roentgenograms are normal if the lesion is mild. With more severe lesions the electrocardiogram shows prominent bifid P waves, signs of left ventricular hypertrophy and sometimes associated right ventricular hypertrophy. Roentgenographically there is prominence of the left atrium and ventricle. When pulmonary hypertension or congestive heart failure supervenes, the pulmonary artery segment and right heart chambers are prominent. Signs of pulmonary venous hypertension are also seen sometimes. Calcification of the mitral valve is rare in children. *Echocardiography* shows an increased velocity of diastolic closure of the anterior mitral leaflet (greater than 170–180 mm/sec) in moderate or severe regurgitation.

Cardiac catheterization and left ventriculography are undertaken only if there is rapid progression of the disease and surgical treatment is contemplated. The cardiac output is normal or decreased in florid lesions. The left atrial pressure is frequently but not always increased. The pulse curve of the left atrium shows a steep rise in early systole to the peak of the "v" wave and is followed by a rapid "y" descent. A diastolic gradient may be measured across the mitral valve even in the absence of mitral stenosis. The left ventricular end-diastolic pressure rises during exercise or in the presence of left ventricular failure. Left ventriculography results in opacification of the left atrium. The degree of opacification is used as a qualitative assessment of the severity of incompetence.

A frequent problem is evaluation of an apical systolic murmur without other signs in patients who have had a mild attack of rheumatic fever or a history of recurrent upper respiratory tract infections. Though many of these patients are considered to have organic mitral insufficiency, the diagnosis is often incorrect. In some the murmur is extracardiac, and sometimes an innocent murmur is transmitted to the apex. Many children with murmurs suggestive of mitral insufficiency lose all evidence of cardiac disease after some years. Patients may require careful follow-up studies for many years before the cause of the murmur becomes apparent. *Untold harm may be done if the patient's activities are reduced on the basis of the presence of a murmur alone.*

During convalescence children with mild cardiac disease often make great improvement, while those with far advanced cardiac disease suffer from the effects of rapid growth. If rheumatic infections recur, the valvular condition may become progressively worse. For prophylactic therapy, see Section 9.

Complications. Severe mitral incompetence may result in cardiac failure. This may be precipitated by progression of the rheumatic process, the onset of atrial fibrillation with rapid ventricular response or subacute bacterial endocarditis. Pulmonary congestion is common, but frank left ventricular failure is unusual. Right-sided heart failure may be accompanied by tricuspid or pulmonary incompetence. Bacterial endocarditis may complicate rheumatic mitral valvular disease, especially when dominant incompetence is associated with moderate stenosis. Occasional atrial or ventricular extrasystoles are well tolerated. First-degree heart block may persist for years after the original rheumatic infection or be due to digitalis therapy. Atrial fibrillation is more common when mitral incompetence is associated with a large hypertensive left atrium.

Treatment. In the majority of patients with mitral insufficiency, prophylaxis against recurrences of rheumatic fever is all that is required, since the lesions are mild and well tolerated. The treatment of complicating heart failure, dysrhythmias and bacterial endocarditis is described elsewhere. Surgical treatment is indicated in a minority who, in spite of adequate medical therapy, suffer from recurrent episodes of heart failure, extreme dyspnea with moderate activity, and progressive cardiomegaly with pulmonary hypertension. Although annuloplasty gives good results in some children and adolescents, the majority require valve replacement.

Mitral Stenosis. Congenital mitral stenosis is described on an earlier page.

Organic mitral stenosis is nearly always rheumatic in origin and results from fibrosis of the mitral ring, commissural adhesions and contracture of the valve leaflets, chordae and papillary muscles. It may take 2 years or more for the lesion to become fully established, although the process may be accelerated in some children. Mitral stenosis is often associated with mitral insufficiency.

Mitral stenosis of critical degree is considered to exist if the valve orifice is reduced to 25 per cent or less of the expected normal. In established lesions the left atrium has difficulty in emptying, which results in hypertrophy and increased pressure in this chamber. The increased pressure results in pulmonary venous hypertension, increased pulmonary vascular resistance and pulmonary hypertension. Right ventricular and atrial dilatation and hypertrophy ensue and are followed by right-sided heart failure.

Generally there is a good correlation between symptoms and severity of obstruction. Patients with mild lesions are asymptomatic. More severe degrees of obstruction are associated with effort intolerance and dyspnea. Critical lesions can result in orthopnea, paroxysmal nocturnal dyspnea and overt pulmonary edema. These symptoms may be precipitated by uncontrolled tachycardia, atrial fibrillation or pulmonary infections. Congestive heart failure is usually associated with moderate or severe pulmonary hypertension. Right ventricular dilatation may result in functional tricuspid incompetence, hepatomegaly, ascites and edema. Hemoptysis may occur, owing to ruptured bronchial or pleurohilar veins and, occasionally, pulmonary infarction. Blood-streaked sputum occurs during episodes of pulmonary edema. Bacterial endocarditis and systemic emboli are uncommon in children.

With severe lesions, cyanosis and a malar flush are seen. The jugular venous pressure is increased in the presence of congestive heart failure, tricuspid valve disease or severe pulmonary hypertension. The heart size is normal with minimal disease. Moderate cardiomegaly is usual with severe mitral stenosis and sinus rhythm, but cardiac enlargement can be great, especially when atrial fibrillation and heart failure supervene. The apical impulse is brief and tapping, and a parasternal right ventricular lift is palpable when pulmonary vascular resistance is high. The principal auscultatory findings are a loud first heart sound, an opening snap of the mitral valve and a long, low-pitched, rumbling mitral diastolic murmur with presystolic accentuation (Fig. 13–64). Severe obstruction is present when (1) the diastolic murmur is long (in the absence of mitral incompetence), (2) the Q-1 interval is long (i.e., time between the Q wave of the electrocardiogram and the first heart sound), and (3) the 2-OS interval is short (i.e., time between aortic valve closure and the opening snap). The mitral diastolic murmur may be absent in congestive heart failure. Presystolic accentuation of the diastolic murmur disappears during atrial fibrillation. An apical systolic murmur may be audible even in the absence of mitral incompetence, and in some is due to complicating tricuspid incompetence. In the presence of pulmonary hypertension, pulmonary valvular closure is accentuated. An early diastolic murmur is usually due to associated aortic incompetence, since pulmonary valvular incompetence is not as common.

Electrocardiograms and *roentgenograms* are normal if the lesion is mild. More severe obstruction is associated with prominent and notched P waves and varying degrees of right ventricular hypertrophy. Moderate or critical lesions are associated with roentgenographic signs of varying degrees of left atrial enlargement, prominence of the pulmonary artery and right heart chambers and a normal or small aorta and left ventricle (Fig. 13–65). Severe obstruction is associated with a redistribution of pulmonary blood flow, so that the apices of the lung show a greater perfusion (i.e., reverse of normal). Serial films of patients with progressive stenosis will show more pulmonary vascular markings at the apices with prominence of the pulmonary veins. Septal lines at the costophrenic angles may also be present. *Echocardiography* shows marked slowing of the diastolic closure of the anterior mitral leaflet (less than 40 mm/sec). Cardiac catheterization quantitates the diastolic gradient across the mitral valve, the degree of pulmonary hypertension and the severity of increase of pulmonary vascular resistance.

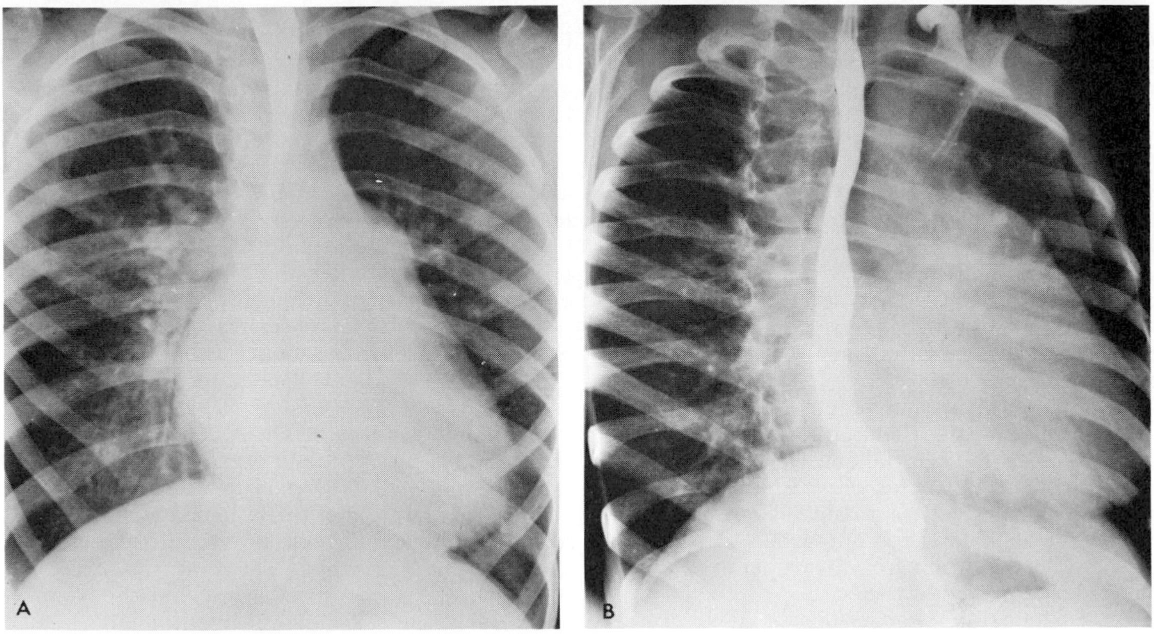

Figure 13–65 *Teleroentgenograms in isolated rheumatic mitral stenosis.* A, *Posteroanterior view showing cardiomegaly and prominent main pulmonary artery. Vascular shadows in lungs due to prominent pulmonary arteries and veins.* B, *Right anterior oblique view showing indentation of esophagus by large left atrium. This patient required mitral valvotomy at age 8 years.*

Treatment. Prophylaxis against recurrences of rheumatic fever and the treatment of cardiac failure and dysrhythmias are similar to those described under Mitral Insufficiency. Surgical treatment is undertaken when there are signs of recurrent pulmonary edema, high pulmonary vascular resistance or systemic emboli. Since extreme valvular distortion and calcification are rare in children, closed mitral valvotomy generally yields good results.

Aortic Insufficiency. In the majority of instances aortic insufficiency results from rheumatic heart disease, but sometimes is associated with congenital cardiovascular lesions (see Coarctation of the Aorta, Aortic Stenosis and Ventricular Septal Defect). In chronic rheumatic aortic insufficiency, sclerosis of the aortic valves results in distortion and retraction of the cusps. Regurgitation of blood results in a volume overload with dilatation and hypertrophy of the left ventricle. Secondary mitral incompetence may follow progressive left ventricular dilatation. Left ventricular failure results in left atrial hypertension. Congestive cardiac failure may occur insidiously or be preceded by bouts of pulmonary edema.

Symptoms are unusual except in gross aortic incompetence. The large stroke volume and forceful left ventricular contractions may result in palpitations. Excessive sweating and heat intolerance are related to vasodilatation. Dyspnea on effort progresses to orthopnea and pulmonary edema. Angina pectoris may occur during heavy exertion. In adolescents with florid incompetence, nocturnal attacks with nightmares, sweating, tachycardia, chest pain and hypertension may occur.

Owing to the reflux of blood through the aortic valve during diastole and to associated vasodilatation, the radial pulses are water-hammer in type and the carotid arteries show bounding Corrigan pulsations. Associated signs of severe aortic insufficiency include capillary pulsations in the lips or fingernails, an audible systolic shock over the peripheral arteries (pistol shot) and systolic and diastolic murmurs over the femoral arteries if pressure is applied to the artery just distal to the stethoscope (**Duroziez's sign**). The systolic blood pressure is elevated, the diastolic lowered.

In severe aortic insufficiency the heart is enlarged, with a left ventricular apical heave. Thrills are absent unless there is an associated aortic stenosis. The typical murmur is early in diastole and is heard over the upper and middle left sternal border with radiation to the apex and to the aortic area. Characteristically it has the hollow, fading quality of a whispered "ping." Generally the murmur is more easily audible in full expiration with the patient leaning forward, or it may be louder in the recumbent position. A systolic ejection murmur sometimes preceded by a click is frequent and is produced by the large stroke volume. An apical presystolic murmur (Austin-Flint) resembling that of mitral stenosis is heard sometimes. It is probably due to interference with valvular function by the large regurgitant blood flow which deflects the aortic cusp of the mitral valve.

The *echocardiogram* shows diastolic mitral valve flutter or oscillation, having a frequency of 30 to 40 cycles per second. This results from the regurgitant jet striking the anterior mitral leaflet.

Roentgenograms show prominence and exaggerated pulsations of the left ventricle and aorta. The electrocardiogram may be normal, but in severe cases reveals signs of left ventricular hypertrophy with prominent P waves.

Cardiac catheterization is seldom necessary and is undertaken only when surgery is contemplated because of a progressive lesion. The degree of elevation of left ventricular end diastolic, left atrial and pulmonary arterial pressures is quantitated, and ascending aortography demonstrates the regurgitant flow across the aortic valve into the left ventricle.

Mild and moderate lesions are well tolerated. Many adolescents with severe regurgitation are symptom-free and tolerate advanced lesions well into the third and fourth decades. Unfavorable signs are the onset of congestive heart failure, recurrent episodes of pulmonary edema or development of angina pectoris.

Treatment consists in prophylaxis against the recurrence of acute rheumatic fever and occurrence of subacute bacterial endocarditis, as well as encouragement to lead as active and normal a life as possible. Surgical treatment (usually valve replacement) is undertaken only when there is progressive deterioration from heart failure, pulmonary edema or angina pectoris.

Aortic Stenosis. Aortic stenosis in children is usually the result of a congenital lesion. Rheumatic aortic stenosis is rare, although some degree of it may be associated with aortic insufficiency. The signs of pure aortic stenosis are described earlier under Congenital Aortic Stenosis.

Tricuspid Valvular Disease. Tricuspid involvement is rare. *Tricuspid insufficiency* is usually functional, being secondary to right ventricular dilatation resulting from severe left-sided lesions. The signs produced by tricuspid insufficiency include prominent pulsations of the jugular veins with a "c-v" wave, systolic pulsations of the liver and a blowing systolic murmur in the fourth and fifth left parasternal spaces which increases in intensity during inspiration. Concomitant signs of mitral or aortic valvular disease with or without atrial fibrillation are frequent. Signs of tricuspid incompetence improve or disappear when heart failure produced by the left-sided lesions is treated.

Acquired tricuspid stenosis is rare. It is usually associated with rheumatic mitral or aortic valvular disease. The signs are increased jugular venous pressure with prominence of the "a" wave, presystolic hepatic pulsation and a rumbling diastolic murmur in the fourth and fifth left parasternal spaces. Hepatomegaly, edema and ascites are present with severe lesions. Cardiac catheterization shows a gradient of pressure across the tricuspid valve.

Pulmonary Valvular Disease. Pulmonary insufficiency is rarely due to organic disease and is usually functional, secondary to pulmonary hypertension or dilatation of the pulmonary artery. Occasionally it complicates severe mitral stenosis (Graham Steell murmur). The murmurs are similar to those of aortic insufficiency, but the peripheral arterial signs are absent in pulmonary insufficiency. Pulmonic stenosis is usually congenital in origin (see earlier).

Endocarditis

Blount, J. G.: Bacterial endocarditis. Am. J. Med. *38*:909, 1965.

Blumenthal, S., Griffith, S. P., and Morgan, B. C.: Bacterial endocarditis in children with heart disease. Pediatrics *26*:993, 1960.

Geraci, J. E.: Antibiotic therapy of bacterial endocarditis. Heart Bull. *12*:90, 1963.

Lerner, P. I., and Weinstein, L.: Infective endocarditis in the antibiotic era. New Engl. J. Med. *274*:199, 1966.

Tan, J. S., Terhune, C. A., Kaplan, S., and Hamburger, M.: Successful two-week treatment schedule for penicillin-susceptible streptococcus viridans endocarditis. Lancet *2*:1340, 1971.

DISEASES OF THE MYOCARDIUM

CONDITIONS CAUSING MYOCARDIAL DAMAGE

The status of the myocardium is the factor which most influences the prognosis of cardiac disease. If, in spite of congenital cardiac malformations, acquired valvular disease or arrhythmias, the myocardium is able to provide satisfactory circulation of blood, the child will be able to maintain adequate nutrition, growth and activity. The myocardium may be affected by infections, mesenchymal diseases, endocrine disorders, metabolic and nutritional diseases, neuromuscular diseases, blood diseases, tumors, hypertension and congenital anomalies. See also Table 13–7.

BACTERIAL INFECTIONS

Diphtheria. The toxin of diphtheria bacilli may produce peripheral circulatory failure or toxic myocarditis. These complications occur from all types of diphtheria, including the cutaneous form. Peripheral circulatory failure occurs within the first 2 weeks of the disease and is associated with a rapid, thready pulse, cold, pale and clammy skin, and hypotension. In addition to therapy for diphtheria (Section 10), these patients are treated for cardiogenic shock.

Toxic myocarditis is characterized by the development of arrhythmia in the form of partial or complete heart block, bundle branch block or extrasystoles. Congestive cardiac failure occurs later and is associated with cardiac enlargement and gallop rhythm. In addition to the arrhythmia, the electrocardiogram shows S-T segment depression and T wave inversion in most leads. The immediate prognosis is grave (about 50 per cent mortality). Treatment (Section 10) includes strict bed rest until all signs of myocarditis have disappeared. Digitalis is reserved for patients with frank congestive heart failure.

Typhoid Fever. Toxic myocarditis may be inferred if there is electrocardiographic evidence of T wave inversion in most leads. This sign may be transient, however, and by itself is of no clinical significance. Cardiac failure is rare, and peripheral circulatory failure is no longer common.

Acute Glomerulonephritis. (Section 15). Myocardial involvement is evidenced by congestive cardiac failure, cardiac enlargement, gallop rhythm, an apical systolic murmur and electrocardiographic abnormalities. Cardiac failure is evidenced by dyspnea and pulmonary congestion, which are soon followed by increased venous pressure and hepatomegaly. It is usually difficult to determine whether cardiac failure contributes to edema in acute nephritis or whether hypervolemia contributes to cardiac failure. In these patients roentgenographic evidence of pulmonary edema is common. The electrocardiogram is frequently normal, but there may be T wave inversion, prolonged electrical systole or signs of left ventricular hypertrophy.

In addition to antihypertensive drugs and diuretics, digitalization is indicated for cardiac failure. The response is good, and digitalis may be discontinued after a week or two.

Other Bacterial Infections. Circulatory involvement in bacterial infections is manifest as peripheral circulatory collapse or toxic myocarditis. The incidence of toxic myocarditis is difficult to gauge because its diagnosis frequently depends on minor pathologic evidence such as cloudy swelling or fatty degeneration. Toxic myocarditis as evidenced by tachycardia, gallop rhythm and cardiac enlargement may complicate pneumonia, bacterial endocarditis and septicemia. The prognosis depends on control of the primary infection.

VIRAL INFECTIONS. Myocarditis complicating such viral infections as measles, chickenpox and mumps is exceedingly rare. It is difficult to gauge the incidence of myocarditis in *poliomyelitis;* hypertension is not uncommon, but cardiac failure is rare. Terminal pulmonary edema may occur. Electrocardiographic abnormalities are not common. Severe myocarditis has been identified with *coxsackievirus B* (Section 10).

PARASITIC AND FUNGAL INFECTIONS. Lesions in the myocardium have been described in association with *histoplasmosis, coccidioidomycosis, toxoplasmosis* and *trichiniasis.* In these conditions the cardiac lesion seldom produces clinical signs of myocarditis. *Actinomycosis* may involve the pericardium and myocardium by direct contiguity as, for example, from a pulmonary abscess. *Hydatid cysts* of the pericardium may be found on routine roentgenograms of the chest and usually produce symptoms only when they rupture. *Schistosomiasis* may produce pulmonary hypertension and cor pulmonale. *Cruz trypanosomiasis* (Chagas' disease) seldom occurs in North America. It may produce acute or subacute myocarditis and sudden death.

MESENCHYMAL DISEASES. *Rheumatic carditis* is described in Section 10 and on the preceding pages of this Section.

The cardiovascular manifestations of *rheumatoid arthritis, disseminated lupus erythematosus, periarteritis nodosa, dermatomyositis* and *scleroderma* are described elsewhere. In *rheumatoid arthritis,* pericarditis is not uncommon. In patients with rheumatoid arthritis and mitral or aortic valvular disease the latter may be due to coincidental or past rheumatic carditis.

ENDOCRINE DISORDERS. *Hyperthyroidism* produces tachycardia, vasodilatation, wide pulse pressure, cardiac enlargement and, rarely, atrial fibrillation. *Cretinism* seldom produces gross cardiac involvement, but the electrocardiogram discloses bradycardia, low voltage of all complexes, but especially of the P and T waves, left axis deviation and prolonged electrical systole. These signs may disappear within a month of adequate thyroid therapy.

METABOLIC AND NUTRITIONAL DISEASES. Among vitamin deficiency diseases, *beriberi* (Section 3) causes the most conspicuous cardiac damage. In patients with malnutrition the deficiencies are often multiple, and it is difficult to separate the cardiac lesion of one nutritional disease from that of another.

NEUROMUSCULAR DISEASES. In the original description of *Friedreich's ataxia,* heart disease was noted in 5 of 6 cases. In most instances cardiac symptoms are masked by the basic disease, which limits physical activities. In some patients, effort intolerance, chest pain and heart failure have been the presenting symptoms. These are due to primary myocardial disease which affects chiefly the left ventricle and results in congestive or obstructive cardiomyopathy. The electrocardiogram shows generalized T wave inversion or signs of left ventricular hypertrophy. Arrhythmias may also occur and consist of atrial tachycardia or fibrillation or extrasystoles. The cardiac silhouette on the chest x-ray reflects the severity of myocardial involvement and shows varying degrees of cardiomegaly, left ventricular prominence and pulmonary congestion.

In *progressive muscular dystrophy* (Section 21) 50 per cent of children have postmortem evidence of myocardial involvement similar to that of the striated muscle. Cardiac symptoms, however, are not common, but the electrocardiogram is frequently abnormal and may reveal tachycardia, abnormalities of the P waves, short P-R interval and abnormal Q and T waves. Minimal evidence of right or left ventricular hypertrophy may also occur, and some patients have congestive heart failure.

BLOOD DISEASES. In infants and children, anemia is the most common blood disease associated with cardiac involvement, as, for example, in leukemia, hemolytic anemias, severe iron deficiency and hemorrhage. Although cardiac output increases when the hemoglobin is below about 7 gm per 100 ml, in infants cardiac enlargement with or without congestive heart failure occurs only with an extreme reduction in hemoglobin to 3 or 4 gm or less. The heart rate is rapid, the pulse pressure is widened, and the venous pressure is increased. An apical or left sternal border systolic murmur is usual, diastolic murmurs may occur in the same areas, and gallop rhythm is common. The electrocardiographic changes include depressed S-T segments and flat T waves. Occasionally minimal signs and symptoms are present when extreme states of anemia have developed gradually.

Treatment is directed toward the cause of the anemia. If blood transfusions are indicated in the presence of cardiomegaly or cardiac failure, small volumes (4 to 5 ml/kg.) of packed cells are preferred. Venous pressure measurements during transfusion may be used as a guide for the rate and volume of transfusion.

TUMORS OF THE HEART. See Section 25.

CARCINOID. Carcinoid of the small intestine may be accompanied by pulmonic and tricuspid valvular disease. (See Section 25.)

CONGENITAL ANOMALIES

ENDOCARDIAL SCLEROSIS
(Endocardial Fibroelastosis)

This condition has been described under a variety of other terms, including fetal endocarditis, endocardial fibrosis, prenatal fibroelastosis and elastic tissue hyperplasia. The term "endocardial sclerosis" is used in this text because it describes the gross appearance of the heart at autopsy and implies no age predilection or causative factor.

No cause has been definitely established. Proposed possibilities include inflammation or infection before or after birth, maldevelopment and inadequate blood supply to the endocardium. Black-Schaffer suggested that the endocardial changes are secondary to myocardial disease which results in cardiac dilatation and subjects the endocardium to a great stretch, which initiates fibroelastic proliferation. The disease may occur in siblings. Although remote infection with coxsackie or mumps viruses has been considered, neither now appears to be a likely etiologic agent. There is a current debate as to whether the disease is primary or secondary to cardiac dilatation produced by cardiomyopathy.

Pathologically there is a white, opaque fibroelastic thickening of the endocardium, especially of the left side of the heart, which frequently obscures the trabeculation of the inner surfaces of the cardiac chamber. The lesion may spread to involve the valves, especially the aortic and mitral ones. There may be coexisting congenital cardiovascular lesions. Microscopically the lesion consists of a fibroelastic thickening of the endocardium which follows the course of the trabecular sinusoids and may result in subendocardial degeneration or necrosis of muscle with vacuolation of muscle fibers. The involved valve leaflets show a myxomatous proliferation with an increase in collagenous elements.

The clinical picture is variable. Most patients are in one of three groups:

1. Young infants, usually less than 6 months of age, who apparently have been in good health until the sudden onset of congestive cardiac failure, which is frequently precipitated by a respiratory infection. The prognosis is poor unless there is a significant response to therapy for cardiac failure.

2. Infants with similar symptoms, but of milder degree and with periods of remission. At some time during the first 2 years of life they may manifest some dyspnea, refusal of feeding, failure to gain weight adequately and recurrent pulmonary infections. There are repeated episodes of congestive cardiac failure, which in many instances can be controlled by digitalis and diuretics.

3. A miscellaneous group in whom valvular lesions or associated congenital cardiovascular defects are predominant.

The majority of patients fall into groups 1 and 2. During episodes of congestive cardiac failure the infant is acutely ill with dyspnea, cough and anorexia. Cyanosis is infrequent, but is sometimes found in the terminal phase or as a sign of associated congenital cardiovascular defects. The jugular venous pressure is elevated, the liver greatly enlarged, and edema of the extremities, sacral area or face may be present. Rales and rhonchi in the lung fields are due to intercurrent pulmonary infection and congestion. The heart is moderately or greatly enlarged, with a normal or left ventricular impulse. Thrills are not common, and murmurs are insignificant. About 25 per cent of patients have a grade I or II blowing systolic murmur down the left sternal border.

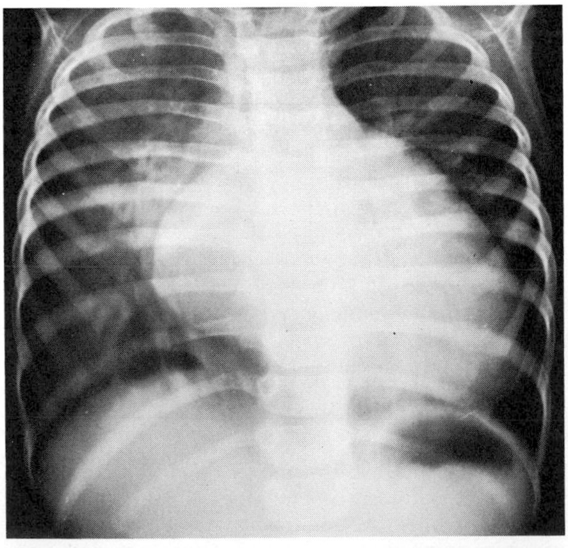

Figure 13–66 *Teleroentgenogram of a 7 month old girl with endocardial sclerosis. The enlarged heart is of an undistinctive contour.*

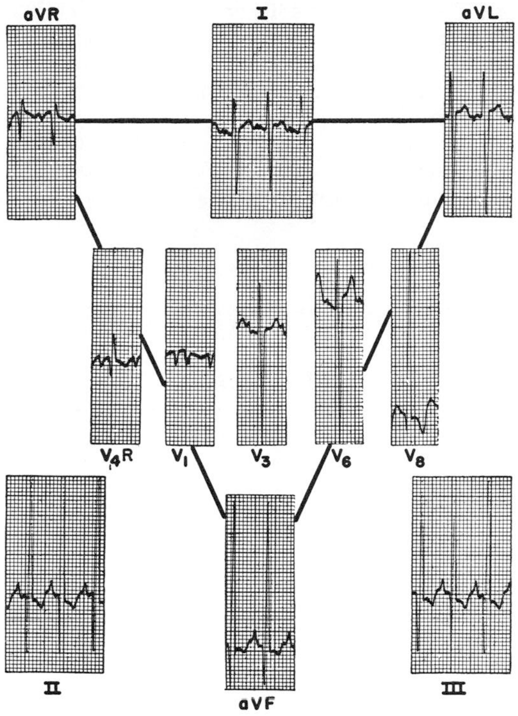

Figure 13–67 *Electrocardiogram of 3 month old girl with endocardial sclerosis. Note the abnormal T waves in leads II, aVF and V_8 and the deep Q and tall R waves in aVF and V_8.*

Roentgenograms confirm the cardiac enlargement (Fig. 13–66). There may be signs of intercurrent pulmonary infection. The *electrocardiogram* is usually abnormal, but not pathognomonic (Fig. 13–67). In the majority of cases tall R waves and inversion of the T waves over the left ventricular surface indicate dominance of the left ventricle. These signs are associated with inversion of the T waves in the standard leads and sometimes with a deep S in the right precordial leads. These electrocardiographic changes may also be seen in primary myocardial disease, gargoylism, glycogen storage disease of the heart, aberrant origin of the left coronary artery from the pulmonary artery, and medial necrosis or calcinosis of the coronary arteries. The outlook has improved recently because of the availability of more potent diuretics and the generally improved management of cardiac failure in infants. Surviving patients remain well, but many have residual signs of cardiomyopathy. In others all abnormal signs disappear; in this group of patients it is difficult to resolve the issue as to whether the original disease was myocarditis or endocardial fibroelastosis.

Treatment is directed toward alleviation of congestive cardiac failure and prevention of intercurrent infections.

CARDIOMYOPATHY

Hypertrophy of unknown origin of either ventricle has been recognized with increasing frequency. The disease may be familial, and the hypertrophy may be massive. The left ventricle is more frequently involved than the right. There are two principal clinical patterns.

OBSTRUCTIVE CARDIOMYOPATHY. Outflow of blood from the left ventricle is obstructed by muscular hypertrophy, producing symptoms and signs which may closely simulate aortic stenosis. In the less frequent right ventricular type the signs may simulate pulmonary stenosis. In other instances the signs mimic those of mitral insufficiency. With left ventricular outflow obstruction a systolic pressure gradient is demonstrable between the left ventricle and aorta. There is great lability of the gradient, however, even from moment to moment. Rapid ejection from the left ventricle occurs in early systole, but with further contraction, obstruction develops to outflow of blood. The severity of obstruction depends on the force of left ventricular contraction and on the volume of the left ventricular cavity. Thus, a postextrasystolic beat does not result in the normally expected increase of arterial pressure. Also, factors which reduce left ventricular systolic volume intensify the gradient, e.g., Valsalva maneuver and inotropic agents, including digitalis. Administration of nitroglycerin or isoproterenol also intensifies the gradient. The compliance of the hypertrophied ventricles is poor.

Many children are asymptomatic and are evaluated because of a heart murmur. In others the clinical picture is dominated by weakness, fatigue, dyspnea on effort, palpitations, angina pectoris, dizziness and syncope. The pulse is brisk because of the early systolic ejection of blood from the ventricle. The heart is enlarged, with a prominent left ventricular lift and double apical impulse. The first and second heart sounds are normal, although paradoxical splitting of the second sound is associated with a large gradient. The rarity of systolic ejection clicks help to differentiate this condition from valvular aortic stenosis. A third sound is not common, but a fourth sound may be audible. The systolic murmur is ejection in type, of medium intensity and heard maximally at the left sternal edge and apex. The *electrocardiogram* shows left ventricular hypertrophy with or without S-T segment depression and T wave inversion (Fig. 13–68). The Wolff-Parkinson-White syndrome or other intraventricular conduction defects may be seen. *Roentgenograms* show cardiomegaly with prominence of the left ventricle and sometimes the right ventricle. The ascending aorta and aortic knob are usually normal. The *echocardiogram* shows asymmetrical ventricular septal hypertrophy and systolic anterior motion of the anterior leaflet of the mitral valve.

The diagnosis is confirmed by *cardiac catheterization,* which demonstrates the unusual gradient described above. Left ventriculography shows encroachment on the left ventricular cavity by the hypertrophied muscle, especially the interventricular septum. The prognosis is unpredictable, especially in the asymptomatic patient; sudden death may occur, presumably from dysrhythmia or sud-

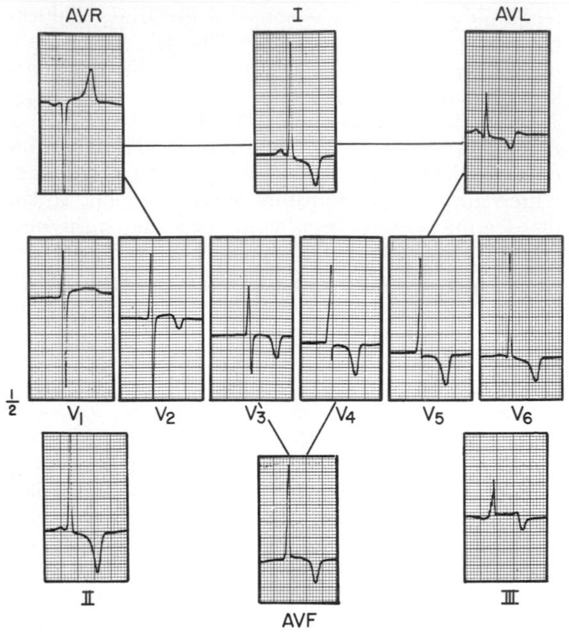

Figure 13–68 Electrocardiogram from 12 year old boy with cardiomyopathy. All chest leads are at half-sensitivity. Although an intraventricular conduction defect is not excluded, the large voltage of R waves in V_5 and V_6, the deep SV_1 and widespread T wave inversion indicate severe left ventricular hypertrophy.

den intensification of the gradient. Treatment is not standardized. Digitalis and nitroglycerin should be used with extreme caution, since they intensify the obstruction. Beta-adrenergic blocking agents (propranolol) have been used successfully. Some prefer surgical incision or resection of the left ventricular outflow tract.

NONOBSTRUCTIVE CARDIOMYOPATHY. In children the nonobstructive type of cardiomyopathy is more common. The enlarged hearts show diffuse hypertrophy, especially of the ventricular septum, and disorganization of the arrangement of muscle bundles. The symptoms are those of chronic congestive heart failure, sometimes with angina pectoris and palpitation. Physical examination reveals cardiac enlargement, nonspecific systolic murmurs and gallop rhythm, but apical murmurs of gross mitral incompetence may be present. Chronic congestive heart failure may result in tricuspid incompetence from right ventricular dilatation. The electrocardiogram usually indicates left ventricular hypertrophy. X-ray films confirm the generalized cardiomegaly, with left ventricular prominence and pulmonary congestion. The prognosis is poor, and treatment is directed toward relief of heart failure.

RESTRICTIVE CARDIOMYOPATHY. This occurs occasionally. The mechanisms producing symptoms are probably related to poor ventricular compliance, so that diastolic filling of the heart is compromised. This results in a clinical picture which closely simulates that of constrictive pericarditis. In its overt form restrictive cardiomyopathy results in dyspnea, edema, ascites, hepatomegaly, increased venous pressure and pulmonary congestion. The heart is mildly or moderately enlarged, and murmurs are nonspecific. The electrocardiogram shows prominent P waves, frequently normal QRS voltage, S-T segment depression and T wave inversion. Roentgenographic examination shows slight or moderate cardiomegaly with poor cardiac pulsations. The prognosis is generally poor. Treatment is directed toward relief of edema with diuretics.

OTHER MYOCARDIAL DISEASES

GLYCOGEN STORAGE DISEASE. The principal type of glycogen storage disease which affects the heart is the generalized form, also known as Pompe's disease or type II (Section 8). The clinical picture is dominated by skeletal muscle weakness, macroglossia and hepatomegaly. Cardiomegaly is massive, but murmurs are insignificant. Pulmonary collapse with secondary infection is common and is related to compression from the large heart. The *electrocardiogram* is characteristic and shows prominent P waves, massive QRS voltage, signs of isolated left or biventricular hypertrophy or intraventricular conduction defects. *Roentgenograms* confirm the striking cardiomegaly with prominence of the left ventricle. The prognosis is poor, and the majority of infants succumb before the age of 2 years. Effective therapy is not available.

GARGOYLISM. In gargoylism (Section 22) the lesion in the heart and great vessels is the same as that in the connective tissue elsewhere in the body. The most pronounced lesions are found in the valves and coronary arteries, but abnormalities in the pericardium and aorta are not uncommon. The heart may be moderately enlarged, with electrocardiographic signs of left ventricular hypertrophy. Cardiac murmurs may result from incompetence and stenosis of the mitral and aortic valves. Sometimes the pulmonary and tricuspid valves are also involved. Coronary arterial disease may result in angina and perhaps explain the not infrequent occurrence of sudden death. The prognosis is poor, and many children succumb before the age of 10 years with heart failure and pulmonary infection.

CALCINOSIS OF THE CORONARY ARTERIES. This is a rare disease of infancy. Familial incidence has been recorded. The coronary arteries are tortuous and calcareous, and the ventricles, especially the left, are hypertrophied. Other blood vessels may be similarly involved. The onset of cardiac failure is sudden; death usually occurs in infancy.

CONGESTIVE HEART FAILURE

In older children the signs and symptoms of congestive heart failure are similar to those in adults. Fatigue, effort intolerance, anorexia, abdominal pain and cough are frequent. In addition to breathlessness at rest, the systemic venous pressure is elevated as gauged by clinical assessment of the jugular venous pressure, the liver is enlarged and tender, and edema may be present. Orthopnea and basal rales are commonly present, and edema usually occurs in dependent portions of the body. Older children may occasionally prefer to lie in the flat position, which causes generalized anasarca. Cardiomegaly is invariably present. Auscultatory findings are those produced by the basic lesion; gallop rhythm is common.

During infancy the presence of congestive heart failure may be more difficult to determine. Symptoms are dominated by tachypnea, feeding difficulties, poor weight gain, excessive perspiration, irritability, weak cry and noisy, labored respiration with costal and subcostal retractions. Flaring of the alae nasi and sternal retractions are frequent. Signs of pulmonary congestion are difficult to interpret, since they may be indistinguishable from those produced by bronchospasm. Pneumonitis with or without collapse of part of the lung is common. Dyspnea and hepatomegaly are nearly always manifest, and cardiomegaly is invariably present. In spite of pronounced tachycardia, gallop rhythm can be recognized frequently. The other auscultatory signs are those produced by the cardiac lesion which resulted in heart failure. A sudden increase in weight which decreases after diuretic therapy is common. A clinical assessment of the jugular venous pressure in infants may be difficult, owing to the shortness of the neck and the difficulty of securing a relaxed state, although it should always be attempted. Edema in infants with cardiac failure is frequently not detectable clinically. When present, the edema may be generalized, involving the eyelids as well as the sacrum, legs and feet.

TREATMENT

The underlying cause of cardiac failure must be removed or alleviated if possible. If the cause is a congenital cardiovascular anomaly amenable to surgery, medical treatment is indicated before the surgical procedure and is continued in the immediate postoperative period. For some diseases, such as hyperthyroidism, hypothyroidism, anemia and beriberi, specific therapy is available, but in the majority of instances only general measures are adaptable.

Bed rest in a comfortable position is essential. Some patients prefer to lie flat, but for most of them breathing is easier in a semireclining position. Initially, sedatives or analgesics may be necessary to produce complete relaxation; the most frequently used drugs are morphine, codeine and the barbiturates.

A *low sodium diet* is efficacious in the treatment of cardiac edema and paroxysmal cardiac dyspnea. The oral intake of sodium should be reduced to 0.5 gm daily; the diet may be made more palatable with a salt substitute. Formulas with a low sodium content are available for infants.

Oxygen administered by any method which is effective and comfortable for the patient will help to relieve dyspnea and cyanosis.

Diuretics relieve the edema and pulmonary congestion of heart failure and therefore are very important in management. Currently available diuretics have a wide range of potency; those most frequently used are furosemide, ethacrynic acid and thiazides. Mercurials are now seldom used, since the newer agents are more effective.

Furosemide and **ethacrynic acid** are extremely potent diuretics and are effective when given orally or parenterally. They act in the renal tubules by inhibiting sodium transport and by interfering with the diluting mechanisms. It has also been shown that a redistribution of blood into the venous pool precedes the diuresis induced by furosemide. With parenteral therapy, the induction of diuresis is rapid (within 30 minutes) and the action short lived (about 4 hours). The usual parenteral dose is 1 mg/kg, although occasionally in resistant patients doses up to 3 mg/kg have been used. One parenteral dose per day usually suffices, although early in the course of therapy the dose can be repeated two or three times in 24 hours if the rapidity of clinical improvement is inadequate. Furosemide is more convenient than ethacrynic acid since the latter must be given intravenously, but furosemide may be administered intramuscularly or intravenously. It is important to measure serum electrolytes during therapy since hypokalemia or hypochloremic alkalosis can be induced with these potent diuretics. Potassium supplementation is advisable because the induced hypokalemia exaggerates signs of digitalis toxicity. The efficacy of therapy is gauged by measuring the urinary volume and by comparison of daily body weights. When a constant weight is reached, it should be maintained. A decrease in venous pressure and hepatic size, with improvement of dyspnea and signs of edema, parallels the diuresis.

Once cardiac failure is compensated, diuretics may be given orally. The usual oral dose of furosemide or ethacrynic acid is 1 mg/kg one or two times daily. In exceptional instances 2–3 mg/kg has been used without apparent ill effect. **Thiazides** are moderately potent diuretic agents. Since they can be given orally (chlorothiazide syrup), they are useful in the long-term management of cardiac failure in infants and children. They act by increasing renal excretion of sodium and chloride with an accompanying volume of water. The usual dose of oral chlorothiazide (Diuril) is 1 to 1.5 gm per square meter of body surface per day. Patients maintained on chlorothiazide should also be given potassium to supplement the usual dietary intake. **Spironolactone** (Aldactone), the aldosterone antagonist, is a useful supplement to the above oral diuretics, especially in patients with resistant peripheral edema. A trial of this agent is warranted in patients who are barely controlled with oral diuretics. It is also considered as a supplement when hypokalemia is difficult to control. *Corticosteroids* generally produce water retention, but are sometimes used in patients whose diuretic-resistant cardiac failure is due to inflammatory disease, e.g., rheumatic carditis.

Cardiac failure which is resistant to therapy or breakdown of response to previously successful management may be due to (1) infection such as reactivation of rheumatic fever, superimposed subacute bacterial endocarditis or intercurrent pulmonary or urinary tract infection, (2) electrolyte imbalance, especially hypokalemia, hypochloremic alkalosis or hyponatremia, (3) development of arrhythmia such as atrial fibrillation with rapid ventricular response, or (4) pulmonary embolism, a rare complication in children. If ascites or pleural effusions produce discomfort, fluid should be removed by paracentesis.

Digitalis should be used in all forms of cardiac failure. The most satisfactory response is obtained in failure due to rheumatic heart disease, paroxysmal tachycardia and myocardial diseases. In general, patients with primary left ventricular failure respond better than those with primary right-sided failure. The response of patients with congestive cardiac failure due to cyanotic congenital cardiovascular disease is unpredictable because hypoxia, acidosis and hypoglycemia may complicate the picture.

Many preparations of digitalis are available, but familiarity with only a few is necessary. The ones most frequently used are digoxin and digitoxin for slow digitalization and maintenance, and lanatoside C (Cedilanid) for rapid digitalization. The dose of digitalis (Section 30) and the rapidity of administration depend on the weight of the patient, the severity of congestive cardiac failure, the type of preparation, and subsequently on the response of the patient.

Digoxin is the form of digitalis used most frequently in pediatric practice because of availabilty in liquid form and the relative ease of control when inadequate or toxic doses have been given. The maximal effect of digoxin occurs about 4 hours after administration; it is excreted within 48 to 72 hours. The recommended dosage schedule is as follows: For *newborn and premature infants,* the digitalizing dose is 0.03 to 0.05 mg/kg, with a daily maintenance of one tenth to one fifth of the digitalizing dose. For *infants beyond the neonatal period, but under 2 years of age,* the oral digitalizing dose is 0.06 to 0.08 mg/kg, with a daily maintenance dose of one fifth to one third of the digitalizing one. In this age group the parenteral digitalizing dose is 0.04 to 0.06 mg/kg, with a daily parenteral maintenance dose of one tenth to one fifth of the digitalizing dose. For *children over 2 years of age* the oral digitalizing dose is 0.04 to 0.06 mg/kg, with a daily oral maintenance dose of one fifth to one third of the digitalizing one. In this age group the parenteral digitalizing dose is 0.02 to 0.04 mg/kg. The author prefers to use a digitalizing dose of 1.5 mg of digoxin per square meter of body surface (see Fig. 30–2) in patients beyond the neonatal period, with the total digitalizing dose not exceeding 2.5 mg. The daily maintenance dose is one fifth to one third of the digitalizing dose. In newborn and premature infants the digitalizing dose is 0.75 mg per square meter of body surface, with a daily maintenance dose of one tenth to one fifth of the digitalizing dose. The *timing of administration* has considerable individual variation. Frequently half of the digitalizing dose is given initially, followed by one fourth of the total dose in 6 to 8 hours, and the remaining fourth is given in another 6 to 8 hours. The daily maintenance dose may be started 12 hours later and is given preferably in two equally divided doses.

The average adequate digitalizing dose of *digitoxin* (oral or intramuscular) for children varies from 0.02 to 0.04 mg/kg. Infants require 0.04 to 0.06 mg/kg, and full-term and premature newborn infants are given 0.015 to 0.03 mg/kg. Owing to the wide variations of these dosage schedules, it may be preferable to calculate the digitalizing dose of digitoxin in older age groups on the basis of 0.75 mg per square meter of body surface (see Fig. 30–2). Full-term and premature newborn infants usually require 0.375 mg per square meter of body surface. The daily maintenance dose of digitoxin is one tenth of the digitalizing dose. The full digitalizing dose is given in divided doses within 12, 24 or 48 hours, depending on the severity of congestive failure. If digitalization is required within 12 hours, half of the digitalizing dose may be given immediately and the remaining half in divided doses over 12 hours. The total dose may be more evenly distributed if 24 or 48 hours are taken for digitalization. The optimal effect of digitoxin occurs 4 to 8 hours after administration, and its excretion is slow (10 to 14 days).

Lanatoside C (Cedilanid) is used for rapid intravenous digitalization; it should be reserved for emergency situations. It begins to act within 3 to 15 minutes after administration, and maximal effects are achieved in about 1 hour; it is excreted within 24 to 36 hours. The digitalizing dose is 0.325 to 0.75 mg per square meter of surface area (see Fig. 30–2). This preparation is seldom used in full-term or premature newborn infants. Cautious redigitalization with digoxin or digitoxin is started about 24 to 36 hours later.

It cannot be overemphasized that *any dosage schedule of any digitalis preparation is only a guide,* since there are individual differences among patients. The dose may need to be modified after part or all of the calculated digitalizing dose has been given. Full-term and premature newborn infants have a distinct intolerance for digitalis preparations. In these patients, digitalization should be controlled by careful and repeated physical examination supplemented by electrocardiography. In some infants the only reliable guide to digitalis intoxication is electrocardiographic evidence of arrhythmia.

The digitalizing dose is effective if the cardiac rate is reduced, the venous pressure and liver size are decreased, dyspnea is relieved and diuresis occurs. Electrocardiographic evidences of digitalis effect include shortening of electrical systole, depression of the S-T segment with T wave inversion and lengthening of the P-R interval. In many patients the difference between an adequate and toxic dose of digitalis is small.

The signs of digitalis toxicity include anorexia, nausea, vomiting, diarrhea, visual symptoms, dizziness, headache and arrhythmias. The arrhythmias include atrial and ventricular extrasystoles, paroxysmal atrial tachycardia with block, atrial flutter or fibrillation, bundle branch block, ventricular tachycardia and intra-atrial block. If signs of digitalis toxicity occur, the drug must be discontinued temporarily, and potassium chloride may be given orally or by intravenous drip if the arrhythmia warrants therapy. The use of digitalis blood levels in the evaluation of digitalis toxicity in the pediatric age group is being investigated.

The convalescent care of children who have suffered from congestive cardiac failure is important. As the child improves, greater freedom of activity may be permitted, and schoolwork may be resumed.

Black-Schaffer, B.: Infantile endocardial fibroelastosis: A suggested etiology. A.M.A. Arch. Path. *63*:281, 1957.

Braunwald, E., Lambrew, C. T., Rockoff, S. D., Ross, J., Jr., and Morrow, A. G.: Idiopathic hypertrophic subaortic stenosis. Circulation *30* (Supp. 4):3, 1964.

Goodwin, J. F.: Disorders of outflow tract of the left ventricle. Brit. Med. J. *2*:461, 1967.

Harris, L. C., and Nghiem, Q. X.: Cardiomyopathies in infants and children. Prog. Cardiovasc. Dis. *25*:255, 1972.

Levine, O. R., and Blumenthal, S.: Digoxin dosage in premature infants. Pediatrics, *29*:1, 1962.

Robinson, S. J.: Digitalis therapy in infants and children. J. Pediatr. *56*:536, 1960.

DISEASES OF THE PERICARDIUM

Congenital malformations of the pericardium are rare. They are chiefly defects of the parietal pericardium and are of little clinical significance. Roentgenographically and electrocardiographically they may simulate pulmonic stenosis.

Pericardial cysts are usually asymptomatic and discovered on roentgenograms of the chest. The cardiopericardial shadow is increased and distorted, depending on the location and size of the cyst. The electrocardiogram is normal. The cysts, which are usually benign, may be removed surgically.

PERICARDITIS

ETIOLOGY. Pericarditis may be primary (rheumatic, viral, postcardiotomy, purulent, traumatic or tuberculous) or an intercurrent manifestation of systemic disease (effusion resulting from congestive cardiac failure, or associated with uremia, rheumatoid arthritis, disseminated lupus, polyarteritis nodosa, primary or secondary neoplastic disease, and hematologic diseases such as leukemia, Cooley's anemia and congenital hypoplastic anemia). Pericarditis may also occur in parasitic and mycotic infections, ulcerative colitis, hypothyroidism, Friedreich's ataxia and glycogen storage disease.

HEMODYNAMICS. The effects on the circulation depend largely on the amount of pericardial fluid, the speed of its accumulation and the myocardial efficiency. Thus, a small amount of fluid in the pericardium with a normal myocardium is compatible with normal cardiovascular dynamics, whereas the rapid accumulation of large amounts of fluid in the pericardium with a normal myocardium may result in cardiac compression or *cardiac tamponade.* Smaller amounts of pericardial fluid with a diseased myocardium may also result in cardiac tamponade, as in acute rheumatic fever. Cardiac compression also occurs in longstanding chronic constrictive pericarditis.

The physiologic abnormality in cardiac compression is inadequate diastolic filling of the ventricles, which results in increased pressure in both atria and in the venous systems. The stroke volume is small and more or less fixed. Cardiac output is maintained by tachycardia, and reflex vasoconstriction maintains the blood pressure.

CLINICAL MANIFESTATIONS. Pain may or may not be present and varies in intensity, location and distribution. Since the lower third of the pericardium is innervated by the phrenic nerve, pain may be referred to the neck or shoulder. The pain may be precordial and pleural when it is aggravated by inspiration and coughing and may be referred to the back. Or it may be precordial, constant and uninfluenced by respiration, but aggravated by rotating the trunk or swallowing. The pain is either sharp or a dull, oppressive, poorly localized ache.

The venous pressure varies with the intrapericardial pressure. If the latter is raised, the venous pressure is elevated, especially during inspiration. Hepatomegaly, ascites and edema may also be present. The pulse is normal and small in volume or paradoxical; it depends on the degree of cardiac compression. A small, rapid pulse is found in patients with a tense pericardium and a low cardiac output. **Pulsus paradoxus** indicates that the pulse becomes smaller or disappears during inspiration; this sign may be confirmed by measuring the blood pressure during the phases of respiration. In the presence of cardiac compression the precordium is quiet to palpation. A large amount of fluid may be detected by percussion, and shifting dullness and by recognizing that the apical impulse is well

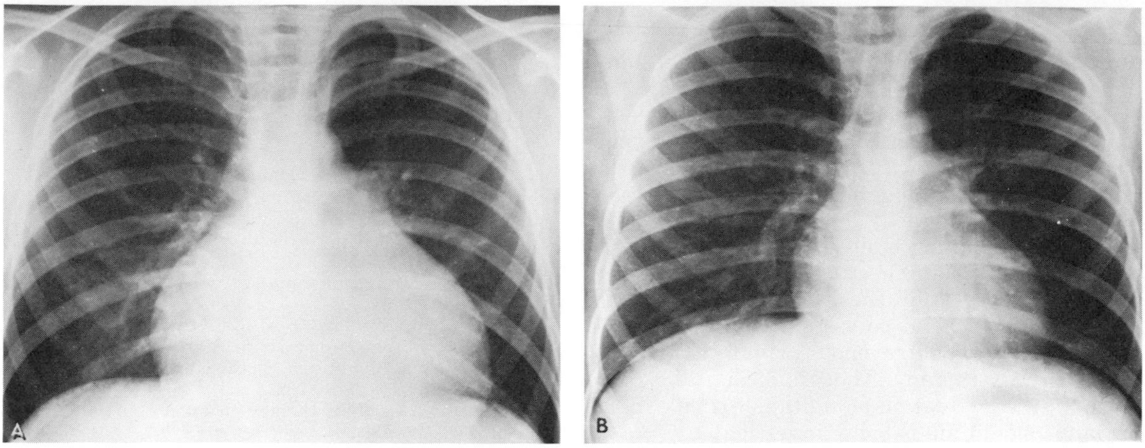

Figure 13–69 *Teleroentgenograms in acute nonspecific pericarditis.* A, *Increase in cardiopericardial shadow due to pericardial effusion. B, One month later after complete recovery.*

within the border of cardiac dullness. The heart sounds may be normal or distant. A pericardial friction rub may be audible even in the presence of large amounts of fluid. The rub is heard anywhere over the heart, but frequently over the lower left sternal border. It is superficial, of varying intensity and does not have any definite relation to the heart sounds.

Pericardial effusion may result in pressure on the left main stem bronchus, with collapse of the left lung resulting in percussion dullness and bronchial breathing at the left base (**Ewart's sign**). Similar signs may occur from secondary pleural effusion.

The findings on *roentgen examination* vary according to the amount of pericardial fluid. In dry pericarditis there are no abnormal findings. If the accumulation is large, the cardiopericardial shadow is enlarged, the normal contours are obscured, and the amplitude of cardiac pulsation is decreased. Other nondiagnostic signs include changes in the shape of the cardiac silhouette with changes in posture, divergent vascular shadows at the base, an acute right cardiophrenic angle and rapid changes in the size of the cardiopericardial shadow. The roentgenographic findings are not pathognomonic and may be simulated closely by acute cardiac dilatation (Fig. 13–69). Pericardial calcification as a result of chronic constrictive pericarditis is rare in children.

The *electrocardiographic* abnormalities are widespread and involve most of the leads. In the acute phase the S-T segment is elevated, and the QRS voltage may be low. As healing progresses the S-T segment becomes isoelectric or depressed, and the T waves are flattened, diphasic or inverted. The graph returns to normal when the pericarditis heals, although T wave inversion may persist for many months after clinical recovery. This electrocardiographic pattern may be transient and localized and may be recognized only with serial tracings.

A simple and reliable method of confirming the diagnosis of pericardial effusion is by *echocardiography.* This detects the separation of the cardiac chambers from the pericardium by echo-free fluid; the amount of fluid may be quantitated in older patients. This method has made obsolete other techniques such as angiocardiography and radioisotope scanning.

In the presence of cardiac compression *cardiac catheterization* reveals an increased pulmonary "capillary" and right atrial pressure. The pulmonary arterial and right ventricular pressures are normal or moderately elevated, and there is a conspicuous dip in the right ventricular pressure curve during early diastole. If the catheter is coiled in the right atrium, the width of the pericardial shadow can be detected.

Cardiac tamponade, whatever the cause, is a medical emergency. If the cardiac output is not maintained during cardiac compression, the patient goes into shock. The intrapericardial pressure must be reduced immediately, usually by pericardiocentesis.

RHEUMATIC PERICARDITIS

Rheumatic pericarditis is usually fibrinous or serofibrinous; a large accumulation of fluid is unusual. The child is usually acutely ill with fever, dyspnea and pericardial pain. The heart is frequently enlarged, and a pericardial friction rub is common. The electrocardiographic changes are as described above. Treatment is directed toward the rheumatic illness as a whole and the relief of pain, and pericardiocentesis is done in the rare instances of cardiac tamponade. Rheumatic pericarditis does not produce serious aftereffects and does not lead to constrictive pericarditis, but there is usually extensive carditis and, therefore, a potentially poor long-term prognosis.

The differential diagnosis of rheumatic pericardial effusion from acute cardiac dilatation is resolved by echocardiography. The essential difference between dry rheumatic pericarditis and other forms of dry pericarditis, such as acute benign pericarditis, is the presence in the former of significant systolic or diastolic murmurs as well as other evidence of acute rheumatic fever.

SEPTIC PERICARDITIS

Septic pericarditis is produced by a variety of bacteria, including *Hemophilus influenzae, Staphylococcus aureus,* streptococci and pneumococci. Foci of infection, usually pneumonia, are frequently present at other sites. The purulent exudate in the pericardium is of varying consistency, and coagulated masses of fibrin and pus are common.

The patients are acutely ill, with fever, pericardial pain and tachypnea. The heart is enlarged, murmurs are insignificant, and a friction rub may or may not be present. The electrocardiographic and radiologic pictures are described above. The diagnosis is confirmed by echocardiography and the causative bacterial agent defined by culture of fluid removed at pericardiocentesis. This procedure may yield only small amounts of pus, owing to the consistency of the exudate and to multiple loculations. Surgical drainage is usually necessary and should be instituted early. This therapy, with the concomitant use of appropriate antibiotics, gives excellent results, and the long-term prognosis is usually good.

ACUTE VIRAL OR IDIOPATHIC PERICARDITIS

This disease frequently follows an upper respiratory tract infection and has an average latent period of 12 days. The onset is usually acute, with fever; pericardial pain and a friction rub are common. Varying amounts of straw-colored pericardial fluid are present, but cardiac compression is rare. The electrocardiogram usually shows the typical pattern of pericarditis.

Although the disease is usually benign without any aftereffects, recurrences, sometimes multiple, have been noted in up to 20 per cent of patients. Symptomatic treatment with aspirin is all that is usually necessary. Corticosteroid therapy may be considered in the severe forms of the disease or in patients with multiple recurrences.

PERICARDITIS IN RHEUMATOID ARTHRITIS

Pericarditis may occur at any stage of rheumatoid arthritis and may precede the typical joint manifestations. Pericardial effusion is rare, and a pericardial friction rub common. Therapy is directed toward the primary disease, since pericarditis improves when the rheumatoid disease is stabilized.

PERICARDITIS IN UREMIA

In the terminal stages of uremia a pericardial friction rub may be heard, or there may be a significant accumulation of pericardial fluid. The diagnosis is confirmed by echocardiography. The fluid resolves with dialysis or after successful renal transplantation.

TUBERCULOUS PERICARDITIS

Tuberculous pericarditis is usually secondary to a lesion in the hilar nodes or in the lung. Pericardial effusion is common and is followed by a fibrotic reaction which may result in constrictive pericarditis. The onset may be insidious or associated with cough, dyspnea, fever, weight loss and night sweats. The diagnosis depends on signs of tuberculosis elsewhere in the body and on recovery of the organism from the sputum, gastric washings or the pericardial fluid. Treatment is that of the tuberculous infection (Section 10). The effusion is cleared more rapidly with added corticosteroid therapy.

CHRONIC CONSTRICTIVE PERICARDITIS

This disease is rare in children. In the majority of instances the cause is unknown, or the disease may follow tuberculosis. Occasionally septic or acute nonspecific pericarditis may be followed by constrictive pericarditis. The hemodynamics and clinical picture are those of chronic cardiac compression and must be distinguished from chronic congestive heart failure and restrictive cardiomyopathy. Atrial fibrillation may occur. If the constriction is severe, pericardiectomy is advised.

POSTOPERATIVE PERICARDITIS

Postoperative pericarditis may follow any direct surgical procedure in the heart. Friction rubs are common during the first 2 weeks after operation. Some patients, however, may have the postcardiotomy syndrome (see earlier pages).

Benzing, G., III, and Kaplan, S.: Purulent pericarditis. Am. J. Dis. Child. *106*:289, 1963.

Cayler, G. G., Taybi, H., Riley, H. D., and Simon, J. L.: Pericarditis with effusion in infants and children. J. Pediatr. *63*:264, 1963.

Nadas, A. S., and Levy, J. M.: Pericarditis in children. Am. J. Cardiol. 7:109, 1961.

DISEASES OF THE BLOOD VESSELS

ANEURYSMS AND FISTULAS

Anuerysms are not common in children and occur most frequently in the aorta in association with coarctation of the aorta, patent ductus arteriosus and Marfan's syndrome and in intracranial vessels (Section 20). They may also occur secondary to an infected embolus, infection contiguous to a blood vessel, trauma, congenital abnormalities of structure, especially of the medial coat, and arteritis, e.g., periarteritis nodosa.

Arteriovenous fistulas may be limited to small cavernous hemangiomas or may be extensive (Sections 23 and 25). The commonest sites for arteriovenous fistulas in infants and children are intracranial, hepatic or in the extremities. They have also been described in other parts of the body, however, especially in vessels in or near the thoracic wall. The fistulas, though usually congenital, may follow trauma or be a manifestation of hereditary hemorrhagic telangiectasia (Rendu-Osler-Weber syndrome).

Cardiovascular manifestations occur only in association with large communications. In these patients arterial blood flows into a low pressure venous system, increasing local venous pressure and decreasing arterial flow beyond the fistula. Systemic arterial resistance falls because of the runoff of blood through the fistula. Compensatory mechanisms include tachycardia and increased stroke volume, so that cardiac output rises. Plasma volume is also increased. Cardiac failure may develop with large arteriovenous fistulas.

The clinical manifestations of arteriovenous fistulas appear to depend primarily on the size of the shunt across the fistula and the associated vasodilatation. Discoloration of the skin, prominence of the superficial vessels and local edema may occur at the site of the fistula or involve a whole extremity. Prominent arterial pulsations and a continuous machinery bruit may be heard over the site of the lesion, especially in the traumatic types. The venous pressure is elevated in an affected extremity, the temperature of the skin may be higher at the site of the lesion, and the venous oxygen saturation distal to the fistula is higher than that of venous blood taken from a similar site on the unaffected side. In extensive fistulas there is left ventricular hypertrophy and dilatation, a widened pulse pressure and congestive heart failure. Arteriograms with the injection of contrast material into an artery proximal to the fistula confirm the diagnosis.

Intracranial arteriovenous fistulas are usually congenital, although they may follow trauma. Congenital fistulas usually involve the Galenic venous system. Neonates with large fistulas suffer heart failure early. Tachypnea, intermittent cyanosis, cardiomegaly and gallop rhythm are frequent, and signs of a high cardiac output state with wide pulse pressure and vasodilatation may be present. It is important to exclude intracranial arteriovenous fistulas in neonates with congestive cardiac failure of obscure cause (Fig. 20–21). In later infancy progressive hydrocephalus or convulsions may occur. Older children suffer from headaches or subarachnoid hemorrhage. Clues to the correct diagnosis include venous engorgement over the scalp and neck as well as cranial bruits. The latter sign is not diagnostic, since bruits may be heard in normal infants, especially over the anterior fontanel.

Hepatic arteriovenous fistulas may be localized or generalized in the liver. In others the fistula is between hepatic artery and ductus venosus or portal vein. Congenital hemorrhagic telangiectasia may be associated with hepatic fistula. Large arteriovenous fistulas are associated with a large cardiac output and heart failure. Hepatomegaly is usual, and systolic or continuous murmurs may be audible over the liver.

Peripheral arteriovenous fistulas normally involve the extremities. These lesions are associated with disfigurement, swelling of the extremity and visible hemangiomas. Only a small minority result in large arterial runoff, so that cardiac failure is not common.

TREATMENT. Surgical extirpation of the fistula is indicated when cardiac enlargement or heart failure occurs. Surgical treatment is difficult in many patients because of the diffuseness of the lesion.

COLD INJURY

(See also Cold Injury of the Newborn, Section 7.)

FROSTBITE. Frostbite may occur in the face or extremities from prolonged exposure to cold. The mechanism of cellular injury is related to intravascular thrombosis or ice crystal formation in the tissues. The skin first becomes red and then pale or, rarely, cyanotic as the arterioles remain in spasm in an effort to preserve body heat. During thawing, hyperemia occurs, and blisters may form on the skin. Gangrene may occur if early relief is not obtained.

Treatment consists in rapidly rewarming the skin of the affected area which is still white. Analgesics are usually necessary. Massage of the damaged area or rubbing with snow or ice is contraindicated. Other therapeutic measures which have yielded equivocal results include anticoagulants (especially heparin), low-molecular-weight dextran, and sympathectomy. Meticulous local care to the injured area is essential. Recovery of an extremity from apparent severe frostbite can be striking and, in the absence of infection, amputation or excision of tissue should be postponed for as long as possible.

CHILBLAINS (PERNIO). This form of cold injury, presumably vascular in origin, consists of a (sometimes blistering) localized erythema which itches, may be painful, and frequently results in swelling and in scabbing ulcerations of the affected areas. The etiologic mechanism is unknown but is probably related to prolonged constriction of peripheral arterioles, manifested by pallor and coldness of the subsequently affected areas, during cold weather, particularly cold, damp weather.

The tops of the ears and tips of the fingers and toes are most frequently affected; the exposed legs of girls wearing skirts and no stockings may also be involved. Without further exposure the lesions usually clear in a week or two but may persist longer.

Avoidance of prolonged chilling or the protection of susceptible areas with woolen caps, gloves and stockings is preventive. A familial susceptibility, ameliorated by the prophylactic use of 500 to 1000 mg of ascorbic acid daily during cold weather, has been reported.

EMBOLISM

Emboli, consisting of bacteria and fibrinous material, usually arise from mural thrombi or vegetations in the heart or large blood vessels, as for example in subacute bacterial endocarditis. Within weeks after bacteriologic cure of bacterial endocarditis, sterile embolization to major vessels may occur; this does not necessarily indicate reactivation of infection. Other, rarer causes of emboli include fat (secondary to trauma) and foreign material such as air introduced accidentally into the vascular system during therapeutic procedures. In patients with atrial or ventricular septal defects, emboli arising in the systemic venous system may pass across the defect and enter the systemic arterial system (*paradoxical embolus*).

When emboli lodge in an artery, the blood flow through the vessel is compromised. If the collateral circulation is inadequate, necrosis or gangrene supervenes; if the collateral circulation is adequate, the emboli may be silent. Thus, an embolus to the arteries of the forearm may not give rise to symptoms and is detected only when the radial or ulnar pulse disappears.

The symptoms and signs produced by arterial emboli depend on their location: e.g., an embolus to the middle cerebral artery may result in hemiparesis; an embolus to the femoral artery may result in ischemia with or without gangrene in the leg. If the emboli are infected, an abscess forms locally.

Treatment consists in eradication of the source of the emboli, e.g., subacute bacterial endocarditis, and in increasing the collateral circulation to the affected area. Surgical therapy such as embolectomy, sympathectomy and amputation may be indicated in specific instances.

Pulmonary embolism is not so frequent in children as in adults. Thrombosis of the calf veins with secondary pulmonary embolism is rare in children. Pulmonary emboli may arise secondary to subacute bacterial endocarditis in patients with a left-to-right shunt and have also occurred in association with ventriculocardiovascular shunts for hydrocephalus. Occasionally pulmonary embolism is seen in older children with chronic rheumatic heart disease and atrial fibrillation. Multiple, small pulmonary emboli have been described elsewhere (see Primary Pulmonary Hypertension, in previous pages).

THROMBOSIS

Frequently *arterial thrombosis* in children is associated with polycythemia secondary to severe cyanotic congenital heart disease. A frequent site for such thrombi is the brain, but they may occur anywhere in the body. They may be precipitated by dehydration.

Venous thrombosis may occur in veins used for prolonged intravenous therapy or in an area surrounding an infective process. The inflammation in the vein (*phlebitis*) is usually local, and the thrombi seldom give rise to emboli.

Any severe illness associated with intense dehydration may be complicated by venous thrombosis. This complication is relatively frequent in infants with severe diarrhea or septicemia and in children with cyanotic congenital heart disease and polycythemia who become dehydrated. The common sites for thrombosis are in the sagittal sinus of the brain and in the renal vein with extension into the inferior vena cava. (See Vascular Disorders of the Central Nervous System [Section 20] and Hemorrhagic Infarction of the Kidney [Section 15].)

SAMUEL KAPLAN

Atherosclerosis

Atherosclerosis is a disease, primarily of large arteries, characterized by plaque-like intimal deposits which contain neutral fat, cholesterol, lipophages and, sometimes, blood or other evidence of hemorrhage. The disease affects arteries supplying the brain, heart and kidneys, and has far-reaching clinical significance, since it ranks among the leading causes of death in the adult population.

Although clinical manifestations of atherosclerosis appear rarely in childhood, the increasing prevalence among adults below the age of 50 of coronary artery disease with its manifestations of angina, infarction and death has led to great interest in and current studies of the possible origin of the parent disease in childhood in relation to living habits and genetic and dietary factors.

EPIDEMIOLOGY. Certain characteristics of individual adults and certain environmental factors appear to be associated with the premature development of atherosclerosis. These so-called risk factors have been shown to apply to the occurrence of clinical manifestations in adults above 30 years of age, but are now under study as applied to children. Of the currently known risk factors, three appear to be of major importance: hyperlipidemia, hypertension and cigarette smoking. An adult 30 years or older, who has one risk factor, has twice the risk of the general population of developing coronary heart disease. Addition of another risk factor doubles that risk. With three risk factors, the risk becomes eight times that of the general population.

PATHOGENESIS. *Fatty streaks* begin to appear in the endothelium of the aorta by 6 months of age; however, these occur in all populations, even in those without significant atherosclerosis among adults. The fate of the fatty streaks is not well established, but animal studies suggest that they may remain unchanged, disappear or ultimately develop into atherosclerotic plaques. The fatty streaks found in coronary arteries at about 15 years of age may be better related to subsequent atherosclerotic plaques than are those in the aorta. *Raised atherosclerotic lesions* may appear in both aorta and coronary arteries before age 20. Their prevalence and extent parallel the frequency of clinical manifestations of atherosclerosis in later life. These raised lesions may narrow the arterial lumen and set the stage for later thrombosis and occlusion. There is little evidence that such advanced lesions regress, even after removal of known predisposing factors.

PREVENTION. Since the first symptom of atherosclerotic heart disease in the adult may be a fatal myocardial infarction, and since what may be precursors of the disease appear in blood vessels in childhood, primary prevention has become an issue for physicians who care for children.

The pediatrician should identify and insofar as possible attempt to prevent the development of any of the three major risk factors (hyperlipidemia, hypertension, cigarette smoking) among his patients. Likewise, he should attempt to eliminate or alleviate these risk factors if already present.

Hyperlipidemia. Identification of children with familial hyperlipidemia (Section 8) is enhanced fourfold by screening (by determination of the level of total serum cholesterol) the children of individuals who have experienced a coronary event before 50 years of age. Serial determinations of lipid fractions at various ages from birth on, combined with analysis of dietary and living habits and personal characteristics, currently being carried out on an investigative basis, may provide clues to predisposing and preventive factors for hyperlipidemia and/or later atherosclerosis. Treatment (see Syndromes with Increased Blood Fat in Section 8) of hyperlipidemia in childhood remains controversial and unsatisfactory. However, appropriate alterations in diet are recommended for children with total serum cholesterol levels above 230 mg/dl.

Hypertension. Hypertension is a well established risk factor, both for coronary and cerebral atherosclerotic disease. All definitions of hypertension are arbitrary, and it is a continuous variable, with prognosis a function of height of either systolic or diastolic pressure, mortality at any age being related to the levels of these pressures.

Since the blood pressure of an adult is reflected in his first-order relatives, and since it has been suggested that this familial aggregation is measurable in childhood, the elicitation of a family history of hypertensive disease may enhance identification of children destined to have hypertension as adults. Such children should have yearly measurements of blood pressure, continued into adult life. If hypertension or its development is identified, appropriate treatment through weight reduction, salt restriction, pharmacologic measures and change of life-style may be indicated.

Cigarette Smoking. There is an established relation between smoking cigarettes and developing coronary atherosclerosis. Persons who have stopped smoking have a decreased mortality from coronary artery disease, depending on the number of cigarettes previously smoked, and on the duration of cessation of smoking. The highest risk occurs among young men who smoke heavily. Therefore, the physician should play an active role in a major effort directed at understanding the motivation to smoke, at persuading smokers to stop, and at convincing adolescents never to begin smoking.

In addition to the above factors predisposing to atherosclerosis, there are probably many not yet identified. However, the influence of environment on occurrence of the disease appears to be a major one. Environmental factors, acting alone or on a genetically susceptible substrate, almost certainly predispose to far more cases of atherosclerosis than do genetic factors alone. In the current state of knowledge, these factors must persist into adult life in order to be significant, but prevention of atherosclerosis in adult life may depend on the pediatrician's helping to identify risk factors as yet unrecognized and in identifying and altering the life-style of those children who have known risk factors. Long-term follow-up studies of such children are of obvious importance. In the meantime, the ruling out of the presence of known risk factors (e.g., hyperlipidemia) may provide reassurance which may be a major contribution to the mental health of those concerned.

MARY JANE JESSE

Armstrong, M. L., Warner, E. D., and Connor, W. E.: Regression of coronary atheromatosis in rhesus monkeys. Circ. Res., *27*: 59, 1970.

Arteriosclerosis: Report by NHLI Task Force on Arteriosclerosis, Washington, D.C., U.S. Government Printing Office, 1971.

Doyle, J. T., Dawber, T. R., Kannel, W. B., et al: The relationship of cigarette smoking to coronary heart disease. The second report of the combined experience of the Albany, N.Y. and Framingham, Mass. studies. JAMA *190*:886, 1964.

Epstein, F. H.: The epidemiology of coronary heart disease—A review. J. Chronic Dis. *18*:735, 1965.

Harold, W. B., and Gordon, T. (ed.): The Framingham Study—An Epidemiological Investigation of Cardiovascular Disease. Monograph, Sec. 1-8; June, 1968; Sec. 9-22: Sept., 1968; Sec. 23: Sept., 1969; Sec. 24: April, 1970; Sec. 25: Sept., 1970; Sec. 26: March, 1971. Bethesda, Md., National Heart and Lung Institute.

Jesse, M. J., Hennekens, C., Ferrer, P., and Blumenthal, S.: Risk factors in progeny of parents with premature myocardial infarction. Circulation *68*:89, 1973.

Kass, E. H., and Zinner, S. H.: How early can the tendency toward hypertension be detected? Millbank Mem. Fund Quart. *47*:143, 1969.

McGill, H. C., Jr., (ed): The geographic pathology of atherosclerosis. Lab. Invest. *18*:465, 1968.

McMillan, G. C.: The onset of plaque formation in arteriosclerosis. Acta Cardiol. *11* (Suppl.):43, 1965.

Mial, W. E., and Oldham, P. D.: The hereditary factor in arterial blood pressure. Br. Med. J. *1*:75, 1963.

Stamler, J., Berkson, D. M., Lindberg, H. A., Hall, Y., Miller, W., Majonnier, L., Levinson, M., Cohen, D. B., and Young, Q. D.: Coronary risk factors. Med. Clin. N. Amer. *50*(1):299, 1966.

Strong, J. P., and McGill, H. C., Jr.: The pediatric aspects of atherosclerosis. J. Atherosclerosis Res. *9*:251, 1969.

Strong, J. P., Richards, M. L., and McGill, H. C., Jr.: On the association of cigarette smoking with coronary and aortic atherosclerosis. J. Atherosclerosis Res. *10*:303, 1969.

HYPERTENSION

Systemic hypertension accompanies a wide variety of acute and chronic illnesses of childhood. Although essential hypertension, which occurs in both children and adolescents, may be a distinct entity, in most instances hypertension in childhood is a secondary manifestation of an underlying disease such as glomerulonephritis or coarctation of the aorta.

Blood pressure increases from infancy through adolescence. It is unclear what level of pressure should be considered distinctly abnormal at a given age. It has been proposed that, if a patient's systolic and/or diastolic pressure is frequently at the 90th percentile for age or at the 95th percentile on one or more occasions, the child should be considered to be hypertensive; however, more studies are needed to substantiate whether this is an appropriate working definition. Until the issue is resolved, most physicians should remain reluctant to investigate or treat young patients whose diastolic blood pressures are less than 90 mm Hg. Figure 13–70 illustrates levels of blood pressure observed in normal children at various ages.

Until recently little attention has been paid by pediatricians to problems of blood pressure in children. Hypertension has always been considered to occur rarely and to be of concern chiefly to pediatric cardiologists and nephrologists. Blood pressure measurements are still infrequently done routinely in patients between 2 and 20 years of age. In the last decade more attention has begun to focus on both hypertension and atherosclerosis in childhood and adolescence. Prevalence data, though sparse, indicate that 1 to 2 per cent of children and up to 11 per cent of adolescents and young adults (< 24 years) have elevated blood pressure according to the criteria already mentioned. Prevalence probably varies from country to country and between races in the same country; e.g., hypertension is commoner in the United States black population than among United States whites. Nonetheless, hypertension appears to be at least as common as congenital heart disease. It therefore seems appropriate for blood pressure to be measured during routine physical examinations performed on children and teenagers. The measurement itself can be made by any person properly trained in the technique.

The past view that essential or idiopathic hypertension is rare in children and that every child or teenager found to have elevated diastolic pressure should be subjected to an extensive diagnostic evaluation in order to eliminate curable forms of underlying disease needs re-examination. Data are accumulating to suggest that idiopathic hypertension certainly occurs in children and may not be at all uncommon in adolescents.

ETIOLOGY. Tables 13–7 and 13–8 summarize causes of potentially curable and incurable forms of hypertension which occur in childhood. Only a few bear discussion here. It is now well known that patients with *Wilms' tumor* may have severe hypertension and even present with hypertensive encephalopathy. The mechanism of the hypertension is not clear, but it may be due to (1) functional narrowing of a renal artery due to compression, (2) compression of the kidney as in the "cellophane wrap" experiment, or (3) direct production of a

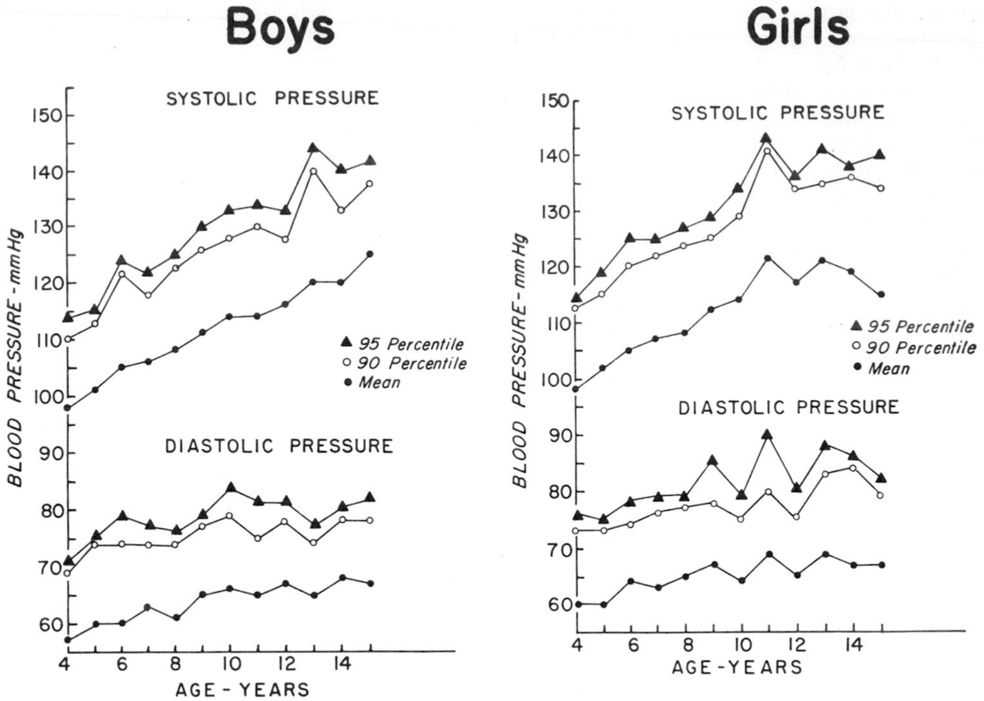

Figure 13–70 Brachial artery cuff blood pressures of 735 normal boys and 738 normal girls from 4 to 15 years of age. Determinations made with children in the supine position. (Adapted from Londe, S.: Clin. Pediatr. 5:71, 1966.)

pressor substance by the tumor. In some situations all three mechanisms may be operative. Hypertension has been reported to recur in the presence of distant metastases, supporting the view that these tumors may sometimes produce a pressor substance which may or may not be renin.

Pheochromocytoma (Section 17) is an unusual curable cause of hypertension in childhood. The observation that hypertension secondary to pheochromocytoma is more often sustained than paroxysmal in children may well be an artifact, since the patients reported probably had their first blood pressure measurements only late in the course of their disease. Familial pheochromocytoma has been erroneously diagnosed as familial dysautonomia and, conversely, patients with *familial dysautonomia* (see The Autonomic Nervous System, Section 20) have been surgically explored for pheochromocytoma. The distinction between these two conditions can be made on clinical grounds and by measuring the excretion of norepinephrine, epinephrine, dopamine and their metabolites in the urine.

Patients with *neuroblastomas* may rarely present with signs or symptoms due to an excess of circulating catecholamines. On occasion they may have marked tachycardia and diastolic blood pressures as high as 120 mm Hg. Any strategically situated intra-abdominal tumor, including a pheochromocytoma, may cause hypertension by either renal artery compression or obstruction of a ureter, with secondary hydronephrosis.

Chronic bilateral pyelonephritis is listed in Table 13–7 as a cause of hypertension, and many physicians infer a cause-and-effect relationship. However, not all patients with chronic pyelonephritis have hypertension, and there is some evidence to suggest that the infection merely unmasks a familial predisposition to essential hypertension.

All the factors which predispose to *essential hypertension* have not yet been elucidated. There is a familial aggregation of persons with high blood pressure, but the role played by genetic as opposed to environmental factors remains unknown. Epidemiologic data from both humans and animals tend to support the hypothesis that essential hypertension is polygenically inherited. Monozygotic twins have pressures that correlate more closely than do those of dizygotic twins who, in turn, have pressures that correlate more closely with each other than do those of nontwin siblings. It has been postulated that a variety of factors, including emotional stress, obesity, excessive salt intake or recurrent urinary tract infections may unmask this presumed inherited predisposition to essential hypertension. Although these speculations are controversial, it is of interest to note, for example, that if one plots the average daily sodium chloride intake against the prevalence of hypertension in different geographic areas of the world and among different races, there appears to be a positive correlation.

Table 13–9 lists conditions which have been noted to be associated with transient or intermittent hypertension in childhood. There is some overlap with conditions listed in Tables 13–8 and 13–9. For example, corticosteroid-induced hypertension is reversible by withdrawal of the steroid, so that it is curable, but its duration may be short or fairly prolonged. The same applies to hypertension as-

TABLE 13–7 POTENTIALLY CURABLE FORMS OF HYPERTENSION IN CHILDREN

Renal
- Unilateral dysplastic kidney
- Unilateral hydronephrosis
- Unilateral pyelonephritis
- Traumatic damage, e.g., constrictive perirenal hematoma
- Renal tumors
- Unilateral multicystic kidney
- Unilateral ureteral occlusion
- Ask-Upmark kidney

Vascular
- Coarctation of the thoracic or abdominal aorta
- Abnormalities of the renal artery (stenosis, arteritis, fibromuscular dysplasia, thrombosis, neurofibromatosis, fistula, aneurysm)
- Renal vein thrombosis

Adrenal
- Neuroblastoma
- Pheochromocytoma
- Cortical hyperplasia (adrenogenital syndrome)
- Cushing's disease
- Primary aldosteronism (hyperplasia or adenoma)

Miscellaneous
- Vascular or unilateral renal parenchymal abnormalities after irradiation
- Ingestion of excessive amounts of licorice
- Administration of glucocorticoids
- Administration of oral contraceptives
- Administration of testosterone

sociated with the use of the *oral contraceptives* in adolescent girls; normotension may not be achieved for 1 to 12 months after withdrawal of these hormone preparations, and hypertensive encephalopathy from their use has been reported. In addition, their use results in changes in the renin-angiotensin-aldosterone system, which can cause confusion in interpretation of laboratory data obtained during a diagnostic evaluation for hypertension. *Pre-eclamptic toxemia* has been listed as a cause of hypertension because, clearly, it may occur in adolescents who become pregnant. The incidence of pre-eclampsia is highest among the disadvantaged, and there appears to be a familial incidence. Current evidence suggests that the renal lesion of pre-eclampsia may be less reversible than previously believed.

Few of the hypertensive mechanisms of the conditions listed in Table 13–9 have been elucidated; an understanding of them might make drug therapy more rational. In addition, neither the incidence of hypertension nor its significance in terms of causing complications is known precisely in all these conditions. *Hypertensive encephalopathy* appears to occur at lower levels of diastolic pressure (110 mm Hg or lower) in acute glomerulonephritis, burns and leukemia. Likewise, patients with unerlying renal disease who rapidly develop hypertension when treated with glucocorticosteroids generally appear to require intensive hypotensive therapy in order to avoid hypertensive seizures.

The current understanding of the physiologic mechanism for regulation of blood pressure is described under that heading in Section 15 and is diagrammed in Figure 5–5.

CLINICAL MANIFESTATIONS. In general, until diastolic blood pressure has been sustained at a high level (> 120 mm Hg) for a relatively prolonged period in those diseases associated with chronic hypertension, the elevation in pressure per se produces no symptoms or signs; only the clinical manifestations of the primary disease may draw the clinician's attention to the hypertension.

When older children or adolescents become

TABLE 13–8 SOME CONDITIONS ASSOCIATED WITH INCURABLE FORMS OF CHRONIC HYPERTENSION IN CHILDREN

Renal
- Chronic glomerulonephritis (all forms including those due to connective tissue diseases)
- Bilateral congenital dysplastic kidneys
- Chronic bilateral pyelonephritis
- Bilateral hydronephrosis
- Polycystic kidneys
- Medullary cystic disease
- Postrenal transplantation (rejection damage)

Vascular
- Surgically irremediable abnormalities of the renal artery
- Surgically irremediable coarctation of the aorta
- Generalized hypoplasia of the aorta

Miscellaneous
- Essential hypertension
- Renal parenchymal damage from irradiation
- Lead nephropathy (late)
- Familial dysautonomia (periodic hypertension)

TABLE 13–9 CONDITIONS ASSOCIATED WITH TRANSIENT OR INTERMITTENT HYPERTENSION IN CHILDREN

Renal
- Acute poststreptococcal glomerulonephritis
- Hemolytic-uremic syndrome
- Anaphylactoid purpura with nephritis
- After genitourinary tract surgery
- After renal transplant (immediate and during episodes of rejection)
- After blood transfusion in patients with azotemia
- Anephric hypervolemia

Miscellaneous
- Administration of corticosteroids (including DOCA and ACTH)
- Administration of oral contraceptives
- Pre-eclamptic toxemia of pregnancy
- Raised intracranial pressure (any cause)
- Hypercalcemia
- Burns
- Guillain-Barré syndrome
- Poliomyelitis
- Leukemia
- Hypernatremia
- Stevens-Johnson syndrome
- Familial dysautonomia
- Mercury poisoning
- Bacterial endocarditis
- Amphetamine overdosage

TABLE 13–10 SOME CLINICAL AND LABORATORY CLUES TO CURABLE FORMS OF HYPERTENSION IN CHILDREN

CAUSE OF HYPERTENSION	HISTORY	PHYSICAL EXAMINATION	READILY AVAILABLE LABORATORY DATA	OTHER STUDIES WHICH MAY BE INDICATED
Coarctation of the aorta				
Thoracic	Nonspecific	Femoral pulses decreased or delayed; higher BP in arms than legs; systolic murmur	None	Cardiac catheterization
Abdominal	Nonspecific	Abdominal bruit may be present; femoral pulses may or not be normal; there may or may not be a significant pressure differential between arms and legs	None	Abdominal angiogram
Renovascular disease	History of trauma to abdomen or flank; pain; hematuria (aneurysm); symptoms of aldosteronism may be present	Bruit in abdomen or flank; café-au-lait spots or other manifestations of neurofibromatosis	Nonspecific unless secondary aldosteronism present (low K, high CO_2, Na may be normal); fast sequence intravenous pyelogram may be abnormal	Abdominal angiogram; measurement of plasma renin activity from both renal veins (ureteral split function studies)
Trauma	Trauma to back or abdomen; hematuria after trauma; closed renal biopsy	May have abdominal bruit or mass	Hematuria; intravenous pyelogram may be helpful	Abdominal angiogram may show fistula, etc.
Unilateral renal parenchymal disease	Symptoms of recurrent urinary tract infection; unexplained fevers; history of trauma to abdomen or flank	Enlarged kidney, if present, may be helpful; costovertebral angle tenderness with acute infection	Urinalysis may be abnormal; intravenous pyelogram abnormal	Abdominal angiogram may demonstrate renal artery stenosis associated with, for example, dysplastic kidney; measurement of plasma renin activity from both renal veins

symptomatic from hypertension, they usually complain of frequent headaches, dizziness and/or changes in vision. If hypertensive encephalopathy is impending or present, vomiting may also be a prominent feature. Seizures, stupor or even coma may also accompany hypertensive encephalopathy. Opinion is divided as to the frequency with which isolated *facial paralysis* occurs as the sole manifestation of systemic hypertension in childhood, but certainly the correlation is strong enough to warrant blood pressure measurement when a child with an isolated facial palsy is seen. Other neurologic manifestations may be present if a cerebrovascular accident has occurred, but such accidents are relatively uncommon sequelae of hypertension in childhood. The heart and kidneys are also target organs for pathologic states resulting from sustained systemic hypertension. Renal function may deteriorate, particularly in the accelerated phase of hypertension, or, alternatively, heart failure may be a presenting manifestation. Rarely, myocardial infarction has been reported in young hypertensives.

It is important to measure blood pressure in any infant or young child who presents with unexplained seizures or heart failure. Patients in this age group cannot communicate symptoms, such as headache, so that their behavior may not be considered abnormal until complications of hypertension are already present. Often, in retrospect, after blood pressure has been lowered, parents of hypertensive infants will comment that their child was previously extremely irritable and indulged in an abnormal degree of head-banging or rubbing. In retrospect again, parents may comment that their infant frequently used to wake screaming at night (when blood pressure tends to be highest) and no longer does so since pressure has been controlled. Retarded growth and hyperactivity have also been reported to accompany hypertension of renovascular origin uncomplicated by renal or heart failure.

The *clinical signs* which can be elicited in a hypertensive child clearly depend upon the underlying cause and the amount of target organ disease present. Patients with mild essential hypertension may have a completely negative history and physical examination except for the blood pressure reading. The important historical and physical findings, as well as the useful laboratory data, in some of the curable forms of hypertension in childhood

TABLE 13–10 SOME CLINICAL AND LABORATORY CLUES TO CURABLE FORMS OF HYPERTENSION IN CHILDREN (*Continued*)

CAUSE OF HYPERTENSION	HISTORY	PHYSICAL EXAMINATION	READILY AVAILABLE LABORATORY DATA	OTHER STUDIES WHICH MAY BE INDICATED
Neuroblastoma	Dependent on site—abdominal mass found by parent; cough, chest pain, dyspnea; spinal cord compression with neurologic signs and symptoms	Abdominal or other masses palpable	Anemia; abnormal cells in marrow; lytic bone lesions; abnormal intravenous pyelogram	Measurement of catecholamines and their metabolites in the urine
Wilms' Tumor	Mass found by parent; fever; abdominal pain; hematuria; rarely seizures	Palpable abdominal mass (usually does not cross midline)	Abnormal intravenous pyelogram	
Pheochromocytoma	Episodes of sweating, flushing or mottling; palpitations or rapid heart beat; episodic headache; weight loss; personality change; polyuria and polydipsia; family history of pheochromocytoma	Tachycardia; flushing; pallor; fever; excess perspiration; palpable tumor; postural hypotension	Hyperglycemia; glucosuria; anemia or polycythemia; leukocytosis; increased cholesterol; reversed A/G ratio; intravenous pyelogram usually not helpful	Measurement of catecholamines and their metabolites in the urine; angiography; measurement of blood catecholamines at various levels in vena cava; pharmacologic tests (i.e., Regitine, histamine, tyramine, glucagon) of limited use
Primary aldosteronism	Periodic muscular weakness; paresthesias; tetany; polyuria; polydipsia; no edema	Muscle weakness; tetany; positive Chvostek's or Trousseau's sign	Serum Na high, K low, CO_2 high; ECG shows hypokalemia, intravenous pyelogram not usually helpful	Abdominal angiography sometimes helpful; measurement of plasma renin activity, aldosterone (urine and/or blood); renin suppression test
Cushing's disease	Retardation of growth and development; weakness; weight gain; easy bruising; change in body habitus	Truncal obesity; buffalo hump; moon facies; hirsutism; red or purple striae	Glucosuria; hyperglycemia; eosinopenia; intravenous pyelogram usually not helpful	Increased plasma cortisol and increased excretion of 17-OHCS in urine

are summarized in Table 13–10. Specific historical and physical findings which should be looked for and recorded in a hypertensive child are mostly those which might point to an underlying cause; e.g., the presence of excessive perspiration, weight loss, personality change, skin mottling and palpitations would all be suggestive of pheochromocytoma. It is extremely important to elicit a history of hypertension, heart disease and stroke in close family members. Parents who say that they have normal blood pressures should be asked when their pressure was last checked, since normotension even a year before does not preclude the subsequent development of hypertension.

In the *physical examination* the cardiovascular system should be carefully checked to determine the presence or absence of pulses and the presence or absence of bruits over the great vessels, in the abdomen or in the flanks. A few minutes of exercise may render a faint abdominal bruit more audible. Heart size should be evaluated and evidence of congestive heart failure sought for. Examination of the optic fundi and classification, using the Keith-Wagener scale of staging, is a mandatory part of the physical examination of a hypertensive patient. The presence of papilledema, hemorrhages or exudates makes treatment urgent.

Although indirect measurements of blood pressure are not entirely accurate, they are even less so if a cuff of incorrect size is used. In general, the bladder of the cuff should cover two thirds of the upper arm without impinging on the antecubital fossa. Cuff size must be determined on an individual basis, not on that of age; the so-called child-size cuff may be far too small for the arm of a well developed 6 year old. The length of the bladder of the cuff is also important, particularly in obese individuals, for whom a bladder of standard length may be too short to encircle the arm and evenly compress the adipose tissue overlying the brachial artery. A cuff larger than the standard adult cuff is available and, on occasions, the cuff made to measure thigh pressure in adults may be the most suitable for an obese adolescent with long arms. The usually recorded large differential between arm and leg pressures is reduced considerably when a cuff which covers two thirds of the thigh is used for measuring leg pressure.

DIAGNOSIS. Once blood pressure has been found to be elevated, it is usual in children and adolescents to rule out all the known curable causes of hypertension in an extensive diagnostic evaluation, particularly if there are no clinical clues to the etiology. Whether this is warranted is open to question, particularly in mildly hypertensive, asymptomatic adolescents with negative physical examinations and a strong family history of hypertension. Experience suggests that in the absence of any clinical or simple laboratory clues to the adrenal forms of hypertension, measurement of catecholamines and their metabolites in the urine, measurement of aldosterone secretion and measurement of plasma cortisol or urinary 17-hydroxysteroids and 17-ketosteroids have been unproductive.

An underlying cause for hypertension is more likely in patients under 10 years of age and in children or adolescents with diastolic pressures over 110 mm Hg; extensive investigation is justified in such patients. In white adolescent boys and black adolescents of both sexes with mild hypertension (diastolic blood pressure < 110 mm Hg), essential hypertension is the usual diagnosis, and a limited diagnostic evaluation may be in order. White adolescent girls with even mild to moderate hypertension usually have some underlying pathology.

Many of the investigative tools used in evaluating the hypertensive child appear in Table 13-11. No attempt will be made to discuss their utility here; the interested reader can consult detailed review articles on the topic. (See references at end of section.) A few points are, however, worth mentioning. A normal rapid-sequence intravenous pyelogram by no means rules out a renovascular lesion; arteriography is the only means by which such lesions can be conclusively excluded. In experienced hands, when the diastolic blood pressure is below 110 mm Hg, the morbidity from abdominal angiography is low. Since bilateral renal artery disease, with or without abdominal aortic coarctation, is not an uncommon finding in hypertensive

TABLE 13-11 DRUGS USED IN TREATMENT

DRUG	SUGGESTED INITIAL DOSE		TIME TO ONSET OF ACTION	
	Oral	*Parenteral*	*Oral*	*Parenteral*
Reserpine (Many trade names)	Patient < 25 kg: 0.02 mg/kg/24 hr in 1-2 doses Patient > 25 kg; 0.25-0.5 mg/24 hr in 1-2 doses	Patient < 25 kg: 0.02 mg/kg/dose IM Patient > 25 kg: 0.5-1.0 mg. total dose	Probably dose-dependent (slow acting, i.e., days rather than hours)	IV – 1 hr IM – ±2 hr
Hydralazine (Apresoline)	0.75 mg/kg/24 hr in 4-6 doses (usually not > 25 mg for first dose)	0.15 mg/kg/dose IV or IM (not to exceed 20 mg)	30-60 mins	IV – may be immediate IM – 15-20 min
Methyldopa (Aldomet)	10 mg/kg/24 hr in 3-4 doses (usually not > 250 mg/dose)	5-10 mg/kg IV (usually not > 375 mg/dose)	6-12 hr	IV – 3 hr
Guanethidine (Ismelin)	0.2 mg/kg/24 hr as a single dose (usually not > 10-20 mg)	Not available	Probably dose-dependent (24-48 hr at low dosage)	–
Diazoxide (Hyperstat)	Not officially available for Rx of hypertension	3-5 mg/kg IV (up to 300 mg)	–	IV ±1 min

youngsters, angiography is particularly useful in defining the extent of the vascular disease.

Ureteral split function studies (Howard, Stamey, Rappaport), performed extensively in hypertensive adults in an effort to determine whether surgical correction of a renovascular lesion is liable to result in improvement or cure of hypertension, are technically difficult in children; the results are, therefore, not always reliable. Catheterization of the renal veins to obtain blood for the measurement of plasma renin activity can easily be performed immediately prior to arteriography, and the predictive value of the renal vein renin ratio for surgical cure of hypertension is probably somewhat better than that of ureteral split function studies. When a renovascular lesion exists in a child and hypertension is present, there is virtually always a cause and effect relationship; predictive tests of the outcome of surgery with respect to blood pressure in isolated renal artery stenosis are probably less important in children than in adults. In children the renal vein renin ratio may have its greatest value when bilateral renal artery or unilateral renal parenchymal disease is present in association with hypertension.

Pheochromocytomas can be located in any site where sympathetic nervous system tissue has existed, but they are usually intra-abdominal. When the diagnosis is suspected on clinical grounds, the safest way of establishing it is by measuring the urinary excretion of catecholamines and their metabolites; the pharmacologic tests for pheochromocytoma have a limited place in the diagnosis of this tumor. A positive phentolamine (Regitine) test in a patient with a suspicious history can be diagnostically helpful, particularly if the patient is in urgent need of treatment. However, both false positive and false negative tests occur, and definite confirmation of the diagnosis is still made only by chemical quantitation of the catecholamines and their metabolites in the urine. In normotensive or mildly hypertensive patients with a history suggestive of pheochromocytoma and without striking abnormalities in catecholamine excretion, the administration of histamine, glucagon or tyramine may provoke massive release of catecholamines by the tumor and be diagnostically useful.

Finally, since pheochromocytomas may be very small and, particularly in children, may be multiple, preoperative localization may be helpful to

OF HYPERTENSION IN CHILDREN*

TIME TO MAXIMUM EFFECT		DURATION OF ACTION		
Oral	*Parenteral*	*Oral*	*Parenteral*	SIDE EFFECTS†
±7–14 days	4–6 hr	Effect may persist for 2–4 weeks when Rx discontinued	IV—6–8 hr IM—10–12 hr	Flushing (parenteral), drowsiness, irritability, depression, nasal stuffiness, bradycardia, diarrhea *Less common:* Parkinson-like state, tremors, nightmares
± 2 hr	10–80 min	1–4 hr	1–4 hr	Tachycardia, headache, nausea, vomiting, rheumatoid syndrome, lupus syndrome *Less common:* Psychic disturbances, peripheral neuropathy
±8 hr	4–6 hr	8–12 hr	8–10 hr (maybe longer)	Drowsiness, irritability, emotional lability, bradycardia, postural hypotension, diarrhea, positive direct Coombs *Less common:* Paradoxical pressor response (parenteral), fever, abnormal liver function tests, "black" tongue, breast enlargement with or without lactation, hemolytic anemia
2–7 days for full therapeutic effect	–	When Rx discontinued, full effect may persist 3–4 days; return of BP to pretreatment level in 1–3 weeks	–	Postural hypotension, postexercise syncope, diarrhea, rising BUN, ptosis of eyelids, impotence, failure of ejaculation
–	Within 5 min	–	5–24 hr	Burning at injection site, chest and abdominal pain, vomiting, tachycardia, hyperuricemia, weight gain, edema

nformation from multiple sources, including personal observations. Not all data well documented.
ther rare side effects occur but are not listed.

the surgeon. As angiographic techniques have improved, localization of tumors by these methods has also improved. In addition, it may be helpful to sample blood at various levels in the vena cava for measurement of plasma catecholamines. A marked step-up in concentration from one site to another may give localizing information.

COURSE AND PROGNOSIS. The course and prognosis of individual hypertensive patients depends upon the nature of their underlying disease. Still and Cottom reported the duration of life and causes of death in 55 patients aged several months to 14 years, all of whom had diastolic blood pressures in excess of 120 mm Hg and either clinical or electrocardiographic evidence of left ventricular hypertrophy at the time of inclusion in the study. Fifty-six per cent of their patients died after an average of 14 months from the time hypertension was recognized. However, 70 per cent of their patients had hypertension secondary to renal disease, and the majority died of uremia; there is no doubt that successful kidney transplantation has since considerably altered the prognosis of such patients. Other authors have reported survival times ranging between 10 and 22 years for a small group of patients under 17 at the time of diagnosis. However, in addition the recent availability of more effective antihypertensive drugs, such as diazoxide, may now have altered the prognosis for life of even severe hypertensives.

Ninety per cent of both children and adults with untreated *malignant hypertension* die within one year of diagnosis. In these patients there is clear evidence that aggressive treatment with antihypertensive drugs prolongs life. Although there are no data concerning the effects on longevity of the treatment of mild, moderate and severe hypertension in children and adolescents, there are data to indicate that lowering blood pressure in adults with moderately severe or severe hypertension prolongs life and delays the onset of cardiovascular, renovascular and cerebrovascular disease.

TREATMENT. To treat hypertension properly it is essential to know the time to onset of action, the time to maximal effect, the duration of action, the mechanism of action and the major side effects produced by the antihypertensive drug used. Some of this information can be found in Table 13–11.

The total daily dose and also the individual doses of antihypertensive drugs can and should be tailored to the needs of the individual patient. Dosage is determined, in most instances, by the hypotensive effect and the side effects which are produced in the individual patient. This is true for both emergency and chronic treatment of hypertension. It should be emphasized that antihypertensive drugs can be titrated against blood pressure over a wide range of doses, provided unacceptable side effects do not supervene. Recognized sources of pediatric drug dosages tend to put erroneous emphasis on fixed dosages of these agents.

In treating hypertension, one aims ideally to achieve normotension throughout the day without incapacitating the patient with drug side effects. Since blood pressure is often higher in the evening than in the morning, one may have to cluster fast-acting, relatively short-acting drugs such as hydralazine during those times of day when pressure is highest. This is easier to achieve in a hospital than in an outpatient setting unless accurate blood pressure measurements can be made several times a day at home. Whether one is treating a hypertensive emergency or chronic hypertension, graphs of blood pressure plotted against the dosages of antihypertensive drugs are invaluable in making therapeutic decisions.

It is most logical to start therapy with one drug and use it until the desired hypotensive effect has been achieved, until unacceptable side effects supervene or until the top of the dose-response curve has been reached. It is, in general, not logical to start treatment with two or three drugs, since one may have no idea which drug is producing a hypotensive effect, and the patient may be exposed to unnecessary side effects.

Hypertensive emergencies are encountered infrequently in pediatric practice. Acute hypertension associated with acute poststreptococcal glomerulonephritis is probably still the most common one in childhood. However, children do present with heart failure, hypertensive encephalopathy, malignant hypertension or Grade III fundi (hemorrhages and exudates); they require prompt, intensive therapy with parenterally administered antihypertensive drugs. In most cases blood pressure need not be lowered precipitously to normotensive levels but can be gradually returned toward normal over a period of days.

There is no good evidence that hypertensive children should be restricted in either their activity or their diet except in specific circumstances; e.g., patients with relatively severe hypertension who are receiving guanethidine may exhibit post-exercise syncope and may have to be restricted in their activity in order to avoid this complication. Restriction of salt and water may be the best method of controlling blood pressure in many azotemic patients.

For technical reasons, renovascular procedures are more difficult and less successful in children than in adults. Nephrectomy is usually either the primary procedure in unilateral stenosis of the renal artery, or it has to be performed as a secondary measure when a revascularization procedure has failed. Autotransplantation of kidneys in patients with renal artery abnormalities has had some success in adults and has been reported in one child.

JENNIFER M. H. LOGGIE

Loggie, J. M. H.: Systemic hypertension in children and adolescents. I. Causes and diagnostic studies. J. Pediatr. *74*:331, 1969.

Loggie, J. M. H.: Hypertension in children and adolescents. II. Drug therapy. J. Pediatr. *74*:640, 1969.

Loggie, J. M. H.: Systemic hypertension in children and adolescents. Pediat. Clin. N. Amer. *18*:1273, 1971.

Stackpole, R. H., Melicow, M. M., and Uson, A. C.: Pheochromocytoma in children: Report of 9 cases and review of first 100 published cases with follow-up studies. J. Pediatr. *63*:314, 1963.

Still, J. L., and Cottom, D.: Severe hypertension in children. Arch. Dis. Child. *42*:34, 1967.

14
DISEASES OF THE BLOOD

DEVELOPMENT OF THE HEMATOPOIETIC SYSTEM

As long as animals remained small and the cells of their bodies had direct access to the surrounding sea water, exchange of gas and nutrients was easily effected by simple diffusion. With the evolution of multicellular and terrestrial organisms came development of a vascular system and hemic fluid. Blood probably originated as a simple saline solution similar to sea water; cellular components with specialized functions must have appeared soon thereafter. Among the principal functions of blood cells are transport of respiratory gases, hemostasis, and phagocytosis and other defense mechanisms. Most advanced organisms have separate lines of blood cells, each concerned with specialized functions.

Blood formation in the human embryo can be recognized as early as the third week after conception. Large, primitive hematopoietic elements are then widely scattered through mesodermal tissues, intimately associated with developing vascular channels. By two months active hematopoiesis is established in the liver, which is the main site of blood formation during the middle portion of fetal life. After about six months hematopoiesis shifts gradually to the medullary spaces, and by birth most blood formation normally takes place in bone marrow.

Active hematopoietic tissue (red marrow) fills the medullary spaces of the bones of infants. During childhood fatty tissue (yellow marrow) gradually replaces hematopoietic tissue in the long bones, so that in the older child and the adult active blood formation is concentrated in ribs, sternum, vertebrae, pelvis, skull, clavicles and scapulas. The yellow marrow of the extremities has the potential for reconversion to active hematopoiesis in response to certain severe hematologic stresses.

Study of the bone marrow provides valuable information in the evaluation of many hematologic diseases. Marrow aspiration is a safe and technically simple procedure. Although the marrow aspiration represents only a minute sample of the entire hematopoietic tissue, in most instances there is a striking uniformity of aspirates taken simultaneously from multiple sites. In the infant the preferred sites for aspiration are the proximal tibia and posterior iliac crest. In older children the posterior iliac crest provides a large marrow-bearing space which is not adjacent to major blood vessels or vital organs. Table 14–1 lists the types and proportions of cells which occur in marrow of normal infants and children.

TABLE 14–1 DIFFERENTIAL COUNTS OF BONE MARROW DURING INFANCY AND CHILDHOOD

AGE	BLASTS	PRO-MYELO-CYTES	MYELO-CYTES AND META-MYELO-CYTES	BANDS AND POLY-MORPHO-NUCLEARS	EOSINO-PHILS	LYMPHO-CYTES	NUCLE-ATED RED BLOOD CELLS	MYELOID/ERY-THROID (M:E) RATIO
Birth	1	2	5	40	1	10	40	1.2/1
7 days	1	2	10	40	1	20	25	2.1/1
6 months to 2 years	0.5	0.5	8	30	1	40	20	2.0/1
6 years	1	2	15	35	1	25	20	2.7/1
12 years	1	2	20	40	1	15	20	3.2/1
Adult	2	2	22	44	2	10	20	3.5/1

The Red Cells

Synthesis of red cells requires a constant supply of amino acids, iron, certain vitamins and other trace nutrients. Production of red cells is regulated by a specific erythroid-stimulating hormone—erythropoietin. This hormone is largely produced or activated in the kidney and is responsive to changes in tissue oxygenation. The principal action of erythropoietin is to induce the differentiation of primitive stem cells into an erythrocytic sequence. The early erythrocyte precursors then undergo several successive cellular divisions. The processes of cellular differentiation which occur as the red cell attains maturity include condensation and extrusion of the nucleus and production of a complement of hemoglobin. Ninety per cent of the dry weight of the mature red cell is hemoglobin.

HEMOGLOBIN

The combustion which is essential to life requires a constant supply of oxygen to the tissues of the body. The capacity of sea water and its internal equivalent, the plasma, to transport dissolved oxygen is limited. The evolutionary development of oxygen-carrying proteins, the hemoglobins, has increased the ability of blood to transport this gas. Further, because of the remarkable way in which hemoglobin combines with and dissociates from oxygen, the entire transport process is accomplished without expenditure of metabolic energy.

Hemoglobin is a complex protein consisting of the iron-containing heme groups and the protein moiety, globin. A dynamic interaction between heme and globin is responsible for the unique physiologic properties of hemoglobin in the reversible transport of oxygen. The hemoglobin molecule is a tetramer; i.e., it is made up of two pairs of polypeptide chains, each chain having a heme group attached to it. The polypeptide chains of each kind of hemoglobin are of chemically different types. For example, the hemoglobin of the normal adult (Hgb A) is made up of two pairs of chains called the alpha (α) and beta (β) polypeptide chains. Hemoglobin A can therefore be represented as $\alpha_2{}^A\beta_2{}^A$. Alpha and beta chains differ from each other in both the number and sequence of amino acids, and their synthesis is directed by separate genes.

The human hemoglobins are not homogeneous. Within the red cells of the embryo, fetus, child and adult, five different hemoglobins may be detected. They can be classified as the embryonic hemoglobins, Gower 1 and Gower 2; the fetal hemoglobin, Hgb F; and the adult hemoglobins, Hgb A and A_2. These variants have different electrophoretic mobilities, which reflect their different chemical structures. The compositions of the polypeptide chains of human hemoglobins are listed in Table 14–2. The time of appearance and quantitative relations between these hemoglobins are determined by complex developmental processes. The relations are depicted in Figure 14–1.

EMBRYONIC HEMOGLOBINS. The blood of early human embryos contains the two slowly migrating hemoglobins called Gower 1 and Gower 2. The Gower hemoglobins contain a unique type of polypeptide chain called the epsilon chain. Hemoglobin Gower 1 has the tetramer structure ϵ_4, and Gower 2, $\alpha_2\epsilon_2$. In embryos of 4 to 8 weeks' gestation the Gower hemoglobins predominate, but by the third month they have disappeared. Another embryonic variant (Hgb Portland-1) has also been described but its structure and significance have not been well defined.

FETAL HEMOGLOBIN. Hemoglobin F contains gamma polypeptide chains, which substitute for the beta chains of Hgb A. Hemoglobin F can be represented as $\alpha_2{}^A\gamma_2{}^F$. It resists denaturation by strong alkali, and the technique of alkali denaturation is usually used for quantitation. After the eighth gestational week it is the predominant hemoglobin, and in the 6 month old fetus constitutes 90 per cent of the total hemoglobin. After this a gradual decline occurs, so that at birth Hgb F averages 70 per cent of the total. Synthesis of Hgb F decreases rapidly postnatally, and by 6 to 12 months of age only a trace is present. Less than 2.0 per cent can be detected by alkali denaturation in older children and adults. Recent studies indicate that there is a heterogeneity of Hgb F due to two types of γ chains. These differ at position #136 of the γ chain by the presence of either a glycine or an alanine residue.

ADULT HEMOGLOBINS. Some Hgb A ($\alpha_2{}^A\beta_2{}^A$) can be detected even in the smallest embryos, and by the sixth month of gestation Hgb A is present to about 5 to 10 per cent. A steady increase follows, so that at term Hgb A averages 30 per cent. By 6 to 12

TABLE 14–2 THE NORMAL HUMAN HEMOGLOBINS

HEMOGLOBIN NAME	FORMULA	COMMENT
Gower 1	$\epsilon_4{}^{Gower\ 1}$	Major embryonic hemoglobins
Gower 2	$\alpha_2\epsilon_2{}^{Gower\ 2}$	Not present after third month of gestation
Fetal (Hgb. F)	$\alpha_2{}^A\gamma_2{}^F$	Predominant hemoglobin throughout fetal life Alkali-resistant
Adult (Hgb. A)	$\alpha_2{}^A\beta_2{}^A$	Major adult hemoglobin
A_2	$\alpha_2{}^A\delta_2{}^{A_2}$	Minor adult hemoglobin Detectable postnatally

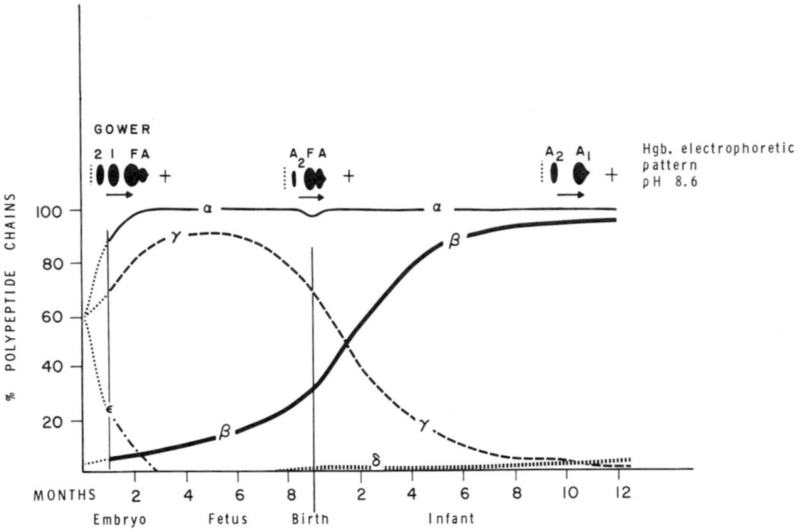

Figure 14-1 *Proportions of the various human hemoglobin polypeptide chains through early life. The hemoglobin electrophoretic pattern typical for each period is also shown. (From H. A. Pearson: J. Pediatr. 69:466, 1966.)*

months of age the normal adult hemoglobin pattern appears. The minor adult hemoglobin component Hgb A_2 contains delta (δ) chains and has the structure of $\alpha_2{}^A\delta_2{}^{A_2}$. It is seen only when significant amounts of Hgb A are also present. At birth less than 1.0 per cent of Hgb A_2 is seen, but by 12 months of age the normal level of 2.0 to 3.4 per cent is attained. Throughout life the proportion of Hgb A to A_2 is about 30 to 1.

NORMAL RELATIONS OF THE VARIOUS HEMOGLOBINS. During fetal life and early childhood there is an inverse relation between the rates of synthesis of gamma and beta chains and, hence, between the amounts of Hgb A and Hgb F. How this reciprocal relation is regulated is uncertain. By borrowing heavily upon the models of microbiologic biochemical genetics, a "switch mechanism" involving regulator genes has been postulated. During fetal life this mechanism facilitates gamma chain synthesis, while beta and delta chain production is repressed. After birth the "switch" is reversed, so that fetal hemoglobin synthesis is inhibited and the adult hemoglobins accumulate. Crucial factors influencing these regulatory mechanisms have not been clearly defined.

ALTERATIONS OF THE HEMOGLOBINS BY DISEASE. The relative proportions of the various hemoglobins are not usually altered by hematologic disease.

Since hemoglobins containing epsilon chains are normally present only very early in intrauterine life, they are largely of theoretic interest. Small amounts of the Gower hemoglobins have been detectable in a few newborn infants with the syndrome of D_1 (13–15) trisomy.

Levels of fetal hemoglobin may be influenced by a variety of factors. In patients heterozygous for β thalassemia (β-thalassemia trait), the postpartum decrease of Hgb F is retarded, and about half of these patients have elevated levels of Hgb F (more than 2.0 per cent) in later life. In homozygous thalassemia (Cooley's anemia) and in hereditary persistence of fetal hemoglobin large amounts of Hgb F are characteristically seen. In patients with major beta chain hemoglobinopathies (Hgb SS, SC, and so on) Hgb F is usually elevated, particularly during childhood. Finally, moderate elevations of Hgb F may be seen in many diseases accompanied by hematologic stress, such as hemolytic anemias, leukemia and aplastic anemia. This is often due to the presence of a small population of red cells which contain increased amounts of Hgb F, and which can be demonstrated by the acid-elution staining technique of Kleihauer and Betke.

The normal adult level of Hgb A_2 (2.4 to 3.4 per cent) is seldom altered. A level of Hgb A_2 exceeding 3.4 per cent is found in most persons with the β-thalassemia trait, and moderate increases have been documented in those with megaloblastic anemias secondary to vitamin B_{12} and folic acid deficiency.

METABOLISM OF THE RED CELL

The nucleated red cell in the bone marrow is able to perform a variety of metabolic functions, including active protein synthesis. After extrusion of the nucleus much of this metabolic capacity is lost, and the mature red cell is unable to synthesize proteins. Although loss of the nucleus makes the red cell a more perfect vessel for oxygen transport, it does impose upon the red cell a finite life span, for the cell cannot replace or repair its vital enzymatic proteins. The mature red cell contains more than 40 enzymes. Many of these are essential for cellular viability, but genetically determined deficiencies of others, such as catalase, do not interfere with normal survival.

The mature red cell is not metabolically inert. Glucose is utilized and lactic acid produced mostly by anaerobic glycolysis (Embden-Meyerhof pathway); about 10 per cent of glucose is metabolized oxidatively through the pentose phosphate path-

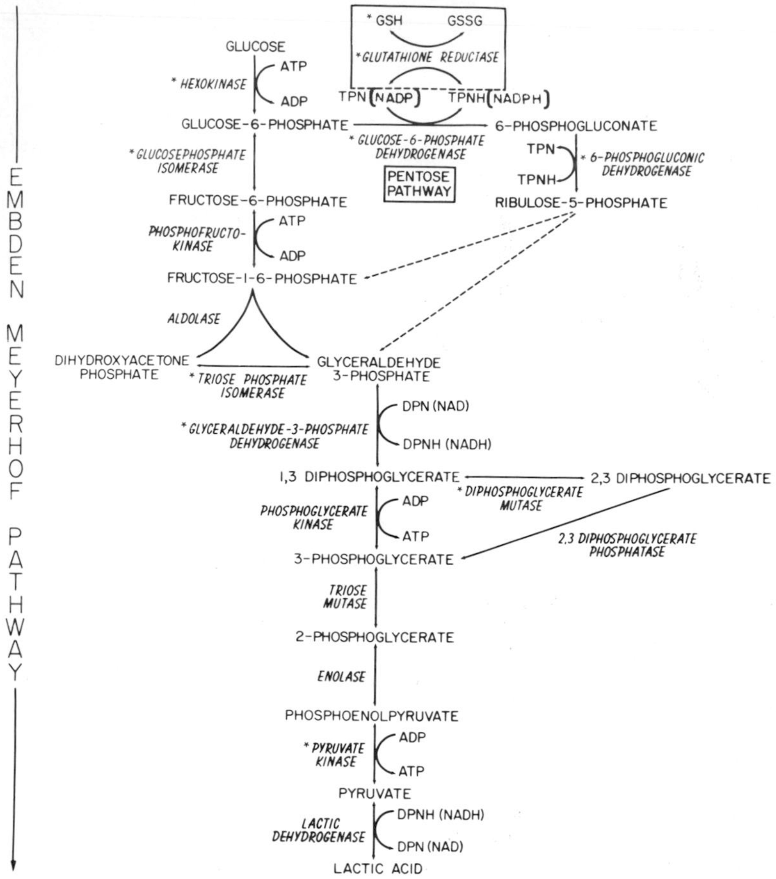

Figure 14–2 *Metabolic pathways of glucose metabolism in the mature red blood cell. Congenital deficiency states have been described for the enzymes indicated by an asterisk (*).*

way. Figure 14–2 depicts these pathways and shows the enzymes essential to metabolism of glucose by the mature red cell. At least four uses for the energy generated by glucose metabolism have been identified as essential for normal cell viability: (1) Maintenance of electrolyte gradients. The principal intracellular cation of the red cell is potassium, while that in the plasma is sodium. There is a constant tendency for sodium to enter the red cell and concomitantly for potassium to leak out. Reversal of these flows and preservation of normal ionic gradients are accomplished by an energy (ATP)-dependent membrane mechanism, the cation pump. When the cation pump fails, sodium and water accumulate within the red cell, causing it to swell and ultimately to hemolyze. (2) Maintenance of the red cell membrane and shape. The red cell membrane is a complex phospholipid structure, and maintenance of these phospholipids consumes energy. Maintenance of the biconcave shape is probably also energy-dependent. (3) Maintenance of heme iron in the reduced (ferrous) form. Oxidative potentials within the red cell may cause oxidation of the iron of hemoglobin. Hemoglobin containing ferric iron (methemoglobin) is ineffective in oxygen transport. If peroxides and other oxidant substances are not inactivated, hemoglobin may be denatured and precipitated. Cells containing such denatured hemoglobin are rapidly removed from the circulation. Protection of the red cell from the detrimental effects of oxidation ultimately depends upon NADPH and NADH. These compounds are constantly regenerated by activities of the glycolytic pathway and pentose shunt. Genetically determined deficiencies of a number of the glycolytic and pentose pathway enzymes have been identified, many of which produce hemolytic states because the energy necessary to perform these vital functions cannot be generated. (4) Maintenance of the levels of organic phosphates such as 2,3 diphosphoglycerate (2,3-DPG) and ATP within the red cells. These compounds actively interact with hemoglobin and have a profound effect upon oxygen affinity.

THE ANEMIAS

Anemia is defined as a reduction of the red cell volume or hemoglobin concentration below the range of values occurring in healthy persons. Table 14–3, on following page, lists the means and ranges for hemoglobin and hematocrit values by age groups of well nourished children.

Although reduction in amount of circulating hemoglobin decreases the oxygen-carrying capacity of the blood, few physiologic disturbances occur until the hemoglobin level falls below 7 to 8 gm/dl. Below this level, pallor becomes evident in skin and mucous membranes. Physiologic adjustments to anemia include tachycardia, increased cardiac output, a shift in the dissociation curve which makes oxygen more readily available to the tissues, and a deviation of blood flow toward vital organs and tissues. Anemia also has an effect upon red cell metabolism. In response to anemia or hypoxia the concentration of 2,3-DPG increases within the red cell. In conjunction with reduced hemoglobin, this causes a "shift to the right" of the oxygen dissociation curve. This shift, by reducing the affinity of hemoglobin for oxygen, results in more complete transfer of oxygen to the tissues. The same shift may also occur at high altitude in response to a decrease in oxygen content of inspired air. When moderately severe anemia develops slowly, surprisingly few symptoms or objective findings may be evident, but weakness, tachypnea, shortness of breath on exertion, tachycardia, cardiac dilatation and congestive heart failure ultimately result from increasingly severe anemia, regardless of its cause.

Anemia is not a specific entity, but is an indication or manifestation of an underlying pathologic process or disease. A useful physiologic classification of the anemias of childhood divides them into two large groups: (1) those resulting primarily from decreased production of red cells or hemoglobin; and (2) those in which increased destruction or loss of red cells is the predominant mechanism. In Table 14–4 (see p. 1111) the important anemias of childhood are classified by these criteria. In every case of significant anemia it is essential to describe the morphologic characteristics of the red cells, to determine the relative importance of defective red cell production and of cell destruction in the genesis of the anemia, and, when possible, to identify the basic etiologic process.

Anemias Resulting from Inadequate Production of Red Cells

These anemias result when the bone marrow is unable to produce sufficient numbers of new red cells to replace those removed from the circulation. A slight reduction in the red cell life span may be present, but generally this is insufficient to cause anemia if hematopoiesis is adequate. Low reticulocyte counts are observed in most anemias of this group.

CONGENITAL PURE RED CELL ANEMIA

(Congenital Hypoplastic Anemia; Diamond-Blackfan Syndrome)

This rare condition usually becomes symptomatic in early infancy. The most characteristic diagnostic feature is a deficiency of red cell precursors in an otherwise normally cellular bone marrow.

ETIOLOGY. A genetic basis is suggested by several instances of familial occurrence. Males and females are affected in equal numbers. Although an ill defined abnormality of tryptophan metabolism has been reported in some children, the biochemical basis for the disease is still uncertain. High levels of erythropoietin are present in serum and urine.

CLINICAL MANIFESTATIONS. Although some of these infants appear pale even in the first few days of life, hematopoiesis must have been generally adequate during intrauterine life. Profound anemia usually becomes evident by 2 to 6 months of age, occasionally somewhat later. Unless blood transfusions are given, the anemia progresses to such severity that heart failure and death occur. The liver and spleen are not enlarged initially. A few cases of pure red cell anemia have been associated with congenital anomalies, including triphalangeal thumbs. Patients with the Turner syndrome phenotype but normal karyotypes have had pure red cell anemia.

LABORATORY DATA. The red blood cells are normochromic and normocytic; there are no morphologic or biochemical abnormalities. The level of Hgb F is increased for age, and thrombocytosis may also be present. The most important feature is the lack of evidence of erythropoietic activity in blood and bone marrow. Reticulocytes are diminished even when the anemia is severe. Red cell precursors are markedly reduced in the marrow,

TABLE 14–3 HEMATOLOGIC VALUES DURING INFANCY AND CHILDHOOD

	HEMOGLOBIN GM/DL %		HEMATOCRIT %		RETIC-ULO-CYTES %	WBC/MM.^{3} %		NEUTROPHILS %		LYMPHO-CYTES %	EOSINO-PHILS %	MONO-CYTES %	NUCLE-ATED RED CELLS
AGE	MEAN	RANGE	MEAN	RANGE	MEAN	MEAN	RANGE	MEAN	RANGE	MEAN (RELA-TIVELY WIDE RANGE)	MEAN	MEAN	/100 WBC
Cord blood	16.8	13.7-20.1	55	45-65	5.0	18,000	(9-30,000)	61	(40-80)	31	2	6	7.0 (3-10)
2 weeks	16.5	13.0-20.0	50	42-66	1.0	12,000	(5-21,000)	40		48	3	9	0
3 months	12.0	9.5-14.5	36	31-41	1.0	12,000	(6-18,000)	30		63	2	5	0
6 mos.-6 yrs.	12.0	10.5-14.0	37	33-42	1.0	10,000	(6-15,000)	45		48	2	5	0
7-12 yrs.	13.0	11.0-16.0	38	34-40	1.0	8,000	(4500-13,500)	55		38	2	5	0
Adult Female Male	14 16	12.0-16.0 14.0-18.0	42 47	37-47 42-52	1.6	7,500	(5-10,000)	55	(35-70)	35	3	7	0

TABLE 14–4 CLASSIFICATION OF THE ANEMIAS

- I. Anemias resulting primarily from inadequate production of red cells or hemoglobin
  - A. Decreased numbers of red cell precursors in the marrow
    - 1. "Pure red cell" anemias
      - a. Congenital pure red cell anemia
      - b. Acquired pure red cell anemias
  - B. Inadequate production despite normal numbers of red cell precursors
    - 1. Anemia of infection, inflammation and cancer
    - 2. Anemia of chronic renal disease
    - 3. Congenital dyserythropoietic anemias
  - C. Deficiency of specific factors
    - 1. Megaloblastic anemias
      - a. Folic acid deficiency
      - b. Vitamin B_{12} deficiency
      - c. Orotic aciduria
    - 2. Microcytic anemias
      - a. Iron deficiency
      - b. Pyridoxine-responsive and X-linked hypochromic anemias
      - c. Lead poisoning
- II. Hemolytic anemias
  - A. Intrinsic abnormalities of the red cell
    - 1. "Structural" defects
      - a. Hereditary spherocytosis
      - b. Hemolytic elliptocytosis
      - c. Paroxysmal nocturnal hemoglobinuria
    - 2. Enzymatic defects (nonspherocytic hemolytic anemias)
      - a. Enzymes of glycolytic pathway; pyruvate kinase, hexokinase and others
      - b. Enzymes of the pentose phosphate pathway and glutathione complex
    - 3. Defects in synthesis of hemoglobin
      - a. Hgb. S, C, D, E, etc., alone and in combination
      - b. Thalassemia
  - B. Extrinsic (extracellular) abnormalities
    - 1. Immunologic disorders
      - a. Passively acquired antibodies (hemolytic disease of the newborn)
        - (1) Rh isoimmunization
        - (2) A or B isoimmunization
        - (3) Other blood group families
      - b. Active antibody formation
        - (1) Idiopathic autoimmune hemolytic anemia; cold agglutinin diseases
        - (2) Symptomatic—lupus, lymphoma
        - (3) Drug-induced
    - 2. Nonimmunologic disorders
      - a. Toxic from drugs, chemicals
      - b. Infections—malaria, clostridium
    - 3. Infantile pyknocytosis

See also anemia in pancytopenias and leukemia.

resulting in myeloid-erythroid ratios of 10:1 to 200:1. In some cases a few pronormoblasts may be present, but not more mature forms. A normal complement of white cells, platelets and megakaryocytes is present. Serum iron is elevated, with a decrease in the iron-binding capacity. Red cell survival is normal.

DIFFERENTIAL DIAGNOSIS. Congenital hypoplastic anemia must be differentiated from other anemias in which there are low peripheral reticulocyte counts. The anemia of the convalescent phase of hemolytic disease of the newborn may, on occasion, be associated with markedly reduced erythropoiesis. This terminates spontaneously at 5 to 8 weeks of age, whereas congenital hypoplastic anemia is not usually recognized before this time. Aplastic crises, characterized by reticulocytopenia and decreased numbers of red cell precursors, may complicate various types of hemolytic disease. These episodes are transient, and evidence of antecedent hemolytic disease is usually present.

COURSE. Unless corticosteroid therapy produces remission of hypoplastic anemia, survival depends upon blood transfusions given as needed, usually at intervals of 4 to 8 weeks. By late childhood affected children may have had a hundred or more transfusions, and hemosiderosis is an inevitable consequence. The liver and spleen enlarge, and secondary hypersplenism with leukopenia and thrombocytopenia may occur. Growth retardation, possibly secondary to hypopituitarism, is usual, and puberty may not occur. Diabetes mellitus due to hemosiderosis is common.

Death usually occurs in the second decade. Chronic congestive heart failure due to ischemic and siderotic myocardial disease is a common terminal event. Despite this grave prognosis, spontaneous remissions occasionally occur, some after very extended periods of dependency upon transfusion.

TREATMENT. When anemia becomes severe, blood transfusions must be given. Corticosteroid therapy is frequently beneficial if begun early; the mechanism of its effect is unknown. Relatively large doses, 2 to 4 mg/kg, of prednisone or its equivalent are administered initially. One to 3 weeks after therapy is begun red cell precursors appear in bone marrow, and then a brisk peripheral reticulocytosis occurs. The hemoglobin may reach normal level in 4 to 6 weeks. The dose of corticosteroid may then be reduced gradually until the lowest effective dose is found. This is often a very small amount, such as 2.5 mg/day of prednisone or less, which may produce no adverse side effects or growth suppression. Intermittent administration every other day or for 3 or 4 consecutive days each week may also be effective. Therapy should be discontinued periodically to determine whether the child is still dependent upon steroids, since most responsive cases ultimately outgrow the dependence on steroid therapy and maintain normal hemoglobin levels indefinitely.

About 25 per cent of patients do not respond to corticosteroid therapy, and transfusions are necessary to sustain life. A large number of other therapies, including all known hematinics, cobalt and testosterone, have had no beneficial effect. Splenectomy is usually of no value, but may decrease the need for transfusion if hypersplenism or iso-immunization has developed. Because of the possibility of spontaneous remission, children refractory to corticosteroid therapy should be maintained as long as possible by transfusions, preferably of freshly drawn, packed red cells.

ACQUIRED PURE RED CELL ANEMIAS

A number of forms of acquired anemia with reticulocytopenia and reduced red cell precursors in the marrow have been described. The cause of most of the acquired instances is uncertain. In some cases in adults a tumor of the thymus has been present, remissions following its removal. Only one association of thymoma and red cell aplasia has been reported in a child. In other cases an erythropoietin-inhibiting antibody has been demonstrated in the plasma, and in still others, antibodies to erythroblasts or plasma inhibitors of heme synthesis. The acquired pure red cell anemias may respond to therapy with corticosteroids, and a trial is indicated in any chronic case.

Administration of large doses of chloramphenicol inhibits erythropoiesis. Reticulocytopenia, erythroid hypoplasia and vacuolated pronormoblasts in the marrow are reversible pharmacologic effects of this drug. (See also Pancytopenias.)

Episodes of acute failure of erythropoiesis may follow a variety of viral infections. During these episodes, there are a marked reduction in circulating reticulocytes (<0.1 per cent) and an elevation of the serum iron level. Bone marrow aspiration shows markedly reduced numbers of erythrocytic precursors. These episodes are self-limited, lasting only 10 to 14 days, and are of no consequence to a child with a normal red cell survival. In a patient with a shortened red cell survival, however, profound anemia may ensue; this is the basis of the so-called aplastic crises of some hemolytic anemias.

ANEMIAS OF CHRONIC INFECTION, INFLAMMATION AND RENAL DISEASE

Anemia complicates a number of chronic systemic diseases associated with infection, inflammation or tissue breakdown. Examples of such conditions include chronic pyogenic infections such as bronchiectasis and osteomyelitis; chronic inflammatory processes such as rheumatic fever, rheumatoid arthritis and ulcerative colitis; and advanced renal disease. Despite diverse underlying causes, the erythrokinetic abnormalities are similar. The red cell life span is moderately decreased, but the principal factor determining the degree of anemia is a relative inability of the bone marrow to fabricate red cells. How these systemic diseases inhibit the marrow activity is not clear, but inadequate production of erythropoietin is not the primary mechanism.

CLINICAL MANIFESTATIONS. Few symptoms are attributable to the moderate degree of anemia usually present; the important symptoms and signs are those of the underlying disease.

LABORATORY DATA. Hemoglobin concentrations usually range from 6 to 9 gm/dl. The red blood cell count and hemoglobin and hematocrit levels are proportionately decreased, resulting in a normochromic and normocytic anemia. Occasionally a modest degree of hypochromia and microcytosis is observed. Reticulocyte counts are normal or low. Leukocytosis is often present. Serum iron is low; however, there is no increase in total iron-binding capacity as in iron deficiency anemia. Rather, a decrease may result in a fairly normal saturation percentage. This pattern of serum iron and iron-binding protein is a regular and valuable diagnostic feature. The bone marrow has normal cellularity. The red cell precursors are adequate, and granulocytic hyperplasia may be present. Increased hemosiderin can often be demonstrated in marrow.

TREATMENT AND PROGNOSIS. Since these anemias are secondary to another disease process, they do not respond to iron or hematinics. Transfusions raise the hemoglobin concentration only temporarily and are rarely indicated. If the underlying systemic disease can be controlled, the anemia corrects spontaneously.

CONGENITAL DYSERYTHROPOIETIC ANEMIAS

These rare, recessively transmitted normocytic or macrocytic anemias display multinuclearity and abnormal chromatin patterns in red cell precursors. Some patients show an abnormal Ham (acidified serum) test.

PHYSIOLOGICAL ANEMIA OF INFANCY

The normal newborn has higher hemoglobin and hematocrit levels than older children and adults. Within the first week of life, a progressive decline in hemoglobin level begins, which persists for approximately six to eight weeks. This decline is generally referred to as a physiological anemia of infancy. The term is a misnomer, for at its nadir the hemoglobin level in the full-term infant rarely falls below 10 gm/dl.

A number of factors are operative. First, there is an abrupt cessation of erythropoiesis with onset of respiration, when arterial oxygen saturation rises from 45 toward 95 per cent. Concomitantly, the high fetal levels of erythropoietin drop to undetectable levels. A shortened survival span of the fetal red cell also contributes to the development of physiological anemia. Further, the sizeable expansion of blood volume which accompanies rapid weight gain during the first three months of life creates a situation which has aptly been described as "bleeding into the circulation." It is likely that among these factors the relative inactivity of bone marrow is the most important determinant of physiological anemia. When the hemoglobin level has fallen to 10 to 11 gm/dl at 2 to 3 months of age, erythropoietin can again be detected and active erythropoiesis resumes. This "anemia" should be viewed as a physiological adaptation to extrauterine life.

The premature infant also develops a physiological anemia; the same factors are operative as in term infants, but they are exaggerated. The decline in hemoglobin level is both more extreme and more rapid. Minimal hemoglobin levels of 7 to 9 gm/dl commonly occur by 3 to 6 weeks of age, and, in very small prematures, levels as low as 5 to 6 gm/dl.

The marginal erythropoietic equilibrium responsible for physiological anemia can aggravate such processes associated with increased hemolysis as erythroblastosis fetalis, hereditary spherocytosis and other congenital hemolytic anemias, which may be associated with severe anemia in the early weeks of life.

Dietary factors may also aggravate physiological anemia. Deficiencies of folic acid or vitamin E superimposed upon the physiological process may result in more severe anemia. On the other hand, unless there has been significant perinatal blood loss, iron deficiency should not be considered as a cause of anemia in the first two months of life.

TREATMENT. As a developmental process, physiological anemia usually requires no therapeutic considerations other than that the diet of the infant contain the essential nutrients for normal hematopoiesis, especially iron, folic acid and vitamin E. A premature infant who is feeding well and growing normally rarely needs transfusion. Occasionally very low hemoglobin levels (< 6 gm/dl) or complicating medical conditions may necessitate small transfusions of packed red blood cells. If so, only enough blood should be given to raise the hemoglobin level to about 8 gm/dl. Larger transfusions are not indicated and may delay spontaneous recovery by suppressing normal erythropoiesis. Administration of iron has no effect upon physiological anemia.

MEGALOBLASTIC ANEMIAS

The megaloblastic anemias all have in common certain abnormalities of red cell morphology and maturation which are diagnostic. The red cells at every stage of development are larger than normal and have a peculiar open, finely dispersed arrangement of nuclear chromatin and an asynchrony between the maturation of nucleus and cytoplasm. Biochemically, there is an increased amount of RNA in proportion to DNA in megaloblastic tissues. Megaloblastic morphology may be seen in a number of conditions, but almost all instances in children result from a deficiency of either folic acid or vitamin B_{12} or from a combined deficiency of them. Both substances are necessary cofactors in the synthesis of nucleoproteins. Megaloblastic anemias are uncommon in the United States.

FOLIC ACID DEFICIENCY
(Megaloblastic Anemia of Infancy)

This disease is caused by a deficient intake or absorption of folic acid. Dietary deficiency is usually compounded by rapid growth or infection, which may increase folic acid requirements. The normal daily requirement is small, having been estimated at 20 to 50 μg per day. Human and cow's milks provide adequate amounts of folic acid. Goat's milk is clearly deficient; folic acid supplementation must be given when it is the main food, and "goat's milk" megaloblastic anemia is still occasionally seen in the United States. In these cases goat's milk has usually been prescribed because of gastrointestinal symptoms ascribed to allergy. Unless supplemented, powdered milk may also be a poor source of this vitamin. Ascorbic acid deficiency probably impairs the availability of dietary folic acid conjugates.

CLINICAL MANIFESTATIONS. Megaloblastic anemia has a peak incidence at 4 to 7 months of age, somewhat earlier than iron deficiency anemia. In addition to the usual features of severe anemia, these infants are irritable, fail to gain weight adequately, and have chronic diarrhea. Thrombocytopenic hemorrhages occur in advanced cases. Concomitant signs and symptoms of scurvy may be present. Prematurity may be a predisposing factor.

LABORATORY DATA. The anemia varies in degree, but is progressive. Because the red blood cell count is disproportionately lower than the hematocrit levels, the anemia is macrocytic. Nevertheless, considerable variations in red cell shape and size are common (Fig. 14–3, *C*). The reticulocyte count is low, but nucleated red cells demonstrating megaloblastic morphology are often seen in the peripheral blood. Neutropenia and thrombocytopenia may be present. The neutrophils are large, with hypersegmented nuclei; more than 5 per cent of the neutrophils will have five or more nuclear segments. Serum folic acid activity, as measured by microbiologic assay, is less than 3 mμg/ml. Levels of iron and vitamin B_{12} in serum are normal or elevated. Formiminoglutamic acid is excreted in the urine, especially after an oral dose of l-histidine. Serum levels of lactic acid dehydrogenase (LDH) are markedly elevated. The bone marrow is hypercellular because of erythroid hyperplasia. Megaloblastic changes are prominent, though some normal red cell precursors may also be present. Large, abnormal neutrophilic forms (giant metamyelocytes) with cytoplasmic vacuolization are seen, as well as hypersegmentation of the nuclei of megakaryocytes.

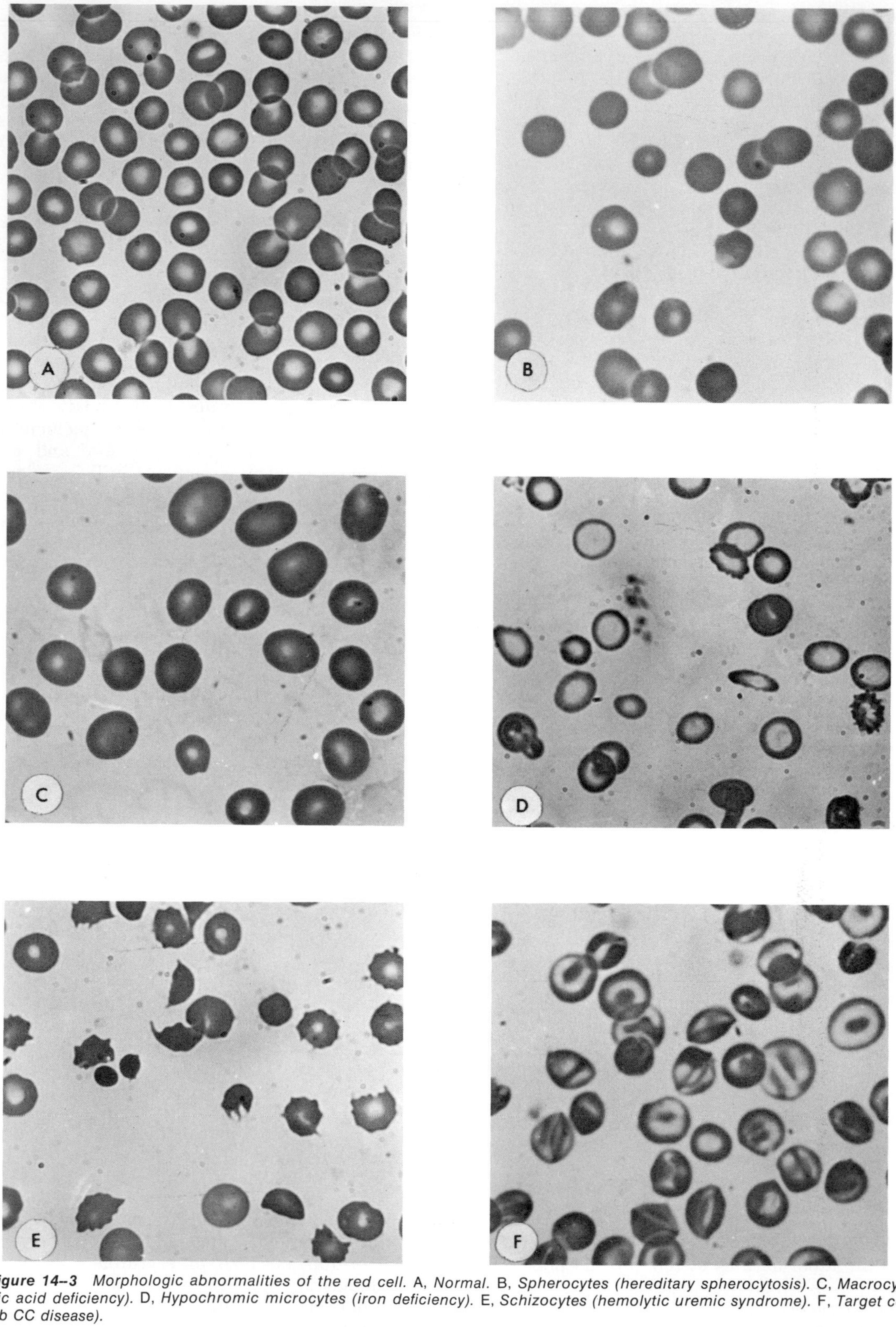

Figure 14–3 *Morphologic abnormalities of the red cell.* A, *Normal.* B, *Spherocytes (hereditary spherocytosis).* C, *Macrocytes (folic acid deficiency).* D, *Hypochromic microcytes (iron deficiency).* E, *Schizocytes (hemolytic uremic syndrome).* F, *Target cells (Hgb CC disease).*

TREATMENT. Initially folic acid may be administered parenterally in a dose of 2 to 5 mg/day. Since a hematologic response can be expected within 72 hours, transfusions are indicated only when the anemia is severe or the child very ill. Folic acid therapy should be continued for 3 to 4 weeks. Satisfactory responses have been obtained with doses of folic acid as low as 50 μg/day. These "physiologic" doses have no effect on primary vitamin B_{12} deficiencies; a therapeutic test using such low amounts may be used, therefore, to differentiate between primary folic acid and vitamin B_{12} deficiencies. If there is a likelihood that juvenile pernicious anemia may be present, or if the anemia recurs after therapy, the prolonged use of folic acid should be avoided, since in pernicious anemia folic acid may produce a partial response of anemia without benefiting the neurologic abnormalities. If signs of scurvy are present, therapeutic doses of ascorbic acid should be given. Antibiotic therapy should be used for superimposed bacterial infection.

Folic Acid Deficiency of Malabsorption Syndromes

Folic acid is absorbed throughout the small intestine, and diffuse inflammatory or degenerative disease of the intestine may markedly impair absorption. Celiac disease, chronic infectious enteritis and enteroenteric fistulas may lead to folic acid deficiency and megaloblastic anemia. (See also Section 11.)

Folic Acid Deficiency Complicating Hemolytic Anemias

Folic acid is necessary for normal hematopoiesis, and it is possible that chronic hemolytic processes may increase the requirement for this vitamin. Frank megaloblastic erythropoiesis may complicate hemolytic anemia, leading to more severe anemia and increased need for transfusion. The bone marrow should be examined for megaloblastic changes if there is an unexplained worsening of chronic anemia or increased transfusion requirements in chronic hemolytic states. Continuous folic acid supplementation is not ordinarily necessary for such patients if their diet is normal.

Folic Acid Deficiency Associated with Anticonvulsants and Other Drugs

Many patients have low serum levels of folic acid during therapy with certain anticonvulsant drugs (e.g. Dilantin, Mysoline), but they usually have no anemia or symptoms. Rarely such patients do have a frank megaloblastic anemia, which responds to folic acid therapy even if administration of the offending drug is continued. Malabsorption of folic acid induced by diphenylhydantoin is the probable mechanism for folate deficiency.

A number of drugs have antifolic acid activity as their primary pharmacologic effect and will regularly produce megaloblastic anemia. Methotrexate and aminopterin prevent the utilization of folic acid by inhibiting its enzymatic reduction to active coenzymatic forms. Pyrimethamine (Daraprim) and pentamidine isethionate, which are used in the therapy of toxoplasmosis and *Pneumocystis carinii* pneumonia, respectively, may induce folic acid deficiency and megaloblastic anemia.

VITAMIN B_{12} DEFICIENCY

In order to be absorbed, dietary vitamin B_{12} must combine with a glycoprotein (intrinsic factor) secreted by the parietal cells of the gastric fundus. The B_{12}–intrinsic factor complex passes to the terminal ileum, where specific absorptive sites exist. In the presence of intrinsic factor and ionic calcium, vitamin B_{12} traverses the intestinal mucosa and enters the blood. Vitamin B_{12} deficiency may therefore result from (1) inadequate intake, (2) lack of secretion of intrinsic factor by the stomach, (3) consumption or inhibition of the B_{12}–intrinsic factor complex, or (4) abnormalities involving the receptor sites in the terminal ileum.

Because vitamin B_{12} is present in many foods, dietary deficiency is rare. Instances have been reported in breast-fed infants whose mothers had deficient diets or pernicious anemia. Since vitamin B_{12} is so ubiquitous, most cases of deficiency stem from failure to absorb the vitamin.

Juvenile Pernicious Anemia

This rare disease is due to inability to secrete gastric intrinsic factor. It differs from the typical disease in adults in that the stomach secretes acid normally and is histologically normal. Consanguinity is common in parents of affected children, and a mendelian recessive inheritance pattern is suggested.

CLINICAL MANIFESTATIONS. The symptoms of juvenile pernicious anemia become prominent at 9 months to 3 years of age. This interval is consistent with exhaustion of the stores of vitamin B_{12} acquired in utero. As the anemia becomes severe, irritability, anorexia and listlessness occur. The tongue is smooth, red and painful. Neurologic involvement is manifested by ataxia, paresthesias, hyporeflexia, Babinski responses, clonus and coma.

LABORATORY DATA. The anemia is macrocytic, with prominent macro-ovalocytosis of the red cells. The neutrophils are large and hypersegmented. In advanced cases neutropenia and thrombocytopenia are seen. Serum vitamin B_{12}, as measured by radioactive techniques or microbiologic assay, is below 100 $\mu\mu$g/ml. Concentrations of serum iron and serum folic acid are normal or elevated. Levels of serum LDH are markedly increased, and excessive amounts of methylmalonic acid are excreted in the urine. Serum antibodies directed against parietal cells or intrinsic factor cannot be detected. Gastric acidity may be reduced initially, but returns to normal when vitamin B_{12} therapy is instituted. Biopsy reveals a normal gastric mucosa, but intrinsic factor activity is absent in the gastric secretion.

Absorption of vitamin B_{12} is usually assessed by the Schilling test, using radioactive vitamin B_{12}. When a normal person ingests a small amount of vitamin B_{12} containing ^{57}Co or ^{60}Co, the radioactive vitamin combines with the intrinsic factor in the stomach secretions and passes to the terminal ileum, where absorption occurs. As the absorbed vitamin is bound to blood proteins and tissues, none is normally excreted in the urine. If a large (1000 μg) dose of nonradioactive vitamin B_{12} is then injected parenterally ("flushing dose"), from 10 to 30 per cent of the previously absorbed radioactive vitamin will appear in the urine. Patients with pernicious anemia excrete 2 per cent or less under these conditions. That malabsorption of vitamin B_{12} is due to lack of intrinsic factor can be confirmed through a modification of the standard Schilling test: 30 mg of intrinsic factor is administered along with the radioactive vitamin; if absence of intrinsic factor is the basis of the B_{12} malabsorption, normal amounts of radioactive vitamin should now be absorbed and flushed out. On the other hand, when vitamin B_{12} malabsorption is due to disease of the ileal receptor sites or other intestinal causes, no improvement in absorption will be seen with intrinsic factor. The Schilling test result will remain abnormal in pernicious anemia, even when therapy has completely reversed the hematologic and neurologic manifestations of the disease.

TREATMENT. A prompt hematologic response follows parenteral administration of vitamin B_{12}. The physiologic requirement for vitamin B_{12} is 1–5 μg/day, and hematologic responses have been observed with these small doses. If there is evidence of neurologic involvement, 1 mg should be injected intramuscularly daily for at least 2 weeks. Maintenance therapy will be necessary throughout the patient's life; monthly intramuscular administration of 1 mg of vitamin B_{12} is sufficient. Attempts at oral therapy are contraindicated.

Vitamin B_{12} Deficiency in Older Children

Vitamin B_{12} malabsorption has been described in late childhood. In some cases atrophy of the gastric mucosa and achlorhydria have been seen; in others the stomach is normal. Malabsorption of vitamin B_{12} may also occur in combination with a familial syndrome of cutaneous moniliasis, hypoparathyroidism and other endocrine deficiencies. The serum contains antibodies against parietal cells and intrinsic factor. The Schilling test result is abnormal, but is corrected by addition of exogenous intrinsic factor. Parenteral vitamin B_{12} should be administered regularly to these patients to prevent the development of megaloblastic anemia.

Vitamin B_{12} Malabsorption Due to Intestinal Causes

A few cases have been reported of familial occurrence of a specific intestinal defect in the absorption of vitamin B_{12}, in some instances associated with proteinuria. Surgical resection of the terminal ileum or such inflammatory diseases as regional enteritis or tuberculosis may also impair absorption of vitamin B_{12}. When the terminal ileum has been removed, life-long parenteral administration should be considered if the Schilling test indicates that vitamin B_{12} is not absorbed. An overgrowth of intestinal bacteria within diverticula or duplications of the small intestine may cause vitamin B_{12} deficiency through consumption of the vitamin or the splitting of its complex with intrinsic factor. In these cases hematologic response may follow broad spectrum antibiotic therapy. Similar mechanisms may operate when the fish tapeworm *Diphyllobothrium latum* infests the upper small intestine. When megaloblastic anemia occurs in these situations, the serum vitamin B_{12} level is low, the gastric juice contains intrinsic factor, and the abnormal Schilling test result is not corrected by the addition of exogenous intrinsic factor.

RARE MEGALOBLASTIC ANEMIAS

Orotic aciduria is a genetically determined defect in nucleoprotein synthesis associated with a severe megaloblastic anemia and crystalluria due to excretion of orotic acid. Physical and mental retardation is frequently present. The anemia is refractory to vitamin B_{12} or folic acid, but responds promptly to administration of the nucleic acid precursor, uridine. Inheritance is autosomal recessive.

A single case of megaloblastic anemia which responded to thiamine (vitamin B_1) therapy has been described.

MICROCYTIC ANEMIAS

IRON DEFICIENCY ANEMIA

Anemia resulting from lack of sufficient iron for synthesis of hemoglobin is by far the most frequent hematologic disease of infancy and childhood. The prevalence of this deficiency is related to certain basic aspects of iron metabolism and nutrition. The body of the newborn infant contains about 0.5 gm of iron in contrast to the iron content of the adult, which is estimated at 5.0 gm. In order to make up this 4.5 gm discrepancy, an average of 0.8 mg of iron must be absorbed each day during the first 15 years of life. To this growth requirement an additional small amount is necessary to balance normal losses through excretion of iron. Accordingly, to maintain a normal positive iron balance in childhood, 0.8 to 1.5 mg of iron must be absorbed each day. As only about 10 per cent of dietary iron is absorbed, a diet containing 8 to 15 mg of iron is necessary for optimal nutrition. During the first years of life, because relatively small quantities of iron-rich foods are taken, it is often difficult to attain these amounts. For this reason the diet should include such foods as infant cereals or cow's milk formulas which have been fortified with iron. At best, the infant is in a precarious situation with respect to iron. Should the diet become inadequate or should abnormal external blood loss occur, anemia ensues rapidly.

ETIOLOGY. A preponderance of the iron of the newborn is contained in the circulating hemoglobin. Low birth weight and significant perinatal hemorrhage are associated with a decreased neonatal hemoglobin mass and store of iron. As the high hemoglobin concentration of the newborn decreases during the first 2 to 3 months of life, considerable iron is reclaimed and stored. (See physiological anemia of infancy.) These reclaimed stores are usually sufficient for blood formation for the first 6 to 9 months of life; but in low-birth-weight infants or with perinatal blood loss, stored iron may be depleted earlier, and dietary sources become of paramount importance. Anemia due solely to inadequate dietary iron is unusual during the first 4 to 6 months, but becomes common from 9 to 24 months of age. Thereafter it is relatively infrequent. The usual dietary pattern observed in infants with iron deficiency anemia is the consumption of large amounts of milk and of carbohydrates, unsupplemented with iron.

Blood loss must be considered a possible cause in every case of iron deficiency anemia, particularly in the older child. Chronic iron deficiency anemia from occult bleeding may be due to a lesion of the gastrointestinal tract such as peptic ulcer, Meckel's diverticulum, polyp or hemangioma. In some geographic areas hookworm infestation is an important cause. It is now recognized that as many as one third of infants with iron deficiency in the United States have chronic intestinal blood loss induced by exposure to a heat labile protein in whole cow's milk. This syndrome was described and defined by Wilson, Lahey and Heiner. With special techniques, loss of 1 to 7 ml of blood in the stools each day is demonstrated. The fecal blood loss is not influenced by iron replacement or transfusion, but can be prevented either by reduction of the quantity of whole cow's milk to 1 pint per day or less, or by using heated or evaporated milk or a milk substitute. This gastrointestinal reaction is not related to enzymatic abnormalities in the mucosa, such as lactase deficiency. Characteristically, involved infants develop anemia which is more severe and occurs earlier than would be expected simply from inadequate intake of iron.

Histologic abnormalities of the mucosa of the gastrointestinal tract are present in advanced iron deficiency anemia, as are significant decreases in intracellular iron-containing enzymes in the mucosal cells. The morphologic changes may be a direct manifestation of tissue deficiency of iron.

CLINICAL MANIFESTATIONS. Pallor is the most important clue to iron deficiency. When the hemoglobin level falls below 5.0 gm/dl, irritability and anorexia are prominent. Tachycardia and cardiac dilatation occur, and systolic murmurs are often present.

The spleen is palpably enlarged in 10 to 15 per cent of cases, and in longstanding ones widening of the diploë of the skull similar to that seen in congenital hemolytic anemias may occur. These changes resolve slowly with adequate replacement therapy. The child with iron deficiency anemia may be obese, or underweight with other evidences of undernutrition. Pica is sometimes prominent. The irritability and anorexia characteristic of advanced cases may reflect deficiency in tissue iron, for with iron therapy striking improvement in behavior frequently occurs before significant hematologic improvement.

LABORATORY DATA. In progressive iron deficiency a fairly definite sequence of biochemical and hematologic events occurs. First, the tissue iron stores represented by liver and bone marrow hemosiderin disappear. Next there is a decrease in serum iron to less than 50 μg/dl. Concomitantly the iron-binding capacity of the serum increases to more than 350 μg/dl and the per cent saturation falls below 15 per cent. As the deficiency progresses, hematologic changes ensue. The red cells become smaller than normal, their hemoglobin content decreases, with mean corpuscular volumes less than 75 μ^3. With increasing severity the red cells become deformed and misshapen. These changes result in the characteristic morphologic findings of microcytosis, hypochromia and poikilocytosis (Fig. 14-3, *D*), without which a diagnosis of significant iron deficiency anemia is untenable. The reticulocyte count is normal or minimally elevated; nucleated red cells may occasionally be seen in the peripheral blood. White blood cell counts are normal. Thrombocytosis, sometimes of a striking degree (600,000 mm^3 to 1,000,000 mm^3) may occur. On the other hand, in a few cases significant thrombocytopenia may be present. The mechanism of these platelet abnormalities is not clear; they return to normal with iron therapy. The bone marrow is hypercellular with erythroid hyperplasia. The normoblasts have scanty, fragmented cytoplasm with poor hemoglobinization. Leukocytes and megakaryocytes are normal. Hemosiderin cannot be demonstrated in marrow specimens by the Prussian blue staining techniques. In about a third of cases occult blood can be detected in the stools.

DIFFERENTIAL DIAGNOSIS. Iron deficiency must be differentiated from other hypochromic microcytic anemias. In lead poisoning the red cells are morphologically similar, but coarse basophilic stippling of the red cells is prominent, and elevations of blood lead, free erythrocyte protoporphyrins and urinary coproporphyrins are seen. The blood changes of thalassemia trait resemble those of iron deficiency, but characteristic alterations in the levels of Hgb A_2 and Hgb F are usually present, whereas they are not in iron deficiency. Thalassemia major with its pronounced erythroblastosis and hemolytic component should present no diagnostic confusion.

TREATMENT. The regular response of iron deficiency anemia to adequate amounts of iron is an important diagnostic as well as therapeutic feature. Oral administration of simple ferrous salts (sulfate, gluconate, fumarate) provides inexpensive and satisfactory therapy. There is no evidence that addition of any trace metal, vitamin or other hematinic substance significantly increases the response to simple ferrous salts. On the other hand, absorption of some iron chelates may be suboptimal. For routine clinical use the physician should familiarize himself with an inexpensive preparation of one of the simple ferrous compounds. The therapeutic dose must be calculated in terms of elemental iron; ferrous sulfate is 20 per cent, and ferrous gluconate is 10 to 12 per cent elemental iron by weight. A daily total of 6 mg/kg of elemental iron in 3 divided doses provides an optimal amount of iron for the stimulated bone marrow to utilize. Doses of elemental iron in excess of 6 mg/kg per day do not result in a more rapid hematologic response. Better absorption may result when medicinal iron is given between meals. Ingestion of large amounts of milk may significantly decrease absorption of iron. Intolerance to oral iron is extremely rare; malabsorption of oral iron is more frequently invoked than documented. A parenteral iron preparation (iron-dextran) is currently available for pediatric use. This is an effective, reasonably safe form of iron when given in a properly calculated dose, but the response to parenteral iron is no more rapid or more complete than that obtained with proper administration of iron orally, and in most cases the indication for parenteral iron therapy is a social one.

While adequate iron medication is given, the family must be educated about the patient's diet, and the consumption of milk should be limited to a reasonable quantity, preferably to 1 pint per day or less. This reduction has a dual effect: the amount of iron-rich foods in the diet is increased; and gastrointestinal blood loss from intolerance to cow's milk proteins is prevented. When the re-education of child and parent is not successful, parenteral iron medication may be indicated.

Within 72 to 96 hours after administration of iron to the anemic child, peripheral reticulocytosis is seen. The height of this response is inversely proportional to the severity of the anemia. Reticulocytosis is followed by a rise in the hemoglobin level, which may increase as much as 0.5 gm/dl/day. Iron medication should be continued for 4 to 6 weeks after blood values are normal. Failures of iron therapy occur when the child does not receive the prescribed medication, when it is given in a form which is poorly absorbed, or when there is continuing unrecognized blood loss. An incorrect original diagnosis of iron deficiency anemia may be revealed by therapeutic failure of iron medication.

Since a rapid hematologic response can be confidently predicted in typical iron deficiency, blood transfusion is indicated only when the anemia is very severe or when superimposed infection may interfere with the response. It is not necessary and may be dangerous to attempt rapid correction of severe anemia by transfusion, owing to associated hypervolemia and cardiac dilatation. Slow administration of packed or sedimented red cells is usually sufficient to raise the hemoglobin to a safe level, at which the response to iron therapy can be awaited. In general, severely anemic children with hemoglobins less than 4 gm/dl should be given only 2–3 ml/kg of packed cells at any one time. If evidence of frank congestive heart failure is present, a modified exchange transfusion employing fresh packed red cells should be considered. Digitalis is usually unnecessary.

Sideroblastic Anemias

The sideroblastic anemias are a heterogeneous group of hypochromic microcytic anemias whose basic defects may be abnormalities of iron or heme metabolism. Serum iron levels are abnormally increased. In the bone marrow ringed sideroblasts are found; these are nucleated red cells with a perinuclear collar of coarse hemosiderin granules.

A form of sideroblastic anemia transmitted as an X-linked recessive trait becomes symptomatic by late childhood. Splenomegaly is usually present.

Some cases of sideroblastic anemia are partially responsive to pyridoxine (vitamin B_6) given in doses of 20 to 500 mg/day, though abnormalities of tryptophan metabolism are inconstantly found and other findings of B_6 deficiency are not observed.

LEAD POISONING

(See also Section 28.)

Lead interferes with iron utilization and hemoglobin synthesis, so that a hypochromic microcytic anemia is a prominent finding in chronic lead poisoning. The red cells are hypochromic and microcytic, with coarse basophilic stippling. Examination of the red cells with the ultraviolet microscope reveals intense fluorescence due to markedly increased levels of free erythrocyte protoporphyrin, for which there are useful screening tests.

RARE TYPES OF HYPOCHROMIC MICROCYTIC ANEMIA

Isolated cases are known of hypochromic microcytic anemia with other abnormalities of iron metabolism; some cases have had defects in iron mobilization or re-utilization. Congenital absence of the iron-binding protein (atransferrinemia) is associated with hypochromic anemia.

Several patients have had refractory hypochromic anemia associated with lymphatic tumors or lymphoid hyperplasia. Correction of the anemia followed removal of the abnormal lymphatic tissue in these cases.

See also Thalassemia.

Hemolytic Anemias

The fundamental basis of the hemolytic anemias is a shortened survival time of the red blood cells. Red blood cells normally spend 100 to 120 days in the circulation; about 1 per cent of red cells (senescent ones) are removed from the blood each day and are replaced by an equal number of new cells released from the bone marrow.

In response to a shortened peripheral survival of red cells, the activity of bone marrow increases. The peripheral reticulocyte count exceeds 2 per cent. Sustained reticulocytosis in conjunction even with an unchanging hemoglobin level is presumptive evidence of a hemolytic disorder. Hyperplasia of the erythropoietic marrow elements occurs, with lowering of the myeloid-erythroid ratio. In the chronic hemolytic processes of childhood, hypertrophy of the marrow may expand the medullary spaces and result in striking roentgenographic changes, particularly in the skull.

Products of red cell breakdown increase with hemolysis. Elevations of unconjugated (indirect) bilirubin accompany many hemolytic states, but if hepatic function is not impaired, readily distinguishable jaundice is unusual, and bilirubin levels may even be normal. Accelerated destruction of red cells increases the quantity of heme pigments excreted in the bile. These products of hemoglobin catabolism can be quantitated by the tedious and unesthetic measurement of fecal urobilinogen. Pigmented gallstones composed of calcium bilirubinate may be formed as early as the fourth year of life, and a chronic hemolytic process should be considered possible in any case of cholelithiasis in childhood, but only about 15 per cent of cases of gallstones in children are a consequence of hemolytic anemia. Plasma concentrations of hemoglobin increase in hemolytic anemias, and the free hemoglobin combines irreversibly with specific binding proteins called haptoglobins. The large haptoglobin-hemoglobin complex is cleared from the circulation by reticuloendothelial activity. In severe hemolytic states the loss of haptoglobin exceeds the synthetic capacity of the liver, and serum haptoglobin is decreased or absent. The level of hemopexin, another plasma protein which binds hemoglobin, is also reduced in hemolytic states. Catabolism of hemoglobin results in formation of carbon monoxide, and quantitation of CO in blood or expired air can provide a dynamic indicator of hemolysis. The assay is difficult, however, and not often employed clinically.

In addition to these indirect indicators of hemolysis, red cell survival can be directly estimated by isotopic techniques. Sodium chromate ($Na_2{}^{51}CrO_4$) and diisofluorophosphate ($DF^{32}P$) are the radioactive compounds most often used as red cell "tags." The ^{51}Cr technique is the most frequently used because of its simplicity. After injection of ^{51}Cr-tagged red cells, blood radioactivity normally decreases to 50 per cent of its initial level in 25 to 35 days (^{51}Cr $T^{1}/_{2}$ or half-life). A shortened red cell survival is likely when the ^{51}Cr $T^{1}/_{2}$ is reduced below 20 days. $DF^{32}P$ is expensive and more difficult to count, but permits an actual measurement of red cell survival. In practice, it is rarely necessary to use these specialized isotopic techniques.

The stimulated normal bone marrow can ordinarily increase its output sixfold to eightfold. By such compensation red cell survival can theoretically be reduced to 15 to 20 days without producing anemia, but most often in childhood chronic hemolysis results in some degree of anemia. Patients with hemolytic anemias of whatever type may have transient episodes of bone marrow failure. These *aplastic crises* are characterized by reticulocytopenia and markedly decreased numbers of red cell precursors in the marrow. Occasionally huge abnormal erythroid precursors ("gigantoblasts") are seen. Profound and life-threatening anemia may develop quickly because the shortened red cell survival is no longer even partially compensated. These episodes of acute marrow failure are self-limited and last 10 to 14 days. Aplastic crises are usually associated with infection, and may occur within a few days in several affected members of a family. They constitute a potentially serious, life-threatening complication of any chronic hemolytic process.

The hemolytic anemias may be divided into two large classes: (1) those with premature destruction due to intrinsic abnormalities of the red cell, and (2) those due to noxious extraerythrocytic factors. Table 14–4 lists the important hemolytic anemias of childhood. In hemolytic states associated with intrinsic defects, red cell survival is short in normal persons receiving a transfusion of the patient's red cells, as well as in patients themselves. In contrast, red cells from patients with anemias due to extrinsic factors have an adequate life span when transfused to a normal recipient.

HEMOLYTIC ANEMIAS DUE TO INTRINSIC ABNORMALITIES OF THE RED CELL

HEREDITARY SPHEROCYTOSIS

(Congenital Hemolytic Anemia; Congenital Acholuric Jaundice)

This is the most common of the hereditary hemolytic states in which there is no abnormality of hemoglobin. The classic features are a congenital and familial hemolytic process associated with splenomegaly and with red cells which are spherical in shape. Typical cases have been reported in most ethnic groups, but the disease is particularly prevalent among persons of northern European origin.

ETIOLOGY. Hereditary spherocytosis is transmitted as an autosomal dominant trait; about 20 per cent of cases are sporadic and presumably represent new mutations. Although the basic defect has not been precisely delineated, its expression is an abnormality of the red cell membrane, which renders these cells unduly permeable to sodium. An increased concentration of intracellular sodium leads to an increased utilization of ATP to drive the so-called cation pump. Premature senescence and destruction of red cells are thought to result from metabolic overwork. Spherocytosis is the morphologic expression of these biochemical abnormalities.

The spleen is intimately involved in the hemolytic process. The splenic circulation imposes a metabolic environment which is particularly stressful to the spherocytic cell, and damage from repeated passages through this unfavorable environment results in their sequestration and destruction. The hemolytic process abates after splenectomy, even though the biochemical and morphologic abnormalities persist.

CLINICAL MANIFESTATIONS. The disease has its onset in infancy and may present in the neonatal period with anemia and hyperbilirubinemia severe enough to require exchange transfusions. The anemia varies considerably in severity during infancy and childhood, but tends to be similar within families. Some patients with relatively severe anemia during the first 6 to 8 months of life show thereafter more satisfactory compensation. Slight jaundice is usually present. Moderate expansion of the marrow cavity of the skull may occur, but not so extreme as in thalassemia or the hemoglobinopathies. After infancy the spleen is almost always palpably enlarged. Although pigmentary gallstones have been reported as early as 4 to 5 years of age, they usually do not develop until late childhood or adolescence. Approximately 75 per cent of untreated patients will ultimately form gallstones. Aplastic crises are the most serious complications which occur during childhood.

LABORATORY DATA. The usual evidences of hemolysis, including reticulocytosis, anemia and hyperbilirubinemia, are present. The characteristic spherocytic red cell is smaller than the normal erythrocyte and lacks the central pallor of the biconcave disk (Fig. 14–3, *B*). This morphologic change may be subtle, and only a relatively small proportion of the cells may be spherocytic. Though there is erythroid hyperplasia in marrow, the red cell precursors are not spherocytic. There are no abnormal hemoglobins.

The basic abnormality of the red cell can be demonstrated by osmotic fragility studies. When red cells are placed in hypotonic saline solutions, water and sodium enter the cells, causing them to swell. The normal red cell of biconcave shape can increase its volume, but the spherical cell already contains the maximum volume for its surface area. Imbibition of small amounts of water causes the spherocyte to rupture. In 10 to 20 per cent of cases of hereditary spherocytosis the abnormality may be demonstrated only if the blood is incubated at 37° C for 24 hours before determining osmotic fragility. The autohemolysis test is also useful in hereditary spherocytosis. When normal blood is incubated under sterile conditions for 48 hours at 37° C, less than 5 per cent of the red cells hemolyze. Red cells of patients with hereditary spherocytosis have markedly increased rates of autohemolysis (15 to 45 per cent). Abnormal autohemolysis can be corrected by the addition of small amounts of glucose to the blood before incubation.

DIFFERENTIAL DIAGNOSIS. Hereditary spherocytosis must be differentiated from other congenital hemolytic states. The family history, blood smear, and studies of osmotic fragility and autohemolysis are of most diagnostic value. Acquired spherocytosis of the red cells is seen in autoimmune hemolytic anemias; here the spherocytosis is more noticeable than in hereditary spherocytosis, and the Coombs test result is usually positive. It may be difficult to differentiate hereditary spherocytosis in the newborn infant from hemolytic disease due to A or B incompatibility when an appropriate blood group incompatibility is coincidentally present. A period of observation may be necessary to clarify the diagnosis.

TREATMENT. Splenectomy invariably produces a clinical cure. Elective splenectomy should be planned for the patient at 4 to 6 years of age. If anemia is severe enough to impair growth or if aplastic crises are frequent, the operation may be considered earlier; an extended period of observation will be indicated before splenectomy can be justified in infancy. Splenectomy prevents gallstones and eliminates the threat of aplastic crises. Hemochromatosis and hepatic failure have been described in adults with hereditary spherocytosis who were not splenectomized. After splenectomy, jaundice and reticulocytosis rapidly disappear, and the hemoglobin attains the normal range, though the spherocytosis and abnormal osmotic fragility become more pronounced. Thrombocytosis may occur in the immediate postoperative period, but anticoagulation therapy is not routinely indicated. The syndrome of overwhelming sepsis after splenectomy is not a frequent threat to older patients with hereditary spherocytosis, but the febrile or infected child after splenectomy should be carefully evaluated. Occasionally in the newborn infant with hereditary spherocytosis, phototherapy or exchange transfusion may be required for control of hyperbilirubinemia.

HEREDITARY ELLIPTOCYTOSIS

Oval or elliptical shape of red cells occurs as a benign, dominantly inherited morphologic curiosity in about 1 in 2000 persons (Fig. 14–4, *E*).

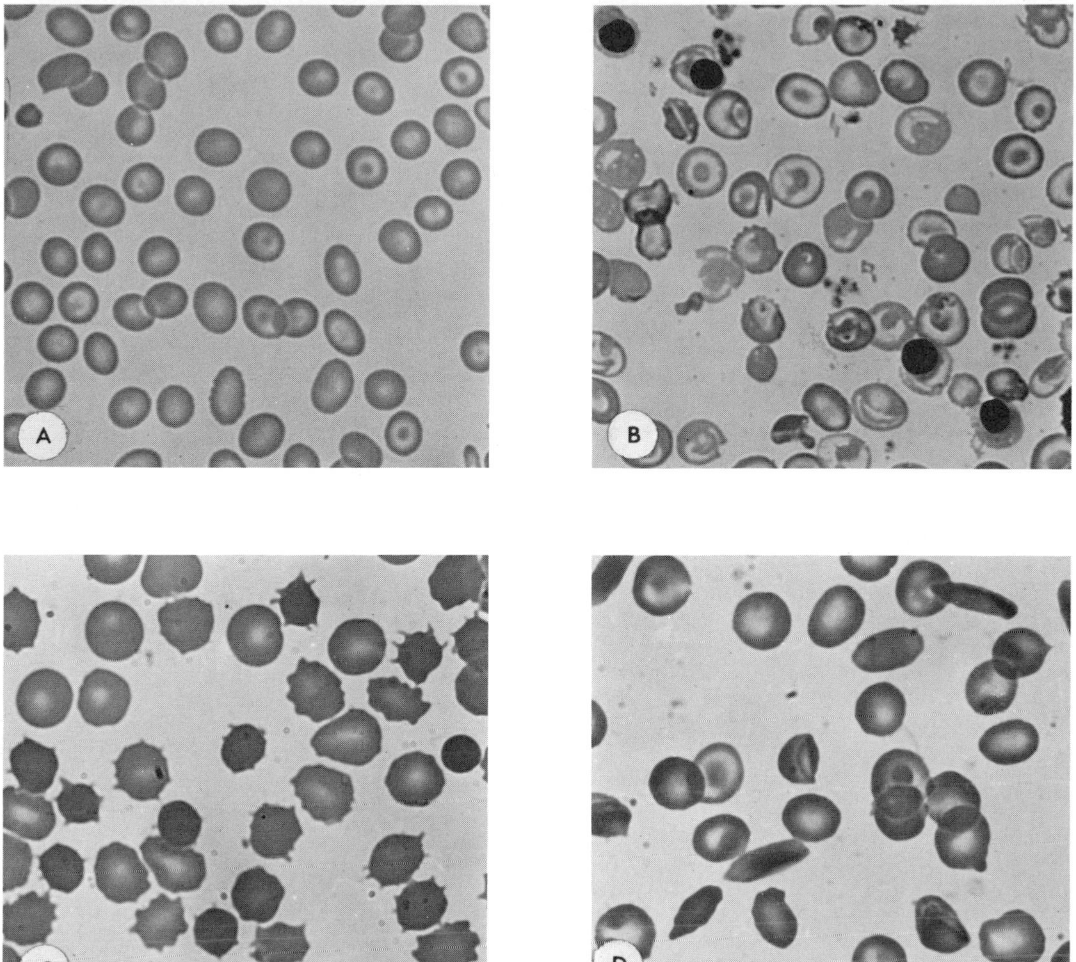

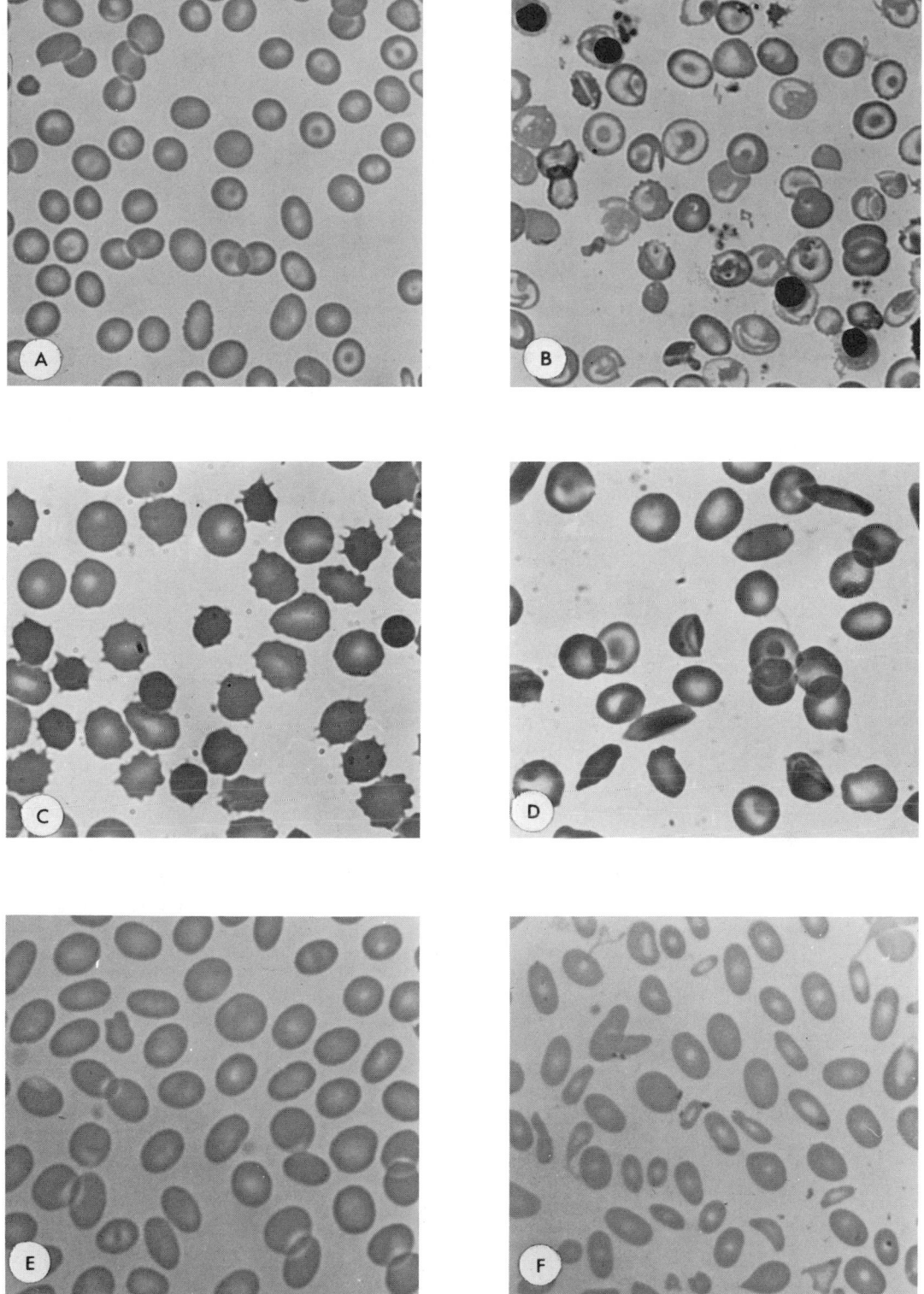

Figure 14–4 *Morphologic abnormalities of the red cell.* A, *Thalassemia trait.* B, *Thalassemia major.* C, *Acanthocytes (a-betalipoproteinemia).* D, *Sickle cells (Hgb SS disease).* E, *Elliptocytes (hereditary elliptocytosis).* F, *Bizarre elliptocytes (hemolytic elliptocytosis).*

Hemolysis is usually mild or absent; however, in about 10 per cent of patients there may be a significant hemolytic anemia.

ETIOLOGY. The cause is uncertain. Family studies of affected children usually reveal one parent with elliptocytosis without hemolysis, while the other parent is normal. A few cases may have represented homozygous inheritance. The gene for elliptocytosis is sometimes linked with the Rh locus. No biochemical abnormality of the red cell has been defined.

CLINICAL MANIFESTATIONS. Hemolytic elliptocytosis may manifest as jaundice in the neonatal period even though characteristic elliptocytosis may not be evident at that time, the blood of the affected newborn showing bizarre poikilocytosis and pyknocytosis. The usual features of a chronic hemolytic process are seen later, manifest by anemia, jaundice, splenomegaly and osseous changes. Cholelithiasis may occur in late childhood, and aplastic crises have been reported.

LABORATORY DATA. The morphology of the red blood cells is the most important diagnostic feature (Fig. 14–4, *F*). Elliptical cells are prominent, but many bizarre poikilocytes, microcytes and spherocytes are also present. The reticulocyte count is greatly increased. Erythroid hyperplasia is present in the bone marrow, but red cell precursors are not elliptical. There is no abnormal hemoglobin.

TREATMENT. Splenectomy decreases the hemolytic component of this disease, although some degree of hemolysis may continue. It should be performed if there is significant chronic hemolysis. The red cell morphology is not corrected by the operation and may be considerably more abnormal in the postoperative period.

OTHER STRUCTURAL DEFECTS

PAROXYSMAL NOCTURNAL HEMOGLOBINURIA

Paroxysmal nocturnal hemoglobinuria is a rare chronic anemia with prominent intravascular hemolysis. The hemolysis is characteristically worse during sleep, and morning hemoglobinuria is a classic finding. The disease is not congenital. It results from an ill defined intrinsic defect of the red cell, which renders it susceptible to hemolysis in an acid medium. In addition to chronic hemolysis, there may be pancytopenia. Pyogenic infection and thrombosis are serious complications. Since a number of cases have followed aplastic anemia, it has been suggested that the same agent causing aplastic anemia may predispose to paroxysmal nocturnal hemoglobinuria. The diagnosis is established by a positive result in the acid hemolysin or thrombin tests, and by markedly reduced levels of red cell acetylcholinesterase activity. Splenectomy is not indicated. Prolonged anticoagulation therapy may be of benefit when thromboses occur.

HEREDITARY STOMATOCYTOSIS

Hereditary stomatocytosis is a rare morphologic abnormality of the red cells, characterized by a mouthlike slit in place of the usual circular area of central pallor. There may be hemolytic anemia. Extreme permeability of the red cell membrane to cations has been observed in one patient. Splenectomy has not been consistently effective, but may be indicated in patients with severe hemolysis.

ACANTHOCYTOSIS

In this rare defect of lipid metabolism the distorted red cells have sharp projections (Fig. 14–4, *C*), but there may be no hemolytic anemia. The striking morphologic changes presumably result from decreased levels of cholesterol and beta-lipoprotein in the serum. (See A-beta-lipoproteinemia, in Sections 8, 11 and 20.)

ENZYMATIC DEFECTS OF THE RED CELLS

Development of techniques for quantitating various red cell enzymes has permitted the identification of a number of specific entities within a group of diseases which have been identified collectively as congenital nonspherocytic hemolytic anemias because of the lack of spherocytes and normal osmotic fragility. Abnormalities of enzymes may involve the major pathways of glucose catabolism, the anaerobic Embden-Meyerhof pathway or the oxidative pentose phosphate shunt (Fig. 14–2).

Biochemical criteria suggested for diagnosis of these diseases include demonstration of a markedly reduced level of enzyme activity in the patient's red cells by specific assay. In addition there should be an increase in glycolytic intermediates which precede the enzyme block and a reduced level of substances dependent upon the enzyme for formation. Assays for the most important enzymes (glucose 6-phosphate dehydrogenase, pyruvate kinase) are widely available; several research laboratories in the United States are able to quantitate all glycolytic enzymes and intermediate compounds.

PYRUVATE KINASE DEFICIENCY

A congenital hemolytic anemia occurs with homozygous manifestations of an autosomal recessive gene which causes either a marked reduction in red cell content of pyruvate kinase or production of an abnormal enzyme with decreased activity. Generation of ATP within the red cell is impaired, and low levels of ATP, pyruvate, and NAD are seen. Concentrations of 2,3-DPG are increased. As a consequence of decreased ATP, potassium leaks from the red cell at a markedly increased rate and its life span is considerably reduced.

CLINICAL MANIFESTATIONS AND LABORATORY DATA. Jaundice and anemia may occur in the neonatal period, and kernicterus has been reported. During later life the severity of the hemolytic component is variable from patient to patient, but pallor, jaundice and splenomegaly are usually present.

Macrocytosis and polychromatophilia in peripheral blood reflect the elevated reticulocyte count. Spherocytes are uncommon, but a few spiculated pyknocytes are usually present. Nonincubated osmotic fragility is normal. Autohemolysis is moderately or markedly increased, but addition of glucose does not regularly correct the abnormality as it does in hereditary spherocytosis.

Diagnosis rests upon demonstration by spectrophotometric assay of marked reductions of pyruvate kinase activity in the red cells. Other red cell enzymes are normal or even elevated. There are no abnormalities of hemoglobin components. The white blood cells have normal pyruvate kinase activity. The heterozygous carriers usually have moderately reduced levels of pyruvate kinase activity.

TREATMENT. Exchange transfusions may be indicated for control of hyperbilirubinemia during the neonatal period. Transfusions of packed red cells may be necessary for severe anemia or for aplastic crises. If the degree of anemia is consistently severe, splenectomy should be performed after 1 or 2 years of age. Although not curative, the operation may be followed by higher hemoglobin levels. The reticulocyte count may be strikingly high (20 to 30 per cent) following splenectomy; deaths due to overwhelming pneumococcal sepsis have followed splenectomy.

DEFICIENCIES OF OTHER GLYCOLYTIC ENZYMES

Development of specific assays for red cell enzymes has permitted the demonstration that congenital nonspherocytic anemias may stem from defects in hexokinase, glucose phosphate isomerase, phosphofructokinase, glyceraldehyde 3-phosphate dehydrogenase, triose phosphate isomerase, and 2,3-diphosphoglycerate mutase, which are transmitted as autosomal recessive traits. Instances of phosphoglycerate kinase deficiency due to an X-linked defect have also been described in a mentally retarded boy.

In these conditions the red cell morphology is not strikingly abnormal except for polychromasia and macrocytosis. Nonincubated osmotic fragility is normal. Splenectomy has not been of regular benefit.

DEFICIENCIES OF ENZYMES OF THE PENTOSE PHOSPHATE PATHWAY AND RELATED COMPOUNDS

The most important function of the pentose pathway, through which about 10 per cent of the glucose utilized by the red cell passes, is to provide NADPH or reduced triphosphopyridine nucleotide (TPNH). NADPH is necessary for conversion of oxidized to reduced glutathione, which is esential for the physiologic inactivation of oxidant compounds such as hydrogen peroxide which accumulate within the red cell. If glutathione or any of the compounds or enzymes necessary for maintaining it in the reduced state are decreased, hemoglobin may become denatured and precipitated into red cell inclusions called *Heinz bodies.* Once Heinz bodies have formed, the red cell is rapidly removed from the circulation; an acute hemolytic process may result.

GLUCOSE 6-PHOSPHATE DEHYDROGENASE (G-6-PD) DEFICIENCY

G-6-PD deficiency, the most important disease in this group, is responsible for two clinical syndromes: an episodic hemolytic anemia induced by infections or certain drugs, and a spontaneous chronic nonspherocytic hemolytic anemia.

Drug-induced Hemolytic Anemia Associated with G-6-PD Deficiency
(Primaquine Sensitivity)

Synthesis of red cell G-6-PD is determined by genes borne on the X chromosome. Diseases involving this enzyme occur, therefore, more frequently in males than in females. About 10 per cent of American black males and 2 per cent of black females have a defect which results in a deficiency of red cell G-6-PD. Italians, Greeks and other Mediterranean, Middle Eastern, African and Oriental ethnic groups also have high frequencies ranging from 5 to 40 per cent. The G-6-PD activity of the homozygous female or the hemizygous male is one tenth to one twentieth of normal. The heterozygous female has an intermediate enzymatic activity, and, as an example of random X chromosome inactivation (Lyon hypothesis), has two populations of red cells; one is normal, the other deficient in G-6-PD activity. The heterozygous female does not, however, have clinical hemolysis after exposure to oxidant drugs. There appears to be considerable variation in the defect among various racial groups; the defect in blacks is less severe than in affected Caucasians. In blacks, enzyme deficiency is invariably associated with an electrophoretically distinct enzyme variant designated A^-, while affected Caucasians have a variant designated B^-. The basic defect appears to be production of an unstable enzyme which becomes inactive much more rapidly than normal.

In the usual pattern of G-6-PD deficiency no evidence of hemolysis is apparent until 48 to 96 hours after the patient has ingested a substance which has oxidant properties. Drugs which have these properties include antipyretics, sulfonamides, antimalarials and naphthaquinolones. The fava bean, a Mideastern dietary staple, is also particularly potent, producing an acute and severe hemolytic syndrome called "favism." The degree of hemolysis varies with the agent and the amount ingested. In severe cases, hemoglobinuria and jaundice are seen and the hemoglobin concentration may decrease 60 to 70 per cent. Even if administration of the responsible drug is continued, recovery is the rule, with evidence of a compensated hemolytic process. Occasionally infection may result in hemolysis. This defect is an important cause of neonatal hyperbilirubinemia and kernicterus in Greek and Chinese newborn infants. Significant hemolysis may occur even when no exposure to drugs can be documented. In black newborns, spontaneous hemolysis may occur in premature, but not term, infants with G-6-PD deficiency. When a pregnant woman ingests drugs such as sulfonamides or naphthalene, they may be transmitted to her G-6-PD-deficient fetus, and severe hemolytic anemia and jaundice may ensue after birth.

LABORATORY DATA. Hemoglobinemia and hemoglobinuria are manifest in severe acute cases. Unstained or supravital preparations of the red cell reveal the multiple small round inclusions called Heinz bodies, which are not visible on Wright-stained blood smears. Because cells containing these inclusions are rapidly removed from the circulation, they are not seen after the first 3 to 4 days of illness. Recovery is heralded by reticulocytosis and increase in hemoglobin concentration.

DIAGNOSIS. Diagnosis is dependent upon direct or indirect demonstration of reduced G-6-PD activity in red cells. By direct measurement, enzyme activity in affected persons is one tenth of normal or less, and the reduction of enzyme is more extreme in Caucasians than in blacks. Satisfactory screening tests are based upon decoloration of methylene blue and upon reduction of methemoglobin. Immediately after a hemolytic episode reticulocytes and young red cells predominate. These young cells have significantly higher enzyme activity than older cells; therefore, testing may have to be deferred for a few weeks before a diagnostically low level of enzyme can be shown.

TREATMENT. Prevention of hemolysis constitutes the most important therapeutic measure. When possible, males belonging to ethnic groups in which there is a significant incidence of G-6-PD deficiency should be tested for the defect before drugs are given which are known to be oxidant. When hemolysis has occurred, supportive therapy may include blood transfusions. Spontaneous recovery is the rule.

Other Hemolytic Anemias Associated with Deficiencies of G-6-PD and Related Substances

A rare form of chronic nonspherocytic hemolytic anemia has been associated with profound deficiency or absence of G-6-PD. The anemia is inherited as an X-linked recessive, and most reported cases have been in males of northern European origin. Chronic hemolytic anemia is maintained, and worsening of the hemolytic process may follow ingestion of oxidant drugs. Splenectomy is of no value. A mild, chronic nonspherocytic anemia has also been reported in association with a genetically determined deficiency of red cell glutathione. 6-Phosphogluconic dehydrogenase deficiency has been associated with drug hemolysis. Hyperbilirubinemia has been related to a deficiency of glutathione peroxidase in several newborn infants.

HEMOGLOBINOPATHIES

The clinically important abnormal hemoglobin syndromes result from single amino acid substitutions in the alpha or beta chains of adult hemoglobin. Although a large number of hemoglobin variants have been described, only a few of these are relatively prevalent.

Tremendous advances have been made in the biochemical characterization of the hemoglobins. Alpha and beta chains consist of about 150 amino acids, and the precise sequence of these amino acids in the polypeptide chains has been defined by a sophisticated analytic technique called "fingerprinting." By means of this technique it is possible to localize precisely and identify single amino acid substitutions which result in the abnormal hemoglobins. (See also Section 8.)

SICKLE CELL HEMOGLOBINOPATHIES

The sickle cell hemoglobinopathies serve as superb models for demonstrating the mechanism of molecular disease, from the levels of gene structure and action to the ultimate clinical syndrome in the patient. The basic defect is a mutant, autosomal gene which causes a valine residue to be substituted for a glutamic acid one in the no. 6 position of a beta polypeptide chain ($\alpha_2\beta_2{}^{6val}$). This minor substitution has profound physiochemical consequences: deoxygenation results in a surface change which facilitates stacking of sickle hemoglobin molecules into monofilaments, which aggregate into elongated crystals, distorting the red cell membrane and forming the sickle cell.

Sickle Cell Trait

Heterozygous occurrence of the sickle gene is associated with a benign clinical course. About 8 per cent of American blacks have the trait; there is a much greater prevalence in parts of Africa. Typical cases also occur in other ethnic groups from Mediterranean and Mid- and Near-Eastern areas. Possession of a sickle gene is believed to confer a degree of resistance to falciparum malaria. The individual red cells of persons with the trait contain a mixture of normal and sickle hemoglobins (Hgb A and Hgb S). The Hgb S proportion varies from 30 to 45 per cent. With these low proportions of Hgb S, sickling does not occur under physiologic conditions. On rare occasions severe hypoxia resulting from shock or flying at high altitudes in unpressurized aircraft may be associated with vaso-occlusive phenomena. Spontaneous hematuria, usually from the left kidney, and hyposthenuria may also occur; but anemia, hemolysis or other clinical abnormalities are not attributable to the uncomplicated sickle trait. The sickle cell trait does not affect longevity. Carriers should avoid situations in which hypoxia may occur, but otherwise do not need to modify their life or activities. The diagnosis has genetic implications, for in families in which both mother and father have sickle cell trait, approximately 25 per cent of the children will have sickle cell anemia.

Sickle Cell Anemia

Sickle cell anemia is a severe, chronic hemolytic anemia occurring in persons homozygous for the sickle gene. The clinical course is marked by episodes of pain due to occlusion of small blood vessels by spontaneously sickled red cells.

CLINICAL MANIFESTATIONS. Manifestations of sickle cell disease do not usually appear until the latter part of the first year of life, because the large amounts of Hgb F present in the red cells of young infants obscure the detection of small amounts of nonfetal hemoglobins. Use of specialized techniques such as agar gel electrophoresis at acid pH is necessary for precise diagnosis in early life. Coincidentally with the postnatal decrease in Hgb F, the concentration of Hgb S rises. Intravascular sickling and evidences of a hemolytic process may then occur. Patients with sickle cell anemia experience episodes which traditionally have been called "crises." These are of several varieties, however, and the "crisis" is not a specific diagnostic entity.

Most frequent are the painful or *vaso-occlusive crises*. These result from occlusion of small blood vessels with distal ischemia and infarction. They may be precipitated by infections or develop spontaneously in any or in many parts of the body. Symmetrical, painful swelling of the hands and feet (hand-foot syndrome) caused by infarction in the small bones of the extremities may be the initial manifestation of sickle cell anemia in infancy. Striking bony destruction with periosteal reaction may be observed radiographically (Fig. 14–5). In older patients the large joints and surrounding parts may become painful and swollen. Severe abdominal pains, resembling those of an acute surgical condition of the abdomen, are often due to infarction in abdominal structures. Strokes due to cerebral occlusion are serious and, if not immediately fatal, may leave hemiplegias. Extensive pulmonary infarction is difficult to differentiate from pneumonia. Vaso-occlusive crises are not associated with pronounced changes in the hematologic picture.

A second type of crisis, seen only in the young patient, is the so-called *sequestration crisis*. For unknown reasons large amounts of blood become acutely pooled in the liver and the spleen. The spleen becomes massively enlarged, and signs of circulatory collapse develop rapidly. If the patient is supported by hydration and by blood transfusion, much of the sequestered blood is remobilized. This sort of episode is a frequent cause of death in the infant with sickle cell disease and occurs in older patients with sickle cell variants in whom splenomegaly persists into later life.

The third well characterized type of crisis is the *aplastic crisis* previously described.

Hyperhemolytic crises are unusual, but may re-

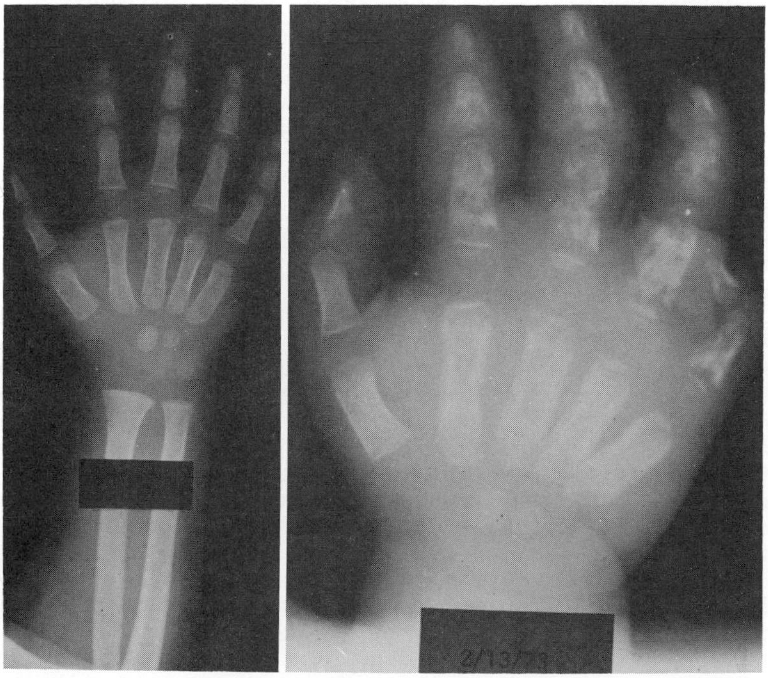

Figure 14–5 *Roentgenographs of infant with sickle cell anemia. Note bony destruction.*

sult when a person with homozygous sickle cell disease, who coincidentally has G-6-PD deficiency, ingests an oxidant drug.

In addition to the acute crises, a wide variety of clinical signs and symptoms result from severe hemolytic anemia and chronic vaso-occlusive disease. Progressive impairment of liver function contributes to the visible jaundice these patients regularly demonstrate. Gallstones have been seen in patients as young as 3 years of age. Renal function is progressively impaired by diffuse glomerular and tubular fibrosis, and the nephrotic syndrome may occasionally occur. The spleen is initially considerably enlarged. Recent studies indicate that although the spleen is clinically enlarged it has markedly reduced phagocytic and reticuloendothelial functions, and there is functional hyposplenism. Later, because of repeated episodes of infarction, the spleen becomes small and fibrotic and is rarely palpably enlarged after 5 to 6 years of age. Persons with sickle cell anemia have a markedly increased susceptibility to pneumococcal meningitis and septicemia, like patients after splenectomy, and this is a common cause of death in the first one to two years of life. In later life, a striking susceptibility to salmonella osteomyelitis is present. Although growth may be initially normal, by later childhood most patients are underweight, and puberty is delayed. As a consequence of the varied and severe problems, many die during the first two decades of life.

LABORATORY DATA. Hemoglobin concentrations range from 6 to 8 gm/dl. A peripheral blood smear usually contains sickled cells (Fig. 14–4, *D*). Observation of spontaneous sickling in capillary blood smears almost always indicates classic homozygous sickle cell disease; it is not observed in the trait and is infrequently present in the sickle cell variants. Target cells, poikilocytes and hypochromia are frequently seen. The reticulocyte count ranges from 5 to 15 per cent, and nucleated red cells and Howell-Jolly bodies are often present. The total white blood cell count is elevated to 15,000 to 25,000 per cu mm with a predominance of neutrophils. The platelet count may be increased; the sedimentation rate is slow. Other changes include abnormal liver function test results, hyperbilirubinemia and diffuse hypergammaglobulinemia. The bone marrow is markedly hyperplastic and shows erythroid predominance.

Study of the red cells and hemoglobin is essential to establish the diagnosis. A usually rapid, simple test to determine the presence of Hgb S is the sickle cell preparation, in which red cells are deoxygenated or exposed to reducing agents such as sodium metabisulfite. Virtually 100 per cent of the red cells can be induced to sickle in both sickle disease and sickle trait; but sickling is more rapid and extreme in the disease state than with the trait. A decreased percentage of sickling occurs only after transfusion or during early infancy. Rapid solubility tests are also available for detection of the presence of Hgb S in red cells. Neither sickling nor solubility tests are genetically definitive, both giving false positive and false negative test results. Electrophoretic examination of hemoglobin is necessary for precise diagnosis. After infancy the red cells of patients with sickle cell anemia contain approximately 90 per cent Hgb S, 2 to 10 per cent Hgb F, and a normal amount of Hgb A_2. No Hgb A is present. Each parent has either the sickle cell trait or one of the sickle variants.

DIFFERENTIAL DIAGNOSIS. Sickle cell disease may be associated with a wide variety of clinical signs and symptoms. The presence of painful joints plus the heart murmurs of anemia may suggest acute rheumatic fever or rheumatoid arthritis. Osteomyelitis and leukemia are occasionally difficult to differentiate. Because of the varied signs and symptoms of sickle cell anemia, it is important to perform electrophoretic studies on black patients.

TREATMENT. No therapy is necessary, except during acute episodes. Administration of extra quantities of vitamins and of hematinics is of no proved value although some centers prescribe folic acid supplements. Prolonged iron therapy is contraindicated. There is no pharmacological treatment of the painful crisis which has proved of consistent value, including the use of infusions of urea. Analgesics such as codeine and phenothiazines are usually sufficient for the discomfort and pain. Dehydration and acidosis should be vigorously corrected. Complicating bacterial infections require appropriate antibiotic therapy. Blood transfusions are not necessary for the usual painful crises, but when pain is prolonged or extreme or when there is extensive involvement of lungs or central nervous system, they are of value. Transfusions of packed red cells are given to dilute the patient's red cells with normal ones. When the proportion of Hgb SS red cells can be reduced to less than 40 per cent by transfusions, vaso-occlusive symptoms will generally abate. Partial exchange transfusions have been suggested. Transfusions are essential in sequestration and aplastic episodes. Splenectomy is not indicated unless recurrent sequestration crises have occurred or hypersplenism can be shown to be present.

OTHER HEMOGLOBINOPATHIES

HEMOGLOBIN C ($\alpha_2\beta_2^{6\ \text{lys.}}$). Hemoglobin C, an abnormal hemoglobin with slow electrophoretic mobility, occurs in about 2 per cent of American blacks. In the heterozygous state (Hgb AC) no anemia or disease is present, although increased numbers of target cells are seen in the peripheral blood. In the homozygous person (Hgb CC disease) a moderately severe hemolytic anemia and splenomegaly are observed. The peripheral blood contains a striking number of target cells (Fig. 14–3, *F*).

HEMOGLOBIN D. Hemoglobin D represents several varieties of abnormal hemoglobin with electrophoretic mobilities similar to that of Hgb S, but with different biochemical and physical properties. Sickling does not occur in Hgb D syndromes. Hgb D has normal solubility and a different mobility from Hgb S in electrophoresis at acid pH. The homozygous state (Hgb DD) is characterized by a mild hemolytic anemia with splenomegaly.

HEMOGLOBIN E ($\alpha_2\beta_2{}^{26\ \text{lys.}}$). Hemoglobin E is prevalent in persons from Southeast Asia, particularly Thailand. The clinical and hematologic findings are similar to those associated with Hgb C.

HEMOGLOBIN S-C DISEASE. When the genes for both Hgb S and Hgb C are present in the same person, a moderately severe anemia with splenomegaly results. Although there are vaso-occlusive episodes, they are usually less frequent and milder than those of sickle cell disease. Aseptic necrosis of the femoral head is an occasional complication and severe eye damage also occurs. The hemoglobin concentration averages 9 to 10 gm/dl. Target cells are numerous, but sickled cells are usually not present. Hemoglobin electrophoresis reveals a nearly equal mixture of Hgb S and Hgb C, with slight elevation of Hgb F. Aplastic and sequestration crises are potential threats to life. Hgb S-C disease does not usually affect growth and is compatible with survival into adult life.

UNSTABLE HEMOGLOBINS

Several varieties of abnormal hemoglobin with amino acid substitutions which cause molecular instability lead to chronic hemolytic processes characterized by intraerythrocytic inclusions (Heinz bodies) and usually by excretion of dark brown urine containing dipyrrolic compounds, often especially pronounced after splenectomy. These anemias are transmitted as autosomal dominant states. A number of variants have been described and assigned the names of their city of origin (Hgb Zürich, Köln, Santa Ana, etc.).

Hemolysis usually becomes evident 3 to 6 months after birth. Jaundice and splenomegaly are regularly found. The abnormal hemoglobin accounts for 30 to 40 per cent of the total. It may or may not be detected by electrophoresis. Heating of hemolysate at 50°C for one hour, however, results in a heavy precipitate of the abnormal hemoglobin, whereas normal hemoglobin is not affected. Heinz bodies may be produced by incubation of whole blood for 48 hours prior to supravital staining. They appear in markedly increased numbers following splenectomy. In one of these variants (Hgb Zürich) hemolysis is precipitated by ingestion of sulfonamides. Splenectomy is of uncertain benefit.

Hemoglobins with Altered Oxygen Affinity

Hemoblobin variants may have altered affinities for oxygen. In some variants decreased affinity results in low arterial oxygen saturation and cyanosis (Hgb Kansas). Hemoglobins with increased oxygen affinity are associated with a familial polycythemia transmitted in an autosomal dominant pattern.

The hemoglobin M syndromes are due to dominantly inherited hemoglobin variants which produce methemoglobinemia. The amino acid substitutions are strategically located near the attachments of heme groups, and internal oxidation of heme iron to the trivalent (ferric) form occurs. The Hgb M diseases are characterized by cyanosis and mild polycythemia. With Hgb M variants resulting from β chain substitutions, such as Hgb M Saskatoon, cyanosis is not seen until 4 to 6 months of age, whereas in α chain variants, such as Hgb M Boston, cyanosis is congenital.

THALASSEMIA

The thalassemias are a group of heritable hypochromic anemias of varying degrees of severity. Although the basic natures of these genetic defects have not been defined, their result is an altered quantity or quality of messenger RNA, leading to deficient synthesis of hemoglobin polypeptide chains. Different types of thalassemia with different clinical and biochemical manifestations are associated with defects in each kind of polypeptide chain (α, β, γ, δ). In contrast to the hemoglobinopathies, no basic chemical abnormality of hemoglobin species lies behind the thalassemias; however, alterations in the amounts of Hgb A_2 and Hgb F may be seen, and Hgb H may be found in certain types of alpha-thalassemia (see below).

The most common genetic variety of thalassemia is associated with impaired production of beta chains and called β-thalassemia. The gene is prevalent in ethnic groups from areas around the Mediterranean Sea, especially in Italy, in Greece and on the Mediterranean islands. About 3–5 per cent of Americans of Italian or Greek ancestry carry a gene for β-thalassemia. The prevalence of β-thalassemia in non-Mediterranean peoples is very low, but typical cases have been documented in many racial groups. Like the sickle cell gene, that of thalassemia appears to be associated with increased resistance to malaria, which may account for its prevalence and geographic distribution. Most cases can be clinically classified as thalassemia major or minor, to correspond in general with a heterozygous or homozygous genotype.

Thalassemia Minor

(β-Thalassemia Trait)

Heterozygous β-thalassemia is associated with mild anemia. The hemoglobin concentration averages 2 to 3 gm/dl lower than normal. The red cells are hypochromic and microcytic and manifest poikilocytosis, ovalocytosis and sometimes basophilic stippling (Fig. 14–4, *A*). The mean corpuscular volume (MCV) is consistently low and averages 69 μ^3. Target cells are present, but usually are not prominent and should not be considered specific for thalassemia. Although a mild decrease in red cell survival can be documented, no overt signs of hemolysis are usually present. The serum iron level is normal or elevated. More than 90 per cent of persons with the β-thalassemia trait have diagnostic elevations of Hgb A_2 to 3.4 to 7.0 per cent. About 50 per cent of affected persons have slight elevations of Hgb F, from 2 to 6 per cent. In a small number of otherwise typical cases normal levels of Hgb A_2, with Hgb F levels ranging from 7 to 15 per cent are found (the so-called high fetal or β-δ thalassemia variant).

Thalassemia Major
(Cooley's Anemia)

Homozygous thalassemia usually becomes symptomatic as a severe, progressive hemolytic anemia during the second 6 months of life. Regularly spaced blood transfusions are necessary to prevent profound weakness and cardiac decompensation due to anemia. In response to severe anemia and hemolysis, hypertrophy of erythropoietic tissue occurs in medullary and extramedullary locations. The bones become thin, and pathologic fractures may occur. Massive expansion of the marrow of the face and skull (Figs. 14–6 and 14–7) produces a typical facies. Pallor, hemosiderosis and jaundice combine to produce a greenish brown complexion. The spleen and liver are enlarged because of extramedullary hematopoiesis and hemosiderosis. In older patients the spleen may reach such proportions that it causes mechanical discomfort and secondary hypersplenism. Growth is impaired in older children, and puberty rarely occurs. Diabetes secondary to pancreatic siderosis is frequent. Cardiac complications such as pericarditis and chronic congestive heart failure are frequent terminal events; death usually occurs during the second decade, but a few patients have survived to their thirties.

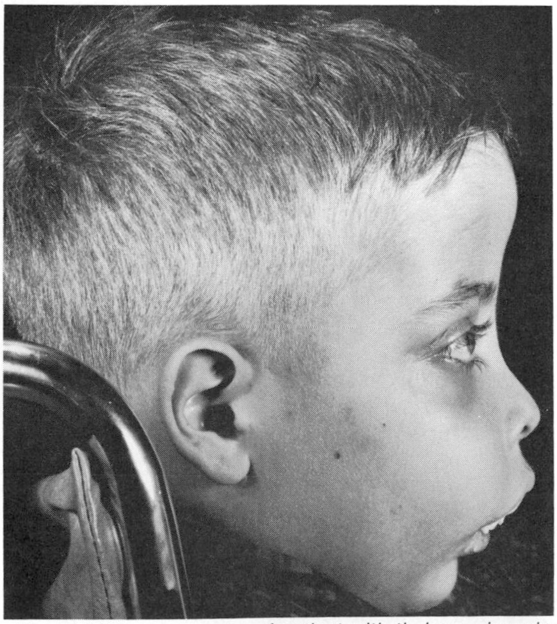

Figure 14–6 *Appearance of patient with thalassemia major (Cooley's anemia). Note the maxillary hyperplasia and resulting dental abnormality.*

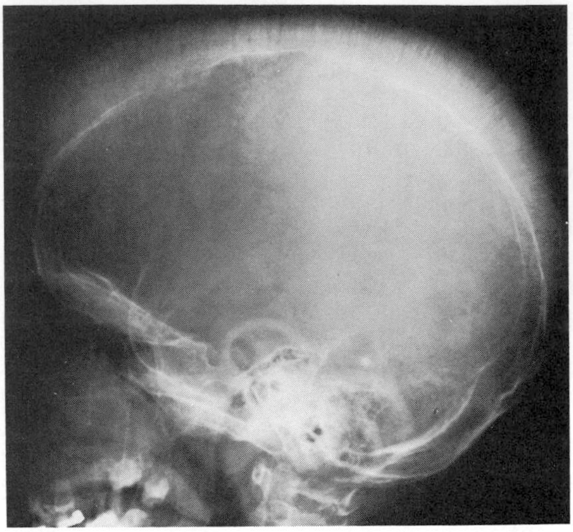

Figure 14–7 *Roentgenogram of skull, showing overgrowth of the maxilla with opacification of the sinuses. The diploic spaces are widened, with prominent vertical trabeculae (hair on end).*

LABORATORY DATA. The red cell changes of thalassemia major are extreme. In addition to severe hypochromia and microcytosis (Fig. 14–4, *B*), many bizarre, fragmented poikilocytes and target cells are present. Large numbers of nucleated red cells circulate, especially after splenectomy. Intraerythrocytic precipitations thought to represent excess alpha chains are also seen after splenectomy. In the usual case the hemoglobin level falls progressively to less than 5 gm/dl unless transfusions are given, but about 10 per cent of patients with homozygous thalassemia can maintain hemoglobin levels of 6 to 8 gm/dl without transfusions. The unconjugated serum bilirubin level is elevated. The concentration of serum iron is high, with saturation of the iron-binding capacity. A striking biochemical characteristic is the presence of large amounts of fetal hemoglobin in the red cells. The level of Hgb F is greater than 50 per cent during the early years of life, but has a tendency to decline with increasing age. Quantitation of fetal hemoglobin is imprecise because of frequent transfusions. Hemoglobin A_2 level is usually less than 3 per cent, but the ratio of Hgb A_2 to Hgb A is markedly increased. Dipyrrolic compounds render the urine dark brown.

TREATMENT. Transfusions are given to maintain the hemoglobin level above 9–10 gm/dl. Keeping the hemoglobin above these levels has striking clinical benefit: it permits normal activity with comfort; it prevents progressive marrow expansion leading to cosmetic problems associated with facial bone changes; and it minimizes cardiac dilatation and osteoporosis. Transfusions of 15 ml/kg of packed cells are usually necessary every 4 to 6 weeks.

Careful crossmatching should be performed to forestall iso-immunization and prevent transfusion reactions. The use of fresh packed red blood cells is desirable. Even with meticulous transfusion techniques, febrile reactions to transfusions are common. These may be minimized with the use of erythrocytes reconstituted from frozen blood.

Hemosiderosis is an inevitable consequence of prolonged transfusion therapy; removal of iron by various chelating agents such as deferoxamine has not been sufficiently effective to warrant routine use in infancy and early childhood. In older patients they may be of benefit, but their use is considered experimental at the present time. Splenectomy is often necessary because of the massive size of the organ or because of secondary hypersplenism, but has no effect on the basic hematologic disease. In a third of patients who have had splenectomy severe, overwhelming sepsis may develop, and for this reason the operation should be performed only for significant indications and should be deferred if possible until after infancy or early childhood.

Other Thalassemic Syndromes

Thalassemia Intermedia

This clinically descriptive term is often assigned to patients with a thalassemia syndrome intermediate in severity between major and minor forms. Jaundice and moderate splenomegaly are present, and the hemoglobin level is 7–8 gm/dl. Transfusions are not regularly necessary.

The genetic make-up of these patients is heterogeneous, for some are apparently homozygous while others are heterozygous for thalassemia genes.

Hemoglobin S-Thalassemia

Combination of a thalassemia gene with that of an abnormal beta-chain hemoglobin results in clinical disease more severe than either trait alone. Hemoglobin S-thalassemia is a moderately severe hemolytic anemia with mild to moderate vaso-occlusive symptoms and significant splenomegaly. The hemoglobin electrophoretic pattern shows a predominance of Hgb S, ranging from 60 to 80 per cent, the remainder being Hgb F and Hgb A. In some instances no Hgb A can be detected, and the electrophoretic pattern is indistinguishable from that of sickle cell disease. In sickle cell anemia, however, the red cells are normocytic, whereas in Hgb S-thalassemia microcytosis with an MCV about 75 μ^3 is present. In addition, in such instances family studies will usually reveal one parent to have thalassemia trait and the other, the sickle cell trait.

Hemoglobin C-Thalassemia and D-Thalassemia

Hemoglobin C-thalassemia and D-thalassemia are mild hemolytic anemias with significant splenomegaly. Hemoglobin electrophoresis reveals that the abnormal hemoglobin, C or D, constitutes more than 60 per cent of the total.

Alpha-Thalassemia

A group of diseases especially prevalent in southeastern Asia and in China resulting from genetically determined blocks in alpha-chain synthesis are called α-thalassemia. There appear to be two distinct types of α-thalassemia, designated α thal-1 and α thal-2. No specific alterations in the proportions of the minor hemoglobins A_2 or F are seen in the heterozygous state. Special techniques may reveal traces of hemoglobin tetramers lacking alpha chains. These are Hgb H (β_4) and Barts (γ_4). In the newborn period, between 5 and 10 per cent of Hgb Barts is found in the blood. It does not persist after 6 months, except occasionally in trace amounts. In the homozygous state, α-thalassemia produces the clinical picture of hydrops fetalis. In these cases the predominant hemoglobin is Hgb Barts, γ_4. This variant has abnormal oxygen dissociation properties which make oxygen unavailable to the tissues under physiologic conditions.

Alpha-thalassemia is also involved in the Hgb H syndromes. These are moderately severe anemias resembling Cooley's anemia. They are characterized, however, by the presence of a fast-moving, unstable hemoglobin component called Hgb H or β_4. The combination of α-thalassemia with genes for beta-chain hemoglobin abnormalities or β-thalassemia results in hematologic diseases which are no more severe than with either trait alone.

Hereditary Persistence of High Fetal Hemoglobin

This interesting condition is associated with very high levels of normal fetal hemoglobin, but with no other abnormalities. It is thought to result from a genetically determined inability to convert from gamma- to beta-chain synthesis at the time of birth. The trait occurs most frequently in blacks, Italians and Greeks. In the heterozygous person the level of Hgb F is 20 to 30 per cent. There is an even distribution of fetal hemoglobin through the red cell population, in contrast to the thalassemias, in which Hgb F content shows variation from cell to cell. Instances of homozygosity for the high fetal gene have been observed. These patients' hemoglobin was completely Hgb F, but no significant anemia or manifestations of hematologic disease were found. When both the high fetal gene and the sickle gene are present in the same person, hematologic manifestations are very mild. The large amount of Hgb F prevents the sickling process.

HEMOLYTIC ANEMIAS DUE TO ABNORMALITIES OF THE RED CELL PRODUCED BY EXTRINSIC FACTORS

A number of agents with capacity to damage red blood cells may lead to their premature destruction. Among the most clearly defined of these are antibodies associated with immune hemolytic anemias. These antibodies, directed against specific intrinsic antigens, so damage the red cell that viability is compromised and rapid destruction ensues. The hallmark of this group of diseases is the positive result of the Coombs test, which detects a coating of immunoglobulin on the red cell surface. The most important immune hemolytic disorder encountered in pediatric practice is hemolytic disease of the newborn (erythroblastosis fetalis), caused by passive transplacental transfer of a maternal antibody active against the red cells of the fetus, which is described elsewhere. (See Section 7.)

AUTOIMMUNE HEMOLYTIC ANEMIAS ASSOCIATED WITH "WARM" ANTIBODIES

In the autoimmune hemolytic anemias abnormal antibodies directed against red cells are produced by the patient himself. The pathogenic mechanism of these disorders is uncertain. One theory postulates the basic cause to be an autonomous proliferation of a forbidden clone of immunologically competent cells which do not have the capacity of recognizing self-antigens. An alternative explanation suggests that drugs or infectious agents in some way alter the red cell membrane so that it becomes "foreign" or antigenic to the host.

Autoimmune hemolytic anemias associated with an underlying disease process such as lymphoma or lupus erythematosus are said to be secondary or symptomatic. In other instances the disease is termed idiopathic because no underlying cause can be found. A number of drugs may act as haptens which combine with proteins of the red cell membrane to form antigenic complexes. Penicillin and certain related drugs and methyldopa are occasionally involved in these drug-induced hemolytic processes. Readministration of the drug may result in a Coombs-positive hemolytic anemia.

CLINICAL MANIFESTATIONS. Anemia may develop acutely, with prostration, pallor, jaundice, and hemoglobinuria. The spleen is usually palpably enlarged, and lymphadenopathy is often present. In secondary cases, manifestations of an underlying disease may be prominent.

LABORATORY DATA. In many cases the anemia is profound, with hemoglobin levels less than 6 gm/dl. Considerable spherocytosis and polychromasia are present on the peripheral smear. More than 50 per cent of the circulating red cells may be reticulocytes, and large numbers of nucleated red cells may be present. Leukocytosis is common. The platelet count is usually normal, but occasionally a concomitant immune thrombocytopenic purpura is present (*Evans syndrome*).

The direct Coombs test result is strongly positive, and free antibody can sometimes be demonstrated in the serum. These antibodies are active at 37° C ("warm" antibodies), and belong to the IgG class. They do not require complement for activity, and may not produce agglutination in vitro. Antibodies from the serum, and those eluted from the red cells, react with many different red cells, including those of the patient. Although they have often been regarded as nonspecific panagglutinins, careful studies have revealed many to have specificity for certain red cell antigens, usually those of the Rh system. A number of such antibodies have had anti-e (hr″) specificity. Since more than 95 per cent of the red cell population have the e antigen, the antibody might be considered a panagglutinin unless careful tests were performed. Sometimes spontaneous agglutination of the patient's own red cells occurs in all testing serums, so that the patient may be mistakenly blood-typed as group AB Rh-positive.

TREATMENT. Transfusions are usually of only transient benefit, but may be necessary because of the severity of the anemia. It may be extremely difficult to find compatible blood; in selecting blood the red cells giving the least positive in vitro reaction by the Coombs technique should be chosen. The mainstays of therapy are the corticosteroids. Prednisone or its equivalent should be administered in a dose of 2.5 mg/kg/day. This should be continued until the evidence of hemolysis disappears, and then the dose is gradually reduced. If relapse occurs, resumption of full dosage may be necessary. The disease tends to remit spontaneously within a few weeks or months. The Coombs test result may remain positive even after hemolysis has subsided. When hemolytic anemia remains severe despite corticosteroid therapy, or if very large doses are necessary to maintain a reasonable hemoglobin level, splenectomy may be beneficial. Immunosuppressive agents have been of some benefit in chronic cases refractory to conventional therapy.

COURSE AND PROGNOSIS. Idiopathic autoimmune hemolytic disease in childhood is usually acute and may be severe, but is self-limited. In infancy the disease may be extremely fulminating, and severe cases have been reported which have been refractory to all treatment, including corticosteroids, immunosuppressive agents, splenectomy and thymectomy. Corticosteroid therapy has permitted most of these patients to be sustained until recovery has occurred; deaths are unusual. In immune hemolytic anemia secondary to lymphoma or lupus erythematosus the status of the basic disease determines the ultimate prognosis.

AUTOIMMUNE HEMOLYTIC ANEMIAS ASSOCIATED WITH COLD ANTIBODIES

Red cell antibodies most active at low temperatures have been called "cold" antibodies. They belong to the IgM class and require complement for activity.

COLD AGGLUTININ DISEASE

Cold antibodies may be present in low levels in normal blood. Following viral infections or mycoplasmal pneumonia, the levels may increase considerably, and occasionally enormous increases may occur, titers of 1/30,000 or greater being recorded. The antibody has specificity for the I antigen and reacts poorly with human cord blood cells possessing the I antigen.

When very high titers of cold antibodies are present, severe episodes of intravascular hemolysis with hemoglobinemia and hemoglobinuria may follow exposure of the patient to low temperatures.

PAROXYSMAL COLD HEMOGLOBINURIA

This form of hemolytic anemia is associated with a specific type of cold antibody, the Donath-Landsteiner hemolysin, which has anti-P specificity. About one-third of cases are associated with either congenital or acquired syphilis.

Treatment consists of transfusions for severe anemia. Chilling of the patient should be avoided.

HEMOLYTIC ANEMIAS OF INTOXICATIONS AND INFECTIONS

In sufficiently large doses, arsenic and phenylhydrazine produce hemolysis in any person.

Hemolytic anemias may complicate a variety of infections. Direct red cell damage by microorganisms or their toxins may be the basis of hemolysis observed in septicemia. Actual parasitism of the red cell occurs in malaria and bartonellosis.

INFANTILE PYKNOCYTOSIS

Infantile pyknocytosis is an acute, self-limited hemolytic anemia occurring during the first 3 months of life. The peripheral blood contains large numbers of characteristically malformed red cells called pyknocytes. These are contracted, densely stained cells with irregular contours and several sharp spinelike projections. A small number of pyknocytes (0.5 to 2.0 per cent) may be present in the blood of normal newborn infants, and premature infants may have as many as 5 per cent. Pyknocytosis must be differentiated from crenation, which is a technical artifact of fixation and staining of blood smears. The cause is uncertain, but the condition does not result from an intrinsic defect; abnormalities of the red cell's environment may be important. Low levels of serum vitamin E have been found in premature infants with a hematologic syndrome resembling infantile pyknocytosis. Some of these infants had G-6-PD deficiency, but this may have been coincidental.

CLINICAL AND LABORATORY DATA. Affected infants frequently become jaundiced during the neonatal period. Pallor and signs of anemia are evident after the second or third week. The spleen and liver are usually enlarged.

The anemia may be severe, with hemoglobin levels as low as 4 to 5 gm/dl, and reticulocytosis is also present. Twenty to 50 per cent of the circulating red cells are pyknocytes. Survival studies reveal that life spans of both transfused red cells and those of the patients are shortened.

TREATMENT. Exchange transfusion may be required in the neonatal period for hyperbilirubinemia. If the anemia becomes severe, transfusions with packed or sedimented red cells may be given. Oral vitamin E (alpha tocopherol) in a dose of 200 mg/day has been of apparent benefit in some cases. Even without therapy the hemolysis abates, and by 4 months or so of age the patients are hematologically normal.

The Red Cells

Harris, J. W., and Kellermeyer, R. W.: The Red Cell. 2nd ed. Cambridge, Harvard University Press, 1970.

Oski, F. A., and Naiman, J. L.: Hematologic Problems in the Newborn. 2nd ed. Philadelphia, W. B. Saunders Company, 1972.

Smith, C. H.: Blood Diseases of Infancy and Childhood. 3rd ed. St. Louis, The C. V. Mosby Co., 1972.

Wintrobe, M. M.: Clinical Hematology. 7th ed. Philadelphia, Lea & Febiger, 1973.

Congenital Pure Red Cell Anemia

Allen, D. M., and Diamond, L. K.: Congenital (erythroid) hypoplastic anemia—Cortisone treated. Am. J. Dis. Child. *102*:416, 1961.

Diamond, L. K., Allen, D. M., and Magill, F. B.: Congenital (erythroid) hypoplastic anemia. Am. J. Dis. Child. *102*:403, 1961.

Anemias of Chronic Infections, Inflammation and Renal Disease

Cartwright, G. E.: The anemia of chronic disorders. Semin. Hematol. *3*:351, 1966.

Physiological Anemia of Infancy

O'Brien, R. T., and Pearson, H. A.: Physiological anemia of infancy. J. Pediatr., *79*:132, 1971.

Megaloblastic Anemias

Dahlke, M. B., and Mertens-Roesler, E.: Malabsorption of folic acid due to diphenylhydantoin. Blood *30*:341, 1967.

Haggard, M. E., and Lockhart, L. H.: Megaloblastic anemia and orotic aciduria. An hereditary disorder of pyrimidine metabolism responsive to uridine. Am. J. Dis. Child. *113*:733, 1967.

Herbert, V.: Megaloblastic Anemias—Mechanism and Management. Chicago, Year Book Medical Publishers, Inc., 1965.

Klipstein, F. A.: Subnormal serum folate and macrocytosis associated with anticonvulsant drug therapy. Blood *23*:68, 1964.

Lampkin, B. C., Shore, N. A., and Chadwick, D.: Megaloblastic

anemia of infancy secondary to maternal pernicious anemia. New Engl. J. Med. *274*:1168, 1966.
Luhby, A. L.: Megaloblastic anemia in infancy. III. Clinical considerations and analysis. J. Pediatr. *54*:617, 1959.
McIntyre, O. R., Sullivan, L. W., Jeffries, G. H., and Silver, R. H.: Pernicious anemia in childhood. New Engl. J. Med. *272*:981, 1965.
Rogers, L. E., Porter, F. S., and Sidbury, J. B.: Thiamine-responsive megaloblastic anemia. J. Pediatr. *74*:544, 1969.

Microcytic Anemia
Committee on Nutrition: Iron balance and requirements in infancy. Pediatrics *43*:134, 1969.
Dallman, P. R., Sunshine, P., and Leonard, Y.: Intestinal cytochrome response with repair of iron deficiency. Pediatrics *39*:863, 1967.
Erlandson, M. E.: Iron metabolism and iron deficiency anemia. Pediat. Clin. N. Amer. *9*:673, 1962.
Horrigan, D. L., and Harris, J. W.: Pyridoxine-responsive anemia: Analysis of 62 cases. Adv. Intern. Med. *12*:103, 1964.
Losowsky, M. S., and Hall, R.: Hereditary sideroblastic anaemia. Brit. J. Haemat. *11*:70, 1965.
Moe, P. J.: Iron requirements in infancy. Longitudinal studies of iron requirements during the first year of life. Acta Paediat. *52* (Suppl. 150):54, 1963.
Naiman, J. L., Oski, F. A., Diamond, L. K., Vawter, G. F., and Shwachman, H.: The gastrointestinal effects of iron deficiency anemia. Pediatrics *33*:83, 1964.
Schulman, I.: Iron requirements in infancy. J.A.M.A. *175*:118, 1961.
Wilson, J. F., Heiner, D. C., and Labey, M. E.: Milk-induced gastrointestinal bleeding in infants with hypochromic microcytic anemia. J.A.M.A. *189*:568, 1964.

Hemolytic Anemias
Dacie, J. V.: The Haemolytic Anemias. 3rd ed. New York, Grune & Stratton, 1970.

Hereditary Spherocytosis
Jacob, H. S.: Hereditary spherocytosis; A disease of the red cell membrane. Semin. Hematol. *2*.139, 1965.
Krueger, H. C., and Burgert, E. O.: Hereditary spherocytosis in 100 children. Mayo Clin. Proc. *41*:821, 1966.
Trucco, J. T., and Brown, A. K.: Neonatal manifestations of hereditary spherocytosis. Am. J. Dis. Child. *113*:263, 1967.

Hereditary Elliptocytosis
Austin, R. F., and Desforges, J. F.: Hereditary elliptocytosis: An unusual presentation of hemolysis in the newborn associated with transient morphologic abnormalities. Pediatrics *44*:196, 1969.
Jensson, O., Jonasson, T., and Olafsson, O.: Hereditary elliptocytosis in Iceland. Brit. J. Haemat. *13*:884, 1967.
Pearson, H. A.: The genetic basis of hereditary elliptocytosis with hemolysis. Blood *32*:972, 1968.

Paroxysmal Nocturnal Hemoglobinuria
Miller, D. R., Baehner, R. L., and Diamond, L. K.: Paroxysmal nocturnal hemoglobinuria in childhood and adolescence. Pediatrics *39*:675, 1967.

Hereditary Stomatocytosis
Zarkowsky, H. S., Oski, F. A., Sha'Afti, R., Shohet, S. B., and Nathan, D. G.: Congenital hemolytic anemia with high sodium, low potassium red cell. New Engl. J. Med. *278*:573, 1968.

Enzymatic Defects of the Red Cell
Beutler, E.: Glucose 6-phosphate dehydrogenase deficiency and nonspherocytic congenital hemolytic anemia. Semin. Hematol. *2*:91, 1965.
Jaffe, E. R.: Hereditary hemolytic disorders and enzymatic deficiencies of human erythrocytes. Blood *35*:116, 1970.

Autoimmune Hemolytic Anemia
Hitzig, W. H., and Massino, L.: Treatment of autoimmune hemolytic anemia in children with azathioprine (Imuran). Blood *28*:840, 1966.
O'Connor, W. J., Vakiener, J. M., and Watson, R. J.: Idiopathic acquired hemolytic anemia in young children. Pediatrics *17*:732, 1956.
Oski, F. A., and Abelson, N. M.: Autoimmune hemolytic anemia in an infant. J. Pediatr. *67*:752, 1965.
Zuelzer, W. W., Mastrangelo, R., Shulberg, C. S., Paulik, M. D., Page, R. H., and Thompson, R. I.: I Autoimmune hemolytic anemia natural history and viral-immunologic interactions in childhood. Am. J. Med. *49*:80, 1970.

Hemoglobinopathies
Diggs, L. W.: Sickle cell crises. Am. J. Clin. Path. *44*:1, 1965.
Nechles, T. F., Allen, D. M., and Finkel, H. E.: Clinical Disorders of Hemoglobin Structure and Synthesis. New York, Appleton-Century Crofts, Inc., 1969.
Pearson, H. A., Spencer, R. P., and Cornelius, E.: Functional asplenia in sickle cell anemia. New Engl. J. Med. *281*:923, 1969.
Pearson, H. A., and Diamond, L. K.: Sickle cell disease. Pediatrics *48*:629, 1971.
Pearson, H. A., and O'Brien, R. T.: Sickle cell testing programs. J. Pediatr. *81*:6, 1972.
Porter, F. S., and Thurman, W. G.: Studies of sickle cell disease: Diagnosis in infancy. Am. J. Dis. Child. *106*:35, 1963.
Scott, R. B.: Sickle cell anemia. Pediat. Clin. N. Amer. *9*:649, 1962.

Thalassemia
Fink, H. (ed.): Problems of Cooley's anemia. Ann. New York Acad. Sci. *165*:1, 1969; *119*:369, 1964.
Weatherall, D.: The Thalassemia Syndromes. 2nd ed. London, Blackwell Scientific Publications, Ltd., 1972.

Infantile Pyknocytosis
Oski, F. A., and Barness, L. A.: Vitamin E deficiency: A previously unrecognized cause of hemolytic anemia in the premature infant. J. Pediatr. *70*:211, 1967.
Tuffy, P., Brown, A. K., and Zuelzer, W. W.: Infantile pyknocytosis. Am. J. Dis. Child. *98*:227, 1959.

POLYCYTHEMIA

(Erythrocytosis)

Polycythemia may be diagnosed when the red cell count, the hemoglobin and hematocrit levels, and the total red cell volume significantly exceed the upper limits of normal. In the older child the levels of hemoglobin and hematocrit which can be considered to represent polycythemia are 16 gm/dl and 55 per cent, respectively, corresponding to a total red cell mass exceeding 35 ml/kg. A decrease in plasma volume, such as occurs in acute dehydration and burns, may result in disproportionately high levels of hemoglobin and hematocrit. In these situations, more accurately designated hemoconcentration rather than relative polycythemia, the actual red cell volume is not increased. Expansion of the plasma volume or rehydration restores the hematocrit to normal levels.

Measurement of the red cell volume by radioisotopic techniques is essential in the differential diagnosis of polycythemia. True polycythemia is characterized by increases of both the red cell and total blood volumes.

SECONDARY POLYCYTHEMIA

Polycythemia may be present in any clinical situation associated with arterial oxygen desaturation. Hypoxia of the kidney results in increased production of erythropoietin. This in turn stimulates increased production of red cells which ultimately results in greatly expanded red cell mass. Cardiovascular defects involving right-to-left shunts and pulmonary diseases interfering with proper oxygenation are the most common causes of secondary polycythemia. Examples of such conditions are cyanotic congenital heart disease, cystic fibrosis, asthma, emphysema and bronchiectasis. Clinical findings usually include cyanosis, hyperemia of sclerae and mucous membranes and clubbing of the fingers. The red blood cell count and hemoglobin and hematocrit values are all increased. Thrombocytopenia may occur. The oxygen saturation of arterial blood is decreased. Living at high altitudes also causes a secondary polycythemia.

More subtle forms of hypoxia may also cause polycythemia. Congenital methemoglobinemia due to a deficiency of NADH-reactive diaphorase may cause familial cyanosis and polycythemia. This condition is transmitted as an autosomal recessive. Dominantly transmitted cyanosis and polycythemia may be associated with the hemoglobins which have altered oxygen affinity (see above). Transient benign polycythemia is said to occur in otherwise healthy adolescents; this syndrome has not been studied sufficiently to determine its frequency or cause.

Polycythemia has also been reported in association with renal tumors and cysts and with vascular tumors of the cerebellum. Excessive red cell production occurs because these tumors secrete erythropoietin.

When the hematocrit exceeds 65 to 70 per cent, periodic phlebotomies may be done, blood being replaced with plasma or saline solution.

POLYCYTHEMIA RUBRA VERA
(Erythremia)

This severe disorder is characterized by polycythemia, leukocytosis, thrombocytosis, and hyperplasia of the bone marrow. Only a few children thought to have this syndrome have been described. Most of these were not studied with modern diagnostic tests; it is uncertain, therefore, whether this disease occurs in childhood.

PLETHORA OF THE NEWBORN

High levels of hemoglobin and hematocrit are characteristic of the newborn infant. The range of normal hemoglobin at birth is 14.7–21 gm/dl, and the hematocrit 45 to 65 per cent. The blood volume of normal term newborns is 70 to 100 ml/kg, and the red cell volume, 40 to 60 ml/kg. Occasionally the blood values of newborn infants significantly exceed these ranges. Some of these plethoric infants have convulsions, respiratory distress, tachycardia, congestive heart failure and hyperbilirubinemia. Hypoglycemia and hypocalcemia may contribute to morbidity of this syndrome. Monozygotic twins with placental vascular anastomosis may have unequal distribution of the circulation, so that one twin is born with anemia and hypovolemia, while the other twin is plethoric. On rare occasions maternofetal transfusion and congenital adrenal hyperplasia may be associated with neonatal polycythemia. Neonatal polycythemia has also been reported to occur with increased frequency in the Down and Beckwith syndromes, and recent reports associate neonatal polycythemia with intrauterine growth retardation in small for gestational age newborns. In most instances no cause can be discovered. When these infants have symptomatic difficulties, phlebotomy in increments of 10 to 15 ml/kg replaced with an equal volume of plasma or normal saline may be indicated to reduce red cell mass and hyperviscosity.

THE PANCYTOPENIAS

Aplasia of bone marrow, or replacement of its hematopoietic elements by other tissue, results in profound depression of all the formed elements of the blood. The clinical manifestations which result are anemia, thrombocytopenic hemorrhage and decreased resistance to infection because of neutropenia. The pancytopenias have traditionally been classified with the anemias, but the consequences of the thrombocytopenia and the neutropenia are much more striking and serious than the anemia. The pancytopenias may be constitutional, often due to ill defined genetic factors, may be acquired as a result of damage to the marrow by a variety of chemical or other agents, or may result from invasion by abnormal tissue. In these conditions underproduction of blood cells is due to hypocellularity or replacement of marrow. Examination of an adequate sample of marrow is essential to diagnosis.

CONSTITUTIONAL APLASTIC PANCYTOPENIA

(Fanconi Syndrome)

The constitutional aplastic anemias are familial disorders inherited on an autosomal recessive basis. About half of affected children have evident congenital anomalies; especially common are microcephaly, microphthalmia and absence of the radii and thumbs (Fig. 14–8); abnormalities of heart and kidney are also relatively common. Some affected children have no serious anatomic defects, but are short in stature and have a peculiar dark pigmentation of the skin and café-au-lait spots, as do most of those with structural anomalies.

Pancytopenia is not usually present at birth or during early infancy. Bruising, the first indication of hematologic disease, is usually observed by 3 to 12 years of age. The consequences of a progressively severe anemia and leukopenia are noted shortly thereafter.

LABORATORY DATA. Severe pancytopenia is evident in peripheral blood. The bone marrow is strikingly hypocellular, with depression of all the cell types and an increase in fatty tissue. Reticulum, plasma and mast cells are prominent. A surgical or needle biopsy of the bone marrow is useful as an adjunct to aspiration, for it provides a large specimen in which to judge cellularity. Analysis of the hemoglobin reveals an increase in the percentage of Hgb F of 5 to 15 per cent. This abnormality may antedate development of marrow aplasia and pancytopenia. Chromosomal studies reveal an abnormally high percentage of chromatid breaks and unusual chromosomal alignments; these also precede frank pancytopenia. The same changes are seen in tissue fibroblast cultures, and offer the possibility of prenatal diagnosis by amniocentesis.

TREATMENT. In addition to symptomatic treatment with blood transfusions and antibiotics, therapy with androgenic steroids is beneficial. Testosterone propionate is given as sublingual tablets in a dose of 1 to 2 mg/kg day to a maximum of 60 mg/day. Alternatively, 400 to 600 mg may be given as an intramuscular injection every 4 weeks. Synthetic androgen derivatives such as oxymetholone and stanozolol are also effective. Relatively small doses of corticosteroids, such as 5 to 10 mg of prednisone or equivalent, are also given. In a majority of instances a hematologic response becomes evident within 2 to 4 months. The marrow develops greater cellularity, and the hemoglobin rises to normal levels. The response of the neutrophils is usually less complete, and platelets may show only a moderate increase in numbers. When the hemoglobin has reached normal levels, it is often possible to reduce the dose of androgen. But if the drug is too rapidly or drastically decreased, relapse occurs. These effective doses of androgen regularly produce signs and symptoms of masculinization, including acne, hirsutism, deepening of the voice, and enlargement of the penis or clitoris. Synthetic androgen derivatives have fewer of these side effects, but some degree of masculinization is probably inevitable. In addition, some of the testosterone preparations have hepatic toxicity. Prior to the advent of testosterone therapy these patients usually died during late childhood of hemorrhage, infection or the complications of multiple transfusions. Experience with androgen therapy is still too recent to know what the ultimate prognosis may now be. Hemorrhagic cysts of the liver (peliosis hepatis) and malignant hepatomas occur with increased frequency in patients receiving prolonged treatment with large doses of androgens. An increased incidence of leukemia has been reported in children with this disease, and in their close relatives.

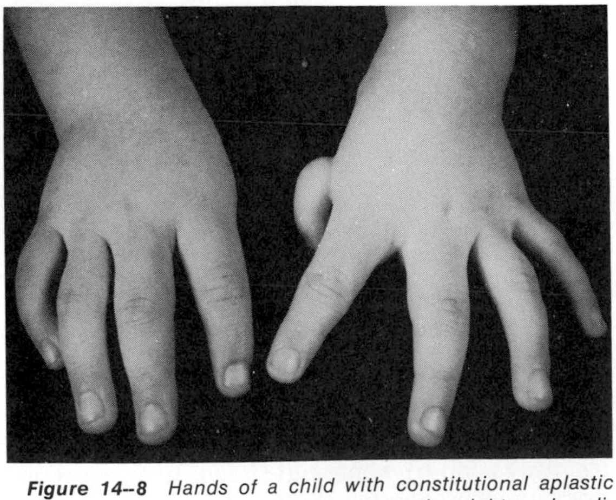

Figure 14–8 Hands of a child with constitutional aplastic pancytopenia. The thumb is absent on the right and rudimentary on the left.

ACQUIRED APLASTIC PANCYTOPENIAS

A number of physical, chemical and infectious agents may severely damage the bone marrow and lead to severe pancytopenia. Some of these agents have the capacity to produce marrow aplasia in any person who is exposed to them in a sufficient dose. Such obligate marrow depressants include ionizing radiation; chemotherapeutic drugs such as nitrogen mustard, 6-mercaptopurine and methotrexate; and certain organic solvents, especially benzene. A second group of agents produce aplastic pancytopenia only in a small, often a remarkably small, number of persons exposed to them. In these latter persons the adverse hematologic reactions must reflect idiosyncrasies. The drug most frequently associated with aplastic pancytopenia is chloramphenicol. It has been estimated that only 1 in 24,000 to 60,000 patients taking chloramphenicol suffers marrow aplasia; nevertheless, the drug is involved in more than half of the drug-related aplastic pancytopenias. Other drugs associated with an appreciable incidence of marrow aplasia are sulfonamides, phenylbutazone and certain anticonvulsants. Severe infections may also produce severe marrow damage, but it is often difficult to decide whether the infection represents cause or effect. A number of cases of marrow aplasia have been described following infectious hepatitis. In about half of cases of aplastic pancytopenia no history of exposure to toxins or other agents can be elicited. These cases are usually designated as idiopathic, although the possibility of an environmental factor or toxin cannot be excluded with certainty.

CLINICAL AND LABORATORY DATA. Hemorrhage secondary to thrombocytopenia is usually the first clinical manifestation. The signs and symptoms of anemia and neutropenia become apparent subsequently. The spleen and lymph nodes are not enlarged. Profound depression of red cells, platelets and neutrophils is present. The level of fetal hemoglobin may be increased. The marrow aspirate is scanty; the particles are fatty, and lymphocytes, plasma cells and reticulum cells predominate. Levels of Hgb F may be elevated above 2 per cent, but reports that this provided prognostic information have not been confirmed.

TREATMENT. The patient must immediately be removed from contact with any potentially toxic drugs or agents. When the onset of the disease is acute, with massive hemorrhage and serious sepsis, aggressive therapy with platelet concentrates and antibiotics is necessary; choice of antibiotic should be based upon bacterial culture and sensitivity tests. In any fully developed case, therapy with testosterone and corticosteroids should be given, as described for constitutional pancytopenia. Because response to these medications may not be evident for 2 to 4 months, an early start is advisable. Recent reviews are far less optimistic about the value of androgens in cases of acquired aplastic pancytopenia. Other forms of therapy are not of regular value. Hematinics are worthless, and splenectomy is hazardous. The value of bone marrow transplantation in aplastic anemia is being actively investigated at the present time. Successful marrow grafts have been obtained between identical twins. Tissue typing has also permitted successful engraftment of aplastic anemia patients with bone marrow from HL-A compatible siblings. Minor incompatibilities necessitate concomitant immunosuppressive therapy. Because of the gravity of this disease, tissue typing of the patients and all available siblings should be performed soon after the diagnosis is established, and consultation should be established with centers where bone marrow transplantation programs are operative.

COURSE. Approximately a third of patients die very quickly as a result of uncontrollable hemorrhage and infection. Pseudomonas and staphylococcal septicemias are frequent causes of death. The remaining two thirds of children have a subacute clinical course. In some of these patients androgen therapy often has a beneficial effect. Half of this group ultimately recover completely; the other half have a chronic course, many succumbing to sepsis and hemorrhage months or years after onset. Leukemia and paroxysmal nocturnal hemoglobinuria have developed in some children after recovery from aplastic anemia.

PANCYTOPENIA DUE TO MARROW REPLACEMENT

Diffuse replacement of marrow space by nonhematopoietic tissue results in peripheral pancytopenia. *Neuroblastoma* is the childhood tumor which most frequently metastasizes to the bone marrow. *Osteopetrosis,* or marble bone disease, is frequently associated with anemia and thrombocytopenia, owing to marrow obliteration; an element of hypersplenism may also be present. *Acute leukemia* occasionally presents with pancytopenia and a reticular appearance of the initially aspirated marrow. Adequate sampling or biopsy of the marrow from other sites will usually provide the proper diagnosis.

Myelofibrosis has occurred in a few infants and children, presenting as severe anemia with abnormal forms (tear drops, ovalocytia) and nucleated red cells, and with liver and spleen enlarged owing to extramedullary erythropoiesis.

TRANSFUSIONS*

The most important indications for transfusions are to restore blood volume and treat shock following acute blood loss and to provide red cells for maintenance of the blood hemoglobin level. An individual component of blood, such as red cells, platelets, plasma or specific plasma proteins, may often be used effectively in place of whole blood.

*See Section 7 for Exchange Transfusion.

INDICATIONS FOR TRANSFUSION

ACUTE HEMORRHAGE

The signs and symptoms accompanying hemorrhage vary with the magnitude and rapidity of the blood loss. When 15 to 20 per cent or more of the circulating blood volume is acutely lost, tachycardia, hypotension and shock may develop, accompanied by weakness, restlessness and syncope. Immediately after acute hemorrhage the hemoglobin or hematocrit level may be deceptively high, but hemodilution soon reduces this to a value reflecting the magnitude of the blood loss. Thrombocytosis and neutrophilia occur within a few hours and reticulocytosis within a few days of an acute bleeding episode. The most common causes of severe acute hemorrhage are trauma and gastrointestinal bleeding from peptic ulcers, Meckel's diverticulum and esophageal varices. In patients with defects of the hemostatic mechanism, exsanguinating hemorrhage may occur from nosebleeds or gastritis.

Severe bleeding in the perinatal period may result in the clinical picture of asphyxia pallida. Pallor, shock, tachycardia and low venous pressures are seen. External hemorrhage may occur from the umbilicus or the gastrointestinal tract. The fetus may bleed before and during birth into the maternal circulation, and fetofetal transfusions between identical twins are not infrequent.

LABORATORY DATA. The anemia of acute blood loss is usually normochromic and normocytic. Depending upon the duration of the hemorrhage and timing of the tests, compensatory reticulocytosis and normoblastemia may be seen. In the newborn infant with hemorrhage, the Coombs test result is generally negative and the level of serum bilirubin low. With loss of blood from fetus to mother, maternal blood will contain cells with Hgb F (Kleihauer technique).

TREATMENT. When possible, local measures to control the hemorrhage should be taken. Whole blood transfusions should be given to restore blood volume and treat shock; 20 ml/kg of blood should be administered initially. The need for additional blood will be guided by the clinical response and by physical and laboratory findings. Plasma or plasma expanders may be used to sustain the patient in shock until blood can be made available, but if the blood loss has been great, red cell replacement will be necessary.

CHRONIC ANEMIAS

In anemias which develop slowly and which stabilize at a level of 6 to 9 gm/dl, remarkably few symptoms may be experienced by the patient. Transfusions are usually not routinely indicated in management. When such anemias result from deficiency of a specific factor such as folic acid or iron, a rapid response will follow replacement therapy. Transfusion is indicated only if the anemia is profound or if infections or other complications are present. No hard and fast rule can be made about the hemoglobin level at which transfusion is recommended. Some children with iron deficiency anemia may have hemoglobin levels of 4 to 5 gm/dl with few signs of clinical or cardiorespiratory distress. A reasonable estimate of the effect of transfusion of packed red cells is given by the following formula:

Increase in Hct =
ml/kg of packed cells transfused.

That is, if 5 ml/kg of packed cells are given, the recipient's hematocrit will rise about 5 per cent. The formula assumes a recipient blood volume of about 75 ml/kg and a hematocrit of about 75 per cent in packed red cells.

In progressive refractory anemias such as thalassemia major and pure red cell anemias, transfusions are necessary to sustain life. Packed or sedimented red cells are preferred for the correction of such chronic anemias. The maximum dose of packed red cells to be given in one transfusion is 15 ml/kg; if signs of congestive heart failure are present, considerably smaller amounts should be used. In extreme anemia with secondary heart failure, multiple small transfusions of 2 to 4 ml/kg of packed red cells may be helpful, or even exchange transfusion. Digitalis and oxygen are of limited value.

PLATELET TRANSFUSIONS

Platelets may be transfused to attain temporary hemostasis in some patients with thrombocytopenic hemorrhage. Although administration of fresh whole blood produces inconsequential rises in the recipient's platelet count, clinical hemorrhage may be controlled. Use of platelet-rich plasma or platelet concentrates prepared from fresh blood drawn in plastic equipment permits attainment of more nearly normal platelet counts. Platelet transfusions are temporarily beneficial in thrombocytopenias due to inadequate production such as hypoplastic pancytopenia and leukemia, but are useless or of only transient value in states characterized by peripheral hyperdestruction of platelets such as idiopathic thrombocytopenic purpura. In addition, isoantibodies to platelet antigens are frequently formed after transfusions of platelets from multiple donors. With successive platelet transfusions, decreasing response is noted.

WHITE BLOOD CELLS

Because of the brief intravascular life span and low concentration of leukocytes in normal blood, transfusions of normal blood have no practical value for the supply of white blood cells. Transient clinical and hematologic benefit in neutropenias has been reported from use of donor blood from patients with chronic granulocytic leukemia who have very high total white blood cell counts. Equipment permitting extraction of large numbers of polymorphonuclear leukocytes from normal donors by continuous plasmapheresis has been reported to be of value in selected cases.

PLASMA AND PLASMA CONCENTRATES

In acute dehydration when the plasma volume is decreased, but the red cell mass is adequate, plasma can be used effectively to expand the blood volume, and to restore circulation and renal blood flow. The usual dose of plasma is 10 ml/kg. The use of fresh plasma and of concentrates of plasma such as factor VIII and fibrinogen preparations for bleeding disorders is described elsewhere. The usual gamma globulin preparations cannot be administered intravenously because they form large reactive aggregates which may produce hypotension and shock.

SPECIAL CONSIDERATIONS

CHOICE OF BLOOD FOR TRANSFUSION

Storage of blood at 4°C results in a decrease in red cell viability which is proportional to the length of storage time. When blood is given for acute hemorrhage, this is of no consequence, but in children who must receive transfusions repeatedly the blood selected should be as fresh as possible.

A citrate-phosphate-dextrose (CPD) mixture has supplanted ACD as the standard anticoagulant, owing to its better maintenance of red cell viability.

Blood for transfusion should be of the same blood group (O, A, B or AB) as the recipient's. The donor red cells should always be tested for compatibility with the recipient's plasma (major crossmatch) by the Coombs technique. Compatibility for the Rh antigens between donor and recipient is desirable. Rh-negative (d/d) persons should never receive Rh-positive blood; the reverse is permissible. Though considerable battlefield experience indicates that the use of so-called universal donor blood (group O Rh-negative blood with a low titer of anti-A and anti-B isohemagglutinins) is safe, with adequate modern blood banking facilities this is rarely necessary except in an emergency.

RISKS OF BLOOD TRANSFUSION

Although modern technology has made blood transfusion a generally safe procedure, a definite risk is involved. Transfusions should be given, therefore, only when the benefit to the patient exceeds the inherent danger of the procedure. It has been estimated that of every 2000 persons receiving a blood transfusion, one dies as a result of the immediate procedure or its consequences. Problems may arise from:

CLERICAL ERRORS. The mislabeling or faulty identification of containers may lead to a patient's receiving the wrong blood. If a type O patient receives type A or B blood, fatal intravascular hemolysis may occur.

RED CELL ISO-IMMUNIZATION. In almost every blood transfusion the donor red cells have some antigenic factor which the recipient does not possess. Many such factors are poor antigens, but some evoke intense antibody formation, the immunized person being at increased risk if another transfusion is given.

HEPATITIS. A small proportion of the normal population are asymptomatic carriers of the agent for homologous serum hepatitis. Even with modern techniques only about one third of donors who can transmit homologous serum hepatitis have demonstrable hepatitis-associated antigen (HAA, Australia antigen) in their blood. There is no way to detect carriers with certainty, nor to inactivate the agent in blood, the risk in pooled plasma being proportional to the number of donors to the pool. Syphilis and malaria can also be transmitted by blood transfusion.

WHITE CELL, PLATELET AND PLASMA PROTEIN IMMUNIZATION. White cells, platelets and some of the serum proteins have polymorphic antigens; multiple transfusions may be associated with development of antibodies against these components.

CIRCULATORY OVERLOAD. Patients with chronic anemia have expanded plasma volume and increased cardiac output; infusion of blood or plasma may precipitate congestive heart failure; rapid administration of large volumes of blood should be avoided.

DEPLETION OF LABILE SUBSTANCES. Storage of blood is associated with loss of platelets and decreasing activities of the labile coagulation factors, such as factor VIII. When massive or exchange transfusions of stored blood are given, a complex disturbance of hemostasis may ensue. Use of fresh blood will avoid these complications. As a general rule, when multiple transfusions are given in a short period of time, every fourth unit of blood should be fresh. Acute citrate toxicity may also occur.

IRON OVERLOAD. Each 500 ml of blood contains about 250 mg of iron. Patients with refractory anemias who require frequent transfusion ultimately have hemosiderosis. Iron is deposited in skin, liver, spleen and other organs, and may interfere with normal function.

REACTIONS TO BLOOD TRANSFUSION

ALLERGIC REACTIONS. These occur in association with 1 to 2 per cent of transfusions. The most common clinical manifestation is urticaria; occasionally wheezing and arthralgia occur. The mechanism of these reactions is not certain, but they may be due to allergenic substances or to antibodies in the donor plasma. The development of urticaria alone does not necessitate discontinuing the transfusion; therapy with antihistamines or corticosteroids is effective in treating or preventing this type of reaction.

FEBRILE REACTIONS. The use of disposable plastic equipment has eliminated most external pyrogenic substances. Sensitization to white cell antigens may produce febrile reactions to transfusions. The use of packed cells, excluding the buffy coat, and liberal use of salicylates may modify these reactions. Use of reconstituted frozen red cells may greatly ameliorate severe febrile reactions. Rarely a unit of blood may be contaminated with bacteria. Severe febrile reactions, shock and death may occur if infected blood is transfused.

HEMOLYTIC TRANSFUSION REACTIONS. Hemolytic reactions result in massive intravascular destruction of red cells, manifest clinically by fever, chills, headache and back pain. These symptoms do not appear when the patient is anesthetized. In severe reactions, shock and acute renal failure may ensue. Hemoglobinemia and hemoglobinuria are usually observed. When a hemolytic reaction is suspected, the transfusion should be *terminated immediately.* Diagnosis is proved by re-examining the blood types of donor cells and the recipient, repeating the crossmatch, and examining plasma and urine for free hemoglobin. A diuresis should be established by fluid therapy and administration of mannitol. Immediate heparinization to combat intravascular coagulation should be considered. The patient generally survives the initial acute episode; if he can be sustained through a period of renal failure, recovery is the rule.

Polycythemia
Michael, A. F., Jr., and Mauer, A. M.: Maternal-fetal transfusion as a cause of plethora in the neonatal period. Pediatrics *28*:458, 1961.
Naeye, R.: Human intrauterine parabiotic syndrome and its complications. New Engl. J. Med. *268*:804, 1963.
Usher, R., Shepard, M., and Lind, J.: The blood volume of the newborn infant and placental transfusion. Acta. Paediat. Scand. *52*:497, 1963; *54*:419, 1965.
Weinberger, M. M., and Oleinick, A.: Congenital marrow dysfunction in Down's syndrome. J. Pediat. *77*:273, 1970.

The Pancytopenias
Bloom, G. E., Warner, S., Gerald, P. S., and Diamond, L. K.: Chromosome abnormalities in constitutional aplastic anemia. New Engl. J. Med. *274*:8, 1966.
Huguley, C. M., Jr., Lea, J. W., and Butts, J. A.: Adverse hematologic reactions to drugs. *In* Brown, E. B., and Moore, C. V. (eds.): Progress in Hematology. Vol. V, p. 105. New York, Grune & Stratton, Inc., 1966.
Li, F. P., Alter, B. P., and Nathan, D. G.: The mortality of acquired aplastic anemia in children. Blood *40*:153, 1972.
Schwartz, E., Bachner, R. L., and Diamond, L. K.: Aplastic anemia following hepatitis. Pediatrics *37*:681, 1966.
Shahidi, N. T., and Diamond, L. K.: Testosterone-induced remission in aplastic anemia of both acquired and congenital types. New Engl. J. Med. *264*:953, 1961.
Shahidi, N. T., Gerald, P. S., and Diamond, L. K.: Alkali-resistant hemoglobin in aplastic anemia of both acquired and congenital types. New Engl. J. Med. *266*:117, 1962.
Thomas, E. D., Buckner, C. D., Storb, R., Neiman, P. E., Fefer, A., Clift, R. A., Slichter, S. J., Funk, D. D., Bryant, J. I., and Lerner, K. E.: Aplastic anaemia treated by marrow transplantation. Lancet *1*:284, 1972.

Transfusions
Bucholz, D. M.: Pediatric transfusion therapy. J. Pediatr., *84*:1, 1974.
Chown, B.: The fetus can bleed. Am. J. Obstet. Gynec. *70*:1298, 1955.
Purugganan, H. B., and Naiman, J. L.: Exchange transfusion in severe iron deficiency anemia prior to emergency surgery. J. Pediatr. *69*:804, 1966.

DISORDERS OF THE LEUKOCYTES

The leukocytes of the blood and their precursors in the bone marrow are easily studied, enumerated and classified. The most important leukocyte functions are concerned with resistance to infection and disposal of products of cellular breakdown. Because characteristic changes occur in many diseases, the white blood cell and differential counts are important as general screening tests. Normal values are listed in Table 14-3.

The leukocytes are divided into two major classes: the granulocytes, consisting of neutrophils, eosinophils and basophils; and the nongranulated lymphocytes and monocytes. White cells have cellular antigens different from those of the erythrocyte.

TYPES OF LEUKOCYTES

NEUTROPHILS. Neutrophils are the predominating type of granulocyte. The nuclei of these cells have 1 to 5 segments, which accounts for their designation as polymorphonuclear leukocytes. They have ameboid motility, chemotaxis and the capacity for active phagocytosis. Their fine cytoplasmic granules have a light purple (neutrophilic) color when stained with Wright's stain. These granules are lysosomes and contain digestive enzymes of several sorts, including proteases, cathepsins and lysozymes. When bacteria or other particles are ingested by neutrophils, degranulation occurs as the enzymes of the granules are discharged into a vacuole formed about the ingested material. The phagocytic process is associated with a burst of metabolic activity and a considerable increase in oxygen consumption. The metabolic burst is associated with hydrogen peroxide formation and a marked increase in activity of the pentose phosphate pathway of glucose metabolism. Aberrations of the biochemistry of phagocytosis and intracellular digestion may result in markedly impaired resistance to disease.

The neutrophils occupy definable compartments or pools within the body. The *mitotic compartment* consists of myeloblasts, promyelocytes and myelocytes of the bone marrow. The *maturation compartment* consists of metamyelocytes and band forms, which are relatively completely differentiated and have lost the capacity to divide, but still reside within the marrow. The *marrow storage compartment* consists of a rapidly mobilizable reserve of mature neutrophils. It has been estimated that it takes 6 to 11 days for a cell to pass through the stages of differentiation from a myeloblast to a mature neutrophil emerging into the peripheral blood.

The neutrophils of the peripheral blood exist in two exchangeable pools of approximately equal size. The *circulating granulocytic compartment* is in equilibrium with a *marginal compartment* consisting of neutrophils sequestered in small blood vessels. Vigorous exercise or injection of epinephrine causes the marginal pool to be mobilized into the circulation. The half-time of granulocytes within the circulation is 6 to 9 hours, after which they enter the *tissue pool*, where they carry out their primary function of phagocytosis. Little is known of their survival in the tissues.

Techniques are available for studying the various neutrophil compartments. The intramedullary mitotic and maturation compartments are generally estimated by examining bone marrow tissue. Hypertrophy of the neutrophilic series is reflected in alterations of the ratio between myeloid and erythroid elements (M/E, or myeloid-erythroid, ratio). The usual M/E ratio of between 2 and 4 to 1 may be markedly increased to between 5 and 10 to 1 in the presence of chronic inflammatory processes. Adequacy of the marrow storage compartment can be estimated from changes in the peripheral leukocyte count after intravenous injection of extracts of bacterial endotoxin or the steroid compound etiocholanolone. Normally a twofold to fourfold increase in the numbers of circulating neutrophils results from such stimulated release of cells from the marrow storage compartment. In states of marrow hypoplasia or failure, no increase occurs. Radioisotopic techniques have been devised for estimating the time required for maturation and release of neutrophils from the marrow, as well as rate of turnover of neutrophils in the blood.

EOSINOPHILS. The eosinophils are characterized by large coarse granules of a prominent red color with Romanowsky stains and by a nucleus with 1 or 2 segments. They normally account for less than 5 per cent of the circulating leukocytes. Eosinophil counts are depressed by high levels of adrenocortical hormones and increased in parasitic and allergic disorders. Eosinophilia may also accompany Hodgkin's disease. A mild increase in eosinophils may be seen in the convalescent period of viral infections. The most pronounced eosinophilia encountered in this country accompanies such diseases as visceral larva migrans and trichinosis, in which actual invasion of the tissue by parasitic helminths occurs. Familial, and presumptively genetic, eosinophilia has been described.

BASOPHILS. These leukocytes are distinguished by coarse, deep blue granules which fill the cytoplasm and obscure the nucleus. They contain large amounts of heparin and histamine. They normally account for less than 1 per cent of the circulating leukocytes. Increases occur in chronic myelogenous leukemia and in generalized mast cell disease.

LYMPHOCYTES. Lymphocytes constitute 30 to 60 per cent of the blood leukocytes. Most are small cells measuring 9 μ in diameter, with a round, dark, blue-black nucleus and scanty blue cytoplasm. Other lymphocytes, probably younger forms, have more abundant blue cytoplasm. Lymphocytes are actively motile, but not phagocytic. The lymphocytes appear to be of two types: One of these has a brief life span, whereas the other is exceedingly long-lived. Small lymphocytes have the capacity to undergo blastic transformation and mitosis when stimulated by phytohemagglutinin. The lymphocytes are intimately involved in various aspects of the immune mechanism, especially in transmission of delayed immunity, and in immunoglobulin synthesis. A pronounced lymphocytosis is characteristic of pertussis and the syndrome of infectious lymphocytosis. In infectious mononucleosis characteristically atypical lymphocytes appear in large numbers. Thymic alymphoplasia is associated with profound lymphopenia and immunoglobulin deficiency. (See also Section 9.)

MONOCYTES. These large phagocytic cells are characterized by a large lobulated nucleus and an abundant gray cytoplasm containing fine azurophilic granules. They normally account for 1 to 5 per cent of the circulating leukocytes, but are increased in such diseases as tuberculosis, systemic mycosis, bacterial endocarditis and certain protozoan infections.

Quantitative Disorders of the Neutrophils

Absolute neutrophil counts vary widely in normal subjects. The relative proportion of neutrophils and lymphocytes in the blood varies with age. Neutrophils predominate at birth, but decrease rapidly in the first few days of life. During infancy they constitute 30 to 40 per cent of the circulating leukocytes. Parity between neutrophils and lymphocytes occurs by about 5 years of age, but the approximately 70 per cent predominance of neutrophils characteristic of the adult is not attained until puberty. In normal healthy children, therefore, from 30 to 70 per cent of the total circulating white blood cells may be neutrophils. In absolute terms they number 2500 to 6000 per $mm.^3$ Levels exceeding this range are designated neutrophilia.

NEUTROPHILIA

Neutrophilia accompanies a wide variety of localized and generalized pyogenic infections as well as some noninfectious inflammatory processes.

Both the total white blood cell count and the proportion of neutrophils increase. In addition, larger numbers of nonsegmented (band) neutrophils and even more immature cells (metamyelocytes and myelocytes) may be seen ("shift to the left"). In general, younger children demonstrate more pronounced responses to infections than adults and manifest higher white cell counts with greater numbers of immature forms. When the total white cell count exceeds 40,000 per mm^3, a "leukemoid" blood picture is said to be present. A presumptive cause is usually evident for leukemoid reactions, such as infection, intoxication, and the like, but occasionally the blood picture may be difficult to differentiate from chronic myelogenous leukemia. The neutrophils in leukemoid reactions have elevated levels of alkaline phosphatase activity, whereas this enzyme is low in chronic myelocytic leukemia. The neutrophilia of infection or inflammation is accompanied by increased activity and hypertrophy of the entire neutrophilic series. On the other hand, the transient neutrophilia accompanying acute stress reflects shifts of previously formed neutrophils between circulating and marginal pools, rather than actual increased production, and is not accompanied by changes in marrow.

NEUTROPENIA

Neutropenia is a reduction below normal of the numbers of circulating neutrophils. This occurs in a substantial number of congenital and acquired diseases and results from either underproduction or peripheral hyperdestruction of neutrophils. When the absolute neutrophil count is less than 1500 per mm^3, the patient becomes unusually susceptible to bacterial infections, especially to those of the skin and respiratory tract. Buccal and rectal ulcerations are also frequently associated.

INFANTILE LETHAL AGRANULOCYTOSIS. This familial disease is characterized by the onset in early infancy of recurrent, severe pyogenic infections, especially of the skin and the lung. Neutrophils are totally absent in the blood or present in reduced numbers; there are absolute monocytosis and eosinophilia. The platelets are normal, and primary anemia is absent. The bone marrow contains markedly decreased numbers of neutrophilic precursors. The neutrophilic series is represented by a few promyelocytes and myelocytes. Lymphocytes and plasmacytes are prominent. The erythrocytic and megakaryocytic elements are normal.

There is no specific or effective therapy. Hematinics, corticosteroids and splenectomy produce no beneficial effect. Although antibiotics may be of temporary value, death frequently occurs during infancy or the first few years of life as a result of overwhelming sepsis. The disease appears to be genetically determined; most pedigrees suggest an autosomal recessive transmission. The basic enzymatic or metabolic defect is unknown.

CHRONIC NEUTROPENIAS. This group of diseases usually produces relatively mild clinical manifestations and is differentiated from the preceding disorder by its relative mildness and sporadic occurrence. The child experiences recurrent pneumonia, pyoderma and mouth ulcerations. The peripheral white blood cell count is decreased, and there is a striking paucity of neutrophils. There is no anemia, and the platelets are normal. Compensatory monocytosis and eosinophilia are usually present. Serum protein studies demonstrate diffuse hypergammaglobulinemia. In the bone marrow there is maturation arrest at the myelocyte or metamyelocyte stage and plasmacytosis, but no alteration of the erythrocytic and megakaryocytic elements. Some of these patients appear to be able to mobilize a neutrophilic response when challenged by significant pyogenic infections.

Infections can be controlled by appropriate antibiotic therapy. Attempts to stimulate granulopoiesis with corticosteroids or other therapy are usually ineffectual. Affected children tend to improve with age and may undergo total remissions in late childhood. Although most cases are sporadic, at least two pedigrees suggesting autosomal dominant inheritance have been described.

ACQUIRED NEUTROPENIA. Decrease in the total white blood cell count and concomitant neutropenia occur in many viral infections, particularly roseola infantum, rubella, rubeola and influenza. Neutropenia is also characteristic of typhoid and paratyphoid infections and brucellosis. In severe pyogenic infections the observation of neutropenia is an ominous prognostic sign, often indicating the overwhelming nature of the disease. In some cases of rheumatoid arthritis and lupus erythematosus, neutropenia also occurs. The pathogenesis of the leukopenia in these diseases is uncertain, but may represent peripheral sequestration or hyperutilization.

Neutropenia results from marrow insufficiency in leukemia, aplastic pancytopenia and disseminated neoplasms such as neuroblastoma. In advanced megaloblastic anemia due to deficiency of vitamin B_{12} or folic acid, neutropenia regularly occurs, possibly owing to ineffective leukopoiesis. On the other hand, an enlarged spleen may filter or sequester large numbers of neutrophils from the circulation. Ionizing radiation and such drugs or chemicals as nitrogen mustard, methotrexate and benzene regularly cause marrow depression and neutropenia in any person receiving them in sufficient amounts.

DRUG-INDUCED NEUTROPENIAS
(Malignant Agranulocytosis)

This syndrome is characterized by a profound reduction of neutrophils in the blood and of their precursors in the bone marrow, accompanied by severe systemic infection. It is usually self-limited, but occasionally lethal.

ETIOLOGY. The drugs or agents which produce this condition do so in a relatively small number of patients, so that an idiosyncrasy would seem to be partly responsible. In some instances, such as in neutropenia associated with aminopyrine, an immunologic basis is probable. This drug acts as a hapten in combination with a protein of the neutrophil, forming an antigenic complex which stimulates formation of a leukocidal antibody. Currently the drug most frequently producing neutropenia is the aminopyrine derivative, dipyrone (Pyralgin). The use of this potentially dangerous drug for its symptomatic effect on fever is inappropriate. Neutropenia following the use of phenothiazines has been attributed to a toxic inhibition of nucleic acid synthesis. Other drugs associated with a significant incidence of neutropenia include thiourea derivatives and sulfonamides. In many cases of neutropenia no cause can be discovered.

CLINICAL MANIFESTATIONS. An abrupt onset with a racking rigor occurs in aminopyrine-induced neutropenia. In other cases the onset may be insidious. Ulcerations of the mouth and rectum, cutaneous infections, and pneumonia are frequent. Despite the absence of neutrophils, the temperature curve is septic, with frequent high spikes. Purulent exudates are not formed, so that the usual physical findings of pyogenic infections may not occur. Death results from overwhelming sepsis in the first week of the disease in about 20 per cent of cases unless antibiotic therapy is effective in treating bacterial infections. Intestinal perforations may occur.

LABORATORY DATA. The total white blood cell count is reduced. Circulating neutrophils are low ($<1000/mm^3$), but a compensatory monocytosis and eosinophilia are frequently present. There is no anemia or thrombocytopenia. Bone marrow changes depend upon the stage of illness. At the height of the disease the marrow is cellular, with normal numbers of erythroid precursors and megakaryocytes, but neutrophilic precursors are reduced. Five to 20 per cent of the nucleated cells may be plasma cells. Recovery is presaged by a return of granulopoiesis in the marrow, which proceeds as a surge of maturation through the several stages of development. Bone marrow examination in this early recovery stage may be misinterpreted as showing a maturation arrest. Four to 5 days after the return of precursors to the marrow, mature neutrophils reappear in the blood. Coincident with their reappearance, prompt defervescence and clinical improvement usually ensue.

TREATMENT. The most important therapeutic measure is immediate discontinuation of any medications which may be causative. Infection should be treated with therapeutic doses of antibiotics, the choice of which should be determined by culture and sensitivity studies; when feasible, bactericidal antibiotics should be used. Prophylactic antibiotics are not indicated. Corticosteroid therapy is not of significant value. Once a patient has acquired neutropenia after administration of a specific drug, that drug or closely related agents should not be administered again. White blood cell transfusions have been used for support during periods of profound neutropenia but are still experimental and of uncertain value owing to their short survival in the circulation.

CYCLIC NEUTROPENIA

This ill defined disease is characterized by periodic episodes of fever and oral ulcerations accompanied by profound neutropenia. Neutropenia persists from 5 to 10 days, after which the white blood cell count returns to normal and the symptoms abate. Such episodes occur at cycles of 14 to 45 days. The bone marrow during the period of neutropenia shows diminished numbers of neutrophilic precursors or maturation arrest. Between episodes the blood and marrow are normal. Therapy is symptomatic and consists of antibiotic treatment of bacterial infections.

TRANSITORY NEUTROPENIA OF THE NEWBORN

Neutrophilia is characteristic of the immediate postnatal period, but with severe infections such as cytomegalic inclusion disease, toxoplasmosis or bacterial sepsis, striking neutropenia may occur. Newborn infants have been described with familial neutropenia and superimposed bacterial infections. In some of these cases the mother has also been neutropenic, suggesting transmission of a humoral inhibitor or antibody from mother to infant. Iso-immunization to neutrophil antigens analogous to Rh sensitization has been suggested as causative, and leukocyte antibodies have been demonstrated in some cases. Bacterial infections usually respond to vigorous antibiotic therapy. The duration of the neutropenia is 4 to 7 weeks.

Inherited Abnormalities of the Leukocytes

Ninety per cent of the neutrophils in the peripheral blood of normal persons have 2 to 4 segments. Only about 5 per cent are unsegmented (bands), and less than 5 per cent have 5 segments. An increase in unsegmented forms, or "shift to the left," usually indicates infection or inflammation, whereas hypersegmentation, or "shift to the right," most commonly occurs in megaloblastic anemias due to folic acid or vitamin B_{12} deficiency.

HEREDITARY HYPOSEGMENTATION (PELGER-HUET ANOMALY). This defect of neutrophilic segmentation is inherited as an autosomal dominant trait. In heterozygous persons more than 90 per cent of circulating neutrophils and eosinophils either are unsegmented or have only two lobes. Despite this abnormal nuclear configuration, their phagocytic capacity is normal, and no predisposition to infection is associated with the trait. The homozygous state may be lethal.

HEREDITARY HYPERSEGMENTATION (UNDRITZ ANOMALY). This rare condition is characterized by predominance of neutrophils with 4 and 5, or even more, segments. The anomaly is inherited as an autosomal trait. No adverse clinical effects are associated with its presence.

MAY-HEGGLIN ANOMALY. This rare, dominantly transmitted anomaly involves the neutrophils and platelets. A majority of the neutrophils contain irregular blue cytoplasmic inclusions similar to Döhle bodies. Döhle bodies consist of precipitated nucleoprotein material and are usually observed in patients with severe systemic infections. In patients with the May-Hegglin anomaly no infection need be present. There may be abnormally large platelets and, at times, thrombocytopenia. The thrombocytopenia responds to splenectomy.

ALDER ANOMALY. In this condition, which is probably transmitted as an autosomal recessive trait, the neutrophilic granulations are larger and stain much more prominently than normal. The granules are distinctly lavender or blue, a circumstance which permits their differentiation from eosinophils. A very small proportion of patients with the Hunter-Hurler syndrome may show somewhat similar granulations in their neutrophils (Reilly bodies).

QUALITATIVE ABNORMALITIES OF THE NEUTROPHILS

A number of syndromes with intracellular defects of the neutrophils display increased susceptibility to infections despite adequate numbers of these cells in the circulation.

Chronic Granulomatous Disease (CGD)

This disease is characterized by a metabolic defect which results in failure of intracellular killing of certain types of bacteria following their phagocytosis by the neutrophils. The disease is in most instances transmitted as an X-linked recessive trait. Occurrence of a few cases in females suggests more than one genetic variety.

The condition becomes manifest in early life with purulent skin lesions and enlarged regional lymph nodes which frequently suppurate. Enlargements of the liver and spleen are nearly always found; pigment-containing granulomas are found in liver, lung and bone. Recurrent bronchopneumonia, empyema and hilar lymphadenopathy often occur.

The disease can be diagnosed by techniques which assess intracellular killing of bacteria by the neutrophils. Neutrophils from normal individuals kill almost all phagocytosed staphylococci or serratia organisms, whereas 80 to 100 per cent of these bacteria remain viable following phagocytosis by the neutrophils of these patients. The neutrophils in CGD also fail to reduce ingested nitroblue tetrazolium dye (NBT), and this property has been used as the basis of a histochemical test to identify patients with this disease. Female carriers of the gene for CGD can be shown to have a heterogeneous population of neutrophils: about half of their cells reduce NBT, while the others are inactive.

The exact biochemical defect in CGD is unsettled. The neutrophils fail to show an increase in pentose phosphate pathway activity and in H_2O_2 production during phagocytosis. The lack of H_2O_2 may be the basis for the failure to kill bacteria such as staphylococci, which do not themselves produce H_2O_2. Streptococci and pneumococci, which do produce H_2O_2, can be killed by the CGD neutrophil.

TREATMENT. High doses of antibiotics with bactericidal activity are indicated for even trivial infections in these patients, and determination of the infecting organism is essential for proper choice of agent. Prompt surgical drainage of abscesses is also indicated. The use of isoniazid and rifamycin (Rifampin), which penetrate leukocytes freely, has been suggested recently as having some benefit. Chronic anemia is common in CGD, but blood transfusions may be hazardous because these patients frequently possess a very rare red cell antigen of the Kell system called K_0. Transfusion almost inevitably leads to iso-immunization. Despite intensive therapy most of these patients die in the first decade of life.

Myeloperoxidase Deficiency

A few patients with increased susceptibility to pyogenic infections and defective intracellular killing of bacteria have been shown to have a defect of the enzyme myeloperoxidase. The NBT test is normal in these individuals.

Chediak-Higashi Disease

This recessively transmitted syndrome includes partial albinism, photophobia, and increased susceptibility to pyogenic infections. The neutrophils contain large greenish brown cytoplasmic inclusions which represent giant abnormal lysosomes, and the cells appear to be engaged in autophagocytic activity.

The granules of eosinophils and basophils are also very large. Peripheral neutropenia is often present, secondary to intramedullary destruction of granulocytes and hypersplenism. The phagocytic cells in this disease have multiple functional defects. Intracellular killing of bacteria is impaired, probably owing to a failure in discharge of lysosomal enzymes into the phagocytic vacuole. In addition granulocyte chemotaxis is impaired.

Patients with the disease have a high incidence of lymphoreticular malignancy and frequently die of sepsis during childhood.

Job Syndrome

This apt term describes patients with multiple recurrent severe cold staphylococcal abscesses of the skin. Some patients may represent a variant of chronic granulomatous disease; in others, the basis for infection is not clear.

Disorders of Leukocyte Chemotaxis

Migration of leukocytes to areas of inflammation and infection depends in part upon the complement system; accordingly, in congenital or acquired deficiency of any of several of the phases of complement, impaired chemotaxis may result in infection. Isolated defects in chemotaxis as a result of cellular abnormalities have also been described.

The Leukemias

Leukemia is a malignant disease due to uncontrolled neoplastic proliferation of leukocyte precursors in blood, bone marrow and reticuloendothelial tissues. Without specific treatment the disease is uniformly fatal in a short period of time.

ETIOLOGY. The cause of leukemia has thus far eluded definition, but there are a number of clues. A genetic predisposition is suggested by a high concordance rate (25 per cent) in identical twins. There is a statistical increase of risk in siblings, but familial occurrence is rare. Certain hereditary conditions which demonstrate chromosomal instability are associated with an increased rate of leukemia, such as the Fanconi aplastic anemia and the Bloom syndrome. Diseases associated with disorders of the immune mechanism, such as agammaglobulinemia and ataxia-telangiectasia, have an increased incidence of leukemia and other lymphoreticular malignancies, and in the Down syndrome the rate of leukemia is increased to 10 to 20 times normal. There is an increased incidence in children of higher socioeconomic backgrounds.

A great deal of interest has been centered on a possible infectious origin; certain animal leukemias are of proved viral origin. Epidemiologic evidence possibly supporting an infectious factor in human leukemia includes the observation of geographic and temporal "clusters" of cases markedly in excess of expected frequency. In addition, virus-like bodies can be demonstrated by electron microscopy in the blood and bone marrow of many leukemic patients. Circumstantial evidence indicates a virus origin for the Burkitt lymphoma, which sometimes terminates in leukemia. Of several hundred reported instances of maternal leukemia during pregnancy, only two infants have been known subsequently to have the disease. The recent observation of leukemic transformation of normal bone marrow engrafted into a leukemic patient strongly suggests the presence and persistence of an oncogenic agent in these patients. The finding of a specific enzyme, reverse transcriptase, in some leukemic tissue suggests an oncogenic RNA virus (oncornavirus).

Leukemia has a striking peak of age of onset in children at 3 to 4 years of age, a phenomenon which was not seen prior to about 1940. There is a slightly increased incidence in males. In blacks the disease seems to be somewhat less common, and the peak of onset at 4 years not so striking.

TYPES OF LEUKEMIA. The leukemias of childhood are classified according to the morphologic characteristics of the abnormal leukemic cells rather than the symptoms or length of survival. During childhood acute leukemias predominate. The abnormal cells of acute leukemia are primitive, undifferentiated forms called "blast" or stem cells. About 80 per cent of cases of childhood leukemia are the acute lymphoblastic type (ALL). In about 15 per cent of cases the disease may be classified as acute granulocytic or myelogenous (AGL); chronic granulocytic leukemia (CGL) accounts for 3 to 5 per cent. Erythroleukemic, eosinophilic, monocytic and plasmacytic varieties are rare. Chronic lymphatic leukemia has rarely been convincingly documented in childhood. Although it is not always possible to classify precisely the type of a given case of acute leukemia, attempts should be made for prognostic purposes. Acute lymphoblastic leukemia frequently responds to chemotherapy, whereas in other acute varieties a response is far less predictable.

CLINICAL MANIFESTATIONS. The presenting signs and symptoms of leukemia result from anemia, neutropenia and thrombopenia, and from diffuse infiltration of organs and tissues.

Anemia of a profound degree is present in about two thirds of patients, with its attendant symptoms of weakness, lassitude and dyspnea. The skin has a peculiar lemon yellow hue. Cardiac dilatation, tachycardia and systolic-flow murmurs are often present. Petechiae and purpura are often the first recognized signs of the disease. Extensive bruising of the legs and large ecchymoses after minor trauma, as well as cutaneous petechiae, are frequently present. Epistaxis and oral and scleral hemorrhages may be prominent. Occasionally hematuria and melena occur. Blood loss may significantly increase the severity of anemia.

Bone and joint pain may be prominent, and leukemia should be considered in the differential diagnosis of children with unexplained bone pain or limp. This pain results from infarction and bone destruction, from subperiosteal hemorrhage and possibly from pressure exerted by hyperplastic neoplastic tissue within the medullary space. Areas of bone destruction and periosteal elevation are seen roentgenographically. A transverse line of radiolucency is frequently seen at the metaphysis of the long bones. Uncommon findings include infiltrations of skin or testes and increased intracranial pressure as a result of meningeal infiltration.

Although leukemia represents an uncontrolled proliferation of abnormal white cells, leukemic cells do not have effective phagocytic function, and pyogenic infections of skin and lung are common. Fever may reflect a hypermetabolic state due to rapid growth and destruction of leukemic tissue; substantial pyrexia usually indicates infection, however, and antibiotic therapy should be instituted upon this premise.

Another prominent group of signs and symptoms of leukemia is due to proliferation of leukemic cells in abdominal viscera and lymph nodes. The testes and kidneys are sometimes diffusely enlarged. The liver and spleen are usually significantly enlarged, and nodular infiltrates of skin occasionally occur, particularly in cases of granulocytic leukemia. The lymph nodes are enlarged and firm, but not painful or tender. Enlargement of mediastinal lymph nodes may produce respiratory obstruction due to pressure on the bronchial tree and anterior mediastinal masses. In about 5 per cent of patients the liver, spleen and lymph nodes are not significantly enlarged.

LABORATORY DATA. The diagnosis of acute leukemia is established on demonstration of leukemic blast cells in blood, bone marrow and other tissues. It cannot be overemphasized that leukemic infiltration of the marrow or other tissues must be shown unequivocally before a diagnosis of this potentially fatal disease can be made.

The accompanying anemia is normochromic and normocytic. The reticulocyte count is low, but a few nucleated red cells may be observed on the peripheral smear. Severe thrombocytopenia is usually present, with platelet counts of less than 20,000 per $mm.^3$ The total leukocyte count is variable. In about half the cases the leukocyte count is within the normal range (7000 to 12,000 per mm^3). Five to 10 per cent of cases demonstrate severe leukopenia (white blood cells less than 3000 per mm^3). In the remaining cases varying degrees of leukocytosis are seen, and markedly elevated white cell counts occur occasionally. The diagnostic circulating cell is the blast cell. In acute lymphoblastic leukemia this is a large cell with scanty blue cytoplasm which contains no granulations. The nuclear chromatin is dispersed in a finely stippled pattern. One or more nucleoli may be seen Occasionally, prominent, sharp, punched-out vacuoles may be seen within the blast cells; these represent degenerative changes. In addition to the blast cells, more mature cells of the lymphocytic series are present. In the 15 per cent of cases of childhood leukemia classified as granulocytic, the leukemic cells correspond to myeloblasts and promyelocytes and many contain primitive granulations. Occasionally red, needle-like, cytoplasmic crystals called Auer rods are present. Special staining procedures utilizing Sudan black and periodic acid–Schiff stains may be useful in differentiating myeloblastic and lymphoblastic varieties. The lymphoblast usually gives PAS-positive and Sudan black-negative reactions, whereas the converse is seen in the myeloblastic variety.

In the stained aspirate of bone marrow the varied, colorful appearance of normal marrow is replaced by monotonous sheets of blast cells. Fat spaces are reduced, and megakaryocytes and erythroid precursors are markedly diminished; the marrow may be so hypercellular that aspiration is unsuccessful. A "dry tap" almost always indicates an abnormal marrow. A specimen suitable for diagnosis can be obtained from the iliac crest with a Silverman or Westerman-Jensen needle or by surgical biopsy. In a small proportion of cases the initial sampling of marrow does not reveal typical findings, but hypoplasia or fibrillar reticulum tissue may be observed. Although aspiration from another site may reveal typical morphology, on rare occasions it may initially be impossible to differentiate between leukemia and aplastic anemia. Since therapy with most antileukemic drugs is disastrous in aplastic anemia, these chemotherapeutic measures should be withheld until an unequivocal histologic diagnosis is made. In these cases of so-called aleukemic leukemia, conventional findings usually become apparent in a short time. In a case of presumed aplastic anemia, if corticosteroids induce a very rapid recovery from pancytopenia, the response is very suggestive of leukemia. Other laboratory findings are relatively unimportant and inconstant. Hyperuricemia may occur, particularly when high white blood cell counts are present, and especially with initiation of chemotherapy. There are no specific or regular chromosomal changes observed in acute leukemia, but peripheral blood and bone marrow cultures frequently reveal aneuploidy.

DIFFERENTIAL DIAGNOSIS. Leukemia should be included in the differential diagnosis of any child with unexplained depression of any of the formed elements of blood, and complete hematologic investigation, including examination of the bone marrow, is mandatory. Diseases sometimes confused with leukemia include idiopathic thrombocytopenic purpura and other forms of thrombocytopenia, scurvy, acute rheumatic fever, rheumatoid arthritis, aplastic anemia, sickle cell disease, osteomyelitis, and infectious mononucleosis and lymphocytosis.

Other malignant processes mimic acute leukemia. About 25 per cent of patients with lymphoma exhibit hematologic changes of acute leukemia during the course of their disease. In disseminated neuroblastoma the marrow may be sufficiently replaced by metastatic disease that morphologic differentiation from leukemia may be difficult. In metastatic neuroblastoma there is a tendency to form syncytia, with a mosaic appearance and occasional pseudorosettes. In addition, most patients with neuroblastoma usually have primary tumor masses in the abdomen or thorax and excrete large amounts of urinary catecholamines.

COURSE AND PROGNOSIS. The course of untreated acute lymphoblastic leukemia of childhood is short. Death from infection or hemorrhage almost always occurs within 6 months. Symptomatic therapy with blood transfusion and antibiotics is of only transient benefit. Before the chemotherapeutic era a few children had spontaneous remissions, with temporary return of the blood and bone marrow to normal status. These remissions usually followed severe infections and were of short duration, survivals for more than 9 to 10 months being remarkable.

The development of specific chemotherapeutic agents for acute leukemia has changed the survival time significantly. In most instances of acute lymphatic leukemia it is possible to induce remissions which may be maintained for prolonged periods. Newer regimens employing multiple chemotherapeutic agents, combined with prophylactic therapy of the central nervous system, have dramatically changed survival patterns. Substantial numbers of children with acute lymphoblastic leukemia are alive and in remission more than 3 years after initial diagnosis. There is mounting optimism that some of these patients may never relapse and thus represent "cures."

Certain patients are unlikely to respond for extended periods: nonwhite children; those with initial white blood cell counts over 35,000/mm^3; and those with large masses in the anterior mediastinum.

TREATMENT. Treatment of acute leukemia must include both supportive and specific modalities. General supportive therapy includes transfusions and antibiotics. Fresh whole blood and platelet concentrates can be given to control hemorrhage and to correct anemia. Infections must be vigorously treated. Antibiotic therapy should be used when bacterial infection is likely, and based upon appropriate cultures and sensitivity tests whenever possible. Pseudomonas, *Escherichia coli* and staphylococcal septicemias are common. Because of their debilitated state and altered resistance, affected children may also become infected by opportunistic agents, such as fungi, *Pneumocystis carinii* and cytomegalovirus.

Chemotherapeutic Agents. The drugs that have been shown to be valuable in the therapy of leukemia are listed in Table 14–5. All are used to induce or to maintain "remissions." The remission is characterized by eradication of recognizable leukemic cells from the blood and bone marrow, restoration of normal hematologic values in the blood, disappearance of leukemic enlargement of liver, spleen and lymph nodes, and return of clinical well-being. It is necessary to attain a remission if life is to be prolonged.

The anti-leukemic drugs can be classified into two groups: first, the remission-inducing agents, which act rapidly in a high proportion of cases, but have effects of short duration; and second, the remission-maintaining agents, which have the capacity to sustain remissions for long periods of time.

Following establishment of the diagnosis of acute lymphoblastic leukemia, therapy with prednisone is administered in a dose of 2.0 mg/kg/day (or 40 mg/M^2/day), and vincristine is given in weekly injections of 1.5 mg/M^2. When there is a high white count or bulky adenopathy, this treatment may result in such rapid lysis of leukemic cells that hyperuricemia leads to precipitation of uric acid crystals in the renal tubules; acute anuria may occur. This complication can be avoided through adequate hydration, alkalinization of urine, and oral administration of allopurinol in a dose of 10 mg/kg day. Acute hyperkalemia may also occur.

Ninety to 95 per cent of children with acute lymphoblastic leukemia treated in this manner will obtain a complete remission within 4 to 6 weeks. Maintenance therapy must then be given, since remissions last for only about 1 to 3 months unless continuous therapy is employed. Longer responses can be attained by the use of combinations of maintenance agents rather than a single drug. Various protocols involving different combinations of drugs, different schedules and routes of administration and different doses have been studied in an attempt to find the best survival and to minimize drug toxicity. Most regimens include some combination of 6-mercaptopurine, cyclophosphamide, methotrexate and cytosine arabinoside. The optimal regimen has probably not yet been defined.

The "prophylactic" treatment of the central nervous system to eradicate foci of leukemic cells appears to be very important in producing increased numbers of long-term survivors. These cells are presumed to be in so-called sanctuaries, protected from systemic drugs which penetrate the cerebrospinal fluid very poorly. Prophylactic therapy consists of 2000 to 2400 r of radiation delivered to the cranium during a 2- to 3-week period. In addition, several doses of methotrexate, 12 mg/M^2, are given

TABLE 14–5 DRUGS USEFUL IN THE TREATMENT OF CHILDHOOD LEUKEMIA

GENERIC NAME	PROPRIETARY NAME AND MANUFACTURER	TYPE OF LEUKEMIA*	ROUTE OF ADMINISTRATION	USUAL DOSAGE	PREDOMINANT TOXICITIES
Induction Agents					
Corticosteroids, e.g., prednisone	Deltasone (Upjohn) Delta-Dome (Dome) Betapar (Parke, Davis) Prednisone (McKesson) Meticorten (Schering)	ALL/AML	Oral	40 mg/M^2/day or 2 mg/kg/day	Cushing syndrome
Vincristine	Oncovin (Lilly)	ALL/AML AML	Intravenous	1.5 mg/M^2/week, or 0.075 mg/kg/ week (maximum 2 mg per dose)	Peripheral neurotoxicity; alopecia; local necrosis on extravasation
L-Asparaginase	Investigative	ALL/AML ?AML	Intravenous	100–500 IU/kg/day or 500–1000 IU/ kg/twice weekly	Anaphylaxis; hypoproteinemia; nausea and vomiting
Daunomycin or adriamycin	Investigative	ALL/AML ?AML	Intravenous		Marrow suppression, alopecia; gastrointestinal irritation
Thioguanine		AML	Intravenous	1.25–2.5 mg/kg/ twice daily	Marrow suppression
Cytosine arabinoside	Cytosar (Upjohn)	AML	Intravenous	50–100 mg/kg/ twice daily	Marrow suppression; nausea and vomiting
Cyclophosphamide	Cytoxan (Mead Johnson)	AML	Intravenous	50–100 mg/kg twice daily	Marrow suppression; nausea and vomiting
Busulfan	Myleran (Burroughs-Wellcome)	CML	Oral	2.0 mg/day	Marrow suppression
6-Mercaptopurine	Purinethol (Burroughs-Wellcome)		Oral	2.5 mg/kg/day	
Maintenance Agents					
6-Mercaptopurine	Purinethol (Burroughs-Wellcome)	ALL/AML AML	Oral	2.5 mg/kg/day	Marrow suppression
Amethopterin	Methotrexate (Lederle)	ALL/AML	a. Oral b. Intravenous c. Intrathecal	a. 1.25–5 mg/day, or 20–30 mg/M^2 twice weekly b. 50–300 mg/M^2 weekly to biweekly c. 0.5 mg/kg, or 12 mg/M^2 (maximum 12 mg) twice weekly until CSF clears	Marrow suppression; nausea and vomiting; gastrointestinal mucosal irritation
Cyclophosphamide	Cytoxan (Mead Johnson)	ALL/AML AML ?CML	a. Oral b. Intravenous	a. 2.5 mg/kg/day or 400 mg/M^2/week b. Variable	Marrow suppression; nausea and vomiting
Cytosine arabinoside	Cytosar (Upjohn)	ALL/AML	Intravenous	Variable	Marrow suppression; nausea and vomiting
Thioguanine		AML	Oral	Variable	Marrow suppression
Vincristine	Oncovin (Lilly)	?AML	Intravenous	1.5 mg/M^2 weekly or biweekly (maximum 2 mg per dose)	Neurotoxicity; alopecia; local necrosis on extravasation

*ALL = acute lymphoblastic leukemia; AML = acute myelogenous leukemia; CML = chronic myelogenous leukemia.

intrathecally in order to reach possible leukemic infiltrates in the spinal meninges. Other programs have used craniospinal radiation or long-term intrathecal methotrexate.

Regimens employing prednisone-vincristine induction, prophylactic CNS therapy, and maintenance therapy with a combination of drugs appear to offer the best chance at present for long-term control of acute lymphoblastic leukemia. Median survival has been extended to more than 3 years, and substantial numbers of children have had initial remissions lasting for more than 3 years. Extrapolation of earlier data suggests that some of these long-term survivors may represent bona fide cures. It is not possible at present to be sure of this, and the ultimate consequences of these very vigorous programs have not been determined. Because of the considerable toxicity implicit in these rigorous programs, they should be directed by individuals with considerable experience. Unless a physician is sufficiently experienced, adequately equipped, and willing and able to devote the necessary attention and time to such programs, he should consider referral of children with leukemia to centers which can assist him with their management.

Investigation is being directed at the possibility of enhancing host resistance to leukemia by various forms of immunotherapy. Such studies, still very preliminary, have utilized repeated vaccinations with BCG or extracts of leukemic cells. Some combination of chemotherapy and immunotherapy may offer the best hope for ultimate control of this disease.

It is very important to identify cases of *acute granulocytic leukemia* (AGL), since the response of this variety to therapy is less predictable; remissions are fewer and shorter. Steroids are often of little value. At the present time the best regimen for inducing and maintaining remissions of AGL appears to be a combination of high dose 6-mercaptopurine or thioguanine and cytosine arabinoside. Because it may be necessary to produce severe aplasia of the marrow before repopulation with normal marrow can occur, the patient may have to be sustained through a relatively long period of hazardous pancytopenia by transfusions of platelets and red blood cells and vigorous antibiotic therapy.

CENTRAL NERVOUS SYSTEM LEUKEMIA

Twenty-five to 50 per cent of children with leukemia develop leukemic infiltration of the meninges. The symptoms and signs are those of increased intracranial pressure, with headache and morning vomiting as frequent initial manifestations. Papilledema and, in longstanding cases, increased head circumference are seen, with spreading of the sutures evident roentgenographically. This complication of acute leukemia usually occurs after a period of successful chemotherapy, but may rarely be present at the onset of the disease. Lumbar puncture reveals increased pressure, somewhat increased protein and a mononuclear pleocytosis of 50 to 5000 per mm^3 of leukemic blast cells. It has been postulated that leukemic cells may be protected from the effects of systemic chemotherapy by the blood-brain barrier, since the levels of these drugs in the spinal fluid are less than one tenth those in the serum.

The complication can be treated effectively by 3 or 4 injections of 12 mg/M^2 of methotrexate into the subarachnoid space by lumbar puncture. This therapy is effective even when the systemic disease has become refractory to methotrexate. Systemic corticosteroids may also be of value. Roentgen therapy in a dose of 400 to 600 r directed to lateral skull ports may also be effective. In some medical centers craniospinal radiation is given. If this complication is not recognized and prompt therapy initiated, ocular palsies and even blindness may ensue. "Prophylactic" treatment of the central nervous system with radiation and intrathecal methotrexate reduces the frequency of this complication to less than 5 per cent of patients.

Intrathecal cytosine arabinoside may also be effective.

COUNSELING THE FAMILY OF THE CHILD WITH LEUKEMIA

There are few situations in pediatric practice in which wise and sympathetic support and counseling are of greater value. (See also pages 142–144.)

The possibility of leukemia should not be discussed unless the diagnosis is unequivocal, and consultation or referral should be considered in any questionable case. If leukemia is present, the parents must be told the diagnosis. The skillful management of the initial interview profoundly affects subsequent relations between family and physician.

The physician must state the diagnosis without equivocation and without using euphemisms. A less positive approach, or expressed doubts of the diagnosis, may raise false hopes in the parents' minds. A number of questions, fears and feelings of guilt are so common in parents that they should be anticipated by the physician. The parents should be told that leukemia is not contagious, so that there is no significantly increased risk to playmates. There is a statistical increase in risk to siblings, but this is not high enough to cause concern except in identical twins. The parents can be told that acts of omission and commission do not cause leukemia, and that there is no known way that the disease could have been prevented. Reassurance can be given that delays in diagnosis do not, in general, affect the long-term results.

A brief explanation of the nature of the disease and its clinical manifestations should be given. The remission should be described and the probability that remissions can be attained in the vast majority of cases of acute lymphoblastic leukemia should be emphasized. A definite prediction of survival should not be given, but it can be stated that remissions often last for many months or years. The fact that most care can be given without admission to a hospital should be emphasized. The family can be advised that the treatment of leukemia is fairly standardized; scientific communications are well developed, so that as definitive therapies are discovered, information is rapidly disseminated to those with special interests. Parents can, therefore, be assured that there is, in general, little to be gained by seeking novel therapy or cures. Finally, the parents can be told that leukemia is not usually associated with pain, and in most instances it is possible to prevent undue suffering.

During the early days of the disease, frequent reassurance and discussions help the entire family, including the siblings, to make the necessary adjustments to the diagnosis and the possibility that the patient may ultimately die. Management and support of the older child or adolescent with leukemia present particular challenges. These children will often themselves learn of their diagnosis from friends or neighbors, and it may be better that they be told by their parents or physician if questions arise.

ACUTE LEUKEMIA IN THE NEWBORN

Leukemia in newborn infants is generally of the acute granulocytic type. They have profound anemia and thrombocytopenia, and markedly elevated white cell counts with large numbers of circulating blast cells are common. There may be nodular leukemic infiltrations of the skin and massive hepatosplenomegaly. Response to chemotherapy has been poor. Leukemia must be differentiated from various neonatal diseases such as syphilis, cytomegalic inclusion disease, toxoplasmosis, rubella and hemolytic disease of the newborn (erythroblastosis fetalis). Newborn infants with the Down syndrome may have a hematologic syndrome indistinguishable from acute granulocytic leukemia and have had remissions of very long duration. It is impossible to say whether this represents a variant of leukemia or an unusual leukemoid reaction. In any case, caution is indicated in diagnosing leukemia in newborns with trisomy 21.

CHRONIC GRANULOCYTIC LEUKEMIA

About 5 per cent of leukemias in children are of the chronic granulocytic variety (CGL). The spleen usually becomes gigantic in size, often descending into the left pelvis. White blood cell counts may exceed 70,000/mm^3, and blast cells, promyelocytes, myelocytes and metamyelocytes, as well as more mature granulocytes, are present in the blood. Nucleated red blood cells and an absolute eosinophilia and basophilia are also observed. The more mature granulocytes in this disease have very low alkaline phosphatase activity, in contradistinction to the high activity of granulocytes in leukemoid reactions. Serum levels of vitamin B_{12} are also very high in this form of leukemia.

Chronic granulocytic leukemia is the only human malignancy in which a characteristic cytogenetic abnormality occurs and has been regularly observed. Peripheral blood and bone marrow culture reveals an abnormal G group chromosome (probably number 22) which has lost material from both long arms; a minute fragment results, called the Philadelphia or Ph chromosome. The circulating lymphocytes do not have the Ph chromosome and so the usual phytohemagglutinin-stimulated blood culture cannot be used to demonstrate it. Although most typical cases of chronic granulocytic leukemia have the Ph chromosome, a number of young children with similar hematologic findings have not had it. An elevated level of fetal hemoglobin and high levels of serum and urine muramidase (lysozyme) are characteristic of this latter variety. Affected patients pursue an acute fulminating clinical course; they do not respond well to therapy.

Chronic granulocytic leukemia may be treated with busulfan (Myleran), a nitrogen mustard derivative. This is given orally in a dose of 1 to 4 mg/day until the white blood cell count drops below 20,000 per mm.[3] Maintenance therapy at a lower dose may then be begun, or the drug discontinued until relapse occurs. Mercaptopurine (6-MP) is also effective. The disease may be controlled for many months or even years, but ultimately large numbers of blast cells appear in the circulation. At this point the disease may be indistinguishable from acute granulocytic leukemia, and death usually occurs in a short time despite further chemotherapy.

GENERAL

Cartwright, G. E., Athens, J. W., Boggs, D. R., and Wintrobe, M. M.: The kinetics of granulopoiesis in normal man. Ser. Haematol. *1*:1, 1965.

Davidson, W. M.: Inherited variations in leukocytes. Brit. Med. Bull. *17*:190, 1961.

Neutropenia

Kauder, E., and Mauer, A. M.: Neutropenias of childhood. J. Pediatr. *69*:147, 1966.

Qualitative Abnormalities of Neutrophils

Johnston, R. B., Jr., and Baehner, R. L.: Chronic granulomatous disease: Correlation between pathogenesis and clinical findings. Pediatrics *48*:730, 1971.

Quie, P. G.: Disorders of phagocyte function. Curr. Probl. Pediatr. *2*:11, 1972.

Leukemia

Aur, R. J. A., Simone, J., Hustu, O., Walters, T., Boulla, L., Pratt, C., and Pinkel, D.: Central nervous system therapy and combination chemotherapy of childhood lymphocytic leukemia. Blood *37*:272, 1971.

Holland, J. F., and Glidewell, O.: Chemotherapy of acute lymphocytic leukemia of childhood. Cancer *30*:1480, 1972.

Thomas, E. D., Bryant, J. I., Buckner, C. D., Clift, R. A., Fefer, A., Johnson, F. L., Neiman, P., Ramberg, R. E., and Storb, R.: Leukaemic transformation of engrafted human marrow cells in vivo. Lancet, *1*:1310, 1972.

HEMORRHAGIC DISEASES

The blood is in dynamic equilibrium between fluidity and coagulation. This balance must be precisely maintained to assure that exsanguination does not result from trivial trauma or that spontaneous thrombosis does not occur. The hemostatic mechanism is complex and involves local reactions of the blood vessels, the several activities of the platelet, and finally the interactions of a number of specific coagulation factors which circulate in the blood. The vascular endothelium is the primary barrier against hemorrhage. When small blood vessels are transected, active vasoconstriction and local tissue pressure control minute areas of bleeding even without mobilization of the coagulation process, but the platelet is essential for maintenance of small blood vessels and of their endothelial stability. Hemostatic defects due to abnormalities of the vessels are manifest by small intracutaneous hemorrhages and petechiae. Hemorrhagic states related to the platelets and the soluble coagulation proteins are more dramatic and urgent.

SCHEMA OF COAGULATION

The classic schema of coagulation, formulated at the turn of the century, pictured coagulation as proceeding in three phases. In phase I a hypothetical substance called thromboplastin was formed by interaction of plasma, platelets and tissue juice. In phase II, prothrombin was converted to thrombin in the presence of thromboplastin and calcium. Finally, in phase III, thrombin converted soluble fibrinogen into the visible fibrin clot. Although this simple scheme, involving only six substances, has been expanded so that a dozen factors have now been defined, retention of the concept of a basic three-phase reaction has considerable merit. Table 14–6 lists the currently recognized coagulation factors and their common synonyms. A comprehensive schema of coagulation is depicted in Figure 14–9.

In phase I, in addition to an increased number of factors, intrinsic and extrinsic systems have been recognized. The intrinsic mechanism involves the successive enzymatic conversion of the inactive forms of factors XII, XI, IX, VIII to their active forms. Active factors VIII and a phospholipid substance (partial thromboplastin) derived from platelets catalyze the successive conversion of inactive factors X and V to active counterparts. The extrinsic mechanism involves the conversion of inactive factor VII to its active state by a substance derived from tissue fluid. In the extrinsic system active factor VII does not require the platelet phospholipid to activate factors X and V. A specific substance which has been identified as thromboplastin probably does not exist.

Phase II of coagulation is concerned with the enzymatic cleavage of inactive prothrombin into active thrombin. This step requires factor II as substrate, as well as active factors X and V and calcium.

Finally, in phase III, thrombin splits two small peptides from the fibrinogen molecule, uncovering reactive sites in the fibrin monomer. These monomers then spontaneously polymerize to form long chains of fibrin. Factor XIII facilitates lateral bonding between fibrin strands to form a stable three-dimensional clot.

TESTS FOR EVALUATION OF THE HEMOSTATIC MECHANISM

Laboratory tests are of considerable value in the diagnosis of hemorrhagic disorders, but the importance of the history, including the family history, and of the physical examination cannot be overemphasized. Significant congenital defects are almost invariably associated with histories of easy bruising or prolonged bleeding after minor injury.

TABLE 14–6 THE COAGULATION FACTORS

INTERNATIONAL NUMBERS	SYNONYMS	COMMENT
I	Fibrinogen	Number rarely used—congenital deficiency known (afibrinogenemia)
II	Prothrombin	Number rarely used—congenital deficiency known
III	Thromboplastin	No specific factor identified
IV	Calcium	Number rarely used
V	Labile factor proaccelerin	Congenital deficiency known (parahemophilia, Owren's disease)
VI	Activated labile factor, accelerin	No longer differentiated from V
VII	Stable factor, SPCA, proconvertin	Congenital deficiency known
VIII	Antihemophilic factor (AHF) or globulin (AHG)	Hemophilia A (classic hemophilia) results from congenital deficiency
IX	Christmas factor, plasma thromboplastin component (PTC)	Hemophilia B results from congenital deficiency
X	Stuart-Prower factor	Congenital deficiency known
XI	Plasma thromboplastin antecedent, PTA	Congenital deficiency known
XII	Hageman factor	No clinical symptoms associated with congenital deficiency
XIII	Fibrin stabilizing factor	Congenital deficiency known

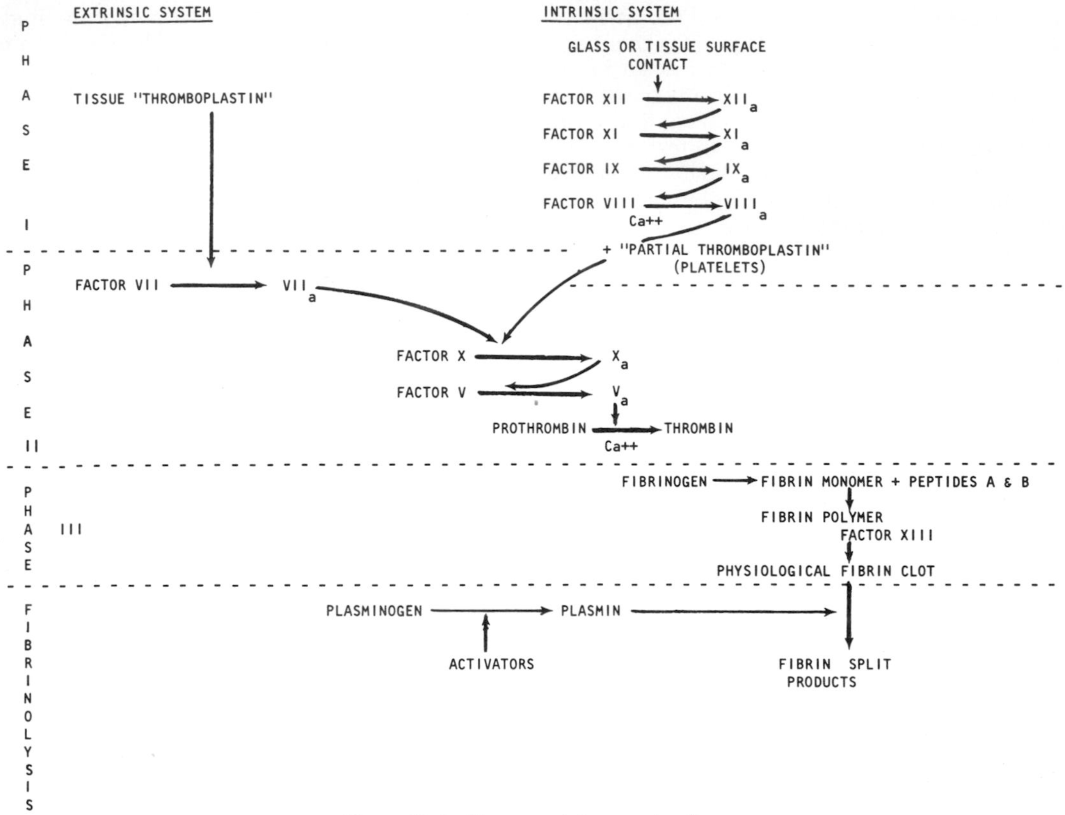

Figure 14–9 *The coagulation mechanism.*

The platelet count, tourniquet test and bleeding time are used to assess the integrity of the small blood vessels. The *tourniquet test* is performed by inflating a blood pressure cuff to a point midway between the systolic and diastolic pressures for 5 minutes. Normally this stress results in fewer than 5 petechiae on an area of skin on the forearm 2.5 cm square. A greater number of petechiae indicates thrombocytopenia, increased fragility, or dysfunction of the small blood vessels. The *Ivy bleeding time* also assesses the vascular and platelet phases of hemostasis. A blood pressure cuff is applied to the arm and inflated to 40 mm Hg, and a stab incision 2 mm long and deep is made with a scalpel blade. At 30-second intervals drops of blood are blotted from the margin of the incision. Normally blood flow stops within 4 to 8 minutes. A *platelet count* or estimation is essential in the evaluation of any patient suspected of having a hemostatic disorder. When the platelet count is less than 40,000 per mm^3, those tests which rely upon platelet function, such as the bleeding time and tourniquet test, usually give abnormal results. Platelet function tests include measurement of clot retraction, glass bead adhesion (Salzman test) and platelet aggregation.

The *whole blood clotting time* tests the entire coagulation mechanism. The interval for a firm blood clot to form in a glass test tube is normally 8 to 12 minutes; if a careful three-tube technique is used, the upper limit of normal is 15 to 19 minutes. The clotting time is a very gross assessment of the hemostatic mechanism, since fairly severe defects may be present in spite of a normal clotting time. The capillary tube clotting time is unreliable.

The three phases of coagulation can be individually assessed by simple, accurate tests. In any hemorrhagic state the adequacy of phase III should be ascertained first. Unless adequate fibrinogen is present, the blood is incoagulable, and the other laboratory tests in which the formation of a visible clot is the end-point give, perforce, abnormal results. Phase III can be evaluated by the *thrombin time,* the time required for plasma to clot after the addition of bovine thrombin. The normal thrombin time is 15 to 20 seconds. Prolongation indicates hypofibrinogenemia or a circulating anticoagulant.

Phase II in its entirety is assessed by the *prothrombin time,* the time taken for plasma to clot after the addition of thromboplastin and calcium. Normal prothrombin time is 12 to 14 seconds. If phase III is intact, a prolonged prothrombin time indicates a deficiency involving factors II, V, VII or X, alone or in combination. Specific assays for all these factors are available. The level of ionized calcium must be less than 2.5 mg/dl in order to interfere with blood coagulation.

Phase I, the most complex part of the coagulation mechanism, can be evaluated by several tests. The *partial thromboplastin time* (PTT) is the time required for clotting of plasma which has been activated by incubation with kaolin, when calcium and platelets or a lipid substitute for platelets (partial thromboplastin) are added. The normal partial thromboplastin time is 25 to 40 seconds. The PTT is a simple, inexpensive and reliable way to assess the adequacy of factors XII, XI, IX and VIII. The *prothrombin consumption time* is a standard prothrombin determination performed on serum instead of plasma. Because prothrombin is used up during coagulation, the serum normally contains little prothrombin, and the serum prothrombin time is prolonged to 35 seconds or greater. Deficiencies of the phase I factors are associated with poor utilization of prothrombin. If the serum prothrombin time does not differ significantly from that obtained with plasma, deficiency of one of the phase I factors is likely.

The *thromboplastin generation* test is the most sensitive of all the tests of phase I. The thromboplastic activity of an incubated mixture of plasma, serum and platelet substrate is estimated at regular intervals. A deficiency of any of the phase I factors will be reflected in an abnormal generation test result. This test can be modified so as to quantitate precisely factors VIII and IX.

There is considerable difference in sensitivity among these tests. For example, a plasma level of factor VIII which is only 1 or 2 per cent of normal is sufficient for a normal clotting time. A level of factor VIII at 3 to 5 per cent of normal produces a normal prothrombin consumption test. The PTT and thromboplastin generation test results become abnormal when the factor VIII level is 15 to 20 per cent of normal or less.

If the PTT, prothrombin consumption or thromboplastin generation test results are abnormal, the way in which they can be corrected identifies the specific deficiency. Normal plasma adsorbed with barium sulfate retains factors VIII and XI. Normal serum contains factors IX and XI. Therefore, if an abnormal test result can be rectified by adsorbed plasma, but not by serum, factor VIII deficiency is proved. If an abnormal result is corrected by serum, but not by adsorbed plasma, factor IX deficiency is present. If both serum and plasma are corrective, factor XI deficiency may be present.

Coagulation Disorders

PHASE I DISORDERS—THE HEMOPHILIAS

The hemophilias are the most common and serious of the congenital coagulation disorders. They are associated with genetically determined deficiencies of factors VIII, IX or XI.

FACTOR VIII DEFICIENCY
(Classic Hemophilia; Hemophilia A)

About 80 per cent of cases of hemophilia are caused by a gene carried on the X chromosome which results in a profound depression of the level of factor VIII in the plasma. Recent studies indicate that there is material present in the circulating blood of hemophiliac patients which is antigenically similar to factor VIII but which is devoid of coagulant activity. The disease is transmitted by asymptomatic female carriers to affected sons. In most instances it is impossible to detect the carrier state by usual laboratory tests, but newer procedures have permitted a diagnosis of the carrier female with better accuracy, permitting reliable genetic counseling in many instances. In 80 per cent of cases the family history is positive. Sporadic cases may represent new mutations. The clinical severity depends upon the level of factor VIII in the plasma, severe cases having less than 1 to 3 per cent of the normal level; the degree of severity tends to be constant within a given family.

CLINICAL MANIFESTATIONS. Since factor VIII does not cross the placenta, a bleeding tendency may be evident in the neonatal period. Hematomas after injections and bleeding from circumcision are common, but many affected newborns exhibit no clinical abnormalities. As ambulation begins, excessive bruising is observed. Large intramuscular hematomas result from minor trauma. A relatively minor traumatic laceration, as of the tongue or lip, which bleeds persistently for hours or days is frequently the event that leads to diagnosis. Ninety per cent of patients with severe disease have had clinical evidence of increased bleeding by 3 to 4 years of age. The hallmark of hemophilia is hemarthrosis. Hemorrhages into the elbows, knees and ankles cause pain and swelling and limit movement of the joint. Repeated hemorrhages may produce degenerative changes, with osteoporosis, muscle atrophy and, ultimately, a fixed, unusable joint. Spontaneous hematuria is a troublesome, but not usually serious, complication. Intracranial hemorrhage and bleeding into the neck constitute life-threatening emergencies.

Patients with levels of factor VIII greater than 5 per cent may not have severe spontaneous symptoms. These patients with "mild hemophilia" may experience only prolonged bleeding following tooth extractions, surgery, or injury.

LABORATORY DATA. The only significant laboratory abnormalities occur in coagulation tests and are due to serious deficiency of factor VIII. The partial thromboplastin time (PTT) is greatly prolonged. Prothrombin consumption is so markedly impaired that the serum and plasma prothrombin times may be similar. The thromboplastin generation test result is grossly abnormal. The abnormal tests can be corrected by normal plasma adsorbed with barium sulfate, but not by serum. In less severe cases only the PTT and thromboplastin generation test result may be abnormal.

TREATMENT. Prevention of trauma constitutes a most important aspect of care for the hemophilic child. During early life the crib and the playpen should be padded, and the child should be carefully supervised while he is learning to walk. As he becomes older, physical activities which do not entail a risk of trauma should be encouraged. It is important that a course between overprotection and permissiveness be followed in the supervision of these patients.

When bleeding episodes occur, replacement therapy is essential to prevent pain, disability or life-threatening hemorrhage. The aim of therapy is to increase the level of factor VIII in the plasma to assure hemostasis. Presently this can be done only by the intravenous infusion of fresh plasma or plasma concentrates.

The factor VIII level can be effectively increased by infusion of fresh or fresh-frozen plasma in a dose of 10 to 15 ml/kg every 12 hours. This regimen maintains a plasma level between 10 and 25 per cent of normal. Because of danger of circulatory overload, no more than 30 ml/kg of plasma should be administered in a 24-hour period.

Therapy of the hemophiliac patient has been considerably facilitated by the development of factor VIII concentrates; these permit fairly precise estimation of the dosage necessary to attain hemostatic levels. By definition, 1 ml of normal plasma contains 1 unit of factor VIII. Because the plasma volume is about 45 ml/kg, it is necessary to infuse 45 units/kg of factor VIII to increase its level in the hemophiliac recipient from 0 to 100 per cent. A dose of 25–50 units/kg of factor VIII is usually given to raise the recipient's level to 50 to 100 per cent of normal. Because the half-life of factor VIII in the plasma is about 8 to 12 hours, repeated infusions can be given as necessary to maintain a desired level of activity. For severe hemorrhage (intracranial, retroperitoneal) or for surgery the level should be increased to 70 to 100 per cent and maintained above 40 per cent for 7 to 10 days. For the usual hemarthroses, many centers employ a single infusion calculated to increase the recipient's level to 70 to 100 per cent of normal; such a level remains above 5 per cent for about 48 hours.

Several factor VIII concentrates are currently available. The most inexpensive of these is cryoprecipitate, which can be prepared in the blood bank from fresh plasma. Two hundred and fifty milliliters of fresh plasma yields one bag of cryoprecipitate, which usually contains 75 to 125 units of factor VIII. One bag of cryoprecipitate per 5 kg. of body weight will raise the recipient's level to about 50 per cent of normal.

Commercial preparations containing large amounts of relatively pure factor VIII are also available. These are dispensed as lyophilized powders in bottles of about 250 units which can be reconstituted just prior to use; they have tremendous utility and convenience. Because of their potency and relatively low protein content they permit rapid restoration of normal hemostatic levels with very small volumes.

Most commercial factor VIII concentrates also contain the anti-A and anti-B isohemagglutinins; when massive amounts of them are given to the blood group A or B individual, hemolysis may occur. Hyperfibrinogenemia may also be seen, owing to their fibrinogen content.

When the hemophiliac child has significant bleeding, local measures should include application of cold and pressure. For ordinary hemarthroses, therapy with plasma or concentrates is administered to raise the factor VIII level to above 50 per cent and to maintain it at least above 5 per cent for 48 to 72 hours. Immobilization is indicated initially, but passive exercises should be begun within 48 hours to prevent joint stiffness and fibrosis. The necessity of aspiration of blood from the joint is somewhat controversial. When the skin overlying the joint is very tense, aspiration of blood, when adequate factor VIII has been given, may provide relief of pain. Replacement therapy is probably the most important part of management of hemarthrosis, since equally good results have been obtained by groups who routinely practice aspiration and by others who do not. Aggressive replacement therapy with factor VIII and careful orthopedic management of hemarthroses can prevent much severe deformity and crippling. When hemorrhage occurs in vital areas such as the brain or neck, or when surgery or dental extractions are contemplated, intensive therapy using factor VIII concentrates is indicated to maintain the plasma level above 75 per cent. Venipunctures should be performed only from superficial veins; aspiration from femoral or internal jugular veins is hazardous.

Factor VIII concentrates have permitted the development of pilot programs for home management or self-treatment of the hemophiliac patient, or even "prophylactic" therapy. There is good evidence that early treatment reduces disability and deformity and probably reduces the amount and duration of replacement treatment necessary for bleeding episodes. Parents, or even the older patient himself, can be trained to give intravenous infusions of concentrates, with substantial decreases in hospitalization and morbidity and with savings in costs.

The major obstacles have been the unavailability and costs of concentrates, and the reluctance of health insurance programs to underwrite costs of this kind of treatment. There is little doubt that home treatment, in conjunction with periodic assessment and counsel from the physician, represents optimal management for the hemophiliac child and his family, and it is to be hoped that this enlightened management will permit the present generation of hemophiliac children to enter adult life without major physical or psychologic crippling.

FACTOR VIII INHIBITORS. A small number of patients with hemophilia become refractory to factor VIII therapy, owing to development of a circulating inhibitor or antibody. The development of inhibitors is not related to the number of plasma transfusions. These inhibitors are IgG globulins and are specifically active against factor VIII. It is virtually impossible to overpower an inhibitor, but when hemorrhage occurs, massive doses of factor VIII concentrates or exchange transfusions with fresh blood should be given and may be of temporary benefit.

FACTOR IX DEFICIENCY
(Christmas Disease; Hemophilia B)

About 15 per cent of cases of hemophilia are due to a genetically determined deficiency of factor IX. This disease is clinically indistinguishable from factor VIII deficiency, and is also transmitted as an X-linked recessive trait. The disease has a wide range of clinical severity, which in general corresponds to the level of factor IX in the serum.

LABORATORY DATA. The partial thromboplastin time (PTT), prothrombin consumption and thromboplastin generation test results are usually abnormal. These *in vitro* abnormalities can be corrected by normal serum, but not by adsorbed plasma.

TREATMENT. Replacement therapy is accomplished by infusions of plasma. Ten to 15 ml/kg should be given every 12 to 24 hours during bleeding episodes. The response to fresh or fresh-frozen plasma is superior to that obtained with stored plasma.

A commercial concentrate containing factors II, VII, IX and X (Konyne) has excellent levels of factor IX—about 250 units per bottle; it can be given in dosage similar to that outlined for factor VIII, although because the half-life of factor IX is about 24 hours, administration may be less frequent. The commercial concentrate appears to be strongly contaminated with the agent for homologous serum hepatitis; it must be used with caution, particularly in patients with liver disease.

FACTOR XI DEFICIENCY
(PTA Deficiency; Hemophilia C)

This usually mild bleeding disorder is inherited as an autosomal dominant trait, and typical cases are seen in both sexes. The usual clinical manifestations are nosebleeds, and excessive hemorrhage and hemarthroses are rare. The PTT, prothrombin consumption and thromboplastin generation test results are abnormal in the more severe cases. Both normal plasma and serum correct the deficiency. Plasma therapy in a dose of 10 to 15 ml/kg every 12 to 24 hours should be given for significant clinical hemorrhage.

FACTOR XII DEFICIENCY
(Hageman Factor Deficiency)

This fascinating condition is due to homozygous occurrence of an autosomal gene which results in a profound deficiency of factor XII. Despite abnormal test results of the first phase of coagulation, these patients have no clinical abnormalities of blood clotting.

VON WILLEBRAND'S DISEASE
(Vascular Hemophilia)

This dominantly inherited disease is complex. It is characterized by a capillary defect manifest by prolonged bleeding time, a deficiency of factor VIII in many cases, and decreased platelet adhesiveness, as demonstrated by the Salzman test. The clinical manifestations are nosebleeds and increased bleeding after trauma or surgery. The tourniquet test result and bleeding time are usually abnormal. Although fresh plasma infusions result in increases in the factor VIII level which are sustained for several days, owing to de novo synthesis, they have an inconsistent effect on the bleeding time. Cryoprecipitate has recently been shown to correct the prolonged bleeding time. It is of interest that the synthesis of factor VIII is controlled by both autosomal (von Willebrand) and X-linked (hemophilia A) genes.

PHASE II DISORDERS

Factors II, V, VII and X are involved in the second phase of coagulation and are designated the *prothrombin complex*. The factors are produced in the liver, and all except factor V require vitamin K for normal synthesis. The laboratory diagnosis of these deficiencies depends upon a prolonged prothrombin time. Significant bleeding does not usually occur until the prothrombin time exceeds 30 to 35 seconds, corresponding to a level of 10 to 15 per cent of normal.

Genetically determined congenital deficiencies of factors II, V and VII have been described, the most common of which is factor V deficiency (parahemophilia, Owren's disease). The clinical manifestations of these deficiencies are mucocutaneous hemorrhages, bleeding into tissues, and hemorrhages after injury. Hemarthroses occur frequently. These deficiencies are refractory to vitamin K therapy, and fresh plasma should be administered for active hemorrhage.

HEMORRHAGIC DISEASE OF THE NEWBORN

Hemorrhagic disease of the newborn is a self-limited bleeding disorder usually occurring on the second or third day of life, and resulting from a deficiency of the coagulation factors dependent upon vitamin K.

The levels of factors II, VII, IX and X are nearly normal in umbilical cord blood, but decline rapidly to reach a nadir at 48 to 72 hours of life. In 0.25 to 0.5 per cent of infants the decline is so extreme that severe hemorrhage may result. Thereafter the levels of these factors slowly increase, but remain below adult values for several weeks. The increase results from absorption of vitamin K from the diet. Cow's milk contains a good level of vitamin K. Breast milk, on the other hand, has quite low levels, and symptomatic hemorrhagic disease of the newborn is much more frequent in breast-fed than formula-fed infants unless vitamin K prophylaxis is given.

CLINICAL MANIFESTATIONS. In most instances hemorrhagic manifestations become evident on the second or third day of life. Melena, bleeding from the navel and hematuria are frequent signs of the disorder. The most serious complications are intracranial hemorrhage and anemic shock.

TREATMENT. Prophylactic administration of vitamin K_1 to the newborn prevents the postnatal decline of the factors of the prothrombin complex and virtually eliminates hemorrhagic disease of the newborn. Preparations of vitamin K_1 are indicated, for they do not have a hemolytic effect as do large doses of synthetic vitamin K analogues. Although vitamin K given to the mother may be beneficial, a therapeutic effect is more certain if the drug is administered to the newborn infant. As little as 25 μg of vitamin K prevents the postnatal decline of the prothrombin complex; the currently recommended dose of 1 mg of vitamin K_1 is safe and effective. Larger doses do not increase the therapeutic effect.

In overt hemorrhagic disease 1 mg of vitamin K_1 should be given by intravenous or intramuscular injection. Clinical hemorrhage usually stops within 2 hours. If intracranial or other serious hemorrhage has occurred, an infusion of 10 to 15 ml/kg of fresh plasma will immediately correct the hemostatic defects. Profound anemia and shock may be corrected by infusions of fresh blood.

Premature infants may experience a complex hemorrhagic state involving multiple coagulation factors as well as platelet abnormalities. Vitamin K therapy is ineffective in correcting the abnormalities, owing to hepatic immaturity. Fresh plasma infusions are indicated if significant hemorrhage occurs.

Vitamin K deficiency rarely occurs after the neonatal period. Intestinal malabsorption of fats and prolonged administration of broad spectrum antibiotics may, however, result in vitamin K deficiency, and cystic fibrosis and biliary atresia may be complicated by disorders of the prothrombin complex. Prophylactic administration of water-soluble vitamin K is indicated in these situations. In the past, certain formulas based on meats or hydrolysates were low in vitamin K, but this deficiency has been corrected. In advanced liver disease, synthesis of the factors of the prothrombin complex may be compromised, owing to hepatocellular damage. Vitamin K therapy is not often effective in correcting the disorders if advanced liver disease is present. The anticoagulant properties of Dicumarol and other coumadin derivatives depend on interference with synthesis of factors II, VII and X. Vitamin K_1 is a specific antidote.

PHASE III DISORDERS

CONGENITAL AFIBRINOGENEMIA. This is a rare hemorrhagic disorder due to homozygous occurrence of an autosomal recessive gene. Despite totally incoagulable blood, these patients usually do not have severe spontaneous hemorrhages or hemarthrosis, but trauma or surgery may be followed by severe bleeding. Therapy with 100 mg/kg of concentrated fibrinogen provides a hemostatic plasma level. Since the plasma half-life of fibrinogen is 5 days, frequent infusions are not necessary. A very high risk of homologous serum hepatitis is attendant upon use of fibrinogen concentrates. Cryoprecipitate also contains fibrinogen, and may be used effectively for replacement therapy.

FACTOR XIII DEFICIENCY (FIBRIN STABILIZING FACTOR). A deficiency of factor XIII is the most recently recognized inherited hemorrhagic disease. Onset is most often in infancy, with bleeding after separation of the umbilical cord stump. Gastrointestinal, intracranial and intra-articular hemorrhages have been the most common clinical manifestations. Routine coagulation studies are normal. Factor XIII deficiency is diagnosed by finding an abnormal solubility of the clot in 5M urea and a short euglobulin lysis time.

Aballi, A.: The actions of vitamin K in the neonatal period. South. Med. J. *58*:48, 1965.

Bahner, R. L., and Strauss, H. S.: Hemophilia in the first year of life. New Engl. J. Med. *275*:524, 1966.

Bennett, B., and Ratnoff, O. D.: Detection of the carrier state for classic hemophilia. New Engl. J. Med. *288*:342, 1973.

Bleyer, W. A., Hakami, N., and Shepard, T. H.: The development of hemostasis in the human fetus and newborn infant. J. Pediatr. *75*:838, 1971.

Dallman, P. R., and Pool, J. G.: Treatment of hemophilia with factor VIII concentrates. New Engl. J. Med. *278*:199, 1968.

Honig, G. R., Forman, E. N., Johnston, G. A., Seeler, R. A., Abildgaard, C. F., and Schulman, I.: Administration of single doses of AHF (factor VIII) concentrates in the treatment of hemophilic hemarthroses. Pediatrics *43*:26, 1969.

Perkins, H. A.: Correction of the hemostatic defects of von Willebrand's disease. Blood *30*:375, 1967.

Pool, J. G., and Shannon, A. E.: Production of high potency concentrates of antihemophilic globulin in a closed-bag system. New Engl. J. Med. *273*:1443, 1965.

Rabener, S. F., and Telfer, M. C.: Home transfusion for patients with hemophilia A. New Engl. J. Med. *283*:1011, 1970.

The Purpuras

The purpuras are a group of diseases in which small hemorrhages occur into the superficial layers of the skin, producing areas of purple discoloration. Minute extravasations of blood about the small vessels are recognized as petechiae; more extensive hemorrhages cause ecchymoses. Bleeding may also occur from the mucous membranes and into other organs and tissues. The purpuras may be classified into two general groups according to platelet count. In *thrombocytopenic purpuras* the platelet count is reduced below 40,000 per mm^3, and hemorrhages are due to this quantitative deficiency. In *nonthrombocytopenic purpuras,* bleeding results from defects in the small blood vessels or from defective platelet function despite their adequate numbers.

NONTHROMBOCYTOPENIC PURPURAS

Platelets are non-nucleated, cellular fragments produced by the megakaryocytes of the bone marrow. The large size of the megakaryocyte reflects its polyploidy. As the megakaryocyte reaches maturity, extreme fragmentation of the cytoplasm occurs, and large numbers of platelets are liberated. They have a life span in the circulation of 7 to 10 days. The platelet has a number of intrinsic antigens, which are distinct from those of the red blood cell, but some are shared by the leukocytes.

The platelets are intimately involved in both the vascular and the clotting aspects of hemostasis. They are necessary for integrity of the vascular endothelium; when small blood vessels are transected, platelets accumulate at the site of injury, forming a hemostatic plug. Platelet adhesion is initiated by contact with extravascular components such as collagen. Release of endogenous ADP causes firm aggregation. Serotonin and histamine liberated during these processes increase local vasoconstriction. Platelets have a phospholipid with partial thromboplastin activity, which makes an important contribution to coagulation. They also transport other blood coagulation factors through adsorption to the platelet surface. Finally, the platelet is necessary for normal clot retraction.

The *normal platelet count* is 150,000 to 400,000 per mm^3. Counts below this range indicate thrombocytopenia, owing either to inadequate production or to excessive destruction or removal of platelets. Inadequate production is almost always due to marrow dysfunction, which decreases the number of megakaryocytes. By contrast, in the thrombocytopenias due to increased destruction, the megakaryocytes are quantitatively normal or increased. The hypomegakaryocytic thrombocytopenias result from aplasia of the marrow or from its infiltration by abnormal or neoplastic tissue. Because of the grave prognosis of such disorders, bone marrow aspiration is indicated in every case of significant thrombocytopenia. Bone marrow aspiration can usually be performed without serious bleeding even in the presence of severe thrombocytopenia, since thromboplastins in marrow juice will usually effect hemostasis.

PURPURA ASSOCIATED WITH NORMAL NUMBERS OF PLATELETS

The most common nonthrombocytopenic purpura is *anaphylactoid purpura,* or *Henoch-Schönlein syndrome* (Section 10), an acute inflammatory process of unknown origin involving the small blood vessels of the skin, joints, gut and kidney. The striking centrifugal distribution of the rash and involvement of the legs and buttocks are characteristic, particularly when combined with arthritis, nephritis or gastrointestinal bleeding. The petechiae must be differentiated from those of early meningococcemia or septicemia due to other microorganisms. Demonstration of bacteria in blood expressed from the cutaneous lesions of septicemia is a valuable method for early diagnosis. Septic emboli cause the petechiae observed in bacterial endocarditis. Toxic vasculitis may produce a hemorrhagic rash as a reaction to drugs such as arsenicals and iodides. Similar findings may occur during viral or rickettsial infections.

The *thrombasthenias,* or thrombocytopathic purpuras, are associated with quantitatively normal platelets with defective function. Abnormal function is reflected in petechiae and excessive bleeding. The abnormality of platelet function may also be revealed by defective clot retraction or by failure of the patient's platelets to support normal thromboplastin generation.

ABNORMALITIES OF PLATELET AGGREGATION

A large number of drugs have the property of inhibiting release of endogenous ADP and preventing platelet aggregation. This abnormality can be demonstrated most easily with a platelet aggregometer. The most important drug having this effect is aspirin, but some antihistamines also inhibit platelet aggregation. The effect is not dose-related; following ingestion of the drug the abnormal platelet function persists for 4 to 6 days. Under usual circumstances the effects of these drugs produce no clinical problems, although prolongation of the bleeding time is frequently seen. If, however, the patient has an underlying bleeding disorder such as hemophilia or undergoes a surgical operation, severe hemorrhage may occur. Aspirin or other drugs which inhibit platelet aggregation are contraindicated in these circumstances. Salicylates and antihistamines may have transplacental effects on the newborn's platelet function.

THROMBOCYTOPENIC PURPURAS

IDIOPATHIC THROMBOCYTOPENIC PURPURA

Idiopathic thrombocytopenic purpura (ITP), the most common of the thrombocytopenic purpuras of childhood, is associated with mucocutaneous bleeding and hemorrhages into tissues. There is a profound deficiency of circulating platelets despite adequate numbers of megakaryocytes in the marrow.

ETIOLOGY. The disease often appears to be related to sensitization by viral infections, for in about 50 per cent of cases there is an antecedent disease such as rubella, rubeola or viral respiratory infection. It seems likely that an immune mechanism is the basis for the thrombocytopenia. Platelet antibodies can rarely be detected in acute cases, probably owing to limitations of current methods. During the early stages of the disease the hemorrhagic manifestations are so acute and generalized that a vasculitis or defect of the capillary endothelium has been postulated.

CLINICAL MANIFESTATIONS. The onset is frequently acute. One to 4 weeks after a viral infection, or without antecedent illness, bruising and a generalized petechial rash occur. Hemorrhages in mucous membranes may be prominent, with hemorrhagic bullae of the gums and lips. Nosebleeds are often severe and difficult to control. The most serious complication is intracranial hemorrhage, which occurs in less than 1 per cent of cases. The liver, spleen and lymph nodes are not enlarged. Except for the signs of bleeding, the patient appears clinically well. The acute phase of the disease associated with spontaneous hemorrhages lasts for only a week or two. Even though thrombocytopenia persists, spontaneous mucocutaneous hemorrhages then subside. In some instances the onset is insidious, with moderate bruising and few petechiae.

LABORATORY DATA. The platelet count is reduced below 20,000 per mm^3, and those tests which depend upon platelet function such as the tourniquet test and bleeding time and clot retraction give abnormal results. The white blood cell count is normal, and anemia is not present unless significant external blood loss has occurred.

Bone marrow aspiration reveals normal granulocytic and erythrocytic series, and numerous megakaryocytes. Some of the latter are immature, with deep basophilic cytoplasm; platelet budding may be scanty, but there is no pathognomonic or diagnostic morphology of the megakaryocytes.

DIFFERENTIAL DIAGNOSIS. Idiopathic thrombocytopenic purpura may be differentiated from aplastic or infiltrative processes of the bone marrow by marrow examination. Significant enlargement of the spleen will suggest primary liver disease with congestive splenomegaly, lipidosis or reticuloendotheliosis. Thrombocytopenic purpura may be an initial manifestation of systemic lupus erythematosus, but this sequence is unusual in children; in adolescents the possibility is greater.

TREATMENT. Idiopathic thrombocytopenic purpura has an excellent prognosis even when no specific therapy is given. Seventy-five per cent of patients recover completely within 3 months, most within 8 weeks. Severe spontaneous hemorrhages and intracranial bleeding are usually confined to the initial phase of the disease. After the initial acute phase, spontaneous manifestations tend to subside. Nine to 12 months after the onset, 90 per cent of affected children have regained normal platelet counts, and relapses are unusual.

Fresh blood or platelet concentrates are of no value or of only transient benefit, owing to the very short survival of transfused platelets, but they may be tried when life-threatening hemorrhage occurs. Corticosteroid therapy is of great value; though it has not decreased the number of chronic cases, it does reduce the severity and shorten the duration of the initial phase.

When the disease is mild and hemorrhages of the retina or mucous membranes are not present, no specific therapy may be indicated. The affected child should be protected from falls or trauma. Bacterial infections should be treated with appropriate antibiotics. Vitamins K and C have no therapeutic effect. Although infusions of plasma have been reported to be occasionally followed by sustained rises of platelet count, the efficacy of plasma therapy in ITP is unproved. In more severe cases, therapy with a corticosteroid, such as prednisone in a dose of 1 or 2 mg/kg, or its equivalent, is indicated. This therapy is continued until the platelet count is normal or for 3 weeks, whichever comes first. At this point, steroid therapy should be discontinued even if the platelet count remains low. Prolonged corticosteroid therapy is not indicated and may, in itself, depress the bone marrow. If thrombocytopenia persists for 4 to 6 months, a second short course of corticosteroid therapy may be given. Splenectomy should be reserved for chronic cases and for the severe ones which do not respond to corticosteroids, in which considerable improvement can be expected in most instances. Only about 2 per cent of cases of ITP in children tend to be chronic and refractory to all therapy.

OTHER THROMBOCYTOPENIC PURPURAS

DRUG-INDUCED THROMBOCYTOPENIAS. A number of drugs may be associated with immune thrombocytopenia. It has been clearly shown that quinidine and apronalide (Sedormid) function as haptens which combine with proteins on the platelet surface and stimulate antibody formation. Administration of these drugs to sensitized persons is followed by severe thrombocytopenia. This syndrome is unusual in pediatric practice because the responsible drugs are rarely prescribed. In any case of thrombocytopenia, however, a careful search for any drug exposure should be made, and the patient removed from contact with potential offenders.

WISKOTT-ALDRICH SYNDROME AND OTHER INHERITED THROMBOCYTOPENIAS. The Wiskott-Aldrich syndrome consists of cutaneous eczema, thrombocytopenic hemorrhage, and increased susceptibility to infection due to an immunologic defect. The disease is transmitted as an X-linked recessive trait. Bloody diarrhea or hemorrhage during the first months of life is usually the initial clinical manifestation. The bone marrow contains a normal number of megakaryocytes, but many have bizarre nuclear morphology. Homologous platelets survive normally when transfused into these patients but autologous platelets have somewhat shortened life span. Wiskott-Aldrich syndrome may represent a unique circumstance in which thrombocytopenia results from abnormal platelet formation or release despite quantitatively adequate numbers of megakaryocytes. The immunologic defect involves macroglobulin (IgM) synthesis, as indicated by absence of isohemagglutinins and low levels of IgM. Splenectomy is contraindicated; it has often been followed by overwhelming sepsis and death when it has been performed. A significant number of patients have developed lymphoreticular malignancies. A few cases have been reported to benefit from administration of transfer factor.

A number of other types of inherited thrombocytopenias have been described. Some are X-linked, and some have autosomal transmission. Responses to therapy, including splenectomy, have usually been disappointing. The mortality of young males splenectomized for presumed ITP is inordinately high, suggesting that, even without other stigmata, X-linked thrombocytopenia may represent a variant of Wiskott-Aldrich syndrome.

THROMBOPOIETIN DEFICIENCY. A single child has been described (Schulman) with chronic thrombocytopenia, presumably resulting from a deficiency of a megakaryocyte maturation factor contained in normal plasma. Plasma infusions repeatedly produced a sustained peripheral rise in the platelet count.

THROMBOCYTOPENIA WITH CAVERNOUS HEMANGIOMA. Some infants with large cavernous hemangiomas of the trunk or extremities have severe thrombocytopenia and other evidence of intravascular coagulation. Histologic and isotopic studies indicate that platelets are trapped and destroyed within the extensive vascular bed of the tumor. The peripheral blood shows thrombocytopenia and red cell fragments, and the bone marrow contains adequate numbers of megakaryocytes. Spontaneous thrombosis within the tumor may lead to obliteration of the vascular channels and spontaneous recovery; radiation therapy in a single dose of 600 to 800 r may accelerate this process, but repeated courses may be necessary. When anatomically feasible, external compression or total excision may be attempted, but surgery may be associated with uncontrollable hemorrhage. Other forms of therapy are usually without effect; corticosteroids may hasten involution and warrant trial. Splenectomy is contraindicated.

NEONATAL THROMBOCYTOPENIA

Thrombocytopenia of the newborn has unique aspects which merit special consideration. Thrombocytopenia may reflect primary systemic diseases of the infant's hematopoietic system or be due to transfer of abnormal factors from the mother.

SEPTIC THROMBOCYTOPENIAS. A variety of fetal and neonatal infections may result in significant thrombocytopenic bleeding. These include virus infections (especially rubella and cytomegalic inclusion disease), protozoal infections such as toxoplasmosis, syphilis, and bacterial infections, especially those caused by gram-negative bacilli. Hemolysis is usually also present in infants with prominent anemia and jaundice. The liver and spleen are considerably enlarged. The bone marrow changes are variable, but reduced numbers of megakaryocytes may be seen.

IMMUNE NEONATAL THROMBOCYTOPENIA. About 30 per cent of infants born of mothers with idiopathic thrombocytopenic purpura (ITP) have thrombocytopenia in the neonatal period, owing to transplacental transfer of antiplatelet antibodies. Infants with neonatal disease have been born of mothers with normal platelet count whose disease has been inactive for many years. Petechiae are not present initially, but appear in a generalized distribution within a few minutes after birth. Bleeding from bowel and kidney and intracranial hemorrhage may occur. In mild cases there may be few abnormal findings. Hepatosplenomegaly is not present. The duration of the thrombocytopenia is 2 to 3 months. Although therapy is not strikingly successful, fresh blood, exchange transfusions or platelet transfusions may be of temporary value. Corticosteroid therapy has not been convincingly beneficial. Because of the self-limited nature of the disease, splenectomy is contraindicated.

When the fetus has platelet antigens which the mother does not have, iso-immunization may occur. If maternal antibodies to fetal platelet antigens reach a sufficiently high titer, they may cross the placenta and produce thrombocytopenia in the fetus. The disease may be familial, and first-born infants are frequently affected. The clinical signs include petechiae and other hemorrhagic manifestations. By use of sensitive tests involving complement fixation, antiplatelet antibodies can be demonstrated in about 50 per cent of cases. Exchange transfusion is temporarily effective in stopping bleeding. If compatible platelets can be obtained (these are most easily procured by plasmapheresis of the mother), these offer specific effective therapy.

When the mother has drug-induced thrombocytopenia, both antibody and drug may cross the placenta and cause neonatal thrombocytopenia.

Corticosteroid therapy and especially exchange transfusions should be considered when bleeding manifestations are severe.

CONGENITAL HYPOPLASTIC THROMBOCYTOPENIA WITH ASSOCIATED MALFORMATIONS. Severe thrombocytopenia has been described as a familial condition associated with aplasia of radius and thumbs, and cardiac and renal anomalies. Severe hemorrhagic manifestations are evident in the first days of life. Hemoglobin levels are normal; leukocytosis has been documented in some cases. The only recognized abnormality of the bone marrow is absence of megakaryocytes.

The combination of anomalies in this disease is identical with that observed in Fanconi's pancytopenia, in which the hematologic abnormalities are not usually observed until the third and fourth years of life. Chromosomes do not show the chromatid breaks and other abnormalities which are found in the Fanconi syndrome. No infants with congenital hypoplastic thrombocytopenia have been reported who developed the full blown Fanconi syndrome, nor have cases of both conditions been observed in the same family.

THROMBOCYTOSIS

(Thrombocythemia)

Platelet counts in excess of 750,000 per mm^3 may be designated as thrombocytosis. Markedly elevated counts may accompany hemorrhage, iron deficiency anemia, hemolytic anemias and primary myeloproliferative disorders. After splenectomy for ITP or hemolytic anemia, the platelet count often rises precipitously and may exceed 1,000,000 per mm^3 10 to 14 days postoperatively. In general, no specific therapy such as anticoagulation is necessary, for thrombosis is extremely rare.

A case of primary thrombocytosis associated with thrombotic episodes and myocardial infarction has been described.

Canales, M. L., and Mauer, A. M.: Sex-linked hereditary thrombocytopenia as a variant of Wiskott-Aldrich syndrome. New Engl. J. Med., *277*:899, 1967.

Lusher, J. M., and Zuelzer, W. W.: Idiopathic thrombocytopenic purpura in childhood. J. Pediat., *68*:971, 1966.

McIntosh, S., and Pearson, H. A.: Isoimmune neonatal purpura. J. Pediat. *82*:1020, 1973.

Schulman, I.: Diagnosis and Treatment: Management of Idiopathic Thrombocytopenic Purpura. Pediatrics *33*:979, 1964.

Schulman, I., Pierce, M., Lukens, A., and Currimbhoy, Z.: Studies on thrombopoiesis. I. A factor in normal human plasma required for platelet production, chronic thrombocytopenia due to its deficiency. Blood *16*:943, 1960.

Spach, M. A., Howell, D. A., and Harris, J. S.: Myocardial infarction with multiple thrombosis in a child with primary thrombocytosis. Pediatrics *31*:268, 1963.

Weiss, H. J., and Aledort, L. M.: The effects of salicylates on the hemostatic properties of platelets in man. J. Lab. Clin. Invest. *47*:2169, 1968.

Wolff, J. A.: Wiskott-Aldrich syndrome: Clinical immunologic and pathologic observations. J. Pediat. *70*:221, 1967.

Zinkham, W. H., Osborn, J. E., and Medearis, D. N., Jr.: Blood and bone marrow findings in congenital rubella. J. Pediat. *67*:985, 1965.

CONSUMPTION COAGULOPATHIES AND FIBRINOLYTIC STATES

Consumption coagulopathy is a unifying concept for a group of conditions associated with disseminated intravascular coagulation. Disseminated intravascular coagulation has been described in a large number of clinical states, including incompatible blood transfusions, cyanotic congenital heart disease, hemangioma with thrombocytopenia, fulminating meningococcemia with Waterhouse-Friderichsen syndrome, purpura fulminans and acute promyelocytic leukemia. In some of these states intravascular hemolysis appears to initiate thrombosis. In others diffuse vasculitis may be the primary abnormality, and an endotoxin may be of primary importance in some. Endotoxic shock appears particularly important in the genesis of disseminated intravascular coagulation. Depletion of the consumable coagulation factors (I, II, V and VIII) may be a consequence of this process. Clinical and pathologic features of some of these syndromes have been compared to those of the generalized Shwartzman reaction. Thrombocytopenia and hemolytic anemia with bizarre red cell changes are often prominent.

THE FIBRINOLYTIC MECHANISM

Fibrinolysis, the process of dissolution of the clot, is an essential physiologic mechanism. This mechanism is complex and involves a number of fairly well defined factors, the most important of which is a fibrinolytic enzyme called plasmin and its inactive precursor plasminogen. Thrombin and a urokinase found in urine are particularly potent in the conversion of inactive plasminogen to its active enzymatic form. The fibrinolytic system is activated at the same time that coagulation occurs, with the result that in diseases associated with diffuse intravascular coagulation, increased fibrinolytic activity of the plasma can often also be found, and fibrin degradation products can be found in the circulation. Increased fibrinolytic activity is demonstrated in the test tube by spontaneous dissolution of the clot on incubation of clotted blood, or by a shortened euglobulin lysis time. Spontaneous fibrinolytic states may on rare occasions be associated with hemorrhagic symptoms. It may be difficult to differentiate these primary fibrinolytic states from consumption coagulopathies, in which fibrinolysis is a secondary phenomenon. In consumption coagulopathies, factors I, II, V and VIII and platelets are usually decreased, whereas in fibrinolytic states platelets are usually normal and the other factors inconstantly affected. Treatment with epsilon aminocaproic acid (EACA) may be of value in fibrinolytic states, but is not indicated in consumption coagulopathies.

HEMOLYTIC-UREMIC SYNDROME

(See also Section 15.)

This acute disease of infancy and early childhood usually follows an episode of acute gastroenteritis. Shortly thereafter signs and symptoms of hemolytic anemia, thrombocytopenia and glomerulonephritis develop. Bilateral renal cortical necrosis may occur, and case fatality rates as high as 30 per cent have been reported. Its sometimes epidemic occurrence suggests that an infectious agent may be involved.

LABORATORY DATA. The hemolytic anemia is associated with characteristically bizarre red cell morphology. Many of the red cells are contracted and distorted, with prominence of spherocytes, burr cells and helmet-shaped forms (Fig. 14–3,*E*). A depressed platelet count despite normal numbers of megakaryocytes in marrow indicates excessive peripheral destruction. Tests of the coagulation mechanism may give abnormal results. Protein, red cells and casts are present in the urinary sediment, and grave renal damage is reflected in oliguria and azotemia. Renal biopsy reveals fibrinoid deposits in small blood vessels and glomeruli, which may represent deposition of fibrin on a diffusely damaged endothelium.

TREATMENT. For management of uremia and anuria, see Section 15. Transfusions are indicated for severe anemia. Corticosteroid therapy has not been convincingly beneficial. Heparin, in doses of 50 to 100 units/kg given intravenously every 4 to 6 hours, may halt intravascular coagulation but does not appear to affect survival or prognosis.

THROMBOTIC THROMBOCYTOPENIC PURPURA

This rare and serious disease has many similarities to the hemolytic-uremic syndrome. Diffuse embolism and thrombosis of the small blood vessels of the brain are evidenced by shifting neurologic signs such as aphasias, blindness and convulsions. The prognosis is grave. Laboratory findings include thrombocytopenia and a hemolytic anemia associated with distorted and fragmented red cells. Treatment has been of dubious success, but large doses of ACTH or corticosteroids and emergency splenectomy have been advocated. Anticoagulant therapy may also be of value.

PURPURA FULMINANS

Purpura fulminans is an unusual disease which usually occurs in the convalescent phase of a bacterial or viral infection. Diffuse symmetrical hemorrhages occur, with prominent inflammatory vasculitis and necrosis of skin and subcutaneous tissues, particularly involving the buttocks and lower extremities. Systemic toxicity may be extreme, and mortality is high. In nonfatal cases large areas of gangrenous skin and muscle may slough, leaving areas requiring plastic surgical repair. The platelet count is normal or low. Fragmented red cells may be seen on blood smear. The levels of consumable coagulation factors, especially of fibrinogen, are decreased. Replacement therapy with fibrinogen and fresh plasma transfusions, as well as high doses of corticosteroids, have appeared to be helpful on occasion. Intravenous administration of heparin, 50 to 100 units/kg (0.5 to 1 mg/kg) every 4 to 6 hours, or the use of dextran infusions may arrest the progression of the cutaneous lesions and correct the coagulation defects.

Abildgaard, C. F., Corrigan, J. J., Seeler, R. A., Simone, J. V., and Schulman, I.: Meningococcemia associated with intravascular coagulation. Pediatrics *40*:78, 1967.

Allen, D. M.: Heparin therapy of purpura fulminans. Pediatrics *32*:211, 1966.

Corrigan, J. J., and Jordan, C. M.: Heparin therapy in septicemia with disseminated intravascular coagulation. New Engl. J. Med. *283*:778, 1970.

Edson, J. R., Krivit, W., White, J. G., and Sharp, H. L.: Intravascular coagulation in acute stem cell leukemia successfully treated with heparin. J. Pediatr. *71*:342, 1967.

Hardaway, R. M., III: Syndromes of Disseminated Intravascular Coagulation. Springfield, Ill., Charles C Thomas, 1966.

Lanzkowsky, P., and McCrory, W.: Disseminated intravascular coagulation as a possible factor in the pathogenesis of thrombotic microangiopathy. J. Pediatr. *70*:460, 1967.

Liberman, E.: Hemolytic uremic syndrome. J. Pediatr. *80*:1, 1972.

MacWhinney, J. B., Jr., Packer, J. T., Miller, G., and Greendyke, R. M.: Thrombotic thrombocytopenic purpura in childhood. Blood *19*:181, 1962.

Rodriguez-Erdmann, F.: Bleeding due to increased intravascular blood coagulation. New Engl. J. Med. *273*:1370, 1965.

THE SPLEEN

The spleen has excited speculations of man since antiquity. Pliny believed it to be the seat of mirth and laughter; Galen pronounced it an organ full of mystery. Although no unique cells or tissues occur within the spleen, their particular arrangements and the anatomic relations are responsible for unique functions. The spleen is a large mass of lymphoid and phagocytic reticuloendothelial cells with a complex network of tortuous capillaries and fenestrated sinusoids. These impart the important properties of a biologic filter to the spleen.

FUNCTIONS. A number of functions can be assigned to the spleen, and some of these are germane to hematologic processes and diseases:

Reservoir Function. In lower animals the spleen is a contractile organ, owing to the presence of considerable smooth muscle in the capsule and trabeculae. In man little muscle is present, and the reservoir function is normally not very great. The spleen does release both factor VIII and platelets following infusion of epinephrine. The normal spleen contains only about 25 ml of blood, but when the spleen enlarges for any reason, its content of blood increases. The sequestration crisis of sickle cell states is an exaggeration of reservoir function.

Hematopoiesis. The spleen is a site of active blood formation during fetal life, but by about 6 months of gestation hematopoiesis disappears unless a condition such as hemolytic disease of the newborn is present. In a few exceptional diseases such as thalassemia and osteopetrosis, hematopoiesis persists or is resumed postnatally. The stimulus for this is not known.

"Culling." This term has been used to describe the ability of the spleen by virtue of its unique circulation and structure to remove damaged or abnormal blood cells from the circulation. This function is clearly demonstrated by the fact that red cells and platelets lightly coated by antibodies are selectively sequestered and destroyed by the spleen. The spleen's activity in destroying spherocytes is another example of culling.

"Pitting." The spleen has the ability to remove structures such as Howell-Jolly bodies or siderotic granules from within the red cell without destroying the cell. The peripheral blood of a person with no spleen contains relatively large numbers of these intracellular inclusions.

Destruction of Old Red Cells. The spleen is probably the principal site of destruction of senescent red cells. This function is easily assumed by other portions of the reticuloendothelial system, however, and red cell life span is not significantly increased in the absence of spleen.

Membrane Effect. The normal spleen is postulated to have an ill defined effect on the red cell membrane. When the spleen is absent, red cells are flatter and thinner than normal, increased numbers of target cells are seen, and osmotic fragility is decreased.

Filtering and Immunologic Functions. Because of the intimate relation of the circulating blood with lymphoid and reticuloendothelial elements within the spleen, this organ plays an important role in primary defense against bacteria which gain access to the circulation. The spleen is especially vital in the immature and nonimmune person, for it constitutes the primary site of clearance of organisms such as pneumococci in the absence of specific antibody. The spleen has a relatively minor role in overall antibody formation so long as the antigen is administered by intramuscular or subcutaneous routes, but the spleen is essential to antibody formation in response to small doses of particulate intravenous antigens.

Hormonal Function. It has been postulated that the spleen produces a hormonal substance ("splenin") which exerts an effect on bone marrow activity. There is little evidence for such a hormone, and "hypersplenism" is better explained on the basis of excessive filtering or culling activities. The spleen can be functionally inactive despite clinical enlargement, as has been demonstrated in young children with sickle cell anemia.

CLINICAL EXAMINATION. Careful and gentle palpation of the relaxed abdomen provides reliable information about the size of the spleen. The tip can be felt at the left costal margin in 5 to 10 per cent of normal children and in a higher proportion of children with viral infections. The spleen must be increased to two or three times average size before it can be regularly felt on physical examination. Lesser degrees of enlargement can be detected radiographically. An enlarged spleen must be differentiated from other masses in the left upper quadrant. Useful physical characteristics which aid in identifying the spleen include concealment of its upper margin by the rib cage, the presence of a palpable notch, and the absence of overlying bowel. When it is impossible to be certain of the identity of a mass, isotopic scanning studies are of great value. Short-lived isotopes such as technetium-99m (^{99m}Tc) may be used to label colloidal particles. When these radioactive colloids are injected intravenously, they are rapidly cleared by reticuloendothelial elements in the liver, spleen and, to a lesser extent, bone marrow. Surface scanning permits definition of the size and configuration of the spleen and liver. This technique has proved of great value in demonstrating anatomic abnormalities of the spleen, for the procedure is noninvasive and produces a very low radiation exposure.

The spleen has vascular, lymphatic and reticuloendothelial components; pathologic processes in-

TABLE 14–7 SOME CAUSES OF SPLENOMEGALY IN CHILDREN

I. *Hematologic diseases*
Hemolytic anemias—due to extramedullary hematopoiesis and reticuloendothelial hyperplasia
A. Congenital hemolytic anemias
B. Hemoglobinopathies and thalassemia
II. *Infections*
A. Bacterial: septicemias; typhoid; endocarditis
B. Viral: infectious mononucleosis
C. Protozoal: malaria, toxoplasmosis
III. *Congestive splenomegaly*
A. Secondary to portal or splenic vein obstruction
B. Secondary to intrahepatic disease—cirrhosis
C. Chronic congestive heart failure
IV. *Infiltrations*
A. Lipidoses—Niemann-Pick, Gaucher's diseases
B. Nonlipid reticuloendothelioses
V. *Cysts*
A. Congenital—epidermoid cysts
B. Acquired—pseudocysts
VI. *Neoplasms*
A. Leukemia and lymphosarcoma
B. Hodgkin's disease
C. Hemangioma and lymphangioma
VII. *Miscellaneous*
A. Rheumatoid arthritis (Still's disease)
B. Lupus erythematosus
C. Cysts

volving any of these systems may be manifested as splenomegaly. Table 14–7 lists important causes of splenic enlargement.

CONGESTIVE SPLENOMEGALY
(Banti Syndrome)

The venous outflow from the spleen may be obstructed within the liver or in the portal or splenic veins. This vascular obstruction produces congestion and ultimately splenomegaly. Liver diseases associated with parenchymal inflammation, fibrosis and vascular constriction include postnecrotic cirrhosis, galactosemia, Wilson's disease, cystic fibrosis and biliary atresia. Septic omphalitis, either primary or following umbilical vein cannulation, may progress to portal vein thrombophlebitis and thrombosis. Rarely, congenital or acquired anomalies of the splenic or portal veins may cause obstruction and secondary splenomegaly. In some areas of the world schistosomiasis and malaria are important causes of splenomegaly.

CLINICAL MANIFESTATIONS. Observation or palpation of an enlarged spleen may be the initial indication of the disease. The enlarged spleen may filter out and destroy increased numbers of blood cells and platelets, resulting in thrombocytopenic hemorrhage and anemia. As a response to portal vein obstruction, collateral circulation develops through the short gastric, esophageal, superficial abdominal and hemorrhoidal veins. In a significant proportion of cases, massive gastrointestinal hemorrhage from ruptured esophageal varices may be the first clinical manifestation of congestive splenomegaly.

LABORATORY DATA. Pancytopenia of varying degrees of severity is seen. The bone marrow shows active hematopoiesis with abundant megakaryocytes. Liver function tests may indicate hepatocellular disease. It is possible to measure portal venous pressure, and injection of radiopaque dyes into the spleen will permit radiologic visualization of the splenic and portal veins. This should usually be done under direct vision, for percutaneous needling may lead to laceration of the splenic capsule.

TREATMENT. The site of obstruction must be determined. If only the splenic vein is involved, splenectomy is curative. In cases in which the portal vein is extensively involved or in which intrahepatic obstruction is present, splenectomy will correct pancytopenia, but will not relieve portal hypertension. Portacaval anastomosis, which in general is preferred to splenorenal shunting in the young child, is indicated when portal hypertension is clearly shown or when bleeding from esophageal varices has occurred. Successful relief of portal hypertension may result in decrease in splenic size and improvement of pancytopenia.

ANOMALIES AND TRAUMA

SPLENIC CYSTS. Cysts of the spleen are of two general types: Epidermoid cysts are lined with stratified columnar epithelium. Pseudocysts, which are presumably of post-traumatic origin, have no epithelial lining and are filled with necrotic material and blood. Diagnosis is suggested by an asymptomatic smooth mass in the left upper quadrant which displaces the stomach medially. Isotopic scans with ^{99m}Tc gelatin colloid clearly indicate that the cystic mass is within the substance of the spleen. Splenectomy is indicated.

ACCESSORY SPLEENS. Multiple and accessory spleens are not uncommon. A large cooperative study found one or more accessory spleens in 229 (16 per cent) of 1413 children subjected to splenectomy for various indications. Of these 229 children 145, or 60 per cent, had only one accessory spleen and 10 had 5 or more. Accessory spleens are usually located close to the hilum or adjacent to the tail of the pancreas.

CONGENITAL ABSENCE OF THE SPLEEN. Absence of the spleen occurs as part of an unusual group of anomalies, including complex abnormalities of the heart and great vessels with severe cyanotic congenital heart disease. Apparent dextrocardia and varying degrees of heterotopia of the abdominal viscera are seen. The condition can be suspected from examination of the blood: target cells, increased numbers of spherocytes, intraerythrocytic inclusions such as Howell-Jolly and Heinz bodies and hemosiderin granules are easily demonstrated. The incidence of overwhelming sepsis appears to be increased in congenital asplenia.

HYPERSPLENISM. Hypersplenism is not a specific diagnosis, but rather a descriptive term for a clinical complex which includes (1) depression of one or more of the cellular elements of the blood; (2) active formation of that element in the bone marrow; (3) an enlarged spleen, which may be due to a large number of causes (Table 14–7); and (4) correction of the hematologic abnormalities by splenectomy. A diagnosis of primary hypersplenism is difficult to establish; other causes of splenomegaly with secondary pancytopenia must be excluded.

FUNCTIONAL ASPLENIA. Occasionally, anatomically enlarged spleens may be devoid of reticuloendothelial activity. This has been most clearly demonstrated in infants and young children with sickle cell anemia. In the great majority of these children ^{99m}Tc scans fail to demonstrate RES activity of the anatomically enlarged organ. Howell-Jolly and Heinz bodies are seen in the blood. Young children with sickle cell anemia are 600 times more likely to develop pneumococcal meningitis and sepsis than their normal peers, and this propensity to infection is, in part, due to defective splenic function. Functional asplenia can be temporarily reversed with transfusion of normal red blood cells; after years autoinfarction ultimately reduces the spleen to a siderofibrotic nubbin.

RUPTURE OF THE SPLEEN. Traumatic injury of the spleen may result from a hard, direct blow to the left flank or left side of the abdomen, such as may occur during automobile accidents or contact sports. If the tear in the splenic capsule is small, the symptoms may be moderate and include left upper quadrant or left shoulder pain and signs of peritoneal irritation due to blood. In more extreme cases, shock may develop rapidly. When the spleen is pathologically enlarged, rupture may occur after relatively minor trauma. This occurs in the newborn infant with hemolytic disease, and in the older child with infectious mononucleosis. Laparotomy and splenectomy are indicated when rupture is suspected or diagnosed. Isotopic scanning has been valuable in demonstrating lacerations and hematomas of the spleen.

SPLENECTOMY

Removal of the spleen is a common operation which is performed for a variety of indications. Primary surgical indications include (1) rupture of the spleen; (2) removal of tumors, cysts or vascular anomalies involving the spleen; (3) when necessary for adequate surgical exposure of the left upper portion of the abdomen; (4) as part of certain shunting procedures; and (5) for relief of mechanical distress due to massive enlargement in thalassemia major or Gaucher's disease.

Hematologic indications include (1) congenital hemolytic states such as hereditary spherocytosis and elliptocytosis, and some cases of nonspherocytic anemias such as pyruvate kinase deficiency; (2) autoimmune hemolytic anemia when chronic and refractory to corticosteroid therapy; (3) chronic idiopathic thrombocytopenic purpura (ITP); and (4) hypersplenism. The results derived from the operation vary considerably with the basic disease process.

OVERWHELMING SEPSIS FOLLOWING SPLENECTOMY. There is general agreement that removal of the spleen alters host resistance and that overwhelming and often fatal meningitis and septicemia are seen with increased frequency in asplenic persons. The consequences and risks vary considerably, depending primarily upon the disease for which splenectomy is performed and to a less extent upon the age of the patient.

The risk of overwhelming sepsis is low (0.5 to 1 per cent) when splenectomy is done for traumatic rupture, hereditary spherocytosis and ITP. A higher incidence of infection is seen when the indication is thalassemia major, or histiocytosis and lipidosis. The risk is inordinately high when there is an underlying disease which in itself has a predisposition to infection, such as the Wiskott-Aldrich syndrome. The risk is somewhat increased in all categories for younger infants and children, but cases have occurred at all ages and regardless of the indication for splenectomy. Severe infections after splenectomy, usually meningitis and septicemia, are characterized by an acute and fulminating course, death frequently occurring within 12 to 24 hours after onset of symptoms. In more than 60 per cent of cases, pneumococci are the responsible agents; *Hemophilus influenzae* and meningococci are responsible for a smaller number of infections. Because of this risk, splenectomy should be performed only for pressing indications, and when possible the operation should be deferred until after 3 to 4 years of age. Prophylactic penicillin has been advocated for the young child during the first year or two after splenectomy, but there are no data adequately assessing the effectiveness of such management.

Crosby, W. H.: Normal functions of the spleen relative to red blood cells; A review. Blood *14*:399, 1959.

Ellis, E. F., and Smith, R. T.: The role of the spleen in immunity. Pediatrics *37*:111, 1966.

Eraklis, A. J., and Feller, R. M.: Splenectomy in childhood: A review of 1413 cases. J. Pediat. Surg. 7:382, 1972.

Eraklis, A. J., Kevy, S. V., Diamond, L. K., and Gross, R. E.: Hazard of overwhelming infection after splenectomy in childhood. New Engl. J. Med. *276*:1225, 1967.

Pearson, H. A., Spencer, R. P., and Cornelius, E.: Functional asplenia in sickle cell anemia. New Engl. J. Med. *281*:923, 1969.

Pearson, H. A., Spencer, R. P., and Touloukian, R.: The binary spleen: A radioisotopic scan sign of splenic pseudocyst. J. Pediatr. 77:216, 1970.

Schulkind, M. L., Ellis, E. F., and Smith, R. T.: Effect of antibody upon clearance of I^{125}-labelled pneumococci by the spleen and liver. Pediat. Res. *1*:178, 1967.

THE LYMPHATIC SYSTEM

The lymphatic system includes the free lymphocytes of the blood and lymph as well as the organized lymphatic structures such as lymph nodes, spleen, Peyer's patches, appendix and tonsils. The origin of lymphocytes is uncertain; some are believed to originate in the embryonic thymus, from which their progenitors migrate to populate other lymphatic tissues. Others, or all, may arise from other tissues such as the lymphoid areas of the gastrointestinal tract, tonsillar area, or the appendix.

The lymph vessels start as small capillaries between the cells of all organs except the brain and the heart. Small lymphatic capillaries join to form progressively larger channels which drain the extremities, trunk and head. The largest of the lymphatic vessels is the thoracic duct, which discharges most of the central return of body lymph into the left subclavian vein.

The lymph channels are characteristically interrupted by lymph nodes. These well defined structures are networks of dilated sinusoids lined by reticuloendothelial elements and surrounded by masses of actively proliferating lymphocytes. The lymph nodes are located in groups, through which the lymphatic drainage of well defined anatomic areas passes. Because of their locations and structure, the lymph nodes function as protective barriers to the spread of infections. They also filter particulate antigens, and the lymphocytes and plasma cells within lymph nodes actively participate in antibody formation.

The superficial lymph nodes are evaluated by palpation. Small nodes can normally be felt in the neck, axillae and groin. Roentgenograms of the chest assess enlargement of the mediastinal lymph nodes. Lymphangiography permits evaluation of the size and structure of the pelvic and retroperitoneal lymph nodes.

The lymph is a clear fluid. It has a protein content intermediate between that of interstitial fluid and plasma and contains a substantial number of small lymphocytes.

DISEASES OF THE LYMPH VESSELS

ACUTE LYMPHANGITIS. This is an inflammation of the lymphatics draining an area of acute infection, usually bacterial. It is manifested as red painful streaks radiating proximally from the infected site. Painful swelling of the regional nodes is also usually present.

LYMPHEDEMA. Lymphedema is a diffuse, permanent pitting edema due to obstruction of the lymph drainage of an area, usually an extremity. Congenital lymphedema occurs in so-called Milroy s disease and as part of the syndrome of gonadal dysgenesis. Acquired lymphedema may result from inflammatory processes or from surgical or radiologic obliteration of lymph nodes or lymph channels.

DISEASES OF THE LYMPH NODES

Enlargement of the lymph nodes occurs in response to a wide variety of infectious, inflammatory and neoplastic processes. Enlargement of a single node or group of nodes is most frequently due to an infection in the area it drains. Generalized lymphadenopathy occurs in many acute infections, especially rubella, rubeola, typhoid, tularemia and infectious mononucleosis. Leukemia, lymphoma and reticuloendotheliosis are sometimes accompanied by striking degrees of lymph node enlargement. Malignant tumors such as neuroblastoma sometimes metastasize to lymph nodes, and large numbers of lipid-bearing histiocytes may be present in the lymph nodes of Gaucher's disease and other lipidoses.

ACUTE LYMPHADENITIS

As a result of cellulitis or other infections, bacteria and toxins and other by-products of acute inflammation are carried in the lymph to regional lymph nodes where an acute inflammatory process occurs. Bacteria may cause abscess formation. Acute cervical adenitis secondary to acute pharyngitis and inguinal lymphadenopathy resulting from infections of the lower extremity are common. The involved nodes become swollen and painful, and the overlying skin is hot and red. Although the primary infectious process is usually obvious, the site of inoculation may not be apparent, as in cat-scratch disease. Mediastinal lymphadenitis secondary to pulmonary infections may produce obstructive symptoms and cough. Mesenteric lymphadenopathy may, on occasion, be associated with crampy abdominal pain simulating appendicitis.

TREATMENT. Antibiotic therapy which is appropriate for the primary infection will benefit the lymphadenitis. When suppuration occurs, needle aspiration or surgical drainage is necessary.

CHRONIC LYMPHADENITIS

Chronic infection or inflammation is frequently associated with hyperplasia of the lymph nodes. Tuberculous infections regularly result in regional lymphadenopathy. Scrofula, or chronic cervical lymphadenopathy, may be secondary to infection of the nasopharynx with bovine tuberculosis. This organism is uncommon in the United States, where chronic lymphadenopathy is more often due to infection by atypical acid-fast organisms. The organisms are trapped in the nodes, where granuloma and caseous necrosis occur. Affected nodes are hard, nontender and frequently matted to adjacent tissues. Biopsy may be necessary to differentiate chronic infections from malignant processes.

LYMPHORETICULAR MALIGNANCIES

Hodgkin's Disease

Hodgkin's disease is a lymphoreticular malignancy with a histologic picture characterized by varying numbers of reticulum cells, lymphocytes, eosinophils and fibrosis, with disruption of normal lymph node architecture. Multinucleated giant cells (Reed-Sternberg cells) constitute a diagnostic and prognostic feature.

ETIOLOGY. The etiology of Hodgkin's disease has eluded detection. Clusters of cases have been interpreted as suggesting that an infectious agent might be involved. The disease is unusual in the first decade of life, but becomes more frequent thereafter.

CLINICAL MANIFESTATIONS. Lymphadenopathy is the commonest presenting feature of Hodgkin's disease. The posterior cervical chain of lymph nodes is most commonly involved, but occasionally axillary, anterior mediastinal, retroperitoneal and inguinal lymph nodes may be primarily affected. The nodes are firm to examination, discrete, and not painful. Diagnosis is based upon histologic examination of an excised lymph node or other tissue showing the characteristic malignant changes.

The management and prognosis of Hodgkin's disease are influenced by three factors: histopathology, clinical stage, and the presence or absence of systemic symptoms. There are four histopathologic classes: lymphocyte predominance, nodular sclerosis, mixed type, and lymphocyte depletion. In general, the more aggressive growths are associated with few lymphocytes, disorderly fibrosis, and many Reed-Sternberg cells. The lymphocyte depletion variety has a particularly poor prognosis. The nodular sclerosis variety predominates in most series of pediatric cases.

Clinical staging of Hodgkin's represents a systematic attempt to determine the extent of dissemination of the disease. In stage I the disease is limited to lymph nodes of a single anatomic region; in stage II the lymph nodes in two contiguous or noncontiguous anatomic regions on the same side of the diaphragm are involved; in stage III disease is present both above and below the diaphragm, but limited to lymph nodes, spleen and Waldeyer's ring; and in stage IV there is such visceral involvement as of lung, liver, bowel, bone and/or bone marrow.

The subclassifications A or B are appended to the anatomic stages in accordance with the presence (B) or the absence (A) of systemic symptoms of fever, night sweats and weight loss greater than 10 per cent of body weight.

Because staging has an important bearing on treatment and prognosis, an extensive examination is carried out, including, in all cases, detailed history and physical examination, chest roentgenogram, skeletal survey, intravenous urogram and bone marrow biopsy. Further specialized procedures may include lymphangiogram and liver scan, and in many centers a laparotomy is performed for diagnostic staging, at which time biopsy specimens are taken from multiple retroperitoneal lymph nodes and from the liver, and splenectomy is performed.

TREATMENT. Radiation therapy is the preferred treatment for stage I and II disease and possibly stage III A. Large doses (4000 to 4500 r) of high voltage radiation are administered to a field which includes all lymph node-bearing areas on the same side of the diaphragm as the presenting tumor. This involves so-called mantle and inverted Y radiation ports.

In stage IV disease, and probably in III B, it is impossible to effect a cure with radiation, but therapy with a combination of chemotherapeutic agents markedly increases duration of useful survival. The frequently used regimen (MOPP) for stage III B and stage IV Hodgkin's disease employs cycles of nitrogen mustard (*M*ustargen), vincristine (*O*ncovin), *p*rednisone and *p*rocarbazine. Given in cycles for 6 months to patients with stage IV Hodgkin's disease, this combination produced complete remissions in 81 per cent, with a median duration of remission greater than 18 months.

COURSE AND PROGNOSIS. Without therapy the course of Hodgkin's disease is relentless and fatal. Treated with extended field radiation, the prognosis of stage I and II A disease is excellent, control and probable cure having been obtained in about 80 per cent of cases. In stages III and IV, with combination chemotherapy substantial numbers of patients are alive and apparently free of disease for up to 6 years. These encouraging results have been obtained by radiotherapists and chemotherapists with experience in the management of these diseases; their consultation should generally be sought.

Non-Hodgkin Lymphomas

The modern classification of the lymphoreticular malignancies exclusive of Hodgkin's disease divides them into two groups, in accord with the predominant cell type. The lymphocytic or lymphoblastic varieties correspond to lymphosarcoma and the histiocytic variety to reticulum cell sarcoma.

ETIOLOGY. The cause of these malignancies is unknown. They occur with markedly increased frequency in diseases involving defects of the immune mechanism, such as Wiskott-Aldrich syndrome and ataxia-telangiectasia. One particular form, the *Burkitt lymphoma of African children,* is the first human malignancy in which evidence for a viral origin or relation is considered convincing.

This tumor has a clinical predilection for the jaws. The histologic picture is characteristic. Sheets of primitive lymphoblasts are interspersed with large, pale, lipid-filled histiocytes. This tumor is prevalent in areas of Africa where climatic conditions are favorable for virus-bearing arthropod vectors; Epstein-Barr (EB) virus can be demonstrated and grown in tissue cultures from these tumors. It is not clear, however, whether or how viruses are related to the more usual cases of lymphoreticular malignancy. Sporadic cases of Burkitt lymphoma have been described throughout the world.

CLINICAL MANIFESTATIONS. Lymph node involvement is the most common initial manifestation. The area most commonly affected is the posterior cervical triangle; next, the axillary and inguinal regions. Mediastinal and retroperitoneal areas may be affected in the absence of superficial involvement. Mediastinal lymphadenopathy may produce respiratory symptoms or cough by compressing the airway. In addition to mechanical symptoms due to the enlarged nodes, systemic manifestations such as fever and weight loss are common constitutional symptoms.

In some centers staging procedures similar to those described for Hodgkin's disease are employed. Extranodal involvement is much more common, however, than in Hodgkin's disease.

In about 20 to 30 per cent of cases the blood and bone marrow may be invaded, with a clinical and hematologic picture indistinguishable from that of acute lymphoblastic leukemia.

TREATMENT. Surgical biopsy is essential to obtain adequate tissue for histologic diagnosis. If complete excision of the affected node is feasible at the time of biopsy, this is advisable, but extensive surgical procedures are not indicated.

These malignancies are sensitive to radiation, which constitutes a mainstay of therapy. In localized disease, cure is possible. Radiotherapy should be given in doses of 3000 to 4000 r. to the primary lesion and to the adjacent lymph node regions. When respiratory symptoms are present, radiation therapy should be administered cautiously, for edema may occur, temporarily aggravating the degree of obstruction. Chemotherapy may be particularly useful in this situation.

In disseminated disease smaller amounts of radiation delivered to the most significant tumor masses are of considerable palliative value.

Chemotherapy is useful in these diseases, and the alkylating agents, nitrogen mustard and cyclophosphamide, are most frequently used. Nitrogen mustard in a total dose of 0.4 mg/kg is administered in 1 or 2 intravenous injections. Care should be exercised, for the drug is vesicant when extravasation occurs. Cyclophosphamide may be given either orally in a daily dose of 2.5 mg/kg or intravenously in a weekly dose of 10 to 15 mg/kg. Nitrogen mustard therapy usually results in prompt relief of constitutional symptoms and reduction in size of the lymph nodes. The clinical improvement following chemotherapy may last for many months. Chemotherapy with multiple agents has proved more effective than single drug therapy. One regimen employs Cytoxan, Oncovin, arabinosylcytosine and prednisone (COAP) in combination.

COURSE AND PROGNOSIS. Without treatment the prognosis is, in general, very grave. With treatment of disease localized at presentation, the outlook is much better; 5-year survival rates of 50 per cent have been reported. In disseminated disease, therapy is often effective in extending comfortable life for many months, and in some cases very long survival may be obtained with aggressive treatment.

HOWARD A. PEARSON, M.D.

Burkitt, D.: Determining the climatic limitations of children's cancer common in Africa. Brit. Med. J. *2*:1019, 1962.

Butler, J. J.: Hodgkin's Disease in Children in Neoplasia in Childhood. Chicago, Year Book Medical Publishers, Inc., 1969, p. 267.

Carbone, P.: Non-Hodgkin's lymphoma: Recent observations on natural history and intensive treatment. Cancer *30*:1511, 1972.

De Vita, V. T., Canellos, G. P., and Moxley, J. H.: A decade of combination chemotherapy of advanced Hodgkin's disease. Cancer *30*:1495, 1972.

Jones, B., and Klingberg, W. G.: Lymphosarcoma in children—A report of 43 cases and a review of the recent literature. J. Pediatr. *63*:11, 1963.

Kaplan, H. S.: Clinical evaluation and radiotherapeutic management of Hodgkin's disease and the malignant lymphomas. New Engl. J. Med. *278*:892, 1968.

Rubin, P.: Updated Hodgkin's disease. A. Introduction; B, Curability of localized disease; C. Advanced disease and special problems. J.A.M.A. *222*:1292, 1972; *233*:49, 164, 1973.

15
THE URINARY SYSTEM

THE KIDNEY

Renal Anatomy

The kidneys are paired organs lying in the abdomen at the level of the first to fourth lumbar vertebrae. They normally lie in the flank at or slightly above the level of the umbilicus and can usually be palpated in the neonate. The kidneys, ureters and bladder are retroperitoneal structures. The external surface of the kidney of the fetus is lobulated; the lobulations gradually disappear as the parenchymal mass expands with age. Each kidney contains 8 to 12 pyramidal lobes. The base of each lobe forms the kidney surface and the apex is the papilla, which enters the collecting system at a minor calyx. Each lobe consists of two principal zones: (1) the cortex, the outer zone, where the glomeruli and the proximal and distal convoluted tubules are located; and (2) the medulla, the inner or deeper zone, where the vasa recta and the descending and ascending limbs of the loop of Henle and the collecting ducts are located. These structures are arranged in a fan-like distribution and funnel toward the tips of the medullary pyramids, where the urine is delivered through the ducts of Bellini (formed by the fusion of many collecting ducts) into the minor calyces. These are subdivisions of the superior and inferior major calyces which unite to form the renal pelvis, from which urine drains into the ureter and is transported by active peristalsis to the bladder.

BLOOD SUPPLY. In proportion to their weight, the kidneys receive the greatest blood flow (20 to 25 per cent of the cardiac output) of any organ.

The renal or main artery of each kidney arises from the aorta; occasionally a kidney may have more than one such artery. The principal branches, termed interlobar arteries, pass dorsally and ventrally to the renal pelvis between the pyramids or lobes. At the junction of cortex and medulla, the interlobar arteries divide to form the arciform arteries which run between the cortex and medulla parallel to the surface of the kidney. The arciform arteries, in turn, divide into the interlobular arteries, which enter the cortex and run perpendicularly to the kidney surface (Fig. 15–1). The interlobular arteries give rise to the afferent arterioles, each of which supplies a glomerulus. About 50 μ before the afferent arteriole enters the glomerulus there is a change in the pattern of the muscle cells of the arteriolar media, and they assume the appearance of secretory cells containing granular deposits believed to be renin. This region, which is at the vascular pole of the glomerulus, is called the *juxtaglomerular apparatus.* Just beyond the point at which the arteriole enters Bowman's capsule, it subdivides into several main branches which in turn branch into a rich network of individual capillary loops. These subsequently reunite to form the *efferent arteriole,* which emerges from the glomerulus at the vascular pole; this arteriole does not have granulated cells. At the vascular pole the renal tubule, in returning to the cortex, makes tangential contact with the afferent arteriole of its own glomerulus. At this area of contact the tubular epithelium adjacent to the arteriole changes. The cells become narrower and their nuclei prominent and crowded together. This region of the tubule is known as the *macula densa.*

The blood supply to *cortical nephrons* is different from that of nephrons situated at the junction of cortex and medulla – the so-called *juxtamedullary nephrons* (Fig. 15–2). The diameter of the efferent

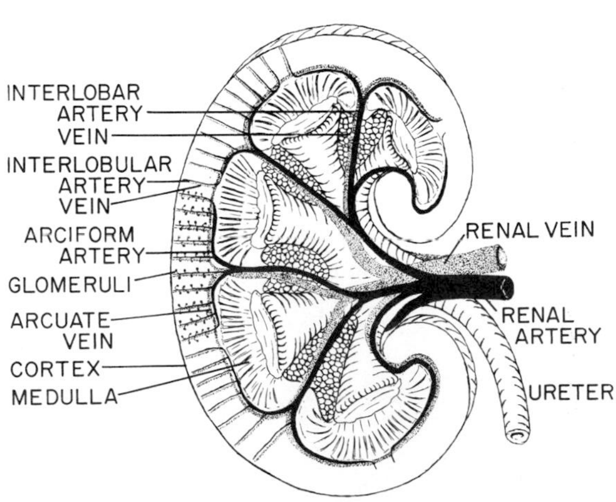

Figure 15–1 *Gross morphology of the renal circulation. (From Pitts, R. F.: Physiology of the Kidney and Body Fluids. 3rd ed. Chicago, Year Book Medical Publishers, Inc., 1974. Used by permission.)*

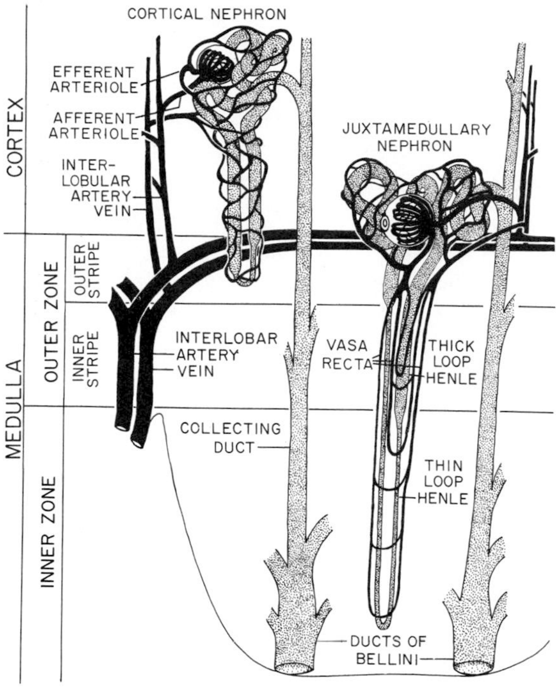

Figure 15–2 Comparison of the blood supplies of cortical and juxtamedullary nephrons. (From Pitts, R. F.: Physiology of the Kidney and Body Fluids. 3rd ed. Chicago, Year Book Medical Publishers, Inc., 1974. Used by permission.)

arteriole of a cortical nephron is slightly less than that of the afferent arteriole, whereas in the juxtamedullary glomerulus the efferent arteriole is slightly larger. The efferent arteriole of the cortical nephron divides into a freely anastomosing network of capillaries which surround proximal and distal convoluted tubules and the cortical parts of Henle's loop and the collecting ducts; there is free communication with the capillary network derived from other nephrons. The walls of these capillaries are extremely thin and are in very close proximity to the membrane surrounding each tubule, the distance between the tubular membrane and the lumen of a capillary being no more than 0.1 μ. The cortical capillaries finally merge to form the interlobular veins.

The efferent arterioles of the juxtamedullary nephrons give off side branches which provide a capillary network for their proximal and distal convoluted tubules. In addition, the efferent arterioles of the juxtamedullary nephrons branch repeatedly and give rise to the *vasa recta.* These are recurrent arterial loops which run parallel to the loop of Henle as it descends through the medulla to the papillae. The vasa recta turn at the bend of the loop and ascend to the juxtamedullary region where they reunite to enter the interlobular vein. The vasa recta function as countercurrent exchangers, as described under Water Balance and Urine Concentration in the following section on Renal Physiology.

The general pattern of venous drainage corresponds to that of the arterial supply.

THE NEPHRON. The functioning unit of the kidney in terms of formation of urine is the nephron, of which there are about one million in each kidney. Each nephron has a number of different anatomic and functional components, which will be discussed separately below. The nephrons whose glomeruli lie in the zone adjacent to the medulla, the so-called juxtamedullary nephrons, differ from the more superficial nephrons in that their loops of Henle extend deep into the medulla, their blood supply is different, and they play a different role in regulation of salt and water excretion. The ratio of cortical to juxtamedullary glomeruli is about 7:1.

THE GLOMERULUS. The glomerulus (average diameter, 110 to 160 μ) is the filtering apparatus of the nephron and, as such, initiates the formation of urine. The adult numbers of glomeruli are present by the time the fetus attains a weight of 2 to 2.5 kg. The glomerulus consists of an intricate spherical-shaped, convoluted capillary network, arising from the afferent arteriole. The walls of the capillaries of this network form a membrane across which the process of filtration occurs. Under electron microscopy (Fig. 15–3) this membrane is seen to have three layers: (1) an inner layer of *endothelial cells* which are continuous with the endothelial cells of the afferent arteriole; (2) the *glomerular basement membrane proper,* which is an uninterrupted highly convoluted membrane about 1200 Å in thickness. It is formed of a glycoprotein consisting of a nonfibrillar collagen-like protein and two different carbohydrate complexes, one a disaccharide and the other a heteropolysaccharide; these are linked with specific amino acid residues in the protein chains. Under the electron microscope the glomerular basement membrane appears as an amorphous matrix, but a layering into a dense central zone and less dense inner and outer zones has been described with the use of certain fixation techniques; (3) an outer layer of large *visceral epithelial cells* with extensive cytoplasmic projections which subdivide into *foot processes* and are in direct contact with the glomerular basement membrane. Covering and between these cytoplasmic extensions is a carbohydrate-rich polyanionic mucoprotein, the negative charge of which is derived primarily from the carboxyl groups of sialic acid. Histochemical techniques with such stains as Alcian blue or colloidal iron are required to demonstrate this material.

In addition to the endothelial and epithelial cells of the glomerular basement membrane, there is a third cell type—the mesangial cell. These cells lie centrally within the glomerulus and have cytoplasmic extensions which are in contact with the endothelial cells. In disease they may extend between the endothelial cell and the glomerular basement membrane. Mesangial cells are believed to function in a manner analogous to cells of the reticuloendothelial system and probably remove macromolecular substances from the circulation.

Bowman's capsule surrounds the glomerulus. Its basement membrane is continuous with the basement membrane of the proximal convoluted tubule and is lined on its inner aspect by the parietal

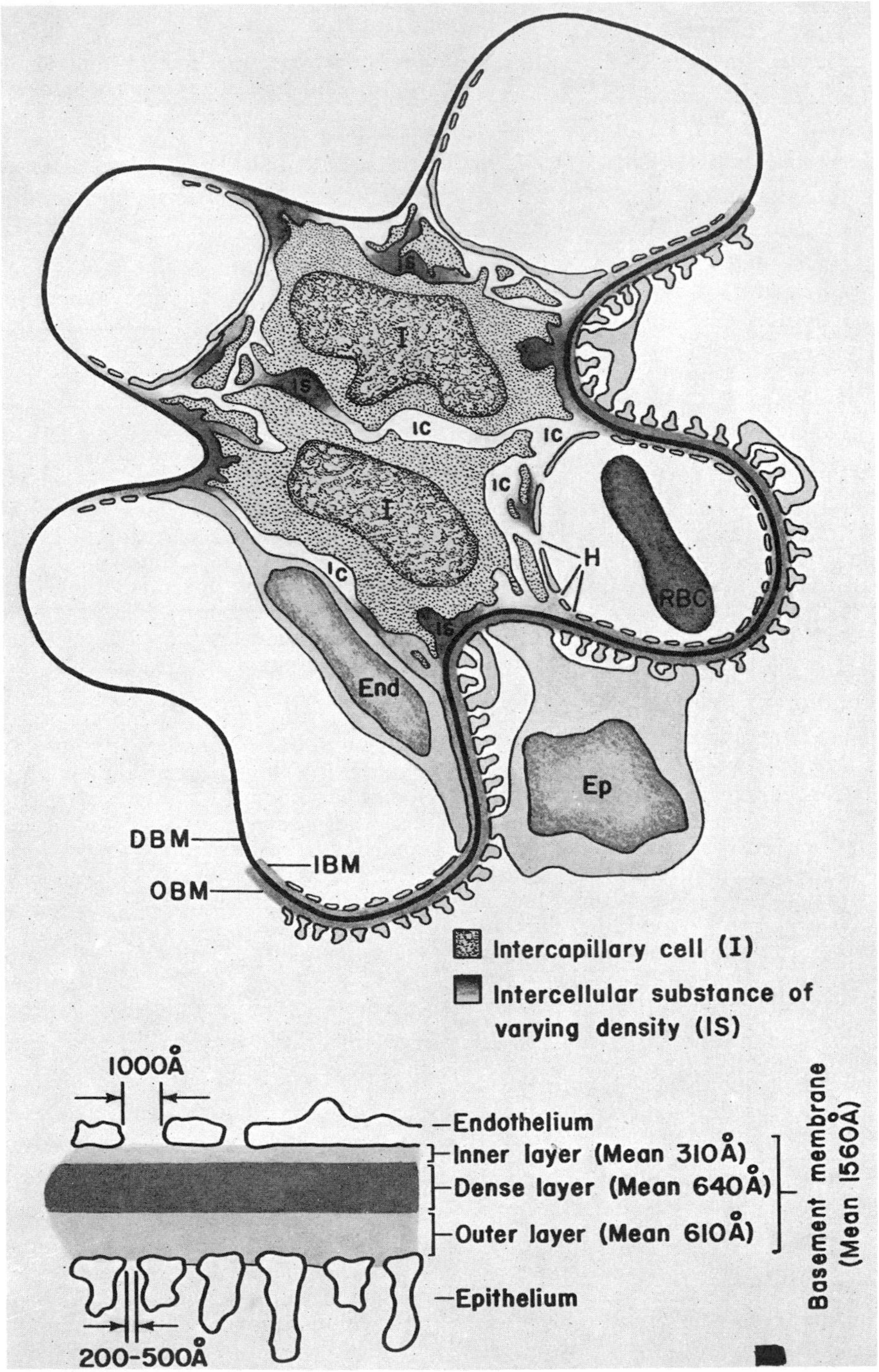

Figure 15–3 Glomerular lobule with its centrolobular region (mesangium). Measurements of the peripheral basement membranes based on a study of rats. Abbreviations: DBM, dense layer of basement membrane (lamina densa); OBM and IBM, outer and inner layers, respectively, of basement membrane; Ep, epithelium; End, endothelium, IC, intercapillary channel; H, holes or gaps in endothelium; RBC, red blood cell. (From Latta, H., Maunsbach, A. B., and Madden, S. C.: J. Ultrastruct. Res., 4:455, 1960.)

epithelial cells. The tubular portion of the nephron begins at an orifice in the capsule usually situated opposite the vascular pole.

THE TUBULES. Distal to the glomerulus, the nephron becomes a tubule, the various segments of which are characterized by their location and histologic appearance; moreover, each segment has distinct physiologic functions. The tubular portions of the nephron are the *proximal convoluted tubule,* the *loop of Henle,* the *distal tubule* and the *collecting duct.* The collecting duct is not, strictly speaking, a part of the nephron, because it arises embryologically from a different source; structurally and functionally, however, it is reasonable to consider it as a part of the nephron. The tubules are enveloped by a continuous basement membrane throughout their length that joins a similar basement membrane covering the parietal layer of Bowman's capsule. The tubular basement membrane provides an uninterrupted framework upon which the tubular epithelium rests.

Proximal Convoluted Tubule. The proximal convoluted tubule has the widest diameter of all the tubular segments and is situated in the cortex. Its epithelium is cuboidal and unicellular in depth; the spherical nuclei are situated at the base (contraluminal) surface of the cell. Although the spaces between the cells are difficult to define by electron microscopy, they play an important role as channels through which solutes and water reabsorbed from the lumen by the cells pass to the peritubular capillaries. There is an abundant luminal brush border which increases the reabsorptive surface of the cells and a tight junction between each of the cells. This luminal junction of the cells is relatively impermeable to solute or water, but it is likely that back-diffusion of reabsorbed solute and water into the tubular lumen occurs via these intercellular junctions. Mitochondria are numerous in the cells of the proximal tubule and are situated principally in the basal two thirds of the cell. The basal surface of each tubular cell (*basal plasma membrane*) has numerous infoldings which bring it into close proximity with the mitochondria of the cell. The peritubular capillaries are in immediate proximity to the tubular basement membrane. As will be discussed under Renal Physiology, the proximal tubular cells are engaged in transporting or reabsorbing large quantities of water and solute from the tubular lumen.

Henle's Loop. Henle's loop is the tubular segment which continues from the final straight segment of the proximal convoluted tubule. The extent of development of Henle's loop varies according to the location of its glomerulus within the cortex. Nephrons whose glomeruli are situated in the outer two thirds of the cortex have short or even an absence of loops; those with glomeruli in the inner third of the cortex have longer loops which descend toward the tips of the papillae.

After descending a variable distance into the medulla, the loop changes direction abruptly and turns back on itself to ascend toward the cortex where it becomes the distal tubule. The epithelium of the *descending limb* of the medullary loop is flat and squamous, and the tubular diameter is considerably less than that of the proximal convoluted tubule. This section is called the *thin segment* of Henle's loop and may be confined to the descending portion, or may form the bend of the loop and continue for a variable distance up the ascending limb. The luminal surface of the cells of the thin segment have short, widely spaced microvilli and only infrequent mitochondria throughout the cellular cytoplasm. The *ascending limb* of the loop has a thicker epithelium, with nuclei situated in the luminal half of the cell, and is referred to as the *thick segment.* Numerous rod-shaped mitochondria occupy the basal half of these cells and short microvilli arise from their luminal surfaces. There are cleft-like infoldings of the basal plasma membrane of the cells of the ascending limb which bring it into intimate contact with the mitochondria.

Distal Tubule and Collecting Duct. The distal tubule continues from the ascending limb of Henle's loop. The initial portion, the *pars recta,* continues in a straight course toward its glomerulus. As the distal tubule passes its glomerulus of origin, it makes contact with the afferent arteriole; this portion is the *macula densa.*

Thereafter, the distal tubule becomes convoluted; the cells are cuboidal and have a dense, coarsely granular cytoplasm consisting of numerous mitochondria. The location of the cell nuclei is apical rather than basal, as they are in the proximal tubule. The luminal surface has numerous short microvilli which are coarser and less abundant than the brush border projections of the cells of the proximal tubule.

The collecting duct is formed by the junction of two or more terminal segments of distal convoluted tubules and receives further branches throughout its course toward the medullary papilla. It has a simple cuboidal epithelium. This is the final segment of the nephron and joins one of the ducts of Bellini which receive urine from other collecting ducts and discharge it into a minor calyx at the papillary tip.

Renal Physiology

GLOMERULAR FILTRATION

Formation of urine begins in the glomerulus, where, in response principally to intraluminal hydrostatic pressure, an ultrafiltrate of plasma is formed by filtration across the glomerular basement membrane. Permeability of this membrane to any given molecule is determined primarily by its molecular weight, although the shape and electrical charge of a molecule may also be a factor in determining the ease with which it is filtered. In general, molecules with a weight over 70,000 are not filtered in appreciable amounts in health; the permeability of the glomerular basement membrane to smaller molecules increases in inverse relation to the molecular weight. Inulin, a fructose polymer with a mean molecular weight of 5000, is completely filtrable, as are smaller molecules; the concentration of these substances is thus virtually the same in the ultrafiltrate as in the plasma. By contrast, the barrier to filtration of substances of larger molecular weight is remarkably efficient. For example, the concentration of protein in the filtrate is less than 2 mg/dl, whereas the concentration within the capillary lumen is approximately 7000 mg/dl.

GLOMERULAR FILTRATION RATE. The volume of the filtrate formed per unit of time, usually expressed as ml/minute, is called the glomerular filtration rate (GFR). About 20 per cent of the total renal plasma flow is filtered; this is called the *filtration fraction.* After about 1 year of age the GFR is approximately 70 ml/min/m^2(71 $\pm$ 5) or 100 liters/m^2/day. Such a volume of filtrate in a healthy child would contain about 850 gm of salt, 100 gm of glucose and 5 gm of calcium.

The rate of glomerular filtration depends on four variables:

1. **The permeability of the glomerular basement membrane** is considered to remain constant under normal conditions, but it is possible that the percentage of the total available capillary bed being used for filtration may vary. In glomerular diseases the permeability of the glomerular basement membrane may be altered. In the nephrotic syndrome, for example, molecules such as proteins, which are normally excluded from the glomerular filtrate, pass through into the filtrate. Such a change in permeability has no effect on the rate of filtration of small molecules since the membrane is normally freely permeable to them, so that their concentration in the glomerular filtrate is the same as in the plasma. Reduced permeability of the glomerular basement membrane is rare; in most disorders affecting the glomerulus the basement membrane becomes, if anything, more permeable. In some glomerular diseases, however, there is a progressive fall in the number of functioning glomeruli that leads to a reduction in the total area of the filtering bed and thus to a decrease in GFR.

2. **Intracapillary hydrostatic pressure** is the major determinant of the rate of glomerular filtration. It is dependent on the systemic aortic blood pressure and on the afferent and efferent arteriolar tone.

3. **The intracapsular hydrostatic pressure** opposes the intracapillary hydrostatic pressure and, under normal circumstances, probably does not have a significant effect on GFR. In circumstances, however, in which the outflow from the tubule is reduced, e.g., acute hydronephrosis, an increase in pressure within Bowman's capsule may contribute to reduction in GFR.

4. **Colloid osmotic pressure** is a function of the plasma proteins and is roughly equivalent to a hydrostatic pressure of 25 to 30 mm Hg. This pressure opposes that of the intracapillary hydrostatic force, which drives fluid through the filtering membrane. Under normal circumstances the plasma colloid osmotic pressure is constant and in health has little effect on the regulation of GFR.

TUBULAR REABSORPTION AND SECRETION

REABSORPTION. Since only a fraction of the fluid and solute filtered at the glomerulus is excreted in the urine, it is evident that during the course of the filtrate through the various segments of the tubule a large portion is reabsorbed and returned to the plasma. This process plays a fundamental role in safeguarding against excessive loss of water, electrolytes and other solutes necessary for life. The kidney regulates both the plasma concentration and total body content of these substances by modifying their rate of reabsorption, and thus the amount excreted, in response to differing circumstances. The renal tubular cells are also able to add to or to secrete into the luminal fluid a variety of molecules, including a number of drugs and their metabolites, and other organic compounds.

Tubular reabsorption or secretion can be either passive (i.e., reabsorption occurs in relation to the electrochemical [e.g., chloride ion] or osmotic [e.g., water or urea] gradient) or active (i.e., by a mechanism that requires the expenditure of energy to transport the substance against an electrochemical or concentration gradient). Energy for the active transport of many substances, notably sodium and potassium, is derived from the cleavage of adenosine triphosphate under the influence of sodium or potassium adenosine triphosphatase.

Active tubular reabsorption is mediated by a number of transport mechanisms, each of which is involved in the transport of a limited number of specific compounds. For example, reabsorption of amino acids involves at least five different mechanisms, one for each of the following groups of amino acids: (1) neutral amino acids; (2) cystine, lysine, arginine and ornithine; (3) imino acids and glycine; (4) dicarboxylic acids; and (5) beta amino acids. There is often competition for the transport site within the group of compounds carried by a given mechanism. If the concentration of one of the substances increases in the tubular fluid, it may reduce by competitive inhibition reabsorption of other substances transported by the same system. Capacity for active transport is limited, and the amount of solute expressed in milligrams per minute which can be reabsorbed or secreted varies for different substances. This maximal tubular reabsorptive or secretory rate is known as the **tubular maximum** or **Tm.** Solutes with a Tm for reabsorption include glucose, sulfate, phosphate, amino acids, lactate, malate, acetoacetate, vitamin C and β-hydroxybutyrate. When the Tm of a compound has been reached, any further amount of it filtered by the glomerulus is excreted and thus lost from the body's supply.

SECRETION. In addition to mechanisms with an absolute limit for reabsorptive capacity, two secretory mechanisms are known to exhibit the same characteristic: (1) a heterogeneous group of compounds, of which many are carboxylic or sulfonic acids (e.g., p-aminohippurate, penicillin, a variety of glucuronides and sulfuric acid esters, acetylated sulfonamides, and urologic contrast media such as Diodrast); and (2) organic bases such as guanidine, choline, hexamethonium and histamine. When the plasma concentration of a substance exceeds the level at which the specific mechanisms for its tubular secretion are functioning at full capacity, additional excretion of that substance in the urine, if any, must be by means of glomerular filtration.

RENAL CLEARANCE OF PLASMA SOLUTES

(Glomerular Filtration Rate)

Substances appearing in the urine are removed from the plasma either by glomerular filtration alone or in combination with tubular secretion. The renal clearance of a solute refers to that volume of plasma which can be considered to be completely cleared of a solute in order to account for the quantity of that solute excreted in the urine during a specified time. Thus if the plasma concentration of a solute is p mg/ml and x mg are excreted/min, it follows that the volume of plasma which is totally cleared of this solute $= \frac{\text{x mg/min}}{\text{p mg/ml}} = \frac{\text{x}}{\text{p}}$ ml/min. This volume is referred to as the clearance of that particular solute (glomerular filtration rate—GFR). Conventionally this is expressed in the following way:

$$\text{Clearance (ml/min)} = \frac{\text{UV}}{\text{P}}, \text{ where}$$

U = urinary concentration of solute (mg/ml)
V = urinary volume (ml/min)
P = plasma concentration of solute (mg/ml)

For solutes with a molecular weight sufficiently low to pass freely through the glomerular basement membrane and which are neither reabsorbed nor secreted by the tubule, the amount excreted in the urine (UV) equals the amount filtered (GFR × P), or GFR × P = UV. Thus, $\text{GFR} = \frac{\text{UV}}{\text{P}}$, i.e., the clearance of such a solute is the same as the GFR. Solutes which are handled in this way by the human kidney and whose clearance $\left(\frac{\text{UV}}{\text{P}}\right)$ may be used as a measurement of the GFR include inulin, other polyfructosans, iothalamate, cyanocobalamin (vitamin B_{12}) and mannitol. Measurement of the inulin clearance is generally considered best for the accurate determination of GFR. Despite the fact that there is minimal tubular secretion of creatinine, measurement of the clearance of endogenous creatinine is the most commonly used means of measuring GFR in clinical practice. Unfortunately, because of the difficulties in measuring the true level of creatinine in plasma, determination of GFR by this technique may be imprecise.

RENAL CONTROL OF CONCENTRATION OF ELECTROLYTES IN PLASMA

SODIUM AND CHLORIDE

The kidneys control the volume and osmolality of the extracellular fluid by the reabsorption of **sodium,** its attendant anions, and water from the glomerular filtrate.

PROXIMAL CONVOLUTED TUBULE. Sixty to 80 per cent of sodium filtered is reabsorbed in the proximal convoluted tubules. This fraction varies with contraction or expansion of the extracellular fluid volume, when a greater or lesser proportion, respectively, will be reabsorbed in this segment. The epithelium of the proximal convoluted tubule permits movement of water and sodium not only from lumen to peritubular capillary, but also from peritubular capillary to lumen. The net rate of sodium reabsorption thus represents the difference between these two fluxes. Sodium enters the tubular cell across the brush border membrane and is extruded from the cell across the lateral or basilar peritubular membrane into the interstitial space, from which it then enters the peritubular capillary. The extrusion of sodium from the cell represents transport against both an electrical and a chemical gradient, since the sodium concentration within the cell is much less than in the surrounding fluid. The first step (the entry of luminal sodium into the tubular cell) and the final step (the passage of sodium from the interstitial space into peritubular capillaries) can be accounted for by passive forces. Normally the concentration of sodium throughout its course in the proximal convoluted tubule remains the same as that in the initial glomerular filtrate. For this to occur, an osmotically equivalent amount of water must be removed at each stage from the lumen. It is likely that sodium is actively transported out of the cell into the intracellular spaces and that water is drawn passively by osmotic forces across the cell, so that the fluid emerging for entry into the peritubular capillaries is iso-osmotic to tubular fluid. The transport mechanism of the proximal convoluted tubule is not able to reduce the luminal concentration of sodium below about 75 per cent of the plasma sodium concentration. This limitation is probably the result of high passive permeability in the region of the tight junctions and intercellular spaces, which leads to a leak back from the peritubular surface to the capillary lumen. When the amount of osmotically active solute in the lumen is high, as in diabetes mellitus, a constraint is imposed on the amount of sodium reabsorbed. Passive reabsorption of water is retarded, and the limiting gradient for sodium transport is attained. This osmotic effect is exerted principally at a site distal to the proximal convoluted tubule, most likely in the loop of Henle.

Reabsorption of **chloride** in the proximal convoluted tubule is not fully understood. It has generally been assumed that its reabsorption is passive down an electrochemical gradient, but the possibility of an active transport system exists, particularly in Henle's loop and in the distal convoluted tubule.

LOOP OF HENLE. As will be discussed later under Water Balance and Urine Concentration, sodium and chloride reabsorption in the ascending limb of the loop of Henle is central to the countercurrent multiplier system which is responsible for development of the medullary hypertonicity required for urine concentration. It is now clear that the loop also is important in the overall control of sodium and water reabsorption. When the load of sodium delivered to the loop of Henle is increased or decreased as a result of changes in the amount reabsorbed in the proximal convoluted tubule, the absolute rate of reabsorption in the loop changes in the same direction as the concentration of the load. Most of an excess load is reabsorbed in Henle's loop. In contrast to water reabsorption in the loop, which occurs in the descending limb, all sodium reabsorption in Henle's loop occurs in the ascending portion.

DISTAL TUBULE AND COLLECTING DUCT. Throughout the distal tubule and collecting duct, sodium is reabsorbed against a large concentration gradient from lumen to plasma; there appears to be no limit to the reduction in luminal sodium concentration that can be reached. On the other hand, in comparison with the proximal convoluted tubule and the loop of Henle, the total capacity for sodium reabsorption is more limited. Thus, if the load of sodium reaching the distal tubule increases significantly, reabsorption does not increase proportionately and the added load is excreted in the urine.

REGULATION OF SODIUM EXCRETION. The regulation of sodium excretion is determined by a number of factors:

Tubular Response to Changes in GFR. As the GFR falls so do the amounts of sodium filtered and reabsorbed. Inasmuch as there is a proportionately lesser decrease in the amount of sodium reabsorbed, a greater percentage of the filtered load is returned to the plasma.

Starling's Forces in the Peritubular Capillary. There is a direct relation between the peritubular capillary colloid osmotic pressure, determined principally by the protein concentration, and the rate of sodium and water reabsorption from the proximal tubule. Peritubular hydrostatic pressure may also act in the regulation of sodium and water reabsorption from the proximal tubule. Increased hydrostatic pressure in the peritubular capillaries may retard reabsorption and vice versa. It is possible that these physical factors may alter the efficiency of sodium transport into the intercellular spaces by regulating the leak from the interstitium back into the tubular lumen.

Osmotic Forces Within the Tubular Lumen. As mentioned earlier, the presence in the lumen of a large amount of solute reduces the net reabsorption of sodium.

Aldosterone and Other Mineralocorticoids. These hormones exert their effects primarily on the distal convoluted tubule. It is likely, however, that they act throughout the nephron in enhancing reabsorption of sodium.

Extracellular Volume. Changes in extracellular volume have an important effect on sodium excretion, principally in the proximal nephron. If the extracellular volume increases, so does the excretion of sodium, and vice versa. The effect is not entirely dependent on changes in GFR nor on aldosterone secretion. It is possible that some of the physical factors mentioned earlier are operative. It has been speculated that a natriuretic hormone may be secreted in response to an increase in extracellular volume.

Distribution of Filtration Within the Kidney. It is likely that preferential perfusion of more superficial nephrons enhances sodium excretion, whereas when juxtamedullary or deep glomeruli are perfused a greater percentage of the filtered sodium is reabsorbed.

POTASSIUM

Urinary excretion of potassium varies widely from a small per cent of the filtered load to amounts in excess of that accountable for by filtration. Hence, potassium can be both reabsorbed and secreted by the tubule.

In the *proximal tubule* reabsorption of potassium is directly influenced by the net reabsorption of fluid, which in turn is dependent on active sodium transport. Thus, factors which increase or decrease sodium reabsorption in the proximal tubule have a similar influence on potassium reabsorption, 50 to 60 per cent of which occurs at that site. Potassium is actively reabsorbed in the *ascending limb of Henle's loop*; fluid in the first part of the distal tubule invariably contains less than 10 per cent of the filtered potassium load. The subsequent handling of potassium by the *distal convoluted tubule* and possibly by the collecting ducts largely determines the amount of potassium excreted in the urine. Under states of maximum potassium conservation, continued reabsorption occurs in the distal tubule; with a normal dietary intake or when excretion is increased for other reasons, secretion of potassium is the net result. The postulate that sodium and potassium transport in the distal tubule are tightly coupled is now doubted. It is more likely that potassium secretion occurs as a passive process driven by electrochemical gradients across the luminal and peritubular membranes of the distal tubular cell.

During *systemic acidosis* there is a reciprocal exchange of hydrogen and potassium at the peritubular membrane of the distal tubular cell, leading to a decrease in the potassium content within the cell and to decreased secretion of potassium by the cell. Conversely, during *alkalosis* hydrogen is exchanged for potassium at the peritubular membrane; the amount of potassium available for secretion increases, and potassium excretion is enhanced. This inverse relation of hydrogen and potassium excretion obtains under a wide variety of circumstances.

Urinary excretion of potassium is increased when there are such conditions as persistent increased intake of potassium, respiratory and metabolic alkalosis, increased amounts of circulating mineralocorticoid hormones, or administration of diuretics such as hydrochlorothiazide and furosemide. Potassium excretion is reduced during respiratory and metabolic acidoses.

WATER BALANCE AND URINE CONCENTRATION

The plasma osmolality remains almost constant at 285–295 mOsm/kg H_2O regardless of day-to-day fluctuations in solute and water intake and in sweat and insensible water loss. This constancy is achieved by regulation of the volume and osmotic pressure of the urine in response to changes in plasma osmolality or volume. A fall in plasma osmolality indicates relative excess of water and leads to an increased volume of urine with an osmolality below that of plasma, thus restoring plasma osmolality to normal. Conversely, when plasma osmolality rises above normal, the volume of urine falls and its osmolality rises above that of plasma. This regulation of urine volume and concentration depends principally on the neurohypophyseal-renal axis. Vasopressin is released by the posterior pituitary gland in response to stimuli from osmoreceptor cells in the hypothalamus, which shrink when the *effective osmotic pressure** of the plasma is elevated. This causes production of concentrated urine of decreased volume, which, in effect, restores solute-free water to the plasma. Vasopressin secretion falls as plasma osmolality is reduced to normal. When plasma hypo-osmolality is present, swelling of osmoreceptors occurs and inhibition of vasopressin release results. This leads to the excretion of an increased volume of urine which is more dilute than plasma, and plasma osmolality rises toward normal. The initiation or inhibition of release of vasopressin is graded. This permits the continuous regulation of urine volume and osmolality necessary to maintain a constant plasma osmolality and minimizes fluctuations which would otherwise occur as a consequence of the normal variations in fluid and solute intake.

The intrarenal events which lead to these changes in urine volume and concentration may be described as follows: Plasma ultrafiltrate formed at the glomerulus is modified during its course along the nephron by two fundamental processes: the selective transport of solute from the tubular lumen, and the passive diffusion of water along an osmotic gradient into the renal interstitial tissue. Diffusion of water occurs in the proximal tubule, the descending limb of Henle's loop, the distal segment and the collecting duct. The proximal tubule and descending loop are freely permeable to water at all times, whereas diffusion of water from the distal tubule and collecting duct occurs only in the presence of vasopressin. Sixty to 80 per cent of filtered sodium is reabsorbed in the proximal convoluted tubule by an active transport mechanism. Water and chloride ion are reabsorbed passively along the electrochemical and osmotic gradient which is created. Thus, the remaining 20 to 40 per cent of filtered water, sodium and chloride is presented to the descending limb of Henle's loop in a concentration isotonic to plasma. This portion of the loop is freely permeable to water and solutes, whereas the epithelium of its ascending limb is relatively impermeable to water. Here sodium and chloride are actively transported out of the lumen, leading to progressive dilution of the urine as it flows back toward the cortex. At any point along its course the transport system of the ascending limb can maintain an osmotic gradient of about 200 mOsm between lumen and medullary interstitium. The consequence of sodium and chloride transport from the ascending limb, with retention of luminal water, is the delivery of a dilute urine to the distal tubule. Furthermore, sodium and chloride removed from the ascending limb of the loop are concentrated in the medullary interstitium. As water diffuses from the permeable descending limb, the concentration of the urine and of the fluid in the medullary interstitium becomes progressively more hypertonic as the medullary papilla is approached. This development of a hypertonic medullary gradient is a consequence of the countercurrent multiplier characteristics of Henle's loop. Although a gradient of only 200 mOsm between lumen and medullary interstitium is maintained at any point along the ascending limb, the outward diffusion of water from the descending limb of the loop and movement of solute from the ascending limb into the interstitium creates a gradient whose osmolality approaches 1200 mOsm/kg at the papillae. Sodium reabsorption continues in the distal convoluted tubule. Depending on whether vasopressin is present, water diffuses into the cortical interstitium, which is isotonic to plasma.

If vasopressin is present, luminal urine will have an osmolality of about 285 as it enters the collecting duct. In the presence of vasopressin the urine

*The effective osmotic pressure is that produced by solutes which do not readily penetrate cell membranes; sodium and chloride are primarily responsible for the effective osmotic pressure of extracellular fluid. In contrast, urea, which contributes to the total plasma osmolality, diffuses readily across cell membranes and thus is relatively ineffective in altering distribution of water between intracellular and extracellular spaces.

becomes progressively more concentrated along the course of the collecting duct as water diffuses into the hypertonic medullary interstitium. By the time the urine enters the minor calyces it has by passive osmotic diffusion achieved the same concentration as the fluid in the hypertonic medullary papilla.

If vasopressin is absent, continued reabsorption of sodium in the distal tubule and collecting duct leads to further dilution of the urine. Since the distal tubule and collecting duct are now impermeable to water, diffusion into the hypertonic interstitium does not occur and a dilute urine is formed.

The major influence of vasopressin on water balance occurs in the distal convoluted tubule where, in a state of antidiuresis, approximately 15 per cent of filtered water is reabsorbed as the luminal urine becomes iso-osmotic. Although urine becomes hyperosmotic in the collecting duct, the actual volume of water reabsorbed in this segment is small.

Water, electrolytes and solutes, such as urea, accumulate in the medulla as a consequence of their removal from the tubular urine during its transit through the loop of Henle and the collecting duct. The vasa recta from the efferent arterioles of the juxtamedullary glomeruli are permeable to water and solute and serve as countercurrent exchangers. The osmolality of the blood in these vessels approaches that of the medullary interstitium at any point during their course through the medulla. Free diffusion of solute from the ascending (outflowing) limbs of the vasa recta into the interstitium and thence into the descending (inflowing) limbs permits recirculation of solute within the medulla and serves to avoid dissipation of the medullary osmotic gradient created by the countercurrent multiplier system of Henle's loop. Some solute and water is, however, removed by these vessels.

The countercurrent exchange system of the vasa recta not only maintains a high concentration of sodium chloride in the medullary interstitium, but also serves to trap urea which diffuses from the collecting duct into the interstitium. In the state of antidiuresis, when urea is the major solute contributing to urine osmolality, the concentration of urea in the urine of the collecting duct is about equal to that in the medullary interstitium. Since urea in the collecting duct is osmotically balanced by that in the surrounding medullary interstitium, its contribution to urine osmotic pressure is above and beyond that attained by osmotic equilibration with the high interstitial concentration of sodium chloride. It also follows that urine osmolality will vary directly with the load of urea presented to the collecting duct. If this load is small the concentrating ability of the kidney may appear to be limited, even though this is not the case.

Several factors other than the presence of vasopressin and the ability of the distal convoluted tubule and collecting duct to respond to it may influence urine osmolality. When GFR falls, a proportionately greater amount of sodium chloride and water is reabsorbed in the proximal tubule, and a smaller volume of hypotonic urine is delivered to the distal tubule and collecting duct. Even in the absence of vasopressin the outward movement of water from these segments may be sufficient to result in some concentration of the small volume of urine ultimately reaching the collecting duct.

The presence of nonreabsorbable osmotically active solutes in the tubular lumen (e.g., glucose in diabetes mellitus) imposes a constraint on the amount of water which can diffuse into the hypertonic medullary interstitium. This not only limits the capacity to concentrate the urine maximally but also leads to increased excretion of sodium, since there is a limit to the gradient against which sodium can be reabsorbed while water remains within the tubular lumen.

ACID-BASE BALANCE

See also Hydrogen Ion and Figure 5–7 under Pathophysiology of Body Fluids, Section 5.

In health the hydrogen ion (H^+) concentration of extracellular fluid is maintained within a narrow range of 35 to 40 mEq/l (pH 7.43 to 7.35). The bicarbonate (HCO_3^-)–carbonic acid (H_2CO_3) buffer system plays the key role in maintaining H^+ concentration within this range. Both components of the buffer pair are regulated by remarkably effective homeostatic mechanisms. Carbonic acid concentration is dependent on plasma PCO_2, which is stabilized by the respiratory system; HCO_3^- concentration is regulated by the kidney. The ratio of HCO_3^- to H_2CO_3 determines the H^+ concentration of extracellular fluid and thus fixes the ratios of the other extracellular buffer pairs.

The kidneys participate in regulation of acid-base balance by maintaining the plasma HCO_3^- level between 24 and 26 mEq/l. This is accomplished by reabsorption of HCO_3^- from the glomerular filtrate and by excretion of acid derived from dietary and metabolic sources. On a normal diet the amount of strong acid (H^+A^-) generated by oxidation of dietary sulfur and phosphorus is 1–2 mEq/kg body weight. In the plasma this acid is buffered by bicarbonate ($H^+A^- + Na^+HCO_3^- \rightarrow Na^+A^- + H_2CO_3 \rightarrow CO_2 + H_2O$), leading to depletion of HCO_3^- stores. To maintain normal acid-base balance, HCO_3^- must be regenerated; this is accomplished in the renal tubule by two principal mechanisms: (1) the excretion of H^+ as titratable acid, by which Na^+ is exchanged for H^+ in the phosphate buffer pair Na_2HPO_4/NaH_2PO_4, and (2) secretion of ammonia (NH_3) produced in the tubular cell from glutamine; NH_3 neutralizes secreted H^+ by combining with it to form ammonium ion (NH_4^+). From 25 to 40 per cent of metabolically derived H^+ is excreted as titratable acid; the rest is excreted, fully neutralized by NH_3, in the form of NH_4^+.

HYDROGEN ION SECRETION. The mechanism by which the kidney regulates plasma HCO_3^- is mediated by the secretion of H^+ into the tubular lumen in exchange for Na^+. The source of H^+ is H_2CO_3, which dissociates into $H^+ + HCO_3^-$ and is formed in the tubular cell by the hydration of CO_2. The enzyme carbonic anhydrase (ca) catalyzes this reaction. Cellular HCO_3^- (remaining after H^+ secretion) and Na^+ (reabsorbed from the lumen in exchange for H^+) then enter the peritubular capillaries. Present evidence suggests that the exchange is not specific and that H^+ secretion may occur in the absence of luminal Na^+. Hydrogen ion secretion is active and occurs against an electrochemical gradient at a transport site on the luminal membrane. Active secretion of H^+ against this gradient is opposed by passive back flux; net H^+ secretion is therefore the amount of H^+ secreted minus the passive back flux. The steepest lumen-to-cell gradient is 1000/1, which is achieved in the collecting duct. Poorly reabsorbed luminal buffers such as phosphate bind H^+ and enhance H^+ secretion, as well as increase the epithelial-luminal H^+ gradient.

Even under conditions of maximal acidification, the minimum urinary pH which can be achieved is 4.0 to 4.5 (about 0.04 mEq H^+/l), so that only a very small quantity of free H^+ is excreted. Accordingly, for net excretion of acid to occur, as it must if acid-base balance is to be maintained, secreted H^+ must either be bound by phosphate buffer and excreted as titratable acid, or buffered by NH_3 to form NH_4^+.

When the plasma HCO_3^- concentration is normal, about 97 per cent of total H^+ secretion is used for HCO_3^- reabsorption (see below). In the adult this amounts to about 3500 mEq H^+/day. The remaining 3 per cent is used to form titratable acid and NH_4^+. Secretion of hydrogen ion for HCO_3^- reabsorption may thus be regarded as a high-capacity system, active mainly in the proximal tubule. Here, because of dissipation of H_2CO_3 into $CO_2 + H_2O$, H^+ secretion operates against a low gradient. Conversely H^+ secretion, which leads to formation of titratable acid and NH_4^+, occurs principally in the distal tubule and collecting duct and is a low-capacity system which operates against a high lumen-to-cellular H^+ gradient.

BICARBONATE REABSORPTION. Tubular capacity to reabsorb HCO_3^- is great, but, if the filtered load is excessive, HCO_3^- will spill into the urine. The plasma concentration of HCO_3^- above which HCO_3^- spills into the urine in normal children over 1 month of age is 24–26 mEq/l. At this level the maximal rate of tubular reabsorption of HCO_3^- is reached. In infants under 1 month of age the level is about 22 mEq/l. The lower threshold is probably the result of the morphologic and functional heterogeneity of the developing nephrons. A urine pH of 6.2 or less indicates that urinary HCO_3^- is negligible. On a normal diet all filtered HCO_3^- is reabsorbed, about 85 per cent in the proximal tubule and the remainder in the distal nephron. During metabolic acidosis, because of increased H^+ secretion, a proportionately greater amount of HCO_3^- is reabsorbed proximally. Carbonic anhydrase in the cells of the proximal tubule is present both in the cytoplasm and along the brush border which is in contact with tubular urine. Bicarbonate which enters the tubule in the glomerular filtrate combines with H^+ secreted by the cell to form H_2CO_3. In accordance with the law of mass action, the carbonic anhydrase of the brush border dissipates accumulation of excess H_2CO_3 by increasing the rate of CO_2 and H_2O production from H_2CO_3. This reduces the gradient against which H^+ must be secreted. The CO_2 and H_2O diffuse into the tubular cell, where, catalyzed by carbonic anhydrase, they again combine to form H_2CO_3. This in turn dissociates to yield H^+ for secretion into the lumen and HCO_3^- for diffusion into peritubular capillaries. (See Figure 5–7.) The transfer of HCO_3^- from cell to peritubular capillaries probably occurs by passive diffusion down an electrochemical gradient. Although HCO_3^- reabsorption is mediated principally by this mechanism of H^+ secretion, it is possible that some HCO_3^- is transferred directly in an ionic form from tubular lumen through the cell to the peritubular capillaries. Such a mechanism may be operative when the filtered load of HCO_3^- is high.

Factors Influencing Bicarbonate Reabsorption. A number of factors cause an increase in the rate of H^+ secretion by the proximal tubule and lead to increased HCO_3^- reabsorption with consequent elevation of plasma HCO_3^-. These include: elevation of plasma pCO_2, hypokalemia, reduction in effective arterial blood volume (e.g., after vomiting, hemorrhage or burns) and administration of mineralocorticoids. On the other hand, H^+ secretion and thus HCO_3^- reabsorption is decreased in states of decreased plasma pCO_2, inhibition of carbonic anhydrase (e.g., by drugs such as acetazolamide and by mineralocorticoid deficiency). Reduction in plasma HCO_3^- may occur in these situations.

Not only does the serum level of K^+ affect tubular H^+ secretion, but the acid-base status also affects K^+ excretion; potassium secretion is increased by alkalosis and depressed during acute acidosis of either metabolic or respiratory origin. Potassium secretion, and hence urinary excretion, is also enhanced by increased alkalinity of the tubular fluid, as may occur when there is a high luminal concentration of HCO_3^-.

HYDROGEN ION SECRETION IN THE DISTAL NEPHRON. The diversion of secreted H^+ into non-bicarbonate buffers such as Na_2HPO_4 and NH_3 is favored when the luminal HCO_3^- concentration and pH are low. Although titration of Na_2HPO_4 to NaH_2PO_4 and formation of NH_4^+ from $NH_3 + H^+$ occur to some extent in the proximal tubule, this is facilitated after bicarbonate reabsorption is complete and the H^+ concentration is increased. The total H^+ secretory capacity of the collecting duct is small, but its capacity to maintain a steep H^+ gradient from lumen to tubular cell enables titration of the Na_2HPO_4 and NH_3 buffers to an extent sufficient that the combined amount of H^+ secreted as NaH_2PO_4 and NH_4^+ is equal to the nonvolatile acid derived from dietary or metabolic sources.

Ammonia can be regarded as a base which in acid solution buffers H^+ to form NH_4^+. As a free base it has no electrical charge and readily diffuses through the tubular cell membrane into the lumen. The charged ammonium ion (NH_4^+) penetrates cellular membranes slowly. These properties are critical to the process of nonionic passive diffusion of NH_3, which underlies tubular secretion of ammonia. Ammonia diffuses passively into acid urine where it combines with H^+ to form NH_4^+ which, because it is relatively nondiffusible, is trapped within the lumen. The rate of ammonia secretion by the tubule is thus directly related to the urine H^+ concentration, i.e., inversely related to urinary pH. The tubular cell adapts to chronic metabolic acidosis by increasing the amount of ammonia formed and diffused into the lumen.

About 90 per cent of the NH_3 formed within the tubular cells is derived from the amide and amino nitrogens of the amino acid glutamine. A small quantity of excreted NH_3 reaches the kidney as NH_3 in renal arterial blood.

REGULATION OF BLOOD PRESSURE

The kidney is important in the regulation of systemic blood pressure. Renin, formed and stored in the juxtaglomerular apparatus of the afferent arteriole, is released into the circulation in response to a fall in the mean arteriolar pressure. Renin catalyzes the conversion of angiotensinogen to angiotensin I. The latter is converted, chiefly in the lung, by the action of angiotensin-converting enzyme to angiotensin II, which is vasoactive and also stimulates the secretion of aldosterone by the adrenal. This enhances sodium reabsorption from the renal tubule and leads to augmentation of the extracellular volume. As discussed earlier, the regulation of renal excretion of sodium depends on many other factors as well. The body's sodium content is a principal determinant of extracellular volume, which is itself important in determining the blood pressure. (See Figure 5–5.)

RED BLOOD CELL PRODUCTION

The kidney is of primary importance in the physiologic control of production of red blood cells. The hormone erythropoietin is produced by the kidney in response to reduced oxygen tension in renal tissue. In the bone marrow erythropoietin acts on stem cells, which are transformed into hemoglobin synthesizing pronormoblasts. Control of red cell production seems to involve a feedback system between the kidney and bone marrow, mediated in one direction by red cell bound oxygen and in the other by erythropoietin. Red cell production is influenced by factors other than erythropoietin, as evidenced by the slow constant rate of erythropoiesis in patients who have received a blood transfusion or who are anephric. An inappropriately high rate of erythropoietin secretion leading to polycythemia occurs in a small percentage of patients with renal neoplasms. This is more common in patients with hypernephroma, but also occurs with Wilms' tumor, some benign renal tumors, cystic renal disease and hydronephrosis.

CALCIUM AND PHOSPHATE HOMEOSTASIS

The kidney also plays a key role in calcium and phosphate homeostasis and in bone metabolism. The ultrafiltrate of plasma formed at the glomerulus contains phosphate and ionized calcium in virtually the same concentrations as in plasma. Renal tubular reabsorption of the filtered calcium and phosphate is influenced by parathyroid hormone, which augments calcium and decreases phosphate reabsorption. Parathyroid hormone also affects renal tubular function by reducing proximal tubular reabsorption of amino acids and bicarbonate. When excess parathyroid hormone is present, *aminoaciduria* and a bicarbonate-wasting form of renal tubular acidosis develops.

Impaired renal tubular reabsorption of phosphate leads to an excessive loss of phosphate in the urine, hypophosphatemia and rickets; this occurs in the hereditary X-linked disorder known as hypophosphatemic or vitamin D-resistant rickets.

Tubular unresponsiveness to parathyroid hormone occurs in the hereditary disorder pseudohypoparathyroidism; this leads to elevation of the plasma phosphate concentration and to hypocalcemia.

The kidney plays another vital role in calcium metabolism which has only recently been defined: the hydroxylation of 25-hydroxycholecalciferol at the 1 position to form 1,25-dihydroxycholecalciferol; this takes place in the cells of the proximal tubule. 1,25-Dihydroxycholecalciferol is the primary physiologic stimulus to absorption of calcium from the gut and to its release from bone. There is also evidence that it plays a role in absorption of phosphate from the gut. Absent or decreased production of 1,25-dihydroxycholecalciferol has been postulated as the basic defect in so-called vitamin D-dependent rickets, and it is undoubtedly a factor of importance in the pathogenesis of renal osteodystrophy. See also Metabolic Disorders with Osseous Lesions in Section 22.

PROSTAGLANDINS

The kidney both synthesizes and metabolizes prostaglandins. One of the renal prostaglandins, PGE_2, may play a role in regulating intrarenal distribution of blood flow, enhancing sodium excretion, and in the poorly understood antihypertensive function of the kidney. The enzymes which metabolize prostaglandins probably protect against the potent vasodilator and diuretic effects of prostaglandins synthesized elsewhere in the body.

GASTRIN

Recent evidence suggests that the kidney plays a principal role in the catabolism of the hormone gastrin. When renal function is impaired, or if the patient is anephric, increased circulatory levels of gastrin can lead to gastric hyperacidity and peptic ulceration.

SOMATOMEDIN

The kidney is probably a site of production of somatomedin, a growth-regulating substance which is produced following stimulation by growth hormone.

DEVELOPMENTAL ASPECTS OF RENAL FUNCTION

Urine formation begins between the ninth and eleventh weeks of fetal life. The role of the fetal kidney in maintaining homeostasis during subsequent gestation is speculative, although experimental studies in a variety of mammals indicate that it is able to dilute and acidify urine, to reabsorb phosphate and to transport organic materials. The placenta is able to meet the excretory needs of the fetus; indeed, in infants with bilateral renal agenesis, the composition of the body tissues does not differ from normal. Immediately following birth, the kidney must replace the placenta as the principal organ responsible for maintaining the homeostasis of body fluids. Fetal renal blood flow and the glomerular filtration rate are quite low, and within the first few days of extrauterine life undergo a dramatic increase. During the first year of life there is a more gradual rise to levels which appear to be comparable to adult values.

Decrease in renal arteriolar vascular resistance and an increase in the fraction of the cardiac output directed to the kidney are principally responsible for the dramatic increase in GFR and renal blood flow which occurs during the first few days after birth and during the first year. Circulation in the medullary and juxtamedullary nephrons develops more rapidly than in the outer cortical nephrons. The rate of tubular development seems to set the pace for overall renal maturation during the first year of life, and postnatal growth of the kidney is principally accounted for by increase in tubular mass. The formation of new glomeruli ceases at a fetal weight of approximately 2100 to 2500 gm.

Values for GFR (determined by inulin clearance) and the effective renal plasma flow (ERPF) (determined by para-aminohippurate clearance) at different stages during the first several years of life are shown in Table 15–1. These are expressed as milliliters per square meter of surface area. Data obtained in the developing guinea pig suggest that the initial increment in GFR (days 1 to 15) is due principally to an increase in the GFR of deep nephrons, whereas the subsequent more gradual rise is accounted for solely by an increase in the filtration rate of superficial nephrons.

TABLE 15–1 GLOMERULAR FILTRATION RATE (GFR) AND EFFECTIVE RENAL PLASMA FLOW DURING THE FIRST THREE YEARS OF LIFE*

AGE	GFR†	ERPF†
Newborn	15	50
3 days	20	77
1–2 weeks	30	
2–4 months	35	135
6 months–1 year	45–50	200–245
1–3 years	50–70	310–380

*Adapted from McCrory, W. W.: Developmental Nephrology. Cambridge, Harvard University Press, 1972.

†Values are expressed as $ml/min/m^2$.

The fraction of the renal plasma flow which is filtered is high in infants (0.32 to 0.34) in comparison to that in adults (0.18 to 0.20). Despite the low GFR value when expressed per unit of surface area, glomerular function is relatively more mature than tubular function. Thus, if a comparison is made between the GFR and the tubular maximum for either glucose reabsorption or secretion of para-aminohippurate, the ratio is higher in infants than in later childhood, suggesting that the GFR is excessive in relation to tubular functional capacity. This phenomenon is called *glomerular-tubular imbalance.* It results in a lower fractional reabsorption in the proximal tubule of many filtered solutes than is the case later in life. This probably accounts for the fact that infants excrete a higher percentage of the filtered load of glucose, phosphate and amino acids than do older children and adults. The threshold for HCO_3^- absorption is also lower in infants (19–21 mEq/l) than in children beyond 6 months of age. Morphologic studies have demonstrated that the ratio at birth of glomerular surface area to proximal tubular volume is high relative to adult values and falls rapidly during the first year.

Ninety-three per cent of normal newborn infants void within 24 hours of birth, and > 99 per cent within 48 hours. The mean value of maximal urine osmolality in the newborn is 600–700 mOsm/l. This does not reflect an inability of the immature kidney to concentrate urine but is rather a consequence of the anabolic state of the infant which results in little of the dietary protein being metabolized and excreted as urea. If a high urea or protein diet is given, the maximal urine concentration approximates that of adults (1200 mOsm/l) within several weeks after birth.

The capacity of the infant's kidney to form a dilute urine is qualitatively the same as in adults, indicating adequate ability to deliver sodium to the diluting segment. Following a water load, however, the absolute rate of urine flow is considerably less than in the mature state, a feature that may make the infant more vulnerable to sudden increases in fluid intake.

The capacity of the neonate's kidney to conserve sodium is good, and although less than in adults, the ability to adapt during infancy is considerable. Since the medullary region is relatively more developed than the cortical zone, the infant is better able to withstand the stress of deprivation of sodium and water than of their excessive loading.

For the first several days of life the infant cannot excrete a strongly acid urine, but by the second week this capacity is comparable to that of older children and adults. During the first year, in comparison with older children, a greater proportion of H^+ is secreted as titratable acid than as ammonium.

Berliner, R. W.: Outline of renal physiology. *In* Strauss, M. B., and Welt, L. G. (eds.): Diseases of the Kidney. Boston, Little, Brown and Company, 1971.

DeLuca, H. F.: The kidney as an endocrine organ involved in calcium homeostasis. Kidney Int. *4*:80, 1973.

de Rouffignac, C.: Physiological role of the loop of Henle in urinary concentration. Kidney Int. *2*:297, 1972.

Dirks, J. H., and Seely, J. F.: Renal tubular function. *In* Downman, C. B. B. (ed.): Modern Trends in Physiology. London, Butterworth & Co., Ltd., 1972.

Earley, L. E., and Daugharty, T. M.: Sodium metabolism. New Engl. J. Med. *281*:72, 1969.

Edelmann, C. M., Jr.: Pediatric nephrology. Pediatrics *51*:854, 1973.

Fried, W.: Erythropoietin. Arch. Intern. Med. *131*:929, 1973.

King, R., and Hansky, J.: Serum-gastrin after renal transplantation. Lancet *1*:169, 1974.

Malnic, G., and Giebisch, G.: Mechanism of renal hydrogen ion secretion. Kidney Int. *1*:280, 1972.

McCrory, W. W.: Developmental Nephrology. Cambridge, Harvard University Press, 1972.

McGiff, J. C., Crowshaw, K., and Itskovitz, D. H.: Prostaglandins and renal function. Fed. Proc. *33*:39, 1974.

Moore, E. S., and Glavez, M. B.: Delayed micturition in the newborn period. J. Pediatr. *80*:867, 1972.

Pitts, R. F.: Physiology of the Kidney and Body Fluids. 3rd ed. Chicago, Year Book Medical Publishers, Inc., 1974.

Sedlin, D. W., and Wilson, J. D.: Renal tubular acidosis. *In* Stanbury, J. B., Wyngaarden, J. B., and Fredrickson, D. S. (eds.): The Metabolic Basis of Inherited Disease. New York, McGraw-Hill Book Co., 1972.

Spitzer, A., and Brandis, M.: Functional and morphologic maturation of the superficial nephrons. J. Clin. Invest. *53*:279, 1974.

Van Wyk, J. J., Underwood, L. E., Lister, R. C., and Marshall, R. N.: The somatomedins. Am. J. Dis. Child. *126*:705, 1973.

Diagnostic Assessment of Structure and Function

A variety of techniques are needed to evaluate the structure and function of the kidneys and other components of the urinary system. Experience and judgment are required not only in choosing which studies should be carried out, but in interpreting and synthesizing the data which have been gathered so that the patient's problem may be defined in a coherent and meaningful way. Few disciplines are as demanding in this respect as is nephrology. In a real sense the skills required are those of a clinician, physiologist, immunologist, pathologist and radiologist.

HISTORY

Important areas which should be explored in the patient's history include the following:

1. Family history of renal disease, deafness, hypertension, renal calculi, structural developmental anomalies of the urinary tract or of any of the syndromes known to have associated abnormalities of the urinary system.
2. Abnormalities or changes in the pattern of micturition; these include increased urinary frequency, nocturnal or daytime enuresis, increased or decreased urine volume, urgency, dribbling, poor urinary stream, dysuria.
3. Changes in the color or smell of the urine.
4. Exposure to nephrotoxic agents or ingestion of potentially nephrotic drugs.
5. Facial and/or generalized edema.
6. Symptoms suggestive of chronic renal failure with its multifaceted manifestations: fatigue, anorexia, nausea, failure to thrive, growth arrest, bone pain, paresthesias, seizures, headache.

PHYSICAL EXAMINATION

The principal physical findings which help in assessing the presence and severity of renal disease include growth retardation, pallor or sallow complexion, tachypnea, dehydration, edema with or without ascites, hypertension, signs of circulatory congestion, enlargement of the kidneys, flank or suprapubic tenderness, abnormalities of external genitalia, and physical features of syndromes known to have associated urinary tract involvement.

DIAGNOSTIC EVALUATION OF URINE AND ITS FORMATION

COLLECTION OF URINE SPECIMEN

With patience and ingenuity it is usually not difficult to obtain a specimen of urine from even the smallest infant. A plastic urine collector bag, the edges of which adhere to the skin around the genitalia, can be used. The perineum and genitalia should be cleansed with soap and water and rinsed thoroughly so that the urine is free of contaminating debris. The collector should be removed as soon as the urine is passed to reduce the likelihood of fecal contamination. Care must be taken to avoid excoriating the skin to which the bag is attached, especially when frequent urine collections are required. Children of 2 years or older will usually void on request, and a midstream specimen can be easily collected. In boys, if the foreskin is easily retractable, this should be done and the glans cleansed, particularly if urine is being collected for culture. Suprapubic aspiration of urine from the bladder, as described in the section on Urinary Tract Infection, may be required in infants, particularly if an infection is suspected; this technique is not without risk.

When it is necessary to perform accurate clearance studies in infants or in children who cannot cooperate, an indwelling flexible urethral catheter of appropriate size with extra holes cut in it may be used.

The technique for collecting urine for culture is outlined in the section on Urinary Tract Infection.

URINALYSIS

This should be done within several hours of obtaining the specimen. It is preferable that the external genitalia be cleansed before voiding. For routine urinalysis the specimen should be kept at body temperature rather than refrigerated, since refrigeration may cause precipitation of phosphates or urates, which makes microscopic examination of the sediment difficult.

The *color* of the urine should be noted. Urine is normally pale yellow or amber. If the urine is almost colorless, it is probably very dilute with a low specific gravity; however, under conditions of osmotic diuresis, as seen for example in diabetes mellitus, the urine may be very pale yet have a high specific gravity, owing to the presence of dissolved solute—in this instance, glucose. The urine may be pink or reddish because of urates, red blood cells, free hemoglobin or, rarely, porphyrins. It may have a pink color following ingestion of beets, blackberries and vegetable dyes used in coloring foods, candies and soft drinks. Phenolphthalein, a constituent of some laxatives, may color the urine pink or red; conjugated bilirubin, orange-red. Blood or free hemoglobin may give a brown or tea color. Indigo blue, an oxidation product of the tryptophan metabolite indican, may cause a blue, non-water-soluble discoloration of the diaper; the urine itself is not colored blue, and the staining of the diaper takes several hours to develop.

The *odor* of urine should be noted. An acetone scent is indicative of ketonuria. In maple syrup urine disease the urine has an odor resembling that of maple syrup. A fecal odor suggests infection with coliform bacteria, as does an ammoniacal odor from the diaper.

The *osmolality or specific gravity* should be measured. An osmometer is used to measure the osmolality. Determination of osmolality following a period of dehydration is the best means of measuring the ability to concentrate urine. Normal children and infants beyond 2 months of age can concentrate urine to over 900 mOsm/l following an overnight fast. The urine specific gravity gives similar information concerning concentrating ability and can be measured by a simple hydrometer, or with a refractometer,* which requires only a drop of urine.

In general there is a direct relation between urine osmolality and specific gravity; however, when there is glucose, protein or a compound such as urographic contrast medium in the urine, the specific gravity may be elevated to a greater extent than the osmolality, since these molecules have a relatively large molecular weight and contribute only slightly to the osmolality.

Screening tests for glucose, ketones, blood and protein should be done. The simplest way to screen for these substances is to use a dipstick.† It should be noted that the dipstick test for glucose is specific for glucose and does not give a positive reaction for other reducing substances. A copper sulfate solution or Clinitest tablet‡§ may be used to detect reducing substances such as galactose which are not identified by the glucose oxidase test. The dipstick test** for proteinuria is sensitive and will detect urinary protein at a concentration of 20 mg/dl or more.

For microscopic examination of the urine sediment, 10 to 12 ml of urine are centrifuged in a clean centrifuge tube at 800 to 1000 rpm for 5 minutes. The supernatant is discarded and the sediment resuspended by brisk agitation in the remaining 0.5 ml at the bottom of the tube. Several drops of the sediment are poured onto a clean glass slide. Depending on the preference of the examiner, a coverslip may or may not be used.

The sediment should be examined for the presence of red and white blood cells, epithelial cells, casts (red cell, white cell, mixed, granular, heme-granular, hyaline), crystals (cystine, uric acid, calcium oxalate, triple phosphate, sulfonamide) and bacteria or yeasts. It is not valid to set precise figures for the number of red or white blood cells per high power microscopic field which should be accepted as normal, because the urine concentration and the thickness of the sediment drop vary. Generally more than five red or white blood cells per high power field (× 250) is considered abnormal. The possibility of urinary contamination with cells from a vaginal discharge should be considered. Rarely hyaline and granular casts, or long cylindrical casts with cells attached to their outer aspect, may be seen in normal urine.

---

*Total Solids Meter—American Optical Corp., Buffalo, N.Y.

†Labstix Reagent Strips—Ames Co., Elkhart, Indiana.

‡Clinitest Reagent Tablets—Ames Co., Elkhart, Indiana.

§The Clinitest tablet contains the same essential ingredients as are present in Benedict's solution—copper sulfate, caustic soda, sodium carbonate and citric acid. A tablet plus 5 drops of urine and 10 drops of water will give a blue, green-yellow or orange-red precipitate, depending on the amount of reducing sugar present.

**Albustix Reagent Strips—Ames Co., Elkhart, Indiana.

The finding of tubular casts is of particular importance since they must by definition arise from the kidney. Their presence in association with an excessive number of red and/or white blood cells is evidence in favor of a renal problem as distinct from a disorder in the lower urinary tract. This is particularly important in patients with pyuria or hematuria.

PROTEINURIA

There are a number of methods for measuring the amount of protein in the urine. The simplest methods for detecting proteinuria are:

1. Urine dipstick,* in which the test paper is impregnated with tetrabromophenol blue buffered to an acid pH; the color of the strip is yellow in the absence of protein, but changes within 10 seconds to a shade of green, depending on the concentration of protein present.

2. The sulfosalicylic acid method, in which 0.5 ml of 3 per cent sulfosalicylic acid is added to an equal volume of urine. The test is positive for protein if the urine becomes turbid; the degree of turbidity is directly related to the protein concentration.

For precise quantitation of the concentration of urinary protein a simple technique is described in the footnote.† Other methods for measuring the amount of proteinuria include the biuret technique and the Lowry technique using the Folin phenol reagent.

If benzalkonium, used to wash the genitalia, contaminates the urine specimen it may result in a falsely positive dipstick test for protein.

In normal infants and children the concentration of protein in urine is less than 20 mg/dl, usually less than 5 mg/dl. The volume of urine changes, depending on fluid intake and concentrating ability of the kidney; thus, when a given quantity of protein is excreted per unit of time, the urine protein concentration will vary, depending on how dilute the urine is. For this reason if proteinuria in excess of 20-30 mg/dl is detected, the *total* quantity of protein excreted over a known period of time should be measured. A 24-hour period is usually selected; the normal value for infants and children is less than 150 mg/24 hr; the great majority excrete less than 50 mg/24 hr. It is generally accepted that the term proteinuria should apply only when the total daily excretion of protein exceeds 150 mg.

In urine from normal resting subjects about 70 per cent of the protein has the electrophoretic mobility of globulins; urinary globulins are usually smaller than plasma globulins and up to half of them are not present in the plasma. They probably originate in the kidney, urinary tract or seminal glands. The rest of the urine protein has the mobility of albumin and is probably identical to plasma albumin. The *Tamm-Horsfall mucoprotein* is an alpha globulin of high molecular weight that is formed in the kidney; it is a principal constituent of the matrix of urinary casts. With exercise, excretion of plasma proteins increases to the extent that they constitute about 85 per cent of the proteins in urine.

In most disorders with increased protein excretion, albumin accounts for 60 to 90 per cent of the protein. This is particularly true in the nephrotic syndrome and other glomerular disorders. In tubular disorders such as the Fanconi syndrome, proteinuria of 500 to 800 mg/24 hr may occur. This "tubular" proteinuria differs from that of glomerular disease in that low molecular weight (10,000 to 20,000) globulins predominate. When hyperglobulinemia is present, e.g., in multiple myeloma or chronic active hepatitis, increased excretion of globulin may also occur.

With the use of sensitive immunologic techniques many of the proteins which are present in normal plasma can be detected in urine from normal subjects and from patients with proteinuria. These proteins include transferrin, ceruloplasmin, IgG, IgA, α_2 macroglobulin, a variety of other plasma globulins and, as mentioned earlier, albumin. From a practical viewpoint, however, it is seldom helpful to determine which particular proteins are present. Immunologic or electrophoretic studies of urinary proteins are of little diagnostic value except in distinguishing tubular from glomerular proteinuria; in the former, globulins predominate, whereas albumin is the principal protein excreted in glomerular diseases.

Depending on the type and severity of injury to the glomerular basement membrane, there is a difference in the molecular weight of the proteins which are filtered and excreted. For example, in the minimal lesion nephrotic syndrome, a condi-

---

*Albustix Reagent Strips—Ames Co., Elkhart, Indiana

†Determination of urine protein content by a quantitative sulfosalicylic acid method:

Reagents: 3 per cent sulfosalicylic acid and distilled water. Procedure: The spectrophotometer is set at wavelength 520 mμ and turned on 30 minutes before determinations are to be made. An Albustix dip test is done on the urine to be tested. Thirty milligrams or less indicate that no dilution of the urine is needed. One hundred to 300 mg per cent indicate that the urine should be diluted 1:1 with distilled water. If the protein concentration is 300 mg per cent or more, a 1:5 or 1:10 dilution should be made.

Into the *standard* or control cuvette, 0.5 ml of distilled water is pipetted; 0.5 ml of 3 per cent sulfosalicylic acid, into the *test* cuvette. Urine, 0.5 ml diluted if necessary as described above, is pipetted into each cuvette and mixed thoroughly. The *standard* is placed into the spectrophotometer and adjusted to zero absorbance. The *test* cuvette is inserted and the optical density is read. The protein concentration is determined from the standard curve. If the urine was diluted 1:1 then the actual protein concentration is double that indicated by the standard curve, etc.

The standard curve is prepared in the following way: Using human or bovine crystalline albumin, solutions are made in distilled water ranging from 5 to 80 mg/dl. A sulfosalicylic acid test is performed, using 0.5 ml of 3 per cent sulfosalicylic acid and 0.5 ml of the standard. Nine different concentrations from 5 to 80 mg/dl (5, 10, 20, etc.) are employed. A plot is made of the optical density versus the protein concentration. The protein concentration of *test* samples can then be determined from this standard curve.

Cipriani, A., and Brophy, D. A.: Method for detecting cerebrospinal fluid protein by photoelectric colorimeter. J. Lab. Clin. Med. *28*:1269, 1943.

Looney, J. M., and Walsh, A. I.: The determination of spinal fluid protein with the photoelectric colorimeter. J. Biol. Chem. *127*:117, 1939.

tion in which glomerular basement membrane injury is so minimal as to be indiscernible by electron microscopic examination, there is preferential excretion of low molecular weight plasma proteins such as transferrin; the clearance of such low molecular weight proteins is greater than that of larger molecular weight ones such as α_2 macroglobulin, to which the glomerular basement membrane remains relatively impermeable. In contrast, when there is more serious damage, the glomerular basement membrane loses its capacity to restrict the filtration of proteins of all molecular weights, and the clearance of both large and small molecular weight proteins increases. Knowledge of such *protein selectivity* has some usefulness in assessing the severity of injury to the glomerular basement membrane.

In assessing the patient with proteinuria it is important to establish whether the proteinuria is *persistent* (i.e., present every day over a period of at least several weeks, throughout the day and independent of changes in posture) or *transient* (i.e., changing in relation to exercise or posture, or present for a limited period of time only). Transient proteinuria occurs in fixed reproducible orthostatic proteinuria (see below), in intercurrent acute febrile illnesses, after administration of epinephrine, following plasma or blood transfusions, in skin diseases and in extensive burns.

When proteinuria is persistent, sequential determination of the 24-hour excretion may be a useful guide to the progress of the condition or to the efficacy of treatment. Quantitative excretion of protein must be evaluated in relation to other measures of renal function. For example, in a disorder with progressive glomerular destruction, a decrease in total urinary excretion of protein may result from a lesser amount of protein being filtered because of reduction in the number of functioning glomeruli; in this context, reduction in excretion of protein could hardly be regarded as a sign of improvement.

Patients with persistent proteinuria may be separated arbitrarily into three groups based on the amount of protein excreted in 24 hours: 150 to 500 mg—mild proteinuria; 500 to 2000 mg—moderate; and over 2000 mg—massive. Massive proteinuria is usually a sign of glomerular disorder, but it may also be seen in congestive heart failure and constrictive pericarditis. Mild proteinuria is seen in some glomerular disorders such as acute poststreptococcal glomerulonephritis, recurrent macroscopic hematuria and hereditary nephritis with deafness (Alport's disease).

Proteinuria may be absent or mild in many important renal diseases. These include polycystic kidney disease, nephronophthisis, analgesic nephropathy, hypercalcemic and hypokalemic nephropathy, most congenital renal anomalies, obstructive uropathy, nephrolithiasis and pyelonephritis.

Tubular proteinuria is usually mild, and the proteins are of low molecular weight. Conditions in which tubular proteinuria is seen include congenital metabolic disorders in which the proximal tubule is affected, chronic heavy metal poisoning, chronic pyelonephritis, analgesic nephropathy, acute intrinsic renal failure, interstitial nephritis, Balkan nephropathy and following renal transplantation.

ORTHOSTATIC (POSTURAL) PROTEINURIA. In most normal individuals the quantity of protein excreted per unit of time is five to fifteen times greater in urine formed in the upright than in the recumbent postion; the protein concentration in the upright position is, however, not above 30 mg/dl, and the total daily excretion of protein is less than 150 mg. In some individuals, however, the protein concentration in urine formed in the upright position is considerably higher and may even reach 150 to 1200 mg/dl. Proteinuria which is present in the upright position but absent when recumbent is called orthostatic or postural proteinuria. Orthostatic proteinuria may be present over a prolonged time (5 to 10 years), in which case it is referred to as fixed and reproducible orthostatic proteinuria.

Although orthostatic proteinuria is seen in some forms of renal disease, most children with this finding are healthy and there is no underlying renal pathology. The sex incidence is equal, and the usual age of detection is during the second decade, when proteinuria is discovered incidentally on routine urinalysis. In at least 50 per cent of patients, the condition is still present 10 years after detection. Currently available data suggest that postural proteinuria may be a normal variant.

A simple test designed to confirm the diagnosis of orthostatic proteinuria is described in the footnote.* Collection of a 24-hour specimen† for total protein excretion can be done before the postural test. With the information gained from these determinations and a routine urinalysis it is possible to be confident of the diagnosis and to reassure the patient and the parents about the prognosis. The routine urinalysis shows a variable protein concentration and no other abnormal findings; the urine formed while the child is recumbent has a protein concentration of 2–25 mg/dl, and the protein concentration in the urine formed while the child is in the upright position is 75–1500 mg/dl; the total 24-

---

*The test is done in the morning. The night before the test the child voids at bedtime and this specimen is discarded. One glass of water is given. Upon wakening in the morning the child voids immediately, preferably before getting out of bed or while sitting on the side of the bed. This specimen is labeled "recumbent specimen." A large glass of water or fruit juice is then given and the child stands with the back arched for 20 to 30 minutes. Then the child voids again and the specimen is saved in a separate container labeled "upright specimen." The arched position may be somewhat uncomfortable. A comparison of the protein concentration in these two consecutive specimens is then made.

†The time to start the collection is not fixed; any convenient 24-hour period may be used. Beginning for example at 8 A.M. the child voids and the specimen is discarded. All urine voided after this time up to and including the specimen voided at 8 A.M. the following day is saved. This completes the collection. The collected urine is refrigerated; it may all be placed in the same bottle.

hour urinary excretion of protein seldom exceeds 1000 mg.

HEMATURIA

By hematuria is meant an abnormal number of red blood cells in the urine. It is difficult to quantify the number of RBC's which are present in normal urine; usually there are less than 5 per high power field (×250) in the sediment of a 10-ml centrifuged fresh specimen; one may arbitrarily consider that hematuria is present when this number is exceeded. When hematuria is of clinical importance, many times this number of RBC's are usually seen. Attempts have been made to quantify the number of red and/or white cells and tubular casts passed during a given interval. A 12-hour Addis count has been widely used in the past for this purpose. In view of the errors inherent in this test it is not reliable in the evaluation of renal disorders in children; a properly done urinalysis provides the necessary information concerning cellular elements and casts excreted.

The term "gross" or "macroscopic" hematuria is used when the urine has a pink or brown color owing to the presence of RBC's; free hemoglobin resulting from hemolysis of excreted RBC's is often also present. Hematuria may also be suspected when the urine has a greenish-brown color. Bright red urine, with or without clots, suggests an extrarenal or lower urinary tract source of bleeding, whereas when the urine is brown or tea-colored, a renal source is more likely. Free hemoglobin which may spill into the urine following acute hemolysis may color the urine reddish brown; more commonly, free hemoglobin arises from lysis of RBC's while in the urine. The indicator strip on the Labstix* dipstick is a sensitive means of detecting hemoglobin, either free or contained in erythrocytes.

Hematuria, especially if only microscopic, does not necessarily represent a disorder of the kidney and/or urinary tract. Microscopic hematuria may be present during a variety of intercurrent unrelated conditions such as viral or bacterial respiratory infections, nonspecific febrile disorders, gastroenteritis with dehydration and following strenuous exercise. Urine may also be contaminated by RBC's from the external genitalia, e.g., urethral meatal ulcer or menstrual blood.

If it is established that RBC's are present in a clean voided urine specimen and are not from the external genitalia, several features are helpful in assessing the significance. If proteinuria is present it usually signifies that the hematuria is clinically important and often suggests a renal source. The second differential feature is the presence or absence of casts, particularly RBC casts. If casts are present the source of the hematuria must be the kidney. The presence of both proteinuria and tubular casts in a patient with hematuria is evidence that the hematuria is renal in origin and most likely the result of a glomerular disorder.

As is the case with proteinuria, the absence of hematuria does not exclude a number of important renal disorders, including, for example, the minimal lesion nephrotic syndrome, nephronophthisis and many of the developmental renal anomalies.

In the initial evaluation of a child with hematuria the following should be done: (1) exclude contamination of urine with blood from external genitalia, (2) determine if proteinuria is present, and (3) examine the sediment for tubular casts. If a renal source of the hematuria is strongly suggested by these steps, the need for extensive radiologic and urologic examination of the lower urinary tract is unnecessary.

Microscopic examination of the sediment, apart from the search for casts, may also be helpful in elucidating the cause of hematuria. Numerous bacteria and pus cells may be present, indicating an acute infection, or specific crystals (e.g., cystine or sulfonamide) may be seen, suggesting that the hematuria results from injury by stone formation in the collecting system.

In evaluating hematuria the tendency often is to focus on the bladder as the source of the bleeding. Indeed, in many hospitals children with hematuria undergo cystoscopic examination as a routine procedure. In most instances this is unnecessary. The cause and site of origin can usually be ascertained by assessing the history and clinical findings, and by microscopic examination of the urine sediment, quantitation of proteinuria and, if necessary, radiologic study of the urinary tract. Multisystem disorders such as systemic lupus erythematosus and anaphylactoid purpura, which may cause renal damage and hematuria, should be excluded by appropriate studies. In some patients with hematuria of renal origin a biopsy may be indicated to establish the diagnosis.

Table 15–2 lists some of the causes of hematuria in children.

ABILITY TO CONCENTRATE URINE

Following a 12-hour period of fluid restriction the normal child can concentrate the urine to 900 mOsm/l or more. The mean value for children 2 years or older is approximately 1100 mOsm/l (range 870–1300 mOsm/kg H_2O). In infants it may be unwise to restrict fluids for a period as long as 12 hours, and the normal values are less well defined. In general, beyond the age of 2 months infants should be able to concentrate urine to a value of 900 mOsm/l or more after fluid deprivation; between 1 week and 2 months of age, an osmolality of 700 or more can be expected. When an impaired ability to concentrate urine is suspected, care should be taken to avoid dehydration, contraction of extracellular fluid volume and weight loss as a consequence of fluid deprivation during the test, as may occur in the face of continued excretion of dilute urine. Tests of urine con-

*Ames Co., Elkhart, Indiana

TABLE 15-2 CAUSES OF HEMATURIA IN CHILDREN

1. *Acute and chronic forms of acquired glomerular injury*—e.g., acute poststreptococcal glomerulonephritis, hemolytic-uremic syndrome, membranoproliferative glomerulonephritis, recurrent macroscopic hematuria with mesangial IgA and IgG deposition (Berger's disease)
2. *Hereditary or familial renal disorders*—e.g., hereditary nephritis with deafness, familial benign recurrent hematuria, polycystic kidney disease
3. *Systemic disorders with vasculitis which may affect the kidney*—e.g., systemic lupus erythematosus, anaphylactoid purpura
4. *Thrombosis of renal vein or artery*
5. *Neoplasm*—e.g., Wilms' tumor
6. *Trauma*
7. *Developmental anomalies*—e.g., obstructive uropathy causing hydronephrosis (minor renal trauma may cause gross hematuria in patients with structural renal anomalies)
8. *Bacterial or viral infection of the urinary tract*
9. *Nephrolithiasis*
10. *Chronic bacteremia*—e.g., subacute bacterial endocarditis, shunt nephritis
11. *Miscellaneous*—e.g., sickle cell anemia, urethral meatal ulcer, malignant hypertension, coagulation disturbances, hematuria following strenuous exercise, drug- or chemical-induced hematuria (e.g., hemorrhagic cystitis due to cyclophosphamide)

centrating ability should be done during the day under close supervision if there is any question of serious impairment of the urine concentrating mechanism.

The ability of the kidney to form a concentrated urine is impaired in a number of different renal disorders. For example, in chronic renal failure, as the glomerular filtration rate declines so does the ability to dilute and to concentrate the urine; the maximum urine concentration, even after fluid restriction, may not exceed that of plasma by more than 150 mOsm/l. Patients with diabetes insipidus also have impaired concentrating ability; here the maximum urine osmolality may be in the range of 60-100 mOsm/l. In disorders in which the renal medulla is damaged, e.g., obstructive uropathy with hydronephrosis or pyelonephritis, the maximum urine concentration is often below the normal range. The details of a simple way to carry out this test are given in the footnote.*

RENAL EXCRETION OF ACID

In most instances it is unnecessary to test by administration of an acid load, such as with ammonium chloride, the capacity of the kidney to acidify the urine and excrete hydrogen ion, since, in children with suspected impairment of renal acidifying capacity, metabolic acidosis is already present, and the urine pH, titratable acidity and ammonium excretion can be determined. In fact, in patients with an impaired ability to excrete hydrogen ion an imposed acid load is not without risk.

In a state of metabolic acidosis, the otherwise normal child should excrete a urine of pH 5.0 to 5.5 or less, with titratable acid and ammonium of approximately 30 and 42 μEq/min/m^2. During the first year of life the titratable acid excretion is approximately 20 per cent higher and the ammonium excretion approximately 20 per cent less than this.

For an oral ammonium chloride loading test the dose is about 5 gm/m^2; the intent is to lower the plasma bicarbonate level 3 to 5 mEq/l to about 18 mEq/l. This test should not be done if the child is already acidotic (actual bicarbonate of 18 mEq/l or less). Plasma HCO_3^- and H^+ concentrations and pCO_2 are obtained 3 to 5 hours after giving the ammonium chloride, and two consecutive urine collections (each of 60-minute duration) are obtained. A urine pH under 5.5 and the values for titratable acid and ammonium excretion mentioned above should be present in the normal child. If there is systemic metabolic acidosis these data can be obtained without administration of ammonium chloride and, indeed, it is not warranted to risk inducing more severe acidosis by giving this acid load.

URINE EXCRETION OF AMINO ACIDS, ELECTROLYTES AND OTHER METABOLITES

Paper chromatographic techniques can be used to detect excessive excretion of amino acids. The references at the end of this section to the book by Scriver and Rosenberg and to the article by Frimpter can be referred to for details. The nitroprusside test* can be used to detect excess cystine excretion as occurs in cystinuria.

Urinary excretion of *calcium* may need to be determined in patients suspected of having idiopathic hypercalciuria, hyperparathyroidism or inadequately controlled distal renal tubular acidosis. Normal urine calcium values are under 5 mg/kg/day (usually <2 mg/kg) while receiving a calcium intake of less than 500 mg/day.

Under some circumstances the daily urine excretion of *sodium* or *potassium* may need to be measured. When the sodium intake is restricted, e.g., below 20 mEq/m^2/day, the kidney can reduce the sodium excretion to very low levels; the urine sodium concentration in this situation may be less than 10 mEq/l.

Excessive urinary loss of sodium during a restricted intake may indicate inadequate adrenal

*Normal diet; N.P.O. after lunch except a dry supper until the test is completed. The child is instructed to void before he goes to bed; this urine is not saved. The first morning specimen is obtained and the time of collection noted; the minimum amount of urine required is 2 ml, but more than 5 ml is preferable. The specimen should not be refrigerated; it should be sent in a sealed container to the laboratory.

*Nitroprusside test reagents: 5 per cent sodium cyanide, fresh saturated solution of sodium nitroprusside. Procedure: To 1 to 2 ml of urine add an equal volume of 5 per cent sodium cyanide; wait 10 minutes. Add 3 to 4 drops of saturated sodium nitroprusside solution. A positive test is indicated by a dark magenta color.

mineralocorticoid secretion or impaired ability of the kidney to conserve sodium. Impaired renal conservation of sodium occurs in chronic renal failure, nephronophthisis and pseudohypoaldosteronism.

In health the urinary excretion of sodium usually reflects the dietary intake; the normal kidney adapts readily to changes in intake of sodium and can excrete up to 250 $mEq/m^2/day$. If the dietary intake is chronically above this level the kidney is able to excrete even higher amounts.

In health the urinary excretion of potassium also depends on the intake, and a range from 20 to 250 $mEq/m^2/day$ may be seen. Potassium excretion in excess of intake occurs in metabolic acidosis, extracellular volume contraction, diuretic therapy, hypercortisonism and administration of a corticosteroid.

Determination of the amount of *chloride* excreted may be helpful in distinguishing the cause of metabolic alkalosis. In metabolic alkalosis owing to volume contraction, the urine chloride concentration is usually < 10 mEq/l; correction of volume contraction by administration of saline is indicated. With potassium depletion the urine chloride concentration is considerably higher, and it is necessary to administer KCl to correct the metabolic alkalosis.

Urinary *oxalate* excretion is elevated in oxalosis—an inherited metabolic disorder associated with calcium oxalate nephrolithiasis—and in a variety of conditions with secondary hyperoxaluria. Normal values of urinary oxalate excretion are <40 mg/24 hr.

CLEARANCE AND REABSORPTION STUDIES

GLOMERULAR FILTRATION RATE

The normal glomerular filtration rate in children over 1 year of age is 70 ± 5 (1 SD) $ml/min/m^2$. This is the value obtained using inulin or iothalamate ^{125}I. The endogenous creatinine clearance measured over a 6- to 24-hour period is used much more frequently to determine the GFR. For a period of this duration, errors introduced by incomplete collection, inaccurate timing and uncertainty concerning complete bladder emptying can be minimized. Values with this technique are usually 10 to 15 per cent less than with inulin. Because of difficulty in the accurate chemical determination of plasma creatinine, especially at levels under 1 mg/dl, there is considerable variation in GFR estimation using the endogenous creatinine clearance measurement. The method for measuring the endogenous creatinine clearance is: (1) collect a 12- or 24-hour urine specimen (discarding the first and including the last specimen of the designated timed collection period), (2) measure the total creatinine excreted during the period, (3) obtain a plasma creatinine value during the period of urine collection, and (4) calculate the GFR as follows:

$$\mathrm{GFR} = \frac{\text{creatinine excreted (mg/min)}}{\text{plasma creatinine (mg/ml)}} = \text{ml/min}$$

The serum creatinine value may be used as a rough guide to the GFR. In children under 2 years of age the normal value is less than 0.5 mg/dl. From 2 years to onset of puberty the normal concentration is under 0.8 mg/dl, and from onset of puberty until maturity the normal value is less than 1.2 mg/dl, usually less than 1.0 mg/dl. The blood urea nitrogen value may also be used as a rough index of the GFR, although it is influenced by factors other than the GFR; the normal value in infants and children is less than 15 mg/dl.

Single injection techniques using either inulin* or iothalamate ^{125}I† have been described; these permit accurate measurement of the GFR without introducing the theoretic and practical difficulties encountered when constant infusion techniques are used in children. The reader is referred for details of these methods to the articles by Harries et al. and Cohen et al. listed in the references.

PHOSPHATE CLEARANCE

As discussed in the section on renal physiology, the renal clearance of a number of solutes can be measured. Other than creatinine or inulin clearance, the phosphate clearance (C) is the one most commonly measured. The C_p is influenced principally by parathyroid hormone. The normal value is under 8.0 $ml/min/m^2$. Values in excess of this may indicate an impaired ability of the proximal tubule to reabsorb phosphate, or the existence of hyperparathyroidism. Values less than 2.0 ml/min occur when phosphorus restriction is severely limited or in hypoparathyroidism.

The tubular reabsorption of solutes such as phosphate which are almost completely freely filtered at the glomerulus, i.e., not protein bound, and whose concentration in the plasma is virtually identical to that in the glomerular filtrate can be calculated in several ways. Using phosphate as an example, the per cent of the phosphate filtered which is reabsorbed by the tubules—i.e., the per cent tubular reabsorption of phosphate or TRP—is determined in the following way:

A. 1. GFR (ml/min) can be measured by endogenous creatinine, inulin or iothalamate ^{125}I clearance.
   2. Filtered phosphate = GFR (ml/min) $\times$ plasma phosphate concentration (mg/ml) = mg/min.
   3. Excreted phosphate is measured for a given time interval.
   4. The per cent TRP, defined as that percentage of

*Inulin 10 per cent—Arnar Stone Laboratories, 601 E. Kensington Rd., Mt. Prospect, Ill.

†Glofil—Abbott Laboratories, P.O. Box 68, Abbott Park, North Chicago, Illinois 60064

the filtered phosphate which is reabsorbed, is thus =

$$\frac{\text{reabsorbed phosphate}}{\text{filtered phosphate}} \times \frac{100}{1}$$

Since the reabsorbed phosphate is the difference between the amount filtered and that excreted, then the per cent TRP =

$$\frac{\text{filtered phosphate (mg/min)} - \text{excreted phosphate (mg/min)}}{\text{filtered phosphate (mg/min)}} \times \frac{100}{1}$$

B. Another way to calculate the per cent TRP is to subtract from 100 per cent the ratio, expressed as a percentage, of the phosphate clearance (ml/min) to the GFR (ml/min), i.e.,

$$\text{per cent TRP} = 100 - \left[\frac{C_p \text{ (ml/min)}}{\text{GFR (ml/min)}} \text{ (expressed as a percentage)}\right]$$

Here the GFR can be measured as the clearance of inulin or as the endogenous creatinine clearance, viz.,

$$\text{per cent TRP} = 100 - \left[\frac{\frac{\text{Up} \times \text{vol}}{P_p}}{\frac{\text{Ucr} \times \text{vol}}{\text{Pcr}}}\right] = 100 - \left[\frac{\text{Up} \times \text{Pcr}}{P_p \times \text{Ucr}}\right]$$

where Up and Ucr are, respectively, the urine phosphate and creatinine concentrations and P_p and Pcr are the plasma phosphate and creatinine concentrations; vol refers to the volume of urine.

The duration of the collection period and the volume of urine specimen need not be recorded when the second method (B) is used for calculation of the per cent TRP.

RADIOLOGIC EXAMINATION OF THE URINARY TRACT*

Radiologic study of the kidney and its collecting system is particularly useful in the diagnosis of developmental structural abnormalities, obstructive uropathy, renal neoplasm, pyelonephritis, vesicoureteral reflux and ureteral or bladder dysfunction. Sequential studies over a period of months or years may also be helpful in evaluating the course of a disorder. The time of appearance and the concentration of contrast medium may be used as an estimate of the adequacy of renal function.

A history of sensitivity to urographic contrast medium or iodine should be sought. On the morning of the study the patient should be given a saline enema containing 5 mg of bisacodyl† per pint. A light breakfast is allowed; infants should be allowed their usual feedings. It is not advisable to reduce the fluid intake before the examination.

A preliminary film of the abdomen is taken to see if the bowel preparation has been adequate and to detect abnormalities such as radiopaque calculi. Following the preliminary film the contrast medium is injected, a full glass of water is given, and the child is asked to void.

For intravenous urography a 60 per cent solution of meglumine diatrizoate* is given intravenously in a dose of 1.5 ml/kg, up to a maximum of 50 ml, within about 1 minute. If renal function is reduced the total dose necessary for visualization of the kidney may be up to 75 ml. A film is taken at 6 minutes after completing the injection in uncomplicated cases; in infants, at 10 minutes because excretion of the dye is slower. The kidneys and collecting system usually are well visualized at this time. The concentration and volume of dye in the bladder can be used to estimate the amount of residual urine left after the voiding 6 to 10 minutes earlier. If the pelvicalyceal system, ureters and bladder are adequately visualized on the 6 to 10 minute film, an additional radiograph may not be needed. A more detailed examination of the bladder is possible 30 to 60 minutes after the injection of contrast medium. If indicated, a kinescopic voiding-cystourethrogram can be done at that time, using the contrast medium which has collected in the bladder. In most instances a postvoiding film is not warranted. Thus, a complete study is usually possible with two or, at most, three films: the preliminary film, the 6 to 10 minute film and, if warranted, the 30 to 60 minute bladder film.

The kinescopic examination is carried out about 30 minutes after the injection of contrast medium to detect such disorders as abnormalities in voiding pattern or in bladder contraction, vesicoureteral reflux, urethral obstruction or retention of urine. The study is carried out as follows: Before the child voids, a kinescopic recording is made of the ureters and kidneys; the child is asked to void and a kinescopic record is made of the bladder area in an anteroposterior projection throughout voiding. If a urethral abnormality is suspected, an oblique projection is used. In either case a spot film is obtained during and immediately after voiding.

A retrograde cystourethrogram may be indicated when there is inadequate visualization of the bladder and urethra, or when there is concern about vesicoureteral reflux or abnormalities of the bladder or urethra. For this purpose the safest and simplest technique is to insert a No. 5 soft plastic feeding tube into the bladder via the urethra and gradually fill the bladder with a 30 per cent solution of the same contrast medium used for intravenous urography. The volume ranges from 40 to 50 ml in an infant to 200 ml in an 8 to 10 year old. The contrast medium is allowed to flow via a standard intravenous infusion set from a sterile bottle raised about 3 feet above the patient. The child is encouraged not to void while the bladder is being filled. Fluoroscopic examination is carried out intermittently during filling to determine the posi-

*This section was prepared with the assistance of Dr. J. Lussier-Lazaroff.

†Dulcolax—Boehringer Ingelheim, Inc., 33 West Tarrytown, Elmsford, N.Y.

*Hypaque—Winthrop Laboratories, Inc., 90 Park Ave., New York, N.Y.

tion of the catheters and to detect passive vesicoureteral reflux; if reflux is noted, a kinescope study is performed to document it. The kinescopic-voiding study and spot films are obtained as described previously.

In patients with hypertension, in whom stenosis of the renal artery is suspected, a rapid sequence intravenous urogram is obtained. In this instance the contrast medium is injected as rapidly as possible, and films, coned down to the renal areas, are obtained immediately and at 1 and 2 minutes to detect differences in the time of appearance of the nephrogram and in visualization of the pelvicalyceal collecting system. A full abdominal radiograph is obtained after 6 or 10 minutes. Renal angiography and isotope studies of the renal blood flow may be indicated in patients with suspected renovascular hypertension.

RENAL BIOPSY

Renal biopsy often enables precise diagnosis and evaluation of severity of an illness, gives information relative to the prognosis and allows the nephrologist to make reasonable decisions concerning treatment of the disorder in question.

Percutaneous renal biopsy should be done only in conditions in which it is suspected that there is a generalized abnormality which is not confined to a localized area of the kidney. The conditions in which renal biopsy is of most help are those which affect the glomeruli principally. These include a number of specific disorders which may share any of the following relatively nonspecific findings: reduced glomerular filtration rate, hematuria and proteinuria. A biopsy may also be helpful in establishing the diagnosis in patients with acute renal failure of unknown etiology and in evaluating the condition of a transplanted kidney. Sequential biopsies may be used to monitor the course of a disorder.

Biopsy is done only after complete evaluation of the patient's problem by means of appropriate clinical, biochemical, bacteriologic and radiologic studies. It should be performed only by someone who has considerable experience with the technique. It is also essential that facilities and personnel be available to prepare the renal tissue for light and electron microscopic study and for immunopathologic examination and skilled interpretation and integration of the clinical and pathologic findings. In infants under 6 months of age, an open rather than a percutaneous biopsy is generally considered safer.

Cohen, M. L., Smith, F. G., Jr., Mindell, R. S., and Vernier, R. L.: A simple, reliable method of measuring glomerular filtration rate using single, low dose sodium iothalamate I^{131}. Pediatrics *43*:407, 1969.

Edelmann, C. M., Jr., Barnett, H. L., Stark, H., Boichis, H., and Rodriguez-Soriano, J.: A standardized test of renal concentrating capacity in infants and children. Am. J. Dis. Child. *114*:639, 1967.

Edelmann, C. M., Jr., Boichis, H., Rodriguez-Soriano, J., and Stark, H.: The renal response of children to acute ammonium chloride acidosis. Pediatr. Res. *1*:452, 1967.

Gilbert, E. F., Khoury, G. H., Hogan, G. R., and Jones, B.: Hemorrhagic renal necrosis in infancy: Relationship to radiopaque compounds. J. Pediatr. *76*:49, 1970.

Goldman, H. S., and Freeman, L. M.: Radiographic and radioisotopic methods of evaluation of the kidneys and urinary tract. Pediat. Clin. N. Amer. *18*:409, 1971.

Harries, J. D., Mildenberger, R. R., Malowany, A. S., and Drummond, K. N.: A computerized cumulative integral method for the precise measurement of the glomerular filtration rate. Proc. Soc. Exp. Biol. Med. *140*:1148, 1972.

Lowry, O. H., Rosebrough, N. J., Farr, A. L., and Randall, R. J.: Protein measurement with the Folin phenol reagent. J. Biol. Chem. *193*:265, 1951.

Manuel, Y., Revillard, J. P., and Betuel, H. (eds.): Proteins in Normal and Pathologic Urine. Baltimore, University Park Press, 1970.

Robinson, R. E., and Glenn, W. G.: Fixed and reproducible orthostatic proteinuria. IV. Urinary albumin excretion by healthy human subjects in the recumbent and upright postures. J. Lab. Clin. Med. *64*:717, 1964.

Scriver, C. R., and Rosenberg, L. E.: Amino Acid Metabolism and Its Disorders. Philadelphia, W. B. Saunders Company, 1973.

Diseases of the Glomerulus

It is clinically useful and, in most instances, theoretically sound to consider renal disease from the standpoint of the primary site of injury or disturbed physiology. Any of the individual components of the nephron (glomerulus, proximal tubule, distal tubule), the interstitial tissue or the renal vasculature may be the principal site of damage or abnormal function. There is, however, a close relationship between the various parts of the nephron, and they in turn are dependent on the integrity of the renal blood supply and interstitium; a disturbance in or pathologic insult to one of these components of the kidney is often reflected in altered structure or function in others. In this section, disorders which affect the glomerulus primarily are discussed.

If diseases of the glomerulus are to be understood, correctly diagnosed and intelligently handled, it is necessary first to consider what is known about the etiology and pathogenesis of the injury, the types of histopathologic change which may be present, the spectrum of clinical and laboratory manifestations, the role of host factors and the natural history of each disorder. Although it is more demanding of the physician, the failure to use an integrated approach and to examine each problem in its entirety is responsible for much of the misunderstanding about glomerular diseases.

ETIOLOGY AND PATHOGENESIS OF GLOMERULAR INJURY. Although in almost all forms of glomerular injury it is impossible to specify precisely the molecular basis of the events leading to the structural and functional changes observed, it is usually possible to group etiologic factors on a general basis.

Hereditary or Familial Factors. Hereditary factors play a role in many forms of glomerular disease. In some, interstitial parenchymal and tubular lesions may develop and progress in parallel with the glomerular lesions. Included are hereditary nephritis with deafness (Alport syndrome), microcystic congenital nephrotic syndrome, benign familial recurrent hematuria and the glomerulopathies of the nail-patella syndrome (hereditary osteo-onychodysplasia) and of Fabry's disease. A complete list of the known heritable conditions in which renal manifestations are present comprises about 50 distinct entities; in many of these, the glomeruli are affected. These conditions are listed in Table 15–7. A complete description of each disorder is not given since many are rare or find expression only in adulthood. Some of the specific forms of hereditary renal disease are discussed later under that heading. Genetic factors are also operative in some patients with the minimal lesion form of the nephrotic syndrome and in some with the hemolytic uremic syndrome.

Immunologic Factors. Although it was suspected since the early 1900's that immune factors are important in the pathogenesis of renal disease, it has been only since the late 1950's that there have been both a delineation of the specific conditions in which they are operative and a clarification of the pathogenesis of immunologic glomerular injury. These advances have resulted from the development and use of immunopathologic techniques to study human renal disease directly and to study experimental models of immunologically induced renal disease in animals, and from the use of the electron microscope in the study of pathologic structural changes.

Several types of immunologic glomerular injury are recognized. The *most common type* results from deposition of antigen-antibody complexes in the glomerulus; these complexes bind complement. During circulation through the glomerulus, they may be sequestered in the mesangium or in a subendothelial position between the endothelium and the glomerular basement membrane; more commonly, however, they penetrate the glomerular basement membrane and are trapped on its epithelial aspect. Neither antigen nor antibody bears any immunologic specificity to glomerular constituents; they are merely trapped in the glomerulus as a consequence of two physiologic processes: filtration and the mesangial trapping of macromolecular aggregates. The principal site of deposition within the glomerulus is related to the size of the complex and the ratio of antigen to antibody. The presence of complement in the complexes and its consequent apposition to glomerular constituents such as mesangium and glomerular basement membrane is of paramount importance in the development of the ensuing lesions. In some diseases with immune complex deposition, the amount of available antigen is limited, e.g., a bacterial antigen may be eliminated by host defense mechanisms or by specific treatment. In such conditions, glomerular deposition of complexes is also limited and damage may be mild or of short duration, e.g., in the nephritis of serum sickness. When there is an unlimited or persistent source of antigen, the host continues to produce antibody, and chronic formation of antigen-antibody complexes results; glomerular deposition persists and progressive glomerular damage may occur, e.g., in untreated systemic lupus erythematosus.

Characteristic of this type of immunologic injury is the electron microscopic finding of discrete masses or lumps in mesangial, subendothelial or epimembranous sites; IgG and β_{1C} globulin are usually identifiable within these deposits by immunopathologic techniques. If *chronic* deposition of complex occurs, the nodules are incorporated into the glomerular basement membrane, which gradually becomes thickened to produce membranous glomerulonephritis. This membranous change or transformation occurs in a variety of unrelated conditions which have in common the production or release of an antigen capable of stimulating antibody production, with the consequent formation of soluble antigen-antibody complexes. Factors of importance in the formation of complexes capable of damaging the glomerulus are the ratio of antigen to antibody in the complex (those with an antigen:antibody ratio of 2:1 are most harmful), the size of the complex (those with a sedimentation coefficient more than 19S have a greater tendency to be trapped) and the type of antibody formed (usually a nonprecipitating antibody of the IgG or IgM class). Diseases in which glomerular deposition of immune complexes occurs include serum sickness, systemic lupus erythematosus, congenital or secondary syphilis, chronic septicemia with bacteria of low virulence (as in infected shunts for hydrocephalus) and *Plasmodium malariae* infestation. In most patients with chronic membranous glomerulopathy, however, the nature and source of the antigen are unknown.

In the *second type of immunologic injury,* host antibodies react with glomerular antigens, usually the glycoprotein moiety of the glomerular basement membrane; they are deposited in a linear, uninterrupted pattern along the endothelial aspect of the glomerular basement membrane. Complement is fixed at the site of this antigen-antibody reaction. The linear pattern of antibody and complement deposition is in contrast to the nodular deposition of immune complexes described above. There are several possible explanations for the development of host antibodies which react with the patient's own glomeruli. These include an alteration in glomerular antigenic structure, possibly as the result of injury, which renders the proteins foreign to the host's antibody-producing cells;

thus, antibodies capable of reacting with glomerular antigens are formed. It is also possible that glomerular antigens previously confined to the glomerulus and without access to antibody-producing sites are released into the circulation from the glomeruli to stimulate antibody production. This response is analogous to that in sympathetic ophthalmia, in which the normal eye can be damaged by antibodies that are formed in response to antigens developed and released because of traumatic injury to the other eye. The patient may also produce antibodies to foreign protein, such as a viral or bacterial antigen, and these antibodies may cross-react with glomerular antigens. Nonrenal host antigens may also be released following injury, and antibodies produced to such antigens may cross-react with glomerular constituents which have similar antigenic determinants.

Although the antiglomerular basement membrane form of injury has been extensively studied in experimental animals, this mechanism is probably operative in less than 10 per cent of human immunologic renal diseases. Included are Goodpasture syndrome, some cases of rapidly progressive glomerulonephritis and some of chronic glomerulonephritis; all are rare in children.

The *third type of immunologic renal injury* involves activation of the complement system by a mechanism independent of the aggregation of immunoglobulin molecules in relation to antigen. In this system, factors either exogenous or present in the patient's serum activate the complement system at the third component, bypassing C1, 4 and 2. Although the final sequence of complement activation leading to release of biologically active compounds is the same here as in the classic system involving C1, 4 and 2, the participation of an antigen-antibody reaction is not needed to initiate the sequence of complement activation after C3. This mechanism operates in chronic hypocomplementemic glomerulonephritis (membranoproliferative glomerulonephritis) and may also be of importance in acute poststreptococcal glomerulonephritis and in the nephritis of systemic lupus erythematosus.

Two other types of immunologic glomerular injury have recently been proposed; each is based on studies of experimentally induced glomerulonephritis in animals: (1) The mesangium has an active phagocytic function, similar to that of other organs of the reticuloendothelial system. Macromolecules with antigenic properties may be trapped and sequestered within the mesangium. The host may produce antibodies to this trapped antigen which react with it; complement is then fixed at the site of this antigen-antibody reaction to the mesangium. (2) The other mechanism is poorly understood and is probably uncommon in humans. It involves deposition of glomerular immunoglobulin without complement. Some classes of immunoglobulin (IgA, E, D) and subgroup 4 of the IgG class do not fix complement. In one example of experimental antikidney (nephrotoxic) serum nephritis, immunoglobulin deposition without complement deposition has been described; likewise, in the glomerulopathy of congenital and secondary syphilis, subepithelial immunoglobulin deposits have been demonstrated without associated complement.

In most known forms of immunologic glomerular injury, the **complement system** is of fundamental importance in the actual mediation of damage. Complement participates in three principal ways: the causation of inflammation by immune adherence of leukocytes and by chemotaxis, damage of biologic membranes, and enhancement of blood coagulation. As discussed earlier, there are two pathways by which the complement system is activated, each leading to generation of biologically active complement fragments and other products, such as kinins, which lead to glomerular damage. The first is the *classic pathway,* in which antibody molecules aggregated in relation to specific antigens interact with the C1q subunit of C1. Of the five classes of immunoglobulin in man – IgG, IgM, IgA, IgD, IgE – only IgM and the first three subgroups (1, 2 and 3) of IgG bind C1q. Following this binding with C1q, C1 is activated and catalyzes the assembly of the C4 and C2 components to form the enzyme C3 convertase (C4,2), which in turn activates the terminal complement components C3 and C5 through C9 with resultant release of biologically active complement products.

In the second or *alternate pathway,* C1, C2 and C4 are bypassed and C3 is activated by a C3 activator enzyme derived from a serum protein called C3 proactivator. This enzyme has an action similar to that of the complement enzyme C3 convertase (C4,2). As in the classic system, the activation of C3 by this alternate route brings the terminal components into action and there is generation of biologically active products. The role of properdin in this alternate pathway is of interest; the properdin system is probably closely related, or possibly identical, to the C3 activator system.

Metabolic or Toxic Factors. Most known nephrotoxic drugs or chemicals damage principally renal tubules or interstitial tissue; glomerular damage is mainly secondary to this initial injury. Certain drugs such as trimethadione, however, may selectively damage the glomeruli and cause increased permeability of the glomerular basement membrane to protein; this may also occur in chronic mercury poisoning. A good example of a glomerular alteration developing in a metabolic disease is seen in diabetes mellitus. An increase in mesangial tissue and thickening of the basement membrane develop early in the disease at a time when there is no clinical evidence of renal disease. Some authors have also proposed that the minimal lesion form of the nephrotic syndrome is due to a disorder of glomerular biochemistry or metabolism. One example cited as supporting evidence of this hypothesis is the fact that the clinical picture and lesions of trimethadione-induced nephrosis resemble those in minimal lesion nephrotic syndrome.

Coagulation Disturbances. The presence of

fibrin or its derivatives at the site of glomerular injury, the detection of fibrin degradation products in serum and urine and the modification by anticoagulation of the course of some glomerular diseases, particularly nephrotoxic nephritis in animals, has led to the hypothesis that altered coagulation mechanisms may be operative in the pathogenesis of some glomerular diseases. It is not established that glomerular fibrin deposition is an initial or important event in human glomerular damage, despite the fact that fibrin and its derivatives are sometimes present in epithelial crescents, in areas of mesangial proliferation or along the glomerular basement membrane. Some authors consider that, although the coagulation mechanism may not be critical in the initial insult, it does participate in progressive glomerular damage. Conditions in which glomerular fibrin deposition is common include anaphylactoid purpura, the membranous nephropathy of systemic lupus erythematosus and proliferative glomerulonephritis with crescents.

Other Factors. There are undoubtedly other causes of glomerular injury. Few if any of them or of those already discussed can be considered as isolated factors, since their actions are often interrelated. For example, immune complex deposition involves complement activation which may enhance blood coagulation locally; this in turn may accentuate glomerular damage. Similarly, in diabetes mellitus, which is primarily a disorder of carbohydrate metabolism, there is evidence of immunoglobulin deposition along glomerular basement membrane in about half the patients. It is likely that this is a secondary event and not of pathogenetic importance, but it is a good example of how interrelated and complex are the factors which may lead to glomerular injury. Finally, there is evidence that a common consequence of glomerular injury, such as increased permeability of the glomerular basement membrane to protein, may in turn have an effect on glomerular function and/or structure.

Idiopathic Factors. The causes of most forms of glomerular injury remain unknown. In children, the most common disorders of this category include the minimal lesion form of the nephrotic syndrome, the nephritis of anaphylactoid purpura, benign recurrent hematuria and some forms of rapidly progressive glomerulonephritis.

HISTOPATHOLOGY OF GLOMERULAR DISEASE. Despite the wide heterogeneity of causes and pathogenetic mechanisms in glomerular injury, the range of possible clinical, laboratory and pathologic responses is limited. Furthermore, although there is a relation between the pathologic lesions, laboratory findings and clinical manifestations, the relationship is often not accurately predictable from knowledge of one or two of them.

In assessment of the pathologic changes in glomeruli by light microscopy, the following points should be considered: (1) Are there abnormal findings? (2) Do the lesions affect all glomeruli (uniglomerular), many of the glomeruli (multiglomerular) or only some, i.e., less than half of the glomeruli (focal)? (3) In affected glomeruli, does the lesion affect the entire glomerulus (diffuse) or is it confined to limited areas (segmental)? (4) Is there evidence that the lesion is recent (acute) or longstanding (chronic)? (5) Is there abnormal lobulation of the glomeruli? (6) Is there cellular proliferation and, if so, which cells are involved—mesangial, endothelial or epithelial? Has proliferation of parietal epithelial cells led to epithelial crescent formation? (7) Is there a reduction in the number of patent capillary loops? (8) Is there an increase in mesangial matrix? (9) Is there an infiltrate of polymorphonuclear leukocytes to indicate inflammation? (10) Is there evidence of necrosis of any part of the glomerulus? (11) Are the glomerular basement membranes thickened? If so, is the thickening uniform or localized? Is it due to proliferation of the mesangial tissue which has extended between the endothelial cells and the glomerular basement membrane proper, or is it due to deposition of material, such as immune complexes, along the epithelial or endothelial aspect of the glomerular basement membrane? (12) Is Bowman's capsule thickened? Are there adhesions between the glomerular tuft and Bowman's capsule? (13) Are the lesions minimal, moderate or severe? (14) Are the interstitial tissue and the blood vessels involved? Are these changes secondary to or independent of the glomerular lesion? Is there periglomerular fibrosis, tubular atrophy or dilatation, interstitial scarring or inflammation?

By evaluating glomerular lesions in the above manner, a description of the pathologic findings is made. It is then possible to assess the severity of the lesions, to decide if they are likely to be self-limited, progressive and amenable to therapy; it is also often possible to identify specific disease entities. *Percutaneous renal biopsy* is the technique used to obtain tissue for these studies.

CLINICAL MANIFESTATIONS OF GLOMERULAR DISEASE. The clinical conditions resulting from glomerular disorders are determined not only by the type of injury, its extent, its severity and its rate of progression, but by host determinants, some of which are unknown, and by factors such as age, state of nutrition, amount of proteinuria and the intake and excretion of fluid and electrolytes.

The major clinical patterns resulting from glomerular injury are listed in Table 15-3. It should be emphasized that they are not mutually exclusive and that, with time, one may supersede another.

LABORATORY MANIFESTATIONS OF GLOMERULAR DISEASE. Apart from laboratory tests which may help in the diagnosis of a specific disease, there are three areas of laboratory investigation which are particularly helpful in the assessment of glomerular involvement: (1) Measurement of glomerular filtration rate; values below normal are reflected in elevation of the blood urea nitrogen and serum creatinine concentrations. When the glomerular

TABLE 15-3 CLINICAL PATTERNS OF GLOMERULAR DISEASE

CLINICAL PATTERN	MANIFESTATIONS
1. Nephrotic syndrome	Generalized edema, proteinuria in excess of 2 gm/m^2/day, reduced serum protein concentration, elevated serum cholesterol; transient microscopic hematuria and hypertension are occasional manifestations
2. Acute glomerulonephritis	Hematuria, oliguria, hypertension, mild edema, circulatory congestion, azotemia
3. Mixed nephritic-nephrotic pattern	A combination of features of (1) and (2)
4. Acute renal failure	Anuria or severe oliguria with fluid, acid-base, and electrolyte disturbances; hypertension, circulatory congestion and edema may be present
5. Chronic renal insufficiency or failure	Growth retardation, anemia, azotemia, metabolic acidosis, hyperphosphatemia, hypocalcemia, renal osteodystrophy, polyuria and polydipsia.
6. Recurrent or persistent hematuria	Episodic gross hematuria with intermittent or persistent microscopic hematuria; moderate proteinuria usually present during episodes of hematuria
7. Asymptomatic proteinuria	Persistent proteinuria in an otherwise apparently healthy child

filtration rate falls below 25 per cent of normal, serum phosphate and uric acid levels may also rise above normal. (2) Measurement of urinary protein excretion; a common response of the glomerulus to a wide variety of injuries is increased permeability of the glomerular basement membrane to macromolecules which are normally excluded from the filtrate. This leads to the excretion of an abnormal amount of protein in the urine. In healthy children the 24-hour protein excretion is less than 150 mg; in the large majority it is less than 30 mg. Persistent values over 150 mg/24 hr are abnormal unless the child has orthostatic proteinuria. An arbitrary but useful division based on the 24-hour excretion is as follows: 150 to 500 mg is considered mild proteinuria; 500 mg to 2 gm, moderate; over 2 gm, massive. (3) Examination of the urine sediment; an abnormal excretion of red blood cells and, if glomerular inflammation is present, of white blood cells, is a common finding in many forms of glomerular injury. These cellular elements may result from renal lesions at sites other than the glomerulus, or from bleeding or inflammation in the ureters and lower urinary tract; their renal source is distinguished by the presence of casts. Red and/or white blood cells may be embedded in the matrix of the cast or it may be hyaline or granular. In most instances the presence of casts reflects not only a renal but actually a glomerular origin of the abnormal sediment.

Germuth, F. G., Jr., and Rodriguez, E.: Immunopathology of the Renal Glomerulus. Immune Complex Deposit and Antibasement Membrane Disease. Boston, Little, Brown and Company, Inc., 1973, p. 227.

Kincaid-Smith, P.: Coagulation and renal disease. (Editorial review.) Kidney Int. *2*:183, 1972.

Lewis, E. J., and Couser, W. G.: The immunologic basis of human renal disease. Pediat. Clin. N. Amer. *18*:467, 1971.

Michael, A. F., Drummond, K. N., Vernier, R. L., and Good, R. A.: Immunologic basis of renal disease. Pediat. Clin. N. Amer. *11*:695, 1964.

West, C. D., Ruley, E. J., Forristal, J., and Davis, N. C.: Mechanisms of hypocomplementemia in glomerulonephritis. Kidney Int. *3*:116, 1973.

THE NEPHROTIC SYNDROME

The nephrotic syndrome results from increased permeability of the glomerular basement membrane to protein. It is characterized by general *edema, hypoproteinemia* with serum albumin levels usually below 2 gm/dl, *hyperlipidemia* with serum cholesterol levels above 220 mg/dl, and excessive *proteinuria,* 2 gm/m^2/24 hr or more. The essential common feature shared by all manifestations of the syndrome is marked proteinuria. A classification of the various causes and types of the nephrotic syndrome is given in Table 15-4. A discussion of the specific clinical entities which are manifested as the nephrotic syndrome is given after the following general comments on the pathogenesis of the principal features.

PROTEINURIA. The excessive excretion of protein results from increased glomerular filtration of protein owing to increased permeability of the glomerular basement membrane. Generally, plasma proteins of low molecular weight such as albumin, immunoglobulin G and transferrin are excreted more readily in the nephrotic syndrome than are proteins of large molecular weight such as the lipoproteins. The relative clearances of the various plasma proteins thus differ in inverse relation to their size or molecular weight, a concept referred to as the selectivity of the proteinuria.

The reduction in serum protein concentration, particularly of the lower molecular weight proteins such as albumin, immunoglobulin G (IgG) and transferrin, is primarily a consequence of loss of protein in the urine. There is also evidence of increased protein catabolism, some of which may take place in the renal tubular cells. In addition to a reduction in the total serum protein concentration, there is a paradoxical increase in the concentration of some proteins of larger molecular weight, particularly of α_2 globulins; the plasma lipoproteins are in this fraction. The plasma calcium concentration may be low as a consequence of the reduced albumin level, since about half of the plasma calcium is bound to albumin; the amount of ionized calcium, however, remains normal.

EDEMA. Although edema is almost always present at some time during the course, it is the most variable of the cardinal features of the nephrotic syndrome. It is certainly the sign which dominates the clinical picture from the parents' point of view. However, it must be regarded as a secondary manifestation whose presence or absence is influenced by a number of factors such as fluid and salt intake; as mentioned before, the primary pathophysiologic event is increased urinary excretion of protein. The precise mechanism of edema formation in the nephrotic syndrome is complex; some of the known factors are: (1) *reduction in plasma colloid osmotic pressure* consequent to the decreased concentration of serum albumin, which is responsible for redistribution of extracellular water, with an increase in the interstitial compartment relative to that in the intravascular compartment; (2) *marked reduction in urinary excretion of sodium* owing to an increase in tubular reabsorption of sodium. The mechanisms which lead to enhanced sodium reabsorption with consequent negligible urinary sodium loss are more complicated than formerly believed. It is clear that there is a distinct elevation in urinary excretion of aldosterone secondary to increased excretion of renin. It is probable that a reduction in intravascular volume resulting from a shift of fluid to the extravascular space is the prime stimulus for an increase in secretion of renin. Decreased plasma colloid osmotic pressure caused by the low plasma albumin concentration has a direct effect on tubular reabsorption of sodium. The interrelation of factors influencing sodium reabsorption in the nephrotic syndrome is very complex and as yet incompletely understood; (3) *retention of water.* Reduction of plasma colloid osmotic pressure and retention of all ingested sodium would not in themselves be sufficient for the development of significant edema in the nephrotic syndrome, even though they might be expected to result in a limited redistribution of fluid from the intravascular to the interstitial space. In order for edema to develop, there must be a retention of water for which there are several explanations. If electrolyte concentrations in body fluids are to remain isotonic in the face of retention of virtually all ingested sodium, water must be conserved. For each 140 mEq of sodium ingested and not excreted, one liter of water must be retained. Normal tonicity is maintained through the secretion of antidiuretic hormone, which leads to reabsorption of water in the distal tubules and collecting ducts and the elaboration of a hypertonic or concentrated urine. That this is the principal explanation for water retention is suggested by the observation that in most nephrotic children in whom the sodium intake is markedly reduced, there is no need to restrict the intake of water, since the ability to excrete water is not impaired.

Other reasons for water retention may exist; a small percentage of nephrotic children continue to retain water to the point of becoming markedly hyponatremic, even when their sodium intake is nil. This may result from inappropriate (in the face of hypotonicity of the plasma) continued release of antidiuretic hormone in response to contraction of the intravascular volume. It is also possible that, as a consequence of a net increase in sodium reabsorption in the proximal tubule together with passive reabsorption of water along an osmotic gradient in this segment, a reduced volume of filtrate is delivered to the ascending limb of the loop of Henle and to the distal convoluted tubules for formation of dilute urine. In such a situation, ingestion of excess water could lead to progressive decrease in plasma osmolality, as a result of the progressive fall in concentration of serum sodium. In nephrotic patients the retention of salt and water does not correct what may be considered a physiologic response to reduced plasma oncotic pressure, contracted intravascular volume and hypertonicity, since the retained fluid escapes into the interstitial space and the patient becomes more and more edematous in direct relation to the amount of ingested sodium and water.

HYPERLIPIDEMIA. Most of the lipid fractions normally found in plasma are elevated in the nephrotic syndrome. There is a variable inverse relation between the degree of hyperlipidemia and the reduction in plasma albumin. Among the possible explanations of the elevated plasma concentration of lipoproteins is their relatively high molecular weight and consequent negligible loss in the urine in comparison with that of albumin. Since lipoproteins play a role in lipid transport, their increase in plasma may also influence lipid levels. A decrease in plasma lipoprotein lipase activity in children with the nephrotic syndrome has also been postulated as a contributing factor to hyperlipidemia.

Albrink, M. J., Hald, P. M., Man, E. B., and Peters, J. P.: The displacement of serum water by the lipids of hyperlipidemic serum. A new method for the rapid determination of serum water. J. Clin. Invest. *34*:1483, 1955.

Cameron, J. S., and White, R. H. R.: Selectivity of proteinuria in children with the nephrotic syndrome. Lancet *1*:463, 1965.

Churg, J., Habib, R., and White, R. H. R.: Pathology of the nephrotic syndrome in children. A report for the international study of kidney disease in children. Lancet *1*:1299, 1970.

Grausz, H., Lieberman, R., and Earley, L. E.: Effect of plasma albumin on sodium reabsorption in patients with nephrotic syndrome. Kidney Int. *1*:47, 1972.

Habib, R., and Kleinknecht, C.: The primary nephrotic syndrome of childhood: Classification and clinicopathologic study of 406 cases. *In* Sommers, S. C. (ed.): Pathology Annual 1971. New York, Appleton-Century-Crofts, Inc., 1971, p. 417.

MINIMAL LESION FORM OF THE NEPHROTIC SYNDROME

(Lipoid Nephrosis, Nephrosis, Idiopathic Nephrotic Syndrome of Childhood)

This form of the nephrotic syndrome is characterized by responsiveness to corticosteroid therapy

TABLE 15–4 CLASSIFICATION OF THE NEPHROTIC SYNDROME IN CHILDHOOD*

DISORDER	ETIOLOGY	AGE OF ONSET	NOTEWORTHY FEATURES	PATHOLOGY
A. Infantile mycrocystic disease	Autosomal recessive	Birth to 3 months	Toxemia of pregnancy; prematurity; placentomegaly	Dilated proximal tubules
B. Minimal lesion nephrotic syndrome	Idiopathic	Usually after 6 months, peak onset 2–5 years	Frequent relapses; usually responds to steroid therapy	Fusion of visceral epithelial foot processes†
C. Focal glomerular sclerosis	Idiopathic	>6 months	Microhematuria; steroid resistance with progressive renal failure may occur	Focal segmental or focal diffuse glomerular sclerosis; tubular atrophy
D. Omniglomerular diffuse mesangial sclerosis	May be familial	<6 months	Progressive uremia	Omniglomerular diffuse mesangial sclerosis; interstitial fibrosis
E. Epimembranous glomerulopathy	1. Idiopathic	All ages	Clinical features of nephrotic syndrome	Thickened glomerular basement membranes with epimembranous deposits; IgG with or without IgM, fibrin and β_{1c} globulin are present in the deposits along the membrane
	2. Congenital syphilis	<6 months	Clinical features of congenital syphilis	
	3. Lupus erythematosus	Children, adolescents	Clinical features of lupus erythematosus	
	4. Malaria	4–8 years	Quartan malaria (*P. malariae*)	An epimembranous glomerulopathy may be present; radiolucent lacunae with splitting of the basement membrane may also occur; IgG, β_{1_C} and IgM deposits are usually present in the glomeruli
F. Membranoproliferative glomerulonephritis	1. Idiopathic	Adolescents	Anemia; hypocomplementemia or normocomplementemia	Large glomeruli; lobulation of tufts; increase in mesangial cells and matrix; subendothelial extension of mesangial matrix; subendothelial or intramembranous electron-dense deposits seen on electron microscopy; glomerular properdin deposition seen in idiopathic form
	2. Lipodystrophy		Generalized or partial lipodystrophy	
	3. Shunt nephritis		Chronic bacteremia; splenomegaly; anemia; hypocomplementemia	
G. Proliferative glomerulonephritis	1. Idiopathic		All 4 etiologies: hematuria; hypertension; azotemia; nephrotic syndrome	Proliferation of mesangial cells; crescents often seen; polymorphonuclear leukocyte
	2. Acute poststrep-			

	tococcal glomerulonephritis 3. Lupus erythematosus		Plus associated features of SLE	infiltration in glomeruli; may have foci of fibrinoid necrosis; on electron microscopy: subendothelial, subepithelial and mesangial deposits in lupus, subepithelial deposits in acute glomerulonephritis
	4. Anaphylactoid purpura		Plus associated features of anaphylactoid purpura	
H. Miscellaneous conditions which occasionally may be associated with the nephrotic syndrome:				
1. Genital anomalies		< 2 years		Glomerular sclerosis and interstitial fibrosis
2. Nephroblastoma		< 2 years		
3. Nail-patella syndrome	Familial	1 case at birth; usually > 3–4 years	Dystrophic nails; absent patellae	Focal glomerular sclerosis; by electron microscopy, lucent areas and collections of collagen fibrils in the glomerular basement membrane
4. Alport syndrome	Familial	Adolescents	Deafness; eye changes	Lucent areas in basement membrane on electron microscopy; interstitial foam cells commonly present
5. Cystinosis	Autosomal recessive	< 5 years	Fanconi syndrome; the nephrotic syndrome in cystinosis is uncommon and occurs as a late feature	Multinucleate giant cell transformation of visceral glomerular epithelium; cystine crystals are deposited in the kidney
6. Hemolytic uremic syndrome	Idiopathic; hereditary and/or environmental factors in some cases	Usually < 2 years	Microangiopathic hemolytic anemia; thrombocytopenia	Subendothelial vacuolation in glomeruli; subendothelial fibrin deposition in smaller renal arteries and arterioles; microangiopathy
I. Drug-induced nephrotic syndrome	Mercury			No abnormalities on light microscopy
	Penicillamine			Deposition of immune complexes along glomerular basement membrane
	Tridione			Fusion of visceral epithelial foot processes

*Dr. Bernard Kaplan assisted in the preparation of this table.
†Similar morphologic changes may be seen in patients with Hodgkin's disease and the nephrotic syndrome.

and by characteristic glomerular findings on histopathologic study, namely, the absence of significant glomerular lesions on examination by light microscopy, the absence of deposition of glomerular immune globulin or complement as evidenced by immunopathologic studies and fusion of the epithelial foot processes without other significant glomerular lesions by electron microscopy.

ETIOLOGY. The etiology is unknown. A nonspecific illness, usually a viral upper respiratory tract infection, often precedes the initial episode and subsequent relapses by a period of 4 to 8 days. This association, however, is considered a precipitating event rather than a specific cause. Rarely, genetic factors appear to be a factor; nephrosis has been observed in siblings and in other relatives.

INCIDENCE. The incidence of new cases from birth to 16 years of age is about 2 per 100,000 population per year in North America. It is rare under 6 months of age and uncommon under 1 year. Most cases have their onset between 2 and 7 years, and there is a slightly higher incidence in males. The minimal lesion disease accounts for 80 to 90 per cent of children with the nephrotic syndrome, whereas in adults the figure is about 30 per cent.

PATHOLOGY AND PATHOGENESIS. The pathologic changes in the kidney are minimal if biopsy is done near the time of onset. The glomeruli are essentially normal by light microscopy, except for occasional areas of prominence of the mesangial matrix; these tend to become more pronounced as the duration of proteinuria increases. Tubular casts contain protein and, at times, hyaline droplets. Electron microscopy demonstrates fusion of the epithelial cell foot processes along the epithelial aspect of the glomerular basement membrane. Immunopathologic studies reveal an absence of deposits of immune globulin or complement components. Although the term, "minimal lesion nephrotic syndrome," is appropriate early in the course, some patients develop progressive sclerosis of the glomeruli if satisfactory control, i.e., cessation of proteinuria, is not achieved.

The pathogenesis of glomerular abnormality is not understood. Extensive search has failed to demonstrate glomerular deposition of immunoglobulins or complement components in most cases, even though occasional mesangial deposition is observed, possibly as a consequence of mesangial protein trapping. It is suspected that a metabolic, biochemical or physicochemical disturbance in the glomerular basement membrane leads to increased permeability to protein, but data are not yet available to support this hypothesis.

CLINICAL MANIFESTATIONS AND COURSE. Edema which has developed over the course of several weeks is the usual presenting manifestation. Sometimes there is a history of transient edema within the preceding months. An antecedent respiratory infection is not uncommon and may on occasion precipitate a relapse. The child may be lethargic or anorexic; a weight gain of 15 to 20 per cent is common and is due to accumulation of edema fluid. The volume of urine is usually decreased and the concentrated urine may appear dark.

The child usually does not appear seriously ill; the most striking feature is generalized edema, often with ascites and pleural effusion. The edema fluid accumulates in dependent sites; after a night's sleep, the face and eyelids or sacral region may be edematous, whereas during the day, swelling of the legs and abdomen is more prominent. The blood pressure is usually normal or even slightly decreased; in some instances, however, it is elevated, probably because of hyperreninemia, leading to excess production of angiotensin. There is a more than usual susceptibility to bacterial infection, possibly at least in part related to the low level of gamma globulin in the plasma. Peritonitis or septicemia, caused by *Diplococcus pneumoniae* or coliform organisms, and cellulitis are the more common infections. Venous or arterial thrombosis is an infrequent but potentially serious complication and is possibly accentuated by steroid therapy. Shock is another infrequent complication and is usually secondary to rapid diuresis induced by aggressive therapy in a patient whose intravascular volume is already contracted.

Untreated patients tend to have a prolonged course characterized by recurrent episodes; in some instances, remission may occur spontaneously or after intercurrent illnesses such as measles.

LABORATORY DATA. Proteinuria in excess of 2 gm/m^2/day, accompanied by a reduction of total plasma proteins with the albumin fraction reduced to less than 2 gm/dl, elevation of α_2 globulins and hyperlipidemia are the characteristic findings. The urine seldom contains red blood cells; oval fat bodies (tubular cells containing lipid) and hyaline casts are seen in the sediment. Proteinuria is highly selective; there is relatively greater clearance of proteins of low rather than of high molecular weight. There is usually an absence of anemia; hemoglobin and hematocrit may even be elevated, owing to hemoconcentration. The white blood cell count is normal or mildly elevated to 10,000–12,000/mm^3. The erythrocyte sedimentation rate may be elevated and, at times, there is a mild azotemia which is usually prerenal in origin as a result of reduced intravascular volume and/or decreased urine flow leading to a reduced clearance of urea. If the child is well hydrated and if hypovolemia is not significant, the glomerular filtration rate is usually normal. The serum level of β_{1C} globulin is normal. The serum sodium concentration is often decreased to 130 to 135 mEq/l.

DIAGNOSIS. The diagnosis is based on the typical clinical and laboratory features, the characteristic findings on renal biopsy and the usual responsiveness to corticosteroid therapy. In addition, there is absence of significant or persistent hypertension, of gross or persistent hematuria, of significant or persistent azotemia and of depression of serum B_{1C} globulin.

Differential Diagnosis. This includes, in particular, other glomerulopathies which clinically are characterized by the nephrotic syndrome. These include:

Idiopathic membranous glomerulopathy, which may present identical clinical findings, except that the usual age of onset is over 10 years and the response to corticosteroids is poor. Proteinuria is less selective and renal biopsy shows thickening of glomerular basement membrane deposits of IgG, with or without β_{1_C} globulin.

Membranoproliferative or hypocomplementemic glomerulonephritis, which is distinguished by a depressed concentration of serum β_{1_C} globulin, hematuria as well as proteinuria, azotemia and, not uncommonly, hypertension. Renal biopsy shows glomerular lobulation and mesangial proliferation. The onset is frequently beyond 10 years of age.

Acute idiopathic proliferative glomerulonephritis with epithelial crescent formation (subacute glomerulonephritis or *rapidly progressive glomerulonephritis),* which is manifested by impressive nephritic as well as nephrotic features, but serum complement levels are usually normal. More than one specific etiologic entity is included under this heading.

Membranous glomerulopathy, which may be associated with systemic disorders such as *lupus erythematosus, malaria* or *syphilis,* is distinguished by the specific features of the respective systemic disease.

Glomerulonephritis of anaphylactoid purpura, which is a proliferative lesion involving primarily the mesangium, with or without epithelial crescent formation. The features of the underlying disease may or may not be present at the time of the nephrotic episode. A nephritic component is common.

Drug- or toxin-induced nephrotic syndrome, which may be secondary to trimethadione therapy, ingestion of mercury, exposure to poison oak or to a bee sting. The clinical and pathologic features may be indistinguishable from the minimal lesion form of the nephrotic syndrome, and diagnosis may be made only by eliciting a history of exposure.

Focal sclerosing glomerulopathy, which may be indistinguishable from the minimal lesion form of the nephrotic syndrome at onset, but is less responsive to therapy and has a poorer prognosis. These patients tend to have more in the way of microscopic hematuria than those with minimal lesion disease. The diagnosis rests on the characteristic changes in biopsies of renal tissue.

Acute poststreptococcal glomerulonephritis may occasionally present clinically as the nephrotic syndrome; the distinguishing features are discussed in the section dealing with this entity.

The nephrotic syndrome in the first year of life includes a group of different disorders which are described later.

TREATMENT. The goal of treatment is reduction in excretion of urinary protein to a normal quantity. To this end, corticosteroids should be given in sufficient dosage for an appropriate length of time. The most frequently used, least expensive and safest drug is prednisone in a dosage of 2 mg/kg (60 mg/m^2)/day, in three or four divided doses, up to a maximum of 60 mg/day. The drug is continued until urine protein excretion has returned to and remained normal for 10 days to 2 weeks. The dose is then tapered to discontinuance over a period of 3 or 4 days. There is no advantage in using a larger dose. In over 90 per cent of patients, the protein excretion returns to normal within 4 weeks, with a mean response time of about 2 weeks. Response may occur as early as 3 or 4 days after beginning prednisone, but if it is not obtained after 1 month of daily treatment, the likelihood of subsequent response to continued therapy falls dramatically. Of those whose protein excretion returns to normal on corticosteroid treatment, only 10 per cent will do so in the second month of daily therapy; the response rate after 2 months is virtually nil. For this reason it is sensible to consider patients with minimal lesion disease as steroid-resistant if protein excretion has not returned to normal after 1 month of treatment, and certainly after 2. Lack of response after 1 month of daily adequate steroid treatment is an indication for reevaluation or change of therapy. If the diagnosis was made on the basis of clinical and laboratory features alone, a renal biopsy should be done at this point to establish the precise diagnosis, since of the different glomerular diseases which may cause the nephrotic syndrome in childhood, only the minimal lesion form should be treated with corticosteroids.

About 30 per cent of children who respond to corticosteroid therapy will not have relapses, but most will have at least one or two. If a tendency to relapse is demonstrated, particularly if the relapse occurs within several months to a year after discontinuance of treatment, an interrupted schedule of administration of prednisone should be given after completion of a daily course repeated as outlined above. A safe and effective interrupted schedule consists of prednisone in a dosage of 60 mg/m^2 on alternate days in a single dose, i.e., every 48 hours, administered in the morning soon after rising. This schedule should be continued for 6 months to 1 year; it reduces the number of relapses to about one third the number which would otherwise occur. An alternate form of interrupted therapy may also be used. It consists of prednisone in a dose of 60 mg/m^2/day given in three or four divided doses for the first three or four days of each week for 6 to 12 months after remission is obtained with daily therapy. Although the relapse rate can be reduced by such regimens, there remain about 20 per cent of children with minimal lesion nephrotic syndrome who relapse. These patients may be treated again with daily administration of prednisone followed as before by an interrupted schedule.

If, however, the side effects of steroid therapy pose a threat to the child's growth and general health, it is possible to reduce the relapse rate by using an oral alkylating agent, such as cyclophosphamide. The dose is 1 to 2.5 mg/kg/day given for a period of 6 weeks to 4 months. Prednisone should be given in addition, as outlined above and continued on an alternate day basis until administration of cyclophosphamide is stopped. The shorter course appears to have less potential for inducing subsequent sterility; however, the relapse rate is higher following the short course. Because of the potential risk of sterility induced by this drug, as well as side effects such as hemorrhagic cystitis and alopecia, it is recommended that it be used only in carefully selected patients and under the direct supervision of a pediatric nephrologist. There is an increased mortality from chickenpox among those who contract it while receiving cyclophosphamide.

Before starting daily treatment with prednisone for either the first attack or for a relapse, it is best, for a number of reasons, to wait 1 to 2 weeks: (1) Spontaneous remission may occur, particularly if the episode has been precipitated by an intercurrent illness. The disadvantages of an unnecessary course of therapy with prednisone may thus be avoided and a delay of this length of time does not influence the ultimate response. (2) Latent bacterial infection which could spread or reactivate during corticosteroid treatment must be excluded, particularly active or inactive tuberculosis and unrecognized urinary tract infection. (3) Marked edema and ascites may make the child uncomfortable, anorexic and unable to move about, and the skin may break down and become infected. If excessive edema can be reduced by diuretics prior to prednisone therapy, the patient's overall condition will probably be better during the course of prednisone therapy. For this purpose, a combination of oral hydrochlorothiazide, 75 mg/m^2/day, and triamterene, 300 mg/m^2/day, given in three divided doses is usually effective over 4 to 7 days and is safe since the diuresis induced is usually gradual. If this attempt at diuresis is ineffective, or if the child's condition warrants a more immediate response, furosemide can be given orally or parenterally in a dosage of 1–3 mg/kg. Because of the danger of contraction of the vascular volume, electrolyte disturbances and shock with intensive diuretic therapy of the nephrotic child, such therapy should be undertaken with extreme caution and preferably in the hospital.

Since the tendency to retain sodium in the nephrotic state is accentuated by steroid therapy, the dietary intake of it should be restricted; an intake of 17 mEq/day (1 gm of sodium chloride) is recommended as long as there is significant edema and proteinuria. Water intake should be limited only if there is progressive accumulation of edema despite dietary restriction of sodium or if there is an impaired ability to excrete a normal intake of water. Clear evidence of dilution of body fluids is indicated by a serum sodium level of 130 mEq/l or less. Physical activity during an attack of the nephrotic syndrome should be as desired and tolerated by the child. Enforced bed rest has been shown to contribute more to prolonging the disability than to the patient's well-being in virtually all disorders of the kidney and urinary tract.

PROGNOSIS. The prognosis for ultimate recovery from the minimal lesion nephrotic syndrome is quite good. Although relapses are common and there is always the danger of an unpredictable event such as sepsis, peritonitis or shock, most children with this condition will respond to treatment and can look forward to a healthy future. For those who have numerous relapses or who cannot be controlled adequately with steroid therapy alone, alkylating agents such as cyclophosphamide or chlorambucil provide the possibility of prolonged remission. The activity of the disease itself tends to lessen after adolescence, and the likelihood of relapse decreases as each year without an attack passes. Unfortunately, perhaps 10 per cent of children with what is considered to be minimal lesion nephrotic syndrome are resistant to steroid therapy. Some of these will respond to long-term treatment with alkylating agents; a few will progress to glomerular sclerosis and renal insufficiency over the course of several years.

Chiu, J., and Drummond, K. N.: Long-term follow-up of cyclophosphamide therapy in frequent relapsing minimal lesion nephrotic syndrome. J. Pediatr. *84*:825, 1974.

Drummond, K. N., Michael, A. F., Good, R. A., and Vernier, R. L.: The nephrotic syndrome of childhood: Immunologic, clinical and pathologic correlations. J. Clin. Invest. *45*:620, 1966.

Heymann, W., Makker, S. P., and Post, R. S.: The preponderance of males in the idiopathic nephrotic syndrome of childhood. Pediatrics *50*:814, 1972.

Kendall, A. G., Lohmann, R. C., and Dossetor, J. B.: Nephrotic syndrome. A hypercoagulable state. Arch. Intern. Med. *127*:1021, 1971.

Rothenberg, M. B., and Heymann, W.: The incidence of the nephrotic syndrome in children. Pediatrics *19*:446, 1957.

Siegel, N. J., Goldberg, B., Krassner, L. S., and Hayslett, J. P.: Long-term follow-up of children with steroid-responsive nephrotic syndrome. J. Pediatr. *81*:251, 1972.

FOCAL GLOMERULOSCLEROSIS

(Focal Sclerosing Glomerulopathy)

This entity may be difficult to differentiate from minimal lesion nephrotic syndrome; children present with the same clinical and laboratory findings except that some of them have microscopic hematuria. About half are resistant to corticosteroid therapy and have progressive glomerular scarring which may lead to renal insufficiency. Early in the course only some glomeruli are scarred; i.e., the lesions are focal, and the scarring may be segmental or involve the entire glomerulus. Since juxtamedullary glomeruli are involved first, renal biopsy may not demonstrate the affected glomeruli if only superficial ones are obtained. There is no evidence of an immune pathogenesis. Although it has been suggested that this disease is an entity distinct from minimal lesion nephrotic syndrome, it is also possible that it is part of the spectrum of this disease and that, for unknown reasons, children who fail to respond to corticosteroid treatment develop focal glomerulosclerosis. It is clear that the finding of focal glomerulosclerosis in a child with the nephrotic syndrome, particularly if detected early in the course of illness, carries with it a high probability of corticosteroid resistance. Some of these patients will, however, gradually respond over a period of three months to a year to treatment with daily cyclophosphamide and alternate day prednisone.

Habib, R.: Focal glomerular sclerosis. Kidney Int. *4*:355, 1973.
Hoyer, J. R., Raij, L., Vernier, R. L., Simmons, R. L., Najarian, J. S., and Michael, A. F.: Recurrence of idiopathic nephrotic syndrome after renal transplantation. Lancet *2*:343, 1972.
Hyman, L. R., and Burkholder, P. M.: Focal sclerosing glomerulopathy with segmental hyalinosis. A clinicopathologic analysis. Lab. Invest. *28*:533, 1973.

IDIOPATHIC MEMBRANOUS GLOMERULOPATHY

(Membranous Glomerulonephritis, Epi- or Extramembranous Glomerulopathy, Membranous Glomerulonephropathy, Extramembranous Glomerulonephritis)

INCIDENCE. Idiopathic membranous glomerulopathy accounts for about 5 per cent of cases of the nephrotic syndrome in children, and is more common in late childhood; about 20 per cent of patients with onset of the nephrotic syndrome after the age of 15 have this condition.

PATHOLOGY. The characteristic pathologic change is uniform thickening of the glomerular basement membrane without inflammation or significant increase in mesangial tissue. The thickening begins with deposition of immune complexes on the epithelial aspect of the membrane, detectable by light and electron microscopic and immunopathologic techniques. The immune complexes appear as discrete nodular masses or bumps projecting from the epithelial surface of the membrane, which extends in a spiked or saw-toothed pattern between the complexes. As the disease progresses, the masses are incorporated into the membrane, which in turn becomes progressively thicker as the formerly discrete nodules are fused or united with each other. Over a period of years there is gradual sclerosis of the glomerulus. The nodular or irregular membranous deposition of immunoglobulin G and of β_{1c} globulin and fibrin or its derivatives is distinctive. In the idiopathic form of membranous glomerulopathy, there is no detectable underlying systemic disorder; the kidney alone appears to be the site of disease, and the nature of the antigen (or antigens) is unknown. In some systemic disorders, such as systemic lupus erythematosus,* parasitemia with *P. malariae** or syphilis, identical pathologic changes may occur and the nephrotic syndrome may be manifest.

*In systemic lupus erythematosus and in *P. malariae* infestation, renal lesions other than membranous glomerulopathy may occur. Lupus glomerulonephritis is discussed later. In parasitemia with *P. malariae,* a distinctive nephropathy with glomerular basement membrane thickening may be detected by electron microscopy. This is the result of increased basement membrane-like material arranged in a plexiform manner in the subendothelial zone and small lacunae within the glomerular basement membrane. Renal disease in patients with *P. malariae* infestation is called quartan malarial nephropathy.

CLINICAL MANIFESTATIONS. The onset is gradual with little in the clinical picture or laboratory findings to distinguish it from minimal lesion nephrotic syndrome. The serum complement level is usually normal, there is marked proteinuria and the urine sediment may contain hyaline casts and a few red blood cells. Renal biopsy is required for precise diagnosis. If proteinuria persists, gradual progressive sclerosis of glomeruli occurs and evidence of renal insufficiency may develop within a decade. A gradual spontaneous remission, however, occurs in about 40 per cent of patients; thus, the indications for therapy with potentially harmful drugs such as cyclophosphamide and azathioprine remain controversial.

TREATMENT. Treatment is directed toward control of the underlying disease when one is identified; the prognosis with respect to the renal involvement is, to a large extent, related to achieving this goal, although in some of the disorders, e.g., *P. malariae* infestation, when significant renal lesions have developed, progression may occur despite control of the underlying disease. Membranous glomerulopathy does not usually respond to corticosteroid therapy, but some patients reduce their protein excretion to normal levels with a prolonged course of cyclophosphamide.

Habib, R., Kleinknecht, C., and Gubler, M. C.: Extramembranous glomerulonephritis in children: Report of 50 cases. J. Pediatr. *82*:754, 1973.
Hendrickse, R. G., Glasgow, E. F., Adeniyi, A., White, R. H. R., Edington, G. M., and Houba, V.: Quartan malarial nephrotic syndrome. Lancet *1*:1143, 1972.
Olbing, H., Greifer, I., Bennett, B. P., Bernstein, J., and Spitzer, A.: Idiopathic membranous nephropathy in children. Kidney Int. *3*:381, 1973.

MEMBRANOPROLIFERATIVE GLOMERULONEPHRITIS

(Hypocomplementemic Glomerulonephritis, Lobular Glomerulonephritis, Mesangioproliferative Glomerulonephritis)

This condition has been increasingly recognized as a cause of glomerular damage in children. The onset is usually in early adolescence, and there is a slightly higher incidence in girls.

The characteristic pathologic feature is proliferation of mesangial cells with an increase in mesangial matrix. The proliferating mesangial tissue extends between the endothelial cells and the glomerular basement membrane, which thus becomes thickened from its inner aspect. This thickening by encroachment of mesangial fibers from its endothelial aspect gives the glomerular basement membrane an appearance of being split or frayed. The number of patent capillary lumina is reduced. The glomeruli are usually very large, and progressive glomerular lobulation and scarring occur.

When the onset is acute, infiltration with polymorphonuclear leukocytes and formation of epithelial crescents may be present. Immunopathologic studies show granular deposition of β_{1C} globulin in proliferating mesangial regions or at the periphery of the glomerular lobules; immunoglobulin G (IgG) is identified in less than half the patients. Properdin deposition is usually present in the same location as the β_{1c} globulin. The complement system is apparently activated via the alternate pathway, possibly by a factor in the plasma in this disease. The finding of properdin in the glomeruli provides support for this hypothesis.

Membranoproliferative glomerulonephritis may be manifest as the nephrotic syndrome or as acute nephritis, a mixed nephritic-nephrotic pattern, asymptomatic proteinuria, chronic renal failure or with recurrent episodes of gross hematuria. Hypertension is common. The glomerular lesions progress slowly, leading to renal insufficiency in at least half the patients. The characteristic laboratory finding is a depression of the third component of complement, but the terminal complement components, C5 to C9, are also decreased; C1, 4 and 2 are not significantly reduced.

There is no consensus about the value of treatment. Some nephrologists believe that treatment with antimetabolic drugs such as azathioprine, particularly in the acute proliferative stage, reduces the glomerular injury and retards the rate of progression.

Habib, R., Kleinknecht, C., Gubler, M. C., and Levy, M.: Idiopathic membranoproliferative glomerulonephritis in children. Report of 105 cases. Clin. Nephrol. *1*:194, 1973.

Michael, A. F., Westberg, N. G., Fish, A. J., and Vernier, R. L.: Studies on chronic membranoproliferative glomerulonephritis with hypocomplementemia. J. Exp. Med. *134* (No. 3, pt. 2): 208s, 1971.

Westberg, N. G., Naff, G. B., Boyer, J. T., and Michael, A. F.: Glomerular deposition of properdin in acute and chronic glomerulonephritis with hypocomplementemia. J. Clin. Invest. *50*:642, 1971.

THE NEPHROTIC SYNDROME IN THE FIRST YEAR OF LIFE

The nephrotic syndrome in infancy may be considered separately because the diseases which cause it at this period are significantly different from those causing it in later life; *minimal lesion nephrotic syndrome* which may begin in the second 6 months of life, is described elsewhere in this Section.

INFANTILE MICROCYSTIC DISEASE (THE CONGENITAL NEPHROTIC SYNDROME; CONGENITAL NEPHROSIS). This autosomal recessive condition is seen most frequently in the Scandinavian countries, particularly in Finland, Proteinuria is usually present from birth but may begin several months later. Toxemia of pregnancy, an enlarged placenta and prematurity are common associated features. The pathognomonic lesion is cystic dilatation of the proximal tubules. The pathogenesis is unknown; there is no evidence of immune mechanisms. No treatment is known to be effective, although measures such as sodium restriction and the provision of a nutritious diet may help to maintain the general state of health. The disease is usually fatal within the first 2 years, but some success has been reported with renal transplantation.

MEMBRANOUS NEPHROPATHY OF CONGENITAL SYPHILIS. The onset of the nephrotic syndrome is within the first 6 months, and other stigmata of congenital syphilis are usually present. The pathologic change is a membranous nephropathy; immunopathologic studies reveal nodular deposits containing immunoglobulin G (IgG) with or without β_{1C} globulin. The pathogenetic basis is immune complex deposition; the antigen presumably is an unidentified component of *Treponema pallidum*. Complete recovery from the nephrotic syndrome and resolution of the renal lesion usually occur in response to antisyphilitic therapy.

MISCELLANEOUS CONDITIONS. Some rare conditions may be associated with or cause the nephrotic syndrome in infancy. These include progressive diffuse glomerulosclerosis, interstitial nephritis, focal glomerulosclerosis, mercury poisoning and nephroblastoma with or without pseudohermaphroditism.

Habib, R., and Bois, E.: Hétérogénéité des syndromes néphrotiques à début précoce du nourrisson (syndrome néphrotique "infantile"). Helv. Paediatr. Acta *28*:91, 1973.

Hallman, N., Norio, R., and Kouvalainen, K.: Main features of the congenital nephrotic syndrome. Acta Paediatr. Scand. *172*(Suppl.): 75, 1967.

Hoyer, J. R., Kjellstrand, C. M., Simmons, R. L., Najarian, J. S., Mauer, S. M., Buselmeier, T. J., Michael, A. F., and Vernier, R. L.: Successful renal transplantation in 3 children with congenital nephrotic syndrome. Lancet *1*:1410, 1973.

Hoyer, J. R., Michael, A. F., Jr., Good, R. A., and Vernier, R. L.: The nephrotic syndrome of infancy: Clinical, morphologic, and immunologic studies of four infants. Pediatrics *40*:233, 1967.

Kaplan, B. S., Bureau, M. A., and Drummond, K. N.: The nephrotic syndrome in the first year of life: Is a pathologic classification possible? J. Pediatr. In press.

OTHER CAUSES OF THE NEPHROTIC SYNDROME IN CHILDHOOD

The nephrotic syndrome may develop in the course of a number of primary glomerular disorders or conditions in which the glomerulus is involved as part of a systemic disease. Since the most common clinical presentation in these disorders is not the nephrotic syndrome, they will not be discussed here; but they include acute poststreptococcal glomerulonephritis, systemic lupus erythematosus, malaria, anaphylactoid purpura, and acute idiopathic proliferative glomerulonephritis with crescents (subacute glomerulonephritis, rapidly progressive glomerulonephritis).

THE NEPHROTIC SYNDROME ASSOCIATED WITH MALIGNANT LYMPHOMAS AND OTHER NEOPLASMS

The nephrotic syndrome, as well as various forms of proliferative glomerulonephritis, may occur in association with a variety of malignant tumors. In some instances a membranous nephropathy is seen on renal biopsy; presumably an immune complex mechanism is involved in which some constituent of the neoplastic tissue serves as an antigen. In other patients, particularly those with reticuloendothelial malignancies such as Hodgkin's disease, the renal lesions are minimal and indistinguishable from those of the minimal lesion nephrotic syndrome.

Hyman, L. R., Burkholder, P. M., Joo, P. A., and Segar, W. E.: Malignant lymphoma and nephrotic syndrome. J. Pediatr. *82*:207, 1973.

ACUTE GLOMERULONEPHRITIS

The term "acute glomerulonephritis" has clinical, laboratory and pathologic implications; it includes a number of distinct entities, in some of which the glomerulus is affected as the primary event and in others of which renal involvement is only one manifestation of a systemic disorder. The clinical and laboratory features of acute glomerulonephritis include. (1) *Oliguria.* The urine volume may fall below 150 ml/m²/day, the amount required for excretion of the minimal possible solute load, below which a diagnosis of oliguric renal failure may be made. (2) *Edema* may be slight and is seldom as marked as in the nephrotic syndrome. The acute nature of the illness does not afford a long enough time for significant quantities of water and salt to be ingested, and the plasma colloid osmotic pressure is not reduced, since the serum protein level is usually within normal limits. (3) *Hypertension* and *circulatory congestion* are common to most forms of acute glomerulonephritis. The cause of the hypertension is not well understood; factors such as increased peripheral resistance because of peripheral arteriolar vasoconstriction and excess renin secretion have been suggested. It appears, however, that retention of sodium and water is of prime importance. Circulatory congestion may be manifested by pulmonary edema and by other features of cardiac overload such as hepatomegaly, distention of the external jugular veins and gallop rhythm. (4) *Hematuria* may cause dark, cloudy urine which is brownish red to light tea-colored. The sediment usually contains red blood cells, plus cells and mixed, granular and red blood cell casts. (5) *Proteinuria* varies from a modest elevation of 30 to 100 mg/dl to "nephrotic" levels of 1000 mg/dl or more. (6) *Azotemia* and other findings are consequent to a reduction in glomerular filtration rate; these include elevation of the blood urea nitrogen, serum creatinine and sometimes of the serum phosphorus and uric acid; the serum calcium level may be depressed consequent to elevation of the serum phosphorus. (7) Frequently there is a mild normochromic *anemia,* with a hemoglobin concentration of 9–11 gm/dl. (8) *Electrolyte and acid-base disturbances* include *hyperkalemia* from reduced urinary excretion of potassium in the face of continued potassium intake and tissue catabolism, hyponatremia resulting from continued water intake in the presence of reduced urine volume and metabolic acidosis, particularly if oliguria is severe. Acidosis may accentuate the hyperkalemia.

The pathologic findings in acute glomerulonephritis depend, to a large extent, on the specific disease entity and will be discussed under the respective disorders; there are, however, common features in most forms, which include polymorphonuclear leukocyte infiltration, cellular proliferation of one or more of the glomerular cell types (endothelial, mesangial or epithelial), increased glomerular size, mesangial edema or increase of mesangial matrix (usually of a fine fibrillar type) and reduction in the number of open capillary loops. In addition, there may be focal infiltration of mononuclear or polymorphonuclear leukocytes in the interstitial areas. The spectrum of clinical, laboratory or pathologic abnormalities owing to acute glomerulonephritis may range from minimal to severe, even though a single disease entity may be present and only one pathogenetic mechanism is operative.

ACUTE POSTSTREPTOCOCCAL GLOMERULONEPHRITIS

Acute poststreptococcal glomerulonephritis is an acute, specific, self-limited glomerulonephritis resulting from a prior pharyngeal or cutaneous infection with a nephritogenic strain of group A beta-hemolytic streptococci. It is the most common form of acute glomerulonephritis and is the human immunologic renal disease about which most is known.

ETIOLOGY AND EPIDEMIOLOGY. The precipitating event is the streptococcal infection, either in the upper respiratory tract or of the skin. Although the clinical pattern of the nephritis is the same following infection at either of these sites, there are a number of important differences, including the types of streptococci involved, epidemiology, age, sex, seasonal incidence, latent period between infection and onset of nephritis and antibody response to the infection. Only certain serotypes of group A beta-hemolytic streptococci, characterized either by their M or T antigens, cause acute poststreptococcal glomerulonephritis. These nephritogenic strains are listed in Table 15–5. The most frequent pharyngeal and skin streptococci

TABLE 15-5 M STREPTOCOCCAL SEROTYPES ASSOCIATED WITH ACUTE NEPHRITIS*

	TYPE OF INFECTION	
	Pharyngitis	*Pyoderma*
Commonest and best confirmed	12	49
Less frequent but good evidence for association	1, 3, 4	2, 55, 57
Probable or possible association	6, 25, 49	31, 52, 56

*Based on data from Wannamaker, L. W.: New Engl. J. Med. *282*:23, 1970.

are M types 12 and 49, respectively. Some of the nephritogenic strains of streptococci which infect the skin are difficult to type on the basis of their M protein antigen but are typeable on the basis of T antigen agglutination. Of these strains, those with the T-14 antigen are the most common.

Acute glomerulonephritis associated with streptococcal respiratory tract infection is more common in temperate or cold climates, has a peak seasonal incidence in winter and spring, affects mainly children of early school age, but older children and adults as well, and follows onset of the streptococcal infection by 9 to 11 days. The ratio of boys to girls affected is about 2:1, despite a lack of difference in the incidence of either streptococcal pharyngitis or impetigo in the two sexes. By contrast, acute glomerulonephritis associated with streptococcal infection of the skin is more common in hot or tropical climates, with a seasonal peak in late summer and early fall; preschool children are most frequently affected, the sex incidence is equal, and the latent period between onset of skin infection and onset of nephritis is 3 weeks or longer. In nephritis associated with either pharyngitis or impetigo, the attack rate, i.e., the percentage of patients who develop nephritis after infection with a nephritogenic serotype is 10 to 15 per cent. Multiple cases tend to occur in families, often within several weeks of each other; second attacks are rare. It is not known whether early treatment of streptococcal impetigo will reduce the attack rate of nephritis, but it appears that early antistreptococcal treatment will reduce the incidence of nephritis associated with streptococcal pharyngitis by about one half. There is also a difference in antibody response to streptococcal antigens following throat and skin infections. Antibodies (anti-NADase) to streptococcal nicotinamide adenine dinucleotidase (alternatively designated streptococcal diphosphopyridine nucleotidase [DPNase]) and, to a slightly lesser extent, to streptococcal deoxyribonuclease B (anti-DNase B) and streptolysin O (ASO) are usually present in nephritis after pharyngitis. In nephritis following impetigo, a vigorous anti-DNase B or antihyaluronidase response is seen, but the ASO and anti-NADase responses are irregular or weak. Thus, there appears to be an advantage in the anti-NADase (anti-DPNase) test for detecting preceding streptococcal infection in acute glomerulonephritis following streptococcal pharyngitis and a definite superiority of the anti-DNase B test in nephritis induced by skin infection.

PATHOGENESIS AND PATHOLOGY. It has been postulated since early in this century that immune mechanisms are of importance in the development of acute poststreptococcal glomerulonephritis. Several observations support this concept: (1) the characteristic latent period between streptococcal infection and the development of nephritis; (2) the depression of serum complement activity; (3) the finding by immunopathologic techniques of immune reactants at the site of glomerular injury; and (4) the marked similarity between the immunopathologic and electron microscopic findings in acute poststreptococcal glomerulonephritis and those in immunologically induced experimental renal disease in animals, particularly the acute serum sickness nephritis seen following injection of a foreign protein.

During the late 1960's it was generally accepted that acute poststreptococcal glomerulonephritis was analagous to serum sickness nephritis as seen in human beings following injection of a foreign protein, such as horse antitetanus serum, or as induced in the experimental animal. Several perplexing problems remain unexplained, however, if this hypothesis is correct. These include: (1) the inability to identify a specific streptococcal antigen at the site of the IgG and β_{1C} globulin deposits in the kidney; (2) the finding by immunopathologic techniques of β_{1C} globulin more frequently than IgG in glomerular deposits; and (3) the complement profile, i.e., marked depression of C3 and terminal components of complement with relative sparing of C1, C4 and C2, together with a marked depression of serum properdin level and deposition of properdin in the glomeruli, suggests the operation of the alternate pathway of complement activation rather than the classic one activated by antigen-antibody complexes. Thus, the earlier hypothesis which favored a glomerular localization of immune complexes containing IgG, β_{1C} globulin and an as yet unidentified streptococcal antigen is confused by more recent observations, which implicate the alternate pathway of complement activation. It is possible that both systems are operative, as has been suggested also for the nephritis of systemic lupus erythematosus.

The pathologic findings are confined largely to the glomeruli, in which initially there are infiltration with polymorphonuclear leukocytes, proliferation of endothelial and mesangial cells, increase in fibrillar mesangial matrix and, infrequently, parietal epithelial crescent formation. The glomeruli appear hypercellular and swollen and the number of open capillary loops is reduced. Electron microscopic or ultrathin light microscopic studies demonstrate, in addition, discrete nodular deposits along the epithelial aspect of the glomerular basement membrane, within the mesangium and in a subendothelial position. Polymorphonuclear leukocytes are often seen adjacent to these deposits. Within 2 to 3 weeks of onset most of these changes begin to resolve; the abnormalities of the mesangial matrix are the last to return to normal. In virtually all children with acute poststreptococcal glomerulonephritis, significant microscopic lesions are no longer detectable by 2 months after onset. Tubular and interstitial changes, consisting of interruptions in the tubular basement membrane and occasional interstitial inflammatory foci, may be present during the acute stages, but these are neither striking nor specific.

CLINICAL MANIFESTATIONS AND COURSE. Although the clinical pattern varies significantly in the degree of severity and in the extent of the various manifestations, from a very mild to an extremely critical disorder, in most instances the clinical pattern and course are fairly characteristic. In many instances a history of pharyngitis or impetigo can be elicited. The onset is usually abrupt, the earliest symptoms being dark-colored urine, mild facial edema and decreased urinary output. Flank or midline abdominal pain, irritability, general malaise and a low-grade fever are common. Acute hypertension may cause headache and other central nervous system manifestations, such as seizures. Symptoms related to circulatory congestion or overload, compounded by hypertension, may also be found. These include dyspnea, tachypnea and a tender, enlarged liver. Less common ways in which acute poststreptococcal glomerulonephritis may present and which may direct attention away from the correct diagnosis, particularly if abnormalities in urine color or sediment are minimal or absent, include the acute onset of seizures due to hypertensive encephalopathy, frank pulmonary edema and circulatory congestion with cardiac decompensation. In these circumstances, hypertension is usually present and should lead the physician to suspect an atypical presentation of acute poststreptococcal glomerulonephritis. Uncommonly the clinical presentation and accompanying laboratory features may be those of the nephrotic syndrome; the history of preceding pharyngeal or skin infection and the presence of hypertension, circulatory overload and the characteristic laboratory findings discussed below should clarify the diagnosis. Urinalyses or β_{1C} globulin levels done on schoolmates and members of patients' families show that an appreciable number of apparently healthy individuals have abnormalities in the urine and reduced β_{1C} globulin levels, suggesting that acute poststreptococcal glomerulonephritis may occur in a subclinical form among individuals exposed to a nephritogenic type of streptococci.

There are usually mild periorbital edema, irritability and hypertension. Signs of circulatory overload such as cardiomegaly, venous distention, hepatomegaly, pulmonary edema and a gallop rhythm may be present. Features of hypertensive encephalopathy include irritability, headache, vomiting, somnolence or generalized seizures. Significant retinal changes due to hypertensive encephalopathy are absent and, if found, should direct attention to the possibility of a more chronic problem.

The acute phase with malaise, oliguria, edema, azotemia, circulatory congestion and hypertension usually lasts from 4 to 10 days. During the first few days, the urine remains dark, and electrolyte and acid-base disturbances, hypertension and circulatory congestion may be prominent problems. Subsequently, urine output increases, there is loss of edema, and blood urea nitrogen and creatinine return to normal levels. Hypertension and circulatory congestion usually resolve at this time, but in some patients elevated blood pressure and modest azotemia may persist for up to 2 weeks following return of the urine volume to normal. Gross hematuria seldom persists beyond the first week, but microscopic hematuria and casts may persist for 1 to 2 months. An increase in hematuria may occur with exercise or with an unrelated intercurrent illness during this time. Within 3 weeks of onset, most children have returned to their usual state of general health and will experience no further problems related to this illness.

LABORATORY MANIFESTATIONS. Laboratory findings include a mild normochromic anemia (hemoglobin = 10 to 11 mg/dl) due largely to hemodilution; mild leukocytosis (WBC = 12,000-15,000/mm^3) with a polymorphonuclear shift to the left; increased erythrocyte sedimentation rate; elevated blood urea nitrogen and serum creatinine levels, with the former being proportionately greater; serologic evidence of preceding streptococcal infection (see Etiology); reduction in serum complement activity with marked reduction in C3 and terminal components, with relative sparing of the early components, C1, C2 and C4; and a decrease in serum properdin. Serum complement remains low for about 10 days and returns to normal within 4 to 5 weeks. In approximately 10 per cent of patients the β_{1C} globulin level is not reduced, even during the first week of illness.

The *urine* is usually tea-colored; microscopic examination reveals numerous red and white blood cells and a mixture of casts, of which erythrocyte and granular are the most common. The urinary excretion of protein is not excessive, usually under 1 gm/24 hr, with a protein concentration of 30-100 mg/dl. Urine volume is reduced during the first 3 to 5 days and may remain low for up to 10 days; anuria may occur. Electrolyte and acid-base disturbances may occur, particularly in the presence of anuria or oliguria. These include hyponatremia owing to fluid overload in the face of reduced urinary output, hyperkalemia with levels from 5.5-9.0 mEq/l, and metabolic acidosis. *Electrocardiographic changes* resulting from hyperkalemia may be present and should be sought in each patient since they reflect potentially serious changes in the electrical activity of the heart which may warrant immediate medical intervention. In approximate relation to the degree of hyperkalemia these changes are:

tall, narrow T waves (5.5 mEq/l); widening of the QRS complex (6.5 mEq/l); decrease in P wave amplitude, increase in P wave duration and prolongation of the P-R interval (over 7 mEq/l). With higher serum concentrations of potassium, the QRS complex merges with the T wave and forms a biphasic sine wave and there may be premature ventricular contractions, supraventricular tachycardia and atrial fibrillation. When the concentration is over 9 mEq/l, ventricular fibrillation may supervene.

Roentgenograms of the chest may show interstitial pulmonary edema, more pronounced in the hilar regions; if there is marked circulatory overload, cardiomegaly and frank pulmonary edema are seen. *Cultures* from the pharynx or skin lesions may not grow group A beta-hemolytic streptococci, since the patient often has received effective antibacterial therapy for the preceding streptococcal illness.

DIAGNOSIS. Although the clinical features of acute poststreptococcal glomerulonephritis may be atypical in a small percentage of patients, the correct diagnosis is readily made in most instances if full consideration is given to all clinical and laboratory features. A renal biopsy is infrequently indicated in cases with unusual clinical and laboratory manifestations. Accuracy in the diagnosis of this and other glomerular disorders is important because of differences in prognosis and treatment.

Differential Diagnosis. This includes most of the conditions which may cause any or all of the principal features of acute poststreptococcal glomerulonephritis; hematuria, edema, hypertension and oliguria. To be considered are: the *hemolytic-uremic syndrome, membranoproliferative glomerulonephritis,* nephritis associated with such systemic disorders as *systemic lupus erythematosus* and *anaphylactoid purpura, focal glomerulonephritis with recurrent hematuria, benign familial hematuria, acute exacerbation of chronic glomerulonephritis, malignant hypertension, idiopathic rapidly progressive glomerulonephritis (omniglomerular diffuse proliferative glomerulonephritis with epithelial crescents), hereditary nephritis, renal trauma, acute renal tubular injury* and *acute hemorrhagic cystitis.* These conditions are discussed elsewhere in this Section and can usually be excluded without difficulty by their own characteristic clinical and laboratory features. In some instances the correct diagnosis can be established only by the pathologic and immunopathologic renal changes visualized in tissue biopsies.

PREVENTION. The relative effectiveness of early antibiotic treatment of nephritogenic streptococcal infections of the pharynx or skin in the prevention of glomerulonephritis has not been established; it is generally considered, however, to be at least 50 per cent. Therefore, members of the patient's family should have appropriate bacterial cultures, and those with documented streptococcal infections should be treated with penicillin or erythromycin. Systemic treatment is superior to local therapy of streptococcal pyoderma. In closed epidemics of nephritogenic streptococcal infection, as, for example, in military establishments, early antibiotic treatment can limit the spread of nephritogenic strains of streptococci.

TREATMENT. Treatment involves diligent management during the acute phase, which usually lasts for 1 to 2 weeks, the approximate time required for the renal lesions to recover spontaneously.

Since the severity of the acute phase is extremely variable and not predictable, the child with a suspected diagnosis of acute glomerulonephritis should be hospitalized and carefully assessed. The major early life-threatening potentials are: (1) acute renal insufficiency, resulting in fluid, electrolyte and acid-base abnormalities; and (2) acute hypertension, which may cause hypertensive encephalopathy and which, when compounded by the consequences of severe oliguria or anuria, may lead to circulatory congestion and pulmonary edema. Present evidence does not support primary myocardial failure as the cause of the circulatory congestion, which appears more likely to be the consequence of salt and water retention and of hypertension.

Treatment of Acute Renal Insufficiency. The treatment of acute renal insufficiency consists in (1) fluid restriction to an amount equal to insensible water loss (about 400 ml/m^2/day) plus urinary output; (2) provision of an adequate number of calories, at least 400/m^2/day, in the form of carbohydrates to minimize endogenous tissue catabolism (if the patient is vomiting or is otherwise unable to be fed orally, fluid and carbohydrate requirements should be met by intravenous administration of 10 to 20 per cent glucose in water); (3) correction of metabolic acidosis by parenteral administration of sodium bicarbonate; and (4) prevention and correction of electrolyte and fluid disturbances.

Hyperkalemia can profoundly affect cardiac depolarization and thus constitute a threat to life. The serum potassium level should immediately be determined in each patient and a baseline electrocardiogram obtained. The potassium intake should be reduced to nil until it is certain that there is an adequate urinary output and that hyperkalemia is not present. If there is evidence of cardiac toxicity in the presence of hyperkalemia, immediate measures should be taken to reduce the concentration of serum potassium. Calcium gluconate should be administered intravenously under direct electrocardiographic monitoring over a period of 15 to 30 minutes; the calcium ion serves to counteract the deleterious effect on cardiac function of the hyperkalemia. An amount of calcium gluconate is given to provide 10 to 15 mg/kg of elemental calcium; a gram of calcium gluconate contains 93 mg of calcium. Correction of metabolic acidosis with sodium bicarbonate also serves to reduce hyperkalemia. Care should be taken, however, not to administer excessive amounts of sodium, particularly when there are circulatory congestion and edema. It may be necessary to repeat administration of calcium gluconate if serious electrocardiographic changes persist during the time required to reduce the elevated plasma concentration of potassium.

For an anuric patient, free of diarrhea, vomiting, volume depletion or dehydration, the fluid requirement is 300-400 ml/m²/day. If oral intake is not feasible, 20 per cent glucose solution should be given at a uniform rate, except during the first several hours, when it may be necessary to infuse more rapidly. Since 20 per cent glucose solution may irritate small veins and lead to occlusion, a large vein or a cutdown may be needed. If the electrocardiographic changes are serious, crystalline insulin, 0.1 unit/kg, may be given intravenously, and the same dose subcutaneously sometime after the glucose infusion has been started, to enhance the effect of glucose infusion in reducing the serum potassium concentration. Blood glucose values should also be monitored to detect hypoglycemia induced by the insulin.

An ion exchange resin (e.g., Kayexalate*) may also be given orally or rectally to aid in the removal of excess potassium. Ten to 25 gm of the resin are suspended in 50 to 100 ml of 5 per cent glucose and water. If given as an enema, it should be retained for 30 to 60 minutes and then rinsed out with isotonic saline. This resin tends to cause constipation and care should be taken to avoid fecal impaction.

It is uncommon for hyperkalemia to be so severe that the preceding measures will not produce an adequate response. On occasion, however, serious hyperkalemia persists and poses a threat to the patient's life. When this is the case, peritoneal dialysis using a potassium-free fluid is an effective means of removing potassium. In the face of severe acidosis, circulatory congestion and hyperkalemia, this may be the best way to re-establish normal electrolyte, acid-base and fluid balance. Hemodialysis is also effective but is seldom required.

Composition of some solutions commercially available for peritoneal dialysis†

1. Inperinol 1.5% (Abbott Laboratories Ltd., P.O. Box 68, Abbott Park, North Chicago, Illinois):

dextrose	15 gm/l	magnesium	1.5 mEq/l
sodium	140.5 mEq/l	chloride	101 mEq/l
calcium	3.5 mEq/l	lactate	44.5 mEq/l

2. Inperinol 4.25%:

dextrose	42.5 gm/l	magnesium	1.5 mEq/l
sodium	140.5 mEq/l	chloride	101 mEq/l
calcium	3.5 mEq/l	lactate	44.5 mEq/l

3. Inperinol 4.25%:

dextrose	42.5 gm/l	magnesium	1.5 mEq/l
sodium	132 mEq/l	chloride	99 mEq/l
calcium	3.5 mEq/l	lactate	35 mEq/l

This last solution, which has a lower sodium concentration, should be used when hypernatremia is a problem, especially after hypertonicity induced by too rapid dialysis or prior administration of hypertonic sodium bicarbonate.

4. Other preparations:
   a.) Dianeal 1.5% (Travenol Laboratories, Inc., Morton Grove, Illinois)
   b.) Dianeal 4.25%
   c.) McGaw peritoneal dialysis solution, either 1.5% or 4.25 per cent (McGaw Laboratories, Division of American Hospital Supply Corp., Glendale, California). This solution substitutes sodium acetate for sodium lactate and may be used if the patient has lactic acidosis: each of these solutions has an electrolyte concentration similar to Inperinol.

If lactic acidosis is present, sodium bicarbonate can also be substituted for sodium lactate. In this case calcium chloride cannot be used in the dialysis solution because a precipitate of calcium carbonate will form. Instead, calcium, as calcium gluconate, should be given intravenously and the plasma level monitored closely.

The technique of peritoneal dialysis in children:

The reader is also referred to the article by Feldman et al. listed in the references.

1. Empty bladder with a No. 5 or No. 8 feeding tube unless it is certain that the bladder has just been emptied.
2. A sterile technique is used.
3. Add 1000 μ heparin to each liter of dialysis solution.
4. Add potassium chloride to a concentration of 4.0 mEq/l if hyperkalemia is not present or has been corrected by prior dialysis.
5. Keep the dialysis solution warmed to 37 to 38°C.
6. Using a sterile aseptic technique, anesthetize the skin and subcutaneous tissue with a local anesthetic at the proposed site of insertion of the peritoneal catheter (Trocath peritoneal dialysis catheter—McGaw Laboratories, Division of American Hospital Supply Corp., Glendale, California).
7. Infuse 25 ml/kg of dialysis solution over a 10- to 15-minute period via a lumbar puncture needle into the peritoneal cavity prior to insertion of catheter.
8. Insert trochar and catheter in midline just below the umbilicus or just lateral to the rectus muscle at the level of the umbilicus after making certain that the liver and spleen are not enlarged. After removing the trochar the catheter is directed toward and into the pelvic cavity.
9. Establish that there is free flow from the catheter and begin the dialysis. About 50 ml/kg of dialysis fluid are used during each cycle. The fluid is run in over 10 to 15 minutes, allowed to equilibrate for 20 to 30 minutes, and then drained over 15 to 20 minutes. With each cycle the peritoneal cavity is drained completely; this may require positioning the patient.
10. An accurate cumulative record of the electrolytes and volume of fluid infused and withdrawn must be kept. If a progressive positive

*Winthrop Laboratories, Aurora, Ontario, Canada, division of Sterling Drug, Inc., 90 Park Avenue, New York, N.Y. 10016.

†Dr. R. W. Chesney assisted in preparing this information concerning peritoneal dialysis.

balance develops, a solution with a higher dextrose concentration may be used. If an excessive negative balance develops, the abdominal cavity should still be drained completely each cycle, but replacement can be made by intravenous administration of 5 to 10 per cent dextrose and water or a solution similar in composition to Ringer's lactate; the decision as to the composition of the replacement solution depends on the plasma electrolyte values and on the state of fluid and electrolyte balance.

11. The dialysis fluid should be cultured several times daily.

12. If marked hyperglycemia occurs, short-acting insulin, 0.1-0.2 μ/kg, should be given intravenously.

13. The total duration of dialysis in most instances is about 48 hours.

Hyponatremia, as a consequence of continued intake or administration of hypotonic fluids in the presence of severe oliguria or anuria, may occur. Restriction of fluids is usually all that is necessary to allow the serum sodium level to return to normal. If, however, the serum sodium is depressed to 120 mEq/l or lower and central nervous system signs of water intoxication are present, 3 per cent sodium chloride solution should be administered intravenously over 15 to 60 minutes in an amount calculated to effect a half-correction of the serum sodium concentration.

Treatment of Acute Hypertension. Acute elevation of blood pressure is an integral feature of acute poststreptococcal glomerulonephritis and must be anticipated and, if present, treated. Blood pressure determinations should be taken at regular intervals of 4 to 6 hours. Judgment is required concerning the level of blood pressure at which treatment is necessary. If there is evidence of hypertensive encephalopathy such as seizures, coma, drowsiness or headache, if there are signs of circulatory congestion and pulmonary edema in association with hypertension, or if the diastolic blood pressure is over 95 mm Hg, treatment is definitely indicated. In the face of an acute hypertensive emergency such as hypertensive encephalopathy with seizures, the drug of choice is diazoxide, 5-10 mg/kg, given intravenously and as rapidly as possible. Intravenous methyldopa, 10-20 mg/kg, may also be used. In less urgent situations the most frequently used and effective drugs are hydralazine, 0.1-0.7 mg/kg, and reserpine, 0.07 mg/kg (maximum dose = 2 mg), given together intramuscularly. This combination may be repeated if the blood pressure does not fall within 2 or 3 hours. More than three injections of reserpine are not recommended, but hydralazine, if effective, may be continued as necessary and may be given either intramuscularly or intravenously over a 5- to 10-minute period. Oral methyldopa, 20-40 mg/kg/day in four divided doses, or a combination of hydrochlorothiazide, 2.5 mg/kg/day, and hydralazine, 2-4 mg/kg/day in three divided doses, can be instituted after parenteral therapy has reduced the blood pressure to levels which are considered safe (diastolic pressure <90 mm Hg; systolic pressure <140). With concomitant hypertension and circulatory congestion, a potent diuretic such as furosemide, 1-5 mg/kg/dose, given by intravenous or intramuscular injection, can relieve both the circulatory congestion and the hypertension; it may also be effective in reducing hyperkalemia.

Circulatory Congestion. This may pose a serious problem because of pulmonary edema and cardiac decompensation. An initial roentgenogram of the chest should be taken to assess the heart size and extent of pulmonary edema; gallop rhythm and hepatomegaly may be present. Treatment consists of restricting the intake of sodium and of fluid, treatment of hypertension, use of parenteral diuretics such as furosemide or ethacrynic acid (1-5 mg/kg/dose) and, in refractory, progressive cases, phlebotomy or dialysis to reduce intravascular volume.

Other Aspects of Treatment. The diet recommended depends on the stage and severity of the illness. In the acute oliguric, edematous, hypertensive phase, restriction in intake of sodium, potassium, protein and fluids is necessary; most of the calories should be provided in the form of carbohydrate and fat. This initial period usually lasts less than a week, and subsequent dietary restriction is usually unnecessary.

If the child feels well and is not at risk there is no advantage to enforced bed rest; ambulation with return to normal activities should be encouraged if the general condition permits. Although increased physical activity may lead to increased urinary sediment, this is of no consequence insofar as the healing of the renal lesions is concerned.

When there is an active pharyngeal or cutaneous streptococcal infection, appropriate cultures should be obtained initially and it should be treated with an appropriate antibiotic.*

PROGNOSIS. The long-term prognosis for acute poststreptococcal glomerulonephritis in children is excellent; complete recovery occurs in close to 100 per cent of children who survive the acute stage. Mortality in the acute phase is the result of disturbances which in virtually all cases are readily amenable to appropriate medical treatment. Exacerbations during the healing phase, i.e., within the first 2 months following onset, occur infrequently, are usually precipitated by an intercurrent acute respiratory illness, are manifested principally by hematuria and are self-limited. Second attacks of acute poststreptococcal glomerulonephritis are rare but may occur following infection with a different nephritogenic streptococcal strain.

Feldman, W., Baliah, T., and Drummond, K. N.: Intermittent peritoneal dialysis in the management of chronic renal failure in children. Am. J. Dis. Child. *116*:30, 1968.

*It is essential to emphasize the great variability in the acute phase of poststreptococcal glomerulonephritis. The above description is mainly that of the moderately severe to severe forms, which are relatively common. In many instances, however, the clinical manifestations may be mild, and all that is required is careful monitoring of blood pressure and fluid intake and, initially, sharp reduction in intake of potassium. But even the patient with a mild onset must be hospitalized, where he can be closely observed during the initial days, as severe manifestations may occur precipitously and should be treated promptly.

Fish, A. J., Herdman, R. C., Michael, A. F., Pickering, R. J., and Good, R. A.: Epidemic acute glomerulonephritis associated with type 49 streptococcal pyoderma. Am. J. Med. *48*:28, 1970.

Jennings, R. B., and Earle, D. P.: Post-streptococcal glomerulonephritis: Histopathologic and clinical studies of the acute, subsiding acute and early chronic latent phases. J. Clin. Invest. *40*:1525, 1961.

Lewy, J. E., Salinas-Madrigal, L., Herdson, P. B., Pirani, C. L., and Metcoff, J.: Clinico-pathologic correlations in acute poststreptococcal glomerulonephritis. Medicine *50*:453, 1971.

McLaine, P. N., and Drummond, K. N.: Intravenous diazoxide for severe hypertension in childhood. J. Pediatr. *79*:829, 1971.

Metcoff, J. (ed.): Acute Glomerulonephritis. Boston, Little, Brown and Company, 1967, p. 437.

Michael, A. F., Jr., Drummond, K. N., Good, R. A., and Vernier, R. L.: Acute poststreptococcal glomerulonephritis: Immune deposit disease. J. Clin. Invest. *45*:237, 1966.

Rammelkamp, C. H., Jr., and Weaver, R. S.: Acute glomerulonephritis. J. Clin. Invest. *32*:345, 1953.

Wannamaker, L. W.: Differences between streptococcal infections of the throat and of the skin. New Engl. J. Med. *282*:23; 78, 1970.

THE NEPHRITIS OF ANAPHYLACTOID PURPURA

The nonrenal aspects of anaphylactoid purpura are discussed in Section 9 under Henoch-Schönlein Vasculitis. About 50 per cent of children with anaphylactoid purpura develop glomerulonephritis, but the number with serious renal involvement is only about 2 to 3 per cent. Severe nephritis is uncommon under the age of 2; thereafter its frequency increases with age.

PATHOGENESIS AND PATHOLOGY. The pathogenesis of the nephritis of anaphylactoid purpura is unknown. Although glomerular deposits of IgG and β_{1C} globulin have been observed, these are inconsistent and do not have the characteristic location or appearance seen in other forms of immune complex injury. Fibrinogen or its derivatives are consistently present at the site of glomerular damage, and there is also mesangial deposition of IgA. It is likely that a localized disturbance in coagulation initiated by unknown mechanisms and leading to fibrin deposition within the glomerulus is an important factor; the lesions may be omniglomerular or focal, segmental or diffuse. The principal site of involvement is the mesangium. In patients with clinical evidence of serious renal disease, a high percentage of glomeruli are affected. Local interstitial inflammation in relation to small arterioles may also be present.

CLINICAL MANIFESTATIONS AND COURSE. In most children the clinical features of the nephritis of anaphylactoid purpura are overshadowed by the skin, joint and gastrointestinal manifestations. Microscopic hematuria and mild proteinuria (less than 500 mg/24 hr) are the usual manifestations; a small but important number, however, may have the clinical features of acute glomerulonephritis: gross hematuria, oliguria, edema and hypertension. If proteinuria is marked, a full-blown nephrotic pattern may be present. In a few patients, florid, proliferative glomerulonephritis may occur and progress to advanced renal failure over a period of 1 to 6 months. The development of the renal manifestations of anaphylactoid purpura late in the clinical course, at a time when other features of the illness are subsiding or have completely disappeared, is not infrequently a cause of concern and may occur as late as 1 or 2 months after the onset of the purpuric cutaneous lesions.

In most cases the nephritis of anaphylactoid purpura is self-limited, becoming inactive within 6 months of onset and leaving no clinically important residual renal damage. There may be minor abnormalities in the urine sediment without significant proteinuria for a more prolonged period, but this usually does not signify progressive renal damage. In most patients with severe nephritis, either progressive renal failure has developed within the first 6 months or a stable state is reached, albeit possibly with compromised renal function.

LABORATORY FINDINGS. These are not specific. There are usually gross or microscopic hematuria and variable proteinuria, in most instances under 1 gm/24 hr. With omniglomerular, diffuse, proliferative involvement, with or without parietal epithelial crescents, the protein excretion is higher, often above 2 gm/day, and the nephrotic syndrome may be manifest. If renal insufficiency is present, the blood urea nitrogen and serum creatinine levels are elevated and disturbances may be seen in electrolyte, acid-base and fluid status. A moderate leukocytosis (WBC = 12,000 to 18,000) with a relative neutrophilia and an elevation in erythrocyte sedimentation rate are common. Elevation of the serum IgA level has been reported; the serum β_{1C} globulin level is normal.

DIAGNOSIS AND DIFFERENTIAL DIAGNOSIS. Manifestations of renal involvement range from asymptomatic microscopic hematuria to acute glomerulonephritis, the nephrotic syndrome or rapidly progressive glomerulonephritis terminating in renal failure. The severity of the nephritis correlates well with the amount of protein excreted.

The principal conditions to be differentiated from the nephritis of anaphylactoid purpura include the *hemolytic-uremic syndrome,* and other conditions such as *systemic lupus erythematosus* in which both vasculitis and nephritis may be associated. In the hemolytic-uremic syndrome, the purpuric areas are not predominantly on the lower extremities and are less discrete, and there is a microangiopathic hemolytic anemia. In systemic lupus erythematosus a cutaneous vasculitis, indistinguishable from that of anaphylactoid purpura, may be present, but other characteristic clinical and laboratory features suggest the diagnosis. In patients who develop nephropathy after other manifestations of anaphylactoid purpura have subsided, it may be difficult to ascertain whether the renal problem is a consequence of anaphylactoid purpura. It is recommended that regular follow-up of patients with anaphylactoid purpura be done for several months in order to exclude the late development of nephritis after other problems have resolved. Biopsy may also exclude other glomerular diseases and can provide valuable information concerning the severity and extent of involvement.

TREATMENT. Since in most instances the

nephritis is minor and self-limited, treatment is usually unnecessary. Treatment measures outlined in the sections on acute poststreptococcal glomerulonephritis, the nephrotic syndrome and acute and chronic renal failure may be needed if similar clinical renal problems present. For those patients with marked proteinuria and evidence of progressive renal failure, or with biopsy-documented omniglomerular, diffuse, proliferative glomerulonephritis, it seems reasonable to treat with azathioprine, 3-4 mg/kg/day, for 6 months to 1 year, in combination with prednisone, 2 mg/kg/day, up to maximum of 60 mg/day. Prednisone should be given daily for 3 to 4 weeks followed by an alternate day regimen for the duration of the azathioprine therapy.

PROGNOSIS. In the majority of instances, the prognosis is excellent. The prognosis in patients with more severe nephritis is less favorable, but may be improved by appropriate treatment.

Allen, D. M., Diamond, L. K., and Howell, D. A.: Anaphylactoid purpura in children (Schönlein-Henoch syndrome). Am. J. Dis. Child. *99*:833, 1960.

Ayoub, E. M., and Hoyer, J.: Anaphylactoid purpura: Streptococcal antibody titers and β_{1C}-globulin levels. J. Pediatr. *75*:193, 1969.

Hurley, R. M., and Drummond, K. N.: Anaphylactoid purpura nephritis: Clinicopathological correlations. J. Pediatr. *81*:904, 1972.

Meadow, S. R., Glasgow, E. F., White, R. H. R., Moncrieff, M. W., Cameron, J. S., and Ogg, C. S.: Schönlein-Henoch nephritis. Quart. J. Med. *41*:241, 1972.

Urizar, R., Michael, A., Sisson, S., and Vernier, R.: Anaphylactoid purpura. II. Immunofluorescent and electron microscopic studies of the glomerular lesions. Lab. Invest. *19*:437, 1968.

HEMOLYTIC-UREMIC SYNDROME

The hemolytic-uremic syndrome is an acute disorder characterized by microangiopathic hemolytic anemia, nephropathy and thrombocytopenia. These features are usually preceded by gastroenteritis, viral respiratory illness or another definable event such as a "flu"-like illness or an immunization.

HISTORY. The syndrome was first recognized as a distinct entity in 1955. Although it is likely that it occurred prior to this time, its characteristic features and the fact that a large and, in some areas, epidemic number of patients have been recognized, suggests that it may be a relatively new disorder, the incidence of which has increased in the past 20 years.

ETIOLOGY. The syndrome has been reported following coxsackie- and arboviral infections, mumps and smallpox immunization, group A beta-hemolytic streptococcal infection and administration of pyran copolymer. In many instances a severe nonspecific gastroenteritis or upper respiratory tract infection precedes onset. Hereditary and environmental factors may both be operative, since the syndrome has occurred in unrelated adopted children living in the same house, in identical twins and in siblings. A rickettsial organism referred to as a microtatobiote has been implicated in some patients, and mycoplasma infections and endotoxemia have been considered as precipitating events. In view of the heterogenous nature of these recognized precipitating events, it is not possible to identify a single cause.

EPIDEMIOLOGY. The syndrome has been recognized predominantly in Caucasians and is uncommon in other racial groups, even those inhabiting the same region. The great majority of patients are children, usually under 5 years of age, although adults have been affected. South Africa, Argentina and California appear to be endemic areas.

PATHOLOGY AND PATHOPHYSIOLOGY. The variability in pathologic changes probably reflects not only differences in severity, extent and stage of development of lesions, but also probably the possibility that different disease entities may have common clinical expression as the hemolytic-uremic syndrome. *Renal microangiopathy* affecting small arterioles and glomerular capillaries is the most consistent change. The endothelial cells of the arterioles are swollen and disrupted with fibrin deposition in the subendothelial and intramural areas. This leads to narrowing and even occlusion of these vessels. Platelet aggregates may occur along the irregular endothelial lining. A variety of *glomerular lesions* have been described, including swelling of endothelial cells, subendothelial and mesangial deposition of an unidentified material with a foamy or vacuolated appearance, fibrinous microthrombi and, less commonly, an acute exudative or proliferative glomerulitis. Patchy or extensive cortical necrosis may occur consequent to compromise of the blood supply by the microangiopathy. Extrarenal findings are inconstant, frequently nonspecific and usually result from the consequences of renal failure. In adults an apparently similar microangiopathy affecting renal, cerebral, splenic and other vessels may occur; this disorder is known as **thrombotic thrombocytopenic purpura,** which is believed to be the adult analogue of the hemolytic-uremic syndrome.

The *pathogenesis* of these lesions is uncertain. Endothelial damage in renal arterioles and glomeruli by a variety of unrelated agents is a possible initiating event. Immune mechanisms are not considered to be operative, since there is no deposition of complement components or immunoglobulins at the site of the arteriolar or glomerular lesions. Nodular deposits of β_{1C} globulin in the mesangium and along the basement membrane have been described in one patient with a marked depression of serum β_{1C} globulin. Although disseminated and localized intravascular coagulation and endotoxin-induced Shwartzman reaction have been invoked in the pathogenesis, the evidence for implication of these processes is tenuous.

The *hemolytic anemia* is Coombs-negative, unassociated with red cell enzyme defect and characterized by fragmented, irregular, anisocytotic red cells, some of which are helmet-shaped or have spur-like projections *(burr cells).* These changes are believed to result from physical stress during passage through narrowed arterioles with irregular or denuded endothelial surfaces. *Thrombocytopenia* probably results from platelet aggregation within damaged vessels or from injury to platelets during passage through them, with subsequent sequestration in reticuloendothelial organs such as the spleen.

CLINICAL MANIFESTATIONS AND COURSE. The onset is abrupt and usually follows within a week an acute "flu"-like illness, gastroenteritis or upper respiratory infection. Marked pallor, bruising or purpura, irritability, lethargy and decreased output of urine (which is darkly colored) usually herald the onset. Mild jaundice, seizures, circulatory congestion and continuing bloody diarrhea simulating that of ulcerative colitis may follow.

The child is anorectic, irritable and pale. Hypertension, edema, splenomegaly, purpura or petechiae and signs of circulatory congestion, such as hepatomegaly, pulmonary edema, cardiomegaly, tachycardia, gallop rhythm and venous distention, may be present. The urinary output is reduced, and the urine may appear dark yellow or tea-colored. In mild cases this acute phase lasts 1 to 2 weeks, and gradual improvement occurs over 1 to 2 months. In severe cases there is more extensive renal damage, with anuria or sustained oliguria, persistent hemolysis leading to severe anemia and progressive renal failure with hypertension. Terminal renal insufficiency may supervene within 2 to 6 months. A more chronic course over a period of 6 to 12 months leading to fixed renal insufficiency or to terminal renal failure is seen in a minority of instances. Occasionally progressive renal failure may follow a temporary remission.

LABORATORY FINDINGS. A severe hemolytic anemia with hemoglobin levels of 5 to 7 gm/dl is common. The red cells have the characteristic features of fragmentation hemolysis: anisocytosis, fragmented and helmet-shaped cells and cells with protruding spikes or burrs (burr cells). The reticulocyte count is elevated. The platelet count may initially be normal, but at some time during the first week, depression to a level below 100,000/mm^3 almost always occurs. There is no consistent change in the white blood cell count or differential, but counts of 15,000-20,000/mm^3 with a predominance of polymorphonuclear leukocytes are not uncommon. The serum lipid concentration may be elevated and, although the serum B_{1C} globulin is usually normal, a decrease in total hemolytic complement may be manifest. The serum sodium concentration is normal, but for unexplained reasons the serum potassium is often decreased despite active hemolysis in the presence of renal insufficiency, a situation which might be expected to lead to hyperkalemia. The blood urea nitrogen and serum creatinine concentrations are usually elevated. There is proteinuria of 1 to 2 gm or more per 24 hours. The sediment is indicative of active glomerular damage, with microscopic or gross hematuria and red blood cell and/or granular casts.

DIAGNOSIS. The triad of severe microangiopathic hemolytic anemia, nephropathy and thrombocytopenia of acute onset following an acute illness is sufficient to permit a diagnosis of the hemolytic-uremic syndrome. Renal biopsy may be helpful if the characteristic arteriolar or glomerular endothelial, subendothelial and mesangial changes are present, but the specificity of these lesions is questioned. Biopsy findings may, however, indicate the extent and severity of the nephropathy and may exclude other disorders which must be considered in the differential diagnosis.

Differential Diagnosis. Other forms of acute hemolytic anemia, such as those of immune pathogenesis or those owing to an intrinsic defect of a red cell enzyme, may initially resemble the hemolytic-uremic syndrome and cause minor abnormalities in the urinary sediment. Thrombocytopenia, nephropathy and hemolytic anemia may be associated with active systemic lupus erythematosus. The anemia in this disease is not microangiopathic, however, and is often Coombs-positive. Patients with systemic lupus erythematosus are also usually older, and other manifestations of the disease are commonly present. Other causes of acute renal failure of either glomerular or interstitial origin may also resemble the hemolytic-uremic syndrome but can usually be differentiated without difficulty.

TREATMENT. The following types of treatment have been proposed but none has been proved to be effective (in view of the risks which they impose, none is recommended): anticoagulation with heparin or dicumarol-like drugs, corticosteroids, cytotoxic agents such as azathioprine or cyclophosphamide, and fibrinolytic therapy with agents such as streptokinase. There is evidence that early peritoneal dialysis in severe cases has reduced the mortality. It is not clear whether this treatment has a beneficial effect by removing some noxious causal agent or whether it simply tides the patient over until spontaneous recovery can occur. Generally, treatment measures should be directed to control of the complications of renal failure and the hematologic manifestations. The most frequently encountered renal problems are oliguria, electrolyte disorders, acidosis, hypertension and fluid overload. Their treatment is discussed in the sections on Acute Renal Failure and Acute Poststreptococcal Glomerulonephritis. If anemia is severe, transfusion with fresh, washed, packed red cells may be necessary. Because of hypertension and circulatory congestion resulting from the renal disorder and the added load that blood transfusion may impose, extreme caution should be exercised when blood transfusion is given. One should not attempt to raise the hemoglobin level above 7-8 gm/dl, but levels of 5 gm/dl or less are usually unsafe. Careful judgment is thus required to balance the risks of profound anemia against those imposed by blood transfusion in an oliguric, hypertensive patient with circulatory congestion. Peritoneal or hemodialysis, or parenteral furosemide may be required to alleviate the circulatory congestion. Bleeding resulting from thrombocytopenia aggravated by uremia may require platelet transfusions and dialysis. The goal of therapy is to provide an adequate time for the spontaneous recovery of renal function and resolution of the microangiopathy. If, despite judicious conservative management, there is progression of the disease and terminal renal failure develops, consideration must be given to institution of chronic dialysis with a view to eventual renal transplantation. As yet there is inadequate experience with the long-term results of renal transplantation in the hemolytic-uremic syndrome to warrant a definite recommendation.

PROGNOSIS. The prognosis appears to vary in different geographic areas, and probably reflects differences in the nature of the disease process and possibly in therapy. The recovery rate in endemic areas such as South Africa approaches 85 per cent, but in North America, where only sporadic cases are seen, the recovery rate is lower.

Gervais, M., Richardson, J. B., Chiu, J., and Drummond, K. N.: Immunofluorescent and histologic findings in the hemolytic-uremic syndrome. Pediatrics *47*:352, 1971.

Gianantonio, C. A., Vitacco, M., and Mendilaharzu, F.: The hemolytic-uremic syndrome. Proc. Third Int. Congr. Nephrol., Washington *3*:24, 1966.

Habib, R., Mathieu, H., and Royer, P.: Le syndrome hemolytique et uremique de l'enfant. Nephron *4*:139, 1967.

Kaplan, B. S., Katz, J., Krawitz, S., and Lurie, A.: An analysis of the results of therapy in 67 cases of the hemolytic-uremic syndrome. J. Pediatr. *78*:420, 1971.

Tune, B. M., Leavitt, T. J., and Gribble, T. J.: The hemolytic-uremic syndrome in California: A review of 28 nonheparinized cases with long-term follow-up. J. Pediatr. *82*:304, 1973.

Vitsky, B. H., Suzuki, Y., Strauss, L., and Churg, J.: The hemolytic-uremic syndrome. A study of renal pathologic alterations. Am. J. Path. *57*:627, 1969.

RECURRENT MACROSCOPIC HEMATURIA WITH FOCAL GLOMERULONEPHRITIS

(Benign Recurrent Hematuria, Focal Nephritis, Focal Proliferative Glomerulitis, Idiopathic Focal Proliferative Nephritis)

This condition is characterized by recurrent episodes of gross hematuria with or without persistent microscopic hematuria, and absence of systemic disease or other known glomerular or nonglomerular causes of hematuria; focal segmental mesangial proliferation is the principal pathologic finding. The etiology is unknown, but episodes of gross hematuria are usually precipitated by nonspecific viral respiratory infections or mild febrile episodes, less frequently by strenuous exercise.

INCIDENCE. The condition occurs throughout childhood, but most cases have their onset after age 2. Although once considered principally a pediatric condition it is now clear that it also occurs in adults. Boys are affected about twice as often as girls.

PATHOLOGY AND PATHOGENESIS. The most characteristic lesion is focal, segmental, mesangial cellular and matrix proliferation of mild severity involving a variable number of glomeruli, usually less than half, but more extensive and severe changes do occur. These include synechiae between glomerular tufts and Bowman's capsule, small epithelial crescents and focal areas of glomerulosclerosis. Characteristically a significant number of glomeruli may appear completely normal by light microscopy, and there is considerable variability in the severity of pathologic lesions in the involved glomeruli. Electron microscopy inconsistently shows mesangial and, less frequently, glomerular basement membrane deposits. Immunopathologic studies also have given variable results. In about half the patients with the clinical and laboratory features of this condition, mesangial deposition of IgA, IgG, IgM, β_{1C} globulin, fibrin and/or properdin have been demonstrated, the most consistent being β_{1C} globulin and IgA. Although these proteins may be deposited in all glomeruli, changes seen by light microscopy are usually confined to a limited number of glomeruli and vary considerably in severity. Positive fluorescence for IgA and β_{1C} globulin has also been demonstrated in renal biopsies done between attacks of gross hematuria. Sequential biopsies over a period of years, during which the patient has repeated episodes of gross hematuria, show no significant change or progression in most instances; in a minority the lesions become worse and there is progressive glomerular destruction with resultant chronic or end-stage renal disease. This latter course is more common in patients with persistent proteinuria between episodes of hematuria and in those with biopsy evidence of extensive mesangial immunoglobulin and β_{1C} globulin deposition or of focal glomerulosclerosis.

The *pathogenesis* of the glomerular lesions in this condition is poorly understood. The differences in immunopathologic findings between patients, and the fact that some patients follow a progressive downhill course, whereas most have a benign one, suggest that several disease entities are included in this syndrome. In some patients there is no evidence that immunologic mechanisms are operative; in others, a variety of immunoglobulins and β_{1C} globulin have been found, particularly in a mesangial location, suggesting immunologic injury. The finding of deposits of IgA in about one third of these patients is of considerable interest, since this immunoglobulin is secreted locally by cells along the respiratory and gastrointestinal tracts and plays a role in local immunity. Mesangial deposits of IgA are seen in anaphylactoid purpura and systemic lupus erythematosus and thus cannot be considered a unique or specific feature of recurrent gross hematuria with focal glomerulonephritis.

CLINICAL MANIFESTATIONS, COURSE AND PROGNOSIS. Most of the attacks of gross hematuria are preceded within 1 to 3 days by a mild, nonspecific viral upper respiratory infection or febrile episode, less often by a bout of strenuous exercise. The onset of hematuria is usually abrupt and unaccompanied by other symptoms. Some patients, however, complain of lethargy or malaise or of abdominal, flank or lower back pain. Hypertension, oliguria and edema are absent. Gross hematuria usually lasts from 2 to 4 days and then clears rapidly. Microscopic hematuria is usually present between episodes of gross hematuria. Many such attacks may occur over a period of 5 to 10 years. The condition clears spontaneously within 5 years in about half of the patients. A progressive course leading to renal insufficiency or sustained hypertension occurs in about 15 per cent of patients, principally in those who have persistent proteinuria between the episodes of hematuria.

LABORATORY FINDINGS. During an attack the urine is red, brown or tea-colored. The presence of red blood cell casts signifies a renal source of the bleeding, The urinary excretion of protein is moderately elevated during episodes of gross hematuria, but seldom exceeds 1.5 gm/24 hr. In most patients the proteinuria disappears as the hematuria subsides. There is no depression of serum β_{1C} globulin or other components of complement, no elevation of antistreptococcal antibody titers or bacteriologic evidence of group A beta-hemolytic streptococcal infection, and no laboratory evidence of a generalized or systemic disease such as systemic lupus eythematosus. A minority of patients show a transient decrease in glomerular filtration rate during episodes, but since the duration is only several days to a week this is of no clinical significance.

DIAGNOSIS AND DIFFERENTIAL DIAGNOSIS. The characteristic clinical picture of recurrent episodes of gross hematuria lasting several days, triggered by a mild nonspecific respiratory or febrile illness or by exercise, with persistent microscopic hematuria between episodes, suggests the diagnosis of idiopathic focal proliferative nephritis. The finding of red blood cell casts in the urine is of particular importance in excluding nonrenal sources of bleeding. The laboratory and renal biopsy findings previously described provide confirmatory evidence.

A renal biopsy should be done in patients in whom this diagnosis is suspected, particularly if there is persistent proteinuria; in addition to confirming the diagnosis and giving prognostic information, it enables exclusion of other more serious and potentially treatable diseases. Other conditions which must be considered include many of the causes of hematuria in children listed in Table 15–2, such as membranoproliferative glomerulonephritis, hereditary nephritis with deafness, benign familial hematuria and chronic glomerulonephritis, each of which can be reactivated by intercurrent illness and cause episodic gross hematuria. These disorders can each be diagnosed on the basis of their own specific features. It is essential to exclude nonglomerular causes of hematuria such as renal tumor, hydronephrosis, trauma, calculus, polycystic kidney disease or other congenital structural or vascular anomaly of the urinary tract. If the diagnosis is in question, particularly if red blood cell casts are not present in the urinary sediment, an intravenous urogram should be done to exclude such conditions. Acute hemorrhagic cystitis of bacterial or viral etiology may present with gross hematuria and abdominal discomfort, with or without other symptoms of urinary tract infection. Extensive unnecessary urologic evaluation, including repeated cystoscopic examinations, is the not infrequent fate of a number of these children because of lack of awareness of benign recurrent hematuria; they should be avoided.

TREATMENT. There is no specific treatment for the renal lesion. Reassurance should be given, since the attacks of gross hematuria are self-limited and the course is benign in the large majority of patients. Bed rest is not indicated, but if the child does not feel well, he may wish to restrict his activity for several days. Even if by avoiding exercise the number of episodes of gross hematuria could be reduced, this would probably not affect the long-term prognosis, and the patient should be encouraged to lead a completely normal life.

Ayoub, E. M., and Vernier, R. L.: Benign recurrent hematuria. Am. J. Dis. Child. *109*:217, 1965.

Berger, J.: IgA glomerular deposits in renal disease. Transplantation Proc. *1*:939, 1969.

Gervais, M., and Drummond, K. N.: L'hematurie recidivante chez l'enfant. L'Union Méd. Canad. *99*:1234, 1970.

Hendler, E. D., Kashgarian, M., and Hayselett, J. P.: Clinicopathological correlations of primary haematuria. Lancet *1*:458, 1972.

Lowance, D. C., Mullins, J. D., and McPhaul, J. J.: Immunoglobulin A (IgA) associated glomerulonephritis. Kidney Int. *3*:167, 1973.

Roy, L. P., Fish, A. J., Vernier, R. L., and Michael, A. F.: Recurrent macroscopic hematuria, focal nephritis, and mesangial deposition of immunoglobulin and complement. J. Pediatr. *82*:767, 1973.

NEPHRITIS IN SYSTEMIC LUPUS ERYTHEMATOSUS

See Section 9 for a general discussion of systemic lupus erythematosus.

It is unclear why the kidneys are affected in only some patients with systemic lupus erythematosus or why, in a given patient with renal involvement, only one of several possible types of pathologic lesion tends to be present. The incidence of renal disease in drug-induced lupus erythematosus is lower than in the idiopathic form; overall, it varies from 60 to 80 per cent, depending on the criteria used to define renal involvement. The lower figure obtains if clinical criteria such as edema, hypertension, nephrotic syndrome, hematuria, proteinuria and azotemia are used; histopathologic, electron microscopic and immunopathologic studies of renal biopsy specimens indicate that there is some form of glomerular abnormality in about 80 per cent of patients. The incidence of nephritis is the same in both sexes.

PATHOLOGY AND PATHOGENESIS. The glomerulus is the principal site of injury in "lupus nephritis." Four distinct forms of involvement may be seen. These are not successive or different stages of a single type of lesion; rather, in most instances each is a separable entity which, for a given patient, is the type of nephritis that he will have throughout the course of the disease. Furthermore, the presence or absence of nephritis and the form which it will take are usually established early in the disease. The four forms are:

Normal Glomeruli by Light Microscopic Examination. No abnormalities are detectable on routine histopathologic study. Immunofluorescent techniques show omniglomerular mesangial deposits of IgG and of β_{1C} globulin in about half these patients; mesangial deposits may also be seen by electron microscopy. Hematuria and proteinuria are absent or minimal, and there is little likelihood of development of a more serious form of nephritis.

Focal Segmental Proliferative Lupus Nephritis (Lupus Glomerulitis). Lesions are confined to only some glomeruli, and only some lobules or segments of these glomeruli are affected. Characteristically there is mesangial hypercellularity with increased mesangial matrix, reduction in patent capillary lumina in affected segments, mild polymorphonuclear infiltration, localized thickening of peripheral capillary basement membranes and, less commonly, some nuclear fragmentation. A mild periglomerulitis may be present. Electron microscopic findings include dense mesangial deposits, with occasional subendothelial or intramembranous deposits in regions where a proliferative reaction is present. Immunopathologic study reveals focal mesangial deposits of IgG and β_{1C} globulin and occasionally of fibrin, IgM, IgA or properdin. Subendothelial and epimembranous deposits are also seen. Even if untreated, these lesions do not tend to progress to a more serious type.

Diffuse Proliferative Lupus Glomerulonephritis. This is the most active and serious form of glomerular injury and constitutes about 20 per cent of cases of lupus nephritis in children. All glomeruli are involved. Characteristic histopathologic features are a marked increase in the mesangial matrix, with obliteration of capillary lumina, necrosis of glomerular nodules, nuclear fragmentation, localized thickening of glomerular basement membranes to give the so-called wire loop appearance, and infiltration with polymorphonuclear leukocytes. There may be epithelial crescent formation, interstitial edema, and local interstitial perivascular inflammation and plasma cell infiltration. Electron microscopy reveals extensive mesangial and subendothelial deposits with marked increase in mesangial matrix. The subendothelial deposits along the glomerular basement membrane correspond to areas of wire loop change seen by light microscopy. Marked deposition of IgG, β_{1C} globulin and fibrin is present, often in a lumpy, lobular pattern, involving the glomerulus diffusely; IgM, IgA and properdin may also be seen. DNA and other nuclear antigens are present at the site of these immune deposits. If untreated, this form progresses rapidly to glomerular destruction within several months.

Membranous Lupus Nephritis. This is the least common form of lupus nephritis in children. It is a chronic, indolent process with little cellular proliferation but with omniglomerular diffuse thickening of the basement membranes. The thickening is the result of subepithelial epimembranous deposits similar to those in idiopathic membranous nephropathy. In comparison with the diffuse proliferative form there is less subendothelial and mesangial deposition. The subepithelial deposits contain IgG, β_{1C} globulin and fibrin; IgM, IgA and DNA may also be present. This form of lupus nephritis progresses slowly and responds slowly, if at all, to treatment.

There is good evidence that the *pathogenesis* of the renal lesions involves deposition of immune complexes. A number of distinct immume complex systems have been identified. Antibodies to nuclear constituents such as native and single-stranded DNA, cytoplasmic constituents, clotting factors, gamma globulins, red blood cell antigens, platelets and various tissue antigens are detectable in the serum of patients with active systemic lupus erythematosus. The formation of DNA/anti-DNA immune complexes which bind complement, and the subsequent deposition of these complexes in the glomerulus, is one of the principal mechanisms of glomerular injury. It is possible that differences between the types of lupus nephritis just described are the result of differences in the immune complex system involved.

CLINICAL MANIFESTATIONS AND COURSE. Renal disease in systemic lupus erythematosus is one of the major causes of morbidity and mortality; thus, it is critical to establish whether it is present. Furthermore, since each of the forms of lupus nephritis has a different natural history and requires different therapy, the particular type of nephritis should be established by renal biopsy.

In focal proliferative lupus glomerulitis there may be microscopic hematuria with red blood cell casts and mild proteinuria. Hypertension, edema and azotemia are uncommon. Usually the renal lesions do not progress and treatment should be aimed primarily at control of the nonrenal manifestations of lupus erythematosus.

In diffuse proliferative lupus glomerulonephritis, the renal manifestations are a major clinical problem. Hypertension, edema, azotemia, microscopic or gross hematuria and moderate or marked proteinuria are usually present; i.e., there is a mixed nephritic-nephrotic picture. If untreated, this form of lupus nephritis progresses over a period of several months to advanced renal failure. In children, aggressive treatment is effective in reversing this course; if started early enough, considerable resolution of the lesion can usually be anticipated.

The nephrotic syndrome is the principal manifestation of membranous lupus nephritis. Microscopic hematuria, hypertension and mild azotemia may also be present. The course is usually chronic, with slow progression to renal insufficiency or gradual response to treatment over a period of months to several years.

LABORATORY FINDINGS. Hematuria with red blood cell casts, pyuria, proteinuria and azotemia are the principal laboratory manifestations. If the nephrotic syndrome is present, hypoproteinemia, particularly hypoalbuminemia, is also present. In patients with active lupus nephritis the level of serum complement, particularly β_{1C} globulin, is low, and the titer of antinuclear antibodies, especially anti-DNA antibodies, is elevated. With treatment, these tend to return to normal levels. An elevated antinuclear antibody titer and depressed serum complement level can be present, however, in the absence of renal involvement.

DIFFERENTIAL DIAGNOSIS. Other forms of renal disease may be present in a patient with systemic lupus erythematosus; specifically, it is essential to exclude urinary tract infection since this may not be clinically apparent and may cause progressive renal destruction or sepsis, while being masked by corticosteroid treatment. Iatrogenic urinary abnormalities may also occur; e.g., cystitis or mucosal ulceration at various sites along the urinary tract may result from treatment with cyclophosphamide or azathioprine.

The diagnosis and differential diagnosis of systemic lupus erythematosus is considered in Section 9. Similar changes in the renal biopsy may be seen in anaphylactoid purpura, subacute bacterial endocarditis, nephritis owing to infected shunts, and other causes of membranous glomerulonephritis; these conditions can be diagnosed by their own particular features.

PREVENTION. No means of prevention of lupus nephritis is known. Likelihood of reactivation or exacerbation of systemic lupus erythematosus can be reduced by avoiding exposure to ultraviolet irradiation, i.e., sunlight. Sudden changes in medication, such as rapid reduction in corticosteroid therapy or withdrawal of azathioprine, should be avoided, since this can reactivate lupus nephritis, and adequate control may subsequently be difficult to achieve.

TREATMENT. The treatment of *focal proliferative nephritis* ordinarily requires only the usual course of prednisone (1–2 mg/kg/day) given for treatment of the underlying disease. Close attention should be paid to urinary and biopsy findings, however, to assess whether progression is occurring.

With *diffuse proliferative lupus nephritis,* active treatment of the renal lesion itself must be undertaken. Doses of prednisone adequate to control nonrenal manifestations are often inadequate to treat this form of nephritis; doses of 2–3 mg/kg/day should be given for 1 to 2 months along with azathioprine in a dose of 3–4 mg/kg/day. The course should be monitored by the usual laboratory and clinical evaluations and by sequential renal biopsies. Attention should be paid to the possible development of steroid-induced hypertension and edema; restriction of salt intake to 1–2 gm/day should be instituted, and antihypertensive and/or diuretic therapy may be needed. Gradual introduction of an alternate-day prednisone regimen by reducing on alternate days the dosage by 5–10 mg/week, while maintaining the same initial dose on the other days, should be started after several months of daily therapy. During the initial treatment period, prednisone is given in three divided doses daily; as treatment proceeds, one should aim for a single dose on the day it is given. Daily azathioprine treatment should be continued for an indefinite time; a gradual reduction to a maintenance dose of 2 mg/kg/day may be attempted after satisfactory control has been achieved. Cyclophosphamide can be used instead of azathioprine.

The treatment of *membranous lupus nephritis* is controversial. Less aggressive treatment is indicated than for diffuse proliferative lupus glomerulonephritis. Long-term azathioprine and alternate-day prednisone therapy have reduced the protein excretion and improved the degree of renal insufficiency in some patients.

PROGNOSIS. Although lupus nephritis is an important cause of morbidity and mortality if untreated, the prognosis with respect to renal involvement is good if adequate treatment is given early. The most dramatic improvement occurs in the diffuse proliferative form, and the least in the membranous type.

Agnello, V., Koffler, D., and Kunkel, H. G.: Immune complex systems in the nephritis of systemic lupus erythematosus. Kidney Int. *3*:90, 1973.

Dujovne, I., Pollak, V. E., Pirani, C. L., and Dillard, M. G.: The distribution and character of glomerular deposits in systemic lupus erythematosus. Kidney Int. *2*:33, 1972.

Pollak, V. E., Pirani, C. L., and Schwartz, F. D.: The natural history of the renal manifestations of systemic lupus erythematosus. J. Lab. Clin. Med. *63*:537, 1964.

Rothfield, N. F.: The kidney in systemic lupus erythematosus. Kidney *5* (No. 2):1, 1972.

Sharon, E., Kaplan, D., and Diamond, H. S.: Exacerbation of systemic lupus erythematosus after withdrawal of azathioprine therapy. New Engl. J. Med. *228*:122, 1973.

GLOMERULONEPHRITIS ASSOCIATED WITH SEPSIS, INFECTED SHUNTS FOR HYDROCEPHALUS OR SUBACUTE BACTERIAL ENDOCARDITIS

Any patient with chronic bacteremia may develop proliferative glomerulonephritis. Conditions commonly associated include coagulase-positive staphylococcal osteomyelitis, shunts for hydrocephalus infected with coagulase-negative staphylococci and subacute bacterial endocarditis owing to a variety of organisms. The pathologic features range from a focal segmental mesangial proliferative glomerulonephritis to severe omniglomerular diffuse proliferative glomerulonephritis with epithelial crescent formation, segmental fibrinoid necrosis, localized thickening of the basement membrane and interstitial infiltration with mononuclear cells. The lesions may be acute and active, or may become chronic with segmental or diffuse glomerular hyalinization and scarring. Immunopathologic study reveals nodular or granular deposits of IgG and β_{1C} globulin, with or without IgM, IgA or fibrin. These deposits are situated along the epithelial aspect of the glomerular basement membrane and within the mesangium. The pathogenesis of these lesions is of the immune complex type, involving antibody of the IgG or IgM type against antigens of the infecting bacteria.

The clinical presentation is usually that of a mixed nephritic-nephrotic type with hematuria, red cell casts, proteinuria, azotemia and hypertension. In infants with infected shunts, the nephrotic syndrome has been a common presentation. In virtually all patients, clinical evidence of bacteremia or sepsis, such as fever and hepatosplenomegaly, precedes the renal manifestations. A positive blood culture can usually be obtained, but urine culture is frequently negative. Normochromic anemia and leukocytosis are present; the serum β_{1C} globulin level is depressed. Immune complex nephritis should be suspected in any patient with chronic bacterial infection who develops an abnormal urinary sediment, proteinuria, azotemia, and/or hypertension. The diagnosis is supported by reduction in serum complement levels; renal biopsy can establish the presence of glomerulonephritis and give valuable information regarding its severity and prognosis.

Treatment consists of appropriate antibiotic therapy for the infecting organism and, in most cases of infected shunts for hydrocephalus, removal of the shunt. The prognosis depends largely on the nature of the underlying disease, which may itself be serious and not amenable to cure. If the infection can be controlled, the renal lesions tend to become inactive. Depending on the severity and extent of the lesions, the renal problem may resolve completely, a stable nonprogressive state of renal insufficiency may result or, less commonly, progressive glomerular destruction leading to chronic renal failure may occur.

Black, J. A., Challacombe, D. N., and Ockenden, B. G.: Nephrotic syndrome associated with bacteraemia after shunt operations for hydrocephalus. Lancet *2*:921, 1965.

Gutman, R. A., Striker, G. E., Gilliland, B. C., and Cutler, R. E.: The immune complex glomerulonephritis of bacterial endocarditis. Medicine *51*:1, 1972.

Levy, R. L., and Hong, R.: The immune nature of subacute bacterial endocarditis (SBE) nephritis. Am. J. Med. *54*:645, 1973.

Stickler, G. B., Myung, H. S., Burke, E. C., Holley, K. E., Miller, R. H., and Segar, W. E.: Diffuse glomerulonephritis associated with infected ventriculoatrial shunt. New Engl. J. Med. *279*:1077, 1968.

TUBULAR DISORDERS

Disorders of renal tubular function include a variety of conditions whose common feature is impairment of one or more specific tubular functions in the absence of an overall decrease in renal function or reduction in glomerular filtration rate. Many of these disorders are hereditary and involve: (1) a primary defect in a transport mechanism for reabsorption of one or more specific solutes from the glomerular filtrate, e.g., cystinuria, renal glycosuria; (2) inability of the tubular cell to respond to normal hormonal stimuli, e.g., pseudohypoparathyroidism, nephrogenic diabetes insipidus; or (3) inability to develop or to maintain a requisite electrical or chemical gradient in order that certain specific physiologic tubular functions may be performed, e.g., distal renal tubular acidosis.

Some tubular disorders are secondary or acquired; such tubular dysfunction might occur (1) during the course of a systemic disease, usually metabolic in nature, in which there is deposition of a metabolic product in the tubules (e.g., cystine crystals in cystinosis) or there is a circulating metabolite which has a toxic effect on the tubule (e.g., fructose-1-phosphate in hereditary fructose intolerance); or (2) as a consequence of an exogenous drug or toxin, e.g., distal renal tubular acidosis from amphotericin B or generalized proximal tubular dysfunction from lead poisoning.

In some conditions, although only tubular function may be affected initially, there is subsequent interstitial or glomerular damage which leads to reduction in glomerular filtration rate; e.g., nephrocalcinosis and interstitial scarring may develop in distal renal acidosis and lead to chronic renal failure; cystine stones may form in cystinuria, leading to obstructive renal damage and increased susceptibility to pyelonephritis.

Hereditary conditions in which tubular dysfunction is present either as a primary or secondary event are listed in Table 15–7 in the section on Hereditary or Familial Disorders.

Table 15–6 lists the causes of distal and proximal renal tubular acidosis and includes hereditary disorders and many of the exogenous toxins or drugs which cause impaired tubular function. Many of the agents which cause proximal renal tubular acidosis may also cause the Fanconi syndrome, which is discussed later in this section.

RENAL TUBULAR ACIDOSIS

See also Acid-Base Balance under Renal Physiology.

Renal tubular acidosis (RTA) is a clinical syndrome of sustained hyperchloremic metabolic acidosis in the absence of a significant reduction in glomerular filtration rate. It results from an impaired ability of the kidney to maintain plasma HCO_3^- levels within the normal range because of defective acidification of urine or impaired reabsorption of bicarbonate. The urine pH is inappropriately high in relation to the metabolic acidosis; there is reduced excretion of titratable acid and ammonia. Two physiologically distinct and some intermediate forms of RTA are recognized; the principal forms are distal renal tubular acidosis (type I, classic type) and proximal renal tubular acidosis (type II).

ETIOLOGY. Distal and proximal renal tubular

TABLE 15–6 CAUSES OF RENAL TUBULAR ACIDOSIS

DISTAL TYPE	PROXIMAL TYPE
Primary	*Primary*
Sporadic, with infantile or later onset	Sporadic, with infantile or later onset
Hereditary, with infantile or later onset	Hereditary, with infantile or later onset
*Secondary**	*Secondary†*
Amphotericin B	Cystinosis
Hyperimmunoglobulinemia	Galactosemia
Renal transplantation	Heavy metals (lead, cadmium)
Medullary nephrocalcinosis due to hypercalcemia, hyperparathyroidism, vitamin D intoxication, etc.	Hereditary fructose intolerance
Toluene sniffing	Primary or secondary hyperparathyroidism
Ehlers-Danlos syndrome	Hyperimmunoglobulinemia
	Vitamin D deficiency rickets
	Wilson's disease
	Lowe syndrome
	Tyrosinosis
	Outdated tetracycline
	Familial nephrotic syndrome with tubular dysfunction
	Leigh syndrome
	Glycogen storage disease, type I
	Renal vascular accidents in the newborn period

*Distal renal tubular acidosis has been reported rarely in other conditions; most of these are listed in the reference articles.

†Many of these disorders cause the Fanconi syndrome of proximal renal tubular dysfunction and are thus associated with generalized aminoaciduria, glycosuria, hyperkaliuria, uricosuria, hypercalciuria and phosphaturia in addition to bicarbonaturia.

acidoses (RTA) occur either as primary abnormalities in urine acidification or as secondary disorders consequent to systemic disease or intoxication. *Primary distal RTA* may be inherited by an autosomal recessive mode, particularly the form expressed in childhood, or by an autosomal dominant mode, the one whose expression is delayed until adulthood, when the incidence is higher in females. Usually, however, the disorder is sporadic and without evidence of hereditary factors.

While *proximal RTA* also occurs as a primary isolated defect, especially in male infants, it is more commonly secondary to a systemic disorder or toxin and is usually associated with other features of impaired proximal tubular transport. Table 15–6 lists some of the known causes of distal and proximal RTA.

PATHOLOGY. In *distal RTA,* a specific pathologic lesion has not been recognized. Nephrocalcinosis, particularly in the medulla, usually develops if adequate control of the acidosis is not achieved. Tubular degeneration and interstitial fibrosis may result from the nephrocalcinosis and from the repeated episodes of hypokalemia that often complicate the course. Nephrocalcinosis and nephrolithiasis may predispose to urinary tract infection and pyelonephritic changes.

In *primary proximal RTA* a specific lesion has not been described. Proximal tubular dilatation and the "swan neck deformity" are seen in some children with proximal RTA and other features of impaired proximal tubular transport. In cystinosis, in which proximal RTA and other features of the Fanconi syndrome are present, cystine crystals are present within the interstitium and there are tubular damage and interstitial scarring; giant cell transformation of the visceral epithelial cells of the glomerulus may occur. Nephrocalcinosis is rarely seen in proximal RTA.

PATHOPHYSIOLOGY. In *distal RTA* the functional defect is an inability to maintain a steep enough H^+ gradient in the distal tubule and collecting duct, by sufficient excretion of titratable acid and ammonium chloride, to permit, by titratable acid and ammonium chloride excretion, regeneration of the HCO_3^- used in buffering nonvolatile acids formed in normal metabolic activity. Consequently the plasma HCO_3^- level remains below normal. The fixed acids are excreted as sodium salts, resulting in a net sodium deficit to which the physiologic response is secondary hyperaldosteronism. This accentuates sodium and chloride reabsorption and potassium loss, especially in the distal tubule; the net result is a negative potassium balance and hypokalemia. The decreased plasma HCO_3^- concentration is accompanied by a corresponding elevation in chloride concentration. Bone buffers, particularly calcium carbonate, modify the severity of the systemic acidosis, but in so doing, excessive amounts of calcium salts are excreted in the urine. Because of the relatively high urine pH and the low urinary excretion of citrate consequent to the systemic acidosis, the calcium salts are not kept in solution in the urine and are deposited to produce nephrocalcinosis and/or lithiasis. The ensuing interstitial medullary damage may interfere with the normal countercurrent multiplier and exchange systems by which the kidney concentrates urine. This situation is aggravated by tubular and interstitial damage caused by episodic or sustained hypokalemia. The net result is impaired concentrating ability and polyuria. A fall in glomerular filtration rate sometimes develops; the physiologic changes which this induces, in concert with the bone changes induced by systemic acidosis, may lead to osteomalacia and/or rickets.

In most patients with distal RTA, the amount of HCO_3^- lost in the urine is small, less than 3 per cent of the filtered load. This persistent slight bicarbonaturia and the inability to maintain a sufficient lumen-to-plasma H^+ gradient results in inability to reduce urine pH below 6.0 even in the face of severe acidosis. In some children there is also a significant reduction in the capacity to reabsorb HCO_3^-, and bicarbonaturia may equal 5 to 10 per cent of the amount filtered; HCO_3^- loss may be quantitatively more important in the pathogenesis of acidosis than impaired excretion of acid.

In *proximal RTA,* the defect is one of reduced proximal tubular HCO_3^- reabsorption owing to a decreased Tm HCO_3^-. At normal plasma HCO_3^- levels, over 15 per cent of filtered HCO_3^- is spilled in the urine. Bicarbonaturia also occurs when mild acidosis is present (HCO_3^- levels of 16–22 mEq/l). Below this level sufficient H^+ can be secreted by the proximal tubule to permit reabsorption of most of the filtered HCO_3^-. At this point bicarbonaturia ceases and, since distal tubular function is intact, generation of a normal H^+ gradient with a urine pH less than 5.5 occurs, with normal net acid excretion as titratable acid and ammonium chloride. Proximal RTA usually occurs as part of a more complex abnormality in the proximal tubules, known as the Fanconi syndrome, which is discussed later.

Potassium loss in proximal RTA, whether or not it is associated with the Fanconi syndrome, results in part from impaired proximal tubular K^+ reabsorption. In addition, the increased amount of HCO_3^- reaching the distal tubule enhances passive K^+ secretion into the lumen at this site. Moreover, raising the serum HCO_3^- level by alkali therapy further increases the amount of HCO_3^- reaching the distal tubule and further augments K^+ secretion. By contrast, in distal RTA, proximal HCO_3^- reabsorption is usually normal at physiologic levels of plasma HCO_3^-, and a significant increment in K^+ loss consequent to therapy is not observed. In fact, many patients with distal RTA do not require potassium supplements to maintain normal serum K^+ levels, providing sustained correction of the metabolic acidosis is achieved. The hypokalemia in either proximal or distal RTA may have profound physiologic consequences. These include impairment in urine concentrating ability, muscle paralysis and predisposition to tetany during correction of acidosis.

Hypercalciuria and resultant hypocalcemia may also occur in proximal RTA, and secondary hyperparathyroidism, induced by the hypocalcemia, may magnify the defects in proximal tubular transport. Thus, correction of hypocalcemia may be an important consideration in the therapy of proximal RTA in that it decreases secretion of parathyroid hormone.

Incomplete or partial forms of RTA have been described in adults. Such patients are clinically well but, when stressed by ammonium chloride loading, they do not develop an appropriately acid urine and may become acidotic. It is not established whether these patients represent examples of the heterozygote state of distal RTA.

Although hyperchloremic acidosis occurs in patients with congenital or acquired deficiency in secretion of aldosterone, the pathogenesis is poorly understood. There is evidence that a proximal type of RTA that is reversible by mineralocorticoid administration is present in at least some of these patients.

CLINICAL MANIFESTATIONS AND COURSE. The clinical features of RTA are linked to the associated electrolyte and fluid disturbances and, in the case of proximal RTA, with abnormalities due to other defects of proximal tubular function of which RTA may be but one manifestation. Furthermore, in systemic or toxic conditions that may cause either proximal or distal RTA, the features of the underlying disorder may overshadow those due only to RTA.

The age of onset of RTA is variable. In infants with the inherited form of *distal RTA* the acidifying defect is usually present at birth, although the correct diagnosis is often not made until several months or even years later. Failure to thrive and polyuria may be present from early infancy. Some patients who present in infancy with what appears to be distal RTA apparently recover spontaneously, but most do not and require alkali therapy throughout life. In some patients with inherited distal RTA the onset is delayed until the third or fourth decade.

Primary proximal RTA, unassociated with the Fanconi syndrome of proximal tubular dysfunction, is more common in boys. The clinical onset is usually in the first 18 months; growth failure and a history of vomiting in early infancy are present. In many patients the defect in HCO_3^- reabsorption is not permanent and after a number of months therapy can be stopped without relapse.

In children RTA is characterized by hyperchloremic metabolic acidosis, which causes marked growth failure, tachypnea, thirst, polyuria and osteomalacia. Dehydration, vomiting, episodic fever, nephrolithiasis secondary to hypercalciuria, muscle weakness or paralysis due to hypokalemia and episodes of severe, life-threatening acidemia (sometimes triggered by an intercurrent illness) are seen. Tetany, muscle cramps and even seizures during correction of acidosis may be a prominent feature in patients with hypocalcemia and/or hypokalemia. Recurrent urinary infections may occur if nephrolithiasis is present.

Correction of acidosis by alkali therapy with or without K^+ supplementation leads to dramatic improvement in the clinical condition, and normal growth resumes. If muscle weakness and polyuria secondary to hypokalemia are present, these are also ameliorated. In patients with distal RTA, it is not uncommon for impaired ability to concentrate urine to persist because of permanent damage caused by nephrocalcinosis and episodes of hypokalemia.

LABORATORY FINDINGS. The cardinal metabolic variations of *distal RTA* are sustained metabolic acidosis with hypocarbia and hyperchloremia in the presence of an inappropriately alkaline urine of pH 6.0 or higher. An elevated serum H^+ concentration (decreased serum pH) may also be present. Hypokalemia, excessive excretion of potassium in the urine, hypercalciuria (over 4 mg/kg/day) and hypocalcemia may be present. In the face of this sustained metabolic acidosis, the net acid excretion (urinary titratable acid, plus ammonia, minus bicarbonate) is decreased. Aminoaciduria, phosphaturia and glucosuria are absent. The plasma level at which bicarbonate spills into the urine is usually normal (23–25 mEq/l); however, some patients with distal RTA have a reduced HCO_3^- threshold. The ability to concentrate urine is often impaired; maximal values of 300–500 mOsm/l after overnight fasting are the rule. Roentgenograms may reveal medullary nephrocalcinosis and decreased bone density.

In *proximal RTA* systemic acidosis with hyperchloremia is also seen. In contrast to distal RTA, the urine may be acid if the plasma HCO_3^- level is sufficiently low for complete reabsorption of HCO_3^-. The urine pH will be above 6.0 because of bicarbonaturia when plasma levels are above the HCO_3^- threshold (usually 17–20 mEq/l); the pH will be appropriately acid with a normal net acid excretion when the plasma HCO_3^- level is below the threshold value. Urinary loss of K^+ is excessive and tends to increase as the plasma HCO_3^- level rises. Impaired ability to concentrate urine is a less prominent feature than in distal RTA; it may, however, occur as a result of tubular damage in some of the disorders with which proximal RTA may be associated and because of hypokalemia. If proximal RTA is associated with the Fanconi syndrome, laboratory features of this condition will also be present. These include generalized aminoaciduria, glucosuria, phosphaturia, uricosuria, tubular proteinuria and hypophosphatemia.

DIAGNOSIS AND DIFFERENTIAL DIAGNOSIS. The diagnosis of *distal RTA* can be established by the presence of an inappropriately alkaline urine (pH > 6.0) in the presence of sustained metabolic acidosis without evidence of significant reduction in functioning renal tissue, i.e., without significant elevation of blood urea nitrogen or serum creatinine. Associated clinical and laboratory features, as described earlier, are usually present. In most instances it is not necessary to perform an ammonium chloride loading test to determine maximal urine acidification, since acidosis is already present, and the procedure is not without risk under these circumstances.

The diagnosis of *proximal RTA* depends on the finding of both a sustained metabolic acidosis and a lowered tubular threshold for HCO_3^-. Thus, although the urine pH may be appropriately acid (pH < 5.5) when the plasma HCO_3^- is very low, an alkaline urine (pH > 6.0) is present when the plasma HCO_3^- is above the patient's threshold value, yet still in a range below the normal level at which bicarbonaturia appears (24–26 mEq/l). This may be verified by actual measurement of the HCO_3^- threshold by sodium bicarbonate infusion or by giving sufficient alkali orally to maintain the serum HCO_3^- level at 20–22 mEq/l, at which level, despite mild metabolic acidosis, the urine pH is inappropriately alkaline and net acid excretion is reduced. The presence of other characteristic laboratory and clinical findings may provide supportive evidence.

In addition to establishing the diagnosis of either proximal or distal RTA or one of their variants, it is necessary to determine whether any of the known predisposing causes of RTA, as listed in Table 15-6, is present. Appropriate historical, clinical and laboratory features of each of these conditions should be sought.

Specific conditions which may cause some of the clinical and laboratory features of RTA include severe diarrhea, small bowel fistula, ingestion of acidifying salts or of the carbonic anhydrase inhibitor acetazolamide, saline infusion, ureterosigmoidostomy, diabetes insipidus, respiratory alkalosis, lactic acidosis, acidosis of prematurity, chronic renal failure and other disorders of metabolism which lead to metabolic acidosis.

PREVENTION. Except in well documented kindreds where genetic counseling may be of value, primary inherited RTA cannot be prevented. In many of the conditions known to be associated with RTA of either proximal or distal type, avoidance of toxic doses of drugs or awareness of the possibility that RTA may develop can permit either prevention or early diagnosis.

TREATMENT. In both distal and proximal RTA the central goal of therapy is to provide sufficient alkali to maintain the plasma HCO_3^- level within the normal range and to correct associated electrolyte disorders, notably hypokalemia. In distal RTA this usually requires administration of sodium bicarbonate ($NaHCO_3$), 1–3 mEq/kg/day in four to six divided doses. The amount required in proximal RTA is much higher, usually 5–15 mEq/kg/day. The amount of potassium required is variable; an initial supplement of 2 mEq/kg/day as potassium chloride should be given, but children with proximal RTA may require 4–10 mEq/kg/day to maintain the serum K^+ within the normal range. Alkali may also be given in the form of sodium and potassium citrate, such as Shohl's solution (140 gm citric acid and 90 gm hydrated crystalline salt of sodium citrate in 1 liter of water) or Polycitra*, either of which is slightly more palatable than sodium bicarbonate or potassium chloride. A mixture of 10 per cent each of sodium and potassium citrate in a sweet syrup provides 1 mEq each of Na^+ and K^+/ml and the equivalent of 2 mEq of HCO_3^-/ml. Oral therapy will not suffice in an acutely ill, severely acidotic, dehydrated child. A reasonable solution for intravenous administration consists of sodium bicarbonate in a concentration of 60–100 mEq/l with potassium chloride in a concentration of 40–60 mEq/l. The amount given should be calculated to correct the base deficit, i.e., to raise the plasma HCO_3^- level to normal over a period of 12 to 24 hours. If the plasma H^+ concentration is elevated, i.e., the pH is decreased, more HCO_3^- than calculated to raise the plasma level to normal will be necessary. Care should be taken to

*Polycitra—Willien Drug Company, Baltimore, Md.

avoid tetany, muscle cramps and seizures, which are likely to develop if the acidosis is corrected too rapidly, especially if hypocalcemia and/or hypokalemia are present. Administration of calcium gluconate in a dose calculated to give about 15 mg of calcium per kg over 1 to 2 hours via a separate intravenous route may be used to prevent or treat hypocalcemia. Water intake as high as 2–5 l/m^2/day may be necessary because of impaired ability to concentrate urine.

It is important to establish whether RTA is temporary or permanent and to exclude or treat any underlying cause. Chronic administration of alkali and potassium supplements and careful surveillance over a lifetime may be required. Adequacy of control should be monitored by periodic evaluation of plasma electrolyte and acid-base status; urinary calcium excretion may also be a useful guide, since hypercalciuria disappears when good control is achieved. Usual vitamin supplements are necessary, and a generous fluid intake, particularly during intercurrent illnesses, should be given to patients with poor ability to concentrate urine.

PROGNOSIS. The prognosis of primary distal RTA is excellent if therapy is begun early and continued in a dosage appropriate to maintain the serum HCO_3^- level and other electrolytes within the normal range. If the diagnosis is not made until renal damage secondary to hypokalemia or nephrocalcinosis has developed, some residual functional damage may persist. Even under these circumstances proper therapy may permit normal life expectancy. A small percentage of infants with primary distal RTA recover spontaneously and require no further therapy. The prognosis in children with primary proximal RTA is less well established, but some appear to recover spontaneously over a period of 4 to 12 months. Control of the acid-base and electrolyte status is not so easy in proximal RTA, and return to completely normal growth and health is less common.

In both proximal and distal RTA the presence of an underlying systemic or toxic condition are of fundamental importance in influencing the ultimate prognosis.

Morris, R. C., Jr.: An experimental renal acidification defect in patients with hereditary fructose intolerance. J. Clin. Invest. *47*:1648, 1968.

Morris, R. C., Sebastian, A., and McSherry, E.: Renal acidosis. Kidney Int. *1*:322, 1972.

Nash, M. A., Torrado, A. D., Greifer, I., Spitzer, A., and Edelmann, C. M.: Renal tubular acidosis in infants and children. J. Pediatr. *80*:738, 1972.

Richards, P., and Wrong, O. M.: Dominant inheritance in a family with familial renal tubular acidosis. Lancet *2*:998, 1972.

Sedlin, D. W., and Wilson, J. D.: Renal tubular acidosis. *In* Stanbury, J. B., Wyngaarden, J. B., and Fredrickson, D. S., (eds.): The Metabolic Basis of Inherited Disease. New York, McGraw-Hill Book Co., 1972, p. 1548.

Stark, H., and Geiger, R.: Renal tubular dysfunction following vascular accidents of the kidneys in the newborn period. J. Pediatr. *83*:933, 1973.

Taher, S. M., Anderson, R. J., McCartney, R., Popovtzer, M. M., and Schrier, R. W.: Renal tubular acidosis associated with toluene "sniffing." New Engl. J. Med. *290*:765, 1974.

FANCONI SYNDROME

The principal features of this syndrome are osteomalacia or rickets, growth retardation, proximal type renal tubular acidosis with bicarbonaturia, glycosuria without hyperglycemia, phosphaturia with hypophosphatemia, generalized aminoaciduria in the absence of elevated plasma levels of amino acids, tubular proteinuria, ketonuria, excessive urinary sodium and potassium excretion, hypokalemia, hypouricemia, variable hypercalciuria and an impaired ability to concentrate the urine which may lead to polyuria. In patients with cystinosis a glomerular lesion may develop and there can be proteinuria in excess of 1 gm/24 hr. In this situation the protein excreted is the same as in other forms of glomerular injury.

The severity of any of these findings varies from patient to patient. There is, however, a common pathogenesis, namely, a complex proximal tubular dysfunction. Depending on which transport mechanisms are principally affected, there is a corresponding failure to reabsorb different substances from the tubular lumen and they consequently appear in the urine.

See Section 22 for a full account of the Fanconi syndrome and of cystinosis.

Spear, G. S., Slusser, R. J., Schulman, J. D., and Alexander, F.: Polykaryocytosis of the visceral glomerular epithelium in cystinosis with description of an unusual clinical variant. Johns Hopkins Med. J. *129*:83, 1971.

NEPHROGENIC DIABETES INSIPIDUS (VASOPRESSIN-RESISTANT DIABETES INSIPIDUS)

See also section on Water Balance and Urine Concentration.

DEFINITION. This is a congenital hereditary disorder in which the kidneys do not respond to antidiuretic hormone (vasopressin). Consequently the urine volume is high and its concentration is persistently hypotonic. The term "nephrogenic" is used to distinguish this condition from diabetes insipidus which is the result of insufficient antidiuretic hormone production and in which the kidney is able to elaborate a concentrated urine when vasopressin is administered.

HISTORY. In North America most patients with nephrogenic diabetes insipidus are descended from the Ulster Scots, who reached Nova Scotia on the ship Hopewell in 1761. Clusters of affected patients are still found in localized areas of New England and the Canadian Maritime provinces.

ETIOLOGY. Nephrogenic diabetes insipidus is probably inherited by an X-linked recessive mode, with a variable degree of expression in heterozygous females.

PATHOLOGY AND PATHOPHYSIOLOGY. No consistent renal pathologic changes have been demonstrated, and it is likely that the disorder is a consequence of an enzymatic or biochemical abnormality in renal tubular function. The disorder, however, is clearly of renal origin; the neurohypophyseal system by which vasopressin is released in response to increased plasma tonicity is intact. Nor is there evidence that an abnormal type of vasopressin is released or that the hormone is inactivated. Unresponsiveness of the distal tubule and collecting duct to vasopressin is believed to be the primary defect.

Vasopressin normally increases the permeability of the distal tubule and collecting duct to water and thus allows passive diffusion of luminal water into the hypertonic medullary interstitium. This increase in permeability to water is mediated by cyclic adenosine—3′, 5′ monophosphate (3′, 5′-AMP). Production of this cyclic nucleotide from adenosine triphosphate (ATP) is catalyzed by adenyl cyclase in the distal tubular and collecting duct cells under the stimulus of vasopressin. It is currently held that in nephrogenic diabetes insipidus this sequence does not obtain because of failure to bind vasopressin at some receptor site or because of defective adenyl cyclase activity; either possibility results in production of inadequate cyclic 3′, 5′-AMP.

Distal tubule and collecting duct permeability to water is reduced and its passive diffusion along an osmotic gradient into the hypertonic interstitium from the lumen is restricted. Since sodium and chloride transport from the ascending limb of Henle's loop and distal tubule is intact, the urine is hypotonic to plasma regardless of the body's need to conserve water. If the capacity to concentrate the urine is thus impaired, and maximal urine osmolality is 80–150 mOsm/l, it follows that a greater urine volume is required to excrete a given solute load than would be the case if the urine osmolality were high, e.g., 800–1200 mOsm/l. At the lower range of urine concentration, e.g., 100 mOsm/l, the volume of urine in which 1 mOsm is excreted is 10 ml, whereas at a urine concentration of 1000 mOsm/l the volume of urine is only 1 ml/mOsm. Thus the solute load is of great importance in determining the requisite volume of urine in a patient with an impaired ability to concentrate the urine. If the fluid intake which is needed to produce the required volume of urine is not provided, the plasma solute concentration, as reflected by the sodium chloride and urea concentrations, will rise. Furthermore, given an inadequate fluid intake in the face of a high obligatory water loss, owing to impaired urine concentrating ability, the patient's total body water decreases and he becomes dehydrated.

CLINICAL MANIFESTATIONS AND COURSE. Nephrogenic diabetes insipidus is present at birth, although it is common for the diagnosis not to be made until some months later. Frequent urination of a large volume of dilute urine, extreme thirst, repeated episodes of dehydration and failure to thrive are the common initial manifestations. The signs of severe dehydration in infancy are often nonspecific; however, loss of skin turgor, constipation, vomiting, otherwise unexplained fever and even convulsions may occur. Growth retardation results from inadequate food intake because of uncontrolled polydipsia, and from general poor health because of dehydration and hypernatremia. These features may have a harmful effect on mental and motor development; the severity of retardation is directly related to the age at which the diagnosis is made and therapy begun. Children who are old enough to express their needs have an insatiable thirst, and the lengths to which they will go to satisfy this need are often extreme. Because of the large urinary volume, which may reach 6–10 liters/m^2/day, there may be dilatation of the renal collecting system and ureters and of the bladder.

Growth and development and general health, however, can be normal if diagnosis is made early and proper treatment is instituted and maintained.

DIAGNOSIS AND DIFFERENTIAL DIAGNOSIS. The clinical and laboratory features described above lead to the suspicion of nephrogenic diabetes insipidus. A family history of a similar disorder in males provides supportive evidence.

The specific feature is failure of the adequately hydrated subject to increase urine osmolality in response to administration of vasopressin. This failure of response differentiates nephrogenic diabetes insipidus from diabetes resulting from insufficient circulating vasopressin from the posterior pituitary. Nephrogenic diabetes insipidus may be suspected when there is persistently hypotonic urine (specific gravity 1.002 to 1.006; osmolality, 80 to 120) in the face of clinical evidence of dehydration or a raised serum sodium concentration or osmolality. The serum chloride concentration is often elevated during periods of dehydration. Hyperuricemia has been described in adults with nephrogenic diabetes insipidus.

Hyposthenuria and failure of the kidney to respond normally to vasopressin may be seen in a number of other conditions; these, however, usually have characteristic features which should preclude errors in diagnosis. They include hypercalcemia, hypokalemia, distal renal tubular acidosis with nephrocalcinosis, postobstructive nephropathy, sickle cell neuropathy, nephronophthisis, uremia, the diuretic phase of recovery from acute renal tubular injury, and amyloidosis. In patients with psychogenic polydipsia, a poor response to vasopressin may be manifest; this, however, is transient, and a normal response can be elicited after several weeks of a normal fluid intake. Polyuria owing to diabetes mellitus should be excluded.

PREVENTION. No means of prevention is known. However, genetic counseling may be of value; mothers and half of the sisters of affected males are carriers of the gene, and the risk of their male children being affected or of their female children being carriers is 1 in 2. A decreased ability to concentrate the urine has been described in women presumed to be carriers, even though overt clinical manifestations may be mild or absent.

TREATMENT. There is no specific treatment. The cornerstone of therapy is the provision of sufficient intake of water to prevent dehydration and to maintain serum osmolality, as expressed by the serum sodium concentration, within normal limits. The fluid intake required to do this may be in the range of 6–10 l/m^2/day. Proper nutrition and an adequate caloric intake must also be given.

Since, as mentioned earlier, an obligatory urine volume of 8 to 12 ml is required to excrete each mOsm of solute, it follows that fluid requirements can be reduced if the solute load is decreased. This requires a greater than usual proportion of dietary calories in the form of carbohydrate and fat. These are metabolized to carbon dioxide and water and thus do not constitute a solute load. The protein and salt intake should be reduced, as should the amount of foods containing phosphorus.

Hydrochlorothiazide and other diuretics, such as ethacrynic acid, which lead to a negative sodium balance when used in combination with a reduced sodium intake have an important role in therapy. They lead to a reduction in urinary volume and to a modest increase in urinary concentration. The mechanism of action of these saliuretic drugs in this disease is not completely understood. The response results in part from the state of sodium depletion they induce, which in turn leads to reabsorption of a greater than normal proportion of filtered sodium and water in the proximal tubule. This alone reduces urine volume; in addition, less filtrate is delivered to the ascending limb of Henle's loop and the distal tubule where urine dilution occurs. A trial of hydrochlorothiazide in a dose of 0.5-1.5 mg/kg/day in combination with a low sodium intake of under 1 mEq/kg/day is warranted; reduction of urinary volume of 40 or 50 per cent may be achieved. Attention should be paid to the possible development of hypokalemia due to the hydrochlorothiazide; potassium supplements of 2–4 mEq/kg/day may be required. It is of interest that chloropropamide, which may be of value in patients with diabetes insipidus resulting from vasopressin insufficiency, is not useful in nephrogenic diabetes insipidus; its mode of action in diabetes insipidus appears to be one of potentiating the effect of vasopressin in the renal tubule.

PROGNOSIS. With early diagnosis and adequate therapy, the prognosis for life and for normal development is good. The condition is, however, not curable, and the problem of ensuring adequate hydration is lifelong.

Bode, H. H., and Crawford, J. D.: Nephrogenic diabetes insipidus in North America—the Hopewell hypothesis. New Engl. J. Med. *280*:750, 1969.

Orloff, J., and Burg, M. B.: Vasopressin-resistant diabetes insipidus. *In* Stanbury, J. B., Wyngaarden, J. B., and Fredrickson, D. S. (eds.): The Metabolic Basis of Inherited Disease. New York, McGraw-Hill Book Co., 1972, p. 1567.

ten Bensel, R. W., and Peters, E. R.: Progressive hydronephrosis, hydroureter, and dilatation of the bladder in siblings with congenital nephrogenic diabetes insipidus. J. Pediatr. *77*:439, 1970.

Ziegler, E. E., and Fomon, S. J.: Fluid intake, renal solute load, and water balance in infancy. J. Pediatr. *78*:561, 1971.

RENAL GLYCOSURIA (RENAL GLUCOSURIA)

This is a specific hereditary defect in tubular glucose transport in which there is a variable amount of glucose excreted in the urine even though the blood glucose level is normal. Glucosuria resulting from impaired glucose reabsorption may also occur in the Fanconi syndrome. However, the term renal glycosuria is used to denote the tubular abnormality in which only glucose transport is affected. The amount of glucose excreted is variable and in children may range from 1 to 30 gm/day. In general, the degree of glycosuria is independent of the diet, although the amount of glucose excreted may increase if more carbohydrate is ingested. Usually all urine specimens contain glucose. The urinary loss of glucose has little effect on blood glucose concentration, and the glucose tolerance curve is either normal or flat. There is no generalized defect in glucose metabolism.

Renal glycosuria is usually detected in the second decade, although it is probably present from birth. It is benign and symptomless except during starvation or pregnancy, when ketosis and dehydration may develop. There appears to be no association with diabetes mellitus. Renal glycosuria may be diagnosed by the consistent finding of glucosuria in conjunction with a normal concentration of blood glucose, when other features of abnormal glucose metabolism are absent. Disorders in which other sugars or reducing substances appear in the urine should be excluded by appropriate chemical tests; these include pentosuria, fructosuria, galactosuria, sucrosuria and maltosuria.

It is likely that the phenotypic expression of renal glycosuria may result from a number of different mutations. One classification proposes two principal forms: types A and B. In type A renal glycosuria the defect in glucose reabsorption is diffuse and involves all nephrons, and there is a uniformly reduced glucose Tm. In type B a variable glycosuria occurs over a range of blood sugar concentrations, but the overall glucose Tm is normal; there appear to be two distinct groups of nephrons which differ in their capacity to reabsorb glucose.

In some families the condition is inherited as an autosomal dominant, in others an autosomal recessive mode is probable.

Krane, S. M.: Renal glycosuria. *In* Stanbury, J. B., Wyngaarden, J. B., and Fredrickson, D. S. (eds.): The Metabolic Basis of Inherited Disease. New York, McGraw-Hill Book Co., 1972, p. 1536.

CYSTINURIA

This defect of amino acid transport affects cells of the renal tubules and gastrointestinal tract. It is inherited as an autosomal recessive. The transport defect involves a group of amino acids: cystine, lysine, arginine, ornithine and cysteine-homocysteine mixed disulfide. Clinically the problem arises from the cystine, which is the least soluble of the group and precipitates in the urine to form calculi. Both sexes are affected, but problems tend to be more serious in the male, possibly because of the differences in urinary tract anatomy which result in a greater likelihood of urethral obstruction by calculi.

Although the transport defect is present from birth, the peak time of diagnosis is the second or third decade. The usual presentation is that of ureteral colic or obstruction. The latter may lead to urinary infection and reduced renal function. Cystine stones form in acid urine, as do uric acid stones, but unlike the latter they are radiopaque. They tend to form in a staghorn pattern and to be recurrent. The simplest diagnostic test is microscopic examination of the urine for the hexagonal-shaped flat cystine crystals. The urine cyanide-nitroprusside test is positive; a positive test also is obtained in homocystinuria and acetonuria. Amino acid chromatography is of value in detecting cystine and the other amino acids, which are excreted in excessive amounts.

The clinical importance of cystinuria derives from the relative insolubility of cystine in urine, where it precipitates to form calculi. Treatment is based on attempts to increase cystine solubility by keeping the urine dilute and alkaline, and by reducing the amount of cystine excretion. At pH 7.5 approximately 300 mg/l of cystine will be in solution. Increasing the urine volume reduces cystine concentration and therefore the likelihood of precipitation. Many cystinuric subjects excrete amounts of cystine in the range of 1 gm and thus require a urine output of 3 to 4 liters to reduce the likelihood of stone formation. It is important to maintain dilution of the urine during the night as well as during the day; thus, several glasses of water should be taken on retiring. Cystine solubility is highest at a urine pH above 7.5, and alkalinizing agents, such as sodium citrate or bicarbonate, should be given to maintain urine pH at or above this level.

D-Penicillamine leads to production of a mixed disulfide of cysteine-penicillamine which is much more soluble than cystine and thus is responsible for a reduction in cystine excretion as such. In patients with recurrent stone formation not controlled by dilution of urine and alkalinization, D-penicillamine may be effective in diminishing the threat of progressive renal damage. This drug, however, has a number of undesirable side effects including allergic reactions and renal damage; it should thus be used with caution and reserved for patients who fail to respond to conservative therapy.

If recurrent stone formation and urinary tract infection can be avoided, progressive renal damage is unlikely and the prognosis is reasonably good.

Crawhall, J. C., and Watts, R. W. E.: Cystinuria. Am. J. Med. *45*:736, 1968.

Thier, S. O., and Segal, S.: Cystinuria. *In* Stanbury, J. B., Wyngaarden, J. B., and Fredrickson, D. S. (eds.): The Metabolic Basis of Inherited Disease. New York, McGraw-Hill Book Co., 1972, p. 1504.

TUBULAR DISORDERS DUE TO ELECTROLYTE DISTURBANCES

The two principal electrolyte disturbances which lead to abnormal tubular function are hypercalcemia and hypokalemia.

Hypercalcemia leads to impaired sodium transport from the ascending limb of Henle's loop and thus causes a disturbance in the medullary countercurrent multiplication system. The renal medulla is less hypertonic than normal, and this results in an impaired ability to concentrate the urine. Hypercalcemia may also lead to a reduction in permeability to water in the distal tubule and collecting duct. The clinical consequences of these disturbances are polyuria and polydipsia. In addition to these effects on tubular function, hypercalcemia may lead to the development of *nephrocalcinosis,* particularly in the medulla, where interstitial scarring results in destruction of nephrons and reduction in the glomerular filtration rate. It is important to know that significant nephrocalcinosis with impaired renal function can be present in the absence of any detectable radiologic evidence of calcium deposition in the kidneys.

The causes of hypercalcemia are numerous and are discussed elsewhere. To avoid the potentially serious renal consequences of hypercalcemia, therapy should be directed toward reduction of the serum calcium level to normal as soon as possible.

Potassium depletion leading to hypokalemia also leads to impairment of urine concentration. The degree of impairment is a function of the duration and severity of the potassium deficit. As in the case of hypercalcemia, reduced tubular permeability to water and/or interference with the countercurrent multiplier and exchange systems probably account for the reduced ability to concentrate urine.

Structural changes consisting of a vacuolar lesion in the proximal and, sometimes, distal tubules, lamination of the tubular basement membranes, swelling of tubular mitochondria and increased interstitial collagen in both cortex and medulla are undoubtedly important in the pathogenesis of the functional changes observed. If potassium depletion is not corrected, these alterations lead to a progressive nephropathy with the development of renal insufficiency.

Epstein, F. H.: Calcium nephropathy. *In* Strauss, M. B., and Welt, L. G. (eds.): Diseases of the Kidney. Boston, Little, Brown and Company, 1971, p. 903.

Hollander, W., Jr., and Blythe, W. B.: Nephropathy of potassium depletion. *In* Strauss, M. B., and Welt, L. G. (eds.): Diseases of the Kidney. Boston, Little, Brown and Co., 1971, p. 933.

HEREDITARY OR FAMILIAL DISEASES

At least 15 per cent of pediatric renal diseases are genetically determined. The number of such known disorders currently approaches 50. Understanding of the pathogenesis is limited or nonexistent in most of these conditions; attempts to classify them on a pathologic basis have left much to be desired. A proposed grouping of these disorders is given in Table 15–7; it is recognized that the list is likely to be incomplete. A discussion of the principal entities follows.

HEREDITARY NEPHRITIS WITH DEAFNESS AND OCULAR ABNORMALITIES
(Alport Syndrome)

This hereditary disease is characterized by progressive renal failure of variable severity (usually more severe in males), high-frequency sensorineural deafness and ocular abnormalities. The dis-

TABLE 15–7 HEREDITARY CONDITIONS IN WHICH RENAL MANIFESTATIONS ARE USUALLY PRESENT*

1. *Conditions in which any of the following are principal manifestations: reduced glomerular filtration rate, hematuria, proteinuria, hypertension*
   - Hereditary nephritis with deafness (Alport syndrome)
   - Benign familial hematuria
   - Nephronophthisis (medullary cystic disease, familial juvenile nephronophthisis)
   - Childhood type polycystic kidney disease
   - Adult type polycystic kidney disease
   - Congenital nephrotic syndrome (infantile microcystic disease)
   - Familial nephrotic syndrome of the minimal lesion type
   - Familial nephrotic syndrome with nephrocalcinosis and tubular dysfunction
   - Diffuse mesangial sclerosis of infancy
   - Familial renal-retinal dystrophy
2. *Disorders in which a renal tubular defect is of principal importance*
   - Renal tubular acidosis
   - Nephrogenic diabetes insipidus
   - Pseudohypoparathyroidism
   - Renal glycosuria
   - Hypophosphatemic rickets (familial vitamin D-resistant rickets with hypophosphatemia)
   - Familial iminoglycinuria
   - Idiopathic Fanconi syndrome with proximal tubular dysfunction
   - Familial hyperglycinuria
   - Essential pentosuria
   - Hartnup disease
   - Liddle syndrome (pseudohyperaldosteronism)
   - Pseudohypoaldosteronism
   - Cystinuria
3. *Systemic metabolic disorders which may lead to renal damage*
   - Cystinosis
   - Fabry's disease (ceramide trihexosidase deficiency)
   - Oxalosis
   - Lipodystrophy
   - Familial Mediterranean fever with amyloidosis
   - Wilson's disease
   - Glycogen storage disease
   - Gout
   - Diabetes mellitus
   - Tyrosinemia
   - Galactosemia

*The renal manifestations of the conditions listed in this table are very diverse. Included are disorders which are expressed in a variety of unrelated ways such as defects in tubular transport, aminoaciduria, structural developmental abnormalities, and diseases of the glomerular basement membrane. In some the renal problem is secondary or of little clinical consequence; in others it is the chief cause of morbidity and/or mortality.

ease has a wide geographic distribution and has been reported in patients of different ethnic and racial backgrounds. It is the most common of the heritable renal diseases.

PATHOLOGY AND PATHOGENESIS. Both glomerular and interstitial lesions develop in parallel. The glomerular lesions initially are focal areas of glomerular basement membrane thickening, with some increase of mesangial cells and matrix. Adhesions to Bowman's capsule and occasional epithelial cell proliferation may occur. Progressive thickening of the glomerular basement membrane leads to omniglomerular sclerosis and hyalinization. Electron microscopic studies have shown increased thickness of the glomerular basement membrane with distortion of the lamina densa. A fibrillar network enclosing clear electron-lucent areas, which contain round granulations, has been described as a characteristic finding in the glomerular basement membrane.

Abnormalities in the interstitial tissue include periglomerular fibrosis, a general increase in fibrous tissue, tubular atrophy and focal mononuclear cell infiltration. Interstitial foam cells, once considered specific, have been recognized in other renal diseases. They are seen in about one third of patients, mainly at the corticomedullary junction.

As the lesions progress the kidney shrinks in size, and an end-stage chronic glomerulonephritis results.

CLINICAL MANIFESTATIONS AND COURSE. The mean age of onset of renal disease is 6 years but it has been noted as early as 5 months. The usual initial presenting feature is hematuria—usually mi-

TABLE 15–7 HEREDITARY CONDITIONS IN WHICH RENAL MANIFESTATIONS ARE USUALLY PRESENT (*Continued*)

Xanthinuria
Hereditary fructose intolerance

4. *Multisystem disorders or syndromes*
   Laurence-Moon-Biedl syndrome
   Fanconi syndrome of multiple congenital anomalies and aplastic anemia
   Lowe syndrome (oculocerebrorenal syndrome)
   DiGeorge syndrome
   Zellweger syndrome (cerebrohepatorenal syndrome)
   Tuberous sclerosis
   Nail-patella syndrome (hereditary onycho-osteodysplasia)
   Prune-belly syndrome (triad syndrome)
   Oral-facial-digital syndrome
   Meckel syndrome (dysencephalia splanchnocystica syndrome)
   Dandy-Walker malformation of the brain
   Autosomal trisomy syndromes D and E
   Von Hippel-Lindau disease
   Jeune's asphyxiating thoracic dystrophy
   Syndrome of hamartomas, nephroblastomatosis, fetal gigantism, and hypoglycemia
   Thymic alymphoplasia
   Russell-Silver dwarfism
   Beckwith-Wiedemann syndrome
   Ehlers-Danlos syndrome
   Cockayne syndrome
5. *Developmental structural abnormalities and tumors* (hereditary factors are not operative in most renal tumors and developmental structural abnormalities of the urinary tract)
   Nephroblastomatosis
   Hypernephroma
   Renal sarcoma
   Unilateral hydronephrosis
   Congenital megaloureter
   Congenital renal and ear abnormalities
   Familial renal agenesis or hypoplasia (bilateral or unilateral)
   Familial renal dysplasia
   Crossed fused renal ectopia
   Familial renal dysplasia with blindness
   Childhood type polycystic kidney disease
   Adult type polycystic kidney disease
   Leopard syndrome (multiple lentigenes)
6. *Miscellaneous*
   Familial urolithiasis, with or without hypercalciuria
   Familial vitamin D-dependent rickets (impaired renal 1-hydroxylation of 25-hydroxycholecalciferol)
   Sickle cell anemia
   Hyperuricemia, renal insufficiency, ataxia and deafness
   Familial deficiency of C_3 (β_{1c} globulin) with glomerulonephritis

croscopic—with red blood cell casts. Transient episodes of gross hematuria may occur, especially in relation to exercise or respiratory infection. About three fourths of patients have mild proteinuria; the 24-hour excretion seldom exceeds a gram. At onset the glomerular filtration rate is usually normal, but with progressive renal damage, azotemia, hypertension and other features of chronic renal failure supervene. The nephrotic syndrome rarely occurs. In most kindreds the course in affected males is more serious than in affected females; terminal uremia tends to develop in the second decade of life. In some families, however, girls are as seriously affected as boys. In one kindred with deafness and hereditary nephritis extending over five generations, none of the 20 affected patients had progression of the neuropathy to uremia.

A sensorineural, high-frequency deafness is present in about half the patients; it usually has its onset in the first decade and is more pronounced in males; the severity is roughly related to that of the nephropathy. The hearing loss is usually progressive; it may be asymmetrical or even unilateral. In some kindreds deafness is not a feature. There may be severe renal disease without deafness, and deafness may be present without renal involvement. Deafness may not be recognized clinically and, for this reason, an audiographic examination may be necessary.

Ocular abnormalities are present in about 10 per cent of patients; the most frequent are cataracts and myopia; lenticonus, keratoconus, nystagmus and microspherophakia also occur.

An apparent variant of Alport syndrome has been described in which hereditary deafness and progressive nephritis are associated with macrothrombocytopathia or giant size platelets. Thrombocytopenia may also be present. There are increased bruising and bleeding from early childhood; the renal and hearing defects appear subsequently.

GENETIC ASPECTS. Several modes of inheritance have been proposed. The most likely is that of an autosomal dominant gene with variable penetrance. Half the sons and half the daughters of either affected parent receive the mutant gene. There is reduced penetrance, thus less likelihood of developing the disease, in boys who receive the gene from their fathers rather than from their mothers. By contrast, penetrance is complete in sons of affected females; affected mothers have an equal frequency of affected and unaffected offspring of both sexes. Although the frequency of renal involvement is less in boys, it is usually more serious in them than in girls. About one half of affected males develop terminal renal failure before age 30. The risk of developing kidney disease, overt or only with microscopic hematuria, if either parent has overt Alport syndrome is given in Table 15–8.

TABLE 15–8 RISK OF DEVELOPING OVERT SIGNS OF KIDNEY DISEASE OR MICROSCOPIC HEMATURIA AMONG OFFSPRING OF PARENTS WITH SYMPTOMATIC ALPORT SYNDROME (EXPRESSED AS A PER CENT)*

AFFECTED PARENT	SONS	DAUGHTERS
Mother	42	45
Father	13	53

*From Preus, M., and Fraser, F. C.: Clin. Genet. *2*:331, 1971.

LABORATORY DATA. Initially there is usually microscopic hematuria with red cell casts; mild proteinuria is present in about three fourths of the patients, and pyuria is relatively infrequent. Serum complement level is normal. With progression of the renal disease, the serum creatinine and blood urea nitrogen values increase and other characteristic changes of chronic renal failure become evident.

DIAGNOSIS AND DIFFERENTIAL DIAGNOSIS. The association of a progressive hereditary renal disease, deafness, ocular abnormalities and compatible changes on renal biopsy suggest the diagnosis of Alport's syndrome. A pattern of autosomal dominant inheritance, and evidence of more serious disease in male family members and of deafness even in relatives without nephritis provides strong supportive evidence. An audiogram, urinalysis and appropriate blood studies should be done on each available family member. Other forms of hereditary or familial renal disease which present with microscopic hematuria should be considered in the differential diagnoses. Of these, benign familial hematuria is important to exclude, since its prognosis is excellent; deafness and progressive renal failure do not occur in this condition.

PREVENTION. Genetic counseling and appropriate contraceptive measures in affected adults will reduce the number of affected children.

TREATMENT. There is no specific therapy for the nephritis. Standard therapeutic measures for renal insufficiency and its complications as outlined in the section on chronic renal failure should be used when specific problems arise. Dialysis or renal transplantation should be carried out when advanced renal failure supervenes.

PROGNOSIS. The prognosis with respect to rate of progression of the renal disease tends to follow a similar pattern in a given kindred. In general, half the affected males will develop terminal renal failure before age 30, often within the first two decades. The remainder progress more slowly, but most eventually reach a state of seriously compromised renal function. Females fare better in general, and in many kindreds have a nearly normal life expectancy despite persistent microscopic hematuria. In some families girls are as seriously affected as boys. The prognosis for those with otherwise terminal uremia has been considerably improved by dialysis and renal transplantation.

GENERAL

Bergsma, D. (ed.): Conference on genetic and cellular bases of congenital renal dysfunction. Birth Defects: Original Article Series *6* (No. 3):1, 1970.

Clarke, J. T. R., Knaack, J., Crawhall, J. C., and Wolfe, L. S.:

Ceramide trihexosidosis (Fabry's disease) without skin lesions. New Engl. J. Med. *284*:233, 1971.
Fraser, D., Kooh, S. W., Kind, H. P., Holick, M. F., Tanaka, Y., and DeLuca, H. F.: Pathogenesis of hereditary vitamin-D-dependent rickets. New Engl. J. Med. *289*:817, 1973.
Frimpter, G. W.: Aminoacidurias due to inherited disorders of metabolism. Parts I and II. New Engl. J. Med. *289*:835; 895, 1973.
Greene, M. L., Marcus, R., Aurbach, G. D., Kazam, E. S., and Seegmiller, J. E.: Hypouricemia due to isolated renal tubular defect. Am. J. Med. *53*:361, 1972.
Senior, B.: Familial renal-retinal dystrophy. Am. J. Dis. Child. *125*:442, 1973.

Alport Syndrome

Ferguson, A. C., and Rance, C. P.: Hereditary nephropathy with nerve deafness (Alport's syndrome). Am. J. Dis. Child. *124*:84, 1972.
Grünfeld, J.-P., Bois, E. P., and Hinglais, N.: Progressive and nonprogressive hereditary chronic nephritis. Kidney Int. *4*:216, 1973.
Hinglais, N., Grünfeld, J.-P., and Bois, E.: Characteristic ultrastructural lesion of the glomerular basement membrane in progressive hereditary nephritis (Alport's syndrome). Lab. Invest. *27*:473, 1972.
Preus, M., and Fraser, F. C.: Genetics of hereditary nephropathy with deafness (Alport's disease). Clin. Genet. *2*:331, 1971.

BENIGN FAMILIAL HEMATURIA

This is a benign hereditary or familial condition usually inherited on an autosomal dominant basis. It is characterized by persistent microscopic hematuria of glomerular origin; episodic macroscopic hematuria is often precipitated by an intercurrent acute respiratory illness. Males and females are affected equally. Proteinuria is absent, except at times during episodes of gross hematuria. There are no other characteristic abnormalities and there is no progression to renal insufficiency. Findings on histopathologic examination are normal, although red blood cells may be seen in Bowman's space. In one kindred, localized areas of thinning of the glomerular capillary basement membrane have been demonstrated by electron microscopy.

It is important to establish the correct diagnosis in this condition in order to exclude other potentially more ominous diseases. In particular, hereditary nephritis with deafness (Alport's syndrome) must be ruled out. (See previous discussion.) Recurrent macroscopic hematuria with focal glomerulonephritis should also be considered; this condition is not familial and can be identified by renal biopsy.

The other causes of hematuria listed in Table 15–2 should also be considered and can be differentiated by their own clinical, laboratory or histopathologic features. The diagnosis of benign familial hematuria is established by exclusion of other similar renal disorders and can only be considered benign after a prolonged observation. An overly aggressive series of investigations, however, is not warranted. The demonstration of casts in the urinary sediment will establish the renal origin of the hematuria. Measurement of the 24-hour urinary excretion of protein, blood urea nitrogen and serum creatinine concentrations and an intravenous pyelogram should be obtained. Urinalyses on family members as well as a careful family history regarding serious renal disease, deafness or ocular abnormalities will help to establish the diagnosis. No treatment is needed and the prognosis is good.

Marks, M. I., and Drummond, K. N.: Benign familial hematuria. Pediatrics *44*:590, 1969.
Rogers, P. W., Kurtzman, N. A., Bunn, S. M., Jr., and White, M. G.: Familial benign essential hematuria. Arch. Intern. Med. *131*:257, 1973.

NEPHRONOPHTHISIS

(Medullary Cystic Disease, Familial Juvenile Nephronophthisis)

Nephronophthisis is a progressive hereditary renal disease characterized pathologically by tubular atrophy, interstitial fibrosis, glomerular sclerosis and medullary cysts and, clinically, by anemia, impaired urinary concentrating ability and renal loss of sodium.

HISTORY. Lack of knowledge of pathogenetic mechanisms in hereditary renal diseases, particularly those in which cysts are present, has made meaningful classification difficult. Some of the cystic disorders are discussed elsewhere in this chapter or are listed in Table 15–9. Some

TABLE 15–9 CONDITIONS IN WHICH RENAL CYSTS MAY BE PRESENT

Hereditary
- Childhood type polycystic kidneys
- Adult type polycystic kidneys
- Nephronophthisis
- Infantile microcystic disease
- Genetic disorders in which renal cysts may occur:*
  - Tuberous sclerosis†
  - Laurence-Moon-Biedl syndrome‡
  - Oral-facial-digital syndrome
  - Meckel syndrome (dysencephalia splanchnocystica syndrome)
  - Dandy-Walker malformation of the brain
  - Zellweger syndrome (cerebrohepatorenal syndrome)
  - Autosomal trisomy syndromes C, D and E
  - Von Hippel-Lindau disease
  - Jeune's asphyxiating thoracic dystrophy

Nonhereditary
- Cystic kidneys with lower urinary tract obstruction
- Multilocular renal cysts
- Medullary sponge kidney§
- Renal dysplasia with cysts (multicystic kidney, multicystic dysplasia)||
- Simple renal cyst¶

*Renal cysts in these conditions are sometimes of no clinical importance.

†Angiomyolipomatous malformation is more common than cysts.

‡Glomerular sclerosis and interstitial fibrosis are prominent features.

§Rare in childhood; calculi in cysts are common; rare familial cases reported.

||Often unilateral; lower urinary tract abnormalities present in 50 per cent of cases.

¶Uncommon in childhood; not bilateral; usually an incidental finding at autopsy.

advance has been made in the understanding of the nephropathy associated with medullary cysts since the description by Smith and Graham in 1945. The term "medullary cystic disease" has been used for the condition in North America, whereas in Europe the designation has been familial juvenile nephronophthisis. It had been assumed that these were separate disorders. While some disagreement persists, it is now generally agreed that the terms describe a single entity which will be referred to here as nephronophthisis. It is likely that the general condition described does include more than one specific entity, each having common clinical and pathologic expressions.

ETIOLOGY. The cause is unknown. Hereditary factors are of importance in many instances.

EPIDEMIOLOGY. Although not a common disease, it has been diagnosed with increasing frequency. There is wide geographic distribution and patients from many ethnic backgrounds have been reported. Both sexes are equally affected.

PATHOLOGY AND PATHOPHYSIOLOGY. Both glomeruli and interstitial tissue are involved. There is progressive interstitial scarring, tubular atrophy with thickening of the tubular basement membranes and periglomerular fibrosis. Medullary cysts are not an essential feature but are present in about two thirds of patients who die in terminal uremia; they vary from microscopic size to 3 or 4 cm in diameter, involve the distal tubule and collecting duct, and are lined with flattened epithelium. The cysts may not be present initially but may develop as the disease progresses. Foci of chronic inflammatory cells may be present in the interstitium. Most glomeruli show progressive sclerosis and hyalinization.

The structural changes in the medullary interstitium probably account for the reduced ability to concentrate urine. Impaired retention of sodium probably results from the osmotic load imposed on surviving nephrons and from the cortical and interstitial fibrosis, which interferes with normal tubular function.

CLINICAL MANIFESTATIONS AND COURSE. There is a spectrum of clinical findings which probably reflects differences in the stage and severity of the illness, the likelihood that more than one specific disease entity is included under this designation and the possibility that differences exist between kindreds in the expression of a single genetic disorder.

Typically the clinical onset is between 5 and 20 years of age. The initial features are polyuria, thirst, and profound anemia. The urine is dilute, the sediment is normal, and proteinuria is usually absent. Hypertension and edema are not present until late in the course. Initially azotemia is mild, with levels of blood urea nitrogen of 20–40 mg/dl. An inability of the kidneys to conserve sodium is often present and, in order to stay in balance, some children require a large dietary intake of salt. Urinary excretion of calcium may also be high and may result in hypocalcemia with episodes of clinical tetany. Severe renal osteodystrophy is not uncommon. Progression to renal insufficiency over a period of 5 to 10 years is the usual course. In some families associated abnormalities may be present; ocular lesions such as retinitis pigmentosa, cataracts, macular degeneration, myopia and nystagmus are the most common.

GENETIC FEATURES. In most families, an autosomal recessive mode of inheritance is likely and a history of consanguinity is not uncommon. In several kindreds an autosomal dominant mode has been documented. Single sporadic cases also occur and probably represent either mutation or the clinical expression of a recessive gene in a homozygous individual.

LABORATORY DATA. There are no specific laboratory changes. Normochromic anemia is out of proportion to the degree of uremia. Unless uremia is advanced, urinary excretion of sodium and calcium is elevated; the serum calcium level is usually low in relation to the degree of phosphate elevation. Marked secondary hyperparathyroidism with attendant osseous changes is not uncommon. Urinalysis is unremarkable except for the low specific gravity. Impaired ability to acidify the urine following an ammonium chloride load has been documented in some patients. Glycosuria and aminoaciduria are usually absent. Routine intravenous urography usually shows poorly functioning, slightly small kidneys; the medullary cysts are seldom seen.

DIAGNOSIS. In the recessively transmitted form, a positive family history is usually not obtained except for the possibility that the parents may be related. The constellation of polyuria, thirst, renal salt wasting, hyposthenuria, normal urinary sediment and absence of edema and hypertension, with or without ocular abnormalities, suggests the diagnosis.

Other causes of polyuria and hyposthenuria should be considered. These include the nephropathies resulting from hypercalcemia or hypokalemia, obstructive uropathy and chronic pyelonephritis. Renal biopsy may not provide a specific diagnosis, since medullary cysts are not always present, or may be missed on a random biopsy. The other characteristic morphologic changes may, however, provide strong support for the diagnosis.

PREVENTION. No means of prevention is known, although genetic counseling, especially for those with the autosomal dominant form, may reduce the likelihood of their having affected offspring.

TREATMENT. There is no specific treatment. Care should be taken to provide an adequate fluid and salt intake, particularly during periods of intercurrent illness when the child may not be well enough to take appropriate amounts himself. As the disease progresses, the amount of renal salt loss decreases and hypertension may develop. The anemia may require occasional transfusions with freshly washed, packed red blood cells. Aggressive treatment of renal osteodystrophy and adequate supplementation of calcium are required. Apart from these measures, standard methods of treating uremia should be used. Dialysis and renal transplantation have a definite role in terminally affected patients.

PROGNOSIS. In most patients a relentless downhill course to terminal uremia takes place over a period of 3 to 10 years; in some kindreds a more slowly progressive course is followed.

Boichis, H., Passwell, J., David, R., and Miller, H.: Congenital hepatic fibrosis and nephronophthisis. Quart. J. Med. *42*:221, 1973.

Herdman, R. C., Good, R. A., and Vernier, R. L.: Medullary cystic disease in two siblings. Am. J. Med. *43*:335, 1967.

Makker, S. P., Grupe, W. E., Perrin, E., and Heymann, W.: Identical progression of juvenile hereditary nephronophthisis in monozygotic twins. J. Pediatr. *82*:773, 1973.

Mongeau, J. G., and Worthen, H. G.: Nephronophthisis and medullary cystic disease. Am. J. Med. *43*:345, 1967.

THE NAIL-PATELLA SYNDROME

(Hereditary Onycho-osteodysplasia)

This disorder is characterized by: (1) multiple osseous abnormalities, including absence or hypoplasia of the patellae, hypoplasia of the proximal radial heads, iliac horns and talipes equinovarus deformities of the feet; (2) flexion contractures of a variety of joints, especially the elbows; (3) hypoplasia, absence, ridging or flatness of the nails, especially those of the thumb and index fingers; (4) ocular abnormalities such as ptosis of the upper eyelids, abnormal pigmentation of the iris, glaucoma, microcornea and strabismus; and (5) renal disease.

The condition is transmitted as an autosomal dominant trait strongly linked to the ABO blood group locus.

The most common initial manifestation of renal involvement is proteinuria; it is present in about half the patients; a mild urinary concentrating defect and/or microscopic hematuria may also be present initially. In the majority of patients with these manifestations of renal involvement there is no associated morbidity; however, in about a fifth of them there is slow progression to renal failure within 5 to as long a period as 25 years, during which the only manifestation may be asymptomatic proteinuria. The nephrotic syndrome is an infrequent complication.

The histopathologic changes consist of focal glomerular basement membrane thickening and increase in mesangial matrix. The tubules of the sclerosed glomeruli become atrophic. Immunopathologic findings are variable; focal deposition of IgM and β_{1_C} globulin along glomerular basement membranes and within arteriolar walls has been described. Electron microscopic findings are probably pathognomonic for the syndrome. There are lucent areas within irregularly thickened glomerular basement membranes; within the lucent areas are fibrils with the characteristic periodicity of collagen.

No specific treatment for the renal disorder is known.

Bennett, W. M., Musgrave, J. E., Campbell, R. A., Elliot, D., Cox, P., Brooks, R. E., Lovrien, E. W., Beals, R. K., and Porter, G. A.: The nephropathy of the nail-patella syndrome. Am. J. Med. *54*:304, 1973.

Hoyer, J. R., Michael, A. F., and Vernier, R. L.: Renal disease in nail-patella syndrome: Clinical and morphologic studies. Kidney Int. *2*:231, 1972.

Morita, T., Laughlin, L. O., Kawano, K., Kimmelstiel, P., Suzuki, Y., and Churg, J.: Nail-patella syndrome. Arch. Intern. Med. *131*:271, 1973.

LIPODYSTROPHY

See also Section 23.

This condition is characterized by atrophy of subcutaneous fat with variable association of other findings such as increased height, enlarged genitalia, skin pigmentation, hirsutism, hepatomegaly, central nervous system disturbances, an abnormal glucose tolerance curve or insulin-resistant diabetes mellitus, hyperlipidemia and, in about 25 per cent of affected persons, progressive renal disease. On the basis of the distribution of the atrophy of subcutaneous fat, both partial and total forms of lipodystrophy are described. In the total form there is a higher incidence of the associated abnormalities, but renal disease occurs with equal frequency in both forms. An absolute distinction between the total and partial forms of lipodystrophy appears unwarranted, since there is considerable overlap in many of the features. Although most cases are sporadic, there are instances of familial involvement, e.g., in one family two siblings—one male, one female—and a first cousin were affected. The mode of inheritance is probably on an autosomal recessive basis.

The renal pathology consists of an active progressive glomerulonephritis with mesangial hypercellularity and increased matrix, thickening of glomerular basement membranes and glomerular lobulation; these lead to eventual chronic sclerosing glomerulonephritis. Electron microscopic studies show mesangial proliferation and thickening of the glomerular basement membrane. Electron-dense deposits within the glomerular basement membrane and mesangium are also seen. Recently immunopathologic studies in several patients have revealed the presence of IgG and β_{1_C} globulin in a nodular or bumpy configuration, suggesting that glomerular immune complex deposits are present; decreased levels of serum complement components have also been reported.

Evidence of renal involvement is usually present within several years of onset of lipodsytrophy. Proteinuria with or without microscopic hematuria is present, the nephrotic syndrome may develop, and progressive decrease in renal function leading to terminal uremia within a period of several years occurs in at least half of those with evidence of renal involvement. Hypertension is a prominent feature.

There is no specific treatment for lipodystrophy nor for its renal manifestations. Successful renal transplantation has been reported in a patient with terminal uremia.

Eisinger, A. J., Shortland, J. R., and Moorhead, P. J.: Renal disease in partial lipodystrophy. Quart. J. Med. *51* (No. 163):343, 1972.

Peters, D. K., Charlesworth, J. A., Sissons, J. G. P., Williams, D. G., Boulton-Jones, J. M., Evans, D. J., Kourilsky, O., and Morel-Maroger, L.: Mesangiocapillary nephritis, partial lipodystrophy, and hypocomplementaemia. Lancet *2*:535, 1973.

FAMILIAL NEPHROTIC SYNDROME

Although it is uncommon, there are occasional families in which more than one member has minimal lesion nephrotic syndrome; it has not been established whether hereditary or environmental influences are operative. In any case, the typical features of the disorder, including responsiveness to corticosteroid therapy, are present.

The nephrotic syndrome may also develop during the course of several clearly hereditary disorders. These include infantile microcystic disease of the kidney (congenital nephrotic syndrome), Alport's disease (hereditary nephritis with deafness) and the nail-patella syndrome. These are discussed elsewhere in this Section.

FAMILIAL NEPHROTIC SYNDROME WITH NEPHROCALCINOSIS AND TUBULAR DYSFUNCTION

Several families have been described in which children present between 3 and 6 years of age with the nephrotic syndrome which is resistant to corticosteroid therapy. Aminoaciduria, glycosuria, renal tubular acidosis, nephrocalcinosis, growth retardation, tetany and renal osteodystrophy are associated findings. Death from renal failure at about 8 years of age has been the usual course.

Burke, E. C., Holley, K. E., and Stickler, G. B.: Familial nephrotic syndrome with nephrocalcinosis and tubular dysfunction. J. Pediatr. *82*:202, 1973.

SICKLE CELL ANEMIA AND THE KIDNEY

The principal renal manifestations are gross or microscopic hematuria and impaired ability to concentrate urine; less common are the nephrotic syndrome, papillary necrosis and progressive renal insufficiency.

A spectrum of pathologic changes, many of which are probably nonspecific, has been described. Characteristically the glomeruli are enlarged and there is dilatation of capillary loops. Glomerular sclerosis develops later, and tubular atrophy and dilatation are seen. Papillary necrosis and interstitial fibrosis have been observed.

Impaired ability to concentrate urine normally is an early and common functional change. This finding is not the result of the anemia per se; the defect is present in patients with the sickle cell trait who are not anemic. To some extent, and temporarily, it is reversible by transfusion with normal red blood cells. This defect worsens with time and becomes no longer reversible by transfusion, suggesting that permanent structural changes supervene. The basis for the concentrating defect is not known; one likely factor is the increased tendency of sickling to occur in a hypertonic medium. Since the medulla is hypertonic relative to plasma, red cells in the vasa recta may have a tendency to sickle. This could reduce medullary blood flow and impair the normal functioning of the countercurrent multiplier system. Episodes of painless gross hematuria or periods of microscopic hematuria occur at some time in about 20 per cent of patients with SS, SA or SC hemoglobinopathy. The explanation of the hematuria is not known but is probably related to congestion and dilatation of papillary vessels, submucosal hemorrhage and, uncommonly, to frank papillary necrosis.

Although both renal failure and the nephrotic syndrome have been reported in conjunction with sickle cell anemia, they are rare in children; it is not certain that there is a causal relation to sickle cell anemia.

OXALOSIS

(Primary Hyperoxaluria)

See also Section 8.

Oxalosis is a rare hereditary disorder in glyoxalate metabolism transmitted by an autosomal recessive mode in which there is hyperoxaluria, calcium oxalate nephrolithiasis, widespread extrarenal deposition of calcium oxalate crystals and progressive renal failure leading to death, usually before adulthood. Two different types have been characterized. (See Section 8.)

Secondary hyperoxaluria may occur in patients with ileal dysfunction. A genetic predisposition to the formation of calcium oxalate renal calculi has also been demonstrated in patients without any evidence of abnormal glyoxalate metabolism; hyperoxaluria is not present in these patients.

In most patients with oxalosis, symptoms from renal calculi occur in the first decade. Progressive renal failure resulting from calcium oxalate deposition and recurrent episodes of nephrolithiasis follow, and death from uremia usually occurs before or during the third decade.

The diagnosis of oxalosis should be considered in patients presenting with recurrent and progressive nephrolithiasis beginning in the first decade. Calcium oxalate calculi are radiopaque. The most consistent and diagnostic laboratory finding is an increased urinary excretion of oxalate in the absence of excess oxalate ingestion or pyridoxine deficiency. Normal children excrete less than 40 mg of oxalate per 24 hours; in primary hyperoxaluria the amount excreted usually exceeds 200 mg/24 hr. As renal failure progresses the amount of oxalate excreted decreases.

There is no specific treatment. Attempts should be made to reduce the formation of oxalate calculi by a copious intake of water in order to dilute the urine.

In view of the extensive extrarenal deposition of calcium oxalate crystals and the likelihood of recurrent calculi in a transplanted kidney, renal transplantation does not appear to be indicated.

Boquist, L., Lindqvist, B., Östberg, Y., and Steen, L.: Primary oxalosis. Am. J. Med. *54*:673, 1973.

Hagler, L., and Herman, R. H.: Oxalate metabolism. I.–V. Am. J. Clin. Nutr. *26*:758; 882; 1006; 1073; 1242, 1973.

HEREDITARY DISORDERS WITH RENAL CYSTS

Cortical and/or medullary renal cysts are relatively common in genetically determined renal disorders. Renal cysts may also occur in developmental abnormalities which are not genetically determined, and there is evidence that cysts can sometimes develop even in previously normal nephrons. The problem of cystic renal disorders is thus a confusing one. There follows a discussion of some of the heritable conditions in which renal cysts are a prominent feature. A more complete list of these disorders, both hereditary and nonhereditary, is given in Table 15–9. Disorders of a nonhereditary nature in which renal cysts occur are described in the section on developmental abnormalities.

CHILDHOOD TYPE POLYCYSTIC KIDNEYS

(Infantile Polycystic Kidney Disease, Infantile Sponge Kidney, Congenital Hepatic Fibrosis with Renal Cysts)

This autosomal recessive disorder affects the kidneys and liver. Its clinical and pathologic features are largely age-related; renal abnormalities are predominant in early infancy, and problems related to the liver assume greater importance in later childhood. In a given pedigree the pattern of disease, i.e., predominantly renal, hepatic or intermediate, and the age of presentation are relatively constant among affected members. It has been suggested that differences in pattern between various age groups reflect different genetic entities; however, since the lesions at different ages are qualitatively identical, although quantitatively different, it seems more reasonable to consider this as a single disease with a spectrum of age-related manifestations.

PATHOLOGY AND PATHOGENESIS. In the newborn infant the kidneys are grossly enlarged and contain innumerable radially arranged fusiform cysts; the kidney has a diffusely spongy appearance on gross examination. The renal pelves, ureters, bladder and urethra are normal. On microscopic examination the cysts are lined by hyperplastic, cuboidal or low columnar epithelium. Glomeruli and remaining interstitial tissue are normal. By microdissection the cysts are seen to represent dilated distal tubules and collecting ducts; there is continuity between the lumina of tubules and cysts. About 90 per cent of tubules are involved in affected infants. In older children the kidneys are less enlarged, the cortex is not extensively involved, and there are more intervening areas of normal parenchyma. In patients presenting at adolescence or later, only 10 to 20 per cent of nephrons may be affected, and the principal finding is dilatation of medullary collecting ducts. At this age the renal lesion is usually an incidental finding of no clinical importance; radiologic examination shows good renal function with tubular ectasia. In the liver there is proliferation, infolding and dilatation of portal bile ducts and ductules with a variable degree of fine periportal and subcapsular fibrosis; all portal triads are involved, and the changes are distributed uniformly throughout the liver. Hepatic lesions are not severe in young infants; however, progressive extensive periportal fibrosis is seen in affected older children and often leads to portal hypertension with esophageal varices and splenomegaly in the second decade.

Pancreatic cysts of no clinical importance are occasionally present. The pathogenesis of the renal and hepatic lesions is unknown. The clinical presentation bears a close relationship to the predominant underlying pathologic change.

CLINICAL MANIFESTATIONS AND COURSE. In affected neonates there is often a history of oligohydramnios and dystocia. The so-called Potter facies may be present. The abdomen is distended and the enlarged kidneys are readily palpable. There may be anuria or oliguria, respiratory distress and gross or microscopic hematuria. Radiologic study shows enlarged flank masses on the plain abdominal film and markedly decreased function by intravenous urography. Contrast medium may be concentrated in collecting ducts and tubules; calyces may be blunted or distorted. In most instances, however, insufficient contrast medium is concentrated in the collecting system to permit its adequate visualization, even though some appears in the bladder. Death from progressive renal failure usually occurs within a period of weeks to months. Older infants and children have proportionately less renal and more hepatic problems, so that in affected adolescents the presenting problem is likely to be the result of portal hypertension, and renal medullary tubular ectasia with or without blunted calyces is found as an incidental abnormality by intravenous urography. The clinical picture of patients presenting between infancy and maturity is determined principally by the degree of renal involvement; this is manifested clinically by enlargement of the kidneys, a variable degree of chronic or progressive renal insufficiency, hypertension and intermittent hematuria.

DIAGNOSIS. The differential diagnosis in the young infant includes other causes of kidney enlargement, abdominal mass and renal failure. These are Wilms' tumor, neuroblastoma, bilateral hydronephrosis, multicystic renal dysplasia and bilateral renal vein thrombosis. Medullary sponge kidney, a benign condition rarely seen in childhood, may require differentiation in an older child whose urogram shows medullary cysts with calyceal distortion. Other hereditary conditions in which renal cysts may occur should be considered as well; most are readily diagnosed on the basis of their own particular features. The diagnosis in older children may be more difficult to establish; the association of hepatosplenomegaly and portal hypertension should suggest the possibility of childhood polycystic kidney disease and an intravenous urogram should be obtained. In some instances liver biopsy may be helpful. A positive family history, particularly if there is a similarly affected sibling, is strong evidence for the disease.

LABORATORY DATA. A variable hematuria with minimal proteinuria may occur, and azotemia and other nonspecific features of chronic renal failure may supervene. Radiologic and liver biopsy findings as discussed earlier may help in establishing the diagnosis.

PREVENTION. The risks of having an affected sibling are one in four.

TREATMENT. There is no specific treatment. Early death from renal failure or respiratory difficulties is the rule in affected infants. In older children with decreased renal function, standard measures for treatment of chronic renal failure may be used, and, if available, dialysis and renal transplantation should be considered. Surgical measures may be necessary to relieve portal hypertension if recurrent esophageal bleeding is a problem.

PROGNOSIS. When clinical manifestations are apparent in early infancy, a short, rapidly fatal course is to be expected. In older children the kidneys are less severely affected and renal failure develops more slowly or not at all. Esophageal varices and other problems of portal hypertension are important in the prognosis; if these can be treated successfully, the outlook is reasonably good.

ADULT TYPE POLYCYSTIC KIDNEYS

This is a hereditable, autosomal dominant disorder with a high degree of penetrance, in which the clinical manifestations seldom have their onset before the third decade. Unlike the childhood form, the cysts are larger and irregular in size and cause marked distortion of the renal outline and calyces. Other segments of the nephron than the collecting ducts may be involved, although, as in the childhood type, this is the principal segment affected. The cysts are lined with flattened epithelium and increase in size with age, leading to progressive renal enlargement. Focal cystic formation in the liver, of no clinical consequence, is present in about one third of patients; aneurysms of cerebral arteries are seen in about 15 per cent of patients. Coarctation of the aorta and cardiac abnormalities such as endocardial sclerosis are rarely associated anomalies. In childhood the condition is usually asymptomatic; however, episodic hematuria, hypertension, renal enlargement and even progressive renal failure have been observed in affected children. The differential diagnosis includes multiple simple cysts, which are irregularly distributed and are separated by zones of uninvolved parenchyma.

There is no specific treatment, and the course is one of progressive renal failure with hypertension; major clinical problems usually do not occur before the fourth or fifth decades.

Bernstein, J., and Kissane, J. M.: Hereditary disorders of the kidney. *In* Rosenberg, H. S., and Bolande, R. P. (eds.): Perspectives in Pediatric Pathology. Chicago, Year Book Medical Publishers, 1973, Vol. I, p. 117.

Blyth, H., and Ockenden, B. G.: Polycystic disease of the kidneys and liver presenting in childhood. J. Med. Genet. *8*:257, 1971.

Lieberman, E., Salinas-Madrigal, L., Gwinn, J. L., Brennan, L. P., Fine, R. N., and Landing, B. H.: Infantile polycystic disease of the kidneys and liver. Medicine *50*:277, 1971.

Murray-Lyon, I. M., Ockenden, B. G., and Williams, R.: Congenital hepatic fibrosis—is it a single clinical entity? Gastroenterology *64*:653, 1973.

ACUTE RENAL FAILURE

Acute renal failure (ARF) is a complex syndrome which results from an acute reduction in or cessation of renal function. It is characterized by anuria or oliguria (less than 180 ml of urine/m^2/24 hr), electrolyte and acid-base disturbances (notably hyperkalemia and metabolic acidosis) and impaired excretion of substances such as creatinine, urea and phosphate.

ETIOLOGY. A large number of unrelated clinical conditions which damage or interfere with the function of one or more of the structural or functional units of the kidney may cause ARF. Table 15–10 lists the clinical conditions and causes of ARF and their commonly associated renal pathologic changes. Chronic renal failure complicated by intercurrent problems such as dehydration, volume contraction, obstruction to urine flow or infection may present as ARF.

PATHOPHYSIOLOGY

Oliguria. Acute renal failure may be classified as prerenal, intrinsic renal or postrenal in origin. Prerenal refers to the reduction in urine volume and retention of waste products which occur during reduction in effective plasma volume or congestive heart failure; it is not the result of actual renal damage. In this situation the urine concentration of sodium is low; it is usually less than 20 mEq/l, and the urea concentration and osmolality are high. The urine volume increases following correction of the underlying disorder. Severe or

TABLE 15–10 CAUSES AND PRINCIPAL RENAL PATHOLOGIC LESIONS OF ACUTE RENAL FAILURE IN CHILDREN

CAUSES OR CLINICAL CONDITIONS	PATHOLOGY
Renal ischemia owing to hemorrhage, hypotension, nephrotoxins, dehydration, anoxia, sepsis, shock	Tubulorrhexis;* renal cortical or papillary necrosis
Renal bacterial infection; sulfonamides; methicillin; aminoglycosides; colistin	Interstitial nephritis
Stomal closure; obstruction by calculi, blood clots, sulfonamide crystals, uric acid crystals	Obstructive nephropathy with or without crystal deposition
Dehydration; sepsis; infant of diabetic mother; cyanotic congenital heart disease	Renal vein thrombosis
Hemolytic-uremic syndrome	Renal microangiopathy; cortical necrosis
Poisoning with diethylene glycol, mercury, carbon tetrachloride	Nephrotoxic necrosis†
Acute poststreptococcal glomerulonephritis; shunt nephritis; subacute bacterial endocarditis; anaphylactoid purpura nephritis; proliferative glomerulonephritis with crescents; acute membranoproliferative glomerulonephritis	Glomerulonephritis

*Tubulorrhexis: disruption of the tubular basement membrane with damage of epithelial cells; affects different segments of random nephrons.

†Nephrotoxic necrosis: epithelial cell damage and desquamation affecting principally the proximal tubule; basement membrane of tubule remains intact

Ischemia results in tubulorrhexis; nephrotoxins may cause tubulorrhexis and/or nephrotoxic necrosis.

prolonged contraction of intravascular volume may cause structural renal damage with resultant intrinsic renal failure.

Acute intrinsic renal failure results from kidney damage of one sort or another. If the principal site of injury is the renal tubule the urine concentration of sodium is often elevated to 50–100 mEq/l; if glomerular injury predominates and tubular function is intact, urine concentration of sodium less than 40 mEq/l may be expected. The urine volume is usually low or nil, although a nonoliguric form of ARF may develop following burns, trauma or methoxyflurane anesthesia. The cause of oliguria in acute intrinsic renal failure has been the subject of much discussion. With severe glomerular damage, reduction of the filtration rate may be assumed. In conditions in which tubular or interstitial changes are prominent, mechanisms such as obstruction of tubular lumina by epithelial debris or casts, interstitial edema, back diffusion of filtrate through damaged tubular epithelium and/or redistribution of renal blood flow with a shift of flow to medullary from cortical regions have been proposed as explanations. In classic acute intrinsic renal failure resulting from tubular damage the course may be divided into three stages: anuric or oliguric, diuretic, and convalescent; the management of these stages differs. In children this classic sequence often does not occur.

Postrenal ARF results from obstruction of urine flow at some point in the pelvicalyceal collecting system or in the ureters.

Hyperkalemia. Hyperkalemia develops because of decreased renal excretion of potassium in conjunction with cellular release of potassium as a result of trauma, hemolysis, infection or hypoxia. Metabolic acidosis, which is often present in ARF, also leads to an increased plasma K^+ concentration because of an intracellular shift of H^+ in exchange for K^+. The cardiotoxic effects of hyperkalemia result from a decreased ratio of intracellular to extracellular K^+.

Sodium and Water. Fluid and sodium overload during reduced excretion of urine may lead to interstitial and pulmonary edema, pleural effusion, hypertension and circulatory congestion. Hyponatremia in ARF is the result of dilution of body fluids as a consequence of excessive intake of water relative to that of sodium.

Acid-Base Balance. Moderate to severe metabolic acidosis with or without increased plasma H^+ concentration (acidemia) is a common finding in ARF and is the consequence of impaired ability of the kidney to eliminate acid in the face of increased production of acid radicals owing to the catabolic state.

Hypertension. Depending on the underlying cause of ARF, the blood pressure may be normal or reduced. Acute hypertension may constitute a major threat since it may result in hypertensive encephalopathy or aggravate circulatory congestion. Hypertension is common in glomerular diseases such as acute poststreptococcal glomerulonephritis and may be seen in other conditions such as the hemolytic uremic syndrome, burns and acute obstructive nephropathy, any of which may lead to ARF. The pathogenesis of the hypertension is poorly understood.

Miscellaneous. Blood urea nitrogen, plasma creatinine and uric acid concentrations are elevated because of reduced excretion. The rate of rise of blood urea concentration varies with the extent of tissue injury and the severity of the catabolic state. Anemia, thrombocytopenia, leukocytosis, impaired carbohydrate tolerance and hyperlipidemia may also occur in ARF.

CLINICAL MANIFESTATIONS. The clinical pattern of ARF is often overshadowed by the manifestations of the precipitating cause. For example, the patient may be in shock as a result of endotoxemia; severely dehydrated with gastroenteritis; jaundiced with carbon tetrachloride poisoning; or having seizures with the hypertensive encephalopathy of acute glomerulonephritis. In the initial assessment one or more of the following may be a precipitating or associated feature: shock, trauma, hemolysis, sepsis, dehydration, intoxication, hemorrhage, hypertension, cardiac arrhythmia due to hyperkalemia, circulatory congestion, metabolic acidosis, congestive heart failure, pelvicalyceal or ureteral obstruction, and/or underlying or preexisting chronic renal disease.

The clinical features related more specifically to ARF include decreased urinary output, edema, drowsiness, the cardiac arrhythmia of hyperkalemia, circulatory congestion and tachypnea as a result of metabolic acidosis. If the underlying disorder, e.g., shock, can be treated successfully, the degree of recovery of renal function is often surprisingly good, even though there may have been severe oliguria for several days to several weeks. In ARF of acute poststreptococcal glomerulonephritis, complete recovery is the rule, providing the electrolyte and acid-base disturbances, circulatory congestion and hypertensive complications are managed satisfactorily.

LABORATORY DATA. The usual findings include hyperkalemia, hyponatremia, metabolic acidosis, elevation of serum concentrations of urea, phosphate, uric acid and creatinine, hypocalcemia and anemia. The urine may contain red blood cells, protein, broad casts and tubular cells. The urinary concentration of sodium is usually low in prerenal ARF and ARF owing to glomerular disease, and elevated in tubular disorders. Electrocardiographic findings indicative of hyperkalemia may be present. Radiologic studies may reveal cardiomegaly, pulmonary congestion, radiopaque calculi, shrunken kidneys or a single enlarged kidney.

DIAGNOSIS AND DIFFERENTIAL DIAGNOSIS. The diagnosis of ARF is based simply on a state of anuria or of oliguria with a urine volume of <180 ml/m^2/24 hr.

It is important to decide if ARF is prerenal, intrinsic renal or postrenal in origin. The presence of congestive heart failure, shock, elevated central venous pressure, dehydration, low urine sodium concentration (less than 20 mEq/l) and high urine osmolality suggests a prerenal cause. The features of intrinsic renal disease have been detailed in prior portions of this Section. Postrenal or obstructive causes include renal calculi, sulfonamide therapy resulting in obstruction by crystal formation and trauma leading to passage of blood clots. Historical, physical and/or laboratory data may provide the necessary information to establish the nature of the precipitating event leading to ARF.

TREATMENT. The first steps are establishment of the underlying cause and securement of baseline laboratory data. The following sequence of investigations is recommended for initial evaluation: general clinical assessment including accurate blood pressure and weight; urinalysis, including electrolytes, pH, osmolality or specific gravity; serum potassium; electrocardiogram; abdominal and chest x-rays; blood studies for Na^+, Cl^-, H^+, pCO_2, HCO_3^-, calcium, phosphorus, urea nitrogen, creatinine and uric acid; hemoglobin, platelet count, white blood cell count and examination of blood smear for fragmented erythrocytes; blood culture; initial bladder catheterization to exclude urethral obstruction and for possible retrograde radiologic studies to establish integrity of the lower urinary tract; and, if circulatory congestion is not present, a test dose of mannitol (0.2 gm/kg intravenously) can be given over 20 to 30 minutes.

If the patient is well hydrated or if circulatory congestion is present, a diuretic such as furosemide (1 mg/kg intravenously) should be used. These steps may help to distinguish potentially reversible intrinsic renal damage, in which mannitol and/or furosemide may induce a temporary diuresis, from intrinsic, potentially irreversible, ARF, in which increase in urinary output rarely occurs. Addition evaluative information should be obtained by continuous collection of urine to determine volume, protein excretion and electrolyte loss. Less urgent blood studies which may be helpful are determination of antistreptolysin O titer, β_{1_C} globulin level and total serum protein concentration. An intravenous pyelogram may be indicated if anuria persists after the patient is out of shock or when circulatory congestion is no longer present, or an isotope renal scan may provide important information without the risks associated with intravenous pyelography. Renal biopsy may be indicated in order to establish the nature and severity of the renal damage. Evidence that a coagulation disturbance is not present should be obtained before this is done.

The indications for each of the above studies must be considered carefully for each patient, since all are not required in every case and in some they may pose an undue risk or expense.

Hyperkalemia and Hyponatremia. See treatment of acute poststreptococcal glomerulonephritis.

Shock and Dehydration. Urgent correction of hypovolemia is indicated irrespective of whether the volume depletion is the result of blood or plasma loss or of dehydration. Twenty ml/kg (about 450 ml/m^2) of plasma or Ringers' lactate solution can be infused rapidly as initial deficit replacement over 15 to 45 minutes; the patient must be carefully monitored. The patient is then reassessed. If the ARF is the result of prerenal failure, an increase in urine output may be anticipated. Maintenance fluids and replacement of remaining electrolyte deficits and of ongoing losses are required. In the absence of an increase in urine output after volume depletion is corrected, a test dose of 20 per cent mannitol, 0.2 gm/kg, intravenously over a 10- to 20-minute period, with or without furosemide, 1 mg/kg intravenously, can be given. Mannitol should not be given to a patient in cardiac failure, nor furosemide if he is hypovolemic. Mannitol and/or furosemide may induce diuresis in reversible intrinsic renal failure.

Metabolic Acidosis. General measures include correction of the catabolic state by treatment of shock, infection and hypoxia and by provision of an adequate caloric intake. At least 300 calories/m^2/day given as carbohydrate or fat are required to minimize endogenous catabolism. During the oliguric or anuric phase 10 to 30 per cent glucose may be given intravenously. With improving renal function, high quality proteins may gradually be introduced. There is evidence that provision of essential amino acids and glucose intravenously may speed recovery and help to maintain an anabolic state.

The specific means for correction of metabolic acidosis is administration of $NaHCO_3$. (See Parenteral Fluid Therapy in Section 5.) Since most preparations of $NaHCO_3$ for intravenous use are very hypertonic (890 mEq Na/l), dilution to 250 to 400 mEq/l is advisable to avoid rapid changes in plasma osmolality.

Fluid and Electrolyte Requirements. A detailed balance sheet of intake and output of all fluids and electrolytes should be kept. This should include losses by vomiting or gastric suction as well as urinary losses, and oral as well as intravenous intake. Such a record is essential to estimate the child's electrolyte and fluid requirements. Maintenance fluids should include replacement of insensible water loss (300–400 ml/m^2/day); this can be given intravenously as 10 to 30 per cent dextrose. Such a concentration of glucose will irritate small veins, and it may be necessary to use a "cut-down" or a larger vein. The fluid can be given orally, if the patient tolerates it. Oral feeding of carbohydrate (as hard candy) and fat can be used to increase the caloric intake. The usual vitamin requirements should be met. Unless the patient is voiding or has a definite sodium deficit, it is unnecessary to give sodium or other electrolytes. Unnecessary administration of sodium increases edema and aggravates circulatory congestion and hypertension.

It is not necessary to use an indwelling urethral catheter to collect urine; rather it should be avoided, because of the risk of infection.

Hypertension. (See treatment of acute poststreptococcal glomerulonephritis).

Dialysis. The indications for peritoneal dialysis or hemodialysis in patients with ARF are: (1) severe metabolic acidosis or acidemia which cannot be safely corrected with $NaHCO_3$; (2) failure of the previously discussed measures to reduce serum potassium concentrations to a safe range; and (3) circulatory congestion, pulmonary edema and marked fluid overload which are threatening survival.

Infection. Bacterial infection accounts for about one third of deaths in ARF. It therefore should be anticipated, diagnosed promptly and treated. Prophylactic antibiotics are not indicated. Unexplained persistent hyperkalemia may be caused by infection. Blood and other potential sites of infection should be cultured. A roentgenogram of the chest may reveal an unsuspected pneumonia. Dosages of antibiotics should be adjusted in the presence of renal failure if their primary route of excretion is via the kidney. This is particularly important in the case of potentially toxic drugs such as the aminoglycoside antibiotics.

Diuretic or Recovery Phase. During recovery from ARF the patient may undergo a period of diuresis. In severe glomerular disease which is improving, although the urine volume may be high, the tubules are usually able to respond to physiologic homeostatic mechanisms, and excessive losses of fluid and electrolytes do not usually occur. In this situation the diuresis represents excretion of excess fluid and electrolytes accumulated during the oliguric phase.

When ARF is the consequence of tubular damage, a marked diuresis may occur as tubular function begins to return. In this instance regenerating tubular epithelium may be unable to respond to the normal stimuli which regulate sodium, potassium and water excretion, and serious depletion as a result of urinary loss may occur. During this time, which may last from a few days to several weeks, adequate replacement of measured fluids and electrolytes should be ensured. At some stage during the diuretic phase an attempt can be made to determine whether normal tubular function is returning by reducing the intake to determine if the tubules respond.

PROGNOSIS. The immediate prognosis in ARF depends largely on the nature and severity of the precipitating event and on the promptness and degree of satisfactory management of the numerous and complex associated problems. The ultimate prognosis insofar as renal function is concerned depends on the type and severity of the renal damage. Although apparent complete clinical recovery occurs in many patients with acute tubular necrosis, about half the patients have residual renal dysfunction, such as impaired urine concentrating ability and/or reduced glomerular infiltration. In some instances these may be of little or no clinical consequence.

Abel, R. M., Beck, C. H., Jr., Abbott, W. M., Ryan, J. A., Jr., Barnett, G. O., and Fischer, J. E.: Improved survival from acute renal failure after treatment with intravenous essential L-amino acids and glucose. New Engl. J. Med. *288*:695, 1973.

Feldman, W., Baliah, T., and Drummond, K. N.: Intermittent peritoneal dialysis in the management of chronic renal failure in children. Am. J. Dis. Child. *116*:30, 1968.

Flamenbaum, W.: Pathophysiology of acute renal failure. Arch. Intern. Med. *131*:911, 1973.

Flores, J., DiBona, D. R., Beck, C. H., et al.: The role of cell swelling in ischemic renal damage and the protective effect of hypertonic solute. J. Clin. Invest. *51*:118, 1972.

Groshong, T. D., Taylor, A. A., Nolph, K. D., et al.: Renal function following cortical necrosis in childhood. J. Pediatr. *79*:267, 1971.

Hall, J. W., Johnson, W. J., Maher, F. T., et al.: Immediate and long-term prognosis in acute renal failure. Ann. Intern. Med. *73*:515, 1970.

Hollenberg, N. K., Adams, D. F., Oken, D. E., Abrams, H. L., and Merrill, J. P.: Acute renal failure due to nephrotoxins. New Engl. J. Med. *282*:1329, 1970.

Kleinknecht, D., Jungers, P., Chanard, J., et al.: Factors influencing immediate prognosis in acute renal failure with special ref-

erence to prophylactic hemodialysis. *In* Hamburger, J., Crosnier, J., and Maxwell, M. H. (eds.) Advances in Nephrology. Vol. 1. Chicago, Year Book Medical Publishers, 1971, p. 207.
Montgomerie, J. Z., Kalmanson, G. M., and Guze, L. B.: Renal failure and infection. Medicine *47*:1, 1968.
Morris, C. R., Alexander, E. A., Bruns, F. J., and Levinsky, N. G.: Restoration and maintenance of glomerular filtration by mannitol during hypoperfusion of the kidney. J. Clin. Invest. *51*:1555, 1972.
Vertel, R. M., and Knochel, J. P.: Nonoliguric acute renal failure. J.A.M.A. *200*:598, 1967.

CHRONIC RENAL FAILURE

Chronic renal failure (CRF) may be defined as a complex of clinical and laboratory disturbances due to a permanent reduction in renal function, of which the essential feature is a decreased glomerular filtration rate. Clinical problems are usually not evident until the GFR is below 20 ml/min/m^2; in preadolescent children with a GFR at this level the blood urea nitrogen is usually above 40 mg/100 ml and the serum creatinine over 1.6 mg/dl. The normal GFR in children over 1 year of age is 70 ± 5 (1 SD) ml/min/m^2. As CRF progresses, the clinical condition deteriorates; this advanced phase is referred to as uremia.

ETIOLOGY. The causes of CRF in children in order of their incidence are: congenital renal and urinary tract malformations, glomerular and hereditary renal diseases. Renal vascular disorders such as the hemolytic-uremic syndrome, arterial or venous thrombosis and papillary or cortical necrosis account for a small percentage of children with CRF.

Congenital anomalies of the kidney and urinary tract tend to produce signs of CRF before age 5 years, whereas glomerular and hereditary renal diseases usually lead to the development of CRF between ages 5 and 15. According to Habib et al., the principal congenital renal and urinary tract abnormalities leading to CRF are renal hypoplasia, with or without dysplasia, and bilateral marked vesicoureteral reflux, with or without lower tract obstruction. The incidence of urinary tract abnormalities is about three times as common in males as in females. The glomerular disorders that most frequently lead to CRF are membranoproliferative glomerulonephritis, focal and segmental glomerulosclerosis and glomerulopathy in such systemic diseases as anaphylactoid purpura and lupus erythematosus. The most common hereditary renal disorders which lead to CRF in children are nephronophthisis, Alport disease, polycystic renal disease, the renal lesion of the Laurence-Moon-Biedl syndrome, cystinosis, oxalosis and the congenital nephrotic syndrome.

PATHOLOGY. The renal pathologic changes in CRF depend on the type of underlying renal disease; these are discussed separately elsewhere in this Section.

PATHOPHYSIOLOGY

Adaptation to Reduction in Number of Nephrons. The observations that (1) clinical evidence of CRF commonly does not develop until reduction of GFR to about 25 per cent of normal, and (2) survival is possible for a prolonged time when GFR is reduced to 2 to 5 per cent of normal, suggest that surviving nephrons are adaptable to the needs of the patient. The most satisfactory explanation of these functional changes is the one proposed by Bricker; this is usually referred to as the intact nephron hypothesis (see reference). As destruction proceeds, each surviving nephron responds in an orderly, predictable manner to the increasing excretory requirements which must be met if homeostasis is to be maintained. Practically speaking, this means that for solutes which are filtered and partially reabsorbed it is necessary for there to be a progressive decrease in the fraction of the filtered load which is reabsorbed as the number of surviving nephrons falls. For example, when the GFR is normal, only 0.5 per cent or less of the filtered sodium is excreted; in contrast, the surviving nephrons of a patient with a GFR of 5 ml/m^2/min excrete 30 to 40 per cent of the filtered sodium.

The precise mechanisms by which modification in tubular function is mediated are poorly understood. In the case of phosphate the mediator of the increased fractional excretion rate is parathyroid hormone. With each decrement in GFR there is a minimal increment in plasma phosphate concentration, which results in a reciprocal decrease in plasma concentration of ionized calcium which, in turn, results in a rise in secretion of parathyroid hormone (PTH). This leads to a reduced rate of tubular phosphate reabsorption and an increment in calcium reabsorption. Consequently the plasma calcium and phosphate concentrations return toward normal levels.

These adaptive changes which surviving nephrons undergo permit a remarkably good balance between intake and excretion of water, solutes and electrolytes. With severe reduction in the number of functioning nephrons, the balance becomes precarious and a sudden increase in intake may not be accompanied by an equivalent increment in excretion. Fluid, solute and electrolytes may then accumulate. The ability to concentrate the urine to an osmolality much above that of the plasma and to conserve sodium is gradually lost as the degree of renal failure progresses. Because of this and the obligatory water and electrolyte losses imposed by the solute diuresis on each surviving nephron, a sudden restriction in intake of fluid or electrolytes may not be followed by a suitable reduction in excretion rate, with the result that deficits leading to volume contraction may occur. Prolonged administration of diuretics in CRF may also lead to salt depletion and volume contraction.

Potassium Disturbances. Excretion of potassium in CRF is remarkably efficient, and an appropriate balance between intake and output is usually maintained. However, acute K^+ loads are poorly tolerated and may result in hyperkalemia. Hyperkalemia may also be induced by an acute catabolic event, such as a bacterial infection or hemolysis; acute metabolic acidosis may accentuate hyperkalemia. Hypokalemia may be a reflection of an inadequate intake of potassium or an excessive loss induced by continuous diuretic therapy.

Acid-Base Balance. A sustained metabolic acidosis is usual in CRF when the GFR is decreased to 15 ml/min/m^2 or less. The acidosis is a reflection of several features. These include: (1) impaired reabsorption of bicarbonate, (2) reduction in urinary excretion of ammonium, and (3) impaired excretion of endogenous or dietary acid metabolites because of reduction in GFR. In order for acid excretion and HCO_3^- regeneration to occur, it is necessary for the acid salt to be filtered so that reclamation of $NaHCO_3$ by physiologic tubular mechanisms can take place.

An appropriately acid urine with a pH less than 5.5 is usual in CRF. Since net urinary acid excretion is less than normal and since a progressively more acidotic state does not usually develop, some other buffering mechanism must maintain the plasma pH at a level compatible with life. Bone salts, notably calcium carbonate, appear to play a vital role as buffers in this regard. The plasma HCO_3^- usually stabilizes at 18-20 mEq/l.

Disturbances of Bone, Calcium and Phosphorus. Profound changes in calcium and phosphorus homeostasis occur in CRF. As noted, the systemic acidosis leads to leaching of bone salts to be used as buffers. Reduction in GFR leads to elevation of plasma phosphate, and this to a reciprocal decrease in the ionized calcium concentration, which in turn is responsible for an increased secretion of parathyroid hormone. (See above.) The hyperparathyroidism also results in excessive reabsorption of bone. Calcium absorption from the gut is decreased, principally as the result of relative vitamin D resistance, and contributes to the development of secondary hyperparathyroidism.

This complex disturbance in calcium, phosphorus and bone metabolism is expressed principally as growth arrest or retardation, hypocalcemia, hyperphosphatemia and hyperparathyroid bone disease. The bony changes are usually referred to as renal or uremic osteodystrophy.

Hematologic Abnormalities. A moderate to severe normochromic anemia is common; the etiology is multifactorial and includes depression of erythropoiesis by uremic toxins and decreased erythropoietin production, shortened red blood cell survival, blood loss and defective utilization of iron.

Abnormalities in the coagulation system may include decreased platelet adhesiveness, prolongation of the bleeding time and reduced activation of platelet factor 3.

Delayed Growth and Sexual Maturation. These distressing complications and their etiology are poorly understood. Renal osteodystrophy is an important cause of growth failure; even when it is absent or controlled, growth is usually retarded. Inadequate caloric intake, poor nutrition and sustained acidosis are believed to be important factors in retardation of growth and sexual maturation.

Neurologic Complications. With advanced renal failure neurologic manifestations may appear. These include confusion and impaired ability to concentrate. Neuromuscular irritability, cramps, seizures and vomiting may also occur. The pathogenesis of these alterations is poorly understood but is believed to be related to accumulation of uremic toxins such as guanidinosuccinic acid, phenolic compounds, methyl guanidine and other metabolites such as urea and uric acid. Disturbances in water and electrolyte balance and altered calcium ion concentration may also play a role. Sudden reduction in the concentration of some of these compounds following hemodialysis may precipitate confusion and seizures in uremic patients. Severe hypertension may be a factor in uremic encephalopathy.

Peripheral neuropathy with impairment of sensory and motor functions may develop in long-standing cases; demyelination of the distal parts of some of the peripheral nerves has been described.

Miscellaneous Metabolic Abnormalities. In addition to the abnormal accumulation of such metabolites as urea, creatinine and uric acid, a number of potentially toxic metabolites such as guanidinosuccinic acid, methyl guanidine and certain phenolic compounds are also retained. They may play a role in such diverse disturbances as altered postheparin lipoprotein lipase activity, reduced platelet adhesiveness, decreased nerve conduction and uremic encephalopathy.

The kidney normally has an important role in degradation of the hormone gastrin; in uremic or anephric patients, plasma levels of gastrin may be elevated and may be causative factors in gastric hypersecretion and peptic ulceration, which occur in some patients.

The principal disturbance in carbohydrate metabolism is an elevation in peak blood glucose level following an oral glucose load, with a delayed return to fasting levels.

CLINICAL MANIFESTATIONS AND COURSE. The discussion here will be confined to the features of CRF; the manifestations of the underlying disease, however, may be identifiable and, when present, must be taken into account in the management of the patient.

The onset is usually gradual, and the initial complaints are often vague or nonspecific. They include lassitude, fatigue, headache, anorexia and nausea. More specific symptoms are polyuria and polydipsia, mild facial puffiness, bone or joint pain, growth retardation, dryness or itchiness of the skin, muscle cramps, localized paresthesia and specific sensory or motor loss indicative of a neuropathy.

As CRF advances, anorexia, nausea, fatigue and lassitude become more pronounced. There may be vomiting, diarrhea (sometimes bloody), confusion, easy bruising, edema and a declining volume of urine. Hypertension, acidosis, fluid retention and anemia may cause symptoms of cardiac failure and circulatory congestion such as tachypnea, shortness of breath and tenderness of the liver and abdomen. Headache is common, and seizures may occur.

Physical findings vary, depending on the severity or stage of CRF. The following may be present: pallor and a sallow, brownish complexion, growth retardation, muscle weakness and wasting, edema, dry or bruised skin with scratch marks from pruritus, systolic and diastolic hypertension, signs of circulatory overload such as pulmonary edema, tachycardia, tachypnea, jugulovenous distention, cardiomegaly, gallop rhythm and ejection systolic murmur, bony deformity with or without tenderness resulting from renal osteodystrophy, characteristic uremic malodorous breath, coated tongue, signs of specific neuropathy such as loss of deep tendon reflexes, of sensation, or of muscle strength, uremic retinopathy with exudates, vascular narrowing and possibly hemorrhages.

The course depends principally on the nature of the underlying disease, which may lead to progressive, inexorable nephron destruction over a relatively short period of several months to a year, or may cause a stable reduction in renal function which does not progress and which may be compatible with an indefinite period of relatively good health. The age at which CRF develops also influences the course, particularly with respect to growth and to the ease with which it is possible to manage the patient's medical problems. When it develops in infancy, impairment of growth will be much more profound than when it occurs in a previously healthy teen-ager; the medical management is also more difficult in younger children.

LABORATORY DATA. The essential features are a reduction in glomerular filtration rate as shown by decreased inulin, iothalamate or creatinine clearance and elevation of the blood urea nitrogen and creatinine concentrations. The extent of reduction in GFR is the major determinant of the severity and of the extent to which other abnormal laboratory findings will be present. These include hyperphosphatemia, hypocalcemia, hyperuricemia, metabolic acidosis, hyperkalemia, hypoproteinemia, normochromic anemia, reduced platelet adhesiveness, prolonged bleeding time and isosthenuria or vasopressin-resistant hyposthenuria. Depending on the cause of CRF, there may be renal salt wasting, proteinuria or an abnormal urinary sediment.

Radiologically there may be such manifestations of circulatory congestion as hypertension, heart failure including cardiomegaly, aortic dilatation, left ventricular hypertrophy, pulmonary edema and pleural effusion. Renal osteodystrophy is most pronounced at such areas of rapid growth as the upper humerus, knees, wrists and lateral aspect of the clavicle. The changes include demineralization, coarsened trabeculation, patchy erosion, thinning or loss of cortex owing to secondary hyperparathyroidism, rachitic changes, retarded bone age, foci of osteosclerosis and, in advanced cases, actual bone deformity, particularly at sites of weight-bearing such as the hips and knees. Changes in the phalanges of the index and middle fingers, best demonstrated by a nonscreen radiograph, are early and sensitive findings.

DIAGNOSIS AND DIFFERENTIAL DIAGNOSIS. It is essential, if possible, to establish the nature of the underlying disease leading to the CRF, since it may be a principal determinant of treatment and of the ultimate prognosis. Conditions which may aggravate a pre-existing state of chronic renal insufficiency include: (1) congestive heart failure; (2) uncontrolled hypertension; (3) hypovolemia resulting from gastrointestinal or urinary losses related to diuretic therapy or impaired ability to conserve fluid and electrolytes in the face of inadequate intake; (4) infection of the urinary tract; (5) obstruction by calculi, stomal closure or uric acid nephropathy; (6) disturbances in concentrations of plasma electrolytes, e.g., hypercalcemia or hypokalemia, which lead to impaired renal function; and (7) nephrotoxicity caused by drugs or other exogenous agents (discussed elsewhere in this Section).

PREVENTION. Prevention of CRF is one of the most challenging problems in pediatric nephrology. Remarkable advances in hemodialysis and renal transplantation have drawn attention away from a fact of fundamental importance: with proper therapy a high proportion of children with CRF need never reach the stage of advanced renal insufficiency which requires these dramatic procedures to prolong life. In this context some of the problems discussed under Diagnosis and Differential Diagnosis, must be considered; these include such diverse features as proper antibacterial agents for treatment of urinary tract infection, avoidance of or cessation of use of nephrotoxic drugs, and use of anti-inflammatory or cytotoxic drugs in specific glomerular diseases; prevention and treatment of nephrocalcinosis or urolithiasis in renal tubular acidosis, hyperuricemia and cystinuria; diagnosis and treatment of obstructive uropathy and control of hypertension.

The principal problems leading to CRF for which at present there are not satisfactory means of prevention include major congenital structural anomalies which seriously compromise renal function at an early age and many hereditary or familial nephropathies whose pathogenesis is poorly understood and for which effective therapy is unavailable. Even in these situations, however, diligent attention to intercurrent or complicating factors which accelerate nephron destruction can preserve sufficient renal function for a relatively long time, during which the child may lead a reasonably normal life.

TREATMENT. Management of CRF demands not only an understanding of the complex pathophysiologic disturbances and the necessary skills in diagnosis and treatment, but, as importantly, an awareness of and a sensitivity in dealing with the tremendous impact that chronic, progressive renal disease has on the life of the patient and his family. Resources other than those which the physician can provide may be needed to deal effectively with these problems. A team approach which uses the talents of the nurse, social worker, dietitian, teacher, and psychiatrist is often effective.

As mentioned, it is important to establish the nature of the disorder which led to CRF and to exclude any intercurrent or potentially reversible problem. The goal is to preserve every functioning nephron for as long a time as possible. Specific treatment for individual conditions which may lead to CRF are discussed elsewhere in this Section. The following discussion of treatment is applicable to most patients with CRF regardless of the underlying disorder.

Diet and Nutrition. Provision of the caloric and nutritional requirements of the child with CRF is a major problem. It is less difficult with mild to moderate renal insufficiency (GFR>15 ml/min/m²), but when there is severe impairment of renal function the child's appetite is poor, nausea and other gastrointestinal complaints are common and constraints on the dietary intake of fluid, phosphorus, electrolytes and nitrogen are imposed by the kidney's impaired excretory ability. Phosphorus is the principal substance which must be restricted; its retention is one of the crucial factors in the pathogenesis of renal osteodystrophy. Decreasing the dietary intake of phosphorus requires restriction of milk and other sources of protein, and they are important for good nutrition. An oral aluminum hydroxide gel* can be used to bind phosphorus in the gut and, when given with the meal, may allow a more liberal phosphorus intake. It is, however, not very palatable, especially to an anorectic patient, and also causes constipation. It can be incorporated into a cookie with a not unpleasant taste, and this may be used not only to reduce absorption of phosphorus but to provide calories in an acceptable form. The recipe for these cookies is given below; each cookie contains the equivalent of 2 Amphojel tablets.†

Amphojel Cookies

1 cup salt free butter
1½ cups white sugar
1½ cups cake flour
3/4 cups cornstarch
1 egg
3 tsp. vanilla or 3 tsp. almond extract or 2 tsp. cinnamon
100 tablets Amphojel powdered (grind in small blender)

Drop batter well apart on an ungreased cookie sheet and press flat with a floured fork. Bake at 350° F until done.

Yield: 50 cookies
1 cookie = 2 tablets

When the GFR falls to 15 ml/min/m² or less, the serum phosphorus level usually begins to rise. Restriction of dietary phosphorus to 200-500 mg/day as well as the administration of oral aluminum hydroxide gel in a dose of 1 or 2 tablets (or the equivalent in liquid form) with each meal may be necessary to keep the plasma phosphorus level below 6 mg/dl. When the blood urea nitrogen level is above 70-80 mg/dl, the child's appetite for nitrogen-containing foods often declines. With the combination of restriction of protein and phosphorus intake and the child's anorexia it is almost inevitable that malnutrition will result; the degree of wasting may be masked by edema. Consequently the diet often is a compromise between what the child will eat and what is optimal in light of the constraints imposed by the altered pathophysiology of CRF. An attempt should be made to supply an adequate caloric intake for growth and to give high quality protein such as that in eggs or calves' liver.

Restriction of milk to decrease phosphorus intake results in reduction of calcium intake. A calcium supplement of approximately 1 gram of calcium/day should be given, either as a calcium salt in a syrup* or as an effervescent tablet† dissolved in water.

Vitamin D supplementation is necessary. The usual requirement is between 2000 and 25,000 units of vitamin D_2 (calciferol) per day. This should be introduced gradually to avoid hypercalcemia. Dihydrotachysterol in a dose of 0.05-0.1 mg/day may be used instead of vitamin D. A normal intake of other vitamins and minerals should be assured.

Sodium, Potassium and Water. In the absence of salt wasting, edema or an abnormal plasma concentration of sodium it is usually not necessary to modify the intake of sodium or water. Measurement of the 24-hour urinary excretion of sodium, chloride and potassium during a time when the dietary electrolyte intake is not restricted may provide useful information about the kidney's ability to excrete electrolytes. It is essential to know the dietary intake of each of these electrolytes during the time of urine collection. In general the thirst mechanism regulates intake of water satisfactorily, and the child's usual intake of salt should be permitted. Vigorous restriction of sodium, particularly during continuous diuretic therapy, can cause extracellular volume contraction and a further decline in GFR. In nephronophthisis excessive urinary excretion of salt is relatively common, so that the intake must be compensatorily high, sometimes in the range of 15-20 gm/day.

When edema is present it is necessary to restrict the intake of sodium, even to as low as 10-15 mEq/day. A low plasma concentration of albumin may contribute to salt and water retention. Congestive cardiac failure due to longstanding hypertension, fluid overload and anemia can ac-

*Aluminum hydroxide-dimethylpolysiloxane compound tablets (Amphojel 65)—Wyeth International, P.O. Box 8616, Philadelphia, Pa. 19101.

†Aluminum hydroxide tablets (Amphojel Preparations)—Wyeth International, P.O. Box 8616, Philadelphia, Pa. 19101.

*Calcium-Sandoz Syrup—Sandoz Pharmaceutical, Division of Sandoz-Wander, Inc., Hanover, N.J. 07936.

†Calcium-Sandoz Forte 500 mg—Sandoz Pharmaceutical, Division of Sandoz-Wander, Inc., Hanover, N.J. 07936.

centuate fluid retention and requires specific therapy such as digitalis, transfusion with washed, packed red blood cells and diuretic therapy.

Attention should be paid to the plasma sodium level, since in advanced uremia the ability to dilute urine may be impaired, and hyponatremia may develop from excessive intake of water. Refractory edema with or without hyponatremia can develop despite restriction of sodium and fluid intake. In such circumstances the use of furosemide or ethacrynic acid either orally or intravenously in a dose of 1-5 mg/kg/day may be helpful. *Each of these drugs is potentially ototoxic and can cause deafness.* Peritoneal dialysis or hemodialysis is effective in removing edema fluid, if other measures fail; they are particularly helpful during circulatory congestion and congestive cardiac failure.

The capacity to excrete potassium remains remarkably adequate even when renal function is severely reduced. Unless the urinary volume is decreased to the extent that fluid is retained, or unless the plasma potassium is above 7.0 mEq/l with accompanying electrocardiographic changes of hyperkalemia, it is generally not necessary to reduce the intake of potassium. Chronic hyperkalemia can usually be tolerated in CRF. A sudden elevation in the concentration of plasma K^+, however, may result in life-threatening hyperkalemia.

Long-term diuretic or antihypertensive therapy with furosemide or hydrochlorothiazide can cause K depletion and chronic hypokalemia; K^+ supplementation may be required. Hypokalemia may also contribute to digitalis toxicity; nausea and vomiting in such a situation may be mistaken for symptoms of CRF.

Metabolic Acidosis. Sodium bicarbonate or citrate in a dose to supply the equivalent of 0.5-2.0 mEq/kg/day of bicarbonate and given in three or four divided doses may be used to treat the metabolic acidosis of CRF. It is not desirable to attempt complete correction of the plasma base deficit; a plasma bicarbonate level of 18-20 mEq/l should be accepted as adequate when the GFR is 15 ml/min/m^2 or less. If sodium bicarbonate or citrate increases edema, calcium carbonate may be used. Severe metabolic acidosis may require dialysis. The possibility of digitalis toxicity resulting from reduction of plasma K^+ levels during dialysis must be recognized. Rapid correction of acidosis may precipitate tetany in a hypocalcemic patient.

Hypertension, Cardiac Failure and Circulatory Congestion. An attempt should be made to maintain the *blood pressure* within the normal range; at times, however, an elevation of 10 to 15 mm Hg in diastolic pressure may have to be accepted. Conservative measures using standard antihypertensive agents with or without sodium restriction, depending on whether there is edema, are usually successful. Hydrochlorothiazide 50-75 mg/m^2/day in combination with either methyldopa 500-750 mg/m^2/day or hydralazine 75-200 mg/m^2/day should be used as initial therapy. Guanethidine 5-25 mg/m^2/day is sometimes effective. Each of these medications should be given in three divided doses. Strict restriction of sodium to a level of 5-10 mEq/day may be necessary in severely oliguric hypertensive patients.

In patients who have hyperreninemia, propranolol 30-120 mg/m^2/day in combination with hydralazine 75-200 mg/m^2/day and a diuretic such as hydrochlorothiazide 50-75 mg/m^2/day may be useful.

The emergency treatment of hypertensive crises with encephalopathy, pulmonary edema or cardiac failure consists in the administration of (1) diazoxide, hydralazine or methyldopa intravenously as outlined in the section on Acute Poststreptococcal Glomerulonephritis, and (2) parenteral administration of furosemide or ethacrynic acid in a dose of 30-90 mg/m^2.

Cardiac failure requires the skillful balancing of several types of therapy. These include: (1) reduction of blood pressure to normal, (2) increasing the hemoglobin concentration to 8 to 9 gm slowly by small transfusions of washed packed red blood cells, (3) decreasing circulatory congestion by restriction of salt and fluids and the use of diuretics such as furosemide, and (4) judicious use of digoxin. Since digoxin is largely excreted by the kidney the dose must be reduced in CRF. The digitalizing dose should be cut to about one half the usual amount; the maintenance dose is reduced to about one quarter and should be given at extended intervals, such as every second or third day. Digitalis is not dialysable, and care must be taken to avoid digitalis toxicity. When cardiac failure becomes life threatening and is not amenable to conservative measures, consideration must be given to instituting peritoneal dialysis or hemodialysis.

Circulatory congestion is best treated by rigid restriction of sodium and fluids and by oral or parenteral administration of furosemide or ethacrynic acid. Since the problems of hypertension, cardiac decompensation and circulatory congestion are interrelated in their pathogenesis, so too are the therapeutic measures used in their treatment. Improvement in one of these circulatory problems by a single treatment measure is often accompanied by parallel improvement in the others.

Renal Osteodystrophy. The principal measures for prevention and treatment are (1) restriction of dietary phosphorus, (2) administration of aluminum hydroxide gel to bind phosphorus in the intestine, (3) provision of supplemental calcium, (4) provision of vitamin D or dihydrotachysterol, (5) control of metabolic acidosis, and (6) provision of a nutritious diet.

Radical measures such as parathyroidectomy to treat hyperparathyroid bone disease are seldom required. If the plasma phosphorus is elevated, calcium supplementation and vitamin D should be used judiciously so that a gradual elevation of plasma calcium to normal is achieved. Metastatic calcification is a complication of hypercalcemia, especially if there is hyperphosphatemia. A reduction in plasma concentration of phosphorus to normal values can usually be achieved by the measures discussed earlier.

Anemia. The chronic normochromic anemia of

CRF is difficult to treat. A hemoglobin level of 7 to 8 gm per cent is compatible with a reasonable state of well-being, and it is unwise to attempt to keep the hemoglobin at normal levels by repeated transfusions. If the hemoglobin level falls below 6 gm per cent the danger of cardiac decompensation resulting from hypoxia and hypertension makes it reasonable to give small (20 to 75 ml) transfusions of fresh packed, washed red blood cells to raise the hemoglobin to 7 or 8 gm per cent. Caution should be exercised to avoid circulatory overload during such transfusions; it is sometimes necessary to withdraw an equivalent volume of blood from the patient.

A normal intake of dietary iron should be assured to avoid iron deficiency anemia. Erythropoiesis may be improved by treatment of underlying infections, regular dialysis and proper nutrition.

Drug Dosage in CRF. The route of excretion of many drugs is via the kidney. Thus, if the dosage is not reduced in CRF, impaired renal function may lead to retention of the drug or its metabolites, with the likelihood that very high blood and tissue concentrations will be reached. It is important to know which drugs are excreted principally by the kidney and to modify the dosage of them in order that toxic concentrations in plasma and tissue are avoided. Should the drug be potentially nephrotoxic, the risk of increasing the degree of renal insufficiency is an extremely serious one. The extent of renal damage varies considerably in patients with CRF, so that the need to reduce either drug dosage or frequency of administration will differ accordingly. The question of drug dosage in CRF is complex and a complete discussion cannot be given here. Table 15–11 lists drugs used in children which are excreted principally by the kidney, the dosages of which must therefore be modified in CRF. More detailed information is available in the reference articles noted below.* The ideal method for determining drug dosage in relation to renal failure is to measure either the rate of disappearance from the plasma following a single dose and thus establish the half-life of the drug or to determine the plasma concentration at any given time in order to know if a safe and therapeutic level is present. For most drugs, however, this is not practicable, and modification in dosage is based on an educated guess which takes into account the degree of renal failure, the extent to which the drug is normally excreted by the kidney, the potential toxicity of the drug if elevated levels are inadvertently reached, and clinical observations which suggest drug toxicity.

Dialysis and Transplantation. Peritoneal dialysis, hemodialysis and renal transplantation are now established, effective forms of therapy for children with advanced renal failure.

*See references for articles by Bennett, Singer, and Coggins (1968, 1973); Jelliffe and Blankenhorn; Lloyd-Mostyn and Reidenberg.

TABLE 15–11 DRUGS, THE DOSAGE OF WHICH SHOULD BE MODIFIED IN CHILDREN WITH RENAL FAILURE

Antimicrobial drugs
Amphotericin B*
Cephaloridine*
Cephalothin
Colistin (colistimethate)*
Trimethoprim-sulfamethoxazole
Gentamicin*
Kanamycin*
Methenamine mandelate†
Neomycin*
Nitrofurantoin†
Aminosalicylic acid†
Penicillins*
Pentamidine
Polymyxin B*
Streptomycin*
Sulfonamides*
Tetracycline
Vancomycin
Sedative, anticonvulsant and analgesic drugs
Acetaminophen†
Aspirin
Phenobarbital
Phenothiazines
Phenylbutazone*†
Primidone
Trimethadione*
Antihypertensive, cardiovascular and diuretic drugs
Acetazolamide†
Digitoxin
Digoxin
Ethacrynic acid†
Guanethidine
Mercurials*†
Methyldopa
Quinidine
Spironolactone†
Thiazides†
Triamterene†
Miscellaneous drugs
Allopurinol*
Aminocaproic acid†
Azathioprine
Chlorpropamide†
Gold salts*†
Insulin
6-Mercaptopurine
Methotrexate
Penicillamine*
Propylthiouracil

*Drugs which are potentially nephrotoxic.
†Drugs which should be avoided or used with great care when the GFR is below 15 ml/m²/day.

The indications for these forms of therapy and the criteria for patient selection have changed dramatically since the techniques were first introduced; it is inevitable that they will continue to change in response to advances in technology, availability of dialysis and transplantation facilities and developments in transplantation biology.

The goal of dialysis and transplantation is to return renal function to normal. Dialysis is used as a means of sustaining the child during the time before transplantation. In children the problems encountered are considerably different from those in adults. They include the important ones of psychosocial and emotional development, physical growth and technical difficulties related to the comparably smaller size of the child.

The decision to begin chronic dialysis or to perform transplantation should be made after careful consideration of the total constellation of problems presented by the child and his family. Ideally decisions concerning these procedures should be made in consultation with a pediatric nephrologist and carried out in a center in which a pediatric nephrology team with all the necessary laboratory facilities and allied professional personnel assumes active responsibility for the ongoing care of the patient.

Dialysis and transplantation should be considered when the conservative measures outlined above are no longer effective. The principal problems that lead to consideration of these forms of treatment are (1) growth arrest; (2) severe renal osteodystrophy; (3) cardiovascular, circulatory, fluid and acid-base disturbances; (4) malnutrition and inadequate caloric intake; and (5) inability to carry out normal activities which are essential for emotional well-being and development.

PROGNOSIS. The prognosis for children with CRF has improved dramatically during the decade 1965 to 1975; few children need die of uremia at this time. However, the goal of complete rehabilitation with normal physical and emotional development is still not achieved in a high proportion of affected children.

Bennett, W. M., Singer, I., and Coggins, C. H.: A practical guide to drug usage in adult patients with impaired renal function. J.A.M.A. *214*:1468, 1970.

Bennett, W. M., Singer, I., and Coggins, C. H.: Guide to drug usage in adult patients with impaired renal function. J.A.M.A. *223*:991, 1973.

Bricker, N. S.: On the meaning of the intact nephron hypothesis. Am. J. Med. *46*:1, 1969.

Bricker, N. S.: On the pathogenesis of the uremic state. An exposition of the "trade-off hypothesis." New Engl. J. Med. *286*:1093, 1972.

DeFronzo, R. A., Andres, R., Edgar, P., and Walker, W. G.: Carbohydrate metabolism in uremia: A review. Medicine *52*:469, 1973.

Feldman, W., Baliah, T., and Drummond, K. N.: Intermittent peritoneal dialysis in the management of chronic renal failure in children. Am. J. Dis. Child. *116*:30, 1968.

Habib, R., Broyer, M., and Benmaiz, H.: Chronic renal failure in children. Causes, rates of deterioration and survival data. Nephron *11*:209, 1973.

Holliday, M. A.: Calorie deficiency in children with uremia: Effect upon growth. Pediatrics *50*:590, 1972.

Jelliffe, R. W., and Blankenhorn, D. A.: Improved method of digitalis therapy in patients with reduced renal function. Circulation *36*(Suppl. 2):150, 1967.

Korman, M. G., Laver, M. C., and Hansky, J.: Hypergastrinaemia in chronic renal failure. Brit. Med. J. *1*:209, 1972.

Lloyd-Mostyn, R. H., and Lord, I. J.: Ototoxicity of intravenous furosemide. Lancet *2*:1156, 1971.

Mauer, S. M., Shideman, J. R., Buselmeier, T. J., and Kjellstrand, C. M.: Long-term hemodialysis in the neonatal period. Am. J. Dis. Child. *125*:269, 1973.

Mawer, E. B., Backhouse, J., Taylor, C. M., Lumb, G. A., and Stanbury, S. W.: Failure of formation of 1,25-dihydroxycholecalciferol in chronic renal insufficiency. Lancet *1*:626, 1973.

McVicar, M., Gauthier, B., and Goodman, C. T.: Uremic neuropathy. Am. J. Dis. Child. *125*:263, 1973.

Potter, D., Belzer, F. O., Rames, L., Holliday, M. A., Kountz, S. L., and Najarian, J. S.: The treatment of chronic uremia in childhood. 1. Transplantation. Pediatrics *45*:432, 1970.

Potter, D., Larsen, D., Leumann, E., Perin, D., Simmons, J., Piel, C. F., and Holliday, M. A.: Treatment of chronic uremia in childhood. II. Hemodialysis. Pediatrics *46*:678, 1970.

Reidenberg, M. M.: Renal Function and Drug Action. Philadelphia, W. B. Saunders Company, 1971.

Slatopolsky, E., and Bricker, N. S.: The role of phosphorus restriction in the prevention of secondary hyperparathyroidism in chronic renal disease. Kidney Int. *4*:141, 1973.

Welt, L. G., Black, H. R., and Krueger, K. K., eds.: Symposium on Uremic Toxins. (Symposia Vol. 7.) Arch. Intern. Med. *126*:773, 1970.

INFECTION OF THE URINARY TRACT

Bacterial infection of the urinary tract may be defined as infection of any part of the urinary tract or the presence of bacteria in the urine. Although it may be simpler to consider the infection as confined to a section of the urinary tract, e.g., the bladder (cystitis) or to involve the kidney (pyelonephritis), for practical purposes it is usually impossible in children to establish whether upper, lower or both areas of the tract are involved.

HISTORY. In the early 1960's two observations led to concern that infections of the urinary tract constituted a major unrecognized health hazard: (1) the discovery of clinically unrecognized chronic pyelonephritis in 2 to 20 per cent of unselected autopsies, and (2) the detection of asymptomatic bacteriuria in about 6 per cent of adult women and in 1 to 2 per cent of apparently healthy female children. These two observations were interpreted as being causally related and led to the frequent employment of sometimes drastic and usually fruitless diagnostic and therapeutic urologic procedures in an attempt to prevent a presumed gradual but relentless development of renal insufficiency resulting from chronic pyelonephritis.

The decade of 1960 to 1970 has provided a perspective which permits the conclusion that the proportion of children with urinary tract infection for whom this ultimately constitutes a serious or life-threatening problem is relatively small, and that surgical procedures are probably indicated only for the relatively small number of children who have repeated infections associated with gross and easily identified structural abnormalities of the urinary tract.

ETIOLOGY. The susceptibility of the urinary tract to infection by organisms which are not ordinarily pathogenic is poorly understood. The bacteria are predominantly coliforms, and the source is usually the patient's own fecal flora. Congenital structural anomalies of the urinary tract, particularly if there is obstruction to urine flow, predispose to urinary tract infection. Other predisposing factors are foreign bodies, indwelling urethral catheter, nephrolithiasis and possibly severe constipation. In some children, however, with anatomic or functional abnormalities such as bladder wall thickening, vesicoureteral reflux or an abnormal voiding pattern, it is likely that these are consequences of urinary tract infection rather than predisposing causes. In most children with urinary tract infection, a significant structural or functional anomaly which could be considered to make the patient susceptible to infection is not present. The consistently higher incidence in girls beyond infancy may result from the short female urethra; it is reasonably well established that the usual route of infection is an ascending one from external genitalia via the urethra to the bladder.

INCIDENCE. The incidence of urinary tract infection in girls is three to four times that in boys except in infancy when the ratio is about equal. In infancy major congenital structural anomalies of the urinary tract probably account for the higher incidence in boys than is the case when they are older. Screening programs in apparently healthy schoolchildren show that at any given time from 1 to 2 per cent of girls have an active urinary tract infection and that in most it is asymptomatic. At some time prior to maturity about 5 per cent of girls will have at least one urinary tract infection.

PATHOGENESIS AND PATHOLOGY. There is little understanding of why in some instances these organisms are able to establish a foothold, multiply and initiate an actual infection. Nor is the mechanism understood by which urine stasis from whatever cause predisposes to infection. In view of the recurrent or persistent nature of this problem in many children, especially in girls, even in the absence of demonstrable anatomic abnormalities, it is probable that unrecognized host factors play an important role in enhancing bacterial colonization in some children and not in others. Acute or chronic inflammation of the bladder—cystitis—secondary to recurrent infection leads to inflammatory changes which may distort the normal anatomic relationships of the ureter in its course through the bladder wall and cause incompetence of the vesicoureteral valve. This may permit reflux of urine into the ureter, especially during voiding, with subsequent ureteral dilatation and access of organisms in infected urine to the upper tract. Infection of the kidney—pyelitis or pyelonephritis—may then develop. Infection of renal parenchyma may also develop via a hematogenous route. This is probably a more common route in infants, particularly when there is a structural anomaly. Several explanations of the peculiar susceptibility of the kidney to organisms which are not usually pathogenic in other areas of the body have been proposed. These include inhibition of activity of normal host defense mechanisms such as the complement system by medullary production of ammonia, and impaired migration of polymorphonuclear leukocytes and phagocytosis because of medullary hypertonicity.

When infection has been established, functional changes may occur. If only the bladder is infected, inflammation causes irritability and spasm of the smooth muscle of the bladder, leading to urgency and urinary frequency. Infection of the renal medulla may interfere with normal mechanisms for urine concentration; polyuria and impaired ability to concentrate the urine may develop.

In acute uncomplicated infection the principal changes are confined to the bladder, whose mucosa becomes edematous and inflamed. Hemorrhage into inflamed areas may occur, leading to the passage of bloody urine. With chronic infection the bladder wall becomes thicker and fibrous tissue may develop. Edema and distortion of the valve orifice and of the intramural portion of the ureter cause valvular incompetence, with reflux of the urine into the ureter. Stasis of infected urine in the ureter results in inflammation and dilatation of the ureter. The kidney is usually infected via the collecting system. Acute and chronic inflammatory changes in the pelvis and medulla develop, interfering with normal structural relationships and function in this region. Calyceal blunting results from the loss of parenchyma by infection and from atrophy caused by the back pressure of urinary reflux. These changes tend to be asymmetric and localized and lead to formation of focal scar tissue. With chronic recurrent episodes of renal infection there is contraction of the entire kidney.

Foci of acute and chronic inflammatory cells are seen in the interstitium, and with time there is an increase in fibrous tissue. In acute fulminating pyelonephritis the kidney is swollen and edematous, and there is a diffuse interstitial infiltrate of polymorphonuclear cells.

CLINICAL MANIFESTATIONS AND COURSE. A large proportion of children with active urinary tract infection are essentially asymptomatic, and when there are complaints, they may not be related to the urinary system.

Urgency, frequency, dysuria, dribbling, nocturnal enuresis or daytime incontinence in a previously dry child and foul-smelling urine are common presenting complaints. Fever, irritability, abdominal pain, loss of appetite or vomiting, inflammation of the mucous membrane of the external genitalia and hematuria are not uncommon. In infants unexplained jaundice, lethargy or an appearance suggestive of sepsis may be present. The appearance of being seriously ill, with high fever, flank pain and leukocytosis, is relatively uncommon. If untreated, the clinical features usually subside within several weeks; however, the infection can persist, and recurrent episodes with similar clinical features and/or the continuance of asymptomatic bacteriuria are common sequelae. In the absence of major structural abnormalities, despite recurrent or chronic infections extending over a period of years, significant renal or ureteral damage is relatively uncommon.

LABORATORY DATA. The diagnosis of urinary tract infection rests primarily on the detection of bacteria in normally sterile urine.

Urine Collection. The external genitalia may harbor bacteria, feces, vaginal secretions containing pus and epithelial cells and, in uncircumcised males, debris under the foreskin. Thus, a randomly voided urine is easily contaminated and often contains bacteria, cells and other material not present in the bladder urine. To avoid confusion in diagnosis which this contamination introduces, it is important that the external genitalia be cleansed, the foreskin be retracted in uncircumcised males and, whenever possible, a midstream specimen obtained. While this is desirable in collection of urine for routine urinalysis, it is essential when the urine is to be cultured. Sterile cotton balls soaked in a nonirritating antiseptic solution such as aqueous benzalkonium chloride 1:1000 may be used to cleanse the genitalia. With the use of sterile precautions, the labia should be separated and the vulva wiped gently from front to back with three or four separate antiseptic-soaked cotton balls. The antiseptic solution should be rinsed off with sterile water. In boys the foreskin should be retracted and the glans and prepuce thoroughly cleansed and then rinsed. The genitalia should then be dried with a sterile absorbent gauze or cotton ball and the child asked to void into a sterile container from which urine for culture and urinalysis can be taken. In infants a sterile urine container may be attached to the penis or vulva following cleansing. If this is done, it is important that frequent checks be made to determine when voiding has occurred and to avoid fecal contamination; the mother can be of help in this task.

Despite the most diligent attempts, it is not uncommon that some contamination of the urine occurs; it is thus essential that the specimen obtained for bacterial culture be plated as soon as possible, preferably within half an hour. If this is not possible it should be refrigerated at 4° C to inhibit multiplication of contaminating bacteria which could lead to a false positive culture. The specimen for culture can be kept at this temperature for 48 hours and then plated without danger of spurious results.

Sometimes it is not feasible to obtain a clean voided urine specimen. For example, the clinical condition of the patient may be so serious that there is insufficient time, sequential urine specimens may be contaminated leading to equivocal or erroneous results, or the child may be uncooperative. In these circumstances urine may be obtained under sterile conditions by urethral catheterization or by direct aspiration of the bladder. This latter technique has been used extensively in infants because in this age group the bladder is higher, i.e., less in the pelvis, and because it is more difficult to obtain uncontaminated voided specimens. The technique is simple and should be done after the baby has not voided for 1 to 2 hours to ensure that the bladder contains urine. The skin is cleansed and the bladder is aspirated just above the symphysis pubis; a 1 or 1½ inch No. 21 needle attached to a sterile syringe is directed slightly downward. Although this technique is widely used and is generally safe, it is not entirely without risk; bladder hemorrhage and perforation of other intra-abdominal structures have occurred.

Urinalysis. Infected urine often has a strong coliform smell. The urine may be faintly clouded, owing to the presence of numerous pus cells. Hemorrhagic cystitis is not an uncommon manifestation of urinary tract infection, particularly in boys; the urine may have a reddish color. The protein concentration is usually less than 100 mg/dl. Alkaline urine suggests the presence of such organisms as the Proteus species, which split urea, leading to the formation of ammonia.

Microscopic examination of the urinary sediment after centrifugation usually shows numerous pus cells in acute urinary tract infection. Red blood cells may also be present. It may be emphasized that an active urinary tract infection can be present without pus cells in the urine; conversely, the finding of pus cells does not necessarily indicate urinary tract infection. For example, pyuria may occur during a febrile illness or with dehydration, and numerous pus cells are often seen in the urine in acute poststreptococcal glomerulonephritis. Innumerable bacteria per high power field are commonly seen in the unstained centrifuged sediment; this finding correlates well with urine bacterial colony counts of more than 100,000 per ml and may, in the absence of bacteriologic culture data, permit a tentative diagnosis of urinary tract infection.

Urine Culture. The importance of obtaining a suitable specimen and either culturing it immediately or refrigerating it has been stressed. Measurement of the number of bacterial colonies in a known volume of urine is of inestimable value in differentiating between infection and bacterial contamination of the clean voided specimen. Infected urine contins over 100,000 colonies per ml; contaminated urine contains fewer, usually in a range under 10,000 colonies per ml. When there is urinary tract infection, a single organism is usually found, whereas it is not uncommon to find two or more different species in contaminated urine.

When the results of a single colony count are equivocal, e.g., if the number of colonies is between 10,000 and 100,000 per ml, the study should be repeated. Falsely positive colony counts are usually due to bacterial contamination from the external genitalia, to delay between urine collection and plating, or to keeping the urine at a temperature which permits contaminating bacteria to multiply. A falsely low colony count in the presence of infection may occur when the urine is dilute or very acid; contamination of the specimen with the cleansing antiseptic can also lead to a negative culture or low colony count. In patients with chronic or indolent infections, the colony count may be less than 100,000 per ml.

Recently the use of an agar-coated slide which can be dipped in the freshly voided urine has gained wide acceptance. It is particularly useful in the pediatrician's office. The number of bacterial colonies on the dip slide after 24 hours' incubation can be estimated by comparison with standard charts; the results correlate closely with colony counts performed in the bacteriology laboratory. Apart from convenience, a further advantage is that, when there is a significant count, a culture of the organism can be taken from the dip slide for precise classification and for antibiotic sensitivity studies. This technique also has value in screening programs for urinary tract infection and in monitoring patients with recurrent infections.

Radiographic Examination. For details of the technique for radiologic assessment of the urinary tract see earlier section on Diagnostic Assessment of Structure and Function.

In patients with urinary tract infection it is essential to assess the anatomic integrity of the urinary tract in order to identify any structural and functional abnormalities and to detect renal parenchymal damage. About 15 per cent of children who undergo radiologic examination at the time of their first recognized urinary tract infection have important urinary tract abnormalities. These include congenital anomalies of the kidney, obstructive lesions at any site along the urinary tract and/or significant vesicoureteral reflux with ureteral dilatation. Of the remaining children studied 1 to 2 months after their first diagnosed urinary tract infection, about 50 per cent have less serious abnormalities, such as irregularity or thickening of the bladder wall, an abnormal or intermittent voiding pattern with or without postvoiding residual, or minimal vesicoureteral reflux. Many of these minor abnormalities result from the acute inflammation and resolve over a period of months, if the urine remains uninfected. The finding of even minor abnormalities, however, is of prognostic importance, since they are associated with recurrences after an adequate course of treatment in about half of the patients, whereas less than 10 per cent of children with an entirely normal radiologic study have a recurrence.

An adequate examination consists of an intravenous pyelogram; if bladder abnormalities or ureteral dilatation are seen or if the history suggests a voiding disturbance, a cine-voiding cystourethrogram may be indicated to evaluate bladder contraction and to exclude lower tract anomalies or vesicoureteral reflux. Retrograde cystourethrography may occasionally be necessary if adequate visualization of the lower tract is not possible by the antegrade route. To allow sufficient time for acute inflammatory changes to disappear it is best to postpone radiologic examination 4 to 6 weeks after treatment is started and the urine is sterile.

Renal Function Studies. In most children with urinary tract infection there are no changes in renal function. If pyelonephritis is present, however, there may be disturbances in function, the extent and severity of which depend on the severity of the renal lesions, on whether or not both kidneys are affected and on the degree of chronicity. In acute pyelonephritis, mild elevation of the blood urea nitrogen and serum creatinine may be present; these usually return to normal with treatment. The most consistent early finding in chronic pyelonephritis is an impaired ability to concentrate the urine. This is a consequence of damage to the renal medulla; progressive interstitial scarring and nephron destruction may occur. The glomerular filtration rate is reduced, and there are persistent elevations of the blood urea nitrogen and serum creatinine, as well as other findings of chronic renal failure. In some instances, as a consequence of tubular dysfunction, there may be impaired ability to conserve sodium.

DIAGNOSIS AND DIFFERENTIAL DIAGNOSIS. The diagnosis rests on the detection of bacteria in the urine, but as noted there are numerous pitfalls which may make it difficult to be certain of the diagnosis. The principal errors result from improper methods of urine collection and handling, which lead to a spuriously positive urine culture. In acute urinary tract infection the colony count is over 100,000 per ml in virtually all cases; contaminated urine has less than 10,000 per ml. In chronic pyelonephritis, however, active infection may be present with colony counts less than 100,000 per ml. The presence of typical symptoms, a significant colony count and pyuria establish the diagnosis; urinary tract infection, however, can be asymptomatic, and pyuria may be absent in the presence of active infection. Radiologic findings may provide supplementary evidence. Since congenital anomalies of the urinary tract predispose to urinary tract infection, which in turn can lead to abnormal radiologic patterns, it may be difficult to be certain of the genesis of some abnormal radiologic findings. Renal vascular accidents in infancy may impair later kidney growth and lead to irregular anatomic development; these changes may be difficult to distinguish from those resulting from chronic pyelonephritis. In the former, ureteral dilatation and reflux are usually absent.

PREVENTION. In patients with recurrent urinary tract infections it may be necessary to give antibacterial drugs in an attempt to prevent or to decrease the number of recurrences. This is particularly important if there is evidence of structural abnormalities with urinary stasis or reflux or if recurrent infections have already caused significant damage to the kidneys or collecting system. (See Recurrent Infections).

TREATMENT

Acute Uncomplicated Infections. The most common organism in acute uncomplicated urinary tract infection is *Escherichia coli;* an excellent therapeutic response is usually obtained with a short-acting sulfonamide such as sulfisoxazole (Gantrisin) in a dose of 100–125 mg/kg/day in four divided doses. Two weeks is an adequate treatment period, there being no difference in the recurrence rate when treatment is continued for a longer time. Ampicillin, 75–150 mg/kg/day, may be used for initial treatment, but it has no advantage over sulfonamides. Therapy with either of these drugs can be started without the results of bacterial antibiotic sensitivity tests. The clinical condition usually improves within several days. A follow-up urine culture should be obtained 1 to 2 weeks after therapy is completed.

In acutely ill children it may not be possible to give oral medication, and a parenteral route may be indicated. If there is no response to intravenously administered sulfisoxazole or ampicillin, if the patient's condition is serious or deteriorating, or if infection with less common organisms such as *Pseudomonas aeruginosa, Klebsiella-Enterobacter* or *Proteus* is present, the choice of antibiotic will depend on bacterial sensitivity studies; alternatively a potent broad spectrum antibiotic active against gram-negative organisms may be used empirically. In this situation, gentamicin 1.0–1.5 mg/kg/day, kanamycin 7–12 mg/kg/day or polymyxin B 1.5–2.5 mg/kg/day may be used. Attention must be paid to possible neurotoxic or nephrotoxic effects of these drugs, particularly when renal function is impaired and a potentially toxic blood concentration of the drug may be reached if usual doses are given. Penicillin G may be effective in *Proteus mirabilis* infections; erythromycin, 30–75 mg/kg/day, with sodium bicarbonate to alkalinize the urine is effective in certain gram-negative infections, such as *Pseudomonas;* nitrofurantoin, 5–7 mg/kg/day, is also a valuable drug, particularly in infections due to *Klebsiella-Enterobacter.* The combination* of sulfamethoxazole and trimethoprim (a folic acid metabolism inhibitor) is an effective medication for the treatment of a wide spectrum of infections due to gram-negative organisms including *E. coli, Proteus* and *Klebsiella-Enterobacter;* it is not effective against *Pseudomonas aeruginosa.* The dosage is that which provides 20 mg/kg/day of sulfamethoxazole (4 mg/kg/day of trimethoprim), given in two divided doses.

Recurrent Infections. There is a great tendency for urinary tract infection to recur even in the absence of major anatomic abnormalities; furthermore, recurrences are often asymptomatic. It is, thus, essential in the management of urinary tract infection to secure a culture of urine every 1 to 4 months for a sufficient time – usually 1 to 2 years – even when the patient is ostensibly well. The choice of antibacterial therapy for recurrences depends on bacterial sensitivity studies; medication should be given for 2 to 4 weeks. If recurrences are frequent, prolonged therapy for periods up to several years may be considered; such a regimen can significantly reduce the number of infections. For this type of prophylactic therapy nitrofurantoin, methenamine mandelate or sulfisoxazole is usually safe and effective. The combination of sulfamethoxazole and trimethoprim is also useful. The dosage of drug required to prevent infection in patients with a demonstrated tendency to recurrence is about one half that recommended for the treatment of active infections; the medication can be effective if given only once or twice a day.

Potentially toxic antibiotics should be avoided, unless clearly warranted by the patient's condition, since, although infection can be temporarily eradicated with such agents, the tendency to recur usually persists.

*Báctrim – Hoffmann-La Roche, Nutley, N. J., Septra – Burroughs Wellcome & Co., Research Triangle Park, N.C.

Abnormal Bladder Function with Intermittent, Prolonged Voiding. This condition, seen almost exclusively in girls, is associated with recurrent urinary tract infection. It is characterized by daytime incontinence or dribbling and the presence of an abnormal voiding pattern demonstrable by cystourethrography. The bladder contracts irregularly, voiding is prolonged and emptying may be incomplete. Involvement of the upper tract and kidneys is uncommon, although minor degrees of vesicoureteral reflux occur. Long term prophylactic antibacterial treatment as discussed previously is indicated, and regular voiding at approximately 2-hour intervals should be encouraged; the latter may be of considerable help in overcoming the daytime incontinence. Urologic procedures such as ureteral reimplantation, meatotomy and urethral dilatation have been shown not to influence the course of this problem favorably. This type of abnormal voiding pattern is most common in patients between 3 and 10 years of age; after puberty an improvement is often noted.

Vesicoureteral Reflux. The treatment of ureteral reflux associated with urinary tract infection remains an unresolved problem. Minor degrees of reflux are seen in about 25 per cent of children with acute urinary tract infection and usually resolve with control of the infection. The difficult question remains concerning the need for surgical intervention such as reimplantation of the ureters or urinary diversion when the reflux persists 6 to 12 months after infection. The patient should be observed for at least 1 year on conservative medical management with prophylactic antibacterial therapy and regularly spaced urine cultures. Surgical therapy should be considered only if there is unequivocal evidence that deterioration of renal function and structural changes in the upper collecting system are taking place as a result of the reflux. In such instances reimplantation of the ureters or diversion of the urinary stream may be necessary; however, results with long-term conservative therapy have been good in the majority of patients, and caution against an aggressive surgical approach is appropriate.

Meatal Stenosis. The role of distal urethral narrowing or meatal stenosis in the pathogenesis of urinary tract infection, particularly when recurrences are common, has been emphasized in the urologic literature. Many children have been subjected to a variety of surgical procedures, such as meatotomy, urethrotomy or urethral dilatation, on the assumption that urethral obstruction was contributory to the development of urinary tract infection. Although such procedures may alter the anatomy of the urethra, it is clear that true meatal stenosis, defined as a pathologic degree of stenosis or narrowing of the urethral meatus, is a *very uncommon* lesion in children with urinary tract infection. Surgical procedures on the urethra do not affect the infection recurrence rate, and operations of any sort for correction of presumed narrowing or stenosis of the urethra or meatus are rarely indicated in children with urinary tract infection.

Severe Structural Abnormalities of the Urinary Tract. Urologic intervention is necessary when there is an obvious structural anomaly, such as a congenital obstruction along the course of the urinary tract which is amenable to surgery. Such conditions are not infrequently complicated by chronic or recurrent infections with organisms which are resistant to most antibacterial drugs. It may be necessary to accept suppression of the infection rather than complete sterilization of the urine in such cases; a prophylactic regimen as discussed above is warranted.

Renal Parenchymal Involvement. Loss of renal tissue, distortion and clubbing of the calyceal system and irregularity of the outline of the kidney may indicate parenchymal damage as a result of bacterial infection. Significant vesicoureteral reflux is a common associated finding. If recurrent infections occur, long-term prophylactic therapy as outlined should be given. Attention should be directed to possible deterioration in renal function and to the development of hypertension. Radiologic reassessment, every 1 to 3 years, may be indicated to determine if the condition is progressive or stable.

General Therapy of Urinary Tract Infection. Symptomatic treatment for dysuria may be needed during the acute infection. A urinary analgesic such as phenazopyridine HCl, 10 mg/kg/day orally in three or four divided doses, may be helpful for acute dysuria; diluting the urine by increasing the fluid intake may also reduce dysuria. Fever may be treated with acetylsalicylic acid in the usual manner.

If there is evidence of upper tract and renal involvement, it is important that, in addition to control of the urinary tract infection, other aspects of renal function such as urine concentrating ability, blood urea nitrogen and serum creatinine be assessed periodically and that attention be paid to the possible development of hypertension, acid-base disturbances, growth failure and other complications of chronic renal insufficiency.

PROGNOSIS. The prognosis for uncomplicated urinary tract infection is excellent if adequate therapy is instituted for the acute infection and if recurrences are promptly recognized and treated. The long-term prognosis is less favorable for patients with significant structural abnormalities complicated by infection and for patients with renal parenchymal damage. Here the underlying abnormality or the damage already present at the time of the first diagnosed urinary tract infection may not be amenable to medical or surgical therapy, even though further deterioration in renal function from the urinary tract infection per se can usually be prevented.

Cohen, M.: Urinary tract infections in children. I. Females aged 2 through 14, first two infections. Pediatrics *50*:271, 1972.

Drummond, K. N., and Forbes, P. A.: Bacterial infections of the urinary tract (female children). *In* Conn, H. F. (ed.): Current Therapy 1973. 25th. ed. Philadelphia, W. B. Saunders Company, 1973, p. 479.

Forbes, P. A., Drummond, K. N., and Nogrady, M. B.: Initial urinary tract infections. J. Pediatr. *75*:187, 1969.

Forbes, P. A., Drummond, K. N., and Nogrady, M. B.: Meatotomy in girls with meatal stenosis and urinary tract intections. J. Pediatr. *75*:937, 1969.

Holland, N. H., and West, C. D.: Prevention of recurrent urinary tract infections in girls. Am. J. Dis. Child. *105*:60, 1963.

Kunin, C. M., and Halmagyi, N. E.: Urinary-tract infections in schoolchildren. II. Characterization of invading organisms. New Engl. J. Med. *266*:1297, 1962.

Kunin, C. M., Zacha, E., and Paquin, A. J.: Urinary-tract infections in schoolchildren. I. Prevalence of bacteriuria and associated urologic findings. New Engl. J. Med. *266*:1287, 1962.

O'Grady, F., and Brumfitt, W. (eds.): Urinary Tract Infection. London, Oxford University Press, 1968, p. 244.

Pryles, C. V., and Eliot, C. R.: Pyuria and bacteriuria in infants and children. Am. J. Dis. Child. *110*:628, 1965.

Saccharow, L., and Pryles, C. V.: Further experience with the use of percutaneous suprapubic aspiration of the urinary bladder: Bacteriologic studies in 654 infants and children. Pediatrics *43*:1018, 1969.

Smellie, J. M.: The disappearance of reflux in children with urinary tract infection during prophylactic chemotherapy. *In* Proceedings of the 4th International Congress on Nephrology, Stockholm, 1969. Vol. 3. Alwall, N., Berglund, F., and Josephson, B., (eds.): Clinical Nephrology, Immunology. Basel, S. Karger AG, 1970, p. 357.

Zinner, S. H., Sabath, L. D., Casey, J. I., and Finland, M.: Erythromycin and alkalinisation of the urine in the treatment of urinary-tract infections due to gram-negative bacilli. Lancet *1*:1267, 1971.

RENAL TUBERCULOSIS

Tuberculosis of the kidney is uncommon in children except as a manifestation of generalized miliary tuberculosis. The rare instances of localized renal tuberculosis produce no symptoms or any or all of the following: fever; emaciation; local pain, tenderness and enlargement; urinary frequency; dysuria and hematuria. Persistently sterile pyuria suggests renal tuberculosis. Tubercle bacilli, which must be differentiated from smegma bacilli, may be identified microscopically. The treatment is that of progressive pulmonary tuberculosis (Table 10–9). Rarely, surgical removal may be indicated for lesions affecting one kidney only.

DEVELOPMENTAL ABNORMALITIES

Developmental abnormalities of the kidney and urinary tract are present in about 10 per cent of people. Some are minor and of no clinical significance; others are major and pose problems to the patient's health and survival. Collectively they account for about 45 per cent of cases of chronic renal failure in childhood; they often have a hereditary basis and are frequently associated with abnormalities in other organ systems. The prognosis is often prejudiced by failure to recognize the anomaly at an early age.

An entirely satisfactory grouping of the developmental abnormalities of the kidney and urinary tract is not yet possible, because little is known of their pathogenesis, and because similar pathologic findings may be seen in conditions which are almost certainly unrelated. One classification which takes into account both clinical and pathologic features is presented in Table 15–12. Although many of these conditions are hereditary, in terms of the number of patients affected, the majority occur sporadically without evidence of genetic influences.

RENAL AGENESIS

Renal agenesis may be unilateral or bilateral, and may occur sporadically or on a hereditary basis.

UNILATERAL RENAL AGENESIS

The incidence of unilateral renal agenesis is about 1 in 2500 live births. The single kidney may be completely normal and without associated abnormalities. These children may have a normal life expectancy without morbidity; it has been suggested that the risk of urinary infection and calculus formation is higher than in patients with two normal kidneys.

Unilateral agenesis may be clinically important for two other reasons: (1) the single kidney may be abnormally formed and there may be associated abnormalities of the urinary collecting system, and (2) there is a notable incidence of extrarenal congenital abnormalities in patients with unilateral agenesis. These include cardiac (ventricular septal defect), nervous system (meningomyelocele), gastrointestinal (strictures, esophageal atresia, tracheoesophageal fistula, imperforate anus), skeletal (vertebral, limb, digital, long bone, rib) and genital anomalies (ipsilateral unicornate uterus, absence of fallopian tube, absence of or hypoplastic testes).

The normal solitary kidney increases in size by compensatory hypertrophy after birth so that by the time the child is several years of age its volume may approach twice the normal one. Inadvertent surgical removal of a solitary kidney following trauma has been reported. Most nephrologists consider that biopsy of a solitary kidney is contraindicated.

TABLE 15–12 DEVELOPMENTAL ABNORMALITIES

Abnormalities in the amount of renal tissue
- Unilateral or bilateral agenesis
- Hypoplasia
- Supernumerary kidneys

Abnormalities in renal location or shape
- Ectopia
- Fusion (horseshoe kidney)

Abnormalities in renal differentiation
- Dysplasia, with or without cysts
- Polycystic renal disease
- Congenital renal neoplasms (nephroblastomatosis, Wilms' tumor)

Renal and urinary tract abnormalities in multisystem disorders or syndromes
- Laurence-Moon-Biedl syndrome
- Fanconi syndrome of multiple congenital anomalies and aplastic anemia
- DiGeorge syndrome
- Zellweger syndrome
- Tuberous sclerosis
- Prune-belly syndrome
- Oral-facial-digital syndrome
- Meckel syndrome
- Dandy-Walker malformation of the brain
- Turner syndrome
- Autosomal trisomy syndromes D and E
- Von Hippel-Lindau disease
- Jeune's asphyxiating thoracic dystrophy
- Thymic alymphoplasia
- Russell-Silver dwarfism
- Syndrome of renal hamartomas, nephroblastomatosis and fetal gigantism
- Beckwith-Wiedemann syndrome
- Congenital renal and ear abnormalities
- Familial renal dysplasia with blindness.
- Cat-eye syndrome
- Ehlers-Danlos syndrome
- Rubinstein-Taybi syndrome
- Cockayne syndrome
- Syndromes with abnormalities of the urinary tract, müllerian ducts, ears and distal extremities

Abnormalities of the collecting system, bladder and/or urethra
- Hydronephrosis due to pelviureteric obstruction
- Hydroureter and megaureter
- Vesicoureteral reflux
- Ureterocele
- Duplication of the kidney and collecting system
- Ectopic ureteral insertion
- Epispadias and bladder exstrophy
- Hypospadias
- Posterior urethral valve
- Other anomalies of the urethra

BILATERAL RENAL AGENESIS
(Potter Syndrome)

This occurs in about one in 3000 births. Seventy-five per cent of those affected are males. Oligohydramnios, amnion nodosum, prematurity, small size for gestational age and breech presentation are common. Extrarenal abnormalities are usually present. These include characteristic facies (wide-set eyes, parrot-beak nose, pliable low-set ears, receding chin); spade-like hands; dry, wrinkled skin; pulmonary hypoplasia or dysplasia; limb abnormalities and ovoid-shaped adrenal glands. Lower urinary tract or genital abnormalities may also be present.

The abnormal facies, although characteristic, is not specific for bilateral renal agenesis. It has been suggested that the oligohydramnios resulting from absent urine formation in utero is important in the pathogenesis of some of the extrarenal anomalies, particularly pulmonary hypoplasia.

About 40 per cent of those affected are stillborn. Those who are liveborn usually die before several weeks of age from renal failure or pulmonary problems.

RENAL HYPOPLASIA

This is a rare anomaly in which the number of renal lobules is reduced to five or less, and the number of calyces is correspondingly low. The kidney is small, the weight being only a fraction of normal, but normal nephron differentiation has occurred. The renal artery is also reduced in size. In the majority of instances both kidneys are involved. Usually there are no associated abnormalities in the urinary collecting system.

In bilateral hypoplasia, the total mass of functioning renal tissue is inadequate to sustain normal growth and development and renal failure with growth arrest ensues. Clinical recognition may be as early as several weeks of age and as late as the second decade. Unilateral hypoplasia may present no clinical problems.

Other more common causes of reduced kidney size which should be differentiated from renal hypoplasia include renal dysplasia, atrophy as a result of reflux or pyelonephritis and renal vascular insult in infancy.

SEGMENTAL HYPOPLASIA
(The Ask-Upmark Kidney)

This is a variant of renal hypoplasia which may be unilateral or bilateral; it is twice as frequent in girls as in boys. There is a reduction in the number of renal lobules, with arrest in development in one or more of them. There are cortical or surface grooves at the site of the undeveloped lobules, and there is ectasia of the calyces which these lobules would have supplied had their growth proceeded normally. At the base of the groove there is a sclerotic fibrous plate in which there are thick-walled tortuous arteries and dilated, thyroid-like epithelium-lined microcysts.

Clinically the principal problem is hypertension, which usually presents at about 10 years of age and which may be refractory to medical management. Resection of the hypoplastic zone or even nephrectomy may be necessary. Hyperrenninemia may be involved in the pathogenesis of the hypertension.

OLIGOMEGANEPHRONIC RENAL HYPOPLASIA

This is a nonhereditary bilateral developmental abnormality in which the kidneys are hypoplastic; there are only five or six renal lobules, the number of nephrons is reduced to about one fifth the usual number, and the diameter of the surviving glomeruli is about twice normal. The surviving tubules are hypertrophic, and the intervening interstitial tissue is fibrotic. There are no associated abnormalities of the urinary collecting system. The condition is more common in boys. Signs of renal failure usually present during the first year of life. There are growth failure, polyuria, thirst, vomiting, fever, dehydration and acidosis. The urinary sediment is normal, but there is moderate proteinuria. Hypertension is uncommon. A stable period without further progression of renal failure often occurs after the first year or two, and the patient's general condition may remain unchanged until toward the end of the first decade, when deterioration in renal function and terminal uremia develop. Such patients can usually be managed satisfactorily during the first decade by the standard measures for treatment of chronic renal failure. When these measures do not suffice, the patients are generally good candidates for dialysis and transplantation.

SUPERNUMERARY KIDNEY

This is a rare abnormality in which there is an extra mass of renal tissue, usually smaller than a normal kidney; it has no connection with the normal kidney and usually lies caudal to it. Ureteral drainage into the normal ureter of the same side is common, but the insertion of the ureter may be ectopic, e.g., into the vagina. The clinical problem is usually one of urinary tract infection; apart from appropriate antibacterial therapy for infection, surgical removal of the extra kidney may sometimes be necessary.

RENAL ECTOPIA

This is a congenital malposition of one or both kidneys. The ectopic kidneys may be displaced but normally lateralized, or there may be crossed ectopia, in which case lateralization is not normal and the ureter from the ectopic kidney crosses the midline before draining into the bladder. The most common site of the unilateral ectopic kidney is the pelvis; the renal mass is often small or dysplastic, with associated abnormalities in arterial supply and ureteral origin or insertion. In crossed ectopia the ectopic kidney is usually caudal to and fused with the normal kidney. Crossed, fused renal ectopia is found in about 1 in 7500 births, has occurred in identical twins and is said to be more common in males than females.

Renal ectopia often causes no clinical problem, except that the ectopic kidney may be more subject to infection; furthermore, if the site of ureteral insertion is abnormal, e.g., into the vagina, there may be a persistent vaginal discharge of urine.

HORSESHOE KIDNEY

This is the most common form of renal fusion; the kidneys are joined inferiorly by an isthmus of renal parenchyma which passes anterior to the aorta and to the inferior vena cava. Some caudal displacement of the fused kidney is common. In this sense the horseshoe kidney could be considered as a form of bilateral renal ectopia with fusion. Usually the nephrons in the parenchyma of the isthmus drain into one or two calyces which, in turn, drain into the pelvis of one of the kidneys. The pelves of each half of the horseshoe kidney and their ureters arise more anteriorly than normal. In children the condition is usually asymptomatic; there is, however, an increased incidence of urinary infection and the kidney may be more susceptible to trauma. Adults rather commonly have episodes of abdominal pain which may be consequent to obstruction of the ureters as they angulate in passing over the isthmus. Horseshoe kidney is one of the renal developmental anomalies of Turner syndrome; an intravenous urogram should be done routinely in this disorder.

RENAL DYSPLASIA

By renal dysplasia is meant a developmental defect in differentiation of nephrogenic tissue which may be partial or total and involve either or both kidneys. Dysplastic tissue in the kidney may include any of the following: mesenchymal stroma, dilated ducts lined by tall columnar epithelium, smooth muscle, cartilage, bone, immature ductules, primitive glomeruli and abundant fibrous tissue. Cysts are common in dysplastic kidneys and may be a prominent feature on gross examination. This admixture of various embryonic elements may alter the organ's shape, so that it bears no resemblance to a kidney. The dysplastic kidney may be abnormally small; however, if cysts are present, the total renal mass may be several times normal size. *Unilateral renal dysplasia with cysts* is the most common cystic renal disorder in infants and children and the most common cause of a unilateral abdominal mass in the newborn. This defect is sometimes referred to as a unilateral multicystic kidney.

In about 90 per cent of patients with renal dysplasia there are other anomalies of the urinary tract. Of these the most common are absence, atresia or obstruction of the ureter. Abnormalities of the lower tract such as *posterior urethral valves* or bladder anomalies are sometimes seen and are more common when renal dysplasia is bilateral. There is no evidence of hereditary or familial factors in the majority of cases, and there is no sex predilection. Renal dysplasia may be seen in some of the multisystem disorders or syndromes listed in Tables 15–7 and 15–12; a number of these disorders are hereditary in nature.

The clinical problems related to renal dysplasia are (1) renal failure in patients with bilateral dysplasia; it may be evident in the newborn period. These infants often have the associated extrarenal features seen with bilateral renal agenesis; (2) abdominal mass which may be unilateral or bilateral in infants with cystic renal dysplasia; (3) obstructive uropathy at any point along the course of the collecting system; (4) hypertension, and (5) urinary infection.

POLYCYSTIC KIDNEY DISEASE

See section on hereditary and familial renal disease.

CONGENITAL RENAL TUMORS

These are rare; however, congenital nephroblastomatosis must be considered in an infant presenting with an abdominal mass. This condition may be familial and is sometimes associated with gigantism and hypoglycemia. See also Section 25 on Neoplasms.

MULTISYSTEM DISORDERS OR SYNDROMES

A variety of renal developmental defects is seen in many of the conditions listed under the above heading in Tables 15–7 and 15–12; they will not be discussed in detail here. Attention is drawn to these disorders so that the reader may be aware that renal anomalies are often present and may be of great clinical importance. Appropriate studies, including radiologic examination of the urinary tract, should be considered in many of these conditions.

The prune-belly syndrome is described as an example of one of these disorders.

PRUNE-BELLY SYNDROME
(Triad Syndrome)

This syndrome consists of deficiency of the abdominal musculature, cryptorchidism and abnormalities of the urinary tract; the most common of those of the urinary tract are cystic renal dysplasia, megaloureter, megacystis and urethral obstruction. Although almost all affected infants are males, females with deficient abdominal musculature and urinary tract anomalies have been observed. It is not definitely established that this is a hereditary condition. The striking male preponderance remains unexplained; however, an X-linked recessive mode of inheritance has been proposed. Urethral obstruction, caused by posterior urethral valves, pinpoint meatal stenosis or atresia of the urethra, is an ominous prognostic sign, since the extent of renal dysplasia is greater when this is present. If urethral obstruction is absent, about one third of patients survive the first several months, but the long-term prognosis is guarded because of the possibility of progressive renal failure resulting from associated bladder, ureteral and renal anomalies. An aggressive surgical approach, including early urinary diversion, does not at this time appear warranted.

BILATERAL RENAL ENLARGEMENT IN THE NEWBORN INFANT

A number of conditions may cause bilateral nephromegaly in the newborn infant and must be considered when enlarged kidneys are found on abdominal examination. Some may not, strictly speaking, be considered as developmental anomalies, but since they develop during the course of gestation, they are listed in Table 15–13.

TABLE 15–13 CONDITIONS IN WHICH THERE IS BILATERAL RENAL ENLARGEMENT IN INFANCY

Bilateral renal cystic dysplasia
Infantile polycystic kidney disease
Bilateral thromboses of renal veins or arteries
Bilateral hydronephrosis owing to obstruction at ureteropelvic junction
Maternal diabetes mellitus
Beckwith-Wiedemann syndrome
Syndrome of nephroblastomatosis, renal hamartomas and fetal gigantism
Bilateral Wilms' tumor
Bilateral mesoblastic nephroma
Nephroblastomatosis (familial or nonfamilial forms)
Conditions with infiltration or accumulation of substances not normally stored in the kidney: glycogen storage disease type I; acute leukemia

CONGENITAL MALFORMATIONS OF THE URINARY COLLECTING SYSTEM, BLADDER AND URETHRA

A heterogeneous group of malformations are included under this heading; they are about three times more common in males than females, are often associated with anatomic or functional obstruction to urine flow and are clinically important because: (1) they account for about 20 per cent of chronic renal failure in children; (2) they are not infrequently associated with renal and extrarenal congenital abnormalities; (3) they predispose to recurrent infection and urolithiasis of the urinary tract; and (4) the prognosis usually depends on early diagnosis and appropriate surgical therapy.

Although some anomalies are hereditary, most occur sporadically. Suspicion should be directed to the existence of one of these anomalies if there is a history of oligohydramnios and if there are such physical findings as abnormal external genitalia, unusually shaped or positioned external ears, anorectal anomalies, spina bifida or a single umbilical artery. In children presenting features of the multisystem disorders or syndromes listed in Tables 15–7 and 15–12, the possibility of these associated urinary tract anomalies should also be considered. The principal means of diagnosis is radiologic examination of the urinary tract by intravenous pyelography, retrograde cystourethrography and/or renal angiography. A complete urologic examination, including a cystoscopic study, may also be required.

Although the clinical features of malformation of the collecting system depend on the nature and severity of the anomaly, the following are common: polyuria with impaired urine concentrating ability, disorders of micturition, recurrent urinary infection and urolithiasis. Hypertension is not a prominent feature. Furthermore, should chronic renal failure develop it usually does so gradually over a period of years, unless there is a major anomaly with severe obstruction.

HYDRONEPHROSIS RESULTING FROM PELVIURETERIC OBSTRUCTION

Obstruction to urine flow at the junction of the renal pelvis and ureter accounts for about one third of the cases of hydronephrosis in childhood. The most common finding is a large dilated extrarenal pelvis; the calyceal system may initially be relatively normal, but it becomes dilated. Persistence of obstruction and recurrent infection may lead to loss and thinning of renal parenchyma.

The most common cause of pelvic ureteric obstruction is some form of intrinsic abnormality of the collecting system. Included are primary stricture at the upper end of the ureter and interruption in the circular coat of smooth muscle at the point of obstruction, which causes a functional obstruction because there is failure to transmit peristaltic waves from the renal pelvis to the ureter. Aberrant extrinsic vessels and kinking of the ureter at the site of the pelviureteric junction may also obstruct urine flow.

In most instances there is no associated vesicoureteral reflux. Pelviureteric obstruction may be bilateral, and there may also be anomalies elsewhere in the urinary tract.

The clinical picture depends on the age of the patient and on the degree of obstruction. In infants the presenting sign is often an abdominal mass. Acute pyelonephritis is common. Occasionally there is intermittent crampy abdominal or loin pain. Hematuria, particularly following minor trauma, is sometimes the initial clinical event in older children. Calculus formation in the dilated pelvis may also occur.

The diagnosis is made by intravenous urography, which shows a dilated renal pelvis, a variable degree of calyceal blunting, loss of renal parenchyma and an abrupt narrowing of the pelvis at the site of obstruction.

Treatment will depend on the degree of obstruction and on whether it is causing symptoms and/or progressive renal damage. A mild to moderate degree of obstruction, even with some calyceal blunting, may represent a stable problem without the likelihood of progressive damage; in such a case periodic radiologic reassessment and regular urine cultures, with appropriate therapy should infection appear, may be indicated for several years to determine the clinical importance of the lesion. On the other hand, if there are severe obstruction, evidence of progressive loss of renal function, recurrent infection and/or or stone formation, or of symptoms related to the obstruction, surgical correction is warranted.

HYDROURETER AND MEGAURETER

The term, *hydroureter,* is used for ureteral dilatation from anatomic obstruction, e.g., at the vesicoureteral junction or in the urethra. The term, *megaureter,* indicates chronic ureteral dilatation without an anatomic obstructing lesion but rather as a result of functional obstruction, because normal ureteral peristalsis with propulsion of urine downward into the bladder does not occur. Depending on the site of the obstruction in a hydroureter and on the competence of the valve at the vesicoureteral junction in either hydroureter or megaureter, there may or may not be associated vesicoureteral reflux. Both hydroureter and megaureter are more common in boys, may be bilateral and may be associated with congenital renal anomalies such as dysplasia or unilateral agenesis. Either may lead to progressive hydronephrosis with reduction in functioning renal tissue and/or to recurrent urinary infection. The child usually presents because of urinary infection, failure to thrive, or polyuria because of impaired urine concentrating ability. Diagnosis is made by intravenous urography, retrograde cystourethrography and/or cystoscopic examination. Treatment involves control of infection, surgical relief of anatomic obstruction and, in selected cases, a diversionary procedure which drains the urine to an ileal loop or to the skin by means of a ureterostomy.

VESICOURETERAL REFLUX

The problem of vesicoureteral reflux in children, whether congenital or acquired, is a difficult one. The basic problem is one of incompetence of the vesicoureteral valve. The normal valve at rest or during voiding is remarkably efficient in that no reflux of urine from bladder to ureter occurs. This is the consequence of several factors, which include active ureteral peristalsis to propel urine from the ureter into the bladder, the length of the intramural portion of the ureter in relation to the diameter of the ureteral orifice (normally about 6:1) and the angle of the ureteral course through the bladder wall, which is usually sufficiently oblique that, when the bladder contracts, the intramural portion of the ureter is occluded.

Abnormal insertion of the ureter into the bladder, congenital ureteral defects such as hydroureter or megaureter, inflammation of the bladder, urethral obstruction or abnormal contraction of the bladder owing to recurrent infection or a congenital or acquired neurologic problem may interfere with the competence of the vesicoureteral valve and lead to reflux of urine from bladder to ureter. Reflux may be present at low intravesical pressures or may occur only during voiding. Furthermore, the reflux may extend only into the lower portion of the ureter without significant ureteral dilatation, or there may be reflux either at rest or during voiding into a widely dilated ureter all the way to the renal pelvis.

Reflux can be demonstrated by retrograde cystography or by cine-voiding cystourethrography using radiographic contrast media. Severe reflux, either passive or during voiding, can lead to parenchymal atrophy and predispose to urinary infection.

The proper management of vesicoureteral reflux is controversial. Minor degrees of reflux often resolve spontaneously with growth or control of urinary infection; good response is also seen with surgical therapy such as ureteral reimplantation. Advocates of medical or surgical therapy can thus justifiably claim good results when dealing with minor or moderate degrees of reflux. The difficulty arises when there is gross incompetence of the vesicoureteral valve, with reflux to the renal pelvis, abnormal bladder contraction, marked dilatation of the ureter (>1 cm diameter throughout its course) and/or absence of ureteral peristalsis. In this situation the results of either medical or surgical therapy, in terms of restoring normal ureteral peristalsis and competence of the vesicoureteral valve, are far from being consistently good.

A reasonable approach to this vexing problem would seem to be to: (1) control urinary infection; (2) establish that an anatomic obstruction at the bladder neck or in the urethra is not present; (3) rule out a neurogenic lesion; (4) encourage frequent voiding, so that the bladder is not distended; (5) assure that the patient does not have fecal impaction and constipation; and (6) observe the patient over a period of 6 months to a year to ascertain if there is progressive loss of renal function or worsening of ureteral dilatation.

A conservative approach to this problem, such as outlined above, will separate those patients who can be managed medically from those who require ureteral reimplantation. Surgical intervention is necessary in only about 15 per cent of children with vesicoureteral reflux. Close cooperation between the pediatric radiologist, nephrologist, and urologist will facilitate selection of those patients who are best managed surgically.

URETEROCELE

Two forms of ureterocele are recognized: simple and ectopic. The **simple ureterocele** is a fusiform dilatation of the intravesical portion of the ureter secondary to stenosis of the ureteric orifice at the trigone of the bladder. The orifice may be only pinpoint in size. The dilatation may become sufficiently severe to cause evagination of the dilated portion of the ureter into the extravesical segment of the ureter adjacent to the bladder; dilatation of the upper ureter, however, with damage to the kidney is seldom seen. The principal problem is urinary infection; sometimes there is flank or loin pain, and calculi may form. Unless there is evidence of progressive ureteral dilatation or of upper tract involvement, a conservative approach to management is recommended; this includes periodic radiologic assessments and regular urine cultures.

Ectopic ureterocele is a condition in which (1) the ureter has an ectopic distal insertion, most commonly into the proximal urethra just below the bladder neck; and (2) its most distal portion bulges into the bladder lumen; here it is covered by a thinned layer of vesical mucosa. This bulge may stretch the trigonal area, so that the normal ureteric orifices are displaced. The ectopic orifice is usually patent and may even allow reflux. Its ureter usually drains the upper pole of a kidney with a double collecting system. This upper renal segment is often abnormal in that it is small, dysplastic or hydronephrotic. The ureter which terminates in the ureterocele is often dilated and tortuous.

The most common clinical presentation is infection of the urinary tract, which usually involves the ectopic dilated ureter. The ureterocele may obstruct the bladder neck and cause urinary retention, or it may prolapse into the urethra and appear in girls as a pink swelling at the urethral meatus. Intravenous urography, retrograde cystourethrography and cystoscopy are useful in the diagnosis. The ureter from the upper abnormal portion of the kidney may visualize poorly and is often dilated. In the bladder the ureterocele appears as a smooth filling defect.

The usual treatment is heminephrectomy with complete excision of the ectopic ureter and uncovering of the ureterocele within the bladder.

DUPLICATION OF THE KIDNEY AND COLLECTING SYSTEM

Duplication of the ureter and renal pelvis is one of the most common congenital anomalies of the urinary tract. The duplication is often bilateral.

The malformation occurs because an accessory ureteric bud arises from the developing ureter to cause an incomplete duplication, or from the wolffian duct when there is complete duplication of the collecting system. These ureteric buds grow into a single undifferentiated metanephric mass, which is destined to develop into the renal parenchyma. Nephrons differentiate in the metanephros in relation to each of the collecting systems. The kidney itself, however, usually remains undivided. The upper system is usually the smaller. The duplicated systems may join above the site of insertion into the bladder. If, however, there is complete duplication of the ureter, the branch draining the upper system usually inserts nearer the bladder neck, i.e., caudal and medial to that of the lower renal segment.

The importance of partial or complete duplication derives from two features: (1) one of the duplicated segments may be functionless and thus not easily recognized, and (2) there is a high incidence of urinary tract infection. Interestingly the ureter of the lower pole, the insertion of which is at a normal site, is more often the one affected by reflux. Pelviureteric obstruction affecting the lower renal segment is not uncommon when there is complete ureteric duplication, and pyelonephritic changes with loss of functioning renal tissue may occur in the lower renal pole.

Surgery may be required in patients with recurrent infection or with problems related to obstruction. Many patients are asymptomatic, and medical therapy of infection may suffice.

ECTOPIC URETERAL INSERTION

Apart from the ectopic ureteral insertion in duplicated collecting systems and in ectopic ureterocele, there is the possibility that the ureter may arise from a single kidney and terminate far from its normal site of insertion. In girls the ureter may insert into the bladder neck, lower urethra or vagina. In boys the ectopic ureter may insert into the posterior urethra, the ejaculatory duct or even the vas deferens. In both sexes the kidney drained by the ectopic ureter is often small or dysplastic. Urinary incontinence or dribbling and recurrent infections are common presenting problems.

EPISPADIAS AND EXSTROPHY OF THE BLADDER

These abnormalities are part of a spectrum of anomalies resulting from failure of midline fusion of the mesodermal structures of the abdominal wall below the umbilicus. They are more common in males than in females. The structures which may be involved are the anterior bladder wall, urethra, genital tubercle, pubic rami and the muscles of the abdominal wall. At one end of the spectrum of these anomalies are minor degrees of episadias involving the penis and distal urethra; at the other is exstrophy of the bladder with failure of fusion of the anterior wall of the bladder. Anomalies of the gastrointestinal tract such as vesicointestinal fistula may be present in more severely affected patients. There is downward displacement of the umbilicus and anterior displacement of the anus in both sexes, the extent depending on the severity of the anomaly. Complete exstrophy is more common than minor degrees of fusion, such as epispadias.

In **epispadias** the proximal urethra and bladder neck are intact; the penis is shortened and there is an upward chordee. The dorsal penile split may be confined to the glans or may extend proximally. The corpora cavernosa are not adherent one to another, as is the case normally. The pubes are often united by a fibrous band but not joined at the symphysis. The testes and other parts of the genital tract are usually intact. In the female the clitoris is separated into two distinct bodies; the vagina is intact; dribbling and urinary incontinence are almost always present. The ability to carry out normal sexual relations depends on the extent of the anomalies; this is especially the case in males, in whom the chordee may present serious limitations. Decisions concerning management should be made in consultation with a urologist and a plastic surgeon.

Exstrophy of the bladder is a more serious problem. The bladder is smaller than normal and its anterior surface lies open on the abdominal wall; its mucosa is continuous laterally with the skin. The mucosa often is polypoid, with glandular metaplasia; the muscular layer is poorly formed. Inguinal and umbilical hernias and rectal prolapse are commonly associated. The ureters traverse the bladder wall at a right angle instead of obliquely. The pelvic ring is incomplete anteriorly, the pubes being widely separated and joined by fibrous tissue behind the urethral strip at the base of the bladder. The male urethra is a broad mucosal strip on the upturned shortened penis. In the female the urethra is very short and the vaginal opening faces anteriorly just below the bladder neck; two separate bodies constitute the clitoris. The uterus is normal.

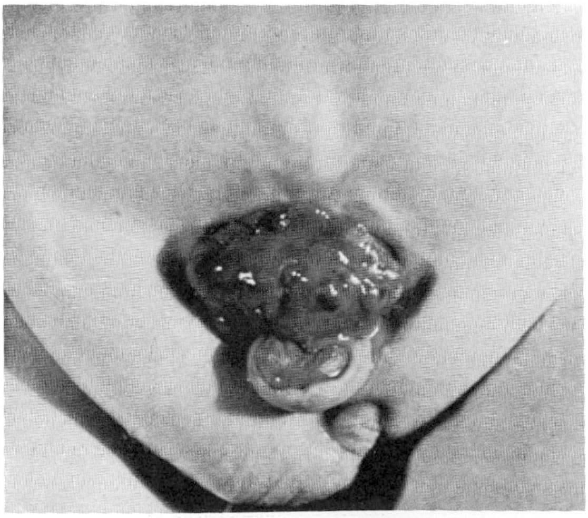

Figure 15–4 Exstrophy of the bladder in a boy 10 years of age. Below the bladder is the dysplastic penis and, below it, the empty scrotum. There is also a right inguinal hernia.

The initial principal clinical problems are urinary incontinence, which leads to excoriation of surrounding tissue, and ulceration of the bladder mucosa. Inguinal and umbilical hernias may also be a problem. Upper tract infection with renal damage is not common. A waddling gait, owing to the abnormalities of the pelvic bones, is usual. Late complications include malignancy of the bladder mucosa in adulthood and difficulty in sexual intercourse, the latter being more of a problem in the male because of the shortened deformed penis. Social problems related to urinary incontinence are also of concern.

Reconstructive therapy designed to allow closure of the bladder and fixation of the pubic ring is the principal goal of surgical treatment. The results are seldom satisfactory. For the first 6 months of life the exposed mucosa should be protected by petrolatum gauze; then reconstructive surgery may be initiated. Some patients with bladder exstrophy have relatively large, flexible bladders which permit reasonable reconstruction; subsequent operations to lengthen the urethra and to prevent vesicoureteral reflux may be required. The majority of patients, however, have small fibrotic bladders which may best be treated by urinary diversion onto the anterior abdominal wall. A urine collection device fastened to the abdominal skin will be required. Reconstruction of the penis and treatment with systemic and/or topical sex hormones may allow development of external genitalia with some semblance of normalcy; unfortunately their capacity to function is in most instances considerably impaired.

Treatment of this serious anomaly requires the skills of orthopedic, plastic and urologic surgeons and of the pediatrician. Furthermore, the impact on the psychosocial development of the child with exstrophy of the bladder and its associated anatomic and functional abnormalities may be profound; attention must be paid to the management of this important aspect of the problem.

HYPOSPADIAS

See Section 18.

POSTERIOR URETHRAL VALVES

Valvular obstruction of the posterior urethra is an important cause of severe urinary obstruction in infants. Since urine formation begins about the twelfth week of gestation, severe irrevocable renal damage owing to this obstruction may be present at birth. The most common type of posterior urethral valve is that in which there is an exaggeration of the normal ridges which extend from the midline dorsal urethral ridge and from the verumontanum to surround the urethra just before the membranous region. The urethra proximal to these valves becomes distended. The bladder wall is trabeculated and thickened, and diverticula may form. Ureteral reflux and hydronephrosis are common. Obstruction to urine flow may be complete or partial.

In most instances the clinical problems are manifest in the first year of life, usually within 3 months after birth. If obstruction is complete, oligohydramnios is common, no urine is passed after birth, and early deterioration is seen. In patients with partial obstruction, failure to thrive, systemic acidosis with renal failure and continuous overflow dribbling rather than a good urinary stream are present. Apart from the problem of renal damage consequent to the obstruction, these children are subject to recurrent urinary infections.

Excretory urography and retrograde cystourethrography are needed to establish the diagnosis. The characteristic proximal ballooning of the urethra is best seen during micturition or attempts to express urine from the bladder. Observation of the infant while he is voiding to note the force of the urinary stream is the most important clinical diagnostic measure.

Early surgical decompression is warranted. A temporary diversionary procedure is recommended, with a definitive operation at a later age to correct the valvular obstruction.

Those presenting in early infancy have more severe obstruction, the extent of renal damage is usually more severe, and the long-term prognosis is only fair. Despite relief of obstruction, the extent of renal parenchymal and ureteric damage is often so severe that irreversible changes have occurred and the prognosis is poor. If the obstruction is less pronounced, the outlook for maintaining renal function sufficient to sustain life is better.

OTHER ANOMALIES OF THE URETHRA

Congenital urethral strictures and *atresia* are rare anomalies. *Distal urethral narrowing* and **meatal stenosis** do occur in both males and females and have been thought to be responsible for recurrent urinary infections, particularly in girls. Narrowing of the distal urethra and meatal stenosis are much less common than some of the urologic literature would lead one to suspect, and care should be taken to avoid overdiagnosis of these conditions. Examination of the urinary stream and a voiding cystourethrogram are helpful in assessing whether these conditions are present and how severe they are.

Acquired meatal stenosis is much more common, especially in males. Here it usually is a complication of a meatal ulcer following circumcision or of diaper dermatitis. Even though the meatus may appear small on physical examination, it is reasonable to assess the strength of the urinary stream and to decide if a significant obstruction is present before recommending surgical correction.

Anterior urethral diverticula or valves and stenosis of the preputial orifice **(phimosis)** may also obstruct urine flow. Acquired phimosis is more common than congenital phimosis and is usually the consequence of ill-advised attempts to retract the infant's foreskin (leading to scarring and stenosis) or of inadequate circumcision.

Bernstein, J.: The morphogenesis of renal parenchymal maldevelopment (renal dysplasia). Pediat. Clin. N. Amer. *18*:395, 1971.

Bernstein, J., and Meyer, R.: Parenchymal maldevelopment of the kidney. *In* McQuarrie, I., (ed.): Brennemann's Practice of Pediatrics. Hagerstown, Md., Harper and Row, 1972, Vol. III, part 2, Chapter 26, pp. 1–30.

Dieker, H., and Opitz, J. M.: Associated sacral and renal malformations. Birth Defects: Original Article Series *5*(No. 3):68, 1969.

Emanuel, B., Nachman, R., Aronson, N., and Weiss, H.: Congenital solitary kidney. Am. J. Dis. Child. *127*:17, 1974.

Feinberg, T., Lattimer, J. K., Jeter, K., Langford, W., and Beck, L.: Questions that worry children with exstrophy. Pediatrics *53*:242, 1974.

Greene, L. F., Feinzaig, W., and Dahlin, D. C.: Multicystic dysplasia of the kidney: With special reference to the contralateral kidney. J. Urol. *105*:482, 1971.

Haslam, R. H. A., Berman, W., and Heller, R. M.: Renal abnormalities in the Russell-Silver syndrome. Pediatrics *51*:216, 1973.

Kanasawa, M., Moller, J., Good, R. A., and Vernier, R. L.: Dwarfed kidneys in children. Am. J. Dis. Child. *109*:130, 1965.

Kissane, J. M.: Congenital malformations. *In* Heptinstall, R. H. (ed.): Pathology of the Kidney. 2nd. ed. Boston, Little, Brown and Company, 1974.

Kissane, J. M.: Development of the kidney. *In* Heptinstall, R. H. (ed.): Pathology of the Kidney. 2nd. ed. Boston, Little, Brown and Company, 1974.

Kohn, G., and Borns, P. F.: The association of bilateral and unilateral renal aplasia in the same family. J. Pediatr. *83*:95, 1973.

Liban, E., and Kozenitsky, I. L.: Metanephric hamartomas and nephroblastomatosis in siblings. Cancer *25*:885, 1970.

Mauer, S. M., Dobrin, R. S., and Vernier, R. L.: Unilateral and bilateral renal agenesis in monoamniotic twins. J. Pediatr. *84*:236, 1974.

Perlman, M., Goldberg, G. M., Bar-Ziv, J., and Danovitch, G.: Renal hamartomas and nephroblastomatosis with fetal gigantism: A familial syndrome. J. Pediatr. *83*:414, 1973.

Pinsky, L.: A community of human malformation syndromes involving the Müllerian ducts, distal extremities, urinary tract, and ears. Teratology *9*:65, 1974.

Rizza, J. M., and Downing, S. E.: Bilateral renal agenesis in two female siblings. Am. J. Dis. Child. *121*:60, 1971.

Rogers, L. W., and Ostrow, P. T.: The prune-belly syndrome. Report of 20 cases and description of a lethal variant. J. Pediatr. *83*:786, 1973.

Rosenfeld, J. B., Cohen, L., Garty, I., and Ben Bassat, M.: Unilateral renal hypoplasia with hypertension (Ask-Upmark kidney). Brit. Med. J. *2*:217, 1973.

Royer, P., Habib, R., Broyer, M., and Nouaille, Y.: Segmental hypoplasia of the kidney in children. Adv. Nephrol. *1*:145, 1971.

Royer, P., Habib, R., Mathieu, H., and Courtecuisse, V.: L'hypoplasie rénale bilatérale avec oligonéphronie. Arch. Franç. Pediatr. *24*:249, 1967.

MISCELLANEOUS CONDITIONS

NEPHROLITHIASIS

(Renal Calculus)

Although renal calculi are less common in children than in adults, they often signal an important underlying disorder for which it may be possible to institute specific therapy. The basic physicochemical events leading to calculus formation are poorly understood, regardless of the underlying disorder.

Nephrolithiasis occurs about twice as frequently in boys as in girls. Renal calculi are more common in some of the developing countries of southeast Asia than in North America. As the standard of living rises, the incidence of calculi appears to decline. The principal causes of nephrolithiasis in children in order of frequency are: (1) urinary infection, notably those associated with stasis; (2) idiopathic; (3) hypercalciuria; (4) cystinuria; and (5) hyperoxaluria (oxalosis).

Cystinuria and oxalosis are uncommon causes of nephrolithiasis in children. They are discussed elsewhere.

Most stones consist principally of calcium oxalate or calcium phosphate, or a mixture of them. Magnesium ammonium calcium phosphate stones occur principally in patients with infections, usually with a urea-splitting organism, especially of the *Proteus* genus. In this situation urinary concentration of ammonia rises as urea is split and the urine becomes alkaline. This favors the precipitation of calculi.

Calculi in *idiopathic nephrolithiasis* usually consist of calcium oxalate; there is no evidence of excessive excretion of any urinary crystalloid. A genetic predisposition to the formation of calcium oxalate stones has been recognized apart from that in patients with hyperoxaluria and hypercalciuria. This condition is probably of polygenic origin and the female appears to be at lesser risk than the male.

It has been suggested that idiopathic hypercalciuria is the result of a primary renal defect in the handling of calcium. Increased intestinal absorption of calcium and secondary hyperparathyroidism have also been observed in some patients. Hypercalciuria occurs in uncontrolled distal renal tubular acidosis, in hypercortisonism or with corticosteroid administration, in hypercalcemia due to a variety of causes and during immobilization for major fractures.

The signs and symptoms of renal calculi include colicky abdominal or flank pain, hematuria, repeated urinary infections, passing of the calculus and, uncommonly, urethral obstruction. When the underlying disorder, e.g., renal tubular acidosis or chronic renal failure owing to oxalosis is present, clinical manifestations of the basic disorder may also be observed.

Evaluation for nephrolithiasis should include: family history; an examination of the urine for red blood cells and for crystals, which may provide a clue to the diagnosis; urine culture; simultaneous determination of urine pH and serum bicarbonate concentration to exclude renal tubular acidosis; determination of blood levels of calcium, phosphorus, alkaline phosphatase and uric acid; chromatographic examination of urine for amino acids; nitroprusside test for cystine; 24-hour urine determination of calcium and oxalic acid excretion; roentgenogram of the abdomen for stones; and chemical analysis of any stones which are passed.

TREATMENT. A high fluid intake should be assured throughout the 24-hour period in order to reduce the concentration of precipitable crystalloids. If there is acute renal colic, an analgesic should be given. Surgical intervention is infrequently warranted, and, given time, the calculus will either pass or be dissolved. Urinary infection, when present, should be treated with appropriate antibacterial drugs.

Specific measures include correction of major

anatomic obstructive lesions; urine acidification with vitamin C, 500 mg q 6 h, and continuous prophylactic antibacterial therapy when calculi are known to be the result of recurrent urinary infection; reduction of calcium intake and administration of hydrochlorothiazide in idiopathic hypercalciuria (oral cellulose phosphate, 5 gm two or three times daily, is effective in adults with this disorder); specific treatment of recognizable causes of hypercalciuria such as renal tubular acidosis; and alkalinization of the urine in patients with cystinuria (penicillamine may also be used).

There is no specific therapy for oxalosis.

HYPERURICEMIC NEPHROPATHY

Although urate and uric acid stones are rare in children, excessive elevation of plasma concentration of uric acid in patients receiving therapy for reticuloendothelial malignancies, sarcomas or acute lymphoblastic leukemia may lead to deposition of uric acid in the renal medullary collecting ducts and cause an obstructive uropathy. Uric acid levels as high as 25-40 mg/dl may occur. Complete anuria is not an uncommon consequence. Fortunately with adequate hydration and alkalinization of the urine by administration of $NaHCO_3$ the precipitated uric acid can usually be dissolved and is excreted. Prophylactic therapy with allopurinol is advised in such patients in order to avoid undue elevation of the plasma uric acid.

Coe, F. L., Canterbury, J. M., Firpo, J. J., and Reiss, E.: Evidence for secondary hyperparathyroidism in idiopathic hypercalciuria. J. Clin. Invest. *52*:134, 1973.

Dent, C. E., and Sutor, D. J.: Presence or absence of inhibitor of calcium-oxalate crystal growth in urine of normals and of stone formers. Lancet *2*:775, 1971.

Passwell, J., Boichis, H., and Cohen, B. E.: Hyperuricemic nephropathy. Am. J. Dis. Child. *120*:154, 1970.

Wenzl, J. E., Burke, E. C., Stickler, G. B., and Utz, D. C.: Nephrolithiasis and nephrocalcinosis in children. Pediatrics *41*:57, 1968.

Williams, H. E.: Nephrolithiasis. New Engl. J. Med. *290*:33, 1974.

RENAL VEIN THROMBOSIS

Thrombosis of the renal vein occurs in two unrelated and distinct contexts in children: in infants as an acute, catastrophic and potentially life-threatening event, and as an associated finding in children with the nephrotic syndrome.

RENAL VEIN THROMBOSIS IN INFANTS

ETIOLOGY. In infancy renal vein thrombosis usually occurs in patients who are already at risk because of conditions such as dehydration, shock, septicemia, cyanotic congenital heart disease, congenital renal anomaly, severe pyelonephritis, or as a consequence of maternal diabetes; infrequently there is no recognized predisposing cause. Three quarters of the patients are less than 1 year of age, and most of these are less than 1 month. Boys and girls are equally affected.

PATHOLOGY AND PATHOGENESIS. The kidney is enlarged, red, tense and friable. Microscopic examination reveals infarction with areas of necrosis. There is interstitial edema and hemorrhage. A thrombus, possibly undergoing organization, obstructs the main renal vein and its branches and may extend into the inferior vena cava. In approximately half the patients thrombosis is bilateral. Thromboses in other organs distant from the kidney are found in about half the patients who die.

The pathogenesis of renal vein thrombosis in infants is probably related to venous stasis secondary to shock, septicemia or dehydration. Fulminant infection of the renal parenchyma may be a factor in initiating the thrombotic process. Thrombocytopenia and extrarenal thrombi suggest that consumptive coagulopathy or disseminated intravascular coagulation may be a feature present in some patients.

CLINICAL MANIFESTATIONS AND COURSE. The sudden appearance in an infant, with one of the predisposing conditions mentioned above, of marked deterioration in the clinical condition, flank mass, oliguria and hematuria is the typical presenting pattern. Fever is not uncommon; edema and hypertension are usually absent. Manifestations of the underlying or predisposing condition are often present. If untreated, the patient's condition usually deteriorates over a period of several days and death ensues.

LABORATORY DATA. Leukocytosis of 12,000-15,000/mm^3 with a shift to the left, thrombocytopenia, moderate azotemia and metabolic acidosis may be present. Radiologic examination reveals an enlarged kidney, which usually does not visualize on intravenous urography. Inferior vena cavagram may demonstrate thrombosis of either or both renal veins and, possibly, thrombosis of the inferior vena cava.

DIFFERENTIAL DIAGNOSIS. The differential diagnosis includes other conditions in which any of the following are present in a seriously ill infant: a flank mass, oliguria or anuria, hematuria and a unilateral nonfunctioning kidney. The clinical conditions to be considered include: renal cortical or papillary necrosis, acute tubular necrosis, unilateral cystic kidney, renal arterial occlusion, renal trauma with perirenal hemorrhage, severe obstructive uropathy, nephroblastoma and neuroblastoma.

PREVENTION. There is no specific means of preventing renal vein thrombosis; however, it may be assumed that correction of the underlying or predisposing illness will diminish the likelihood of its development. Of special importance is the avoidance of dehydration in a seriously ill infant.

TREATMENT. The most important aspect of treatment is correction or management of the underlying disorder. Bacteriologic culture of the blood, urine and cerebrospinal fluid should be obtained if septicemia is suspected, and appropriate antibacterial treatment should be instituted. Rehydration and measures to correct shock are essential. There remains controversy about the value of heparin in renal vein thrombosis, since the above supportive measures may suffice. If there is evidence of thrombocytopenia or other features suggesting widespread intravascular coagulation, the patient may be heparinized with the intent to maintain the clotting time longer than 20 minutes. In the past the diagnosis of renal vein thrombosis was an indication for immediate nephrectomy; however, results with conservative treatment justify a nonsurgical approach, except for bilateral involvement or associated inferior vena caval thrombosis, when a thrombectomy is indicated as soon as the patient's condition permits. Angiography or intravenous urography should be done only when the patient is adequately hydrated and not in shock.

PROGNOSIS. The prognosis depends to a large extent on the severity of the underlying condition and on whether the thrombosis is bilateral. If the patient's general condition and underlying problem can be managed for several days, there is a reasonable possibility of survival. Recovery of renal function on the affected side is then not uncommon; this is a compelling reason to avoid nephrectomy, if at all possible. Renal tubular dysfunction has been reported following recovery from renal vein thrombosis in infancy.

Belman, A. B., Susmano, D. F., Burden, J. J., and Kaplan, G. W.: Nonoperative treatment of unilateral renal vein thrombosis in the newborn. J.A.M.A. *211*:1165, 1970.

Mauer, S. M., Fraley, E. E., Fish, A. J., and Najarian, J. S.: Bilateral renal vein thrombosis in infancy: Report of a survivor following surgical intervention. J. Pediatr. *78*:509, 1971.

Renfield, M. L., and Kraybill, E. N.: Consumptive coagulopathy with renal vein thrombosis. J. Pediatr. *82*:1054, 1973.

Stark, H.: Renal vein thrombosis in infancy: Recovery without nephrectomy. Am. J. Dis. Child. *103*:430, 1964.

RENAL VEIN THROMBOSIS AND THE NEPHROTIC SYNDROME

It is not established whether renal vein thrombosis is the cause or a complication of the nephrotic syndrome. Nor is it understood how renal vein thrombosis in otherwise healthy subjects may lead to the development of the nephrotic syndrome.

The association of renal vein thrombosis and the nephrotic syndrome has been recognized since 1840. The incidence in adults with the nephrotic syndrome is about 5 per cent; a much lower incidence is seen in children.

PATHOLOGY AND PATHOGENESIS. In about one third of patients the thrombosis is bilateral or there is thrombosis of the inferior vena cava. Thromboses at extrarenal sites are not uncommon. The affected kidney is initially enlarged, tense and congested; subsequently fibrosis may lead to contraction and reduction in mass. A number of specific entities known to cause the nephrotic syndrome have been associated with renal vein thrombosis; their specific features are detectable in the kidney whose renal vein is thrombosed as well as in the uninvolved kidney. These include membranous nephropathy, congenital nephrosis, minimal lesion nephrotic syndrome, focal glomerulosclerosis and amyloidosis. The specific features of renal vein thrombosis are superimposed on the changes seen in these conditions and include interstitial edema and congestion, with foci of polymorphonuclear and round cell infiltration, interstitial fibrosis, tubular atrophy, margination of polymorphonuclear leukocytes in capillary lumina, glomerular capillary loop ectasia with stasis of blood and microthrombi.

The pathogenesis of renal vein thrombosis and its relation to the nephrotic syndrome are poorly understood. In view of the heterogeneity of the nephrotic disorders in which renal vein thrombosis may occur, it is reasonable to assume that in most instances the thrombosis is a complication of the nephrotic syndrome rather than its cause. Furthermore, there is a tendency for both arterial and venous thromboses in patients with the nephrotic syndrome, and extrarenal thromboses are not less common than renal vein thrombosis. This propensity to thromboembolic phenomena in nephrotic patients may be due to a hypercoagulable state, i.e., an increase in certain of the clotting factors and thrombocytosis, and possibly may be accentuated by corticosteroid or diuretic therapy or by bed rest. The alternate possibility remains that renal vein thrombosis may be a cause of the nephrotic syndrome by the release of host renal antigen, which in turn is responsible for the development of immune complex membranous nephropathy.

CLINICAL MANIFESTATIONS AND COURSE. Renal vein thrombosis may be clinically silent in a nephrotic patient. More commonly there are symptoms of low back or flank pain. The affected kidney may be tender and slightly enlarged. If there is bilateral involvement or inferior vena caval obstruction there may be a drastic worsening in the clinical state with increasing edema of the lower extremities. Hypertension is not uncommon and may develop in a previously normotensive nephrotic patient. The acute phase is influenced by whether there is bilateral renal vein and/or inferior vena caval involvement, which increases the morbidity and mortality considerably. The ultimate course is mainly dependent on the nature of the underlying disorder.

LABORATORY DATA. There are no specific laboratory manifestations of renal vein thrombosis. Microscopic or gross hematuria may develop, and the urinary excretion of protein may increase. Radiographic study reveals a slightly enlarged kidney with less function than on the uninvolved side. Inferior vena cavagram may reveal thrombosis of the inferior vena cava or a clot extending into its lumen from the affected vein. Absence of normal venous blood flow from the affected side may also be seen. Renal biopsy may, in addition to providing confirmatory evidence for the diagnosis, give information concerning the basic glomerular pathology.

PREVENTION. Appropriate treatment of the nephrotic syndrome with a view to reducing the protein excretion to normal, and measures designed to reduce the relapse rate, may reasonably be expected to decrease the incidence of renal vein thrombosis.

TREATMENT. Anticoagulation with heparin is the generally accepted therapy for renal vein thrombosis. Some advocate thrombectomy in addition to anticoagulation; it appears to be particularly important when there is bilateral and/or inferior vena caval involvement. There is no particular reason to discontinue whatever therapy of the nephrotic syndrome was being given prior to development of thrombosis, but aggressive antidiuretic therapy should be stopped.

PROGNOSIS. The prognosis of treated unilateral renal vein thrombosis is good, particularly if measures to treat the nephrotic syndrome itself are successful. With bilateral or inferior vena caval involvement the prognosis is much worse, although early diagnosis, surgical intervention and anticoagulation therapy increase the survival rate. The long-term prognosis is influenced by the nature of the primary renal disease.

Duffy, J. L., Letteri, J., Cinque, T., Hsu, P. P., Molho, L., and Churg, J.: Renal vein thrombosis and the nephrotic syndrome. Am. J. Med. *54*:663, 1973.

Kendall, A. G., Lohman, R. C., and Dossetor, J. B.: Nephrotic syndrome: A hypercoagulable state. Arch. Intern. Med. *127*:1021, 1971.

Lieberman, E., Heuser, E., Gilchrist, G. S., et al.: Thrombosis, nephrosis, and corticosteroid therapy. J. Pediatr. *73*:320, 1968.

Moore, H. L., Katz, R., McIntosh, R., Smith, F., Michael, A. F., and Vernier, R. L.: Unilateral renal vein thrombosis and the nephrotic syndrome. Pediatrics *50*:598, 1972.

Schwartz, M. M., and Lewis, E. J.: Immunopathology of the nephrotic syndrome associated with renal vein thrombosis. Am. J. Med. *54*:528, 1973.

VIRAL CYSTITIS

(Acute Hemorrhagic Cystitis)

Acute hemorrhagic cystitis of viral etiology is a self-limited benign disease which is most common in school-age males. There is evidence that adenovirus types 11 and 21 may be causative in some patients. The symptoms are those of acute cystitis of bacterial origin. The most common presenting complaint is sudden onset of gross hematuria. Microscopic examination of the urine reveals numerous red and white blood cells. Urine culture is negative. The usual duration of symptoms and hematuria is about 4 days.

Mufson, M. A., Belshe, R. B., Horrigan, T. J., and Zollar, L. M.: Cause of acute hemorrhagic cystitis in children. Am. J. Dis. Child. *126*:605, 1973.

Numazaki, Y., Kumasaka, T., Yano, N., Yamanaka, M., Miyazawa, T., Takai, S., and Ishida, N.: Further study on acute hemorrhagic cystitis due to adenovirus Type 11. New Engl. J. Med. *289*:344, 1973.

TRAUMA TO THE URINARY TRACT

KIDNEY

The most common causes of renal injury are participation in sports and automobile accidents. In the latter, multiple injuries involving head, chest, limbs and other abdominal organs may temporarily direct attention away from renal trauma. Gross hematuria is the most frequent manifestation; clots in the renal pelvis and ureter may cause renal colic, and there may be oliguria as a result of obstruction. Intravenous urography should be done as soon as possible; this may demonstrate the site of injury, extravasation of contrast medium into the perirenal region, clots in the renal pelvis or ureteral obstruction, or there may be nonvisualization of a pole of the kidney. Delay in carrying out the intravenous urogram can be dangerous because, if there is continued renal bleeding, it is critical to know the site and extent of injury. Renal isotope scan and arteriography may also be useful, particularly if there is nonvisualization of the kidney on the urogram.

In most instances a conservative approach is warranted. Attention should be given to the replacement of blood loss and to recognition and treatment of infection and obstruction. Indications for exploring a renal injury are limited mainly to rapid deterioration from extensive loss of blood or to removal of an infected hematoma. The extravasation of urine from the kidney into the surrounding area is itself a matter of little consequence. A progressive increase in the size of a perinephric hematoma may be an indication for surgical drainage, particularly if it causes displacement of the kidney. The incidence of nephrectomy should be less than 4 per cent. Hypertension is an important complication; it occurs in about 15 per cent of patients and may be manifest in the immediate days or weeks following trauma or may not appear until several months to years later.

Minor renal trauma may cause hematuria in children with underlying developmental abnormalities of the urinary tract, in particular in those who have obstructive uropathy with hydronephrosis.

BLADDER AND URETHRA

Rupture of the bladder is a relatively common complication of a fractured pelvis; about 10 per cent of patients with a ruptured bladder have an associated tear of the posterior urethra.

Rupture of the urethra can be suspected if there is failure to pass urine and if there is blood at the urethral meatus. Introduction of a urethral catheter in such patients can aggravate the urethral tear, which in posterior urethral rupture is often only partial. Instead of immediately inserting a catheter in an attempt to drain the bladder, observation for 12 to 24 hours is recommended to determine whether the bladder will distend or the patient will void spontaneously. If the latter occurs, there is the possibility of spontaneous repair.

Insertion of a catheter in suspected cases of urethral rupture increases the possibility of introducing infection and may sever a residual strand of mucosal tissue bridging the margins of the tear. If the bladder distends, suprapubic drainage can be instituted. After several weeks the urethra can be inspected by an experienced endoscopist to determine the site of urethral rupture. An important and often late complication is a urethral stricture. Foreign body reaction and infection caused by an indwelling catheter increase the likelihood of late urethral structure.

Mitchell, J. P.: Trauma to the urinary tract. New Engl. J. Med. *288*:90, 1973.

NEUROGENIC BLADDER

Neurogenic bladder is an important and complex problem; the most common cause in children is myelomeningocele, which occurs in approximately 3 of every 1000 births. The size and site of the spinal defect bears little relation to the disorder of the urinary tract, except that cranial, cervical and thoracic lesions are less likely to be associated with bladder dysfunction than are lumbar or sacral defects.

Bladder dysfunction secondary to upper motor neuron lesions is characterized by spasticity, involuntary contractions, trabeculation, small capacity and initiation of urination by reflex stimulation. The neurogenic bladder in disturbances of lower motor neurons, such as poliomyelitis, tends to be smooth walled and have a large capacity. Anal tone is lax. Such bladders are flaccid and without sensation, and there is usually a large residuum of urine. A mixed upper and lower motor neuron pattern is seen in children with myelomeningocele. There is usually distention of the bladder with continuous overflow dribbling. Urinary infection and vesicoureteral reflux are relatively common.

Diversionary procedures to channel urine to an ileal loop or cutaneous ureterostomy have been used to prevent damage to the upper urinary tract and kidney from back pressure. Recently regular catheterization with a clean stainless steel catheter has been found effective in enabling a good degree of urinary continence without infection of the bladder and in avoiding development of upper tract damage. For this purpose an artificial perineal urethra is created in boys. Since there is usually absence of sensation in this region, the technique is not unpleasant or painful.

ENURESIS

(See also Section 2.)

Enuresis or involuntary emptying of the bladder beyond the age when bladder control should have been established may be nocturnal or diurnal; the former is the more common. Nocturnal enuresis is present in about 10 to 15 per cent of otherwise normal 5 year old children and in about 1 per cent of normal 15 year old ones. It is slightly more common in boys. There is a familial tendency. Nocturnal enuresis usually has no organic basis and is due to delayed maturation of bladder control or to emotional factors. Separation from the family, death of a parent and birth of a sibling are examples of events which may precipitate nocturnal enuresis in a previously continent child.

Organic disorders which may cause nocturnal enuresis include nocturnal epilepsy, urinary tract infection, increased urinary volume in diabetes mellitus, diabetes insipidus, obstructive uropathy and chronic renal failure and other conditions in which the ability to concentrate urine is impaired. Appropriate tests to exclude organic causes of enuresis should be carried out.

The initial examination of the child with nocturnal enuresis should include an evaluation of possible psychogenic factors, a complete physical examination, routine urinalysis and measurement of the urine specific gravity after an overnight fast. If there is reason to suspect an underlying organic disorder, appropriate blood and urine studies should be carried out, including an intravenous urogram. These studies are warranted in a minority of patients with nocturnal enuresis.

A number of schemes for dealing with nocturnal enuresis not associated with organic disease have been devised. The important point to remember is that in the final analysis the condition is benign and self-limited, and steps should be taken to eliminate the emotional impact of this problem on the child. The following are a few simple guidelines for the management of the child with nocturnal enuresis: (1) avoid ingestion of fluids after supper; (2) void before retiring; (3) rouse the child to void before the mother retires; (4) counsel the parents to avoid emotional reaction in regard to whether the child does or does not wet the bed on a given night (there must be no shame or guilt associated with enuresis; it would seem that the more the child wishes to be dry the more likely he is to fail; a matter-of-fact attitude toward success or failure should be adopted); and (5) drug therapy should not be considered in children under 6 years of age and should not be continued beyond 8 weeks.

Imipramine for enuresis. The Medical Letter *16*(No. 5):22, 1974.
Marshall, S., Marshall, H. H., and Lyon, R. P.: Enuresis: An analysis of various therapeutic approaches. Pediatrics *52*:813, 1973.

RENOVASCULAR HYPERTENSION

Unilateral renal ischemia is a well recognized cause of systemic hypertension. Although the pathogenesis of the elevated blood pressure is complex, the principal mechanism appears to involve the renal angiotensin system. *Congenital stenosis of a renal artery* or one of its branches is a rare cause of hypertension in childhood. Renal ischemia leading to renovascular hypertension is usually acquired, occurring for example following renal trauma, when the renal artery is constricted. Narrowing of the renal artery may occur in neurofibromatosis and result in hypertension.

Unilateral developmental or acquired renal parenchymal lesions are a more frequent cause of hypertension than are disorders of the renal artery or one of its branches. The pathogenesis of hypertension in these lesions probably also involves the renin angiotensin system, but it is often difficult to substantiate this even by differential determinations of renin in blood from the renal veins.

When renovascular hypertension is suspected, a rapid sequence intravenous pyelogram should be obtained. An isotope scan using technetium-99 may be helpful in demonstrating a reduction in blood supply to one of the kidneys. Renal angiography is required for visualization of the renal vasculature to determine the site of a renal arterial constriction or lesion.

Comparison of the renin concentrations in the renal vein of each kidney should be obtained when a unilateral lesion is suspected. In children the most reliable way of establishing a renal arterial lesion responsible for hypertension is angiography.

Selection of therapy is influenced by the nature of the problem. Conservative management with antihypertensive medication should be tried initially; a combination of hydralazine, hydrochlorothiazide and propranolol is often effective. If there is unequivocal localized arterial narrowing, reconstructive vascular surgery, or resection of the renal segment supplied by a narrowed subdivision of the main artery, may be carried out. Nephrectomy is seldom indicated and, in any event, should not be done unless it has been demonstrated that control of the hypertension is not possible with antihypertensive medications.

See also Figure 5-5 and discussion of hypertension in Section 13.

TABLE 15-14 NEPHROTOXIC COMPOUNDS*†

Nephrotic syndrome

- Gold salts
- Mercurial diuretics
- Miscellaneous compounds containing mercury
- Paramethadione
- Penicillamine
- Perchlorate
- Probenecid
- Tolbutamide
- Trimethadione

Nephrogenic diabetes insipidus

- Amphotericin B
- Demeclocycline
- Lithium carbonate
- Methoxyflurane
- Propoxyphene

Fanconi syndrome

- Cadmium
- Lead
- Lysol
- Mercury
- Nitrobenzene
- Outdated tetracycline
- Salicylate
- Uranium

Interstitial nephritis with or without papillary necrosis

- Amidopyrine
- Bunamiodyl (papillary necrosis only)
- p-Aminosalicylate
- Penicillins (especially methicillin)
- Phenacetin
- Phenylbutazone
- Salicylate
- Sulfonamides

Renal vasculitis with or without glomerular capillary involvement

- Hydralazine
- Isoniazid
- Sulfonamides
- Any of the numerous other drugs which may cause a hypersensitivity reaction

Nephrocalcinosis or nephrolithiasis

- Allopurinol
- Ethylene glycol
- Methoxyflurane

Miscellaneous renal manifestations including proteinuria, hematuria, oliguria, tubular necrosis and renal failure

- Arsenic
- Bacitracin
- Cadmium
- Carbon tetrachloride
- Cephaloridine
- Cephalothin
- Colistin
- Copper
- Ethylene glycol
- Gentamicin
- Gold salts
- Iron
- Kanamycin
- Mercury
- Neomycin
- Pentamidine
- Polymyxin B
- Streptomycin
- Sulfonamides
- Tetrachlorethylene
- Vancomycin
- Viomycin

*Dr. Sean O'Regan assisted in the preparation of this table.

†The agents are grouped according to the principal site of injury or manifestation.

TOXIC NEPHROPATHY

A wide variety of compounds may damage the kidney. In many instances the damage is transient and reversible if exposure to the noxious agent is stopped. Table 15–14 lists the most common nephrotoxins, grouped according to the principal site of injury or the clinical picture they induce. For a more exhaustive list of agents which are potentially damaging to the kidney the reader is referred to the references at the end of this section. In addition, Table 15–11, which lists drugs whose dosages should be modified in children with reduced renal function, and Table 15–6, which lists the causes of renal tubular acidosis, should be consulted.

Kovnat, P., Labovitz, E., and Levinson, S.: Antibiotics and the kidney. Med. Clin. N. Amer. 57:1045, 1973.
Schreiner, G. E.: Toxic nephropathy due to drugs, solvents and metals. Progr. Biochem. Pharmacol. 7:248, 1972.

TUMORS OF THE KIDNEY AND URINARY TRACT

See Section 25.

16
METABOLIC DISORDERS

DIABETES MELLITUS

Diabetes mellitus is a common disorder of energy metabolism which results from an absolute or functional deficiency of insulin. Insulin deficiency leads to impairment of glucose transport, to a decrease in storage and synthesis of lipid, and to a decrease in synthesis of protein. These biochemical alterations lead to specific acute and chronic clinical features.

INCIDENCE. Diabetes mellitus occurs in all races and in all geographic areas. Its geographic prevalence varies widely, in some measure in relation to differences in gene frequencies, but likely more in relation to nutritional and other environmental factors. Epidemiologic studies are in general agreement that about 1 per cent of adults in the United States are known to have diabetes, and that a comparable number, as may be determined by screening procedures, have asymptomatic carbohydrate intolerance, or "chemical diabetes." The prevalence of diabetes increases with age and body weight. Diabetes occurs in approximately 1 of 2500 children under 15 years of age and 1 of 1000 school-age children, with no sex preference. It is very uncommon in infancy. The prevalence of known diabetes increases from 8 per 1000 adults in the age range from 25 to 44 years to over 60 per 1000 in those over 60 years of age. About 4 per cent of persons known to have diabetes have had the onset of clinical features before they were 15 years of age. The frequency with which children may have asymptomatic chemical diabetes is not known, but it is probably less common than in adults. Screening of siblings with diabetes has disclosed that 12 to 25 per cent have asymptomatic carbohydrate intolerance. Diabetes ranks eighth as a cause of death in the United States. It is probably the most common serious endocrine problem occurring in children.

GENETICS. There is overwhelming evidence that most cases of diabetes mellitus are genetically determined. The mode of genetic transmission, however, is still uncertain, as there is no specific genetic marker. It is probable that hyperglycemia is many steps removed from the primary genetic abnormality, and it may be that patients with diabetes mellitus do not represent a homogeneous genetic disorder, but rather a group of diseases sharing insulin deficiency and hyperglycemia. If the latter is the case, it is not surprising that the results of genetic studies do not permit clear mendelian interpretation.

Autosomal recessive transmission has been most frequently proposed, in which case one would anticipate the eventual development of diabetes in 100 per cent of children of two diabetic parents and of identical twins of diabetics. Cooke et al. found overt diabetes in only 4.4 per cent of children of two diabetic parents, and felt that only 25 per cent would eventually become diabetic. On the other hand, Kahn et al., after serial testing of a large group of offspring of two diabetic parents, found that 8.8 per cent had overt diabetes and that 45 per cent of those with normal body weight and 62 per cent with obesity had chemical diabetes. Given the rate of appearance of chemical diabetes in these children, they predicted that 100 per cent would eventually develop carbohydrate intolerance.

Twin studies may be similarly interpreted. Using an abnormal glucose tolerance test as the diagnostic criterion, White found a 48 per cent concordance for overt diabetes in identical twins, in contrast to 2 per cent in nonidentical twins. Then-Berg found 65 per cent concordance in monozygotic twins, 22 per cent in dizygotic twins. When only monozygotic twins over 43 years of age are considered, the concordance rises to almost 100 per cent. Notwithstanding such studies indicating that in some families diabetes seems to follow simple autosomal recessive transmission, some have suggested that diabetes is best explained on a multifactorial or polygenic basis. It is proposed that there are several genes that may affect carbohydrate metabolism and that an accumulation or association of genetic defects would lead to increasing biochemical and clinical alterations. The expression of these genetic disturbances is proposed to be greatly influenced by a variety of environmental factors, such as diet, body weight, emotional stress, and so forth.

The need for a genetic understanding of diabetes cannot be overemphasized. The discovery of a genetic marker is a requirement for the success of any future program of prevention or successful interruption of progression of diabetes prior to the onset of the earliest clinical abnormalities.

DIAGNOSIS. In diabetes energy metabolism is affected in a variety of ways, but the diagnosis continues to rest upon definition of an abnormality in metabolism of glucose. Although it presents a number of problems, the oral glucose tolerance test (GTT) remains the best single diagnostic criterion. The use of the GTT in large surveys does not divide normal people sharply into two distinctly different groups, one "normal" and the other "diabetic or prediabetic"; consequently, statistical criteria must be invoked to define abnormal responses.

Several slightly different diagnostic criteria have been proposed, all based on studies of adult populations. Table 16–1 compares the criteria of Mosenthal and Barry, of Fajans and Conn, and of the United States Public Health Service. Danowski has recommended that the results of the GTT be expressed as a single value derived from summing the individual points in the curves.

It is probable that criteria for interpretation of the GTT in adults are not entirely applicable to children. The few studies carried out on normal children are summarized in Table 16–2. Variables that must be considered in the interpretation of the results include the size and route of glucose administration, type of blood specimen examined (venous or capillary; whole blood, plasma, or serum), and method of assay for glucose. The dose of glucose most commonly used in children is 1.75 gm/kg, with a maximum dose of 100 gm. Slightly higher glucose loads (2.5 gm/kg) have generally been used in children under 3 years of age. In the study of obese children some investigators have used a dose of glucose calculated for ideal rather than actual body weight.

The glucose load is generally administered as a 20 per cent aqueous solution. This occasionally results in nausea and vomiting. Carbonated glucose loads (such as Glucola) have greater acceptability and have become popular. It is usually recommended that 75 gm of glucose in carbonated solution be considered equivalent to 100 gm in aqueous solution. Glucose concentrations in plasma and serum are essentially identical. The concentration of glucose in whole blood is lower than that in plasma, however, owing to the "dead space" contributed by red blood cell membranes. For normal hematocrit levels, the glucose concentration in plasma is about 14 per cent higher than that in whole blood. There is little difference between concentrations of glucose in capillary and in venous whole blood in measurements made in fasting subjects, but from 1/2 to 2 hr after glucose loading the capillary concentration is higher, by a variable amount (10 to 30 mg/dl).

The most specific and precise technique in general use for determination of glucose concentration in biologic fluids is the glucose-oxidase method, which measures true glucose concentration. This method does not lend itself to automation. The use in an AutoAnalyzer of the Somogyi-Nelson filtrate, with copper, ferricyanide or toluidine reagents will usually yield results which are 5 to 10 mg/dl higher than true glucose concentration.

The glucose tolerance test is rarely necessary for diagnosis of diabetes in the child. The finding of glucosuria and hyperglycemia (glucose concentrations over 120 mg/dl fasting or over 160 mg/dl 2 hr postprandial) should establish a diagnosis of diabetes mellitus if other diabetogenic conditions can be ruled out. Factors which may adversely affect glucose utilization include acute and chronic illness, starvation, excess of growth hormone, administration of cortisone, epinephrine or glucagon, and liver disease or uremia. Acute stress, such as fever, trauma, surgery, encephalitis or psychologic factors, may produce transient carbohydrate intolerance. Patients who have displayed glucosuria and hyperglycemia under such circumstances should be followed with serial glucose tolerance tests to ascertain whether chemical diabetes may be present. Some investigators recommend high carbohydrate intake for 3 days prior to studies of glucose tolerance. In well children we have found it unnecessary to alter the usual dietary pattern.

STAGES OF DIABETES. Among patients with diabetes the degree of impairment of carbohydrate metabolism may vary greatly, as it also may within the same patient under varying circumstances. Patients may be broadly categorized as prediabetic, as having chemical diabetes or as having overt diabetes. It has long been generally held that carbohydrate intolerance is invariably progressive in children and that children have overt diabetes only. Recent studies indicate that neither of these concepts is true; in children, as in adults, carbohydrate intolerance may for years remain static at the chemical diabetes level or may slowly or rapidly progress to overt diabetes.

TABLE 16–1 COMPARISON OF CRITERIA FOR AN ABNORMAL ORAL GLUCOSE TOLERANCE TEST*

SAMPLE	MOSENTHAL AND BARRY, (100 gm†)	FAJANS AND CONN (1.75 gm/kg†)	EIGHT CONSULTANTS TO U.S. PUBLIC HEALTH SERVICE, (100 gm†)	
Fasting			110	(1 point)
1 hour (or maximum value)	150	160	170	(1/2 point)
1 1/2 hours		140		
2 hours	100	120	120	(1/2 point)
3 hours			110	(1 point)
Criteria for abnormal test	Greater than both values	Equal to or higher than all three values	Equal to or higher than at least three values, or equal to or higher than fasting and 3-hour values, or a total of 2 points	

*Whole blood values by a "true sugar" method, as mg/dl.
†Dosage of oral glucose.

TABLE 16-2 ORAL GLUCOSE TOLERANCE TESTS IN NORMAL CHILDREN

INVESTIGATOR		PICKENS ET AL.		COLE		DRASH		ROSENBLOOM	
Age group		1–14 yr		0–12 yr		4–16 yr		1½–12 yr	
Number		200		159		55		54	
Fluid		Capillary whole blood		Capillary whole blood		Capillary whole blood		Venous plasma	
Method		Somogyi–Nelson		Auto Analyzer		Glucose oxidase		Auto Analyzer	
Glucose load		1.75 gm/kg		variable		1.75 gm/kg		1.75 gm/kg	
		X	+2 SD	X	+2 SD	X	+2 SD	X	+2 SD
Time	0	82*	110	72	83	78	112	86	104
(min.)	30	135	193	119	160	138	208	143	204
	60	112	170	108	149	121	189	113	157
	120	101	141	94	130	101	150	102	134
	180	84	124	76	105	75	118	83	119
	240	–	–	–	–	77	110	80	107

*Glucose in mg/dl. X = mean; SD = standard deviation.

Prediabetes. Theoretically all persons who eventually develop diabetes pass through a prediabetic stage between onset of or commitment to diabetes and its overt manifestations. Identical twins of patients with diabetes, or offspring of two diabetic parents, can be specifically assigned to this diagnostic category if we assume that diabetes is transmitted as an autosomal recessive condition. In all other cases it is a retrospective diagnosis. Glucose intolerance is not present at this stage, and there are no other specifically identifiable diagnostic abnormalities. On the other hand, examination of blood vessels in muscle biopsies has been reported to show an elevated incidence of hypertrophy of basement membrane in patients with overt or chemical diabetes, and in biochemically normal close relatives of diabetic persons. These observations suggest either that the microangiopathic changes characteristic of diabetes may be a basic genetic expression of the disease or that there are biochemical alterations antedating glucose intolerance which can induce vascular damage. Elevation of the concentration of free fatty acids (FFA) in blood has been observed by some investigators in the prediabetic and subclinical diabetic stages. This observation has no diagnostic usefulness but may be of some importance in understanding the progression of the disease.

Chemical Disorders

Subclinical Diabetes. In subclinical diabetes the response to the usual glucose tolerance test is normal, but that to a glucose tolerance test carried out with the patient receiving cortisone is abnormal. The implication is that stress is a factor in the emergence of clinical diabetes. This interpretation is supported by the finding that temporary glucose intolerance is associated with physical trauma, emotional stress, infection and pregnancy in persons with subclinical diabetes. Women who develop mild glucose intolerance during pregnancy frequently give birth to unexpectedly large babies which have the clinical features of infants of mothers with overt diabetes. The cortisone-glucose tolerance test has not been adequately evaluated for its diagnostic or prognostic value in children.

Latent Diabetes. The patient with latent diabetes is asymptomatic and may have a normal fasting blood glucose concentration; but there are postprandial hyperglycemia and a clearly abnormal glucose tolerance test. The widespread use of the multichanneled AutoAnalyzer has detected many such patients who were being medically evaluated for other reasons.

The identification of children with chemical diabetes is an important initial step in the development of a better understanding of the relationship between mild carbohydrate intolerance, overt diabetes and the development of vascular "complications." To attempt to identify children with chemical diabetes through widespread glucose tolerance testing of healthy populations is obviously inappropriate; but screening of close relatives of diabetic patients can be expected to result in the detection of individuals with carbohydrate intolerance. From 15 to 35 per cent of siblings of diabetic children who require insulin have been reported to have chemical diabetes. Overt diabetes is reported to occur in 3 to 9 per cent of siblings of diabetics. The difference between the incidences of chemical and of overt diabetes in siblings of diabetic patients indicates that for possibly as many as 60 per cent of such patients the stage of chemical diabetes is a relatively stable one rather than leading rapidly to more severe carbohydrate intolerance.

Overt Diabetes. In overt diabetes fasting and postprandial hyperglycemia are regularly present. Characteristic symptoms occur, and therapeutic intervention is needed to prevent further metabolic decompensation. We and others have found that at the time of onset of clinical diabetes the following conditions are to be expected: basal plasma insulin levels are significantly below normal, but insulin is present; the response of endogenous insulin to the administration of glucose, tolbutamide, glucagon or arginine is extremely blunted when compared with the responses of normal children or of adults; the rates of disposal of glucose are prolonged; the concentrations of all lipid fractions in serum are usually elevated, including those of total lipids, triglycerides, cholesterol, cholesterol esters, phospholipids and free fatty acids

(FFA); lipoprotein electrophoresis is regularly abnormal in those children with ketosis; and increases in the concentrations of both beta and prebeta lipoprotein are common. In our experience the concentration of alpha lipoprotein is also increased. Less frequently, chylomicra are detected. These lipid abnormalities are regularly reversible to within the normal range with a few weeks on adequate doses of insulin. Basal levels of growth hormones in serum are within normal limits; elevation of growth hormone levels after provocative stimulation, or random variation as determined by frequent sampling over a 24-hr period, has been reported to be excessive. Cortisol production rates are normal in diabetic children without acidosis, but are elevated in those with severe acidosis or coma. Serum osmolality may be moderately to markedly elevated, owing principally to glucose, but hypernatremia may also be a factor. An appreciation of the hyperosmolar component is important in the initial parenteral fluid therapy of children with diabetic acidosis.

PATHOGENESIS. Diabetes mellitus occurs when there is a functional deficiency in circulating insulin. This may occur through several distinctly different mechanisms. The traditional view is that it results from a deficiency of synthesis and/or release of insulin from the beta cells of the pancreas, in which case the concentration of insulin in the peripheral circulation would be zero or low, and the usual response to challenge with insulinogenic agents would be absent or grossly blunted. This is precisely the situation in the child with symptomatic diabetes. In adult diabetics, however, or in children with chemical diabetes, insulin levels may be higher and the responses to stimulation may be greater than normal. There are three possible explanations:

Defective Insulin Molecule Concept. O'Brien has proposed that certain forms of diabetes may result from the production of a biologically defective insulin molecule. Such a molecule would be detected by immunoassay as "insulin" but have decreased biologic activity. The discovery of proinsulin, the naturally occurring, immediate precursor of insulin, may fit into this concept. Proinsulin, a single-stranded, cross-linked polypeptide, is found in the general circulation of normal subjects in very minimal concentration or not at all. It is found in increased concentration in obesity and in some cases of islet cell adenoma. Proinsulin is measured along with insulin by current immunoassay techniques, but probably has less than 20 per cent of the biologic activity of insulin itself. Studies to date do not suggest that the "hyperinsulinism" commonly seen in maturity-onset diabetes can be explained on the basis of large amounts of proinsulin in the circulation.

Sluggish Insulin Release Concept. In the normal individual the ingestion or injection of insulinogenic compounds such as glucose, sulfonylurea compounds, amino acids or glucagon leads very rapidly to release of insulin from the pancreas. There is evidence that in patients with maturity onset type of diabetes, a basic defect is an impairment in insulin release following glucose challenge, which allows the concentration of glucose to rise more rapidly and to higher levels than normal. This may secondarily be followed by excessive insulin release, which may explain the reactive hypoglycemia seen not uncommonly in the early phase of maturity-onset diabetes.

Insulin Resistance Concept. In acromegaly, in Cushing syndrome and in patients with pheochromocytoma, specific hormones, elaborated in excess, effectively antagonize the action of insulin at one or several biochemical sites. Most patients with diabetes have no clinically apparent features that suggest excesses of hormone antagonists to insulin, but the possibility that subtle increases in pituitary or adrenal hormones may be involved in the etiology of diabetes cannot be completely eliminated at this time. Growth hormone (GH) continues to be of special interest in this regard. Growth hormone levels are frequently elevated in overt diabetes, particularly in juvenile diabetics under poor control. There is conflicting evidence on GH levels in asymptomatic chemical diabetics. Our studies of chemical diabetes in children indicated normal growth hormone levels both in the basal state and following stimulation.

Other factors that may effectively interfere with the action of insulin at the cell membrane include a material extracted by Vallance-Owen from serum of diabetics, which antagonizes insulin action in vitro and is known as synalbumin. It is considered by some as a specific genetic marker for diabetes; others feel that the antagonist is an artifact of extraction.

A highly specialized form of insulin antagonism occurs in patients with lipoatrophic diabetes. The antagonist, the so-called lipid mobilizing factor, is probably either pituitary or hypothalamic in origin.

In obesity, which is commonly associated with hyperinsulinism and frequently with carbohydrate intolerance, insulin resistance probably results from an increase in adipose tissue mass, as well as from enlargement of individual adipocytes. Weight reduction frequently leads to improvement in tolerance for carbohydrate and to reduction in insulin concentration. Several investigators, studying both lean and obese subjects, have provided evidence that the primary defect in many patients with mild diabetes is peripheral resistance to the action of insulin. Such patients frequently have circulating insulin levels appreciably higher than normal. A further connection between hyperinsulinism and progressive carbohydrate intolerance may be seen in the fact that children of normal weight, whose mild, asymptomatic chemical diabetes has been detected by surveys of diabetic families, have hyperinsulinemic responses to glucose challenge. As such children become overtly diabetic, their insulin response mechanism eventually fails completely. Also, obese children who have marked hyperinsulinism become less capable of maintaining high insulin output as carbohydrate intolerance progresses.

Diabetes is reported to be more common in children who have had congenital rubella. Pancreatitis may rarely result in diabetes, specific examples occurring occasionally in mumps. Diabetes may be a late complication of cystic fibrosis. Levels of antibodies to coxsackievirus B have been reported to be elevated in children with recently diagnosed diabetes. The question of autoimmunity in the etiology of diabetes has not been adequately assessed. Diabetes occurs in increased incidence with such "autoimmune" endocrine diseases as Hashimoto's thyroiditis and Addison's disease. Antibodies to thyroid, adrenal and gastric tissues are found in approximately 15 per cent of children with diabetes mellitus and are found in increased incidence and titers in families of such children. Antibodies to insulin, which are found regularly after a few weeks of exogenous insulin therapy, have not been reported in new diabetics, but the possibility that antibodies to islet cell tissue may lead to inflammation and eventual destruction of islet cells has not been excluded.

PATHOPHYSIOLOGY. The classic clinical features of diabetes mellitus in the child include polyuria, polydipsia, polyphagia and weight loss, which directly reflect a declining capacity to synthesize and release insulin in response to ingestion of food. The rate of progression of the symptoms varies with the rate of decline in the response of the beta cell to stimulation. Increased demands for insulin, such as occur with intercurrent infections, emotional stress, trauma, pregnancy and obesity, will "uncover" the diabetic diathesis somewhat earlier than might otherwise have occurred.

In maturity-onset diabetes either moderate deficiency of biologically effective insulin or a delay of insulin release will result in carbohydrate intolerance as evidence of impairment of peripheral uptake of glucose. Ketosis is not a problem because the quantity of circulating insulin is adequate to inhibit excessive fat mobilization. In the child with diabetes, on the other hand, the biochemical alterations stem from a more complete deficiency of insulin. Marked insulin deficiency produces a metabolic state similar to that of starvation. There are: (1) decreased synthesis of protein, lipid and glycogen; (2) inhibition of peripheral glucose uptake; (3) reversal of the glycolytic pathway, with active hepatic production of glucose from amino acids despite the presence of hyperglycemia; (4) active mobilization of fats from adipose tissue, leading to marked elevations in the concentration of total lipids, cholesterol, triglycerides and free fatty acids in plasma; and (5) development of ketoacidosis.

Postprandial hyperglycemia is one of the early biochemical signs of diabetes as the responsiveness of the islet cell begins to decline. There are no clearly discernible symptoms until plasma levels exceed the renal threshold for glucose (about 160 mg/dl), when glucosuria develops. Glucosuria is initially intermittent but eventually becomes persistent. Further decline in insulin production leads to interruption of lipid synthesis and to increased mobilization of fat from adipose tissue. When the rate of release of free fatty acids from peripheral adipose tissue exceeds the rate of free fatty acid utilization, ketones accumulate in excess. Long-chain acetyl CoA radicals accumulate; metabolism through the citric acid cycle is slowed; and there is shunting to production of acetoacetate and beta-hydroxybutyrate. Ketone bodies may be oxidized by peripheral tissues, but the quantity produced soon exceeds capacity. Since the renal threshold for ketones is quite low, urinary losses occur early.

Insulin-deficiency diabetes represents a state of extreme catabolism. Energy requirements can be met only at the expense of a prodigious loss of calories. For example, a normal 10 year old child has a caloric requirement of about 2000 calories per day, of which approximately 50 per cent or 1000 calories would be derived from carbohydrate. The development of diabetes in such a child might easily lead to polyuria of 5 liters per day, with a mean urinary glucose concentration of 5 per cent. To meet this loss of 250 gm of glucose, equivalent to 1000 calories, the child would need to double his carbohydrate intake. Since this would only lead to further hyperglycemia and glucosuria, we can expect increases in fluid and food intake to stabilize the nutritional status only temporarily. The development of ketonemia and ketonuria results in rapid decompensation. The need for ketones to be excreted with cations (Na, K, NH_4+) results in further depletion of water and in acidosis. If therapy is not promptly initiated, impairment of consciousness and coma will follow. Coma is probably a consequence of several factors, including acidosis, hyperosmolality, cerebral dehydration and diminished cerebral oxygen utilization.

NATURAL HISTORY. The classic symptoms of onset of diabetes in the child include polyuria, polydipsia and polyphagia. Weight loss, fatigue, irritability and moodiness may also be seen. The onset may occur at any age from infancy through adolescence. The duration of symptoms prior to diagnosis is less than 30 days in half the children and less than 2 weeks in 20 per cent. The most common symptom is polyuria, often expressed as nocturia or as enuresis in a previously toilet-trained child. Concern about possible urinary tract infection may lead to the correct diagnosis.

Mild ketosis occurs in 20 to 40 per cent of newly diagnosed patients. Severe diabetic ketoacidosis and coma are now uncommon presenting features, owing to generally improved pediatric care and increased awareness of the possibility of diabetes on the part of both physicians and parents. Those children who do present severe metabolic derangement are most commonly younger (often under 2 years old), have had a more rapidly progressive illness, and may have intercurrent infection as a complicating or precipitating problem. Such patients typically have vomiting, dehydration, fever and progressive somolence and central nervous system depression.

About half of newly diagnosed patients will give a clinical history which exceeds 30 days in duration, and a small number may have a history compatible with mild carbohydrate intolerance for a period of months or years. Approximately 5 per cent of our new patients have a history and course quite comparable to that seen in maturity-onset diabetes. Such children are frequently obese.

Diabetes in the child evolves through several fairly clearly recognizable phases. These include the initial acute metabolic derangement, initial stabilization, remission, intensification and permanent diabetes. The general principles of basic management are the same in each stage, but certain features, notably insulin dosage, must be adjusted to meet changing demands.

Metabolic Derangement. Either at the time of initial acute metabolic derangement or with later development of ketoacidosis, insulin requirements may be relatively high. Why periods of relative insulin resistance occur is not known, but the mechanism is probably a combination of high concentrations of insulin antagonists (such as growth hormone, epinephrine and cortisone) and the inhibiting effect of acidosis and elevated free fatty acid concentration on the action of insulin. With correction of acidosis, dehydration and hyperglycemia, insulin requirements promptly fall. In the child with newly diagnosed diabetes there is an additional decline in insulin requirement that may merge imperceptibly into the first. More often this occurs 1 to 3 months following diagnosis and is referred to as a remission, or the "honeymoon" phase.

Remission. Approximately 90 per cent of new patients will have a spontaneous decline in insulin requirement to less than 50 per cent of the dose established following initial metabolic correction and stabilization. In a small number of children (3 to 5 per cent), insulin administration may be completely discontinued for some period of time. In such patients glucosuria and hyperglycemia do not occur after meals, but the glucose tolerance test remains abnormal, and the response of the insulin level, although improved over that seen at the time of diagnosis, remains below normal. These observations clearly suggest that for the first several months following diagnosis, the pancreas can and does produce some insulin in response to food ingestion. The duration of this state of remission is variable, from weeks to several months or, rarely, for several years. The period of remission is usually a trouble-free time, except for the difficulty created in acceptance of the diagnosis of diabetes on the part of both patients and parents. The major management concerns are the prevention of hypoglycemia in the early phase, as insulin requirements fall, and the later recognition of increasing insulin needs with intercurrent infections or stress and with spontaneous termination of the remission phase. Unlike other workers, we have found no evidence that the mode of early therapy has any significant effect on the completeness of the remission phase, or on its duration.

Intensification. Within several months of clinical onset, and following the remission phase, there is usually a gradual increase in insulin requirement which leads eventually to a state of "total diabetes." The termination of remission may be acute, possibly associated with infection, ketoacidosis or development of adolescence. In most children complete loss of islet cell function occurs within 2 to 6 years following diagnosis. This stage is determined by the absence of endogenously produced insulin in the circulation or in the pancreas, with histologic evidence of islet cell destruction.

Factors Affecting Carbohydrate Homeostasis. The developmental phases of diabetes in the child reflect the changing availability of endogenous insulin. A number of other factors may acutely or chronically alter glucose homeostasis. Exercise increases the rate of glucose utilization and may produce hypoglycemia. Irregularity of food intake leads to excessive fluctuation of blood glucose concentration and increases the likelihood of episodes of hypoglycemia. Both infection and physical or emotional stress produce insulin resistance and may lead rapidly to diabetic ketoacidosis if proper therapy is not initiated.

When hypoglycemia occurs from whatever cause (excessive insulin administration, avoidance of meals, exercise), there is a counterregulatory response, which includes release of growth hormone, ACTH, cortisone and epinephrine. This response blunts the actions of insulin and the utilization of both glucose and free fatty acids, with the result that there is a transitory phase of insulin resistance. If hypoglycemia is inadvertently induced frequently or on a continuing basis, extreme difficulty in management may result. (See Somogyi phenomenon, below.)

Remission during the early stages of diabetes is common; remission two or more years after diagnosis is extremely rare. Adolescent girls may have hysterical reactions which are misinterpreted as hypoglycemic episodes and suggest that insulin requirements are falling. In such patients a progressive decrease in insulin dosage, which is interpreted by the patient and parent as evidence for improving diabetes, will lead to ketoacidosis if not interrupted. The only true late remission we have seen is in patients who have developed concomitant endocrine deficiency diseases such as hypothyroidism, Addison's disease or hypopituitarism. Such events are rare, but must be considered in the evaluation of patients with declining insulin requirements.

Growth and Development. Insulin is a growth hormone. In synergy with pituitary growth hormone, insulin stimulates the uptake of amino acids into individual cells, supports a positive nitrogen balance and stimulates cell division and increased cell growth. In the absence of insulin, basic growth processes are adversely affected.

The quality of growth in the child with diabetes is of importance both from the point of view of general health and nutrition and as an indicator of adequacy of management. At the time of diagnosis, most children are appreciably underweight but are of normal or above average height. Prior to the availability of insulin, severe growth failure was characteristic of the child with diabetes. During the years when therapy was carried out with multiple injections of regular insulin daily, a form of dwarfism was common which included growth retardation, obesity, hepatomegaly and retarded emotional and sexual development (Mauriac syndrome). With the advent of intermediate and long-acting insulin preparations, this form and degree of dwarfism became uncommon. A number of longitudinal studies, however, document some impairment of rates of both linear growth and adolescent development in children with diabetes. There is no doubt that extremely poor control of diabetes is associated with growth failure, but it is less clear that there are significant differences in growth between groups of patients who are rigidly controlled and those in whom a more liberal approach to management is employed.

Convulsions and the Diabetic Child. Epilepsy is reported to occur more commonly than expected in children with diabetes. The expected incidence among children is 0.7 per cent, whereas an incidence of 10 per cent has been reported in children with diabetes. The differentiation of insulin-induced hypoglycemia from idiopathic epilepsy may be difficult, and the use of anticonvulsants in children with hypoglycemic seizures may appear to decrease the frequency and severity of seizures; but the appropriate approach is obviously to adjust the insulin dose so as to avoid hypoglycemia. We use an approach to management that includes prevention of hypoglycemia as a primary objective; we do not find that there is an unusual incidence of epilepsy among our diabetic patients.

Intellectual Capacity and School Achievement. There is no evidence that the biochemical abnormalities of diabetes have a direct effect on either intellectual function or emotional development. There are, however, several secondary considerations which may adversely affect school achievement. Newly diagnosed patients and adolescents (and their families) often find it difficult to accept the diagnosis of diabetes and the restraints which management imposes. The rebellion phase of adolescence may be exaggerated and associated with declining interest in school achievement. In the child with poorly controlled diabetes, fatigue, inattention and irritability may be common, owing to inadequate sleep due to nocturia and owing to loss of calories in glucosuric polyuria. Recurrent hypoglycemia may lead to deterioration of school performance. Readjustment of insulin dose and of time of food intake will readily correct this problem.

MANAGEMENT. The management of the child with diabetes mellitus must be concerned with the day-to-day prevention or control of symptoms resulting from metabolic abnormalities and with the prevention, if possible, of the late vascular complications which are the major cause of morbidity and mortality. Most investigators agree that a therapeutic program which does not control the overt symptoms of diabetes is inadequate and probably associated with an increased rate of complications, but there is appreciably less agreement as to whether therapeutic programs directed toward rigid normalization of blood glucose fluctuation are more effective in preventing complications than are less rigid approaches.

The juvenile diabetic has characteristically been considered "unstable" or "brittle" and an unusually difficult management problem. This reputation is unwarranted and results at least partly from application to the child of standards for control of the adult diabetic. The child's energy requirements vary greatly from those of the sedentary adult. Energy is expended in bursts associated with sporadic, unscheduled and frequently extreme exercise. It is not surprising that blood glucose levels in children with diabetes vary more from moment to moment than those of individuals who lead basically quiet, scheduled lives. A willingness to accept these variations and to focus attention upon the problems of the whole child is an important element in the success of working with the child with diabetes and his family.

Specific objectives of management should include elimination of all overt symptoms of diabetes, prevention of ketoacidosis, prevention of hypoglycemia, maintenance of normal growth and development, participation in full activity appropriate to age, assumption by the child of increasing responsibility for management decisions and the development in the child of an informationally accurate and psychologically mature understanding of the disease and its consequences. These objectives can be readily achieved in the majority of children without insistence upon the complete normalization of glucose metabolism. That is not to say that freedom from glucosuria may not be a desirable or obtainable goal. It is possible that aglucosuria can or could be achieved in many diabetic children by a program involving multiple daily injections of insulin and rigid control of food ingestion and of activities, in an emotional climate in which rewards and punishment were a daily feature of the parent-child-physician relationship. The critical question is unresolved whether the achievement of this intensity of control will improve the outcome, when compared with a therapeutic program which is less rigid but no less concerned about the health of the child and his future.

Insulin. The daily administration of insulin is required in almost all children with diabetes. Many insulin preparations are available; they are listed in Table 16–3. Insulin is available in forms for rapid action (regular or crystalline, and Semi-Lente), for intermediate action (NPH, Lente, and globin), and for long action (PZI and Ultra-Lente). Heretofore, insulin has been supplied in two concentrations, 40 units/cc (U40) and 80 units/cc (U80); henceforth, insulin will be available in a single concentration only: 100 units/cc (U100). An additional change expected in commercial insulin is the marketing of much more highly purified

TABLE 16-3 FORMS OF INSULIN COMMERCIALLY AVAILABLE

INSULIN PRODUCT	APPROXIMATE HYPOGLYCEMIC EFFECT IN HOURS		
	Onset	*Peak*	*Duration*
Rapid Action—Short Duration			
Regular (unmodified, zinc crystalline)	½	2–4	6–8
Semi-Lente	½	2–4	10–12
Intermediate in Rapidity of Action—Relatively Long Duration			
NPH (isophane)	2	8–10	28–30
Lente (70% Ultra-Lente and 30% Semi-Lente)	2	8–10	20–26
Globin	2	8–16	Up to 24 hours
Delayed Action—Long Duration			
Protamine zinc (PZI)	4–8	14–20	24–36
Ultra-Lente	4–8	14–24	36 or more

preparations, which may minimize the problems of insulin allergy and of local reactions to insulin injection.

The uses of particular forms of insulin result as much from personal preference as from scientific evidences of their superiority, except that the long-acting insulin preparations are rarely used in children because of the danger of hypoglycemia during sleep. Our preference is for regular and NPH insulins. In most cases Lente and NPH are directly interchangable.

At the time of diagnosis patients may require from 0.5 to 3.0 units of insulin/kg/day, depending upon the severity of metabolic derangement. As gross metabolic abnormalities are corrected, insulin requirements fall rapidly. The total insulin dose is calculated counting 1 unit for each unit of NPH or Lente and 0.33 unit for each unit of regular or Semi-Lente insulin. During the phase of remission many children require less than 0.5 units/kg/day. As endogenous insulin production wanes several months later, the insulin requirement gradually rises to a mean dose in the phase of total diabetes of 0.8 units/kg/day in the preadolescent and about 1.1 unit/kg/day in the adolescent.

Most new patients are started on a combination of NPH and regular insulins, given together before breakfast. The doses are adjusted to eliminate all symptoms of diabetes and to minimize glucosuria, without attempting to eliminate glucosuria completely. In most preadolescents, as they move into the remission period, regular insulin can be discontinued and a single injection of NPH given once daily. Adolescents, however, appear to be better controlled on a combination of NPH and regular insulins. The dose of regular insulin is usually 25 to 30 per cent of the dose of NPH, but may be considerably higher in some patients.

Some diabetologists recommend routinely that children with diabetes be given at least two injections of insulin daily. Their regimens usually involve a combination of an intermediate and a short-acting insulin preparation before breakfast and an intermediate or combination of intermediate and short-acting insulin before the evening meal. We have not found this approach necessary routinely, but it is useful in patients who are adequately controlled during the daytime hours but have marked nocturnal hyperglycemia and glucosuria. In the patient who has recurrent hypoglycemia at night but inadequate control during the day, it is essential to decrease the morning dose of NPH insulin. If hyperglycemia during the day cannot be adequately controlled by increasing the morning dose of regular insulin, the problem may be resolved by moving 25 to 30 per cent of the morning NPH dose to the late afternoon. In the patient whose insulin requirement exceeds 1.5 units/kg/day, splitting the dose is generally useful and may result in a decrease in total insulin requirement. Periodic clinical evaluation of the adequacy of insulin therapy emphasizes general health, physical growth and development, activity level and emotional well-being. Biochemical evaluations may be concerned with the fasting and/or postprandial glucose concentrations, fasting blood lipid concentration and urinary glucose concentration. We do not find that random or periodic blood glucose determinations are of much value in assessing adequacy of control.

Urinary glucose concentrations, as determined by the two-drop Clinitest method, are the basic tool used to guide changes in therapy. Urine specimens are routinely checked for glucose four times daily: before breakfast, lunch and dinner, and before a bedtime snack. The reliability of the information obtained is improved if the specimens are second voidings. This testing may be supplemented periodically by quantitative glucose analysis of a 24-hour urine collection. In the majority of patients 24-hour urinary glucose losses of less than 25 gm (100 calories) can be readily achieved. Insulin dosage is gradually adjusted (every 1 to 2 weeks unless there are acute problems) in order to diminish the degree of glucosuria without inducing hypoglycemia. An adjustment involving 10 per cent of the total dose is usually safe. The dose of regular insulin is increased if hyperglycemia and glucosuria are excessive in late morning and early afternoon. The dose of NPH is increased for excessive glucosuria later in the day or overnight. If, in children receiving insulin once a day, such simple changes in dosage are not effective, then splitting of the dose may be necessary, as indicated above.

Complications of Insulin Therapy

HYPOGLYCEMIA. Hypoglycemia is the major complication of insulin therapy. Severe hypoglycemia may lead to generalized convulsions, irreversible central nervous system damage and death. Whether mild, recurrent hypoglycemic episodes may damage the brain in some degree is not clear, but the transient interruption of activities and mental processes associated with hypoglycemia can and should be avoided by careful adjustment of insulin dose and food intake. Hypoglycemia presents various symptoms, depending upon the rate, degree and duration of fall of glucose concentration. There are also individual idiosyncrasies in expression of hypoglycemia. Mild hypoglycemia is usually expressed as anxiety, change in mood, inattention, headache, blurred vision, hunger or abdominal pain. With more severe hypoglycemia, symptoms of epinephrine discharge usually predominate, including tachycardia, profuse perspiration, tremulousness and headache. With advanced hypoglycemia there are disorientation, slurred speech, uncontrolled aggressive behavior, somnolence and focal or generalized neurologic changes, such as hemiparesis or grand mal seizures.

Most children quickly learn to recognize the early signs of hypoglycemia and its management. At the first signs of hypoglycemia, foods with a high content of readily available glucose should be taken promptly. Orange juice with 1 to 2 tablespoons of table sugar is very effective, as are many carbonated beverages (not *diet* varieties), hard candy and sugar cubes. If the child is disoriented or combative, it is preferable first to give 1 mg of crystalline glucagon intramuscularly and then to provide food as the child begins to respond. In the convulsing or unconscious patient glucagon may be given, or preferably 50 per cent dextrose intravenously as soon as possible, at a dose of 0.5 to 1.0 ml/kg. If hypoglycemia has been particularly severe or prolonged, it may take several hours or days for neurologic function to return fully to normal.

INSULIN ALLERGY. Commercial insulin is derived from beef or pork sources and contains about 8 per cent impurities. Although antibodies to insulin are regularly demonstrable in the patient's serum after a few weeks on insulin therapy, significant allergic reactions to insulin are remarkably uncommon, occurring in 2 to 3 per cent of cases. Most such reactions take the form of local erythema, induration and pruritis at the site of injection and can be controlled by the use of antihistamines or by switching to insulin of a different source (say, pure pork). More serious allergic reactions are rarely encountered; generalized hives, asthma or anaphylactic shock may require the temporary use of steroids and desensitization, in addition to immediate therapy. It is hoped that the availability of more highly purified insulin preparations (single component or "single peak" insulin) will minimize the problems of insulin allergy as well as hypertrophy and atrophy.

PROBLEMS OF LOCAL INJECTION. Much more common and bothersome than local allergic reactions are the development of localized subcutaneous lipid hypertrophy ("insulin tumors") and the loss of subcutaneous adipose tissue (insulin atrophy). These problems are primarily cosmetic but may lead to anxiety and psychologic problems, particularly in adolescent girls. Their causes are not well understood and there is no reliable therapy. The hypertrophic or atrophic area will usually gradually return to normal over a period of months or years. It is probably best to avoid these areas when injecting insulin. There have, on the other hand, been recent reports of successful filling-in of atrophic areas by injection of regular "single peak" insulin directly into the involved area.

INSULIN RESISTANCE. It is probable that some degree of insulin resistance occurs in all diabetics on chronic insulin therapy. The antibodies which readily develop to commercial insulin probably bind injected insulin locally, as well as in the circulation, and result in some change in timing of release and action, as well as necessitating a modest increase in dose. Such marked resistance as to require more than 200 units daily is rare in children. If infection, ketoacidosis, or unusual stress cannot account for unusual insulin requirements, a switch to a purified insulin preparation, splitting of the insulin dose, or administration of an adrenal steroid may be effective in lowering the insulin need. Whatever measures are taken, there is usually an eventual disappearance of resistance.

The Somogyi Phenomenon. Somogyi described the progressive deterioration of diabetic control in patients receiving increasing doses of insulin and showed that these patients were markedly overinsulinized, with symptomatic or inapparent hypoglycemia followed by reactive hyperglycemia and frequently by ketonuria. The findings of progressive hyperglycemia, glucosuria and ketonuria were interpreted as indicating a need for more and more insulin, but the patients became worse rather than better.

This is not an uncommon problem in the diabetic child and frequently results when attempts are made to eliminate glucosuria completely. When a child with persistent or recurrent marked hyperglycemia and ketonuria is receiving more than 1.5 units/kg of insulin, with or without overt symptoms of hypoglycemia, this problem should be suspected. It can be diagnosed by establishing that there are recurrent episodes of hypoglycemia followed by a spontaneous reactive hyperglycemia. The necessary study requires hospitalization and hourly samples of blood for glucose level. A slow reduction in the total dose of insulin and/or splitting of the dose is usually effective in management.

Oral Agents. There are two general types of compounds that may be effective in the management of patients with mild diabetes mellitus. The sulfonylurea compounds act primarily, if not exclusively, by stimulating the release of insulin from the pancreas. The biguanides may lower blood glucose concentration either as intracellular enzyme poison, inhibiting oxidative phosphorylation and increasing the rate of glucose utilization or, more likely, through partial inhibition of glucose absorption from the gastrointestinal tract. Probably less than 5 per cent of children with diabetes would receive any potential therapeutic benefit from either of these compounds. In the light of recent reports raising questions about the long-term safety and efficiency of these compounds in the chronic therapy of diabetes, their use in children probably should be limited to investigative studies.

Nutrition and Diet. Everyone agrees that nutrition is important in the overall management of the patient with diabetes, but there remain widely divergent views on the type of diet which should be recommended. In addition to supplying all necessary nutritional ingredients for normal growth, development and activity, it is to be hoped that the chosen diet would minimize excessive fluctuations in daily glucose concentration, maintain blood lipid concentrations within normal limits, and impede the development and progression of cardiovascular pathology. It is not clear that there is a single diet which will meet these criteria. It is probable that diet, like the use of insulin, must be tailored to meet individual needs. We currently recommend a diet composed of 50 per cent carbohydrate, 30 per cent fat and 20 per cent protein. Approximately 65 per cent of the carbohydrate is derived from slowly absorbed starches and 35 per cent from the more rapidly absorbed disaccharides and monosaccharides, such as sucrose, lactose, glucose and fructose. The fat component of the diet is restricted modestly, with particular restriction of cholesterol and saturated fats, and with some increase in unsaturated fats. The increase in protein and limitation of saturated fats make it necessary to supplement lean meat with skimmed milk, fish and chicken. The caloric recommendations are those adequate to maintain normal growth and avoid obesity. As a general rule, the estimate of 1000 calories + 100 calories/year of age is a useful starting point. The child's appetite or hunger is a more useful indication of adequacy of intake than any predetermined formulas, increased food intake being allowed according to appetite, at mealtimes and at specified snacks, so long as excessive weight gain does not occur. With appropriate consideration for the individual family's food preferences and eating habits, the distribution of calories is approximately 20 per cent at breakfast, 40 per cent at lunch, and 40 per cent at dinner. Scheduled snacks are recommended in midmorning and midafternoon and at bedtime. Many older children prefer not to take a midmorning snack. Dietetic foods are to be avoided, with the exception of low calorie carbonated beverages.

Diabetic Ketoacidosis. Diabetic ketoacidosis is the most important cause of acute mortality and serious morbidity in the child with diabetes. Its genesis is discussed above. Patients with diabetic ketoacidosis present dehydration, abdominal pain, vomiting, fever, Kussmaul respiration, somnolence or coma, in addition to the signs and symptoms of whatever infection or other stressful situation may be precipitating the ketoacidotic state. In addition to hyperglycemia, glucosuria, ketonemia and ketonuria, such patients have a metabolic acidosis, with depressed blood pH, CO_2 content and bicarbonate concentration. The blood lipids are elevated. There is invariably a total body deficit of sodium and potassium, but the serum concentration of these cations may be normal, high or low.

The treatment of diabetic ketoacidosis should be directed simultaneously toward correction of (1) the basic metabolic defect, (2) the acidosis, and (3) the dehydration. Administration of crystalline insulin is essential, in large enough amounts and frequently enough to promote glucose uptake and utilization and to prevent further mobilization of free fatty acids. Depending upon the degree of acidosis, insulin therapy is initiated with 1.0 to 2.0 units/kg of regular insulin, given either all intravenously or half intravenously and half subcutaneously. Insulin administration is repeated as necessary, but not less often than every 6 hours during the first day of therapy.

Fluid therapy is designed to correct dehydration, to replace depleted electrolytes and to correct acidosis. The degree of dehydration is estimated clinically, and the calculated fluid deficit is administered during the first 8 hours of intravenous therapy. During the first hour Ringer's lactate solution is given at a rate of 20 ml/kg. This is then replaced by a solution containing not less than 80 mEq/l of sodium. Depending upon the degree of acidosis, this may be physiological saline solution or Ringer's lactate solution diluted with an equal part of distilled water, or some other fluid containing sodium bicarbonate and sodium chloride. If the patient's serum has a CO_2 content below 12 mEq/l, sodium bicarbonate is administered over a 3- to 8-hour period according to the following formula:

$$\text{Sodium bicarbonate dose (mEq)} = 0.6 \times \text{body weight in kg} \times (15\ \text{mEq} - \text{observed } CO_2 \text{ content})$$

This schedule provides partial correction of acidosis, allowing complete correction to occur in response to insulin therapy and rehydration. The above dose of sodium bicarbonate should not be given more acutely, owing to the danger of excessive osmotic changes.

Glucose is added to the infusion in 5 per cent concentration when the blood glucose level falls below 300 mg/dl. Potassium should be added to the initial solution at a concentration of 20 to 30 mEq/l.

During the remaining 16 hours of the first day of therapy for diabetic ketoacidosis, intravenous fluid is delivered at a rate calculated to supply normal 24-hour requirements plus any continuing losses from glucosuria, vomiting, or diarrhea. A solution of 5 per cent glucose in 0.2 per cent NaCl with added potassium is an adequate replacement solution under most circumstances. By the end of the first day of treatment most children can begin to receive oral alimentation, with clear fluids to be followed by a soft diet.

Hyperosmolar Diabetic Coma. Hyperosmolar diabetic coma is a recently recognized syndrome, occurring infrequently in the child with diabetes, characterized by marked hyperglycemia and hyperosmolality, marked dehydration, coma and little or no acidosis. The absence of acidosis is not understood. Therapy is similar to that for ketoacidosis; the rate of correction of dehydration should be slower, however, in order to prevent rapid osmotic changes which may further disturb central nervous system function. The mortality in this syndrome is very high, approximating 50 per cent in most series.

The "Brittle" Diabetic. The majority of children with diabetes present no great management problems for the physician, the patient, or his family. In every large series of diabetic patients, however, there are a few who have repeated hospitalizations for recurrent ketoacidosis and coma. In our experience, most such patients have the "Somogyi phenomenon" and respond well to readjustment of the insulin regimen. A few patients cannot be explained on this basis; they are usually adolescent girls with serious psychologic problems, and frequently stem from families which have difficulty in psychologic adjustment and in resolution of problems. Following acute emotional stress these patients may rapidly decompensate from reasonable diabetic control to ketoacidosis. The mechanism probably relates to excessive release of epinephrine and/or growth hormone, resulting in mobilization of glucose and free fatty acids and insulin resistance. Adrenergic-blocking agents have been used with some success in the treatment of these children. A more appropriate and generally more successful approach is to involve both patient and parents in psychotherapy. Long-term therapy may be required.

Emotional Adjustment. There is no evidence that the child with diabetes mellitus has any specific psychologic make-up prior to diagnosis or that the metabolic abnormalities produce specific behavioral alterations. On the other hand, there is ample evidence that psychologic disturbances are more common in children with diabetes than among children generally. This is not surprising. Any chronic, serious illness in a child puts the entire family under emotional and often financial stress. From the point of view of its potential for psychologic stress, diabetes has some particularly trying features: it is genetic in origin, which may arouse feelings of guilt in one or both parents; the approach to management may utilize a system of rewards and punishments which induce guilt in the patient when he breaks the rules or becomes ill; the child is frequently expected to assume mature responsibility for daily management decisions before he has either the intellectual understanding or emotional maturity to make such decisions; and the eventual disabilities of diabetes are of such magnitude as to induce a sense of hopelessness and despair about the future. It is most important for the physician to be sensitive to these problems in order to cope with them early. For children and families having troubles, psychiatric assistance should be obtained before it becomes mandated by severe behavioral disturbances in the child. It is a tribute to the personal emotional strength of children and their families that most survive the stresses of growing up with diabetes without sustaining permanent emotional scars.

PROGNOSIS. Vascular disease is the major problem facing the patient with diabetes and is of two types: microangiopathy and arteriosclerosis. Various manifestations of these pathologic processes account for 75 per cent of the mortality in patients with diabetes.

The microangiopathic lesions reflect a pathologic process rather unique to diabetes mellitus and lead to proliferative retinopathy and blindness, to Kimmelstiel-Wilson disease and progressive renal failure, to obstructive peripheral arterial disease, and to neuropathies affecting various peripheral nerves. Retinopathy develops in 63 per cent of juvenile diabetics by 30 years of age and in 88 per cent by 50 years; and nephropathy is found in 18 per cent by 30 years and in 37 per cent by 50 years, according to Joslin Clinic studies.

The atherosclerosis of the diabetic is apparently not pathologically differentiated from that seen in the general population, but affects the patient at an earlier age and leads to high morbidity and mortality from myocardial infarction, renal disease, hypertension and cerebrovascular accidents. Approximately 50 per cent of all diabetic patients die of myocardial infarction.

The life expectancy for the patient with diabetes is approximately two thirds that of the general population having the same age as the patient at the time of diagnosis. For example, the life expectancy of the boy who develops diabetes at 10 years of age is for 43.6 additional years, whereas normal 10 year old males can expect 59 years. The expectation for additional life is 35.4 years for the male who develops diabetes at 20 years, 49.5 years for the nondiabetic.

The relationship between "control" of diabetes and the development of complications remains an area of disagreement. There is no therapeutic modality which is known to prevent complications. Poorly controlled diabetics may have about two and a half times the mortality rate of well controlled patients, but comparisons of patients who are moderately well controlled with those very well controlled provide little evidence for differences in rate of development of or mortality from vascular disease.

In the experimental animal chronic hyperglycemia may lead to high concentrations of sorbitol in various tissues, and may result in vascular damage. This recent finding of possibly major importance is the first clear indication of a direct relationship between hyperglycemia and vascular injury. Whether this process is of clinical importance in the child or adult with diabetes mellitus has not been firmly established. If it proves to be so, a more vigorous attempt to achieve normoglycemia in the patient with diabetes may be indicated.

Notwithstanding the acute problems of day-today management and the ultimately high incidence of vascular complications, the child with diabetes should be expected to achieve a satisfying and productive place in society. The physician should encourage both the child and his family to plan for a future that will challenge the patient's innate capabilities to the maximum.

THE DIABETES MELLITUS SYNDROME IN THE NEWBORN INFANT

A few instances of a transient state of diabetes mellitus developing in the neonatal period, persisting for weeks or months and terminating apparently in complete recovery, have been reported. Clinically the syndrome fulfills the diagnostic requirements: viz., hyperglycemia, glycosuria and clinical control with exogenous insulin. It is most likely to occur in infants less than 6 weeks of age whose birth weight was low for gestational age. The onset may be sudden, with severe dehydration, polyuria, fever and metabolic acidosis; if the condition is not treated with insulin and supportive therapy, brain damage or death may result. Ketonuria may not occur; if present, it is usually mild. Ketonemia may exist in the absence of ketonuria in the neonatal period. Occasionally transient hypoglycemia in the newborn may precede the development of transient diabetes mellitus. Infection has not seemed to be an important instigating factor. The management is that of diabetes mellitus, but extreme care must be taken to avoid hypoglycemia and to determine when administration of insulin is no longer required. By contrast with the true disease, complete recovery occurs and, so far as is known, is permanent.

True diabetes mellitus is also rare in newborn infants, but it does occur. Differentiation from the transient state can be made only after sufficient time has elapsed to determine whether the diabetic state is permanent.

ALLAN DRASH

Berson, S. A., and Yalow, R. S.: Insulin "antagonists" and insulin resistance. *In* Ellenberg, M., and Rifkin, H. (eds.): Diabetes Mellitus: Theory and Practice. New York, McGraw-Hill Book Company, 1970, p. 388–423.

Bunnell, C. E., and Monif, G. R.: Interstitial pancreatitis in the congenital rubella syndrome. J. Pediatr. *80*:465, 1972.

Camerini-Davalos, R. A., Oppermann, W., Velasco, C., and Cole, H. S.: Abnormalities at the stage of chemical asymptomatic diabetes. Metabolism *22*:219, 1973.

Cerasi, E., and Luft, R.: The prediabetic state, its nature and consequences—A look toward the future. Diabetes *21* (suppl. 2):685, 1971.

Cooke, A. M., Fitzgerald, M. F., Malins, J. M., and Pyke, D. A.: Diabetes in children of diabetic couples. Brit. Med. J. *2*:674, 1966.

Danowski, T. S., Aarons, J. H., Hydovitz, J. D., and Wingest, J. P.: Utility of equivocal glucose tolerances. Diabetes *19*:524, 1970.

Drash, A.: Diabetes mellitus in childhood: A review. J. Pediatr. *78*:919, 1971.

Drash, A., Field, J. B., Garces, L. Y., Kenny, F. M., Mintz, D., and Vazquez, A.: Endogenous insulin and growth hormone response in children with newly diagnosed diabetes mellitus. Pediatr. Res. *2*:94, 1968.

Fajans, S. S.: Diagnostic tests for diabetes mellitus. *In* Williams, R. H. (ed.): Diabetes. New York, Paul B. Hoeber, Inc., 1960, pp. 397–399.

Fajans, S. S., Floyd, J. C., Pek, S., and Conn, J. W.: The course of asymptomatic diabetes in young people as determined by levels of blood glucose and plasma insulin. Trans. Ass. Amer. Phys. *82*:211 1969.

Gamble, D. R., and Taylor, K. W.: Seasonal incidence of diabetes mellitus. Brit. Med. J. *3*:631, 1969.

Goldstein, D., Drash, A., Gibbs, J., and Blizzard, R. M.: Diabetes mellitus: The incidence of circulating antibodies against thyroid, gastric, and adrenal tissue. J. Pediatr. *77*:304, 1970.

Goodkin, G.: How long can a diabetic expect to live? Nutr. Today *6*:21, 1971.

Jackson, W. P. U.: Diabetes mellitus in different countries and different races. Prevalence and major features. Acta Diabetol. Lat. *7*:361–401, 1970.

Kahn, C. B., Soeldner, J. S., Gleason, R. E., Rojas, L., Camerini-Davalos, R. A., and Marble, A.: Clinical and chemical diabetes in offspring of diabetic couples. New Engl. J. Med. *281*:343, 1969.

Knowles, H. C., Jr., Guest, G. M., Lampe, J., Kessler, M., and Skillman, T. G.: The course of juvenile diabetes treated with unmeasured diet. Diabetes *14*:239, 1965.

Larsson, Y., and Sterky, G.: Long-term prognosis in juvenile diabetes mellitus. Acta Paediatr. *51*:1–76, Supplement 130, 1962.

Monif, G. R.: Can diabetes mellitus result from an infectious disease? Hosp. Practice *8*:124, 1973.

Mosenthal, H. P., and Barry, E.: Criteria for an interpretation of normal glucose tolerance tests. Ann. Intern. Med. *33*:1175, 1950.

National Center for Health Statistics: Characteristics of Persons with Diabetes, United States, July 1964–June 1965. Washington, D.C., U.S. Public Health Service Publication 1000, Ser. 10, No. 40, October, 1967.

Neel, J. V.: Current concepts of the genetic basis of diabetes mellitus and the biological significance of the diabetic predisposition. *In* Ostman, J. (ed.): Diabetes: Proceedings of the Sixth Congress of the International Diabetes Federation. Amsterdam, Excerpta Medica Foundation (supplement), 1969, pp. 68–78.

O'Brien, D.: Evidence for an abnormal insulin in diabetes mellitus. *In* Proceedings of the First International Symposium on Early Diabetes. New York, Academic Press, Inc. 1970.

Pickens, J. M., Burkeholder, J. M., and Womack, W. N.: Oral glucose tolerance test in normal children. Diabetes *16*:11, 1967.

Reaven, G., Olefsky, J., and Farquhar, J.: Does hyperglycemia or hyperinsulinemia characterize the patient with chemical diabetes? Lancet *1*:1247, 1972.

Remein, Q. R.: A current estimate of the prevalence of diabetes mellitus in the United States. Ann. N.Y. Acad. Sci. *82*:229, 1959.

Remein, Q. R.: The genetics of diabetes mellitus. *In* Ellenberg, M., and Rifkin, H. (eds.): Diabetes Mellitus: Theory and Practice. New York, McGraw-Hill Book Company, 1970, pp. 564–581.

Remein, Q. R., and Wilkerson, H. L.: The efficiency of screening tests for diabetes. J. Chron. Dis. *13*:6–21, 1961.

Rosenbloom, A., Guthrie, R., and Drash, A.: Chemical diabetes mellitus in the child. Metabolism *22*:209–422, 1973.

Rubin, H. M., Kramer, R., and Drash, A.: Hyperosmolality complicating diabetes mellitus in childhood. J. Pediatr. *74*:177, 1969.

Salans, L., Knittle, J., and Hirsch, J.: The role of adipose cell size and adipose tissue insulin sensitivity in the carbohydrate intolerance of human obesity. J. Clin. Invest. *47*:153, 1968.

Siperstein, M. D., Unger, R. H., and Madison, L. L.: Studies of muscle capillary basement membranes in normal subjects,

diabetics, and prediabetic patients. J. Clin. Invest. *47*:1973, 1968.
Somogyi, M.: Exacerbation of diabetes by excess insulin action. Amer. J. Med. *26*:169, 1959.
ThenBerg, H.: The genetic aspect of diabetes mellitus. (Foreign letter, Berlin.) J.A.M.A. *112*:1091, 1939.
The University Group Diabetes Program: A study of the effect of hypoglycemic agents on vascular complications in patients with adult-onset diabetes. Diabetes *19* (suppl. 2):747–830, 1970.
Unger, B., Stocks, A., Martin, F., Whittengham, S., and Mackay, S.: Intrinsic factor antibody, parietal cell antibody and latent pernicious anemia in diabetes mellitus. Lancet *2*:415, 1968.
Vallance-Owen, J.: Synalbumin insulin antagonism. Diabetes *13*:241, 1964.
West, K. M., and Kalbfleische, J. M.: Influence of nutritional factors on prevalence of diabetes. Diabetes *20*:99, 1971.
White, P.: The inheritance of diabetes. Med. Clin. N. Amer. *49*:857, 1965.
White, P., and Graham, C.: The child with diabetes. *In* Marble, A., White, P., Bradley, R., and Kroll, L. (eds.): Joslin's Diabetes Mellitus. Philadelphia, Lea & Febiger, 1971, p. 339.

HYPOGLYCEMIA

Hypoglycemia is a state in which there is an abnormally low level of blood glucose, the principal circulating hexose and physiologically the most important one. The normal fasting blood glucose level is lower in infants than in children. Hypoglycemia is especially common in the newly born infant, affecting 3 of every 1000 live-born full-term infants and 43 of every 1000 premature infants. It is more apt to occur in infants of mothers with toxemia and in association with hypothermia in the newborn. Infants who are small for gestational age and the smaller of twins of discordant weight are markedly predisposed to hypoglycemia during the newborn period.

The precise definition of hypoglycemia in the newborn period is still unsettled, but it is generally agreed that if two determinations of glucose level in whole blood fall below 30 mg/dl in the full-term infant or below 20 mg/dl in the premature infant, such findings are definitely pathologic. After 72 hours of age, the blood glucose level is normally over 40 mg/dl, and in older infants and children fasting levels below 50 mg/dl may be considered hypoglycemic.

The diagnosis and management of hypoglycemia in the newborn are discussed in Section 7.

PHYSIOLOGIC CONSIDERATIONS. Glucose may be derived directly from dietary intake by intestinal absorption, by conversion of other hexoses after absorption (galactose, fructose), by hydrolysis of polyglucose units (maltose, starch, glycogen) or by combinations of these processes (lactose, sucrose). Glucose can also be derived from dietary or endogenous amino acids, but there is no *net* synthesis of glucose from exogenous or endogenous lipids.

Figure 16–1 depicts in simplified form some of the pathways of glucose metabolism. Although free glucose may passively diffuse through most cell membranes, it is usually taken up from the lumen of the intestinal tract by the mucosal cells, from the lumen of the renal tubules by their epithelial cells, or from the blood stream by various parenchymal cells against a concentration gradient. Such an active process requires energy and is brought about by the phosphorylation of glucose, using ATP and either hexokinase or glucokinase. Once within the cells, the glucose-6-phosphate may be metabolized or may be hydrolyzed to glucose, which is then free to diffuse out of the cell again. The main routes of metabolism are as follows: (1) The Embden-Meyerhof pathway of anaerobic glycolysis converts the 6-carbon glucose to 3-carbon acids (pyruvic and lactic) with a small release of energy. (2) The pentose-phosphate shunt, which is initiated by the enzyme glucose-6-phosphate dehydrogenase, yields ribose among other sugars or joins the Embden-Meyerhof scheme at the level of glyceraldehyde-3-phosphate. The reduction of NADP along this pathway is important for lipid synthesis and for the maintenance of glutathione in the reduced form. (3) Glucose is also converted to glucose-1-phosphate, which is in equilibrium with galactose-1-phosphate. Glycogen is the form in which glucose units are stored and is in equilibrium with circulating glucose via the pathways depicted.

The ultimate product of glycolysis is pyruvic acid. After the addition of carbon dioxide or after oxidization to acetyl coenzyme A, it enters the citric acid cycle (tricarboxylic acid or Krebs cycle). Acetyl coenzyme A can also be used in the synthesis of fatty acids, cholesterol and steroid hormones or to form the ketone bodies (acetone, acetoacetic acid and beta-hydroxybutyric acid). The enzymes of the citric acid cycle are found in the mitochondria within the cells, where most of the energy resident in glucose is released and captured in the form of ATP. It is in the citric acid cycle that many amino acids are in equilibrium with glucose. By transamination or oxidation, glutamic acid is converted to alpha-ketoglutaric acid, aspartic acid to oxaloacetic acid, and alanine to pyruvic acid.

The process of gluconeogenesis involves overcoming the thermodynamically unfavorable reaction which changes pyruvic acid to phosphoenolpyruvic acid. This is accomplished, as illustrated in Figure 16–1, by transfer of pyruvic acid from the cytosol to the mitochrondrion. Once within the mitochondrion, pyruvic acid is converted to either oxaloacetic acid or malic acid, both of which can then diffuse out into the cytosol, where they are in equilibrium with each other. Once in the cytosol, oxaloacetic acid is converted to phosphoenolpyruvic acid by phosphoenol-pyruvate carboxykinase, one of the key enzymes in the gluconeogenic pathway.

Many of the enzyme systems involved in the me-

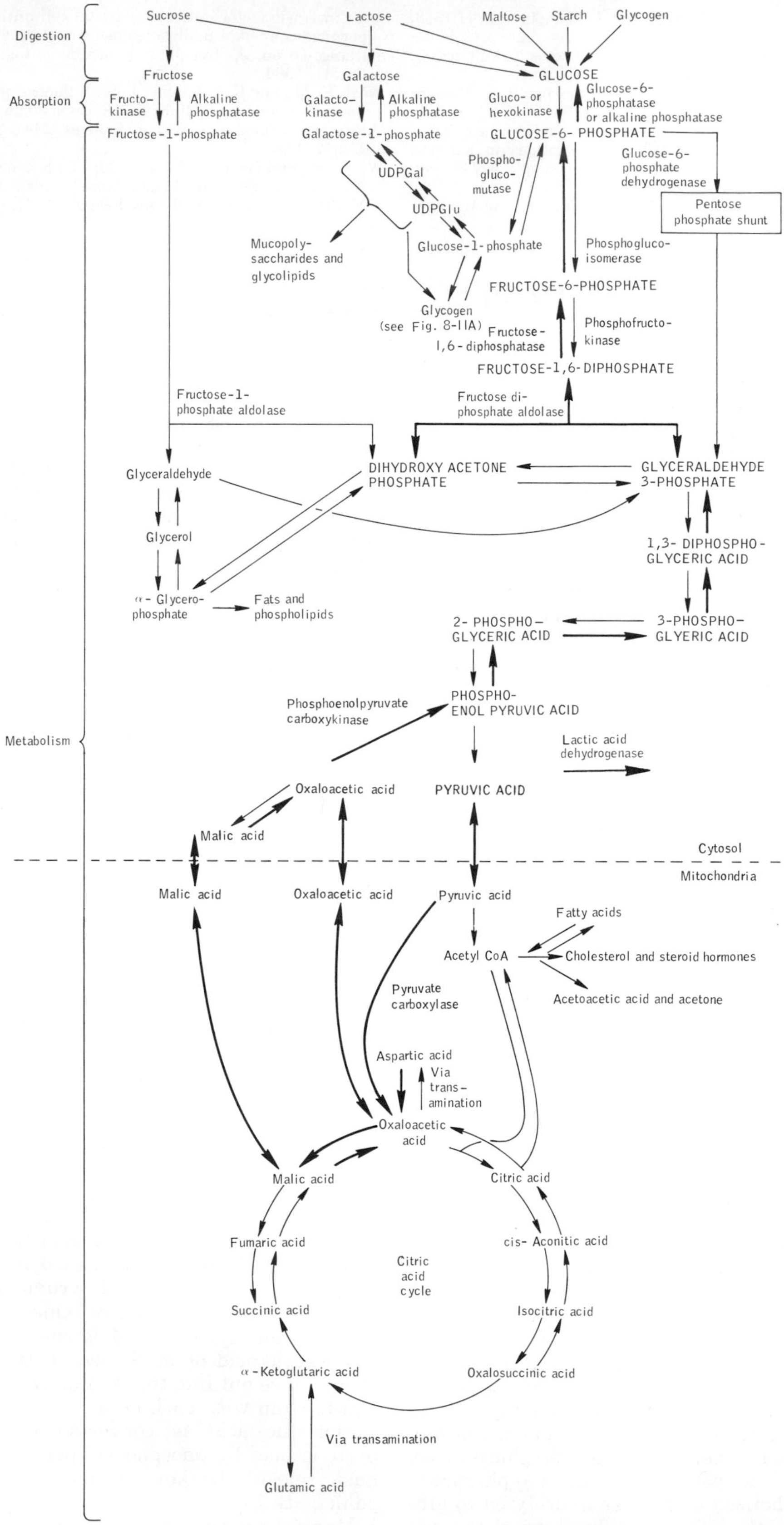

Figure 16–1 *The metabolism of glucose. The compounds of the Embden-Meyerhof pathway are indicated in capital letters. The pathway for gluconeogenesis is indicated by heavy arrows.*

TABLE 16-4 CLASSIFICATION OF HYPOGLYCEMIAS

A. With hyperinsulinism
  1. Beta-cell tumors
  2. Beta-cell adenomatosis
  3. Nesidioblastosis
  4. Beta-cell hyperplasia
    a. In association with hypopituitarism
    b. Infant of diabetic mother
    c. Infant with erythroblastosis fetalis
    d. Beckwith syndrome
    e. Leprechaunism
    f. Etiology unknown
  5. Teratoma containing pancreatic tissue
  6. Functional beta-cell secretory defect
B. With hepatic enzyme deficiencies
  1. Glucose-6-phosphatase
  2. Amylo-1,6-glucosidase
  3. Phosphorylase kinase
  4. Glycogen synthetase
  5. Fructose-1-phosphate aldolase
  6. Fructose-1,6-diphosphatase
  7. Pyruvate carboxylase
  8. Galactose-1-phosphate uridyl transferase
  9. Maple syrup urine disease
C. With endocrine deficiencies
  1. Pituitary
    a. Isolated growth hormone deficiency
    b. Isolated ACTH deficiency
    c. Panhypopituitarism
      1. With hypoinsulinism
      2. With hyperinsulinism
  2. Adrenal
    a. Addison's disease
    b. Congenital adrenal hypoplasia
    c. Congenital adrenal hyperplasia
    d. Familial glucocorticoid deficiency
    e. Adrenal medullary unresponsiveness
D. Ketotic hypoglycemia
E. Due to drugs and toxins
  1. Ethyl alcohol
  2. Salicylates
  3. Sulfonylureas
  4. Propranolol
  5. Jamaican vomiting sickness
F. Other
  1. Hepatic damage
    a. Reye syndrome
    b. Leukemia
  2. Malabsorption
  3. Renal glycosuria
  4. Malnutrition
    a. Kwashiorkor
    b. Low phenylalanine diet
  5. Extrapancreatic neoplasms

Hypoglycemia in the neonate may be caused by many of the conditions listed above as well as by other less well delineated factors (see Section 7).

tabolism of glucose are under hormonal control. The mechanisms and exact sites of action of the various hormones have been the subject of intensive investigation in recent years. Insulin is known to increase the activity of glucokinase, to increase permeability of the cell membrane for glucose and to facilitate removal of glucose from the circulation and to increase its utilization. Glucagon stimulates hepatic phosphorylase, resulting in increased glycogen breakdown and hyperglycemia. Epinephrine acts in the same manner as glucagon and also reduces peripheral utilization of glucose. Many of these hormones stimulate the enzymatic formation of cyclic 3′,5′ AMP, a compound which has many physiologic and pharmacologic effects. The enzymatic sites of action of growth hormone, corticotropin and glucocorticoids, all of which produce hyperglycemia, are through similar mechanisms. One of the effects of glucocorticoids is to promote gluconeogenesis via amino acids.

CAUSES OF HYPOGLYCEMIA

In a complicated system such as the metabolism of glucose, there are numerous loci where aberrations of control can lead to hypoglycemia. These defects in the control mechanisms may involve inborn errors of metabolism, alterations of endocrine balance and exogenous drugs and toxins (Table 16-4). Since hypoglycemia may result from a wide variety of factors, and since rational treatment and prognosis depend upon the nature of the disorder, it is essential to determine its cause.

HYPERINSULINISM

BETA CELL ADENOMA. Functioning beta cell adenoma of the pancreas is a rare lesion, now reported in about 50 children. In most instances onset of symptoms has occurred after 4 years of age, but in 11 instances hypoglycemia was manifest during the neonatal period. Symptoms may be severe and unremitting or may be mild and intermittent. The adenoma is usually solitary but may be multiple or associated with adenomatosis. In adults approximately 10 per cent of beta cell tumors are malignant, but in children malignancy is rarer.

BETA CELL HYPERPLASIA AND BETA CELL NESIDIOBLASTOSIS. Hyperinsulinism occurs more frequently in the absence of a discrete beta cell tumor. In patients with beta cell hyperplasia or nesidioblastosis, the hypoglycemia most often begins in the first weeks or months of life and is usually severe and intractable. It has been suspected for many years that many affected infants had hyperinsulinism, but their condition was called *idiopathic hypoglycemia of infancy* before assays for insulin were available. Examinations of the resected pancreas from such patients by conventional histochemical techniques reveal that approximately one third have *beta cell hyperplasia* and an occasional one has diffuse adenomatosis or nesidioblastosis of the beta cells. When, however, a histochemical technique specific for insulin (pinacyanole metachromasia) is utilized, most of the previously designated "normal" pancreases also exhibit a surplus of beta cells, scattered either singly or in small groups. These are separate from the islets, most often seen around the walls of small ducts or in the glandular acini. It is believed that the pancreatic duct cell is the primordial cell of the pancreas from which duct, acinar and islet cells arise when appropriately stimulated (hence the term nesidioblast meaning "islet builder"). The cause for islet cell hyperplasia or nesidioblastosis is not known; nor is it known if the condition is primary or secondary.

Nesidioblastosis has been reported as a familial disorder in association with multiple endocrine adenomatosis; it usually presents in adult life but may begin during childhood. In addition to oversecretion of insulin, there may be elevated glucagon and/or gastrin levels.

LEUCINE SENSITIVITY. Administration of L-leucine to normal children produces a small rise in the level of insulin in the blood, with a concomitant decrease of approximately 10 mg/dl in the level of glucose. Many children with hyperinsulinism exhibit marked sensitivity to leucine, with a fall of glucose to hypoglycemic levels. Patients with beta cell adenoma, islet cell hyperplasia or nesidioblastosis usually, but not always, exhibit an exaggerated response to leucine. Leucine is a direct stimulator of beta cell secretory activity. There is increasing evidence that most leucine-sensitive children with hypoglycemia have increased numbers of beta cells in pancreatic tissue examined by appropriate techniques. It is not known, however, whether at least in some instances the increase in beta cells is due to a primary functional aberration of the cell in its response to leucine. Familial instances of such leucine-sensitive children are known.

In other conditions in which hypersecretion of insulin occurs in response to glucose, patients may also be leucine-sensitive. Children with obesity, including Prader-Willi syndrome and the Laurence-Moon-Biedl syndrome, patients with lipodystrophy, adults with acromegaly and normal individuals pretreated with chlorpropamide have a markedly increased secretion of insulin in response to leucine. In the obese individual, however, the depression of blood glucose level is the same as for normal persons, indicating increased resistance to the effects of insulin.

HYPERINSULINISM IN ASSOCIATION WITH PANHYPOPITUITARISM. This has recently been recognized as a discrete entity. Hypoglycemia usually has its onset during the first days of life. In spite of deficiency of growth hormone, ACTH and TSH, serum insulin levels are inappropriately elevated for the level of glucose. Hyperplasia of the beta cells has been found in some patients. The hypopituitarism appears to be hypothalamic in origin, but the cause for the hyperinsulinism is obscure.

NEWBORN INFANTS OF DIABETIC AND PREDIABETIC MOTHERS. These infants frequently exhibit hyperplasia of the beta cells of the islets of Langerhans. Increased insulin content of the pancreas and increased insulin levels in blood have been found in such infants; hypoglycemia is common and often symptomatic. The disorder is thought to be caused by exposure of the fetus to maternal hyperglycemia.

OTHER HYPOGLYCEMIAS. In newborn infants with moderate or severe *erythroblastosis fetalis* clinical manifestations of hypoglycemia and blood glucose levels under 30 mg/dl occur with some frequency. Hyperplasia of the pancreatic islets has been observed in many infants dying with this disorder; it is not so marked as that which occurs in infants of diabetic mothers, and eosinophilic infiltrations are usually not present. The insulin content of the pancreas is increased and insulin levels in blood and urine are increased. The stimulus which leads to the hyperplasia of the islet cells is not known. The condition is ordinarily transitory, but hypoglycemia has been reported in two siblings at 7 and 25 months of age, presumably as a late sequel of severe erythroblastosis fetalis.

The use of blood containing acid citrate dextrose (ACD) for exchange transfusion of affected infants may lead to a hypoglycemic response which is delayed for 2 to 3 hours after completion of the transfusion. The high level of glucose in ACD blood corrects any initial hypoglycemia but causes an increased secretion of insulin which may provoke a precipitous fall of blood glucose. Careful monitoring of glucose levels should continue beyond the period of exchange.

Hyperplasia of the pancreatic islets has also been observed in *Beckwith syndrome.* This disorder is characterized by macroglossia, visceromegaly (large kidneys, liver and pancreas), and umbilical defects, including omphalocele. Cytomegaly of the adrenal fetal cortex and a wide variety of other minor defects are common features of the disorder. Hypoglycemia occurs in the first days of life and usually disappears spontaneously after a few weeks or months.

Hypoglycemia associated with a marked increase in the size and number of islets has been observed in *leprechaunism (Donohue syndrome).*

Teratomas, especially mediastinal and sacrococcygeal, frequently contain pancreatic tissue. Asymptomatic hypoglycemia and an increased level of insulin were detected in a 5 year old boy with a mediastinal teratoma. This may occur more often than heretofore suspected.

Most infants with hyperinsulinism do not come to surgery; it is not firmly established, therefore, that increased numbers of beta cells are invariably present in these patients. A deranged homeostatic mechanism leading to increased responsiveness of the islet cells remains a possible cause of hypoglycemia. It is even possible that *functional hyperinsulinism* is a primary defect leading to increased numbers of beta cells.

HEPATIC ENZYME DEFICIENCIES

GLYCOGENOSES. *Deficiency of glucose-6-phosphatase* leads to severe hypoglycemia in the fasting state and 4 to 6 hours after meals. This is the most important enzyme involved in the breakdown of glycogen into free glucose, and its deficiency leads to accumulation of glycogen and to hepatomegaly (see Glycogenoses, Section 8). Even after a short period of fasting, rather than yielding a normal release of glucose, the glycogen is metabolized via the Emden-Myerhof pathway, with release of pyruvic and lactic acids (Fig. 16–1). As a consequence, the hypoglycemia is associated with metabolic acidosis. Affected patients may have levels of glucose as low as 10 mg/dl and of lactate as high as 200 mg/dl.

Affected patients are not, as a rule, mentally retarded or excessively prone to convulsions even at these low concentrations of glucose. It is believed that their brains adapt to the utilization of amino acids, free fatty acids, and/or lactate and pyruvate.

When there is *deficiency of debranching enzyme (amylo-1,6-glucosidase)*, glycogen can be degraded only up to branch points in the molecule. The decreased production of glucose from the liver leads to hypoglycemia, but this is largely compensated for by increased gluconeogenesis. Marked hepatomegaly and growth failure are common; spontaneous improvement occurs at puberty.

Children with *deficiency of phosphorylase kinase* manifest hepatomegaly, mild muscular weakness, growth retardation and mild hypoglycemia. Glycogen is slightly increased in liver (10 per cent compared to normal <5 per cent) and in muscle (1.5 per cent compared to normal <1 per cent). Nevertheless, considerable degradation of glycogen occurs since injection of glucagon results in an appropriate rise in the level of blood glucose. In contrast to all other hepatic enzymatic defects resulting in hypoglycemia, which are inherited in an autosomal recessive fashion, this defect is inherited as an X-linked trait. Heterozygous females may manifest enlargement of the liver in childhood. The signs and symptoms of this disorder disappear at puberty.

In the very rare instances of *deficiency of glycogen synthetase*, only small amounts of glycogen can be synthesized in the liver. In this disorder, severe hypoglycemia occurs after an overnight fast.

HEREDITARY FRUCTOSE INTOLERANCE. The ingestion of fructose leads to abnormally elevated blood levels of fructose (fructosemia) in two conditions: One of these, *benign fructosemia*, also known as fructosuria, is an asymptomatic disorder resulting from a deficiency of fructokinase. The other disorder, known as *hereditary fructose intolerance*, is a serious disorder of infancy and one of the easily treated causes of hypoglycemia. (See also Section 8.)

The clinical symptoms of hypoglycemia in hereditary fructose intolerance are associated with other systemic manifestations. Affected infants do not exhibit symptoms until fructose is added to the diet. The infant then becomes anorexic, vomits and fails to thrive. Hypoglycemic manifestations include drowsiness during feeding, excessive sweating, pallor, rolling of the eyes, twitching and convulsions. Jaundice and hepatosplenomegaly develop and may be the presenting manifestations. Renal tubular involvement may result in glycosuria, aminoaciduria, proteinuria and acidosis. A low blood glucose concentration may be masked by elevated levels of fructose, unless the measurement is made by the glucose oxidase method. If not recognized and treated, the disorder may be fatal. The development of an aversion to fruits and other fructose-containing foods or to sucrose results in the spontaneous amelioration of symptoms and may account for survival into childhood before recognition of the disorder.

This is a genetic disorder transmitted in an autosomal recessive manner. The primary defect is a structural mutation of one of the two isozymes of aldolase, the so called liver type. This enzyme normally reacts with both fructose-1-phosphate and fructose-1,6-diphosphate. The muscle type of aldolase which remains in the liver reacts more readily with the diphosphate than the monophosphate; accordingly, the accumulation is primarily of fructose-1-phosphate.

The mechanism of the hypoglycemia is not known. It has been suggested that accumulation of fructose-1-phosphate may inhibit hepatic enzymes involved in the release of glucose.

FRUCTOSE-1,6-DIPHOSPHATASE DEFICIENCY. Hypoglycemia, acidosis and hepatomegaly are the characteristic hallmarks of this disorder; these findings are also typical of Type I glycogen storage disease (glucose-6-phosphatase deficiency). Fasting hypoglycemia may be severe or moderate and frequently has its onset in the newborn period. Episodes of dyspnea, tachypnea and hypotonia may occur and there is progressive hepatomegaly. Increased plasma levels of lactate, pyruvate, free fatty acids, ketones, alanine and uric acid are present. The five reported pedigrees have been of Dutch, German and Italian ancestry; the error appears to be inherited as an autosomal recessive trait.

Administration of glucagon results in a hyperglycemic response in the fed state but not in the fasting state. Glucose, galactose, maltose and lactose can be utilized, or stored as glycogen and then metabolized, since the glycogenolytic pathway is intact. On the other hand, fructose, glycerol and alanine cannot be converted to glucose and lead to lactic acidosis. The cause of the hypoglycemia is not certain but it is postulated that glycogenolysis is inhibited by accumulation of triose phosphates.

PYRUVATE CARBOXYLASE DEFICIENCY. Severe hypoglycemia with lactic acidosis has been reported in a neonate with deficiency of one of the two enzymatic activities of pyruvate carboxylase normally found in liver. The defective activity was for the low Km (high substrate affinity) component, and the infant was responsive to thiamine. It is not known how thiamine enhanced disposal of pyruvate and corrected lactic acidosis.

Mild hypoglycemia has been noted in some patients with *Leigh syndrome (subacute necrotizing encephalomyelopathy)*, a disorder also presumably due to a defect in pyruvate carboxylase. This enzyme has been found markedly reduced late in the course of Leigh syndrome, but it is not known whether this is a consequence or cause of the disorder.

Alanine, lactate and pyruvate equilibrate with each other, and are all elevated when there is deficiency of pyruvate carboxylase (Fig. 16–1).

GALACTOSEMIA. Hypoglycemia may be one of the clinical manifestations of galactosemia (galactose-1-phosphate uridyl transferase deficiency). (See also Section 8.) The low levels of glucose may be readily overlooked unless specific methods are utilized for its measurement, since concurrently elevated levels of galactose are measured by nonspecific reducing methods such as the Nelson-Somogyi and ferricyanide procedures. Hypoglycemia may occur after ingestion of milk, or during the course of a galactose tolerance test; blood glucose may fall to as low as 10 mg/dl. The mechanism responsible for the hypoglycemia is not completely understood; it has been suggested that the toxic amounts of galactose-1-phosphate and dulcitol found in this disorder not only cause renal damage, cataracts and cerebral damage, but also interfere with glucose release from the liver by inhibition of phosphoglucomutase and glucose-6-phosphatase.

MAPLE SYRUP URINE DISEASE. Fasting hypoglycemia has been observed in patients with this disorder. This appears to be related to a defect in gluconeogenesis from amino acids.

ENDOCRINE DEFICIENCIES

Cortisol and growth hormone are two of the principal hormones antagonistic to insulin and are necessary to maintain glucose homeostasis. Symptomatic hypoglycemia, especially after fasting, occurs in 10 to 20 per cent of patients with *isolated deficiency of growth hormone* or with *panhypopituitarism.* Prolonged and profound hypoglycemia in the neonatal period may be the first clue to severe hypopituitarism. The hypoglycemia appears to result from an inadequate supply of endogenous gluconeogenic substrates. For example, concentrations of amino acids 2 to 4 hours after a meal are markedly reduced. The hepatic gluconeogenic enzyme system is normal. When there is deficiency of both ACTH and growth hormone, replacement therapy with both cortisol and growth hormone is necessary to restore carbohydrate metabolism to normal. It is noteworthy that "ketotic" hypoglycemia has been described in patients with isolated deficiency of ACTH or of growth hormone.

Children with failure to thrive or *maternal deprivation syndrome* may first present to the physician with an episode of seizure or coma resulting from severe hypoglycemia. Deficiencies of ACTH and/or of growth hormone have been incriminated but they probably only aggravate the already deficient gluconeogenic substrates present in these patients.

Fasting hypoglycemia is a frequent concomitant of *Addison's disease* but is an uncommon presenting manifestation. In *congenital virilizing adrenal hyperplasia,* hypoglycemia has been noted only rarely. On the other hand, hypoglycemia is frequently the presenting manifestation in the newborn with *congenital adrenal hypoplasia* and in children with *familial glucocorticoid insufficiency* (see Section 17). The increased pigmentation which is almost invariably associated with the latter disorder is an important diagnostic clue.

Patients with hypopituitarism generally have decreased insulin release, but a subgroup of patients has been identified who have *hyperinsulinism* in association with deficiencies of growth hormone, ACTH and TSH. (See Section 17.)

Adrenal medullary unresponsiveness has been thought to be the cause of hypoglycemia in some children. Recent evidence indicates that failure to increase levels of epinephrine in response to hypoglycemia is a concomitant of the entity known as ketotic hypoglycemia.

KETOTIC HYPOGLYCEMIA

Ketotic hypoglycemia is the most common cause of hypoglycemia in childhood, accounting for more than half of all cases. Onset is usually between 18 months and 5 years of age, with spontaneous remission by 9 to 10 years of age. Boys are affected twice as often as girls, and low birth weight is a common characteristic of affected children. The attacks are episodic, most apt to occur in the morning, and frequently associated with ketonuria. Episodes seem to be related to periods of illness, vomiting or deprivation of food. Between attacks, affected children are in good health but tend to be small and thin. Hypoglycemic episodes respond promptly to administration of glucose.

Between attacks, carbohydrate tolerance tests give normal results. Hypoglycemia can be precipitated by prolonged fasting (18 to 24 hours) or by feeding a low-calorie, high-fat, low-carbohydrate (ketogenic) diet. Ketonuria frequently occurs under these conditions but is not a specific finding, since it may occur in normal children during fasting; moreover, unlike adults, about 20 per cent of normal children have blood glucose levels below 40 mg/dl after a 24-hour fast. Children with ketotic hypoglycemia usually do not respond to administration of glucagon with appropriate rises in blood glucose during either spontaneous or induced episodes of hypoglycemia; by contrast, one study found 49 of 52 normal children to have a greater than 10 mg/dl rise in glucose following administration of glucagon after a 24-hour fast. Failure to respond to glucagon reflects depletion of hepatic glycogen, but it may also be noted occasionally in fasted normal children and is not diagnostic. Between hypoglycemic episodes, the response to glucagon is normal, indicating normal hepatic glycogenolysis. During hypoglycemic episodes or during prolonged fasting, levels of insulin are appropriately low for the level of glucose. Insulin levels are normal after overnight fasting or after glucose tolerance tests made between attacks.

The precise mechanism of ketotic hypoglycemia is unsettled. The underlying defect is probably present at birth but does not become manifest until the child is stressed with caloric deprivation. Evidence suggests that hypoglycemia may be due to a deficient supply of endogenous gluconeogenic amino acids. Concentrations of plasma alanine are abnormally low in these children under basal and fasting conditions; infusions of alanine restore the hypoglycemic blood glucose level to normal without altering concentrations of pyruvate or lactate. The cause for the hypoalaninemia in these patients is unknown. Patients with deficiency of pituitary or adrenocortical hormones are also deficient in the same substrate; it is not surprising, therefore, that "ketotic" hypoglycemia has been reported in these conditions.

There have been reports of children with an inability to increase their plasma levels of epinephrine (*adrenal medullary hyporesponsiveness*) when they are subjected to hypoglycemia. This aberration was earlier thought to be a distinct cause of hypoglycemia, but increasing evidence indicates that affected patients have many of the clinical features of patients with ketotic hypoglycemia and that the two conditions are the same. In normal persons during hypoglycemic episodes excretion of epinephrine in the urine and levels in plasma are increased 5 to 20 fold above euglycemic levels. In children with ketotic hypoglycemia, both urinary excretion and rises in plasma levels of epinephrine are deficient when hypoglycemia is induced either by insulin or by a ketogenic diet. The cause for this effect is not known, nor is it settled whether it is specific for ketotic hypoglycemia or a primary or secondary effect. Many affected children also exhibit a subnormal response of endogenous cortisol level to hypoglycemia. Adrenomedullary and adrenocortical hyporesponsiveness are independent of each other, and it has been suggested that the primary defect may be in the hypothalamus or in delayed maturation of adrenal medullary synthesis of epinephrine.

DRUGS AND TOXINS

Ingestion of ethyl alcohol precipitates hypoglycemia in normal adults after a fast of 2 to 3 days, but in persons in whom the gluconeogenic reserve is decreased the hypoglycemic potential of alcohol is revealed after only 12 hours or so of fasting. The hypoglycemia is not mediated by an increase in insulin secretion and is not responsive to glucagon administration. It has been shown that ethanol itself, and not congeners or denaturants, is responsible for the hypoglycemia; the effect appears to result from suppression of hepatic gluconeogenesis and reduction of hepatic glucose output.

Young children are unusually susceptible to alcohol and may develop profound, disabling and even lethal hypoglycemic coma within an hour of drinking a leftover cocktail. There are reports of 28 instances of children developing hypoglycemia following ingestion of alcoholic beverages or substances containing alcohol; in one case the hypoglycemia was induced in a 6 month old febrile infant by sponging with alcohol. Convulsions were frequent, and 7 children died. The prevalence of this cause of hypoglycemia is much greater than the number of reported cases would indicate. Immediate intravenous administration of glucose corrects the condition; relapse is uncommon and continued administration of glucose is rarely necessary.

Salicylates and related compounds such as acetaminophen may cause hypoglycemia. This effect does not appear to be mediated through increased release of insulin, but it is possible that these drugs interfere with enzyme systems involved in glucose homeostasis.

Therapy with sulfonylureas during the last trimester of pregnancy has resulted in life-threatening hypoglycemia in newborn infants within hours of birth. Chlorpropamide, acetohexamide and tolbutamide have all been incriminated. Sulfonylureas cross the placenta and stimulate secretion of insulin from fetal islets. Intravenous glucose may be required continuously for as long as 4 days. Exchange transfusion has also been effective in treatment.

Propranolol, a beta-adrenergic blocking agent, has caused hypoglycemia in children who have been fasted in preparation for surgery or who have been on diminished oral intakes because of illness. In such instances, tachycardia and sweating may not be manifest, owing to the effect of the drug.

Jamaican vomiting sickness results from ingestion of "bush tea" made from unripe fruits of the ackee, which is grown in Jamaica. This disorder is characterized by severe vomiting, prostration, drowsiness, convulsions, hypoglycemia and coma, with blood glucose levels as low as 10 mg/dl. The mortality rate is high, death occurring within 24 hours. There are severe hepatic changes, including depletion of liver glycogen and fatty degeneration. The agent responsible is the plant toxin hypoglycin A, an unusual amino acid whose chemical structure is α-amino-methylenecyclopropylpropionic acid. Hypoglycin A is a specific inhibitor of isovaleryl CoA dehydrogenase, and leads to increased concentrations of isovaleric acid with some features of isovaleric acidemia. (See Section 8.) Accumulation of branched pentanoic acids may account for the fact that some patients with the illness fail to respond even to massive infusions of glucose.

OTHER CAUSES OF HYPOGLYCEMIA

HEPATIC DAMAGE. Severe hepatic damage may disturb the metabolism of carbohydrates sufficiently to produce hypoglycemia. Hepatotoxic agents, such as phosphorus, halogenated hydrocarbons (carbon tetrachloride) and hydrazine, may be responsible for hypoglycemia. Extensive infiltration of the liver by neoplastic cells, fibrous tissue, granulomas or fat may also lead to hypoglycemia, as may acute and chronic infectious hepatitis in the terminal stages. The mechanisms are not completely understood, but the hypoglycemia probably results from failure to store glycogen, impaired release of glucose into the blood stream, and decreased net synthesis of glucose from amino acids.

Reye syndrome is characterized by encephalopathy and fatty degeneration of the viscera; blood glucose levels below 25 to 30 mg/dl are common in younger children. Serum insulin levels are normal, and blood glucose levels are not increased by administration of glucagon. The hypoglycemia appears to be secondary to decreased hepatic glucose production; it is easily managed by infusion of glucose but such treatment appears to have little influence on the outcome.

On rare occasions, hypoglycemia occurs in patients with *leukemia*. The cause is not known; it has been suggested that reduced levels of glucose-6-phosphatase in the liver infiltrated by leukemia may play a role.

IMPAIRED INTESTINAL ABSORPTION OF GLUCOSE. Unlike most adults, children and especially infants may exhibit lowering of the blood glucose level when carbohydrate is withheld for 24 to 48 hours. However, fasting is rarely by itself a cause of clinical hypoglycemia; it may be a precipitating factor when other defects that may cause hypoglycemia are present. This may be the case when the level of blood glucose is lowered by impaired intestinal absorption accompanying chronic diarrhea, celiac disease or the edematous phase of the nephrotic syndrome. There are several specific defects in the intestinal absorption of sugars (See Section 11) such as of glucose and galactose, of sucrose and isomaltose, and of lactose, which are characterized by diarrhea, but they do not lead to significant hypoglycemia. Delayed absorption of glucose occurs in hypothyroidism, but is rarely of sufficient magnitude to lead to hypoglycemia.

RENAL GLYCOSURIA. Glycosuria due to defective tubular reabsorption of glucose occurs in a variety of clinical entities. It occurs as an isolated hereditary condition, in combination with glycinuria, in the de Toni-Fanconi syndrome, and in some patients with lead poisoning. It is rare that any of these conditions leads to hypoglycemia.

OTHER. Mild hypoglycemia is a complication of *kwashiorkor*, in which it may be secondary to impaired gluconeogenesis.

Hypoglycemia has occurred in *phenylketonuric* children when dietary restriction of phenylalanine has been too severe during the course of treatment. In these instances general malnutrition has been thought to be the principal factor causing the hypoglycemia.

Hypoglycemia has been observed repeatedly in association with some *extrapancreatic tumors*. The tumors are usually large mesodermal neoplasms (sarcomas) arising in the abdominal or thoracic cavity. The majority of reported patients have been adults; the phenomenon has been observed in a 5 year old child with Wilms' tumor and in two infants with congenital neuroblastoma. Hypoglycemia due to tumor is probably underdiagnosed, since fasting blood glucose levels are not determined routinely in children with tumors; its mechanism is unsettled.

Though the residuum of instances in which no cause for hypoglycemia can be established has decreased markedly in recent years, new pathogenetic causes continue to be discovered. A defect in glycerol metabolism has recently been found to account for hypoglycemia and ketonuria in a young child. Other recent reports of unique and bizarre symptom complexes with hypoglycemia suggest that much remains to be learned concerning glucose homeostasis.

CLINICAL MANIFESTATIONS OF HYPOGLYCEMIA

There is no constant relationship between blood glucose levels and the development or severity of symptoms of hypoglycemia in different patients or even in the same patient at different times. The rate of fall of blood glucose seems to be an important determining factor for the appearance of symptoms; a rapid fall is especially likely to produce symptoms. Even at extremely low blood levels of glucose, children manifest great variability in their responses. Some become conditioned to repeated hypoglycemic episodes or to hypoglycemia of long duration, so that they have few or no symptoms. This is evidenced by children with type I glycogenosis (von Gierke's disease). The symptoms of hypoglycemia are derived chiefly from disturbances of the central nervous system. Neural tissue has little stored carbohydrate and, unlike other tissues, cannot utilize sugars other than glucose, so that it is dependent upon a continuous and adequate supply of blood glucose to maintain its normal functions. There is evidence that neural tissue can utilize free fatty acids or amino acid as sources of energy; this is thought to be the case in children with prolonged hypoglycemia who are asymptomatic.

Hypoglycemic symptoms are protean, but often produce more or less characteristic patterns in individual patients. Sweating, pallor, fatigue, hunger, tachycardia and nervousness occur as a result of excessive secretion of epinephrine in response to the hypoglycemia. Central nervous system dysfunction is manifested by headache, irritability, negativism, alterations in behavior, drowsiness, mental confusion, psychotic behavior, seizures and coma.

In newborn and young infants, recognition and evaluation of symptoms may be difficult except as the possibility of hypoglycemia is considered. Convulsions are often the first recognized manifestation, but irritability, poor feeding, lethargy, excessive drowsiness, eye-rolling, sweating and twitching are more common symptoms. Even with very low glucose levels, hypoglycemic symptoms may be absent in the neonate. It has been recently recognized that young infants with hypoglycemia may manifest cardiomegaly and even heart failure, which remit promptly with elevation of the blood level of glucose.

DIAGNOSIS OF HYPOGLYCEMIA

Two distinct problems are posed: (1) the detection of hypoglycemia, and (2) the determination of its cause. Many children exhibit clinical manifestations on one or more occasions which suggest hypoglycemia, but hypoglycemia can be demonstrated in them only under specific conditions. In others, hypoglycemia is readily demonstrated by blood glucose determinations. Once hypoglycemia is established, it is essential to determine the cause. There is no routine approach for the study of patients with manifestations of hypoglycemia; individualization in the choice of diagnostic procedures is essential.

One must evaluate the information garnered from the history and physical examination before undertaking exhaustive tests of carbohydrate function. Since many of the causes for hypoglycemia are genetically determined, a family history of other affected persons or of consanguinity may be pertinent. The initial episode of hypoglycemia caused by ingestion of alcohol or other toxins can usually be identified by the history. The infant with galactosemia usually has other clinical manifestations to suggest the diagnosis before hypoglycemia is suspected. A history of aversion to fruits and sweets, and the occurrence of gastrointestinal manifestations as well as those of hypoglycemia following ingestion of foods containing fructose should suggest hereditary fructose intolerance. Aggravation of hypoglycemic symptoms by meals rich in protein suggests leucine sensitivity and hyperinsulinism.

Hepatomegaly should alert one to the hepatic causes of hypoglycemia. Growth failure directs attention to pituitary hypofunction, whereas manifestations of Addison's disease lead to consideration of adrenal hypofunction. The association of large tumors in the thoracic or abdominal cavity with hypoglycemia should suggest a causative relation. The presence of acidosis points to a deficiency of one of the hepatic enzymes.

Hypoglycemic episodes which follow periods of undereating or of vomiting and which have their onset after 1 to 2 years of age are suggestive of ketotic hypoglycemia. Once the acute episode is over, all the usual tolerance tests are normal, and it generally requires a period of prolonged fasting (18 to 24 hours) to provoke hypoglycemia.

One of the most difficult differentials is to distinguish the child with a functioning islet cell tumor. Levels of insulin in other conditions may not be clearly elevated. In the presence of abnormally low glucose levels, however, plasma insulin should normally be suppressed; levels as low as 7 to 15 μU/ml, therefore, may be indicative of hyperinsulinism. The leucine and tolbutamide tests are very useful for unmasking states of insulin hypersecretion. Once hyperinsulinism is established, a trial of therapy with diazoxide may serve as a useful mode of treatment as well as of diagnosis. Most patients with functioning beta cell tumors will not respond to diazoxide and laparotomy is then usually necessary to establish the diagnosis.

LABORATORY DATA. Tests for the evaluation of carbohydrate metabolism (Table 16–5) are usually performed after an overnight fast except in young infants, for whom a 6-hour period is adequate. Oc-

TABLE 16–5 TOLERANCE TESTS FOR THE EVALUATION OF CARBOHYDRATE METABOLISM

COMPOUND	ROUTE		TIME TO OBTAIN SAMPLES (MINUTES)	CRITICAL MEASUREMENTS
L-Alanine	Oral	500 mg/kg	0,30,60,90	Glucose and lactate
	IV	250 mg/kg (as 10% solution in sterile pyrogen-free water)	0,10,20,30,45,60 90	
Glucose	Oral	1.75 gm/kg	0,30,60,90,120, 180,240,300	Glucose and insulin
	IV	0.4 gm/kg (as 10 to 20% solution over 4 min. period)	0,5,10,20,30,40, 50,60	
Galactose	Oral	1.75 gm/kg	0,30,60,90,120	Glucose and lactate
Glycerol	Oral	1 gm/kg	0,10,20,30,45,60,90, 120	Glucose and lactate
Fructose	Oral	0.5 gm/kg	0,30,45,60,90	Glucose, phosphate and lactate
	IV	0.25 gm/kg (as 10% solution over 4 min. period)	0,10,20,30,45,60,90,120	
L-Leucine	Oral	150 mg/kg (as 2% solution or slurry)	0,15,30,45,60,90,120	Glucose and insulin
	IV	75 mg/kg (as 2% solution in 0.45% NaCl)	0,10,20,30,45,60,90	
Glucagon	IM	30 μg/kg (1 mg maximum)	0,15,30,45,60,90,120	Glucose and lactate
Tolbutamide	IV	20 mg/kg (1 gm maximum) (over 1 min. period)	0,5,10,20,30,45, 60,90,120	Glucose and insulin

IV = intravenous; IM = intramuscular.

casionally, owing to the severity of the hypoglycemia, shorter periods of fasting are indicated. When the expected response of a given test is a lowering of the blood glucose level, the fasting glucose level should be 50 mg/dl or higher to permit a sufficient differential in glucose levels for comparative purposes. The patient should be in reasonably good nutritional state and free of fever when a test is performed.

It is important that appropriate analytic methods be used to determine the concentration of glucose. Glucose is measured specifically when glucose oxidase or one of the other enzymatic methods is used, whereas methods depending upon reduction are not specific for glucose. It is also important to consider that values for serum or plasma levels of glucose are approximately 15 per cent higher than those obtained when whole blood is utilized.

A number of tests have evolved for the study of the patient with hypoglycemia. Some are of little value and others of importance only in the delineation of specific disorders. The appropriate use of these tests is based on a knowledge of carbohydrate metabolism and the purposes for which the tests were designed. Precise diagnosis of some hypoglycemic conditions requires measurements of lactate, ketones, growth hormone or cortisol, or assay of specific enzyme activities.

Levels of insulin should be measured in all hypoglycemic patients. The fasting level is rarely above 10 μU/ml. A level above 10 μU/ml in plasma with a blood glucose under 50 mg/dl is abnormal and suggests hyperinsulinism.

The *glucagon tolerance test* is a useful procedure to study the ability of the liver to release glucose into the circulation from stored glycogen. The *epinephrine tolerance test* has been replaced by the safer glucagon test. Normally a rise of blood glucose of 25 to 50 mg/dl. should occur within 15 to 45 minutes. Failure of an adequate response may be due to depletion of liver glycogen by starvation or hepatic disease. It may be necessary to test the patient in both the fed and fasting state. For example, in glucose-6-phosphatase deficiency, there is no rise in glucose level following administration of glucagon in either the fasting or fed state, whereas in debrancher deficiency the response is normal postprandially but not after fasting. Children with ketotic hypoglycemia exhibit an inadequate response to glucagon during the hypoglycemic episode or after a 24-hour fast, but respond normally between attacks.

The *galactose tolerance test* should not be used for the diagnosis of galactosemia, since it may induce severe hypoglycemia; direct assay of uridyl transferase activity is the appropriate diagnostic method. Infusion of galactose provokes a rise in the level of lactate in patients with glucose-6-phosphatase deficiency but not with other conditions.

The *fructose tolerance test* is primarily of use in the detection of hereditary fructose intolerance and of fructose-1,6-diphosphatase deficiency. Administration of fructose to patients results in a decrease of blood glucose to hypoglycemic levels and a rise in the level of blood fructose. In addition, the level of serum inorganic phosphorus is decreased, the concentration of lactic acid is increased, and the insulin level remains unchanged. For this test the blood glucose level must be measured by the glucose oxidase method, since the total concentration of reducing sugar remains relatively constant.

The *leucine tolerance test* is used to determine whether this amino acid provokes an exaggerated release of insulin. It is helpful in unmasking hypersecretory states (see above). Normal children exhibit a small but significant rise in concentration of insulin in blood and a decrease of approximately 10 mg/dl in concentration of glucose. In some pathologic states, a marked rise in level of insulin is accompanied by a profound fall in level of glucose, as in leucine-sensitive hypoglycemia. In other conditions, such as obesity, a marked rise in the level of insulin is associated with only a normal decline in level of blood glucose.

The *tolbutamide tolerance test* measures the ability of the pancreas to release insulin, as determined by the degree and duration of the hypoglycemic response. In normal children the blood glucose level falls about 20 to 40 per cent within 20 to 30 minutes and returns to normal within 60 to 90 minutes. In hypoglycemic patients there is an exaggerated response in the increase of insulin level and in the decrease of glucose level. The increase in level of insulin in response to tolbutamide is quite rapid and can be easily missed if blood levels are not obtained early. Infants with hyperinsulinism of any etiology may exhibit a profound and prolonged response to tolbutamide.

The *alanine tolerance test* is useful for evaluating gluconeogenesis. In normal individuals administration of L-alanine results in an increase in blood levels of glucose if the patient has been suitably fasted and hepatic glycogen stores are depleted. Patients with deficiency of fructose-1,6-diphosphatase do not exhibit a rise in blood glucose; instead, the already elevated level of lactate is increased further.

The *glycerol tolerance test* may be utilized for the same purpose as alanine.

TREATMENT OF HYPOGLYCEMIA

During a hypoglycemic attack the child should under no circumstances be left unattended. The immediate symptoms may be relieved by the administration of glucose, but it should be kept in mind that hypoglycemia of either the organic or functional type may be only temporarily abated by the administration of glucose and may rebound to hypoglycemic levels as the release of additional insulin is evoked. In such situations frequent feedings of small amounts of carbohydrates are advisable until the patient is stabilized.

For some conditions glucagon in a dose of 1 mg intramuscularly is usually effective in terminating a hypoglycemic episode. This form of therapy is a useful emergency measure which parents can be trained to utilize in the home. It is *not* effective in the glycogenoses, in other hepatic disease or in ketotic hypoglycemia. Even when it is effective, it should be followed by the oral administration of sugar in some readily absorbable form acceptable to the child.

When the cause of the hypoglycemia is established, treatment should be related to it.

Patients with ketotic hypoglycemia do well with a program of frequent feedings (4 or 5 meals a day) of a diet high in protein and in carbohydrate. During periods of illness and fasting, high carbohydrate liquids should be offered at frequent intervals. Patients with deficiencies of specific hepatic enzymes may require special dietary management to remove offending foodstuffs. Children with pituitary or adrenocortical insufficiency require replacement therapy with the appropriate hormones.

The most difficult patients to manage have been those with hyperinsulinism. Diazoxide, a non-diuretic benzothiodiazine, has proved to be a remarkably effective agent in controlling hypoglycemia in these patients. The drug acts primarily by suppressing insulin release. The usual dose is 10 mg/kg/day, given orally in two divided doses; the dose range has been 5 to 20 mg/kg/day. The most common side effect is hypertrichosis, particularly of the back, extremities and face. Once the drug is discontinued, the hypertrichosis disappears. The majority of children with hyperinsulinism of any etiology other than adenoma respond satisfactorily. Failure to respond suggests a functioning adenoma, though there have been occasional patients with proven adenomas who have responded quite satisfactorily to diazoxide. On the other hand, some patients with beta cell hyperplasia or nesidioblastosis have failed to respond. Patients who fail to respond to treatment with diazoxide should be explored for an adenoma. If none is found, a subtotal pancreatectomy will frequently be helpful in reducing the frequency and severity of hyperglycemic attacks. In the event of recurrence of hypoglycemia after pancreatectomy, another course of diazoxide is indicated, since the drug may then be effective. The occasional refractory patient may require corticosteroids, repeated attempts at surgical control, or even Streptozotocin, a potent diabetogenic antibiotic used primarily to treat carcinoma of the pancreatic islet cells (still under investigation).

A significant number of patients with hyperinsulinism exhibit spontaneous remissions. The hypoglycemic episodes become less frequent and fasting glucose levels gradually rise. Diazoxide may be discontinued and the patient remain asymptomatic. Some such patients still exhibit leucine-sensitivity. Patients with ketotic hypoglycemia characteristically remit by 10 years of age.

Brain damage is a frequent concomitant of hypoglycemia. The earlier in life the onset of hypoglycemia and the more protracted and profound its course, the more likely is brain damage a sequel. It is usually manifested by mental retardation, learning and behavior problems, ataxia and/or seizures. The electroencephalogram is usually abnormal during hypoglycemic episodes and may remain abnormal between seizures. Even after hypoglycemia is in remission, abnormal EEG tracings and seizures may persist; such normoglycemic seizures require treatment with anticonvulsant agents.

Psychologic guidance of the hypoglycemic child and his family is of paramount importance.

ANGELO M. DIGEORGE
VICTOR H. AUERBACH

Abbasi, A., and Power, L.: Insulin and insulin-like activity in extracts of tumors associated with hypoglycemia. Diabetes *22*:762, 1973.

Baerentsen, H.: Neonatal hypoglycemia due to an islet-cell adenoma. Acta Paediatr. Scand. *62*:207, 1973.

Baker, L., Kaye, R., Root, A. W., and Prasad, A. L. N.: Diazoxide treatment of idiopathic hypoglycemia of infancy. J. Pediatr. *71*:494, 1967.

Balsam, M. J., Baker, L., Bishop, H. C., Hummeler, K., Yakovac, W. C., and Kaye, R.: Beta cell adenoma in a child with hypoglycemia controlled with diazoxide. J. Pediatr. *80*:788, 1972.

Brunette, M., Delvin, E., Hazel, B., and Scriver, C. D.: Thiamine-responsive lactic acidosis in a patient with deficient low-Km pyruvate carboxylase activity in liver. Pediatrics *50*:702, 1972.

Buist, N.R.M., Campbell, J. R., Castro, A., and Brant, B.: Congenital islet cell adenoma causing hypoglycemia in a newborn. Pediatrics *47*:605, 1971.

Chaussain, J. L.: Glycemic response to 24 hour fast in normal children and children with ketotic hypoglycemia. J. Pediatr. *82*:438, 1973.

Christensen, N. J.: Hypoadrenalinemia during insulin hypoglycemia in children with ketotic hypoglycemia. J. Clin. Endocrinol. *38*:107, 1974.

Colle, E., and Ulstrom, R. A.: Ketotic hypoglycemia. J. Pediatr. *64*:632, 1964.

Collipp, P. J.: Hypoglycemia and leukemia. Pediatrics *46*:788, 1970.

Combs, J. T., Grunt, J. A., and Brandt, I. K.: New syndrome of neonatal hypoglycemia: Association with visceromegaly, macroglossia, microcephaly and abnormal umbilicus. New Engl. J. Med., *275*:236, 1966.

Cornblath, M., Pildes, R. S., and Schwartz, R.: Hypoglycemia in infancy and childhood. J. Pediatr. *83*:692, 1973.

Cornblath, M., and Schwartz, R.: Disorders of Carbohydrate Metabolism in Infancy. Philadelphia, W. B. Saunders Company, 1966.

Danks, D. M.: Childhood hypoglycemia, as a sequel of erythroblastosis fetalis. Acta Paediatr. Scand. *58*:369, 1969.

DiGeorge, A. M., Auerbach, V. H., and Mabry, C. C.: Leucine-induced hypoglycemia. III. The blood glucose depressant action of leucine in normal individuals. J. Pediatr. *63*:295, 1963.

Dodge, P. R., Mancall, E. L., Crawford, J. D., Knapp, J., and Paine, R. S.: Hypoglycemia complicating treatment of phenylketonuria with a phenylalanine-deficient diet. New Engl. J. Med. *260*:1104, 1959.

Ehrlich, R. M., and Martin, J. M.: Tolbutamide tolerance test and plasma-insulin response in children with idiopathic hypoglycemia. J. Pediatr. *71*:485, 1967.

Falorni, A., Fracassini, F., Mass-Benedetti, F., and Amici, A.: Glucose metabolism, plasma insulin, and growth hormone secretion in newborn infants with erythroblastosis fetalis compared with normal newborns and those born to diabetic mothers. Pediatrics *49*:682, 1972.

Glasgow, A. M., Cotton, R. B., and Dhiensiri, K.: Reye syndrome. III. The hypoglycemia. Am. J. Dis. Child. *125*:809, 1973.

Goodall, McC., Cragan, M., and Sidbury, J.: Decreased epinephrine excretion in idiopathic hypoglycemia. Am. J. Dis. Child. *123*:569, 1972.

Grover, W. D., Auerbach, V. H., and Patel, M. S.: Biochemical studies and therapy in subacute necrotizing encephalomyelopathy (Leigh's syndrome). J. Pediatr. *81*:39, 1972.

Haworth, J. C., and Coodin, F. J.: Idiopathic spontaneous hypoglycemia in children. Report of seven cases and review of the literature. Pediatrics *25*:748, 1960.

Haymond, M. W., Karl, I. E., Feigin, R. D., DeVivo, D., and Pagliara, A. S.: Hypoglycemia and maple syrup urine disease: Defective gluconeogenesis. Pediatr. Res. *7*:500, 1973.

Honicky, R. E., and dePapp, E. W.: Mediastinal teratoma with endocrine function. Am. J. Dis. Child. *126*:650, 1973.

Huijing, F.: Genetic defects of glycogen metabolism and its control. Ann. N.Y. Acad. Sci. *210*:290, 1973.

Joassin, G., Parker, M. L., Pildes, R. S., and Cornblath, M.: Infants of diabetic mothers. Diabetes *16*:306, 1967.

Johnson, J. D., Hansen, R. C., Albritton, W. L., Worthemann, U., and Christiansen, R. O.: Hypoplasia of the anterior pituitary and neonatal hypoglycemia. J. Pediatr. *82*:634, 1973.

Koffler, H., Schubert, W. K., and Hug, G.: Sporadic hypoglycemia: Abnormal epinephrine response to the ketogenic diet or to insulin. J. Pediatr. *78*:448, 1971.

Levin, B., Snodgrass, G. J. A. I., Oberholzer, V. G., Burgess, E. A., and Dobbs, R. H.: Fructosaemia. Observations on seven cases. Am. J. Med. *45*:826, 1948.

Loridan, L., Sadeghi-Nejad, A., and Senior, B.: Hypersecretion of insulin after the administration of L-leucine to obese children. J. Pediatr. *78*:53, 1971.

Loutfi, A. H., Mehrez, I., Shahbender, S., and Abdine, F. H.: Hypoglycaemia with Wilms' tumour. Arch. Dis. Child. *39*:197, 1964.

McBride, J. T., McBride, M. C., and Viles, P. H.: Hypoglycemia associated with propranolol. Pediatrics *51*:1085, 1973.

Molsted-Pedersen, L., Trautner, H., and Jorgensen, K. R.: Plasma insulin and K values during intravenous glucose tolerance test in newborn infants with erythroblastosis foetalis. Acta Paediatr. Scand. *62*:11, 1973.

Moss, M. H.: Alcohol induced hypoglycemia and coma caused by alcohol sponging. Pediatrics *46*:445, 1970.

Nordmann, Y., Schapira, F., and Dreyfus, J. C.: A structurally modified liver aldolase in fructose intolerance: Immunologic and kinetic evidence. Biochem. Biophys. Res. Commun. *31*: 884, 1968.

Pagliara, A. S., Karl, I. E., DeVivo, D. C., Feigen, R. D., and Kipnis, D. M.: Hypoalaninemia: A concomitant of ketotic hypoglycemia. J. Clin. Invest. *51*:1440, 1972.

Pagliara, A. S., Karl, I. E., Haymond, M., and Kipnis, D. M.: Hypoglycemia in infants and childhood. Part I. J. Pediatr. *82*:365; Part II. 558, 1973.

Paliara, A. S., Karl, I. E., Keating, J. P., Brown, B. I., and Kipnis, D. M.: Hepatic fructose-1,6-diphosphatase deficiency. A cause of lactic acidosis and hypoglycemia in infancy. J. Clin. Invest. *51*:2115, 1972.

Parks, J. S., Baker, L., Vaidya, V., Moshang, T., Jr., and Bongiovanni, A. M.: Hyperinsulinism and hypoglycemia in hypopituitary children. Abstracts Endo. Soc., 1973, p. A-166.

Schiff, D., Aranda, J. V., Colle, E., and Stern, L.: Metabolic effects of exchange transfusion. II. Delayed hypoglycemia following exchange transfusion with citrated blood. J. Pediatr. *79*:589, 1971.

Schutt-Aine, J. C., Drash, A. L., and Kenny, F. M.: Possible relationship between spontaneous hypoglycemia and "maternal deprivation syndrome." Case Reports. J. Pediatr. *82*:809, 1973.

Schwartz, J. F., and Zwiren, G. T.: Islet cell adenomatosis and adenoma in an infant. J. Pediatr. *79*:232, 1971.

Seltzer, H. S.: Drug-induced hypoglycemia. A review based on 473 cases. Diabetes *21*:955, 1972.

Shapiro, M., Sincha, A., Rosenmann, E., and Shafrir, E.: Hypoglycemia associated with neonatal neuroblastoma and abnormal responses of serum glucose and free fatty acids to epinephrine injection. Israel J. Med. Sci. *2*:705, 1966.

Slone, D., Taitz, L. S., and Gilchrist, G. S.: Aspects of carbohydrate metabolism in kwashiorkor: with special reference to spontaneous hypoglycaemia. Brit. M. J. *1*:32, 1961.

Snyder, R. D., and Robinson, A.: Leucine-induced hypoglycemia. Am. J. Dis. Child. *113*:566, 1967.

Tanaka, K., Isselbacher, K. J., and Shih, V.: Isovaleric and α-methylbutyric acidemias induced by hypoglycin A: Mechanism of Jamaican vomiting sickness. Science *175*:69, 1972.

Tietze, H. U., Zurbrügg, R. P., Zuppinger, K. A., Joss, E. E., and Käser, H.: Occurrence of impaired cortisol regulation in children with hypoglycemia associated with adrenal medullary hyporesponsiveness. J. Clin. Endocrinol. *34*:948, 1972.

Underwood, L. E., van den Brande, J. L., Antony, G. J., Voina, S. J., and van Wyk, J. J.: Islet cell function and glucose homeostasis in hypopituitary dwarfism: Synergism between growth hormone and cortisone. J. Pediatr. *82*:28, 1973.

Vance, J. E., et al.: Familial nesidioblastosis as the predominant manifestation of multiple endocrine adenomatosis. Am. J. Med. *52*:211, 1972.

Yakovac, W. C., Baker, L., and Hummeler, K.: Beta cell nesidioblastosis in idiopathic hypoglycemia of infancy. J. Pediatr. *79*:226, 1971.

Woolf, L. I.: Inherited metabolic disorders: Galactosemia. Adv. Clin. Chem. *5*:1, 1962.

17
THE ENDOCRINE SYSTEM

DISORDERS OF THE HYPOTHALAMUS AND PITUITARY GLAND

The pituitary gland and the hypothalamus consist of seven or more separate functional units working in concert to maintain endocrine homeostasis. Certain conditions heretofore classified as disorders of the pituitary gland really have a hypothalamic origin. Recent advances in the isolation and synthesis of hypothalamic hormones (factors) have permitted more precise delineation of many endocrinologic conditions. The techniques for differentiation between hypopituitary and hypothalamic aberrations are rapidly becoming available for general clinical application, and new therapeutic approaches are in sight.

The pituitary gland is attached by a stalk to the median eminence of the brain and consists of a posterior lobe (neurohypophysis) and an anterior lobe. The differing connections of each lobe to the hypothalamus reflect their different embryologic origins. The posterior lobe is derived from the infundibulum of the diencephalon and has direct neural connections via a large tract of fibers originating in the supraoptic and paraventricular nuclei of the anterior hypothalamus, whereas the anterior lobe develops from ectoderm of the stomadeum (Rathke's pouch) and is controlled by hypothalamic secretions. The nerve endings of a variety of hypothalamic nerve fibers liberate neurohormones into the capillaries of the median eminence, from which they are carried by the portal vessels to the pituitary gland. Accordingly, the median eminence is the final common pathway of all releasing factors. Fetal rests of the original connection of Rathke's pouch with the primitive oral cavity may persist in postnatal life; tumors developing from such rests are known as craniopharyngiomas and are the most common tumor arising in the region of the pituitary gland during childhood.

FUNCTION

Anterior Lobe. The anterior pituitary consists of at least six different types of secretory cells which synthesize and secrete a variety of protein hormones. These hormones act either on other endocrine glands or directly on a wide variety of body cells to affect almost every organ. The pituitary gland itself is under the control of hypothalamic secretions, each of which regulates specific pituitary target cells. Hypothalamic secretions are of two types, those which release pituitary hormones (releasing hormones) and those which inhibit secretion of pituitary hormones (inhibitory hormones). Pituitary hormones which lack feedback control from the product of a target gland (growth hormone, prolactin and melanocyte-stimulating hormone) require hypothalamic inhibitors and stimulators for their control. Only hypothalamic stimulators are known for corticotropin, thyrotropin, luteinizing hormone and follicle-stimulating hormone, since inhibition is effected by target gland hormones (corticosteroids, thyroxine and sex steroids).

Growth hormone (HGH) is a protein with 188 amino acids. Unlike other pituitary hormones, it is species-specific; only primate growth hormone is effective in man. All the growth hormone currently used to treat HGH-deficient children is obtained from human pituitaries laboriously collected at autopsy. The hypothalamic-releasing hormone (GH-RH) has yet to be isolated. On the other hand, the inhibiting hormone (GH-IH) has been isolated, characterized and synthesized; it consists of 14 amino acids and has been named *somatostatin.* Preliminary studies with this hormone have established that it can suppress secretion of growth hormone in man, and it is hoped that it may be useful in the management of diseases associated with excess secretion, such as acromegaly, gigantism and diabetic angiopathy, particularly retinopathy.

Deficiency of growth hormone results in dwarfism, and an excess in gigantism or acromegaly. It is now established that growth hormone stimulates skeletal and protein anabolism via the production of a class of intermediary hormones named *somatomedins* (formerly known as sulfation factor). Somatomedins are peptides with molecular weights about one third that of growth hormone and appear to be synthesized in the liver and kidney. How many such substances exist, their structures, the manner in which they are formed and their physiologic roles remain to be determined. Defects in this class of potent insulin-like substances probably account for some types of growth disorders; pure somatomedins might prove to be potent therapeutic agents. Growth hormone-deficient children have low levels of somatomedins, which return to normal during treatment with HGH.

Random levels of growth hormone in normal children may be quite low for much of the day and fail to distinguish between normal and growth hormone-deficient patients. Hence, a variety of provocative tests have evolved for clinical evaluation of pituitary growth hormone reserves. Both insulin-induced hypoglycemia and intravenous infusion of arginine evoke prompt rises in serum HGH in normal patients. Recently a single oral dose of L-dopa (500 mg) has proved to be a reliable stimulus of growth hormone secretion, circumventing the need for intravenous infusion or the risk of dangerous hypoglycemia. L-Dopa crosses the blood-brain barrier and probably increases hypothalamic levels of dopamine, which stimulates growth hormone-releasing hormone and, in turn, stimulates growth hormone secretion. This test is becoming the preferred test to evaluate growth hormone secretory reserve. If the results are abnormal, the provocative tests with insulin and/or arginine are indicated. After 3 to 6 months of age, a definite cycle develops, with sharp rises of growth hormone levels during deep sleep. A single normal growth hormone level 45 to 90 minutes after onset of sleep is strong indication that growth hormone deficiency is not present, whereas a low level requires provocative tests. A short period of exercise strenuous enough to make the patient breathless is also a potent stimulator of growth hormone secretion and can be used as a screening test to rule out growth hormone deficiency.

Prolactin (HPr) has only recently been separated from growth hormone in man and established as a separate molecule. Prolactin activity had for many years been ascribed to growth hormone because the ratio in the pituitary of growth hormone to prolactin (between 100 and 500 to 1) hampered its isolation. With pure prolactin available, a specific and sensitive radioimmunoassay has been developed, and data concerning levels in normal and aberrant physiologic states are being accumulated. The only established role for prolactin is the initiation and maintenance of lactation. Stimulation of the nipple is a potent physiologic stimulus to prolactin secretion. Mean serum levels in children and fasting adults of both sexes are about 5–20 ng/ml. Grossly elevated levels occur in full term neonates and during pregnancy. Extremely high levels of prolactin occur in amniotic fluid (10,000 ng/ml in the first trimester and 1000 ng/ml at term); neither its source nor its function is known.

Prolactin is controlled primarily by prolactin-inhibiting factor (PIF). There is evidence for the existence of a prolactin-releasing factor (PRF), but neither PIF nor PRF has been isolated or characterized. Chlorpromazine increases and L-dopa decreases serum prolactin, presumably by altering catecholamine levels in the hypothalamus, with resultant decrease or increase in prolactin-inhibiting factor. Thyrotropin-releasing factor also increases prolactin levels, but its action is directly on the pituitary gland. These drugs are useful in the functional evaluation of prolactin secretion in man and allow the differentiation of pituitary defects from hypothalamic defects.

Prolactin is pathologically elevated with section of the pituitary stalk, in certain pituitary tumors and in a variety of hypothalamic disorders. Elevated levels of both TSH and prolactin occur in primary hypothyroidism. Failure of an increase in prolactin following administration of throtropin-releasing factor (TRF) is the hallmark of primary pituitary disease.

Thyrotropin (TSH) is a glycoprotein with a molecular weight of about 26,000. TSH increases iodine uptake, iodide clearance from the plasma, iodotyrosine and iodothyronine formation, thyroglobulin proteolysis and release of thyroxine and triiodothyronine from the thyroid. Deficiency results in inactivity and atrophy of the thyroid, and excess results in hypertrophy and hyperplasia. A sensitive radioimmunoassay for TSH in serum aids in the study of clinical problems.

The thyrotropin-releasing factor (TRF), which stimulates release of TSH, was the first hypothalamic hormone to be isolated, characterized and synthesized; it is a tripeptide ([pyro] Glu-His-Pro-NH_2). Thyroxine and triiodothyronine inhibit TSH secretion by blocking the action of TRF upon the pituitary cell. Surprisingly, TRF also stimulates the release of prolactin, in males as well as in females. Synthetic TRF is now available for clinical studies and has already proved to be a useful diagnostic compound for testing pituitary reserve of TSH and prolactin. Through such studies it is possible to discriminate between the hypothalamic and pituitary origins of many disorders.

Corticotropin (ACTH) is a single unbranched chain of 39 amino acids, which acts primarily on the adrenal cortex. It produces changes in adrenal structure, chemical composition and enzymatic activity, and stimulates the release of cortical steroid hormones. Although corticotropin-releasing hormone (CRH) was the first hypothalamic hormone to be demonstrated, attempts at its isolation in sufficient quantities to permit its characterization have been unsuccessful. Radioimmunoassays exist for ACTH in plasma, but their general clinical application has been limited because they require prior extraction of plasma. A new redox bioassay, capable of measuring femtogram (10^{-15}) levels in 10 μl samples of plasma, appears to offer great promise. By this assay, the mean level of circulating ACTH is 30 pg/ml at 9 A.M. and 8 pg/ml at 10 P.M. The normal newborn infant has a mean level of 63 pg/ml in the morning.

Melanocyte-stimulating hormone (MSH) consists of two separate peptides. One, α-MSH, contains 13 amino acids and is identical to the first 13 amino acids of ACTH, but has no corticotrophic activity. The second peptide, β-MSH, consists of 22 amino acids and shares a sequence in common with both α-MSH and ACTH. In man β-MSH is the chief pigmentary hormone, and there is evidence that it is synthesized in the same cell as ACTH. There is good correlation of plasma levels of ACTH and β-MSH when the steroid feedback mechanism is interfered with, as in Addison's disease and in Cushing's disease. On the other hand, insulin-induced hypoglycemia provokes release of ACTH but not of β-MSH. Evidence exists for separate hypothalamic-releasing (MRH) and -inhibiting hormones (MRIH).

Gonadotropic hormones include two specific glycoproteins: luteinizing hormone (LH) and follicle-stimulating hormone (FSH). Each is made up of two subunits, an α subunit and a β subunit. The α subunits of these two hormones as well as of TSH are very similar; specificity of hormone action is endowed by the β subunit, which is different for each of these three hormones. FSH stimulates follicular development in the ovary and gametogenesis in the testis. LH promotes luteinization of the ovary and Leydig cell function of the testis. Highly specific and sensitive radioimmunoassays for FSH and LH are now generally available. Both hormones are measurable in the plasma of prepubertal children.

Hypothalamic control of gonadotropic hormones has long been known, and it was generally accepted that there were separate releasing hormones for FSH and LH. Luteinizing hormone-releasing hormone (LRH), a decapeptide, has been isolated and synthesized. This substance leads to the release of both LH and FSH, and it is now proposed that there may be only one gonadotropin-releasing hormone. Increasing availability of LRH for clinical studies is resulting in important new insights into dysfunctions of the hypothalamic-pituitary-gonadal axis. Thus far, LRH has not proved to be as effective as TRF in differentiating between hypothalamic and pituitary disorders.

Posterior Lobe. The posterior lobe of the pituitary is part of a functional unit known as the neurohypophysis, which consists of (1) the neurons of the supraoptic and paraventricular nuclei of the hypothalamus; (2) their axons, which form the pituitary stalk; and (3) the posterior lobe of the pituitary.

The neurohypophysis is the source of *arginine vasopressin* (antidiuretic hormone or ADH) and *oxytocin*; both are octapeptides, differing in only two amino acids. These hormones are produced by a process of neurosecretion in the hypothalamic nuclei. There is strong evidence that a protein (*neurophysin*) with an affinity for these two hormones is also secreted, that it acts as a transporter of the hormones down the pituitary stalk and that it is with neurophysin that they are stored in the neurohypophysis. Since neurophysin is easier to measure by radioimmunoassay than ADH, it may provide a direct index of vasopressin levels in plasma.

HYPOPITUITARISM

Here we shall discuss only those hypopituitary states associated with deficiency of growth hormone. Affected children have usually been referred to as pituitary dwarfs, a designation best avoided when possible. Isolated deficiencies of thyrotropin, corticotropin and gonadotropin are covered in other sections.

ETIOLOGY

Congenital Defects. Aplasia or hypoplasia of the pituitary without abnormalities of the skull and brain is rare. More often developmental abnormalities of the pituitary are associated with such defects as anencephaly, holoprosencephaly (cyclopia, cebocephaly, orbital hypotelorism) and septo-optic dysplasia. Most information has been deduced from postmortem observations, and limited data are available concerning function of the pituitary in these conditions. For example, hypoplasia of the pituitary in anencephalics has long been recognized, but recent observations reveal a large residuum of normal pituitary function and suggest that the hypoplasia may be secondary to the hypothalamic defect. Now that the techniques are available to directly stimulate the pituitary with hypothalamic-releasing hormones, it is possible to determine if the defect resides in the pituitary or in the hypothalamus. Many of these conditions are lethal early in life, but partial defects may occur in siblings. A child has been reported with isolated deficiency of growth hormone and mild hypotelorism who had two siblings with holoprosencephaly and hypopituitarism. Instances of simple cleft lip and palate without other defects have been associated with pituitary insufficiency.

Blind children who are short should be suspected of having *septo-optic dysplasia.* In this condition, the optic nerves are hypoplastic and the fundus exhibits hypoplastic discs with typical double rims and sparse retinal vessels. Air encephalography usually reveals absence of the septum pellucidum and dilatation of the chiasmatic cistern. The hormonal deficiency may involve only growth hormone or may result in panhypopituitarism, including diabetus insipidus. The defect in this condition is believed to reside in the hypothalamus.

Destructive Lesions. Any lesion which damages the anterior pituitary or hypothalamus may cause cessation of growth. Since such lesions are not selective, multiple pituitary hormonal deficiencies are usually observed. The most common lesion responsible for this condition is the craniopharyngioma; less often hypothalamic tumors, tuberculosis, sarcoidosis, toxoplasmosis and aneurysms are causes for hypothalamic-hypophyseal destruction. These lesions are frequently associated with detectable roentgenographic changes. Diabetes insipidus has been a well known complication of the reticuloendothelioses, but only recently has it been established that deficiency of growth hormone and other pituitary hormones may occur in almost half of affected children. Enlargement of the sella or deformation or destruction of the clinoid processes usually indicates a tumor. Intrasellar or suprasellar calcifications are usually indicative of a craniopharyngioma. Trauma, especially basilar fractures, traction at delivery, anoxia and hemorrhagic infarction may also damage the pituitary, its stalk or the hypothalamus.

Idiopathic Hypopituitarism. More than half of patients with hypopituitarism have no demonstrable lesion of the pituitary or hypothalamus and the cause is not known. In the past it was assumed that the functional defect was in the pituitary, but it is increasingly apparent that the defect is more frequently in the hypothalamus. Approximately half of children with growth hormone deficiency also have deficiencies of other pituitary hormones. The multiple deficiency may be manifest in infancy, or there may be progressive development of the various deficiencies; for example, a child with initially only growth hormone deficiency may eventually exhibit deficiencies of TSH and ACTH. Most often hypopituitarism is sporadic, but affected siblings are not uncommon.

In the other half of children with idiopathic hypopituitarism, growth hormone deficiency occurs as an isolated defect and is often familial. Autosomal recessive inheritance is most common, but autosomal dominant inheritance has also been noted. Puberty may be markedly delayed, but it does occur spontaneously.

CLINICAL MANIFESTATIONS.

In Patients Without Demonstrable Lesion of the Pituitary. The hypopituitary child is usually of normal size and weight at birth. The retardation of growth has a variable onset; in about half of affected children the retardation of growth is noticed by 1 year of age. In others there may be a regular but slow growth in height, with the increments always below those of coevals, or periods of lack of growth may alternate with short spurts of growth. Delayed closure of the epiphyses permits growth beyond the time when normal persons cease to grow.

The head is round, and the face short and broad. The frontal bone is prominent, and the bridge of the nose depressed and saddle-shaped. The nose is small, and the nasolabial folds are well developed. The eyes are somewhat bulging. The mandible and the chin are underdeveloped and infantile, and the teeth, which erupt late, are frequently crowded. The neck is short and the larynx small. The voice is high-pitched and remains high after puberty. The genitalia are usually undeveloped. The extremities are well proportioned, the hands and feet being small. The genitalia are small for the child's age, and sexual maturation may be delayed or absent. Facial, axillary and pubic hair is usually absent; the hair of the scalp is fine. Symptomatic hypoglycemia, usually after fasting, occurs in 10 to 15 per cent of children with panhypopituitarism, as well as with isolated growth hormone deficiency. Intelligence is usually normal. The physical peculiarities of affected children influence their emotions and behavior as they grow older, and they may become shy and retiring.

In Patients with Demonstrable Lesion of the Pituitary. The child is normal initially, and manifestations similar to those seen in the idiopathic pituitary dwarf gradually appear and progress. When complete or almost complete destruction of the pituitary gland occurs, severe manifestations of pituitary insufficiency are present. Atrophy of the adrenal cortex, thyroid and gonads results in loss of weight, asthenia, sensitivity to cold, mental torpor and absence of sweating. Sexual maturation fails to take place, or regresses if already present. Thus, there may be atrophy of the gonads and genital tract with amenorrhea and loss of pubic and axillary hair. There is a tendency to hypoglycemia and coma. Growth ceases. Diabetes insipidus may be present early, but tends to improve spontaneously with progressive destruction of the anterior pituitary.

If the lesion is an expanding tumor, symptoms such as impaired vision, ocular disturbances, pathologic sleep, mental retardation and other neurologic signs may be present.

The growth failure frequently antedates the neurologic signs and symptoms, especially in patients with craniopharyngiomas. In other patients the neurologic manifestations may precede the endocrinologic, or evidence of pituitary insufficiency may first appear after surgical intervention.

LABORATORY DATA. The diagnosis of growth hormone deficiency rests upon demonstration of absent or subnormal reserve of pituitary HGH. Random serum or plasma levels of growth hormone, levels during sleep and levels following exercise are useful screening tests. A level over 10 ng/ml usually excludes growth hormone deficiency, but low levels must be studied further by provocative tests utilizing L-dopa and/or insulin-arginine. Great care must be taken in the administration of insulin to patients with hypopituitarism because of their decreased ability to overcome hypoglycemia. Decreased growth hormone responses also may occur in children with primary hypothyroidism or with emotional deprivation; following correction of the underlying disorder, growth hormone levels return to normal.

Once deficiency of HGH is established, it is necessary to determine the integrity of the remainder of the pituitary-hypothalamic axis. When there is deficiency of thyrotropin, serum levels of thyroxine and TSH are low. A normal rise in TSH and prolactin following stimulation with thyrotropin-releasing factor places the defect in the hypothalamus, whereas absence of response localizes the defect in the pituitary. In most patients with idiopathic multiple anterior pituitary hormone deficiency, there is a normal response to TRF, indicating that the primary deficiency is in the hypothalamus and the deficiency of pituitary hormone is secondary. An elevated random level of plasma prolactin in the hypopituitary patient is also strong evidence that there is a defect in the hypothalamus rather than in the pituitary.

Decreased urinary corticosteroid and plasma cortisol levels indicate deficiency of corticotropin. Insulin-induced hypoglycemia provokes a rise in cortisol levels by stimulating ACTH release; measurements of cortisol levels, therefore, during the provocative test for growth hormone with insulin provide information concerning corticotropin reserve. Metyrapone also may be used as an indirect indicator of corticotropin production. Serum FSH and LH levels may be decreased even below the ordinarily low prepubertal levels.

ROENTGENOGRAPHIC EXAMINATION. The long bones are slender and poor in minerals, the centers of ossification appear late, and the epiphyseal clefts remain open. The fontanels may remain open beyond the second year and, intersutural wormian bones may be found. The sella turcica may be abnormally small, but a normal sellar volume does not exclude the diagnosis. Roentgenograms of the skull are most helpful when there is a destructive or space-occupying lesion causing the hypopituitarism. A history of nausea, vomiting, loss of vision, headache or increase in circumference of the head suggests increased intracranial pressure. Enlargement of the sella, especially ballooning with erosion, strongly suggests a tumor and may require a brain scan, encephalography or arteriography for localization.

DIFFERENTIAL DIAGNOSIS. The causes of growth disorders are legion; only those which most closely mimic hypopituitarism are considered here.

Children with *Laron syndrome* have all the clinical findings of those with idiopathic hypopituitarism, but plasma levels of growth hormone are elevated, somatomedin is low and there is failure of response to administration of HGH. It appears that the primary disorder may be defective somatomedin production. In many instances an autosomal recessive mode of inheritance is suggested, but sporadic cases have been noted.

Primary hypothyroidism is usually easily distinguished on clinical grounds. Responses to growth hormone provocative tests may be subnormal, however, and enlargement of the sella may be present. Elevated levels of TSH clearly establish the diagnosis, and these secondary changes disappear following treatment with thyroid hormone.

Turner syndrome must always be considered in short girls. When this is associated with the usual characteristic congenital deformities, the diagnosis is not difficult, but in other instances there may be few characteristic findings other than shortness of stature. Chromosomal analysis is necessary to establish the diagnosis.

Emotional deprivation may lead to severe retardation of growth and mimic hypopituitarism. Although the mechanisms whereby sensory and emotional deprivation interfere with growth are not fully understood, some degree of functional hypopituitarism may be indicated by decreased pituitary response to metyrapone administration and by inadequate rise of growth hormone levels in response to provocative stimuli. Appropriate history and careful observations reveal disturbed mother-child or family relations which provide clues to diagnosis. Emotionally deprived children frequently have perverted or voracious appetites, are excessively passive or aggressive, and are borderline or dull-normal in intelligence. When child-rearing practices are altered or when the child is placed in a more stimulating environment, improved growth rates and rapid return of pituitary function to normal are noted. During this period of catch-up growth, separation of the sutures and other evidence of tumor cerebri may occur; these changes should not be mistaken for a space-occupying lesion.

In *primordial dwarfism* the growth retardation begins during intrauterine life, is present at birth and is frequently associated with other minor or major defects. This is a heterogeneous group with diverse causative factors. Growth hormone levels are normal. African pygmies in the rain forests of Equatorial Africa superficially resemble pituitary dwarfs but have normal levels of growth hormone and of somatomedin. They do not respond to HGH administration, and it seems that they have peripheral unresponsiveness to growth hormone.

The most frequent growth problem encountered by the pediatrician is the apparently normal child who is below the third percentile in height but who has a normal growth velocity. When skeletal maturation is below the chronologic age but is consistent with height age, the condition is referred to as *constitutional delay in growth.* In these children, growth potential is adequate; adult height and puberty will be achieved later than average. If skeletal maturation is consistent with chronologic age, the condition is known as *genetic short stature.* Other family members with short stature will be commonly found and the growth potential is limited. Growth hormone studies in these two groups of children are normal.

PROGNOSIS. Prognosis for life depends upon the causative factor, and whether it can be eradicated. In the absence of an anatomic lesion the affected person may reach old age.

Prognosis of ultimate height is difficult, since continued growth is possible long after the usual age of adolescence, owing to the persistence of open epiphyses. Sexual maturation may also take place 10 to 20 years later than in normal persons. Catch-up growth is frequently observed in children who have had surgical treatment of a craniopharyngioma or other tumor in the hypothalamic area. Surprisingly, growth may occur even in the absence of demonstrable HGH. Growth appears to be dependent on the presence of somatomedin, since plasma levels are normal. The stimulus for somatomedin production in these patients is unknown.

TREATMENT. In patients with demonstrable organic lesions, treatment should be directed to the underlying disease process.

Replacement of the essential hormonal deficiencies is possible. Administration of growth hormone has been successful in increasing the growth velocity of at least 80 per cent of growth hormone-deficient children, whereas it has failed to alter growth rates in most other conditions of deficient growth. A variety of dosage regimens have been used, but 1 to 2 mg by intramuscular injection two or three times a week is usually effective. Maximal growth response occurs during the first year of treatment; the rate may reach twice that expected for chronologic age, whereas, by the third year of treatment, it averages less than one and a half times that expected for age. Almost half the treated patients develop antibodies to human growth hormone; in some instances this accounts for diminished effectiveness of the hormone.

The hormone is available in only limited amounts owing to the inadequate supply of human pituitary glands, from which the hormone is extracted. One pituitary yields about 5 mg of growth hormone; accordingly, many children with hypopituitarism cannot be treated with HGH. Certain anabolic agents such as oxandrolone, used with due care not to accelerate skeletal maturation more rapidly than linear growth, appear to be useful substitutes for growth hormone.

Replacement with hydrocortisone is indicated if hypoglycemia or proved adrenal insufficiency is present, and treatment with thyroid hormone is indicated when there is secondary hypothyroidism. The doses of these hormones should be kept as small as possible.

DIABETES INSIPIDUS
(Arginine Vasopressin Deficiency)

Diabetes insipidus is characterized by polyuria and polydipsia and results from lack of the antidiuretic hormone, arginine vasopressin. Destruction of the supraoptic and paraventricular nuclei or division of the supraoptic-hypophysial tract above the median eminence results in permanent diabetes insipidus. Transection of the tract below the median eminence or removal of just the posterior lobe may result in transitory polyuria, but release of hormone into the median eminence prevents occurrence of diabetes insipidus. Vasopressin acts directly on the distal tubules and collecting ducts of the kidney to facilitate reabsorption of water. Vasopressin deficiency may be total or only partial, giving varying degrees of polydipsia and polyuria.

ETIOLOGY. Any lesion which damages the neurohypophysial unit may result in diabetes insipidus. Tumors of the suprasellar and chiasmatic regions, particularly craniopharyngiomas and optic gliomas, are common causes; the symptoms of increased intracranial pressure may accompany those of diabetes insipidus or may follow years later. Approximately 25 to 50 per cent of patients with the reticuloendothelioses manifest diabetes insipidus as a consequence of infiltration of abnormal histiocytes in the hypothalamus and pituitary. Deficiency of growth hormone is found in the majority of patients with the reticuloendothelioses who manifest diabetes insipidus. Encephalitis, sarcoidosis, tuberculosis, actinomycosis and leukemia are occasional etiologic agents. Injuries to the head, especially basal skull fractures, may produce diabetes insipidus immediately or only after a delay of several months. Operative procedures in the region of the pituitary or hypothalamus may result in transitory or permanent diabetes insipidus.

In a minority of instances, diabetes insipidus is hereditary. Autosomal dominant and X-linked recessive modes of transmission are known; affected males with either type are indistinguishable. In the genetic forms of the disorder, there is marked reduction of the neurosecretory cells of the supraoptic and paraventricular nuclei. Diabetes insipidus also occurs as a part of a rare genetic recessive disorder in which it is associated with juvenile diabetes mellitus, optic atrophy and perceptive hearing loss. In the Brattleboro strain of rat, diabetes insipidus is transmitted as an autosomal recessive trait; the neurosecretory cells are normal or hypertrophied, suggesting that the basic defect is in the synthesis of the peptide hormone.

In many instances, no specific cause can be found; some of these may represent genetic forms of the disease. Since diabetes insipidus may be the first recognizable sign of an intracranial tumor and may antedate neurologic signs by years, periodic re-evaluation is required for a long time.

CLINICAL MANIFESTATIONS. Polydipsia and polyuria are the outstanding symptoms of diabetes insipidus. In families with the hereditary disorder the polyuria is noted in early infancy. The infant cries excessively and will be dissatisfied when additional milk is offered, but is quieted when given water. Hyperthermia, rapid loss of weight and collapse are common in infancy. Vomiting, constipation and growth failure may be observed. Dehydration in early infancy may result in brain damage and mental deficiency. In the familial forms of vasopressin deficiency, there is wide variability in symptomatology. Severity tends to increase with age, some affected members being asymptomatic until adolescence. Many affected families accept polydipsia and polyuria as a family habit and do not seek medical attention, or may even prefer the symptoms to injections of vasopressin.

In a child who has acquired bladder control, enuresis may be the first symptom. The excessive thirst is a disturbing symptom and interferes with play, learning and sleep. Children with diabetes insipidus do not perspire, and their skin is dry and pale. Anorexia is a common symptom; there is a preference for carbohydrates.

Other signs and symptoms depend on the primary lesion; thus, patients with tumors in the region of the hypothalamus may have disturbance of growth, progressive cachexia or obesity, hyperpyrexia, sleep disturbance, sexual precocity or emotional disorders. Lesions initially causing diabetes insipidus may progress and eventually destroy the anterior pituitary. In such instances the symptoms of diabetes insipidus tend to ameliorate or disappear completely.

LABORATORY DATA. The daily volume of urine may be 4 to 10 liters or more. The urine is pale or colorless; the specific gravity varies from 1.001 to 1.005, with a corresponding osmolality of 50 to 200 mOsm/kg water. Serum osmolality is normal with adequate hydration. During periods of severe de-

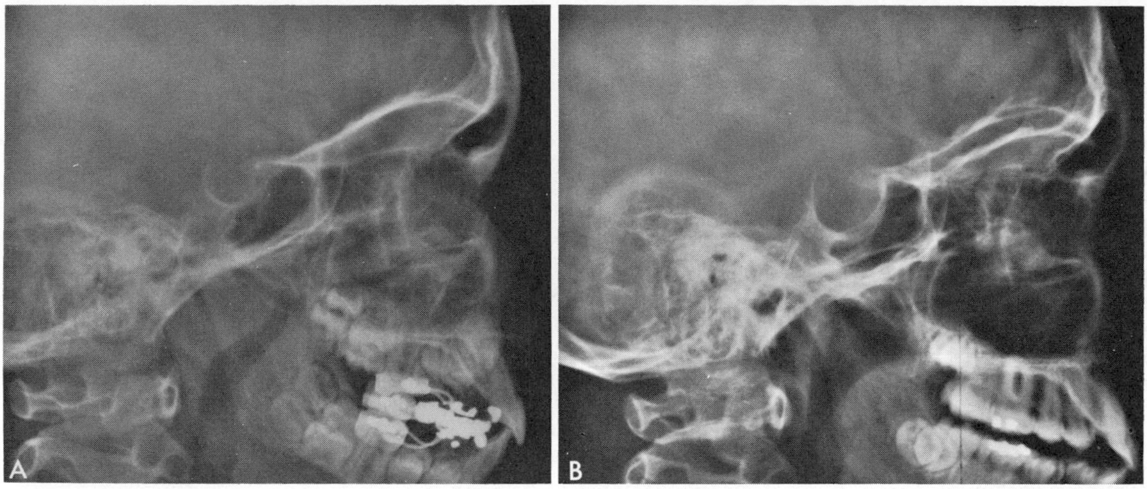

Figure 17–1 *A, Radiograph of skull of 9 year old boy with polydipsia, polyuria, nocturia and enuresis. Urine specific gravity was 1.016 after water deprivation. Growth was normal, and the sella turcica was considered radiologically to be at upper limit of normal, but was probably enlarged. Over the ensuing 6 months the symptoms of diabetes insipidus abated. B, The patient returned at 14 years of age because of growth failure and delay in sexual maturation. Studies revealed a deficiency of growth hormone, gonadotropins, corticotropin and thyrotropin. Note enlargement and thinning of the sella turcica, but absence of intrasellar or suprasellar calcification. Neurologic and ophthalmologic examinations were normal. There was exacerbation of diabetes insipidus with administration of hydrocortisone and thyroxine. Surgery revealed a large craniopharyngioma.*

hydration, the specific gravity may rise to 1.010 and the osmolality to 300. Other renal function studies are normal. Plasma and urine levels of arginine vasopressin are low, but assays are not generally available and confirmation of the diagnosis still rests on application of one of the many water deprivation tests which have been proposed. During water deprivation, patients must be closely observed to prevent surreptitious intake of water on the one hand and to avoid severe and rapid development of dehydration on the other hand. In patients with severe deficiency, a period of dehydration (rarely more than 6 hours) rapidly leads to elevation of plasma osmolality, while urine osmolality characteristically remains below plasma levels. Administration of exogenous vasopressin quickly raises urine osmolality. When the polyuria is mild and the deficiency incomplete, urine osmolality may exceed that of plasma and the response to vasopressin is attenuated.

A highly sensitive radioimmunoassay is capable of measuring as little as 0.1 pg/dl of arginine vasopressin (AVP). Adults deprived of water for 12 to 25 hours had levels ranging from 1.3 to 8.3 pg/dl (mean, 3.7 pg/dl); after water-loading, levels were consistently less than 1.2 pg/dl. AVP levels were undetectable in patients with diabetes insipidus.

Roentgenograms of the skull may reveal such evidence of an intracranial tumor as calcifications, enlargement of the sella turcica, erosion of the clinoid processes or increased width of the suture lines. Roentgenograms of the skull or other bones in patients with the reticuloendothelioses may reveal areas of rarefaction.

DIFFERENTIAL DIAGNOSIS. Polydipsia, polyuria and impaired concentration are common manifestations in patients with hypercalcemia or potassium deficiency. In the young male infant, nephrogenic diabetes insipidus must be differentiated from congenital or inherited types of vasopressin deficiency; failure of response to exogenous vasopressin (Pitressin) is a critical differential criterion.

Compulsive water drinking (psychogenic polydipsia) is rare but may easily be confused with diabetes insipidus. Such persons are usually able to produce a concentrated urine when fluids are withheld. Occasionally, however, diagnosis is difficult because continued polydipsia lowers the maximal urinary concentrations achievable following dehydration or even following infusion of hypertonic saline solution. As a rule, a urine concentration greater after dehydration than after administration of vasopressin alone indicates the ability to secrete vasopressin. On the other hand, if administration of vasopressin produces a urinary concentration substantially more concentrated than dehydration alone, vasopressin secretion is deficient. This rule seems to apply no matter how low or high urinary concentration may be.

Defects in urinary concentration also occur in a variety of chronic renal disorders. Familial nephrophthisis, in particular, can mimic diabetes insipidus. Elevated plasma levels of urea and creatinine, anemia, and isotonic rather than hypotonic urine are characteristics of primary renal disease.

After the diagnosis of diabetes insipidus has been established, the underlying process must be determined.

PROGNOSIS. Diabetes insipidus itself rarely threatens life but it may signify a serious underlying condition. Diabetes insipidus may be only transitory following trauma or surgical intervention in the region of the hypothalamus or pituitary. In the reticuloendothelioses spontaneous remission occasionally occurs, whereas in other patients it may remain as the only residuum after longstanding remission of the primary condition. One should be aware that amelioration of clinical diabetes insipidus may herald the development of anterior pituitary insufficiency. The prognosis of patients with a brain tumor depends upon the site of the lesion and upon the type of neoplastic cell. Occasionally disturbances of the thirst center accompany diabetes insipidus and seriously complicate the management of problems of water balance.

TREATMENT. The causative factor deserves first consideration in the treatment. Patients with uncomplicated diabetes insipidus may go untreated for years without apparent harm other than the inconvenience of polyuria and polydipsia, so long as they have an intact thirst mechanism and are allowed free access to water. Several effective preparations are available for symptomatic treatment. The most satisfactory is Pitressin tannate in oil, a long-acting preparation, which provides relief for 24 to 72 hours when 0.5 to 1.0 ml is administered. The dose must be determined for the individual patient and should not be repeated until symptoms recur. Since the Pitressin tannate is a viscous oil, careful attention must be given to resuspension by warming under a hot water faucet and shaking vigorously before injecting. Injections should be made deep intramuscularly with a 1-inch 20- to 22-gauge needle. Pitressin may also be administered as snuff or nose drops intranasally, or synthetic lysine-8-vasopressin may be administered as a liquid nasal spray; these forms are less satisfactory because they require frequent administration and cause local irritation.

Many patients respond very satisfactorily to oral administration of chlorpropamide. Though this agent has no antidiuretic effect itself, it potentiates the action of suboptimal amounts of vasopressin. In responsive patients, an effect is noted within 24 to 48 hours. Hypoglycemia is a frequent side effect of treatment, particularly in children with anterior pituitary insufficiency, but a decrease in the dose usually averts this problem. An initial dose of 20 mg/kg/day in two divided doses should be reduced to the minimum effective level.

Chlorpropamide is especially useful in those patients who also have hypodipsia from associated involvement of the thirst center, since it appears to restore drinking behavior to normal as well as controlling the diabetes insipidus.

Great care must be taken with patients with diabetes insipidus who are comatose, undergoing surgery or receiving intravenous fluids for any reason. If the patient is receiving Pitressin or chlorpropamide, the clinical manifestations of inappropriate vasopressin secretion follow (see below) unless the total fluid allotment is kept low; serum sodium must be monitored twice daily.

Nephrogenic Diabetes Insipidus
(Vasopressin-insensitive Diabetes Insipidus)

This disorder closely mimics vasopressin deficiency, but levels of the hormone in plasma and urine are normal. Affected patients show no antidiuresis even with large doses of vasopressin, and there is deficient renal medullary production or release of cyclic AMP. Administration of vasopressin does result in increased cortisol levels, indicating that at least one extrarenal effect of vasopressin is intact and that the end-organ resistance is probably limited to the kidney. The disorder occurs primarily in males as an X-linked dominant trait. Heterozygous females are usually asymptomatic but may exhibit a variable defect in concentration, which is probably explained by the Lyon hypothesis of sex-chromosome inactivation.

The onset is shortly after birth, the symptoms being those of diabetes insipidus. In addition to polyuria and polydipsia, unexplained fever, irritability, vomiting, constipation and failure to thrive are common. Fluid restriction or elevated environmental temperature may result in hyperpyrexia, rapid loss of weight and peripheral collapse. Growth is retarded, and mental development may be impaired.

Hyperelectrolytemia and azotemia are almost constant findings in early infancy, but tend to subside later in life. The urine has a low specific gravity, which may rise to about 1.010 during severe dehydration. Administration of vasopressin fails to induce antidiuresis and has no effect on the volume or specific gravity of urine.

Treatment consists in administration of water at frequent intervals in amounts sufficient to prevent dehydration and fever. It is almost impossible to maintain normal serum electrolyte levels without giving a low solute diet, which is justifiable in early life even if growth is retarded.

Diuretics, particularly the thiazides, paradoxically reduce the polyuria. The precise mechanism of action is still unsettled, but the beneficial effect of these drugs appears to be to decrease free water clearance. Chlorothiazide or hydrochlorothiazide, in three divided doses totaling 0.1 gm/M^2/day, has been used successfully when coupled with low solute diets. Since refractoriness to therapy and bone marrow toxicity have been observed, these drugs should be used with caution and administered only to patients with severe manifestations of the disorder.

INAPPROPRIATE SECRETION OF ANTIDIURETIC HORMONE
(Hypersecretion of Vasopressin)

The syndrome of inappropriate antidiuretic hormone secretion (SIADH) is now recognized as one of the most common aberrations of arginine vasopressin (AVP) secretion. In this condition, plasma levels of arginine vasopressin are normal, but are inappropriately high for the concurrent osmolality of the blood and are not suppressed by further dilution of body fluids.

ETIOLOGY. The syndrome is being increasingly observed in a variety of clinical conditions, particularly those involving the central nervous system, including meningitis, encephalitis, brain tumor and abscesses, subarachnoid hemorrhage, Guillain-Barré syndrome and head trauma. Pneumonia, tuberculosis, acute intermittent porphyria, use of positive pressure respirators, and certain drugs such as vincristine also produce the syndrome. The mechanism of the disturbed regulation of vasopressin in these conditions is not fully understood, but in many instances it is clear that there is direct involvement of the hypothalamus. The syndrome has been observed in patients with malignant tumors of the pancreas, duodenum and thymus and particularly in oat cell carcinoma of the lung. In these instances, the tumor presumably synthesizes and secretes vasopressin, the syndrome disappearing when the tumor is removed. In very rare instances no cause for the syndrome has been found.

The syndrome has also occurred during chlorpropamide therapy for diabetes mellitus, presumably owing to the known effect of potentiation of vasopressin by this drug. Patients with diabetes insipidus treated with Pitressin or chlorpropamide readily develop the syndrome during periods of excessive ingestion of fluids or during intravenous fluid therapy.

CLINICAL MANIFESTATIONS. The syndrome is probably most often latent and asymptomatic and explains the long known observations that serum sodium levels may be low in common conditions such as pneumonia, tuberculosis and meningitis. Careful attention to fluid replacement in patients with conditions known to be associated with the syndrome may prevent the development of overt symptoms.

The clinical manifestations are attributable to hypotonicity of body fluids and are those of water intoxication. If the serum sodium is not below 120 mEq/L, there may be no symptoms. Early, there is loss of appetite followed by nausea and sometimes by vomiting. Irritability and personality changes, including hostility and confusion, may occur. When the serum sodium falls to less than 110 mEq/L, neurologic abnormalities and/or stupor are common and convulsive seizures may also occur. Skin turgor and blood pressure are normal and there is no evidence of dehydration.

Serum sodium and chloride concentrations are low, whereas serum bicarbonate usually remains normal. Despite low serum sodium, there is continued renal excretion of sodium. The serum is hypo-osmolar, but the urine is less than maximally dilute and its osmolality is greater than appropriate for the tonicity of the serum. Renal and adrenal function are normal.

TREATMENT. Specific treatment of the underlying disorder (meningitis, pneumonia) is followed by spontaneous remission. Treatment of the hyponatremia consists simply of *restriction of fluids.* Sodium should be made available to replace the sodium loss. Hypertonic saline solution is usually of little benefit, however, since even large sodium loads are excreted in the urine. In instances of severe water intoxication, with convulsions or coma, hypertonic saline solution is indicated to increase osmolality and to control the central nervous system manifestations.

HYPERPITUITARISM

Hypersecretion of pituitary hormones is a normal finding in conditions in which deficiency of a target organ gives decreased hormonal feedback, such as occurs in primary hypogonadism and hypoadrenalism. In primary hypothyroidism, pituitary hyperfunction and hyperplasia can be so marked that the sella may enlarge and erode and there may be, on rare occasions, evidence of increased intracranial pressure. Such changes are not to be confused with primary pituitary tumors and they rapidly disappear when the underlying thyroid condition is treated.

Primary hypersecretion of pituitary hormones is usually associated with a suspected or proved neoplasm of the pituitary; it is extremely rare in childhood. The principal hormone-secreting tumors are the eosinophilic adenoma (growth hormone), basophilic adenoma (ACTH) and chromophobe adenoma (prolactin). There is mounting evidence that these tumors may, at least in some instances, arise secondarily to a primary defect in the hypothalamus, with stimulation of the pituitary by hypothalamic releasing factors. Any pituitary tumor may cause pituitary insufficiency by compression of functioning pituitary tissue.

PITUITARY GIGANTISM AND ACROMEGALY

In young persons with open epiphyses, overproduction of growth hormone results in gigantism; in persons with closed epiphyses, acromegaly results. Often some acromegalic features are seen with gigantism, even in children and adolescents; after closure of the epiphyses, the acromegalic features become more prominent.

ETIOLOGY. Pituitary gigantism is rare and is the result of excessive secretion of growth hormone by the pituitary. The cause is most often an eosinophilic adenoma, but gigantism has been observed in a 2½ year old boy with a hypothalamic tumor. Because of the rarity of the tumor, few children with eosinophilic adenomas have had extensive evaluation of pituitary function by currently available techniques. Tumors in many adults with acromegaly as well as in a 5 year old child have responded with changes in growth hormone levels following administration of provocative or suppressive agents. These data suggest that in some patients gigantism and acromegaly may begin as a hypothalamic disturbance, resulting in hypertrophy and hyperplasia and, ultimately, in tumors of somatotrophic cells.

CLINICAL MANIFESTATIONS. In most of the recorded cases, the abnormal growth became evident at puberty, but the condition has been established as early as 5 years of age. Giants may grow to a height of 8 feet or more. Acromegaly consists chiefly in enlargement of the distal parts of the body, but manifestations of abnormal growth actually involve all portions. The circumference of the skull increases, the nose becomes broad and the tongue is often enlarged, with coarsening of the facial features. The mandible grows excessively and the teeth become separated. The fingers and toes grow chiefly in thickness. There may be dorsal kyphosis. Fatigue and lassitude are early symptoms. Delayed sexual maturation or hypogonadism may occur. Signs of increased intracranial pressure appear later; visual loss may be demonstrable only on careful examination of visual fields.

LABORATORY DATA. Growth hormone levels are elevated at all times and may occasionally be as high as 400 ng/ml. Random fluctuations are common, with no increase in secretion during deep sleep. There is usually no suppression of growth hormone levels by the hyperglycemia of a glucose tolerance test. There may be no response, normal responses or paradoxical responses to various other stimuli. For example, L-dopa may paradoxically decrease growth hormone levels. Surprisingly, administration of TRF results in increased growth hormone levels in some acromegalics, and in a 5 year old giant resulted in a threefold increase in levels of growth hormone. Detailed evaluation of each child is indicated, because the results of such studies not only increase insight into pathologic mechanisms but also provide clues to therapeutic management.

Adenomas may compromise other anterior pituitary function through growth or cystic degeneration. Secretion of gonadotropins, TSH and/or ACTH may be impaired. Prolactin levels may be elevated, and in one instance it was established that the tumor contained secreting lactotropin and somatotropin cells.

Roentgenograms of the skull may reveal enlargement of the sella turcica and of the paranasal sinuses. Tufting of the phalanges and increased heel pad thickness are common. Osseous maturation is normal.

DIFFERENTIAL DIAGNOSIS. In the differential diagnosis hereditary tall stature must be considered. In this condition there is usually abnormal height in one or both parents or in close relatives. Such tall persons are well proportioned and free of signs of increased intracranial pressure. Abnormal growth during preadolescence in obese children is a temporary state; though such children may become tall, they do not attain the height of giants. Children with precocious puberty are often unusually tall, but do not develop into giants, since their epiphyses close early and growth ceases prematurely. Patients with tall stature associated with untreated thyrotoxicosis, hypogonadism and Marfan syndrome are easily distinguished clinically and have normal levels of growth hormone. Gigantism and increased growth hormone levels may occur in some patients with lipodystrophy, but absence of subcutaneous fat is a characteristic finding; there is increasing evidence for disordered hypothalamic function in this condition. Cerebral gigantism, a condition which is far more common than pituitary gigantism, can usually be differentiated on clinical grounds (see below).

TREATMENT. Treatment is difficult and controversial. If there is evidence of increased intracranial pressure, surgical intervention is indicated. In the absence of ocular symptoms such as choked discs and constricted visual fields, irradiation, either conventional or with high energy proton beams, may be an effective form of therapy. The administration of L-dopa may be helpful, but further experience with this agent is required to evaluate its usefulness as an adjunct to conventional forms of therapy. Therapy with chlorpromazine was not successful in lowering growth hormone levels in an affected 17 year old girl.

CEREBRAL GIGANTISM

This disorder, like pituitary gigantism, is characterized by rapid growth; growth hormone levels in the serum are not elevated, however, and evidence suggests a cerebral defect for the pathogenetic mechanism. Birth weight and length are above the ninetieth percentile in most affected infants, and macrocrania may be noted. Growth is rapid, and by 1 year of age all affected infants are over the ninety-seventh percentile in height. Accelerated growth continues for the first 4 to 5 years, and then a normal rate is observed. Puberty usually occurs at the normal time, but may occur slightly early. The hands and feet are large, with thickened subcutaneous tissue. The head is large and dolichocephalic, the jaw prominent; there is hypertelorism, and the eyes have an antimongoloid slant. Clumsiness and awkward gait are characteristic, and affected children have great difficulty in sports, in learning to ride a bicycle and in other tasks requiring coordination. Mental retardation is almost always associated; it may vary considerably in degree but is not progressive.

Radiographs reveal a large skull, a high orbital roof, a sella of normal size but slightly posterior inclination and an increased interorbital distance. Osseous maturation is consistently advanced and compatible with the patient's height. Growth hormone levels are normal, and 17-ketosteroids are only slightly increased. Abnormal electroencephalograms are common, and pneumoencephalography frequently reveals a dilated ventricular system.

The cause of the disorder is unknown, and it is not clear whether all patients with this syndrome have the same defect. It may be that this syndrome is caused by a hypothalamic defect, but to date none has been demonstrated.

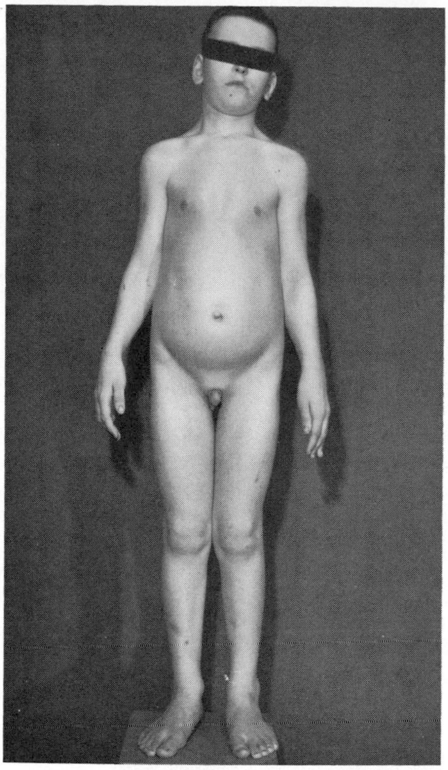

Figure 17–2 *Cerebral giantism in an 8 year old boy. Height age was 12 years; bone-age, 12 years; IQ, 60; abnormal electroencephalogram. Note prominence of forehead and jaw and the large hands and feet. Sexual development was consistent with chronologic age. Hormone studies were normal except for slightly elevated 17-ketosteroids. Adult height was 208 cm (6ft 10 in); normal sexual development. He wears size 18 shoes.*

PRECOCIOUS PUBERTY

PHYSIOLOGY OF PUBERTY. The hypothalamus, pituitary and gonads are active and interacting many years before appearance of the secondary sex characteristics associated with puberty. Low but measurable levels of FSH and LH are present throughout childhood and rise slowly during the prepubertal years. An active hypothalamic-pituitary-gonadal interaction is present prior to puberty, as demonstrated by the finding of elevated gonadotropins in patients with Turner syndrome or with anorchia, compared to normal children of the same age. The prepubertal gonad is capable of responding to stimulation; administration of human chorionic gonadotropin to prepubertal boys results in marked increases in testosterone levels. The factors which influence the onset of puberty are being unraveled, but the mechanisms remain obscure. Prior to puberty, very small amounts of gonadal steroids are able to suppress the hypothalamus and pituitary. With the onset of puberty, the hypothalamic "gonadostat" becomes progressively less sensitive to the suppressive effects of sex steroids on gonadotropin secretion. Consequently LH and FSH increase and stimulate the gonad, and a new level of interaction is achieved. This decrease in hypothalamic sensitivity is thought to be an important change associated with puberty. In girls at puberty a sharp rise in FSH precedes the sharp increase in plasma estradiol; in boys LH rises prior to the sharp increase in testosterone. There is solid evidence that FSH and LH act synergistically to promote changes in the gonad at puberty.

A second critical event occurs in middle or late puberty, at least in girls, and involves cyclicity and ovulation. At this time a positive feedback develops whereby rising levels of estrogen cause a distinct midcycle increase (rather than decrease) of LH. Prior to midpuberty, this ability of estrogen to release LH is not found. Other changes known to occur at the onset of puberty include an increase in LH release during sleep and increased ability of the pituitary to release LH in response to LRF administration. An abrupt change in adrenocortical secretion of androgen also occurs at puberty, but the mechanisms involved are unknown.

The average age of girls at the onset of puberty in the United States is 11 to 12 years; about 95 per cent of girls have at least one sign of puberty by the age of 13.5 years. The breast bud is usually the first sign of puberty and the interval to menarche is 2 to 2½ years but may be as long as 6 years. In boys the average age of onset of puberty is about 6 months later than in girls, and the development of adult sex characteristics takes about 4 years. Peak height velocity is attained about 2 years earlier in girls (always preceding menarche) than in boys. There are, however, wide variations in the sequence of changes involving growth spurt, breast, pubic hair and genital development. Onset of puberty is more closely correlated with osseous maturation than with chronologic age and does not take place until a certain level of skeletal maturation is achieved. Genetic and environmental factors also affect onset of puberty. During the past century, the onset of puberty has occurred one year earlier every 25 calendar years in the industrial countries.

Precocious puberty is difficult to define because of the marked variation in the age at which puberty begins normally. Onset of puberty before 8½ years of age in girls and 10 years in boys may be considered as precocious, but these are arbitrary guidelines.

Precocious pubertal development may be divided into true precocious puberty and precocious pseudopuberty. True precocious puberty is always isosexual and indicates not only precocity of the secondary sexual characteristics, but also an increase in the size and activity of the gonads. In precocious pseudopuberty, some of the secondary sex characteristics appear, but the gonads do not mature and there is no activation of normal pituitary-hypothalamic-gonadal interplay. In this latter group, the sex characteristics may be isosexual or heterosexual and will be discussed later. (See

Adrenocortical Hyperfunction, the Ovary, and the Testis, this Section).

TRUE PRECOCIOUS PUBERTY

Precocious Puberty Without Other Pathologic Findings (Constitutional)

In about 80 to 90 per cent of girls and about 50 per cent of boys with precocious puberty no causative factor can be found. Presumably the normal hypothalamic mechanism which initiates puberty is precociously activated. In many affected children there are electroencephalographic abnormalities, suggesting a primary cerebral abnormality as the cause of the disorder. The condition occurs far more frequently in girls and is usually sporadic. In males the disorder may be familial; the usual pattern of transmission is as a sex-limited autosomal dominant trait transmitted only by affected males to half their sons. An X-linked form, transmitted only by unaffected females, has also been reported.

CLINICAL MANIFESTATIONS. The clinical course is extremely variable. Affected children may complete sexual maturation rapidly or slowly; manifestations may remain stationary or even regress, only to resume development later. Sexual development may begin at any age. In girls the first sign is development of the breasts; pubic hair may appear simultaneously, but more often appears later. Development of the external genitalia, the appearance of axillary hair and the onset of menstruation follow. The early menstrual cycles may be more irregular than with normal puberty. Menarche has been observed within the first year of life. The initial cycles are usually anovulatory, but pregnancy has been reported as early as $5\frac{1}{2}$ years of age.

In boys there are enlargement of the penis and testes, appearance of pubic hair, acne and frequent erections. The voice deepens, and linear growth is accelerated. Spermatogenesis has been observed as early as 5 or 6 years of age, and nocturnal emissions may occur. Testicular biopsies have shown all elements of the testes to be stimulated. If the precocity is complete, various degrees of spermatogenesis are present; even if it is incomplete, the interstitial cells are present.

In both girls and boys there is advancement of growth in height and weight and of osseous maturation. The increased rate of ossification results in early closure of epiphyses, so that ultimate stature is less than it would have been otherwise. Approxi-

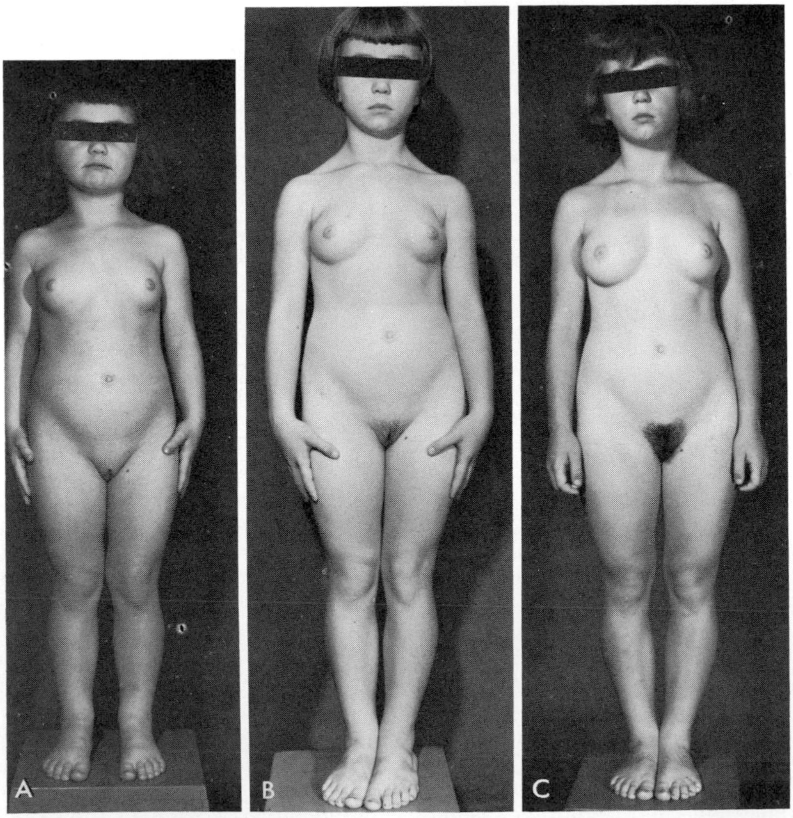

Figure 17–3 *Idiopathic precocious puberty. Patient at (A) $3\frac{11}{12}$, (B) at $5\frac{8}{12}$ and (C) at $8\frac{1}{2}$ years of age. Breast development and vaginal bleeding began at $2\frac{1}{2}$ years of age. Osseous age was $7\frac{1}{2}$ years at $3\frac{11}{12}$, and 14 years at 8 years of age. Repeated estrogen assays have varied between 12 and 132 mouse units. Urinary gonadotropins were not demonstrable until the child was 5 years of age. 17-Ketosteroids varied between 1.6 and 2.1 mg/24 hr during the first 5 years of life. Intelligence and dental age are normal for chronologic age. Growth was completed at 10 years; ultimate height was 142 cm (56 in).*

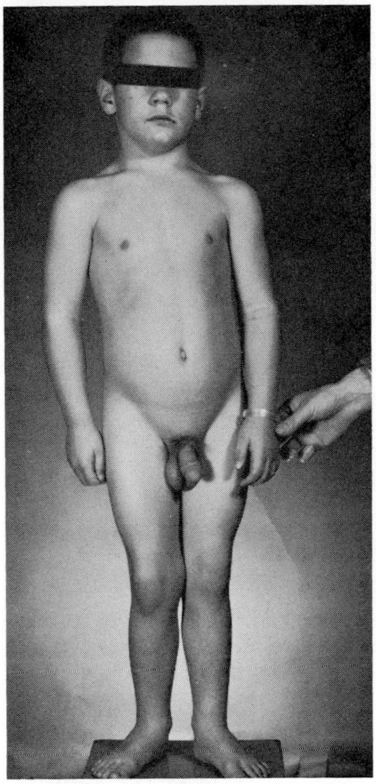

Figure 17–4 Precocious puberty without a demonstrable lesion in a 3½ year old boy. Height age was 5 years and bone-age 8 years. Urinary gonadotropins were demonstrable; 17-ketosteroids, 1.9 mg/24 hr. Note well developed testes; testicular biopsy revealed Leydig cells and well developed tubules with adult spermatogonia. At 5 years of age the boy had a height age of 10 years and osseous maturation of 14 years. Growth ceased at 9 years; ultimate stature was 148.6 cm (58½ in). He had no neurologic abnormalities, and was bright-normal in intelligence and well adjusted emotionally.

mately one third of patients do not achieve a height of 152 cm (5 feet) as adults. Dental age and mental development, however, are usually compatible with chronologic age.

LABORATORY DATA. Radioimmunoassays of plasma FSH and LH may be elevated for the age of the patient. There is considerable overlap, however, with levels in normal children of the same age, and particularly in the early course gonadotropin levels are of limited value in diagnosis. Urinary 17-ketosteroids may be normal or only slightly elevated. Plasma testosterone (in boys) and estradiol (in girls) are usually elevated to a level consistent with the stage of puberty and osseous maturation. Stained vaginal smears reveal cornification and other estrogenic effects. Electroencephalographic abnormalities may be present. Osseous maturation is advanced and consistent with the stage of pubertal development.

DIFFERENTIAL DIAGNOSIS. In girls, lesions of the central nervous system, tumors of the ovaries, feminizing adrenocortical tumors, McCune-Albright syndrome and accidental ingestion of estrogens must be considered in the differential diagnosis. A carefully obtained history, a complete physical examination and appropriate laboratory studies usually resolve the diagnosis. A pelvic examination under anesthesia or pelvic pneumography may be indicated in selected cases to determine whether there is an ovarian tumor. Early, true precocious puberty may be impossible to differentiate from premature thelarche when breast development is the only manifestation. Gonadotropins may be normal or only slightly elevated. A period of follow-up may be necessary to establish the diagnosis.

In boys cerebral lesions, the adrenogenital syndrome, a Leydig cell tumor and a gonadotropin-

TABLE 17–1 CONDITIONS CAUSING PRECOCIOUS PUBERTY

A. True Precocious Puberty
  1. Cerebral lesions
      Brain tumors, pineal tumors, postencephalitic scars, tuberous sclerosis, hydrocephalus, hypothalamic hamartomas
  2. McCune-Albright syndrome
  3. Associated with untreated hypothyroidism
  4. Silver syndrome
  5. Gonadotropin-producing tumors
      Hepatomas, hepatoblastomas, chorionepitheliomas, teratomas
  6. Administration of gonadotropins
  7. Therapy of virilizing adrenal hyperplasia
  8. Idiopathic (constitutional, functional)
    a. Sporadic
    b. Familial (male)

B. Precocious Pseudopuberty
  Females
    Isosexual (feminization)
      1. Ovarian tumors
        a. Granulosa cell tumor
        b. Theca cell tumor
        c. Teratoma
      2. Autonomous functional cyst of ovary
        a. McCune-Albright syndrome
      3. Adrenocortical tumor
      4. Medications (estrogens)
    Heterosexual (virilization)
      1. Congenital adrenal hyperplasia
      2. Adrenocortical tumor
        a. Testosterone-secreting tumor
      3. Arrhenoblastoma
      4. Androgen-producing teratoma
      5. Medications (androgens)
  Males
    Isosexual (masculinization)
      1. Congenital adrenal hyperplasia
      2. Adrenocortical tumor
      3. Leydig cell tumor
      4. Teratoma (containing adrenocortical tissue)
      5. Medications (androgens)
    Heterosexual (feminization)
      1. Adrenocortical tumor
      2. Medications (estrogens)

C. Partial Precocious Puberty
  Premature adrenarche (pubarche)
  Premature thelarche

producing hepatoma must be considered diagnostic possibilities. In the *adrenogenital syndrome* the testes are small relative to the degree of sexual maturation. A *Leydig cell tumor* can usually be detected on physical examination, and a *hepatoma* usually causes hepatomegaly.

When there is no evidence of a cerebral lesion from the initial examination, the child must be carefully and repeatedly observed for several years before the possibility of an intracranial lesion can be excluded.

TREATMENT. Treatment consists essentially in psychologic management of patient and family. A detailed explanation to the parents with the reassurance of the harmlessness of the condition is imperative. They should also be told that the precocious manifestations will persist, but that by the age of 10 to 14 years the child will not be different from other children. Such children should also be guarded against abuses that could result in pregnancy. The few data available indicate that these patients have a normal reproductive span and that menopause takes place within the usual time.

Medroxyprogesterone acetate has been used to treat children with precocious puberty; it results in cessation of menses and regression of breast development in girls and will depress testosterone levels in boys. On the other hand, growth and skeletal maturation usually continue unabated and side effects are common, including suppression of the pituitary-adrenal axis, cushingoid manifestations and alterations of testicular histology. These considerations markedly limit the usefulness of this agent. Safe and effective therapy has yet to be devised.

Precocious Puberty with Polyostotic Fibrous Dysplasia and Abnormal Pigmentation

(McCune-Albright Syndrome)

When fibrous dysplasia of the skeletal system is associated with patchy cutaneous pigmentation and endocrine dysfunction, the clinical association is referred to as McCune-Albright syndrome. The most common endocrine disturbance is sexual precocity, but hyperthyroidism or Cushing syndrome may also occur. The condition occurs most often in girls but has been reported in 8 boys.

For many years the disorder was presumed to reside in the hypothalamus, but more recent data suggest that endocrine disorders in this syndrome may result from autonomous hyperfunction of the peripheral target glands. For example, it is now established that the hyperthyroidism in this condition does not differ from classic Graves' disease and is not hypothalamic in origin; TSH is suppressed and LATS may be present. In both reported instances of associated Cushing syndrome the lesion was bilateral nodular adrenocortical hyperplasia; in one the plasma levels of ACTH were found to be low. Studies of the sexual precocity in 3 girls found suppressed levels of FSH and LH and markedly elevated plasma levels of estradiol and estrone; functioning ovarian cysts were found, and surgical excision resulted in return to normal of the levels of estrogen. It is still questionable whether hypothalamic dysfunction may have initiated the sequence of events leading to autonomous ovarian or adrenal lesions.

The average age of menarche in affected girls is about 3 years, but vaginal bleeding has occurred as early as 4 months of age and secondary sex characteristics at 6 months. The Cushing syndrome has occurred in early infancy, antedating the sexual precocity. The onset of hyperthyroidism is in most instances between 3 and 12 years, though it has occurred as early as 9 months. Gynecomastia and acromegalic features have occasionally been observed. In one patient growth hormone levels were markedly elevated and were not suppressed during a glucose tolerance test.

In view of these new findings, it can no longer be assumed that the precocity is central in origin; accordingly, all patients must be thoroughly investigated. Elevated FSH and LH levels will suggest a hypothalamic etiology, but suppressed levels point to a functional ovarian lesion that may require surgical intervention. The Cushing syndrome requires adrenalectomy; the hyperthyroidism is treated as in any other patient with Graves' disease. Prognosis is favorable for longevity, but deformities may result from the bony lesions and repeated pathologic fractures. The osseous lesions become static in adult life.

Precocious Puberty Resulting from Organic Brain Lesions

ETIOLOGY. A wide variety of lesions of the central nervous system have been associated with sexual precocity. How these lesions activate the hypothalamic mechanisms which initiate puberty is not known, but they all involve the hypothalamus by scarring, invasion or pressure. Tumors are among the more common lesions and include pinealomas, optic gliomas, suprasellar teratomas, neurofibromas, astrocytomas, ependymomas and hypothalamic hamartoma, a benign nodule composed of nerve cells and attached to both the mammillary bodies and tuber cinereum. Postencephalitic scars, tuberculous meningoencephalitis, hydrocephalus and tuberous sclerosis have all, on occasion, been etiologic factors.

Some of these tumors grow slowly and produce no signs other than precocious puberty. Accordingly, a child who is considered intially to have precocious puberty without a lesion may eventually exhibit signs of increased intracranial pressure and be found to have a tumor. Other hypothalamic signs or symptoms such as diabetes insipidus, hyperthermia, obesity, cachexia and unnatural crying or laughing may suggest the possibility of an intracranial lesion. A history of convulsions, retarded mental development or other neurologic signs should also suggest a lesion of the central nervous system.

CLINICAL MANIFESTATIONS. An intracranial

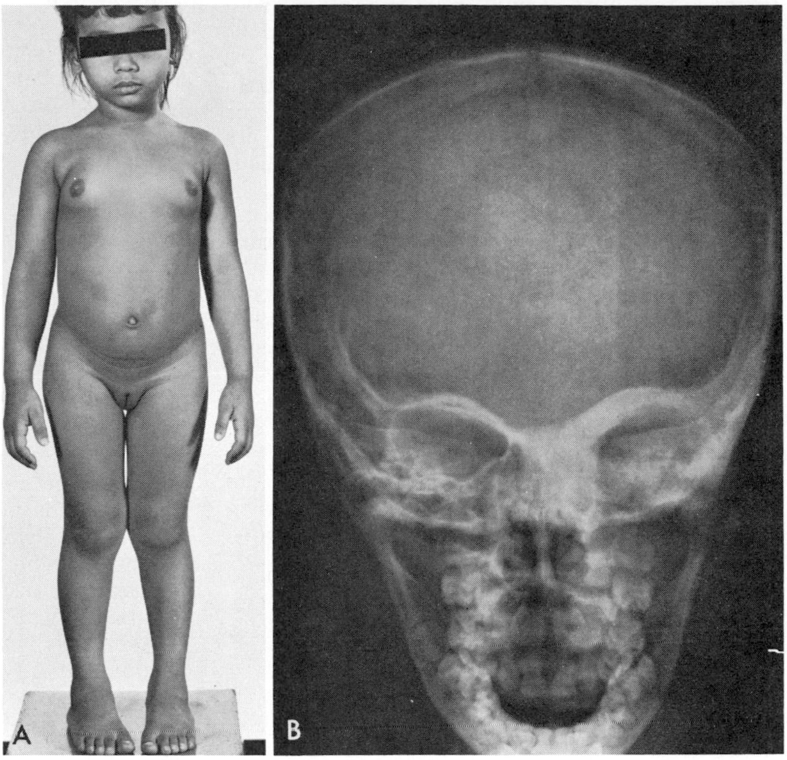

Figure 17–5 *Precocious puberty associated with polyostotic fibrous dysplasia (McCune-Albright syndrome) in a girl $4\frac{1}{2}$ years of age; at this time her height age and osseous age were normal. Menarche at 4 years.* A, *Note bilateral breast development, hyperpigmented spots on abdomen and prominence of left side of face.* B, *Roentgenograms revealed fibrous dysplasia in the distal end of the left ulna and thickening of the bones about the left orbit and the maxillary portion of the frontal bones.*

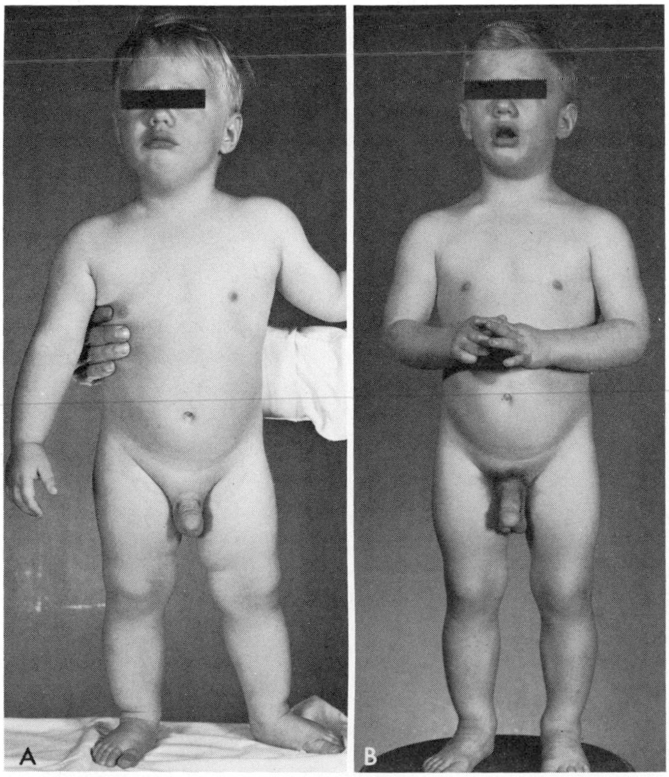

Figure 17–6 *Precocious puberty with central nervous system lesion. Photographs at* (A) *$1\frac{1}{2}$ and* (B) *$2\frac{1}{2}$ years of age. Accelerated growth, muscular development, osseous maturation and testicular development were consistent with the degree of secondary sexual maturation. Urinary gonadotropins were repeatedly negative, 17-ketosteroids usually 2 to 3 mg/24 hr. In early infancy he began having frequent episodes of rapid, purposeless spells; later in life he had episodes of uncontrollable laughing with ocular movements. At 7 years he exhibits emotional lability, aggressive behavior and destructive tendencies. Although a hypothalamic disorder has been suspected, repeated studies have failed to reveal a space-taking lesion.*

tumor is the cause of precocious puberty in about 40 per cent of boys but only 10 per cent of girls; the diagnosis of idiopathic precocious puberty can be made with less confidence in boys, therefore, than in girls. The precocity is always isosexual, and the endocrine pattern and laboratory findings are identical with those observed in children without demonstrable organic lesions.

Roentgenographic examination of the skull, electroencephalographic studies and brain scans are essential parts of the examination. Pneumoencephalography is indicated in all boys with true precocious puberty when no specific cause can be found. Whenever there are any neurologic manifestations suggesting a space-taking lesion, cerebral angiography, pneumoencephalography or ventriculography may be required to localize the lesion.

TREATMENT. Therapy depends on the nature and location of the lesion. Surgical decompression followed by roentgen therapy is usually indicated when removal of the tumor is not possible.

Syndrome of Precocious Puberty and Hypothyroidism

Onset of puberty is usually delayed and generally does not occur until epiphyseal maturation has reached 12 to 13 years of age in children with untreated hypothyroidism. Precocious puberty in a child with untreated hypothyroidism and a prepubertal bone age presents, therefore, a striking appearance and a paradoxical association. There have been only several dozen reported instances, but the phenomenon appears to be not uncommon. Among 54 carefully studied children with primary hypothyroidism, half had varying degrees of isosexual development in advance of their osseous maturation.

All affected patients had severe hypothyroidism of long duration and the usual manifestations were present, including retardation of growth and of osseous maturation. The etiology of the hypothyroidism has been varied and includes lymphocytic thyroiditis, thyroidectomy and overtreatment with antithyroid drugs.

A preponderance of the reported instances involved girls, probably reflecting the higher incidence of hypothyroidism in females. A significant number have also had Down syndrome; this may be related to the known association of this disorder with thyroid autoimmune disorders. Sexual maturation usually includes breast development in girls and testicular enlargement in boys. There is a paucity of the adrenarchal changes of puberty, as reflected in sparse or absent pubic and axillary hair. Menstrual bleeding is a frequent feature, even in girls with minimal breast development. Enlargement of the sella turcica, galactorrhea, excessive pigmentation and papilledema were present in some. In all instances, treatment with thyroid hormone resulted in regression of sexual precocity.

Plasma levels of TSH and prolactin are markedly elevated. LH and FSH levels are also elevated; the precise mechanism responsible for this is unknown. Thyrotropin-releasing factor is presumably markedly elevated, but in normal individuals it does not cause release of LH and FSH. Whatever the deranged hypothalamic-pituitary regulating mechanism may be, it rapidly returns to normal upon treatment with thyroid hormone.

Syndrome of Congenital Asymmetry, Short Stature and Elevated Gonadotropins
(Silver Syndrome)

Silver syndrome consists of short stature, congenital hemihypertrophy, normal genitalia and slightly to moderately increased excretion of gonadotropins. Affected children have low birth weight, even though born at term, a small mandible and shortened and incurved fifth fingers. Osseous maturation is delayed and is consistent with the height-age. Urinary and serum levels of gonadotropins may be increased despite lack of sexual development; other laboratory studies give normal results. The cause of the disorder is unknown.

In spite of the short stature and retarded osseous development, a few of these children have undergone precocious sexual maturation, presumably as a result of early production of gonadotropins.

Heterogeneity of this disorder is suggested by reports of Silver syndrome with a variety of chromosomal aberrations.

Gonadotropin-secreting Tumors

HEPATIC TUMORS. Eight instances of isosexual precocious puberty associated with hepatoblastoma or hepatoma have been recorded. All have involved males, the age of onset varying from 8 months to 7 years. An enlarged liver or mass in the upper quadrant should suggest the diagnosis. Testicular histology reveals interstitial cell hyperplasia and absence of spermatogenesis. The tumor cells produce an ectopic gonadotropin which stimulates precocious maturation of the testes. In one instance, the gonadotropin was proved to be identical with human chorionic gonadotropin. Plasma levels of alpha-fetoprotein may also be elevated. These two biochemical markers are useful for following the effects of therapy. Treatment for these tumors is the same as that for other carcinomas of the liver. All recorded patients with this condition survived less than a year.

OTHER TUMORS. Choriocarcinomas arising in the pineal body may secrete chorionic gonadotropin and cause sexual precocity. This is not to be confused with the situation which occurs with most pineal tumors, in which the sexual precocity is the result of involvement of the hypothalamus. (see above). In the prepubertal female choriocarcinomas have occurred principally in the ovary. Sexual development is produced by stimulation of the opposite ovary. These tumors are highly malignant; cachexia may accompany the sexual precocity. The diagnosis is readily established if the urine contains large amounts of chorionic gonadotropin and there is a positive pregnancy test. Owing to the rarity of these tumors, none has been studied by modern techniques and the gonadotropin has not been definitively characterized.

Recent development of a sensitive and specific radioimmunoassay for human chorionic gonadotropin (HCG) should facilitate diagnosis and identification of the gonadotropin. By this assay, one third of patients with seminoma and one half of those with embryonal carcinoma have HCG production. In adults it is one of the more common hormones ectopically produced by nontrophoblastic neoplasms. No systematic studies of childhood tumors have been conducted thus far.

INCOMPLETE (PARTIAL) PRECOCIOUS DEVELOPMENT

Isolated manifestations of precocity without development of other signs of puberty are not unusual; development of the breasts and growth of sexual hair are the two most common.

PRECOCIOUS THELARCHE (SIMPLE DEVELOPMENT OF BREASTS). Precocious development of breasts may occur without any other pubertal changes. It most often manifests between the first and third years of life, and the enlargement may involve only one breast or one breast more than the other. The breast development may progress, remain stationary or regress. Most often this is a benign abnormality; it may be familial in some instances. Growth and osseous maturation are normal; menarche occurs at the normal time. The usual tests for urinary estrogens are negative and there is no cornification of vaginal epithelium, but plasma levels of estradiol may occasionally be increased. Plasma levels of gonadotropins and urinary 17-ketosteroids are normal. It is thought that the condition is caused by secretion of small, and perhaps transient, amounts of estrogens by the ovaries. Since enlargement of breasts may be the first sign of pseudoprecocious or of true puberty, a prolonged period of observation is indicated in all instances.

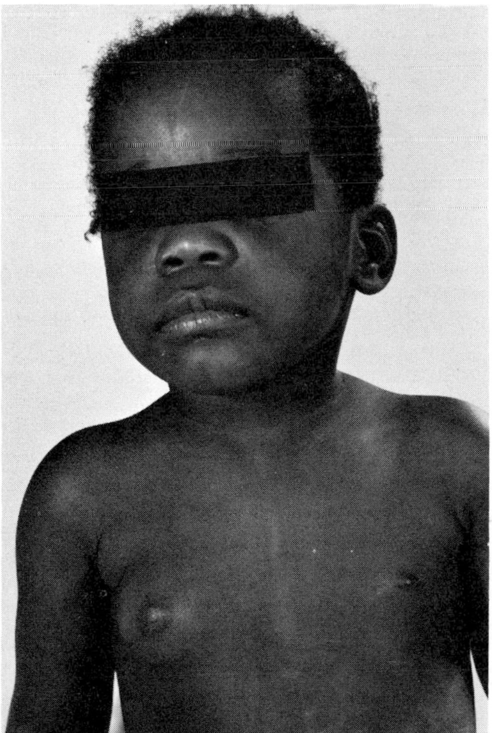

Figure 17–7 Premature thelarche. Simple hypertrophy of the breasts in a 23 month old girl. No demonstrable urinary estrogens or gonadotropin. Normal genitalia and growth. The disparity in size of the breasts is a common finding in this condition as well as in normal puberty.

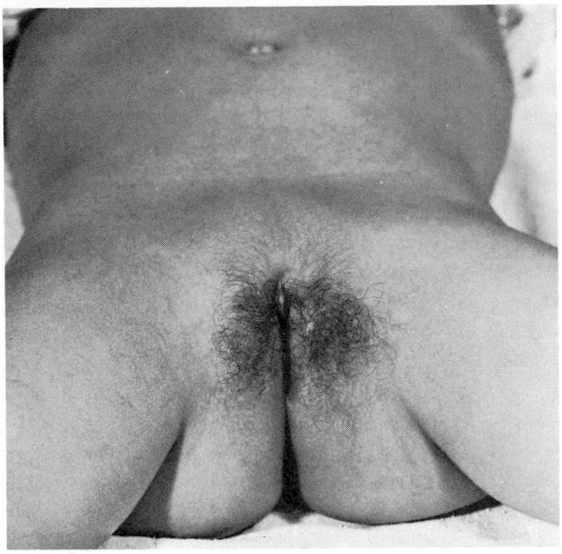

Figure 17–8 Premature adrenarche (pubarche). Isolated development of sexual hair in a 6 year old girl with cerebral palsy. Urinary 17-ketosteroids varied between 1.5 and 3.4 mg/24 hr.

PREMATURE ADRENARCHE (SIMPLE DEVELOPMENT OF SEXUAL HAIR). The appearance of sexual hair at an early age without any other evidence of maturation has been termed *premature adrenarche.* It occurs much more frequently in girls than in boys. Hair appears first on the labia majora, then in the pubic region and, finally, in the axilla. Affected children are taller than average, and their osseous age is generally 1 to 4 years in advance of their chronologic age. Urinary 17-ketosteroids and plasma testosterone levels may be slightly increased beyond values normal for age, but there is no evidence of true virilization. Gonadotropin levels are usually normal. When this disorder occurs in children with cerebral damage, as it often does, the child is usually small for his chronologic age and osseous maturation is not advanced.

This condition appears to result from premature activation of the adrenal cortex, with secretion of adrenal androgens before the pituitary gonadotropic mechanism becomes activated. The reason for the relatively frequent association of the disorder with cerebral damage is not known. Premature adrenarche must be differentiated from early true precocious puberty, adrenal cortical tumors and adrenal hyperplasia. Parents should then be assured that this condition is a harmless variation of development.

The terms *premature pubarche* and *premature adrenarche* have in the past been used interchangeably; it is now suggested that the term "premature pubarche" be reserved for children who have no detectable increase in androgens and whose condition seems to represent inordinate sensitivity of sexual hair follicles to androgen.

MEDICATIONAL PRECOCITY

This type of pseudopuberty is included here to emphasize that a variety of medicaments can induce the appearance of secondary sexual characteristics which may be confused with precocious puberty. A careful history to exclude accidental exposure to or ingestion of sex hormones is of paramount importance. Precocious pseudopuberty in both boys and girls accidentally ingesting stilbestrol has been reported. Exogenous estrogens may induce an intense, dark brown color to the areola of the breasts which is not usually seen in endogenous types of precocity. The precocious changes disappear after cessation of administration of the exogenous hormones.

GENERAL

Rimoin, D. L., and Schinike, R. N.: Genetic Disorders of the Endocrine Glands. St. Louis, The C. V. Mosby Co., 1971.

Saxena, B. B., Beling. C. G., and Gandy, H. M.: Gonadotropins. New York, John C. Wiley & Sons, Inc., 1972.

Schally, A. V., Arimura, A., and Kastin, A. J.: Hypothalamic regulatory hormones. Science *179*:341, 1973.

Wilkins, L.: The Diagnosis and Treatment of Endocrine Disorders in Childhood and Adolescence. 3rd ed. Springfield, Ill., Charles C Thomas, 1965.

Williams, R. H.: Textbook of Endocrinology. 5th ed. Philadelphia, W. B. Saunders Company, 1974.

Hypopituitarism

Aceto, T. Jr., et al.: Collaborative study of the effects of human growth hormone in growth hormone deficiency. I. First year of therapy. J. Clin. Endocrinol. Metab. *35*:483, 1973.

Braunstein, G. D., and Kohler, P. O.: Pituitary function in Hand-Schüller-Christian disease: Evidence for deficient growth hormone release in patients with short stature. N. Engl. J. Med. *286*:1225, 1972.

Brook, C. G. D., Sanders, M. D., and Hoare, R. D.: Septo-optic dysplasia. Brit. Med. J. *2*:811, 1973.

Finkelstein, J. W., Kream, J., Ludan, A., and Hellman, L.: Sulfation factor (somatomedin): An explanation for normal growth in the absence of immunoassayable growth hormone in patients with hypothalamic tumors. J. Clin. Endocrinol. Metab. *35*:13, 1972.

Frohman, L. A., Aceto, T., and MacGillivray, M. H.: Studies of growth hormone secretion in children: Normal, hypopituitary and constitutionally delayed. J. Clin. Endocrinol. Metab. *27*:1409, 1967.

Goodman, H. G., Grumbach, M. B., and Kaplan, S. L.: Growth and growth hormone. II. A comparison of isolated growth-hormone deficiency and multiple pituitary-hormone deficiencies in 35 patients with idiopathic hypopituitary dwarfism. New Engl. J. Med. *278*:57, 1968.

Hall, R., et al.: Action of growth hormone-release inhibitory hormone in healthy men and in acromegaly. Lancet *2*:581, 1973.

Holdaway, I. M., Rees, L. H., and Landon, J.: Circulating corticotropin levels in severe hypopituitarism and in the neonate. Lancet *2*:1170, 1973.

Johnson, J. D., et al.: Hypoplasia of the anterior pituitary and neonatal hypoglycemia. J. Pediatr. *82*:634, 1973.

Kaplan, S. L., Grumbach, M. M., Triesen, H. G., and Costom, B. H.: Thyrotropin-releasing factor (TRF) effect on secretion of human pituitary prolactin and thyrotropin in children and in idiopathic hypopituitary dwarfism: Further evidence for hypophysiotropic hormone deficiencies. J. Clin. Endocrinol. Metab. *35*:825, 1972.

Kenney, F. M., Guyda, H. J., Wright, J. C., and Friesen, H. G.: Prolactin and somatomedin in hypopituitary patients with "catch-up" growth following operations for craniopharyngioma. J. Clin. Endocrinol Metab. *36*:378, 1973.

Klachko, D. M., Winder, N., Burns, T. W., and White, J. E.: Traumatic hypopituitarism occurring before puberty: Survival 35 years untreated. J. Clin. Endocrinol. Metab. *28*:1768, 1968.

Lacey, K. A., Hewison, A., and Parkin, J. M.: Exercise as a screening test for growth hormone deficiency in children. Arch. Dis. Child. *48*:508, 1973.

Laron, Z., Pertzelan, A., and Mannheimer, S.: Genetic pituitary dwarfism with high serum concentration of growth hormone. A new inborn error of metabolism? Israel J. Med. Sci. *2*:152, 1966.

Laron, Z., and Saul, R.: Penis and testicular size in patients with growth hormone insufficiency. Acta Endocrinol. *63*:625, 1970.

Merimee, T. J., Rimoin, D. L., Cavalli-Sforza, L. C., Rabinowitz, D., and McKusick, V. A.: Metabolic effects of human growth hormone in the African pygmy. Lancet *2*:194, 1968.

Merimee, T. J., Rimoin, D. L., and Cavalli-Sforza, L. L.: Metabolic studies in the African pygmy. J. Clin. Invest. *51*:395, 1972.

Hyperpituitarism

AvRuskin, T. W., Sau, K., Tang, S. and Juan, C.: Childhood acromegaly: Successful therapy with conventional radiation and effects of chlorpromazine on growth hormone and prolactin secretion. J. Clin. Endocrinol. Metab. *37*:380, 1973.

Costin, G., Fefferman, R. A., and Kogut, M. D.: Hypothalamic gigantism. J. Pediatr. *83*:419, 1973.

Guyda, H., Robert, F., Colle, E., and Hardy, J.: Histologic, ultrastructural and hormonal characterization of a pituitary tumor secreting both HGH and prolactin. J. Clin. Endocrinol Metab. *36*:531, 1973.

Mabry, C. C., Hollingsworth, D. R., Upton, G. V., and Corbin, A.: Pituitary-hypothalamic dysfunction in generalized lipodystrophy. J. Pediatr. *82*:625, 1973.

Milunsky, A., Cowie, V. A., and Donoghue, E. C.: Cerebral gigantism in childhood. A report of two cases and a review of the literature. Pediatrics *40*:395, 1967.

Musa, B. U., Paulsen, C. A., and Conway, M. J.: Pituitary gigantism. Am. J. Med. *52*:399, 1972.

Poznanski, A. K., and Stephenson, J. M.: Radiographic findings in hypothalamic acceleration of growth associated with cerebral atrophy and mental retardation (cerebral gigantism). Radiology *88*:446, 1967.

Sotos, J. F., Dodge, P. R., Muirhead, D., Crawford, J. D., and Talbot, N. B.: Cerebral gigantism in childhood. New Engl. J. Med. *27*:109, 1964.

Spense, H. J., Trias, E. P., and Raiti, S.: Acromegaly in a 9½-year-old boy. Am. J. Dis. Child. *123*:504, 1972.

Tzagouris, M., Genge, J., and Herrold, J.: Increased growth hormone in partial and total lipoatrophy. Diabetes *22*:388, 1973.

Diabetes Insipidus

Barlow, E. D., and DeWardener, H. E.: Compulsive water drinking. Quart. J. Med. *52*:235, 1959.

Bartter, F. C., and Schwartz, W. B.: The syndrome of inappropriate secretion of antidiuretic hormone. Am. J. Med. *42*:790, 1967.

Baumann, G., Lopex-Amor, E., and Dingman, J. F.: Plasma arginine vasopressin in syndrome of inappropriate antidiuretic hormone secretion. Am. J. Med. *52*:19, 1972.

Bode, H. H., Harley, B. M., and Crawford, J. D.: Restoration of normal drinking behavior by chlorpropamide in patients with hypodipsia and diabetes insipidus. Am. J. Med. *51*:304, 1971.

Braverman, L. E., Mancini, J. P., and McGoldrick, D. M.: Hereditary idiopathic diabetes insipidus. A case report with autopsy findings. Ann. Intern. Med. *63*:503, 1965.

Bretz, G. W., Baghdassarian, A., Graber, J. D., Zacherle, B. J., Norum, R. A., and Blizzard, R. M.: Coexistence of diabetes mellitus and insipidus and optic atrophy in two male siblings. Am. J. Med. *48*:398, 1970.

Coggins, C. H., and Leaf, A.: Diabetes insipidus. Am. J. Med. *42*:807, 1967.
Crawford, J. D., Kennedy, G. C., and Hill, L. E.: Clinical results of treatment of diabetes insipidus with drugs of the chlorothiazide series. New Engl. J. Med. *262*:737, 1960.
Fichman, M. P., and Brooker, G.: Deficient renal cyclic adenosine 3′, 5′-monophosphate production in nephrogenic diabetes insipidus. J. Clin. Endocrinol. Metab. *35*:35, 1972.
Husain, M. K., Fernando, N., Shapiro, M., Kagan, A., and Glick, S. M.: Radioimmunoassay of arginine vasopressin in human plasma. J. Clin. Endocrinol. Metab. *37*:616, 1973.
Linshaw, M. A., Sey, M., DiGeorge, A. M., and Gruskin, A. B.: A potential danger of oral chlorpropamide therapy: Impaired excretion of a water load. J. Clin. Endocrinol. Metab. *34*:562, 1972.
Miller, M., Dalakos, T., Moses, A. M., Fellerman, H., and Streeten, D. H. P.: Recognition of partial defects in antidiuretic hormone secretion. Ann. Intern. Med. *73*:721, 1970.
Miller, M., and Moses, A. M.: Urinary antidiuretic hormone in polyuric disorders and in appropriate ADH syndrome. Ann. Intern. Med. *77*:715, 1972.
Miller, V. I., and Campbell, W. G., Jr.: Diabetes insipidus as complication of leukemia: Case report with literature review. Cancer *28*:666, 1971.
Rallison, M. L., and Tyler, F. H.: Treatment of diabetes insipidus in children with lysine-8-vasopressin. J. Pediatr. *70*:122, 1967.
Robertson, G. L., Bhoopalam, N., and Zelkowitz, L. J.: Vincristine neurotoxicity and abnormal secretion of antidiuretic hormone. Arch. Intern. Med. *132*:717, 1973.
Rosenbloom, A. L.: Chlorpropamide in diabetes insipidus in childhood. Curr. Ther. Res. *13*:671, 1971.
Schotland, M. G., Grumbach, M. M., and Strauss, J.: The effect of chlorothiazides in nephrogenic diabetes insipidus. Pediatrics *31*:741, 1963.
Weissman, P. N., Shenkman, L., and Gregerman, R. I.: Chlorpropamide hyponatremia. Drug induced inappropriate antidiuretic hormone activity. N. Engl. J. Med. *284*:65, 1971.

Precocious Puberty

Aarskog, D., and Tveteraas, E.: McCune-Albright syndrome following adrenalectomy for Cushing's syndrome in infancy. J. Pediatr. *73*:89, 1968.
Barnes, N. D., Hayles, A. B., and Ryan, R. J.: Sexual maturation in juvenile hypothyroidism. Mayo Clin. Proc. *48*:849, 1973.
Beas, F., Zurbrugg, R. P., Leibow, S. G., Patton, R. G., and Gardner, L. I.: Familial male sexual precocity: Report of the eleventh kindred found, with observations on blood group linkage and urinary C_{19}-steroid excretion. J. Clin. Endocrinol. Metab. *22*:1095, 1962.
Braunstein, G. D., Boidson, W. E., Glass, A., Hull, E. W., and McIntire, K. R.: *In vivo* and *in vitro* production of human chorionic gonadotropin and alpha-fetoprotein by a virilizing hepatoblastoma. J. Clin. Endocrinol. Metab. *35*:857, 1972.
Braunstein, G. D., Vaitukaitis, J. L., Carbone, P. P., and Ross, G. T.: Ectopic production of human chorionic gonadotropin by neoplasms. Ann. Intern. Med. *78*:39, 1973.
Bruton, O. C., Martz, D. C., and Gerard, E. S.: Precocious puberty due to secreting chorionepithelioma (teratoma) of the brain. J. Pediatr. *59*:719, 1961.
Camacho, A. M., Williams, D. L., and Montalvo, J. M.: Alterations of testicular histology and chromosomes in patients with constitutional sexual precocity treated with medroxyprogesterone acetate. J. Clin. Endocrinol. Metab. *34*:279, 1972.
Cook, C. D., McArthur, J. W., and Berenberg, W.: Pseudoprecocious puberty in girls as a result of estrogen ingestion. New Engl. J. Med. *248*:671, 1953.
Costin, G., Kershnar, A. K., Kogut, M. D., and Turkington, R. W.: Prolactin activity in juvenile hypothyroidism and precocious puberty. Pediatrics *50*:881, 1972.
Curi, J. F. J., Vanucci, R. C., Grossman, H., and New, M.: Elevated serum gonadotropins in Silver's syndrome. Am. J. Dis. Child. *114*:658, 1967.
Ferrier, P., Shepard, T. H., II, and Smith, E. K.: Growth disturbances and values for hormone excretion in various forms of precocious sexual development. Pediatrics. *28*:258, 1961.
Ferrier, P. E., and Ferrier, S. A., Silver's syndrome: Report of a case with chromosomal and dermatoglyphic study. J. Pediatr. *70*:438, 1967.
Fine, G., Smith, R. W., Jr., and Pachter, M. R.: Primary extragenital choriocarcinoma in the male subject. Am. J. Med. *32*:776, 1962.
Hertz, R.: Accidental ingestion of estrogens by children. Pediatrics *21*:203, 1958.
Hung, W., Milhorat, T. H., Nelson, K. B., and August, G. P.: Sexual precocity as the only sign of a brain tumor in a 9-year-old boy. Am. J. Dis. Child. *121*:524, 1971.
Jenner, M. R., Kelch, R. P., Kaplan, S. L., and Grumbach, M. D.: Plasma estradiol in prepubertal children, pubertal females, and in precocious puberty, premature thelarche, hypogonadism, and in a child with a feminizing ovarian tumor. J. Clin. Endocrinol. Metab. *34*:521, 1972.
Kulin, H. E., and Reiter, E. O.: Gonadotropins during childhood and adolescence: A review. Pediatrics *51*:260, 1973.
List, C. F., Dowman, C. E., Bagchi, B. K., and Bebin, J.: Posterior hypothalamic hamartomas and gangliogliomas causing precocious puberty. Neurology, *8*:164, 1958.
Nitzan, M., Laron, Z., Pertzelan, A., and Scharf, A.: McCune-Albright syndrome with sexual precocity in a boy. Helv. Paediat. Acta. *28*:61, 1973.
Root, A. W.: Endocrinology of puberty. I. Normal sexual maturation. J. Pediatr. *83*:1, 1973.
Root, A. W.: Endocrinology of puberty. II. Aberrations of sexual maturation. J. Pediatr. *83*:187, 1973.
Rosenfield, R. L.: Plasma 17-ketosteroids and 17-beta hydroxysteroids in girls with premature development of sexual hair. J. Pediatr. *99*:260, 1971.
Sigurjonsdottir, T. J., and Hayles, A. B.: Precocious puberty. A report of 96 cases. Am. J. Dis. Child. *115*:309, 1968.
Silverman, S. H., Migeon, C., Rosemberg, E., and Wilkins, L.: Precocious growth of sexual hair without other secondary sexual development: "Premature pubarche," a constitutional variation of adolescence. Pediatrics *10*:426, 1952.
Stool, S., and Cohen, P.: Silver's syndrome. Syndrome of congenital asymmetry, short stature, and altered patterns of sexual development. Am. J. Dis. Child. *105*:199, 1963.
Thamdrup, E.: Precocious Sexual Development. A Clinical Study of 100 Children. Springfield, Ill., Charles C Thomas, 1961.
Visser, H. K. A.: Some physiological and clinical aspects of puberty. Arch. Dis. Child. *48*:169, 1973.
Wolman, L., and Balmforth, G. V.: Precocious puberty due to a hypothalamic hamartoma in a patient surviving to late middle age. J. Neurol. Neurosurg. Psychiat. *26*:275, 1963.

DISORDERS OF THE THYROID GLAND

GENERAL CONSIDERATIONS

The main function of the thyroid gland is to synthesize thyroxine (T_4) and triiodothyronine (T_3). Iodine is essential for the production of these hormones; the daily requirement has been estimated to be about 40 to 100 μg. The daily intake in North America varies from 240 to more than 700 μg. Regardless of the chemical form upon ingestion, iodine eventually reaches the thyroid gland as iodide. Thyroid tissue has a special avidity for this element and is able to trap, transport and concentrate it for synthesis of thyroid hormone.

Before trapped iodide can react with tyrosine it must be oxidized; this reaction is catalyzed by thyroidal peroxidase. The thyroid cells also elaborate a specific thyroprotein, a globulin with approximately 120 tyrosine units. After iodination of tyrosine to form monoiodotyrosine and diiodotyrosine, 2 molecules of diiodotyrosine couple to form 1 molecule of thyroxine, or 1 molecule of diiodotyrosine and 1 of monoiodotyrosine combine to form triiodothyronine. It is uncertain whether a coupling enzyme exists. Once formed, hormones are stored as thyroglobulin in the lumen of the follicle (colloid) until ready to be delivered to the body cells. Thyroglobulin (Tg) has a molecular weight of about 660,000 and under normal conditions is detectable in the blood of most individuals at nanogram levels. T_4 and T_3 are liberated from thyroglobulin by activation of proteases and peptidases.

The metabolic potency of T_3 is three to four times that of T_4, and its clinical significance may be greater than that of T_4. In addition to being secreted by the thyroid, T_3 is derived by deiodination of T_4 in peripheral tissues. There is evidence that T_4 has intrinsic hormonal activity and is not simply a prohormone for T_3. Reliable methods to measure the level of T_3 directly in blood have only recently been developed; its concentration is 1/50 that of T_4. The thyroid hormones increase the metabolic processes of the body by increasing basal consumption of oxygen, but the mechanism of this calorigenic effect is uncertain. There are other widespread biochemical effects, such as stimulation of protein synthesis and effects on carbohydrate, lipid and vitamin metabolism.

The circulating thyroid hormones (T_4 and T_3) are firmly bound to thyroxine-binding proteins; the most important is thyroxine-binding globulin (TBG); of lesser significance are thyroxine-binding prealbumin (TBPA) and albumin. Since the concentration or binding capacity of TBG is altered in many clinical states, it must be considered in the interpretation of T_4 or T_3 levels.

The thyroid is regulated by thyroid-stimulating hormone (TSH), a glycoprotein produced and secreted by the anterior pituitary. This hormone activates proteolytic enzymes in the thyroid gland to effect release of thyroid hormones. TSH is composed of two noncovalently bound subunits (chains): an alpha (hTSH-α), and a beta subunit (hTSH-β). The free subunits as well as TSH can be measured in blood by specific radioimmunoassays. TSH synthesis and release are, in turn, stimulated by thyroid-releasing hormone (TRH) which is synthesized in the hypothalamus and secreted into the pituitary. TRH is a simple tripeptide which has been commercially synthesized and is now available for clinical use. In states of decreased production of thyroid hormone, TSH and presumably TRF are increased. An excess of TRF or of TSH results in hypertrophy and hyperplasia of thyroid cells, increased trapping of iodine and increased synthesis of thyroid hormones. Exogenous thyroid hormone or increased thyroid hormone synthesis inhibits TSH production.

THYROID HORMONE STUDIES

SERUM THYROXINE AND TRIIODOTHYRONINE. For many years, measurement of the protein-bound iodine (PBI) served as a useful estimate of thyroxine in blood. The method is not specific; many compounds containing iodine produce elevated PBI levels for variable periods ranging from a few days to many years. Of special interest is iophenoxic acid (Teridax), an agent formerly used for cholecystography, which has been estimated to elevate the PBI for more than 30 years. This agent can also cross the placenta; many years after its ingestion by the mother it will produce elevated PBI levels in her offspring which persist, in turn, for many years.

The PBI test has been replaced by more specific measurements of thyroxine. The competitive binding method of measuring thyroxine, T_4(D), is the major method in current use for measuring T_4. A radioimmunoassay for T_4,T_4(RIA), has been introduced recently, which will probably replace other methods. T_4(RIA) requires no extraction, is highly specific for thyroxine, and can be performed on as little as 25 μl. of blood. Normal levels of thyroxine during the first weeks of life are higher than subsequently; these age-related variations must be taken into consideration in interpreting results (see Table of Normal Values, Appendix).

Triiodothyronine also can be conveniently and reliably measured in serum by radioimmunoassay. The T_3(RIA) is rapidly becoming an important adjunct to diagnosis of thyroid disorders. Levels are low in cord blood (under 50 ng/dl) but by 3 days of age the levels are similar to those in older children and adults (100 to 170 ng/dl); levels vary somewhat with the radioimmunoassay used.

SERUM THYROXINE-BINDING GLOBULIN (TBG). Estimation of TBG levels is frequently necessary because TBG is increased or decreased in a variety of clinical situations, with effects on the levels of thyroxine. TBG is increased in pregnancy, in the newborn period, by estrogens (oral contraceptives), by perphenazine and in acute intermittent porphyria; it is decreased by androgens, anabolic steroids, prednisone, in the nephrotic syndrome and by major illness or surgical stress. Diphenylhydantoin (Dilantin) does not lower the level of TBG but displaces thyroxine from its binding sites, an effect which leads to decreased T_4 levels. Such patients may be euthyroid in spite of low or elevated thyroxine levels because the total concentration of unbound (free) hormone is normal. Decreased or increased levels also occur as a genetic trait in some families.

A variety of methods have been developed to measure TBG or TBG-binding capacity; the most commonly used method is one of the many variations of the resin triiodothyronine uptake test, RT_3U. At best, it is a screening test with which to interpret T_4 results; it should never be used as an autonomous test of thyroid function. The product of the serum T_4 concentration and the T_3 uptake (thyroxine-resin T_3 index or T_4-RT_3 index) correlates closely with free T_4 concentration in serum. This index is increased in hyperthyroidism, decreased in hypothyroidism, and normal in euthyroid patients with abnormalities in the concentration of TBG. It is important that the clinician be aware of normal values for a given laboratory since T_4 and T_3 uptakes are often determined by a variety of kit methods and the index is calculated and expressed differently in different laboratories. A radioimmunoassay method to measure TBG has recently been developed.

THYROTROPIN. Thyrotropin is readily measured by a radioimmunoassay method, TSH(RIA), which is rapidly becoming generally available for clinical studies. It is one of the most sensitive tests for the detection of hypothyroidism. Normal levels are less than 10 μU/ml; levels over 20 μU/ml indicate hypothyroidism and values between 10 and 20 μU/ml suggest decreased thyroid reserve.

Administration of thyrotropin-releasing hormone (TRH) is rapidly becoming a standard test to distinguish hypothalamic (TRH) deficiency from pituitary (TSH) deficiency, to test pituitary TSH reserve and to confirm questionable instances of thyrotoxicosis. In normal subjects, intravenous administration of TRH (3–4 μg/kg) increases baseline levels of TSH to peak values of 10–30 μU/ml in 30 to 90 minutes. In thyrotoxicosis there is no rise of serum levels of TSH in response to TRH because the elevated level of thyroxine blocks the effect of TRH on the pituitary. Low levels of TSH in a hypothyroid patient may indicate either pituitary or hypothalamic failure. A normal response to TRH localizes the defect in the hypothalamus.

IN VIVO RADIOISOTOPE STUDIES. With the advent of markedly improved direct tests of thyroid function, the usefulness of radioiodine uptake studies has decreased. The iodine-trapping or concentrating mechanism of the thyroid can be evaluated by the radioactive isotopes—^{131}I, with a half-life of 8 days, or ^{123}I, with a half-life of 13 hours. Present technology allows doses of radioiodine that are only a fraction of those formerly used (0.1–0.5 μci). Technetium-99M is a particularly useful radioisotope for children since, in contrast to iodine, it is trapped but not organified by the thyroid and has a half-life of only 6 hours. Thyroid scanning may be indicated to detect ectopic thyroid tissue, to evaluate thyroid nodules and to assess presence of thyroid tissue in questions of thyroid agenesis. These studies should be performed with technetium-99M as pertechnetate since it has the advantages of lower radiation exposure and high quality scintigrams. Use of radioactive iodine in children should be limited to investigative studies concerning kinetics of iodine metabolism or of turnover of hormones and their precursors.

DEFECTS OF THYROXINE-BINDING GLOBULIN

Abnormalities in the level of TBG are not associated with clinical disease and do not require treatment. They are discussed here because aberrations of TBG levels may be a source of diagnostic confusion and errors.

TBG deficiency occurs as an X-linked dominant disorder. Affected patients are euthyroid. TBG is absent or low, T_4 is low and levels of RT_3U are high. Heterozygous females have intermediate levels of TBG, low normal levels of T_4 and high normal levels of RT_3U. Homozygous females have not been reported, but an affected XO female has been discovered. Absence of TBG from the cord blood of an affected male indicates that it does not cross the placenta. A rare instance of total deficiency of TBG in a normal woman established that TBG is not necessary for normal pregnancy. There also appears to be an autosomal dominant form of the disorder in which there is partial deficiency of TBG. A family has been reported in which 4 males with TBG deficiency also had neurologic and mental defects. This may represent a fortuitous association of two different X-linked mutant genes.

Elevated TBG also occurs as an X-linked dominant disorder. Affected patients are euthyroid. The nature of the regulatory genetic defect which results in a single operon overproducing this protein is unknown. TBG and T_4 levels are elevated and RT_3U levels are low.

Levels of TSH and free T_4 are normal in euthyroid patients with either deficient or elevated TBG. A study of appropriate relatives in the family pedigree is usually necessary to establish the genetic origin of the aberrant level of TBG.

HYPOTHYROIDISM

Hypothyroidism results from deficient production of thyroid hormone. The disorder may be manifest very early in life. When symptoms appear after a period of apparently normal thyroid function, the disorder may either be truly "acquired" or only appear so as a result of one of a variety of congenital defects in which the manifestation of the deficiency is delayed. The term "cretinism" is often used synonymously with congenital hypothyroidism; any other use is best avoided.

CONGENITAL HYPOTHYROIDISM

All the congenital causes of hypothyroidism, whether sporadic or familial, goitrous or nongoitrous, will be discussed together. In many of these conditions, the deficiency of thyroid hormone is severe and symptoms develop in the early weeks of life. In others, lesser degrees of deficiency occur and manifestations may be delayed for months or even years.

TABLE 17–2 CLASSIFICATION OF HYPOTHYROIDISM

A. Deficiency of TRF
   1. Isolated
   2. Multiple hypothalamic deficiencies (e.g., idiopathic hypopituitarism)

B. Deficiency of TSH
   1. Isolated
   2. Multiple pituitary deficiencies (e.g., craniopharyngioma)

C. Deficiency of Thyroid Hormone
   1. Aplasia, hypoplasia or ectopia of thyroid
      a. Developmental defects (thyroid dysgenesis)
      b. Maternal radioiodine
      c. Maternal autoimmune disease?
   2. Defective synthesis of thyroid hormone (goitrous hypothyroidism)
      a. Iodide-trapping defect
      b. Iodide-organification defects
         1. Absent peroxidase
         2. Defective binding
         3. Pendred syndrome
      c. Iodotyrosine coupling defect
      d. Iodotyrosine deiodination defect
      e. Thyroglobulin synthesis defect
   3. Iodine deficiency (endemic cretinism)
   4. Damage to thyroid gland
      a. Autoimmune disease (lymphocytic thyroiditis)
      b. Cystinosis
   5. Maternal ingestion of medications (neonatal goiter)
      a. Iodides
      b. Propylthiouracil, methimazole
   6. Iatrogenic
      a. Thyroidectomy
      b. Drugs (iodides, lithium, cobalt, propylthiouracil, methimazole, para-aminosalicylic acid)

D. End-organ Defect
   1. TSH unresponsiveness
   2. Thyroid hormone unresponsiveness

ETIOLOGY. *Developmental defects* of the thyroid gland are the most common causes of congenital hypothyroidism; the condition is referred to as *thyroid dysgenesis.* Rudiments of thyroid tissue may be found in the majority of patients when carefully searched for by sensitive scanning techniques. The thyroid rudiment is most often found in an ectopic location anywhere from the base of the tongue to the normal position in the neck. Little is known of the factors which interfere with normal migration and development of the thyroid gland. The disorder is usually sporadic and rarely affects more than one member in a family. Congenital hypothyroidism has been observed in only one of monozygotic twins, suggesting that a deleterious factor operated during intrauterine life; the onset of hypothyroidism in the second twin may, however, be delayed. In one of another pair of identical twins hypothyroidism associated with an inadequate thyroid in the normal position was diagnosed at 4 months of age; in the second twin an ectopic thyroid did not lose adequate function until 4 to 6 years of age. The disorder has been noted occasionally in siblings; both males and females have been affected, suggesting the possibility of recessive inheritance in some instances.

Lingual thyroid represents the most extreme form of failure of migration of the thyroid gland; the ectopic thyroid tissue may provide adequate amounts of thyroid hormone for many years or it may fail during childhood. Hypothyroidism usually results when a lingual thyroid is surgically removed from a euthyroid patient, since the majority have no other thyroid tissue. Lingual thyroid has been associated with thyroglossal duct cysts and with a family history of other thyroid disorders. In one family, 2 siblings had lingual thyroids and a third sibling had hypoplasia of one lobe of a normally situated thyroid.

It has been suggested that autoimmunity may cause developmental thyroid defects, and a family has been reported in which 6 siblings with congenital hypothyroidism were born to a mother with lymphocytic thyroiditis. No consistent relationship, however, has been established between fetal thyroid disease and maternal autoantibodies. Deficiency of fetal TSH has also been proposed as a possible cause of defective thyroid development. Though possible deficiencies in early fetal life cannot be excluded, TSH is always elevated postnatally.

Radioiodine. Radioiodine administered during pregnancy for treatment of cancer of the thyroid or of hypothyroidism has been reported as a cause of damage to the fetal thyroid in eight instances. In most instances of hypothyroidism resulting from this cause, pregnancy was not suspected at the time of administration of ^{131}I. Great caution must be utilized whenever radioiodine is administered to women of child-bearing age. The fetal thyroid gland is capable of trapping iodine by 12 weeks and of synthesizing thyroid hormone by 14 to 15 weeks. In one instance, ^{131}I was administered to the mother at 14 weeks of gestation for treatment of thyroid carcinoma; the athyreotic infant had a tracheal stricture at the site of the thyroid, T_4 and T_3 were undetectable in cord serum and TSH was markedly elevated (340 μU/ml). This is clear evidence that fetal hypothyroidism occurs and that maternal thyroid hormones do not cross the placenta in significant amounts late in pregnancy. Administration of radioactive iodine to lactating women is also contraindicated, since it is readily excreted in milk.

Thyrotropin Deficiency. Deficiency of TSH and hypothyroidism may occur in any of the conditions associated with developmental defects of the pituitary or hypothalamus or in children with idiopathic hypopituitarism (see Pituitary Disorders, above). More often in these conditions, the deficiency of TSH is secondary to a deficiency of thyrotropin-releasing factor (hypothalamic hypothyroidism). With administration of TRF, TSH increases, indicating a primary hypothalamic defect.

Isolated deficiency of TSH is rare and has been reported only about 20 times, mostly in adults. In three instances, it was associated with pseudohypoparathyroidism (see below, this Section). Isolated TSH deficiency might also be primary, or secondary to TRF deficiency.

Thyrotropin Unresponsiveness. A congenitally nongoitrous hypothyroid boy of a consanguineous mating has been reported with an elevated level of biologically active TSH and normal ^{131}I uptake. Absence of response to thyrotropin was shown in vivo and in metabolism of thyroid tissue in vitro, indicating an impaired ability of the thyroid to respond to TSH.

Thyroid Hormone Unresponsiveness. Three out of 6 siblings of a consanguineous marriage have been reported with goiter, deaf-mutism, stippled epiphyses and clinical euthyroidism, in whom laboratory data suggested both hyper- and hypothyroidism. Levels of T_4, T_3, free T_4, free T_3, and radioiodine uptake were normal. Levels of TSH were normal or slightly elevated. Conversion of T_4 to T_3 was normal. These and extensive other studies indicated tissue resistance to the effect of thyroid hormone at the cellular level, possibly an abnormal receptor. The severity of the syndrome decreases with the passing of time.

Partial target organ resistance has been reported in another child with a goiter and learning disability but without deafness or skeletal changes.

Defective Synthesis of Thyroxine. Congenital hypothyroidism may be due to a variety of defects in the biosynthesis of thyroid hormone. The presence of a goiter is the hallmark of these defects and the condition is termed goitrous hypothyroidism or goitrous cretinism. They are genetically determined and in most instances transmitted in an autosomal recessive manner. The following defects have been identified:

Iodide-trapping Defect. Only 7 instances of this defect have been reported. A goiter is present, but in contrast to all the other defects, the uptake of radioiodine is low. The salivary glands and stomach also lack ability to concentrate iodide. The biochemical defect is unknown, but deficiency of iodide permease is a possibility. A partial defect has been described in two siblings of a consanguineous mating; hypothyroidism presented at 2 months of age.

Iodide Organification Defect. After iodide is trapped by the thyroid, it is rapidly oxidized by H_2O_2 and thyroid peroxidase and is incorporated into tyrosine. In this defect, iodide is not organified and it may be rapidly discharged from the thyroid by administration of perchlorate. Three different organification defects have now been characterized:

1. complete absence of peroxidase activity occurs in a severe form of goitrous hypothyroidism.
2. failure of a prosthetic hematin group to bind to thyroidal apoperoxidase, in euthyroid goitrous patients.
3. Pendred syndrome, in which goiter and nerve deafness accompany deficient organification but the biochemical defect is unknown.

Coupling Defect. After iodine is incorporated into tyrosine in thyroglobulin to form iodotyrosine, an intramolecular rearrangement occurs, leading to coupling of iodotyrosines to form diiodothyronines. Owing to the complexity of this reaction, a heterogeneity of defects is likely, but little is known of the biochemical aberrations involved. It has been proposed that errors may involve defects in an unidentified coupling enzyme system or an abnormality in the steric configuration of the thyroglobulin molecule.

Deiodinase Defect. Free monoiodotyrosine and diiodotyrosine are normally deiodinated within the thyroid or in peripheral tissues by a deiodinase. The iodine thus liberated is then reutilized in synthesis of hormone. Patients with deiodinase deficiency have large amounts of monoiodotyrosine and diiodotyrosine in blood and in urine. The constant loss of iodine from the thyroid and in the urine leads to hormone deficiency and goiter.

Defect of Thyroglobulin Synthesis. Patients with this disorder release from the thyroid into the blood stream iodinated proteins or polypeptides which are calorigenically inactive. Owing to the complexity of thyroglobulin synthesis, this category almost certainly has diverse etiologies.

In some patients there is genetic absence of thyroglobulin synthesis. As a consequence, there is iodination of inappropriate proteins, mainly albumin, and very little thyroxine biosynthesis. There is a high production rate of iodohistidines which are not deiodinated but are excreted in urine and may serve as a clue to detection of defective thyroglobulin synthesis. Some reported cases of defects of "coupling" or of abnormal iodinated compounds in serum and thyroid have probably been the result of defects in thyroglobulin synthesis.

CLINICAL MANIFESTATIONS. Congenital hypothyroidism is about three times as common in girls as in boys. It is recognized only rarely at birth, since the signs and symptoms are usually not sufficiently developed. It can be suspected and the diagnosis established during the early weeks of life if the initial but less characteristic manifestations are recognized. Cretins may be significantly heavier at birth than normal newborn infants, but, owing to the great variation in birth weights, there is little diagnostic value to this observation. Unusual prolongation of physiologic icterus, owing to delayed maturation of glucuronide conjugation, may be the earliest sign. Feeding difficulties, especially sluggishness, lack of interest, somnolence and choking spells during nursing, are often present during the first month of life. Respiratory difficulties, owing in part to the large tongue, include apneic episodes, noisy respirations and nasal obstruction. These infants cry little, sleep much, have poor appetites and are generally sluggish. There may be constipation, which does not usually respond to treatment. The abdomen is large, and an umbilical hernia is usually present. The temperature is subnormal, and the skin, par-

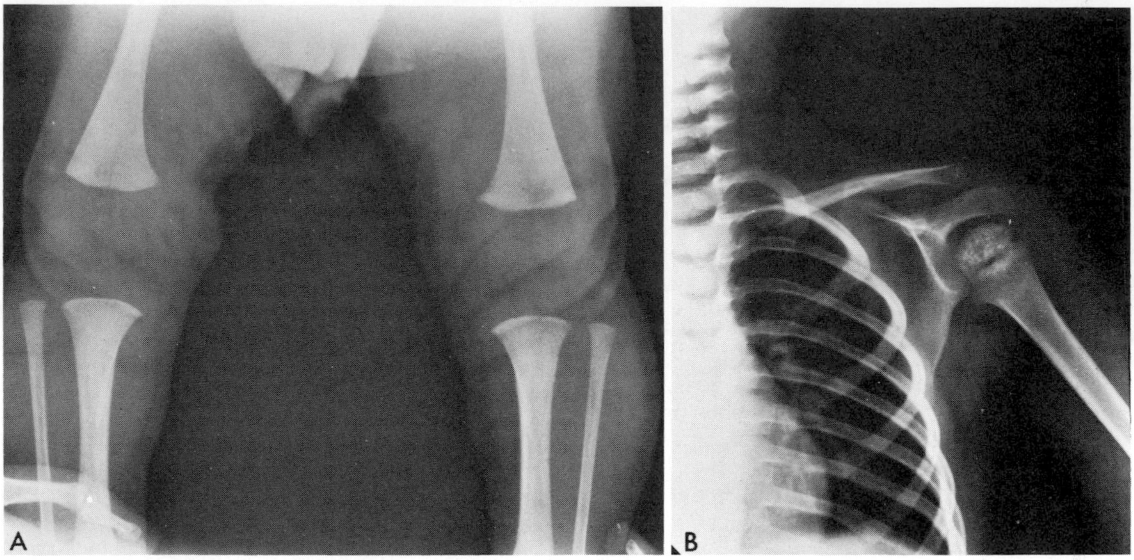

Figure 17–9 Congenital hypothyroidism. A, Absence of distal femoral epiphysis in a 3 month old cretin who was born at term. This is evidence for the onset of the hypothyroid state during fetal life. B, Epiphyseal dysgenesis in the head of the humerus in a 9 year old girl who had been inadequately treated with thyroid.

ticularly of the extremities, may be cold and mottled. The pulse is slow; heart murmurs and cardiomegaly are common. Anemia is often present and is refractory to treatment with hematinics. Since symptoms appear gradually, the diagnosis is often delayed.

These manifestations progress; retardation of physical and mental development becomes greater during the following months, and by 3 to 6 months of age the clinical picture is fully developed. When there is only a partial deficiency of thyroid hormone, the symptoms may be milder, the syndrome incomplete and the onset delayed.

The child is stunted in growth, the extremities being short, and the head seems large. The anterior and posterior fontanelles are widely open; observation of this sign at birth may serve as an initial clue for early recognition of congenital hy-

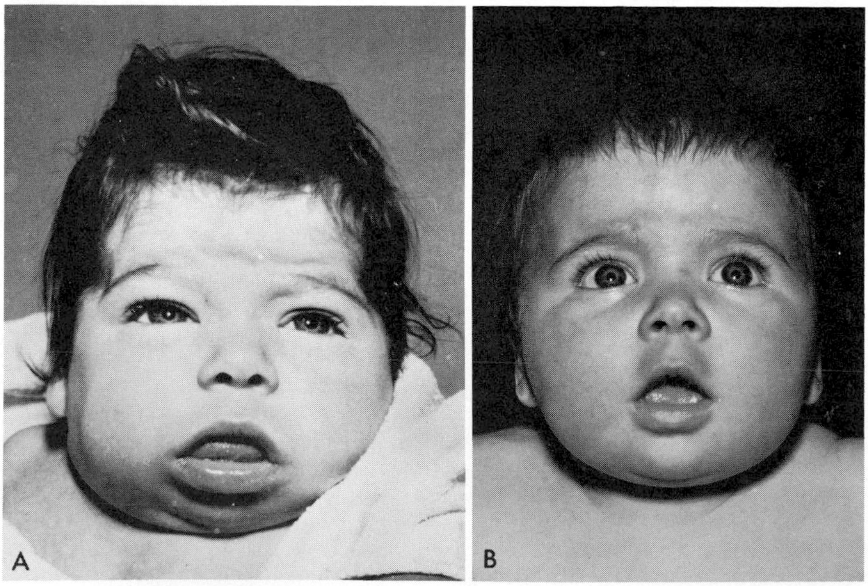

Figure 17–10 Congenital hypothyroidism in an infant 6 months of age. The infant fed poorly in the neonatal period and was constipated. She had a persistent nasal discharge and a large tongue, was very lethargic, and had no social smile and no head control. A, Note puffy face, dull expression, hirsute forehead. Serum cholesterol, 172 mg/dl; alkaline phosphatase, 4.8 Bodansky units; negligible uptake of radio-iodine. Osseous development was that of newborn. B, Four months after treatment with U.S.P. thyroid. Note decreased puffiness of face, decreased hirsutism of forehead and alert appearance.

pothyroidism. Only 3 per cent of normal newborn infants have a posterior fontanelle larger than 0.5 cm. The eyes appear far apart, and the bridge of the broad nose is depressed. The palpebral fissures are narrow and the eyelids swollen. The mouth is kept open, and the thick and broad tongue protrudes from it. Dentition is delayed. The neck is short and thick, and there may be deposits of fat above the clavicles and between the neck and shoulders. The hands are broad and the fingers short. The skin is dry and scaly, and there is little perspiration. Myxedema manifests itself, particularly in the skin of the eyelids, of the back of the hands and of the external genitalia. Carotenemia may cause a yellow discoloration of the skin, but the scleras remain white. The scalp is thickened, and the hair is coarse, brittle and scanty. The hairline reaches far down on the forehead, which usually appears wrinkled, especially when the infant cries.

The muscles are usually hypotonic. In rare instances generalized muscular hypertonia has been observed (*Debré-Sémélaigne syndrome*). Affected children may have an athletic appearance due to pseudohypertrophy of the muscles. Its pathogenesis is unknown; nonspecific histochemical and ultrastructural changes found in muscle biopsies return to normal with treatment. The syndrome has been observed in siblings of a consanguineous mating.

The mental development of cretins is usually retarded. They appear lethargic and are late in sitting and standing. The voice is hoarse, and they do not learn to talk. The degree of physical and mental retardation increases as they become older. Sexual maturation is delayed or does not take place at all. Precocious sexual maturation is an occasional complication.

LABORATORY DATA. Retardation of osseous development can be shown roentgenographically at birth in a high percentage of cretins and indicates some deprivation of thyroid hormone during intrauterine life. For example, the distal femoral epiphysis, normally present at birth, is often absent. In untreated patients there is an increasing discrepancy between chronologic age and osseous development. The epiphyses often have multiple foci of ossification (epiphyseal dysgenesis); deformity ("beaking") of the 12th thoracic or 1st or 2nd lumbar vertebra is common. Roentgenograms of the skull show large fontanelles and wide sutures; intersutural bones (wormian bones) are common. The sella turcica is often enlarged and round; in rare instances, there may be erosion and thinning. Delays in formation of dental buds and in eruption of teeth may be seen. Cardiac enlargement or pericardial effusion may be present.

In children over 2 years of age, the serum level of cholesterol is usually elevated if hypothyroidism is severe. Values over 400 mg/dl are not unusual. A greater impairment in the excretion of cholesterol than in its synthesis is thought to account for this finding.

Serum T_4 and T_3 levels are low or borderline. In the evaluation of newborn infants special attention must be given to the normal range of values for this period in life. (See Appendix.) Hypothyroidism should be suspected if the T_4 (by displacement analysis) is below 9.8 μg/dl during the first 2 weeks or below 8.2 μg/dl during the second 2 weeks of life. If the defect is primarily in the thyroid, serum TSH levels exceed 20 μU/ml after 72 hours of age, and levels of 100 μU/ml or more are commonplace.

Low levels of TSH in hypothyroid patients suggest pituitary or hypothalamic defect and indicate a TRF stimulation study. Levels of growth hormone and responses to provocative stimuli may be abnormally low in primary hypothyroidism but return to normal after treatment with thyroid.

Technetium scanning may be indicated to determine whether there is any thyroid tissue. Patients with goitrous hypothyroidism may require extensive evaluation, including radioiodine studies, perchlorate discharge tests, kinetic studies, chromatography and studies of thyroid tissue if the biochemical nature of the defect is to be determined.

The electrocardiogram may show low voltage P and T waves with diminished amplitude of QRS complexes. The electroencephalogram frequently shows low voltage.

DIFFERENTIAL DIAGNOSIS. Careful plotting on a growth chart of lengths and heights of all infants and children is essential; deceleration of growth velocity frequently provides the first clue to the diagnosis. Once it has been considered, diagnosis is not difficult, since direct tests of thyroid function have been markedly improved and become generally available. Familiarity with those conditions which alter test results, such as alterations in TBG, is essential.

PROGNOSIS. Without treatment, cretins may die of respiratory obstruction or intercurrent infections, and those who live become mentally deficient dwarfs. Treatment with thyroid hormone results in normal linear growth, osseous maturation and sexual development. Mental development, however, is much less predictable. Thyroid hormone is critical for normal cerebral development both in the late months of fetal life and in early months of postnatal life. Hence, the diagnosis must be made early in life and effective treatment initiated promptly in order to minimize irreversible brain damage. Only about half of infants with hypothyroidism who are treated adequately by 3 months of age will achieve an intelligence quotient of 90 or more. In general, the more profound the deprivation of the thyroid hormone in the early months of life, the poorer is the prognosis for mental development. There is evidence, in fact, that in completely athyreotic infants impairment of cerebral development often begins in utero. There is no conclusive evidence that treatment of the pregnant woman with huge doses of thyroid hormone to enhance transplacental transfer of protective levels of hormone to the hypothyroid fetus is effective. When clinical evidence of hypothyroidism is delayed in onset, the outlook for normal mental development is much better; children who acquire hypothyroidism after 2 years of age and are treated appropriately have a good prognosis for mental development.

TREATMENT. Regardless of the etiology of the hypothyroidism, replacement therapy with thyroid hormone is indicated and effective. Sodium-L-thyroxine given orally has the advantage over sesicated thyroid of being a stable preparation with a long shelf life and constant biologic activity. It has been estimated that normally 30 to 50 per cent of circulating thyroxine undergoes peripheral deiodination to become triiodothyronine. Under normal conditions, most circulating T_3 is derived from T_4 rather than directly from the thyroid gland. Hence, treatment with sodium-L-thyroxine provides both T_4 and T_3. In infants the initial dose is 50 μg/day, which may be increased to 100 μg/day 2 to 4 weeks later. This dose may be sufficient for 1 to 2 years, after which it should be increased to 150 to 200 μg/day. Older children may be treated initially with 100–150 μg/day; only rarely is more than 200 μg/day required. Prompt treatment of the young infant is essential to avoid residual or further brain damage.

Levels of both T_4 and T_3 should be monitored and maintained within the normal range. It was formerly thought that when thyroxine was used for replacement therapy, levels of T_4 should be maintained slightly elevated to compensate for the deficiency of T_3, but this is not necessary; provision of normal levels of T_4 ensures normal levels of T_3. After catch-up growth is complete, careful attention to the growth rate is an excellent clinical index of adequacy of therapy. Parents should be forewarned of changes in behavior and activity to be expected with therapy, and special attention must be given to any developmental or neurologic deficits.

JUVENILE HYPOTHYROIDISM

(Acquired Hypothyroidism)

The development of hypothyroidism in a child who previously was euthyroid may be due to a wide variety of factors. A congenitally hypoplastic thyroid gland may furnish amounts of hormone sufficient for the first few years, but the deficiency may become manifest when demands on the gland are increased by rapid growth of the body. Accordingly, any or all of the etiologic causes of congenital hypothyroidism must be considered. In congenital defects clinical manifestations may present as in patients with acquired lesions.

Complete or subtotal thyroidectomy for thyrotoxicosis or cancer may result in hypothyroidism, as may removal of an anomalous thyroid when it constitutes the sole source of thyroid hormone. For example, when the thyroid is ectopically placed at the base of the tongue (lingual thyroid), it is often the only thyroid tissue. Likewise, the entire thyroid gland may consist of a midline nodule mistaken for a thyroglossal duct cyst and excised.

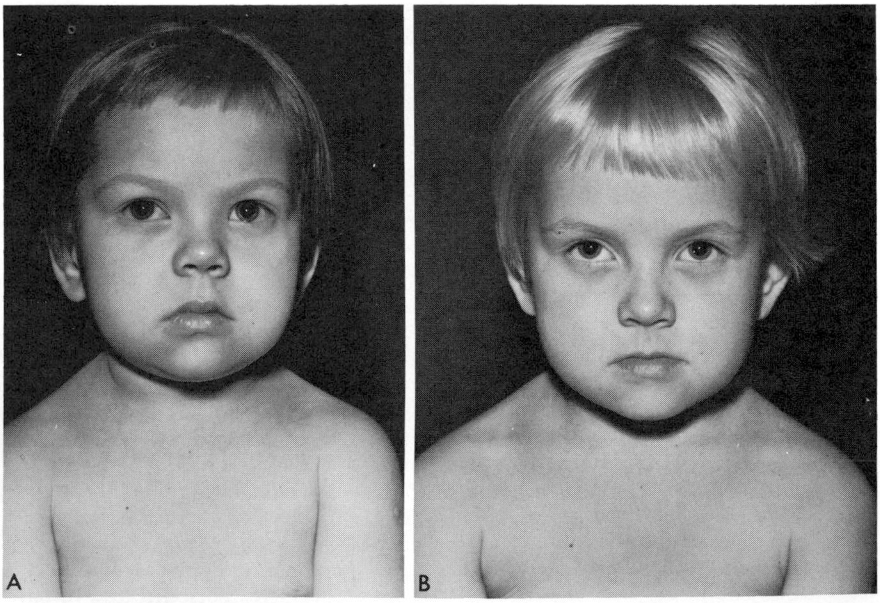

Figure 17–11 Acquired hypothyroidism in a girl 6 years of age. She was treated with a wide variety of hematinics for refractory anemia for 3 years. She had almost complete cessation of growth, constipation, and sluggishness of 3 years' duration. Height age was 3 years; bone age, 4 years. She had a sallow complexion, and immature facies with a poorly developed nasal bridge. A, *Serum cholesterol, 501 mg/dl; alkaline phosphatase, 1.8 Bodansky units; radio-iodine uptake, 7 per cent at 24 hours; PBI, 2.8 μg/dl.* B, *After therapy for 18 months. Note nasal development, increased luster and decreased pigmentation of hair and maturation of face. Height age was 5½ years; bone age, 7 years. There was decided improvement in her general condition. Menarche occurred at 14 years; ultimate height was 61 inches. She graduated from high school. She was well controlled with 200 μg of sodium-L-thyroxine daily.*

Overt hypothyroidism has been observed in 23 per cent of a group of children with cystinosis; the thyroid appears particularly susceptible to the toxic action of cystine.

Hypothyroidism in association with a goiter may be caused occasionally by chronic infectious processes or by the protracted ingestion of medications such as iodides or cobalt. Acquired hypothyroidism, however, most often results from lymphocytic thyroiditis, which may or may not be associated with a goiter. (See below.)

The clinical manifestations depend upon the age of the child at onset and upon the extent of dysfunction. The later in life hypothyroidism is acquired, the less will be the impairment of growth and development. Nevertheless, myxedematous changes of the skin, constipation, sleepiness and a mental decline may be manifest at any age. Cessation or retardation of growth in a child whose growth has previously been normal should always alert one to the possibility of hypothyroidism. (Fig. 17–2). Obese children are frequently, but usually erroneously, considered to have hypothyroidism. Most obese children have warm moist skin, a ruddy complexion and normal thyroid function.

Diagnostic studies and treatment are the same as described for congenital hypothyroidism.

GOITER

A goiter is an enlargement of the thyroid gland. Persons with enlarged thyroids may have normal function of the gland (*euthyroidism*), thyroid deficiency (*hypothyroidism*) or overproduction of the hormones (*hyperthyroidism*). Goiter may be congenital or acquired, endemic or sporadic.

The goiter most often results from increased secretion of pituitary thyrotropic hormone in response to decreased circulating levels of thyroid hormones. Thyroid enlargement may also result from infiltrative processes which may be inflammatory or neoplastic. Goiter in patients with thyrotoxicosis is caused by the long-acting thyroid stimulator (LATS).

CONGENITAL GOITER

Congenital goiter is usually sporadic and may result from the administration of antithyroid drugs and/or iodides during pregnancy for the treatment of thyrotoxicosis. Iodides are included in many proprietary preparations used to treat asthma; these preparations must be avoided during pregnancy, for they have ofttimes been an unexpected cause of congenital goiter. Goitrogenic drugs and iodides cross the placenta and interfere with synthesis of thyroid hormone in the fetus. Most of the infants are euthyroid but a few have evidence of hypothyroidism, which is rarely permanent. Administration of thyroid hormone generally hastens the disappearance of the goiter. Enlargement of the thyroid at birth may occasionally be sufficient to cause respiratory distress which interferes with nursing and may even cause death.

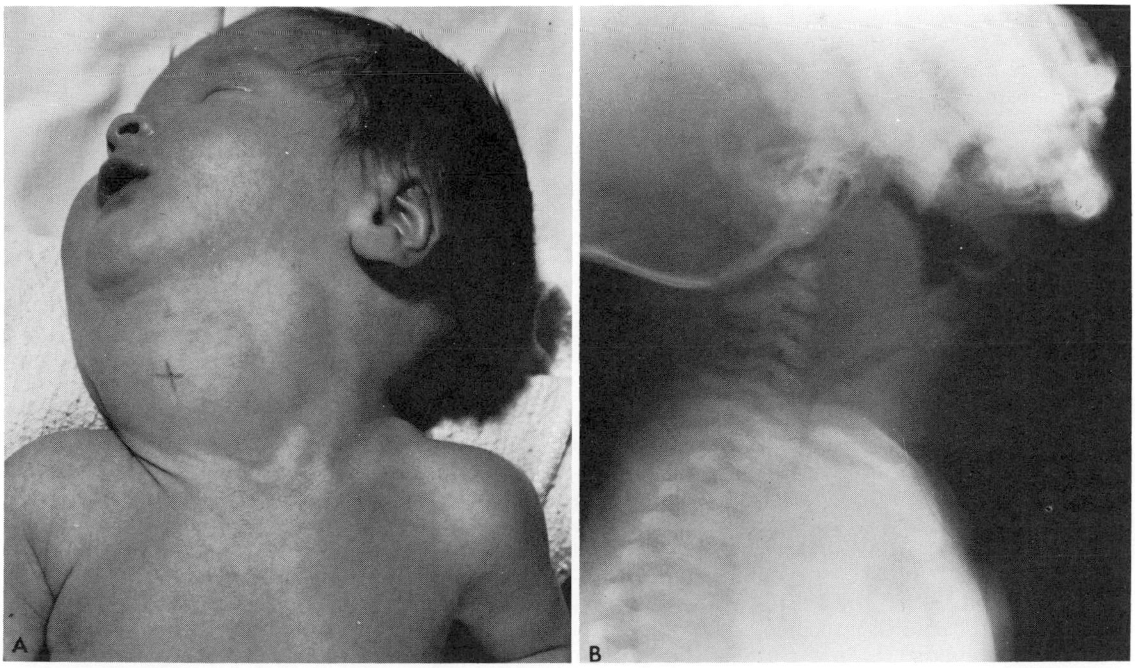

Figure 17–12 Congenital goiter in infancy. A, Large congenital goiter in an infant born to a mother with thyrotoxicosis who had been treated with iodides and methimazole during pregnancy. B, A 6 week old infant with increasing respiratory distress and cervical mass since birth. Operation revealed a large goiter which almost completely encircled the trachea. Note anterior deviation and posterior compression of the trachea. Partial thyroidectomy completely relieved the symptoms. No cause for goiter was found. It is apparent why a tracheotomy is not adequate treatment for these infants.

The head may be maintained in extreme hyperextension. When respiratory obstruction is severe, partial thyroidectomy rather than tracheotomy is indicated.

Goiter is almost always present in the congenitally hyperthyroid infant. These goiters are usually not large; the infant manifests clinical symptoms of hyperthyroidism, and the mother often has a history of Graves' disease.

When no causative factor is identifiable, a defect in synthesis of thyroid hormone must be suspected. Study of this group of infants is complex. If the infant is hypothyroid, it is advisable to treat immediately with thyroid hormone and to postpone more detailed studies for later in life. Since these defects are transmitted by recessive genes, precise diagnosis is important for sound counseling.

Iodine deficiency as a cause of congenital goiters is rapidly diminishing but persists in isolated endemic areas (see below). More important is the recent recognition that severe iodine deficiency early in pregnancy may cause neurologic damage during fetal development even in the absence of goiter.

When the "goiter" is lobulated, asymmetrical, firm or large to an unusual degree, a teratoma within or in the vicinity of the thyroid must be considered in the differential diagnosis. (See Section 25.)

ENDEMIC GOITER AND CRETINISM

The association between deficiency of iodine and the prevalence of goiter and/or cretinism has been recognized for over half a century. If there is a moderate deficiency of iodine, the demand can be satisfied by increased efficiency in synthesis of thyroid hormone. Iodine liberated in the tissues is returned rapidly to the gland, which resynthesizes the hormone at a higher rate then normal. This increased activity is achieved by compensatory hypertrophy and hyperplasia. Thus, the demand of the tissues for thyroid hormone is satisfied. In geographic areas where deficiency of iodine is severe, decompensation and hypothyroidism may result.

Sea water is rich in iodine, and the iodine content of fish and shellfish is also high. Endemic goiter is therefore rare in populations living along the sea. Iodine is deficient in the water and native foods in the Pacific West and the Great Lakes areas of the United States. Deficiency of dietary iodine is even greater in certain Alpine valleys, the Himalayas, the Andes, the Congo and the Highlands of New Guinea. In areas such as in the United States, where iodine is provided in foods from other areas and in iodized salt, endemic goiter has disappeared. Iodized salt in the United States contains 0.01 per cent of potassium iodide and provides excellent prophylaxis. In New Guinea it has been shown that a single intramuscular injection of 4 ml of iodinated poppy seed oil provides prophylactic effects lasting more than 4 years.

CLINICAL MANIFESTATIONS. If the deficiency of iodine is mild, the enlargement of the thyroid does not become noticeable except when there is an increased demand for the hormone. This is true during periods of rapid growth, as in adolescence and during pregnancy. In regions of moderate iodine deficiency, goiter may be observed in schoolchildren. It may disappear when maturity is reached and reappear during pregnancy or lactation. Iodine-deficient goiters are more common in girls than in boys. Where iodine deficiency is severe, as in the hyperendemic Highlands of New Guinea, nearly half the population have large goiters, and endemic cretinism is common.

Serum thyroxine or PBI levels are often low in endemic goiter, though clinical hypothyroidism is rare. This is true in New Guinea, the Congo, the Himalayas and South America. Despite low serum levels of thyroid hormone, serum TSH concentrations are often only moderately increased. It has been found recently that in such patients circulating levels of T_3 are elevated. Moreover, T_3 levels are also elevated in those patients with normal T_4 levels, indicating a preferential secretion of T_3 by the thyroid in this disease.

Endemic cretinism has been recognized for centuries and only in geographic association with endemic goiter. On the other hand, endemic goiter may occur in the absence of endemic cretinism. For many years there was great confusion concerning the pathogenesis of endemic cretinism. It is now recognized that the confusion was caused by including in the term "endemic cretinism" two very different but overlapping syndromes. The "nervous" syndrome is characterized by ataxia, spasticity, deaf-mutism and mental retardation. These "cretins" may be normal in stature and may have little or no impairment of thyroid function. The "myxedematous" syndrome is characterized by marked delays in growth and in sexual development, and by mental retardation and myxedema. Neurologic examination is normal. The term "endemic cretinism" continues to be used for both syndromes because the geographic distribution of both is the same and because both disappear from the population when iodine prophylaxis is introduced. The frequency of the two types varies among different populations; in New Guinea the "nervous" type occurs almost exclusively, whereas in the Northeastern Congo the "myxedematous" type predominates.

Recent evidence from New Guinea strongly suggests that in the "nervous" type a deficiency of iodine has damaged the developing nervous system quite apart from its role in the synthesis of thyroid hormone, the damage occurring in the first trimester of pregnancy even before the fetal thyroid has developed.

The etiology of the "myxedematous" type is less certain. About 25 per cent have goiters, but enlargement of the gland is minimal. Serum thyroid hormone levels are low, and TSH levels are markedly elevated. Thyroid scans are normal and preclude cryptothyroidism. There is marked delay in osseous maturation, which indicates that hypothyroidism appears around birth or during the first months of life. It is hypothesized that iodine deficiency in conjunction with an unknown toxic factor (goitrogen in food?) may alter thyroid function during fetal and neonatal life.

SPORADIC GOITER

Sporadic goiter is a descriptive term which encompasses goiters developing from a variety of etiologic factors; patients are usually euthyroid but may be hypothyroid. The most common cause of sporadic goiter is lymphocytic thyroiditis (below). Intrinsic biochemical defects in the synthesis of thyroid hormone are almost always associated with goiter (above); the occurrence of the disorder in siblings, the onset in early life, and the possible association with hypothyroidism (goitrous hypothyroidism) are important clues to diagnosis. When there are no affected siblings and the derangement is sufficiently mild so that compensatory hypertrophy of the thyroid maintains a euthyroid state, diagnosis is more difficult.

IODIDE GOITER. A small percentage of patients treated with iodide preparations for prolonged periods develop goiters. Iodides are commonly included in cough medicines and asthmatic proprietary mixtures for their expectorant effect. The goiter is firm and diffusely enlarged, and in some instances hypothyroidism may develop. In normal subjects, acute administration of large doses of iodine inhibits the organification of iodine and the synthesis of thyroid hormone (Wolff-Chaikoff effect). This effect is short-lived and does not lead to hypothyroidism. When iodide administration continues, an autoregulatory mechanism in normal persons limits iodine trapping. This permits the level of iodide in the thyroid to fall and organification to proceed normally. In patients with iodide-induced goiter this escape does not occur owing to an underlying abnormality of biosynthesis of thyroid hormone. Subjects most susceptible to the development of iodide goiter are those with lymphocytic thyroiditis or with a subclinical inborn error in thyroid hormone synthesis, and those who have been treated with radioactive iodine for thyrotoxicosis.

Lithium carbonate also causes goiters; it is currently widely used as a psychotropic drug. Lithium competes with iodide; the mechanism producing the goiter and/or hypothyroidism is similar to that described above for iodide goiter. Lithium and iodide also act synergistically to produce goiter; their combined use should be avoided.

Prolonged administration of para-aminosalicylic acid or cobalt and externally applied resorcinol have caused goiter. Discontinuation of contact with the causative agent results in regression of the goiter.

SIMPLE GOITER (COLLOID GOITER). About one third of children with euthyroid nontoxic goiters have simple goiters, a condition of unknown etiology, not associated with hypothyroidism or hyperthyroidism and not caused by inflammation or neoplasia. The condition predominates in girls and has a peak incidence before and during the pubertal years. Histologic examination of the thyroid either is normal or reveals variable follicular size, dense colloid and flattened epithelium. The goiter may be small or large. It is firm in consistency in half the patients and is occasionally asymmetrical or nodular. There is a difference between serum levels of PBI and thyroxine iodide of more than 2.0 μg in almost half the patients. Levels of TSH are normal or low; scintiscans are normal; thyroid antibodies are absent. Differentiation from lymphocytic thyroiditis may not be possible without a biopsy, but biopsy is ordinarily not indicated. Therapy with thyroid hormone may be indicated to avoid progression to a large multinodular goiter. Untreated patients should be re-evaluated periodically. This condition must be differentiated from lymphocytic thyroiditis (below).

ADENOMATOUS GOITER. Rarely a firm goiter with a lobulated surface and palpable solitary nodules is encountered. Because malignancy cannot be ruled out, surgical exploration is indicated. Areas of cystic change, hemorrhage and fibrosis may be present. Follicles vary in size; epithelium is flat or cuboidal, and there may be papillary infoldings. A fetal pattern characterized by small follicles and absent colloid may also occur. Full replacement therapy with thyroid hormone is indicated.

PENDRED SYNDROME

(Goiter and Congenital Deafness)

This syndrome of congenital deafness and goiter is transmitted in an autosomal recessive fashion and is not to be confused with the deaf-mutism seen in endemic cretinism, nor with the minor impairment of hearing which may be found in severely hypothyroid persons. The hearing loss is usually severe and present at birth, although it may not be recognized until later. It is most pronounced in the higher frequencies, is of the perceptive type and exhibits recruitment. The goiter generally appears at puberty or later but may be present in early childhood; it may be barely detectable or may be pronounced. Initially the goiter is soft and diffuse; it tends to become nodular in adult life. Most affected persons are clinically euthyroid, but hypothyroidism may ensue even during childhood. Affected persons are otherwise normal.

Administration of perchlorate causes a significant discharge of iodide from the thyroid gland, indicating a defect in organification. The biochemical defect is not known. There does not appear to be a deficiency in iodide peroxidase or iodotyrosine synthesis nor any defect in binding to apoenzyme. Lifelong substitution treatment with thyroid hormone is indicated to prevent development or progression of the goiter.

INTRATRACHEAL GOITER

One of the many ectopic locations of thyroid tissue is within the trachea. The intraluminal thyroid is beneath the tracheal mucosa and is frequently continuous with the normally situated extratracheal thyroid. The thyroid tissue is susceptible to goitrous enlargement, which involves the normally situated as well as the ectopic thyroid. When there is obstruction of the airway associated with a goiter, it must be ascertained whether the obstruction is extratracheal or endotracheal. If obstructive manifestations are mild, administration of sodium-L-thyroxine (100–300 μg/day) will usually cause the goiter to decrease in size. When symptoms are severe, surgical removal of the endotracheal goiter is indicated.

THYROIDITIS

Lymphocytic Thyroiditis
(Hashimoto's Thyroiditis; Autoimmune Thyroiditis)

Lymphocytic thyroiditis is the most common cause of thyroid disease in children and adolescents and accounts for many of the enlarged thyroids formerly designated incorrectly as "sporadic" goiter or "adolescent" goiter. It also is the most common cause of juvenile hypothyroidism, with or without goiter. Its incidence may be as high as 1 per cent in schoolchildren.

ETIOLOGY. An autoimmune mechanism is responsible for the disorder. There is a genetic predisposition to the development of thyroid autoimmunity, but the basic stimulus or immunologic defect is not known. The condition is characterized histologically by lymphocytic infiltration of the thyroid. Early in the course of the disease, there may be only hyperplasia; this is followed by infiltration of lymphocytes and plasma cells between the follicles, and by atrophy of the follicles. Lymphoid follicle formation with germinal centers is almost always present, whereas the degree of atrophy and of fibrosis of the follicles varies from mild to moderate.

CLINICAL MANIFESTATIONS. The disorder is four to seven times more frequent in girls than in boys. It may occur during the first 3 years of life but becomes sharply more common after 6 years of age and reaches a peak incidence during adolescence. The goiter may appear insidiously and vary in size from slight to marked. In the majority of children, the thyroid is diffusely enlarged, firm and nontender. In about a third of the patients, the gland is lobular and may seem to be nodular. Most affected children are clinically euthyroid and asymptomatic; in some there may be symptoms of pressure in the neck. Some children have clinical signs of hypothyroidism, while others who appear clinically euthyroid have laboratory evidence of hypothyroidism. A few children have manifestations suggestive of hyperthyroidism, such as nervousness, irritability, increased sweating or hyperactivity, but results of laboratory studies are not those of hyperthyroidism. Occasionally the disorder may coexist with Graves' disease. Ophthalmopathy may occur in lymphocytic thyroiditis in the absence of Graves' disease.

The clinical course is variable. The goiter may become smaller or disappear spontaneously, or it may persist unchanged for years while the patient remains euthyroid. A significant percentage of patients who are euthyroid initially gradually exhibit hypothyroidism over the course of months or years. It is now clear that lymphocytic thyroiditis is the cause of most instances of nongoitrous juvenile hypothyroidism.

Familial clusters of lymphocytic thyroiditis are common; the incidence in siblings and/or parents of affected children may be as high as 25 per cent. The concurrence within families of individuals with lymphocytic thyroiditis, "idiopathic" hypothyroidism and Graves' disease provides cogent evidence for a basic relationship among these three conditions. The disorder has been noted in association with many of the other autoimmune disorders more often than expected by chance alone. These include idiopathic adrenal atrophy (Schmidt syndrome), pernicious anemia and diabetes mellitus. A definite association of lymphocytic thyroiditis also occurs in patients with certain chromosomal aberrations, particularly Turner syndrome and Down syndrome. The pathogenetic mechanisms for these associations is not known.

Since thyroid antibodies cross the placenta, it has been suspected that they may cause fetal thyroid damage and congenital cretinism. Though no such relationship has been established, a remarkable family has been reported in which a mother with lymphocytic thyroiditis gave birth to 6 children with congenital hypothyroidism.

LABORATORY DATA. The definitive diagnosis can be established by open biopsy of the thyroid; needle biopsies are generally less satisfactory. These procedures are rarely indicated for clinical purposes alone. An affected parent or sibling is an important diagnostic clue. Thyroid function tests are usually normal, though the slightly elevated level of TSH in some euthyroid individuals exposes a hypothyroid state. The fact that many patients with lymphocytic thyroiditis do not have elevated levels of TSH indicates that the goiter may be caused by the lymphocytic infiltrations. Approximately half the patients have a difference of more than 2 μg/dl between the levels of PBI and of thyroxine iodine. In half the patients, thyroid scans reveal irregular and patchy distribution of the radioisotope, and in about 60 per cent or more of patients the administration of perchlorate results in a greater than 10 per cent discharge of iodide from the thyroid gland. The tanned red blood cell agglutination test for thyroid antibodies is positive in half the patients. Titers as low as 1:4 are suspicious, and titers over 1:16 are diagnostic. In general, levels in children are lower than those in adults with lymphocytic thyroiditis, and repeated measurements are indicated in questionable instances since titers may increase later in the course of the disease. When other techniques, such as immunofluorescent ones, are used to measure thyroid antibodies, these will be found in most patients with lymphocytic thyroiditis.

Antithyroid antibodies may be found also in almost half the siblings of affected patients and in a significant percentage of the mothers of children with Down syndrome or Turner syndrome without demonstrable thyroid disease. They are also found in a significant number of children with diabetes mellitus and with a variety of other autoimmune disorders.

DIFFERENTIAL DIAGNOSIS. It is not possible to distinguish lymphocytic thyroiditis from simple goiter (above) on clinical grounds alone. The signs and symptoms are usually identical. In both conditions, a difference of greater than 2 μg/dl between PBI and thyroxine iodine levels is a common finding. The finding of a positive antibody titer clearly points to lymphocytic thyroiditis, whereas a negative titer does not rule it out unless immunofluorescent techniques are used. An elevated level of TSH points to lymphocytic thyroiditis since patients with simple goiter have normal or low levels.

TREATMENT. If there is evidence of hypothyroidism, replacement treatment with sodium-L-thyroxine (100–250 μg daily) is indicated. The goiter slowly decreases in size, but antibody levels remain unchanged. It may be advisable to treat euthyroid patients also, since in the natural course of the disease some patients develop hypothyroidism and a multinodular goiter. Since the disease may be self-limited in some instances, the need for continued therapy requires re-evaluation. Untreated patients should be maintained under surveillance.

Other Causes of Thyroiditis

Specific conditions such as tuberculosis, sarcoidosis, mumps and cat scratch disease are rare causes of thyroiditis.

Acute suppurative thyroiditis is infrequent, usually being preceded by a respiratory infection or being secondary to trauma. Abscess formation may occur. Recurrent episodes and/or the detection of a mixed bacterial flora suggest that the infection arises from a thyroglossal duct remnant. Exquisite tenderness of the gland, swelling, erythema, dysphagia and limitation of head motion are characteristic findings. Systemic manifestations are often but not invariably absent. Scintigrams of the thyroid often reveal decreased uptake in the affected areas. Thyroid function is usually normal, but thyrotoxicosis owing to escape of thyroid hormone has been encountered in a child with suppurative thyroiditis due to Aspergillus. When suppuration occurs, incision and drainage and administration of antibiotics are indicated.

HYPERTHYROIDISM

Hyperthyroidism results from excessive secretion of thyroid hormone and, with few exceptions, is due to diffuse toxic goiter (Graves' disease) during childhood. Other rare causes of hyperthyroidism which have been observed in children include toxic uninodular goiter (Plummer's disease), hyperfunctioning thyroid carcinoma, thyrotoxicosis factitia and acute suppurative thyroiditis. Hyperthyroidism is a frequent concomitant of McCune-Albright syndrome; in one instance LATS was detected in serum, and in two other instances plasma TSH was suppressed, indicating that the hyperthyroidism is not hypothalamic in origin. TSH-secreting pituitary tumors, presumably increased TRF secretion, choriocarcinoma, hydatidiform mole and struma ovarii have caused hyperthyroidism in adults but have not as yet been recognized as causes in children. In the newborn period hyperthyroidism may occur as a transitory phenomenon or as classic Graves' disease.

GRAVES' DISEASE

ETIOLOGY. There is substantial evidence that immune factors participate in the pathogenesis of Graves' disease and perhaps are essential to the initiation of the disorder. Enlargement of the thymus, splenomegaly, lymphadenopathy, infiltration of the thyroid gland and of retro-orbital tissues with lymphocytes and plasma cells, and peripheral lymphocytosis are common findings in Graves' disease. About 50 per cent of patients have a circulating long-acting thyroid stimulator (LATS) which is an IgG immunoglobulin. The role of LATS in the pathogenesis of the disorder is unsettled. LATS may be a mediator of the disorder, but other antibodies have also been demonstrated in the stroma and basement membrane of the follicles of the thyroid in Graves' disease. There is poor correlation between the presence of LATS in serum and exophthalmos, and it is probably not responsible for the ophthalopathy. There is increasing evidence for distortions in cell-mediated immunity in this disorder, and there are those who believe this is the primary defect. Whether these are all secondary changes or in some way initiate the disorder remains unknown.

Other evidence for an autoimmune basis for Graves' disease is its coexistence with lymphocytic thyroiditis in the same gland. Like lymphocytic thyroiditis, Graves' disease is often associated with other autoimmune disorders such as pernicious anemia, idiopathic adrenal insufficiency, myasthenia gravis and disseminated lupus erythematosus. Antithyroglobulin and other autoantibodies are frequently found in patients with Graves' disease as well as in other members of their families.

CLINICAL MANIFESTATIONS. About 5 per cent of all patients with hyperthyroidism are less than 15 years of age and, of these, 20 per cent are less than 10 years of age; the peak incidence occurs during adolescence. The disease is being increasingly recognized in early infancy apart from the transitory condition which occurs in infants of thyrotoxic mothers (see below); Graves' disease has had its onset between 6 weeks and 2 years of age in 12 children born to mothers without a history of hyperthyroidism. The incidence is about five times higher in girls than in boys.

The clinical course is highly variable but is in general not so fulminant as in many adults. Symptoms develop gradually and the usual interval between onset and diagnosis is 6 to 12 months. The earliest signs in children may be emotional disturbances accompanied by motor hyperactivity. They become irritable and excitable and cry easily. Their schoolwork suffers, and their restlessness, which may resemble that of chorea, causes conflicts. Tremor of the fingers can be noticed if the arm is extended. There may be a voracious appetite combined with loss of or no increase in weight. The thyroid is enlarged, visible and palpable, and bruits may be audible over it. Exophthalmos is noticeable in the majority of patients, but is rarely severe. *Graefe's sign* (lagging of the upper eyelid as the eye looks downward), *Moebius' sign* (inability of convergence) and *Stellwag's sign* (retraction of the upper eyelid and infrequent blinking) may be present. The skin is smooth and flushed, and there is excessive sweating. Muscular weakness is uncommon but may be so severe as to result in falling spells. Tachycardia, palpitation, dyspnea and cardiac enlargement and insufficiency cause discomfort and may endanger the patient's life. Atrial fibrillation is a rare complication. Mitral regurgitation, probably resulting from papillary muscle dysfunction, is the cause of the apical systolic murmur present in some patients. The systolic blood pressure and the pulse pressure are increased. Children with hyperthyroidism are usually tall; their osseous development is advanced for their age, but sexual maturation is not altered.

Thyroid "crisis" or "storm" is a form of hyperthyroidism manifested by an acute onset, hyperthermia and severe tachycardia and restlessness. There may be rapid progression to delirium, coma and death. "Apathetic" or "masked" hyperthyroidism is another variety of hyperthyroidism characterized by extreme listlessness, apathy and cachexia. A combination of both forms may also occur. These symptom complexes are rare in children.

LABORATORY DATA. Levels of both thyroxine and triiodothyronine are usually increased, and thyrotropin levels are low. In some patients the level of T_4 may be normal and only the level of T_3 elevated, a situation which is termed *T_3 toxicosis*. After treatment of hyperthyroidism, the level of T_4 may be low even though the patient is clinically euthyroid. In such patients, T_3 levels may be normal. More extensive investigation is rarely necessary if the clinical manifestations are characteristic. For borderline cases, evaluation of the response to TRH may be necessary. Elevated levels of LATS may be found in only half the patients. Very young children with Graves' disease often have advanced skeletal maturation and craniostenosis.

DIFFERENTIAL DIAGNOSIS. Diagnosis is rarely difficult once it has been considered. Patients with lymphocytic thyroiditis may, on occasion, present manifestations of hyperthyroidism and must be differentiated by appropriate laboratory studies. The clinical pattern of pheochromocytoma may resemble hyperthyroidism, but the elevation of blood pressure is greater, the level of thyroid hormones is within the normal range, and that of catecholamines is elevated.

TREATMENT. There is no consensus as to the preferred method of treatment. Some prefer subtotal thyroidectomy; others, including ourselves, elect a trial of medical therapy before considering surgery. Most pediatric endocrinologists and radiotherapists avoid the use of radioactive iodine to treat children except for the exceptional patient in whom medical treatment is not feasible and operation is contraindicated or refused.

The recommended antithyroid drugs are propylthiouracil and methimazole (Tapazole). These compounds inhibit incorporation of trapped inorganic iodide into organic compounds and thus produce a progressive decrease in the synthesis of thyroid hormone. Toxic reactions occur with about equal frequency with both drugs. The initial dose of propylthiouracil is 100 to 150 mg, three times daily, and that of methimazole is 10 to 15 mg, three times daily. Subsequently the dose is increased or decreased as indicated. Smaller initial doses should be used in early childhood. Overdosage can lead to a hypothyroid state. Clinical response becomes apparent in 2 to 3 weeks, and adequate control in 1 to 3 months. The dose of the medication is then reduced to the minimal level that will maintain the child in a euthyroid state.

The drug should be continued for 2 to 3 years; then it should be discontinued slowly. Approximately 75 per cent of children will have a permanent remission after an average treatment period of 36 months; if a relapse occurs, it will usually appear within 3 months, and almost always within 6 months after therapy has been discontinued. Therapy may be resumed in case of a relapse. In pubertal children it is advisable to continue treatment throughout early adolescence.

The most common toxic reactions are urticarial skin rashes, leukopenia, fever, arthritis or arthralgia. In most instances these reactions are transitory even with continued use of the drug. More serious reactions such as agranulocytosis, hepatitis or a lupus-like syndrome are uncommon. These reactions have been noted with both propylthiouracil and methimazole, in about the same incidence, but changing from one drug to the other may avert the undesirable effect. For unusually hypersensitive patients, it is probably best to treat by thyroidectomy.

Operation is indicated when adequate cooperation for medical management is not possible or when adequate trial of medical management has failed to result in permanent remission. Subtotal thyroidectomy, a rather safe procedure, is performed only after the patient has been brought to a euthyroid state. This may be accomplished with propylthiouracil or methimazole over a 2- to 3-month period. After a euthyroid state has been attained, 5 drops of a saturated solution of potassium iodide per day are added to the regimen for 2 weeks before operation in order to decrease the vascularity of the gland. Complications of surgical treatment are rare and include hypoparathyroidism (transient or permanent) and paralysis of the vocal cords. The incidence of hyperthyroidism or hypothyroidism depends upon the extent of the surgery. With an extensive thyroidectomy, the incidence of recurrence may be low but that of hypothyroidism may exceed 50 per cent.

The ophthalmopathy remits gradually and usually independently of the hyperthyroidism.

CONGENITAL HYPERTHYROIDISM

When hyperthyroidism has its onset in the newborn period, the condition is usually transitory, remitting within a 3-month period. Infants with transient hyperthyroidism have long-acting thyroid-stimulating hormone (LATS) in their circulation and their mothers have a history of active or recently active Graves' disease. Remission of the condition is paralleled by disappearance of LATS in the infant. The condition is thought to be caused by transplacental passage of LATS or other maternal factors as yet unidentified. High levels of LATS in the mother during pregnancy are a good predictor of neonatal thyrotoxicosis. Unlike Graves' disease at every other age, the sex incidence of the transitory variety affects males as often as females. Occasionally the condition does not remit but persists for several years or longer. This group of patients appear to have typical Graves' disease and frequently have an impressive family history of Graves' disease. In some infants there appears to be a blending of LATS transfer from the mother with autonomous Graves' disease of infantile onset.

The clinical course is variable. Many of the infants are premature; the majority, but not all, have goiters. The infant is extremely restless, irritable and hyperactive and appears anxious and unusually alert. The eyes are widely opened and appear exophthalmic. There may be extreme tachycardia and tachypnea, and the temperature is elevated. In severely affected infants, there is progression of symptoms; weight loss occurs despite a ravenous appetite, hepatomegaly increases, and jaundice may become manifest. Cardiac decompensation is common. The condition resolves in 6 to 12 weeks, but the infant may die if therapy is not instituted promptly. The serum level of thyroxine is markedly elevated. Advanced bone age, frontal bossing and cranial synostosis are common, especially in those infants with persistent clinical manifestations of hyperthyroidism.

Treatment consists in administration of Lugol's solution (1 drop every 8 hours) and propylthiouracil (10 mg every 8 hours). If the thyrotoxic state is severe, parenteral fluid therapy, digitalization and propranolol (2 mg/kg/day) may be indicated.

CARCINOMA OF THE THYROID

Carcinoma of the thyroid is a rare lesion in children. The cause is unknown, but about 80 per cent of 227 patients in whom an attempt was made to obtain a history were found to have had irradiation during infancy to the neck and adjacent areas for such benign conditions as "enlarged" thymus, hypertrophied tonsils and adenoids, hemangiomas, nevi, acne, eczema and "cervical adenitis." Irradiation for thymic enlargement in infancy has been found to carry a 4 per cent risk of thyroid carcinoma and an approximately 30 per cent risk of thyroid nodularity. A recent report of follicular carcinoma in a young adult who had received radioactive iodine for diagnostic purposes at 4 and 12 years of age should remind us to be wary in the use of these isotopes in children.

Girls are affected twice as often as boys. The average age at diagnosis is 9 years, but the onset may be as early as the first year of life. A painless nodule in the thyroid is the first evidence of disease in about one fourth of the children. Cervical lymph node involvement is usually present at the time of the initial diagnosis and is often bilateral. The lungs are the most common site of metastases beyond the neck. There may not be any clinical manifestations referable to them; roentgenographically they appear as diffuse miliary or nodular infiltrations, principally in the basal portions. They may be mistaken for tuberculosis, histoplasmosis or sarcoidosis. Other sites of metastases include the mediastinum, long bones, skull and axilla. On rare occasions the carcinoma may be functional and produce symptoms of hyperthyroidism.

Histologically the carcinomas are usually papillary, follicular or mixed differentiated tumors. The neoplasm frequently grows slowly and may even remain dormant for years; undifferentiated neoplasms, however, may have a rapidly fatal course. The case fatality rate is approximately 20 per cent; death usually occurs in the first postoperative year.

The treatment of proved carcinoma of the thyroid is controversial. Some recommend thyroidectomy (hemithyroidectomy with removal of the isthmus if the disease is unilateral), dissection of any enlarged cervical nodes and postoperative roentgen therapy. Others recommend total thyroidectomy and regional dissection of lymph nodes, even though there is no evidence of involvement of them. Inoperable tumors should be removed as completely as possible along with any normal thyroid tissue, in preparation for the possible use of radioiodine. Radioiodine should be used only when the lesion cannot be completely removed surgically and when the cancerous tissue is capable of concentrating therapeutic doses. Regression of extensive pulmonary metastases has been observed to follow the use of radioiodine. Adriamycin, a new antitumor antibiotic, appears to offer some benefit for patients with progressive and refractory metastatic disease.

All patients with a differentiated carcinoma

should also be treated with thyroid hormone in doses sufficient to suppress thyrotropin on the possibility that tumor remnants which are thyrotropin-dependent may regress.

SOLITARY THYROID NODULE

Solitary nodules of the thyroid are uncommon in children. Since about 40 to 50 per cent are caused by carcinoma, however, every identified nodule must be surgically removed. The benign lesions are usually single or multiple adenomas, though lymphocytic thyroiditis and even thyroid abscess have presented as solitary nodules. Children with these lesions are generally euthyroid, and thyroid function studies are normal. Thyroid scans show irregular or decreased uptake.

On very rare occasions, thyroid nodules may be functioning and produce hyperthyroidism (Plummer's disease). The uptake of radioisotope is concentrated in the nodule ("hot" nodule), and thyroid function studies indicate that the nodule is functioning autonomously. Such nodules may secrete T_3 preferentially; hence, T_4 levels may be normal, whereas T_3 levels are elevated (T_3 toxicosis).

A suppressible functioning nodule in a euthyroid child has been reported only once.

MEDULLARY CARCINOMA

This distinctive carcinoma of the thyroid arises from the parafollicular cells (C cells) of the thyroid and accounts for about 10 per cent of all thyroid malignancies. The tumor is pleomorphic in appearance, and there are sheets of spindle or small cells with eosinophilic granular cytoplasm. Deposition of amyloid is invariably present in the stroma and calcification is common. The most common symptom is goiter or a palpable thyroid nodule. In about a third of patients radiographs of the neck reveal dense, conglomerate, homogeneous calcification in the thyroid. Metastases to regional lymph nodes and to liver are common and these too may calcify. Death may result, but long survivals are not uncommon. This tumor is usually transmitted as an autosomal dominant.

Since these tumors arise from the cells which secrete calcitonin, they are rich in this hormone and circulating levels of calcitonin are consistently elevated. Normal levels of calcitonin, either basal or after calcium infusion, usually do not exceed 1.0 ng/ml as measured by a sensitive radioimmunoassay method, whereas levels in patients with tumors are commonly 25 to 50 ng/ml. Measurement of calcitonin levels in relatives of affected individuals is a useful procedure to uncover occult tumors. In this way, tumors too small to be found by palpation or by scanning have been detected. These tumors also elaborate other specific biochemical markers, particularly histaminase and dopa decarboxylase. In addition, elevated levels of prostaglandins, serotonin and ACTH have been detected in tumors and in serum of some patients and have accounted for the diarrhea or for the Cushing syndrome which is occasionally manifested. Monitoring the levels of calcitonin and/or histaminase is useful for diagnosing metastatic lesions and for following the course of disease after operation.

Treatment consists of total thyroidectomy, since the tumor is usually present in both lobes. Diagnosis of medullary thyroid carcinoma should always lead one to search for other associated tumors, pheochromocytoma in particular.

SIPPLE SYNDROME. In some families medullary carcinoma of the thyroid is associated with pheochromocytoma and parathyroid hyperplasia. Penetrance for the various components of the syndrome is high. When pheochromocytomas are found, they are frequently bilateral and may even be multiple. The parathyroid glands may reveal only hypercellularity or may manifest chief-cell hyperplasia. Hypercalcemia may or may not be present. The hyperparathyroidism is probably the result of the same genetic defect responsible for the thyroid carcinoma and for the pheochromocytoma; it does not seem to be secondary to the elevated calcitonin level, since elevated parathormone has been found in patients with normal levels of calcitonin. A primary defect involving the neural crest can account for all the findings in the syndrome.

MUCOSAL NEUROMA SYNDROME. Some patients with medullary carcinoma have multiple mucosal neuromas or neurofibromas; these most often occur on the tongue, buccal mucosa, lips and conjunctiva. Peripheral neurofibromas and café-au-lait patches may be present, and intestinal neuromas or ganglioneuromas are frequent. In addition, these patients may be tall, exhibit arachnodactyly and present a Marfan-like appearance. Scoliosis, pectus excavatum, pes cavus and muscular hypotonia are common. The eyelids may be thickened, the lips patulous, the jaw prognathic. In the complete syndrome, pheochromocytoma and hyperparathyroidism are also present.

It is not clear whether Sipple syndrome and the mucosal neuroma syndrome are a single genetic entity. In any case, interfamilial variability seems to occur, since in some large pedigrees with Sipple syndrome there may be no individuals with mucosal neuromas.

GENERAL

AvRuskin, T. W., Braverman, L. E., and Crigler, J. F.: Thyroxine-binding globulin deficiency and associated neurological deficit. Pediatrics *50*:628, 1972.

AvRuskin, T. W., Tang, S. C., Shenken, L., Mitsuma, T., and Hollander, C. S.: Serum triiodothyronine concentrations in infancy, childhood, adolescence and pediatric disorders. J. Clin. Endocrinol. Metab. *37*:235, 1973.

Carakushansky, G., Cardenus, L. E., and Gardner, L. I.: Transplacental passage and persistence in serum for 6 9/12 years of iophenoxic acid (Teridax) in a child. Pediatrics *44*:1020, 1969.

Gharib, H.: Triiodothyronine. Physiological and clinical significance. J.A.M.A. *227*:302, 1974.

Hodgson, S. F., and Wahner, H. W.: Hereditary increased thyroxine-binding globulin capacity. Mayo Clin. Proc. *47*:720, 1972.

Lieblich, J. M., and Utiger, R. D.: Triiodothyronine in cord serum. J. Pediatr. *82*:290, 1973.

Nusynowitz, M. L., Clark, R. F., Strader, W. J., Estrin, H. M., and Seal, U. S.: Thyroxine-binding globulin deficiency in three families and total deficiency in a normal woman. Am. J. Med. *50*:458, 1971.

Treves, S., and Crigler, J. F.: Diagnostic use of Iodine-131 in children. Safety and utility compared to other tests. Pediatrics *51*:929, 1973.
Williams, R. H. (ed.): Textbook of Endocrinology. 5th ed. Philadelphia, W. B. Saunders Company, 1974.

Hypothyroidism

Andersen, H. J.: Studies of hypothyroidism in children. Acta Paediatr. *50* (Suppl. 125), 1961.
Ashkar, F. S., Miller, R., Smoak, W. M., III, and Cleveland, W. W.: A new rapid technique for the localization of abnormalities in migration of the thyroid gland. J. Pediatr. *78*:870, 1971.
Bode, H. H., Danon, M., Weintraub, B. D., Maloof, F., and Crawford, J. D.: Partial target organ resistance to thyroid hormone. J. Clin. Invest. *52*:776, 1973.
Chan, A. M., Lynch, M. J. G., Bailey, J. D., Ezrin, C., and Fraser, D.: Hypothyroidism in cystinosis. A clinical, endocrinologic and histologic study involving sixteen patients with cystinosis. Am. J. Med. *48*:678, 1970.
Cross, H. E., Hollander, C. S., Rimoin, D. L., and McKusick, V. A.: Familial agoitrous cretinism accompanied by muscular hypertrophy. Pediatrics *41*:413, 1968.
French, F. S., and Van Wyk, J. J.: Fetal hypothyroidism. J. Pediatr. *64*:589, 1964.
Green, H. G., Gareis, F. J., Shepard, T. H., and Kelley, V. C.: Cretinism associated with maternal sodium iodide I^{131} therapy during pregnancy. Am. J. Dis. Child. *122*:247, 1971.
Greig, W. R., Hendersen, A. S., Boyle, J. A., McGirr, E. M., and Hutchison, J. H.: Thyroid dysgenesis in two pairs of monozygotic twins and in a mother and child. J. Clin. Endocrinol. Metab. *26*:1309, 1966.
Hayek, A., Bauman, R. A., and Crawford, J. D.: ^{99m}Tc-pertechnetate for detection of cryptic thyroid tissue in childhood hypothyroidism. J. Pediatr. *79*:466, 1971.
Klein, A. H., Meltzer, S., and Kenny, F. M.: Improved prognosis in congenital hypothyroidism treated before age three months. J. Pediatr. *81*:913, 1972.
Little, G., Meador, C. K., Cunningham, R., and Pittman, J. A.: "Cryptothyroidism." The major cause of sporadic "athyreotic" cretinism. J. Clin. Endocrinol. Metab. *25*:1529, 1965.
Lowrey, G. H., and others: Early diagnostic criteria of congenital hypothyroidism. A comprehensive study of forty-nine cretins. A.M.A. J. Dis. Child. *96*:131, 1958.
MacGillivray, M. H., Aceto, T., Jr., and Frohman, L. A.: Plasma growth hormone responses and growth retardation in hypothyroidism. Am. J. Dis. Child. *115*:273, 1968.
Miyai, K., Azukizawa, M., and Komahara, Y.: Familial isolated thyrotropin deficiency with cretinism. New Engl. J. Med. *285*:1043, 1971.
Moncrief, M. W., and McArthur, R. G.: Hypothyroidism in one of monozygotic twins. Postgrad. Med. J. *44*:423, 1968.
Neel, J. V., Carr, E. A., Beierwaltes, W. H., and Davidson, R. T.: Genetic studies on the congenitally hypothyroid. Pediatrics *27*:269, 1961.
Neinas, F. W., Groman, C. A., Devine, K. D., and Woolner, L. B.: Lingual thyroid. Clinical characteristics of 15 cases. Ann. Intern. Med. *79*:205, 1973.
Orti, E., Castells, S., Quazi, Q. H., and Inamdar, S.: Familial thyroid disease: Lingual thyroid in two siblings and hypoplasia of a thyroid lobe in a third. J. Pediatr. *78*:675, 1971.
Retetoff, S., DeGroot, L. J., Bernard, B., and DeWind, L. T.: Studies of a sibship with apparent hereditary resistance to the intracellular action of thyroid hormone. Metabolism *21*:723, 1972.
Shopsin, B., Shenkman, L., Blum, M., and Hollander, C. S.: Iodine and lithium-induced hypothyroidism. Am. J. Med. *55*:695, 1973.
Smith, D. W., and Popich, G.: Large fontanels in congenital hypothyroidism: A potential clue toward earlier recognition. J. Pediatr. *80*:753, 1972.
Spiro, A. J., Beilin, R. L., and Finkelstein, J. W.: Cretinism with muscular hypertrophy. (Kocher-Debré-Sémélaigne syndrome). Histochemical and ultrastructural study of skeletal syndrome. Arch. Neurol. *23*:340, 1970.
Stanbury, J. B., Rocmans, P., Buhler, U. K., and Ochi, Y.: Congenital hypothyroidism with impaired thyroid responsiveness to thyrotropin. New Engl. J. Med. *279*:1132, 1968.

Goitrous Cretinism

Bax, G. M.: Typical and atypical cases of Pendred's syndrome in one family. Acta Endocrinol. *53*:264, 1966.
Burrow, G. N., Spaulding, S. W., Alexander, N. M., and Bower, B. F.: Normal peroxidase activity in Pendred's syndrome. J. Clin. Endocrinol. Metab. *36*:522, 1973.
Fraser, G. R.: Association of congenital deafness with goiter (Pendred's syndrome). A study of 207 families. Ann. Hum. Genet. *28*:201, 1965.
Gattereau, A., Bernard, B., Bellabarba, D., Verdy, M., and Brun, D.: Congenital goiter in four euthyroid siblings with glandular and circulating iodoproteins and defective iodothyronine synthesis. J. Clin. Endocrinol. Metab. *37*:118, 1973.
Illum, P., Kiaer, H. W., Hvidberg-Hansen, J., and Sondergaard, G.: Fifteen cases of Pendred's syndrome. Congenital deafness and sporadic goiter. Arch. Otolaryngol. *96*:297, 1972.
Lissitzky, S., et al.: Congenital goiter with impaired thyroglobulin synthesis. J. Clin. Endocrinol. Metab. *36*:17, 1973.
Medeiros-Neto, G. A., Bloise, W., and Ulhoa-Cintra, A. B.: Partial defect of iodide trapping mechanism in two siblings with congenital goiter and hypothyroidism. J. Clin. Endocrinol. Metab. *35*:370, 1972.
Riesco, G., Bernal, J., and Sanchez-Franco, F.: Thyroglobulin defect in a human congenital goiter. J. Clin. Endocrinol. Metab. *38*:33, 1974.
Savoie, J. C., Massin, J. P., and Savoie, F.: Studies of mono- and diiodohistidine. II. Congenital goitrous hypothyroidism with thyroglobulin defect and iodohistidine-rich iodoalbumin production. J. Clin. Invest. *52*:116, 1973.
Stanbury, J. B.: Familial goiter. *In* Stanbury, J. B., Wyngaarden, J. B., and Fredrickson, D. S. (eds.): The Metabolic Basis of Inherited Disease. 3rd ed. New York, McGraw-Hill Book Company, Inc., 1972.
Valenta, L. J., Bode, H., Vickery, A. L., Caulfield, J. B., and Maloof, F.: Lack of thyroid peroxidase activity as a cause of congenital goitrous hypothyroidism. J. Clin. Endocrinol. Metab. *36*:830, 1973.

Goiter

Chamberlain, J. L., III: Thyroid enlargement probably induced by cobalt. J. Pediatr. *59*:81, 1961.
Delange, F., Ermans, A. M., Vis, H. L., and Stanbury, J. B.: Endemic cretinism in Idjwi Island (Kivu Lake, Republic of the Congo). J. Clin. Endocrinol. Metab. *34*:1059, 1972.
Galina, M. P., Avnet, N. L., and Fanhorn, A.: Iodides during pregnancy. An apparent cause of neonatal death. New Engl. J. Med. *267*:1124, 1962.
Martin, M. M., and Renato, R. D.: Iodide goiter with hypothyroidism in two newborn infants. J. Pediatr. *61*:94, 1962.
Patel, Y. C., Pharoah, P. O. D., Hornabrook, R. W., and Hetzel, B. S.: Serum triiodothyronine, thyroxine and thyroid-stimulating hormone in endemic goiter: A comparison of goitrous and nongoitrous subjects in New Guinea. J. Clin. Endocrinol. Metab. *37*:783, 1973.
Pharoah, P. O. D., Buttfield, I. H., and Hetzel, B. S.: Neurological damage to the foetus resulting from severe iodine deficiency during pregnancy. Lancet *1*:308, 1971.
Ramalingaswami, V.: Endemic goiter in Southeast Asia. New clothes on an old body. Ann. Intern. Med. *78*:277, 1973.
Randolph, J., Grunt, J. A., and Vawter, G. F.: The medical and surgical aspects of intratracheal goiter. New Engl. J. Med. *268*:457, 1963.

Thyrotoxicosis

Darby, C. P.: Three episodes of spontaneous thyroid storm occurring in a nine-year-old child. Pediatrics *30*:927, 1962.
Hung, W., Wilkins, L., and Blizzard, R.: Medical therapy of thyrotoxicosis in children. Pediatrics *30*:17, 1962.
Kogut, M. D., Kaplan, S. A., Collipp, P. J., Tiamsic, T., and Boyle, D.: Treatment of hyperthyroidism in children. New Engl. J. Med. *272*:217, 1965.
McKendrick, T., and Newns, G. H.: Thyrotoxicosis in children: A follow-up study. Arch. Dis. Child. *40*:71, 1965.

Hyperthyroidism

Amrheim, J. A., Kenny, F. M., and Ross, D.: Granulocytopenia, lupus-like syndrome, and other complications of propylthiouracil therapy. J. Pediatr. *76*:54, 1970.
Brody, J. I., and Greenberg, S.: Lymphocyte dysfunction in thyrotoxicosis. J. Clin. Endocrinol. Metab. *35*:574, 1972.
Farid, N. R., Munro, R. E., Row, U. V., and Volpe, R.: Rosette inhibition test for the demonstration of thymus-dependent lymphocyte sensitization in Graves' disease and Hashimoto's thyroiditis. New Engl. J. Med. *289*:1111, 1973.

Hayles, A. B.: Problems of childhood Graves' disease. Mayo Clin. Proc. *47*:850, 1972.
Hayles, A. B., Chaves-Carballo, E., and McConahey, W. M.: The treatment of hyperthyroidism (Graves' disease) in children. Mayo Clin. Proc. *42*:218, 1967.
Hollingsworth, D. R., Mabry, C. C., and Eckerd, J. M.: Hereditary aspects of Graves' disease in infancy and childhood. J. Pediatr. *81*:446, 1972.
Hulazun, J. F., Anst, C. S., and Lukens, J. N.: Thyrotoxicosis associated with aspergillus thyroiditis in chronic granulomatosis disease. J. Pediatr. *80*:106, 1972.
McKenzie, J. M.: Neonatal Graves' disease. J. Clin. Endocrinol. *24*:660, 1964.
Perry, L. W., and Hung, W.: Atrial fibrillation and hyperthyroidism in a 14-year-old boy. J. Pediatr. *79*:668, 1971.
Pompa, B. H., Cloutier, M. D., and Hayles, A. B.: Thyroid nodule producing T_3 toxicosis in a child. Mayo Clin. Proc. *48*:273, 1973.
Reynolds, J. L., and Woody, H. B.: Thyrotoxic mitral regurgitation. Am. J. Dis. Child. *122*:544, 1971.
Riggs, W., Jr., Wilroy, R. S., Jr., and Etteldorf, J. N.: Neonatal hyperthyroidism with accelerated skeletal maturation, craniosynostosis, and brachydactyly. Radiology *105*:621, 1972.
Samuel, S., Gilman, S., Maurer, H. S., and Rosenthal, I. M.: Hyperthyroidism in an infant with McCune-Albright syndrome: Report of a case with myeloid dysplasia. J. Pediatr. *80*:275, 1972.
Smith, C. S., and Howard, N. J.: Propranolol in treatment of neonatal thyrotoxicosis. J. Pediatr. *83*:1046, 1973.
Solomon, D. H., and Chopra, I. J.: Graves' disease—1972. Mayo Clin. Proc. *47*:803, 1972.
Wilroy, R. S., Jr., and Etteldorf, J. N.: Familial hypothyroidism including two siblings with neonatal Graves' disease. J. Pediatr. *78*:625, 1971.

Lymphocytic Thyroiditis
Clayton, G. W., and Johnson, C. M.: Struma lymphomatosa in children. J. Pediatr. *57*:410, 1960.
Doniach, D., Nilsson, L. R., and Roitt, I. M.: Autoimmune thyroiditis in children and adolescents. Acta Paediatr. *54*:260, 1965.
Fialkow, P. J.: Autoimmunity and chromosomal aberrations. Am. J. Hum. Genet. *18*:93, 1966.
Greenberg, A. H., Czernichow, P., Hung, W., Shelley, W., Winship, T., and Blizzard, R. M.: Juvenile chronic lymphocytic thyroiditis: Clinical, laboratory and histologic correlations. J. Clin. Endocrinol. Metab. *30*:293, 1970.
Goldsmith, R. E., McAdams, A. J., Larsen, P. R., MacKenzie, M., and Hess, E. V.: Familial autoimmune thyroiditis: Maternal-fetal relationship and the role of generalized autoimmunity. J. Clin. Endocrinol. Metab. *37*:265, 1973.
Humbert, J. R., Gotlin, R. W., Hostetter, G., Sherrill, J. G., and Silver, H. K.: Lymphocytic (auto-immune, Hashimoto's) thyroiditis. Arch. Dis. Child. *43*:80, 1968.
Hung, W., Chandra, R., August, G. P., and Altman, P. R.: Clinical, laboratory, and histologic observations in euthyroid children and adolescents with goiters. J. Pediatr. *82*:10, 1973.
Leboeuf, G., and Bongiovanni, A. M.: Thyroiditis in childhood. Adv. Pediatr. *13*:183, 1964.
Ling, S. M., Kaplan, S. A., Weitzman, J. J., Reed, G. B., Custin, G., and Landing, B. H.: Euthyroid goiters in children: Correlation of needle biopsy with other clinical and laboratory findings in chronic lymphocytic thyroiditis and simple goiter. Pediatrics *44*:695, 1969.
Loeb, P. B., Drash, A. L., and Kenny, F. M.: Prevalence of low-titer and "negative" antithyroglobulin antibodies in biopsy-proved juvenile Hashimoto's thyroiditis. J. Pediatr. *82*:17, 1973.
Monteleone, J. A., Danis, R. K., Tung, K. S. K., Ramos, C. V., and Peden, V. H.: Differentiation of chronic lymphocytic thyroiditis and simple goiter in pediatrics. J. Pediatr. *83*:381, 1973.
Saxena, K. M., and Crawford, J. D.: Juvenile Lymphocytic thyroiditis. Pediatrics *30*:917, 1962.
Solomon, I. L., and Blizzard, R. M.: Autoimmune disorders of endocrine glands. J. Pediatr. *63*:1021, 1963.
Winter, J., Eberlein, W. R., and Bongiovanni, A. M.: The relationship of juvenile hypothyroidism to chronic lymphocytic thyroiditis. J. Pediatr. *69*:709, 1966.

CARCINOMA OF THE THYROID
Forsman, P. J., and Jenkins, M. E.: Medullary carcinoma of the thyroid with Marfan-like body habitus. Pediatrics *52*:188, 1973.
Gotlieb, J. A., and Hill, C. S., Jr.: Chemotherapy of thyroid cancer with Adriamycin. N. Engl. J. Med. *290*:193, 1974.
Keiser, H. R., Beaven, M. A., Doppman, J., Wells, S., Jr., and Buja, L. M.: Sipple's syndrome: Medullary thyroid carcinoma, pheochromocytoma and parathyroid disease. Ann. Intern. Med. *78*:561, 1973.
Kirkland, R. T., Kirkland, J. L., Rosenberg, H. S., Harberg, F. J., Librik, L., and Clayton, G. W.: Solitary thyroid nodules in 30 children and report of a child with a thyroid abscess. Pediatrics *51*:85, 1973.
Levin, D. L., Perlia, C., and Tashjian, A. H.: Medullary carcinoma of the thyroid gland: The complete syndrome in a child. Pediatrics *52*:192, 1973.
Pilch, B. Z., Kahn, R., Ketcham, A. S., and Henson, D.: Thyroid cancer after radioactive iodine diagnostic procedures in childhood. Pediatrics *51*:898, 1973.
Pincus, R. A., Reichlin, S., and Hempel-Mann, L. H.: Thyroid abnormalities after radiation exposure in infancy. Ann. Intern. Med. *66*:1154, 1967.
Rosenbloom, A. L.: Functioning solitary nodule of the thyroid in a child. J. Pediatr. *82*:491, 1973.
Sussman, L., Librik, L., and Clayton, G. W.: Hyperthyroidism attributable to a hyperfunctioning thyroid carcinoma. J. Pediatr. *72*:208, 1968.
Williams, E. D., Brown, C. L., and Doniach, I.: Pathological and clinical findings in a series of 67 cases of medullary carcinoma of the thyroid. J. Clin. Path. *19*:103, 1966.
Winship, T., and Rosvoll, R. V.: Childhood thyroid carcinoma. Cancer *14*:734, 1961.

DISORDERS OF THE PARATHYROID GLANDS

For many years parathyroid hormone (PTH) was considered to be the principal hormone regulating calcium homeostasis. During the past decade another hormone, calcitonin, synthesized in the thyroid gland, has been found to be involved with calcium metabolism. A role for vitamin D in calcium homeostasis has been recognized for half a century, but its function as a hormone and its relationship to PTH are just being clarified.

PARATHYROID HORMONE. The principal function of PTH is to raise the concentration of calcium in plasma. This is achieved by increasing absorption of calcium from the intestine and by increasing resorption of bone. These effects may not be direct ones but are probably achieved indirectly by regulating the synthesis of 1,25-dihydroxycholecalciferol (Fig. 17–10). PTH also has two separate renal actions: it increases urinary excretion of phosphate, and it decreases urinary excretion of calcium. Calcium ions (with magnesium ions) reg-

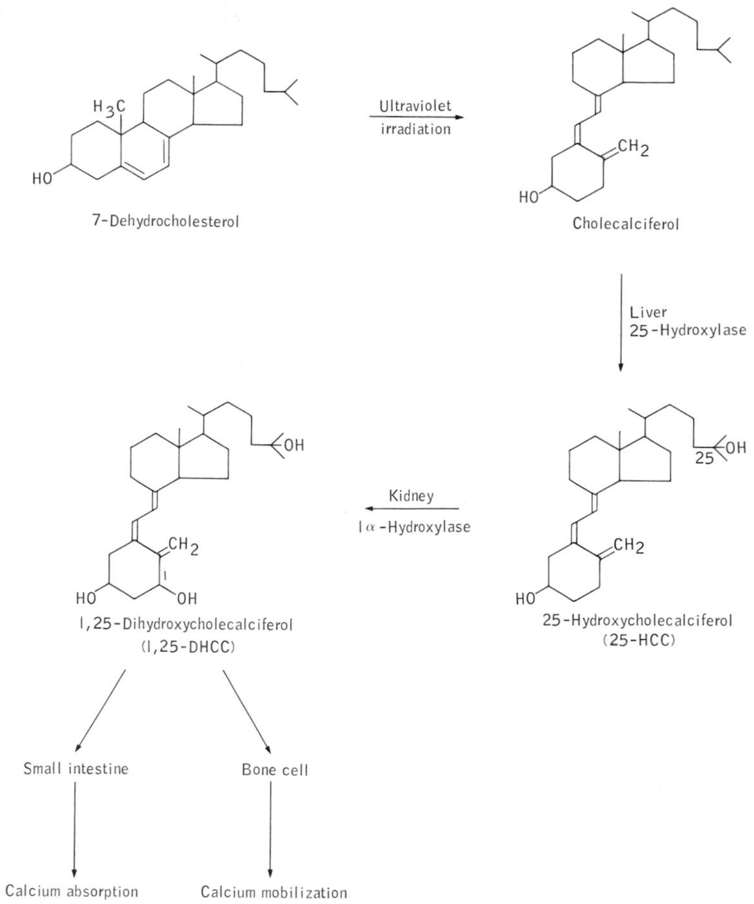

Figure 17–13 *Scheme of 1,25-DHCC synthesis. (25-HCC is now frequently designated as 25-OH-D_3, and 1,25-DHCC as 1,25-$(OH)_2$-D_3.)*

ulate both the synthesis and secretion of parathyroid hormone. The effects of PTH on bone and kidney are mediated through binding to specific receptors on the membrane of target cells and subsequent activation of the adenylate cyclase system. Cyclic AMP, in turn, binds to specific intracellular receptor proteins which mediate the hormone effect.

PTH is an 84 amino acid chain, but the biologically active property of the hormone resides in the first 34 residues. In the parathyroid gland, a proparathyroid hormone (mol. wt. $\geqslant$ 11,000) is synthesized which is converted by specific enzymatic cleavage to parathyroid hormone (mol. wt. = 9500). It is not known if the proparathyroid molecule is released from the gland into the blood. PTH (1-84) is the major circulating species of PTH; it is converted in the circulation to COOH-terminal and NH_2-terminal (C and N) fragments. The N fragment has a faster turnover rate than the C fragment and hence occupies a smaller pool. There is also evidence the gland itself contains enzymes which can cleave PTH to C and N fragments. Discrepancies in the results of radioimmunoassays from numbers of laboratories are now recognized to be due in part to the fact that differing assays for PTH have different specificities for the various immunoactive species of PTH in serum or plasma.

VITAMIN D. For many years vitamin D has been known to be essential to maintain calcium homeostasis. On the other hand, its metabolism, its mode of action at the molecular level and its relationship to parathormone have remained elusive until recently. Its native form, cholecalciferol (vitamin D_3), is formed in the skin from a precursor by the action of ultraviolet light; it is now clear that cholecalciferol is hydroxylated in the liver and other tissues to 25-hydroxycholecalciferol (25-HCC)* (Fig. 17–13). This is the major compound in the circulation with vitamin D activity (approximately 20-30 ng/dl), but it must be further hydroxylated to form the physiologically active compound 1,25-dihydroxycholecalciferol (1,25-DHCC*). Hydroxylation in the 1 position occurs exclusively in the kidneys and appears to be regulated and stimulated via parathormone rather than directly by the concentration of calcium in blood. There is also evidence suggesting that decreased levels of phosphate result in increased synthesis of 1,25-DHCC even in the absence of the parathyroids.

Circulating levels of 1,25-DHCC are about 1/250th those of 25-HCC. This potent "vitamin"

*Revised terminology may assign the following designations: 25-HCC now 25-OH-D_3; 1,25-DHCC now 1,25-$(OH)_2$-D_3.

has all the characteristics of a sterol hormone. It localizes in the nuclei of specific target cells, primarily in intestine and bone. It binds initially to a cytosol receptor, is subsequently transported to nuclear chromatin and induces synthesis of specific mRNA which could code for specific functional proteins. It is believed that the calcium-binding protein in the mucosal cells of the intestine is regulated in this fashion by 1,25-DHCC. This new information is providing new insights into clinical disorders involving calcium, parathyroids and rachitic conditions, though the full story of vitamin D is yet to be unfolded. Synthetic 1α-hydroxycholecalciferol is being used clinically and is equipotent with 1,25-DHCC, to which it is presumably converted in the body.

CALCITONIN. Calcitonin was discovered in 1961; it lowers the levels of both calcium and phosphate in plasma. In birds, amphibians and teleost fishes, calcitonin is synthesized in a discrete structure known as the ultimobranchial body, derived from cells which arise in the neural crest and migrate to become incorporated with the last pharyngeal pouch. In mammals these cells move caudally and become incorporated into the thyroid gland as the parafollicular cells. The hormone is a polypeptide consisting of 32 amino acids and can be measured in plasma by a sensitive and specific radioimmunoassay.

The physiologic role of calcitonin remains uncertain. Medullary carcinoma of the thyroid, which is clearly established as arising from the parafollicular cells, results in marked hypersecretion of calcitonin. In spite of the markedly increased levels of calcitonin, plasma calcium levels are usually normal and there are no overt skeletal abnormalities. With recent improvements in the radioassay for calcitonin, there is increasing evidence that the hormone is of physiologic importance in man. Plasma levels rise with intravenous infusions of calcium and fall after EDTA infusions. Oral administration of calcium produces a much smaller response. The mean basal level of calcitonin is approximately 200 pg/dl.

HYPOPARATHYROIDISM

ETIOLOGY. The normal level of PTH in cord blood is low (approximately 100 pg/dl), and it doubles by the sixth day to reach a level nearly that of normal infants and children. Hypocalcemia is common between 12 and 72 hours of life, especially in premature infants, in infants with asphyxia at birth, and in infants of diabetic mothers *(early neonatal hypocalcemia)*. (See also Section 7.) After the second to third day and during the first week of life, the type of feeding is also a determinant of the level of serum calcium *(late neonatal hypocalcemia)*. The role played by the parathyroids in these hypocalcemic infants remains to be clarified, though functional immaturity of the parathyroids has often been invoked as pathogenetic. In a group of infants with *transient idiopathic hypocalcemia* (1 to 8 weeks of age) serum levels of parathormone were significantly lower than in normal infants. It is possible that the functional immaturity is a manifestation of a delay in development of the en-

TABLE 17–3 ETIOLOGIC CLASSIFICATION OF HYPOCALCEMIA

A. Parathormone (PTH) Deficiency
   1. Congenital aplasia or hypoplasia of parathyroids
      a. With thymic and other III-IV arch defects
      b. With chromosomal abnormalities
      c. Isolated defect
   2. Transient hypofunction
      a. Early neonatal hypocalcemia
      b. Late neonatal hypocalcemia
      c. Maternal functioning adenoma
      d. Other
   3. Familial sex-linked hypoparathyroidism
   4. Idiopathic hypoparathyroidism
      a. Autoimmune hypoparathyroiditis
         1. Isolated
         2. Associated with other autoimmune disorders and/or mucocutaneous candidiasis
      b. Congenital hypoplasia
   5. Surgical removal or damage to parathyroids
   6. Ineffective parathyroid hormone (pseudoidiopathic hypoparathyroidism)
   7. Parathyroid hormone unresponsiveness
      a. Defect in generation of cyclic AMP (Type 1 pseudohypoparathyroidism)
      b. Defect in reception of cyclic AMP signal (Type 2 pseudohypoparathyroidism)

B. Calcitonin Excess?
   1. Medullary carcinoma of thyroid

C. Vitamin D Deficiency
   1. Inadequate irradiation
      Clothing, housing, smog, climate
   2. Dietary deficiency
   3. Malabsorption
      a. Deficiency of bile salts (liver disease)
      b. Deficiency of calcium-binding protein (gluten-sensitive enteropathy)
      c. Intestinal bypass operations
   4. Depletion
      (bile fistulas)
   5. Increased inactivation
      (chronic therapy with diphenylhydantoin and/or phenobarbital)
   6. Impaired synthesis of 25-DHCC
      (severe hepatic disease)
   7. Impaired synthesis of 1,25-DHCC
      a. Renal failure
      b. Renal tubular disease?
      c. Genetic deficiency of 1-hydroxylase (vitamin D-dependent rickets)

D. Magnesium Deficiency
   1. Sex-linked congenital malabsorption
   2. Other malabsorption syndromes

E. Inorganic Phosphate Excess
   1. Poisoning
   2. Initial therapy of leukemia

zymes which convert glandular PTH to secreted PTH; other mechanisms are possible.

Transient hypocalcemia also occurs in infants born to *mothers with hyperparathyroidism.* It appears that the hypocalcemia in such infants results from suppression of the fetal parathyroids by exposure to elevated levels of calcium in maternal serum. Rarely hypocalcemia may persist for weeks or months, but normal functional activity is eventually established. Mothers of infants with presumed transient hypoparathyroidism of unknown etiology should routinely have measurements of calcium, phosphorus and parathormone.

Congenital permanent hypoparathyroidism usually results from *aplasia* or *hypoplasia of the parathyroid glands.* Frequently there are other developmental defects, particularly of structures arising from pharyngeal pouches III and IV; aplasia or hypoplasia of the thymus (see Section 9), right-sided aortic arch with or without other cardiovascular abnormalities, and absence of the isthmus of the thyroid are among the more commonly associated defects. Micrognathia and abnormalities of the ears are occasional external clues. The disorder is usually sporadic and the cause is unknown, though in one family it appears to have resulted from a dominant gene. Radiographs of the chest for visualization of the thymus should be routinely obtained in the study of infants with tetany. Primary hypoparathyroidism without abnormality of the thymus has been reported in an infant with ring chromosome 18 and in another with a ring chromosome 16.

Familial congenital hypoparathyroidism also occurs; since all affected infants have been males, it appears to be transmitted by a sex-linked recessive gene. The nature of the defect is not known; it does not appear to be associated with other congenital defects.

Removal or damage of the parathyroid glands may occur as a complication of thyroidectomy *(surgical hypoparathyroidism).* Hypoparathyroidism has developed even when the parathyroid glands have been identified and left undisturbed at the time of operation. This, presumably, is the result of interference with the blood supply or of postoperative edema and fibrosis. Symptoms of tetany may occur abruptly postoperatively and be permanent or temporary. In some instances symptoms develop insidiously and go undetected until months after thyroidectomy. Occasionally the first evidence of surgical hypoparathyroidism may be the development of cataracts. All patients subjected to thyroidectomy should be carefully studied to determine the status of parathyroid function.

Idiopathic hypoparathyroidism may be acquired at any age. In many of the reported patients who were adults when the diagnosis was established clinical manifestations had begun in childhood. The cause is unknown, but an autoimmune mechanism is suggested by the demonstration that over a third of such patients have parathyroid antibodies. This assumption is further supported by the frequent association of hypoparathyroidism with other disorders believed to have a similar origin, such as Addison's disease, lymphocytic thyroiditis and pernicious anemia. Alopecia areata, ovarian failure and steatorrhea may also occur concurrently with idiopathic hypoparathyroidism. None

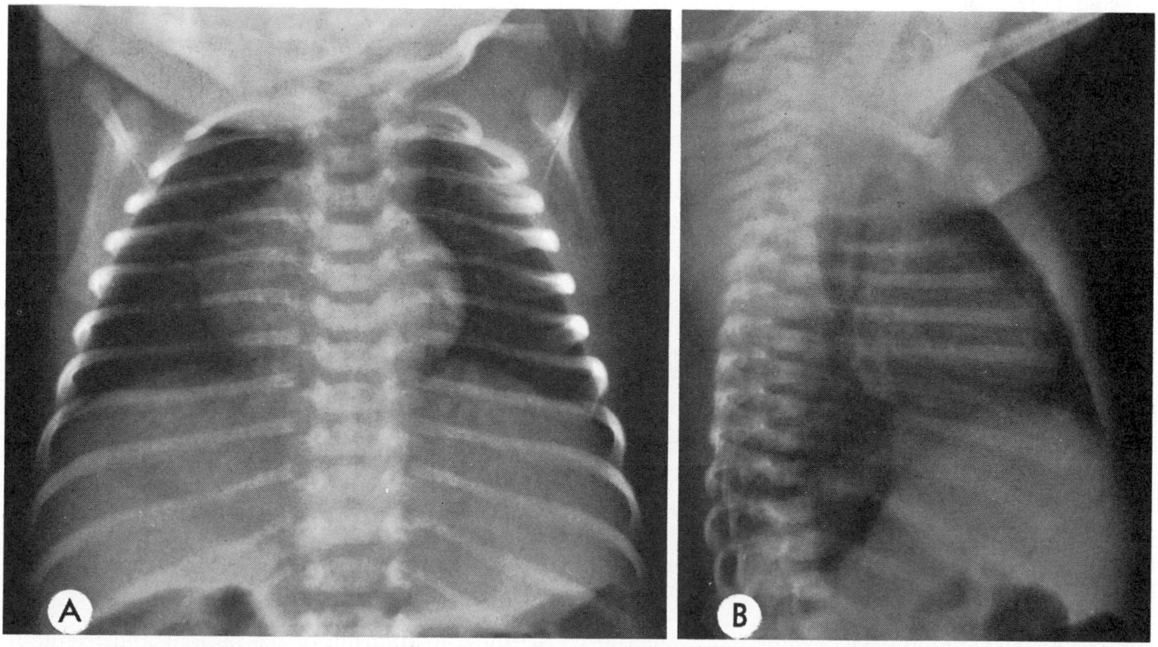

Figure 17–14 *Congenital absence of parathyroid glands; roentgenograms of chest exposed at 6 days of age reveal no evidence of thymus.* A, *The mediastinum is narrow;* B, *the substernal area is radiolucent. (From Kirkpatrick and DiGeorge:* Am. J. Roentgenol., 103*:32, 1968.)*

of these are secondary to the hypocalcemia; all are probably autoimmune in origin. The steatorrhea may lead to magnesium deficiency and complicate the management of the hypocalcemia. Addison's disease and hypoparathyroidism may occur in the same patient or may alternate in members of the same family. Mucocutaneous moniliasis occurs frequently in patients with idiopathic hypoparathyroidism or Addison's disease; there is abundant evidence that it is not the cause of the endocrinopathy. An inherited abnormality of the immunologic mechanism probably accounts for all these findings. At autopsy no parathyroid tissue is demonstrable.

Some patients with idiopathic hypoparathyroidism with onset of symptoms past infancy may manifest some of the congenital defects which originate in pharyngeal pouches III and IV. This suggests that these patients may have had *hypoplasia* or *dysgenesis of the parathyroids* with eventual failure of parathyroid function during childhood or later in life. Such patients would not be expected to have circulating antiparathyroid antibodies nor to have other associated autoimmune disorders.

Pseudoidiopathic hypoparathyroidism is the term used to describe a recently recognized cause of hypoparathyroidism. A young adult has been reported who had the onset of tetany at 8 years of age and all the laboratory findings of idiopathic hypoparathyroidism. He exhibited a normal response to administration of PTH. His serum was found to contain normal to high levels of immunoreactive parathyroid hormone by several assay systems. It appears that this patient's endogenous parathyroid hormone lacks biologic effect, possibly owing to a defect in the conversion of proparathyroid hormone to parathyroid hormone in the gland or to a defect in the peripheral conversion of a secreted, precursor form of PTH to an active form.

CLINICAL MANIFESTATIONS. There is a spectrum of parathyroid deficiencies with clinical manifestations varying from no symptoms to those of complete and longstanding deficiency. Mild deficiency may be revealed only by appropriate laboratory studies. Muscular pain and cramps are early manifestations, which progress to numbness, stiffness and tingling of the hands and feet. There may be only positive Chvostek and/or Trousseau signs, or there may be laryngeal and carpopedal spasms. Convulsions with loss of consciousness may occur at intervals of days, weeks or months. These may begin with abdominal pain, followed by tonic rigidity, retraction of the head and cyanosis. Hypoparathyroidism is frequently mistaken for epilepsy. Headache, vomiting, increased intracranial pressure and papilledema may be associated with convulsions and may suggest a brain tumor.

The teeth erupt late and irregularly. Enamel formation is irregular, and the teeth may be unusually soft. The skin may be dry and scaly, and the nails of the fingers and toes may have horizontal lines. Manifestations of a wide variety of other disorders which are not a direct consequence of parathyroid hormone deficiency may also be seen. Mucocutaneous candidiasis often antedates the development of hypoparathyroidism; the monilia infection most often involves the nails, the oral mucosa, the angles of the mouth and less often the skin. Patients with hypoparathyroidism may also have abnormal loss of hair, manifested as thinning or patchy loss or as complete alopecia.

Cataracts in patients with longstanding untreated disease are a direct consequence of hypoparathyroidism; other ocular disorders such as keratoconjunctivitis may also be associated. Manifestations of Addison's disease, lymphocytic thyroiditis, pernicious anemia, hepatitis and primary gonadal insufficiency may also occur in association with those of hypoparathyroidism.

Permanent physical and mental deterioration occurs if initiation of treatment is delayed for a long time.

LABORATORY DATA. The serum calcium level is low (5 to 7 mg/dl) and the phosphorus elevated (7 to 12 mg/dl). The serum phosphatase level is normal or low. The level of magnesium is normal but should always be checked in hypocalcemic patients (see below). Parathyroid hormone in serum is low, even in the presence of hypocalcemia. Roentgenograms of the bones reveal rarely an increased density limited to the metaphyses, suggestive of heavy metal poisoning, or an increased density of the lamina dura. Roentgenograms of the skull may reveal calcifications in the basal ganglia. There is a prolongation of the Q-T interval on the electrocardiogram, which disappears when the hypocalcemia is corrected. Electroencephalographic tracings usually reveal widespread slow activity; the tracings return to normal after the serum calcium has been within the normal range for a few weeks unless irreversible brain damage has occurred or unless the parathyroid insufficiency is associated with epilepsy. When hypoparathyroidism occurs concurrently with Addison's disease, the serum level of calcium may be normal, but hypocalcemia appears after effective treatment of the adrenal insufficiency.

TREATMENT. Emergency treatment for tetany consists in intravenous injections of 5 to 10 ml of a 10 per cent solution of calcium gluconate at the rate of 0.5 to 1 ml/minute. Initially either vitamin D or dihydrotachysterol should also be administered. Since dihydrotachysterol acts more rapidly, it is preferable in the early stages of treatment and may be given in doses of 1 to 4 ml daily. Foods with a high phosphorus content, such as milk, eggs and cheese, should be reduced in the diet.

Maintenance therapy consists in oral administration of vitamin D in daily doses of 50,000 to 150,000 IU. During the period of stabilization some patients require supplemental calcium, which can be given orally in the form of calcium gluconate or calcium lactate (3 to 9 gm/day).

Clinical evaluation of the patient and frequent determinations of the serum calcium level are indicated in the early stages of treatment in order to determine the dosage requirements of vitamin D and of calcium. Maintenance treatment must be continued indefinitely. If vitamin D therapy is discontinued, the serum calcium level may remain normal for months; hence, a permanent remission cannot be assumed until there has been an adequate period of observation. If hypercalcemia occurs, vitamin D should be discontinued and resumed at a lower dose after the serum calcium level has returned to normal. In cases of long standing, repair of cerebral and dental changes is not likely. Pigmentation, lowering of the blood pressure or weight loss may indicate adrenal insufficiency, which requires specific treatment.

DIFFERENTIAL DIAGNOSIS. *Magnesium deficiency* must be considered in patients with unexplained hypocalcemia. A small number of infants have been reported who developed tetany and seizures during the early weeks of life and who exhibited both hypocalcemia and hypomagnesemia. Administration of calcium proved ineffective, but administration of magnesium promptly corrected both the calcium and magnesium levels. Oral supplements of magnesium are necessary to maintain levels of magnesium in the normal range. The cause for the low levels of magnesium is believed to be an inborn defect leading to impaired intestinal absorption. Since the disease seems to affect only boys, a recessive sex-linked gene appears responsible. (See also Section 7.)

Hypomagnesemia also occurs in malabsorption syndromes and has been noted in granulomatous colitis. Patients with idiopathic hypoparathyroidism may have concurrent steatorrhea and low magnesium levels.

It is not clear how the low levels of magnesium lead to hypocalcemia. There is no evidence for decreased absorption or for excessive renal loss of calcium. Synthesis of 1,25-dihydroxycholecalciferol and localization in the intestine occur normally in the magnesium-depleted chick. On the other hand, both low and elevated levels of PTH have been reported in patients with primary magnesium deficiency. The skeleton appears to be unresponsive to PTH during magnesium depletion. The most recent experimental evidence in chicks suggests that the magnesium depletion may directly affect bone metabolism, resulting in a reduction in release of calcium from the mineral phase of bone and leading to hypocalcemia.

Poisoning with inorganic phosphate leads to hypocalcemia and tetany. Infants poisoned with large doses of inorganic phosphates, either in the form of laxatives or enemas, have developed sudden onset of tetany, with serum calcium levels below 5 mg/dl and markedly elevated levels of phosphate. Symptoms are quickly relieved by intravenous administration of calcium. The mechanism of the hypocalcemia is not clear.

Hypocalcemia may occur early in the course of treatment of *acute lymphoblastic leukemia.* It is usually associated with hyperphosphatemia (resulting from destruction of lymphoblasts), which is probably the primary cause of hypocalcemia.

PSEUDOHYPOPARATHYROIDISM

(Albright's Hereditary Osteodystrophy)

In this syndrome, in contrast to the situation in idiopathic hypoparathyroidism, the parathyroid glands are normal or hyperplastic histologically, and they can synthesize and secrete parathyroid hormone. Serum levels of parathyroid hormone are increased when the patient is hypocalcemic. The primary defect is a failure of the end-organs, particularly of the kidney and skeleton, to respond to parathormone. Administration of parathormone fails to raise the serum level of calcium or to lower the serum level of phosphorus.

In the majority of patients, there is an inability of parathyroid hormone to evoke an increase in intracellular cyclic AMP (*pseudohypoparathyroidism, Type I*), and urinary cyclic AMP excretion after hormone administration is markedly deficient. Very recently a condition (*pseudohypoparathyroidism, Type II*) has been recognized in which parathormone normally activates intracellular cyclic AMP, the urinary excretion of which is elevated both in the basal state and after stimulation. It has been suggested that the defect here lies in an inability of the target cells to respond to the intracellular cyclic AMP signal.

In addition to clinical and chemical findings similar to those of idiopathic hypoparathyroidism, patients have a short, stocky build and a round face. Growth failure may be striking. There is brachydactylia; the first, fourth and fifth metacarpals are most often involved, and the first and fifth metatarsals are also often affected. As a result, the index finger may be longer than the middle finger. There may be other skeletal abnormalities, such as short and wide phalanges, bowing, exostoses, thickening of the calvaria and general demineralization of the bones. These patients frequently have calcium deposits and metaplastic bone formation subcutaneously. Mental retardation is common, as are calcifications of the basal ganglia and lenticular cataracts.

In some patients with pseudohypoparathyroidism, the resistance to PTH appears to be limited to the kidneys, the bones being normally responsive to the elevated levels of circulating hormone. As a result, in addition to the skeletal changes described above, these patients exhibit subperiosteal resorption, osteitis fibrosa and, in children, widening and irregularity of the epiphyseal plates. The condition has been termed *pseudohypohyperparathyroidism* by some, but *pseudohypoparathyroidism with osteitis fibrosa* appears to be a less confusing designation.

There also are patients who have the usual anatomic stigmata of pseudohypoparathyroidism but in whom the serum calcium and phosphorus levels are normal. The term *pseudopseudohypoparathyroidism* has been used to describe these patients. However, transition from the normocalcemic to the hypocalcemic form has been observed, and there are pedigrees with normocalcemic and hypocalcemic forms in different members. The disorder has been regarded as X-linked dominant, but females appear to be more severely affected than males; a family exhibiting both the normocalcemic and hypocalcemic forms of the syndrome as well as male-to-male transmission has been reported. Further clarification of the genetics is required and heterogeneity in the mode of inheritance is possible.

Hypothyroidism has been frequently noted in association with pseudohypoparathyroidism, and in 6 of those reported there was selective deficiency of TSH.

Diagnosis rests on the demonstration of failure of occurrence of the normal increase in urinary cyclic AMP after intravenous infusion of 200 U of parathyroid extract (8 U/kg in infants). This test can also be used to reveal latent pseudohypoparathyroidism in persons at genetic risk who have no other signs of the condition. Failure of the level of serum calcium to rise after 3 days' administration of intramuscular parathyroid hormone (200 U/day) is also indicative of resistance to the hormone.

HYPERPARATHYROIDISM

Excessive production of parathyroid hormone may result from a primary defect of the parathyroid glands such as an adenoma or idiopathic hyperplasia *(primary hyperparathyroidism).*

More often the increased production of parathyroid hormone is a compensatory phenomenon, usually aimed at correcting hypocalcemic states of diverse origins (*secondary hyperparathyroidism*). In vitamin D-deficient rickets and in the malabsorption syndromes intestinal absorption of calcium is deficient, but hypocalcemia and tetany are averted by increased activity of the parathyroid glands. In chronic renal disease, hyperphosphatemia and the consequent hypocalcemia result in compensatory hyperparathyroidism with increases in serum levels of parathyroid hormone. In rare instances, if stimulation of the parathyroids is sufficiently intense and protracted, the glands become autonomous in their secretion of parathyroid hormone. This situation is known as *tertiary hyperparathyroidism.*

PRIMARY HYPERPARATHYROIDISM

Primary hyperparathyroidism is uncommon in children and is usually due to a single *adenoma.* Symptoms generally begin after 10 years of age.

There have been about 20 kindreds with 3 or more members with hyperparathyroidism. In such instances of *familial hyperparathyroidism* most affected members are adults, but children have been involved in about a third of the pedigrees. Some affected patients in these families are asymptomatic and are revealed only by careful study. In some kindreds there is a high frequency of peptic ulcer with islet cell tumors. In other pedigrees there is an association with medullary carcinoma of the thyroid and pheochromocytoma (see above, this Section). In familial hyperparathyroidism, the adenomas are apt to be multiple and, in some patients, the parathyroid may reveal only hyperplasia. The gene follows an autosomal dominant mode of transmission with a high degree of penetrance.

Another form of familial hyperparathyroidism consists of *primary hyperplasia of the parathyroids in infancy.* The condition has its onset in the early weeks of life and may have a rapidly fatal course if diagnosis is delayed. Of the 11 reported cases, there were affected siblings in two families and there was parental consanguinity in two other families, suggesting an autosomal recessive mode of inheritance.

Production of *ectopic PTH* has been demonstrated in a variety of nonendocrine tumors in adults, including those arising in lung, kidney, cervix, ovary, parotid gland and reticulum cell sarcoma. Hypercalcemia and hypophosphatemia are usually the diagnostic clue to the condition. Hypercalcemia without hypophosphatemia frequently occurs in other malignancies, especially carcinoma of the breast, in the absence of elevated PTH levels. The cause for the hypercalcemia in these patients is not known.

A few infants born to mothers with hypoparathyroidism inadequately treated during pregnancy were presumed to have *fetal hyperparathyroidism.* The manifestations involved the bones primarily and were transitory.

CLINICAL MANIFESTATIONS. At all ages the clinical manifestations of hypercalcemia of any cause include muscular weakness, anorexia, nausea, vomiting, constipation, polydipsia, polyuria, loss of weight and fever. Calcium may be deposited in the renal parenchyma, resulting in nephrocalcinosis and progressively diminished renal function. Renal calculi, noted in 12 of 46 children with adenoma, may be manifested by renal colic and hematuria. Osseous changes may be responsible for pain in the back or extremities, disturbance of gait, deformities, fractures and tumors. There may be decrease in height from compression of vertebrae and the patient may become bedridden.

Abdominal pain is occasionally a predominant manifestation and may be associated with acute pancreatitis. There have been four instances of parathyroid crisis in children, manifested by serum calcium greater than 15 mg/dl and progressive oliguria, azotemia, stupor and coma. In infants, failure to thrive, poor feeding and hypotonia are common. Mental retardation, convulsions and blindness may occur as sequelae.

LABORATORY DATA. The serum calcium is elevated; 39 of 45 children with adenomas had levels over 12 mg/dl. The hypercalcemia is more severe in infants with parathyroid hyperplasia; concentrations between 15 and 20 mg/dl are common and values as high as 30 mg/dl have been reported. Ionic (ultrafiltrable) calcium levels are often elevated even when serum calcium is borderline or only slightly elevated. The serum phosphorus level is reduced to about 3 mg/dl or less, and the level of serum magnesium is low. The urine may have a low fixed specific gravity and serum levels of nonprotein nitrogen and uric acid may be elevated. In patients with adenomas who have skeletal involvement serum phosphatase is elevated, whereas in infants with hyperplasia the levels of alkaline phosphatase may be normal even when there is extensive involvement of bone.

Radioimmunoassay for parathyroid hormone is technically difficult; problems of interpretation arise because results may vary markedly from one laboratory to another, depending on the antibody used. Assays of samples of thyroid venous blood for PTH are more reliable because intact hormone is assayed before fragmentation occurs in the periphery. Calcitonin levels are normal. Acute hypercalcemia can stimulate calcitonin release, but with prolonged hypercalcemia, hypercalcitoninemia does not occur.

The most consistent and characteristic roentgenographic findings are resorption of subperiosteal bone, best seen along the margins of the phalanges of the hands. In the skull there may be gross trabeculation or a granular appearance resulting from focal rarefaction; absence of the lamina dura may be noted. In more advanced disease, there may be generalized rarefaction, cysts, tumors, fractures and deformities. Radiographs of the abdomen may reveal renal calculi or nephrocalcinosis. In infants with parathyroid hyperplasia, cupping and fraying at the ends of the long bones and ribs may suggest rickets, and severe demineralization and pathologic fractures are common.

DIFFERENTIAL DIAGNOSIS. *Hypercalcemia* of any origin results in a similar clinical pattern and must be differentiated from hyperparathyroidism. A low serum phosphorus level in association with hypercalcemia is usually diagnostic of primary hyperparathyroidism. Pharmacologic doses of corticosteroids lower the serum calcium level to normal in patients with hypercalcemia from other causes, but generally do not affect the calcium level in patients with hyperparathyroidism. This may be a useful test in differential diagnosis. *Vitamin D intoxication* can be excluded by history, by a normal level of serum phosphorus and by roentgenographic evidence of increased bone density. *Idiopathic hypercalcemia* of infancy may be easily confused with hyperparathyroidism; however, the serum phosphorus level is normal or slightly elevated and, roentgenographically, the increased bone density of idiopathic hypercalcemia contrasts strikingly with the rarefaction of primary hyperparathyroidism. *Hypophosphatasia,* especially when severe, is frequently associated with mild to moderate hypercalcemia. The serum phosphorus level is normal, and that of alkaline phosphatase is depressed. Roentgenograms of the bones may reveal complete disappearance of the zone of provisional calcification and lack of calcification of the metaphyseal bone.

Prolonged immobilization may lead to hypercalcemia and occasionally to decreased renal function, hypertension and encephalopathy. Hypercalcemia is being increasingly recognized in children with *leukemia*; the mechanism is unknown; in one instance it appeared that the leukemic cells produced a PTH-like substance. The hypercalcemia of *sarcoidosis* results from abnormal sensitivity to vitamin D, which leads to increased absorption of calcium. In rare instances, parathyroid adenoma or hyperplasia has been reported to coexist with sarcoidosis. Elevated serum calcium levels have also been observed in patients with *hypervitaminosis A,* in *thyrotoxicosis,* in *subcutaneous fat necrosis* and in malignant disease with *osseous metastases.* Administration of *thiazide diuretics* to hypoparathyroid patients treated with vitamin D can lead to hypercalcemia.

Familial benign hypercalcemia has recently been recognized in four generations of a family. It is characterized by mild hypercalcemia (11.9 mg/dl mean serum calcium level in children), normal or low serum phosphate, low urinary calcium excretion and normal levels of parathyroid hormone by immunoassay. Ionized calcium is elevated in proportion to the serum calcium. The disorder has an autosomal dominant mode of inheritance. Its cause is not known but it has been proposed that there may be an abnormality of the receptor mechanism for secretion of parathormone in regulation of calcium ions.

Hypercalcemia in patients with *familial pheochromocytoma* is usually due to hyperparathyroidism. A 12 year old boy has been reported, however, whose calcium level returned to normal after removal of the pheochromocytoma, suggesting that the tumor itself may have produced a calcium-affecting factor.

TREATMENT. Surgical exploration is indicated in all instances. All glands should be carefully inspected; if an adenoma is discovered, it should be removed. If there is only generalized hyperplasia, subtotal parathyroidectomy should be performed. The patient should be carefully observed postoperatively for the development of hypocalcemia and tetany; intravenous administration of calcium gluconate may be required for a few days. The serum calcium level then gradually returns to normal, and, under ordinary circumstances, a diet high in calcium and phosphorus needs to be maintained for only several months after operation.

Arteriography and selective venous sampling with radioimmunoassay of parathyroid hormone have been successfully applied for preoperative localization and for differentiation of a single adenoma from hyperplasia in adults. These procedures are particularly advisable before re-exploration in cases of persistent or recurrent hyperparathyroidism.

PROGNOSIS. The prognosis is good if the disease is recognized early and there is appropriate surgical treatment. When extensive osseous lesions are present, permanent deformities may persist; when renal disease has occurred, the prognosis is less hopeful. A search for other affected family members is indicated.

Arnaud, C. D.: Parathyroid hormone: Coming of age in clinical medicine. Am. J. Med. *55*:577, 1973.

Aurbach, G. H., Mallette, L. E., Patten, B. M., Heath, D. A., Doppmann, J. L., and Bilezikian, J. P.: Hyperparathyroidism: Recent studies. Ann. Intern. Med. *79*:566, 1973.

Bergman, L., and Hagberg, S.: Primary hyperparathyroidism in a child investigated by determination of ultrafiltrable calcium. Am. J. Dis. Child. *123*:174, 1972.

Berliner, B. C., Shenker, I. R., and Weinstock, M. S.: Hypercalcemia associated with hypertension due to prolonged immobilization. (An unusual complication of extensive burns). Pediatrics *49*:92, 1972.

Blizzard, R. M., Chee, D., and Davis, W.: The incidence of parathyroid and other antibodies in the sera of patients with idiopathic hypoparathyroidism. Clin. Exp. Immunol. *1*:119, 1966.

Bohnen, R. F., Jubiz, W., Rallison, M., Stevens, L. E., and Tyler, F. H.: Sarcoidosis and autonomous parathyroid hyperplasia. J.A.M.A. *217*:1385, 1971.

Bronsky, D., Kushner, D. S. Dubin, A., and Snapper, I.: Idiopathic hypoparathyroidism and pseudohypoparathyroidism: Case reports and review of the literature. Medicine. *37*:317, 1959.

Bronsky, D., Kiamko, R. T., Moncada, R., and Rosenthal, I. M.: Intrauterine hyperparathyroidism secondary to maternal hypoparathyroidism. Pediatrics. *42*:606, 1968.

Daum, F., Rosen, J. F., and Boley, S. J.: parathyroid adenoma, parathyroid crisis, and acute pancreatitis in an adolescent. J. Pediatr. *83*:275, 1973.

Deftos, L. J., Powell, D., Parthemore, J. G., and Potts, J. T., Jr.: Secretion of calcitonin in hypocalcemic states in man. J. Clin. Invest. *52*:3109, 1973.

DiGeorge, A. M.: Congenital absence of the thymus and its immunologic consequences, concurrence with congenital hypoparathyroidism. *In* Bergsma, D. and Good, R. A. (eds.): Birth Defects. Original Article Series, No. 1. New York, The National Foundation; 1968, Vol. IV.

Drezner, M., Neelon, F. A., and Lebovitz, H. E.: Pseudohypoparathyroidism Type II. A possible defect in the reception of the cyclic AMP signal. New Engl. J. Med. *289*:1056, 1973.

Fairney, A., Jackson, D., and Clayton, B. E.: Measurement of serum parathyroid hormone, with particular reference to some infants with hypocalcemia. Arch. Dis. Child. *48*:419, 1973.

Fanconi, A., and Prader, A.: Transient congenital idiopathic hypoparathyroidism. Helv. Paed. Acta. *22*:342, 1967.

Fisher, G., and Skillern, P. G.: Hypercalcemia due to hypervitaminosis A. J.A.M.A *227*:1413, 1974.

Foley, T. P., Jr., Harrison, H. C., Arnaud, C. D., and Harrison, H. E.: Familial benign hypercalcemia. J. Pediatr. *81*:1060, 1972.

Foster, G. V., Byfield, P. G. H., and Gudmondsson, T. V.: Calcitonin. Clin. Endocrinol. Metab. *1*:93, 1972.

Frame, B., Hanson, C. A., Frost, H. M., Block, M., and Arnstein, A. R.: Renal resistance to parathyroid hormone with osteitis fibrosa. "Pseudohypohyperparathyroidism." Am. J. Med. *52*:311, 1972.

Goldbloom, R. B., Gillis, D. A., and Prasad, M.: Hereditary parathyroid hyperplasia: A surgical emergency of early infancy. Pediatrics *49*:514, 1972.

Hartenstein, H., and Gardner, L. I.: Tetany of the newborn associated with maternal parathyroid adenoma: Report of the seventh affected family. New Eng. J. Med., *274*:266, 1966.

Kodichek, E.: The story of vitamin D from vitamin to hormone. Lancet *1*:325, 1974.

Lee, J. B., Tashjian, A. H., Streeto, J. M., and Frantz, A. G.: Familial pseudohypoparathyroidism. Role of parathyroid hormone and thyrocalcitonin. New Engl. J. Med., *279*:1179, 1968.

Levitt, M., Gessert, C., and Finberg, L.: Inorganic phosphate (laxative) poisoning resulting in tetany in an infant. J. Pediatr. *82*:479, 1973.

Marx, S. J., et al.: Familial hyperparathyroidism. Mild hypercalcemia in at least nine members of a kindred. Ann. Intern. Med. *78*:371, 1973.

Marx, S. J., Hershman, J. M., and Auerbach, G. D.: Thyroid dysfunction in pseudohypoparathyroidism. J. Clin. Endocrinol. Metab. *33*:822, 1971.

Neiman, R. S., and Li, H. C.: Hypercalcemia in undifferentiated leukemia. Possible production of a parathormone-like substance by leukemic cells. Cancer *30*:1972.

Nolan, R. B., Hayles, A. B., and Woolner, L. B.: Adenoma of the parathyroid gland in children. Report of case and brief review of the literature. A. M. A. J. Dis. Child., *99*:622, 1960.

Nusynowitz, M. L., and Klein, M. H.: Pseudoidiopathic hypoparathyroidism. Hypoparathyroidism with ineffective parathyroid hormone. Am. J. Med. *55*:677, 1973.

Olambiwonnu, N. O., Ebbin, A. J., and Frasier, D. S.: Primary hypoparathyroidism associated with ring chromosome 18. J. Pediatr. *80*:833, 1972.

Parfitt, A. M.: Thiazide-induced hypercalcemia in vitamin D-treated hypoparathyroidism. Ann. Intern. Med. *77*:557, 1972.

Peden, V. H.: True idiopathic hypoparathyroidism as a sex-linked recessive trait. Am. J. Hum. Genet. *12*:323, 1960.

Reddy, C. R., et al.: Studies on mechanisms of hypocalcemia of magnesium depletion. J. Clin. Invest. *52*:3000, 1973.

Roof, B. S., Carpenter, B., Fink, D. J., and Gordan, G. S.: Some thoughts on the nature of ectopic parathyroid hormones. Am. J. Med. *50*:686, 1971.

Stanbury, S. W.: Azotaemic renal osteodystrophy. Clin. Endocrinol. Metab. *1*:267, 1972.

Swinton, N. W., Clerkin, E. P., and Flint, L. D.: Hypercalcemia and familial pheochromocytoma. Correction after adrenalectomy. Ann. Intern. Med. *76*:455, 1972.

Vainsel, M., Vandevelde, G., Smulders, J., Vosters, M., Hubain, P., and Loeb, H.: Tetany due to hypomagnesaemia with secondary hypocalcaemia. Arch. Dis. Child. *45*:254, 1970.

Weinberg, A. G., and Stone, R. T.: Autosomal dominant inheritance in Albright's hereditary osteodystrophy. J. Pediatr. *79*:997, 1971.

DISORDERS OF THE ADRENAL GLANDS

GENERAL CONSIDERATIONS

The adrenal gland is composed of two endocrine systems, the medullary and the cortical systems. Mesodermal cells contribute to the development of the adrenal cortex, the gonads and the liver; these three tissues are active in steroid metabolism in the fetus. The presence of common primordial cells in the adrenal and gonad helps to explain why they have in common certain enzymes involved in steroid synthesis and why an inborn defect in one tissue may also involve the other.

Beginning about the seventh week of gestation, the primordium of the adrenal cortex is invaded by sympathetic neural elements. About a week later these cells begin to differentiate into the chromaffin cells capable of synthesizing and storing catecholamines, though the methyl transferase which converts norepinephrine to epinephrine does not develop until later in gestation.

In a fetus of 2 months the adrenals are larger than the kidneys, but from the fourth month the kidneys grow rapidly, becoming about twice as large as the adrenals by the end of the sixth month.

At birth the adrenal gland is one third the size of the kidney, and the combined weight of both glands is 7 to 9 gm in the full-term infant.

The adrenal cortex in the fetus and the newborn infant is composed of two histologically distinct components: an outer portion, the true cortex, and a more central portion, known as the "fetal cortex." At birth this fetal cortex makes up about 80 per cent of the gland. Within a few days after birth, it begins to involute, undergoing a 50 per cent reduction by 2 weeks of age and disappearing completely by about 6 months of age. This inner fetal zone of the adrenal cortex produces primarily dehydroepiandrosterone. The pattern of steroid metabolism in the fetus and newborn is distinctly different from that in later infancy.

The true cortex consists of three zones. In the zona glomerulosa, situated beneath the capsule, there is an alveolar arrangement of the cells; in the broader zona fasciculata the columns of cells are radially arranged; in the zona reticularis the cells form a network next to the medulla.

ADRENAL CORTEX. The adrenal cortex secretes various steroid compounds essential to life. The known compounds can be divided into several general categories:

Glucocorticoids. These steroids have a 21-carbon structure and are also referred to as 17-hydroxycorticosteroids or simply as corticosteroids. The principal one is cortisol, which is also known as compound F or hydrocortisone. Cortisone (compound E) is another member of this group.

Glucocorticoids affect the metabolism of most tissues. They attach to specific intracellular receptor proteins which then bind to the cell nucleus to influence RNA and protein synthesis. In many tissues, glucocorticoids have a catabolic effect, resulting in increased degradation of protein; primarily affected are muscles, skin and connective, adipose and lymphoid tissues. On the other hand, glucocorticoids are anabolic in the liver, where they stimulate a number of enzymes, increase protein and glycogen content and enhance its capacity for gluconeogenesis. Glucocorticoids were so named because of their ability to conserve glucose at the expense of other substrates. Hence, patients with cortisol excess (e.g., Cushing syndrome) have increased glucose production, whereas those with deficiency of cortisol (Addison disease) have decreased gluconeogenesis, with hypoglycemia. Insulin and androgens have effects antagonistic to glucocorticoids. Some of the actions of catecholamines and glucagon are facilitated by glucocorticoids.

The 17-hydroxycorticosteroids are excreted in urine and the amounts can be measured chemically. Cortisol itself is excreted in the urine in amounts less than 1 per cent of the adrenal production. Urinary levels of 17-hydroxycorticosteroids and cortisol, when expressed, respectively, as mg or μg per gram of creatinine, are comparable in children and adults and are useful indices of adrenocortical function. Plasma cortisol may be measured by a variety of techniques; methods using competitive protein-binding and radioimmunoassay are replacing all others. Levels of cortisol in plasma vary according to the time of day, since after the first few years of life there is a well developed circadian rhythm which follows that of corticotropin.

Measurement of ACTH in plasma is not yet generally available for routine studies, though radioimmunoassays have recently been shown capable of measuring levels as low as 10 pg/ml. Indirect means must be used to test for pituitary reserve of ACTH. Metyrapone, which inhibits 11-β-hydroxylation by the adrenal, is administered. Because of the effect of this drug, there is decreased secretion of cortisol and increased secretion of 11-deoxycortisol. This latter compound can be measured either directly or indirectly, both in urine and in plasma. When there is deficiency of corticotropin, levels of 11-deoxycortisol fail to rise.

Many synthetic analogues of cortisone and hydrocortisone are available. Derivatives with an additional double bond in ring A are known as prednisone and prednisolone. They are three to four times as potent in anti-inflammatory and carbohydrate activity as the natural steroids, but have less effect on salt and water retention. Halogenated derivatives have different effects; 9-alpha-fluorohydrocortisone is approximately fifteen times as active as hydrocortisone in anti-inflammatory activity, but is more than twenty times as active in salt and water retention. Triamcinolone (delta-1,9-alpha-fluoro, 16 alpha-hydroxyhydrocortisone) is approximately five times as potent as hydrocortisone, and beta-methasone and dexamethasone are approximately twenty-five times as potent; none of them is thought to affect the retention of water and electrolytes. These analogues are usually used in pharmacologic doses for their anti-inflammatory or immunosuppressive properties.

Aldosterone. A potent mineralocorticoid, aldosterone is the 18-aldehyde of corticosterone and is produced primarily in the zona glomerulosa of the adrenal cortex. Its secretion is regulated by activation of the renin-angiotensin system. Renin is a proteolytic enzyme which acts upon renin substrate to yield the inactive decapeptide, angiotensin I. A converting enzyme in the lungs then immediately changes angiotensin I to the biologically active octapeptide, angiotensin II. Angiotensin II is a potent pressor agent, fifty times more potent than norepinephrine. One of its main actions is directly on the adrenal cortex to stimulate the secretion of aldosterone.

In good health and on a normal dietary intake, ACTH plays a minor role in regulation of aldosterone secretion but under some conditions, as in anephric man, it may have a more significant effect. On the other hand, potassium may be of equal importance to the renin-angiotensin system in the regulation of aldosterone secretion. In studies of aldosterone secretion, dietary potassium and sodium should be rigidly controlled.

Sodium deprivation is a potent stimulus to secretion of aldosterone. Changes in intake of sodium result in small changes in blood volume, arterial pressure and renal blood flow. These changes are sensitively monitored by the juxtaglomerular cells on the renal afferent arterioles, which form the receptor site or volume receptor. Activation of the juxtaglomerular apparatus results in increased output of angiotensin II followed by increased secretion of aldosterone.

The principal action of aldosterone is the maintenance of electrolyte equilibrium, which in turn contributes to the stabilization of blood volume and blood pressure. Aldosterone controls sodium reabsorption (and hence water reabsorption) in the distal tubule of the kidney.

Aldosterone can be measured in urine by double isotope dilution or by radioimmunoassay. Aldosterone and renin activity in plasma can also be measured by radioimmunoassay.

Androgens. Dehydroepiandrosterone, androstenedione and testosterone are representative of this group. These hormones are capable of increasing retention of nitrogen, potassium, phosphorus and sulfate. They promote growth and have an androgenic effect, properties which are most conspicuous under pathologic conditions when adrenal hyperplasia or adrenal tumors induce precocious growth and development of secondary male sex characteristics. There is evidence that the adrenal androgens are partly responsible for the development of axillary and pubic hair in the female.

Metabolized adrenal androgens are excreted in the urine as 17-ketosteroids. Their measurement can be accepted as an index of the production of adrenal androgens in the female. In the male approximately one third of the urinary 17-ketosteroids can be attributed to testicular and two thirds to adrenal androgens. In children prior to 8 to 10 years of age the urinary excretion of these substances is small, but there is a constant increase throughout adolescence until adult levels are reached. Under pathologic conditions increased production of adrenal androgens is reflected in increased secretion of urinary 17-ketosteroids.

ADRENAL MEDULLA. The principal hormones of the adrenal medulla are the physiologically active catecholamines: dopamine, norepinephrine and epinephrine. The sequence of reactions representing the biosynthetic route is depicted in Figure 17–15. Catecholamine synthesis also occurs in brain, in sympathetic nerve endings, and in chromaffin tissue other than in the adrenal medulla. The principal metabolites of the catecholamines excreted in the urine are vanilmandelic acid, or VMA, metan-

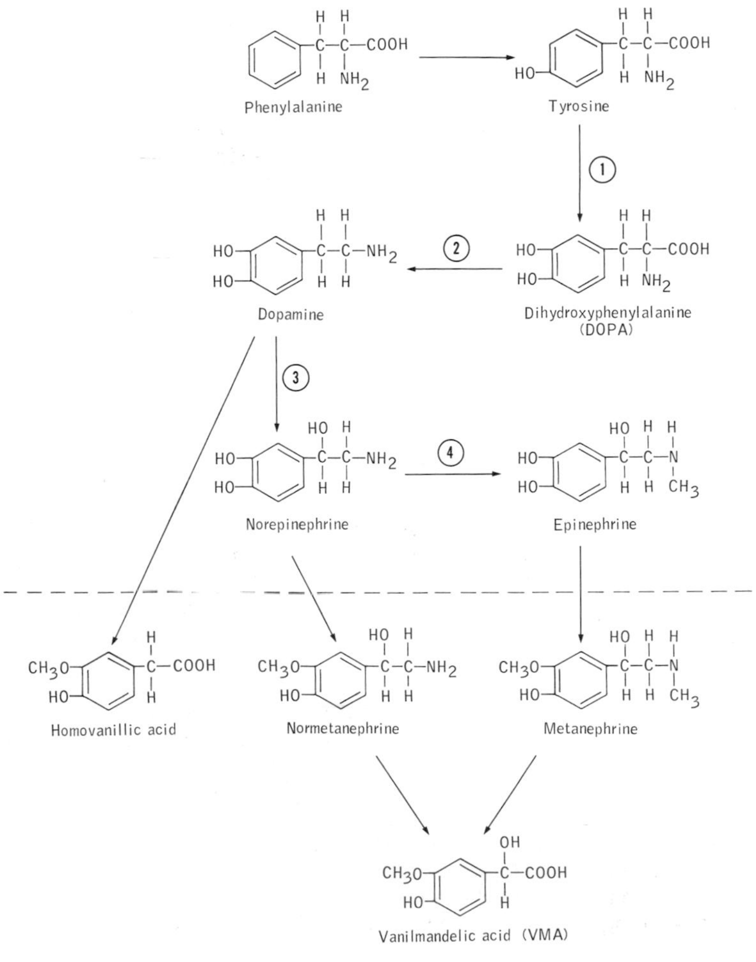

Figure 17–15 *Biosynthesis (above dotted line) and metabolism (below dotted line) of the catecholamines: norepinephrine and epinephrine.*
1. *Tyrosine hydroxylase*
2. *Dopa decarboxylase*
3. *Dopamine-β-oxidase*
4. *Phenylethanolamine-N-methyl transferase*

ephrine and normetanephrine. The relatively large amount of VMA excreted in urine and its relative ease of chemical estimation have made its determination the method of choice for the detection of functioning tumors of the adrenal medulla.

The proportions of epinephrine and norepinephrine in the adrenal vary at different ages. In early fetal stages there is practically no epinephrine, and even at birth norepinephrine is predominant. In adults, norepinephrine makes up only 10 to 30 per cent of the total pressor amines in the medulla. Both epinephrine and norepinephrine raise the mean arterial blood pressure. Norepinephrine accomplishes this without changing the cardiac output. By increasing peripheral vascular resistance, it increases systolic and diastolic blood pressures with only a slight reduction in the pulse rate. Epinephrine increases the pulse rate and, by decreasing the peripheral vascular resistance, decreases the diastolic pressure. The hyperglycemic and calorigenic effects of norepinephrine are much less pronounced than those of epinephrine.

ADRENOCORTICAL INSUFFICIENCY

Deficient production of cortisol and/or aldosterone may result from a wide variety of congenital or acquired lesions of the hypothalamus, pituitary or adrenal cortex (Table 17–4). Depending upon the pathologic lesions, symptoms may be severe or mild, may become manifest abruptly or insidiously, may begin in infancy or later, and may be permanent or temporary.

ETIOLOGY

Corticotropin Deficiency. Congenital hypoplasia or aplasia of the pituitary is almost always associated with secondary hypoplasia of the adrenals, as well as with other hormonal deficiencies. These congenital defects are usually associated with abnormalities of the skull and brain such as anencephaly and holoprosencephaly. Recent studies in such infants have revealed that there is a considerable residuum of pituitary function, and the hypoplasia of the pituitary is probably secondary to the hypothalamic defect and deficiency of corticotropin-releasing factor (CRF). Isolated deficiency of corticotropin is a rare lesion in all ages, occurring in association with deficiency of growth hormone in patients with idiopathic hypopituitarism; indirect evidence suggests that the deficiency in these patients is secondary to deficient CRF. Destructive lesions of the pituitary, particularly craniopharyngioma, are the most common causes of corticotropin deficiency in childhood. In rare instances, autoimmune hypophysitis has been suggested as a possible cause for corticotropin deficiency.

Primary Adrenal Aplasia or Hypoplasia. Aplasia and hypoplasia have been noted in the same patient or in different siblings. The disorder appears to be a defect of organogenesis without any demonstrable disturbance of pituitary function. Corticotropin is present, and the adrenal defect involves both cortisol and aldosterone. Histologic examination of the hypoplastic adrenal cortex in most patients with this disorder reveals disorganization and cytomegaly, findings not present in the adrenals from corticotropin-deficient infants. The condition occurs predominantly in males, and on two occasions has been reported in half brothers with different fathers, establishing an X-linked form of inheritance. Much less frequently both male and female siblings are affected, suggesting

TABLE 17–4 ETIOLOGIC CLASSIFICATION OF ADRENAL CORTICAL HYPOFUNCTION

A. Corticotropin-releasing Factor Deficiency
  1. Hypothalamic defects (e.g., anencephaly, holoprosencephaly)
  2. Idiopathic (e.g., idiopathic hypopituitarism)

B. Corticotropin Deficiency
  1. Pituitary hypoplasia or aplasia
  2. Destructive lesions of pituitary (e.g., craniopharyngioma)
  3. Autoimmune hypophysitis?

C. Primary Adrenal Hypoplasia or Aplasia
  a. X-linked
  b. Autosomal recessive
  c. Sporadic

D. Familial Glucocorticoid Deficiency

E. Inborn Defects of Steroidogenesis
  1. Congenital adrenal hyperplasia
    a. Lipoid adrenal hyperplasia (desmolase defect)
    b. 3-β-Hydroxysteroid dehydrogenase deficiency
    c. 21-Hydroxylase deficiency
  2. Isolated defects of aldosterone synthesis
    a. 18-Hydroxylation deficiency
    b. 18-Dehydrogenation deficiency

F. Unresponsiveness to Mineralocorticoids
  1. Pseudohypoaldosteronism

G. Destructive Lesions of Adrenal Cortex
  1. Granulomatous lesions (e.g., tuberculosis)
  2. Autoimmune adrenalitis (idiopathic Addison's disease)
    a. Isolated
    b. Associated with other autoimmune endocrinopathies or mucocutaneous candidiasis (e.g., Schmidt syndrome)
  3. Neonatal hemorrhage
  4. Acute infection (Waterhouse-Friderichsen syndrome)

H. Iatrogenic
  1. Abrupt cessation of exogenous corticosteroids or corticotropin
  2. Removal of functioning adrenal tumor
  3. Adrenalectomy for Cushing's disease
  4. Drugs
    a. Aminoglutethimide
    b. Mitotane (o,p′-DDD)
    c. Metyrapone

I. Fetal Adrenal Suppression
  1. Maternal Cushing syndrome

an autosomal recessive inheritance. It is not clear if sporadic cases are genetically transmitted.

Familial Glucocorticoid Deficiency. This form of chronic adrenal insufficiency is characterized by isolated deficiency of glucocorticoids and elevated levels of corticotropin in association with normal aldosterone production. As a consequence, the salt-losing manifestations of most other causes of adrenal insufficiency do not occur. Instead, patients present primarily with hypoglycemia, seizures and pigmentation. The disorder affects both sexes equally and appears to be inherited in an autosomal recessive manner. Histologically there appears to be marked adrenocortical atrophy with relative sparing of the zona glomerulosa. The defect is not known. It has been suggested that the unresponsiveness of the adrenal cortex may be due to failure of membrane attachment or to failure of activation of adenyl cyclase by corticotropin, but there is evidence that the adrenocortical defect may result from a degenerative process; perhaps the syndrome is a heterogenous one.

Inborn Defects of Steroidogenesis. The most common causes of adrenocortical insufficiency in infancy are the salt-losing forms of congenital adrenal hyperplasia. About half the infants with the 21-hydroxylase defect, all infants with lipoid adrenal hyperplasia, and most infants with deficiency of 3-β-hydroxysteroid dehydrogenase manifest salt-losing symptoms in the newborn period. In these defects there is a deficiency in the synthesis of both cortisol and aldosterone.

Isolated Deficiency of Aldosterone. This occurs much less commonly; it is due to a defect either in the 18-hydroxylation of corticosterone or in the dehydrogenation of 18-hydroxycorticosterone (Fig. 17–16). In these patients, aldosterone secretion rate is decreased, especially considering the state of sodium depletion, whereas 17-ketosteroids, cortisol and pregnanetriol are normal. There is no unusual pigmentation, and clinical manifestations are primarily those of salt loss. Some adaptation or compensation appears to occur, since amelioration of the salt-losing manifestations is evident with increasing age.

Pseudohypoaldosteronism. About a dozen infants have been described with a salt-losing syndrome despite normal adrenocortical and renal function. Secretion and urinary excretion rates of aldosterone are elevated and remain so after salt supplementation. Administration of DOCA or aldosterone does not correct the urinary sodium loss. Elevated renin activity in plasma indicates that the hyperaldosteronism is secondary to hyperactivity of the renin-angiotensin system. The pathophysiology remains unclear, though an unresponsiveness of the distal tubule to aldosterone has been the usual explanation.

Destructive Lesions of Adrenal Cortex. In older children one of the more common causes of adrenal insufficiency is a destructive lesion of the adrenal gland; the condition is referred to as *Addison disease.* Tuberculosis was once the most frequent cause of Addison disease but this is no longer the case. Histoplasmosis, coccidioidomycosis, torulosis, mycosis fungoides, amyloidosis and metastatic malignancies have been identified as causative agents in adults, but not in children, in whom in most instances "idiopathic atrophy" is noted. The adrenal glands may be so small that they are not visible at autopsy, and only remnants of tissue are found in microscopic sections. Usually, however, the medulla is not destroyed, and there is lymphocytic infiltration in the area of the former cortex and in the medulla. About half the affected patients have antibodies against adrenal tissue, which suggests that the adrenocortical insufficiency results from an *autoimmune adrenalitis.*

Patients with idiopathic Addison's disease are exceptionally prone to a variety of other conditions known or believed to be autoimmune in origin. The principal associated disorders are hypoparathyroidism, pernicious anemia, hypo- and hyperthyroidism, lymphocytic thyroiditis, diabetes mellitus, vitiligo and abnormal gonadal function. A wide variety of other conditions also may occur in association with Addison disease, particularly alopecia areata, subacute hepatitis, neurologic disorders, including Schilder's disease and spastic paraplegia, and chronic mucocutaneous candidiasis. These conditions may have their onsets before Addison disease or years later except for the candidiasis, which almost always occurs first.

Idiopathic Addison's disease often occurs in siblings, particularly when it is associated with other autoimmune disorders. The genetics is not clear, since the primary underlying immunologic defect is not known; heterogeneity of the syndrome is likely. An autosomal recessive mode of inheritance appears most likely, however, especially in children. Heterogeneity within families is also common; e.g., one sibling may have adrenal insufficiency and another hypoparathyroidism.

Hemorrhage into Adrenal Glands. This may occur in the neonatal period as a consequence of difficult labor or of asphyxia. The hemorrhage may be sufficiently extensive to result in death from exsanguination or from hypoadrenalism. Often the hemorrhage is asymptomatic initially and is identified by later calcification of the adrenal. On rare occasions, gradual impairment in function resulting from progressive fibrosis or cystic changes may culminate in adrenocortical insufficiency in infancy or childhood.

Waterhouse-Friderichsen Syndrome. This is a characteristic state of shock resulting from bacterial infection and is usually associated with hemorrhage into the adrenal glands. The syndrome has been recognized most often in patients with fulminating meningococcemia, but it also occurs with septicemia caused by other organisms. The various lesions, including the adrenal hemorrhage, have been attributed to a generalized Schwartzman reaction. Although the circulatory collapse in patients with this syndrome has been attributed to impaired adrenocortical function, in most patients blood levels of corticoids are appropriately ele-

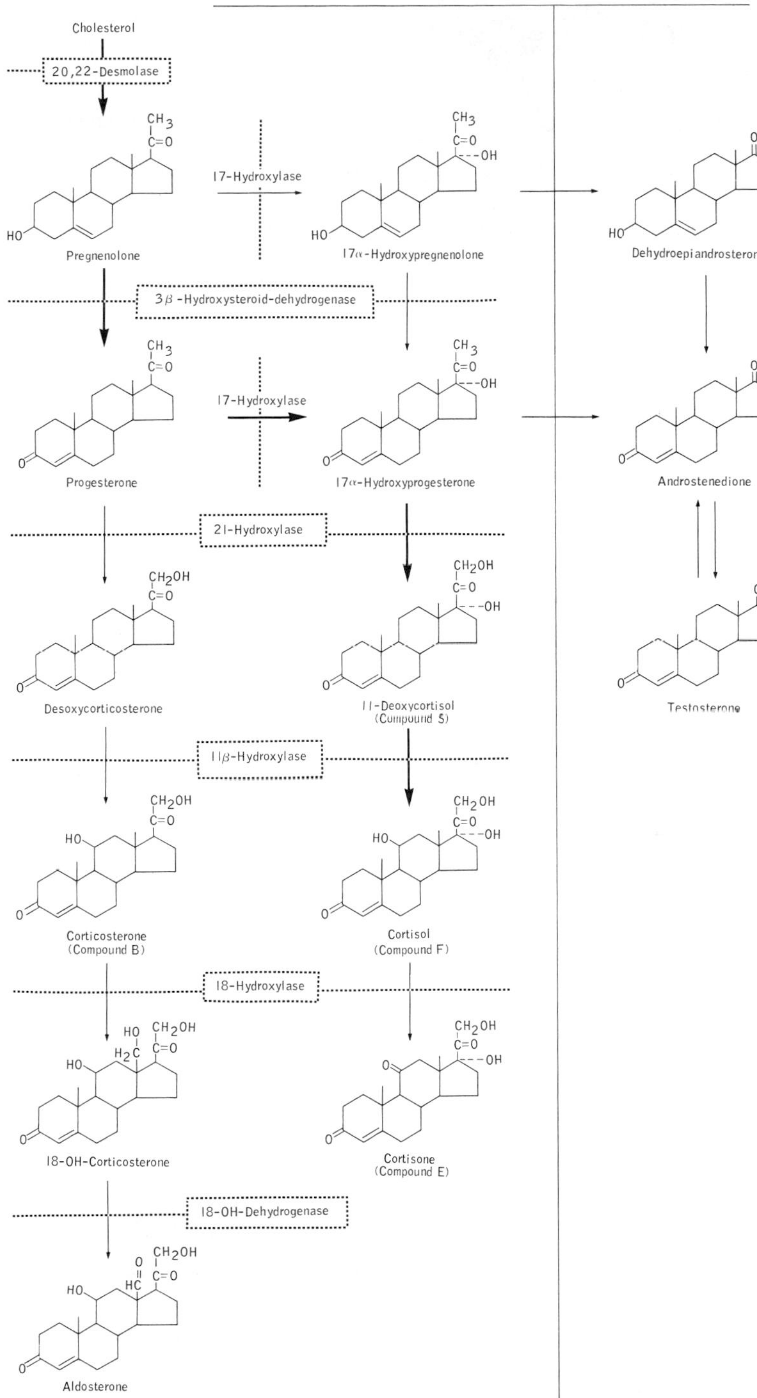

Figure 17–16 *The synthesis of hydrocortisone is shown to the left of the vertical line. The heavy arrows indicate the principal pathway, and the light arrows show alternate pathways of steroid genesis. The enzymatic defects which cause virilizing adrenal hyperplasia and the defects in aldosterone synthesis are shown by horizontal dotted lines. Vertical dotted lines show the defect in 17-hydroxylation. To the right of the vertical line are the predominant adrenal androgens which lead to peripheral conversion to testosterone.*

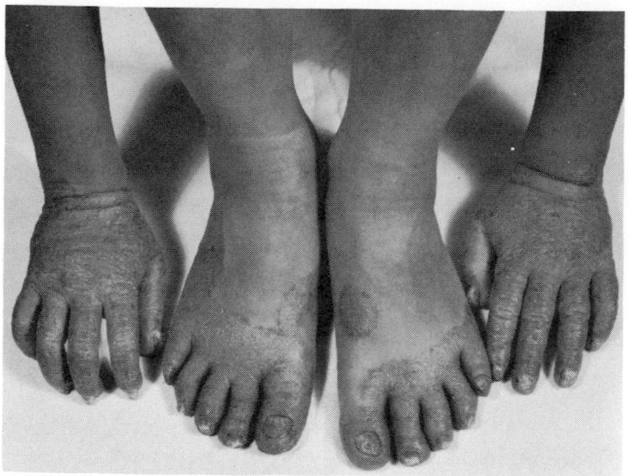

Figure 17–17 Chronic mucocutaneous candidiasis in a boy with Addison disease. Candida infection was first noted on the tongue and buccal mucosa at 9 months; fingernails were first involved at 2 years of age. The lesions have resisted treatment and progressed to involve hands, feet and other cutaneous areas. Addison disease developed at 8 years of age; no other endocrinopathies have developed by 15 years of age.

vated. On the other hand, in some children with hemorrhagic adrenals at autopsy, serum levels of corticoids were undetectable. It appears that the circulatory collapse is, in most instances, the result of the severe toxemia, but it may be aggravated by adrenal insufficiency.

Abrupt Cessation of Administration of Corticotropin or a Corticosteroid. This may result in adrenal insufficiency. Symptoms are most likely to occur after these substances have been given in large doses for a long time to patients who are subsequently subjected to stressful situations such as severe infections or surgical procedures. Administration of these substances results in impaired pituitary or adrenocortical function, and these effects may sometimes persist for a long time after treatment is discontinued.

CLINICAL MANIFESTATIONS. The age of onset of symptoms and the clinical manifestations depend upon the specific etiologic factor involved. In patients with adrenal hypoplasia, defects in steroidogenesis, or pseudohypoaldosteronism, symptoms begin shortly after birth and are characterized by manifestations of salt loss. There are failure to thrive, vomiting, lethargy, anorexia and dehydration; these may be followed by circulatory collapse and death.

In older children with Addison's disease, the onset is usually more gradual and is characterized by muscular weakness, lassitude, anorexia, loss of weight, general wasting and low blood pressure. Abdominal pain may simulate an acute abdominal process, and there may be an intense craving for salt. If the condition is not recognized and treated, *adrenal crisis* may supervene. The patient suddenly becomes cyanotic, the skin is cold and the pulse weak and rapid. The blood pressure falls, and respirations are rapid and labored. In the absence of immediate and intensive therapy, a rapidly fatal course ensues. Crises can also be precipitated in patients with inadequately treated chronic adrenal insufficiency by infection, trauma, excessive fatigue or drugs such as morphine, barbiturates, laxatives, thyroid hormone or insulin.

Increased pigmentation of the skin should always alert the clinician to the possibility of adrenocortical insufficiency. This manifestation occurs in those conditions in which there is deficiency of cortisol and excessive secretion of MSH and corticotropin, as in primary adrenal hypoplasia, familial glucocorticoid deficiency and Addison's disease. Pigmentation may be first apparent on the face and hands and is most intense around the genitalia, umbilicus, axillae, nipples and joints. Scars and freckles may be especially pigmented. Areas of depigmentation may be interspersed with dark areas. The exposed areas of the skin are the most intensely affected, and failure of disappearance of a tan may be the first clue to the condition. In the buccal muscosa, the pigmentation is usually bluish brown.

The presenting manifestations may be those of hypoglycemia, particularly in the neonate with congenital adrenal hypoplasia. Patients with adrenocortical insufficiency are deficient in gluconeogenetic substrates; the hypoglycemia may be associated with ketosis, therefore, and confused with ketotic hypoglycemia. (See Section 16.)

In young children with familial glucocorticoid deficiency, salt-losing manifestations do not occur and the symptoms are primarily increased pigmentation and hypoglycemia. Symptoms may begin

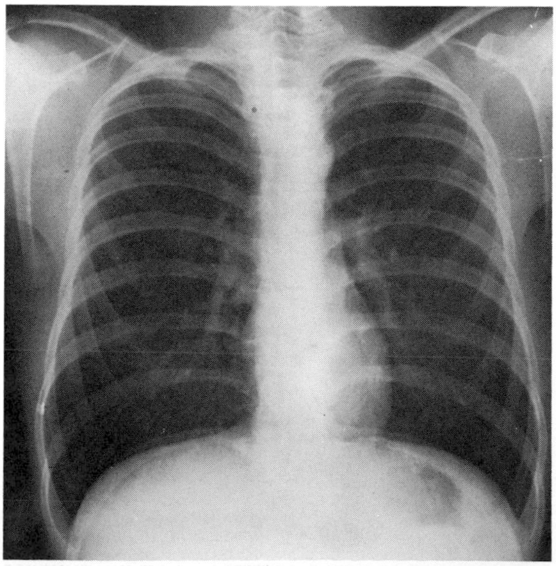

Figure 17–18 Addison disease in a 10 year old boy. On admission he was dehydrated; there was bronzing of the skin and hypotension. Note the microcardia characteristics of untreated Addison disease. Hypoparathyroidism developed subsequently. One sibling had hypoparathyroidism and superficial moniliasis, and another died of Addison disease.

shortly after birth, and almost always by 5 years of age. Many affected children have had other treatment for seizures before their hypoglycemic cause was recognized.

In patients with deficiency of corticotropin, pigmentation does not occur. Hypoglycemia may be manifest, but salt-losing is uncommon, presumably owing to residual ability of the adrenal to secrete aldosterone.

In those conditions known to have a genetic basis, it is important to evaluate fully the adrenocortical function of siblings.

LABORATORY DATA. When salt-losing manifestations are present, the concentrations of sodium and chloride in the serum are usually low, and that of potassium is elevated. There is an increase in the urinary excretion of sodium and chloride and a decrease in that of potassium. The nonprotein nitrogen level in plasma is elevated if there is dehydration. Hypoglycemia may be striking, or not become manifest until after prolonged fasting. The circulating eosinophils may be increased in number. When hemorrhage, adrenal cysts or tuberculosis is the causative factor, roentgenograms of the abdomen may reveal calcifications in the area of the adrenals. A small and narrow roentgenographic shadow of the heart reflects hypovolemia. Electrocardiographic changes are related to potassium levels. The electroencephalogram may show absence or a greatly decreased content of low-voltage, fast-frequency waves.

The most definitive test is the measurement of urinary or plasma levels of corticosteroids before and after the administration of corticotropin. Resting levels of corticosteroids are low and there is no increase after administration of corticotropin. In occasional instances, normal resting levels which do not increase after administration of corticotropin indicate the absence of adrenocortical reserve. A low initial level followed by a significant response to corticotropin may indicate adrenal insufficiency secondary to endogenous insufficiency of corticotropin. When corticotropin deficiency is suspected (as in hypothalamic and pituitary disorders), residual reserve of pituitary corticotropin can be evaluated by using metyrapone (q.v.). Patients with corticotropin deficiency show little response to this test. The ideal specific test would be to measure plasma cortisol and corticotropin simultaneously, but plasma ACTH determinations are not as yet generally available for clinical use.

Measurement of urinary 17-ketosteroids is necessary in infants suspected of adrenocortical insufficiency in order to establish or exclude the diagnosis of congenital adrenal hyperplasia. Aldosterone secretion is low in salt-losing congenital adrenal hyperplasia, in adrenal hypoplasia and in Addison's disease, but its measurement is rarely needed for diagnosis. Measurement of aldosterone is necessary in infants suspected of an isolated defect of aldosterone synthesis (where it is low) and in infants suspected of pseudohypoaldosteronism (where it is usually elevated). In patients with familial glucocorticoid deficiency, aldosterone levels are normal and rise appropriately to salt deprivation.

TREATMENT. Treatment for acute adrenal insufficiency or for crises must be instituted immediately and must be vigorous. Intravenous fluids should consist of 5 per cent glucose in isotonic saline solution to correct the hypoglycemia and the sodium loss. Concomitantly a water-soluble form of hydrocortisone, such as hydrocortisone hemisuccinate, should be given intravenously. High levels may be achieved instantaneously in this manner and large doses can be used safely. As much as 25 mg for infants and 75 mg for older children should be given intravenously at 6-hour intervals for the first 24 hours. These doses may be reduced during the next 24 hours if progress is satisfactory. A salt-retaining hormone should be added to maintain electrolyte balance; desoxycorticosterone acetate (DOCA) in oil may be used in doses of 1 to 5 mg daily intramuscularly. After the first 48 hours, if oral intake is satisfactory, the intravenous fluids may be discontinued and the corticosteroid may be given orally as cortisol in doses of 5 to 20 mg at 8-hour intervals. Further reduction can then be accomplished until maintenance levels and a stable clinical situation are achieved. The daily administration of DOCA is continued throughout this period of treatment.

Once the acute manifestations are under control, most patients require chronic replacement therapy for their deficiencies of aldosterone and cortisol. The cortisol may be given orally in daily doses of 10 mg for infants to 40 mg for adolescents; the daily dose should be divided and administered at breakfast and in the evening. During situations of stress, such as periods of infection or operative procedures, the dose of hydrocortisone should be increased. The daily injections of the salt-retaining hormone, desoxycorticosterone acetate, can be replaced by monthly injections of a long-acting preparation, desoxycorticosterone pivalate, which may be given intramuscularly every 3 or 4 weeks. Or it may be replaced by the salt-retaining hormone, fluorohydrocortisone, which is administered orally in doses of 0.05 to 0.1 mg daily.

Overdosage with DOCA or fluorohydrocortisone results in hypertension and may lead to cardiac enlargement and edema because of excessive retention of sodium chloride and water; excessive loss of potassium may produce weakness or paralysis.

Patients with primary corticotropin deficiency or with familial glucocorticoid deficiency do not require a salt-retaining hormone since their ability to secrete aldosterone is intact. On the other hand, patients with primary defects in aldosterone synthesis do not require cortisol; a salt-retaining hormone may be required, but in milder forms the addition of salt to the diet is adequate to maintain homeostasis. In patients with pseudohypoaldosteronism, administration of DOCA does not correct the urinary sodium loss; therapy must consist of supplementation with sodium chloride. The disorder is self-limited and treatment may be discontinued after 1 to 2 years. In newborn infants with adrenal hemorrhage, vitamins K and C and transfusions with whole blood may be indicated.

Patients with Addison's disease must be closely observed for the development of other endocrine disorders. Appropriate counseling is indicated for disorders known to have a genetic basis.

ADRENOCORTICAL HYPERFUNCTION

Four syndromes are attributable to hyperadrenocorticism: the *adrenogenital syndrome, Cushing syndrome, hyperaldosteronism* and *feminization* (Table 17–5).

ADRENOGENITAL SYNDROME

Congenital Adrenal Hyperplasia

PATHOGENESIS. When the adrenogenital syndrome is associated with congenital adrenal hyperplasia, it is caused by an inborn defect in the biosynthesis of adrenal corticoids. Five different enzymatic defects in this pathway are known (Fig. 17–16), but only some of these are characterized clinically by virilization, the others not permitting excessive androgen secretion. The deficiency of cortisol results in increased secretion of corticotropin, which in turn leads to adrenocortical hyperplasia and overproduction of intermediary metabolites. Each defect is inherited as an autosomal recessive trait. The incidence of the condition varies in different populations but is probably on the order of 1 in 15,000 births. The Yupik eskimos have an unusually high incidence, 1 in 500 live births, of the salt-losing form of the disease.

Deficiency of 21-Hydroxylase. This accounts for over 90 per cent of affected patients. Two clinical variants occur: in the salt-losing forms, the enzymatic defect is presumed complete, with deficiencies of both cortisol and aldosterone; in the nonsalt-losing form, a less complete enzymatic defect, with ensuing hyperplasia of the adrenal cortex, is felt to result in production of sufficient cortisol and aldosterone to avert manifestations of salt loss. Some aspects of this matter are still in dispute; the pathogenetic mechanisms are undoubtedly more complex than set forth here. In any case, each defect is genetically specific; if one form occurs in a family, subsequently affected infants will almost always have the same form. In both variants, excessive production of androgen results in pseudohermaphroditism in the female and in pseudoprecocious puberty in the male.

Deficiency of 11-β-Hydroxylase. This is the second most frequent enzymatic defect causing this syndrome. Of the 50 or so reported cases, most have been adults or children several years old and little is known of their steroid production early in life. Clinical and laboratory findings have been somewhat heterogeneous, but characteristically there are present in the urine large amounts of compound S, the immediate precursor of cortisol. Excessive production and urinary excretion of desoxycorticosterone (DOC) also occurs and accounts for the hypertension which is characteristic of this enzymatic defect. The elevated levels of DOC prevent salt-losing symptoms in spite of suppression of aldosterone secretion. In the only young infant studied, there appeared to be a defect in conversion of compound S to cortisol but not in conversion of DOC to corticosterone. (See Figure 17–16.) This suggests that there may be two 11-β-hydroxylating systems, at least in infancy. As is the case for deficiency of 21-hydroxylase, females have ambiguous genitalia and males are virilized.

Deficiency of 3-β-Hydroxysteroid Dehydrogenase (3-β-HSD). This has been reported in only 13 patients. Deficiency of both cortisol and aldosterone occurs in this defect. Salt wasting is usual, but incomplete defects without salt-losing

TABLE 17–5 CLASSIFICATION OF ADRENAL CORTICAL HYPERFUNCTION

A. Excess Androgen (Adrenogenital Syndrome)
    1. Congenital adrenal hyperplasia
        a. 21-Hydroxylase defect
        b. 11-Hydroxylase defect
        c. 3-β-Hydroxysteroid dehydrogenase defect (females)
    2. Tumor
        a. Carcinoma
        b. Benign adenoma
            1. Isolated testosterone secretion

B. Excess Cortisol (Cushing Syndrome)
    1. Bilateral adrenal hyperplasia
        a. Hypothalamic origin (Cushing's disease)
        b. Pituitary corticotropin-producing tumor
        c. Nodular hyperplasia
        d. Extra-adrenal corticotropin-producing tumor
        e. Exogenous corticotropin
    2. Tumor
        a. Carcinoma
        b. Benign adenoma

C. Excess Mineralocorticoid (Hypertensive Hypokalemic syndrome)
    1. Primary hyperaldosteronism
        a. Adrenal hyperplasia
            1. Congenital aldosteronism
            2. Familial glucocorticoid-suppressible aldosteronism
        b. Tumor
            1. Carcinoma
            2. Benign adenoma
    2. Desoxycorticosterone excess
        a. Adrenal hyperplasia
            1. 11-Hydroxylase defect
            2. 17-Hydroxylase defect
        b. Tumor
            1. Carcinoma

D. Excess Estrogen (Adrenal Feminization Syndrome)
    1. Tumor
        a. Carcinoma
        b. Adenoma

E. Mixed Hypercorticism
    1. Tumor

manifestations have been reported. Females are only slightly virilized at birth; males are usually incompletely virilized and manifest hypospadias. The enzyme is required for the biosynthesis of testicular hormones; its absence in fetal testes probably explains the incomplete virilization of males during fetal life.

Lipoid Adrenal Hyperplasia. This has been reported in 17 patients. Failure of conversion of cholesterol into pregnenolone is due to absence of one of the three enzymes needed for this conversion, presumably the desmolase. There is marked accumulation of lipids and cholesterol in the adrenal cortex, with total failure of synthesis of any adrenal steroids. The enzymatic defect in the adrenal is also present in the testis, preventing synthesis of testicular hormones. As a consequence, males are completely feminized, females exhibiting no genital abnormality. Salt-losing manifestations are usual, and most infants have died in early infancy. Because urinary 17-ketosteroids are not elevated in this form of adrenal hyperplasia, affected infants are apt to be confused with those with adrenal hypoplasia. For example, a phenotypic female infant with salt-losing manifestations at 2 months of age, who was felt to have "Addison disease," developed inguinal testes at 6½ years of age with an XY karyotype; these findings led to the diagnosis of lipoid adrenal hyperplasia. In another instance, an incomplete enzymatic defect led to partial masculinization of a male infant who did not exhibit hypoadrenalism until 7 months of age.

17-Hydroxylase Deficiency. This defect has been described in only 7 adult patients. There is deficiency of cortisol synthesis, the major adrenal corticosteroid being corticosterone (Fig. 17–16). Deoxycorticosterone is also increased and leads to hypokalemic alkalosis and hypertension. Urinary 17-ketosteroids and estrogens are absent; as a consequence, affected females exhibit no secondary sexual characteristics, and amenorrhea and absence of sexual hair are common. When the enzymatic defect occurs in the genotypic male, the fetal testis is also involved and ambiguous genitalia are expected. Males have hypospadias, cryptorchidism and a rudimentary vagina. Patients with this defect must be considered in the differential diagnosis of primary hypogonadism in females or of pseudohermaphroditism in males. (See below, this Section.)

CLINICAL MANIFESTATIONS. Over 90 per cent of patients with congenital adrenal hyperplasia have the defect in 21-hydroxylation and exhibit virilization. About 50 per cent of the affected patients have the compensated variant of the disorder and do not exhibit salt losing. These are described first.

Patients Without Salt Losing. In the *male* the main clinical manifestations are those of premature isosexual development. The infant usually appears normal at birth, but signs of sexual and somatic precocity may appear within the first half-year of life or develop more gradually, becoming evident at 4 or 5 years of age or later. Enlargement of the penis, scrotum and prostate, appearance of pubic hair, and development of acne and of a deep voice are noted. The muscles are well developed, and the bone age is advanced for the chronologic age. Owing to premature closure of the epiphyses, growth stops relatively early, and the adult stature is stunted.

The testes are normal in size, so that they appear relatively small in contrast to the enlarged penis. Occasionally ectopic adrenocortical cells are present in the testes of patients with adrenal hyperplasia; these cells may become hyperplastic just as the adrenal glands do and produce enlargement of the testes. Spermatogenesis does not take place. Mental development is usually normal, but the abnormal physical development may result in behavioral problems.

In the *female* congenital adrenal hyperplasia results in female pseudohermaphroditism (Fig. 17–19). Since the disorder of steroidogenesis begins early in fetal life, there is almost always evidence of some degree of masculinization at birth. It is manifest by enlargement of the clitoris and variable degrees of labial fusion. The vagina has a common opening with the urethra (urogenital sinus). The clitoris may be so enlarged that it resembles a penis, and, since the urethra opens below this organ, a mistaken diagnosis of hypospadias and cryptorchidism is often made. Occasionally the urogenital sinus extends to the tip of the phallus, and the genitalia resemble those of a cryptorchid male. The severity of the virilization is in general greater in infants who are salt-losers than in those who are not. The internal genital organs are those of a normal female.

After birth the masculinization progresses. Pubic and axillary hair develops prematurely, acne appears, and the voice assumes a masculine quality. These girls are tall for their age, ossification is advanced for their age, and they show good muscular development and, in general, have the body build of a boy. Although the internal genitalia are female, breast development and menstruation do not occur unless the excessive production of androgens is suppressed by adequate treatment.

A number of such virilized female pseudohermaphrodites whose condition was not diagnosed until adult life have been erroneously reared as males. These patients have behaved in every way as males, including having sexual intercourse; some have had satisfactory marriages.

With the *11-hydroxylase defect* salt-losing manifestations do not occur. Most patients are hypertensive, though several have been normotensive or have had intermittent hypertension only. The disorder has been diagnosed only rarely early in life, but one affected infant did not have hypertension during the first year of life. Virilization occurs in all patients and is as severe as with the 21-hydroxylase defect.

Patients With Salt Losing. In patients with the salt-losing variant, symptoms begin shortly after birth. There is failure to regain birth weight, progressive weight loss and dehydration. Vomiting is a prominent symptom and anorexia intervenes. Disturbances in cardiac rate and rhythm may

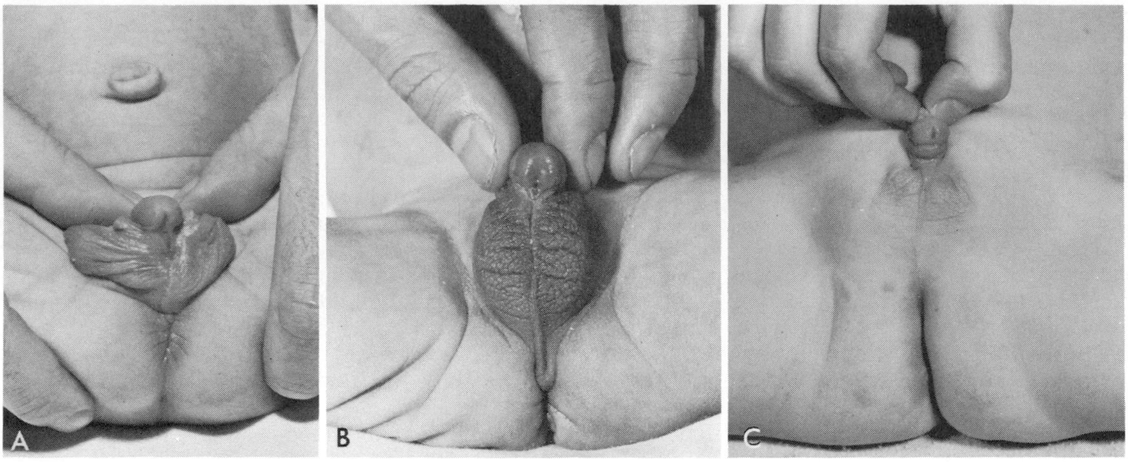

Figure 17–19 *Three female pseudohermaphrodites with untreated congenital adrenal hyperplasia. All were erroneously assigned male sex at birth, and each had normal female sex-chromosome complement. Infants A and B were salt-losers and were diagnosed in early infancy. Infant C was referred at 1 year of age because of bilateral cryptorchidism. Note completely penile urethra; such complete degrees of masculinization in females with adrenal hyperplasia are not extremely rare; most such infants are salt-losers.*

occur, with cyanosis and dyspnea. Without treatment, progression of symptoms to collapse and death usually occur within a few weeks.

In females the virilization of the external genitalia in an infant with the above manifestations directs attention to the correct diagnosis. In the male, on the other hand, the genitalia are normal and the clinical manifestations are more apt to be interpreted as signs of pyloric stenosis, intestinal obstruction, heart disease, cow's milk intolerance or other causes of failure to thrive. As a consequence, the diagnosis is established more frequently in females than in males, though the disorder affects both sexes equally.

The familial homogeneity of each variant suggests two different genetic defects of the 21-hydroxylating system. Under conditions of stress or sodium deprivation, the salt-losing tendency may be provoked in compensated patients. This may account for intermediate cases of late onset of salt loss.

Patients with the *3-β-hydroxysteroid dehy-*

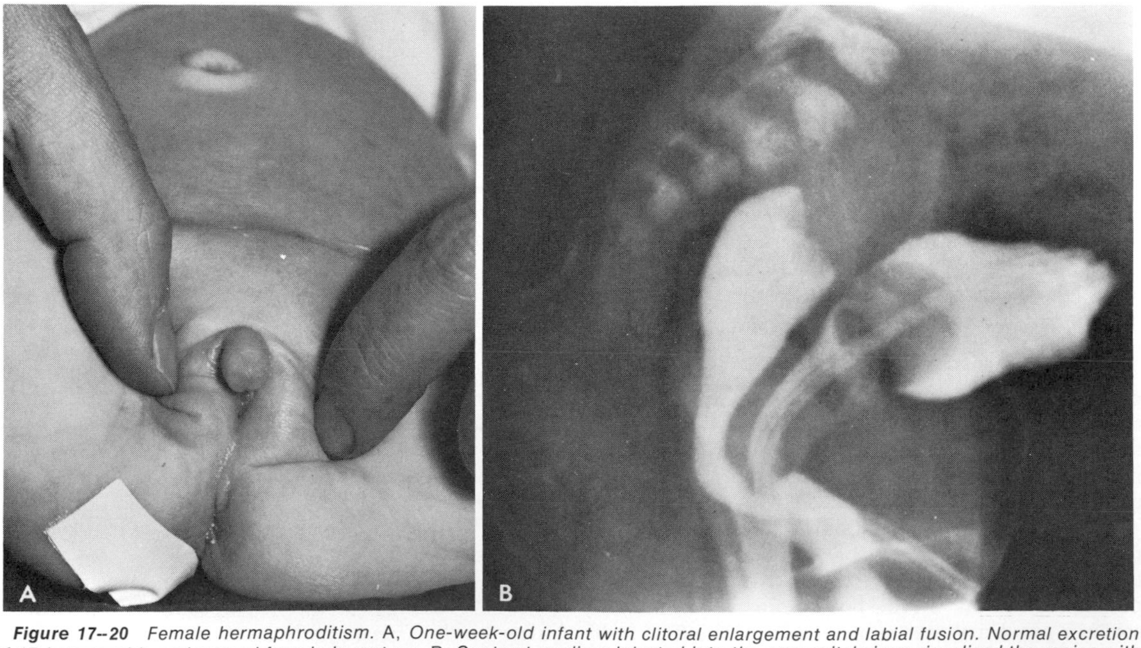

Figure 17–20 *Female hermaphroditism. A, One-week-old infant with clitoral enlargement and labial fusion. Normal excretion of 17-ketosteroids and normal female karyotype. B, Contrast medium injected into the urogenital sinus visualized the vagina with indentation of the cervix as well as the urinary bladder. The mother had received progesterone during the first trimester of pregnancy; this agent is a rare cause of masculinization of the female fetus.*

drogenase defect are usually salt losers, but are less virilized. Enlargement of the clitoris may be mild and escape detection. Labial fusion is usually present; a female with normal genitalia has been observed. In the male, varying degrees of hypospadias may occur, with or without bifid scrotum and/or cryptorchidism.

LABORATORY DATA. These three enzymatic defects are characterized by levels of urinary 17-ketosteroids higher than normal for the age of the patient. Owing to the somewhat normally elevated 17-ketosteroid levels during the first few days of life (2 to 3 mg/day), there may be difficulty in diagnosis at this time, and repeated determinations may be indicated. Examination of the urine for the dominant steroids is necessary for identification of the enzymatic defect. In the 21-hydroxylase defect, 17-hydroxyprogesterone and pregnanetriol predominate. Increased excretion of compounds S and DOC are characteristic of the 11-hydroxylase defect, whereas pregnanetriol is only moderately increased. Steroids with the Δ^5-3-β-OH configuration characterize the 3-hydroxysteroid dehydrogenase defect. In this latter defect, pregnanetriol is low initially, but after the first few months of life values may rise as a consequence of hepatic 3-β-hydroxy steroid dehydrogenase activity. Plasma levels of many steroids can now be measured by radioimmunoassay; their determinations are increasingly helpful in diagnosis.

Blood levels of cortisol and urinary excretion of its metabolites are usually normal in the compensated variant of 21-hydroxylase deficiency but do not increase further upon stimulation with ACTH. Cortisol is usually low in the salt-losing defects. Serum levels of ACTH are increased. A large part of the virilization is caused by increased levels of testosterone; the excess 17-hydroxyprogesterone is partially diverted to androstenedione which, in turn, is converted to testosterone in the periphery (Fig. 17–16).

Plasma renin activity is elevated, especially in infants with the salt-losing form of the disease. In the 21-hydroxylase deficiency, plasma levels of progesterone, 17-hydroxyprogesterone and 21-deoxycortisol are markedly elevated.

Affected females are chromatin positive and have an XX karyotype; males have a normal XY chromosome constitution. Injection of contrast medium into the urogenital sinus of female pseudohermaphrodites usually demonstrates vagina and uterus.

Salt losers have low serum concentrations of sodium and chloride and elevated levels of potassium and nonprotein nitrogen. Elevation of the serum potassium level may be responsible for electrocardiographic abnormalities.

DIAGNOSIS. A history of congenital adrenal hyperplasia in an infant or child should always alert one to the diagnosis in subsequent siblings. The salt-losing form of the disorder must be suspected in any infant who fails to thrive and especially in female infants with ambiguous external genitalia. When virilization occurs postnatally, in either the male or female, a virilizing adrenocortical tumor must be considered in the differential diagnosis.

An adrenal tumor may be palpable or suggested by displacement of the adjacent kidney as demonstrated by pyelography. Urinary 17-ketosteroid excretion is elevated with congenital hyperplasia and with cortical tumors, but very high values favor the diagnosis of a neoplasm. Large amounts of urinary pregnanetriol are highly suggestive of adrenal hyperplasia. A therapeutic test with a corticosteroid is a reliable differential procedure; administration of cortisone or one of its analogues quickly reduces excretion of urinary 17-ketosteroids to normal levels in patients with congenital adrenal hyperplasia, but does not do so in those with a virilizing tumor. Cortisone, by inhibiting secretion of corticotropin, reduces the excessive stimulation of the adrenals in patients with hyperplasia, whereas adrenocortical tumors are not subject to pituitary regulation.

In males with virilization an interstitial cell tumor of the testis and true precocious puberty must also be considered in differential diagnosis. In true precocious puberty, gonadotropins may be elevated. The urinary 17-ketosteroid level is never above normal adult values; pregnanetriol is not found in the urine; the testes are usually well developed; and interstitial cells may be seen in biopsy specimens.

Females with this condition must be differentiated from those with other causes for ambiguity of the external genitalia. Only in this condition, however, are urinary 17-ketosteroids elevated. Males with 3-β-hydroxysteroid dehydrogenase defect may be confused with female pseudohermaphrodites, owing to lack of normal virilization of the external genitalia. These male patients are chromatin-negative and do not have elevated urinary pregnanetriol levels; they are thus easily differentiated from the chromatin-positive female pseudohermaphrodite.

TREATMENT. Hydrocortisone is effective in inhibiting excessive production of adrenal androgens and in stemming the progressive virilization. The maintenance dose may be administered orally as follows: 10 to 20 mg/day to children under 5 years of age; 20 to 30 mg/day to children between 5 and 12; 30 to 50 mg/day after 12 years of age. These doses should be divided into 2 or 3 daily administrations. Such amounts suppress excessive secretion of androgens without producing undesirable effects. Analogues of hydrocortisone or cortisone are effective in suppressing adrenal androgens, but do not provide complete physiologic replacement; they are therefore contraindicated in the treatment of adrenal hyperplasia. Repeated determinations of the urinary excretion of 17-ketosteroids and pregnanetriol and careful measurements of growth are important guides in determining the adequacy of dosage.

Patients who have a disturbance of electrolyte regulation ("salt losers") must have a high salt intake and receive desoxycorticosterone acetate in addition to hydrocortisone. Dehydrated infants

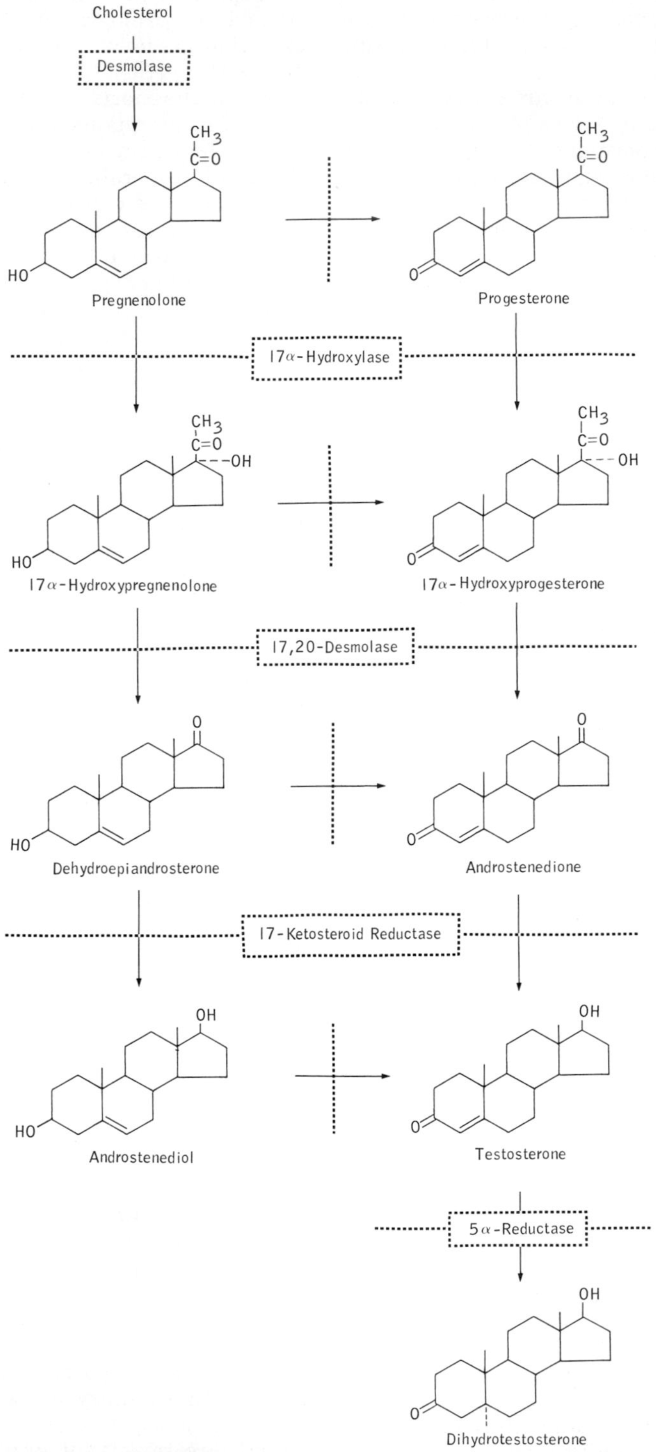

Figure 17–21 *Biosynthesis of androgens. Dotted lines indicate enzymatic defects associated with male pseudohermaphroditism. Vertical dotted line indicates defect in 3β hydroxysteroid dehydrogenase.* *(See page 1360.)*

may require 4 to 8 gm of sodium chloride for adequate replacement therapy during the first 24 hours. DOCA, 2 to 4 mg, should be given daily by intramuscular injection. Once control has been achieved, maintenance doses must be determined, after which we prefer the subcutaneous implantation of pellets of DOCA for long-term maintenance. When the pellets are exhausted, usually in a year, oral therapy is instituted with fluorohydrocortisone, in once daily doses of 0.05 to 0.1 mg. This medication is continued indefinitely in salt losers. With this regimen additional sodium chloride is usually not required, but patients are allowed free access to the salt shaker.

The administration of hydrocortisone must be continued indefinitely in *all* patients. Increased doses are indicated during periods of stress such as infection or surgery, or during periods of decreased salt intake; this is true not only of salt losers but also of all patients, including those with the 11-hydroxylase defect, since they all have defective adrenal reserve.

The enlarged clitoris of female infants usually requires surgical correction; a good age for this elective surgery is 9 months to a year. Total clitorectomy is usually performed; some prefer reduction clitoroplasty. Parents should be reassured that it has been established that complete sexual gratification, including orgasm, can be achieved in the absence of the clitoris. The menarche may occur at the appropriate age, but in perhaps as many as half of affected girls there is significant delay and it is not exceptional for adolescents past 16 not to have begun menstruating. The delay in menarche is probably related to factors in treatment leading to suboptimal control.

Nonsalt losers, particularly males, are frequently not diagnosed until 3 to 7 years of age, at which time osseous maturation may be 5 years or more in advance of chronologic age. Institution of treatment results in deceleration of growth and osseous maturation to more nearly normal rates in some children; in others, especially if the bone age is 12 years or more, spontaneous puberty may occur, therapy with hydrocortisone having suppressed production of adrenal androgens and permitted release of pituitary gonadotropins if the appropriate level of hypothalamic sensitivity is present.

Virilizing Adrenocortical Tumor

Tumors of the adrenal cortex may result in masculinization in girls and pseudoprecocious puberty in boys. Hypertension is common, and manifestations of Cushing syndrome may be present concurrently with virilization.

In males the symptoms are usually the same as those occurring with congenital adrenal hyperplasia. It is virtually impossible to differentiate the two conditions on clinical grounds. *In females* virilizing tumors of the adrenal cause masculiniza-

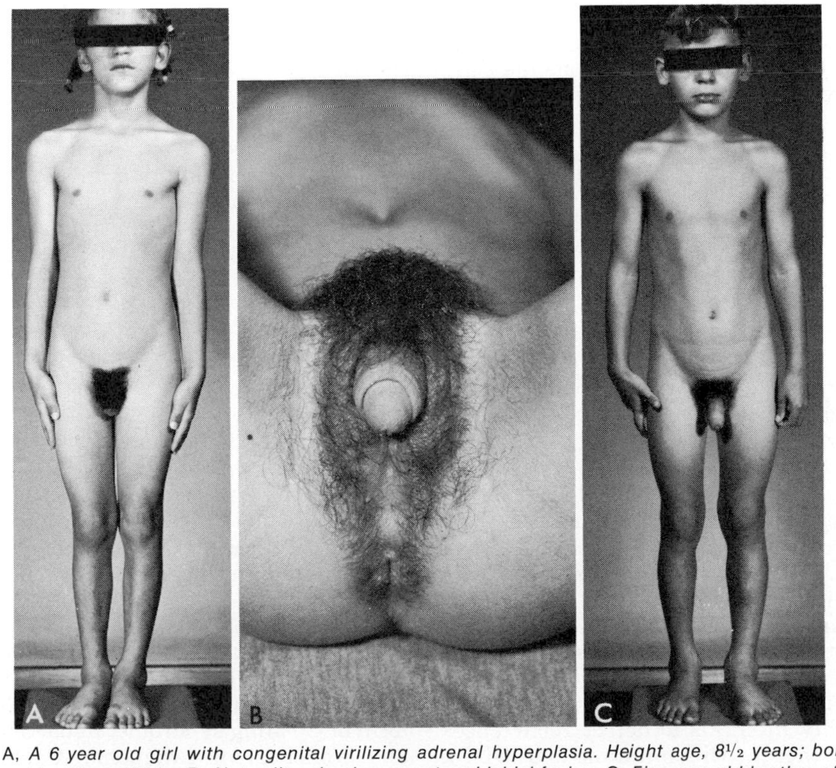

Figure 17–22 A, *A 6 year old girl with congenital virilizing adrenal hyperplasia. Height age, 8½ years; bone-age, 13 years; urinary 17-ketosteroids, 50 mg/24 hr.* B, *Note clitoral enlargement and labial fusion.* C, *Five year old brother of girl in* A *was not considered abnormal by parents. Height age, 8 years; bone-age, 12½ years; urinary 17-ketosteroids, 36 mg/24 hr.*

tion of a previously normal female, whereas congenital hyperplasia is almost always associated with genital abnormalities at birth. There have been a few instances of congenital adrenal hyperplasia in which virilization had its onset postnatally, and an adrenal adenoma is known to have caused intrauterine virilization manifest by clitoral enlargement and mild labial fusion.

Tumors of the adrenal (both with or without Cushing syndrome) have been associated with hemihypertrophy in 10 children, usually during the first few years of life. These tumors are also associated with Beckwith syndrome and other congenital defects, particularly genitourinary tract and central nervous system abnormalities and hamartomatous defects.

Urinary 17-ketosteroids are usually increased, occasionally only modestly but more often markedly, and may exceed 100 mg/day. Recently adrenal adenomas have been recognized which secrete testosterone without significant amounts of adrenal androgens. For example, a 20 month old virilized girl has been reported to have normal levels of 17-ketosteroid excretion but levels of testosterone equivalent to those found in early puberty in males. Assay of testosterone production is essential to the investigation of virilized patients. Selective venous sampling may be indicated to localize small tumors. Roentgenographic studies may reveal calcification in the tumor or displacement of a kidney during pyelography.

The differential diagnosis of virilizing adrenal hyperplasia and adrenal cortical tumor is discussed above.

The treatment is surgical; a transperitoneal approach is usually recommended. Some of these neoplasms are highly malignant and metastasize widely, but cure with regression of the masculinizing features may follow removal of less malignant encapsulated tumors.

A neoplasm of one adrenal may be responsible for atrophy of the other one, owing to excessive production of cortical hormones by the tumor and suppression of the expected stimulation of the normal gland by ACTH. Consequently adrenal insufficiency may follow surgical removal of the tumor. This situation can be avoided by giving 100 mg of cortisone daily, starting on the day of operation and continuing for 3 or 4 days postoperatively. It may also be necessary to give corticotropin concurrently with cortisone to reactivate the atrophied gland. Adequate quantities of water, sodium chloride and glucose must also be provided. On rare occasions the tumors are bilateral and in at least five instances the contralateral adrenal was absent; in such instances, replacement therapy must be continued indefinitely.

The recurrence rate of these tumors is high. Urinary excretion of 17-ketosteroids returns to normal postoperatively if removal of the tumor is complete. The 17-ketosteroid level should be measured at monthly intervals to detect recurrences early. Intensive therapy with mitotane (o,p′-DDD), an isomer of DDD, is indicated for inoperable tumors and for recurrences. This agent can induce regression of metastases and of abnormal steroid excretion, but no cures have been recorded.

CUSHING SYNDROME

Cushing syndrome, a characteristic pattern of obesity in association with hypertension, is the result of maintenance of abnormally high blood levels of hydrocortisone owing to hyperfunction of the adrenal cortex.

ETIOLOGY. The adrenal lesion in infants is often a *functioning tumor,* which is usually a malignant cortical carcinoma; only rarely is it a benign cortical adenoma or bilateral nodular cortical hyperplasia. Patients with cortical tumors often exhibit a mixed form of hypercorticism, owing to overproduction of such other steroids as androgens, estrogens and aldosterone.

Over 50 per cent of cortical tumors occur in children 3 years of age or less and 85 per cent occur in children age 7 years or less.

Spontaneous occurrence of *bilateral hyperplasia* of the adrenal glands is referred to as *Cushing disease.* This condition, formerly thought to be rare in children, is being detected with increasing frequency. Of the 36 reported patients, 75 per cent were over 7 years of age. When Harvey Cushing described the entity in 1932, he attributed it to a basophilic adenoma of the pituitary, but such tumors, if they occur in childhood, are rarely demonstrable before treatment is initiated. The initiating factor for the adrenal hyperplasia is not known; a hypothalamic disturbance is suspected. There is increased secretion of corticotropin, loss of its normal circadian rhythm and relative resistance to suppression of its secretion by glucocorticoids. The failure of growth hormone levels to rise during sleep, even when the disease is in remission, gives additional evidence of hypothalamic dysfunction.

It is possible that overstimulation of the pituitary by the hypothalamic defect may be the cause of pituitary tumors. Enlargement of the sella prior to treatment is extremely rare in children, whereas 7 per cent of adults with Cushing disease show this. The tumors found consist principally of chromophobe cells. In patients with normal-sized sellas, pituitary tumors may appear after adrenalectomy, even in children, and it appears that adrenalectomy may favor the progression or the development of such tumors. These tumors produce increased levels melanocyte-stimulating hormone as well as ACTH; intense pigmentation of the skin and mucous membranes heralds their development.

Bilateral hyperplasia of the adrenals may also occur as a result of production of *ectopic production of ACTH* or of material with ACTH-like activity. In adults, a variety of tumors have caused this form of Cushing syndrome, in particular thymoma and bronchogenic carcinoma. Cushing syndrome has been associated with an islet cell tumor of the

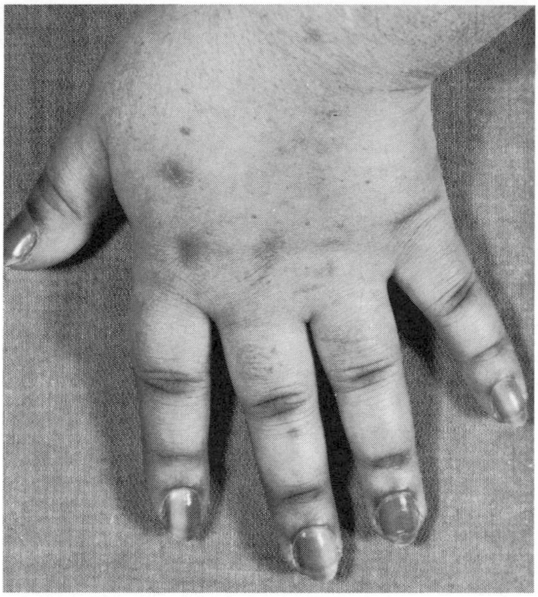

Figure 17–23 Pigmentation of skin in a 12 year old girl with postadrenalectomy pituitary tumor. Note pigmentation of nails and skin folds. Adrenalectomy was performed for Cushing syndrome due to bilateral adrenal hyperplasia, when the girl was 10 years of age. Pigmentation, headaches and enlargement of the sella turcica developed 1 year after adrenalectomy.

pancreas in a 2 year old boy, with neuroblastoma or ganglioneuroblastoma in several children and with a hemangiopericytoma arising from the cerebral tentorium in a 7 year old boy.

Prolonged exogenous administration of corticotropin or hydrocortisone or its analogues results in a clinical pattern identical to the spontaneous disorder and is frequently referred to as *cushingoid syndrome.*

CLINICAL MANIFESTATIONS. Symptoms may begin in the neonatal period or anytime thereafter.

The syndrome has been recognized in infants under a year of age on at least 35 occasions. Early in life girls outnumber boys 3 to 1, and adrenocortical tumors (carcinoma, adenoma and nodular hyperplasia) are the usual causative lesions. The disorder appears to be more severe and the clinical findings more flagrant than later in life. The face is rounded, the cheeks are prominent and flushed (moon facies). The chin is doubled, there is a buffalo hump, and generalized obesity is common. Signs of abnormal masculinization occur frequently, owing to the androgen production of tumors; accordingly, there may be hypertrichosis on the face and trunk, pubic hair, acne, deepening of the voice and, in girls, enlargement of the clitoris. Growth is impaired and length is usually below the third percentile; when significant virilization is present, growth may be normal or even accelerated. Hypertension is common and may lead to heart failure. There is increased susceptibility to infection, which may lead to fatal sepsis. Although infants with Cushing syndrome are monstrous in appearance, they are generally very fragile. Occasionally the condition may be associated with hemihypertrophy or other congenital defects.

In older children bilateral hyperplasia of the adrenals is the most common lesion and the sex incidence is equal. In addition to obesity, short stature is a common presenting feature. Gradual onset of obesity and deceleration or cessation of growth may be the only early manifestations. Purplish striae on the hips, abdomen and thighs are common. Pubertal development may be delayed, or amenorrhea may occur in girls of menarcheal age. Weakness, headache, deterioration in schoolwork and emotional lability may be prominent clinical features. Hypertension is usually present. Renal stones have occurred both in older children and in infants.

LABORATORY DATA. Polycythemia, lymphopenia and eosinopenia are common. The glucose tolerance test may be diabetic in spite of elevated levels of insulin. Levels of serum electrolytes are usually normal, but on occasion potassium may be decreased.

Corticosteroids in blood and urine are usually elevated, but these levels may fluctuate widely from day to day, and repeated determinations may be required to establish the diagnosis. In the majority of patients with Cushing syndrome, the normal diurnal rhythm in levels of plasma cortisol is abolished, and measurements of the levels at 8 A.M., and 8 P.M. may be useful, except in children under 3 years of age, in whom the circadian rhythm is not always established. Urinary 17-ketosteroids may be increased, particularly in virilized patients; very high levels usually indicate adrenal carcinoma.

Special studies are frequently necessary to establish the definitive diagnosis or to differentiate hyperplasia from tumor. Multiple tests may be necessary, particularly in those children with adrenal hyperplasia who have only moderate symptomatology. The dexamethasone suppression test has been devised for this purpose. Administration of 0.5 mg of dexamethasone every 6 hours for 2 days results in suppression of urinary excretion of corticosteroids in normal persons, but not in patients with Cushing syndrome. The same test with a larger dose, 2 mg every 6 hours for 2 days, results in suppression in patients with Cushing disease owing to bilateral adrenal hyperplasia, but not in those with adrenocortical tumors. The test has given both false positive and false negative results. Moreover, the test was devised for use in adults and further experience is needed in children to establish the optimal dose of dexamethasone for differentiation of normal subjects from those with Cushing disease. Studies in adults have recently indicated that the reliability of the dexamethasone test is significantly improved when free cortisol excretion is measured.

Osseous maturation is usually moderately retarded but may be normal; in virilized children the bone age is apt to be advanced. Osteoporosis is common and is most evident in roentgenograms of the spine. Pathologic fractures may be noted. The pituitary sella is usually normal. Diminution of muscle mass and increased deposition of adipose tissue may be noted in roentgenograms of the extremities. The thymic shadow is absent because involution occurs, owing to excessive cortisol. Adrenal tumors occasionally have calcifications and frequently cause displacement of the kidney on the affected side.

DIFFERENTIAL DIAGNOSIS. Cushing syndrome is frequently suspected in children with obesity, particularly when there are striae and hypertension. Differential diagnosis is complicated by the frequent occurrence of elevated urinary concentrations of corticosteroids secondary to obesity alone. Children with simple obesity are usually tall, whereas those with Cushing syndrome are short or decelerating in growth rate. The excretion of urinary corticoids is rapidly suppressed by oral administration of low doses of dexamethasone in persons with uncomplicated obesity.

TREATMENT. Treatment of Cushing syndrome is primarily surgical. If the lesion is benign cortical adenoma, unilateral adrenalectomy is indicated. Such adenomas are occasionally bilateral and the treatment of choice is subtotal adrenalectomy. In either instance, an excellent therapeutic result is achieved by removal of the tumor. Adrenocortical carcinomas, on the other hand, frequently metastasize, especially to the liver and lungs, and the prognosis may be unfavorable in spite of removal of the primary lesion. Rarely, the tumors are bilateral and total adrenalectomy is required. It is often impossible to differentiate benign and malignant tumors by histologic appearance alone.

The optimal treatment of bilateral adrenal hyperplasia (Cushing disease) is generally considered to be total adrenalectomy. After subtotal adrenalectomy, the remaining segment of the adrenal frequently undergoes hyperplasia, and symptoms recur. In some patients after adrenalectomy, there is enlargement of the sella and appearance of chromophobe adenomas even with adequate replacement therapy with cortisol. Slight increase in pigmentation may occur after adrenalectomy and is of no clinical import, but intense melanosis is generally a harbinger of a pituitary tumor *(Nelson syndrome)*. Large doses of hydrocortisone pre- and postoperatively have been recommended to avert the possibly too rapid withdrawal of endogenous cortisol.

Management of patients undergoing adrenalectomy requires adequate and pre- and postoperative replacement therapy with a corticosteroid. Tumors which produce corticosteroids usually lead to atrophy of the opposite adrenal, and replacement with both cortisol and corticotropin may be required. Patients with adrenal hyperplasia must be carefully watched after adrenalectomy for the development of pituitary tumor. Periodic examination of the pituitary fossa and of the ocular system are indicated. Postoperative complications have included sepsis, pancreatitis, thrombosis, poor wound healing and sudden collapse, particularly in infants with Cushing syndrome. Substantial catch-up growth occurs but adult height is often compromised.

EXCESS MINERALOCORTICOID SECRETION

The principal mineralocorticoid secreted by the adrenal is aldosterone. Increased secretion may result from a primary defect of the adrenal (primary hyperaldosteronism) or from factors which activate the renin-angiotensin system (secondary hyperaldosteronism). When excess mineralocorticoid secretion occurs, hypertension or hypokalemia is usually present, except in those patients who have secondary hyperaldosteronism.

Desoxycorticosterone is a precursor of aldosterone, with only about one thirtieth the sodium-retaining potency of aldosterone (see Fig. 17–3), and overproduction of desoxycorticosterone occurs in two different defects of adrenal steroidogenesis. The first of these is a defect in 11-hydroxylation, which also leads to androgen excess and presents clinically as the hypertensive form of the adrenogenital syndrome (see above). The second defect involves 17-hydroxylation, and presents as hypogonadism in the female and as male pseudohermaphroditism in the male since the defect impairs the synthesis of androgens and estrogens as well as of adrenal steroids.

PRIMARY ALDOSTERONISM

ETIOLOGY. Primary hyperaldosteronism occurs most often in the third and fourth decades of life and is rare in childhood. The most common cause in affected adults is a functioning adrenocortical tumor (aldosteronoma). Such tumors have been found in children, the youngest being a 3 year old child. In other children, hyperaldosteronism has been associated with adrenal hyperplasia of unknown origin; the term *congenital aldosteronism* has been used to describe this condition. Demonstration of low renin levels provides strong supportive evidence for a primary adrenal defect; this was the case in the instances in which it was measured. Since most patients improved after resection of the adrenal, it is presumed that the adrenal disorder is primary in these children. Clinical manifestations always include hypertension; it is usually severe and leads to retinopathy and cardiomegaly.

CLINICAL MANIFESTATIONS. Besides hypertension, excess production of mineralocorticoids may produce polydipsia, polyuria, nocturia, paresthesias, visual disturbance, intermittent paralysis, tetany, fatigue and muscle weakness and discomfort. The severe growth retardation and muscular weakness which may occur are probably caused by potassium depletion.

The urine is neutral or alkaline, and the kidneys lose their ability to concentrate urine normally. The serum pH, carbon dioxide content and sodium concentrations are elevated, and the serum potassium, chloride and magnesium levels are decreased. Tetany occurs in spite of normal serum levels of calcium. Urinary excretion of 17-ketosteroids and 17-hydroxycorticosteroids is within normal limits, but urinary excretion of aldosterone is increased. The abnormalities of renal function are attributed to "clear-cell nephrosis," a lesion characteristic of chronic hypokalemia.

Differentiation of children with functioning adrenal adenomas from those with adrenal hyperplasia can be established only by exploratory laparotomy.

DIFFERENTIAL DIAGNOSIS

Secondary Hyperaldosteronism. Secretion of aldosterone is increased in conditions in which there are low body sodium, excessive accumulation of potassium, and/or dehydration; it is a normal homeostatic response. Hyperaldosteronism also occurs in many common disorders such as the nephrotic syndrome, congestive cardiac failure and cirrhosis of the liver. Since the extracellular fluid volume is increased in these conditions, the increased aldosterone excretion is paradoxical and its mechanism unknown. Increased secretion of aldosterone may also occur in conditions in which renin is increased, such as in stenosis of the renal artery and in malignant or essential hypertension.

In patients with hypertension and increased excretion of aldosterone, it may be difficult to separate primary from secondary hyperaldosteronism. Urinary aldosterone levels are, in any case, only moderately increased and it is essential to the diagnosis of primary aldosteronism to demonstrate relative unresponsiveness to the restriction and administration of sodium. The most important diagnostic finding is the level of serum renin during sodium restriction. In secondary hyperaldosteronism, serum renin is high or rises during a low-salt diet, whereas in primary adrenal hypersecretion of aldosterone, the renin-angiotensin system is suppressed.

Bartter Syndrome. This is characterized by hypochloremia, hypokalemic alkalosis and growth failure. The blood pressure is normal, however, and there is increased secretion of renin as well as of aldosterone. Renal biopsy reveals hyperplasia of the juxtaglomerular apparatus. The elevated levels of renin have been attributed to diminished effective blood volume, but other studies indicate that excess renin production may be the primary event. It has been demonstrated that the erythrocytes of patients with Bartter syndrome have an abnormal transport mechanism; a similar defect in the juxtaglomerular cells has been proposed as a cause for the excessive renin production.

Pseudohypoaldosteronism. This is also characterized by increased urinary aldosterone and elevated secretion rates of aldosterone. However, affected infants exhibit salt-wasting symptoms, hyponatremia and hyperkalemia. Elevated plasma renin activity indicates that the hyperaldosteronism is secondary to hyperactivity of the renin-angiotensin system.

Familial Glucocorticoid Suppressible Aldosteronism. This condition of unknown cause closely mimics primary hyperaldosteronism. It has been described in three kindreds and in a single patient. The finding that some patients have affected parents suggests an autosomal dominant mode of transmission. As is the case for primary hyperaldosteronism, affected patients have hypertension, mild alkalosis, hypokalemia and increased levels of aldosterone which are not altered by restriction or excess of sodium. Plasma renin activity is low. Administration of dexamethasone (1 mg/24 hr) results in marked suppression of aldosterone and in the disappearance of the hypertension. This dramatic response to glucocorticoid suppression emphasizes the importance of a trial of such therapy in hypertensive patients with hyperaldosteronism.

Differentiation of children with functioning adrenal adenomas from those with adrenal hyperplasia can be established only by exploratory laparotomy.

TREATMENT. Removal of an aldosteronoma results in cure. The electrolyte abnormality is usually corrected within 10 days, but the blood pressure may not return to normal for several months after operation. In instances of congenital aldosteronism bilateral adrenalectomy is indicated; the results are excellent. Adrenal replacement therapy is, of course, required.

FEMINIZING ADRENAL TUMORS

Adrenocortical tumors associated with excessive production of estrogens and feminization have been recorded in many males, but only 4 patients were children. In these, gynecomastia was the initial clinical manifestation, appearing between 2 and 7 years of age. Growth and development may be normal, or virilization may be present as evidenced by acne, deep voice, phallic enlargement and advanced osseous maturation. Hypertension is common in adults, but has not been observed in children. The demonstration of abnormally high concentration of urinary estrogens and, in some instances, of 17-ketosteroids supports the diagnosis. The tumor may be a benign adenoma or a carcinoma. Gynecomastia regresses after removal of the tumor, and hormone values return to normal.

An instance of an adrenal tumor causing feminization (isosexual precocity) in a $5\frac{1}{2}$ year old girl has also been recorded. In this child there was no clinical evidence of Cushing syndrome or of virilism; 17-ketosteroids as well as estrogens were in the adult range.

EXCESSIVE SECRETION OF CATECHOLAMINES

PHEOCHROMOCYTOMA

The pheochromocytoma, a catecholamine-secreting tumor, arises from the chromaffin cells. The most common site of origin is the adrenal medulla; tumors may develop, however, anywhere along the abdominal sympathetic chain and are particularly apt to be located near the aorta at the level of the inferior mesenteric artery or at its bifurcation. They also appear in the periadrenal area, the urinary bladder or ureteral walls, the thoracic cavity and the cervical region. Less than 5 per cent of reported instances have been in children. Tumors vary in size from about 1 to 10 cm in diameter; they are found more often on the right side than on the left. In 20 per cent of affected children the adrenal tumors are bilateral, and in 30 per cent tumors are found both in the adrenal and in extra-adrenal areas or only in an extra-adrenal area.

Pheochromocytoma is frequently inherited as an autosomal dominant trait. In affected families the ages of patients at the time of diagnosis have varied from the first to the fifth decade of life; more than half the patients have had multiple tumors.

Pheochromocytoma is frequently associated with other syndromes or tumors. Approximately 5 per cent of patients with pheochromocytoma have neurofibromatosis. Sporadic as well as familial instances of pheochromocytoma have been noted in patients with von Hippel-Lindau disease. Kinships have been reported in which some affected members also have asymptomatic islet cell adenomas, and some in which members with pheochromocytoma are asymptomatic, although urinary concentration of catecholamines is elevated.

Pheochromocytoma also may coexist with medullary carcinoma of the thyroid and parathyroid disease; this association is known as *Sipple syndrome.* Some patients with these two tumors may also have multiple mucosal neuromas. The neuromas appear early in life and affect primarily the tongue and lips; they may also affect the gingival, buccal or conjunctival mucosa (See above, this Section.).

These syndromes are all inherited in a dominant fashion; in a single kindred there may be individuals with only a limited number of the manifestations and some with complete expression of the syndrome.

CLINICAL MANIFESTATIONS. These are the result of excessive secretion of epinephrine and norepinephrine; the variability of the clinical picture is related to the quantitative variations in their secretion. All patients have hypertension at some time. The hypertension is usually sustained, but it may often be *paroxysmal.* Paroxysms should particularly suggest pheochromocytoma as a diagnostic possibility. When there are paroxysms of hypertension, the attacks are usually infrequent at first, but become more frequent and eventually give way to a continuous hypertensive state. Between attacks of hypertension the patient may be free of symptoms. During attacks the patient complains of headache and palpitation, and pallor, vomiting and sweating are noticed. Convulsions and other manifestations of hypertensive encephalopathy may occur. In severe cases precordial pains radiate into the arms, and pulmonary edema and cardiac and hepatic enlargement may develop. The child has a good appetite but does not gain weight, and severe cachexia may develop. Polyuria and polydipsia can be sufficiently severe to suggest diabetes insipidus. Growth failure may be striking. The blood pressure may range from 180 to 260 systolic and 120 to 210 diastolic, and the heart may be enlarged. Ophthalmoscopic examination may reveal papilledema, hemorrhages, exudate and arterial constriction.

LABORATORY DATA. The urine contains protein, a few casts and, occasionally, glucose. Gross hematuria suggests that the tumor is in the bladder wall. In many instances the basal metabolic rate may be as high as +50 or +60. Polycythemia is occasionally noted.

The most direct and specific test is the demonstration of increased urinary excretion of catecholamines or of VMA (3-methoxy-4-hydroxymandelic acid), a major metabolite of epinephrine and norepinephrine (Fig. 17–15). The daily urinary excretions of catecholamines and VMA by normal children increase with age; when adjusted to surface area, they are equivalent to those of adults. There is a direct relation between the concentrations of catecholamines in the tumor and in the urine. Norepinephrine is increased in the urine in all patients; when epinephrine is also increased, it strongly suggests that the tumor is adrenal in location. Pharmacologic tests using adrenergic blocking agents or histamine have been utilized for diagnosis; they are not as reliable as determinations of VMA and are now rarely indicated.

DIFFERENTIAL DIAGNOSIS. The various causes of hypertension in children must be considered, such as renal disease, coarctation of the aorta, acrodynia, thallium intoxication, hyperthyroidism, Cushing syndrome, congenital adrenal hyperplasia and essential hypertension. A nonfunctioning kidney may result from compression of a ureter or of a renal artery by a pheochromocytoma. With paroxysmal hypertension, the diagnosis of familial dysautonomia must also be considered. Urinary excretion of VMA is low in familial dysautonomia, owing to a defect in release rather than in synthesis of catecholamines. Cerebral disorders, diabetes insipidus, diabetes mellitus and hyperthyroidism must also be considered in the differential diagnosis. Hypertension in patients with neurofibromatosis may be caused by renal vascular involvement as well as by concurrent pheochromocytoma.

Neuroblastoma, ganglioneuroblastoma and ganglioneuroma frequently produce catecholamines. Secreting neurogenic tumors commonly produce hypertension, excessive sweating, flushing, pallor, rash, polyuria and polydipsia. Diarrhea may also be associated with these tumors, particularly with ganglioneuroma, and may at times be sufficiently persistent to suggest the "celiac syndrome."

TREATMENT. Localization of the tumor is often difficult; only rarely can it be discovered by palpation. Pyelography may reveal the location of the tumor, but often it is located only by surgical exploration. Retroperitoneal gas insufflation, aortography or venous catheterization and sampling of blood at different levels for catecholamine determinations are only rarely necessary to localize the tumor. Since these tumors are often multiple, especially in children, a thorough transabdominal exploration of all the usual sites of localization offers the best insurance for locating all of them. Removal of the tumor(s) results in cure. Although these tumors often appear malignant histologically, only rarely has malignancy been unequivocally established, as demonstrated by the metastasis to lymph nodes of hormonally active chromaffin cells. The operation is not without danger, because an extreme rise of blood pressure may result from massive discharge of hormone during the operative manipulation. Shock from a precipitous drop of blood pressure during operation or within the first 48 postoperative hours is also a danger. These risks can be lessened by the proper preoperative preparation of the patient, by careful monitoring during surgery and by continuous postoperative surveillance. The urinary excretion of VMA should be determined after operation as a measure of the completeness of the surgical removal. Prolonged follow-up is indicated, since functioning tumors at another site may become manifest many years after the initial operation. Examination of relatives of affected patients may reveal other persons harboring unsuspected tumors. In one family with 10 affected individuals the highest blood pressures and urinary concentrations of catecholamines were found in the children, whereas some of the affected adults were normotensive and had only moderately elevated urinary concentrations of catecholamines and VMA.

OTHER CATECHOLAMINE-SECRETING NEURAL TUMORS

Elaboration of excessive catecholamines is not exclusive to pheochromocytomas, but frequently occurs with other neurogenic tumors (neuroblastoma, ganglioneuroblastoma and, less frequently, ganglioneuroma). As a consequence, many of the systemic manifestations characteristic of pheochromocytoma may be seen in patients with other tumors of neural origin. Hypertension, excessive sweating, flushing, pallor, rash, polyuria and polydipsia are the most common findings. Chronic diarrhea may be the only symptom, or it may occur in association with other manifestations. Diarrhea is rarely a prominent manifestation in patients with pheochromocytoma, and the biochemical basis for this symptom in patients with neural tumors is not known. Diarrhea is more apt to occur in association with ganglioneuromas, but it may occur with ganglioneuroblastoma or neuroblastoma. Benign adrenal cortical hyperplasia with Cushing disease has been observed in children with these neural tumors; the secretion of an ACTH-like hormone by the tumor is a likely but not proved explanation. An 18 month old girl has been reported who had a ganglioneuroblastoma as well as an adrenocortical adenoma in each adrenal.

A high percentage of patients with these tumors have increased excretion of dopa, dopamine, norepinephrine, normetanephrine, homovanillic acid and vanilmandelic acid (VMA). Patients with pheochromocytoma usually excrete only epinephrine, norepinephrine, their methoxy analogues and VMA (Fig. 17–15). Elevated excretion of homovanillic acid generally indicates malignant pheochromocytoma or other malignant neural tumors, but it has been noted also with benign pheochromocytoma. Differentiation on a biochemical basis between neuroblastomas, ganglioneuroblastomas and benign ganglioneuromas is not possible. Repeated determinations of VMA and catecholamines, and particularly of norepinephrine and dopamine, are helpful in detecting recurrences and in assessing the effectiveness of therapy. Excretion of these compounds returns to normal if the tumor is completely removed.

A few catecholamine-secreting glomic tumors (chemodectomas) arising in the carotid or jugular bodies have been observed. Whether the cells comprising these tumors are neural in origin is unsettled.

CALCIFICATION WITHIN THE ADRENAL

Calcification within the adrenal glands may occur in a wide variety of situations, some serious and others of no obvious consequence. Adrenal calcifications are often detected as an incidental finding in radiographic studies of the abdomen in infants and children. One may elicit a history of anoxia or trauma at birth. Hemorrhage into the adrenal at or immediately after birth is probably the common factor which leads to subsequent calcification. Though it is advisable to assess the adrenocortical reserve of such patients, there is rarely any functional disorder.

Neuroblastomas, ganglioneuromas, cortical carcinomas, pheochromocytomas and cysts of the adrenal gland may each be responsible for calcifications, particularly if hemorrhage has occurred within the tumor. Calcification in such lesions is almost always unilateral.

The most common infection associated with calcifications within the adrenal is tuberculosis, and the patient usually has the clinical manifestations of Addison disease. Calcifications may also develop in the adrenal glands of children who recover from the Waterhouse-Friderichsen syndrome; such patients are usually asymptomatic.

Infants with *Wolman syndrome,* a rare lipid storage disease, have extensive bilateral calcifications of the adrenal glands. The clinical manifestations include hepatosplenomegaly, gastrointestinal symptoms, and failure to thrive; rapid clinical deterioration and death by 3 to 4 months of age are the usual course. The lipids stored in the affected tissues are cholesteryl esters and triglycerides. Deposition of lipids is especially heavy in the adrenal, but the cause of the calcifications is not known. The disorder is recessively transmitted. It is probable that the patients who have been reported to have had adrenal calcifications in association with Niemann-Pick disease have had this form of xanthomatosis.

GENERAL

Baxter, J. D., and Forsham, P. H.: Tissue effects of glucocorticoids. Am. J. Med. *53*:573, 1972.

Franks, R. C.: Urinary 17-hydroxycorticosteroid and cortisol excretion in childhood. J. Clin. Endocrinol. Metab. *36*:702, 1973.

Johannisson, E.: The foetal adrenal cortex in the human. Its ultrastructure at different stages of development and in different functional states. Acta Endocrinol. Supp. 130, 1968.

Tyler, F. H., and West, C. D.: Laboratory evaluation of disorders of the adrenal cortex. Am. J. Med. *53*:664, 1972.

Villee, D. B.: The development of steroidogenesis. Am. J. Med. *53*:533, 1972.

Visser, H. K. A.: The Adrenal Cortex. Arch. Dis. Child. *41*:2; 113, 1966.

Wilkins, L.: The Diagnosis and Treatment of Endocrine Disorders in Childhood and Adolescence. 3rd ed. Springfield, Ill., Charles C Thomas, 1965.

Williams, G. H., and Dluhy, R. G.: Aldosterone biosynthesis. Am. J. Med. *53*:595, 1972.

Adrenal Cortical Insufficiency

Blizzard, R. M., and Gibbs, J. H.: Candidiasis: Studies pertaining to its association with endocrinopathies and pernicious anemia. Pediatrics *42*:231, 1968.

Blizzard, R. M., and Kyle, M.: Studies of the adrenal antigens and antibodies in Addison's disease. J. Clin. Invest. *42*:1653, 1963.

Boyd, J. F., and McDonald, A. M.: Adrenal cortical hypoplasia in siblings. Arch. Dis. Child. *35*:561, 1960.

Camacho, A. M., Kowarski, A., Migeon, C. J., and Brough, A. J.: Congenital adrenal hyperplasia due to a deficiency of one of the enzymes in the biosyntheses of pregnenolone. J. Clin. Endocrinol. *28*:153, 1968.

Castells, S., Fikrig, S., Inamdar, S., and Orti, S.: Familial moniliasis, defective delayed hypersensitivity and adrenocorticotropic hormone deficiency. J. Pediatr. *79*:72, 1971.

Clayton, B. E., Edwards, R. W. H., and Renwick, A. G. C.: Adrenal function in children. Arch. Dis. Child. *38*:49, 1963.

David, R., Golan, S., and Drucker, W.: Familial aldosterone deficiency, enzyme defect, diagnosis and clinical course. Pediatrics *4*:403, 1968.

Ehrlich, R. M.: Ectopic and hypoplastic pituitary with adrenal hypoplasia; Case report. J. Pediatr. *51*:377, 1957.

Green, W. L., and Ingbar, S. H.: Decreased corticotropin reserve as an isolated pituitary defect. Arch. Intern. Med. *108*:945, 1961.

Hintz, R. L., Menking, M., and Sotos, J. F.: Familial holoprosencephaly with endocrine dysgenesis. J. Pediatr. *72*:81, 1968.

Hung, W., Migeon, C. J., and Parrott, R. H.: A possible autoimmune basis for Addison's disease in three siblings, one with idiopathic hypoparathyroidism. Pernicious anemia and superficial moniliasis. New Engl. J. Med. *269*:658, 1963.

Kelch, R. P., Kaplan, S. L., Biglieri, E. G., Daniels, G. H., Epstein, C. J., and Grumbach, M. M.: Hereditary adrenocortical unresponsiveness to adrenocorticotropin hormone. J. Pediatr. *81*:726, 1972.

Kenny, F. M., Reynolds, J. W., and Green, O. C.: Partial 3β-hydroxysteroid dehydrogenase (3β-HSD) deficiency in a family with congenital adrenal hyperplasia: Evidence for increasing 3β-HSD activity with age. Pediatrics *48*:256, 1971.

Kerenyi, N.: Congenital adrenal hypoplasia. Report of a case with extreme adrenal hypoplasia and neurohypophyseal aplasia drawing attention to certain aspects of etiology and classification. Arch. Path. *71*:336, 1961.

Kersh, A. K., Roe, T. F., and Kogut, M. D.: Adrenocorticotropic hormone unresponsiveness: Report of a girl with excessive growth and review of 16 reported cases. J. Pediatr. *80*:610, 1972.

Kirkland, R. T., Kirkland, J. L., Johnson, C. M., Horning, M. G., Librik, L., and Clayton, G. W.: Congenital lipoid adrenal hyperplasia in an eight-year-old phenotypic female. J. Clin. Endocrinol. Metab. *36*:488, 1973.

Kreines, K., and DeVaux, W. D.: Neonatal adrenal insufficiency associated with maternal Cushing syndrome. Pediatrics *47*:516, 1971.

Margaretten, W., and McAdams, A. J.: An appraisal of fulminant meningococcemia with reference to the Shwartzman phenomenon. Am. J. Med. *25*:868, 1958.

Migeon, C. J., Kenny, F. M., Hung, W., and Voorhees, M. L.: Study of adrenal function in children with meningitis. Pediatrics. *40*:163, 1967.

Moshang, T., Rosenfield, R. L., Bongiovanni, A. M., Parks, J. S., and Amrhein, J. A.: Familial glucocorticoid insufficiency. J. Pediatr. *82*:821, 1973.

Qazi, Q. H., and Thompson, M. W.: Incidence of salt-losing form of congenital virilizing adrenal hyperplasia. Arch. Dis. Child. *47*:302, 1972.

Rappaport, R., Dray, F., Legrand, J. C., and Royer, P.: Hypoaldostéronism congénital familial par défant de la 18-OH-déhydrogénase. Pediatr. Res. *2*:456, 1968.

Sperling, M. A., Wolfsen, A. R., and Fisher, D. A.: Congenital adrenal hypoplasia: An isolated defect of organogenesis. J. Pediatr. *82*:444, 1973.

Søvik, O., Oseid, S., and Vidnes, J.: Ketotic hypoglycemia in a four-year-old boy with adrenal cortical insufficiency. Acta Paediatr. Scand. *61*:465, 1972.

Steiker, D. D., Bongiovanni, A. M., Eberlein, W. R., and Leboeuf, G.: Adrenocortical and adrenocorticotropic function in children. J. Pediatr. *59*:885, 1961.

Turkington, R. W., and Stempfel, R. S.: Adrenocortical atrophy and diffuse cerebral sclerosis (Addison-Schilder's disease). J. Pediatr. *69*:406, 1966.

Adrenal Cortical Hyperfunction

Bacon, G. E., and Lowrey, G. H.: Feminizing adrenal tumor in a six-year-old boy. J. Clin. Endocrinol. *25*:1403, 1965.

Bongiovanni, A. M.: Disorders of adrenocortical steroid biogenesis. The adrenogenital syndrome associated with congenital adrenal hyperplasia. *In* Stanbury, J. B., Wyngaarden, J. B., and Fredrickson, D. S. (eds.): The Metabolic Basis of Inherited Disease. 3rd ed. New York, McGraw-Hill Book Company, Inc., 1972.

Bricaire, H., et al.: A new male pseudohermaphroditism associated with hypertension due to a block of a 17α-hydroxylation. J. Clin. Endocrinol. Metab. *35*:67, 1972.

Brook, C. G. D., Bambach, M., Zachmann, M., and Prader, A.: Familial congenital adrenal hyperplasia. Helv. Paediatr. Acta *28*:277, 1973.

Burkinshaw, J. H., O'Brien, D., and Pendower, J. E. H.: Cushing's syndrome associated with an islet-cell tumor of the pancreas in a boy aged two years. Arch. Dis. Child. *42*:525, 1967.

Burr, I. M., Sullivan, J., Graham, T., Hartman, W. H., and O'Neill, J.: A testosterone-secreting tumour of the adrenal producing virilization in a female infant. Lancet *2*:643, 1973.

Dahms, W. T., Gray, G., Vrana, M., and New, M. I.: Adrenocortical adenoma and ganglioneuroblastoma in a child. Am. J. Dis. Child. *125*:608, 17973.

Eddy, R. L., et al.: Cushing's syndrome: A prospective study of diagnostic methods. Am. J. Med. *55*:621, 1973.

Fraumeni, J. F., Jr., and Miller, R. W.: Adrenocortical neoplasms with hemihypertrophy, brain tumors, and other disorders. J. Pediatr. *70*:129, 1967.

Gabrilove, J. L., Sharma, D. C., Wotiz, H. H., and Dorfman, R. I.: Feminizing adrenocortical tumors in the male. A review of 52 cases including a case report. Medicine *44*:37, 1965.

Giebink, G. S., Gotlin, R. W., Biglieri, E. G., and Katz, F. H.: A kindred with familial glucocorticoid-suppressible aldosteronism. J. Clin. Endocrinol. Metab. *36*:715, 1973.

Godard, C., Riondel, A. M., Veyrat, R., Megevand, A., and Muller, A. F.: Plasma renin activity and aldosterone secretion in congenital adrenal hyperplasia. Pediatrics *41*:883, 1968.

Grim, C. E., McBryde, A. C., Glenn, J. F., and Gunnells, J. C.: Childhood primary aldosteronism with bilateral adrenocortical hyperplasia. Plasma renin activity as an aid to diagnosis. J. Pediatr. *71*:377, 1967.

Haicken, B. N., Schulman, N. H., and Schneider, K. M.: Adrenocortical carcinoma and congenital hemihypertrophy. J. Pediatr. *33*:284, 1973.

James, V. H. T., Landon, J., Wynn, V., and Greenwood, F. C.: A fundamental defect of adreno-cortical control in Cushing's disease. J. Endocrinol. *48*:15, 1968.

Jones, H. W., and Verkauf, B. S.: Congenital adrenal hyperplasia: Age at menarche and related events at puberty. Am. J. Obstet. Gynec. *109*:292, 1971.
Kenny, F. M., Hashaida, Y., Askari, A., Sieber, W. H., and Fetterman, G. H.: Virilizing tumors of the adrenal cortex. Am. J. Dis. Child. *115*:445, 1968.
Klecker, R. L., and Roth, J. B.: Visceral neurofibromatosis and hypertension in childhood. Pediatrics *53*:417, 1974.
Klevit, H. D., Campbell, R. A., Blair, H. R., and Bongiovanni, A. M.: Cushing's syndrome with nodular adrenal hyperplasia in infancy. J. Pediatr. *68*:912, 1966.
Krieger, D. T., Krieger, H. P., and Soffer, L. J.: Cushing's syndrome associated with a suprasellar tumor. Acta. Endocrinol. *47*:185, 1964.
Loridan, L., and Senior, B.: Cushing's syndrome in infancy. J. Pediatr. *75*:349, 1969.
Lubitz, J. A., Freeman, L., and Okun, R.: Mitotane use in inoperable adrenal cortical carcinoma. J.A.M.A. *223*:1109, 1973.
McArthur, R. G., Cloutier, M. D., Hayles, A. B., and Sprague, R. G.: Cushing's disease in children. Findings in 13 cases. Mayo Clin. Proc. *47*:379, 1972.
Migeon, C. J., Green, O. C., and Eckert, J. P.: Study of adrenocortical function in obesity. Metabolism *12*:718, 1963.
Modlinger, R. S., Nicolis, G. L., Krakoff, L. R., and Gabrilove, J. L.: Some observations on the pathogenesis of Bartter's syndrome. New Engl. J. Med. *289*:1022, 1973.
Mosier, H. D., Jr., Smith, F. G., and Schultz, M. A.: Failure of catch-up growth after Cushing's syndrome in childhood. Am. J. Dis. Child. *124*:251, 1972.
New, M. I., and Peterson, R. E.: Aldosterone in childhood. Adv. Pediatr. *15*:111, 1968.
New, M. I., Siegal, E. J., and Peterson, R. E.: Dexamethasone-suppressible hyperaldosteronism. J. Clin. Endocrinol. Metab. *37*:93, 1973.
Penny, R., Olambiwonnu, N. O., and Frasier, S. D.: Precocious puberty following treatment in a six-year-old male with congenital adrenal hyperplasia: Studies of serum luteinizing hormone (LH), serum follicle-stimulating hormone (FSH) and plasma testosterone. J. Clin. Endocrinol. Metab. *36*:920, 1973.
Proesmans, W., Geussens, H., Corbeel, L., Eckels, R.: Pseudohypoaldosteronism. Am. J. Dis. Child. *126*:510, 1973.
Raiti, S., Grant, D. B., Williams, D. I., and Newns, G. H.: Cushing's syndrome in childhood: Post-operative management. Arch. Dis. Child. *47*:597, 1972.
Randolf, J. D., and Hung, W.: Reduction clitoroplasty in females with hypertrophied clitoris. J. Pediatr. Surg. *5*:224, 1970.
Simopoulis, A. P., Marshall, J. R., Delea, C. S., and Bartter, F. C.: Studies on the deficiency of 21-hydroxylation in patients with congenital adrenal hyperplasia. J. Clin. Endocrinol. Metab. *32*:438, 1971.
Snaith, A. H.: A case of feminizing adrenal tumor in a girl. J. Clin. Endocrinol. Metab. *18*:318, 1958.
Strickland, A. L., and Kotchen, T. A.: A study of the renin-aldosterone system in congenital adrenal hyperplasia. J. Pediatr. *81*:962, 1972.
Vazquez, A. M., and Kenny, F. M.: Hypertension secondary to excessive deoxycorticosterone implants or 9-alpha fluorocortisol in salt-losing congenital adrenal hyperplasia. J. Pediatr. *81*:549, 1972.
Zachmann, M., Völlmin, J. A., New, M. I., Curtius, H. C. H., and Prader, A.: Congenital adrenal hyperplasia due to deficiency of 11β-hydroxylation of 17α-hydroxylated steroids. J. Clin. Endocrinol. Metab. *33*:501, 1971.

Pheochromocytoma and Other Neural Tumors

Carman, C. T., and Brashear, R. E.: Pheochromocytoma as an inherited abnormality. Report of the tenth affected kindred and review of the literature. New Engl. J. Med. *263*:419, 1960.
Cone, T. E., and Pearson, H. A.: Malignant pheochromocytoma. Report of a case in a 12-year-old girl. Pediatrics *32*:531, 1963.
Gitlow, S. E., Bertani, L. M., Greenwood, S. M., Wong, B. L., and Dziedzic, S. W.: Benign pheochromocytoma associated with elevated excretion of homovanillic acid. J. Pediatr. *81*:1112, 1972.
Hamilton, J. R., Radde, I. C., and Johnson, G.: Diarrhea associated with ganglioneuroma. New findings related to the pathogenesis of diarrhea. Am. J. Med. *44*:453, 1968.
Keiser, H. R., Beauen, M. A., Doppman, J., Wells, S., Jr., and Buja, L. M.: Sipple's syndrome: Medullary thyroid carcinoma, pheochromocytoma, and parathyroid disease. Ann. Intern. Med. *78*:561, 1973.
Kogut, M. D., and Kaplan, S. A.: Systemic manifestations of neurogenic tumors. J. Pediatr. *60*:697, 1962.
Sarosi, G., and Doe, R. P.: Familial occurrence of parathyroid adenomas, pheochromocytoma and medullary carcinoma of the thyroid with amyloid stroma (Sipple's syndrome). Ann. Intern. Med. *68*:1305, 1968.
Schimke, R. N., Hartman, W. H., Prout, T. E., and Rimoin, D. L.: Syndrome of bilateral pheochromocytoma, Medullary thyroid carcinoma and multiple neuromas. A possible regulatory defect in the differentiation of chromaffin tissue. New Engl. J. Med. *279*:1, 1968.
Smith, A. A., and Dancis, J.: Catecholamine release in familial dysautonomia. New Engl. J. Med. *277*:61, 1967.
Stackpole, R. H., Melicow, M. M., and Uson, A. C.: Pheochromocytoma in children. Report of 9 cases and review of the first 100 published cases with follow-up studies. J. Pediatr. *63*:315, 1963.
von Studnitz, W., Kaser, H,. and Sjoerdsma, A.: Spectrum of catechol amine biochemistry in patients with neuroblastoma. New Engl. J. Med. *269*:232, 1963.
Voorhess, M. L.: Urinary catecholamine excretion by healthy children. I. Daily excretion of dopamine, norepinephrine, epinephrine and 3-methoxy-4-hydroxymandelic acid. Pediatrics *39*:252, 1967.
Wise, K. S., and Gibson, J. A.: Von Hippel-Landau's disease and pheochromocytoma. Brit. Med. J. *1*:441, 1971.

Adrenal Calcification

Crocker, A. C., Vawter, G. F., Neuhauser, E. B. O., and Rosowsky, A.: Wolman's disease: Three new patients with recently described lipidosis. Pediatrics *35*:627, 1965.
Hill, E. E., and Williams, J. A.: Massive adrenal haemorrhage in the newborn. Arch. Dis. Child. *34*:178, 1959.
Jarvis, J. L., and Seaman, W. B.: Idiopathic adrenal calcification in infants and children. Am. J. Roentgenol. *82*:510, 1959.
Stevenson, J., MacGregor, A. M., and Connelly, P.: Calcification of the adrenal glands in young children. A report of three cases with a review of the literature. Arch. Dis. Child. *36*:316, 1961.

DISORDERS OF THE GONADS

MATURATION IN BOYS. The main hormonal product of the testis is testosterone. It is produced in the Leydig cells, which have many enzymes in common with cells of the adrenal cortex. Defects have now been described in each of the steps leading to the biosynthesis of testosterone (Fig. 17–16). Because testosterone is important in normal virilization of the XY fetus, each of these defects has produced some degree of male pseudohermaphroditism. Defects in synthesis of testosterone are even more clearly evident at puberty when normal masculinization fails to occur. These defects are all genetic and almost surely all autosomal recessive, though information is as yet limited for some defects, such as 17,20-desmolase deficiency.

Within specific target cells, testosterone is converted by 5α-reductase to dihydrotestosterone, another potent androgen (Fig. 17–21). There appears to be differential binding of these two androgens in different cells and differences in functional activity. It now appears that in the male fetus at the critical time of masculinization (8 to 12 weeks) these two androgens have distinct and separate function. The recent discovery of patients with deficiency of 5α-reductase has clearly demonstrated that testosterone is necessary for wolffian differentiation, whereas dihydrotestosterone is necessary for masculinization of the external genitalia. Evidence from these same patients suggests that growth of facial hair and prostate may also be dependent upon dihydrotestosterone.

In prepubertal boys, plasma levels of testosterone are low and not different from levels in girls. The level of testosterone rises sharply during puberty, particularly in stage 3 (generally after 12 years of age). The size of the testis increases slightly between 6 and 12 years of age, even before testosterone rises; thereafter, growth of the testis is markedly accelerated. Pubic hair growth, acne, voice change and axillary hair growth correlate with the rising levels of testosterone. Estradiol and adrenal androgens also increase during puberty. In the early stages of puberty, a nocturnal rise of plasma testosterone occurs 40 to 80 minutes after onset of sleep, owing to a slightly earlier sharp rise in the level of LH.

The ability of the prepubertal testis to secrete testosterone can be assessed by the administration of chorionic gonadotropin (HCG), which stimulates the testis in a manner analogous to luteinizing hormone (LH). After administration of HCG for 1 to 3 days, levels of testosterone rise in all stages of puberty; after administration for 2 to 6 weeks, adult levels of plasma testosterone are achieved.

Progressive maturation of the testis occurs under the influence of gradually rising levels of gonadotropins. The normally low levels of FSH and LH begin to rise slowly around the age of 6 to 8 years; there is slight growth of the testis during this period. A sharper rise in the levels of FSH and LH occurs at the beginning of puberty. Plasma levels of FSH increase only to midpuberty, whereas plasma levels of LH continue to rise until about 17 years of age. The somatic changes of puberty and the rising levels of testosterone correlate best with the levels of LH.

It is now clear that the hormonal changes described above are initiated by maturation of the hypothalamus, a process still poorly understood. The key physiologic change at puberty is a decreasing sensitivity of the hypothalamus to the negative feedback effects of the sex steroids. This change is presumably associated with increasing synthesis and release of gonadotropin-releasing factor(s). There also occurs increasing sensitivity of the pituitary to luteinizing hormone-releasing hormone (LHRH). Administration of LHRH to the prepubertal child results in a smaller release of LH than occurs when LHRH is administered during puberty. Thus, the events of puberty and gonadal maturation are associated with stepwise maturation, first in the hypothalamus, then in the pituitary and, finally, in the gonad.

There are wide variations in the clinical pattern of pubertal changes. In 95 per cent of boys enlargement of the genitalia begins between 9½ and 13½ years, reaching maturity between 13 and 17 years. In a small minority of normal boys puberty begins after 15 years of age. In 50 per cent of boys, pubic hair is present by 11 years of age, and by 13 to 17½ years it is equivalent in amount to that of normal adult females. In some boys pubertal development is completed in less than 2 years, whereas in others it may take longer than 4½ years. The adolescent growth spurt occurs later in boys than in girls at corresponding levels of sexual maturation; for example, the peak velocity of change in height is not attained in boys until the genitalia are well developed, whereas in girls the growth rate is usually at its maximum when the nipple and areola have developed but before there is any other significant breast development.

MATURATION IN GIRLS. The most important es-

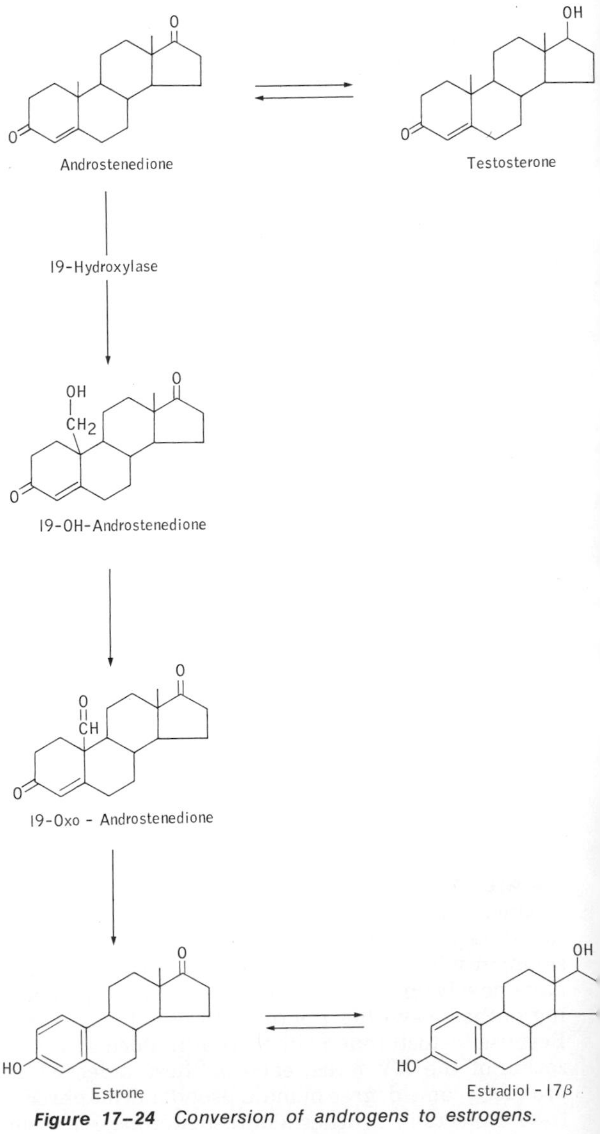

Figure 17–24 *Conversion of androgens to estrogens.*

trogens produced by the ovary are estradiol-17β(E_2) and estrone (E_1); estriol is a metabolic product of these two, and all three estrogens may be found in the urine of mature females. Estrogens also arise from androgens, both in the adrenal and in the testis; the pathway for this conversion is shown in Figure 17–24. (This conversion explains why in certain types of male pseudohermaphroditism feminization occurs at puberty, in 17-ketosteroid reductase deficiency, for example, the enzymatic block results in markedly increased secretion of androstenedione, which is converted in the peripheral tissues to estradiol and estrone; these estrogens, in addition to that directly secreted by the testis, result in normal breast development in XY hermaphrodites with testes.) The ovary also synthesizes progesterone, a progestational steroid; both the adrenal cortex and testis synthesize progesterone as a precursor for other adrenal and testicular hormones.

Plasma levels of estradiol increase slowly but steadily with advancing sexual maturation and correlate well with clinical evaluation of pubertal development, skeletal age and rising levels of FSH. Levels of LH do not rise until secondary sexual characteristics are well developed. Estrogens, like androgens, inhibit secretion of both LH and FSH (negative feedback). It now appears, however, that in females estrogens also provoke the surge of LH secretion which occurs in the midmenstrual cycle. The capacity for this positive feedback is another maturational milestone of puberty. The average age at menarche in American girls is 12½ to 13 years, but the range of normal is wide, and 1 to 2 per cent of normal girls have not menstruated by 16 years of age. Menarche generally correlates closely with skeletal age.

DIAGNOSTIC AIDS. Rapid advances have been made in recent years not only in a better understanding of the hypothalamic-pituitary-gonadal interactions involved with puberty but also in the clinical diagnosis of aberrations of pubertal development. This has been made possible by markedly improved assays for FSH, LH, testosterone and estradiol, which can be measured in small amounts of blood. As these assays become increasingly available, the burdensome collection of 24-hour specimens of urine for hormone assay should become less necessary. With LHRH it is now also possible to differentiate between primary pituitary and hypothalamic defects in hypogonadotropic patients.

THERAPEUTIC AIDS. When the naturally occurring estrogens are administered orally, they are rapidly destroyed by gastrointestinal and liver enzymes; accordingly, they are usually administered as conjugates or esters. The most widely used oral preparations are equine conjugated estrogens (e.g., Premarin) and ethinyl estradiol. Diethylstilbestrol, the most important synthetic estrogen, is not a steroid, but it is effective orally and seems to be metabolized along the same pathway as the natural estrogens. Androgens are generally administered as long-acting esters (enanthate, cyclopentylpropionate, or phenylacetate) because of their potency and steady response. Oral preparations, such as methyltestosterone or fluoxymesterone, do not produce as potent an androgenic response.

Hypofunction of the Testes

Testicular hypofunction may be primary in the testis (primary hypogonadism) or may be secondary to deficiency of pituitary gonadotropic hormones (secondary hypogonadism). Patients with primary hypogonadism have elevated levels of urinary gonadotropin; those with secondary hypogonadism have low or absent levels. Accordingly, hypogonadism may be classified as hypergonadotropic or hypogonadotropic.

HYPERGONADOTROPIC HYPOGONADISM

(Primary Hypogonadism)

Here only those conditions of decreased androgen production are considered which occur in males who were normally virilized during intrauterine life. Other defects of androgen production involving the fetal testis and resulting in male pseudohermaphroditism are discussed with hermaphroditism (below, this Section).

ETIOLOGY. *Congenital anorchia* is found in a few per cent of boys with bilateral cryptorchidism who are otherwise normal. In this condition it is presumed that a noxious factor damaged the fetal testes of the chromosomal male some time after sexual differentiation had taken place. When testicular function fails before the seventh to fourteenth week of fetal life, normal male somatic differentiation does not take place and an intersex results.

A syndrome of *rudimentary testes* has been described in which the testes are exceedingly small; it appears to be inherited as an autosomal or X-linked recessive trait. The etiology is unknown. *Atrophy* of the testes may follow damage to the vascular supply when there has been unskillful manipulation of the testes during surgical procedures for correction of cryptorchidism or as a result of bilateral torsion of the testes. *Acute orchitis* in pubertal or adult males with mumps may also damage the testes; usually only the reproductive function of the testes is impaired. The routine immunization of all prepubertal males with mumps vaccine should prevent this complication.

Cyclophosphamide, an immunosuppressive drug, has been reported to cause testicular atrophy in children and oligo- and azoospermia in adults. It appears that most prepubertal children treated with this agent have normal levels of FSH and LH both during treatment and up to 5 years after treatment has been discontinued. Some treated children followed into adult life have moderately elevated gonadotropin levels, suggesting that the testes may have been damaged. More information is needed concerning the long-range consequences of the use of this agent in children.

In *germinal cell aplasia (Del Castillo syndrome),* sexual maturation occurs normally, Leydig cells are normal and testosterone secretion is normal. The testes are small, however, and the seminiferous tubules are small and devoid of germ cells. Azoospermia and infertility are the rule. The disorder has affected brothers, but the mode of transmission is not clear. FSH levels are elevated; LH levels normal. These findings support the current hypothesis that the germ cells produce a specific inhibitor of FSH.

The term hypogonadism has been widely used to describe children with a variety of syndromes of multiple malformations. In many instances it simply refers to cryptorchidism, a small phallus or a scrotal anomaly. For many of these syndromes, little is known concerning the function of the testes, though both hyper- and hypogonadotropic hypogonadism has been established in some instances.

Varying degrees of hypogonadism also occur in a significant percentage of patients with chromosomal aberrations such as Klinefelter syndrome and in the XY Turner phenotype. These are discussed below under separate headings.

CLINICAL MANIFESTATIONS. The clinical manifestations of hypogonadism are noted only at puberty or subsequently. Secondary sex characters fail to develop. Facial, pubic and axillary hair is scant or absent; there is neither acne nor regression of scalp hair, and the voice remains high-pitched. The penis and the scrotum remain infantile and may almost be obscured by pubic fat; the testes are small or absent. Fat accumulates in the region of the hips and buttocks and sometimes also in the breasts and on the abdomen. The epiphyses close late in life, resulting in long extremities. The span is several inches longer than the height, and the measurement from the symphysis pubis to the soles of the feet is much greater than from the symphysis pubis to the vertex. This clinical state is also known as *eunuchism,* and the proportions of the body are described as "eunuchoid."

DIAGNOSIS. Levels of serum FSH and, to a lesser extent, of LH are elevated above age-specific normal values. These elevated levels indicate that even in the prepubertal child there is an active hypothalamic-gonadal feedback relationship. After the age of 11 years, levels of FSH and LH rise significantly, reaching the postmenopausal range. Plasma testosterone levels are normally low in prepubertal children, rising during puberty to ultimately attain adult levels. During puberty, levels correlate better with testicular size and stage of sexual maturation than with age. In patients with primary hypogonadism, testosterone levels remain low at all ages, and there is no rise following administration of human chorionic gonadotropin (HCG), whereas in normal males, administration of HCG results in a significant rise in plasma testosterone at all stages of development.

XY TURNER PHENOTYPE

The term "male Turner syndrome" has been applied to males who resemble females with Turner syndrome in respect to certain anomalies which occur in both conditions. These boys have normal karyotypes. Moreover, this syndrome also occurs in girls with normal karyotypes. Affected patients, both boys and girls, have been identified by a variety of designations, which include Turner phenotype with normal chromosomes, XY Turner phenotype (boys), XX Turner phenotype (girls), Ullrich-Turner syndrome, Ullrich syndrome, familial Turner phenotype, pseudo-Turner syndrome, male Turner syndrome and Noonan syndrome.

The most common abnormalities consist of short stature, webbing of the neck, pectus carinatum or pectus excavatum, cubitum valgum, congenital heart disease and a characteristic facies. Hypertelorism, epicanthus, an antimongoloid palpebral slant, ptosis, micrognathia and ear abnormalities are common. Other abnormalities such as clinodactyly, hernias and vertebral anomalies occur less frequently. The phenotype differs from true Turner syndrome in the following respects: (1) Mental retardation is much more common. (2) The cardiac defect is most often pulmonary valvular stenosis or atrial septal defect, whereas coarctation of the aorta is rare; the reverse situation is seen in true Turner syndrome. (3) There is a wide spectrum of gonadal defects varying from severe deficiency to apparently normal sexual development. Males frequently have cryptorchidism and small testes; they may be hypogonadal or normal. Females may have a normal or late puberty or fail to develop at all.

The cause is not known. Thyroglobulin antibodies are found in a significant percentage of patients, and hypothyroidism may contribute to growth failure and delayed development in some children. Chromosomes appear normal. Though the disorder is usually sporadic, affected siblings of the same and different sexes have been reported. Partial expression of the syndrome is often present in first degree relatives. In some families the disorder appears to be transmitted from mothers to sons and daughters, which suggests a sex-linked dominant inheritance; male-to-male transmission has also been reported, suggesting an autosomal dominant gene with variable expressivity. These observations suggest that the disorder is heterogeneous; counseling is therefore difficult.

KLINEFELTER SYNDROME

ETIOLOGY. Approximately 1 in 750 newborn males has an XXY chromosome complement. Accordingly, Klinefelter syndrome is slightly more common than Down syndrome. The incidence approximates 1 per cent among the mentally retarded, preferentially among patients with an IQ above 50, and among children admitted to psychiatric hospitals or referred to psychiatric clinics. The chromosomal aberration may result from meiotic nondisjunction of an X chromosome during parental gametogenesis or from mitotic nondisjunction in the zygote. Increased maternal age is a predisposing factor to meiotic nondisjunction and to this syndrome.

The XXY complement is the most common chromosomal pattern in persons with Klinefelter syndrome; some have mosaic patterns, such as XY/XXY, XY/XXYY, XO/XY/XXY and XX/XXY. On rare occasions, occurrence of more than two X chromosomes may result in Klinefelter variants who have XXXY, XXXYY, XXXXY, XXXXXYY, XXY/XXXY, XXY/XXXXY and XXYY karyotypes. It is noteworthy that even with as many as four X chromosomes, the Y chromosome determines a male phenotype.

CLINICAL MANIFESTATIONS. The diagnosis is rarely made prior to puberty, owing to the paucity or subtleness of clinical manifestations in childhood. Since behavioral or psychiatric disorders may often be apparent long before defects in sexual development, the condition should be considered in all boys with mental retardation as well as in children with psychosocial, learning or school adjustment problems. Affected children may be nervous, immature, excessively shy or aggressive; they may engage in antisocial acts. Problems often first become apparent after the child begins school. The patients tend to be tall, slim and underweight and to have relatively long legs; but body habitus can vary markedly. The testes tend to be small for age, but this sign may become substantially apparent only after puberty, when normal testicular growth fails to occur. There is a tendency for the phallus to be smaller than average, and cryptorchidism and/or hypospadias occur in a few patients.

Pubertal development may be delayed, and some degree of androgen deficiency is usually noted, though some patients may undergo almost normal masculinization. About 40 per cent of adults have gynecomastia; facial hair is decreased and most shave less than daily. Azoospermia and infertility are usual, though rare instances of fertility are known. Height tends to be increased. There is an increased frequency of antisocial behavior and delinquency. There is also an increased incidence of pulmonary disease, varicose veins and cancer of the breast.

In adults with *XY/XXY mosaicism,* the features of Klinefelter syndrome are decreased in severity and frequency. Though little is known of children with mosaicism, it is presumed that they may have a better prognosis for virilization, fertility and psychosocial adjustment. The *XXYY male* does not have a phenotype sufficiently distinctive from the XXY patient to permit a clinical differential. Adults with the XXYY chromosome constitution tend to be taller than the average XXY patient.

Klinefelter Variants. When the number of X chromosomes exceeds two, the clinical manifestations are more severe and the degree of mental retardation and the impairment of virilization are greater. Indeed, the rare *XXXXY variant* of Klinefelter syndrome is sufficiently distinctive to be detected in childhood. Affected patients are severely retarded, and many have large malformed ears, a short neck and a typical facies with wide-set eyes which have a mild mongoloid slant, epicanthus, strabismus, a wide, flat upturned nose and a large open mouth. The testes are small and may be undescended, the scrotum is hypoplastic, and the penis is very small. Defects suggestive of Down syndrome, such as short incurved terminal fifth phalanges, single palmar creases, hypotonia and other skeletal abnormalities, including defects in the carrying angle of the elbows and restricted supination, are common. The most frequent radiographic abnormalities are radio-ulnar synostosis or dislocation, elongated radius, pseudoepiphyses, scoliosis or kyphosis, coxa valga and retarded osseous age. Most patients with such extensive changes have an XXXXY chromosome karyotype; the mosaic patterns, XXXY/XXXXY, XXXY/XXXXY/XXXXXY and XXXY/XXXXY/XXXXYY have also been observed. Patients with XXXY syndrome or with mosaic pattern with only three X chromosomes tend to have less extensive changes.

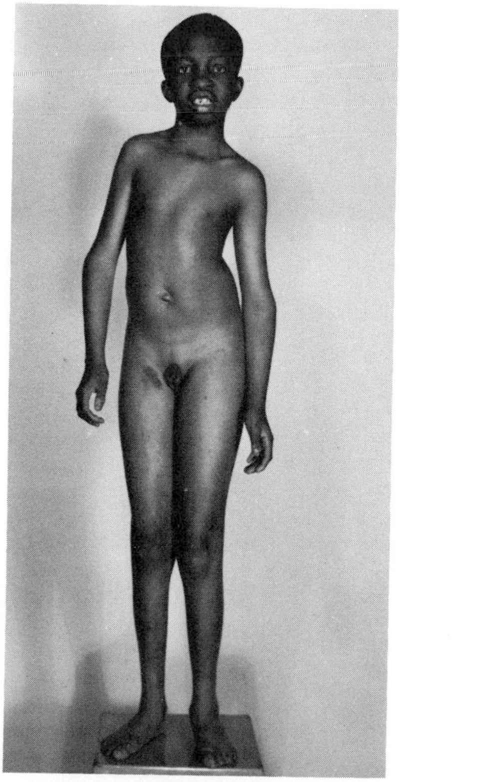

Figure 17–25 *A 12 year old boy with XXXY/XXXXY mosaicism, who has prognathism, epicanthal folds, scoliosis, very small testes, severe mental retardation, clinodactyly and radial-ulnar synostoses.*

LABORATORY DATA. Buccal smears should be examined in all patients suspected of Klinefelter syndrome, particularly those attending child guidance, psychiatric and mental retardation clinics; the number of X chromosomes can be deduced from the number of sex-chromatin bodies. All chromatin-positive boys should have complete study of chromosomes, in order that mosaics such as XY/XXY and patients with the XXYY constitution may be identified.

Gonadotropin levels are usually elevated by the time of puberty, but they may be normal, depending upon the amount of testicular androgen produced. Plasma testosterone levels in men with Klinefelter syndrome are low or low normal.

Testicular biopsy before puberty may reveal only a deficiency or absence of germinal cells. After puberty the seminiferous tubular membranes are hyalinized, and there is adenomatous clumping of Leydig cells. Azoospermia is characteristic; only rarely is spermatogenesis sufficient to permit fertility.

TREATMENT. Replacement therapy with one of the long-acting testosterone preparations should be initiated at 11 to 12 years of age. The cyclopentylpropionate ester may be used in a dose of 50 mg injected intramuscularly every 3 weeks initially. This dose can then be increased by 50 mg increments every 6 to 9 months until a maintenance dose for adults (250 mg every 3 weeks) is achieved. For older boys the initial dose and increments can be larger, to achieve more rapid virilization.

XX MALES

Approximately 50 males have been detected with an XX chromosome constitution. These individuals have a male phenotype, testes and no evidence of ovarian or müllerian duct tissue; they appear, therefore, to be distinct from the XX true hermaphrodite (below). This disorder is tentatively classified as a variant of Klinefelter syndrome, since the histologic features of the testes are essentially the same in two conditions. The incidence of hypospadias, cryptorchidism, gynecomastia and hormonal status is also the same as for Klinefelter syndrome. Only about 20 per cent of reported patients have been prepubertal, the condition usually coming to medical attention in adult life because of hypogonadism or gynecomastia.

Several explanations have been proposed for the findings; these are the same as are used to explain XX true hermaphroditism. The first possibility is that undetected mosaicism is present; indeed, in some otherwise XX males a small number of Y-bearing cells have been detected. To rule out this possibility in presumed XX males, repeated cultures of blood and testicular cells, including quinacrine staining (for fluorescent Y) of fresh, frozen sections, is indicated. For those individuals who appear not to have mosaicism, it has been theorized that male-determining genes have been translocated from the Y chromosome to the X chromosomes or autosomes. Male-determining genes are located on the short arm of the Y chromosome and would not be expected to show fluorescence with quinacrine; such translocations have not as yet been detected. Autosomal inheritance of a male-determining gene has been proposed, especially for the pattern of inheritance observed in one affected family.

XYY MALES

The XYY male does not have hypogonadism; his condition is discussed here for easy comparison with the XXY and the XX male syndromes.

Approximately 1 per 1000 newborn males have an XYY chromosome pattern. Thus far, in a small number of children detected at birth as part of routine screening programs and followed prospectively, no abnormal physical, intellectual or behavioral characteristics have been detected. When this disorder was first discovered in adults, studies of XYY individuals in mental or penal institutions led to a popular stereotype of affected individuals as having deviant behavior manifested by physical aggressiveness and violence. It now appears that though the rate with which XYY individuals are found in mental or penal settings may be as high as 20 times the incidence of the condition in the newborn, studies not biased by behavioral ascertainment do not show deviant behavior to be a prominent feature.

The XYY adult also has few phenotypic manifestations. He tends to be taller than average and is more likely to have severe nodulocystic acne. Dermatoglyphics do not differ significantly from XY males. In affected persons genital abnormalities have been noted, but cryptic mosaicism, such as XO/XYY, is a possibility in these instances. Prolonged PR intervals on electrocardiography and radioulnar synostosis appear to occur more often than in the general population. No clear-cut endocrine abnormalities have been found. Why XYY individuals are more apt to be found in mental or penal institutions is not certain at this time, though it is possible that the XYY genotype results in an abnormality of neural development which may favor deviant behavior in some persons. The nature and extent of such an association are yet to be determined. This condition poses a serious dilemma for counseling of parents of affected infants or children discovered to have this sex chromosome complement. The risks for the child may not be trivial; neither do they appear as dire as thought a few years ago.

HYPOGONADOTROPIC HYPOGONADISM

(Secondary Hypogonadism)

In hypogonadotropic hypogonadism there is deficiency of follicle-stimulating hormone (FSH) and/or of luteinizing hormone (LH). The primary defect may be in the anterior pituitary, or in the hypothalamus as a deficiency of gonadotropin-releasing hormone (LHRH). The testes are normal but remain in the prepubertal state owing to lack of stimulation by gonadotropins. The classification of these disorders is in active evolution, because synthetic LHRH has recently become available.

ETIOLOGY

Hypopituitarism. Patients with deficiency of growth hormone frequently have an associated deficiency of one or more of the other pituitary hormones. (See above, this Section.) The most frequently associated deficiency is that of gonadotropin. In patients with organic lesions in or near the pituitary (e.g., craniopharyngiomas), the gonadotropin deficiency is pituitary in origin. On the other hand, in many patients with "idiopathic" or "familial" hypopituitarism, it now appears that the defect is in the hypothalamus; administration of LHRH to these patients indicates that the pituitary is capable of response. In some patients, in whom the rise of FSH and LH in response to acute administration of LHRH has been impaired or absent, more intensive stimulation produced a response. These findings suggest that the pituitary cells responsible for gonadotropin production can release hormone into the circulation if appropriately stimulated.

Isolated Deficiency of Gonadotropin. This may also result in delayed puberty and hypogonadism. A heterogeneous group of disorders remains to be delineated; in most instances the defect appears to be hypothalamic rather than pituitary. The most clearly defined disorder in this category is *Kallmann syndrome* or *hypogonadotropic hypogonadism and anosmia.* Persons with this syndrome fail to develop sexually, or exhibit only minimal development at puberty. Inability to smell is present from early childhood, but it is usually not discovered except on direct questioning. Both FSH and LH remain at prepubertal levels in adult life. Agenesis of the olfactory lobes of the brain accounts for the anosmia. No histologic lesion has been defined, but it had long been presumed that a hypothalamic defect is the cause for the gonadotropin deficiency, and this has now been confirmed. Administration of LHRH to affected patients has produced increases in FSH and LH. The responses have been minimal; it is not yet clear whether this reflects chronic understimulation or an associated defect in the pituitary.

Other somatic defects have been observed in some patients with Kallman syndrome, particularly cryptorchidism, congenital deafness, harelip or cleft palate and renal abnormalities. Familial occurrences have suggested that the disorder is transmitted by a sex-linked gene, but male-to-male transmission has recently been observed, and it is now thought to be an autosomal domimant defect. The expression is variable; in some kindreds there are anosmic individuals without, as well as with, hypogonadism; in other kindreds there are individuals with only harelip or cleft palate, or with only hypogonadism or anosmia. The incidence of hyposomia in affected families is not known; more males than females have been recognized with the syndrome. Genetic heterogeneity remains a major possibility.

Isolated deficiency of LH has been observed in patients with the *fertile eunuch syndrome.* Failure of the Leydig cells to mature at puberty is accompanied by delayed pubertal development. The testes may be normal in size, however, and spermatogenesis may occur. A good response to administration of chorionic gonadotropin reveals the presence of normal Leydig cell precursors. Serum and urine FSH concentrations are normal, whereas those of LH are undetectable. Fertility has occasionally been noted, but evidence suggests that testicular androgen is necessary for completely normal spermatogenesis. This rare syndrome has been observed in brothers.

Other Syndromes. Syndromes in which the hypogonadism is the result of gonadotropin hormone deficiency have not been evaluated by up-to-date techniques, and the sites of their defects are unknown. In the recessively inherited *Laurence-Moon-Biedl syndrome,* hypogonadism occurs in both males and females, but its incidence is unknown. On occasion the hypogonadism is primary, but deficiency of gonadotropic hormones has been found in brother and sister. Several syndromes of *ataxia and hypogonadotropic hypogonadism* have been reported and appear to have distinctive genetic origins. *Ichthyosis and male hypogonadism* has been described in several families. In one kindred of 10 males in four generations, the hypogonadotropic hypogonadism and ichthyosis were also associated with anosmia and mild mental retardation. In the *multiple lentigines syndrome,* an autosomal dominant disorder, delayed puberty has been observed in about 25 per cent of affected patients. An 18 year old male with this syndrome and delayed puberty had deficiency of FSH and LH and anosmia, suggesting a hypothalamic defect.

DIAGNOSIS. Physiologic delay of puberty is extremely difficult to differentiate from hypogonadotropic hypogonadism, since in both conditions gonadotropin levels remain low after the usual age of puberty. The diagnosis should always be considered if puberty is delayed beyond 16 or 17 years of age. The detection of other pituitary deficits, the discovery of anosmia by careful questioning and the eliciting of a history of other family members with hypogonadism are important clues in diagnosis. Measurement of plasma levels of LH and of testosterone during sleep may be helpful in detecting boys with delayed puberty who are on the verge of spontaneous puberty, inasmuch as augmentation of LH secretion during sleep has its onset in early puberty. In hypogonadotropic hypogonadism there is persistent absence of a sleep-associated rise in LH secretion.

TREATMENT. Administration of chorionic gonadotropin induces satisfactory development of secondary sex characters by stimulating the Leydig cells. The recommended dose is 4000 to 5000 IU three times weekly for 6 weeks. After discontinuation of therapy a period of observation for evidence of regression is necessary to establish the diagnosis. If puberty regresses, the patient has secondary hypogonadism, whereas if puberty continues to progress, the patient has had physiologic delay of maturation. Several such courses may be necessary to exclude the diagnosis of physiologic delayed adolescence. When the diagnosis of secondary hypogonadism is established, maintenance therapy with androgen is initiated.

Pseudoprecocity Resulting from Tumors of the Testes

Functional tumors of the testis are rare causes of sexual pseudoprecocity. Such tumors arise from the Leydig cells. These cells are sparse before puberty and tumors derived from them are more common in the adult; about 50 cases in children have been reported, including one of identical twins. Leydig cell tumors are usually benign.

The clinical manifestations are the same as in other causes of puberty in the male; onset is usually between 4 and 6 years of age. Gynecomastia has occurred in 5 patients. The tumor of the testis can usually be readily palpated; the contralateral unaffected testis is normal in size for the age of the patient.

Urinary 17-ketosteroids are only slightly or moderately increased, but testosterone levels are markedly elevated. FSH and LH levels are suppressed. Treatment consists in surgical removal of the affected testis. Progression of virilization ceases and partial reversal of the signs of precocity may occur.

There are few other causes of testicular enlargement to be considered in the differential diagnosis. In untreated congenital adrenal hyperplasia, the testes will rarely contain ectopic adrenal cortical cells, giving rise to bilateral testicular enlargement; treatment with corticosteroids suppresses adrenocortical activity and the testes return to normal size. In boys with unilateral cryptorchidism, the contralateral testis is about 25 per cent larger than normal for age. The enlargement of the testes which occurs in boys with true precocious puberty is bilateral and symmetrical. A 10 year old boy has been reported with markedly enlarged testes (four times the volume in a normal adult) in whom extensive study failed to reveal any abnormality; the condition has been termed "benign bilateral testicular enlargement."

Gynecomastia

Gynecomastia, or the occurrence of mammary tissue in the male, is a common condition. It occurs in most newborn males as a result of stimulation by maternal hormones. This effect is transient, disappearing in a few weeks.

During pubertal development, approximately two thirds of boys develop varying degrees of subareolar hyperplasia of the breasts. These changes occur concomitantly with rising levels of testosterone. At the same time, levels of estrogen increase only slightly, though estradiol levels are higher in those boys who manifest gynecomastia. *Physiologic pubertal gynecomastia* may involve only one breast, and it is not unusual for both breasts to enlarge at disproportionate rates or at different times. Tenderness of the breast is frequent but transitory. Spontaneous regression may occur within a few months; it rarely persists longer than 2 years. Treatment usually consists in reassurance of the boy and his family of the physiologic and transient nature of the phenomenon. Surgical removal of the breast is rarely indicated; when enlargement is striking and persistent and causes serious emotional disturbance to the patient, removal may be justified.

Several kindreds have been reported in which gynecomastia has occurred in many males without apparent endocrinopathy. Such instances of *familial gynecomastia* are probably inherited as a male-limited autosomal dominant trait.

Occasionally, hypertrophy of the breasts in boys is spectacular, closely resembling female breasts; such instances usually fail to regress. The etiology is not known, but in one instance the condition has been attributed to *hyperleydigism.* Testosterone levels were slightly above the upper range for normal adult males; it has been speculated that in this boy there was unresponsiveness of the negative feedback mechanism or an abnormal threshold set in the hypothalamus.

When gynecomastia occurs in young children, an exogenous source of estrogens must be sought. Exposure to small amounts of estrogens by inhalation, percutaneous absorption or ingestion has caused gynecomastia, either accidentally or therapeutically. Increased pigmentation of the nipple and areola should suggest this cause.

There are a number of other pathologic conditions which cause gynecomastia. It may be associated with interstitial cell tumors of the testis or with feminizing tumors of the adrenal. It occurs in Klinefelter syndrome and with other types of testicular failure (hypergonadotropic states). It is a common finding in certain types of male pseudohermaphroditism, particularly in Reifenstein syndrome, in the testicular feminization syndrome and in patients with the 17-ketosteroid reductase defect. In adults, gynecomastia has frequently occurred with liver cirrhosis, with digitalis therapy of congestive failure, with bronchogenic carcinoma and with administration of a variety of nonsteroidal therapeutic agents.

Hypofunction of the Ovaries

Hypofunction of the ovaries may be due to congenital failure of development or to postnatal destruction (primary or hypergonadotropic hypogonadism) or to lack of stimulation by the pituitary (secondary or hypogonadotropic hypogonadism). Many chronic diseases may result in the latter type.

HYPERGONADOTROPIC HYPOGONADISM

(Primary Hypogonadism)

It has become increasingly possible to diagnose hypergonadotropic hypogonadism prior to puberty, but with the exception of Turner syndrome most affected patients have no clinical manifestations prior to puberty.

TURNER SYNDROME

(Gonadal Dysgenesis)

In 1938 Turner described a syndrome consisting of sexual infantilism, webbed neck and cubitum valgum in adult females. It was subsequently demonstrated that such women have elevated levels of urinary gonadotropins and that the gonads consist of rudimentary elongated streaks containing no germinal elements and consisting of whorls of connective tissue suggestive of ovarian stroma.

PATHOGENESIS. In 1959 it was demonstrated that patients with Turner syndrome have a single X chromosome; they have a 45, XO chromosome constitution. The X chromosome is more often maternal than paternal, but unlike the situation in Klinefelter syndrome, maternal age does not influence the occurrence of Turner syndrome. Most cases probably arise from nondisjunction or anaphase lag in the zygote. A large prospective study found evidence for a seasonal pattern, two thirds of all births with nondisjunction occurring between May and October.

The XO disorder occurs in about 1 in 3000 liveborn females, an incidence much lower than that of Klinefelter syndrome. It appears that the majority (over 95 per cent) of all XO conceptions are aborted; an examination of abortuses reveals that 3 to 5 per cent are XO. Mosaicism (XO/XX) among patients with Turner syndrome is 25 per cent, a proportion higher than with any other aneuploid state, whereas the mosaic Turner constitution is rare among the abortuses. These observations indicate preferential survival for mosaic forms.

Other types of mosaics, such as isochromosome for the long arm, deletion of the short arm, and rings of the X chromosome, are much less common.

Primordial germ cells are present in the gonadal ridges of aborted XO fetuses up to 3 months of gestational age, but disappear thereafter. The number of germ cells in the normal fetus declines rapidly at about 5 months of gestation and then continues to decrease at a slower rate after birth. It seems therefore, that in the XO patient a normal process may be hastened and exaggerated. The streak gonads usually consist of only connective tissue; on occasion a few germ cells may be found to explain the rare occurrence of a limited degree of sexual maturation.

CLINICAL MANIFESTATIONS. In the past the diagnosis was generally not suspected until childhood or at puberty when sexual maturation failed to occur. It is now clear that most XO patients are recognizable at birth, owing to the presence of edema of the dorsum of the hands and feet and loose skin folds in the nape of the neck. Significantly low birth weight and short stature are common. Clinical manifestations in childhood include webbing of the neck, a low posterior hairline, small mandible, prominent ears, epicanthic folds, high arched palate, a broad chest presenting the illusion of widely spaced nipples, cubitum valgum and hyperconvex fingernails. Stature is almost always below the third percentile; an adult height of more than 58 inches is rare. With increasing age, pigmented nevi become more prominent. At the usual time of puberty, sexual maturation fails to occur.

Associated congenital defects are common and should suggest the diagnosis of Turner syndrome. Coarctation of the aorta is the most frequent cardiovascular lesion, but hypertension of unknown etiology and other congenital heart defects may occur. Rupture of a dissecting aortic aneurysm is a rare complication. Approximately half the patients have abnormal urograms, horseshoe kidney and malrotation being the most common anomalies. Hearing and cognitive problems are more common than in the general population.

In the *XO/XX mosaic* the abnormalities are attenuated and fewer. The affected newborn usually has no recognizable findings. Webbing of the neck,

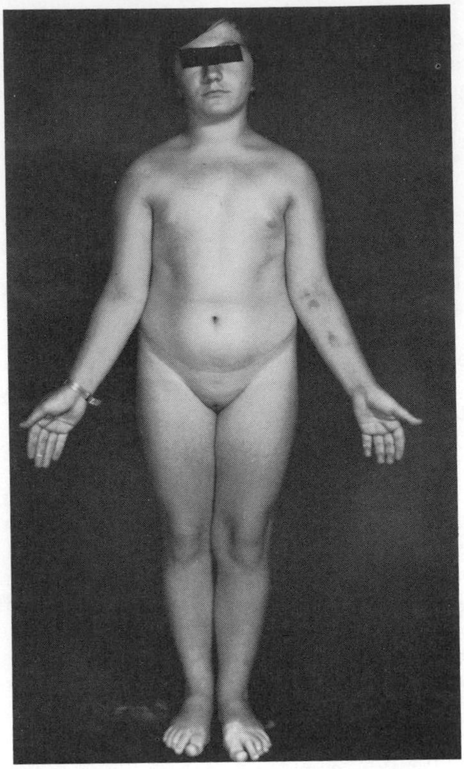

Figure 17–26 Turner syndrome. Gonadal dysgenesis in a 15 year old girl exhibiting failure of sexual maturation, short stature, cubitus valgus and a goiter. There is no webbing of the neck. Karyotype revealed XO/XX sex chromosome complement, and urinary gonadotropin was over 96 mouse units/24 hr. PBI was 3.2 μg/dl and T4 was 2.2 μg/dl. Biopsy of the thyroid revealed lymphocytic thyroiditis.

coarctation of the aorta and edema of hands and feet are infrequent. Short stature is almost as frequent as in the XO patient and may be the only manifestation.

Failure of sexual maturation is usually complete in both the XO and XO/XX adolescent. Occasional patients exhibit varying degrees of breast development and even menstruation. Such patients are more likely to be XO/XX mosaics. Fertility has been reported twice in XO patients; mosaicism remains a possibility even though not detected in the tissues examined.

LABORATORY DATA. Chromosomal analysis should be performed in all suspected patients. The sex-chromatin pattern is normally negative, but occasional XO/XX patients and patients with abnormal X chromosomes could be overlooked. Unusually large sex-chromatin bodies are seen in patients with an isochromosome of the X chromosome, and smaller than normal sex-chromatin bodies suggest a deletion of one of the X chromosomes.

Plasma levels of gonadotropins, particularly of FSH, may be elevated above those of age-matched controls, even in infancy. In prepubertal children, occasional levels of FSH may not be clearly abnormal, owing to the overlap with the range of normal values. After 10 years of age, plasma levels are markedly elevated and approximate menopausal levels. At puberty the release of FSH and LH is pulsatile; this probably accounts for day-to-day variability in plasma levels. Urinary gonadotropins are clearly elevated after 10 to 12 years of age but are less helpful in prepubertal children. Urinary excretion of estrogens and plasma levels of estradiol are very low. Growth hormone secretion in response to provocative stimuli is normal.

Roentgenographic studies may reveal cardiovascular or renal abnormalities. The most common skeletal abnormalities are shortening of the fourth metatarsal and metacarpal bones, epiphyseal dysgenesis in the joints of the knee and elbow, inadequate osseous mineralization, scoliosis and spina bifida occulta.

Patients with Turner syndrome have a higher than expected incidence of chronic lymphocytic thyroiditis, and a high percentage of patients and other family members have significant titers of antibodies to thyroglobulin.

TREATMENT. Replacement therapy with estrogens to initiate and sustain sexual maturation may be deferred until the age 13 to 15 years in order to avoid early closure of the epiphyses. An oral estrogen is administered daily for six months or until menstrual bleeding occurs. Thereafter, cyclic estrogen-progestogen therapy may be given in the form of one of the sequential contraceptive regimens. Stilbestrol is contraindicated, since it is suspected of provoking endometrial carcinoma in these patients.

XX PURE GONADAL DYSGENESIS

Phenotypic females have been found with gonadal lesions identical to those in XO patients but without the somatic features of Turner syndrome; their condition is termed "pure gonadal dysgenesis." Those with an XY karyotype are also designated as having the Swyer syndrome. The disorder is discussed below, with male pseudohermaphroditism; here we discuss only those with the XX chromosome constitution. These two conditions are quite distinct entities; in no instance have XX and XY gonadal dysgenesis been reported in the same family.

The disorder is rarely recognized in children because the external genitalia are normal, no other abnormalities are visible and growth is normal. At puberty sexual maturation fails to take place. Plasma and urinary gonadotropin levels are elevated. Epiphyseal fusion is delayed, resulting in a eunuchoid habitus.

Affected siblings, parental consanguinity and failure to uncover mosaicism (even in the streak gonads) all point to autosomal recessive inheritance. Two families have been reported in which all affected individuals were deaf, suggesting there may be two distinct genetic entities. Tumors of the gonads have not been reported in these patients. Treatment consists of replacement therapy with estrogens.

MIXED GONADAL DYSGENESIS

Patients with this conditon may be considered as part of a spectrum between XO females and XY males. All patients are chromatin negative and the majority are XO/XY mosaics, with varying proportions of each cell line in different individuals. In instances where only XY or XO cell lines have been found it is suspected that mosaicism may have gone undetected. The cytogenetic defect probably occurs early in embryogenesis.

The phenotype is rather characteristic and can be related to the mixture of XO and XY cell lines. The presence of some cells with a Y chromosome always results in some virilization; on occasion the phenotype may be male, but in most instances the genitalia are ambiguous and a unilateral testis is present. A vagina and an infantile uterus are present, and there are usually bilateral fallopian tubes, though there may be only one. A streak gonad is usually present on the side contralateral to the testis. The streak gonad differs somewhat from that in Turner syndrome; in additon to wavy connective tissue there are often tubular or cordlike structures, occasional clumps of granulosa cells and frequently mesonephric or hilus cells. The somatic signs of Turner syndrome are commonly present.

Puberty occurs at the normal time, with virilization; growth of the phallus may be striking. Adult height is greater than in Turner syndrome, particularly if none of the stigmata of Turner syndrome are present. The discrepancy between normal Leydig cell function at puberty and failure of complete genital masculinization during fetal life, as well as the persistence of müllerian ducts, could be explained by a delay in maturation of the fetal testis.

Gonadal tumors, particularly gonadoblastomas, have been reported frequently in patients with mixed gonadal dysgenesis. Analysis of these cases reveals that these patients with mixed gonadal dysgenesis are often less virilized at birth, are more apt to have normal stature, undergo little or no virilization at puberty and are the only ones with breast development. In addition, the majority of patients with tumors have fewer stigmata of Turner syndrome and an XY karyotype. These observations suggest that many of the patients reported as instances of mixed gonadal dysgenesis with tumor are more akin to pure XY gonadal dysgenesis, and that the true incidence of tumors in patients with mixed gonadal dysgenesis may not be so high as formerly thought.

XX TURNER PHENOTYPE

Girls with a phenotype resembling that of Turner syndrome, but with normal sex chromosomes, constitute a separate entity which is described above, with XY Turner syndrome.

OTHER OVARIAN DEFECTS

An increasing number of other young women are being found who have "streak" gonads which may contain no or only occasional germ cells. No chromosomal abnormality is found; gonadotropins are increased. Streak gonads ("ovarian hypoplasia") occur in girls with ataxia-telangiectasia and in some young women with autoimmune Addison disease. The similarity of the "ovaries" in a variety of clinical conditions suggests that several pathogenetic mechanisms may interfere with normal gonadal development.

Cyclophosphamide has produced ovarian failure in a prepubertal child and frequently causes amenorrhea in young adult women. In such women there is marked depletion of ova. Further experience is required to determine the long-range consequences of use of this agent on ovarian function and on reproductive capacity. These side effects should receive due consideration when this drug is being considered for use in children with nonmalignant conditions.

HYPOGONADOTROPIC HYPOGONADISM

(Secondary Hypogonadism)

Hypofunction of the ovaries can result from failure to secrete normal levels of gonadotropins. The defect may be in the anterior pituitary, but as is the case for the male, there is increasing evidence for a hypothalamic defect in a significant proportion of such hypogonadal females.

ETIOLOGY

Hypopituitarism. Destructive lesions in or near the pituitary almost always result in impaired secretion of gonadotropins as well as of other pituitary hormones. In patients with idiopathic hypopituitarism, however, the defect is most often in the hypothalamus. In these patients, administration of LHRH results in increased plasma levels of FSH and LH, and administration of TRF provokes a rise in the plasma level of TSH, establishing the integrity of the pituitary gland.

Isolated Deficiency of Gonadotropins. This is a heterogeneous group of disorders which is only now being sorted out with the help of LHRH. Isolated pituitary deficiency of FSH has been documented, but in most patients the pituitary is normal and the defect resides in the hypothalamus.

Several sporadic instances of anosmia with hypogonadotropic hypogonadism have been reported. Anosmic hypogonadal females have also been reported in kindreds with Kallman syndrome, though hypogonadism more frequently affects the males in these families.

A variety of autosomal recessive disorders such as the Laurence-Moon-Biedl and multiple lentigines syndromes also appear in some instances to include gonadotropic hormone deficiency.

DIAGNOSIS. The diagnosis is not difficult in patients with other deficiencies of pituitary tropic hormones. On the other hand, it is difficult to differentiate isolated hypogonadotropic hypogonadism from physiologic delay of puberty. Repeated measurements of FSH and LH, particularly during sleep, may be helpful in heralding the onset of puberty if rising levels are demonstrated.

POLYCYSTIC OVARIES

(Stein-Leventhal Syndrome)

This syndrome is characterized by amenorrhea, hirsutism, obesity and sterility. The ovaries are enlarged and covered by a condensation of collagen which gives the appearance of a "thickened capsule." Beneath this layer are many small follicular cysts. This disorder accounts for many more instances of virilism than do ovarian tumors. Since the disorder commonly begins at puberty or shortly thereafter, the diagnosis should be considered in adolescent girls with menstrual irregularities and hirsutism. In married women the most frequent complaint is infertility. The enlarged ovaries can often be detected by combined rectal and abdominal palpation.

The cause of the disorder is unsettled, but certain abnormalities in pituitary-ovarian function can be demonstrated. Basal levels of LH in plasma are moderately elevated during the follicular phase of the cycle; levels of FSH are consistently depressed. The elevated level of LH can be suppressed by estradiol, indicating a normal negative feedback mechanism. The secretion of estradiol is decreased, whereas rates of production of testosterone and androstenedione are significantly elevated. The increase in ovarian androgens is presumed to result from the elevated levels of LH. Deficiency of secretion of FSH and abnormal follicular maturation are thought to be the central pathogenetic features.

Bilateral wedge resections of the ovaries result in normal ovulatory menstrual cycles in 70 to 80 per cent of patients. It is believed that this in some way relieves the suppression of FSH and restores normal follicular maturation. Since success of therapy is often of short duration, this form of therapy may be deferred until the patient wishes to become pregnant. For young girls, therapy with clomiphene citrate is probably preferable.

SEX CHROMOSOME ABNORMALITIES WITHOUT GONADAL DEFECTS

A variety of sex chromosomal abnormalities have been uncovered which are not associated with defects in the gonads. These are of interest to the pediatrician primarily because mental retardation may occur in affected patients.

XXX FEMALES. The XXX chromosomal constitution is the most frequent X chromosomal abnormality in females, occurring in almost 1 per 1000 live-born females. Affected infants are not usually recognized but frequently have minor anomalies, particularly clinodactyly, epicanthal folds and wide-set eyes. As with XYY males, little is known of the natural history of this condition, since large numbers of affected persons have only recently been discovered in screening studies of the newborn. Past experience with XXX females has been biased, since most patients were found among the institutionalized mentally retarded. Affected adult females have been found, however, who are completely normal, including having normal fertility. Of a group of 9 triple-X females identified at birth, only 1 was clearly retarded at a year of age. Further follow-up of such patients is required to determine the full spectrum of pathology.

XXXX AND XXXXX FEMALES. About 17 females with four X and 6 with five X chromosomes have been described. All have been mentally retarded except for one of the XXXX girls. Commonly associated defects are epicanthal folds, hypertelorism, clinodactyly, simian crease, radioulnar synostosis and congenital heart disease.

Pseudoprecocity Due to Lesions of the Ovary

Most of the functioning lesions of the ovary in children are neoplasms, the majority of which synthesize estrogens; a few of them synthesize androgens. Infrequently a lesion produces both estrogens and androgens, or a given lesion may produce estrogenic manifestations in one patient and androgenic ones in another. Thus, the rare Sertoli-Leydig cell tumor of the ovary has caused isosexual precocity in some girls and masculinization in others.

ESTROGENIC LESIONS OF THE OVARY

These lesions cause isosexual precocious sexual development, but account for only a small percentage of all instances of precocity.

GRANULOSA-THECA CELL TUMOR

In childhood the most common neoplasm of the ovary with estrogenic manifestations is the granulosa-theca cell tumor. These tumors have variable proportions of granulosa and theca cells; in childhood the granulosa cell is dominant, and tumors which consist almost completely of theca cells (thecoma) are extremely rare. In spite of variable morphology, these tumors produce similar clinical manifestations because they actively synthesize estrogen. Which of the two cells is the site of estrogen synthesis is still unsettled.

CLINICAL MANIFESTATIONS. The tumor has been observed in a newborn infant, but most often clinical manifestations do not appear until after 2 years of age. The breasts become enlarged, rounded and firm, and the nipples are prominent. Axillary and pubic hair appears, and total body growth is accelerated. The external genitalia resemble those of a normal girl at puberty, and the uterus is enlarged. A white vaginal discharge is followed by irregular or cyclic menstruation. Ovulation, however, does not occur; the sexual development is of the pseudoprecocious variety.

A mass in the lower portion of the abdomen is readily palpable in most patients by the time sexual precocity is evident. The tumor may be small, however, and escape detection even by careful rectal and abdominal examination.

Association of these tumors with ascites and hydrothorax has been observed in children; it is more likely to occur with the thecoma. Such manifestations, known as *Meigs syndrome,* should not be confused with metastases and, hence, the primary tumor mistakenly considered inoperable.

Plasma estradiol levels are markedly elevated; in one 9 year old girl with a granulosa cell tumor, the level was 413 pg/dl, in contrast to levels of under 100 pg/dl for fully mature adult females or children with idiopathic precocious puberty. Urinary estrogens are also usually markedly elevated, whereas both urinary and plasma levels of gonadotropins are suppressed. Urinary 17-ketosteroids are normal or only slightly elevated and of little value in diagnosis. Osseous development is moderately advanced.

The tumor should be removed as soon as the diagnosis is established. The mortality rate is approximately 20 per cent; recurrences are known up to 25 years after removal of the tumor. Vaginal bleeding immediately after removal of the tumor is common. Signs of precocious puberty abate and may disappear within a few months after operation. The secretion of estrogens returns to normal postoperatively.

THECA-LUTEIN CYST

Ovarian cysts are common in childhood, but most are nonfunctioning and hence not feminizing. Ovarian cysts are also commonly encountered in the ovaries of children with constitutional sexual precocity. In such instances the cyst is a secondary event; it is not the cause of sexual precocity, and removal of it does not alter the course of sexual precocity. By contrast, removal of a cyst has on rare occasions resulted in regression of sexual precocity. In such instances the theca-lutein cyst is believed to be functional and to be the cause of the sexual precocity. Three children with McCune-Albright syndrome have been reported with such functional cysts as the cause of their sexual precocity. Clinical manifestations are the same as for other causes of isosexual precocity. Laboratory findings are similar to those of children with granulosa-theca cell tumors; estrogens are elevated above normal adult levels and gonadotropins are suppressed.

ANDROGENIC LESIONS OF THE OVARY

Virilizing ovarian tumors are rare at all ages, but particularly so in prepubertal girls. The most common lesion is the arrhenoblastoma, which has been reported as early as 4 years of age. The clinical features are the same as for virilizing adrenal tumors and include acne, hirsutism and clitoral enlargement. Urinary 17-ketosteroids may be normal or only slightly increased. In a recently reported young adult with an arrhenoblastoma, plasma levels of testosterone were markedly elevated; surprisingly, the tumor was responsive to dexamethasone suppression and to stimulation by ACTH and HCG. Now that testosterone-secreting adrenal adenomas are also known, virilizing tumors present a difficult differential diagnosis which may require selective venography.

Hermaphroditism

(Intersexuality)

Hermaphroditism in man implies a discrepancy between the morphology of the gonads and of the external genitalia. It is now well established that many chromosomal aberrations can result in ambiguity of the external genitalia; these conditions are discussed elsewhere in this section. Here we discuss those conditions of aberrant sexual differentiation imposed on the XX or XY genotype (female and male pseudohermaphrodites). An increasing number of such conditions can now be explained, owing to advances in the understanding of normal sexual differentiation. The category known as true hermaphroditism, with few exceptions, is still a poorly understood, heterogeneous group of disorders.

EMBRYONIC SEXUAL DIFFERENTIATION. In normal differentiation, the final form of all sexual structures is consistent with a normal complement of the sex chromosomes (XX or XY). The Y chromosome determines sexual differentiation only to the point of forming the fetal testis, which begins around the fifth to sixth week of intrauterine life. In the XX fetus, essentially the same bipotential embryonic cells which form the testis develop into an ovary considerably later, at about the 12th week. Further male differentiation from gonadal sex into phenotypic sex requires elaboration of several hormones by the fetal testis. Masculinization of the fetus begins at about 8 weeks. Absence of these hormones during this critical period results in failure of masculinization.

It is now clear that the fetal testis secretes two hormones during this period of masculinization (8 to 12 weeks). The first of these is testosterone. This has been established indirectly by correlation with cytodifferentiation of the Leydig cells and directly by measurement of testosterone concentration of fetal testes and plasma. It appears that testosterone acts directly to initiate virilization of the wolffian ducts into the epididymis, vas deferens and seminal vesicle. Testosterone also serves as the prohormone for another effective metabolite, dihydrotestosterone, the androgen which causes virilization of the urogenital sinus and the external genitalia.

The second hormone produced by the fetal testis has been termed the müllerian-inhibiting factor; it appears to be nonsteroidal in structure and is produced only during fetal life. In the presence of this substance, müllerian ducts regress, whereas without it they persist. It can be said, therefore, that maleness is imposed upon a basic female fetus by the hormones of the fetal testis. An appreciation of these basic principles greatly enhances our understanding of various types of hermaphroditic conditions.

FEMALE PSEUDOHERMAPHRODITISM

In the female pseudohermaphrodite, the genotype is XX and the gonads are ovaries, but the external genitalia are virilized. Since there is no müllerian-inhibiting factor, the uterus, tubes and ovaries are present. Since the mechanisms involved in normal female differentiation are considerably less complex than those required for male differentiation, the varieties and causes of female pseudohermaphroditism are fewer. It results in most instances from the exposure of the female fetus to excessive androgens during intrauterine life, and the changes consist principally of virilization of the external genitalia (clitoral hypertrophy and labioscrotal fusion).

CONGENITAL ADRENAL HYPERPLASIA. This is by far the most common cause of the condition. Females with the 21-hydroxylase and 11-hydroxylase defects are the most highly virilized, though minimal virilization also occurs with the 3β-hydroxysteroid dehydrogenase defect. Salt losers tend to have greater degrees of virilization than nonsalt losers. The masculinization may be so intense as to result in a completely penile urethra and may mimic a male with cryptorchidism.

MASCULINIZING MATERNAL TUMORS. In a dozen instances the female fetus has been virilized during fetal life by a maternal androgen-producing tumor. In one instance the lesion was a benign, adrenal adenoma, but all others were ovarian tumors, particularly arrhenoblastomas, luteomas and Krukenberg tumors. Maternal virilization may be manifested by enlargement of the clitoris, acne, deepening of the voice, decreased lactation, hirsutism and elevated 17-ketosteroids. In the infant there is enlargement of the clitoris of varying degrees and often labial fusion. In all instances of unexplained female pseudohermaphroditism the level of plasma testosterone should be measured in the mother of the patient.

ADMINISTRATION OF ANDROGENIC DRUGS TO WOMEN DURING PREGNANCY. This can result in female pseudohermaphroditism. Testosterone and 17-methyltestosterone have been reported to be the masculinizing agents in some instances. The greatest number of cases, however, have resulted from the use of certain progestational compounds for the treatment of threatened abortion. Within the past decade most of these progestins have been replaced by nonvirilizing ones; accordingly, this form of female pseudohermaphroditism has become less frequent.

Infants with female pseudohermaphroditism have been reported for whom no masculinizing agent could be identified. In such instances the disorder is usually associated with other congenital defects, particularly of the urinary and gastrointestinal tracts. No etiologic factors are known.

MALE PSEUDOHERMAPHRODITISM

In the male pseudohermaphrodite the genotype is XY, but the external genitalia are incompletely virilized, ambiguous or completely female. When gonads can be found, they are invariably testes. Because of the complexity of the process of normal virilization in the fetus, it is not surprising that many varieties of male hermaphroditism have been delineated.

DEFECTS OF STEROID BIOSYNTHESIS. In the most common forms of adrenal hyperplasia (21-hydroxylase and 11-hydroxylase deficiencies) males are highly virilized. In some of the less common forms, the adrenocortical defect is shared by the fetal testis, with deficient production of fetal androgen and failure of normal virilization (Fig. 17–21). Males with *3β-hydroxysteroid dehy-*

drogenase deficiency have varying degrees of hypospadias, with or without bifid scrotum and/or cryptorchidism. Affected infants develop salt-losing manifestations shortly after birth.

The male infant with *lipoid adrenal hyperplasia* is usually considered to be a normal female infant until salt-losing symptoms intervene. The fetal testis is unable to synthesize the androgen needed for normal virilization. In at least one instance it appears that a partial defect resulted in a partially masculinized male with ambiguous genitalia and delayed onset of salt-losing symptoms.

The *17-hydroxylase deficiency* has thus far been detected in only 3 males. The genitalia are ambiguous, with hypospadias, cryptorchidism and a rudimentary vagina. The phallus may be so small as to suggest a female phenotype, and at least one patient was reared to adult life as a female. Because of the overproduction of DOC and corticosterone, hypertension and hypokalemic acidosis are characteristic, though in one less severely affected male, the blood pressure was normal in early life. With failure of adrenal and testicular synthesis of androgens, puberty does not occur and the patient remains eunuchoid. Absence of müllerian duct remnants indicates that fetal production of müllerian-inhibiting substance is normal. The diagnosis can be suspected after puberty on the basis of low levels of 17-ketosteroids, of 21-hydroxycorticoids and of plasma androgens. To establish the diagnosis before puberty, it is necessary to determine secretion rates of DOC, corticosterone, cortisol and compound S.

DEFICIENCY OF STEROID 17,20-DESMOLASE. A kindred has been reported in which two first cousins and a maternal "aunt" had ambiguous external genitalia and an XY constitution, with a defect in testosterone secretion. Biochemical studies established a deficiency of the enzyme which cleaves the side-chain of 17α-hydroxypregnenolone and 17α-hydroxyprogesterone (Fig. 17–21). As a consequence, there was deficiency of testosterone and of dehydroepiandrosterone (DHA). The enzymatic deficiency also involved the adrenal, since ACTH administration failed to increase DHA excretion. The inguinal testes in these patients revealed no specific abnormalities; there were no müllerian structures in the two cousins. The defect was probably incomplete, since one would anticipate complete feminization with the total absence of testosterone. This diagnosis can be suspected in male pseudohermaphrodites with histologically normal testes who fail to exhibit a rise in plasma level of testosterone following stimulation with HCG. The mode of transmission is not clear; both X-linked and autosomal recessive inheritance are possible.

DEFICIENCY OF 17-KETOSTEROID REDUCTASE. A defect in testicular 17-ketosteroid reductase has been identified as a cause of male pseudohermaphroditism in 4 patients. Affected patients were completely feminized and reared as females until virilization, primary amenorrhea and, in some patients, gynecomastia occurred at puberty. A shallow vagina is present, but no cervix or uterus. The defect in testosterone synthesis results in low plasma levels of testosterone and in marked accumulation of its precursor, androstenedione (Fig. 17–21). The testis also produces increased rates of estrone. The testicular tubules are small, with a fibrotic lamina propria, and spermatogenesis is arrested at early stages. Marked Leydig cell hyperplasia is present. The defect has been detected only in adults. In prepubertal children the disorder would be easily confused with the testicular feminization syndrome, but it could be suspected if there were no rise in testosterone following a course of human chorionic gonadotropin. In one family the occurrence in siblings with first cousin parents suggests autosomal recessive transmission. Removal of the defective testis prevents or halts virilization. Replacement therapy with estrogens is indicated.

DEFICIENCY OF 5α-REDUCTASE. Twenty-two male pseudohermaphrodites (XY) have been investigated in 12 families from a village in the Dominican Republic. Affected patients have a small phallus, bifid scrotum, urogenital sinus with perineal hypospadias, and blind vaginal pouch. Testes are normal histologically and there are no müllerian structures. At puberty masculinization occurs normally, but beard is scanty and the prostate is small. Plasma levels of testosterone are normal but 5α-dihydrotestosterone is markedly reduced. These findings are consistent with studies in animals which show that wolffian differentiation depends on testosterone, whereas masculinization of the external genitalia depends on the availability of dihydrotestosterone during the critical period of fetal masculinization. Growth of facial hair and of the prostate also appear to be dihydrotestosterone dependent. The disorder is inherited as a male-limited autosomal recessive; the biochemical defect has been demonstrated in the clinically normal female. The next disorder described almost surely represents additional examples of this defect.

PSEUDOVAGINAL PERINEOSCROTAL HYPOSPADIAS (PPSH). This disorder is characterized by a phallus of intermediate size with a ventral urethral groove and a perineal urethral meatus in an otherwise normal male. There is a perineal opening which ends blindly and resembles a vagina (pseudovagina). The scrotum is cleft and resembles labia majora, which may contain normal testes. Müllerian duct structures are absent; the epididymis, vas deferens and seminal vesicles are normal. The phallus has usually been mistaken for an enlarged clitoris, and most affected patients have been reared as females. At puberty, virilization is normal for a male, and plasma testosterone and urinary 17-ketosteroids are in the normal range for males. Breasts do not develop. It appears that the effect of a defect in virilization was limited to fetal life. Occurrence in brothers and consanguinity in parents is evidence for an autosomal recessive mode of transmission. This entity was described before the 5α-reductase defect was recognized; though activity of this enzyme has not been reported for patients with the PPSH syndrome, it appears likely that the two conditions are one and the same.

TESTICULAR FEMINIZATION SYNDROME. This is one of the more common forms of male pseudohermaphroditism. These XY patients appear female at birth and are invariably reared accordingly. The external genitalia are female; the vagina ends blindly in a pouch, and the uterus is absent. The gonads are testes which consist largely of seminiferous tubules. They are usually intra-abdominal, but may descend into the inguinal canal. At puberty there is normal development of breasts and the habitus is female, but menstruation does not occur and sexual hair is often absent. Psychosexual orientation of such persons is entirely female.

The testes of affected adult patients produce normal male levels of testosterone. It is firmly established that the absence of androgenic effects is due to a striking resistance to the action of endogenous or exogenous testosterone at the peripheral cellular level. It appears that affected patients are able to convert testosterone to 5α-dihydrotestosterone, the biologically active androgen at the cellular level. Current evidence suggests that the defect is in the androgen receptor mechanism, probably a deficiency of cytosol receptor. Such a defect has been established in an analogous testicular feminization syndrome of the mouse and rat. Failure of normal male differentiation during fetal life reflects the defective response to testicular androgens at that time.

In adults, amenorrhea is the usual presenting symptom. Prepubertal children with this disorder are often recognized when inguinal masses prove to be testes, or when a testis is unexpectedly found during herniorrhaphy in an apparent female. Examination of a buccal smear is indicated for any female with an inguinal hernia, since 1 to 2 per cent will prove to have this syndrome.

The disorder is inherited, the gene being transmitted by the female carrier; half of her XY offspring are affected, and half of her daughters are carriers. Maternal aunts are frequently affected. It is unsettled whether the trait is X-linked recessive or male-limited autosomal dominant. In prepubertal children the condition must be differentiated from other types of XY male pseudohermaphroditism in which there is complete feminization. These include XY pure gonadal dysgenesis (Swyer syndrome), true agonadism and the testicular 17-ketosteroid reductase defect.

Affected patients should always be reared as females. The testes should be removed, since after the age of 30 about a fourth of the patients develop some sort of gonadal tumor, usually a germinoma. Some recommend not removing the testes until after puberty and completion of secondary sexual development, but a testicular tumor has been found in an affected 18 month old infant. To relieve parental anxiety and to avoid adverse effects on psychosexual orientation of the child, we recommend that the testes be removed as soon as they are discovered. Replacement therapy with estrogens is then indicated at the time of puberty.

INCOMPLETE TESTICULAR FEMINIZATION. In this disorder patients exhibit some degree of masculinization and at birth may have enlargement of the phallus and labioscrotal fusion. The vagina ends blindly and the uterus is absent. Testes are present in the inguinal canal or in the labioscrotal folds. At puberty, breast development occurs as well as axillary and pubic hair. The hereditary pattern is the same as for the testicular feminization syndrome, but the "complete" and "incomplete" forms have not been reported in the same family. It is presumed that these patients have a lesser degree of insensitivity to androgens than those with the complete syndrome, but the precise biochemical defect is not known.

XY GONADAL AGENESIS SYNDROME. In this rare syndrome the external genitalia manifest slight ambiguity and are more nearly female. There are hypoplasia of the labia, some degree of labioscrotal fusion, a small clitoris-like phallus, a perineal urethral opening and usually no vagina. There is no uterus, and no gonadal tissue can be found. At the time of puberty, there is no sexual development and gonadotropins are elevated. Most patients have been reared as females. It is presumed that testicular tissue was present in the fetus for a period long enough to inhibit müllerian duct development, but that its Leydig cell function was minimal.

The disorder described may be considered an extreme form of *anorchia*, a condition in which the testes are absent but there is a complete male phenotype. In this latter condition it is presumed that tissue with fetal testicular function was present at the crucial period of genital differentiation but that sometime later it was damaged. In at least one young child with the XY gonadal agenesis syndrome in whom no testis could be found on exploration, there was a significant rise in testosterone after stimulation with human chorionic gonadotropin, indicating that some functional Leydig cells were present. Two siblings with the disorder have been reported; the syndrome may have a genetic basis.

XY PURE GONADAL DYSGENESIS (SWYER SYNDROME). Patients with this condition have a completely female phenotype, including vagina, uterus and fallopian tubes, but they have streak gonads devoid of germ cells. There are no other associated defects; growth is normal. At puberty there is primary amenorrhea and failure of breast development. There may be hilar cells in the gonad capable of producing some androgens; accordingly, some virilization, such as clitoral enlargement, may occur after puberty.

Pathogenetically the condition is readily explained by assuming destruction of the testis very early in fetal life. This would prevent masculinization as well as production of müllerian inhibiting factor; the development of uterus, tubes and female external genitalia would follow.

The streak gonads may undergo neoplastic changes, possibly more often and earlier than in the testicular feminization syndrome. The gonads should, therefore, be removed before puberty. The disorder appears to be inherited as an X-linked recessive or as an autosomal dominant limited in expression to the male sex.

Pure gonadal dysgenesis also occurs in XX individuals. (See above, this Section.)

REIFENSTEIN SYNDROME. In childhood this inherited disorder is characterized by severe perineal hypospadias and by small testes, which may be found in the scrotal sac or may be cryptorchid. The phallus is usually normal in size, and affected patients are usually considered male. After puberty, hypogonadism is evident and varying degrees of gynecomastia appear. There is lack of facial hair and voice change. Female escutcheon, azoospermia and infertility are usual. The testes are smaller than normal, but larger than those in patients with Klinefelter syndrome. Histologic examination reveals varying amounts of tubular sclerosis, hyalinization and Leydig cell hyperplasia. The defect is not known, but defective development of the external genitalia is thought to result from deficient secretion of androgen by a fetal testis capable of inhibiting müllerian duct differentiation. The mode of inheritance is either X-linked or autosomal dominant limited to males; this disorder can be suspected in prepubertal boys with similarly affected brothers, uncles or male cousins. Management involves surgical correction of the hypospadias and of the gynecomastia, with replacement therapy with androgens at puberty.

UTERINE-HERNIA SYNDROME. Patients with this disorder are phenotypic males and are invariably reared accordingly. They are usually detected when surgical correction of an inguinal hernia in an otherwise normal male discloses uterus and uterine tubes. The degree of müllerian development is variable and may be asymmetrical. Testicular function, including spermatogenesis, may be normal. The disorder is thought to result from an isolated deficiency of müllerian-inhibiting factor by the fetal testis. The disorder may not be so rare as the small number of reported cases suggests. In a family with 2 affected siblings, the testes were bilaterally cryptorchid, in close approximation to the fallopian tubes. An affected adult with bilateral cryptorchidism has had bilateral gonadoblastoma.

OTHER MANIFESTATIONS. There are other XY male pseudohermaphrodites, with much variability of the external and internal genitalia and with varying degrees of phallic and müllerian development. Testes may be histologically normal or rudimentary, or there may only be one. Some of the reported cases may belong to one of the above categories, but have not been adequately studied by the newer techniques. Since ambiguity of the genitalia is associated with a wide variety of chromosomal aberrations, these must always be considered in the differential. The most common condition in this category is the XO/XY syndrome. (See above, this Section.) It may be necessary to examine a variety of tissues in order to establish the mosaic condition. There are also a large number of complex genetic syndromes, many resulting from single gene mutations, which are associated with varying degrees of ambiguity of the genitalia, particularly in the male. These entities must be identified on the basis of the associated extragenital malformations.

PSEUDOHERMAPHRODITISM AND WILMS' TUMOR. About a dozen XY male pseudohermaphrodites are reported to have developed Wilms' tumors, usually in the first 2 years of life. Some patients also had glomerulonephritis, the nephrotic syndrome, aniridia and/or gonadoblastomas. The reason for these associations is not understood, but they are consistent with the increasingly recognized relationship between oncogenesis and certain types of congenital malformations, particularly those involving the genitourinary tract.

TRUE HERMAPHRODITISM

In true hermaphroditism both ovarian and testicular tissue are present either in the same or in opposite gonads. The clinical features may include any of those described for the other types of hermaphroditism. The phenotype may be male or female; usually there is ambiguity of the external genitalia.

Examination of the chromosomes of 119 true hermaphrodites has disclosed 50 per cent to be XX, 20 per cent to be XY and only 30 per cent to be mosaics. Mosaicism may be difficult to establish, requiring study of many different tissues; its possibility can never be completely eliminated. On the other hand, some instances of XX true hermaphroditism have been very intensively investigated, with no evidence found of a Y chromosome. The cause for true hermaphroditism in XX patients is unknown; it has been proposed that in such patients one of the X chromosomes may contain genes controlling testicular function which are normally found on the Y chromosome. Another proposal is that one of the X chromosomes has a mutant male derepressor gene which functions like an active Y chromosome. The most common mosaic conditions have been XO/XY, XX/XXY and XX/XY.

Patients with XX/XY mosaicism are of special interest, and the best understood of patients with true hermaphroditism. Of the 12 reported cases, 9 are known to be whole body chimeras; that is, they were derived from more than one zygote. This has usually been established by blood group studies. The presence of both paternal alleles for some blood groups and of both maternal alleles for other blood groups is clear evidence for chimerism. A variety of mechanisms are possible, including fusion of early zygotes, or double fertilization of a double-nucleated ovum.

DIAGNOSIS AND MANAGEMENT. The diagnosis of the child with hermaphroditism depends upon a thorough review of the numerous mechanisms which may lead to the condition. Screening tests for examination of sex chromatin and for fluorescence of the Y chromosome must always be supplemented by complete chromosomal analysis. It is important to know in which conditions mosaicism is a possibility and to establish the chromosomal constitution in tissues other than blood, such as in skin and any tissues removed at biopsy or surgical exploration.

Studies of adrenal hormones, 17-ketosteroids and pregnanetriol are indicated to exclude the common varieties of the adrenogenital syndrome. Less common defects such as the 17-hydroxylase defect and the testicular defect in 17-ketosteroid reductase require more elaborate hormonal studies; experience with these two conditions in young children is limited and diagnosis may be difficult. For all XX patients, a detailed search for the source of virilization should be undertaken. Urethrovaginogram or endoscopic examination is indicated to establish whether vagina and/or cervix exist in those patients with ambiguous external genitalia.

Surgical exploration is indicated for the majority of male pseudohermaphrodites and true hermaphrodites. Appropriate biopsies and removal of gonadal and accessory tissue are frequently indicated, depending upon the condition.

The assignment of sex of rearing should be settled as early in life as possible. The decision is based largely on the possibilities for correction of the ambiguous genitalia and not on the chromosomal constitution. Female pseudohermaphrodites should almost always be reared as females even when highly virilized. Male pseudohermaphrodites who are totally or significantly feminized should also be reared as females. It is more feasible to reconstruct the external genitalia to create a functional female, particularly when a vagina is already present, than to create a functional male phallus. The management of the potential psychologic upheaval that such problems can generate in patient and/or family is of paramount importance and requires physicians with sensitivity and training and experience in this field. Once the appropriate sex of rearing has been established, parents should be left with no ambiguity in their minds as to the sex of the child.

In some mammals the female exposed to androgens prenatally or in early postnatal life will exhibit aberrant sexual behavior in adult life. Girls who have undergone fetal masculinization from congenital adrenal hyperplasia or from maternal progestin therapy have no such problems in sexual identity, though during childhood they may appear to prefer male playmates and activities to girl playmates or to feminine play with dolls in mothering roles.

ANGELO M. DIGEORGE

GENERAL

August, G. P., Grumbach, M. M., and Kaplan, S. L.: Hormonal changes in puberty: III. Correlation of plasma testosterone, LH, FSH, testicular size, and bone age with male pubertal development. J. Clin. Endocrinol. Metab. *34*:319, 1972.

Grady, H. G., and Smith, D. E.: The Ovary. Baltimore, The Williams & Wilkins Company, 1963.

Judd, H. L., Parker, D. C., Siler, T. M., and Yen, S. S. C.: The nocturnal rise of plasma testosterone in pubertal boys. J. Clin. Endocrinol. Metab. *38*:710, 1974.

Morris, J. M., and Scully, R. E.: Endocrine Pathology of the Ovary. St. Louis, The C. V. Mosby Company, 1958.

Overzier, C.: Intersexuality. New York, Academic Press, 1963.

Penny, R., Olambiwonnu, O., and Frasier, S. D.: Serum gonadotropin concentrations during the first four years of life. J. Clin. Endocrinol. Metab. *38*:320, 1974.

Roth, J. C., Grumbach, M. M., and Kaplan, S. L.: Effect of synthetic luteinizing hormone-releasing factor on serum testosterone and gonadotropins in prepubertal, pubertal and adult males. J. Clin. Endocrinol. Metab. *37*:680, 1973.

Williams, R. H.: Textbook of Endocrinology. 5th ed. Philadelphia, W. B. Saunders Company, 1974.

Winter, J. J. D., Taraska, S., and Faiman, C.: The hormonal response to HCG stimulation in male children and adolescents. J. Clin. Endocrinol. Metab. *34*:348, 1972.

Hypofunction of Testes

Böök, J. A., Eilon, B., Halbrecht, I., Komlos, L., and Shabtay, F.: Isochromosome Y [46, X, i (Yq)] and female phenotype. Clin. Genet. *4*:410, 1973.

Borgaonkar, D. S., Mules, E., and Char, F.: Do the 48, XXYY males have a characteristic phenotype? Clin. Genet. *1*:272, 1970.

Bowen, P., and others: Hereditary male pseudohermaphroditism with hypogonadism, hypospadias, and gynecomastia (Reifenstein's syndrome). Arch. Intern. Med. *62*:252, 1965.

Caldwell, P. D., and Smith, D. W.: The XXY (Klinefelter's) syndrome in childhood: Detection and treatment. J. Pediatr. *80*:250, 1972.

Carakushansky, G., Neu, R. L., and Gardner, L. I.: XYY with abnormal genitalia. Lancet *2*:1144, 1968.

Court Brown, M. W.: Males with an XYY sex chromosome complement. Review article. J. Med. Genet. *5*:341, 1968.

DeGrott, G. W., Faiman, C., and Winter, J. S. D.: Cyclophosphamide and the prepubertal gonad: A negative report. J. Pediatr. *84*:123, 1974.

Dekaban, A. S., Parks, J. S., and Ross, G. T.: Laurence-Moon syndrome: Evaluation of endocrinological function and phenotypic concordance and report of cases. Med. Ann. District Columbia. *41*:687, 1972.

DeLaChapelle, A.: Nature and origin of males with XX sex chromosomes. Am. J. Hum. Genet. *24*:71, 1972.

DeLaChapelle, A., and Hortling, H.: Cytogenetical and clinical observations in male hypogonadism. Acta Endocrol. *44*:165, 1963.

Ewer, R. W.: Familial monotropic pituitary gonadotropin insufficiency. J. Clin. Endocrol. *28*:783, 1968.

Faiman, C., Hoffman, D. L., Ryan, R. J., and Albert, A.: The "fertile eunuch" syndrome: Demonstration of isolated luteinizing hormone deficiency by radioimmunoassay technique. Mayo Clin. Proc. *43*:661, 1968.

Hook, E. B.: Behavioral implications of the human XYY genotype. Science *179*:139, 1973.

Howard, R. P., Sniffen, R. C., Simmons, F. A., and Albright, F.: Testicular deficiency: A clinical and pathologic study. J. Clin. Endocrinol. Metab. *10*:121, 1950.

Kasdan, R., Nankin, H. R., Troen, P., Wald, N., Pan, S., and Yanaibara, T.: Paternal transmission of maleness in XX human beings. New Engl. J. Med. *288*:539, 1973.

Levy, E. P., Pashasyan, H., Fraser, F. C., and Pinsky, L.: XX and XY Turner phenotypes in a family. Am. J. Dis. Child. *120*:36, 1970.

Medeiros-Neto, G. A., et al.: Characterization of the LH response to luteinizing hormone-releasing hormone (LH-RH) in isolated and multiple tropic hormone deficiencies. J. Clin. Endocrinol. Metab. *37*:972, 1973.

Meisner, L. F., and Inhorn, S. L.: Normal male development with Y chromosome long arm deletion (Yq-). J. Med. Genet. *9*:373, 1972.

Naftolin, F., and Harris, G. W.: Effect of purified luteinizing hor-

mone-releasing factor on normal and hypogonadotropic anosmic men. Nature (London) *232*:496, 1971.
Najjar, S. S., Takla, R. J., and Nassar, V. H.: The syndrome of rudimentary testes: Occurrence in five siblings. J. Pediatr. *84*:119, 1974.
Noonan, J. A.: Hypertelorism with Turner phenotype. A new syndrome with associated congenital heart disease. Am. J. Dis. Child. *116*:373, 1968.
Nora, J. J., and Sinha, A. K.: Direct familial transmission of the Turner phenotype. Am. J. Dis. Child. *116*:343, 1968.
Nora, J. J., Torres, F. G., Sinha, A. K., and McNamara, D. G.: Characteristic cardiovascular anomalies of XO Turner syndrome, XX and XY phenotype and XO/XX Turner mosaic. Am. J. Cardiol. *25*:639, 1970.
Nowakowski, H., and Lenz, W.: Genetic aspects of male hypogonadism. Recent Progr. Hormone Res. *17*:53, 1961.
Palutke, W. A., Chen, Y., and Chen, H.: Presence of brightly fluorescent material in testes of XX males. J. Med. Genet. *10*:170, 1973.
Reinfrank, R. F., and Nichols, F. L.: Hypogonadotropic hypogonadism in the Laurence-Monn syndrome. J. Clin. Endocrol. *24*:48, 1964.
Rimoin, D. L., Borgaankar, D. S., Asper, S. P., and Blizzard, R. M.: Chromatin-negative hypogonadism in phenotypic men. Am. J. Med. *44*:225, 1968.
Roth, J. C., Kelch, R. P., Kaplan, S. E., and Grumbach, M. M.: FSH and LH response to luteinizing hormone-releasing factor in prepubertal and pubertal children, adult males and patients with hypogonadotropic and hypergonadotropic hypogonadism. J. Clin. Endocrinol. Metab. *35*:926, 1972.
Santen, R. J., and Paulsen, C. A.: Hypogonadotropic eunuchoidism. I. Clinical study of the mode of inheritance. J. Clin. Endocrinol. Metab. *36*:47, 1973.
Siggers, D. C., and Polani, P. E.: Congenital heart disease in male and female subjects with somatic features of Turner's syndrome and normal sex chromosomes (Ullrich's and related syndromes). Brit. Heart J. *34*:41, 1972.
Sparkes, R. S., Simpson, R. W., and Paulsen, C. A.: Familial hypogonadotropic hypogonadism with anosmia. Arch. Intern. Med. *121*:534, 1968.
Swanson, S. L., Santen, R. J., and Smith, D. W.: Multiple lentigenes syndrome: New findings of hypogonadotrophism, hyposmia, and unilateral renal agenesis. J. Pediatr. *78*:1037, 1971.
Valentine, G. H., McClelland, M. A., and Sergovich, F. R.: The growth and development of four XYY infants. Pediatrics *48*:583, 1971.
Vesterhus, P., and Aarskog, D.: Noonan's syndrome and autoimmune thyroiditis. J. Pediatr. *83*:237, 1973.
Volpe, R., Metzler, W. S., and Johnston, M. W.: Familial hypogonadotropic eunuchoidism with cerebellar ataxia. J. Clin. Endocrol. *23*:107, 1963.
Wieland, R. G., Folk, R. I., Taylor, J. N., and Hamwi, G. T.: Studies of male hypogonadism. I. Androgen metabolism in a male with gynecomastia and galactorrhea. J. Clin. Endocrol. *27*:763, 1967.
Winter, J. S. D., and Faiman, C.: Serum gonadotropin concentrations in agonadal children and adults. J. Clin. Endocrinol. Metab. *35*:561, 1972.
Zarate, A., Kastin, A. J., Soria, J., Canales, E. S., and Schally, A. V.: Effect of synthetic luteinizing hormone-releasing hormone (LH-RH) in two brothers with hypogonadotropic hypogonadism and anosmia. J. Clin. Endocrinol. Metab. *36*:612, 1973.

Tumors of the Testes

Camin, A. J., Dorfman, R. I., McDonald, J. H., and Rosenthal, I. M.: Interstitial cell tumor of the testis in a seven-year-old child. Am. J. Dis. Child. *100*:389, 1960.
Engel, F. L., and others: Clinical, morphological and biochemical studies on a malignant testicular tumor. J. Clin. Endocrol. *24*:528, 1964.
Martin, M. M., Canary, J. J., and Balsamo, P. A.: Virilizing tumor of the testis in one twin. J. Clin. Endocrol. *22*:345, 1962.
Nisula, B. C., Loriaux, D. L., Sherins, R. J., and Kulin, H. E.: Benign bilateral testicular enlargement. J. Clin. Endocrinol. Metab. *38*:440, 1974.
Savard, K., and others: Clinical, morphological and biochemical studies of a virilizing tumor of the testis. J. Clin. Invest. *39*:534, 1960.

Gynecomastia

Goldfine, I., Rosenfeld, R. L., and Landau, K. L.: Hyperleydigism: A cause of severe pubertal gynecomastia. J. Clin. Endocrinol. Metab. *32*:751, 1971.
Green, M.: Gynecomastia and pseudoprecocious puberty following diethylstilbestrol exposure. Am. J. Dis. Child. *95*:637, 1958.
Laron, Z.: Breast development induced by methandrostenolone (Dianabol). J. Clin. Endocrinol. Metab. *22*:450, 1962.
Nydick, M., Bustos, J., Dale, J. H., Jr., and Rawson, R. W.: Gynecomastia in adolescent boys. J.A.M.A. *178*:449, 1961.
Wallach, E. E., and Garcia, C.: Familial gynecomastia without hypogonadism: A report of three cases in one family. J. Clin. Endocrinol. *22*:1201, 1962.

Hypofunction of the Ovaries

Carneiro, I. J., Voorhess, M. L., Schlegel, R. J., and Gardner, L. I.: XX/XO mosaicism in nine preadolescent girls with short stature as presenting complaint. Pediatrics *38*:972, 1966.
Collins, E.: The illusion of widely spaced nipples in the Noonan and the Turner syndromes. J. Pediatr. *83*:557, 1973.
Davidoff, F., and Federman, D. D.: Mixed gonadal dysgenesis. Pediatrics *52*:725, 1973.
Eller, E., Frankenberg, W., Puck, M., and Robinson, A.: Prognosis in newborn infants with X chromosomal abnormalities. Pediatrics *47*:681, 1971.
Friedrich, U., and Nielsen, J.: Chromosome studies in 5,049 consecutive newborn children. Clin. Genet. *4*:333, 1973.
Hecht, F., and MacFarlane, J. P.: Mosaicism in Turner's syndrome reflects the lethality of XO. Lancet *2*:1197, 1969.
Larget-Piet, L., Pignier, J., Berthelot, J., Ayache, P., Bourdon, P., and Larget-Piet, A.: Syndrome 48, XXXX chez une enfant de 5 ans. Pédiatric. *28*:433, 1972.
Larget-Piet, L., et al.: Syndrome 49, XXXXX chez une fille de 5 ans. Ann. Genet. *15*:115, 1972.
Lemli, L., and Smith, D. W.: The XO syndrome: A study of the differentiated phenotype in 25 patients. J. Pediatr. *63*:577, 1963.
Lindsten, J.: The Nature and Origin of X Chromosome Aberrations in Turner's Syndrome. A Cytogenetical and Clinical Study of 57 Patients. Stockholm, Almqvist & Wiksells, 1963.
Moore, K. L.: The Sex Chromatin. Philadelphia, W. B. Saunders Company, 1966.
Nakashima, I., and Robinson, A.: Fertility in a 45, X female. Pediatrics *47*:770, 1971.
Portmann, U. V., and McCullagh, E. P.: Developmental defects following irradiation of the ovaries in a child. J.A.M.A. *151*:736, 1953.
Spitz, I. M., et al.: Isolated gonadotropin deficiency. A heterogenous syndrome. New Engl. J. Med. *290*:10, 1974.
Strader, W. J., Wachtel, H. L., and Lindberg, G. D.: Hypertension and aortic rupture in gonadal dysgenesis. J. Pediatr. *79*:473, 1971.
Tagatz, G., Fialkow, P. J., Smith, D., and Spadoni, L.: Hypogonadotropic hypogonadism associated with anosmia in the female. New Engl. J. Med. *282*:1326, 1970.
Warne, G. L., Fairley, K. F., Hobbs, J. B., and Martin, F. I. A.: Cyclophosphamide-induced ovarian failure. New Engl. J. Med. *29*:1159, 1973.

Tumors of the Ovary

Ammann, A. J., Kaufman, S., and Gilbert, A.: Virilizing ovarian tumor in a 2½-year-old-girl. J. Pediatr. *70*:782, 1967.
Campbell, P. E., and Danks, D. M.: Pseudoprecocity in an infant due to a luteoma of the ovary. Arch. Dis. Child. *38*:519, 1963.
Eberlein, W. R., Bongiovanni, A. M., Jones, I. T., and Yakovac, W. C.: Ovarian tumors and cysts associated with sexual precocity. *J. Pediatr.* *57*:484, 1960.
Faber, H. K.: Meigs' syndrome with thecomas of both ovaries in a 4-year-old girl. *J. Pediat.* *61*:769, 1962.
Tucci, J. R., Zäh, W., and Kalderon, A. E.: Endocrine studies in arrhenoblastoma responsive to dexamethasone, ACTH and human chorionic gonadotropin. Am. J. Med. *55*:687, 1973.

Hermaphroditism

Alexander, D. S., and Ferguson-Smith, M. A.: Chromosomal studies in some variants of male pseudohermaphrodites. Pediatrics *28*:758, 1961.
Armendares, S., Buentello, L., and Frenk, S.: Two male sibs with uterus and fallopian tubes. A rare, probably inherited disorder. Clin. Genet. *4*:291, 1973.
Benirscke, K., Naftolin, G., Gittes, R., Khuder, G., and Yen, S. S. C.: True hermaphroditism and chimerism. Am. J. Obstet. Gynec. *113*:449, 1972.
Bergada, C., Cleveland, W. W., Jones, H. W., Jr., and Wilkins, L.: Gonadal histology in patients with male pseudohermaphrodi-

tism and atypical gonadal dysgenesis: Relation to theories of sex differentiation. Acta Endocrol. *40*:493, 1962.

Bongiovanni, A. M.: The adrenogenital syndrome with deficiency of 3β-hydroxysteroid dehydrogenase. J. Clin. Invest. *41*:2086, 1962.

Bongiovanni, A. M., DiGeorge, A. M., and Grumbach, M. M.: Masculinization of the female infant associated with estrogenic therapy alone during gestation: Four cases. J. Clin. Endocrinol. *19*:1004, 1959.

Bricaire, H., et al.: A new male pseudohermaphroditism associated with hypertension due to a block of 17α-hydroxylation. J. Clin. Endocrinol. Metab. *35*:67, 1972.

Bullock, L. P., and Bardin, W.: Androgen receptors in testicular feminization. J. Clin. Endocrinol. Metab. *35*:935, 1972.

Corey, M. J., Miller, J. R., MacLean, J. R., and Chown, B.: A case of XX/XY mosaicism. Am. J. Hum. Genet. *19*:378, 1967.

Ferguson-Smith, M. A.: X-Y Chromosomal interchange in the aetiology of true hermaphroditism and of XX Klinefelter's syndrome. Lancet *2*:475, 1966.

Goebelsmann, U., et al.: Male pseudohermaphroditism due to testicular 17β-hydroxysteroid dehydrogenase deficiency. J. Clin. Endocrinol. Metab. *36*:867, 1973.

Haymond, M. W., and Weldon, V. V.: Female pseudohermaphroditism secondary to a maternal virilizing tumor. J. Pediatr. *82*:682, 1973.

Imperato-McGinley, J., Guerrero, L., Gautier, T., and Peterson, R. E.: An unusual inherited form of male pseudohermaphroditism. A model of 5α-reductase deficiency in man. Abstracts, Society of Clinical Investigators, Atlantic City, N.J., 1974.

Jeffcoate, S. L., Brooks, R. V., and Prunty, F. T. G.: Secretion of androgens and oestrogens in testicular feminization: Studies in vivo and in vitro in two cases. Brit. J. Med. *1*:208, 1968.

Jones, H. W., Ferguson-Smith, M. A., and Heller, R. H.: Pathologic and cytogenetic findings in true hermaphroditism. Obstet. Gynec. *25*:435, 1965.

Josso, N.: Permeability of membranes to the Müllerian-inhibiting substance synthesized by the human fetal testis in vitro: A clue to its biochemical nature. J. Clin. Endocrinol. Metab. *34*:265, 1972.

Jost, A.: A new look at the mechanisms controlling sex differentiation in mammals. Johns Hopkins Med. J. *130*:38, 1972.

Kirkland, R. T., Kirkland, J. L., Johnson, C. M., Horning, M. G., Librik, L., and Clayton, G. W.: Congenital lipoid adrenal hyperplasia in an eight-year-old phenotypic female. J. Clin. Endocrinol. Metab. *36*:488, 1973.

Morris, J. M., and Mahesh, V. B.: Further observations on the syndrome, "testicular feminization." Am. J. Obstet. Gynec. *87*:731, 1963.

New, M. I.: Male pseudohermaphroditism due to 17α-hydroxylase deficiency. J. Clin. Invest. *49*:1930, 1970.

Novak, D. J., Lauchlan, S. C., McCawley, J. C., and Faiman, C.: Virilization during pregnancy. Case report and review of literature. Am. J. Med. *49*:281, 1970.

Opitz, J. M., Simpson, J. L., Sarto, G. E., Summit, R. L., New, M., and German, J.: Pseudovaginal perineoscrotal hypospadias. Clin. Genet. *31*:1, 1971.

Parks, G. A., Dumars, K. W., Limbeck, G. A., Quinlian, W. L., and New, M. I.: "True agonadism": A misnomer? J. Pediatr. *84*:375, 1974.

Pergament, E., Heimler, A., and Shah, P.: Testicular feminization and inguinal hernia. Lancet *2*:740, 1973.

Reyes, F. I., Winter, J. J. D., and Faiman, C.: Studies on human sexual development. I. Fetal gonadal and adrenal sex steroids. J. Clin. Endocrinol. Metab. *37*:74, 1973.

Rivarola, M. A., Saez, J. M., Meyer, W. J., Kenny, F. M., and Migeon, C. J.: Studies of androgens in the syndrome of male pseudohermaphroditism with testicular feminization. J. Clin. Endocrol. *27*:371, 1967.

Rivarola, M. C., Bergadá, C., and Cullen, M.: HCG stimulation test in prepubertal boys with cryptorchidism, in bilateral anorchia and in male pseudohermaphroditism. J. Clin. Endocrinol. Metab. *31*:526, 1970.

Rosenberg, H. S., Clayton, G. W., and Hsu, T. C.: Familial true hermaphroditism. J. Clin. Endocrinol. Metab. *23*:203, 1963.

Saez, J. M., Morera, A. M., DePeretti, E., and Bertrand, J.: Further in vitro studies in male pseudohermaphroditism with gynecomastia due to a testicular 17-ketosteroid reductase defect (compared to a case of testicular feminization). J. Clin. Endocrinol. Metab. *34*:598, 1972.

Sarto, G. E., and Opitz, J. M.: The XY gonadal agenesis syndrome. J. Med. Genet. *10*:288, 1973.

Shanfield, I., Young, R. B., and Hume, D. M.: True hermaphroditism with XX/XY mosaicism: Report of a case. J. Pediatr. *83*:471, 1973.

Siiteri, P. K., and Wilson, J. D.: Testosterone formation and metabolism during male sexual differentiation in the human embryo. J. Clin. Endocrinol. Metab. *38*:113, 1974.

Spear, G. S., Hyde, T. P., Gruppo, R. A., and Slusser, R.: Pseudohermaphroditism, glomerulonephritis with the nephrotic syndrome, and Wilms' tumor in infancy. J. Pediatr. *79*:677, 1971.

Wilkins, L., Jones, H. W., Jr., Holman, G., and Stempfel, R. S., Jr.: Masculinization of the female fetus associated with administration of oral and intramuscular progestins during gestation; non-adrenal female pseudohermaphroditism. J. Clin. Endocrinol. Metab. *18*:559, 1958.

Zachmann, M., Völlmin, J. A., Hamilton, W., and Prader, A.: Steroid 17, 20-desmolase deficiency. A new cause of male pseudohermaphroditism. Clin. Endocrinol. *1*:369, 1972.

18
THE GENITAL ORGANS

MALE GENITAL ORGANS

EXAMINATION OF THE EXTERNAL GENITAL ORGANS

The external genitalia should be inspected for cleanliness, color, configuration, size, and symmetry or relation in position of one organ to another. Whether the penis is erectile, the opening from which urine flows, and the size of the external urethral meatus should also be noted. In instances of ambiguity, in order to determine the opening from which a child voids, it is sometimes necessary to probe suspected apertures with a sterile catheter.

Palpation of the testes is most successful when the examiner's hands and the examining room are warm. The location, size and consistency are determined. The examiner should attempt to "milk down" testes which are in the inguinal canal. If testes cannot be felt, one of the following maneuvers may result in their descent; the boy sits with his hips and knees in flexion and with his heels on the examining table, just in front of his buttocks; then he grunts. Examination is most effective when the child is not anticipating it; on occasion it may be wise to depend on the findings of a parent in the home. Examination while the child is bathing in a tub of warm water may be particularly revealing.

The skin of the external genitalia is normally more pigmented than that of other parts of the body. This increased pigmentation is particularly notable in black and Latin babies.

Swelling of the scrotum is common in the newborn. It is more severe in infants delivered from a breech presentation; after a few days the edema disappears.

The size of the penis varies. It may be erect when the urinary bladder is full. The foreskin of the newborn infant cannot be retracted. Testes are palpable in the normal newborn male and are frequently not equal in size. The prostate is not palpable.

ANOMALIES OF THE PENIS

AMBIGUITY OF THE EXTERNAL GENITALIA. The external genitalia may be sufficiently ambiguous at birth to preclude the confident assignment of sex. The phallus may be larger than a clitoris, but smaller than a penis, and is often bound down by chordee. The urethra may open along the shaft of the phallus or on the perineum, or be part of a common outlet for the urethra and the vagina (urogenital sinus). Gonads may or may not be palpable. The male infant with hypospadias and undescended testes cannot be distinguished from the virilized female infant who has labioscrotal fusion and clitoral enlargement. A wide variety of factors may cause such genital abnormalities. In all instances investigation is required immediately after birth, prior to assignment of sex of rearing. See Section 17 for differential diagnosis.

Anomalous development of the penis may vary from the clinically insignificant disorder of *torsion of the penis* to the catastrophic condition of penile agenesis. Total *absence of the penis* has been reported at least 36 times; it may occur as an isolated defect, but is frequently associated with other genitourinary and lower intestinal abnormalities. The newborn male with agenesis of the penis should be assigned a female sex shortly after birth; with appropriate surgery and endocrine therapy, a satisfactory and functional (but sterile) female phenotype is possible. Duplications such as *double penis* or *bifid penis* are almost always associated with other defects, particularly with double bladder, exstrophy of cloaca and imperforate anus. Transposition of scrotum and penis *(retroscrotal penis)* is a rare and correctable defect.

A small penis is of concern to parents, but the size of the normal penis varies markedly, and true *micropenis* is uncommon. In most instances, growth during puberty results in a satisfactorily functional organ. For the occasional child with severe micropenis, the topical application of 1 per cent testosterone cream usually results in satisfactory growth of the organ. The *penis of an obese boy* often appears pathologically small because it is partially covered by suprapubic fat. If the physician retracts the fat, he can readily demonstrate to parents and boy that the penis is of normal size. An unusually large penis is usually a manifestation of precocious puberty, but is infrequently brought to the attention of the physician until pubic hair has also made its appearance.

HYPOSPADIAS. In about 1 in 125 infants the urethral orifice is on the ventral surface of the penis. In the majority (87 per cent) the defect is minimal (coronal or glandular hypospadias); in the remainder, the urethral opening is on the shaft (penile) or on the perineum (penoscrotal). There is often chordee or ventral bowing of the penis, and there may be stenosis of the external urethral meatus. Cryptorchidism is an associated defect in approximately 8 per cent of patients.

First-degree relatives of patients with hypospadias are five to ten times more likely than the general population to have hypospadias; the data suggest a multifactorial etiology. In the majority of instances, the cause is not known; a relative deficit of fetal androgen has been postulated. Occasionally hypospadias may be caused by progestins administered to the mother during pregnancy. In a minority of instances, hypospadias, especially when associated with cryptorchidism, may reflect hermaphroditism, may be due to an abnormality of an autosomal chromosome, or may be an associated defect in one of many complex syndromes such as the Smith-Lemli-Opitz, leopard, hypertelorism-hypospadias, cerebrohepatorenal or cryptophthalmos syndromes.

Surgical correction of chordee should usually be made by 2 years of age. Definitive urethroplasty should be performed before the boy enters school so that it will be possible for him to urinate in the standing position. Since the foreskin is used in the repair, boys with hypospadias should not be circumcised.

EPISPADIAS. In this genital anomaly the opening of the urethra is on the dorsal surface of the penis. The condition occurs in about one in 30,000 infants. The urethral opening may be small and situated just behind the glans; in the more extreme varieties a fissure extends the entire length of the penis. This latter type frequently occurs in combination with exstrophy of the bladder. Milder degrees of epispadias occur in the Ellis-van Creveld syndrome. Treatment is surgical.

OTHER ANOMALIES

Phimosis. Phimosis is a narrowing of the preputial opening so that the prepuce cannot be retracted. Rarely there is no opening. The prepuce may be of normal length or elongated. When the opening of the prepuce is small, urination can be accomplished only by straining; the urine is passed in drops or in a small stream. If adhesions are not present, urine accumulates beneath the foreskin.

Treatment by retraction or stretching with forceps is often sufficient, or the preputial orifice may be widened by incision; in severe forms, circumcision is indicated. A redundant prepuce without phimosis is not an indication for circumcision.

Paraphimosis. In *paraphimosis* the prepuce, after retraction beyond the corona, cannot readily be replaced. The circulation in the glans is interrupted by the constriction; edema, bluish discoloration and even gangrene may ensue. Pain and dysuria are usually severe. The accident usually follows retraction of the prepuce by the patient or by mother or nurse when cleansing the penis. Cold compresses should be applied to reduce the swelling, and then an effort should be made to draw the foreskin forward into the normal position. The glans should be well oiled, steadily compressed, and the constricting prepuce pulled forward. If the paraphimosis cannot be corrected in this manner, incision of the constricting ring of skin may be required. If the foreskin is unduly narrow, circumcision should be performed after the inflammation has subsided.

A condition similar to that of paraphimosis may be produced if the patient ties a string around the penis or slips a ring or other object over it.

ABNORMALITIES OF THE TESTES

It is estimated that when a testis is not palpable, there is a 3 per cent likelihood that it is congenitally absent; one testis may be absent (monorchia) or both (anorchia). In such instances, gel-filled silicone prostheses may be implanted.

About 30 instances of duplication of the testis have been noted. Duplication must be differentiated from crossed ectopia, in which the testis originates on one side and migrates to the contralateral scrotum. Common complications are hernia, torsion and hydrocele. Pain in the scrotum or abdomen may occur.

A *saddle anomaly* of the scrotum is a characteristic feature of the *Aarskog syndrome*. The scrotum tends to be cleft or bifid, and the scrotal folds extend ventrally around the base of the penis.

UNDESCENDED TESTES
(Cryptorchidism)

Maldescent of the testis is a common abnormality, but diagnosis of the condition may be difficult, and many aspects of its management are controversial. There are two types of undescended testes: those which are ectopic and those which are incompletely descended.

The *ectopic testis* is one which, having progressed down the inguinal canal and passed through the external ring, has been diverted to become lodged in the perineum, in the pubopenile area or in the femoral area. The testis which lies somewhere along the normal path of descent without ever having been in the scrotum is designated as *undescended, cryptorchid* or *incompletely descended.* Difficulty in diagnosis arises when a hyperactive cremaster muscle retracts the testis which has descended into the scrotum. Such *retractile testes* are intermittently in the scrotum; at other times they are in the inguinal canal or within the abdomen. It is usually possible to "milk" such testes into the scrotum, but other techniques of examination are often necessary to establish that the testis is retractile (see above). These mobile organs become less retractile with advancing years and will eventually reside in the scrotum. The condition is normal and requires only reassurance.

The testes are undescended in approximately 3 per cent of full-term and 30 per cent of premature infants at birth. Most such testes descend in the first weeks or months of life; thereafter, spontaneous descent rarely occurs before puberty. A significant number of testes will be stimulated to descend at puberty by testicular androgens. When the testes remain undescended past puberty, the seminiferous tubules do not develop; infertility results when the condition is bilateral, though androgen secretion is usually unimpaired. The percentage of cryptorchid testes which descend spontaneously and their ultimate functional status are unsettled.

During about the first 5 years of life the histologic appearance of the undescended testis is similar to that of its scrotal mate; thereafter the rate of development of the undescended testis begins to lag. The significance of such changes, particularly as to future potential for fertility, is unknown.

Undescended testes usually occur as an isolated defect, but significant abnormalities of the upper urinary tract have been found in about 13 per cent of patients with this defect. The undescended testis is often one of the characteristic defects of boys with syndromes known to occur in both sexes. Examples are the Smith-Lemli-Opitz, Willi-Prader, and pseudo-Turner (male Turner) syndromes, the syndrome of absence of abdominal muscles, and others. Maldescent may occur as a manifestation of certain types of inherited hypogonadism such as Reifenstein syndrome. In some instances, failure of normal descent is an indication that the testis is defective in other ways. It is often difficult to determine whether *testicular dysgenesis* which is observed histologically is congenital or a consequence of the maldescent. Another manifestation of the defective nature of cryptorchid testes is their proclivity for development of tumors. Tumors may develop even in testes which have undergone orchidopexy during childhood, but most likely in the late teen years or early 20's; the incidence is quite low.

There is general agreement that orchidopexy is the preferred method of treatment when there is no reasonable doubt that the testis is incapable of descent. Opinions differ, however, concerning the advisability of initial therapy with gonadotropin to determine whether the testis can be caused to descend into the scrotum. Approximately 20 per cent of undescended testes will descend with such therapy. When this is the case, it is assumed that descent would have occurred at puberty under the influence of endogenous gonadotropins.

Our current plan of therapy in the established case is to initiate gonadotropin therapy at about 4 to 5 years of age. Human chorionic gonadotropin is administered intramuscularly in five doses of 4000 units given on alternate days. If the testis does not descend, orchidopexy is performed. When a hernia is present, hormone therapy is not used, but a potential hernia does not contraindicate the use of HCG.

FAILURE OF DEVELOPMENT OF THE VAS DEFERENS

Failure of the vas deferens to develop may occur as an isolated congenital defect. The disorder is not recognized until adulthood, when the patient presents with infertility. Virility is unimpaired and spermatogenesis may occur, but there is lack of transport of spermatozoa from the testes; aspermia is found upon analysis of semen. Absence of the vas deferens may be suspected upon careful palpation of the testes and spermatic cords; ipsilateral agenesis of the kidney is commonly associated. The diagnosis is established by surgical exploration. Failure of development of the vas deferens accounts for the infertility of most adult males with *cystic fibrosis;* the cause for maldevelopment of the vas in this condition is uncertain; it may be analogous to the obstruction and obliteration which occur in ducts of the pancreas.

ACQUIRED DISEASE

TORSION OF THE TESTIS. Increased mobility of the testis may result in an axial twist with ensuing torsion of the spermatic cord and interference with its blood supply. Torsion of the spermatic cord almost always results in infarction and necrosis of the testis if it is not corrected within 24 hours of occurrence. The condition may be present at birth or occur at any age; it is usually unilateral, but may be bilateral. The pathogenesis is not clear; it is believed that there is usually an underlying anatomic abnormality, such as a long mesorchium and an abnormal reflection of the tunica vaginalis; this defect is usually bilateral.

The *clinical manifestations* are variable. In the neonatal period there are often no symptoms, and the presenting evidence is reddish or bluish discoloration of the scrotum with enlargement and tenseness of the testis. It is not possible to transilluminate the mass. Systemic manifestations are rare in infants. Beyond infancy the boy may complain initially of a slight discomfort in the swollen testis; later there are intense pain, exquisite tenderness, lower abdominal pain, fever, nausea and vomiting. A prior history of trauma is not uncommon. When the torsion occurs in an undescended testis, diagnosis is more difficult. The disorder is frequently incorrectly diagnosed as epididymitis or orchitis, owing to the similarity in clinical manifestations; in these conditions, Prehn's sign is positive (i.e., elevation of the scrotum relieves the pain), whereas with torsion Prehn's sign is negative.

Treatment is immediate surgical exposure and untwisting of the torsion and fixation of the testis to the scrotal tissues. An abnormally mobile contralateral testis should be similarly fixed to scrotal tissues at the time of operation. The affected testis should be removed only when severe necrosis is apparent, since even when there is bluish black discoloration some return of function may occur. When there is doubt as to the diagnosis, it is preferable to operate rather than delay, since orchitis is rare in childhood. A 70 per cent salvage rate can be achieved when the disorder is treated within 10 hours of its onset; acute scrotal pain should always, therefore, be assessed immediately.

Torsion of one of the appendages of the testis also occurs, most often of the hydatid of Morgagni. The presenting symptom is acute onset of unilateral scrotal pain; the clinical course may be similar to that in torsion of the spermatic cord. Treatment consists in surgical removal of the necrotic appendix testis.

BALANOPOSTHITIS. Inflammation of the prepuce (posthitis) and glans (balanitis) is often associated with phimosis. It may follow injury by masturbation or other means, or it may occur as a complication of urethritis. The prepuce becomes red and edematous, and itches; the meatal orifice is narrowed, and there is a purulent secretion from the inflamed mucous membrane. There are dysuria and cystitis; hydronephrosis may be a complication in severe cases. Ordinarily the inflammation lasts but a few days. An appropriate antibiotic should be administered and cold compresses applied. Rarely, splitting of the foreskin or circumcision is necessary.

STENOSIS OF EXTERNAL URETHRAL MEATUS. An abnormally small external urethral meatus is relatively common; occasionally it is responsible for obstructive uropathy.

The cause of the defect is not definitely established. Since circumcised infants often have urethral meatal ulcers in association with diaper rashes, and since small meatuses are seen with any frequency only in men circumcised in childhood, it is assumed that the strictures are secondary to ulcerations.

If a boy is found to have a small external urethral meatus, it is imperative that he be observed during micturition; a thin or weak stream due to a constricted meatus is an indication for an intravenous pyelogram and for meatotomy.

CIRCUMCISION

Although circumcision is the operation most commonly performed on male infants in the United States, the medical indications for this procedure are not established. It has been noted that carcinoma of the cervix is uncommon in Jewish women (circumcised husbands) and that carcinoma of the penis is rare among men who were circumcised in infancy. A direct relationship is not proved.

The optimal time for circumcising the neonate is early on the first or after the seventh day of life. At these ages the available prothrombin is at the normal level. The operation should be performed by a physician. Circumcision is contraindicated in infants with anomalies of the external genitalia, since the foreskin may be needed for plastic surgery.

ANGELO M. DIGEORGE

Aarskog, D.: Intersex conditions masquerading as simple hypospadias. Birth Defects: Original Article Series *8*:122, 1971.

Abramovich, D. R.: A possible cause of glandular hypospadias in man. Arch. Dis. Child. *49*:66, 1974.

Altman, L. B., and Malament, M.: Carcinoma of the testis following orchidopexy. J. Urol. *97*:498, 1967.

Bender, L., Printz, L., and Presman, D.: Torsion of the hydatid testis: A review of thirteen cases. Pediatrics *42*:531, 1968.

Felton, L. M.: Should intravenous pyelography be a routine procedure for children with cryptorchidism or hypospadias? J. Urol. *81*:335, 1959.

Johnston, J. H.: The undescended testis. Arch. Dis. Child. *40*:113, 1965.

Lattimer, J. K., Smith, A. M., Dougherty, L. J., and Beck, L.: The optimum time to operate for cryptorchidism. Pediatrics *53*:96, 1974.

Kaplan, E., and others: Reproductive failure in males with cystic fibrosis. New Engl. J. Med. *279*:65, 1968.

Leape, L. L.: Torsion of the testis. Invitation to error. J.A.M.A. *200*:669, 1967.

Lilienfeld, A. M., and Graham, S.: Validity of determining circumcision status by questionnaire as related to epidemiological studies of cancer of the cervix. J. Nat. Cancer Inst. *21*:713, 1958.

Michaelis, E., and Mortier, W.: Association of hypertelorism and hypospadias—the BBB syndrome. Helv. Paediat. Acta *27*:575, 1972.

Ochsner, M. G., Brannan, W., and Goodier, E. H.: Absent vas deferens associated with renal agenesis. J.A.M.A. *222*:1055, 1972.

Papadatos, C., and Moutsouris, C.: Bilateral testicular torsion in the newborn. J. Pediatr. *71*:249, 1967.

Richart, R., and Benirscke, K.: Penile agenesis. Report of case, review of the world literature, and discussion of pertinent embryology. Arch. Path. *70*:252, 1960.

Salle, B., Hedinger, C., and Nicole, R.: Significance of testicular biopsies in cryptorchidism in children. Acta Endocrinol. *58*:67, 1968.

Sugarman, G. I., Rimoin, D. L., and Lachman, R. S.: The facial-digital-genital (Aarskog) syndrome. Am. J. Dis. Child. *126*:248, 1973.

Sweet, R. A., Schrott, H. G., Kurland, R., and Culp, O. S.: Study of the incidence of hypospadias in Rochester, Minnesota, 1940–1970 and a case-control comparison of possible etiologic factors. Mayo Clin. Proc. *49*:52, 1974.

Weiss, C.: Ritual circumcision. Comments on current practices in American hospitals. Clin. Pediat. *1*:65, 1962.

Wyatt, J. K., and Mundy, H. B.: Torsion of the testicle: A clinical review of 20 cases. Canad. Med. Ass. J. *107*:971, 1972.

Young, H. H., II, Cockett, A. T. K., Stoller, R., Ashley, F. L., and Goodwin, W. E.: The management of agenesis of the phallus. Pediatrics *47*:81, 1971.

FEMALE GENITAL ORGANS

The female reproductive system undergoes several periods of physiologic change before reaching maturity. Prerequisite to interpretation of the findings on pelvic examination in young females is an appreciation of the dynamics of hormonal and morphologic interaction.

In *early intrauterine life* the secretion of the fetal gonad and not the maternal hormonal environment is responsible for differentiation and development of the genital system. Differentiation always tends to proceed along female lines in the absence of a male gonad. The embryonic testis is the only

TABLE 18–1 AVERAGE 24-HOUR URINARY EXCRETION RATES OF SEX-RELATED HORMONES IN NORMAL FEMALES FROM INFANCY TO MATURITY

	NEWBORN	1–6 YEARS	7 YEARS TO PUBERTY	MATURE ADULT
Total Estrogens	1 μg/24 hr (first week)	0.5–1 μg/24 hr	1–8.5 μg	4–60 μg/24 hr
Pregnanediol	0–0.5 mg/24 hr	0–0.5 mg/24 hr	0.2–1 mg/24 hr	0.5–7 mg/24 hr
17-Ketosteroids	1 mg/24 hr (first 3 wks = 1–2.5 mg)	1 mg/24 hr	5 mg/24 hr	6–15 mg/24 hr
17-Hydroxysteroids	0	0.5–3 mg/24 hr	1.5–8 mg/24 hr	3–12 mg/24 hr
Pregnanetriol	0	0.06 mg/24 hr	0.3–1.5 mg/24 hr	1–2 mg/24 hr
Pituitary gonadotropins	0	0	Less than 6 mouse uterine units/24 hr	6–50 MUU/24 hr

source of the nonsteroidal organizer which suppresses the müllerian system and stimulates development of the wolffian. If the fetal gonad is ovary, if the fetal gonads are absent (Turner syndrome), or if the embryonic testis is deficient in production of this organizer (male pseudohermaphroditism), the genitalia will be phenotypically female.

In *late intrauterine life* the high levels of female sex hormones normally produced by the fetoplacental unit induce feminizing changes in the breast and in the female genitalia. Exposure of the female fetus to androgenic hormones may produce virilization of the external genitalia. Androgens will not cause suppression of the müllerian ducts, that being a function of the testicular organizer. The association of normally developed internal genitalia with virilized external genitalia is found in fetal congenital adrenal hyperplasia, and as an effect of maternal androgenic drugs or of masculinizing tumors.

In the *immature female* the lack of estrogen greatly increases susceptibility of the external genitalia to infection and to effects of trauma; these are responsible for most of the genital disorders in prepubertal girls. In *adolescence*, menstrual problems are the most common concern and stem from imbalance in the estrogen-progesterone cycle. The levels of hormones found in normal female children are indicated in Table 18–1.

METHOD OF EXAMINATION

Pelvic examination can be performed at any age. Anesthesia is rarely necessary. The likelihood and implications of psychic trauma have been overemphasized, the attitude and approach of the physician having much to do with the reactions of the child. Confidence, gentleness and reasonable alacrity are major assets. The essentials of examination include inspection, with ample separation of the labia, and bimanual palpation, which is performed rectally. Endoscopy is included when conditions require visualization of the upper vagina and cervix. Firm pressure applied to the lateral aspects of the labia majora will expose the hymenal orifice with no discomfort, but the hymen itself is highly sensitive to touch. The posterior vaginal fornix is so short in the immature female that the cul-de-sac is almost nonexistent; accordingly, a palpating finger in the vagina cannot be advanced high enough to outline pelvic structures, even under anesthesia. The uterus may be felt and outlined and the adnexal structures explored more definitively on rectal examination. The uterus lies horizontally in midposition and is approximately 2.5 cm in length during the prepubertal years, with the cervix much longer in proportion to the corpus than in adults. Under normal conditions the tubes and ovaries cannot be felt.

A small plastic pipet with an aspirating bulb and with a tip somewhat longer than that of an average medicine dropper is easily inserted into the hymenal orifice for collection of vaginal secretions or discharge. A cotton swab moistened with saline may also be used, but it is more traumatic if the aperture is small, and contamination from the vulvar region is more likely than with the pipet. The aspirate is adequate for smear, culture, pH and cytologic examination.

For visualization of the vagina and cervix, a vaginoscope, a Kelly cystoscope or a tiny speculum is necessary. Makeshift instruments, such as an otoscope or a nasal speculum, are totally inadequate. The anxious child may reject this portion of the examination. Her general behavior or her reaction to the earlier phases of examination will indicate whether endoscopy can or should be done at any given moment. Sedation may be necessary or, in exceptional instances, general anesthesia.

DOUBTFUL SEX AND ANOMALIES OF THE EXTERNAL GENITALIA

Problems involving *sexual ambiguity* in the newborn infant must be dealt with promptly and knowledgeably. Alarmed parents need to be informed convincingly that an accurate diagnosis can always be reached and that appropriate plans for the future can be made with confidence. Information derived from the family history, from the history of the pregnancy, particularly in regard to maternal drug therapy, from the physical examination of the infant, from a buccal smear and from the determination of level of 17-ketosteroids will provide a correct diagnosis in most cases of sexual ambiguity in the newborn period. A positive buccal smear broadly differentiates virilization resulting from administration of androgens to the mother and female pseudohermaphroditism owing to congenital adrenal hyperplasia (CAH) from male pseudohermaphroditism with partial masculinization of the external genitalia. The 17-ketosteroid levels are elevated in CAH, normal in nonadrenal virilization. The normal increase in fetal adrenal activity characteristic of late intrauterine life may persist for two or three weeks after birth. If the 17-ketosteroid values are not definitive in the first days of life, an increase in urinary pregnanetriol excretion in excess of 1 mg/day confirms the diagnosis of CAH. Exploratory laparotomy will be necessary in rare instances when true hermaphroditism is suspected. (See Section 17.)

Because of their close embryologic relationships developmental anomalies of the genital tract may be associated with or mistaken for anomalies of the urinary system. *Ectopic ureter* usually has its terminus just inside the vaginal vault. A cystic mass appearing at the introitus is more commonly an ectopic ureter with a blind terminus than a vaginal or Gartner's duct cyst. *Imperforate hymen* may also appear as a bulging cystic mass at the vaginal introitus if it is distended with mucous secretions. Whether mucocele is associated or not, imperforate hymen should be incised to allow for drainage as soon as the diagnosis is made. Complete *absence of vagina* is rare and often accompanied by rudimentary development of the uterus; operations for correction of this malformation should not be performed until after maturity. *Labial agglutination* resulting from irritation or inflammation of the labia minora can be distinguished from imperforate hymen or absent vagina by the characteristic livid line of agglutination extending vertically down the center of the membrane of closure. Labial agglutination is self-limited, disappearing as puberty approaches and estrogen levels rise. The agglutination encourages pocketing of urine, with irritation and infection. Application of an estrogenic cream induces cornification of the epithelium, and spontaneous separation will usually occur. If not, the edges can easily be separated with a small well lubricated probe.

VULVOVAGINITIS

Vaginal discharge of a thick mucoid secretion is physiologic in the newborn and derives from cervical glands stimulated by estrogen. A small amount of bleeding owing to endometrial shedding may accompany the discharge. Both are transient and disappear within two weeks, when gestational hormones have been metabolized and excreted. Leukorrhea is also physiologic in young girls, beginning a year or more before the menarche when ovarian function starts and estrogen secretion is as yet unopposed by progesterone. Parental concern is the main problem; fears should be allayed but other treatment avoided.

BACTERIAL VULVOVAGINITIS. Almost any of the infectious or irritating agents may cause inflammation of the anestrogenic epithelium. Establishment of organisms from upper respiratory tract, skin or gastrointestinal tract occurs mainly when trauma such as friction or scratching is added to simple contamination. *Nonspecific infections* with mixed bacterial cultures of the coliform-aerogenes group are most common. They tend to be low grade, chronic and very difficult to eradicate permanently. They may be associated with a vaginal foreign body or with pinworm infestations, in which case removal of the cause and local treatment are curative. *Specific infections* in which pure cultures of pneumococci, streptococci, staphylococci, proteus, Shigella or other organisms are found are generally more acute in onset and more responsive to treatment. A purulent discharge is common to all of these, except that streptococci produce a discharge which is more likely to be serosanguineous or frankly bloody.

Gonococcal infections require smear and culture for diagnosis. Intense redness and swelling of the vulva and vagina and thick purulent vaginal discharge occur, but are not themselves pathognomonic. Upper genital infections are exceedingly rare in prepubertal children.

VIRAL INFECTIONS. No age group is immune to genital infection with herpes simplex. Maternal herpes poses a grave threat to the newborn infant, in whom herpes simplex infection may be very serious. Viremia occurs in the neonate soon after the superficial lesions appear, and damage to internal organs, such as the liver and brain, may be fatal. (See Section 10.) Condylomata are occasionally seen in young girls. These are of viral origin and not venereal.

MONILIAL VAGINITIS. This may occur in the newborn period when the estrogen-stimulated epithelium is rich in glycogen. The infection is rare in the prepubertal years except in children with diabetes mellitus or those on prolonged antibiotic therapy. *Trichomonal* infestations are seen infrequently before puberty.

TREATMENT. Hygienic measures, mild soaps rather than detergents, clean cotton panties and local application of an estrogenic cream will clear most nonspecific infections in 10 to 12 days. Estrogens can be given orally to cornify the epithelium and increase local tissue resistance; suppositories are rarely necessary. Infections with specific organisms are treated in accordance with their sensitivity to antibiotics. Procaine penicillin 600,000 units, given on three successive days, is effective treatment for gonococcal infection; reculture after treatment is essential to the detection of resistant strains of this organism. Monilial vaginitis responds to ointments containing such fungicides as nystatin. Gentian violet as a 1 per cent aqueous solution is effective but messy. The possibility of diabetes mellitus should be kept in mind and the blood sugar evaluated. Metronidazole (Flagyl) is the most effective agent currently available for treatment of trichomonas infestation, but the oral preparation is applicable only to girls weighing over 45 kg (100 lb). The topical preparation should be used in smaller girls.

LICHEN SCLEROSUS ET ATROPHICUS

This disorder may involve the entire vulvar and perianal regions. The tissues appear white and thinned out and are often excoriated by scratching. It is believed to be an inflammatory process, but the specific etiology is not known. The gross appearance closely resembles leukoplakia, but differences are evident on biopsy. Lichen sclerosus et atrophicus is characterized by superficial hyperkeratosis, marked atrophy of the rest of the epidermis, loss of the rete pegs and a specific sclerotic change in connective tissue just beneath the epidermis. It is not neoplastic in behavior and tends to disappear at puberty or shortly thereafter; surgical intervention other than for biopsy should be avoided. This restraint should be emphasized, because local treatment with ointments containing estrogens, hydrocortisone or vitamins A and D may provide only minimal relief from pruritus; parents may need repeated reassurances of the benign nature and self-limited course of the condition.

VAGINAL BLEEDING

Conditions commonly associated with this symptom in prepubertal girls include severe vaginitis (particularly streptococcal), foreign body, trauma, prolapsed urethra, precocious puberty and neoplasm.

TRAUMATIC INJURIES. These heal well with minimum scarring and do not interfere with future reproductive functions. Injuries resulting from rape require special handling. Secretions aspirated from the vagina and collected from the clothing should be examined immediately for gonococci, for spermatozoa and for acid phosphatase, which is found in high concentration in semen. Administration of penicillin is advisable as prophylaxis against venereal disease.

PROLAPSE OF THE URETHRAL MUCOSA. This appears as a mulberry mass protruding from and completely occluding the vagina. The mucosa becomes devitalized below the meatal margin and bleeds readily. The treatment is surgical excision at the line of demarcation.

SARCOMA BOTRYOIDES. Although rare, sarcoma botryoides is so rapidly progressive that diagnosis by biopsy must be made without delay. Lesions may arise in multifocal sites along the course of the cervix and vagina, with early involvement of all regional tissues by local invasion. Wide removal of pelvic organs has resulted in a few cures, but the prognosis is generally poor. Radiotherapy and chemotherapy are ineffectual. (See also Section 25.)

PRECOCIOUS PUBERTY. A cause for vaginal bleeding, precocious puberty is also accompanied by changes in secondary sex characteristics. Constitutional precocity is the most common type and accounts for approximately 90 per cent of the cases reported in girls between the ages of 2½ and 9 years. Central nervous system, ovarian, adrenal and thyroid disorders account for a small percentage of isosexual precocity in the female. These are discussed in Section 17.

MENSTRUAL DISORDERS IN ADOLESCENCE

Normal menstruation is dependent upon the functional integrity of: (1) the hypothalamus together with influences from higher centers; (2) the anterior pituitary; (3) the ovary; and (4) the uterus. The complexities of the processes involved in achieving full sexual maturation are such that menstrual irregularities are to be regarded as physiologic during the first few postmenarcheal years.

DELAYED MENARCHE. In the United States the mean age at normal menarche is 12.3 years, with a range of 9 to 17 years. Age differences for this event are attributed to general health and nutrition, heredity, climatic environment and psychosocial development. Whatever the stimulus, activation of the hypothalamus is clearly the force directly responsible for initiation of menstruation and ultimately for regulation of the fully mature ovulatory cycle. The anterior pituitary gland is capable of producing follicle-stimulating hormone (FSH) and luteinizing hormone (LH) in prepubertal girls, but secretion of pituitary gonadotropic hormones is inhibited until the hypothalamus stimulates release of humoral substances (releasing factors) from the median eminence. Ample laboratory and clinical evidence for these relationships may be seen in destructive lesions of the hypothalamus which hasten the onset of puberty, and in transplantation of the pituitary gland from prepubertal rats to adult hypophysectomized female hosts. Harris showed that the newborn or prepubertal pituitary under the influence of the adult hypothalamus was capable of supporting estrus; in some cases pregnancies occurred.

Delay in the menarche beyond the 16th year warrants diagnostic survey. Exclusion of systemic, metabolic or anatomic defects is the first step. Obesity, malnutrition or psychosomatic disorders may play an important role. A buccal smear should be examined to determine nuclear sex. If any of the examinations suggest genetic or physiologic aberration, further studies are indicated. The need for adequate evaluation before resorting to hormone therapy is emphasized by findings of recent surveys in which modern cytogenetic and hormonal assays have been employed. Such studies show that 40 per cent of the cases of primary amenorrhea extending into late adolescence are the result of genetic abnormalities. Of these, the most frequently encountered are various types of gonadal dysgenesis, the triple-X syndrome, isochromosomal abnormalities, testicular feminizing syndrome and, less frequently, true hermaphroditism.

DYSFUNCTIONAL UTERINE BLEEDING. The symptoms characteristic of this disorder are irregular, protracted or excessive vaginal bleeding. It is due primarily to imbalance in secretion of the hormones that normally control menstrual function and to variability in responsiveness of the target organs in adolescence. With rare exceptions the cycles are anovulatory. The hypothalamic-pituitary-gonadal-uterine axis may take as little as a few months or as long as five years to achieve reciprocal balance and full maturation. Ovulation occurs in only about 3 per cent of women during the first six months of menstrual experience and in only about 18 per cent by the end of the first year. Anovulatory cycles may be considered normal for the first one to three years after the menarche, irrespective of the chronologic age of the patient. This is known as the period of relative infertility.

Dysfunctional uterine bleeding is self-limited for the majority of adolescents but not for all. Complete physical and pelvic examinations are necessary to rule out systemic, metabolic and local organic causes, including pregnancy. Hypothyroidism accounts for only about 5 per cent of cases of menstrual dysfunction in adolescence; appropriate treatment is usually curative. On the other hand, if thyroid function is normal, the empiric use of thyroid preparations is ineffectual and in this age group may be especially deleterious. Hematologic causes for dysfunctional uterine bleeding are rare, but excessive menstrual flow is occasionally the first symptom of thrombocytopenic purpura.

Treatment. If no organic causes are found, menstrual irregularities in adolescent girls should be treated expectantly with a high protein diet and vitamin and iron supplements. Bleeding sufficient to lower the hemoglobin or serum iron levels requires more active treatment. Since the cycles are anovulatory, the endometrium reflects persistent estrogen stimulation and lack of progesterone. Administration of potent oral progestins within the last 5 to 7 days of the cycle is capable of inducing secretory changes in the endometrium. This, in turn, results in a more normal physiologic response to withdrawal of hormonal support and more controlled withdrawal bleeding. Treatment is repeated for three successive cycles. The timing of administration of the progestational agent is extremely important. If given too early in the cycle, it will inhibit ovulation and delay the normal occurrence of this event. When maturation is complete and cycles are ovulatory, the menstrual irregularities are usually corrected.

Instances of severe bleeding present special problems. Control can usually be achieved by administration of larger doses of progestational agents such as Provera (medroxyprogesterone acetate), 10 to 30 mg every 6 hours, until bleeding ceases. Dilatation and curettage may be necessary in some cases for control of hemorrhage and in the minority of cases which fail to respond to conservative management.

DYSMENORRHEA. Abdominal discomfort, cramping in nature, backache and leg ache associated with menstruation are extremely common. The term *primary dysmenorrhea* is applied to these symptoms when they are severe enough to interfere with normal activity and when endometriosis, infection and other pelvic disease causing *secondary dysmenorrhea* are not present. No specific etiology of primary dysmenorrhea is known, but contributory factors are well recognized. The symptoms do not usually appear with the first few menstrual cycles. Instead, they tend to be associated with ovulatory cycles, although this is not invariable. Vascular changes associated with menstrual flow provide the most convincing explanation for the local discomfort. Alternate vasoconstriction and vasodilatation of the vessels of the endometrial bed induce local ischemia, edema, necrosis and slough. Psychic factors, tension and anxiety can accentuate the local symptoms and are entirely responsible for associated autonomic nervous system symptoms of nausea, vomiting, pallor, sweating and, occasionally, syncope when these appear. The pain is often misinterpreted as an indication of pelvic disease and a portent of future reproductive difficulties.

Treatment. Pelvic examination is essential to exclude pelvic abnormalities. An explanation of the physiology of menstruation is reassuring; participation in all regular activities and good hygiene should be encouraged. In severe cases suppression of ovulation using progestogens for several months is usually effective. Psychotherapy may occasionally be necessary; surgical procedures are rarely warranted.

ADENOSIS AND ADENOCARCINOMA OF THE VAGINA

Tumors of the female genital tract, both benign and malignant, may appear in children of all ages, including the newborn. These are discussed in detail in Section 25. Attention is directed here toward a specific neoplasm of the vagina or lower genital tract encountered in young females whose mothers ingested diethylstilbestrol or related nonsteroidal synthetic estrogens during pregnancy.

Herbst and his associates first demonstrated the significant association between maternal treatment with these chemicals and the occurrence of lesions in female offspring exposed to them in intrauterine life.

The use of stilbestrol in an attempt to prevent loss of pregnancy was relatively common, beginning with the mid-forties and ending with the mid-fifties. The risk of tumor development in the exposed offspring appears to be small. Herbst and his associates have established a Registry of Clear-Cell Adenocarcinoma of the Genital Tract in Young Females, to which, as of June 1, 1972, 91 cases had been reported. In order of frequency the primary sites of these tumors may be vaginal, cervical or endocervical. The time of appearance is most commonly at puberty, when ovarian hormonal stimulation is established. Vaginal discharge and bleeding are the most frequent symptoms, but as many as 15 per cent of patients found have been asymptomatic. The malignant lesions, whether vaginal or cervical, may be polypoid, nodular or papillary. Some are friable or hemorrhagic. Vaginal cytology (Pap smear) is considerably less reliable for detection of these tumors than for diagnosis of squamous cell carcinoma of the cervix. Screening procedures should include pelvic examination with inspection of the vagina and cervix, rectovaginal palpation for delineation of nodular lesions and upper transverse ridges of the vagina, and vaginal and cervical smears for cytologic examination. In all patients showing any abnormal areas, biopsy must be done.

Treatment of choice is wide local excision. Radiotherapy appears less effective, but has been used in relatively advanced cases.

MEDICOSOCIAL PROBLEMS OF ADOLESCENCE

Social changes of recent years have affected no segment of society more prominently than the adolescent subculture. This is not surprising given the widespread changes in attitudes regarding sexual behavior. The education provided for young people with respect to sexuality and family life continues to be fraught with controversies and inadequacies. Of major concern are alarming increases in venereal disease, in teen-age pregnancies, and in late abortions with their complications. The medical and general health aspects of these conditions present special problems in adolescent patients, owing both to their chronologic age and to psychologic conflicts, which are reflected in a high incidence of nutritional disorders and dangerous delays in seeking medical care. Legal restrictions regarding treatment of minors without first obtaining parental consent exist in many parts of the country and complicate the medical management in this group of patients.

VENEREAL DISEASE (See also section 10.)

Gonorrhea. Gonorrhea leads the list of reportable infectious diseases in incidence. The Center for Disease Control estimated that 2.5 million cases of gonorrhea occurred in 1971. The increasing incidence of this infection at the rate of approximately 15 per cent per year gives evidence of an epidemic out of control. Alarmingly, the most rapid increase in rate is among young persons. One in every five of the newly infected is under 20 years of age.

Even more frequently in the female than in the male lower genital tract gonorrhea may be asymptomatic or become asymptomatic after a brief bout of urinary frequency, dysuria and discharge. Even when symptoms of upper genital tract infection appear, adolescent patients are often reluctant to seek medical care. Procrastination at this stage is likely to result in tubo-ovarian damage, in infertility and in life-threatening rupture of tubo-ovarian abscess; total abdominal hysterectomy and bilateral salpingo-oophorectomy may be necessary for management.

Early treatment of uncomplicated gonorrhea is highly effective. Delays due to adolescent fears of disclosure may be tragic. In this country 24 of the 50 states have enacted legislation permitting the physician to treat minors infected with venereal disease without first obtaining parental consent, but legal restrictions regarding treatment of minors have not been dealt with uniformly.

Treatment regimens recommended by the United States Public Health Service in 1972 are as follows:

1. If the patient is not allergic to penicillin, probenecid, 1 gm orally, followed in 1/2 hour by 4.8 million units of aqueous procaine penicillin intramuscularly.
2. If the patient is allergic to penicillin and not pregnant, tetracycline, 1.5 gm, followed by 0.5 gm four times a day for 4 days; or, spectinomycin dihydrochloride pentahydrate, 4 gm in a single intramuscular injection.
3. If the patient is allergic to penicillin and pregnant, erythromycin 1.5 gm orally, followed by 0.5 gm four times a day for 4 days.

Syphilis. Syphilis is currently fourth in incidence among reportable infectious diseases. Rates for primary and secondary infections increased 8 per cent in 1970 and 15 per cent in 1971. Cases are concentrated into urban foci, so that the epidemic should be amenable to eradication through aggressive case finding and treatment.

PREGNANCY AND BIRTH CONTROL. The incidence of pregnancies in teen-agers continues to rise. The actual number of cases is unknown, owing to unreported spontaneous or induced abortions, but the total is currently estimated to be well in excess of 600,000 adolescents annually in the United States. Late prenatal registration of uninformed or frightened teen-agers is commonplace. As a consequence, valuable time is lost in correction of nutritional deficiencies, anemia and other disorders. The rate at which education is interrupted is high, and few communities have provided either classes for continuing education or adequate counseling for individuals or groups. The main obstetric complication is pre-eclampsia-eclampsia. The consistently high incidence of this disorder in teen-agers appears to be related to inadequate prenatal care and poor nutritional status. The rate of premature delivery is also high. This may have some bearing upon the slightly higher incidence of mental retardation reported for offspring of adolescent mothers. Jorgensen has shown that an adolescent-centered obstetric clinic emphasizing preventive care and peer group interaction can lower obstetric risks and simplify management problems.

Postpartum family planning is exceedingly important for these young mothers. Experience has shown that continued sexual activity is the rule and that the rate of repetition of adolescent pregnancy is very high. Claman's survey of 315 unwed mothers found 38 per cent to have two or more children. In 1971 both the American Academy of Pediatrics and the American College of Obstetricians and Gynecologists recommended that "the teen-age girl whose sexual behavior exposes her to possible conception should have access to medical consultation and the most effective contraceptive advice and methods consistent with her physical and emotional needs; the physician so consulted should be free to prescribe or withhold contraceptive advice in accordance with the best medical judgment in the best interests of his patient." The request for contraceptive advice must be dealt with on an individual basis; an urgent consideration is that in the case of a minor seeking contraceptive advice, counseling regarding both the physiologic and the social aspects of sexual function and sexuality should have an important place in planning and in management.

ELSIE R. CARRINGTON

Ballard, W. M., and Gold, E. M.: Medical and health aspects of reproduction in the adolescent. Clin. Obstet. Gynec. *14*:338, 1971.

Bishop, P. N. F.: Intersexual states and allied conditions. Brit. Med. J. *1*:1255, 1966.

Capraro, V. J.: Sexual assault of female children. (Monograph on Pediatric and Adolescent Gynecology.) Ann. N.Y. Acad. Sci. *142*:817, 1967.

Carrington, E. R.: Laboratory examination of the pediatric gynecologic patient. Ann. N.Y. Acad. Sci. *142*:623, 1967.

Ditkowsky, S. F., Falk, A. B., Baker, N., and Schaffner, M.: Lichen sclerosus et atrophicus in childhood. Am. J. Dis. Child. *91*: 52, 1956.

Donovan, B. T., and Harris, G. W.: Neurohumoral mechanisms in reporduction. Brit. Med. Bull. *11*:93, 1955.

Fetterman, D. D.: Disorders of sexual development. New Engl. J. Med. *277*:351, 1967.

Gray, L., and Kotcher, E.: Vaginitis in childhood. Am. J. Obstet. Gynec. *82*:530, 1961.

Harris, G. W.: Neural Control of the Pituitary Gland. London, Edward Arnold, Ltd., 1955.

Herbst, A. L., Kurman, R. J., Scully, R. E., and Poskancer, D. C.: Clear-cell adenocarcinoma of the genital tract in young females. Registry report. New Engl. J. Med. *287*:1259, 1972.

Huffman, J. W.: The Gynecology of Childhood and Adolescence. Philadelphia, W. B. Saunders Company, 1968.

Jones, H. W., Jr., and Heller, R. H.: Pediatric and Adolescent Gynecology. Baltimore, The Williams & Wilkins Co., 1966.

Jorgensen, V.: Clinical report on Pennsylvania Hospital's adolescent obstetric clinic. Am. J. Obstet. Gynec. *112*:816, 1972.

Lascàno, E. F., Montes, L. F., and Mazzini, M. A.: Tissue changes in lichen sclerosus et atrophicus in children following local application of oestrogens. Brit. J. Dermatol. *76*:496,1964.

McArthur, J. W.: Functional disorders of menstruation in adolescence. New Engl. J. Med. *249*:361, 1953.

Millar, J. D.: The national venereal disease problem. J. Reprod. Med. *11*:111, 1973.

Oppel, W. C., and Royston, A. B.: Teen-age births: Some social, psychological and physical sequelae. Am. J. Pub. Hlth. *61*:751, 1971.

Philip, J.: Primary amenorrhea: A study of 101 cases. Fertil. Steril. *16*:795, 1965.

Southam, A. L.: Disorders of menstruation. Clin. Obstet. Gynec. *9*:779, 1966.

Southam, A. L., and Richart, R. M.: The prognosis of adolescents with menstrual abnormalities. Trans. Am. Ass. Obstet. Gynec. *76*:43, 1965.

Wallace, H. M.: Venereal disease in teenagers. Clin. Obstet. Gynec. *14*:338, 1971.

White, J. G.: Fulminating infection with herpes simplex virus in premature and newborn infants. New Engl. J. Med. *269*:455, 1963.

19
CONVULSIVE DISORDERS

Convulsive phenomena are common in children and occur with a wide variety of disorders of the central nervous system. Seizures may be classified according to (1) their cause or pathogenesis (see Table 19–1), (2) their clinical manifestations, and (3) their electroencephalographic pattern.

INCIDENCE. Consideration of the relative incidence of the various causative factors at different ages is frequently helpful in arriving at a correct diagnosis and in evaluating prognosis.

Convulsions are far more common during the first 2 years than at any other period of life. Intracranial birth injuries, including the effects of anoxia and hemorrhage and congenital defects of the brain, are the most frequent causes of convulsions in very young infants. In the latter part of infancy and in early childhood acute infections (extracranial and intracranial) are the most frequent causes. Far less frequent causes in infants are tetany, idiopathic epilepsy, hypoglycemia, brain tumors, renal insufficiency, poisoning, asphyxia, spontaneous intracranial hemorrhage and thrombosis, postnatal trauma and others listed in Table 19–1.

By midchildhood acute extracranial infections have become an infrequent cause of convulsions, whereas idiopathic epilepsy, first appearing as an important cause of convulsions about the third year of life, is the most common factor. Other causes in the postinfancy period are congenital defects of the brain, residual cerebral damage from earlier trauma, infection, lead poisoning, brain tumors, acute or chronic glomerulonephritis, certain degenerative diseases of the brain and drug ingestion.

ACUTE OR NONRECURRENT CONVULSIONS

CONVULSIONS IN THE NEWBORN INFANT. A clinical seizure at any age is associated with a paroxysmal burst of electrical activity within the central nervous system. In the newborn infant the electrical activity of the cerebral hemispheres is poorly developed, but subcortical rhythms are present. Mass myoclonic movements have been said to occur in utero, but the tonic and clonic movements that characterize grand mal seizures are rarely apparent during the first several weeks of life. The low incidence of grand mal seizures reported during the neonatal period probably reflects both the poor development of the cerebral hemispheres and lack of uniformity in recognizing or classifying seizures or their equivalents. The electroencephalogram, though not so informative as later in infancy and childhood and technically difficult to obtain, may be the only objective means of detecting a seizure in some instances.

After an episode of acute anoxia, a convulsion in the newborn may take the form of a tonic spasm preceded by a few clonic jerks. The electroencephalogram becomes flattened. Focal seizures may be associated with irregular jerky movements and nystagmus or staring, pallor and hypotonia. Paroxysmal bursts of multiple spike and slow wave discharges appear on the electroencephalogram. In some instances the respirations become slow and irregular, with periods of apnea and a feeble cry. The neck becomes rigid, the pupils dilate, and the child drools. Alteration of the electroencephalogram may also occur in association with slight movements of the fingers, toes or eyelids, with a change in color or with chewing.

The presence of a seizure suggests a cerebral insult and should alert the physician to various causative factors, particularly those which can be altered favorably. The possible maternal use of drugs should be considered. A disorder of amino acid metabolism should be sought or excluded through chromatographic examination of urine or serum. A clinical trial of pyridoxine or examination of the urine for maple syrup urine disease may be lifesaving. (See Section 8.)

The prognosis for the newborn infant who has a seizure is best if the episode is early in onset, of brief duration, and associated with no other disease state. Tremors occurring during the first day of life seem to have the best prognosis, if the child's subsequent neonatal course is entirely normal. The outlook is poor if the heart rate is consistently slow or if symptoms of any kind persist for more than 72 hours. Although convulsions are rarely the only manifestation of a bacterial infection, this possibility cannot be excluded by examination alone.

TABLE 19–1 ETIOLOGIC CLASSIFICATION OF CONVULSIVE DISORDERS

I. Acute or nonrecurrent forms

"Febrile convulsions" (e.g. at onset of acute extracranial infections or in association with high environmental temperatures)

Intracranial infections (e.g. acute meningitis, encephalitis, sinus thrombophlebitis, cerebral abscess, tetanus, malaria, typhus fever)

Intracranial hemorrhage (e.g. from birth or other trauma, hemorrhagic disease, rupture of defective vessels, sickle cell disease)

Toxic:

1. Convulsant drugs (e.g. aminophylline, antihistamines, camphor, propoxyphene, pentylenetetrazol, phenothiazine, hexachlorophene, corticosteroids, strychnine and thujone)
2. Tetanus
3. Lead encephalopathy
4. Shigellosis, salmonellosis

Anoxic (e.g. sudden severe asphyxia, inhalation anesthesia)

Metabolic or nutritional (e.g. acute hypocalcemic and hypomagnesemic tetany, hyponatremia and hypernatremia, alkalosis, therapeutic hypoglycemia, pyridoxine deficiency, phenylketonuria, copper deficiency (Menkes), maple syrup urine disease, hyperammonemia, argininuria, argininosuccinic aciduria, hyperlysinemia, tyrosinemia, glycinemia)

Organic acidurias (propionic, lactic, green acyl dehydrogenase deficiency)

Acute cerebral edema (e.g. in acute glomerulonephritis or allergic edema of the brain)

Brain tumor

Miscellaneous (porphyria, systemic lupus erythematosus)

II. Chronic or recurrent forms

Epilepsy:

1. Idiopathic (primary, cryptogenic, essential or genuine epilepsy)
   - a Hereditary or genetic type
   - b Nongenetic or acquired idiopathic type (?)
2. Organic (secondary or symptomatic epilepsy—with residual brain damage from previous focal or diffuse injuries)
   - a Post-traumatic (e.g., from direct laceration of brain tissue)
   - b Posthemorrhagic (e.g., from injury at birth or later, from hemorrhagic diseases, pachymeningitis, rupture of miliary aneurysm)
   - c Postanoxic (e.g., from severe asphyxia neonatorum)
   - d Postinfectious (e.g., following encephalitis, meningitis, sinus thrombophlebitis or abscess)
   - e Post-toxic (e.g., kernicterus, encephalopathy following lead, arsenic or other chronic poisoning)
   - f Degenerative (e.g., "idiopathic atrophy," cerebromacular degeneration, encephalitis periaxialis diffusa, intracranial neurofibromatosis, incontinentia pigmenti)
   - g Congenital (e.g., cerebral aplasia, porencephaly, tuberous sclerosis, hydrocephalus, vascular anomalies such as the Sturge-Weber type and arteriovenous aneurysms)
   - h Parasitic brain disease (cysticercosis, toxoplasmosis, syphilis)
   - i Posthypoglycemic injury
3. Sensory (reading, touch, light, sound, music, self-induced)

Epilepsy-simulating states:

Narcolepsy and cataplexy

Hysteria ("psychogenic epilepsy")

Tetany:

1. Hypocalcemic (e.g., idiopathic, postoperative, neonatal, vitamin D deficiency, deficient intestinal absorption)
2. Of alkalosis (e.g., vomiting, administration of bicarbonate, hyperventilation)

Hypoglycemic states:

1. Hyperinsulinism (e.g., tumor or hyperplasia of islets of Langerhans)
2. Hypopituitarism (e.g., deficiency of adrenocorticotropic, thyrotropic and growth hormones)
3. Adrenocortical insufficiency
4. Hepatic disorders (e.g., von Gierke's disease)
5. Miscellaneous (e.g., leucine-induced, idiopathic ketotic)

Uremia

"Cerebral" allergy

Cardiovascular dysfunction or syncopal attacks (e.g., simple fainting attacks, Stokes-Adams syndrome, hyperactive carotid sinus reflex)

Migraine

Treatment and management of the newborn infant with seizures involve primarily adequate supportive care. This includes prevention of shock, maintenance of an adequate airway, and sedation appropriate to the infant's needs. Diazepam and phenobarbital are the most widely used anticonvulsive agents.

ACUTE CONVULSIONS IN INFANTS AND CHILDREN. The causes of acute convulsive attacks in children are extremely varied (Table 19–1). Any type of seizure may occur as a transient manifestation of acute disease involving the brain, but generalized tonic and clonic convulsions similar to the grand mal attack of epilepsy are by far the most common. Practically all seizures resulting from extracranial disorders are of this type.

Approximately 3 to 5 per cent of children have *febrile convulsions,* most of which occur after the first 6 months of life, but within the first 2 to 3 years. The incidence decreases up to 6 to 8 years, after which such seizures are rare. Males are more often affected than females, and there appears to be an increased susceptibility in some families.

DIAGNOSIS. In the latter part of infancy and in the first few years of childhood most of the convulsions which occur merely represent an initial symptom of an acute benign febrile illness. A child who has had a convulsion should, however, be examined for the possibility of some other cause. Such disorders as tetany, lead encephalopathy, intracranial injury, hemorrhage or tumor, poisoning with a convulsant drug, hypoglycemia, asphyxia, cerebral sinus thrombosis (associated with cyanotic congenital heart disease or cachexia), acute nephritis and epilepsy should be considered. The age of the child should be taken into account in the consideration of causative factors (see above).

A carefully taken history of any previous attacks, of immediately preceding symptoms such as hyperirritability, fever, muscular cramps, headache, vomiting or dizziness, of a possible dietary deficiency, of poisoning of any kind, of cranial injury, of a hemorrhagic tendency, of exposure to infection or of a familial predisposition to seizures is invaluable for orientation.

Complete physical examination and thorough neurologic appraisal are essential, with special attention to features which may point to specific causes for seizures. For example, depigmented areas resembling a white mountain ash leaf or the lesions of adenoma sebaceum suggest the diagnosis of tuberous sclerosis. Other dermatologic findings which may be helpful include port wine hemangiomata of the face and adjacent areas (Sturge-Weber), irregular hyperpigmented areas or subcutaneous nodules (neurofibromatosis), bronzed skin (Addison's disease), eczematoid areas (untreated PKU), or the butterfly rash of the nose and cheeks (systemic lupus erythematosus). Inspection of the eyegrounds may give the first clue to the nature of the primary illness by revealing an optic neuritis or choking of the disks. These may occur in the presence of an expanding intracranial lesion (tumor, cyst, hemorrhage or abscess), acute hydrocephalus or severe encephalitis. Such examination may also reveal the presence of retinal hemorrhages, suggesting intracranial bleeding from trauma or a blood dyscrasia. Albuminuric retinitis may furnish the first clue to the presence of subacute or chronic nephritis. There may be slight choking of the optic disks in acute nephritis with arterial hypertension. Chorioretinitis is suggestive of toxoplasmosis, but is not diagnostic of it. The reddish areas of degeneration in the macular region in cerebromacular degenerative disease and the choroidal tubercles of miliary tuberculosis are highly characteristic.

Determinations of serum calcium, blood sugar and urea nitrogen levels will aid in the diagnosis of hypocalcemic tetany, hypoglycemia and acute nephritis, respectively. Coexisting hypertension, albuminuria and cylindruria are evidences of nephritis. Roentgenograms may show the "lead line" of lead poisoning in the long bones, multiple recent or healed fractures in the battered child syndrome, or thinning of the skull and separation of the sutures in the presence of an expanding intracranial lesion. Examination of the urine for coproporphyrin and for type III uroporphyrin (Watson test) may reveal evidence of lead intoxication or of acute intermittent porphyria.

If the primary disease is infectious, it should be ascertained whether the infection is extracranial (febrile or prefebrile convulsions) or intracranial. It is necessary to determine whether an intracranial infection is meningitis, encephalitis, abscess, sinus thrombophlebitis or tetanus. Certain other infectious diseases, such as typhus fever, shigellosis, salmonellosis and malaria, may occasionally cause convulsions; in some instances the convulsions are related to disturbances of water and electrolyte balance. (See Hyperelectrolytemia, Section 5.)

TREATMENT. For the control of "febrile" convulsions, which occasionally occur at the onset of acute extracranial infections, a sedative dose of phenobarbital (3 mg per kg) and reduction of the elevated body temperature usually suffice.

If the convulsion is prolonged or if the child has a second convulsion before he recovers fully from the first, more vigorous anticonvulsant treatment is indicated. Appropriate treatment for shock and for the primary condition must of course be provided.

Seizures secondary to electrolyte disturbances require special therapy. (See Section 5.) After other causes for seizures have been excluded as well as it is possible to do so, a clinical trial of pyridoxine may be indicated in young infants. (See Section 3.)

PROGNOSIS. When a seizure results from some physical or metabolic disturbance, the prevention of recurrent convulsions is dependent upon eradication or control of the underlying disease.

After a single febrile seizure the family can be reassured that the probability of chronic epilepsy is not great. The occurrence of more than one febrile seizure increases the probability of subsequent spontaneous nonfebrile convulsions. There is a relatively high probability that idiopathic epilepsy will develop in children who have more than five febrile convulsions in a 12-month period, single seizures which last for more than an hour, or persistent electroencephalographic abnormalities. (Note that the electroencephalogram of a child who has had a febrile convulsion may be abnormal as long as a week afterward.) Approximately 25 per cent of epileptic children have a history of febrile seizures.

There are sharp differences of opinion concerning the advisability of daily anticonvulsant treatment for the child who has had one or more febrile convulsions. Some recommend that daily anticonvulsant therapy be maintained for 2 to 4 years after a single seizure and others that anticonvulsant therapy be withheld until after the first afebrile seizure. The reasons given for daily treatment are: (1) that a significant number of young adults who develop psychomotor seizures have a history of "febrile" convulsion; and (2) that data collected by Lennox suggest that febrile seizures do not recur if a serum level of phenobarbital higher than 15 μg/ml is maintained, intermittent administration of phenobarbital being ineffective. The reasons against continuous prophylactic therapy are: (1) that 3 to 5 per cent of all children would be treated for at least two years if such a program were carried out; and (2) that the administration of full therapeutic amounts of phenobarbital is needed to maintain the level of 15 μg/ml.

Our position is that daily anticonvulsant therapy as usually prescribed does not seem to reduce the number or duration of febrile convulsions. Therefore, as long as the physician feels that a child has febrile convulsions, such therapy is not indicated. When convulsions recur with little or no evidence of infection, or if the electroencephalogram is significantly abnormal 2 weeks or more after the last seizure, a therapeutic trial of daily anticonvulsant therapy may be indicated.

An infant or young child who has had one or more febrile seizures is entitled to more prompt antipyretic measures (such as aspirin or tepid sponges) and *anti-infectious* therapy than might otherwise seem indicated. Some physicians give phenobarbital prophylactically to such infants during a febrile episode. If anti-infectious or anticonvulsant therapy is prescribed, the physician must observe the child closely for the possibility that a serious infection such as meningitis may be masked.

CHRONIC OR RECURRENT CONVULSIONS

EPILEPSY

The terms *epilepsy* (from the Greek *epilépsia,* a seizure) and *recurrent convulsive disorder* can be used interchangeably. These terms designate a variable symptom complex characterized by recurrent, paroxysmal attacks of unconsciousness or impaired consciousness, usually with a succession of tonic or clonic muscular spasms or other abnormal behavior. If a cause of the patient's seizures cannot be found, he may be said to have *idiopathic* or *cryptogenic epilepsy;* if a cerebral abnormality is demonstrable, *organic* or *symptomatic epilepsy.*

Because many persons, from prejudice or ignorance, feel that a person with epilepsy will somehow fail to make an adequate social adjustment, some physicians are reluctant to use the term "epilepsy" in discussing the problem with parents. Although its use, even with gentle and dispassionate explanation of its meaning, may be immediately alarming to parents or patient, an affected family should know the term and how it applies to them. This is part of the physician's responsibility as he educates the family toward living more comfortably with a chronic illness. The family's ability and desire to acquire information about a chronic illness is variable, along with the rate at which information can be assimilated. Too much information on a single visit is undesirable. Orientation should be a continuing process, especially during the early period of medical supervision.

IDIOPATHIC EPILEPSY. Although in the majority of instances the cause of recurrent seizures cannot be established, it would seem probable that some specific genetic defect in cerebral metabolism is responsible in many of the afflicted children.

Electroencephalographic tracings, particularly during sleep, show generalized abnormalities in 90 per cent of children with idiopathic seizures. Often there are focal electrical abnormalities on the electroencephalogram which migrate from one area to another as evidenced by variations in serial examinations. These are rarely associated with anatomic defects. Lennox pointed out that electroencephalographic abnormalities (cerebral dysrhythmias) are more likely to be found in parents and siblings of affected children than in the population at large. The most frequent abnormality to be found in otherwise unaffected relatives is the spike-wave discharge.

ORGANIC EPILEPSY. A variety of genetically determined conditions (Table 19–1) are associated with seizures. These disorders may have abnormalities demonstrable anatomically (e.g., congenital ectodermoses) or biochemically (e.g., phenylketonuria). In addition, convulsions may occur after cerebral damage acquired in the prenatal, natal or postnatal period. Neurologic examination of such children frequently shows a motor handicap of central nervous system origin (cerebral palsy) and mental retardation. These patients almost always have electroencephalographic abnormalities.

The recognition of genetically determined conditions is important for several reasons: (1) Cerebral damage in younger siblings of affected patients may be prevented in certain instances by prompt and effective therapy (e. g., leucine-induced hypoglycemia, phenylketonuria, kernicterus). (2) Indefinite signs and symptoms in siblings may be more readily recognized (e. g., tuberous sclerosis, cerebromacular degeneration, neurofibromatosis). (3) Identification of an organic cause of the seizures is important prognostically; in general, control of such seizures is less satisfactory and social adjustment of the child less adequate than in children with idiopathic seizures.

CLINICAL MANIFESTATIONS

Grand Mal Seizures. These seizures may be preceded by a momentary aura, but fewer than a third of epileptic children can give a definite description of such an experience. In some instances a preliminary, localized spasm or twitching of muscles may precede a generalized seizure. This is often referred to as a "motor aura," or warning. Vague prodromal symptoms or signs, such as irritability, intestinal disturbances, headache and mental dullness, may forewarn patients or their parents of impending motor seizures. The period intervening is usually short, but may be hours or even a day or two.

Grand mal seizures are generalized convulsions, usually with tonic and clonic phases of the muscular spasms. The onset of the paroxysm is abrupt, and the tonic spasm may occur simultaneously with loss of consciousness. The patient, if sitting or standing, falls to the ground. His face suddenly becomes pale, the pupils dilate, the conjunctivas become insensitive to touch, the eyeballs roll upward or to one side, the face is distorted, the glottis is closed, the head may be thrown backward or to one side, the abdominal and chest muscles are held rigidly, and the limbs are contracted irregularly or stiffen out. As the air is forced out of the lungs through the glottis by sudden contraction of the diaphragm and the intercostal muscles, a short, startling cry may be heard. The tongue may be severely bitten as a result of the rapid contraction of the jaw muscles. Micturition and less frequently defecation may follow the sudden forceful contraction of the abdominal muscles. As the tonic phase of the seizure continues, facial pallor is quickly followed by suffusion and this, in turn, by cyanosis, occasionally severe, owing to arrest of all respiratory movements. At the end of this phase, which usually lasts not more than 20 to 40 seconds, the clonic phase sets in and lasts for variable periods of time.

The patient may awaken from his postconvulsive sleep with a severe, generalized headache and in a state of confusion. He may go about in a semidazed or stuporous state in which he may perform more or less automatic acts without being able to recollect what he has experienced. These postparoxysmal or postictal reactions are interpreted as malfunctioning of neurons which have not yet recovered from the effects of the seizure. These may be so severe as to result in prolonged automatism, in transient paresis or, more rarely, in hemiplegia or other paralytic manifestations of focal injury or hemorrhage.

A grand mal seizure may occur at night (*nocturnal epilepsy*) without the patient's being aware of it. A bitten tongue or lip, headache, blood on his pillow or a bed wet with urine may be the only clue. Generalized motor seizures tend to be predominantly tonic during infancy, although the clonic feature is always present to some degree.

So-called secondary symptomatology, which pertains chiefly to personality traits such as egocentricity, shallowness, religiosity and chronic negativism, and which is considered by some to be characteristic of epilepsy, is much less prominent in children than in adults. When such personality traits are manifest, they usually represent the patient's response, over a long time, to psychogenically injurious attitudes of other people toward him and his disability. These traits are not to be attributed to the disease itself or confused with the transient behavior disturbances of psychomotor attacks. Similar personality disturbances develop frequently for the same general reasons in children with any chronic handicapping condition.

Petit Mal Seizures. These seizures consist in a transient loss of consciousness. There may be such minor manifestations as an upward rolling of the eyes, moving of the lids, drooping or rhythmic nodding of the head, or slight quivering of the trunk and limb muscles. Clinical evidence of petit mal rarely appears before 3 years of age, and frequently disappears by the time of puberty. Girls are more often affected than boys. Intellectual development is rarely impaired in children who have only simple, staring petit mal seizures. Attacks of this type last less than 30 seconds and are most frequently described by parents or other associates of the child as "dizzy spells," "absences," "lapses" or "fainting turns." The patient rarely falls, but usually drops articles he may have in his hand or mouth. If the child, for example, is performing an act such as writing or reading at the onset, he will suddenly discontinue it, and then resume it when the seizure is ended. He may not be aware of having had a convulsion. Such seizures vary in frequency from one or two a month to as many as several hundred a day. After hyperventilation or exposure to a blinking light a child may have a typical episode. Individual petit mal seizures may, in rare instances, become progressively prolonged and gradually resemble a mild form of grand mal. Prolonged episodes of confusion, inappropriate action and loss of ability to speak or understand (*petit* *mal status*) are rare and can be distinguished from psychomotor seizures only by an electroencephalogram during the attack.

Pyknolepsy (Pyknoepilepsy; "Myriad Spells"). Pyknolepsy is the designation used by Adie for a clinical state in which mild petit mal seizures suddenly appear in great numbers in otherwise normal children between the ages of 3 and 10 years. Such episodes recur over a period of months or years, then cease spontaneously and permanently without impairment of the victim's mentality. The electroencephalograms of such patients are typical of petit mal epilepsy. There is little justification for setting this condition apart as a separate clinical entity.

Psychomotor Seizures. Psychomotor seizures are the most difficult to recognize and among those more difficult to control. They consist in purposeful but inappropriate motor acts, which are repetitive and often complicated. Most frequently a slight aura may manifest itself in a young child by a shrill cry or an attempt to run for help. The seizure itself often consists in a gradual loss of postural tone. For example, the child may extend one arm and make a slow half-turn to one side while falling slowly to the ground. He often has vasomotor changes, such as circumoral pallor. After a 1- to 5-minute episode of unconsciousness the child may resume his normal activity. Often the child is drowsy or sleeps for a short time after the spell. There are usually no tonic or clonic movements. Fugue states or episodes of confusion, which may resemble petit mal, are rarely noted in children. A normal electroencephalogram, except at the time of psychomotor seizure, is not uncommon. Treatment is similar to that of grand mal seizures.

Focal Seizures. These seizures may be sensory or motor in type (*jacksonian epilepsy*), depending upon the location of the focal area of abnormal neuronal discharge. Focal seizures may occasionally occur in the absence of organic lesions. Localized sensory attacks which give rise to a variety of symptoms are rare in children. Unilateral motor or jacksonian attacks, though not infrequently preceded by a brief tonic phase, are typically clonic, indicating their origin in the motor cortex. The muscles most frequently involved in a jacksonian seizure are the ones most specialized for voluntary movements, as in the hand, face and tongue, less often those of the foot and trunk.

As might be expected from the relation of the areas of representation of the various muscle groups in the precentral gyrus, a focal motor seizure beginning in one member spreads or extends to others according to a fixed pattern, e.g., from thumb to fingers, to wrists, to arm, to face and then to the leg on the same side ("jacksonian march" of muscle spasms). When such an attack is of brief duration and remains localized to one area, consciousness may not be disturbed. When its spread is extensive and rapid, however, consciousness is lost, and a generalized convulsion follows, indistinguishable from a typical grand mal seizure.

Infantile Myoclonic Seizures. This convulsive seizure has also been called "infantile spasm," "lightning major" and "jackknife epilepsy." Unlike true petit mal seizures, these episodes occur before 2 years of age and involve more than a single group of muscles. The most common type of mass myoclonus is a sudden dropping of the head and flexion of the arms. The attack may be repeated several hundred times a day. The electroencephalographic changes consist of random high-voltage slow waves and spikes (*hypsarrhythmia*) and suggest a diffuse, disorganized state. It is one of the most characteristic encephalographic patterns and probably represents the response of the immature brain to a profound disturbance.

On the basis of age and developmental ability at the time of onset, an infant with myoclonic seizures may be placed in one of two groups. If his developmental level has never been normal or the seizures occur before 4 months of age, a congenital cerebral defect (Table 19–1) or other organic cause is most likely, and significant developmental retardation is to be expected. If the infant appeared to progress normally until 6 months of age or more before the hypsarrhythmia is detected, an unrecognized encephalitis or an underlying defect in cerebral metabolism may be responsible. The outlook is unfavorable; only about 10 per cent of the infants in this group retain intellectual ability within the normal range.

Usually the infantile myoclonic seizures disappear spontaneously before the fourth year of life; other seizures may occur subsequently. Often the children in the second group have good motor ability, but poor adaptive and language abilities for their chronologic age. This has made the evaluation of treatment, such as with corticotropin, difficult.

A therapeutic trial with corticotropin, a corticosteroid or pyridoxine is indicated. In a number of instances such therapy, when started early, has appeared to produce improvement in the clinical status and in the electroencephalographic pattern. At present, however, a cause-and-effect relation is speculative, since spontaneous improvement, though infrequent, does occur.

Myoclonic and Akinetic Seizures. Myoclonic jerks or involuntary muscular contractions may occur in conjunction with other manifestations of epilepsy, including loss of consciousness, or they may occur alone. A single group of muscles is usually affected. A patient may have a normal electroencephalogram while he is having myoclonic jerks involving one side or extremity. The origin of the seizure is presumed to be subcortical in such instances.

An akinetic seizure is associated with a sudden generalized loss of postural tone and therefore differs from single or repeated myoclonic jerks. These seizures in young children may resemble infantile myoclonic seizures and are sometimes called motor petit mal, jackknife or akinetic seizures. The electroencephalogram usually reveals a spike and wave pattern of less than 3 per second (*petit mal variant*).

Minor motor seizures are often a symptom of degenerative disease or other central nervous system disorders, and may be difficult to control.

Self-induced Seizures. It is possible for some children to induce petit mal or grand mal seizures by overbreathing, by watching a blinking light, or by some other form of learned behavior. Self-induced seizures should be distinguished clinically from other types of convulsions because drug therapy alone is usually unsatisfactory. After a child has learned to draw attention to himself in this manner it is difficult to alter this defensive mechanism. Complex family problems probably underlie this kind of behavior. Therapy in the form of behavioral modification has been successful in some instances.

DIAGNOSIS

Electroencephalography. Three types of rhythms have been described in the electroencephalogram of the normal human adult. The most common one, the alpha rhythm, consists of regular sinusoidal waves, which occur at frequencies of 8 to 12 per second, with a voltage of 20 to 60 microvolts when recorded from the scalp. The second most common one is the beta rhythm, most prominent in the frontal cortex, with lower amplitude and a frequency of 13 to 32 per second. The least common is the gamma rhythm, which arises from the frontal lobes and consists of a more rapid rate, 33 to 55 per second, with waves of extremely low voltage. Slower waves (theta, 5 to 7 per second, and delta, 1 to 4 per second) are not present in normal adults during the waking state.

The interpretation of the electroencephalograms of infants and children is more difficult than of those of adults because of the presence of slow rhythms (3 to 8 per second) in normal children. Cortical rhythm is poorly developed in the newborn infant. As he matures, the electroencephalogram shows random 3- to 7-per-second waves and some low-voltage faster activity. Gradually the basic rhythm becomes more regular, and by 6 years of age the pattern is made up principally of 5- to 7-per-second waves, and by 10 years alpha waves, 8 to 12 per second, predominate. During childhood 14- and 6-per-second positive spikes (ctenoids) are commonly found in presumably healthy subjects. During adolescence some slow wave activity, 4 to 8 per second, is not uncommon and may be incorrectly interpreted if adult standards are used.

Sleep without the use of a hypnotic, hyperventilation for 2 minutes, pentylenetetrazol (Metrazol), artificially induced fever, the vasopressin (Pitressin) test and flickering light serve to bring out latent abnormalities in the electroencephalogram and may on occasion produce a seizure. Of these, sleep and hyperventilation are most frequently used in cooperative subjects.

When there is clinical evidence of a convulsive disorder, an electroencephalogram should be obtained in practically all instances. Documentation of spike-wave or other characteristic patterns may prove valuable for orientation during long-term management.

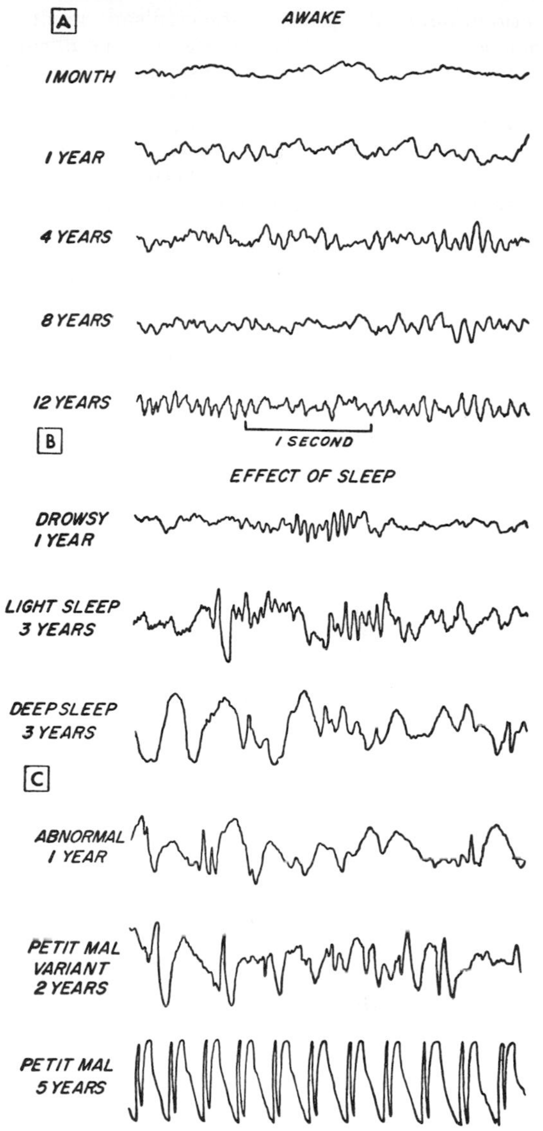

Figure 19–1 *Electroencephalograms of infants and children.* A, *Tracings from comparable areas of the scalp illustrating variations with age of electrical activity in the motor cortex; all were secured during a quiet phase just before sleep.* B, *The effects of sleep, variations of patterns in normal children; compare with tracings in* A *and* C. C, *Abnormal waves.*

Abnormal Waves. Lack of stability of the central nervous system is associated with electroencephalographic abnormalities. If a cell membrane is damaged, the break or leak results in excessive or prolonged release of energy (excessive depolarization). In humans repair of the leak (repolarization) probably depends upon a chemical reaction involving "high energy" phosphate compounds, which respond quickly in order to re-establish the gradient of potassium and sodium across the cell wall. If excessive release of energy from a damaged or leaking cell occurs, neighboring cells become involved, and alterations in many cells and their connections may take place. Anticonvulsant medications probably act by stabilizing the cell membrane so that excessive, repetitive discharges are less likely to occur.

Most patients with frequent *grand mal seizures* have definite abnormalities in their electroencephalograms in the intervals between seizures. These consist of random spike discharges, diffuse high-voltage slow waves or a pattern not consistent with the child's chronologic age. An electroencephalogram obtained during a grand mal seizure shows multiple high-voltage spike discharges. After the seizure there are asymmetries between the two hemispheres and diffuse slowing.

Patients with seizures other than grand mal have a variety of electroencephalographic abnormalities. The most easily recognized one is that of *infantile myoclonic seizures* with its high-voltage, 1- to 2-per-second, spike and wave pattern, the so-called hypsarrhythmia (hyps = high and lofty). The record gives the impression of complete disorganization.

During *petit mal attacks* there is characteristically a 3-per-second spike and wave pattern.

A constant asymmetry of one area compared to its counterpart on the opposite side may be significant, especially if the electrical activity shows phase reversal of slow waves. Shifting foci are more common in children than in adults and indicate a functional disturbance rather than an anatomic lesion.

Absence of electrical activity over an area suggests a large lesion such as a subdural collection of fluid or an abscess. Serial electroencephalograms of children with hydrocephalus show a disturbance of function as the process progresses.

After cerebral insults such as trauma, encephalitis, cerebral thrombosis and prolonged seizures, electrical activity may be slow for a time and may be roughly correlated with the child's clinical course.

Metabolic disorders, such as hypoglycemia, hyperthyroidism and adrenal insufficiency, alter cortical activity; the clinical significance of these changes is not clear.

Various types of cerebral dysrhythmia may occur for short times between clinical seizures. The occurrence of abnormal discharges of short duration, such as a single wave and spike formation or a short series of spikes similar to those in grand mal seizures, without clinical manifestations has given rise to the designation of subclinical or larval seizures. These subclinical bursts may at times foretell the onset of clinical seizures.

Roentgenography. A roentgen examination of the skull is considered an essential part of the diagnostic appraisal in search for such abnormalities as intracranial calcifications, erosion of the base or increased densities, which may indicate reasons for seizures. A hammered-silver pattern of the cranium is present so commonly that by itself it is not considered abnormal. Routine pneumoencephalography in the epileptic child is not necessary, since space-filling lesions without localizing peripheral neurologic changes which justify surgical exploration are an uncommon cause of convulsions in children.

Other Studies. The decision to perform laboratory examinations other than the routine urinalysis, blood cell count and tuberculin test should be based on leads obtained from the medical history, the physical examination and the clinical course. Examination of the cerebrospinal fluid need not be routine, but it may provide additional information when diagnostic considerations include lead poisoning, certain instances of mental deterioration and encephalitis.

When hypoglycemia (Section 16), nephritis (Section 15), lead poisoning (Section 28), and tetany (Section 19) are considered possible causes of convulsions, appropriate diagnostic steps are obviously indicated.

TREATMENT OF RECURRENT CONVULSIONS

Management of the Individual Seizure. Practically all that should be done for a patient during an attack is to protect him from bodily injury. This necessitates constant supervision in severe cases. At the beginning of a major seizure, clothing about the neck should be loosened. The patient should then be turned on his side so that he does not aspirate his pooled secretions. He should be observed carefully for changes in color; administration of oxygen is indicated during prolonged convulsions. Any injury to the tongue and other tissues of the oral cavity during a convulsion is most apt to occur at the onset. Since subsequent injury is not very likely and because additional damage often results from crude efforts, the family should be counseled against placing a stick or other object between the teeth.

Status Epilepticus. If a series of grand mal convulsions occurs before the patient has fully recovered, the prolonged seizure is termed status epilepticus. The intervals between individual convulsions may be so short that the seizures are virtually continuous. During status the muscular contractions may appear to be one-sided or to shift from one group of muscles to another. This does not constitute a true focal (jacksonian) seizure.

The most common cause of status epilepticus is discontinuance of previously continuous daily anticonvulsant medication; often this has occurred within less than 2 weeks.

Drug treatment consists in prompt administration of phenobarbital sodium intramuscularly (average doses, 60 mg at 6 months of age to 120 mg at 2 to 3 years, or 5 to 6 mg per kg.; maximum single dose is 200 mg). If the convulsion is not controlled within 15 minutes, the initial dose should be repeated. If the convulsion has been partially controlled by this time, half the initial dose should be given. Subsequent administrations may be necessary. The rhythmic contraction of a single group of muscles after a severe convulsion does not require additional therapy. Sedative therapy should be limited to a single agent. If the convulsions are not controlled by a total dose of phenobarbital of 15 mg per kg within 60 minutes, the possibility of some organic lesion such as encephalitis, metabolic disturbance or vascular accident should be considered. The administration of a small dose of phenobarbital (less than 2 to 3 mg per kg) to a child in status should be avoided, because it is likely to be inadequate and subsequent control may then be difficult.

The dangers of intravenously administered barbiturates and of inhalation anesthesia are similar to those of anesthetizing an excited child. Such procedures are rarely necessary and, when indicated, should be performed by an experienced anesthesiologist. Laryngeal spasm and even sudden death may occur if treatment is too vigorous.

Experience with diazepam (Valium, see Drug Table) indicates that it is effective in the treatment of status epilepticus. Each ampule of the preparation contains 10 mg in 2 ml of solution for intravenous administration. The solution should not be diluted and should be administered slowly (0.5 ml per minute). The usual dose is 5 to 10 mg, and no more than 6 ml (30 mg) is recommended. Within 1 minute the effect of the drug is usually apparent both clinically and in the electroencephalogram. The limbs become hypotonic, the rate of respiration decreases, the pupils first dilate and later decrease in size, and nystagmus often develops. Excessive salivation and hiccupping may occur. Although the child usually remains quiet, he will respond to painful stimuli. The corneal reflex may be diminished or absent. The effect of the drug lasts from ½ to 3 hours, but drowsiness may be present in some children for as long as 18 hours.

The principal advantage of diazepam is the prompt control of the convulsion. The anxiety of parents, nurses and physicians, which often complicates management, is alleviated early. Disadvantages are that the underlying cause may be masked (e.g., infection, lead encephalopathy) and definitive therapy delayed. Sudden death, which has occurred after the intravenous administration of barbiturates for the treatment of grand mal status, has not yet been reported in children after the administration of diazepam. Its side effects are not fully known. Tolerance tends to occur after the administration of diazepam intravenously on three or four occasions, so that increasing amounts must be administered to regain the initial effect.

We prefer to inject small amounts of isotonic saline before and after the injection of diazepam through the same intravenous needle. Extravasated diazepam is a local irritant; loss of an extremity has been reported (Pediatrics *53*:112, 1974).

Administration of oxygen is indicated during prolonged convulsions, and administration of 5 per cent glucose in 0.45 per cent saline solution intravenously may shorten the recovery time.

A quiet and calm atmosphere, reassurance and avoidance of unnecessary annoyance to the patient are important factors in general management, especially during the recovery phase.

Continuous Therapy of the Epileptic Child. The aims of treatment are to reduce the number of seizures, to encourage the child to function at a level commensurate with his natural endowment, and to promote his acceptance at home and in the community on the basis of his capabilities. The responsibilities of the physician include diagnostic and therapeutic services for the child, information and counsel for the parents, and guidance to the community and the school. The success of the physician at each level will often affect both the number of the seizures and the child's adjustment. There are a number of limiting factors, such as the duration and severity of symptoms, the kind of seizures, the presence of a genetic factor, the presence of complicating cerebral lesions, and the capacity of the patient and his family to cooperate.

If the patient or his family has been unduly frightened by laboratory studies, folk tales or by reading poorly selected medical information, additional explanations (education) by the physician will be necessary. Usually, however, the medical management is relatively easy after the diagnosis of an idiopathic convulsive disorder has been established.

Orientation of the Child. The attitude of the child toward his disease generally reflects that of his parents. It is usually desirable for the child to be present during conferences with the parents. Even if the medical terms are puzzling, the child will sense the philosophy of the physician. If it combines realism with optimism, long-term benefits can be expected. Parents are often poorly equipped to explain a long-term illness to a child. By giving the parents and the child a chance to ask questions in each others' presence, many doubts and fears can be resolved. Attempts to disguise the existence of seizures are unwise and often harmful.

The questions of the child are apt to be related to activity in school, sports, and the like, or to the duration of therapy. Most children are pleased to find that their participation in regular activity is encouraged. The usual restrictions against riding a horse alone or swimming except when attended by a responsible adult are readily accepted. Participation in competitive sports, in which injury to the child or others is possible, must be decided on an individual basis. Seizures during an athletic activity are rare in children who are otherwise well controlled.

The duration of therapy is not predictable. It is preferable to continue medication for a long time even if the dose of the drug is small. A workable rule is to continue medication until the electroencephalogram is consistently normal; it can be repeated annually. It is difficult for both the child and his parents to begin treatment again should seizures recur.

It is usually better to leave discussion about discontinuation of medication until the child has been without seizures for a year. To give the parent or the child an estimate is unwise, because it will seem to them a form of penal sentence. Early in the course of treatment it is enough for the child to know that he may not always have to take medication. Later, if he can lead an otherwise normal life, he will be willing to accept this minor inconvenience.

After the diagnosis of an idiopathic convulsive disorder has been made, return visits to the physician every 2 to 4 weeks may be helpful. Additional questions, the possibility of additional history, information about environmental factors, physical findings and drug toxicity may be dealt with appropriately at these times.

Orientation of the adolescent. Although the behavioral changes of a boy or girl with a convulsive disorder during adolescence are similar to those of unaffected children, they are more likely to be brought to the attention of the physician. Unexplained tearfulness, hostility, clumsiness, inattention (particularly in school), forgetfulness, increased sibling rivalry, antiauthoritarianism and overreaction (by adult standards) to petty annoyance are often part of normal adolescent behavior, but may in a boy or girl with a convulsive disorder be attributed to medication or to the disease. If the physician has previously discussed the increasing need for independence during adolescence, his reassurance after development of symptoms is more likely to be successful. It may be helpful to have the child's teachers and a psychologist work together toward finding a realistic educational program.

The child with epilepsy wants to be "normal," to be independent, to be accepted and admired by his peers, and to achieve status symbols which are sometimes unrealistic. To achieve these goals, the adolescent with a convulsive disorder may test the fantasy that there is nothing wrong with him and refuse or forget to take his medication. If a seizure occurs, his "forgetfulness," personality change (depression) and recurrent seizures may lead to unnecessary hospitalization and unjustified diagnostic procedures. These experiences may further delay the development of an independent, self-sufficient person. In some instances one or both parents may be reluctant to give up control of the child. The patient who has had little opportunity to exercise judgment in activities of daily life is likely to use his handicap as a shield.

Orientation of the Parents. Among the pertinent questions asked of the physician by the parents after the diagnosis of epilepsy has been established are these: Will punishment of the child cause a seizure? What of the child's future? Is his mental development likely to be retarded by the disease? Will mental deterioration occur? Will his life be shortened by it? Should he attend school? Should he marry and have children? As the physician helps the family to understand the general problem, the following points are fundamental:

1. The seizure is a symptom and, unless it is associated with clinical evidence of shock (peripheral vascular collapse), it will rarely produce irreversible damage to the central nervous system.
2. If the child gains excessive attention by having seizures, control by medication alone is likely to be difficult.
3. In most instances, avoidance of emphasis on the recurrence of seizures is helpful.
4. Restoration of confidence, in both the parents and the child, is important. The adults need to feel that they are competent and capable persons who meet their responsibilities appropriately.
5. If the child receives medication in the proper amount, therapy should in no way influence his mental ability or personality or cause him to become a drug addict.
6. It is best to rear the child in a normal fashion. To reward or to punish him differently only because he has seizures leads to behavioral difficulties.
7. The patient needs an environment which will allow him to compete successfully at his own level.

With some parents it is prudent for the physician to say in effect to the parents, "You give the medication and handle the child in a normal fashion, and I will worry about the spells." As members of the family become more mature in their attitudes, they will become more receptive to consideration of any important underlying difficulties such as previously unrecognized mental retardation, behavioral difficulties, inappropriate placement in school, and intrafamily conflicts.

Orientation of the Community. If educational facilities appropriate to his needs are available, the child should attend school close to his own home and participate in activities to which he is naturally inclined. It is the duty of the physician, the nurse and the social worker who are acquainted with the problem to do everything possible to improve the attitude of the public toward the epileptic patient and his disease. Nearly every intelligent epileptic child sooner or later encounters attitudes toward him of pity and oversolicitousness or of disgust and horror. These are likely to be a source of constant anxiety unless he is able to acquire an adequate philosophy.

Drugs. Since the introduction of bromides for the treatment of epilepsy by Leacock in 1858, drug therapy has been the choice and usually the only form of treatment. The tendency to rely upon medication alone was encouraged by the introduction of phenobarbital in 1912. Subsequently dietotherapy came into use when it was discovered that fasting, the ketogenic diet and reduction of the water intake all tended to prevent epileptic seizures. Since the demonstration by Merritt and Putnam in 1938 that sodium diphenylhydantoinate (Dilantin) was effective in the treatment of some patients not controlled by phenobarbital, the tendency to depend mainly upon drug therapy has again increased.

The successful management of the epileptic child requires determination of the most appropriate anticonvulsant drug or combination of drugs for him as well as the most appropriate dosages. To achieve this result, a systematic program for a trial of the various anticonvulsant drugs is necessary; a

TABLE 19–2 SUGGESTED SCHEDULE FOR A THERAPEUTIC PROGRAM IN EPILEPSY

Unless there is a specific contraindication, the administration of phenobarbital, 3 mg/kg/day, in 2 or 3 divided doses to every child with grand mal psychomotor, petit mal, infantile myoclonic or mixed seizures is the treatment of choice.

Example: 20 kg (44 lb) × 3 mg/kg = 60 mg daily; one 30-mg tablet on arising and one at bedtime

Grand mal, psychomotor, and mixed seizures

After 2 weeks if the seizures are not controlled, increase phenobarbital to 5 mg/kg/day in 2 or 3 divided doses. Unless status occurs, devote efforts to the improvement of environmental factors and avoid changes of medication.

After another 2 weeks if seizures are not controlled, **continue phenobarbital** and **add** Dilantin, 2-3 mg/kg/day, in 1 or 2 divided doses.

Example: 20 kg (44 lbs) × 3 mg/kg = 60 mg; one 30-mg capsule of Dilantin on arising and one at bedtime

(Alternate) 20 kg (44 lbs) × 2.5 mg/kg = 50 mg or 1 tablet at bedtime

After the third 2 weeks, if grand mal or psychomotor seizures are not adequately controlled, continue phenobarbital, 5 mg/kg/day, and increase Dilantin to 5-6 mg/kg/day.

After the fourth 2 weeks, Dilantin can again be increased to 7-8 mg/kg/day, but never to more than 300 mg daily in the pediatric age range.

Petit mal

Continue phenobarbital, 3 mg/kg/day, and if seizures are not controlled, add Zarontin, 250 mg (1 capsule) daily. Each succeeding week, if petit mal seizures continue, add 1 capsule (250 mg) of Zarontin to the daily dose (2 or 3 divided doses) until tolerance is reached or spells disappear (not more than 6 capsules daily). If the petit mal spells are associated with a motor component which involves muscles below the neck, add Dilantin in doses of 2-3 mg/kg/day. Medications should be given together. The administration of medications twice daily (on arising and at bedtime) is most desirable because it is least likely to be forgotten and because other children may swallow tablets if they are left at an available site.

Infantile myoclonic seizures

If infantile myoclonic seizures have been of recent origin, the administration of corticotropin (ACTH-gel, 5-10 units daily for 2 weeks) is suggested in addition to phenobarbital, 3 mg/kg/day.

If infantile myoclonic seizures continue or if the electroencephalogram continues to show a hypsarrhythmia, the corticotropin is discontinued, and pyridoxine, 10-15 mg/kg/day orally for 2 weeks, is prescribed in addition to phenobarbital, 3 mg/kg/day.

If there is no improvement either clinically or in the electroencephalogram, the phenobarbital is continued. Although there is no convincing evidence that steroid therapy is beneficial, it is our practice to administer corticotropin again, and to increase the amount by 5-10 units each week until 50 units daily is reached and maintained for 30 days. If 50 units of ACTH-gel for 30 days is not effective in changing the electroencephalogram to an apparently normal pattern, the administration of ACTH is reduced to 10 units weekly and discontinued within several weeks. A corticosteroid such as prednisone (Meticorten), 0.5 mg/kg/day, may be substituted for the corticotropin. If the patient does not respond to the administration of corticotropin or a corticosteroid, supportive care is continued. Although a variety of anticonvulsant medications has been suggested, phenobarbital, 3-5 mg/kg/day in 2 divided doses, seems to be most helpful.

---

suggested schedule to determine an adequate therapeutic program is shown in Table 19–2. A change in the dose of a medication or from one medication to another should usually not be made more frequently than every 2 weeks.

Phenobarbital. Phenobarbital in tablet form is the drug of choice for prolonged use in the average patient with grand mal epilepsy. Its virtues are its relative effectiveness, its comparative harmlessness in therapeutic doses for a prolonged time, its ease of administration and its low cost. Doses range from 8 mg (1/8 grain) 1 to 3 times daily for an infant to 100 mg (1½ grains) 1 to 3 times daily for an older child. It may also be prescribed on a weight basis with an initial dose of 3 mg. per kg. per day in 2 divided doses, with gradual increases to the required maintenance dose. More than 6 mg. per kg. per day may result in drowsiness. The concentration of phenobarbital and other anticonvulsant medications in the serum and other tissues can be measured accurately by the use of gas-liquid chromatography. Because lack of compliance (failure of the child to receive the prescribed amounts of medication) is a frequent cause of poor seizure control, determination of serum levels on one or more occasions is highly desirable. Unless this possibility is seriously considered, less effective or more expensive drugs may be substituted prematurely. Serum levels of 15 to 25 μg/ml are within the therapeutic range.

Two weeks after a child has received phenobarbital in a therapeutic dose on a regular basis, the serum value tends to remain constant. This stable state can be identified by obtaining serum specimens prior to the administration of a morning medication and 3 hours later. A significant variation between the concentrations in the two specimens is strong evidence that the administration of the drug has been irregular. If two or more anticonvulsant drugs are administered on a regular basis, the concentration of each in the serum may be less than would be expected on the basis of single usage of either one. Serum levels of phenobarbital often increase to 30 to 60 μg/ml without apparent alteration of mental or motor functions.

Occasionally a child will have an idiosyncrasy to

phenobarbital. A maculopapular eruption on the skin and mucous membranes, excessive drowsiness and fever may be signs of sensitivity or overdosage. These soon disappear without permanent harm if the dose is reduced or if the drug is withdrawn. Rarely, and particularly when attacks are primarily petit mal, a patient appears to be made worse by phenobarbital and has petit mal variants or psychomotor attacks. In such an event Dilantin may also be administered. Rarely, it is necessary to discontinue phenobarbital, which should always be done gradually, and to substitute another drug.

Mebaral. Mephobarbital (Mebaral) is a barbiturate of value in some cases. The dose is approximately double that recommended for phenobarbital.

Dilantin. The only drugs which rival the barbiturates in the control of grand mal seizures are certain hydantoin compounds, such as diphenylhydantoin sodium, U.S.P., also known as phenytoin sodium (Dilantin). They are administered to older children in capsules and to younger ones in tablet form crushed in a little food or fruit juice. Doses range from 25 mg (1/2 tablet) 1 or 2 times daily in infants to as much as 100 mg once or twice daily in older children. The drug may also be prescribed in an initial dose of 3 mg/kg/day in 2 doses, with gradual increases to the required maintenance dose. More than 8 mg/kg/day may result in toxic manifestations. The chief advantage of hydantoin compounds over the barbiturates is that they act as efficient anticonvulsants without producing excessive drowsiness. One of these should be given a trial, therefore, whenever grand mal seizures are not adequately controlled by phenobarbital alone in nondepressing doses. Replacement should be made gradually, however, since sudden changes may result in increased convulsive reactivity. Serum levels of 15 to 30 μg/ml of hydantoin are usually within the therapeutic range. Somewhat lower levels may be satisfactory.

Painless, nonhemorrhagic hypertrophy of the gums usually follows the administration of Dilantin. It usually requires no special treatment other than good dental hygiene. If it becomes unattractive cosmetically, another drug should be substituted.

Ataxia and drowsiness may occur if the initial dose is too large, if the dose is increased too rapidly or if the total daily dose exceeds about 8 mg/kg/day. Serious toxic reactions such as nausea or vomiting, erythema or a morbilliform eruption and nervous manifestations such as tremor of the hands, ataxia, diplopia with nystagmus, paralytic manifestations and mild psychoses are relatively uncommon, and disappear after reduction of the dose, usually to about two thirds of its former level. *Dilantin should not be administered to infants and young children in the form of a suspension because most parents are not able to administer the small dose accurately.*

Chemical and roentgenographic evidences of rickets (Section 22) have been associated with the administration of Dilantin. In our experience correction of dietary factors and reduction of the Dilantin level in the serum to the currently accepted therapeutic range have been associated with prompt improvement. Most reported instances have occurred among patients in institutions who had received medication for long periods of time. Although adequate intake of vitamins and balanced diets are difficult to assess in these settings, nutritional factors and the relatively high dosage schedules employed probably account for most of the reported cases. These instances emphasize the need for periodic review of dietary habits, recent weight gain and loss, and other evidences of mental and physical growth. In an institution, children unable to make their needs known may require especially careful medical supervision.

Tridione. Trimethadione (Tridione) (3,5,5-trimethyloxazolidine 2,4-dione) is an effective drug for the treatment of petit mal epilepsy in doses of 0.3 gm (5 grains) 1 to 4 times daily. The drug may also be prescribed on a weight basis with an initial dose of 25 mg/kg/day in 2 to 4 doses, which may be gradually increased if necessary to 80 mg/kg/day. Tridione may increase the occurrence of grand mal attacks, if they also exist, and the additional administration of a barbiturate or hydantoin is indicated. Excessive doses or prolonged use of Tridione may result in photophobia, hemeralopia (day blindness), drowsiness, nausea, skin eruptions or nephrosis. Such manifestations tend to disappear after withdrawal of the drug. Several fatalities from aplastic anemia have been reported in patients receiving Tridione regularly for several months. When it is given for more than a short time, periodic blood cell counts should be obtained, and the drug discontinued if any abnormality is found.

Paradione. Paradione is less toxic than Tridione, but also less effective. The dosage is similar to that of Tridione.

Zarontin. Ethosuximide (Zarontin) is probably a more useful agent for the treatment of petit mal seizures than is Tridione. Side effects have been reported to follow the administration of Zarontin, but usually disappear if the amount of medication is decreased. These effects include nausea, dizziness, drowisness, rash and hiccups. The symptoms are unlikely to return if the drug is readministered, beginning with a lower dose, which is then increased gradually to a maintenance level lower than the preceding one. The occurrence of a blood dyscrasia following the administration of Zarontin is unusual. A white blood cell and differential count should be obtained before starting therapy, after 1 month, and then every 3 to 6 months. Routine examination of the urine at these times is also desirable.

Because many children with petit mal seizures can be controlled by phenobarbital alone, the administration of Zarontin is suggested only when necessary in addition to phenobarbital or Mebaral. Occasionally a child with more than one type of convulsion may have an increased number of seizures after Zarontin has been administered.

The recommended starting dose is one capsule (250 mg) daily for a week. If necessary, the daily number of capsules is increased by 1 each week, until a total of 6 capsules daily is reached (2 capsules, 3 times daily). The drug may also be prescribed by weight, 20 to 40 mg/kg/day. Serum levels of 20 to 40 μg/ml are often required. If the administration of the capsule is impractical in young children, the drug may be readily dissolved in 1 to 2 ounces of fluid, and its taste disguised by 8 to 10 drops of calcium cyclamate (Sucaryl), an artificial sweetener.

Mysoline. Mysoline (primidone) (5-phenyl-5-ethyl-hexahydropyrimidine-4:6-dione) is used in the treatment of grand mal and psychomotor seizures. It may be used alone or in combination with other drugs and does not depress hematopoietic activity. The chief side effects—drowsiness, ataxia and dermatitis—can be minimized by starting with small amounts (125 mg) at bedtime and by increasing the dose slowly at 7- to 10-day intervals to a maximum dose of 250 mg, 3 times daily. In patients receiving both mysoline and phenobarbital the serum will contain both primidone and a breakdown product, paraethylmalonic acid (PEMA), but the principal correlate of seizure control seems to be the concentration of phenobarbital.

Diazepam (Valium). (See also Drug Table in Section 30.) The administration of diazepam orally (1 to 10 mg 3 times a day, as tolerated) for the treatment of convulsive disorders is under study. Preliminary indications are that some children, particularly those with petit mal who have been refractory to Zarontin and other agents, do respond favorably. In many instances tolerance occurs after 3 to 14 days of therapy. If the dosage is further increased, undesirable side effects may occur, such as drowsiness, ataxia and slurred speech.

Children who have seizures associated with degenerative disease of the central nervous system often tolerate diazepam well. The dosage schedule must be adjusted individually. We have found that the oral administration of diazepam with phenobarbital and Dilantin is a useful combination in some instances.

Carbamazepine (Tegretol) Tegretol (200-mg tablets, only) has been widely used for relief of pain, primarily for trigeminal neuralgia. Clinical data suggest that this drug may also help to control seizures (particularly of the psychomotor type). Its use in the United States has been limited to investigational purposes. Often observed side effects include dizziness, drowsiness, nausea, vomiting and ataxia. Serious side effects, which have been reported in adults, may reflect the severity of the conditions for which it has been prescribed. The starting dose of 100 mg (1/2 tablet) 2 to 3 times daily with or without other medications can be increased to 400 mg (2 tablets) 2 to 3 times daily in adolescence. Maintenance of serum level of 3 to 10 μg/ml is usually associated with control of seizures. If the administration of the drug is successful, the principal advantage is the lack of sedation.

The Ketogenic Diet. Fasting causes cessation of grand mal seizures in a majority of epileptic children, the effect usually manifesting itself shortly after ketosis has appeared on the third day. A strongly ketogenic diet has a comparable anticonvulsive effect after ketosis has developed. Stringent restriction of the liquid intake, even when the diet is nonketogenic, results in cessation of grand mal seizures in most of those patients who respond favorably to fasting or the ketogenic diet. Establishment of a negative water balance, by restricting the intake or increasing the output, intensifies the anticonvulsive effects of the ketogenic regimen. Administration of alkaline salts in sufficient amount to neutralize the acidogenic effect of fasting or of the ketogenic diet abolishes the anticonvulsive action, whereas administration of inorganic acids or acid-forming salts fortifies or intensifies such action. The ketogenic diet has been used for petit mal and grand mal epilepsy.

The use of the ketogenic diet is limited because of the practical difficulties of adhering consistently to a restricted dietary intake and because of the possibility of attendant emotional disturbances. It may be helpful for children who have frequent seizures which are not controlled by moderate doses of one or more of the anticonvulsant drugs; in such instances the diet may often be used in conjunction with them. The child and his family must be willing and able to accept the dietary regimen without emotional conflict. Owing to the various difficulties of the diet, it is no longer widely used. The use of medium chain triglycerides has been suggested.

PROGNOSIS. The prognosis of a convulsive disorder depends upon any coexisting mental retardation, physical handicaps, possible organic disease, and the adequacy of medical and environmental management. The results of therapy are generally not satisfactory in infants and young children with infantile myoclonic seizures.

The tendency to repeated seizures, with or without apparent organic cause, is found in some families, but the possibility of a convulsive disorder occurring in siblings or in offspring of affected persons is impossible to assess accurately. In a general discussion it may be helpful to stress that residual effects of a convulsion are rare, and to note the observation of Yannet that children with convulsions who had parents with a history of a convulsive disorder were better adjusted and had fewer seizures than those whose parents had not had seizures.

Although it is probable that a severe prolonged seizure of one or more hours may deplete available stores of glucose and interfere with oxygenation and thus cause secondary cerebral changes, there is reason to believe that the usual convulsive episode does not cause irreversible damage. Convulsions followed by permanent hemiplegia are probably more often the result of a vascular accident which occurred before the seizure than to injury during it. In such instances, there are likely to be recurrent convulsions which are more difficult to control than those of idiopathic epilepsy.

Grand mal seizures tend to become more numerous unless the course is modified by therapy. On the other hand, a number of patients with unquestioned idiopathic grand mal epilepsy appear to undergo spontaneous cessation of seizures after adequate treatment. Epileptic patients who are otherwise normal seldom die or sustain serious injuries as a result of their disorder. Patients who are well controlled medically rarely have seizures during participation in athletic activities.

The prognosis for mental development in young epileptic patients or for mental deterioration in older patients was formerly gloomy, chiefly because opinion was based largely upon experiences with the more severe cases in public institutions. Collins and Lennox found the intelligence quotients of 100 children and 200 adults in private practice to average 109, with ranges of 52 to 153 for the former and of 47 to 139 for the latter. The intelligence quotients of those with evidence of cerebral damage before the first seizure averaged 10 points lower than of those with idiopathic epilepsy. The highest scores were found in those with essentially normal electroencephalograms and in those with typical petit mal activity, the lowest in those having both grand mal and psychomotor attacks. With proper treatment most epileptic patients with normal mentality can be expected to maintain it.

DISORDERS SIMULATING EPILEPSY

(Including So-called Epileptic Equivalents)

NARCOLEPSY. Narcolepsy is a syndrome characterized by recurrent diurnal attacks of irrepressible sleep, usually precipitated by a sudden emotional change. It is rare in children and is said to be more frequent in boys than in girls.

Narcolepsy has been classified according to origin into "idiopathic" and "symptomatic" groups. Wilson further subdivided the latter group into 6 categories: toxic-infective, e.g. postencephalitic; circulatory; post-traumatic; endocrine; neoplastic; and psychopathologic.

The attacks resemble those of epilepsy in their brevity, in their abruptness of onset and in their paroxysmal and involuntary nature. The overpowering sleep of narcolepsy may come on suddenly while the patient is engaged in some activity such as talking, walking or driving. He then ceases what he is doing and falls "in a heap." The "sleep" is usually shallow, and the patient is easily aroused. The disturbance apparently has no relation to the physiologic need for sleep. Regular nocturnal sleep is normal. The patient exhibits mental alertness rather than somnolence after he has been aroused.

The disorder tends to be chronic, but spontaneous improvement and cure are more common than in epilepsy. The amphetamines have proved much more effective than ephedrine. Dosage for a child should be the minimal amount which will produce the desired effect.

ABDOMINAL EPILEPSY. Otherwise unexplained recurrent episodes of abdominal pain, nausea, and vomiting have on occasion been considered to be a manifestation of epilepsy. Some epileptic children with psychomotor or grand mal seizures do have abdominal pain just prior to the onset of a convulsion, but abdominal pain as the only overt manifestation of epilepsy must, if it does occur, be extremely rare. Recurrent abdominal pain associated with headache, but without nausea or vomiting, has also been attributed to migraine (see below). If abdominal epilepsy is to be accepted as a diagnostic designation, the criterion for its application in a given case should be quite restrictive. The following clinical pattern would probably be acceptable to most critical observers: recurrent episodes of abdominal pain, with or without associated headache, but without twitching or convulsive movements, somnolence as a postictal manifestation, an abnormal electroencephalogram, and relief from the attacks of abdominal pain with anticonvulsive therapy.

BREATH-HOLDING. See Psychologic Disorders, Section 2. These spells, comparatively common in early childhood, are sometimes associated with tonic and clonic movements.

HYSTERICAL FITS. These can resemble true epileptic seizures in a superficial way. They are fairly easily distinguished by a number of characteristics. There is usually a typical neurotic background. Between attacks the patient may exhibit motor or sensory disturbances which do not follow the true neural patterns, and the gag reflex may be absent. Dilatation of the pupils and pallor of the skin and mucous membranes rarely accompany an attack. Loss of consciousness is superficial and variable. Sphincter control is not lost, and bodily injury from the seizure does not occur. Crying, moaning and disconnected talk throughout the attack, which may last half an hour or longer, are common. Hysterical patients, like other neurotic children with behavior problems, frequently have some abnormalities in the electroencephalogram. The treatment of hysterical seizures is that of the underlying psychologic disorder.

SYNCOPE. Synocopal attacks of various types due chiefly to transient cerebral anemia are frequently complicated by slight tonic and clonic convulsive reactions of short duration confined mostly to the face and arms. The most common form in early life is the *simple fainting spell,* which is brought on reflexly in certain children by a simple procedure such as removal of a sliver or insertion of a needle into the skin, or by a sudden fright while in a standing or sitting posture. The susceptibility to fainting appears to be related to defective reflex regulation of the vascular system, which manifests itself as a sudden relaxation of the visceral venous system with bradycardia and a fall in blood pressure. Placing the patient in a horizontal position or with the head tilted downward at a 45-degree angle will tend to shorten the period of unconsciousness. When it is necessary to subject a child known to faint easily to some painful test or treatment, it is advisable to have him lie on a table during the procedure. Vigorous crying before and during such a procedure as taking a blood sample tends to prevent fainting. In an older child active gripping of some object and voluntary contraction of the abdominal muscles have the same effect.

In the *Stokes-Adams syndrome,* which occurs in heart block (Section 13), a short convulsive reaction often accompanies the syncopal attack. The seizure appears within 10 to 20 seconds after the onset of asystole. Similar syncopal attacks have been reported in patients as a result of *paroxysmal tachycardia,* and attacks occur fairly frequently after muscular effort in young children with certain congenital anomalies of the heart, such as the tetralogy of Fallot.

A *hyperactive carotid sinus reflex* manifests itself by episodes of unconsciousness with or without brief tonic and clonic convulsive attacks. This condition is extremely rare. Pressure over the carotid sinuses in the anterior cervical region causes a slowing or temporary arrest of the pulse in persons subject to attacks. Associated with the asystole are symptoms of faintness, weakness, loss of consciousness and finally the convulsive reaction.

APNEIC EPISODES DURING SWIMMING. These episodes, especially in competitive events, have, in rare instances, been responsible for sudden loss of consciousness and at times for clonic movements. Such attacks presumably have been observed most frequently in adolescent boys, and more often in association with the breast stroke than with other forms of swimming. Even expert underwater swimmers can, by forced hyperventilation before submerging, so deplete the body of carbon dioxide that hypoxia may produce unconsciousness before the respiratory center initiates a breath. Perhaps, in somewhat the same way, an overwhelming desire to attain a competitive goal may dominate the urge to breathe. When respiration cannot be restarted by prompt artificial respiration, it is presumed that ventricular fibrillation has occurred.

MIGRAINE (HEMICRANIA). (See also Section 20.) Migraine has long been regarded as being akin in some respects to epilepsy. The two frequently occur in the same family. Occasionally attacks of migraine are replaced by typical epileptic seizures. Its paroxysmal nature, its chronicity and its genetic features make migraine resemble idiopathic epilepsy. This has given rise to the unfortunate use of the designation "sensory epilepsy" for migraine. In true visual seizures of epileptic patients the eye symptoms are much shorter in duration than they are in migraine and are bilateral.

HENRY W. BAIRD

General Education

Baird, H. W.: The Child with Convulsions. A Guide for Parents, Teachers, Counselors, and Medical Personnel. New York, Grune & Stratton, 1972.

Baird, H. W., and Borofsky, L. G.: Infantile myoclonic seizures. J. Pediatr. *50*:332, 1957.

Baird, H. W., and Garfunkel, J. M.: Electroencephalographic changes in children with artificially induced hyperthermia. J. Pediatr. *48*:28, 1956.

Barrow, R. L., and Flaving, H. D.: Epilepsy, and the Law. New York, Harper and Row, 1966.

Borofsky, L. G., Louis, S., Kutt, H., and Roginsky, M.: Diphenylhydantoin: Efficacy, toxicity, and dose-serum level relationships in children. J. Pediatr. *81*:995, 1972.

Brown, J. K.: Convulsions in the newborn period. Develop. Med. Child Neurol. *15*:823, 1973.

Forster, F. M., Paulsen, W. A., and Baughman, F. A.: Clinical therapeutic conditioning in reading epilepsy. Neurology *19*:717, 1969.

Generoso, G., and Barlow, C.: Juvenile migraine, presenting as an acute confusional state. Pediatrics *45*:628, 1970.

Jasper, H. H., Ward, A. A., and Pope, A.: Basic mechanisms of the epilepsies. Boston, Little, Brown and Company, 1969.

Kales, A., and Kales, J. K.: Sleep Disorders. Recent findings in the diagnosis and treatment of disturbed sleep. N. Engl. J. Med. *290*:487, 1974.

Lennox, W. G., and Lennox, M. A.: Epilepsy and Related Disorders. Boston, Little, Brown and Company, 1960.

Livingston, S.: Comprehensive Management of Epilepsy in Infancy, Childhood and Adolescence. Springfield, Ill., Charles C Thomas, 1972.

Millichap, J. G.: Febrile Convulsions. New York, The Macmillan Company, 1968.

Prensky, A. L., Raff, M. C., Moore, M. J., and Schwab, R. S.: Intravenous diazepam in treatment of prolonged seizure activity. New Engl. J. Med. *276*:997, 1967.

Princhard, J. S., Gauk, E. W., and Kidd, L.: Mechanism of seizures associated with breath-holding spells. New Engl. J. Med. *268*:1436, 1963.

Rodin, E. A.: The Prognosis of Patients with Epilepsy. Springfield, Ill., Charles C Thomas, 1968.

Schneider, S., and Mace, W.: Dangers of intravenous diazepam, loss of limb following intravenous diazepam. Pediatrics *53* :112, 1974.

Svensmark, O., and Buchthal, F.: Diphenylhydantoin and phenobarbital serum levels in children. Am. J. Dis. Child *108*:82–87, 1964.

Verret, S., and Steele, J. C.: Alternating hemiplegia in childhood: A report of eight patients with complicated migraine beginning in infancy. Pediatrics *47*:675, 1971.

Woodbury, D. M., Penny, J. K., and Schmidt, R. P.: Antiepileptic drugs. New York, Raven Press, 1972.

TETANY

Tetany is a state of hyperexcitability of the central and peripheral nervous system resulting from abnormalities of the concentrations of ions in the fluid bathing the nerve cells and peripheral nerves. The specific ionic abnormalities causing this state are decreases of H^+ (alkalosis), of Ca^{++}, or of Mg^{++}. There are obvious interrelations: a decrease in H^+ may precipitate tetany at concentrations of Ca^{++} or Mg^{++} which might otherwise be above the threshold for manifest tetany; and a decrease of K^+ can prevent the development of tetany despite low Ca^{++} concentrations, whereas a rising K^+ can precipitate tetany in a patient with low Ca^{++}. There is thus a range of ionic concentrations at which tetany can be either latent or manifest. Latent tetany is defined as the condition in which mechanical or electrical stimulation of motor nerves or ischemia is required in a degree sufficient to produce the motor response characteristic of tetany.

The serum calcium as usually determined measures both Ca^{++} and undissociated calcium proteinate. The major serum protein which complexes calcium is the albumin fraction. Ca^{++} can be measured, but this procedure is not usually available for clinical diagnostic purposes. At normal concentrations of serum albumin about 50 to 55 per cent of the total calcium is ionized Ca^{++}, i.e., 5.0 to 5.5 mg/dl. When the serum albumin level is reduced, the total serum calcium is decreased without a decrease in Ca^{++}; a rough rule of thumb states that the total serum calcium falls 0.8 mg/dl for each decrease of serum albumin by 1 gm/dl. A patient with nephrosis whose serum albumin concentration is 1 gm/dl might therefore have a total serum calcium concentration between 7.5 and 8.0 mg/dl without reduction of Ca^{++}. (See Figure 30–3.)

At physiologic concentrations of H^+ and K^+, tetany may develop at Ca^{++} concentrations of less than 3.5 mg/dl and will almost always be manifest at Ca^{++} concentrations less than 2.5 mg/dl. If serum albumin concentrations are normal, these levels correspond to total serum calcium concentrations of approximately 7 mg/dl and 5 mg/dl, respectively.

The normal serum magnesium level ranges between 1.8 and 2.5 mg/dl, of which about 75 per cent is Mg^{++}. A reduction of total serum magnesium to less than 1.0 mg/dl may be associated with hyperexcitability of the nervous system.

MANIFEST TETANY. The classic signs of peripheral hyperexcitability of motor nerves are spasms of the muscles of the wrists and ankles (carpopedal spasm) and of the vocal cords (laryngospasm). In carpopedal spasm the wrists are flexed, with extension of the fingers and adduction of the thumbs over the palms, the so-called obstetric position. The feet are extended and adducted. These muscular spasms can be quite painful. Laryngospasm causes inspiratory obstruction, with a high-pitched inspiratory crow; apnea may result. The sensory manifestations are paresthesias, particularly numbness and tingling of the hands and feet. The manifestation of motor excitability of the central nervous system is a convulsion. The convulsions are usually generalized but may be localized to one side of the body. They are often brief but recurrent. Between seizures the patient may be apparently conscious, but after a prolonged series of convulsions a postictal state may result. In young infants convulsions are frequently the only evidence of the hyperexcitability of the nervous system.

LATENT TETANY. Carpopedal spasm may be induced in latent tetany through the production of ischemia of the motor nerves by cutting off the arterial supply with a tourniquet *(Trousseau's sign)*. The usual test employs a blood pressure cuff on the arm, inflated above the systolic blood pressure for 3 minutes. With a positive test the typical pattern of carpal spasm develops.

In tetany motor nerve impulses can be elicited by mechanical tapping, whereas this is not possible under normal physiologic conditions. The facial nerve can be stimulated by tapping anterior to the external auditory meatus. Contraction of the orbicularis oculi occurs with a twitch of the eye, or of the orbicularis oris with a twitch of the upper lip or entire mouth (*Chvostek's sign*). The peroneal nerve can be stimulated by tapping it as it passes over the head of the fibula. A positive *peroneal sign* is dorsiflexion and abduction of the foot.

The motor nerves can also be stimulated by electrical stimulation. *Erb's sign* is a positive response to electrical stimulation with galvanic currents of amperage less than that required to stimulate the motor nerves under normal physiologic conditions.

Another manifestation of reduced Ca^{++} concentration is a prolonged Q-T interval on the electrocardiogram. This may be difficult to interpret unless the Q-T interval is carefully calibrated for variations in heart rate.

ALKALOTIC TETANY. This is very rare in infants and young children. Tetany can be induced through spontaneous overventilation, which produces respiratory alkalosis. Such hyperventilation is most often of psychogenic origin. In patients with low Ca^{++} concentrations tetany may be precipitated by overventilation or by a metabolic alkalosis following administration of sodium bicarbonate. (The metabolic alkalosis resulting from loss of gastric juice owing to pyloric obstruction is rarely associated with tetany.) This phenomenon has been seen in patients with renal disease who have been protected from the consequences of a low Ca^{++} concentration by concurrent metabolic acidosis, in whom correction of the acidosis has caused tetany and convulsions. The treatment of alkalotic tetany due to hyperventilation involves rebreathing in a bag or balloon in order to increase pCO_2.

HYPOCALCEMIC TETANY

DISORDERS OF PARATHYROID FUNCTION. The most common disorder of parathyroid function is transient physiologic hypoparathyroidism of the newborn infant, sometimes referred to as *neonatal hypocalcemia.* Clinically, infants with transient hypoparathyroidism of the newborn can be separated into two groups, one with early hypocalcemia, during the first 36 hours of life, usually before the baby starts to feed, and a second group with iatrogenic hypocalcemia due to high phosphate load, which develops only after the infant has for a number of days been taking a feeding based on cow's milk. The onset of symptoms in the second group is most commonly between 5 and 10 days of life; clinical manifestations have occasionally appeared as late as 6 weeks of age. Both forms are presumed to result from physiologically inactive parathyroid glands which fail to respond normally to low Ca^{++} concentrations. Besides a relative lack of parathyroid hormone output, there may be in the newborn period a partial refractoriness of the target cells to parathyroid hormone. The relative hypoparathyroidism of the newborn has been attributed to the increased serum calcium of the fetus, which reflects a calcium gradient across the placenta. In addition, mild maternal hyperparathyroidism, which may be physiologic during pregnancy, would augment the inhibition of fetal parathyroids by calcium ion. Occasional cases of transient hypoparathyroidism in infants have been associated with clinical hyperparathyroidism in the mother. Physiologic hyperparathyroidism has been indicated by increased parathyroid hormone levels found during pregnancy, and may be more intense in the diabetic woman.

The infants at greatest risk for early hypocalcemia are low-birth-weight infants, both prematurely born and small for gestational age, infants born of diabetic mothers, and infants who have been subjected to prolonged difficult deliveries. The incidence of hypocalcemia in prematurely born infants is extremely high, particularly in those with respiratory distress. It is difficult to evaluate the role of hypocalcemia in the morbidity and mortality in such infants. In infants born of diabetic mothers and those who have been subjected to difficult labors, hypocalcemia should be suspected as one of the possible causes of convulsions. Diagnosis can be made only by determination of serum calcium concentrations. Treatment requires the intravenous injection of 10 per cent calcium gluconate in a dosage of about 2 ml/kg (18 mg Ca/kg). This must be given slowly, with monitoring of the cardiac rate to prevent excessive concentrations of calcium in the right auricle, which might inhibit the rhythmic electrical activity of the sinus node. It is important that the calcium gluconate solution not extravasate, since it causes tissue necrosis and calcification. For the same reason this solution *must not be given intramuscularly*. The intravenous dose of calcium gluconate can be repeated at 6- to 8-hour intervals until calcium homeostasis becomes stable, or the calcium gluconate can be added to a constant intravenous infusion.

The hypocalcemia which results following feeding of high phosphate milks can occur in both full-term and prematurely born infants and in infants whose clinical histories have been benign. The physiologic mechanism involves intake of a high phosphate food in relatively large volume. This leads to an elevated serum phosphate, owing to the relatively high tubular reabsorption of phosphate and the physiologically low glomerular filtration rate of the newborn. The elevated serum phosphate depresses serum calcium through deposition of calcium in bone. The normal physiologic response would be an increased output of parathyroid hormone, which would both increase the solubilization of bone mineral and increase urine phosphate output by blocking tubular reabsorption of phosphate. This would restore serum levels of both calcium and phosphate to the normal range. If the infant's parathyroid glands are not yet able to respond with such an increase of parathyroid hormone, the level of serum calcium progressively falls and symptomatic hypocalcemia may result.

The most important manifestation of hypocalcemia in infants is the convulsive seizure. Typical tetany (carpopedal spasm) is not usually seen. Laryngospasm with cyanosis and apneic episodes may occur. In addition to the characteristic signs of increased excitability of the nervous system, there may be nonspecific symptoms such as poor feeding, vomiting and lethargy rather than irritability. These clinical signs suggest sepsis; serum calcium determinations should be made in addition to other diagnostic studies in infants in whom sepsis is suspected. Rarely, bradycardia with heart block is noted. A prolonged Q-T interval on the electrocardiogram suggests hypocalcemia. A serum calcium concentration below 7 mg/dl establishes the definitive diagnosis. Because of the pathogenesis of the disorder, as described above, the serum phosphate level is increased, sometimes as high as 10 to 12 mg/dl. The urea nitrogen concentrations are not elevated, which distinguishes this condition from the hyperphosphatemia of severe renal dysfunction. It must be remembered in evaluating hyperphosphatemia that normal newborn infants receiving cow's milk feedings have serum phosphate concentrations of 6 to 8 mg/dl and that the concentrations in prematurely born infants may be even higher.

For the convulsing infant the initial treatment is the intravenous injection of 10 per cent calcium gluconate, 2 ml/kg, with the precautions given above. Following this, specific treatment aims at reduction of the serum phosphate. Breast-fed infants rarely if ever develop hypocalcemia since human milk is a low phosphorus food. Human milk is not, however, generally available as a substitute for cow's milk. Even so-called "humanized" infant foods prepared from dialyzed whey of cow's milk are considerably higher in phosphate than human milk. The absorption of phosphate from the food can be suppressed, however, by adding to the formula a great excess of calcium, which precipitates as calcium phosphate in the lumen of the gut. When a soluble calcium salt is added to the milk feeding to achieve a calcium to phosphorus ratio of 4:1, this purpose is achieved. Calcium lactate powder or calcium gluconate is advised for this purpose. We have preferred calcium lactate powder and have not found that its addition to milk produces any important gastrointestinal disturbances. Calcium lactate is 13 per cent calcium, so that 770 mg of the powder must be added for each 100 mg calcium needed; calcium gluconate is 9 per cent calcium, so that 1100 mg of this salt represents 100 mg calcium. A soluble preparation of calcium gluconate is available (syrup of Neo-Calglucon), which contains 92 mg calcium per teaspoonful, but this is a less desirable method of adding calcium and has caused diarrhea in the amounts necessary. Calcium chloride may cause gastric irritation and hyperchloremic acidosis.

Sample Calculation. An infant is taking a volume of prepared infant feeding estimated to contain 300 mg P and 450 mg Ca. To achieve a 4:1 ratio of Ca to P, 750 mg calcium must be added to make a total calcium intake of 1200 mg. This requires addition of 6 gm calcium lactate powder to the total feeding or 1 gm per feeding given every four hours. Since the salt must be dissolved in the milk, calcium lactate tablets are not to be used for this purpose (the compressed tablets are quite insoluble even if fragmented). An example of the effects of this treatment is shown in Table 19–3. As the serum phosphorus level decreases, the serum calcium returns to normal and may even rise to somewhat hypercalcemic levels. At this point, the calcium supplement is reduced in steps, but should not be stopped abruptly since the serum phosphorus may rise precipitously and the calcium concentration fall again to levels producing tetany. In most infants restoration of normal calcium homeostasis and presumably normal parathyroid responsiveness results in one to two weeks. Occasionally a more prolonged period of calcium salt supplementation is needed, so that the treatment must be individualized by serial measurements of calcium and phosphate concentrations. If there is poor response to treatment, the calculations should be checked to determine whether sufficient calcium salt is being added, and the feeding given the baby should be examined to see if the calcium lactate or gluconate has been completely dissolved. If no errors are found and the therapeutic response is inadequate, the diagnosis of congenital hypoparathyroidism should be entertained, or in older infants, vitamin D deficiency or an abnormality of absorption or metabolism of vitamin D.

Congenital absence of the parathyroids can occur either in association with aplasia of the thymus *(DiGeorge syndrome)* or as an isolated parathyroid aplasia. Such patients present with the same symptoms as infants with transient physiologic hypoparathyroidism, but respond incompletely to the simple treatment outlined above and have relapsing hypocalcemia which requires more definitive treatment. In total parathyroid deficiency, substitution for parathyroid hormone of pharmacologic amounts of vitamin D or vitamin D analogs is required. We prefer to use dihydrotachysterol, which at pharmacologic doses is more potent than vitamin D in the correction of hypocalcemia; it is also more rapidly inactivated in the body, so that it is not stored as is vitamin D and does not have so much cumulative toxicity. In the young infant 0.05 to 0.1 mg of dihydrotachysterol should be given daily and the dose adjusted by determination of serum calcium concentrations, which should be returned to levels of about 9 to 10 mg/dl. If vitamin D is used, doses of 10,000 to 20,000 units may be necessary. As the child grows, the dosage of either steroid must be increased as indicated by serum calcium concentrations. The problem of hypoparathyroidism in older children is discussed elsewhere. (See Section 17.)

HYPOCALCEMIA AND TETANY OWING TO VITAMIN D DEFICIENCY OR ABNORMALITIES OF VITAMIN D METABOLISM. When vitamin D deficiency was a common problem in infancy, this type of tetany was also common. The age of onset was usually between 3 and 6 months of age, since this amount of time is necessary for the depletion of the infant's stores of vitamin D; on the other hand, if the mother is vitamin D deficient, hypocalcemia owing to vitamin D deficiency in the infant may occur within the first week of life. Nutritional vitamin D deficiency and tetany are now rare, but vitamin D deficiency will develop in an occasional breast-fed infant whose mother is not aware that human milk is deficient in vitamin D and who does not give the infant supplementary vitamin D.

Hypocalcemia may also be due to failure of normal metabolism of vitamin D. It is now known that vitamin D undergoes two hydroxylation steps, first in the liver and secondly in the kidney, before becoming the metabolically active 1,25-dihydroxy

TABLE 19–3 EXAMPLES OF TREATMENT OF TRANSIENT PHYSIOLOGIC HYPOPARATHYROIDISM OF NEWBORN INFANTS WITH SUPPLEMENTARY CALCIUM

AGE	SERUM LEVELS (mg/dl)			TREATMENT	
(Days)	*Ca*	*P*	*Mg*	*Diet*	*Ca:P Ratio*
				I. Baby McC.	
10	6.9			Standard infant feeding	1.5
12	7.1	9.2	0.86	Calcium lactate supplement	4
14	9.2	8.3	0.91		
19	14.0	3.0	1.64	Supplement discontinued	1.5
22	6.9	8.8	0.77	Calcium lactate supplement	3
32	10.7	6.2	1.80		
				II. Baby O.	
8	5.2			Standard infant feeding	1.5
9	5.0	10.5			
11	6.1			Calcium lactate supplement	4
14	9.4	5.7			
16	12.6	3.6			2.5
26	10.0	7.6		Standard infant feeding	1.5
38	10.5	7.4			

*Formula based on cow's milk.

vitamin D_3. Infants with liver disease such as neonatal hepatitis, cytomegalic inclusion body disease or atresia of the bile ducts may show manifestations of vitamin D deficiency with hypocalcemia because of failure of liver metabolism of vitamin D. In the instance of atresia of the bile ducts, malabsorption of vitamin D may also contribute to the problem. In the genetic defect of vitamin D metabolism called vitamin D dependent rickets, in which there is probably failure of the 1-hydroxylation step in the kidney, affected infants may present with hypocalcemia. Vitamin D deficiency can also result from steatorrhea due to pancreatic lipase deficiency or to intrinsic intestinal mucosal disorders. In recent years a number of cases of rickets and osteomalacia have been found to be associated with the treatment of convulsive disorders by large doses of combined anticonvulsant drugs, principally phenobarbital, diphenylhydantoin and primidone. These patients may present with hypocalcemia as well as with skeletal changes. The mechanism whereby these drugs interfere with vitamin D action is unknown.

Patients presenting with tetany resulting from vitamin D deficiency or failure of normal metabolism of vitamin D can be given initial symptomatic relief by intravenous injection of 10 ml of 10 per cent calcium gluconate, with the usual precaution of monitoring heart rate to prevent too rapid injection. The definitive treatment is vitamin D, and this should be given in amounts adequate to achieve a rapid physiologic effect. One mode of therapy is to give a large load of vitamin D, 600,000 units, in a single dose or divided into several doses over a 24-hour period. For this purpose a highly concentrated vitamin D preparation is needed. The common solution of vitamin D in propylene glycol (Drisdol) 10,000 units/gm is not suitable for this type of therapy since the large volume of propylene glycol would be depressant. An alternative method of therapy would be to give 10,000 units of vitamin D daily for three weeks. These large doses of vitamin D given orally will be effective in true vitamin D deficiency. If there is impaired vitamin D absorption or a defect in the metabolism of vitamin D, larger doses may be required. The active metabolites of vitamin D, 25-hydroxy vitamin D and 1,25-dihydroxy vitamin D, are not yet available for use in treatment, but the hypocalcemia of hepatic disorders or of vitamin D dependent rickets will respond to large doses of vitamin D. Treatment must be individualized and patients closely monitored to avoid vitamin D intoxication. (See also Section 22.)

HYPOMAGNESEMIC TETANY

Hypomagnesemia has been reported as a cause of tetany in association either with low serum calcium levels or even with normal serum calcium concentrations. In the transient physiologic hypoparathyroidism of the newborn, low serum magnesium concentrations may accompany the hyperphosphatemia and hypocalcemia (Table 19–3). This hypomagnesemia usually responds to treatment directed at reducing the serum phosphate concentrations. Occasionally infants with severe hypomagnesemia will require specific magnesium therapy. This can be given by intramuscular injection of 0.2 ml/kg of a 50 per cent solution of $MgSO_4 \cdot 7H_2O$ (25 per cent solution of $MgSO_4$). This treatment will raise serum Mg concentrations into the normal range within an hour and should maintain adequate concentrations for several hours. Often no further therapy is needed. The mechanism of this transient hypomagnesemia is not clear.

See also Hypomagnesemia in the Newborn, Section 7.

HAROLD E. HARRISON

Bakwin, H.: Tetany in newborn infants. Am. J. Dis. Child. *54*:1211, 1937.

Gardner, L. I.: Tetany and parathyroid hyperplasia in the newborn infant. Influence of dietary phosphate load. Pediatrics *9*:534, 1962.

Harrison, H. E.: Hypoparathyroidism. Mod. Treatm. *7*:636, 1970.

Harrison, H. E., Lifshitz, F., and Blizzard, R. M.: Comparison between crystalline dihydrotachysterol and calciferol in patients requiring pharmacologic vitamin D therapy. New Engl. J. Med. *276*:894, 1967.

Paunier, L., Radde, I. C., Kooh, S. W., Cowen, P. E., and Fraser, D.: Primary hypomagnesemia with secondary hypocalcemia in an infant. Pediatrics *41*:385, 1968.

Richens, A., and Rose, D. J. F.: Disturbance of calcium metabolism by anticonvulsant drugs. Brit. Med. J. *4*:73, 1970.

Tsang, R. C., Light, I. J., Sutherland, J. M., and Kleinman, L. I.: Possible pathogenetic factors in neonatal hypocalcemia of prematurity. J. Pediatr. *82*:423, 1973.

20
THE NERVOUS SYSTEM

EVALUATION OF THE CHILD WITH NEUROLOGIC DISEASE

HISTORY—THE SYMPTOMATOLOGY OF NEUROLOGIC DISORDERS

The neurologic evaluation should include a thorough pediatric history, with special attention to the time involved in the evolution of the illness, which may provide important clues regarding the category of neurologic disorder. A static course with disability dating from early infancy suggests a congenital malformation or a lesion acquired in the perinatal period. It is important, however, to be aware that even in static brain lesions new symptoms tend to emerge as the brain matures; the expression of a brain lesion as a disorder of a particular function cannot become apparent until the child reaches the age at which that function normally appears. Steady progression of disability with loss of previously acquired functions is seen in degenerative brain diseases and in chronic encephalitis, uncompensated hydrocephalus and brain tumors. Arrest of development generally precedes loss of function in progressive brain disease in infancy. Sudden disability followed by gradual improvement is characteristic of cerebral vascular diseases. Episodes of exacerbation followed by partial remission are seen most commonly in the demyelinating diseases. A careful developmental history provides the data needed to place the infant or the young child into one of these disease categories. In the older child a history of school performance should be added and should be documented whenever possible with reports from the teacher. Deterioration in school performance, loss of interest, irritability and emotional lability are common symptoms of cerebral dysfunction in later childhood.

Unsteadiness of gait, limping, stumbling, falling, clumsiness, floppiness and tightness of muscles and loss of skill in handwriting are all symptoms of motor dysfunction, but the history should never be relied upon for the localization of motor disorders. This can be accomplished only by neurologic examination.

Children rarely complain of sensory deficits, so that these often go unnoticed until quite severe. Absence of visual following, random searching eye movements and a tendency to look directly at bright lights without evidence of discomfort suggest severe visual defects in the infant. In the older child, loss of visual acuity manifests itself by a tendency to walk into objects and to hold objects close to the eyes for inspection. Unilateral vision loss usually is asymptomatic even in the school-age child until formal testing of vision is carried out. A lack of response to sounds suggests severe hearing loss in the young child, but is easily confused by parents and others with the inattention of the retarded or autistic child. Partial hearing loss may express itself only as absence of speech or delay in its development, which may also be the presenting complaint in retardation or autism. Repeated injuries of which the child fails to complain suggest loss of pain sensation.

The history is especially important in the diagnosis of paroxysmal disorders of the nervous system, such as seizures, syncope and paroxysmal vertigo. Such attacks may occur at infrequent intervals; between attacks the child may be entirely well. The decision regarding special diagnostic studies or therapy, therefore, may have to depend on historical data alone. The events that precede an attack may provide important clues. Anxiety, excitement, pain or crying are common events preceding syncopal attacks but are rarely seen prior to seizures. Exposure to unusual sensory stimuli such as flickering lights (e.g., while watching television) may precipitate seizures. The older child with seizures may be able to relate a warning sensation or aura. The state of the patient during an attack should be ascertained as completely as possible. Was he unconscious, in a state of confusion or lucid? Were there convulsive movements and, if so, were they lateralized? Was he incontinent of urine or feces? Was recovery rapid, or was there a prolonged period of sleep or drowsiness? In infancy and early childhood manifestations of seizures may be so slight as not to be mentioned by parents unless specific inquiry is made. This is especially true of infantile myoclonic seizures. The momentary head, trunk and arm flexion, characteristic of these seizures, is often dismissed as a normal startle response or as colic.

Vertigo—the sensation that the environment is turning or tilting—is easily misinterpreted in the young child who is unable to describe this sensation. The outward manifestations of an attack include unsteadiness, vomiting, fright and unwillingness to move the head, which may be kept rigidly in one position. The child with vertigo remains lucid throughout the attack in contrast to the child with epilepsy.

The correct diagnosis of headache is largely dependent on a careful history. Facts that should be ascertained are time of occurrence of head pain, localization, quality (throbbing, dull, sharp, pressing or bandlike) and associated symptoms such as nausea, vomiting or visual disturbance. Headache that occurs principally after the child arises from bed and is associated with vomiting and drowsiness should alert the physician to the possibility of increased intracranial pressure.

THE NEUROLOGIC EXAMINATION

A careful neurologic examination is essential for the correct localization of neurologic illness; it is a challenging task in the potentially uncooperative young child. The confidence of the child is secured by being gentle and informal and by making the procedure interesting to the patient. Uncomfortable tests, such as the funduscopic examination and sensory testing, should be postponed to the last portion of the examination. Much can be learned by observing the child at play or while walking or running. A portion of the examination can be carried out with the child sitting comfortably and securely on the mother's lap. The examination of the newborn infant, of the child with psychiatric disorder, and of the comatose patient present special problems which are discussed separately. The following observations should be made and recorded in the usual neurologic examination:

ASSESSMENT OF THE CHILD'S BEHAVIOR AND MENTAL STATUS

Important aspects of behavior are the child's ability to relate to others, his level of activity (is he hyperactive?), attention span (does he move quickly from one stimulus to another without adequate exploration of any?), and mood (is he depressed, euphoric or labile?). His ability and/or willingness to cooperate with the examination and the appropriateness of his responses to various situations provide important clues.

Speech functions are divided into expressive speech (talking) and receptive speech (understanding). Expressive speech is tested by informal observation of the child's spontaneous verbal productions for fluency, vocabulary and grammatical structure, and by more formal assessment of his ability to name objects and to repeat phrases verbatim. Understanding of speech is tested by having the child carry out verbal commands. An 18 month old child should be able to point out body parts; the normal 5 year old can carry out three-stage commands. Isolated disorders of central speech mechanisms are referred to as aphasias. Several types of aphasia can be distinguished. In expressive (Broca's) aphasia the patient is unable to speak, or his speech is sparse and labored in telegraphic style. Understanding of verbal commands is preserved. In receptive (Wernicke's) aphasia there is loss of comprehension of speech. The patient speaks fluently, but with little content. He uses empty words such as "that thing," circumlocutions, or made-up words (neologisms). The ability to repeat verbatim is impaired in both types of aphasia. In global aphasia both receptive and expressive speech are affected. Aphasia usually implies a lesion in the dominant temporal lobe. It must be distinguished from speech disorders secondary to hearing loss and from dysarthria, which refers to speech defects resulting from dysfunction of muscles of articulation.

Ability to read is tested by use of graded reading paragraphs. An isolated inability to read in a child of otherwise normal intellectual functions is referred to as dyslexia. The neurologic examination should include an assessment of writing, drawing and copying of shapes. For example, the drawing of a man tests the ability to control a pencil, to produce recognizable shapes, and to arrange shapes in space in proper proportions. As a rough approximation, a 4 year old child should be able to draw a figure with four recognizable parts, a 5 year old with eight recognizable features. Ability to draw shapes can also be tested by having the child copy geometric figures, such as circle and cross (3 years), square (4 years), and triangle and diamond (5 years). Inability to draw objects in a child with otherwise normal motor functions and with good ability to recognize shapes is referred to as apraxia. This type of defect is seen in patients with lesions of a parietal lobe. It also occurs as a transient maturational lag in early school-age children with learning disabilities.

Handedness should be noted. Normally, clear preference for one hand in writing, eating and reaching is established by age 3 years. Delayed development of handedness is found in children with mental slowness and with learning disorders. Right-handed children have left cerebral dominance for speech. However, the dominant hemisphere cannot be predicted for left-handed children, since more than 50 per cent of them also have speech localization in the left hemisphere. Memory can be tested by giving the child a list of four or five object words which he has to repeat 5 minutes later. Testing of arithmetic ability such as counting, addition and subtraction is helpful in the assessment of the child with possible mental slowness. While all aspects of intellectual function may be depressed in mental retardation, the understanding of abstract mathematical concepts tends to be especially poor. Formal psychologic testing often is helpful.

MOTOR EXAMINATION

The motor examination requires an understanding of the organization of the motor system (Fig. 20–1). Voluntary movements are dependent on intactness of pathways that include at least two motor neurons, upper and lower. The axons of the upper motor neurons, whose cells of origin are in the motor cortex, form the *pyramidal tract,* which passes via the internal capsule and brain stem to the spinal cord. The pyramidal tract fibers cross to the opposite side in the lower medulla and synapse on anterior horn cells in the spinal cord. The anterior horn cells or lower motor neurons send their axons via peripheral nerves to muscle. Each lower motor neuron innervates a group of muscle fibers, up to several hundred in some of the large muscles of the extremities. A lower motor neuron and the group of muscle fibers it innervates are known as a motor unit. The basic motor pathway (Fig. 20–1) is influenced by a number of other centers, which as a group are known as the *extrapyramidal motor system.* These include the basal ganglia and the cerebellum. The function of the extrapyramidal motor system includes the control of repetitive motor acts and the coordination of movements. In general, lesions of the upper motor neuron or of the extrapyramidal motor system interfere with voluntary motor activities without interrupting involuntary and reflex motor functions. In many instances, such lesions result in enhancement of involuntary and reflex motor activity, owing to release from central inhibitory influences. Lesions of the lower motor neuron lead to loss of both voluntary and involuntary motor activities. In addition, the denervation of muscle leads to atrophy and to spontaneous activity of individual muscle fibers, which is known as fibrillation. Fibrillations are visible only in the tongue, where they lead to worm-like movements. Coarse, irregular twitches, due to simultaneous contraction of entire motor units, are known as fasciculations, and are seen primarily in diseases involving the anterior horn cells.

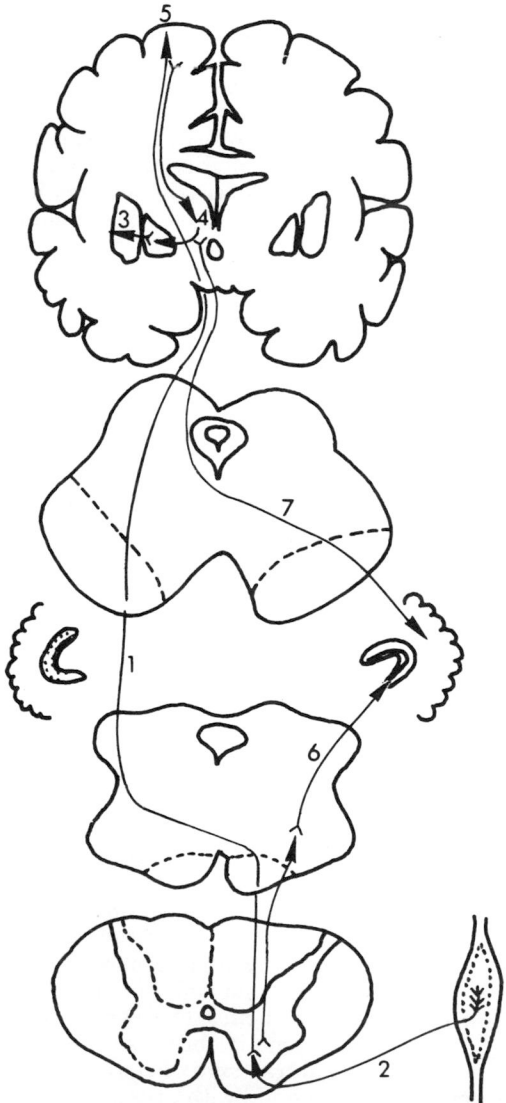

Figure 20–1 *Schematic representation of the more important motor pathways. 1 = upper motor neuron; 2 = lower motor neuron; 3 = basal ganglia, which send efferent fibers to the thalamus (4), which in turn influences the motor cortex (5). 6 = descending fibers from cerebellum influencing motor neuron activity in spintal cord. 7 = ascending fibers from cerebellum, which act on motor cortex via the thalamus.*

It is usually possible to localize a motor lesion in upper or lower motor neurons or in the extrapyramidal motor system by the following simple clinical tests:

ASSESSMENT OF MUSCLE STRENGTH. The strength is tested informally in the younger child. Ability to stand up from the lying position is a good test of back, hip and proximal leg muscles. Walking on tiptoes and on heels tests the gastrocnemius-soleus and the tibialis anterior, respectively. Shoulder muscles are tested by supporting and/or lifting the child with the examiner's hands in the child's axillae. Intercostal muscles can be assessed by observing spontaneous respirations and by asking the child to blow out a match. In the older child, strength is tested separately in individual muscle groups; it is graded on a 0–5 scale as follows.

0 = no movement
1 = movement with gravity eliminated
2 = full range against gravity
3 = movement against slight resistance
4 = movement against moderate resistance
5 = normal strength

Muscular weakness occurs with lesions of both upper and lower motor neurons, but it is usually absent in extrapyramidal disorders. Upper motor neuron lesions produce more severe weakness in the extensor muscles of the upper limbs and in the flexors of the legs. Diseases of the peripheral nerve result in distal weakness; most muscle diseases affect proximal muscles.

ASSESSMENT OF MUSCLE BULK. Atrophy of muscle is marked in lower motor neuron lesions; it is less striking in diseases of upper motor neurons.

Fasciculations should always be looked for in atrophic muscles, since their presence tends to localize the lesion in the anterior horn cells. Both upper and lower motor neuron lesions interfere with growth of the affected extremity. Excessive muscle bulk or muscular hypertrophy is usually due to increased muscular activity. It occurs normally in athletes and abnormally in muscle diseases with myotonia and in disorders of the adrenogenital system. Pseudohypertrophy refers to enlargement of muscles that are weak. It is usually the result of infiltration of muscle with fat, such as occurs in muscular dystrophy, or to distention of muscle by an abnormal substance, such as glycogen in type II glycogenosis (Pompe's disease).

ASSESSMENT OF MUSCLE TONE. This is estimated by the resistance to passive movement of an extremity. It varies from atonia and hypotonia through normal tone to rigidity. Diminished muscle tone occurs in lower motor neuron diseases and also in some extrapyramidal disorders, especially those of the cerebellum. Rigidity is defined as an increase in resistance throughout passive movement of a joint; it occurs in disorders of the basal ganglia. It must be distinguished from spasticity or increased resistance to passive movement which gives way suddenly (clasp-knife effect). Spasticity is a sign of upper motor neuron disease.

TESTS OF FINE MOTOR COORDINATION. Impairment of skilled movements is found in disorders of upper motor neurons and in cerebellar diseases. It can be assessed informally by watching the child manipulate toys, control a pencil or dress himself. A more formal test consists of rapid alternating supination and pronation of the hands. Irregular and slow performance of this test is seen in children with cerebellar disease. Incoordination of gait or ataxia also occurs characteristically with cerebellar lesions. In diseases of the cerebellar hemisphere the patient tends to reel to the side of the lesion. When cerebellar involvement is diffuse or confined to the midline vermis, the child may stagger to either side. Mild degrees of gait ataxia can be brought out by asking the child to walk a line with heel to toe, or by having him hop on one foot.

INVOLUNTARY MOVEMENTS. These occur principally in diseases of basal ganglia and of the cerebellum. They are usually absent during complete relaxation, especially during sleep; they are brought out by attempts to maintain a given posture or to carry out a skilled motor act. *Tremor* is defined as a rapid, regular, repetitive involuntary movement, usually of the distal extremities. A fine tremor of the outstretched hands is seen in anxiety and in thyrotoxicosis. A similar, somewhat more coarse tremor occurs as a benign genetically determined trait. A more proximal tremor of the outstretched arms and wrists (wing-beating tremor) is seen in Wilson's disease. Tremor that becomes more marked on approach of the target is known as intention tremor; it is a sign of cerebellar disorder. It can be observed in the young child when he is reaching for a toy. In the older child it is brought out by the finger to nose test, in which the child touches the examiner's finger and his own nose alternately.

Three characteristic disorders of movement—chorea, athetosis and dystonia—are seen in *diseases of the basal ganglia:*

Chorea consists of irregular jerking and writhing movements, often in proximal muscles such as the tongue, face, neck and shoulder. These may be quite violent and may cause the child to fling his arms or to suddenly drop an object he is holding. Gait is irregular, with sudden lurching to the side; walking may be impossible when chorea is severe. Mild chorea is to be distinguished from tic, which is a stereotyped sudden movement, always involving the same muscle group. Tic can be voluntarily inhibited by the patient for a short period of time.

Athetosis is a slow writhing movement, often more marked in the distal extremities, consisting of alternating supination-pronation and flexion-extension of the limbs.

Dystonia is a tendency toward hyperextension of joints, brought out especially when the patient tries to walk. Typically there is plantar flexion of the feet, hyperextension of the legs, extension and pronation of arms, arching of the back and extension and rotation of the neck.

All extrapyramidal movement abnormalities are accentuated during emotional stress and disappear during sleep. Failure to appreciate these features may lead to the erroneous impression that there is a psychiatric disorder.

EXAMINATION OF REFLEXES. The tendon reflexes are elicited by stretching of a tendon, usually by a quick tap with a reflex hammer. They provide evidence of the intactness of a particular *reflex arc* which includes: sensory nerve endings in tendon, sensory nerve fibers, spinal cord, motor neuron and muscle. The tendon reflexes are decreased or absent in disorders of peripheral nerves or muscle and in diseases that affect the spinal cord or brain stem at the level of the reflex arc. The intactness of specific segments of the neuraxis can be determined as follows.

Reflex	*Central Segment*
Jaw jerk	pons
Biceps jerk	C5-6
Supinator jerk	C5-6
Triceps jerk	C6,7,8
Knee jerk	L3-4
Ankle jerk	S1-2

A nervous or anxious patient may have difficulty relaxing sufficiently for demonstration of the tendon reflexes. Distraction of the patient by having him squeeze with one hand may produce the necessary relaxation. Hyperactivity of tendon reflexes, especially when associated with clonus, is a sign of upper motor neuron disease.

Several superficial reflexes can be elicited by stroking the skin. The plantar reflex is produced by a firm stroke against the lateral aspect of the sole, moving from the heel forward. A normal response consists of flexion of the toes. The abnormal re-

TABLE 20–1 DISEASES OF THE NEUROMUSCULAR SYSTEM

	UPPER MOTOR NEURON	BASAL GANGLIA	CEREBELLUM	ANTERIOR HORN CELLS	PERIPHERAL NERVE	MUSCLE
Strength	Decreased	Normal	Normal	Decreased	Decreased	Decreased
Muscle tone	Spasticity (usually)	Hypotonia or rigidity	Hypotonia	Hypotonia	Hypotonia	Normal or hypotonia
Coordination	Decreased	Decreased	Decreased	Normal	Normal	Normal
Involuntary movements	None	Chorea, athetosis or dystonia	Intention tremor	Fasciculations	None	None
Tendon reflexes	Hyperactive	Normal	Decreased	Absent or decreased	Absent or decreased	Decreased
Babinski sign	Present	Absent	Absent	Absent	Absent	Absent
Sensory deficit	Usually present	Absent	Absent	Absent	Present	Absent

sponse or positive Babinski sign consists of extension of the great toe, often associated with fanning of the other toes. It is indicative of pyramidal tract dysfunction when present beyond age 2 years. The abdominal reflexes consist of contraction of the abdominal muscles following stroking of the overlying skin. Their absence suggests either a lesion of the spinal cord segment that is stimulated (T10-L1), or a central motor lesion. The cremasteric reflex, which consists of ascent of the testis upon stroking the skin of the medial thigh, is absent in lesions involving the L1–2 segment. The anal reflex, elicited by stroking the perianal skin, tests intactness of the lower sacral segments.

Table 20–1 summarizes the clinical abnormalities in various categories of neuromuscular disease.

SENSORY EXAMINATION

This is necessarily limited in the infant and young child. Response to pain can be tested by observation of withdrawal and of emotional reaction to pinprick. This maneuver tests intactness of peripheral pain fibers and of pain pathways up to the level of the thalamus. In the evaluation of unilateral sensory impairment it has to be remembered that there is an overlap of innervation from the two sides near the midline. A sensory defect which ends abruptly at the midline is due to hysteria or malingering, rather than to neurologic disease. Function of posterior column pathways in the spinal cord is tested by asking the child to identify direction of passive movement of a joint (position sense) and by response to the vibration of a tuning fork placed on a bony prominence such as the lateral malleolus. Intactness of the sensory cortex is determined by a number of sensory discrimination tests. They include identification of objects placed into the hand (stereognosis), ability to recognize numbers drawn onto the skin (graphesthesia), response to simultaneous stimulation of two points, and bilateral simultaneous stimulation.

EXAMINATION OF CRANIAL NERVES AND THEIR CENTRAL CONNECTIONS

The cranial nerves innervate the eye muscles, facial muscles and muscles of deglutition, and they carry somatosensory fibers from the face and fibers from the special sensory organs. In testing muscles innervated by cranial nerves the same principles apply as in the examination of motor function in the extremities. Motor abnormalities in muscles supplied by cranial nerves may be due to lower motor neuron, upper motor neuron or extrapyramidal disorders, as is the case in those supplied by spinal nerves.

CRANIAL NERVE I (OLFACTORY NERVE). Ability to identify odors such as peppermint or coffee is determined for each nostril separately. Chronic rhinitis rather than neurologic disease is the most common cause of *anosmia.*

CRANIAL NERVE II (OPTIC NERVE). *Vision* is frequently affected in children with neurologic disease. In the toddler, rough assessment of acuity is possible through observation of the response to a small object, such as a bread crumb. The Snellen picture charts may be used for preschool children. The young child is normally myopic; 20/20 vision is reached at age 6 years. A gross evaluation of visual fields is possible as soon as the infant develops good visual fixation and the ability to follow visually. A test object such as a reflex hammer or a red block is gradually moved into the field of vision. The child fixes on the object as soon as he sees it. In the older child, visual fields are tested by confrontation. The child is asked to close one eye and to fix with the other on the nose of the examiner who confronts him. The examiner's finger or another test object is gradually moved into the field of vision, and the child reports when he first sees it. Formal perimetry is possible by school age. The course of visual pathways from the different retinal areas is indicated schematically in Figure 20–2.

Homonymous hemianopsia, in which the defect involves the temporal field of one eye and the nasal fields of the opposite eye, is seen in lesions of the optic radiations or of the visual cortex. The cerebral lesion is opposite the side of the field defect. A homonymous upper quadrant defect is indicative of a lesion in the temporal lobe white matter, through which the optic radiation fibers from the inferior portion of the retina pass on their way to the visual cortex.

Bitemporal hemianopsia implies a lesion in the region of the optic chiasm, most often in children with a craniopharyngioma.

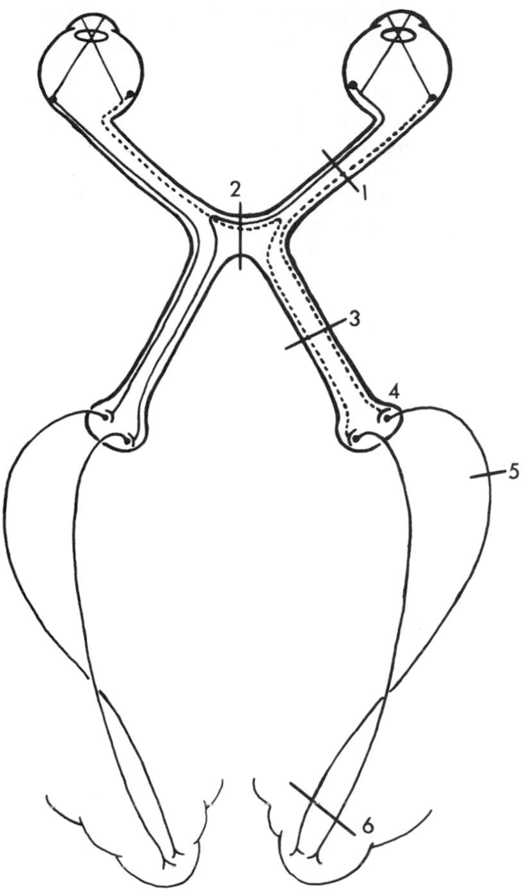

Figure 20–2 *Schematic representation of visual pathways. 1 = optic nerve. Lesions in this location causes unilateral visual loss. 2 = optic chiasm. Lesion results in bitemporal hemianopsia, owing to interruption of fibers to the nasal half of both retinae. 3 = optic tract. Lesion causes homonymous hemianopsia, owing to interruption of temporal fibers on the same side and of nasal fibers on the opposite side. 4 = lateral geniculate body. 5 = optic radiation. Fibers are widely separated and partial lesions are common. The fibers from the lower part of the retina pass in the white matter beneath the temporal cortex; this accounts for the frequency of homonymous upper quadrant anopsia in temporal lobe lesions. 6 = visual cortex. Lesions may cause partial or complete homonymous hemianopsia.*

Funduscopic examination is always included in a complete neurologic evaluation. A pale optic nerve head with sparsity of capillary vessels on the disc indicates optic atrophy. In papilledema the optic disc is hyperemic, the optic cup is obliterated, and the disc may protrude forward into the vitreous. The retinal veins are distended, and venous pulsations are absent. Hemorrhage may be present on the disc or adjacent to it. The appearance of papilledema may be indistinguishable from inflammation of the optic disc or papillitis. However, in papilledema visual acuity tends to be preserved until late, whereas it is lost early in papillitis.

CRANIAL NERVE III. This nerve carries the pupilloconstrictor fibers and innervates all the extraocular muscles except the lateral rectus and superior oblique. Pupillary asymmetry at rest may be due to unilateral visual loss, a midbrain lesion, 3rd nerve palsy, or a lesion of cervical sympathetic nerves. (See Horners' syndrome, this Section.) In unilateral visual loss, the pupil on the affected side is dilated, and the light reflex is diminished or absent when the affected eye is exposed to light. However, the pupil constricts normally when the opposite (seeing) eye is stimulated (consensual light reflex). In lesions of the 3rd nerve or of its cells of origin in the upper midbrain, the pupil of the affected side is dilated, and both direct and consensual light reflexes are lost. In addition to pupillary dilatation, third nerve palsy causes deviation of the eye down and out as a result of unopposed action of the two remaining eye muscles: the superior oblique and the lateral rectus. There also is ptosis, caused by paralysis of the voluntary portion of levator palpebrae.

CRANIAL NERVE IV. This nerve innervates the superior oblique muscle only. An isolated palsy, which is rare, causes inability to turn the affected eye downward when it is in the adducted position.

CRANIAL NERVE VI. Palsy of the 6th nerve results in inability to abduct the eye on the affected side. The lesion has to be distinguished from convergent strabismus. In strabismus, eye movements generally are full when each eye is tested alone; the abnormality is evident only when both eyes are open. Patching of the good eye for a time may be necessary before the child becomes able to abduct the squinting eye.

ABNORMALITIES OF EYE MOVEMENTS SECONDARY TO SUPRANUCLEAR LESIONS. Brain stem lesions may result in abnormalities of eye movements, owing to disruption of the fibers connecting the various oculomotor nuclei. In internuclear ophthalmoplegia the patient is unable to adduct either eye during visual following movements, but adduction during convergence is usually preserved. In skew deviation, one eye is elevated with respect to the other in all directions of gaze. Lesions of the upper brain stem in the pineal region cause paralysis of upward gaze. Paralysis of conjugate lateral gaze may be due to a lesion in the pons on the same side, but more commonly it is caused by a cortical lesion, involving the gaze centers in the frontal or the occipital cortex on the opposite side. In a cortical lesion, only voluntary eye movements are affected. Reflex eye turning, such as may be induced by vestibular stimulation, is preserved.

Lesions involving cerebellar and vestibular pathways produce rhythmic jerking of the eyes known as *nystagmus.* Most forms of nystagmus have a slow and a fast component. In nystagmus due to dysfunction of cerebellum or of cerebellar connections in the brain stem, the nystagmus becomes more marked when the eyes are deviated laterally; the slow component is always toward the midline. This type of nystagmus is seen in intoxication with certain drugs such as diphenylhydantoin and the barbiturates. It may also occur with structural lesions of the cerebellum or brain stem, and it is often present in children with cerebellar tumors. The nystagmus tends to be more coarse and of greater amplitude when the eye is deviated to the side of the tumor.

Nystagmus due to cerebellar or brain stem disorders has to be distinguished from nystagmus caused by labyrinthine dysfunction and from congenital nystagmus. Labyrinthine nystagmus often varies with head position, tends to have a rotary component, is most obvious at rest when the patient is not fixing on any object, and is associated with vertigo and nausea. It occurs acutely following trauma to the labyrinth or inflammation (labyrinthitis). Congenital nystagmus is pendular at rest, with irregular jerking when the eyes are deviated to the sides. It is usually associated with poor visual acuity and is thought to be due to failure of development of visual fixation in infancy.

CRANIAL NERVE V. The trigeminal nerve conveys sensation, including touch and pain, from the entire face except for a small area at the angle of the mandible. Its upper (ophthalmic) division is tested by the corneal reflex. The 5th nerve also has a motor component which innervates the muscles of mastication. Unilateral paralysis causes deviation of the jaw to the side of the lesion. The intactness of the segmental arc involving the muscles of mastication is tested by means of the jaw jerk. A brisk jaw jerk or jaw clonus implies a bilateral upper motor neuron lesion.

CRANIAL NERVE VII. The facial nerve is frequently affected in childhood as a result of congenital anomalies, birth injury, inflammation (Bell's palsy) and tumor. It innervates all the facial muscles except the levator palpebrae. Mild weakness is made evident by asking the child to show his teeth; it can be detected in the infant by watching facial movements during crying. The palpebral fissure is larger on the side of the weakness. In addition to motor fibers, the facial nerve carries parasympathetic fibers to the lacrimal and salivary glands and a sensory branch which transmits taste sensation from the anterior two thirds of the tongue. Lacrimation, salivation and taste are affected only in lesions of the proximal portion of the nerve in its course through the facial canal in temporal bone. Taste is tested by placing salt or sugar on the outstretched tip of the tongue by means of a cotton applicator and having the patient indicate by head nods whether he has the appropriate taste sensation. Peripheral facial nerve weakness has to be distinguished from weakness owing to a central (corticobulbar) lesion. In weakness of facial muscles due to a central nervous system lesion, the upper face is less severely affected and the patient continues to be able to wrinkle his forehead. There is often associated weakness of arm, hand and leg on the same side.

CRANIAL NERVE VIII. This consists of auditory and vestibular divisions. Hearing can be tested grossly in the young child by observing his response to the noise made by the rubbing together of fingers or by the crinkling of a piece of paper; in the older child, by asking him to identify whispered words. Formal audiometry is indicated in any child with suspected hearing or speech disorder, since partial deafness, especially for high tones, is easily missed by gross clinical testing. Vestibular dysfunction is rare in childhood but should be suspected in a child with episodic vertigo, staggering and vomiting, especially when there is associated labyrinthine nystagmus. It can be confirmed by caloric testing with cold water. The normal response consists of deviation of the eyes to the side of stimulation. A more comfortable test consists of rotation of the child, while he is held upright under the arms by the examiner. If vestibular functions are intact this results in ocular deviation to the direction of rotation.

CRANIAL NERVES IX AND X. Dysfunction of these nerves produces difficulty in swallowing and in phonation. There is palatal paralysis, which can be observed by inspection of the soft palate and uvula when the patient says "ah." The gag reflex is diminished or absent. Secretions can be seen pooling in the oropharynx, and the patient drools excessively. With unilateral lesions the voice is nasal or hoarse; bilateral lesions cause aphonia and stridor.

CRANIAL NERVE XI (SPINAL ACCESSORY). This nerve innervates the sternocleidomastoid and trapezius muscles. Paralysis causes weakness in head rotation toward the opposite side, and in elevation of the shoulder on the affected side.

CRANIAL NERVE XII (HYPOGLOSSAL). Lesions of this nerve produce paralysis of tongue movements and atrophy and fibrillations of the tongue. In unilateral involvement the tongue is deviated to the side of the lesion on attempted protrusion.

Lesions of the 9th, 10th and 12th cranial nerves have to be distinguished from impairment of swallowing, phonation and tongue movement resulting from bilateral central nervous system (corticobulbar) disorders. The latter lesions, known collectively as *pseudobulbar palsy,* are manifested by difficulty in swallowing, slurred speech and impaired control of emotional expression with inappropriate laughing and crying. Patients with pseudobulbar palsy have brisk reflex responses involving the bulbar muscles, including a brisk gag reflex. This type of deficit is common in children with spastic cerebral palsy.

EXAMINATION OF THE CRANIUM

The neurologic examination includes inspection of the skull for symmetry and shape and measurement of head circumference. Abnormalities of shape, especially when associated with palpable bony ridges, suggest craniosynostosis. Auscultation over the skull or over the eyes may reveal a cranial bruit. This is a normal finding up to about age 6 years. In the older child it suggests the possibilities of a cerebral vascular malformation or of increased intracranial pressure. Percussion of the skull gives a sound resembling that of a cracked pot—Macewen's sign—when the cranial sutures are separated because of increased intracranial pressure.

EXAMINATION OF THE AUTONOMIC NERVOUS SYSTEM

A limited number of clinical tests can be used to assess intactness of the autonomic nervous system. These include measurement of blood pressure and of body temperature, including diurnal variations. Absence of sweating can be determined by painting a portion of the skin with iodine and covering it with starch powder. The starch fails to turn dark blue in areas of anhydrosis. Parasympathetic function is tested by the Mecholyl test: A 2 per cent solution of methacholine (Mecholyl) is instilled into one conjuctival sac. This produces constriction of the pupil in patients with parasympathetic disorders such as familial dysautonomia. Disorders of the parasympathetic innervation of the bladder result in urinary retention and in incomplete emptying of the bladder. The cystometrogram is a helpful diagnostic test in partial lesions.

NEUROLOGIC EXAMINATION OF THE INFANT

At birth the human nervous system functions largely at a subcortical (brain stem and spinal cord) level. As a result, cortical functions cannot be tested adequately; even major cerebral defects may go unnoticed. An understanding of this limitation is of great importance. One should be extremely cautious in giving a prognosis regarding future intellectual function from the neurologic findings in the neonatal period. Indirect evidence of major cerebral defect can at times be obtained from measurement of head size. A head circumference more than 3 standard deviations below the normal for gestational age suggests a defect in brain growth which will usually be permanent. Major malformations of the cerebrum can sometimes be detected by transillumination of the skull with a bright flashlight equipped with a soft rubber cuff. A totally darkened room is essential. Complete transillumination in which a light beam applied to the occiput can be seen shining through the globes of the eyes is indicative of hydranencephaly. Less marked transillumination is seen in subdural effusions and in extreme hydrocephalus. A localized area of increased transillumination, usually unilateral, is found in porencephaly. During the first year of life intracranial pressure can be assessed clinically by palpation of the anterior fontanelle. Normally the fontanelle is soft and slightly depressed when the infant is in the sitting position. The fontanelle is tense and bulging in the infant with increased intracranial pressure; it is sunken with dehydration or with destructive brain lesions which lead to low intracranial pressure. Chronic increase in intracranial pressure is manifested by abnormal head enlargement.

REFLEXES. A large number of reflex patterns, mediated by brain stem and spinal cord mechanisms, are found in the newborn infant and during the first few months of postnatal life. These responses are stereotyped; they are always present in the normal infant, but may be less brisk when he is sleepy or recently fed. Absence of reflex responses indicates general depression of central or peripheral motor functions; asymmetric responses suggest focal motor lesions, either peripheral or central. As the infant matures the neonatal reflexes disappear in a predictable order as voluntary motor functions supersede them. Abnormal persistence of these reflexes is seen in infants with general developmental lag or with central motor lesions; age of appearance and disappearance of certain of the reflexes is shown in Table 20–2.

The *Moro reflex* (Fig. 20–3) is elicited by placing the infant supine upon the examining table, his head supported by the examiner's hand. The support is withdrawn suddenly, and the head is allowed to fall backward for 10 to 15 degrees. The reflex consists of extension of the trunk and extension and abduction followed by flexion and adduction of the arms, with less regular participation of the legs. The *stepping reflex* consists of movements of progression which are elicited when the infant is held upright and inclined forward with soles of feet touching a flat surface. For demonstration of the *placing reflex* the infant is held erect, and the dorsum of one foot is drawn along the under edge of a table top. The response consists of flexion followed by extension of the leg that is stimulated.

Several *postural reflexes* can be easily observed in the infant. The *tonic neck reflex* (Fig. 20–3) is elicited by rapidly turning the head of the supine infant to one side. The response consists of extension of the arm and leg on the side to which the face is turned, and flexion of the limbs on the opposite side (fencing posture). Tonic neck patterns are normally prominent in the 2 to 4 month old infant. Persistence of the response past age 6 to 9 months occurs with central motor lesions, especially in infants with spastic cerebral palsy. The *neck righting reflex* consists of rotation of the trunk in the direction in which the head of the supine infant

TABLE 20–2 REFLEXES OF NEONATES

REFLEX	AGE AT WHICH REFLEX USUALLY APPEARS	AGE AT WHICH REFLEX IS NORMALLY NO LONGER OBTAINABLE
Moro	Birth	3 months
Stepping	Birth	6 weeks
Placing	Birth	6 weeks
Tonic neck	2 months	6 months
Neck righting	4–6 months	24 months
Landau	3 months	24 months
Parachute reaction	9 months	Persists
Sucking and rooting	Birth	4 months awake 7 months asleep
Palmar grasp	Birth	6 months
Plantar grasp	Birth	10 months
Adductor spread of knee jerk	Birth	7 months

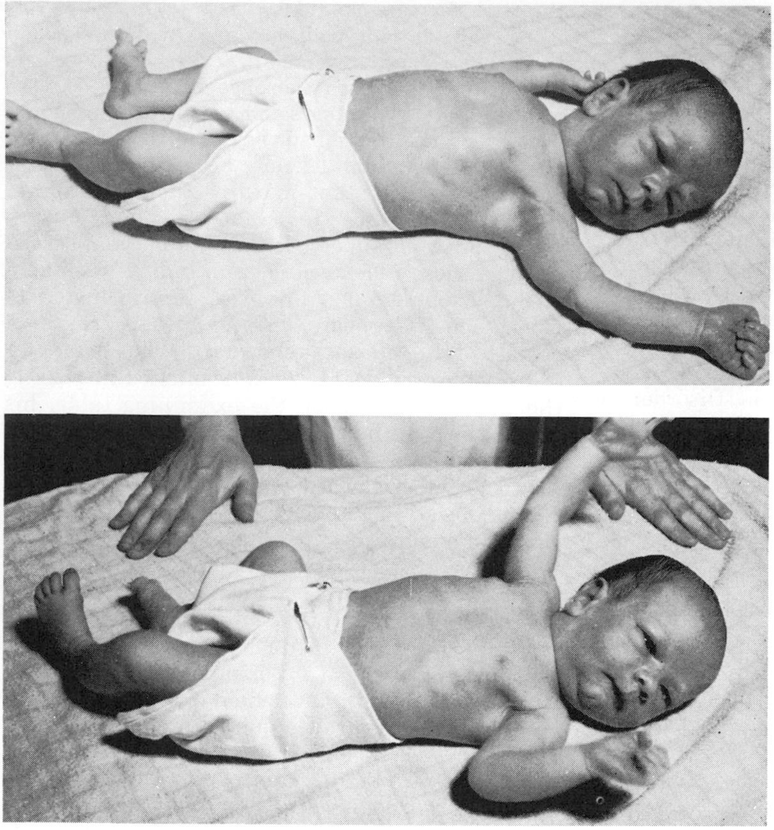

Figure 20–3 *Upper photograph shows a spontaneous tonic neck reflex. Lower photograph shows the Moro reflex.*

is turned. It is absent or decreased in infants with spasticity. *The Landau reflex* is demonstrated by supporting the infant in the prone position with the examiner's hand beneath the abdomen. A normal response consists of extension of head, trunk and hips. Flexion of trunk and hips occurs when the examiner flexes the head. The *parachute reflex* consists of extension of arms, hands and fingers when the infant, suspended in prone position, is suddenly allowed to fall for a short distance onto a soft pad.

The sucking reflex is initiated by stroking the lips. Stroking of the cheek produces the rooting reflex, which consists of turning of the mouth toward the stimulus. The *grasp reflexes* are elicited by light pressure on the palms or on the soles of the feet. The *tendon reflexes* are generally present in the normal neonate, but only the knee jerk may be easily obtainable. Very brisk tendon jerks may be a normal finding and may be accompanied by adductor spread of the knee jerk and by unsustained ankle clonus. Spontaneous clonus of arms, legs and feet is seen in infants with cerebral disorders. Absence of tendon reflexes suggests a neuromuscular disorder, such as Werdnig-Hoffmann disease. The *Babinski sign* is not helpful in infancy, since both flexion and extension of toes may be normally obtained.

ASSESSMENT OF MOTOR FUNCTIONS. This includes careful observations of spontaneous activity, which should be symmetrical. Consistent fisting of hands with adduction of thumbs is abnormal and is suggestive of a central motor lesion. Maintained opisthotonus is evidence of severe spasticity; it is rarely seen in neonatal meningitis except in the terminal stage; it is common in severe kernicterus and may be seen in a variety of other conditions, including congenital toxoplasmosis and maple syrup urine disease and in poisoning, as, for example, with the phenothiazines and strychnine. Scissoring of legs as a result of increased tone in adductors of the hips is a sign of spasticity. Diminished muscle tone is seen in infants with diffuse cerebral dysfunction and in peripheral neuromuscular diseases. Hypotonic infants tend to lie in the frog-leg position, with arms abducted at the shoulders. There is head lag and absence of contraction of shoulder muscles (absent traction response) when the supine infant is pulled to the sitting position. Rapid tremors of the limbs (jitteriness) are seen in infants with metabolic disturbances such as hypoglycemia or hypocalcemia, but may also occur without obvious cause. They have to be distinguished from the slower and often focal intermittent clonic movements that are characteristic of seizure activity in infancy.

The quality of *the infant's cry* can be of diagnostic help. The cry is high pitched in the infant with increased intracranial pressure, hoarse in cretinism, feeble in the infant with Werdnig-Hoffmann disease, and of cat-like quality in a baby with deletion of the short arm of chromosome 5 (cri du chat syndrome).

EXAMINATION OF THE CRANIAL NERVES. This examination presents few special problems in the neonate. The presence of vision is indicated by blinking in response to a bright light. Visual following can usually be demonstrated in the normal full-term infant. Its presence is one of the few signs of cerebral cortical function in the immediate neonatal period. A light or the examiner's face, moved slowly 9 to 12 inches from the child's eyes, is an adequate stimulus. Visual following movements of the infant are irregular and poorly sustained. The eyes tend to move conjugately, but intermittent disconjugate eye movements may occur normally. The presence of full lateral eye movements can be ascertained by rotation of the infant's head, which results in deviation of the eyes to the side opposite the rotation. The pupils of the newborn infant should be approximately equal in size and should respond to bright light. Corneal reflexes are well developed. Funduscopic examination is easily carried out in a dark room with the infant sucking on a nipple. The optic disc is normally pale, because of the poor development of the fine capillary vessels on the nervehead. Preretinal hemorrhages are seen in about 10 per cent of normal neonates. Chorioretinitis is a manifestation of congenital toxoplasmosis, cytomegalic inclusion disease, generalized herpes simplex infection and congenital syphilis. Acute chorioretinitis presents as gray indistinct retinal masses with pigmented borders. After a few weeks the center of the lesion takes on a white punched-out appearance.

A gross determination of hearing can be made. The normal infant startles to a sudden loud noise. Response to more subtle auditory stimuli consists of a change in spontaneous motor activity. Facial movements are assessed most easily when the child is crying. The neonate has a good gag reflex and well coordinated swallowing movements. The tongue should be inspected. An atrophic tongue with fibrillations is seen in Werdnig-Hoffmann disease. The tongue is large and may protrude in infants with cretinism, mongolism, glycogen storage disease of muscle and Beckwith syndrome.

A careful developmental evaluation becomes part of the neurologic examination of the infant after the first month of life. Developmental milestones are given on pages 49 and 50.

NEUROLOGIC EVALUATION OF THE CHILD WITH PSYCHIATRIC DISEASE

(Hysteria)

Older children and adolescents with psychiatric disorders may present with symptoms and signs mimicking neurologic disease. Problems in differential diagnosis arise especially in *hysteria.* The history is helpful, since the system review of the hysterical patient usually reveals a large variety of previous symptoms. Some are fairly characteristic, including a sensation of compression of the throat (globus hystericus) and recurrent abdominal pain without associated positive physical findings. The patient tends to relate symptoms and disabilities in a matter-of-fact, detached manner, an emotional state referred to as "la belle indifférence." Common manifestations easily confused with neurologic dysfunction include hysterical blindness, spasm of convergence, gait disturbance, paralysis, sensory loss, seizures and urinary retention.

Hysterical blindness can usually be distinguished from true visual loss by the absence of funduscopic findings and by preservation of pupillary constriction to light and of the opticokinetic nystagmus. Differentiation from cortical blindness, such as may occur transiently after head injury or after cerebral angiography, may be difficult. Hysterical visual field defects tend to be concentric, with general constriction of the fields in both eyes. Characteristically, the absolute size of the visual fields on a screen remains the same no matter at what distance from the screen the field is tested. Demonstration of this type of "tunnel vision" is very helpful, since it cannot be explained on the basis of any organic lesion.

Spasm of convergence tends to be of sudden onset, usually during some traumatic experience such as a difficult school examination. The child complains of blurring of vision or double vision, and on examination it is noted that the eyes are disconjugate, both in the adducted position. Reassurance and suggestion usually lead to rapid improvement.

Hysterical gait disturbances usually are in the form of astasia abasia, i.e., an inability to stand or to walk without any evidence of neurologic deficit when the patient is tested in the lying position. The gait of the hysteric with astasia abasia is bizarre, with extreme lurching to the sides, requiring exquisite balancing acts to prevent a fall. It has to be distinguished from cerebellar gait ataxia, in which the patient walks on a wide base and has great difficulty maintaining balance.

Hysterical paralysis is distinguished from true paralysis by presence of normal muscle tone, normal tendon reflexes and negative Babinski signs. *Hoover's sign* is helpful in unilateral paralysis involving the legs. The examiner places his hand under the heel of the paralyzed leg and then asks the patient to raise the normal leg against resistance. In hysteria forceful raising of the normal leg leads to downward pressure of the "paralyzed" leg against the examiner's hand: no such pressure occurs in true paralysis.

Hysterical sensory loss, when unilateral, ends exactly at the midline, whereas sensory loss due to an organic lesion shades into normal about 2.5 cm short of the midline, owing to overlapping bilateral innervation of the midline areas. Anesthesia in glove and stocking distribution is commonly the result of hysteria. It has to be distinguished from sensory neuropathy, in which the transition from abnormal to normal is more gradual. A useful maneuver is to test repeatedly, each time shifting the point at which testing is begun. As one starts higher, the boundary of the hysterical sensory loss also moves upward. Occasionally the child with hysteria can be tricked into reporting a touch he feels as "yes" and ones he supposedly does not feel as "no" during testing with eyes closed. The anesthetic side may shift from left to right or vice versa when the patient is moved from supine to prone. The Japanese illusion may be used to bring out left-right confusion in unilateral anesthesia. The patient is asked to cross his arms, oppose the palms, and clasp his fingers. The clasped hands are then rotated inward and the arms extended. This maneuver makes it very difficult for the patient to tell right fingers from left.

Hysterical seizures may be difficult to distinguish from epilepsy, unless they are witnessed by a competent observer. The seizure activity tends to be bizarre, often with rhythmic thrusting and writhing of the trunk. Tongue biting, apnea and incontinence are absent. The eyes tend to be held forcibly closed.

Hysterical urinary retention may present a difficult problem in differential diagnosis. It has to be distinguished from bladder paralysis secondary to spinal cord lesions. The cystometrogram is normal when urinary retention is due to hysteria.

SPECIAL DIAGNOSTIC PROCEDURES

LUMBAR PUNCTURE. This procedure provides much valuable information when it is carefully performed. It is contraindicated in patients with increased intracranial pressure caused by a space-occupying lesion, and in the presence of an untreated clotting defect. The puncture should not be done through an area of infected skin. If possible, the child should be kept from struggling during the tap; local procaine infiltration is helpful for this, even in the infant. The young child should be allowed to suck on a pacifier; sedation may be necessary later in childhood. The puncture is performed in the lateral recumbent position except in the neonate, for whom the sitting position may be preferable. The neck and back are held flexed by an attendant. Careful cleansing of the skin is essential, but drapes are unnecessary. The needle should not be inserted above the L2–3 interspace; L3–4 is the preferred site. A sharp needle with stylet should be used. Omission of the stylet may increase the chance of carrying a fragment of skin into the spinal canal, which may lead to formation of a spinal epidermoid tumor. The needle is advanced slowly, care being taken to stay exactly in the midline, the tip of the needle pointed slightly cephalad. In the small child, it often is not possible to feel the change in resistance that occurs as the dura is penetrated and the subarachnoid space is entered. It therefore is necessary to remove the stylet repeatedly during advance of the needle, until the cerebrospinal fluid drips out. A bloody tap usually occurs when the needle is advanced too far.

Cerebrospinal fluid pressure should be measured whenever it is possible to obtain relaxation. The pressure measurement is most accurate when legs and neck are extended prior to the reading. The normal opening pressure varies from 60 to 160 mm of water.

The color of the fluid should be compared with that of distilled water against a white background. Xanthochromia—a yellow tint—is always abnormal beyond the neonatal period. It may be due to elevation of spinal fluid protein or to accumulation of bilirubin. The latter usually implies recent subarachnoid hemorrhage, but it may also be seen in the absence of CNS lesions in patients with hyperbilirubinemia. The fluid looks cloudy in the presence of more than about 100 leukocytes/mm^3. Bloody spinal fluid may be the result of a traumatic tap, or it may be the result of a recent subarachnoid hemorrhage. To distinguish between these two, the fluid should be centrifuged and the supernatant inspected. In subarachnoid hemorrhage, the supernatant is xanthochromic, and equal amounts of blood are present in successive fractional specimens of fluid. In a bloody tap the supernatant is clear or only faintly yellow, and the amount of blood decreases in successive tubes.

Normally the spinal fluid contains no red blood cells and at most 5 leukocytes/mm^3, except in the newborn infant, in whom up to 500 red cells and up to 15 leukocytes, including granulocytes, may be insignificant. Later in childhood, predominance of granulocytes most often indicates bacterial infection. Occasionally it may be seen during the early phase of acute viral meningitis. Elevation in lymphocytes is seen in a large variety of illnesses in which meningeal irritation and inflammation are factors.

The normal protein content of lumbar spinal fluid in childhood is between 10 and 30 mg/dl except in the first weeks of infancy, when values up to 100 mg/dl are accepted as normal. By age 3 months the protein should be below 30 mg/dl. Elevation in protein is usually due to increased permeability of meningeal vessels; occasionally it is the result of obstruction to spinal fluid circulation, with decrease in resorption of protein. Elevations in the concentration of protein are seen in many neurologic disorders, including brain and spinal cord tumors, degenerative brain diseases and inflammatory diseases of the central nervous system and of peripheral nerves.

Elevation in spinal fluid globulins is detected by immunoelectrophoresis. Normally about 30 per cent of total protein in spinal fluid is represented by globulins, 6 to 8 per cent by gamma globulins. When electrophoresis is not available, the colloidal gold curve may be used as a general measure; a "first zone" colloidal gold curve implies elevation in globulins. Increased gamma globulin values or a first zone colloidal gold curve, in the absence of general elevation in spinal fluid protein, is of considerable diagnostic value. This finding is associated with only a few illnesses, which include multiple sclerosis, subacute sclerosing panencephalitis, neurosyphilis and postinfectious encephalomyelitis. Measurement of measles antibody titer in spinal fluid is an important diagnostic aid when subacute encephalitis is suspected; a measurable titer is found only in subacute sclerosing panencephalitis.

The glucose concentration of spinal fluid is normally about one half that of blood glucose. The ratio between spinal fluid and blood glucose values rather than the absolute value of the former is of importance. A low ratio is seen in bacterial meningitis, fungal meningitis, meningeal tumor and, rarely, in aseptic meningitis.

Spinal fluid should always be cultured for bacteria and, when indicated, for fungi, acid-fast bacilli and viruses. When meningitis is suspected, the fluid is centrifuged and a gram-stained smear of the sediment is examined. An excellent method of spinal fluid preparation for morphologic examination is as follows: A drop of liquid albumin is added to an aliquot of spinal fluid, and the mixture is spun in a cytocentrifuge. The sediment is allowed to dry and is then stained with Wright's stain. Histiocytes and tumor cells as well as normal leukocytes can be readily identified in such a preparation.

SUBDURAL TAP. This procedure is helpful to rule out subdural effusion in infancy. Indications for its performance include unexplained excessive head growth, a bulging anterior fontanelle and positive transillumination of the skull. The scalp hair must be shaved and strict aseptic precautions observed. The head is firmly held by an attendant. A blunt, short-beveled No. 20 needle with a stylet is used. The needle is introduced in the lateral angle of the fontanelle or in the coronal suture, at least 2 cm lateral to the midline: it is advanced perpendicular to the scalp surface. A popping sensation usually is experienced when the dura is penetrated. The needle should be advanced slowly, never more than 1.5 cm from the scalp surface, and the stylet should be removed repeatedly to determine whether a fluid-filled space has been reached. If intracranial pressure is not elevated, it is advisable to hold the head in a somewhat dependent position during the tap, so that flow is aided by gravity. Care has to be taken to avoid to and fro movements of the needle, which could lead to laceration of the meninges or cerebral cortex.

Subdural fluid is xanthochromic, bloody or reddish brown in color, depending on the age of the effusion and the amount of admixed blood. The protein content of the subdural fluid is always elevated, usually above 100 mg/dl. At times a fairly copious amount of clear fluid with low protein content is obtained. This is subarachnoid fluid, whose presence usually is of no pathologic significance. In general, the protein content of subarachnoid fluid obtained over the convexities is about twice that obtained from a lumbar tap.

Subdural fluid should be removed slowly, with no more than 15 ml taken from one side at any one tap. Rapid removal of large quantities may cause shock or intracranial hemorrhage from sudden shift of the intracranial structures. The opposite side should always be tapped when subdural fluid is found; subdural effusions in infancy are bilateral in 80 per cent of cases. Following the tap a pressure dressing is applied and the infant is placed in a semi-erect position in an infant seat to diminish the chance of prolonged leakage from the puncture site.

VENTRICULAR TAPS. These taps should not be performed by the pediatrician, except in cases of life-threatening increase in intracranial pressure when a neurosurgeon is not immediately available. The needle is introduced as for a subdural tap but is inclined slightly forward, toward the nasion. The needle is advanced until ventricular fluid is obtained, usually less than 4 cm from the surface when intracranial pressure is elevated because of ventricular obstruction. The procedure carries the risk of intracerebral or ventricular hemorrhage, and it always leads to some damage to cerebral cortex.

ELECTROENCEPHALOGRAPHY. Electroencephalography (EEG) provides a measure of the electrical activity of the cerebral cortex. Normally, fairly regular wave forms predominate. They are classified according to their frequency as delta waves (1–3/sec), theta waves (4–7/sec), alpha waves (8–12/sec) and beta waves (13–20/sec). During maturation the brain waves gradually become more regular and increase in frequency. Theta and delta waves are normally seen during waking periods in the infant and young child. By age 10 years the normal background rhythm in the waking state consists largely of alpha and beta activity. Slower waves are normal during sleep. Spike discharges, which may replace or be superimposed on the basic brain waves, are indicative of a lowered seizure threshold. They are an important confirmatory sign in the child with a suspected seizure disorder. Metabolic and inflammatory diseases of cerebral cortex tend to be associated with generalized high voltage slow wave (delta) activity. Focal structural lesions of cerebral cortex, such as brain abscesses or brain tumors, cause localized slow wave activity.

BRAIN SCAN. Brain scan is of value for detection of certain focal brain lesions. A radioactive material, usually technetium-90, is injected intravenously, and radioactivity over the skull is counted after a fixed time interval. The test material tends to accumulate in areas of brain where the blood-brain barrier is defective, especially in tumors and surrounding brain abscesses. Positive uptakes are also seen with encephalitis and with subdural hematoma. Cerebral infarcts secondary to vascular occlusion often result in a positive brain scan starting about one week after the infarction; there is a reversion to normal in three or four weeks.

ELECTROMYOGRAPHY. Electromyography is useful in the differential diagnosis of neuromuscular disease. A needle is inserted directly into the muscle to record the electrical activity; normal muscle is electrically silent at rest. Spontaneous discharges of single muscle fibers at rest, known as fibrillation potentials, are indicative of denervation. During normal muscular contraction, groups of muscle fibers in a motor unit are activated in unison. The resulting electrical activity is known as a motor unit potential. Decrease in size of motor unit potentials is seen in primary diseases of muscle. In diseases of peripheral nerves the motor units are decreased in number, but they often are of abnormally large size, as a result of collateral innervation of denervated muscle fibers. Nerve conduction velocity measurements are helpful in the confirmation of peripheral nerve disorders. Maximum conduction velocity is decreased in inflammatory and metabolic diseases of peripheral nerves, especially when the myelin sheaths of the nerve fibers are affected.

MUSCLE BIOPSY. This is frequently necessary to establish the diagnosis of a specific neuromuscular disease.

NEURORADIOLOGIC EXAMINATION. *Skull radiographs* are valuable to identify intracranial calcifications, craniosynostosis, skull fractures or bony defects. They may also provide information regarding the presence of increased intracranial pressure. Elevated pressure in the child causes separation of the cranial sutures. In longstanding increased intracranial pressure, the posterior clinoid processes are eroded, the sella turcica may be flattened and enlarged, and the convolutional impressions on the inner table of the skull are accentuated, resulting in a "beaten silver" appearance. This variegated pattern of the skull by itself is not necessarily evidence of increased intracranial pressure, nor of any demonstrable abnormality.

Structural abnormalities of the brain can often be diagnosed by *pneumoencephalography.* The procedure is carried out in the sitting position, after the child is heavily sedated or anesthetized. Air or oxygen is introduced via a lumbar puncture needle in fractional amounts of 5 to 10 ml. The entire ventricular system and the subarachnoid spaces are outlined by the air. The procedure is safe when it is carried out by experienced personnel. It carries a high risk only in patients with increased intracranial pressure owing to a space-occupying cerebral lesion. *Ventriculography,* in which air is introduced via a direct ventricular tap, is preferable when such a lesion is suspected. *Cerebral angiography* may be superior to air encephalography for the diagnosis of some space-occupying intracranial lesions, or it may be needed in addition to an air study. It is the definitive test for the study of cerebral vascular disorders, including arteriovenous malformations, arterial occlusions and venous thrombosis. In the child, the procedure is carried out most easily and safely via an arterial catheter introduced into one of the femoral arteries.

Myelography is an important procedure in the diagnosis of mass lesions situated in or encroaching upon the spinal cord. It should be carried out only when an experienced radiologist is available. Either iophendylate (Pantopaque) or air is used as contrast material. The injection is made through a lumbar spinal needle when possible. Pantopaque myelography carries a small but definite risk of meningeal reaction to the injected material, which may result in incapacitating and occasionally fatal arachnoiditis.

Brazelton, T. B., Scholl, M. L., and Robey, J. S.: Visual responses in the newborn. Pediatrics *37*:284, 1966.

Denny-Brown, D.: Handbook of Neurological Examination and Case Recording. Cambridge, Harvard University Press, 1965.

Dodge, P. R., and Porter, P.: Demonstration of intracranial pathology by transillumination. Arch. Neurol. *5*:594, 1961.

Fois, A.: Clinical Electroencephalography in Epilepsy and Related Conditions in Childhood. Springfield, Ill., Charles C Thomas, 1963.

Hurley, P. J., and Wagner, H. N.: Diagnostic value of brain scanning in children. J.A.M.A. *221*:877, 1972.

Lorber, J., and Granger, R. G.: Cerebral cavities following ventricular puncture in infants. Clin. Radiol. *14*:98, 1963.

Norris, F.: The EMG; A Guide and Atlas for Practical Electromyography. New York, Grune & Stratton, 1963.

Paine, R. S., and Oppe, T. E.: Neurologic examination of children. Clinics in Developmental Medicine. Vol. 20–21. London, William Heinemann, Ltd., 1966.

Raimondi, A.: Pediatric Neuroradiology. Philadelphia, W. B. Saunders Company, 1972.

Shaywitz, B. A.: Epidermoid spinal cord tumors and previous lumbar puncture. J. Pediatr. *80*:638, 1972.

Widell, S.: On the cerebrospinal fluid in normal children and in patients with acute abacterial meningo-encephalitis. Acta Paediatr. Suppl. 115, 1958.

THE COMATOSE CHILD

CLINICAL ASSESSMENT. Evaluation of the comatose child should provide certain critical information in a minimum of time: Is circulation adequate? Is there a patent airway with sufficient respiratory exchange? Is intracranial pressure elevated, and, if so, is the elevation great enough to be life-threatening? Is there a focal neurologic deficit which might indicate a localized, surgically remediable brain lesion? Is the coma likely to be due to remediable metabolic disease?

The *vital signs*—pulse, respiration and blood pressure—provide information regarding adequacy of circulation and airway and they may give clues to the diagnosis. The pulse is often slow and blood pressure elevated when intracranial pressure is high. Hyperventilation is usually the result of metabolic acidosis, but it may also indicate respiratory alkalosis due to abnormal stimulation of the medullary respiratory center such as may occur in salicylate poisoning, hepatic coma or Reye syndrome. Periodic breathing and irregular (ataxic) breathing are signs of medullary dysfunction. They often precede complete apnea.

The *pupillary reactions* should be assessed when the patient is first seen, and at frequent intervals thereafter. Unilateral dilatation with decrease in the light reflex usually is secondary to 3rd nerve damage by tentorial herniation of the brain (Fig. 20–4). It often is an indication for emergency medical or surgical measures to reduce intracranial pressure. A dilated pupil may also be due to eye trauma, or it may be a transient postictal finding following a grand mal convulsion. Bilateral fixed dilated pupils often, but not invariably, imply irreversible brain stem damage when present for more than 5 minutes. The pupils may be unreactive in reversible coma resulting from poisoning by sedative or atropine-like drugs, and in hypothermia. Dilated, unreactive pupils may also be due to previous local instillation of mydriatics. Pinpoint pupils are seen in poisoning with opiates, during barbiturate coma and with pontine lesions.

Eye movements in comatose patients are tested by the doll's head maneuver. The head is quickly rotated to one side, then to the other. The eyes show conjugate deviation to the side opposite the direction of head rotation. Absence of this response in a comatose patient implies dysfunction of brain stem or of oculomotor nerves. Deviation of the eye down and laterally is frequently seen in association with pupillary dilatation in 3rd nerve dysfunction owing to tentorial herniation. Sixth nerve palsy is usually due to increased intracranial pressure; it does not carry as ominous a prognosis as does 3rd nerve dysfunction.

Funduscopic examination should be carried out to determine whether papilledema is present. Mydriatics should not be used, since they interfere with pupillary reactions, which are invaluable for the clinical assessment of the comatose patient. The absence of papilledema does not rule out increased intracranial pressure of recent onset, since papilledema takes 24 to 48 hours to develop. Distention of retinal veins and absence of venous pulsations are early signs of elevated intracranial tension. Preretinal hemorrhages usually are the result of subarachnoid or subdural bleeding.

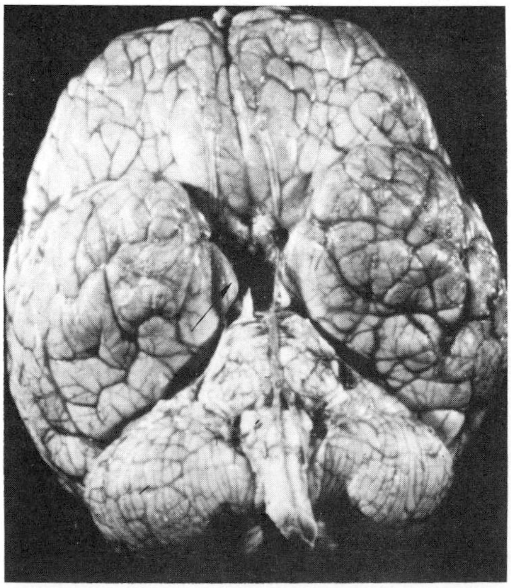

Figure 20–4 *Tentorial herniation secondary to diffuse cerebral edema. The arrow points to the portion of temporal lobe that has herniated through the tentorium. A groove, produced by the tentorial edge, is clearly visible. The third nerve is just below and medial to the area of herniation.*

Assessment of motor functions includes observations of spontaneous activity, posture and response to noxious stimuli. In deep coma, primitive postural reflex patterns emerge as cortical control over motor functions is lost. In "decorticate posturing" the arms are flexed on the chest, hands are fisted and legs extended. This position is seen in severe, diffuse dysfunction of the cerebral cortex. "Decerebrate posturing" is characterized by rigid extension and pronation of arms and extension of legs, often in response to painful stimulation. It is a sign of dysfunction at the level of the midbrain. When decerebrate posturing is unilateral, it is often caused by tentorial herniation, in which case there may be associated contralateral paralysis of the 3rd nerve.

Hemiplegia can be diagnosed even in the deeply comatose patient. The paretic leg lies in external rotation. It moves less than the opposite leg, both spontaneously and in response to pain. The paretic extremity drops more limply when it is picked up and allowed to fall.

Grading of stage of coma is helpful in charting the course of the patient. The following stages are used:

Stage I—stupor. The patient can be roused for brief periods, during which he may be able to make simple verbal and voluntary motor responses. Stupor may alternate with *delirium,* which is a state of mental confusion and motor excitement.

Stage II—light coma. The patient cannot be roused, even with painful stimuli. He may moan and make semipurposeful avoidance movements.

Stage III—deep coma. Painful stimuli now fail to produce a response, or they lead to extension and pronation of arms (decerebrate posturing).

Stage IV—patient is flaccid and apneic. All brain stem functions are lost. Some spinal reflexes may be preserved. The use of artificial ventilation has made it possible to maintain circulation after all brain function is irreversibly lost. The term *brain death* has been applied to this state. The criteria for brain death are as follows: (1) absence of all cerebral function, including pupillary responses, spontaneous respiratory efforts and all but local spinal reflexes for a period of at least 24 hours; (2) total absence of brain waves on at least two EEG recordings obtained at 24-hour intervals; (3) certainty that absence of brain functions is secondary to conditions other than drug intoxication or hypothermia. Termination of resuscitative efforts is justified when each of these three conditions has been appropriately accounted for.

DIFFERENTIAL DIAGNOSIS. Information gained

TABLE 20–3 DIFFERENTIAL DIAGNOSIS OF COMA

NO FOCAL SIGNS		FOCAL SIGNS	
Normal Pressure	*Increased Pressure*	*Normal Pressure*	*Increased Pressure*
Most metabolic encephalopathies	Some metabolic encephalopathies (lead poisoning, water intoxication, Reye syndrome, severe anoxia)	Vascular disease (cerebral artery occlusion)	Trauma (subdural, epidural or intracerebral hemorrhage, cerebral contusion)
Drug intoxication			Brain tumor
CNS infection (meningitis, encephalitis)	CNS infection (meningitis, encephalitis)	CNS infection (encephalitis)	CNS infection (brain abscess, subdural empyema, encephalitis)
Trauma (concussion)	Trauma (subdural hemorrhage in infants, subarachnoid hemorrhage)	Trauma (cerebral contusion)	
Epilepsy (postictal state)	Brain tumor (midline tumors)	Epilepsy (postictal state with Todd's paralysis)	Vascular disease (arteriovenous malformation)
	Hydrocephalus		

during the examination will usually make it possible to place the patient into one of four categories, depending on whether intracranial pressure is elevated and on whether there are focal neurologic signs. Table 20–3 provides the likely diagnostic possibilities in each category.

Laboratory studies which may be needed include determinations of blood sugar, serum electrolytes, blood gases, BUN, liver function tests and toxicology screening. A lumbar puncture is usually necessary to rule out bacterial meningitis. This procedure carries the risk of tentorial herniation in the patient with increased intracranial pressure, especially when a focal brain lesion is present. Neurosurgical consultation should be obtained prior to performance of a spinal tap in a child with increased intracranial pressure and focal neurologic signs. Proper diagnosis of the comatose child with focal signs usually requires cerebral angiography.

MANAGEMENT. The comatose child requires meticulous attention to respiratory status. The child should not be placed flat on his back, but rather should be kept on his side or in a semiprone position to minimize the danger of aspiration of saliva or of vomitus. Frequent suctioning of secretions is essential. The comatose patient should never be left unattended.

Moderately severe hypoxia may not be clinically evident; therefore, repeated determinations of blood gases are necessary. Hyperventilation may also occur and may lead to respiratory alkalosis. It is important to remember that the electrolyte changes in respiratory alkalosis, including increased serum chloride and decreased bicarbonate values, resemble those of metabolic acidosis. The distinction can be made only by measurement of pH.

Intravenous fluid therapy in the comatose child must be carefully monitored by repeated determinations of serum electrolytes. The most common mistake is overhydration, which may result in water intoxication; frequently the child in coma is unable to cope with what would be a moderate water load at other times. This is thought to be the result of dysfunction of the hypothalamus, with inappropriate secretion of antidiuretic hormone (ADH). The patient with inappropriate ADH secretion excretes scant quantities of concentrated urine in the face of hypervolemia and hyponatremia. Attention to urine output alone may give the erroneous impression that the child is dehydrated. Fatal cerebral edema may result if administration of hypotonic solutions is continued. The treatment of inappropriate ADH secretion is simple; it consists only of fluid restriction until serum electrolytes and osmolality return to normal.

Prompt therapeutic intervention may be lifesaving in the comatose patient with marked increase in intracranial pressure. This is especially so when evidence of tentorial herniation is present. When increased intracranial pressure is due to hydrocephalus or to ventricular obstruction by tumor, it is relieved most quickly and effectively by ventricular tap. Several medical measures are available for reduction of the increased intracranial pressure caused by brain swelling. In an emergency situation, osmotic diuretics are used. These agents lead to decrease in brain volume and to lowering in pressure within minutes of the start of infusion. Mannitol (1 to 2 gm/kg) and urea (0.5 to 1 gm/kg) administered rapidly by vein are most effective. A urinary catheter should be in place to prevent overdistention of the bladder by the induced diuresis. The effect of these agents is transient, rarely lasting over 6 hours. The effectiveness decreases markedly on repeated usage. High doses of synthetic corticosteroids are useful for more prolonged control of cerebral edema. Dexamethasone, 0.2–0.4 mg/kg, IV initially, followed by 0.1 to 0.2 mg/kg IM every 6 hours, is commonly employed. A therapeutic response is usually seen within 6 hours after the start of steroids. Stools must be checked for occult blood, and serum electrolytes have to be carefully monitored while the child is receiving steroids. The above measures are nonspecific and should not replace or delay definitive therapy of the underlying disease, when this is available.

Adequate nutritional intake must be assured when coma is prolonged. Nasogastric or nasojejunal feeding should be initiated as soon as the acute phase of the illness has subsided. Blenderized house diet makes an excellent feeding mixture, which is often tolerated better than many artificial formulas.

A definition of irreversible coma: Report of the Ad Hoc Committee of the Harvard Medical School to examine the definition of brain death. J.A.M.A. *205*:337, 1968.
Goldberg, M.: Hyponatremia and the inappropriate secretion of antidiuretic hormone. Am. J. Med. *35*:293, 1963.
Plum, F., and Posner, J. B.: The Diagnosis of Stupor and Coma. Philadelphia, F. A. Davis Co., 1966.

DISEASES OF THE NERVOUS SYSTEM

STATIC AND DEVELOPMENTAL LESIONS

The majority of the neurologic disabilities in childhood result from congenital malformations or from brain damage in the perinatal period and are usually nonprogressive. Knowledge concerning their etiology is often incomplete, and any classification is at best only partly satisfactory. The following classification is based on presumed time of onset of the defect, on the structures involved, and on etiology when known.

I. *Developmental defects of the nervous system (congenital malformations)*
  A. *Closure defects of the neural tube*
    Anencephaly
    Encephalocele
    Myelomeningocele and the Arnold-Chiari malformation
    Spina bifida occulta
    Dermal sinus
    Neurenteric cyst
  B. *Defects in the differentiation and growth of the cerebral hemispheres*
    Chromosomal defects (See other sections)
    Morphologic syndromes with mental retardation (see Appendix)
    Holoprosencephaly (arhinencephaly)
    Agenesis of corpus callosum
    Porencephaly and hydranencephaly
    Lissencephaly
    Polymicrogyria
    Microcephaly
    Megalencephaly
  C. *Defects in development of cerebrospinal fluid circulation—(congenital hydrocephalus)*
    Aqueductal stenosis
    The Dandy-Walker malformation
    "Communicating" hydrocephalus
  D. *Developmental defects of brain stem*
    Moebius syndrome
    Spasmus nutans
II. *Perinatally acquired cerebral lesions*
  A. *Intrauterine and neonatal infections of the nervous system*
    1. Congenital syphilis
    2. Congenital toxoplasmosis
    3. Cytomegalic inclusion disease
    4. Neonatal herpesvirus infection
    5. Other viral encephalitides
    6. Neonatal bacterial meningitis
  B. *Perinatal anoxic encephalopathy*
  C. *Cerebral trauma incident to birth*
    Intraventricular hemorrhage (not necessarily traumatic, see also Section 7)
    Intracerebral hemorrhage and cerebral contusion
    Subarachnoid hemorrhage
    Subdural hemorrhage
  D. *Neonatal metabolic encephalopathies*
    Bilirubin encephalopathy (kernicterus)
    Hypoglycemic encephalopathy
    The aminoacidurias
    Cretinism

DEFECTS OF CLOSURE OF THE NEURAL TUBE

These developmental anomalies are best understood through consideration of the normal formative stages of the nervous system as indicated in Figure 20–5. In the human the first evidence of development of neural tissue occurs at about 20 days' gestation, at which time a distinct depression, the neural groove, appears in the dorsal ectoderm of the embryo (Fig. 20–5 *A*). Over the next few days this groove quickly deepens, and the two margins of the groove become apposed and fuse. This fusion results in formation of the neural tube; it begins near the center of the embryo and progresses cephalad and caudad. By about 23 days' gestation the neural tube is complete, except for an opening at each end, the anterior and posterior neuropores (Fig. 20–5 *B*). Failure of closure of the anterior neuropore causes anencephaly and encephalocele; a closure defect of the posterior neuropore leads to spina bifida and meningomyelocele. The term *rachischisis* is sometimes used for very widespread spinal closure defects involving most or all of the dorsal, lumbar and sacral regions.

ANENCEPHALY. Anencephaly is evident immediately at birth; there is absence of the membranous skull as well as of the cerebral hemispheres. Brain stem and basal nuclei may be well formed and are visible at the base of the skull. The infants are either stillborn or die within a few days of birth.

A mother who has had one anencephalic infant has a recurrence risk of one of the closure defects of

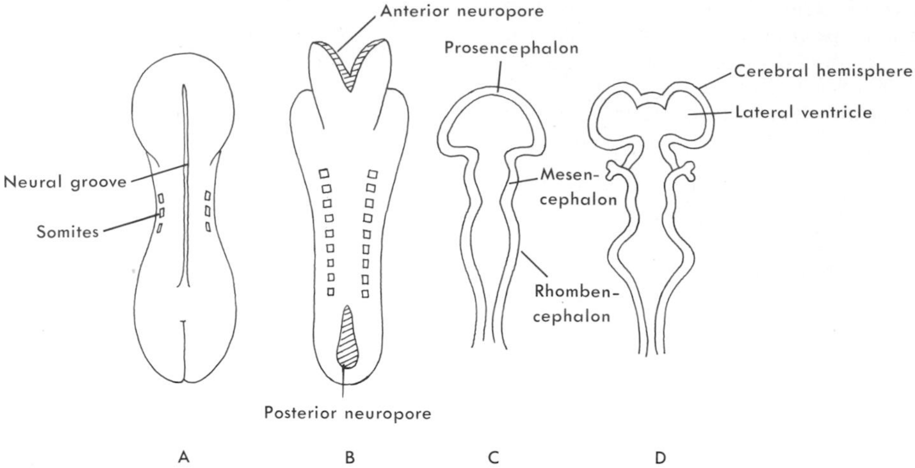

Figure 20–5 Early developmental stages of the human central nervous system. A, *Dorsal view of embryo at 20 days' gestational age. The future nervous system is indicated by a midline depression, the neural grooves.* B, *23 days' gestational age. The neural groove has closed dorsally, except for openings at either end (the anterior and posterior neuropores), to form the neural tube.* C, *Cephalic portion of the embryo, 28 days' gestational age. The cerebral hemispheres are represented by a single midline structure, the prosencephalon.* D, *36 days' gestational age. Paired lateral ventricles and cerebral hemispheres have formed. The outlines of the ventricular system, including the third ventricle, aqueduct of Sylvius and fourth ventricle, are discernible.*

the neural tube of about 10 per cent for each subsequent pregnancy. Ultrasound scanning of the uterus shows absence of the skull in the anencephalic fetus as early as 16 to 18 weeks' gestation, in time for therapeutic abortion. This innocuous examination should be given to any mother who is known to be at risk. Measurement of alpha-fetoprotein content in amniotic fluid may also be of help in intrauterine diagnosis. This protein is elevated in the amniotic fluid of the anencephalic fetus and of the fetus with a spinal closure defect.

ENCEPHALOCELE. Encephalocele consists of a herniation of brain and meninges through a defect in the skull, resulting in a sac-like structure. When the defect contains only meninges it is referred to as a *cranial meningocele.* About 75 per cent of encephaloceles occur in the occipital area; the remainder are parietal, frontal and nasopharyngeal.

Encephalocele usually is obvious at birth as a midline skull defect through which a large pedunculated or sessile mass protrudes. The nasopharyngeal encephaloceles form an exception, in that there is no externally visible anomaly. The child may present with nasal airway obstruction or with cleft palate. Inspection of the nasal passages shows a smooth, round mass projecting downward. A frontal encephalocele may extend into the orbit and may present as proptosis of one eye.

The differential diagnosis of encephalocele from cranial meningocele is made by palpation and transillumination of the mass, and by pneumoencephalography. The latter shows associated hydrocephalus in approximately two thirds of infants with encephalocele. Nasopharyngeal encephalocele has to be differentiated from nasal polyp.

Therapy of encephalocele consists of surgical repair of the defect, unless there is a major associated malformation of the brain which is severe enough to preclude the possibility of meaningful survival. The associated hydrocephalus frequently requires a shunt operation. The prognosis is good in cranial meningocele, with normal intellectual and motor function in 60 per cent of affected infants; it is guarded in occipital encephalocele, with only about a 10 per cent chance of normal intelligence.

SPINA BIFIDA WITH MENINGOMYELOCELE. This is a midline defect of skin, vertebral arches and neural tube, usually in the lumbosacral region. It is one of the most common developmental anomalies of the nervous system; the incidence ranges from 0.2 to 4.0 per 1000 births in different population groups; the highest incidence is reported in the Welsh and Irish. Little is known about the etiology of meningomyelocele. There appears to be an etiologic linkage with anencephaly. Women who have had a child with either anencephaly or meningomyelocele may expect a higher than average incidence of either in subsequent pregnancies (see above). Each defect has been observed following administration of aminopterin during the first month of pregnancy.

Meningomyelocele is evident at birth as a skin defect over the back, bordered laterally by bony prominences of the unfused neural arches of the vertebrae. The defect is usually covered by a transparent membrane which may have neural tissue attached to its inner surface. Cerebrospinal fluid leaks from this membrane initially, but soon after birth drying of the membrane tends to decrease its permeability. As cerebrospinal fluid accumulates the membrane begins to bulge, and it may eventually form a large sac, unless surgical closure of the defect is carried out. In almost all cases, meningomyelocele is associated with a defect of the brain stem and cerebellum known as the *Arnold-Chiari malformation* (Fig. 20–6). This consists of malde-

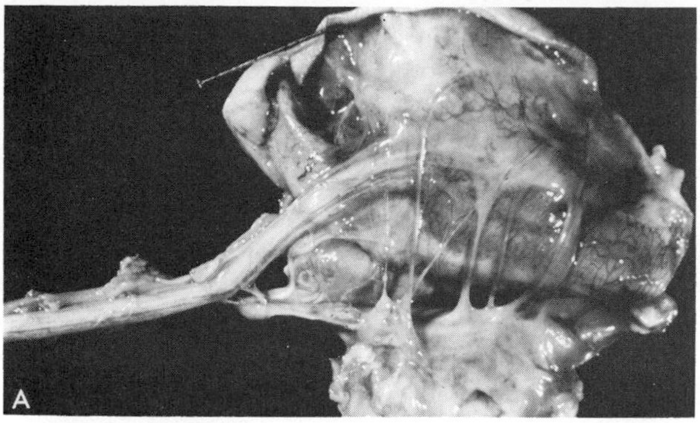

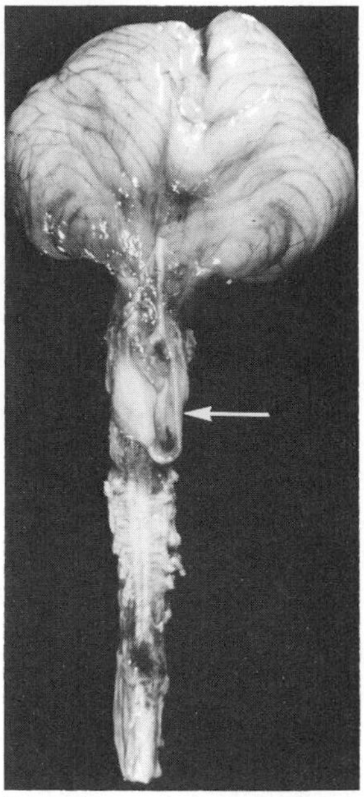

Figure 20–6 Meningomyelocele and Arnold-Chiari malformation. A, Characteristic deformity of the spinal cord. The normally formed thoracic spinal cord (left side of figure) gradually becomes flattened; the lumbar cord is represented by a plate-like structure which is firmly adherent to the surrounding skin. The lumbar spinal nerves can be seen to emerge from the malformed neural plate. B, Arnold-Chiari malformation, same case. The medulla oblongata and fourth ventricle (arrow) show marked downward displacement. The malformed cerebellum is visible above.

velopment and downward displacement into the cervical spinal canal of parts of cerebellum, 4th ventricle and medulla oblongata. A number of other developmental anomalies of neural tissue, including aqueductal stenosis and arrest of migration of cerebral neurons, may coexist. Hydrocephalus develops in about 90 per cent of affected children as a result of the Arnold-Chiari malformation or of the aqueductal stenosis.

Neurologic assessment of the infant with meningomyelocele should be carried out soon after birth to determine the severity of the functional defect. The upper level of spinal cord dysfunction can usually be detected by observing the response to pinprick over legs and trunk. Functional integrity is present when the sensory stimulus leads to limb movements and to arousal and crying. Stimulus-induced movement of limbs without change in the infant's behavior is of little significance, since it may be due to reflexes in spinal cord segments that have no functional connection with higher centers. Defective innervation of bladder is indicated by urinary dribbling; that of the perianal region, by a patulous anal sphincter and lack of anal reflex. The denervated limbs are flaccid and areflexic. Deformities such as talipes equinovarus and dislocated hips are often present. The Arnold-Chiari malformation may lead to medullary and lower cranial nerve dysfunction, including difficulty in swallowing, stridor and atrophy of tongue.

Optimal therapy of meningomyelocele consists of prompt surgical closure of the skin defect, preferably within 48 hours after birth, to prevent meningeal infection. Wide excision of the membranous covering is contraindicated, since the membrane may contain functioning neural tissue. After closure of the defect the infant must be carefully observed for development of hydrocephalus, which is treated surgically when indicated. A variety of urinary diversion operations, including construction of an ileal loop bladder and ureterostomy, are used for infants with bladder dysfunction. Orthopedic procedures are sometimes helpful to correct the hip and foot deformities but should be considered only when the child has some chance of useful function of his lower extremities. An organized plan for management by a specialized multidisciplinary clinical group is essential.

The prognosis depends on the extent of the motor deficit present at birth, on involvement of bladder innervation and on the presence of associated cerebral anomalies. In the infant with total paralysis of legs and of urinary bladder, the outlook is poor even with optimal medical care. The majority of such infants die during early childhood from complications of therapy for hydrocephalus and from chronic renal failure. The remainder are severely restricted by their motor disability, and 50 per cent of them are mentally retarded. The presence of advanced hydrocephalus at birth also carries a poor prognosis. Children with lesser degrees of involvement may lead successful lives. This is especially true for those with spina bifida and meningocele without evidence of neurologic deficit at birth. In the severely affected infant, the decision as to whether to carry out operative procedures or whether to allow the disorder to take its natural course presents serious ethical problems. Unoperated, over 90 per cent of these infants die prior to age 1 year.

SPINA BIFIDA OCCULTA. This consists of a defect of the vertebral arch with failure of posterior fusion of the vertebral laminae and often with absence of the spinous processes. The anomaly is most common at L5 and S1 levels but it may affect any portion of the vertebral column. There may be associated anomalies of vertebral bodies, such as hemivertebrae. The overlying skin and subcutaneous tissues may be normal, or they may show abnormal tufts of hair, telangiectasia or subcutaneous lipoma. Spina bifida occulta is an isolated, insignificant finding in about 20 per cent of all spines examined roentgenographically. A small percentage of affected infants have functionally significant developmental defects of the underlying spinal cord and spinal roots.

As is the case with meningomyelocele, the neurologic deficit may be manifest as motor and sensory disturbances in the lower extremities and/or disturbances of the bladder and bowel sphincters. Unilateral foot deformity and weakness of foot muscles are the most common defects. Smallness of the foot, trophic ulcers and pes cavus occur. These may be associated with sensory loss, especially in L5 and S1 distribution. Bladder sphincter disturbance is seen in about 25 per cent of infants with neurologic involvement and leads to urinary incontinence, dribbling and recurrent urinary infections. It usually is associated with weakness of the anal sphincters and with sensory impairment in the perineal region. The neurologic impairments may gradually worsen, especially during the adolescent growth phase.

The differential diagnosis includes spinal cord tumor, poliomyelitis, developmental defects of the spine such as diastematomyelia, and foot deformities. Diagnostic studies should be limited to roentgenograms of the spine unless there is progressive neurologic impairment. In that case myelography, either with iophendylate (Pantopaque) or with air is performed to rule out associated surgically remediable defects. Lipoma is especially common; it has been found on surgical exploration in about 40 per cent of children with neurologic impairment associated with spina bifida occulta; a dermoid cyst has been present in about 5 per cent. These tumors should be removed, if this can be achieved without damage to neural structures.

DIASTEMATOMYELIA. Diastematomyelia is a fissure or cleft of the spinal cord, usually in the lumbar region, and is often transfixed by a bony or fibrous septum. This septum prevents the normal ascent of the spinal cord in the vertebral canal as the child grows. Tethering of the spinal cord in the vertebral canal may lead to progressive neurologic deficit. Progressive flaccid paraparesis, weakness of one leg or bladder dysfunction may occur. There frequently are associated anomalies, including spina bifida with meningomyelocele, spina bifida occulta, dermal sinus and hemivertebrae. Cutaneous hemangioma, lipoma or a tuft of hair may overlie the site of the spinal defect.

The diagnosis can often be made by radiographic demonstration of a bony spicule in the spinal canal. Myelography further delineates the abnormality. Surgical exploration and resection of the abnormal bone and fibrous tissue is indicated when the lesion is discovered in infancy or in early childhood.

DERMAL SINUS. Dermal sinus is a small midline closure defect which is of importance primarily because the sinus may be a route of entry of bacteria into the subarachnoid space, leading to recurrent meningitis. It usually is located in the lumbosacral area but may occur at any level of the spine or in the midline of the cranium. Its point of origin on the skin is visible as a dimple, often surrounded by a tuft of hair or by a small hemangioma. The low sacral defects known as *pilonidal dimples or sinuses* usually end blindly without communication with the subarachnoid space and are therefore rarely significant. Sinus tracts above that level should be surgically explored and closed.

NEURENTERIC CYST. These rare lesions arise from incorporation of entodermal tissue in the developing neural tissue of the early embryo. They consist of epithelial-lined tracts and cysts which protrude into the spinal canal. Their most common site is in the thoracic and lower cervical regions. Neurologic dysfunction results from compression of the spinal cord by the cystic mass.

The symptoms and signs are those of spinal cord tumor. Some children present with infection of the subarachnoid space, which may lead to recurrent or chronic meningitis. The diagnosis can sometimes be suspected from examination of an anterior view of the spine, which may show a rounded, midline defect in one of the vertebral bodies through which the neurenteric tract gains entry to the spinal canal. In other cases, these lesions have been entirely intraspinal without any associated bony defect. The diagnosis then depends on myelography and on pathologic examination of tissue removed at surgery. Therapy consists of surgical excision of the cyst.

Alter, M.: Anencephalus, hydrocephalus and spina bifida. Epidemiology with special reference to a survey in Charleston, S.C. Arch. Neurol. *7*:411, 1962.

Brock, D. J. H., and Sutcliffe, R. G.: Alpha-fetoprotein in the antenatal diagnosis of anencephaly and spina bifida. Lancet *2*:197, 1972.

Campbell, S., et al.: Anencephaly: Early ultrasonic diagnosis and active management. Lancet *2*:1226, 1972.

Holcomb, G. W., Jr., and Matson, D. D.: Thoracic neurenteric cyst. Surgery *35*:115, 1954.

Ingraham, F. D.: Spina bifida and cranium bifidum. Papers reprinted from the New England Journal of Medicine with addition of a comprehensive bibliography. Boston, Massachusetts Medical Society, 1944.

Laurence, K. M.: The recurrence risk in spina bifida cystica and anencephaly. Develop. Med. Child Neurol. Suppl. 13, 1967, p. 75.

Lorber, J.: Results of treatment of myelomeningocele. Develop. Med. Child Neurol. *13*:279, 1971.

Matson, D. D.: Neurosurgery of Infancy and Childhood. Springfield, Ill., Charles C Thomas, 1969.

Matson, D. D., and Jerva, M. J.: Recurrent meningitis associated with lumbosacral dermal sinus tracts. J. Neurosurg. *25*:288, 1966.

Sheptak, P. R., and Susen, A. F.: Diastematomyelia. Am. J. Dis. Child. *113*:210, 1967.

Sieben, R. L., Hamida, M. B., and Shulman, K.: Multiple cranial nerve deficits associated with the Arnold-Chiari malformation. Neurology *21*:673, 1971.

Swinyard, C. A.: The Child with Spina Bifida. New York, Association for the Aid of Crippled Children, 1971.

Thiersch, J. B.: Therapeutic abortions with a folic acid antagonist, 4-amino-pteroylglutamic acid administered by the oral route. Am. J. Obstet. Gynec. *63*:1298, 1952.

DEFECTS IN THE DIFFERENTIATION AND GROWTH OF THE CEREBRAL HEMISPHERES

The future cerebrum makes its appearance as a recognizable structure in the human embryo at about 28 days' gestation, when the anterior end of the neural tube shows a globular expansion, *the prosencephalon* (Fig 20–5 *C*). Over the next several days the prosencephalon cleaves into two lateral expansions which represent the beginnings of the cerebral hemispheres and of the lateral ventricles (Fig. 20–5 *D*). The walls of the ventricles at this stage are formed by a germinal layer of actively dividing cells, the neuroblasts. Newly formed neuroblasts migrate away from the ventricular wall toward the surface of the primitive cerebral hemisphere, where their accumulation leads to formation of the cerebral cortex. The first arrivals form the lower cortical layers, and later arrivals migrate past them to form the upper layers. Differentiation of neuroblasts leads to formation of neurons and of glial cells. Migrating neuroblasts tend to maintain contact with the ventricular lumen through cellular processes which steadily increase in length, and which eventually make up the axons of the subcortical white matter. Axons crossing from one hemisphere to the other in the future corpus callosum first appear during the third month of gestation; the formation of the corpus callosum is complete by the fifth month. At about that time, the surface of the cerebral cortex begins to show identations which are progressively elaborated during the last trimester until at term the major cerebral sulci and gyri are clearly delineated.

The brain of the term infant contains the full adult complement of neurons, but its weight is only about one third that of the adult. The postnatal increase in weight is the result of myelination of subcortical white matter, of elaboration of neuronal processes, both dendrites and axons, and of increase in glial cells. Myelination of subcortical white matter and elaboration of dendritic branches of cortical neurons are largely postnatal events, as is illustrated in Figure 20–7.

As a general principle, abnormal influences occurring prior to the sixth month of gestation tend to affect development of the gross structure of the brain and to diminish total neuronal number. Pathologic influences in the perinatal period tend to have more subtle effects, such as retardation of myelination and decrease in elaboration of dendrites. Loss of brain substance due to destructive lesions may occur in the late fetal and early infancy periods, either alone or in combination with developmental defects.

HOLOPROSENCEPHALY. Holoprosencephaly is an early developmental defect of brain in which there is failure to form paired cerebral hemispheres. The cerebrum is made up of an unpaired sphere, and the lateral ventricles are represented by a single midline cavity. Usually there is associated *arrhinencephaly*—absence of olfactory bulbs and tracts, cleft lip, and microphthalmia or cyclopia. Occasionally holoprosencephaly occurs in trisomy 13–15; in other instances the etiology is unknown. Severe mental and motor defects are usually present, and the children rarely survive past infancy.

AGENESIS OF THE CORPUS CALLOSUM. This is a developmental anomaly in which the major fiber tracts that connect the two cerebral hemispheres are absent. Rarely, partial agenesis of the corpus callosum is transmitted by recessive inheritance; most cases are of unknown etiology. *Two clinical syndromes are recognized:* (1) The patient has normal intellectual and motor functions, and the malformation manifests itself only as an inability to transfer information from one cerebral hemisphere to the other. For example, the patient, if right-handed, may have difficulty in naming objects placed into the left hand, since this requires transfer of information from right sensory cortex to the speech areas in the left cerebral hemisphere. (2) More commonly, agenesis of the corpus callosum is associated with other developmental defects of cerebrum including failure of migration of neurons and hydrocephalus. These children present in infancy with severe seizures, developmental retardation, abnormal head enlargement and often hypertelorism. The diagnosis is made by pneumoencephalography (Fig. 20–8).

PORENCEPHALY. Porencephaly is a defect in the cerebral mantle resulting in a cyst-like expansion of the lateral ventricle, which may extend up to the pia-arachnoid membrane.

Porencephaly is occasionally due to a primary defect in development of the cerebral mantle, in which case it tends to be bilateral, with replacement of the temporoparietal areas by fluid-filled spaces. Affected infants present with total amentia. More commonly, porencephaly is unilateral and is secondary to local damage of the cerebrum during the late fetal or early infancy period. Cerebral vascular occlusion, encephalitis and needle-puncture of the brain have been implicated as possible etiologic factors. Depending on the location of the porencephaly, the child may have spastic hemiparesis, hemisensory defects or homonymous hemianopsia. Contrary to what one might expect, the skull may expand laterally and be thinner on the side of the porencephaly. These changes appear to be the result of fluid waves in the porencephalic cavity set up by choroid plexus pulsations.

Transillumination of the skull is of great value in the diagnosis of porencephaly and should always be performed in the infant with unexplained hemiparesis. The differential diagnosis includes chronic subdural effusion, in which skull transillumination is also positive. The differentiation can be made by subdural tap and by pneumoencephalography. Shunt surgery may be indicated in the rare instance when porencephaly is associated with abnormal head enlargement and with progressive motor deficit.

HYDRANENCEPHALY. Hydranencephaly is defined as a congenital absence of the cerebral hemi-

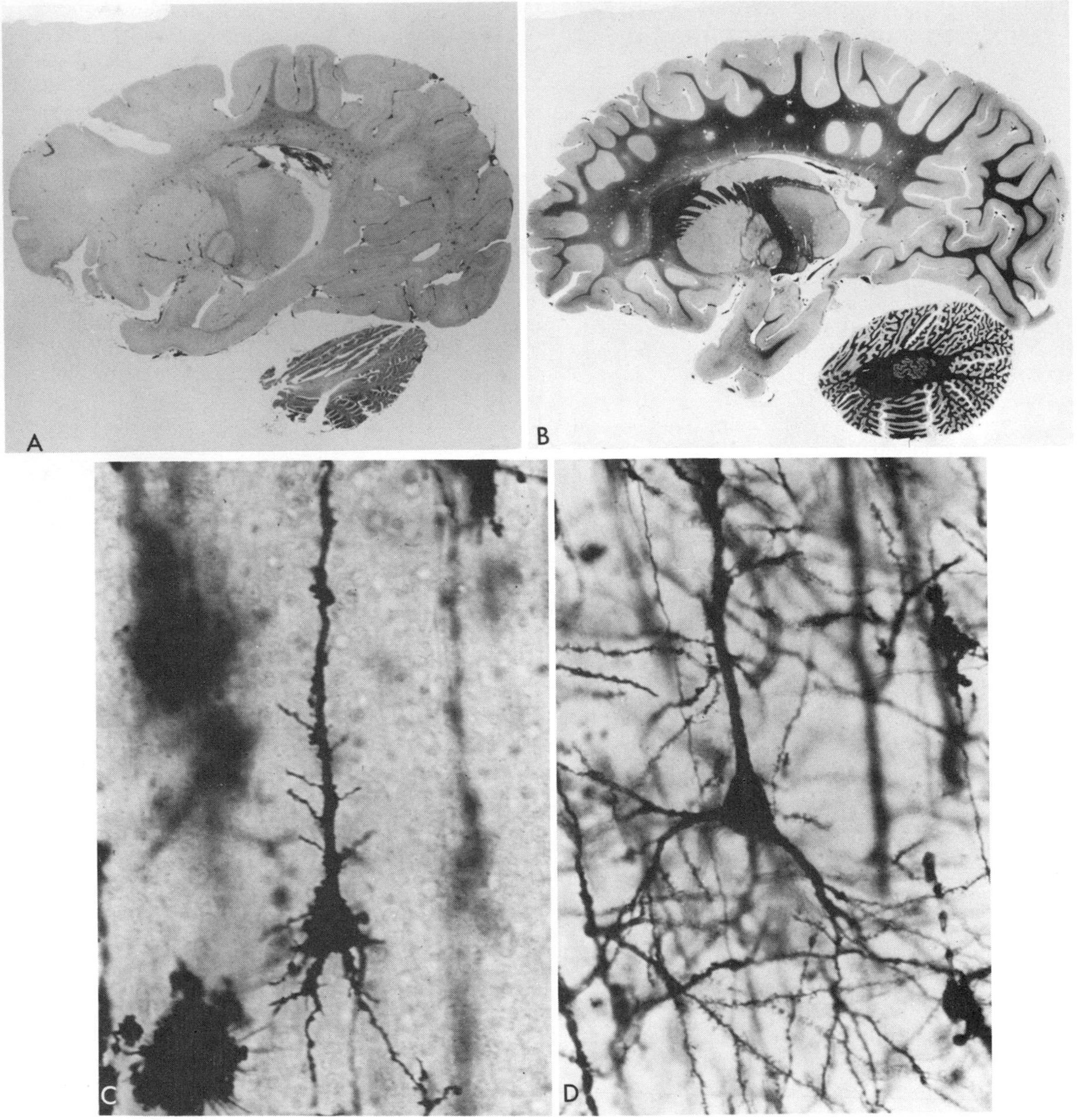

Figure 20–7 *A and B, Sagittal sections of brain stained with myelin stain. A, The brain of a newborn shows little myelin in the subcortical white matter. B, The brain of a 9 month old shows extensive myelination, especially in the primary visual, somatosensory and motor areas. C and D, Single cortical pyramidal neurons stained by the Golgi method to show dendritic development. C is from frontal cortex of a newborn, D from the same area in a 4 year old child, showing marked increase in length and complexity of dendritic branching. (× 100.)*

spheres. The cerebrum is replaced by a large, fluid-filled cavity. The brain stem and basal ganglia are well formed, and rudiments of frontal and occipital cortex may be present. The etiology is unknown. Failure of development of the cerebral arteries and destruction of brain by severe intrauterine infection have been suggested as possible etiologic factors.

The hydranencephalic infant may look remarkably normal at birth. Head size is normal or slightly enlarged. All the normal neonatal reflex patterns may be present. However, the infant does not have visual following, and later in infancy there is complete failure of voluntary motor and intellectual development. Seizures may occur. The diagnosis is suggested by total transillumination of the skull (Fig. 20–9). A similar clinical picture may be seen in advanced congenital hydrocephalus and with extensive bilateral subdural effusions. The diagnosis should be confirmed by cerebral angiography, which shows absence of the major cerebral vessels. The prognosis is hopeless, and early institutional placement is indicated.

LISSENCEPHALY. This is a defect in migration of

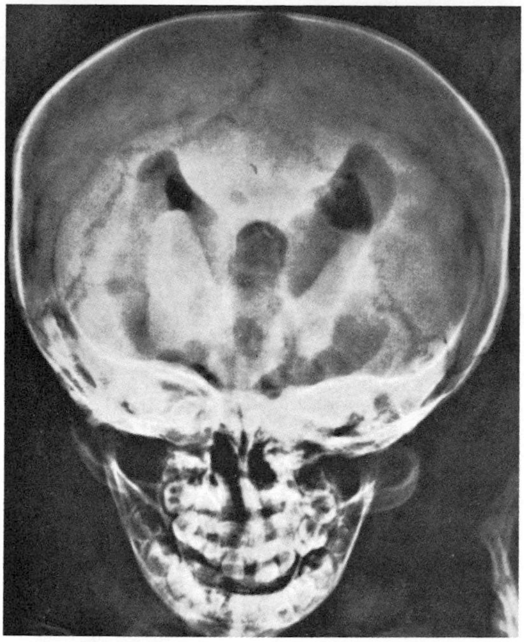

Figure 20–8 *Agenesis of the corpus callosum. Ventricles are dilated, and the lateral ventricles widely separated.*

cerebral neurons in which cortical gyri fail to develop. The surface of the cerebral hemispheres is smooth; microscopic examination shows absence of the normal cortical cell layers and persistence of groups of neurons in the subcortical white matter. The clinical picture is that of severe mental retardation. The diagnosis can be made only at autopsy.

POLYMICROGYRIA. Polymicrogyria is another defect in neuronal migration; a great excess of poorly developed cerebral gyri is formed. The abnormality has been found in association with intrauterine cytomegalovirus infection, but in most cases the etiology is obscure. Severe mental retardation is always present. The diagnosis is made at autopsy.

MICROCEPHALY. This is a defect in the growth of the brain as a whole, resulting in a head size more than three standard deviations below the norm. Developmental abnormalities and destructive processes affecting the brain during the fetal and early infancy periods may lead to this defect. The more important known causes are listed in Table 20–4.

The pathologic examination of the microcephalic brain always shows a decrease in total brain weight, which may be as low as 25 per cent of normal. The number and complexity of cortical gyri may be diminished. The frontal lobes are most severely stunted, and the cerebellum is often disproportionately large. In microcephaly due to perinatal or postnatal disorders there may be neuronal loss and gliosis in the cerebral cortex.

The most severe degree of microcephaly tends to occur in the recessively inherited form. These children have marked backward sloping of the forehead and disproportionately large ears. Motor development often is remarkably good, but mental retardation becomes progressively more evident as the children mature. It often is profound, necessitating institutional care.

The various conditions listed in Table 20–4 have to be considered in the differential diagnosis of the microcephalic infant or child. A backward-sloping forehead, large ears or a history of parental consanguinity suggests the diagnosis of hereditary microcephaly. The possibility that microcephaly might be due to maternal phenylketonuria should always be tested by performance of an amino acid chromatogram or ferric chloride test on the mother's urine. Skull x-rays (Fig. 20–10), lumbar puncture and serologic tests are useful in the diagnosis of microcephaly secondary to intrauterine infection. Diffuse cerebral calcifications are frequently found in congenital toxoplasmosis, while periventricular calcifications are more prevalent in cytomegalovirus disease.

Microcephaly must be distinguished from small head size secondary to synostosis of sagittal and coronal sutures. In craniosynostosis a palpable ridge is present in the region of the prematurely closed suture, and there is evidence of increased intracranial pressure, including papilledema and increase in convolutional markings on skull radiographs.

None of the forms of microcephaly are treatable. However, correct diagnosis is very important for genetic counseling, since some disorders presenting as microcephaly are hereditary, whereas others are clearly sporadic in occurrence.

MEGALENCEPHALY. In this rare developmental defect excessive growth of brain occurs during infancy and is responsible for abnormally rapid enlargement of the head. Remarkably large brains, weighing up to 2800 grams, have been reported.

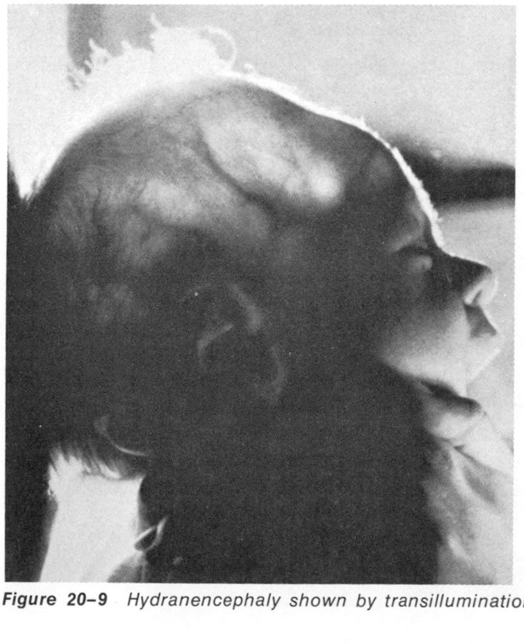

Figure 20–9 *Hydranencephaly shown by transillumination.*

TABLE 20–4 CAUSES OF MICROCEPHALY

DEFECTS IN BRAIN DEVELOPMENT	INTRAUTERINE INFECTIONS	PERINATAL AND POSTNATAL DISORDERS
Hereditary (recessive) microcephaly	Congenital rubella	Intrauterine or neonatal anoxia
Mongolism and other autosomal trisomy syndromes	Cytomegalovirus infection	Severe malnutrition in early infancy
	Congenital toxoplasmosis	
Fetal ionizing radiation	Congenital syphilis	
Maternal phenylketonuria	Neonatal herpes virus infection	
Seckel's dwarfism		
Cornelia de Lange syndrome		
Rubinstein-Taybi syndrome		
Smith-Lemli-Opitz syndrome		

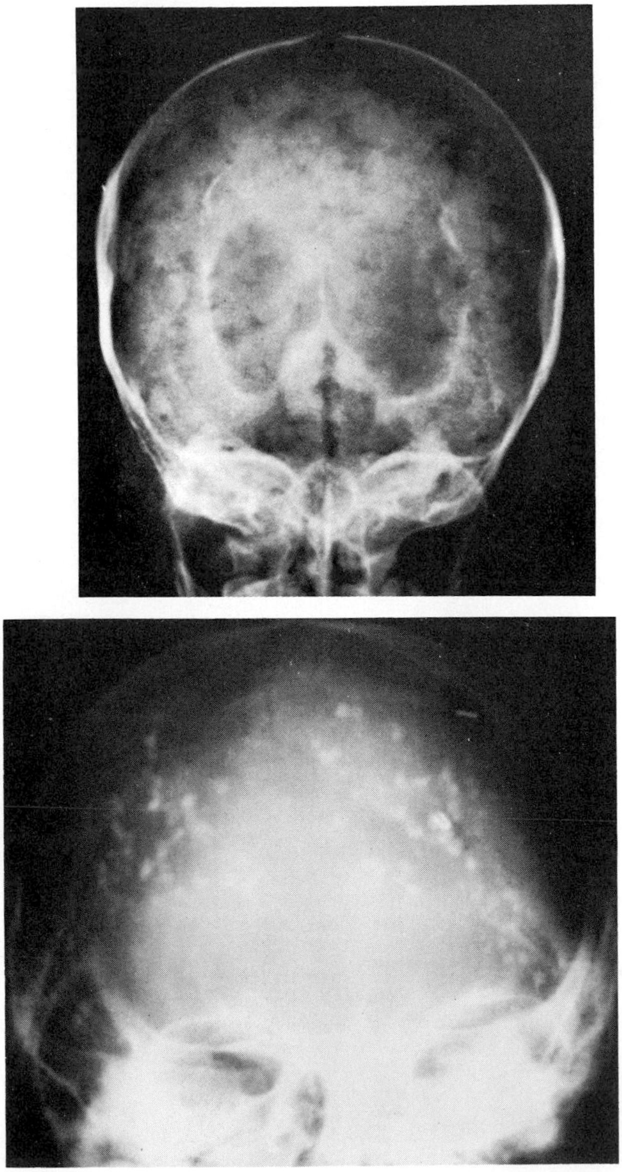

Figure 20–10 A, *Periventricular calcification and hydrocephalus following cytomegalic inclusion disease in the newborn.* B, *Diffuse intracerebral calcifications following congenital toxoplasmosis.*

The excessive brain weight is usually due to overgrowth of glial cells rather than of neurons. The condition is often of unknown etiology, but similar excessive growth of brain may occur in Hurler syndrome in Tay-Sachs disease and in metachromatic leukodystrophy. Affected infants usually have considerable developmental delay in addition to large head size. Signs of increased intracranial pressure are absent. Differentiation from hydrocephalus is made by pneumoencephalography or by cerebral angiography. The prognosis is guarded, since severe mental deficiency is common.

Baron, J., et al.: The incidence of cytomegaloviruses, herpes simplex, rubella and toxoplasma antibodies in microcephalic, mentally retarded and normocephalic children. Pediatrics *44*:932, 1969.

Bishop, K., Connolly, J. M., Carter, C. H., and Carpenter, D. G.: Holoprosencephaly. J. Pediatr. *65*:406, 1964.

DeMyer, W.: Megalencephaly in children. Clinical syndromes, genetic patterns, and differential diagnosis from other causes of megalocephaly. Neurology *22*:634, 1972.

Freeman, J. M., and Gold, A. P.: Porencephaly simulating subdural hematoma in childhood. Am. J. Dis. Child. *107*:327, 1964.

Haberland, C., and Brunngraber, E.: Micropolygyria: A histopathological and biochemical study. J. Ment. Defic. Res. *16*:1, 1972.

Hamby, W. B., Krauss, R. F., and Beswick, W. F.: Hydranencephaly: Clinical diagnosis. Presentation of seven cases. Pediatrics *6*:371, 1950.

Hansen, H.: Epidemiological considerations on maternal hyperphenylalaninemia. Am. J. Ment. Defic. *75*:22, 1970.

Koch, F. P., and Doyle, P. J.: Agenesis of the corpus callosum. Report of eight cases in infancy. J. Pediatr. *50*:345, 1957.

Lorber, J., and Granger, R. G.: Cerebral cavities following ventricular puncture in infants. Clin. Radiol. *14*:98, 1963.

Menkes, J. H., Philippart, M., and Clark, D. B.: Hereditary partial agenesis of corpus callosum. Arch. Neurol. *11*:198, 1964.

Murphy, D. P., Shirlock, M. E., and Doll, E. A.: Microcephaly following maternal pelvic irradiation for interruption of pregnancy. Am. J. Roentgenol. *48*:356, 1942.

Osburn, B. I., Silverstein, A. M., Prendergast, R. A., et al.: Experimental viral-induced congenital encephalopathies. I. Pathology of hydranencephaly and porencephaly caused by bluetongue vaccine virus. Lab. Invest. *25*:197, 1971.

Penrose, L. S. Microcephaly. Folia Hered. Path. *5*:79, 1956.

Yakovlev, P. I., and Wadsworth, R. C.: Schizencephalies. A study of congenital clefts in the cerebral mantel; Clefts with fused lips. J. Neuropath. Exp. Neurol. *5*:169, 1946.

Yu, J. S., and O'Halloran, M. T.: Children of mothers with phenylketonuria. Lancet *1*:210, 1970.

HYDROCEPHALUS

DEFINITION. The term "hydrocephalus" is applied to any condition in which enlargement of the ventricular system occurs as a result of an imbalance between production and absorption of cerebrospinal fluid (CSF). CSF pressure is usually elevated in progressive hydrocephalus, but occasionally it may be normal or nearly so.

PATHOPHYSIOLOGY AND ETIOLOGY. A brief consideration of normal CSF dynamics is necessary for an understanding of hydrocephalus. CSF production depends largely on the active transport of ions, especially sodium, across the specialized epithelial membrane of the choroid plexus into the ventricular cavities. Water follows passively to reestablish osmotic equilibrium; the net result is the accumulation of fluid in the cerebral ventricles. This fluid circulates via the aqueduct of Sylvius and the 4th ventricle and gains access to the subarachnoid spaces through the foramina of Luschka and Magendie. It is reabsorbed into the venous circulation from the subarachnoid spaces over the brain, to some extent from those over the spinal cord, and from the ependymal lining of the ventricles. The circulation of CSF is shown schematically in Figure 20–11.

Hydrocephalus is almost always due to interference with the circulation and absorption of CSF. Rarely, it is due to overproduction of fluid. Excessive fluid production is best documented in papilloma of the choroid plexus, a tumor which actively secretes CSF.

Two anatomic types of hydrocephalus are distinguished: (1) In *obstructive hydrocephalus* there is interference with circulation of CSF within the ventricular system itself. As a result, ventricular fluid cannot gain ready access to the subarachnoid spaces. Enlargement of the ventricular system occurs proximal to the site of obstruction. (2) In *communicating hydrocephalus* CSF pathways inside the ventricular system are open and ventricular fluid is able to move freely into the spinal subarachnoid space. Interference with absorption of CSF is due either to occlusion of the subarachnoid cisterns around the brain stem, or to obliteration of subarachnoid spaces over the convexities of the brain. The entire ventricular system becomes uniformly distended. A number of congenital and acquired conditions may lead to hydrocephalus (Table 20–5).

Obstructive Hydrocephalus. This most commonly is due to *congenital aqueductal stenosis.* The aqueduct of Sylvius is narrowed or is replaced by multiple small channels or "forks" which end blindly (Fig. 20–12). In a small number of cases aqueductal stenosis is transmitted as a sex-linked

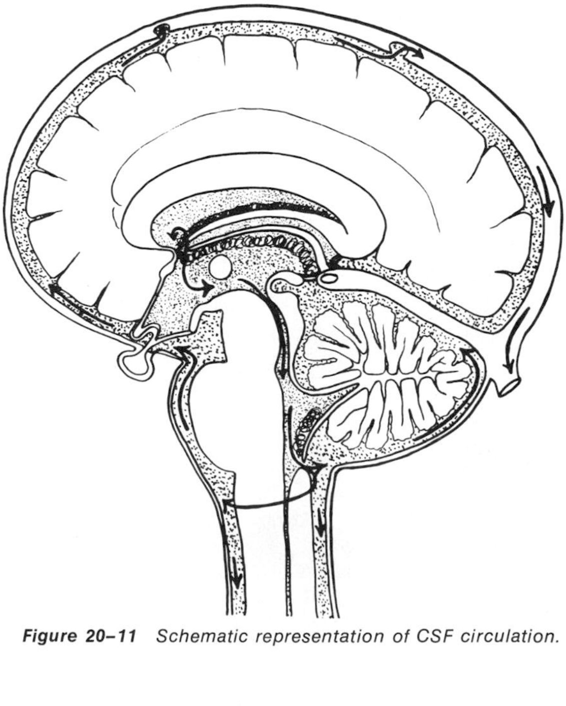

Figure 20–11 *Schematic representation of CSF circulation.*

TABLE 20-5 CAUSES OF HYDROCEPHALUS

OBSTRUCTIVE HYDROCEPHALUS	COMMUNICATING HYDROCEPHALUS
Aqueductal stenosis Congenital Acquired (post-infectious) Midline brain tumors Vein of Galen malformation Posterior fossa subdural hematoma Dandy-Walker malformation	Arnold-Chiari malformation Postinfectious (meningitis, toxoplasmosis, cytomegalic inclusion disease) Secondary to subarachnoid hemorrhage Secondary to excessive production of CSF (papilloma of choroid plexus) Diseases of connective tissue (Hurler syndrome, achondroplasia) Vitamin A intoxication

recessive trait. It may also be a residuum of inflammatory lesions in the periaqueductal region. Experimental evidence in several animal species implicates fetal virus infection, especially mumps virus, as an etiologic factor. Occasionally obstructive hydrocephalus is due to compression of the aqueduct by an extrinsic lesion posterior to the brain stem such as congenital aneurysm of the vein of Galen and posterior fossa subdural hematoma. The latter occurs as a birth injury; the bleeding is secondary to traumatic rupture of veins bridging from the surface of the cerebellum to the transverse sinuses. The diagnosis of posterior fossa subdural hematoma has to be considered in infants who develop hydrocephalus during the first few postnatal weeks, especially when there is a history of difficult birth. The *Dandy-Walker malformation* is a congenital defect of midline cerebellar structures in which hydrocephalus is caused by atresia of the foramina of Luschka and Magendie. When obstructive hydrocephalus is acquired postnatally, it is often due to brain tumors which compress or extend into the ventricular system.

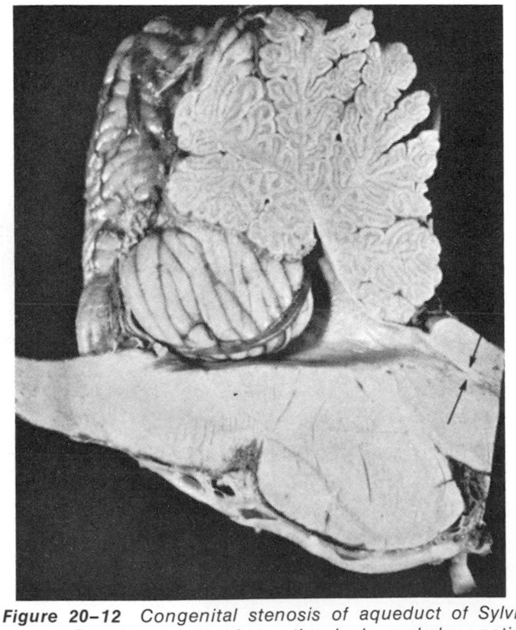

Figure 20-12 Congenital stenosis of aqueduct of Sylvius (arrows). Despite severe obstructive hydrocephalus, patient lived to sixth decade as a self-supporting person.

Communicating Hydrocephalus. Often of unknown etiology, this occurs in the *Arnold-Chiari malformation,* in which it is due to obstruction of subarachnoid pathways around the brain stem by downward displacement of the medulla oblongata and of the cerebellum. Communicating hydrocephalus may occur as a sequel to bacterial meningitis, toxoplasmosis, cytomegalic inclusion disease and subarachnoid hemorrhage. In these conditions, hydrocephalus results from obliteration of subarachnoid spaces by fibrous tissue reaction to meningeal inflammation or to hemorrhage. Hydrocephalus may complicate *Hurler syndrome* because of fibrous tissue proliferation in the subarachnoid spaces. In *achondroplasia* hydrocephalus is probably due to underdevelopment of the occipital skull. The posterior fossa is abnormally small, and this may lead to interference with circulation of CSF in the subarachnoid spaces at the base of the brain. *Vitamin A intoxication* is a rare cause of communicating hydrocephalus; the mechanism by which excessive vitamin A intake leads to hydrocephalus is unknown.

INCIDENCE. The incidence of congenital hydrocephalus varies in different populations. This is especially true for hydrocephalus associated with meningomyelocele, the incidence of which varies from about 4.0 per 1000 births in some parts of Wales and of Northern Ireland, to about 0.2 per 1000 in the Japanese. The incidence of all other forms of hydrocephalus is nearly 1 per 1000. Aqueductal stenosis is found in about one third of all hydrocephalic children.

CLINICAL MANIFESTATIONS. Signs and symptoms of hydrocephalus depend on the time of onset and on the severity of the imbalance between CSF production and resorptive capacity. Abnormal enlargement of the head is an invariable feature of congenital hydrocephalus and of hydrocephalus that has its onset in infancy. In the most severe cases of congenital hydrocephalus there is massive enlargement of the head during the fetal period, which precludes normal delivery of the infant. In milder forms the head is of normal size at birth but then grows at an excessive rate. Serial measurements of head circumference are essential for early diagnosis and for assessment of rate of progression. The skull is distended in all directions, but especially in the frontal area. Occipital expansion is seen in the Dandy-Walker malformation as a result of massive dilatation of the 4th ventricle. The huge, fluid-filled 4th ventricle can be demonstrated by occipital transillumination of the skull. Infants with rapidly progressive hydrocephalus have a large, bulging anterior fontanelle and palpable separation of cranial sutures. Apparently normal fontanelle tension, however, does not rule out the diagnosis. Separation of the cranial sutures leads to a resonant note on percussion of the skull (Macewen's or "cracked pot" sign). The scalp veins are often dilated, and the scalp skin is thin and shiny. The cry becomes high pitched as intracranial pressure rises. In severe infantile hydrocephalus the eyes are often deviated downward ("setting sun" sign). Optic atrophy, resulting from compression of the optic nerve and chiasm, occurs in chronic, untreated cases.

When the onset of hydrocephalus is late in childhood, there may be no appreciable enlargement of the head. Instead, the child has evidence of increased intracranial pressure with chronic papilledema. Combined spasticity and ataxia affecting the legs more than the arms is common, as is urinary incontinence. Progressive decline in mental activity occurs. Higher cortical functions such as judgment and reasoning tend to be affected disproportionately, while speech is often preserved, resulting in rather characteristic empty chatter. There is little correlation between degree of hydrocephalus and intellectual dysfunction. Some children with a hugely dilated ventricular system and a thin cerebral mantle have normal intelligence.

LABORATORY STUDIES. Neuroradiologic investigation is essential for the differentiation of hydrocephalus from other disorders that cause abnormal enlargement of the head, and to identify the site of obstruction to CSF flow. Pneumoencephalography is the preferred procedure in older infants or children in whom intracranial pressure is normal or only mildly elevated. Ventriculography is indicated for the young infant and in the presence of significantly increased intracranial pressure. Ventriculography should include radiographs taken with the child's head in a dependent position to visualize the aqueduct of Sylvius, the 4th ventricle and the subarachnoid spaces.

Air contrast studies tend to exacerbate active hydrocephalus, and they may cause decompensation of previously arrested hydrocephalus. This is an important consideration in the child with mild hydrocephalus, in whom an air study may precipitate the need for surgical intervention. Cerebral angiography may be the preferred initial study in such a child.

The cerebrospinal fluid should always be examined, to rule out chronic meningeal infection as a cause of the hydrocephalus and to determine whether CSF protein is elevated.

DIFFERENTIAL DIAGNOSIS. A number of conditions other than hydrocephalus cause abnormal enlargement of the cranial vault in infancy. Megalencephaly mimics hydrocephalus in most respects. However, signs of increased intracranial pressure are absent in megalencephaly and mental defect is more profound. Chronic subdural effusion in infancy may lead to significant head enlargement. Characteristically, the maximum expansion of the skull is in the parietal areas, rather than frontally as in hydrocephalus. Transillumination of the skull is positive in the frontoparietal regions in chronic subdural effusions and is negative in all but extreme cases of hydrocephalus, in which the cortical mantle is virtually absent. Ventricular enlargement occurs secondary to cerebral atrophy in degenerative and metabolic brain diseases. The head size is normal or small in such infants.

The possibility that hydrocephalus may be secondary to midline brain tumor always has to be considered. Cerebellar, pineal region and third ventricular tumors are likely to produce head enlargement in the absence of focal neurologic signs. Brain tumor has to be considered especially when enlargement in head size is very rapid in a previously normal infant, and when papilledema is present. An underlying cerebral neoplasm can be ruled out only by careful neuroradiologic study, which is mandatory prior to initiation of therapy for hydrocephalus.

THERAPY. The treatment of hydrocephalus has improved in recent years but continues to present many formidable problems. Ideally, the goal is to re-establish equilibrium between CSF production and resorption; however, the various means employed have been only partly successful. Acetazolamide in a dose of 50–75 mg/kg/day diminishes CSF production by about one third and is useful in cases of mild, slowly progressive hydrocephalus. Choroid plexectomy is a surgical method for decreasing CSF production. However, it carries a significant operative mortality, is associated with injury to cerebral cortex and is not always effective.

In obstructive hydrocephalus the site of obstruction can sometimes be bypassed. The Torkildsen shunt is a bypass operation for aqueductal stenosis: a plastic tube is used to connect one lateral ventricle with the cisterna magna and the spinal subarachnoid spaces. The operation is not successful in infants, since these spaces are as yet poorly developed. At present, the most widely used and successful treatments depend on shunting of the excess fluid into some extracranial body compartment. The ventriculo-atrial shunt returns the ventricular fluid directly into the blood stream through a tube that runs from one lateral ventricle via a jugular vein to the right atrium. A one-way valve is inserted in the tubing to prevent reflux of blood into the ventricular system. Complications with this type of shunt are numerous; they include bacterial colonization of the shunt (especially with *Staphylococcus albus*), kinking, plugging or separation of the shunt tubing, pulmonary emboli and nephritis. Shunt infection is the most common serious complication. It may cause recurrent episodes of septicemia or ventriculitis. In either case, cure of the infection requires removal of the shunt in addition to antibiotic therapy. Plugging of the shunt tubing is especially apt to occur when CSF protein is elevated. Growth of the head, neck and chest necessitates repeated shunt revisions during early childhood. Ventriculoperitoneal shunts have less serious complications, but they become more easily occluded. The lumbo-ureteral shunt is little used now, since it requires removal of one kidney. A drainage tube from the spinal subarachnoid space is attached to the ureteral stump. This shunt is useful only in communicating hydrocephalus. It carries the danger of meningitis whenever the child has a bladder infection, and a considerable risk of hyponatremia and dehydration from the direct drainage of CSF into the urinary bladder.

Careful initial evaluation is essential to determine whether a shunt operation is needed, or whether spontaneous arrest of hydrocephalus has occurred. In general, a shunt is not indicated in hydrocephalic infants whose head growth has become arrested or is progressing at or below the normal rate.

When a successful shunt has been established it usually has to be maintained for the life of the patient. Such a child needs careful medical supervision for early detection of evidences of shunt malfunction. Acute shunt failure in the older child causes rapidly progressive increase in intracranial pressure, with headache, vomiting and stupor, progressing to coma. Chronic shunt malfunction may result in school failure, lethargy and deterioration of gait. Repeated intelligence tests are useful for the early detection of decline in mental functions.

PROGNOSIS. The prognosis of infantile hydrocephalus has been significantly but not dramatically improved by introduction of shunt operations. Untreated, 50 to 60 per cent of infants with hydrocephalus succumb to the disorder itself or to intercurrent illnesses. If the process becomes arrested, about 40 per cent are of near-normal intelligence. With good and continued neurosurgical and medical management about 70 per cent can be expected to live beyond infancy; of these, about 40 per cent will retain intellectual capability, and about 60 per cent will have significant intellectual and motor handicaps. The prognosis of infants with both hydrocephalus and meningomyelocele is considerably worse.

Ameli, N. O.: Arrest of development and Dandy-Walker malformation. Brain *89*:459, 1966.

Drachman, D. A., and Richardson, E. P.: Aqueductal narrowing, congenital and acquired. Arch. Neurol. *5*:552, 1961.

Fokes, E. C.: Occult infections of ventriculo-arterial shunts. J. Neurosurg. *33*:517, 1970.

Foltz, E. L., and Shurtleff, D. B.: Five-year comparative study of hydrocephalus in children with and without operation (113 cases). J. Neurosurg. *20*:1064, 1963.

Gilles, F., and Shillito, J.: Infantile hydrocephalus: Retrocerebellar subdural hematoma. J. Pediatr. *76*:529, 1970.

Hagberg, B., and Naglo, A. S.: The conservative management of infantile hydrocephalus. Acta Paediatr. Scand. *61*:165, 1972.

Hagberg, B., and Sjorgen, I.: The chronic brain syndrome of infantile hydrocephalus. Am. J. Dis. Child *112*:189, 1966.

Hart, M. N., Malamud, N., and Ellis, W. G.: The Dandy-Walker Syndrome: A clinical-pathological study of 28 cases. Neurology *22*:771, 1972.

Huttenlocher, P. R.: Treatment of hydrocephalus with acetazolamide. Results in 15 cases. J. Pediatr. *66*:1023, 1965.

Johnson, R. T., and Johnson, K. P.: Hydrocephalus following viral infection: The pathology of aqueductal stenosis developing after experimental mumps virus infection. J. Neuropath. Exp. Neurol. *27*:591, 1968.

Laurence, K. M., and Coates, S.: The natural history of hydrocephalus. Detailed analysis of 182 unoperated cases. Arch. Dis. Child. *37*:345, 1962.

Milhorat, T. H.: Hydrocephalus and the Cerebrospinal Fluid. Baltimore, The Williams & Wilkins Company, 1972.

Noonan, J. A., and Ehmke, D. A.: Complications of ventriculovenous shunts for control of hydrocephalus. Report of three cases with thromboemboli to the lungs. New Engl. J. Med. *296*:70, 1963.

Ransohoff, J., Shulman, K., and Fishman, R. A.: Hydrocephalus. A review of etiology and treatment. J. Pediatr. *56*:399, 1960.

Russell, D. S.: Observations on the pathology of hydrocephalus. Special Report No. 265. Medical Research Council. London, Her Majesty's Stationery Office, 1949.

Scarff, J. E.: Treatment of hydrocephalus: An historical and critical review of methods and results. J. Neurol. Neurosurg. Psychiat. *26*:1, 1963.

Schick, R. W., and Matson, D. D.: What is arrested hydrocephalus? J. Pediatr. *58*:791, 1961.

Stauffer, U. G.: "Shunt nephritis": Diffuse glomerulonephritis complicating ventriculoatrial shunts. Develop. Med. Child Neurol. *22*(Suppl.):161, 1970.

Woodard, W. K., Miller, L. J., and Legant, O.: Acute and chronic hypervitaminosis A in a 4 month old infant. J. Pediatr. *59*:260, 1961.

Yashon, D.: Prognosis of infantile hydrocephalus, past and present. J. Neurosurg. *20*:105, 1963.

DEFECTS IN DEVELOPMENT OF BRAIN STEM

MOEBIUS SYNDROME. Congenital nuclear aplasia falls within this category; there is absence or maldevelopment of cranial nerve nuclei and of the nerves originating from them. The 7th nerves are affected most frequently, but most of the cranial nerves may be involved. The most severely affected children have ptosis, complete ophthalmoplegia, inability to close the eyes, immobility of face and difficulty with chewing and swallowing. There often are associated congenital anomalies, including absence of pectoralis muscles and clubfoot deformities. The expressionless face and constant drooling may give the erroneous impression of mental defect. When lid closure is defective, it is important to protect the corneas by use of artificial tears and by taping the eyelids at night.

SPASMUS NUTANS. This is a disorder of eye movements which is peculiar to infancy and usually is first noted between ages 4 and 12 months. It consists of intermittent rapid pendular nystagmoid movements, often confined to one eye, and, when bilateral, almost always more prominent on one side. About 80 per cent of the infants have intermittent head nodding. The etiology is unknown, and there have been no reported pathologic studies. Insufficient lighting and relative absence of visual stimuli for the infant to fix on have been implicated as possible etiologic factors without convincing evidence. Spontaneous improvement always occurs.

Spasmus nutans has to be distinguished from searching nystagmus due to decreased visual acuity and from hereditary congenital nystagmus. In congenital nystagmus the eye movement abnormality is bilaterally symmetrical, with pendular movements when the eyes are at rest, giving way to jerk nystagmus on attempted lateral gaze.

Hoefnagel, D., and Biery, B.: Spasmus nutans. Develop. Med. Child. Neurol. *10*:32, 1968.

Van Allen, M. W., and Blodi, F. C.: Neurologic aspects of the Moebius syndrome. Neurology *10*:249, 1960.

PERINATALLY ACQUIRED CEREBRAL LESIONS

Damage to the central nervous system in the perinatal period is a major cause of intellectual handicap and of nonprogressive motor disorders. In part, this is related to the unusual stresses to the infant incident to birth, in part to the peculiar susceptibility of the immature central nervous system to injury by a variety of agents. Cerebral anoxia, traumatic injury to brain, infection, hyperbilirubinemia, hypoglycemia, hypothyroidism and the inborn errors of amino acid metabolism are important causes of brain damage in the infant. The reaction of the immature brain to these agents differs markedly from the effects on the mature central nervous system.

Cerebral anoxia in the infant, contrary to that in the older child or adult, frequently causes selective damage to subcortical structures rather than to cortical neurons; especially is this the case in the premature infant, in whom the subcortical white matter is particularly vulnerable. The resulting brain lesion, periventricular leukomalacia, is frequently demonstrated at autopsy of premature infants who have had repeated anoxic episodes. The basal ganglia also are susceptible to anoxic damage in the neonate. Pathologically one finds loss of neurons in basal ganglia and abnormal deposition of myelin to replace them, giving with myelin stains a marbled appearance, "status marmoratus," to the basal ganglia.

Meningeal infection in the neonate results in cerebritis and cerebral vasculitis much more frequently than it does later in life, and these account for brain damage in the majority of survivors. Viral infection, including rubella, cytomegalovirus, herpesvirus and coxsackievirus, and infection with toxoplasma are more likely to involve brain in the fetus and neonate than in the older person. The reaction in the nervous system usually is one of widespread necrosis of tissue.

Elevation in the blood level of indirect reacting (unconjugated) bilirubin above 15–20 mg/dl causes damage in selected structures of the neonatal brain. The basal ganglia and cranial nerve nuclei in the lower brain stem, including those of the 8th nerve, are especially vulnerable. The most prominent acute pathologic change is yellow staining of the affected nuclei (kernicterus) owing to breakdown of the blood-brain barrier and deposition of bilirubin in the damaged tissues. The chronic lesion consists in loss of nerve cells, gliosis and defective myelination.

Severe neonatal hypoglycemia (Section 16) may cause diffuse necrosis of cortical neurons and damage to cerebellum. However, these lesions are uncommon, and it is generally assumed that the immature brain is less sensitive to damage by hypoglycemia than is the mature one.

A number of metabolic diseases lead to cerebral dysfunction by interference with the normal developmental events in postnatal brain; these include congenital hypothyroidism (cretinism) and the large group of inborn errors of amino acid metabolism, of which phenylketonuria is the most common. Myelination of subcortical white matter and the elaboration of dendrites and of synaptic connections between nerve cells are the two most important developmental events in postnatal brain (Figs. 20–6 and 20–7). They are most likely to be disturbed in the metabolic encephalopathies of the infant. Defective myelination has been well demonstrated in phenylketonuria and in maple sugar urine disease. Both the elaboration of cortical dendrites and myelination appear to be inhibited in cretinism.

One of the major problems in neonatal pediatrics is the paucity of early clinical evidences of CNS lesions in many infants damaged in the perinatal period. The infant may initially appear to improve, with cerebral dysfunction becoming manifest only as he matures. Intellectual handicaps, ranging from severe mental defect to mild learning disabilities, are common sequelae of neonatal brain damage. In some damaged infants motor deficits predominate, and there may be relative preservation of intellectual functions. (See Cerebral Palsy.) Others may develop seizures, sometimes a year or more after the initial insult. Since the mental and motor manifestations of cerebral damage may not appear until much later, it often is difficult to ascribe them with certainty to events that occurred in the neonatal period. As a result, the etiology in many children with static cerebral lesions is either unknown or conjectural.

Anderson, J. M., Milner, R. D. G., and Stritch, S. J.: Effects of neonatal hypoglycemia on the nervous system: A pathological study. J. Neurol. Neurosurg. Psychiat. *30*:295, 1967.

Banker, B. Q., and Larroche, J. C.: Periventricular leukomalacia of infancy: A form of neonatal anoxic encephalopathy. Arch. Neurol. *7*:386, 1962.

Berman, P. H., and Banker, B. Q.: Neonatal meningitis. A clinical and pathological study of 29 cases. Pediatrics *38*:6, 1966.

Diamond, I., et al.: Kernicterus: Revised concepts of pathogenesis and management. Pediatrics *38*:539, 1966.

Eayrs, J. T., and Horn, G.: The development of cerebral cortex in hypothyroid and starved rats. Anat. Rec. *121*:53, 1955.

Norman, R. M.: Etat marbré of the corpus striatum following birth injury. J. Neurol. Neurosurg. Psychiat. *10*:12, 1947.

Prensky, A. L., Carr, S., and Moser, H. W.: Development of myelin in inherited disorders of aminoacid metabolism. Arch. Neurol. *19*:552, 1968.

Rosman, N. P., et al.: The effect of thyroid deficiency on myelination of brain. Neurology *22*:99, 1972.

Towbin, A.: Central nervous system damage in the human fetus and newborn infant. Am. J. Dis. Child. *119*:529, 1970.

CEREBRAL PALSY

(Little's Disease)

Cerebral palsy is defined as any nonprogressive central motor deficit dating to events in the prenatal or perinatal periods. It is one of the commonest crippling conditions of childhood; there are almost 300,000 affected children in the United States alone. It is not a clearly defined disease, but rather a group of disorders of varied cause.

ETIOLOGY. The relationship of cerebral palsy to neonatal anoxia was first established by Little in 1843. Recent studies indicate that more than one third of children with cerebral plasy weighed less than 2500 gm at birth. The most likely etiologic event in these infants is cerebral anoxia; mechanical trauma to the brain at birth is also a cause, especially in those with spastic hemiplegia. Congenital malformations of brain and cerebral vascular occlusions during fetal life appear to account for a smaller percentage. Kernicterus, an important cause of cerebral palsy prior to the introduction of exchange transfusion for neonatal hyperbilirubinemia, is now relatively uncommon wherever good obstetric and pediatric care are practiced.

PATHOLOGY. The most severely disabled children are apt to have widespread cerebral atrophy, often with cavity formation in subcortical white matter. Atrophy of basal ganglia is found when rigidity and extrapyramidal movement disorders were present during life. With hemiplegia, there are often atrophy and gliosis of the opposite cerebral hemisphere; this is often confined to the areas supplied by the middle cerebral artery, suggesting the probability of arterial occlusion. Porencephaly occurs in some cases. In milder forms of cerebral palsy the brain may appear grossly normal, but is often reduced in weight. The subcortical white matter tends to be sparse, suggesting that some nerve fibers may have been destroyed by the initial cerebral insult.

CLINICAL MANIFESTATIONS. The clinical classification of patients with cerebral palsy is based on the nature of the observed motor deficit. The following simple classification is useful.

1. *Spastic cerebral palsy*
   Quadriplegia
   Paraplegia
   Hemiplegia
   Monoplegia
2. *Extrapyramidal cerebral palsy*
   Choreoathetosis
   Dystonia
3. *Atonic cerebral palsy*
   Atonic diplegia
   Congenital cerebellar ataxia
4. *Mixed types*

Spastic Cerebral Palsy. This is the most common type of palsy. Early manifestations are those of reflex hyperexcitability and abnormal persistence of neonatal reflexes. Hyperactivity of the grasp reflex leads to tight fisting of the hands. Tonic neck reflexes are often obligatory and may continue to be present long after the normal age of disappearance. Vertical suspension of the infant leads to extensor postures, with arching of back and rigid extension, and adduction and internal rotation of legs. When hip adduction is marked it leads to crossing (scissoring) of the legs. The severely spastic infant may have arching of the back and scissoring even at rest. Tendon reflexes are brisk, often with sustained ankle clonus. A positive Babinski sign is helpful in the diagnosis after age 2 years. Spasticity and rigidity become more evident as the child matures and often lead to abnormal postures of limbs and to contractures. Heel cord contractures, limitation in abduction and external rotation of the hips, and limitation in extension and supination of the forearms are common. Pseudobulbar palsy is present when spasticity is bilateral; it accounts for the swallowing difficulties and excessive drooling of these children.

In *spastic quadriplegia* all four limbs are involved. There usually is associated mental defect. Pseudobulbar palsy is prominent, and convulsions are common. *Diplegia* refers to a motor deficit that affects all four limbs but is much more severe in the lower extremities than in the upper ones. The involvement of hands may be minimal, expressing itself only in clumsiness in grasping and, later in life, in awkwardness of hand movements. Evidence of pseudobulbar palsy may be absent or may be limited to a brisk jaw jerk. Intelligence is often normal or borderline, but apraxias are common and may lead to difficulties in learning to draw and to form letters. More than 50 per cent of children with diplegia have had low birth weights.

In *spastic paraplegia,* a rare form of cerebral palsy, only the lower extremities are affected. The possibility of a spinal cord lesion must always be carefully considered in the child who has spasticity confined to the legs.

Spastic hemiplegia accounts for about one third of children with cerebral palsy. There often is homonymous hemianopsia and a hemisensory deficit on the side of the hemiplegia. The posture of the affected arm is quite characteristic: maintained flexion and pronation of the forearm and flexion of the wrist. The gait of these children is characterized by limping, often with circumduction of the affected leg. The intellectual level depends largely on whether the brain lesion is confined to one hemisphere. Convulsions early in life decrease the likelihood of normal intellectual development.

Monoplegia, spastic weakness confined to one limb, is rare. Careful examination will usually disclose an asymmetric diplegia or hemiplegia with one limb more severely affected than the other.

Extrapyramidal Cerebral Palsy. This is manifest as hypotonia in early infancy and by choreoathetoid movements and dystonia later in childhood. Diagnostic identification is unusual until after age 6 months; abnormal posturing of hands when the infant attempts to reach for an object is an early sign. When choreoathetosis is associated with deafness it is almost always the result of kernicterus. The combination of motor handicap and absence of speech function caused by deafness may give an erroneous impression of severe mental retardation; intellectual capacity can be surmised only after prolonged and careful study.

Atonic Diplegia. Atonic diplegia is a diagnostic term designating hypotonia and motor disability due to central nervous system damage. Severe mental defect is usual. The tendon reflexes are easily obtainable and may be quite brisk, in contrast to the pattern in hypotonia due to peripheral neuromuscular diseases. Some degree of spasticity in later childhood is common.

Congenital Cerebellar Ataxia. This is a rare form of cerebral palsy. Hypotonia and hypoactive tendon reflexes are present in infancy. Usually by the second year, intention tremor and gait ataxia are present. Nystagmus is uncommon. There may be associated mental defect, usually of mild degree.

DIFFERENTIAL DIAGNOSIS. *Spastic cerebral palsy* has to be distinguished from the leukodystrophies. In doubtful cases a spinal tap may provide helpful diagnostic information; spinal fluid protein is almost always elevated in the leukodystrophies, but not in cerebral palsy. The possibility that spastic weakness may be due to hydrocephalus or to subdural effusion should be considered whenever head size is large or when signs of increased intracranial pressure are present. Rarely, a slowly growing tumor of a cerebral hemisphere may be confused with the hemiplegic form of cerebral palsy. In brain tumor the disability is always progressive, and signs of increased intracranial pressure are usually present. Spinal cord lesions, including birth injuries to the cervical cord, tumors and congenital malformations should be considered when spasticity and weakness are limited to the muscle groups below the neck. Spastic diplegia is sometimes confused with muscular dystrophy; heel cord contractures and weakness of legs occur in both. Spasticity, however, is absent in muscular dystrophy, and the tendon reflexes are normal or reduced. In doubtful and early cases measurement of serum enzymes, especially of creatine phosphokinase, is helpful; creatine phosphokinase is always increased in the Duchenne form of muscular dystrophy. Atonic diplegia must be distinguished from a number of neuromuscular diseases of infancy, including Werdnig-Hoffmann disease and benign congenital hypotonia. The presence of mental defect and the preservation of tendon reflexes in atonic diplegia usually make clinical differentiation possible. Congenital cerebellar ataxia must be differentiated from a number of slowly progressive cerebellar degenerations. Early in the course the distinction from ataxia telangiectasia may be especially difficult; children with this illness are often diagnosed as having cerebral palsy. The presence of more than one child with motor deficit in the same family should always alert the physician to the likelihood of a disease other than cerebral palsy; there is no such entity as "familial cerebral palsy."

PROGNOSIS. The outlook for the child with cerebral palsy depends to a large extent on the presence and severity of associated intellectual handicaps. Good adjustment can be made even with fairly severe motor deficits as long as intellectual capacity is good. The reaction of the family to the child is of great importance, as is the availability of adequate educational and therapeutic facilities.

The long-term management and therapeutic approaches are discussed on pages 130–142. The prevention of cerebral palsy constitutes a great challenge to the pediatrician. Much has been accomplished in the prevention of kernicterus through therapy of neonatal hyperbilirubinemia. Meticulous care of low-birth-weight infants may reduce the number of children with spastic diplegia. Careful attention to the respiratory status of the infant and prompt therapy of apneic episodes appear to be especially important.

Crothers, B., and Paine, R.: The Natural History of Cerebral Palsy. Cambridge, Harvard University Press, 1959.

Ford, F. R.: Cerebral birth injuries and their results. Medicine *5*:121, 1926.

McDonald, A. D.: The aetiology of spastic diplegia. A synthesis of epidemiological and pathological evidence. Dev. Med. Child Neurol. *6*:277, 1964.

Mitchell, R. G.: The prevention of cerebral palsy. Dev. Med. Child Neurol. *13*:137, 1971.

Myers, R. E.: Atrophic cortical sclerosis with status marmoratus in the perinatally damaged monkey. Neurology *19*:1177, 1969.

Plum, P.: Aetiology of athetosis with special reference to neonatal asphyxia, idiopathic icterus and ABO-incompatibility. Arch. Dis. Child. *40*:376, 1965.

Towbin, A.: The Pathology of Cerebral Palsy. Springfield, Ill. Charles C Thomas, 1960.

Twitchell, T. E.: The neurological examination in infantile cerebral palsy. Dev. Med. Child Neurol. *5*:271, 1963.

HEADACHE AND VERTIGO

HEADACHE

Recurrent head pain is a common, frequently benign symptom late in childhood and in adolescence; in the young child it is unusual, and more often indicative of serious underlying disease. Headache may stem from any of the pain-sensitive structures of the head, including all the tissues covering the cranium, the intracranial blood vessels, the cranial nerves that carry sensory fibers (V, IX, X), the upper cervical nerves and the meninges near the base of the brain. The brain itself, the calvarium and the meninges overlying the cerebral hemispheres are insensitive to pain.

The following is a useful classification of the various types of headache.

1. *Vascular headache*
   Migraine
   Headache secondary to fever
   Hypertensive headache
2. *Headache related to epilepsy*
3. *Headache secondary to changes in intracranial pressure*
   Brain tumor headache
   Low CSF pressure headache
4. *Tension headache*
5. *Headache related to psychiatric disease*
6. *Headache due to eye strain*
7. *Nasal sinus pain*

MIGRAINE is a common cause of vascular headache in a child.

Pathogenesis. Migraine is incompletely understood. The aura preceding the onset of head pain is thought to be due to abnormal constriction of intracranial arteries, with localized transient ischemia of cerebral tissue. The headache itself is secondary to vasodilatation of cranial vessels, especially those of the scalp. Pain fibers in the vessel walls are stimulated by the abnormal vascular distention and pulsations.

Clinical Manifestations. A positive family history is present in over two thirds of the patients, and a dominant inheritance pattern is suggested in many families. The onset is usually late in childhood or in early adolescence. In some instances there is a history of repeated vomiting in infancy, suggesting that the attacks may start at a time when the child is unable to verbalize his symptoms. Classically an attack of migraine is preceded by an aura, which often consists of transient visual disturbance, but which may include a variety of other fleeting neurologic disabilities. The visual aura consists of scintillating scotomata and of zigzag lines ("fortification phenomena") which move slowly across the visual field. Less commonly, the aura consists of diplopia due to oculomotor nerve palsy (ophthalmoplegic migraine) or of transient hemisensory loss, hemiparesis or aphasia. Within minutes or at most a few hours the aura is followed by throbbing unilateral head pain and by nausea and vomiting. Sleep usually terminates an attack. The frequency of attacks varies greatly even in the same patient; stress appears to increase the number of attacks. Partial forms, in which there is no aura, and atypical attacks with bilateral head pain and without vomiting are probably considerably more common than is the classic migraine described above.

Differential Diagnosis. The diagnosis of migraine can usually be made from the history in combination with the absence of any positive findings on careful funduscopic, physical and neurologic examination. Fever may produce a similar throbbing head pain secondary to peripheral vasodilatation and increased cerebral blood flow. Hypertension should always be ruled out. Congenital cerebrovascular malformations are a rare cause of vascular headache. They usually produce an audible cranial bruit over the head or eyes. Headache due to increased intracranial pressure is ruled out by funduscopic examination and by skull radiographs.

Laboratory Studies. These are of little value. Occasionally it may be necessary to obtain skull x-rays, a brain scan and an electroencephalogram to supplement the clinical evaluation. More extensive evaluations, such as cerebral angiography, should be avoided.

Treatment. Therapy is often only partially satisfactory. Vasoconstrictors such as ergotamine and caffeine taken at the very onset of symptoms may abort an attack; ergotamine tartrate (Cafergot) is widely used. The dosage in a child over age 10 years is one tablet at the first sign of an attack, repeated twice at 30-minute intervals if necessary. Simple analgesics, such as aspirin, may be as effective and should be tried first. Maintenance therapy with phenobarbital sometimes prevents attacks, but is justifiable only if attacks are frequent and incapacitating. Accurate diagnosis and reassurance that the child has a benign condition is often more helpful than drugs. Potentially dangerous medications such as methysergide and narcotics are to be strictly avoided.

HEADACHE AS A SYMPTOM IN EPILEPSY. Headache may occur as part of the aura preceding a grand mal seizure, or as a postictal event. In autonomic seizures headache may be a striking part of the attack itself. Other autonomic disturbances, such as pallor, tachycardia or pupillary dilatation, are easily overlooked. It has been suggested that headache may be the only manifestation of a seizure. This concept is difficult to prove. The presence of electroencephalographic abnormality in a child with recurrent head pain is of little help, since abnormal EEG records are also common in children with classic migraine, especially at the time of the attack.

HEADACHE SECONDARY TO INTRACRANIAL PRESSURE CHANGES. This head pain is probably the result of stretching and deformation of cerebral vessels and of meninges. Brain tumor headache often occurs following changes in head position, such as after arising from sleep. Morning headache in a child should always arouse the suspicion of brain tumor. There may be associated vomiting, often with minimal nausea, and followed by a feeling of well-being. The location of head pain is a good localizing sign in brain tumor. Headache due to posterior fossa tumor is almost always occipital.

Low pressure headache is usually due to a persistent CSF leak after spinal tap. It may also be seen after traumatic meningeal tears with CSF fistula. The pain appears almost immediately on assumption of the upright position, and it is relieved by lying down. This type of headache following lumbar puncture is best treated by bed rest, preferably in the prone position.

TENSION HEADACHE. This is thought to be due to persistent contraction of neck and temporalis muscles, leading to localized ischemia of these structures. It is often described as a dull, steady pain, increasing as the day advances, and relieved after sleep. In its classic form it is rarely seen prior to adolescence.

HEADACHE RELATED TO PSYCHIATRIC DISEASE. Headache is a rather common symptom of depression in childhood. This type of headache is described as continuously present, in contrast to organic head pain which is almost always intermittent. The facial expression of the depressed child with headache bespeaks suffering. Speech may be reduced to a whisper. Poor appetite, constipation and insomnia are frequent associated findings. Failure to recognize this syndrome often leads to performance of extensive and potentially harmful diagnostic procedures.

EYE STRAIN. Eye strain is often implicated as a cause of headache, and glasses are prescribed for relief. There is little evidence in support of such an association. Occasionally, prolonged reading by a child with a refractive error may lead to tension headache.

BENIGN PAROXSYMAL VERTIGO IN CHILDHOOD

This syndrome has its onset in young children, usually between 1 and 4 years of age. It is thought to be secondary to a disturbance in vestibular function. During a typical attack the child suddenly becomes unsteady on his feet and appears frightened; he may clutch his parent. The older child may be able to describe a rotational experience. There is no change in state of consciousness, and after a few minutes the child returns to his former healthy state. The condition is self-limited, tending to subside over a period of 2 or 3 years. Benign paroxsymal vertigo is often misdiagnosed as epilepsy, and anticonvulsant drugs are prescribed unnecessarily. The preservation of normal alertness during the attack is the most important differential point from epilepsy.

Cold water caloric tests may show diminished or absent vestibular response in one or both ears. Audiograms and electroencephalographic tracings are normal. A trial on dimenhydrinate (Dramamine) is indicated when the attacks recur frequently.

Graham, J. H., et al.: Fibrotic disorders associated with methysergide therapy for headache. New Engl. J. Med. *274*:360, 1966.

Holguin, J., and Fenichel, G.: Migraine. J. Pediatr. *70*:290, 1967.

Koenigsberger, M. R., Chutorian, A. M., Gold, A. P., and Schvey, M. S.: Benign paroxysmal vertigo of childhood. Neurology *20*:1108, 1970.

Malmquist, C. P.: Depressions in childhood and adolescence. New Engl. J. Med. *284*:955, 1971.

Pearce, J.: Migraine. Springfield, Ill., Charles C Thomas, 1969.

Waters, W. E.: Headache and the eye. Lancet *2*:1, 1970.

Wolff, H. G.: Headache and Other Head Pain. New York, Oxford University Press, 1963.

THE NEUROCUTANEOUS SYNDROMES

These syndromes, also known as phakomatoses and ectodermal dyplasias, include congenital lesions of the skin and of the central nervous system, often in association with ocular and visceral abnormalities. Several clearly distinct syndromes are recognized.

TUBEROUS SCLEROSIS

(See also other Sections.)

This disorder, a major cause of mental defect and of intractable convulsions, is inherited as a dominant trait, with wide variation in expression. About 50 per cent of cases appear to be new mutations. In the fully developed disease lesions are encountered in numerous organs, including brain, skin, eyes, kidneys, heart, bones and lungs.

The characteristic cerebral lesions are sclerotic patches (tubers) scattered throughout the cortical gray matter: They consist of astrocytes and bizarre giant cells, some of which have the staining characteristics of neurons. In addition, there may be multiple small tumor nodules in a periventricular distribution, made up of fibrous glia, giant cells and blood vessels. These lesions, though present at birth, tend to enlarge gradually, and may form tumor masses which may bulge into the lateral ventricles. Calcium is often deposited in the lesions, and may be visible roentgenographically, usually after age 1 year. Occasionally a paraventricular tumor undergoes malignant transformation into an astrocytoma or glioblastoma.

Convulsions are the most common clinical sign of brain involvement and occur in more than 90 per cent of patients. Myoclonic seizures may occur during the first year of life; grand mal and psychomotor seizures predominate later. Mental defect, varying from mild to severe, is present in 60 to 70 per cent of patients. Behavior disorders, especially hyperactivity and destructiveness, are common. Focal neurologic signs such as hemiparesis or hemianopsia are rare. They suggest the possibility of malignant transformation in a paraventricular tumor, in which case headache and papilledema related to ventricular obstruction are usually present.

Adenoma sebaceum is the most characteristic skin lesion of tuberous sclerosis. It consists of small bright red or brownish nodules in a butterfly distribution on the nose and cheeks. Histologically these lesions consist of a mixture of fibrous tissue and blood vessels. They usually appear between 2 and 5 years of age and, by late childhood, are found in more than 80 per cent of patients. Hypopigmented skin macules on arms, legs and trunk are usually present from birth; they may be oval or irregular in outline, and a few millimeters to several centimeters in diameter (Fig. 20–13 *A*). The presence of these skin lesions in an infant with infantile spasms strongly suggests the diagnosis of tuberous sclerosis. Other skin manifestations include slightly raised, indurated areas of skin, usually over the back (shagreen patches), and gingival and periungual fibromas.

Benign tumors made up of a mixture of fibrous tissue, fat, blood vessels and smooth muscle, often partly cystic, are found in numerous organs, especially kidneys, heart, liver, spleen and lungs. The renal tumors are present in about 80 per cent of patients and may cause renal failure by compression of the ureters or of the renal pelvis. Rhabdomyoma of the heart is an uncommon but important complication of tuberous sclerosis, manifest clinically by progressive cardiac failure, arrhythmias or sudden death. Small tumor nodules and cystic malformations throughout the lungs may lead to recurrent pneumothorax. About 50 per cent of patients have retinal lesions, visible on funduscopic examination as white or yellow raised areas, often near the edge of the optic disc. These are malformations in the nerve fiber layer of the retina, consisting primarily of glial fibers and malformed retinal neuroglial cells. Such lesions usually do not impair vision.

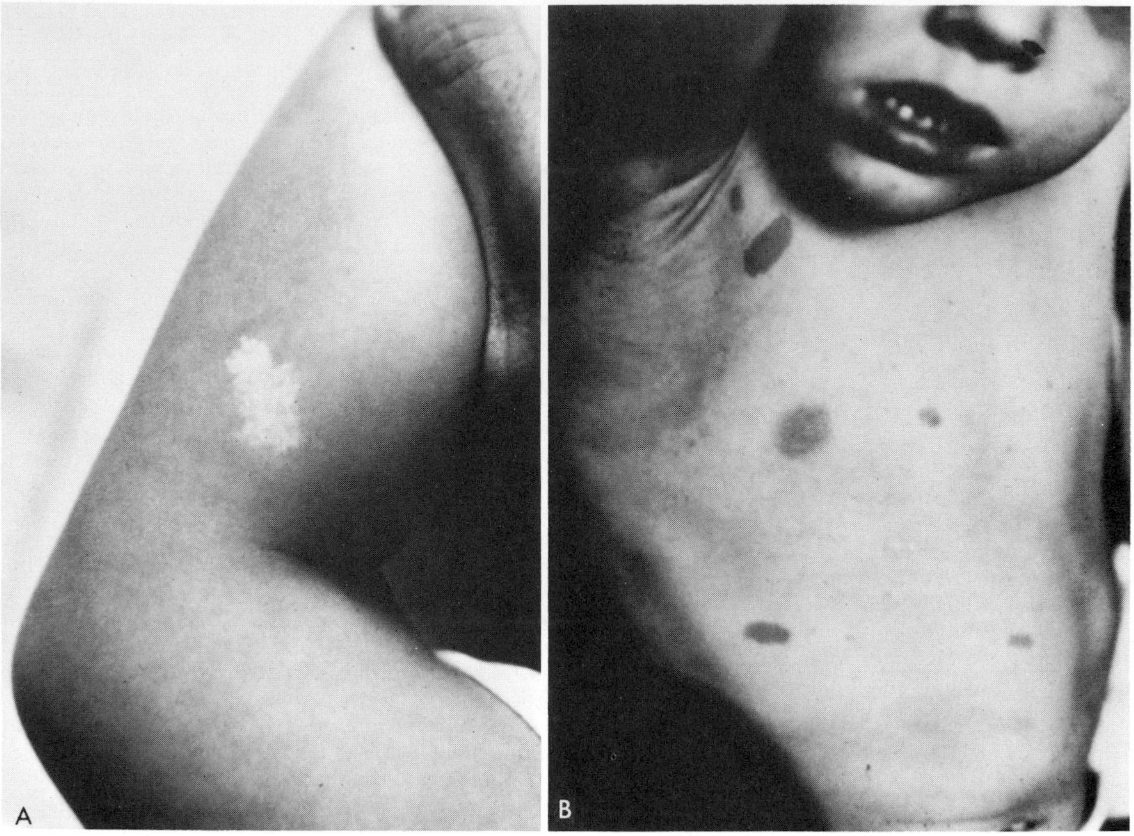

Figure 20–13 A, *Hypopigmented macule of tuberous sclerosis.* B, *Café-au-lait spots in neurofibromatosis.*

Roentgenograms of long bones may disclose areas of sclerosis and of rarefaction, especially in metacarpal and metatarsal bones.

The *prognosis* is extremely variable. Patients with mild involvement may have a full productive life. Institutional care is required for those with severe mental deficiency. Early death may be due to status epilepticus, brain tumor, renal failure or tumor of the heart.

Proper *management* includes treatment of seizures and assessment of intellectual function as a guide to an appropriate educational program. Methylphenidate hydrochloride (Ritalin) or dextroamphetamine may be helpful for control of hyperactivity in the young child with tuberous sclerosis. Surgical excision of tumors is indicated only if they are symptomatic. Genetic counseling is essential. Both parents should be carefully examined for stigmata, including those of skin, retina and brain (roentgenogram of skull). Evidence of tuberous sclerosis in one parent suggests a 50 per cent likelihood of occurrence in subsequent children; a new mutation can be assumed if both parents are free of stigmata.

NEUROFIBROMATOSIS
(von Recklinghausen's Disease)

See also other sections.

Neurofibromatosis is transmitted as an autosomal dominant trait, but new mutations are common and have been estimated to account for about 50 per cent of cases. Manifestations are extremely varied. The skin is involved in the great majority of patients. Café au lait spots, irregularly shaped areas of increased skin pigmentation, are a hallmark of the disease (Fig. 20–13 *B*). Though a few such spots are commonly found in otherwise normal persons, the presence of more than six which are greater than 1.5 cm in diameter is pathognomonic of neurofibromatosis. In addition, there tends to be freckling, especially in the armpits, and general hyperpigmentation of skin.

Cutaneous and subcutaneous neurofibromas are common, often making their appearance in late childhood or in adolescence. These are thought to arise from the Schwann cells of peripheral nerves. The cutaneous tumors tend to form multiple soft pedunculated masses (molluscum fibrosum). The subcutaneous ones are usually palpable as soft nodules attached to the larger peripheral nerves. Less common are plexiform neuromas, which are large infiltrative tumors; they cause considerable disfigurement, usually involving the face or one extremity. Sarcomatous degeneration of one or more neurofibromas occurs in about 10 per cent of patients; it is rare in childhood.

Neurofibromas on cranial or spinal nerve roots may lead to a variety of neurologic symptoms. Tumor of the 8th nerve (acoustic neuroma) causes tinnitus, nerve deafness, loss of corneal reflex, vertigo, ataxia and signs of increased cranial pressure. Neurofibroma involving a spinal root may be manifest as an extramedullary spinal cord tumor. There is also increased incidence of other types of neural tumors, such as glioma of the optic nerve and optic chiasm, meningioma and pheochromocytoma.

A large variety of associated congenital malformations have been described, including congenital bowing and pseudarthrosis of the tibia, cysts of long bones, overgrowth of bone and of soft tissue, scoliosis, megalencephaly and malformation of the greater wing of the sphenoid bone. The latter is associated with pulsating exophthalmus. Mild impairment in intellectual functions is common, but severe mental defect rarely occurs. Convulsions occur in about 5 per cent of patients. Life expectancy is essentially normal; the increased incidence of brain tumors and sarcomas is the principal risk.

The diagnosis of neurofibromatosis is based on the physical findings. Confirmation by biopsy of one of the subcutaneous nodules may be necessary if cutaneous manifestations are lacking. A careful family history and examination of immediate family members is essential in determining whether the disease occurs as a dominant trait or whether the propositus represents a new mutation. The family should be advised that the offspring of any patient with neurofibromatosis has a 50 per cent chance of inheriting the disorder. Therapy is limited to excision of tumors which produce pain or impairment in function, and of rapidly growing masses in which malignant transformation is suspected.

STURGE-WEBER DISEASE
(Encephalotrigeminal Angiomatosis)

Sturge-Weber disease occurs sporadically without known hereditary factors. The basic lesion is a congenital capillary hemangioma which involves skin of the face and cervical area, mucous membranes, meninges and choroid, usually unilaterally. The skin angioma ("nevus flammeus" or "portwine stain") is in the trigeminal distribution, most commonly in the ophthalmic division, but it may extend more widely over cervical segments. In the meninges the malformation often is confined to the pial vessels in the occipitoparietal areas. Sluggish flow of blood in malformed pial vessels leads to anoxic injury in underlying cerebral cortex. The clinical manifestations of cortical damage include convulsions, mental defect and hemiparesis or hemianopsia on the side opposite that of the lesion. Subarachnoid hemorrhage rarely occurs. Calcifications in the damaged cortical layers may become visible radiologically even in infancy and nearly always by late childhood (Fig. 20–14). They are often curvilinear and double contoured ("railroad track pattern") and are pathognomonic in a child with facial nevus. Angioma in the choroid may lead to buphthalmos in infancy or to glaucoma in childhood.

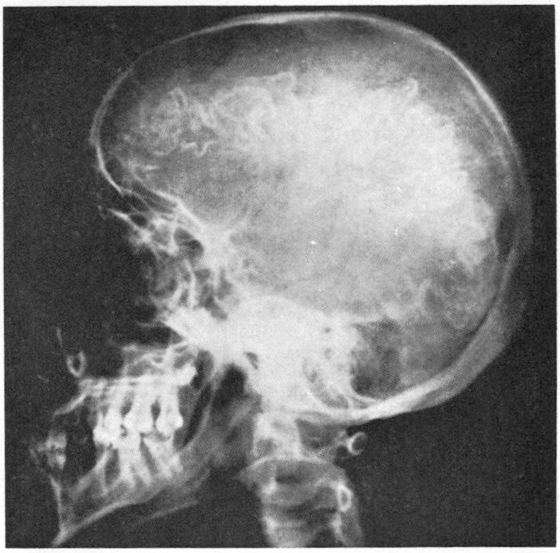

Figure 20–14 *Unusually extensive calcification in Sturge-Weber disease.*

Management of the child with Sturge-Weber disease is determined by clinical manifestations; e.g., anticonvulsant drugs for seizures, physiotherapy for paretic limbs, and periodic eye examination for early detection of glaucoma. Local resection of the cerebral cortical lesion may be indicated when severe convulsions are refractory to medication. A covering cream may be used on the face for cosmetic purposes.

VON HIPPEL-LINDAU DISEASE

This disorder is often included as one of the neurocutaneous disorders, although the skin is not involved. Retinal angiomas are associated with hemangioblastoma of the cerebellum and frequently with such other tumors as hemangioma of spinal cord, hypernephroma and cystadenomas of multiple visceral organs. Dominant inheritance has been demonstrated in several families. Symptoms include visual loss and evidences of cerebellar and spinal cord dysfunction, but these usually do not appear until adolescence or later life.

Alexander, G. L., and Norman, R. M.: The Sturge-Weber Syndrome, Bristol, John Wright and Sons, 1960.

Cooper, J. R.: Brain tumors in hereditary multiple system hamartomatosis (tuberous sclerosis). J. Neurosurg. *34*:194, 1971.

Crowe, F. W., Schull, W. J., and Neel, J. V.: Multiple Neurofibromatosis. Springfield, Ill., Charles C Thomas, 1956.

Fienman, N. L., and Yakovac, W. C.: Neurofibromatosis in childhood. J. Pediatr. *76*:339, 1970.

Gold, A. G., and Freeman, J. M.: Depigmented nevi: The earliest sign of tuberous sclerosis. Pediatrics *35*:1003, 1965.

Hurwitz, S., and Braverman, I. M.: White spots in tuberous sclerosis. J. Pediatr. *77*:587, 1970.

Lagos, J. C., and Gomez, M. R.: Tuberous sclerosis; Reappraisal of a clinical entity. Mayo Clinic Proc. *42*:26, 1967.

Peterman, A. F., et al.: Encephalotrigeminal angiomatosis (Sturge-Weber disease). Clinical study of 35 cases. J.A.M.A. *167*:2169, 1958.

Pitt, M. J., Mosher, J. F., and Ederken, J.: Abnormal periosteum and bone in neurofibromatosis. Radiology *103*:143, 1972.

DEGENERATIVE BRAIN DISEASES

The outstanding characteristic of these illnesses is a history of progressive loss of previously acquired intellectual, motor and sensory functions. Most of them are genetically determined, usually on an autosomal recessive basis; specific enzymatic defects have been demonstrated in some. Identification of carrier states (heterozygotes) as well as intrauterine diagnosis is now possible by enzymatic assays in several of the disorders. A number of the cerebral degenerations, however, cannot be specifically categorized, and effective therapy is lacking for most of them.

Classification is usually based on subdivision into the disorders which principally affect cerebral gray matter and those which affect the white matter. Subdivisions are based, at least in part, on the functional systems involved, e.g., the basal ganglia and the spinocerebellar system. Dementia and seizures are the predominant early manifestations in the gray matter diseases, whereas deterioration in motor function, manifest by spasticity, hypotonia or ataxia, are the early signs of degenerations involving the white matter. Eventually, however, the entire nervous system tends to become affected in both varieties, and, in general, the end stage clinical picture of all the disorders is similar: the child becomes totally helpless, with loss of all intellectual and voluntary motor functions.

The following is a useful classification:

I. *Degenerations of cerebral gray matter*
- A. Neuronal storage diseases
  - 1. Ganglioside storage diseases
    - Tay-Sachs disease
    - Generalized gangliosidosis
  - 2. Storage diseases with accumulation of sphingolipids other than ganglioside
    - Infantile Gaucher's disease
    - Niemann-Pick disease
    - Farber's disease (lipogranulomatosis)
  - 3. Other neuronal storage diseases
    - Late infantile and juvenile cerebromacular degeneration (Bielschowsky, Spielmeyer-Vogt and Batten)
    - Glycogen storage disease of heart, muscle and CNS (Pompe's disease)
- B. Degenerations of gray matter without neuronal storage
  - Alper's disease
  - Leigh's disease
  - Kinky hair (Menkes') disease
  - Subacute sclerosing panencephalitis (SSPE)

II. *Degenerative disorders of cerebral white matter*
- A. The leukodystrophies
  - Metachromatic leukodystrophy (sulfatide lipidosis)
  - Krabbe's disease (cerebroside lipidosis)
  - Sudanophilic leukodystrophies
  - Canavan's disease
- B. Demyelinating diseases
  - Schilder's disease
  - Multiple sclerosis
  - Neuromyelitis optica

III. *System degenerations*
- A. Spinocerebellar and cerebellar degenerations
  - Friedreich's ataxia and its variants
  - Ataxia-telangiectasia
  - Bassen-Kornzweig syndrome
  - Refsum's disease
- B. Basal ganglia degenerations
  - Wilson's disease (hepatolenticular degeneration)
  - Dystonia musculorum deformans
  - Huntington's chorea

DEGENERATIONS OF CEREBRAL GRAY MATTER

Neuronal Storage Diseases

These diseases are characterized by accumulation of lipid substances in cerebral neurons. In most instances the stored material is a sphingolipid; in some, a ganglioside. The sphingolipids are normal components of all cell membranes. Gangliosides are complex sphingolipids, which are normally present in high concentration in neurons; their function is unknown. Neuronal lipid storage is due to deficiency of specific enzymes which normally degrade the sphingolipids. In general, the substrate of the defective enzyme is stored in the cells.

A brief review of the chemistry of the sphingolipids is necessary for an understanding of the neuronal lipid storage diseases. The simplest sphingolipids are made up of the base, sphingosine, and a fatty acid. The resulting compound is referred to as ceramide. In the more complex sphingolipids, a variety of side chains are added to the ceramide molecule. The compounds of ceramide are of particular importance in neuronal lipid storage disease. See diagram at top of following page.

The terminology of Svennerholm is generally used to classify the gangliosides. In this system, the letter G refers to ganglioside; M, D or T refers to the number of sialic acid groups (mono-, di-, or trisialic acid), and the subscript (1, 2 or 3) refers to the number of hexosides in the molecule. Tetrahexosides are assigned the number 1; trihexosides, the number 2, dihexosides, the number 3.

Ganglioside Storage Diseases

At least five illnesses in this category are recognized; they can be differentiated on the basis of clinical findings, age of onset and specific enzyme assays. Each of them is transmitted on an autosomal recessive basis. The salient features are summarized in Table 20–6. The enzymatic defect in each disorder affects all body cells, but functional derangement appears to be limited to the central nervous system in all except generalized gangliosidosis, in which visceral and osseous lesions occur in association with cerebral degeneration. In each disorder, specific diagnosis is possible by assay of the affected enzyme in white blood cells. Heterozygous carriers of the trait can be identified on the basis of partial deficiency of the enzyme. Intrauterine diagnosis can be established by enzyme assay of cultured amniotic fluid cells.

TAY-SACHS DISEASE. Infantile cerebromacular

ceramide-P-choline = sphingomyelin (see Niemann-Pick disease)
ceramide-glucose = glucocerebroside (see Infantile Gaucher Disease)

ceramide-glucose-galactose-acetylgalactosamine-galactose = normal ganglioside (GM_1)
|
sialic acid

ceramide-glucose-galactose-acetylgalactosamine = Tay Sachs ganglioside (GM_2)
|
sialic acid

degeneration is by far the commonest of the gangliosidoses. It is most frequently found in children of Eastern European Jewish (Ashkenazi) ancestry; the incidence of the carrier state among Ashkenazi Jews is estimated to be 2.7 per cent, about 10 times higher than that in other population groups. The clinical findings of the disease are quite characteristic. At 2 to 6 months of age a previously well infant becomes apathetic and loses interest in his surroundings. There is progressive loss of acquired motor functions and of visual ability. An exaggerated startle response to noise (hyperacusis) is an early sign. Progressive spasticity with hyperreflexia and decerebrate posturing, feeding difficulties and emaciation occur in the late stages of the illness, and the head may become abnormally large. Grand mal, tonic or myoclonic seizures are seen. The most characteristic feature is the cherry red spot of the macula; this is a bright red area in the region of the fovea, surrounded by a grayish-white rim (Fig. 20–15). The latter is due to lipid accumulation in the surrounding retinal ganglion cells. The cherry red spot is not pathognomonic; it may also occur in Niemann-Pick and Sandhoff disease (Table 20–6).

Routine laboratory examinations are not helpful in the diagnosis. The cerebrospinal fluid protein is usually normal, but there may be an increase in cerebrospinal fluid enzymes, including lactic dehydrogenase and glutamic oxaloacetic transaminase. The basic defect is virtual absence of the enzyme hexosaminidase A from all body tissues. Measurement of this enzyme in serum, amniotic fluid cells or white cells has become the definitive diagnostic measure. Deficiency of hexosaminidase A results in marked accumulation of GM_2 ganglioside in all neurons, including those in the peripheral autonomic nervous system. GM_2 gangliosides, which normally make up only 1 to 3 per cent of total brain gangliosides, account for more than 90 per cent in patients with Tay-Sachs disease. Pathologically the accumulation of ganglioside is visible by light microscopy as marked ballooning of neurons. By electronmicroscopy the ganglioside is seen as discrete intracellular concretions with a characteristic lamellar structure. Neuronal degeneration and gliosis are marked in infants who survive for several years.

There is no therapy for Tay-Sachs disease. The prognosis is hopeless, and death usually occurs

TABLE 20–6 GANGLIOSIDE STORAGE DISEASES

DISEASE	ENZYME DEFECT	AGE AT ONSET	CHARACTERISTIC PHYSICAL FEATURES
Tay-Sachs disease (GM_2 gangliosidosis, type 1)	Absence of hexosaminidase A	3–6 mos	Hyperacusis, dementia, seizures, cherry red spot of macula, blindness, macrocephaly
Sandhoff disease (GM_2 gangliosidosis, type 2)	Absence of hexosaminidase A and B	3–6 mos	Same as Tay-Sachs disease
Juvenile GM_2 gangliosidosis (GM_2 gangliosidosis, type 3)	Partial deficiency of hexosaminidase A	2–6 yr	Dementia, ataxia, spasticity, seizures
Generalized gangliosidosis (GM_1, gangliosidosis, type 1)	Absence of β-galactosidase A, B and C	In utero or early infancy	Hepatosplenomegaly, Hurler-like features and bone changes, failure of intellectual and motor development
Juvenile GM_1 gangliosidosis (GM_1 gangliosidosis, type 2)	Absence of β-galactosidase B and C	6 mos–2 yr	Spasticity, ataxia, dementia

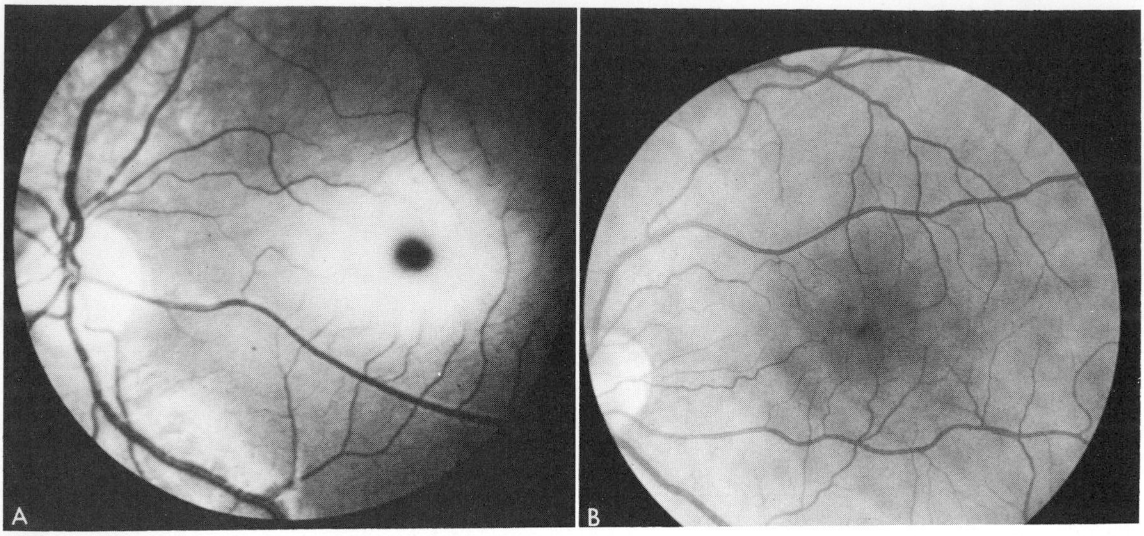

Figure 20–15 *A, Cherry red spot of the macula in Tay-Sachs disease. B, Normal macula for comparison.*

prior to age 4 years. Efforts should be made to prevent the birth of an affected fetus. Heterozygous carriers in populations known to be at risk can be identified by serum assay of hexosaminidase A. Diagnostic aminocentesis should be offered when both parents are known to be heterozygotes. It should be carried out at about 18 weeks' gestation, in time for safe therapeutic abortion of an affected fetus.

OTHER GANGLIOSIDE STORAGE DISEASES. See Table 20–6.

Late Infantile and Juvenile Cerebromacular Degenerations

These disorders are the second most common group of degenerative disorders of the cerebral gray matter. Onset is between ages 1 and 3 years in the late infantile form *(Bielschowsky syndrome)* and usually between 5 and 7 years in the more common juvenile variety *(Spielmeyer-Vogt* or *Batten's* disease). As yet, it is unknown whether the two represent variants of the same illness or different genetic defects. Transmission of these disorders is on an autosomal recessive basis.

Pathologically there is distention of neurons with material that has the staining characteristics of lipofuscin. Electronmicroscopy shows curvilinear and lattice-like neuronal cytoplasmic inclusions. Neuronal involvement is widespread and includes cells in the anterior horn of the spinal cord and in the peripheral autonomic ganglia. Lipofuscin-like material also accumulates in other organs, especially in the thyroid gland and in sweat glands.

The illness often starts with progressive loss of vision. Ophthalmologic changes vary among affected families; they may consist of retinitis pigmentosa, pigmentary degeneration of the macular region or simple optic atrophy. The electroencephalogram may be abnormal, with diffuse spike-wave activity, long before the onset of neurologic deterioration. Grand mal or myoclonic seizures and symptoms of dementia may appear 1 to 3 years after onset of visual loss. The child becomes hyperactive and irritable. There is deterioration of speech, often characterized by peculiar stammering, slurring and repetition of words. Cerebellar ataxia, tremor, rigidity, spastic paralysis and complete dementia are manifest late in the course. Progression is slow, and the patient may survive into adolescence or early adult years; the course is relatively slower the later the onset.

The diagnosis should be suspected in a child with the combination of progressive visual loss, seizures and mental deterioration. Ganglioside storage diseases, which may present with identical clinical findings, can be ruled out by assay of hexosaminidase or beta-galactosidase in white cells. Ballooned ganglion cells laden with lipofuscin can be seen in biopsies of rectal tissue. Electronmicroscopic examination of muscle or of sweat glands will reveal characteristic electron-dense bodies similar to those found in neurons.

Aronson, S. M., and Volk, B. W. (eds.): Cerebral sphingolipidoses. A Symposium on Tay-Sachs Disease and Allied Disorders. New York, Academic Press, Inc., 1962.

Carpenter, S., Karpati, G., and Andermann, F.: Specific involvement of muscle, nerve and skin in late infantile and juvenile amaurotic idiocy. Neurology *22*:170, 1972.

Fawcett, J. S., et al.: On the natural history of late infantile cerebromacular degeneration. Neurology *16*:1130, 1966.

Jervis, G. A.: Juvenile amaurotic idiocy. A.M.A. J. Dis. Child. *97*:663, 1959.

Landing, B. H., Silverman, F. N., et al.: Familial neurovisceral lipidosis. Am. J. Dis. Child. *108*:503, 1964.

Milunsky, A., Littlefield, J. W., et al.: Prenatal genetic diagnosis. New Engl. J. Med. *283*:1370; 1441; 1498; 1970.

O'Brien, J. S., et al.: Generalized gangliosidosis. Am. J. Dis. Child. *109*:338, 1965.

O'Brien, J. S., Okada, S., et al.: Tay-Sachs disease. Detection of heterozygotes and homozygotes by serum hexosaminidase assay. New Engl. J. Med. *283*:15, 1970.

Zeman, W., and Dyken, P.: Neuronal ceroid-lipo-fuscinosis (Batten's disease): Relationship to amaurotic family idiocy. Pediatrics *44*:570, 1969.

Degeneration of Gray Matter Without Neuronal Storage

ALPER'S DISEASE. Alper's disease is a syndrome resulting from degeneration of gray matter in infancy; it is unlikely that it is a single entity. Pathologic changes in brain are nonspecific; there are widespread loss of neurons and gliosis in cerebral cortex and in cerebellum. The most prominent symptoms are recurrent seizures and dementia. Several siblings may be affected, suggesting a recessive pattern of inheritance.

LEIGH'S DISEASE. *Subacute necrotizing encephalomyelopathy* is a metabolic brain disease which leads to widespread cerebral damage, especially in the brain stem. It is inherited on an autosomal recessive basis.

Pathologic changes in the brain consist of degeneration of neural structures and capillary proliferation in a characteristic distribution surrounding the 3rd ventricle, the aqueduct of Sylvius and the 4th ventricle. The lesions are strikingly similar to those of thiamine deficiency (Wernicke's) encephalopathy. It is possible that Leigh's disease is secondary to an inborn error in thiamine metabolism. (See also Section 8.)

Onset is usually in infancy; it may be subacute, with vomiting, weight loss, weakness, seizures and stupor, or the course may be more chronic, with developmental arrest, loss of vision and dementia. Nystagmus and extraocular palsies are common. Both spastic weakness due to upper motor neuron degeneration and flaccidity due to spinal cord and peripheral nerve involvement are seen. Irregular respirations, periodic hyperventilation and sudden apnea are late manifestations. The course often is one of repeated exacerbations and remissions, a feature which may be of aid in differentiation from other cerebral degenerations of infancy. Death may occur within a few weeks of onset, or the child may survive many years. Therapy with massive doses of thiamine has been advocated, but results are inconclusive.

KINKY HAIR DISEASE. *Menkes' syndrome* is a sex-linked recessive abnormality in copper metabolism in which severe cerebral degeneration and arterial changes lead to death in infancy.

Pathologic changes include widespread cerebral degeneration with loss of cerebral cortical neurons; gliosis and cysts replace the most severely damaged areas. Extensive vascular changes include fragmentation of the elastica and intimal thickening. The basic defect appears to be in the intestinal absorption of copper, leading to profound copper deficiency. (See Section 8.)

Inadequate gain in weight and hypothermia are manifest from birth, and there appears to be an unusual susceptibility to sepsis. The scalp hair initially is normal, but it rapidly becomes sparse and brittle. Microscopically the shaft has a twisted appearance (pili torti). Seborrheic dermatitis is common. Profound developmental retardation becomes evident within the first few months of life and may be accompanied by myoclonic seizures. Most of the reported infants have died within the first year.

Laboratory studies are necessary for definitive diagnosis. Radiographs of long bones show changes that resemble those of scurvy. Serum copper and ceruloplasmin values are low. Parenteral copper therapy is indicated, but it is unlikely to prevent cerebral damage unless instituted in early infancy.

SUBACUTE SCLEROSING PANENCEPHALITIS (SSPE). This disease, though of viral etiology, is included among the cerebral degenerative disorders because of its chronic course and absence of clinical evidences of infection. The incidence varies from 1 to 4 per million in different geographic areas; a high incidence has been found in the southeastern United States.

Pathologic changes in brain include perivascular lymphocytic infiltrates, intranuclear viral inclusions in neurons and glial cells, widespread loss of cortical neurons and gliosis. A measles-like virus has been grown from cerebral tissue. It is thought that the disease is secondary to measles virus which gains entrance into the brain during acute measles infection and becomes adapted to chronic intracellular propagation in the nervous system. Cerebral degeneration becomes apparent at an average of 7 years after primary measles infection.

Clinical manifestations appear between ages 2 and 21 years, with peak incidence between 8 and 14 years. The first manifestations are those of progressive decline in higher cerebral functions, especially school failure, subtle personality changes and emotional lability. Generalized myoclonic jerks, recurring at regular intervals of several seconds, are characteristic. Barely noticeable at first, they eventually become so severe that ambulation is hampered. Grand mal seizures also may occur. In the late stages the child becomes demented and is bedridden, with generalized rigidity.

Changes in the cerebrospinal fluid include elevated gamma globulin values, a first zone colloidal gold curve, and a measurable measles antibody titer. CSF protein concentration and cell count are often normal. Measles antibody titer in serum is usually above 1:128 by the complement fixation method. The electroencephalographic pattern is fairly characteristic, consisting of regularly repeated bursts of generalized high voltage slow wave complexes.

Therapeutic trials with a number of antiviral agents have not produced convincing results. The disease is almost always fatal, usually within two years of onset, but rare instances of prolonged spontaneous remission have been reported.

Blackwood, W., Buxton, P. H., Cummings, J. N., et al.: Diffuse cerebral degeneration of infancy (Alper's disease) Arch. Dis. Child. *38*:193, 1963.

Danks, D. M., et al.: Menkes' kinky hair syndrome. An inherited defect in copper absorption with widespread effects. Pediatrics *50*:188, 1972.

Detels, R., et al.: Further epidemiologic studies of subacute sclerosing panencephalitis. Lancet *2*:11, 1973.

Katz, M., et al.: Subacute sclerosing panencephalitis: Isolation of a virus encephalitogenic for ferrets. J. Infect. Dis. *121*:188, 1970.

Pincus, J. H.: Subacute necrotizing encephalomyelopathy (Leigh's disease): A consideration of clinical features and etiology. Dev. Med. Child. Neurol. *14*:87, 1972.

Sever, J. L., and Zeman, W. (eds.): Measles virus and subacute sclerosing panencephalitis. Neurology *18* (pt. 2): 1, 1968.

DEGENERATIVE DISORDERS OF CEREBRAL WHITE MATTER

In most of these diseases there is faulty formation or excessive breakdown of myelin. Myelin, one of the major components of cerebral white matter, consists of proteolipid membranes that are wrapped around axons in concentric layers. Myelination markedly increases the speed and efficiency of conduction of nerve impulses; it is essential for normal function of the mammalian nerve system. In the human, myelination of the axons in subcortical white matter is largely a postnatal event; maximal formation occurs within the first year of life. Diseases in which there is faulty formation of central myelin therefore tend to have their onset during infancy; they present clinically as arrest of normal motor development, or as progressive disturbance of gait, weakness, spasticity and ataxia.

Two groups of cerebral white matter degenerations have been distinguished. In one, characterized as the *leukodystrophies,* there are enzymatic defects in myelin lipid metabolism, which lead to excessive tissue deposition of a normal component of myelin lipids or of breakdown products of myelin. The clinical disorders include *metachromatic leukodystrophy* and *Krabbe's disease.* The second group, known as the *demyelinating diseases,* result from the degeneration of previously normal myelin, which is caused by an unknown exogenous factor. *Multiple sclerosis, neuromyelitis optica,* and *Schilder's disease* belong in this group.

The Leukodystrophies

METACHROMATIC LEUKODYSTROPHY. *Sulfatide lipidosis* is the most common of the white matter degenerations in childhood. It is transmitted on an autosomal recessive basis.

The basic defect in metachromatic leukodystrophy is deficiency of the enzyme aryl sulfatase A in brain and other tissues. This enzyme normally splits the sulfate group from ceramide-galactose-sulfate or sulfatide, a normal component of the myelin lipids. Large amounts of sulfatide accumulate in the white matter and can be identified on light microscopy by the metachromatic (reddish brown) staining with toluidine blue. Similar deposits are found in peripheral nerves. There is diffuse demyelination of white matter tracts throughout the nervous system, most extensive in tracts which myelinate late.

Clinical manifestations usually appear at about age 1 year, but onset may be later in childhood. Initially there is a disturbance in gait, and the child may be unable to learn to run or to walk stairs. In the early stage, spasticity of limbs, hyperreflexia and extensor plantar responses are noted. Though most of the tendon reflexes are brisk, the ankle jerks may be diminished or absent, owing to involvement of peripheral nerves. Flaccid weakness and atrophy of distal muscles, especially in the lower extremities, occur when peripheral nerve involvement is severe. Eventually the child becomes bedridden and demented. Death usually occurs prior to the age of 10 years.

Definitive diagnosis depends on demonstration of absent or significantly reduced activity of aryl sulfatase A in one or more body tissues. Renal tubule cells from urinary sediment, white blood cells or cultured fibroblasts are suitable for this analysis. A rapid but inaccurate screening test is the demonstration of metachromatic material in urinary sediment stained with toluidine blue. Dysfunction of the gallbladder, resulting from storage of sulfatide in its wall, can be demonstrated by failure of filling on attempted oral cholecystography. Conduction velocity in peripheral motor and sensory nerves is decreased. The increased concentration of cerebrospinal fluid protein may be of aid in distinguishing leukodystrophy from the much larger group of nonprogressive motor deficits, classified as cerebral palsy. Differentiation is of considerable importance for genetic counseling and for prognostic purposes. Intrauterine diagnosis of metachromatic leukodystrophy is possible by measurement of aryl sulfatase A in cultured cells from the amniotic fluid; the test should be offered to prospective parents who are both known to be carriers of the abnormal gene.

KRABBE'S DISEASE. *Cerebroside lipidosis,* or *globoid leukodystrophy,* is transmitted on an autosomal recessive basis. The pathologic changes in brain consist of diffuse lack of myelin in white matter and of accumulation of peculiar multinucleated giant cells (globoid cells). Chemical study of the white matter discloses an increased ratio of cerebroside (ceramide galactose) to sulfatide (ceramide-galactose-sulfate), but usually there is no absolute increase in the quantity of cerebroside. These changes are thought to be secondary to an inherited defect in cerebroside metabolism, with deficiency of galactocerebrosidase activity.

The illness becomes evident in early infancy with progressive rigidity, hyperreflexia and swallowing difficulties, and with failure of normal motor and intellectual development. Peripheral nerve involvement may lead to hypotonia; death usually occurs within 2 years. The diagnosis is established by assay of galactocerebrosidase in peripheral white blood cells. Spinal fluid protein is elevated, and peripheral nerve conduction velocity is slowed. The parents of a child with proved Krabbe's disease should be advised that there is a 25 per cent chance that any subsequently born child will be affected. Intrauterine diagnosis is possible by enzymatic assay of cultured amniotic fluid cells.

Several other forms of leukodystrophy are as yet incompletely defined and usually are diagnosable only by postmortem examination of the brain.

Canavan's Disease (Spongy Degeneration of the Cerebral White Matter). This is transmitted on an autosomal recessive basis. The characteristic pathologic change is diffuse vacuolization of the brain in the deep cortical layers and in subcortical white matter, apparently secondary to excessive accumulation of water in glial cells and in myelin. Clinical manifestations appear in early infancy with poor head control, blindness, optic atrophy, rigidity, hyperreflexia and progressive macrocephaly. The last may suggest the diagnosis of hydrocephalus or of subdural effusion. The ventricular system, however, is normal in size or only mildly dilated. Death occurs within 5 years.

The Sudanophilic Leukodystrophies. These derive their name from the accumulation in white matter of breakdown products of myelin, especially neutral fats, which stain positively with Sudan stains. Included in this group is *Pelizaeus-Merzbacher disease,* which is transmitted by sex-linked recessive inheritance. The onset is in infancy, with nystagmus and head nodding, followed by progressive ataxia, spasticity and choreoathetosis. Progression is slow, with survival into adulthood. Clinical differentiation from cerebral palsy may be difficult. *Sudanophilic leukodystrophy with adrenal insufficiency* has been described; it is also transmitted on a sex-linked recessive basis. Onset is toward the end of the first decade, with progressive spasticity and dementia. Increased pigmentation of skin and other evidences of Addison's disease develop after onset of the neurologic disorder.

Austin, J.: Studies in globoid (Krabbe) leukodystrophy. Arch. Neurol. *9*:207, 1963.

Austin, J., et al.: Metachromatic leukodystrophy. Arch. Neurol. *18*:225, 1968.

Banker, B. Q., Robertson, J. T., and Victor, M.: Spongy degeneration of the central nervous system in infancy. Neurology *14*:981, 1964.

Hoefnagel, D., et al.: Addison's disease and diffuse cerebral sclerosis. J. Neurol. Neurosurg. Psychiat. *30*:56, 1967.

Leroy, J. G., et al.: Infantile metachromatic leukodystrophy. Confirmation of a prenatal diagnosis. New Engl. J. Med. *288*:1365, 1973.

Norman, R. M., et al.: Pelizaeus-Merzbacher disease: A form of sudanophil leucodystrophy. J. Neurol. Neurosurg. Psychiat. *29*:521, 1966.

Percy, A. K., and Brady, R. O.: Metachromatic leukodystrophy: Diagnosis with sample of venous blood. Science *161*:594, 1968.

Suzuki, Y., and Suzuki, K.: Krabbe's globoid cell leukodystrophy: Deficiency of galactocerebrosidase in serum, leukocytes, and fibroblasts. Science *171*:73, 1971.

The Demyelinating Diseases

These illnesses, which include Schilder's disease, multiple sclerosis and neuromyelitis optica, occur sporadically without known genetic factors. It is not clear whether they are separate entities or different manifestations of the same pathologic process. Transitional forms have been described. In all three there is breakdown of myelin in the central nervous system without involvement of the myelin of the peripheral nerves. A perivascular lymphocytic inflammatory reaction is present in the areas of demyelination, suggesting the possibility of an autoimmune disorder or of a viral infection; definite evidence for either possibility is lacking.

SCHILDER'S DISEASE. *Diffuse sclerosis* may occur at any age but is most common in late childhood. A positive diagnosis usually is possible only at autopsy; there is diffuse demyelination of the central white matter with relative sparing of subcortical U fibers. Lipid breakdown products of myelin accumulate in the areas of demyelination. The pathologic picture resembles that of the sudanophilic leukodystrophies, except for the presence of perivascular lymphocytic infiltrates. The neurologic findings are extremely varied. Cortical blindness, optic neuritis, spastic hemiplegia, paraparesis, cortical deafness, aphasia and seizures have been described in the early phase. Late manifestations include dementia and coma. Occasionally there are signs of increased intracranial pressure, with papilledema secondary to cerebral swelling. The course may be acute and death may occur within a few weeks of onset, or the illness may be protracted over several months or years. Rarely, there is partial remission or a relapsing course. The cerebrospinal fluid may be normal, or there may be an increase in protein and lymphocytes. The differential diagnosis includes brain tumor, viral encephalitis, subacute sclerosing panencephalitis (SSPE) and the leukodystrophies.

MULTIPLE SCLEROSIS. *Disseminated sclerosis* is a chronic cerebral disorder characterized by remissions and exacerbations and by multifocal lesions. The disease is uncommon in childhood; in about 1 per cent of cases the onset is before age 15 years. The pathologic changes in the brain consist of scattered foci of demyelination in cerebral white matter, often in a perivenous distribution with associated perivascular lymphocytic infiltrates. The lesions may occur in brain stem and spinal cord as well as in the central white matter.

Cerebellar ataxia is the most common presenting sign in childhood or adolescence, followed by spastic weakness (which is often asymmetric), optic neuritis and diplopia. The optic neuritis tends to be retrobulbar in type. There is loss of vision without at first any funduscopic changes. Temporal pallor of the optic discs indicative of optic atrophy develops over subsequent weeks or months. The onset may be acute or subacute over several weeks. Recovery from acute episodes may initially be complete or nearly so, but after repeated attacks the patient is left with fixed neurologic deficits, often including spastic paralysis and ataxia. Intellectual functions are preserved until late in the course. The clinical diagnosis is based on (1) the presence of multiple neurologic deficits that cannot be due to a single anatomic lesion, and (2) the relapsing course. A definite clinical diagnosis cannot be established at the time of the first attack. The differentiation from hysteria may be difficult initially, especially when there is visual disturbance without objective eye findings. The spinal fluid may be normal, or there may be an increase in gamma globulin which is responsible for a positive first zone colloidal gold curve. A pleocytosis, with up to 100 lymphocytes/mm^3 may occur during acute exacerbations.

Treatment of acute exacerbations of multiple sclerosis with short courses of ACTH has a slight but statistically significant beneficial effect. ACTH gel is given intramuscularly, 40–80 units per day for 2 weeks; the dose is then tapered and discontinued over the subsequent week. Physiotherapy is of help in patients with spastic weakness. Careful bladder care and therapy of urinary tract infections are essential when spinal cord involvement results in bladder dysfunction. The prognosis of multiple sclerosis is guarded but not hopeless. Exacerbations may be infrequent, and there may be symptom-free intervals of many years' duration.

NEUROMYELITIS OPTICA. *Devic's disease* probably is a variant of multiple sclerosis in which demyelination occurs in the optic nerves and in the spinal cord. The only reason for separation from multiple sclerosis is that there may be a single attack without later exacerbations. However, a relapsing course with eventual involvement of other white matter tracts is also possible. The illness starts acutely, usually with eye pain followed by loss of vision, which may affect one or both eyes. Funduscopic examination may reveal swelling and hyperemia of the optic disc, distended retinal veins and peripapillary hemorrhages; in some instances the fundi initially appear normal. The onset of spinal cord involvement is also acute, at times with fever, back pain and nuchal rigidity. It usually follows the visual loss by several days, but may precede it. A level of sensory involvement on the trunk can be demonstrated; it is usually in the thoracic area. Initially the legs are weak, flaccid and areflexic, and the plantar responses are absent or flexor. The bladder is distended. After a few days the involved extremities become spastic and the tendon reflexes become hyperactive, with clonus at the ankles and with a positive Babinski sign.

The spinal fluid may be normal, or there may be pleocytosis; polymorphonuclear cells may be present initially. Myelography may be necessary to rule out acute compression of the spinal cord, especially by spinal epidural abscess. This study is usually normal in neuromyelitis optica, but there may be partial obstruction to movement of the dye at the level of the cord lesion secondary to edema of the spinal cord. Dexamethasone in high doses for a period of 5 to 7 days during the acute illness may be helpful in the prevention of pressure necrosis of the edematous segment of the spinal cord. The prognosis for return of vision is good, but some degree of persistent paraparesis and bladder dysfunction can be expected.

Gall, J. C., Jr., et al.: Multiple sclerosis in children: Clinical study of 40 cases with onset in childhood. Pediatrics *21*:703, 1958.

Kennedy, C., and Carter, S.: Relationships of optic neuritis to multiple sclerosis in children. Pediatrics *28*:377, 1961.

Low, N. L., and Carter, S.: Multiple sclerosis in children. Pediatrics *18*:24, 1956.

Rose, A. S., et al.: Cooperative study in the evaluation of therapy in multiple sclerosis: ACTH vs. placebo – Final report. Neurology *20*:1, 1970.

Salguero, L. F., Itsabashi, H. J., and Gutierrez, N. B.: Childhood multiple sclerosis with psychotic manifestations. J. Neurol. Neurosurg. Psychiat. *32*:572, 1969.

Suzuki, K., and Grover, W. D.: Ultrastructural and biochemical studies of Schilder's disease. J. Neuropath. Exp. Neurol. *29*:392, 1970.

Walsh, F. B.: Neuromyelitis optica. An anatomical-pathological study of one case. Clinical studies of three additional cases. Bull. Johns Hopkins Hosp. *56*:183, 1935.

THE CEREBELLAR AND BASAL GANGLIA DEGENERATIONS

In this category are included a number of illnesses in which spinocerebellar pathways or basal ganglia are selectively involved in a degenerative process. Most of these diseases are genetically determined. In a few, metabolic error has been defined with accumulation of a substance that has differential toxicity for specific functional groups of neurons, but the etiology of the majority is unknown.

The Spinocerebellar Degenerations

FRIEDREICH'S ATAXIA. This is the term applied to a rather heterogeneous group of disorders which have in common onset in late childhood or adolescence of progressive cerebellar and spinal cord dysfunction. Almost certainly one is dealing with more than one distinct illness. As new knowledge has accumulated, several disorders such as ataxia-telangiectasia and the Bassen-Kornzweig syndrome have been clearly separated from Friedreich's ataxia. It is likely that there will be further subdivisions as underlying metabolic disturbances are defined. In most families, so-called Friedreich's ataxia is transmitted on an autosomal recessive basis. A few families with similar abnormalities, but usually somewhat later in onset, have dominant inheritance.

Pathologic changes include degeneration of spinocerebellar, posterior column and corticospinal tracts. In addition, there often are necrosis and degeneration of cardiac muscle fibers.

The clinical history is that of a progressive gait disturbance, followed by incoordination of the upper limbs. Initially, associated skeletal deformities, including a highly arched foot (pes cavus) (Fig. 20–16), hammer toes and scoliosis, may attract more attention than the neurologic disabilities. Occasionally the child presents in cardiac failure, with cardiomegaly and cardiac arrhythmia. Clinical signs of cerebellar disorder include gait ataxia, dysarthria, intention tremor and, less commonly, nystagmus. In addition, patients with Friedreich's ataxia usually have evidence of corticospinal tract dysfunction and of peripheral neuropathy. The former leads to a positive Babinski sign; the latter, to loss of tendon reflexes and to distal weakness and muscle atrophy. The combination of ataxia, Babinski sign and absent ankle jerks is almost pathognomonic of the disease. Sensory loss occurs especially in the feet, with position and vibration senses most severely affected.

Several related syndromes are recognized which cannot be clearly separated from Friedreich's ataxia. Hyperreflexia and spasticity, rather than areflexia and muscle atrophy, are seen in some families. Some patients have onset of areflexic ataxia and pes cavus in infancy, with very slow progression; this is consistent with a normal life span. This condition, known as the *Roussy-Lévy syndrome,* is transmitted on a dominant basis.

The diagnosis is almost totally dependent on the

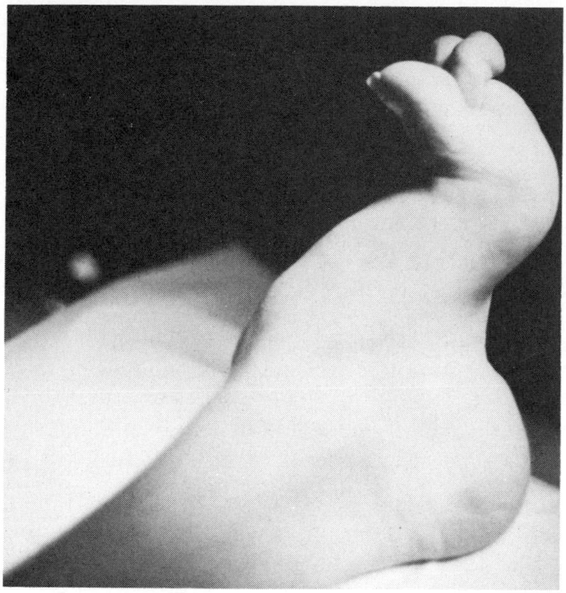

Figure 20–16 *Pes cavus in a 12 year old child with Friedreich's ataxia.*

clinical findings. Laboratory examinations are negative, except for electrocardiographic changes suggestive of myocarditis and, in some instances, slowing of peripheral nerve conduction velocity owing to peripheral neuropathy. There is no effective treatment. Extensive orthopedic surgical procedures, especially those requiring prolonged confinement to bed, should be avoided. The disease tends to be relentlessly progressive; the gait ataxia usually precludes independent walking by early adult years. Death in childhood is almost always secondary to myocardial failure.

ATAXIA-TELANGIECTASIA. This is a complex disorder in which a specific immunologic dysfunction is associated with progressive cerebellar degeneration, telangiectasis of bulbar conjunctiva and skin, and an increased likelihood of malignancy. The disease is transmitted on an autosomal recessive basis. Affected children have immunologic deficits, including a decrease in delayed hypersensitivity, which suggests early thymic dysfunction. It is unknown whether there is any causal relationship between the immunologic disorder and the cerebellar degeneration. Pathologic changes in the nervous system tend to be limited to degeneration in the cerebellum and in the spinocerebellar tracts.

Clinical manifestations may be subdivided into those caused by central nervous system dysfunction, skin changes and immunologic disorders. The neurologic manifestations usually begin in infancy. Affected children learn to walk late and their gait is always ataxic. Late in childhood there is progressive dysarthria, nystagmus, intention tremor and choreoathetosis. The tendon reflexes are diminished or absent. A peculiar abnormality of the eye movements is characteristic, the child being unable to move the eyes on command, while involuntary movements are retained. The skin changes, usually evident by age 5 years, consist of telangiectasias over the bulbar conjunctiva (Fig. 20–17), along the nasolabial folds, over the external ears and along flexor creases of the extremities. Clinical evidences of immunologic deficiency are variable. Some of the children have severe recurrent sinus, ear and pulmonary infections from early childhood, but some never suffer from increased susceptibility to infection. Tonsillar tissue is diminished or absent, and there usually are no palpable lymph nodes. The illness runs a slowly progressive course. The neurologic deficits often lead to scoliosis in late childhood, and by early adolescence independent ambulation becomes impossible. Mild dementia is seen during the late stages of the illness. Death usually occurs in adolescence or in early adulthood as a result of pulmonary failure, infection or malignancy. The incidence of several tumors, especially lymphomas and brain tumors, is increased.

Laboratory findings include, in varying combinations, a decrease or absence of serum IgA and IgE proteins, a decrease in the number of small circulating lymphocytes, and decrease or absence of delayed hypersensitivity reactions to intradermal injection of mumps or candida antigens. The skin sensitization reaction to dinitrochlorobenzene is usually absent. These tests are helpful in the differential diagnosis from Friedreich's ataxia and from the ataxic form of cerebral palsy, which are easily confused with ataxia-telangiectasia during the early stages. The neurologic manifestations of these illnesses usually differ sufficiently to aid in the differentiation. A positive Babinski sign is present in Friedreich's ataxia, but not in ataxia-telangiectasia. Friedreich's ataxia tends to be of later onset and the eye movement abnormalities seen in ataxia-telangiectasia are absent.

Therapy is limited to the prompt treatment of the associated infections; replacement therapy with gamma globulin does not appear to be helpful. The parents should be informed of the 25 per cent recurrence risk in subsequently born children.

ABETALIPOPROTEINEMIA (ACANTHOCYTOSIS: THE BASSEN-KORNZWEIG SYNDROME). This is a rare, recessively inherited disease in which malabsorption of fat and abetalipoproteinemia are associated

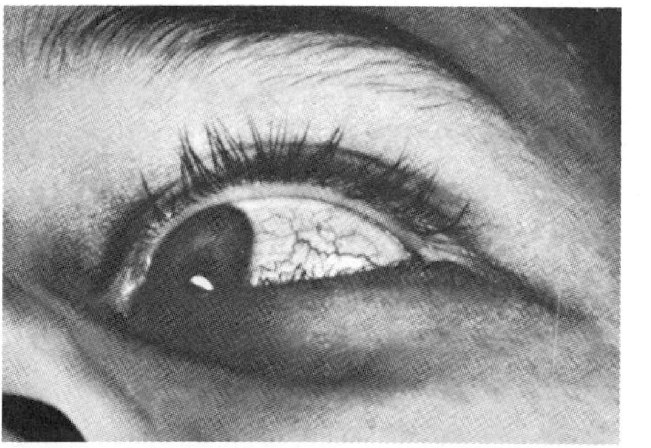

Figure 20–17 *Ataxia-telangiectasia. Arterial telangiectasis on bulbar conjunctiva.*

with progressive cerebellar ataxia and pigmentary degeneration of the retina. The onset is in infancy with the manifestations of intestinal malabsorption. Ataxia, which is slowly progressive, appears later in childhood; the retinal degeneration becomes evident during adolescence. The clinical pattern may resemble that of Friedreich's ataxia, including the Babinski sign, distal sensory loss, areflexia, scoliosis and pes cavus.

Low density lipoproteins are absent or markedly reduced in serum, and carotene, vitamin A and cholesterol values are also low, the last below 60 mg/dl. Lipid droplets (triglycerides) can be seen in the intestinal mucosa obtained by peroral biopsy. The red blood cells have multiple spiny projections, a feature which accounts for the term acanthocytosis as well as for the low sedimentation rate. As yet it is unknown whether the defect in the synthesis of low density lipoproteins is the basic abnormality. Therapy at present is limited to supplementary administration of the fat-soluble vitamins, including A, D and E.

REFSUM SYNDROME. Refsum syndrome is another rare form of hereditary ataxia which deserves mention because it has a known metabolic basis and an effective therapy. The onset is late in childhood or adolescence, with progressive cerebellar ataxia, distal weakness and sensory loss due to polyneuritis, retinitis pigmentosa, deafness and ichthyosis. The metabolic abnormality consists of inability to oxidize phytanic acid (3,7,11,15 tetramethylhexadecanoic acid), which accumulates in serum and in body tissues. The cerebrospinal fluid protein is elevated. Therapy with a diet low in foods containing phytanic acid, i.e., exclusion of all green vegetables, has resulted in improvement in the neurologic deficit.

MYOCLONIC ENCEPHALOPATHY OF CHILDHOOD. Kinsbourne syndrome is a rare neurologic disorder of unknown etiology which has its onset between ages 1 to 3 years. It is characterized by irregular, rapid jerking movements of limbs and trunk (myoclonus) and by similar chaotic, irregular jerking of the eyes (opsoclonus). In addition there is gait ataxia, intention tremor and nystagmus. Several recorded cases have had associated occult *neuroblastoma,* and removal of the tumor has resulted in striking improvement in the neurologic state. In children without tumor and in those with inoperable neoplasms, therapy with ACTH may induce remissions.

Boder, E., and Sedgwick, R. P.: Ataxia-telangiectasia: Familial syndrome of progressive cerebellar ataxia, oculocutaneous telangiectasia, and frequent pulmonary infection. Pediatrics *21*:526, 1958.

Boyer, S. H., Chisolm, A. W., and McKusick, V. A.: Cardiac aspects of Friedreich's ataxia. Circulation *25*:493, 1962.

Critchley, E. M. R.: The genetic basis of hereditary ataxias. J. Roy. Coll. Physicians Lond. *4*:88, 1969.

Farquhar, J. W., and Ways, P.: Abetalipo-proteinemia. *In* Stanbury, J. B., Wyngaarden, J. B., and Frederickson, D. S. (eds.): The Metabolic Basis of Inherited Disease. New York, McGraw-Hill Book Co., 1966.

Greenfield, J. C.: The Spino-Cerebellar Degenerations. Springfield, Ill., Charles C Thomas, 1954.

Herndon, J. H., Jr., Steinberg, D., and Uhlendorf, B. W.: Refsum's disease: Defective oxidation of phytanic acid in tissue cultures derived from homozygotes and heterozygotes. New Engl. J. Med. *281*:1034, 1969.

Kinsbourne, M.: Myoclonic encephalopathy of infants. J. Neurol. Neurosurg. Psychiat. *25*:271, 1962.

McFarlin, D. E., Strober, W., and Waldman, T. A.: Ataxia-telangiectasia. Medicine *51*:281, 1972.

Moe, P. G., and Nellhaus, G.: Infantile polymyoclonus-opsoclonus syndrome and neural crest tumors. Neurology *20*:756, 1970.

Degenerations of the Basal Ganglia

WILSON'S DISEASE. Hepatolenticular degeneration is a recessively inherited disorder of copper metabolism which leads to injury of liver and of basal ganglia. Pathologic changes in the brain include cavitation, gliosis and neuronal degeneration in basal ganglia, which is most severe in the putamen. Similar changes may occur in the cerebral cortex, especially in frontal lobes. The pathogenesis of Wilson's disease is not completely understood. A defect in the synthesis of the copper-carrying protein, ceruloplasmin, explains many of the findings. Decreased protein binding of serum copper appears to lead to increased leakage of copper into the tissues. Copper poisoning is a plausible explanation for the hepatic, basal ganglia and renal tubular damage. See also Sections 8 and 11.

Clinical Manifestations. The onset may be manifest by subacute or chronic hepatic failure in early childhood. Neurologic abnormalities generally do not appear until later in childhood or adolescence; they may precede or follow clinical evidence of liver disease. The diagnosis of Wilson's disease should be considered in any child past 8 years of age who develops a motor disorder or unexplained mental changes. A peculiar flapping tremor of the shoulders and wrists (wing-beating tremor) is characteristic but is not always present. Instead there may be dysarthria, choreoathetoid movements or rigidity. Dysfunction of the bulbar musculature tends to occur early and leads to an immobile grinning facial expression, drooling and dysarthria. Rarely, there is spasticity, hemiparesis or a positive Babinski sign. It is important to remember that Wilson's disease may present with mental changes in the absence of any other neurologic changes. Emotional lability, progressive school failure and frank psychotic states may occur. The most important physical finding is the Kayser-Fleischer ring of the cornea, a greenish yellow rim near the limbus, often most evident superiorly and inferiorly. It is due to deposition of copper in Descemet's membrane and is seen only in Wilson's disease and in exogenous copper poisoning. It is usually visible, but, if not, it should be searched for by slit lamp examination.

Laboratory Data. The diagnosis is confirmed by determination of ceruloplasmin (the copper-carrying protein) in blood and by measurement of urinary copper excretion. A serum ceruloplasmin value less than 50 per cent of normal suggests the diagnosis, but a normal value does not rule it out. Urine copper values are usually above 200 μg/24 hr, as they may also be in hepatic cirrhosis from other causes. Excretion increases following administration of penicillamine; this is a helpful diagnostic test in doubtful cases. Serum copper concentrations tend to be lower than normal, owing to a decrease in the fraction bound to ceruloplasmin. Other laboratory findings include generalized aminoaciduria, low serum concentration of uric acid, and glycosuria; all result from renal tubular damage. In addition, there usually is chemical evidence of liver disease.

Prognosis. The prognosis of untreated Wilson's disease is poor, with a fatal outcome usually within 5 years after onset. Early treatment, directed at removal of excessive copper stores from tissues, has greatly improved the outlook.

Therapy. Various chelating agents have been used, but penicillamine, at a dosage of 1 to 2 gm per day by mouth, is most effective. Allergic reactions, including fever, rash and leukopenia, unfortunately are common. Penicillamine is a pyridoxine antimetabolite, and supplemental pyridoxine should be given during long-term therapy. A diet low in copper is a valuable adjunct to penicillamine therapy. Foods to be avoided include liver, shellfish, nuts and chocolate.

DYSTONIA MUSCULORUM DEFORMANS (TORSION DYSTONIA). Dystonia occurs in a number of static and progressive brain diseases. The static disorders are perinatal brain injuries and postencephalitic syndromes; the progressive ones include Wilson's disease, Huntington's chorea and several other rare degenerative brain disorders. In addition to these diseases, there is a clinical entity characterized by dystonia as an isolated, genetically determined abnormality.

The term *dystonia musculorum deformans* is applied to this disorder. Inheritance may be on a dominant or a recessive basis, the latter especially among East European (Ashkenazi) Jews. The pathogenesis of torsion dystonia is obscure, and there are no consistent pathologic lesions in the brain. A biochemical rather than a structural lesion of the basal ganglia appears to be responsible. Torsion dystonia has its onset during childhood or early adolescence in the recessive group, usually somewhat later in families with dominant inheritance. Progression tends to be rapid, with grotesque distortion of limbs (Fig. 20–18) and incapacitation within a few years of onset. Intelligence is preserved, and there is no evidence of disorder of the pyramidal motor system. Wilson's disease should be ruled out by appropriate laboratory tests. There are no other helpful laboratory studies. A few patients with dystonia musculorum deformans have responded to therapy with L-dopa; haloperidol has occasionally been helpful. Stereotactic thalamotomy produces dramatic but often transient improvement.

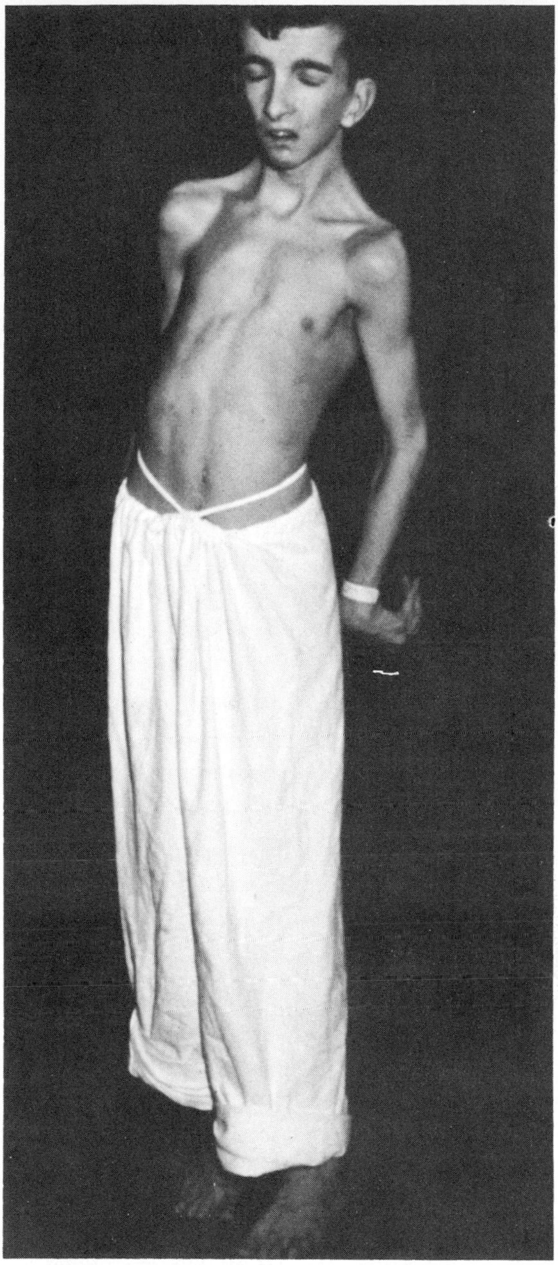

Figure 20–18 Hyperextension of back and abnormal posture of limbs in a patient with dystonia.

HUNTINGTON'S CHOREA. Huntington's chorea is a dominantly inherited degeneration of the basal ganglia, especially of the caudate nucleus, manifest clinically by dementia, irregular dancing gait and choreiform movements. Onset usually is in middle age. The disease, however, may begin in childhood with learning disorders, seizures and rigidity, or with chorea. In the latter instance, it must be differentiated from Sydenham's chorea and from Wilson's disease. In addition, there is a syndrome of dominantly inherited *benign chorea* which does not lead to dementia or to marked incapacitation. The diagnosis of Huntington's chorea in childhood usually is possible only if a parent has the fully developed disease. L-Dopa may cause chorea in an asymptomatic person who is a carrier of the gene for Huntington's chorea; this test has been used as an aid in early diagnosis. At present, there is no effective therapy. Genetic counseling is important, since any offspring of an affected person has a 50 per cent chance of developing this tragic disorder.

Byers, R. K., and Dodge, J. A.: Huntington's chorea in children. Neurology *17*:587, 1967.

Denny-Brown, D.: Hepatolenticular degeneration (Wilson's disease). New Engl. J. Med. *270*:1149, 1964.

Eldridge, R. (ed.): The torsion dystonias (dystonia musculorum deformans). Neurology *20* (part 2), 1970.

Goldstein, N. P., et al.: Wilson's disease (hepato-lenticular degeneration). Treatment with penicillamine and changes in hepatic trapping of radioactive copper. Arch. Neurol. *24*:391, 1971.

Klawans, H. L., Paulson, G. W., Ringel, S. P., and Barbeau, A.: Use of L-dopa in the detection of presymptomatic Huntington's chorea. New Engl. J. Med. *286*:1332, 1972.

Markham, C. H., and Knox, J. W.: Observations on Huntington's chorea in childhood. J. Pediatr. *67*:46, 1965.

Oliver, J., and Dewhirst, K.: Childhood and adolescent forms of Huntington's chorea. J. Neurol. Neurosurg. Psychiat. *32*:455, 1969.

O'Reilly, S.: Problems in Wilson's disease. Neurology *17*:137, 1967.

Pincus, J. H., and Chutorian, A.: Familial benign chorea with intention tremor: A clinical entity. J. Pediatr. *70*:724, 1967.

Sternlieb, I., and Scheinberg, I. H.: Prevention of Wilson's disease in asymptomatic patients. New Engl. J. Med. *278*:352, 1968.

Tu, J., et al.: DL-Penicillamine as a cause of optic axial neuritis. J.A.M.A. *185*:83, 1963.

Walshe, J. M.: The physiology of copper in man and its relation to Wilson's disease. Brain *90*:149, 1967.

NEOPLASMS OF THE BRAIN

GENERAL CONSIDERATIONS. Next to the leukemias, brain tumors are the commonest type of neoplasm in children. Incidence is highest during the second half of the first decade, but they may occur at any age, including early infancy. The incidence of the various cerebral neoplasms and their location differ greatly from those observed in the adult. Tumors of the cerebellum are most common and account for about 40 per cent of the total. Tumors in other posterior fossa structures, including the brain stem and the 4th ventricle, make up about 15 per cent. Suprasellar lesions, which include craniopharyngiomas, optic pathway gliomas and gliomas of the hypothalamus, also are relatively common and account for another 15 per cent. Tumors of the cerebral hemisphere, the ventricles and the meninges account for the remainder. In about 80 per cent of neoplasms in children, the basic cell is glial in origin. The remainder are craniopharyngiomas, teratomas, hemangiomas, sarcomas and meningiomas. Metastatic tumors to the brain are rare in childhood.

Most brain tumors occur sporadically and are of unknown cause. Several of the early childhood tumors, including teratomas and craniopharyngiomas, result from congenital malformations. An increased incidence of certain intracranial neoplasms is seen in the neurocutaneous syndromes. Irradiation of the brain increases the incidence of cerebral sarcomas.

CLINICAL MANIFESTATIONS. The clinical manifestations in childhood are largely those of increased intracranial pressure, because the majority of the tumors are in the posterior fossa and midline structures where a mass lesion will lead to early obstruction to CSF circulation. An important exception is the brain stem glioma which, although in a midline location, rarely leads to increased intracranial pressure.

The manifestations of increased intracranial pressure vary somewhat with age. In infancy there is abnormal enlargement of the head. Brain tumor should always be considered in the differential diagnosis of hydrocephalus. Later in childhood marked expansion of the skull is no longer possible, and the increased intracranial pressure produces symptoms by compression of brain, meninges and cerebral vessels. Headache is a common early symptom, characteristically occurring shortly after the child arises from bed, or following changes in head position at other times of day. As pressure rises, headache becomes more severe and prolonged, but it is rarely continuous. The site of the pain has some localizing value. It tends to be suboccipital with posterior fossa tumors and may be lateralized to the side of the lesion in tumors of the cerebral hemisphere. Vomiting is common. It becomes projectile eventually and is characteristically unaccompanied by nausea. It is due to compression of the medulla and is therefore most severe in tumors of the posterior fossa. Drowsiness and stupor are rather late signs, and are most likely secondary to pressure on the midbrain. Compression of vagal nuclei in the medulla leads to slowing of the pulse. Blood pressure is frequently elevated. Papilledema is almost always present, but is less likely in early infancy. Several intracranial structures are especially susceptible to damage by increased intracranial pressure. Sixth nerve palsies are common and lead to blurring of vision and to diplopia; damage to optic nerves causes diminished visual acuity and may result in total blindness in longstanding cases. Important shifts of brain substance may also occur: inferior portions of cerebellum, i.e., the inferior vermis and the cerebellar tonsils, may herniate downward through the foramen magnum, producing the syndrome of tonsillar herniation. This is especially apt to occur with posterior fossa tumors. It is manifested by neck stiffness and often by a head tilt toward the side of herniation. Respirations become irregular and may suddenly cease, owing to compromise of the respiratory centers in the medulla. Forceful neck flexion must be carefully avoided, since it may lead to further compression of the medulla and sudden respiratory arrest. Supratentorial lesions, especially the laterally located ones, may lead to tentorial herniation.

The diagnostic study and management of brain tumor presents many special problems which fall outside the scope of pediatrics. However, the pediatrician needs to be thoroughly familiar with the presenting symptoms and signs, since he is likely to be the first to evaluate the child. The differential diagnosis includes a number of common and benign syndromes, even school phobia. The pediatrician also has an important role in the pre- and postoperative care of children with brain tumors, especially those with tumors in the suprasellar region which may lead to severe disorders of fluid and electrolyte balance. Perhaps most important, he can provide much support and comfort to parents during the course of a very trying illness.

INFRATENTORIAL NEOPLASMS

Four types of neoplasm are commonly found in the posterior fossa. Cerebellar astrocytoma and medulloblastoma are of approximately equal incidence and together account for about 65 per cent of the tumors in this location. Brain stem gliomas account for about 20 per cent and ependymomas of the 4th ventricle for about 10 per cent. Acoustic neuromas and meningiomas in this area are rare in childhood.

CEREBELLAR ASTROCYTOMA. This is usually a cystic tumor that tends to arise near the midline, but often extends into one cerebellar hemisphere. It may occur throughout childhood, but maximum incidence is from 3 to 8 years. Manifestations of increased intracranial pressure occur early and may be the only changes. More commonly, signs of unilateral cerebellar dysfunction are superimposed. These include hypotonia and intention tremor on the side of the lesion and nystagmus which is of greater amplitude when the child attempts to look toward the side of the tumor. Gait ataxia may be present, often with a tendency to veer toward one side. Somnolence occurs eventually, owing to compression of the brain stem. Pressure on vital structures in the brain stem appears to account for peculiar seizure-like states which occur at times and which have been referred to as "cerebellar fits." They are characterized by loss of consciousness with extensor rigidity, neck retraction, dilatation of pupils and respiratory irregularity. Such attacks are cause for immediate investigation.

Early diagnosis is aided by brain scan, which localizes the tumor in the majority of instances. Roentgenograms of the skull may show lateralized thinning and bulging of the occipital bone on the side of the lesion in addition to the nonspecific signs of increased intracranial pressure. Rarely, calcifications are visible in the tumor. Ventriculography or vertebral angiography may be needed to localize the tumor in doubtful cases. Therapy is by surgical excision. Expert surgical management results in close to 90 per cent long-term survivals. Though the majority of these appear to be cures, late recurrence is possible. Radiation therapy is used only for recurrent tumor or when the tumor is not completely resectable.

MEDULLOBLASTOMA. Medulloblastoma is a midline cerebellar tumor which is made up of undifferentiated small round cells. It grows extremely rapidly, has a tendency to seed along the entire cerebrospinal axis, and is one of the few brain tumors that may metastasize to extraneural tissues. The peak incidence is from 3 to 5 years, with boys affected about twice as frequently as girls. It is not possible to differentiate this tumor reliably from cerebellar astrocytoma on the basis of history or clinical examination. However, statistically the tumor is more likely to occur in the younger child, especially in a boy who has a history of rapidly progressive signs of increased intracranial pressure. There often is gait ataxia without any lateralizing signs. Roentgenograms of the skull show evidence of increased intracranial pressure, but no focal abnormalities. The brain scan is often negative. Vertebral angiography and/or ventriculography are usually necessary to localize the tumor.

Therapy consists in surgical excision of accessible tumor followed by focal radiation to the posterior fossa and low dose radiation to the entire neuraxis. After completion of a course of radiation, chemotherapy may be advisable. A simple and well tolerated program consists of alternate weekly intravenous injections of vincristine and Cytoxan; these are continued for 12 to 18 months. The prognosis of medulloblastoma, which is hopeless with surgical therapy alone, is improved somewhat with the use of combined treatment. A 20 to 30 per cent cure rate has been achieved with surgery plus radiation. As yet, it is not known whether the addition of chemotherapy results in a significant increase in cures. In general, the outlook is hopeful if the child has no evidence of recurrence 18 months after his initial surgery.

EPENDYMOMA. Ependymoma in the posterior fossa arises from the ependymal lining of the floor of the 4th ventricle. Upward extension into the ventricle causes early obstruction to CSF flow. The symptoms and signs are those of increased intracranial pressure. Cranial nerve palsies and positive Babinski signs may be present, owing to infiltration of the brain stem. These tumors may calcify and the diagnosis can occasionally be made by visualization of calcification in the area of the 4th ventricle on a lateral roentgenogram of the skull. Surgical excision of accessible tumor often results in transient improvement. Total surgical removal, however, is rarely possible. Postoperatively, radiation therapy is given to the posterior fossa. There are few long-term survivors.

GLIOMA OF THE BRAIN STEM. Pontine glioma has its peak incidence from ages 6 to 8 years. The clinical history and physical findings are almost pathognomonic. They consist of progressive appearance of multiple bilateral cranial nerve palsies, in combination with pyramidal tract signs (hyperreflexia and Babinski sign) and ataxia. Usually there is no evidence of increased intracranial pressure. All the cranial nerves may be affected, with 7th and 6th nerve palsies being most common. The diagnosis is established by pneumoencephalography, which shows a smooth posterior displacement of the 4th ventricle and aqueduct of Sylvius as a result of enlargement of the pons. The diagnosis can usually be made on the basis of the clinical picture in conjunction with pneumoencephalography and vertebral angiography. The tumors cannot be removed surgically, and therapy consists of local radiation. Most of the children die within 18 months of diagnosis, but a few long-term survivors have been reported.

SUPRATENTORIAL NEOPLASMS

CRANIOPHARYNGIOMA. Craniopharyngioma is the most common tumor of the sellar and suprasellar regions in childhood. It is of special pediatric interest, owing to the numerous problems in management associated with hypothalamic and pituitary dysfunctions. The tumor is congenital in origin, arising from squamous epithelial cell rests of the embryonic Rathke pouch. It often has a large cystic component; the growth characteristics are those of a benign neoplasm.

Symptoms may appear at any time during childhood and adolescence and include: (1) growth failure, (2) progressive visual loss, and (3) symptoms of increased intracranial pressure. These may occur singly or in any combination. The diagnosis should be considered whenever there is an arrest of linear growth after a period of normal gain in height. Other endocrine abnormalities are rare initially. Diabetes insipidus occurs *preoperatively* in less than 10 per cent. Puberty is delayed in the older child. The visual impairment classically consists of bitemporal hemianopsia. However, asymmetric field defects, unilateral blindness and bilateral decrease in visual acuity may be manifest. Funduscopic examination reveals optic atrophy or papilledema. Roentgenographs of the skull are of considerable diagnostic aid; calcifications in a supra- or intrasellar location are found in about 80 per cent of the craniopharyngiomas that present during childhood (Fig. 20–19). The sella turcica may be ballooned or distorted. The bone age is often retarded.

The location of the craniopharyngioma makes therapy a formidable problem. Cure by complete surgical removal is possible, but this requires both unusual surgical skill and meticulous postoperative care. Therapy with cortisone acetate is initiated on the day prior to operation, at a dosage of about 40 mg/M^2/day and is continued for at least two weeks postoperatively. Supplementary hydrocortisone is given intravenously during the operation. Postoperatively fluid intake is carefully matched to output; diabetes insipidus occurs almost invariably and must be controlled by replacement therapy. A marked decrease in urine output often occurs on the second or third postoperative day, owing to inappropriate release of antidiuretic hormone. It is essential that fluids are restricted during this period to prevent water intoxication and cerebral edema. Serum electrolytes must also be carefully monitored, and imbalances corrected. Occasionally there is persistent hypernatremia, owing to damage to the hypothalamic thirst regulating mechanism. With expert management a satisfactory result can be achieved in approximately 60 per cent of patients. Aspiration of the tumor cyst, followed by radiation of the tumor has been proposed as an alternate method of therapy, but as yet there is little information on long-term results.

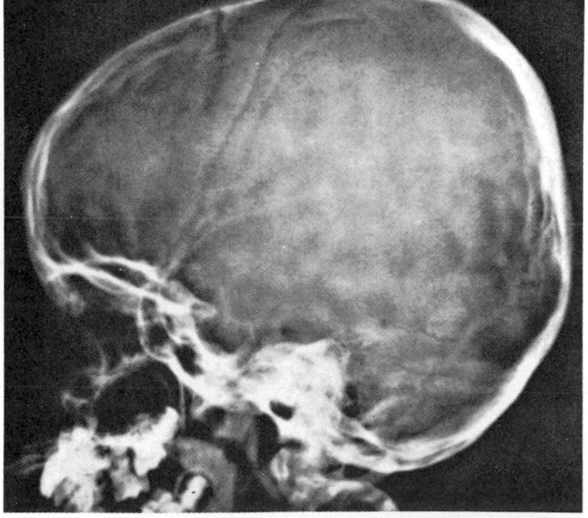

Figure 20–19 Craniopharyngioma in a boy 8 years of age. Note fluffy suprasellar calcification, enlarged sella turcica, digital markings of skull, and early sutural separation.

GLIOMAS OF THE OPTIC PATHWAYS. These occur with increased frequency in patients with neurofibromatosis. They present with unilateral or bilateral visual loss. Extension of the tumor into the orbit may cause proptosis. Evidences of hypothalamic dysfunction and of increased intracranial pressure appear late. A surgical cure can be achieved when the tumor is confined to one optic nerve, but those involving the optic chiasm are inoperable. However, these lesions progress very slowly and survival without treatment may be as long as 20 years. Radiation therapy has been advocated.

HYPOTHALAMIC GLIOMAS. These occur mainly in infants, in whom they produce a very characteristic syndrome of emaciation, *the diencephalic syndrome of infancy.* Tumors of the hypothalamus occurring later in childhood usually present as precocious puberty. These children also tend to be excessively large for age. They may have increased intracranial pressure owing to extension of the tumor into the 3rd ventricle, and visual loss owing to involvement of the optic chiasm. Various types of tumor are seen, including hamartomas, gliomas, ectopic pinealomas and teratomas.

TUMORS OF THE CEREBRAL HEMISPHERES

In childhood tumors of the cerebral hemispheres may be of several histologic types, including astrocytoma, oligodendroglioma, ependymoma, glioblastoma and sarcoma. The symptoms and signs depend on the location and on the growth characteristics of the tumor. Low-grade hemispheral tumors such as astrocytomas or oligodendrogliomas may initially cause convulsions without any other abnormalities. These lesions often become partially calcified, a possibility warranting radiographs of the skull as part of the diagnostic study of a child with seizures. As the tumors enlarge, they tend to produce spastic hemiparesis, hemisensory defects or hemianopsia. Symptoms of increased intracranial pressure appear late. The more malignant tumors, such as the glioblastomas, present with rapidly progressive increase in intracranial pressure and with focal neurologic signs, including hemiparesis, hemianopsia, aphasia and unilateral choreoathetoid movements. Accurate localization is achieved by brain scan, electroencephalography and cerebral angiography. Hemispherical tumors in childhood are rarely curable. However, partial removal of the more benign types may lead to many years of symptom-free life.

NEOPLASMS IN THE PINEAL REGION. These are uncommon in childhood, but they deserve mention in view of their characteristic clinical presentation. They result in early compression of the upper midbrain, which is manifest by paralysis of upward gaze and by pupillary dilatation with diminution in the light reflex *(Parinaud syndrome)*. Hydrocephalus is due to obstruction of the posterior 3rd ventricle and the aqueduct. The lesions cannot be removed surgically, but palliation can be achieved by a shunt operation, which is followed by radiation of the tumor.

Developmental tumors, referred to as *epidermoids, dermoids* and *teratomas,* may occur in the pineal region and elsewhere along the midline. Epidermoids contain only stratified squamous epithelium; dermoids are made up of all skin structures, including hair and sebaceous glands. The teratomas contain mesodermal and endodermal tissues as well. Occasionally the latter may be diagnosable roentgenographically by the visualization of bones or of teeth in the tumor. These developmental tumors may form large cysts filled with sebaceous secretions and desquamated skin. Depending on location, complete surgical removal may be possible.

CHOROID PLEXUS PAPILLOMAS. Papillomas are most common prior to age 3 years. They usually arise from choroid plexus of the lateral ventricle. Focal neurologic signs are rare. Increased production of CSF and obstruction to CSF flow by the tumor mass leads to early hydrocephalus. This tumor needs to be considered in the differential diagnosis of any child with hydrocephalus of obscure etiology. It usually is readily apparent on a pneumoencephalogram or ventriculogram. Complete surgical removal is possible and leads to cure of the associated hydrocephalus.

PSEUDOTUMOR CEREBRI

As the name implies, this condition produces symptoms and signs that mimic those of brain tumor. The increased intracranial pressure is caused by diffuse cerebral edema.

Pseudotumor cerebri may occur as a complication of hypoparathyroidism and of galactosemia. It is occasionally seen during corticosteroid therapy, especially while the dose is being tapered off or after it has been discontinued. It may also follow the administration of tetracycline or high doses of vitamin A. The majority of cases are of obscure etiology; obese adolescent girls are especially apt to acquire this condition.

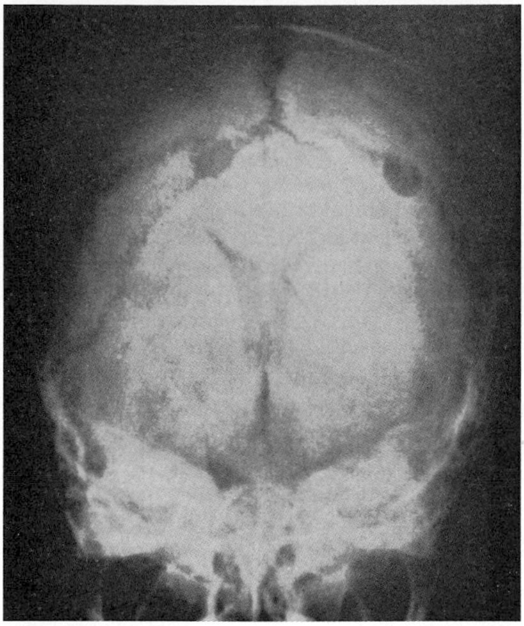

Figure 20–20 *Benign increased intracranial pressure or pseudotumor in a boy 4 years of age. Sutures are separated, but ventricles are small and unshifted. Note trephine openings.*

The clinical presentation is with headache, morning vomiting, papilledema and sometimes a 6th nerve palsy. Somnolence may occur but is rarely marked. Signs of focal neurologic disease are absent. A child with this combination of symptoms and signs usually requires special neuroradiologic studies—either cerebral angiography or ventriculography—to rule out a focal mass lesion. The diagnosis of pseudotumor cerebri should be suspected in a child with increased intracranial pressure in whom these studies fail to show a mass or an enlargement of the ventricular system. The lateral ventricles may be reduced in size due to compression by the edematous brain (Fig. 20–20). The CSF is normal except for a low protein content in some instances.

The elevation in intracranial pressure may persist for several months, but it always subsides eventually. The chief danger is that of damage to optic nerves from chronic compression. No treatment is needed in mild cases. Patients with severe increase in pressure may be helped by repeated removal of CSF via lumbar puncture. Adrenocortical steroid therapy is very effective, but relapse may occur when therapy is discontinued. Weight reduction is indicated when the child is obese.

Banna, M., et al.: Craniopharyngioma in children. J. Pediatr. *83*:781, 1973.

Bray, P. F., Carter, S., and Taveras, J. M.: Brain stem tumors in children. Neurology *8*:1, 1958.

Chutorian, A. M., et al.: Optic gliomas in children. Neurology *14*:83, 1964.

Gareis, F. J., and Johnson, J. A.: Inanition in infants associated with diencephalic neoplasms. Am. J. Dis. Child. *109*:349, 1965.

Greer, M.: Benign intracranial hypertension. Neurology *12*:472, 1962; *14*:469, 1964; and *15*:382, 1965.

Lassman, L. P., et al.: Sensitivity of intracranial gliomas to vincristine sulfate. Lancet *1*:296, 1965.
Lysak, W. R., and Svien, H. J.: Long-term follow-up on patients with diagnosis of pseudotumor cerebri. J. Neurosurg. *25*:284, 1966.
Matson, D. D.: Neurosurgery of Infancy and Childhood. Springfield, Ill., Charles C Thomas, 1969.
Matson, D. D., and Crigler, J. F., Jr.: Radical treatment of craniopharyngioma. Ann. Surg. *152*:699, 1960.
McFarland, D. R., et al.: Medulloblastoma—a review of prognosis and survival. Brit. J. Radiol. *42*:198, 1969.
Rose, A., and Matson, D. D.: Benign intracranial hypertension in children. Pediatrics *39*:227, 1967.
Wilson, Ch. B.: Medulloblastoma. Current views regarding the tumor and its treatment. Oncology *24*:273, 1970.

INTRACRANIAL MASS LESIONS SECONDARY TO INFECTION

Pyogenic infections may lead to abscess formation within the brain or to effusions or purulent exudates in subdural or epidural spaces. In each of these conditions intracranial pressure is increased, owing to a local mass effect. When signs of infection are absent, as they may be, differentiation from brain tumor and from other conditions which cause increased intracranial pressure may be difficult.

BRAIN ABSCESS

Pyogenic abscess of the brain is now seen most commonly in children with cyanotic congenital heart disease. This peculiar susceptibility appears to be directly related to the presence of a right to left shunt which eliminates the normal filtering of venous blood by the capillary bed of the lungs. In addition, the hypoxic brain appears to be an especially good culture medium for the anaerobic bacteria that are usually found in such lesions. Somewhat less than half of brain abscesses in childhood are secondary to infection in other locations. Some occur by intracranial extension of infection from mastoids, paranasal sinuses and skull. This sequence of events was much more common prior to the widespread use of antibiotics. Occasionally brain abscess is metastatic from a lung abscess, empyema or endocarditis. It rarely is a complication of bacterial meningitis or of a penetrating injury to the skull. In a significant number of children there is no history of any major preceding infection. The organisms found in brain abscess include microaerophilic or anaerobic streptococci, *Staphylococcus aureus,* pneumococcus, proteus and *Hemophilus influenzae.*

Clinical evidence of infection may be absent throughout the entire course of the illness. When present, it usually consists of low-grade fever and stiffness of the neck. Focal neurologic signs depend on the location of the abscess. Focal seizures and hemiparesis occur in abscess of the cerebral hemisphere. Temporal lobe abscess, which may complicate mastoiditis, causes aphasia if the dominant side is involved. Cerebellar abscess, also usually secondary to mastoiditis, results in ataxia and nystagmus. Evidence of increase in intracranial pressure is almost always present. Headache, vomiting, irritability and drowsiness may be the presenting symptoms, and papilledema is usually present. The course is usually subacute over a period of weeks. Untreated, the child eventually becomes comatose. Death results from rupture of the abscess with overwhelming meningitis or from tentorial or cerebellar herniation.

Leukocytosis and elevated sedimentation rate may or may not be present. Brain scan and the electroencephalogram are the two most valuable initial laboratory tools. The brain scan is almost always positive; it may show a ring-shaped area of increased uptake of radioactive material corresponding to the capsule of the abscess. In supratentorial abscesses the EEG shows a prominent slow wave focus in the area of the lesion. Cerebral angiography is usually needed to define the extent and location of the abscess. Lumbar puncture is of limited diagnostic help and should be avoided when intracranial pressure is high. The CSF is sterile, unless the abscess has ruptured. The protein content usually is elevated, and white blood cells may be present, with lymphocytes predominating. A roentgenogram of the chest is essential to look for a suppurative lesion of the lungs.

As soon as a tentative diagnosis of brain abscess is made, broad spectrum antibiotic therapy should be initiated. Surgical drainage of the abscess is performed when it is felt to be clearly localized. It may be an emergency procedure in the comatose child with markedly increased intracranial pressure. Excision of the abscess, including its capsule, is advocated by some neurosurgeons. The most common sequel is the occurrence of seizures for which continuous anticonvulsant therapy usually is needed.

SUBDURAL AND EPIDURAL EMPYEMA

Collections of pus in the subdural or epidural spaces have become relatively rare since the introduction of antibiotics. They usually are secondary to frontal sinusitis or to infections of the scalp and skull. The purulent exudate acts as a space-occupying lesion, compressing the underlying brain. In addition, there is thrombophlebitis of the cortical veins that pass through the infected subdural space; interference with venous drainage leads to severe cerebral swelling. The course is subacute, with fever, severe headache, lethargy, convulsions and hemiparesis. Papilledema is present, and there may be rapid progression to coma and to tentorial herniation. The differential diagnosis includes brain abscess and cortical vein thrombosis. Cerebral angiography is needed to establish the diagnosis; it shows an avascular mass overlying one cerebral hemisphere, and shift of the midline cerebral structures to the opposite side. Therapy consists of prompt surgical drainage followed by appropriate antibiotic coverage.

SUBDURAL EFFUSION COMPLICATING MENINGITIS

This disorder is thought to be peculiar to infancy. The peak incidence is at age 4 to 6 months; it is rarely recognized beyond 1 year of age. Subdural effusion may be associated with any of the bacterial meningitides, but occurs most often following *Hemophilus influenzae* meningitis. It seems probable that there are small collections of fluid in the subdural spaces in most persons with meningitis. The great majority of them, however, are insignificant and resorb spontaneously. The incidence of large collections which cause significant increase in intracranial pressure and which require therapy is much smaller, and probably less than has been thought to be the case in recent years.

The pathogenesis of subdural fluid collections after meningitis is incompletely understood. Initially the fluid is an inflammatory exudate. The arachnoid membrane in the infant is a poor barrier to the spread of infection into the subdural space. Subdural fluid obtained early in the course of meningitis often is purulent and bacteria may be grown from it. Several mechanisms appear to act to maintain and enlarge the fluid collection after the infection has been controlled. As the subdural space becomes expanded, there may be rupture of small bridging veins. The occurrence of repeated hemorrhage into the space is suggested by the fact that the fluid frequently is bloody. Transudation of fluid from inflamed capillary vessels may also be important. The protein composition of subdural fluid is that of a transudate of plasma. The formation of large collections of fluid is aided by the distensibility of the skull of the infant. Longstanding effusions lead to the formation of vascular membranes, which become especially well developed along the outer wall of the subdural space. These membranes are friable, and capillary bleeding may occur from their surface.

It is difficult to identify symptoms that are clearly related to the presence of postmeningitic subdural effusions. Convulsions, vomiting, irritability and persistent drowsiness may occur, but are also seen in infants with meningitis that is not complicated by effusion. Physical findings in infants with subdural effusions include persistent fever, a bulging anterior fontanelle and abnormal head enlargement. The most definitive finding is the presence of positive transillumination of the skull. The diagnosis is confirmed by subdural tap, which should be performed on both sides since effusions are bilateral in over two thirds of cases. Treatment is directed toward prevention of large fluid collections, which may damage brain by compression. Repeated subdural taps are indicated in infants with bulging fontanelle or abnormal head enlargement. Taps are repeated every 24 to 48 hours, always bilaterally if fluid collections have been demonstrated on both sides. It is not necessary to tap small collections which are not associated with increased intracranial pressure. Too many taps may actually worsen the problem by causing bleeding into the subdural spaces. Small collections subside spontaneously. If large quantities of high protein or bloody fluid continue to accumulate after two weeks of repeated tapping, the subdural spaces should be surgically drained via bilateral burr holes. Surgical excision of subdural membranes has been advocated but it has not been proved that this improves the outcome.

Farmer, T. W., and Wise, G. R.: Subdural empyema in infants, children and adults. Neurology *23*:254, 1973.

Gitlin, D.: Pathogenesis of subdural collections of fluid. Pediatrics *16*:345, 1955.

Hitchcock, E., and Andreadis, A.: Subdural empyema: A review of 29 cases. J. Neurol. Neurosurg. Psychiat. *27*:422, 1964.

Liske, E., and Weikers, N. J.: Changing aspects of brain abscess. Neurology *14*:294, 1964.

Matson, D. D., and Salam, M.: Brain abscess in congenital heart disease. Pediatrics *27*:772, 1961.

McKay, R. J., Jr., Ingraham, F. D., and Matson, D. D.: Subdural fluid complicating bacterial meningitis. J.A.M.A. *152*:387, 1953.

Raimondi, A. J., Matsumo, S., and Miller, R. A.: Brain abscess in children with congenital heart disease. J. Neurosurg. *23*:588, 1965.

Tefft, M., Matson, D. D., and Neuhauser, E. B. D.: Brain abscess in children. Radiologic methods for early recognition. Am. J. Roentgenol. *98*:675, 1966.

ACUTE TOXIC ENCEPHALOPATHY AND THE REYE SYNDROME

The label "acute toxic encephalopathy" has been applied to a clinical syndrome in which depression in state of consciousness occurs acutely without apparent cause. The history is that of a previously well child who lapses into stupor and coma, often with associated convulsions. The cerebrospinal fluid may be under increased pressure but is otherwise normal.

In 1963 Reye et al. reported the presence of abnormal liver function and pathologic changes in the liver and other visceral organs in a group of children with "acute toxic encephalopathy." Since then, it has been found that hepatic dysfunction occurs in a majority of children who fall within the toxic encephalopathy group. A rather distinct, easily recognizable clinical syndrome has emerged and is referred to as *Reye syndrome.*

PATHOLOGY AND PATHOPHYSIOLOGY. The pathologic changes in Reye syndrome consist of marked fatty infiltration of liver cells in the form of small lipid droplets, and similar but less intense fatty infiltration in the proximal tubules of the kidneys, in myocardium and in other visceral organs. Electronmicroscopy of the liver shows evidence of mitochondrial damage. Inflammatory changes are lacking. The brain is markedly edematous, and there may be widespread neuronal necrosis, often in a distribution suggestive of anoxic damage.

Little is known about the pathogenesis of this syndrome. The pathologic findings suggest the action of a hepatotoxin or of a general cellular poison. However, none has been identified to date. The neurologic dysfunction may be in part secondary to ammonia intoxication, but is not entirely explained by it.

INCIDENCE. This disorder is emerging as one of the more common causes of death in childhood. Small epidemics have occurred at the time of influenza B outbreaks, and a few instances of simultaneous involvement of more than one child in a family have been reported.

CLINICAL MANIFESTATIONS. The clinical history is remarkably constant. The illness may occur at any time during childhood from infancy to adolescence. It almost always follows an acute viral infection. The prodromal illness has been identified as influenza type B in a large proportion of cases, and as chickenpox in a smaller number. The child appears to be recovering from the initial disease, but then has recurrent vomiting which may last for 24 to 48 hours. Toward the end of this period stupor and delirium supervene. The child rapidly lapses into coma, with or without associated convulsions. There are no focal neurologic signs, but there are general hyperreflexia and a positive Babinski sign. Hyperventilation is characteristic. Decerebrate rigidity and dilation of pupils occur in the most severely affected children, as does evidence of increased intracranial pressure, including papilledema. Terminally, signs of tentorial herniation of the brain supervene, with appearance of 3rd nerve palsy, followed by respiratory arrest. Clinical evidence of liver disease is limited to mild hepatomegaly. There is no jaundice. Survivors make a rapid recovery, often within 2 or 3 days. Residual disability is uncommon.

Laboratory findings are largely limited to chemical evidence of hepatic dysfunction. SGOT and LDH are markedly elevated, and the liver-dependent blood clotting factors such as prothrombin are diminished. Serum bilirubin is normal or only mildly elevated. Early in the course blood ammonia is always increased. Hypoglycemia is common in young children. Mild evidence of renal dysfunction, including elevation in blood urea nitrogen and generalized aminoaciduria, occur inconstantly, and respiratory alkalosis is frequently present. The peripheral white blood count may be as high as $40,000/mm^3$, with predominance of granulocytes.

DIFFERENTIAL DIAGNOSIS. The differential diagnosis includes a number of toxic and metabolic disorders, including drug poisoning, especially with salicylates, hypoglycemic encephalopathy, hepatic coma due to acute hepatitis, and acute water intoxication. The possibility of anoxic brain damage secondary to a seizure has to be considered when convulsions occur early in the course. Sudden obstruction to CSF flow by an intraventricular tumor may cause a similar clinical picture, as may the occasional case of encephalitis without spinal fluid pleocytosis. Chemical evidence of hepatic dysfunction, including ammonia intoxication, is of great value for the rapid differentiation of Reye syndrome from most other severe, acute encephalopathies. Acute hepatitis can usually be excluded by the absence of jaundice and by the presence of a palpable liver.

TREATMENT. Therapy consists of supportive measures, including administration of 10 per cent glucose and electrolyte solution by vein. Overhydration has to be carefully avoided, since it may exacerbate cerebral edema. Synthetic corticosteroids such as dexamethasone in high doses and intravenous mannitol or urea, 1 gm/kg, appear to be of value for the treatment of increased intracranial pressure due to cerebral edema. Anticonvulsant drugs are indicated when seizures complicate the illness. Care should be taken not to administer drugs such as acetylsalicylic acid or phenothiazines which may exacerbate the cerebral and hepatic dysfunctions. Strict attention to respiratory status is important. Assisted ventilation is indicated in the severely affected child. Despite use of these measures, there has been a high mortality rate which has varied from 40 to 80 per cent in different series. The prognosis is especially poor in children under age 2 years and when the clinical course is complicated by convulsions. Vigorous treatment for ammonia intoxication either by exchange blood transfusion or by peritoneal dialysis may further improve the chance of survival; the number of children so treated is as yet, however, insufficient for any definite conclusions.

Huttenlocher, P. R.: Reye's syndrome: Relation of outcome to therapy. J. Pediatr. *80*:845, 1972.

Huttenlocher, P. R., Schwartz, A. D., and Klatskin, G.: Reye's syndrome: Ammonia intoxication as a possible factor in the encephalopathy. Pediatrics *43*:443, 1969.

Lyon, G., Dodge, P. R., and Adams, R. D.: The acute encephalopathies of obscure origin in infants and children. Brain *84*:680, 1961.

Partin, J. C., Schubert, W. K., and Partin, J. S.: Mitochondrial ultrastructure in Reye's syndrome (encephalopathy and fatty degeneration of the viscera). New Engl. J. Med. *285*:1339, 1971.

Pross, D. C., Bradford, W. D., and Krueger, R. P.: Reye's syndrome treated with peritoneal dialysis. Pediatrics *45*:845, 1970.

Reye, R. D. C., Morgan, G., and Baral, J. Encephalopathy and fatty degeneration of the viscera. Lancet *2*:749, 1963.

CEREBRAL VASCULAR DISEASES

This group of illnesses is characterized by the precipitous onset of signs and symptoms of neurologic dysfunction. They may be subdivided into two categories: *intracranial hemorrhage* and *vascular occlusion.*

INTRACRANIAL HEMORRHAGE

See also Section 7.

Spontaneous intracranial hemorrhage in childhood usually results from the rupture of a congenital vascular lesion such as an arteriovenous malformation or an arterial aneurysm. Hemorrhage from a vascular malformation or an aneurysm has to be differentiated from intracranial bleeding secondary to blood coagulation defects and from traumatic hemorrhage. Intracranial bleeding occurs occasionally in hemophilia and in idiopathic thrombocytopenia and may be a terminal event in leukemia. Traumatic hemorrhage may be especially difficult to distinguish in the small child for whom a history of overt head trauma may be lacking.

ARTERIOVENOUS MALFORMATIONS. These may occur in any part of the brain; they consist of large arterial feeding vessels, a mass of dilated communicating channels and large draining veins that carry arterialized blood. The larger malformations may produce symptoms in infancy without hemorrhage. This is especially true of malformations involving the posterior cerebral artery and the great vein of Galen; the arteriovenous shunt may be so large as to cause congestive heart failure and polycythemia. Enormous saccular dilatation of the vein of Galen may also lead to hydrocephalus in infancy, owing to obstruction of the aqueduct of Sylvius. The majority of arteriovenous malformations, however, are clinically silent for a number of years, then suddenly cause symptoms as a result of rupture of one of the communicating vessels, leading to subarachnoid and intracerebral hemorrhage.

Sudden severe headache, drowsiness and nuchal rigidity due to subarachnoid hemorrhage and focal neurologic signs from damage of brain tissue at the site of the hemorrhage are the most common presenting signs. Detection of an intracranial bruit is a helpful confirmatory sign, especially after age 4 or 5. When intracranial bleeding is massive, the child rapidly lapses into coma. Funduscopic examination may show retinal and preretinal hemorrhages. Occasionally the history is that of repeated episodes of headache and focal convulsions, which probably represent recurrent minor episodes of bleeding.

The diagnosis is confirmed by the presence of bloody or xanthochromic CSF. Cerebral angiography is essential for determination of the exact location and extent of the lesion (Fig. 20–21). Arteriovenous malformations that are superficially located in the cerebral cortex may be amenable to complete surgical excision. Ligation of feeding arteries alone usually is of limited effectiveness.

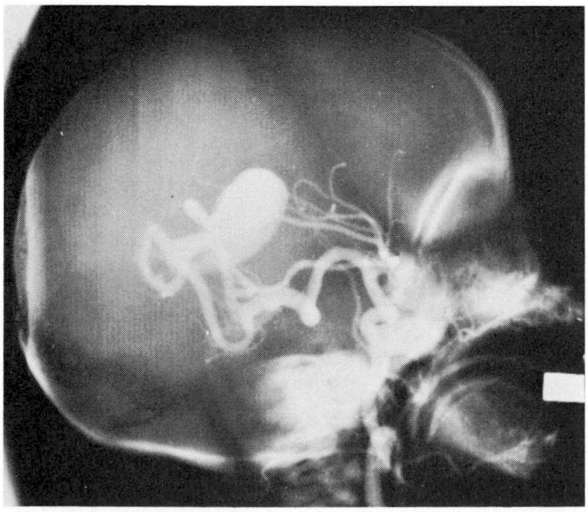

Figure 20–21 Intracranial arteriovenous fistula and aneurysm in a 2 week old infant who presented with cardiac failure. Note the large feeding vessels.

INTRACRANIAL ARTERIAL ANEURYSMS. These aneurysms are usually due to *congenital malformations* in the media of arterial walls at points of bifurcation. The incidence is higher than usual in association with coarctation of the aorta and with polycystic disease of the kidney. The most common sites are the anterior communicating and anterior cerebral arteries, and the terminal branching of the internal carotid artery. Occasionally aneurysms form at sites of damage to cerebral arteries by infection *(mycotic aneurysms).*

Intracranial arterial aneurysms are rarely diagnosed in childhood. Though the defect is almost always a congenital one, it is not apt to be manifest until early adult years. Symptoms of intracranial aneurysms are mainly those of subarachnoid and intracerebral hemorrhage from rupture of the aneurysm. The typical history is that of a previously well child who suddenly develops excruciating headache and then lapses into stupor and coma. Nuchal rigidity and preretinal hemorrhage are evidences of subarachnoid bleeding. Third nerve palsies are common after rupture of an aneurysm of the carotid artery; hemiparesis, with rupture of a middle cerebral artery aneurysm. The cerebrospinal fluid is bloody and xanthochromic and is under increased pressure. Cerebral angiography is needed for definitive diagnosis. Surgical ligation or clipping of the aneurysm is indicated, if this is judged to be possible. The mortality of unoperated ruptured aneurysms is about 50 per cent. Rebleeding may occur up to many years later in survivors.

CEREBRAL VASCULAR OCCLUSIONS

Occlusive cerebral vascular disorders include arterial occlusions, either thrombotic or embolic, and venous occlusions which are due to thrombosis or thrombophlebitis in cerebral veins.

ARTERIAL OCCLUSIONS (ACUTE INFANTILE HEMIPLEGIA). Occlusion of cerebral arteries is uncommon in childhood, but occurs with increased frequency in late infancy, from 1 to 3 years of age. It is due to thrombosis or embolism in one of the major cerebral arteries, usually the internal carotid or middle cerebral artery. Thrombosis in the extracranial (cervical) portion of the internal carotid artery may be caused by localized vasculitis from spread of tonsillar infection or cervical adenitis, or by local trauma, especially from a pencil point or other sharp object pushed into the region of the tonsillar fossa. The cause is less often evident in occlusions of the intracranial vessels. Local arteritis, atherosclerosis and fibromuscular hyperplasia of the vessel wall have been implicated, often without histologic proof. Thrombocytosis has been associated, but it is not known that it has a causal relationship to the thrombosis. Systemic illnesses which may be complicated by arterial occlusions in childhood include sickle cell disease, lupus erythematosus, periarteritis nodosa and cyanotic heart disease. Infants under age 2 years with cyanotic congenital heart disease, who have both polycythemia and iron deficiency, are especially prone to cerebral artery occlusion. The possibility of cerebral embolus has to be considered in the older child with congenital heart disease.

The clinical manifestations of cerebral vascular occlusion in childhood resemble those of stroke in the adult. However, in the child there often is a preceding acute febrile illness. The child may be found to be hemiparetic when he awakens from sleep. In other instances, progressive weakness is noted over a period of several hours. The child may remain lucid; aphasia is common when the dominant hemisphere is affected. Convulsions, which may be either focal or generalized, occur frequently during the acute phase. There is no evidence of increased intracranial pressure, and the CSF remains normal. The diagnosis may be confirmed by cerebral angiography, if it is performed early. Recanalization of the occluded vessel occurs rapidly, and arteriography a few weeks after the onset may show a normal vascular system.

The differential diagnosis of cerebral artery occlusion includes a postictal paralysis (Todd's) when the acute illness is complicated by convulsions. Encephalitis has to be considered, but can usually be ruled out if the child remains fairly alert and if there are no inflammatory changes in the CSF.

Therapy is limited to treatment of definable underlying conditions such as infection. The prognosis for recovery of speech functions is good, but almost always there is some residual hemiparesis. Spasticity tends to develop over a period of weeks or months. Recurrent seizures are common, especially following acute hemiplegia in infancy. Many of these children are left with mild intellectual impairment and behavioral abnormalities.

VENOUS OCCLUSIONS. Thrombosis of cerebral veins occurs principally as a complication of severe dehydration and as an extension of local infection into cerebral veins. Several clinical symptoms are recognizable, depending on the portion of the venous system that has become occluded:

Sagittal Sinus Thrombosis. This is a rare complication of severe dehydration, especially in the infant with diarrhea. Obstruction of the sinus leads to cerebral swelling, which produces signs of increased intracranial pressure, including stupor, coma, dilated scalp veins and bulging anterior fontanelle. When thrombosis extends into the cortical veins there may be widespread hemorrhagic infarction of the brain. Seizures and quadriparesis may occur. The clinical diagnosis can rarely be made with certainty. The clinical picture may mimic encephalitis and various metabolic encephalopathies, especially water intoxication in the dehydrated infant who has been rehydrated too rapidly.

Lateral Sinus Thrombosis. This is a complication of neglected otitis media and mastoiditis. Obstruction to the sinus results from septic thrombophlebitis. There may be chills and fever, or the onset may be insidious with signs of increased intracranial pressure. Focal neurologic signs are usually absent. This condition has become rare following the widespread use of antibiotics for the treatment of otitis media.

Cavernous Sinus Thrombosis. This follows infection of the face, orbit or nasal sinuses. Pyogenic infections of the nose are a common source. The infection spreads via anastomoses of the facial vein with the ophthalmic veins, which drain directly into the cavernous sinus. Onset is with high fever, drowsiness and proptosis of the eye on the affected side. Within hours or at most one or two days, the veins of the lid become distended and chemosis develops. There is paralysis of one or more of the ocular muscles. Funduscopic examination reveals blurring of the disc margins and engorgement of retinal veins. Untreated, the thrombophlebitis spreads to the other side via the circular sinus, and this is usually followed by fatal intracranial extension.

The *diagnosis* of cerebral venous thrombosis is based to a large extent on the clinical findings. CSF examination is of little help. CSF pressure is usually elevated; the fluid may be bloody and it may show white cells and an elevated protein content. Cerebral angiography is of value in localizing the site of obstruction.

TREATMENT. Therapy of cerebral vein thrombosis consists of intravenous administration of appropriate antibiotics in full dosage, when thrombosis is secondary to infection. Localized collections of pus should be drained surgically. Life-threatening increase in intracranial pressure may be treated with mannitol or dexamethasone. Anticoagulant therapy is not indicated, since it may worsen hemorrhage into infarcted brain areas.

Bickerstaff, E. R.: Aetiology of acute hemiplegia in childhood. Brit. Med. J. *2*:82, 1964.

Brown, P.: Septic cavernous sinus thrombosis. Bull. Johns Hopkins Hosp. *109*:68, 1961.

Gold, A. P., Ransohoff, J., and Carter, S.: Vein of Galen malformation. Acta Neurol. Scand. *8* (Suppl.):1964.

Greer, M.: Benign intracranial hypertension—1. Mastoiditis and lateral sinus obstruction. Neurology *12*:472, 1962.

Isler, W.: Acute Hemiplegias and Hemisyndromes in Childhood. Clinics in Developmental Medicine, Nos. 41/42. Philadelphia, J. B. Lippincott Co., 1971.

Levine, O. R., Jameson, A. G., Nelhaus, G., and Gold, A. P.: Cardiac complications of cerebral arteriovenous fistula in infancy. Pediatrics *30*:563, 1962.

Matson, D. D.: Intracranial arterial aneurysms in childhood. J. Neurosurg. *23*:578, 1965.

Pool, J. L., and Potts, D. G.: Aneurysms and Arteriovenous Anomalies of the Brain; Diagnosis and Treatment. New York, Paul B. Hoeber, 1965.

Solomon, G. E., et al.: Natural history of acute hemiplegia of childhood. Brain *93*:107, 1970.

Tyler, H. R., and Clark, D. B.: Incidence of neurological complications in congenital heart disease. Arch. Neurol. Psychiat. *77*:17, 1957.

HEAD INJURY

Craniocerebral trauma is one of the major causes of serious disability and death in childhood. About 200,000 children per year are admitted to United States hospitals for observation and treatment following head injury. A much larger number are seen by the local physician and observed at home. The difficult decision as to whether a potentially life-threatening head injury requires hospitalization frequently has to be made by the practicing pediatrician.

MINOR HEAD TRAUMA

A closed head injury usually can be assumed to be insignificant when the initial blow to the head is not followed by unconsciousness; the child can usually be followed at home without special diagnostic study. Dizziness, nausea, occasional vomiting and headache may be seen during the first 24 to 48 hours after minor head trauma. They are not cause for alarm unless they are accompanied by marked or progressive lethargy. Even after apparently mild head trauma the parents should be instructed to check the child at least once during the first night to make certain that he is rousable. This is of importance, since intracranial hemorrhage, especially into the subdural space, occasionally follows apparently trivial head trauma.

CONCUSSION

This is defined as a head injury which is immediately followed by a period of unconsciousness. Concussion is not associated with any obvious pathologic changes in brain. It is assumed to be due to disturbance in function of the brain stem caused by sudden jarring. After a concussion the patient has loss of memory for the events surrounding the injury. Memory loss for what preceded the injury is termed retrograde amnesia; memory loss for occurrences after the injury is known as antegrade amnesia. In general, the duration of unconsciousness and the extent of retrograde amnesia show a good correlation to the severity of injury. Retrograde amnesia diminishes during recovery, but it never disappears completely.

Concussion implies a significant blow to the head, with sufficient distortion of intracranial structures to make severance of intracranial vessels a possibility. Following a concussion the child should be carefully observed for delayed evidences of intracranial hemorrhage. A baseline neurologic examination should be obtained, including a check for pupillary size and reaction to light, funduscopic examination, and assessment of reflexes for symmetry and for presence of a Babinski sign. In the infant, tension of the fontanelle should be assessed and the head size measured. It is advisable to obtain roentgenograms of the skull, to rule out skull fractures. Not every child with concussion needs to be treated in the hospital. Close observation at home may be sufficient, if the initial evaluation fails to indicate any neurologic abnormality and if the child has regained a normal state of alertness.

SKULL FRACTURE

The radiographic demonstration of a skull fracture provides important information regarding the site of injury, but does not per se imply serious underlying brain injury. The likelihood of intracranial hemorrhage must of course be recognized. A fracture that crosses the middle meningeal artery groove should alert one to the possibility of epidural hemorrhage. Occipital skull fracture may be associated with posterior fossa hemorrhage (see below). Basal skull fractures may lead to leakage of CSF into the middle ear with bulging of the tympanic membrane, and to otorrhea, if the tympanic membrane is ruptured. Rhinorrhea, or escape of CSF from the nose, occurs with fractures through the cribriform plate. Basal skull fractures may lead to meningitis by spread of organisms from the nose or ear. Prophylactic use of one of the penicillins is justifiable for basal skull fracture with rhinorrhea or otorrhea. Linear fractures require no specific therapy. Depressed fractures should be surgically elevated, unless depression is minimal. Occasionally surgical closure of dural defects is necessary to control CSF leakage.

Skull fractures in infancy may lead to progressively enlarging defects of the skull (spreading fractures) over a period of months or years. These are due to entrapment of the meninges in the fracture line. Large meningeal cysts may form and may have to be surgically resected.

SEVERE HEAD INJURY

This should be assumed when the child fails to awaken within some minutes after the accident. Structural damage to brain tissue has to be expected in such a patient. This may take the form of contusion or bruising of brain, usually either at the site of the blow (coup) or opposite the site (contracoup). Actual *laceration* of brain tissue and meninges may occur, often with associated intracerebral, subarachnoid and subdural hemorrhage. Intracranial pressure may increase rapidly, both as a result of hemorrhage and of edema of injured tissue.

The acute management of the child with severe head injury presents a challenging problem. Generally the child is comatose. The first priorities are ascertainment that the patient has adequate blood pressure, that the airway is patent and that respirations are well maintained. Movement of the patient should be avoided until it has been demonstrated that there are no serious injuries such as fractures of the spine or of other major bones. Prompt neurologic assessment should be carried out, as summarized for the comatose patient. This is repeated at frequent intervals until the patient's condition is stable. Neuroradiologic studies and/or neurosurgical intervention may be indicated when there is progressive deepening of coma or when signs of tentorial herniation appear. The medical management of the child who remains comatose following severe head injury is that of coma from any cause. Medical management of cerebral edema, usually by use of dexamethasone, is an important adjunct to the therapy of severe head trauma.

EPIDURAL HEMORRHAGE

This is usually secondary to severance of the middle meningeal artery, most often as a result of a fracture crossing the artery's groove in the skull. Fracture is less likely in the infant or small child with epidural hemorrhage in whom bleeding is frequently venous, from dural veins. The characteristic history of epidural hemorrhage is that of a patient who awakens from a concussion and who, after a brief lucid interval, lapses into coma again. This is rapidly followed by signs of tentorial herniation, unless therapy is promptly instituted. If the initial injury is severe enough to cause cerebral contusion, the lucid interval is absent, and there is progressively deepening coma. Surgical evacuation of blood from the epidural space is lifesaving and will lead to complete recovery, if it is done promptly.

When epidural hemorrhage is venous in origin, the course is less rapid and is clinically indistinguishable from that of subdural hematoma. Hemorrhage into the epidural space of the posterior fossa may follow trauma to the occiput, with or without fracture. The bleeding is from the lateral sinus or from tributary veins. The child becomes progressively drowsy after a lucid interval. Vomiting and irregular respirations occur early, owing to compression of the brain stem. A hematoma in the posterior fossa may lead to hydrocephalus from compression of the aqueduct and the 4th ventricle; this lesion is a possibility in the infant who develops hydrocephalus following a traumatic delivery.

SUBDURAL HEMATOMA

Subdural hematoma may be acute or chronic. Chronic subdural hematoma is most common in infancy; it presents special problems, which are discussed below.

ACUTE SUBDURAL HEMATOMA. This is almost always associated with meningeal tears and with contusion and hemorrhage in the underlying brain. It has to be thought of in the child with severe head trauma who remains in deep coma and has evidence of progressively increasing intracranial pressure. Prognosis is guarded even when the collection of blood is removed promptly, because there is usually severe injury to the brain.

CHRONIC SUBDURAL HEMATOMA. In the child, as in the infant, there is gradual leakage of blood from torn frontal or parietal cortical veins which traverse the subdural space in their course to the sagittal sinus. The initial injury may be minor, usually a concussion from which the child at first appears to recover. Within days or sometimes weeks of the injury the child develops signs of increased intracranial pressure, including headache, vomiting, drowsiness, unsteadiness of gait and 6th nerve palsy. Hemiparesis and convulsions may occur. Papilledema is usually present. The initial injury may have been forgotten, and the first consideration may be of brain tumor. Coma and signs of tentorial herniation develop in neglected cases. The diagnosis is confirmed by cerebral angiography, which shows an avascular space between the superficial cerebral vessels and the inner table of the skull. Brain scan may show increased uptake of radioactive material in the area of the hematoma. The EEG may show lower amplitude on the affected side, but this is not a reliable finding. Surgical evacuation of the chronic subdural hematoma in the older child usually results in cure.

CHRONIC SUBDURAL HEMATOMA IN THE INFANT. This occurs with maximum incidence from ages 2 to 6 months. In about 25 per cent of the infants, there is a history of birth trauma, and about an equal number have a history of postnatal head injury. In a significant number of infants there is no clear history of trauma, even when there are distinct evidences of such injuries as fractures of long bones, ribs and the skull. (See battered child syndrome, p. 107.) The evolution of chronic subdural hematoma in infancy is as follows: The initial clot liquefies and leads to movement of water into the subdural space to maintain osmotic equilibrium. Repeated small hemorrhages occur from rupture of bridging veins, which are put under stress as the subdural space enlarges. The infant's skull readily expands in response to increase in intracranial pressure. As a result, very large collections of fluid may form. The fluid is initially bloody. It gradually clears and becomes straw-colored; it has a high protein content in the chronic state. Chronic subdural effusions become encapsulated by vascular inner and outer membranes. The outer membrane may become quite thick and occasionally calcifies (Fig. 20–22).

Presenting symptoms include repeated vomit-

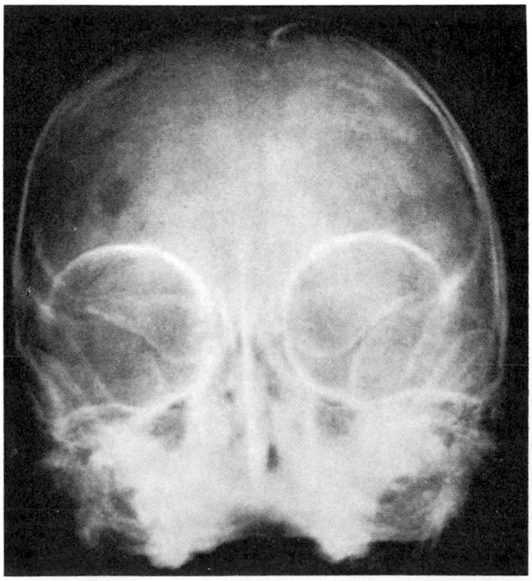

Figure 20–22 Calcified subdural membrane in a microcephalic retarded child. Right subdural hematoma drained in infancy (note trephine), left side not explored. Calcified membrane discovered years later.

ing, failure to gain weight, unexplained fever, irritability, drowsiness and convulsions. Focal neurologic signs are rare; rather, one finds evidences of increased intracranial pressure, including a bulging fontanelle and mild head enlargement. Biparietal prominence of the skull is characteristic, in contrast to hydrocephalus, in which the prominence tends to be frontal. Transillumination of the skull is increased after liquefaction of the initial hematoma has occurred. Funduscopic examination reveals retinal hemorrhages in more than half of the infants.

The diagnosis is made by subdural tap or by cerebral angiography. Initially, therapy consists of repeated subdural taps, but surgical drainage is frequently required. The prognosis depends on the degree of cerebral damage that occurred at the time of the initial trauma, as well as on the duration and size of the subdural effusion at the time therapy was initiated. The outcome is satisfactory in about 60 per cent of patients. Mental defects, convulsions and quadriparesis are the most common residuals.

POST-TRAUMATIC SYNDROMES

The brain of the child shows remarkable capacity for recovery from acute injury. Good functional recoveries have been reported in children who remained comatose for over one month. Post-traumatic epilepsy occurs in about 10 per cent of survivors from severe head injury and usually has its onset within one year after the trauma. The most common residuals are minor changes in behavior and in learning. Headache and dizziness are rather frequent complaints. Hydrocephalus may develop when there was subarachnoid hemorrhage.

DeVivo, D. C., and Dodge, P. R.: The critically ill child: Diagnosis and management of head injury. Pediatrics *48*:129, 1971.

Ingraham, F. D., and Matson, D. D.: Subdural hematoma in infancy. J. Pediatr. *24*:1, 1944.

Mealey, J., Jr.: Pediatric Head Injuries. Springfield, Ill., Charles C Thomas, 1968.

Richardson, F.: Some effects of severe head injury. A follow-up study of children and adolescents after protracted coma. Dev. Med. Child. Neurol. *5*:471, 1963.

Shulman, K., and Ransohoff, J.: Subdural hematoma in children. The fate of children with retained membranes. J. Neurosurg. *18*:175, 1961.

Taveras, T. M., and Ransohoff, J.: Leptomeningeal cysts of the brain following trauma with erosion of the skull: A study of 7 cases treated by surgery. J. Neurosurg. *10*:233, 1953.

Till, K.: Subdural hematoma and effusion in infancy. Brit. Med. J. *3*:400, 1968.

DISEASES OF THE SPINAL CORD

GENERAL CONSIDERATIONS. Diseases of the spinal cord are uncommon in childhood, but prompt recognition of them is of great importance, since there is often compression of the cord. Early diagnosis and treatment may avoid permanent paraplegia and incontinence.

Compression of the spinal cord results in a variety of characteristic symptoms and signs; these include, with varying frequency and depending upon the location of the spinal lesion: localized back tenderness, pain and immobility, scoliosis, and bladder dysfunction, manifest initially as frequency and urgency and followed by distention and incontinence. The most common motor manifestation is disturbance of gait, initially with a limp, which may progress to paraplegia. When the lesion involves the cervical cord there may be quadriparesis, usually with muscle atrophy, areflexia and hypotonia in the upper limbs and hyperreflexia and spasticity in the legs. In general, flaccid weakness and areflexia are found at the level of the lesion, with spasticity below that level. In acute lesions, however, the paralysis is flaccid throughout, owing to spinal "shock." A sensory level on the trunk identified by pinprick and touch is indicative of spinal cord disease and establishes the approximate site of the lesion. Often the actual lesion is several segments above the upper extent of sensory impairment.

NEOPLASMS OF THE SPINAL CORD

When spinal cord dysfunction evolves in a subacute or chronic manner, it is most often due to a neoplasm. Gliomas, including astrocytomas and ependymomas, are the most common types. Neuroblastoma is next in frequency; it is the most likely cause of spinal cord compression in the infant. In lymphoma, the spinal cord may be compressed by tumor masses in the epidural space. Spinal neurofibroma may be associated with generalized neurofibromatosis. Various developmental lesions, including teratoma, lipoma and neurenteric cysts, account for most of the remaining spinal cord tumors in childhood. Spinal cord compression occurs occasionally with chronic hemolytic anemia as a result of extramedullary hematopoiesis in the extradural space.

Careful neurologic examination of the child with unexplained limp or bladder dysfunction is essential for early diagnosis of spinal tumors. Radiographs of the spine may provide helpful information; with slowly growing tumors, the spinal canal is widened in the area of the lesion and there is bony erosion, especially of the pedicles. Defects of the neural arches are found in developmental tumors. The lumbar spinal fluid is xanthochromic and high in protein content, when there is obstruction of the spinal subarachnoid space. Myelography is needed to localize the exact level and extent of the tumor, and whether it is extrinsic to or within the spinal cord.

Intrinsic spinal cord tumors may be difficult to distinguish from *syringomyelia,* a spinal cord disease of unknown cause with cavitation in the center of the cord, usually in the cervical area. Atrophy of hand muscles and loss of pain sensation in the upper limbs are the most common clinical findings.

Prompt surgical exploration is indicated in most types of spinal cord tumor. Local irradiation is the therapy of choice in spinal cord compression secondary to lymphoma.

ACUTE SPINAL CORD LESIONS

SPINAL CORD TRAUMA. Spinal cord trauma in childhood most often is the result of breech deliveries, automobile accidents and diving injuries. It usually is associated with fracture or dislocation of vertebrae. Dislocations are especially common at the C1–2 level in association with fracture of the odontoid process, at the lower cervical level and at T12–L1. Complete cord transsection at the upper cervical level leads to rapid death from respiratory paralysis. Less severe injury at this level causes quadriparesis and often respiratory embarrassment, which requires assisted ventilation. It is very important to avoid movement of such a patient. When this is absolutely necessary it must be accomplished en bloc. If possible, the patient should be kept in the supine position, on a firm support. Gentle neck traction is helpful during transportation of the patient with cervical spine injury. Complete loss of function below the level of the lesion lasting for over 24 hours is almost always permanent. Surgical exploration of the damaged area, to have any chance of success, must be carried out within the first few hours.

ATLANTOAXIAL (C1-2) DISLOCATION (FIG. 20–23). This may occur without a clear history of trauma, especially in patients with congenital malformations of the spine or with metabolic bone diseases such as the chondrodystrophies. Flexion of the neck causes compression of the cervical cord in such patients. The history is that of progressive weakness and gait disturbance. There is spastic paresis of arms and legs, without dysfunction of cranial nerves. The lesion is treatable and must be distinguished from spastic cerebral palsy and from the leukodystrophies and demyelinating diseases. Therapy consists of reduction of the dislocation by neck traction, followed by immobilization of the neck.

SPINAL EPIDURAL ABSCESS. This is a localized accumulation of pus in the spinal epidural space, usually posterior to the cord in the thoracic area. It may be an acute abscess, usually staphylococcal in origin or subacute from extension of tuberculous osteomyelitis of the spine. Exquisite pain and percussion tenderness are present over the site of the abscess, and the spine is held rigidly extended. Signs of spinal cord dysfunction, including paraparesis, loss of bladder and bowel control and a sensory level on the trunk, evolve rapidly. Systemic evidence of infection may be absent. The diagnosis is occasionally made at lumbar puncture, when pus under pressure is obtained before the dura is penetrated. Myelography may be necessary to document the presence of spinal cord compression. Spinal epidural abscess represents a neurosurgical emergency; prompt drainage of the abscess may prevent permanent paraplegia.

VASCULAR ANOMALIES OF THE SPINAL CORD. These include arteriovenous malformations, venous angiomas and telangiectasia. These lesions may cause sudden spinal cord dysfunction, if there is rupture of an abnormal blood vessel, with hemorrhage into the spinal cord or into the spinal subarachnoid space. Nuchal rigidity occurs when subarachnoid hemorrhage is massive. Recurrent, acute exacerbations and partial remissions are characteristic. The cerebrospinal fluid may be bloody, or the protein content may be elevated. Myelography is usually diagnostic, by demonstrating tortuous, dilated vascular channels. At times, the presence of a vascular anomaly may be suspected from the presence of a portwine stain (nevus flammeus) covering the skin in a segmental distribution corresponding to the level of the vascular malformation. Surgical removal of vascular

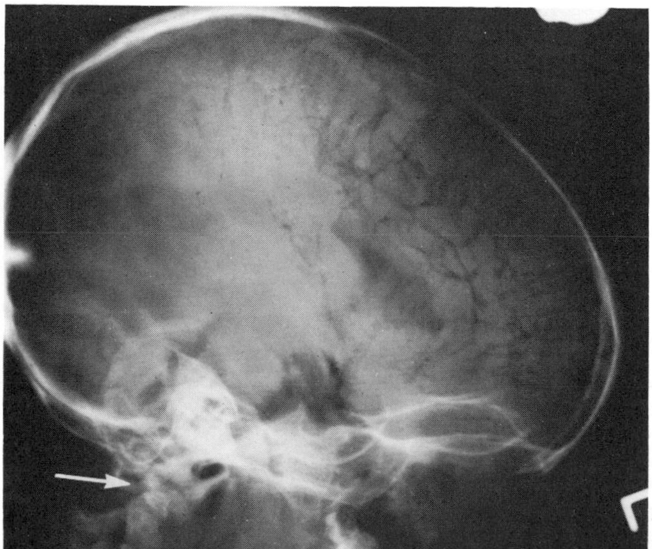

Figure 20–23 *The patient, a 4 year old child with progressive paraparesis, was initially thought to have cerebral disease for which she had diagnostic studies, including a pneumoencephalogram. A lateral radiograph at the time of pneumoencephalography, obtained during flexion of the neck, showed atlantoaxial dislocation (arrow), which proved to be the cause of the neurologic disability.*

anomalies of the spinal cord has been attempted, but is not often successful.

TRANSVERSE MYELOPATHY. Often misdesignated transverse myelitis, transverse myelopathy is a syndrome in which segmental spinal cord dysfunction appears rapidly, usually within hours, without evidence of a compressive lesion or of hemorrhage. In some instances the disorder is secondary to demyelinating disease. In others, there is segmental necrosis of the cord, probably as a result of vascular occlusion. Occlusion of the anterior spinal artery is a likely cause when posterior column functions (position and vibration senses) are spared. The onset of transverse myelopathy may be preceded by a mild febrile illness, or it may be sudden in a previously healthy child. Localized back pain at the site of the lesion is usually present, but is much less severe than in spinal epidural abscess. This is followed by paraparesis, a sensory level and inability to void. The CSF is usually normal, but there may be mild elevation in protein content and in cell count. Myelography may be needed to rule out compressive lesions. Corticosteroid therapy has been used, with equivocal results. Partial recovery of function is usual.

CHRONIC CARE OF THE PARAPLEGIC CHILD

Children who survive acute spinal cord diseases are frequently left with paraplegia and bladder dysfunction. The paraplegia is initially flaccid, but spasticity develops gradually, often with appearance of painful flexor spasms. These are especially common in poorly cared for paraplegics with decubitus ulcers. Stimulation of pain fibers in the areas of skin breakdown leads to activation of flexor reflexes in the severed spinal cord segments. Frequent turning, use of an air mattress and physiotherapy are important aspects of management which may prevent both decubitus ulcers and flexor spasms. The urinary bladder of the acutely paraplegic patient is atonic and becomes massively distended unless catheter drainage is instituted. Chronically, the bladder may become spastic with frequent partial reflex emptying. Chronic urinary tract infection from inadequate drainage and calciuria from immobility lead to renal and bladder calculi, unless they are properly treated.

Alexander, E., Jr., Masland, R., and Harris, C.: Anterior dislocation of first cervical vertebra simulating cerebral birth injury in infancy. Am. J. Dis. Child. *85*:151, 1953.

Matson, D. D.: Neurosurgery of Infancy and Childhood. Springfield, Ill., Charles C Thomas, 1969.

Paine, R. S., and Byers, R. K.: Transverse myelopathy in childhood. Am. J. Dis. Child. *85*:151, 1953.

Rand, R. W., and Rand, C. W.: Intraspinal Tumors of Childhood. Springfield, Ill., Charles C Thomas, 1960.

Rowland, L. P., Shapiro, J. H., and Jacobson, H. G.: Neurological syndromes associated with congenital absence of the odontoid process. Arch. Neurol. Psychiat. *80*:286, 1958.

Tarlov, I. M.: Spinal cord injuries—early treatment. Surg. Clin. N. Amer. *35*:2, 1955.

DISORDERS OF THE AUTONOMIC NERVOUS SYSTEM

The autonomic nervous system provides neural control over a large variety of vegetative functions such as heart rate, blood pressure, temperature regulation, micturition and intestinal motility. It consists of two large divisions, sympathetic and parasympathetic, whose actions are often but not invariably antagonistic. The highest level of integration of autonomic functions occurs in the hypothalamus. From there central parasympathetic and sympathetic pathways descend to the brain stem and spinal cord.

Parasympathetic nerve fibers leave the central nervous system via the cranial nerves and via the sacral spinal nerves. These fibers synapse in peripherally located parasympathetic ganglia, from where the peripheral fibers in turn are distributed to the visceral organs as follows:

Nerves in which parasympathetic fibers travel	*Organ innervated*
Cranial III	Sphincter of pupil
VII	Submaxillary and sublingual glands
IX	Parotid gland
X	Esophagus, bronchi, lungs, heart, stomach, pancreas, small intestine, proximal colon
Sacral ($S_2 - S_4$)	Distal colon, rectum, bladder, external genitalia

Stimulation of the parasympathetic nerves releases acetylcholine at the nerve terminals. The actions of this system can be explained entirely in terms of local pharmacologic effects of acetylcholine and can be reproduced by administration of such parasympathomimetic drugs as methacholine (Mecholyl) and pilocarpine and blocked by atropine and atropine-like drugs. Examples of parasympathetic effects include constriction of the pupils, salivation, bronchial constriction, slowing of the heart rate, gastric secretion of hydrochloric acid, stimulation of peristalsis and micturition.

Sympathetic nerve fibers leave the central nervous system only at the spinal level and travel with the thoracic and upper two lumbar spinal nerves. They synapse in peripheral sympathetic ganglia and are distributed to the visceral organs and to blood vessels, hair follicles, sweat glands and adrenal medulla. Stimulation of the sympathetic nervous system releases norepinephrine at most of the peripheral nerve endings; exceptions are the sweat glands, where the neurohumoral substance is acetylcholine, and the adrenal medulla, where it is epinephrine. Many of the effects of sympathetic nervous system stimulation can be reproduced by administration of norepinephrine or of such sympathomimetic drugs as amphetamine and ephedrine. These actions are blocked by adrenergic blocking agents such as phenoxybenzamine (Dibenzyline). Examples of the effects of sympathetic nervous system stimulation include pupillary dilatation, constriction of blood vessels, acceleration of heart rate, sweating, pilo-erection and bronchodilatation.

Autonomic nervous system functions are disturbed in a large number of systemic and neurologic illnesses, many of which are discussed elsewhere. The following outline includes disorders in which abnormalities of the autonomic nervous system are most prominent.

1. *Developmental defects*
   Familial dysautonomia (Riley-Day syndrome)
   Hirschsprung's disease
2. *Tumors*
   Neuroblastoma
   Ganglioneuroma
   Pheochromocytoma
   Hypothalamic tumor—the diencephalic syndrome of infancy
3. *Poisonings*
   Atropinism
   Botulism
4. *Injuries to autonomic nerves*
   Horner syndrome
   Adie syndrome
5. *Inflammatory disorders of autonomic nerves*
   Autonomic neuropathy
   Postinfectious polyneuritis (Guillain-Barré syndrome
6. *The "psychosomatic" disorders*
   Cushing-Rokitansky ulcer
   Curling ulcer

FAMILIAL DYSAUTONOMIA

The Riley-Day syndrome is a genetically determined disturbance in autonomic and peripheral sensory functions. The disease is transmitted as a simple recessive gene. It is most common in Ashkenazi Jews, among whom the frequency of the carrier state is estimated at about 1 per cent.

Neuropathologic findings are sparse and are confined to the peripheral sensory system. The taste buds (fungiform papillae) of the tongue are absent or decreased in number. The peripheral nerves have a deficit in the number of small unmyelinated fibers, which normally carry pain, temperature and taste sensations, and of the large myelinated fibers, which carry afferent impulses from muscle spindles. These abnormalities are not always present, and the autonomic nervous system usually has no pathologic changes. Disturbed autonomic function is reflected in a number of metabolic abnormalities. The plasma of about 25 per cent of children with the disease shows no dopamine-beta-hydroxylase, the enzyme which catalyzes the conversion of dopamine to norepinephrine. Vanillylmandelic acid (VMA), an excretion product of norepinephrine, is usually diminished in the urine of patients, and homovanillic acid (HVA), a metabolite of dopamine, is increased. The cerebrospinal fluid level of HVA is also elevated.

Clinical manifestations of the disease are prominent in infancy. Swallowing movements are poorly coordinated, leading to gagging, vomiting and aspiration of food. Excessive bronchial secretions and repeated aspiration contribute to recurrent bouts of pulmonary infection with eventual chronic pulmonary failure. Evidences of autonomic disturbances include excessive salivation and sweating, decrease or absence of tear formation, marked blotching of the skin during excitement, urinary incontinence, labile hypertension and orthostatic hypotension, and defective temperature regulation with periodic fevers. Clinical manifestations of peripheral sensory dysfunction consist of absence of taste sensation, diminished or absent pain sense leading to repeated skin trauma and to asymptomatic fractures, and absence of corneal sensation. The latter, together with the defect in tear formation, increases the susceptibility to corneal ulceration. Tendon reflexes are diminished or absent, probably as a result of defective formation of muscle spindle afferent fibers. The central nervous system is usually affected; the manifestations include mental defect, dysarthria, clumsiness and emotional lability.

LABORATORY DATA. Roentgenograms of the chest show atelectasis and pulmonary infiltrates similar to the changes in cystic fibrosis. The Mecholyl test for denervation hypersensitivity of the pupil (a fresh 2 per cent solution of Mecholyl is instilled into one conjunctival sac, the other eye serving as a control) is positive; constriction of the pupil appears within 10 minutes. There is no response to the histamine skin test (0.05 ml of a 1:1000 solution of histamine is injected intradermally), which is normally characterized by a red flare and pain at the injection site. Urinary VMA is decreased; HVA is increased. Slow intravenous infusion of norepinephrine produces an exaggerated pressor response. The hypotensive response to infusion of Mecholyl is increased.

The differential diagnosis of familial dysautonomia includes other causes of "failure to thrive" in infancy, chronic pulmonary diseases in childhood, congenital universal indifference to pain and congenital sensory neuropathy.

Treatment is directed toward control of the recurrent respiratory infections, prevention of corneal ulceration by use of artificial tears, and protection from injuries related to lack of pain sensation. Recently, bethanecol (Urecholine) has been used to increase tear formation. Genetic counseling is an important part of the management.

The prognosis of the child with familial dysautonomia is poor. A majority succumb to the illness prior to adulthood, usually from chronic pulmonary failure.

DIENCEPHALIC SYNDROME OF INFANCY

This is one of the definable causes of failure to thrive. It is usually due to glioma of the anterior hypothalamus, but the same syndrome may also occur with inflammatory or destructive lesions in this region. The infants have a number of endocrine and central autonomic disturbances secondary to hypothalamic dysfunction. The most striking clinical findings are extreme emaciation, in spite of apparently adequate food intake, and a hypermetabolic state with overactivity and "hyperalertness." The autonomic disturbances consist of excessive sweating, easy flushing of the skin, tachycardia and vomiting. Evidences of endocrine abnormality include increased linear growth, advanced bone age and excessive size of hands and feet. Late in the course the infants develop abnormal enlargement of the head, optic atrophy and searching nystagmus secondary to visual loss. The syndrome may occur at any time from 3 months to 4 years of age.

Soft tissue roentgenograms of the extremities show complete absence of the normal subcutaneous fat shadow. There may be fasting hypoglycemia. Pneumoencephalography is the definitive diagnostic test. It usually shows evidence of an intrinsic tumor in the area of the hypothalamus. Therapy is generally unsatisfactory, but long-term remissions have been induced by radiation therapy.

INJURY TO AUTONOMIC NERVES

HORNER SYNDROME. This refers to a lesion of the cervical sympathetic nerve fibers; it is usually unilateral. These fibers are especially prone to injury, owing to their long intra- and extracranial course. Central sympathetic neurons descend in the lateral medulla and spinal cord to the upper thoracic spinal level. Preganglionic cervical sympathetic fibers then leave the spinal cord in the upper thoracic ventral spinal roots and pass upward in the paravertebral sympathetic chain. The majority of fibers synapse in the superior cervical ganglion and then follow the course of the common carotid artery in the neck. Sudomotor and vasomotor fibers travel in close relation to the external carotid artery to be distributed to the skin over the face; fibers innervating the pupil and the upper eyelid (oculosympathetic fibers) follow the internal carotid and ophthalmic arteries to the orbit. The Horner syndrome may be due to lesions at any of these anatomic levels, i.e., at the medulla oblongata, cervical or upper thoracic spinal cord, posterior mediastinum or neck. A partial syndrome in which only the oculosympathetic fibers are affected is seen with lesions near the internal carotid artery or in the orbit.

The clinical manifestations of the Horner syndrome consist of ptosis due to weakness of the levator palpebrae muscle, meiosis due to dysfunction of pupillodilator fibers and absence of sweating over the ipsilateral face. In congenital Horner syndrome there is heterochromia iridis as a result of failure in pigmentation of the iris on the affected side.

Pharmacologic tests are of some help in differentiating Horner syndrome caused by a central nervous system lesion from that caused by a peripheral sympathetic lesion. Instillation of a 4 per cent solution of cocaine into the conjunctival sac normally produces dilatation of the pupil by potentiation of the effect of locally released norepinephrine. This response is absent in the Horner syndrome associated with a peripheral sympathetic lesion, whereas it is preserved in a lesion involving central sympathetic pathways. Instillation of a 1:1000 solution of epinephrine normally produces no pupillary reaction, but will result in dilatation of the pupil in Horner syndrome caused by a peripheral sympathetic lesion. The results of these tests may be equivocal, when the Horner syndrome is incomplete. A search for tumor or other compressive lesion is indicated in any patient who develops Horner syndrome. This should include careful palpation of the neck and of the supraclavicular areas, and roentgenograms of the chest and the cervical spine. Horner syndrome per se does not produce any significant disability and requires no therapy.

ADIE SYNDROME. The Adie syndrome is a disorder of the parasympathetic innervation of the iris of unknown etiology, which usually first appears in young adults but may occasionally occur in childhood. The affected pupil is large and reacts little or not at all to light, but will often react slowly to accommodation. Patients with Adie's pupil often have hyporeflexia, especially absence of the knee jerks. Occasionally there is associated anhidrosis over the trunk. The Adie pupil is hypersensitive to locally instilled parasympathomimetic agents, and instillation of 2 per cent Mecholyl into the conjunctival sac produces brisk contraction. The Adie syndrome is essentially a benign condition, and no therapy is necessary. Prompt recognition of this entity may spare the patient from unnecessary diagnostic studies.

INFLAMMATORY DISORDERS OF AUTONOMIC NERVES

The peripheral autonomic nervous system is occasionally involved in inflammatory diseases of nerve. In postinfectious polyneuritis (Guillain-Barré syndrome), autonomic dysfunction may represent a clinically significant complication. Evidences of autonomic disturbance include postural hypotension, hypertension, unexplained tachycardia, sweating and urinary retention. Urinary excretion of VMA may be increased.

A few cases of isolated *acute autonomic neuropathy* have been reported. Such patients have acute onset of diminished pupillary reaction to light, dryness of mouth, hypohydrosis, urinary retention and vomiting. Recovery is gradual over a period of weeks or months. The condition must be distinguished from atropinism and from botulism.

PSYCHOSOMATIC DISORDERS

It has long been known that lesions of the central nervous system may induce visceral abnormalities through stimulation of central autonomic pathways. A striking example is the *Cushing-Rokitansky ulcer* of the stomach or duodenum which occurs in children with posterior fossa tumor, often a few days after surgical resection of the neoplasm. Gastric ulceration in these children probably is due to abnormal stimulation of vagal (parasympathetic) nuclei in the medulla, which leads to increased gastric hydrochloric acid secretion. Nonspecific stress may lead to overactivity of hypothalamic parasympathetic centers with the same end result of gastric and duodenal ulceration and hemorrhage. This complication has been observed with special frequency in patients suffering from extensive burns (*Curling ulcer*).

It has been suggested that less specific stresses of life may be causative factors in the formation of gastric and duodenal ulcers as well as in the etiology of a number of other disorders such as ulcerative colitis, asthma and essential hypertension. However, proof of cause-effect relationships has been inconclusive, and the concept of psychosomatic illnesses has contributed little to our understanding of these systemic disorders.

Aguayo, A., Nair, P., and Bray, G.: Peripheral nerve abnormalities in the Riley-Day syndrome. Arch. Neurol. *24*:106, 1971.
Axelrod, F. B.: Treatment of familial dysautonomia with bethanecol (Urecholine). J. Pediatr. *81*:573, 1972.
Dancis, J., and Smith, A. A.: Familial dysautonomia. New Engl. J. Med. *274*:207, 1966.
Esterly, N., Cantoline, S. J., Alter, B. P., et al.: Pupillotonia, hyporeflexia and segmental hypohydrosis: Autonomic dysfunction in a child. J. Pediatr. *73*:852, 1968.
Loggie, J. M. H., and Van Maanen, E. F.: The autonomic nervous system and some aspects of the use of autonomic drugs in children. J. Pediatr. *81*:Part I, 205; Part II, 432, 1972.
Mitchell, P. L., and Meilman, E.: The mechanism of hypertension in the Guillain-Barré syndrome. Am. J. Med. *42*:986, 1967.
Poznanski, A. K., and Manson, G.: Radiographic appearance of the soft tissues in the diencephalic syndrome of infancy. Radiology *81*:101, 1963.
Riley, C. M., and Moore, R. H.: Familial dysautonomia differentiated from related disorders. Pediatrics *37*:435, 1966.
Russel, A.: A dicencephalic syndrome of emaciation in infancy and childhood. Arch. Dis. Child. *26*:274, 1951.
Smith, A. A., and Dancis, J.: Catecholamine release in familial dysautonomia. New Engl. J. Med. *277*:61, 1967.
Thomashefsky, A. J., Horowitz, S. J., and Feingold, M. H.: Acute autonomic neuropathy. Neurology *22*:251, 1972.
Weinshilboum, R. M., and Axelrod, J.: Reduced plasma dopamine-hydroxylase activity in familial dysautonomia. New Engl. J. Med. *285*:938, 1971.

PETER R. HUTTENLOCHER

21
NEUROMUSCULAR DISEASES

NEUROPATHIES AND MUSCULAR DISORDERS

Disorders of the peripheral motor and sensory systems are known collectively as the neuromuscular diseases. These illnesses involve one or more of the structures concerned with the segmental spinal reflex arc; these are the anterior horn cells, motor nerve fibers, neuromuscular junction, muscle, and sensory nerve fibers from muscle and tendons (Fig. 21–1). Interference with this reflex arc leads to depression of tendon reflexes, which is characteristic of all neuromuscular diseases. In addition, weakness and muscle atrophy usually are present.

The following is a useful classification of the more common disorders:

1. *Anterior horn cell diseases*

   Werdnig-Hoffmann disease
   Poliomyelitis (Section 10)
   Other viral infections (Section 10)

2. *Polyneuropathies*

   Postinfectious polyneuritis (Guillain-Barré syndrome, Section 10)
   Diphtheritic polyneuritis (Section 10)
   Toxic neuropathies (heavy metal poisoning, Section 28), drug-induced neuropathies, metabolic diseases with polyneuropathy (Table 21–2)
   Hypertrophic interstitial neuritis (Dejerine-Sottas)
   Charcot-Marie-Tooth disease (peroneal muscular atrophy)
   Congenital sensory neuropathy
   Congenital indifference to pain

3. *Mononeuropathies*

   Congenital ptosis
   Oculomotor nerve palsy (Tolosa-Hunt syndrome)
   Sixth nerve palsy (Duane syndrome)
   Facial palsy (Bell's palsy)
   Erb's palsy (Section 7)
   Peroneal palsy
   Sciatic nerve injury

4. *Diseases of the neuromuscular junction*

   Myasthenia gravis

5. *Diseases of Muscle*

   Inflammatory diseases of muscle

   Polymyositis
   Myositis ossificans

   Endocrine myopathies

   Hyperthyroid myopathies
   Hypothyroid myopathy
   Steroid myopathy

   Congenital defects of muscle

   Absence of muscle
   Congenital torticollis
   Congenital myopathies (central core disease and nemaline myopathy)

   Myotonia

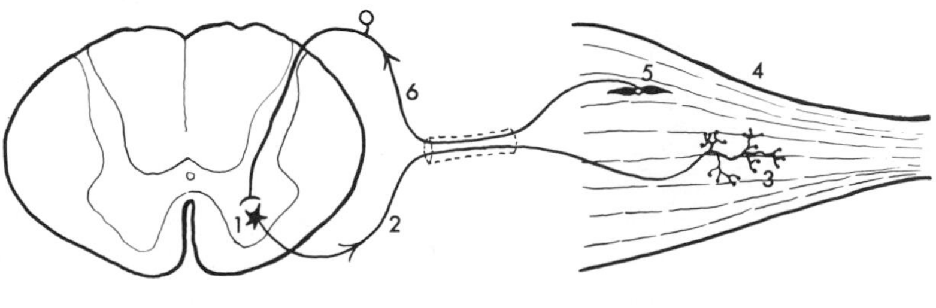

Figure 21–1 *Schematic representation of the structures that make up the neuromuscular system. 1 = anterior horn cell; 2 = motor nerve fiber; 3 = motor end-plate on muscle; 4 = muscle; 5 = sensory receptor in muscle (muscle spindle); 6 = sensory nerve fiber.*

Myotonia congenita (Thomsen's disease)

Periodic paralyses

Hyperkalemic form (adynamic episodica hereditaria)
Hypokalemic form
Paroxysmal myoglobinuria
McArdle's disease (Section 8)

The muscular dystrophies

Pseudohypertrophic form (Duchenne)
Congenital muscular dystrophy
Facioscapulohumeral form
Limb-girdle form
Ocular myopathy
Myotonic dystrophy

ANTERIOR HORN CELL DISEASES

The anterior horn cells are selectively affected in poliomyelitis and occasionally by infection with other viruses including the coxsackie and echoviruses. Degeneration of the anterior horn cells as an inherited disorder occurs primarily in infancy.

INFANTILE SPINAL MUSCULAR ATROPHY. *Werdnig-Hoffmann disease* is transmitted as a recessive trait. The etiology is obscure. The primary pathologic change consists of atrophy of anterior horn cells in the spinal cord and of motor nuclei in the brain stem (Fig. 21–2). Atrophy of motor nerve roots and of muscle occurs secondarily.

Onset is prior to age 2 years and often occurs in utero. Rare instances of a similar illness with onset later in childhood have been described. The early manifestations are weakness and hypotonia of the proximal and distal limbs, intercostal and bulbar muscles. The legs tend to lie in a frog-leg position, with hips abducted and knees flexed (Fig. 21–3). The diaphragms are relatively spared. Their maintained function in the presence of weakness of the intercostal muscles results in characteristic paradoxical breathing, with inward movement of the chest on inspiration. Extraocular muscles are unaffected, and eye movements are well preserved even in the late stages. Fibrillations usually are visible in the tongue. Tendon reflexes are almost always absent. Mental development is normal, and the bright look of these infants is in striking contrast to their lack of motor activity. Initially the infants tend to be obese. In the late stages swallowing becomes impossible. Death results from respiratory failure and from aspiration of food. Infants with onset in utero usually die prior to age 2 years. Those with later onset may survive for some years, occasionally to adulthood.

The *diagnosis* of Werdnig-Hoffman disease is based largely on the clinical findings. Electromyography often shows evidence of denervation of muscle, including fibrillation potentials and fasciculations. Muscle biopsy shows groups of muscle fibers in varying stages of degeneration, each group representing muscle cells innervated by a single motor neuron. Spinal fluid values, nerve conduction measurements and serum enzyme values are within normal ranges.

The *differential diagnosis* of Werdnig-Hoffmann disease includes a large number of less common conditions in which hypotonia and weakness occur in infancy. The term "floppy infant" is often used to refer to the group of disorders in which hypotonia is prominent (Table 21–1).

Disorders of the central nervous system presenting with hypotonia can usually be differentiated from the peripheral neuromuscular diseases by the presence of decreased alertness and visual responsiveness, and by the preservation of tendon reflexes. Special studies, including spinal fluid examination, nerve conduction velocity measurements, serum enzyme determinations and muscle biopsy, may be needed to distinguish Werdnig-Hoffmann disease from disorders of peripheral nerves or of muscle. There are a small number of hypotonic infants who cannot be placed into the classification of Table 21–1. These infants appear normally alert. Tendon reflexes are depressed but usually not completely absent. Laboratory investigations, including muscle biopsy, are unrevealing. Hypotonia and

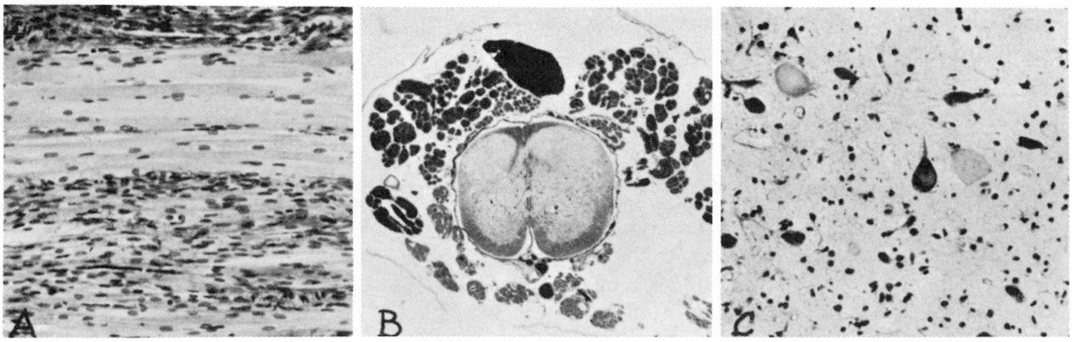

Figure 21–2 Werdnig-Hoffmann disease. A, *Fascicular atrophy of muscle.* B, *Pallor of ventral roots.* C, *Degenerating motor neurons.*

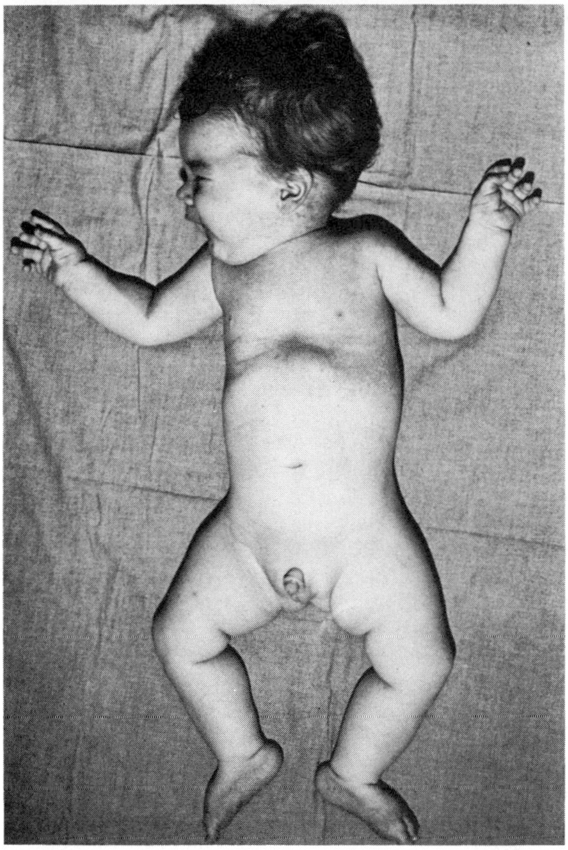

Figure 21–3 *Typical posture of the infant with Werdnig-Hoffmann disease.*

weakness gradually improve in most of these infants. Such diagnostic labels as *benign congenital hypotonia* and *amyotonia congenita* have been used. However, it is unlikely that this group represents a single disease entity.

Brandt, S.: Werdnig-Hoffmann's Infantile Progressive Muscular Atrophy. Copenhagen, Ejnar Munksgaard, 1950.

Byers, R. K., and Banker, B. Q.: Infantile muscular atrophy. Arch. Neurol. *5*:140, 1961.

Chambers, R., and MacDermot, V.: Polyneuritis as a cause of "amyotonia congenita." Lancet *1*:397, 1957.

Dubowitz, V.: The Floppy Infant. London, William Heinemann, Ltd., 1969.

Eden, A. N.: Guillain-Barré syndrome in a 6 month old infant. Am. J. Dis. Child. *102*:224, 1961.

Garvie, J. M., and Woolf, A. L.: Kugelberg-Welander syndrome (hereditary spinal muscular atrophy). Brit. Med. J.: *1*:1458, 1966.

Paine, R. S.: The future of the "floppy infant." A follow-up study of 133 patients. Dev. Med. Child Neurol. *5*:115, 1963.

Rabe, E. F.: The hypotonic infant. J. Pediatr. *64*:422, 1964.

Walton, J. N.: Amyotonia congenita. A follow-up study. Lancet *1*:1023, 1956.

POLYNEUROPATHIES

Involvement of multiple peripheral nerves is found in many systemic diseases, intoxications and infections. In addition, there are a number of genetically determined illnesses in which degeneration of peripheral nerves is the primary abnormality. These conditions are discussed in detail below. The more common causes of polyneuropathy are listed in Table 21–2.

The *clinical manifestations of polyneuropathy* include weakness, muscular atrophy, loss of tendon reflexes and sensory impairment. The distal limbs—feet and hands—are affected first and there is gradual proximal progression as the disorder becomes more severe. Motor fibers are more severely affected than sensory ones in some polyneuropathies, including lead poisoning, the Guillain-Barré syndrome and Charcot-Marie-Tooth disease. Gait disturbance with foot drop is an early manifestation in these illnesses. Fairly selective damage to sensory fibers occurs in diabetes mellitus and in some of the genetically determined neuropathies. All types of sensation, including

TABLE 21–1 DISEASES INCLUDED IN THE DIAGNOSTIC TERM, THE "FLOPPY INFANT," AND CHARACTERIZED BY PERSISTENT HYPOTONIA

CENTRAL NERVOUS SYSTEM DISORDERS	SPINAL CORD DISEASES	DISEASES OF PERIPHERAL NERVE	DISEASES OF THE NEUROMUSCULAR JUNCTION	MUSCLE DISEASES
Atonic diplegia	Spinal cord trauma	Polyneuritis (Guillain-Barré syndrome)	Myasthenia gravis	Congenital muscular dystrophy
Congenital cerebellar ataxia	Werdnig-Hoffmann disease	Familial dys-autonomia		Myotonic dystrophy
Kernicterus		Congenital sensory neuropathy		Glycogen storage disease of muscle and heart (Pompe)
Chromosomal defects				Central core disease
Oculocerebrorenal syndrome (Lowe)				Nemaline myopathy
Cerebral lipidoses				Mitochondrial myopathies
Prader-Willi syndrome				

TABLE 21–2 THE MORE COMMON POLYNEUROPATHIES

POISONING	DRUG TOXICITY	INFECTIONS	METABOLIC DISORDERS	DEGENERATIVE DISEASES
Lead	Vincristine	Diphtheria	Diabetes mellitus	Hypertrophic interstitial neuritis
Mercury	Isoniazid		Uremia	Charcot-Marie-Tooth disease
Thallium	Nitrofuran	Guillain-Barré syndrome	Porphyria	Congenital sensory neuropathy
Arsenic		Leprosy	Thiamine deficiency	Metachromatic leukodystrophy
			Vitamin B_{12} deficiency	Krabbe's disease
			Refsum's disease	Leigh's disease
				Spinocerebellar degenerations

pain, touch, temperature, position and vibration sense, are impaired, often in a "stocking and glove" distribution. Injured sensory nerve endings may become abnormally sensitive to stimulation, and innocuous stimuli may be interpreted as being painful (hyperpathia), while tingling or "pins and needles" sensations may occur in the absence of stimulation. Loss of sensory and autonomic innervation results in trophic changes in skin and nails and occasionally in loss of toes and fingers. Remarkable recovery from polyneuritis may follow removal of the offending agent, owing to the capacity of peripheral nerves, in contrast to central neural pathways, to regenerate after injury.

The *pathologic changes* in some peripheral neuropathies consist of patchy loss of the myelin sheath of the nerve fibers (segmental demyelination); in other instances degeneration of the axons appears to be the primary process. In chronic neuropathies there often is considerable fibrous tissue reaction, which may result in palpable enlargement of the affected nerves.

Measurement of nerve conduction velocity is the most helpful diagnostic aid. Decrease in conduction velocity is seen exclusively in disorders of peripheral nerve and is especially striking when demyelination is a prominent pathologic finding. Biopsy of the sural nerve may also be useful in confirming the diagnosis, except in predominantly motor neuropathies, in which this sensory nerve may be spared. Neither of these measures, however, provides information regarding the specific cause of the neuropathy. The recognizable toxic and metabolic causes listed in Table 21–2 must, when possible, be identified by toxicologic and other special tests. A careful family history and examination of family members are important for the diagnosis of the genetically determined polyneuropathies. Included in this group are hypertrophic interstitial neuritis, Charcot-Marie-Tooth disease (peroneal muscular atrophy) and several forms of sensory neuropathy.

HYPERTROPHIC INTERSTITIAL NEURITIS (Dejerine-Sottas). This is an uncommon, recessively inherited disease that has its onset in late infancy or early childhood. Motor development may be slow from the start. Later in childhood there is progressive gait disturbance, with foot drop and ataxia caused by loss of position sense. Associated findings include pes cavus and scoliosis. Eventually, but rarely during childhood, the peripheral nerves become palpably enlarged. The disease is slowly progressive and permits a normal life span. The CSF protein content is usually elevated, a finding of some value in differentiation from other neuropathies and from diseases of muscle.

CHARCOT-MARIE-TOOTH DISEASE. *Peroneal muscular atrophy* is a motor neuropathy that disproportionately affects the nerves to the legs. Inheritance is usually on a dominant basis. Onset is during late childhood or adolescence, with pes cavus, foot drop and peroneal myatrophy. The distal wasting of the legs gives the characteristic "stork leg" appearance. Foot drop leads to a high "steppage" gait. The intrinsic hand muscles are affected eventually. Mild distal sensory impairment may be present. Progression is slow, and the disease rarely becomes severe enough to preclude ambulation. The CSF is normal.

CONGENITAL SENSORY NEUROPATHY. This is inherited on a recessive basis. The abnormality is usually noted in late infancy when the child fails to respond to painful stimuli applied to the hands or feet. These children tend to bite and otherwise injure their fingers. Ulceration and progressive loss of digits are common. All sensory modalities are affected, with distal limbs involved more severely than proximal. Anhydrosis may be present and may be manifest by recurrent fevers. Other associated abnormalities include mental retardation, deafness and retinitis pigmentosa. The differential diagnosis includes hereditary ectodermal dysplasia, the Lesch-Nyhan syndrome (Section 8), infantile autism, the Riley-Day syndrome (Section 20), and congenital indifference to pain.

CONGENITAL INDIFFERENCE TO PAIN. This is a rare syndrome in which absence of appropriate responses to painful stimuli is found as an isolated abnormality. Other sensory modalities are intact. Failure to appreciate pain leads to repeated minor skin trauma and to burns. Acute surgical abdominal disorders and fractures may go undetected for a long time. In some patients, absence of pain response has been associated with anhydrosis and mental defect. The anatomic basis of congenital indifference to pain is unknown. The condition is distinguished from congenital sensory neuropathy by the universal absence of pain sensation, and by the preservation of touch, position, vibration and temperature sense.

Baxter, D. W., and Olszewski, J.: Congenital universal indifference to pain. Brain *83*:381, 1960.
Byers, R. K., and Taft, L. T.: Chronic multiple peripheral neuropathy in childhood. Pediatrics *20*:517, 1957.
Dyck, P. J., and Lambert, E. H.: Lower motor and primary sensory neuron diseases with peroneal muscular atrophy. 1. Neurologic, genetic and electrophysiologic findings in hereditary polyneuropathies. Arch. Neurol. *18*:603, 1968.
Landwirth, J.: Sensory radicular neuropathy and retinitis pigmentosa. Pediatrics *34*:519, 1964.
Linarelli, L. G., and Prichard, J. W.: Congenital sensory neuropathy. Am. J. Dis. Child. *119*:513, 1970.
Pinsky, L., and DiGeorge, A. M.: Congenital familial sensory neuropathy with anhydrosis. J. Pediatr. *68*:1, 1966.

MONONEUROPATHIES

Defects involving single peripheral nerves may be congenital or secondary to inflammation, trauma or injection of irritant materials.

CONGENITAL PTOSIS. Congenital ptosis is probably secondary to faulty innervation of the levator palpebrae muscle. It is often transmitted by dominant inheritance. Drooping of one or both eyelids is noted in the neonatal period and persists throughout life. The ptosis is rarely complete. Occasionally movements of the jaw will elevate the ptotic eyelid. This finding, referred to as "jaw winking" (Marcus Gunn phenomenon) is due to aberrant innervation of the levator palpebrae, with an admixture of 3rd and 5th cranial nerve fibers.

Congenital ptosis has to be differentiated from myasthenia gravis, brain stem lesions and ocular myopathy. Surgical correction for cosmetic reasons is indicated when the defect is severe.

THE TOLOSA-HUNT SYNDROME. *Oculomotor nerve palsy* consists of painful, unilateral paralysis of one or more oculomotor nerves (usually the 3rd) of unknown etiology. The onset is acute, with retro-orbital pain and diplopia, and usually with ptosis and mydriasis on the affected side. Gradual improvement always occurs, but there may be repeated attacks. Aneurysm of the internal carotid artery and parasellar neoplasms have to be ruled out by appropriate studies; carotid angiography is usually required. A rapid therapeutic response to adrenocortical steroids is said to be characteristic.

SIXTH NERVE PALSY. This may occur as an isolated congenital anomaly. There is inability to abduct the eye on the affected side. The abducens muscle may be replaced by a fibrous band that also prevents full adduction of the eye. Attempted adduction leads to retraction of the globe (Duane syndrome). The differentiation of congenital 6th nerve palsy from convergent strabismus may be difficult. In strabismus, however, the squinting eye can be shown to move fully after a period of patching.

SEVENTH (FACIAL) NERVE PALSY. This may be congenital or acquired later in life.

Congenital Facial Nerve Palsy. This palsy often is partial, with selective weakness of muscles innervated by the mandibular branch, resulting in paralysis of the lower lip and the angle of the mouth. The unopposed action of the opposite lower facial muscles pulls the mouth toward the normal side (Fig. 21–4). The cosmetic defect tends to be quite mild, but there may be associated congenital anomalies.

Bell's Palsy. Bell's palsy refers to 7th nerve paralysis of sudden onset and usually of obscure etiology. Otitis media and herpes zoster of the geniculate ganglion have been implicated in a few

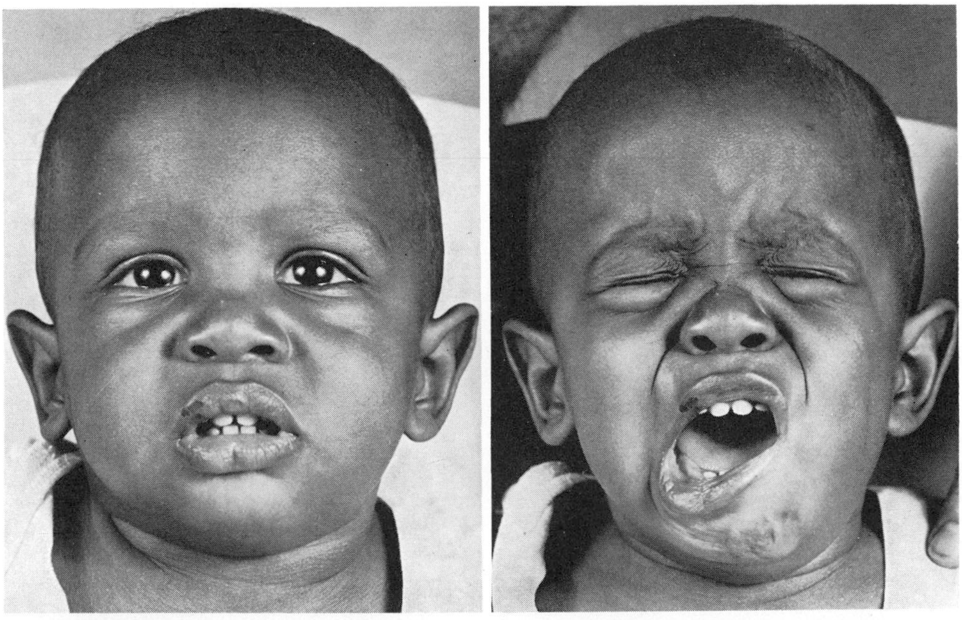

Figure 21–4 *Congenital paralysis of left inferior angle of mouth.* A, *At rest, face is symmetrical.* B, *During crying the left labial angle does not depress, and* right *facial palsy may be misdiagnosed.*

instances. The condition occurs with increased frequency in children with hypertension and with diabetes mellitus. The facial weakness appears over a few hours, occasionally with associated pain in the ear on the affected side. The face is pulled toward the normal side; the nasolabial fold on the affected side is flattened, and the child is unable to close the eye. Attempted closure leads to upward deviation of the eye (Bell's sign). Loss of taste may occur over the anterior two thirds of the tongue, and there may be hyperacusis owing to involvement of the nerve to the stapedius muscle. Occasionally, recurrent attacks of 7th nerve weakness of obscure etiology occur in association with edema of the lips, a condition known as *Melkersson syndrome.*

The *differential diagnosis* of Bell's palsy includes tumor involving brain stem or temporal bone, basal skull fracture, otitis media and mastoiditis. Therapy consists of protection of the cornea on the affected side by taping the eye in a closed position or by instillation of artificial tears into the conjunctival sac. ACTH and corticosteroids have been used to reduce inflammatory swelling of the facial nerve in Bell's palsy; there is some evidence that this form of therapy improves the outcome. Prednisone, 40 mg/day is given for three days and the dose is then tapered over a one-week period. Untreated, the incidence of permanent residual weakness is between 10 and 20 per cent.

TRAUMA TO PERIPHERAL NERVES. Trauma occurs rather frequently at birth (Erb's palsy, Section 7). Later in infancy or childhood peripheral nerves may be injured by pressure such as may occur from an improperly applied cast or IV board or from failure to position the limbs properly in a comatose child. The *peroneal nerve* is most frequently affected. Damage to this nerve leads to foot drop and to sensory impairment over the lateral aspect of the leg and the dorsum of the foot. *Radial nerve* injury causes wrist drop. Paralysis of intrinsic hand muscles with claw-hand deformity is present in *ulnar nerve* palsy.

Sciatic nerve injury by faulty intramuscular injection in the buttock is an important cause of mononeuropathy in early childhood. When this nerve is severely injured in the gluteal region, there is paralysis of knee flexion and of all movements below the knee as well as anesthesia over the foot and over the lateral aspect of the lower leg.

Pressure neuropathies usually recover as long as the nerve is protected from repeated compression. Lacerations of peripheral nerves require surgical exploration and suture of the severed nerve ends. Surgical exploration and lysis of adhesions has been recommended for postinjection injuries of the sciatic nerve when there is no evidence of improvement three months after the injury. Permanent sciatic nerve damage in early childhood results in considerable disability, including arrest of growth of the affected limb.

Adour, K. K., et al.: Prednisone treatment for idiopathic facial paralysis (Bell's palsy). New Engl. J. Med. *287*:1268, 1972.
Gilles, F. H., and French, J. H.: Postinjection sciatic nerve palsies in infants and children. J. Pediatr. *58*:195, 1961.
Hoefnagel, D., and Penry, J. K.: Partial facial paralysis in young children. New Engl. J. Med. *262*:1126, 1963.
Lloyd, A. V. C., Jewitt, D. E., and Still, J. D. L.: Facial paralysis in children with hypertension. Arch. Dis. Child *41*:292, 1966.
McHugh, H. E., Sowden, K. A., and Levitt, M. N.: Facial paralysis and muscle agenesis in the newborn. Arch. Otolaryngol. *89*:157, 1969.
Manning, J. J., and Adour, K. K.: Facial paralysis in children. Pediatrics *49*:102, 1972.
Paine, R. S.: Facial paralysis in children. Pediatrics *19*:303, 1957.
Pape, K. E., and Pickering, D.: Asymmetric crying facies and other congenital anomalies. J. Pediatr. *81*:21, 1972.
Terrence, C. F., and Samaha, F. J.: The Tolosa-Hunt syndrome (painful ophthalmoplegia) in children. Dev. Med. Child Neurol. *15*:506, 1973.

DISEASES OF THE NEUROMUSCULAR JUNCTION

There are several disorders in which muscular weakness is caused by a defect in neuromuscular transmission. Normal transmission of the nerve impulse to muscle involves three steps: (1) release of acetylcholine at terminal nerve endings; (2) action of acetylcholine at receptor sites in the muscle membrane, which leads to depolarization of this membrane; and (3) removal of the released acetylcholine through hydrolysis by the enzyme cholinesterase. Blockade of neuromuscular transmission may result from interference with any of these steps.

Several toxins, such as those of botulinus and of the tick, act by preventing release of acetylcholine (step 1). At step 2 the action of acetylcholine at receptor sites is blocked by curare; at step 3 cholinesterase inhibitors interfere with the removal of released acetylcholine. Accumulation of acetylcholine leads to dysfunction by persistent depolarization of the muscle membrane (depolarized block). Paralysis due to cholinesterase inhibition occurs in poisoning with organic phosphate insecticides (Section 28) and in overdosage of anticholinesterase drugs such as neostigmine. The most important disease of neuromuscular transmission is myasthenia gravis.

MYASTHENIA GRAVIS. Myasthenia gravis is uncommon in childhood, but its prompt recognition is of great importance, since proper therapy may be lifesaving. Despite extensive study, there is no certainty regarding the etiology of the disease. Neuromuscular blockade by a circulating curare-like substance and faulty release of acetylcholine at nerve terminals have both been implicated. It is possible that the disease is due to immunologic dysfunction. There are a high incidence of thymic hyperplasia and of thymoma, the frequent presence of circulating antimuscle antibodies, and an increased incidence of myasthenia in patients with lupus erythematosus. Three myasthenic syndromes are recognized in childhood: *transient neonatal myasthenia gravis, persistent neonatal myasthenia gravis,* and *juvenile myasthenia gravis.*

Transient Neonatal Myasthenia Gravis. This is seen only in infants whose mothers have myasthenia. The disease in the mother may be very mild and earlier unrecognized. The infant is weak and hypotonic, with poor suck, feeble respiratory effort and ptosis. Untreated, these infants may die within hours or days after birth or they may gradually improve. Recovery is complete within two to four weeks.

Persistent Neonatal Myasthenia Gravis. This presents in the neonatal period with symptoms that are identical to the transient form, but here there is no indication of myasthenia in the mother. More than one sibling may be affected. The disease persists throughout life. The eyelids and extraocular muscles tend to be most severely affected.

Juvenile Myasthenia Gravis. This usually has its onset after age 10 years; girls are affected six times as often as boys. Ptosis and double vision, owing to weakness of extraocular muscles, are the most common presenting complaints. Neck, facial, bulbar and intercostal muscles also are frequently affected. Paralysis of virtually all muscles occurs in the most severe form. A striking feature of the weakness is its amelioration after rest, and its exacerbation on repetitive movement. Sudden, life-threatening exacerbations known as myasthenic crises may occur during intercurrent infections or during stresses such as minor surgical procedures.

The diagnosis is based on the characteristic distribution of weakness and on the demonstration of progressive weakness on repetitive or sustained muscular contractions. The latter can often be brought out by having the patient maintain upward gaze, which leads to progressively increasing ptosis. Confirmation of the diagnosis is obtained by observation of the response to anticholinesterase drugs. Edrophonium chloride (Tensilon), 0.2 mg/kg IV, or neostigmine, 0.04 mg/kg IM, may be used. Increase in strength after intravenous edrophonium chloride is almost immediate but lasts for less than 5 minutes. A more prolonged response is obtained with neostigmine. Atropine sulfate, 0.01 mg/kg, should be readily available during performance of the neostigmine test and should be given if the patient develops evidence of excessive parasympathetic stimulation, such as abdominal cramps, salivation or bradycardia. Electrical testing of neuromuscular transmission is a helpful adjunct to the diagnosis; there is progressive decrease in muscle response on repetitive stimulation of nerve at low rates. The possible presence of thymoma should be explored radiologically.

Anticholinesterase drugs are effective therapeutic agents in myasthenia gravis. Pyridostigmine bromide (Mestinon) is the least toxic. The beginning dose is about 30 mg orally every 4 hours in the older child, and 5 mg every 4 hours for the infant. Neostigmine (Prostigmin) or ambenonium chloride (Mytelase) may be used instead of or in addition to pyridostigmine. The dosage of the anticholinesterase drug is gradually increased until the weakness is controlled or until symptoms of parasympathetic stimulation occur. These include lacrimation, salivation, vomiting, diarrhea, abdominal cramps and bradycardia. Further increase in dosage may be dangerous and may actually exacerbate weakness, owing to excessive accumulation of acetylcholine at the neuromuscular junction, which leads to depolarized block (see above). At times it may be difficult to be certain whether increase in weakness is due to worsening of the myasthenia or to overdosage of anticholinesterase drugs. The Tensilon test is very helpful in the differentiation, since Tensilon will improve the myasthenic symptoms, but will transiently increase weakness owing to excess of anticholinesterase drugs. The parents of a child with myasthenia gravis should be warned of the possibility of sudden exacerbation at times of stress and of the need for immediate medical attention in such an event. If possible, the therapy of severe myasthenia should be supervised at a center where physicians with wide experience in the management of this disease are available. Intermittent assisted ventilation and tracheotomy may be needed. Thymectomy or corticosteroid therapy may be indicated in intractable, severe myasthenia.

The prognosis of myasthenia gravis in childhood is somewhat better than it is in later life. With optimum therapy most children with myasthenia gravis can lead near-normal lives. Complete remissions occur in about 25 per cent of affected children.

Brunner, N. G., Namba, T., and Grob, D.: Corticosteroids in management of severe, generalized myasthenia gravis. Neurology *22*:603, 1972.

Mackay, R. I.: Congenital myasthenia gravis. Arch. Dis. Child. *26*:289, 1951.

Millichap, J. G., and Dodge, P. R.: Diagnosis and treatment of myasthenia gravis in infancy, childhood and adolescence. Neurology *10*:1007, 1960.

Osserman, K. E., and Genkins, G.: Studies in myasthenia gravis: Review of a twenty-year experience in over 1200 patients. Mt. Sinai J. Med. (N. Y.) *38*:497, 1971.

Teng, P., and Osserman, K. E.: Studies in myasthenia gravis: Neonatal and juvenile types. A report of 21 and a review of 188 cases. J. Mt. Sinai Hosp. (N. Y.) *23*:711, 1956.

DISEASES OF MUSCLE

Skeletal muscle is affected in a large number of degenerative, metabolic and inflammatory disorders. Degeneration of muscle fibers occurs in most of these, and, in the chronic state, there often is replacement of muscle by fibrous connective tissue and fat. Proximal muscles tend to be affected more severely than distal ones, and lower extremities more than the upper. As a result, children with diseases of muscle often have a waddling gait, are unable to run and have difficulty climbing stairs and standing up from the sitting position. The tendon reflexes are usually depressed in proportion to the degree of weakness. There are no sensory abnormalities.

Measurement of serum enzyme activity, especially that of creatine phosphokinase (CPK) often is a helpful laboratory test in the differential diagnosis of muscle disease. This enzyme, which catalyzes the reaction: phosphocreatine + ADP $\longrightarrow$ creatine + ATP is present primarily in brain and muscle tissues. Excessive leakage of the enzyme into the extracellular spaces and into blood occurs in several diffuse muscle diseases, especially in the muscular dystrophies. Serum lactic dehydrogenase and glutamic-oxaloacetic transaminase are also often elevated in muscle disease, but the wide distribution of these enzymes in other tissues, including liver, makes these tests less specific. A muscle biopsy is usually needed for the definitive diagnosis of muscle disease.

INFLAMMATORY DISEASES OF MUSCLE. Inflammation of muscle occurs in a number of infectious illnesses, especially in trichinosis (Section 10), toxoplasmosis and coxsackievirus infections. It also is a component of the collagen diseases Section 9, including dermatomyositis, lupus erythematosus, polyarteritis nodosa and rheumatoid arthritis. Diffuse inflammation of muscles as an isolated abnormality of unknown cause is known as polymyositis.

Polymyositis. Polymyositis presents with progressive, principally proximal, muscular weakness and pain. The neck muscles are frequently affected, and the child may have difficulty lifting his head or supporting it in the upright position. Laboratory evidence of inflammation includes elevation of sedimentation rate and of the white blood cell count, but their absence does not rule out the diagnosis. The serum enzymes are usually elevated. Muscle biopsy shows degeneration and attempted regeneration of muscle fibers and lymphocytic infiltration. The differentiation from childhood muscular dystrophy and from dermatomyositis may be difficult. It is not clear whether polymyositis represents a forme fruste of dermatomyositis. However, the histologic appearance of muscle is somewhat different in the two conditions. Evidence of vasculitis, which is prominent in childhood dermatomyositis, is usually absent in polymyositis. The prognosis is somewhat better in polymyositis. Therapy with corticosteroid hormones frequently leads to remission, but relapse may occur following steroid withdrawal.

Myositis Ossificans Progressiva. This is a rare progressive disease of connective tissue and muscle, of unknown etiology. The illness has been described in siblings, including identical twins, and in successive generations. An autosomal dominant pattern of inheritance with variable expression has been suggested. Boys are more commonly affected, at a ratio of two to three to one.

Pathologic changes depend on the age of the lesions. During the early stages localized areas of edema and inflammatory cell infiltrates are found in muscle and tendons. Later, granulation tissue replaces the areas of inflammation and, eventually, sheets of cartilage and of bone are laid down in involved areas.

About 75 per cent of affected children have congenital malformations, most commonly microdactyly and ankylosis of phalanges of the great toes; there may also be small thumbs, polydactyly, incurving of digits, webbing of toes, deformity of the ears, deafness and absence of teeth. The same anomalies may occur in relatives who do not develop the progressive connective tissue and muscle lesions. Age of onset of these lesions varies from birth to late childhood. A typical lesion evolves through three stages: (1) a localized, often hot and tender doughy swelling of soft tissue, possibly following mild local trauma; (2) after a few days the early evidences of inflammation subside, and the affected area becomes indurated; and (3) the final stage is ossification of the lesion. New lesions appear periodically, especially over the cervical and dorsal regions. Torticollis, owing to lesions in the sternocleidomastoid, may be the initial feature. Eventually there is widespread ossification of tendons and fascia. The spine and the joints of the extremities become ankylosed (Fig. 21–5). The masseter and mandibular joints are likely to be affected, leading to difficulty in chewing. Spicules of bone may be extruded through the skin. Severe incapacitation and death from respiratory failure often occurs in the early adult years; cases of sur-

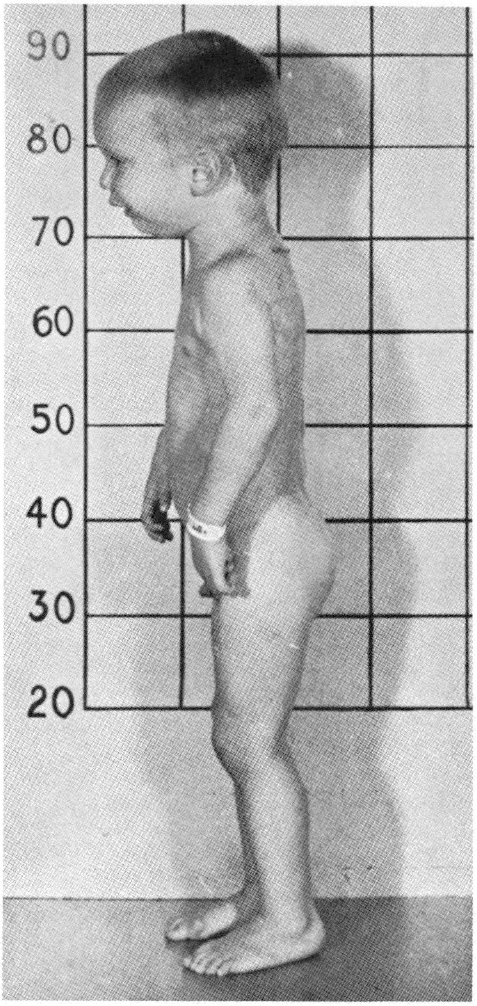

Figure 21–5 *Myositis ossificans progressiva. No radiographically demonstrable calcification, but typical histologic changes. Note posture and rigidity of neck and back.*

vival to old age have been reported. The incidence of osteosarcoma is increased.

The same process may at times remain localized to one area, usually following definite trauma to soft tissue *(myositis ossificans circumscripta)*. Widespread calcification of muscle also may occur in chronic polymyositis and dermatomyositis.

Laboratory studies are of little help in the diagnosis. Serum calcium, phosphate and alkaline phosphatase values are normal, as are those of creatine phosphokinase and the other serum enzymes. Analysis of the bone in the soft tissues has not shown any difference from normal bone.

Therapy often is unsatisfactory; corticosteroids and ACTH have been reported to decrease the rate of progression in a few cases. It is doubtful, however, whether they have a significant effect on the eventual outcome.

ENDOCRINE MYOPATHIES. Muscular weakness, at times severe, occurs in a number of endocrine disorders, these require consideration in the differential diagnosis of progressive weakness of obscure etiology.

Hyperthyroid Myopathy. This is an uncommon complication of thyrotoxicosis. Ptosis, bifacial weakness and proximal weakness of limb muscles are manifestations. Some of the usual signs of hyperthyroidism may be masked by the weakness. Tachycardia, excessive sweating and enlargement of the thyroid gland, however, are manifest. The tendon reflexes remain brisk, in contrast to all other forms of myopathy. The weakness improves slowly after correction of the hyperthyroid state.

Hypothyroidism. Hypothyroidism in the infant is associated with weakness and hypotonia. In the older child with myxedema there is weakness, slowness of muscular contraction and relaxation, and at times muscular hypertrophy (Debré-Sémélaigne syndrome). The combination of weakness and muscular hypertrophy may lead to the erroneous diagnosis of muscular dystrophy.

Corticosteroid Myopathy. This may complicate Cushing's disease, but is seen more commonly during therapy with high doses of synthetic steroids. Weakness is most marked in the hip girdle muscles, leading to a waddling gait and to difficulty in standing and in climbing stairs. The knee jerks are depressed. Muscle wasting may be marked. Myopathic changes may be seen in muscle tissue, but they are usually mild, even when weakness is profound. Recovery after discontinuance of steroid therapy is slow, taking months.

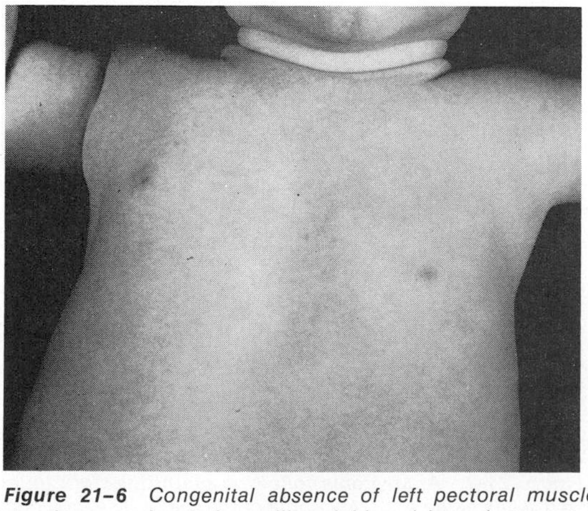

Figure 21–6 Congenital absence of left pectoral muscle. Note absence of anterior axillary fold and low placement of nipple.

Hyperparathyroidism. Hyperparathyroidism leads to weakness and hyporeflexia, which appear to be secondary to hypercalcemia; they are readily reversed after correction of the metabolic abnormality by parathyroidectomy.

CONGENITAL DEFECTS OF MUSCLE

Congenital Absence of Muscle. Failure of muscle development may be widespread, leading to immobility of multiple joints, a condition known as arthrogryposis multiplex congenita (Section 22). More commonly, congenital absence is limited to one muscle. Absence of the sternal head of the pectoralis major is a frequent isolated anomaly (Fig. 21–6). Occasionally syndactyly is found on the same side. (See Poland Syndrome, Section 29.) Absence of the pectoral muscle is found with increased frequency in children with muscular dystrophy. Congenital absence of abdominal muscles is often associated with anomalies of the urinary tract. (See Prune-Belly Syndrome, page 1247.)

Congenital Torticollis. Torticollis or wry neck is due to shortening or contracture of the sternocleidomastoid muscle on one side. The head is tilted toward the side of the contracture and the chin is turned toward the opposite side (Fig. 21–7). Considerable resistance is encountered to attempts to correct the deviation. A firm mass may be palpable in the involved sternocleidomastoid muscle. The cause of this condition is unclear; birth trauma has long been incriminated. However, torticollis has occasionally been observed at cesarean section, suggesting a prenatal cause in at least some cases.

The differential diagnosis of congenital torticollis includes head tilt secondary to malformation of the cervical spine, such as occurs in the Klippel-Feil anomaly, and fracture or dislocation of cervical vertebrae. Roentgenograms of the cervical spine should be obtained to rule these out. In the older child head tilt may also occur secondary to strabismus, dystonia, posterior fossa or cervical cord tumor, myositis ossificans, cervical adenitis or hiatus hernia. Most infants with congenital torticollis improve with simple muscle-stretching exercises. Persistent torticollis leads to asymmetric development of the face and skull (Fig. 21–7) and may have to be treated with surgical section of the affected muscle to assure a good cosmetic outcome.

Congenital Myopathies. This group includes several rare inherited disorders in which weakness and hypotonia are present from infancy. (See the "floppy infant," Table 21–1.) The correct diagnosis of these disorders is important from a prognostic standpoint. In general, the outlook for a normal life span and useful existence is good in contrast to that of the hypotonic infant with Werdnig-Hoffmann disease or with congenital muscular dys-

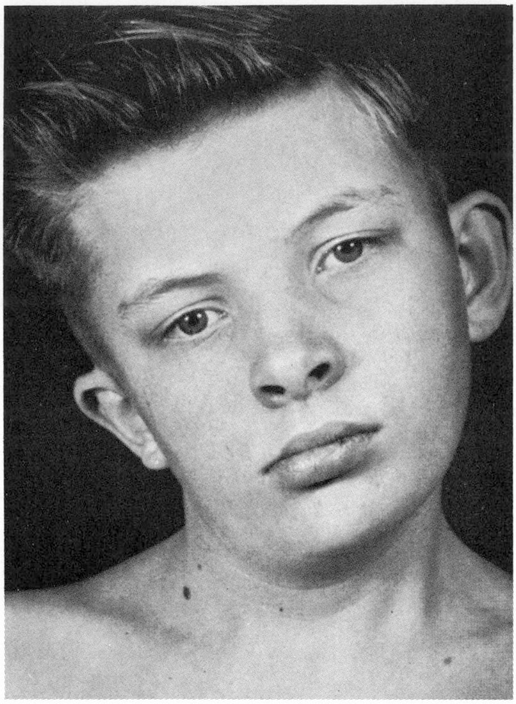

Figure 21–7 Congenital torticollis, untreated until age of 12 years. Note wryneck and deformity of face.

trophy. The identification of the congenital myopathies is dependent on study of biopsies of skeletal muscle.

Central Core Disease. In central core disease the center of each muscle fiber shows abnormal, homogenous staining. Electronmicroscopy shows a marked decrease of mitochondria and of sarcoplasmic reticulum in the central portion of the affected fibers.

Nemaline Myopathy. Nemaline myopathy derives its name from the presence of thread-like structures within muscle cells. Electronmicroscopy indicates that these are the result of abnormalities of the Z bands of myofibrils.

Several myopathies have been described in which alteration of muscle mitochondria is the most prominent finding. In *megaconial myopathy* the mitochondria are abnormally large. In *pleoconial myopathy* they are increased in number. The latter condition presents with weakness and hypotonia in infancy and with episodic weakness later in childhood.

MYOTONIA. Myotonia is a symptom of a variety of muscle diseases, including myotonic dystrophy, the hyperkalemic form of familial periodic paralysis and glycogen storage disease of muscle. It is defined as abnormal slowness in relaxation of muscle following voluntary or induced muscular contraction. Clinically it manifests itself by inability to relax the hand grip, and by visible maintained contraction following direct stimulation of a muscle by sharp tap (Fig. 21–8 *A*). The latter is demonstrated by tapping a superficial muscle group such as the tongue or the thenar eminence with a reflex hammer. The presence of myotonia is confirmed by electromyography, which shows persistence of muscle action potentials following relaxation of voluntary contraction (myotonic discharges).

Myotonia Congenita (Thomsen's Disease). This is a disorder in which myotonia occurs as an isolated finding. It is transmitted by dominant inheritance. The disease may be manifest in infancy as slow swallowing and gagging, owing to failure of normal relaxation of oropharyngeal muscles. Later in childhood, inability to release a firm hand grip may attract attention. The muscles tend to become stiff when the child first attempts to carry out a motion. This stiffness gradually subsides when the movement is repeated a few times. For example, a patient with myotonia congenita may have difficulty initiating the act of walking. The first few steps tend to be slow and awkward. After a few seconds of practice the gait becomes normal, or nearly so. These symptoms are worse during emotional upset and on exposure to cold. Strength is normal and muscles are well developed, often unusually large, giving the child an athletic appearance.

The diagnosis is based on the clinical and electromyographic demonstration of myotonia. Serum enzymes are normal. The only histologic alteration is hypertrophy of muscle fibers.

Differentiation from myotonic dystrophy is based on the absence of muscle weakness or atrophy and on the lack of dystrophic changes in biopsies of muscles. Therapy with procainamide or quinidine sulfate lessens the myotonia and is indicated when there is significant functional im-

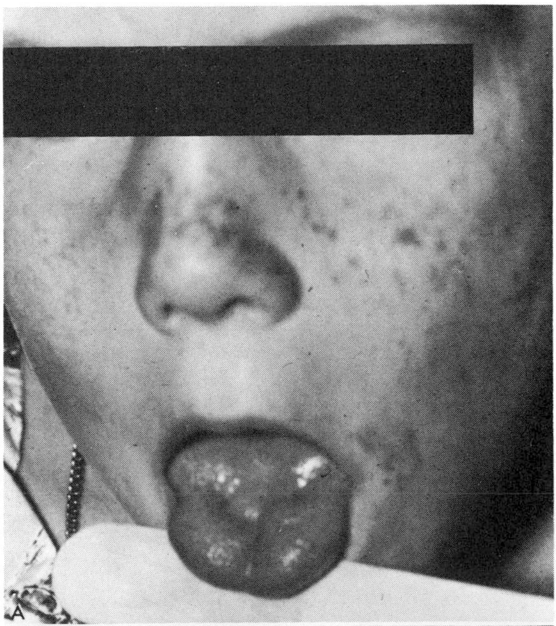

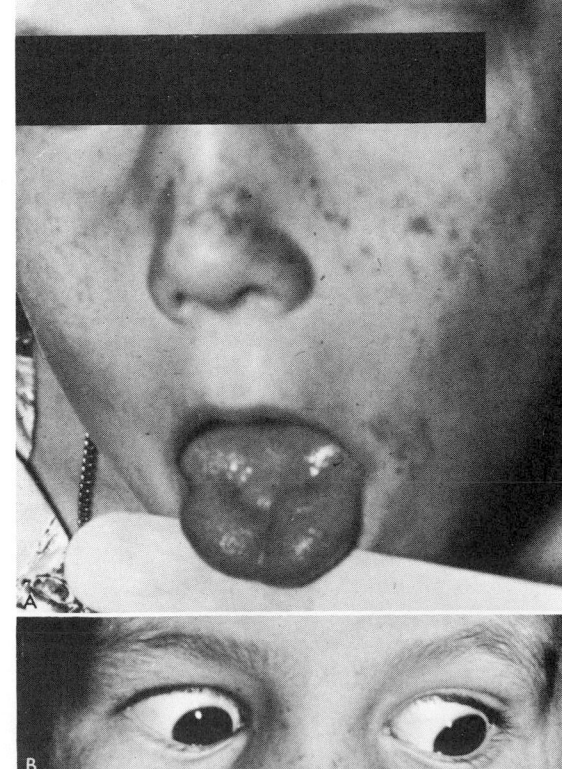

Figure 21–8 A, Myotonia following tap of the right tongue with a reflex hammer. B, Myotonia of the eyelid. The lid remains contracted when the child is asked to look down. The child has the hyperkalemic form of familial periodic paralysis.

pairment. The disorder is benign and may improve with age.

THE PERIODIC PARALYSES. In this group of illnesses weakness occurs intermittently with complete or nearly complete recovery of muscle strength between attacks. The group includes muscle phosphorylase deficiency (McArdle's disease, Section 8) in addition to the conditions discussed here.

Hyperkalemic Periodic Paralysis. *Adynamia episodica hereditaria* or *paramyotonia* is transmitted as a dominant trait, with more severe expression in the male. Onset is during early childhood and sometimes in infancy. Rest after strong exertion appears to precipitate paralytic episodes. Weakness develops rapidly. The legs are most severely affected; muscles of respiration are usually spared. Attacks rarely last for more than a few hours. Myotonia is common and may persist between attacks. It tends to be most marked in the eyelids, resulting in lid lag when the patient is asked to look downward. (Fig. 21–8 *B*).

During the attack the serum concentration of potassium is often elevated, but repeated measurements during several episodes may be necessary to demonstrate it. An oral potassium load of 2 to 3 gm may be used to precipitate an attack, but should be given only when an EKG monitor is available. Acetazolamide is effective in preventing recurrent paralysis. The most severely affected patients eventually develop mild persistent weakness and dystrophic changes in muscle.

Hypokalemic Periodic Paralysis. *Familial periodic paralysis* also is transmitted in a dominant manner; the symptoms are more severe in males. Onset is somewhat later than in the hyperkalemic form; the first attacks usually occur in late childhood or early adolescence. Large, predominantly carbohydrate meals or rest after strong exertion may precipitate the paralysis. Typically the patient wakes up paralyzed in the morning following a day of heavy exercise capped by a large evening meal. During the attack the limbs are flaccid and areflexic. The muscles of respiration may be affected. An attack may last longer than 24 hours. Serum potassium values are usually low, in the 2 to 3 mEq/l range, during the paralytic phase. The basic defect is unknown. Patients with repeated severe attacks eventually develop fixed weakness and dystrophic changes in muscle. Therapy during an attack consists of oral administration of potassium chloride, beginning with a dose of 2 to 3 gm. Acetazolamide is effective in reducing the frequency of attacks.

Paroxysmal Myoglobinuria. Idiopathic myoglobinuria includes a heterogeneous group of clinical entities in which attacks of paralysis and associated myoglobinuria occur spontaneously or following strenuous exercise. Dominant and sex-linked inheritance has been described in different families. The affected muscles, often of the calf and thigh, become painful and swollen during an attack. The urine becomes dark red or brown. The myoglobinuria may cause renal tubular necrosis, with death from renal failure.

The diagnosis is confirmed by demonstration of myoglobin in urine. A positive benzidine test in urine free of red cells suggests the presence of myoglobin, especially when a concomitant serum sample is clear (free of hemoglobin). Definite differentiation from hemoglobin is accomplished by spectrophotometry. Paroxysmal myoglobinuria must be distinguished from McArdle's disease (Section 8) and from the myoglobinuria which may occur in a normal person following severe unaccustomed exertion or following crushing injury of muscle. Myoglobinuria after heavy exertion occurs occasionally in pseudohypertrophic (Duchenne) muscular dystrophy.

Treatment consists of bed rest, assisted ventilation when necessary, and hydration to minimize the danger of renal injury.

THE MUSCULAR DYSTROPHIES. The muscular dystrophies are a group of disorders of genetic origin in which gradual degeneration of muscle fibers occurs. Their classification is based on age of onset, rate of progression of weakness, distribution of muscular involvement and mode of inheritance.

Pseudohypertrophic Muscular Dystrophy. The *childhood* or *Duchenne* form of muscular dystrophy is the commonest of this group of muscle diseases, with an incidence of about 0.14/1000 children. In its classic form it occurs only in boys. A history of sex-linked inheritance is obtained for about 50 per cent of propositi. The remainder occur sporadically and appear to represent mutations. The diagnosis is rarely made prior to age 3 years. However, a history of slow motor development with late onset of sitting, walking and running is usually obtained, indicating a much earlier onset. Waddling gait, difficulty in climbing stairs and hypertrophy of calf muscles are the common presenting findings. Occasionally muscles other than the calf, including deltoid, brachioradialis and tongue, are increased in bulk. The term "pseudohypertrophy" is used; early in the disease the hypertrophied muscles have considerable strength, but later the enlarged muscles are often weak since much of the increased bulk is due to fatty infiltration. The hypertrophic calf muscles are stronger than the anterior leg muscles, and this accounts for the frequent presence of toe walking and contracture of the heel cords. Weakness of pelvic girdle muscles results in the characteristic waddling, lordotic gait and in difficulty in arising from the floor. The child with moderately severe muscular dystrophy demonstrates Gowers' sign: in getting up from the floor he first rolls to the prone position, kneels, and then raises himself to standing by pushing with his hands against shins, knees and thighs (Fig. 21–9). Weakness of shoulder girdle muscles can be brought out by lifting the child with the examiner's hands under the axillae. He will slip through the examiner's hands rather than support himself by adducting the arms. Eventually the child becomes unable to lift his arms above his head. Profound muscle atrophy occurs in the late stages. Ambulation usually becomes impossible by age 12 years, and death occurs prior to age 20 years in 75 per cent of patients. Cardiomyopathy is

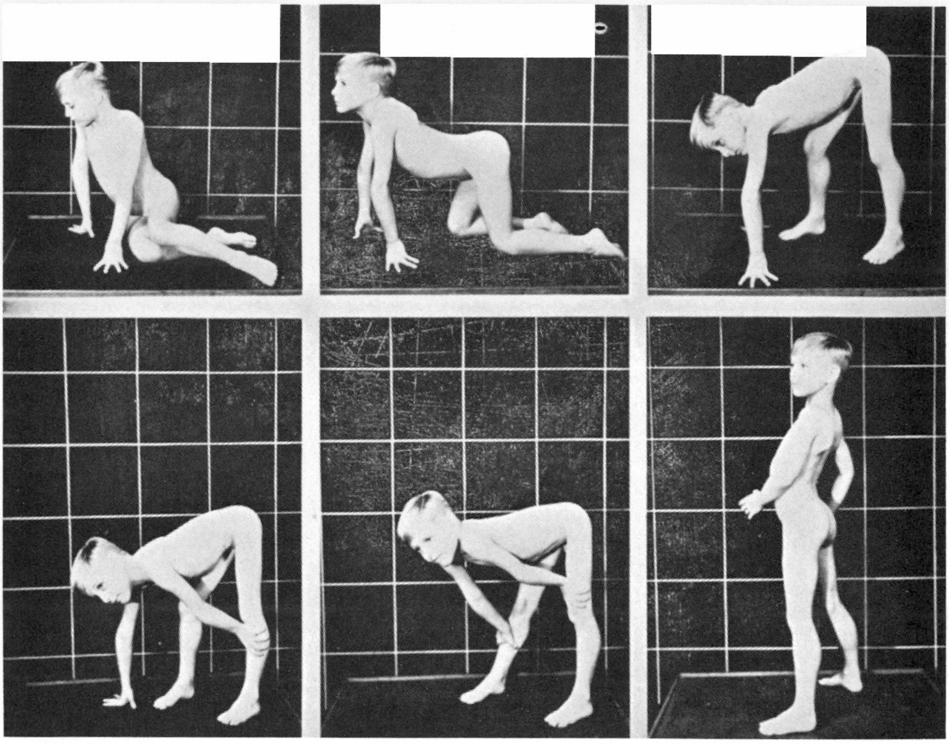

Figure 21–9 A child 7 years of age with pseudohypertrophic muscular dystrophy, showing characteristic manner of rising from the floor. The last picture shows the standing position with the severe lordosis.

present in the majority of patients and occasionally is the cause of sudden death. There are instances of sex-linked pseudohypertrophic muscular dystrophy in which onset is in late childhood and survival is prolonged. Mild mental defect is a commonly associated abnormality in the Duchenne form of muscular dystrophy. The mean IQ of children with Duchenne muscular dystrophy is about 20 points below the normal mean, and frank mental defect is present in about 25 per cent.

The *differential diagnosis* of Duchenne muscular dystrophy includes the late infantile form of Werdnig-Hoffmann disease and a number of diseases of muscle such as the endocrine myopathies, glycogen storage disease of muscle and polymyositis. Occasionally the presence of heel cord contractures and of toe walking leads to the erroneous diagnosis of cerebral palsy. However, the spasticity and hyperreflexia found in cerebral palsy are absent in muscular dystrophy.

The *diagnosis* of Duchenne muscular dystrophy is confirmed by measurement of serum enzymes, by electromyography and by muscle biopsy. The serum enzymes, especially CPK, are increased as much as ten times normal, more so in infancy prior to appearance of clinical weakness. Electromyography shows myopathic changes consisting primarily of a decrease in amplitude and duration of motor unit potentials. Histologic changes in muscle include degeneration of muscle fibers, with variation in fiber size and central nuclei, and replacement of muscle fibers by fat and by connective tissue. The diagnosis of muscular dystrophy can be established at birth by measurement of CPK levels; intrauterine diagnosis is as yet not possible. Identification of female carriers of the disease by laboratory tests cannot be achieved with certainty. There is mild to moderate elevation of serum CPK in 60 to 80 per cent of known carriers; this is more likely to occur during childhood than later in life.

There is no effective treatment for childhood muscular dystrophy. The children should be kept active and in an ambulatory state as long as possible. Very strenuous exercise is to be avoided, since it may hasten the breakdown of muscle fibers. Occasionally surgical lengthening of the heel cords may improve ambulation. Prolonged bed rest, however, after orthopedic procedures may hasten muscle atrophy. Genetic counseling is an important aspect of management. When there is a pattern of sex-linked inheritance, male siblings of an affected child have a 50 per cent chance of being afflicted; the sisters have a 50 per cent chance of being carriers.

Congenital Muscular Dystrophy. An autosomal recessive disorder, this is a cause of hypotonia and weakness in infancy and should be considered in the differential diagnosis of the "floppy infant" (Table 21–1). The onset is in utero. Occasionally, profound muscle atrophy, contractures and limitation of joint movements are present at birth. Clinically the differentiation from Werdnig-Hoffmann disease is difficult. Fasciculations of the tongue, a common finding in Werdnig-Hoffmann disease, however, do not occur in congenital muscular dystrophy. The tendon reflexes are depressed, but usually not completely absent. Muscles of respiration, including the diaphragms, are affected. The most severely ill infants die of respiratory failure prior to age 1 year; milder forms may be compatible with prolonged survival. Serum enzymes are not so consistently elevated as in Duchenne muscular dystrophy. Dystrophic changes in muscle can be seen in tissue biopsies.

Facioscapulohumeral Muscular Dystrophy. This is a mild form of dystrophy which is transmitted on an autosomal dominant basis. Onset is usually in the second decade, with weakness and atrophy of facial and shoulder girdle muscles. The face is expressionless; forceful eye closure and whistling are not possible. The illness progresses slowly and is compatible with a normal life span. The diagnosis is based on the clinical findings and on the pattern of inheritance. Biopsy of affected muscles shows dystrophic changes. The serum CPK may be normal or mildly elevated.

Limb-Girdle Muscular Dystrophy. This is a term applied to a heterogeneous group of patients with slowly progressive muscular dystrophy. Onset may be in later childhood or adolescence or in adulthood. The pelvic girdle muscles are most commonly affected. The disorder is usually transmitted on an autosomal recessive basis.

Ocular Myopathy. This is a dystrophic process that affects principally the extraocular muscles. Onset is usually during childhood or adolescence, with progressive ptosis and limitation of eye movements; occasionally the weakness extends to facial and neck muscles. No clear inheritance pattern has been established. This disorder must be differentiated from myasthenia gravis and from cranial nerve palsies resulting from a tumor in the brain stem.

Myotonic Dystrophy. Usually thought to have its onset in adulthood, myotonic dystrophy has recently been found to begin in infancy and childhood in a significant proportion of patients. The illness is transmitted on an autosomal dominant basis. It is of interest that patients with onset in childhood almost always have an affected mother, suggesting that a factor in the intrauterine environment influences the severity of expression. Hypotonia and poor sucking ability may be present at birth. Developmental delay is noted later in infancy, as is mental retardation. In early childhood muscle weakness and atrophy are found principally in the facial, jaw and temporalis muscles; bilateral ptosis is common. Myotonia may be demonstrated by percussion of muscle, by electromyography or by the child's inability to relax a hand grip (see above). Weakness and atrophy of limb muscles, often distal in distribution, become evident in late childhood and adolescence. Cataracts, baldness and testicular atrophy are characteristic of the adult form of the disease.

The diagnosis of myotonic dystrophy is based on the demonstration of myotonia, along with the characteristic distribution of weakness, history of dominant inheritance, and demonstration of dystrophic changes on muscle biopsy. The prognosis of the childhood form of the disease must be guarded. Mental defect is usually present, and the muscle weakness is apt to be a second major handicap by the time the patient reaches adulthood. Treatment with procainamide or quinine is indicated in the occasional patient in whom myotonia is severe enough to lead to functional impairment.

PETER R. HUTTENLOCHER

Byers, R. K., Bergman, A. B., and Joseph, M. C.: Steroid myopathy. Pediatrics *29*:26, 1962.

Dodge, P. R., Gamstorp, I., Byers, R. K., and Russell, P.: Myotonic dystrophy in infancy and childhood. Pediatrics *35*:3, 1965.

Dowben, R. M., Vawter, G. F., et al.: Polymyositis and other diseases resembling muscular dystrophy. Arch. Intern. Med. *115*:584, 1965.

Drachman, D. H.: Ophthalmoplegia plus. Arch. Neurol. *18*:654, 1968.

Dubowitz, V.: Intellectual impairment in muscular dystrophy. Arch. Dis. Child. *40*:296, 1965.

Engel, W. K., et al.: Central core disease—an investigation of a rare muscle cell abnormality. Brain *84*:167, 1961.

Favara, B. E., Vawter, G. F., et al.: Familial paroxysmal rhabdomyolysis in children. Am. J. Med. *42*:196, 1967.

Frame, B., et al.: Myopathy in primary hyperparathyroidism. Ann. Intern. Med. *68*:1022, 1968.

Gonatas, N. K., Shy, G. M., and Godfrey, E. H.: Nemaline myopathy: The origin of nemaline structures. New Engl. J. Med. *274*:535, 1966.

Harper, P. S., and Dyken, P. R.: Early-onset dystrophia myotonica. Evidence supporting a maternal environmental factor. Lancet *1*:53, 1972.

Illingworth, R. S.: Myositis ossificans progressiva (Munchmeyer disease). Arch. Dis. Child. *46*:264, 1971.

Jackson, C. E., and Strehler, D. A.: Limb-girdle muscular dystrophy: Clinical manifestations and detection of preclinical disease. Pediatrics *41*:495, 1968.

Layzer, R. B., Lovelace, R. E., and Rowland, L. P.: Hyperkalemic periodic paralysis. Arch. Neurol. *16*:455, 1967.

Lockhart, J. D., and Burke, F. G.: Myositis ossificans progressiva. Report of a case treated with corticotropin (ACTH) Am. J. Dis. Child. *87*:626, 1954.

McArdle, B.: Familial periodic paralysis. Brit. Med. Bull. *12*:226, 1956.

Najjar, S. S., and Nachman, H. S.: Kocher-Debré-Sémélaigne syndrome: Hypothyroidism with muscular "hypertrophy." J. Pediatr. *66*:901, 1965.

Pearson, C. M.: The periodic paralyses: Differential features and pathological observations in permanent myopathic weakness. Brain *87*:391, 1964.

Ramsey, I.: Thyrotoxic muscle disease. Postgrad. Med. J. *44*:385, 1968.

Resnick, J. S., Engel, W. K., Griggs, R. C., and Stam, A. C.: Acetazolamide prophylaxis in hypokalemic periodic paralysis. New Engl. J. Med. *278*:582, 1968.

Shy, G. M., Gonatas, N. K., and Perez, M.: Two childhood myopathies with abnormal mitochondria. 1. Megaconial myopathy. 2. Pleoconial myopathy. Brain *89*:133, 1966.

Shy, G. M., and Magee, K. R.: A new congenital nonprogressive myopathy. Brain *79*:610, 1956.

Smith, H. L., Amick, L. D., and Johnson, W. W.: Detection of subclinical and carrier states in Duchenne muscular dystrophy. J. Pediatr. *69*:67, 1966.

Thompson, C. E.: Polymyositis in children. Clin. Pediatr. *7*:24, 1968.

Vignos, P. J., Jr., Bowling, G. F., and Watkins, M. P.: Polymyositis. Effect of corticosteroids on final results. Arch. Intern. Med. *114*:263, 1964.

Zellweger, H., Afifi, A., McCormick, W. F., and Mergner, W.: Severe congenital muscular dystrophy. J. Dis. Child. *114*:591, 1967.

Zundel, W. S., and Tyler, F. H.: The muscular dystrophies. New Engl. J. Med. *273*:537; 596, 1965.

22
THE BONES AND JOINTS

The disturbances of the skeleton are divided here somewhat arbitrarily into two subsections: Skeletal Defects and Pediatric Orthopedics. In the first subsection are grouped various anatomic defects, many of which are genetically determined. Some develop in utero, some after birth. For the majority of them there is no therapy, but there are exceptions, e.g., the craniosynostoses, the funnel chest deformities associated with cardiorespiratory embarrassment, and basilar impression (platybasia) associated with compression of the brain stem.

The section entitled Pediatric Orthopedics includes the skeletal disturbances likely to be the joint concern of the pediatrician and the orthopedic surgeon. The remediable congenital dislocations and deformities are included in this division.

SKELETAL DEFECTS

Defects in Ossification of the Skull

ANENCEPHALY
(Acrania)

See Section 20.

CRANIOSYNOSTOSIS

Premature closure of one or more sutures of the skull results in deformity of the head and may cause damage to the brain and the eyes.

ETIOLOGY. Congenital craniosynostosis originates in embryonic life for unknown reasons and may be associated with other skeletal defects. In other instances craniosynostosis may be postnatal, as in rickets, hypophosphatasia, idiopathic hypercalcemia and other disorders. Early recognition of the congenital synostoses is important, since some may be responsible for damage to the brain, and in all instances there will be some degree of cranial deformity.

PATHOLOGY. In the normal newborn infant the bones of the cranium are separated, but soon after birth the definitive sutures are established. The edges of the flat bones are separated by fibrous tissue in which growth takes place perpendicular to the line of the suture. When a suture is obliterated, growth ceases and fibrous tissue disappears. Premature closure leads to deformity because growth of the vault is restricted at right angles to the involved suture and compensatory growth takes place in the regions where the sutures are open. The definitive sutures, such as the coronal, sagittal and lambdoid, begin to close after the thirtieth year.

CLINICAL FORMS. When the *sagittal suture* is closed prematurely, the head becomes long and narrow *(scaphocephaly),* and a bony ridge often marks the obliterated suture. Males are affected more often than females. Associated ocular or neurologic abnormalities are rarely related to the abnormality of the suture.

Closure of the *coronal suture* results in severe deformity *(oxycephaly, acrocephaly),* with involvement of the face and the orbits. The roof of the orbit is depressed, exophthalmos develops, and there may be strabismus, nystagmus, papilledema, optic atrophy and loss of vision. The complications are more severe in those patients in whom *both coronal sutures* are obliterated or in whom other sutures are involved. Other malformations such as cardiac anomalies, choanal atresia or defects of the elbow and knee joints may also be present. Syndactylism is the most frequently associated anomaly (see below). A familial form of closure of the coronal sutures associated with hemolytic jaundice has been reported.

Acrocephalosyndactyly (Apert syndrome) is a disorder consisting of pointing of the head anteriorly (acrocephaly), abnormalities of the sutures and syndactyly of the hands and sometimes of the feet. It has been observed in more than one generation and is thought to be transmitted on an autosomal dominant basis.

Acrocephalopolysyndactyly (Carpenter syndrome) has certain similarities to the Apert syndrome and to the Laurence-Moon-Biedl syndrome (Section 17). In addition to the acrocephaly, the syndrome is characterized by a peculiar facies, brachysyndactyly of the fingers, preaxial polydactyly, and syndactyly of the toes, hypogenitalism, obesity and mental retardation. It is transmitted on an autosomal recessive basis.

Craniofacial dysostosis (Crouzon's disease) is a syndrome characterized by acrocephaly, a beak-shaped nose, hypoplastic maxilla, short upper and protruding lower lips, hypertelorism, exophthalmos and external strabismus. This disorder is transmitted as a dominant hereditary trait with variable expressivity.

DIFFERENTIAL DIAGNOSIS. Oxycephaly must be distinguished from a familial form of high skulls in which premature closure of the sutures does not take place. In microcephaly the head is small, owing to failure of the brain to grow; there are no evidences of increased intracranial pressure. The vault is symmetrical. Although the anterior fontanel closes early, the sutures are not obliterated.

Roentgenograms of the skull in craniosynostosis reveal an abnormally shaped head and secondary changes in the bones of the face and in the floor of the skull, depending on the suture or sutures involved. The involved suture may be obliterated or marked by a thin lucent line, but there is frequently thickening of bone along the suture and bony bridging (Fig. 22–1).

PROGNOSIS. Closure of the sagittal suture is rarely associated with complications except for the cosmetic ones of a long narrow head. In other congenital forms of craniosynostosis there may be compression of the brain or cranial nerves, which requires surgical treatment. In rare instances premature synostosis occurs as a hereditary trait which results only in deformity of the skull without compression of the brain.

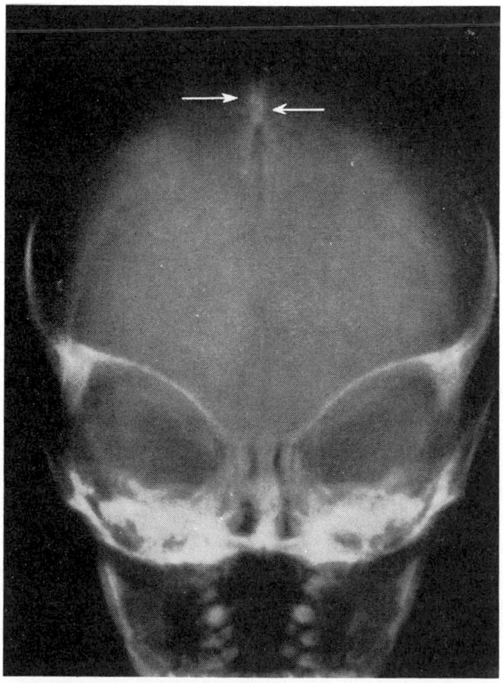

Figure 22–1 Craniosynostosis. The sagittal suture is narrow and bridged by bone (arrows). The skull was elongated in its anteroposterior dimension.

TREATMENT. When the lesion, e. g., coronal or multiple synostoses, is one which may result in significant cerebral or visual damage, surgical intervention in early infancy may lessen or avoid such damage. There is lack of evidence to support the decision to repair isolated sagittal synostosis except for cosmetic or psychologic reasons. Surgical treatment consists in linear craniectomy along the prematurely closed suture. Since there is rapid growth of the brain during the first 6 months of life, surgery will be most effective when performed soon after birth. Secondary closure of one or more of the cranial sutures occurs months after birth and only rarely requires surgical treatment.

BASILAR IMPRESSION

(Occipitalization of the Atlas; Platybasia)

This condition may be primary or secondary. In *primary* basilar impression, which is perhaps better designated as occipitalization or assimilation of the atlas, there is a congenital malformation, with encroachment upon the upper cervical vertebral canal and posterior cranial fossa. The first and second occipital segments and the first and second cervical vertebrae may all be fused into one bony mass, similar to the fusion or failure of segmentation of the cervical vertebrae below the second one in the Klippel-Feil syndrome.

Secondary basilar impression occurs when disease has softened the cranial bones to such an extent that they no longer suffice to support the weight of the head. This may occur in rickets and certain forms of osteomalacia. The posterior cranial fossa is encroached upon as the cranial vertex approaches the occiput. Flattening of the base of the skull (platybasia or an increased basal angle) is at times associated with basilar impression.

With either primary or secondary basilar impression the medulla may be kinked over the odontoid process of the second cervical vertebra, with resultant pressure upon the spinal tracts. Localized thickening of the dura at the craniovertebral junction is frequently associated with these bony anomalies and contributes to constriction of the brain stem.

The encroachment of the osseous structures upon the brain stem may be relieved in some instances by surgical means.

HYPERTELORISM

This condition, characterized by an abnormally large distance between the eyes and an apparent broadening of the root of the nose, is a nonspecific sign and not a disease entity. It is often associated

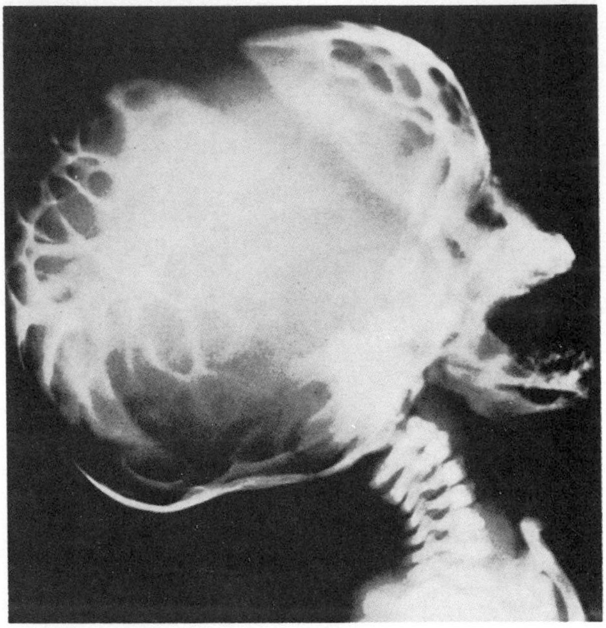

Figure 22–2 *A typical example of lacunar skull (age, 18 days). Note the arborizing patterns of bony ridges which sharply delineate and separate rounded defects from one another. This patient had a large lumbosacral meningocele. (Vogt and Wyatt:* Radiology, *Vol. 36, 1941.)*

with mental deficiency and may be combined with other congenital defects. Mild forms occur in otherwise normal children. The lesser wings of the sphenoid bone are overdeveloped, the greater wings relatively small. Hypertelorism can be transmitted through several generations. The diagnosis is made by determining the distance between the pupils, rather than by inspection alone. Epicanthic folds may result in an appearance similar to hypertelorism, but the interpupillary distance is normal. In Waardenburg syndrome, for example, there is **dystopia canthi**, with lateral displacement of the lacrimal points.

PARIETAL FORAMINA

These are irregularly shaped congenital defects with well defined margins symmetrically placed on each side of the posterior third of the sagittal suture. They can be felt, but frequently their presence is discovered roentgenographically. They may be transmitted through several generations or occur sporadically in otherwise normal persons. At times they are associated with other congenital defects of skeleton, eye, central nervous system or heart. They must be distinguished from defects of the skull associated with meningoencephalocele or from defects caused by the reticuloendothelioses, infection, multiple myeloma or malignant metastases. Parietal foramina do not cause discomfort, and no treatment is indicated.

LACUNAR SKULL

This cranial anomaly is characterized by defects in the vault in the form of shallow depressions or deep cavitations extending to the outer surface and occurring mainly in the frontal or parietal areas. The thinned areas of bone are lined by dura and bordered by ridges of osseous tissue. The outer surface of the skull is smooth, but the inner table is rough, and on the irregular surface are many interlacing columns of bone surrounding oval depressions covered with a parchment-like membrane or a thin layer of bone. The roentgenographic appearance is diagnostic and shows diminution in the thickness of the skull bones and variations in their density as irregular patches of rarefaction, or lacunae, separated by ridges of increased density (Fig. 22–2). Differentiation must be made from the generalized "hammered-silver" or "digital impression" appearance of the skull bones, which is observed on occasion without any apparent explanation for it and in other instances in association with increased intracranial pressure.

Meningocele is the most frequently associated defect. Lacunar skull can be detected in roentgenograms of about half the infants with meningocele or myelomeningocele. When a meningocele is associated with a lacunar skull, progressive hydrocephalus is a frequent complication. As the cranium enlarges, the bony ridges become thin and the lacunae disappear.

Deformities of the Vertebrae, Scapulae and Sternum

KLIPPEL-FEIL SYNDROME. In this syndrome there is a reduced number of cervical vertebrae, or there are multiple hemivertebrae fused into one osseous mass. Basilar impression, spina bifida, scoliosis, torticollis, Sprengel's deformity or other malformations may be associated. The neck is short, the hairline low. The motion of the neck is limited. In severe cases neurologic complications may develop.

CONGENITAL ABSENCE OF CAUDAL SPINE (SACRAL AGENESIS). The clinical picture varies in cases of agenesis of the caudal vertebrae. If the first sacral vertebra is present, the bony ring of the pelvis is complete, and the weight of the trunk is transmitted normally. If the sacrum is completely missing and the iliac bones are in direct contact, the transverse diameter of the pelvis is diminished, the buttocks are flattened, and their cleft is short. Muscular atrophy of the legs is particularly notable below the knees. Dislocation of the hip, clubfoot, spina bifida, arthrogryposis, renal anomalies and fecal incontinence are additional manifestations. Roentgenograms reveal the extent of the skeletal anomaly. A syndrome of anomalies of the lower spine and of the lower extremities has been observed in children of diabetic mothers ("caudal dysplasia [regression] syndrome").

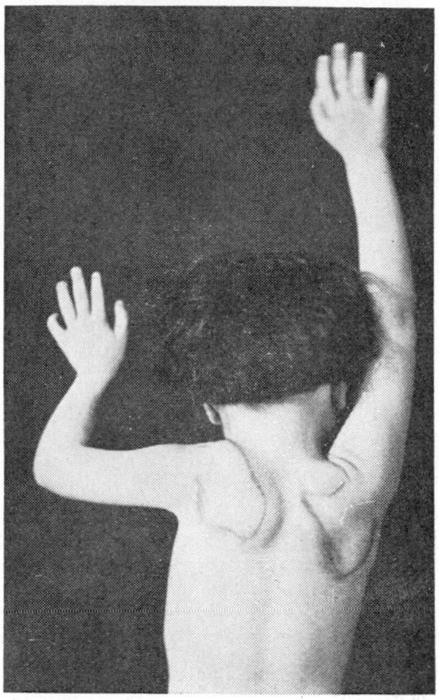

Figure 22–3 Sprengel's deformity, showing inability to raise the arm completely on the affected side.

SPRENGEL'S DEFORMITY. In this congenital deformity (Fig. 22–3) one or both scapulae are in a high position, with the lower angle turned toward the spine. Sometimes a bridge of bone unites the spine to the scapula (omovertebral bone). The arm on the affected side cannot be raised above a right angle with the body, and the head is inclined toward this side. Scoliosis is present. Sprengel's deformity may occur with the Klippel-Feil syndrome.

DEFORMITIES OF THE STERNUM. The halves of the sternum may remain separated *(fissure of the sternum). Pigeon breast* consists in a prominence of the sternum and the cartilaginous parts of the ribs, with lateral depressions of the thorax. A short sternum is a common manifestation of trisomy-18.

PECTUS EXCAVATUM (FUNNEL CHEST). Funnel chest, or indentation of the lower part of the sternum, may be rachitic in origin or the result of chronic obstruction to respiration. In most instances, however, the condition is congenital. The reason for the defect is not apparent in all instances, but in some it is due to a short central tendon of the diaphragm. The manubrium sterni is at the normal level, but the inferior parts are depressed and the xiphoid may approach the vertebral bodies. The volume of the lung may be decreased and the heart displaced to the left. There are often no symptoms, but respiration may be paradoxic, since contraction of the diaphragm exerts a pull on the xiphoid and the costal cartilages. The patient may appear round-shouldered, hollow-chested, thin and underdeveloped. The deformity can have untoward psychologic effects on the child. Surgical improvement may be attempted for cosmetic reasons if the deformity is severe, or if compression causes pulmonary embarrassment.

Deformities of the Extremities

Severe deformities of the extremities are often associated with malformations not compatible with life. Surviving children with extensive defects of the limbs were rarities until the epidemic of partial and total absence of limbs (reduction malformations) resulting from maternal ingestion of the drug thalidomide. Since rehabilitation of patients with such limb defects has become an important problem, knowledge of the terminology is necessary. Minor limb defects are frequent. They may be harmless variations of development or indicators of more serious anomalies of other organ systems.

Absence or extensive reductions of limbs present at birth are often called *congenital amputations.* This term should be reserved for secondary intrauterine destruction of limbs that were originally

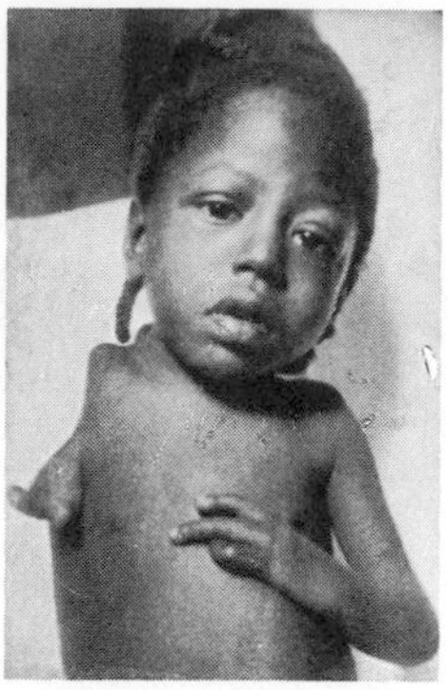

Figure 22–4 Phocomelia and partial adactylia in a girl $3\frac{1}{2}$ years of age.

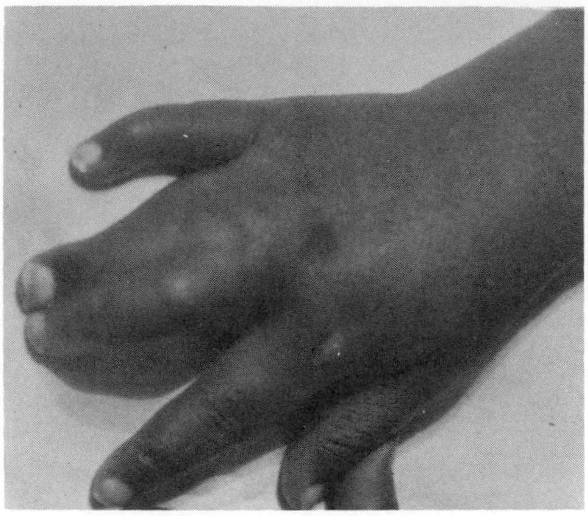

Figure 22–6 Syndactyly.

formed as normal anlagen. Limb defects due to primary inhibition of development or growth are better called *reduction malformations.* Such malformations frequently have terminal fingers or nails, indicating that no true amputation has occurred.

Amelia means absence of limbs. *Hemimelia* (absence of a portion) is commonly used for defects of the distal parts of the extremities such as absence of forearm and hand or lower leg and foot. *Phocomelia* signifies a great reduction in size of proximal parts of the limb, resulting in an approach of distal parts toward the trunk (Figs. 22–4 and 22–5). In complete phocomelia the hand or foot seems to spring directly from the trunk. *Acheiria* and *apodia* are terms for absence of a hand or foot; *adactylia,* for absence of digits; and *aphalangia,* for absence of phalanges. Individual bones may be absent. Absence of the humerus or ulna is rare; absence of the radius is usually associated with club-hand. Absence of the fibula is more frequently encountered than absence of the femur or tibia. As a rule, it is combined with pes valgus. Absence of the patella is indicated by a transverse fold of the skin in front of the knee joint during extension. It is often associated with iliac horns and deformity of the radial head.

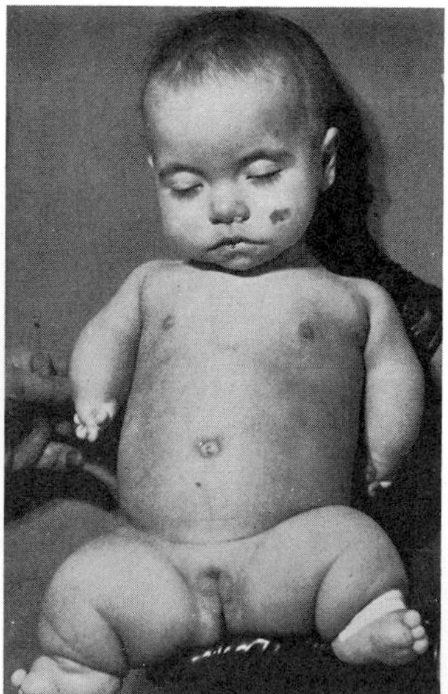

Figure 22–5 Partial phocomelia in an infant 11 months of age; picture taken at autopsy.

Polydactyly (supernumerary fingers or toes) may be found in a single member of a sibship, but there are pedigrees in which polydactyly is inherited as a dominant trait. Polydactyly is sometimes associated with other malformations (see Chondro-ectodermal Dysplasia, later, this Section).

Syndactyly (Fig. 22–6), union of fingers or toes, may consist in fusion of the bones or webbing of the skin *(zygodactyly).* Syndactyly most frequently involves the third and fourth fingers and the second and third toes. It is often seen in children with multiple malformations (acrocephalosyndactyly), but it may also occur in children who otherwise are entirely normal. In the latter, syndactyly is often hereditary.

Split hand and split foot (lobster claw) are deep clefts in the anterior part of the hand or foot, and the fingers and toes have different degrees of syndactyly. The foot appears split in the area where

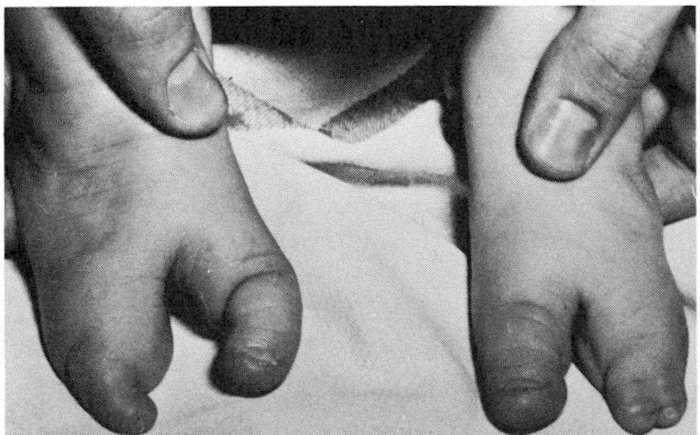

Figure 22–7 Split feet (lobster claws) in a child whose mother, maternal aunt and maternal grandfather had similar malformations.

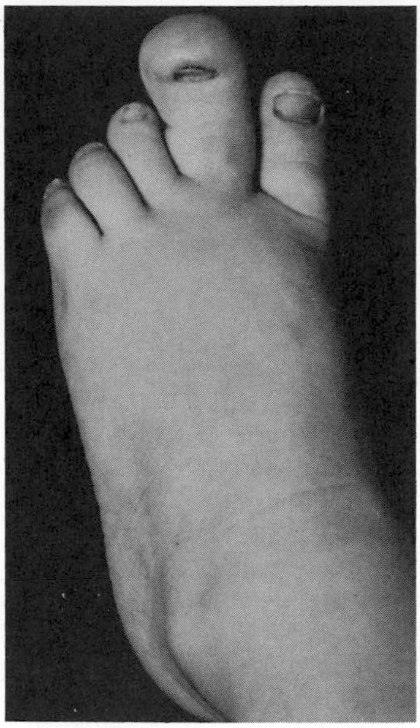

Figure 22-8 Macrodactylia.

the second or third toe should be. The parts of the foot which lie on either side of the cleft are fused into masses in which terminal digits can be recognized (Fig. 22-7). Many pedigrees are known in which this malformation is inherited as a dominant trait. *Brachydactyly,* abnormal shortness of fingers and toes resulting from lack or reduction in size of a phalanx or metacarpal bone, may be genetically determined. It may be seen in pseudohypoparathyroidism, pseudopseudohypoparathyroidism and Turner syndrome. *Clinodactyly,* incurving of the little finger, may be inherited as a dominant trait. It is also often seen in the Down syndrome. *Camptodactylia,* permanently flexed fingers, can be transmitted as a dominant trait; it also occurs in trisomies D and E (Section 6). *Macrodactylia* is a hypertrophy of one or several fingers and toes (Fig. 22-8). It may be a manifestation of neurofibromatosis.

A variety of skeletal defects, of which absence of thumbs and radii is common, occur at times in association with a congenital hypoplastic anemia (Section 14), congenital heart disease and other syndromes.

Generalized Skeletal Defects

ACHONDROPLASIA
(Chondrodystrophy)

Achondroplasia is a disorder of cartilage which begins in prenatal life and leads to a specific type of dwarfism. The long bones are most severely affected, so that disproportionate dwarfism becomes manifest with growth.

ETIOLOGY. Genetic factors play a leading role, most pedigrees suggesting a dominant mode of transmission. Sporadic cases occur frequently; they should be attributed to new mutations. Advanced parental (probably paternal) age has been considered a possible factor. Males and females are equally affected.

PATHOLOGY. The basic process is a disturbance of endochondral ossification caused by an inability of the epiphyseal plate to produce a sufficient amount of columnar cartilage. The result is deficient growth of bones of endochondral formation. The rows of columnar cartilage lack parallel arrangement and are of unequal length. The line of preparatory ossification is irregular. The bone trabeculae are short and thick and lack normal orderly arrangement. Sometimes a transverse vascular strip of connective tissue, which originates in the periosteum, grows between the epiphysis and the diaphysis, adding another obstacle to longitudinal growth. If this strip affects only one side of the bone, bowing occurs with growth. Periosteal ossification is little affected, so that transverse growth of bone is not greatly disturbed. As a result, the bones appear thick.

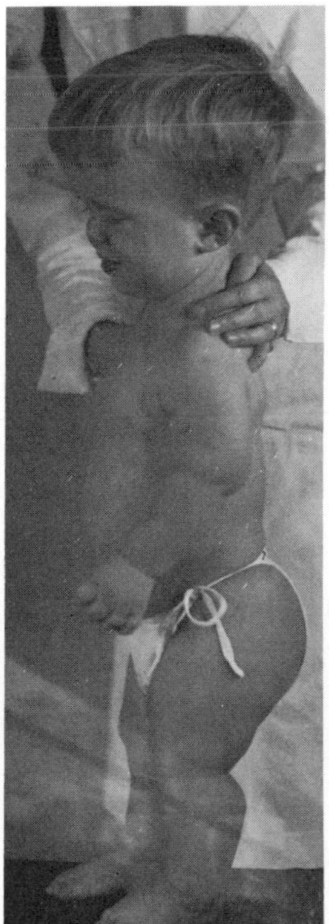

Figure 22-9 Achondroplasia in a child. Note the relatively large head, the saddle nose and brachycephaly, the short extremities and the lordosis with forward tilting of the pelvis.

The epiphyseal cartilage, which is underdeveloped in the longitudinal direction, may extend well beyond the shaft in the transverse direction, creating a mushroom-like enlargement. Hypoplasia of the cartilage may be seen in the transverse as well as in the longitudinal direction, in which case the enlargement of the metaphysis is less pronounced. Owing to insufficient cartilaginous growth, the base of the skull is short, but the bones of the cranial vault, which are of membranous origin, continue to grow. This disproportionate growth results in a typical profile characterized by a depressed nasal bridge and a bulging forehead.

CLINICAL MANIFESTATIONS. The chief characteristic of achondroplasia is the combination of short extremities with a head that is often somewhat enlarged (and in all instances seems even relatively larger than it is) and a trunk approximating normal size. The limbs are often curved, and their epiphyseal junctions enlarged and prominent. The proximal portions of the extremities are most severely affected; the hands, which are short and broad, may not reach the hips. The relatively large head exhibits a prominent forehead, flattening of the bridge of the nose, and a forward projection of the mandible; hydrocephalus is sometimes present. The chest is of normal length, but narrow in the anteroposterior dimension, and beading of the ribs and flaring of the costal margins are generally noticeable.

The thoracic kyphosis and the lumbar lordosis are usually accentuated. Protrusion of the abdomen and the gluteal region results in a characteristic posture. The deformed pelvis in affected women may be an obstacle to delivery, often necessitating cesarean section. The gait is waddling. Extension of the joints may be impeded by the irregular shape of the epiphyses. The skin is loose and may form transverse folds and pads. The muscular development is good. The mentality is usually normal.

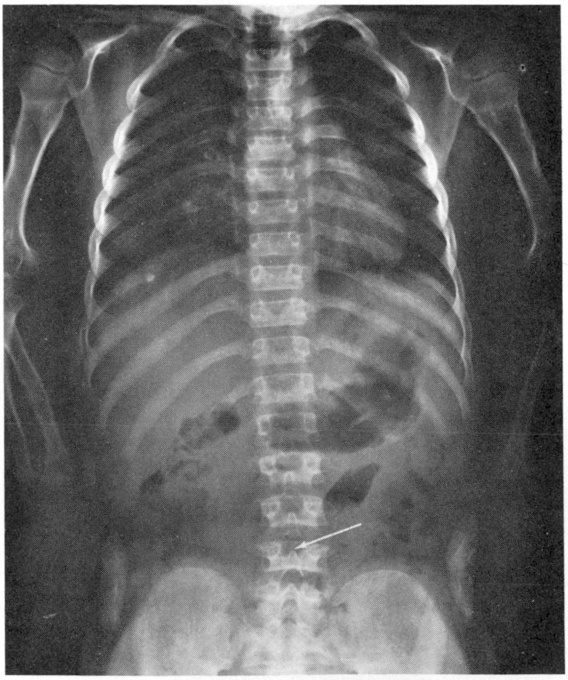

Figure 22–10 *Achondroplasia. The length of the upper extremities may be compared with the length of the trunk. The small interpediculate distances of the lumbar vertebrae (arrow) and the narrow sacrum are evident.*

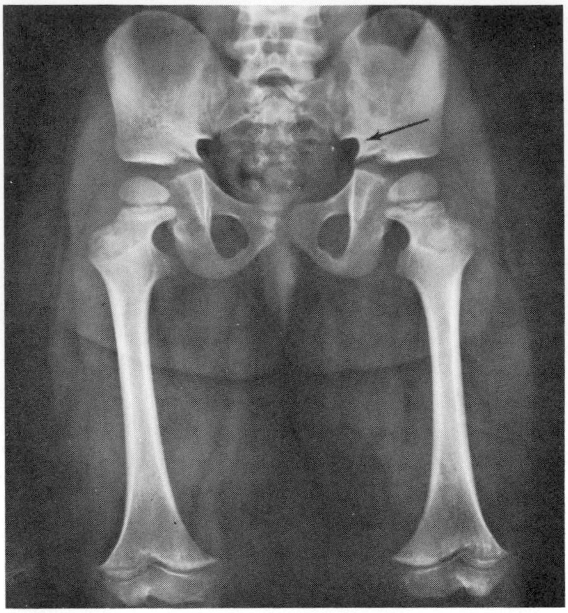

Figure 22–11 *Achondroplasia. The sacrum articulates low on the ilia. The sciatic notch is small (arrow), and the roof of the acetabulum is broad and flat. Flaring of the distal end of the short femurs is evident.*

DIAGNOSIS. The thickness of the bones and their irregular epiphyseal ends as seen in the roentgenogram make the diagnosis possible even in the newborn infant. The bones of the extremities are short and broad and have a mushroom-like broadening at the ends of the shafts. The fibula is often longer than the tibia. Curving may be seen in various places. At the epiphyseal ends of the shafts are such irregularities as cupping, fraying and spurs. The mineral content is good throughout the bones, and there are no periosteal changes. Ossification of the epiphyses and of the carpal and tarsal bones is not delayed, but their outlines are irregular though smooth. The metacarpal, metatarsal and phalangeal bones are also short and thick and have irregularities at their epiphyseal ends (Fig. 22–11). On the lateral view the base of the skull appears short. The bones of the vault bulge on all sides beyond the base.

The alterations of the bones of the pelvis and of the lumbar spine are important in diagnosis. The height of the iliac bones is diminished in the region of the acetabulum, so that the acetabular roof is flat and broad, and the sciatic notch is small. There is a decrease in the interpediculate distances of the lumbar vertebrae as a manifestation of the small spinal canal. The vertebral bodies are usually of normal height, but occasionally a wedge-shaped vertebra is present. Herniation of intervertebral disks is common.

The depressed bridge of the nose may suggest syphilis or cretinism. *Syphilis* can be ruled out by the roentgenogram and by serologic tests; normal mental development and normal serum concentration of protein-bound iodine rule out *cretinism.* A superficial examination of the roentgenograms may suggest *rickets;* however, the intensive calcification of the irregular epiphyses is characteristic of achondroplasia, and the serum calcium, phosphorus, and alkaline phosphatase levels are normal.

Other forms of micromelia can be distinguished by clinical examination or the roentgenogram. The legs of children with *osteogenesis imperfecta* or *osteopsathyrosis* may become shortened and deformed after repeated fractures, but the bones are long and slender. *Hypophosphatasia* resulting in congenital micromelia can be mistaken for achondroplasia in the neonatal period, but the deficiency of ossification and the low serum phosphatase value establish the diagnosis.

PROGNOSIS AND TREATMENT. Many children with a specific type of achondroplasia, (thanatophoric dwarfism), die in utero or soon after birth. Those who survive usually have good general health, and their mental development is satisfactory. Their height rarely exceeds 140 cm (55 inches).

No specific treatment is known. Early orthopedic correction of developing deformities may improve the appearance.

OTHER CHONDRODYSPLASIAS

A variety of skeletal disorders which clinically resemble achondroplasia in some respects and the mucopolysaccharidoses in others have been observed in several generations of some kinships. These disorders, usually not noticeable at birth, manifest themselves during the first years of childhood and result in variable degrees of shortness of stature. Roentgenographically the irregularities are most apparent in the epiphyses, but the diaphyses are not entirely spared.

SOME DOMINANTLY INHERITED CHONDRODYSPLASIAS

The following four systemic skeletal disorders are inherited as dominant traits; there are many intermediate forms which are not readily classified.

SPONDYLOEPIPHYSEAL DYSPLASIA. This syndrome was in the past considered a variant of achondrodysplasia. It differs in several ways, but especially in that the infant appears to be normal at birth, and the evidence of dwarfism is not apparent for several years. Other differences are the lack of involvement of the head and face and the more extensive changes in the epiphyses in spondyloepiphyseal dysplasia. The epiphyses are small, irregular and fragmented (Fig. 22–12). The vertebral bodies are somewhat flattened and have a tendency to be biconvex. By midchildhood the affected person has an outward appearance simulating that of achondrodysplasia, with short extremities and lordosis; the head, how-

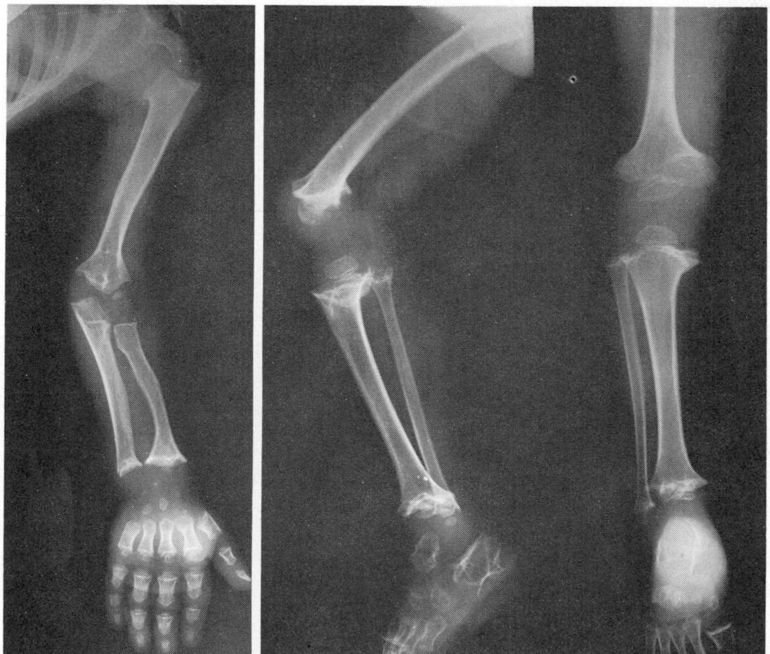

Figure 22–12 *Spondyloepiphyseal dysplasia.*

ever, though relatively large, is not abnormal. A congenital spondyloepiphyseal dysplasia has been described in which myopia and retinal detachment may develop.

MULTIPLE EPIPHYSEAL DYSPLASIA. (Fairbank's disease). A variety of terms describe irregularities of ossification, which are largely seen in the epiphyses; differences evident at the moment appear to be largely in degree of involvement, but it is not unlikely that distinct entities may eventually be separated out from the general category. Roentgenographic changes in the epiphyses vary from stippling to an appearance of almost complete destruction. In the hips the roentgenographic appearance may resemble that of aseptic necrosis (see Legg-Calvé-Perthes disease). The vertebral pattern is normal or nearly so. Shortness in stature is variable, and in later life arthritic changes are common.

METAPHYSEAL DYSOSTOSIS. The principal involvement is in the metaphyses of the long bones. Roentgenographically the ends of the bones appear frayed, irregular and widened, resembling the osseous changes of rickets. The serum levels of phosphorus, calcium and phosphatase, however, are within normal limits. The child is short in stature and bowlegged.

DYSCHONDROSTEOSIS. In this disorder the forearms and the lower legs are principally affected, while the proximal portions of the skeleton appear to be normal or less involved (mesomelia). The radius is particularly bowed, often curving around the ulna. A bayonet-like volar displacement of the dorsum of the hand against the forearm is a prominent feature (Madelung's deformity).

RECESSIVELY INHERITED CHONDRODYSPLASIAS

DIASTROPHIC DWARFISM. At birth the appearance is that of achondroplasia because of the shortness of the extremities, but characteristically there are clubfoot and often contractures of other joints, cleft palate and ear deformities. During childhood, scoliosis, kyphosis and dislocations develop, and the clubfeet and flexion of knees and hips become more pronounced.

CHONDRO-ECTODERMAL DYSPLASIA (ELLIS-VAN CREVELD SYNDROME). The combination of chondrodysplasia, ectodermal dysplasia, polydactyly and congenital heart disease is a rare syndrome. The bones of the extremities are short and thick, and the terminal phalanges of the fingers and toes and the nails are dystrophic. The distal long bones are most severely affected. There is a sixth finger on the ulnar side of each hand. Dentition is defective, but the sweat glands and the skin are normal.

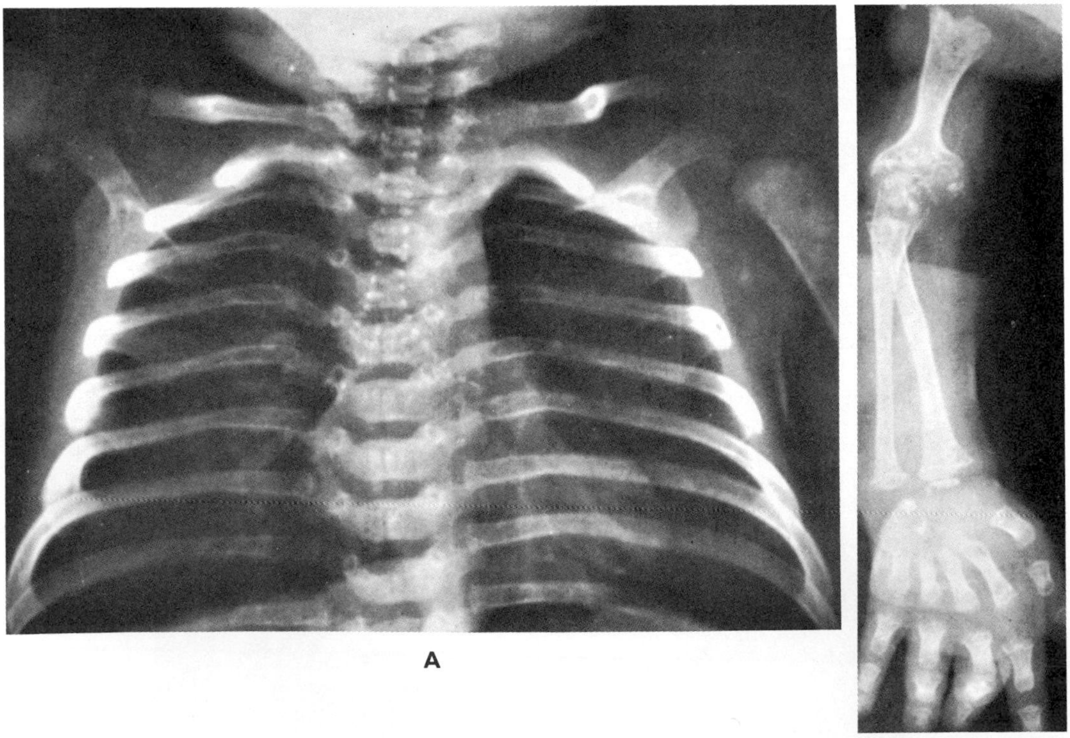

Figure 22–13 *Chondrodystrophia calcificans congenita.* A, *Diffuse calcification of the laryngeal, tracheal and bronchial cartilages. In early infancy the infant had significant dyspnea, presumably due to a constricted tracheobronchial tree.* B, *Shortening of humerus. Numerous calcifications in the area of the elbow joint. Contractures of finger joints.*

Stillbirth or death in early infancy is common. This syndrome has been identified among the Amish of Lancaster County, Pennsylvania.

ASPHYXIATING THORACIC DYSTROPHY (JEUNE SYNDROME). Asphyxiating thoracic dystrophy is a descriptive term applied to a dysplasia of the skeleton characterized by very short ribs, slight shortening of the long bones, polydactyly and cleft-like lesions in the acetabulum and in the metaphyses of the long bones. The skull and the spine appear to be normal. The thorax is narrow and relatively immobile, air exchange is limited, and the patient's course is complicated by repeated respiratory infections. This condition was first reported by Jeune in siblings; both males and females are affected. Some of these patients survive childhood and develop renal complications.

CHONDRODYSTROPHIA CALCIFICANS CONGENITA. (CONRADI'S DISEASE). This rare form of chondrodysplasia has a typical roentgenographic appearance. The carpal and the tarsal bones are replaced by numerous small but distinctly calcified spots scattered about the affected areas. They represent deposits of calcium in cartilage. The epiphyses may be stippled with similar small calcium deposits. The limbs are often short, particularly in their proximal segments Contractures are not rare, and cataracts are often present. Calcifications may also occur in the tracheal cartilages (Fig. 22–13) and be responsible for respiratory embarrassment. The severe form of this syndrome is transmitted on a recessive basis; a mild form of stippled epiphyses is dominantly transmitted.

MUCOPOLYSACCHARIDOSES

The mucopolysaccharidoses comprise a group of diseases which have in common disorders in the metabolism of mucopolysaccharides and which are separated by genetic, clinical and biochemical characteristics. Classification is still in flux, many subgroups being distinguished. Hurler syndrome is the prototype of these disorders.

The mucopolysaccharides comprise much of the ground substance of connective tissue; they are present in mucous secretions; and one, heparin, is found in the circulation, where it exerts an anticoagulative effect. Chemically they are long, linear polymers consisting of substituted glucose and galactose residues. They contain nitrogen in the form of glucosamine and galactosamine as well as carboxylic acid groups and sulfate molecules esterified to either one of the hydroxyl groups or bound to the amine groups.

The various compounds which are excreted, such as chondroitin A or B, hyaluronic acid, keratosulfate and heparitin sulfate, are all mucopolysaccharides whose structures are known. The acidic groups of the mucopolysaccharides react characteristically with dyes such as toluidine blue, or Alcian blue. This reaction is used clinically in the detection of these disorders. Some of the enzymology concerning these compounds is known, and a specific enzyme dysfunction is under investigation.

HURLER SYNDROME

(Gargoylism; Dysostosis Multiplex)

This disorder is a metabolic disturbance which affects both skeleton and soft tissues. Although the metabolic disturbance is present at birth, most of the manifestations develop in postnatal life. The fully developed disease is characterized by cloudy corneas, hepatosplenomegaly, mental deficiency, skeletal changes and dwarfism. Both sexes may be affected. The disorder is genetically determined, and inherited as an autosomal recessive trait. The basic metabolic disturbance results in accumulation of an abnormal intracellular material which affects the cells and structure of many organs. The nature of the stored substances is inadequately defined, but they are thought to be acid mucopolysaccharides. Specifically, chondroitin sulfate B and heparitin sulfate are found in abnormal amounts in the urine.

CLINICAL MANIFESTATIONS. The skull is frequently malformed and may be scaphocephalic, oxycephalic or enlarged. Closure of the anterior fontanel may be delayed. The supraorbital ridges are prominent, and the bridge of the nose is depressed. A profuse nasal discharge is usually present because of the deformed pharynx, which is often blocked by lymphoid tissue. The tongue is enlarged, and the neck short. There is a kyphosis in the dorsolumbar region (Fig. 22–14, *A*). The heart is frequently enlarged, and a systolic murmur can be heard (Section 13). Dyspnea occurs on slight exertion; cyanosis, in advanced stages. The abdomen is prominent; the spleen and liver are enlarged; and an umbilical hernia is frequently present. Externally the sex organs appear normal, but sexual maturation does not occur. The joints have limited extensibility, particularly in the fingers. The appearance of the hands is characteristic (Fig. 22–14, *B*): the breadth is greater than the length, the fingers are maintained in a "clawing" position, and the fourth and fifth fingers are incurved. Coxa valga and genu valgum of a moderate degree may be present. The combination of the clawlike hands, the large head, the grotesque facies and deformed limbs accounts for the designation "gargoylism." The thickness of the skin contributes to the characteristic picture. Corneal opacities and mental retardation are prominent manifestations. In the white blood cells abnormal granulations *(Reilly bodies)* may be found. Increased amounts of mucopolysaccharides are present in the urine. A diagnostic spot test is available which is based on the detection of chondroitin sulfuric acid on paper chromatograms by toluidine blue.

DIAGNOSIS. The stunted growth, the thickness of the skin and the mental retardation suggest cre-

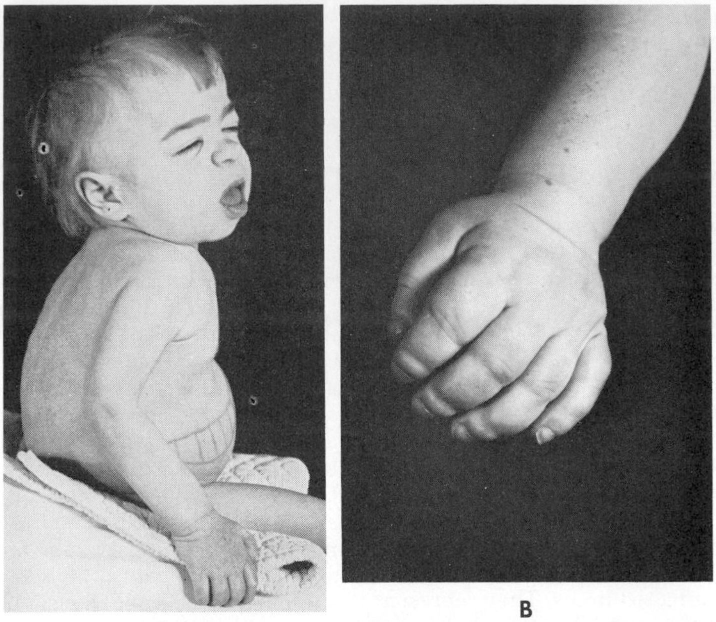

B

A

Figure 22–14 A, *Hurler syndrome in a child 2 years of age, showing coarse features, depressed nasal bridge, kyphosis and stunting of growth; also outline of the enlarged liver. Child had corneal opacity and was mentally deficient.* B, *Typical spadelike hand.*

tinism, but the laboratory data and the roentgenographic changes are adequate for differentiation. Roentgenographically the sella turcica is often elongated and the mandibular condyles are concave. The changes of the spinal column are best seen in the lateral view. The vertebral bodies are short in the sagittal direction, their anterior and posterior outlines appear concave, and the spinous processes are directed downward. The first or second lumbar vertebra is small and displaced backward, resulting in deformity of the spine (Fig. 22–15, *A*). The lower ribs are club-shaped. The humerus is long and thick; the ulna and radius, short and thick. Their epiphyseal ends and their epi-

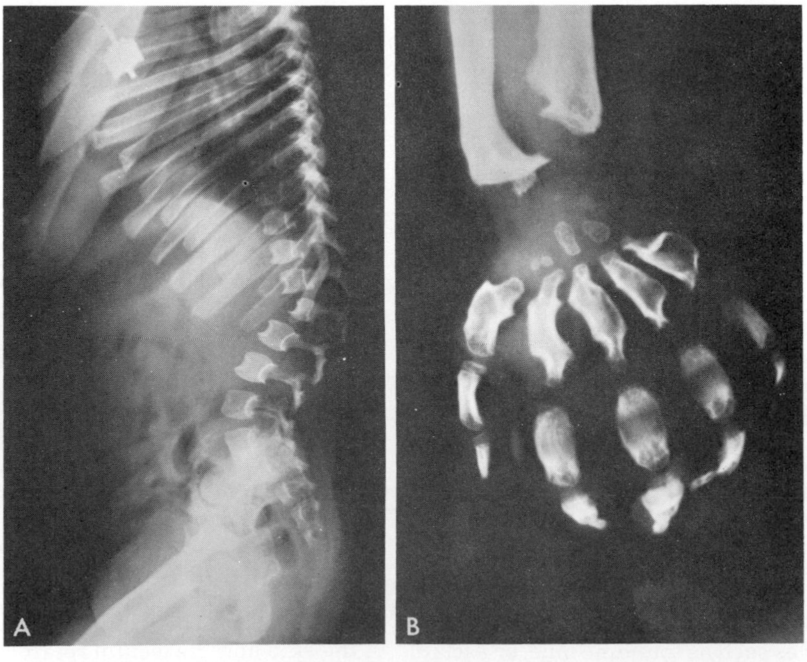

Figure 22–15 *Hurler syndrome.* A, *Lateral view of spinal column;* B, *hand.*

physyses have irregular outlines. The metacarpal bones are bottle-shaped, the basal phalanges cylindrical (Fig. 22–15, *B*). The femur, tibia and fibula are moderately thickened, and their epiphyses are angular.

PROGNOSIS AND TREATMENT. The prognosis is unfavorable, since the patients remain retarded in mental and physical development. Orthopedic treatment may aid in correcting the deformity of the spine.

HUNTER SYNDROME

This syndrome is characterized by a physical resemblance to Hurler syndrome, but the disease is inherited as a sex-linked recessive. Mental deterioration is slower, and clouding of the cornea is rare. Progressive deafness is frequent. Chondroitin sulfate B and heparitin sulfate are found in the urine.

SANFILIPPO SYNDROME

This form is characterized by less severe somatic alterations, but mental retardation is profound. It is inherited as an autosomal recessive. Heparitin sulfate is found in the urine in large amounts.

MORQUIO'S DISEASE

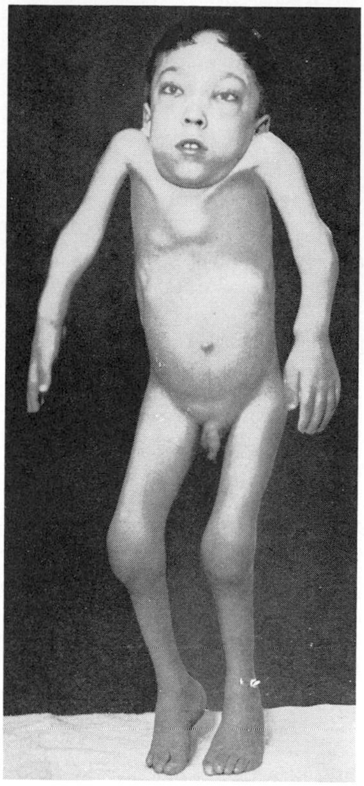

Figure 22–16 Morquio's disease.

This chondrodystrophy is genetically determined. Consanguinity of the parents and also of the paternal grandparents was reported in the family described by Morquio. A recessive mode of transmission is suggested; in one unusual sibship the disorder was transmitted as a sex-linked recessive trait. (See Section 6). Sporadic cases have also been described. Abnormal amounts of keratosulfate may be found in the urine.

CLINICAL MANIFESTATIONS. Development appears to be normal until the infant begins to walk. The face and the skull are only slightly affected, but the neck is short (Fig. 22–16). In contrast to achondroplasia (above), the spine and the chest become severely deformed. Fusion of cervical vertebrae and platybasia may occur. The thorax is short and broad because the vertebrae are flat; the anteroposterior diameter is increased, and the sternum protrudes. There are an exaggerated thoracic kyphosis of the spine and scoliosis of a varying degree. The abdomen protrudes; genital development is normal. The relatively long arms extend to the knees. The hands and fingers are long and soft. Genu valgum and flat feet are present. The joints are enlarged; the muscles and ligaments are flaccid; the gait is waddling. The osseous manifestations are unlike those of the Hurler syndrome. The mentality is usually normal.

DIAGNOSIS. There is an external resemblance to rickets, but the absence of hypophosphatemia and the roentgenographic appearance of the bones exclude rickets. In Morquio's disease basilar invagination and occipitalization may be present in addition to anomalous segmentation of the cervical vertebrae. The vertebrae are flattened, and their cranial and caudal surfaces are uneven. The shafts of the long bones are of normal length and shape. The outlines of their epiphyseal ends are irregular, with flattening in some places and abnormal projections in others. The epiphyses are of irregular shape and sometimes fragmented. The ends of the metacarpal bones resemble those seen in typical achondroplasia.

PROGNOSIS AND TREATMENT. As far as physical development is concerned, the prognosis is unfavorable, since the deformities progress and become more pronounced. There is no specific treatment. Orthopedic treatment may prevent or correct the deformities to some extent.

SCHEIE SYNDROME

This form is characterized by physical changes resembling those of Hurler syndrome, but intelligence is not impaired. Excessive amounts of chondroitin sulfate B are found in the urine.

POLYDYSTROPHIC DWARFISM
(Maroteaux-Lamy Syndrome)

The clinical manifestations, which include growth retardation, lumbar kyphosis, sternal protrusion and genu valgum, develop after 2 years of age. The facial features are coarse, and hepatosplenomegaly is present in most cases. There is no mental retardation. The patients excrete large amounts of chondroitin sulfate B.

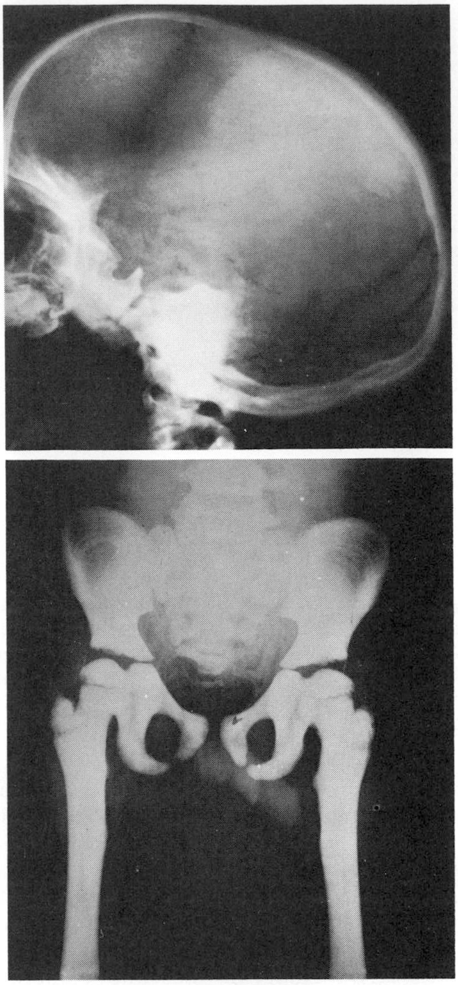

Figure 22–17 Osteopetrosis of skull, pelvis and femurs.

MUCOLIPIDOSES

In certain cases both mucopolysaccharide and lipid metabolism are abnormal. The clinical and roentgenologic pictures may resemble in some respects those of Hurler syndrome. Involvement may be present at birth. Classifications of mucolipidoses have been attempted.

OSTEOPETROSIS

(Albers-Schönberg Disease; Marble Bones)

Osteopetrosis is a rare disorder characterized by hard and brittle bones.

ETIOLOGY. In the majority of cases the mode of inheritance appears to be recessive, but a milder dominant form occurs. Males and females are equally affected.

PATHOLOGY. The cortex of the bones, as well as the trabeculae, is thickened. Endochondral ossification is disturbed by lack of resorption of cartilaginous intercellular ground substance. Islands of this partly calcified ground substance, which under normal conditions is replaced by bone, persist and are found in the shafts of the bones. The trabeculae are unusually crowded and numerous. At the ends of the long bones, as well as in the scapulae and pelvic bones, zones of increased and decreased density alternate. The medullary cavity is reduced in volume, and the marrow may contain abnormal cells or fibrous tissue. The foramina for the cranial nerves are often constricted by an overgrowth of bone. The chemical composition of the bones is normal.

CLINICAL MANIFESTATIONS. This condition probably always begins in utero, although clinical symptoms may be absent in infancy. Brittleness predisposes the bones to fracture, and roentgenograms taken on occasion of a fracture often reveal the underlying process for the first time. Although the fractures, as a rule, heal satisfactorily, deformities frequently develop. The head is square and somewhat enlarged, and deformities of the chest and spine may be present. Vision is usually disturbed early in life and diminishes progressively; the movements of the eyes may be impaired. Cataracts and optic atrophy may develop. There may be progressive deafness. The teeth develop abnormally and have a tendency to decay. The patient often has a hypochromic anemia, and in the final stage of the disease, a myelophthisic one. Hepatosplenomegaly and enlargement of the lymph nodes have been observed. Osteomyelitis is a frequent complication, particularly in the mandible or maxilla. General growth is retarded, and some of the patients are dwarfed. The mentality is normal, but chronic illness, blindness or deafness may interfere with intellectual development.

DIAGNOSIS. Roentgenographic demonstration of increased density of the entire skeleton is diagnostic. No distinction can be made between cortex and marrow. The bones of the base of the cranium are thick and dense; those of the vault are less affected (Fig. 22–17). The long bones, particularly the femur and tibia, are club-shaped, and transverse bands are seen near their ends. Bandlike stratification may also be found in the os ilium and in the scapula. Skeletal maturation is normal.

Localized sclerotic processes as seen in *syphilis* and *sclerosing osteitis* are easily distinguished from osteopetrosis. A generalized *osteosclerosis* may result from fluorine poisoning, but in such cases calcification of muscles and ligaments is also often present. Cranial alterations in idiopathic hypercalcemia resemble those of osteopetrosis, as do those in craniometaphyseal dysplasia.

PROGNOSIS AND TREATMENT. The prognosis is unfavorable in the majority of cases observed during childhood. Accidental detection of osteopetrosis in a number of apparently healthy adults is evidence that the disorder may exist for a long time without causing significant symptoms.

There is no treatment. The complications are treated symptomatically.

PYKNODYSOSTOSIS

This is a form of osteosclerosis combined with delayed closure of the fontanels, separated cranial sutures and hypoplasia of the terminal phalanges. It may be confused with osteopetrosis, because the bones are denser than usual on the roentgenogram and they fracture with slight trauma.

OSTEOGENESIS IMPERFECTA

This disease is characterized by increased fragility of the bones, which are easily fractured by slight trauma. Patients with this disorder usually have blue scleras and flaccid ligaments; some of them become deaf in later life.

In severe cases, fractures occur in utero, and the infant is born with deformities *(osteogenesis imperfecta congenita).* In other instances, fractures do not occur until several years after birth and the tendency to fracture disappears after puberty *(osteopsathyrosis, osteogenesis imperfecta tarda).* This latter form usually has a milder course, but often occurs repeatedly in the same family or sibship. Whether the two forms are identical is under debate.

ETIOLOGY. The disorder is determined before birth. Osteopsathyrosis is often transmitted as a dominant hereditary trait, but the different manifestations (blue scleras, fragility of the bones, deafness, and the like) may show intrafamilial variability in penetrance or expressivity (Section 6). The congenital form is usually not repeated in families, although rarely it may alternate with the late form (osteopsathyrosis). Recessive inheritance has been infrequently demonstrated.

PATHOLOGY. Osteogenesis imperfecta is a systemic disease whose manifestations are considered to be due to a defect of the mesenchyme and its derivatives (scleras, bones and ligaments).

The cortex is invariably diminished in thickness, owing to disturbed formation of periosteal bone. Inactivity of the patient contributes to the atrophy of the bones. Osteoblastic activity is defective. The generalized mesenchymal involvement in the congenital form of the disease is demonstrable in sections of the skin and scleras by a failure of the reticulum to differentiate into mature collagen. In some cases the abnormally thin scleras allow the underlying pigment to show through. In others, increased transparency, but not thinness, of the sclera is observed. Occasionally cataract, coloboma and embryotoxon are associated with this disorder. Deafness may be due to otosclerosis or labyrinthine disturbance.

CLINICAL MANIFESTATIONS. In *osteogenesis imperfecta congenita* fractures may occur in utero,

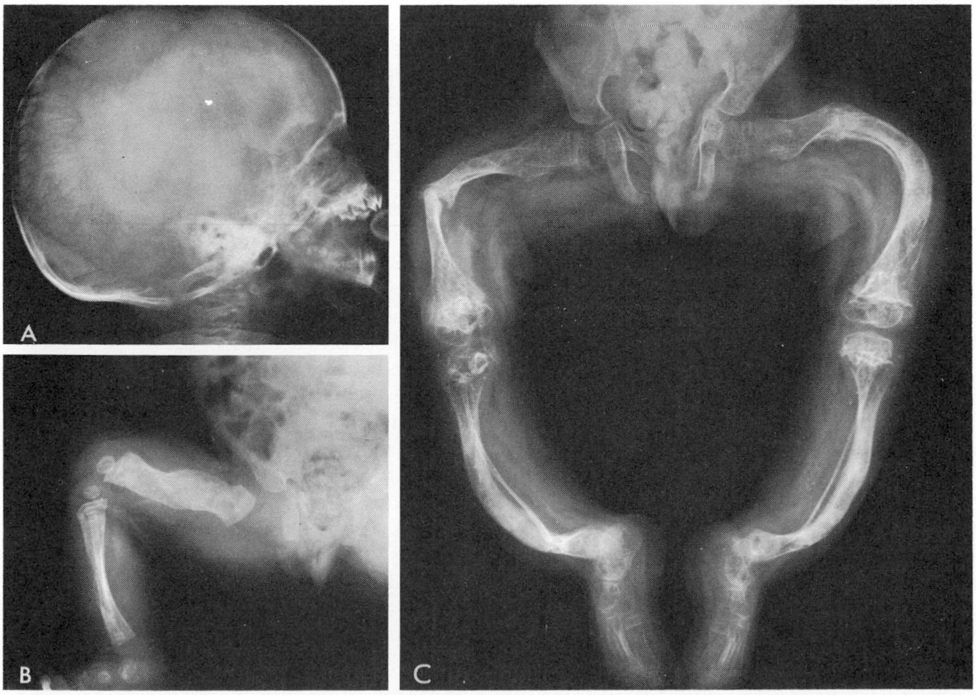

Figure 22–18 *Osteogenesis imperfecta.* A, *Skull showing wormian bones.* B, *Roentgenogram of leg at birth.* C, *Roentgenogram of legs at 5 years of age.*

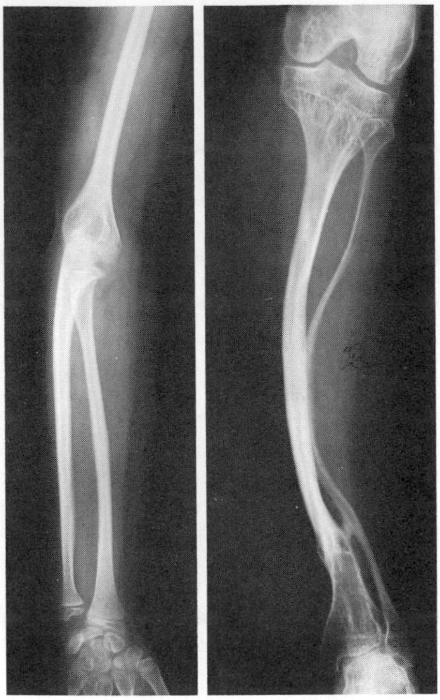

Figure 22–19 Osteopsathyrosis.

and the infant is born with deformities, since the bones generally heal in abnormal positions. Fractures may also occur during delivery. The skull has wide membranous spaces between the bones of the vault, and crackling is often felt on pressure. Many wormian bones are found within the occipital, parietal and temporal bones (Fig. 22–18). The eyes are often prominent, the scleras blue. Dental changes *(dentinogenesis imperfecta)* may be prominent. The neck is short. The chest and the spine are deformed in severe cases. Many children with the severe congenital form die soon after birth. In those who survive, fractures of the extremities may result from otherwise inconsequential trauma. Callus usually forms rapidly, and the process of healing is considered satisfactory. The callus, however, is often replaced by inferior bone which is prone to bend and fracture. Most of the fractures occur in the legs, where bizarre deformities develop.

Serum levels of calcium and phosphorus are within normal ranges.

In *osteopsathyrosis (osteogenesis imperfecta tarda)* the child appears normal at birth, and fractures usually do not occur until after the first year of life. There is great variation in the time of the first fracture. Occasionally osteopsathyrosis is so severe that it resembles the congenital form in the development of early and numerous fractures; in the majority of instances, however, only a moderate number of fractures occur, and the fragility ceases with puberty. The bones of the extremities are long and slender (Fig. 22–19); most of the fractures are in the legs. Healing takes place rapidly, but deformities may develop. As a rule, all the affected members of a family can be recognized by their blue scleras. Only about two thirds of the members with blue scleras suffer from increased fragility of the bones, and only about one fourth from deafness. The flaccidity of the ligaments and muscles may result in repeated dislocations. Deafness is usually a late manifestation and is rare in children.

A clear distinction between osteogenesis imperfecta congenita and tarda cannot always be made, and intermediate forms may be encountered.

DIAGNOSIS. In roentgenograms of the newborn infant with *osteogenesis imperfecta congenita* the unbroken bones are thin, but otherwise normal. The previously fractured bones appear irregularly thickened, curved or angulated; the epiphyseal ends are usually normal. The skull is characterized by thinness of the bones and by osseous islands, the wormian bones, which are separated from each other by numerous sutures of irregular shape. The mineral content of the bones seems reduced, but the bone age corresponds to the child's chronologic age. As the child grows older and the processes of fracturing and healing continue, the shafts of the bones assume grotesque shapes.

In *osteopsathyrosis,* roentgenograms show the unbroken long bones to be slender and elongated. Their epiphyses are normal in appearance. Improper healing of fractures may result in deformities; demineralized areas are frequent.

The diagnosis of osteogenesis imperfecta and of osteopsathyrosis is easier if there are blue scleras; and in osteopsathyrosis there is usually a family history. *Achondroplasia* and osteogenesis imperfecta result in micromelia, but otherwise the two disorders have little in common. In the former the bones are thick and short, and the epiphyseal ends irregular. *Hypophosphatasia* in the newborn may resemble osteogenesis imperfecta congenita, but is readily recognized (see later, this Section) by the low serum phosphatase value and by the rachitic appearance of the bones.

PROGNOSIS AND TREATMENT. Many children with *osteogenesis imperfecta congenita* are stillborn or die soon after birth. Those who survive usually become severely deformed.

Children with the late form, *osteopsathyrosis,* may also become deformed, but the deformities can be lessened by orthopedic treatment. Frequently the patients can live fairly normal lives. The prospects of developing deafness and of transmitting the disorder to offspring, however, must be considered in relation to the prognosis.

Many treatments for osteogenesis imperfecta have been recommended, but there is no agreement on their effectiveness. Good nutrition and correct treatment for the fractures are essential.

Miscellaneous Disorders

CLEIDAL AND CLEIDOCRANIAL DYSOSTOSES

This congenital syndrome is characterized by defects or absence of the clavicles and often by delay of ossification of the skull. The defect is usually transmitted as a dominant trait; some sporadic cases, in which inheritance cannot be proved, are regarded as new mutations. Males and females are equally affected. The defective bones are mostly membranous in origin. The ends of the clavicles, which are often also missing, are derived from cartilage, however, and other bones of cartilaginous origin may also be affected.

CLINICAL MANIFESTATIONS. The entire clavicle may be absent, or the sternal and acromial ends may be present but disconnected. Sometimes the two ends are fairly well developed and joined by a narrow fibrous strip, simulating the appearance of a fractured clavicle on the roentgenogram.

In serious clavicular defect the shoulders can be approximated in front to a remarkable degree (Fig. 22–20). The muscles which are normally attached to the clavicle may also be defective. At birth ossification of the calvarial bones is so delayed that the fontanels are excessively large and the sutures widely open. Large bosses develop in the frontal, parietal and occipital regions, and the skull assumes a globular shape, at times with a "hot cross bun" type of deformity, owing to depressions along the coronal and sagittal sutures. As the patient grows older, ossification of the calvarial bones progresses slowly, but the fontanels may remain open until adulthood. The sutures frequently close with interposition of wormian bones. The facial bones are underdeveloped, and the sinuses may be absent. The palate is usually highly arched and, in some cases, cleft. The dentition is irregular. Congenital *cranial dysostosis* may occur without anomalies of the clavicle. Deformities of the vertebrae and of the bones of the fingers and toes and delayed ossification of the pubic bones have also been observed. In hereditary cases the cleidal and the cleidocranial forms have alternated in the same sibship. The patients are usually short of stature, but their mentality and general health may be unaffected.

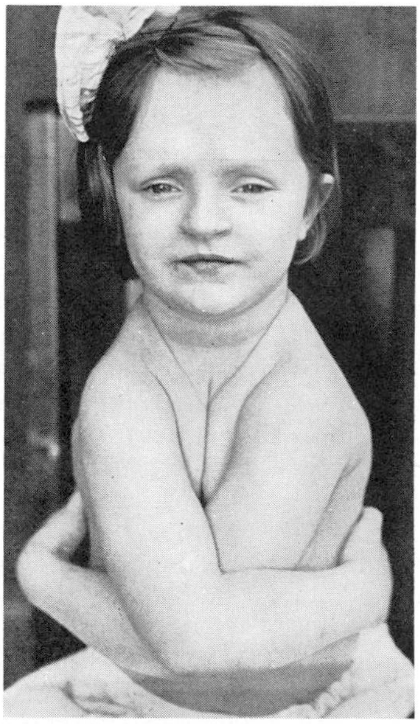

Figure 22–20 Cleidocranial dysostosis in a 5 year old girl. (Cook: Arch. Pediatr., *Vol. 51, 1934.)*

DIAGNOSIS. Roentgenograms reveal absence of all or part of the clavicles and a lack of ossification of the cranial and pelvic bones, particularly of the pubic bones. The delayed ossification of the calvaria may suggest hydrocephalus or cretinism.

PROGNOSIS AND TREATMENT. The defects rarely cause discomfort or disability. Occasionally a clavicular fragment may press on nerves and cause pain; removal of the disturbing fragment is indicated.

ARACHNODACTYLY

(Marfan Syndrome; Dolichostenomelia)

Arachnodactyly, abnormal length of the extremities, particularly of the fingers and toes, is a congenital anomaly which is frequently combined with luxation of the lens (Marfan syndrome) and other malformations.

ETIOLOGY. The disorder is considered a general "mesodermal dystrophy." The syndrome is inherited as a dominant trait. There are sporadic cases which are probably the result of new mutations.

CLINICAL MANIFESTATIONS. The patients tend to be tall and slender, and their extremities are long and thin (Fig. 22–21). The phalanges, metacarpals and metatarsals are unusually long; the fingers are often termed "spider fingers." The muscles are flaccid, so that the joints are hyperextensible except when the syndrome is combined with arthrogryposis. The skull is long and narrow, the palate high. The external ears are frequently deformed. Luxation of the lens may be combined with cataract, megalocornea, coloboma and other defects of the eye. Myopia, strabismus and nystagmus are frequently present. There may be scoliosis or kyphosis. Deformities of the chest and cardiovascular disease develop as the children grow older. Cardiac hypertrophy, valvular deformities, aortic cystic medionecrosis, aortic aneurysm (sometimes dissecting) and other anomalies have been found at autopsy. Imperfect lobation of the lungs, renal ectopy, dislocation of the hips and other malformations are also occasionally as-

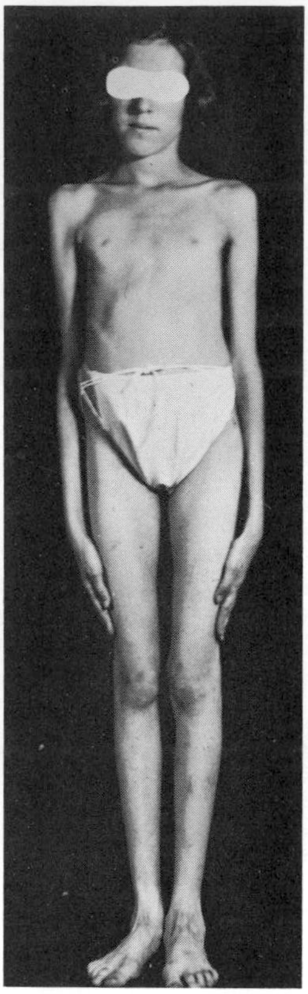

Figure 22–21 Arachnodactyly.

sociated with the syndrome. The mentality is normal in the majority of instances.

PROGNOSIS AND TREATMENT. Respiratory disease is common, but the prognosis depends chiefly upon the cardiac lesions. Some children reach maturity and transmit the disorder to some of their offspring.

Appropriate treatment of the deformities of the spine and of the eye defects is required.

Ectopia lentis and skeletal changes resembling arachnodactyly have been found associated with homocystinuria (Section 8), a metabolic disorder attributed to autosomal recessive inheritance.

MULTIPLE EXOSTOSES

(Osteochondroma; Diaphyseal Aclasis; Dyschondroplasia; Ecchondrosis Ossificans)

In this disorder hard, irregular prominences appear in the region of the metaphyses of bones. The condition is hereditary in the majority of instances, a dominant mode of transmission being the rule. If a person appears to be "skipped" in a pedigree, roentgenographic examination may reveal small exostoses that have escaped external inspection. A sporadic instance may represent a new mutation, or the patient may belong to a family in which the disorder had not been noticed before. Males are affected more severely than females.

PATHOLOGY. The exostoses consist of spongy bone covered by a layer of compact bone and a shell of hyaline cartilage. The excrescence enlarges by endochondral, periosteal and perichondral ossification. Exostoses develop only on parts of the skeleton previously cartilaginous. They develop from intraperiosteal or subcortical cartilaginous rests, whereas the enchondromas sometimes associated with them arise from cartilaginous islands situated in the spongiosa. Exostoses occur chiefly on the long bones, but occasionally the base of the skull, the vertebral column, the ribs, the scapulae and the pelvis are affected.

CLINICAL MANIFESTATIONS. Although exostoses are frequently present at birth, they are usually not noticed before the second year of life, when osseous elevations become prominent near the ends of bones. Growth of the affected bones is retarded, and deformities may develop. The radius is often longer than the ulna and bends around the end of this bone, resulting in ulnar deviation of the entire hand. Genu valgum and pes planus frequently develop. The exostoses are usually bilateral and often symmetrical. Occasionally a large exostosis may interfere with movement of a joint or press on nerves or blood vessels.

DIAGNOSIS. On the roentgenogram, exostoses appear as small or large spurs (Fig. 22–22), which originate within the metaphysis and always grow away from the epiphysis. The structure of the entire metaphysis is abnormal; it is broad and may be irregularly ossified.

PROGNOSIS AND TREATMENT. Exostoses are not malignant; rarely they may be transformed into chondrosarcomas. Exostoses become quiescent when growth of the patient is complete. Surgical intervention may be required for limitation of movement or for the relief of pressure symptoms on nerves or blood vessels.

OLLIER'S DISEASE

(Chondrodysplasia; Dyschondroplasia)

This malformation of the ends of the shafts is characterized by the presence of nonossified cartilage in the metaphyses and adjacent diaphyses of long bones. The disorder is usually unilateral, but occasionally lesser changes of the same sort are found on the opposite side. Facial asymmetry is sometimes present. There is no evidence that this disorder is genetically determined.

PATHOLOGY. The cartilaginous islands consist of hyaline cartilage upon which bone is deposited. The cells are larger and more irregularly distributed than usual. The cartilage is calcified in parts of its periphery, but it does not ossify normally.

CLINICAL MANIFESTATIONS. There is a gradual onset of symptoms during the first few years of life. It may be noticed that one limb is shorter than the other, or an external deformity may appear near a joint. In many instances the disease affects the arm

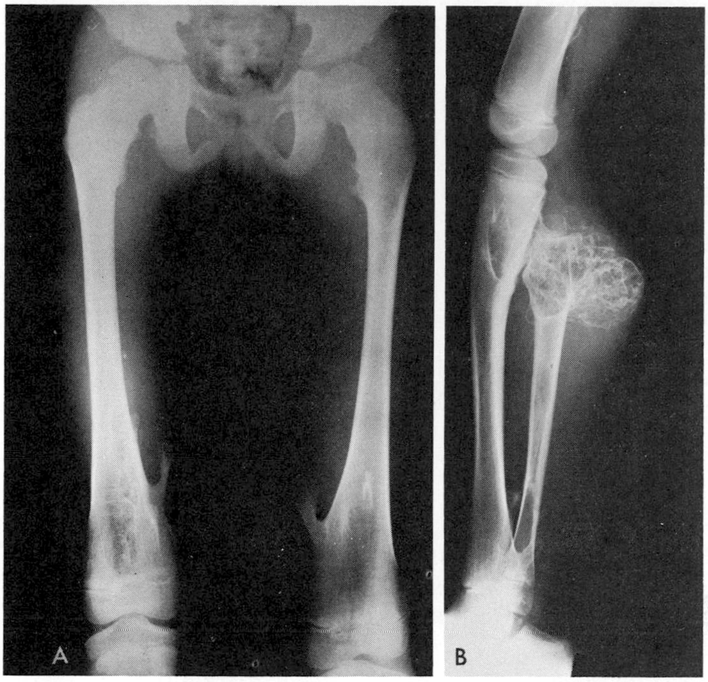

Figure 22–22 A, *Exostoses of both femurs.* B, *Large exostosis or osteochondroma in the fibula of the same patient.*

and the leg of the same side, and the pelvic and facial bones may also be involved. There may be deformity, shortening of the limbs and limitation of movement. The process is not inherently painful, but use of the deformed extremities may cause discomfort.

DIAGNOSIS. The disorder is easily recognized when the lesions are unilateral. In roentgenograms the upper end of the humerus, for example, may appear thickened, and the cortex of the diaphysis defective, with linear areas of rarefaction in the metaphysis and extending into the diaphysis. The distal ends of other long bones may have similar defects; the epiphyses are also affected (Fig. 22–23).

PROGNOSIS AND TREATMENT. The process is not progressive, but shortening of affected bones becomes manifest as the rest of the body increases in size. Infrequently sarcoma has developed in an affected bone. Fractures may occur in the rarefied areas. Orthopedic treatment for the correction of malformations and the prevention of further deformities is indicated.

MELORHEOSTOSIS

This skeletal disorder is a form of hyperostosis which begins in infancy or childhood and progresses slowly on one side of the bones of a single extremity. Enlargement, swelling and curving of the fingers or toes, and pain and deformity of the proximal bones of the same limb are clinical manifestations. Roentgenograms reveal a characteristic hyperostosis limited to one side of the bone. Melorheostosis is probably a developmental disorder, but infection and disturbance of sympathetic vasomotor control have also been considered possible causative factors.

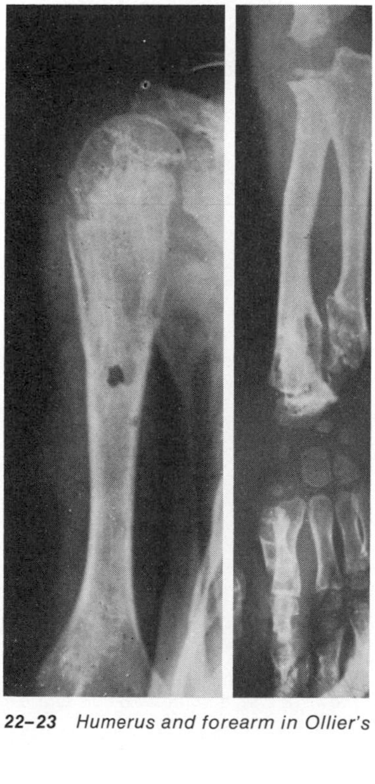

Figure 22–23 *Humerus and forearm in Ollier's disease.*

PROGRESSIVE DIAPHYSEAL DYSPLASIA

(Camurati-Engelmann's Disease)

This disorder is a developmental anomaly that can be transmitted as a dominant trait. It is characterized by thickening of the cortices of the long bones and by neuromuscular dystrophy. The dystrophy is responsible for general wasting of muscles and a peculiar waddling gait. In some instances there is also thickening of the flat bones, including those of the skull.

Roentgenographically there is thickening of the cortex of the diaphyses of the long bones with irregular narrowing of the medullary canal. The metaphyses and epiphyses are not involved, in contrast with osteopetrosis.

FIBROUS DYSPLASIA OF BONE

(Osteitis Fibrosa Disseminata; Polyostotic Fibrous Dysplasia; Osteodystrophia Fibrosa)

Fibrous dysplasia may affect one or many bones of the skeleton. In polyostotic cases the distribution tends to be unilateral; if both sides are involved, one side is affected more than the other. Fibrous dysplasia is probably due to a developmental error of early embryonic life, but there is no proof that the disorder is hereditary. The lesion consists of a fibrous matrix studded with trabeculae of immature bone with varying degrees of calcification. Monostotic cases may be free of symptoms or show only a local swelling. Sometimes a fracture, pain, or a functional impairment leads to recognition of the disease. If several bones of a limb are affected, clinical complaints are more frequent, and bowing and fractures are common manifestations. Flat bones sometimes become distended into tumor-like masses, while long bones become shortened, curved and thickened. Roentgenographic changes include diffuse and cyst-like lesions, sclerosis, evidence of fractures and abnormal outlines of the bones (Fig. 22–24). Sclerosis with thickening is the usual form of involvement of the bones of the orbit and face (Fig. 22–25). In the severest form of the disease several limbs may be involved, and the skull, vertebral column and pelvis may be included in the pathologic process. In such cases the osseous changes are often associated with brown pigmentation of the skin and with precocious osseous development and precocious puberty, which is seen more often in girls than in boys (McCune-Albright syndrome, Section 17). The serum levels of calcium and phosphorus are normal, but the serum phosphatase is elevated. Fibrous dysplasia may also be associated with arteriovenous fistulas, particularly in the extremities.

ARTHROGRYPOSIS

The term "arthrogryposis" denotes congenital contraction of joints in flexion. It usually occurs

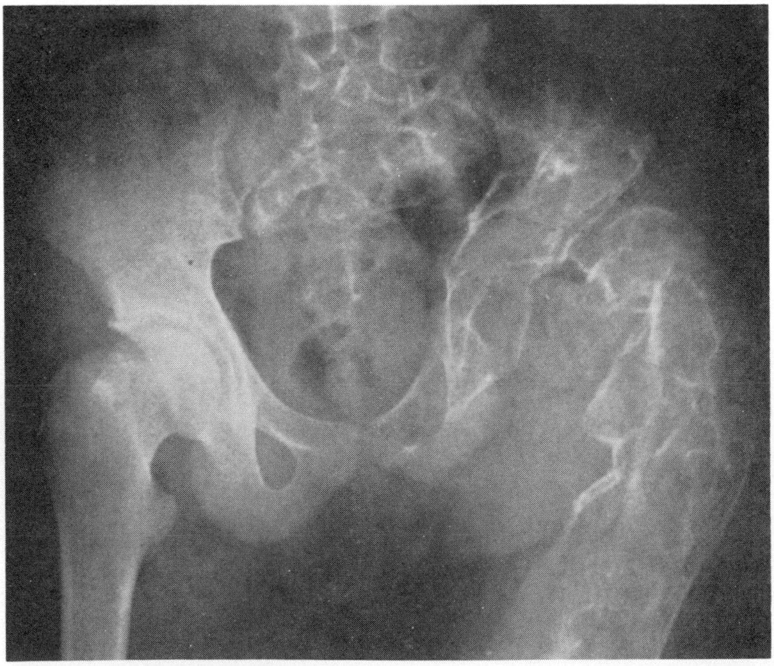

Figure 22–24 *Osteitis fibrosa disseminata. Roentgenogram showing extensive fibrous dysplasia of the sacrum, left ilium and femur. Note the irregular demineralization and expansion of the cortex. (Stauffer, Arbuckle and Aegerter:* J. Bone Joint Surg., *Vol. 23, 1941.)*

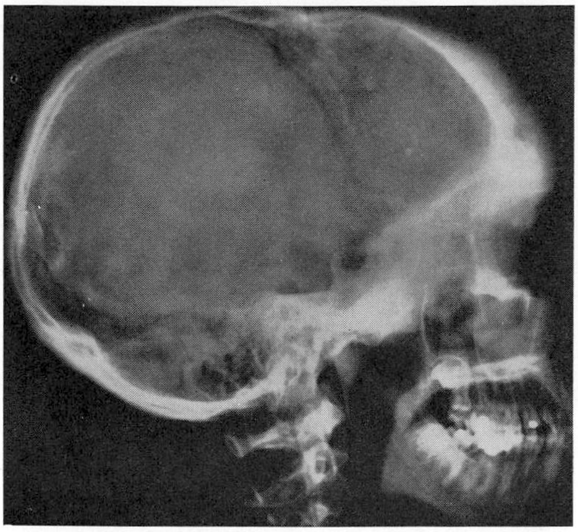

Figure 22–25 *Fibrous dysplasia. The bones at the base of the skull are opaque and markedly thickened. The paranasal sinuses, except for the right maxillary sinus, are obliterated, and the left orbit is distorted. The patient is 17 years of age. (From Aegerter, E., and Kirkpatrick, J. A., Jr.:* Orthopedic Diseases. *3rd ed. 1968.)*

alone, but may be associated with other malformations, such as arachnodactyly, premature synostoses of the bones of the skull, and many etiologically heterogeneous forms.

PATHOLOGY. The pathologic changes involve thick, inelastic articular capsules and atrophic muscle fibers with some fibrosis and fatty infiltration. Degeneration in the cells of the anterior horns of the spinal cord is found in typical arthrogryposis multiplex congenita.

CLINICAL MANIFESTATIONS. *Arthrogryposis multiplex congenita* is the term used for a special form of this disorder in which there is a congenital stiffness of one or more joints associated with a hypoplasia of the attached muscles. It is the result of incomplete fibrous ankylosis. Dislocation of the hips and of other joints is common. Since ankylosis of some joints occurs in extension, the term "arthrogryposis" is not entirely justified, and *multiple congenital articular rigidities,* a name also used, is more adequate. The disorder has been attributed to prolonged intrauterine pressure, but the frequent association with such malformations as defects of the palate or vertebrae and absence of the sacrum and fibula indicates origin early in embryonic life before intrauterine pressure becomes a teratogenic factor.

The disorder appears sporadically, but familial cases have been observed. The arms are rotated inward; the thighs, outward. The elbows and knees, which are described as cylindrical, are usually ankylosed in extension, although fixation of the knees in flexion also occurs. The wrists and fingers are flexed, and club feet are present. Certain muscle groups may be underdeveloped or absent. The skin appears thickened, and there may be dimples in the skin near the joints. Roentgenograms show only atrophy of the bones and small muscles. Some arthrogryposes are associated with diastrophic dwarfism or with congenital muscular dystrophy.

TREATMENT. Treatment consists in massage, passive movements, gradual correction of deformities by splints and plaster casts, and orthopedic surgery.

HEMIHYPERTROPHY

In hemihypertrophy, a congenital malformation, one side of the body is larger than the other (Fig. 22–26).

ETIOLOGY. The most credible explanation of this malformation is a faulty cell division of the zygote, resulting in two daughter cells of unequal size; it has been considered a form of incomplete twinning. Females are more often affected than males, the right side of the body more frequently than the left.

CLINICAL MANIFESTATIONS. The difference in the two sides is usually greatest in the extremities, the genitalia and the trunk. Facial and palatal inequality may also be present. The paired internal organs are sometimes of unequal size. In true hemihypertrophy the bones of the larger side are longer and thicker than their counterparts. There may be a difference in maturation as seen roentgenographically in the centers of ossification. There may be associated malformations such as aniridia, polydactyly, hypospadias, cryptorchidism, nevi and hemangiomas. Instances of association with Wilms's tumor and adrenal or hepatic neoplasms have been reported. The mentality may be normal, but retarded development has been observed.

DIFFERENTIAL DIAGNOSIS. Differentiation from *hemiatrophy* may be difficult, but hemiatrophy is

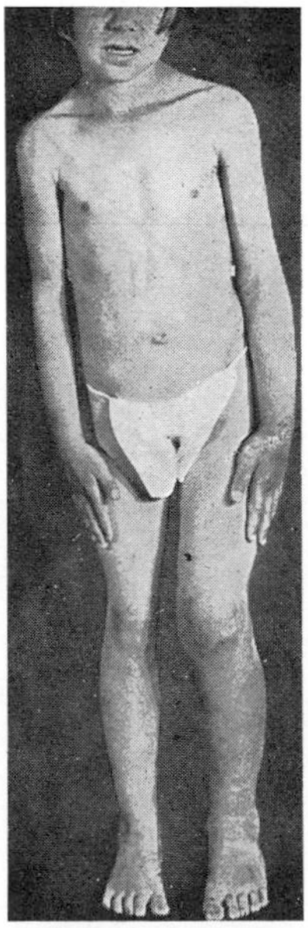

Figure 22–26 *Hemihypertrophy in a girl 4 years of age. The hypertrophy was of the entire left side of the body, including the face, teeth and tongue.*

frequently associated with such neurologic lesions as paralysis and athetosis. A congenital arteriovenous fistula may result in overgrowth of one extremity, and a similar effect can be caused by a low-grade nondestructive infection near an epiphysis. In *Milroy's disease* the soft tissues only are involved. *Recklinghausen's neurofibromatosis* can result in hypertrophy of an entire limb. In children who have had intrauterine growth retardation, one side may be smaller than the other (hemidystrophy). Such children show slow postnatal growth and associated malformations, but no tendency to tumor formation has been noted.

PROGNOSIS AND TREATMENT. The differences in the 2 sides often become less as the child grows older. Treatment is symptomatic; orthopedic corrections should be instituted early in life.

HYPERTROPHIC PULMONARY OSTEOARTHROPATHY

This condition, sometimes termed "Marie-Bamberger disease" or "hippocratic fingers," occurs in association with chronic pulmonary conditions and with congenital cyanotic heart disease. The lesions are an ossifying periostitis, effusion into the joints, erosion of the cartilages and hypertrophy of the soft tissues. In mild cases there is only clubbing of the fingers, the nails being broad and curved both transversely and longitudinally. In well developed cases there is also enlargement of the ends of the long bones and of the hands and feet, with pain and swelling of the joints. Clubbing of the fingers does not appear until several weeks to a year or longer after development of the causative disease.

A hereditary type of clubbing of the fingers, not dependent upon circulatory or pulmonary disease, has been described.

JOSEF WARKANY
JOHN A. KIRKPATRICK, JR.

GENERAL

Birth Defects, Original Article Series Parts III and IV. New York, National Foundation—March of Dimes, 1969.

Warkany, J.: Congenital Malformations, Notes and Comments. Chicago, Year Book Medical Publishers, Inc., 1971.

Craniosynostosis

Hemple, D. J., Harris, L. E., Svien, H. J., and Holman, C. B.: Craniosynostosis involving the sagittal suture only; Guilt by association? J. Pediatr. *58*:342, 1961.

Park, E. A., and Powers, G. F.: Acrocephaly and scaphocephaly with symmetrically distributed malformations of the extremities. Am. J. Dis. Child. *20*:235, 1920.

Temtamy, S. A.: Carpenter's syndrome: Acrocephalopolysyndactyly. J. Pediatr. *69*:111, 1966.

Basilar Impression

Chamberlain, W. E.: Basilar impression (platybasia). Yale J. Biol. Med. *11*:487, 1939.

Lacunar Skull

Vogt, E. C., and Wyatt, G. M.: Craniolacunia (Lückenschädel). Radiology *36*:147, 1941.

Malformations of the Extremities

Frantz, C. H., and O'Rahilly, R.: Congenital skeletal limb deficiencies. J. Bone Joint Surg. *43*-A: 1202, 1961.

Klippel-Feil Syndrome

Shoul, M. I., and Ritvo, M.: Clinical and roentgenological manifestations of the Klippel-Feil syndrome. Am. J. Roentgenol. *68*:369, 1952.

Congenital Absence of Caudal Spine

Blumel, J., Evans, E. B., and Eggers, G. W.: Partial and complete agenesis or malformation of the sacrum with associated anomalies; Etiologic and clinical study with special reference to heredity; A preliminary report. J. Bone Joint Surg., *41*-A:497, 1959.

Passarge, E., and Lenz, W.: Syndrome of caudal regression in infants of diabetic mothers. Pediatrics *37*:672, 1966.

Achondroplasia

Caffey, J.: Achondroplasia: *In* I. McQuarrie (ed.): Brennemann's Practice of Pediatrics. Hagerstown, Md., W. F. Prior Company, Inc., 1957, Vol. 4, Chap. 28.

Silverman, F. A.: Differential diagnosis of achondroplasia. Radiol. Clin. N. Amer. *6*:223, 1968.

Chondro-ectodermal Dysplasia

Ellis, R. W. B., and Van Creveld, S.: A syndrome characterized by ectodermal dysplasia, polydactyly, chondrodysplasia and congenital morbus cordis. Arch. Dis. Child. *15*:65, 1940.

McKusick, V. A., Eldridge, R., Hostetler, J. A., et al.: Dwarfism in the Amish. II. Bull. Johns Hopkins Hosp. *116*:285, 1965.

Mucopolysaccharidoses

Hurler, G.: Ueber einen Typ multipler Abartungen, vorwiegend am Skelettsystem. Z. Kinderh. *24*:220, 1919.

McKusick, V. A.: Heritable Disorders of Connective Tissue. 3rd ed. St. Louis, The C. V. Mosby Company, 1966.

Morquio, L.: Sur une forme de dystrophie osseuse familiale. Arch. Méd. Enf. *32*:129, 1929.

Noorden, G. K., Zelliwveger, H., and Ponsetti, I. V.: Ocular findings in Morquio-Ulrich's disease, with report of two cases. Arch. Ophthalmol. *64*:585, 1960.

Strauss, L.: The pathology of gargoylism: Report of a case and review of the literature. Am. J. Path. *24*:855, 1948.

Mucolipidoses

Spranger, J. W., and Wiedemann, H. R.: The genetic mucolipidoses. Humangenetik *9*:113, 1970.

Cleidal and Cleidocranial Dysostosis

Anspach, W. E., and Huepel, R. C.: Familial cleidocranial dysostosis (cleidal dysostosis); Preosseous and dentinal dystrophy. Am. J. Dis. Child. *58*:786, 1939.

Osteopetrosis

Clifton, W. M., and Frank, A.: Osteopetrosis (marble bones). *In* McQuarrie, I. (ed.): Brennemann's Practice of Pediatrics. Hagerstown, Md., W. F. Prior Company, Inc., 1957, Vol. 4, Chap. 23, Section 2.

Elmore, S. M.: Pycnodysostosis: A review. J. Bone Joint Surg. *49*-A:153, 1967.

Osteogenesis Imperfecta

Follis, R. H.: Osteogenesis imperfecta congenita: A connective tissue diathesis. J. Pediatr. *41*:713, 1952.

Multiple Exostoses

Jaffe, H. L.: Hereditary multiple exostosis. Arch. Path. *36*:335, 1943.

Ollier's Disease

Ollier, M.: De la dyschondroplasie. Bull. Soc. Chir. Lyon *3*:22, 1899.

Melorheostosis

Hall, G. S.: A contribution to the study of melorheostosis: Unusual bone changes associated with tuberous sclerosis. Quart J. Med. *12*:77, 1943.

Progressive Diaphyseal Dysplasia

Neuhauser, E. B. D., Schwachman, H., Wittenborg, M., and Cohen, J.: Progressive diaphyseal dysplasia. Radiology *51*:11, 1948.

Arthrogryposis

Drachman, D. B., and Banker, B. Q.: Arthrogryposis multiplex congenita. Case due to disease of the anterior horn cells. Arch. Neurol. *5*:77, 1961.

Stern, W. G.: Arthrogryposis multiplex congenita. J.A.M.A. *81*:1507, 1923.

Hemihypertrophy

Miller, R. W., Fraumeni, J. F., and Manning, M. D.: Association of Wilms's tumor with aniridia, hemihypertrophy and other congenital malformations. New Engl. J. Med. *270*:922, 1964.

Ward, J., and Lerner, H. H.: A review of the subject of congenital hemihypertrophy and a complete case report. J. Pediatr. *31*:403, 1947.

Osteitis Fibrosa Disseminata

Albright, F., Butler, A. M., Hampton, A. O., and Smith, P.: Syndrome characterized by osteitis fibrosa disseminata, areas of pigmentation and endocrine dysfunction, with precocious puberty in females; Report of five cases. New Engl. J. Med. *216*:727, 1937.

McCune, D. J., and Bruch, H.: Osteodystrophia fibrosa; Report of a case in which condition was combined with precocious puberty, pathologic pigmentation of skin and hyperthyroidism, with review of literature. Am. J. Dis. Child. *54*:806, 1937.

PEDIATRIC ORTHOPEDICS

RESPONSE OF BONE TO LOCAL AND GENERAL DISTURBANCES

Bones grow in length by new formation at the physis or growth plate and in width or diameter by appositional growth at the deepest layer of the periosteum. Neither growing nor mature bone is a solid substance of inert matter, but a living tissue composed of constantly changing molecules, responsive and changeable. "Tagged" calcium molecules in a particular bone at one examination may be in another bone at a subsequent examination or may have been excreted. Perhaps bone would remain relatively constant in its component molecules, and perhaps a certain calcium molecule deposited in bone would remain stationary for an indefinite time, except that both environmental conditions and bones are changing continuously, even in the normal person, and these changes are accentuated during infectious and metabolic diseases and starvation.

Traumatic, nutritional, metabolic, endocrine, neurologic, infectious, circulatory and mechanical factors all cause changes in chemical and physical characteristics of bone. For example, increase in circulation, such as that caused by traumatic or hemangiomatous arteriovenous shunts or by a local inflammation, as in rheumatoid arthritis, may cause increased growth in length. Some bone tumors retard growth. Interference with nerve supply to an extremity retards both linear and cross-sectional growth; complete inactivity causes atrophy and demineralization, and damage to a physis disrupts growth or causes its total cessation.

RELATION OF INTRAUTERINE POSITION TO ORTHOPEDIC DISTURBANCES

Congenital malformations are considered earlier in this section.

Different etiologic factors can be responsible for identical structural defects in the fetus. In the rat, for example, congenital cleft palate may be genetic in origin or may result from infection, poisoning or vitamin deficiencies in the pregnant mother rat. It seems possible also that intrauterine posture can produce cleft palate in man. The "*position of comfort*" of the newborn with severe brachygnathia suggests this possibility. When the mandible is extremely small or posteriorly subluxated, it may be accompanied by cleft palate. The tongue, which is rarely, if ever, proportionately small, must be accommodated in the nasopharynx, since the mouth does not provide ample space for it.

Normally the fetus floats freely for the first half of the gestational period. After this time it begins to impinge on the uterine wall, and the mother translates these collisions as "feeling life." The fetus becomes increasingly restricted and less able to change position in relation to its mother.

The intrauterine position can be reconstructed after birth by "folding" the infant into his most comfortable position. Infants subjected to stretching of joint capsules as they become flexed in the uterus are likely to be fretful in the unaccustomed position in which they find themselves after birth. When such an infant is "folded," his fretting may cease, and he may fall asleep in his "position of comfort."

"Positions of comfort" are of infinite variety. They include hands hyperflexed along the forearms or grooving the thorax, heads indented by an arm, feet pressed tightly against the tibias, and many others. Reconstruction of the "position of comfort" may possibly explain some instances of club feet, torticollis, dislocated elbows, and asymmetries, as well as other deformities.

After the first week of life the relaxation diminishes rapidly but selectively. Muscles and joint capsules which were not stretched or strained during fetal life retain considerable pliancy throughout infancy, whereas those affected by fetal position may be restricted in their range of motion. Perhaps the jaw which was pressed against the sternum cannot be opened wide, and the thighs of an infant whose hip joint capsule was stretched cannot be abducted. In other stretched joints this stiffness is present for only a few months, but in the jaw and in the hips it may last longer, in part because the muscles closing the mouth are stronger than those opening it, and those adducting the hip are stronger than those abducting it.

THE FOOT

NORMAL FOOT. The normal foot of the infant appears grossly abnormal if judged by adult standards. It is fatter and wider than that of the adult. Fat pads create a fullness which suggests flatfoot; there is seldom a distinct longitudinal arch and never a transverse one. This pattern is accentuated by the normally soft and pliant muscles. The line of the Achilles tendon may be moderately angulated laterally and the foot slightly everted.

PRONATION (FLATFOOT). The term *flatfoot* as applied to the infant most often indicates that the medial longitudinal arch does not *look* as high as the parents or physician would like to see it. Most often there is no abnormality.

To decide whether the foot of a child is normal requires careful *examination* of its component parts and evaluation of its functional status. If the child with the suspected flatfoot will stand on his toes, a definite longitudinal arch will usually appear. Next the child is asked to stand on his heels with the front of the foot off the floor. If these maneuvers are successfully accomplished, there is high probability that the feet are developing within normal limits.

The joints are examined by checking their motions. The ankle joint moves in dorsiflexion and plantar flexion, the joints of the foot in eversion and inversion. After the physician has examined a few children with normal feet he will have learned the normal range of motion. The length of the heel cord must be tested with the knee straight and the foot inverted; then when the ankle is dorsiflexed, the lateral border of the foot should make an acute angle with the tibia of 80 degrees or less. A short heel cord is an abnormality and requires treatment.

The muscles which activate the joints are as follows: tibialis anticus, to produce dorsiflexion and inversion; tibialis posticus, to produce plantar flexion and inversion; peroneus tertius, to produce dorsiflexion and eversion; peroneus longus and brevis, to produce plantar flexion and eversion; and gastrocnemius and soleus, to produce plantar flexion. The child should carry out each of these motions actively, and the strength of the muscles should be tested. The range and strength of extension and flexion at the metatarsophalangeal joints should be carefully examined, since the integrity of the anterior arch depends on the flexibility of these joints.

The dorsalis pedis and posterior tibial pulses are palpated, and the Achilles tendon and plantar reflexes tested. Sensation is checked on the dorsal and plantar surfaces.

If this systematic examination reveals no abnormalities, the feet are "normal," and no treatment for the "flatfoot" is required. Specifically, so-called orthopedic shoes with Thomas heels are not indicated.

Occasionally a child will complain of pain or fatigue in the feet after play, and neither the examination described nor a roentgenographic examination of the foot will reveal any abnormality. *Foot strain* is the usual cause of such complaints, and exercises to improve the tone of the muscles supporting the foot are indicated. The young child should be instructed to walk "tiptoe" for 5 to 10 minutes daily; the older one, to stand slightly pigeon-toed with the weight thrown on the lateral border of the foot for 5 to 10 minutes daily. Mechanical support for the arch is not required *and is contraindicated in the absence of abnormal findings.*

PIGEON TOE. Pigeon toe is a frequent complaint. There are three common causes for toeing-in. *Metatarsus adductus* consists in adduction of the forefoot with no deformity of the hindfoot. It is the most common of the congenital foot deformities and is frequently associated with congenital dysplasia of the hip. Treatment is required as early as possible and before the infant walks. The deformity is easily corrected by passive stretching, reverse shoe, or casts and wedging, depending on its severity. It rarely recurs.

The second most common cause of pigeon toe is *inward tibial torsion.* A line drawn from the anterior-superior iliac spine through the center of the patella normally intersects the second toe when the foot is held at a right angle to the tibia and when the forefoot is held neither abducted nor adducted. In tibial torsion this line intersects the fourth or fifth toe or a point lateral to the fifth one. Tibial torsion is always associated with a tibial bow. It requires no treatment such as braces, bars or shoe wedging, but is corrected as the extremity grows. Tibial torsion is frequently associated with metatarsus adductus; the latter should be corrected as described above. Some degree of pigeon toe will persist until growth has corrected the tibial torsion, when the toeing-in will be self-corrected. External rotation bars are unnecessary in the treatment of inward tibial torsion.

The third cause of pigeon toe is *inward femoral torsion.* For examination the child is placed supine, and the legs are inwardly rotated and then outwardly rotated at the hips. Normally, inward rotation is about 30 degrees and outward rotation 60 degrees. In inward femoral torsion the inward rotation will approach 90 degrees, the patellae will face each other, and outward rotation is practically nonexistent. No treatment is required; correction usually does not occur with growth, but the patient develops an outward tibial torsion which compensates for the inward femoral torsion.

CLUBFOOT. The usual so-called congenital clubfoot is a secondary deformity of the foot and ankle. The most frequent deformity is that of *equinovarus,* in which the foot is in plantar flexion and deviates medially. More than 95 per cent of congenital club feet are of the equinovarus type. Next most frequent is the deformity of *calcaneovalgus,* in which the foot is dorsiflexed and deviated laterally. Many children are born with the positional abnormality of equinovarus or calcaneovalgus. If the foot can be passively brought into the opposite position, the infant does not have a clubfoot and requires only simple exercises for correction of the deformity. The primary type of congenital clubfoot is rare and results from absence of muscles or bones or of fusion of bones. *The foot which cannot be passively overcorrected is a clubfoot and requires orthopedic treatment.* Conservative treatment with casts and wedgings or the Denis Browne splint is preferred. Forcible manipulation and surgery are usually unnecessary, but occasionally lengthening of the heel cord will be required, after forefoot wedging.

SHOES. Before he begins to walk, it is unnecessary for an infant to wear shoes; so long as walking is limited to carpeted floors, the shoes should be the softest obtainable, usually of the moccasin type. Later, when the feet need protection against the pounding received on hard floors and pavements, somewhat thicker soles become desirable. These should be as pliable as possible, since stiff-soled shoes limit the range of foot motion and therefore impede development of the supporting muscles. It is essential that the shank be flexible, the leather soft and the last straight or swung in. The basic requirements for new shoes during the growth period are adequate width and adequate length. The big toe should be a thumb's width from the end of the shoe in the weight-bearing position. The width of the shoe should be enough so that with the child in the weight-bearing position the leather over the widest part of the forefoot is sufficiently loose to permit a small amount of leather to be picked up when it is pinched. The so-called orthopedic shoe should be restricted to pathologic conditions. Under no circumstances should it be used for the normal foot.

THE LEG

BOWLEG AND KNOCK-KNEES. In most instances bowleg and knock-knees cannot be explained on any pathologic basis. If such acquired lesions as rickets and such congenital abnormalities as achondroplasia can be ruled out, they should be considered to be developmental variants even though the apparent deformity may be severe. It can be expected that they will be corrected by growth within the limits of genetic potential. Wedges in the shoes have no effect on bowleg or knock-knee. Braces are used only in deformities in which the collateral ligaments of the knees are becoming stretched; they do not correct the deformity and are used only to prevent further relaxation of ligaments. A single anteroposterior roentgenogram of the knees should be obtained in patients with severe bowleg or knock-knee.

In developmental bowleg a record should be kept of measurements of the distance between the medial aspects of the knees when the medial malleoli are held against each other. In knock-knee the distances between the malleoli are measured when the medial aspects of the knees are held against each other. For either deformity serial tracings of the legs may be made on long sheets of paper.

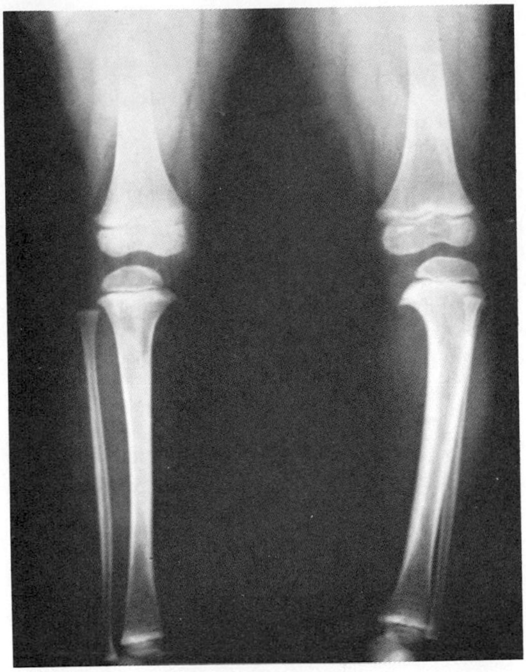

Figure 22–27 Blount's disease. The medial aspect of the proximal end of the left tibia is irregular and "beaked." There is also minimal involvement of medial aspects of the proximal tibial epiphyseal center. As a consequence of the proximal tibial deformity, there was abnormal weight bearing, which in turn was responsible for the thickening shown in the medial cortex of the left tibia. The right tibia is normal.

Blount's disease, or tibia vara, is an acquired lesion of the proximal tibial metaphysis and epiphysis; it results in bowleg because of retardation of growth of this medial portion of the tibia. The cause is unknown. Roentgenographically there is irregularity of the medial aspect of the tibial epiphyseal center and tibial metaphysis with the formation of a beaklike projection (Fig. 22–27). Treatment may require bracing and frequently osteotomy, depending on the severity of the process and the degree of the deformity.

CONGENITAL GENU RECURVATUM. Hyperextension of the knee is not unusual in the newborn infant and may be the result of positioning in utero. It is usually corrected spontaneously within the first few weeks of life. Persistence for more than several weeks requires splinting in slight flexion to permit shortening of the posterior capsule of the knee joint.

THE HIP

CONGENITAL DYSPLASIA OF THE HIP

Congenital dysplasia of the hip is defined as abnormal development of the hip joint, the acetabulum, femoral head, capsule and other soft tissues. The head of the femur may be partially dislocated from the shallow acetabulum (congenital subluxation of the hip), or it may be completely dislocated (congenital dislocation of the hip).

The cause of congenital dysplasia of the hip is unknown. Abnormal development of the joint caused by fetal position or by genetic factors, and abnormal relaxation of the capsule and ligaments of the joint by hormonal factors have been suggested.

Congenital subluxation of the hip is much more frequent than congenital dislocation. In many infants with congenital subluxation, during the first

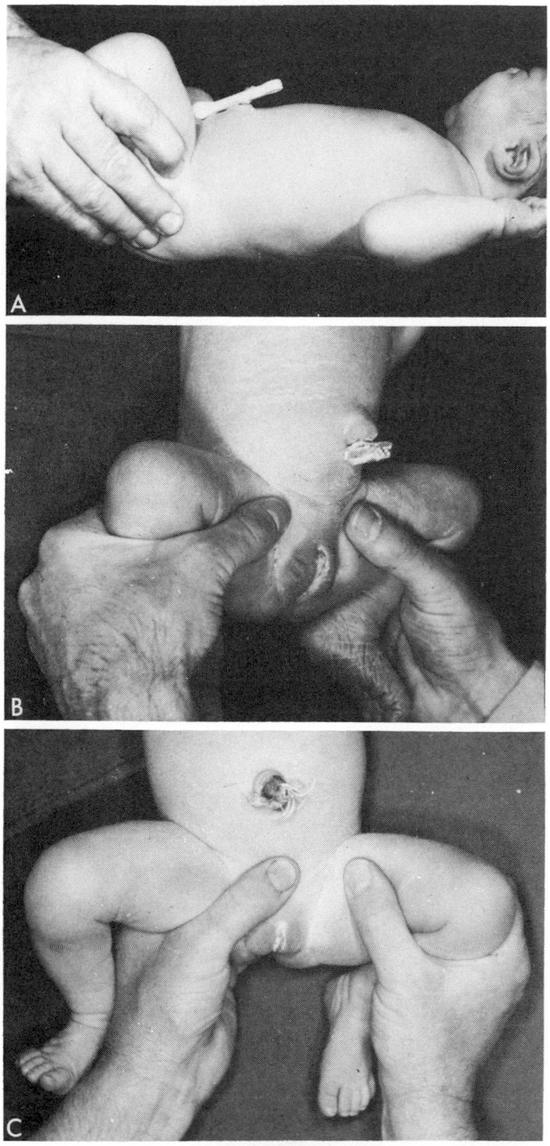

Figure 22–28 A, *The newborn child is laid on its back with the hips and knees flexed, and the middle finger of each hand is placed over each greater trochanter.* B, *The thumb of each hand is applied to the inner side of the thigh opposite the lesser trochanter.* C, *In a doubtful case the pelvis may be steadied between a thumb over the pubis and fingers under the sacrum while the hip is tested with the other hand.*

week after birth the head of the femur may be made to dislocate from the acetabulum by Barlow's modification of Ortolani's maneuver (Fig. 22–28).

The test is made in two parts: The baby is placed on its back with the legs pointing toward the examiner. The hips are flexed to a right angle and the knees are fully flexed. The middle finger of each hand is placed over the greater trochanter (Fig. 22–28 *A*) and the thumb of each hand is applied to the inner side of the thigh opposite the position of the lesser trochanter (Fig. 22–28 *B*). The thighs are carried into mid-abduction, and forward pressure behind the greater trochanter is exerted by the middle finger of each hand in turn while the other hand holds the opposite femur and pelvis steady. If the femoral head slips forward into the acetabulum the hip has been dislocated. If there is no movement of the femoral head the hip is not dislocated. This completes the first part of the test. The second part of the test consists in applying pressure backward and outward with the thumb on the inner side of the thigh. If the femoral head slips out over the posterior lip of the acetabulum and back again immediately the pressure is released, the hip is "unstable"—that is to say, the hip is not dislocated but is dislocatable.

In a doubtful case the stability of each joint can be further tested with the pelvis firmly held between a thumb on the pubis and fingers under the sacrum (Fig. 22–28 *C*).

As the femoral head moves with Barlow's maneuver into or out of the acetabulum, a "click" of entry or of exit may be felt by the examiner (Ortolani's sign).

In congenital subluxation of the hip there may be no limitation of abduction in the first few weeks of life, but by 3 to 6 weeks, as secondary shortening of the adductor muscles occurs, abduction of the flexed hip will be limited (Fig. 22–29). When the normal infant is on his back with his hips flexed to a right angle with the trunk, the thighs can be abducted passively until the knees nearly reach the examining table. In unilateral dysplasia the limitation of abduction is obvious when the involved side is compared with the normal. When abduction of both hips does not permit the knees to nearly touch the examining table, bilateral dysplasia must be suspected and roentgenograms obtained. *The hips should be flexed and abducted on every visit of the infant to the physician's office, because limitation of abduction may appear even after the fourth or fifth month of age.*

Shortening of the leg is absent or minimal in congenital subluxation of the hip, and asymmetry of skin folds is of little or no value in diagnosis. An anteroposterior roentgenogram of the subluxated hip often shows: (1) An increased slope of the acetabular roof. Normally the angle which the roof of the acetabulum makes with a horizontal line drawn through the centers of the acetabular epiphyses is less than 40 degrees. (2) Slight lateral and cephalic displacement of the upper end of the femur. A true anteroposterior roentgenogram of the pelvis with the hips in a neutral position (not abducted or adducted, nor inwardly or outwardly

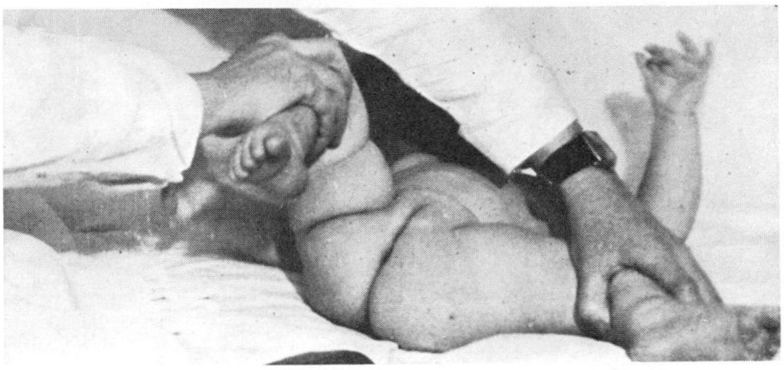

Figure 22–29 Limitation of abduction is an early sign of congenital dislocation of the hip. Note restriction in abduction of right leg.

rotated) is essential to evaluation of differences between the two hips (see Fig. 22–30).

Coleman's criteria for the diagnosis of congenital dysplasia of the hip are (1) presence of Ortolani's sign, (2) an acetabular angle above 40 degrees, (3) lateral displacement of the upper end of the femur, or (4) persistent limitation of abduction of the flexed hip. Any one of these findings indicates need for treatment of the abnormal hip.

Treatment of congenital subluxation of the hip consists of maintenance of abduction of the hips until the hip is normal clinically and roentgenographically. In infants in whom Ortolani's sign is elicited by Barlow's maneuver during the first week after birth, simple double diapering is usually adequate to reconstruct the dysplastic hip. But if Ortolani's sign persists past the third week or if limited abduction of the hip is found later, more adequate splinting is necessary (Fig. 22–31). Usually the hip is normal by the third month if adequate treatment is begun in the first week of life.

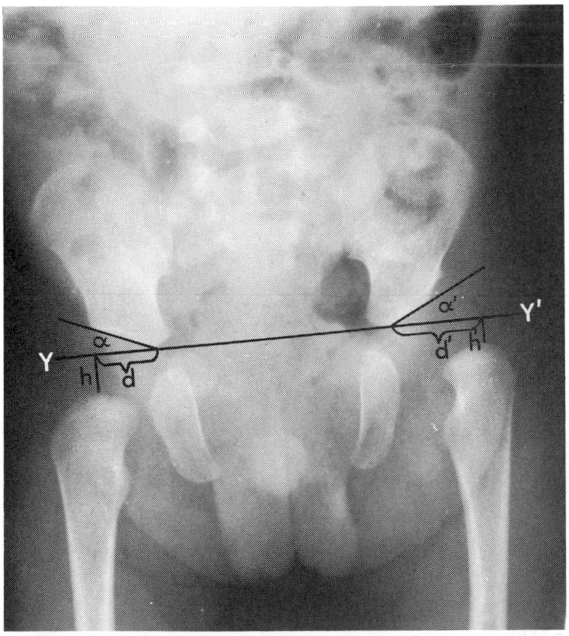

Figure 22–30 Hilgenreiner's method for identification of dysplasia of the hip prior to ossification of the capital femoral epiphysis. α' is greater than α, indicating greater obliquity of the acetabular roof. d' is greater than d, indicating lateral displacement of the femur. h is greater than h', indicating cephalic displacement of the femur. These relations indicate dysplasia of the patient's left hip.

In infants who have limitation of abduction, whether or not Ortolani's sign has been present earlier, abduction splinting applied by an orthopedist is necessary. The splint must be carefully applied so that forcible abduction is avoided; otherwise the vascular supply to the femoral capital epiphysis may be compromised.

If treatment is not carried out *in congenital dysplasia of the hip with subluxation,* one of three things may occur: (1) The dysplastic hip may become normal because of the abduction produced by the normal diaper. (2) The hip may remain partially dislocated, the acetabulum shallow and the head of the femur slightly deformed. The patient usually has no symptoms until later in life, when degenerative changes may develop in the mechanically imperfect hip. (3) The partially dislocated (subluxated) hip may rarely go on to complete dislocation, in which case the patient will have the signs of a congenital dysplasia of the hip with dislocation.

In congenital dysplasia of the hip with dislocation, the dislocation may be present at birth or very rarely may develop in an untreated, partially dislocated hip. The head of the femur is usually dislocated posterosuperiorly. It may be dislocated anteriorly, however, in which case the diagnosis is more difficult. In posterosuperior dislocation, abduction is limited; Ortolani's sign may be present in reverse. As Barlow's maneuver is started, when the flexed hip is abducted, the head of the femur may slip back into the acetabulum, and a "click of entry" will be felt; then as the flexed hip is adducted, a "click of exit" will be felt. There is shortening of the leg, which is best demonstrated with the infant lying flat on his back and with his hips flexed to 90 degrees, a difference in the level of the knees indicating shortening of one thigh. Telescoping is present; alternating push and pull on the flexed thigh moves the head of the femur back and forth on the side of the ileum. Normally the femoral artery in the groin is palpated against the head of the femur; when the head is dislocated, the artery is not so easily palpated as on the normal side. The inguinal crease is deeper than on the normal side; the greater trochanter is palpated more

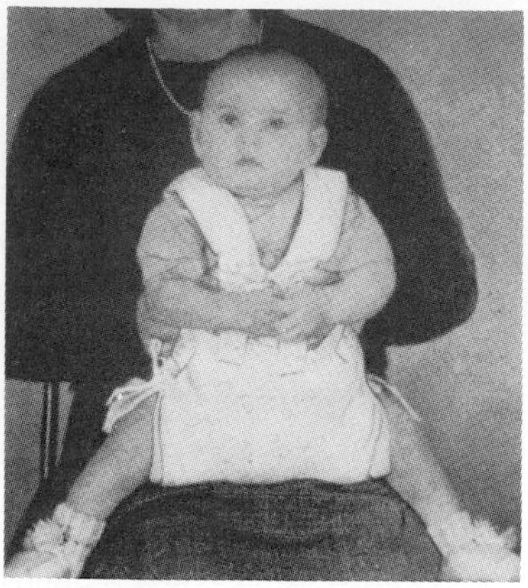

Figure 22–31 The Fredjka abduction splint for treatment of congenital subluxation of the hip. The splint is discontinued when roentgenographic and clinical studies demonstrate ossification of the acetabular roof and a stable hip joint. Use of the splint is usually required for several months. It should not be used before the infant is three months old. (Hart, V. L.: Congenital Dysplasia of the Hip Joint and Sequelae. Courtesy of Charles C Thomas, Springfield, Ill., 1952.)

cephalad than on the normal side. Straight-leg raising is greatly increased on the side with the dislocation. When the baby is turned face down on the examination table, the buttock on the involved side is flatter and wider than the normal one.

When the child can stand, if he stands on the abnormal leg, the pelvis drops on the normal side (Trendelenburg's sign). When he walks, his trunk dips when he puts weight on the involved leg, the so-called going-downstairs limp. Bilateral dislocation of the hip causes a "duck waddle" gait. Lumbar lordosis is increased when the child stands. If a line is drawn from the umbilicus to the ischial tuberosity (Nélaton's line), the trochanter will be palpated above the line.

If the head of the femur is dislocated anteriorly rather than posterosuperiorly, abduction of the flexed hip will be limited. The inguinal crease will not be so deep as on the normal side, and though shortening will be present, it will be minimal. Telescoping also will be much less than if the hip were dislocated posterosuperiorly. When the child starts to walk, although a limp will be present, it will not be very obvious, and the lumbar spine, instead of having increased lordosis, will be flattened.

The roentgenogram of the dislocated hip will demonstrate obvious dislocation; even in the early months of life before the capital epiphysis is ossified, the upper end of the femur does not point into the acetabulum (Fig. 22–32).

Treatment of congenital dysplasia of the hip with dislocation is usually by closed reduction of the hip and maintenance of the reduction by adequate immobilization, usually in a hip spica cast. If diagnosis is delayed beyond 12 to 18 months, closed reduction may not be possible, and operative reduction will be necessary. The later the diagnosis is made and treatment started, the poorer the prognosis for a normal hip.

The emphasis in respect to congenital hip dysplasia should be on early diagnosis. The most important clinical findings are Barlow's signs in the first week of life and limitation of abduction of the flexed hip thereafter. Since limitation of abduction may not appear early, it is essential that the physician abduct the flexed hips of the infant on every visit during the first year of life.

ACQUIRED DISEASES OF THE HIP

A variety of lesions of the hip, especially in their initial stage, may produce similar symptoms. These include trauma, acute and chronic infections, Perthes's disease and slipped epiphysis. The common presenting symptoms are those of *synovitis*: limp and pain in the hip, or, frequently, *pain referred to the knee.*

INFECTION. Infection is usually manifest systemically by fever and signs of toxemia, as well as by such local signs as muscle spasm, tenderness, swelling and pain on attempted passive motion of the joint. Acute suppurative synovitis is not uncommon. Paracentesis should be done for diagnosis when infection is suspected. Recovery of pus demands immediate surgical drainage.

TRAUMA. This is the most frequent cause of suddenly acquired limp and pain in the hip or knee *(synovitis of the hip)* which brings the child to the physician. Often the trauma has been so slight that it was overlooked or perhaps never known to the parents. A few hours later the joint is full of fluid and painful.

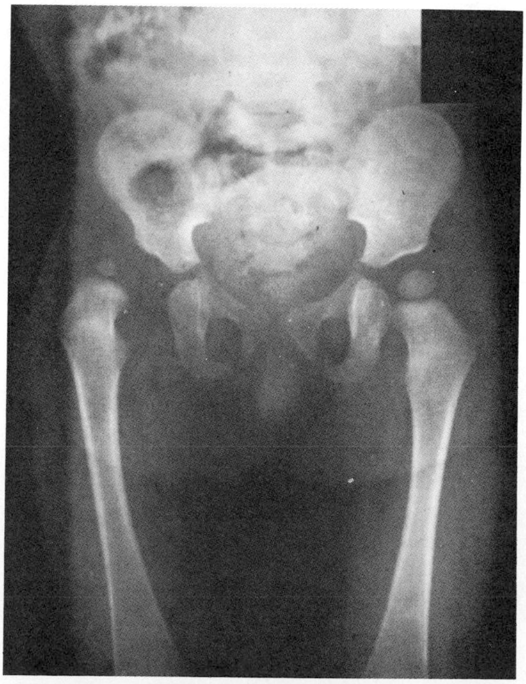

Figure 22–32 Untreated congenital dislocation of the right hip, demonstrating superior and lateral displacement of the underdeveloped femoral head and capital epiphysis, underdevelopment of the acetabulum and an increase in the slope of the acetabular roof.

Examination may reveal limitation of motion, muscle spasm and swelling of the joint. Motion is tested in three planes: flexion and extension, abduction and adduction, and inward and outward rotation, and compared with that of the normal side. When limitation of motion is due to muscle spasm, the range of motion gradually increases as gentle pressure is maintained against the leg and the muscle becomes fatigued. Swelling of the joint is demonstrated by placing the thumb over the femoral artery where it crosses the inguinal ligament and the other four fingers posteriorly over the buttock opposite the position of the thumb. In this way the joint with the soft tissue anterior and posterior to it is grasped between the thumb and fingers. When the hip joint is swollen, it will feel thicker than the normal one *(Gill's sign).*

It is impossible to distinguish the joint lesion of trauma from that of early Perthes's disease before radiologic changes have become manifest. If roentgenographic examination is negative, the child should be put to bed for 3 or 4 days. If the spasm persists, the child should have Buck's traction on both legs for 3 weeks. If the signs of spasm have then disappeared, as they usually will have if trauma has been the cause, gradually increasing activity is allowed. If spasm persists, traction is continued for another 3 weeks, when the roentgenographic examination is repeated. The characteristic changes of Perthes's disease will usually have appeared by then.

PERTHES' DISEASE. Legg-Calvé-Perthes disease is an aseptic necrosis of the capital femoral epiphysis causing signs and symptoms of synovitis as described above, followed by characteristic radiologic changes.

The cause is unknown. Males between the ages of 4 and 10 years are most frequently affected; infrequently the disease is bilateral. Three stages are usually described, each lasting about 9 months to a year. The first stage is one of aseptic necrosis; roentgenographically there may be no change during the first weeks, after which a relative opacity of the epiphysis becomes evident. The second stage consists in revascularization, and the epiphysis becomes mottled and fragmented (Fig. 22–33). In the third stage there is reossification, and serial films demonstrate gradual re-formation of the head of the femur. The principle of treatment is avoidance of weight bearing, by any of several methods. The head of the femur tends to flatten and becomes mushroom-shaped, causing incongruity between head and acetabulum with degenerative changes later in life. The main prognostic factors as far as the eventual shape of the head of the femur is concerned are the age of the child at time of onset, the amount of involvement as shown roentgenographically, and whether dislocation of the hip or some other predisposing condition has been present in the past; sickle cell disease and corticosteroid therapy, for example, may cause circulatory changes in the head of the femur. In recent years, besides limitation of weight bearing, surgical intervention has been advocated in order to maintain the spherical shape of the femoral head; the merits of surgery have not been proved.

SLIPPED EPIPHYSIS. This occurs typically in the adolescent. In its early stages it is characterized by the signs and symptoms of synovitis. The cause is unknown, but the condition occurs mostly in the "overlarge" child. The onset is insidious and characterized by pain in the knee, so that hip disease may not be suspected even though the child limps. Roentgenographic examination will reveal widening of the epiphyseal line or displacement posteriorly and inferiorly of the femoral capital epiphysis. This is shown on the lateral projection, but not always on the anterior-posterior one. The anterior bowing of the neck which occurs as the "slip" progresses makes subsequent therapy difficult, so that early diagnosis is of great importance.

The principle of treatment is arrest of the slipping, which can be attained by immobilization of the hip in a spica cast, or more surely, surgically,

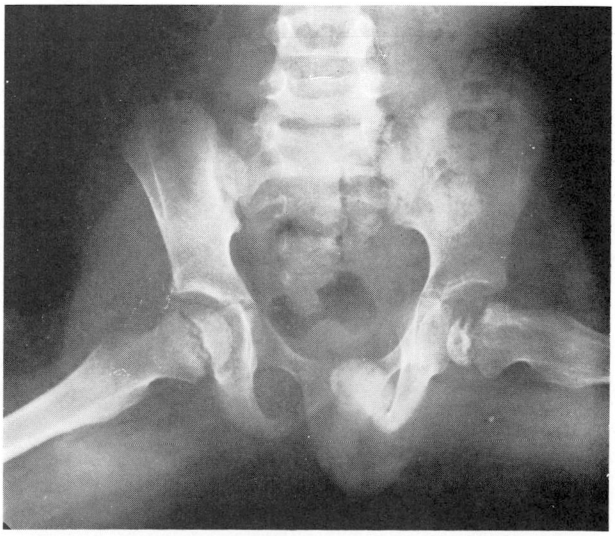

Figure 22–33 *Legg-Calvé-Perthes disease of the left hip in a boy 6 years of age. The presenting complaints were limp and pain in the left knee. The lateral roentgenogram reveals sclerosis of the femoral capital epiphyseal center, which is also fragmented and flattened. The "joint space" is wider than normal. At this stage there is little deformity of the neck of the femur.*

by internal fixation of the epiphysis to the metaphysis of the neck of the femur.

THE SPINE

SPONDYLOLISTHESIS. In this condition there is an anterior displacement of a lumbar vertebra, usually the fifth, associated with a bilateral defect in the *pars interarticularis.* The cause is unknown. In children under 10 years of age spondylolisthesis usually does not cause symptoms and is an incidental finding on a roentgenogram. If serial roentgenograms show that the vertebral body continues to be displaced forward, spinal fusion is indicated. Symptoms may appear in the adolescent. Pain in the low back is occasionally referred to the sciatic area, and there is an increasing lumbar lordosis. When such symptoms are present, a brace should be provided, and spinal fusion will be indicated if the symptoms persist or if the slipping progresses. Frequently the earliest sign of nerve root irritation is spasm of the hamstring muscles with limited "straight-leg raising."

SCOLIOSIS. Scoliosis is a lateral curvature of the spine. It is most commonly caused by a short leg, and will be overcorrected by putting a lift under the short leg or by bending toward the convex side of the curve. Such a curve is termed a *functional scoliosis* and does not become structural. Functional scoliosis may also be caused by muscle spasm secondary to trauma.

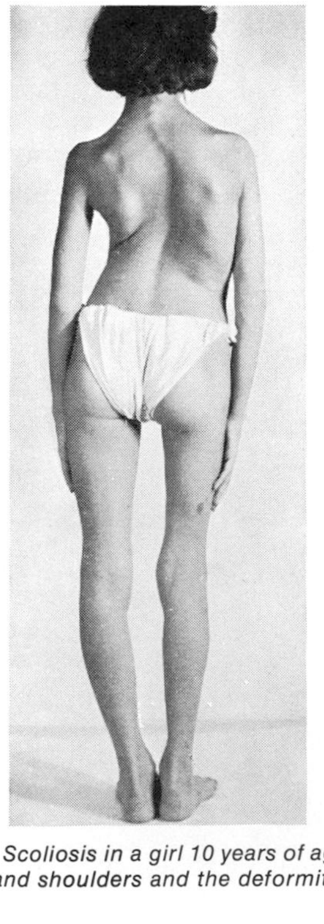

Figure 22–34 *Scoliosis in a girl 10 years of age, showing the tilt of the pelvis and shoulders and the deformity of the thorax.*

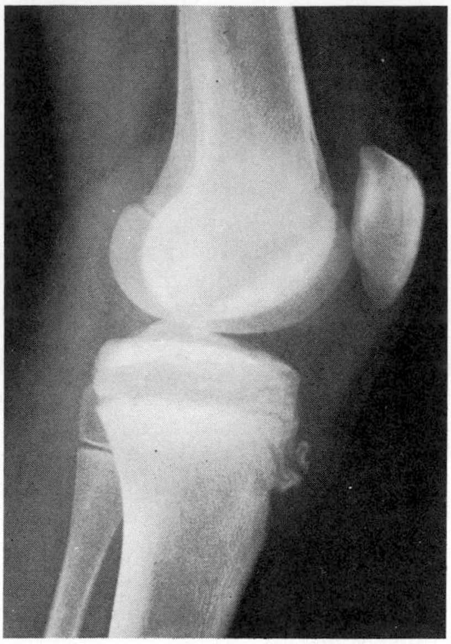

Figure 22–35 *Osteochondrosis of tibial tubercle (Osgood-Schlatter disease) in a boy 13 years of age. Roentgenogram shows irregular ossification of tibial tubercle and associated thickening of infrapatellar tendon. The roentgenographic examination is often normal in this condition.*

A fixed scoliosis not overcorrectable by bending is termed a *structural scoliosis.* It may be caused by such lesions as hemivertebra, fusion of ribs, absence or paralysis of muscles, neurofibromatosis, or vertebral destruction by infection or tumor; most often it is idiopathic. Idiopathic scoliosis occurs most frequently in adolescent girls and requires treatment. The prognosis for excellent results of treatment has been greatly improved in recent years with the use of the Milwaukee brace, and with improved methods of mechanical correction of the curve, followed by spinal fusion.

OSTEOCHONDROSIS

Several different entities were classified in the past as osteochondrosis because of similarities in roentgenographic appearance. Aseptic necroses of the capital femoral epiphysis *(Perthes' disease)* (see above), of a metatarsal head *(Freiberg's disease),* or of the tarsal navicular *(Köhler's disease)* are not uncommon and cause pain in the involved area and frequently limping and possibly subsequent deformity.

Scheuermann's disease of the spine, probably a developmental abnormality, causes kyphosis (round back) and frequently requires bracing to lessen pain and to prevent deformity. *Osgood-Schlatter disease* of the tibial tuberosity (Fig. 22–35), almost certainly caused by chronic trauma to the tibial tuberosity as a result of overuse of the quadriceps muscle, causes pain and swelling and should be treated by immobilizing the knee in a walking cast for 6 weeks. If not treated it will usually persist until the epiphyseal line of the upper end of the tibia has closed. *Sever's disease* of the apophysis of the os calcis is analogous to Osgood-Schlatter disease and results from traction on the apophysis by the tendo Achillis. It, too, should be treated by immobilization for 6 weeks if the symptoms warrant.

SUBLUXATION OF HEAD OF RADIUS

Subluxation of the head of the radius occurs frequently in children 2 to 5 years of age; it is rare after 9 years of age. The child has usually been forcibly jerked by the hand by a taller person while the elbow is in full extension; the subluxation occurs with an audible snap.

The symptoms include immediate but usually not persistent pain in the elbow, an inability to supinate the forearm, and a tendency to hold the elbow in slight flexion. Palpation and roentgenograms of the elbow do not reveal any abnormality, and there is no edema. The diagnosis is confirmed by the easy reduction of the subluxation. This is accomplished by firmly grasping the hand of the affected arm and holding the elbow with the thumb of the other hand pressed against the head of the radius while forcibly supinating the forearm beyond the point of obstruction. The click of the return of the radial head to position is usually followed by immediate recovery of painless function.

INFECTIONS OF THE BONES AND JOINTS

ACUTE INFECTIOUS ARTHRITIS

This condition is most common in the first 6 months of life. It is usually preceded by an infection elsewhere in the body, often in the upper respiratory tract. The causative organism is usually one of the common pyogens, such as the staphylococcus, streptococcus, pneumococcus, or *H. influenzae* and, less commonly, the gonococcus, meningococcus, typhoid bacillus or one of the salmonella group of organisms. The shoulder, hip and other large joints are most commonly affected, but any joint may be involved. Pyogenic arthritis will result in rapid destruction of cartilage and ankylosis of the joint if diagnosis and treatment are delayed.

CLINICAL MANIFESTATIONS. The onset is sudden, with systemic symptoms of sepsis. Local swelling appears rapidly, with muscular rigidity and intense pain on motion of the joint, and, if untreated, is followed quickly by suppuration. When the hip is affected, it may become dislocated with astonishing rapidity.

DIFFERENTIAL DIAGNOSIS. Acute suppurative arthritis must be differentiated from *acute osteomyelitis.* In acute suppurative arthritis even slight motion of the joint is painful, whereas in osteomyelitis the joint may be moved without pain if done carefully. In suppurative arthritis there is ring tenderness around the joint; in osteomyelitis the tenderness is localized to the metaphysis. In the hip the differentiation cannot be made. The roentgenogram may be of no value in early diagnosis. *Rheumatic fever* rarely occurs in infancy and often involves more than one joint; a prompt response to salicylate therapy is suggestive of rheumatic fever. When an acute pyogenic infection of a joint is suspected, the joint should be aspirated and any material obtained cultured. A blood culture should also be obtained.

TREATMENT. The principle of treatment is immediate drainage of the joint. Emergency drainage can be obtained initially by paracentesis of the joint, but when, by smear or culture, the diagnosis of suppurative arthritis is established, prompt surgical drainage of the joint should be done. Appropriate antibiotic therapy is essential (see Osteomyelitis, below).

OSTEOMYELITIS

This disease occurs most often between 5 and 14 years of age and twice as frequently in boys as in girls. In infants under 2 years of age acute hematogenous osteomyelitis differs in many respects from that in older children.

ETIOLOGY AND PREDISPOSING FACTORS. The causative organism in the majority of instances is the hemolytic *Staphylococcus aureus,* though most of the other pathogenic bacteria may also be responsible. Primary lesions are often demonstrable and include furunculosis, impetigo, infected chickenpox and burns, and vaccinations.

PATHOLOGY. Osteomyelitis begins as a hematogenous abscess in the metaphysis, and then, if uninterrupted, the abscess ruptures subperiosteally and spreads along the shaft of the bone *under the periosteum.* The infection then penetrates to the bone marrow. The deep layer of the separated periosteum forms a shell of new bone around the infected shaft. The pieces of dead bone are known as sequestra, and the new bone formed by the periosteum as the involucrum. Sinuses may form between the sequestra and the skin surface. In the hip the metaphyseal abscess ruptures into the joint and creates a suppurative arthritis.

CLINICAL MANIFESTATIONS. The onset is usually abrupt, with fever, malaise, and pain with sharply localized tenderness in the bone *at the metaphysis.* Shortly thereafter swelling and redness over the affected bone may be present. These signs appear earlier in infants than in older children. The patient is toxic and extremely weak and irritable.

When osteomyelitis follows an infection which has been treated with an antibacterial agent, the clinical course may be modified sufficiently so that the true nature of the lesion may not be suspected until it is well advanced. In addition, inadequate antibacterial therapy of an acute osteomyelitic infection may temporarily abolish the clinical manifestations, but permit the infection to continue in a suppressed state only to become evident days or weeks later.

DIAGNOSIS. There is a leukocytosis of 15,000 to 25,000 cells or more, and the blood culture is usually positive. Roentgenographic examination does not reveal the process for at least 5 days in small children; in older children this period may be as long as 8 to 10 days. At this time there is rarefaction of the involved area, and soon there is evidence of the formation of involucrum.

DIFFERENTIAL DIAGNOSIS. Rheumatic fever, leukemia, primary or metastatic neoplasm, sprain, cellulitis, erysipelas and scurvy are likely to require differentiation. The presence of great toxicity and localized pain suggests osteomyelitis. Usually this is enough to distinguish the condition from *rheumatic fever,* but a history of involvement of other joints is indicative of the latter disease, as is the response to salicylates. *Scurvy* produces painful and tender swelling along the shaft of the bone, but roentgenograms of the long bones should be diagnostic. See also Acute Infectious Arthritis.

PROGNOSIS. The mortality rate from acute pyogenic infections of the bones has decreased since the availability of specific antibacterial agents. The rate is lower in newborn infants than in older infants and children, as is the incidence of chronic and metastatic lesions. Both the course and prognosis depend on early institution of appropriate therapy and continuance of it for an adequate time.

TREATMENT. Like acute pyogenic arthritis, osteomyelitis should be handled as a medical and orthopedic emergency. As soon as one or two specimens have been obtained for blood culture, intravenous antibiotic therapy is initiated. In children under 3 years of age either penicillin-resistant staphylococci or gram-negative organisms are likely to be found, so that therapy should be initiated both with a penicillinase-resistant agent such as methicillin or nafcillin or clindamycin and with

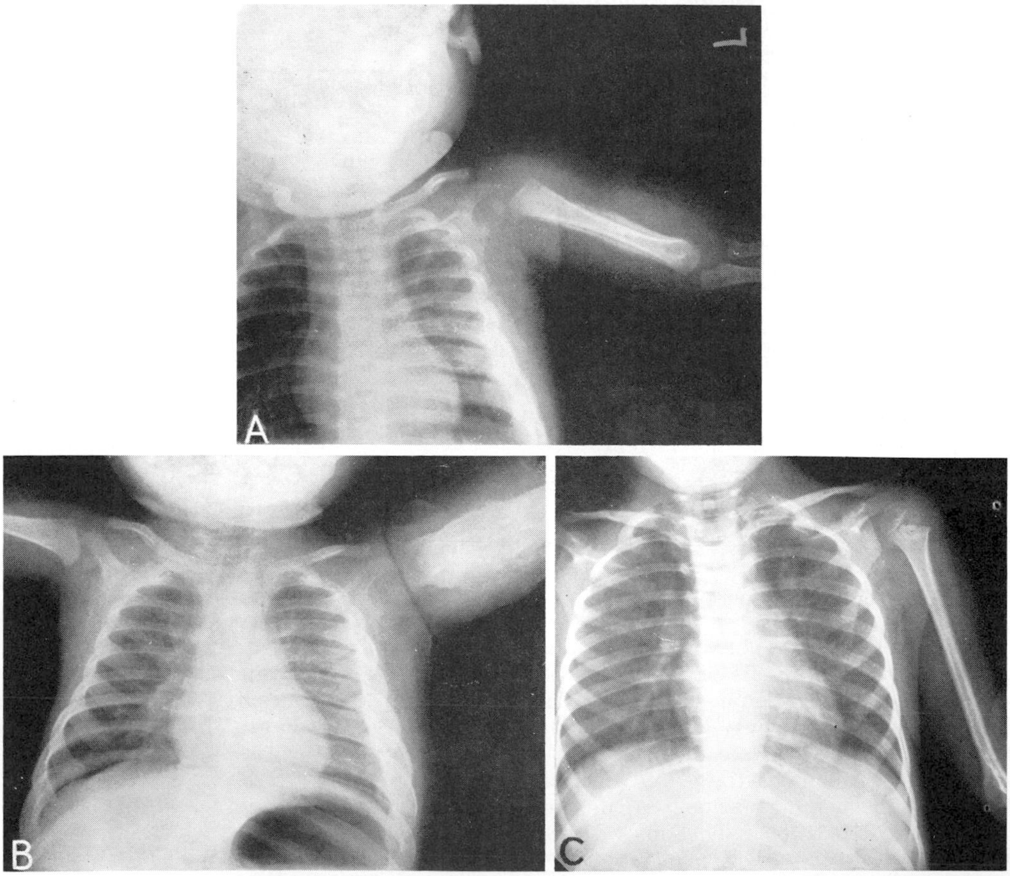

Figure 22–36 *Infantile cortical hyperostosis.* A, *Subperiosteal calcification of left lower ribs and left humerus. No evidence of bone destruction. The infant was moderately ill with an upper respiratory tract infection and was somewhat listless. The only localized finding was a disinclination to use the left arm, but there was no paralysis of it.* B, *Increase in subperiosteal calcification of left ribs and humerus developed within 1 month. There is similar involvement of lower right ribs and of facial bones. Evidence of illness has mostly disappeared at the time this roentgenogram was made.* C, *One and a half years later there is no evidence of the cortical disturbance.*

ampicillin, which will be effective against *H. influenzae*. In the newborn infant kanamycin or gentamicin is substituted for ampicillin. In children over 3 years of age ampicillin need not be used until or unless cultures indicate. Penicillin G may be used alone when and if cultures have recovered an organism sensitive to it. Intravenous therapy is continued until acute systemic manifestations of infection have subsided; oral therapy is thereafter maintained in full doses for 3 to 4 weeks.

Local treatment of choice for early osteomyelitis is immediate surgical drainage of the metaphysis, though some clinicians illogically prefer to wait 24 to 48 hours to evaluate the response to antibiotic therapy. When the abscess has ruptured into the subperiosteal space, chronic osteomyelitis is the inevitable sequel. Watching and waiting in such a situation is attended with considerable risk.

INFANTILE CORTICAL HYPEROSTOSIS

This lesion, also known as Caffey's disease, is a hyperplasia of subperiosteal bone (Fig. 22-36) over which there is a soft tissue swelling and at times a brawny discoloration of the skin. The cause is unknown. It has been observed in the fetus. Hyperostoses have been observed in the calvarium, mandible, clavicles, scapulas, ribs and the long bones of the extremities, including the metatarsals. The mandible and clavicles appear to be most frequently affected. The clinical features vary considerably, but the symptoms are not severe as a rule. Fever, usually of a low degree, tenderness, hyperirritability, pseudoparalysis, dysphagia, pleurisy, anemia, increased sedimentation rate and elevated serum phosphatase level have been observed in variable combinations.

Duration of clinical activity has been observed for as long as 9 months. No treatment has been effective. Recovery has occurred in all reported instances. Residual deformity is infrequent; bridging of the bones of the forearms has been reported.

Hypervitaminosis A may simulate infantile cortical hyperostosis in certain respects. In hypervitaminosis A the ulnas and one or more metatarsals, other than the first, have been the bones most frequently involved; the mandibles and other flat bones are apparently not affected. This distribution plus a history of excessive ingestion of vitamin A serves to distinguish this entity.

TUBERCULOSIS

TUBERCULOUS LESIONS OF THE BONES AND JOINTS. These lesions are hematogenous in origin, usually stemming from a pulmonary focus, which may not be demonstrable. There is usually only a single osseous lesion. The bones most frequently involved are the head of the femur (hip), the vertebrae and those of the fingers and toes.

TUBERCULOUS DACTYLITIS. Dactylitis occurs most frequently in early childhood and involves one or more of the phalanges, the metacarpal bones or the corresponding bones of the feet. The medullary canal of the involved bone becomes caseous; the cortex, thinned and expanded; and the periosteum, thickened. The entire digit develops a spindle-shaped, hard, red swelling as the soft tissues are affected. The process is comparatively painless, but it lasts many months and may leave a permanent deformity. The differential diagnosis is chiefly from the dactylitis of congenital syphilis, which is more often multiple and symmetrical. Dactylitis may also occur in sickle cell anemia and in coccidioidomycosis.

The involved region should be put at rest with a splint or cast, and operation is indicated if an abscess develops.

TUBERCULOUS SPONDYLITIS

(Pott's Disease)

This tuberculous osteitis originates in the body of one or more vertebrae, destroys the bone and spreads to all the tissues of the articulation. The spinous process and arches are unaffected. Kyphosis is most common in mid-dorsal lesions. Some scoliosis may accompany the kyphosis if the lesion is disproportionately unilateral.

The lower dorsal part of the spine is most likely to be involved, with the lumbar and the cervical segments next in order of frequency. Paraplegia may occur when the upper dorsal or cervical region is affected, but is rarely associated with involvement below the mid-dorsal region. *Psoas abscess* is a complication of caries in the lumbar vertebrae. A *cold abscess* in the cervical vertebrae may open into the pharynx (retropharyngeal abscess) or above the clavicle; one originating opposite the lower cervical or upper dorsal vertebrae may rupture into the pleura or penetrate to the scapula, but often it gravitates and points above Poupart's ligament.

CLINICAL MANIFESTATIONS. Symptoms are insidious in onset, the earliest being irritability. Persistent or intermittent pain may occur over the distribution of the spinal nerves arising adjacent to the affected vertebrae. This pain is increased by pressure on the head, but not by pressure over the lesions. Muscular rigidity splints the back, and the child assumes a position which will best take the weight from the diseased spine and prevent jarring. He may avoid bending to reach an object on the floor, may walk stiffly or carefully on his toes, or may prefer to lie on his abdomen and to rest frequently across a chair or over his mother's lap. With cervical involvement the child may hold his head stiffly or support it with his hand.

DIFFERENTIAL DIAGNOSIS. *Rickets* produces kyphosis of greater length and uniformity, which is unaccompanied by rigidity and disappears when the patient is prone. *Nontuberculous scoliosis* is seldom accompanied by rigidity or pain. *Hip joint disease* may be suspected when lameness is the result of lumbar tuberculosis, but in the latter there is no limitation of movement of the hip except in the presence of psoas abscess, when extension will be limited. *Acute nontuberculous osteomyelitis of the vertebrae* can be distinguished by its greater toxicity, leukocytosis and fever. In addition, the roentgenographic findings are usually well established in a tuberculous lesion of the vertebrae when symptoms first become manifest, whereas they are not likely to be demonstrable during the first few days of an acute pyogenic osteomyelitis. The *Klippel-Feil* syndrome may be confused with tuberculosis of the cervical spine, but is readily distinguishable by roentgenogram.

PROGNOSIS. The reparative process may not begin for 1 to 3 years, but in carefully treated cases recovery with ankylosis and little or no deformity can be expected in the majority of instances. Paraplegia often disappears completely.

TREATMENT. Traditionally, therapy consisted in continuous extension on a Bradford frame until there was no evidence of active infection, and then spinal fusion. Early surgical eradication of the tuberculous abscess in conjunction with specific antimicrobial therapy is now the accepted treatment.

TUBERCULOSIS OF THE HIP
(Tuberculous Coxitis)

This is the most common tuberculous involvement of the joints. The disease may begin in the synovial membrane, but usually starts as an osteitis of the femoral epiphysis, followed by a tuberculous arthritis and finally by an abscess resulting in destruction of the femoral head.

CLINICAL MANIFESTATIONS. Usually the first symptom is a slight lameness which is likely to be intermittent, occurring when the patient first gets out of bed and after exercise. It may disappear for days or weeks at a time. Pain may be present at this stage or may develop later and is usually referred to the knee or the inner side of the thigh. As destruction of the joint proceeds, the thigh is flexed and adducted, and the rotation which initially was outward becomes inward. Swelling about the hip increases, and an abscess may form from which pus may discharge anteriorly to the joint or be disseminated in other directions. Absorption of the head and neck of the femur may take place without evidence of suppuration.

DIFFERENTIAL DIAGNOSIS. Distinction must be made from *osteochondrosis of the femoral head* (Legg-Calvé-Perthes disease), which occurs in the same age group, but limits abduction to a greater extent than it does extension and in which roentgenographic changes do not extend beyond the femoral capitular epiphysis. In tuberculous coxitis the acetabulum may also be affected. The two conditions may be indistinguishable in the early stage, and the clinical course must be relied upon to differentiate them. A negative tuberculin reaction is of great value. The insidious onset of tuberculous coxitis serves to distinguish it from *rheumatic fever* and *acute arthritis.*

PROGNOSIS. After abscess formation the disease may last 2 to 4 years or longer. When treatment is begun in the first few weeks of the disease, the inflammation may cease entirely before the joint itself is attacked, but in the majority of cases the joint is finally ankylosed.

TREATMENT. Treatment consists of bed rest, traction on the leg to reduce muscle spasm and specific antibacterial therapy. Surgical eradication of the abscess may be considered in selected cases in conjunction with antibacterial therapy. Arthrodesis of the joint is often necessary.

MULTIPLE TRAUMATIC SKELETAL LESIONS IN EARLY LIFE

(The Battered-Child Syndrome; See also Section 2)

Traumatic lesions of the bones are relatively common in infants and small children and often are not associated with clinical manifestations proportionate to their severity or at times even sufficient to call attention to them. Frequently they are recognized only through roentgenographic examination performed for some unrelated reason. In some instances the trauma is accidental and may or may not be known to the parents; on other occasions they may be hesitant to disclose the possibility of trauma. In some instances the trauma is inflicted willfully by an adult, usually a parent, often in a burst of temper. When there are rather frequently repeated assaults, the radiographic examination of the skeleton reveals multiple traumatic osseous lesions in different stages of healing. This clinical pattern has been termed the battered-child syndrome. It is a significant cause of failure to thrive, of disability and even of death. Nearly all the patients are under 3 years of age, and the majority are less than 1 year.

The skeletal lesions reflect certain characteristics of growing bones. The periosteum is not firmly attached in infancy and is easily elevated by hemorrhage; periosteal new bone formation is active. Epiphyseal separation and displacement are readily achieved. There may also be fractures of the metaphysis or diaphysis, at times with significant deformity. When there are multiple lesions, they are apt to be in varying stages of healing, indicative of recurrent episodes of trauma and suggestive of a psychopathic situation within the home. Subdural hematomas are frequently found in association with the skeletal lesions and contribute to the failure of the infant to thrive.

At times the diagnosis is suggested by limitation of motion or use of an extremity, or by pain on manipulation. Ecchymoses and other evidences of soft tissue injury are not so common in infants as they are under similar circumstances in older children.

The history is often not helpful, either because the parents are unaware of the accidents or because they choose not to disclose them. The differential diagnosis includes scurvy, congenital syphilis, cortical hyperostosis, osteogenesis imperfecta and neoplasm; if the injury is in the region of a joint, it may simulate suppurative arthritis.

Orthopedic management will be required in the cases of epiphyseal separation or of fractures. Psychosocial management is discussed in Section 2.

JOHN LACHMAN

Helfer, R. E., and Kempe, C. H. (eds.): The Battered Child. Chicago, University of Chicago Press, 1968.

Staheli, L. T., Church, C. C., and Ward, B. H.: Infantile cortical hyperostosis (Caffey's disease). J.A.M.A. *203*:384, 1968.

METABOLIC DISORDERS WITH BONE LESIONS

Differential diagnosis and management of metabolic bone disease depend upon clear understanding of the principles of osteogenesis. Essentials for the formation and maintenance of bone include an appropriate organic matrix (osteoid) and suitable concentrations of calcium and phosphorus in extracellular fluid. Most bones are endochondral, arising in cartilaginous models. Growth, mineralization and systematic removal of cartilage are therefore determinants of skeletal form and composition.

Chondrocytes and osteoblasts synthesize cartilage and osteoid, respectively. The principal component of each of these matrices is collagen; small amounts of mucopolysaccharide, chiefly chondroitin sulfate, are also present. What determines calcification is not known. Neither epiphyseal cartilage nor osteoid can be distinguished chemically from tendon, fascia or ear cartilage, none of which normally mineralizes.

The first perceptible mineral deposit in cartilage is amorphous tricalcium phosphate ($Ca_3(PO_4)_2$), which gradually accumulates hydroxyl ions to become crystalline hydroxyapatite. In osteoid, apatite crystals (and presumably their antecedent, tricalcium phosphate) are first seen in the light zones of the periodic bands characteristic of collagen fibers. During crystalline growth a close orientation with the underlying fibers persists. The fiber surface appears to create a micro-environment favorable to crystallization. Whether this involves adsorption, chelation or an enzyme-dependent reaction is presently obscure.

Alkaline phosphatase is abundant not only in areas of osteoid formation, but also wherever collagen synthesis is active, as in healing wounds. In phosphatase deficiency (see Hypophosphatasia, below) osteoid is formed but does not mineralize normally.

Although apatite can be formed at very low concentrations of calcium and phosphate, mineralization of osteoid at a rate commensurate with normal bone growth requires an adequate supply of *both* ions. Howland and Kramer found that rickets ensued when the product of serum calcium and phosphorus (in milligrams per deciliter, or mg/dl) was less than 30. Subnormal Ca × P products usually

TABLE 22–1 SKELETAL EFFECTS OF METABOLIC DISORDERS

I. Disorders affecting formation or maintenance of bone matrix
  - A. Nutritional
    - Scurvy
    - Protein deficiency
    - Caloric deficiency
  - B. Endocrine
    - Hypothyroidism
    - Hyperthyroidism
    - Hyperadrenalism (Cushing syndrome)
    - Side effects of corticosteroid therapy
  - C. Metabolic and genetic
    - Osteoporosis of disuse
    - Hypophosphatasia
    - Hyperphosphatasia
    - Osteogenesis imperfecta
    - Gargoylism (and other mucopolysaccharidoses)
    - Osteopetrosis
    - Achondroplasia and other chondrodysplasias

II. Disorders affecting mineralization of bone matrix
  - A. Nutritional
    - Rickets due to vitamin D deficiency
    - Malabsorptive states
      - Celiac disease, cystic fibrosis, biliary atresia
  - B. Endocrine
    - Hypoparathyroidism
    - Hyperparathyroidism
  - C. Renal tubular dysfunction with losses of minerals
    - Hypophosphatemic vitamin D-resistant rickets (renal hypophosphatemia)
    - Hypocalcemic vitamin D-resistant rickets
    - Fanconi syndrome (renal hypophosphatemia with renal glycosuria and aminoaciduria)
    - Lignac syndrome (Fanconi syndrome with cystinosis)
  - D. Chronic metabolic acidosis
    - Renal tubular acidosis
    - Oculocerebrorenal syndrome (Lowe)

III. Complex disorders of bone, affecting both matrix and mineralization
  - A. Hyperparathyroidism
    - Local osteolytic activity and hypophosphatemia
  - B. Chronic renal failure
    - Decreased calcium absorption and secondary hyperparathyroidism

reflect hypophosphatemia, since calcium is closely regulated by the parathyroids.

Since the solubility of apatite varies inversely with pH, demineralization has been attributed to chronic acidosis. Respiratory acidosis does not affect bone, perhaps because the high concentration of bicarbonate in interstitial fluid decreases the solubility of calcium. In chronic renal insufficiency it is impossible to dissociate the effects of acidosis from those of other chemical disturbances. In diabetes mellitus and in acute renal failure the duration of acidosis is too brief to affect bone significantly. In untreated renal tubular acidosis, hyperphosphaturia is pronounced; it is probably this feature of the disease, rather than depression of pH, that is responsible for osteomalacia.

Synthesis and destruction of osteoid are continuous throughout life. The *amount* of bone present at any given time is the resultant of these two processes; the *morphology* of bone is determined by remodelling. Continuous removal of mineral from resorbing surfaces and redeposition of it in newly formed osteoid effect a slow redistribution of skeletal calcium and phosphate. Since metabolic factors causing loss of calcium or phosphate from body fluids lead to osteomalacia by compromising the mineralization of continuously synthesized osteoid, it is not necessary to postulate accelerated destruction to account for the appearance of bone lesions.

There is a direct osteolytic action of parathyroid hormone, but the mechanism is not defined. This effect is presumably mediated through the osteoclasts, which increase in numbers and in apparent activity when the parathyroids are stimulated or when exogenous parathyroid hormone is given. Removal of osteoid accompanies demineralization and results in increased excretion of mucopolysaccharide and hydroxyproline. Parathyroid hormone also has an indirect effect on bone through inhibition of renal tubular phosphate reabsorption, which causes a decrease in the concentration of serum phosphorus.

The skeletal effects of metabolic disorders, considered in terms of these critical factors, are as shown in Table 22–1.

CALCIFEROL

Recent studies of vitamin D have shown that the parent compound (endogenous cholecalciferol or exogenous ergocalciferol) must undergo two hydroxylations to develop maximal physiologic activity. The first hydroxylation is accomplished by a hepatic microsomal hydroxylase; the rate is regulated by the end-product. The second hydroxylation occurs in the kidney; its rate is inversely proportional to the concentration of ionized calcium in serum or tissue fluid, and is also regulated by parathyroid hormone. The final product of this regulated biosynthesis is 1-25-dihydroxycholecalciferol, which is currently regarded as a hormone rather than a vitamin. A specific hereditary defect in renal 25-hydroxylase has been identified as the cause of one form of refractory rickets (see below). Both hepatic and renal rickets probably result, in part, from hydroxylation defects. Renal rickets can be cured with 1-25-dihydroxycholecalciferol. A synthetic analog, 1-α-OH-cholecalciferol, has equivalent biologic activity and promises to be therapeutically useful.

REFRACTORY RICKETS

Since vitamin D deficiency has become a rarity in the United States and many other countries, most rickets presently seen is of endogenous origin and is resistant to the usual intake of vitamin D (400 to 1000 IU per day). Rickets refractory to vitamin D occurs in association with several complex disorders; these include the relatively common hypophosphatemic variety of vitamin D-resistant rickets and the rare hypocalcemic form, Fanconi syndrome, cystinosis, renal tubular acidosis, Lowe syndrome and renal osteodystrophy, each of which is described in this section. Rickets may also develop in the malabsorption syndromes if defective intestinal absorption of vitamin D is not compensated by the administration of relatively large doses in water-miscible preparations, or in extreme situations parenterally.

HYPOPHOSPHATEMIC VITAMIN D-RESISTANT RICKETS

In this clinical entity, rickets resistant to unusually large doses of vitamin D is the only obvious manifestation; the condition is commonly called "refractory rickets." It occurs in familial and sporadic forms, which are clinically and chemically indistinguishable.

ETIOLOGY. Cartilage from untreated patients will calcify in normal serum, and intravenous infusions of phosphate result in rapid mineralization of rachitic lesions in vivo; the osteoid appears, therefore, to have its usual potential for apatite deposition. Serum calcium concentration is nearly always normal, but hypophosphatemia is characteristically severe and intractable; the resulting Ca $\times$ P product is in the rachitic range (below 30).

Intestinal absorption of calcium is low before treatment and increases after very large doses of vitamin D. It has been postulated that the parathyroids, stimulated by calcium deficit, are continuously hyperactive, sustaining the serum level of calcium by withdrawing it from bone and by suppressing renal tubular reabsorption of phosphate. Phosphate clearance is increased even in the presence of hypophosphatemia, a finding consistent with compensatory hyperparathyroidism. When calcium is given intravenously, tubular reabsorption of phosphate increases promptly, as does the concentration of serum phosphorus. This effect, presumably due to parathyroid suppression, is interpreted as evidence that phosphaturia is a secondary phenomenon. There are several objections, however, to the notion that an intestinal absorptive defect is primary: (1) since serum calcium in untreated patients is nearly always normal, there is no evident "feedback" stimulus to the parathyroids; (2) although massive vitamin D therapy frequently causes hypercalcemia, the serum level of phosphorus usually remains low, and hyperphosphaturia persists; (3) the roentgenographic appearance of the bones is not consistent with hyperparathyroidism; e.g., such changes as cysts, subperiosteal erosion and fraying of the terminal phalanges are absent; and (4) since tubular phosphate reabsorption can be increased by calcium infusion even in the absence of the parathyroids, this test is not diagnostic of hyperparathyroidism.

Refractory rickets was originally classified in the group of intrinsic renal tubular defects, which includes nephrogenic diabetes insipidus, renal glycosuria, renal tubular acidosis. Fanconi syndrome, Lowe syndrome, cystinuria and glycinuria. The concept that hypophosphatemia depends on a primary incapacity of the tubules to reabsorb phosphate does not readily explain diminished intestinal absorption of calcium. If a tubular defect exists, it must be relative, since reabsorption of phosphate can be decreased by injection of parathyroid hormone and increased by infusion of calcium.

EPIDEMIOLOGY. Refractory rickets is often familial. Some family members without obvious disease may be found to have mild involvement on careful clinical and radiographic examination; others have hypophosphatemia without demonstrable bone lesions. Roentgenography, however, is an insensitive indicator, and too few chemical or histologic examinations have been made to permit the conclusion that apparently nonrachitic members of the kindreds studied have normal bones.

Genetic analysis indicates a sex-linked dominant mode of inheritance, with complete penetrance of hypophosphatemia, but irregular expressivity of disease. Hypophosphatemic males have rachitic changes more often than their female counterparts, and their serum phosphorus concentrations are slightly lower. Whether persons with sporadic refractory rickets can transmit the disease to their offspring is unknown.

CLINICAL MANIFESTATIONS. The general health of the child is unaffected, and the muscular hypotonia prominent in vitamin D-deficiency rickets is absent. Typical lateral bowing deformities of the legs appear during the second year; other rachitic stigmata such as frontal bossing, costochondral beading, enlarged wrists and dental defects are usually present, but easily missed. Sitting deformities (anterior bowing of the femora and tibiae) attest to the early onset of disease, but are rarely noticed by parents. Linear growth is retarded.

The roentgenographic appearance is indistinguishable from that of vitamin D-deficiency rickets. The serum phosphorus level is low and usually responds only partially to otherwise successful therapy. The serum calcium level is characteristically within the normal range. Rarely, however, it is low, and the untreated patient may have tetany. Plasma electrolyte composition is otherwise normal. Alkaline phosphatase is elevated in active disease and decreases during successful treatment. Aminoaciduria is an inconstant finding; it disappears after therapy in some instances, as it does in deficiency rickets.

DIAGNOSIS. Nonrachitic bowing is differentiated by roentgenography. In familial cases the history may be diagnostic. If the intake of vitamin D has been adequate and malabsorption is not suggested by nutritional status and description of stools, refractory rickets is probable. When the primary disorder is renal tubular acidosis, Fanconi syndrome or Lowe syndrome, the general health is severely affected. When rickets is the sole manifestation, failure to respond to moderate doses of vitamin D establishes the diagnosis of refractory rickets.

When 1500 to 3000 IU of vitamin D are given daily, a month is necessary to determine the presence or absence of effect. This time can be shortened by giving 600,000 IU in a single dose; in simple vitamin D deficiency chemical improvement occurs within a few days and perceptible roentgenographic changes within two weeks. Rarely it may be necessary to repeat the dose after two weeks. This procedure requires close supervision, preferably in the hospital, to avoid the dangers of overdosage. If improvement occurs, the high tissue level of vitamin D established suffices for four to five months, after which the usual supplement may be instituted. Infection during the observation period may negate the test.

TREATMENT. Since resistance to vitamin D in this disorder unfortunately does not protect against its toxic effects, the large doses required for healing may cause anorexia, hypercalcemia, polyuria and renal damage. Therapy, therefore, requires a compromise in determining a dose which will promote maximal healing with minimal risk of renal damage.

Oral supplementation with phosphate reduces the amount of calciferol required for healing, by partially compensating for renal phosphate losses. Children treated with both calciferol and phosphate show better growth and fewer episodes of hypercalcemia then those given calciferol alone. Glorieux and his associates have found that the $P_{50}O_2$ of erythrocytes (an index of their capacity to release oxygen in peripheral tissues) is low in hypophosphatemia and improves with treatment. This may account for some of the favorable effects of the oral phosphate regimen. A mixture of sodium monohydrogen and dihydrogen phosphates in a molar ratio of 4:1 provides an appropriately buffered solution. This may be prescribed as $NaH_2PO_4 \cdot H_2O$, 18 gm, and $Na_2HPO_4 \cdot H_2O$, 145 gm, with water to make 1000 ml. This solution provides 2 gm of phosphorus per deciliter. Proprie-

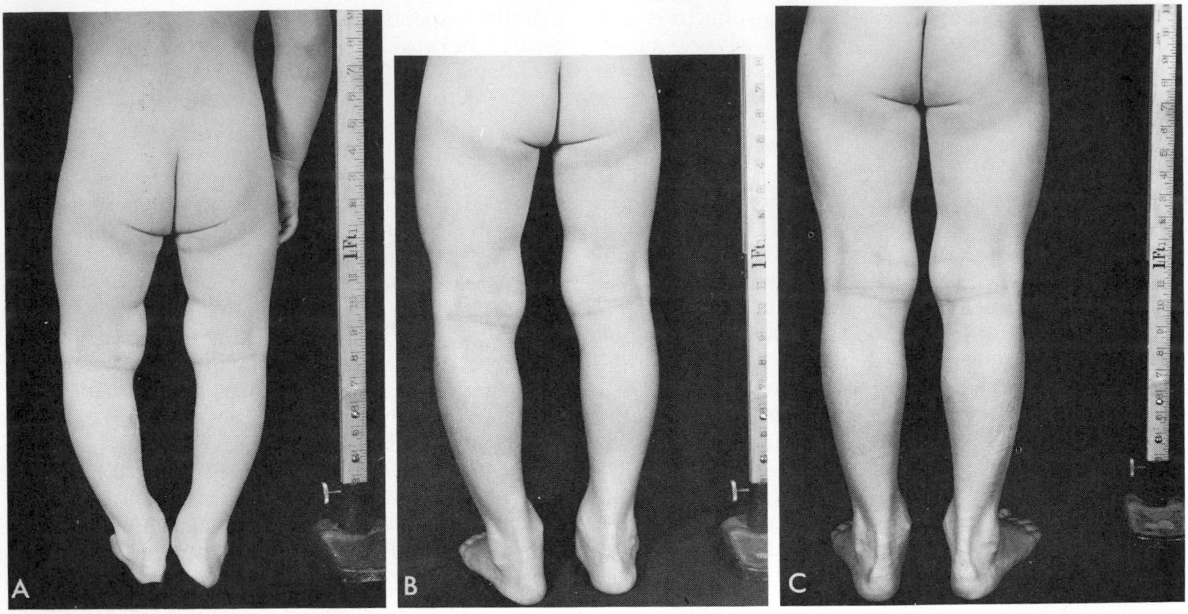

Figure 22–37 *Refractory rickets.* A, *Untreated, age 3 years.* B, *Age 6 years, after vitamin D, 50,000 units per day for 3 years.* C, *Age $7\frac{1}{2}$ years, after corrective osteotomy of left tibia.*

tary ("phosphosoda") preparations are also available. Most patients will tolerate 2.0 gm of phosphorus per day; best results are achieved by scheduling small doses at frequent intervals; e.g., 0.3 gm six times daily is better tolerated and sustains serum phosphate more evenly than 0.6 gm three times daily.

A reasonable initial dose of calciferol is 25,000 IU per day (0.625 mg). If no healing is seen within six to eight weeks, the dose must be increased. Serum calcium concentration must be measured at monthly intervals, and parents should be warned that anorexia, thirst and polyuria may be signs of hypercalcemia.

If deformities are pronounced before treatment is begun, corrective osteotomy may be necessary (Fig. 22–37); mineralization should first be augmented by treatment. Administration of vitamin D should then be discontinued two weeks before operation and resumed only when the patient is ambulatory; immobilization may otherwise cause dangerous hypercalcemia.

HYPOCALCEMIC VITAMIN D-RESISTANT RICKETS

(Pseudodeficiency Rickets)

This form of vitamin D-resistant rickets has been separated from the much more common variety described above. Clinically and radiographically the two are similar. In contrast to the low serum concentration of phosphate in the hypophosphatemic variety, which is only partially corrected by administration of large doses of vitamin D, the concentration of phosphate in the hypocalcemic variety is within the normal range, or nearly so, and the concentration of calcium is abnormally low. Tetany can usually be demonstrated in its latent phase, and seizures may occur. Serum chloride and alkaline phosphatase values are high, and aminoaciduria is increased. The hypocalcemia form appears to be transmitted as an autosomal dominant pattern in contrast to the sex-linked inheritance of hypophosphatemic refractory rickets. A specific defect in renal 1-hydroxylase has been found; minute doses of 1-25-dihydroxycholecalciferol are curative.

The daily dose of vitamin D should be adjusted so that the serum concentration of calcium is maintained within the normal range. The bone lesions disappear with such therapy, and in contrast to the situation in the hypophosphatemic form, growth in stature approximates normal expectancy. This feature suggests that stunting in hypophosphatemic rickets may be due to an inadequate supply of phosphorus for bone metabolism.

FANCONI SYNDROME

(Refractory Rickets Associated with Multiple Defects of the Renal Tubules; de Toni-Debré Fanconi Syndrome)

Aminoaciduria, renal glycosuria, hypophosphatemia and hyperphosphaturia characterize Fanconi syndrome. Proteinuria, hyposthenuria and acidosis are often present; hypokalemia may occur in conjunction with acidosis. The disorder causes dwarfing and rickets resistant to vitamin D.

ETIOLOGY. The cause of Fanconi syndrome is not clear. Both familial and sporadic cases occur. In some instances the syndrome accompanies other disorders, including heavy metal poisoning (lead, uranium, cadmium), cystinosis, glycogenosis, hereditary fructose intolerance, galactosemia, tyrosinosis, Wilson's disease and multiple myeloma. It may occur in adults. A degradation product of outdated tetracycline can cause a reversible form of the disease.

PATHOGENESIS. The basic defect may be resistance to several effects of vitamin D, since large doses of vitamin D reduce fecal calcium, partially restore tubular transport of amino acids, glucose and phosphate, and improve acidosis and hypokalemia. Intestinal absorption of calcium, consistently low in simple refractory rickets, is not always depressed in multiple tubular dysfunction. As in simple refractory rickets, the chemical derangements of Fanconi syndrome may occur without evident bone involvement.

The characteristic histologic changes occur in the proximal tubules, which are shorter than normal and are connected to the glomeruli by an abnormally narrow segment ("swan's neck"). Vacuolization of distal tubular cells is a less specific finding and may be the result of depletion of potassium.

Changes in the plasma and urine in Fanconi syndrome result from decreased tubular reabsorption of phosphate, glucose, amino acids and, in some instances, water. Urinary ammonia and titratable acidity are insufficient to prevent loss of fixed base. Hypophosphatemia and acidosis are both conducive to the development of rickets. Since acidosis is inconstant and its amelioration does not result in healing, its role in rachitogenesis is apparently minor.

CLINICAL MANIFESTATIONS. Characteristically, the infant appears normal at birth; symptoms appear after the first six months of life, when growth failure, weakness, dehydration and fever may appear. Dehydration is often associated with polyuria and vomiting. Constipation is common.

The bony abnormalities of rickets appear despite adequate intake of vitamin D and may dominate the clinical pattern if the systemic manifestations are mild. Linear growth is restricted. The skeletal changes may be those of renal osteodystrophy late in the course of the illness, when renal failure supervenes.

LABORATORY DATA. Serum analysis reveals low phosphorus and normal calcium values initially and, in some instances, hyperchloremic acidosis and hypokalemia. As renal function fails, the serum phosphorus level increases along with that of nonprotein nitrogen, and calcium may fall to tetanic levels. Alkaline phosphatase is elevated if active rickets is present. The urine contains glucose and excessive amounts of 10 or more amino acids; excretion of them may cease with renal failure. The pattern of excretion of amino acids may vary in different patients, but is consistent for the individual. Organic aciduria appears to reflect the same tubular defect which causes aminoaciduria.

Urinary ammonia and titratable acidity may be low, and excretion of bicarbonate high in proportion to the acidosis. Urinary pH may be relatively high. Proteinuria is inconstant.

DIAGNOSIS. Since aminoaciduria, diminished tubular reabsorption of phosphate and elevated serum levels of alkaline phosphatase are present in other forms of rickets, they are not diagnostic. Demonstration of renal glycosuria in the presence of stunting and refractory rickets indicates multiple tubular dysfunction. Hyperchloremic acidosis and hypokalemia, if present, are corroborative. Glucose tolerance tests have caused severe and occasionally fatal shocklike reactions, probably by shifting potassium into cells during glycogen deposition in patients already hypokalemic.

TREATMENT. When an underlying cause is identified, it should be appropriately treated. Rickets and osteomalacia respond to large doses of vitamin D (5000 to 50,000 units daily). The dose should be individualized as suggested above for simple refractory rickets, beginning perhaps with a dose of 5000 units daily, with frequent adjustment to the response obtained; 2000 to 10,000 units per day is often sufficient. Hypercalcemia must be scrupulously avoided; additional calcium, however, may be required under unusual circumstances (see above). For correction of acidosis and hypokalemia a mixture of sodium and potassium citrate is appropriate. A liter of flavored syrup containing 100 gm of each salt provides 2 mEq of cation per ml. The dose is approximately 5 mEq/kg/day; it should be adjusted by periodic determinations of serum bicarbonate. Potassium should be included even if hypokalemia is not present, since sodium loading may otherwise cause depletion of potassium. In several instances renal tubular acidosis and glycosuria have responded to therapy with calciferol alone. Electrolyte supplementation should therefore be deferred until the effects of vitamin D have been observed for a few weeks. When renal failure supervenes, therapy must be re-evaluated in terms of the capacity to excrete sodium and potassium.

Although temporary improvement may be gratifying, most patients survive only a few years. The cause of death is usually chronic renal failure and uremia. When the disease begins in late childhood, the course may be more benign, and when effective treatment of an underlying disorder is possible, it may significantly ameliorate the renal lesion.

HEPATIC RICKETS

Rickets associated with liver disease has usually been attributed to a failure of absorption of dietary calciferol, secondary to demonstrable or presumptive steatorrhea. It now appears that inadequate hydroxylation of calciferol may be of equal or greater importance. Treatment with large doses of aqueous dispersions of ergocalciferol, or with parenteral injections at intervals of one to three months, has been helpful.

CYSTINOSIS

(Lignac Syndrome; Fanconi Syndrome with Cystinosis)

Cystinosis was first recognized at autopsy in 1903 and was established as a clinical entity by

Lignac in 1924. This disorder is characterized by the clinical pattern of Fanconi syndrome as described above, with the added presence of cystine crystals in various tissues of the body. Some investigators consider Fanconi syndrome and cystinosis to be variants of the same disorder. Certainly some of the cases reported as Fanconi syndrome in the past may have had undetected deposition of cystine crystals. It is clear, however, that Fanconi syndrome occurs without cystinosis.

PATHOGENESIS. The pathogenesis of cystinosis is unknown. It has been proposed that the renal defect may be due to the nephrotoxic activity of cystine. The deposition of cystine crystals in the tissues has been attributed to aberrant cystine metabolism, but an enzymatic defect has not been demonstrated.

The characteristic pathologic lesion is the deposition of cystine in the reticuloendothelial system, especially apparent in the liver, spleen, lymph nodes and bone marrow. Cystine deposits also occur in the renal tubular cells and in the cornea and conjunctiva. Changes in renal tubular morphology are similar to those described for Fanconi syndrome. The crystals are most readily demonstrated in the cornea and in the bone marrow. The cornea may be normal on gross and ophthalmoscopic examination, but examination by slit-lamp biomicroscopy reveals a myriad of highly refractile bodies. Occasionally the crystals may be seen in the peripheral white blood cells, but more often they can be demonstrated in bone marrow aspirates, or in lymph node or renal tissue obtained by biopsy. Fixing or staining procedures which dissolve the cystine crystals should be avoided. Granular and circinate irregularities in the peripheral pigmentation of the retina may be seen funduscopically as early as 5 weeks of age. They antedate the appearance of crystals by several months.

CLINICAL MANIFESTATIONS AND LABORATORY FINDINGS. Other than those of crystal deposition, these are similar to those described for Fanconi syndrome. Photophobia and a preference or craving for meat and other protein foods may also be noted and should suggest cystinosis as a diagnostic possibility.

TREATMENT. In general, this is the same as that for Fanconi syndrome. The use of penicillamine has been proposed; its efficiency is undetermined. Few children live beyond 8 years of age.

RICKETS ASSOCIATED WITH RENAL TUBULAR ACIDOSIS

(Lightwood Syndrome; Albright Syndrome)

This disorder is characterized by metabolic acidosis, hyperchloremia, inability to form an adequately acid urine, hypercalciuria and sometimes hypokalemia. There appear to be two distinct clinical types: the infantile form (Lightwood syndrome) is self-limited; the persistent form of the disease has a later onset with rickets or osteomalacia.

ETIOLOGY. Hydrogen ion clearance is inadequate; i.e., the urine pH, though low at times, is always higher than is appropriate for the plasma bicarbonate. This results in excessive excretion of bicarbonate and increased tubular reabsorption of chloride. Associated losses of sodium and potassium may lead to acidosis and hypokalemia. Potassium deficit is probably the cause of hyposthenuria. Hypercalciuria, another aspect of fixed base loss, is readily reversed by administration of alkali; if it is allowed to persist, nephrocalcinosis and nephrolithiasis ensue. Susceptibility to these serious complications is increased by the absence of urinary citrate, a constituent which normally forms a soluble complex with calcium. Diminished tubular reabsorption of phosphate results in hypophosphatemia and rickets.

Although the chemical pattern of the disease can be simulated by giving carbonic anhydrase inhibitors, no deficiency of the enzyme has been established.

CLINICAL MANIFESTATIONS. In infancy the principal manifestations are nonspecific and include anorexia, vomiting, constipation, apathy, irritability and weakness. Death may result from dehydration and acidosis. Rickets and nephrocalcinosis do not occur in the infantile form.

Later in childhood the presenting complaints may be similar, or may relate to growth retardation, bony deformities or pathologic fractures. Terminal renal insufficiency may result from nephrocalcinosis. Roentgenograms reveal rickets and, in later stages, nephrocalcinosis.

EPIDEMIOLOGY. Although familial cases occur, the mode of inheritance has not been defined.

TREATMENT. The mixture of sodium and potassium citrate recommended for Fanconi syndrome (100 gm of each per liter of vehicle) is satisfactory; the dose should be regulated by appropriate serum analyses. Calcium supplementation may be necessary during the initial period of rapid remineralization, but is not indicated thereafter. After acidosis has been corrected the vitamin D requirement is not elevated; conversely, even large doses are ineffectual in the presence of acidosis.

See also in Section 15, Tubular Dysfunctions Associated with Generalized Renal or Urinary Tract Disease.

LOWE SYNDROME

(Oculocerebrorenal Dystrophy)

This rare affliction is characterized by mental retardation, glaucoma, organic aciduria, aminoaciduria, and diminished renal production of ammonia. Hypotonia and areflexia appear in the latter half of the first year of life along with generalized hyperactivity. Cataracts are usually present. Febrile episodes are frequent, probably as a result of dehydration. Some patients have metabolic acidosis and rickets. Large doses of vitamin D are ineffectual unless calcium and sodium supplements are also provided.

The disease is inherited in a sex-linked partially dominant pattern; so far the fully manifest syndrome has been observed only in males. The female carrier may have lenticular opacities.

RENAL OSTEODYSTROPHY

(Renal Rickets)

Bone lesions resulting from chronic glomerular and tubular insufficiency were previously designated as renal rickets. This term, however, obscures the complex nature of the disorder and misrepresents the roentgenographic appearance.

ETIOLOGY. Renal hypoplasia, polycystic disease of the kidney, hydronephrosis, pyelonephritis and chronic glomerulonephritis are the commonest causes of reduction in effective renal mass. Acidosis and hyperphosphatemia result from tubular and glomerular hypofunction. Intestinal absorption of calcium is depressed, perhaps owing to failure of the kidney to effect the final hydroxylation of cholecalciferol. Extreme hypocalcemia is unusual, however, since the combination of acidosis and secondary hyperparathyroidism sustains a higher calcium concentration than would be predicted from the observed hyperphosphatemia. The $Ca \times P$ product is usually elevated and may exceed 100. Tetany is rare. Compensatory hyperparathyroidism may be detected by typical roentgenographic changes, by the microscopic appearance of bone in biopsy or necropsy material and by direct examination of the glands at autopsy. Such studies have made it clear that secondary hyperparathyroidism is variable in degree and that its role in the production of osteodystrophy may at times be minor.

Calcium deficiency and acidosis reduce the rate of mineralization in growing bone; hyperparathyroidism, when present, causes erosion and cyst formation. The microscopic appearance combines the features of osteomalacia (undermineralized osteoid) and osteitis fibrosa cystica (erosion of bone substance). Either may predominate. Areas of osteosclerosis also may occur, especially in the vertebral bodies; this phenomenon has not been explained.

CLINICAL MANIFESTATIONS. Growth failure, anemia and general debility are the usual presenting complaints, preceding the appearance of bone deformities. In the patient presented in Figure 22–38 osteodystrophy was apparent within a year of the onset of uremia; in most instances the interval is longer. Skeletal involvement may create extremely severe functional and cosmetic handicaps, including bowing, knock-knee, frontal bossing and dental defects. Bone pain may be crippling. Roentgenograms reveal demineralization, coarsening of the trabecular pattern and usually subperiosteal rarefaction. When growth is minimal, the wide, clear epiphyseal zones of rickets are absent, being replaced by areas of ragged, chaotic erosion. Osteosclerosis of the axial skeleton may be seen. At autopsy the bones are generally soft, osteoclasts are abundant, and the proportion of ash to organic matrix is low. Azotemia is combined with the chemical changes in the serum mentioned above, and the concentration of alkaline phosphatase is increased. Hypertension, polyuria and isosthenuria are often present.

DIAGNOSIS. This is seldom difficult. In primary hyperparathyroidism the foregoing clinical and chemical disorders may supervene when renal failure complicates the terminal stage, but this entity is extremely rare in childhood, fewer than 25 cases having been reported. No other condition is known to produce the combination of biochemical and morphologic changes described.

TREATMENT. Previous therapeutic plans were based on restriction of dietary protein and phosphate and on provision of supplementary alkali. Oral administration of aluminum hydroxide and of a cation exchange resin to remove phosphate and potassium has also been recommended. These measures reduce azotemia and hyperphosphatemia; healing of bone lesions occasionally follows correction of metabolic acidosis, but results are seldom satisfactory.

More recently, the use of vitamin D in large doses has led to remarkable clinical and roentgenographic improvement in bone lesions and in suppression of secondary hyperparathyroidism. This regimen increases calcium absorption and promotes mineralization of bone through mechanisms presently obscure. The dose of vitamin D ranges from 25,000 to 250,000 units per day; after healing, 10,000 units per day may suffice. Good results ensue despite persistent acidosis, hyperphosphatemia and uremia. Close chemical and roentgenographic control is essential; as in refractory rickets, hypercalcemia is an indication of overdosage of vitamin D. Dihydrotachysterol is as effective as calciferol, the dose in milligrams being the same for each sterol. One milligram of calciferol (vitamin D_2) contains 40,000 units. Restriction of phosphate is apparently unnecessary and has in fact been found to exaggerate osteomalacia.

If correction of acidosis is desired, sodium citrate (10 mEq/gm) or sodium bicarbonate can be given, starting with 5 mEq/kg/day. Supplementary calcium should be provided, since tetany may otherwise ensue when the serum pH is increased in the presence of hyperphosphatemia. Calcium lactate (8 gm = 1 gm of calcium) may be given in fruit juice or ginger ale. It may be necessary to add potassium citrate in order to prevent hypokalemia. The high phosphate and solute contents of cow's milk make it particularly unsuitable for patients with renal disease.

IDIOPATHIC HYPERCALCEMIA

Osteosclerosis, best seen in the metaphyses, is the skeletal hallmark of iodiopathic hypercalcemia. When the diaphyses are also involved, the long bones may mimic osteopetrosis.

In 1952 Lightwood described a syndrome comprising hypercalcemia and failure to thrive. The original patients appeared to have a relatively mild disorder, self-limited and reversible when administration of calcium and vitamin D was discontinued. Fanconi and Schlesinger then reported

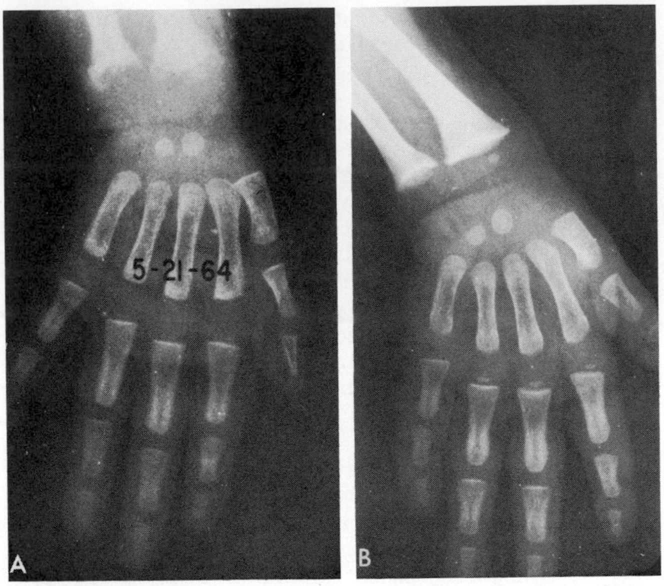

Figure 22–38 Renal osteodystrophy. A, Age 16 months. Calciferol, 400 units a day since early infancy. Serum: calcium, 9.5 mg/dl., phosphorus, 5 mg/dl.; pH, 7.35; blood urea nitrogen, 30 mg/dl. Intravenous pyelogram showed renal hypoplasia. B, Healing after 7 weeks of therapy with calciferol, 25,000 units a day. Hypercalcemia ensued after 3 months; 5000 units a day thereafter sustained healing without hypercalcemia.

seriously affected infants, and a wide spectrum of severity was soon apparent. Hypercalcemia, "elfin" facies (combining prominent epicanthal folds, retroussé nose, long overhanging upper lip without Cupid's bow, wide mouth, receding chin and misshapen ears), mental retardation, hypertension and nephrocalcinosis characterize the disease in its most severe form. Irritability, anorexia, constipation and polyuria are nonspecific features presumably due to hypercalcemia. Hypercalcemic patients absorb a higher proportion of dietary calcium than normal infants.

Between 1953 and 1955 more than 200 cases were seen in Great Britain. At the same time fewer than 10 patients were reported in the United States. Dietary supplementation of vitamin D assured most British babies an intake of 2000 to 3000 units per day, or approximately five to six times the American average. When the British intake was reduced to 400 units per day, hypercalcemia promptly became a rarity. It has therefore been concluded that the disease represents chronic vitamin D intoxication resulting from variable individual tolerance of the sterol.

In 1961 Williams, Barrat-Bayes and Lowe described the association of supravalvular aortic stenosis, mental retardation and peculiar facies. By 1963, when several more reports of this syndrome has appeared, Black and Bonham-Carter recognized the facies as that of idiopathic hypercalcemia, and in reviewing autopsy material of the latter condition found descriptions of stenotic lesions of the aorta and renal arteries. Beuren and his associates noted similar facies and vascular lesions in German infants whose mothers had received several massive doses of vitamin D (500,000 units) during pregnancy. Friedman and Roberts then showed a high incidence of arterial stenoses in rabbits whose mothers had been given large doses of vitamin D.

It thus appears that vitamin D in excess of individual tolerance produces a variety of aberrations in form (vascular, facial, skeletal) and function (hypercalcemia, hypertension, growth retardation, mental retardation, and so forth). The nature and extent of the lesions produced and their reversibility depend on the time of exposure to the agent. Early severe damage may cause permanent morphologic changes which remain after recovery from hypercalcemia.

TREATMENT. Administration of vitamin D must be discontinued; this requires scrutiny of the whole diet to avoid unsuspected supplements in milk, cereals or other foods. A low calcium diet is achieved by substituting a meat-base formula for milk or use of decalcified milk (available in Great Britain as Locasol). Cortisone, 10 to 25 mg/day (or equivalent amounts of prednisolone), reduces intestinal absorption of calcium and has produced prompt improvement. Sodium ethylenediaminetetraacetate administered parenterally (sodium versenate) is rapidly effective but dangerous. Sodium sulfate (orally) has also been effective in reducing absorption of calcium, but it may cause hypernatremia. When hypercalcemia has been corrected, the usual calcium intake can be gradually resumed. Most patients are soon able to maintain normal serum calcium concentrations with vitamin D restriction, but they remain sensitive to calciferol; in some instances exacerbations have followed exposure to sunlight. Osteosclerosis and facial deformities may be corrected by growth if the disease is recognized and treated early in infancy. Reversibility of vascular lesions has not been proved, and mental retardation is said to be permanent.

OSTEOPOROSIS IN MALNUTRITION

Caloric deficit can retard both skeletal growth and bone age. When dietary protein is especially deficient, as in kwashiorkor, both general and local rarefaction of bone may be seen in addition to delayed "bone age." The designation "osteoporosis" implies that the fundamental defect lies in osteoid synthesis rather than in apatite formation. This supposition has not been confirmed by chemical analyses. Osteoporosis attributed to protein deficit also occurs in Cushing s syndrome and in chronic hepatic diseases. In severely ill patients it may be difficult to separate the effects of malnutrition from those of inactivity, the latter resulting in *osteoporosis of disuse.*

HYPOPHOSPHATASIA
(Low Phosphatase Rickets)

Hypophosphatasia, first described by Rathbun in 1948, is characterized by abnormal mineralization of bone, diminished serum and tissue alkaline phosphatase activity and increased urinary excretion of phosphorylethanolamine and decreased excretion of hydroxyproline. The serum phosphorus level is normal, but calcium may be elevated in severely affected infants. Bone samples from patients do not mineralize in normal serum, indicating a defect in the synthesis of matrix. Teree and Klein also found that bronchial mucus was unusually viscid in infants who died after repeated episodes of pneumonia. The disorder appears to be inherited as a simple recessive trait. It is of interest that heterozygous relatives may be clinically well with serum phosphatase levels as low as those of affected infants.

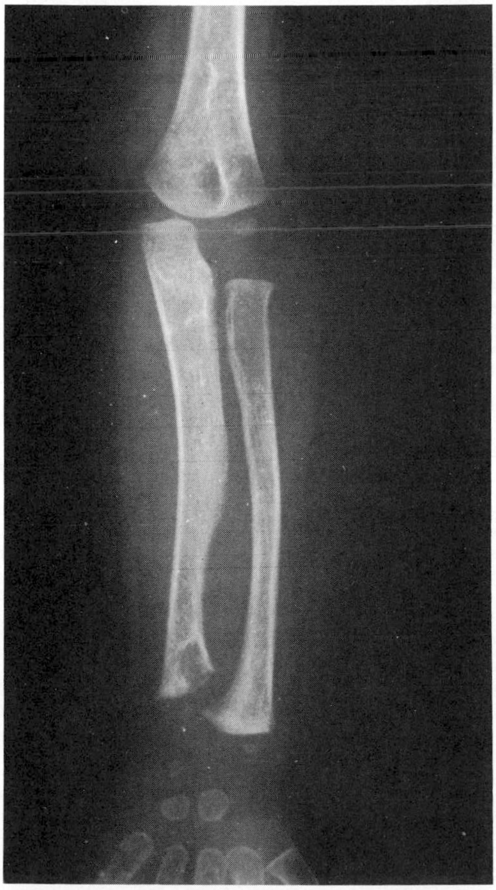

Figure 22–39 *Hypophosphatasia. Infant at age of 19 months; Ca, 10.2 mg/dl; P, 6.3 mg/dl; alkaline phosphatase, 0.7 B-L units. Dwarfing and loss of teeth noted. Long bones show both diffuse and localized rarefaction.*

CLINICAL MANIFESTATIONS. These vary widely in severity. They may be present at birth, appear in infancy or remain inapparent until later. Symptoms such as anorexia, irritability, vomiting, seizures, recurrent episodes of cyanosis or pneumonia are seen in infants. In older children the initial signs may be orthopedic deformities such as genu valgum, growth failure or premature loss of deciduous teeth (Fig. 22–39).

Roentgenograms of the bones reveal changes similar to those of rickets (Fig. 22–40). There is disappearance of the zone of provisional calcification owing to defective mineralization of osteoid tissue, which may extend well into the diaphysis. In severely affected infants the skull is soft, and the fontanels and sutures appear large, owing to large areas of uncalcified osteoid. Paradoxically, cranial synostosis is common in survivors. In older children the osseous lesions are less notable.

When the disorder starts early in infancy, it is usually severe, and a fatal outcome is the rule. Less severely affected patients may have a normal life expectancy, and gradual improvement of the osseous lesions may occur. Vitamin D, even in large doses, has no therapeutic value and may be harmful by producing severe hypercalcemia. Cortisone has been reported to benefit some patients, but is usually ineffective. An instance has been reported of favorable response to a high phosphate intake.

HYPERPHOSPHATASIA
(Hyperostosis Corticalis Deformans Juvenilis)

The manifestations of this rare disease include pain in the bones, fever, hypochromic anemia and severe bowing deformities. The level of serum alkaline phosphatase is persistently elevated (130 King-Armstrong units in Swoboda's first case). There is cortical thickening of the bones and diminished density. The trabecular architecture is chaotic; osteoblasts are abundant. In one of the few examples thus far reported an osteoma arising from a rib was found in the chest. Symptomatic improvement without radiographic changes has been achieved with prednisolone.

WILLIAM H. BERGSTROM
LYTT I. GARDNER

GENERAL

Fanconi, G.: Physiology and pathology of calcium and phosphate metabolism. Adv. Pediatr. *12*:307, 1962.

Fourman, P.: Calcium Metabolism and the Bone. Philadelphia, F. A. Davis Company, 1963.

Fraser, D., and Salter, R. B.: The diagnosis and management of the various types of rickets. Pediatr. Clin. N. Amer. *5*:417, 1958.

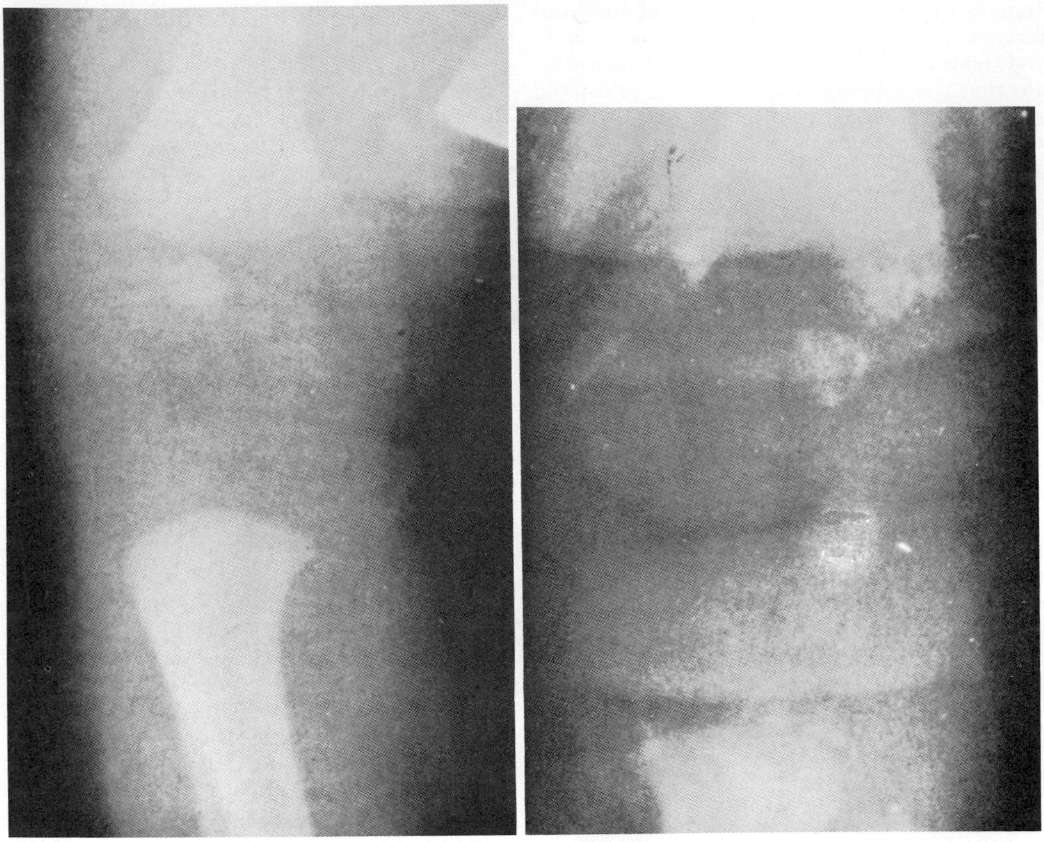

A **B**

Figure 22–40 *Evolution of osseous changes in hypophosphatasia. Roentgenograms of knee at 7 days* (A) *and at 4 months* (B) *of age. Serum alkaline phosphatase values 0.5 to 2.0 Bodansky units. (From T. M. Teree and L. Klein: Hypophosphatasia:* J. Pediatr., *72:41, 1968. Reproduced through the courtesy of The C. V. Mosby Company.)*

Stanbury, J. B., Wyngaarden, J. B., and Frederickson, D. S.: The Metabolic Basis of Inherited Disease. 3rd ed. New York, McGraw-Hill Book Company, Inc., 1972.

Osteogenesis

McLean, F. C., and Urist, M. R.: Bone, Fundamentals of the Physiology of Skeletal Tissue. Chicago, University of Chicago Press. 3rd ed. 1968.

Neuman, W. F., and Neuman, M. W.: The Chemical Dynamics of Bone Mineral. Chicago, University of Chicago Press, 1958.

Calciferol

DeLuca, H. F.: Vitamin D: A new look at an old vitamin. Nutr. Rev. *29*:179, 1971.

Hypophosphatemic Vitamin D-Resistant Rickets

Harrison, H. E.: Mechanisms of action of vitamin D. Pediatrics *14*:285, 1954.

West, C. D., Blanton, J. C., Silverman, F. N., and Holland, N. H.: Use of phosphate salts as an adjunct to vitamin D in the treatment of hypophosphatemic vitamin D refractory rickets. J. Pediatr. *64*:469, 1964.

Winters, R. W., Graham, J. B., Williams, T. F., McFalls, V. W., and Burnett, C. H.: A genetic study of familial hypophosphatemia and vitamin D-resistant rickets, with a review of the literature. Medicine *37*:97, 1958.

Glorieux, F. H., Scriver, C. R., Reade, T. M., Goldman, H., and Roseborough, A.: Use of phosphate and vitamin D to prevent dwarfism and rickets in X-linked hypophosphatemia. New Engl. J. Med. *287*:481, 1972.

Hypocalcemic Vitamin D-Resistant Rickets

Fraser, D., Kooh, S. W., Kind, H. P., Holick, M. F., Tanaka, Y., and DeLuca, H. F.: Pathogenesis of hereditary vitamin D-dependent rickets. New Engl. J. Med. *289*:817, 1973.

Prader, A., Illig, R., and Heierli, E.: Eine besondere Form der primären vitamin-D-resistenten Rachitis mit Hypocalcämie und autosomal-dominantem Erbgang: die hereditäre Pseudo-Mangelrachitis. Helv. Paediatr. Acta *16*:452, 1961.

Soriano, J. R., Einhorn, A., Stark, H., and Edelmann, C. M., Jr.: Deficiency type rickets due to decreased sensitivity to vitamin D. J. Pediatr. *68*:227, 1966.

Refractory Rickets with Multiple Tubular Dysfunction

Dent, C. E.: Rickets and osteomalacia from renal tubular defects. J. Bone Joint Surg. *34-B*:266, 1952.

Harrison, H. E.: The Fanconi syndrome. J. Chronic Dis. *7*:346, 1958.

Leaf, A.: The Syndrome of Osteomalacia, Renal Glycosuria, Aminoaciduria, and Hyperphosphaturia (the Fanconi Syndrome). *In* Stanbury, J. B., Wyngaarden, J. B., and Frederickson, D. S. (eds.): The Metabolic Basis of Inherited Disease. 2nd ed. New York, McGraw-Hill Book Company, Inc., 1966.

Schneider, J. A., Wong, V., and Seegmiller, E.: The Early Diagnosis of Cystinosis. J. Pediatr. *74*:114, 1969.

Refractory Rickets with Renal Tubular Acidosis

Albright, F., Burnett, C. H., Parson, W., Reifenstein, E. C., Jr., and Roos, A.: Osteomalacia and late rickets. Medicine *25*:399, 1946.

Smith, L. H., Jr.: Renal tubular acidosis. *In* Stanbury, J. B., Wyngaarden, J. B., and Frederickson, D. S. (eds.): The Metabolic Basis of Inherited Disease. 2nd ed. New York, McGraw-Hill Book Company, Inc., 1966.

Refractory Rickets Associated with Lowe's Syndrome

Lowe, C. U., Terry, M., and MacLachlan, E. A.: Organic-aciduria, decreased renal ammonia production, hydrophthalmos, and mental retardation: A clinical entity. Am. J. Dis. Child. *83*:164, 1952.

Renal Osteodystrophy

Burke, E. C., Stickler, G. B., and Rosevear, J. W.: Renal Osteodystrophy in two siblings. Am. J. Dis. Child. *105*:478, 1963.

Dent, C. E., Harper, C. M., and Philpot, G. R.: The treatment of renal-glomerular osteodystrophy. Quart. J. Med. *30*:1, 1961.

Fraser, D., and Salter, R. B.: The diagnosis and management of the various types of rickets. Pediatr. Clin. N. Amer. *5*:417, 1958.

Stanbury, S. W., and Lumb, G. A.: Metabolic studies of renal osteodystrophy. Medicine *41*:1, 1962.

Rickets in Steatorrhea

Parsons, L. G.: Celiac disease: Rachford Memorial Lecture. Am. J. Dis. Child. *43*:1293, 1932.

Osteoporosis in Nutritional Deficiency

Teng, C. T., and others: Liver diseases and osteoporosis in children. J. Pediatr. *59*:684, 1961.

Jones, P. R. M., and Dean, R. F. A.: The effects of kwashiorkor on the development of the bones of the knee. J. Pediatr. *54*:176, 1959.

Talbot, N. B., Sobel, E. H., McArthur, J. W., and Crawford, J. D.: Functional Endocrinology from Birth Through Adolescence. Cambridge, Harvard University Press, 1952.

Idiopathic Hypercalcemia

Smith, D. W., Blizzard, R. M., and Harrison, H. E.: Idiopathic hypercalcemia. A case report with assays of vitamin D in the serum. Pediatrics *24*:258, 1959.

Taussig, H. B.: Possible injury to the cardiovascular system from vitamin D. Ann. Intern. Med. *65*:1195, 1966.

Hypophosphatasia

Bartter, F. C.: Hypophosphatasia. *In* Stanbury, J. B., Wyngaarden, J. B., and Frederickson, D. S. (eds.): The Metabolic Basis of Inherited Disease. 2nd ed. New York, McGraw-Hill Book Company, Inc., 1966.

Bongiovanni, A. M., Album, M. M., Hope, J. W., Root, A. W., Marino, J., and Spencer, D. W.: Studies in hypophosphatasia and response to high phosphate intake. Am. J. Med. Sci. *255*:3; 163, 1968.

Teree, T. M., and Klein, L.: Hypophosphatasia, clinical and laboratory studies. J. Pediatr. *72*:41, 1968.

Hyperphosphatasia

Swoboda, W.: Hyperostosis corticalis deformans juvenilis (hyperphosphatasia). Helv. Paediatr. Acta, *13*:292, 1958.

23

THE SKIN

The skin is a complex organ system in dynamic equilibrium with the internal milieu; it serves important physical, biochemical, physiologic and psychologic functions. Unlike most other organ systems, the skin must constantly respond to changes in both the external and the internal environment. An understanding of the anatomy, chemistry and physiology of the skin during its developmental phases will enhance understanding of its disorders in the infant and child.

The skin of the newborn infant differs in certain structural and functional respects from that of the adult. The epidermis is thin, particularly the transitional and keratinous layers. The adult capillary pattern in the skin slowly proliferates as the skin surface grows. Vasomotor tone of the peripheral circulation during the immediate neonatal period reflects the hemodynamic changes occurring in the cardiopulmonary, umbilical and other major vessels after birth. There is a tendency toward extravasation of fluid within the dermis, with the easy blister formation seen in primary bacterial infections and in mast cell disease. The sebaceous and apocrine glands, which function transiently under the influence of maternal hormones during the neonatal period, are incompletely developed. The eccrine sweat glands, though their function can be demonstrated with local injections of cholinergic agents, do not respond to the stimulus of heat because of incomplete development of the nervous system; full responsiveness may be delayed for two to two and a half years. During the first few days of life, the surface pH is elevated (6.34), presumably influenced by the vernix caseosa and amniotic fluid. After removal of the vernix, the pH remains high for several days, declining to a more acid surface pH (3.4) with increasing postnatal age.

A major function of the skin is to provide an extensive physical barrier at the interface between the baby and its environment. Other functions include prevention of percutaneous absorption, preservation of the internal environment, and prevention of transepidermal water loss to the external environs. The epidermal barrier to percutaneous absorption resides within the compact outer keratinous layer of the epidermis. The entry of exogenous material into the dermis is primarily the result of diffusion through the stratum corneum, a small contribution being made by the dermal appendages. Aside from its function as a physical barrier, little is known regarding the mechanism by which the skin maintains the internal environment or prevents transepidermal water loss. The local application of an aqueous solution of Neo-Synephrine produces vasoconstriction in preterm infants; this suggests an abnormality in barrier function. There is limited capacity in the newborn infant to promote water loss through the epidermis when he is compared with the infant a few weeks older. This is in part owing to functional impairment of the eccrine sweat glands, but other poorly understood factors may also be operative. Generalized cutaneous disease significantly increases transepidermal water loss and may lead to secondary changes in hemodynamics.

The clinical appearance of the newborn skin varies from generalized erythema to reticular mottling; the changes reflect instability and sensitivity in vascular adjustment to extrauterine conditions. Little is known of how immaturity of the autonomic and peripheral nervous systems contributes. The immaturity of the peripheral nervous system is well indicated, however, by the difficulty with which histamine induces an axon reflex response in premature infants.

DEVELOPMENT OF THE SKIN AND APPENDAGES DURING EMBRYONIC LIFE

The epidermis arises from ectoderm, the dermis and hypodermis from mesoderm. The pluripotential cells of the epidermis later give rise to the sudoriferous glands (apocrine and eccrine sweat glands), the pilosebaceous complex and the nails. The specific mechanisms which regulate differentiation of epidermal cells are not known, but they are early interdependent with dermal mesenchyme. Once their differentiation has started, epidermal cells can function as an organized unit in the absence of underlying dermis.

By the end of the first month of fetal development, the epidermis consists of two layers of cells: a protective peritrichial outer layer (periderm) and an inner layer, the stratum germinativum, which contains the parent cells of epidermis and dermal appendages (pilosebaceous, sudoriferous and nail structures).

Angiogenesis in skin occurs in the second fetal month as an extension of a plexus of subcutaneous vessels.

The first evidence of epidermal melanogenesis is found early in the third fetal month as silver-staining dendritic cells appear adjacent to the basement membrane or within the three-layered epidermis. These melanoblasts form a more complicated dendritic pattern, become intercalated among the epithelial cells of the basal and intermediate layers of the epidermis and begin to produce melanin by the fifth month. Melanogenesis within the melanocytes proceeds at a high rate through the sixth and seventh months. The melanin produced is transferred to the surrounding basal epidermal cells by the dendrites where it is preferentially distributed in the perinuclear region. During the final fetal month, the pattern of pigment distribution begun in the sixth and seventh months is intensified, culminating in the pigment pattern present at birth. Neither numbers nor regional distribution of melanocytes differentiates skin of various races; differences in pigmentation result from quantitative differences in production of melanin. Pigmentary abnormalities may result from faulty function, migration, localization or concentration of melanocytes in the skin (*dermal melanocytosis*) or be associated with other developmental defects (*Peutz-Jeghers syndrome, multiple lentigines with electrocardiographic abnormalities, Albright syndrome, neurofibromatosis*).

By the third fetal month, the proliferating stratum germinativum extends into the dermis and differentiates into the epidermal ridges, the pilosebaceous apparatus and the sudoriferous glands. Beneath some of the clusters, epithelial and mesenchymal cells aggregate to form hair follicle bulbs and dermal papillae. Failure of development at this stage results in *atrichia congenita.* Functional pilary appendages appear from the third to the fourth month. Other clusters of epithelial cells extend deeper and form coils and tubules which, together with vascular elements of the underlying mesenchyme, form eccrine and apocrine glands. In *congenital anhidrotic ectodermal defect,* the sweat glands fail to develop.

By the third month, the posterior limiting sulcus of the nail bed is established as an invagination of the epidermis. The nails arise from the wedge of basal-like cells which grow proximally by the tenth week of development into the deeper tissues of the phalanx in the region of the future terminal interphalangeal joint. As early as 13 weeks, differentiation commences with formation of the matrix, the nail plate evolving until 30 to 32 weeks of development. The nail bed serves no function in the developing nail. Until about the 20th week of development there is a prominent granular layer, which disappears as the nail plate grows distally over the nail bed.

After the fifth intrauterine month, the periderm slowly disappears and is replaced by the stratum corneum. A number of congenital keratinizing abnormalities result from faulty development of epithelial cells at this stage (*ichthyosis* and *ichthyosiform erythrodermas*). In the last trimester of intrauterine life the newly formed stratum corneum is covered by vernix caseosa.

The components of the dermis arise from undifferentiated mesenchyme with the formation of a delicate argyrophilic reticulum by the fibroblasts during the third fetal month. Individual fibers of this newly formed reticulum increase in number and thickness to form collagen bundles. Structural alterations at this stage result in *cutis hyperelasticum* (Ehlers-Danlos disease) or *focal dermal hypoplasia* (Goltz syndrome). The elastic fibers, whose origin is still uncertain, do not appear until about the sixth month. Developmental defects of elastic tissue formation produce *cutis laxa* (generalized elastolysis). Fetal subcutaneous fat, which is highly cellular, becomes apparent at the third month of uterine life and persists into the neonatal period. Biochemical alteration of fetal fat may result in unusual nonedematous hardening of the skin (*subcutaneous fat necrosis* or *sclerema neonatorum*).

The skin is composed of three distinct structural compartments (the epidermis, dermis and subcutaneous tissue) with interrelated functions. The epidermis contains basal or germinative keratinocytes, melanocytes and Langerhans' cells. The constituents of the dermis are the dermal connective tissue (90 per cent of which is collagen), reticulin, elastic tissue fibers, amorphous ground substance, cellular components (fibroblasts, mast cells, histiocytes), blood and lymphatic vessels, in a network of neurologic structures with special functions and cellular components. The subcutaneous tissue is highly active metabolically, and consists of fat cells, fibrous tissue, nerves, vessels, reticuloendothelial cells and transient white blood cells.

The epithelial cells of the epidermis are replenished from the basal layer (stratum germinativum). The cells of the stratum germinativum express their pluripotentiality after experimentally induced damage, being able on demand to reproduce appendageal structures, possibly excluding hair. Epithelial cells arising from the stratum germinativum become displaced into the overlying prickle cell layer, where subsequently, in the more superficial layers, keratohyaline granules form in cytoplasm. Ultimately all the internal structures of these epithelial cells are lost except the fibrous protein, keratin. The "turnover time" (t/o) for this process is normally about 28 days; in psoriasis and in congenital ichthyosiform erythroderma (nonbullous type) the t/o time is approximately 72 hours.

Even after embryonal differentiation of the epidermal cells has occurred, dermis and epidermis remain strongly interdependent. An inflammatory reaction in the dermis may produce an alteration in epidermal kinetics (scaling) or result in blister formation. Scaling can be distinguished microscopically as hyperkeratosis (increase in the thickness of the stratum corneum, as in ichthyosis vulgaris), parakeratosis (abnormal keratinization with retention of pyknotic nuclei, as in psoriasis) or dyskeratosis (individual cell keratinization, as in keratosis follicularis). Abnormal keratinization may also be caused by heritable alterations in function of the keratinocyte. A generalized form of

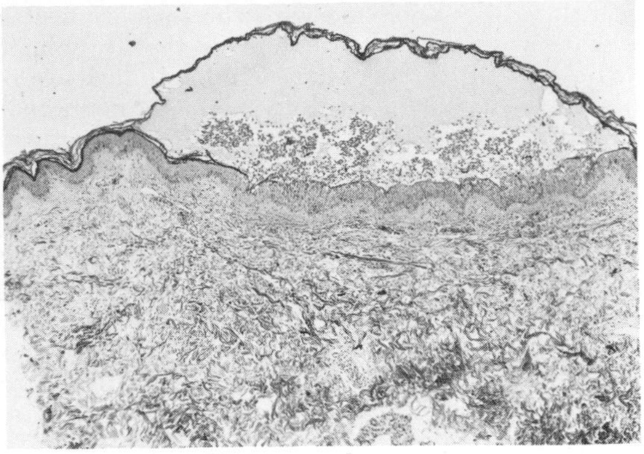

Figure 23–1 Subcorneal blister of impetigo showing superficial location of blister. (× 50.)

hyperkeratosis (*congenital ichthyosiform erythroderma*) and a localized form (*epithelial nevus* and *acrokeratosis verruciformis of Hopf*) are inherited recessively; other generalized forms (*ichthyosis* and *ichthyosiform dermatoses*) may be inherited either dominantly or recessively.

Blisters may be classified in accordance with the location of the blister within the skin and by histopathologic type, in accordance with specific changes due to the different forces which may produce the blister; for example, (1) subcorneal (impetigo, toxic epidermal necrolysis), as in Fig. 23–1; (2) intraepidermal (spongiotic, with increase in intercellular fluid, as seen in allergic contact dermatitis) (Fig. 23–2); (3) loss of intercellular cohesion (acantholytic, due to alteration of tonofibrils with dissolution of desmosomal attachments between cells, as seen in some viral infections and pemphigus) (Fig. 23–3); (4) epidermal-dermal separation (tension type, as seen in erythema multiforme) (Fig. 23–4). Observations of the dynamics of blister formation at the ultrastructural level permit more precise classification on anatomic interrelationships. Light and electron microscopy indicate that blisters at any anatomic locations are associated with morphologic alterations of cells (Fig. 23–5).

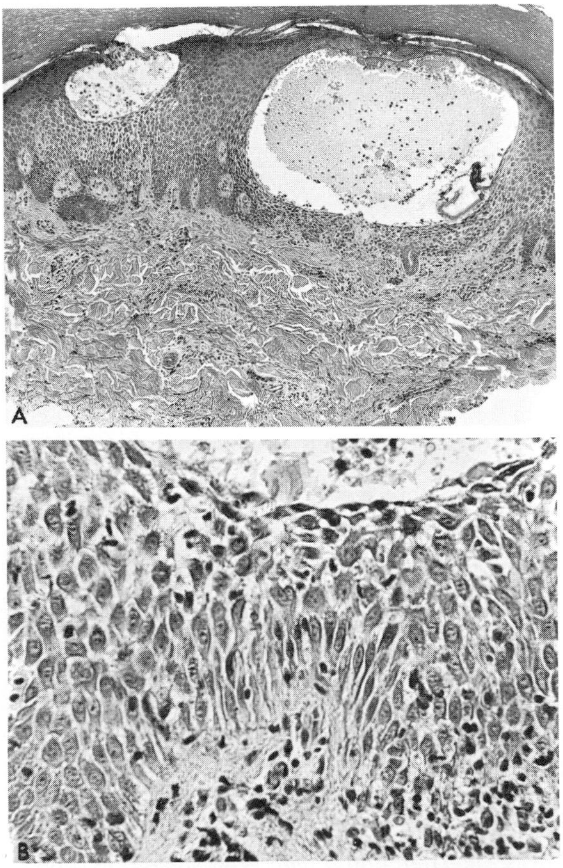

Figure 23–2 Spongiotic blister in lesion of allergic contact dermatitis. A, Intercellular edema and vesicle formation. × 50. B, "Stretching" of intercellular bridges by intercellular edema (spongiosis). (× 250.)

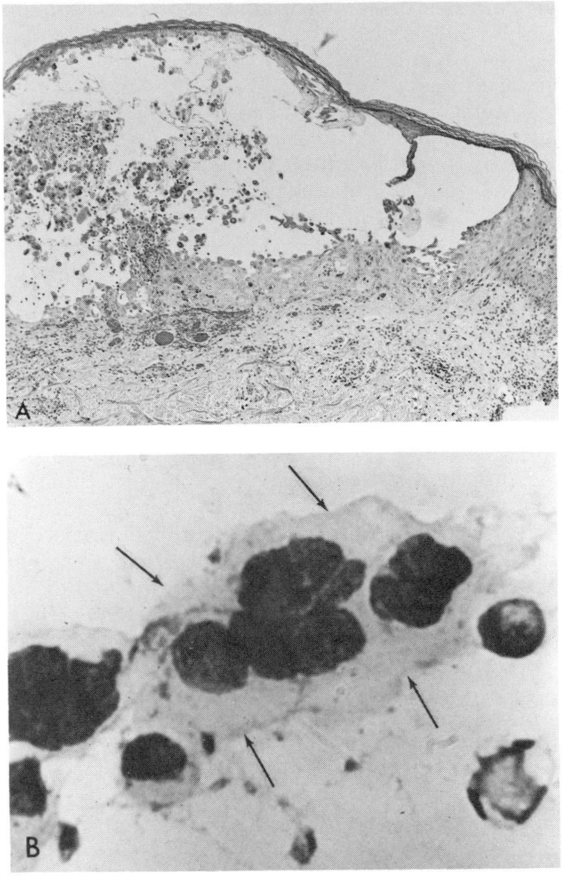

Figure 23–3 Acantholytic blister of herpetic infection. A, Loss of intercellular bridges and epithelial giant cells. B, Exfoliative cytology, showing diagnostic multinucleated epithelial giant cells and margination of nuclear chromatin in varicella-zoster infection.

Pathophysiologic changes in the cutaneous system may result from cutaneous disease or reflect participation of the skin in a systemic disorder. The spectrum of skin changes is so variable that diagnostic confusion is common. Evaluation of the dynamics of the process through correlation of history and clinical appraisal with histopathology helps to determine the primary disease.

Generalized abnormalities or local disturbances in other organ systems may alter the metabolism of skin; examples are the excessive secretion of sodium chloride by eccrine sweat glands in cystic fibrosis, the hyperpigmentation in Addison's disease or the abnormalities of hair in argininosuccinic aciduria. The skin may participate in such diverse systemic abnormalities as the porphyrias, certain disturbances in lipid metabolism, the reticuloendothelioses, mast cell disease, neurofibromatosis of von Recklinghausen, McCune-Albright syndrome, tuberous sclerosis, various diseases of connective tissue, lymphomas, syphilis and other infections, to name only a few conditions in which changes in the skin and its appendages may be diagnostic.

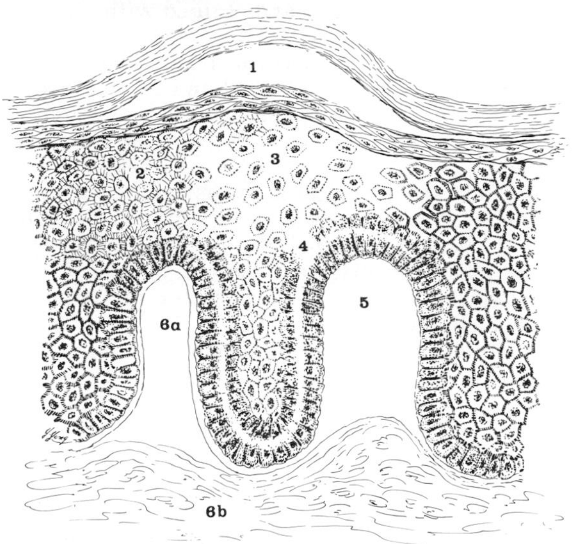

Figure 23-5 *Diagrammatic illustration, showing various anatomic sites and types of blister formation:* (1) subcorneal *(impetigo–intraepidermal);* (2) spongiotic *(allergic contact dermatitis–intraepidermal);* (3) acantholytic *(varicella-zoster, herpes virus hominis–intraepidermal);* (4) suprabasalar *(epidermolysis bullosa simplex, pemphigus–intraepidermal);* (5) intermembrane space *(epidermolysis bullosa letalis–epidermal-dermal interface);* (6) subepidermal *((a) erythema multiforme, (b) epidermolysis bullosa dystrophica–profound connective tissue changes in dermis).*

DIAGNOSTIC METHODS

A variety of procedures may help to confirm a diagnostic impression or establish a diagnosis. Most are easily accomplished and can, with a little practice, be carried out by most physicians.

BIOPSY. Biopsy of the skin is accomplished easily with a 3 to 4-mm punch after local anesthesia. It is important that a *representative early lesion* be selected for biopsy. Suturing of the biopsy site is not essential, but the cosmetic effect is better. Experience is important in evaluation of histologic sections of skin. Tumors will be familiar to most general pathologists, but the inflammatory diseases of skin occasionally present major diagnostic difficulty, even to the dermal pathologist of wide experience.

DIRECT MICROSCOPIC EXAMINATION

Examination for Fungi. Hairs or scales from scrapings are placed on a glass slide, covered with a drop of Amann's chloroactophenol, covered by a cover slip, gently heated and examined microscopically; scales should also be inoculated on Sabouraud's and Litman's media.

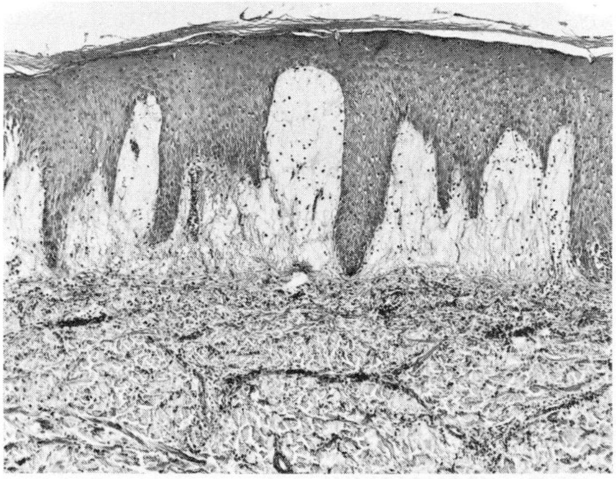

Figure 23-4 *Tension type blister of erythema multiforme, demonstrating separation at dermal-epidermal junction.* (× 75.)

Examination for Bacteria. Smears and cultures for bacteria should be done from exudative lesions. Material from the moist surface is smeared on a glass slide and stained with Gram stain. Material for culture should be obtained from encrusted, moist lesions and, if not plated directly, should be plated in conservation media. Special media are required if there is suspicion of gonococcal infection (chocolate agar incubated in high carbon dioxide environment) or of infection due to beta-hemolytic streptococci (sheep's blood agar).

Examination of Scrapings for Acari. In suspected scabies, scrapings should be obtained from a lesion in the interdigital area or on the flexural surface of the wrist. The roof of the vesicle or burrow is removed with a No. 15 Bard-Parker blade, placed on a glass slide, covered with a coverslip and examined for the mite or ova with the low power magnification of the microscope.

Direct microscopic examination of the hair to determine gross morphology and growth phase is useful in distinguishing hair defects in a large number of syndromes. Additional observations on the hair shaft may be made by examining the hair with polarizing lenses, x-ray diffraction, amino acid analysis, scanning and electron microscopy.

CYTODIAGNOSIS. Cytological changes in some blisters and tissue imprints from infiltrative lesions of the skin or tumors may be useful adjuncts to diagnosis.

The roof of a fresh unruptured blister is reflected, using sharp iris scissors. The roof and the base of the blister are gently scraped with the blade of a No. 15 Bard-Parker scalpel; the material obtained is spread thinly on a clean glass slide, fixed in methyl alcohol and stained with Giemsa stain.

Tissue imprints may be made from a biopsy specimen. The specimen is bisected and the cutaneous surface gently smeared on a clean, dry glass slide. The material is fixed and stained as described above.

The blisters in varicella, zoster and herpes simplex infections are associated with diagnostic types of multinucleated epithelial giant cells. In acantholytic blistering diseases (pemphigus) many isolated epithelial cells with characteristic features may be observed.

IMMUNOFLUORESCENT EXAMINATION. On biopsy specimens frozen in liquid nitrogen direct or indirect immunofluorescence techniques may demonstrate immunoglobulins bound to tissue in vivo or circulating immunoglobulins specific for elements of skin. The technique is useful in some blistering diseases (dermatitis herpetiformis, pemphigus vulgaris, bullous pemphigoid) and in lupus erythematosus.

DARKFIELD EXAMINATION. Examination of serum from suspected syphilitic lesions with the darkfield microscope to demonstrate *Treponema pallidum* is essential to the diagnosis of early syphilis. In preparing material from a skin lesion for darkfield examination, the examiner wears rubber globes or surgical gloves for his protection. The lesion to be examined is firmly abraded with a gauze square to remove the surface epidermis. The abraded area is held firmly between the thumb and forefinger and the serous exudate touched to a clean, dry glass slide and examined under oil in the darkfield microscope. The spirochetes may also be shown in specially stained tissue section, but this exercise is impractical and often unrewarding.

WOOD'S LIGHT EXAMINATION. Examination of the skin with monochromatic ultraviolet (365 nm) is a useful diagnostic aid. Some ringworm infections of the scalp (*Microsporum canis, M. audouini*) give a greenish white fluorescence; some bacterial infections (*Corynebacterium minitisimum, Pseudomonas aeruginosa*) give coral red fluorescence; and abnormalities of pigment distribution (freckles, hypomelanosis of tuberous sclerosis, Albright syndrome) may have characteristic fluorescence or the lack of it.

SKIN OF THE NEONATE

TRANSIENT LESIONS

Some transient skin lesions are seen during the neonatal period. Their significance lies in recognition of them for what they are, which permits appropriate counseling of parents.

CUTIS MARMORATA. This is characterized by mottling of the skin conforming to the dermal vascular pattern. It is a physiologic response to environmental cooling, and reflects the immaturity of the neurovascular system.

HARLEQUIN COLOR CHANGE. This is characterized by a red appearance of the dependent half of the skin of the reclining infant, with a sharp line of demarcation at the midline. This vascular phenomenon is seen more frequently in infants with low birth weight; episodes last from 10 seconds to 20 minutes, and usually cease by the end of the first week of life.

CAPILLARY NEVI. *Nevus flammeus* is characterized by the appearance of macular vascular lesions ranging in color from pink to deep purplish red. Some remain unchanged throughout life (see Nevi, below); others similar in appearance, located in the nape of the neck, glabella and eyelids, may be transient. Most lesions of the eyelids will disappear by the end of one year, the glabellar lesions at a somewhat slower rate; only about one half of the nuchal lesions disappear by the end of the first year.

TRAUMATIC ASPHYXIA (COMPRESSION SYNDROME). Compression of the chest and abdomen during delivery may result in localized cyanosis of the head, and rarely of the neck and upper part of the trunk, which is not relieved by otherwise adequate oxygenation. Vascular damage in the involved areas produces petechiae and ecchymosis of the skin and subconjunctival hemorrhages. No therapy is required for the skin involvement itself, nor are any residuals related to it.

ERYTHEMA TOXICUM (URTICARIA NEONATORUM). Erythema toxicum is a transient eruption of unknown origin characterized by discrete erythematous areas 5 to 15 mm in diameter with yellowish or whitish hive-like elevations in the center resembling flea bites. The lesions appear suddenly in the first two days of life and disappear spontaneously by the ninth day. They are located predominantly on the trunk and buttocks. Infrequently the lesions become pustular. Histopathologically there is edema in the upper corium associated with a predominantly perivascular cellular infiltrate consisting mainly of eosinophilic leukocytes. The pustules are located in the subcorneal or intraepidermal layers. A Giemsa-stained smear from a pustule shows a large number of eosinophils.

Staphylococcal infection must be differentiated. No treatment is necessary.

DEFLUVIUM. Defluvium of the newborn is a physiologic form of diffuse loss of hair; it begins and is completed in the first two to three months of life in all infants. Loss of hair is first noted in the occipital and frontal areas; it may begin suddenly, progress rapidly and be completed in a few weeks, or it may be so gradual as to escape notice.

MILIA NEONATORUM. These are pearly white, evanescent, pinhead-sized papules which occur on the faces of approximately 40 per cent of newborn infants and disappear within a few weeks. Widespread persistent milia may occur in association with other congenital abnormalities (orofacial-digital syndrome, Marie Unna hypotrichosis). Histopathologically they are cysts filled with keratinous debris and are located superficially in the dermis. No treatment is required.

ACNE NEONATORUM. This syndrome represents a true acne vulgaris occurring in an infant presumably genetically predisposed by end-organ hypersensitivity. Typical lesions of acne are seen occasionally, predominantly in male infants, during the first three months of life. In another group of infants, with no preference for males, acne lesions develop after the neonatal period and up until about 2 years of age. Lesions typical of acne, consisting of erythematous follicular papules, papulopustules, and comedones, appear usually on the cheeks, but the forehead and chin may also be involved (Fig. 23-6). Occasionally the pilosebaceous inflammatory reaction may be so severe as to produce a nodulocystic lesion which, on resolution, results in a pitted scar. In most instances, treatment is not required; the disease is mild and the duration short. In rare instances, however, where the eruption is severe and protracted, local treatment is indicated., as in adolescent acne. (See later discussion in this Section.)

PERIANAL DERMATITIS. Perianal dermatitis in the neonatal period (see Diaper Dermatitis) is a reaction to irritation, characterized by erythematous dermatitis and superficial erosion. The lesions will tend to disappear if diapers are removed promptly after a bowel movement. In some infants perianal dermatitis is related to gastrointestinal intolerance to cow's milk or other foods. In an infant whose perianal area is unusually susceptible to irritation, Lassar's paste may be used as a protective film after each change of diaper. In stubborn inflammatory reactions the application after each diaper change of an emollient base such as hydrophilic petrolatum, U.S.P. XVIII, containing 0.5 to 1.0 per cent hydrocortisone (alcohol) is helpful.

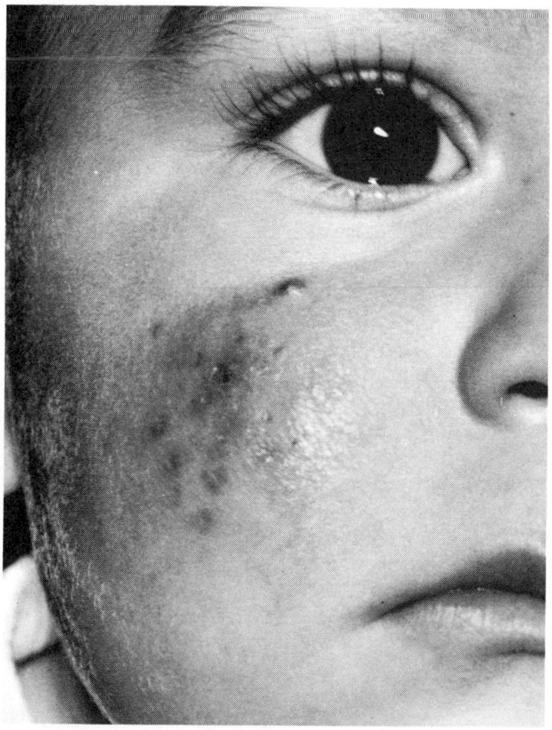

Figure 23-6 Acne neonatorum in 9 month old male infant showing inflammatory lesion and pitted scarring.

MILIARIA (SWEAT RETENTION SYNDROME; PRICKLY HEAT). Miliaria is a transient inflammatory disease of the skin of infants caused by mechanical obstruction of the sweat ducts. It occurs primarily in hot humid environments. Histopathologic sections show keratin plugs at various levels of the sweat duct.

The clinical appearance of the skin lesions depends on the level of obstruction of the duct. Superficial plugging produces a blister with watery contents (*miliaria crystallina*). *Miliaria pustulosa* follows within 24 to 48 hours as a result of polymorphonuclear invasion of the vesicle of miliaria crystallina. In *miliaria rubra* an erythematous, papulovesicular lesion is produced by deep plugging of the duct. The eruption occurs most commonly on the cheeks, neck, trunk and diaper area.

In differential diagnosis, erythema toxicum and yeast and pyogenic infections must be distinguished. They can be differentiated easily by the demonstration of eosinophils in erythema toxicum and of yeast or bacteria in the latter on direct microscopic examination of Giemsa-stained smears.

Effective management consists of preventing the lesions by control of environmental temperature and by avoidance of excessive clothing. Symptomatically the child may be made more comfortable by a cool environment and frequent cooling baths.

SUCKING BLISTERS. These small blisters (0.5 to 1.5 cm) appear transiently on the radial surface of the forearm, the dorsum of the thumb or index finger, and the central portion of the upper lip. They are presumed to occur in utero as the result of vigorous sucking by the infant. They rapidly resolve during the neonatal period and no new blisters appear. No therapy is required.

PERMANENT AND LIFE-THREATENING LESIONS

Besides the transient and generally inconsequential skin lesions characteristic of the neonatal period, there are a number of conditions which require differentiation because they may be either persistent or threats to life. These conditions may be categorized according to their morphologic and histologic characteristics as follows: blistering diseases, keratinizing abnormalities, diseases of pigmentation, developmental abnormalities, diseases of the subcutaneous tissue and diseases affecting the dermis.

Blistering Diseases

The mechanism of blister formation is not well understood. Blisters form as the result of: (1) infection (bacterial, viral or spirochetal); (2) congenital defects in which minor mechanical trauma produces blisters (*epidermolysis bullosa*); (3) infiltrative disease in the dermis (*mast cell disease*); (4) diseases of unknown etiology in which blisters

TABLE 23-1 BLISTERING DISEASES IN THE NEONATE

NAME OF DISEASE	CAUSE	ANATOMIC SITE OF BLISTER	MODE OF INHERITANCE	ASSOCIATED SKIN CHANGES
Nonscarring				
1. Sucking blister	Trauma	Epidermal-dermal junction (IMS)	None	None
2. Infection:				
a. Bacterial—Impetigo of the newborn (pemphius neonatorum)	Staphylococcus or Streptococcus	Subcorneal	None	None
Toxic epidermal necrolysis	Staphylococcus	Subcorneal	None	Generalized erythema
b. Viral	Herpes simplex, varicella	Intra-epidermal (acantholytic)	None	None
c. Spirochetal	*T. pallidum*	Epidermal-dermal junction	None	None
3. Epidermolysis bullosa simplex	Trauma	Intra-epidermal (basal cell)	Dominant	Localized abscesses of skin
4. Epidermolysis bullosa hereditaria letalis(Herlitz)	Trauma	Epidermal-dermal junction (IMS)	Recessive	Loss of nails
5. Bullous congenital ichthyosiform erythroderma	Trauma	Intra-epidermal	Dominant	Generalized erythema and hyperkeratosis
6. Pachyonychia congenita	Trauma	Intra-epidermal	Dominant	Dystrophic nails, hyperkeratotic skin lesions, oral leukokeratoses
7. Acrodermatitis enteropathica	Trauma	Intra-epidermal	X-linked	Hair loss, dystrophic nail changes, stomatitis
8. Incontinentia pigmenti		Intra-epidermal	X-linked	Pigmentation and/or hyperkeratotic lesion
9. Mast cell disease	Trauma	Epidermal-dermal junction	Unknown	Generalized infiltration of skin
Scarring				
Epidermolysis bullosa				
a. Dystrophic dominant	Trauma	Beneath epidermal-dermal junction with degeneration of connective tissue	Dominant	Scarring, milia, loss of nails
b. Dystrophic recessive	Trauma	Same as above	Recessive	Oral and ocular mucous membranes
c. Dystrophic acquired	Trauma	Same as above		

occur as one of the expressions of the disease (*acrodermatitis enteropathica, incontinentia pigmenti*); and (5) some keratinizing abnormalities (*congenital ichthyosiform erythroderma, bullous type,* or *pachyonychia congenita*) (Table 23–1).

Infections in the Neonatal Period

Colonization of the newborn skin by bacteria is usually uneventful. The bacterial flora of the normal skin includes transient organisms, which may be cultured at one time or another, and resident organisms which multiply freely on the skin. The resident flora of children differs from that of adults and includes Sarcina, gram-positive facultative anaerobic bacilli which are mainly spore formers, Neisseria and nonhemolytic streptococci. Establishment of the normal flora of the skin apparently begins about the fourth day of life. Colonization by staphylococci may begin in the first few hours after delivery. The introduction of group 2 staphylococci, or group A streptococci, may result in bacterial infection of the umbilical stump and adjoining abdominal wall, or in paronychial infection of the skin around the nail fold.

The skin of infants and children differs from that of adults in its resistance and in its response to pathogenic staphylococci and streptococci. The high frequency of primary pyogenic infection of the skin in children reflects altered resistance, and the ease of blister production with pus-forming organisms indicates an altered response, which may be due to immaturity of the skin or to biochemical factors. The clinical patterns produced by infection of the skin are extremely variable.

The characteristic bullous response of the skin to staphylococcal and occasionally to streptococcal infection may occur in two different morphologic forms in the first few weeks of life (*impetigo of the newborn* and *toxic epidermal necrolysis*).

IMPETIGO OF THE NEWBORN. Pemphigus neonatorum generally starts between the fourth and tenth days of life. Easily ruptured bullous lesions appear on a slightly erythematous base on any part of the body, but most commonly on the face, hands and exposed areas. There is also a predilection for the diaper area in male infants. The blisters rupture and form crusts, and new bullae form; the entire cutaneous surface may become involved. Although constitutional symptoms are at first absent, septicemia may occur. The diagnosis can be established by a smear and by culture of exudate.

Vigorous local and systemic antibiotic treatment should be started. Laboratory tests for the antibiotic sensitivity of the causative agent must be initiated as a guide to any necessary subsequent modification of therapy. Outbreaks of this type of infection in newborn nurseries can usually be traced to carriers among personnel. A prophylactic and treatment regimen should be followed. (See Section 7.)

TOXIC EPIDERMAL NECROLYSIS. This has been described under a variety of names such as scalded-skin syndrome, dermatitis exfoliativa neonatorum and Ritter's disease. This syndrome is an acute reaction of the skin, involving formation of flaccid bullae, a painful exfoliative erythroderma and a systemic reaction.

In infants, hemolytic staphylococci of several group 2 phage types have been isolated from "primary areas" of the disease, but cultures from the erythematous areas have been sterile. In older children the syndrome may be produced by drug hypersensitivity or by systemic viral infections such as measles, herpes simplex or cytomegalic inclusion disease. In biopsies of early lesions the histopathologic changes are indistinguishable from those of dermatitis exfoliativa neonatorum; they consist of reversal of staining properties of the stratum corneum and stratum malpighii, with intraepidermal or subepidermal separation and a minimal dermal inflammatory reaction.

The skin changes usually start suddenly with perioral erythema and crusting, which are followed by a tender, sensitive, generalized erythema within 24 to 48 hours. A systemic reaction with fever (38 to 40° C, or 101 to 104° F) and a moderate leukocytosis may occur. The epidermis quickly becomes separated by fluid, in poorly circumscribed areas of various sizes. These superficial blisters may be easily wiped off, and the erythematous skin in nonblistered areas may be removed by light rubbing (Nikolsky's sign), leaving a moist surface. Individual erythematous areas merge, giving the skin a scalded appearance (Fig. 23–7). Denuded areas dry quickly, and within a few days the involved skin becomes dry and scaling; it returns to normal within 7 to 10 days. Involvement of mucous membranes is insignificant. Some infants may have one or more bullous lesions of impetigo, but others have no lesions prior to the appearance of generalized exfoliation.

Refusal of feeding is an early sign of systemic illness and is followed by vomiting, prostration, abdominal distention and, occasionally, jaundice. Diarrhea with mucoid green stools may be associated with shock. A fatal illness may last less than 36 hours.

Though the appearance of toxic epidermal necrolysis is rather distinctive, several other diseases may have a superficial resemblance. Erythema multiforme in the newborn might be confused initially, but it does not have the rapid evolution or pain and has a different histopathologic picture. The skin changes in boron poisoning may be similar in appearance, but are usually associated with neurologic disturbances and renal failure. In epidermolysis bullosa blisters appear at sites of trauma, with slow progression and a different histopathologic pattern.

A semisynthetic penicillin should be administered initially, since penicillin-resistant organisms are frequently found. Isolation in an incubator protects the painful skin and permits temperature and humidity control. The danger of absorption of toxic preparations through the damaged skin may be considerable; soap substitutes containing hexachlorophene should be avoided. The loosened areas of skin should be debrided, the skin cleansed with a solution of benzalkonium chloride 1:10,000 and an ointment applied containing polymyxin and bacitracin. Fluid and electrolyte balance must be maintained. In older children in whom sensitization to a drug is considered a likely cause of toxic epidermal necrolysis, systemic administration of a corticosteroid may be indicated. During the scaling stage of regression an emollient ointment such as hydrophilic petrolatum, U.S.P. XVIII, with 20 per cent distilled water is useful.

SPIROCHETAL INFECTIONS. Vesiculobullous lesions, particularly on the palms and soles, may be seen in congenital syphilis. The presence of erythematous, infiltrated papular skin lesions, mucosal involvement, lymphadenopathy and hepatosplenomegaly suggests a treponemal infection. (See Syphilis, Section 10.)

VIRAL INFECTIONS. Infections caused by the viruses of herpes simplex, varicella or variola-vaccinia may produce vesiculobullous lesions in the newborn infant if the mother has the infection at the time of delivery and is in the phase of viremia. Infection may also occur in an infant who has no passively transferred antibodies if he has extraneous contact with the virus. The clinical appearance of the lesions resembles that seen in any primary infection with the virus. A Giemsa-stained smear, skin biopsy and appropriate viral studies will establish the diagnosis.

Infections After the Neonatal Period

After the neonatal period, the most common skin infections are caused by group 2 staphylococci or group A beta-hemolytic streptococci; these are the primary pyodermas, which include impetigo, ecthyma, folliculitis, furunculosis (furuncles and carbuncles), eccrine sweat gland infections (periporitis), paronychial infections and erysipelas. Infections caused by *Pseudomonas aeruginosa, Mycobacterium tuberculosis* and other organisms occur uncommonly.

In secondary pyodermas, streptococcal and staphylococcal infection may complicate a wide variety of pre-existing skin lesions, most frequently atopic dermatitis, allergic contact dermatitis and seborrheic dermatitis. The possibility of such infection must be continually in mind, for infected lesions of eczema may show only crusting, without purulent discharge, cellulitis, lymphangiitis or lymphadenitis. The smear and culture of chronic eczematized lesions for bacteria are essential to management.

IMPETIGO CONTAGIOSA. This is a superficial infection of the skin caused by beta-hemolytic streptococci, group A, or by coagulase-positive hemolytic *Staphylococcus aureus.* There are vesicular or pustular lesions which rapidly become exudative and crusted. Pathologically the same subcorneal blister in the epidermis occurs whether infections are caused by streptococci or staphylococci. The stratum granulosum usually remains intact and forms the base of the blister. The blister fluid is filled with numerous polymorphonuclear leukocytes. There are perivascular inflammation and dilatation of the capillaries in the upper portion of the dermis.

The earliest skin changes consist of a blister, with serum which rapidly becomes cloudy. The blisters are prone to early rupture, with the formation of yellowish, nonadherent crusts surrounded by erythema. The individual lesions vary in size from a few millimeters to several centimeters. There is a tendency for central clearing and peripheral spreading, with the development of circles, arcs or serpiginous morphology (Fig. 23–8). The infection occurs most commonly on the face, less frequently on the extremities and trunk. Removal of crusts leaves a weeping surface from which bacteria can readily be recovered; the disease is autoinoculable. The morphology does not differentiate between the causative organisms, but regional lymphadenopathy may occur more frequently with streptococcal infection.

The yield of streptococci on culture may be incorrectly low unless precautions are taken to offset the tendency of *Staphylococcus aureus* to overgrow streptococci. The phage type of staphylococcus found in both pure and mixed impetigo is most commonly group 2 type 71. The earlier the lesion is cultured, the more likely streptococci are to be found, whereas staphylococci are most commonly isolated from older lesions. It is suggested that the staphylococcus is often a secondary invader. Elevated ASO titers may be found in patients with staphylococcal impetigo, with no history or culture of streptococci in the throat.

Glomerular nephritis (see Section 15) is a

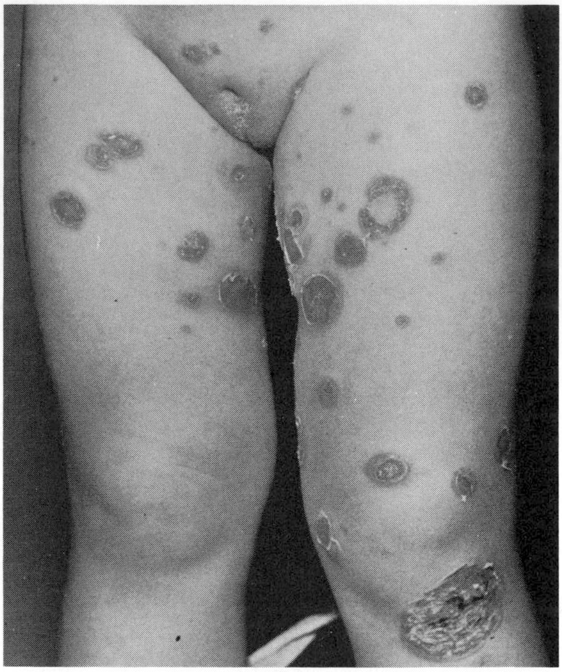

Figure 23–8 Impetigo, showing vesiculobullous lesions and crusting. Some lesions have cleared centrally and spread peripherally, simulating a ringworm infection.

frequent complication of skin infection caused by group A streptococci. It most commonly follows impetigo, but may also follow secondarily infected eczematous dermatitis. The nephritogenic strains causing skin infection have different serotypes from those producing pharyngitis and nephritis. Nephritis following skin infection has its peak incidence in late summer and early fall, whereas nephritis and rheumatic fever following streptococcal pharyngitis occur chiefly in winter and spring. The incidence of positive streptococcal throat cultures is usually no higher in patients with either staphylococcal or streptococcal impetigo than in the general population. The incidence of nasal carriage of staphylococcus is high, however, in patients with staphylococcal impetigo, and in most instances the same phage type can be found in both nose and skin.

Systemic antibiotic therapy is indicated since nephritogenic strains of beta-hemolytic streptococci appear to play a significant role in impetigo. Penicillin is the drug of choice in streptococcal infections. A semisynthetic penicillin may be preferred for treatment, since over 50 per cent of the staphylococci recovered from skin infections are resistant to penicillin G. Epidemics of bacterial infection complicated by nephritis sometimes occur which demand prophylactic use of penicillin in a defined population.

Local antibacterial treatment may control the infection if properly carried out. Crusts should be gently scrubbed off with cotton, using water and a soap substitute containing hexachlorophene. Then an antibiotic ointment containing bacitracin and neomycin is applied. To prevent autoinoculation, a soap substitute containing hexachlorophene is suggested for general cleansing, and the use of an ointment containing neomycin and bacitracin in the nares and beneath the fingernails is helpful.

ECTHYMA. Ecthyma is a superficial pyogenic infection of the skin caused by either staphylococci or streptococci, involving both the epidermis and dermis, and ultimately resulting in scarring. It differs from impetigo in the superficial ulceration of the epidermis and in involvement of the dermis. The vessels in the epidermis are dilated at the periphery of the erosion and are frequently thrombosed near the center; beneath the degenerating epithelium the connective tissue may be necrotic and contain numerous polymorphonuclear leukocytes.

The primary lesion is a pustule which ruptures after several days. The patient is usually first seen with a crusted lesion; the crust is adherent peripherally and when removed leaves a small ulceration. The lesions may be multiple and vary in size from 0.5 to 2.0 cm. In the course of several weeks the lesions heal, leaving a scar with hyperpigmentation at the border. Lesions occur most frequently on the lower extremities below the knees. As with impetigo, the disease is infectious and autoinoculable. The patient should be investigated and treated as for impetigo. Usually local treatment is all that is necessary in staphylococcal infection.

BACTERIAL INFECTION OF APPENDAGEAL STRUCTURES OF THE SKIN. Infection with staphylococci results in a variable clinical picture, depending on the anatomic site of invasion and the depth of infection; infections occur in the pilosebaceous apparatus (folliculitis, furuncle, carbuncle), in eccrine sweat glands (periporitis and multiple sweat gland abscesses), or in apocrine sweat glands (hidradenitis suppurativa). Differences between the adnexal infections depend mainly on the anatomic distributions of the structures. Follicular infections occur at any age; eccrine gland infections are seen most frequently during infancy; apocrine sweat gland infections occur at puberty. The pathologic picture is similar and may vary from a periductal or perifollicular inflammatory process to dermal necrosis with abscess formation deep in the dermis or in the subcutaneous tissue.

Folliculitis. Folliculitis is a superficial staphylococcal infection of the hair follicle. Usually there are multiple erythematous pustules centered about individual hair follicles. The individual infection is often self-limited and, if unscratched, dries up and forms a crust. Because they itch, lesions are scratched and the infection is disseminated.

A furuncle is a deeper staphylococcal infection of the hair follicle, producing an area of central necrosis. Furuncles are usually solitary but may occur in successive crops (*furunculosis*). A *carbuncle* is a group of closely connected follicular infections with still deeper involvement of the hair follicles and penetration into the subcutaneous tissue. Deep follicular infection produces a red, extremely tender papule which becomes a pustule, with a central core which may be expressed 3 to 4 days after onset of the infection. Furuncles occur wherever there are hair follicles, but are most common on the buttocks, extremities and scalp. Infections in the central portion of the face constitute a threat to life because of the possibility of cavernous sinus thrombosis.

Periporitis and Multiple Sweat Gland Abscesses. These are superficial and deep infections of the eccrine sweat glands, which may occur in a few follicles or be generalized. The individual eccrine infections resemble those seen with folliculitis and furunculosis except that hairs cannot be found in the central portion of the inflammatory process. The severest form of infection is most commonly seen in infants under 1 year of age, in whom the infection may be progressive, old lesions regressing and new ones appearing as in chronic furunculosis.

Hidradenitis Suppurativa. This is an acute staphylococcal infection of the apocrine sweat glands, which are found on the female breast, in the inguinal regions and around the genitalia, in the axillae and in the perianal region and buttocks. It is most common during the pubertal and postpubertal periods. Infection occurs most often in the axillae and is often mistaken for furunculosis. An erythematous, tender, solitary, deep-seated nodule appears that develops into an abscess, which may rupture spontaneously and resolve or become persistent. New nodules develop, and if lesions persist, a chronic, deep-seated infection with discharging sinuses and intercommunicating tracts and scar tissue develops.

Treatment. Isolated lesions of the adnexa of the skin should be treated with intermittent hot surgical soaks until the lesions localize and drain. Local antibiotics are indicated; systemic antibiotics are not usually necessary unless the infection occurs in the central area of the face. Surgical intervention is contraindicated owing to the possibility of dissemination of the staphylococci and because scarring is increased. After localization of the infection the fluctuant area is opened or aspirated to allow drainage.

In recurrent infections a search for systemic causes such as abnormalities of immune mechanisms should be made, along with an epidemiologic survey of persons in the patient's environment. Prophylactic measures are indicated, as for impetigo, and the epidemiologic survey should include nasopharyngeal cultures of the family members and phage typing of the staphylococci isolated. All members of an involved family should use a soap substitute containing hexachlorophene and rinse their hands with 70 per cent alcohol. An ointment containing neomycin and bacitracin may be used in the nostrils, under the fingernails and in the perianal area. There is no clear evidence that staphylococcal vaccines or toxoids are helpful. Patients should be advised to avoid sharing towels and washcloths with other members of the family.

Treatment of isolated infections is generally satisfactory, but widespread sweat gland infections with abscesses present special problems. In hidradenitis suppurativa, in addition to the routine management outlined above, the chronic sinus tracts should be marsupialized. In longstanding areas with scarring and multiple sinus tracts, block excision is necessary.

PSEUDOMONAS INFECTIONS. In septicemia due to *Pseudomonas aeruginosa,* skin lesions consisting of yellowish green pustules with a surrounding zone of erythema often appear suddenly. The pustules discharge a mucoid material with a characteristic fruity odor and subsequently become necrotic, leaving a punched-out ulcer which slowly enlarges. Occasionally large necrotic lesions produced by an endotoxin of the organism will appear as the first cutaneous lesion. (See also Section 10.)

TUBERCULOSIS OF THE SKIN. Cutaneous tuberculosis is rare in the United States. The tubercle bacillus may invade the skin directly through an abrasion (primary infection), by continuity from an underlying tuberculous lesion such as that of a lymph node, or by hematogenous distribution. Cutaneous lesions such as tuberculides and erythema nodosum may also be produced by circulating antigens of the tubercle bacillus. (For erythema nodosum, see Section 9.)

In *primary tuberculous lesions* tubercle bacilli invade the skin or mucous membrane through abrasions; the intact skin is not vulnerable. The resemblance of the primary lesion to a syphilitic chancre is at times striking. The common sites are the lip, nose, chin, extremities and genital region; there is an accompanying involvement of the regional lymph nodes to complete the primary complex. The initial lesion may occur as a dark red papule, as a small crusted ulcer with an elevated border or as a small plaque. Tubercle bacilli may be found in the skin lesion and in the lymph nodes; the histologic findings are those of tuberculosis. Excision of the primary lesion and of the lymph nodes is indicated if they are in appropriate sites. Antibacterial therapy is indicated in all instances. (See Section 10.)

Lupus Vulgaris. Lupus vulgaris frequently begins in childhood as numerous pinpoint- to pinhead-sized, grouped or disseminated, reddish, yellowish or brownish flat papules. Gradually they enlarge to form tubercles or nodules which, in turn, coalesce into variously shaped and sized pustules. As extension continues slowly, the older lesions may disappear, leaving a scaly, atrophic scar, or they may ulcerate, crust and eventually heal with a residual scar. The disease is chronic and may persist into adult life with considerable disfigurement.

Scrofuloderma. Scrofuloderma begins in one or more lymph nodes or in bone and extends to the surface to involve the skin in a tuberculous process. When lymph nodes are involved, they are initially swollen and painful, but later undergo caseation and suppuration and form sinuses which discharge a caseous, sanious fluid. The resultant skin involvement appears as an oval or linear ulceration, with violaceous, undermined edges and an uneven base with pale, flabby granulations. The surface may be crusted.

The lesions of *lichen scrofulosus* are pinhead-sized, firm, yellowish brown or reddish nodules. The nodules coalesce into coin-sized patches and are situated chiefly on the trunk. They may be accompanied by slight itching. The course is chronic, though the prognosis is favorable.

Tuberculides. These are thought to be caused by reactivity to the antigens of the tubercle bacillus, the most common lesion in children being the papulonecrotic tuberculide. The lesions, which appear in crops, are pea-sized or smaller, firm, bluish red papules, crusted at the summit. When the crust is removed, there is a crater-like depression. Search should be made for the primary tuberculous focus, which is usually in the lungs.

Treatment. Treatment of tuberculosis of the skin consists in improving the general health by means of fresh air, sunshine, vitamin D and an adequate diet. Antimicrobial therapy is indicated in all instances in children irrespective of apparent activity of other lesions. (See Section 10.)

ATYPICAL MYCOBACTERIAL INFECTION. Atypical mycobacterial infections of the skin are caused by *M. marinum* or *balnei,* an acid-fast bacillus antigenically related to *M. tuberculosis.* Where this organism gains entrance into traumatized skin it may produce chronic infection. It grows in warm, nonchlorinated swimming pools or aquaria.

Histopathologically there is a nonspecific granulomatous infiltrate in which the organisms may be found. The skin lesions appear 3 to 6 weeks after a self-healing abrasion; brownish red papules develop, which coalesce to form a nodule, often on the elbows or knees. The nodule may, in turn, become a crusted ulcer, which may persist for months. The nodules are usually but not invariably single. Regional lymphadenopathy is minimal or absent. In differential diagnosis, primary tuberculosis must be considered.

Prophylaxis consists in chlorination and in covering the cement surfaces of swimming pools with porcelain tile. The granulomas usually regress spontaneously within a few months; the organism is only moderately sensitive to streptomycin and is resistant to para-aminosalicylic acid and isoniazid.

Conditions in which Blisters Are Induced by Trauma

EPIDERMOLYSIS BULLOSA. This comprises a group of genetically transmitted skin diseases characterized by blister formation at the site of trauma. The only point of similarity among the syndromes is the trauma-blister sequence; postblister scarring and the genetic determinants vary, and the histologic level of blister formation differs.

Epidermolysis Bullosa Simplex (EBS). This form is transmitted as an autosomal dominant trait. The blisters, which may be present at birth or deferred until the infant begins to crawl, range from a few millimeters to several centimeters in diameter and arise as the result of extremely variable degrees of trauma to the skin. The blisters are superficial, separation occurring in the epidermis within minutes of trauma. The accumulation of fluid within the damaged space results in blister formation within a few hours or less. Microscopic examination of the early stage of blister reveals changes at the level of the basal cell. The intraepidermal location of the blister precludes scarring unless secondary bacterial infection occurs.

Recurrent Bullous Eruption of the Hands and Feet. Weber-Cockayne disease is transmitted as a recessive trait and usually occurs in the first year or two of life, though it may be delayed until adolescence. The blisters appear on both the plantar and dorsal surfaces of the feet at the sites of maximum trauma. Large accumulations of hyperkeratotic skin accumulate over the roof of the blisters. The level of blister formation is the same as in epidermolysis bullosa simplex.

Epidermolysis Bullosa Hereditaria Letalis (Herlitz). This disorder usually presents at birth with large erosions on the legs or feet with oozing surfaces, or with large, tense or flaccid blisters on a nonerythematous base. The dermis is often thin, and subcutaneous vessels may easily be observed through the skin. The skin around the mouth and the oropharyngeal mucous membranes may be involved; the vermilion border is usually spared. The blisters increase in number, rupture and leave large denuded areas (Fig. 23–9). There is no evidence of altered immunologic responses. Fluid and electrolyte loss and secondary bacterial infections usually result in early death. Occasionally children survive, with general development secondarily retarded. Microscopic examination of fresh blisters reveals blister formation at the dermal-epidermal junction. Electron microscopic examination shows the separation to lie within the intermembrane space [IMS] (between the basement membrane and the plasma membrane of the basal cell).

The *scarring* varieties of epidermolysis bullosa are divided into dominant and recessive types:

Dominant Dystrophic Epidermolysis Bullosa. The dominant dystrophic form is intermediate in severity, varying between the simplex type (EBS) and the recessive form. The blisters are subepidermal and usually result in a thin scar. Mucous membranes may be involved, and the nails may become atrophic or thickened and clawlike. Microscopic examination of early blisters shows blister formation beneath the basement membrane with varying degrees of connective tissue degeneration in the upper portion of the dermis.

Recessive Dystrophic Epidermolysis Bullosa. The recessive form is the most severe and destructive form compatible with life. The appearance of blisters at sites of trauma is followed by slow healing; blisters between fingers and toes result in fusion of the digits; involvement of the esophagus ultimately leads to stricture formation. Repeated cycles of blistering and secondary infection produce wide areas of superficial and hypertrophic scarring. Oral and ocular complications are not uncommon in severely affected children. The microscopic changes are similar to those seen in the dominant dystrophic variety.

Epidermolysis Bullosa Acquisita. There is a third type of scarring bullous disease which is classified as "acquired" epidermolysis bullosa when there is no evidence of hereditary transmission. Clinical manifestations appear after infancy and consist of noninflammatory blisters primarily on the skin or interphalangeal joints, knees and elbows, and scars at the site of healed blisters.

The greatest problem in diagnosis is to distinguish between the types of epidermolysis bullosa, but in differential diagnosis several other blistering diseases must also be considered (dyskeratosis congenita, acrodermatitis chronica enteropathica, incontinentia pigmenti, bullous syphiloderm, toxic epidermal necrolysis and impetigo of the newborn).

Treatment. Treatment of all variants is directed toward minimizing trauma. After blisters have appeared, efforts are directed toward preventing secondary bacterial infection. Systemic administration of large doses of corticosteroids may diminish the frequency of blister production in epidermolysis bullosa hereditaria letalis and in recessive dystrophic epidermolysis bullosa.

DYSKERATOSIS CONGENITA. This is a rare disease, probably transmitted as an X-linked recessive trait. It is characterized by a reticulated hyperpigmentation on the face, trunk and arms, atrophy of skin on the dorsa of the hands and feet, leukokeratosis on the oral mucosa, dystrophic nail changes, and subepidermal blisters at the sites of trauma.

Infiltrative Diseases with Blister Formation

MAST CELL DISEASE (URTICARIA PIGMENTOSA). Mast cell infiltration of the skin characterizes a chronic disease of unknown origin in which there are blisters, pigmented maculopapules, nodules or thickened skin (Fig. 23–10). It is usually present at birth or appears in the first two years of life. Mast cell disease may be classified according to distribution of mast cells in the skin as (1) solitary *mastocytoma,* (2) *urticaria pigmentosa* with or without blisters, or (3) *diffuse mast cell infiltration (mastocytosis)* with systemic involvement. The histopathologic changes are distinctive and consist of an infiltrate of mast cells in the upper part of the dermis. The epidermis is usually normal in appearance except for some increase in melanin in the basal layer. In the bullous variety there are intracellular edema and vesicle formation.

Transient urticaria or blisters may appear at birth or shortly thereafter. Initially urticarial lesions, blisters or orange-brown macules resembling a lipid deposit in the skin may be present, alone or in combination. In diffuse mast cell disease the entire skin is thickened, with a "parchment-like" yellow color and a fine, papular "Scotch-grained" surface with exaggerated skin lines. Scratching in affected areas produces a wheal and flare (Darier's sign). The urticarial and

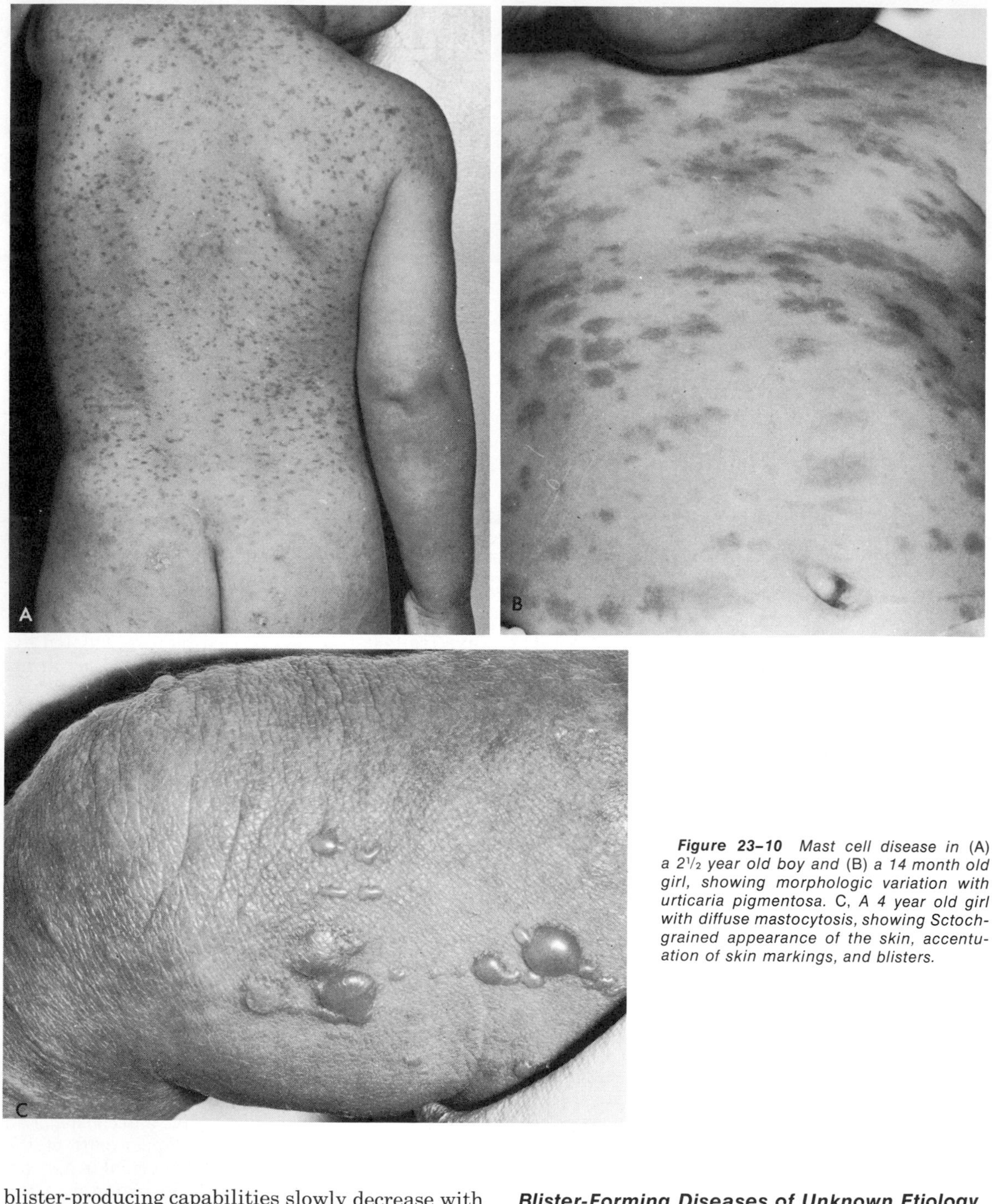

Figure 23–10 Mast cell disease in (A) a 2½ year old boy and (B) a 14 month old girl, showing morphologic variation with urticaria pigmentosa. C, A 4 year old girl with diffuse mastocytosis, showing Sctoch-grained appearance of the skin, accentuation of skin markings, and blisters.

blister-producing capabilities slowly decrease with approach of puberty. Cystic changes of the bone are present occasionally in urticaria pigmentosa, and widespread organ involvement is the rule in diffuse mastocytosis.

In differential diagnosis of solitary mastocytoma, juvenile xanthogranuloma and xanthoma must be distinguished; in the blistering form, dermatitis herpetiformis must be distinguished.

No treatment is known to be effective. In the vesiculobullous stage the local application of a broad spectrum antibiotic may prevent secondary bacterial infection.

Blister-Forming Diseases of Unknown Etiology

ACRODERMATITIS CHRONICA ENTEROPATHICA. This is a chronic, often fatal disease of unknown origin, possibly transmitted as a recessive trait. Onset may be as early as the first month of life, but it usually occurs later in infancy. It is characterized by a vesiculo-pustulo-bullous eruption symmetrically arranged on the extremities and around the mouth and anal areas, by loss of hair and by diarrhea (Fig. 23–11).

A biopsy of the skin is not diagnostic. The blisters are located intraepidermally and contain

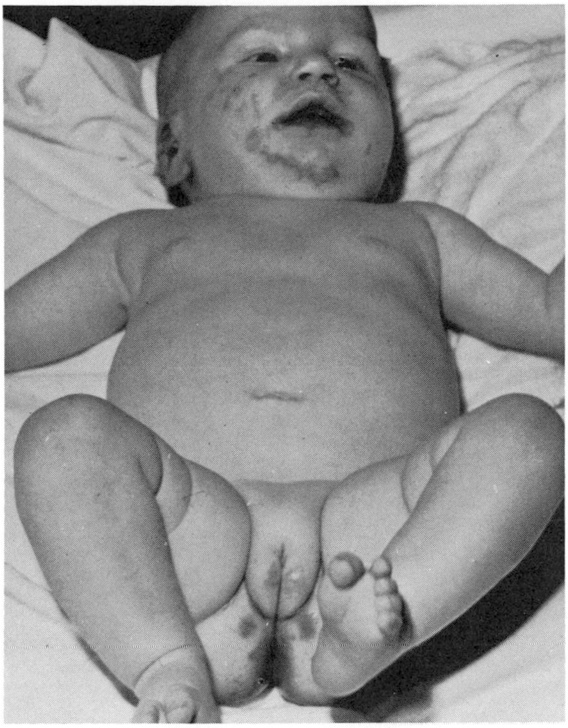

Figure 23–11 Acrodermatitis chronica enteropathica in a 4 month old infant, showing the characteristic periorificial involvement. A male sibling had died with the disease.

polymorphonuclear leukocytes and eosinophils. There is a diffuse infiltrate in the papillary bodies and in the upper portion of the dermis, with perivascular round cell infiltration in the mid-dermis. Chronic scaly lesions are characterized by acanthosis, hyperkeratosis and a dermal inflammatory infiltrate.

The blisters appear on normal skin and evolve to form eczematous patches; in a few weeks they become crusted and form erythematous psoriasiform plaques. Loss of hair occurs early; paronychial and dystrophic nail changes are usually present. The eruption may wax and wane, the gastrointestinal disturbance paralleling the skin changes, or the disease may become progressively more severe and the infant become apathetic and cachectic. Response to parenteral administration of fat suggests a basic defect of fatty acid metabolism.

Untreated, the disease runs a chronic course with partial remissions, progressive malnutrition and death within 1 to 3 years of onset. Remissions may often be obtained by treatment with diiodohydroxyquinoline (Diodoquin) given daily for long periods of time. On occasion a child who fails to respond to this drug will respond to iodochlorohydroxyquinoline (Entero-Vioform). Secondary monilial and bacterial infections should be treated specifically.

INCONTINENTIA PIGMENTI. This disorder of hyperpigmentation may be present at birth, and usually exhibits three distinct phases: vesiculobullous inflammatory, hyperkeratotic and pigmentary. It appears almost exclusively in girls and is probably transmitted as sex-linked dominant. In addition to the cutaneous changes, there are multiple ectodermal and mesodermal defects.

The histopathologic pattern varies with the stage of the disease. In the vesiculobullous stage, there is intercellular edema with vesicle formation and a mixed inflammatory infiltrate in the dermis. In the hyperkeratotic stage, there are proliferation of epithelial cells and hyperkeratosis. In the final stage the epidermis appears essentially normal except for the diminution of pigment in the lower epidermal layers and for large amounts of melanin in the melanophages in the upper portions of the dermis.

The skin changes are present at birth or appear shortly thereafter. The only evidence of the disease may be bizarre asymmetrical whorls or bands of macular brownish pigment on the extremities or trunk, or it may progress from an inflammatory reaction with blisters to a stage in which the vesicles are replaced by keratotic lesions (Fig. 23–12). The inflammatory or hyperkeratotic lesions ultimately disappear, leaving macular pigmentation at the site of previous activity. Abnormalities of the eyes, hair and teeth, epilepsy, mental deficiency and cardiac abnormalities have been associated.

During the inflammatory phase the morphologic changes may suggest an eczematous dermatitis (atopy), epidermolysis bullosa, dermatitis herpetiformis or bullous urticaria pigmentosa; melanocytic nevus must be considered in the pigmentary stage, and epithelial nevus in the keratotic stage.

No treatment is indicated except in the blister phase, when application of a broad spectrum antibiotic is indicated to prevent secondary bacterial infection.

DERMATITIS HERPETIFORMIS. This is an uncommon papulovesicular dermatitis of unknown etiology characterized by pruritus, erythema and grouped lesions varying from urticarial papules to tense blisters, with a predilection for the lumbar area and extremities (Fig. 23–13). It occurs usually in otherwise healthy male infants or children. A significant incidence of small bowel enteropathy has been reported in adults. The histopathologic changes consist of a diagnostic accumulation of eosinophilic leukocytes in the tips of the individual dermal papillae.

In differential diagnosis, juvenile bullous pemphigoid and erythema multiforme need be considered. In each, the clinical appearance of the eruption is similar, but mucous membrane involvement is more common than in dermatitis herpetiformis. In pemphigus vulgaris, mucous membrane lesions are common, but the flaccid blisters usually appear on normal skin. Histopathologically a subepidermal split at the epidermal-dermal junction is the earliest change in juvenile bullous pemphigoid. In erythema multiforme the subepidermal blister occurs in conjunction with a perivascular infiltration in the dermis. The changes in pemphigus vulgaris are characterized by an intraepidermal blister and acantholysis.

The administration of sulfapyridine or sulfones

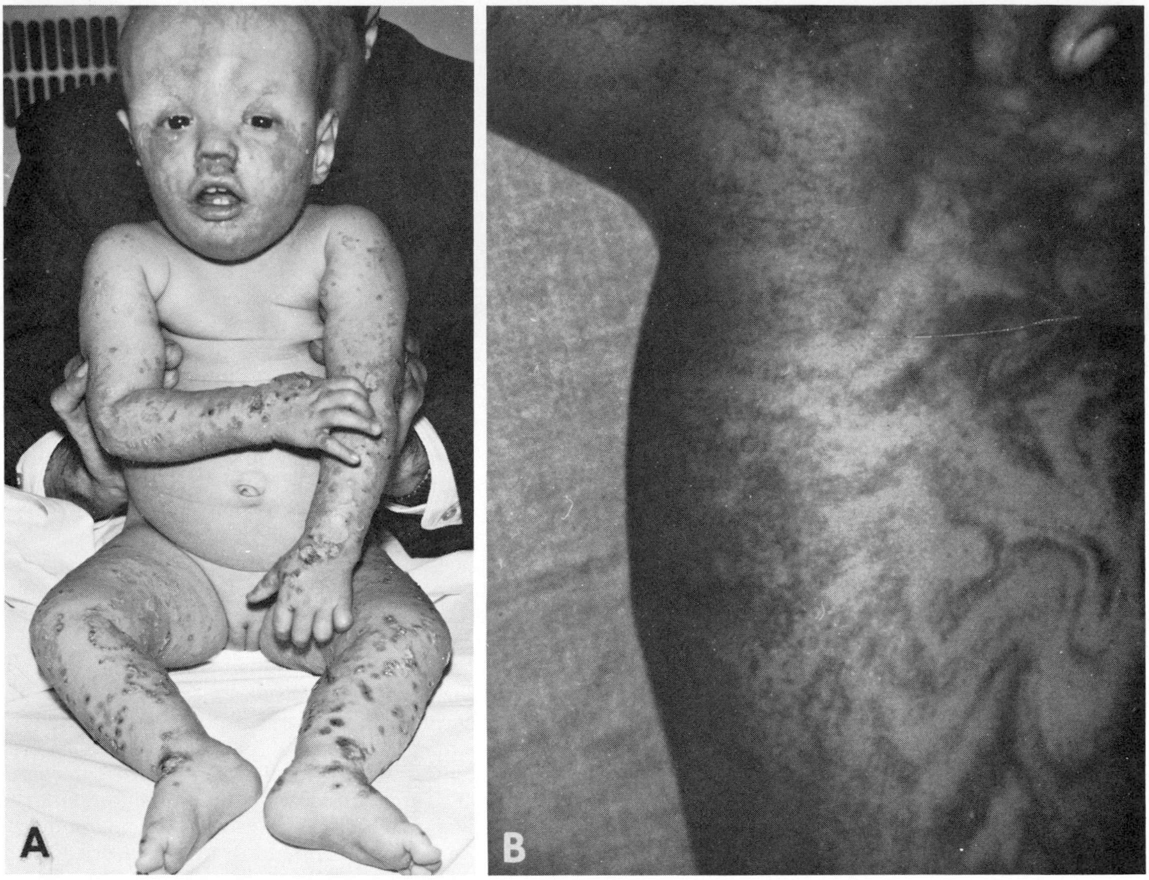

Figure 23–12 *Incontinentia pigmenta.* A, *Papulovesicular and hyperkeratotic papules arranged in bizarre gyrate configuration in infant at 11 months of age; she had craniosynostosis and skin lesions at birth; a younger male sibling has similar skin changes and developmental defects.* B, *Final hyperpigmented stage.*

(dapsone) are usually effective in suppressing blister formation. The dosage required is variable (1–2 gm/day for sulfapyridine; 100–200 mg/day for dapsone). The possibility of side effects with both drugs requires close surveillance. Corticosteroids may be required orally for control if drug intolerance develops.

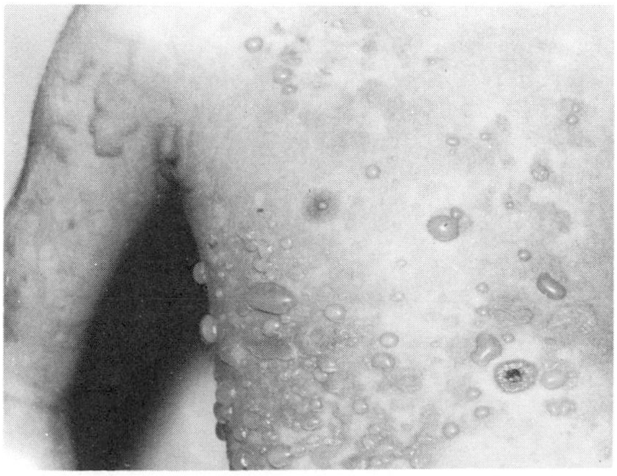

Figure 23–13 *Dermatitis herpetiformis in a 5 year old boy, showing multiform lesions.*

ERYTHEMA MULTIFORME. Erythema multiforme is an acute inflammatory disease of hypersensitivity origin, involving the skin and mucous membranes in a life-threatening major form (*eruptive fever with stomatitis and ophthalmia, Stevens-Johnson syndrome*) and a less severe minor form. It may be induced by many precipitating factors, ranging from drugs to viral infection. The condition is characterized by the sudden appearance of a morphologically variable eruption, consisting of macular and hive-like patches of erythema, blisters and a distinctive urticarial lesion with a dusky center and a bright red raised border (iris lesions) on the palms, soles, trunk and extremities. Mucous membrane blisters which lead to superficial erosion occur commonly; occasionally they may be the only manifestation of the disorder.

The histopathologic changes consist of an allergic vasculitis and subepidermal blister formation. The minor form runs its course in 2 to 3 weeks. The mucous membrane lesions may be treated with a quaternary ammonium compound mouthwash (Cepacol) after meals and at bedtime, followed by the application of triamcinolone in Orabase. Systemic treatment is not usually necessary, but an antihistamine may hasten recovery.

Keratinizing Abnormalities with Blisters

Congenital ichthyosiform erythroderma (epidermolytic hyperkeratosis) and *pachyonychia congenita* may also have blister formation in addition to other abnormalities. (See this Section below.)

Keratinizing Abnormalities

The hereditary keratinizing abnormalities comprise a group of unrelated diseases and syndromes in which there is generalized dryness and scaling of the skin. Ichthyosis and the ichthyosiform dermatoses may be considered to be the result of altered epithelial cell maturation. Normally the basal cells reproduce at a steady rate, transit through the epidermis being characterized by the loss of nuclei and the formation of the keratinous layer. Disruption of the balance between cell proliferation and the elimination of keratin, through increased production or through decreased shedding, results in a thickened stratum corneum. The congenital abnormalities of keratinization (*keratodermas*), relatively uncommon as a group, consist of a number of clinical entities which can be distinguished by genetic, clinical and histopathologic characteristics. Variability in phenotypic expression of the abnormality may cause some difficulty in differentiation.

"HARLEQUIN FETUS." This is a descriptive term for the fetus with the most severe form of ichthyosis, in which the skin is encased in a thickened, fissured, keratinous covering producing a grotesque morphologic appearance (Fig. 23–14). Movement and suckling are limited by the keratinous shell and virtually all affected infants die within the first few hours or days of life. X-ray diffraction studies indicate an abnormal structural protein. Until this rare disease is more clearly defined, the possibility that it may represent an extreme phenotypic variant of lamellar ichthyosis or sex-linked ichthyosis cannot be excluded. This differentiation is important in genetic counseling.

"COLLODIAN MEMBRANE." In the newborn infant, this probably represents the phenotypic expression of more than one genotype. It consists of cellophane-like covering which fissures and exfoliates shortly after birth. Affected infants may develop either nonbullous congenital ichthyosiform erythroderma (lamellar ichthyosis) or X-linked ichthyosis (Fig. 23–15). Occasionally the membrane is shed completely in the neonatal period and the skin appears normal thenceforth.

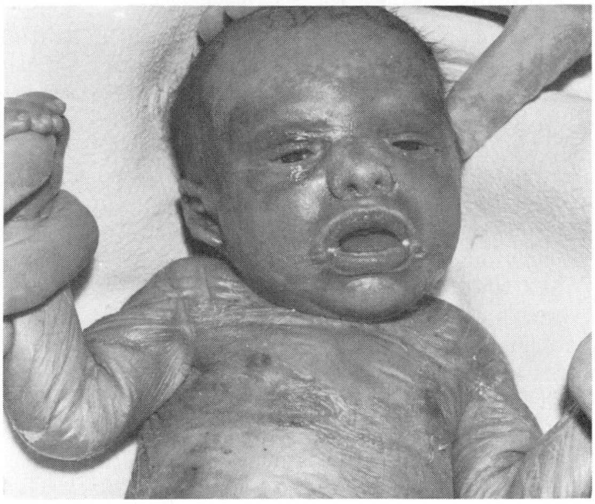

Figure 23–15 *Collodion-like membrane in a newborn female infant who later had lamellar ichthyosis.*

ICHTHYOSIS VULGARIS. Ichthyosis vulgaris is characterized by generalized dryness, keratosis pilaris and increased markings on the palmar and plantar skin. It is the most common variety of ichthyosis but is seldom seen before the age of 3 months. This disease is inherited as an autosomal dominant trait. Frequency is difficult to determine because the manifestations may be so mild; a minimal estimate is on the order of 1 in 1000 persons. Atopic manifestations are observed in approximately 50 per cent of the patients, but this association does not seem to alter the clinical picture of ichthyosis. Involvement of the flexural surfaces is rare. The palmar surfaces of the hands and soles of the feet have increased markings. The scaling on the trunk is more prominent on the back than on the abdomen. Follicular keratoses are common, appearing primarily on the proximal lateral aspects of the arms and legs. The scales are small, fine and white, and there is striking diminution in the severity of scaling with increasing age. Warm weather has a beneficial effect. The histologic features are hyperkeratosis with a diminished or absent granular layer. Studies of cellular kinetics indicate a normal rate of cell turnover, the defect being prolonged retention of the stratum corneum.

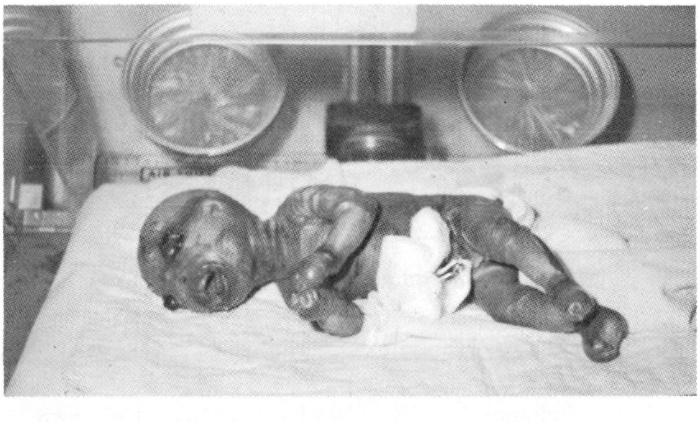

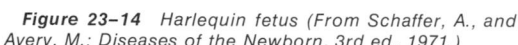

Figure 23–14 *Harlequin fetus (From Schaffer, A., and Avery, M.: Diseases of the Newborn, 3rd ed., 1971.)*

The skin can be kept in as good condition in winter as in summer by a technique of hydration followed by lubrication. The hydrophilic keratin may be hydrated by soaking baths once or twice a day, followed by the application of a water-in-oil ointment (20 per cent distilled water in hydrophilic petrolatum, USP XVIII). An aqueous solution of propylene glycol (40 to 60 per cent) may also produce decreased scaling when used beneath an impervious plastic covering at night.

SEX-LINKED ICHTHYOSIS VULGARIS. This is the commonest form of ichthyosis in the first three months of life. The frequency is estimated at 1 in 6000 males. Genetic studies have indicated that the locus for X-linked ichthyosis and the locus for the Xg blood groups are probably close together on the short arm of the X chromosome. A collodian membrane may be present at birth. Generalized scaling often commences in the first week of life, and though the process remains more or less generalized, the areas of involvement will vary with time. Children characteristically have thick scales on the scalp, with grayish, dirty-appearing hyperkeratotic changes on the sides of the face and neck, whereas in adults the abdomen, legs and the popliteal fossae are most frequently affected. The palms and soles are normal. The scales are typically large and grayish, and are shed episodically. The histologic features are striking hyperkeratosis, increased thickness of the stratum granulosum, normal to acanthotic epidermis and a perivascular inflammatory infiltrate in the dermis. The defect in keratinization is similar to that in ichthyosis vulgaris. The characteristic skin change of the X-linked variety is the large scale, with prominent localization to the neck, but the hallmark of X-linked ichthyosis is the demonstration of deep corneal opacities by slit-lamp examination. There may be improvement during warm weather. The treatment is the same as for ichthyosis vulgaris.

Ichthyosis-like Dermatoses

The ichthyosis-like dermatoses may be grouped according to the presence or absence of varying degrees of erythema and/or blisters at birth, type of scale, mode of inheritance, associated findings and histology. The variable phenotypic expressions of the various genotypes has led to a long, confusing list of ichthyosiform dermatoses, which probably reflects nothing more than the relative infrequency of a few distinct types. Brocq originally described congenital ichthyosiform erythroderma (CIE), which histologic and genetic studies have shown to be two separate entities, bullous and nonbullous congenital ichthyosiform erythroderma. The bullous variety has been renamed *epidermolytic hyperkeratosis* because there are vacuolated cells in the epidermis; the nonbullous type has been designated lamellar ichthyosis. The ichthyosis-like dermatoses also include a variety of syndromes in which there is generalized scaling (Table 23–2).

CONGENITAL ICHTHYOSIFORM ERYTHRODERMA, NONBULLOUS TYPE (LAMELLAR ICHTHYOSIS). This rare congenital abnormality is inherited as an autosomal recessive trait and characterized by a collodian-like membrane which covers the entire cutaneous surface at birth. Typically the infant is completely enveloped in a thin, dry, shining epidermal layer which is brownish yellow and resembles a collodion coating. There is eversion of the eyelids. The membrane cracks within a few hours, and thin sheets of scales peel off, leaving an erythematous base; the scales reform, and the process is repeated. After the neonatal period and throughout life, the ichthyotic scaling persists; it may be widespread or become localized to the flexural surfaces. The large, grayish brown scales are adherent in the center with slightly raised edges (Fig. 23–16). Aggravation of the ichthyosis during warm weather has been reported. The process of abnormal keratinization persists throughout life, with large coarse scales covering most of the body.

Ichthyosis linearis circumflexa is considered to be a variant of this disease, characterized by an erythematous scaling skin evident at birth or during the first year of life, hyperkeratotic lesions on the flexural surfaces of the arms and legs, and numerous serpiginous lesions with raised erythematous hyperkeratotic borders on the trunk and proximal portions of the extremities. Skin changes may be

TABLE 23–2 ICHTHYOSIS-LIKE SYNDROMES

	ONSET	INHERITANCE	CARDIO-VASCULAR	MUSCULO-SKELETAL	NEURO-LOGIC	EYE	META-BOLIC	HAIR
Conradi syndrome	NB	Rec	+	+	+	+	0	0
Netherton syndrome	NB	Rec	0	0	0	0	+ (amino-aciduria)	+
Refsum syndrome	Ch	Rec	0	+	+	+	+	+
Rud syndrome	Inf	Unk	0	+	+		0	+ (alopecia)
Sjögren-Larsson syndrome	NB	Rec	+	0	+	+	0	0
Tay syndrome	NB	Rec	0	0	+	0	0	+
Psoriatic erythroderma	NB	Dom	0	0	0	0	0	0

Ch —Childhood Inf —Infancy Rec —Recessive
Dom—Dominant NB —Newborn Unk—Unknown

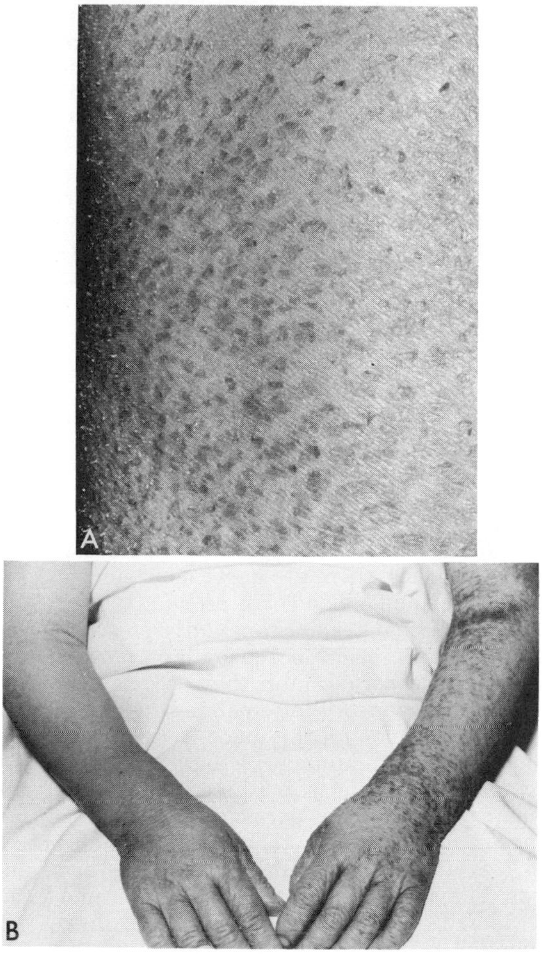

Figure 23–16 A, *Lamellar ichthyosis in a* $2^1/_2$ *year old child who had a collodion type of covering and erythema at birth. Note the characteristic central adherence of the "potato chip" type of scale.* B, *Unilateral response to treatment with vitamin A acid ointment on the right, and absence of response on the left.*

associated with assorted defects of the hair shaft.

Histologically there is a dense, homogeneous, thickened keratin layer, with scattered parakeratotic nuclei. The epidermis is of normal thickness or moderately acanthotic with a distinct granular layer. Keratotic plugs are observed in the pilosebaceous orifices. There is a mild inflammatory infiltrate in the dermis. There is no histologic evidence of a persistent epitrichial layer. Studies of cellular kinetics indicate an increased rate of cell turnover; this, coupled with a maturation defect in the keratinization process, accounts for the scaling.

Treatment with antimetabolites (methotrexate) has been reported to be useful, but is as yet experimental. Topical application of vitamin A acid in a 0.05 to 1.0 per cent lotion or cream is less hazardous and may be helpful.

CONGENITAL ICHTHYOSIFORM ERYTHRODERMA, BULLOUS TYPE (EPIDERMOLYTIC HYPERKERATOSIS). The main features of the bullous type of congenital ichthyosiform erythroderma are present at birth and consist of hyperkeratosis, blisters and erythema. The disease is inherited as an autosomal dominant trait. A thick, scaly mantle covers the skin at birth, but is shed almost immediately, leaving a raw surface. The skin gradually becomes dry and scaly again and assumes the changes characteristic of this disorder. The erythema is less vivid than in nonbullous congenital ichthyosiform erythroderma. It is most obvious on the face, neck and body folds, but may be generalized. It may be most noticeable only when the thickened keratin is removed. The ichthyotic changes vary from slight dryness to dark brown, verrucoid elevated ridges (*ichthyosis hystrix*) resembling porcupine skin. The scalp is covered with thick, greasy, seborrhea-like scales. Hairs, nails, eyes, teeth and mucous membranes appear normal. The blisters appear spontaneously on any part of the body except the palms, soles and mucous membranes. Episodes of blister formation are frequently associated with secondary bacterial infection and may be accompanied by temperature elevation. Blisters are usually generalized but may appear only in areas subjected to trauma. The palms and soles are usually slightly erythematous and scaly.

Histologically there is a thickened, verrucous, loosely laminated, horny layer, with an accentuated granular layer and characteristic replacement of the cytoplasm by clear spaces. Electron microscopy has shown an inappropriate accumulation of large numbers of subcellular organelles in the "clear" spaces. These changes result in increased cellular metabolism and an increased turnover time like those of nonbullous CIE (lamellar ichthyosis). In the dermis, blood vessels are slightly dilated and there is perivascular round cell infiltration. Intracellular and intercellular edema gives the epidermis a characteristic reticular pattern in histologic sections. Collections of coarse keratohyaline granules are seen beneath the stratum corneum.

The hydration and lubrication treatment technique described for ichthyosis vulgaris is helpful in removing accumulated keratotic debris. The local application of vitamin A acid as in nonbullous CIE may also be useful.

Smears and cultures should be taken from infected blisters and local or systemic antibacterial treatment instituted in accordance with in vitro sensitivity of the isolated pathogen to antibiotics. Prevention of secondary bacterial infection may be accomplished by routine cleansing with a soap substitute containing hexachlorophene and the application of a broad spectrum antibiotic ointment on the broken blisters. Hexachlorophene should be used sparingly, if at all, in infants.

A less severe *variant* is distinguished by the absence of blisters, with the hyperkeratotic papules and verrucoid ridges localized to the flexural surfaces of the arms and legs and the remainder of the skin usually little involved. In some instances the changes may be generalized and indistinguishable from those of the bullous variety of the disease except for the absence of blister formation. In addition, localized forms exist in which the hyperkeratotic lesions appear in linear form resembling linear nevi, or localized to the palms and soles, simulating keratosis palmaris et plantaris. In these variants the histologic features are indistinguishable from epidermolytic hyperkeratosis. The treatment is the same as for the generalized form.

OTHER ICHTHYOSIS-LIKE DERMATOSES. The presence of generalized scaling resembling that of ichthyosis at birth may cause difficulty in differentiating these rare syndromes from ichthyosis and the ichthyosiform dermatoses just described (Table 23–2).

Conradi Syndrome (Chondrodystrophia Congenita Punctata). (See also Section 22.) Generalized or localized erythema with a thick white adherent scale with a distinctive whorled pattern occurs in approximately 25 per cent of the infants affected with this recessively transmitted syndrome. Anomalies affecting bone, joint, lens and occasionally the cardiovascular or central nervous systems may occur; nails and hair are normal. The keratoderma of the palms and soles, as well as the scaling and erythema, decrease with age but may be followed by follicular atrophy. Hyperpigmentation resembling the pattern seen in incontinentia pigmenti may follow resolution.

Netherton Syndrome. This consists of generalized erythema and scaling resembling nonbullous congenital ichthyosiform erythroderma (lamellar ichthyosis) or one of its morphologic variants (ichthyosis linearis circumflexa) and atopic manifestations (asthma, allergic rhinitis). After 6 months of age, "bamboo hairs" appear on the scalp and are associated with increased fragility of the hair shaft. Aminoaciduria may be present and persist, though the hair abnormalities clear at puberty.

Refsum Syndrome (Heredopathia Atactica Polyneuritiformis). This is a rare metabolic abnormality related to phytanic acid degradation. There are generalized ichthyosis, retinitis pigmentosa, peripheral neuropathy, progressive nerve deafness and elevated levels of protein in cerebrospinal fluid. It is transmitted as an autosomal recessive trait.

Rud Syndrome. Rud syndrome is characterized by oligophrenia, epilepsy and ichthyosis. Associated anomalies may consist of dwarfism, partial gigantism, structural defects of the hands and feet, nerve deafness, hypoplastic or absent teeth and eye defects. The cutaneous changes vary from generalized scaling to a clinical picture resembling ichthyosis vulgaris.

Sjögren-Larsson Syndrome. This is characterized by generalized ichthyosis and erythema involving the face and flexural surfaces of the palms and soles, in association with neurologic and ophthalmologic abnormalities. It is transmitted as an autosomal recessive trait. The histologic findings in a skin biopsy are similar to those in lamellar ichthyosis (nonbullous CIE).

Tay Syndrome. Tay syndrome is characterized by generalized erythema and scaling at birth, hair abnormalities associated with increased fragility, a progeric appearance and mental and physical retardation. In early childhood the erythema disappears and the scaling is localized to the face, trunk and extensor surfaces of the extremities, with keratoderma of the palms and soles.

Psoriasiform Erythroderma. This is characterized by generalized lobster-red erythema with a generalized hyperkeratotic scale at birth. It is considered to be a congenital form of psoriasis.

Other Defects in Keratinization

PACHYONYCHIA CONGENITA. This rare disease is transmitted as a dominant trait and characterized by remarkable thickening of the nails and by keratinizing abnormalities of the skin, hair and mucous membrancs.

Histopathologically the hyperkeratotic lesions have an intact stratum granulosum, parakeratosis and acanthosis; there are keratinous plugs in follicular and some eccrine orifices.

The nail changes are constantly present. A yellowish discoloration of the nails is noted during the neonatal period; later they become characteristically thickened. White patches resembling leukoplakia develop on the mucous membranes, and there are noninflammatory bullous lesions, predominantly on the feet. Blisters become less frequent with time, but persistent keratotic patches appear, and follicular keratotic lesions also occur on the lateral, proximal aspects of the arms and legs. The abnormalities of the nails become so accentuated that the wearing of shoes is uncomfortable and manual dexterity is impaired (Fig. 23–17). Less commonly there may be involvement of the nasal mucosa, tympanic membrane or cornea. Epidermolysis bullosa may be considered in differential diagnosis because of blister formation and nail thickening, but the persistence of keratotic patches at former sites of blisters and the leukokeratosis of mucous membranes serve as differentiating features. The nails should be removed and the nail matrix destroyed.

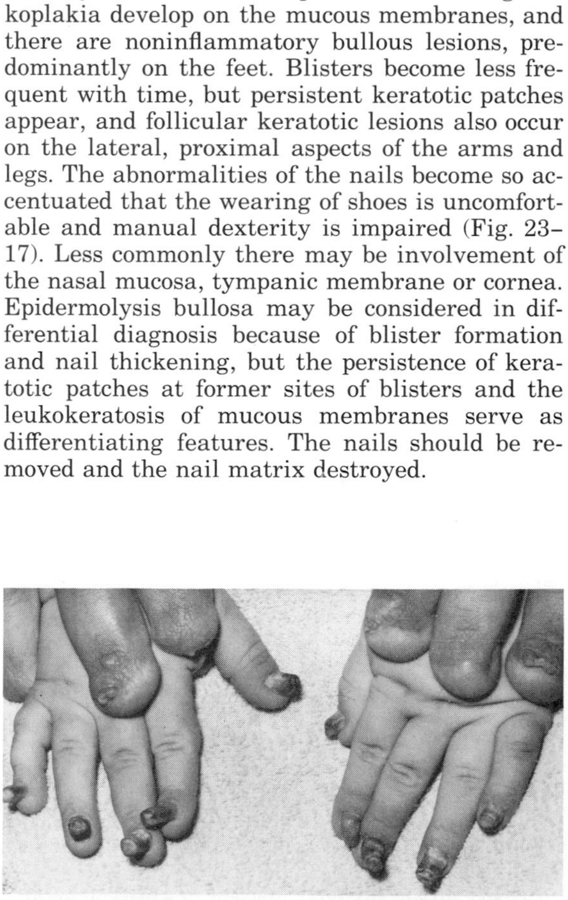

Figure 23–17 Pachyonychia congenita in a 2 year old boy. Note father's fingernails after surgical removal of distal portion of fingers.

CONGENITAL ICHTHYOSIS OF THE PALMS AND SOLES (KERATOSIS PALMARIS ET PLANTARIS; TYLOSIS OF PALMS AND SOLES). This is characterized by hyperkeratosis and by hyperhidrosis. It is usually transmitted as a dominant trait.

Histopathologically there is excessive keratosis associated with hyperplasia of the prickle cell layer and with elongation of the papillae.

The skin of the palms and soles may appear normal at birth or become erythematous and scaly during the neonatal period. More commonly the thickening of the skin appears later in the first year of life and progresses with variable degrees of thickening of the palms, soles and flexural surfaces of the fingers and toes. The changes stop abruptly at the lateral and medial borders of the hands and feet and at the flexural folds on the wrists.

Treatment is essentially the same as for ichthyosis; in addition, ointments or plasters containing a keratolytic agent (salicylic acid) are useful for severe hyperkeratosis.

KERATODERMA OF PALMS AND SOLES AND PREMATURE PERIODONTOCLASIA (PAPILLON-LEFÈVRE SYNDROME). This is differentiated from other keratinizing abnormalities of the palms and soles by premature periodontoclasia and calcification of the dura. It is transmitted as an autosomal recessive trait. Histologically there is acanthosis with a striking hyperkeratosis, and a perivascular inflammatory round cell infiltrate in a somewhat thinned dermis. The gingivae show a striking perivascular inflammatory infiltrate and edema, with destruction of the epithelial attachment and a degeneration of the periodontal fibers.

The hyperkeratotic changes on the palms and soles usually appear around the fourth and fifth years of life concurrently with periodontal involvement of the deciduous dentition, but the skin changes may appear earlier. The palmar and plantar involvement is characterized by varying degrees of hyperkeratosis, with sharp margination at the lateral borders. The hyperkeratosis is most frequently diffuse in the involved areas, but may also be patchy or punctate. As in ichthyosis, there may be exacerbation in the winter, with painful fissures. The development and eruption of deciduous teeth are normal, but with the appearance of hyperkeratosis the gingivae become red, swollen and boggy, and bleed easily. The formation of deep pockets of periodontal pus is accompanied by bad breath. The teeth rapidly become mobile and are shed by the fourth or fifth year of age. The mucous membranes then become normal, but the process is repeated when the permanent dentition erupts. When all the permanent teeth are lost, the gingivae return to normal and tolerate dentures well. Roentgenograms of the skull may show calcium deposits in the attachments of the tentorium and choroid plexus by the age of 4 or 5 years. No known treatment alters the course of the periodontoclasia. The hyperkeratotic lesions on the palms and soles are helped with the same technique of hydration and lubrication as described above for ichthyosis.

MAL DE MELEDA. This is a congenital symmetrical hyperkeratosis of the palms, soles, elbows and knees, and the dorsa of hands and feet. The disease is transmitted as a recessive trait; it is common on the island of Meleda in the Adriatic Sea.

Histopathologically there is severe hyperkeratosis, as well as hyperplasia of the prickle cell layer with acanthosis. The stratum lucidum is increased and the granular layer is prominent over the interpapillary portion of the prickle cell layer.

The first changes consist of erythema of the palms and soles within the first two years of life, followed by horny thickening which is characteristically surrounded by a dusky erythematous zone. This hyperkeratosis slowly spreads to involve the dorsa of the hands and feet, the extensor surfaces of forearms and legs and the elbows and knees. Hyperhidrosis and dystrophic changes of the nails also occur.

Treatment is not satisfactory; the same measures may be used as for congenital ichthyosis of the palms and soles.

ACROKERATOSIS VERRUCIFORMIS OF HOPF. A rare, localized epithelial nevus, this is transmitted as a dominant trait. It is characterized by asymptomatic symmetrical, flat, wart-like papules 2 to 4 mm in diameter located predominantly on the dorsa of the hands and feet. They may be present at birth or appear during infancy. Papules on the wrists, ankles, palms and soles, as well as ichthyotic changes of the skin, may also appear later, usually at puberty. The nails may be opaque and brittle, with vertical, linear striations.

Histopathologically the epidermis is thickened, with hyperkeratosis and accentuated granular layer with some parakeratosis. The dermis appears normal.

In differential diagnosis, juvenile flat warts must be considered. No known treatment is effective.

LICHEN SPINULOSUS. This is a rare keratinizing abnormality of unknown cause characterized by patches of horny spines involving primarily the hair follicles; there is a mild inflammatory reaction.

Histopathologically there is widening of the orifices of the hair follicle and sweat ducts, which are filled with keratotic plugs. Keratotic accumulations occur independently of either pilar or sweat units. Sebaceous glands are atrophic or absent. There is an inflammatory infiltrate around the vessels in the dermis.

The skin lesions, which appear in crops, consist of slightly erythematous patches with spiny projections. The erythematous phase is transient, but the spiny papules persist. The eruption is usually asymptomatic.

In differential diagnosis, pityriasis rubra pilaris, keratosis pilaris, lichen scrofulosus and phrynoderma must be distinguished.

Treatment during the inflammatory phase consists in the application of an anti-inflammatory agent (0.5 per cent hydrocortisone) in an emollient base; in the keratotic phase a keratolytic agent (salicylic acid) in an emollient base is indicated.

PHRYNODERMA. Phrynoderma is a cutaneous

expression of severe vitamin A deficiency, characterized by a dry, roughened skin with acuminate, follicular horny papules and dome-shaped keratotic papules. Skin lines are exaggerated, producing a wrinkled appearance. The eruption is usually generalized, but may appear in local areas of chronic trauma to the skin.

In differential diagnosis, pityriasis rubra pilaris, keratosis pilaris, lichen scrofulosus and lichen spinulosus must be distinguished.

Treatment consists of supplementation of the diet with vitamin A.

PITYRIASIS RUBRA PILARIS. This is a rare, slightly inflammatory keratinizing abnormality which may be transmitted as an autosomal dominant trait. It is characterized by horny follicular, acuminate papules which coalesce into scaling patches. There are acquired and familial types; the latter appears in infancy or childhood.

Histopathologically there is keratosis around the hair follicles and in the stratum corneum above the dermal papillae and plugging of the follicles; in the dermis there is perivascular and perifollicular and inflammatory infiltration.

The skin changes appear slowly; when established, they are usually symmetrical and include seborrheic scaling on the scalp, erythema of the face, hyperkeratosis of the palms and soles, and eventually circumscribed, scaling patches on the face, trunk and extremities. Follicular papules tend to persist on the proximal portion of the phalanges.

In differential diagnosis, phrynoderma, keratosis pilaris and lichen spinulosus should be distinguished.

The disease can be cleared with large doses of vitamin A by mouth, though there is no evidence of vitamin A deficiency. Local treatment consists of hydration and lubrication as in ichthyosis.

KERATOSIS FOLLICULARIS (DARIER'S DISEASE). This is an uncommon abnormality of keratinization transmitted as an autosomal dominant trait. It is characterized by the appearance of flesh- to tan-colored scaling papules which appear primarily on the trunk during childhood. As the disease progresses, the face, scalp and intertriginous areas may become involved. Histopathologically acantholysis and individual cell keratinization (dyskeratosis) with formation of intraepidermal spaces are characteristic.

Large doses of vitamin A (200,000 to 300,000 units per day) will produce clearing in 3 to 4 weeks but may be associated with toxicity. The local application of vitamin A acid (0.05 to 0.1 per cent) in a lotion or cream base is safe and usually effective.

ACANTHOSIS NIGRICANS. This is a distinctive type of epidermal change characterized by hyperkeratosis and pigmentation distributed primarily on the neck, axillary spaces, genitocrural region and, occasionally, the flexural surfaces of the arms and legs; it may be present at birth, transmitted as an autosomal dominant trait (benign acanthosis nigricans), or may occur during adolescence (pseudoacanthosis nigricans) secondary to obesity or drug ingestion (corticosteroids or nicotinic acid). Malignant acanthosis nigricans, though similar in appearance and distribution, occurs in adults and is associated with a high incidence of internal cancer. In spite of the similarity in morphologic appearance, transition between the two forms does not occur and each may be regarded as a separate disease.

In the benign form skin lesions may be present at birth but usually develop during childhood. The earliest skin changes consist of a brownish pigmentation, with thickening of the epidermis producing a velvety appearance. The appearance of the earliest changes around the neck suggests that the skin has not been properly cleansed; skin changes progress slowly to the time of puberty and remain stationary thereafter or, in some instances, regress. A wide variety of developmental abnormalities may be associated (endocrinopathy, neurofibromatosis and mental deficiency).

Treatment with vitamin A acid cream 0.05 per cent may be helpful. In pseudoacanthosis nigricans, removal of secondary factors results in resolution of the skin changes.

SEBORRHEIC DERMATITIS. Seborrheic dermatitis is a chronic, recurrent inflammatory reaction of the skin transmitted genetically and characterized by a tendency to a dermatitic reaction in the scalp and intertriginous areas, vulnerability to secondary bacterial and yeast infections in the affected areas, and oily skin during adolescence.

Histopathologically the lesion is not diagnostic; it consists of intermittent parakeratosis and variable acanthosis, intercellular edema, some inflammatory cells in the epidermis, and mild perivascular inflammatory infiltrate in the dermis.

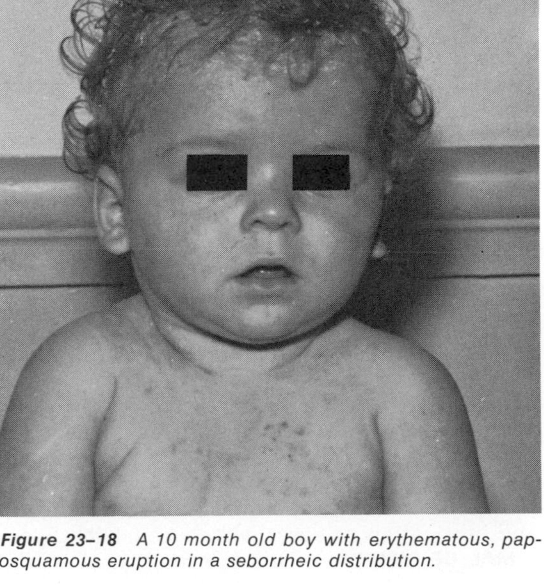

Figure 23–18 A 10 month old boy with erythematous, papulosquamous eruption in a seborrheic distribution.

The most common expressions of seborrheic diathesis in infants and children in order of frequency are (1) "cradle cap," (2) intertriginous eruption beginning in the genitocrural fold of the diaper area (Fig. 23–22), (3) dermatitis in the auriculocephalic fold, (4) blepharitis, (5) otitis externa, and (6) exfoliative erythroderma (Leiner's disease).

Cradle Cap. Common in infancy, cradle cap varies considerably in severity. It is characterized by adherent, yellowish, scaling or crusted patches of plaques on the scalp; when it is extensive, the forehead may also be involved. Similar eruptions may also be located on the lid margins, external ears, genitocrural folds or postauricular areas. There may be mild inflammatory changes.

Leiner's Disease. Erythroderma desquamativa is characterized by an exfoliative erythematous eruption which starts in any of the areas mentioned above and progresses to become generalized (Fig. 23–19). In some infants the generalized exfoliative dermatitis starts within a week or two of birth and is associated with diarrhea, bacterial infections (usually gram-negative), wasting and death; in a familial type of Leiner's disease there is a deficiency of the opsonic activity of the C-5 component of complement (Miller).

In differential diagnosis the following diseases should be distinguished: psoriasis, Letterer-Siwe disease and tinea capitis.

Treatment of the scalp consists of daily shampoos followed by application of a local preparation containing sulfur (2 per cent), salicylic acid or coal tar (5 to 10 per cent) alone or in combination (Pragmatar). The dermatitic reaction in the other areas responds promptly to the local application of 0.5 to 1.0 per cent hydrocortisone cream alone or in combination with 2 per cent sulfur. Administration of fresh plasma to infants with C-5 dysfunction may be lifesaving.

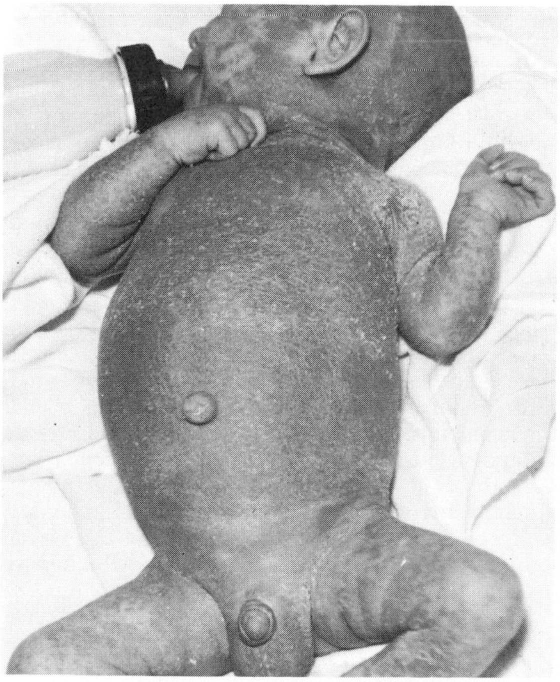

Figure 23–19 *Seborrheic diathesis in an infant at 2 months of age; dermatitis started in genitocrural fold and became generalized (Leiner's disease).*

Pigmentary Abnormalities

Alteration of the normal pattern of pigmentation of the skin may result from abnormal distribution or altered function of melanocytes. It may be caused by a genetic abnormality, be the result of nutritional (kwashiorkor) or endocrine (congenital Addison's disease) abnormalities, or be induced by transplacental transfer of hormones. Pigmentary abnormalities may be classified as localized or diffuse. Variations in the normal coloring of the skin may also be produced by the absorption of heavy metals (lead, bismuth), ingestion of precursors of vitamin A (carrots, squash, sweet potatoes or egg yolk), from inborn errors in metabolism (ochronosis) or from phototherapy used to reduce hyperbilirubinemia (bronze baby syndrome). Localized or generalized errors in melanogenesis may produce absence of or decrease in pigment (tuberous sclerosis, ataxia-telangiectasia, Chédiak-Higashi disease, Waardenburg syndrome, Vogt-Koyanagi-Harada syndrome, phenylketonuria, partial albinism and vitiligo, incontinentia pigmenti achromians), or an increase in pigment (Peutz-Jeghers syndrome, McCune-Albright syndrome, neurofibromatosis, pigmented nevi, generalized hereditary lentiginosis and incontinentia pigmenti).

LOCALIZED HYPERPIGMENTED LESIONS. Circumscribed flat brown spots of variable size ranging from small (lentigenes) to large (café-au-lait spots) may be the presenting cutaneous sign of significant disease.

Neurofibromatosis (von Recklinghausen's Disease). (See also Section 20.) Neurofibromatosis characteristically presents as multiple café-au-lait patches of pigmentation. Sharply demarcated tan patches measuring 1 cm or more may appear in the first weeks or months of life and are fully developed by 5 years of age. The more classic features of neurofibromatosis are often not present before puberty; six or more café-au-lait patches presume the diagnosis of neurofibromatosis. Such pigmented patches may provide a clue to the correct diagnosis in infants with glaucoma or skeletal anomalies at birth or shortly thereafter.

McCune-Albright Syndrome. (See also Section 17.) This includes bone lesions and endocrine dysfunction leading to precocious puberty, primarily in females, but occasionally in males; it is commonly associated with brownish macular patches with serrated or irregular jagged borders. Differentiation between macular brown patches of von Recklinghausen's disease and McCune-Albright syndrome may be difficult because of similarity in morphology, but giant pigment granules are seen in melanocytes and keratinocytes from affected areas in the former but not the latter.

Lentigo (Freckles). Lentigines are brown-to-black macular lesions up to 0.5 cm in diameter appearing on the skin or mucous membranes. They appear most frequently in childhood but may appear at any age, with no relation between the appearance of lentigines and exposure to the sun. They are made up of collections of normal melanocytes located just above the basement membranes.

Several syndromes associated with systematized distribution of lentigines in association with multisystem disease have been described. These include: (1) electrocardiographic abnormalities in patients in whom pigmented lesions appear during the first year of life; (2) lentigines at birth in patients with nystagmus and mental retardation transmitted as an autosomal dominant trait; and (3) association with congenital deafness and discrete dysraphia, possibly transmitted as an irregular dominant with X-chromosomal hereditary determination.

Dermal Melanocytosis (Mongolian Spot, Nevus of Ota, Nevus of Ito). This is characterized by a poorly circumscribed macular blue-black area present at birth. Histologically the lesion is composed of clusters of spindle-shaped melanocytes scattered throughout the mid-dermis. In *mongolian spot* the pigmentation is most commonly located in the lower part of the back around the buttocks in a black, Polynesian or Oriental infant. The pigmentation usually diminishes and disappears by early childhood. In the *nevus of Ota* (papulodermal melanocytosis) hyperpigmentation is localized to the skin around the eye, sclera, cornea, iris and the periorbital tissues. The discoloration of the skin may involve the shoulder and neck areas alone (*nevus of Ito*). In the latter two diseases, the pigmentation persists throughout life.

Blue nevus is a type of dermal melanocytosis in which the collection of melanocytes produces a flat or dome-shaped blue-black lesion which usually appears on the face or extremities early in life, grows to 2 to 3 mm in diameter and then remains stationary in size. Its importance lies in the possible confusion with melanoma. Excisional biopsy is the treatment of choice.

Peutz-Jeghers Syndrome. This is characterized by brown-to-black lentigines distributed primarily around the mouth, on both sides of the hands, and especially on the dorsal surfaces of the fingers. The pigmented lesions on the mucous membranes are always present and persist throughout life, though there is some fading with age. It is transmitted as an autosomal dominant trait and is always associated with intestinal polyposis.

Incontinentia Pigmenti. (See above, this Section.) Bizarre macular brownish whorls and swirls may be the only manifestation of this disease.

Nevi. In a broad sense, nevi are local excesses, congenital in origin, of one or more normal components of the skin. *Pigmented nevi* (nevus cell nevi, or moles) consist of proliferative aggregates of normal melanocytes. They are hereditarily determined and may be classified, depending on morphologic and histologic criteria, as lentigo, junctional, compound and dermal nevi, and benign juvenile melanoma. The development of pigmented nevi is a dynamic process, the early macular lesion being of junctional type, later evolving into compound nevi with both junctional and dermal activity, and finally into mature nevi with only intradermal changes. In some compound nevi in childhood there is rapid evolution, with the histologic appearance of active growth suggestive of neoplastic change, but these tumors are benign and are called benign juvenile melanoma.

Nevus cell nevi vary considerably in their morphology and degree of pigmentation; several different clinical types may be recognized: (1) macular lesions, (2) slightly elevated papules, (3) papillomatous lesions, (4) dome-shaped papules which may or may not be pigmented or contain hairs, and (5) pedunculated lesions. Less common forms of nevus cell nevi are the halo nevus and the giant pigmented nevus (bathing trunk nevus); malignant degeneration is frequent in the latter.

Junctional Nevi. Junctional nevi are flat, sharply circumscribed, brown-to-black lesions found anywhere on the skin. Their special importance lies in the possibility that they may undergo melanomatous degeneration, though the risk is small; most persons have or have had one or more junctional nevi. Microscopically groups of nevus cells are found intraepidermally. Surgical removal is indicated if there is evidence of unusual activity such as increase in the pigmented area, scaling, crusting or inflammation. Pathologic evaluation is mandatory; if malignancy is suspected, consultation with a dermatologic pathologist should be sought, owing to difficulties in evaluating the nature of these pigmented nevi.

Compound and Intradermal Nevi. These are extremely variable in their morphology and color. Most of the slightly elevated lesions, and some of the papillomatous lesions, are compound nevi; most of the papillomatous lesions and nearly all the dome-shaped and pedunculated lesions are intradermal nevi. They vary in color from flesh-colored or pink with little brownish pigment to brown or black. They vary in size from a few millimeters to extensive involvement, with a tendency toward the dermatome distribution of the giant pigmented nevus (bathing trunk nevus). In these giant nevi the involved area is pigmented, hairy and frequently verrucous. This variety of nevus is important because it tends to undergo melanomatous degeneration. The *halo nevus* is a variant of a compound or intradermal nevus, which is surrounded by depigmented cells. Over a period of several months, involution of the nevus occurs, leaving a depigmented patch which may also slowly disappear. This process often extends to other nevi simultaneously or successively. Treatment of small compound or intradermal nevi is indicated for cosmetic reasons, if they are in locations where they may be frequently irritated, or if there is suspicion of melanomatous degeneration. Excision is the treatment of choice. When cosmetic considerations are paramount, a shave excision gives an excellent cosmetic result; it is a safe procedure if controlled histologically. Because of its tendency to neoplastic degeneration, giant pigmented nevus should be removed, if feasible, by a plastic surgeon.

Benign Juvenile Melanoma. This occurs most frequently between the ages of 3 and 13 years. It is characterized by the appearance of a smooth, dome-shaped, circumscribed, firm, nonhairy, pink or purplish red asymptomatic nodule, most frequently on the face. The tumors may vary in size from a few millimeters to several centimeters in diameter. Histologically juvenile melanoma is a compound nevus, but because of the pleomorphism of the cells and the frequency of inflammatory infiltrate, the histologic picture closely resembles that of an invasive melanoma. In spite of this resemblance to melanoma, the experienced pathologist can usually make the distinction. In differential diagnosis, juvenile xanthogranuloma, granulomatous insect bite reaction, keloid or a solitary nodule of urticaria pigmentosa are suggested. Since the natural history of these tumors is unknown and because they usually present a cosmetic problem, simple excision is recommended. Recurrences may be anticipated if the tumor is not completely removed.

LOCALIZED DECREASE IN PIGMENTATION. A decrease in skin pigmentation is classified as amelanotic (total absence of melanin pigment—albinism), hypomelanotic (decrease in normal melanin pigmentation—tuberous sclerosis), or depigmented (loss of previously existing melanin—postinflammatory) according to the degree of decrease of melanocytic function. Generalized dilution of pigment of skin (hypomelanosis), hair and eye color is a feature of phenylketonuria.

Albinism. (See also Section 8.) Albinism is a genetically transmitted metabolic defect of melanocytes of the skin, hair and choroid in which they are relatively or absolutely incapable of producing melanin.

Absence of pigment produces a pinkish white appearance of the skin at birth in the Caucasian, whereas in the nonwhite person freckle-like, pigmented macules are scattered over the skin. The hair is fine and white. The iris is pink in the Caucasian and pale blue in the nonwhite person. Ocular manifestations include photophobia, lacrimation and nystagmus, and less often retinitis pigmentosa, cataracts and color blindness. In one variation of albinism the melanocytes produce small amounts of pigment. In another variant the skin is considerably lighter than normal, but the iris is blue, and photophobia and nystagmus are present.

Treatment consists in the prophylactic use of ultraviolet screening preparations to protect against sunburn.

Partial Albinism (Piebaldism). This is transmitted as a dominant trait and characterized by circumscribed areas of depigmentation in which the melanocytes give a negative dopa reaction. The patches of depigmentation are present at birth; in most instances a white forelock is present.

In differential diagnosis, vitiligo, nevus achromicus, nevus anemicus and Waardenburg syndrome need be considered. *Nevus anemicus* appears as a pale, mottled macular patch in which the vascular defect, rather than loss of pigment, is the cause for the pale color. It usually appears on the trunk and is frequently present in patients with neurofibromatosis. *Nevus achromicus* consists of a hypopigmented, irregularly shaped, streaky appearing, macular hypopigmented patch. It may be small or cover a large part of the body and is present at birth.

Incontinentia Pigmenti Achromians. This is a pigmentary disorder consisting of generalized asymmetric hypopigmented macules arranged in a "whorled or marble-cake" configuration on the face, trunk and extremities. It is most probably transmitted as an autosomal dominant trait. Biopsy from a hypomelanotic area shows a reduced number of melanin granules in the basal layer of the epidermis. This disorder is in no way related to incontinentia pigmenti.

Waardenburg Syndrome. This includes a fusion of the eyebrows, loss of pigment in the iris and fundus, white forelock and localized patches of hypopigmentation. The patches of hypopigmentation may be sufficiently large as to make differentiation between this syndrome and partial albinism difficult.

Chédiak-Higashi Syndrome. This syndrome is a lethal variety of partial albinism transmitted as an autosomal recessive trait. It is characterized by photophobia, pale optic fundi, granular inclusions in leukocytes of blood and bone marrow, repeated pyogenic infections and terminal hepatosplenomegaly.

Vitiligo. Vitiligo may be an acquired disorder as well as a hereditary one. It is characterized by patchy, progressive loss of pigment due to failure of the melanocytes to produce pigment. Histopathologically the changes are indistinguishable from partial albinism. The halo nevus is a variant in which the depigmented area surrounds a pigmented nevus.

In differential diagnosis, piebaldness, postinflammatory depigmentation, leprosy and pinta must be distinguished.

Treatment is unsatisfactory.

Tuberous Sclerosis. (See also Section 20.) Hypomelanotic macules varying in size from a few millimeters to several centimeters frequently appear on the trunk and extremities as the first clinical evidence of tuberous sclerosis.

Developmental Abnormalities of Skin

Abnormalities of Blood Vessels and Lymphatics

Hamartomatous growths of the vessels are composed of blood vessels, of lymph vessels or of combinations of the two.

VASCULAR NEVI. Vascular nevi are the most common dermal tumors manifest at birth or during the neonatal period. The benign vascular tumors may be divided clinically and pathologically into capillary types (nevus flammeus and nevus vasculosus), cavernous types and mixed types, in which capillary and cavernous components are both present in the same tumor.

Nevus Flammeus (Port-wine Stain). Nevus flammeus appears as a flat, irregular erythematous patch of variable size present at birth; its significance depends mainly on its location. Lesions are especially common on the back of the neck and face, but may appear anywhere. The slightly erythematous patches present on the eyelids and in the glabellar area of the newborn infant, which undergo spontaneous resolution, should not be confused with the persistent patches of nevus flammeus.

Involvement of the skin in the distribution of the fifth cranial nerve has special significance because of the frequency of vascular abnormalities in the ipsilateral cerebral hemisphere. (See Sturge-Weber Syndrome, Section 20.) Many methods of treatment, including superficial radiation, tattooing and cryotherapy, have produced indifferent results. A cosmetically acceptable cover (Covermark) is recommended for lesions in exposed areas.

Nevus Vasculosus (Strawberry Mark). This is the most common of the vascular nevi; it is a sharply demarcated, erythematous, raised tumor which is usually present at birth or may appear during the first month of life. The earliest sign may be a blanched area in the skin preliminary to the appearance of the vascular nevus. Small vascular ectasias then arise within the pale zone, become raised, and finally develop the typical appearance of hemangioma. A blanched area around the small erythematous papule or larger vascular tumor is a useful prognostic sign, for it often marks the limits of future growth. During early infancy there is proliferation of endothelial cells and capillary proliferation, but when growth ceases, fibrosis replaces the capillaries, and shrinking of the tumor results. The growth pattern during the first 6 to 8 months of life is variable (Fig. 23–20); the tumors usually disappear spontaneously.

Cavernous Hemangioma. This consists of a subcutaneous collection of vessels with normal, but bluish, overlying skin; nevus vasculosus may also be present (mixed vascular nevus). Histologically there are in the lower dermis and subcutaneous tissue large, irregular vascular spaces filled with blood. In the mixed variety there are histologic changes of both the capillary nevus of the nevus vasculosus type and cavernous hemangioma. These tumors also tend to regress without treatment, but are more likely than nevus vasculosus to involute incompletely; in tumors in which there is arteriovenous shunting, involution does not occur.

In rare instances a cavernous or mixed type hemangioma may undergo such tremendous increase in size as to interfere with function. Complications include severe anemia due to an increase in

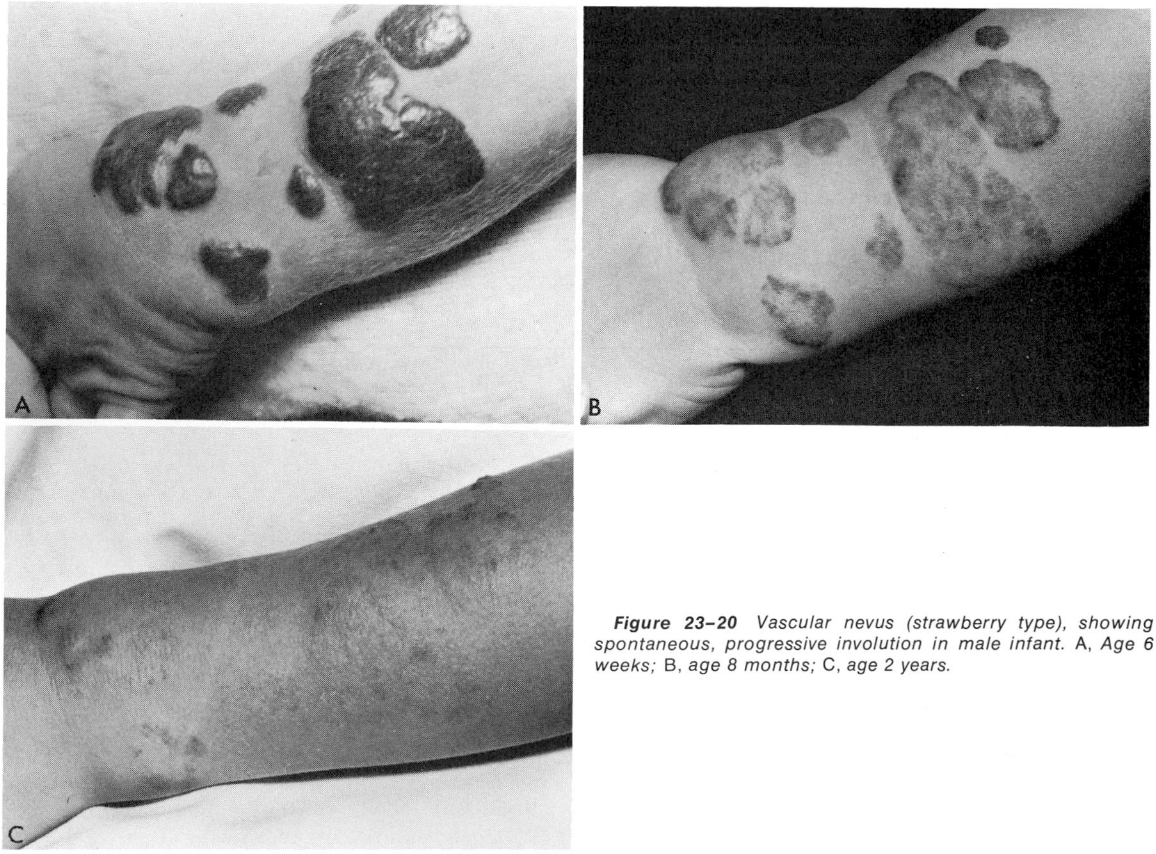

Figure 23–20 *Vascular nevus (strawberry type), showing spontaneous, progressive involution in male infant.* A, *Age 6 weeks;* B, *age 8 months;* C, *age 2 years.*

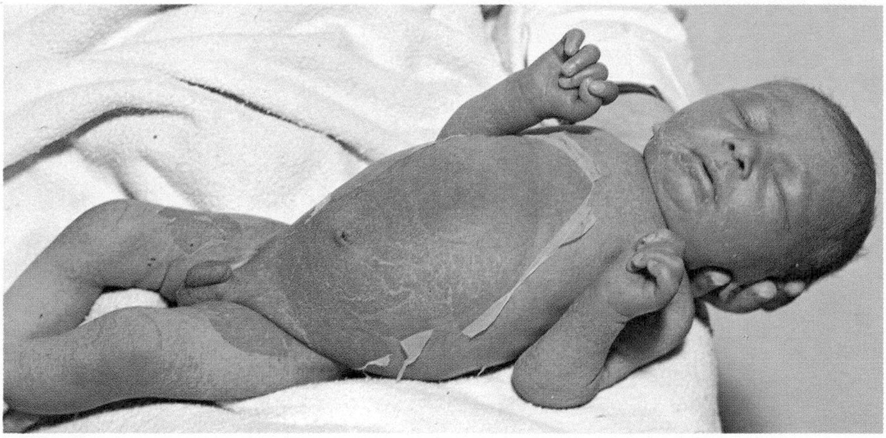

Figure 23–7 *Toxic epidermal necrosis (dermatitis exfoliativa, Ritter's disease) in a newborn infant, showing erythema, edema and exfoliation at site of subcorneal blisters (see p. 1521).*

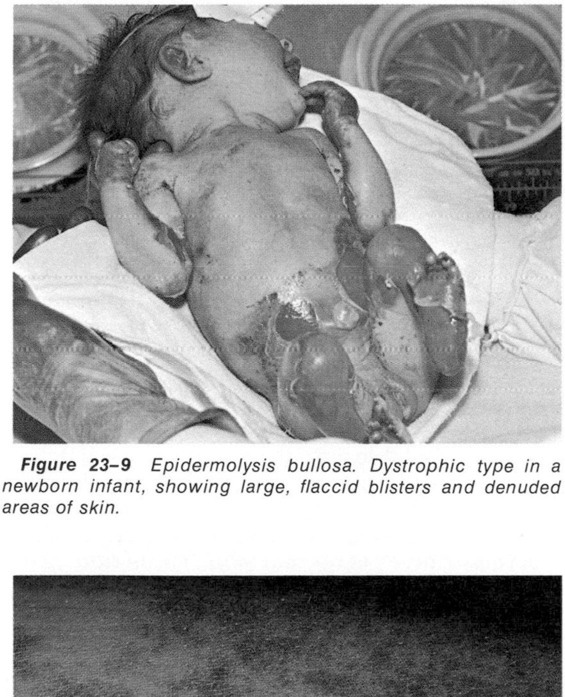

Figure 23–9 *Epidermolysis bullosa. Dystrophic type in a newborn infant, showing large, flaccid blisters and denuded areas of skin.*

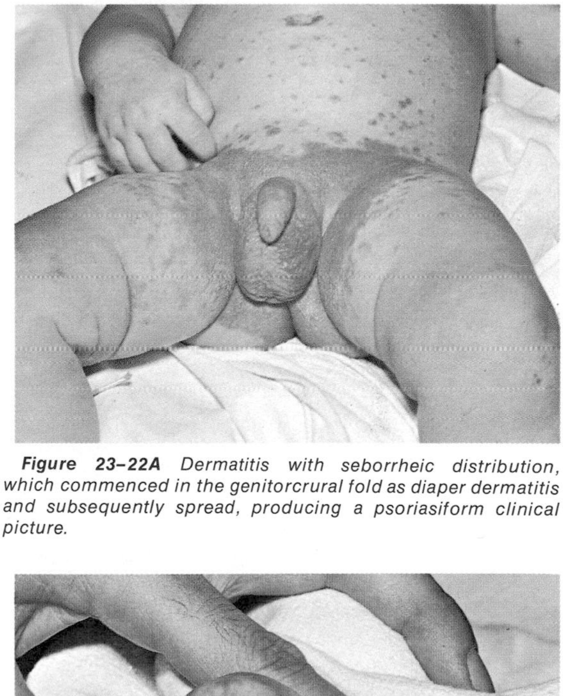

Figure 23–22A *Dermatitis with seborrheic distribution, which commenced in the genitorcrural fold as diaper dermatitis and subsequently spread, producing a psoriasiform clinical picture.*

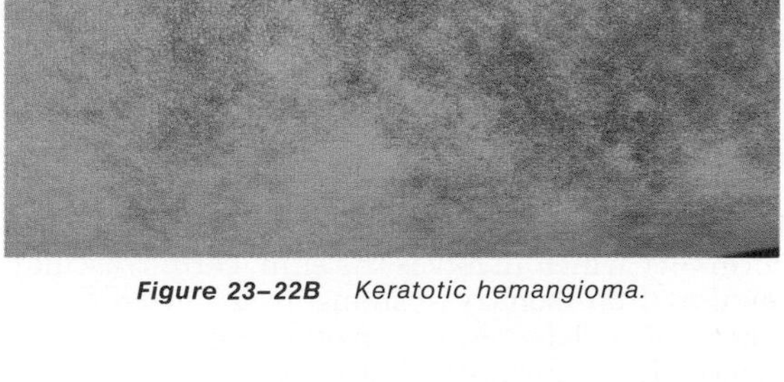

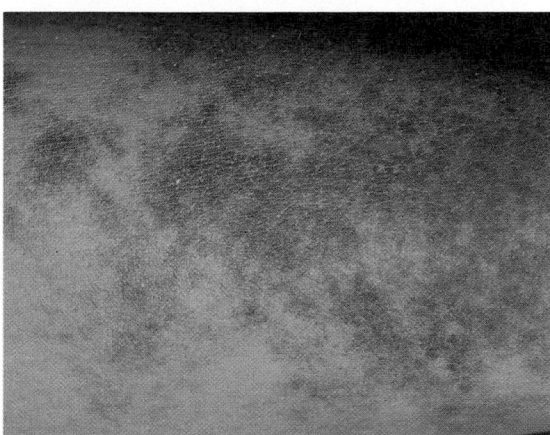

Figure 23–22B *Keratotic hemangioma.*

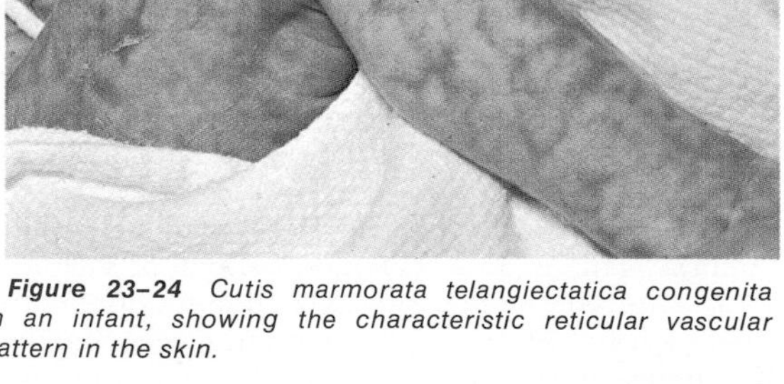

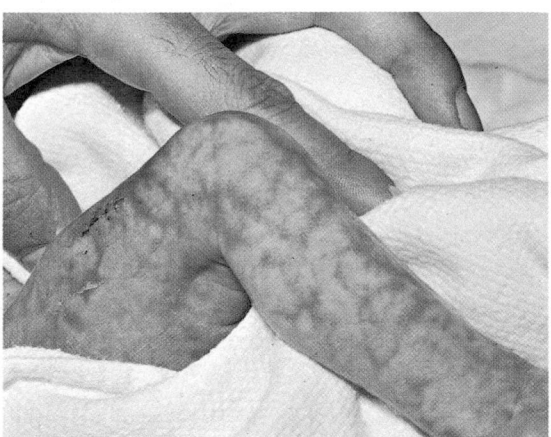

Figure 23–24 *Cutis marmorata telangiectatica congenita in an infant, showing the characteristic reticular vascular pattern in the skin.*

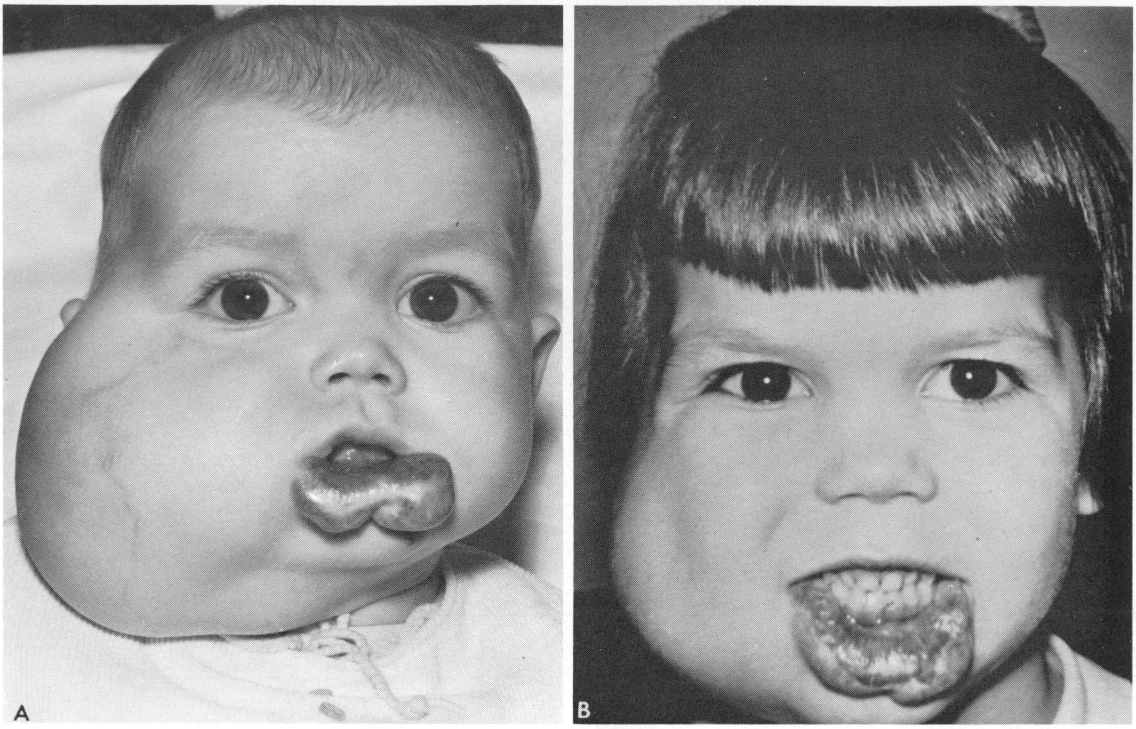

Figure 23–21 *A, Vascular nevus (cavernous type) in an 8 month old girl which progressed alarmingly in a 7 month period from a 3-cm. tumor in the right preauricular area; the increase in size was associated with progressive severe anemia. B, The tumor at age 4½ years, showing spontaneous regression, with scarring and eversion of the lower lip.*

volume of blood within the tumor, a coagulopathy with thrombocytopenia (Kasabach-Merritt syndrome) due to sequestration of platelets and other defects in coagulation (Factors II, V and VII, and hypofibrinogenemia). Treatment of extensive hemangiomas has been frustrating; administration of prednisone (20 to 30 mg each day) for 8 to 12 weeks and administration of fresh blood or platelet-rich transfusions is indicated in instances of severe petechial or ecchymotic manifestations. Complications and long-term sequelae preclude treatment by radiation or by injection of sclerosing agents. In those instances in which angiosarcomatous degeneration occurs, complete excision of the entire vascular abnormality is indicated (Fig. 23–21).

Blue Rubber Bleb Nevus. This is a variant of cavernous hemangioma in which there are innumerable bluish cavernous hemangiomas distributed over the skin surface. In addition to the cutaneous lesions, there may be hemangioma in the intestinal tract and in other internal organs.

Maffucci Syndrome. In the Maffucci syndrome the combination of cavernous hemangiomas and dystrophy of cartilage causes bizarre deformities of the extremities.

Keratotic Vascular Nevus (Verrucous Hemangioma). This is an uncommon persistent variant of a capillary or cavernous hemangioma in which epithelial hyperplasia occurs secondarily. Histologically the typical lesions have a papillary surface with hyperkeratosis, parakeratosis, subepidermal dilated vessels and capillary-like vessels in the dermis extending into subcutaneous tissue (Fig. 23–22). The deep dermal and subcutaneous vascular involvement precludes superficial removal of the lesion. The clinical picture varies from nonkeratotic, erythematoviolaceous, compressible retiform vascular lesions to hyperkeratotic patches which often become secondarily infected after trauma. Lesions are most common on the lower extremities either singly or in multiple patches with intervening areas of normal skin. These tumors do not regress spontaneously and become increasingly hyperkeratotic. If removal is indicated, it should be accomplished surgically.

Angiokeratoma of Mibelli. Another variety of purplish black raised patch is the angiokeratoma of Mibelli which may be distinguished from keratotic vascular nevi by the fact that it appears to be made up of confluent individual lesions (Fig. 23–23). Histologically this tumor differs from the keratotic vascular nevus in the presence of vascular channels within the epithelial layer itself as well as in the superficial portions of the dermis. Treatment is surgical removal when cosmetic considerations justify it.

ANGIOKERATOMA CORPORIS DIFFUSUM (FABRY). This is an extremely rare, widespread vascular abnormality which involves the skin, cardiovascular, renal and pulmonary systems. It is caused by absence of or a defect in the enzyme ceramide trihexosidase. It is transmitted as a sex-linked trait. Histopathologically the capillaries supplying the

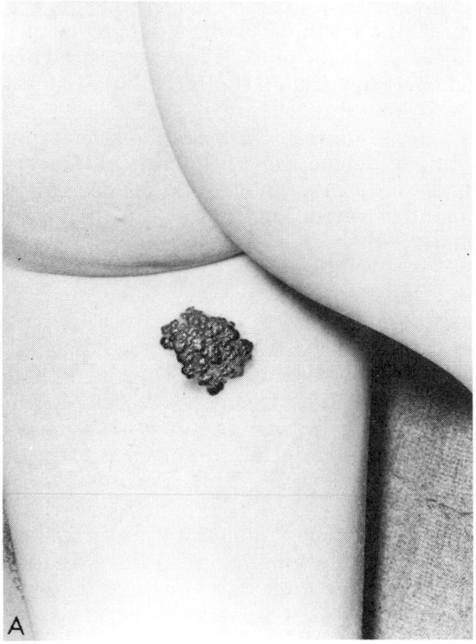

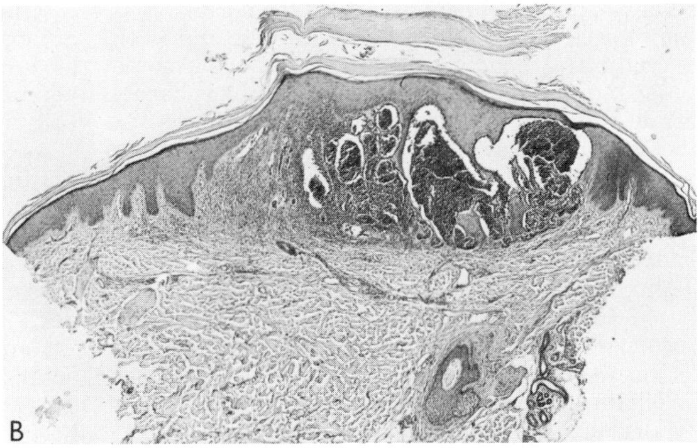

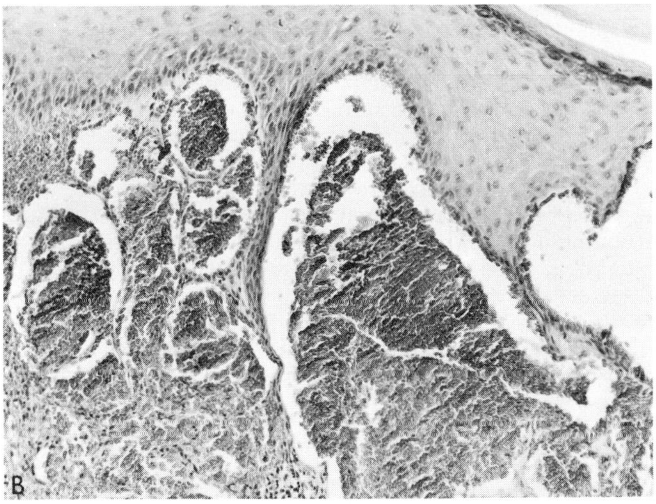

Figure 23–23 *A, Angiokeratoma (Mibelli). B demonstrates vascular channels in the epithelium and superficial portions of the dermis.*

papillae are dilated, forming large vascular spaces filled with thrombi just below the epidermis. Similar changes are found in other organ systems. The skin lesions are purplish black maculopapules varying in size from 1 to 2 mm and located predominantly on the lower portion of the trunk and the thighs. The signs and symptoms relate to almost every organ system of the body. General deterioration begins with a breakdown in cell wall glycolipids which ultimately results in renal failure. In differential diagnosis, pain and swelling of extremities need to be distinguished from rheumatic fever.

CUTIS MARMORATA TELANGIECTATICA. A rare abnormality of the superficial vessels of the dermis, this is of unknown origin. The skin changes are present at birth or shortly after and consist of a peculiar red reticulated pattern producing a striking marbled effect (Fig. 23–24). Histopathologically there are a large number of capillaries, some with thick elastic fibers in their walls, in the dermis and subdermis.

Involvement may be generalized or localized to the extremities, with normal-appearing skin between the reticulated areas. Ulcerations and scarring may occur as a consequence of the vascular changes.

In differential diagnosis, physiologic cutis marmorata needs to be considered.

No treatment is necessary, as a rule. The prominent vascular markings usually slowly regress over a period of years, but may persist. Ulcers should be treated with a local antibiotic to prevent secondary bacterial infection.

ATAXIA-TELANGIECTASIA. (See also Section 20.) This is a rare disease characterized by oculocutaneous telangiectasia, progressive cerebellar ataxia, peculiar eye movements and frequent sinopulmonary infections. It is transmitted as an autosomal recessive trait.

Histopathologically there are telangiectatic vessels in the upper corium and in the cerebellum.

Ataxia is evident by 1 to 1½ years of age, and the telangiectasia appears by about the age of 5 years on the temporal and nasal sides of the bulbar conjunctiva and slowly progresses to involve the eyelid, malar areas, ears, chest, popliteal and antecubital fossae and dorsum of the hands.

In differential diagnosis familial hemorrhagic telangiectasia must be distinguished. Treatment of the skin lesions is not indicated.

SPIDER ANGIOMA. Spider telangiectasis occurs as a localized capillary dilatation of pre-existing blood vessels and is occasionally associated with the development of new vessels in the dermis. It is characterized by a red nonpulsatile macule with fine radiating blood vessels which give the lesion a spider-like configuration. Spider angioma is barely visible initially, but gradually becomes more distinct and may present as a cosmetically disturbing red spot on the face or on the dorsa of the hands and fingers. Angiomas may be single or multiple. An arteriovenous shunt may be confused diagnostically, but its pulsatile central papule serves to distinguish it. Treatment consists in destruction of the central dilated vessels with fine needle electrosurgery. If properly done, this procedure should not result in scarring.

HEREDITARY HEMORRHAGIC TELANGIECTASIA. This is an uncommon familial disease characterized by numerous telangiectasias of the skin and mucous membranes. (See also Section 11.)

Histopathologically the epidermis is normal, and in the papillary and subpapillary zones of the dermis are lake-like vascular dilatations. The vessels are made up of a single row of endothelial cells without muscular or elastic tissue.

The telangiectasias are nonpulsatile, spider-like, bright red maculopapular lesions, 2 to 3 mm in diameter. They occur initially on the mucous membranes and are most frequently manifest by nosebleeds in children; after maturity they appear on the skin.

In differential diagnosis, ataxia-telangiectasia must be distinguished.

Abnormalities of Lymphatic Vessels

Malformation of the lymphatic vessels may result in localized or diffuse cutaneous abnormalities comparable in most respects to hemangiomas. The varying clinical expression of lymphatic involvement is dependent on their size, depth and site of involvement.

Circumscribed lymphangioma is the most common variety of lymphangioma and may be present at birth or appear in early childhood. The lesions consist of small, grouped, thick-walled vesicles which exude a serous exudate when excised. Solitary, circumscribed dermal or subcutaneous nodules may appear, indicating involvement of more deeply placed lymphatic vessels. Cavernous lymphangioma is the result of large cystic dilatation of the lymphatic vessels in the dermis, subcutaneous tissue and intramuscular septa. Treatment of all varieties of lymphangioma is surgical except for the cavernous type which is impractical because of the wide lymphatic involvement.

Other Developmental Abnormalities

EPIDERMIS, DERMIS AND DERMAL APPENDAGES. Circumscribed malformations of the skin of congenital origin may arise as the result of defects in any of the components of the skin (epidermis, sebaceous glands, hair follicles, apocrine or eccrine sweat glands, smooth muscle and connective or elastic tissue).

Epidermal Nevi. These may be classified according to their clinical and histologic features as *verrucous nevi,* in which there is a brownish verrucoid overgrowth of epithelial cells distributed in a linear configuration.

Nevus Unius Lateris. This is an erythematous scaling linear dermatitis with clinical features resembling psoriasis or an eczematous dermatitis.

Treatment of verrucous nevi is unsatisfactory. Occasionally, when they are located on exposed areas, surgical removal of the epidermis and underlying dermis may be necessary.

Connective Tissue Nevi. These nevi are characterized by flesh-colored, yellowish patches with accentuation of the poral orifices (shagreen patch) in the lumbosacral area. It may be an isolated phenomenon or occur in association with tuberous sclerosis. In the differential diagnosis, elastic tissue nevus need be considered. No treatment is necessary.

Congenital Aplasia. Congenital aplasia of the skin is a localized developmental failure believed to be transmitted as a recessive trait or as an incomplete dominant. It is characterized by the presence of single or multiple atrophic or ulcerative lesions 2 to 3 cm in diameter on the scalp. Histopathologically the epidermis is atrophic; the dermis and subcutaneous fat are hypoplastic, with decreased or absent dermal appendages; and the lesion is covered by a single layer of epithelial cells. Spontaneous epithelialization is rapid, so that treatment is usually not necessary. Application of a broad spectrum antibiotic may prevent secondary bacterial infection.

Cutis Verticis Gyrata. In this disorder the skin of the scalp is folded on itself, giving a corrugated appearance; it is associated with disorders of the central nervous system.

Congenital Anhidrotic Ectodermal Defect. This is a hereditary developmental abnormality characterized by aplasia or hypoplasia of eccrine sweat, sebaceous and mucous glands, pilar structures and tooth buds.

Histopathologically there is thinning of the epiderm and dermis. Eccrine sweat glands are absent or may be rudimentary. There is thinning of the epithelial layer in the respiratory mucous membranes and hypoplasia of the underlying mucous glands.

Affected infants appear normal at birth, but they do not perspire. In early infancy an otherwise unexplained fever which is directly related to high environmental temperature may provide a clue to early diagnosis. At this time confirmatory diagnostic evidence can be secured from a roentgenogram of the jaws, which will show no or deficient dental structures.

Chronic rhinitis and pharyngitis are common. The hair of the scalp is very fine and sparse and grows slowly. Dentition is delayed or may be absent; when present, the incisors are widely spaced and the canines are conical. Characteristic alteration of the face occurs as early as 11 months and consists of prominent frontal bosses and a saddle-shaped nose (Fig. 23–25). In differential diagnosis, congenital syphilis and chondroectodermal dysplasia must be distinguished.

Treatment is symptomatic.

Hidrotic Ectodermal Defect. This is transmitted as a dominant trait and is characterized by hypotrichosis, hyperpigmentation, dystrophic nails and hyperkeratosis of palms and soles. Hair may be partially or completely absent at birth; when present, it is fine and easily fractured. The nails may be thin or thickened, striated, rough or completely absent. Palms and soles are hyperkeratotic, and there is hyperpigmentation on the extensor surfaces of the elbows, axillae, areolar area of the breasts, umbilicus and the interphanalgeal joints.

In differential diagnosis the anhidrotic type of ectodermal defect must be distinguished.

Sebaceous Nevus. This is characterized by yellowish, dome-shaped nodular lesions distributed primarily on the face. It consists of sebaceous glands of varying degrees of maturity.

Nevus Sebaceus of Jadassohn. A common organoid nevus present at birth and comprised of all elements of the skin, this is characterized by the presence on the hairy area of the scalp of round, linear or crescentic, well demarcated, yellowish to orange, flat or slightly raised patches devoid of normal hairs, though vellus hairs may be present. Because the nevus is made up of skin appendages that change with age, there is a characteristic overdevelopment of the normal constituents of the skin, and papillomatous changes occur on the surface of the nevus at puberty (Fig. 23-26). In some patients basal cell carcinoma may appear. Rarely, nevus sebaceus may be associated with developmental abnormalities of the eye or of the cardiovascular or nervous systems. The cosmetic appearance of the bald patch and the possibility of secondary neoplastic degeneration make excision of the nevus the treatment of choice.

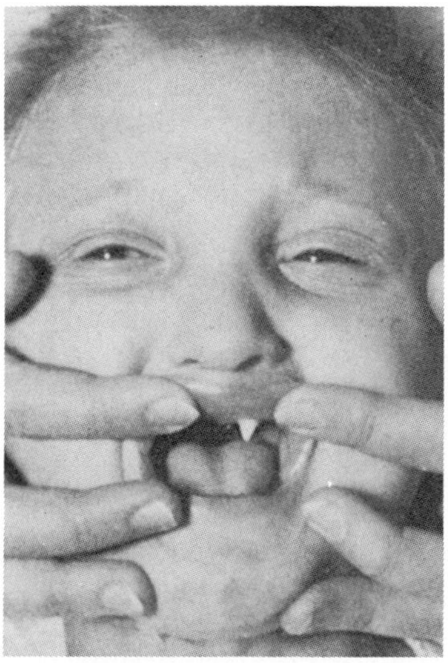

Figure 23-25 *Congenital anhidrotic ectodermal defect showing characteristic facies and tooth dysplasia.*

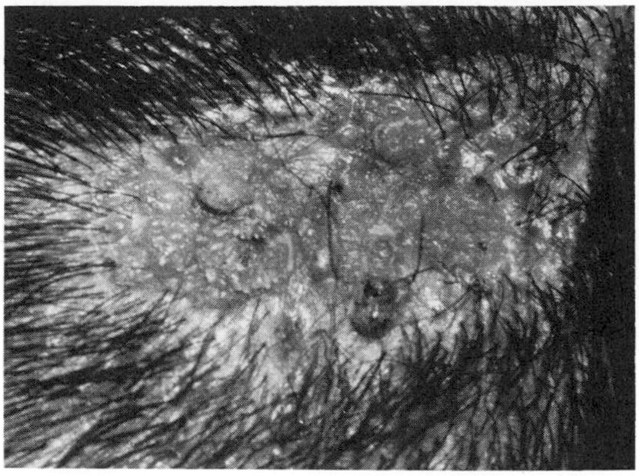

Figure 23-26 *Nevus sebaceus of Jadassohn, showing verrucoid hyperplasia of the skin during adolescence.*

In differential diagnosis, *nevus syringocystadenosus papilliferus* needs consideration. This abnormality arises from the apocrine sweat glands and may also undergo neoplastic degeneration (basal cell) later in life. Excision is the treatment of choice.

Nevus Pilosus. This presents with an unusual number of mature hairs in an abnormal location. They may be cosmetically significant on exposed areas; they may be removed permanently by electrolysis after childhood.

Embryologic Developmental Errors. These may result in a variety of pits, fistuli or tags which may produce only a minor defect or be associated with other developmental abnormalities. Some are listed in Table 23-3.

ABNORMALITIES OF THE MUCOUS MEMBRANES

Grooved Tongue. Deep furrows on the surface of the tongue are apparently inherited as a dominant characteristic; this is seen in approximately 0.5 per cent of persons. In Down syndrome it is acquired by friction of the tongue over the teeth in characteristic tongue-sucking.

Congenital Fistula of the Lip. A rare developmental abnormality probably transmitted as an autosomal dominant trait, the fistulous tracts are located symmetrically on either side of the midline of the transitional area of the mucous membranes of the lip. A clear mucoid fluid usually exudes from the mucous glands of the lip. The fistulous tracts should be excised.

Hypertrophied Frenulum Syndrome. This consists of an abnormally developed frenulum with a pseudocleft in the upper lip, tongue and palate, mental retardation, trembling and syndactyly. It is probably transmitted as a dominant autosomal trait.

Hereditary Gingival Fibromatosis. This is characterized by firm, enlarged gingival tissue over the crowns of permanent teeth. It usually becomes evident with the eruption of the permanent incisors. Hypertrichosis may be associated with the syndrome. It is probably transmitted as a dominant autosomal trait. Excision is usually as-

TABLE 23-3 SKIN PITS, FISTULAS AND TAGS OF THE EARS, LIP AND NECK

DISEASE	CLINICAL MANIFESTATIONS	INHERITANCE	ASSOCIATED ABNORMALITIES
Congenital fistulas of lip	Uni-or bilateral pits or fistulas of lower lip, near midline of vermilion border	None	Occasional cleft lip or cleft palate
Congenital auricular fistulas	Preauricular pits and/or fistulas	Autosomal dominant	Occasionally, multiple anomalies of face and ears
Treacher Collins syndrome	Preauricular tags and/or fistulas	Autosomal dominant	Hypoplastic nose cartilage and fistula-like mouth, coloboma, occasionally skeletal and cardiac abnormalities
Goldenhar syndrome	Bilateral auricular tags and fistulas	None	Epibulbar desmoids, malar hypoplasia, receding chin
Auricular appendages	Tags on preauricular skin	None	Occasionally, other ear and face defects
Branchiogenic fistulas	Lower portion of neck, anterior to original external mastoid	Autosomal dominant	None
Thyroglossal fistula	Upper third of neck near midline	None	None

sociated with regrowth, whereas regression usually follows dental extraction.

Leukokeratosis. Leukokeratosis is an asymptomatic, whitish thickening of the mucous membranes which is transmitted as an autosomal dominant trait in Caucasians. Irregular, thickened whitish plaques with a verrucoid surface appear most commonly in the mouth at birth or at any time up to adolescence. No treatment is necessary.

Fordyce's Spots. Fordyce's spots of the mucous membranes of the cheeks and lips are a common, asymptomatic developmental abnormality of ectopic sebaceous glands. They first appear in the preadolescent period and are characterized by discrete yellowish papules. They occur in approximately 50 per cent of children under 11 years of age. No treatment is necessary.

Transitory Benign Plaque. Transitory benign plaque of the mucous membrane of the mouth is a recurrent, asymptomatic alteration characterized by fleeting, sharply circumscribed, erythematous patches about 0.5 cm in diameter which spread to form a ring with a yellowish white border and then fade only to reform at a different spot. The tongue is the site of predilection, but the buccal, gingival and labial mucosa may be involved. No treatment is necessary.

DEVELOPMENTAL ABNORMALITIES OF HAIR. These are indicated in the following table, which also includes abnormalities of hair acquired through trauma or other conditions:

I. Congenital anatomic defects
  - Congenital alopecia
  - Monilethrix
  - Pili torti
  - Pili annulati
  - Trichorrhexis nodosa
  - Woolly hair
  - Trichorrhexis invaginata

II. Loss of hair due to alterations of growth cycle (hypotrichosis)
  - Defluvium of the newborn
  - Inflammation (second-degree thermal burn, kerion, alopecia areata, bacterial infection, seborrhea)
  - Fever
  - Roentgen radiation (low dosage)
  - Syphilis
  - Drugs (thallium, folic acid antagonists, vitamin A toxicity)
  - Endocrine (hypothyroidism)
  - Systemic disease (dermatomyositis, systemic lupus erythematosus)

III. Fracture of the hair shaft
  - Trauma (hair twisting, compulsive brushing or combing)

IV. Epilation
  - Trichotillomania
  - Marginal alopecia

V. Scarring
  - Congenital dermal defect
  - Severe infection (bacteria, kerion)
  - Third-degree thermal burn
  - Roentgen radiation (high dosage)
  - Discoid lupus erythematosus

Variations in structure, function or distribution of the scalp hair may occur as isolated phenomena or be associated with various ectodermal defects or as part of multisystem diseases.

Congenital Alopecia. Congenital alopecia is an abnormality in the production of hair usually transmitted as a dominant trait, but occasionally as a recessive. It is characterized by complete absence of hair or poor growth of it on the scalp; eyebrows and eyelashes are also frequently in-

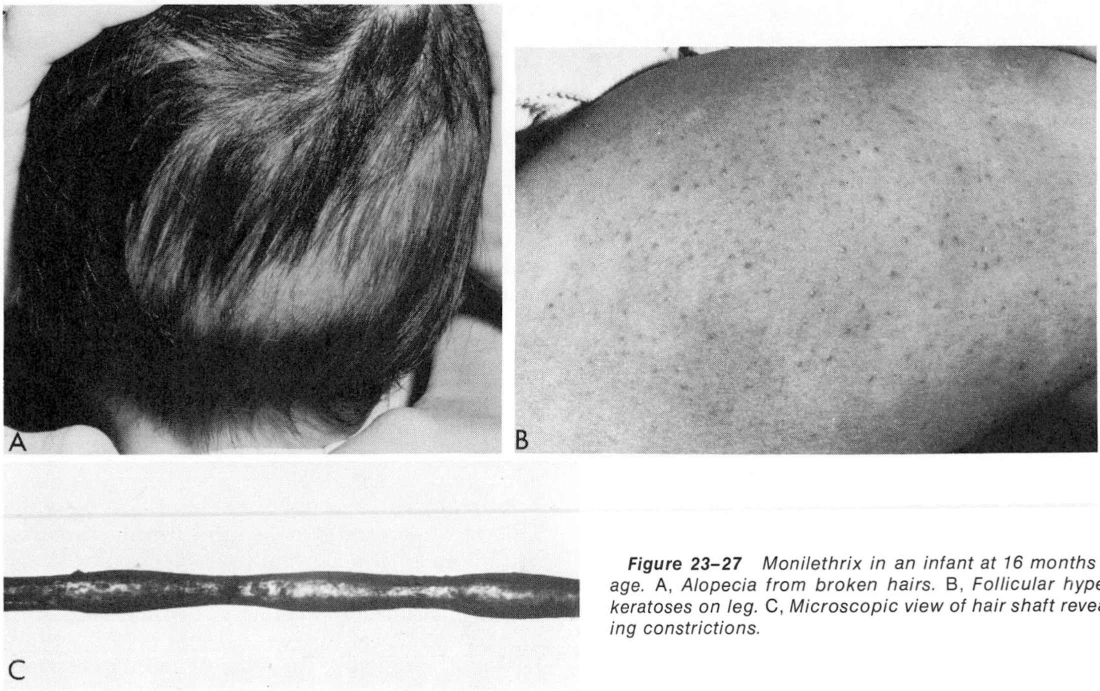

Figure 23–27 *Monilethrix in an infant at 16 months of age.* A, *Alopecia from broken hairs.* B, *Follicular hyperkeratoses on leg.* C, *Microscopic view of hair shaft revealing constrictions.*

volved. Histopathologically hair follicles are absent or hypoplastic, and sebaceous glands and arrectores pilorum muscles are hypoplastic.

In some families the infants are practically bald at birth, whereas in others the hair is normal, but later falls out and is replaced by a scanty growth. The abnormality has been associated with webbed fingers, cataracts and Friedreich's ataxia. It must be differentiated from the hidrotic and anhidrotic types of ectodermal dysplasia in children with scanty hair.

Monilethrix. Monilethrix is characterized by constriction of the hair of the scalp at regular intervals, by fracture of the hair shafts and by follicular keratoses. It is inherited as a dominant trait. Abnormal excretion of amino acids in urine may occur. Histopathologically, under direct examination, the fusiform swelling of the hair, which occurs at intervals of approximately 1 mm, is normal in appearance but the medulla is absent; the cortex is diminished, and the cuticle is thickened at the constrictions. The pilar orifices contain hyperkeratotic plugs (Fig. 23–27). In the differential diagnosis, pili torti, trichorrhexis nodosa, tinea capitis and trichotillomania must be considered. There is no treatment, but the frequency of fractures may be diminished by avoiding combing and brushing as much as possible. In some instances, the hair abnormality remains throughout life, whereas in others spontaneous recovery may occur in puberty or there may be progressive improvement through adult life.

Pili Torti. Pili torti is characterized by twisting of the shaft of the hair on its axis and by increased fragility at the twisted sites. The defect appears in families and may be inherited as an autosomal dominant or recessive trait. Concurrent pili torti and nerve deafness have been reported. The hair appears dry and lusterless, and areas of stubble appear where the hair has been broken off (Fig. 23–28). The cosmetic aspects are especially obvious in girls. There is no treatment, but the frequency of fractures may be diminished by avoidance of combing and brushing the hair as much as possible.

Pili Annulati. This is a rare abnormality of the hair characterized by alternate pigmented and depigmented areas at intervals of approximately 1 mm, producing a ringed appearance. It is probably inherited as an irregular dominant trait. The abnormality is asymptomatic and does not require treatment.

Trichorrhexis Nodosa. This is characterized by nodular swellings through the hair shaft which produce increased fragility. Microscopically the nodes represent a partial fracture of the shaft, producing the appearance of two brooms pushed end to end. Abnormal excretion of amino acids in urine has been reported.

Woolly Hair. Woolly hair is characterized by short, woolly, tightly curled hairs in localized patches or generalized on the scalp. The woolly hair may be present at birth or appear during the first two years of life. Associated ectodermal abnormalities have been reported. It is transmitted as an autosomal dominant trait or, in some families, as a sex-linked trait.

Trichorrhexis Invaginata (Bamboo Hairs). This occurs in the Netherton syndrome. Short fragile hairs are first observed during the first year of life in association with nonbullous congenital ichthyosiform erythroderma (lamellar ichthyosis)

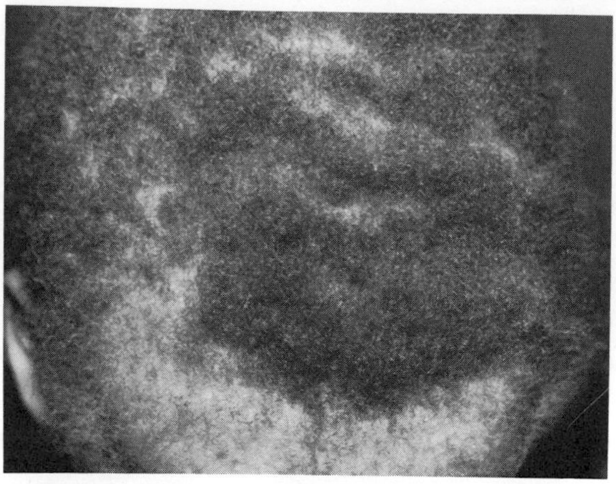

A

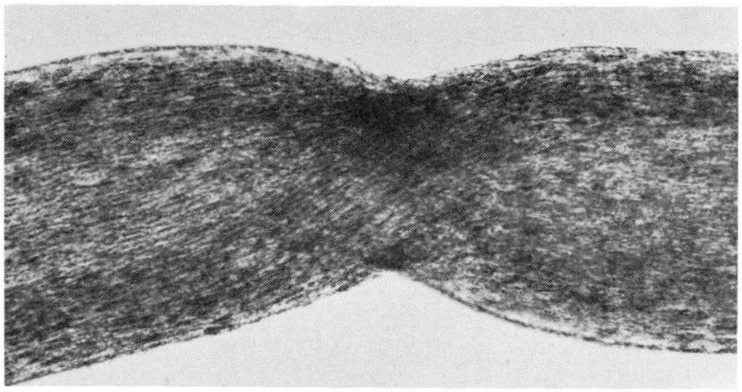

B

Figure 23–28 A, *A 5 year old Caucasian boy with short, "kinky" hairs; fracture of the hairs precluded hair cutting.* B, *Microscopic examination showing twisting of the hair shaft (KOH preparation). (× 250.)*

and an atopic diathesis. The hair defect is seen histologically as a cup-like defect with the distal portion of the shaft inserted in a cup formed by the proximal portion of the hair shaft. (See also elsewhere, this Section.)

DEFECTS OF THE NAILS. A variety of congenital and familial defects of the nails occur during the neonatal period, either as isolated abnormalities or as expressions of generalized disorders. Defects may involve the nail plate, bed or paronychial area and result in changes varying from the total absence of the nail plate to thickening, discoloration, striation, splitting, fragmentation or discoloration. Associated conditions include: epidermolysis bullosa, incontinentia pigmenti, conjunctional ectodermal defect, nail patella syndrome, dyskeratosis congenita, acrodermatitis enteropathica and pachyonychia congenita.

DEVELOPMENTAL DISORDERS OF THE SUBCUTANEOUS TISSUE. Several uncommon disorders of the subcutaneous tissue may occur during the neonatal period and cause confusion in differential diagnosis. The changes may be localized (as in subcutaneous fat necrosis) or generalized (edema of the newborn, sclerema neonatorum). In these disorders, the skin has a thickened feel on palpation. Of these uncommon diseases, subcutaneous fat necrosis is the most common; sclerema neonatorum and edema neonatorum are rare. *Nevus lipomatosus cutaneus superficialis* consists of small yellowish or skin-colored papules or nodules, arranged in groups or in a linear manner on the buttocks or thighs; it may be seen as a type of lipomatous nevus.

Edema of the Newborn. Sclerema edematosum (scleredema) is a rare disorder of unknown cause seen in weak newborn and especially in premature infants; it is characterized by widespread pitting edema of the extremities and trunk and by pallor and lividity of the skin. Most infants so affected do not survive, but the edema may subside spontaneously if the general condition of the infant improves. Histopathologic examination reveals engorgement of the vessels in the corium, with some perivascular infiltration and edema of the dermis and underlying muscles. In differential diagnosis sclerema and scleredema of Buschke must be considered. No specific therapy is known.

Subcutaneous Fat Necrosis of the Newborn. This is an uncommon benign disorder occurring equally in both sexes and characterized by sharply circumscribed indurated lesions of the skin and underlying tissue of variable size, appearing in the first few weeks of life in otherwise healthy infants. Histopathologically the earliest changes consist of endothelial swelling and a perivascular inflammatory infiltrate followed by necrosis of the subcutaneous fat and a dense granulomatous and inflammatory infiltrate containing foreign body type giant cells with needle-like crystals. The lesions generally appear near the end of the first week of life, but may appear as late as the sixth week. The onset is not associated with constitutional symptoms. Lesions vary in size from 1 or 2 up to 10 or more cm; they are hard and plaque-like and do not pit on pressure. Although they may appear anywhere, they are located most commonly on the posterior portion of the trunk, buttocks, thighs, cheeks, arms and feet. The skin overlying the plaque may have a slightly livid discoloration. Small lesions may be freely movable over underlying structures. The borders of the lesions are sharply defined, and the plaques are slightly elevated above the normal skin. The hard plaque slowly softens after 6 to 8 weeks, and complete resolution usually occurs within several months. During the stage of resolution the mass may be misdiagnosed as an abscess. Calcification of some lesions may occur, but widespread calcification of such indurated areas would suggest hypercalcemia. No treatment is indicated, and under no circumstances should the mass be incised. The disease must be differentiated from nodular nonsuppurative panniculitis, which is usually associated with tender nodules in the skin and splenomegaly, and from lipogranulomatosis (Farber).

Sclerema Neonatorum. Sclerema neonatorum is an uncommon alteration of the subcutaneous fat in weak premature infants or in term infants with severe systemic, especially diarrheal, disease. It should be regarded as a physical sign and not as a disease entity. It is characterized by a rapidly spreading, waxy-appearing, cool, leathery change in the skin, with purplish mottling; the skin feels adherent to underlying structures. The histologic picture is similarly that of subcutaneous fat necrosis of the newborn, but usually has a less intense inflammatory infiltrate and fewer foreign body giant cells. The process frequently commences on the legs and gradually spreads in the course of a few days to involve the entire cutaneous surface. Immobility of the face produced by this cast-like solidification of the subcutaneous tissue makes feeding difficult. Death usually occurs within a few days or weeks, though recovery has been reported. The process must be differentiated from edema neonatorum. Treatment, in general, is supportive and specifically directed at the underlying disease.

Absence of Adipose Tissue. The absence of subcutaneous fat results in two clinically distinct syndromes of unknown origin, partial and total lipodystrophy.

Partial Lipodystrophy. This is characterized by the symmetrical loss of fat from the face with or without disappearance of fat also from the arms, chest, abdomen and hips, but with normal distribution on the lower extremities. The ratio of affected females to males is approximately 4:1. The cause is unknown. The only histologic change observed is the absence of subcutaneous fat in affected areas, normal epidermis and dermis lying directly on fascia or muscle. The clinical onset is most often between 5 and 15 years of age, but may be as early as the first year. There is an insidious loss of subcutaneous fat from the face without inflammatory reaction or symptoms. Slow progression may occur, with involvement of the neck, arms, chest and abdomen. Normal or even increased fat deposition may persist over the legs, but fat loss becomes complete on the face. These patients have a strikingly cadaverous appearance. Aside from the fat loss, the majority appear well, but renal disorders, disturbances of central nervous system function, hepatomegaly, hyperlipemia and disordered glucose metabolism have been associated. These features, which suggest total lipodystrophy, are more evident in the older patient. There is no known treatment.

Total Lipodystrophy. This is characterized by the complete loss of adipose tissue, generalized hyperpigmentation and hypertrichosis, which may be present at birth. It is a multisystem disease regularly associated with liver abnormalities and commonly with other variable features, including increased height, advanced bone maturation, hirsutism, pigmentation, prominence of muscles, abdominal protuberance, penile or clitoral enlargement, anatomic or functional disturbances of the central nervous system, neuropathy, cardiomegaly, insulin-resistant hyperglycemia, hyperlipemia and hypermetabolism. The ratio of affected females to males is 2:1. The disorder is transmitted as an autosomal recessive trait. The disease may be apparent at birth or may commence during childhood. The clinical appearance of the child is similar to that of patients with partial loss of fat, but because the condition is generalized, the striking contrast between affected and unaffected areas is absent, and the diagnosis may not be so apparent. Generalized pigmentation is common. Accentuated pigmentation in the axillary areas may be associated with the velvety verrucoid skin changes of acanthosis nigricans. A moderate degree of hirsuties may be present. Scalp hair may be abundant and may become curly concurrently with the loss of fat. An insulin-antagonizing and fat-mobilizing property has been found in the urine.

There is no known treatment for this disease.

In differential diagnosis, leprechaunism needs to be considered. Affected infants usually suffer from severe infection and die in infancy.

Cold Panniculitis. Chilblain is characterized by the appearance of warm erythematous indurated plaques appearing within hours of the exposure to cold. It is most commonly seen in infants and young children on the cheeks. The histologic findings are confined to the dermis and subcutaneous fat and consist of a perivascular inflammatory infiltrate of lymphocytes, polymorphonuclear leukocytes and histiocytes. Treatment is not necessary, since the inflammatory panniculitis resolves spontaneously in about two weeks.

DEVELOPMENTAL DISORDERS AFFECTING THE DERMIS. Developmental, metabolic and inflammatory diseases involving the dermis result in a variety of unrelated diseases.

Lipoid Proteinosis. This is a rare metabolic disturbance transmitted as a recessive trait. A structureless hyaline material made up of a carbohydrate-protein complex is deposited in affected skin and mucous membranes as an extracellular mantle around vessels of the dermis and as a diffuse infiltrate in connective tissue. Lipids appear as the lesions become more advanced.

The skin lesions may be present at birth, but usually develop later. They characteristically consist of yellowish white papules which may coalesce into plaques or nodules. Yellowish verrucoid lesions also occur on the extensor surface of the elbows, knees and hands. Subsequently there is extensive involvement of the mucous membrane of the tongue, lips, oral cavity, pharynx, larynx and rectal area. The infiltration of the vocal cords precludes speaking above a whisper as the child grows. Aplasia or hypoplasia of teeth is commonly associated.

In differential diagnosis, the xanthomas do not have the woody feel of the tongue found in this disorder.

The course of the disease is usually benign and no treatment is necessary, but tracheotomy may be required for extensive infiltration of the vocal cords.

Cutis Hyperelastica and Cutis Laxa. These have similar nomenclature and some common clinical features; the essential alteration is in elastic tissue fibers in both diseases. The possibility of an associated alteration of collagen has not been completely excluded in either disease.

Cutis Hyperelastica. Ehlers-Danlos syndrome

is a quantitative heritable abnormality of elastic tissue transmitted as an incomplete dominant trait. It is usually present at birth and is characterized by hyperelasticity and fragility of the skin and hyperextensibility of the joints. Light microscopy and electron microscopy reveal a striking increase in the number of elastic fibers of normal morphology. Slight trauma produces in the fragile skin large lacerations which are impossible to suture and which heal with scars resembling cigarette paper. Minor trauma may also frequently produce large hematomas. Small nodules (pseudotumors) may be found on the skin at the sites of traumatic hemorrhage and consist of inflammatory infiltrate with foreign body giant cells or connective tissue proliferation with large numbers of vessels. Some nodules become calcified. The hemorrhagic tendency may suggest hemophilia, pseudotumors and neurofibromatosis, but the other classic features of the disease should make differentiation easy. Avoidance of trauma to the skin by protection of the lower portions of the legs and bony prominences with foam rubber is useful. Closure of lacerations is impossible with single sutures and is difficult with mattress sutures, but can be accomplished by use of adhesive butterflies.

Cutis Laxa (Generalized Elastolysis). This is a generalized degenerative disease of elastic tissue fibers present at birth and inherited as a recessive trait. There are hypertrophy and laxity of the skin and underlying connective tissue which result in the skin hanging in folds and presenting a picture of premature senility. Histologic changes include a striking granular degeneration of elastic tissue fibers leading to their complete disappearance in some areas. There is a striking increase in the acid mucopolysaccharide content of the dermis.

The skin is soft, doughy and inelastic, lies in folds on the face, neck, chest and abdomen, and droops over the eyelids and around the mouth. The pulmonary, genitourinary and gastrointestinal systems may be involved in the generalized elastic tissue alteration. When the disease is not limited to the skin, the systemic involvement may be incompatible with life. There is no known treatment for the basic defect, but appearance may be improved with plastic surgery.

Elastosis Perforans Serpiginosa. Perforating elastoma is an elastic tissue disorder characterized by asymptomatic or keratotic papules arranged in annular or acriform pattern appearing primarily on the nape of the neck, face or extremities during adolescence (Fig. 23–29). Histologically there is epidermal predisposition toward perforation, with channels extending from the dermis to the skin surface. Special stains for elastic tissue show hyperplasia of elastic tissue fibers in the dermis below the perforating channels. The significance of this disorder is its occasional association with other disorders (Marfan syndrome, osteogenesis imperfecta, Ehlers-Danlos disease, Rothmund-Thomson syndrome).

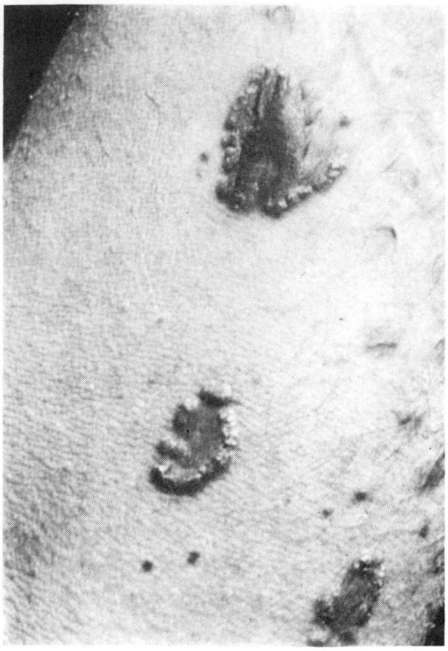

Figure 23–29 *Elastosis perforans serpiginosa.*

Focal Dermal Hypoplasia (Goltz syndrome). This is a hereditary abnormality of ectodermal and mesodermal derivatives in the skin and other organs. The histologic findings in the skin consist of a strikingly thinned dermis, with fat lying just beneath the epidermis. The characteristic cutaneous findings consist of atrophy in areas in which there is herniation of fat through the absent dermis. There may be patches of general aplasia, or blisters may form.

Mucopolysaccharidoses. These have been classified into distinct syndromes by virtue of their phenotypic, genetic and biochemical characteristics. They are characterized by mucopolysacchariduria and by deposits of polysaccharides in various tissues. The cutaneous lesions consist of generalized thickening of skin, which is taut and inelastic and feels bound down to the underlying structures, or of isolated nodules or plaques.

Lipogranulomatosis. Farber's disease is a rare form of lipidosis, manifest within the first few months of life. It follows a progressive course in which tenderness and swelling of the extremities are accompanied by dysphonia, a systemic reaction with temperature elevation, generalized joint involvement, nodules and infiltrated plaques in the skin, and cardiopulmonary and central nervous system involvement (Fig. 23–30). The early skin lesions are slightly erythematous nodules which become ill defined plaques with a predisposition for the extremities.

Granuloma Annulare. This is a self-limited inflammatory process of unknown cause characterized by papules or nodules on the extremities. The primary lesion is a slightly erythematous or yellowish red, waxy-appearing papule which slowly increases in size and clears in the center, or a group of papules may form a ring. Single lesions are the rule, but occasionally disseminated lesions appear on the extremities (Fig. 23–31).

Histopathologically there is a distinctive area of coagulation necrosis in the upper portion of the dermis surrounded by a radially arranged infiltrate composed of epitheloid, lymphocytic, plasma and connective tissue cells.

In differential diagnosis the annular lesions of sarcoid (rare in children), rheumatic nodules and the skin lesions associated with juvenile rheumatoid arthritis should be considered.

The disease is usually self-limited, and in many instances the lesions regress rapidly. In persistent lesions local application of triamcinolone in a 0.05 per cent cream under a plastic film or injection of it (5 mg/ml) into the lesion will produce prompt regression.

Pityriasis Lichenoides et Varioliformis Acuta. Mucha-Habermann syndrome is an asymptomatic inflammatory disease of the skin of unknown origin. In its more severe or acute form, papules, vesicles and papulonecrotic lesions appear in crops over a period of weeks or months. The lesions may resemble those of smallpox or varicella, but heal without scarring. In the milder form a few brownish red papules appear in crops on the trunk and extremities and slowly resolve. In both instances new lesions recur with diminishing frequency as the disease disappears.

In the acute phase the histologic picture is essentially that of a lymphocytic vasculitis, which damages the vessel wall and leads to necrosis of the overlying dermis and epidermis. The vasculitis differs from allergic vasculitis in the absence of neutrophils and in the fibrinoid deposits within and around the blood vessels. Varicella is most often confused clinically, but the short duration, contagiousness and constitutional symptoms of varicella serve to differentiate it. The multinucleated epithelial giant cells found at the base of a blister in varicella are diagnostic. Treatment is not necessary in most instances, owing to the self-limited nature of the disease. Corticosteroids may be useful in the severe form.

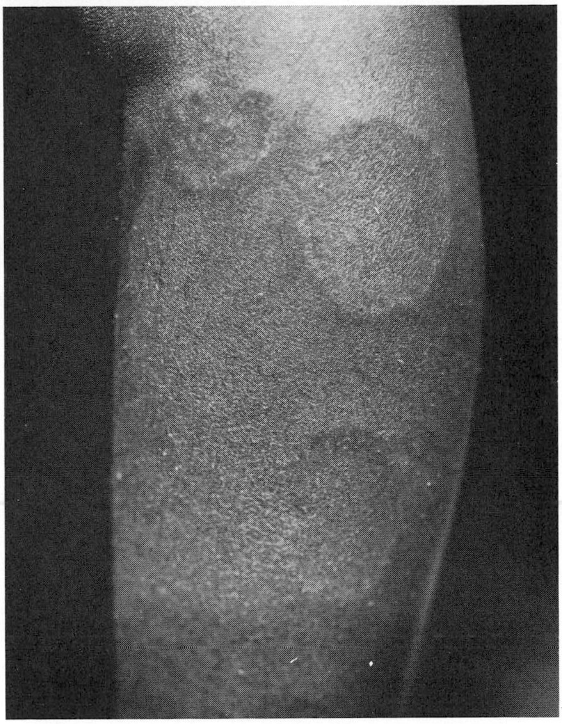

Figure 23–31 Granuloma annulare in a 5 year old child, showing multiple, distinctive, annular lesions.

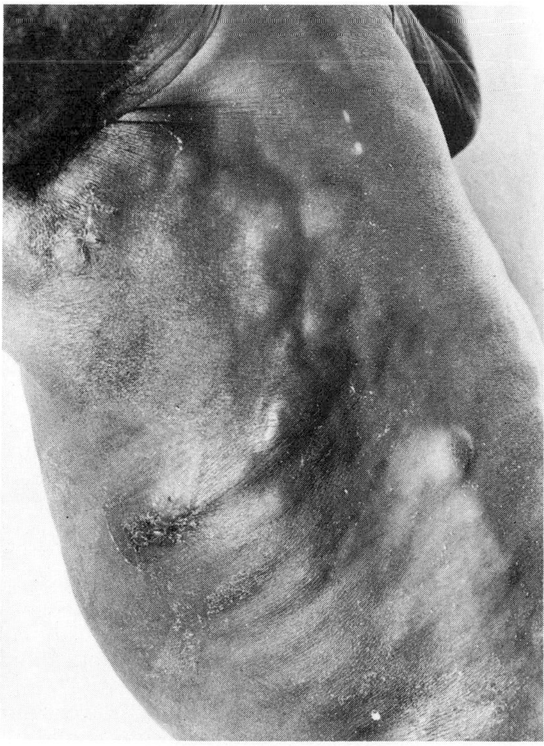

Figure 23–30 Lipogranulomatosis in a cachetic infant at 4 months of age, demonstrating nodular plaques in the skin of the back.

Lichen Sclerosus et Atrophicus. This is a primary atrophic process of unknown origin which frequently involves the vulva, perineum, shoulders and lumbosacral areas. It has been reported in males, but occurs most frequently in females. Histologically there is atrophy of the epidermal layer, with edema and homogenization of the upper third of the dermis. The skin lesions consist of atrophic white maculopapules, varying from 1 to 3 mm in diameter, with a small central horny plug. They are frequently grouped together to form patches, but the diagnostic discrete papules can be seen at the border of the lesions. Blisters may occasionally form on the patches. Pruritus is a common symptom, and painful fissures are often present in the perianal and vulvar lesions. The skin changes may persist for years or may regress spontaneously. The patches of confluent papules may resemble localized scleroderma (morphea). Relief of symptoms may be obtained by the use of a corticosteroid cream (1 per cent hydrocortisone). Topical estrogen creams are useful also in the genital area, but may produce side effects associated with percutaneous absorption.

Diaper Dermatitis. Diaper dermatitis is a cutaneous reaction localized to the area ordinarily covered by the diaper. A variety of morphologic changes are produced by multiple causative factors. The histopathologic changes vary with the causative factor:

I. Predisposing factors
   A. Inheritance of a reactive skin that is easily irritated
   B. Inherited seborrheic diathesis with a propensity for irritation in the anal and genitocrural folds and vulnerability to secondary yeast and bacterial infections
   C. Atopic diathesis
   D. Systemic disease such as syphilis, acrodermatitis chronica enteropathica (Fig. 23–11) and Letterer-Siwe disease may produce a lowering of skin resistance
II. Activating factors
   A. Maceration caused by continuous contact with a wet diaper and intensified by the moist heat produced by an impervious rubber or plastic cover
   B. Retention of sweat caused by keratotic plugging of orifices of eccrine glands, secondary to A
   C. Contact factors, including allergic (e.g., sensitization to fluorochrome dyes in detergent soaps, or to plastic diaper covers) and primary irritants (e.g., feces, or ammonia in decomposed urine).
   D. Maternal factors, such as failure to carry out instructions or overassiduousness in cleansing the affected areas
   E. Infection (e.g., yeast, bacterial, syphilitic, viral) (Fig. 23–32)
   F. Mechanical irritation in areas of friction or from pressure

Morphologic changes vary from diffuse erythema, in which the skin has a parchment-like appearance, to nodular infiltrated lesions (granuloma gluteale infantum) which may become vesicular, pustular or bullous.

Prevention consists in prompt changing of diapers after urination and in appropriate cleansing of the skin with each change of diaper, particularly after bowel movements, in elimination of an impervious diaper cover, covering with only one diaper, in application of a protective paste (Lassar's paste), and in using diapers rinsed in a quaternary ammonium compound (Roccal 1:3000).

Treatment should be guided by a careful evaluation of the history of onset and of the morphology and localization of the lesions. Seborrheic lesions are treated with 0.5 per cent hydrocortisone ointment; yeast infections are sponged with benzalkonium chloride 1:3000 and then covered with Vioform cream alone, or in combination with 0.5 per cent hydrocortisone or with nystatin (Mycostatin ointment); bacterial infections should be cleansed with an unscented white soap, and a broad spectrum antibiotic ointment such as neomycin, bacitracin and polymyxin should be applied. Contact dermatitis is treated with 0.5 to 1.0 per cent hydrocortisone ointment.

Exposure of the uncovered diaper area to dry heat, as from an electric light, is especially helpful and can be done to advantage during naps.

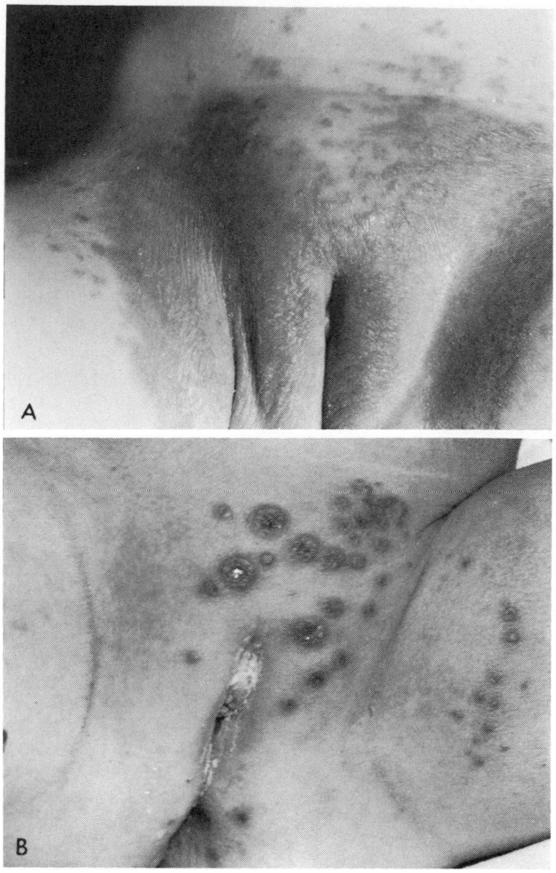

Figure 23–32 *A, Diaper dermatitis caused by yeast infection, showing characteristic vesicular pustules; the organisms were demonstrated by direct microscopic examination (potassium hydroxide preparation). B, Staphylococcal infection in the diaper area secondary to sweat retention.*

ALLERGIC DISORDERS

Cutaneous expressions of the hypersensitivity state include contact dermatitis, atopic dermatitis, drug allergy, granulomatous vasculitis, allergy of infection (reactions to fungi, bacteria, viruses, protozoa) and allergy of infestation (parasites and insects).

CONTACT DERMATITIS. Contact dermatitis is an acute inflammatory reaction of the skin which may be divided into two categories: (1) reactions which occur on first contact in all subjects and are usually produced by chemicals; and (2) reactions which occur only in persons who have been previously sensitized. Contact dermatitis is the most common type of dermatitis in children from 2 to 12 years of age; atopic dermatitis is more common during infancy. The causative agents (excluding medications) in order of frequency are weeds and vines (usually poison ivy) (Fig. 23–33), the ether-soluble portion of airborne allergens, toys, cosmetics and chemicals in clothing and shoes.

Histopathologically contact dermatitis is characterized by intercellular edema, exocytosis and intraepidermal vesicle formation, with a mild perivascular inflammatory infiltrate. A primary

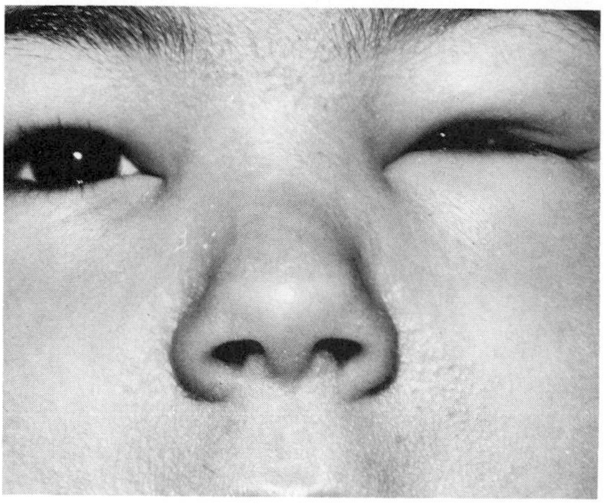

Figure 23–33 A 6 year old boy with allergic contact dermatitis (Rhus toxicodendron), showing erythema, edema and vesicles 72 hours after contact.

irritant reaction is differentiated from allergic reactions by the migration of polymorphonuclear leukocytes through the epidermis and into the vesicles, whereas in the allergic reaction lymphocytes predominate. The skin response to a contact allergen depends on the level of sensitivity, varying from erythema with edema to blister formation. If additional contact is eliminated, the dermatitis is self-limited and regresses in approximately two weeks. In dermatitis produced by contact with weeds the eruption frequently appears in a linear streak at the site of a brushing contact. Characteristically the eruption occurs on exposed areas, but the allergen may be carried to covered areas by the hands.

In differential diagnosis, nummular eczema and photosensitivity must be distinguished. Correlation of the history with responses to patch tests will frequently establish the causative allergen.

Treatment of all acute contact dermatitis is the same, irrespective of the cause. It consists in elimination of contact. Corticosteroids are the most effective agents for reducing the inflammatory reaction and lessening subjective reactions. Depending on the extent of involvement, they should be used locally or systemically. They are most effective when their administration is started prior to blister formation. For local treatment, 0.5 to 1.0 per cent hydrocortisone in a hydrophilic ointment is used. Systemic treatment is indicated only in children with widespread dermatitis; it may be given in full therapeutic doses for 5 to 7 days and stopped without fear of recurrence of the dermatitis, if contact with the allergen has been eliminated, or of adrenocortical suppression.

Prophylaxis is best accomplished by avoidance of contact. When poison ivy is the allergen, the child should be taught to recognize the vine. Thorough cleansing of the skin with soap and water within minutes of contact will prevent dermatitis. Hyposensitization may be tried by preseasonal treatment with the oral preparation of the ether-soluble fraction of *Rhus toxicodendron* (Hollister-Stier). The antigen is administered daily by mouth in capsules in increasing doses and decreasing dilution, starting two to three months before expected contact.

NUMMULAR ECZEMA. Nummular eczema is a common cutaneous reaction pattern characterized by round, papulovesicular patches. It is often an expression of atopic reactivity, but also occurs without family history of major hypersensitivity and without skin test evidence of atopic reactivity.

Histopathologically the lesion is not diagnostic and presents intercellular edema with slight endothelial swelling of the vessels in the dermis and a mild perivascular inflammatory infiltrate.

The individual patches are distinctively circinate, measuring from one to several centimeters in diameter. The lesions remain constant in size and location, occasionally clearing centrally. They are erythematous, palpably infiltrated and extremely pruritic (Fig. 23–34). The primary lesions are papulovesicles, which later ooze and become crusted. The eruption often waxes and wanes; it tends to remain localized to hands and feet, but may be generalized. In differential diagnosis, tinea corporis, allergic contact dermatitis and pruritus hiemalis must be distinguished.

In treatment, allergic inhalants, ingestants and contact agents need be regarded as causative possibilities and eliminated when indicated. Irrespective of the stage of the dermatitis, the most effective local treatment is the application of 0.5 to 1.0 per cent hydrocortisone (alcohol), 0.05 to 0.25 per cent triamcinolone cream or 0.025 per cent 17-valerate of betamethasone in a cream base. The addition of 1 to 3 per cent iodochlorhydroxyquino-

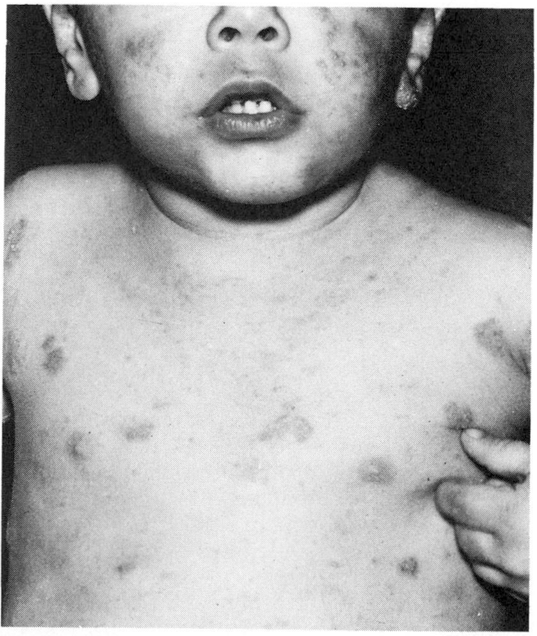

Figure 23–34 Nummular eczema in a 15 month old child, showing scattered, pruritic, patchy, eczematous lesions.

line (Vioform) to the steroid cream may enhance its effectiveness. Antihistamines are of doubtful value, but some phenothiazines (such as promethazine [Phenergan] 6.25 to 12.5 mg 3 to 4 times a day) may help to control itching.

DRUG ALLERGY. Drug allergy may be caused by diverse organic and inorganic substances which form conjugates with body protein and in this form act as allergens, producing a reaction of hypersensitivity. Such reactions may occur in breast-fed infants from maternally administered drugs. The underlying factors which determine the capacity to become sensitized are unknown. Children who have inherited the atopic diathesis may be expected to have allergic reactions more frequently than others.

The histopathology of skin changes in drug allergy is not specific for individual drugs. Changes include endothelial swelling of the dermal blood vessels and a perivascular infiltrate of eosinophils, histiocytes and lymphocytes. The epidermal changes may be minimal or profound, with subepithelial blister formation.

The morphology of the eruption varies greatly and may be that of practically any type characterized by sudden onset. Of the drugs used in pediatric practice, penicillin is most likely to produce an urticarial or erythema multiforme type of reaction; sulfonamides, novobiocin and barbiturates are apt to produce a maculopapular eruption; aspirin, most likely to produce angioneurotic edema of the face; phenothiazine derivatives and tetracyclines (Declomycin), to give photosensitivity reactions (see below).

In diagnosis, the history and biopsy may be helpful.

The only satisfactory treatment is elimination of the drug; depending upon the severity of the reaction, this may be sufficient. The antihistaminic drugs are useful for relief of itching and for suppression of urticaria. Corticosteroids should be given in full therapeutic dosage for any severe generalized eruption. In widespread bullous involvement antibiotic therapy is indicated; previously administered ones, however, should not be selected. Local therapy in blistering reactions should include a wide spectrum antibiotic ointment to prevent secondary bacterial infection.

ABNORMAL RESPONSES OF SKIN TO ULTRAVIOLET LIGHT

Exposure of the skin for a sufficient time to the ultraviolet portion of the spectrum (296 to 400 nm) may produce a normal sunburn reaction or an abnormal cutaneous response. The normal response following exposure to sunlight consists of immediate pigmentation, produced mostly by the longer wavelengths of ultraviolet. After a latent period of about 8 hours the wavelengths around 300 to 320 nm produce the erythema of sunburn, followed in several days by the pigmentation of delayed melanogenesis. After repeated exposures epidermal thickening, compacted stratum corneum and hyperpigmentation occur.

TABLE 23–4 ABNORMAL RESPONSES OF SKIN TO ULTRAVIOLET LIGHT

I. Abnormal responses of skin to ultraviolet light
  A. Ultraviolet rays of wavelengths 280–320 mμ
    1. Recurrent summer eruptions
      a. Polymorphic light eruptions
      b. Hydroa vacciniforme
    2. Xeroderma pigmentosum
  B. Ultraviolet rays primarily of wavelengths longer than 320 mμ
    1. Erythropoietic protoporphyria
    2. Cockayne syndrome
    3. Urticaria solare
    4. Hartnup's disease
II. Abnormal responses of skin to ultraviolet rays in conjunction with photoactive substances
  A. Substances administered systemically
    1. Sulfonamides
    2. Barbiturates
    3. Phenothiazine derivatives (chlorpromazine, Phenergan)
    4. Tetracyclines (Declomycin)
  B. Substances applied locally
    1. Furocoumarins (lime, parsley, parsnips, figs)
    2. Berloque (perfumes)
    3. Halogenated salicylanilides (soap)
III. Skin diseases flared by ultraviolet exposure
  A. Lupus erythematosus
  B. Pellagra

Abnormal cutaneous responses to ultraviolet (Table 23–4) are characterized by morphologic changes ranging from urticarial to eczematous reactions. These untoward cutaneous reactions may depend upon unknown factors (polymorphic light eruption), upon metabolic abnormalities (porphyrins, tryptophan), upon the ingestion or local application of photoactive agents such as phenothiazines, tetracyclines and halogenated salicylanilides, or upon specific reactivity to ultraviolet exposure in some diseases (lupus erythematosus).

POLYMORPHIC LIGHT ERUPTION. This is a recurrent erythematous dermatitis of unknown origin which appears on areas of the skin exposed to light in March or April in the north temperate zone and disappears spontaneously in August or September. The eruption is usually preceded by burning and itching shortly after exposure. Within hours pruritic, erythematous, urticaria-like papules appear on the exposed areas of the face, arms and hands. Subsequently the papules become confluent, forming relatively persistent plaques (Fig. 23–35). Less commonly, eczematous patches with vesiculation appear as a morphologic variant. Tanning proceeds normally, and the skin returns to normal during the winter.

In differential diagnosis, lupus erythematosus, Hartnup disease and the porphyrias must be distinguished.

Therapy consists of the prophylactic use of sunscreens, such as 10 to 15 per cent PABA in hydrophilic ointment or red veterinary petrolatum with titanium dioxide (RV Paque). (See Protective Effect, below.) The antimalarial drugs such as chloroquine or hydroxychloroquine (Plaquenil) are

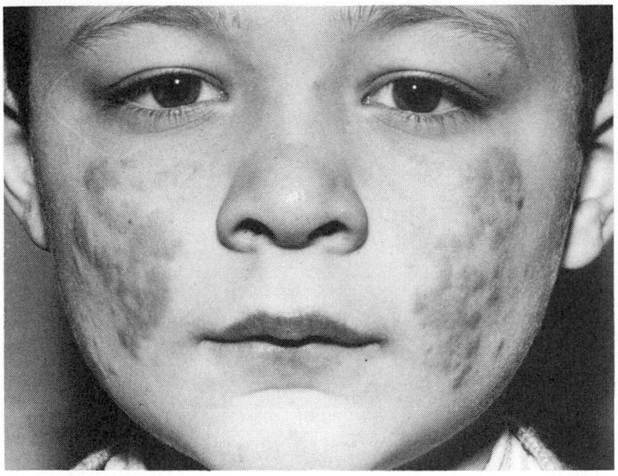

Figure 23–35 *Polymorphic light eruption in 8 year old boy simulating lupus erythematosus; lesions characteristically flared with ultraviolet exposure in early summer and cleared in late summer.*

useful in treatment. Careful control is necessary because of the danger of drug toxicity. If the antimalarial drugs are used, ophthalmologic examination should precede treatment, and evaluation at three-month intervals should be done because of the dangers of ocular toxicity.

THE PORPHYRIAS. (See also Section 8.) The porphyrias are a heterogeneous group of diseases characterized by the excretion either of porphyrins or of porphyrin precursors in the urine or stools.

Congenital Porphyria. This is an extremely rare disorder of porphyrin metabolism characterized by blister formation on areas of skin exposed to light and the excretion of very large amounts of coproporphyrin and uroporphyrin. Hemolytic anemia and red teeth are usually present. Transmission is probably autosomal recessive.

Erythropoietic Protoporphyria. This is a relatively uncommon abnormality of porphyrin metabolism characterized by photosensitivity in childhood, abnormal excretion of porphyrins in urine, and slightly elevated fecal excretion of protoporphyrins. The skin changes include erythema, edema and itching of the exposed parts of the skin following brief exposure to sunlight. The reaction may be precipitated through window glass.

Hydroa Aestivale and **Hydroa Vacciniforme.** These are photosensitive disturbances associated in most instances with erythropoietic protoporphyria. The aestivale variety consists of polymorphic skin lesions; the vacciniforme variety has been associated with blister formation and scarring. Histologically the lesions resemble those of erythrocytic protoporphyria and consist of necrosis of the epidermis and adjacent dermis, with surrounding edema and a diffuse perivascular inflammatory infiltrate. Summer prurigo of Hutchinson may be differentiated by normal porphyrins. The variations in the results of monochromatic exposures to light suggest that these patients do not represent a homogenous group.

Treatment consists of the avoidance of direct sunlight and of the prophylactic use of sunscreens which eliminate all ultraviolet (benzophenones and para-aminobenzoic acid).

HARTNUP DISEASE. (See also Section 8.) This photosensitive skin reaction is caused by an abnormality in tryptophan metabolism transmitted as an autosomal recessive trait. The cutaneous picture resembles pellagra. Oral nicotinamide treatment is beneficial.

COCKAYNE SYNDROME. This syndrome is characterized by a photosensitive dermatitis, dwarfism, musculoskeletal anomalies, intracranial calcifications, hepatosplenomegaly, senile facies and ophthalmologic abnormalities. Neurologic defects appear during the second year of life. The photosensitivity of the skin is marked by erythema, scaling and crusting, followed by hyperpigmentation and scarring.

In differential diagnosis, progeria, Bloom syndrome, Rothmund-Thomson syndrome, ataxia-telangiectasia and dyskeratosis congenita should be considered. Photosensitivity of the skin is a useful differential diagnostic point, for ultraviolet sensitivity is not found in progeria, is rare in dyskeratosis congenita, occurs occasionally in the Rothmund-Thomson syndrome, and is expected in Bloom syndrome and ataxia-telangiectasia.

BLOOM SYNDROME. This is a heritable dermatosis characterized by telangiectatic erythema of the face, photosensitivity, small stature and a low birth weight for gestational age. The differential diagnosis includes such diseases as might be confused with Cockayne syndrome.

POIKILODERMA CONGENITA. Rothmund-Thomson syndrome is a rare hereditary dermatosis characterized by an initial inflammatory reaction followed by telangiectases, pigmentation and atrophy and, in some instances, alteration of hair growth, juvenile cataracts, congenital bone defects and photosensitivity. The syndrome is probably transmitted as a recessive trait.

Skin changes may be present at birth, but generally erythema and edema of the face appear during the first six months of life. Soon the extensor and later the flexural surfaces of the extremities and the buttocks become involved. The process progresses slowly, and by the fifth year the erythematous phase subsides, leaving punctate areas of atrophy, telangiectasia and hyperpigmentation. Many patients have absent or sparse eyebrows and eyelashes as well as areas of alopecia or diminished hair on the scalp.

No treatment is known to be effective.

XERODERMA PIGMENTOSUM. Malignant freckles is a rare, hereditary skin disease of the early years of life and is the result of defective repair replication of the DNA molecule. It is characterized by large freckles, areas of cutaneous atrophy, keratoses, photophobia and conjunctivitis. Multiple skin cancers develop, which lead to early death. The disease is inherited in a simple recessive manner. Relatives of affected children frequently have a tendency to intense freckling.

Histopathologically atrophy alternates with acanthosis and hyperkeratosis. Much melanin is deposited in the basal cell layer, with basophilic degeneration of the collagen, disappearance of the elastic fibers and thinning of the dermis. The capillaries are relatively few; large venules are common. The earliest symptom is photophobia. Erythema of the conjunctiva occurs on the first exposure of the infant to direct sunlight and recurs on subsequent exposures. Erythema of the skin exposed to direct sunlight is rapidly followed by intense freckling. After a few months or years, telangiectases and atrophy appear in the freckled areas; warty, hard keratoses and multiple malignant skin tumors follow shortly. The tumors may be squamous cell carcinomas, sarcomas, basal cell carcinomas and even melanomas; death usually occurs in the adolescent years.

Therapy consists of protection from ultraviolet light and removal of malignant neoplasms when they appear. The prognosis is poor.

PAPULOSQUAMOUS ERUPTIONS

PITYRIASIS ROSEA. Pityriasis is an acute, self-limited disease, probably infectious in origin. It is characterized by the appearance of pinkish, oval scaling lesions distributed mostly on the trunk. Histopathologically there is a nonspecific dermatitic reaction consisting of intercellular edema, exocytosis and a perivascular inflammatory infiltrate of lymphocytes, histiocytes and occasional polymorphonuclear leukocytes and plasma cells.

In the majority of instances the first sign is a solitary, erythematous papule on the trunk which enlarges peripherally and clears centrally (the herald lesion) (Fig. 23–36). Occasionally there is a mild prodrome of headache, malaise, pharyngitis and lymphadenitis. Within five to 14 days an erythematous eruption similar to the original lesion, except that the macules are smaller and follow the lines of skin cleavage, appears both on the trunk and on proximal portions of the arms and legs. In some instances the morphology of the eruption may be predominantly papulovesicular. The disease is rare in the first year of life.

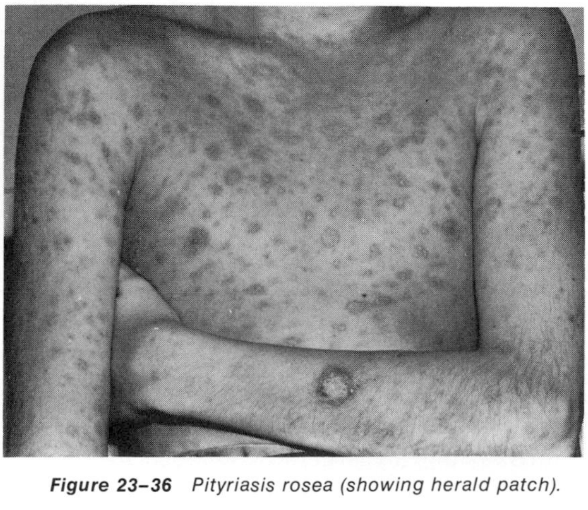

Figure 23–36 *Pityriasis rosea (showing herald patch).*

In differential diagnosis the primary lesion must be differentiated from tinea corporis; the scaling lesion, from guttate psoriasis and seborrheic dermatitis; and the papulovesicular eruption, from nummular eczema.

Treatment is symptomatic in mild cases and consists of a local application of a cream containing solution of coal tar (10 per cent) and salicylic acid (2 per cent) or an anti-inflammatory cream of 0.5 per cent hydrocortisone. In addition, an erythema-producing dose of ultraviolet seems to have an ameliorating effect.

In children with severe pruritus and extensive eruptions, oral administration of a corticosteroid for five to seven days is occasionally justified.

PSORIASIS. Psoriasis is a chronic, recurrent disease of unknown origin transmitted as an autosomal, irregularly dominant trait and characterized by sharply circumscribed scaly patches. The histopathologic picture characteristically reveals parakeratosis, a diminished or absent granular layer, acanthosis, papillomatosis with thinned suprapapillary plate, mild perivascular infiltrate and microabscesses in the epidermis. On the other hand, morphologically characteristic skin lesions frequently have a nonspecific dermatitic reaction.

Psoriasis is not common in children under 6 years of age and in comparison with the disease in adults is usually atypical in its morphology and course. Evidence of the disease is often limited to single or multiple sharply circumscribed, erythematous, scaling patches on the scalp or to fine, pitted stippling of all or most of the nails, without skin changes (Fig. 23–37). At times an erythematous papular eruption appears suddenly and becomes scaly within seven to 14 days. In many instances the eruption is transient and clears completely, leaving only the suspicion that it was psoriasis; sooner or later the typical changes seen in adults appear, which consist of chronic circumscribed patches with a micaceous scale.

The lesions must be differentiated from those of pityriasis rosea, seborrhea, secondary syphilis and drug eruptions; in addition, the scalp lesion must be distinguished from seborrhea and tinea capitis.

Response in young children is usually prompt to treatment with 5 to 10 per cent solution of coal tar and 2 per cent salicylic acid in hydrophilic ointment. Intertriginous involvement responds promptly to an anti-inflammatory cream (0.025 per cent triamcinolone), owing to the ease of percutaneous absorption in this anatomic area. Scalp lesions may be treated with 2 to 4 per cent salicylic acid ointment or 10 per cent solution of coal tar in olive oil, or the 17-valerate of betamethasone (Valisone) in a cream base may be effective. Recalcitrant patches may be managed with 20 per cent oil of cade, 10 per cent sulfur and 5 per cent salicylic acid in petrolatum.

PITYRIASIS ALBA. This is a chronic, slightly inflammatory disease of unknown origin which is characterized by patchy scaling and hypopigmentation on the face.

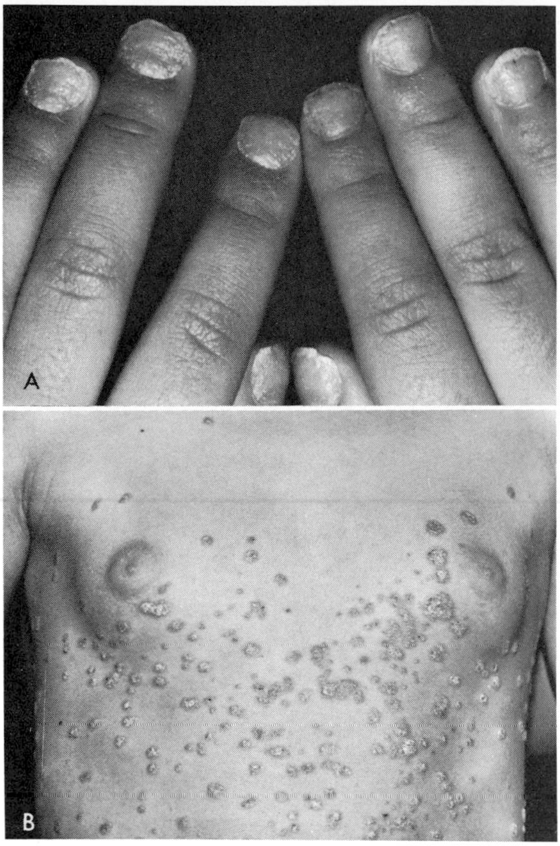

Figure 23–37 A, *Psoriasis of the nails, showing characteristic pits in all nails. The skin was clear, but psoriatic skin lesions appeared later.* B, *Psoriasis of 3 weeks' duration in an 11 year old child, showing erythematous, scaling papules.*

Histopathologically the changes are mild and consist of parakeratosis, acanthosis and spongiosis and a predominantly lymphocytic perivascular infiltrate in the upper corium.

There may be one or more sharply circumscribed, slightly erythematous, scaling hypopigmented patches on the cheeks, chin and forehead. Untreated lesions persist for many months; there are no symptoms.

Differential diagnosis includes vitiligo and postinflammatory depigmentation.

Regression can be produced by a variety of local therapeutic preparations such as 2 per cent salicylic acid in hydrophilic petrolatum, a broad spectrum antibiotic such as Neosporin or perhaps most effectively by an anti-inflammatory agent (0.5 per cent hydrocortisone).

LICHEN STRIATUS. Lichen striatus is an asymptomatic inflammatory eruption of unknown origin occurring principally in children. It is characterized by rapid appearance, usually on the extremities, of a nonsegmental linear papular eruption.

The histopathologic changes are not characteristic; there are perivascular inflammatory infiltrate, intercellular edema in the prickle layer and some hyperkeratosis.

Initially the eruption consists of discrete, erythematous, lichenoid papules in linear patterns. These rapidly coalesce to form a scaly dermatitic reaction (Fig. 23–38). The eruption usually regresses spontaneously though it may occasionally persist for a long time. Linear ectodermal nevus, the lesions of lichen planus, psoriasis and verruca occurring at sites of trauma (as in a scratch) should be differentiated.

Resolution of the lesion can be hastened by local application of 0.05 per cent triamcinolone cream beneath a plastic covering.

LICHEN NITIDUS. This is an inflammatory disease of unknown origin characterized by an asymptomatic papular eruption on the flexor surfaces of the wrists, elbows, hands, genitalia or abdomen.

Histopathologically the infiltrate consists of lymphocytes, epithelioid cells and occasional giant cells limited to papillary and subpapillary areas of the dermis.

The papules are pinhead in size, slightly raised, slightly erythematous or waxy and semitranslucent, suggestive of deep-seated vesicles. They do not coalesce. The lesions usually remain localized, but they may be widely distributed and may occur along scratch marks.

In differential diagnosis flat warts and lichen scrofulosus should be distinguished.

FUNGUS INFECTIONS

The dermatomycoses are caused by highly specialized fungi, the dermatophytes. In their para-

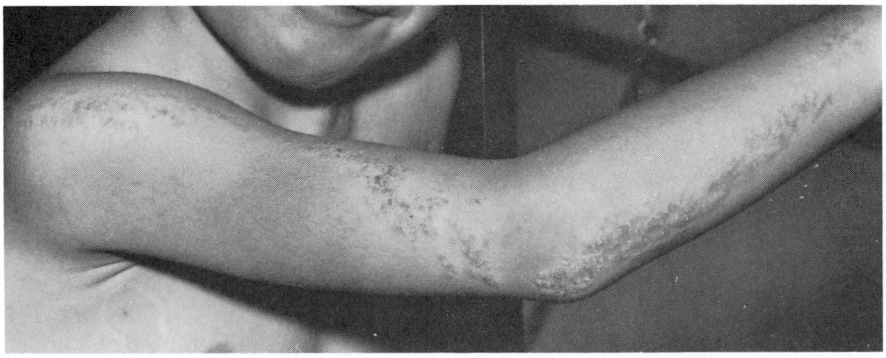

Figure 23–38 *Lichen striatus in a $2\frac{1}{2}$ year old boy, showing the range of morphologic variation from lichenoid papules proximally to confluent eczematous patches distally.*

sitic phase their growth is restricted to the keratinized structures. In children these organisms produce morphologically distinct diseases of the skin, mucous membranes and dermal appendages.

Tinea Capitis (Ringworm of the Scalp)

ETIOLOGY. Tinea capitis is caused by species of the genera Microsporum and Trichophyton. The source of infection varies: *M. audouini, T. tonsurans, T. violaceum, T. sulfureum* and *T. schoenleini* are transmitted from person to person; *M. canis, T. mentagrophytes* and *T. verrucosum* are contracted principally from animals; *M. gypseum* is acquired from soil. In the United States most epidemics are caused by *M. audouini.*

CLINICAL MANIFESTATIONS. The clinical lesion varies from scaly, circumscribed patches resembling seborrhea to patchy, scaling areas of alopecia with broken hairs (Fig. 23–39). Generally the infection is asymptomatic, but a severe inflammatory reaction may occur (kerion), which represents hypersensitivity of the host to the invading organism. *Trichophyton schoenleini* infection produces a specific type of host response (favus) characterized by a peculiar mousey odor and cup-shaped, yellowish brown crusts (scutula); it produces scarring and permanent alopecia.

DIAGNOSIS. Examination of the scalp with a Wood's light (which emits monochromatic ultraviolet [365 nm]) is a rapid, useful method for screening children with suspected infection. Only *M. audouini* and *M. canis* infections respond with typical greenish white fluorescence. Hairs infected by *T. schoenleini* produce variable fluorescence, whereas other trichophyton infections are not fluorescent. Falsely positive or falsely negative fluorescence of hairs may result from the use of local medications. Direct microscopic examination of affected hairs in a 10 per cent solution of potassium hydroxide or in chlorolactophenol is necessary for positive diagnosis; culture is required for identification of species.

Alopecia areata, trichotillomania, monilethrix and loss of hair from inflammatory lesions must be considered in differential diagnosis.

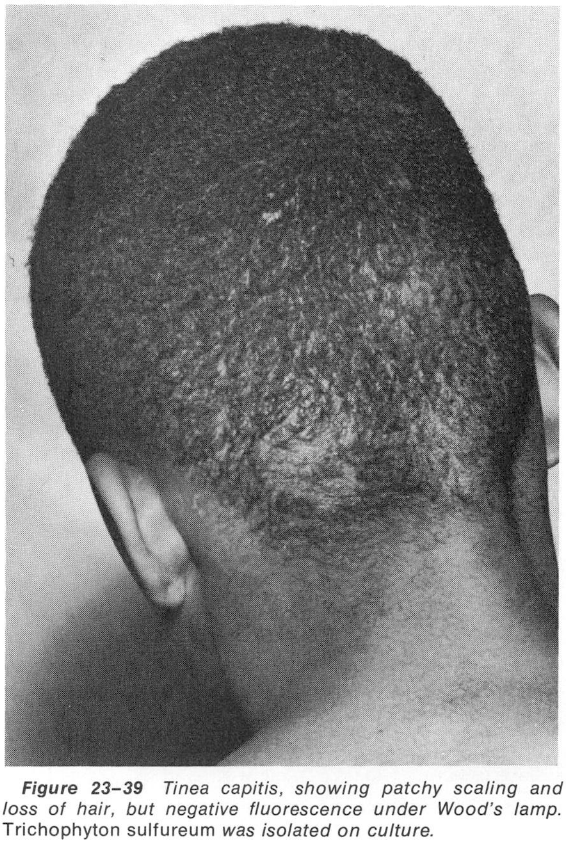

Figure 23–39 Tinea capitis, showing patchy scaling and loss of hair, but negative fluorescence under Wood's lamp. Trichophyton sulfureum *was isolated on culture.*

PREVENTION. Transmission of infection from person to person (*M. audouini* and Trichophyton species) is possible for the duration of the disease. Fortunately there are significant host factors which do not permit easy infection of contacts.

TREATMENT. Oral administration of griseofulvin has revolutionized the treatment of infections of the scalp by all species of dermatophytes. A dose of 20 mg/kg/day (10 mg/lb/day) for 7 to 10 days results in cure in the majority of instances. The dose may rarely need to be doubled or quadrupled.

Local therapy is probably not necessary, but the application of a strong antifungal ointment such as Whitfield's ointment, U.S.P. XVIII (12 per cent benzoic acid and 6 per cent salicylic acid), is advisable. Criteria for cure should include a negative direct microscopic examination and a negative culture. Fluorescence alone is unreliable as a criterion of cure, since some fluorescence may be lasting even in the absence of demonstrable mycelia.

Tinea Corporis

Infection on the skin is caused by species of genera Trichophyton, Microsporum and Epidermophyton through close contact with infected animals or human beings. Generally the lesion is a round or oval, erythematous scaling patch which spreads peripherally and clears centrally. The spreading border is rather intensely inflamed and may become vesiculated (Fig. 23–40).

A direct microscopic examination of scales from the periphery of a lesion will serve to differentiate the fungus infection from pityriasis rosea, nummular eczema, pityriasis alba, psoriasis and seborrheic dermatitis. The scalp should always be examined for evidence of infection when the glabrous skin is infected.

TREATMENT. The local treatment of choice is Whitfield's ointment, U.S.P. XVIII (6 per cent benzoic acid and 3 per cent salicylic acid). If local treatment fails, griseofulvin in a daily dose of 20 mg/kg (10 mg/lb) for 10 to 14 days in combination with local therapy will usually clear the infection.

Tinea Cruris

Infection of the skin in the genitocrural region is rare in the preadolescent; it is most frequently caused by *E. floccosum* and *T. rubrum.* The re-

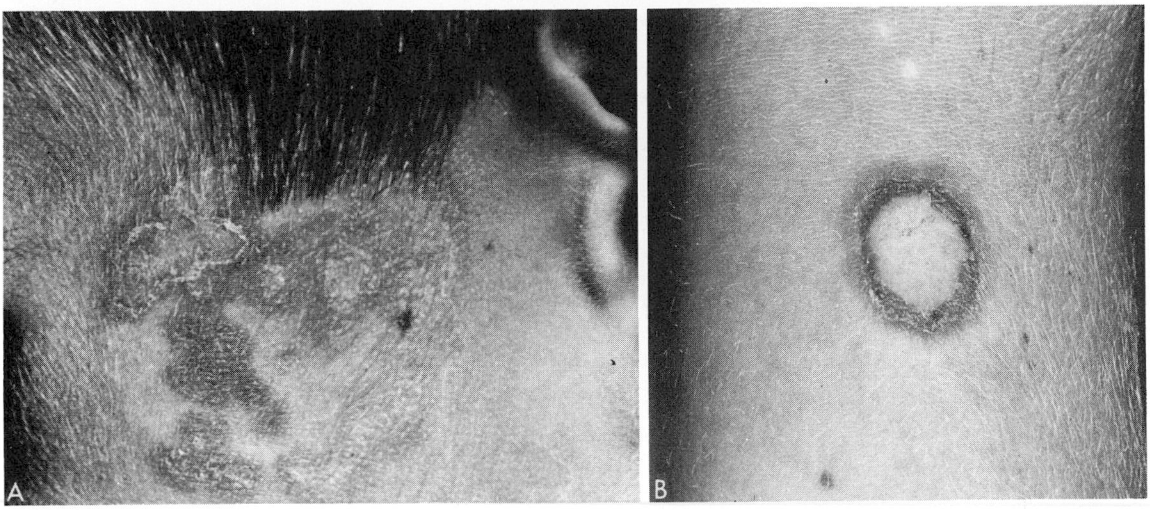

Figure 23–40 *Tinea corporis.* A, M. audouini *infection of skin in 5 year old boy who also had a patch of fluorescent hairs on the scalp which were demonstrated under the Wood's lamp.* B, T. granulosum *infection from pet mice on forearm of 6 year old boy, showing vesicles at border.*

sponse of the skin to the invading organism is similar to that to *T. corporis,* with central clearing and peripheral spreading. The infection remains localized, however, to the medial proximal aspect of the thigh and crural fold, but the skin of the scrotum may be involved in males. The intertriginous area should also be examined for evidence of infection. In differential diagnosis seborrheic psoriasis, seborrheic dermatitis and localized neurodermatitis should be considered.

The infection will in most instances respond promptly to an oil-in-water base (hydrophilic ointment, U.S.P. XVIII) containing 2 per cent salicylic acid and 5 per cent benzoic acid.

Tinea Pedis (Athlete's Foot)

Infection of the intertriginous areas between the toes or on the plantar surface of the feet is usually caused by *E. floccosum, T. rubrum* and *T. interdigitale.*

Although infection occurs most frequently in adolescents and adults, dermatophytic infections occasionally occur in preadolescent children. The lesions may vary from maceration and fissuring between the toes to patches with pinhead-sized vesicles on the plantar surface.

Candidiasis and nocardiosis (erythrasma) between the toes may produce lesions indistinguishable from those of tinea infections. A direct microscopic examination of scrapings will serve to differentiate them. Tissue infected with Nocardia will characteristically produce a coral red fluorescence when examined under Wood's lamp.

Local treatment of choice is Whitfield's ointment, U.S.P. XVIII. Therapy with griseofulvin has not been very effective in chronic recurrent fungal infections between the toes.

Tinea Versicolor

Tinea versicolor is a benign, chronic superficial fungus infection caused by *Malassezia furfur.* It is common and world-wide, occurring most frequently in adults in temperate climates, but with frequency in younger age groups in the tropics. Pathologically there are abundant short blunt mycelia and spores in the horny layer of the skin. The clinical picture is characterized by pigmented or hypopigmented maculopapular spots, patches or large confluent areas (Fig. 23–41), with an inapparent scale which may be easily demonstrated by light scratching. Infection occurs most frequently on the trunk, but may also appear on the neck, face and proximal portions of the arms and legs. In infants there is a tendency to involvement of the face and diaper areas. The epidemiology of the infection is not completely understood, but there is a familial susceptibility, enhanced by glucocorticoid hormones (in Cushing's disease or iatrogenic hyperadrenal states). In differential diagnosis, localization of the infection to the face may suggest pityriasis alba, vitiligo or seborrheic dermatitis, from which it can usually be distinguished by the

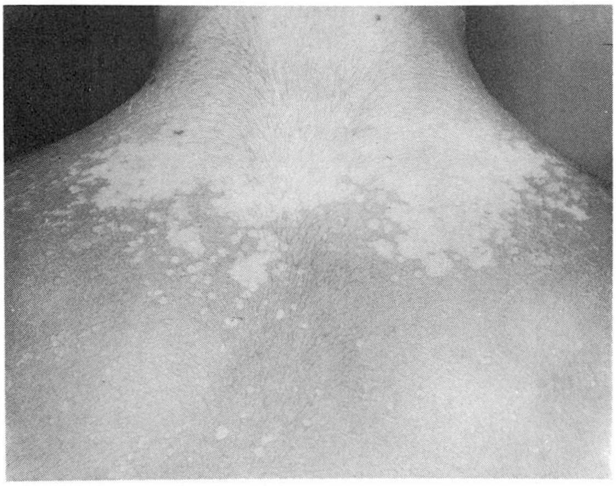

Figure 23–41 *Tinea versicolor in an 11 year old boy, showing discrete and confluent, hypopigmented areas. The patient's father had a similar infection.*

presence of organisms on the direct microscopic examination of a scale in potassium hydroxide.

Almost any mild antifungal preparation is effective in the management of the infection, but recurrence is common. A preparation of 2 per cent salicylic acid and 5 per cent benzoic acid in 20 per cent distilled water in hydrophilic ointment, U.S.P. XVIII, applied once or twice daily, is effective. A suspension of selenium sulfide (Selsun) applied in a thin layer after bathing is also effective, but this preparation should not be applied in the anogenital region because of the likelihood of irritation.

Candidiasis (Moniliasis)

A yeast-like fungus which can be recovered from the intestinal tract and mucous membranes of normal persons may cause infection of the mouth (thrush), nails (paronychia), vagina and intertriginous areas and, occasionally, systemic infection. Oral thrush is relatively common in newborn infants, including otherwise healthy ones. After this age moniliasis is practically nonexistent in healthy persons. Infections are usually caused by *Candida albicans,* but may be produced by *C. tropicalis, C. stellatoidea, C. paropsilosis* and *C. guilliermondii.* In children with debilitating disease (hypoparathyroidism, hypoadrenalism, acrodermatitis chronica enteropathica, immunologic incompetence, Letterer-Siwe disease) such infections may be widespread and persistent.

Intertriginous moniliasis involving the genitocrural fold, gluteal fold, axillae and umbilicus is characterized by a sharply circumscribed, erythematous, moist surface with scattered, superficial satellite pustules. The infection is most frequently confused with a pyoderma because of the pustules, but organisms can be differentiated easily on direct microscopic examination or by culture on Sabouraud's medium. The infection can usually be cleared rapidly by sponging the area with 1:5000 benzalkonium chloride (U.S.P.) three times a day followed by local application of a cream containing nystatin (Mycolog) or amphotericin B (Fungizone).

PARONYCHIAL INFECTION. This is characterized by erythema and swelling of the paronychial area and horizontal ridging of the nails after the infection has been established for several months. It is seen most frequently on the thumbs of infants and children who are finger-suckers. Paronychial infection due to yeast must be differentiated from infection due to staphylococci. The infection is best treated by soaking the involved fingers in 1:5000 benzalkonium chloride, to be followed by application of 2 per cent salicylic acid in a 30 per cent alcohol solution. In order to cure infection of the thumb, it should be protected from being sucked.

In widespread cutaneous infection accompanying underlying systemic disease, the infection does not remain localized to the intertriginous areas or mucous membranes, but spreads over the trunk, face, scalp and extremities (Fig. 23–42). The cutaneous lesions may be sharply demarcated or confluent, forming hyperkeratotic scaling patches which may resemble dermatophytic infections. Unless the underlying disease can be controlled, treatment of the cutaneous infection is not curative, but will diminish the severity of the infection. Local treatment with an antimonilial agent (amphotericin B or nystatin) is usually the most effective treatment.

MONILIAL GRANULOMA. This is an unusual response to yeast infection which occurs usually in infancy or early childhood. In contrast to the usual superficial invasion of the skin, the inflammatory process extends into the corium. The oral mucosa, face, scalp, nails and paronychial areas are usually involved. The initial lesion is an inflammatory papule covered by an adherent, yellowish brown crust surrounded by erythema. These papules become hornlike plaques which, on removal, leave bleeding granulation.

VIRAL INFECTIONS

WARTS. Warts are small benign tumors of the skin or adjoining mucous membrane; they occur predominantly during the preschool and adolescent periods. They are caused by a specific viral agent, about 50 $m\mu$ in diameter, which grows within the nucleus of epithelial cells and produces hyperplasia. The elementary body is indistinguishable from that of polyoma virus morphologically, but there does not appear to be an antigenic relationship. Warts have been classified according to morphology and location of the tumor, but it appears they are all produced by the same agent.

Histopathologically there are acanthosis and hyperkeratosis; the proliferation of the prickle cell layer is accentuated in the central part of the tumor. With special staining for deoxyribonucleic acid and by diligent search, specific intranuclear inclusions can be found.

Common Warts. Common warts are raised circinate lesions with a pitted, keratinized surface and a semitranslucent base, measuring 3 to 10 mm in diameter. Thrombosed capillary tufts are frequently seen as black pinpoint spots. They are commonly situated on the fingers and dorsa of the hands, but may appear anywhere on the glabrous skin.

Plantar Warts. Plantar warts are, as the result of pressure, practically flat. They are often painful on weight bearing and may be inapparent because of an overlying callosity. If the callus is carefully pared away, the features of the common wart are observed. Early lesions may resemble deep-seated vesicles. Multiple warts are not uncommon and may be grouped to create a mosaic pattern.

Flat Warts. Flat warts appear as small (1 to 6 mm), flat, flesh-colored papules on the dorsa of the hands and on the face. They have a tendency to appear in a linear distribution at the sites of scratches.

Filiform Warts. These are single fine projections (5 to 10 mm in length) with keratinized tips

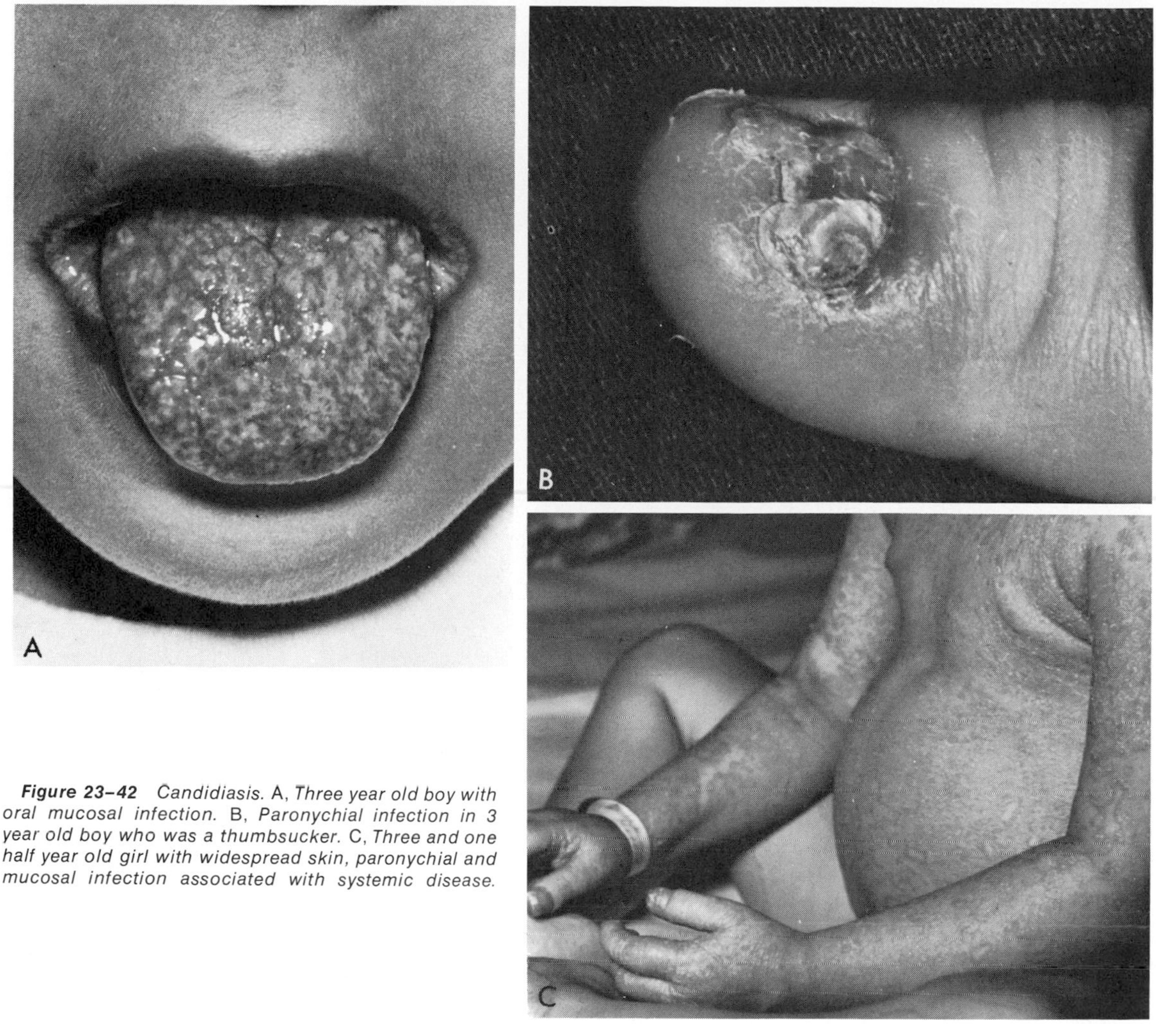

Figure 23–42 Candidiasis. A, Three year old boy with oral mucosal infection. B, Paronychial infection in 3 year old boy who was a thumbsucker. C, Three and one half year old girl with widespread skin, paronychial and mucosal infection associated with systemic disease.

and a sessile base. Groups of these single projections are called *digitate warts.* These warts are uncommon in children.

Mucous Membrane Warts. These are usually multiple, frequently confluent, pinkish or flesh-colored, nonkeratinizing, finger-like projections which occur in the moist areas around the anus, genitalia, mouth and, occasionally, the eye. These warts are common in the preschool period.

In differential diagnosis, plantar verruca must be distinguished from a foreign body reaction on the sole of the foot with overlying callosity or from a localized area of abnormal keratinization (inverted corn) with overlying callosity. Lichen planus, lichen nitidus, and the papules of keratosis follicularis on the dorsum of the hands must be distinguished from flat warts.

Treatment of warts is not uniformly successful and depends upon local destruction, and at times apparently upon "suggestion." Treatment must be individualized according to the type and location of the wart and to the experience of the therapist. In preschool and adolescent age groups consideration must be given to the possible effects of painful, emotionally traumatic methods. Some type of therapeutic suggestion is sufficient to produce clearing in 30 to 50 per cent of infections. Cryotherapy (liquid nitrogen) and electrosurgery are locally destructive, nonscarring measures, and in experienced hands are effective in 75 to 85 per cent. Podophyllin, a poison, is the treatment of choice in mucous membrane lesions; careful application of 20 per cent podophyllin in compound tincture of benzoin is necessary to minimize the severe inflammatory reaction produced on the surrounding normal mucous membrane.

MOLLUSCUM CONTAGIOSUM. Molluscum contagiosum is a small benign tumor of the skin which occurs predominantly in the preschool and adolescent periods. It is caused by a specific brick-shaped virus (300 by 220 mμ) which grows within the cytoplasm of epithelial cells.

Histopathologically there is a localized proliferation of the prickle cells which pushes down into the dermis like an inverted mushroom. The cytoplasmic inclusion of molluscum can be identified easily within the epithelial cells of the central portion of the tumor. The skin lesions are characteristically waxy papules varying in size from 2 to 10 mm with a central umbilication; they may be found at any dermal site except on the palms and soles. Spontaneous resolution of papules often occurs in association with an inflammatory reaction which resembles a pustule.

In differential diagnosis flat warts, nonpigmented dermal type nevi, and xanthogranuloma must be distinguished. Expression of the molluscum body by squeezing the papule with opposing fingernails is diagnostic. Treatment is simple and effective; the molluscum body is shelled out by pricking the base with a scalpel (No. 11) or an acne stylet.

PARASITIC DISEASES

Some parasitic infestations of human beings may be limited to the skin; in others cutaneous lesions may be associated with systemic disease. The more common parasitic disorders are described in Section 10.

INSECT BITES. The important role of some of the arthropods in transmission of disease has tended to minimize interest in the cutaneous reaction to the bites of insects. Local reactions may result from bites of many kinds of insects, including mosquitoes, fleas, lice, bedbugs and flies.

The skin reaction to the bite of an insect is due to hypersensitivity and is species-specific. There is little or no reaction in a nonsensitized person, whereas in the sensitized one there may be either an immediate or a delayed reaction or a combination of the two. The characteristic response of the sensitized skin to the bite is the immediate appearance of an evanescent, urticarial type of papule surrounded by an erythematous flare; pruritus is prominent. This reaction usually subsides within an hour and is followed within a few hours by a delayed, more persistent, erythematous, severely pruritic papule.

PAPULAR URTICARIA (LICHEN URTICATUS). This chronic, recurrent, pruritic papulovesicular eruption is caused by sensitization to salivary polypeptides conveyed in the bites of fleas, lice, mites, mosquitoes or bedbugs (Fig. 23–43). The eruption associated with flea bites characteristically appears with a centrifugal distribution during the summer months. The bites from bedbugs are most commonly seen on the ankles, buttocks, knees and shoulders, but may appear on any part of the body.

Histopathologically there are varying degrees of intercellular edema, including vesicle formation, vasodilatation and perivascular infiltration by many eosinophils, histiocytes and lymphocytes in the middle and lower dermis. In chronic lesions there may be a lymphoma-like pattern.

The skin lesion is biphasic; the initial wheal is evanescent and is followed by an extremely pruritic inflammatory papule or papulovesicle. In the patient's efforts to obtain relief from the itch, the papule is excoriated and frequently becomes secondarily infected. Most lesions are on the extremities. In differential diagnosis, pyoderma, varicella, scabies and pediculosis must be distinguished.

Treatment depends on the determination of the source of infestation. One should be aware of the longevity of lice in damp areas. Elimination of fleas from an animal's sleeping quarters can be attained by use of a spray containing phosphorothioate (Dursban). For satisfactory treatment, fleas or bedbugs must be eliminated from the environment. Carpets, cracks and crevices in the floor, overstuffed furniture and bedding may be sprayed with a perimeter spray containing phosphorothioate (Diazinon, Dursban). It may be necessary to have the house fumigated by an experienced exterminator. A dog may be treated effectively with Tritox dip (Pitman-Moore), and cats with a rotenone or pyrethrum powder. Repellents such as 6-12 or Off are useful in protecting the child from bites. Symptomatic relief can be accomplished by use of 0.5 to 1.0 per cent hydrocortisone cream, or its equivalent.

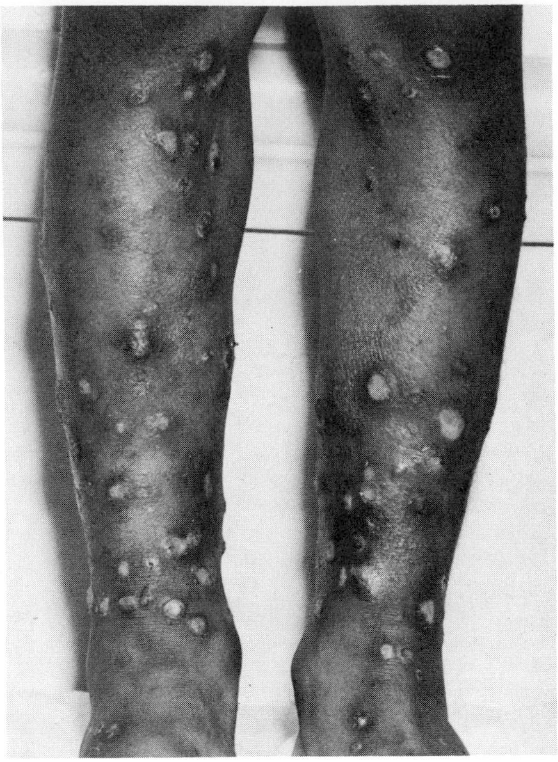

Figure 23–43 Papular urticaria caused by flea sensitivity, with secondary pyoderma (ecthyma).

PEDICULOSIS. Two species of lice produce infestation of the scalp, body and pubic area in man; only pediculosis of the scalp has practical significance in pediatric practice.

Pediculosis capitis is a chronic infestation of the scalp and hair and occasionally of the eyelids by *Pediculus humanus* var. *capitis.* It feeds on blood and perishes within two to three days after removal from the host. As the eggs (nits) hatch, they become glued to the hairs and reach maturity within two to three weeks.

The skin lesions are at first minimal, consisting of slight erythema and a purpuric spot at the site of feeding; repeated exposure results in sensitization, and an inflammatory papule appears at the site of each bite, to be followed by a severe pruritic reaction, secondary infection and occipital and posterior cervical lymphadenopathy. In all instances of pyoderma of the scalp, the possibility should be considered that pediculi are the initiating factor.

Treatment with a 2%-benzyl benzoate-20%-benzocaine emulsion or with gamma benzene hexachloride (Kwell) is effective. One application at night followed by shampoo in the morning is sufficient to produce a cure in most instances. Infection of the eyelids may be successfully treated with an ophthalmologic ointment containing 0.25 per cent physostigmine (Eserine ointment). Examination of the remainder of the family for infestation is essential.

SCABIES. This chronic infestation is caused by burrowing of the impregnated female mite (*Sarcoptes scabiei* var. *hominis*) into the skin. She lays a few eggs each day for several weeks in her burrow; the larvae developing from the ova emerge on the surface as adults; the female becomes impregnated and starts a new cycle. In this invasive process a burrow is formed which appears as a tiny, straight or tortuous linear elevation. As this repetitive process continues, sensitization occurs within a month or so after infestation, with the production of symptoms. After the latent period a pruritic papulovesicular eruption appears, with a striking predisposition for the interdigital spaces, palms, flexural surfaces of the wrists, anterior axillary folds, waistline, areolar area of girls and penis of boys (Fig. 23–44). In infants, vesiculobullous lesions are common, and are frequent on the face and feet.

Histopathologically the mite, ova and feces may be found in a burrow in the stratum corneum. After sensitization there is a mild inflammatory reaction, with intracellular edema and vesicle formation in the prickle cell layer. There are vascular dilatation, perivascular infiltration and edema of the upper portion of the dermis.

Diagnosis may be difficult because the typical lesions are altered by excoriation or secondary infection; it is dependent upon demonstration of a mite from a burrow in the skin.

Treatment by the following plan is effective within 48 hours: a prolonged hot soaking bath is followed by two applications of 15% benzyl benzoate emulsion or Kwell lotion at intervals of 12 hours, and by a second bath 12 hours after the last application. The medicine is applied to the face in infants with facial lesions, but otherwise to the entire skin surface from the neck down. Following this regimen, secondary bacterial infection should be treated with a broad spectrum antibiotic ointment, and 0.5 per cent hydrocortisone cream should be applied to counteract the irritative reaction.

Canine scabies (*Sarcoptes scabiei* var. *canis*) may be transmitted from young dogs to children. The areas involved most commonly are those in contact with infested animals. Mites cannot be demonstrated in the skin, since the female does not burrow into the skin of the unnatural host. Treatment of dog and child is the same as for the human variety of mites.

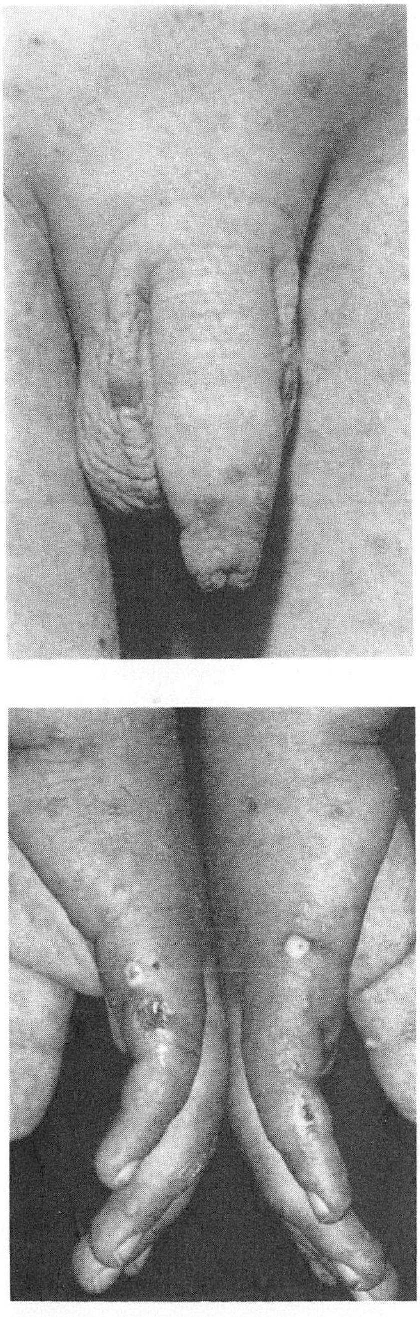

Figure 23–44 Scabies. (From Korting, G. W.: Diseases of the Skin in Children and Adolescents, 1969.)

CREEPING ERUPTION (CUTANEOUS LARVA MIGRANS). This is a distinctive clinical entity caused by the migration of a nematode parasite through the skin. Infestations caused by *Ancylostoma braziliense* (cat hookworm) or *A. caninum* (dog hookworm) occur along the Gulf Coast and the Eastern Seaboard from Virginia to Florida.

The infestation is characterized by the appearance of a pruritic red papule at the point of invasion of the skin. As the larva moves through the upper layers of the epidermis it produces a raised erythematous serpiginous linear lesion (Fig. 10–65); eczematous changes with vesicle formation, scaling and finally complete resolution of the inflammatory process ensue. The infestation may last for months as the parasite meanders through the skin.

The treatment of choice is oral thiabendazole (two doses of 25 mg/kg, one after the evening meal and the other after breakfast the next morning, for 2 to 3 days). Gastric irritation with nausea is a frequent complication.

ACNE VULGARIS

Acne vulgaris is an inflammatory disease of the pilosebaceous unit, with peak incidence in midadolescence. Occasional comedones and inflammatory lesions accompany the emotional, endocrinologic and anatomic changes of adolescence so commonly as to suggest a physiologic rather than a pathologic event. On the other hand, acne is commonly of sufficient severity as to require treatment.

HISTOPATHOLOGY. The relationships between the clinical lesion and the histologic changes are known. The first change observed in the involved pilosebaceous apparatus is a hyperkeratotic thickening of the epithelium of the duct of the sebaceous gland before it joins the follicular canal. It has been proposed that an acnegenic factor in sebum precipitates this change, but neither this nor the alteration of the sebaceous gland duct has been proved to be the initial event in induction of acne. Extension of the keratotic plug to the follicular canal and the skin surface results in the appearance of a comedone. The retention of sebum and a concurrent inflammatory change combine to produce an inflammatory reaction and the papulopustular lesion. Leakage of irritating follicular contents (free fatty acids) into the dermis increases the intensity of the inflammatory reaction. Post-acne scarring is determined by the severity and depth of the inflammatory response: deep and extensive inflammation causes a saucerized scar, whereas local destruction of the pilosebaceous unit results in pitted scars (Fig. 23–45).

ENDOCRINE FACTORS. Endocrine factors have important roles in acne, but the mechanisms of their participation are obscure. Androgenic stimulation at puberty initiates sebaceous gland development. Studies have failed to show differences in hormonal physiology between normal individuals and patients with acne. The absence of acne in castrates and its precipitation by androgens suggest that androgens play a permissive role in preparing the follicular epithelium to react in the presence of an acnegenic agent. Several hormones or hormone-like substances may aggravate acne: ACTH, testosterone, gonadotropins, anabolic agents and corticosteroids (Fig. 23–6). The premenstrual exacerbation of acne in some individuals is not adequately explained, since physiologic levels of progesterone have no effect on sebaceous glands.

SEBACEOUS GLANDS. The association of oily skin and acne is well known. The rate of excretion of sebum by sebaceous glands is higher than normal in patients with acne or those who have had acne, and the degree of seborrhea and the severity of the acne are directly related. These observations and the fact that seborrhea persists after the acne clears suggest that sebum plays a central but not fully defined role in the pathogenesis of acne.

BACTERIOLOGY. Infection by pyogenic organisms is not a primary problem in acne but the normal resident flora is an important factor in pathogenesis. The bacteriology of the acne lesion consists predominantly of resident organisms: *C. acnes* and *S. epidermidis,* alone or in combination. Organisms from patients with acne have been shown to have lipolytic activity (lipase) which converts the lipid mixture secreted by sebaceous glands to free fatty acids. Differences between *C. acnes* and *S. epidermidis* in their ability to split triglycerides of shorter chained fatty acids suggest

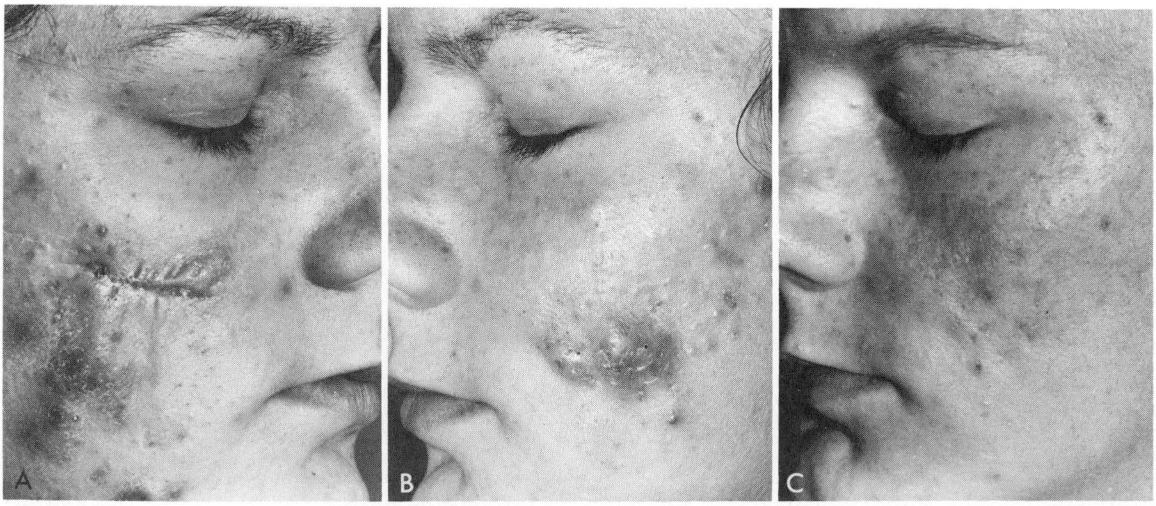

Figure 23–45 *Nodulocystic lesions in 18 year old girl.* A, *Treated by incision and drainage.* B, *Before treating by stilet incision and drainage and intralesional steroids.* C, *After treatment (1 week).*

that *C. acnes* may be of primary importance in the pathogenesis of acne.

These findings may correlate with the clinical observation that some antibiotics cause amelioration of acne; in particular, tetracyclines decrease the concentration of free fatty acids on the skin surface without affecting the concentration of total fatty acids or the rate of sebum secretion. This observation supports the concept that free fatty acids in sebum play a major role in the pathogenesis of acne, inasmuch as they are produced largely by lipolytic activity of the normal bacterial flora.

GENETIC FACTORS. Clinical experience suggests that genetic factors predispose to susceptibility to acne. There is a high degree of concordance in identical twins. The distribution of acne in some families suggests simple dominant transmission, but inheritance is more likely multifactorial.

PROVOCATIVE FACTORS. When appropriate predisposing factors are present, diet, emotions, climate, drugs and external factors provoke the development of acne.

Diet. The role of dietary factors has been greatly exaggerated, but some authorities still believe that carbohydrates and fats in general (and specifically chocolate and nuts), including cola drinks, precipitate exacerbations of acne. Specific foods may occasionally aggravate acne, but proof is lacking that patients with acne respond uniformly to these foods.

Psychologic Factors. Emotional stress plays a minor part in the overall pathogenesis of acne, but in clinical practice many observations of exacerbation of existing acne with emotional stress provide convincing proof of a relationship. A preliminary evaluation of the patient's personality and his attitude toward the acne is made at the first interview. Subsequently, the extent to which emotional stress is influencing the course of the acne can be determined.

Climate. In temperate climates, acne is a year-round problem in many patients, but it regularly worsens during the winter months. Whether this results from lack of exposure to ultraviolet light or from increased adrenocortical activity is not known. In tropical or subtropical areas, the effects of heat and humidity may convert mild or moderate acne into a severe form (tropical acne).

External Factors. Habitual manipulation of the skin by rubbing, squeezing, application of occlusive cosmetics of the pancake type and of hair pomades will aggravate existing acne. Contamination of skin by mineral oil, chlorinated hydrocarbons, crude petroleum and insoluble cutting oils may precipitate acne. Topical corticosteroids applied under an occlusive dressing may aggravate existing acne or precipitate activity in a predisposed individual.

CLINICAL FEATURES. The variation in morphology and course of the pilosebaceous inflammatory reaction in acne is so great that a classification based on the presence of comedones, papulopustules or cystic forms serves no useful purpose. On the other hand, a severe variant (acne conglobata) appearing almost exclusively in males in late adolescence requires consideration. It is a chronic suppurative variant of acne vulgaris characterized by burrowing abscesses, draining sinus tracts and severe scarring. It runs a chronic course and may be associated with systemic signs (temperature elevation and leukocytosis) and systemic symptoms (malaise and arthralgia).

Acne is most severe in the 14 to 17 year age group in girls, and between 16 and 19 years in boys. The incidence and severity decrease rapidly in the second and third decades, though activity may persist into the fourth or fifth decades or exceptionally past the age of 50 years. Rarely, the characteristic lesions of acne appear on the cheeks of infants (acne neonatorum). (See Section 7.) Acne neonatorum is considered a true acne in a highly predisposed individual; these children invariably have recurrences of acne during adolescence.

TREATMENT. Acne in the adolescent should never be dismissed as "part of growing up." At the first interview, it is important to obtain full cooperation of the patient by establishing adequate rapport. The patient should be given a brief, comprehensible explanation of what acne is and of the principles on which treatment is planned. Misinformation regarding causation and significance should be dispelled. The patient must understand that something can be done, but that improvement is slow and that therapy may need careful and continuous attention over a period of months or years. Appropriate and consistent care will greatly ameliorate the severity of acne and lessen the risk of subsequent scarring.

Treatment of acne takes account of its multifactorial pathogenesis. Control of endocrine factors, sebaceous gland activity and the bacterial flora of the sebaceous gland are the desired goals in the systemic, topical and physical management of acne in the following regimen:

1. Cleansing of the face with soap and water on arising, after school and at bedtime. A soap substitute containing sulfur and salicylic acid (Fostex) may be more effective than soap.
2. After each washing, application of a lotion containing sulfur and salicylic acid (Sulforcin, Fostril). The frequency of application depends upon the degree of dryness produced.
3. Ultraviolet (cold quartz or hot quartz) irradiation at weekly intervals to increase peeling of stratum corneum.
4. Removal of comedones and pustular lesions with a comedo extractor. The stylet attached to the extractor is effective in securing drainage of nodulocystic lesions and produces less pain and a better cosmetic result than incision and drainage with a scalpel. After evacuation, infiltration of the lesion with triamcinolone (3.33 mg/ml) produces rapid resolution of the inflammatory nodule (Fig. 23–45).
5. Roentgen therapy will suppress sebaceous gland activity, but it is mentioned only to condemn it. The beneficial effect is transient, and the hazards are significant.
6. Abrasive material incorporated in powder or soap is not necessary.
7. Removal of superficial pitted scars can be accomplished successfully by a variety of plastic planing procedures (sandpaper, stainless steel rotary brush and shaving techniques). These procedures are not recommended during the active phase of the disease and not during adolescence.

In selected patients *systemic therapy* of resistant pustular, nodulocystic acne with antibiotics is justified; the tetracyclines are the drugs of choice, in doses of 250 mg four times a day for 4 days, 250 mg three times a day for 3 days, 250 mg twice a day for a week, and then 250 mg daily as indicated. Although estrogenic hormones will sometimes alter the course of resistant acne in the male, their use is not recommended in the adolescent child. In the girl with severe, uncontrollable premenstrual flare of her acne, treatment with oral estrogen (Premarin) in doses of 0.60 to 1.25 mg per day beginning 7 to 10 days premenstrually and continued until the beginning of menstrual flow may be tried.

PSYCHOCUTANEOUS DISORDERS

Emotional factors are involved in diseases of the cutaneous system to varying degrees. They play a primary role in localized neurodermatitis, trichotillomania and in some instances of chronic urticaria and alopecia areata; and a secondary role in such widespread, chronic, disfiguring diseases of the skin as ichthyosis vulgaris, epidermolysis bullosa or congenital ichthyosiform erythroderma; and collaborative or potentiating roles in atopic dermatitis and psoriasis, wherein the basic problem may be accentuated by triggering emotional factors. Assessment of the role of emotional state is an essential part of the dermatologic management of cutaneous problems. In every instance some psychologic guidance is needed, and in some cases psychiatric therapy may be required.

LOCALIZED NEURODERMATITIS. This chronic, extremely pruritic eruption is characterized by circumscribed patches of various sizes, in which the skin is thickened and the normal skin lines are exaggerated. It occurs infrequently in children. Histologically there is hyperkeratosis with regular thickening of the epithelial layer. There is a mild inflammatory infiltrate in the upper portion of the dermis, and the picture may closely simulate the changes of chronic psoriasis.

Characteristically the disorder begins with intermittent pruritis on the elbows, knees, ankles, or less often at other sites, without any skin changes.

As a result of persistent rubbing and scratching, the characteristic changes appear in the skin.

In differential diagnosis, psoriasis may cause confusion because of the appearance of lesions on elbows or knees. The lesions of localized neurodermatitis may be multiple, but usually only one is present.

When there is persistence or recurrence of localized neurodermatitis, the need for psychiatric help should be considered. In many instances, the lesions and pruritus persist beyond resolution of the emotional stress, owing to changes in the skin. Local treatment is useful and consists of the application of a keratoplastic agent (2 to 10 per cent coal tar) in hydrophilic ointment or 0.05 per cent hydrocortisone cream. In addition, a phenothiazine drug (promethazine) may help to control itching.

ALOPECIA. Alopecia may be classified broadly as (1) scarring, with permanent loss of hair, and (2) nonscarring, with transient loss of hair.

Marginal Alopecia. This is a type of hair loss at the margins of the frontal, temporal and parietal areas of the scalp often caused by the continuous traction of the "pony tail" or tight hair braiding. The hair loss is typically symmetrical, triangular in shape and anterior to and just above the ears. It may, of course, occur anywhere on the scalp, depending on the hairdo.

The process is usually reversible, but if the stress is continued for a long time, the hair follicles may atrophy, and the loss of hair may be permanent.

Alopecia Areata. This is a nonscarring type of baldness in which single or multiple circumscribed patches of hair are suddenly lost from the scalp. Histologically there is a perivascular, inflammatory infiltrate involving the vessels in the lower portion of the corium. The hair bulbs are reduced in size, and the shaft contains keratin. Initially the skin has a slightly erythematous appearance, and there may be scattered broken hairs superficially resembling the stubble seen in trichotillomania. The scalp is primarily involved, but at times the eyebrows, eyelashes and hair on other parts of the body may be lost. The first patch is usually 2 or 3 cm in diameter and may enlarge. Several areas of alopecia may appear simultaneously or consecutively and may become confluent. In rare instances all hair is lost within a few weeks. The alopecia may persist for many months, or there may be prompt regrowth followed by subsequent recurrences. There is a high incidence of emotional aberrations in affected children, and it has been suggested that alopecia areata is a psychocutaneous disturbance.

In differential diagnosis, trichotillomania, tinea capitis and discoid lupus erythematosus must be distinguished.

Treatment. Psychiatric guidance may be indicated. Systemic therapy with a corticosteroid will usually reverse the process, but the effect is usually transient, and the hair falls out again when treatment is discontinued. A more practical method is the intralesional injection of triamcinolone (3.33 mg/ml) in single patches or the continuous application of 0.05 per cent triamcinolone beneath an impervious plastic film cap.

TRICHOTILLOMANIA. Trichotillomania is an emotional disorder in which the hair becomes the target of expression and is either pulled out or twisted off. The scalp is the most frequent site of involvement; less often the eyebrows and pubic hairs may be pulled out. There are usually no subjective symptoms, and the child frequently denies manipulating the hair. The hair loss is usually in a readily accessible area and results in one or more irregular patches of alopecia of variable size (Fig. 23–46). The patchy alopecia is characterized by a "migrating" loss of hair, with an advancing border at one side and the stubble of regrowing hair at the other. The coarse stubble of regrowing hair in the area of involvement is the hallmark of this disturbance. Trichotillomania must be differentiated

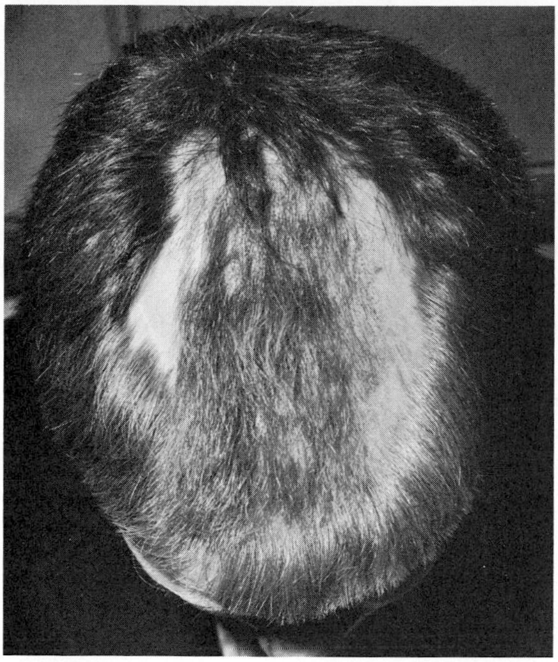

Figure 23–46 Trichotillomania in a 10 year old child, showing typical "migrating" type of hair loss.

from alopecia areata, tinea capitis and patchy hair loss in the occipital area caused by rubbing on the bed, and from that seen in thumb-suckers who simultaneously manipulate the hair gently. Trichotillomania is an indication for psychiatric guidance.

TUMORS OF THE SKIN

Tumors of the skin (see also Section 25) are uncommon in infancy and childhood. Some benign tumors appear clinically and histologically aggressive in childhood, possibly as the result of growth stimulus during this period. In general, such tumors appear less neoplastic with time, as with most hemangiomas and in benign juvenile melanoma, but malignant melanoma or angiosarcoma may rarely occur. Among the uncommon conditions which should be borne in mind are Gardner syndrome, connective tissue tumors, pilomatrixoma, nevoid basal cell carcinoma syndrome and basal cell carcinoma.

GARDNER SYNDROME. (See also Sections 25 and 29.) This is transmitted as an autosomal dominant trait and is characterized by cystic skin lesions, fibrous tissue tumors, multiple polyposis of the colon, osteomatosis and dental anomalies.

NEVOID BASAL CELL CARCINOMA SYNDROME. This may appear early in childhood and is characterized by the appearance of multiple basal cell cancers, palmar and plantar pits, jaw cysts, ectopic calcification and skeletal anomalies. It is transmitted as an autosomal dominant trait. Histologically the skin tumors show the characteristic features of basal cell carcinoma. Clinically they may be flesh-colored or pigmented pearly papules which appear during the first few years and continue to appear throughout life. There is a predilection for the face, head and neck, but many tumors occur also on the trunk, abdomen and extremities. They behave as neoplastic tumors, slowly increasing in size, and finally producing a classic rodent ulcer with bleeding and crusting. Asymptomatic pinhead-sized pits in the palms and soles are a hallmark of the syndrome, but they do not appear until after adolescence. When the tumors appear on the face, they must be differentiated from the periorbital eccrine sweat gland tumors and trichoepithelioma. Treatment of the tumors should be conservative, with electrocoagulation and curettage as the tumors arise. Treatment should be undertaken first in the critical areas around the eyelids.

BASAL CELL CARCINOMA. This is a neoplastic tumor rare in childhood, which may occur occasionally on the face or scalp. Basal cell epitheliomatous degeneration of pre-existing organoid lesions (nevus sebaceus of Jadassohn) is not uncommon. Histologically there is basal cell proliferation and invasion of the dermis by basal cells in nests and cords and with adenoid patterns. The tumor is characterized by a pearly-appearing papule with or without melanin pigment or prominent vascular markings. Pigmented lesions may resemble melanoma; benign juvenile melanoma may also have a semitranslucent appearance and needs to be differentiated.

CONNECTIVE TISSUE TUMORS. See Tumors of Soft Tissues, Section 25.

JUVENILE XANTHOGRANULOMA. Nevoxanthoendothelioma is a transient benign tumor of unknown origin which presents in the first two years of life. The lesions are reddish yellow to brown; they vary in size from papules to nodules and may appear singly, grouped or generalized. There is a predilection for the face, scalp and extremities (Fig. 23–47). Involvement may rarely occur in other tissues such as the eye, pericardium, liver, lung or tonsils.

Histopathologically the epidermis overlying the ill defined infiltrated area is atrophic. The infiltrate may extend to the lower portion of the dermis and consists of lipophagic histiocytes, giant cells and scattered foci of lymphocytes, plasma and eosinophilic cells. These changes represent a benign reactive process involving histiocytic cells which show xanthomatization.

In differential diagnosis the solitary tumors of urticaria pigmentosa and xanthoma should be considered.

Treatment is usually not necessary, but regression may be hastened by infiltration of the lesions with triamcinolone, injectable (5 mg/ml).

PYOGENIC GRANULOMA. Pyogenic granuloma is a rapidly growing vascular tumor which occurs at the site of an injury to the skin and bleeds profusely on slight trauma. The growth is bright red or purplish and may be crusted or moist. It may form a pedunculated or sessile tumor, up to a centimeter or so in diameter.

Histopathologically it consists of newly formed capillaries; there are numerous microorganisms and an infiltrate consisting of mast and plasma

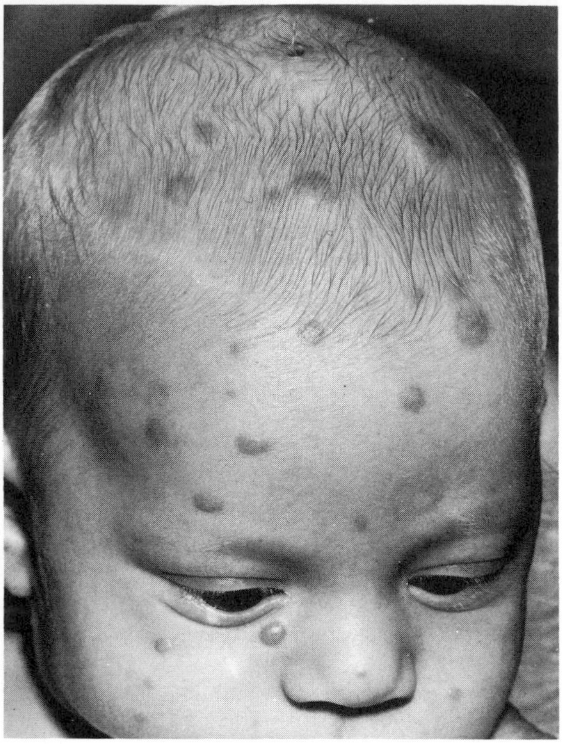

Figure 23-47 Juvenile xanthogranuloma in an infant 10 months of age, with multiple lesions simulating urticaria pigmentosa.

cells and leukocytes and, later, fibroplastic proliferation.

In differential diagnosis, hemangioma, hemangiosarcoma and melanoma must be distinguished.

Surgical excision is not indicated, since removal of the tumor electrosurgically with destruction of its vascular supply will prevent recurrence.

JUVENILE ELASTOMA. Nevus elasticus is a nevus of elastic tissues with onset in childhood and is transmitted as an autosomal dominant trait. Spotty, dense, sclerotic changes (osteopoikilosis) have been reported at the ends of the femora, tibiae and humeri.

Histologically the elastic fibers in the subepidermal region are greatly increased in number and size, but otherwise normal. The skin changes consist of single or multiple, flat, yellowish plaques with a tendency to localization in the lumbosacral area. In differential diagnosis the connective tissue patches (shagreen) of epiloia need to be differentiated.

ADENOMA SEBACEUM. This is the cutaneous expression of tuberous sclerosis (epiloia) (see Section 20), which is characterized clinically by mental deficiency and epilepsy and transmitted as an autosomal dominant trait. Multiple benign tumors may be found in brain and retina (gliomas), heart (rhabdomyomas) and kidneys (angiomyolipomas). Histologically the misnamed papules on the face consist of fibrosis, dilatation of capillaries and atrophy of the sebaceous glands. The skin changes are characterized by the presence of oval hypopigmented macules at birth and the later appearance of skin-colored or yellowish red papules, located primarily on the medial aspects of the cheek and nose (Fig. 23-48); they are frequently associated with telangiectasis. Subungual fibromas frequently develop; thickened connective tissue patches (shagreen) appear by predilection in the lumbosacral area. The course of the disease is variable, depending on the extent of involvement; life span may be shortened. If the papules and patches of adenoma sebaceum are cosmetically disturbing, they can be satisfactorily removed by shaving off the lesions flush with the skin surface and lightly desiccating the base to control bleeding.

CUTANEOUS MENINGIOMAS. These are uncommon, benign, solitary tumors of the skin, probably derived from ectopic arachnoidal cells. The histologic appearance of the tumor is identical to that of intracranial meningiomas, with psammoma bodies scattered through the tumor. Clinically a nondiagnostic, infiltrated, freely movable skin-colored patch is located on the scalp or trunk.

CALCIFYING EPITHELIOMA OF MALHERBE. Pilomatrixoma is a benign, freely movable subcutaneous nodule most commonly found on the face, neck and arms. Histologically there is a circumscribed mass of bands and sheets of epithelial cells in the dermis or in the subcutaneous fat tissue, surrounded by compressed collagen. Keratin may be found in some areas; a high percentage of the tumors undergo calcification and ossification. It is generally accepted that this tumor arises from primitive epidermal germ cells which are differentiating toward hair matrix cells. It is usually single, but two or more may appear during infancy or early adolescence. They usually remain asymptomatic, but occasionally become inflamed. They are most frequently confused clinically with keratin cysts. Surgical excision is the treatment of choice.

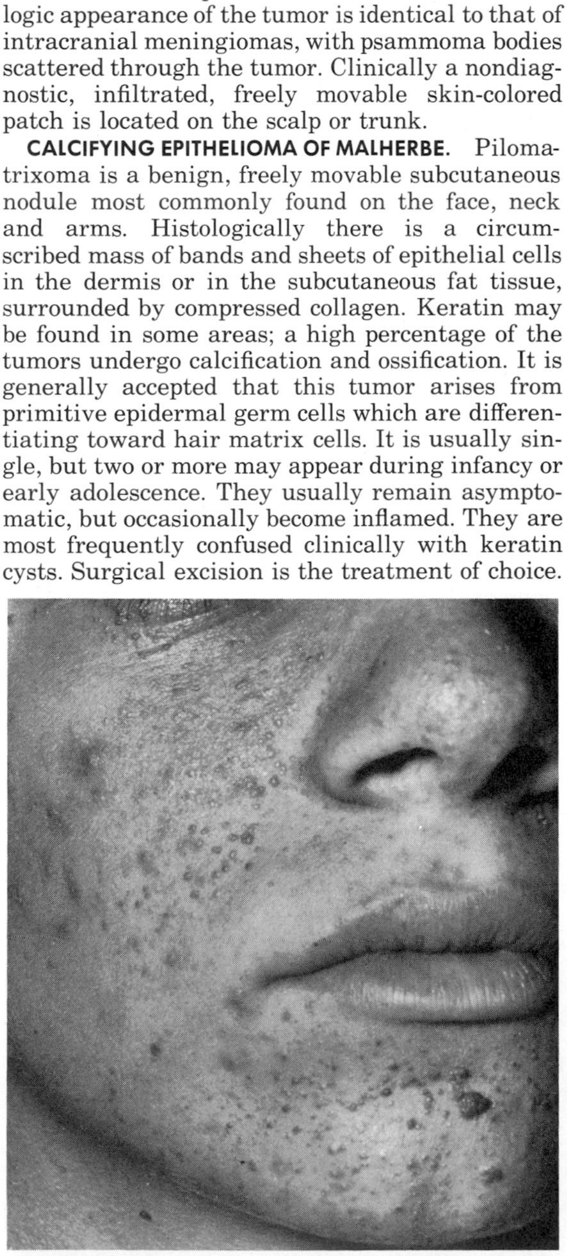

Figure 23-48 Adenoma sebaceum, showing scattered erythematous papules in a 12 year old boy.

Pharmacologic Basis for Local Therapy

The introduction of effective antibacterial, antifungal and anti-inflammatory agents and advances in formulation have revolutionized topical therapy. Such therapy should be planned to fit the problem at hand. The principal considerations are the choice of active ingredients, the vehicle, an esthetically acceptable preparation and detailed instructions for use. In medications for local application, concentration of the active agent in the vehicle is a primary consideration, whereas total quantity of the drug applied is of no importance unless the drug is absorbed through the skin and is applied over large areas.

Absorption of drugs through the normal intact skin is negligible, but absorption may be significant and produce systemic effects when the surface barrier membrane is damaged by the denudation of a dermatitic process through scratching or by the application of an impervious occlusive covering. Consideration of percutaneous absorption is, therefore, particularly important in pediatric practice. For example, boric acid powder applied to inflamed skin can be absorbed and produce boron poisoning; ointments or powders containing mercury under similar circumstances can result in acrodynia. Application of corticosteroids topically over large surfaces of the skin has not produced undesirable side effects except for fluid retention with local use of 9-alpha fluorohydrocortisone (Florinef) and dermal atrophy following longstanding use of other fluorinated corticosteroids (triamcinolone acetonate, 17-valerate of betamethasone, etc.). The covering of locally applied steroids by an occlusive plastic dressing enhances the therapeutic effect but also increases absorption and the danger of adrenocortical suppression. This method of treatment, in any case, is usually not practical for infants and small children, owing to their resistance to being bandaged.

The following effects can be accomplished by the application of therapeutic agents to an abnormal skin surface:

CLEANSING. Local treatment, to be effective, must be preceded by proper cleansing to remove crusts, scales and previously applied medication. This may be accomplished by gently scrubbing with cotton or gauze moistened with a white non-scented soap (Basis) or soap substitute (Lowila).

ANTIPRURITIC EFFECT. Except for the local anesthetic agents (lidocaine-containing ointments), there is no medication administered locally or orally which is specifically effective in the relief of pruritus. Control of itching depends on reduction of the inflammatory reaction.

ANTI-INFLAMMATORY EFFECT. This effect is accomplished by vasoconstriction and by the anti-exudative effect of hydrocortisone or one of its analogues. Using vasoconstriction as a parameter of absorption, the acetate is the best absorbed salt of corticosteroids. A number of synthetic glucocorticosteroids (triamcinolone, fluocinolone, and betamethasone) may be more effective in specific instances of disease when applied locally. The effect may be enhanced by polyethylene film occlusion, but at the risk of adrenocortical suppression if used over a large area. Occasional dermal atrophy or striae may occur as complications of this type of treatment. When used intralesionally they may produce dermal atrophy and rarely calcium deposits in the atrophic area. The atrophy is usually reversible, but may be permanent.

ANTIBACTERIAL EFFECT. Antibiotics should be selected which are not likely to be used systemically and which presumably have a low incidence of sensitization. An ointment (bacitracin, neomycin, polymyxin B) or cream (polymyxin B, gramicidin and neomycin) meets these criteria and has broad spectrum coverage. Because of their sensitizing capacities, sulfonamides, penicillin, streptomycin and the furan derivatives should not be used topically. A soap substitute containing hexachlorophene (pHisoHex) is useful in decreasing or eradicating an abnormal bacterial flora in selected patients, but the possibility of percutaneous absorption and toxicity when used on denuded skin or in the neonate must be carefully weighed.

ANTIFUNGAL EFFECT. In tinea capitis the fungistatic effect of griseofulvin has revolutionized treatment. In superficial fungus infections of the skin, however, a modification of Whitfield's formulation (2 to 4 per cent salicylic acid, and 5 to 10 per cent benzoic acid in hydrophilic petrolatum) is still preferred for local treatment. In moniliasis, local applications of nystatin (Mycolog), amphotericin B (Fungizone), a quaternary ammonium compound (benzalkonium chloride 1:10,000) or iodochlorhydroxyquinoline (Vioform) are highly effective; aqueous gentian violet 0.5 to 1.0 per cent is effective but unsightly.

ANTIPARASITIC EFFECT. A lotion or cream containing gamma benzene hexachloride (Kwell) or 20 per cent benzylbenzoate is effective for scabies; for pediculosis Kwell lotion is preferred. Modern insect repellents such as 2-ethyl, 1-3 hexanediol (6–12, OFF) are useful in the prevention of insect bites.

EMOLLIENT EFFECT. A dry, scaly skin results from decreased water-holding capacity of the keratinous layer. Lubrication may be obtained by soaking in plain water followed by the application of a greasy ointment (hydrophilic petrolatum, U.S.P. XVIII) to impede water loss. The technique of hydration and lubrication is useful in avoiding the drying of skin during cold weather.

PROTECTIVE EFFECT. Protection from sunburn may be accomplished by the application of a vehicle containing a mechanical barrier (titanium dioxide) or a chemical light screen (para-aminobenzoic acid or benzophenone) in an appropriate vehicle Pre-sun or Solbar. Protection from the macerating effect of moisture can be induced by the application of a greasy water in oil ointment (hydrophilic petrolatum, U.S.P. XVIII) or the local use of a paste (Lassar's paste).

KERATOPLASTIC EFFECT. The distillation products of wood, coal and bituminous shales, vitamin A and glucocorticosteroids tend to diminish epithelial proliferation and hyperkeratosis and to promote a return to normal keratinization. Coal tar is a complex mixture containing phenols, benzene, toluenes, naphthalene, creosote, anthracenes and fluorescent substances. Wood tars do not contain the anthracene compounds, which are carcinogenic to the skin of mice, but they exert less keratoplastic effect. Notwithstanding the carcinogenicity of coal tar for the skin of experimental animals, cancer has not been attributed to therapeutically applied coal tar products. Folliculitis and photosensitivity to coal tar occur as undesirable side effects. Caution should be exercised in applying coal tar to areas exposed to light. The tars are generally used in ointment or cream vehicles in concentrations from 2 to 10 per cent; undiluted tar may be used in certain instances.

KERATOLYTIC EFFECT. Salicylic acid in concentrations of 2 to 5 per cent is the most frequently used agent to remove hyperkeratotic scales. It is useful in plaster form (40 per cent) for the removal of thickened keratotic lesions such as warts.

VEHICLES. The vehicle itself may have some therapeutic effect through its physical properties. In the past, pharmacologically active agents were applied to the skin in powders, lotions, emulsions, ointments or pastes, or in solution on compresses or in baths. The formulations of the newer cream and ointment bases provide for a wide range of applicability and have largely replaced other types of vehicles.

COMPRESSES AND BATHS. Wet dressings and baths have time-proved usefulness in the treatment of acute dermatitis, especially for the removal of crusts and scales. The antiexudative, anti-inflammatory, vasoconstrictive and antibacterial properties of potassium permanganate, Burow's solution, and the like, are minimal in comparison with those of the corticosteroid preparations and specific antibacterial agents.

Medicated baths containing emulsions of oils (cottonseed, mineral oil) or tars (coal or wood) alone or in combination are useful in the treatment of dry skin (Lubath, Alpha Keri) or in keratinizing abnormalities in which a keratoplastic effect is desired (Zetar Emulsion).

PASTES. Ointment bases occlude the skin surface and impede the loss of water. Retention of water in the keratotic layer results in increased percutaneous absorption. The most occlusive ointment bases are mixtures of hydrocarbons (petrolatum) and mixtures of palmitic, stearic and oleic acid glycerides (lard). Pastes are defined as having 30 to 50 per cent solids in a greasy ointment base; they are now rarely used as vehicles. Owing to its physical properties, Lassar's paste, however, is an effective protective agent for the skin in the diaper area of the infant with readily irritated skin.

Some of the newer ointment vehicles have a greasy consistency and can be properly selected to accomplish certain therapeutic purposes. Occlusiveness of the various ointment bases is directly related to their water miscibility. The following are listed in decreasing order in respect to their occlusive potential: petrolatum, lard, hydrophilic petrolatum, hydrophilic ointment, polyethylene glycol ointment. Owing to their effective occlusiveness, petrolatum, lard and hydrophilic petrolatum should not be used on acute inflammatory lesions.

There are many ointment vehicles available under different proprietary names; here only those contained in the United States Pharmacopeia are listed.

Hydrophilic ointment, U.S.P. XVIII, an oil-in-water emulsion, is a water-washable or vanishing cream type of base. It is relatively nonocclusive and may be used as a vehicle in acute dermatitic reactions. A semisolid emulsion can be obtained by adding 20 per cent distilled water; it can be used in place of a lotion on weeping dermatitic lesions.

Hydrophilic petrolatum, U.S.P. XVIII, is a water-in-oil emulsion. It is the classic "cold cream" type base. Its cooling effect results from the evaporation of the aqueous phase after application to the skin.

Polyethylene glycol ointment, U.S.P. XVIII, is a mixture of polymerized polyethylene glycols. It is water soluble and is easily washed off.

ACKNOWLEDGMENT

Clinical and microscopic photography for this section was done by Gerald Pearlman, Staff Photographer, Department of Dermatology, Temple University School of Medicine, Philadelphia.

C. F. Burgoon, Jr.

Burgoon, C. F., Jr., (ed.): Symposium on Pediatric Dermatology, Pediatr. Clin. N. Amer., Philadelphia, 1956.
Burgoon, C. F., Jr. (ed.): Symposium on Pediatric Dermatology, Pediatr. Clin. N. Amer., Philadelphia, 1961.
Butterworth, T., and Strean, L. P.: Clinical Genodermatology. Baltimore, The Williams & Wilkins Co., 1962.
Fitzpatrick, T. B., Arndt, K. A., Clark, W. H., Eizen, A. Z., Van Scott, E. J., and Vaughan, J. H.: Dermatology in General Medicine. New York, McGraw-Hill Book Co., Inc., 1971.
Gedde-Dahl, J., Jr.: Epidermolysis Bullosa. Baltimore, The John Hopkins Press, 1971.
Graham, J. H., Johnson, W. C., and Helwig, I. B.: Dermal Pathology. New York, Harper and Row, 1972.
Jacobs, A. H. (ed.): Symposium on Pediatric Dermatology. Pediatr. Clin. N. Amer., 1971.
Korting, G. W.: Diseases of the Skin in Children and Adolescents. American edition translated by Curth, W. and Curth, H. W., Philadelphia, W. B. Saunders Company, 1970.
Leider, M.: Practical Pediatric Dermatology. 2nd ed. St. Louis, The C. V. Mosby Co., 1961.
Lever, W. F.: Histopathology of the Skin. Philadelphia, J. B. Lippincott Co., 1967.
Montgomery, H.: Dermatopathology. Vols. I and II. New York, Hoeber Medical Division, Harper and Row, 1967.
Perlman, H. H.: Pediatric Dermatology. Chicago, Year Book Medical Publishers, 1960.
Rook, A., Wilkinson, D. S., and Ebling, F. J. G.: Textbook of Dermatology. Vols. I and II. 2nd ed. Philadelphia, F. A. Davis, 1971.
Solomon, L. M., and Esterly, N. B.: Neonatal Dermatology. Philadelphia, W. B. Saunders Company, 1973.

24
PEDIATRIC OPHTHALMOLOGY

EYES OF THE NEWBORN INFANT

The eye and the brain achieve maximal postnatal growth rates during the first year and continue at a rapid but decelerating rate until the third year. Growth continues at a slower rate until puberty, after which additional growth is negligible. Various parts of the eye grow disproportionately at different times. In general, the structures of the anterior part of the eye grow proportionately less than those of the posterior portion.

At birth the eye is three quarters of adult size. The orbital margin is circular rather than oval. The diameter of the cornea is 10 mm (it is 12 mm in the adult). The sclera is thin, giving a bluish tint. The lacrimal gland is small and is capable of producing tears at birth. The macula is completely developed shortly after birth; the fovea continues to be further differentiated for about 16 weeks. The angle of the anterior chamber contains mesodermal tissue, in some cases until the third postnatal month.

The eyes of the newborn infants remain closed most of the time in the early postnatal days and are sensitive to light. The infant sees at birth and is able to fixate points of contrast in the visual field. An optokinetic response has been recorded in infants ranging between 1½ hours and 5 days of age which was equivalent to approximately 20/670 on the usual Snellen chart. By the end of 2 weeks the infant is able to give more sustained attention to large objects and to follow them in some measure with his gaze. By 4 or 5 weeks he can attend smaller objects, and by 8 to 10 weeks follows a moving object through a motion of 180 degrees. He turns his head away from bright light. There is a gradual increase in visual acuity, binocular vision, ocular motility, convergence and conjugate movements.

Characteristically in the fundus of the newborn infant, especially in the premature one, the nerve head has a grayish pallor, and there is absence of pigment and frequently a grayness in the periphery of the retina; the veins and arteries are more nearly alike in size and color than in the adult. Remnants of the hyaloid artery and of the pupillary membrane may occasionally be observed. Retinal hemorrhages have been observed in as many as 25 per cent of newborn infants, but they absorb promptly and only rarely leave any permanent effect.

EXAMINATION OF THE EYE

The infant or child with complaints referable to the eye is likely to have one or more of the following: (1) deformity; (2) injury; (3) redness, pain, watering or photosensitivity; (4) visual disturbance such as subnormal vision or double vision; or (5) reading disability.

General inspection of the eyes can be performed best in a room without direct or intense illumination. Simple toys which make a little noise are helpful in attracting the gaze in various directions to permit preliminary evaluation of muscular adequacy. A small flashlight is useful in detecting strabismus by observing the position of the corneal reflexes, while covering with the hand first one eye and then the other.

The **eyelids** are examined for crusts, ulceration of the margins and position of the lacrimal puncta. When pressure with the index finger over the lacrimal sac expresses mucopurulent material through the puncta, it is indicative of obstruction of the nasolacrimal duct and infection of the tear sac. The ability to open and close the lids should be tested. Ptosis is a common defect characterized by drooping of the eyelid; it is due to weakness of the levator muscle.

The **conjunctiva** is examined for color, smoothness, thickness, secretion, injection, follicles and papillae, and for the presence of a foreign body. The ability to evert the upper lid skillfully should be acquired. The child is asked to look down at his toes; the examiner then grasps the lashes with his right thumb and index finger; he pulls the lid downward and away from the globe, placing a probe, or his other index finger, at the upper level of the tarsal plate. The right fingers pull the eyelid upward and slightly outward, over the finger or probe. The lid is kept everted by holding the thumb against the brow and reminding the child to keep looking downward. Foreign bodies are usually found in the concavity just above the margin of the lid.

The **sclera** is examined for blueness, which indicates thinness. The intraocular pressure can be estimated by palpation with both index fingers through the skin of the lid above the tarsus. It can be measured accurately with a tonometer or a special applanation tonometer during local (tetracaine, proparacaine, 0.5 per cent) or general anesthesia.

The **cornea** is examined for luster, ulceration, foreign body, blood vessels and scars. The diameter of the cornea should be appraised. Megalocornea is a benign condition to be differentiated from an enlarged cornea; the latter is part of generalized enlargement of the globe in congenital glaucoma. Microcornea is often associated with other congenital anomalies. Keratoconus is not common in children except in the Down syndrome.

The **anterior chamber** is assessed for depth by estimating the distance between the cornea and the iris. Cellular activity may be observed with the aid of brilliant illumination and magnification such as is provided by a corneal microscope.

The **iris** should be examined for color and surface markings and for reaction to light and to accommodation. The last is tested by observing both pupils in equal light while the patient looks at a distant object and then at the examiner's finger. Adhesion of the iris to the cornea or the lens should be looked for.

The clarity of the **lens** can be examined by the ophthalmoscope with a plus 10 lens at a point 10 cm from the patient's eye.

EXAMINATION OF THE OCULAR FUNDI. Dilatation of the pupil is essential for adequate examination of the fundus, especially in children who tend either to watch the ophthalmoscope light or to look around the room. Dilatation can be done quickly and effectively with 1 drop of 10 per cent phenylephrine (Neo-Synephrine) or 0.5 per cent tropicamide (Mydriacyl). Homatropine 5 per cent is also effective, but atropine is not safe for the newborn infant except in oil or ointment form, which prevents rapid absorption from the nasal mucous membrane. Cyclopentolate (Cyclogyl) (0.5 and 1.0 per cent) is an excellent cycloplegic agent. The lens and vitreous are examined for opacities. The nerve head is examined for shape, color, nature of its margins, type of cupping and evidence of edema. The macula should be examined routinely, but requires dilatation of the pupil. Some lesions of the macula in children are pathognomonic and aid in establishing the diagnosis in otherwise puzzling conditions. Each vein and artery should be followed from the disk to the periphery. Much more of the fundus can be seen if the child is directed to look up, down, right and left as the corresponding portions of the fundus are examined. One should not hesitate to examine children under satisfactory sedation or with general anesthesia if the information desired is of sufficient importance. If the examination is made during anesthesia, it is essential to have forceps to steady and move the globe, which rolls upward during light anesthesia.

VISUAL TESTS. Testing of visual acuity can be accomplished after 3 years of age by the use of a Snellen E chart, consisting of rows of the letter E in various sizes corresponding to the regular visual test chart. The E's have their "fingers" pointing upward, right, down and left. Cooperation is obtained more easily by having the child place his fingers on the chart itself, indicating the position of the "fingers" of a few of the E's; the chart is then moved 20 feet away, and the child is asked to continue to show which way the "fingers" point by extending his own fingers in the same direction. It is often helpful to have the parent instruct the child at home in the method of "playing the E game." Other charts with familiar pictures of various sizes are useful for smaller children, but are less accurate.

Before the age of 2 years visual acuity can be tested by the response of the child to a small toy or similar object of interest such as keys or his mother's bracelet. His ability to watch a light with each eye separately is a gross screening measure. Normal pupillary responses to light may be present in cerebral blindness. If the child loses interest or behaves badly when one eye is covered but cooperates well when the other eye is covered vision is probably reduced considerably in the first eye. In cases of strabismus, it is essential to determine which eye is preferred for visual fixation of the target or whether the eyes freely alternate.

The field of vision can be tested by the confrontation method until the child is old enough to cooperate in the use of a perimeter. With patience and a projection-type of perimeter, accurate visual fields can be mapped at a relatively early age.

Color blindness can be tested by use of colored wools or having a child trace numbers on an Ishihara or American Optical Color Chart with his finger. Defective color vision is not uncommon in the male, but is rare in the female. "Color ignorance" refers to inability to tell shades of color; this condition responds somewhat to education.

Subnormal dark adaptation is difficult to test in young children. Vitamin A deficiency is the only causative condition amenable to treatment. Retinitis pigmentosa and choroideremia are characterized by night blindness with reduced peripheral vision.

Examination by the Child's Physician. Routine examinations of the eyes should include: (1) the use of a Snellen E or letter chart (see above); (2) examination of motility of the eyes by checking rotations and the near-point of convergence and movements with the cover test described under Strabismus; and (3) examination of the media and fundi with an ophthalmoscope.

Visual screening tests of children in offices and in schools have proved to be effective. The Atlantic City eye test* can be done rapidly, provides adequate information, does not require a skilled examiner or extensive equipment and is readily interpreted. It tests visual acuity and muscle balance and provides a rough test for refractive error. After testing the visual acuity with the Snellen chart, a +1.75 lens is placed before each eye. If the child can then read the 20/20 line on the chart, he fails the test, and has hyperopia. Muscle balance is checked by the use of a green rectangle in which a red dot should be seen. If the red dot is outside the rectan-

*Obtainable from William Freund, 1415 Pacific Ave., Atlantic City, N.J. 08401.

gle, the child has more than 1 prism diopter of hyperphoria or more than 4 prism diopters of esophoria or exophoria.

Examination by an Ophthalmologist. Infants and children should be examined by an ophthalmologist whenever an ocular abnormality is noted. Children do *not* "grow out" of strabismus. The optimal schedule for examination by an ophthalmologist is (1) in the neonatal period; (2) before entering school (age 4 years); and (3) at intervals of 2 years beginning at puberty. In addition, examination is indicated whenever vision for either distance or nearness is defective; whenever strabismus is noted, since poor vision from disuse is usually not easily correctable after the sixth year of life; and at any sign or symptom of disease of the eye.

Cycloplegics traditionally include atropine, 0.5 to 1.0 per cent (in an ointment or oil rather than solution to lessen absorption from the nasal mucosa), and, in children over 12 years of age, homatropine, 5 per cent. Cyclopentolate (Cyclogyl) is now, however, the one of choice at all ages. It is almost as effective as atropine, acts more rapidly, and paralyzes accommodation for only 24 hours, as compared with 5 days for atropine and scopolamine.

DYSLEXIA

Children are frequently examined by the ophthalmologist because of reading difficulties. Children with average or superior intelligence who exhibit reading problems based on defects in visual interpretation of symbols and who have adequate function of peripheral sensory mechanisms are said to have *dyslexia*—primary, specific or developmental *reading disabilities.* Secondary reading disabilities also exist and may be the result of slow maturation, emotional disturbances, environmental situations, uncontrolled seizure disorders or organic brain damage.

Surveys have shown a relatively high incidence of cerebral dysfunction, farsightedness, exophoria, fusional difficulties, convergence insufficiency, crossed dominance and inability to maintain binocular fixation in retarded readers; but children with similar disabilities may be excellent readers, and it is evident that there are additional factors to be considered in the child with a reading disability.

Children with reading disabilities may have difficulty in perceiving letters or words in their proper order. Questions are raised about mirror vision far more often than it occurs. Children may experiment with reversals of letter order while learning to read, just as they use toys in unexpected ways, but if true mirror vision occurs, it is very rare.

Problems in visual perception are best handled first by an ophthalmologic examination to detect or exclude organic disease, and then in cooperation with the orthoptic technician, who will determine the degree of visual sensorimotor coordination. If a problem is found, every effort should be made to improve the ocular status prior to remedial reading. If a careful examination indicates no ocular problem, children with reading problems should be referred for remedial reading to qualified professional personnel for highly individualized instruction. Visual associations can be augmented in useful ways through auditory, tactile, and a kinesthetic input. (See also pages 123–126.)

REFRACTIVE ERRORS

Most children are born farsighted, about 5 per cent are nearsighted, and 20 per cent have practically no refractive error.

HYPEROPIA (FARSIGHTEDNESS). The hyperopic eye is shorter than normal, so that the focused image falls posterior to the retina. Hyperopia over 4 diopters is considered abnormal in children; in hyperopia of lesser degree the power of accommodation is sufficient to supplement the refracting power, but its constant use may cause fatigue and ocular discomfort. The total refractive error is determined under atropine or Cyclogyl cycloplegia. Refraction is indicated in children with poor vision, lack of interest in reading or looking at picture books, headache, eye discomfort, strabismus, corneal disease or inflammations of the lid. Proper lenses provide correction adequate for distinct vision and prevention of fatigue.

MYOPIA (NEARSIGHTEDNESS). The myopic eye is longer than normal, so that the focused image falls anterior to the retina. There is poor vision for distant objects, and accommodation does not improve it. Proper lenses for full correction of the refractive error should be worn for best vision, and re-examination is ideally performed semi-annually for the first few years and then annually. Children of myopic parents should be examined at an early age owing to a hereditary tendency.

ASTIGMATISM. In astigmatism there is a difference in the refractive power of the various corneal meridians of the eye, owing to a slight irregularity in the spherical shape of the eyeball. The child may appear to be a careless reader because a distorted image is obtained. Symptoms include headache, eye pain, fatigue, nervousness and conjunctival injection. Astigmatism may be combined with myopia or hyperopia; slight astigmatism is extremely common. Cylindric or spherocylindric lenses provide an optical correction for the defect. Slight degrees of astigmatism often do not require correction; moderate degrees usually require glasses for reading, movies, television, and so forth; severe degrees require that glasses be worn constantly.

Paralysis of accommodation may be due to diphtheritic paralysis of the ciliary muscle or to other neurologic conditions.

DISORDERS OF EYEBALL AND ADNEXA

Diseases of the *orbit* may be classified as developmental, inflammatory, vascular, traumatic, neoplastic, or secondary to a systemic defect. The eyeball responds to changes in orbital volume by appearing pushed forward (exophthalmos, proptosis), by being sunken (enophthalmos) or by being displaced vertically.

The method of examination involves inspection, palpation, auscultation and roentgenography. The use of retrobulbar air and contrast media may be of special help. The Hertel exophthalmometer is valuable in quantitating the degree of exophthalmos for comparison of serial measurements.

DEVELOPMENTAL ABNORMALITIES. Structural anomalies of the bony orbit, dermoid cysts, teratomas, encephalocele, and microphthalmos with cyst are included among the developmental abnormalities. Craniostenosis may be responsible for deformities of the orbit, usually with loss of depth anteroposteriorly. Reduction in orbital volume may result in proptosis; exotropia, papilledema and optic atrophy are other possible sequelae.

INFLAMMATION. Acute inflammatory orbital disease is usually secondary to inflammation in adjacent structures, except for penetrating orbital injuries. The most common sources of orbital infection are sinuses, teeth, eyelids and face. Edema of the lids and proptosis may occur in the child without definite orbital disease, particularly in paranasal sinus disease (ethmoiditis). Orbital cellulitis is usually associated with severe inflammation, proptosis, lid rigidity and immobility of the eyeball. Allergic reactions about the lids may simulate orbital disease.

Chronic inflammatory disease of the orbit is relatively common; it is observed with chronic sinusitis, osteomyelitis, pseudotumors, tuberculosis and fungal and parasitic infections. *Cavernous sinus thrombosis* may occur as a rare sequel to orbital cellulitis. Severe pain, edema of the lid and conjunctiva, proptosis, immobility of the eye, papilledema, decreased vision and severe general toxicity are the principal manifestations of this complication.

TRAUMA. Traumatic injuries to the orbit may result from blunt or penetrating injuries; examination should include a search for retained foreign bodies. Blowout fractures of the floor of the orbit may be caused by a sharp blow. Routine roentgenograms frequently fail to demonstrate a fracture; laminograms may be required. All penetrating injuries to the orbit demand evaluation of the central nervous system to determine whether the brain has been injured by perforation of the posterior orbital wall. Orbital hemorrhage and infection are common with penetrating injuries and must be treated as emergencies.

VASCULAR DISEASE. Primary orbital vascular abnormalities are uncommon, as are varices, pulsating exophthalmos from carotid–cavernous sinus fistula and aneurysm. Hemangioma is the most common vascular tumor and can usually be removed surgically through a lateral orbitotomy.

TUMORS. Rhabdomyosarcoma is the most common primary malignant orbital tumor in children. Glioma of the optic nerve is usually associated with von Recklinghausen's disease; it grows slowly, producing loss of vision with gradually increasing proptosis. Meningioma and carcinoma of the paranasal sinuses occur less commonly in children than adults. Dermoid cysts are benign encapsulated tumors which are relatively common in the region of the orbit. Their growth is slow in early life, but accelerated at puberty. Other benign orbital tumors include cholesteatoma, angioma, fibroma and neurofibroma.

ORBITAL CHANGES SECONDARY TO SYSTEMIC DISEASE. Exophthalmos secondary to thyroid disease is uncommon in children. The Hand-Schüller-Christian syndrome includes exophthalmos. Proptosis secondary to orbital hemorrhage may be seen with blood dyscrasias and scurvy. Leukemia and neuroblastoma may produce proptosis through orbital hemorrhage and infiltration.

CONGENITAL OCULAR ABNORMALITIES. Congenital defects of the eye occur in two primary ways: (1) those that are presumably genetic in origin and interfere with embryonal development, e.g., microphthalmos, colobomata, cataract and dermoid tumor; or (2) those that are due to intrauterine inflammation, e.g., chorioretinopathies (toxoplasmosis and cytomegalic inclusion disease), corneal scars (syphilis) and cataract (German measles).

Colobomata characteristically arise from a failure of fusion of embryonic tissue. Failure of regression of vascular tissue is most commonly seen as a remnant of the hyaloid artery or a persistence of the tunica vasculosa lentis. *Congenital cataracts* develop at any time during the formation of the lens, which occurs about the sixth or seventh week of gestation. Congenital cataracts may be unilateral or bilateral, or in any stage of development from minimal involvement to complete opacification. *Microphthalmos* varies in degree, may involve one or both eyes, and may be accompanied by such conditions as cataract, aniridia, irideremia, colobomata, somatic abnormalities and meningoencephalocele. Microphthalmos is often determined by a recessive gene, but may appear as a dominant trait. When *aniridia* is not on a familial basis, but appears to be a new mutation, the concurrence of Wilms's tumor must be considered. Deficiencies in visual function are frequently associated with anatomic anomalies.

Congenital defects of the choroid and retina are visible ophthalmoscopically. Colobomata of the uveal structures may be located inferiorly or inferior-nasally. They may be unilateral or bilateral and may also involve the iris, choroid or optic nerve singularly or in combination. Central macular pigmentary lesions are often caused by toxoplasmosis and cytomegalic inclusion disease. Other congenital lesions of the choroid or retina include drusen, aneurysm, optic nerve malformation, medullated nerve fibers and macular degenerations. Persistence of the tunica vasculosa lentis or persistent hyperplastic vitreous must be differentiated from congenital cataract and retrolental fibroplasia.

EXTERNAL DISEASE OF THE EYE

CONGENITAL ANOMALIES OF THE LIDS. The most common congenital conditions of the lids are epicanthus and blepharoptosis. Blepharophimosis (small opening), dystrichiasis (misdirection or extra rows of lashes) and colobomata are occasionally seen.

Epicanthus is common and is produced by a fold of skin extending downward from the brow to the nose, obscuring the medial canthus. It is always bilateral and frequently produces an apparent asymmetry of the eyes suggesting strabismus. Epicanthus usually disappears as the nasal bridge develops and the face broadens.

Blepharoptosis results from a defect or a paresis of the levator palpebral muscle. The condition is more commonly unilateral, but often bilateral. It may be familial. Sometimes it is associated with paresis of the superior rectus muscle. Surgical correction is frequently required by age 5 years and is accomplished by resecting the levator muscle.

DISEASES OF THE LIDS. The skin of the lids may be involved in a variety of conditions affecting the skin elsewhere in the body. Edema of the lids may be due to local or general disease. Allergy is a common cause. Infections of the skin, paranasal sinuses, orbit, tear sac or eyeball may produce edema. Hemorrhage into the lids results in ecchymosis and is of particular importance; when it appears 24 to 48 hours after a head injury, it suggests the possibility of basal skull fracture.

Emphysema of the lids usually denotes a fracture of the medial wall of the orbit (lamina papyracea), permitting communication with the nasal cavity (ethmoid sinus). The lids are swollen, and on palpation there is a sensation of crepitation.

Hordeolum (sty) is common in children and is nearly always due to staphylococcal infection. Vaccine appears at times to be helpful in treatment of persistent recurrences. *Acute chalazion* responds to anti-inflammatory measures, but if a lump remains after 2 months, excision of the granuloma is required. *Ectropion* is an outward turning of the lid margin, and *entropion* is an inward turning.

Benign neoplasms include papillomas, hemangiomas, dermoid cysts, nevi, lymphangioma and lipoma. Non-neoplastic growths that may be found on the lids are xanthoma, molluscum contagiosum and milium. These growths may be excised if they interfere with function or become unsightly. Malignant tumors of the lid are rare in children.

Blepharitis is an inflammation which principally involves the margins of the eyelids and the skin around the base of the cilia. Redness, scales, crusts and ulcerations may be present. The eyelashes are often matted by cellular debris and exudate and sometimes may cease to grow satisfactorily. Seborrhea is a common cause, alone or complicated by secondary infection. Treatment of seborrhea of the scalp and brows is important for improvement of the marginal blepharitis.

TABLE 24–1 DIFFERENTIAL DIAGNOSIS OF OCULAR INFLAMMATION IN CHILDREN

ACUTE CONJUNCTIVITIS	ACUTE KERATITIS	ACUTE UVEITIS	CONGENITAL GLAUCOMA
Common	Common, often secondary to trauma	Not common	Not common
Mucopurulent discharge	Lacrimation, but no discharge	Lacrimation	Lacrimation
Foreign body sensation	Pain, photophobia and foreign body sensation	Pain and photophobia	Photophobia
Conjunctival redness only	Perilimbal injection	Redness at limbus	Minimal congestion
Vision normal	Vision reduced	Vision reduced	Vision poor
Pupil normal	Pupil normal or smaller	Pupil small, irregular	Pupil small
Cornea clear	Cornea hazy or gray	Cornea usually clear	Cornea hazy or quite cloudy
Anterior chamber normal	Anterior chamber normal	Anterior chamber cloudy	Anterior chamber deep
Ocular tension normal	Ocular tension normal	Ocular tension normal to low	Ocular tension elevated

THE LACRIMAL APPARATUS. Epiphora due to a congenital obstruction of the nasolacrimal duct is common. Dacryocystitis may result from obstruction of long standing. Pressure over the tear sac, combined with "drops" to control infection, is usually successful in opening the duct. Probing may be required, if conservative means fail, and is generally successful. In the event of repeated failures, however, a new opening from the tear sac to the nasal cavity may be required. Absence of the puncta or accessory puncta is rare.

THE CONJUNCTIVA. *Chemosis* is edema of the bulbar conjunctiva and results from trauma, local irritation, allergic reactions or trichinosis. *Hyperemia* of the conjunctiva is caused by local irritations such as foreign bodies, dust, exposure to bright light, coryza or allergy. *Subconjunctival hemorrhage*, manifested by bright or dark red patches on the bulbar conjunctiva, may be the result of injury or inflammation. It may occasionally result from severe sneezing or coughing, or may be a manifestation of a blood dyscrasia.

Symblepharon is a cicatricial attachment of the conjunctiva of the lid to the eyeball; the lower lid is usually affected. It follows operation or injuries, especially burns from lye, acids or molten metals. It may interfere with motion of the eyeball and cause diplopia. The band should be separated and the raw surfaces kept from uniting during healing. Grafts of oral mucous membrane may be necessary.

Acute conjunctivitis, characterized by redness, chemosis and mucopurulent discharge, is common in children and particularly in newborn infants. The instillation into the eyes of prophylactic silver nitrate frequently produces in the newborn infant a chemical irritation, with a purulent discharge lasting 24 to 48 hours. Gonorrheal conjunctivitis of the newborn must be considered in differential diagnosis.

Gonorrheal conjunctivitis is manifested by an acute, copious, purulent discharge which begins within 3 to 5 days after birth. The conjunctiva becomes red and chemotic, and the lids are so swollen that separating them is very difficult. When there has been premature rupture of the membranes, infection may be present at birth. The term *ophthalmia neonatorum* applies to any acute conjunctivitis in the newborn infant. When smears and cultures indicate gonorrheal infection, therapy includes systemic penicillin and frequent local instillation of a chemotherapeutic agent.

Acute purulent conjunctivitis is more frequently caused by staphylococcus, streptococcus, pneumococcus, *Hemophilus influenzae* and Koch-Weeks bacilli, and usually responds promptly to antimicrobial therapy.

Vernal conjunctivitis is characterized by papillary hypertrophy of the palpebral conjunctiva and tends to occur principally in warm weather. Allergy plays a role in its origin. Symptoms include lacrimation, itching and photophobia. The upper palpebral conjunctivae contain hard, flattened papillae. In the *bulbar form* the conjunctiva adjacent to the limbus contains gelatinous elevations. The conjunctiva is congested and exhibits stringy, mucoid secretions that contain eosinophils. Vernal conjunctivitis responds to topical corticosteroid medication.

Inclusion blennorrhea is a viral infection transmitted in a variety of ways. The infant can be infected during birth by organisms in the maternal genital tract. During childhood, infection from contaminated swimming pools is relatively common. The neonatal lesion resembles gonococcal conjunctivitis at the outset, but it does not appear until 5 to 7 days after birth. These viral infections are effectively treated with a sulfonamide.

Epidemic keratoconjunctivitis is caused by adenovirus type 8 and is transmitted by direct contact. Initially there is a sensation of a foreign body beneath the lids and itching and burning. Edema and photophobia develop rapidly, and large oval follicles appear within the conjunctiva. There are frequently preauricular adenopathy and a pseudomembrane on the conjunctival surface. Blurring of vision results from subepithelial corneal infiltrates, which usually disappear, but have been known to reduce permanently the visual acuity. When epidemic keratoconjunctivitis occurs in children under the age of 2 years (and sometimes up to 5 years), 50 per cent of patients have systemic findings consisting of fever, sore throat, and malaise, with occasional otitis media or diarrhea. Symptoms are usually milder than in pharyngoconjunctival fever. Corneal changes are rare.

Pharyngoconjunctival fever is characterized by marked febrile symptoms, lymphadenopathy and severe follicular conjunctivitis. It is frequently epidemic.

Chronic catarrhal conjunctivitis can develop from repeated attacks of acute conjunctivitis and may be associated with chronic infections of the lids, chronic dacryocystitis, irritants, and viral warts at the lid margin. The conjunctiva is red and thickened, and there is a mild discharge. There is a scratchy, burning and heavy sensation about the lids. Determination and elimination of the cause are often difficult.

Vaccinia of the lids or conjunctiva may occur as a result of an accidental inoculation. Single or multiple ulcers with gray necrotic material are characteristic. The great danger is corneal involvement, which can produce dense scarring and visual loss.

DISEASES OF THE CORNEA

The cornea has attained most of its growth at birth and therefore appears relatively large in comparison to other structures. The transverse diameter is 10 mm at birth and attains adult size (12 mm) during the first year of life. Any abnormal increase in size is an urgent cause for ophthalmologic consultation. Corneal haze or opacity accompanied by photophobia and lacrimation is a characteristic sign of congenital glaucoma. Corneal lesions may be classified as superficial or deep keratitis, or as corneal ulcers when there is demonstrable loss of substance. Inflammatory lesions of the cornea appear as grayish infiltrations or opacities, accompanied by circumcorneal redness, pain, photophobia and lacrimation. Inflammatory lesions may be bacterial, viral or fungal and are frequently secondary to trauma.

Interstitial keratitis is a chronic cellular infiltration of the deeper layers of the cornea without ulceration. It is frequently associated with uveitis, corneal opacities and corneal vascularization. Congenital syphilis is the most frequent cause; tuberculosis and leprosy are less frequent ones. The lesion may be acute or chronic; in the acute form the cornea has a characteristic "salmon pink patch."

Phlyctenular keratoconjunctivitis appears as a small, gray, discrete, elevated lesion at the corneal limbus. Extreme photophobia and lacrimation make examination difficult. The lesion has been attributed to undernutrition and to tuberculosis.

VIRAL KERATITIS. Dendritic keratitis, which may be caused by herpesvirus, is the most troublesome of corneal viral infections. It is manifest as a dendritic, tree-like staining figure on the cornea accompanied by photophobia and lacrimation. Not infrequently it follows trauma, especially if corticosteroid drops have been used for any length of time. Combined antibiotic-steroid eyedrops for ordinary external inflammatory disease of the eye are to be avoided unless there is a clear-cut indication for their use.

Corneal ulcers are always a cause for immediate concern and may result from traumatic lesions which become secondarily infected. Many organisms are capable of producing an infected ulcer, but the most troublesome is *Pseudomonas aeruginosa.* Fungi may be recovered from chronic corneal ulcers. Scarring or perforation due to corneal ulceration is an important cause of blindness throughout the world and is estimated to be responsible for 10 per cent of blindness in this country.

Vitamin A deficiency, abnormalities of the fifth cranial nerve and exposure can cause severe corneal changes. Trachoma, which is highly prevalent in North Africa and the Middle East, is probably the commonest cause of blindness in that area, producing severe corneal and conjunctival scarring, as well as lid deformities which lead to the rubbing of eyelashes against the eyeball.

THE PUPIL

In the *Adie syndrome* one pupil is myotonic and is larger than its mate; the Achilles and patellar reflexes are often absent. The slow contracture of the pupil in response to continuous direct light is characteristic. The pupil remains contracted for a long time after the light stimulation has been removed. The normal pupil fails to contract to 2.5 per cent methacholine (Mecholyl), whereas the involved pupil does. The cause of the syndrome is not known. No treatment is required.

Horner syndrome consists of unilateral miosis, apparent enophthalmos, narrow palpebral fissure and absence of facial sweating and represents a disturbance in the cervical sympathetic chain. The pupil fails to dilate with cocaine, but does dilate with epinephrine 1:1000, which ordinarily has no effect on the normal pupil.

LEUKOCORIA (WHITE PUPIL). A white pupillary reflex in a child is indicative of a serious disorder; examination under general anesthesia is frequently indicated. The differential diagnosis includes cataract, retrolental fibroplasia, persistent primary hyperplastic vitreous, retinoblastoma, severe intraocular infection and exudative retinopathy (Coats's disease, see below).

DISORDERS OF THE LENS

Congenital cataracts are relatively common, but do not always cause significant visual disturbance. They are usually bilateral and often genetically determined. Maternal rubella (Section 10) is a common cause; galactosemia and hypocalcemia are less frequent ones. Cataracts may develop secondary to such intraocular diseases as uveitis, retinitis pigmentosa, retinal detachment or retrolental fibroplasia, or may represent the toxic effect of certain drugs and chemicals or the long-term administration of corticosteroids. Traumatic cataracts may develop from a direct blow or a penetrating injury. The lens opacity often becomes manifest rapidly and may be complicated by pain, inflammation and glaucoma.

Dislocation of the lens may be associated with arachnodactyly (Weill-Marfan syndrome), Marchesani syndrome, homocystinuria or trauma.

The opacities vary considerably in density and morphology. They can be observed through a +10 diopter lens with the ophthalmoscope held at a distance of approximately 10 cm from the eye.

Other ocular abnormalities are frequently associated with congenital cataract such as microphthalmos, nystagmus, amblyopia, strabismus, corneal changes, aniridia, dislocation of the lens, and choroidal and retinal diseases. In addition, a high percentage of affected children may be mentally retarded or have associated disturbances of the cardiovascular, renal, skeletal or central nervous system, skin, muscles or endocrine glands.

The surgical results with congenital cataract are not as good as with the cataracts of adults. The high percentage of associated defects, including mental retardation and nystagmus, makes the prognosis guarded as to eventual visual function. In cases of maternal rubella, operation should be postponed until the age of 2 years, since activation of virus may occur if the operation is done earlier.

It is generally agreed that children with cataracts who have corrected vision of 20/50 or better should not be operated upon. If one eye is normal, a complete cataract in the other eye should be left alone until the patient is older. After the removal of a unilateral cataract, binocular visual function is possible only with a contact lens or with a prosthetic lens placed within the eye.

In borderline cases with moderate involvement of both eyes, one must be guided by the child's ability to progress in schoolwork and to function socially. The ultimate decisions as to management must rest jointly with the ophthalmologist and the pediatrician.

GLAUCOMA

Infantile congenital glaucoma is characterized by increased intraocular pressure; it may be present at birth or become manifest in the first 3 years of life. It may be transmitted in an autosomal recessive manner. Congenital glaucoma may be associated with other congenital anomalies, which include aniridia (a vestigial root of iris remaining), pigmentary glaucoma (degeneration of pigment epithelium of iris), the Axenfeld syndrome (anomalous iris angle), the Sturge-Weber syndrome, neurofibromatosis, the Marfan syndrome and the Lowe syndrome.

The earliest and most constant symptom is tearing, which must be differentiated from that due to congenital obstruction of the nasolacrimal duct. Corneal clouding associated with tears in Descemet's membrane is also an early sign. Photophobia may render ordinary examination difficult, since the avoidance of light is extreme. Increased intraocular pressure is the principal sign; accurate measurement must be made under general anesthesia. Cupping of the optic disk may occur early. Enlargement of the eye to a corneal diameter in excess of 12 mm and a deep anterior chamber are significant. Repeated measurements of tension may be necessary to differentiate glaucoma from congenital megalocornea.

Treatment of infantile glaucoma is surgical, involving goniotomy, trabeculotomy, or trabeculectomy; the abnormally high insertion of the iris or membrane must be incised. Repeated surgical procedures are frequently required, using a special lens to view the iris angle.

Surgery should be performed as soon as the diagnosis is made; nearly 80 per cent of cases are evident by 3 months of age. The earlier the disease becomes manifest, the less favorable is the prognosis. Surgery leads to normal tension in about 75 per cent. Long-term visual results are not good despite normal tension.

STRABISMUS

(Cast; Squint; Cross-eye; Walleye; Tropia; Heterotropia)

Strabismus is an imbalance of the extraocular muscles. It is of considerable importance in pediatric practice, for it often results in functional loss of vision known as *amblyopia ex anopsia* (poor vision from disuse and absence of fusion). Owing to the cosmetic blemish, psychologic problems may arise. Parents should never be told to "wait and let the child outgrow crossed eyes."

Transient overconvergence or pseudostrabismus does occur, but the differential diagnosis should be the responsibility of the ophthalmologist. Infants with suspected strabismus should be referred to the ophthalmologist as soon as it is noticed. Strabismus may be congenital, and is familial in about 50 per cent of cases. Strabismus is frequently observed in cerebral palsy, in children born prematurely, and with many central nervous system abnormalities.

Few people have completely "normal" muscle balance (orthophoria); most have a tendency for the eyes to deviate in or out, up or down (heterophoria). A person with a *phoria* can keep his eyes straight by exerting effort to maintain fusion. A patient with a *tropia* frequently manifests an actual visible deviation, since the visual axes are not parallel. Some children have a phoria which at times becomes a tropia (or true deviation); this accounts for the parents' observation that the eyes are straight except under such circumstances as fatigue, illness, or for near or distant vision. Fusion may be possible in some fields of gaze, but impossible in others. For example, the child may see singly when he looks straight ahead or downward, but double when he looks upward. He therefore does all he can to avoid looking up.

Two conditions may give the appearance of strabismus when it is not there, or accentuate it when it is: epicanthal folds and the relative position of the eyeballs in the orbit. The latter represents a disparity between the anatomic axis and the visual axis.

Though there is wide variation in the manifestations of strabismus, there are general categories that are helpful to identify in planning the man-

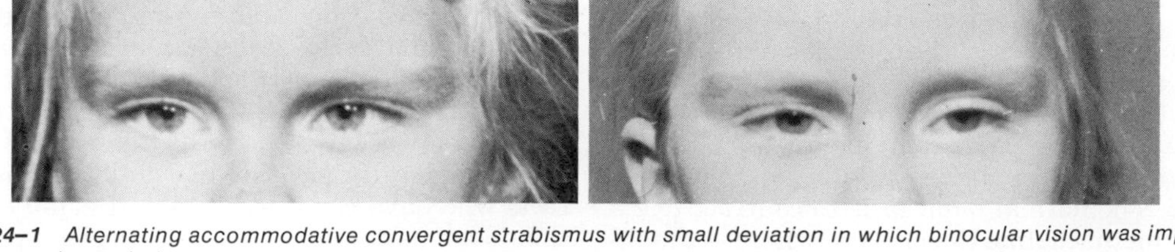

Figure 24–1 *Alternating accommodative convergent strabismus with small deviation in which binocular vision was improved by orthoptic exercise techniques.*

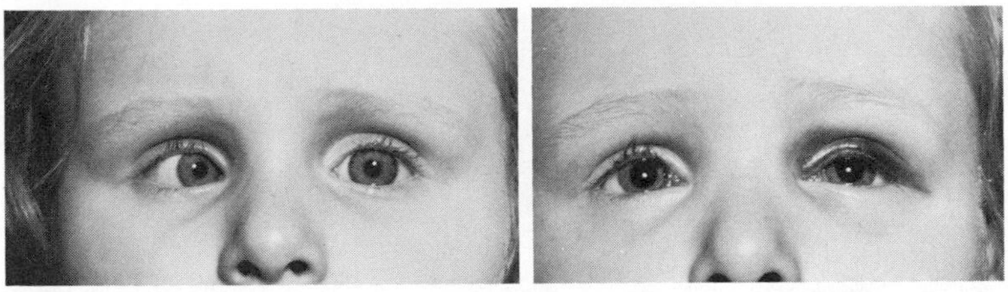

Figure 24–2 Alternating convergent strabismus corrected by surgery. Strabismus may be corrected by corrective lenses, orthoptic exercises or surgery or a combination of the 3 procedures. The early treatment of strabismus is emphasized, since best results are obtained when correction is undertaken before the age of 5 years.

agement of each case. *Paralytic (noncomitant) strabismus* is due to paralysis of a muscle. The eyes are straight except when they are moved in the direction of the paralyzed muscle. Double vision may be present in this case, or the child may in time learn to suppress the vision in the affected eye. Suppression in children under the age of 5 years frequently results in some degree of amblyopia. In *nonparalytic (comitant) strabismus,* which is the usual type, all the muscles are capable of rotating the eyeball as they should, but they do not work together. Both eyes are in the same relative position irrespective of the direction of gaze.

There are lateral, vertical and mixed lateral and vertical types of strabismus. Paralysis of one of the vertically acting muscles may initiate the lateral imbalance. The child sees two images, one above the other and close together. He makes every attempt to avoid double vision. He may tilt his head, close one eye or allow one eye to deviate in or out in order to get the two images together or so far apart that they do not bother him. During this transient period of double vision the child may stumble, fall, overreach or otherwise appear awkward. He may be fussy and difficult to manage. This is the ideal time to start covering one eye. The procedure makes an alternator out of what would probably be a monocular squinter, and so promotes the development of good vision in each eye.

In *monocular* strabismus one eye deviates permanently, while the other eye is always being used. The deviating eye not used for definitive seeing fails to develop good central vision *(amblyopia ex anopsia)*. Amblyopia in this case implies that the eye is organically sound; the fundus appears normal. As previously noted, central vision is not fully developed at birth. The suppression of the image in the deviating eye will not permit central vision to develop normally. Peripheral vision, however, remains good. The nonstrabismic eye develops normally, and the child has no evidence of poor vision until this eye is covered; then the disparity in vision between the two eyes is striking. Patching of the good or fixating eye is essential. This must be done *constantly* for weeks or months, and care must be taken that the improved vision does not decrease when the patch is taken off.

Alternating strabismus is a condition in which either eye may be used for fixation while the other eye deviates. Since each eye is used part of the time for definitive seeing, vision is developed more or less equally in both eyes, and there may be no necessity for patching either eye. These children do not have double vision, since they suppress the image in the nonfixing eye. Neither do they have binocular vision with depth perception, but they do not miss it since they have never had it. Operation is usually required, and the prognosis is generally good.

Accommodative strabismus depends upon the relation between convergence and accommodation, both of which are controlled by the third cranial nerve and are called upon to function at the same time. A high degree of hyperopia necessitates excessive accommodation, with accompanying overconvergence. Myopia is more likely to be associated with divergent strabismus. Accommodative esotropia may disappear during cycloplegia, and corrective lenses keep the eyes straight by relieving the stimulus for excessive accommodation-convergence. Good vision should be maintained in both eyes, but this is not automatically done in many cases. It is therefore sometimes necessary to use occlusion as well as glasses.

STRABISMUS AND CEREBRAL PALSY. Children with cerebral palsy may have a variety of ocular palsies and, as a result, may have double vision in some directions of gaze. Esotropia is more common (46 per cent) than exotropia (8 per cent). It is

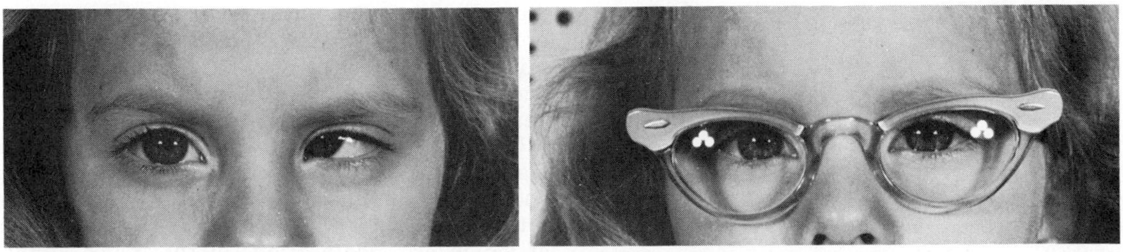

Figure 24–3 Accommodative convergent strabismus straightened by corrective lenses.

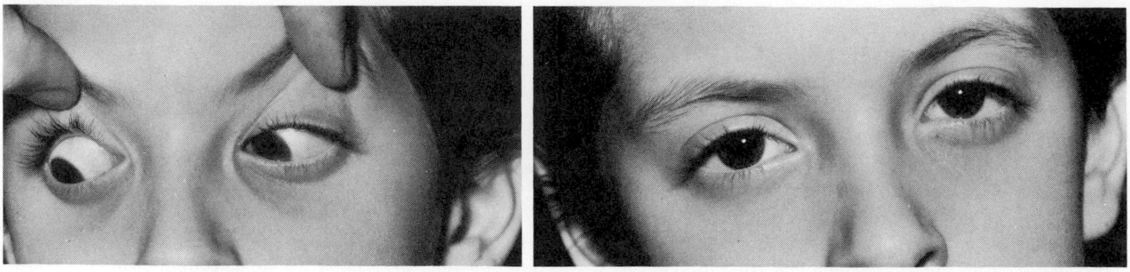

Figure 24–4 Right head tilt associated with paresis of left superior oblique muscle.

desirable to remedy double vision as soon as possible, especially since many of these children have severe problems in locomotion and since improved cosmetic appearance may help in general social development. In cases of persistent esotropia with one eye deviating, patching the good eye to prevent amblyopia is indicated, although this may be rendered difficult by other problems. Children with cerebral palsy commonly have refractive errors, nystagmus, paralysis of conjugate gaze, blepharoptosis, cataracts, optic atrophy, defects of visual fields, aphasia and dyslexia, and such developmental ocular defects as microphthalmos, pupillary abnormalities, aniridia and colobomata.

METHODS OF TESTING FOR STRABISMUS. In very young infants one can tell whether the eyes are straight by observing the position of the light reflexes on the corneas when a light is held before the face. Each reflex should be in the center of the pupillary space or at corresponding points in the two corneas, such as the corneoscleral junction nasally on one eye and temporally on the other.

For older children the screen or cover test is the best one; it is carried out by having the child look at or fixate a distant target while a narrow card is used to cover first one eye and then the other. Absolutely straight eyes *(orthophoria)* make no movement whatever when the card is moved. If crossing *(esotropia)* is present, each eye will move outward to fix on the light. If the eyes are divergent *(exotropia)*, each eye will jump inward to fix on the light. One watches only the eye that is just being uncovered. Measurement of the amount of deviation is obtained by holding prisms base-out or base-in before the eyes during the cover test. When the proper prism is found, no movement of either eye occurs.

The ocular rotations and the ability to converge should also be tested. The near point of convergence is measured by bringing a small object of interest to the child slowly toward his nose. This near point should be within 10 cm of the base of the nose. When the rotations are tested, one should note the relative motility with both eyes opened and with each eye closed.

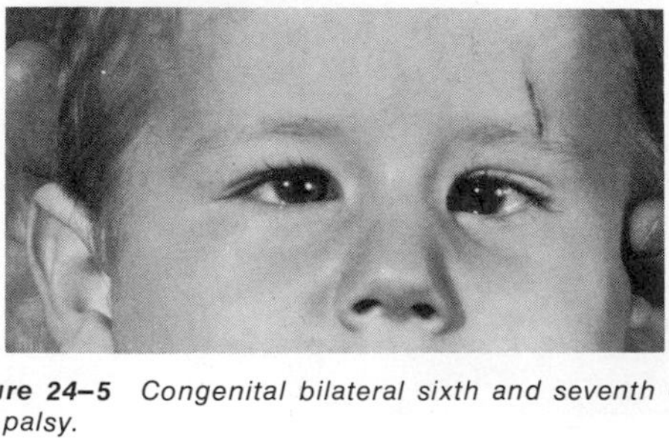

Figure 24–5 Congenital bilateral sixth and seventh cranial nerve palsy.

A light may be used as a target of fixation. An accommodative target is preferable, since the child must attempt to focus; the stimulation of the accommodative mechanism may reveal an accommodative esotropia. Simple toys, preferably those that move or create a gentle noise, are particularly useful in attracting the attention of young children. Sudden movements, loud noises and holding the child's head are to be avoided; rather, the light or toy should be slowly moved from one position to another. Small children should sit on a parent's lap. Quiet observation of the youngster prior to examination frequently reveals considerable information. During the examination the parent and office nurse should not talk or move about the room; a child's attention, once distracted, may not be regained at that session.

TREATMENT. *Parents should know that practically all deviating eyes can be straightened by corrective lenses, miotic therapy, orthoptics, surgery, or some combination of them, and that the straightening should be accomplished at the earliest possible time.*

Treatment of amblyopia ex anopsia should begin as soon as possible and must be carried out before the age of 6 years if vision is to be restored, and may be continued until the age of 10 years if necessary. A large number of children with strabismus have some degree of amblyopia; it has been estimated to occur in 5 per cent of the population. In a child with strabismus one may infer that amblyopia is present if one eye is invariably used for fixation of an object. At 1 year of age amblyopia may be eliminated within a few weeks by patching the good eye. The longer amblyopia persists, the more difficult it is to eradicate. Amblyopia should be prevented rather than treated. Good results are obtained in 80 per cent of children from 2 to 4 years of age, but in only 40 per cent of those from 4 to 7 years of age.

Orthoptics and Pleoptics. The techniques and training methods for adjusting binocular vision, visual perception and ocular motility are known as orthoptics. A series of complex instruments, many of which are modifications of the major amblyoscope, are used for both diagnosis and therapy. Diagnostic orthoptic procedures have become established as a valuable aid to the ophthalmologist; there are, however, variations in opinion about the benefits to be obtained from orthoptic therapy. It is useful in children with intermittent divergence and in the postoperative management of children to assist in the development of fusional amplitude. In children with pure alternating strabismus of significant degree, orthoptic treatment is usually unrewarding and may be a source of emotional fatigue.

A new method, pleoptics, has been developed for eccentric fixation (vision other than through the central macula), which may be effective in rehabilitating visual disturbances that heretofore had not been correctable in children of 8 years or older. Amblyopia is always present in cases of eccentric fixation.

Operative Treatment. Glasses can correct only a portion of the deviation in accommodative esotropia. *Surgical correction* will be necessary for those children who do not respond to the wearing of glasses or to exercises, or for those with residual esotropia. A high percentage of patients with strabismus, particularly if it is convergent, will eventually require surgery, and it is the only successful treatment for a marked alternating strabismus. Monocular strabismus of even moderate degree should be operated upon as early as possible after treatment has overcome amblyopia. Divergent strabismus offers less cosmetic blemish, and surgical treatment is often delayed. Excellent cosmetic results can usually be obtained and binocular vision developed.

Not infrequently multiple surgical procedures are required for strabismus, but the majority of uncomplicated cases can be corrected with two procedures. The ophthalmic surgeon aims for functional results (binocular stereo vision), but in cases of refractory amblyopia he must be satisfied with cosmetically straightened eyes.

INJURIES

About one third of all blindness in children results from trauma, usually avoidable. Such injuries are caused by air rifles, arrows, darts, stones and missile-throwing toys, sticks, sharp tools, explosives and strong chemicals. Small abrasions and superficial foreign bodies causing acute pain should prompt immediate consultation with a physician; unfortunately, some injuries do not produce pain, bleeding, sensitivity to light or blepharospasm, and often are ignored, e.g., intraocular foreign bodies, traumatic iritis, perforating wounds, dislocation of the lens and detachment of the retina. The end-results of injuries to the eye indicate that treatment should be the responsibility of the ophthalmologist from the outset.

Ecchymosis and edema are signs of injury to the *eyelids.* Ecchymosis (black eye) is usually of no great importance, except when the eyeball is involved. Blood from a basal skull fracture may appear under the bulbar conjunctiva a day or so after the injury.

Lacerations of the eyelid are generally more extensive than they appear externally. A small wound on the skin surface may not reflect the extent of the laceration of the tarsus. With any history of injury, prompt and complete examination of the lids, conjunctiva, cornea and sclera is necessary, even if general anesthesia is required. One or two sutures properly placed in the lid margin may obviate the necessity for extensive plastic repair at a later date, and even blindness may be avoided by prompt suturing of perforating wounds.

Slight *abrasions of the corneal surface* can be revealed by application of moistened fluorescein strips (sterile paper impregnated with fluorescein).

Large lacerations of the cornea and sclera require proper appositional suturing after excision of any free uveal tissue, vitreous or damaged lens tissue. Large wounds with escape of vitreous and with hemorrhage into the eye involve the choroid and retina. Detachment of the retina may occur. Frank infection is surprisingly infrequent. Emergency treatment should consist of instillation of a sterile atropine solution and application of a sterile pad. No ointment should be applied to the eyeball. After repair of the globe, atropine, a topical steroid-antibiotic solution and rest in bed are indicated until the true status of the eye can be determined.

Perforating wounds of the globe are always dangerous, even though the eye looks white and is not painful. Even small perforations may be complicated by *sympathetic ophthalmia.*

A *foreign body* on the cornea or conjunctiva is usually responsible for sudden onset of pain with lacrimation and with congestion of the conjunctiva. Most foreign bodies can be located by examination with a good light and a magnifying lens. Irregularities on the corneal surface may indicate the location of the foreign body. If a foreign body is suspected, but not found, the eye should be examined roentgenographically. The instillation of 0.5 per cent tetracaine will facilitate examination as well as removal of the foreign body. It is wise to be certain that the anesthesia is complete and that the patient is relaxed enough to remain motionless. Foreign bodies that are not embedded may be removed by gently touching them with a moistened, cotton-tipped applicator. Embedded foreign bodies requiring instrumentation should be removed by an ophthalmologist.

Burns of the eye should be irrigated and covered with a bland oil or ointment and the eye bandaged. Initially, burns from acid appear to be more severe than those from alkali, but the latter are usually more serious. In powder burns the particles, when accessible, should be removed as soon as possible by copious irrigations. Tetracaine may be used to relieve the pain. Reparative operations may be necessary after the acute stage.

Ultraviolet burns of the cornea produce extensive loss of the cells of the corneal epithelium, causing pain, photophobia and blepharospasm. Treatment consists in dilatation of the pupil with homatropine, 5 per cent, and the frequent application of tetracaine ointment, 0.5 per cent. Both eyes should be kept closed until healing has taken place, which generally requires 24 to 48 hours.

INTERNAL DISEASES OF THE EYE

The *uveal tract* is the vascular inner coat of the eye composed of the iris, ciliary body and choroid. Iritis may occur alone or in conjunction with infection of its contiguous structure, the ciliary body, as iridocyclitis. Pain, photophobia and lacrimation are characteristic early symptoms.

All children with *acute anterior uveitis* deserve extensive investigation. The cause may be obscure, but the most common causes are rheumatoid arthritis, sarcoidosis and trauma; uveitis may also be secondary to a corneal lesion, such as an ulcer or herpetic keratitis.

Posterior uveitis is an inflammatory lesion of the choroid, but it invariably involves the retina. The cause of posterior uveitis may also remain obscure, but the more common causes are toxoplasmosis, tuberculosis, syphilis, brucellosis, parasitic infestation and cytomegalic inclusion disease. Uveitis may also be a manifestation of septicemia.

Sympathetic ophthalmia is a rare inflammatory response of the normal eye following perforating trauma to the other eye in which there has been a prolapse of uveal tissue. It may occur weeks or even months after the accident. A hypersensitivity phenomenon involving uveal pigment is the most probable cause.

Endophthalmitis is usually a blood-borne infection; the initial manifestations may be retinitis and involvement of the vitreous and the uveal tract. It occurs with a variety of infections, such as meningitis, scarlet fever, measles and subacute bacterial endocarditis. It usually leads to blindness.

Panophthalmitis is an inflammation of all the structures of the eye and is frequently suppurative. It produces pain, severe congestion of the eyeball, eyelids and orbit, and loss of vision. Management includes symptomatic measures and systemic antibiotic therapy until it is safe to enucleate the globe.

Nevoxanthoendothelioma is a granulomatous lesion of the iris, which appears as a slightly raised yellowish mass. It is the most common cause of spontaneous bleeding in the anterior chamber of children. Blood in the anterior chamber may result in secondary glaucoma, which may require surgery. The lesion responds to small doses of radiation.

RETINA

Defects of the choroid and retina can be plainly seen through a dilated pupil by means of an ophthalmoscope. The appearance of the choroid is determined to some degree by the density of the retinal pigment layer. In albinism and in the blond fundus, the choroidal vasculature is most prominent. In the darkly pigmented eye the choroidal vessels are less easily visible, except when sclerotic. Choroideremia, or absence of the choroid, is a rare, genetically determined defect. Colobomata involving the choroid and retina occur inferiorly and are usually associated with coloboma of the iris. Other congenital lesions of the choroid and retina include large "rock candy" drusen, aneurysms, malformations of the optic disk, medullated nerve fibers and hereditary macular degenerations.

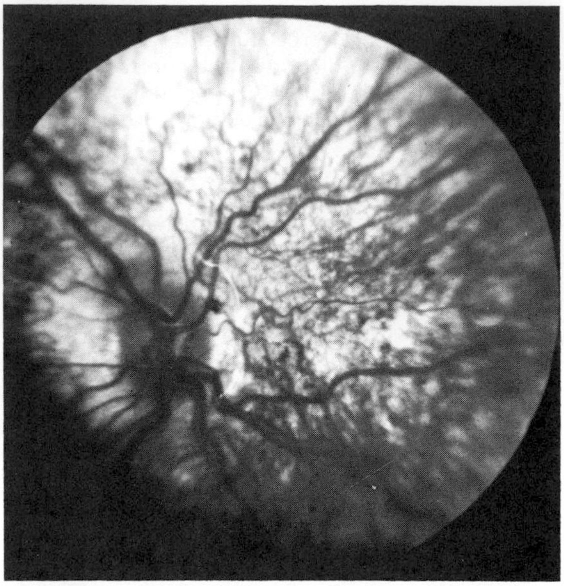

Figure 24–6 *Rubella retinopathy, illustrating pigment mottling.*

There may be characteristic retinal changes with certain systemic diseases (see Medical Ophthalmology). In leukemia there may be hemorrhages with white centers, dilatation and tortuosity of the veins, and exudation. In rare instances in uncontrolled diabetic children the retinal vessels appear to be filled with cream (lipemia retinalis). In chronic nephritis and in hypertension there may be edema about the disk and adjacent retina accompanied by flame-shaped hemorrhages.

CHORIORETINITIS. Chorioretinitis occurs with syphilis, tuberculosis, toxoplasmosis, cytomegalic inclusion disease, histoplasmosis, fungus infection, nematode infestation and septic infections. There is a reduction or loss of vision in the part of the field corresponding to the areas involved. These are at first yellowish, with ill-defined margins; later there is organization, leaving atrophic areas that are whitish with pigmented margins. Vitreous opacities may be associated. The prognosis depends upon the location of the inflammation and the response to therapy. Treatment should include rest, injections of foreign protein, corticosteroids and whatever specific measures may be directed against the cause.

RETINAL DETACHMENT. A detached retina is more common in older persons, but it may be observed in children, in whom there is frequently a history of trauma or a family history of retinal detachment or of other congenital ocular or systemic conditions. Retinal detachment can be primary, with a retinal tear and liquefied vitreous behind the detached area, or it can be secondary, in which case the subretinal exudate originates from some disturbance in choroidal or retinal circulation. The secondary form of retinal detachment may be associated with uveitis, parasitic disease, hypertensive disease, collagen disease and diabetes mellitus. Retinal detachment is usually symptomless except for a decided loss of acuity in the visual field corresponding to the detached portion.

RETROLENTAL FIBROPLASIA. This occurs most commonly in premature infants treated with high concentrations of oxygen during the early days of life. The active stage of the disease is first manifest in constriction of the retinal vessels, followed by dilatation and tortuosity. Hemorrhages may occur, and neovascularization is sometimes visible, especially at the periphery of the fundus. As the lesion progresses, neovascularization becomes more obvious and the peripheral retina appears clouded. A vitreous haze may be present. At this stage, spontaneous regression is possible; but peripheral retinal detachment next develops, which may progress to involvement of the entire retina. Detachment leads to the cicatricial stage and to complete loss of vision. The retina may be reduced to the appearance of a white fibrous sheath on the posterior surface of the lens.

The disease does not necessarily run a complete course, but may become arrested at an earlier stage, with some residual vision. "Dragged" disks, nystagmus, microphthalmos and myopia are often present in arrested cases.

The relationship between retrolental fibroplasia and the use of oxygen in treatment of the respiratory distress syndrome or other conditions is well established. Retrolental fibroplasia is not likely if ambient oxygen levels are held to 40 per cent or less of inspired air, but such levels may be insufficient to relieve anoxia in distressed infants, and close attention to the arterial pO_2 may be necessary.

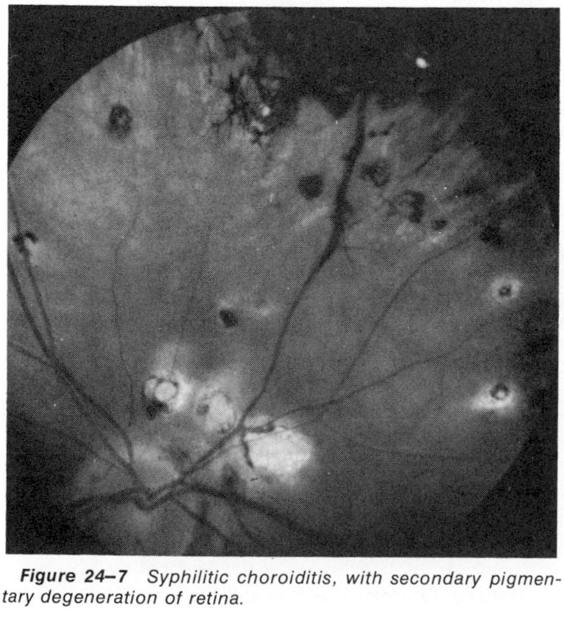

Figure 24–7 *Syphilitic choroiditis, with secondary pigmentary degeneration of retina.*

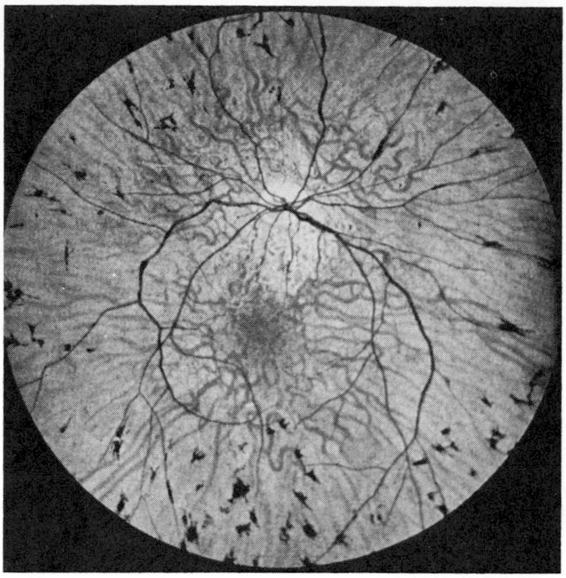

Figure 24–8 *Retinitis pigmentosa.*

Whenever an infant receives oxygen therapy in the early postnatal period, the eyes must be examined at frequent intervals to detect the early signs of the condition. Examination of the retina for vasoconstriction can provide an excellent clue as to the oxygen levels to which the infant is exposed, inasmuch as constricted retinal vessels are an early sign of oxygen toxicity. The constricted vessels may relax and dilate during ophthalmoscopy, so that as early as 10 to 15 minutes after removal of the infant from the incubator, the vessels may be nearly normal in caliber. If oxygen levels are reduced at this time, permanent retinal damage may be avoided. If vasospasm persists after 20 minutes in room air, some degree of retrolental fibroplasia is more likely ultimately to occur. Thorough ophthalmoscopy by an experienced physician is advisable at the time of discharge of premature infants who have received oxygen therapy and again when they are 6 months old.

JUVENILE RETINOSCHISIS. This is a sex-linked hereditary degenerative disease of the retina in which there is a splitting of the retina into two layers. The condition is bilateral and may be noted during infancy. The progress is slow, and visual loss may not result for many years. A retinal cyst must be considered in the differential diagnosis.

RETINAL DEGENERATIONS. These may be divided into central and peripheral forms. Changes are rarely present at birth, but may be noted during study of the child with "failure to thrive" or the child who ceases to develop normally. Retinal

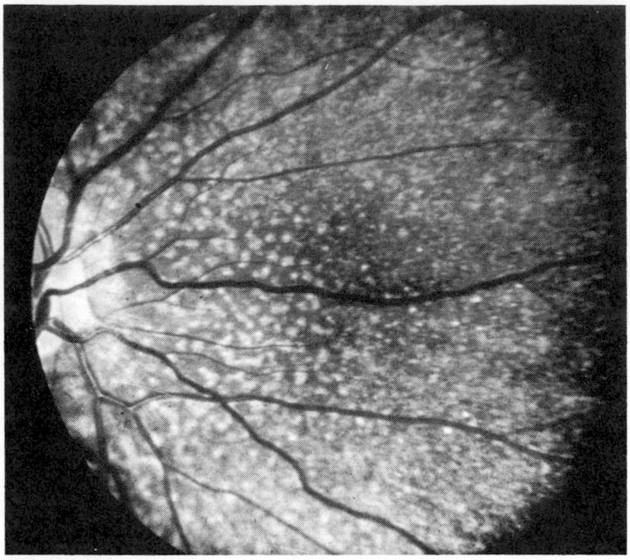

Figure 24–9 *Retinitis punctata albecens, associated with constricted visual fields and night blindness.*

degenerations are associated with a number of the degenerative encephalopathies (Section 20).

EXUDATIVE RETINOPATHY (COATS'S DISEASE). Coats's disease is an exudative process beneath the retina associated with telangiectases and recurrent retinal hemorrhages. It is usually unilateral, occurs most commonly in male children, and results in detached retina with severe loss of vision.

HEREDOMACULAR DEGENERATION. A number of hereditary retinal macular dystrophies are characterized by bilateral degenerative changes in the macular area *without* degenerative changes in the

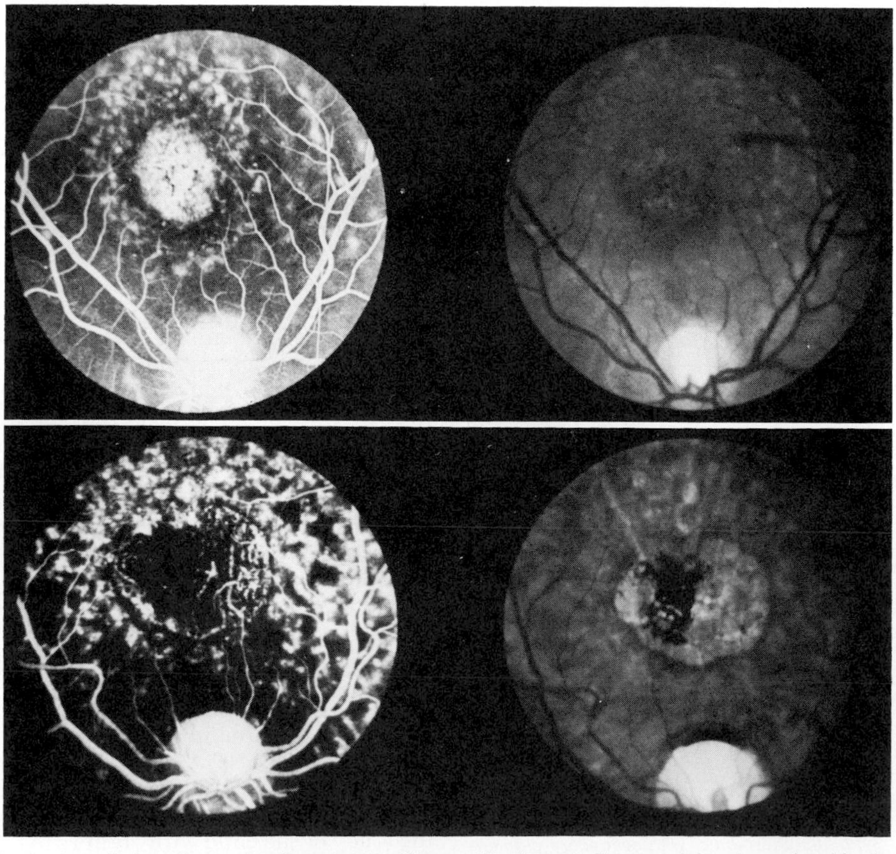

Figure 24–10 *Juvenile heredomacular degeneration (Stargardt's disease). Fluorescein angiography aids visualization.*

central nervous system. They may appear at any age from infancy to adult life. A loss of central vision is the primary problem.

PERIPHERAL RETINAL DEGENERATION. Peripheral pigmentary degeneration occurs with a large group of diseases, which include Friedreich's ataxia and Laurence-Moon-Biedl syndrome. *Retinitis pigmentosa* and the closely related *retinitis punctata albescens* are classic examples of peripheral retinal degeneration. Night blindness is the first symptom; daytime vision and central vision remain good. Peripheral sight gradually deteriorates until the patient is reduced to "gun-barrel" vision.

RETINOBLASTOMA. Retinoblastoma is a malignant tumor of the retina. It generally occurs before the fifth year, most commonly in the earlier years. Strabismus or unilateral nystagmus may be an early sign. The tumor is frequently first noted through a white reflex produced in the pupillary area, the "amaurotic cat's eye" appearance. The tumor is highly malignant and usually metastasizes by direct extension into the optic nerve and brain. It is bilateral in about a third of cases. Enucleation is indicated when the tumor is unilateral; for bilateral involvement the less severe eye is vigorously treated by radiation and triethylenemelamine, and the more involved eye is excised.

About 6 per cent of retinoblastoma are familial; the mode of inheritance in these cases is autosomal dominant. The frequency with which the gene becomes manifest in persons carrying it (penetrance) varies from 20 to 95 per cent in different families and is most frequently stated to be about 80 per cent. Normal parents with one affected child and no history of other cases in the family have a 4 to 7 per cent chance of producing more offspring with retinoblastoma. If normal parents have two or more affected children, one of them is established as a probable carrier, so that the risk of future children carrying the gene will be 50 per cent for each child, and the proportion of children developing retinoblastoma will be determined by the penetrance of the gene in that particular family. The same considerations obtain in the case of the survivor of retinoblastoma of established hereditary occurrence. Survivors of bilateral "sporadic" retinoblastoma produce clinically affected offspring in 50 per cent of cases. Only 10 per cent of survivors of unilateral sporadic retinoblastoma produce clinically affected children.

ANOMALIES OF THE OPTIC NERVE. Some of the anomalies of the optic nerve may resemble papilledema and present difficult problems in differentiation. Pseudopapilledema is usually seen in hyperopic (farsighted) eyes. The disk margins are blurred and may be elevated. The physiologic cupping may be absent.

Medullated nerve fibers are a common finding at the disk margin; normally, they stop at the nerve head. These nerve fibers may extend as white, feathery patches from the disk onto the retina in any direction.

Drusen appear ophthalmoscopically as highly refractile, yellow, glistening, round bodies on or within the optic nerve head. They may give the disk an irregular, scalloped appearance.

The hyaloid vessels may persist as black, wavy lines from the disk, owing to failure of resorption during embryonic life.

Colobomata of the optic nerve, which result from inadequate closure of the fetal fissure, cause considerable distortion of the optic disk. Pits in the optic disk and choroidal pigment crescents at the disk margin may also be seen rather commonly; they do not impair visual function.

THE OPTIC NERVE. Diagnosis of lesions of the optic nerve can be difficult, since many normal variations resemble organic changes. The optic disk of the infant may appear pale in comparison with that of an older child. Infants' eyes are difficult to examine, however, and one must be certain that pressure is not exerted on the eyeball which can produce blanching of the disk.

Pallor of the disk does not always signify optic atrophy. Optic atrophy implies functional loss of vision, which is not always easy to document. In the differentiation of the suspected "blind child" the electroretinogram is useful in differentiating cerebral from ocular blindness.

Papilledema (choked disk) in its fully developed form with marked elevation, hemorrhages at the disk margin and large distended veins is not difficult to recognize. Early papilledema, however, can easily be mistaken for structural blurring of the disk margins as well as for other congenital changes such as medullated nerve fibers and hyaline bodies. Choked disk is always a matter for concern; increased intracranial pressure of whatever cause must be the first consideration.

OPTIC NEURITIS. This is often bilateral in children. Rapid loss of central vision with or without papilledema is pathognomonic. Demyelinating diseases, inflammatory diseases of the eye or orbit and encephalomyelitis must be considered in the causation of optic neuritis. When the inflammatory area occurs behind the disk, it is known as *retrobulbar neuritis*, and the disk may appear normal.

OPTIC ATROPHY. This is characterized by pallor of the disk, loss of disk substance, and loss of visual function. It may be primary, as in congenital optic atrophy, or secondary, following optic neuritis, longstanding papilledema, central nervous system degenerative disorders, congenital glaucoma or tumor of the optic nerve. Unilateral optic atrophy may be the first sign of glaucoma.

HYGIENE OF THE EYE

Proper illumination minimizes "eyestrain" and increases reading efficiency. There is no proof that poor lighting causes organic eye disease, but it definitely accelerates the onset of eye fatigue. Children should be encouraged to read in a good light (100 to 150 watts) which comes from behind and does not produce reflected glare. Fluorescent light, when it flickers, has been known to increase symptoms of discomfort and fatigue in some persons. Printed matter should be held at least 14 inches from the eye, and the print should not be too small. It is wise to have the book tilted to prevent reflection from glossy paper. Good posture while reading should be encouraged.

Television is not harmful to the eyes, though it frequently brings on symptoms of fatigue and "eyestrain." The child should sit at least 10 to 12 feet from the screen in a room which has some general illumination, and the picture should be sharply focused. The poor content of the programs is of more concern than is any possible deleterious effect on the eyes. Allowing a child to watch television while wearing a patch over one eye is sometimes effective in the treatment of amblyopia ex anopsia (see above).

There need be no restriction of children's reading because of refractive errors or muscular imbalance.

SIGHT-SAVING CLASSES AND SCHOOLS FOR BLIND CHILDREN

Sight-saving and training classes have been established in public and in private schools for children whose vision is reduced to such an extent that they cannot meet the requirements of the ordinary school curriculum. The training consists chiefly in following the regular school curriculum through books printed in large type on suitable contrast backgrounds so that ocular failure is minimized. Special attention is given to lighting and reading posture. With such a regimen children with limited but not complete loss of vision can be adequately educated. Books with large print are provided by the National Aid to the Visually Handicapped.* These promote self-help in partially sighted children.

The cooperative system for educating partially sighted children is recommended, rather than placing them in schools for the blind or in special schools where they are grouped with children with other handicaps, such as deafness or cerebral palsy. Even placement in segregated classes in public schools adds its stigma. The cooperative plan places the partially seeing children with the normally seeing children in regular classrooms. Projects requiring concentrated eye work by the partially sighted children are conducted in separate, specially equipped classrooms. The psychologic advantages of this plan are tremendous, just as the term "semisighted" is preferable to "semiblind."

When vision has been reduced to 10/200 or less, it is almost impossible for the child to continue in sight-training classes, and he should then be enrolled in a school for the blind. Here he is taught one of the touch systems of reading. Emphasis is placed on the teaching of manual arts and the development of a sense of independence and self-sufficiency. Those schools in which the curriculum includes instruction for the parents as to how they may participate in the training of their visually handicapped child are the most effective ones.

Children who have never had vision do not miss it and may be content with their condition. They should be treated socially as normal children and neither pitied nor rejected. Parents often regard a blind infant with awe and must be helped to adjust to and manage the situation constructively and intelligently.

*3201 Balboa St., San Francisco, Calif. 94121.

MEDICAL OPHTHALMOLOGY

Ocular findings are of interest and significance in a wide variety of medical conditions of children. The most important disorders include the following.

HYPERTENSION. In the early stages there may be no observable ocular change. Generalized constriction and irregular narrowing of the arterioles are usually the first changes in the fundus. Other alterations include retinal edema, flame-shaped hemorrhages, "cotton-wool patches" and papilledema. These changes are reversible if the disease process can be eliminated in the early stages, but in hypertension of long standing the changes are irreversible and simulate those of arteriosclerotic disease. Hypertension in the child should alert the physician to renal disease, pheochromocytoma, collagen diseases and cardiovascular disorders, such as coarctation of the aorta.

RENAL RETINOPATHY. Renal and other hypertensive retinopathies are often indistinguishable; pallor of the disk and macular star formations are more commonly associated with nephritis.

CYANOSIS OF THE RETINA. This may occur with congenital heart diseases, chronic pulmonary insufficiency, or other disorders responsible for cyanosis. The conjunctival vessels may be congested and dark. The retinal veins are dark, tortuous and dilated, and the retina appears cyanotic at times, with scattered hemorrhages.

SUBACUTE BACTERIAL ENDOCARDITIS. Retinopathy is present in 40 per cent of cases during the course of the disease; the lesions include hemorrhages, Roth spots (white areas surrounded by hemorrhage), papilledema and, rarely, embolic occlusion of the central retinal artery.

BLOOD DISORDERS

Primary and Secondary Anemias. Retinopathy in the form of hemorrhages and "cotton-wool patches" generally occurs only when the red blood cell count drops to 2 million or below. Vision will be affected if a hemorrhage is present in the macular area. The hemorrhages may be light and feathery or dense and preretinal.

Polycythemia Vera. The retinal veins are dark, dilated and tortuous. Retinal hemorrhages, retinal edema and papilledema may be observed.

(*Text continued on page 1599*)

TABLE 24–2 OCULAR CHANGES IN DEVELOPMENTAL PEDIATRIC SYNDROMES

DISEASE	OCULAR MANIFESTATION	SYSTEMIC MANIFESTATION	INHERITANCE*
Abeta-lipoproteinemia (acanthocytosis; Bassen-Kornzweig)	Pigmentary degeneration of retina	See Sections 8 and 11	A–R
Achromatopsia	Amblyopia, nystagmus and photosensitivity; visual acuity often 20/200; total absence of color discrimination; failure with Sloan achromatopsia test; absent photopic ERG		A–R
Acrocephalo-polysyndactyly (Carpenter syndrome)	Lateral displacement of inner canthi and/or inner canthal folds	See Section 22	A–R
Acrocephalo-syndactyly (Apert)	Exophthalmos, exotropia, optic atrophy, partial ophthalmoplegia and cataracts	See Section 22	A–R
Albinism (oculocutaneous)			
Complete albinism	Iris is thin, pink or pale blue; a characteristic orange reflex from the pupil occurs when light rays penetrating the pigment-deficient membranes of the eye are reflected back to the observer's eye; prominent choroidal vessels with poorly defined fovea; nystagmus, head-nodding and frequently myopic astigmatism and strabismus; marked photophobia; the eyelashes and eyebrows are white	White hair and brows; two distinct genotypes depending on presence or absence of tyrosinase; tyrosinase absent in complete albinism	A–R
Modified complete albinism	Slight pigmentation, some yellow pigment flecks at pupillary border; minimal to absent red reflex; may be nystagmus, photophobia and myopia; choroidal vessels prominent	Tyrosinase positive; in Caucasians, no phenotypic difference between tyrosinase positive and negative; in Blacks, slight pigmentation, golden hair, with tendency to hyperkeratoses and freckling in exposed areas of skin	A–R
Ocular albinism	Marked deficiency of pigment in iris and choroid, nystagmus and myopic astigmatism; iris of female carrier is frequently translucent	Normal pigmentation elsewhere	X–R
Amish albinism	At birth complete albinism with blue translucent irides and albinotic fundal reflex; nystagmus and photophobia; increasing pigmentation with age	White hair and skin at birth; increasing pigmentation with yellow hair and normal skin which tans; biochemically gives intermediate reaction between tyrosinase positive and negative	A–R

*A–R = autosomal recessive; X–R = X-linked recessive; A–D = autosomal dominant; X–D = X-linked dominant.

Table 24–2 continued on following page.

TABLE 24-2 OCULAR CHANGES IN DEVELOPMENTAL PEDIATRIC SYNDROMES *(Continued)*

DISEASE	OCULAR MANIFESTATION	SYSTEMIC MANIFESTATION	INHERITANCE*
Albinism with deafness	Typical ocular changes	Typical albinism with nerve deafness	X–R
Albright syndrome (polyostotic fibrous dysplasia; McCune-Albright syndrome)	Unilateral proptosis, visual field defects, papilledema, optic atrophy	See Sections 18 and 22	A–D?, most cases sporadic
Alkaptonuria and ochronosis	Scleral pigmentation most marked at recti muscle insertions	See Section 8	A–R
Alpers' diffuse cerebral degeneration	Cortical blindness	Hyperkinesis; seizures; rigidity; opisthotonos	A–R
Alport syndrome	Cataracts, anterior lenticonus, spherophakia	Nerve deafness; hemorrhagic nephritis	A–D, with anomalous segregation
Alstrom's disease	Retinitis pigmentosa and cataract	Nerve deafness; diabetes mellitus in childhood and obesity	A–R
Aicardi syndrome	Large, discrete areas of chorioretinopathy, microphthalmos	Spasms and toxic seizures in female infants; defects of corpus callosum, cortical heterotopia; dorsal vertebral anomalies; characteristic EEG and mental retardation	A–D, lethal in the male
Amaurotic Family Idiocy Tay-Sachs disease (GM_2 ganglioside storage disease)	Cherry red spot in macula, optic atrophy, gradual onset of ophthalmoplegia, visual loss to blindness	See Sections 8 and 20	A–R
Late infantile form of amaurotic familial idiocy (Batten-Bielschowsky)	Dark red spot on macula, optic atrophy	See Section 20	A–R
Juvenile amaurotic familial idiocy (Batten-Mayou Vogt-Spielmeyer)	Reddish brown spot in macula, peripheral retinal degeneration, nystagmus, gradual visual loss to blindness	See Section 20	A–R
Late juvenile or adult form of amaurotic familial idiocy (Kufs')	No visual loss, and fundi may be normal or show mild retinal pigmentary changes	See Section 20	A–R
Generalized gangliosidosis (GM_1)	Cherry red spot in half of patients	See Section 20	A–R
Aminopterin-induced syndrome	Shallow orbital ridge from severe hypoplasia of frontal bone, broad nasal bridge and epicanthus, prominent eyes.	Generalized congenital hypoplasia; cleft palate and low set ears; partial syndactyly and hypotonia; aminopterin or methotrexate used as abortifacient during first trimester	Teratogenic
Amyloidoses, hereditary	Sheet-like hyaline vitreous opacities, visual loss, exophthalmos, ophthalmoplegia,	Peripheral neuropathy; chronic gastrointestinal symptoms; hoarseness;	A–R

TABLE 24–2 OCULAR CHANGES IN DEVELOPMENTAL PEDIATRIC SYNDROMES *(Continued)*

DISEASE	OCULAR MANIFESTATION	SYSTEMIC MANIFESTATION	INHERITANCE*
	corneal dystrophy from amyloid, conjunctival amyloidosis, pupils small and irregular	autonomic dysfunction; occurs with high frequency in Portuguese	
Aniridia	Complete or partial absence of iris; associated with coloboma in family; nystagmus, hypoplasia of macula, glaucoma, cataract	Cerebellar ataxia and oligophrenia reported; Wilms' tumor occurs with sporadic aniridia, but usually not familial	A–D A–R sporadic
Anophthalmos or microphthalmos	Small rudimentary globe deep in orbit	Polydactyly; craniofacial and brain malformations	A–D A–R X–R
Ataxia-telangiectasia (Louis-Bar syndrome)	Telangiectatic bulbar conjunctiva in medial and lateral canthi, nystagmus, ocular motor apraxic movement, frequent loss of optokinetic response, strabismus and poor convergence	See Section 20	A–D
Basal Cell Nevus Syndrome	Strabismus, cataract, iris coloboma, hypertelorism; synophrys	Basal cell nevi over upper torso; prone to carcinoma; mental deficiency; odontogenic cysts of mandible; misshapen teeth; bifid ribs	A–D
Bonnevie-Ullrich (Turner phenotype)	Cataract and ptosis; varying sexual development, genetic heterogeneity; occurs in both males and females	See Section 17	Chromosomal Heterogeneous
Cataract, congenital	Cataracts of all forms	See text and index for diseases associated with cataract	Depends on specific entity
Cerebral Sclerosis Group			
Pelizaeus-Merzbacher disease (diffuse cerebral sclerosis)	Nystagmus, optic atrophy	See Section 20	X–R (infancy) A–D (late form)
Krabbe's disease (globoid cell sclerosis)	Optic atrophy, nystagmus	See Section 20	A–R
Scholz' disease (subacute diffuse cerebral sclerosis)	Cortical blindness, nystagmus	Generalized CNS deterioration, beginning at age 8 to 10; intermediate between Pelizaeus-Merzbacher and Krabbe See Section 20	A–R?
Cerebrohepatorenal syndrome (Zellweger syndrome)	Bilateral congenital glaucoma, partial cataracts and epicanthi	See Sections 15 and 29	A–R
Charcot-Marie tooth (progressive neuromuscular atrophy)	Reduced vision, nystagmus and optic atrophy	See Section 21	A–R
Chediak-Higashi syndrome	Partial albinism, diminished uveal and retinal pigmentation with photophobia and	See Section 14	A–R

Table 24–2 continued on following page.

TABLE 24–2 OCULAR CHANGES IN DEVELOPMENTAL PEDIATRIC SYNDROMES *(Continued)*

DISEASE	OCULAR MANIFESTATION	SYSTEMIC MANIFESTATION	INHERITANCE*
	nystagmus; histologic examination of the eyes has shown papilledema, lymphocytic infiltration of the optic nerve, and leukocytes containing the typical metachromatic inclusion granules in the limbal area, iris and choroid		
Cockayne syndrome	Cataract, pigmentary degeneration and optic atrophy	See Section 23	A–R ?
Congenital alopecia	Bilateral cataracts	Congenital absence or extremely poor development of hair of the scalp, trunk, pubic region and eyebrows; Friedreich's ataxia, obesity, hyperhidrosis and syndactyly	A–D
Conradi's disease (chondrodystrophia calcificans congenita)	Bilateral cataract, optic atrophy and hypertelorism	See Sections 22 and 29	A–R
Chromosomal Abnormality syndromes			
Cri-du-chat syndrome Partial deletion of short arm of chromosome number 5 (5p–)	Hypertelorism, epicanthus, strabismus	See Section 6	Usually sporadic, occasional translocation
Partial deletion of #4 short arm (4 p–)	Iris coloboma	Cleft palate; hypospadias	Sporadic
Partial deletion of long arm #18 (18 q–)	Optic disc pallor, nystagmus, tapetoretinal degeneration	Psychomotor retardation with microcephaly; prominent chin	Sporadic or familial translocation
Partial deletion of #18 short arm (18 p–)	Hypertelorism, epicanthal fold, ptosis, strabismus	Short stature; webbed neck; mental retardation	Sporadic or familial translocation
Partial deletion of D long arm and ring D (Dq –)	Epicanthal folds, ptosis, hypertelorism, microphthalmia, iris, coloboma, retinoblastoma	Mental retardation, microcephaly; small chin; facial asymmetry	Sporadic
Cat-eye syndrome	Microphthalmia, coloboma, partial irideremia, absent macular areas, pale disks	Anal atresia; pre-auricular skin tags; umbilical hernia	Extra small chromosome, sporadic or familial
Trisomy-13	Microphthalmos, enophthalmos, corneal opacity, cataract, retinal dysplasia with cartilage, hypoplastic optic nerve and iris coloboma	See Section 6	Usually sporadic, rarely inherited as translocation
Trisomy-18	Blepharoptosis, corneal opacity, short palpebral fissures and epicanthal folds	See Section 6	Usually sporadic, rarely

TABLE 24–2 OCULAR CHANGES IN DEVELOPMENTAL PEDIATRIC SYNDROMES *(Continued)*

DISEASE	OCULAR MANIFESTATION	SYSTEMIC MANIFESTATION	INHERITANCE*
			inherited as translocation
Trisomy-21 (Down syndrome; Mongolism)	Mongoloid slant to palpebral fissures, epicanthus, cataract, Brushfield's spots, strabismus, and acute keratoconus with corneal hydrops	See Sections 2 and 6	Usually sporadic, 5 per cent due to familial translocation
Turner syndrome (45 X-0; mosaic variants)	Ptosis, color blindness, cataracts, strabismus, epicanthus, blue sclera, nystagmus	See Section 17	Sporadic
Klinefelter syndrome (XXY, XXXY, XXXXY)	Hypertelorism, epicanthus, strabismus, Brushfield's spots, myopia	See Section 17	Sporadic
Cornelia de Lange syndrome	Long curly eyelashes, bushy eyebrows and synophrys, strabismus, myopia, optic atrophy, proptosis	See Section 20	Unknown
Crouzon's disease (craniofacial dysostosis)	Exophthalmos, exotropia, optic atrophy, hypertelorism, and cataracts	See Section 22	A–D
Cryptophthalmia	Fusion of eyelids, unilateral or bilateral; microphthalmos	Deformity of pinnae; atresia of auditory canal; malformed teeth; spina bifida; syndactyly; abnormal hairline	A–R
Cystic fibrosis	Dilated dark, tortuous retinal veins, retinal hemorrhages	See Section 11	A–R
Cystinosis (Fanconi syndrome with renal tubular defects)	Cystine crystals seen in cornea and conjunctiva with corneal microscope; peripheral retinal pigmentary degeneration	See Section 22	A–R
Diabetes mellitus	Rapid change in refractive error, cataract, retinal microaneurysms, retinopathy, retinitis proliferans, retinal detachment	See Section 16	Familial, modes of inheritance obscure
Dyskeratosis congenita syndrome	Blepharitis, ectropion, nasolacrimal obstruction or atresia of lacrimal ducts	Hyperpigmentation of the skin; leukoplakia; nail dystrophy; sparse hair; pancytopenia and testicular atrophy; see Section 23	X–R
Ectodermal dysplasia (Marshall's type)	Congenital or juvenile cataracts which may spontaneously absorb, myopia.	See Section 23	A–D
Ectodermal hypohidrotic dysplasia (anhidrotic)	Tear deficiency leading to keratitis and photophobia, cataracts and microphthalmia	See Section 23	X–R
Ehlers-Danlos syndrome	Epicanthic folds, blue sclera, keratoconus, subluxation of lens and retinal detachment	See Section 23	A–D

Table 24–2 continued on following page.

TABLE 24-2 OCULAR CHANGES IN DEVELOPMENTAL PEDIATRIC SYNDROMES *(Continued)*

DISEASE	OCULAR MANIFESTATION	SYSTEMIC MANIFESTATION	INHERITANCE*
Fabry's disease (angiokeratoma corporis diffusum)	Whorl-like corneal opacities are characteristic, corkscrew tortuosity of veins in posterior pole, spoke-like lens opacities in 50 per cent, dilated, sausage-shaped conjunctival vessels, and periorbital edema	See Section 23	X–R
Falls-Kertesz syndrome	Distichiasis of all four lids and partial ectropion of lower lids	Chronic lymphedema of both lower extremities (Milroy's type) and pterygium colli	A–D
Familial blepharophimosis	Epicanthus inversus, lateral displacement of inner canthi with short palpebral fissures and bilateral ptosis; strabismus and nystagmus may occur	Possible generalized hypotonia	A–D
Familial dysautonomia (Riley-Day syndrome)	Tear deficiency, corneal anesthesia, ulceration and corneal scarring	See Section 20	A–R
Fanconi syndrome with pancytopenia	Strabismus, ptosis, nystagmus, microphthalmos	See Section 14	A–R
Farber disease (disseminated lipogranulomatosis)	Grayish area posterior pole, with cherry red spot and diffuse pigmentary mottling, granulomata in and around eye	See Section 8	A–R
Flynn-Aird syndrome	Severe myopia, bilateral cataracts, retinitis pigmentosa	Bilateral nerve deafness; dental caries; kyphoscoliosis; skin atrophy; baldness; muscle wasting; mental retardation; ataxia and seizures	A–D
Franceschetti syndrome (Treacher Collins syndrome; mandibulofacial dysostosis)	Lid coloboma, microphthalmia, antimongoloid slanting of lids	See Section 22	A–D
Fraser syndrome	Cryptophthalmos, hypertelorism and lacrimal duct defects	See Section 29	A–R
Freeman-Sheldon syndrome (whistling face or craniocarpotarsal dystrophy)	Deep-set eyes, blepharophimosis, ptosis, strabismus, and epicanthus	See Section 29	A–D
Galactosemia	Cataract, bilateral	See Section 8	A–R
Gaucher's disease			
Infant form	Visual defect, strabismus	See Section 8	A–R
Adult form	Wedge-shaped pinguecula, conjunctival pigmentation; reddish spot in macula may be present	See Section 8	A–R

TABLE 24–2 OCULAR CHANGES IN DEVELOPMENTAL PEDIATRIC SYNDROMES *(Continued)*

DISEASE	OCULAR MANIFESTATION	SYSTEMIC MANIFESTATION	INHERITANCE*
Goldenhar syndrome (oculoauriculo-vertebral)	Epibulbar dermoid involving conjunctiva and cornea	External ear deformity or absence which may be associated with deafness; preauricular cutaneous appendages; mandibular hypoplasia; occipitalization of atlas	Not known
Goltz syndrome	Strabismus, coloboma and/or microphthalmos	Areas of hypoplasia and altered pigmentation of skin; dystrophic nails, enamel hypoplasia and syndactyly; only females affected, presumed lethal in male	?
Granulomatous disease (chronic) of childhood	Pleomorphic, atrophic chorioretinal lesions, blepharitis, conjunctivitis and keratitis	See Section 9	X–R
Hallerman-Streiff (dyscephalia mandibulo-oculo-facialis)	Bilateral microphthalmia and bilateral congenital cataracts which may resorb spontaneously, blue sclera, nystagmus	Small stature; brachycephaly; malar hypoplasia; micrognathia; small parrot beak nose; skin atrophy over nose and scalp; sparse hair; hypoplasia of teeth and hypotrichosis	A–D ?
Hallgren's disease	Retinitis pigmentosa	Congenital nerve deafness, vestibular ataxia; mental retardation and psychosis	A–R
Hartnup disease	Nystagmus, photophobia, strabismus	See Section 8	A–R
Hemophilia Factor VIII deficiency (classic hemophilia; hemophilia A)	Orbital, hemorrhage, subconjunctival hemorrhage	See Section 14	X–R
Factor IX deficiency (Christmas disease; hemophilia B)	15 per cent show ocular changes similar to factor VIII deficiency	See Section 14	X–R
Hereditary benign intraepithelial dyskeratosis (Witkop-Von Sallmann syndrome)	Foamy gelatinous plaques on a hyperemic bulbar conjunctiva at nasal and temporal limbus may be noted by age 1 yr; corneal dyskeratosis can lead to severe visual loss	Soft white folds and plaques involving mucosal surface of mouth, tongue, tonsils and palate	A–D with high degree of penetrance
Hereditary cerebellar ataxia with optic atrophy—(Behr syndrome)	Nystagmus, atrophy of papillomacular bundle and external ophthalmoplegia	Ataxia, and loss of coordination; pyramidal tract signs (increased tendon reflexes, positive Babinski); mental deficiency; vesical sphincter weakness	A–R ?
Homocystinuria	Dislocated lenses, cataract, secondary glaucoma, peripheral cystic degeneration of retina	See Section 8	A–R

Table 24–2 continued on following page.

TABLE 24–2 OCULAR CHANGES IN DEVELOPMENTAL PEDIATRIC SYNDROMES *(Continued)*

DISEASE	OCULAR MANIFESTATION	SYSTEMIC MANIFESTATION	INHERITANCE*
Hooft's disease (hypolipidemia syndrome)	Tapetoretinal degeneration resembling retinitis pigmentosa; extinguished ERG	Onset by age 2 yr; red skin lesions on face and limbs; white nails, abnormal teeth and mental retardation	A–R
Hyperlysinemia	Subluxation of lens, spherophakia and strabismus	See Section 8	A–R
Hyperphosphatasia, hereditary (juvenile Paget's disease)	Optic atrophy and angioid streaks with macular changes, blue sclera may be observed	See Section 22	A–R
Hypophosphatasia	Band-shaped keratopathy and calcific deposits in conjunctiva; exophthalmos, papilledema and optic atrophy reported	See Section 22	A–R
Ichthyosis			
Congenital ichthyosis	Ectropion and keratopathy; congenital cataracts may occur	See Section 23	A–R
Lamellar ichthyosis	Ectropion	See Section 23	A–R
Ichthyosis and cataracts	Cortical cataracts	Same as congenital ichthyosis	A–R
Ichthyosis vulgaris	Ichthyosis of lids, scales on lashes, punctate keratitis, corneal erosions and stromal opacities; lens changes	See Section 23	A–D
Bullous ichthyosiform erythroderma	Scales on lashes	Similar to congenital ichthyosis, but exhibiting bullae	A–D
X-linked ichthyosis	Ocular changes as in ichthyosis vulgaris	Similar to ichthyosis vulgaris, but palms and soles normal	X–R
Infantile subacute necrotizing encephalomyelopathy (Leigh syndrome)	Optic atrophy, nystagmus, intermittent ptosis, miosis	See Section 8	A–R
Incontinentia pigmenti (Bloch-Sulzberger)	Strabismus, corneal opacities, cataract, persistent hyperplastic primary vitreous	See Section 23	X–D ? lethal in male?
Jeune syndrome (thoracic asphyxiating dystrophy)	Loss of visual acuity and peripheral field, retinal degeneration with diminishing ERG	See Section 22	A–R
Kearns syndrome (external ophthalmoplegia, pigmentary degeneration and cardiomyopathy)	Chronic progressive external ophthalmoplegia, pigmentary degeneration of the retina with abnormal ERG	Cardiomyopathy; weakness of facial and laryngeal muscles; weakness of trunk and extremity musculature; deafness; small stature; EEG changes and high CSF protein	A–D
Keratosis palmoplantaris with corneal lesions (Richner-Hanhart)	Herpetiform lesions of the cornea and photophobia	See Section 23	A–R

TABLE 24–2 OCULAR CHANGES IN DEVELOPMENTAL PEDIATRIC SYNDROMES *(Continued)*

DISEASE	OCULAR MANIFESTATION	SYSTEMIC MANIFESTATION	INHERITANCE*
Klippel-Feil syndrome	Congenital strabismus, bilateral Duane's retraction syndrome	See Section 22	A–R ? A–D ? (irreg.)
Lawrence-Moon-Biedl syndrome	Retinitis pigmentosa, optic atrophy, strabismus	Obesity; polydactyly; hypogenitalism; mental retardation	A–R
Leber's congenital amaurosis	Blindness with normal fundi; may develop retinitis pigmentosa appearance later	Mental retardation; epilepsy or neurologic disorders	A–R, probably more than a single genetic entity
Leber's hereditary optic atrophy	Central scotoma, bilateral, not concurrent with eventual disk pallor, especially of papillomacular bundle	Vertigo, but usually normal	X–R, A–R, heterogeneous
Lipoid proteinosis (Urbach-Wiethe)	Yellowish white, beadlike lesions on eyelid margins	See Section 23	A–R
Lowe syndrome (oculocerebrorenal)	Congenital cataracts and glaucoma	See Section 22	A–R
Macular dystrophies	Macular degenerations	Varied. See text and Section 20	Varied
Mannosidosis	Small cloudy opacities beneath anterior lens capsule, optic disks pale, with blurred margins	See Section 8	A–R
Marfan syndrome	Dislocated lens, spherophakia, nystagmus, exotropia	See Section 22	A–D
Marinesco-Sjögren syndrome	Bilateral congenital cataract, horizontal or rotary nystagmus	Oligophrenia and spinocerebellar ataxia; similar to Sjögren syndrome (q.v.)	A–R
Meckel syndrome	Microphthalmos, anophthalmos, cataract, partial aniridia, sclerocornea, cryptophthalmos, retinal dysplasia and hypoplasia of the optic nerve	Occipital encephalocele; polycystic kidneys; polydactyly; congenital heart disease; abnormal genitalia; normal chromosomes	A–R
Metachromatic leukodystrophy	Nystagmus, strabismus, cherry red spot in macula, optic disk pallor	See Section 20	A–R
Microphthalmos, corneal dystrophy, mental retardation and spasticity	Microphthalmos, corneal dystrophy (lattice) and pupillary changes	Mental retardation; spasticity and seizures	A–D ?
Mieten syndrome	Corneal opacities, nystagmus and strabismus	See Section 29	A–R
Milroy's disease (chronic hereditary lymphedema)	Ptosis, glaucoma, distichiasis and strabismus	See Section 14	A–D
Moebius syndrome	Bilateral, unequal involvement of 6th and 7th nerves with frequent contracture of medial recti	See Section 20	A–D, varying expressivity

Table 24–2 continued on following page.

TABLE 24-2 OCULAR CHANGES IN DEVELOPMENTAL PEDIATRIC SYNDROMES *(Continued)*

DISEASE	OCULAR MANIFESTATION	SYSTEMIC MANIFESTATION	INHERITANCE*
Mucopolysaccharidoses			
Hurler syndrome (gargoylism MPS I)	Corneal clouding, ptosis, strabismus and thickened eyelids, glaucoma; pigmentary degeneration of retina occurs	See Sections 22 and 29	A–R
Hunter syndrome (MPS II)	Cornea usually clear, but mild clouding may be seen by slit lamp; pigmentary degeneration of retina often seen	Similar to Hurler syndrome, but only mild mental change(?); defect only in males	X–R
Sanfilippo syndrome (MPS III)	No specific eye change; genetic heterogeneity	See Section 22	A–R
Morquio syndrome (MPS IV)	Corneal clouding may occur, but cornea usually grossly clear; retinal pigmentary changes may be observed	See Section 22	A–R
Scheie syndrome (MPS V)	Corneal clouding, but central area less severely affected	See Section 22	A–R
Maroteaux-Lamy syndrome (MPS VI)	Corneal clouding begins in early life	See Section 22	A–R
β-Glucuronidase deficiency	Corneal clouding	See Section 22	A–R
Muscular dystrophy with external ophthalmoplegia	Bilateral ptosis and extraocular muscle paresis progressing to immobility	See Section 21	A–D
Myotonia congenita (Thomsen's disease)	Sudden closure of eyelids results in inability to open lids for several seconds; esotropia rare	See Section 21	A–D, A–R
Myotonic dystrophy (Steinert's disease)	Bilateral cataracts beginning as subcapsular opacities progressing to total opacities, ptosis and pigmentary retinopathy	See Section 21	A–D, variable expressivity
Nail patella syndrome (hereditary osteo-onychodysplasia)	Dark, "clover leaf" pigmentation of iris, cataract, ptosis, keratoconus, microcornea and microphakia	See Section 29	A–D
Niemann-Pick disease	Reddish brown spot in macula; visual loss not complete	See Section 8	A–R
Norrie's disease	Blindness shortly after birth; persistent hyperplastic primary vitreous; corneal opacity cataract; phthisis bulbi	Mental retardation; deafness; CNS degenerative changes	X–R
Oculocerebral syndrome with hypopigmentation	Microcornea, myopia, optic atrophy, cloudy vascularized corneas and nystagmus	Hypopigmentation spasticity; athetosis and mental retardation	A–R
Oculodentodigital dysplasia (Meyer-Schwickerath)	Microphthalmia, congenital glaucoma and iris anomalies	See Section 29	A–D

TABLE 24–2 OCULAR CHANGES IN DEVELOPMENTAL PEDIATRIC SYNDROMES *(Continued)*

DISEASE	OCULAR MANIFESTATION	SYSTEMIC MANIFESTATION	INHERITANCE*
Osteogenesis imperfecta (Van Der Hoeve syndrome)	Blue sclera, anterior segment defects and keratoconus; cataract and ectopia lentis are rare	See Section 22	A–D, A–R ?
Osteopetrosis (Albers-Schönberg)	Cranial nerve palsies and blindness from marrow compression of foramina	See Section 22	A–R
Infantile form	Pigmentary degeneration of the retina; optic atrophy	See Section 22	A–R
Oxycephaly	Exophthalmos, zonular cataracts, nystagmus, and optic atrophy	See Section 22	A–D
Pachyonychia congenita	Corneal thickening and cataracts	See Section 23	A–D
Peter syndrome	Central corneal leukoma, central defect of Descemet's membrane and a shallow anterior synechia with peripheral anterior synechia, cataract	Skeletal anomalies and developmental defects of the gastrointestinal tract and central nervous system; hydrocephalus and mental retardation	A–R
Phakomatoses (hamartoses)			
Sturge-Weber syndrome	Congenital glaucoma, angiomatous formation in choroid, retinal detachment	See Section 20	Unknown
Von Hippel-Lindau	Angiomatous lesion in peripheral retina associated with dilated, tortuous vessels	See Section 20	A–D
Tuberous sclerosis (Bourneville's disease)	Retinal hamartomas	See Section 20	A–D ?
Neurofibromatosis (von Recklinghausen)	Neurofibromatous lesion of retina, iris or lids	See Sections 20 and 23	A–D
Wyburn-Mason (angiomatosis of midbrain retina)	Markedly enlarged retinal vessels; may involve orbit and optic nerve	Angiomatous lesions of midbrain	?
Pierre Robin syndrome	Congenital glaucoma, retinal detachment, esotropia	Micrognathia; cleft palate; glossoptosis	No known genetic etiology; rarely X–R
Porphyria, acute intermittent	Optic neuritis, bilateral ptosis, partial third nerve paralysis and visual disturbances	See Section 8	A–D
Prader-Willi syndrome	Strabismus	See Section 29	No known genetic etiology
Pseudoxanthoma elasticum	Angioid streaks, hemorrhage in macula	See Section 29	A–R
Radial aplasia-thrombocytopenia. (absent radius syndrome)	Strabismus	See Section 14	A–R

Table 24–2 continued on following page.

TABLE 24–2 OCULAR CHANGES IN DEVELOPMENTAL PEDIATRIC SYNDROMES *(Continued)*

DISEASE	OCULAR MANIFESTATION	SYSTEMIC MANIFESTATION	INHERITANCE*
Refsum syndrome (heredopathia atactica polyneuritiformis)	Atypical pigmentary retinal degeneration, night blindness and diminished vision, cataracts.	See Sections 20 and 23	A–R
Retinitis pigmentosa	Night blindness, narrowed arterioles, bone corpuscle-shaped pigment deposits, optic atrophy, ring scotoma	Deafness; mutism; mental retardation; high arched palate	A–D, A–R, X–R
Retinitis punctata albescens	Related to retinitis pigmentosa; numerous small yellow dots scattered over retina; may also contain pigment	Deaf-mutism described	A–R, X–R
Rieger syndrome	Hypoplasia of anterior stromal leaf of iris with iridotrabecular adhesions inserted in corneal periphery; microcornea, corneal opacity and pupillary anomalies occur; glaucoma is common	Hypodontia, myotonic dystrophy and mental deficiency; hypertelorism found in one fourth of patients	A–D
Rothmund syndrome (poikiloderma atrophicans vasculare)	Bilateral cataracts developing in 3rd to 5th year; corneal dystrophy	See Section 23	A–R
Rubinstein-Taybi syndrome (broad thumb and toe syndrome)	Epicanthus, strabismus, refractive error, cataract, coloboma, ptosis, long eyelashes and hypertrichosis	See Section 29	No known genetic etiology
Schwartz syndrome	Blepharophimosis, myopia and long eyelashes in irregular rows	See Section 29	A–R
Sickle cell disease Hemoglobin SS	Venous tortuosity, arteriolar and venous occlusion, chorioretinal scars, comma-shaped conjunctival capillaries	See Section 14	A–R
Hemoglobin SC	Arteriovenous abnormality extending into vitreous (sea fan), vascular occlusion and chorioretinal scars	See Section 14	A–R
Sieman syndrome	Congenital cataracts	Hypoplasia or atrophy of skin	A–R
Sjögren-Larsson syndrome	Pigmentary retinal degeneration (30 per cent)	See Section 23	A–R
Sjögren syndrome	Bilateral congenital cataracts, nystagmus, microphthalmos and detached retina	Oligophrenia	?

TABLE 24–2 OCULAR CHANGES IN DEVELOPMENTAL PEDIATRIC SYNDROMES *(Continued)*

DISEASE	OCULAR MANIFESTATION	SYSTEMIC MANIFESTATION	INHERITANCE*
Smith-Lemli-Opitz syndrome	Bilateral ptosis, epicanthus, strabismus	See Section 29	A–R
Spondylo-epiphyseal dysplasia, congenital	Myopia and retinal detachment	See Section 22	A–D
Spongy degeneration of the white matter. (Canavan's disease)	Optic atrophy and nystagmus, cherry red spot in macula	See Section 20	A–R
Stickler syndrome (progressive arthro-ophthalmopathy)	Progressive myopia, retinal detachment, secondary glaucoma	Pain and stiffness of joints with bony enlargement; deafness and kyphosis	A–D
Sulfite oxidase deficiency	Bilateral dislocated lenses	See Section 8	A–R
Tangier disease	Fine, dotted, stromal opacities in cornea	See Section 8	A–R
Unverricht-Lafora's disease (progressive familial myoclonus epilepsy)	Cherry-red spot and retinitis pigmentosa-like pigmentation reported; visual loss, Lafora bodies (inclusion bodies) reported in retina, brain and spinal cord	See Section 20	A–R
Usher syndrome	Retinitis pigmentosa	Nerve deafness; mental retardation; high arched palate and epilepsy	A–R
Von Gierke's disease	Retinal changes consisting of discrete, nonelevated, round yellow flecks in macular area; no visual impairment	See Section 8	A–R
Waardenburg syndrome	Lateral displacement of lower puncta and inner canthus, blepharophimosis heterochromia and hyperplasia of eyebrows medially	Deafness; white forelock and a broad nasal root; see also Sections 22 and 29	A–D, varying penetrance
Weill-Marchesani syndrome	Spherophakia, ectopic lens, myopia, possible glaucoma	See this Section	A–R
Wilson's disease (hepatolenticular degeneration)	Kayser-Fleischer ring, sunflower cataract	See Sections 11 and 20	A–R
Xeroderma pigmentosa	Eyelids exposed to direct sunlight develop large freckles followed by telangiectases and atrophic areas which become warty and undergo malignant degeneration; photophobia and conjunctivitis	See Section 23	A–R

This table adapted from Punnett, H. H., and Harley, R. D.: Genetics in pediatric ophthalmology. *In* Harley, R. D.: *Pediatric Ophthalmology.*

TABLE 24–3 COMMON OCULAR THERAPEUTIC AGENTS*

Irrigating solution:	
For ocular irrigation: physiologic saline solution	
	GM OR ML
Astringent solution:	
Zinc sulfate	0.065
Epinephrine (1:1000)	4.00
Zephiran chloride (1:20,000)	30.00
One drop in each eye every 3 hours	
Local anesthetics:	
Proparacaine hydrochloride (Ophthaine, Ophthetic)	0.5%
Tetracaine hydrochloride (Pontocaine)	0.5%
Cocaine hydrochloride	0.5%, 2%, 5%
Procaine hydrochloride	1%, 2%
Lidocaine hydrochloride (Xylocaine)	2%
Parasympatholytic drugs (mydriatic or cycloplegic):	
Homatropine hydrobromide	5%
Tropicamide (Mydriacyl)	0.5% or 1%
Atropine sulfate (in ointment)	0.5% or 1%
Cyclopentolate hydrochloride (Cyclogyl)	0.5% or 1%
Parasympathomimetic drugs:	
Pilocarpine hydrochloride	1 to 4% solution
Carbachol (Carcholin)	0.75 or 1.5%
Echothiophate iodide (Phospholine Iodide)	0.06% or 0.12%
Sympathomimetic drug:	
Phenylephrine hydrochloride (Neo-Synephrine)	5% or 10%
Dyes:	
Fluorescein sodium ophthalmic solution. (sterile paper strip or sterile solution in single-dose container)	2%
Antimicrobial and chemotherapeutic agents:	
Sulfisoxazole (Gantrisin)	4% solution and ointment
Sodium sulfacetamide (Sod-Sulamyd)	10% or 15% solution and ointment
Chloramphenicol (Chloromycetin)	Prepared in ointment or powder to be reconstituted
Neomycin sulfate (Mycifradin)	Ointment or solution
Frequently combined with other drugs to widen the spectrum of activity, as in Neosporin, which contains neomycin, polymyxin and bacitracin	
Adrenal corticosteroids:	
Corticosteroids are frequently prescribed in combination with an antibiotic to reduce the inflammatory response. *Corticosteroids may be dangerous in herpes simplex keratitis, and their use in any condition for an extended time is not desirable except under the direction of an ophthalmologist.* Glaucoma may occur with prolonged use.	
5-Iodo-2-deoxyuridine (I.D.U.):	
This drug may be useful in the early epithelial stages of herpex simplex keratitis when begun early and used every hour.	

*All the solutions listed are packaged in a sterile state in plastic squeeze bottles and are not readily contaminated.

Hemorrhagic Disorders. Retinal hemorrhages may be seen in any of the bleeding disorders. Spontaneous hemorrhages may be expected in those with thrombocytopenia.

Leukemia. The veins are characteristically dilated, with sausage-shaped constrictions. Hemorrhagic exudates and white-centered hemorrhages are common during the severe stage. Exophthalmos occurs from orbital hemorrhage and leukemic infiltrations.

DIABETES MELLITUS. The most common ocular complications of diabetes mellitus are in the fundi. Changes also occur in the iris, lens, optic nerve and extraocular muscles. Sudden changes in the refractive error may be the first sign of diabetes. The earliest retinal changes are punctate hemorrhages and capillary microaneurysms. The hemorrhages are characteristically small and round. Later the veins become dilated and somewhat tortuous. Small, yellow, waxy exudates appear, first in the macular area and later scattered over the posterior portion.

Contracture of the scar tissue at sites of hemorrhage may lead to irreversible changes and visual loss. From 60 to 75 per cent of juvenile diabetics suffer a severe retinopathy within 20 years or so. Minute, so-called snowflake cataracts are relatively common, and extensive opacification of the lens occurs occasionally. These changes may occur early in the disease.

Lipemia retinalis is a spectacular ophthalmoscopic finding during the uncontrolled phase of diabetes. The vessels appear as though the blood had been replaced by cream.

GENETICALLY DETERMINED DISEASES WITH OCULAR MANIFESTATIONS. These are listed in Table 24–2.

ENDOCRINE DISEASES. Hyperthyroidism, hypoparathyroidism and hyperparathyroidism are discussed in Section 17.

DISEASES RELATED TO NUTRITIONAL DEFICIENCIES. See Vitamin A Deficiency, Hypervitaminosis A, deficiencies of vitamin B and Scurvy in Section 3.

DISEASES OF CONNECTIVE TISSUE. See Section 10.

OPHTHALMIC PHARMACOLOGY

Table 24–3 lists ocular therapeutic agents in common use.

ROBISON D. HARLEY

Apt, L.: Diagnostic Procedures in Pediatric Ophthalmology. Boston, Little, Brown and Company, 1964.

Francois, J.: Heredity in Ophthalmology. St. Louis, C. V. Mosby Company, 1961.

Harley, R. D. (Ed.): Pediatric Ophthalmology. Philadelphia, W. B. Saunders Company, 1974.

Liebman, S., and Gellis, S.: The Pediatrician's Ophthalmology. St. Louis, C. V. Mosby Company, 1966.

Ophthalmic Staff of the Hospital for Sick Children: The Eye in Childhood. Chicago, Year Book Medical Publishers, Inc., 1967.

Scheie, H. G., and Albert, D. M.: Adler's Textbook of Ophthalmology. Philadelphia, W. B. Saunders Company, 1969.

25

NEOPLASMS AND NEOPLASTIC-LIKE LESIONS

Although less than 2 per cent of malignant neoplasms occur in children, cancer, including leukemia, is now the leading cause of death from disease in children beyond infancy in the United States. Between the ages of 1 and 14 years it is responsible for about 12 per cent of all deaths. Although the increasing importance of cancer as a cause of death in children is in large part related to the decline in death rates from infectious and other diseases, there is some evidence to indicate an absolute as well as a relative increase in its incidence.

The incidence of cancer among children is higher during the first 5 years of life than during either of the two ensuing quinquennia. The frequency of malignant neoplasms during the first 5 years of life probably reflects the embryonal nature of certain of the more common tumors encountered in this period, e.g., Wilms' tumor, neuroblastoma and possibly even acute leukemia. Such embryonal neoplasms tend to mimic structures normally present during active organogenesis and appear to be derived from cells which have never matured. They may be present at birth or may arise postnatally from cells which have not attained complete maturation.

The embryonal origin of certain neoplasms of early life is undoubtedly responsible for differences between these tumors and the more common malignant neoplasms encountered in adults. The rapidity of progress of many of the neoplasms of children as compared with those of adults is probably related to the growth characteristics of embryonic tissues. As a result of this rapid growth, the clinical manifestations of certain neoplasms in infants and children may be those of an acute infectious process, with few or none of the classic signs of malignancy encountered in adults. With the exception, however, of the two most common types of neoplasms encountered in early life, i.e., acute leukemia and tumors of the central nervous system, most malignant neoplasms in infants or children manifest themselves by the presence of an abnormal solid mass, which may attain a large size in a brief time. Characteristically, even large tumors are not associated with significant anemia, loss of weight or cachexia.

Benign tumors are far more common in early life than malignant ones, and many of them are hamartomas rather than true neoplasms.

Hamartomas are tumor-like, non-neoplastic malformations characterized by localized overgrowth of one or more tissues indigenous to the site in which they arise. They thus comprise such diverse lesions as hemangiomas and lymphangiomas, diffuse lipomatoses, rhabdomyomas of the heart and the tubers in the central nervous system of persons with tuberous sclerosis. Some of them, notably the hemangiomas, may spontaneously regress and ultimately disappear. Although initially non-neoplastic, infrequently a true neoplasm may develop within a hamartoma, e.g., a glioma may arise in a tuberous focus in tuberous sclerosis.

Malignant neoplasms of almost all types have been reported during early life, but their common sites of origin differ sharply from those in adults. For example, the hematopoietic system, central and sympathetic nervous systems (including eye and adrenal medulla), soft tissues, bone and kidney are the common sites of origin of malignant tumors in infants and children; common epithelial tumors of adults, such as carcinomas of the skin, lung, stomach, breast and uterus, are rare in early life.

The natural course and the therapeutic response of tumors in infants and children cannot always be predicted accurately on the basis of experience with neoplasms in adults. For example, encapsulation of a neoplasm is often considered to be indicative of benignancy in adults, but in children Wilms' tumor and even neuroblastoma are initially encapsulated. Increased cellularity, invasion of adjoining tissues and the presence of mitotic figures are commonly associated with malignancy in adults, yet their occurrence in hemangiomas in infants is entirely compatible with a benign clinical course. Conversely, some "benign" tumors may, in early life, because of their location and continued growth, be responsible for death even in the absence of metastases, e.g., mediastinal lymphangiomas.

Although the results of therapy are still far from satisfactory, when one compares the probability of cure of an infant with a Wilms' tumor or even a neuroblastoma with that of an adult with such a common malignant neoplasm as carcinoma of the lung, the results are certainly encouraging. Moreover, with few exceptions, rates of "cure" rather than simple "survival rates" can be determined for such malignant neoplasms in infants and children as Wilms' tumor, neuroblastoma and rhabdomyosarcoma. If after removal of the tumor, metastases or recurrences have not taken place after a period of time equivalent to the age of the patient at the time of removal plus 9 months, the probability of recurrence is only slight (Collin's law). In general, the prognosis is equally good if there is no evidence of recurrence or metastasis two years after removal of such a malignant neoplasm.

Every solid mass in an infant or child should be regarded as a malignant neoplasm until proved otherwise. Needless palpation of a suspected neoplasm should be avoided, and the mass should be removed as soon as is consistent with adequate clinical evaluation and preparation of the patient for operation; usually this period should not exceed 24 to 48 hours. As a general rule, treatment by other than surgical excision should not be instituted until an unequivocal diagnosis has been established by histologic study. With certain neoplasms, most notably the neuroblastoma, cures can sometimes be effected even in the presence of recognizable metastases. Therapy is best designed and the patient's progress followed in a center accustomed to dealing with cancer in children. Observance of these principles should prevent a number of needless deaths from cancer in infants and children.

Although the *causes of neoplasms in early life* remain unknown, certain observations in recent years provide clues to further understanding of some of the factors which may play a role in the development of neoplasms in infants and children.

The importance of therapeutic irradiation of the head, neck and chest in early life in the subsequent development of carcinoma (and less frequently adenoma) of the thyroid is now established. Although irradiation is not the sole etiologic factor, the incidence of carcinoma of the thyroid in persons receiving therapeutic irradiation to the thymus is approximately 100 times the expected rate. There also appears to be an increased incidence of leukemia in children so irradiated. Osteosarcoma and other types of malignant neoplasms may follow curative radiotherapy of retinoblastomas. Benign tumors, in addition to adenomas of the thyroid, have also been observed following therapeutic irradiation, e.g., neurofibroma and, more frequently, osteochondroma. As many as 10 per cent of persons receiving therapeutic doses of irradiation for Wilms' tumor or neuroblastoma before the age of 3 years have osteochondromas after latent periods up to 10 years or longer. Less frequently a malignant mesenchymal neoplasm has followed such therapeutic irradiation.

Other factors also play a role in the development of malignant neoplasms in early life. For example, the administration of stilbestrol to pregnant women to prevent abortion has been implicated as the cause of adenocarcinoma of the vagina in their daughters, 14 to 22 years later.

Certain chromosomal abnormalities are accompanied by an increased frequency of leukemia. In two genetically transmitted diseases characterized by chromosomal fragility (Bloom syndrome and Fanconi's aplastic anemia), the probability of developing leukemia, usually in adolescence or early adult life, is about one in 10. The probability that a child with Down syndrome (trisomy-21) will develop leukemia is about one in 200, or approximately 15 times the expected rate. It should be recognized, however, that a transient leukemoid reaction simulating congenital leukemia occurs with some frequency in infants with the Down syndrome and may disappear spontaneously.

The relationship of immune disorders to malignant neoplasms is becoming increasingly apparent. The probability of children with such genetically transmitted immunodeficiency diseases as ataxia-telangiectasia, Wiskott-Aldrich syndrome, Bruton's type of agammaglobulinemia and Chediak-Higashi syndrome developing a malignant neoplasm, usually a malignant lymphoma, is estimated to be about 2 to 10 per cent.

Malignant neoplasms other than those of the lymphoreticular system occur with increased frequency in association with some congenital malformations which are apparently not genetically determined. For example, children with aniridia, almost always of the sporadic type, are at increased risk for the development of Wilms' tumor. Hemihypertrophy is accompanied not only by an increase in the frequency of Wilms' tumor, but also of adrenocortical carcinoma and carcinoma of the liver; rarely hemihypertrophy has developed after the occurrence of a Wilms' tumor. These same neoplasms occur with some frequency in association with Beckwith-Wiedemann syndrome. Such isolated facts should provide further insight into the causes of a variety of neoplasms in early life.

MATERNAL AND FETAL TRANSMISSION OF NEOPLASMS. Rarely a woman with far advanced neoplastic disease, especially malignant melanoma, may transmit the process to her offspring. Probably somewhat more frequently a maternal neoplasm metastasizes to the placenta without other involvement of the fetus.

Placental chorioepithelioma may be responsible for widespread metastases in the fetus, which may not be apparent for several weeks or months after birth. The placental growth may invade the uterine wall and be responsible for a maternal neoplasm; in some instances it is apparently discharged from the uterine cavity without residual maternal disease.

Neuroblastoma in the fetus with extensive hepatic metastases may be responsible for a hydropic placenta containing metastatic tumor, but metastases to the mother have not been seen.

Placental chorioangioma, a benign hemangioma of the placenta, may be responsible for hydrops fetalis or for transient neonatal thrombocytopenia and multiple petechiae. The hydrops is probably the result of hypoproteinemia caused by loss of protein from the tumor. The pathogenesis of the thrombocytopenia is presumably similar to that which occurs with other giant hemangiomas.

TUMORS OF THE HEAD AND NECK

These are a heterogeneous group, some of which are true neoplasms and others hamartomas or malformations. Some of them are peculiar to this region, e.g., thyroglossal duct and branchial cleft cysts. Others, such as teratomas, neuroblastomas, rhabdomyosarcomas and lymphangiomas, occur not only in the head and neck, but also in a number of other sites. Owing to their location, complete removal of a cervical tumor is sometimes impossible, and even a non-neoplastic lesion such as a cystic lymphangioma or a diffuse neurofibroma may infrequently be responsible for death. Of the malignant neoplasms, lymphomas, neuroblastomas and rhabdomyosarcomas are the most common, and recognition of their occurrence in this region as primary rather than as metastatic neoplasms is of obvious importance in their management.

The occurrence of a single enlarged cervical lymph node or a group of persistently enlarged nodes presents a common diagnostic problem in infants and children. The differential diagnosis includes cervical lymphadenitis, including infection with an atypical strain of mycobacterium or, less commonly today, with the tubercle bacillus, cat-scratch disease, the reticuloendothelioses, malignant lymphoma, and metastatic malignant neoplasms such as carcinoma of the thyroid, neuroblastoma arising in the cervical region and lymphoepithelioma. The majority of cervical lesions will prove to be inflammatory rather than neoplastic, and a definitive diagnosis based on surgical excision and histologic examination should not be attempted until a reasonable length of time has elapsed. After 3 or 4 weeks, if the lymphadenopathy has remained stationary or has increased, the nodes feel hard on palpation, the tuberculin reaction is negative, there is no serologic evidence of infectious mononucleosis or toxoplasmosis, and there is no recognizable source or history of any focus of infection to account for the enlarged nodes, excisional biopsy is indicated. This should be preceded by roentgenographic examination of the cervical region, since certain malignant neoplasms, notably the neuroblastoma, may have areas of calcification.

TUMORS OF THE NOSE, SINUSES, PHARYNX, EAR AND ORAL CAVITY

Nasal polyps are the most common tumors in the nose and paranasal sinuses. The other lesions described below are rare, but are important in the differential diagnosis, since some of them may be confused clinically with nasal polyps and have a different prognosis. Embryonal rhabdomyosarcoma occurs in these areas in children with sufficient frequency to warrant consideration in the differential diagnosis of a tumor of the upper air passages.

Nasal polyps are not true neoplasms, but are chronic, inflammatory pedunculated masses of edematous mucosa arising from the turbinates or accessory sinuses. Many of them are probably allergic in origin; they occur with unusually high frequency in children with cystic fibrosis. They contribute to chronic nasal obstruction and discharge, and at times to headache. The polyps appear as single or multiple, white to pale pink, relatively avascular, edematous masses. They are apt to recur after removal, unless the basis for their origin can be controlled.

Juvenile nasopharyngeal angiofibroma is a relatively rare neoplasm occurring almost entirely in males, usually between 10 and 20 years of age. The most frequent manifestations are those of nasal obstruction and epistaxis; the bleeding is usually intermittent and is sometimes alarmingly profuse, often necessitating nasal packing for its control. The tumor, which usually arises high on the lateral wall of the nasopharynx, may obstruct one or both posterior nasal orifices and often protrudes into the nasal cavity. Continued growth may be responsible for a variety of deformities, e.g., downward and forward displacement of the soft palate, replacement of the maxillary sinus and the subsequent development of a subcutaneous mass, or exophthalmos as a result of invasion of the orbit.

The tumor is nonencapsulated and has a sessile or somewhat pedunculated base. It consists of a fibrous matrix and numerous vascular spaces of varying size and shape with walls of variable thickness. It is benign in that it does not metastasize, but recurrences following attempted removal are common. Severe hemorrhage may occur during removal or may develop postoperatively. Excision following adequate exposure is the treatment of choice; both transantral and transpalatine approaches have been advocated.

Olfactory neuroepithelial tumors (olfactory neuroblastomas) are rare malignant neoplasms, especially in children; they originate in the olfactory mucous membrane high in the nasal fossa. Unilateral nasal obstruction and epistaxis are the most common initial manifestations; in some instances there is a history of recurrent "nasal polyps." The neoplasm may be responsible for unilateral exophthalmos or swelling at the root of the nose. It may invade the paranasal sinuses, hard palate, intraorbital tissues, bones of the skull and the brain. Metastases may occur, sometimes after a period of several years, and involve especially the bones, lungs and cervical lymph nodes. The tumor is apt to be radiosensitive, but not radiocurable. It is probably best treated by a combination of surgery and irradiation and possibly chemotherapy.

Histologically the neoplasm is composed of sheets of undifferentiated cells with round or oval nuclei divided into incomplete lobules by slender vascular septa of connective tissue. Pseudorosettes similar to those in neuroblastoma and occasionally true rosettes may be present.

Teratomas may arise in the base of the skull, in the roof of the pharynx, in the hard or soft palate or in the base of the tongue and project into the mouth, nose or cranial cavity. The more complex ones, in which both intracranial and extracranial masses are sometimes connected to each other through a defect in the basisphenoid, are present at birth; the infants seldom survive beyond the neonatal period. Some of the well differentiated teratomas projecting from the mouth contain structures resembling fetal parts and have been referred to as *epignathi.*

The less complex tumors, sometimes referred to as dermoids or *"hairy polyps,"* are often pedunculated structures composed of a central core of adipose tissue containing plaques of cartilage and mucous glands and covered by stratified squamous epithelium. The relation of these tumors to the complex teratomas is not clear. It is possible that some of those which arise in the region of the tonsil may represent malformations derived from the branchial arches and not true neoplasms. More than half of them occur in infants under 1 year of age, in whom they may be responsible for respiratory distress and attacks of coughing and cyanosis. The tumor sometimes can be readily seen or may be detected on lateral roentgenograms of the nasopharynx as an osseous or soft tissue density depressing the soft palate. These less complex lesions usually occur in the absence of other malformations. If they are removed surgically, the prognosis is excellent.

Chordomas (p. 1643) of the base of the skull may project into the nasopharynx, or the initial manifestations may be those of an intracranial tumor. Owing to their location, surgical removal is difficult.

Osteoma. See page 1640.

Papillomas are rare benign epithelial tumors composed of irregular polypoid masses. They may be single or multiple; they arise from the nasal mucosa more often than from the paranasal sinuses. Clinically they may be confused with nasal polyps. Repeated recurrences are common, and malignant transformation has been reported.

Adenomas are rare benign tumors arising from the glands of the mucous membrane of the nasal cavity and paranasal sinuses. They are most frequently located in the nasal cavity and ethmoidal region; those in the latter site may erode the cribriform plate. The symptoms are related to nasal obstruction or swelling; nasal bleeding is common. There is frequent local recurrence, and the prognosis must be guarded because of the difficulty of complete removal.

Mixed tumors of salivary gland origin (p. 1605) may arise in the mucous membranes of the nose, paranasal sinuses or the palate. Palatal tumors commonly arise from the posterolateral portion of the hard palate and project into the floor of the nasal cavity and maxillary sinus. The symptoms are those of nasal obstruction. Difficulty in swallowing may be noted in association with palatal tumors. The tumors may be well circumscribed and erode the adjoining bone or may be poorly circumscribed invasive lesions. Clinical or pathologic differentiation of benign and malignant tumors may be difficult or impossible. Metastases are infrequent. Surgical removal is the treatment of choice, but some of these tumors, especially those in which the epithelial elements predominate, may respond to irradiation.

Carcinoma of the nasopharynx or of the *tonsil* may be a poorly differentiated epidermoid growth; it has been referred to as a transitional cell carcinoma or a lymphoepithelioma. A distinction between such neoplasms and lymphosarcomas arising in the lymphoid tissue of the nasopharynx may be difficult. The primary neoplasm in the nasopharynx may be a diffuse, infiltrative, nonulcerated lesion. The initial manifestation is often that of tender unilateral cervical lymphadenopathy with or without trismus and/or torticollis. A palpable nasopharyngeal mass may be present, or the diagnosis may be made only by the presence of metastases in a cervical lymph node. Under such circumstances careful search for the primary tumor should be made, if necessary under general anesthesia. Treatment is by irradiation and chemotherapy.

Nasal glioma is a rare non-neoplastic lesion composed of neuroglia and occasionally some neurons. It is usually manifest at birth as a smooth, round, firm, nonpulsatile mass over the bridge of the nose. It is often located somewhat lateral to the midline and may extend to the inner canthus of one eye. The overlying skin is apt to be faintly red to purple, and the lesion has often been mistaken for a hemangioma. Infrequently the mass is intranasal and simulates a nasal polyp. Rarely both an intranasal and an extranasal mass are present; the two usually communicate through a defect in the nasal bone.

Nasal gliomas should be differentiated from encephaloceles, since removal of the latter may lead to meningitis. In contrast to encephaloceles, only about 25 per cent of nasal gliomas have an intracranial communication.

Heterotopic pharyngeal brain tissue, although non-neoplastic, may be life-threatening to the newborn infant. Respiratory distress and dysphagia are usually present from birth. The mass, which is covered by mucosa, may extend from the roof of the nasopharynx to the level of the esophagus, displacing the larynx and tongue anteriorly; intracranial extensions of the mass have not been reported. In three of the nine reported cases there was a cleft palate. In contrast to nasal gliomas, pharyngeal brain tissue may also contain mature ependymal elements, including choroid plexus structures. Usually the mass can be successfully resected.

Congenital macroglossia is discussed in Section 11.

Lymphangiomas of the tongue occur predominantly on the dorsum anteriorly. They vary from isolated, pinhead-sized cystic structures to diffuse lesions which infiltrate the entire tongue with resultant macroglossia, and even extend into surrounding structures such as the lips and cheeks. They may be present at birth or may not appear until adult life; more than one third of them are present before 6 years of age. Clinically they are manifest by recurrent episodes of glossitis and swelling of the tongue, the surface of which is studded with irregular gray and pink nodules. Macroglossia may be so extreme as to preclude containment of the bulky tongue within the oral cavity. In the absence of symptoms no active therapy may be necessary, but in some patients local excision, wedge resection or hemiglossectomy may be indicated.

Hemangioma of the tongue may be localized or diffuse. It is a less frequent cause of macroglossia than is lymphangioma, from which it may be distinguished by its deep red color and tendency to bleed.

Neurofibroma may be responsible for unilateral macroglossia. It usually develops before the age of 3 years and is often associated with neurofibromas of the skin and *café au lait* spots. It is usually noncompressible and relatively avascular. Surgical excision may be difficult, since these neoplasms tend to be nonencapsulated and to extend to the floor of the mouth.

The mucosal neuroma syndrome is usually a sporadic mutation but may be inherited as a dominant trait. Oral and labial neuromas are variable in their time of onset but may be the first manifestation of this syndrome, which also includes medullary carcinoma of the thyroid with an amyloid stroma, pheochromocytoma and intestinal ganglioneuromatosis; incomplete expressions of the mutant gene may occur.

Mucosal neuromas are sometimes present at birth or within the first few years of life. They involve principally the lips and tongue but may also occur on the buccal, gingival, nasal or conjunctival mucosa. Lingual lesions appear as multiple pink, pedunculated nodules on the anterior aspect of the tongue. Both lips are apt to be diffusely enlarged, and the jaw may be prognathic because of soft tissue swelling. Thickened lid margins may cause a "sleepy" appearance, and the corneal nerves are often enlarged. Histologically the neuromas suggest plexiform neurofibromas or amputation neuromas and need be treated only for cosmetic reasons.

The body habitus is apt to be arachnodactylic, and pes cavus or excavatum, kyphosis, lax joints and hypotonia are sometimes present. The ocular and cardiovascular manifestations of the Marfan syndrome, however, are absent.

Diarrhea is sometimes the initial complaint in this syndrome. It may be caused by a medullary carcinoma of the thyroid secreting serotonin (5-hydroxytryptamine) or prostaglandin, or by autonomic dysfunction as a result of diffuse ganglioneuromatosis of the bowel. The latter may be so extensive as to produce a roentgenographic appearance suggesting ulcerative colitis; in other instances dilatation of the bowel may simulate Hirschsprung's disease; diverticulosis has been present in some patients.

The presenting complaint is often that of a mass in the neck, viz., a medullary carcinoma of the thyroid with amyloid stroma. These tumors do not usually appear until the late teens. They comprise less than 10 per cent of all carcinomas of the thyroid, but almost all the familial carcinomas of this gland. They are derived from the parafollicular or C-cells of the thyroid and may elaborate not only calcitonin but also other hormonally active substances such as prostaglandins and ACTH. The tumor is characteristically multifocal in origin and consists of sheets or nests of round to spindle-shaped cells devoid of follicles or papillary formations. Fibrous septa divide the groups of neoplastic cells into lobules of varying size. Masses of amyloid in the stroma or within the nests of cells may become calcified. The neoplasm tends to metastasize to regional lymph nodes early, but long-term survival may occur. The lesion is best treated by surgical excision. Terminally the lungs, liver and bones are common metastatic sites.

Pheochromocytomas occurring in this syndrome usually do not appear until later childhood or adult life. More than half of them are bilateral, but metastases are rare. They are best treated surgically. The intestinal ganglioneuromatosis is usually too diffuse to be surgically corrected, but recognition of its manifestations in this syndrome may avert needless laparotomy.

Any infant or child with multiple mucosal neuromas should be followed throughout adult life for the possible development of pheochromocytoma or medullary carcinoma of the thyroid, and the presence of either such neoplasm should elicit a careful family history.

Granular cell myoblastoma is discussed on page 1635.

Epulis is a term commonly used for any tumor-like growth of the gums, many of which are reactive rather than neoplastic. They are pedunculated or sessile growths which may recur after removal, but do not metastasize.

Congenital epulis is a soft, spherical mass most commonly located on the margin of the upper gum in the incisor region. It occurs almost exclusively in female infants and is usually noticed at birth or shortly afterward. It is usually a solitary tumor, but sometimes two or three masses are present. Histologically it consists of large polyhedral cells with lightly staining granular cytoplasm; scattered nests of paradental epithelium are sometimes present. It probably represents a non-neoplastic hamartomatous malformation.

The *lingual thyroid* is a mass in the region of the foramen cecum at the base of the tongue which must be differentiated from a thyroglossal duct cyst. It represents residual thyroid tissue along the course of the primitive thyroglossal duct; in some instances there may be complete failure of descent of the thyroid, in which case removal of the lingual thyroid is followed by hypothyroidism.

Rhabdomyosarcoma of the head and neck is primarily a disease of infancy and childhood; more than three fourths of affected persons are not more than 12 years of age and one third of them are under 6 years; infrequently the tumor is present at birth. The orbit and the eyelid are the most frequent sites in the head and neck; this tumor is the most common primary malignancy of the orbit in children. Orbital neoplasms usually present with unilateral proptosis, whereas those arising in the lids are apt to be responsible for a palpable, nontender mass, which may be mistaken for a chalazion. Rhabdomyosarcomas arising in the nasopharynx, tongue, palate or elsewhere in the mouth, hypopharynx or maxillary sinus, as well as those originating in the region of the mandible, occiput or salivary gland, usually present as a mass or with signs and symptoms which lead to the detection of a mass; if the tumor grows freely into a cavity, the resultant mass often assumes a grape-like configuration *(sarcoma botryoides).* The neoplasm may also arise in the middle ear or mastoid and be responsible for "otitis media," a polypoid mass in the external auditory canal, a bloody discharge and cranial nerve palsies.

Most of these tumors are embryonal rhabdomyosarcomas, the alveolar and especially the pleomorphic types being much less common. The lungs, lymph nodes and bones are the most frequent sites of metastases. The prognosis is grave, but has been vastly improved by the combined use of surgery, irradiation and chemotherapy; in one series 14 of 19 patients were living with no evidence of disease after two or more years. Orbital lesions have the best prognosis and have sometimes been treated by irradiation and chemotherapy, without enucleation.

Retinal Anlage Tumor. See page 1641.

TUMORS OF THE MAJOR SALIVARY GLANDS

These tumors, uncommon in infants and children, arise more often in the parotid than in the submaxillary gland. The most common tumor of the major salivary glands in early life is the hemangioma of the parotid, a lesion which is rare beyond infancy. *Other benign tumors* include papillary cystadenoma lymphomatosum (Warthin tumor), fibromatoses, lipomas, lymphangiomas, neurilemmomas and neurofibromas; almost all mixed tumors in children are benign.

Malignant neoplasms are most often epithelial in origin, mucoepidermoid carcinoma being the most common. Undifferentiated carcinoma has been seen in infancy, whereas, in the pediatric age period, adenocarcinomas, including adenoid cystic carcinoma and acinic cell carcinoma, as well as squamous cell carcinomas, have been observed almost entirely in older children and adolescents. Sarcoma of the major salivary glands is rare; embryonal rhabdomyosarcoma of the parotid has been observed in infancy (p. 1637).

Occasionally differentiation of a neoplasm from *chronic parotitis* may be difficult, but a history of repeated swelling of the gland, often bilateral, suggests the possibility of an inflammatory rather than a neoplastic process (Section 11); in such instances, if histologic diagnosis is deemed necessary, biopsy of the mass is preferable to total excision, since it is much less apt to be followed by paralysis of the facial nerve.

Mikulicz's disease, although predominantly a disease of adult women, may occur in childhood and may be responsible for painless enlargement of a salivary gland simulating a neoplastic process (Section 11).

Hemangioma of the parotid or, less frequently, of the submaxillary gland is the most common tumor of the salivary glands in early life. It usually manifests itself as a bluish preauricular swelling at or shortly after birth, sometimes with an associated hemangioma of the overlying skin. There may be an alarming increase in size during the first several months of life; subsequently there may be little or no growth. Spontaneous regression may take place, as is true of many of the rapidly growing hemangiomas of the skin in infants. If one can be reasonably certain on clinical grounds that the mass is a hemangioma, a conservative, nonoperative approach of watchful waiting is indicated. If a biopsy is indicated, again a conservative attitude will usually suffice. If surgical excision proves necessary, particular care must be taken to avoid the facial nerve, which is more superficially located in the infant than in the adult. In spite of their cellularity and lack of encapsulation, these tumors are benign.

Mixed tumors of salivary glands are uncommon in children. The neoplasm may arise in the parotid or less frequently in the submaxillary gland. It usually presents as a round firm mass behind the ramus of the mandible. The tumor should be treated by removal of the entire gland or by total lobectomy if located in the parotid gland. Metastases are almost nonexistent during childhood.

Mucoepidermoid carcinomas, although less common than mixed tumors, are the most frequent type of malignant neoplasm of the salivary glands in children. Most often the initial manifestations appear after the age of 5 years. The tumor arises in the parotid more often than in the submaxillary gland. Recurrence or persistent growth of the neoplasm after initial excision, as well as metastases to regional lymph nodes, occurs in 20 to 30 per cent of the children, but widespread metastases are rare. There is poor correlation between the histologic pattern of these neoplasms and biologic behavior.

Undifferentiated carcinoma usually arises in the parotid, tends to be far more malignant than the mucoepidermoid carcinoma and to occur at an earlier age; it may be present at birth. It is apt to grow rapidly, to recur soon after removal and to metastasize to the regional lymph nodes and to the lungs.

Adenoid cystic carcinoma (cylindroma), a rare type of adenocarcinoma, is occasionally encountered in the parotid or submaxillary gland in older children. It is relatively slow-growing; it may recur years after excision and be responsible for distant metastases in adult life.

Acinic cell carcinoma is a specific type of adenocarcinoma which usually arises in the parotid gland. It is usually not encountered until late childhood or adolescence. It is a low-grade carcinoma which may recur repeatedly and, at least in adults, occasionally gives rise to widespread metastases.

TUMORS OF THE NECK

A *thyroglossal duct cyst* may be located anywhere from the base of the tongue at the foramen cecum to the isthmus of the thyroid gland along the course followed by this gland in its descent into the neck. Usually the duct atrophies; when it does not do so, a cystic swelling may appear superficially, usually in the midline of the neck just below the hyoid bone. The swelling usually develops as a painless, progressively enlarging and movable mass; it may appear at any age. The cyst moves upward when the tongue is protruded or during swallowing. It may become infected and may rupture spontaneously. Recurring inflammation or a discharging fistula causes the patient to seek medical attention. The discharge is intermittent and slight except when activated by infection.

The differential diagnosis of such a midline mass includes an epidermal inclusion cyst, a lymph node which may be near enough to the midline to cause confusion, and the thyroglossal duct cyst. True differentiation can be made only after excision of the mass.

The cyst and the entire tract, including the midportion of the body of the hyoid bone, must be *completely excised to the base of the tongue.* Surgical removal should be undertaken only when an existing infection is under control.

The *branchial cleft cyst* (lateral cervical cyst) is located anterior to the sternocleidomastoid muscle, but, in contrast to the thyroglossal duct cyst, not in the midline. The branchial cleft cyst represents a remnant of a right or left branch of a branchial cleft. Although the cyst may not be recognized until adolescence, it or its anlage has been present since birth. It grows slowly, is oval-shaped and may become extremely large. It is usually smooth, fluctuant and moderately movable and may be attached to the skin. The cyst is sometimes mistakenly diagnosed as an abscess and incised.

The branchial cleft remnant may occur only as a sinus from which small amounts of mucus may be expressed. The course of the sinus, as with the cyst, is upward from above the lower third of the sternocleidomastoid muscle, traversing between the bifurcation of the carotid vessels to empty into the piriform sinus on either side. Any remnant of this pathway may persist. Total excision is the therapy of choice.

Adenomas of the thyroid are rare in children. They are encapsulated neoplasms which do not invade normal tissue or metastasize. They are usually solitary, but multiple adenomas may be present. The presenting complaint is that of a mass in the region of the thyroid without evidence of dysfunction of the gland. Any nodule in the thyroid should be removed and examined histologically; differentiation of benign adenoma and carcinoma, however, is not always possible.

Carcinoma of the thyroid and *congenital goiter* are discussed in Section 17.

Teratomas of the neck may be located within or outside the thyroid. The neoplasms are usually present at birth and may be so large as to obstruct the airway. They consist of solid and cystic areas containing a variety of well differentiated tissues.

Cervical thymic masses may result from failure of the normal descent of the thymus on one side of the neck or from growth of a nodule of thymic tissue which has become separated from the main gland and has remained in the neck. A small nodule of thymic tissue near or even within the lower pole of the thyroid and separate from the remainder of the thymus is a common incidental finding at necropsy in infants; infrequently it attains sufficient size as to present as a cervical mass.

Thymic cysts are rare; they may be located in the neck or in the anterior mediastinum or extend into both regions. They are usually first detected in early childhood along a line extending from the angle of the jaw to the suprasternal notch. They are benign unilocular or more often multilocular cysts containing a cloudy or brown fluid in which there may be multiple yellow granules. Histologically the cysts are lined by flattened, squamous, cuboidal or cylindrical epithelial cells, some of which may be ciliated. Thymic tissue with Hassall's corpuscles is present in the wall. The lesion is non-neoplastic and is probably a developmental defect related to a branchial cyst.

Hygroma colli. See page 1631.

Malignant lymphoma. See Section 14.

Cervical neuroblastoma. See page 1619.

Rhabdomyosarcoma of the head and neck. See page 1637.

TUMORS OF THE MEDIASTINUM

Mediastinal masses in infants and children are relatively common. If malignant lymphomas are excluded, most of which are accompanied by manifestations in addition to those referable to the mediastinum, approximately three fourths of the mediastinal masses are neurogenic or teratomatous neoplasms or non-neoplastic cysts, e.g., duplications of the esophagus and neurenteric or bronchogenic cysts. Approximately 25 per cent of mediastinal masses in infants and children are malignant as compared with 15 per cent of those in adults. Tumors arising in the anterior mediastinum are predominantly teratomas, whereas most of those originating in the posterior mediastinum are neurogenic neoplasms; masses confined to the mid-mediastinum are usually lymphomas or non-neoplastic cysts.

Approximately two thirds of the infants and children with a mediastinal mass are symptomatic; in the others the lesion is a chance finding on a roentgenogram of the chest. Cough, dyspnea, stridor and pain are the most frequent manifestations and are especially apt to occur with teratomas, malignant neoplasms of any type and with nonneoplastic cysts; vascular tumors and benign neurogenic ones are often unassociated with respiratory symptoms.

Mediastinal teratomas are located in the anterior mediastinum, usually in its superior aspect. Many of them apparently arise in the thymus. Rarely they arise within the pericardial sac and simulate a congenital cardiac lesion. Many are benign cystic neoplasms, commonly referred to as *dermoid cysts,* which are cystic variants of the more solid teratomas. Symptoms may not be apparent until adult life. Dyspnea, cyanosis and cough may be manifestations, and expectoration of hair and sebaceous material may occur if the tumor perforates into a bronchus. Infection of the cystic mass may produce symptoms simulating a pneumonic process. Rarely the neoplasm extends into the suprasternal or supraclavicular area. Compression of the superior vena cava causes dilation of the veins of the head, neck and upper part of the thorax. Roentgenographic examination reveals a circumscribed mass extending from the anterior mediastinum into one hemithorax; when teeth or skeletal elements are demonstrable roentgenographically, the nature of the mass is established.

The teratomas may be composed of one or more cysts; less frequently they are predominantly solid tumors. The cysts contain sebaceous material, hair or mucoid material. Histologically almost any type of tissue may be present, especially in the solid neoplasms. Malignant teratomas, nearly all of which occur in males, are usually solid or finely cystic tumors containing actively proliferating, poorly differentiated tissue in addition to more mature elements; metastatic lesions may resemble the primary tumor or consist only of embryonal carcinoma. Mediastinal teratomas should be surgically removed.

Thymomas are rare in children. In adults they sometimes accompany or precede the development of myasthenia gravis. This association is extremely rare in children, as is the association of thymoma with aregenerative anemia. Thymomas may be asymptomatic and discovered only roentgenographically, or they may be responsible for vague retrosternal pain, cough, dyspnea or signs of compression of the superior vena cava. They are usually encapsulated and composed of an admixture of lymphoid and epithelial cells; typical Hassall's corpuscles are rare. True thymomas are usually benign; occasionally they infiltrate and implant on the pleura.

Mediastinal seminomas are predominantly tumors of young adult males but do occur in teenage boys. They may be responsible for cough or pain in the chest, but many are asymptomatic and are discovered by chance roentgenographically in the anterior mediastinum. Grossly the tumor may be encapsulated or may invade or surround one or more of the great vessels; in some instances the gross appearance may suggest a thymic cyst, and the wall of any such cyst should be carefully examined for the presence of this tumor. Histologically they resemble their counterpart in the testis, consisting of sheets of relatively uniform medium to large cells in a fibrovascular stroma. A lymphoid infiltrate, often with germinal centers, is present and there are usually epithelioid granulomas. If other germinal elements are excluded by careful histologic study of multiple sections, the prognosis is excellent; cures have been attained even after metastasis. In the absence of a palpable mass in a testis, orchiectomy or testicular biopsy is not indicated; the necessity of performing lymphangiography to exclude retroperitoneal involvement is doubtful. Treatment is by total surgical excision if possible, possibly followed by irradiation to the mediastinum, supraclavicular, infraclavicular and low cervical lymph nodes.

Thymic enlargement in children is more often caused by a *teratoma* arising within this organ than by a thymoma. By far the most common causes of a pathologically enlarged thymus, however, are leukemia, lymphosarcoma and Hodgkin's disease; in such cases there is usually but not invariably an accompanying enlargement of the mediastinal lymph nodes.

Thymolipoma is a rare tumor occurring predominantly in children 10 to 15 years of age. It may be responsible for cough, dyspnea and pain, or it may be discovered by chance on a roentgenogram of the chest. The tumor, which is benign and is apt to attain a large size, is located in the anterior portion of the mediastinum. It is encapsulated and composed of an admixture of fat and thymic tissue. A relation between thymolipomas and mediastinal lipomas has been suggested.

Angiomatous lymphoid hamartoma (benign lymphoid hamartoma) usually presents as a mass in the mid-mediastinum at the hilus of one lung. It may, however, arise in the anterior or posterior mediastinum; about one fourth of the reported instances have been extrathoracic in location, e.g., in the neck, retroperitoneum, axilla, pectoralis or muscles of the upper extremity. The tumor occurs predominantly in young adults; about 10 per cent of affected persons are less than 15 years of age. Although almost always an asymptomatic mass, it may be responsible for failure of growth, severe hypochromic anemia refractory to treatment with iron, hypergammaglobulinemia and low-grade fever; these manifestations disappear after removal of the mass. The tumor, which often reaches a rather large size, is well circumscribed or encapsulated. It is composed of lymphoid tissue devoid of normal sinusoids and contains evenly distributed follicles, the centers of which may bear a superficial resemblance to Hassall's corpuscles. The lesion has been confused with a thymoma, but it is probably not a true neoplasm. It is benign, and recurrences or metastases do not occur.

Lymphangioma of the mediastinum is usually associated with a cervical hygroma (p. 1631). Less frequently the tumor is confined to the mediastinum, where it may assume a bizarre shape and attain a large size in the absence of any clinical manifestations. The tumor is usually a multilocular cystic structure. It may arise anywhere in the mediastinum, but most frequently originates anteriorly. Chylothorax is an infrequent but serious complication.

Mediastinal hemangiomas are rare and occur principally in infants and children. Although predominantly located in the anterior mediastinum, these tumors may arise posteriorly and involve the spinal cord, with resultant neurologic manifestations. The patients may be asymptomatic or complain of pain or dyspnea. The diagnosis is rarely established prior to thoracotomy. The tumor, which is usually cavernous in type, is best treated surgically. Rarely it has been responsible for death in early infancy as a result of rupture into the pleural cavity.

Mediastinal lipomas usually originate in the anterior mediastinum, often at the cardiophrenic angle. They may be unassociated with any clinical manifestations or may be responsible for pain and dyspnea. The tumors, although encapsulated, tend to grow extensively through the mediastinum and may reach an enormous size before giving rise to symptoms. They should be surgically excised.

Lipomas may also arise in the subpleural fat and project into the pleural cavity, the cervical region or through an intercostal space. They may sometimes be identified by their radiolucency and may be suspected when there is extrathoracic extension of a mediastinal mass.

Fibromatosis of the mediastinum may be localized or may occur in conjunction with similar changes in the cervical region or in the retroperitoneum. These are fibrous, infiltrative tumors which tend to grow slowly and almost never metastasize. They may encase the vena cava and be responsible for the superior vena cava syndrome.

Mesenchymomas are rare in the mediastinum, but both benign (p. 1634) and malignant (p. 1638) types have been observed in children. Even "benign" tumors composed of an admixture of mature mesenchymal elements may be so infiltrative as to be responsible for death.

Rhabdomyosarcoma (p. 1637) of the mediastinum is a rare, highly malignant neoplasm, usually located in the anterior portion of the mediastinum.

Mediastinal lymphosarcoma is apt to be responsible for respiratory difficulty and cough, sometimes associated with superior vena caval obstruction, pleuritic pain, pleural effusion and/or fever. Extension into the cervical region may already have occurred when the patient is first seen. Roentgenographic examination reveals the presence of mediastinal masses, which usually originate in the mid-mediastinum but have frequently extended into the anterior mediastinum by the time clinical manifestations are present; in some instances the neoplasm originates in the thymus as an anterior mediastinal mass. The incidence of leukemic development in children with lymphosarcoma is very high, and meningeal involvement occurs in almost half of those who develop leukemia; infrequently it may precede the development of leukemia.

Neuroblastoma. See page 1619.

Ganglioneuroma. See page 1620.

Neurilemmoma. See page 1636.

Neurofibroma. See page 1636.

Thymic cysts. See page 1606.

TUMORS OF THE HEART

Neoplasms of the heart are rare in all age groups. The majority are histologically benign, but their location may be responsible for death. Some of the neoplasms, e.g., myxomas, are apt to produce clinical manifestations at any age period in which they occur, but are usually encountered in adults. Some, however, such as fibromas, occur predominantly in infants and children, in whom they may be responsible for sudden death.

The diagnosis of a primary neoplasm of the heart is usually not suspected during life; death sometimes occurs suddenly with no previous symptoms of cardiovascular disease. In some instances, however, clinical manifestations referable to the cardiovascular system are present, and, through such studies as angiocardiography and coronary arteriography, the diagnosis may be established during life. Tumors such as myxomas of the atrium and intrapericardiac teratomas may be successfully treated surgically, and even intramural fibromas have been excised.

In addition to the lesions described below in separate paragraphs, a variety of other neoplasms or neoplastic-like lesions have been described in the heart of an infant or child. *Lymphangioma* of the heart may occur as an isolated lesion or in association with an extracardiac hygroma. It may be a polypoid mass projecting from the epicardial surface or a diffuse infiltrative lesion with resultant thickening of the wall of the left ventricle by innumerable cystic spaces. Bleeding into a diffuse myocardial lymphangioma may be responsible for sudden death. Hemopericardium has occurred, even during the neonatal period, as a result of rupture of an epicardial *hemangioma,* and massive hemorrhagic pericardial effusion has occurred in an infant with *juvenile xanthogranulomas* involving the skin and the epicardium. *Plexiform neurofibroma, intracardiac lipoma, epicardial cyst* and *epidermoid cysts* have also been seen in infants and children; the last arise in the atrial septum immediately above the tricuspid valve. The relation of the epidermoid cysts to benign or malignant intracardiac teratomas arising in a somewhat comparable location is not clear.

Rhabdomyomatous malformation of the heart (congenital rhabdomyoma) is not a true neoplasm and possibly represents a hamartomatous malformation. It is found predominantly in infants and children, about 60 per cent of affected persons being less than a year of age. It is often associated with tuberous sclerosis. (See p. 1619.) Usually the cerebral lesions so characteristic of tuberous sclerosis are not apparent in infants with rhabdomyomatous malformations of the heart who die during the first two or three months of life; of those who survive more than a few years, most will have other stigmata of tuberous sclerosis.

The myocardial lesions often are not responsible for any symptoms and are discovered incidentally at necropsy. Occasionally they are responsible for sudden death or for massive cardiomegaly and cardiac failure.

The cardiac lesions are usually multiple and are fairly well demarcated, yellowish brown, firm, elastic nodules of varying size. Histologically these are composed of tremendously enlarged cardiac muscle fibers which appear as empty, somewhat irregular tubes whose walls, although extremely thin, may still contain longitudinal and cross striations. A few granules of glycogen may be present within these otherwise empty, enlarged muscle fibers, but the bulk of their content is dissolved out by the usual fixatives. Many of the nuclei lie against the walls of the empty fibers, but some are centrally located with radially arranged cytoplasmic strands, producing the so-called spider cells.

Myxoma of the heart, the most common primary cardiac neoplasm in adults, is rare in children. It usually arises from the region of the foramen ovale in the left atrium and projects as a polypoid, smooth or lobulated mass into the cavity of the atrium, where it may obstruct the mitral orifice. Rarely it extends through the foramen ovale and produces neoplastic masses in both atria.

The clinical manifestations are often bizarre and include the sudden onset of dyspnea, fainting spells or cyanosis. Adams-Stokes syndrome may occur, and the lesion may be responsible for sudden death. Embolic phenomena in any location, but especially cerebral ones, are common. The clinical manifestations may closely simulate those of rheumatic heart disease with mitral stenosis or insufficiency, but without any history of rheumatic fever. The sedimentation rate may be elevated, and leukocytosis and some degree of anemia are present in about one fourth of the patients. Splinter hemorrhages and other embolic phenomena may simulate bacterial endocarditis. Alterations in its nature or disappearance of the murmur with change of position or relief of symptoms following such a change suggests the possibility of an intracavitary tumor. As a rule, the diagnosis of an intracavitary tumor can be established by demonstration of a filling defect, usually in the left atrium. Operation is the treatment of choice; the patient can be cured.

Fibroma of the heart is a rare solitary tumor which is usually located in the wall of the left ventricle. It is sometimes associated with extracardiac anomalies and has been observed with the Beckwith-Wiedemann syndrome. The tumor may be responsible for sudden death. The mass is often several centimeters in diameter; it is a well circumscribed but nonencapsulated ovoid mass (Fig. 25–1). Histologically it is composed of interweaving bundles of spindle-shaped fibroblasts associated with a variable amount of collagen and elastic fibers. Occasional foci of calcification may be present, and strands of cardiac muscle fibers are often incorporated within the tumor, especially in its peripheral portion.

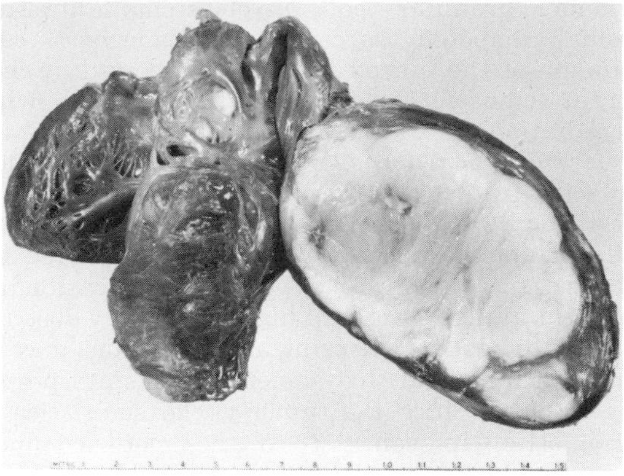

Figure 25–1 *Fibroma of the right ventricle in a 4 year old girl. Almost the entire lateral wall of the right ventricle is occupied by the tumor. A small atrial septal defect above and to the left of the tumor is filled with cotton.*

Benign mesothelioma of the node of Tarawa is a rare, minute, primary tumor of the posterior part of the atrioventricular node. It may occur in children or adults and is always responsible for partial or complete heart block, sometimes accompanied by the Adams-Stokes syndrome. The tumor, which may be demonstrable only histologically, is probably derived from primitive epicardial (mesothelial) cells. These form varying numbers of tubules lined by a single or multiple layers of cuboidal cells. A homogeneous pink material is frequently present. Varying degrees of squamous metaplasia may occur in the tubular lining cells.

Primary malignant neoplasms of the heart in children are extremely rare; most of them are rhabdomyosarcomas. Differentiation of primary from metastatic rhabdomyosarcoma of the heart may be difficult or impossible.

TUMORS OF THE LARYNX

Papillomas of the larynx (Section 12) are the only tumors which occur at this site with any degree of frequency. In infants subglottic hemangiomas, though rare, are important lesions which may be overlooked at laryngoscopy and even at necropsy. *Pseudosarcomas* (p. 1634) may occur in the larynx, trachea or bronchi, and their recognition as benign, non-neoplastic lesions is of obvious importance. In addition to these tumors and neurofibromas, isolated instances of lymphangioma, granular cell myoblastoma, fibrosarcoma, rhabdomyosarcoma and epidermoid carcinoma of the larynx have been reported in children; some of the last have developed following irradiation of laryngeal papillomas.

Hemangioma of the larynx is a rare tumor which affects girls more often than boys. Clinical manifestations are apparent during the first 6 months of life in approximately 90 per cent of affected infants, and inspiratory stridor is occasionally present at birth. Signs of high respiratory obstruction with stridor, wheezing and retractions may be intermittent and are sometimes misinterpreted as "croup." Since the tumor is characteristically subglottic, in contrast to the more common hemangioma on or above the vocal cords of adults, hoarseness is usually absent. Cutaneous hemangiomas are present in only about half of affected infants. Lateral roentgenograms often reveal a discrete tumor in the subglottic area. Laryngoscopically the tumor characteristically appears as a soft, pink to bluish subglottic mass, but because of its diffuseness and the absence of distinct discoloration, the true nature of the mass may not be appreciated and it may be regarded simply as subglottic edema or stenosis. Even at postmortem examination the lesion may not be recognized macroscopically; histologic examination of the subglottic region should be a routine procedure. Biopsy of the mass is contraindicated when the diagnosis is reasonably well established by history and laryngoscopic examination. Tracheotomy may be necessary. Irradiation or the use of corticosteroids has been advocated but the tumor may regress spontaneously.

Neurofibromas of the larynx are rare. They are usually solitary lesions; only 10 to 20 per cent are accompanied by other stigmata of multiple neurofibromatosis. In infants and children, however, a number of them have been plexiform neurofibromas (p. 1636) and possibly were the initial manifestations of von Recklinghausen's disease. They are usually submucosal masses located at the level of the aryepiglottic folds and the ventricular bands. Clinical manifestations, which may begin in early infancy, are those of any slowly growing benign tumor of the larynx, e.g., hoarseness, stridor, cough and dyspnea. Recurrence following removal is rare.

TUMORS OF THE TRACHEA, BRONCHI AND LUNGS

Primary neoplasms of the trachea, bronchi or lungs are rare in children, although pulmonary metastases from various sites are relatively common. Whenever a pulmonary tumor is demonstrated, it is mandatory to search for a primary extrapulmonary lesion. Removal of a suspected malignant neoplasm from any site should be preceded by roentgenographic examination of the chest in search for pulmonary metastases.

Papillomas of the trachea or bronchi are rare, and most of them are complications of laryngeal papillomas (Section 12), the lesions tending to occur especially around a tracheotomy wound.

Tracheobronchial papillomatosis is a rare and usually late complication of laryngeal papillomas. The bronchial papillomas may occur with laryngeal papillomas or may follow them after many years. Rarely the papillomas are confined to the tracheobronchial tree and lungs, the larynx being spared. The papillary tumors grow slowly and extend into the alveolar spaces. The involved bronchi expand into cystic cavities containing bulky papillomatous masses which may contain columnar ciliated as well as squamous epithelium. The lesions, which have been erroneously interpreted as carcinoma, do not metastasize and are probably of multicentric origin rather than implants from an initial primary tumor. Clinically they are characterized by recurrent hemoptysis; with a preceding history of laryngeal papillomas, hemoptysis should suggest the possibility of tracheobronchial papillomatosis. Roentgenographic examination reveals areas of nodular density and cavitation within the lungs and, with the history of hemoptysis, may lead to an erroneous diagnosis of tuberculosis. The cavities may become secondarily infected. Treatment should be conservative; if a symptomatic lesion must be excised, no more pulmonary parenchyma than is absolutely necessary should be removed.

Bronchogenic cysts are non-neoplastic lesions most frequently encountered in adults, in whom they are often asymptomatic. In the pediatric age period, especially in infants, they are more apt to be associated with manifestations of bronchial obstruction, e.g., periodic episodes of dyspnea, wheezing, stridor, cough and cyanosis. These may begin early in life, even during the neonatal period, and are sometimes accompanied by recurrent attacks of pneumonia. The cyst, which only rarely communicates with the tracheobronchial tree, is typically located near the carina anterior to the esophagus, but may be lateral to the trachea at a somewhat higher level, in the wall of the esophagus or elsewhere in the mediastinum. It is characteristically manifest roentgenographically as a sharply circumscribed, dense, round or oval mass arising in the mid-mediastinum and displacing the esophagus posteriorly and laterally; only rarely is an air-fluid level present. Occasionally no mass has been detected roentgenographically, and failure to remove the cyst has proved lethal.

Bronchial adenoma is a low-grade carcinoma which presents as a firm, spherical tumor projecting into the lumen of the trachea or one of the larger bronchi. The tumor extends through the bronchial wall; the extrabronchial portion may be larger than the intraluminal one. Cough, wheezing and recurrent episodes of pneumonia, sometimes with hemoptysis, are the usual manifestations. Affected children are sometimes treated for bronchial asthma for years before the neoplasm is discovered. Bronchial obstruction and repeated infections may lead to bronchiectasis. Tracheal neoplasms may be unaccompanied by roentgenographic changes, but bronchial tumors, which are more common, are usually associated with emphysema, atelectasis or a pulmonary infiltrate in the area supplied by the affected bronchus. Histologically the neoplasm may resemble a carcinoid (p. 1613) or, much less frequently, resembles an adenoid cystic carcinoma (cylindroma); rarely a polypoid tumor is a true adenoma composed of distinct glands lined by tall cylindrical epithelium and filled with mucus. The tumor should be surgically resected, even if lobectomy or pneumonectomy is required. Although in adults the cylindromatous neoplasm has proved to be more malignant than the carcinoid, in children metastases to regional lymph nodes have been observed in both types. In general, the prognosis is good even if regional lymph nodes are involved.

Pulmonary arteriovenous fistulas (cavernous hemangiomas of the lung) are solitary or multiple lesions associated with telangiectases in other parts of the body in about half of the patients, and in more than half of affected persons there is a family history of hemorrhagic telangiectasia (Rendu-Osler-Weber disease, Section 11). The clinical manifestations are cyanosis, which may be present at birth or appear in early childhood, dyspnea, polycythemia and clubbing of the fingers and toes; repeated epistaxes are common. A systolic or continuous murmur may be audible over the lesion, and the diagnosis of congenital heart disease may be considered. Roentgenographically the lesion is usually demonstrable as a homogeneous density of variable size and shape continuous with the hilar vascular shadows. The lesion should be excised.

Hamartomas of the lung in the pediatric age period are almost all cystic adenomatoid malformations. The so-called chondromatous hamartomas are extremely rare in children; they are usually small subpleural nodules composed predominantly of cartilage. Between the lobules of cartilage are clefts lined by bronchial epithelium and surrounded by loose connective tissue, fat and smooth muscle fibers.

Lymphangiomas and *hemangiomas* are rare types of hamartomas of the lung. Lymphangioma usually involves only a single lobe. Hemangioma of the lung is sometimes multicentric, involving both lungs.

Cystic adenomatoid malformation of the lung is discussed in Section 12.

Fibrosarcoma of a bronchus is an extremely rare neoplasm which tends to occur in children and young adults; almost half of affected persons are less than 15 years of age. Cough, dyspnea, fever and repeated episodes of atelectasis and lower respiratory tract infections are common. Metastases in children are almost nonexistent; some of the reported instances probably were pseudosarcomas (p. 1634) which would have responded satisfactorily to local bronchoscopic excision. If the diagnosis of fibrosarcoma is firmly established, however, lobectomy or pneumonectomy is indicated.

Leiomyomas, neurilemmomas or *neurofibromas* which arise in the pulmonary parenchyma are rare and usually asymptomatic. Roentgenographically any of these appears as a well circumscribed, spherical, homogeneous density. In contrast, intrabronchial leiomyomas and neurofibromas are responsible for cough, fever, atelectasis and recurrent lower respiratory tract infections. Lobectomy is the treatment of choice.

Leiomyosarcomas may arise in the trachea, bronchi or pulmonary parenchyma. These are usually responsible for symptoms such as cough and dyspnea, sometimes accompanied by pain in the chest. In children, in whom these neoplasms are extremely rare, there may be local extension into a pulmonary vein; metastases rarely occur. Treatment is by excision, including lobectomy or pneumonectomy if necessary for complete removal of the mass.

Postinflammatory tumors of the lung are rare. Symptoms are apt to be mild, e.g., a moderate cough. Hemoptysis, which is common in adults, is infrequent in children. There is usually a history of a preceding respiratory infection. Roentgenographically the lesion is a solitary, sharply circumscribed, lobulated mass, infrequently with central cavitation. Histologically the tumor is composed of spindle-shaped cells, often arranged in whorls or interlacing bundles, vascular channels, nests of foam cells and an infiltrate of inflammatory cells, predominantly plasma cells. The tumor is probably not true neoplastic growth, but is important because it may be confused clinically with tuberculosis or a malignant growth. Pathologically it may be erroneously interpreted as a neurofibroma or even a fibrosarcoma. The relation of these tumors with those described as *sclerosing hemangiomas* of the lung is not clear, but the two may represent the same lesion.

Bronchogenic carcinoma is extremely rare in early life, but has been reported even in infants. The initial manifestations may be referable to the primary neoplasm, e.g., cough, dyspnea and pain in the chest, or to metastatic foci. The neoplasm may be large and bulky and may replace most of the affected lung, displace the mediastinum to the opposite side, obliterate the pleural space and even extend into the intercostal spaces; a primary focus within a bronchus is unusual. Metastases occur in lymph nodes, the opposite lung, bone and a variety of other sites; the brain, liver and adrenals are usually spared. Histologically undifferentiated epidermoid and adenocarcinomas have been described.

TUMORS OF THE GASTROINTESTINAL TRACT

Tumors of the gastrointestinal tract may be symptomless or may be manifest by abdominal pain, intestinal obstruction (especially intussusception), hemorrhage, or rarely by a palpable mass. With the exception of the juvenile polyp, no tumor of the gastrointestinal tract can be considered common in children, but both benign and malignant neoplasms do occur.

Juvenile polyps are common tumors of the gastrointestinal tract in early life. They are much more common in the first than in the second decade, but are infrequent during the first year of life. The polyps are usually located in the rectum, less frequently in the sigmoid colon and uncommonly in the more proximal colon, the small intestine or the stomach. They are usually solitary, but occasionally several polyps may be scattered through the bowel, especially in the colon.

The common clinical manifestation is bleeding from the rectum, small amounts of bright red blood being passed with or after defecation. The continuous loss of even small amounts of blood over a period of several months may be responsible for hypochromic anemia. Abdominal pain may occur, but intussusception is infrequent. Occasionally the polyp prolapses through the anus and is spontaneously extruded.

These are benign tumors with an entirely different histologic pattern from the common polypoid lesion of the bowel in adults, from the polyps in multiple familial polyposis and from those in the Peutz-Jeghers syndrome. There is no evidence that the juvenile polyp undergoes malignant transformation; occasionally they may disappear spontaneously. Treatment consists in removal of a solitary polyp, usually at sigmoidoscopy. If additional polyps are demonstrated, they should be removed only if they are responsible for symptoms.

Multiple familial polyposis is a rare condition characterized by the presence of innumerable sessile and pedunculated tumors in the rectum and colon. It should not be confused with scattered juvenile polyps, which are benign and do not predispose to the development of carcinoma, nor with the Peutz-Jeghers syndrome, in which the polyps involve predominantly the small intestine. The disease is transmitted as a mendelian dominant trait with incomplete penetrance; approximately one third of the cases appear to be sporadic. The clinical manifestations are usually diarrhea and bleeding; they usually appear in the teen-age period. If untreated, these patients almost all develop carcinoma, many prior to 15 years of age. Treatment, therefore, consists in total colectomy.

Peutz-Jeghers syndrome is a rare condition inherited in a dominant manner and characterized by intestinal polyps and deposits of pigment, especially in the lips and buccal mucosa, but sometimes also in the skin of the face and in the palmar and plantar surfaces of the fingers and toes. The polyps are usually multiple and may be located in the stomach, colon and rectum, small bowel or in all these sites. The clinical manifestations referable to the polyps are those of recurrent transient intussusception, gastrointestinal bleeding and hypochromic anemia. The polyps, which are considered to be hamartomas, contain glands lined by cells of all types normally found in the affected part of the gastrointestinal tract. Cystic dilatation of the glands is common, and the polyps often contain strands of smooth muscle. In general, treatment should be conservative, with removal of only those polyps which are responsible for symptoms. The development of carcinoma, presumably from these polyps, is infrequent, but has occurred, especially in the duodenum.

Gardner syndrome is inherited as an autosomal dominant trait and is characterized by the presence of multiple polyps of the colon and rectum, multiple osteomas involving especially the facial bones, multiple epidermoid cysts, fibromatous growths (desmoids) which tend to develop in incisional scars on the abdomen after intestinal surgery, and mesenteric and retroperitoneal fibrosis. The polyps, which may develop in infancy or not until adult life, are multiple but usually scattered; there may be polyps elsewhere in the gastrointestinal tract. There is a striking tendency to malignant transformation of the colonic polyps. Intestinal manifestations are often preceded by one or more of the other stigmata of the syndrome, the presence of which should lead to a thorough investigation for the possibility of intestinal polyposis. The disease is not simply a variant of multiple familial polyposis.

Benign "lymphomas" of the rectum and anal canal are small polypoid lesions composed of aggregates of lymphocytes containing germinal centers. They are usually solitary, sessile lesions located in the lower third of the rectum. The lymphoid tissue comprising the mass usually does not extend beyond the submucosa and is covered by intact mucosa. The most frequent clinical manifestation is rectal bleeding. The lesions are not related to malignant lymphomas and are probably inflammatory in origin. Treatment, if any, should be nothing more than simple excision.

Lymphoid hyperplasia of the colon is a benign, non-neoplastic condition which is most frequently associated with rectal bleeding. It probably represents the response of lymphoid tissue of the bowel to a variety of stimuli. Roentgenographically it is characterized by small, uniform, umbilicated polypoid lesions involving all or part of the colon; rarely the small intestine or even the stomach may be involved. The umbilication of the lesions as well as the young age of the patients, most of whom are less than 2 years of age, should differentiate these changes from those of multiple familial polyposis, with which this condition has occasionally been confused. Lymphoid hyperplasia of the small intestine may be associated with hypogammaglobulinemia, splenomegaly and enlarged tonsils.

Lymphosarcoma is the most common malignant neoplasm of the gastrointestinal tract in early life. The tumor usually arises in the small intestine, especially the ileum; it may originate in the colon, appendix or even the stomach. The presenting complaint is usually crampy abdominal pain, often accompanied by vomiting and a palpable mass; the mass may be the neoplasm or an intussusception. Morphologically a segment of the bowel may be diffusely infiltrated by neoplastic cells with resultant thickening of the wall and superficial ulceration of the mucosa, or a polypoid mass may project into the lumen of the bowel. Metastases may be widespread throughout the abdominal organs. The prognosis is grave, but not hopeless. Some cures have been obtained by surgical removal of the affected segment of bowel and the regionally involved lymph nodes; the survival rate is probably improved by subsequent irradiation and chemotherapy.

Carcinoma of the colon is rare in children; it may occur as a complication of multiple familial polyposis (see above) or of prolonged chronic ulcerative colitis. The incidence of carcinoma is greater in those who develop chronic ulcerative colitis in childhood rather than in adult life, and malignancy occasionally develops in childhood.

Rarely carcinoma of the colon occurs in infancy or childhood in the absence of known predisposing factors. It is more common in the rectum and distal colon than in the proximal large bowel. The symptoms are similar to those in adults. Abdominal pain, vomiting, constipation, loss of weight and blood in the stools are the most common symptoms; a mass is palpable in more than half of the affected children. In contrast to adults, in whom most of the neoplasms are fairly well differentiated adenocarcinomas, almost half of those in children are poorly differentiated neoplasms with signet ring cells. The prognosis is grave, but apparent cures have been effected, especially when the tumor is well differentiated.

Carcinoma of the stomach is also rare in children; it has occurred with ataxia-telangiectasia in the late teens. The presenting complaints are apt to be those of pain, vomiting and loss of weight; a palpable abdominal mass is present in about three fourths of the patients. The prognosis is very grave, probably in part because of the delay in diagnosis.

Carcinoids (argentaffin tumors) occur in less than 0.2 per cent of appendices removed from children under 14 years of age. The tumor is usually located in the distal end of the appendix, where it presents as a firm, yellow mass arising deep in the mucosa, infiltrating the muscularis and often extending to the serosa. It is usually an incidental finding observed in an appendix removed for some other reason. Infrequently the mass may be located more proximally in the appendix and be responsible for obstruction of the lumen and acute appendicitis. Although appendiceal carcinoids are indistinguishable morphologically from malignant carcinoids arising elsewhere in the gastrointestinal tract, those in the appendix rarely metastasize. If, as is usually true, the tumor is less than 2 cm in diameter, and there are no grossly recognizable metastases, simple appendectomy is adequate treatment; this is true regardless of the location of the tumor in the appendix and regardless of histologic evidence of peritoneal involvement or lymphatic invasion.

Rarely a carcinoid may arise in a Meckel's diverticulum or in the ileum; in the ileum it is a rare cause of intussusception.

The *malignant carcinoid syndrome,* which consists of valvular disease of the right side of the heart, sudden flushing of the skin, an unusual type of patchy, changing cyanosis, frequent watery stools and "asthmatic attacks," is predominantly a disease of adults; it may, however, have its onset during childhood. It is caused by a carcinoid in the ileum which has metastasized to such an extent as to be responsible for the presence of a large accumulation of neoplastic tissue; the metastases usually involve the liver, but may be confined to the mesenteric lymph nodes. The manifestations result from excessive amounts of serotonin (5-hydroxytryptamine) in the blood and tissues; the diagnosis can be confirmed by the demonstration of excessive amounts of its metabolite, 5-hydroxyindoleacetic acid, in the urine. Some of these patients survive for many months or even years in spite of extensive inoperable metastatic disease.

Hemangiomas of the intestine are extremely rare, but have been observed in all age groups. They may be diffuse infiltrating lesions involving a segment of the bowel with resultant thickening of the wall and narrowing of the lumen or may be localized and project into the lumen. They are sometimes multiple and may be associated with hemangiomas elsewhere, e.g., in the stomach, liver, bladder, renal pelves and skin. The manifestations are those of intestinal obstruction, hemorrhage, pain or intussusception; only rarely is there a palpable mass.

Leiomyosarcomas have been observed in the stomach, small intestine and colon of children; their benign counterpart, the *leiomyoma,* has been reported as arising from these sites as well as from the esophagus and from a Meckel's diverticulum. Estimation of the biologic behavior of smooth muscle tumors based upon their histologic characteristics is extremely difficult, but with the exception of tumors arising in the stomach, recurrences or metastases in children are rare. The neoplasms, regardless of their site of origin in the enteric canal, are usually firm, circumscribed but nonencapsulated tumors. Those arising in the stomach may be responsible for gross bleeding and a palpable mass, whereas those arising in the small intestine are apt to be manifest by signs of intestinal obstruction; tumors of the small bowel are rarely palpable, but they may serve as the lead point for an intussusception. Tumors of the large intestine may reach a large size and be responsible for obstruction and a palpable mass.

Teratoma of the stomach is an extremely rare benign lesion usually encountered in infants less than 1 year of age. In addition to a palpable mass, there may be severe anemia secondary to bleeding. The tumor may herniate into the thorax through the esophageal hiatus.

TUMORS OF THE LIVER

Metastatic neoplasms of the liver are more frequent than primary ones and may originate from a variety of tumors. They are usually not responsible for any manifestations other than hepatomegaly.

Primary neoplasms of the liver in infants and children, the majority of which are malignant, occur with sufficient frequency that they must be considered in the differential diagnosis of a mass in the upper part of the abdomen. Some of them can be successfully treated surgically.

Infantile hemangioendothelioma is the common vascular tumor of the liver in infants; cavernous hemangiomas similar to those encountered in adults are rare. The tumors are commonly multicentric within the liver, and extrahepatic hemangiomas are present in some instances. The multiplicity of the lesions and the active proliferation of vessels within them may suggest a malignant neoplasm, but they are probably simple vascular hamartomas rather than true neoplasms and are comparable to the cellular hemangiomas so common in the skin of infants.

Clinical manifestations are commonly present in the first weeks of life. An abdominal mass is often the only presenting complaint, but anemia and rarely ascites and jaundice may be present. In some instances cardiomegaly and congestive heart failure may lead to an erroneous diagnosis of congenital heart disease; cardiovascular manifestations have been attributed to arteriovenous shunts within the tumor. Fatal hemorrhage may occur spontaneously or after biopsy. The solitary tumors are probably best treated surgically. Multicentric tumors of the liver may regress spontaneously. If treatment is necessary, irradiation and/or the administration of corticosteroids may be beneficial; signs of cardiac failure may be an indication for ligation of the hepatic artery.

Adenomas are rare, solitary circumscribed neoplasms composed of hepatic cells. There are no bile ducts or portal triads. There is no associated cirrhosis. The adenoma should be differentiated from the adenomatous hyperplastic nodules associated with hepatic damage. Differentiation from carcinoma may be difficult or impossible, and the diagnosis is often indefinite until sufficient time has elapsed to ensure that a recurrence is not likely. The tumor should be widely excised.

Focal nodular hyperplasia of the liver is a rare tumor the exact nature of which is not known. It is probably not a true neoplasm. The initial complaint is usually related to abdominal enlargement or to a palpable mass; at times there is discomfort in the upper part of the abdomen.

The lesion, which is almost always solitary, may be pedunculated or located deep within the liver. It is sharply demarcated from the adjacent hepatic tissue; toward the center of the mass a stellate zone of connective tissue is present, from which bands of collagen radiate peripherally. The lesion is benign and does not warrant a radical surgical procedure. It should, however, be resected if this can be easily accomplished.

Mesenchymal hamartomas of the liver are cystic masses which are usually manifest during infancy. The presenting complaint is that of an upper abdominal mass, which may increase rapidly in size owing to the accumulation of fluid in it. The tumor is usually located near the lower margin of the right lobe of the liver, to which it is sometimes attached by a pedicle. It may project into the pelvis and can often be outlined roentgenographically. The tumor can usually be identified grossly by its multicystic appearance (Fig. 25–2). It is poorly demarcated from the adjoining hepatic parenchyma. Histologically it consists of connective tissue containing cystic spaces, many of which may have no demonstrable lining cells. Small numbers of hepatic cells and bile ducts are present, especially about the periphery of the lesion. The tumor is benign, but should be excised.

Congenital solitary hepatic cysts are nonneoplastic malformations which are only rarely responsible for a palpable abdominal mass. The cyst is initially lined by biliary epithelium, but it may become partially or completely denuded. The lumen contains a mucoid material.

Carcinoma of the liver in the pediatric age period occurs in two distinct forms: *hepatoblastoma* and *hepatoma.* These tend to occur at different ages and are distinct morphologically and probably pathogenetically. The prognosis is grave in both. Both types are more common in males. Generalized demineralization of the skeleton occasionally occurs with either one, as may hyperlipemia. Alpha$_1$-fetoglobulin may be present in the serum and viscera with either type, but especially with hepatoblastoma; cystathioninuria may also occur with either type. Isosexual precocious puberty in the male with elevated levels of urinary gonadotropins is a rare manifestation of carcinoma of the liver, usually a hepatoblastoma. Hepatomas occasionally appear to complicate other hepatic disease, such as neonatal hepatitis, galactosemia, glycogen storage

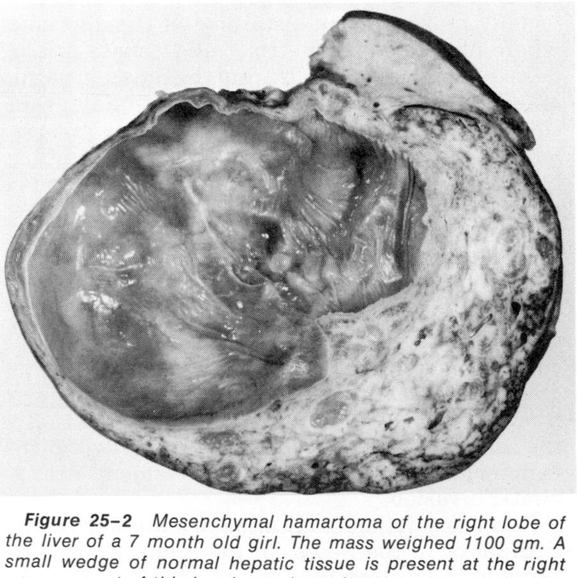

Figure 25–2 Mesenchymal hamartoma of the right lobe of the liver of a 7 month old girl. The mass weighed 1100 gm. A small wedge of normal hepatic tissue is present at the right upper aspect of this hemisected specimen.

disease, tyrosinosis, biliary cirrhosis secondary to atresia of the bile ducts, and may develop after prolonged treatment with methyltestosterone. Hepatoblastomas appear to bear no relation to pre-existing hepatic disease.

Metastases from hepatoblastoma or hepatoma occur principally in the lungs, liver, abdominal lymph nodes and bones. Cure of either type of tumor is rare, but has been effected by resection, including lobectomy.

Hepatoblastomas are more common in the pediatric age period than are hepatomas. They occur almost entirely in the first 3 years of life and may be present at birth. The initial manifestation is hepatomegaly with abdominal enlargement. Roentgenographic examination occasionally reveals mottled amorphous calcification within the tumor. Morphologically the hepatic neoplasm is usually solitary, but at times it is accompanied by multiple smaller nodules of neoplastic tissue. Histologically the tumor consists of discrete hepatic parenchymal cells resembling those of the fetal liver, but not arranged in the normal lobular pattern. Bile canaliculi may be present, and the neoplastic cells may contain glycogen and fat. Foci of extramedullary hematopoiesis are usually present. In addition, more primitive dark-staining cells arranged in sheets or ribbons, sometimes forming acini, pseudorosettes or papillary structures, may be present, and in some there are also primitive mesenchymal elements with varying degrees of differentiation. Osteoid, bone, cartilage and islands of squamous epithelial cells with distinct keratinized pearls may be present.

Hepatomas tend to occur after 5 or 6 years of age. Progressive abdominal enlargement sometimes accompanied by a definite mass is common. A history of anorexia, nausea, loss of weight and intermittent abdominal pain is more frequent than with hepatoblastoma. The neoplasm may be solitary, or there may be multiple nodules. Histologically the tumors are predominantly hepatocellular carcinomas similar to those encountered in adults; cholangiocarcinomas and mixed hepatic cell and cholangiocarcinomas are rare. The tumors consist of broad trabeculae of neoplastic cells containing variable amounts of fat, glycogen and bile. The trabeculae are separated from each other by sinusoids lined by endothelium.

Teratoma of the liver is rare; it is usually recognizable at or shortly after birth. It tends to have a bizarre lobated structure and contains a variety of tissues foreign to the liver, which are derived from multiple germ layers, e.g., skin, brain, bone, intestinal glands.

Mesenchymomas of the liver are composed of a mixture of mesodermal elements, i.e., angiomatous, fibrous and undifferentiated mesenchymal tissue. Epithelial elements are usually absent. Although those occurring in the liver usually appear to be malignant, some have been successfully resected.

Sarcoma of the liver is rare. The neoplasms are often undifferentiated and are classified with difficulty. Embryonal rhabdomyosarcomas may arise in the liver or in the common bile duct.

Sarcoma botryoides of the common bile duct occurs principally in males. Clinical manifestations of icterus, fever and a tender liver may simulate infectious hepatitis. The tumor may extend beyond the confines of the greatly dilated common bile duct and compress the duodenum. Metastases may be widespread.

Ectopic adrenal tissue may occur beneath the hepatic capsule, and rarely benign or malignant adrenocortical tumors may arise in the liver. The diagnosis of such an *adrenal rest tumor* within the liver probably should not be made unless evidences of adrenocortical hyperfunction are present and the hormones are identified within the tumor.

TUMORS OF THE SPLEEN

Primary splenic tumors are rare in any age period, splenic enlargement usually being part of a systemic disease such as leukemia, hemolytic anemia, lipidosis or infection or the result of increased venous pressure (Section 14).

Splenic cysts are rare. In children epidermoid cysts and pseudocysts are more frequent than parasitic ones resulting from echinococcal infection. *Pseudocysts* of the spleen are secondary to old trauma or infarction. Their walls are composed of fibrous or granulation tissue with no specific lining cells. Certain cysts that have been interpreted as pseudocysts, however, may well have been true or "neoplastic" ones, the lining cells of which were destroyed by trauma and hemorrhage.

Epidermoid cysts of the spleen, though rare, are the most common type of true cysts in the spleen in children (Fig. 25-3). They are usually large solitary structures, sometimes with smaller satellite cysts about them. They contain clear or chocolate-

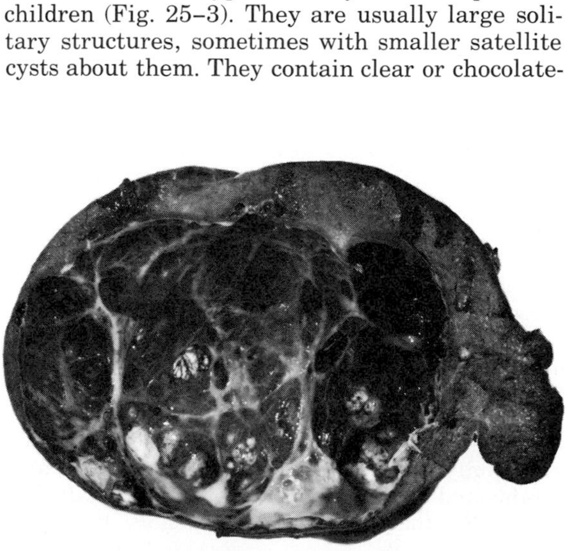

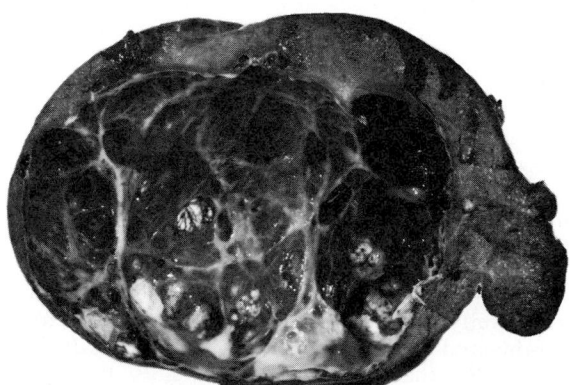

Figure 25-3 *Epidermoid cyst of the spleen from a girl 8 years old. The spleen weighed 600 gm. This cut surface reveals the trabeculated wall of the cyst, the lumen of which contained at least 335 ml of turbid brown fluid. The cyst was lined by cells which varied from cuboidal to squamous; intercellular bridges were present, but there was no keratinization.*

colored fluid that usually includes cholesterol. Their walls are trabeculated and consist of fibrous tissue lined in some areas by nonkeratinized squamous epithelial cells. Intercellular bridges are present, but there are no skin appendages. In some areas the lining cells are absent or resemble mesothelium. They occur predominantly in girls more than 5 years of age, in whom they are responsible for an asymptomatic mass in the left upper quadrant of the abdomen. Roentgenographic examination reveals a large, rounded, homogeneous density displacing the stomach to the right and the splenic flexure of the colon downward.

Hemangioma and *lymphangioma* are extremely rare causes of splenomegaly in children; they may be incidental findings at autopsy in adults. Thrombocytopenia, purpura, anemia and a deficiency of fibrinogen have been observed in an infant with a giant hemangioma of the spleen.

Splenomas (splenic hamartomas) are rare, usually solitary, tumors most often found incidentally at autopsy in elderly adults. The tumors are solid, well circumscribed but not encapsulated structures within the splenic parenchyma, sometimes producing a bulge on the surface. They may differ from the surrounding spleen only by their consistency or paler color. Histologically they are composed of lymphoid tissue, red pulp and sinusoids, often with considerable fibrosis. Tumors composed predominantly of lymphoid tissue may simulate malignant lymphoma, from which they may be differentiated by the presence of numerous sinusoids.

TUMORS OF THE PANCREAS

Adenoma of the islets of Langerhans (Section 16) may be functional or nonfunctional. About one third of the reported children with functional (hypoglycemia) tumors have been less than 2 years old. Beta cell tumors are usually small, tan or pink circumscribed masses which may be multicentric. Histologically they consist of cords or ribbons of cells embedded in a prominent fibrillary or hyaline stroma; areas of calcification may be present.

Carcinoma of the pancreas is rare in children but has been reported as early as 3 months of age. The presenting complaints are abdominal pain and/or a palpable mass. Icterus, anorexia, vomiting and loss of weight are other manifestations. The tumor may arise from the ducts or the islets of Langerhans; determination of the cell of origin may be enhanced by electron microscopy. Carcinoma of islet cell origin is only rarely responsible for hypoglycemia in infants and children. Metastases are especially apt to involve the regional lymph nodes, liver and lungs.

Cystadenoma of the pancreas is rare in any age group, but especially so in children. It is responsible for a large abdominal mass which may displace the kidneys posteriorly and the colon anteriorly. If the tumor is located in the head of the pancreas the duodenum is compressed and its curve widened. The neoplasm is a coarsely lobulated, multilocular cystic mass. The cysts are lined by cuboidal and flattened epithelium. Papillary projections into the cysts are occasionally present. The tumor is benign and should be removed surgically.

Multiple endocrine adenomatosis (Wermer syndrome) is characterized by hyperplasia or neoplasia of multiple endocrine glands, most often the parathyroids, pancreatic islets and pituitary. It is probably inherited as an autosomal dominant trait. Although it usually manifests itself in the third or fourth decade, chemical findings compatible with hyperparathyroidism have been found in a child in an affected family prior to the age of 10 years. The endocrine tumors may or may not be functional and any combination of glands may be involved, as a result of which the manifestations are protean. Within a family, however, the disorder often manifests itself in a fairly consistent manner.

Clinical manifestations vary considerably and are related to the anatomic lesions, especially those of the parathyroids, pancreatic islets and pituitary. Hyperfunction may be limited to a single endocrine system for many years, but hyperparathyroidism, the clinical manifestations of which are usually quite mild, ultimately appears in most affected persons. The endocrine tumors are apt to be multicentric, and either beta or non-beta cell tumors of the pancreatic islets are almost as common as parathyroid lesions. The islet cell tumors may be responsible for hypoglycemia or for excessive secretion of gastrin. Carcinoma of the islets may occur, but in spite of metastases this is only infrequently the cause of death. There may be acidophilic hyperplasia or adenomas of the pituitary with acromegaly or, more often, nonfunctional chromophobe adenomas.

Zollinger-Ellison syndrome is a phenotypic variant of Wermer syndrome characterized by peptic ulcers, which are often multifocal and refractile to therapy; peptic ulcers are present in more than half of those with Wermer syndrome and are often responsible for the initial complaints. They are presumably the result of islet cell tumors or hyperplasia, which causes excessive secretion of gastrin and an increase of gastric acid production. There may be frequent watery diarrhea, with severe water and electrolyte loss and hypokalemia. The peptic ulcers may be located in the duodenum, jejunum, prepyloric region and/or even the esophagogastric junction. They are responsible for bleeding and epigastric pain and occasionally for perforation. Roentgenographically, in addition to the ulcer(s), there are giant gastric rugae, a large, atonic stomach, distention of the duodenum and often of the small bowel, with hyperperistalsis, rapid transit and an edematous intestinal mucosa.

Surgical exploration for islet cell tumors causing peptic ulcers should include mobilization of the head and tail of the pancreas and resection of the neoplasm if it occupies the body or tail of the pancreas and is not widespread. Multiple regional lymph nodes should be removed for diagnostic purposes. Removal of the pancreatic tumor is usually unsuccessful because of its multifocal nature. If the diagnosis of an islet cell tumor can be established histologically either from a primary or a metastatic site in a person with this syndrome, total gastrectomy is probably the treatment of choice, even in children. This may result in disappearance of metastatic lesions.

Pseudocysts of the pancreas are discussed in Section 11.

TUMORS OF THE KIDNEY

Wilms' tumor (nephroblastoma) is one of the most common abdominal neoplasms of early life; approximately two thirds appear before the age of 4 years. Although authentic Wilms' tumors do occur in the neonatal period, almost all the tumors reported as such at this early age have been leiomyomatous hamartomas of the kidney; either of these occurring at birth may be accompanied by polyhydramnios. Bilateral renal involvement is uncommon; when it occurs it is usually detectable at the time of the initial diagnosis; otherwise, the second tumor usually appears within a year or so. Wilms' tumor occurs with increased frequency in children with aniridia, hemihypertrophy and Beckwith-Wiedemann syndrome and probably in those with fused kidneys. The incidence of Wilms' tumor with bilateral aniridia has been reported as high as 1:73 as contrasted with the usual rate of 1:50,000 to 1:100,000 and conversely, Wilms' tumors have occurred in as many as 7 of 28 children under 4 years of age hospitalized with aniridia. The aniridia accompanying Wilms' tumor is almost always of the sporadic type and is apt to be associated with other congenital defects, e.g., cataracts, mental retardation and genitourinary anomalies, including cryptorchidism.

The presenting complaint is usually that of an abdominal mass. Abdominal pain and fever may be the first manifestation. Hematuria is relatively infrequent and, contrary to earlier opinions, is probably not a poor prognostic sign. Physical examination reveals a firm, nontender mass in the renal area which may extend down into the iliac fossa but usually does not cross the midline. Hypertension, the pathogenesis of which is not always clear, may be present.

Roentgen examination reveals a soft tissue density which is apt to displace the intestine toward the opposite side. Calcification is infrequent; when present it is apt to be dense and curvilinear, in contrast to the stippled appearance common in a neuroblastoma. Pyelography, preferably including an inferior vena cavagram, usually reveals distortion of the renal pelvis; displacement or extension of the tumor into the inferior vena cava is sometimes apparent. In some instances the kidney on the affected side cannot be visualized by intravenous pyelography. The pyelographic findings are not pathognomonic of a Wilms' tumor but instead indicate the presence of an intrarenal mass. Probably the most important reason for obtaining pyelograms is the demonstration of the presence and apparent normality of the opposite kidney.

Macroscopically the tumor usually presents as a bulky circumscribed mass replacing much of the affected kidney and covered externally by the thin renal capsule. With continued growth, however, there may be invasion of the renal pelvis and/or veins and extension beyond the capsule into the perirenal fat, adrenal, diaphragm or colon. On section the tumor bulges beyond the surface of the adjoining kidney (Fig. 25–4). It is yellowish gray and soft, friable or semiliquid as a result of multiple areas of necrosis; it often contains myxomatous areas and foci of hemorrhage. Areas of necrosis may be responsible for cysts containing clear or hemorrhagic fluid. The renal pelvis is usually elongated and distorted, and occasionally masses of neoplastic tissue extend into its lumen. Careful search should be made for islands of neoplastic tissue in the remainder of the affected kidney since there is some evidence to indicate that such multicentric or metastatic lesions affect the prognosis adversely. Metastases occur principally in lymph nodes, lung and liver.

The histologic pattern is variable. There are often broad sheets or cords of undifferentiated mesenchymal cells within which are scattered epithelial-lined tubules; rarely the latter, if incompletely differentiated, may resemble the pseudorosettes of a neuroblastoma. Abortive glomeruli are sometimes present. Bands of loose, more differen-

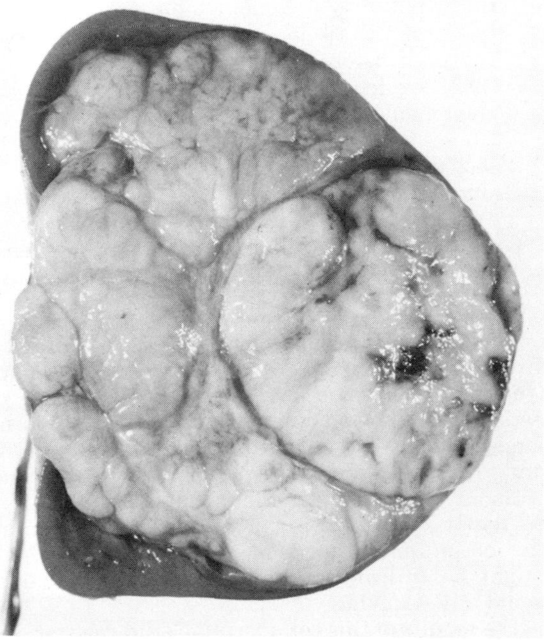

Figure 25–4 *Wilms' tumor of the left kidney from a boy 10 months old. The major part of the kidney is replaced by the lobulated tumor. A small segment of the distorted renal pelvis may be seen at the lower pole.*

tiated mesenchymal tissue tend to divide the more cellular areas into coarse lobules, and within these bands smooth and skeletal muscle or, less frequently, bone or cartilage may be present. There is some evidence to suggest that those patients in whom the neoplasm is predominantly epithelial have a better prognosis.

The basic treatment is prompt (but not emergency) radical nephrectomy performed under optimal conditions, usually within 24 to 48 hours after discovery of the mass. Undue palpation of the tumor should be avoided. Preoperatively, roentgen films of the chest should be obtained and the presence and apparent normality of the opposite kidney established by pyelography. Compatible blood should be available if needed for transfusion during operation. At the time of surgery, which should be by the transabdominal approach, the contralateral kidney should be carefully inspected and palpated, the abdominal viscera investigated for evidence of neoplasm and extent of the tumor marked by radiopaque clips.

An attempt to determine optimum therapy is currently being conducted by the National Wilms' Tumor Study. The patients are grouped as follows:

Group I: The tumor is limited to the kidney and is completely resected.

Group II: The tumor extends beyond the kidney but is completely resected; e.g., there has been penetration beyond the capsule, involvement of peri-aortic lymph nodes or infiltration of renal vessels outside the kidney, but there is no apparent tumor beyond the margins of resection.

Group III: There is residual nonhematogenous tumor confined to the abdomen. This includes those patients in whom biopsies have been taken of the tumor, in whom the tumor has ruptured before or during surgery, in whom there are local peritoneal implants, nodal involvement beyond the periaortic chain, or in whom the tumor cannot be completely resected.

Group IV: There are hematogenous metastases, e.g., to the lungs, liver, bone or brain.

Group V: There is bilateral renal involvement either apparent at operation or appearing subsequently.

The treatment of all patients entered into the study is randomized. All patients in Group I are treated by excision and the administration of actinomycin D and vincristine; irradiation is no longer routinely used. All patients in Groups II and III are treated by excision, irradiation, actinomycin D and vincristine. Randomization is currently employed in an attempt to determine the optimum duration of chromotherapy which might be utilized in order to effect cure and to avoid any sequelae.

The results of this collaborative study are not yet available, but the improvement in prognosis following excision, irradiation and chemotherapy has been striking. In one series apparent cures were obtained in 47 of 53 patients who had no demonstrable metastases on admission and in 18 of 31 of those with metastases. With rare exceptions, if a child with a Wilms' tumor is alive and well with no evidence of recurrence or metastatic disease two years after removal of the tumor, a cure has been effected. Such patients should be followed indefinitely, however, for the possible development of subsequent neoplasms secondary to the effects of irradiation.

Leiomyomatous hamartomas of the kidney (congenital mesoblastic nephroma of infancy) are clinically and radiologically similar to Wilms' tumor. Macroscopically the tumors do not have the areas of necrosis often present in Wilms' tumor, and the cut surfaces are firm, smooth and not lobulated, but have a whorl-like pattern similar to that of a uterine leiomyoma. Histologically they consist of interweaving bundles of smooth muscle and fibroblastic tissue, embedded within which are nests of relatively normal-appearing renal tubules and glomeruli. There is no evidence that these tumors metastasize, and even local recurrence is extremely rare. They are benign lesions and should be treated by nephrectomy alone. It is probable that almost all renal tumors recognized in the neonatal period and reported as Wilms' tumors belong in this category.

Renal cell carcinoma, the common malignant neoplasm of the kidney in adults, is extremely rare in children. It is usually first manifest in midchildhood by intermittent painless gross hematuria and an abdominal or flank mass and/or pain. The absence of a well formed pseudocapsule and the presence of vascular invasion are poor prognostic signs.

Lymphomas of the kidney are usually bilateral and associated with other evidences of *lymphosarcoma* or *leukemia.* Leukemic involvement of the kidney may take the form of nodular masses or of diffuse infiltration of both kidneys, the leukemic cells being most numerous in the cortices.

The extreme enlargement of the kidneys and the striking elongation of the pelves, infundibula and calices can be demonstrated roentgenographically. In spite of the extensive involvement of both kidneys, renal function is usually preserved. Regression of the renal enlargement usually occurs after relatively small doses of irradiation.

Angiolipoleiomyoma is a noncapsulated tumor which characteristically occurs in association with *tuberous sclerosis.* The tumors are usually multiple and involve both kidneys. They are present in about 40 per cent of children with tuberous sclerosis and in 75 per cent of those 15 years of age or older. Although clinical manifestations referable to the tumors have occurred as early as 15 years of age in conjunction with tuberous sclerosis, they are often only incidental findings at necropsy.

Angiolipoleiomyoma occurs infrequently in persons without other evidences of tuberous sclerosis; in such instances the tumor is usually a solitary one. Bleeding into the substance of the tumor or into the perinephric tissue may be responsible for pain and, at times, hematuria and a palpable mass.

The tumor, which is identical in persons with and without tuberous sclerosis, is composed of varying amounts of adult adipose tissue, smooth muscle and atypical vessels. They are probably hamartomas rather than true neoplasms, but in extremely rare instances in adults, metastases have been recorded.

Other renal lesions which have been encountered in persons with *tuberous sclerosis* include multiple small cysts lined by prominent cuboidal or columnar epithelium, multiple papillary adenomas and glomerular inclusions of fat and of epithelial-like cells resembling those of the convoluted tubules.

Hemangioma of the kidney may be asymptomatic or may be responsible for painless hematuria or for bleeding associated with pain as a result of the passage of clots or of interstitial hemorrhage. Only about 5 per cent of these rare tumors occur in infants and children. The lesions may consist of solitary or multiple soft dark red nodules, or there may be diffuse involvement of most of one kidney. The tumors, which are more often cavernous than capillary, are located anywhere in the kidney, e.g., in a calyx, the renal pelvis, the medulla or even the cortex. Occasionally they are large enough to be detected by urography. If responsible for symptoms, they are best treated surgically.

Lindau's disease is characterized by the presence of cysts or adenomas of kidney, cysts of the pancreas and hemangiomas of the retina, cerebellum, brain stem or spinal cord. A familial history may be elicited, some members of the family having only retinal angiomatosis (*von Hippel's disease*), some only angiomas of the central nervous system, and some the complete syndrome. Although visual impairment may develop during late childhood, manifestations referable to the central nervous system usually do not appear until adult life.

Teratoma of the kidney, in contrast to a Wilms' tumor, contains derivatives of all three germ layers. It is an extremely rare tumor which may occur in association with multiple congenital anomalies.

TUMORS OF THE ADRENAL

Neuroblastoma is one of the most common malignant neoplasms in infants and children. Although more than half of them arise from the adrenal or from the retroperitoneal sympathetic chain, the neoplasm may originate at any site along the sympathetic chain, e.g., in the posterior mediastinum, pelvis or cervical sympathetic ganglia; the tumor may also arise from other derivatives of neural crest origin, such as the dorsal root ganglia. Neuroblastoma is primarily a disease of early life; one fourth of the affected persons have their initial manifestations during the first year of life and three fourths before the age of 5 years. It is the most common malignant neoplasm to be identified at birth, and metastases may even be present at this time.

The presenting manifestation of a neuroblastoma arising in the adrenal or in the neighboring sympathetic ganglia is usually an abdominal mass. It often crosses the midline, in contrast to Wilms' tumor. Roentgen examination reveals a soft tissue mass which displaces the kidney on the affected side downward and laterally; focal areas of calcification are often present. Intravenous pyelography characteristically reveals displacement rather than distortion of the renal pelvis; occasionally, as with Wilms' tumor, the pelvis is not visible on the affected side.

Intrathoracic neuroblastomas are almost always located in the posterior portion of the mediastinum at any level and may be responsible for cough, dyspnea and pain in the chest. A mass may be responsible for separation of the posterior portions of the ribs and some narrowing and erosion of them. In a number of instances, owing to extradural extensions of the mass, there are manifestations referable to compression of the spinal cord. *Pelvic neuroblastomas* usually produce a demonstrable mass which in some instances simulates a sacrococcygeal teratoma. They may be responsible for urinary or rectal obstruction. *Cervical neuroblastomas* usually do not reach a large size before being recognized. They are apt to present as a hard, lobulated mass involving the posterior triangle of the neck or extending both anterior and posterior to the sternocleidomastoid muscle. In some instances fine stippled areas of calcification within the mass are demonstrable roentgenographically.

The majority of patients with neuroblastoma have metastases when the tumor is first recognized. In some instances the presenting complaint is referable to metastases rather than to the primary tumor, e.g., massive hepatomegaly, especially in young infants, or cervical or axillary lymphadenopathy. Persistent pain and fever may occur with osseous metastases even in the absence of roentgenographic changes and may simulate rheumatic fever or rheumatoid arthritis. Involvement of retrobulbar soft tissues, probably secondary to osseous metastases, may be responsible for proptosis and/or ecchymosis of the upper eyelids. One or more bluish subcutaneous nodules may precede other complaints, especially during the neonatal period. Infrequently, only the metastatic disease is apparent during life, no primary site being identified.

The majority of patients with neuroblastoma have elevated levels of catecholamines or of one or more of their derivatives in the urine. There is some evidence to suggest that this may not occur with tumors which arise in the dorsal root ganglia. Relatively few patients with neuroblastoma, however, initially present with signs of functional endocrine activity such as flushing, perspiration, tachycardia and headache. Intractable diarrhea is an uncommon manifestation. Measurements of the urinary excretion of catecholamines and of their metabolites, e.g., 3-methoxy-4 hydroxymandelic acid (VMA) and homovanillic acid (HVA) may be of diagnostic significance and may also be helpful in the demonstration of residual, recurrent or metastatic disease. Cystathioninuria may also be a diagnostic aid but is less reliable.

Uncommonly acute cerebellar encephalopathy may precede, follow or occur concomitantly with the discovery of a neuroblastoma. There are ataxia, weakness of the extremities and oculogyric crises unaccompanied by pleocytosis in the cerebrospinal fluid and with little or no fever. The cerebellar signs may disappear following removal of the tumor, but mental retardation may persist. Although the mechanism responsible for this association is not clear, patients with acute cerebellar encephalopathy should probably be investigated for the possible presence of an inapparent neuroblastoma.

Metastases of neuroblastoma occur by way of the lymphatic and blood streams; regional and distant lymph nodes, the skeletal system and the liver are the most frequent sites of metastatic spread. Pulmonary metastases occur in only about 10 per cent of patients. Osseous metastases are often bilateral; a unilateral lesion may lead to an erroneous diagnosis of a primary neoplasm of the bone. The roentgenographic changes in the skeleton are characterized by areas of destruction and proliferation of new bone, which may closely simulate the appearance of Ewing's tumor, of eosinophilic granuloma of bone or of skeletal involvement in leukemia. There may be extensive mottling of the cranial bones and separation of the sutures, owing to increased intracranial pressure from metastatic invasion of the dura mater. Neoplastic cells are frequently demonstrable in smears of the bone marrow, even in the absence of roentgenographic changes in the bones themselves.

The neuroblastoma is initially an encapsulated neoplasm, but it soon infiltrates adjoining tissues and, if arising in the adrenal or neighboring sympathetic ganglia, may surround the aorta, inferior vena cava, ureter or renal pedicle and render complete surgical removal impossible (Fig. 25–5). Areas of hemorrhage and necrosis are commonly present, as are minute flecks of calcium. Histologically there may be varying degrees of differentiation toward mature ganglion cells or, less frequently, toward chromaffin cells. The least differentiated neoplasms may be misinterpreted as lymphosarcomas, but additional sections of the same tumor will usually reveal better differentiated areas of neoplastic cells embedded in a haphazard manner within a delicate fibrillary tissue or arranged as pseudorosettes. Less frequently, immature or mature ganglion cells or even chromaffin cells may be present.

The prognosis for the child with a neuroblastoma is dependent upon a number of factors, e.g., extension of the neoplasm across the midline and the extent of maturation of the tumor as determined histologically. The poorer prognosis related to abdominal tumors as contrasted with cervical or mediastinal ones is probably largely dependent upon the more advanced stage of the disease at the time of diagnosis. Age appears to be the single most important factor with respect to prognosis. The over-all survival rate is in the range of 30 per cent and increases to about 70 per cent in those under 2 years of age. Infants less than 1 year of age, even with metastases to the liver, skin and/or bone marrow but without roentgenographic changes in the bones, have good chances of survival. Cures in the presence of demonstrable osseous metastases have been observed infrequently, even in children over 2 years of age.

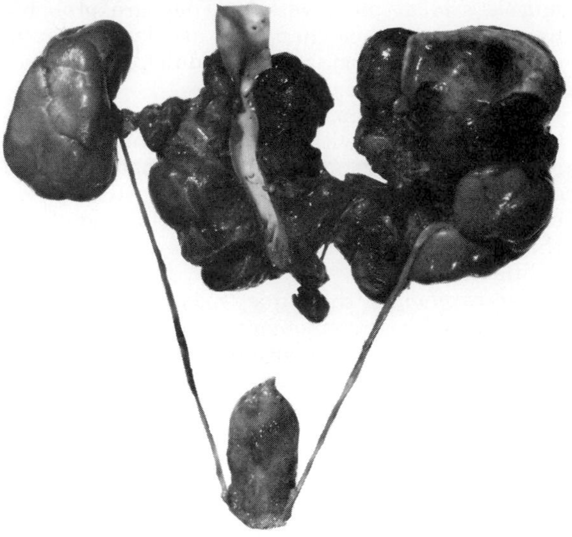

Figure 25–5 Posterior view of a neuroblastoma arising from the right adrenal and displacing the kidney downward and laterally. The tumor crosses the midline and surrounds the aorta and inferior vena cava. (From Arey, J. B.: Pediat. Clin. N. Amer., Vol. 10, 1963.)

Complete surgical removal of the primary tumor is the treatment of choice, but even incomplete removal may be followed by a cure; irradiation is probably indicated if all the tumor is not removed. Chemotherapy, especially with vincristine sulfate and cyclophosphamide (Cytoxan) may cause striking regression of the tumor and relief of symptoms in children with widespread disease, but its role in the treatment of those with more localized disease has yet to be established. Certainly the known adverse effects of irradiation and the possibly still unknown effects of chemotherapy must be considered in evaluating the optimum therapy for any patient with this unpredictable neoplasm, in which even spontaneous cures may take place.

Ganglioneuromas are benign tumors which arise in the sympathetic ganglia in the posterior mediastinum, retroperitoneum, pelvis or neck or in the adrenal. Rarely they arise in other sites such as the skin, tongue, pharynx or gastrointestinal tract; in the last site they may be diffuse rather than encapsulated and be accompanied by symmetric hypertrophy of the various layers of the affected intestinal segment. Although the majority of them are discovered before the age of 20 years, and most in the first decade, they tend to occur at a slightly older age than the neuroblastoma. Rarely they are associated with von Recklinghausen's disease or with the multiple mucosal neuromata syndrome (p. 1604). Neoplasms arising in the retroperitoneum or cervical region are apt to be responsible for a palpable mass, but many of the patients with posterior mediastinal ganglioneuromas are asymptomatic, and the tumors are found only by roentgenographic examination of the chest. In some instances dumbbell-shaped tumors extend through the intervertebral foramina into the spinal canal and are responsible for manifestations referable to compression of the spinal cord. Mature ganglioneuromas, as well as ganglioneuroblastomas and neuroblastomas, may be endocrinologically functioning neoplasms with resultant hypertension, tachycardia, fever, sweating, pallor and increased excretion of catecholamines (Section 17). Chronic diarrhea with frequent watery, foul-smelling stools, failure to thrive, abdominal distention, hypokalemia and flushing of the skin accompany some neural tumors, especially those in which there is partial or complete differentiation toward ganglion cells. Urinary excretion of catecholamines and their metabolites is increased and falls to normal after removal of the neoplasm, and diarrhea ceases. The mechanism responsible for the diarrhea is not known.

The tumors are characteristically circumscribed and encapsulated, but may be so densely adherent to adjoining structures as to preclude complete removal. Histologically they are composed of mature ganglion cells, occurring singly or in groups, and set in a matrix composed of large numbers of neurites with Schwannian sheaths which occasionally are myelinated. Distinct palisading of the nuclei is sometimes present, making the pattern similar to that of a neurilemmoma (p. 1636).

Partially differentiated ganglioneuromas are composed of incompletely differentiated ganglion cells, with or without mature ganglion cells, but without truly undifferentiated neuroblastic elements. The prognosis appears to be somewhat better than with one composed of undifferentiated neuroblasts; metastases, however, may occur, in contrast to the fully differentiated ganglioneuroma.

Ganglioneuroblastomas are malignant neoplasms composed of undifferentiated neuroblasts and of partially or completely differentiated ganglion cells. Although the prognosis may be somewhat better than that of the pure neuroblastoma, metastases may occur.

Pheochromocytoma. See Section 17.

Adrenal cortical tumors. See Section 17.

OTHER RETROPERITONEAL TUMORS

Retroperitoneal neoplasms are associated with a palpable mass in about nine tenths of affected infants and children, and in most of them the mass or enlargement of the abdomen is the initial complaint. Infrequently no mass is palpable.

About half of abdominal masses which necessitate operative intervention in infants and children are derived from the kidney or adjacent structures; hydronephrosis, neuroblastoma and Wilms' tumor are the most frequent; in the newborn infant a unilateral multicystic kidney is the most common abnormal mass. A variety of other benign and malignant tumors, however, must be included in the differential diagnosis. These include retroperitoneal teratoma, lymphosarcoma, ganglioneuroma, lipoma, liposarcoma, fibrosarcoma, rhabdomyosarcoma, benign and malignant mesenchymoma, hemangioma and hemangiopericytoma.

Retroperitoneal teratomas are often discovered in the first months of life, about one third of them appearing in the first year. The presenting complaint is usually abdominal enlargement and a palpable mass. The neoplasm usually arises high in the retroperitoneal region, close to the pancreas, kidney and root of the mesentery. It may present on either side of the abdomen or cross the midline. Roentgen examination often reveals spotty areas of mineralization or even distinct teeth or bones. Intravenous pyelography usually reveals displacement of the kidney and ureter on the affected side; mild hydronephrosis may be present as a result of ureteral compression. Operative removal may be very difficult because of the large size and extensive attachments of many of these neoplasms to adjoining structures, but prompt removal is the treatment of choice. With rare exceptions these neoplasms are well differentiated and benign.

Occasionally a teratoma arising in the presacral region extends upward into the retroperitoneal tissue and presents as a mass in the pelvis or lower part of the abdomen, *with or without an associated external mass in the sacrococcygeal region.* Such neoplasms, which may be responsible for intestinal or urinary obstruction, are almost always attached to the coccyx or to the lowermost part of the sacrum. Although the incidence of malignancy appears to be higher in these than in the usual retroperitoneal teratomas, most of them are benign.

Retroperitoneal fetus in fetu (*intraperitoneal teratoma*) is a monozygotic twin included within its host during development. In contrast to the retroperitoneal teratomas, these are included within an amnion-like sac which projects into the peritoneal cavity and is attached by a pedicle to the upper retroperitoneal tissues near the origin of the superior mesenteric artery. The mass has a vertebral axis, indicative of the earlier primitive streak, often accompanied by an appropriate arrangement of other organs or limbs with respect to this axis.

Sacrococcygeal teratomas arise from the region of the coccyx or lowermost part of the sacrum. They are probably derived from the primordial, totipotential cells of the primitive knot (Hensen's node) which, during embryonic life, finally comes to rest in the region of the coccyx. These tumors are three or four times more frequent in girls than in boys, and there is a significant increase in the incidence of twinning in families of persons with sacrococcygeal teratomas. At least three fourths of the tumors are apparent at birth, usually presenting as a mass at the tip of the coccyx extending externally in the midline or into one or both buttocks. Large tumors, which may exceed the size of the infant's head, displace the coccyx posteriorly and the anus anteriorly. Occasionally the mass is responsible for urinary or intestinal obstruction, but, in contrast to large myelomeningoceles, they are not responsible for neurologic defects in the extremities.

Rectal examination usually discloses a readily palpable mass posterior to the rectum, which is sometimes encircled by it. Roentgenographic examination usually reveals a soft tissue density in the pelvis, sometimes with displacement of the coccyx posteriorly. Areas of calcification or actual bone are demonstrable in about half of the tumors. In contrast to sacral chordomas, roentgenographic evidence of destruction of the sacrum is rare; when present, it is indicative of a malignant neoplasm. Occasionally spina bifida or lumbosacral anomalies are also present.

The differential diagnosis includes meningocele or meningomyelocele; pressure on such a sac will cause the fontanel to bulge, or, if this is closed, crying or straining should increase tension within the mass. Neurogenic tumors, e.g., neuroblastoma and ganglioneuroma, may be clinically indistinguishable from a sacrococcygeal teratoma. Chordomas are rare in children; they are responsible for destruction of the sacrum and only rarely extend into the buttock. Papillary ependymoma (below) may present as a mass in the sacrococcygeal region. Cystic lymphangiomas and hemangiomas may simulate sacrococcygeal teratoma, as may duplication of the hind gut. Occasionally a sacrococcygeal teratoma presents as a red, inflamed mass or as a draining sinus and thus simulates an infected pilonidal sinus.

The neoplasms are connected to the lowermost part of the sacrum or to the coccyx; the coccyx should always be removed with them. Rarely the tumor extends into the vertebral canal. The tumors are usually well circumscribed solid masses containing multiple cystic structures. Histologically they contain a vast array of tissues; fat, neural elements, smooth and skeletal muscle, bone, cartilage and intestinal and bronchial elements are the most frequent. Teratomatous elements such as pancreatic islets or adrenocortical tissue are sometimes present and may, rarely, produce functional manifestations.

Most sacrococcygeal teratomas are benign, and cures are sometimes obtained even after one or more recurrences. Most of the tumors discovered before 2 months of age consist only of mature or less often of immature fetal elements and are associated with an excellent prognosis, whereas those appearing later usually contain embryonal carcinomatous areas and are highly malignant. Tumors present at birth but not excised until after 4 months of age are more apt to be malignant than those removed earlier. Symptoms of bowel or bladder dysfunction increase the probability that the neoplasm is malignant. Tumors detected after 5 years of age, as in adults, may be benign or malignant. Recurrences or metastases, if they occur, usually do so within two years after operation.

Tumors of the soft tissues of the retroperitoneum include benign and malignant tumors derived from adipose tissue or from multiple mesenchymal elements, fibromatoses, vascular tumors, lymphomas and malignant neoplasms derived from skeletal muscle. They may be bulky masses indistinguishable from the more common retroperitoneal neoplasms.

Papillary ependymoma is a rare cause of a mass in the soft tissues overlying the sacrococcygeal region. Clinically it may suggest a pilonidal cyst or sinus. The tumor may arise in the cauda equina and extend through a bony defect or through the sacral foramen into the soft tissues. It may arise from an extradural remnant of the filum terminale, i.e., the coccygeal medullary vestige. The tumor is usually a lobulated, well circumscribed mass which may, however, extend into the perirectal tissue and be attached to or even destroy the sacrum. Histologically it consists of papillary projections covered by cuboidal or columnar cells with apically located nuclei. The underlying stroma of the papillary projections reveals varying degrees of myxomatous tissue which stains positively with mucicarmine and the periodic acid-Schiff technique. Excision is the treatment of choice. Recurrences and metastases to the inguinal lymph nodes and even to the lungs may occur many years after initial therapy.

Retroperitoneal lymphangiomas are large cystic tumors which may occur independently or in conjunction with similar tumors in the mesentery.

Retractile sclerosing mesenteritis is predominantly a lesion of middle-aged adults but has been observed as early as 6 years of age. It occurs predominantly in males. Abdominal pain is usually the presenting complaint, and there may be a palpable mass. The site and extent of mesenteric involvement are variable and are characterized by thick plaques of fibroadipose tissue which may compress the adjoining bowel. Histologically the lobules of adipose tissue in the mesentery are more or less replaced by bands of exuberant fibrous tissue infiltrated by varying numbers of foamy histiocytes, lymphocytes, plasma cells and even neutrophils. The lesion is probably not neoplastic. A relationship between it and *retroperitoneal xanthogranuloma,* which is also rare in childhood, as well as with *idiopathic retroperitoneal fibrosis,* has been suggested but not proved.

Retroperitoneal lipoma, liposarcoma, mesenchymoma, hemangioma, hemangiopericytoma, lymphoma and *rhabdomyosarcoma* are described elsewhere in this Section. (See Index.)

TUMORS OF THE BLADDER AND PROSTATE

Neoplasms of the bladder or prostate are rare in infants and children. Most of them are malignant, rhabdomyosarcoma being the most frequent type.

Leiomyosarcoma, neurofibrosarcoma, lymphosarcoma and neuroblastoma are extremely rare. So also is the common epithelial tumor of the bladder in adults, i.e., transitional cell carcinoma; this is a papillary tumor which is usually of low-grade malignancy in children.

Benign tumors include leiomyomas, neurofibromas, hemangiomas and pheochromocytomas. *Leiomyomas* may be attached to the posterior urethra or to the trigone and be responsible for urinary obstruction and infection. *Neurofibromas* may be isolated or part of generalized neurofibromatosis and may cause diffuse induration of the bladder, ureteral orifices and urethra, even in the early weeks of life; occasionally they contain ganglion cells. *Hemangiomas* are responsible for hematuria; they may also involve the rectum and cause rectal bleeding. *Pheochromocytomas* may be responsible for sustained hypertension and paroxysms characterized by an abrupt rise of blood pressure, headache, palpitation and nervousness, often occurring immediately after urination. An extremely rare but sometimes progressive papillary vascular tumor has been referred to as a "hamartoma," but its exact classification is not clear. The following discussion will be limited to rhabdomyosarcoma.

About half the *rhabdomyosarcomas of the bladder* in children are recognized within the first two years of life; rarely the tumor is present at birth. It is more common in boys than in girls. Urinary obstruction, incontinence, urinary tract infection and strangury are common manifestations, the last being comparable to the pain resulting from impaction of a stone in the posterior urethra; hematuria is a late occurrence. An excretory urogram reveals dilatation of the upper urinary tract, sometimes with wide separation of the distal ureters, and lobulated filling defects in the bladder.

The neoplasm usually arises from the region of the trigone. It originates as a pedunculated mass in the submucosa, occasionally involving the most superficial muscle layer. As it grows it becomes more sessile, obstructs the ureteral ostia and assumes a grape-like configuration (*sarcoma botryoides*), the polypoid projections of which may obstruct the urethral orifice. In girls, protrusion of the mass through the urethral meatus may fill the entire introitus and simulate sarcoma botryoides arising from the vagina; at times extension of a primary vaginal lesion into the bladder may make the exact site of origin difficult to determine. Histologically the polypoid submucosal masses consist of myxomatous tissue containing scattered elongate and stellate cells with a few neutrophils and lymphocytes; a more compact zone of cells, the cambium layer, is often present immediately beneath the epithelium. Because of its edematous appearance, the presence of inflammatory cells and the sparcity of recognizable neoplastic elements, superficial biopsies taken early in the course of the disease may erroneously be interpreted as inflammatory rather than neoplastic. A clue to the rhabdomyoblastic origin of the tumor may be provided by the presence of a cambium layer and of scattered round cells with sharply defined cell boundaries and bright acidophilic cytoplasm. Slim, spindle-shaped cells with eosinophilic cytoplasm may be present and if the nucleus is located near one end, enlargement of the cell here produces a "tadpole" appearance. Cross striations are often difficult or impossible to identify.

Rhabdomyosarcoma of the bladder tends to grow by diffuse superficial infiltration, with deep extensions occurring only relatively late. Metastases to regional lymph nodes and distant sites tend to be delayed; most patients die with only local recurrence. Because of the diffuse nature of the spread of the tumor, however, subtotal cystectomy is usually ineffective in eradicating the local disease. Treatment thus consists of total cystectomy, including excision of the bulbomembranous urethra in the male and perhaps of the vagina in the female. This should be followed by chemotherapy; if residual tumor is demonstrable even histologically at the margins of the resected specimen, irradiation to the local site probably should also be employed. Survival rates with localized disease should approximate 60 to 70 per cent.

Rhabdomyosarcoma of the prostate is less common than is that of the bladder. The tumor is a bulky, nodular mass composed largely of undifferentiated mesenchymal tissues (Fig. 25–6). Because of the more gradual onset of signs of obstruction, and the tendency of the tumor to involve deep structures early, including regional lymph nodes

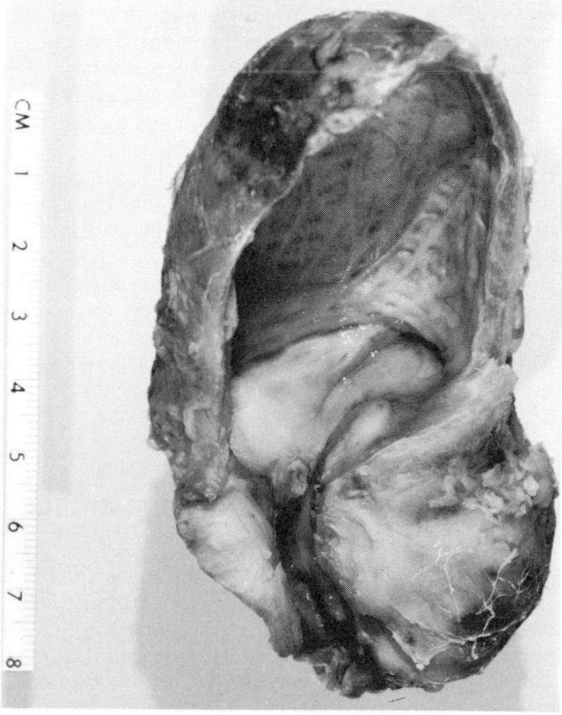

Figure 25–6 Rhabdomyosarcoma of the prostate from a boy 3 years old. The bulky mass displaces the urethra posteriorly and to the right and is beginning to protrude into the lumen of the trabeculated bladder.

and vessels, distant metastases to lungs, bones and bone marrow, liver and brain tend to occur earlier than with tumors of the bladder. The prognosis is even more grave, but some survivals can be expected. Therapy consists of radical prostatectomy followed by chemotherapy. Irradiation to the local tumor site is also indicated if tumor tissue is demonstrated at the lines of resection of the excised specimen.

TUMORS OF THE TESTIS AND PARATESTICULAR STRUCTURES

Malignant or potentially malignant testicular neoplasms in infants and children are usually of germ cell origin; the most common ones are infantile embryonal carcinoma and teratoma. Testicular tumors of nongerm cell origin, e.g., tumors of specialized gonadal stroma, are rare but are relatively more common in infants than in adults. A testicular mass is occasionally the initial manifestation of a malignant lymphoma, but most instances of lymphomatous involvement of the testis are one manifestation of disseminated disease. The testes are usually infiltrated by leukemic cells in acute leukemia.

Paratesticular tumors are extremely rare in infants and children. An intrascrotal, extratesticular tumor resembling a pseudomucinous cystadenoma of the ovary has been described in a child; an intrascrotal, extratesticular hemangioma involving the scrotal septum, in an infant. A cystic teratoma of the tunica albuginea has also been observed, and we have seen an epidermoid cyst in this site and a papillary mesothelioma arising in a hernial sac. Tumors of the epididymis are almost nonexistent in early life, though melanotic ectodermal tumors have been seen in infants. Other than such rare exceptions, paratesticular tumors in persons less than 20 years of age are almost always *rhabdomyosarcomas.* The presenting complaint is usually that of swelling of a few weeks duration, the nature of which may be obscured by an accompanying hydrocele. Orchiectomy, excision of retroperitoneal lymph nodes and chemotherapy constitute the treatment of choice. If the nodes are involved, irradiation should also be employed. The prognosis is good if there are no metastases in the nodes.

TESTICULAR TUMORS OF GERM CELL ORIGIN

Embryonal carcinomas or teratomas of the testis in infants and children occur predominantly during the first few years of life; the tumor may be apparent at birth. The presenting complaint is usually painless enlargement of the testis; occasionally this is accompanied by or is erroneously interpreted as a hydrocele.

There are certain noteworthy differences between testicular neoplasms of infants and children and those of adults. Seminoma, the most common testicular neoplasm in adults, is extremely rare in children, as is choriocarcinoma. The probability that a tumor may develop in an undescended testis in an adult is about 10 to 14 times greater than in a normally located testis; such a striking difference is not apparent in the pediatric age group. In general, the prognosis for infants and children with testicular neoplasms is considerably better than that for adults.

Infantile embryonal carcinoma (orchioblastoma; yolk sac tumor; endodermal sinus tumor; Teilum's tumor) is one of the most common testicular neoplasms occurring in early life; it probably represents a malignant variant of a teratoma. The majority occur in the first two years of life; rarely it is present at birth. The presenting complaint is usually that of painless unilateral scrotal swelling, often of less than 6 months' duration. Initially it may be considered to be a hydrocele.

The mass is usually ovoid, corresponding to the shape of the testis. The tunica albuginea is almost always intact, but the mediastinum testis is usually involved; invasion of the epididymis is infrequent. On section the tumor usually replaces most of the testis. It is light tan to gray, rather soft, friable and sometimes mucoid. Histologically a variety of features are often present in the same tumor, i.e., papillary projections, acinar or tubular epithelial lined spaces and solid sheets of undifferentiated cells. Many of the cells are vacuolated and may contain mucin, glycogen or fat. Occasionally mature teratomatous tissue is in continuity with the embryonal carcinoma.

The tumor is probably best treated by removal of the testis and spermatic cord and dissection of the retroperitoneal lymph nodes; if neoplastic tissue is identified in the lymph nodes, the entire periaortic chain should probably be irradiated; chemotherapy may also be indicated under these circumstances. Metastases occur both to the retroperitoneal lymph nodes and by way of the bloodstream. The metastatic lesions resemble the primary tumor histologically. The prognosis is good for boys under 2 years of age but not so favorable in older children; almost all deaths occur within the first 18 months after diagnosis.

Most *testicular teratomas* of early life are discovered during the first few years of life, sometimes at birth; rarely there are bilateral tumors. The presenting complaint is usually that of painless enlargement of the testis. Growth of the tumor may not be as rapid as with an embryonal carcinoma, and the interval between the discovery of the mass and therapy thus tends to be somewhat longer. Macroscopically these tumors are circumscribed and usually replace most of the testis. They vary from solid structures containing multiple minute cysts to grossly multicystic lesions; rarely they are composed of only a solitary cyst. Histologically a wide variety of tissues are usually present, representative of all three germ layers. The cysts are commonly lined by epidermis, respiratory, neural and intestinal epithelium. Glial tissue is often abundant and may contain foci of necrosis and calcification. Structures resembling retina, the pigmented ciliary body, salivary gland and pancreas may be present in addition to lymphoid tissue, smooth muscle, cartilage, bone, adipose tissue and fibrous tissue. The more immature tissues may contain multiple mitoses, and occasional foci resemble embryonal carcinoma.

Testicular teratomas in early life, in contrast to those in adults, are usually benign. Even in the presence of immature elements, metastases to the retroperitoneal lymph nodes, lungs and liver are rare and occur principally in later childhood. In young children the malignant neoplasm usually is characterized by embryonal carcinomatous elements. Simple orchiectomy is probably the treatment of choice, especially for those discovered during the first year of life. If definite embryonal carcinomatous areas are present, however, excision of the retroperitoneal lymph nodes is indicated.

TESTICULAR TUMORS OF NONGERM CELL ORIGIN

In any age group these are much less common than tumors of germ cell origin. They consist of a heterogeneous group of neoplasms, only two of which are specifically gonadal in origin: interstitial cell tumors and androblastomas.

Tumors of specialized gonadal stroma (testicular and ovarian). The specialized stroma of the gonads, i.e., the endocrinologically active portion of the ovaries and testes, is derived from a common embryologic source, the mesoderm of the urogenital ridge. Tumors of this specialized stroma, whether located in testes or ovaries, are thus capable of reproducing all the endocrinologically active portion of the gonads of both sexes. They may contain Sertoli cells and their ovarian homologues, the granulosa cells, as well as Leydig cells and their ovarian counterparts, the theca cells. Varying degrees of luteinization of the specialized ovarian cells may occur.

A variety of endocrinologic disturbances may be associated with tumors of such specialized stroma, whether they are located in the testis or in the ovary. Attempts have been made to classify them on the basis of their endocrinologic function. Such a classification is unsatisfactory, however, since some of these tumors are inactive, whereas others may give rise to both androgenic and estrogenic substances; a morphologic classification is, in general, more applicable.

Interstitial (Leydig) cell tumor. See Section 17.

Androblastomas (tumors of specialized gonadal stroma; gonadal stromal tumor; Sertoli cell tumor; granulosa-theca cell tumor of the testis). These are rare tumors derived from the specialized stroma of the gonad and thus capable of reproducing the supporting tissues of the gonads of both sexes. They are characterized by a variety of histologic patterns ranging from an epithelial form having a close resemblance to normal Sertoli cell tubules or to granulosa cells to a form consisting largely of fibroblast-like cells. Elements resembling luteinized cells of the corpus luteum or interstitial cells of the testis may also be present. Though predominantly tumors of adults, significant numbers have occurred in infants less than 1 year of age, and the tumor may be present at birth. The presenting complaint is usually painless swelling of the testis, infrequently accompanied by gynecomastia. Metastases have occurred rarely in adults; they are even more rare in children.

The tumors in children are usually relatively small and are circumscribed, firm, gray-white to yellow, solitary masses confined to the testis. Histologically some of the tumors are almost entirely epithelial, but most of them consist of varying admixtures of epithelial and fibrous elements. Epithelial elements are present in some areas in almost all the tumors. They are often arranged in a tubular manner, with radially directed cells, simulating the appearance of the prepubertal testis. The cells, however, may be arranged in a cyst-like pattern, suggesting graafian follicles, or in sheets and cords of small, cuboidal epithelial cells resembling those of a granulosa cell tumor of the ovary. In some instances there are nests of cells with abundant acidophilic cytoplasm which resemble luteinized cells or Leydig cells. The fibrous elements consist of bands of spindle-shaped cells with elongated nuclei and somewhat acidophilic cytoplasm interspersed between the tubular elements or scattered haphazardly through the tumor. Mitotic figures are sometimes present. Little or none of the material stains positively with the periodic acid-Schiff technique, in contrast to the abundance of such deposits in embryonal carcinomas.

The tumors appear to recapitulate the structures formed by the specialized stroma of either the testis or ovary, and thus are the homologues of the ovarian arrhenoblastomas (p. 1627) and granulosa cell tumors (Section 17). They do not contain cells characteristically believed to be of germ cell origin, in contrast to the gonadoblastoma (p. 1628), though cells closely resembling primitive germ cells are occasionally present.

Sertoli cell adenomas are benign tumors which frequently occur in the testes of persons with the testicular feminizing syndrome, in whom a variety of other testicular tumors may also be encountered, especially after puberty. Sertoli cell adenomas are sometimes bilateral. The individual lesion may be minimal or it may reach a large size and completely replace a gonad; in such a case it has been misinterpreted as a well differentiated Sertoli-Leydig cell tumor of the ovary. It is devoid of germ cells and consists of uniform tubules lined by Sertoli cells, with variable numbers of Leydig cells in the intertubular tissue. The tumors are benign and without demonstrable endocrine effects. They may represent hyperplasia of testicular tubules and be comparable to the smaller, nonneoplastic *tubular adenomas which are frequently found in cryptorchid testes* as minute, solitary or multiple discrete nodules composed of well differentiated Sertoli cells.

TUMORS OF THE OVARY

Though ovarian tumors are relatively infrequent during the pediatric age period, a variety of neoplasms and non-neoplastic cysts originating in or about the ovaries may be responsible for clinical manifestations. Teratomas, usually benign cystic ones, comprise only 10 to 15 per cent of ovarian neoplasms in adults, but are by far the most common tumor of the ovary in children. Non-neoplastic cysts, i.e., follicular, lutein or simple ovarian cysts, are second in frequency. Infrequently, a follicular or theca-lutein cyst of moderate to large size is apparently responsible for signs of precocious puberty (Section 17). Much more often, however, precocious puberty resulting from ovarian disease is caused by a granulosa-theca cell tumor (Section 17). Precocious puberty is only rarely caused by a malignant chorioepithelioma within an embryonal carcinoma or teratoma of the ovary. Pseudomucinous and serous cystadenomas and cystadenocarcinomas, the most common ovarian neoplasms of adults, are rare in children; when they do occur, they usually occur in older children.

The other primary ovarian neoplasms discussed here are rare in early life. Secondary involvement of the ovaries of children by neoplastic disease is usually from a lymphomatous process. Infrequently non-neoplastic lesions such as paro-varian cysts and hydatids of Morgagni are responsible for clinical manifestations during childhood.

The most common manifestations referable to an ovarian tumor in an infant or child are those of abdominal pain and/or tumor. Pain is a more common complaint in children than in adults; it may be mild to moderate and persist for a considerable time. In a number of instances, however, the tumor manifests itself by an acute attack or recurrent episodes of abdominal pain, often accompanied by nausea and vomiting and closely simulating acute appendicitis. Such attacks usually result from *torsion of the ovarian pedicle,* which is more common in infants and children than in adults; it may occur with any type of ovarian mass and rarely may take place with an apparently normal ovary. Torsion of the ovarian pedicle may be followed by infarction and hemoperitoneum. In the absence of torsion an ovarian tumor usually presents as a mass in the lower part of the abdomen or as gradual enlargement of the abdomen, with or without apparent discomfort. Rarely abdominal distention is present at birth as a result of rupture of an ovarian cyst. In the case of functional tumors the initial manifestations are apt to be those of sexual precocity or, much less frequently, of virilism or of a combination of these.

Teratoma of the ovary, the most common ovarian neoplasm of children, is usually a cystic structure, the so-called *dermoid cyst* or *benign cystic teratoma.* Ovarian teratomas have been observed as early as 16 months of age. In addition to the clinical manifestations described above, there is rarely an associated hemolytic anemia which responds only to removal of the neoplasm. Roentgen examination frequently reveals areas of calcification in bones or teeth. Hydronephrosis and hydroureter secondary to obstruction by the mass may occur.

Macroscopically a cystic ovarian teratoma is usually a globular, unilocular cyst filled with sebaceous material; it commonly contains hair. At one point in the wall a sessile mass often projects into the lumen. This mound of tissue is covered by thick squamous epithelium beneath which are numerous hair follicles, sebaceous glands, adipose tissue and sometimes bone and teeth. The remainder of the lining of the cyst is usually smooth, but is sometimes granular, shaggy and ulcerated, in which case the wall is apt to be thickened and fibrotic and contain areas of calcification.

Histologically the tumors contain a variety of well differentiated tissues. Ectodermal elements, especially stratified squamous epithelium, sebaceous glands, hair follicles and often sweat glands are common. Other tissue elements may include those of neural, osseous, muscular, fat and endodermal origins. The wall of the cyst may be ulcerated and have a chronic inflammatory reaction with numerous foamy macrophages and foreign body giant cells.

Much less frequently ovarian teratomas are predominantly solid structures with multiple small cysts. These *solid teratomas* are usually unilateral and encapsulated; extension beyond the capsule with adherence to adjoining structures and peritoneal implants may, however, be apparent at the time of surgery. If composed entirely of mature tissues, such tumors are usually benign. Sometimes, however, they are *teratocarcinomas* which contain moderate to large amounts of a wide variety of primitive tissues reminiscent of the developmental stages of the embryo; an undifferentiated cellular stroma containing structures resembling embryonic neural epithelium is common. The degree of differentiation of the tumor appears to have some bearing on the prognosis. Mature solid teratomas may be accompanied by peritoneal implants of neuroglial tissue and still have an excellent prognosis. Even teratocarcinomas which have ruptured before or during surgery are sometimes followed by maturation of the seeded cells and the development of a secondary mature intraperitoneal teratoma and multiple neuroglial implants, still with a good prognosis (Fig. 25–7). In general, however, highly undifferentiated teratocarcinomas which have extended beyond the capsule and adhered to adjoining structures, or those with metastases or recurrences, have a grave prognosis, as do those containing germinal elements such as embryonal carcinoma or chorioepithelioma. Teratocarcinomas of the ovary, as well as of the testis, may be accompanied by elevated concentration of alpha-fetoprotein in the serum, but its level need not correspond with the extent of the tumor.

Bilateral ovarian teratomas are infrequent in children in contrast to an incidence of over 10 per cent in adults.

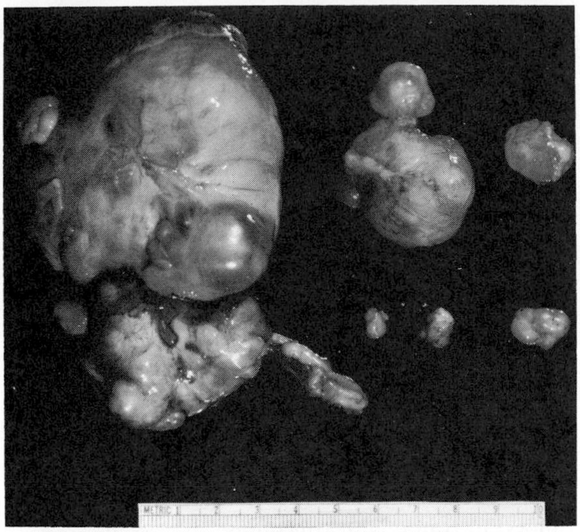

Figure 25–7 *Implants of teratoma on diaphragmatic surface removed from a girl 10 years old. A "solid" ovarian teratoma containing a variety of elements, many of which were immature neuroectodermal tissue, had been removed a year before. The masses shown here contained a variety of tissues, not all neuroglial, almost all of which were well differentiated. She is living and well almost 6 years later.*

The prognosis for children with cystic ovarian teratomas is good. Treatment should consist only of simple oophorectomy or, if possible, excision of the neoplasm, sparing any intact ovarian tissue on the affected side. Solid teratomas should be treated by salpingo-oophorectomy if confined to the ovary; more radical surgery may be indicated if there is extension of the tumor.

Dysgerminoma (germinoma), the ovarian counterpart of the seminoma, is believed to arise from the sexually undifferentiated cells of the primitive gonad. As many as 7 per cent of the tumors are discovered in the first decade and 40 per cent in the first two decades of life. The neoplasm is usually hormonally inactive. Sometimes, however, it has been described in patients with genital hypoplasia, in virilized phenotypic females, in Turner syndrome and even with precocious pseudopuberty; probably many if not all the tumors associated with such changes have been gonadoblastomas rather than pure dysgerminomas.

The neoplasm is usually a unilateral, solid, rounded mass with a smooth or coarsely lobulated surface. On section multiple yellow patches of necrosis may be present. Histologically its appearance is similar to that of the testicular seminoma. The neoplasm is usually one with a low degree of malignancy, but it may infiltrate locally, spread to the opposite ovary and regional lymph nodes and be responsible for peritoneal implants, ascites or even distant metastases; highly malignant dysgerminomas are apt to contain other germinal elements, e.g., embryonal carcinoma or chorioepithelioma.

A pure dysgerminoma confined to one ovary in a child should probably be treated by unilateral salpingo-oophorectomy followed by a lymphangiogram; if there is no evidence of metastasis, no further therapy is indicated, but the patient should be followed carefully. With spread of the tumor bilateral salpingo-oophorectomy, hysterectomy and dissection of the iliac lymph nodes may be indicated, followed by irradiation. The tumor is radiosensitive, and, if other germinal elements are not present, the prognosis is good.

Embryonal carcinoma of the ovary is a rare neoplasm histologically similar to the testicular tumor of this name. It is probably of germ cell origin and tends to occur in young persons. It is soft and friable, with multiple cystic spaces and areas of hemorrhage and necrosis. The prognosis is much graver than that of the testicular ones. The tumor is usually radioresistant, and treatment, which is often unsuccessful, consists of removal of all visible tumor followed by combined chemotherapy. The tumor is usually unilateral; removal of the unaffected ovary or uterus probably does not enhance survival.

Tumors of specialized gonadal stroma (testicular and ovarian). See page 1625.

Granulosa-theca cell tumor. See Section 17.

Sertoli-Leydig cell tumors (arrhenoblastomas; testicular tubular adenomas of Pick; ovarian androblastomas) are rare neoplasms comparable to the testicular tumors of specialized gonadal stroma. They occur predominantly during the reproductive period and only rarely have been observed in children. They are characteristically masculinizing tumors; but they may have no endocrine effects or may even be accompanied by estrogenic manifestations, e.g., isosexual precocious puberty. Virilizing manifestations have been noted before 12 years of age, and a nonfunctional tumor has been described as early as 4 years. Aldosteronism with precocious puberty has been observed in a 9 year old girl.

The neoplasm is usually a slowly growing one involving only one ovary. It may be firm or soft, is frequently lobulated and occasionally is polycystic. Histologically the pattern varies considerably. The well differentiated areas consist of distinct tubular structures lined by Sertoli cells, with or without Leydig cells in the intertubular tissue. Neoplasms exhibiting an intermediate degree of differentiation may assume a bewildering array of patterns. The Sertoli cells may be arranged as broad anastomosing trabeculae or as solid nests of cells; small cystic spaces resembling the Call-Exner bodies of the granulosa cell tumor are sometimes present. The intervening tissue consists of Leydig cells, spindle cells and hyalinized collagen. The least differentiated neoplasms may bear little or no resemblance to the foregoing patterns, but resemble a sarcoma or even a carcinoma. In contrast to the frequent absence of endocrinologic manifestations in persons with well differentiated tumors, masculinization is usually apparent in those with the less differentiated neoplasms.

Well differentiated Sertoli-Leydig cell tumors are usually benign, but local recurrences or peritoneal spread probably occurs in about 25 per cent of the less differentiated tumors. Treatment for an apparently localized tumor in a child may perhaps be limited to unilateral salpingo-oophorectomy. In older persons in whom maintenance of reproductive ability is no longer important, however, total hysterectomy with bilateral salpingo-oophorectomy is indicated.

Gynandroblastoma (sex cord–mesenchyme tumors of indeterminate or mixed cell type) is a rare ovarian tumor of specialized gonadal stroma which contains distinct cords or tubules of Sertoli cells as well as definite granulosa cell elements; varying numbers of Leydig cells, thecal cells and luteinized cells may also be present, but germinal cells are absent, in contrast to the gonadoblastoma; differentiation from other tumors of specialized gonadal stroma may be difficult or even impossible. It may be responsible for evidences of androgenic or estrogenic activity or both or may simply be responsible for a palpable mass. Gynandroblastomas are usually benign.

Sex cord tumor with annular tubules is a rare ovarian tumor which may be the first clue to the diagnosis of Peutz-Jeghers syndrome, in which other ovarian tumors may also occur. When associated with this syndrome the tumors are characteristically small (sometimes being visible only microscopically), multiple and, at times, bilateral; whenever available, the ovaries of patients with this syndrome should be carefully examined for the presence of such tumors. Discovery of such a tumor should be followed by a careful family history and search among relatives for pigmentation and intestinal polyps. In those patients in whom the diagnosis of Peutz-Jeghers syndrome has not been proved the tumor may reach a considerable size. The tumor is believed to arise from granulosa cells which grow in a pattern more characteristic of Sertoli cells. It is composed of rounded epithelial nests containing eosinophilic hyaline bodies. The nuclei of the epithelial cells are typically palisaded along the periphery of the nests and their cytoplasm is abundant, pale and often rich in fat; elongated structures resembling prepubertal testicular tubules may be present. The nests of cells lie within an ovarian type of stroma in which foci of lutein cells may be present. There may be extensive fibrosis and hyalinization of the stroma and calcification of the epithelial nests. The tumor, which is apparently benign, may be associated with endometrial hyperplasia.

Lipid cell tumors (adrenal rest tumors; masculinovoblastomas; Leydig [hilus] cell tumors; luteomas) are extremely rare ovarian tumors composed of nests of polyhedral cells with clear cytoplasm containing abundant lipid and resembling the cells of the adrenal cortex, Leydig cells or theca-lutein cells. Since morphologic differentiation of these cells may be impossible, the term "lipid cell tumor" is applied to the entire group.

Although there may be no endocrine effects, characteristically there is masculinization. In some instances in which the tumor has occurred before puberty there has been isosexual precocious puberty.

The neoplasm may reach a large size or may be so small that it is not detected upon physical examination. Metastases have been reported with both functioning and nonfunctioning tumors. In children the tumor should probably be removed by unilateral salpingo-oophorectomy.

Ovarian fibromas and thecomas are extremely rare in children; most of the thecomas described in children have contained nests of granulosa cells and are probably better classified as granulosa-theca cell tumors. Differentiation of ovarian fibromas and thecomas may be only arbitrary; those fibromas which contain discrete nests of large, pale, polyhedral cells with abundant cytoplasm filled with fat are classified as thecomas. Thecomas are almost always unilateral and responsible for manifestations similar to those of granulosa-theca cell tumors. Meigs syndrome of ascites and hydrothorax has been observed with granulosa cell tumors, fibromas and thecomas.

Sclerosing stromal cell tumors of the ovary are rare neoplasms which tend to occur in the second and third decades. They are solitary, grayish white, rather poorly demarcated tumors which usually replace most of the ovarian tissue on the affected side. Histologically they are characterized by striking vascularity and a variegated, pseudolobular pattern produced by admixtures of cellular, densely fibrous and edematous tissue; in the cellular areas there is considerable variation in the size and shape of the cells; spindle-shaped cells and rounded cells with clear cytoplasm are haphazardly arranged within the cellular areas. There is as yet no proof that any of these tumors is malignant or hormonally active.

NEOPLASMS ASSOCIATED WITH DYSGENETIC GONADS

Gonadoblastomas are rare neoplasms occurring almost exclusively in dysgenetic gonads. A variety of other neoplasms may arise in such gonads. The tumor may originate in a gonadal streak, in a cryptorchid, dysgenetic testis or in a gonad of undetermined origin. About one-fourth of the tumors are bilateral and somewhat less frequently they are demonstrable only histologically. These tumors occur most frequently in phenotypic females, many of whom are virilized. About one fifth are found in phenotypic males, almost all of whom have cryptorchidism, hypospadias and female internal secondary sex organs. There is strong evidence of the production of androgens by some of these tumors.

Histologically the tumor is composed of discrete aggregates of germ cells with large nuclei, similar to those in a dysgerminoma, with smaller cells resembling immature Sertoli and granulosa cells; nests of Leydig or lutein cells are often present in the stroma, especially in persons over 16 years of age. The immature Sertoli and granulosa cells may surround circular spaces containing hyaline eosinophilic material and superficially simulating Call-Exner bodies or they may surround individual germ cells or nests or cords of such cells. Calcification is common and may be extensive enough so as to be demonstrable roentgenographically.

The germ cells may penetrate beyond the confines of the isolated nests of cells and result in a dysgerminoma which contains germ cells, an infiltrate of lymphocytes and even a granulomatous reaction. In some instances there may be massive overgrowth of dysgerminomatous elements so that the nests of cells are easily overlooked; any dysgerminoma accompanied by endocrine disorders or located in a dysgenetic gonad should be carefully examined for nests of specialized gonadal stromal cells. Occasionally other germinal tumors may occur in a gonadoblastoma, e.g., embryonal carcinoma or teratoma.

Malignant change in a gonadoblastoma may occur as early as the first decade; since the tumor arises in an expendable gonad, it should be removed as soon as detected.

TUMORS OF THE VAGINA AND UTERUS

Sarcoma botryoides is a descriptive term referring to the grape-like configuration assumed by *embryonal rhabdomyosarcomas* (p. 1637). Other tumors may rarely present a similar appearance, including infantile carcinoma of the vagina (below) or benign vaginal polyps.

Embryonal rhabdomyosarcoma, presenting as sarcoma botryoides, is the most common neoplasm of the lower urogenital tract of infants and children. It may arise in the vagina, bladder or even the labium majus. Rhabdomyosarcomas arising in the prostate may extend into the bladder and produce a similar appearance. Similar neoplasms occur in the common bile duct, anus, nasopharynx, oropharynx, middle ear and maxillary antrum.

The vaginal tumor usually manifests itself during the first four years of life and may be present at birth. The initial manifestation may be a bloody vaginal discharge but often is that of a mass protruding from the vagina. The neoplasm arises from the vagina and may extend into the cervix, vulva or urethra as well as into the urinary bladder and pelvis; with extensive involvement it may be impossible to determine the primary site. The tumor may metastasize both by the lymphatic and blood streams. Histologically it resembles its homologue in the urinary bladder.

The prognosis is not so hopeless as formerly believed. Treatment consists of removal of the vagina and uterus, leaving the ovaries; more extensive tumors may necessitate more radical surgery. Surgical removal should be followed by chemotherapy and perhaps irradiation.

Infantile carcinoma of the vagina is a rare neoplasm which grossly and clinically may simulate sarcoma botryoides. It usually appears in the first two years of life and is responsible for vaginal bleeding or discharge and/or a friable, polypoid vaginal mass. The tumor is usually considered as mesonephric in origin, but an origin from primitive germ cells is possible. It bears histologic resemblance to the embryonal carcinoma of the infantile testis or ovary (pp. 1624, 1627).

Adenocarcinoma of the vagina in adolescents and young women 14 years of age or more occurs especially in daughters of mothers who have received stilbestrol during pregnancy; benign adenosis of the vagina is also unusually frequent in girls and young women who have had similar fetal exposure. The tumor is manifest by prolonged or persistent irregular vaginal bleeding, which is apt to be considered anovulatory bleeding. Young women with persistent vaginal bleeding should have careful vaginal inspection to exclude the presence of a neoplasm. Histologically the tumor consists of tubules and glands lined by clear cells containing glycogen and "hobnail" cells; clear cells also occur in solid nests. It is probably of müllerian rather than mesonephric origin and may be radiosensitive.

Carcinoma of the uterus in infants and children is rare. In contrast to those in adults, the tumors are usually adenocarcinomas of the cervix, some of which have been interpreted as mesonephric in origin. They are responsible for a watery or purulent vaginal discharge and bleeding. The prognosis is poor, probably partly because of delay in diagnosis.

A *benign papilloma* of the cervix is a rare cause of vaginal bleeding. The tumor may have a polypoid configuration and a central core of loose myxoid tissue and suggest a sarcoma botryoides. It should be completely excised and all the fragments carefully examined. The patient probably should be followed at frequent intervals even if it is interpreted as histologically benign.

Hymenal polyps are benign, non-neoplastic, rounded tags or finger-like pedunculated lesions; they arise from the dorsal part of the hymen and protrude from the vulva. They are composed of a rather vascular stroma covered by well differentiated squamous epithelium. They are present in about 6 per cent of newborn female infants examined on the first or second day of life; they require no treatment, since they disappear spontaneously within a few weeks after birth.

Squamous cell *carcinoma of the vulva* has been observed in a girl 4 years of age.

TUMORS OF VASCULAR ORIGIN

These are the most common tumors of early life. Most of them are probably hamartomas rather than true neoplasms, and most are benign. They may occur in any organ, but there are sites of predilection: the skin and subcutaneous tissue (Section 23), skeletal muscle, liver, salivary gland, larynx and bone.

Capillary hemangiomas (nevus vasculosus; strawberry mark) are discussed in Section 23.

Cavernous hemangiomas are poorly circumscribed, blue or purple elevated tumors which tend to extend more deeply into the subcutaneous tissues than do the capillary hemangiomas. They consist of numerous cystic vascular spaces containing blood. Mixed forms of cavernous and capillary hemangiomas are common; in such lesions regression of the cavernous elements may be slower and less constant than that of the superficial capillary elements. Cavernous elements which do not regress spontaneously are probably best treated by surgical excision. Cavernous hemangiomas may occur in sites other than the skin, e.g., in bone, liver and the tongue. In skeletal muscles they manifest themselves as a diffuse mass, sometimes accompanied by pain; the mass decreases in size with elevation of the part. Foci of calcification may be demonstrable by roentgenographic examination.

A *giant hemangioma,* usually of the skin or subcutaneous tissue, but infrequently a visceral one, may be accompanied by thrombocytopenia, bleeding and a consumptive coagulopathy. This is most often seen in the first year of life with a large, rapidly growing cavernous hemangioma, but may occur at a later date in children with multiple hemangiomas that do not involute. Treatment, if necessary, has included the administration of corticosteroids, platelet transfusions, replacement of clotting factors, the use of anticoagulants and/or irradiation. *Diffuse hemangiomas* of an extremity may be associated with hypertrophy of the part and of the associated bone.

Nevus venosus (nevus flammeus, port-wine mark). See Section 23.

Cirsoid aneurysms (racemose hemangioma, congenital arteriovenous fistula) are rare lesions consisting of a pulsating mass of dilated tortuous arteries, veins and capillaries. Arteriovenous aneurysms of the brain may be responsible for cardiac failure and death in the first week of life; a bruit may or may not be audible. The diagnosis may be established by selective arteriography. Pulmonary arteriovenous fistulas are apt to be part of the Rendu-Osler-Weber disease.

Hereditary hemorrhagic telangiectasia (Rendu-Osler-Weber disease). See Section 11.

Angiomas of the retina (von Hippel's disease) may be associated with cerebellar angiomas, cysts of the pancreas and adenomas of the kidney (Lindau's disease, Section 19).

Sturge-Weber syndrome. See Section 19.

Glomus tumor is a small, circumscribed red to blue tumor usually located in the dermis and subcutaneous tissue, especially of the extremities. Infrequently it arises in the ligaments, periosteum, phalanges or joint capsules. Only about 7 per cent of glomus tumors manifest themselves before 16 years of age, but the tumor may be present at birth. Multiple tumors are present in about one fourth of affected infants and children; pain is relatively uncommon in children, in contrast to adults. The tumors consist of congeries of capillaries sheathed by distinct cuboidal epithelial-like cells or pericytes. Infiltrative growth is more frequently associated with tumors which have their origin during childhood than in adulthood. The tumor is benign. It will not regress spontaneously and recurs if incompletely excised.

Kaposi's sarcoma, which involves males predominantly, is extremely rare in early life. Among the reported instances in infants and children almost half have occurred in African blacks. The onset is characterized by the appearance of one or more bluish to red nodules of variable size in the skin, usually of the extremities, or by a maculopapular rash. Intractable edema of an extremity may precede or accompany the appearance of the lesions of the skin. In black African children the initial manifestation may be referable to involvement of lymph nodes.

Histologically the lesions are characterized by anastomosing capillaries with endothelial proliferation, accompanied by an interstitial proliferation of fibroblasts; the latter may predominate and simulate a fibrosarcoma.

The course of the disease may be fulminant, with the appearance of innumerable nodules in the skin and viscera, and death in less than two years. More frequently, however, the disease persists for many years. The tumors may respond to systemic chemotherapy.

Hemangiopericytomas are rare in all age groups, and only about 10 per cent are first manifest before 16 years of age. They are composed of capillaries surrounded by pericytes, but without the organoid pattern characteristic of the glomus tumor. Rarely there are multiple tumors. Clinically the neoplasm rarely appears to be vascular; even in histologic sections reticulin stains may be necessary to identify the vascularity.

These tumors usually arise in the subcutaneous tissue, but occasionally in such sites as skeletal muscle, the retroperitoneum, tongue and brain. Differentiation of benign and malignant hemangiopericytomas may be difficult or impossible, but those present at birth are usually benign and those arising in deep sites such as the retroperitoneum and muscles of the thigh are apt to be malignant. They should be radically excised.

Low-grade angiosarcomas are rare neoplasms which usually arise in the soft tissues, sometimes within a diffuse hemangioma of an extremity or a tumor in bone. The lesion may be manifest at birth or not until late childhood. Histologically it consists of anastomosing vascular channels lined by atypical-appearing endothelial cells; multiple papillary projections extend into the lumens of the vessels. Local excision is usually curative.

Poorly differentiated angiosarcomas are highly cellular tumors in which the vascular component may not be prominent, rendering identification difficult. They may metastasize by the lymphatic and blood streams and should be treated by wide surgical excision and, possibly, irradiation.

Lymphangiomas, which are less common than

hemangiomas, are also probably malformations (hamartomas) rather than true neoplasms. They may also contain other mesodermal elements, e.g., smooth muscle, adipose tissue, foci of lymphocytes and hemangiomatous areas. They may be present at birth or not be apparent until later. The most common locations are in the neck and extremities. The tumors are benign, but because of their infiltrative tendency, recurrences after attempted surgical removal are common.

Lymphangioma of the tongue. See Section 11.

Lymphangioma circumscriptum is a rare condition characterized by small groups of vesicles composed of dilated lymphatics in the superficial dermis. It may be present at birth or begin in infancy or childhood.

Diffuse lymphangiomas are poorly circumscribed tumors occurring in the skin, mucous membranes or muscles. They are usually congenital. In the tongue and lips they are responsible for macroglossia and macrocheilia, respectively. Diffuse lymphangioma of an extremity is responsible for one form of elephantiasis *(elephantiasis lymphangiectatica)*. It may involve an entire extremity or only a portion, e.g., the fingers or foot; there may be associated hypertrophy of the bone as well as of the soft tissues of the length as well as the girth of the extremity. Histologically the dilated lymphatic channels may be obscured by abundant fibrous tissue. The more localized lesions should be treated by surgical excision, but recurrences are frequent. Treatment of the more diffuse lesions is apt to be unsatisfactory.

Cystic lymphangiomas (cystic hygromas) are most frequently encountered in the neck *(hygroma colli)* and in the axillae, but may also occur in the inguinal and retroperitoneal regions. In the cervical region they may extend into the mediastinum, and rarely mediastinal hygromas may occur in the absence of a cervical component. *Mesenteric cysts* are simply cystic lymphangiomas of the mesentery, and many omental cysts are lymphangiomas. *Sacral hygromas* may simulate lipomas or sacrococcygeal teratomas; they are sometimes connected with the spinal canal. Enlargement of cystic lymphangiomas may occur by enlargement of the individual cysts, by formation of new cysts or by hemorrhage into the cysts.

Hygroma colli is the most common type of cystic lymphangioma. It is usually demonstrable at birth as a soft, poorly defined mass, often in the posterior cervical triangle; many of the tumors can be transilluminated. Periodic fluctuations in the size of the mass are common; rapid increase in size is often associated with hemorrhage into the cystic spaces. The size of the cervical component of a cervicomediastinal hygroma is greatly influenced by crying or by the phase of respiration. The tumors are often asymptomatic, but respiratory difficulty or difficulty in swallowing may occur.

The tumor may surround vessels and nerves, making surgical excision difficult. They are usually lobulated, thin-walled, multilocular cystic structures; the cysts may be independent of one another or may communicate freely. The contents usually consist of clear colorless fluid, but this may be xanthochromic or bloody.

Cystic lymphangiomas should be treated for cosmetic purposes, as well as to prevent such complications as hemorrhage into the lumens of the cyst, infection and mediastinal compression. Surgical excision is the treatment of choice.

Angiomatosis is an uncommon disorder characterized by the presence of multiple hemangiomas or lymphangiomas in various sites, especially the bones, skin and subcutaneous tissues and the spleen. It is more common in females. The lesions in the skin may be evident at birth or not until childhood or adolescence. Clinical manifestations are variable and are dependent upon the sites and extent of involvement. Massive chylous effusions, especially *chylothorax,* are relatively common. In some instances there may be a rash overlying the affected hemithorax, which waxes and wanes with the effusion. Multiple osteolytic defects in the bones are among the most common manifestations and may involve any of the bones. Lesions of the skin and subcutaneous tissue may resemble cavernous hemangiomas or lymphangiomas. The prognosis is dependent upon the extent and sites of involvement; the lesions are often progressive, and, especially if chylous effusions are present, the outlook must be guarded.

TUMORS OF THE SKIN

Squamous cell and *basal cell carcinomas* are extremely rare in children, occurring especially in persons with xeroderma pigmentosum, in whom melanomas may also occur.

Multiple nevoid basal cell carcinoma syndrome is inherited on an autosomal dominant basis, with a high degree of penetrance but variable expressivity. Not all features of the disorder need be present, and even the tumors of the skin are found in only about one half of the affected persons. These are flesh-colored to pale brown, firm, painless papules occurring especially on the face, neck, back and thorax. They usually appear about the time of puberty but may occur in infancy. Multiple cysts of the jaw are one of the more constant features of the syndrome. They often initially appear during the first decade and may be responsible for swelling of the jaw or dull pain. They may involve either jaw, but more often the mandible; they vary from microscopic size to several centimeters in diameter. They may displace adjoining teeth. There are various osseous anomalies, especially splayed and/or bifurcated ribs and kyphoscoliosis. Other features include frontal and temporoparietal bossing, lamellar calcification of the falx cerebri and ocular anomalies. Calcified ovarian fibromas and lymphangiomas of the mesentery have been seen in some affected adults. Shortening of the fourth metacarpals and absence of significant phosphorus diuresis after intravenous administration of parathyroid hormone have suggested a relation of this syndrome to *pseudohypoparathyroidism. Medulloblastoma,* usually appearing in the first two years of life, seems to be part of the syndrome, and its occurrence is an indication for a careful family history.

The tumors of the skin arise in the basal layer of the epidermis and in the upper part of the hair follicles. They resemble the usual basal cell carcinomas, except for their multiplicity, for their occurrence at a young age, for their development in areas not especially exposed to sunlight, and for their more frequent association with an inflammatory infiltrate and with minute areas of calcification. The cysts of the jaw have been classified as *primordial cysts* or odontogenic keratocysts. They may contain a misplaced tooth and, if uninfected, are lined by a uniform layer of stratified squamous epithelium covered by a thin layer of keratin. Recurrence following curettage is common, possibly from adjacent microcysts.

Epidermoid cysts are spherical, benign tumors often located in the skin of the neck, face or scalp; they are probably derived from congenital ectodermal rests and are not true neoplasms. The wall of the cyst is lined by a thin layer of stratified squamous epithelium, and the lumen contains cornified debris; in some instances the epithelial lining is largely destroyed and is replaced by a foreign-body giant cell type of reaction. Skin appendages are often present in the wall of the cyst.

Epidermoid cysts in the calvarium are demonstrable roentgenographically as sharply demarcated defects surrounded by dense sclerotic bone.

Pigmented nevi in infants and children are usually clinically benign. They may be present at birth as large, rough, dark brown or black areas, as in the "bathing trunk" nevus. Smaller nevi may first be noted in infancy, childhood or even adult life at almost any site. They may be smooth or papillary, light brown to almost black, and may contain hair.

Certain nevi, especially in children, may suggest a malignant melanoma. These have been referred to as *epithelioid cell* and *spindle cell nevi (juvenile melanomas).* They tend to be purplish red rather than dark brown, hairless, and somewhat more elevated than the usual nevi in children. They occur most frequently on the cheek as small, protuberant, red or pink lesions which may grow rapidly and suggest a pyogenic granuloma. They may recur if incompletely excised, but are benign lesions which should be treated by conservative surgical measures.

Owing to their frequency, removal of all nevi is not feasible. Those on the genitalia, palms of the hands and soles of the feet, as well as those in other sites which are subjected to repeated irritation, probably should be removed before puberty. The occurrence of increasing pigmentation, ulceration or rapid growth of a nevus is an indication for surgical excision of the growth with a wide margin of intact skin.

Halo nevi are characterized by a central reddish brown papular nevus surrounded by a ring of depigmented skin. The average age at the time of their occurrence is 17 or 18 years, but they may be noted as early as 5 years. The nevus precedes the depigmentation and ultimately may spontaneously disappear, leaving a residual depigmented area. Histologically these are usually compound nevi with distinct nests of nevus cells in the junctional zone and in the superficial dermis, associated with a heavy infiltrate of lymphocytes, histiocytes and occasional plasma cells. The adjoining epidermis is amelanotic and constitutes the "halo." The inflammatory infiltrate should not be interpreted as evidence of malignancy, and, as with most nevi in children, these are almost always benign.

Balloon cell nevi contain a preponderance of large, pale, finely vacuolated cells. Although these cells may occur in nodular aggregates, they are usually diffusely distributed among the conventional nevus cells. Although balloon cells may be encountered in some malignant melanomas, their presence in an otherwise histologically benign nevus does not increase its malignant potential.

Malignant melanoma is rare before puberty, but may be present at birth. It may occur in association with xeroderma pigmentosum. About one fourth of the noncongenital, malignant melanomas in children have arisen in giant nevi. The risk of malignancy developing in a giant nevus is probably relatively high; such melanomas in children are almost uniformly fatal and cerebral metastases are common. In contrast, the 3-year survival rate, without recurrence, for other melanomas in children is about 25 per cent. Widespread malignant melanoma in the pregnant woman may metastasize to the placenta and fetus.

Neurocutaneous melanomatosis is a rare congenital disorder characterized by the development of melanotic tumors of the skin, leptomeninges and central nervous system. The dermal lesion is usually a giant nevus, especially one in the occipital or nuchal region. The leptomeningeal and neural lesions vary from pigmented areas, usually in a perivascular location, that do not distort the architecture of the brain to massive neoplastic thickening of the leptomeninges, with resultant hydrocephalus and neuraxial infiltrates. Rarely the leptomeningeal and neuraxial lesions occur in the absence of apparent dermal ones. The rare presence of neurofibromatous areas in the dermal nevus may link this syndrome with von Recklinghausen's disease.

Blue nevi are usually smooth, firm, blue or bluish black nodules occurring on the face, buttocks or dorsum of the feet or hands. The lesion contains cells similar to those in a Mongolian spot, but typically these occur in clumps and wavy groups. Although usually a relatively small lesion, blue nevus rarely may reach a large size, extending through the dermis into the underlying fascia and muscle. *Cellular blue nevi* have been misinterpreted as malignant, but even metastases to regional nodes are extremely rare.

The *nevus of Ota* is usually a macular pigmented

area located on the side of the face and often involves the sclera; the ocular muscles and retro-orbital fat may also be involved. Its histologic appearance may be that of a Mongolian spot or of a blue nevus, sometimes of the cellular type.

Cutaneous leiomyomas are solitary or multiple small nodules in the skin, especially on the extensor surfaces of the extremities. They are sometimes present from birth or early childhood. They may be tender and painful. The tumors are circumscribed and consist of interlacing bands or cords of smooth muscle fibers. They may be quite vascular. The tumors are benign and should be excised.

Dermatofibrosarcoma protuberans is a slowly growing invasive tumor arising in the dermis. It begins as one or more hard, painless nodules which slowly coalesce, protrude from the skin and may ulcerate. The fibroblastic tissue within the neoplasm tends to form irregular strands and whorls. The tumor may recur locally over a period of many years, but metastases are rare.

TUMORS OF SKIN APPENDAGE ORIGIN

Tumors of skin appendage origin are usually benign, but histologically they may suggest a variety of malignant neoplasms. The classification of a number of them is still disputed. Only a few of them are described here.

Calcifying epitheliomas (pilomatrixomas) are relatively common, hard, sharply demarcated benign tumors of the skin which may arise at any site, especially in the face or arms. Clinically they are usually confused with epidermoid cysts, and histologically they may be misinterpreted as carcinoma. They are probably derived from cells which are differentiating toward hair matrix cells.

Syringocystadenoma papilliferans usually occurs as a single verrucous plaque, most frequently on the scalp. Areas of crusting may be present on its surface. Histologically the overlying epithelium is thickened, hyperkeratotic and distorted into wart-like protrusions. The tumor consists of closely packed papillary projections, covered by two layers of epithelial cells, which extend into the lumens of ducts. There is often a dense inflammatory infiltrate.

Syringomas occur as hundreds of soft, slightly elevated, yellowish pinhead-sized nodules, especially about the eyelids, chest, neck and thighs. They occur predominantly in females and develop at puberty. Histologically they consist of numerous small cystic ducts located in the dermis. These are benign.

Cylindromas (turban tumors) are multiple benign growths which are often familial. They occur predominantly on the scalp of females, usually appearing at puberty or in young adult life. They usually appear initially on the forehead as smooth, firm, freely movable, painless nodules. They increase in number and size throughout life, so that ultimately the entire scalp may be covered by a lobulated mass of lesions. They are nearly always benign and are best treated by surgical excision.

Trichoepithelioma (epithelioma adenoides cysticum) also usually occurs in females at puberty. It is frequently familial. Multiple, small, discrete yellow to pink nodules appear on the face and occasionally on the upper part of the trunk. The tumor is derived from hair follicles and may contain areas closely simulating basal cell carcinoma.

Nevus sebaceus is a circumscribed, slightly raised, firm yellow plaque usually occurring on the scalp or face; it may be present from birth. It is composed of large numbers of sebaceous glands.

Adenoma sebaceum. See Section 20 and angiolipoleiomyoma, page 1618.

TUMORS OF THE SOFT TISSUES

Neoplasms arising from muscle, fat and connective tissue comprise a miscellaneous but important group of tumors of early life. They may arise at almost any site and vary from benign neoplasms such as the lipoma to highly malignant sarcomas; the latter may be so undifferentiated as to preclude accurate determination of the cell of origin. They may occur at any age. The most frequent manifestation is a visible or palpable mass. Clinical differentiation of benign and malignant neoplasms is often impossible. Every solid mass should be considered malignant until proved otherwise by histologic examination of the excised mass.

Lipomas in children are rare, but they may occur in the soft tissues at any site; rarely they are familial. Those in the central nervous system may occupy a defect in the corpus callosum or be intramedullary lesions of the spinal cord; in either site they are usually inoperable lesions which are sometimes continuous with a subcutaneous lipoma. These, as well as the tumor-like masses of fat which sometimes are associated with a meningocele or myelomeningocele *(lipomeningocele* or *lipomyelomeningocele),* are probably malformations and not true neoplasms. Any child with a lipoma of the head or midline of the back should be studied for the presence of an associated bony defect and of an intracranial or intraspinal lipoma.

Lipomas arising in the retroperitoneum or mediastinum may reach a huge size. From the latter site they may penetrate an intercostal space and present externally. A child with a thoracic lipoma should have roentgenograms to exclude the presence of an intrathoracic tumor. A lipoma in the buttock may simulate a sacrococcygeal teratoma. Lipomas may be radiolucent; rarely they contain foci of calcification. Malignancy developing in a pre-existing lipoma is almost nonexistent.

Subcutaneous lipomas are rare in children. Rarely they are multiple and present at birth. They are benign encapsulated tumors which usually grow slowly but progressively and should be excised.

Retroperitoneal lipomas are rare; they may attain a huge size and be responsible for progressive abdominal enlargement. They usually arise in the perirenal region, but may arise from the mesentery. Roentgenographically they are relatively radiolucent and may contain foci of calcification.

Lipoma of the parotid gland is encapsulated and is often attached to the deep lobe of the gland.

Hibernomas are rare tumors composed of brown fat, i.e., immature adipose tissue similar to that of the hibernating glands of animals. They are usually superficial, benign tumors.

Diffuse lipomatosis is probably a hamartomatous malformation rather than a true neoplasm. It consists of infiltrative, nonencapsulated masses of adult adipose tissue growing diffusely in the soft tissues. It may manifest itself at birth as enlargement of an extremity, sometimes accompanied by extensive deformities of adjoining bones, or at times as an ill-defined tumor of skeletal muscle. Owing to its infiltrative nature, complete removal of the mass may be difficult or impossible, and recurrences are common, but the lesion is benign and does not metastasize.

Lipoblastoma is a rare tumor which affects only infants and young children, usually before the age of 3 years. It is probably a developmental defect resulting from proliferation of lipoblasts in the postnatal period. The tumor most commonly involves the soft tissues of the extremities but may arise in the neck, trunk, retroperitoneum or mediastinum. Usually it is a circumscribed mass *(benign lipoblastoma),* less often a diffuse growth *(benign lipoblastomatosis).* The most characteristic feature is the lobular arrangement of the fat cells, the individual lobules being separated by septa of varying thickness. Dilated, plexiform vessels are commonly present in the septa. The fat cells in the lobules vary from mature ones to small lipoblasts with a "signet-ring" appearance. Other polyhedral lipoblasts may be multivacuolated, and there may be cells resembling those of a hibernoma. Poorly differentiated spindle or stellate cells embedded in a myxoid stroma may be present, especially at the periphery of the lobules. In isolated areas the tumor may closely resemble a low-grade myxoid liposarcoma. The tumor is benign and recurrences, which are infrequent, occur principally with the diffuse type.

Histiocytic tumors (fibrous xanthomas; histiocytomas; sclerosing hemangiomas) comprise a rather ill defined group of neoplasms or neoplastic-like lesions, which usually involve the skin and subcutaneous tissue, synovia and tendon sheaths, and less frequently other sites, including skeletal muscle and lung. The tumor is painless, usually does not exceed 2 or 3 cm in diameter, is well circumscribed, firm and gray to yellow. It is composed predominantly of histiocytes and fibroblasts. Scattered lymphocytes and plasma cells, deposits of hemosiderin and multinucleated cells, including Touton giant cells, may also be present. There are variable amounts of lipid in the cells. When the tumor consists almost entirely of histiocytes with a large amount of acidophilic cytoplasm, differentiation from the reticuloendothelioses may be difficult. When it is composed predominantly of fibroblasts, it may closely resemble, if not be identical with, a dermatofibrosarcoma protuberans.

These tumors are essentially benign, although they may recur if incompletely excised. A rare malignant variant has been described.

Giant cell tumors of tendon sheath origin (benign synoviomas) may represent one type of histiocytic tumor. These are small, firm tumors which arise from a tendon sheath or less often from an articular capsule. They are most frequent on the flexor surfaces of the fingers; less often they occur on the toes. They are benign, but may recur if incompletely removed. They are rare in children.

Pseudosarcomatous fasciitis is a lesion which is probably inflammatory and not neoplastic and which is of importance principally because it may be misinterpreted as a malignant neoplasm. It occurs predominantly in the subcutaneous tissue, especially in an arm; less frequently it arises in such sites as skeletal muscle, breast or the tracheobronchial tree. The tumor, which may appear during infancy, usually grows rapidly and, at least in children, is apt to be painless. It usually does not exceed a few centimeters in diameter, is nonencapsulated and is apt to be adherent to the surrounding tissues. Histologically it consists of a peculiar myxoid fibroblastic tissue with many capillaries and some inflammatory cells toward its periphery; these are usually predominantly lymphocytes and macrophages. The lesion invades the surrounding tissue and may contain considerable numbers of normal mitotic figures. Direct invasion of an adjoining lymph node is possible, but metastases do not occur. The lesion is usually cured by simple excision.

Myxomas are rare tumors in children. Although probably capable of arising in almost any site, they are located most frequently in the superficial soft tissues, the bones, especially the maxilla, and the heart. The tumors, which may be apparent at birth, are non-encapsulated and may recur and produce extensive destruction of the tissues in which they are located. They do not metastasize. Treatment is by wide excision.

Benign mesenchymomas (mixed mesodermal tumors) are rare tumors composed of an admixture of differentiated mesenchymal elements, most often fat, smooth muscle and blood vessels. The tumors are usually solitary and well circumscribed but not encapsulated; if located in muscle they infiltrate extensively. They occur predominantly in the skin, subcutaneous tissue and muscles of the extremities, but may arise in almost any site, including the mediastinum, retroperitoneum or viscera. They may be present at birth or appear during infancy or childhood. The tumors, many of which are probably hamartomas, may recur, but are essentially benign and do not metastasize.

Leiomyomas only rarely arise from the soft tissues of infants and children, but occur somewhat more frequently in the viscera, e.g., the bladder, lung, gastrointestinal tract and kidney. They are well circumscribed tumors which should be excised.

Fetal rhabdomyomas are rare benign tumors

which occur predominantly in males in the first three years of life. The tumor may be present at birth and infrequently grows rapidly. It arises in the subcutaneous tissue, especially of the posterior auricular region, and presents as a nontender, fluctuant to rubbery, freely movable mass. It is moderately well circumscribed. It consists of bundles of immature muscle fibers containing myofibrils, haphazardly arranged with undifferentiated mesenchymal cells in a mucoid ground substance. The more differentiated elements tend to predominate at the periphery of the tumor. Differentiation from embryonal rhabdomyosarcoma may be difficult. It is enhanced by the superficial location, circumscribed nature and evidence of maturation at the periphery of the fetal rhabdomyoma, as well as its more uniform cell population, less hyperchromatic nuclei and the paucity of mitotic figures. It should be treated by local excision.

Granular cell myoblastoma is a rare tumor in infants and children. It is usually solitary, but may be multiple. The site of origin is most commonly in the skin and subcutaneous tissue and the tongue, less frequently in the vulva, muscles or even a bronchus. It is composed of large granular cells; the overlying epithelium of the skin or tongue characteristically reveals pseudoepitheliomatous hyperplasia. The cell of origin is not clearly established, but it may be neural rather than muscular. These tumors are benign in children.

Tumoral calcinosis is a rare disorder of unknown cause, distinct from calcinosis universalis or circumscripta. The onset is usually in the first or second decade. Siblings may be affected, and an association with pseudoxanthoma elasticum has been described. The serum calcium value is usually normal, but that of serum phosphate may be elevated. Clinically there are large, nodular, periarticular deposits of calcium, especially about the hips, shoulders and elbows, and at times smaller deposits elsewhere. Histologically the masses are composed of multicystic spaces filled with deposits of calcium and phosphorus and separated from each other by fibrous septa containing macrophages, multinucleated giant cells and chronic inflammatory cells. The general health of the affected persons is usually unimpaired.

Fibrous hamartoma of infancy is a benign tumor of the skin and deep subcutaneous tissues which occurs almost exclusively in infants under 2 years of age and most frequently involves the region of the shoulder or an upper extremity. It may be present at birth and be adherent to the overlying skin. Histologically it consists of fibroblastic connective tissue, islands of cellular mesenchymal tissue with an organoid pattern and adipose tissue. It should be excised.

Juvenile fibromatosis may be located in diverse anatomic sites, but most frequently in skeletal muscle, fascia (including that of the hands and feet) and subcutaneous tissue. Most of them are solitary, nonencapsulated, infiltrative lesions which grow rather slowly and are responsible for a palpable mass; in children, about 10 per cent are multiple. They almost never metastasize, but often recur if incompletely excised; infrequently they infiltrate so extensively as to necessitate mutilating operative procedures and may be responsible for death. In general they are composed of well differentiated fibroblastic tissue forming considerable amounts of collagen.

Desmoids are *fibromatoses* of the musculoaponeurotic sheaths. Although their neoplastic nature is not universally accepted, their clinical behavior, with infiltration of surrounding tissue, continued growth and repeated recurrences, is certainly that of a neoplasm of low-grade malignancy. It does not, however, metastasize. These tumors are uncommon in early life, but may be present at birth. They arise from such diverse sites as the abdominal wall, the shoulder girdle, thigh and neck. They are usually poorly circumscribed and may recur even after apparently complete excision. Treatment is by wide excision.

Fibromatosis of the plantar and palmar fascia, though rare, is of importance in children principally because it may be misinterpreted as fibrosarcoma and needless amputation performed.

Palmar fibromatosis is the basic lesion responsible for Dupuytren's contracture; this is extremely rare in children, and when it does occur in early life, is usually not associated with the presence of tumor-like nodules.

Fibromatosis of the plantar fascia is usually unassociated with contractures and manifests itself as single or multiple nodular swellings sometimes accompanied by pain. Rarely a nodule may be present in the sole of the foot at birth. These lesions are nonencapsulated firm masses only infrequently adherent to the overlying dermis. Histologically they consist of closely packed, spindle-shaped cells in considerable amounts of mature collagen. As a rule, few or no mitoses are present, but infrequently the nuclei are somewhat bizarre. Occasionally the pattern may simulate that of fibrosarcoma, but malignant neoplasms of fibroblastic origin are rare in this site. The lesion is benign, and if the diagnosis is established by biopsy and the patient is asymptomatic, no further treatment need be instituted. Recurrence may follow incomplete removal; if symptoms are present, the entire plantar fascia should be removed.

Juvenile aponeurotic fibroma is a rare tumor which occurs predominantly in infants and children and may be present at birth. Although usually arising in the palm, it may occur in the foot and presumably at any site among muscles and tendons. It presents as a firm, painless tumor not fixed to the overlying skin and not responsible for contractures. Although nonencapsulated and invasive, in older children it tends to be somewhat more compact and to be stippled with areas of calcification which are demonstrable roentgenographically. Histologically it consists of numerous plump, oval nuclei of uniform appearance lying in a pink-staining matrix. All the cells appear to be oriented in one direction, in contrast to the interweaving pattern in other fibromatoses. The tumor is benign, but infiltrates fat and skeletal muscle and is apt to recur after limited excision. Localized removal and not amputation is the treatment of choice.

Digital fibromatoses generally first appear in early infancy as one or more firm masses on the lateral or dorsal surfaces of the fingers or toes. The tumors are often multiple. Histologically the lesions are nonencapsulated and consist of interdigitating bands of fibrous connective tissue with abundant collagen. Mitotic figures are infrequent. The tumor should be removed by wide excision; amputation of the digit is indicated only for very advanced lesions.

Congenital generalized fibromatosis is an extremely rare condition characterized by the presence of multiple small, firm, spherical or ovoid tumors of the subcutaneous and muscular tissues as well as of the viscera and the osseous system. Numerous nodules are characteristically present at birth. The lesions vary from microscopic dimensions to several centimeters in diameter and may contain roentgenographically demonstrable foci of calcification. They are widely distributed over the body, possibly with some predilection for the shoulder girdle, arms, lower back, gluteal region and thighs. Some of the superficial tumors may resemble hemangiomas or, histologically, neurofibromas. Visceral involvement is characteristically widespread and may be responsible for varied manifestations, which include intestinal obstruction, diarrhea as a result of innumerable polypoid growths of the small and large intestines, and respiratory disturbances. Death often occurs in early infancy. In a few instances in which the number of detectable nodules has been limited, survival has followed removal of them. Spontaneous regression of osseous defects as well as of multiple more superficial masses has been observed.

TUMORS OF NERVE SHEATH ORIGIN

There is confusion about the nomenclature of tumors of nerve sheath origin and the relation of these tumors to neurofibromatosis. The neurilemmoma usually occurs as an isolated, encapsulated tumor, but occasionally there are associated stigmata of multiple neurofibromatosis. Neurofibromas are characteristically not well circumscribed or encapsulated and, though they also may occur as solitary growths, are much more commonly part of multiple neurofibromatosis.

Neuromas are not true neoplasms, but consist of proliferative masses of Schwann cells, axon fibers and connective tissue which develop at the proximal end of a severed nerve. They may be extremely painful.

Neurilemmomas (schwannoma, neurinoma) are benign, solitary, encapsulated tumors which arise from the peripheral, sympathetic or cranial nerves. *Acoustic neuromas,* the commonest neurilemmomas of cranial nerves, are rare in children. Peripherally located tumors are not likely to become as large as those in the posterior mediastinum or retroperitoneum. The tumor may be solid or partially cystic.

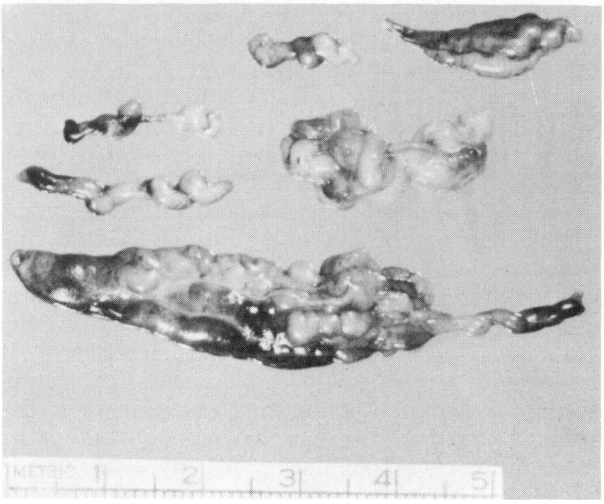

Figure 25–8 *Plexiform neurofibroma removed from the neck of a girl 4 years old. Note the irregularly enlarged, tortuous nerves.*

Neurofibromas may occur as solitary tumors, but are often associated with multiple neurofibromatosis (Section 20). The tumor may be firm or cystic. It is usually painless, but relatively large tumors in an enclosed space, e.g., the ulnar nerve at the elbow, may cause pain. *Plexiform neurofibromas* may first manifest themselves during infancy or, more frequently, during childhood. The affected nerves are elongated, tortuous and enlarged, appearing as a tangled mass of worms (Fig. 25–8). They may occur as isolated lesions, but are often accompanied by other stigmata of multiple neurofibromatosis. Plexiform neurofibromas may be a part of *elephantiasis neuromatosa,* in which diffuse fibrous thickening of the skin and subcutaneous tissue may be associated with hypertrophy of the bone. *Intraspinal neurofibromas* may occur singly or in association with multiple neurofibromatosis. The tumors may be entirely intraspinal or may penetrate an intervertebral foramen and produce a paravertebral mass.

Vascular neurofibromatosis may be responsible for coarctation of the abdominal aorta or aneurysm or stenosis of one or both renal arteries with resultant hypertension.

SARCOMAS OF SOFT TISSUES

These malignant mesenchymal neoplasms, situated in the connective tissue, muscle and fat of the nonparenchymatous tissues, probably comprise 10 to 20 per cent of malignant neoplasms in infants and children. They usually present as a mass which has grown rapidly; accelerated growth, however, does not occur with all such neoplasms and may also be manifest by benign tumors. Sarcomas may differentiate toward skeletal or smooth muscle or toward fat or fibrous tissue, but in highly undifferentiated neoplasms it may be impossible to determine the line of differentiation, if indeed it exists; infrequently there are several cell types, producing a mesenchymoma.

In general, treatment of sarcomas of soft tissues is by excision, with removal of a substantial margin of surrounding normal tissue; the edges of the resected specimen should be examined histologically to determine the adequacy of removal. Inadequate removal of sarcomas of even low-grade malignancy, as well as of some benign tumors, is followed by recurrence; there is no convincing evidence that the malignancy of the recurrent tumor is increased.

In discussing treatment of malignant tumors of soft tissues and of bone, as well as those of many other sites, it should be recognized that advances are occurring rapidly and are often encouraging. Current methods described here may already be superseded by more appropriate ones. *Following a prompt, accurate diagnosis, it is essential that a center accustomed to treating cancer in children plan the therapy and follow the patient's course.*

Rhabdomyosarcoma is the most common malignant neoplasm of soft tissues encountered in the pediatric age period. It is somewhat more frequent in males than in females. At least three different histologic types of rhabdomyosarcoma are described; some neoplasms contain morphologic features of more than one type.

Pleomorphic rhabdomyosarcoma is predominantly a lesion of the extremities of adults. It is a poorly demarcated, invasive neoplasm. *Alveolar rhabdomyosarcoma* tends to occur in adolescents and young adults and involves especially the muscles of the extremities and trunk, the perineal, perianal and perirectal areas and the orbital region. It is characterized by alveoli lined by one or more layers of cells which are closely applied to their walls, with single and multinucleated cells lying free in the lumens (Fig. 25–9). Such neoplasms may be misinterpreted as carcinoma, lymphoma, malignant melanoma or even neuroblastoma. *Embryonal rhabdomyosarcoma* occurs predominantly in infants and children and arises principally in the head and neck, lower genitourinary tract, pelvis and extremities. It is apt to be poorly differentiated, containing stellate cells and long, thin, spindle-shaped cells with bright acidophilic cytoplasm. Cross striations are relatively infrequent.

Sarcoma botryoides is an embryonal rhabdomyosarcoma which, because of its location just beneath the mucous membrane of a hollow viscus or the serosal surface of a body cavity, assumes a grape-like or polypoid configuration. The term describes the gross appearance of a tumor and not its histologic character; rarely other tumors may produce a similar botryoid configuration. The term is commonly used in the literature and is retained here to refer only to rhabdomyosarcomas, which may arise in the head and neck, the lower genitourinary tract or the common bile duct. Ulceration of the overlying epithelium with secondary infection, coupled with the edematous appearance of the mass, may lead to an erroneous diagnosis of an inflammatory rather than a neoplastic lesion.

Rhabdomyosarcomas are apt to recur locally, and metastases are relatively frequent in regional lymph nodes, lungs and bones. Most recurrences occur within two years of the diagnosis. For tumors of the orbit, nasopharynx and middle ear some would advocate only chemotherapy and irradiation. Prompt surgical extirpation combined with irradiation and chemotherapy is the treatment of choice at any other site. The prognosis following

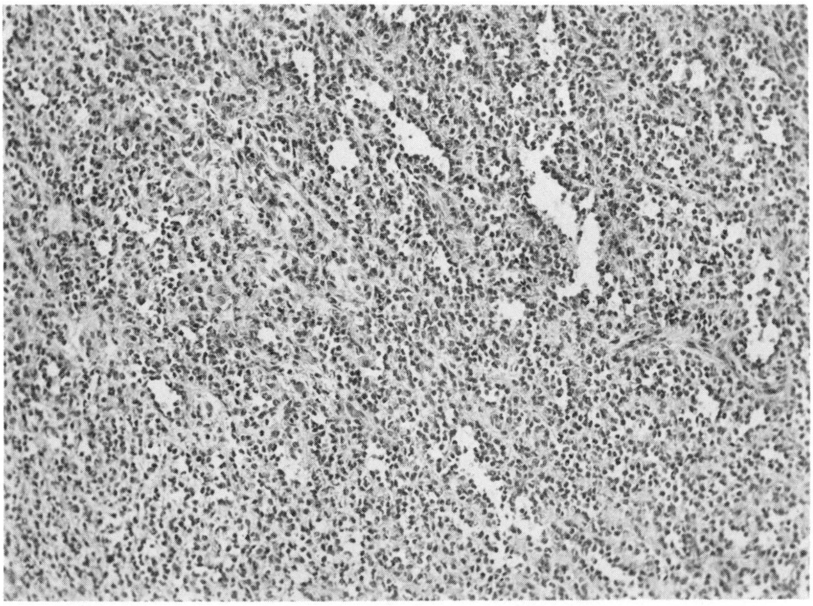

Figure 25–9 *Alveolar rhabdomyosarcoma. Multiple irregular spaces are lined by one or more layers of cells, some of which have been cast off into the lumens.*

such combined therapy has been greatly improved, and some patients with incompletely resected tumors may recover.

Fibrosarcomas may be present at birth. They are composed of spindle-shaped cells accompanied by reticulin fibers. It should be recognized that a variety of other cells, including lipoblasts and histiocytes, are capable of forming fibroblastic tissue and that neoplasms containing such tissue should not be considered fibrosarcomas. Low-grade fibrosarcomas may be difficult or impossible to differentiate from juvenile fibromatoses, and identification of the potential for metastasizing may be impossible. These tumors are locally invasive and should be widely excised with a generous margin of intact tissue; metastases occur in less than 10 per cent of affected children.

Neurofibrosarcomas (malignant schwannomas) may occur as solitary tumors or in conjunction with multiple neurofibromatosis. Most children with such neoplasms have other stigmata of von Recklinghausen's disease, but only a minority of those with multiple neurofibromatosis have sarcomas during childhood. The incidence is unknown; it has been estimated as less than 5 per cent and as high as almost 30 per cent. Children and young adults less than 30 years of age are more often affected than older adults.

An enlarging mass, sometimes accompanied by pain, is usually the initial manifestation. The tumor usually develops in the deep, soft tissues adjacent to neurofibromatous tissue. Rarely neurofibrosarcomas differentiate in some areas into rhabdomyosarcomas and are referred to as malignant *"Triton"* tumors (Fig. 25–10). The prognosis, with or without such differentiation, is grave.

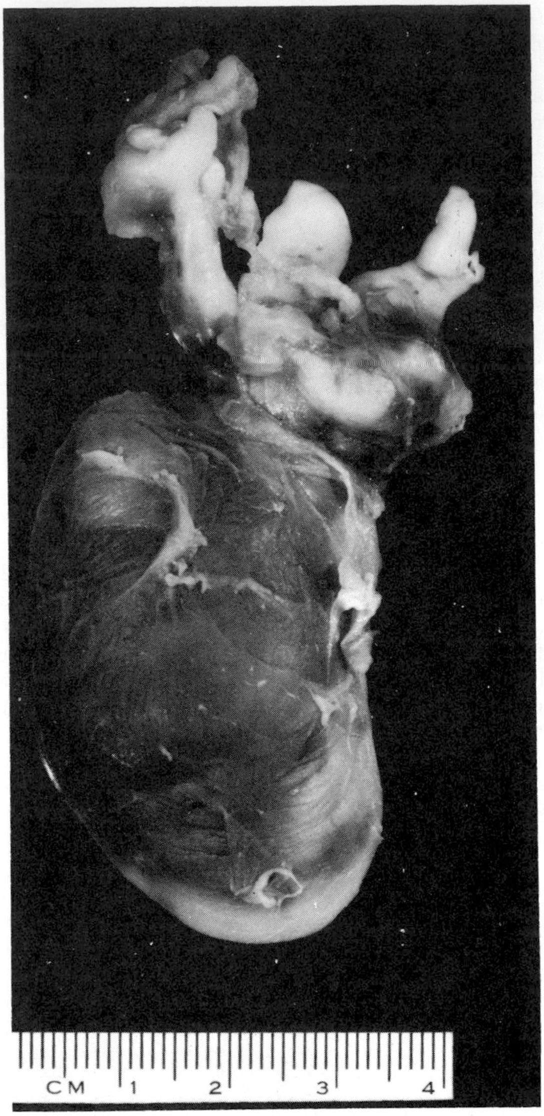

Figure 25–10 *Neurofibrosarcoma of the neck arising in association with a plexiform neurofibroma in a girl 12 years old with von Recklinghausen's disease. Enlarged tortuous nerves are seen above the solid neoplasm. The tumor is a malignant schwannoma containing rhabdomyosarcomatous elements (malignant "Triton" tumor).*

Synovial sarcomas are uncommon during childhood. They usually arise in the para-articular tissues, especially about the hand or knee. The initial manifestation may be localized pain, point tenderness or a palpable mass. Roentgenographic examination may disclose areas of calcification. Macroscopically the neoplasm often appears encapsulated, but histologically there is commonly evidence of proximal extension along fascial planes. Recurrences are apt to occur, sometimes after an interval of several years. Metastases are chiefly to the lungs; involvement of the regional lymph nodes occurs in about one fourth of the patients. The prognosis is grave. Because of the delayed appearance of recurrences, 5- and 10-year "cures" must be accepted with reservations.

Clear-cell sarcomas of tendons and aponeuroses are rare neoplasms occurring principally in the region of the foot and knee; they are intimately bound to tendons or aponeuroses. They are usually small, slow-growing and painless and are not fixed to the overlying skin. Histologically they have a uniform pattern of nests of pale cells with an epithelioid appearance. Repeated local recurrence and eventual metastases are common, especially to the regional lymph nodes and to the lung.

Liposarcomas are rare in early life; rarely the tumor is present at birth. The neoplasms are commonly found within muscles or superficially attached to them and occur in a variety of sites, including the extremities, neck, mediastinum, retroperitoneum and even the pharynx. They are usually low-grade myxoid liposarcomas which may recur but do not metastasize. Treatment is by wide excision.

Malignant mesenchymomas contain two or more malignant mesenchymal elements; fibrosarcomatous tissue is not one of them. These are rare tumors, but may be present at birth. Although most of them arise in the skeletal soft tissues, they may occur in almost any site, including the mediastinum, retroperitoneum, liver, ileum, orbit, nasopharynx and spinal canal. Grossly, they often appear to be partially or completely encapsulated, but histologically they are usually found to be invasive. They are often variegated in structure, and the larger lesions are apt to contain multiple areas of necrosis. Metastases may occur by way of the lymphatic and blood streams. Apparent cures have been effected even in the presence of metastases to regional lymph nodes, especially in infants. Most of the congenital neoplasms have behaved in a benign manner.

Leiomyosarcomas of the soft tissues are rare in the pediatric age period; differentiation of these from benign leiomyomas may be difficult. Recurrence sometimes takes place after an interval of several years. The tumors are infiltrative and should be widely excised.

Epithelioid sarcoma is a rare tumor, possibly of histiocytic origin. About one third of those reported have occurred in the first two decades of life, sometimes as early as 4 years of age. It occurs especially in the soft tissues of the hand, forearm and pretibial regions. It tends to grow in a nodular or multinodular manner along the fascia and tendons, usually presenting as a slow-growing, indurated nodule in the subcutaneous tissue. Ulceration of the overlying skin may occur, and the lesion is often interpreted as a draining abscess. Histologically it consists of nodular masses of large, deeply acidophilic polygonal cells admixed with plump, spindle-shaped cells. Extensive deposits of birefringent collagen may be present. The nodular character of the tumor, often with central necrosis, and a chronic inflammatory infiltrate at the periphery may lead to an erroneous diagnosis of a chronic granulomatous inflammatory process. Metastases usually do not occur until after local recurrence. They involve especially the lungs or pleura and skin, especially of the scalp. Treatment is by wide local excision and possibly radiation.

Alveolar soft part sarcomas occur predominantly in the muscles of the extremities, especially the thigh, more commonly in girls than in boys. The tumor is usually a slowly growing one which may metastasize 15 years or more after removal of the primary neoplasm. The histogenesis is unknown. Histologically it is characterized by a pseudoalveolar arrangement of the neoplastic cells in relation to delicate endothelial-lined vascular channels and septa; the cells may contain crystalline deposits which stain positively with PAS after digestion with diastase. The tumor should be widely excised and combined chemotherapy probably should be given. These are indolent growths, and survival may be relatively long, even after metastases appear. The current probability of cure, however, is slight.

Extraosseous chondrosarcoma and osteosarcoma are extremely rare, especially in children. They arise in the soft tissues, especially of the extremities, and are not attached to bone. Their behavior is similar to that of their counterparts in bone. They should be differentiated from mesenchymomas, approximately one fourth of which contain osteoid or bone, and from other neoplasms of soft tissues which may contain metaplastic bone, e.g., neurofibrosarcoma and synovial sarcoma. Of greater importance, however, is the differentiation of extraskeletal osteosarcoma from either myositis ossificans circumscripta or progressiva.

NEOPLASMS OF BONE

A variety of benign and malignant neoplasms of bone have been described in children in addition to non-neoplastic lesions which clinically and roentgenographically simulate true neoplasms. Diagnosis and treatment of suspected neoplasms of bone require *clinical, roentgenographic* and *histologic* studies.

BENIGN NEOPLASMS AND NEOPLASTIC-LIKE LESIONS

Osteochondromas (osteocartilaginous exostoses) may be solitary or multiple. They are probably anomalies of development rather than true neoplasms. Multiple exostoses are discussed in Section 22. The solitary osteochondroma is one of the most common of the benign osseous tumors. It is most frequently located at or near the ends of the long bones, especially the lower end of the femur or upper end of the tibia, but may arise from any bone which is preformed in cartilage. It is usually manifest in childhood or adolescence by a bony protuberance; occasionally pain may result from a fracture through its stalk or from the development of an overlying bursitis. The tumor consists of a bony mass near the epiphysis which protrudes in the direction of the shaft and is covered by a cap of cartilage. Growth of the mass tends to cease at or before cessation of skeletal growth, when the cap of cartilage may disappear, leaving only the residual outgrowth of bone *(osteoma).* Malignant transformation of an osteochondroma usually does not occur until after cessation of skeletal growth and is more apt to occur with multiple exostoses; the resultant neoplasm is usually a parosteal sarcoma. About 5 per cent of patients with *multiple exostoses* can be expected to have malignant neoplasms from one or more sites. Surgical resection of the tumor should be performed whenever feasible as a prophylactic measure against malignancy.

Enchondromas are benign cartilaginous tumors arising within the metaphyses of cylindrical bones, especially those of the hands and feet. Skeletal *enchondromatosis* refers to the presence of such tumors in multiple sites; when the involvement is predominantly unilateral, the condition is referred to as *Ollier's disease* (Section 22); when there are associated vascular malformations, it is referred to as *Maffucci syndrome.*

Solitary enchondromas tend to occur at a later age than does enchondromatosis. The initial symptoms are often pain and swelling following a pathologic fracture. Roentgenograms reveal a well circumscribed area of rarefaction within the bone, with or without expansion of it and attenuation of the overlying cortex; dense stippled foci representing areas of calcification are commonly present. There is usually no periosteal formation of new bone unless infraction of the cortex has occurred. Histologically the tumors consist of lobules of atypical hyaline cartilage, the matrix of which may have undergone a myxomatous change. Treatment of solitary enchondroma consists in curettage, and the introduction of bone chips or a bone graft if necessary.

Solitary enchondromas in the small bones of the hands or feet are almost always benign; those in the metaphysis of a large cylindrical bone, in the middle third of any bone or in a flat bone are more apt to be chondrosarcomas. Histologic differentiation of benign from malignant tumors may be difficult or impossible.

Benign chondroblastomas are rare tumors derived from young cartilage cells. They occur predominantly in adolescent males and characteristically involve the epiphyseal end of a long bone. The neoplasm is manifest by pain which is often referred to the neighboring joint. Roentgenographically the lesion appears as a rarefied mottled focus arising in the epiphysis, but sometimes extending into the adjoining metaphysis; it tends to be encircled by a narrow line of increased density. Histologically it consists of cellular areas of compact, round or polyhedral cells, deposits of hyaline cartilaginous matrix, myxoid material and collagen. Irregular masses of calcium are usually present, and there may be small amounts of osteoid. Multinucleated giant cells may be present; the tumor has been misinterpreted as a giant cell tumor, chondrosarcoma or osteosarcoma. Treatment consists in curettage with instillation of bone chips; there may be recurrences.

Chondromyxoid fibroma is closely related to the chondroblastoma. It is a rare benign tumor usually encountered in the metaphysis of one of the long bones of the extremities. Pain and, less often, swelling are common manifestations. Although many different bones have been affected, the upper end of the tibia and lower end of the femur are most commonly involved. The lesion appears as an eccentrically located, expansile, rarefied area in the metaphysis; the borders tend to be scalloped and well defined by a narrow band of opaque sclerotic bone. In small bones the roentgenographic appearance may be that of an expansile, pseudotrabeculated cyst occupying the entire width of the bone. Histologically the tumor consists of lobulated masses of closely packed cells embedded in a myxoid matrix; the matrix may undergo extensive fibrosis, and in some areas recognizable cartilaginous matrix may be formed by the neoplastic cells. The tumor, though rare, is of importance because it may be confused with a malignant tumor, especially a chondrosarcoma. Curettage followed by the instillation of bone chips may suffice for therapy, but may be followed by recurrence, especially in children. Complete removal of the tumor by resection which includes the tumor bed is the treatment of choice.

Osteomas are benign tumors of osseous tissue which arise in the bones of the face or skull and may project from the surface or extend into the orbit or paranasal sinuses. Their presence, if associated with multiple soft tissue tumors, should lead to a careful examination of the gastrointestinal tract for the presence of polyps, as a part of Gardner syndrome (p. 1612).

Osteoid osteoma has been reported in every bone but occurs most frequently in the lower extremity, especially in the femur. The predominant symptom is pain, often with localized tenderness; swelling and, rarely, slight local heat and redness may also be present. Roentgenograms may not demonstrate a distinctive lesion in the early stages. Characteristically a small radiolucent area is surrounded by a zone of sclerotic bone which may extend well beyond the lesion and may obscure the area of radiolucency. In some instances the central nidus may be radiopaque and thus not be visible within the dense peripheral sclerotic bone.

The tumor consists of a central nidus of sharply circumscribed osteoid tissue with varying degrees of mineralization. The dense peripheral zone noted on the roentgenogram consists of reactive, nonneoplastic bone. The tumor is benign and can be cured by complete removal of the nidus; incomplete removal is followed by recurrence of symptoms.

Benign osteoblastoma (osteogenic fibroma, giant osteoid osteoma) is a rare neoplasm composed of a fibrous matrix with areas of osteoblastic activity, osteoid tissue and bone. It occurs predominantly in children and young adults and involves especially the neural arches of the vertebral column, flat bones and bones of the hands and feet. Roentgenographically it is a well circumscribed lesion which may expand and attenuate the cortex; its inner border may be limited by a zone of sclerotic bone. Although the lesion is clinically benign, its histologic features may simulate those of an osteosarcoma as well as of a variety of neoplastic and nonneoplastic lesions of bone.

Nonosteogenic fibroma, a benign tumor whose neoplastic nature is in doubt, usually occurs near the end of the diaphysis of one of the long bones, especially in the leg. The lesion may be asymptomatic, or pain, sometimes interpreted as arthritis, may occur. Roentgenograms reveal a rarefied, trabeculated lesion with a sharply outlined margin of sclerotic bone; the lesion is usually eccentrically located within the bone. The tumor consists of bundles of spindle-shaped connective tissue cells with no attempt at the formation of bone. Abundant hemosiderin pigment, multinuclear giant cells, foam cells and collagen may be present. The lesion can be successfully treated by curettage, but often heals spontaneously.

Subperiosteal cortical defect is probably closely related to nonosteogenic fibroma. It is a common, sometimes multiple or symmetrical lesion involving especially the lower end of the femur or the upper end of the tibia of children. It apparently erodes the bone from without, in contrast to the nonosteogenic fibroma, which develops on the inner surface of the cortex. It is a benign lesion which may heal spontaneously.

Giant cell reparative granuloma occurs either centrally in the jawbones or peripherally as a giant cell epulis. The central lesions cannot be differentiated histologically from the osseous lesions of hyperparathyroidism.

Cherubism usually appears in children 3 to 5 years of age as hard, symmetrical swellings of the mandible and/or maxilla accompanied by submandibular lymphadenopathy. It is probably inherited as an autosomal dominant trait. Histologically it may be indistinguishable from central giant cell reparative granuloma.

Neurofibromas may involve the bones directly, with extensive destruction and deformity. *Multiple neurofibromatosis* may be associated with skeletal abnormalities such as scoliosis, pseudarthrosis, skeletal enlargement of part or of an entire extremity, or a defect in the wall of the orbit with unilateral pulsating exophthalmos.

Giant cell tumors are rare in childhood, since they characteristically occur in the ends of long bones after closure of the epiphyses. The majority of lesions interpreted as such are probably solitary unicameral cysts.

Hemangiomas may occur as primary osseous lesions or in association with hemangiomas in adjoining soft tissues. Primary osseous hemangiomas are located especially in the vertebrae but occur in other sites. Roentgenographically they may appear as pseudotrabeculated, cystic expansile lesions. In the skull a so-called sunray appearance may be noted on the roentgenogram. Hemangiomas may involve two or more adjoining vertebral bodies and produce a vertical striated appearance; collapse of the vertebrae with pressure on the spinal nerve rootlets may be responsible for symptoms.

Massive osteolysis (disappearing bone) occurs predominantly in otherwise healthy children and young adults; it is characterized by gradual absorption of one or more bones over a period of years. Almost any bone may be involved. The disease usually progresses until one or more of a group of bones have entirely or partially disappeared, after which the condition stabilizes. Rarely it results in death. The cause is unknown. Histologically there is striking proliferation of thin-walled vessels in the bone and in the fibrous tissue which replaces it. The vascular channels usually contain red blood cells *(hemangiomatosis)*, but sometimes appear to be lymphatics *(lymphangiomatosis)*. The lesion differs from an ordinary hemangioma, which as a relatively localized process may destroy but does not completely dissolve bone. It is probably closely related to *angiomatosis*, but differs from classic instances of the latter in the absence of extraosseous lesions, in the unicentric nature of the osseous lesions and in the roentgenographic appearance of lysis of affected bone(s) rather than of multiple osteolytic defects.

Unicameral (solitary) cysts are common lesions in the metaphyses of long bones, especially in the upper ends of the tibia and the humerus and lower end of the femur. They rarely occur after closure of the epiphyseal line. The lesion is often symptomless until pain occurs after a pathologic fracture.

The lesion probably begins in the metaphysis, and growth of the bone displaces it away from the epiphyseal plate. It causes central rarefaction of bone, often with a pseudotrabecular pattern; the defect is usually no wider than the adjacent metaphysis, although expansion of the shaft may occur. The cortex is attenuated and may be infracted. The roentgenographic appearance may be similar to that of such conditions as fibrous dysplasia, enchondroma or eosinophilic granuloma. In contrast to the giant cell tumor and benign chondroblastoma, it does not cross the epiphyseal plate.

The lesions are cystic and contain blood or fluid, which is often xanthochromic. The cyst is lined by a small amount of nonspecific vascular connective tissue containing deposits of hemosiderin, lipid-laden macrophages and multinucleated giant cells.

Treatment consists in curettage and packing with bone chips. Spontaneous healing may occur, especially after a pathologic fracture, but treatment is usually indicated.

Aneurysmal bone cysts are probably not true neoplasms. They may involve almost any bone, but especially the vertebrae and the long bones of the extremities. The presenting complaint is usually pain, at times associated with a palpable mass; neurologic manifestations may be present with lesions of the vertebrae. Roentgenographically they appear as cystic expansile lesions which, especially in the long bones, tend to extend beyond the normal contour of the bone and produce a saccular, aneurysmal-like protrusion. Multiple incomplete septa are often visible within the radiolucent area. The expanded lesion is usually outlined by a thin shell of periosteal new bone, but rupture of this may occur with extension of the process into the adjoining soft tissues. Macroscopically the cysts contain bloody fluid and soft, hemorrhagic or reddish brown tissue. Histologically they consist of pools of blood separated by septa of connective tissue; giant cells, hemorrhages and newly formed bone may be present within the septa. Treatment is indicated because of the tendency of the lesion to progress. Curettage, surgical resection and/or irradiation have been successfully employed; the possibility of the development of a malignant neoplasm following irradiation must be recognized.

Melanotic neuroectodermal tumor of infancy (retinal anlage tumor) is a rare tumor which occurs in infants. A mass or swelling is usually present before the age of 6 months. The tumor arises predominantly in the maxilla, especially in the anterior portion, less frequently in the mandible and rarely in such sites as the scalp in the region of the anterior fontanel, in the subcutaneous tissue of the deltoid region, in the posterior mediastinum or in the epididymis. Roentgenographic examination reveals an expansile, rarefied lesion in the affected bone. Urinary excretion of VMA is sometimes elevated. The tumor is benign, although invasive. Recurrences following removal are rare.

Adenoameloblastoma is a benign, nonrecurrent lesion which occurs most frequently in girls in the second decade of life, usually in the maxilla in the region of an incisor or cuspid; it is *not* a variant of the ameloblastoma.

Myxomas. See page 1634.

Eosinophilic granuloma. See page 1650.

Epidermoid cyst. See page 1632.

MALIGNANT TUMORS OF BONE

By far the most frequent primary malignant tumors of bone are the osteosarcoma and Ewing's tumor, the majority of which occur between 10 and 25 years of age; males are affected more frequently than females. Osteosarcoma characteristically involves the metaphyseal end of a long bone, whereas Ewing's tumor involves the shaft, but roentgenographic differentiation of these neoplasms is not always possible. Of greater importance, however, is the fact that many, if not all, of the roentgenographic features of these tumors may be duplicated by non-neoplastic lesions of bone. Accordingly, treatment of lesions suspected of being malignant should not be instituted until an unequivocal diagnosis is established by histologic study of the tumor. Moreover, the pathologist is limited in his ability to establish a diagnosis on the basis of histologic studies alone. For example, an actively growing callus about a fracture may closely simulate the histologic appearance of an osteosarcoma, yet correlation of the material obtained at biopsy with the roentgenographic findings may clearly indicate the true non-neoplastic nature of the process. *Thus, the pathologist must evaluate all pertinent clinical, roentgenographic and surgical data before he arrives at a diagnosis.*

Osteosarcoma (osteogenic sarcoma) is more common than Ewing's tumor. It usually begins at the lower end of the femur or the upper end of the tibia or humerus, but may arise at other sites. The presenting complaint is commonly that of pain and swelling of the affected part, which the patient may attribute to trauma.

Roentgenographic studies reveal varying degrees of destruction of bone and of new bone formation. Codman's triangle is a radiopacity at the end of the tumor where the periosteum has been elevated. Neither this finding nor the perpendicular striations of new bone in the subperiosteal neoplasm ("sunray appearance") are always present, nor are they pathognomonic of an osteosarcoma. The level of serum alkaline phosphatase may be elevated.

The neoplasm occupies the medullary cavity and penetrates the cortex to the subperiosteal zone; penetration of the periosteum into adjoining soft tissues may also occur. Histologically the appearance is varied, but consists essentially of atypical mesenchymal cells with varying degrees of formation of collagen, typical or atypical osteoid tissue and true bone. Cartilaginous areas and areas of myxomatous tissue may be present. Osteosarcoma commonly metastasizes to the lungs, although other organs may also be involved; osseous metastases are rare. Amputation appears to offer the best possibility of cure, but the case fatality rate is high. In one series an exceptional 5-year survival rate of 19 per cent has been recorded. Recently the use of one or more chemotherapeutic agents has given encouraging results in the control of metastases and probably should be utilized postoperatively in all patients; such therapy can be administered only in a hospital equipped with facilities to control the adverse side effects of the treatment.

Ewing's tumor may involve the same bones as does osteosarcoma; in addition, there is relatively frequent involvement of the flat bones and the ribs. The initial complaints are often similar to those associated with an osteosarcoma; fever and leukocytosis may occur with either tumor, but are more likely to be associated with Ewing's tumor.

Roentgenographically there is a mottled area of rarefaction, often associated with increased density and periosteal formation of new bone (Fig. 25–11). The latter may be deposited in layers, resulting in an "onion-skin" appearance, but this finding is often absent and may appear in association with other osseous lesions. The roentgenographic appearance may closely simulate that of osteomyelitis, osteosarcoma, eosinophilic granuloma of bone or metastatic neuroblastoma.

Gross examination of an affected bone usually reveals more extensive neoplastic involvement than was demonstrable roentgenographically. His-

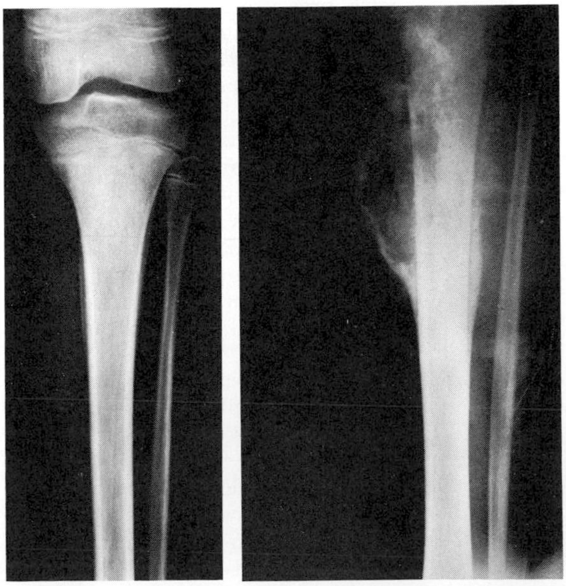

Figure 25–11 *Roentgenograms of a Ewing's tumor of the tibia. A, The initial film revealed only slight periosteal proliferation. B, Roentgenogram taken 3 months later reveals cortical destruction and proliferation of new bone, the latter assuming a "sun-ray" appearance in some areas.*

tologically the tumor consists of sheets of uniform round or oval nuclei with little or no cytoplasm. The neoplastic cells do not form new bone. Extensive areas of hemorrhage and necrosis are commonly present. The histologic appearance may simulate that of a malignant lymphoma or a metastatic neuroblastoma, and every attempt should be made to exclude the presence of an extraosseous primary lesion.

Ewing's tumor usually involves a single bone when first recognized, but ultimately many bones may be affected. Metastases to the lungs are also common. Treatment currently consists in supervoltage irradiation and chemotherapy rather than amputation. The 5-year survival rate should be in the vicinity of 25 per cent or possibly more; occasionally apparent cures have been effected after the development of metastases.

Primary reticulum cell sarcoma of bone often arises in a long bone and may simulate Ewing's tumor both roentgenographically and histologically. Metastases to lymph nodes occur more frequently than in Ewing's tumor, and osseous metastases are infrequent. Irradiation and chemotherapy probably constitute the treatment of choice; recurrences and metastases sometimes occur years after the initial treatment.

Chondrosarcoma is rare in children. It usually arises from the bones of the trunk or the upper ends of the humerus, femur or tibia. The clinical course is less rapid than that of osteosarcoma, and the prognosis, when amputation can be performed, is somewhat more favorable.

Primitive multipotential primary sarcoma of bone is rare in comparison to classic osteosarcoma and Ewing's tumor. It is most common in the second and third decades, but may occur as early as 2 years of age. It occurs about equally in the two sexes and may occur in long or flat bones, the most common site of origin being the femur. Histologically it consists of sheets of undifferentiated cells interspersed among other neoplastic elements such as those of Ewing's sarcoma, osteosarcoma, chondrosarcoma and reticulum cell sarcoma. The presence of numerous pseudorosettes may suggest the diagnosis of metastatic neuroblastoma; other areas may simulate metastatic adenocarcinoma. Metastases occur not only to the lungs, but also to other bones; in a series of 25 patients there were only 5 survivors. The neoplasm is of importance because of the diagnostic problems it presents and because it affords some appreciation of the interrelations of various types of tumors which are usually considered to be distinct clinicopathologic entities, e.g., osteosarcoma, Ewing's tumor and chondrosarcoma.

Fibrosarcoma (p. 1638) may arise within the medullary cavity of a bone (central fibrosarcoma), commonly the lower end of the femur, or peripherally from the periosteum, and erode the adjacent bone. It differs from osteosarcoma and parosteal sarcoma in that there is no tendency to formation of even atypical osteoid, cartilage or bone. Roentgenographically the underlying bone may appear intact, or there may be areas of cortical destruction; the margins of the neoplasm are usually poorly defined. Amputation is usually the preferred treatment but wide local resection may be successful with some of the smaller and less anaplastic tumors in the extremities and in the mandible. The tumor, especially in adults, may be secondary to prior irradiation. The 5-year survival rate is only about 30 per cent.

Multiple myelomas are extremely rare in children. Roentgenographically they may simulate metastatic neuroblastoma, Ewing's tumor, acute leukemia, multiple eosinophilic granulomas, Hand-Schüller-Christian or Letterer-Siwe disease. Survival in children is usually shorter than in adults, most children dying within a year after the diagnosis is established.

Chordomas, or tumors derived from remnants of the notochord, are rare in children. Although not strictly neoplasms of bone, they invade and destroy bone at their site of development, usually the sacrococcygeal region or base of the skull. They are locally invasive tumors which usually cannot be successfully removed; metastases are unusual. Some chordomas in children have been reported as responding to irradiation.

Ameloblastomas (adamantinomas) are epithelial tumors presumably derived from remnants of the enamel organ. They occur more frequently in the mandible than in the maxilla. Tumors arising in the maxilla may obliterate the antrum and bulge into the orbit, nasal cavity or mouth. Roentgenographically they are usually expansile, well circumscribed lesions, but they may penetrate into adjoining tissues. Recurrences following curettage are frequent, but metastases are rare. Craniopharyngiomas (Section 20) may have the histologic appearance of an ameloblastoma, and tumors of similar appearance have been reported in the tibia.

JAMES B. AREY

GENERAL

Marsden, H. B., and Steward, J. K. (eds.): Tumours in Children. New York, Springer-Verlag, 1968.

Wells, H. G.: Occurrence and significance of congenital malignant neoplasms. Arch. Path. *30*:535, 1940.

Sutow, W. W., Vietti, T. J., and Fernbach, P. J. (eds.): Clinical Pediatric Oncology. St. Louis, The C. V. Mosby Co., 1973.

Postradiation Neoplasia

Tefft, M., Vawter, G. F., and Mitus, A.: Second primary neoplasms in children. Am. J. Roentgenol. *103*:800, 1968.

Other Factors Predisposing to Cancer

Kersey, J. H., Spector, B. D., and Good, R. A.: Primary immunodeficiency—Cancer registry. Int. J. Cancer *12*:333, 1973.

Lanier, A. P., Noller, K. L., Decker, D. G., Elveback, L-R., and Kurland, L. T.: Cancer and stilbestrol. A follow-up of 1,719 persons exposed to estrogens in utero and born 1943-1959. Mayo Clinic Proc. *48*:793, 1973.

Rosner, F., and Lee, S. L.: Down's syndrome and acute leukemia: Myeloblastic or lymphoblastic? Report of forty-three cases and review of the literature. Am. J. Med. *53*:203, 1972.

Maternal and Fetal Transmission of Neoplasms

Anders, D., Kindermann, G., and Pfeifer, U.: Metastasizing fetal neuroblastoma with involvement of the placenta simulating erythroblastosis. Report of two cases. J. Pediatr. *82*:50, 1973.

Sweet, L., Reid, W. D., and Roberton, N. R. C.: Hydrops fetalis in association with chorioangioma of the placenta. J. Pediatr. *82*:91, 1973.

Tumors of the Nose, Sinuses, Pharynx, Ear and Oral Cavity

Apostol, J. V., and Frazell, E. L.: Juvenile nasopharyngeal angiofibroma. A clinical study. Cancer *18*:869, 1965.

Cohen, A. H., and Abt, A. B.: An unusual cause of respiratory obstruction: Heterotopic pharyngeal brain tissue. J. Pediatr. *76*:119, 1970.

Donaldson, S. S., Castro, J. R., Wilbur, J. R., and Jesse, R. H., Jr.: Rhabdomyosarcoma of head and neck in children. Combination treatment by surgery, irradiation, and chemotherapy. Cancer *31*:26, 1973.

Pick, T., Maurer, H. M., and McWilliams, N. B.: Lymphoepithelioma in childhood. J. Pediatr. *84*:96, 1974.

Ringertz, N.: Pathology of malignant tumors arising in the nasal and paranasal cavities and maxilla. Acta Otolaryng. Suppl. 27, 1938.

Schimke, N.: Multiple mucosal neuromata syndrome. *In* Lynch, H. T. (ed.): Skin, Heredity, and Malignant Neoplasms. Flushing, New York, Medical Examination Publishing Co., Inc., 1972.

Yeh, S.: A histological classification of carcinomas of the nasopharynx with a critical review as to the existence of lymphoepitheliomas. Cancer *15*:895, 1962.

Tumors of the Major Salivary Glands

Galich, R.: Salivary gland neoplasms in childhood. Arch. Otolaryng. *89*:878, 1969.

Krolls, S. O., Trodahl, J. N., and Boyers, R. C.: Salivary gland lesions in children. A survey of 430 cases. Cancer *30*:459, 1972.

Tumors of the Mediastinum

Heimburger, I. L., and Battersby, J. S.: Primary mediastinal tumors of childhood. J. Thorac. Cardiovasc. Surg. *50*:92, 1965.

Pachter, M. R., and Lattes, R.: Mesenchymal tumors of the mediastinum. Cancer *16*:74; 95; 108, 1963.

Schantz, A., Sewall, W., and Castleman, B.: Mediastinal germinoma. A study of 21 cases with an excellent prognosis. Cancer *30*:1189, 1972.

Talerman, A., and Amigo, A.: Thymoma associated with aregenerative and aplastic anemia in a five-year-old child. Cancer *21*:1212, 1968.

Tung, K. S. K., and McCormack, L. J.: Angiomatous lymphoid hamartoma. Report of five cases with a review of the literature. Cancer *20*:525, 1967.

Tumors of the Heart

Fine, G., and Morales, A.: Mesothelioma of the atrioventricular node. Arch. Path. *92*:402, 1971.

Prichard, R. W.: Tumors of the heart. Review of the subject and report of one hundred and fifty cases. A.M.A. Arch. Path. *51*:98, 1951.

Reddy, J. K., Schimke, R. N., Chang, C. H. J., Svoboda, D. J., Slaven, J., and Therou, L.: Beckwith-Wiedemann syndrome. Wilms' tumor, cardiac hamartoma, persistent visceromegaly, and glomeruloneogenesis in a 2-year-old boy. Arch. Path. *94*:523, 1972.

Tumors of the Larynx

Ferguson, C. F., and Flake, C. G.: Subglottic hemangioma as a cause of respiratory obstruction in infants. Ann. Otol. *70*:1095, 1961.

Gibbs, N. M., Taylor, M., and Young, A.: Von Recklinghausen's disease in the larynx and trachea of an infant. J. Laryng. *71*:626, 1957.

Norris, C. M., and Peale, A. R.: Sarcoma of the larynx. Ann. Otol. *70*:894, 1961.

Walsh, T. E., and Beamer, P. R.: Epidermoid carcinoma of the larynx occurring in two children with papilloma of the larynx. Laryngoscope *60*:1110, 1950.

Tumors of the Trachea, Bronchi and Lungs

Anderson, A. E., Buechner, H. A., Yager, I., and Ziskind, M. M.: Bronchogenic carcinoma in young men. Am. J. Med. *16*:404, 1954.

Arean, V. M., and Wheat, M. W., Jr.: Sclerosing hemangiomas of the lung. A case report and review of the literature. Am. Rev. Resp. Dis. *85*:261, 1962.

Condon, V. R., and Phillips, E. W.: Bronchial adenoma in children. A review of the literature and report of three cases. Am. J. Roentgenol. *88*:543, 1962.

Giampalmo, A.: The arteriovenous angiomatosis of the lung with hypoxaemia. Acta Med. Scand. *139*(Suppl. 248):1, 1950.

Guida, P. M., Fulcher, T., and Moore, S. W.: Leiomyoma of the lung. Report of a case. J. Thorac. Cardiovasc. Surg. *49*:1058, 1965.

Moore, R. L., and Lattes, R.: Papillomatosis of larynx and bronchi. Case report with 34-year follow-up. Cancer *12*:117, 1959.

Webb, W. R., and Hare, W. V.: Primary fibrosarcoma of the bronchus. Am. Rev. Resp. Dis. *84*:881, 1961.

Tumors of the Gastrointestinal Tract

Canby, J. P., and Mehlop, F. H.: Ulcerative colitis in children. Am. J. Gastroent. *42*:66, 1964.

Capitanio, M. A., and Kirkpatrick, J. A.: Lymphoid hyperplasia of the colon in children. Roentgen observations. Radiology *94*:323, 1970.

Field, J. L., Adamson, L. F., and Stoeckle, H. E.: Review of carcinoids in children. Functioning carcinoids in a 15-year-old male. Pediatrics *29*:953, 1962.

Horn, R. C., Jr., Payne, W. A., and Fine, G.: The Peutz-Jeghers syndrome (gastrointestinal polyposis with mucocutaneous pigmentation): Report of a case terminating with disseminated gastrointestinal cancer. Arch. Path. *76*:29, 1963.

McKusick, V. A.: Genetic factors in intestinal polyposis. J.A.M.A. *182*:271, 1962.

Michaels, D. L., Go, S., Humbert, J. R., Dubois, R. S., Stewart, J. M., and Ellis, E. F.: Intestinal nodular hyperplasia, hypogammaglobulinemia, and hematologic abnormalities in a child with a ring 18 chromosome. J. Pediatr. *79*:80, 1971.

Middelkamp, J. N., and Haffner, H.: Carcinoma of the colon in children. Pediatrics *32*:558, 1963.

Roth, S. I., and Helwig, E. B.: Juvenile polyps of the colon and rectum. Cancer *16*:468, 1963.

Wafne, A.: Gardner's syndrome. *In* Lynch, H. T. (ed.): Skin, Heredity, and Malignant Neoplasms. Flushing, New York, Medical Examination Publishing Co., Inc., 1972.

Tumors of the Liver

Edmondson, H. A.: Differential diagnosis of tumors and tumorlike lesions of liver in infancy and childhood. A.M.A. Am. J. Dis. Child. *91*:168, 1956.

Finklestein, J. Z., Higgins, G. R., Faust, J., and Karon, M.: Serum fetoprotein and malignancy in children. Cancer *30*:80, 1972.

Meadows, A. T., Naiman, J. L., and Valdes-Dapena, M.: Hepatoma associated with androgen therapy for aplastic anemia. J. Pediatr. *84*:109, 1974.

Misugi, K., Okajima, H., Misugi, N., and Newton, W. A., Jr.: Classification of primary malignant tumors of liver in infancy and childhood. Cancer *20*:1760, 1967.

Murthy, A. S. K., Vawter, G. F., Kopito, L., and Rossen, E.: Biochemical studies on liver tumors of children. Arch. Path. *96*:48, 1973.

Nikaidoh, H., Boggs, J., and Swenson, D.: Liver tumors in infants and children. Clinical and pathological analysis of 22 cases. Arch. Surg. *101*:245, 1970.

Stanley, R. J., Dehner, L. P., and Hesker, A. E.: Primary malignant mesenchymal tumors (mesenchymoma) of the liver in childhood. An angiographic-pathologic study of three cases. Cancer *32*:973, 1973.

Whelan, T. J., Jr., Baugh, J. H., and Chandor, S.: Focal nodular hyperplasia of the liver. Ann. Surg. *177*:150, 1973.

Tumors of the Spleen

Berge, Th.: Splenoma. Acta Path. Microbiol. Scand. *63*:333, 1965.

Griscom, N. T.: Huge splenic cysts. Am. J. Dis. Child. *109*:224, 1965.

Wexler, L., and Abrams, H. L.: Hamartoma of the spleen. Angiographic observations. Am. J. Roentgenol. *92*:1150, 1964.

Tumors of the Pancreas

Cathcart, R. S., III, Webb, C. M., and Othersen, H. B., Jr.: Zollinger-Ellison syndrome in a seven-year-old boy. A case report. Surgery *66*:401, 1969.

Gundersen, A. E., and Janis, J. F.: Pancreatic cystadenoma in childhood. Report of a case. J. Pediatr. Surg. *4*:478, 1969.

Rimoin, D. L., and Schimke, R. N.: Genetic Disorders of the Endocrine Glands. St. Louis, The C. V. Mosby Co., 1971.

Tsukimoto, I., Watanabe, K., Lin, J-B., and Nakajuvia, T.: Pancreatic carcinoma in children in Japan. Cancer *31*:1203, 1973.

Tumors of the Kidney

Bogdan, R., Taylor, D. E. M., and Mostofi, F. K.: Leiomyomatous hamartoma of the kidney. A clinical and pathologic analysis of 20 cases from the Kidney Tumor Registry. Cancer *31*:462, 1973.

Cassady, J. R., Tefft, M., Filler, R. M., Jaffe, N., and Hellman, S.: Considerations in the radiation therapy of Wilms' tumor. Cancer *32*:598, 1973.

D'Angio, G. J.: Management of children with Wilms' tumor. Cancer *30*:1528, 1972.

Filippi, G., and McKusick, V. A.: The Beckwith-Wiedemann syndrome (the exomphalus-macroglossia-gigantism syndrome). Report of two cases and review of the literature. Medicine *49*:279, 1970.

Fu, Y-S., and Kay, S.: Congenital mesoblastic nephroma and its recurrence. An ultrastructural observation. Arch. Path. *96*:66, 1973.

Margolis, L. W., Smith, W. B., Wara, W. M., Kushner, J. H., and De Lorimer, A. A.: Wilms' tumor—An interdisciplinary treatment program with and without Dactinomycin. Cancer *32*:618, 1973.

Pratt-Thomas, H. R., Spicer, S. S., Upshur, J. K., and Greene, W. B.: Carcinoma of the kidney in a 15-year-old boy. Unusual histologic features with formation of microvilli. Cancer *31*:719, 1973.

Price, E. B., Jr., and Mostofi, F. K.: Symptomatic angiomyolipoma of the kidney. Cancer *18*:761, 1965.

Tumors of the Adrenal

Bray, P. F., Ziter, F. A., Lahey, M. E., and Myers, G. G.: The coincidence of neuroblastoma and acute cerebellar encephalopathy. J. Pediatr. *75*:983, 1969.

Evans, A. E., D'Angio, G. J., and Randolph, J.: A proposed staging for children with neuroblastoma. Children's Cancer Study Group A. Cancer *27*:374, 1971.

Konrad, P. N., Singher, L. J., and Neerhout, R. C.: Late death from neuroblastoma. J. Pediatr. *82*:80, 1973.

Stella, J. G., Schweisguth, O., and Schlienger, M.: Neuroblastoma. A study of 144 cases treated in the Institut Gustave-Roussy over a period of 7 years. Am. J. Roentgenol. *108*:324, 1970.

Voorhess, M. L.: Neuroblastoma with normal urinary catecholamine excretion. J. Pediatr. *78*:680, 1971.

Other Retroperitoneal Tumors

Conklin, J., and Abell, M. R.: Germ cell neoplasms of sacrococcygeal region. Cancer *20*:2105, 1967.

Donnellan, W. A., and Swenson, O.: Benign and malignant sacrococcygeal teratomas. Surgery *64*:834, 1968.

Spark, R. B., Yakovac, W. C., and Wagget, J.: Retractile sclerosing mesenteritis. Case report. Clin. Pediatr. *10*:119, 1971.

Wolff, M., Santiago, H., and Duby, M. M.: Delayed distant metastasis from a subcutaneous sacrococcygeal ependymoma. Case report, with tissue culture, ultrastructural observations, and review of the literature. Cancer *30*:1046, 1972.

Tumors of the Bladder and Prostate

Tefft, M., and Jaffe, N.: Sarcoma of the bladder and prostate in children. Rationale for the role of radiation therapy based on a review of the literature and a report of fourteen additional patients. Cancer *32*:1161, 1973.

Tumors of the Testis and Paratesticular Structures

Abell, M. R., and Holtz, F.: Testicular neoplasms in infants and children. I. Tumors of germ cell origin. Cancer *16*:965, 1963.

Holtz, F., and Abell, M. R.: Testicular neoplasms in infants and children. II. Tumors of non-germ cell origin. Cancer *16*:982, 1963.

Mostofi, F. K.: Testicular tumors. Epidemiologic, etiologic and pathologic features. Cancer *32*:1186, 1973.

Pierce, G. B., Bullock, W. K., and Huntington, R. W., Jr.: Yolk sac tumors of the testis. Cancer *25*:644, 1970.

Tumors of the Ovary

Asadourian, L. A., and Taylor, H. B.: Dysgerminoma. An analysis of 105 cases. Obstet. Gynec. *33*:370, 1969.

Breen, J. L., and Neubecker, R. D.: Ovarian malignancy in children, with special reference to the germ-cell tumors. Ann. New York Acad. Sc. *142*:658, 1967.

Chalvardjian, A., and Scully, R. E.: Sclerosing stromal tumors of the ovary. Cancer *31*:664, 1973.

Favara, B. E., and Franciosi, R. A.: Ovarian teratoma and neuroglial implants on the peritoneum. Cancer *31*:678, 1973.

Finklestein, J. Z., Higgins, G. R., Faust, J., and Karon, M.: Serum fetoprotein and malignancy in children. Cancer *30*:80, 1972.

Huntington, R. W., Jr., and Bullock, W. K.: Yolk sac tumors of the ovary. Cancer *25*:1357, 1970.

Morris, J. McL., and Scully, R. E.: Endocrine Pathology of the Ovary. St. Louis, The C. V. Mosby Co., 1958.

Scully, R. E.: Sex cord tumor with annular tubules. A distinctive ovarian tumor of the Peutz-Jeghers syndrome. Cancer *25*:1107, 1970.

Wisniewski, M., and Deppisch, L. M.: Solid teratomas of the ovary. Cancer *32*:440, 1973.

Tumors Associated with Dysgenetic Gonads

Scully, R. E.: Gonadoblastoma. A review of 74 cases. Cancer *25*:1340, 1970.

Tumors of the Vagina and Uterus

Allyn, D. L., Silverberg, S. G., and Salzberg, A. M.: Endodermal sinus tumor of the vagina. Report of a case with 7-year survival and literature review of so-called "mesonephromas." Cancer *27*:1231, 1971.

Borglin, N. E., and Selander, P.: Hymenal polyps in newborn infants. Acta Paediatr., Suppl. *135*:28, 1962.

Greenwald, P., Barlow, J. J., Nasca, P. C., and Burnett, W. S.: Vaginal cancer after maternal treatment with synthetic estrogens. New Engl. J. Med. *285*:390, 1971.

Huffman, J. W.: The Gynecology of Childhood and Adolescence. Philadelphia, W. B. Saunders Company, 1968.

Talerman, A.: Sarcoma botryoides presenting as a polyp on the labium majus. Cancer *32*:994, 1973.

Tumors of Vascular Origin

Bill, A. H., Jr., and Sumner, D. S.: A unified concept of lymphangioma and cystic hygroma. Surg. Gynec. Obstet. *120*:79, 1965.

Dabska, M.: Malignant endovascular papillary angioendothelioma of the skin in childhood. Clinicopathologic study of 6 cases. Cancer *24*:503, 1969.

Fost, N. C., and Esterly, N. B.: Successful treatment of juvenile hemangiomas with prednisone. J. Pediatr. *72*:351, 1968.

Najman, E., Fabecic-Sabadi, V., and Temmer, B.: Lymphangioma in the inguinal region with cystic lymphangiomatosis of bone. J. Pediatr. *71*:561, 1967.

Stern, L., Ramos, A. D., and Wiglesworth, F. W.: Congestive heart failure secondary to cerebral arteriovenous aneurysm in the newborn infant. Am. J. Dis. Child. *115*:581, 1968.

Tumors of the Skin and Skin Appendages

Forbis, R., Jr., and Helwig, E. B.: Pilomatrixoma (calcifying epithelioma). Arch. Dermat. *83*:606, 1961.

Gorlin, R. J., and Sedano, H. O.: The multiple nevoid basal cell carcinoma syndrome revisited. *In* Lynch, H. T. (ed.): Skin, Heredity, and Malignant Neoplasms. Flushing, New York, Medical Examination Publishing Co., Inc., 1972.

Lerman, R. I., Murray, D., O'Hara, J. M., Booher, R. J., and Foote, F. W., Jr.: Malignant melanoma of childhood. A clinicopathologic study and a report of 12 cases. Cancer *25*:436, 1970.

Skov-Jensen, T., Hastrup, J., and Lambrethsen, E.: Malignant melanoma in children. Cancer *19*:620, 1966.

Slaughter, J. C., Hardman, J. M., Kempe, L. G., and Earle, K. M.: Neurocutaneous melanosis and leptomeningeal melanomatosis in children. Arch. Path. *88*:298, 1969.

Tumors of Soft Tissues

Chung, E. B., and Enzinger, F. M.: Benign lipoblastomatosis. An analysis of 35 cases. Cancer *32*:482, 1973.

Dehner, L. P., Enzinger, F. M., and Font, R. L.: Fetal rhabdomyoma. An analysis of nine cases. Cancer *30*:160, 1972.

Enzinger, F. M.: Fibrous hamartoma of infancy. Cancer *18*:241, 1965.

Lafferty, F. W., Reynolds, E. S., and Pearson, D. H.: Tumoral calcinosis. A metabolic disease of obscure etiology. Am. J. Med. *38*:105, 1965.

Moscovic, E. A., and Azar, H. A.: Multiple granular cell tumors ("myoblastomas"). Case report with electron microscopic observations and review of the literature. Cancer *20*:2032, 1967.

Stout, A. P.: Juvenile fibromatoses. Cancer *7*:953, 1954.

Stout, A. P., and Lattes, R.: Tumors of the Soft Tissues. Second Series, Fascicle I. Washington, D.C., Armed Forces Institute of Pathology, 1967.

Tumors of Nerve Sheath Origin

Fienman, N. L., and Yakovac, W. C.: Neurofibromatosis in childhood. J. Pediatr. *76*:339, 1970.

Klecker, R. L., and Roth, J. B.: Visceral neurofibromatosis and hypertension in childhood. Pediatrics *53*:417, 1974.

Sarcomas of Soft Tissues

Brasfield, R. D., and Das Gupta, T. K.: Von Recklinghausen's

disease: A clinicopathological study. Ann. Surg. *175*:86, 1972.
Enzinger, F. M., and Shiraki, M.: Alveolar rhabdomyosarcoma. An analysis of 110 cases. Cancer *24*:18, 1969.
Jaffe, N., Filler, R. M., Farber, S., Traggis, D. G., Vawter, G. F., Tefft, M., and Murray, J. E.: Rhabdomyosarcoma in children. Improved outlook with a multidisciplinary approach. Am. J. Surg. *125*:482, 1973.
Lieberman, P. H., Foote, F. W., Jr., Stewart, F. W., and Berg, J. W.: Alveolar soft-part sarcoma. J.A.M.A. *198*:1047, 1966.
Mackenzie, D. H.: Synovial sarcoma. A review of 58 cases. Cancer *19*:169, 1966.
Soule, E. H., and Enriquez, P.: Atypical fibrous histiocytoma, malignant fibrous histiocytoma, malignant histiocytoma, and epithelioid sarcoma. A comparative study of 65 tumors. Cancer *30*:128, 1972.
Soule, E. H., Mahour, G. H., Mills, S. D., and Lynn, H. B.: Soft tissue sarcomas of infants and children: A clinicopathologic study of 135 cases. Mayo Clin. Proc. *43*:313, 1968.
Sutow, W. W., Sullivan, M. P., Ried, H. L., Taylor, H. G., and Griffith, K. M.: Prognosis in childhood rhabdomyosarcoma. Cancer *25*:1384, 1970.
Woodruff, J. M., Chernik, N. L., Smith, M. C., Millett, W. B., and Foote, F. W., Jr.: Peripheral nerve tumors with rhabdomyosarcomatous differentiation (malignant "Triton" tumors). Cancer *32*:426, 1973.

Tumors of Bone

GENERAL

Aegerter, E., and Kirkpatrick, J. A., Jr.: Orthopedic Diseases. 3rd ed. Philadelphia, W. B. Saunders Company, 1968.
Dahlin, D. C.: Bone Tumors. 2nd ed. Springfield, Ill., Charles C Thomas, 1970.
Lichtenstein, L.: Bone Tumors. 4th ed. St. Louis, The C. V. Mosby Co., 1972.

BENIGN TUMORS

Abrams, A. M., Melrose, R. J., and Howell, F. V.: Adenoameloblastoma. A clinical pathologic study of ten new cases. Cancer *22*:175, 1968.
Allen, M. S., Jr., Harrison, W., and Jahrsdoerfer, R. A.: "Retinal anlage" tumors. Melanotic progonoma, melanotic adamantinoma, pigmented epulis, melanotic neuroectodermal tumor of infancy, benign melanotic tumor of infancy. Am. J. Clin. Path. *51*:309, 1969.
Borello, E. D., and Gorlin, R. J.: Melanotic neuroectodermal tumor of infancy—A neoplasm of neural crest origin. Report of a case associated with high urinary excretion of vanilmandelic acid. Cancer *19*:196, 1966.
Dehner, L. P.: Tumors of the mandible and maxilla in children. I. Clinicopathologic study of 46 histologically benign lesions. Cancer *31*:364, 1973.
Hamner, J. E., III., and Ketcham, A. S.: Cherubism: An analysis of treatment. Cancer *23*:1133, 1969.
Rahimi, A., Beabout, J. W., Ivins, J. C., and Dahlin, D. C.: Chondromyxoid fibroma: A clinicopathologic study of 76 cases. Cancer *30*:726, 1972.
Sapp, J. P.: Ultrastructure and histogenesis of peripheral giant cell reparative granuloma of the jaws. Cancer *30*:1119, 1972.

MALIGNANT TUMORS

Hutter, R. V. P., Foote, F. W., Jr., Francis, K. C., and Sherman, R. S.: Primitive multipotential primary sarcoma of bone. Cancer *19*:1, 1966.
Jaffe, N., Farber, S., Traggis, D., Geiser, C., Kim, B. S., Das, L., Frauenberger, G., Djerassi, I., and Cassady, J. R.: Favorable response of metastatic osteogenic sarcoma to pulse high-dose methotrexate with citrovorum rescue and radiation therapy. Cancer *31*:1367, 1973.
Maeda, K., Abesamis, C. M., Kuhn, L. M., and Hyun, B. H.: Multiple myeloma in childhood: Report of a case with breast tumors as a presenting manifestation. Am. J. Clin. Path. *60*:552, 1973.
Rosen, G., Wollner, N., Tan, C., Wu, S. J., Hajdu, S. I., Cham, W., D'Angio, G. J., and Murphy, M. L.: Disease-free survival in children with Ewing's sarcoma treated with radiation therapy and adjuvant four-drug sequential chemotherapy. Cancer *33*:384, 1974.

26

UNCLASSIFIED DISEASES

SUDDEN UNEXPECTED DEATH IN INFANCY

(Crib Death, Cot Death)

As other causes for postneonatal deaths of infants have diminished, particularly in more medically sophisticated countries, sudden unexpected death in infancy has become an increasingly prominent public health problem. There are now estimated to be about 10,000 crib deaths annually in the United States.

The incidence of crib death varies remarkably little throughout the world. Figures range from 1.2/1000 livebirths in a United States rural area and small middle class community to 3.1/1000 livebirths in a typical large city. In Ireland the rate is reported to be 2.5 and in East Germany 2.6/1000 livebirths.

The now generally accepted definition of crib death was agreed upon at the Second International Conference on Causes of Sudden Death in Infants. It is "the sudden and unexpected death of an infant who was either well or almost well prior to death and whose death remains unexplained after the performance of an adequate autopsy." If this definition is not strictly adhered to, the issue becomes clouded, since at least 15 per cent of sudden unexpected infant deaths will be found due to lesions which are disclosed only by necropsy.

Clinically, little is known about the manner of death. Most of these infants die at home, in the night and unobserved. Rarely, however, an infant is actually being watched at the time of death; as the event is described by those who have been present, the otherwise apparently healthy infant suddenly turns blue, stops breathing, and becomes limp. There is no cry and no struggle.

Most crib deaths involve infants 2 to 4 months of age; few occur in infants more than 6 months of age. Disproportionate numbers have been born prematurely, and more males than females are affected. The majority have had trivial symptoms, such as a cold, in the day or days preceding death; position in sleep seems to be irrelevant.

There is little difference in the rate of occurrence of crib deaths between summer and winter months in subtropical and temperate climates; in parts of the world where seasonal temperature differences are great, however, far more deaths occur during the winter than the summer. This observation has led to the suspicion that cold weather may be in some way implicated. A few observers have noted a higher incidence on weekends than on weekdays. It is generally agreed that most crib deaths occur between midnight and 9 o'clock in the morning, suggesting that a substantial period of sleep may be part of the ultimate mechanism.

Social and economic factors in the background of the infant are of some importance. Children of minority groups and lower socioeconomic classes, wherever they may be, consistently experience more crib deaths than those of the well-to-do. This is true of the blacks of Philadelphia and New York City, of the immigrants from India and Ireland living in England, and of the American Indians in Seattle. There is a higher rate among illegitimately born children than among those with legal fathers. The homes of affected infants are often overcrowded; many are foster homes. The mothers are, as a rule, younger than those of unaffected infants and are of significantly higher parity. The general standard of maternal care is often poor, and affected families visit pre- and postnatal clinics less frequently than do other families.

Deaths of this type do recur within families; the rate among siblings of affected infants is four to seven times that for the population at large; the data, however, do not suggest as yet any coherent mendelian interpretation.

There appear to be "near-misses," infants within the susceptible age who almost die, suddenly and unexpectedly, but whose lives are apparently saved by timely intervention. Various resuscitative measures have reportedly been successful, including different forms of tactile stimulation as well as mouth-to-mouth breathing. Some infants thus rescued go on to live normal lives, whereas others succumb to similar episodes a few days after the first. Detailed medical investigation of the survivors usually fails to reveal any abnormality.

The mechanism of sudden infant death is unknown. Some theories held in the past have been disproved, such as that these deaths were due to accidental suffocation by bed clothing, to hypoparathyroidism, or to cervical spinal epidural hemorrhage. The consensus now is that this type of death represents the instantaneous interruption of some basic physiologic function, and great interest has been expressed in the possibility of a sudden malfunction of central control for respiration and/or cardiac action, resulting in apnea and/or extreme bradycardia.

If such central failure is responsible, it is likely that there are predisposing factors which make the infant unusually vulnerable. There are morphologic, virologic and immunologic evidences of viral infection in a significant number of these infants. Sleep may be another predisposing factor, since it depresses both respiratory and cardiac activity.

Recurrent episodes of spontaneous protracted sleep-induced apnea have now been shown to occur in otherwise well infants. Such episodes have been established as preceding some instances of typical sudden death; in at least two such instances autopsies revealed no disease process which could have caused the death. In another study, histologic studies of the walls of small pulmonary arteries of a series of affected infants showed thickening similar to that seen in the vessels of young children who had lived at a high altitude, suggesting that the infants had been subjected to chronic hypoxia. Accordingly, apneic episodes may be responsible for death in some instances of crib death; a number of research projects are currently in progress to explore that possibility.

Two other current hypotheses are worthy of mention: One is that these infants are obligate nose-breathers who die during an upper respiratory infection because their nasal passages are occluded, and they are unable to breath through their mouths. The other thesis attributes death to a sudden spasm of the larynx. There is as yet no substantial evidence to support either of these views.

Physicians must be concerned about their responsibilities to the families of infants who die suddenly and unexpectedly. The feelings of loss on the part of parents and their concern that they have at least partial responsibility for the death of their child may persist for a long time and cause them immeasurable unhappiness. The pediatrician or family physician has an obligation to investigate each episode as thoroughly as possible, including seeing that an adequate necropsy is performed, and then, in the typical instance, of assuring the parents that nothing they did or did not do was in any way responsible for their infant's death. Parent groups* have done much to alleviate this suffering on the part of parents through personal contacts and through the dissemination of educational literature.

MARIE VALDES-DAPENA

INFORMATION FOR PARENTS

Facts About Sudden Infant Death Syndrome. U.S. Department of Health, Education, and Welfare, Public Health Service, DHEW Publication No. (NIH)72-225. Bethesda, Maryland, National Institutes of Health, 1972.

GENERAL

Bergman, A., Beckwith, J. B., and Ray, C. G.: Sudden Infant Death Syndrome. The Proceedings of the Second International Conference on Causes of Sudden Death in Infants, Seattle, Washington, February, 1969. Seattle, University of Washington Press, 1970.

Frogatt, P., Lynas, M. A., and Marshall, T. K.: Sudden unexpected death in infants ("cot death"). Report of a collaborative study in Northern Ireland. Ulster Med. J. *40*:116, 1971.

Kraus, J. F., and Borhani, N. O.: Post-neonatal sudden unexplained death in California, a cohort study. Am. J. Epidemiol. *95*:497–510, 1972.

Steinschneider, A. L.: Prolonged apnea and the sudden infant death syndrome: Clinical and laboratory observations. Pediatrics *50*:646–654, 1972.

Urquhart, G. E. D., and Grist, N. R.: Virological studies of sudden, unexplained infant deaths in Glasgow 1967–70. J. Clin. Path. *25*:443, 1972.

Valdes-Dapena, M. A.: Sudden and unexpected death in infancy: A review of the world literature 1954–1966. Pediatrics *39*:123, 1967.

**Addresses of Parent Groups*

The National Foundation for Sudden Infant Death, Inc., 1501 Broadway, New York, N.Y. 10036

The Guild for Infant Survival, 6822 Brompton Road, Baltimore, Md. 21207

AMYLOIDOSIS

Amyloidosis is much less common in children than in adults. Its pathogenesis remains obscure. Electron microscopic, immunoelectrophoretic and biochemical studies suggest that amyloid consists of fine fibrils of protein produced by reticuloendothelial cells and deposited in a ground substance composed of abnormal mucopolysaccharides. When the deposition of amyloid is advanced, involved organs become enlarged, rubbery and pale. Liver, spleen, kidneys, adrenals, heart and gastrointestinal tract are the most frequent sites of deposition, but fibrils may be found in any organ, including the media and adventitia (sometimes the intima) of blood vessels. Several tests exist for recognition of amyloidosis, one of which involves the intravenous injection of Congo red; if 60 per cent or more of dye is removed rapidly from the circulation, the result is considered positive, but final diagnosis must rest on biopsy of involved tissue, in which such stains as Congo red produce with amyloid a green birefringence seen with the polarizing microscope.

Classifications of amyloidosis have been based on so-called types of amyloid, but the disorder is perhaps best categorized clinically as primary or secondary.

Amyloidosis not accompanying other diseases is logically, if perhaps temporarily, called *primary* and includes several rare heredofamilial disorders. *Familial amyloidosis with polyneuropathy* produces peripheral neuropathy, trophic skin lesions, especially of the lower extremities, vitreous opacities, and occasionally hepatosplenomegaly. Inheritance is dominant. The condition affects young adults and, only rarely, children. *Familial Mediterranean fever* is found primarily in ethnic groups originating from the Mediterranean area. It is included among the periodic diseases. Clinically there are bouts of fever and of abdominal or chest pain and recurrent joint pains; ultimately renal amyloidosis gives rise to proteinuria, the nephrotic syndrome and kidney failure. Inheritance is autosomal recessive. A history of family members having repeated laparotomies because of recurrent abdominal pain is not unusual. Rectal or gingival biopsy may permit a diagnosis of amyloidosis. Because amyloid may be found very early in association with familial Mediterranean fever, it is not felt to be a secondary phenomenon.

Other conditions in which amyloidosis may be "primary" include *heredofamilial urticaria, deafness and neuropathy, familial cutaneous amyloidosis* and *familial amyloid-producing thyroid carcinoma.*

Secondary amyloidosis was more common when antibiotic therapy was not available for such chronic diseases as osteomyelitis, bronchiectasis and tuberculosis. It has been reported also to complicate rheumatoid arthritis, ulcerative colitis and regional ileitis. It occurs in adults with multiple myeloma and Hodgkin's disease, but rarely in children with such disorders.

There is no treatment at present for the conditions associated with primary amyloidosis. Treatment of secondary amyloidosis depends on control of the basic disorder. It has been suggested that corticosteroids may augment amyloid formation, but this is not proved.

SYDNEY S. GELLIS

Cohen, A. S.: Amyloidosis. New Engl. J. Med. *277*:522, 528, 628, 1967.

Heller, H., Sohar, E., Gafni, J., and Heller, J.: Amyloidosis in familial Mediterranean fever: An independent genetically determined character. Arch. Intern. Med. *107*:539, 1961.

Muckle, T. J., and Wells, M.: Urticaria, deafness and amyloidosis: New heredo-familial syndrome. Quart. J. Med. *31*:235, 1962.

Sagher, F., and Shannon, J.: Amyloidosis cutis: Familial occurrence in three generations. Arch. Derm. *87*:171, 1963.

SARCOIDOSIS

Sarcoidosis, a chronic, multisystem disease of obscure origin, occurs in children, but is uncommon below the age of 10 years. Weight loss, fever, abdominal pain and anorexia are the most frequent of an otherwise variable pattern of signs and symptoms related to the organs and tissues involved.

The *pathologic abnormalities* noted in sarcoidosis simulate those observed in chronic granulomatous diseases, especially tuberculosis. *Mycobacterium tuberculosis* has not been demonstrated in the lesions, and most patients with sarcoidosis do not have dermal reactions to tuberculin.

The *epidemiology* is obscure. Blacks are more commonly affected than Caucasians, and most patients, regardless of race, have come from rural communities in the southeastern United States.

The lung is the organ most frequently affected; pulmonary involvement is widely variable in its extent and characteristics, including parenchymal infiltrates, miliary nodules, and hilar and paratracheal lymphadenopathy (Fig. 26–1). Hepatic involvement, skin lesions and uveitis or iritis occur frequently. Uveoparotid fever has been described, with painless swelling of the parotid or salivary glands, fever and uveitis. Multiple cystic lesions in

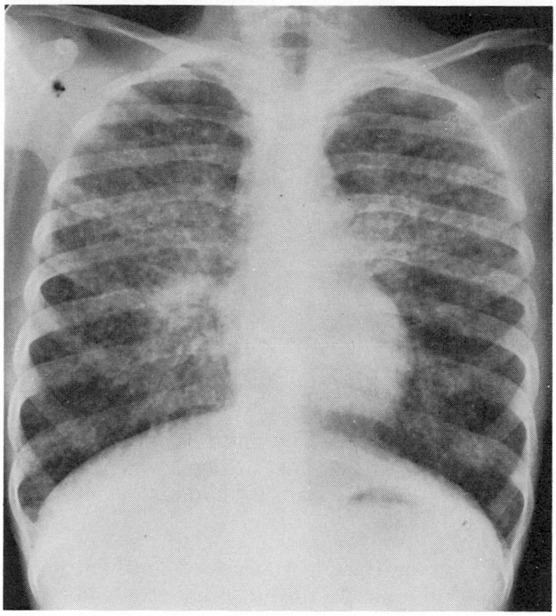

Figure 26–1 *Sarcoidosis in a white girl 10 years of age. Note the widely disseminated peribronchial infiltrations and multiple small nodular densities, the overaeration of the lungs, and the hilar adenopathy.*

the bones of the hands and feet have been noted in some patients, as has disseminated sarcoidosis involving most of the viscera. Characteristic features of the rare cases in children under 1 year of age are arthritis, skin lesions and eye involvement. The arthritis, which can be confused with rheumatoid arthritis, is manifest as large, painless, boggy synovial and tendon sheath effusions with little limitation of motion.

Sarcoidosis is commonly associated with hyperproteinemia, hyperglobulinemia, hypercalcemia, hypercalciuria and eosinophilia.

There are no specific diagnostic tests. The Kveim test, consisting of the formation of a granuloma several weeks after intradermal injection of material from a sarcoid lesion, is positive in the majority of active cases; biopsy of affected areas provides the most valuable diagnostic study.

Owing to its protean manifestations, the *differential diagnosis* of sarcoidosis is extremely broad and includes tuberculosis, the various pulmonary mycoses and inflammatory ocular lesions such as phlyctenular conjunctivitis.

Treatment is symptomatic and supportive. Corticosteroids may suppress the acute manifestations, especially the inflammatory ocular lesions and the hypercalcemia.

The natural history of sarcoidosis in children is not well established. Some cases show spontaneous recovery after a prolonged illness of several months to several years, but others may develop chronic changes, including progressive and obstructive lung disease. Eye involvement may lead to blindness.

FLOYD W. DENNY

Jasper, P. L., and Denny, F. W.: Sarcoidosis in children. J. Pediatr. *73*:499, 1968.
Kendig, E. L.: Disorders of the Respiratory Tract in Children. 2nd ed. Philadelphia, W. B. Saunders Company, 1972, Chap. 45.
Longcope, W. T., and Freiman, D. G.: A Study of sarcoidosis. Medicine *31*:1, 1952.
North, A. F., Fink, C. W., Gibson, W. M., Levinson, J. E., Schuchter, S. L., Howard, W. K., Johnson, N. H., and Harris, C.: Sarcoid arthritis in children. Am. J. Med. *48*:449, 1970.
Proceedings of the International Conference on Sarcoidosis. Am. Rev. Resp. Dis. *84* (part 2), 1961.
Siltzback, L. E.: Sarcoidosis and Mycobacteria. Am. Rev. Resp. Dis. *97*:1, 1968.

THE HISTIOCYSTOSIS SYNDROMES

(Eosinophilic Granuloma of Bone, Schüller-Christian and Letterer-Siwe Syndromes, Reticuloendothelioses)

The histiocytosis syndromes, identified by the foregoing diagnostic terms, present a wide spectrum of clinical pictures in which the underlying common denominator is the development of granulomatous lesions with histiocytic proliferation. The clinical expression appears to be a reactive phenomenon, the triggering mechanism for which is unknown, and may range from an isolated, slow-growing lesion, particularly in the medullary cavity of bone, to aggressive, widely disseminated disease with fatal outcome.

Separate diagnostic terms were originally suggested for the different forms of the disease. The defense for the "unitarian" concept derives from an inductive study of the histology of the various lesions, from the realization that many patients who eventually have generalized disease initially had only a localized lesion, and that an occasional patient will demonstrate the complete sequence of clinical involvement.

Failure to identify the cause of the granulomatous process or the true biologic setting for its development has allowed the unsatisfactory nomenclature to persist. For the moment, therefore, it is reasonable to use the traditional terms, readily acknowledging their arbitrary nature. Hence, "eosinophilic granuloma of bone" is applied to patients with lesions in bone only; "Schüller-Christian syndrome" or "Hand-Schüller-Christian syndrome" to those with chronic, slowly progressing involvement resulting chiefly in symptoms from lesions in bone; and "Letterer-Siwe syndrome" to patients with a pattern of deeper, more rapid, visceral spread, often involving bones as well.

ETIOLOGY. Consideration of the cause of the histiocytosis syndromes must begin by specifying what the disease process *is not.* It is not hereditary or familial. It is not contagious and not transplantable to animals, and no microorganisms have been recovered from mature lesions by standard bacteriologic, fungal or viral isolation techniques. The process is not a true neoplasm, as shown by its potentiality for spontaneous resolution and its heterogeneous cellularity. Present knowledge allows one only to postulate that the granuloma lies in a borderland zone. It represents a response, perhaps because of a special reactivity in the susceptible patient, to a stimulus assumed to be exogenous, stopping short of the development of full malignancy. The role of the host in determining the final picture is suggested by the influence of age (younger patients tend to have more disseminated lesions), by the wide variation in the extent of involvement, and by the consistent predominance of males in each clinical group. In a few infants, skin lesions have been present at birth.

PATHOLOGY. The microscopic picture of the lesions, whether in solitary foci or in disseminated disease, is that of a nodular or spreading infiltration, invariably containing numerous large histiocytes. Accompanying these characteristic cells may be variable numbers of other reactive elements, such as eosinophils, neutrophils and, less characteristically, lymphocytes and plasma cells. There is a tendency for the more rapidly developing and disseminated lesions to be more heavily histiocytic, whereas the isolated lesion in bone is notable for its high eosinophil population. An accurate prognosis cannot be made from the histology alone. The histiocyte may show giant cell formation, and may develop vacuolated cytoplasm. One can occasionally find masses of histiocytes which have become markedly lipidized, for obscure reasons, with greatly increased cholesterol content (especially in bone, dura, thymus and skin), but this does not imply any true relation to the constitutional lipidoses. In involuting phases the lesions are gradually replaced by fibrosis. Proliferative, destructive, xanthomatous and sclerosing features may coexist in the same lesion. In the severely affected child, tissues in all regions of the body may become involved, but marrow, skin, lymph nodes, lung, liver and meninges are the common sites. The pathologic diagnosis of these disorders is, in part, one of exclusion, and it is necessary to correlate the tissue findings with the clinical data before accepting the "idiopathic" nature of the granuloma being studied.

CLINICAL MANIFESTATIONS. The assignment of a patient to a particular category among the histiocytosis syndromes is somewhat arbitrary. It is useful to note, however, that in the majority of affected children there is a natural progression for some months, followed by stabilization of their disease at a certain level. Most of the clinical pictures can be assigned to one of five general categories.

1. About half of the patients have *lesions only in bone.* From one to a dozen or so lytic defects may be present; the skull, legs, spine and pelvis are the areas most commonly involved. In this group the first symptoms typically occur at the age of 4 to 7 years, and consist of bone pain, local swelling or irritability. The process usually subsides within one to two years from the time of onset. Such children will ordinarily be classified as having "eosinophilic granuloma of bone."

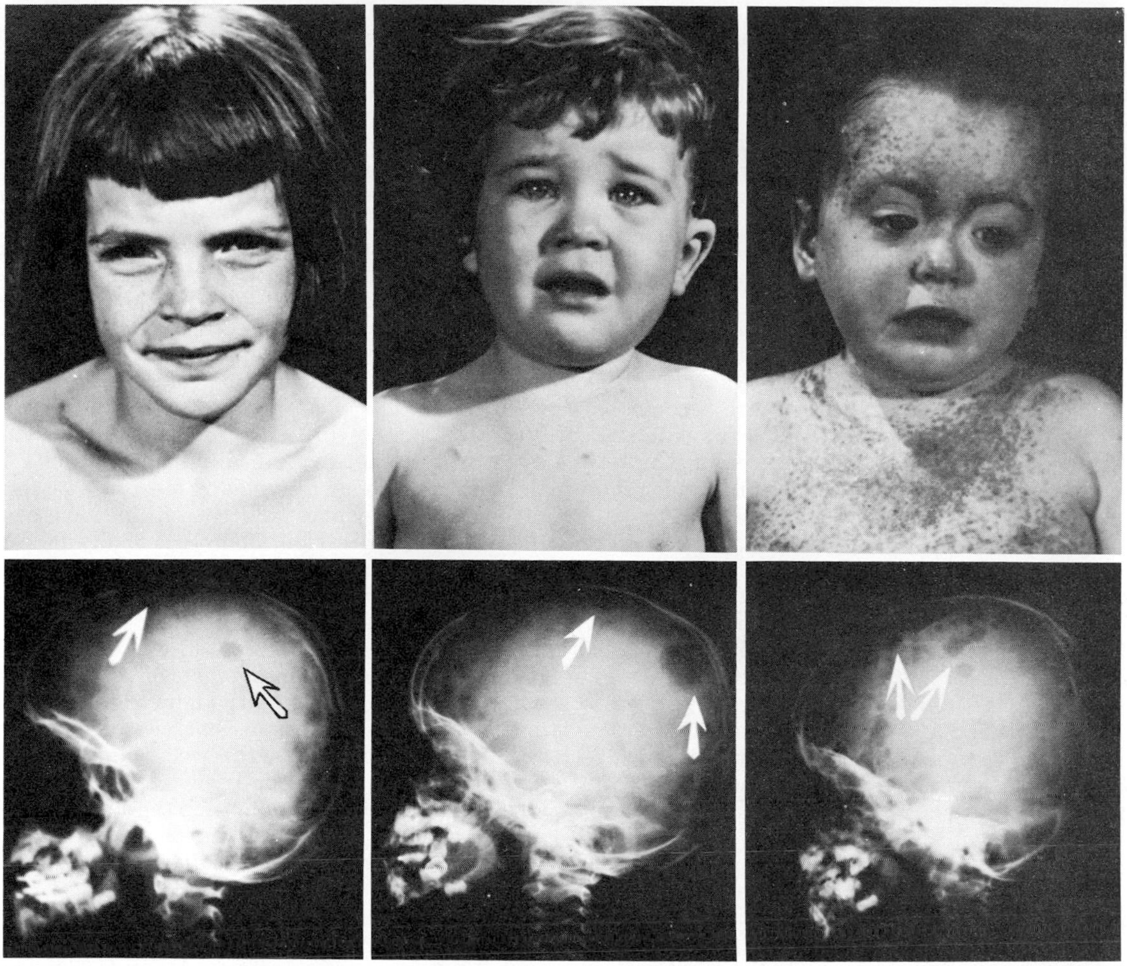

Figure 26–2 Common clinical patterns. Girl on left *did not progress beyond brief involvement with isolated bone lesions which could be categorized as eosinophilic granuloma, and had good recovery.* Girl in middle *had several dozen bone lesions, a papular skin eruption, scalp "seborrhea," stomatitis, vaginitis, pulmonary infiltration and diabetes insipidus. The diagnostic term Schüller-Christian syndrome is applicable here. Her disease responded well to chlorambucil therapy.* Girl on right *had extensive bone disease, plus a febrile course, anemia, severe skin eruption, generalized adenopathy, hepatosplenomegaly, pulmonary infiltration, and a fatal outcome in spite of antitumor chemotherapy. This patient fits the category of Letterer-Siwe syndrome.*

Early biopsies of bone lesions from all three patients showed a similar type of histiocytic granuloma.

2. A second, smaller group, if followed through the full course of the disease, will have *osseous lesions and minor additional involvement,* including anemia, limited eruptions on the skin or mucous membranes, and, infrequently, an invasive process in the pituitary-hypothalamic area which produces diabetes insipidus. This pattern is most common in the child whose illness begins at 2 to 3 years of age. The use of the term "Schüller-Christian syndrome" is appropriate here.

3. A third, more extensive form, which is relatively common, has *osseous lesions and moderate visceral involvement.* These children, who frequently manifest their illness at 1 to 2 years of age, may have papular skin lesions, a seborrhea-like eruption on the scalp and in the ear canals, stomatitis, pulmonary infiltrations, mild general adenopathy, some hepatomegaly, and invasion around the orbits, middle ears and pituitary area. The process usually continues to be active for several years and then may subside spontaneously. Some patients in this group die from complicating infections or from late effects of the intracranial involvement. Almost all these children, when first seen, have extension of the disease beyond the osseous lesions. The problems in nomenclature are demonstrated by such patients, who would be listed as having Schüller-Christian syndrome by some authors. The term "Letterer-Siwe syndrome" is also acceptable here, owing to its implication of a deeper penetration of the pathologic process.

4. The most serious clinical problem occurs in the infant who rapidly exhibits *major visceral involvement.* This pattern, also a common one, characteristically appears during the first year of life. Within a few months there may be significant hepatomegaly and splenomegaly, widespread pulmonary infiltration, adenopathy, marrow failure, fever and debilitating infection. Roentgenograms of the chest may reveal a granular appearance in the pulmonary parenchyma, or an extensive "miliary" type of infiltration. There is a variety of skin

lesions, including a diffuse papular eruption of vesicular nature in the younger patient, a scaly and petechial dermatitis (especially on the forehead and trunk), and a moist, denuded involvement in intertriginous areas. An inflamed and pruritic eruption about the anal and vaginal orifices is common. In the mouth one may find gingival hypertrophy, inflammation, necrosis and retraction, with resultant loss of teeth. In some patients the osseous lesions are demonstrable on the roentgenogram, although they are usually not the source of the first symptoms; in others, osseous lesions as such are not evident, but in biopsy or autopsy studies a diffuse involvement of the medullary cavity may be demonstrated. A fatal outcome is to be expected when this picture becomes advanced, deaths being attributed to exhaustion, toxicity, marrow depletion and septicemia. The term "Letterer-Siwe syndrome" has been used for these patients.

5. Occasional patients have *atypical involvement,* with extreme progression in only one area, such as in the lungs (with cyst formation and/or pneumothorax), cervical lymph nodes or liver. Whenever the familiar osseous lesions are absent or not notable, a more thorough study of the histopathology is needed to rule out other diseases. For example, a number of syndromes of familial reticuloendotheliosis have been described which resemble the Letterer-Siwe syndrome superficially. In these syndromes there are characteristically significant involvement of the central nervous system, including pleocytosis of the spinal fluid, such hematologic abnormalities as leukopenia, lymphocytosis or eosinophilia (with erythrophagocytosis evident in bone marrow and lymph node specimens), alteration of serum globulins, and a rapid, fatal course unaffected by corticosteroids or antitumor therapy.

LABORATORY DATA. There is no diagnostic serologic or immunologic test for these syndromes. Laboratory studies show only the nonspecific effects to be expected because of the organ or tissue involvement. Anemia is common, and leukocytosis may occur; the bone marrow is normal until the histiocytic proliferation has become widespread. Serum protein levels are usually normal, as are those of the serum lipids. The roentgenographic appearance of lesions in bones and lungs, although not completely specific, often provides the first clue to the nature of the disease and allows the progress of the disease to be followed with some accuracy. Biopsy studies are mandatory.

TREATMENT. There is no specific treatment. A number of therapeutic measures suppress the granuloma, but appear to succeed only when favorable host factors are present simultaneously. Individual lesions of bone, troublesome skin eruptions and large lymph nodes are benefited by radiotherapy. This is especially useful for inducing rapid involution of bone lesions which threaten to produce pathologic fractures, as in the spine and femora. Relatively small doses (400 to 600 r at depth) usually suffice. If there is diabetes insipidus, early radiotherapy to the pituitary-hypothalmic area may eliminate interference with nerve tracts before irreversible nerve cell damage occurs. Pitressin replacement therapy is indicated as long as there is evidence of clinical deficit. Radiation therapy to visceral lesions, such as those in the lungs, liver and spleen, is not helpful. Antibacterial agents do not suppress the basic process.

At present, antitumor chemotherapy holds the greatest promise for eventual control of the granulomatous process; clinical investigations are under way in a number of medical centers. Corticosteroids provide useful support, but are not sufficient as the only medication. More definite suppressing action has been observed with the alkylating agents (including nitrogen mustard and cytoxan, but, more specifically, chlorambucil). In the child with bone lesions and moderate visceral involvement they may induce a striking slowing of the clinical progression, and occasionally be considered lifesaving. Unfortunately the patient who has early severe visceral spread of the disease seems to receive only temporary aid. Vinblastine and vincristine are additional medications of definite value. Folic acid antagonists have rarely produced favorable results. Although no single agent, or combination, has been discovered which consistently gives good results, the well planned use of presently available, partially successful drugs is to be encouraged. In addition, these patients receive great assistance from a program of general supportive care, which includes blood transfusions, antibiotic therapy, radiotherapy and orthopedic care as indicated.

Allen C. Crocker

Avery, M. E., McAfee, J. G., and Guild, H. G.: The course and prognosis of reticuloendotheliosis (eosinophilic granuloma, Schüller-Christian disease and Letterer-Siwe disease); A study of forty cases. Am. J. Med. *22*:636, 1957.

Crocker, A. C.: The histiocytosis syndromes. *In* Fitzpatrick, T. B., Arndt, K. A., Clark, W. H., Jr., Eisen, A. Z., Van Scott, E. J., and Vaughan, J. H. (eds.): Dermatology in General Medicine. New York, McGraw-Hill Book Company, 1971, p. 1328.

Crocker, A. C.: The histiocytosis syndromes. *In* Gellis, S. S., and Kagan, B. M. (eds.): Current Pediatric Therapy 6. Philadelphia, W. B. Saunders Company, 1973, p. 375.

Green, W. T., and Farber, S.: "Eosinophilic or solitary granuloma" of bone. J. Bone Joint Surg. *24*:499, 1942.

Miller, D. R.: Familial reticuloendotheliosis: Concurrence of disease in five siblings. Pediatrics *38*:986, 1966.

Oberman, H. A.: A clinicopathologic study of 40 cases and review of the literature on eosinophilic granuloma of bone, Hand-Schüller-Christian disease and Letterer-Siwe disease. Pediatrics *28*:307, 1961.

PROGERIA

(Hutchinson-Gilford Progeria Syndrome)

The Hutchinson-Gilford progeria syndrome has been reported in 60 patients since first described in 1886 by Sir Jonathan Hutchinson. Data are insufficient to verify either an autosomal recessive or autosomal dominant mode of inheritance. It has been frequently diagnosed erroneously in conditions resembling it, (e.g., Cockayne's syndrome, Hallerman-Streiff syndrome) despite a remarkably constant phenotype. Features *always* present once the condition has become apparent are: short stature; weight decrease disproportionate to height; failure to complete sexual maturation; diminished subuctaneous fat; head disproportionately large for face; micrognathia; prominent scalp veins; generalized alopecia; prominent eyes; "plucked-bird appearance"; delayed and abnormal dentition; pyriform thorax; short, dystrophic clavicles; "horse-riding" stance; wide-based, shuffling gait; coxa valga and thin limbs with prominent, stiff joints. Features *frequently* present are: skin which may be thin, taut, dry, wrinkled, brown-spotted in various areas, or "sclerodermatous" over lower abdomen, proximal thighs and buttocks; prominent superficial veins; decreased sweating; absent eyebrows and eyelashes; persistent patent anterior fontanelle; "sculptured," beaked nasal tip; midfacial, nasolabial faint cyanosis; thin lips; protruding ears; absent ear lobes; thin, high-pitched voice; dystrophic nails; progressive radiolucency of terminal phalanges.

Children with progeria are usually considered to be normal as infants but may have findings ("scleroderma," midfacial cyanosis, and "sculptured nose") suggesting the syndrome at birth. Profound growth failure develops during the first year of life. The characteristic facies, alopecia, loss of subcutaneous fat, abnormal posture, stiffness of joints, and bone and skin changes become apparent during the second year. Motor and mental development are normal.

There are no demonstrable abnormalities of thyroid, parathyroid, pituitary or adrenal function. There is insulin resistance, abnormal collagen, increased metabolic rate, and variable abnormalities of serum lipids. Growth hormone responses are normal.

Although progeric patients develop atherosclerosis and die of cardiac or cerebral vascular disease between 7 and 27 years of age, with a median age of 13.4 years at death, many other features (cataracts, presbycusis, presbyopia, arcus senilis, osteoarthritis, or senile personality changes) associated with aging are absent.

F. L. DeBusk

DeBusk, F. L.: The Hutchinson-Gilford progeria syndrome. J. Pediatr. *80*:697, 1972.

Villee, D. B., Nichols, G., Jr., and Talbot, N. B.: Metabolic studies in two boys with classical progeria. Pediatrics *43*:207, 1969.

FAILURE TO THRIVE

The term "failure to thrive" has come to be used for infants and children who, without superficially evident cause, fail to gain and often lose weight. This situation is observed most often in infants, but also occurs later in childhood. It has occurred frequently among institutionalized children, especially those who were retarded.

ETIOLOGY. Most instances of failure to thrive result from psychosocial circumstances, not always apparent, which adversely affect the child's intake, absorption or utilization of food. Emotional deprivation and physical neglect or abuse, including the withholding of food (see Neglect and Abuse of Children, Section 2), are commonly associated. Failure to thrive, with malabsorption, has been reported as unduly frequent among children with autism and adults with schizophrenia. Sometimes the emotional or physical deprivation of the child is related to a physical handicap, such as cerebral palsy or cleft palate, or to difficult behavior owing to temperament (q.v.) or other causes. The syndrome may also result from obscure organic abnormalities, as well as from overt or easily discoverable diseases in which growth failure occurs. For many children who experience a period of failure to thrive with no ascertainable organic or environ-

TABLE 26–1 SOME SUPERFICIALLY OBSCURE CAUSES OF FAILURE TO THRIVE AND SCREENING TESTS FOR THEM

CAUSE	SCREENING TESTS
Environmental	
Inadequate intake of food	History; observation in hospital
Emotional deprivation	History; observation in hospital
Environmental disruptions	History; observation in hospital
Rumination (Section 2)	Observation in hospital
Organic	
Central nervous system abnormalities	Neurologic examination; developmental assessment; transillumination of skull; brain scan
Intestinal malabsorption	Observation in hospital; stool fat
Cystic fibrosis of the pancreas	Sweat test
Intestinal parasites (rarely a cause in temperate climates)	Stool for ova and parasites
Partial cleft palate	Physical examination; observation of feeding
Chronic heart failure	Physical examination; roentgenogram of chest
Endocrine disorders	Construction of growth chart; blood test for thyroid function; films for bone age
Idiopathic hypercalcemia	Serum calcium
Turner syndrome (girls)	Buccal smear
Other chromosomal disorders	Chromosomal analysis in patients with peculiar facies or multisystem defects
Renal insufficiency	Urinalysis; blood urea nitrogen
Renal tubular disorders	Urinalysis; urinary amino acid screen
Chronic infection (usually tuberculous or mycotic)	Tuberculin test; chest roentgenogram; temperature pattern in hospital
Chronic inflammation (e.g., rheumatoid arthritis)	Physical examination
Malignancies (especially of kidney, adrenal, brain)	Roentgenograms of abdomen, chest; intravenous urography; brain scan

mental cause, retrospective analysis indicates the likelihood of psychosocial origin. Table 26–1 lists some of the psychosocial and organic conditions with which failure to thrive has been observed.

CLINICAL MANIFESTATIONS. The clinical picture may be simply failure to gain weight or to grow at the expected rate. More characteristically there are also signs of developmental retardation and of physical and emotional deprivation, such as apathy, poor hygiene, intense eye contact with people, withdrawing behavior, and disorders of food intake which may be manifest as anorexia, voracious appetite or pica. Vomiting, regurgitation, diarrhea and general neuromuscular spasticity or hypotonia may be concurrent.

DIAGNOSIS AND DIFFERENTIAL DIAGNOSIS. Hospitalization for study and treatment provides opportunity for quantitation of factors governing the net caloric intake (food intake, vomiting, stools), and for observation of interactions of the child, especially during feeding and play, with his mother, with health personnel and with other children. Hospitalization frequently leads to dramatic improvement in weight gain and in social responses. This occurrence provides evidence that environmental factors are causative and usually renders unnecessary any exhaustive and expensive search for hidden organic disease.

History-taking by different interviewers at different times is often helpful in turning up psychosocial problems which are inapparent or unexpressed at the initial interview. Information from friends, relatives and neighbors may reveal unsuspected adverse factors in the child's family environment.

Construction and study of a growth chart and of a developmental flow sheet may identify the point in time when the child began to fail to thrive, and may be useful in uncovering the environmental or physical factors responsible. On the other hand, if growth has been steady, though below the expected level (e.g., always just below the third percentile), such diagnoses as constitutional short stature, hypopituitarism or chromosomal abnormality must be considered.

If history and/or physical examination suggest disturbances in any particular organ systems, appropriate diagnostic study is warranted. This should begin with screening tests and proceed in detail only as these are positive. Routine blood counts and urinalyses will serve as screening tests for the hematologic and renal systems. Extensive study to rule out most or all possible underlying organic lesions is justified only if the initial data base (Section 5) has failed to provide clues pointing to a specific environmental or organic etiology; *in addition*, there should be demonstrated failure of a favorable response to hospitalization. It should be noted that children chronically deprived of food may have stools consistent with malabsorption when an adequate dietary intake is initiated. They gain weight, however, and resume a normal stool pattern after some weeks or months. Some organic causes of failure to thrive are listed in Table 26–1.

PREVENTION. Prevention of environmental causes of failure to thrive rests chiefly on the successful application of social measures such as education for parenthood, encouragement of couples to have only as many children as they are economically and emotionally capable of supporting (this may be none for some), discouragement of unwanted or irresponsible parenthood, reduction of social stresses which weaken the family relationship, and creation and maintenance of a social structure which will provide maximum nurturance of infants and children. The role of the physician and other health personnel in prevention of failure to thrive lies in early recognition of the syndrome and of the characteristics and circumstances of parents which may lead to it. These include general immaturity, drug addiction or abuse, irresponsible or antisocial behavior, dislike of children, low tolerance for stress, emotional instability, economic stress, marital discord, single parenthood, and sometimes severe temporary stresses such as family tragedies, which may lead to temporary failure to thrive in an otherwise healthy environment. Early counseling and adequate direct support in the care of the threatened child will often prevent the development of failure to thrive in these situations.

TREATMENT. A temporary change of environment, such as hospitalization for necessary evaluation, may be sufficient to relieve the tension in family patterns of interaction to the extent that, with advice, counseling and support from a social worker or family service agency, adjustments can be made which will ensure adequate care of the child when he returns to his home. If not, temporary or permanent placement in a foster home may be necessary. Identified organic disease should be treated appropriately.

Giulio J. Barbero
R. James McKay

Barbero, G. J., and Shaheen, E.: Environmental failure to thrive: A clinical view. J. Pediatr. *71*:5, 1967.

Smith, C. A., and Berenberg, W.: The concept of failure to thrive. Pediatrics *46*:661, 1970.

27
RADIATION INJURY

The possibility of untoward biologic effects of radiation is of special interest in relation to the child, for these effects may be most serious in growing tissues. By judicious limitation of roentgen procedures during childhood a margin of safety for unavoidable radiation exposure later in life can be preserved.

Ionizing radiation produces injury in the same manner regardless of the type of particle or ray emitted. The variation is quantitative rather than qualitative. Absorption of energy may cause molecules in the path of the radiations to become ionized. In attaining stability these molecules may form substances which alter, temporarily or perhaps permanently, biochemical processes within the cell or its environment. These effects upon cellular structures provide an explanation for the deaths of persons exposed to ionizing radiations, for the death of certain cancer cells treated with roentgen rays, for genetic mutations and for the production of cancer as a late effect of exposure to radiations.

Susceptibility of tissues to roentgen rays is, generally speaking, greater in the more rapidly mitosing and the more undifferentiated cells. Owing to an abundance of this type of tissue in the abdomen, a patient is more likely to have radiation sickness from roentgen therapy to this region than from comparable exposure elsewhere.

DOSAGE FACTORS. Radiation absorption increases with the volume of the child's body exposed, with prolongation of exposure or with an increase in amperage or voltage. Absorption decreases in relation to the effectiveness of filters used and with an increase in distance between the patient and the roentgen tube.

Adverse acute effects of roentgen rays are diminished when the total dose is administered in several exposures separated by sufficient time for recovery from the subclinical effects of each. Repeated exposures may produce pathologic effects not manifest until years later. Some of the chemical changes produced in cells by roentgen rays are irreversible, and may lie dormant until aging, infection, hormonal alterations or further exposure to toxic agents makes them manifest.

The young infant may be more susceptible to the effects of roentgen rays than is the adult. Moreover, even if there are no essential differences in susceptibility, his longer life span provides more time for such changes to develop.

The roentgen dosage from fluoroscopy generally exceeds that required for roentgenograms. A standard chest film, for example, involves about 0.02 rads, whereas chest fluoroscopy, using an old machine, might expose the child to 20 rads—a 1000-fold difference. Roentgen rays in low doses do not have a stimulative action on cells.

EARLY EFFECTS OF IRRADIATION. Exposure of the entire body to 100 roentgens usually produces illness in man. A dose of about 450 roentgens will cause death in 50 per cent of exposed persons. Higher doses can be tolerated if only a part of the body is exposed. Death results within hours to days when the entire body is exposed to the overwhelming dosage of an atomic bomb.

Symptoms of radiation sickness, which vary with the exposure, are malaise, fever, nausea, vomiting and diarrhea. Leukopenia develops rapidly, and in more severe instances thrombocytopenia may appear within a week. When the initial symptoms are not severe, they are followed by a temporary period of well-being. Epilation begins about two weeks after the exposure. The leukopenia increases susceptibility to infection, and the low platelet count predisposes to hemorrhage. When autopsy does not reveal the cause of death, one can only assume that the radiation injury was responsible for lethal "cytochemical changes." If the patient survives for six weeks, death is not likely from these effects of radiation.

Only a small percentage of deaths caused by an atomic explosion can be attributed to radiation effects alone; thermal and blast injuries account for most of them. Traumatic injuries do not heal effectively in persons with radiation sickness.

Therapy for radiation sickness resulting from exposure of the entire body is not very effective. Prophylactic administration of broad-spectrum antibiotics may diminish mortality. Transfusions of stored blood have not reduced the mortality in experimental animals nor altered the bleeding diathesis; transfusion of stored blood is therefore indicated only when the deficiency of red blood cells justifies it.

LATE EFFECTS OF IRRADIATION. Within the decade following the detonations of the atomic bombs in Japan there was a significant rise in the incidence of leukemia in those who were within 1500 meters of the hypocenter (the spot on the ground immediately under the center of an air burst). An increase in leukemia rates has been observed at doses as low as 20 to 49 rads among Hiroshima survivors of all ages. Children under 10 years of age at the time of the bombing were more susceptible to leukemogenesis than were older persons. Those under 10 years when exposed have also exhibited a substantially higher frequency than usual of other cancers when they reached the ages of 16 to 31 years, a possible portent of a still greater excess as the group enters the age period when cancer is more common. There has been an excess of thyroid neoplasia.

In Britain and in the United States, in utero exposures to diagnostic irradiation have been reported to increase the relative risk of death from cancer before 10 years of age by about 50 per cent. No such effect was found among children exposed in utero to the atomic bomb.

Among persons exposed in utero to radiation from the Hiroshima atomic bomb (beginning at 10 to 19 rads) before the 18th week of gestation, small head circumference occurred with excessive frequency. The effect increased in frequency and severity with increasing dose. Mental retardation occurred in those exposed to doses of 50 rads and above, and affected the majority exposed before the 18th week of gestation to 150 rads or more. The observations at low doses are not directly applicable to medical radiology because of the possible influence of (1) neutrons in the Hiroshima explosion and (2) interactions with nutritional deprivation and infection following the bomb explosion.

Complex chromosomal abnormalities are still found in the peripheral lymphocytes of atomic-bomb survivors more than 25 years after exposure, including those who were in utero—even in the first trimester—but not among persons conceived after the explosion. On the basis of animal experimentation, there is no doubt that point mutations occurred, but no effect could be demonstrated among the 75,000 first-generation offspring examined.

Small lenticular opacities of the posterior capsule of the lens have developed in 85 per cent of those who epilated soon after the bomb explosion; the lesions are asymptomatic. Only 10 of the thousands of survivors have grade III or IV radiation-induced cataracts.

Radiation-induced premature aging has been described in animals, characterized by early senescence and death in middle age from diseases that ordinarily beset the elderly members of the species. It has not been conclusively demonstrated in man.

That therapeutic doses of partial-body radiation may predispose to cancer is indicated by reports of a greater incidence of leukemia among adults treated for ankylosing spondylitis and of thyroid tumors among persons treated in early infancy for thymic enlargement. That repeated small doses of radiation to the entire body may predispose to leukemia is indicated by the increased occurrence of this disease among radiologists in the past.

Effects of exposure of parts of the body include temporary sterility, dermatitis, bone and skin tumors and developmental defects in the teeth. There are several reports of arrest in bone growth in children who received cancericidal doses of roentgen rays.

RADIOISOTOPES. Radioisotopes provide approaches to diagnosis, therapy and investigative studies. Hazards are comparable to those of roentgen rays, but the total amount of radiation is much less because of the small doses used. Biologic effects continue until the radioisotopes are excreted or until they disintegrate.

PREVENTIVE MEASURES. Exposures to ionizing radiation should be limited to situations in which commensurate benefits are expected. The average *whole-body* exposure of the general population, based on the genetically significant dose, should not exceed 0.17 rem per year, according to the Federal Radiation Council. The limit for occupational exposure of individuals (as contrasted with the population average) is 0.5 rem per year. Physicians and radiology technicians fall into this category. No limits have been defined for the *partial-body* radiation received by patients during radiography. The potentials for delayed somatic illnesses produced by partial-body radiation are not known, but it is thought that radiation changes within somatic cells are *incompletely* additive throughout life.

The child of today is likely to have repeated exposures to ionizing radiations, and there is a possibility that his tolerance may be dissipated. The pediatrician should limit as much as possible the exposure of his patients (and himself) to the emanations of roentgen-ray machines and radioisotopes, but should not refrain from using them for essential diagnostic and therapeutic procedures. The patient's gonads should be shielded whenever possible. When a roentgen examination is needed, a film study should be obtained initially whenever possible. Subsequent fluoroscopic examination can be made if it is still required.

The duration of fluoroscopy can be shortened if no conversation is conducted during the examination. The machine should be operated only while the physician can use his eyes most effectively, i.e., after he has adapted to the dark and while he is thinking only of the picture before him—*not while he is trying to interpret the findings.* The field under study must be kept as small as possible by reducing the shutter opening to a minimum. The machine should be operated with the most effective filter available, with the roentgen-ray tube at the greatest possible distance from the patient, and with the lowest amperage and kilovoltage permitting adequate examination. Electronic amplification of the fluoroscopic image, image intensification, permits fluoroscopy at very low levels of radiation. The method is particularly adaptable to the examination of children because the room need not be darkened. Thus, the patient is more apt to be cooperative and the examination is shortened. A pregnant woman should *not* enter a fluoroscopy or therapy room.

Roentgen therapy should never be used except when the indications are unmistakable or the risk justified, as, for example, in the treatment of malignant tumors. Extreme care must be exercised to avoid unnecessary damage to osseous growth centers and tooth buds.

Roentgen ray machines should be checked at least once a year for leakage which might be a hazard to personnel. The physician should wear his lead apron and gloves whenever the machine is in operation and should not expose unshielded parts of his body to the radiation beam.

Robert W. Miller

Hempelmann, L. H.: Risk of thyroid neoplasms after irradiation in childhood. Science *160*:159, 1968.
Ishimaru, T., Hoshino, T., Ichimaru, M., Okada, H., Tomiyasu, T., Tsuchimoto, T., and Yamamoto, T.: Leukemia in atomic bomb survivors. Hiroshima and Nagasaki, 1 October 1950–30 September 1966. Radiat. Res. *45*:216, 1971.
Jablon, S., and Kato, H.: Childhood cancer in relation to prenatal exposure to atomic-bomb radiation. Lancet *2*:1000, 1970.
Jablon, S., Tachikawa, K., Belsky, J. L., and Steer, A.: Cancer in Japanese exposed as children to atomic bombs. Lancet *1*:927, 1971.
Miller, R. W.: Delayed radiation effects in atomic-bomb survivors. Science *166*:569, 1969.
Miller, R. W., and Blot, W. J.: Small head size following in utero exposure to atomic radiation. Lancet *2*:784, 1972.
Report of the Advisory Committee on the Biological Effects of Ionizing Radiation: The Effects on Populations of Exposure to Low Levels of Ionizing Radiation. Washington, D.C., National Academy of Sciences–National Research Council, 1972.
United Nations Scientific Committee on the Effects of Atomic Radiation to the General Assembly: Ionizing Radiation: Levels and Effects. Vols. I and II. New York, United Nations Publ. E. 72.IX. 17, 1972.

28

POISONING FROM FOOD, CHEMICALS, DRUGS AND METALS

FOOD POISONING

The "food poisoning syndromes" are characterized by local gastroenteric disturbances, at times further complicated by systemic disease, owing to absorption of the etiopathologic agent through the gastrointestinal tract. They may also be due to systemic reflection of the gastrointestinal pathology, or to altered metabolism or physiology. The causes of food poisoning may be outlined as follows:

A. Contamination of foods with known poisons
   1. Organic chemicals
   2. Microorganisms
      a. Bacteria and fungi per se
      b. Chemical metabolites of microorganisms (exo- and endotoxins and mycotoxins)
   3. Plant poisons
      a. Primitive plants; mushrooms, bryophytes, thallophytes (i.e., mosses, lichens, sprouts)
   4. Animal and insect poisons
B. "Poisoning" due to altered food substances (i.e., spoiled foods, eggs, cheese, meats, rancid oils)
C. "Poisoning" due to altered host responses (i.e., altered host responses to foods containing tyramines, tryptamines and certain cheeses, nuts, mushrooms and fish)
D. Intolerance ("poisoning") to exotic foods (i.e., moray eels, shellfish, frog's legs, chilies, mushrooms)

Food can be poisoned or contaminated at any point in the ecologic food chain. Contamination may be present in the soil or seed or plants. Marine and terrestial animals may be poisonous themselves or have fed on plant material poisonous to man. Food poisoning may be due to treatment of seeds, plants or foodstuffs with insecticides, pesticides, and weedicides such as lead arsenate, mercurials and organophosphorus. Poisons may also be introduced during preservation, packaging or canning, e.g., mercurial fungicides and zinc, cadmium or tin containers.

Contamination of food may occur at the source from insecticides, such as lead arsenate, or from preservatives or fungicides, such as formaldehyde or copper sulfate. Lead arsenate may be on fruits and vegetables in sufficient quantity to produce symptoms of acute or chronic poisoning. Foods may become contaminated after packaging; the container or its lining may dissolve in the food or enter into a chemical reaction with it. At times foods have been placed in containers previously used for mixing arsenic sprays or lead paints. Insect powders have been added to foods when mistaken for baking powder or flour. Silverware cleaned with cyanide polish has produced poisoning. Ingestion of the flesh of cattle and fowl that have fed on fruits and vegetables heavily contaminated with arsenic may also cause poisoning. Atropine poisoning may occur from the ingestion of rabbit meat; rabbits have a species tolerance for atropine, but their meat may contain considerable amounts of atropine materials from ingested plants.

Natural foodstuffs contain large numbers of toxic components, such as lathyrogens, pressor amines, azoglycosides and labile sulfur compounds. Of particular interest are the osteolathyrogens such as γ-glutamyl-β-aminopropionitrile, which is found in sweet pea *(Lathyrus odoratus)* seeds and induces skeletal deformities and aortic rupture, probably by interfering with normal maturation of collagen fibers. Neurolathyrism in man may be caused by β-N-oxalyl-L-α,β-diaminopropionic acid, a neurotoxin identified in *Lathyrus sativus* seeds. Histamine, tyramine, norepinephrine, serotonin and other pressure amines occur in foods such as bananas, pineapples, cheese and wine. Consumption of such foods by patients taking monoamine oxidase-inhibiting drugs may produce serious hypertensive crises. Cycad nuts, widely used as human food in tropical and subtropical areas, contain methyl asoxymethanol, which is removed by bleaching in water.

Bacterial contamination of foods usually takes place between the time of preparation and the time of consumption. A large variety of organisms may produce poisoning. Two general types of bacterial toxins are known: the exotoxins freed into the external medium, which cause disease without association of living bacteria at the time of ingestion; and the endotoxins, which are formed within the bacterial cell after invasion of the host.

BOTULISM

Botulism is an often fatal intoxication due to the ingestion of food containing *Clostridium botulinum,* an anaerobic spore-former. The source of the infection is chiefly home-canned foods, especially underprocessed, nonacid meat, fish and vegetables. Six distinct serotypes A to F are known. A, B and E are of most concern to man; C and D produce disease in birds and certain animals; D may infect domestic cattle. E is found more commonly in foods of marine origin, particularly in the Baltic Sea and the Great Lakes of North America. The spores show varied heat resistance. The toxins are not heat-stable and can be completely destroyed by thorough cooking (80° C for 10 minutes).

SYMPTOMS. Some patients may have an acute digestive disturbance with nausea, vomiting and sometimes diarrhea, abdominal pain and distention, and difficulty in urinating. Central nervous system symptoms develop in 12 to 48 hours and are due to the curare-like action of the toxin on the motor end-plate. Decreased synthesis of acetylcholine, both in vivo and in vitro, has been observed with small amounts of A or B toxin. Acetylcholine and nicotine may still cause muscle contraction in botulinum poisoning, but fail to do so in curare poisoning. There may be a somewhat characteristic triad consisting in the absence of pupillary reflex, a peculiar dry, rough surface of the tongue, and progressive respiratory paralysis. Anorexia, weakness, dizziness, diplopia, ptosis of the eyelids, strabismus, and difficulty in breathing, swallowing and talking are common. Death may occur in 1 to 8 days. Diagnosis may be confirmed by serologic demonstration of toxin in the blood.

TREATMENT. In addition to lavage and catharsis, specific antitoxin, up to 50 ml, should be given intravenously as early as possible after testing for sensitization. Parenteral fluid therapy should be continued during the acute phase. In acute severe paralytic respiratory failure, resuscitation, maintenance on a respirator, and the use of hyperbaric oxygen are advocated. The botulinus toxins have a relatively short half-life and do not fix firmly in tissues; hence, it is important that supportive therapy be continued until paralysis abates.

STAPHYLOCOCCAL AND OTHER BACTERIAL POISONING

Some strains of staphylococci produce heat-stable enterotoxins in pastry and other starchy foods, whereas other strains may develop a soluble, heat-labile enterotoxin in such foods as salads, chicken, ham and beef in hash, or in gelatin, whipped cream and custards, especially when prepared in large quantities some time before consumption. These foods are particularly susceptible to becoming infected unless caution is taken in their preparation and refrigeration. The poisons may be preformed and left in the food, as with exotoxins, or formed in situ by organisms still in the food, as with endotoxins.

SYMPTOMS. The symptoms of staphylococcal poisoning appear suddenly within 1 to 6 hours after the ingestion of contaminated food and include severe nausea and vomiting, with retching, abdominal pain, acute prostration and diarrhea. There may be blood and mucus in the stools. The temperature may or may not be elevated. There is frequently sweating, hypotension and shock. The course of the poisoning is usually limited to 12 to 24 hours. Staphylococcal poisoning should always be suspected when an entire family or a large group of people become ill about the same time.

Clostridium botulinum and *Staphylococcus aureus* are the only food poisoning organisms for which causative exotoxins have been unequivocally demonstrated, but several other species have been implicated in illnesses in which leukocytosis and elevated temperature are usually absent and, hence, the disease differs from the known enteric infections. The spores of *C. perfringens* are heat-resistant and may produce symptoms of mild malaise, abdominal pain and diarrhea, often without vomiting, 8 to 24 hours after ingestion. Food poisoning due to *Bacillus cereus* and pathogenic halophiles is similar to *C. perfringens* poisoning, but the food is usually heavily infected and the organisms are found in large numbers. Large populations, particularly in Japan, have been infected with uncooked fish containing large quantities of gram-negative pleomorphic rods originally called *Pseudomonas enteriditis.* Food poisoning from the enterococci such as *Streptococcus fecalis* has not been clearly established.

TREATMENT. If the patient is seen within the first few hours, a saline cathartic may be given. Food should be withheld until the diarrhea is controlled. The important measures, however, are supportive ones. Fluids should be administered intravenously to combat dehydration and shock as well as any acidosis.

CHOLERA

Although the disease is bacterial in origin, inclusion under diseases due to *bacterial toxins* is justified as the disease is caused by the endotoxins elaborated by the organisms *Vibrio cholera,* serotypes Inaba, Ogawa and Hikojima, and the *Vibrio el tor.* The crystallized enterotoxin (molecular weight, 84,000) has six subunits (molecular weights, approximately 15,000) which also have the toxicity of the parent toxin. The cholera toxin acts by stimulating the production and release of cyclic adenosine monophosphate in mucosal cells, which in turn cause water loss. The loss is not, as once believed, the result of a primary disturbance of absorption of sodium and glucose.

Voluminous "rice water stools," high in electrolytes (especially potassium) and low in proteins are due to increased permeability of the mucosa to water and injury to electrolyte-balance regulations of the bowel mucosa.

The action of cholera toxin is blocked by indomethacin or aspirin inhibition of prostaglandin synthesis (PGF_2d from arachidonic acid).

The organism requires an alkaline medium for incubation, in vitro growth, toxin production and tissue invasiveness; accordingly, fasting favors invasion and establishment of the disease. Hence, eating of noninfected food to keep gastric secretion active is a preventive measure in endemic areas.

MYCOTOXIC POISONING

Food poisoning may also be due to toxic metabolites from fungi which occur in certain geographic areas. These mycotoxins are metabolites of fungi, produced during their life cycle.

ASPERGILLUS AND PENICILLIUM SPECIES. These produce **aflatoxins** of B1, B2, G1, G2, and M types, which may be a cause of Indian childhood cirrhosis. Circumstantial evidence includes the following: aflatoxins have been found in cereal grains used as postweaning diets and in breast milk, in the urine of patients, and in liver biopsy tissues.

CLAVICEPS PURPURA (ERGOT FUNGI). Rye, barley, oat, wheat, or Asian bhajra (*Pennisetum typhoideum* Hubb) flour may be infected. The alkaloids produced are ergotoxin, ergotamine and ergometrine. Following ingestion, injection or application to mucous membranes, all act centrally to produce hallucinations, neuritis, tremors, convulsions, vomiting, diarrhea, dizziness and coma ("Holy Fire" epidemics), with vascular damage and coagulation with resulting dry gangrene. Ergot is present in certain proprietary abortifacients. The dose required to produce an abortion may cause death.

FUNGI IMPERFECTI. Eating of grains (*Paspalum scrobiculatum*) contaminated with *fungi imperfecti,* produces giddiness, hallucinations, delirium and tremors, vomiting and convulsions. Boiling of the grains and husks destroys the mycotoxins.

HETEROSPORIUM SPECIES. Ingestion of the grain Indian ragi (*Eleusine coracana* Gaertn) infected with the fungus *Heterosporium* has caused severe nausea, vomiting and death due to cardiac arrest.

MUCOURACAE SPECIES. Ingestion of *Physalis moongensis, alba* and wheat grains infected with the fungus, results in severe vomiting of central origin; vomitus may contain red blood cells. Regurgitation of *Escherichia coli* into the upper gastrointestinal tract during vomiting is not the cause of the vomiting. Epidemics may occur. The mycotoxin is heat stable. Treatment includes the antifungal antibiotic hamycin orally, as the ingested fungus continues to elaborate the mycotoxin.

RHIZOPUS NIGRICANS VAR. THIRUM. This fungus produces a heat-stable, hydrophilic mycotoxin, rhizotoxin. Ingestion of apparently normal-looking grains of Asian bhajra (*Pennisetum typhoideum* Hubb) whose core is infected with the fungus causes a syndrome (Sassoon Hospital syndrome) characterized by polyuria and secondary polydipsia, resulting in fluid and electrolyte imbalance and renal failure. Transmammary passage occurs, and nursing babies are affected. The polyuria does not respond to antidiuretic hormone. The antifungal antibiotic hamycin given orally is effective in killing the mycelium in the gut, which may continue to elaborate the toxin.

CHEMICAL AND DRUG POISONING

GENERAL CONSIDERATIONS. In the United States accidents and poisonings account for the largest number of deaths in the pediatric age group, more than the next seven causes of fatalities combined. Poisoning is now the most common medical emergency in children.

Over 3000 fatal poisonings occur each year in persons of all ages; one third occur in children under the age of 15, and approximately four fifths of these are in children of 1 to 4 years. Nonfatal poisonings are estimated to be 100 to 150 times the number of reported fatalities; hence, poisoning may account for over one million illnesses a year in the United States. Poisoning is more frequent in boys than in girls under the age of 5 years. The frequency and causes of poisoning vary in different sections of the country and between rural and metropolitan populations. Fatal poisonings from petroleum products are most frequent in the Southern states and in the nonwhite population; lye poisoning also occurs mostly in the Southern states and in rural communities. The most frequent causes of poisoning in children under 5 years of age in frequency order are aspirin, soaps, detergents, cleansers, bleaches, vitamins, minerals—including iron—insecticides (excluding mothballs), plants, polishes and waxes, hormones, tranquilizers and other analgesics and antipyretics.

Since the establishment of the National Clearing House for Poison Control Centers, little change in the causes of poisoning from year to year has been noted. Seasonal variation in respect to aspirin, plants, petroleum products and pesticides remains about the same. There is a tendency for younger children to ingest common household products and older children to ingest medicines. The reduction in deaths under the age of 5 years is in large part due to a decrease in number of deaths from aspirin and salicylate poisoning. Further reduction in deaths resides primarily in educational and preventive efforts by responsible physicians and parents.

PREVENTION OF POISONING. The majority of cases of accidental poisoning in childhood are preventable. The responsibility for prevention lies not only with the parents, but also with the child's physician.

In the home parents have a primary responsibility to keep medicines and poisons out of the reach of the naturally curious child. Highly poisonous substances should be labeled and locked in cabinets; all medicines and poisonous chemicals should be properly discarded when they are no longer needed. Poisons should never be stored with foods. All medicines and chemicals should be kept in their original containers, which should be properly labeled. Three fourths of poisonings from household medications occur because the medicine was not returned to its usual storage place and the products were "in sight." The physician and the pharmacist, by meticulous attention to accurate prescription writing and compounding, may prevent many cases of poisoning. Prescriptions containing poisonous drugs should be written for small quantities sufficient only for the immediate medical need. Proprietary medicines should be properly labeled with instructions and precautions about administration to children. Particular attention to the dangers of medication in "candy" form is imperative, since it is responsible for as much as 87 per cent of the cases of aspirin poisoning. *Fatal* aspirin poisoning is, however, more often due to ingestion of tablets for adult use. Forty one per cent of childhood poisonings occur in the kitchen, 21 per cent in the bathroom, 12 per cent in the bedroom and 26 per cent elsewhere.

Parents fail to realize that a number of common household substances are poisonous; legislation requiring manufacturers to declare the presence and the nature of the hazardous ingredients on the labels of household products is essential. Caution must be taken in the storage of many household products such as bleaches, polishes and insecticides which, as a group, account for approximately half of the poisonings from household materials in both the United States and England. These substances are often stored in cabinets under sinks and are easily accessible to the young child. Poisonings are more frequent in families in which the mother is employed away from the home. The physician should instruct parents to purchase medicines and household products whenever possible in containers with safety lock caps that cannot be removed by small children.

Safety instructions to parents should become a routine part of pediatric care when the infant is about 6 months of age. (See Section 4.)

DIAGNOSIS OF POISONING. Acute poisoning may simulate many acute diseases such as peritonitis, intestinal obstruction, appendicitis, acute diarrheal disease, tetany, meningitis or encephalitis. When adequate evidence cannot be found for the symptoms of an acutely ill child, poisoning should be considered. Symptoms occurring in several persons after ingestion of food from the same source are strongly suggestive of food poisoning.

The action of many poisons may be characteristic. Gastrointestinal disorders with vomiting, diarrhea and abdominal pain occur commonly in metallic, acid, alkali, veratrum and bacterial poisonings. Convulsions are characteristic of poisoning by central nervous system stimulants such as camphor, picrotoxin and strychnine and by poisons producing anoxia from methemoglobin formation. Central nervous system depressants, such as alcohol, atropine (initial effect is stimulation), chloral hydrate, barbiturates, opiates, chloroform and others causing anoxia, may produce coma. Dilated pupils suggest poisoning from atropine, nicotine (late), cocaine and ephedrine. Pinpoint pupils may be due to opiates, physostigmine, muscarine and nicotine (initial). Caustic alkalis produce lesions of the mucous membranes of the mouth and skin. The odor of some poisons is characteristic; e.g., kerosene, gasoline, turpentine, acetone, alcohol, the classic "bitter almond" smell of cyanide poisoning, and the garlic odor noted on the breath in cases of arsenic or phosphorous poisoning. In addition, turpentine and eucalyptol may impart an odor of violets to the urine.

Mercury poisoning tends to cause pronounced proteinuria; poisoning by other metals, boric acid and phenol derivatives, a moderate proteinuria. Intense cyanosis and dyspnea suggest poisoning by carbon monoxide, cyanide, strychnine, aniline derivatives or botulism. Cherry red mucous membranes are seen with carbon monoxide poisoning, whereas chlorates cause a chocolate brown discoloration.

Methemoglobinemia. This is caused by many poisons and deserves special attention, since the resulting anoxia may lead to death or serious disturbance of vital functions. Nitrites, aniline derivatives, acetanilid, pyridium, dinitrophenol, methyl alcohol and potassium chlorate are the poisons which most commonly produce methemoglobinemia. (See also Section 14.) Relatively small amounts of methemoglobin (15 per cent of the total hemoglobin) may produce recognizable cyanosis, which is usually more gray than blue and often not associated with dyspnea.

The symptoms of methemoglobinemia are those of anoxia and are related to the concentration of methemoglobin in the blood. A concentration of 15 per cent produces only cyanosis, particularly acrocyanosis; one of 20 per cent causes mild fatigue and cyanosis, whereas 30 to 40 per cent may produce weakness, tachycardia, nausea and generalized pains. Concentrations over 40 per cent cause weakness, tachycardia, confusion and coma, and death may occur.

Hypoglycemia. This may occur in a variety of chemical intoxications, and symptoms attributed to the drug action may in fact be due to severe hypoglycemia. Hypoglycemia has been noted in toxic hepatitis due to herbal poisoning, in acute alcohol intoxication, in salicylate intoxication, in the late phase of kerosene poisoning, and in organic phosphate poisoning.

Identification of Poisonous Agent. Attempts should always be made to identify the poison. If the child is known to have ingested some household substance or drug, knowledge of its use may be of value in diagnosis. If the specific contents are not listed on the label, the container or bottle should be obtained and information about its contents sought from the prescribing druggist, poison control center or manufacturer. If this information is not available, the residual gastric contents should be analyzed. Emergency treatment should not be delayed until an analysis can be done, but the first emesis or initial lavage specimen and a specimen of urine should be saved for analysis, a procedure legally compulsory in certain countries. Analysis and the clinical picture may be complicated by the fact that many household products and prescriptions contain several potentially poisonous ingredients. Approximately 50 per cent of poisonings are due to such medications as salicylates (especially aspirin), laxatives, sedatives and cough preparations; cleaning, polishing and sanitizing agents such as bleaches, lyes, furniture polishes and cleaning fluids are responsible for at least 25 per cent, and petroleum products, including kerosene, produce 10 to 20 per cent.

GENERAL TREATMENT OF POISONING. The treatment of acute poisoning is always an emergency. Time cannot be taken initially to analyze the poison ingested, and most emergency treatment is, of necessity, symptomatic. Procedures generally to be followed and always to be considered are (1) removal of the poison, (2) prevention of further absorption of the yet unabsorbed poison, (3) administration of an antidote, and (4) general or specific supportive and symptomatic treatment. At times it is necessary to give a specific antidote in order to neutralize or detoxify the poison "in vivo" or "in situ" before removal of the poison is attempted.

REMOVAL OF POISON. Poisons on the external surface of the body and in the nasal and oral cavities should be removed by copious irrigation with water. Acids should be neutralized with weak bases, and alkalis with weak acids. If toxic oils are present, organic solvents should be applied, and removed with a mild soap solution. Orally ingested poisons may be removed by inducing emesis or by gastric lavage. Lavage is contraindicated with corrosive and highly irritant poisons because of danger of perforation. Certain drugs, e.g., opium, are absorbed in the intestines and resecreted back into the stomach for several days; for these, intermittent gastric lavage with water and a retention lavage with an oxidizing agent such as potassium permanganate 1:5000 solution may be helpful. Immediate induction of vomiting may be lifesaving and can be carried out by the parents before the physician's arrival. Emesis may be induced after oral administration of 15 ml of syrup of ipecac or powdered mustard in lukewarm water; stimulation of the posterior pharynx with the finger may facilitate the response. The child should be held with his head dependent to avoid aspiration. Ipecac syrup may be sold without prescription in 30 ml amounts. A dose of 15 ml will induce vomiting in over 95 per cent of children if food is present in the stomach or if water has been given. At least 85 per cent of the gastric volume may be emptied in 10 to 30 minutes. A second dose of 15 ml may be given if vomiting does not occur in 15 to 30 minutes. Other drug emetics are usually ineffective and may intensify the depressing action of some poisons. Emesis should never be induced in a comatose patient or after ingestion of caustic alkali or kerosene. Lavage is also not without danger. In corrosive poisoning the esophagus may be perforated; in strychnine ingestion the stimulation of a lavage tube may induce a fatal convulsion, and in kerosene poisoning, lavage, improperly done, may cause aspiration and pneumonia.

Gastric aspiration should be performed with caution. The child should be properly restrained, with his head slightly dependent and his face turned to one side. The gastric contents should be removed with a well lubricated, large-bore (28 French or larger) catheter, using an Ewald aspirating bulb. Small amounts of lavage solution (150 to 200 ml of potassium permanganate [1:5000 solution in water]) should be introduced intragastrically and aspirated as many times as necessary to remove all traces of the poison. Lavage should be continued as long as the returning aspirate is pink (potassium permanganate is decolorized when it oxidizes the poison). Two to 4 liters of solution should be used. Water, weak salt and sodium bicarbonate solutions may be used until a more suitable solution is available.

Activated charcoal mixed with water will absorb large amounts of certain drugs such as strychnine, morphine and atropine, mercuric and arsenic compounds, pentobarbital and malathion by mechanical and electrochemical adsorption. Tannic acid also precipitates alkaloid and metallic poisons, and strong tea may be used. Magnesium oxide suspensions are of value in mineral acid poisoning. Potassium permanganate 1:5000 solution will oxidize various organic poisons.

Administration of Antidote. Antidotes for poisons are of two types: (1) chemical agents which by direct combination render the poison innocuous or unabsorbable, and (2) physiologic agents which counteract the effects of poisons after absorption. Specific chemical and physiologic antidotes are not available for all poisons.

Milk and egg white are more or less specific chemical antidotes for metallic poisons. Strong tea, tannic acid and dilute iodine solutions are effective against alkaloids.

Sodium formaldehyde sulfoxalate, if given immediately, is effective in the treatment of mercury poisoning. Nitrites and sodium thiosulfate have a specific action in cyanide poisoning. Nitrites convert hemoglobin into methemoglobin and cyanmethemoglobin (thus sparing the vital respiratory enzyme, cytochrome oxidase), which reacts with the sodium thiosulfate to form innocuous thiocyanates. Methylene blue is indicated in methemoglobinemia for its reducing action; it is itself oxidized to a colorless leuko-compound. Ascorbic acid given intravenously may also be effective. Methylene blue is of questionable value in sulfhemoglobinemia and in large doses may produce further methemoglobin. Epinephrine, strychnine, picrotoxin and inhalations of oxygen and carbon dioxide may be indicated when central nervous system depression and anoxia are present. Stimulant and convulsive poisons demand sedation.

Gastric lavage may be followed by a large dose of a saline cathartic to hasten removal of poisons from the gastrointestinal tract. Catharsis is contraindicated in severe phosphorus poisoning when bloody diarrhea and desquamation of the intestinal mucosa are present. Magnesium sulfate may produce severe central nervous system depression because the rate of absorption of magnesium from the bowel may exceed the rate of excretion, particularly if there is oliguria or renal damage.

British anti-lewisite (BAL, 2,3-dimercaptopropanol) deserves special mention because of its remarkable effect on some metallic poisons. The toxic action of the metallic ions, particularly mercury and arsenic, is thought to be due to their chemical combination with important tissue sulfhydryl groups, with inactivation of essential enzyme systems. The administration of BAL can reverse the inhibiting action of antimony, bismuth, chromium, nickel, copper and zinc on the sulfhydryl enzymes. BAL is ineffective in poisoning caused by tellurium, thallium or vanadium. Under certain conditions, it may augment the toxic effects of lead and may actually hasten death in poisoning due to cadmium and selenium.

Undesirable side effects are common with administration of BAL. These are lacrimation, salivation, nausea, vomiting, headache, pain in teeth, a burning sensation of the lips, mouth, throat and eyes, sweating, generalized muscular aching with tingling of the extremities, a sense of constriction in the chest, tachycardia, fever and agitation. Toxic symptoms begin within 10 to 15 minutes after injection and gradually subside within 1 to 2 hours. (For dosage schedule of BAL see Treatment of Arsenic and Mercury Poisoning, see below, this Section.)

Certain metallic poisonings, particularly lead, mercury and iron, have responded to treatment with ethylenediaminetetraacetic acid (EDTA), a synthetic polyamino acid. Various soluble salts of this compound, such as calcium disodium versenate, have the property of forming with divalent and trivalent metal ions virtually nonionized metal complexes (chelates). The chelate is less toxic than the ionized metal and is excreted in the urine. Increase in the excretion of lead and mercury results without increase in toxicity. Toxic reactions of chelating compounds have not been clearly defined.

An exchange transfusion may be of value in certain poisonings. Exchange transfusions should be considered for poisoning with methyl salicylate, boric acid, paranitraniline, chlorinated hydrocarbons, benzene, chlorate and bromate, copper sulfate, cyanide, dicoumarin, ferrous sulfate, naphthalene, phenol and thiocyanates. Hemodialysis is of value when (1) the poison is distributed in an accessible body compartment and is diffusible through a cellophane membrane, and (2) the toxicity is related to the concentration of the poison in the blood. Hemodialysis may be of value in poisoning with barbiturates, salicylates, radioactive calcium, tritium, bromide, thiocyanate, ammonia and strontium. Little value would be expected when the poison is a protein-binding one.

Supportive Therapy. Excessive manipulation of the child must be avoided at all times, and medications, particularly stimulants and sedatives, should be administered with caution. Overtreatment may cause more damage than the poison itself. General supportive therapy is frequently more effective than removal of the poison or administration of specific antidotes. The type of supportive therapy required is dependent upon the actions of the poison involved. All organ systems of the body may be affected by poisons, and toxicity of one system may seriously affect other vital functions; e.g., respiratory depression may be secondary to central nervous system intoxication.

The nervous system is exceptionally vulnerable to the toxic action of poisons, but the symptomatology is variable. Evidence of stimulation or depression is usually noted. Stimulation results in convulsions, restlessness, confusion and delirium. Sedation is frequently indicated, but must be administered with caution to avoid depression. Sedation also masks many signs and symptoms, making evaluation of the patient's condition difficult. Depression of the central nervous system is the most dangerous complication of poisoning. It is manifested by lethargy, stupor and coma. Central nervous system depression and coma may be primary, in which case the action of the poison is directly on the nervous system, or secondary as a result of shock, destruction of tissues, or of cardiac, hepatic or renal failure. Prompt, intensive therapy is mandatory and is directed toward stimulation of the central nervous system and support of other systems affected.

The respiratory system is affected by many poisons, and the patient must be observed for evidence of respiratory depression, obstruction, pulmonary edema and pneumonia. Tachypnea may result from central nervous system stimulation and produce respiratory alkalosis. Artificial respiration, administration of oxygen and maintenance of a patent airway may be imperative.

Involvement of the cardiovascular system is frequent. Peripheral circulatory collapse may occur and must be combated by intravenous administration of saline and glucose solutions, plasma or blood and possibly sympathomimetic vasoconstricting agents. Cardiac failure may occur initially or later, and disturbances of the heart rate and rhythm require emergency treatment.

Some poisons cause intense gastrointestinal irritation, with severe vomiting and diarrhea. Replacement of water and electrolyte loss by parenteral fluid therapy is imperative. Nausea, pain and abdominal distention may be severe. Poisons affect the kidney either by direct toxic action or by the production of shock with renal ischemia. The most important aspect of therapy is administration of appropriate amounts of fluids and electrolytes which will maintain homeostasis of the intracellular and extracellular fluid compartments. The extent of renal damage varies from mild involvement to acute tubular necrosis. If metabolic equilibrium is maintained by the judicious use of fluids containing electrolytes, glucose and protein, severe renal damage may be reversible. Hypertension from renal or peripheral vascular involvement is frequent. Urinary retention may also result from bladder atony or vesical neck spasm, and repeated catheterizations or the insertion of an indwelling catheter may be necessary in case of possible reabsorption of certain toxins from the bladder.

The extent of liver involvement in poisoning varies from minimal damage to severe necrosis. Supportive therapy is primarily the provision of a diet adequate in protein and carbohydrate and low in fat, with vitamin supplementation. The extent of recovery is variable, but considerable regeneration of liver cells does occur. A serious manifestation of hepatic toxicity is depletion of prothrombin; vitamin K administration is indicated prophylactically.

Disturbance of fluid and electrolyte balance is associated with many poisonings. The types, amounts and methods of administration of fluids and electrolyte-containing solutions must be selected for the individual case. The following are general considerations:

1. Administration of total fluids in amounts adequate to meet the daily body requirements.
2. Avoidance of water intoxication, hyperelectrolytemia or hypoelectrolytemia resulting from administration of inadequate or excessive amounts of water or electrolyte-containing solutions.
3. Correction of any potassium or calcium imbalances.
4. Maintenance of an adequate caloric and vitamin intake. For children oral feedings are preferable if they can be retained.

The control of body temperature is frequently impaired, and avoidance of hyperthermia or hypothermia is important. In barbital and opiate poisonings the depressant action of these drugs is intensified by hypothermia, which affects the enzymatic detoxifying capacity of the liver.

The child who is poisoned may be susceptible to infection, and use of antimicrobial agents should be considered, but not instituted routinely. Antibiotic therapy is indicated for the prevention of secondary bacterial infection in poisoning by kerosene and other hydrocarbons that produce chemical pneumonitis.

The child may often be in severe pain, which must be alleviated because pain itself contributes to the stress-shock syndrome. In planning the management of the child who has been poisoned, the need for competent, continuous nursing care must never be overlooked.

CHEMICAL POISONING

In each case of poisoning, efforts should be made to identify the toxic agent. The chemical constituents of many medicinal, household and chemical products are recorded on the labels, and this practice must become increasingly common. If the chemical composition is not recorded, it may be obtained from the manufacturer or textbooks of toxicology. Information about new or unusual poisons and their pharmacologic action, as well as the composition of commercial products, is available through Poison Control Centers. Further information is available from the National Clearing House of Poison Information Centers, Department of Health, Education, and Welfare, Accident Prevention Division, Washington, D.C.

It is impossible to include in a pediatric textbook all known toxic chemical substances. In the following section a number of potentially toxic chemical compounds are listed; included are general classes of chemicals (alphabetically arranged) with associated signs and symptoms of toxicity and recommended therapy. A more extensive List of Chemicals follows the general list immediately below, and includes individual chemical compounds. Many chemicals are now assigned commercial or trade names, and, in general, these are used rather than the chemical nomenclature. Synonyms are also listed.

1. **Abrin.** The toxic albumin found in jequirity beans *(Abrus precatorius)*. Ricin is a related toxic albumin found in castor beans *(Ricinus communis)*. The beautiful scarlet jequirity bean with a black "eye" at the hilus is used for necklaces, belts, bead bags, moccasins and slippers, rosaries, brooches, earrings and eyes for dolls

and grotesque animal ornaments. One bean thoroughly chewed may cause fatal poisoning. Toxic material causes hemolysis of red blood cells at extreme dilutions. In acute poisoning, vomiting, diarrhea and circulatory collapse may occur. Symptoms may be delayed 1 to 3 days. Hemolysis, hemorrhages and edema of the gastrointestinal tract occur.

TREATMENT. Gastric lavage followed by catharsis and treatment for shock are indicated, and alkalinization of the urine if hemoglobinuria is present.

2. **Acids, Corrosives and Acid-like Substances.** Corrosive acids (e.g., H_2SO_4, HCl, HNO_3, oxalic) produce irritation, blistering and destruction of mucous membranes within a few moments after ingestion. Lesions may be brown or black, except with nitric and picric acids, which produce yellow stains. Severe burning pain in the mouth, pharynx and abdomen followed by bloody vomiting and diarrhea may occur. Shock followed quickly by death occurs in approximately half of the patients. Esophageal stricture occurs in the majority of patients who recover.

TREATMENT. Water, milk or beaten eggs should be given immediately and repeated to dilute any free acid. Milk and the raw white of eggs neutralize acids by forming inert metaproteins. Gastric lavage, if performed, should be done with a soft latex tube. It is not without danger at any stage and probably should not be performed later than 1/2 hour after ingestion. Later, perforation of the esophagus or stomach may occur. For more detailed treatment see Section 11.

3. **Alcohols and Glycols.** *Methyl alcohol.* The ingestion of 30 to 60 ml may be fatal. The metabolic products, formic acid or formaldehyde, inhibit cellular metabolism, particularly retinal glycolysis and respiration. Toxic and degenerative changes occur in the liver, kidneys, heart and brain. Optic atrophy may follow recovery from acute poisoning. Ethyl alcohol delays competitively the metabolism of methyl alcohol to formaldehyde, since it has a greater affinity for the involved enzyme systems. There may be a delay in onset of symptoms of several hours to as long as 2 days.

TREATMENT. Gastric lavage should be done promptly and repeated over a period of 24 to 48 hours, since methanol may continue to be resecreted into the stomach. Intravenous administration of large amounts of alkali is indicated to combat severe acidosis due in part to organic acids, which may increase 20- to 40-fold in the urine. Potassium should be administered to correct hypokalemia. Peritoneal dialysis can reduce the blood level of methanol to practically zero in 24 hours.

Ethyl alcohol. Signs and symptoms include, first a release of lower centers from the inhibition of higher cortical centers; apparent stimulation is followed by generalized depression of the central nervous system. Fatalities occur at blood alcohol concentrations above 0.3 to 0.5 per cent.

	BLOOD CONCENTRATION
Mild intoxication	0.05 – 0.15%
Moderate intoxication	0.15 – 0.3 %
Severe intoxication	0.3 – 0.5 %
Coma	Above 0.5%

Fatal dose for an adult is 300 – 400 ml

TREATMENT. Gastric lavage is the first step. Further treatment varies with the severity of poisoning and is usually unnecessary if the patient can be roused. Adequate respiratory function should be maintained, with attention to maintenance of the airway, prevention of aspiration, and the use of respiratory stimulants and mechanical ventilation if necessary. Appropriate intravenous therapy will prevent dehydration and electrolyte imbalance from developing. Since the glycogenolytic system is inhibited, intravenous fluids should contain 5 to 10 per cent glucose to prevent the hypoglycemia which may account for the residual brain damage occasionally seen after severe intoxication in small children. Since alcohol is soluble and freely diffusible in water, peritoneal and hemodialysis should be effective in case of urgent need for prompt removal of alcohol from the body. The addition of 40 units of crystalline insulin to 500 ml of Ringer-lactate solution with glucose has been recommended as an enhancing mechanism for metabolic degradation of alcohol.

Ethylene glycol, diethylene glycol. These substances are metabolized to oxalic acid (see Oxalates and Oxalic Acid). Central nervous system depression, shock and anuria may occur within a few hours, and respiratory failure and pulmonary edema occur within 24 hours.

TREATMENT. Lavage, catharsis and calcium gluconate.

4. **Aluminum and Zinc Salts.** Aluminum and zinc salts are used as astringents, deodorants and antiseptics. Symptoms include burning pain in the mouth and throat, vomiting, watery or bloody diarrhea, anuria, hepatic damage, collapse and convulsions.

TREATMENT. Immediate dilution with water or milk followed by repeated gastric lavage (see 2 and 49). In poisoning with zinc salts, EDTA, 50 mg/kg intramuscularly or 15 mg/kg intravenously, is recommended.

5. **Amphetamine, Privine, Ephedrine and Related Drugs.** Acute poisoning from ingestion, inhalation, injection or application to mucous membranes produces nausea, vomiting, chills, cyanosis, nervousness, irritability, insomnia with confused cognition, and fever. Repetitive administration, as in addiction, leads to a paranoid psychosis-like condition. Blurred vision, mydriasis, altered ocular reflexes, spasms, convulsions, coma and respiratory failure may follow.

TREATMENT. Lavage and catharsis are indicated. Administration of barbiturates may be followed by severe depression. The solubility and renal tubular maximum value and ionization of the amphetamine radical in the blood can be increased by acidification of the blood; this should be followed by forced diuresis.

6. **Aniline, Dimethylaniline, Nitroaniline, Toluidine and Nitrobenzene, Acetophenetidin, Acetanilid.** These dyes are used in paints, paint removers, printing inks and cloth-marking inks and as solvents. Aniline poisoning of infants may occur from dye materials recently stamped on diapers or shirts. Paranitraniline is found in some yellow and orange wax crayons. A roentgenogram of the abdomen may show the opaque pieces of crayon in the intestine. Intense methemoglobinemia is produced by all these compounds. Symptoms include cyanosis, headache, shallow respiration, dizziness, hypotension, convulsions and coma. Hemolytic anemia may occur later. Five to 20 gm of acetanilid may be fatal; a single dose of 0.5 to 5.0 gm produces sweating, chills, gastric irritation, tinnitus, hypotension and circulatory collapse. Chronic exposure leads to urinary papilloma and papillocarcinoma.

TREATMENT. Removal of poison from skin, repeated gastric lavage followed by catharsis. Oxygen, transfusion, exchange transfusion and methylene blue are of value.

7. **Antimony.** After ingestion, nausea, vomiting and severe diarrhea occur. Anemia, eosinophilia, hemoglobinuria and hematuria may be present.

TREATMENT. See 9.

8. **ANTU** *(Alphanaphthylthiourea).* ANTU produces pulonary edema and pleural effusion in animals by a toxic vasodilatory action on capillaries, and by increasing lymph flow. It is thought to be relatively nonpoisonous to man; more than 1 pound of a 20 per cent mixture has been ingested without producing symptoms.

9. **Arsenic.** Arsenic poisoning may be acute, subacute or chronic. Arsenic compounds may be absorbed from the gastrointestinal tract, lungs and skin. Arsenic inactivates sulfhydryl-containing enzymes and inhibits cellular respiration. It is stored in the tissues for a long time and is excreted slowly in the urine and feces. The more soluble salts may produce death quickly. In *acute poisoning* symptoms usually occur within ½ to 1 hour after ingestion. If arsenic is ingested with a meal, there may be delay as long as 12 hours. There are feelings of intense burning and constriction of the pharynx and larynx, dysphagia and intense gastric pain. Persistent and projectile vomiting occurs; stomach contents may contain flakes or grains of unabsorbed arsenical compounds or may be colored with yellow sulfide of arsenic; the vomitus soon becomes bilious. A severe bloody diarrhea may become so copious and watery as to resemble the "rice water" stools of cholera. Arsenic poisoning may be mistaken for cholera in tropical countries, where neither is rare. Hematuria, proteinuria and oliguria follow. Eventually shock develops, with cardiovascular and respiratory failure accompanied by severe pulmonary edema and by hemorrhagic spots due to the capillary injury. Terminal convulsions and coma occur.

Subacute or chronic poisoning. If the patient survives the acute phase, there may be residual symptoms such as multiple neuritis, myelitis and hypoplastic anemia. Alopecia, dermatitis, macular erythema and pigmentation of the skin may also occur. In chronic arsenic poisoning due to ingestion of small amounts of arsenic over a period of time the development of symptoms is insidious, with weakness, languor, anorexia, occasional nausea and vomiting, and constipation or diarrhea. Later, coryza, nasal and conjunctival congestion, edema of the lower eyelids, stomatitis, salivation and a garlic-like odor to the breath are present. The early symptoms may be followed by or associated with any of the residual signs of involvement of the nervous system, the liver or the hematopoietic and epithelial tissues that occur in patients surviving acute poisoning. Pigmentation, hyperkeratosis of the soles and palms and exfoliative dermatitis are sometimes striking.

TREATMENT. Even though symptoms of acute arsenic poisoning are present, intensive and repeated lavage is indicated. If the patient is seen early, repeated lavage with a freshly prepared mixture of ferric hydroxide and magnesium oxide is said to be of value, through converting the arsenic into insoluble ferric arsenite, which is relatively innocuous. Intensive intravenous hydration therapy is necessary. Sedation and morphine for pain are advisable.

BAL should be given promptly. The recommended intramuscular dose is 2.5 to 5 mg/kg; the larger amount is approximately half of the toxic dose, so that undesirable side effects are frequent (see above for toxic reactions). For mild arsenic reactions each subsequent injection should provide 2.5 mg of BAL per kg. Four injections are given on the first day and 4 injections on the second day, 2 on the third day, and 1 injection on each of the following 10 days, or until recovery. For severe arsenic reactions each injection should provide 3 mg/kg. On the first and second days 6 injections are given each day at intervals of 4 hours; on the third day 4 injections are given, and subsequently, until recovery, 2 injections are given daily. For reactions to gold, dosage schedules are essentially the same.

Treatment should also be directed toward support of the damaged nerve, liver and kidney tissues.

10. **Aspidium, Male Fern.** Aspidium is an oleoresin of *Dryopteris filix mas,* and is used as a vermifuge. The active principal, filicic acid, may produce vomiting, diarrhea, abdominal pain, headache, colored or blurred vision owing to a pharmacologic affinity for the optic nerve, tremors, abortion, collapse, convulsions and death in respiratory failure. If recovery occurs, dullness and blindness may persist for weeks.

TREATMENT. Gastric lavage followed by catharsis, and general supportive measures for respiratory paralysis and fluid and electrolyte imbalance. Castor oil and other oily cathartics should be avoided.

11. **Asterol.** A commercial fungicidal agent used against tinea infections. It has been reported to produce generalized muscular contractions. The sensorium is clear. There may be rotatory nystagmus and mydriasis.

TREATMENT. Supportive.

12. **Atropine.** Active alkaloid of a number of the Solanaceae, which include *Datura stramonium* (Jimson weed, thorn apple), *Hyoscyamus niger* (henbane), *Datura arborea* (angel's trumpet), *Solanum nigrum* (black or deadly nightshade), *Solanum pseudocapsicum* (Jerusalem cherry), *Solanum dulcamara* (true bittersweet) and *Dubosia* (cork woods in New South Wales and Queensland). Severe poisoning may occur in children from the therapeutic use of atropine, homatropine and scopolamine, and after conjunctival or nasal instillation, especially in infants; from the eating or chewing of the leaves of plants which contain belladonna alkaloids; and from eating the meat of rabbits which have eaten belladonna leaves (in rabbits no poisoning occurs owing to the presence of the enzyme atropinase, which is absent in man). Symptoms develop promptly after ingestion. Dryness and burning of the mouth, thirst and difficulty in swallowing and talking occur. The vision is blurred, and photophobia is prominent. The skin is dry, hot and flushed. A rash occurs over the face, neck and upper part of the trunk, and desquamation may follow. In infants and small children the temperature may rise as high as 107° F. The pupils are widely dilated; the pulse becomes weak and rapid, though this may not occur in infants; the blood pressure is elevated; and there may be palpitation, urinary urgency and difficult micturition. There may also be restlessness, excitability, confusion, weakness, muscular incoordination, giddiness and mild delirium, suggesting an acute psychosis. In infants the outstanding manifestations may be extreme abdominal distention, rapid respirations and distinct discomfort. Symptoms may persist for several hours or days, and the initial phase of excitement may be followed by depression with circulatory collapse, respiratory failure and death. Diagnosis is often difficult; the rash, fever, tachycardia and delirium may suggest the onset of scarlet fever. The subcutaneous injection of 0.1 to 0.3 mg/kg of acetylbetamethylcholine (Mecholyl) or of 0.02 to 0.06 mg/kg of physostigmine may be of diagnostic value. If salivation, sweating, lacrimation and intestinal hyperactivity do not occur after its injection, atropine poisoning may be present.

TREATMENT. Administration of water, milk or universal antidote should be followed by repeated gastric lavage and measures to reduce high fever. Short-acting barbiturates may control excitement and delirium. Physostigmine, given intramuscularly or subcutaneously in repeated doses, will antagonize or reverse the peripheral and central effects of atropine. Neostigmine has also been used, but is less effective. Morphine should not be used, because it enhances central respiratory depression produced by atropine and belladonna alkaloids.

13. **Barbiturates.** Five to six times the average hypnotic doses are toxic. The depressant action of barbiturates is due to an inhibition of the pyruvic-oxidase system. Symptoms vary with the rapidity of action and the duration of the effect of the various compounds, and include somnolence, stupor, contracted pupils, coma, fall in blood pressure, respiratory and circulatory depression and occasionally pulmonary edema. In some instances there are hyperexcitability and confusion.

TREATMENT. The intensity of therapy should be adjusted to the degree of depression. Careful evaluation of the reflex responses and the cardiocirculatory and respiratory states should be made before institution of therapy. Short-acting barbiturates may produce death within an hour. Long-acting barbiturates may have depressing effects for 4 or 5 days. Lavage, saline catharsis, establishment of an unimpeded airway, artificial respiration, and oxygen are indicated. Hemodialysis or peritoneal dialysis will facilitate removal of the drug. Alkalinization of blood and urine will increase the solubility of barbiturates and effect better renal excretion. Diuresis may be encouraged through the use of mannitol or ethacrynic acid.

Following return to a conscious state the patient should be kept under continual observation, owing to the possibility of relapse due to cyclic recirculation of the barbiturate between the central nervous system and peripheral adipose depots. The release of barbiturate from the brain, with return to consciousness, may occur through its deposition in peripheral adipose tissue, from which it can be mobilized again to affect the brain. The temporary return to consciousness is called the "lucid interval" of barbiturate poisoning.

Analeptics such as bemegride (Megimide), methylphenidate (Ritalin) and ethamivan (Emivan) are capable of causing arousal and return of consciousness in lightly narcotized patients, and in deeply narcotized patients who cannot be aroused they may produce a variable degree of elevation in reflex activity as well as help to maintain blood pressure. The repeated administration of picrotoxin intravenously in the comatose patient may avoid further respiratory failure and lessen the depth of coma, but does not produce arousal or return to consciousness. Intravenous glucose and saline solutions facilitate excretion of the drug and aid the liver in its detoxification. But, owing to the low ventilatory exchange, administration of large amounts of fluids too rapidly may lead to pulmonary edema. Maintenance of body temperature is of great importance.

14. **Barium Salts.** The carbonate, hydroxide and chloride salts are used as pesticides; the sulfide, in depilatories. The barium ion produces stimulation of all muscle cells. After ingestion, tightness of the muscles of the face and neck, vomiting and diarrhea, muscular tremors, weakness, difficulty in breathing, cardiac irregularity, convulsions and death, from cardiac or respiratory failure, occur, the action being mediated probably through the release of acetylcholine and by a disturbance of sodium and calcium ion metabolism.

TREATMENT. Ten milliliters of 10 per cent sodium sulfate should be injected slowly intravenously every 15 minutes until symptoms subside. Gastric lavage may be performed with such a solution or with 5 per cent magnesium sulfate, to convert the barium salt into the relatively inert sulfate. Thirty grams of sodium sulfate in 250 ml of water may be administered orally following lavage, and given again in one hour. Procainamide and nitroglycerin may be needed to counter cardiac arrhythmia and ischemia.

15. **Benzene Derivatives.** *Benzene.* Ingestion or inhalation of benzene fumes produces central nervous system depression. Principal clinical findings are coma and anemia. In mild poisoning, dizziness, weakness, euphoria, headache, nausea, vomiting, tightness in the chest and staggering occur. In severe poisoning visual blurring, tremors, shallow rapid respiration, paralysis, unconsciousness and convulsions ensue. Violent excitement or delirium may precede unconsciousness. Chronic poisoning from inhalation produces headache, anorexia, drowsiness, nervousness, pallor, anemia, petechiae and abnormal bleeding.

TREATMENT. Gastric lavage followed by catharsis. Great care should be taken to avoid aspiration. Epinephrine and ephedrine may induce ventricular fibrillation and should not be given.

Naphthalene. Common ingredient of moth repellents. Naphthalene produces hemolysis of red blood cells, resulting in hemoglobinuria and hematuria. Liver necrosis may occur. Symptoms from acute poisoning following ingestion or inhalation are nausea, vomiting, diarrhea, oliguria, anemia, jaundice and pain on urination. Excitement, coma and convulsions may occur. Mental confusion and visual disturbances may occur after inhalation of fumes. Hemoglobinuria, albuminuria and casts may be present (Section 14).

TREATMENT. Gastric lavage followed by catharsis. Blood transfusions for anemia and exchange transfusion may be of value.

Turpentine. One half ounce may cause fatal poisoning. Turpentine produces severe abdominal burning, nausea and vomiting. Diarrhea, pain on urination, unconsciousness, shallow respiration, bronchopneumonia and convulsions occur. Anemia, hemoglobinuria, hematuria, albuminuria and glycosuria may be present.

TREATMENT. Lavage should be performed carefully to avoid aspiration. Mineral oil may allay gastric irritation. General supportive measures, especially for prevention and treatment of pulmonary edema and anuria, and exchange transfusion are indicated.

16. **Bismuth.** Poisoning from injectable bismuth compound is rare. Both bismuth subnitrite and nitrate may be converted to nitrite through the action of intestinal flora (see nitrites, 57). Bismuth produces a metallic taste, stomatitis, violet-black lines on the gums and "bismuth breath" (possibly owing to tellurium contamination). Diarrhea, hypotension and renal failure may occur.

TREATMENT. Gastric lavage with demulcents should be done, and intramuscular BAL given. If BAL is not available, 0.5 gm of 10 per cent sodium thiosulfate may be given intravenously.

17. **Boric Acid and Borate Salts.** Boric acid may produce toxic symptoms when ingested or used as a wet dressing or as an ointment on large areas of injured skin, as in burns, diaper rashes or eczema. The mortality rate in infants is about 70 per cent. Excretion of boric acid from the body is slow, and cumulative action may occur. Symptoms include nausea, vomiting, abdominal pain and diarrhea. A maculopapular, urticarial or scarlatiniform rash occurs; the soles and palms are red. Desquamation follows in a few days. The mucous membranes are intensely congested. In infants signs of meningeal irritation may occur. Convulsions, delirium and coma follow. Albuminuria and azotemia may occur.

TREATMENT. Symptomatic. Exchange transfusion or hemodialysis may be lifesaving. Universal antidote may help to delay absorption of the poison taken by mouth.

18. **Bromate.** Potassium bromate is used as a neutralizer in hair permanents. Ingestion, because of contact with gastric HCl, results in release of hydrogen bromate. Vomiting, diarrhea, abdominal pain, oliguria, lethargy, coma, convulsions and shock may occur.

TREATMENT. Gastric lavage followed by catharsis. Sodium thiosulfate solution is recommended: 100 to 500 ml of a 1.0 per cent solution, intravenously. It acts to reduce the highly toxic bromate ion to bromide. The same solution may be used also for gavage, but it should not be left in the stomach, since highly toxic hydrogen sulfide may be formed with gastric acid. Exchange transfusion or hemodialysis may be indicated, especially in the treatment of anuria.

19. **Bromides.** Bromides depress the central nervous system and may produce delirium and hallucinations. Nasolacrimopharyngeal irritation, bromide halitosis, maculopapular eruptions, loss of neuromuscular coordination and impotence have been reported.

TREATMENT. The chloride ion, particularly ammonium chloride, may expedite elimination of bromide; 5 to 8 gm/day in divided doses is recommended for adults. Intake of fluids should be generous.

20. **Cadmium.** Cadmium may be dissolved from plated pitchers and ice trays by such acid-containing foods as citrus fruit juices. Symptoms are manifest within approximately 1/2 hour and include nausea, vomiting, cramps and occasionally diarrhea, accompanied by general weakness. Pulmonary edema with pneumonitis and aspermia have been reported. Recovery is usually rapid, within less than 24 hours.

TREATMENT. General supportive and sedative therapy is indicated. Edathamil calcium disodium given orally for a week may reduce the elevated cadmium level in the blood in cases of chronic poisoning. BAL will increase the concentration of cadmium in the urine, producing destructive tubular changes, and should not be used.

21. **Carbon Disulfide.** Inhalation of fumes or ingestion of the liquid produces central nervous system depression, with coma and terminal convulsions. Recovery may be followed by permanent damage to the central nervous system (extrapyramidal, with parkinsonism) or the peripheral nerves. Absence of corneal reflex is said to be highly characteristic of chronic poisoning. The blood may show moderate lymphocytosis, marked monocytosis, and occasionally eosinophilia.

TREATMENT. Supportive.

22. **Carbon Monoxide.** The symptoms of carbon monoxide poisoning are predominantly those of anoxia of varying degrees, with severe headache, weakness, dizziness, dimness of vision, nausea, vomiting, collapse, coma, intermittent convulsions and failing respiration. The symptoms depend upon the concentration of carboxyhemoglobin in the blood. A cherry red color is particularly noticeable on the lips and fingernails. Permanent residual damage to the central nervous system may occur if the anoxia is profound or prolonged.

Blood containing more than 40 per cent carboxyhemoglobin remains bright red after diluting 1 drop with 5 ml of 1 per cent ammonium hydroxide and adding 10 mg of sodium hydrosulfite. Normal blood becomes brown or brown-black. Normal blood, diluted 1:10 with water, will turn dark green when an equal volume of 10 per cent sodium hydroxide is added, whereas blood containing carbon monoxide retains a light red color for several minutes. Two dark spectroscopic bands, between 500 and 600 $m\mu$ are observed with 0.2 per cent dilution of normal blood as well as with carboxyhemoglobin; however, the addition of a few drops of ammonium sulfide will cause the two bands produced by normal oxyhemoglobin to fuse, while those produced by carboxyhemoglobin remain unchanged.

Carbon monoxide has 200 to 240 times greater affinity for hemoglobin than does oxygen, and carbon monoxide interferes with the release of oxygen from hemoglobin; death may occur quickly because of tissue anoxia. Toxicity may be delayed 4 to 6 hours after exposure; firemen are advised not to go to sleep for 6 hours after exposure. In adults, cigarette smoking increases the carbon monoxide inhaled by 3 to 10 per cent. Persons in ill health are particularly susceptible to carbon monoxide poisoning; low hemoglobin levels are quickly saturated with carbon monoxide. Susceptibility of children is increased by their higher metabolic rate and greater oxygen demand.

TREATMENT. Carbon monoxide can be removed almost completely from the blood in 30 minutes if oxygen in high concentration with not greater than 5 per cent carbon dioxide is administered. Controlled hypothermia has been effective in experimental animals; however, it is contraindicated if barbiturate poisoning is also present. Artificial respiration should be continued until normal breathing is resumed. Administration of methylene blue is dangerous, since it decreases the oxygen-carrying capacity of the blood.

23. **Chenopodium (Wormseed Oil).** Ten to 12 drops of oil of chenopodium may produce toxic symptoms and death. The symptoms are dizziness, tinnitus, impaired vision, vomiting, profound depression and unconsciousness and, in more severe cases, diarrhea, muscular twitchings and convulsions. Glycosuria has been observed. If the patient survives the acute symptoms, deafness may be present for a few days to a month. Damage to the liver is manifested by jaundice; injury to the kidney by hematuria and albuminuria.

TREATMENT. Saline catharsis, stimulants, oxygen and copious amounts of oral and parenteral fluids are required.

24. **Chlorobenzene Derivatives.** A large number of chlorobenzene derivatives are found in household solvents, insecticides, fungicides, sprays, waxes, paint solvents and cleansers. These agents, used as dusts, wetting powders and solutions for spraying, are stable and fat-soluble. Their toxicity increases in organic fat solvents. The volatile halogenated hydrocarbons are very toxic. Absorption may be through contaminated food, by inhalation, by transconjunctival or percutaneous routes (especially in organic solvents, such as indican derivatives) and death may occur within an hour. For treatment, see chlorinated insecticides, 25.

25. **Chlorinated Insecticides.** These consist of the *chlorobenzene derivatives:* DDT, TDE, DFDT, Methoxychlor, Dimite, DMC, Neotran, Ovotran, Dilan; *the chlorinated camphenes* such as toxaphene; and the *indan derivatives,* Chlordane, heptachlor, Aldrin, Dieldrin, Endrin and Diendrin. Aldrin and Endrin are more toxic than chlorinated insecticides like DDT, the fatal dose of which is 0.5 gm per kg. These are fat-soluble, highly stable insecticides used as dusts, wetting powders and solutions in organic solvents. Most toxic is Aldrin. Skin absorption of indan derivatives in organic solvents may be fatal within an hour. One to 3 gm of these derivatives produces severe symptoms and may be fatal. Symptoms are nausea, vomiting, intestinal spasms, pharyngolaryngismus, pulmonary edema and neurologic signs such as hyperexcitability, tremors, ataxia and convulsions, beginning within 30 minutes to 6 hours. Central nervous system depression with respiratory failure is the

cause of death; no direct effect on the cholinesterase system occurs. Recovery is more likely if convulsions are delayed.

TREATMENT. Gastric lavage with large volumes of water; egg whites should be given to absorb the poison, and followed by catharsis. The skin should be scrubbed with soap and water to remove contamination. Oils increase absorption. Convulsions may be controlled with barbiturates, intramuscularly or intravenously. Stimulants should be avoided, and epinephrine is contraindicated.

26. **Chromates.** Chromate salts are highly irritating and destructive to tissues. The hexavalent ones produce penetrating, nonhealing ulcers called "chrome holes." After ingestion, dizziness, intense thirst, abdominal pain, vomiting, shock and oliguria or anuria occur. The poison is also absorbed through respiratory inhalation and through the skin. Chronic poisoning produces an eczematous dermatitis, periostitis and hepatic and renal injury.

TREATMENT. Gastric lavage followed by catharsis; administration of magnesium or calcium carbonate (to form magnesium or calcium chromates); and supportive fluid therapy.

27. **Cleaning Solutions.** Chemical constituents of various types: *automobile paint cleaners* (free alkali, alkali salts, detergents, soap); *brush cleaners* (aromatics, halogenated hydrocarbons, alcohols, paraffins); *carbon cleaners* (aromatics, halogenated hydrocarbons, alcohols, paraffins); *dry cleaners for clothes* (halogenated hydrocarbons, alcohols, paraffins); *glass and furniture cleaners* (ammonium hydroxide, methyl alcohol, sodium hydroxide, detergents, soap); *grease removers* (usually contain paraffins such as kerosene, hydrocarbons, gasoline or free alkali, alkali and salts, detergents, soap); *gun cleaners* (nitranilines); *metal cleaners* (nitric acid, sulfuric acid, cyanides); *silver polish* (silver nitrate, free alkali, alkali salts); *radiator (automobile) cleaning compounds* (free alkali, alkali salts, detergents, soap); *straw hat cleaners* (oxalic acid); *toilet and drain cleaners* (hydrochloric acid, sulfuric acid, sodium sulfate, sodium hydroxide, sodium carbonate); *typewriter cleaners* (aromatics, halogenated hydrocarbons, and paraffins).

28. **Cocaine.** The alkaloid contained in the leaves of *Erythroxylon coca* is a benzoyl methyleczonine. Toxicity develops quickly after oral ingestion, hypodermic injection or local application of cocaine or its derivatives to mucous membranes. Symptoms are excitability, restlessness, confusion, delirium, hyperactive reflexes, rapid pulse, elevated blood pressure, widely dilated pupils and exophthalmos. Sensory hallucinations, paresthesias and muscular spasms occur. Nausea and vomiting are due to central stimulation. Death is preceded by Cheyne-Stokes respiration and convulsions. Chronic poisoning (addiction) causes hallucinations and a change of personality. Repetitive use as a nasal snuff causes a nonhealing perforation of the nasal septum.

TREATMENT. See 73. The patient should be catheterized to prevent reabsorption of cocaine from the bladder.

29. **Coniine.** Toxic component of the parsley family. These include poison hemlock *(Conium maculatum,* associated with the death of Socrates) and water hemlock *(Cicuta maculata* and other Cicuta species) containing coniine or propylpyridimine (Conium species) or cicutoxin (Cicuta species). Coniine produces peripheral muscular paralysis similar to that of curare; Cicuta causes gastroenteric symptoms of nausea, vomiting and diarrhea, with death due to cardiorespiratory failure. Increasing muscular weakness, paralysis and respiratory failure occur.

TREATMENT. Gastric lavage followed by catharsis, artificial respiration and oxygen.

30. **Cosmetics.** *Deodorants* (aluminum salts); *depilatories* (barium or sodium sulfide); *freckle removers* (bichloride of mercury, bismuth, ammoniated mercury); *skin foods and creams* (mercury, salicylic acid); *hair sprays* (synthetic and natural resins). Inhalation of some sprays produces diffuse pulmonary granulomatous lesions.

Some 70,000 cosmetic preparations are or have been marketed under individual names, and it is estimated that at least 1000 new cosmetics appear each month. Poison Control Centers may have details.

31. **Cough Medicines.** These commonly contain antibiotics, antihistamines, chloroform, codeine, ephedrine sulfate and related compounds, opium derivatives and barbital derivatives.

32. **Cyanide.** Acute cyanide poisoning from ingestion of the salt or inhalation of hydrocyanic acid produces giddiness, flushing, hyperpnea, headache, palpitation, cyanosis, hypertonia and unconsciousness, with asphyxial convulsions resulting in death within a few seconds to minutes. Death may be delayed as long as 3 hours. The odor of oil of bitter almonds on the breath is diagnostic. There is a cherry red color of blood and mucosae owing to formation of cyanmethemoglobin. Symptoms may be confused with those of nitrobenzene poisoning, which produces methemoglobinemia with cyanosis. Potassium cyanide causes a less severe form of poisoning, with gastric irritation, pain, vomiting and cyanosis, followed by coma and death; silver cyanide (from silverware polish) has caused severe nonfatal gastroenteritis.

TREATMENT. Specific, prompt treatment is indicated, in this toxicologic emergency. Poisoning following inhalation of cyanide gas should be treated with amyl nitrate inhalation immediately and repeated every 5 minutes unless blood pressure falls. Clothing should be removed and the skin washed with soap and water. Artificial respiration and oxygen should be given. Ten milliliters of 3 per cent sodium nitrite solution should be administered intravenously at a rate of 2.5 to 5 ml per minute; if the systolic blood pressure falls below 80 mm Hg, it should be stopped. After administration of sodium nitrite, 50 ml of a 25 per cent solution of sodium thiosulfate should be given intravenously at a rate of 2.5 ml per minute. The sodium nitrite produces methemoglobin, which can combine with the cyanide ion to form cyanmethemoglobin. The sodium thiosulfate is injected slowly to convert the cyanide released by dissociation of cyanmethemoglobin to thiocyanate, catalyzed by the enzyme rhodanase. One per cent solution of methylene blue intravenously may be of some value. Dicobalt acetate forms a direct complex with the cyanide ion.

33. **Daphne (Daphnin).** Ingestion of the bright red berries or other parts of *Daphne mezereum* and *alpina* produces abdominal pain, vomiting, bloody diarrhea, weakness, convulsions and renal damage.

34. **Darnel.** *Lolium temulentum* (darnel) is a grassy weed whose seeds resemble wheat. Their contamination with a fungus yields a mycotoxin. Flour contaminated with infected darnel seeds, and bread made with such flour, may produce vertigo, staggering, vomiting, visual disturbances, burning pain in the mouth and prostration.

35. **Detergents.** Detergents lower surface tension and denature protein; if inhaled, they produce pulmonary irritation and exudation with edema. If enzymes are present in the detergent preparation, they will increase toxicity through their proteolase and amylase actions on mucous and tissue proteins. *Cationic* detergents include benzethonium chloride (Phemerol), Benzalkonium chloride (Zephiran), Methylbenzalkonium chloride (Dia-

parene), and cetyl pyridinium chloride (Ceepryn chloride); they destroy bacteria and are used as skin cleansers, on surgical instruments, cooking equipment, sick room supplies and diapers. Ingestion of 1 to 3 gm may be fatal. Symptoms are vomiting, collapse, convulsions and coma, with death within a few hours. *Anionic surfactant* detergents include sodium tripolyphosphate, fatty acid amides, tetrasodium pyrophosphate, sodium-o-phosphate, sodium silicate-sulfate or carbonate; they are alkaline and burn mucous membranes. Certain polyphosphates produce hypocalcemia. Nonionic detergents include polyether sulfates, polyethylene glycol, and alkyl or aryl ethers; these cause mild to moderate mucocutaneous irritations.

TREATMENT. Gastric lavage should be done immediately and thoroughly, using ordinary soap solutions for cationic detergent poisoning, and demulcents for gastric irritation. Convulsions and respiratory distress require anticonvulsants, oxygen and appropriate supportive measures.

36. **Digitalis.** Poisoning occurs most commonly from medicinal preparations. Digitalis glucosides, however, are contained in a large number of plants. Symptoms of poisoning occur within 1/2 to 6 hours after ingestion of large doses and are usually initiated by nausea and vomiting of reflex origin. Electrocardiographic changes are present in about two thirds of overt poisonings. Overdosage of digitalis during therapeutic administration of the drug produces first anorexia, followed soon by nausea and vomiting. These symptoms may become manifest over a period of several days; if large doses have been given, the vomiting may occur without preceding episodes of nausea. Excessive salivation and diarrhea may appear, often accompanied by abdominal discomfort and pain. Cardiac arrhythmias, particularly extrasystoles of ventricular origin, and paroxysmal tachycardia may also occur. Bradycardia may result from the direct action of digitalis on the sinoatrial pacemaker or the atrioventricular conduction system or from loss of potassium from the myocardium. Death may occur from ventricular fibrillation. Headaches, fatigue, drowsiness and malaise may occur, along with blurred vision and disturbances of visual field (scotomata) and color vision. Mental symptoms of confusion, disorientation, hallucinations and even convulsions and coma have been described. Eosinophilia, cutaneous rashes and coagulopathies may occur.

TREATMENT. When poisoning is due to accidental ingestion, prompt gastric lavage is indicated, but when it results from continued overdosage, lavage will not be helpful. Adequate fluids should be given to facilitate excretion, but diuretics may be dangerous, owing to excessive extraction of potassium from the tissues. This may lead to a removal of the protective effect of potassium against the digitalis toxicity, and has been termed "diuretic redigitalization." Absolute bed rest should be enforced until clinical and electrocardiographic evidence of toxicity to the heart has disappeared. Nothing more is indicated if the pulse is slow or even if there is a heart block, but when there is ventricular tachycardia, emergency treatment is required to avoid ventricular fibrillation.

The disturbance in rate and rhythm may be modified, at least transiently, by one or more of the following drugs: atropine, potassium salts, magnesium salts, procainamide, quinidine, diphenylhydantoin, and sodium salts of EDTA (ethylenediaminetetraacetic acid). These are largely symptomatic and supportive therapeutic attempts to control the mechanism of heart beat until he body can eliminate the glucoside. Potassium is probably most useful and may be given as potassium chloride, the dose to be monitored by blood levels and electrocardiograms.

Rarely, magnesium sulfate is useful; 5 to 10 ml of a 10 per cent solution may be given intravenously for an immediate effect; it should be followed by oral administration of quinidine sulfate, 60–120 mg every 2 to 3 hours for 2 or 3 days. If the child is vomiting, intramuscular injection of quinidine is required. Calcium or corticosteroids are contraindicated, owing to their effects on potassium metabolism.

37. **Dinitro-ortho-cresol and Dinitrophenol.** Derivatives of phenol and cresol are used as insecticides and herbicides. They inhibit phosphate synthesis and result in increased cellular respiration. *Acute poisoning* from skin contamination, ingestion or inhalation produces fever, prostration, thirst, nausea and vomiting, excessive perspiration and difficulty in breathing. Later, anoxia, cyanosis, muscular tremors and coma occur. *Chronic poisoning* produces skin eruption, neuritis, hepatic and renal damage and injury to the bone marrow.

Urine which darkens rapidly on contact with air may contain dinitrophenol or 2-amino-4-nitrophenol.

TREATMENT. Induction of emesis with ipecac or thorough lavage with saturated bicarbonate solution should be done, followed by catharsis. Control of body temperature, oxygen and support of respiration are required. Intravenous glucose to support increased metabolic activity is advisable.

38. **Esters, Aldehydes and Ethers.** ***Dimethylsulfate*** is caustic to mucous membranes of the eyes, nose, throat and lungs. Inhalation produces pulmonary edema. Symptoms of intense irritation and erythema of the eyes, severe lacrimation, and chemosis occur after inhalation, skin absorption or ingestion. Cough and edema of the tongue, lips, larynx and lungs follow. The corrosive action is similar to that of sulfuric acid; dimethylsulfate in the presence of water hydrolyzes to methyl alcohol and sulfuric acid.

TREATMENT. Copious washing of contaminated mucous membranes and skin surfaces, and bronchodilators are indicated for laryngobronchial spasm.

Tri-ortho-cresyl-phosphate. The ortho form is toxic. The agent is used as a lubricant, fireproofer and plasticizer in coating plastics. Food may become contaminated. Symptoms are due to demyelination and to inhibition of cholinesterase, which produce weakness and paralysis of distal muscles, often manifested by wrist or foot drop. Death from respiratory paralysis may occur. Symptoms may be delayed several weeks, and degenerative changes in the muscles and spinal cord may be observed at autopsy.

TREATMENT. Gastric lavage followed by saline cathartics and support of respiration are necessary. Atropine is indicated to counteract the anticholinesterase effect.

Acetaldehyde, metaldehyde and paraldehyde. Paraldehyde and metaldehyde are thought to degrade to acetaldehyde in the body. Toxicity is related to limited oxidation of acetaldehyde. Acetaldehyde vapors cause severe irritation of mucous membranes, cough, pulmonary edema and narcosis. Ingestion causes nausea, vomiting, diarrhea, abdominal pain, flushing of the face, throbbing headache and hypotension (all attributable to vasodilatation); dyspnea, sweating, thirst, a sense of constriction of the chest and a feeling like that of anaphylactic shock also occur, with narcosis and respiratory failure. Paraldehyde produces deep and prolonged sleep, and metaldehyde causes nausea, severe vomiting, abdominal pain, muscular rigidity, convulsions, and death from respiratory failure.

TREATMENT. Copious washings of material from mucous membranes and gastric lavage, followed by saline catharsis. Artificial respiration is necessary.

39. **Favism.** Ingestion of *Vicia fava* (broad beans, horsebean) or inhalation of the dust of such beans may produce severe hemolytic anemia with jaundice, particularly in children and in those probably made hypersensitive by previous contact. The mechanism by which hemolysis is brought about is related to a defect in the glucose-6-phosphate dehydrogenase system of the erythrocytes (Section 14).

TREATMENT. Severe hemolytic anemia may require transfusions, along with alkalinization of the blood and urine, and supportive corticosteroid therapy.

40. **Fish Poisoning.** Several varieties of fish contain physiologically active substances poisonous to man. Some are dangerous throughout the year, others only during the spawning season. Fish may also become contaminated with pathogenic or saprophytic organisms (salmonella, typhoid, staphylococci). Fish poisoning (ichthyotoxism) may be due to eating of Tetraodontidae (puffers) or of the Diodontidae (porcupine fish). The Clupeidae (herring family), particularly *Clupea thrissa* and *venonosa*, and the Scarus (parrot fish) may also contain poisons. Some varieties of sturgeon (Acipenseridae), pike (Esocidae) and barbel (species of Barbus) have poisons in their reproductive organs during the spawning season. An alkaloid-like substance, fugin, present in puffers and certain other fish produces headaches, restlessness, salivation, vomiting, paralysis, cyanosis, and dilatation of the pupils, followed by convulsions and coma. Recovery may be temporary or leave prolonged residuals such as paresis, nerve palsies and sensory paresthesias, in the form of reversed temperature sensation.

TREATMENT. Gastric lavage, with symptomatic and supportive measures as indicated for respiratory failure and convulsions.

Scromboid fish poisoning is not uncommon in Japan, and occurred recently in the United States. With poor refrigeration, normal marine bacterial flora act on the fish meat, converting histidine to histamine and other toxins (including saurine), to produce scombrotoxins. Tuna (Scombroidei) was involved in the recent outbreak; similar symptoms may be caused by nonscombroid fishes. Symptoms occur within 1 hour after consumption and last up to 8 to 12 hours and include nausea, vomiting, diarrhea, abdominal cramps; flushing, headache, urticaria and a burning sensation in the mouth. These are attributable partially to the histamine in the scombrotoxin complex.

TREATMENT. Antihistaminics to counter the histaminoid toxicity, and sympathomimetics for bronchospasm have been advocated. Steroids may be of value.

41. **Fluoride.** Fluoride poisoning occurs through contamination of baking powder, from insecticides or rodenticides, or from inhalation of fluoride dust or gases. Fluoride salts and compounds are rapidly absorbed and slowly excreted. They are protoplasmic poisonings, inhibiting cellular enzyme action, especially glycolysis. Poisoning produces severe nausea and vomiting, owing to local gastroenteric mucosal irritation, and diarrhea and collapse within a few hours. If illness persists, there are excessive salivation, dilated pupils, thready pulse, shallow and unlabored respirations and weak heart tones. Cyanosis due to fluoromethemoglobinemia is not uncommon. Signs and symptoms are due to a disturbance of calcium metabolism, leading to paralysis of the muscles of diglutition, to carpopedal spasms and to muscular spasms of the extremities. Irritability, tonic and clonic convulsions and hypotension with death from cardiorespiratory failure ensue. Chronic poisoning leads to thickening of the cortex of bone, to calcification of tendons ("crippling fluorosis") as a result of calcium-binding, and to replacement of hydroxyapatite by fluoroapatite, and to mottling of newly forming or erupting teeth.

TREATMENT. Immediate lavage with 1.0 per cent calcium chloride, calcium hydroxide, or calcium carbonate prevents absorption by forming insoluble calcium fluoride; if calcium chloride is not available, copius quantities of milk may be given, after lavage with warm water. Intravenous calcium chloride or calcium gluconate may also be of value. Treatment is largely symptomatic and supportive. Exchange transfusion may be indicated.

42. **Fluoroacetate.** Fluoroacetate blocks aerobic metabolism at the citric acid level of the Krebs cycle by forming fluorocitric acid. It increases membrane permeability and breaks down the blood-brain barrier, leading to the rapid onset of cerebral and pulmonary edema. Very small doses may be fatal for children, and 300 mg may be fatal for an adult. Symptoms are prompt, vomiting, apprehension, stupor and generalized convulsions occurring within 6 hours. Carpopedal spasm may be present. Respiratory and cardiac irregularity and failure may occur.

TREATMENT. Lavage and catharsis are indicated. Cardiac and central nervous system symptoms may be modified by administration of 0.1 to 0.5 ml per kg of acetate such as glycerol monoacetate injected intramuscularly at hourly intervals. An overdose of monoacetate may lead to nervous system depression and death. Calcium may be of value for tetanic manifestations. Digitalization for cardiac irregularities is of little value. Fluid therapy should be cautious because of cardiac and respiratory stress.

POISONS

43. **Formaldehyde.** Formaldehyde is a general protoplasmic poison. It is a protein precipitant which preserves and hardens tissues. The gas is now infrequently used as a fumigant. Exposure to the gas produces intense conjunctivitis and irritation of the respiratory tract, often with resulting coryza, bronchitis and pneumonia. Ingestion of formaldehyde is followed by severe irritation of the mucosa of the mouth, throat and intestinal tract, intense abdominal pain, vomiting and diarrhea. Formaldehyde depresses the central nervous system, producing vertigo, depression and coma. Convulsions are rare. Oxidation of formaldehyde by the body produces formic acid and a resultant acidosis and renal damage. The tissues of the gastroenteric tract are white, hardened and parchment-like, with severe mucus exudation.

TREATMENT. Lavage should be carried out using 0.2 per cent ammonia water (1 teaspoonful of strong ammonia water diluted with 1 pint of water), ammonium acetate (3 teaspoonfuls in 1 pint of water), 1 per cent ammonium carbonate, egg whites or universal antidote. Ammonium salts convert formaldehyde to methenamine. The acidosis and impending shock must be treated, and respiratory stimulants may be indicated.

44. **Hydrocarbons (Kerosene, Furniture Polish Solvent Distillate and Gasoline).** As the amount of these petroleum distillates ingested exceeds 10 ml, the toxicity increases tremendously; furniture polish is the most toxic. These agents produce over 200 deaths a year in children in the United States. The routes for toxicity are aspiration or ingestion, inhalation and transcutaneous absorption, in decreasing order of severity. Within 15 minutes to an hour after ingestion of most hydrocarbons, symptoms of nausea, vomiting, cough and central nervous system stimulation may occur. Kerosene produces a gastroenteritis and acute chemical toxic hepatitis; gasoline usually does not. The hydrocarbons are readily ab-

sorbed and are excreted by the lungs, but aspiration due to choking, gagging, vomiting and attempts at gastric lavage is the chief route for pulmonary toxicity. Vertigo, fever, drowsiness, confusion and coma result. Levels of consciousness may be more closely related to blood glucose levels than to direct action of hydrocarbons on the central nervous system. Methemoglobin formation is common. Bronchitis or pneumonia from aspiration of hydrocarbons may develop within the first 24 hours, or be delayed. Death is primarily due to hepatocellular failure, with hypoglycemia, pulmonary edema and pneumonitis as contributory causes; severe pulmonary involvement may itself be lethal. Inhalation of gasoline produces intense burning sensation in the throat and lungs within a few minutes after exposure, and bronchopneumonia may develop rapidly.

TREATMENT. It is advisable not to induce vomiting in hydrocarbon poisoning, since the frequency of pulmonary complications is thought to be greater. Lavage carefully done is advisable, extreme caution being taken to avoid aspiration. The administration of mineral oil will reduce absorption of ingested kerosene. When only small amounts have been taken, catharsis with saline purgatives is indicated, and lavage is usually not necessary. General supportive measures, oxygen, transfusion for methemoglobinemia, and carbon dioxide stimulation may prevent development of secondary bacterial pneumonia.

45. **Hydrocarbons (Halogenated).** ***Carbon tetrachloride.*** A nonflammable volatile solvent, used as a cleaner in floor waxes and in fire extinguishers. Ingestion of 3 to 5 ml may be fatal. Exposure to an atmosphere containing 45 to 100 parts per million may produce symptoms. Symptoms occur quickly after inhalation or ingestion or from skin absorption. Signs of central nervous system depression, such as dizziness, confusion and unconsciousness, occur. Respiratory and cardiac irregularity and collapse occur. Recovery may be followed in a few days or up to 2 weeks by evidence of jaundice (hepatocellular), albuminuria, and anuria. Ethyl alcohol potentiates the toxicity. Carbon tetrachloride in small amounts directly suppresses hepatic mitochondrial activity; larger doses produce a hepatitis with fatty degeneration, and release sympathetic neurohormones, which in turn cause constriction of liver sinusoids and produce anoxia of liver cells. Adrenergic blocking agents can prevent liver necrosis but not fatty infiltration in poisoned animals.

TREATMENT. General supportive measures, artificial respiration and gastric lavage followed by catharsis. A high carbohydrate intake is advisable. Dimercaprol (BAL) protects hepatic sulfhydryl enzyme systems. A clinical trial with one of the adrenergic blocking agents may be desirable as soon as acute nervous system symptoms subside. Sympathomimetic amines are contraindicated, as they may induce myocardial fibrillation.

Methyl bromide, methyl chloride. These gases are used as refrigerants and fumigants. They may be present with carbon tetrachloride in fire extinguishers. Toxic tissue effects are similar to those of carbon tetrachloride except that bronchopneumonia and pulmonary edema are more common. The substances are metabolized to methyl alcohol and hydrobromic or hydrochloric acid in the body. Acute poisoning from inhalation, ingestion or skin absorption produces nausea, vomiting, vertigo, weakness, oliguria, drowsiness, hypotension, coma and convulsions. Pulmonary edema develops and progresses for several hours. In mild poisoning the symptoms may not develop for several hours. Vesiculation of the skin may be present where contact has occurred.

TREATMENT. As for carbon tetrachloride, with special measures for pulmonary edema.

Trichloroethane. This solvent may be present in rug, wall and clothing cleaners. Symptoms are severe depression of the central nervous system followed by evidence of myocardial, hepatic and renal injury. Recovery may be rapid after removal of the poison; late jaundice occurs rarely.

TREATMENT. As for carbon tetrachloride.

Tetrachloroethane. Occasionally present in household cleaners, it is the most poisonous of the halogenated hydrocarbons. Death from acute poisoning may occur quickly and leave evidence of congestion of the lungs, kidneys, brain and gastrointestinal tract. Symptoms of acute poisoning are intense irritation of the eyes and nose, headache, nausea, cyanosis and central nervous system depression appearing over a period of 1 to 4 hours. After recovery, jaundice, anuria and uremia may be present.

TREATMENT. As for carbon tetrachloride.

Ethylene chlorohydrin. Used as a cleaning solvent and also to speed the germination of seeds and potatoes. It is treacherous because it is odorless and relatively nonirritating to mouth or nasal pharynx. Ingestion or inhalation results in pulmonary edema, vascular damage, direct toxic action on cardiac muscle and depression of the nervous system followed by damage to the liver and kidneys. Symptoms are those of respiratory and circulatory failure.

Chlorinated naphthalene and chlorinated diphenyl (Halowax, Arochlor). These substances are used as high-temperature dielectrics for electrical equipment. Chronic poisoning produces acneiform lesions, drowsiness, hepatic injury and coma.

TREATMENT. As for carbon tetrachloride.

46. **Iodine.** The toxic effects of iodine are due largely to its corrosive action on the gastrointestinal tract. Iodine is highly reactive and combines readily with starch, proteins and fats in the digestive tract. Ingestion is followed by reflex vomiting, burning, abdominal pain, and bloody diarrhea. Shock may result from fluid loss, and death may occur in 1 to 48 hours. The diagnosis is obvious from the brownish staining of the mucous membrane and the lips and angles of the mouth, and the blue color of the vomitus or lavaged material.

Acute anaphylactic hypersensitivity to iodinated substances used in diagnostic radiography may result in shock and death. Chronic iodism is characterized by acneiform and erythematous rashes, frontal headaches, chronic catarrh, salivation and gastrointestinal symptoms.

TREATMENT. Lavage with soluble starch solutions or a combination of sodium thiosulfate (5 per cent) and albumen (egg white). Intravenous fluid is indicated to avert dehydration and shock.

47. **Iron (Ferrous Salts).** The oral ingestion of 2 to 4 gm of soluble iron salts (ferrous sulfate, gluconate) may be fatal in 50 per cent of cases. Iron toxicity may also occur in hemosiderosis. Excessive iron in the intestines overwhelms the mucosal mechanism for absorption; free iron is released from apoferritin complexes and exceeds the capacity of the plasma and tissue proteins to bind iron. Toxic effects ensue. The serum iron concentration is helpful in diagnosis, but does not necessarily correlate with symptoms or prognosis.

The principal life-threatening pathophysiologic effects are hemodynamic alterations producing shock and associated central nervous system depression. Early symptoms are due to gastrointestinal irritation and hemorrhagic necrosis of gastrointestinal mucosa, producing vomiting and shortly thereafter diarrhea, often bloody. Direct hepatic damage may occur. Pallor, drowsiness, lethargy and coma may develop as early as 15 to 30 minutes after ingestion or may be delayed for several hours. The hemodynamic alterations are due to the action of vasodepressor materials, most likely ferritin. Acidosis occurs, probably owing in part to accumulation of lactic and citric acids.

If coma and shock do not ensue, recovery is likely. Fatal cases are invariably among patients who are semicomatose or comatose and in shock. In animals respiratory failure due to metabolic acidosis appears to be the direct cause of death. Fibrous stricture of the pylorus may occur in patients who survive. Deposition of iron in tissues may lead to hemosiderosis in lungs, liver, kidneys and heart, and to isolated thrombotic disorders.

TREATMENT. Lavage with sodium bicarbonate may have two useful actions. Insoluble ferrous carbonate may be formed; but it may be more important that, at pH 6.0 or above, the chelating agent deferoxamine has an equimolar binding capacity for iron.

Deferoxamine, a sideramine derived from *Actinomycetes* and composed of trihydroxamic acid, has proved to be of value in experimental animal toxicity and in acute poisoning in children. Theoretically, 100 mg of deferoxamine combines with 9.3 mg of trivalent iron and removes iron from transferrin, hemosiderin and ferritin. Deferoxamine forms a nontoxic, unabsorbable complex with iron in the intestinal tract and competes for the iron of ferritin and hemosiderin in the tissues; the resultant complex is readily excreted in the urine. It partially removes the iron from transferrin, but iron in cytochromes and hemoglobin is unaffected.

Because the pH of the gastric and duodenal secretions is acid, excess deferoxamine, 5 to 10 gm in 200 ml of water, should be given by gavage. The intravenous dose may vary between 500 and 1500 mg (in 50 to 250 ml of 5 per cent glucose); the amount required is related to the variable amount of free iron in the plasma and tissues. Administration should be slow, and the patient should be observed for restlessness, flushing, tachypnea, tachycardia, circumoral pallor and hypotension, since both deferoxamine and the iron-deferoxamine complex have a hypotensive action, probably mediated through release of histamine. Shock should be treated vigorously. The organic acidosis should be corrected, preferably with sodium bicarbonate rather than with sodium lactate.

The chelating agents, BAL (British anti-lewisite), EDTA (ethylenediaminetetraacetic acid) and DTPA (diethylenetriaminepentacetic acid), can detoxify absorbed iron and remove it from the body by the renal route, but experience has shown that they have not significantly reduced mortality.

48. **Lathyrism.** Consumption of the grains of *Lathyrus sativa* as the major part of the diet may result in a disease characterized by gradual or subacute onset of severe pains in the calf, which extend to the thighs, and to motor hyperreflexia and a positive Babinski sign. Terminal involvement of vesical and rectal function occurs. There is no sensory involvement. The disease has been attributed to the low tryptophan content of the diet, as well as to a toxic amino acid, beta-(N) oxalyl amino L-alanine. Intrathecal injection of this amino acid reproduces the paraplegia in primates, but not oral consumption as in man. A mycometabolite may be involved; the disease does not occur if the grains are parboiled or fully boiled. Treatment with a diet rich in proteins, amino acids (especially tryptophan) and vitamins (including vitamin A and related carotenes) has been recommended.

49. **Lye and Corrosive Alkalis.** Potassium hydroxide, sodium hydroxide, potassium carbonate, sodium carbonate, sodium phosphate and sodium silicate are corrosive alkalis. Ammonia and ammonium hydroxide may also produce corrosive tissue actions. These substances produce intense local irritation of the mouth, pharynx, esophagus and stomach, vomiting and abdominal cramps, and a severe mucoid and bloody diarrhea which leads to collapse. Sudden exposure to concentrated fumes of ammonia can lead to sudden death as a result of vagal syncope. Perforation of the esophageal or gastric wall may occur within a relatively few hours. Recovery is invariably associated with scarring of the esophagus and with stenosis unless proper precautions are taken.

TREATMENT. Lavage with copious volumes of dilute vinegar, lemon juice or weak acids. Instillation of several ounces of olive oil or flour paste after lavage may be of value. Vomiting should not be induced in corrosive alkali poisoning. If an hour or more has elapsed since ingestion, lavage should be avoided, and only aspiration of the thick accumulated secretions from the pharynx should be performed. Small quantities of olive oil should be given at frequent intervals, with morphine for the intense pain. Moist oxygen is helpful in exposure to ammonia vapor. A liquid diet and parenteral fluids are necessary, owing to the dysphagia. Stricture of the esophagus may at times be avoided by use of corticosteroids and early dilation. See Section 11.

50. **Meadow Saffron (Colchicum autumnale).** Colchicine is present in the leaves and seeds, which may be eaten in salad. Symptoms occur 3 to 6 hours after ingestion, with abdominal discomfort, irritation, thirst and violent uncontrollable vomiting, and purging with bloody diarrhea. A sensation of precordial compression with vertigo, precordial muscular twitchings and spasm with cyanosis and collapse from exhaustion and dehydration follow. Death is due to respiratory paralysis.

TREATMENT. Lavage and saline catharsis with tannic acid to neutralize the alkaloid colchicine are indicated. Dehydration and shock must be treated.

51. **Mercury.** (See also Acrodynia, in this Section.) Inorganic mercury, usually ingested by children in the form of mercury bichloride tablets, is a protein precipitant. Mercury produces severe, painful lesions of an ashen gray color on the mucous membranes of the mouth, throat, stomach and intestines. In the stomach it causes intense gastric pain, and vomiting of grayish mucus and bloody mucosal shreds within a short time. The prognosis is improved if the interval between ingestion and vomiting is short and if there is extensive vomiting. If mercury reaches the small intestine, a severe, profuse, bloody diarrhea occurs, and gangrenous colitis develops. Mucosal shreds may be passed. Profound shock due to circulatory collapse soon follows. If the patient survives the acute phase, severe symptoms of systemic toxicity appear within a few hours and last for many days. Damage to the renal capillaries and tubules is responsible for the albuminuria, hematuria and excretion of casts. Diuresis sometimes occurs initially, owing to the faulty reabsorption of water by damaged renal tubules, but eventually there is oliguria and anuria, with tremors and convulsions in severe cases. Widespread capillary hemorrhages and transudation of protein and fluid from the blood stream result in circulatory failure and shock. Toxicity results from inactivation of cellular enzymes through complexing of sulfhydryl groups by mercury. Fumes of metallic mercury and dermal contact with metallic mercury may cause poisoning. Chronic poisoning results in salivation, a brownish blue line on the gums, loss of teeth, cutaneous erythematous eczema, nephritis, tremors and pancytopenia.

TREATMENT. Immediate and repeated lavage with raw egg white or milk provides protein for precipitation by the mercury. BAL is particularly effective. The SH groups of BAL are more attractive to mercury than the SH groups of enzyme systems; accordingly, mercury is removed by chelation with BAL. It should be given intramuscularly as promptly as possible, since experimentally it is less effective after extensive tissue damage has occurred. The initial dose should be 5 mg/kg, followed in 1 to 2 hours by a dose of 2.5 mg/kg. After 2 to 4 hours the latter dose should be repeated, and in severe cases a fourth one should be administered within the first 12 hours after the first injection. On the second day two injections may be given, each of 2.5 mg/kg. On the third day only one dose of 2.5 mg/kg is necessary.

Sodium formaldehyde sulfoxalate is said to reduce soluble mercuric salts to the insoluble monovalent (mercurous) form and the perchlorate to the metallic ion of mercury. The stomach is lavaged with 250 ml of a 5 per cent solution. From 100 to 250 ml, depending upon the age of the child, are then left in the stomach. This procedure is followed by intravenous administration of 50 to 200 ml of a 10 per cent solution. Lavage with 10 ml of 10 per cent sodium hypophosphite containing 2.5 ml of hydrogen peroxide and diluted to 100 ml is also of value. Sodium hyposulfite, chalk, freshly precipitated ferrous hydroxide, milk of magnesia, starch paste or N-acetyl-D,L-penicillamine may be used orally. After lavage, attention should be given to maintenance of a normal composition of the body fluids; one half isotonic Ringer's or polyionic solutions should be given parenterally to maintain body fluids and to produce a copious diuresis in order to protect the kidneys from high concentrations of mercury. Such therapy should be continued unless edema and oliguria develop. Prognosis depends upon the amount of mercury taken, the interval between ingestion and lavage, and the degree and duration of kidney damage. The immediate removal of ingested mercury is of utmost importance since absorption is rapid. In **organic mercurial poisoning** the principal agents involved are methyl, phenyl and alkyl compounds. These are formed from metallic mercury by a biodegradation process which takes place in rivers, lakes and sea waters contaminated with inorganic mercury. Poisoning may be endemic, as reported in the Kumato Prefecture of Japan, where 111 inhabitants who ate fish from sea waters near Minamata Bay developed **Minamata disease.** Illness was due to methyl mercury and was characterized by neurologic signs and symptoms, including sensory changes in peripheral and perioral nerves, disturbances of hearing, constriction of visual fields, impaired motor involvement, speech disturbances, tremors and absence of deep tendon reflexes. In late stages cerebellar ataxia, contractions and spastic paraplegia may occur. High concentrations of methyl mercury were found in hair, blood and urine of the patients.

TREATMENT. Penicillamine and alpha-mercaptopropionylglycine, and tetracyclines combine organic mercurials and have been advocated. Dimercaprol, effective in inorganic poisoning, is not effective in organic poisoning, and may be dangerous.

52. **Milk Sickness.** "Trembles" occurs in animals from eating the rayless goldenrod or the white snakeroot, which contain toxic substances (tremetol). In man the ingestion of milk products or the flesh of poisoned animals produces nausea, vomiting, constipation, jaundice (hepatocellular type) and oliguria and anuria. The tongue becomes dark red and tremulous; the cheeks are flushed and the lips red. Abdominal pain and muscular weakness with convulsions may occur. Deaths have been reported.

53. **Monk's Hood Root (Wolfsbane) and Larkspur.** The fresh leaves and roots of these plants contain aconite. Absorption occurs readily and may result in instantaneous death, probably from paralysis of the heart. Symptoms result from stimulation and then paralysis of peripheral nerves and of the heart; they include tingling in the mouth, stomach and skin (most important diagnostic feature), excessive salivation, nausea, vomiting and diarrhea. The pulse is slow and feeble, with cardiac arrhythmia, and there are dyspnea, weakness, impaired speech, unconsciousness and convulsions. Death usually follows in 2 to 6 hours.

TREATMENT. Prompt lavage with potassium permanganate, 1:5000, should be followed by saline catharsis and administration of tannic acid, and artificial respiration, oxygen, atropine for bradycardia or procainamide for arrhythmias, and respiratory stimulants when indicated.

54. **Mountain Laurel (Andromedotoxin).** Ingestion of young shoots and leaves produces salivation, lacrimation and nasal discharge. Vomiting, convulsions, slowing of pulse, lowering of blood pressure and paralysis may occur.

TREATMENT. See 77.

55. **Mushroom. Amanita muscaria (Fly amanita).** This mushroom contains both the parasympathomimetic alkaloid muscarine and an atropine-like alkaloid causing central nervous symptoms (mycetismus nervosus). It produces severe gastrointestinal symptoms soon after ingestion, followed shortly by profuse perspiration, salivation, miosis, delirium, hallucinations, convulsions and coma. The pharmacologic action of muscarine resembles that of acetylcholine. Mild degrees of intoxication occur, and there may be individual susceptibility, especially to hepatocellular damage; jaundice, ketosis and renal failure with anuria and uremia may occur.

TREATMENT. Lavage with potassium permanganate followed by saline catharsis, with administration of tannic acid or activated charcoal, is imperative. Atropine should be given hypodermically and repeated. Thioctic acid 300 mg in glucose by slow intravenous injection is of value.

Amanita phalloides (Death Cup, Destroying Angel). This mushroom is extremely toxic, containing several toxins not completely identified; the mortality rate in human poisoning is 60 to 100 per cent. Symptoms may be delayed 6 to 16 hours after ingestion, when there are sudden, severe abdominal cramps followed by vomiting and diarrhea, with mucous and bloody stools (mycetismus choleriformis). The intoxication is prolonged, and jaundice develops in 2 to 3 days, indicating severe degenerative changes in the liver. The kidney is involved, and direct toxic action on the heart may result in cardiac failure and death within 5 to 8 days.

TREATMENT. Immediate lavage, enemas and saline catharsis are indicated. Dehydration and shock must be treated. Atropine should be given until complete atropinization occurs. The degree of toxic tissue changes may be ameliorated by large amounts of glucose, plasma and blood intravenously. Hemodialysis is recommended. Carbohydrates in large quantities may protect the liver. The use of artificial respiration following succinylcholine, or of chlorpromazine has been advocated.

56. **Nicotine.** The toxicity and rapidity of action of nicotine are comparable to those of cyanide. It produces first stimulation then paralysis of the parasympathetic ganglia; symptoms are initially cholinergic and then anticholinergic. The local caustic action produces nausea, salivation, abdominal pain, vomiting (both peripheral and central in origin) and diarrhea. After absorption there are headache, dizziness, visual and hearing disturbances, mental confusion and intense weakness with tremors; death may follow within a few minutes. Respira-

tory stimulation, elevated blood pressure and slow pulse are also early manifestations, followed by cardiac arrhythmia and dyspnea. Later there are pinpoint pupils and a curare-like action on the skeletal and respiratory muscles. Respiratory and circulatory failure is followed by convulsions and death.

TREATMENT. Lavage with tannic acid, strong coffee or tea for ingested poison. Atropine appears useful for the initial parasympathetic toxicity, and neostigmine for the late anticholinergic effects, along with caramephen diethazine hydrochloride. Nicotine on the skin should be thoroughly washed off. Owing to the rapid destruction of nicotine in the body, death can be averted if primary attention is directed toward prevention of respiratory failure. Artificial respiration and oxygen should be continued until normal breathing is resumed or the heart has stopped. Epinephrine, caffeine and the like are not ordinarily indicated unless respiratory failure develops.

57. **Nitrites.** Medications such as bismuth subnitrite, amyl nitrite, sodium nitrite or spirit of glyceryl trinitrate may be taken accidentally by children. Therapeutic use of bismuth subnitrite may result in formation of nitrites by bacterial decomposition in the intestines. Cyanosis in infants due to poisoning with water containing nitrates has been described. Water seeping from barnyards heavily laden with bacteria and dissolved nitrogenous materials may become increasingly purified by passage through the soil, but certain soil bacteria oxidize the ammonia and other nitrogenous compounds to nitrates. The solution of nitrates, free of coli organisms, may enter subsurface channels leading directly into wells used for drinking purposes. Ingestion of such water in milk formulas may result in conversion of the nitrates to nitrites by gastrointestinal organisms. Flushing of the skin, fall in blood pressure, severe methemoglobinemia, cyanosis and dyspnea develop. Syncope and respiratory failure may occur.

TREATMENT. Lavage should be followed by saline catharsis, particularly in bismuth subnitrite poisoning. When syncope occurs, epinephrine and other vasopressor agents should be avoided. A deep Trendelenburg position of the body and passive movements of extremities may facilitate return of venous blood to the heart. Transfusions and oxygen may be indicated for the methemoglobinemia, and methylene blue is of value.

58. **Nutmeg.** One teaspoonful of powdered nutmeg may produce severe toxic symptoms. Narcosis with periods of delirium and excitability may occur within 1 to 6 hours.

59. **Oils.** Most of the nonvolatile hydrocarbon oils are nontoxic. Ingestion, however, may be associated with vomiting and aspiration into the lungs. Pulmonary complications are more intense with vegetable and animal oils.

TREATMENT. Emetics should not be given. Lavage should be done with care, avoiding emesis.

60. **Opiates.** Several natural alkaloids of opium, particularly morphine and codeine, and some synthetic narcotics cause toxic effects in infants and children. Poisoning occurs as a result of excessive therapeutic administration from accidental ingestion, from the milk of a nursing mother who has ingested opium, or from the feeding of small quantities of opium to children to keep them asleep, as occurs in some communities. Manifestations of opiate poisoning consist of transient excitation, followed by depression of all central nervous system functions. Vomiting may result from vagal stimulation. Acute anaphylactoid reactions and convulsions may be seen. Children and the elderly are more prone to poisoning, owing to limited hepatic detoxification mechanisms. Somnolence, coma and respiratory depression, often severe, may be noted. Pinpoint pupils occur, but are not diagnostic of opiate poisoning.

TREATMENT. Prompt, vigorous treatment is mandatory and should be directed to the prevention of anoxia and further respiratory depression. Oxygen and artificial respiration may be indicated, and the airway must be kept patent. Gastric lavage should be done with potassium permanganate 1:5000, which oxidizes morphine to oxydimorphine, or with tannic acid or activated charcoal. Permanganate solution should be left in the stomach and intestines, since morphine is excreted into the gastrointestinal tract, where residual potassium permanganate may act upon it.

Three specific opiate antagonists are available: N-allylnormorphine (Nalline), L-3 hydroxy-N-allylmorphinan tartrate (Lorfan), and naloxone (Narcan). The latter is preferred because of its lack of agonistic action. All three drugs have specific antagonistic actions against all opiates, natural and synthetic. They are ineffective against other central nervous system depressants such as phenobarbital; Nalline and Lorfan will produce the toxic effects of opiates if used in situations other than opiate poisoning. The drugs should be administered intravenously as rapidly as possible. See Table 30–1 and package inserts for dosages.

61. **Oxalates and Oxalic Acid.** Local irritation followed by severe corrosion is produced by ingested oxalic acid. Both the acid and its salts are rapidly absorbed, and death occurs quickly. Absorbed oxalate combines with the ionized calcium of the blood, producing hypocalcemia leading to muscular twitchings, laryngospasm, tetany and convulsions. The heart stops beating in diastole. If recovery from the acute phase occurs, renal tubular necrosis may follow, with proteinuria, hematuria, anuria, and renal failure. Besides local irritant or corrosive action, the absorbed poison has a direct toxic action on the central nervous system.

TREATMENT. Lavage with 1:5000 potassium permanganate should be followed by a 5 per cent calcium chloride, chalk or lime solution. Calcium gluconate or calcium chloride intravenously is of value if signs of tetany are present. Alkalis and bicarbonates should not be given, since they form more readily absorbable salts with oxalic acid.

62. **Phenols (Carbolic Acid, Cresol, Creosote, Creolin, Lysol, Resorcinol and Pyrogallol).** Phenol may produce symptoms leading to death within a few minutes, dependent upon the surface from which the substance is absorbed. Death (lethal dose is 8 to 15 gm) usually occurs within 24 hours from respiratory failure. Initial symptoms are severe, painful local corrosion of mucous membranes and severe vomiting. Phenol precipitates proteins of the mucous membranes, and penetrates into the tissues, where it acts as a protoplasmic poison. In contact with skin or mucous membranes, it forms ulcers which are initially painful, later anesthetic. Widespread capillary damage, medullary depression and shock occur quickly. Fleeting excitement may occur, followed by unconsciousness. Other symptoms are low blood pressure, cold sweat, hypothermia, oliguria, albuminuria and hemoglobinuria. Urine (and diapers) may turn dark green on exposure to air, owing to reduction of hydroquinone and pyrocatechols, which are oxidation products of carbolic acid.

TREATMENT. The drug must be removed promptly before absorption occurs. Lavage with olive oil or other vegetable oils provides a solvent for the phenol. Emetics are usually ineffective, owing to the anesthetic effect of phenol on the gastric mucosa, and are contraindicated. Neither alcohol nor mineral oil should be used; alcohol facilitates absorption, and mineral oil is a poor solvent for phenol. After lavage several ounces of olive oil should be left in the stomach. Copious parenteral fluid administration should be instituted to protect the kidneys. The acidosis responds promptly to intravenous administration of sodium bicarbonate or sixth-normal sodium lactate. Artificial respiration should be performed when respiratory failure occurs.

63. **Phenolphthalein.** Phenolphthalein is present in many candy cathartics (Analax, Ex-lax, Phenolax and cathartic chewing gum). Children have been known to eat more than a box of the tablets. Apparently, large amounts of phenolphthalein can be ingested without serious results. The range of toxic doses is not known. Severe toxic reactions may be manifest in hypersusceptible persons. A violent cathartic action results several hours later. A bright red skin eruption and swelling of the eyelids may occur, resembling the Stevens-Johnson syndrome. The urine appears bright red, if alkaline, and the diagnosis may be established easily through detection of a pink color in lavaged material, in stool, or in urine, upon the addition of alkali. High fever, meningismus, hemiplegia, albuminuria, oliguria and respiratory and cardiac failure have been attributed to phenolphthalein poisoning.

TREATMENT. General supportive treatment is indicated. If violent catharsis is present, and dehydration and acidosis ensue, parenteral fluid therapy should be administered. Activated charcoal should be given repeatedly to absorb the phenolphthalein. Castor oil may be given to speed removal of phenolphthalein from the gut in a "therapeutic catharsis." Kaolin and other constipating agents are contraindicated, since they will enhance retention and further toxicity of phenolphthalein in the bowel.

64. **Phenothiazines (prochlorperazine [Compazine], promazine [Sparine], perphenazine [Trilafon] and others).** The major toxic symptoms are motor: dystonia (incoordinated spasmodic movements producing torticollis, retrocollis, opisthotonos, trismus and oculogyric crises); dyskinesia (rhythmic movements of jaws, tongue, swaying and rocking of the body); akathisia (inability to sit still); rigidity; and tremor. Other symptoms include nasal congestion, xerostomia, palpitation, postural hypotension, drowsiness and hypothermia, and, in postpubertal males, difficulty in ejaculation. Large doses may produce seizures, and patients with brain damage are particularly susceptible. Permanent neurologic damage has been noted in patients with previous evidence of brain damage. Chronic use may result in jaundice of the toxic hepatocellular and obstructive type, in blood dyscrasias (especially leukopenia), in dermatitis, and in an abnormal patchy gray-blue pigmentation. Chlorpromazine raises the blood cholesterol level and increases the toxicity of alcohol and morphine.

TREATMENT. Lavage. Diphenhydramine hydrochloride (Benadryl) may be effective in treatment of extrapyramidal symptoms; sympathomimetic amines are indicated for central depression and hypotension.

65. **Phosphorus, Inorganic.** Red phosphorus is considered nonpoisonous and nonabsorbable; it contains 0.1 to 0.6 per cent yellow phosphorus, however, and may therefore cause toxicity. Yellow phosphorus is highly poisonous, producing severe tissue destruction. Yellow or white phosphorus is used in rodent and insect poisons, in fireworks and in the manufacture of fertilizer. Zinc phosphide used in rat poisons releases phosphine on contact with water. Symptoms of acute poisoning occur within 1 to 2 hours. Nausea, bilious hemorrhagic vomiting (luminescent in the dark), diarrhea and a garlic odor of the breath and excreta may be noted. Coma may occur within 24 to 48 hours. If recovery from the acute phase occurs, symptoms may return in 2 to 6 days, with nausea, vomiting, diarrhea, jaundice, a large tender liver (acute yellow atrophy), shock, oliguria, and multiple hemorrhages from mucosal and serous surfaces. Abortion may occur in pregnant women, and late neurologic signs are frontal headache, impairment of vision and hearing, and paralysis. Phosphorus causes second- to third-degree burns on contact with the skin.

TREATMENT. Acute poisoning should be treated by gastric lavage with large amounts of 0.1 per cent copper sulfate, which acts as an antidote by forming an insoluble copper phosphide. Activated charcoal absorbs inorganic phosphorus. Potassium permanganate, 1:5000, or 2 per cent hydrogen peroxide tends to convert elemental phosphorus to less toxic phosphoric acid and phosphates. Mineral oil cathartics or absorbable fats or oils should not be used; the latter promote further absorption of the phosphorus. Supportive measures include treatment for dehydration, acidosis and shock, and subsequently a high carbohydrate diet and amino acids, orally or parenterally, to protect the liver from serious injury. When there has been liver damage, such treatment should be continued until there is evidence that function has returned.

66. **Phosphorus, Organic.** Phosphate ester insecticides should never be used in homes. All are anticholinesterase compounds with initial muscarinic, followed by nicotinic, activity and direct actions on the central nervous system. There are three main types of organic phosphate insecticides: the nitrophenyl thiophosphates, the alkyl pyrophosphates and the phosphoramides. They vary in distribution in tissues and in duration of action. The phosphoramide compounds have no cerebral action, acting entirely by peripheral inhibition of cholinesterase. The alkyl pyrophosphates are rapidly hydrolyzed in the body to nontoxic metabolites. The thiophosphates are more stable and are detoxified slowly. Potentiation may occur between two organophosphates, ethyl-P-nitrophenyl benzenthionophosphonate (EPN) and malathion, belnav and malathion, or guthion and dipterex. Accidents are possible when small amounts of potentiating compounds are present in the daily diet. Moreover, certain drugs of the phenothiazine type potentiate the toxic effect of organophosphates. The importance of long-term consumption of pesticide-contaminated foods is not known, but acute poisoning from contamination of grain has occurred, as in the "Follidol poisoning" in Southern India.

Most of these compounds are several times more toxic than nicotine. One drop of parathion in the eye may be fatal. Malathion is probably the least toxic; 1 gm, however, may be fatal. Symptoms are prompt (within 30 minutes) and may continue for 24 to 48 hours. They include increased secretions (such as sweat, saliva, tears and bronchial fluids), nausea, vomiting, diarrhea with the typical odor of organophosphates, miosis, blurred vision, retinopathy and retinal hemorrhages, bronchiolar spasms and pulmonary edema. Ataxia, vertigo, tremors, muscular weakness, fibrillation, fasciculation, finger and mouth twitching, muscular paralysis, cyanosis, dyspnea, chest constriction, stupor, coma and convulsions may also occur. Blood dyscrasias with porphyrins in blood and urine, and chromolachrymorrhea (red-stained tears) have occurred.

TREATMENT. Artificial respiration to maintain ventilatory exchange is indicated. Wash all insecticide off the skin and mucous membranes. Atropine is helpful, but its action is limited to antagonization of the excess acetylcholine accumulated as a result of decreased cholinesterase activity. In severe poisoning, atropine should be given intravenously and should be repeated at 5- to 10-

minute intervals until signs of atropinization occur. Hyperatropinization and toxicity should be avoided, especially since the neuromuscular actions and tremors of hyperatropinization resemble those of organophosphate poisoning. Residual incoordination and tremors due to overuse of atropine may occur.

In severe organic phosphate poisoning the specific cholinesterase reactivator, 2-pyridine aldoxime methiodide (2-PAM), should be given. Doses of 1 gm intravenously have been found to be effective in adults. 2-Pyridine aldoxime ethanesulfonate (P2S) has been shown to be just as effective as 2-PAM iodide and has the advantage of being water soluble. Reflexes are restored within 20 minutes. Morphine, barbiturates and respiratory depressants should be avoided.

67. **Rotenone (Derris Root, Cubeb).** An insecticide frequently mixed with pyrethrum powder. The lethal dose is probably large. Solutions or powder may be absorbed from the lungs or gastrointestinal tract. Symptoms are predominantly respiratory. There is an acceleration in the respiratory rate followed by a decrease; death occurs from respiratory failure. Evidence of gastric irritation such as nausea and vomiting may occur, which may partly reflect central emetic action as well. Symptoms occur promptly within a few minutes to an hour.

TREATMENT. Lavage, catharsis and supportive measures are used; oils and oily cathartics are contraindicated, since they increase the solubility and absorption of the poison.

68. **Salicylates (Methyl Salicylate, Salicylic Acid, Sodium Salicylate, Acetylsalicylic Acid and a Variety of Proprietary Ointments and Medications Containing Either Salicylic Acid or Salicylates).** Prolonged excessive or accidental ingestion of salicylates may result in severe poisoning. Absorption may occur from the mouth, gastrointestinal tract and skin. The peak action occurs about 4 hours after a single toxic dose and may last longer than 18 hours. Rarely, effects of poisoning may persist for 10 days. Methyl salicylate and salicylic acid produce symptoms rapidly. Both cause severe gastrointestinal irritation with nausea and vomiting and colicky abdominal pain. Local painful lesions are caused by the caustic action of the acid, while systemic intoxication may lead to a scarlatiniform or bullous rash, with pruritis. Intoxication may occur from the use of salicylic acid powder or ointment on large, open, weeping skin lesions. The toxic dose is usually in excess of 0.15 gm per kg.

Initial symptoms are respiratory. Respiratory stimulation occurs via the vagus. There is an increase in the respiratory minute volume without necessarily an increase in rate, but with a characteristic and marked prolongation of the expiratory phase, leading to a decrease in the pCO_2. The resulting respiratory alkalosis leads to cerebral symptoms of apathy, confusion, coma and an increase in cerebrospinal fluid pressure. Renal compensation follows, producing an increase in bicarbonate in the urine, a decrease in urine chloride, with corresponding rise in plasma chloride and a decrease in serum base. Renal compensation thus leads to loss of base from the body, predominantly sodium. In addition, salicylates appear to disturb the metabolism of carbohydrate. An unusually striking and persistent ketosis is associated with or soon follows early symptoms of toxicity. The ketoacidosis produces further base depletion through the kidney, and a true metabolic acidosis may be superimposed upon the respiratory alkalosis. Thus, diagnosis of the electrolyte disorder cannot be made merely by determination of the carbon dioxide content of the blood. Measurement of the pH of the blood is of value when correlated with other findings. Salicylates have an inhibiting effect on the formation of prothrombin by the liver, leading to purpuric manifestations. Renal and hepatic dysfunction impair detoxification and elimination of excess salicylates and prolong toxicity. Hypersensitivity to salicylates, with cutaneous, bronchopulmonary or angiotic-anaphylactoid features, is well known. Dehydration in uncomplicated salicylate poisoning in a well child is usually not striking; salicylate poisoning often occurs, however, in children who are ill, and the dehydration produced may be moderate to severe, with marked hyperthermia. Fever and dehydration may enhance toxicity of salicylates. Vertigo, tinnitus, deafness, blurred vision, retinal hemorrhages and amblyopia, central nervous system effects of restlessness, apprehension, garrulity, hallucinations, and tremors followed by mental disturbances ("salicylate jag") and convulsions and coma may occur. Anorexia, vomiting, sweating, pallor or flushing, cyanosis, tetany, numbness and tingling of the face, lips and extremities, and bleeding from any area of the body may occur. Laboratory findings of diagnostic value are acetonuria and a falsely positive test result for diacetic acid with ferric chloride. Diacetic acid produces with ferric chloride a burgundy color in urine, whereas salicylates produce a violet to a deep purple color. Boiling of acidified urine will volatilize the diacetic acid, producing a negative ferric chloride test result in the absence of salicylate. Salicylates can give a false positive result for "sugar" in urine tested by Fehling's or Benedict's reagents. Later evidences of toxicity may consist of erythematous, scarlatinaform, pruritic, eczematous or desquamative skin lesions. Salicylates may also impair coagulation, leading to a hemorrhagic diathesis.

TREATMENT. Gastric lavage or induction of emesis to remove salicylates from the gastrointestinal tract, followed by correction of dehydration and acidosis, requires appropriate fluid therapy. Correction of hyperthermia with external cooling, and elimination of the poison with a "forced alkaline diuresis" or with peritoneal or hemodialysis is indicated. Potassium will be given for hypopotassemia, and vitamin K or prothrombin infusions for the hemorrhagic coagulopathy of salicylism.

69. **Santonin.** The high solubility of santonin in bile and alkaline solutions causes rapid absorption from the upper intestine and leads to rapid development of toxic symptoms. An unknown product is formed which, when excreted, is an aid in diagnosis, since it produces a yellow color in acid urine and a pink color in alkaline urine. Toxic symptoms are manifested initially by transitory blue vision and later by yellow vision (xanthopsia). Other symptoms include headache, vomiting and confusion; with large doses there may be abdominal pain, diarrhea and bloody urine. The skin is cold and clammy and covered with perspiration. A fall in body temperature, a skin rash, tremors, cardiac and respiratory depression and convulsions develop.

TREATMENT. Immediate lavage should be followed by saline catharsis. Oily demulcents or oily cathartics are contraindicated, since they enhance the absorption of poison. Intramuscularly administered barbiturates may be used for convulsions.

70. **Shellfish.** Most shellfish poisoning in the United States is due to contamination by staphylococci or to allergic sensitivity. In some localities during certain seasons (summer and fall) mussels and clams may contain powerful neurotoxins. The origin of the poison is thought to be a dinoflagellate in the bodies of the clams. The poison is not destroyed by heating. Three general types of involvement occur: (1) gastroenteritis with nausea, vomiting and diarrhea; (2) nervous symptoms (paresthesias, tremors and convulsions), diffuse erythema, urticaria, angina and dyspnea; and (3) a paralytic

form in which symptoms simulate those of curare poisoning with respiratory paralysis.

TREATMENT. Induction of emesis, lavage and maintenance of respiration. Prostigmine methylsulfate (1:2000 solution) intravenously has been recommended.

71. **Sodium Hypochlorite.** Bleaching solutions contain sodium hypochlorite, 3 to 6 per cent in water. Their action is similar to that of sodium hydroxide in high concentrations. Acid secretions in the stomach release irritating hypochlorous acid. Fifteen to 30 ml orally may be fatal for children. Inhalation of hypochlorous acid fumes produces pulmonary irritation, coughing and choking, laryngobronchial spasm, and pulmonary edema. Ingestion causes irritation and corrosion of mucous membranes. Edema of the pharynx and larynx may be intense.

TREATMENT. Repeated lavage with sodium bicarbonate or sodium thiosulfate solution. Administration of a saline cathartic is advisable. Acid antidotes should never be used.

72. **Solanine (Solanism).** Symptoms of poisoning may follow ingestion of sprouted potatoes containing an alkaloid, solanine, found in or near the peel. Species of solanum (black nightshade, bittersweet) also contain the poison. Vomiting, diarrhea, colicky pains, headaches, depression, pain in the rectum, suppression of urine, and collapse occur within a few hours. Hallucinations and coma are sometimes present.

73. **Strychnine.** Strychnine is a powerful central nervous system stimulant. It produces little local gastrointestinal reaction, and the first symptoms are those of nervous system stimulation. At first a stiffness of the face and neck muscles occurs, followed by hyperactive reflexes of all muscles, and later by muscular twitchings and spinal convulsions. A characteristic position of the body occurs due to the action of the stronger groups of muscles. The back is arched in a position of opisthotonos; the legs are adducted and extended, and the feet turned in; the fists are clenched and the facial muscles are tightly contracted, producing risus sardonicus; there is exophthalmos and mydriasis. Involvement of the muscles of respiration produces respiratory arrest with resultant cyanosis. The patient usually remains conscious and is in severe pain. After such a convulsion, which lasts a minute or more, there is a period of relaxation with depression and, in some instances, unconsciousness due to apnea and anoxemia. In 10 to 15 minutes another spinal convulsion occurs. Medullary paralysis, due to excessive stimulation or anoxemia, follows the second to fifth convulsion.

TREATMENT. Lavage should not be done during convulsive attacks. Recurrence of convulsions must be prevented. Large doses of short-acting barbiturates should be given intravenously and repeated if necessary; sodium phenobarbital and amytal are effective. The dose should be sufficient to prevent or stop convulsions and keep the patient asleep, but not to depress respiration or blood pressure. Anesthesia may be necessary temporarily until a barbiturate can be given. All types of stimuli should be avoided. Lavage with 2 per cent tannic acid or strong tea binds the alkaloid. Maintenance of respiration, using an artificial respirator, with a muscle relaxant such as *d*-tubocurarine or gallamine triethiodide initially, and mephenesin during the phase of recovery is recommended.

74. **Thallium.** Thallium acetate has been administered orally to produce depilation in the treatment of ringworm of the scalp and locally as a depilatory for cosmetic purposes, but owing to the danger of serious toxic effects such use is to be condemned. The initial acute gastrointestinal symptoms, which usually result from accidental ingestion, occur 12 to 24 hours after ingestion. There is severe, paroxysmal abdominal pain with vomiting and diarrhea, necrosis of hepatic and renal cells, proteinuria, oliguria and anuria. Hemorrhage, desquamation of the mucosa, and eosinophilia may be present. The late effects of acute or chronic poisoning are predominantly on the nervous system. Peripheral neuritis with paralysis, optic atrophy, tremors, ataxia, hallucinations, convulsions and coma occur. Alopecia is common and is attributed to a toxic effect on the sympathetic nervous system. In chronic poisoning thallium accumulates in the skin and hair.

TREATMENT. Essentially the same as for arsenic (9), but BAL is of limited value. Gastric lavage with 1 per cent potassium-iodide and oral administration of potassium iodide with diuretics has been tried.

75. **Thiocyanate Insecticides.** These agents, which contain methyl and ethyl thiocyanates, induce coma, cyanosis, dyspnea and tonic convulsions. Respiratory difficulty may occur.

TREATMENT. Skin contamination should be removed by scrubbing with soap and water. Gastric lavage with tap water and saline catharsis are advisable. Renal and hepatic injury may occur later. Hemodialysis is recommended, as renal tubular damage retards the efficacy of forced diuresis.

76. **Veratrine.** An alkaloid obtained from *V. cevadilla* (sabadilla), a false hellebore plant, all parts of which are poisonous, especially the roots. Cevadine is crystallized veratrine. Sabadilla dusts and sprays and extracts of sabadilla are used as insecticides and pediculicides. Ingestion produces violent vomiting by a central action on the nodose ganglion of the vagus, diarrhea, intense burning and generalized muscular weakness. Muscular and autonomic nervous system reactions are similar to those from pyrethrum and nicotine.

TREATMENT. See 56.

77. **Veratrum.** Veratrum and Zygadenus are found in hellebore *(Veratrum album, viride* or *californicum). Zygadenus venenosus,* the death camass, contains similar nitrogenous compounds. Ingestion of these plants produces nausea, severe vomiting, diarrhea, muscular weakness, paresthesias, hiccups, salivation, sweating, visual disturbances, bradycardia and low blood pressure. Very large doses may produce hypotension, which has been the basis of its use as an antihypertensive drug. In digitalized patients, veratrum alkaloids will induce arrhythmia and ventricular fibrillation.

TREATMENT. Gastric lavage followed by saline catharsis, tannic acid, and activated charcoal to adsorb the alkaloid. Atropine is of value to block the fall of blood pressure and the bradycardia. Sympathomimetic vasopressors may be needed for severe hypotensive episodes.

78. **Warfarin (Dicoumarin) (3-Alpha-acetonyl benzyl-4-hydroxycoumarin).** A rodenticide found in Dethmor, Rax Powder, D-con and other products. Available in 1:200 concentration in cornstarch and used as a rat bait in 1:400 concentration in cornmeal. The dicumarol action inhibits prothrombin formation, but it is more potent than dicumarol. Absorption of other coumarins is slow and irregular, and especially of bishydroxycoumarin. Twenty-four to 48 hours may elapse before any effect is noted; the absorption and action of warfarin is faster and more complete. Elimination is slow. The action is chiefly on the synthesis of prothrombin, with a gradual depression of prothrombin levels in the blood leading to spontaneous hemorrhages in skin and mucous membranes, hematuria, hematemesis, melena and liver hemorrhage. The action may persist for 10 days.

TREATMENT. Gastric lavage and catharsis should be instituted. Vitamin K in large doses should be given intravenously. Whole blood transfusions or exchange transfusion may also be needed.

79. **Zinc Stearate Powder.** A severe irritation of the

respiratory mucous membranes is produced by aspiration of the zinc stearate powder in talcum powder, resulting in congestion, hyperemia, edema, and obstruction of bronchioles with mucus. Bronchopneumonia is common in infants who survive the first day or two, and may be followed by intrapulmonary fibrosis or a diffuse microgranulomatosis of the lungs. Choking, coughing, cyanosis and signs of suffocation tend to develop immediately.

TREATMENT. Aspiration of the powder and accumulated secretions by bronchoscopy is worthy of trial, but it is not likely to be effective because of the adhesive quality of the powder. Administration of oxygen is important, and there may be an added advantage in giving it in combination with helium. Powders containing zinc stearate should *never* be used for infants and small children.

LIST OF CHEMICALS

The following list includes individual chemical compounds, alphabetically arranged, with an appended numeral referring to the class (see above) with which they are associated; e.g., Chloroethane (46) is referred to Hydrocarbons (Halogenated).

Abrin, 1
Acetaldehyde (ethyl aldehyde), 38
Acetanilid (N-phenylacetamide), 6
Acetic acid, concentrated, 2
Acetoarsenite (Paris green), 9
Acetone, 3
Acetophenetidin (phenacetin), 6
Acetylene tetrachloride (tetrachloroethane), 45
Acetylsalicylic acid (aspirin), 68
Acid. See particular acid.
Acid-like substances, 2
Aconite (aconitine), 53
Alcohol, 3
Alcohol, ethyl (ethanol, grain alcohol, neutral spirits), 3
Aldehydes, 38
Aldrin (Compound 118), 25
Alkalis, corrosive, 49
Allethrin (Allyn cinerin), 56
Allyl-isopropylacetyl-carbamide (Sedormid), 13
Allyn cinerin (Allethrin), 56
Aluminum salts, 4
Amanita, 55
p-Aminophenol, 6
Aminopyrine (amidopyrine), 6
Ammonia (ammonium hydroxide), 49
Ammoniated mercury, 51
Ammonium hydroxide (ammonia), 49
Amobarbital (Amytal), 13
Amphetamine, 5
Amyl nitrite, 57
Amytal (amobarbital), 13
Andromedotoxin, 54
Aniline (phenylamine), 6
Antihistaminics, 13
Antimony, 7
Antipyrine, 6
ANTU, 8
Arochlor, 45
Arsenates and arsenites, 9
Arsenic trioxide (white arsenic), 9
Aspidium, 10
Aspirin (acetylsalicylic acid), 68
Asterol, 11
Atropine, 12
Barbital (Veronal), 13
Barbiturates, 13
Barium salts, 14
Benadryl, 13
Benzalkonium chloride (Zephiran), 35
Benzene (benzol), 15
Benzene hexachloride (hexachlorocyclohexane), 25
Benzethonium chloride (Phemerol), 35
Benzine, 44
Benzol (benzene), 15
Beta-naphthol (β naphthol), 62
Bichloride of mercury (mercuric chloride, corrosive sublimate), 51
Bismuth, 16
Bismuth subnitrate, 57
Boracic acid (boric acid), 17
Borate salts, 17
Borax (sodium tetraborate), 17
Boric acid (boracic acid), 17
Boron, 17
Bromate, methyl, 45
Bromate salts, 18
Bromides, 19
Brown Mixture (contains tartar emetic), 7
Butacaine, 28
Cadmium salts, 20
Calcium hypochlorite (chlorinated lime), 71
Calomel (mercurous chloride), 51
Campho-phenique, 62
Camphor (gum camphor), 62
Camphor tar (naphthalene, naphthene), 15
Carbitol, 3
Carbolic acid (phenol, hydroxybenzene), 62
Carbon bisulfide (carbon disulfide), 21
Carbon monoxide, 22
Carbon tetrachloride (perchloromethane), 45
Castrix, 73
Catechol (pyrocatechol), 62
Caustic potash (potassium hydroxide), 49
Caustic soda (sodium hydroxide), 49
Ceepryn chloride (cetyl pyridinium chloride), 35
Cetyl pyridinium chloride (Ceepryn chloride), 35
Chenopodium oil (wormseed oil), 23
Chloral hydrate, 13
Chlordane (Compound 1068), 25
Chloride, methyl, 45
Chlorinated camphene (Toxaphene, Compound 3956, octachlorocamphene), 25
Chlorinated diphenyl, 45
Chlorinated insecticides, 25
Chlorinated lime (calcium hypochlorite), 71
Chlorinated naphthalene, 45
Chlorine water, 49
Chloroacetic acid, 42
Chloroaniline, 6
Chlorobenzene, 24
Chlorobutanol, 13
Chloroethane (ethyl chloride), 45
Chloroform (trichloromethane), 45
Chlorohydrin, ethylene, 45
Chloronitrobenzene, 6
Chromate salts, 26
Chromic acid, 2
Cicutoxin, 73
Cleaning solutions, 27
Clorox, 71
Cobalt salts, 2
Cocaine, 28
Codeine, 60
Colchicum autumnale, 50
Compound 42 (Warfarin), 78
Compound 118 (Aldrin), 25
Compound 1068 (Chlordane), 25

JOHN A. ANDERSON
MANDAYAM J. NARASIMHAN, JR.

Arena, J. M.: Poisoning: Toxicology–Symptoms–Treatments. 3rd ed. Springfield, Ill., Charles C Thomas, 1973.
Gleason, M. N., Gosselin, R. E., Hodge, H. C., and Smith, R. P.: Clinical Toxicology of Commercial Products. 3rd ed. Baltimore, The Williams & Wilkins Company, 1969.
Goodman, L. S., and Gilman, A.: The Pharmacological Basis of Therapeutics. 4th ed. New York, The Macmillan Company, 1970.
Hardin, J. W., and Arena, J. M.: Human Poisoning from Native and Cultivated Plants. Durham, N. C., Duke University Press, 1973.

ACRODYNIA

(Pink Disease; Swift's Disease; Feer's Disease; Erythredema; Dermatopolyneuritis)

Acrodynia (the term, derived from the Greek, denotes painful extremities) is a syndrome consisting of many unusual symptoms which, in the well established case, are so distinctive that there is practically no differential diagnosis. There are few clinical conditions in which extreme and persistent misery is such a prominent part of the clinical picture.

HISTORY. In 1828 an outbreak of pink disease in France was attributed to arsenical poisoning, whereas in 1903 Selter of Solingen described this disease and called it a trophodermatosis. Feer of Zurich, whose name is attached to the disease in Europe, did not know that such a clinical entity existed until the early 1920's, when he described his interpretation of it as "Vegetative Neurose des Kleinkindes." The condition had been recognized in Australia as early as 1890 as "pink disease," but it was not until 1914 that Swift's paper brought it into focus as a distinct clinical entity under the name "erythredema." The disease had been observed and commented upon as early as 1915 by Bilderback in Oregon, but there was nothing in British or American literature on the condition in the United States until Bilderback and Byfield independently published articles describing it in 1920.

ETIOLOGY AND EPIDEMIOLOGY. Acrodynia is principally a disease of infancy and early childhood. In the United States it has become uncommon, as it apparently has in other parts of the world where it once was relatively common, especially in England and Australia. Formerly it was attributed to multiple vitamin deficiencies and to a virus.

From the studies of Warkany and Hubbard and of others, it now seems that most and perhaps all cases of acrodynia represent the clinical response to repeated ingestion of or contact with mercury. Whether this response is the result of chronic poisoning or is an unusual reaction occasioned by other factors is not clear. Since only a fraction of the infants and children exposed to mercury for periods of time apparently adequate for the development of acrodynia acquire the disease, the possibility exists that the disease is the result of a sensitization to mercury followed by a hypersensitive state.

The frequency with which unusual amounts of mercury are demonstrated in urine would seem to be highest in areas where mercurial medications are or have been widely prescribed. In the southern United States and in England, teething powders and lotions have been a principal source of mercury, whereas in France and Switzerland, vermifuges have been a more common source. Other reported sources of mercury include calomel, mercurial ointments, diaper rinses, paints, wallpaper, and even absorption from dental fillings. The possibility of accidental ingestion of mercurials is another factor.

PATHOLOGY. Many of the changes such as degeneration, chromatolysis and demyelinization of peripheral nerves are attributed to mercurial toxicity associated with semistarvation and malnutrition.

CLINICAL MANIFESTATIONS. The natural course of acrodynia is prolonged, extending from several months to a year. There are all grades of severity. The child becomes listless; he is no longer interested in play and is restless and irritable. Generalized, inconstant rashes, which are protean, recur from time to time. Early the tips of the fingers, toes and nose acquire a pinkish color, and later the hands and feet become a dusky pink, with patchy areas of ischemia and cyanotic congestion. This shades off at the wrists and ankles; the extremities are cold and clammy. These changes in the extremities are the most distinctive features of the syndrome, being different from those of any other disease occurring in children, and are responsible for the term "pink disease." Frequently the cheeks and the tip of the nose acquire a scarlet color.

As the disease becomes established, the sweat glands are enormously dilated and enlarged, and perspiration is profuse; at times the infant may be drenched, necessitating frequent changes of clothing. Secondary infection may lead to a severe pyoderma. There is desquamation of the soles and palms, which, though usually superficial, may be severe and recur during the course of the disease. The fingers and toes appear edematous; the swelling is due to hyperplasia and hyperkeratosis of the skin. An outstanding symptom is constant pruritus with excruciating pain in the hands and feet (Fig. 28–1). Children will rub their hands together for hours, and older children will complain of a severe burning sensation.

The nails become dark and frequently drop off. Occasionally gangrene of the toes and fingers develops, and trophic ulcers may result from the constant rubbing of the hands and feet. The hair tends to fall out and is often pulled out by the child. The vascular and trophic changes in the extremities and the cutaneous pruritus are neurologic in origin.

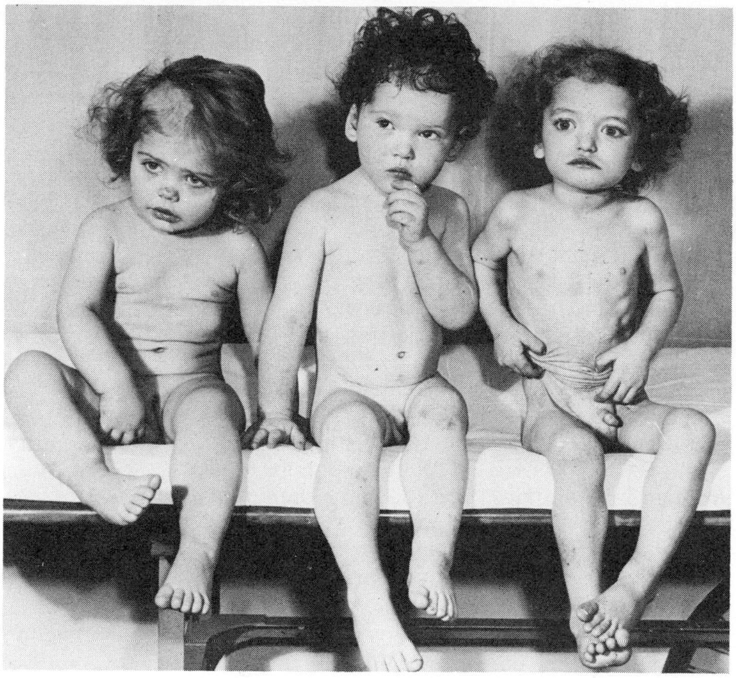

Figure 28–1 Three children with acrodynia. They have constant pruritus, patchy areas of ischemia on legs and arms; acral pinkish blue discoloration of hands, feet, mouth and nose; patchy loss of hair; and a rash on arms and legs and trunk. All had hypertension, hypotonicity, irritability, polyuria, polydipsia and anorexia. The child on the right had malnutrition and severe hypoelectrolytemia.

In more than 60 per cent of the patients there is photophobia without evidence of local inflammation of the eyes. The children shield their eyes or bury their faces in their pillows. The lax ligaments and hypotonia permit the children to assume unusual positions (Fig. 28–2), and they often lie for hours with their heads between their legs. The so-called salaam position is frequently assumed, often with constant rubbing motions of the hands and feet, owing to the pain and itching.

In extreme cases the teeth may be lost; necrosis of the jaw bones frequently follows. Initially the gums appear normal except for a slightly deeper red color; later they become inflamed and swollen. Salivation then becomes pronounced, and the saliva often flows from the mouth in a constant stream. Anorexia is prominent, but because of the excessive perspiration large quantities of water are consumed. There may be diarrhea, and prolapse of the rectum is a frequent complication. The blood pressure and pulse rate may be increased significantly. Fever is usually not present unless there is some complication such as a urinary tract infection or bronchopneumonia.

Nervous symptoms are an important part of the syndrome and include peripheral ones such as neuritis, and central ones such as mental apathy and irritability. Early in the disease the tendon reflexes may be normal or increased, but later they disappear. There is not a true motor paralysis, but because of the soft, flabby musculature the child has no desire to walk and is hypotonic, listless and hypomotile. Many of the symptoms and signs suggest involvement of the vasomotor mechanism. The severe pain prevents normal sleep. There is no time when a child with acrodynia appears happy or comfortable; he does not play or smile, but appears dejected and melancholic, a picture of abject mis-

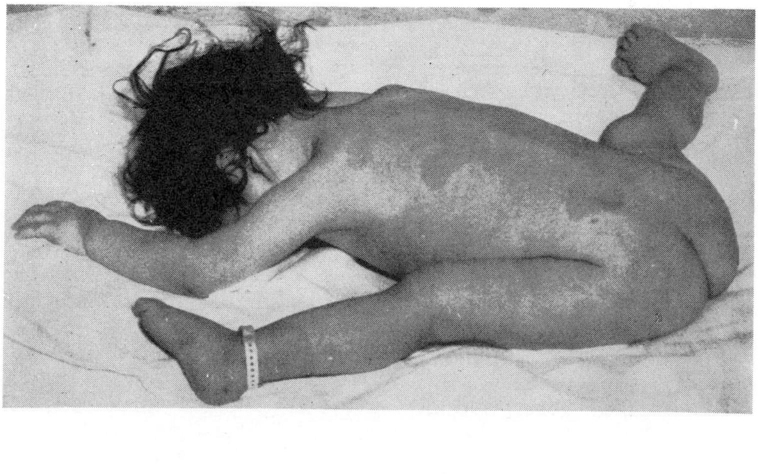

Figure 28–2 Extreme hypotonia and photophobia in an infant with acrodynia. This bizarre position may be maintained for hours.

ery. The sympathovasomotor dysfunction, the hyperhidrosis, trophic changes, and photophobia indicate an autonomic dysfunction, a form of selective dysautonomia, as the basis, with hypersensitivity to mercurials as the most probable cause of acrodynia.

LABORATORY DATA. There are no characteristic morphologic changes of the blood or significant changes in the cerebrospinal fluid. There may be proteinuria, but the only characteristic urinary finding is the presence of mercury.

PROPHYLAXIS. There is little or no need for mercurial medications in pediatric practice, and they should be avoided whenever possible. It is most important that one be alert for possible contacts with mercury in various household and industrial preparations.

TREATMENT. There is probably no more difficult problem in pediatrics than the management of an infant with severe acrodynia. The extreme restlessness, irritability and pain are not readily allayed. Barbiturates are usually not so effective as paraldehyde administered rectally in olive oil (5 to 10 ml). Symptomatic relief has also been reported from the use of tolazoline hydrochloride (Priscoline) in doses of 12.5 mg at intervals of 4 to 6 hours.

BAL (British anti-lewisite; 2,3-dimercaptopropanol) has been used therapeutically, apparently with good effect in some instances and especially when administration was begun early in the disease. The recommended plan of treatment is 3 mg per kg every 4 hours for 48 hours, then every 6 hours for 24 hours, followed by administration at intervals of 12 hours for 7 days. The drug is administered intramuscularly in a 10 per cent solution. Toxic effects of BAL have been observed (see Table 30–1).

Penicillamine (N-acetyl-D,L-penicillamine) has been used with apparent beneficial effect in chronic mercury poisoning, including acrodynia, and has the advantage over BAL that it is administered orally. Tetracyclines can bind inorganic mercury in experimental animals.

The diet should contain generous amounts of proteins, minerals and vitamins, especially those of the B-complex group, including nicotinamide and thiamine. Frequently anorexia is so great that feeding must be by gavage.

Owing to the profuse sweating, thirst is usually prominent, and, in contrast to the frequent refusal to eat, the child will usually take relatively large quantities of fluids. Severe deficits in serum electrolytes (sodium, potassium, and chloride) may occur; oral as well as intravenous replacement may be required. Insofar as possible, fluid intake should be oral rather than parenteral.

The child should be kept as clean as possible to minimize the chances of secondary pyogenic skin infections. Frequent alcohol rubs may aid in this respect in addition to being soothing. The clothing should be light, preferably of cotton, and should be changed frequently when perspiration is profuse.

It is obvious that the family must be made aware of the nature of the illness and of its prolonged course if they are to be expected to play their part successfully.

J. B. Bilderback*
John A. Anderson

Bilderback, J. B.: Group of cases of unknown etiology and diagnosis. Northwest Med. *19*:263, 1920.
Bilderback, J. B.: Acrodynia, J.A.M.A. *84*:495, 1925.
Bilderback, J. B.: Acrodynia, Swift's disease. Northwest Med. *31*:161, 1932.
Bivings, L.: Acrodynia: A summary of BAL therapy reports and a case report of calomel disease. J. Pediatr. *34*:322, 1949.
Byfield, A. H.: A polyneuritic syndrome resembling pellagra-acrodynia (?) seen in very young children: Report of cases. Am. J. Dis. Child. *20*:347, 1920.
Editorial: New source of mercury poisoning. New Engl. J. Med. *269*:926, 1963.
Fanconi, G., and Botsjtejn, A.: Die feersche Krankheit (Akrodynia) und Quecksilbermedikation. Helvet. Paediat. Acta *3*:264, 1948.
Feer, E.: Die spezifische vegetative Neuropathie des Kleinkindes (kindliche Akrodynia). Schweiz. Med. Wchnschr. *65*:977, 1935.
Hirschman, S. Z., Feingold, M., and Boylen, G.: Mercury in house paint as a cause of acrodynia. Effect of therapy with N-acetyl-D,L-penicillamine. New Engl. J. Med. *269*:889, 1963.
Peterson, J. C., and Laughmiller, R.: Acrodynia: Treatment with adrenolytic drugs. Acta Paediat. *43*:517, 1954.
Smith, A. D. M., and Miller, J. W.: Treatment of inorganic mercury poisoning with N-Acetyl-D, L-penicillamine. Lancet *1*:640, 1961.
Swift, H.: Erythroedema. in Transactions of the Tenth Session, Australasian Medical Congress. Auckland, New Zealand, 1914, p. 547.
Warkany, J.: Acrodynia—Postmortem of a disease. Am. J. Dis. Child. *112*:147, 1966.
Warkany, J., and Hubbard, D. M.: Adverse mercurial reactions in form of acrodynia and related conditions. Lancet *1*:829, 1948.
Weston, W.: Acrodynia. Arch. Pediat. *37*:513, 1920.

*Deceased.

INCREASED LEAD ABSORPTION AND LEAD POISONING

Of children in the United States 1 to 6 years of age, 10 per cent or more have absorbed significantly increased amounts of lead. Abnormally high absorption is most prevalent in old housing in both rural and urban areas. Most children with increased lead absorption give evidence of disturbed heme synthesis, but few have clear-cut symptoms of plumbism.

Acute encephalopathy is the most severe form of disease. Chelation therapy substantially reduces lead poisoning mortality, but 50 per cent or more of the survivors of encephalopathy treated *after* the onset of symptoms sustain *severe* permanent brain damage. Prognosis following less severe but recurrent *symptomatic* bouts of plumbism is also poor. These observations emphasize the need to detect and treat children who are in the early states of increased lead absorption in the hope of preventing permanent neurologic sequelae. Where there have been effective screening programs, the incidence of new cases is decreasing.

DEFINITIONS. "Normal" exposure to lead is generally defined as consisting of lead found in uncontaminated food, water and air. "Undue" lead exposure refers to exposure to additional nondietary sources, the most important of which are particulate lead in household dust, in soil and in paints. The current and recent levels of lead absorption in various groups of children can be estimated on the basis of their mean blood lead levels. For normally exposed groups in uncontaminated areas, the mean concentrations of lead are generally 15 to 20 μg/dl of whole blood (range 10 to 35 μg). For groups with undue exposure to nondietary sources, the mean blood lead levels generally range from 30 to 50 μg/dl. In study of the individual, serial measurements are essential. Ordinarily the term "increased lead absorption" implies sustained levels above 50 μg/dl. The individual's blood lead concentration is related to the risk of toxicity, but the measurement of lead in body fluids does not directly measure toxicity. "Lead poisoning" signifies *both* increased lead absorption *and* metabolic, functional or clinical evidence of toxicity. The total lead burden of the body is the amount in all tissues, including bone.

PATHOPHYSIOLOGY AND EPIDEMIOLOGY. The body's total lead burden is divided into two major components—that in bone and that in soft tissues. The amounts and proportions of lead sequestered in bone increase with age, under conditions of normal exposure. The time of residence of lead in soft tissues is about 1 month, whereas its residence when incorporated into bone is about 25 years. Lead sequestered in bone is essentially removed from the active metabolic pool, and the toxicity of lead is related to changes in the small mobile soft tissue pool.

Lead may inhibit heme synthesis at a number of steps, but the effects are reversible and slowly disappear after excessive intake ceases. In adults, the level of hemoglobin falls as the blood lead level rises above 60 μg/dl. A high proportion of developing erythroblasts in the marrow show basophilic stippling, but basophilic stippling is an inconstant feature in smears of peripheral blood. Severe acute lead poisoning may be associated with the Fanconi syndrome (generalized renal aminoaciduria, mellituria and hyperphosphaturia, with hypophosphatemia), owing to acute proximal renal tubular injury. This, too, is reversible after several weeks. Late lead nephropathy characterized by hyperuricemia, with or without gout, has been reported as a sequel of chronic childhood plumbism only in Australia.

Tenfold or greater increases over normal exposures to lead are required to raise soft tissue levels from normal to levels associated with acute clinical manifestations. A three- to fivefold increase is sufficient to disturb heme synthesis. Children with radiologic evidence of increased storage of lead in bone show very slow rates of decline in blood lead concentrations and in abnormal levels of heme metabolites after separation from sources of excess lead. In general, the period required for return of levels in soft tissues to near normal ranges is at least twice the length of the period of increased intake. Spontaneous urinary excretion of lead is generally less than 50 μg/day; it may or may not be increased in clinically manifest cases of acute poisoning.

Balance studies in children suggest that 15 to 20 per cent of dietary lead is retained, with an unknown but probably substantial fraction incorporated into growing bone. An FAO/WHO panel has recommended that dietary lead intake be set at less than 5 μg/kg/day. Experimental studies in weanling rodents suggest that absorption, retention and toxicity of lead are enhanced by deficiencies in dietary iron, calcium and possibly magnesium.

Assimilation of airborne lead through the respiratory tract has been studied extensively in adults, but not in children. The fraction of particulate lead suspended in air that is retained in the pulmonary bed depends on the size of the particles. It is estimated that about 30 to 40 per cent of particles under 2 μ in diameter reach the pulmonary bed and are retained. At currently prevalent airborne lead levels (under 2 μg Pb/M^3), the amount assimilated by the respiratory route is probably small in comparison to alimentary intake. Airborne lead settles and accumulates on the surface of the soil, where it may significantly contribute to total intake in toddlers. The powdering of paint from the surfaces of old buildings and the lead from automotive exhausts are major contributors to the lead content of surface soil and dust, but their relative contributions are not precisely known. Exposure to dust may account for a large proportion of those children whose blood lead levels remain in the range from 30 to 50 μg/dl.

Children may have multiple sources of exposure to lead, most of which are singly negligible. The total daily diet generally contains less than 100 μg, though in an infant a diet containing a preponderance of canned items may produce some increase in dietary intake. On the other hand, a gram of street dust in urban areas may contain from 1500 to 2500 μg of lead, and multilayered chips of old lead pigment paints may contain 20,000 to 100,000 μg/cm^2 of exposed surface. Lead paints are found in both interior and exterior paints, and especially in houses built and painted before 1950. According to the 1970 United States census, 30 million such dwellings are still in use, about one fourth in deteriorated condition. Sporadic cases of clinical plumbism have been traced to other sources of very high concentrations of lead besides old paint. These unusual sources include: (1) lead shot, fishing weights and leaded jewelry swallowed and retained in the stomach, where lead is slowly dissolved over a period of weeks; (2) juices conveyed or stored in improperly lead-glazed earthenware; (3) chewing on lead type or toys; (4) lead nipple shields; (5) soft drinking water stored in lead-lined cisterns; (6) lead-soldered vessels used in cooking; and (7) burning casings of storage batteries. In addition, children who remain in old houses during the removal of old lead paint by burning and scraping may show sharp rises in lead absorption for periods of several months.

CLINICAL MANIFESTATIONS. During the course of chronically increased lead absorption, there may be recurrent acute symptomatic episodes. Milder episodes may abate spontaneously. The syndrome of lead colic is characterized in children by hyperirritability, anorexia, decreased play activity and sporadic vomiting and constipation. Affected patients may have iron deficiency or lead-induced anemia or both. Loss of recently acquired developmental skills also occurs. Colic may be observed at blood lead levels as low as 60 μg/dl, though children with blood lead levels up to 250 μg/dl may appear clinically well.

Acute encephalopathy is usually manifested by the sudden onset of persistent vomiting, ataxia, impairment of consciousness, coma and seizures. In acute lead encephalopathy massive cerebral edema is present, though the classic signs of increased intracranial pressure may not be found. Subtle premonitory behavioral changes may not be appreciated by physician or parent or they may be attributed to other causes. Acute encephalopathy is most common during the summer months in children 1 to 3 years of age. In affected patients, blood lead concentrations almost always exceed 100 μg/dl and usually exceed 150 μg/dl. If acute lead encephalopathy is suspected, the diagnosis can usually be made without resort to lumbar puncture, which is very risky. If examination of the cerebral spinal fluid becomes essential for differential diagnosis, the least amount of fluid required ought to be obtained (several drops), which will in affected children show mild pleocytosis, mild to moderate increase in protein and increased cranial pressure. Affected patients may also show inappropriate secretion of antidiuretic hormone, partial heart block and profoundly impaired renal function.

The term "chronic encephalopathy" is sometimes applied to less acute but nevertheless severe central nervous system manifestations more commonly recognized after 2 to 3 years of age. These include seizure disorders, hyperkinetic and aggressive behavior disorders, developmental regression and progressive loss of speech. Evidence of acutely increased intracranial pressure is absent. These chronic encephalopathic manifestations may occur either as sequelae of acute encephalopathy or in relation to current excessive intake.

Sequelae of encephalopathy include seizure disorders, impaired mentation and hyperkinetic behavior disorders. Seizures and altered behavior tend to abate during adolescence, but intellectual deficits persist. Blindness and hemiparesis are restricted to the most severe cases. Treatment reduces mortality but may have little influence on the occurrence of these residual central nervous system effects. Recently, subclinical plumbism has come under suspicion as one of the etiologic factors in the syndrome of minimal brain damage. Impaired learning and hyperactivity can be produced in very young animals with doses of lead producing no other clinical effects. Data on children suggest that sustained blood lead levels over 50–60 μg/dl during the early preschool years, even without symptoms, may produce deficits identified later. Considerably more research is needed to establish the range of tissue lead levels in children which may cause subtle but permanent central nervous injury.

Peripheral neuropathy as a sign of lead poisoning, manifested in adults primarily by motor weakness in the distal muscles of the arms and legs, is rare in children.

DIAGNOSIS. In view of the nonspecific nature of the clinical features of the above syndromes, laboratory evidence of increased lead absorption and deranged heme synthesis is needed to establish the diagnosis of lead poisoning. There are no satisfactory means of making a retrospective diagnosis of prior plumbism in older children in whom sequelae of plumbism are suspected.

Physical examination in plumbism generally reveals little or nothing abnormal unless gross hyperirritability, seizures, ataxia and/or coma are present. Emphasis must be placed, therefore, on environmental and behavioral history, environmental sampling and laboratory data. Behavioral changes, isolated seizures and self-limited episodes of vomiting during the recent past may represent episodes of plumbism, particularly if the child lives in or visits an old house, if his mother is unavailable to him much of the time, and if a history of pica for any substance is obtained. Recent changes of address, recent renovations in the home and time spent unsupervised or with babysitters and relatives should be ascertained. Persistent pica is particularly associated with inadequate mothering. Mothers may be unavailable to affected children because they are working or preoccupied with their own personal and emotional problems or with the arrival of a new infant in the family. Pica also occurs in retarded children. Information regarding the above is essential in planning the details of management appropriate for each case. Whenever an index case is found, other housemates aged 1 to 5 years should also be examined.

Laboratory evaluation requires at least one index of tissue lead (CaEDTA mobilization test) or of current lead absorption (blood lead) and at least one index of metabolic effect (free erythrocyte protoporphyrin [FEP], δ-aminolevulinic acid dehydratase activity in blood [ALA-D], or 24-hour urine output of δ-aminolevulinic acid [ALA-U] or of coproporphyrin [CP-U]). These metabolic indices predict the lead content of soft tissues better than do blood lead levels. In emergencies in which these tests are not immediately available and where acute lead encephalopathy is a diagnostic possibility, the findings of a strongly positive qualitative CP-U test, of many stippled erythroblasts in bone marrow and of glycosuria and hypophosphatemia indicate presumptive plumbism. Radiopaque flecks in the intestinal tract signify recent ingestion of foreign matter containing lead; these are found in about one third of the examinations of children with pica for paint. Broad bands of increased density at the metaphyses of the long bones usually signify increased storage of lead in bone, but radiographs of long bones may sometimes be normal or equivocal in very acute and severe plumbism. Because the level of lead in blood is labile, confirmation by other tests is essential in making the diagnosis secure. Microfluorometric tests for FEP (normal range: 20 to 75 μg/dl of red cells) are the most useful. Twenty-four hour collections of urine are necessary for measurement of ALA-U and CP-U in asymptomatic children, since tests on random samples of urine may give very misleading results. As the concentration of lead in blood rises above 30–50 μg/dl, the levels of FEP, ALA-U, CP-U and chelatable lead increase exponentially, and ALA-D is uniformly decreased to less than 15 to 20 per cent of normal. FEP levels up to five times normal (250 μg/dl) may signify either iron deficiency or subclinical plumbism. If the FEP levels exceed 500 μg/dl, plumbism is present, with or without iron deficiency. FEP levels over 250 μg/dl indicate blood lead levels over 50–60 μg/dl, as does a response to the CaEDTA mobilization test of more than 1 μg Pb excreted in a 24-hour collection of urine for each mg CaEDTA administered, following a single intramuscular injection of CaEDTA (25 mg/kg). The diagnostic CaEDTA mobilization test *should not be used in patients with symptoms* of plumbism.

Short-term responses to treatment may be followed by direct measurement of urinary lead output or indirectly with ALA-U or ALA-D measurements. FEP tends to decline more slowly, though it too can fluctuate with chelation therapy. FEP tests in children show good day-to-day stability and serve well as indicators of the chronic level of lead absorption; on the other hand, the measurement is quickly responsive to marked changes in lead absorption. The levels of blood lead, serum iron and total iron-binding capacity, in conjunction with FEP, serve to differentiate between iron deficiency and increased lead absorption. Blood and urine to be examined for lead content must be collected with special equipment. There is a risk of contamination in obtaining blood samples by fingerprick for microchemical determination of lead levels. Measurements of blood levels or of chelatable lead are essential, inasmuch as local laws and regulations for the abatement of housing hazards are currently tied directly to the measurement of lead. Plumbism is a reportable condition.

TREATMENT. Major emphasis in treatment is placed on the identification of hazardous environmental lead sources and the separation of the child from them. In the past, most attention has been given to interior paint, though the lead content of exterior paint may be greater. Affected children should be removed from the home during the burning and scraping of paints containing lead pigment.

Most children being examined in current screening programs have blood lead levels ranging from 30 to 50 μg/dl, with normal to moderately elevated levels of FEP. Pica is not necessarily implicated where levels stabilize in this range. Correction of iron deficiency, if present, and a change from dry sweeping to damp cleaning methods to reduce dust in the home are advised. Such children, particularly those under 3 years of age, should be tested periodically to determine the trend of lead absorption.

In children with FEP greater than 150–250 μg/dl and blood lead levels greater than 50–60 μg/dl, there is a greater probability that the child eats paint and that there is stress within the family. In most such cases, long-term follow-up by a social worker or agency and by the physician are indicated. For asymptomatic children in this group there are no clearly defined criteria for the use of chelation therapy. At present, it is prudent to restrict its use to patients showing metabolic abnormalities (FEP over 250 μg/dl).

Parenteral courses of CaEDTA should be limited to three to five days, at a dose of 50 mg/kg/day. Oral treatment with CaEDTA is contraindicated. Oral D-penicillamine is effective, but the drug is currently classed in the United States by the FDA as investigational when used for lead poisoning. Chelation therapy prior to the onset of symptoms may lessen the risk of permanent brain injury.

Symptomatic plumbism (colic, seizures, acute encephalopathy) should be promptly treated with chelating agents if presumptive laboratory tests are distinctly positive. The onset and clinical course of encephalopathy are unpredictable. Colic and seizures may either abate spontaneously or be the immediate prelude to frank encephalopathy. Accordingly, the risk of delay outweighs by far the risk of a few days of chelation therapy. If the blood level of lead or the output of lead in urine during the first 24 hours of therapy is subsequently found to be normal or only slightly elevated, treatment should be stopped and the presumptive diagnosis reconsidered.

In acute encephalopathy higher doses are indicated than those given above, owing to the higher levels of lead in tissues. The following regimen combines BAL and CaEDTA. Four hours after a priming dose of BAL (4 mg/kg, intramuscularly) BAL 4 mg/kg every 4 hours and CaEDTA 12.5

mg/kg every 4 hours are given intramuscularly, for five days. In less severe cases or those which show immediate clinical improvement, the total daily dose may be decreased by one third after 72 hours. If repeated courses are needed, the reduced total daily dosage (CaEDTA, 50 mg/kg/day, and BAL, 15 mg/kg/day) is safer and adequate. If the patient becomes anuric, CaEDTA but not BAL should be temporarily withheld. (CaEDTA is a nonmetabolizable drug excreted exclusively by the kidney.) Side effects of CaEDTA include hypercalcemia, rising blood urea nitrogen and renal injury. Side effects of BAL include vomiting, hypertension and tachycardia. Side effects of both drugs require careful evaluation, since some of them are also features of acute lead encephalopathy. BAL may occasionally evoke intravascular hemolysis in patients with severe G-6-PD deficiency.

Fluid and electrolyte management are also important in treatment of lead encephalopathy. After an initial priming infusion of 10 per cent dextrose in water (and mannitol, if necessary) to establish urine flow, continuous intravenous infusion should be restricted to basal requirements and a minimal estimate of the amounts required for replacement of losses due to vomiting, dehydration and activity associated with seizures. It is prudent to manage parenteral fluids initially in the same manner in mildly symptomatic cases and in asymptomatic cases with very high tissue lead levels until the trend of the clinical course becomes clear. The use of enemas to remove lead from the lower bowel should not be permitted to delay treatment.

Seizures may be controlled initially with diazepam and thereafter with repeated doses of paraldehyde until the patient's state of consciousness is much improved. As the dose of paraldehyde is lowered, long-term anticonvulsant therapy with diphenylhydantoin or phenobarbital is started.

Patients should be followed at least until school age in order to prevent recurrences and to assess the degree of residual brain damage, which may not become evident until several years after an acute episode. Some survivors of encephalopathy may require either special school placement or institutionalization, despite early therapy.

The occurrence of increased lead absorption and lead poisoning in children is not likely to diminish further until existing old housing is either replaced or maintained more adequately than at present. The effect, if any, of a recent decision to reduce the lead content of gasoline may become evident in several years.

J. JULIAN CHISOLM, JR.

Chisolm, J. J., Jr.: The use of chelating agents in the treatment of acute and chronic lead intoxication in childhood. J. Pediatr. *73*:1, 1968.

Chisolm, J. J., Jr.: Pica; Acute lead poisoning and asymptomatic increased lead absorption. *In* Gellis, S. S., and Kagan, B. M. (eds.): Current Pediatric Therapy. 6th ed. Philadelphia, W. B. Saunders Company, 1973, pp. 32–33 and 746–748.

Chisolm, J. J., Jr.: Management of increased lead absorption and lead poisoning in children. New Engl. J. Med. *289*:1016, 1973.

Emmerson, B. T.: The clinical differentiation of lead gout from primary gout. Arthritis Rheum. *11*:623, 1968.

Granick, S., Sassa, S., Granick, J. L., Levere, R. D., and Kappas, A.: Assays for porphyrins, δ-aminolevulinic-acid dehydratase, and porphyrinogen synthetase in microliter samples of whole blood: Applications to metabolic defects involving the heme pathway. Proc. Nat. Acad. Sci. *69*:2381, 1972.

Lead, Airborne Lead in Perspective. Washington, D.C., National Research Council–National Academy of Sciences, 1972.

Low level lead toxicity and the environmental impact of cadmium. Environmental Health Perspectives, Experimental Issue No. 7, May, 1974.

Lourie, R. S., Layman, E. M., and Millican, F. K.: Why children eat things that are not food. Children *10*:143, 1963.

Perlstein, M. A., and Attala, R.: Neurologic sequelae of plumbism in children. Clin. Pediatr. *5*:292, 1966.

Sayre, J. W., Charney, E., Vostal, J., et al.: House and hand dust as a potential source of childhood lead exposure. Am. J. Dis. Child. *127*:167, 1974.

29
MORPHOLOGIC SYNDROMES

Multiple physical abnormalities may be the consequence of a *single* localized defect in early morphogenesis resulting in *secondary* anomalies by the time of birth. An example is the combination of meningomyelocele, clubfoot and hydrocephalus; the initiating *primary* defect is incomplete early closure of the neural tube. For such disorders the diagnosis is usually an anatomic one, and counseling as to the risk of recurrence is empiric. *Multiple primary* major and minor defects within one or more systems pose the broader question of diagnosis of a specific syndrome disorder. If the clinician can recognize a concise syndrome, he can utilize past knowledge relative to natural history, management and recurrence risk for that disorder. Some of the many such syndromes are listed in the following table.

KEY TO USE OF TABULAR LISTING OF SYNDROMES

The formulation of the following tabular listing of morphologic syndromes is based on the concept that individual defects are rarely pathognomonic, but that identification of two or more anomalies may provide a diagnostic core pattern for a particular syndrome. Thus, for each syndrome a core pattern of two or more clinically detectable abnormalities has been selected which is highly suggestive or even diagnostic of that syndrome *as contrasted to all other recognized conditions.* For example, webbed neck is not included under XO (Turner) syndrome because it is not one of the more frequent features, and simian crease was not included in any of the core patterns because it is a feature of many syndromes and therefore is of limited value in differential diagnosis. For each disorder, in addition to the core pattern of defects, small stature and mental deficiency are listed if they are part of the syndrome; the etiology or mode of genetic determination is listed if known; a representative reference (literature) is added as a source of more complete information, and the page reference to a description in this text is noted. Below the number of each syndrome in the left hand column of the table the numbers in parentheses indicate the listed syndromes which merit special consideration in the differential diagnosis.

The grouping of syndromes is based on the systems involved, the type of abnormality and, in the case of chromosomal aberrations, the etiology. Within each group the order of presentation is determined principally by clinical similarities. The groups in order of listing are as follows:

I. Bone and connective tissue dysplasias
 A. Connective tissue disorders
 B. Mucopolysaccharidoses
 C. Osteochondrodystrophies
II. Chromosomal imbalance syndromes
III. Miscellaneous patterns of malformation
 A. Predominantly facial defects
 B. Unusually small stature with associated defects
 C. Senile-like appearance with associated defects
 D. Joint dysplasia with associated defects
 E. Broad thumb with associated defects
 F. Deafness with associated defects
 G. Neurologic disorders with associated defects
 H. Muscular disorders with associated defects
 I. Hematopoetic disorders with associated defects
 J. Other disorders
IV. Hamartoses
V. Ectodermal dysplasias

The reader is cautioned that the core patterns were selected as leads to aid in the diagnosis of each syndrome, rather than to describe it, and that not all patients with a given disorder will have all the anomalies of the core pattern. Nor are all syndromes of multiple defects included in these tables; the author has listed only those which appear to be well defined syndromes of *multiple primary* defects. The reader is further cautioned that vague or partial similarity is insufficient for a diagnosis. The table is only a guide; specific diagnosis must rest on careful correlation of the patient's signs with the total picture of the syndrome as derived from study of the appropriate references. Genetic counsel should be rendered only after a careful assessment of the family history; many patients with a single altered gene have a fresh mutation which does not increase the risk that the parents will have another affected child. For example, about 85 per cent of children with achondroplasia, an autosomal dominant disorder, are born of normal parents. Likewise, the possibility must be kept in mind that multiple primary defects may have an infectious rather than a genetic origin, as in the rubella syndrome.

ALPHABETICAL LISTING

The following alphabetical listing may assist the reader in more readily finding a particular syndrome in the following table:

BONE AND CONNECTIVE TISSUE DYSPLASIAS: A. CONNECTIVE TISSUE DISORDERS

The connective tissue disorders are so categorized because the basic problem appears to be in fibrous tissue and its derivatives. Relative laxity of joints, bluish sclerae and inguinal hernias are rather nonspecific and may be found as features of Syndromes 2 through 5. Abnormality in blood vessels may lead to serious vascular disease in conditions 2, 3, 4 and 6.

SYNDROME	*DIAGNOSTIC MANIFESTATIONS* Facial	Limbs	Other	Mental Defic.	Short Stature	Genetic Trans-mission	Refer-ence
1. Contractural arachnodactyly (2)	"Crumpled" ears	Arachnodactyly; joint contractures				Aut. Dom.	10
2. Marfan syndrome (1,3)*†	Subluxation of lens	Arachnodactyly	Aortic dilatation			Aut. Dom.	3
3. Homocystinuria (2)*†	Subluxation of lens; malar flush	Osteoporosis	Venous thromboses	+/−		Aut. Rec.	3
4. Ehlers-Danlos syndrome†		Hyperextensible joints	Hyperextensible skin; poor wound healing with thin scar; subcutaneous nodules			Aut. Dom.	3
5. Osteogenesis imperfecta†	Bluish sclerae; odontogenesis imperfecta	Fragile bones	+/−Deafness		+/−	Aut. Dom.; rare Aut. Rec.	3
6. Pseudoxanthoma elasticum	Angioid retinal streaks	Thickened yellowish skin in flexural areas	Arterial medial degeneration with hemorrhagic tendency			Aut. Rec.	3
7. Fibrodysplasia ossificans progressiva (myositis ossificans)†		Short hallux +/− short thumb	Fibrous dysplasia in muscle and subcutaneous tissues leading to mineralization		+/−	Aut. Dom.	3

BONE AND CONNECTIVE TISSUE DYSPLASIAS: B. MUCOPOLYSACCHARIDOSES

The mucopolysaccharidoses are categorized together on the basis of excess tissue storage and urinary excretion of mucopolysaccharides. Clinically, all tend to produce some coarsening of the facial features. Other manifestations are broadening and altered configuration of bone, joint limitation, corneal opacity, hepatosplenomegaly, mental deterioration and cardiovascular changes—all features of the prototype, Hurler syndrome. The age of onset may be a helpful clinical clue in these disorders. With the exception of G_{M1} gangliosidosis, which is listed here because of clinical similarity, even though it is not a mucopolysaccharidosis, these disorders seldom become clinically manifest until *after* birth.

SYNDROME	*DIAGNOSTIC MANIFESTATIONS*			Mental Defic.	Short Stature	Genetic Trans-mission	Refer-ence
	Facial	Skeletal	Other				
8. G_{M1} gangliosidosis (generalized gangliosidosis)†	Coarse facies; hypertrophy of alveolar ridges at birth	Kyphosis in early infancy	Renal dysfunction	?+	+	Aut. Rec.	6
9. Hurler syndrome (MPS type I) (10,11)*†	Coarse facies; cloudy cornea, early	Stiff joints by 1 yr; kyphosis by 1-2 yr	Valvular heart disease	+	+ Onset, 6-18 mo	Aut. Rec.	3
10. Hunter syndrome (MPS type II) (9, 11)*†	Coarse facies; clear cornea	Stiff joints; kyphosis, rare	Deafness develops	+	+ Onset, 2-4 yr	X-linked Rec.	3
11. Maroteaux-Lamy syndrome (MPS type VI) (9, 10)*†	Mildly coarse facies; cloudy cornea, early	Stiff joints, kyphosis			+ Onset, 1-3 yr	Aut. Rec.	3
12. Morquio's disease (MPS type IV) (19, 20, 25)*†	Mildly coarse facies; cloudy cornea, usually after 5 yr	Mildly stiff joints; vertebrae become flattened; severe kyphosis			+ Onset, 1-3 yr	Aut. Rec.	3

*The numbers in parentheses refer to syndromes listed in this table which merit special consideration in the differential diagnosis.

†Syndrome is described in text; see index for location.

Table continued on following page

BONE AND CONNECTIVE TISSUE DYSPLASIAS: B. MUCOPOLYSACCHARIDOSES *(Continued)*

SYNDROME	*DIAGNOSTIC MANIFESTATIONS* Facial	Skeletal	Other	Mental Defic.	Short Stature	Genetic Trans-mission	Refer-ence
13. Sanfilippo syndrome (MPS type III) (14)*†	Mildly coarse facies; clear cornea	Mildly stiff joints, no kyphosis		+		Aut. Rec.	3
14. Scheie syndrome (MPS type V) (13)*†	Broad mouth; cloudy cornea	Stiff joints by 5-8 yr; no kyphosis				Aut. Rec.	3

BONE AND CONNECTIVE TISSUE DYSPLASIAS: C. OSTEOCHONDRODYSPLASIAS

SYNDROME	*DIAGNOSTIC MANIFESTATIONS* Craniofacial	Limbs	Other	Mental Defic.	Short Stature	Genetic Trans-mission	Refer-ence
15. Achondrogenesis (16)	Low nasal bridge	Very short limbs	Vertebrae not mineralized	Early lethal	++	?Aut. Rec.	27
16. Thanatophoric dwarfism (15)	Large cranium; low nasal bridge	Short limbs	Flat vertebrae	Early lethal	++	?Aut. Rec.	27
17. Achondroplasia (18)*†	Low nasal bridge +/−macrocephaly	Short limbs, short hands and feet, limited elbow extension	Caudal narrowing of spinal canal; short ileum with sacroiliac notch		+	Aut. Dom.	4
18. Hypochondroplasia (17)	Near normal	Short limbs	Caudal narrowing of spinal canal		+	Aut. Dom.	32
19. Metatropic dwarfism (12)*	Normal facies	Short limbs; small epiphyses; metaphyseal flare	Severe early kyphoscoliosis; flattened vertebrae		+	?Aut. Rec.	4
20. Camptomelic syndrome	Flat facies	Bowed tibiae with skin dimpling	Hypoplastic scapulae, short vertebrae	Usually early lethal	+	?	20

21. Diastrophic dwarfism*†	Hypertrophied or cystic auricular cartilage; cleft palate	Short limbs; short 1st metacarpal; joint limitations with clubfoot			+	Aut. Rec.	4
22. Ellis-van Creveld syndrome (chondroectodermal dysplasia)*†	Neonatal teeth, hypoplasia of teeth	Short distal limbs; polydactyly; nail hypoplasia	Small thorax; cardiac defect		+	Aut. Rec.	4
23. Thoracic asphyxiant dystrophy (24)*†	Normal facies	Short limbs; short hands; +/− polydactyly	Constricted small thorax +/− renal disease		+	Aut. Rec.	4
24. Spondyloepiphyseal dysplasia (pseudoachondroplasia)*†	Normal facies	Postnatal onset of short limbs; irregular epiphyses and metaphyses; limited elbow extension	Short trunk; lumbar lordosis		+	Aut. Dom.	3
25. X-linked spondyloepiphyseal dysplasia*	Normal facies	Onset of epiphyseal irregularity at 5-10 yr.	Short trunk due to flattening of vertebrae		+ (late)	X-linked Rec.	4
26. Multiple epiphyseal dysplasia†	Normal facies	Short fingers; epiphyseal hypoplasia; metaphyseal flaring	Joint limitation; eventual osteoarthritis of hip		+	Aut. Dom.	4
27. Metaphyseal dysostosis, dominant type (28)*†	Normal facies	Bowlegs; irregular, wide metaphyses	Variable limitation in full extension of fingers		+	Aut. Dom.	4
28. Cartilage-hair hypoplasia (21)*†	Fine, sparse hair; normal facies	Mild bowing of legs; wide, slightly irregular metaphyses	+/− Intestinal malabsorption		+	Aut. Rec.	3
29. Multiple exostoses (30)†	Normal facies	Diaphyseal outgrowths leading to limb deformities	+/− Short metacarpals		+/−	Aut. Dom.	4
30. Langer-Giedion syndrome (29, 31)	Bulbous nose	Exostoses, cone-shaped phalangeal epiphyses	Loose skin in infancy	+	+/−	?	19
31. Trichorhinophalangeal syndrome (30)	Bulbous nose	Cone-shaped phalangeal epiphyses	Sparse hair		+/−	Aut. Dom. & ?Aut. Rec. type	15
32. Conradi-Hünermann type of chondrodysplasia punctata (33)	Low nasal bridge	Limb asymmetry	Early punctate epiphyseal mineralization		+/−	Aut. Dom.	30

*The numbers in parentheses refer to syndromes listed in this table which merit special consideration in the differential diagnosis.
†Syndrome is described in text; see index for location.

Table continued on following page

BONE AND CONNECTIVE TISSUE DYSPLASIAS: C. OSTEOCHONDRODYSPLASIAS *(Continued)*

SYNDROME	*DIAGNOSTIC MANIFESTATIONS* Craniofacial	Limbs	Other	Mental Defic.	Short Stature	Genetic Trans-mission	Refer-ence
33. Rhizomelic type of chondrodysplasia punctata (32)	Low nasal bridge	Short proximal limbs	Early punctate epiphyseal mineralization	+	+	Aut. Rec.	30
34. Hypophosphatasia†	Delayed closure of fontanels +/− craniosynostosis; early loss of deciduous teeth	Bowing of legs; poor and irregular mineralization, especially at metaphyses			+	Aut. Rec.	4
OSTEOPETROSES							
35. Hyperphosphatasia with osteoectasia	Macrocranium	Broad diaphyses	Hyperphosphatasia		+	Aut. Rec.	31
36. Camurati-Engelmann syndrome	May have sclerosis, base of skull	Broad diaphyses	Weak; leg pains			Aut. Dom.	29
37. Craniometaphyseal dysplasia of Pyle (38, 39)	Frontal bulge	Genu valgus; metaphyseal flare	+/− Weakness			Aut. Rec.	16
38. Craniometaphyseal dysplasia, dominant type (39)	Wide prominent nasal bridge	Metaphyseal flare	Development of deafness			Aut. Dom.	16
39. Frontometaphyseal dysplasia of Gorlin (37, 38)	Prominent supra-orbital ridges	Metaphyseal flare; joint contractures				?	16
40. Osteopetrosis, severe (Albers-Schönberg disease) (41)*†	Thick calvaria with cranial nerve compression; +/− macrocephaly	Dense, thick, fragile bones	Secondary pancytopenia, splenomegaly		+/−	Aut. Rec.	3

41. Osteopetrosis, mild (40)	Dense calvaria	Moderately dense bone liable to fracture +/−osteomyelitis				Aut. Dom.	3
42. Pyknodysostosis of Maroteaux and Lamy (43, 44)*†	Tooth anomalies; delayed closure of fontanels; facial bone hypoplasia	Osteosclerosis; shortening of distal phalanges			+	Aut. Rec.	4
43. Pyknodysostosis of Stanesco (42)*	Brachycephaly with thin cranium; facial bone hypoplasia	Osteosclerosis; relatively short upper arms			+	Aut. Dom.	4
44. Cleidocranial dysostosis (42)*†	Delayed closure of fontanels with frontal bossing; late eruption of teeth		Defect of outer clavicle		+	Aut. Dom.	4
			CRANIOSYNOSTOSES WITH OR WITHOUT SYNDACTYLY				
45. Crouzon's disease (craniofacial dysostosis)*†	Proptosis with shallow orbits; maxillary hypoplasia; craniosynostosis					Aut. Dom.	4
46. Pfeiffer syndrome (47)	Brachycephaly	Broad thumbs; mild syndactyly		+/−		Aut. Dom.	6
47. Saethre-Chotzen syndrome (46)	Brachycephaly; ptosis; prominent ear crus	Mild syndactyly		+/−		Aut. Dom.	8
48. Apert syndrome (acrocephalosyndactyly) (46, 47–49)*†	Craniosynostosis; irregular midfacial hypoplasia; and hypertelorism	Syndactyly; broad distal thumb and toe		+		Aut. Dom.	4
49. Carpenter syndrome (48, 123)*†	Craniosynostosis; midfacial hypoplasia; lateral displacement of inner canthi	Polydactyly; syndactyly	Obesity	+	+/−	Aut. Rec.	4

*The numbers in parentheses refer to syndromes listed in this table which merit special consideration in the differential diagnosis.
†Syndrome is described in text; see index for location.

Table continued on following page

BONE AND CONNECTIVE TISSUE DYSPLASIAS: C. OSTEOCHONDRODYSPLASIAS *(Continued)*

SYNDROME	DIAGNOSTIC MANIFESTATIONS: Craniofacial	Limbs	Other	Mental Defic.	Short Stature	Genetic Trans-mission	Refer-ence
OTHER SKELETAL DYSPLASIAS							
50. Aminopterin-induced syndrome	Cranial dysplasia with broad nasal bridge; low-set ears			?	+		4
51. Nail-patella syndrome		Patella hypoplasia; nail hypoplasia	Iliac horns; scoliosis			Aut. Dom.	4
52. Dyschondrosteosis of Leri-Weill†		Short forearms with Madelung deformity +/−short lower leg			+	Aut. Dom.	4
53. Albright's hereditary osteodystrophy (pseudohypopara-thyroidism) (59, 55)*	Rounded facies	Short metacarpal bones, especially 4th	Obesity; hypocalcemia and/or extraskeletal mineralization	+	+	? X-Linked Dom.	4
54. Acrodysostosis	Low nasal bridge; maxillary hypoplasia	Short hands and feet with peripheral dysostosis		+	+	?	25
55. Marchesani syndrome (53)*†	Small spherical lens	Brachydactyly			+	Aut. Rec.	4
56. Beal syndrome of auriculo-osteodysplasia	Long fused ear lobes	Radial head elbow dysplasia	Large prominent scapulae		+	Aut. Dom.	9

CHROMOSOMAL IMBALANCE SYNDROMES

The following chromosomal abnormalities give rise to particular patterns of multiple defects which allow for clinical recognition. They are grouped together to aid the clinician in deciding which patients clearly merit chromosomal study for confirmatory diagnosis and genetic counsel.

SYNDROME	DIAGNOSTIC MANIFESTATIONS: Craniofacial	Limbs	Other	Mental Defic.	Short Stature	Genetic Trans-mission	Refer-ence
57. XYY syndrome	Long head; prominent glabella	Tend to be tall	Poor coordination; aberrant behavior	+/−		XYY	12
58. XXY syndrome		Long legs	Hypogenitalism; hypogonadism; behavioral aberrations	+/−		XXY	11
59. XXXXY (61, 107, 123)*†	Inner epicanthic fold and/or upslanting of palpebral fissures	Limited elbow pronation; low dermal ridge count on fingertips (mostly low arches)	Hypogenitalism	+	+	XXXXY	4
60. Penta-X (61)*†	Upward slant to palpebral fissures	Small hands; clinodactyly of 5th finger	Patent ductus arteriosus	+	+	XXXXX	4
61. Down syndrome (mongolism) (59, 60, 108)*†	Upward slant to palpebral fissures; flat facies	Short hands; clinodactyly of 5th finger	Hypotonia	+	+/−	21 Trisomy	4
62. 18 Trisomy (63, 124)*†	Microstomia; short palpebral fissure	Clenched hand, 2nd finger over 3rd; low arches on fingertips	Short sternum	+	+	18 Trisomy	4
63. 13 (D_1) Trisomy (62, 65, 94, 106)*†	Defects of eye, nose, lip and forebrain of holoprosencephaly type	Polydactyly; narrow, hyperconvex fingernails.	Skin defects, posterior scalp	+	+	13 Trisomy	4
64. Schmid-Fraccaro syndrome (cat-eye syndrome)	Hypertelorism with slight downslanting of palpebral fissures, coloboma of iris and/or preauricular fistula		Anal atresia	+/−		Small extra chrom.	4

*The numbers in parentheses refer to syndromes listed in this table which merit special consideration in the differential diagnosis.
†Syndrome is described in text; see index for location.

Table continued on following page

CHROMOSOMAL IMBALANCE SYNDROMES *(Continued)*

SYNDROME	DIAGNOSTIC MANIFESTATIONS			Mental Defic.	Short Stature	Genetic Trans-mission	Refer-ence
	Craniofacial	Limbs	Other				
65. **Chromosome No. 4 short-arm deletion syndrome (63, 106)***†	Short philtrum and nasal septum; ocular hypertelorism +/− prominent glabella; low-set simple ear with preauricular dimple; +/− cleft lip and palate		+/− Midline scalp defects	+	+	#4 p-	4
66. **Cri du chat syndrome**†	Epicanthic folds and/or slanting palpebral fissures, microcephaly with round facial contour		Cat-like cry in infancy	+	+	#5 p-	4
67. **Chromosome No. 18 long-arm deletion syndrome**†	Midfacial hypoplasia; atretic or narrow ear canal	High frequency of whorl digital pattern		−	+	#18 q-	4
68. **Chromosome No. 18 short-arm deletion syndrome**	Ptosis eyelid or epicanthal folds; prominent auricles	Small hands and feet		−	+	#18 p-	6
69. **Chromosome No. 13 long-arm deletion syndrome (63)**	Eye defect; microcephaly with high nasal bridge	Thumb hypoplasia	Hypospadias	−	+	#13 q-	6
70. **Chromosome No. 21 long-arm deletion syndrome**	Downslanting palpebral fissures; large malformed external ears; micrognathia			+	+	#21 q-	4
71. **XO (Turner) syndrome (122)***†	Heart-shaped facies; prominent ears	Congenital lymphedema or its residua	Broad chest with widely spaced nipples; low posterior hairline	+/−	+	XO	4

MISCELLANEOUS PATTERNS OF MALFORMATION: A. PREDOMINANTLY FACIAL DEFECTS

SYNDROME	*DIAGNOSTIC MANIFESTATIONS* Craniofacial	Limbs	Other	Mental Defic.	Short Stature	Genetic Trans-mission	Refer-ence
72. Treacher Collins syndrome (mandibulofacial dysostosis) (73)*†	Malar and mandibular hypoplasia; downslanting palpebral fissures	Defect of lower eyelid	Malformation of external ear			Aut. Dom.	4
73. Goldenhar syndrome (72)*	Malar hypoplasia	Epibulbar dermoid and/or lipodermoid +/− other eye defect	Malformed ear with preauricular tags			Unknown ? Aut. Rec.	4
74. Pierre Robin syndrome†	Micrognathia	Glossoptosis	Cleft palate			?	4
75. Hypoglossia-hypodactyly syndrome	Hypoglossia; micrognathia	Hypodactyly				?	18
76. Lip fistula and cleft lip (91)*	Lower lip fistulas (pits)	Cleft lip and/or cleft palate				Aut. Dom.	4
77. Familial blepharophimosis	Lateral displacement of inner canthi	Inverted inner canthal fold	Ptosis of eyelids			Aut. Dom.	4

MISCELLANEOUS PATTERNS OF MALFORMATION: B. UNUSUALLY SMALL STATURE WITH ASSOCIATED DEFECTS

SYNDROME	Craniofacial	Limbs	Other	Mental Defic.	Short Stature	Genetic Trans-mission	Refer-ence
78. Silver syndrome (Russell-Silver syndrome)†	Triangular hypoplastic facies with downturning mouth	Skeletal asymmetry; clinodactyly of 5th finger			+	?	4
79. Bloom syndrome (85)	Cutaneous photosensitivity; telangiectatic erythema; malar hypoplasia		Chromosomal breakage in vitro		+	Aut. Rec.	4

*The numbers in parentheses refer to syndromes listed in this table which merit special consideration in the differential diagnosis.
†Syndrome is described in text; see index for location.

Table continued on following page

MISCELLANEOUS PATTERNS OF MALFORMATION: B. UNUSUALLY SMALL STATURE WITH ASSOCIATED DEFECTS *(Continued)*

SYNDROME	*DIAGNOSTIC MANIFESTATIONS*			Mental Defic.	Short Stature	Genetic Trans-mission	Refer-ence
	Craniofacial	Limbs	Other				
80. Seckel syndrome	Facial hypoplasia; prominent nose; microcephaly	Multiple minor joint and skeletal abnormalities		+	+	Aut. Rec.	4
81. Coffin hypoplastic nail syndrome	Coarse facies (mild)	Hypoplastic distal phalanges with hypoplastic nails	+/− Hypotrichosis	+	+	?	13
82. Cornelia de Lange syndrome	Synophrys (continuous eyebrows); thin down-turning upper lip	Small or malformed hands and feet; proximal thumb	Hirsutism	+	+	?	4
83. Robert syndrome (154)	Midfacial defect +/− cleft lip and palate	Hypomelia	Hypotrichosis	+	++	Aut. Rec.	6
84. Hallerman-Streiff syndrome (86)*†	Microphthalmia and cataracts; small pinched nose; micrognathia	Thin skin over nose; hypotrichosis			+	? Aut. Dom.	4
85. Dubowitz syndrome (79)	Shallow supra-orbital ridges; ptosis		Infantile eczema	+	+	? Aut. Rec.	17

MISCELLANEOUS PATTERNS OF MALFORMATION: C. SENILE-LIKE APPEARANCE WITH ASSOCIATED DEFECTS

	Facial	Cutaneous	Other	Mental Defic.	Short Stature	Genetic Trans-mission	Refer-ence
86. Progeria (84, 87)*†	Facial bone hypoplasia	Alopecia; thin skin with atrophy of subcutaneous adipose	Straight femoral neck, short distal phalanges, premature atherosclerosis		+	?	4
87. Cockayne syndrome (86)*	Retinal degeneration	Hypotrichosis; photo-sensitivity; thin skin; diminished subcutaneous adipose	Impaired hearing	+	+	Aut. Rec.	4
88. De Sanctis-Cacchione syndrome (xerodermic idiocy) (152)	Microcephaly		Sun-sensitive xeroderma pigmentosa; hypogonadism	+	+	Aut. Rec.	23
89. Rothmund-Thomson syndrome (poikiloderma congenita) (149)*†	Development of cataracts	Development of poikiloderma	Other features of ectodermal dysplasia		+/−	Aut. Rec.	4

MISCELLANEOUS PATTERNS OF MALFORMATION: D. JOINT DYSPLASIA WITH ASSOCIATED DEFECTS

SYNDROME	DIAGNOSTIC MANIFESTATIONS: Craniofacial	Limbs	Other	Mental Defic.	Short Stature	Genetic Trans-mission	Refer-ence
90. Familial dwarfism with stiff joints (92)*	Hyperopia	Stiff joints			+	Aut. Dom.	4
91. Popliteal web syndrome (76)*	Lower lip pits; cleft palate	Popliteal web				? Aut. Rec. or Aut. Dom.	4
92. Stickler's progressive arthro-ophthalmopathy (92)*	Progressive myopia; retinal detachment	Joint limitation from childhood; +/− arachnodactyly	Sensorineural deafness			Aut. dom.	4
93. Larsen syndrome	Flat facies	Multiple joint dislocations; short metacarpals				?	4

MISCELLANEOUS PATTERNS OF MALFORMATION: E. BROAD THUMB WITH ASSOCIATED DEFECTS (48, 49)

SYNDROME	Craniofacial	Limbs	Other	Mental Defic.	Short Stature	Genetic Trans-mission	Refer-ence
94. Rubinstein-Taybi syndrome (63, 95, 96)*	Slanting palpebral fissures; maxillary hypoplasia; microcephaly	Broad thumbs and toes		+	+	?	4
95. Leri's pleonosteosis (94, 96)*	Upward slant to palpebral fissures	Broad thumb in valgus position; joint limitation with partial flexion of fingers				Aut. Dom.	3
96. Taybi otopalatodigital syndrome (94, 95)*	Cleft soft palate; microstomia	Broad distal digits, "tree-frog-like"	Deafness, conductive	+/−	+	? X-linked	4
97. Mohr syndrome (118)	Cleft tongue	Partial duplication of hallux	Deafness, conductive		+/−	? Aut. Rec.	4

*The numbers in parentheses refer to syndromes listed in this table which merit special consideration in the differential diagnosis.
†Syndrome is described in text; see index for location.

Table continued on following page

MISCELLANEOUS PATTERNS OF MALFORMATION: F. DEAFNESS WITH ASSOCIATED DEFECTS

	Craniofacial	Limbs	Other	Mental Defic.	Short Stature	Genetic Transmission	Reference
98. Rubella syndrome†	Cataract		Deafness; patent ductus arteriosus	+/−	+/−		4
99. Waardenburg's syndrome†	Lateral displacement of inner canthi and puncta		Partial albinism; white forelock; heterochromia of iris; vitiligo; +/− deafness			Aut. Dom.	4

MISCELLANEOUS PATTERNS OF MALFORMATION: G. NEUROLOGIC DISORDERS OTHER THAN MENTAL DEFICIENCY, WITH ASSOCIATED DEFECTS

	Neurologic	Other	Mental Defic.	Short Stature	Genetic Transmission	Reference
100. Ataxia-telangiectasia†	Development of ataxia	Telangiectasia; frequent upper respiratory tract infections		+	Aut. Rec.	4
101. Biemond syndrome	Ataxia	Short 4th metacarpal			Aut. Dom.	4
102. Marinesco-Sjögren syndrome	Cerebellar ataxia; hypotonia	Cataracts; sparse hair	+	+	Aut. Rec.	4
103. Sjögren-Larsson syndrome	Spasticity, especially of legs	Ichthyosis	+	+	Aut. Rec.	4
104. Menkes syndrome	Progressive cerebral deterioration with seizures	Twisted, fractured, stubby hair	+	+	X-Linked Rec.	4

105. Möbius syndrome	Expressionless facies; ocular palsy		+/–Club foot; syndactyly	+/–	+/–	? Probably Variable	6
106. Meckel-Gruber syndrome (63, 65)	Encephalocele		Polydactyly; polycystic kidney	+	+	Aut. Rec.	6

MISCELLANEOUS PATTERNS OF MALFORMATION: H. MUSCULAR DISORDERS WITH ASSOCIATED DEFECTS

	Craniofacial	Limb and Other	Muscle Dysfunction				
107. Prader-Willi syndrome (59, 123)*†	+/–Upward slant to palpebral fissures	Small hands and feet; obesity from late infancy; hypogenitalism; diabetes mellitus	Hypotonia, especially in early infancy	+	+	?	4
108. Cerebrohepatorenal syndrome (61, 109)*	High forehead; flat facies	Hepatomegaly; death in early infancy	Hypotonia	?+	+	? Aut. Rec.	4
109. Lowe syndrome (oculocerebrorenal syndrome) (108)*†	Cataract	Renal tubular dysfunction	Hypotonia	+	+	X-Linked Rec.	4
110. Myotonic dystrophy of Steinert*	Cataract	Hypogonadism	Myotonia with muscle atrophy; weakness	+/–		Aut. Dom.	4
111. Rieger syndrome*	Hypodontia; iris dysplasia		Myotonic dystrophy	+/–		Aut. Dom.	4
112. Freeman-Sheldon "whistling face" syndrome (113)*	Hypoplastic alae nasi	Club feet	Mask-like "whistling face"		+/–	? Aut. Dom.	4
113. Schwartz syndrome (112)*	Blepharophimosis	Joint limitation	Myotonia		+	? Aut. Rec.	4
114. Abdominal muscle deficiency syndrome		Renal and urinary tract dysplasia; cryptorchidism	Abdominal muscle hypoplasia			?	4

*The numbers in parentheses refer to syndromes listed in this table which merit special consideration in the differential diagnosis.
†Syndrome is described in text; see index for location.

Table continued on following page

MISCELLANEOUS PATTERNS OF MALFORMATION *(Continued)*
H. MUSCULAR DISORDERS WITH ASSOCIATED DEFECTS *(Continued)*

	Craniofacial	Limb and Other	Muscle Dysfunction	Mental Defic.	Short Stature	Genetic Trans-mission	Refer-ence
115. Poland syndrome	Unilateral syndactyly of hand	+/− Unilateral hypoplasia to absence of nipple	Unilateral absence of pectoralis minor			?	4

MISCELLANEOUS PATTERNS OF MALFORMATION:
I. HEMATOPOIETIC DISORDERS WITH ASSOCIATED DEFECTS

		Limbs	Other	Mental Defic.	Short Stature	Genetic Trans-mission	Refer-ence
116. Fanconi syndrome of pancytopenia and multiple defects (151)*†		Hypoplastic thumb and/or radius	Hyperpigmentation; development of pancytopenia	+/−	+	? Aut. Rec.	4
117. Radial aplasia-thrombocytopenia syndrome*†		Radial aplasia	Thrombocytopenia with megakaryocytopenia; +/− cardiac defect			Aut. Rec.	4

MISCELLANEOUS PATTERNS OF MALFORMATION:
J. OTHER DISORDERS

	Craniofacial	Limbs	Other	Mental Defic.	Short Stature	Genetic Trans-mission	Refer-ence
118. Orofacialdigital syndrome (97, 119)*	Hypoplasia of alae nasi; oral frenula and clefts	Digital asymmetry		+/−		Dom. ? Lethal in male	4
119. Mieten syndrome (118)*	Narrow nose; corneal opacity	Flexion contracture of elbow		+	+	? Aut. Rec.	4

120. Oculodentodigital syndrome	Narrow nose; microphthalmos; +/− glaucoma; enamel hypoplasia	Camptodactyly of 5th fingers				? Aut. Rec.	4
121. Holt-Oram syndrome (cardiac-limb syndrome)		Upper limb defect, especially of thumb and radius	Cardiac septal defect; narrow shoulders			Aut. Dom.	4
122. Turner-like syndrome (Noonan syndrome) (71, 125, 146)*†	Webbing of posterior neck		Pectus excavatum; cryptorchidism; pulmonic stenosis	+/−	+	?	4
123. Laurence-Moon-Biedl syndrome (49, 59, 107)*†	Retinal pigmentation	Polydactyly	Obesity	+	+/−	Aut. Rec.	4
124. Smith-Lemli-Opitz syndrome	Anteverted nostrils and/or ptosis of eyelid	Syndactyly 2nd and 3rd toes	Hypospadias; cryptorchidism	+	+	? Aut. Rec.	4
125. Aarskog syndrome (122, 126)	Hypertelorism	Small hands and feet	Scrotal "shawl" above penis		+	Dom., ? Aut. vs. X-linked	7
126. Opitz syndrome (125, 127)	Hypertelorism; +/− cleft palate		Hypospadias			Dom., ? Aut. vs. X-linked	22
127. Opitz-Frias syndrome (G syndrome)	Hypertelorism (mild)		Swallowing problems; hypospadias			? X-linked Rec.	21
128. Fraser syndrome	Cryptophthalmos (lids fused); defect of auricle		Genital anomaly			? Aut. Rec.	4
129. Cerebral gigantism†		Large hands and feet	Large size in early life; poor coordination	+/−		?	4
130. Hypercalcemia, peculiar facies, supravalvular aortic stenosis†	Full lips; small nose with anteverted nostrils		+/− Hypercalcemia in infancy; supravalvular aortic stenosis	+	+	?	4

*The numbers in parentheses refer to syndromes listed in this table which merit special consideration in the differential diagnosis.
†Syndrome is described in text; see index for location.

Table continued on following page

MISCELLANEOUS PATTERNS OF MALFORMATION *(Continued)*

	Craniofacial	Limbs	Other	Mental Defic.	Short Stature	Genetic Trans-mission	Refer-ence
131. Leprechaunism (Donohue syndrome)	Full lips		Adipose deficiency; extreme growth deficiency with large hands and feet; enlarged phallus; hirsutism, especially face	?	+	Aut. Rec.	4
132. Berardinelli's lipodystrophy		Tall stature and muscle hypertrophy; phallic hypertrophy; lipoatrophy; hepatomegaly and hyperlipemia		+/−		Aut. Rec.	4
133. Pachydermoperiostosis	Coarse, thick skin	Clubbing	Hyperhidrosis of hands and feet			Aut. Dom.	24
134. Distichiasis-lymphedema syndrome	Double row of eyelashes	Congenital lymphedema of legs	Epidural spinal cysts			Aut. Dom.	26

HAMARTOSES

The hamartoses are a group of diseases in which there is an organizational defect leading to abnormal admixture of tissues, often with a tumor-like excess of one or more tissues. Included are hemangiomas, melanomas, including altered skin pigmentation, fibromas, lipomas, adenomas, and some strange admixtures which create nosological confusion such as the "adenoma sebaceum"—which are not derived from sebaceous glands—in tuberous sclerosis. Certain hamartomatous lesions are liable to grow locally or metastasize, a low-risk phenomenon in some of these diseases such as the Peutz-Jeghers syndrome, but a major risk in others such as Gardner syndrome. Altered morphogenesis other than hamartoma occurs in some of these conditions, notably the altered facies of the basal cell nevus syndrome and syndactyly in Goltz syndrome.

SYNDROME	*DIAGNOSTIC MANIFESTATIONS*			Mental Defic.	Short Stature	Genetic Trans-mission	Refer-ence
	Craniofacial	Skeletal	Other				
135. Sturge-Weber syndrome (136)†	Flat hemangioma of face, most commonly trigeminal in distribution		Hemangiomas of meninges with seizures	+/−		?	4

136. Klippel-Trenaunay-Weber syndrome (135)		Limb hypertrophy, asymmetric	Variable hemangiomas	+/−		?	5
137. Maffucci syndrome		Enchondromatosis	Cavernous hemangiomas			?	1
138. Von Hippel-Lindau syndrome†	Retinal angiomas		Cerebellar hemangioblastoma			Aut. Dom.	1
139. Riley syndrome†	Macrocephaly; pseudopapilledema		Cutaneous hemangiomas			? Aut. Dom.	4
140. Gardner syndrome (141)*†		Osteomas	Polyposis of colon; fibromatous growths in scars; epidermal cysts			Aut. Dom.	4
141. Peutz-Jeghers syndrome (140)*†	Mucocutaneous spotty pigmentation, especially lips		Intestinal polyposis			Aut. Dom.	4
142. Linear nevus sebaceus syndrome	Midfacial nevus sebaceus		+/− Seizures		+/−	?	6
143. Tuberous sclerosis (adenoma sebaceum)†	Hamartomatous pink to brownish facial skin nodules	+/− Bone lesions	Seizures	+/−		Aut. Dom.	1, 2
144. Neurofibromatosis†		+/− Bone lesions	Neurofibromas; café-au-lait spots			Aut. Dom.	1,2
145. Multiple neuroma syndrome	Neuromas of tongue, lips	Arachnodactyly tendency	+/− Thyroid carcinoma; +/− pheochromocytoma			Aut. Dom.	14
146. Multiple lentigines (Leopard syndrome) (122)	Mild hypertelorism		Multiple lentigines; pulmonic stenosis; deafness		+/−	Aut. Dom.	28
147. Basal cell nevus syndrome†	Broad facies	Rib anomalies	Basal cell cutaneous nevi	+		Aut. Dom.	4
148. McCune-Albright syndrome†		Polyostotic fibrous dysplasia	Irregular skin pigmentation; sexual precocity, female			?	4
149. Goltz syndrome (focal dermal hypoplasia), mainly female (89)*	Dental anomalies	Cutaneous syndactyly	Poikiloderma with focal dermal hypoplasia		+/−	Dom.	4
150. Incontinentia pigmenti, mainly in female†	+/− Dental defect		Irregular skin pigmentation in fleck, whorl or spidery form; +/− patchy alopecia	+/−		Dom.	4

*The numbers in parentheses refer to syndromes listed in this table which merit special consideration in the differential diagnosis.
†Syndrome is described in text; see index for location.

Table continued on following page

HAMARTOSES *(Continued)*

SYNDROME	DIAGNOSTIC MANIFESTATIONS: Craniofacial	Skeletal	Other	Mental Defic.	Short Stature	Genetic Transmission	Reference
151. Dyskeratosis congenita syndrome (116)*		Nail dystrophy	Hyperpigmentation; leukoplakia; development of pancytopenia; +/− hemangiomas		+/−	? Aut. Rec.	4
152. Xeroderma pigmentosa (88)	Sun-sensitive atrophic and pigmentary skin changes		Actinic skin tumors			? Aut. Rec.	1

ECTODERMAL DYSPLASIAS

The ectodermal dysplasias, so categorized because the abnormal tissues were predominantly derived from embryonic ectoderm, include hypoplasia of skin and its derivatives plus defects of nails, teeth and lens or sensorineural deafness. The most common type is anhidrotic ectodermal dysplasia. The other types are called hidrotic ectodermal dysplasias since they do not have serious defects in sweating.

SYNDROME	DIAGNOSTIC MANIFESTATIONS: Facial	Nails	Other	Mental Defic.	Short Stature	Genetic Transmission	Reference
153. Hypohidrotic ectodermal dysplasia†	Peg-shaped teeth; partial anodontia; midfacial hypoplasia		Hypoplasia to aplasia of sweat glands; hyperthermia; alopecia			X-linked Aut. Dom., Aut. Rec.	6
HIDROTIC ECTODERMAL DYSPLASIAS†							
154. Ectrodactyly-ectodermal dysplasia-cleft lip (EEC) syndrome (83)	Cleft lip, hypo- and microdontia	Ectrodactyly	Sparse hair; thin hyperkeratotic skin			? Aut. Dom.	6
155. Marshall type	Cataract; midfacial hypoplasia		Deafness			Aut. Dom.	2

156. Robinson type (157)*	Peg-shaped teeth	Hypoplastic nails	Deafness		Aut. Dom.	4
157. Feinmesser type (156)*		Rudimentary nails	Deafness		? Aut. Rec.	4
158. Pili torti and deafness			Deafness; hair twisted, fine and short		? Aut. Rec.	4
159. Enamel hypoplasia and curly hair	Enamel hypoplasia	+/−Nail dystrophy	Hair thick and curly		Aut. Dom.	4
160. Clouston type		Nail dystrophy	Dyskeratotic thick palms and soles	+/−	Aut. Dom.	4
161. Basan type		Thin, fragile nails	Smooth palms and soles		Aut. Dom.	4

*The numbers in parentheses refer to syndromes listed in this table which merit special consideration in the differential diagnosis.
†Syndrome is described in text; see index for location.

DAVID W. SMITH

REFERENCES

General

1. Butterworth, T., and Strean, L. P.: Clinical Genodermatology. Baltimore, The Williams & Wilkins Company, 1962.
2. Gorlin, R. J., and Pindborg, J. J.: Syndromes of the Head and Neck. New York, McGraw-Hill Book Company, Inc., 1964.
3. McKusick, V. A.: Heritable Disorders of Connective Tissue. 3rd ed. St. Louis, The C. V. Mosby Company, 1966.
4. Smith, D. W.: Recognizable Patterns of Human Malformation. Philadelphia, W. B. Saunders Company, 1970.
5. Warkany, J.: Congenital Malformations. Chicago, Year Book Medical Publishers, 1971.
6. Holmes, L. B., et al.: Mental Retardation, An Atlas of Diseases with Associated Physical Abnormalities. New York, The Macmillan Company, 1972.

Specific Disorders

7. Aarskog, D.: A familial syndrome of short stature associated with facial dysplasia and genital anomalies. J. Pediatr. 77:856, 1970.
8. Bartsocas, C. S., Weber, A. L., and Crawford, J. D.: Acrocephalosyndactyly type III: Chotzen's syndrome. J. Pediatr. 77:267, 1970.
9. Beals, R. K.: Auriculo-osteodysplasia. J. Bone Joint Surg. *49-A*:1541, 1967.
10. Beals, R. K., and Hecht, F.: Delineation of another heritable disorder of connective tissue. J. Bone Joint Surg. *53-A*:987, 1971.
11. Caldwell, P. D., and Smith, D. W.: The XXY syndrome in childhood. J. Pediatr. *80*:250, 1972.
12. Cleveland, W. W., Arias, D., and Smith, G. F.: Radioulnar synostosis, behavioral disturbance, and XYY chromosomes. J. Pediatr. *74*:103, 1969.
13. Coffin, G. S., and Siris, E.: Mental retardation with absent fifth fingernail and terminal phalanx. Am. J. Dis. Child. *119*:433, 1970.
14. Gorlin, R. J., et al.: Multiple mucosal neuromas. Cancer *22*:293, 1968.
15. Gorlin, R. J., Cohen, M. M., and Wolfson, J.: Tricho-rhino-phalangeal syndrome. Am. J. Dis. Child. *118*:595, 1969.
16. Gorlin, R. F., Spranger, J., and Koszalka, M. F.: Genetic craniotubular bone dysplasias and hyperostoses. Birth defects *4*:79, 1969.
17. Grosse, R., Gorlin, J., and Opitz, J. M.: The Dubowitz syndrome. Z. Kinderheilk. *110*:175, 1971.
18. Hall, B. D.: Aglossia-adactylia. Birth Defects 7:233, 1971.
19. Hall, B. D., et al.: Langer-Giedion syndrome. Birth Defects Vol. 17, 1974.
20. Hoefnagel, D., et al.: Camptomelic dwarfism. Lancet *1*:1068, 1972.
21. Little, J. R., and Opitz, J. M.: The G syndrome. Am. J. Dis. Child. *121*:505, 1971.
22. Opitz, J. M., Summitt, R. L., and Smith, D. W.: The BBB syndrome, familial telecanthus with associated congenital anomalies. Birth Defects *5*:86, 1969.
23. Reed, W. B., May, S. B., and Nickel, W. R.: Xeroderma pigmentosum with neurological complications. Arch Derm. *91*:224, 1965.
24. Rimoin, D. L.: Pachydermoperiostosis. New Engl. J. Med. *272*:923, 1965.
25. Robinow, M., et al.: Acrodysostosis. Am. J. Dis. Child *121*:195, 1971.
26. Robinow, M., Johnson, G. F., and Verhagen, A. D.: Distichiasis-lymphedema. Am. J. Dis. Child. *119*:343, 1970.
27. Saldino, R. M.: Lethal short-limbed dwarfism: Achondrogenesis and thanatophoric dwarfism. Am. J. Roentgenol. Radium Ther. Nucl. Med. *112*:185, 1971.
28. Sommer, A., et al.: A family study of the Leopard syndrome. Am. J. Dis. Child. *121*:520, 1971.
29. Sparkes, R. S., and Graham, C. B.: Camurati-Engelmann disease. J. Med. Genet. *9*:73, 1972.
30. Spranger, J. W., Opitz, J. M., and Bidder, U.: Heterogeneity of chondroplasia punctata. Humangenetik *11*:190, 1971.
31. Thompson, R. C., et al.: Hereditary hyperphosphatasia. Am. J. Med. *47*:209, 1969.
32. Walker, B. A., et al.: Hypochondroplasia. Am. J. Dis. Child. *122*:95, 1971.

30
APPENDIX

Table 30–1: Table of Drugs*
(Including doses, generic and trade names, contraindications for use, warnings, precautions, adverse reactions, and how the drugs are supplied)

Dosage listed in the following table is not specifically intended for premature and newborn infants unless so indicated.

All doses are average doses and are approximate. Variability of response may require alteration of dosage. Doses based on different criteria (body weight, surface area, etc.) frequently do not correspond.

To change the dose per kilogram to the dose per pound, divide the dose by 2.2 (or, more conveniently, by 2). To change the dose in g*/kg to gr*/lb, multiply the dose in g/kg by 7.

Drugs recognized as essential are included in *The Pharmacopeia of the United States.* These are the "blue ribbon" drugs. *The National Formulary* includes drugs of demonstrated value. These compendia (USP XIX and NF XIV, official July 1, 1970) recognize only *essential* and *valuable* drugs. The designations USP and NF have been added to drugs of this table to identify such drugs.

Generic names are derived from (a) United States Adopted Names (USAN), (b) USP Diction-

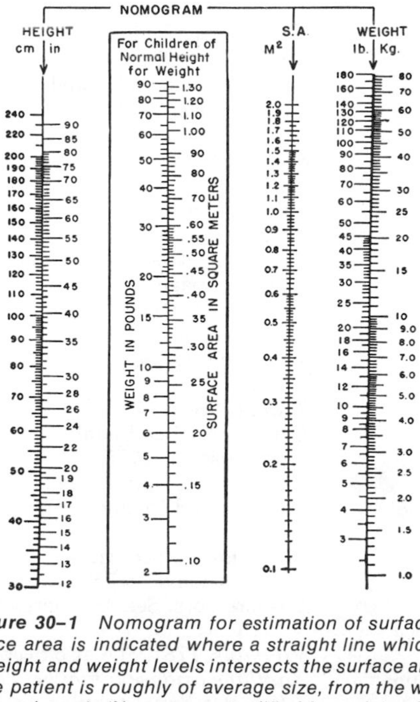

Figure 30–1 *Nomogram for estimation of surface area. The surface area is indicated where a straight line which connects the height and weight levels intersects the surface area column; or the patient is roughly of average size, from the weight alone (enclosed area). (Nomogram modified from data of E. Boyd by C. D. West.)*

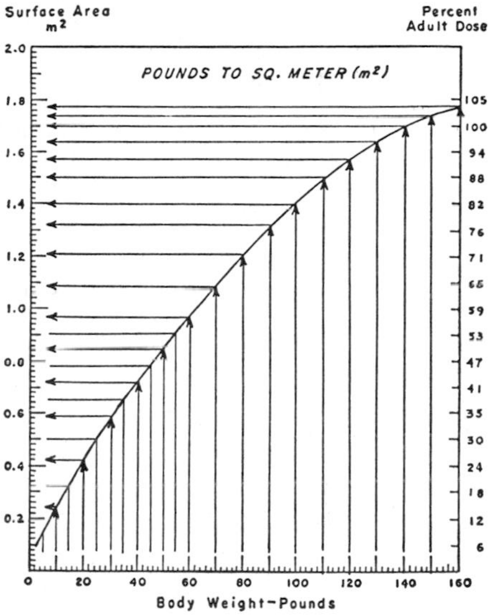

Figure 30–2 *Relations between body weight in pounds, body surface area and adult dosage. The surface area values correspond to those set forth by Crawford et al. (1950). Note that the 100 per cent adult dose is for a patient weighing about 140 pounds and having a surface area of about 1.7 square meters. (From N. B. Talbot et al.:* Metabolic Homeostasis—A Syllabus for Those Concerned with the Care of Patients. *Cambridge, Harvard University Press, 1959.)*

*Throughout this table, grams is abbreviated as g; gr is the abbreviation for an antiquated measure in the apothecaries system, i.e., grains. The metric system of weights and measures was adopted by the USP in 1890 to replace the apothecaries system.

ary of Drug Names, No. 10. Rockville, Maryland, United States Pharmacopeial Convention, 1972, (c) Ibid. Supplement, 1973, and (d) Ibid. Supplement, 1974.

Mixtures of two or more active drugs are generally not included.

Many drugs released since 1962 have not been sufficiently tested in children to permit precise recommendations regarding dosage. Such drugs (see Therapeutic Orphans, Section 5) may be listed with restrictions on use in children or may be given with adult dosage only; many drugs of little importance have been omitted.

See package inserts for restrictions on use during pregnancy. Some teratogens are discussed in Section 7.

The drugs in Table 30–1 are listed alphabetically in various categories indicated by italics below. To locate specific drugs, see the appropriate diagnostic or therapeutic category, or consult the Index, which lists all the drugs in the table.

DRUGS

TABLE 30–1 *(Continued)*

DRUG, HOW SUPPLIED	DOSAGE, ROUTES, CONTRAINDICATIONS AND WARNINGS *
ACIDIFIERS	
Ammonium chloride, NF *Available as:* Tablets: 0.3 g, and (enteric coated) 0.5 and 1 g Solutions and syrups Vials: 5 mEq/ml	Dose: 75 mg/kg/24 hr; 2 g/M^2/24 hr; divide into 4 doses (O) **Caution:** May produce acidosis by continued use; not to be used in liver disease; use with caution in infants
Ascorbic acid, USP *Available as:* Tablets: 25, 50, 100, 250, 500 mg, and 1 g Capsules: 25, 100, 250 and 500 mg, and 1 g Drops: 50 mg/0.6 ml Solution (for injection): 100 and 250 mg/ml	Dose: 0.5 g with each dose of methenamine mandelate **Caution:** Solutions stronger than 10% may decompose, with production of CO_2 under high pressure; wrap ampoule while opening. Ascorbic acid and penicillin G are incompatible; do not mix
Calcium chloride, USP (See Calcium salts)	
Methionine, NF (Amurex, Pedameth, Uranap) *Available as:* Powder: envelopes, 2 g Tablets: 0.25 and 0.5 g Capsules: 200 and 500 mg Liquid: 75 mg/5 ml	Dose for urinary tract infections: 250 mg/kg/24 hr; 8 g/M^2/24 hr; divide into 3–4 doses (O) Dose for ammoniacal dermatitis: 200 mg/24 hr, in single dose (O) **Contraindication:** Liver disease **Caution:** Not on empty stomach
ADRENAL STEROIDS (See Endocrines)	
ADRENERGIC BLOCKING AGENTS (See Phentolamine, Propranolol, and Cardiovascular Drugs [antihypertensives])	
ADRENERGICS	
Amphetamine sulfate (Benzedrine sulfate)	Dose: 5–20 mg/24 hr; 15 mg/M^2/24 hr; divide into 3 doses or as prolonged-action single dose (O)
Amphetamine phosphate (many trade names) *Available as:* Tablets: 5 and 10 mg, and (prolonged action) 15 mg.	15 mg/M^2/dose (IM or slowly IV as analeptic); repeat prn **Contraindications:** Agitated prepsychotic patients; those taking monoamine oxidase inhibitors (or 2 weeks after); hyperthyroidism **Caution:** Use with caution in hypersensitivity to sympathomimetics, in severe hypertensive or cardiovascular disease **Warning:** Tolerance to anorectic effects; do not increase; advise need for care in operation of vehicles or machinery; may alter insulin requirements when used as anorectic **Overdose:** See Section 28
Dextroamphetamine sulfate, USP (Dexedrine sulfate and many other trade names) *Available as:* Tablets: 5 mg Capsules (prolonged-action): 5, 10, and 15 mg	Dose: 2–15 mg/24 hr; 10 mg/M^2/24 hr; divide into 3 doses or as prolonged-action single dose (O) Dose (minimal brain dysfunction): not recommended for this use under age 3 years; age 3–5 years, 2.5 mg/24 hr (O) initially, increased at weekly intervals by 2.5 mg to gain optimal response (range 2.5–40 mg); age 6 years and older, double the above dose (range 2.5–40 mg) Dose (narcolepsy): age 6–12 years, 5 mg/24 hr (O) initially, increased by

*For individual drugs, see general index. *Consult package inserts.*

Key: M^2, dose per square meter of body surface; IM, intramuscular; ITh, intrathecal; IV, intravenous; O, oral; R, rectal; SC, subcutaneous; Subl, sublingual; T, topical.

Table continued.

TABLE 30–1 (*Continued*)

DRUG, HOW SUPPLIED	DOSAGE, ROUTES, CONTRAINDICATIONS AND WARNINGS*
Elixir: 5 mg/5 ml	5 mg at weekly intervals to optimum response (range 5–60 mg); 12 years and older, double the above (range 5–60 mg) Dose (obesity): not recommended under 12 years of age Dose (analeptic, in central depression): 0.2–0.5 mg/kg, or 6–15 mg/M^2; single dose (IV or IM, slowly); repeat at 30 minute intervals; when conscious (O) **Contraindications:** See Amphetamine sulfate **Caution:** See Amphetamine sulfate
Ephedrine sulfate, USP *Available as:* Tablets and capsules: 25 and 50 mg Capsules (delayed action): 30 and 60 mg Syrups: 20 mg/5 ml (USP); others 11 and 15 mg/5 ml Injection: 25 and 50 mg/ml	Dose: 3 mg/kg/24 hr; 100 mg/M^2/24 hr; divide into 4–6 doses (O, SC, or IV) **Caution:** Insomnia, headache, nervousness, palpitation, (arrhythmias on digitalis therapy), precordial pain, nausea, sweating, urinary retention; may potentiate theophylline or aminophylline toxicity
Epinephrine, USP (Adrenalin and many other trade names) *Available as:* Aqueous solution, 1:1000: Ampules, 1 ml; Syringe (disposable), 1 ml; Vials, 30 ml; bottles, 30 ml Aqueous solution, 1:100: Bottles, 5 ml Suspension, 1:200 (Sus-Phrine): Vials, 5 ml; Ampules, 0.5 ml Suspension, 1:400 (Asmolin): Vials, 10 ml In oil, 1:500: Ampules, 1 ml	Dose for asthma or tolerance test: 0.01 ml/kg/dose of aqueous 1:1000 solution (maximum, 0.5 ml); 0.3 ml/M^2/dose; repeat every 4 hr prn (SC) Dose for asthma: aqueous solution 1:100 given only by nebulizer prn; suspension 1:200, 0.004 ml/kg/dose, or 0.125 ml/M^2/dose, repeat every 8–12 hr (SC); suspension 1:400, double dose for suspension 1:200; in oil 1:500, 0.01–0.02 ml/kg/dose, or 0.3–0.6 ml/M^2/dose, daily or every 12 hr (IM) **Caution:** Overdosage **Contraindications:** Glaucoma; shock; during anesthesia with halogenated hydrocarbons or cyclopropane; in organic brain damage; in cardiac dilatation or coronary insufficiency; phenothiazine intoxication **Warnings:** Use with caution in cardiovascular disease, hypertension, hyperthyroidism, long standing bronchial asthma and emphysema; avoid IV injection (hypertension and cerebrovascular hemorrhage); peripheral vasoconstriction may produce pulmonary edema (nitrites or alpha blocking agents may counteract effect); use with large dose of digitalis, mercurials, other drugs, may dispose to cardiac arrhythmias, not recommended; with care in diabetes **Precautions:** Protect from light; do not use if brown in color or precipitated; readily destroyed by alkali and oxidants; may be potentiated by tricyclic antidepressants, some antihistamines (see package insert), and sodium L-thyroxine **Adverse reactions:** Transient headache, palpitations, anxiety with usual dosage; necrosis at site of repeated local injections
Isoproterenol hydrochloride, USP (Isuprel hydrochloride, Norisodrine hydrochloride, Proterenol hydrochloride) *Available as:* Tablets: 10 and 15 mg (Subl or R); 15 and 30 mg (prolonged-action) Solutions: vials, 1:200 or 1:100 Nebulizer: pressurized mist, 1:400 Injection: 200 μg/ml (1:5000)	Dose: 5–10 mg (Subl or R); repeat 3–4 times every 24 hr (maximum 300 mg); IV use possible (see text or package insert) **Contraindication:** With epinephrine (may produce arrhythmia) **Caution:** Careful dosage adjustment in hyperthyroidism, heart failure or limited cardiac reserve, sensitivity to sympathomimetics
Isoproterenol sulfate, NF (Norisodrine sulfate) *Available as:* Powder: 10 and 25%, in cartridges for inhalation	Dose: 1:200 or 1:400, 1–2 inhalations; powder by inhalation **Contraindication:** With epinephrine (may produce arrhythmia) **Caution:** Careful dosage adjustment in hyperthyroidism, heart failure or limited cardiac reserve, sensitivity to sympathomimetics

*For individual drugs, see general index. *Consult package inserts.*

Key: M^2, dose per square meter of body surface; IM, intramuscular; ITh, intrathecal; IV, intravenous; O, oral; R, rectal; SC, subcutaneous; Subl, sublingual; T, topical.

TABLE 30–1 ***(Continued)***

DRUG, HOW SUPPLIED	DOSAGE, ROUTES, CONTRAINDICATIONS AND WARNINGS
Tablets: 10 mg Solution: 0.2% (1:500), pressurized for inhalation; 1% (10 mg/ml) Suppositories: 5 mg	
Levarterenol bitartrate, USP, norepinephrine bitartrate (Levophed bitartrate) *Available as:* Solution: 0.2% (2 mg/ml), for injection	Dose: 1 ml 0.2% solution (0.1% base) in 250 ml diluent; drip at 0.5 ml/min to give 2 μg (base)/min (IV); 2 μg/M²/min (IV); titrate dose with blood pressure **Contraindication:** During cyclopropane and halothane anesthesia; hypertension **Caution:** Headache, hypersensitivity, bradycardia; slough results from extravascular leakage; treat extravasated area quickly, infiltrating with phentolamine solution (5–10 mg in 15 ml saline solution) **Warning:** Not with MAO inhibitors, imipramine, or triptylene drugs
Mephentermine sulfate, NF (Wyamine sulfate) *Available as:* Injection: 15 and 30 mg/ml Syringe (disposable): 30 and 60 mg	Dose: 0.4 mg/kg, or 12 mg/M², as single dose (O, IM, or slowly IV); repeat prn or by slow drip (0.1%) **Contraindications:** Hemorrhagic shock, concealed hemorrhage, phenothiazine hypotension
Metaraminol bitartrate, USP (Aramine bitartrate) *Available as:* Solution: 10 mg/ml, for injection	Dose: 0.1 mg/kg, or 3 mg/M², as single dose (SC or IM) Intravenous: 1/10 of above dose as single dose; 0.4 mg/kg, or 12 mg/M² by IV drip, diluting each mg in 25 ml isotonic saline solution or 5% glucose; adjust rate to maintain blood pressure **Caution:** Cyclopropane anesthesia; thyroid or heart disease, diabetes
Methoxamine hydrochloride, USP (Vasoxyl) *Available as:* Solution: 10 and 20 mg/ml, for injection	Dose: 0.25 mg/kg, or 7.5 mg/M², as single dose (IM); 1/3 of IM dose for IV dose (slowly) **Caution:** Severe hypertension, hyperthyroidism
Phenylephrine hydrochloride, USP (Neo-Synephrine hydrochloride and many other trade names) *Available as:* Capsules: 10 and 25 mg Elixir: 5 mg/5 ml Solution: 2 and 10 mg/ml, for injection	Dose: 0.1 mg/kg, or 3 mg/M², as single dose (SC or IM); 1 mg/kg/24 hr, or 30 mg/M²/24 hr, divided into 6 doses (O) **Caution:** Severe hypertension, cardiac disorders, hyperthyroidism, hyperglycemia
ADRENOCORTICOTROPIN (ACTH) (See Endocrines)	
ANALEPTICS (central nervous system stimulants)	
Amphetamine sulfate (See Adrenergics)	
Caffeine and sodium benzoate injection, USP *Available as:* Solution: 0.25 and 0.5 g, for injection	Dose: 8 mg/kg/dose (maximum, 500 mg); 250 mg/M²/dose; repeat every 4 hr prn (SC, IV, or IM) **Toxicity:** See Poisons, Section 28 **Caution:** In jaundiced infant, uncouples bilirubin-albumin (kernicterus)
Dextroamphetamine sulfate (See Adrenergics)	
Ephedrine sulfate (See Adrenergics)	
Methylphenidate hydrochloride, USP (Ritalin hydrochloride)	

Table continued.

TABLE 30–1 (*Continued*)

DRUG, HOW SUPPLIED	DOSAGE, ROUTES, CONTRAINDICATIONS AND WARNINGS *
Available as: Tablets: 5, 10, and 20 mg Solution: 10 mg/ml, for injection	Dose (minimal brain dysfunction): 6 years and older, 5 mg (O) before breakfast and lunch, initially; increase by 5–10 mg (O) weekly (maximum 60 mg/24 hr) to effective dose; reduce or discontinue with aggravation of symptoms or with adverse reaction; discontinue periodically to reevaluate, or if no improvement in 1 mo **Contraindications:** Convulsive disorders, hypersensitivity, glaucoma **Caution:** Use cautiously with pressor agents; may cause gastrointestinal symptoms, headache, rash, angina, cardiac arrhythmia, hypertension **Overdose:** Vomiting, hallucinations, agitation, tremors, convulsions, coma (CNS effects); sweating, flushing, mydriasis, headache, hyperpyrexia (sympathetic NS effects) **Warning:** Should not be used under age of 6 yr; monitor growth; discontinue with seizures; not for severe depression
ANALGESICS (NARCOTIC)	
Codeine phosphate, USP *Available as:* Tablets: Many sizes Cough syrups: Often contain 10 mg/5 ml Tubex (disposable): 30 and 60 mg, for injection	Dose for pain: 3 mg/kg/24 hr, or 100 mg/M²/24 hr; divide into 6 doses (O or SC) Dose for cough: 1/3–1/2 of dose for pain **Warning:** May be habit-forming **Caution:** Side effects like morphine (large doses) **Toxicity:** See Opiates, Section 28
Diphenoxylate hydrochloride with atropine sulfate (Lomotil) *Available as:* Tablets: 2.5 mg diphenoxylate HCl and 0.025 mg atropine sulfate Liquid: the above in 5 ml **NB:** This antidiarrheal agent has narcotic potential; not designed for analgesia primarily	Dose (of diphenoxylate HCl): Adults, 15–20 mg/24 hr, divided into 3 or 4 doses (O); 2–5 yr old, 6 mg/24 hr (O), divided into 3 doses; 5–8 yr old, 8 mg/24 hr (O), divided into 4 doses; 8–12 yr old, 10 mg/24 hr (O), divided into 5 doses **Contraindications:** Not for less than 2 yr old, or with hypersensitivity to diphenoxylate or atropine; not for jaundiced patient **Warnings:** With caution in young child; with MAO inhibitors may produce hypertensive crisis; with liver disease may precipitate hepatic coma **Precautions:** Addiction to diphenoxylate theoretically possible; subtherapeutic dose of atropine added, to discourage overdosage; must observe contraindications, warnings, precautions for use of atropine (q.v.); may produce atropinism in children, even at recommended dosage **Adverse effects:** Atropine effects (see atropine); abdominal discomfort, nervous symptoms, CNS depression, nausea, vomiting, angioedema, pruritus also reported (see package insert)
Meperidine hydrochloride, USP (Demerol hydrochloride) *Available as:* Tablets: 50 and 100 mg Elixir: 50 mg/5 ml Ampules: 0.5 ml, 1 ml, 1.5 ml, and 2 ml, all containing 50 mg/ml Vials: 50 and 100 mg/ml Syringes (disposable): 75 and 100 mg/ml Tubex (disposable): 25, 50, 75, and 100 mg Powder (vials): 15 g	Dose: 6 mg/kg/24 hr (maximum, 100 mg/dose), or 175 mg/M²/24 hr; divide into 6 doses (O, IM, or SC) **Contraindications:** Intracranial lesions causing increased pressure, auricular flutter, bronchial asthma; with or within 2 wk of monoamine oxidase inhibitors, isoniazid, or derivatives; hypersensitivity **Warning:** May be habit-forming; for overdosage, see Opiates, Section 28 **Caution:** In abdominal pain or asthma; may aggravate convulsions, cause urinary retention, or produce allergic reactions
Methadone hydrochloride, USP (Adanon hydrochloride, Althose, Amidone hydrochloride, Dolophine hydrochloride) *Available as:*	Dose for analgesia: 0.7 mg/kg/24 hr, or 20 mg/M²/24 hr; divide into 4–6 doses (O or SC) Dose for antitussive effect: 1/4 of analgesic dose (O) Dose for detoxification or maintenance of addicts: See package insert **Warning:** May be habit-forming

*For individual drugs, see general index. *Consult package inserts.*

Key: M², dose per square meter of body surface; IM, intramuscular; ITh, intrathecal; IV, intravenous; O, oral; R, rectal; SC, subcutaneous; Subl, sublingual; T, topical.

TABLE 30–1 *(Continued)*

DRUG, HOW SUPPLIED	DOSAGE, ROUTES, CONTRAINDICATIONS AND WARNINGS
Tablets: 2.5, 5, 7.5, and 10 mg Elixir: 5 mg/5 ml Syrup: 1.66 mg/5 ml Solution: 10 mg/ml, for injection	**Caution:** May cause nausea, vomiting, dizziness, dry mouth, euphoria, depression, pulmonary edema; hypersensitivity may occur **Toxicity:** See Opiates, Section 28
Morphine sulfate, USP (paregoric contains 0.4 mg morphine/ml) *Available as:* Tablets: 8, 10, 15, and 30 mg Solution (suitable salts): 8, 10, and 15 mg/ml for injection Syringe (disposable): 8, 10, and 15 mg	Dose for analgesia: In general use, 0.1–0.2 mg/kg/dose (SC), with maximum 15 mg; preoperative, see Section 5, Preoperative and Postoperative Care **Toxicity:** See Opiates, Section 28
Paregoric, USP (camphorated opium tincture) *Available as:* Tincture: 0.4 mg morphine/ml	Dose for analgesia: 0.25–0.5 ml/kg/dose (O); smaller dose may be offered initially; increase to analgesic dose as maximum Other considerations: As for morphine sulfate, above
ANALGESICS (NON-NARCOTIC) AND ANTIPYRETICS	
Acetaminophen, N-acetyl-*p*-aminophenol, USP (Liquiprin, Tempra, Tylenol, and many other trade names) *Available as:* Tablets: 325 mg (scored, Tylenol); 120 mg (chewable, Tempra) Syrup or elixir: 120 mg/5 ml Drops: 60 mg/0.6 ml	Dose: under 1 yr, 60 mg; 1–3 yr, 60–120 mg; 3–6 yr, 120 mg; 6–12 yr, 240 mg; single dose repeated every 4–6 hr (O); 0.7 g/M^2/24 hr, divided into 4–6 doses (O)
Aspirin, acetylsalicylic acid, USP *Available as:* Tablets: 60, 81, 200, 300, and 600 mg Suppositories: 60, 200, 300, and 600 mg; also in other forms	Dose (antipyretic): 65 mg/kg/24 hr (maximum, 3.6 g/24 hr); or 1.5 g/M^2/24 hr; divide into 4–6 doses (O or R); avoid overdosage, particularly in infants Dose (to obtain blood salicylate level of 20 mg/dl): 3 g/M^2/24 hr (O) **Caution:** Salicylism, especially in infants
Dipyrone (Narone, Pyralgin and many other trade names) *Available as:* Tablets: 0.5 and 0.65 g Liquid: 0.5 g/5 ml Pediatric drops: 0.25 g/ml Injection: 0.5 g/ml	Only for serious and life threatening situations when other drugs are ineffective or contraindicated Dose (adult): Not to exceed 0.5–1 g/dose (No more than 3 g/24 hr) Dose (children): (brief use) 250–500 mg/dose, repeated in 3–4 hrs only if necessary; not to exceed in 24 hrs, 1 g (up to 6 yr) or 2 g (6–12 yr); if possible, *avoid* this drug; it is an *aminopyrine* derivative **Warning:** This drug may cause fatal agranulocytosis **Caution:** Use only in conditions in which it is specifically indicated and in which other less toxic drugs have proved ineffective or are not tolerated; potential benefit must be weighed against the possibility of fatal agranulocytosis, which has been reported after short-term use, intermittent use, and after long-term use; use should be as brief as possible **Precautions:** Frequent white blood cell and differential counts should be carried out, but agranulocytosis may occur precipitously without prior warning; discontinue at the first evidence of any alteration of the blood count or sign of agranulocytosis, or at the first indication of sore throat or sign of other infection in the mouth or throat (pain, swelling, tenderness, ulceration).
Propoxyphene hydrochloride, USP (Darvon) and **napsylate** (Darvon-N) *Available as:* Capsules (hydrochloride): 32 and 65 mg	Dose (hydrochloride): Adult, 65 mg or 40 mg/M^2, as single dose (O); repeat every 4 hr, as needed Dose (napsylate): 1½ times the above dose **Contraindications:** Hypersensitivity to propoxyphene **Warnings:** May produce psychic or, less often, physical dependence or

Table continued.

DRUGS

TABLE 30-1 (*Continued*)

DRUG, HOW SUPPLIED	DOSAGE, ROUTES, CONTRAINDICATIONS AND WARNINGS*
Tablets (napsylate): 100 mg Suspension (napsylate): 50 mg/5 ml	tolerance; may impair mental function for complicated or hazardous tasks; not recommended for use in children **Precautions:** CNS depression may potentiate effects of other CNS depressants; confusion, anxiety, tremors reported when given with orphenadrine **Adverse reactions:** Dizziness, sedation, nausea, vomiting, especially in ambulatory patients; other effects (see package insert) **Toxicity:** See opiates, Section 28
Salicylamide (Amid-Sal, Dropsprin, Raspberin, Salamide, Salicim, Salrin) *Available as:* Tablets: 300 and 600 mg Suspension: 65 mg/ml (325 mg/5 ml) **Note:** Salicylamide has been replaced with acetaminophen in Liquiprin	Dose (antipyretic-analgesic): 65 mg/kg/24 hr, or 1.5 g/M²/24 hr; divide into 6 doses (O) **Caution:** Sensitivity to salicylates; may cause nausea, vomiting, drowsiness, hyperventilation, rash
ANTHELMINTICS	
Bephenium hydroxynaphthoate, USP (Alcopara) *Available as:* Granules (packets): 5 g (equivalent to 2.5 g base)	Dose: Under 23 kg, 5 g/24 hr; over 23 kg and adult, 10 g/24 hr; divide into 2 doses (O); bitter taste may be disguised in carbonated beverages, flavored milk, orange juice; withhold food for 2 hr after use for *Ancylostoma duodenale,* may repeat in a few days, if necessary; for *Necator americanus,* treat for 3 days in a row **Caution:** Nausea, vomiting and diarrhea may occur; correct electrolyte imbalance before use; careful use in hypertension **Precautions:** Support debilitated, anemic or dehydrated patient before therapy; may produce brief hypotension in hypertensives **Adverse reactions:** In a few patients, nausea, vomiting or diarrhea
Diethylcarbamazine citrate, USP (Hetrazan) *Available as:* Tablets: 50 mg Syrup: 120 mg/5 ml	Dose (filariasis): 6 mg/kg/24 hr, or 150 mg/M²/24 hr; divide into 3 doses (O); treat 7–10 days Dose (ascariasis): 15 mg/kg/24 hr, or 500 mg/M²/24 hr (O); single daily dose for 4 consecutive days **Caution:** May cause headache, malaise, weakness, nausea, vomiting, many reactions from filaricidal action
Gentian violet, methyl rosaniline chloride, USP *Available as:* Tablets: 15 and 30 mg, and (enteric coated) 10 and 30 mg Solutions: to order Powder	Dose (oral moniliasis): Apply 0.25% aqueous solution (T), for 3-day courses Dose (oxyuriasis): Use coated tablets, 2 mg/kg/24 hr, or 50 mg/M²/24 hr; divide into 2–3 doses/24 hr (O); treat 7–10 days, with 7–10 days rest between treatments **Caution:** Caustic, not to be chewed; may cause nausea, vomiting (purple), diarrhea, abdominal pains; use with caution in cardiac, hepatic, renal or gastrointestinal disease
Piperazine salts (piperazine citrate, USP) (Antepar citrate, and others) *Available as:* Tablets: 250 and 500 mg Wafers: 500 mg Syrup: 500 mg/5 ml	Dose is expressed as hydrous base Dose (oxyuriasis): Up to 7 kg, 250 mg; 7–14 kg, 500 mg; 14–27 kg, 1 g; over 27 kg, 2 g; or 1 g/M²; once daily for 7 consecutive days (O) Dose (ascariasis): Up to 14 kg, 1 g; 14–23 kg, 2 g; 23–45 kg, 3 g; over 45 kg, 3.5 g; or 2 g/M²; once daily for 2 consecutive days (O) **Contraindications:** Patients with predisposition to grand or petit mal epilepsy **Caution:** Vomiting, blurred vision, muscle weakness, urticaria, with large doses
Pyranthel pamoate, USP (Antiminth) *Available as:* Oral suspension: 250 mg/5ml	Dose (ascariasis and enterobiasis): in children and adults, 11 mg/kg (O), as a single dose (Maximum 1 g), with or without food (no purge) **Precautions:** Minor transient elevations of SGOT; use with caution in pre-existing liver dysfunction.

*For individual drugs, see general index. *Consult package inserts.*

Key: M², dose per square meter of body surface; IM, intramuscular; ITh, intrathecal; IV, intravenous; O, oral; R, rectal; SC, subcutaneous; Subl, sublingual; T, topical.

TABLE 30-1 (*Continued*)

DRUG, HOW SUPPLIED	DOSAGE, ROUTES, CONTRAINDICATIONS AND WARNINGS
	Adverse Reactions: Anorexia, nausea, vomiting, gastralgia, adbominal cramps, diarrhea and tenesmus transient elevation of SGOT; headache, dizziness, drowsiness, and insommia; rashes
Pyrvinium pamoate, USP (Povan) *Available as:* Tablets (coated): 50 mg (base) Suspension: 50 mg (base)/5 ml	Dose: 5 mg/kg (as base), or 150 mg/M^2; single doses (O) **Caution:** Colors stools red; nausea, vomiting, cramping; suspension and chewed tablets stain; tablets to be swallowed whole; *not for aspirin sensitive patient* (coated tablets contain tartrazine)
Quinacrine hydrochloride, USP	See Antiprotozoan drugs, below
Tetrachloroethylene, USP *Available as:* Capsules: 0.2, 0.5, 1, 2.5, and 5 ml, veterinary preparation of USP purity	Dose: 0.1 ml/kg (maximum, 5 ml), or 3 ml/M^2; single dose (O) **Caution:** Avoid fats or alcohol (drug vehicle); toxic reactions rare—dizziness, nausea, drowsiness
Thiabendazole, USP (Mintezol) *Available as:* Tablets (chewable): 500 mg Suspension: 500 mg/5 ml	Dose: 50 mg/kg/24 hr (maximum, 3 g/24 hr), or 1.3 g/M^2/24 hr; divided into 2 doses (O); for *enterobiasis,* repeat above dose in 7 days, or if not practical, give above dose on 2 successive days; for *intestinal parasitoses* (singly or in combinations), above dose on 1 day or 2 successive days; for *cutaneous larva migrans,* above dose on 2 successive days, to be repeated if lesions active after 2 days; for *trichinosis,* above dose on 2–4 successive days; experience with *ascariasis uncinariasis, trichuriasis,* and *strongyloidiasis* limited for children under 15 kg **Warning:** Patients receiving this drug should be cautioned against engaging in hazardous occupations requiring complete mental alertness, e.g., operating machinery or driving a motor vehicle **Caution:** Gastrointestinal symptoms, dizziness, headache, fatigue, pruritus; rarely tinnitus, collapse, abnormal ocular sensations, numbness, hyperglycemia, xanthopsia, enuresis, cephalin flocculation and SGOT rises (transitory); odor to urine, crystalluria; transient leukopenia; hypersensitivity (Stevens-Johnson syndrome) may occur and be fatal **Precautions:** Support debilitated, anemic or dehydrated patient prior to treatment; caution with hepatic or renal dysfunction **Adverse reactions;** See package insert
ANTIASTHMATICS (See also Bronchodilators)	
Cromolyn sodium (Aarane, Intal) *Available as:* Capsules: 20 mg	Dose: Adults and children over 5 yr; 80 mg/24 hr by insufflation; divide into 4 doses **Note:** Not to be swallowed or used under 5 yr of age **Contraindication:** Hypersensitivity to the drug **Warning:** Not for treatment of an acute attack of asthma, especially status asthmaticus; consideration should be given to decreasing the dosage or discontinuing the administration of the drug in patients with impaired renal or hepatic function; eosinophilic pneumonia has been reported rarely (if this occurs, the drug should be discontinued); because of the possibility that adverse effects of the drug could become apparent only after many years, a benefit-risk consideration of the long term use is particularly important in children. **Precautions:** Cough and/or bronchospasm may follow inhalation; patients with cromolyn sodium induced bronchospasm may not be able to continue its administration despite prior use of bronchodilators; asthma may recur if drug is reduced below the recommended dosage, or discontinued. **Adverse reactions:** Maculopapular rash and urticaria reported to have cleared promptly upon withdrawing the drug; cough and/or bronchospasm may occur

Table continued.

TABLE 30–1 (*Continued*)

DRUG, HOW SUPPLIED	DOSAGE, ROUTES, CONTRAINDICATIONS AND WARNINGS *
ANTIBIOTICS	
ANTIBIOTICS, GENERAL	
Amoxicillin (See Penicillins, below)	
Ampicillin (See Penicillins, below)	
Bacitracin, USP (1 mg = 50 units) *Available as:* Powder (ampules): 2000, 10,000, and 50,000 units Tablets: 2500 and 5000 units	Dose (systemic infections): For premature infants, 900 units/kg/24 hr; in full-term newborn infants to age of 1 yr, 1000 units/kg/24 hr, or 30,000 units/M^2/24 hr; divide into 2–3 doses (IM); not longer than 10–12 days Dose (enteric infections): Premature infants, 1000 units/kg/24 hr; older infants and children, 2000 units/kg/24 hr, or 60,000 units/M^2/24 hr; divide into 4 doses (O) **Caution:** Nephrotoxicity, anorexia, nausea, rashes, local irritation; store solution at 4° C; use within 24 hr after mixing
Benzathine penicillin G (See Penicillins, below)	
Carbenicillin disodium (See Penicillins, below)	
CEPHALOSPORINS	
Cefazolin sodium (Ancef, Kefzol) *Available as:* Injection: 250 and 500 mg and 1 g	Dose (adults): Mild infections, 0.75–1.5 g/24 hr, divided into 3 doses (IM or IV); moderate or severe infections; 1.5–4 g/24 hr, divided into 3–4 doses IM or IV Dose (children): Mild to moderately severe infections, 25–50 mg/kg/24 hr or 1.25 g/M^2/24 hr **Contraindications:** In patients with sensitivity to cephalosporin drugs (see Cephaloglycin, below) **Warnings:** With great caution in penicillin allergic patients; safety for use in premature and infants under 1 mo of age not established **Cautions:** Overgrowth of nonsusceptible organisms with prolonged use; lower dose with renal impairment; false positive reaction for glucose with copper salts **Adverse reactions:** Hypersensitivity (fever, rash, pruritus, eosinophilia); blood (neutropenia, leukopenia, thrombocytopenia, positive direct and indirect Coombs test); hepatic and renal (transient rise in SGOT, SGPT, BUN, alkaline phosphatase); gastrointestinal symptoms; oral candidiasis; pain and phlebitis at sites of injection
Cephaloglycin, NF (Kafocin) *Available as:* Capsules: 250 mg	Dose: Not recommended under 1 yr of age (insufficient data) Dose: (Over age 1 yr): for usual infections, 25 mg/kg/24 hr, or 0.6 g/M^2/24 hr; divide into 4 doses (O); for more severe infections, double the above dose (maximum, 2 g/24 hr); for urinary tract infection in adult, 1 g/24 hr (2 g/24 hr if severe), divided into 4 doses (O); for urinary tract infection in child over 1 yr old, 25–50 mg/kg/24 hr, or 0.6–1.2 g/M^2/24 hr, divided into 4 doses (O); insufficient data to establish dose or safety under 1 year of age—not recommended **Contraindication:** In patients with known allergy to cephalosporin group of antibiotics **Warning:** In penicillin-allergic patients, cephalosporin C derivatives should be used with great caution, owing to clinical and laboratory evidence of partial cross-allergenicity of the penicillins and the cephalosporins; there are instances of patients who have had reactions to both drugs (including fatal anaphylaxis after parenteral use); a patient who has demonstrated some form of allergy, particularly to drugs, should receive antibiotics cautiously and then only when absolutely necessary; positive Coombs tests and elevations of SGOT and SGPT may occur

*For individual drugs, see general index. *Consult package inserts.*

Key: M^2, dose per square meter of body surface; IM, intramuscular; ITh, intrathecal; IV, intravenous; O, oral; R, rectal; SC, subcutaneous; Subl, sublingual; T, topical.

TABLE 30–1 (*Continued*)

DRUG, HOW SUPPLIED	DOSAGE, ROUTES, CONTRAINDICATIONS AND WARNINGS
	Caution: Patients should be followed carefully for side effects or unusual manifestations of drug idiosyncrasy; if an allergic reaction occurs, the drug should be discontinued and the patient treated with appropriate agents (e.g., epinephrine, antihistamines, pressor amines, or corticosteroids); prolonged use may result in the overgrowth of resistant organisms; administer with caution in the presence of impaired renal function; under such conditions careful clinical observation and laboratory studies should be made because minimal safe dosage may be lower than that usually recommended; false-positive reaction for glucose in the urine may occur (observed with tests for reducing substances, but not with tests using glucose oxidase) **Adverse reactions:** *Gastrointestinal*—most frequently diarrhea, with nausea, vomiting, dyspepsia, and abdominal pain also occurring; *hypersensitivity*—allergies in the form of rash and urticaria have been observed, usually subsiding upon discontinuation of the drug; *other reactions* have included genital and anal pruritus, genital moniliasis, vaginitis and vaginal discharge, dizziness, fatigue and headache; eosinophilia has been reported.
Cephalexin, USP (Keflex) *Available as:* Capsules: 250 and 500 mg Oral suspension: 125 and 250 mg/5 ml Drops: 100 mg/ml	Dose: For mild to moderate infections, 25–50 mg/kg/24 hr, or 0.75–1.5 g/M²/24 hr; divide into 4 doses (O); for severe infections double the above dose **Contraindication:** Cephalexin is contraindicated in patients with allergy to the cephalosporin group of antibiotics **Warning, caution, and adverse reactions:** See Cephaloglycin, above
Cephaloridine, NF (Loridine) *Available as:* Ampules: 0.5 and 1 g	Dose (adults): For mild infection, 0.75–1.5 g/24 hr or 0.45–0.9 g/M²/24 hr; for moderate infection, 1.5–3.0 g/24 hr or 0.85–1.75 g/M²/24 hr; for moderately severe infection, 2–4 g/24 hr or 1.15–2.3 g/M²/24 hr; divide into 3 doses (IM or IV) or continuous IV; for acute gonorrhea, 2 g/single dose (IM); for early syphilis, 0.5–1.0 g/24 hr (IM), daily for 10–14 days Dose: Not recommended for premature infants and full-term infants under 1 month of age Dose (children): For mild to moderate infections, 30–50 mg/kg/24 hr (maximum, 4 g/24 hr), or, 0.9–1.5 g/M²/24 hr; divide into 3 doses, given IM deep, for unusual infection or IV by slow injection or continuous drip, for extremely serious infections; for *severe infections,* 100 mg/kg/24 hr (maximum, 4 g/24 hr), or 2.3 g/M²/24 hr; divided into 4 doses, given as above, refrigerate freshly made solutions, discarding after 96 hr **Contraindications:** Hypersensitivity to this drug or cephalothin (Keflin), azotemia; not for oral use (poorly absorbed) **Warning:** Caution in administration of this or other antibiotics to allergic patients (particularly to drugs); give only for absolute necessity; anaphylaxis is rare; doses not to exceed 4 g/24 hr (nephrotoxicity); close observation or hospitalization, if known or suspected renal impairment; with evidence of renal impairment (casts, proteinuria, falling urinary output, rising BUN or creatinine levels), use with caution and in reduced dose; use with caution when given with other potential nephrotoxic antibiotics **Caution:** Protect from light; do not mix with other antibiotics; full 10-day course for streptococcal treatment; darkfield examination of lesions and at least 3 monthly serologic tests for syphilis in gonorrheal patients; superinfection with resistant organisms may occur; safety for premature infants under 1 mo of age not established and no use recommended; urticaria, skin rash and itching (3% of patients); eosinophil rise (1% of patients), leukopenia, transaminase elevations, alkaline phosphatase rise, acute tubular necrosis, renal failure and death have occurred (possibly greater in seriously ill given more than recommended dose); rare gastrointestinal symptoms; local pain, phlebitis rare; may produce positive Coombs test and positive tests for reducing substances in urine (see Cephaloglycin)

Table continued.

TABLE 30–1 (*Continued*)

DRUG, HOW SUPPLIED	DOSAGE, ROUTES, CONTRAINDICATIONS AND WARNINGS*
Cephalothin sodium, USP (Keflin) *Available as:* Ampules: 1 and 4 g, sterile	Dose (adults): Most infections, 2 g/24 hr, divided into 4 doses; severe infections, 3–4 g/24 hr, divided into 4–6 doses; life-threatening infections, 12 g/24 hr, divided into 6 doses Dose (children): For most infections, 80–160 mg/kg/24 hr, or 3 g/M²/24 hr; divide into 4 doses, given IM (deep) or IV (slow push or continuous drip); for severe infections, may need double above dose; for life-threatening infections or lowered resistance, 80–225 mg/kg/24 hr (maximum 12 g/24 hr), or 2.5–7 g/M²/24 hr; divide into 4–6 doses, given as above; with moderately severe *oliguria,* 120 mg/kg/24 hr (maximum), or 3.5 g/M²/24 hr (maximum); divide into 4–6 doses, given as above; with *anuria,* loading dose, 120 mg/kg, or 3.5 g/M², maintenance dose 1/6–1/2 of loading dose; single dose or divided into 2 doses or into 2–3 doses if dialysis is performed, in each case IM or IV, as above; for *peritoneal dialysis,* up to 6 mg/dl dialysis fluid; store solution in refrigerator not more than 48 hr; add to IV solutions (5% D/W or isotonic saline) with pH between 4.0 and 7.0 **Caution:** May produce neutropenia, eosinophilia, allergic reactions, rash, anaphylaxis, positive Coombs test in azotemia or in newborn infant if mother treated; positive urinary reducing agents to copper salts; irritating IM (pain, induration) and IV (phlebitis); overgrowth of nonsusceptible organisms may occur; SGOT, BUN, alkaline phosphatase may rise
Cephapirin sodium (Cefadyl) *Available as:* Injection: 1 g(IV or IM)	Dose (adult): For skin, soft tissue, most urinary tract infections, 2–3 g/24 hr; for more serious infections, 4–6 g/24 hr; for very serious infections (life threatening), up to 12 g/24 hr; divide into 4–6 doses (IV or IM); with reduced renal function (serum creatinine above 5 mg/dl), 7.5–15 mg/kg/dose; for patients to be dialysed, give dose just prior to dialysis, with repeated doses every 12 hours (IV or IM) Dose (children): 40–80 mg/kg/24 hr, divided into 4 doses (IV or IM) **Note:** Under age 3 mo consider relative benefit/risk; not extensively studied in infants **Contraindications, warnings, precautions, and adverse reactions:** See Cephaloglycin, above, and package insert
Chloramphenicol, USP (Amphicol, Chloromycetin, Mychel), **chloramphenicol palmitate, USP, and chloramphenicol sodium succinate, USP** *Available as:* Capsules: 50, 100, and 250 mg Suspension (palmitate): 150 mg/5 ml Sodium succinate: Vials, 1 g (IV only), 100 mg/ml	Dose: In premature and full-term newborn infants (up to 2 wk), 25 mg/kg/24 hr; over 2 wk, 50 mg/kg/24 hr, or 1.5 g/M²/24 hr; double dose for severe infections; give in divided doses, at 6 hr intervals (O), or continuous (IV) **Warning:** Serious and even fatal aplastic anemia, hypoplastic anemia, thrombocytopenia and granulocytopenia (long- or short-term therapy); blood studies should be done during treatment; not to be used when less dangerous agents will be effective; not to be used for trivial infections or to prevent bacterial infections, or in known sensitivity to it; danger of high levels in hepatic or renal disease **Caution:** Adjust newborn infant's dose by frequent blood levels (10–20 μg/ml) to avoid "gray syndrome"; see package insert for limitations **Note:** Chloramphenicol solution, also available, is "Not for Pediatric Use"
Clindamycin hydrochloride, USP, palmitate hydrochloride and **phosphate, NF** (Cleocin hydrochloride, palmitate hydrochloride and phosphate) *Available as:* Capsules: 75 and 150 mg Oral solution: 75 mg/5 ml Injection: 150 mg/ml	Dose (adult): Mild to moderate infection, 0.6–1.2 g/24 hr; severe infection, 1.2–2.7 g/24 hr; divide into 3 or 4 doses (O, IM or IV) Dose (children): *Hydrochloride:* for mild or moderate infection, 8–12 mg/kg/24 hr; for severe infection, 16–20 mg/kg/24 hr *Palmitate hydrochloride:* for mild infection, 8–12 mg/kg/24 hr; for moderate infection, 13–16 mg/kg/24 hr; for severe infection, 17–25 mg/kg/24 hr *Phosphate:* for mild infection 8–12 mg/kg/24 hr; for moderate infection, 15–25 mg/kg/24 hr; for severe infection 25–40 mg/kg/24 hr

*For individual drugs, see general index. *Consult package inserts.*

Key: M², dose per square meter of body surface; IM, intramuscular; ITh, intrathecal; IV, intravenous; O, oral; R, rectal; SC, subcutaneous; Subl, sublingual; T, topical.

DRUGS

TABLE 30-1 (*Continued*)

DRUG, HOW SUPPLIED	DOSAGE, ROUTES, CONTRAINDICATIONS AND WARNINGS
	Generally: for mild to moderate infection, 350 mg/M²/24 hr; for severe infection 450 mg/M²/24 hr, divide into 3 or 4 doses (O, IM or IV) **Contraindications:** Sensitivity to clindamycin or lincomycin **Warnings:** May cause severe diarrhea (blood, mucus) necessitating discontinuance; not for treatment of meningitis; not to be administered with erythromycins **Precautions:** In allergic and atopic patients; periodic liver tests and blood counts with prolonged use; may produce overgrowth of resistant organisms (yeasts); use with caution in severe renal, hepatic or metabolic disease; caution with curare type drugs. **Adverse reactions:** Hypersensitivity (rash, urticaria, Stevens-Johnson syndrome, anaphylaxis); liver (jaundice and abnormal function tests); blood (transient neutropenia and eosinophilia, agranulocytosis and thrombocytopenia)
Cloxacillin (See *Penicillins,* below)	
Colistin (Coly-Mycin) (See *Polymyxins,* below)	
Dicloxacillin (See *Penicillins,* below)	
ERYTHROMYCINS	
Erythromycin and salts, USP and NF (E-Mycin, Erythrocin, Ilotycin, Pediamycin and others) *Available as:* Tablets (enteric coated): 125, and 250 mg; and (chewable) 200 mg Suspension: 200 mg/5 ml Drops (O): 100 mg/2.5 ml (dropperful calibrated) Sterile: 250 and 500 mg, 1 g powder (IV) Suppositories: 125 mg	Dose: *Oral,* 30–50 mg/kg/24 hr, or 0.9–1.5 g/M²/24 hr; divide into 4–6 doses (O); *parenteral,* 10–20 mg/kg/24 hr, or 300–600 mg/M²/24 hr; divide into 2–3 doses (IV); for *rheumatic fever prophylaxis,* two doses of 250 mg/24 hr (O); for *primary syphilis,* 30–40 g in divided doses for 10–15 days Dose *(severe infection)*: Double above doses **Caution:** Hypersensitivity to this drug; overgrowth of nonsusceptible organisms; care in liver disease **Warning:** Inadequate to treat syphilis in utero; IM route not recommended (pain, necrosis) **Adverse reactions:** Gastrointestinal symptoms; rashes, urticaria, anaphylaxis
Erythromycin estolate, NF (Ilosone) *Available as:* Tablets: 500 mg Tablets (chewable): 125 and 250 mg Capsules: 125 and 250 mg Liquid: 125 and 250 mg/5 ml Suspension: 125 and 250 mg/5 ml Drops: 100 mg/ml (calibrated at 25 and 50 mg)	Dose (adult): 1 g/24 hr; for severe infection, up to 4 g or more/24 hr; divide into 4 doses (O) Dose (children): 30–50 mg/kg/24 hr or 0.9–1.5 g/M²/24 hr; divide into 4 doses (O); for severe infections, double the dose; for *rheumatic fever prophylaxis,* 500 mg/24 hr, divided into 2 doses; for *primary syphilis,* 20 g in divided doses for 10 days **Contraindications:** Sensitivity to the drug; not reliable for treatment of syphilis in utero **Warnings:** Hepatic dysfunction occurs, with or without jaundice, chiefly in adults; esoinophilia and leukocytosis occur; nausea, vomiting, abdominal cramps **Precautions:** Use with care in liver disease (drug excreted by liver) **Adverse reactions:** See Erythromycin, above
Gentamicin sulfate, USP (Garamycin) *Available as:* Solution: 10 mg/ml (pediatric) and 40 mg/ml, for injection	Dose (adult): 3 mg/kg/24 hr, divided into 3 doses (IM or IV); for life-threatening infections, up to 5 mg/kg/24 hr, reduced to 3 mg/kg/24 hr as indicated, divided into 3 or 4 doses (IM or IV) Dose (children): 3–5 mg/kg/24 hr or 125 mg/M²/24 hr, divided into 3 doses (IM or IV) Dose (infants): 6 mg/kg/24 hr, divided into 2 or 3 doses (IM or IV); for premature or full term neonate (under 1 week of age), divide into 2 doses (IM or IV) Duration of treatment: Usually 7–10 days; if longer, monitor renal, auditory and vestibular function; with impaired renal function, reduce dose **Contraindication:** Sensitivity to this drug **Warnings:** Watch closely for ototoxicity, more likely with renal impairment or nitrogen retention; avoid serum concentrations above 12 μg/ml;

Table continued.

DRUGS

TABLE 30-1 (*Continued*)

DRUG, HOW SUPPLIED	DOSAGE, ROUTES, CONTRAINDICATIONS AND WARNINGS *
	avoid concurrent use of neurotoxic or nephrotoxic drugs or potent diuretics **Adverse reactions:** nephrotoxic (oliguria, rising BUN or serum creatinine); neurotoxic (auditory, vestibular, numbness, tingling, twitching, convulsions); others (rises in SGOT, SGPT, bilirubin; falling calcium; blood dyscrasias; fever, splenomegaly; see package insert)
Hetacillin (See *Penicillins*, below)	
Kanamycin sulfate, USP (Kantrex) *Available as:* Capsules: 0.5 g Solution: 37.5 mg/ml, 250 mg/ml, 333 mg/ml, for injection	Systemic infections: IM preferably or very slowly IV (avoid in severe renal insufficiency); see package insert. Dose (premature and full-term newborn infants to 1 yr): 15 mg/kg/24 hr; divide into 2 doses (IM) Dose (older infants and children): 6–15 mg/kg/24 hr, or 150–450 mg/M²/24 hr; divide into 2 doses (IM) Dose (for suppression of intestinal bacteria): In *hepatic coma,* 8–12 g/24 hr, in divided doses (O); to *cleanse large bowel,* 1 g/hr for 4 hr, then 1 g/6 hr for 36 to 72 hr (O). Dose (inhalation): Add 1 ml (250 mg/ml) to 3 ml physiologic saline, 2–4 times/24 hr **Contraindications:** Sensitivity to this drug; prior administration of this or other ototoxic drug if other effective therapy available; not for long term therapy; not for oral route (intestinal obstruction) **Precautions:** Potentially nephrotoxic, ototoxic (see package insert for details). Avoid concurrent use of other nephrotoxic drugs. Risk of ototoxicity is increased with potent diuretics (avoid); with intraperitoneal use during recovery from anesthesia, neuromuscular paralysis with respiratory depression; danger with concomitant use of anesthesia and muscle-relaxing drugs; with prolonged use, danger of overgrowth of nonsusceptible organisms **Adverse reactions:** Nephrotoxicity (cells and casts, azotemia, oliguria); ototoxicity (tinnitus, vertigo, deafness); other (local irritation from injection, skin rash, fever, headache, paresthesias); with oral use, malabsorption syndrome, nephrotoxicity, ototoxicity
Lincomycin hydrochloride, USP (Lincocin) *Available as:* Capsules: 250 and 500 mg Syrup: 250 mg/5 ml Solution: 300 mg/ml, for injection	Dose: Not for infants under 1 mo of age; for adults, see package insert Dose (oral): For *mild to moderately severe infections,* 30 mg/kg/24 hr, or 0.9 g/M²/24 hr; divide into 3–4 doses (O); nothing but water by mouth 2 hr before and after administration; for *severe infections,* double above dose (O) Dose (intramuscular): For *mild to moderately severe infections,* 10 mg/kg/24 hr, or 0.3 g/M²/24 hr; single dose (IM); for *severe infections,* repeat dose every 12 hr (IM) Dose (intravenous): 10–20 mg/kg/24 hr, or 0.3–0.6 g/M²/24 hr; divide into 2–3 doses (IV) **Contraindications:** Hypersensitivity to this drug or clindamycin; not for infants under 1 mo of age **Warnings:** May cause severe diarrhea (blood, mucus), necessitating discontinuance of drug **Caution:** In patients with history of asthma or significant allergies; may result in overgrowth of nonsusceptible organisms, particularly yeasts; antimonilial treatment if used concomitant with monilial infections; not recommended in liver disease; neuromuscular blocking agent (large doses), additive with curare type drugs **Adverse reactions:** Gastrointestinal (glossitis, stomatitis, pruritus ani, nausea, vomiting, diarrhea, enterocolitis [see warning]); blood (neutropenia, leukopenia, agranulocytosis, thrombopenic purpura, aplastic anemia, pancytopenia); skin, mucous membranes (rashes, urticaria,

*For individual drugs, see general index. *Consult package inserts.*

Key: M², dose per square meter of body surface; IM, intramuscular; ITh, intrathecal; IV, intravenous; O, oral; R, rectal; SC, subcutaneous; Subl, sublingual; T, topical.

TABLE 30–1 (*Continued*)

DRUG, HOW SUPPLIED	DOSAGE, ROUTES, CONTRAINDICATIONS AND WARNINGS
	exfoliative and vesiculobullous dermatitis, vaginitis); liver (altered function tests, jaundice); rapid infusion (hypotension, cardiopulmonary arrest)
Methicillin (See *Penicillins,* below)	
Nafcillin (See *Penicillins,* below)	
Neomycin sulfate, USP (Mycifradin sulfate, Neobiotic) *Available as:* Tablets: 0.5 g Oral suspension: 125 mg/5 ml Vials: 0.5 g (0.35 g base) Vials (T): 5 and 10 g (lg = 0.7 g of neomycin base)	Dose (infectious diarrhea, with pathogenic *E. coli*): For adults, 3 g/24 hr; for children, 50 mg/kg/24 hr; for adults and children, 1.7 g/M²/24 hr; divide into 4 doses (O) a day for 3 days Dose (hepatic coma): For adults, 4–12 g/24 hr; for children or adults, 2.5–7 g/M²/24 hr; give in divided doses (O) for 5–6 days; in chronic hepatic failure, give the smaller dose for an indefinite period Dose (preoperative): For adults and children, 90 mg/kg/24 hr or 2.5 g/M²/24 hr, divided into 6 doses (O), for 3 days; initial dose to follow saline cathartic Dose (urinary tract infection, *in adults only*): 15 mg/kg/24 hr (maximum 1g), divided into 4 doses (IM); for not more than 10 days; use in infants and children (IM) not recommended **Contraindications:** Hypersensitivity to the drug; in intestinal obstruction **Warnings:** Deafness may follow oral use, may increase in severity weeks after discontinuance; more likely with renal insufficiency, prolonged use, or parenteral route; audiometry advisable before and during therapy (discontinue drug for tinnitus or hearing loss); monitor renal function; do not give other nephrotoxic or neurotoxic or ototoxic drugs concurrently; *get informed consent to use;* more toxic in premature infant or other neonate; overgrowth of nonsusceptible organisms may occur **Precautions:** See warnings, above; avoid potent diuretics; examine urine daily for protein, casts, cells; BUN before and every other day during therapy; audiometry before and twice weekly during therapy
Oxacillin sodium (See *Penicillins,* below)	
Paromomycin sulfate, NF (Humatin sulfate) *Available as:* Equivalent of base: Capsules: 250 mg Syrup: 125 mg/5 ml	Dose (for intestinal amebiasis), as base: 25 mg/kg/24 hr for 5 days, or 0.75 g/M²/24 hr for 5 days; divided into 3 doses (O) Dose (dysentery): Double amebiasis dose up to 7 days; divide into 3–4 doses (O); if *severe,* up to 4 times amebiasis dose **Caution:** Course of treatment should not exceed 10 days; potential nephrotoxicity from absorption; overgrowth of non-susceptible organisms, diarrhea, nausea common; headache, vertigo, skin rashes, abdominal pain, and vomiting may occur
PENICILLINS	
Amoxicillin (Amoxil, Larocin) *Available as:* Capsules: 250 and 500 mg Oral suspension: 125 mg/5 ml and 250 mg/5 ml Drops (pediatric): 50 mg/ml	Dose (for infections of ear, nose, throat, genitourinary tract, skin and soft tissues): In adults, 750 mg/24 hr; in children under 20 kg (over 20 kg, treat as adult), 20 mg/kg/24 hr; for children and adults, 450 mg/M²/24 hr; divide into 3 doses (O); for severe infections among the above, or for lower respiratory infections, double the dose; for gonorrhea, 3 g as a single dose (O) **Contraindications:** See Penicillin G **Warnings:** See Penicillin G **Precautions:** See Penicillin G; in patients with gonorrhea, if syphilis is suspected or possible, make darkfield examination before therapy and serologic tests monthly for at least 4 months
Ampicillin, anhydrous, trihydrate, and sodium, USP (Alpen, Amcill,	Dose (under 40 kg): For *moderately severe infections,* 50–100 mg/kg/24 hr, divided into 3–4 doses (O, IM, or IV); for *severe infections,* 200 mg/kg/24

Table continued.

DRUGS

TABLE 30–1 (*Continued*)

DRUG, HOW SUPPLIED	DOSAGE, ROUTES, CONTRAINDICATIONS AND WARNINGS*
Omnipen, Penbritin, Polycillin, Principen, Totacillin) *Available as:* Tablets (chewable): 125 mg Capsules: 250 and 500 mg Oral suspension: 125 and 250 mg/5 ml Drops: 100 mg/ml Sterile powder: 125, 250, and 500 mg; 1 and 2.5 g	hr, divided into 4 doses (O, IM, or IV); for *very severe infections,* doses of as much as 400 mg/kg/24 hr have been successfully and often given, but this dose has not yet been approved for the package insert Dose (over 40 kg and adults): For *moderate infections,* 1–2 g/24 hr, divided into 4 doses (O, IM, or IV); for *severe infections,* up to 8–14 g/24 hr, divided into 4 doses (O, IM, or IV) **Note:** With parenteral route, use within 1 hr of reconstitution; if by direct IV, give slowly (5 min); avoid prolonged IV drip, owing to 10% loss of activity in 4 hr **Contraindications:** Sensitivity to any penicillin; penicillinase-producing organisms; infectious mononucleosis (rash) **Caution:** Allergic patients; periodic renal, hepatic and hematopoietic tests; care in newborn use; superinfections with resistant organisms may follow use; skin, gastrointestinal, anaphylactic reactions, SGOT rise, eosinophilia; sodium represents 6.2% sodium ampicillin or 2.7 mEq Na/g **Adverse reactions:** see Penicillin G
Carbenicillin disodium, USP (Geopen, Pyopen) and **carbenicillin indanyl sodium** (Geocillin) *Available as:* Tablets: equivalent to 382 mg of carbenicillin Sterile powder: 1 and 5 g, for injection after solution	Dose (adult, oral): For *E. coli* or *Proteus mirabilis* infection, 1–2 tablets, four times daily; for *Pseudomonas* infection, 2 tablets, 4 times daily Dose (children, oral): No dosage established as yet Dose (adult, parenteral): For *urinary tract infections* (severe), 200 mg/kg/24 hr (IV); for *severe systemic infection,* 300–400 mg/kg/24 hr (if due to *Proteus* or *E. coli*) or 400–500 mg/kg/24 hr (if due to *Pseudomonas,* given (IV) in divided or continuous dosage; reduce dose with renal insufficiency (see package insert); probenecid enhances blood levels Dose (children, parenteral): For *urinary tract infection,* 50–100 mg/kg/24/hr (if due to *Proteus* or *E. coli*) or 50–200 mg/kg/24 hr (if due to *Pseudomonas*), in divided doses every 4–6 hr (IM or IV); for *severe systemic infection,* 300–400 mg/kg/24 hr (if due to *Proteus* or *E. coli*) or 400–500 mg/kg/24 hr (if due to *Pseudomonas*), in divided doses (IM or IV) or continuously (IV); data insufficient to establish a dose for children with renal insufficiency Dose (neonatal): For *severe infection,* initial dose 100 mg/kg, followed by 225 mg/kg/24 hr (if under 2000 g weight) or by 300 mg/kg/24 hr (if over 2000 g weight); given IM or IV; after 7 days (if under 2000 g) or 3 days (if over 3000 g), increase to 400 mg/kg/24 hr; gentamicin may be given concurrently to sepsis suspect until cultures and sensitivities are known **Contraindications:** See Penicillin G **Warnings:** See Penicillin G; watch for hematuria as sign of renal impairment (adjust dose) **Caution:** With prolonged therapy check renal, hepatic and hematopoietic systems; emergence of resistant organisms may cause superinfections; discontinue with bleeding manifestations, more likely in renal impairment; 1 g equivalent to 4.7 mEq Na; refrigerate prepared solutions; discard after 72 hr **Adverse reactions:** *Hypersensitivity reactions:* skin rashes, pruritus, urticaria, drug fever and anaphylactic reactions *Gastrointestinal disturbances:* Nausea *Hemic and lymphatic systems:* As with other penicillins, anemia, thrombocytopenia, leukopenia, neutropenia and eosinophilia may occur *Blood, hepatic, and renal studies:* As with other semi-synthetic penicillins, SGOT and SGPT elevations (particularly in children) *CNS:* As with other penicillins, convulsions or neuromuscular irritability could occur with excessively high serum levels *Other:* Pain at the site of injection *Uremic patients* receiving high doses may have hemorrhagic manifestations associated with abnormalities of coagulation tests such as clotting time and prothrombin time

*For individual drugs, see general index. *Consult package inserts.*

Key: M^2, dose per square meter of body surface; IM, intramuscular; ITh, intrathecal; IV, intravenous; O, oral; R, rectal; SC, subcutaneous; Subl, sublingual; T, topical.

TABLE 30–1 (*Continued*)

DRUG, HOW SUPPLIED	DOSAGE, ROUTES, CONTRAINDICATIONS AND WARNINGS
	Vein irritation and phlebitis: From undiluted solution directly injected into the vein
Cloxacillin sodium, USP (TegoPen) *Available as:* Capsules: 250 mg Oral solution: 125 mg/5 ml	Dose (up to 20 kg): 50 mg/kg/24 hr; double dose for severe infections Dose (over 20 kg and adults): For *mild-moderate infections,* 1 g/24 hr, or 0.6 g/M²/24 hr; for *more severe infections,* 2 g/24 hr, or 1.2 g/M²/24 hr; divide into 4 doses (O); for *very severe infections,* larger and more frequent doses **Contraindications:** See Penicillin G **Caution:** See Penicillin G **Adverse reactions:** Gastrointestinal (nausea, flatulence, loose stools); hypersensitivity (rashes, wheezing, sneezing, eosinophilia); rises in SGOT and SGPT; see also penicillin G
Dicloxacillin sodium, USP (Dynapen, Pathocil, Veracillin) *Available as:* Capsules: 125 and 250 mg Oral suspension: 62.5 mg/5 ml Injection: 250 mg	Dose: *In mild to moderate infections* in adults and children over 40 kg, 500 mg/24 hr; in children under 40 kg, 12.5 mg/kg/24 hr; in *severe infections,* double above doses; divide into 4 doses (O); give 1–2 hr a.c. **Contraindications:** History of allergy to penicillin or to this drug; neonatal dose not established **Caution:** In asthma or allergies, may cause skin rash, pruritus, urticaria, drug fever, eosinophilia, gastrointestinal disturbances, elevated SGOT, positive cephalin flocculation test; with long-term therapy periodically assess hepatic, renal and hematopoietic function
Hetacillin and hetacillin potassium (Versapen and Versapen-K) **Note:** 1 g of hetacillin potassium contains 2.6 mEq of potassium *Available as:* Capsules: 225 and 450 mg Oral suspension: 112.5 and 225 mg/5 ml Drops: 112.5 mg/ml (calibrated) Solution: IV, 225, 450 and 900 mg; IM, 225 and 450 mg, with lidocaine	Dose (mild to moderate infection): Over 40 kg, 900 mg/24 hr; less than 40 kg, 22 mg/kg/24 hr, or 600 mg/M²/24 hr; divided into 4 doses (O, IV, or IM) Dose (more severe infection): Over 40 kg, 1.8 g/24 hr; less than 40 kg, 45 mg/kg/24 hr, or 1.4 g/M²/24 hr; divide into 4 doses, initiate IV or IM **Contraindications:** As for ampicillin and penicillin G **Warning:** As for ampicillin and penicillin G **Caution:** Oral preparation should not be relied on in patients with severe illness or with nausea, vomiting, gastric dilatation, cardiospasm, or intestinal hypermotility; in such instances a parenteral drug should be used; see also ampicillin; in dogs, epinephrine vasopressor action is enhanced; IV solutions must be used within 6 hr after reconstitution **Adverse reactions:** Skin rashes and urticaria frequently; few cases of exfoliative dermatitis and erythema multiforme; elevations in one or more liver function tests; see also ampicillin and penicillin G
Methicillin sodium, USP (Celbenin, Staphcillin) *Available as:* Solution: 1, 4, and 6 g (1 g is equivalent to 900 mg base), for injection	Dose (IM): For adults, 4–6 g/24 hr, divided into 4–6 doses (IM); for infants and children, 100 mg/kg/24 hr, divided into 4 doses (IM) Dose (IV): For adults, 4 g/24 hr, divided in 4 doses (IV); for infants and children, no specific dosage recommended as yet (see Therapeutic Orphans) **Contraindications:** See penicillin G below **Warnings:** See penicillin G below **Precautions:** See penicillin G below; frequent examination of blood levels advisable in infants **Adverse reactions:** In patients with allergies or asthma; may cause skin rash, urticaria, pruritus, overgrowth of nonsusceptible organisms, transient neutropenia, bone marrow depression, renal impairment; in prolonged therapy do periodic assessment of renal, hepatic and hematopoietic function; avoid mixing with other drugs
Nafcillin sodium, USP (Unipen) *Available as;* Tablets (coated): 500 mg Capsules: 250 mg Oral solution: 250 mg/5 ml For injection: Reconstituted, 250 mg/ml	Dose (oral): For *adults* with *mild to moderate* infections, 1–3 g/24 hr or 0.6–1.8 g/M²/24 hr, divided into 4–6 doses (O); for *adults* with *severe* infections, 4–6 g/24 hr or 2.3–3.5 g/M²/24 hr, divided into 4–6 doses (O); for *children* with *streptococcal, pneumococcal* infections, 25 mg/kg/24 hr or 0.75 g/M²/24 hr, divided into 4 doses (O); for *children* with *staphylococcal infections,* double the above dose; for *neonates,* 30–40 mg/kg/24 hr, divided into 3–4 doses (O); give oral doses 1–2 hours before meals Dose (intravenous): For usual infections in *adults,* 3 g/24 hr, divided into 6 doses (IV); for usual infections in *infants and children,* 60 mg/kg/24 hr or 1.8 g/M²/24 hr, divided into 6 doses (IV); for *severe* infections, double the above doses

Table continued.

TABLE 30–1 (*Continued*)

DRUG, HOW SUPPLIED	DOSAGE, ROUTES, CONTRAINDICATIONS AND WARNINGS*
	Dose (intramuscular): For usual infections in *adults*, 2 g/24 hr, divided into 4 doses (IM); for *severe infections*, give 1½ times the above dose, divided into 6 doses (IM); in *infants and children*, 50 mg/kg/24 hr or 1.2 g/M^2/24 hr, divided into 2 doses (IM); in *neonates*, 20 mg/kg/24 hr, divided into 2 doses (IM) **Contraindications, warnings, precautions, and adverse reactions:** See Penicillin G below
Oxacillin sodium, USP (Bactocill, Prostaphlin) *Available as:* Capsules: 250 and 500 mg Oral solution: 250 mg/5 ml Solution: 250, 500 mg, and 1 and 2 g, for injection	Dose (for mild to moderate infections of skin, soft tissues or upper respiratory tract): In adults and children more than 40 kg, 2–3 g/24 hr, divided into 4–6 doses (O, IV, or IM); in children less than 40 kg, 50 mg/kg/24 hr or 1.5 g/M^2/24 hr, divided into 4 doses (O, IV, or IM); give oral doses 1–2 hr before meals; in *prematures and newborn infants*, limited experience demands caution in administration, frequent evaluation of function of organ systems **Contraindications, warnings, precautions, and adverse reactions:** See Penicillin G and methicillin
Penicillin G: **(Benzyl penicillin G)** **Potassium penicillin G, USP** (1 mg = 1595 units) **Sodium penicillin G, NF** (1 mg = 1667 units) *Available as:* Many forms and preparations	Dose (premature and full-term newborn infants): 60,000 units/kg/24 hr; divide into 2 doses (IM or IV) Dose (older children): 25,000–50,000 units/kg/24 hr, or 0.5–1 g/M^2/24 hr; divide into 4–6 doses (O, IM, IV, or SC): if (O), then ½ hr a.c. or 2 hr p.c. Dose (severe infections (e.g., meningitis)): 200,000–400,000 units/kg/24 hr (IV) Dose (rheumatic fever prophylaxis): 200,000 units, twice daily (O) Doses (other): See index for specific infections **Note:** If either Na^+ or K^+ effect is feared (large doses IV), order particular salt desired; each million units of potassium penicillin G yields 1.68 mEq potassium (65.8 mg); each million units of sodium penicillin G yields 1.68 mEq sodium (38.7 mg); dilute well and give slowly **Contraindications:** Hypersensitivity to any penicillin (see cross reactivity with cephalosporins) **Warnings:** Serious or fatal anaphylactic reactions may occur, more commonly after parenteral administration or in patients with multiple allergies; severe reactions to penicillin may occur in patients allergic to cephalosporins; history of allergies essential prior to administration; treat allergic or anaphylactic reactions with pressor amines, antihistamines, corticosteroids, as indicated (see Section 9) **Precautions:** Use with care in patients with allergies and/or asthma; with prolonged therapy make periodic examination of renal and hematopoietic systems; streptococcal infection should have adequate duration of treatment and follow-up cultures (see Section 10); with high doses, care must be given to potassium or sodium content of drug administered, especially if renal or cardiac function is impaired (monitor electrolyte levels); growth of nonsusceptible organisms may occur with prolonged use; sensitivity of staphylococcal isolates must be determined; appropriate surgical management of infections should accompany penicillin therapy; in treatment of gonorrhea, if primary or secondary syphilis is suspected, appropriate diagnostic procedures should be done, with monthly serologic tests for at least 4 months; after treatment of syphilis, clinical and serologic examinations should be repeated at 6 month intervals for at least 2 or 3 years (see Section 10) **Adverse reactions:** Hypersensitivity reactions range from urticarial and maculopapular eruptions to exfoliative dermatitis and Stevens-Johnson syndrome; serum-sickness–like reactions include chills, fever, arthralgia, prostration; blood disturbances (hemolytic anemia, leukopenia, thrombocytopenia), neuropathy, and nephropathy are rare, usually with high dose intravenous administration; electrolyte im-

*For individual drugs, see general index. *Consult package inserts.*

Key: M^2, dose per square meter of body surface; IM, intramuscular; ITh, intrathecal; IV, intravenous; O, oral; R, rectal; SC, subcutaneous; Subl, sublingual; T, topical.

TABLE 30–1 (*Continued*)

DRUG, HOW SUPPLIED	DOSAGE, ROUTES, CONTRAINDICATIONS AND WARNINGS
	balances (see above) may give potassium intoxication (especially in patients with renal impairment) or sodium excess (edema, congestive failure); the Jarisch-Herxheimer reaction may occur in patients treated for syphilis
Penicillin G, benzathine, USP (Bicillin, Permapen) (1 mg = 1211 units) *Available as:* Sterile suspension: 300,000 and 600,000 units/ml Disposable syringe: 600,000; 1.2 million, and 2.4 million units	Dose: 0.6–1.2 million units (IM) Dose: For rheumatic fever prophylaxis, 1.2 million units once a month (IM) **Contraindications:** See penicillin G **Caution:** See penicillin G
Penicillin G, procaine, USP (1 mg = 1009 units) *Available as:* Sterile suspension: 300,000 units/ml (0.3 g/ml) 500,000 units/ml (0.5 g/ml) 600,000 units/ml (0.6 g/ml) Syringe (disposable): 300,000 and 600,000 units, 1.2 and 2.4 million units With aluminum stearate: 300,000 units/ml (0.3 g/ml)	Dose: 0.5–1 million units/M^2/24 hr, or 0.5–1 g/M^2/24 hr, in a single dose (IM); avoid in newborn infants **Contraindications, caution, warning, adverse reactions:** See penicillin G
Penicillin V, phenoxymethyl penicillin, USP (Compocillin V, Pen-Vee, V-Cillin, others) (1 mg = 1695 units) *Available as:* Tablets and capsules: 125 mg (200,000 units) 250 mg (400,000 units) 300 mg (500,000 units) 500 mg (800,000 units) Suspension or oral solution: 90 mg (150,000 units)/5 ml 125 mg (200,000 units)/5 ml 180 mg (300,000 units)/5 ml 250 mg (400,000 units)/5 ml Drops: 90 mg/ml 125 mg/0.6 ml Wafers (chewable): 125 mg (200,000 units) 250 mg (400,000 units)	Dose: 25,000–50,000 units/kg/24 hr, or 0.5–1 g/M^2/24 hr, divided into 4 doses daily (O); for *rheumatic fever prophylaxis,* 125 mg twice daily (O) **Contraindications, caution, warning, adverse reactions:** See penicillin G
Penicillin V potassium, phenoxymethyl penicillin potassium, USP (Compocillin-VK, Ledercillin VK, Pen-Vee K, Ro-cillin VK, Uticillin VK, V-Cillin K, Veetids) (1 mg = 1530 units) *Available as:* Tablets: 125 mg (200,000 units) 250 mg (400,000 units) 500 mg (800,000 units) Tablets (prolonged action): 250 mg (400,000 units)	Dose: Same as penicillin V, above **Contraindications, caution, warning, adverse reactions:** See penicillin G

DRUGS

Table continued.

TABLE 30–1 *(Continued)*

DRUG, HOW SUPPLIED	DOSAGE, ROUTES, CONTRAINDICATIONS AND WARNINGS*
Liquids (solutions and suspensions): 125 mg (200,000 units)/5 ml 250 mg (400,000 units)/5 ml	
Probenecid (Benemid) *Available as:* Tablets (scored): 0.5 g (See also p. 1775)	Given *with penicillin therapy:* for adults and children over 50 kg, 2 g/24 hr, divided into 4 doses; for children 2–14 yr (less than 50 kg), initial 25 mg/kg or 0.7 g/M^2/kg (single dose); with maintenance 40 mg/kg/24 hr or 1.2 g/M^2/24 hr, divided into 4 doses **Contraindications:** Hypersensitivity to this drug; children under 2 yr of age; not recommended in persons with known blood dyscrasias or uric acid kidney stones. **Precautions:** Decreases the renal excretion of conjugated sulfa drugs; plasma concentrations of the latter should be determined from time to time; a reducing substance may appear in the urine **Adverse reactions:** Headache, gastrointestinal symptoms (e.g., anorexia, nausea, vomiting), urinary frequency, hypersensitivity reactions (including anaphylaxis, dermatitis, pruritus, and fever), sore gums, flushing, dizziness, and anemia have occurred; also hemolytic anemia which in some instances could be related to genetic deficiency of glucose-6-phosphate dehydrogenase in red blood cells; nephrotic syndrome, hepatic necrosis, and aplastic anemia occur rarely
POLYMYXINS	
Colistin sulfate and colistimethate sodium, USP, polymyxin E (Coly-Mycin S and Coly-Mycin M) *Available as:* Oral suspension (Coly-Mycin S): 25 mg/5 ml Solution (Coly-Mycin M Intramuscular): 75 mg/ml (contains dibucaine hydrochloride (Nupercaine)), for injection IM only Solution (Coly-Mycin M Parenteral): 10 and 75 mg/ml, for IV and ITh injection	Dose: For *bacterial enterocolitis,* 3–5 mg/kg/24 hr, or 90–150 mg/M^2/24 hr, divided into 3 doses (O); for *systemic infections* (normal renal function), 2.5–5 mg/kg/24 hr, or 75–150 mg/M^2/24 hr, divided into 2–4 doses (IM or IV); avoid IM preparation for IV use **Contraindications:** Sensitivity to this drug **Warning:** Maximum daily dose 5 mg/kg/24 hr with normal renal function; transient neurologic disturbances may occur (circumoral paresthesia, tingling of extremities, pruritus, vertigo, dizziness, slurring of speech); patient should not drive or operate hazardous machinery while receiving drug; reduced dose may alleviate these effects; overdosage may cause renal insufficiency, muscle weakness, apnea **Precautions:** Use with care in patient with possible impairment of renal function; monitor urinary output, BUN and serum creatinine levels; owing to neuromuscular blocking effect, should be used only with greatest caution concomitantly with antibiotics (kanamycin, streptomycin, polymyxin, neomycin) or other drugs (ether, tubocurarine, succinylcholine, gallamine, decamethonium, sodium citrate) having similar effects (treat apnea with assisted ventilation, oxygen, and calcium injection) **Adverse reactions:** Respiratory arrest reported after IM injection; impaired renal function increases risk (monitor closely, especially in infant or young child)
Polymyxin B sulfate, USP (Aerosporin sulfate) (1 mg = 10,000 units) *Available as:* Tablets: 50 mg Tablets (soluble): 25 mg Sterile suspension: 50 mg/vial	Dose (enteric infections): 10–20 mg/kg/24 hr, or 250 mg/M^2/24 hr; divided into 3–4 doses (O) Dose (systemic infections): By *intramuscular* route, 1.5–2.5 mg/kg/24 hr, (maximum, 200 mg/24 hr, or 120 mg/M^2/24 hr), divided into 4 doses (IM, deep); by *intravenous* route, 2.5 mg/kg/24 hr (maximum, 200 mg/24 hr), as single infusion or divided into 2 infusions (give dose in 1–1½ hr) Dose (renal impairment): 1.5 mg/kg/24 hr (IV or IM)

*For individual drugs, see general index. *Consult package inserts.*

Key: M^2, dose per square meter of body surface; IM, intramuscular; ITh, intrathecal; IV, intravenous; O, oral; R, rectal; SC, subcutaneous; Subl, sublingual; T, topical.

TABLE 30-1 (*Continued*)

DRUG, HOW SUPPLIED	DOSAGE, ROUTES, CONTRAINDICATIONS AND WARNINGS
	Dose (intrathecal [in addition to systemic doses]): Avoid local anesthetic in solution; under age 2 yr, 2 mg every day for 3–4 days, then 2.5 mg every other day or initially and every other day; over age 2 yr and adults, 5 mg every day for 3–4 days, then 5 mg every other day; in susceptible infections continue for at least 2 wk after CSF is sterile and sugar normal **Contraindications:** Hypersensitivity to this drug **Warning:** Give IM or ITh to hospitalized patient only, so that supervision can be constant; may result in overgrowth of non-susceptible organisms, including fungi **Precautions:** Same as for colistin above **Adverse reactions:** Same as for colistin above; other reactions include signs of meningeal irritation with intrathecal therapy (fever, headache, stiff neck), with increased cells and protein in CSF; drug fever, urticaria, severe pain with IM injection, and thrombophlebitis at site of IV injection
Procaine penicillin G (See above)	
Rifampin, USP (Rifadin, Rimactane) *Available as:* Capsules: 300 mg	Dose: In primary tuberculosis, 10–20 mg/kg (not to exceed 600 mg/24 hr), given as a single dose once daily (O) in conjunction with at least one other antituberculous agent; in *Neisseria meningitidis* carriers, the same dose for 4 consecutive days; not recommended for under 5 yr of age **Contraindications:** Hypersensitivity reaction to any of the rifamycins **Warning:** Has produced liver dysfunction; there have been fatalities associated with jaundice in patients with liver disease or receiving rifampin concomitantly with other hepatotoxic agents; since an increased risk may exist for individuals with liver disease, benefits must be weighed carefully against the risk of further liver damage; periodic liver function monitoring is mandatory; possibility of rapid emergence of resistant meningococci restricts use to short-term treatment of asymptomatic carrier state; **not to be used for treatment of meningococcal disease** **Caution:** Increases the requirements for anticoagulant drugs of the coumarin type; if used together, it is recommended that daily prothrombin times be performed until dose of anticoagulant is established; urine, feces, saliva, sputum, sweat and tears may be colored red-orange **Adverse reactions:** Heartburn, epigastric distress, anorexia, nausea, vomiting, gas, cramps, and diarrhea; headache, drowsiness, fatigue, ataxia, dizziness, inability to concentrate, mental confusion and visual disturbances; muscular weakness, fever, pains in extremities and generalized numbness; pruritus, urticaria, skin rashes, eosinophilia, sore mouth and sore tongue; thrombocytopenia, transient leukopenia and decreased hemoglobin; elevation in BUN and serum uric acid; transient abnormalities in liver function tests (elevations of serum bilirubin, BSP, alkaline phosphatase and serum transaminases)
Spectinomycin dihydrochloride penthydrate (Trobicin) *Available as:* Injection: 2 and 4 g, IM only, 400 mg/ml	Dose (male): for urethritis (GC), 2 g IM (deep); may divide into 2 sites; for proctitis, treatment failure and geographic area of resistant organisms, double dose for urethritis Dose (female): Double dose for the male urethritis **Contraindications:** Hypersensitivity to this drug **Warnings:** Not effective in the treatment of syphilis; used in high doses for short periods of time to treat gonorrhea may mask or delay the symptoms of incubating syphilis; patients treated for gonorrhea should be closely observed clinically, with serologic follow-up for at least 3 months if syphilis is suspected; safety for use in infants and children has not been established **Precautions:** Usual precautions with atopic individuals; monitor to detect development of resistance by *N. gonorrhoeae* **Adverse reactions:** Soreness at the injection site, urticaria, dizziness, nausea, chills, fever and insomnia; reduction in urinary output
Streptomycin sulfate, USP *Available as:* Syrup: 250 mg/5 ml Solution: 0.4 and 0.5 g/ml, for injection Tubex (disposable): 0.5 and 1 g	Dose (premature and full-term newborn infants): 20–30 mg/kg/24 hr; divide into 2 doses (IM); decrease with decreased urinary output; give not more than 10 days Dose (general use [older children]): 40 mg/kg/24 hr, or 1 g/M²/24 hr, divided into 2 doses (IM); give up to 10 days, with *renal depression,* give ½–¾ of above dose

Table continued.

DRUGS

TABLE 30–1 (*Continued*)

DRUG, HOW SUPPLIED	DOSAGE, ROUTES, CONTRAINDICATIONS AND WARNINGS*
Vials (powder): 1 and 5 g	Dose (tuberculosis): 20 mg/kg/24 hr, as a single dose (IM); when used as an aerosol 300 mg/2 ml dose, repeat 4 times daily Dose (intrathecal): 1 mg/kg/day, diluted to 5 mg/ml Dose (intraperitoneal, intrapleural, intra-articular): 50 mg/ml **Contraindications:** Sensitivity to this drug **Caution:** Observe and test auditory and vestibular function, nephrotoxicity; may cause optic nerve dysfunction, paresthesias of lips and extremities, allergic reactions (skin, eosinophilia, drug fever, blood dyscrasias), CNS depression (stupor, flaccidity, coma, respiratory depression); intrathecal use—cervical pain, headache, malaise, convulsions; reduce dose with renal excretory impairment; overgrowth of nonsusceptible organisms may occur
TETRACYCLINES	
Chlortetracycline hydrochloride, NF (Aureomycin) **Chlortetracycline calcium** *Available as:* Capsules: 250 mg Solution: 500 mg (IV)	Dose: As for tetracycline, below **Contraindications, caution:** See tetracycline
Demeclocycline and demeclocycline hydrochloride, NF, demethylchlortetracycline (Declomycin) *Available as:* Capsules: 75 and 150 mg Tablets: 75, 150, and 300 mg Syrup: 75 mg/5 ml Suspension: 75 mg/5 ml Drops: 60 mg/ml	Dose: 10 mg/kg/24 hr, or 0.3 g/M²/24 hr; divide into 2–4 doses (O) **Contraindications:** See tetracycline **Caution:** See tetracycline
Doxycycline and doxycycline hyclate, USP (Vibramycin) *Available as:* Hyclate: Capsules: 50 and 100 mg Vials (IV): 100 and 200 mg Monohydrate: For oral solution: 25 mg/5 ml	Dose (for weight less than 45 kg): Initially, 4.4 mg/kg/24 hr, divided into 2 doses (O); for maintenance, 1/2 of above dose, single or divided into 2 doses (O) Dose (more than 45 kg and adults): Initially, 200 mg divided into 2 doses (O); maintenance, 1/2 of above dose, single or divided into 2 doses (O) **Contraindications:** Sensitivity to this drug **Warning:** Hepatic toxicity with excessive dosage or renal impairment with standard dosage (lower dose and do serum level determinations with renal impairment); see tetracycline caution (below) for other dangers—bone, tooth, increased intracranial pressure, photosensitivity **Caution:** Overgrowth of nonsusceptible organisms, gastrointestinal symptoms, vaginitis, dermatitis, glossitis, stomatitis, proctitis, onycholysis, discoloration of nails, elevation of SGOT or SGPT, anemia, neutropenia, eosinophilia may occur; discontinue use with severe adverse reaction
Methacycline hydrochloride, NF (Rondomycin) *Available as:* Capsules: 150 and 300 mg Syrup: 75 mg/5 ml	Dose: 12 mg/kg/24 hr, or 350 mg/M²/24 hr; divide into 2–4 doses, given 2 hr pc or 1 hr ac **Contraindications:** See tetracycline **Caution:** See tetracycline
Minocycline hydrochloride, USP (Minocin, Vectrin) *Available as:* Capsules: 50 and 100 mg Syrup: 50 mg/5 ml Vials: 100 mg	Dose (adult): Initial, 200 mg; maintenance, 200 mg/24 hr, divided into 2 doses (O or IV) Dose (children): Initial, 4 mg/kg; maintenance, 4 mg/kg/24 hr, divided into 2 doses (O or IV) **Note:** Avoid rapid IV infusion **Contraindications, warnings, precautions, adverse reactions:** See tetracycline

*For individual drugs, see general index. *Consult package inserts.*

Key: M², dose per square meter of body surface; IM, intramuscular; ITh, intrathecal; IV, intravenous; O, oral; R, rectal; SC, subcutaneous; Subl, sublingual; T, topical.

TABLE 30–1 (*Continued*)

DRUG, HOW SUPPLIED	DOSAGE, ROUTES, CONTRAINDICATIONS AND WARNINGS
Oxytetracycline, NF, and oxytetracycline hydrochloride, USP (Terramycin) *Available as:* Capsules: 125 and 250 mg Syrup: 125 mg/5 ml Pediatric drops: 5 mg/drop IM (ampules and vials): 50 and 125 mg/ml IV: 250 and 500 mg	Dose: As tetracycline (below); also given as aerosol, 50 mg/ml twice daily, in 10% propylene glycol **Contraindications:** See tetracycline **Caution:** See tetracycline
Tetracycline, USP, its salts, NF and complexes (Achromycin, Bristacycline, Kesso-Tetra, Panmycin, Robitet, Tetracyn, Tetrex, and others) *Available as:* Tablets: 50 and 250 mg Capsules: 50, 100, 125, 250, and 500 mg Suspension: 125, 250, and 500 mg/5 ml Syrup: 125 mg/5 ml Drops: 100 mg/ml Calibrations: 5 mg/drop, or 25 and 50 mg Vials: IM (local anesthetics added): 100 and 250 mg IV: 100, 250, and 500 mg	Dose (newborn infants): Not recommended; 100 mg/kg/24 hr, divided into 2 doses (O); or 10–15 mg/kg/24 hr, divided into 2 doses (IV) Dose (older infants and children): 25–50 mg/kg/24 hr, or 0.6–1.2 g/M²/24 hr, divided into 4 doses (O), given 1 hr before feedings; or 10–25 mg/kg/24 hr (not more than 250 mg/injection), divided into 2–3 doses (IM); or 10–15 mg/kg/24 hr, divided into 2 doses (IV) Dose (children over 40 kg and adults): For moderate infections, 1 g/24 hr, divided into 4 doses (O); for severe infections, double this dose (O); for moderate infections, 200–300 mg/24 hr, divided into 2–3 doses (IM); for severe infections, 500 mg/24 hr, divided into 2 doses (IM) Dose (adult): 1 g/24 hr; divided into 2 doses (IV) (maximum, 2 g/24 hr) **Contraindications:** Sensitivity to tetracyclines or additives (see labels of containers) **Warnings:** *The use of drugs of the tetracycline class during tooth development (last half of pregnancy, infancy, and childhood to the age of 8 yr) may cause permanent discoloration and enamel hypoplasia of the teeth (yellow-gray-brown),* more commonly during long-term use but also following repeated short-term courses; *tetracyclines, therefore, should not be used in this age group unless other drugs are not likely to be effective or are contraindicated;* usual oral or parenteral doses may lead to excessive systemic accumulation and possible liver toxicity; photosensitivity in patients exposed to direct sunlight or ultraviolet light (discontinue at the first evidence of skin erythema); may cause an increase in BUN (in patients with significantly impaired function, higher serum levels of tetracycline may lead to azotemia, hyperphosphatemia, and acidosis) **Usage in newborns, infants, and children:** (See above "Warnings" about tooth development); tetracyclines form a stable calcium complex in bone; decrease in the fibula growth rate has been observed in prematures; tetracyclines are present in the milk of lactating women taking it **Precautions:** May result in overgrowth of nonsusceptible organisms, including fungi; if used in the treatment of gonorrhea, a darkfield examination should be made of any lesions suggestive of syphilis before treatment is started and serologic tests for syphilis should be made monthly for at least 4 months afterwards; with long-term therapy, periodic laboratory evaluation of organ systems, including hematopoietic, renal, and hepatic studies should be performed; *infections due to group A beta-hemolytic streptococci should be treated for a minimum of 10 days;* bacteriostatic drugs may interfere with the bactericidal action of penicillin (avoid giving tetracyclines in conjunction with penicillin.) **Adverse reactions:** *Gastrointestinal* (anorexia, nausea, vomiting, diarrhea, glossitis, dysphagia, enterocolitis, and inflammatory lesions [with monilial overgrowth] in the anogenital region); skin (maculopapular and erythematous rashes, photosensitivity); *renal* (rise in BUN, apparently dose related); *hypersensitivity* (urticaria, angioneurotic edema, anaphylaxis, anaphylactoid purpura, pericarditis, and exacerbation of systemic lupus erythematosus); *bulging fontanels in young infants,* which disappear rapidly when drug discontinued; *blood* (hemolytic anemia, thrombocytopenia, neutropenia, eosinophilia); when given over prolonged periods, tetracyclines have been reported to produce brown-black microscopic discoloration of thyroid glands (no abnormalities of function known); *other* (see Fanconi syndrome due to outdated tetracycline)
Vancomycin hydrochloride, USP (Vancocin)	Dose: In premature and newborn infants, 10 mg/kg/24 hr, divided into 2 doses (IV); in older infants and children, 40 mg/kg/24 hr, or 1.2 g/M²/24

Table continued.

DRUGS

TABLE 30-1 (*Continued*)

DRUG, HOW SUPPLIED	DOSAGE, ROUTES, CONTRAINDICATIONS AND WARNINGS*
Available as: Solution: 500 mg (50 mg/ml), sterile	hr, by daily continuous (IV) or divided into 2–4 doses **Contraindications:** Sensitivity to this drug **Warnings:** Ototoxic and nephrotoxic; avoid in renal insufficiency, or in patients with previous hearing loss, if possible (monitor blood levels); tinnitus may precede deafness, which may progress despite cessation of therapy **Precautions:** With renal impairment monitor auditory function and blood levels; all patients need periodic hematologic studies, urinalyses, and studies of renal and hepatic function; irritating to tissues (necrosis on IM injection, thrombophlebitis at IV site), with severe pain; minimize thrombophlebitis by use of *dilute solutions* (at least 200 ml) and rotation of sites of infusion. **Adverse reactions:** Nausea, chills, fever, urticaria and macular rashes; eosinophilia and anaphylactoid reactions; overgrowth of nonsusceptible organisms
ANTIFUNGAL DRUGS	
Amphotericin B, USP (Fungizone) *Available as:* Solution: 50 mg (mix with 5% D/W; pH above 5.0), for injection	Dose: For test dose, 0.1 mg/kg/24 hr (IV) in 6 hr; increase to 1 mg/kg/24 hr (IV), or 30 mg/M²/24 hr (IV) (give over 6–8 hr period) Intrathecal: See package insert **Contraindications:** Sensitivity to this drug unless condition is life-threatening and amenable only to this drug **Caution:** *Under no circumstances should a total daily dose of 1.5 mg/kg be exceeded* **Warning:** When amphotericin B is the only effective treatment for a potentially fatal disease, its dangers must be weighed against the possible life-saving effect; primarily for progressive and potentially fatal fungal infections; not for less severe fungal infections (see package insert) **Precautions:** Prolonged therapy usually necessary; side effects common and some are potentially dangerous; parenteral use only in hospitalized patients with severe infections, or with close clinical observation; corticosteroids to be used concomitantly *only if necessary* to control drug reactions; use nephrotoxic antibiotics or antineoplastic agents only with great caution; monitor renal function at least weekly; reduce dose or discontinue if BUN exceeds 40 mg/dl; follow blood counts; hypomagnesemia reported; after interruption of medication for over 7 days, reinitiate treatment with lowest level of dose **Adverse reactions:** Intolerance common at less than full therapeutic dosage; aspirin and antihistamines may help; alternate day treatment may diminish anorexia and phlebitis; small doses of corticosteroid given just before or with amphotericin infusions may help control febrile reactions; addition of heparin (small dose) to infusion may minimize thrombophlebitis; extravasation irritating; *common reactions* include fever, malaise, chills, headache, anorexia, nausea, vomiting, weight loss, pain and cramps in muscles, abdominal pain, pain at infusion site with thrombophlebitis, anemia, hypokalemia, and impaired renal function, which may be permanent; *less common* are anuria, cardiovascular effects, coagulation defects, blood cell disturbances, neurologic defects (including tinnitus and hearing loss), anaphylactic reactions, and liver failure (see package insert)
Flucytosine (Ancobon) *Available as:* Capsules: 250 and 500 mg	Dose (for cryptococcus, candida): 50–150 mg/kg/24 hr, or 1.5–2.25 g/M²/24 hr, divided into 4 doses (O); give each dose over 15 minute interval (to avoid nausea); if elevated BUN or creatinine or other signs of renal impairment, give initial dose at lower level **Contraindications:** Hypersensitivity to the drug **Warnings:** Extreme caution with impaired renal function (assay blood levels to determine the adequacy of renal excretion in such patients);

*For individual drugs, see general index. *Consult package inserts.*

Key: M², dose per square meter of body surface; IM, intramuscular; ITh, intrathecal; IV, intravenous; O, oral; R, rectal; SC, subcutaneous; Subl, sublingual; T, topical.

TABLE 30–1 ***(Continued)***

DRUG, HOW SUPPLIED	DOSAGE, ROUTES, CONTRAINDICATIONS AND WARNINGS
	with extreme caution with bone marrow depression (monitor hepatic function and hematopoietic system); see package insert **Precautions:** Before therapy, hematologic and renal status should be determined (close monitoring essential); liver enzyme levels (alkaline phosphatase, SGOT, SGPT) at frequent intervals during therapy, as indicated **Adverse reactions:** Nausea, vomiting, diarrhea, rash, anemia, leukopenia, thrombopenia, and elevation of hepatic enzymes, BUN and creatinine; less frequently reported were confusion, hallucinations, headache, sedation and vertigo
Gentian violet, methylrosaniline chloride, USP	See Anthelmintics, above
Griseofulvin, USP (microsize) (Fulvicin-U/F, Grifulvin V, Grisactin) *Available as:* Tablets (scored): 125, 250, and 500 mg Capsules: 125 and 250 mg Suspension: 125 mg/5 ml	Dose: 10 mg/kg/24 hr, or 300 mg/M²/24 hr, divided into 2–4 doses (O); widespread lesions may require 450–600 mg/M²/24 hr, reducing dose to usual levels with response **Contraindications:** Hypersensitivity to this drug, porphyria, hepatocellular failure **Warning:** Safety for prophylaxis not established **Precautions:** Patients should have periodic monitoring of organ system functions, including hematologic, hepatic and renal; possibility of cross-reactivity with penicillin in allergic patients; may be photosensitizing (avoid sun or other intense light); barbiturates depress activity of griseofulvin (adjust dose) **Adverse reactions:** Rashes, urticaria or angioedema may require discontinuance of therapy; paresthesias with extended therapy; occasional gastrointestinal and neurologic effects (see package insert); rare proteinuria or leukopenia (discontinue for agranulocytosis)
Griseofulvin (regular size) (Fulvicin, Grifulvin, Griseofulvin-Ayerst) *Available as:* Tablets (scored): 250 and 500 mg Suspension: 250 mg/5 ml	Dose: Double the dose of griseofulvin, microsize **Contraindications:** As for griseofulvin, microsize **Caution:** As for griseofulvin, microsize
Nystatin, USP (Mycostatin, Nilstat) *Available as:* Tablets: 500,000 units Suspension (O or T): 100,000 units/ml	Dose: In premature and full-term newborn infants, 400,000 units, divided into 4 doses (O); in older infants and children, 1–2 million units/24 hr, divided into 4 doses (O); in *oral moniliasis,* 4 times daily (T) **Contraindication:** Hypersensitivity to this drug **Caution:** May produce diarrhea and gastrointestinal distress
ANTIPYRETICS (See *Analgesics* (nonnarcotic) and *Antipyretics*)	
ANTITUBERCULOSIS DRUGS	
Aminosalicylic acid, *p*-aminosalicylic acid (PAS), NF (Pamisyl, Para-Pas, Parasal), **Salts of PAS: Sodium potassium, and calcium** *Available as:* Acid: Tablets: plain, enteric coated, effervescent: 0.3, 0.5, 1 and 2 g Crystals Powder Resin: 8 g Calcium salt: Tablets: 0.5 g Potassium salt: Tablets: 0.5 g Powder	Dose: PAS, 0.3 g/kg/24 hr, or 8 g/M²/24 hr, divided into 3 doses pc (O); PAS salts, increase dose by 25% **Caution:** Do not use solutions older than 24 hr or if darker than when prepared; may cause nausea, vomiting, abdominal pain, diarrhea, goiter (hypothyroidism), electrolyte disturbances, hypersensitivity, albuminuria, hematuria, skin reactions, lymphadenopathy, fever, jaundice, hepatomegaly, eosinophilia, blood dyscrasias, fatal hepatic damage, fever, crystalluria **Note:** 1 g sodium salt yields 109 mg Na; urine reduces copper reagents

Table continued.

TABLE 30–1 (*Continued*)

DRUG, HOW SUPPLIED	DOSAGE, ROUTES, CONTRAINDICATIONS AND WARNINGS*
Sodium salt: Tablets: 0.5, 0.69, and 1 g Granules: 454 g Powder: To be reconstituted, 0.93 and 1 g/5 ml Vials (dry): Reconstituted, 100 mg/ml	
Cycloserine (Seromycin) *Available as:* Capsules: 250 mg	Dose: For initial 2 wk course, 10 mg/kg/24 hr, or 300 mg/M²/24 hr, divided into 2 doses (O); for maintenance, titrate dose to yield blood level of 20–30 μg/ml **Contraindications:** Hypersensitivity to this drug, epilepsy, emotional disturbances, renal impairment, concurrent ingestion of alcohol **Warnings:** Discontinue or reduce dose for CNS effects (see package insert); toxicity closely related to blood levels (above 30 μg/ml), potentiated (convulsion) in alcoholism; monitor blood, renal and hepatic functions and blood level of drug; dosage and safety not established for children **Precautions:** Establish sensitivity of organism to be treated; keep blood level below 30 μg/ml; use anticonvulsant drugs or sedatives for CNS effects (see package insert) **Adverse reactions:** Chiefly CNS (see above and package insert); allergic rashes occur; serum transaminase may rise
Ethionamide, USP (Trecator) *Available as:* *Tablets: 250 mg*	Dose (adult): 0.5–1 g/24 hr Dose (children): 12–15 mg/kg/24 hr (maximum 750 mg/24 h), or 300–600 mg/M²/24 hr; use highest tolerated dose; divide into three doses (O) **Contraindications:** Hypersensitivity to this drug **Precautions:** For use when organism is not susceptible to primary therapy; examine blood, urine, and hepatic and renal function at regular intervals **Adverse reactions:** Anorexia, metallic taste, vomiting, sialorrhea, diarrhea, weight loss, jaundice, SGOT elevation, headache, neuritis, depression, acne, rash, exfoliative dermatitis
Isoniazid, USP (many trade names) *Available as:* Tablets and capsules: 50, 100, and 300 mg Syrup: 50 mg/5 ml Solution: 100 mg/ml, for injection	Dose: For conversion of tuberculin test with no manifest disease and "prophylaxis," 15 mg/kg/24 hr, or 450 mg/M²/24 hr, divided into 2 or 3 doses (O or IM); for therapy of active disease, meningitis (tuberculous), miliary, 20 mg/kg/24 hr, or 0.6 g/M²/24 hr, divided into 2 or 3 doses (O or IM) **Contraindication:** Hypersensitivity to this drug, including drug-induced hepatitis **Warnings:** Hepatitis may occur; monitor patients on prophylactic regimens at monthly intervals, discontinuing drug if hepatic damage is detected; defer prophylactic treatment if acute hepatic disease is present **Precautions:** Discontinue drug for hypersensitivity reaction (along with all drugs concomitantly given); if isoniazid to be given again, begin with small doses and gradual increases; monitor patients with convulsive disorders, hepatic diseases, or renal disease with special care; periodic ophthalmoscopic examination recommended **Adverse reactions:** Usually only with higher doses, especially in "slow inactivators"; *neurologic* (peripheral neuropathy, convulsions, toxic encephalopathy, optic neuritis or atrophy, toxic psychosis); *gastrointestinal* and *hepatic* (nausea, vomiting, rises in SGOT and SGPT, bilirubinuria, hepatitis with or without jaundice); *hematologic* (agranulocytosis, hemolytic or aplastic anemia, thrombocytopenia, eosinophilia); *hypersensitivity* (rash, vasculitis, fever); *metabolic* (pyridoxine deficiency, hyperglycemia, acidosis, gynecomastia); *others* (see package insert)
Rifampin (see Antibiotics, above)	
Streptomycin (see Antibiotics, above)	

*For individual drugs, see general index. *Consult package inserts.*

Key: M², dose per square meter of body surface; IM, intramuscular; ITh, intrathecal; IV, intravenous; O, oral; R, rectal; SC, subcutaneous; Subl, sublingual; T, topical.

TABLE 30–1 (*Continued*)

DRUG, HOW SUPPLIED	DOSAGE, ROUTES, CONTRAINDICATIONS AND WARNINGS
Viomycin sulfate, USP (Viocin sulfate) *Available as:* Powder (injection): 1 and 5 g (diluted to 150, 200, 250, and 400 mg/ml)	Dose (intramuscular only): In adult, 2 g/24 hr every third day, divide into 2 doses (IM); for child, 40 mg/kg/24 hr every third day, 1.2 g/M²/24 hr every third day, divided into 2 doses (IM); lower dose with impaired renal function **Caution:** Toxic antibiotic not for routine use; skin reactions (treat with antihistaminics or discontinue use), renal irritation (severe with pre-existing renal damage), electrolyte disturbances, ECG changes; overgrowth of nonsusceptible organisms; careful observation for allergic reactions, albuminuria and cylinduria, eosinophilia, edema and increase of weight (fluid), abnormal renal function, dizziness, hearing loss (audiometric testing prior to and at regular intervals during use); consult literature
ANTIVIRAL DRUGS	
Amantadine hydrochloride, NF (Symmetrel) *Available as:* Capsules: 100 mg Syrup: 50 mg/5 ml	Dose: 1–9 yr, 4–8 mg/kg/24 hr (not more than 150 mg/24 hr), divided into 2–3 doses (O); 9–12 yr, 200 mg/24 hr, divided into 2 doses (O); for known exposure, give 10-day course; for possibly repeated, unknown exposure, give 30-day course; for possibly repeated, uncontrolled, and unknown exposure, up to 90-day course **Contraindications:** Known sensitivity to this drug; not for prophylaxis of any viral infection except for influenza A_2; *not for treatment of any disease* **Warnings:** Seizures may increase in patients with convulsive disorders; congestive failure may develop in patients with heart disease; monitor closely clinically **Precautions:** May potentiate anticholinergic effects of other drugs (see package insert); adjust dose carefully in renal or heart disease **Adverse reactions:** Depression, psychosis, congestive failure, orthostatic hypotension, urinary retention reported; rarely, convulsions, leukopenia, neutropenia; many others (see package insert)
CHEMOTHERAPEUTICS	
SULFONAMIDES	
Phthalylsulfathiazole, NF (Cremothalidine, Sulfathalidine) *Available as:* Tablets: 0.5 g Suspension: 1 g/5 ml	Dose (presurgery): Initial, 125 mg/kg/24 hr; for maintenance, 125 mg/kg/24 hr (maximum, 8 g/24 hr), or 4 g/M²/24 hr; divide into 3, 4, or 6 doses (O) Dose (ulcerative colitis): 0.05–0.1 g/kg/24 hr (maximum, 8 g/24 hr); divide into 3, 4, or 6 doses (O) **Contraindications, warnings, precautions, adverse reactions:** See sulfadiazine
Salicylazosulfapyridine, NF (Azulfidine) *Available as:* Tablets: 0.5 g Tablets (enteric coated): 0.5 g	Dose: Initial (usual), 75–150 mg/kg/24 hr, or 2.3–4.5 g/M²/24 hr, divided into 4, 6, or 8 doses (O); initial (severe colitis), 37.5–150 mg/kg/24 hr, or 1.2–4.5 g/M²/24 hr, divided into 3, 4, or 6 doses (O); maintenance, 40 mg/kg/24 hr, or 1.25 g/M²/24 hr, divided into 4 doses; for recurrence of symptoms increase to previously effective dose **Contraindications:** See sulfadiazine
Succinylsulfathiazole (Sulfasuxidine) *Available as:* Tablets: 0.5 g Powder: 454 g (bulk)	Dose: 0.25 g/kg/24 hr, or 8 g/M²/24 hr; divide into 6 doses (O) **Contraindications:** Intestinal obstruction; see sulfadiazine **Warnings, precautions, adverse reactions:** See sulfadiazine
Sulfadiazine or sodium salt, USP (or combinations of sulfonamides) *Available as:* Tablets: 60, 250, 300, and 500 mg Tablets (chewable): 300 mg Suspension: 0.5 g/5 ml Solution (sodium): 0.25 g/ml, for injection	Dose (oral, over age 2 mo): Initial, ½ of 24 hr dose; maintenance, 150 mg/kg/24 hr (maximum, 6 g/24 hr), or 4 g/M²/24 hr; divide into 4–6 doses/24 hr (O) Dose (parenteral, over age 2 mo): Initial, ½ of 24 hr dose; maintenance, 100 mg/kg/24 hr, or 2.25 g/M²/24 hr; divide into 3 doses/24 hr (SC 5% solution) or into 4 doses/24 hr (IV) Dose (rheumatic fever prophylaxis): Under 30 kg, 0.5 g/24 hr (O); over 30 kg, 1 g/24 hr (O) **Note:** Sodium represents 8.4% of sodium sulfadiazine or 3.65 mEqNa/g **Contraindications:** Sensitivity to sulfonamides; under age 2 mo except con-

Table continued.

TABLE 30–1 (*Continued*)

DRUG, HOW SUPPLIED	DOSAGE, ROUTES, CONTRAINDICATIONS AND WARNINGS*
	genital toxoplasmosis; pregnancy at term and nursing period (kernicterus) **Warnings:** Safety in pregnancy not established; *hypersensitivity reactions* may be fatal (agranulocytosis, aplastic anemia, other blood dyscrasias, renal and hepatic damage, CNS changes, skin eruptions, Stevens-Johnson syndrome); monitor patient closely, respecting clinical condition, blood counts, and urinalysis (see package insert) **Precautions:** Give with caution to patients with impaired renal or hepatic function or with severe allergy or asthma; may produce hemolytic anemia in patients with G6PD deficiency; maintain adequate fluid intake to prevent crystalluria and stone formation **Adverse reactions:** Most commonly, anorexia, nausea, vomiting, gastric distress; *blood dyscrasias* (agranulocytosis, aplastic anemia, thrombocytopenia, leukopenia, hemolytic anemia, purpura, hypoprothrombinemia and methemoglobinemia); *hypersensitivity* (rashes, erythema multiforme [Stevens-Johnson], exfoliative dermatitis, epidermal necrolysis [Lyell syndrome] with corneal damage, photosensitization, anaphylaxis, serum sickness syndrome, drug fever, myocarditis, polyarteritis nodosa, LE phenomenon); *gastrointestinal* (above, and diarrhea, malabsorption, stomatitis, hepatitis, pancreatitis); *neurologic* (see package insert); *renal* (crystalluria, hematuria, proteinuria, nephrotic syndrome); *metabolic* (goitrogenic, hypoglycemia); for other details see package insert
Sulfamethizole, NF (Sulfurine, Thiosulfil, others) *Available as:* Tablets (scored): 0.25, 0.5, and 1 g Suspension: 0.25 and 0.5 g/5 ml	Dose (oral): See sulfadiazine **Contraindications, warnings, precautions, adverse reactions:** See sulfadiazine
Sulfamethoxazole, NF (Gantanol and many other trade names) *Available as:* Tablets (double scored): 0.5 g Suspension: 0.5 g/5 ml	Dose: Initial, 60 mg/kg/24 hr (maximum, 2 g), or 1.2 g/M²/24 hr, as single dose (O); for maintenance, above dose divided into 2 doses (O) **Contraindications, warnings, precautions, adverse reactions:** See sulfadiazine
Sulfamethoxazole and trimethoprim (See trimethoprim and sulfamethaxazole, below)	
Sulfisoxazole, and acetyl sulfisoxazole, USP (Gantrisin and many other trade names) *Available as:* Tablets (scored): 0.5 g Syrup (acetyl): 0.5 g/5 ml Lipo-Gantrisin (acetyl): 1 g/5 ml Solution (diolamine): 400 mg/ml, for injection	Dose: Initial (O), give ½ of daily maintenance dose; for maintenance (O), 150 mg/kg/24 hr (not more than 6 g/24 hr, or 4 g/M²/24 hr), divided into 4–6 doses (O); initial (parenteral), 50 mg/kg, or 1.2 g/M²; maintenance (parenteral), 100 mg/24 hr, or 2.4 g/M²/24 hr, divided into 3 (SC) or 4 (IV, IM) doses; not more than 5 ml (400 mg/ml) at any one site (IM) **Contraindications:** As for sulfadiazine **Warnings:** As for sulfadiazine **Precautions:** As for sulfadiazine **Adverse reactions:** As for sulfadiazine
Trimethoprim and sulfamethoxazole (Bactrim, Septra) *Available as:* Tablets: 80 mg of trimethoprim and 400 mg of sulfamethoxazole	Dose (adult): 4 tablets daily, divided into 2 doses (O); adjust dose for renal impairment; if creatinine clearance above 30 ml/min, give above dose; for 15–30 ml/min, give one half above dose; if below 15 ml/min, use of drug not recommended **Note:** Not recommended under 12 yr **Contraindications:** Hypersensitivity to trimethoprim or sulfonamides; pregnancy and nursing

*For individual drugs, see general index. *Consult package inserts.*

Key: M², dose per square meter of body surface; IM, intramuscular; ITh, intrathecal; IV, intravenous; O, oral; R, rectal; SC, subcutaneous; Subl, sublingual; T, topical.

TABLE 30–1 (*Continued*)

DRUG, HOW SUPPLIED	DOSAGE, ROUTES, CONTRAINDICATIONS AND WARNINGS
	Warnings: Same as for sulfadiazine, as regards sulfamethoxazole; trimethoprim may cause decreased hematopoiesis, thrombopenia and purpura (with thiazides concurrently); do frequent blood counts, discontinuing if significant reduction of formed elements occurs **Precautions:** Use with care in impaired renal or hepatic function, with possible folate deficiency and with severe allergy or bronchial asthma; in G6PD-deficient individuals, hemolysis may occur; adequate fluid intake to prevent crystalluria and stone formation; urinalyses with careful microscopic examination and renal function tests should be performed, particularly with impaired renal function **Adverse reactions:** *Blood* (agranulocytosis, aplastic anemia, megaloblastic anemia, thrombopenia, leukopenia, hemolytic anemia, purpura, hypoprothrombinemia and methemoglobinemia); *allergic* (erythema multiforme, Stevens-Johnson syndrome, generalized skin eruptions, epidermal necrolysis, urticaria, serum sickness, pruritus, exfoliative dermatitis, anaphylactoid reactions, periorbital edema, conjunctival and scleral injection, photosensitization, arthralgia and allergic myocarditis); *gastrointestinal* (glossitis, stomatitis, nausea, emesis, abdominal pains, hepatitis, diarrhea and pancreatitis); *neurologic* (headache, peripheral neuritis, mental depression, convulsions, ataxia, hallucinations, tinnitus, vertigo, insomnia, apathy, fatigue, muscle weakness and nervousness); *miscellaneous* (drug fever, chills and toxic nephrosis with oliguria and anuria, periarteritis nodosa and LE phenomenon; goiter production, diuresis and hypoglycemia have occurred rarely); *cross-sensitivity* may exist with acetazolamide and the thiazides.
OTHER CHEMOTHERAPEUTICS	
Furazolidone, (Furoxone) *Available as:* Tablets (scored): 100 mg Suspension: 16.7 mg/5 ml	Dose: 6 mg/kg/24 hr, or 200 mg/M²/24 hr; divide into 4 doses (O) **Contraindications:** Not for use in infants under 1 mo old; hypersensitivity to this drug; use of monoamine oxidase inhibitors (use with caution); ingestion of alcohol discloses disulfiram-like effect **Precautions:** Orthostatic hypotension and hypoglycemia may occur **Adverse reactions:** May cause hemolytic anemia in G6PD deficient patients; rashes and gastrointestinal symptoms (see package insert)
Methenamine mandelate, USP (Mandacon, Mandelamine) *Available as:* Tablets: 0.25, 0.5, and 1 g Tablets (enteric coated): 0.25, 0.5, and 1 g Granules: 0.5 and 1 g Suspension: 250 mg/5 ml Suspension (Forte): 500 mg/5 ml	Dose: 0.1 g/kg/24 hr initially, then 0.05 g/kg/24 hr (maximum, 3 g/24 hr), or 3 g/M²/24 hr initially, then 1.5 g/M²/24 hr; divide into 3 doses (O) **Contraindication:** Renal insufficiency **Precautions:** Dysuria at high dosage; urine must be acid–if acidification contraindicated or unobtainable (urea-splitting organisms), the drug is not recommended **Adverse reactions:** Occasional gastrointestinal upset or skin eruption
Methenamine hippurate (Hiprex, Urax) **Note:** Safe dosage not established for children under 6 yr of age *Available as:* Tablets (scored): 1 g	Dose: 40 mg/kg/24 hr, or 1.2 g/M²/24 hr; divide into 2 doses (O) **Contraindications:** In renal insufficiency, severe hepatic disease, severe dehydration; as sole agent in parenchymal infections with systemic symptoms **Caution:** Maintain acid urine; perform liver function studies periodically; may cause gastrointestinal symptoms, dysuria, rash
Nalidixic acid, NF (Neg-Gram) *Available as:* Tablets: 250 and 500 mg (O) Suspension: 250 mg/5 ml	Dose: Over 3 mo. of age, 50 mg/kg/24 hr, or 1.5 g/M²/24 hr; divide into 4 doses (O); over 12 yr, 4 g/24 hr, divided into 4 doses **Contraindications:** Hypersensitivity to this drug; convulsive disorder **Warnings:** CNS effects include convulsions, increased intracranial pressure, toxic psychosis, usually from overdosage or with predisposing factors **Precautions:** Periodic blood, renal and hepatic test if drug given for more than 2 weeks; avoid exposure to sun (photosensitization); resistant organisms may emerge rapidly; leads to reducing substances in urine, may give false values for 17-keto and ketogenic steroids **Adverse Reactions:** *See package insert; neurologic* (see above); *hypersensitivity* (rashes, angioedema, eosinophilia, photosensitivity)

Table continued.

TABLE 30–1 *(Continued)*

DRUG, HOW SUPPLIED	DOSAGE, ROUTES, CONTRAINDICATIONS AND WARNINGS*
Nitrofurantoin, USP (Furadantin, Macrodantin, others) *Available as:* Tablets (scored): 50 and 100 mg Capsules (Macrocrystals): 25, 50 and 100 mg Oral suspension: 25 mg/5 ml Sterile for injection (sodium): 180 mg (dry) (60 mg/ml)	Dose: Up to 7 kg, 6 mg/kg/24 hr; 7–11 kg, 50 mg/24 hr; 12–21 kg, 100 mg/24 hr; 22–31 kg, 150 mg/24 hr; 32–40 kg, 200 mg/24 hr; or 150 mg/M^2/24 hr; divide into 4 doses (O); reduce to 1/2 of above dosage if continued beyond 10–14 days; after another 10–14 days reduce to 1/4 of above Dose (macrocrystals): 6 mg/kg/24 hr (maximum, 400 mg/24 hr), or 150 mg/M^2/24 hr (O); divide into 4 doses (O) **Contraindications:** Anuria, oliguria, *infants* under 1 mo **Warnings:** Safety not established for use in patients under 12 years old; may produce hemolytic anemia in G6PD deficient patient or newborn **Precautions:** Peripheral neuropathy may occur (may become severe or irreversible); various conditions may predispose (see package insert) **Adverse reactions:** Nausea, emesis, diarrhea (may respond to reduced dosage); *hypersensitivity* (skin eruptions, angioedema, pulmonary infiltrates, pleural effusion, eosinophilia reported); chills, fever, jaundice, others (see package insert); pain at site of intramuscular injection
ANTICHOLINERGICS (See Cholinergic blocking agents)	
ANTICHOLINESTERASES (See Cholinesterase inhibitors)	
ANTICOAGULANTS	
Heparin sodium, USP (1 mg = 120 or more USP units) *Available as:* In thousands of units: Ampules and vials: 1, 5, 7.5, 10, 15, 20 and 40/ml Syringes (disposable): 20/ml Tubex (disposable): 1, 5, 7.5, 10, 15, and 20 ml Tablets (Subl) (potassium): 1500 units Protamine sulfate (antidote): Ampules and vials: 10 mg/ml	Dose: Initial, 50 units/kg (IV, drip); maintenance, 100 units/kg added and absorbed every 4 hr (IV, drip), or 20,000 units/M^2/24 hr, continuous dosage; titrate dose to yield 20–30 min clotting time or 2–3 times preheparin clotting time **Antidote:** Protamine sulfate (IV, drip)—1 mg for each 1 mg heparin in previous 4 hr **Contraindications:** Bleeding tendency (hemophilia, purpura, jaundice, postoperative oozing of blood, etc.), subacute bacterial endocarditis, intracranial or hidden hemorrhage, ulcerative lesions (hidden), shock, hypersensitivity to this drug **Caution:** Monitor clotting time; may cause fever, skin rashes, nasal congestion, asthma, anaphylaxis, alopecia
ANTICONVULSANTS (See Section 19 for details)	
Acetazolamide (See Diuretics)	
Amphetamine sulfate (See Adrenergics)	
BARBITURATES (For other barbiturates see Sedatives and hypnotics)	
Mephobarbital, NF (Mebaral) *Available as:* Tablets: 30, 50, 100, and 200 mg	Dose: 1 1/2–2 times dose of phenobarbital **Contraindications:** See phenobarbital **Caution:** See phenobarbital
Metharbital, NF (Gemonil) *Available as:* Tablets (scored): 100 mg	Dose: Initial (O), for infants and small children, 50–100 mg 1–3 times daily; for adults, 100 mg 1–3 times daily **Contraindications:** See phenobarbital **Caution:** See phenobarbital

*For individual drugs, see general index. *Consult package inserts.*

Key: M^2, dose per square meter of body surface; IM, intramuscular; ITh, intrathecal; IV, intravenous; O, oral; R, rectal; SC, subcutaneous; Subl, sublingual; T, topical.

TABLE 30–1 (*Continued*)

DRUG, HOW SUPPLIED	DOSAGE, ROUTES, CONTRAINDICATIONS AND WARNINGS
Phenobarbital and phenobarbital sodium, USP (Luminal) *Available as:* Tablets: 8, 15, 30, 60, and 100 mg Capsules (prolonged action): 60 and 100 mg Elixir: 20 mg/5 ml Solution (sodium): 25, 50, 125, 150, and 300 mg/ml, for injection Syringes (disposable): 50, 100, and 130 mg	Dose: For *sedation,* 2 mg/kg/24 hr, or 70 mg/M²/24 hr, divided into 4 doses (O or R); for *anticonvulsant* use, 3.5 mg/kg/dose (IM), or 125 mg/M²/dose (IM); may be given in dilute solution *slowly* IV **Contraindications:** In severe hepatic or renal dysfunction, porphyria, hypersensitivity to barbituric acid derivatives **Warnings:** May be habit forming; sudden withdrawal of drug may precipitate convulsions or status epilepticus **Precautions:** Use with care in debilitated patient and with pulmonary disease **Adverse reactions:** Uncommon with small doses; with large single doses drowsiness may persist 24 hr or more; occasional vertigo, nausea, hebetude, headache; delirium, stupor, ataxia usually from overdosage; cutaneous eruptions (usually transient); megaloblastic anemia in a few patients after prolonged therapy (responds to folic acid or vitamin B_{12} but such therapy may precipitate seizures) **Toxicity:** See Section 28
Bromides *Available as:* Three bromides tablets: Total: 0.45 and 0.9 g Bromides syrup: Total: 1.2 g/5 ml Three bromides elixir: Total: 1.2 g/5 ml	Dose: As anticonvulsant, 50–100 mg/kg/24 hr, or 1.5–3 g/M²/24 hr; divide into 3 doses every 8 hr (O) Maximum blood level: 200 mg/dl **Caution:** Acne, rash, granuloma, ataxia, lethargy, and psychosis
Dextroamphetamine (See Adrenergics)	
Diazepam (Valium) (See Tranquilizers, and Section 19)	
Diphenhydramine hydrochloride (Benadryl) (See Antihistaminics)	
HYDANTOINS	
Diphenylhydantoin and diphenylhydantoin sodium (See Phenytoin, below)	
Phenytoin and phenytoin sodium, USP, (diphenylhydantoin and diphenylhydantoin sodium, USP (Dilantin and Dilantin Sodium, and many other trade names) *Available as:* Tablets: 100 mg Tablets (chewable): 50 mg Capsules: 30, 100, and 250 mg 100 mg (prolonged action) 100 mg (in oil) Suspension: 30 and 125 mg/5 ml Solution: 50 mg/ml, for injection	Dose: 3–8 mg/kg/24 hr, or 250 mg/M²/24 hr; give as single dose or divide into 2 doses (O, IM, or IV slowly) **Contraindications:** Hypersensitivity to hydantoin products; in sinus bradycardia, heart block, Adams-Stokes syndrome (see package insert) **Warnings:** Abrupt withdrawal may precipitate status epilepticus; not indicated in seizures due to hypoglycemia or other easily identifiable and correctable causes; metabolism may be altered by concomitant administration of other drugs **Precautions:** Early toxicity with impairment of hepatic function; a few patients have genetic impairment in metabolism of drug; lymph node hyperplasia may occur, generally reversible (substitute another drug, if possible); discontinue drug for skin eruption (resume drug cautiously if eruption not exfoliative, purpuric, or bullous—if milder eruption recurs, further use contraindicated. **Adverse reactions:** *Neurologic* most common (nystagmus, ataxia, slurred speech, confusion, dizziness, twitching, headache); *gastrointestinal* (nausea, vomiting, constipation); *dermatologic* (scarlatiniform and morbilliform rashes [sometimes with fever], and more serious eruptions such as bullous, exfoliative, purpuric types, lupus erythematosus or Stevens-Johnson syndrome); *hematologic* (thrombocytopenia, leukopenia, granulocytopenia, agranulocytosis, pancytopenia, megaloblastic anemia [usually responding to folic acid], and lymphadenopathy); *gingival hypertrophy* common; *others* (see package insert); cardiovascular collapse with rapid intravenous use (see package insert)

Table continued.

TABLE 30–1 (*Continued*)

DRUG, HOW SUPPLIED	DOSAGE, ROUTES, CONTRAINDICATIONS AND WARNINGS*
Ethotoin, ethyl phenylhydantoin (Peganone) *Available as:* Tablets (scored): 250 and 500 mg	Dose: 80 mg/kg/24 hr, or 2.5 g/M^2/24 hr; divide into 4 doses **Caution:** Withdraw therapy with liver damage or marked depression of blood count; blood counts, urinalyses at onset of therapy and monthly intervals; liver function tests with clinical suggestion of hepatic disorder; caution if given with phenacemide (paranoid symptoms); less gastric distress (nausea, vomiting) when given after meals; may cause fatigue, insomnia, dizziness, headache, diplopia, nystagmus, numbness, rash, fever, diarrhea, chest pain; ataxia and gingival hypertrophy rarely, lymphadenopathy, lupus erythematosus syndrome (remitting on drug withdrawal)
Mephenytoin, NF, methyl phenylethylhydantoin (Mesantoin) *Available as:* Tablets: 100 mg	Dose: 3–15 mg/kg/24 hr, or 100–450 mg/M^2/24 hr; divide into 3 doses/24 hr (O) **Caution:** Discontinue use with untoward reactions: (1) skin rash, (2) blood dyscrasias, (3) CNS effects; do WBC differential (neutrophils) before therapy, at 2 wk (on low dosage), and 2 wk (on full dosage), monthly for 1 yr, then every 3 mo; counts every 2 wk if neutrophils drop to 2500–1600/mm^3; stop drug for count of 1600/mm^3 or less; instruct patient and/or parents of symptoms and signs of agranulocytosis; keep under close observation
Magnesium sulfate (See Laxatives, below)	
OXAZOLIDINES	
Paramethadione, USP (Paradione) *Available as:* Capsules: 150 and 300 mg Solution: 300 mg/ml	Dose: Under age 2 yr, 0.3 g/24 hr; 2–6 yr, 0.6 g/24 hr; over 6 yr and adults, 0.9 g/24 hr; adjust subsequent doses by response (O) **Contraindications:** See trimethadione **Caution:** See trimethadione
Trimethadione, USP (Tridione) *Available as:* Capsules: 300 mg Tablets (Dulcet): 150 mg Solution: 200 mg/5 ml	Dose (initial daily): In infants, 300 mg; at age 2 yr, 600 mg; at age 6 yr, 900 mg; at age 13 yr, 1200 mg Dose (maintenance): 40 mg/kg/24 hr, or 1 g/M^2/24 hr; divide into 3–4 doses (O) **Contraindications:** Not ordinarily to be used with severe hepatic or renal impairment or blood dyscrasias **Caution:** In diseases of the retina or optic nerve; withdraw if the following are encountered: scotomas, persistent or increasing albuminuria, jaundice or other signs of hepatitis, lupus-like manifestations or lymphadenopathy, total number of neutrophils of 2500/mm^3 or below, or skin rash; may cause "glare phenomenon" (relieved with dark glasses), drowsiness (relieved with amphetamines), leukopenia, blood dyscrasias (including fatal aplastic anemia), nephrosis, grand mal seizures, hair loss; avoid concurrent use of other drugs known to cause toxic effects or use with extreme caution; strict medical supervision during initial treatment period, laboratory tests of blood and urine at monthly intervals, more frequent when WBC count is less than 3000/mm^3
Paraldehyde (See Sedatives and hypnotics, below)	
Phenacemide, phenacetylcarbamide (Phenurone) *Available as:* Tablets (scored): 500 mg Tablets (enteric coated): 300 mg	Dose (for age 5–10 yr): Initial dose, 0.75 g/24 hr, divided into 3 doses; 2nd wk, add 0.25 g on arising; 3rd wk, may add 0.25 g at bedtime (O) **Caution:** Ordinarily should not be used unless other anticonvulsants have been found ineffective; may cause psychic changes, hepatitis, skin rash, gastrointestinal disturbances, nephritis; extreme caution in patients who previously have shown personality disorders (alert patient and family to possibilities of suicide and psychoses and to report same); use with

*For individual drugs, see general index. *Consult package inserts.*

Key: M^2, dose per square meter of body surface; IM, intramuscular; ITh, intrathecal; IV, intravenous; O, oral; R, rectal; SC, subcutaneous; Subl, sublingual; T, topical.

TABLE 30–1 (*Continued*)

DRUG, HOW SUPPLIED	DOSAGE, ROUTES, CONTRAINDICATIONS AND WARNINGS
	caution if history of liver dysfunction (death reported) or if history of allergy, particularly in association with use of other anticonvulsants; withdraw drug if the following are encountered: severe or exacerbated personality changes, jaundice or other signs of hepatitis, marked depression of blood count, abnormal urinary findings; laboratory tests should be performed: complete blood counts before use, at monthly intervals for 1 yr, and (if no abnormalities) at extended intervals (follow total numbers of cellular elements; leukopenia [4000/mm^3], aplastic anemia, and death have occurred); liver function tests before and during therapy, urine examinations at regular intervals
Phenothiazines (See Tranquilizers, below)	
Primidone, USP (Mysoline) *Available as:* Tablets (scored): 50 and 250 mg Oral suspension: 250 mg/5 ml	Dose: *Wk* / *Adults and children over 8 yr* / *Children under 8 yr* 1 — 250 mg hs — 125 mg hs 2 — 250 mg bid — 125 mg bid 3 — 250 mg tid — 125 mg tid 4 — 250 mg qid — 125 mg qid Continue weekly increments; dose not to exceed 2 g/24 hr, or 1.25 g/M^2/24 hr; divide into 2–4 doses (O) **Caution:** May cause megaloblastic anemia (rare) (responding to folic acid while continuing drug); minor and infrequent: gastrointestinal symptoms, drowsiness, fatigue, hyperirritability, emotional disturbance, dizziness, ataxia, diplopia, nystagmus, morbilliform rashes; persistent or severe effects—withdraw drug
Quinacrine hydrochloride (See Antiprotozoan Drugs, below)	
SUCCINAMIDES	
Ethosuximide, USP (Zarontin) *Available as:* Capsules: 0.25 g Syrup: 250 mg/5 ml	Dose (initial): Under 6 yr, 0.25 g/24 hr (O); over 6 yr, 0.5 g/24 hr; divide into 2 doses (O) Dose (continued): Increase only as necessary; add 0.25 g every 4–7 days **Contraindications:** History of sensitivity to succinimides **Warnings:** Blood dyscrasias reported, some fatal (monitor); may produce abnormal renal and liver function tests (use with caution in renal or hepatic disease, with periodic monitoring); systemic lupus erythematosus reported; may impair mental function for driving or other hazardous activities (caution accordingly) **Precautions:** May increase grand mal seizures when used alone in mixed types of epilepsy; change dose gradually (abrupt withdrawal may precipitate petit mal status) **Adverse reactions:** *Gastrointestinal* (anorexia, nausea, vomiting, pain, diarrhea, weight loss); *hematologic* (leukopenia, agranulocytosis, pancytopenia, eosinophilia); *neurologic* (drowsiness, headache, dizziness, euphoria, hiccups, irritability, lethargy, fatigue, ataxia, emotional disturbances, insomnia, night terrors, paranoia, depression, suicidal tendencies); *dermatologic* (pruritic rashes, urticaria, Stevens-Johnson syndrome, lupus erythematosus); *other* (myopia, gum hypertrophy, hirsutism); see package insert
Methsuximide, NF (Celontin) *Available as:* Capsules: 0.15 and 0.3 g	Dose: Initial, 0.3 g/24 hr for 1 wk (O); for increase, 0.3 g/24 hr/wk for 3 wk to 1.2 g/24 hr (O) **Contraindication:** Sensitivity to this drug **Warnings:** As for ethosuximide, above **Precautions:** Withdraw drug slowly on appearance of unusual depression, aggressiveness or other behavioral alterations; change dose slowly (see ethosuximide); may increase frequency of grand mal seizures in some patients (see ethosuximide, above) **Adverse reactions:** See ethosuximide, above, and package insert
Phensuximide, NF (Milontin) *Available as:*	Dose: 1–3 g/24 hr; divide into 2–3 doses (O) **Caution:** Evaluate patient, blood and urine studies regularly; when dis-

Table continued.

TABLE 30–1 (*Continued*)

DRUG, HOW SUPPLIED	DOSAGE, ROUTES, CONTRAINDICATIONS AND WARNINGS *
Capsules: 0.25 and 0.5 g Suspension: 300 mg/5 ml	continuing drug, do so gradually; may cause gastrointestinal symptoms (anorexia, vomiting), CNS symptoms (drowsiness, dizziness), microscopic hematuria, granulocytopenia, aplastic anemia, skin reactions
ANTIDOTES (See also Adrenergics, Analeptics, Antihistaminics, Calcium salts, Cholinesterase inhibitors, Sedatives—barbiturates; see also Section 28 for details)	
Atropine sulfate (See Cholinergic blocking agents, below)	
Biperiden, biperiden hydrochloride or lactate, NF (Akineton) *Available as:* Tablets (scored): 2 mg Ampules: 5 mg/ml	Dose (for drug-induced extrapyramidal reactions): 0.04 mg/kg, or 1.2 mg/M²; give as single dose (IM); repeat in 1/2 hr if needed, not more than 4 doses in 24 hr **Caution:** In glaucoma; may cause dry mouth, blurred vision, drowsiness, decreased urinary flow, disorientation, euphoria, gastric irritation, postural hypotension
Charcoal, activated, USP *Available as:* Powder, (USP)	See Section 28
Deferoxamine mesylate, USP (Desferal mesylate) *Available as:* Sterile (for injection): 500 mg	Dose (parenteral only); Initial, 20 mg/kg, or 0.6 g/M², with 1/2 initial dose given every 4 hr (2 doses); for subsequent doses, 1/2 of initial dose every 4–12 hr (depending on clinical response), not to exceed 6 g/24 hr (adult) or 3.5 g/M²/24 hr; IM (preferred) in *all patients not in shock,* or by slow infusion (IV) not to exceed 15 mg/kg/hr (IV), or 0.45 g/M²/hr (IV), *only for patients in cardiovascular collapse;* discontinue IV and give IM as soon as clinical condition permits **Contraindications:** Contraindicated in patients with severe renal disease or anuria, since drug and chelate that it forms with iron are excreted primarily by the kidney **Warning:** Long-term administration has been associated with cataracts in dogs and humans; no ocular abnormalities by slit lamp in a few patients treated for acute iron intoxication **Caution:** Flushing of the skin, urticaria, hypotension, shock (rapid intravenous injection); *give intramuscularly or by slow intravenous infusion;* pain and induration at the site of injection; long-term therapy, allergic-type reactions (cutaneous wheal formation, generalized itching rash, anaphylactic reaction), blurring of vision, abdominal discomfort, diarrhea, leg cramps, tachycardia and fever
Dimercaprol, USP, British anti-lewisite (BAL) *Available as:* Solution: 100 mg/ml (10% in oil), for injection	Dose: For arsenic, mercury, and gold poisoning (mild) (IM): 1st day, 2.5 mg/kg every 4 hr (6 injections); 2nd day, 2.5 mg/kg every 6 hr (4 injections); 3rd day, 2.5 mg/kg every 12 hr (2 injections); each of following 10 days (or until total recovery), 2.5 mg/kg each day (1 injection); increase dosage 25% for severe poisoning **Caution:** See Section 28
Edetate calcium disodium, calcium disodium edathamil, EDTA calcium disodium, USP (Calcium Disodium Versenate) *Available as:* Ampules: 200 mg/ml Tablets: 500 mg	Dose: Not to exceed 70 mg/kg/24 hr, or 1.7 g/M²/24 hr; divide into 2 doses (IV), diluted to 0.2–0.4% solution; give up to 5-day course, with intervals of 2 days between additional repeat courses, if needed **Contraindications:** Do not give during anuria **Warnings:** Capable of producing toxic and potentially lethal effects; dosage schedule should be followed; never exceed recommended dosage; avoid rapid infusion in lead encephalopathy (intramuscular route preferred); do not give oral drug if lead in GI tract

*For individual drugs, see general index. *Consult package inserts.*

Key: M², dose per square meter of body surface; IM, intramuscular; ITh, intrathecal; IV, intravenous; O, oral; R, rectal; SC, subcutaneous; Subl, sublingual; T, topical.

TABLE 30-1 (*Continued*)

DRUG, HOW SUPPLIED	DOSAGE, ROUTES, CONTRAINDICATIONS AND WARNINGS
	Precautions: May (like severe acute lead poisoning) produce proteinuria and microscopic hematuria; monitor urinalysis daily, and discontinue therapy if proteinuria and hematuria worsen or if large epithelial cells appear in urine; monitor renal function (BUN before and during therapy); monitor cardiac rhythm **Adverse reactions:** Renal tubular necrosis the principal toxic effect; see package insert, and Lead poisoning, Section 28
Edetate disodium, USP (Endrate disodium) *Available as:* Solution: 150 mg/ml, for injection	Dose: 50 mg/kg, or 1.5 g/M^2; single dose (IV), slowly over 3–4 hr **Caution:** Concentration not to exceed 7 mg/ml; avoid extravasation; frequent serum calcium levels (ready calcium gluconate solution in syringe), urinalyses; with caution in tuberculosis and metastatic calcification (embolization); may cause hypocalcemic convulsions, cardiac and respiratory collapse, reduced prothrombin time, thrombophlebitis, hypotension, chills, fever, back pain, muscle cramps, vomiting, urinary urgency, gastrointestinal symptoms, genitourinary reactions (See calcium disodium edetate)
Levallorphan tartrate, NF (Lorfan) *Available as:* Solution: 1 mg/ml, for injection	Dose: In newborn infants, 0.02 mg/kg, as a single dose (IV, IM or SC), repeat if needed; in premature infants, 0.05 mg (IV or IM) **Contraindications:** Respiratory depression; narcotic addiction (may produce withdrawal symptoms) **Warnings:** Ineffective against and may potentiate respiratory depression due to barbiturates, anesthetic agents, or other drugs or pathologic causes; see also Opiates, Section 28 **Precautions:** If used in absence of narcotic, may produce rather than relieve respiratory depression; repeated doses lose effect, produce respiratory depression **Adverse reactions:** Dysphoria, miosis, pseudoptosis, lethargy, dizziness, drowsiness, gastric upset, sweating; pallor, nausea, sense of heaviness in limbs; in high doses psychotomimetic (weird dreams, hallucinations, disorientation, feelings of unreality); in *asphyxia neonatorum,* irritability and increased crying may occur
Methylene blue, USP *Available as:* Solution: 10 mg/ml (1%), for injection	Dose: In methemoglobinemia, 2 mg/kg/dose, or 50 mg/M^2/dose; give over 5-min period (IV)
Methylphenidate hydrochloride, USP (Ritalin hydrochloride) (See Analeptics, above)	
Nalorphine hydrochloride, NF (Nalline) *Available as:* Solution (for neonatal use): 0.2 mg/ml, for injection Solution: 5 mg/ml, for injection	Dose: 0.1 mg/kg/dose (IV or IM); may repeat in 15 min **Caution:** See Opiates, Section 28
Naloxone hydrochloride, USP (Narcan) **Note:** The package insert describes usage in newborns; despite this, it is *not recommended* in neonates or children *Available as:* Solution: 0.4 mg/ml, for injection	Dose: 0.005 mg/kg, or 0.25 mg/M^2, as a single dose (IV, IM or SC); may repeat IV within 2–3 min, if needed (IM and SC are reasonably absorbed); repeat 2–3 times if required (see also Section 7) **Contraindications:** In patients known to be hypersensitive to this drug **Warning:** Administer cautiously to persons known or suspected to be dependent on narcotics; abrupt and complete reversal of narcotic effects may precipitate acute abstinence syndrome; after use keep under continued surveillance and repeated doses should be administered, as necessary, since the duration of action of some narcotics may exceed that of naloxone; not effective against respiratory depression due to nonnarcotic drugs; should bleeding occur following use, a complete coagulation workup, including PTT, is indicated **Adverse reactions:** Rarely nausea and vomiting in postoperative patients in doses higher than those recommended

Table continued.

TABLE 30–1 *(Continued)*

DRUG, HOW SUPPLIED	DOSAGE, ROUTES, CONTRAINDICATIONS AND WARNINGS*
Penicillamine, USP (Cuprimine) *Available as:* Capsules: 250 mg	Dose: In infants over 6 mo and young children, 250 mg (O), as a single dose (in fruit juice); in older children and adults, 1 g/24 hr (O), divided into 4 doses; dose based on urinary copper excretion; may increase to 4–5 g/24 hr **Caution:** Routine urinalysis, WBC, differential, Hb, platelet count every 3 days (4 wk), every 7–10 days (3 mo), then monthly; frequent liver and kidney function tests; careful observation with renal disease; take temperature nightly first few months; observe skin and mucous membranes for allergic reactions; discontinue drug if fever or reaction in skin or above tests indicate; reinstitute small dose, gradually increase to full dosage; may need systemic adrenocorticosteroid for toxicity (second or third time); discontinue drug with bleeding into skin; may cause nephrotic syndrome, elevated sedimentation rate, liver dysfunctions, eosinophilia, monocytosis and leukocytosis, thrombopenia and leukopenia, fatal granulocytopenia; examine eyes for cataracts before and twice yearly during drug therapy; give pyridoxine (25 mg daily); discontinue sulfurated potash or resin when iron is administered
Pralidoxime chloride, USP (Protopam chloride) *Available as:* Tablets: 0.5 g Sterile: 1 g	Dose: 25–50 mg/kg, or 0.6–1 g/M^2, as 5% solution (IV, slowly) (IM or SC not preferred); repeat every 10–12 hr if needed **Contraindications:** Poisoning by the carbamate insecticide Sevin; in patients receiving morphine, theophylline and derivatives, succinylcholine, reserpine and phenothiazine-type drugs **Precautions:** Intravenous administration should be slow, preferably by infusion (may otherwise produce tachycardia, laryngospasm and muscular rigidity); blood levels increased with renal impairment (adjust dose in renal insufficiency); use with great caution in treating organophosphate overdosage in myasthenia gravis (may precipitate a myasthenic crisis); when *atropine* and pralidoxime are used together, signs of atropinism may appear unexpectedly early, especially if large doses of atropine have preceded the administration of pralidoxime
Protamine sulfate, USP *Available as:* Solution: 10 mg/ml, for injection	Heparin antidote (See Anticoagulants, above)
ANTIEMETICS	
ANTIHISTAMINICS (See Antihistaminics, below)	
Diphenidol hydrochloride, NF (Vontrol) *Available as:* Tablets: 25 mg Suppositories (contain benzocaine): 25 and 50 mg Solution: 20 mg/ml, for injection	Dose: For 6 mo of age or 12 kg or more, not more than 5 mg/kg/24 hr, or 150 mg/M^2/24 hr; divide into 6 doses (O or R); for IM, 60% of above dose; IV and SC not recommended for children **Contraindications:** Anuria, hypotension **Caution:** In glaucoma, pylorospasm or stenosis, obstructing gastrointestinal or genitourinary lesions, sinus tachycardia; drowsiness, dizziness, auditory and visual hallucinations, confusion can occur; avoid operation of machinery; patients under hospital or comparable supervision
TRANQUILIZERS (See Tranquilizers, below)	
Trimethobenzamide hydrochloride, NF (Tigan) *Available as:* Capsules: 100 and 250 mg Suppositories (contain benzocaine): 200 mg Solution: 100 mg/ml, for injection	Dose: 15 mg/kg/24 hr, or 450 mg/M^2/24 hr, divided into 3 or 4 doses (O, R); IM not recommended for children; R not recommended for newborn infants **Caution:** Drowsiness (prohibit motor operation), obscures gastrointestinal diagnoses, sensitivity to "-caine" anesthetics (suppositories), parkinsonism-like reactions, hypotension, rare reports of blood dyscrasias, other reactions

*For individual drugs, see general index. *Consult package inserts.*

Key: M^2, dose per square meter of body surface; IM, intramuscular; ITh, intrathecal; IV, intravenous; O, oral; R, rectal; SC, subcutaneous; Subl, sublingual; T, topical.

TABLE 30–1 ***(Continued)***

DRUG, HOW SUPPLIED	DOSAGE, ROUTES, CONTRAINDICATIONS AND WARNINGS
ANTIEPILEPTICS (See Anticonvulsants, above)	
ANTIFUNGAL DRUGS (See Antibiotics and Chemotherapeutics)	
ANTIHELMINTICS (See Anthelmintics, above)	
ANTIHISTAMINICS	**Contraindications:** Hypersensitivity to the particular drug **Caution:** All antihistaminics produce undesired effects; be familiar with each drug prescribed, read package insert and pharmacology text; choose and use only a few; may produce many effects: CNS (sedation [avoid motor vehicle operation], excitation, insomnia, nervousness, convulsions, death); autonomic imbalance (dryness of mucous membranes, blurred vision, urinary retention, tachycardia, hypotension); gastrointestinal disturbances (anorexia, vomiting, diarrhea, pain); blood dyscrasias (pancytopenia, agranulocytosis, thrombocytopenia); additive effects with depressant drugs **Toxicity:** See Section 28
Brompheniramine maleate, NF (Dimetane) *Available as:* Tablets (scored): 4 mg Tablets (prolonged action): 8 and 12 mg Elixir: 2 mg/5 ml Solution: 10 and 100 mg/ml, for injection	Dose: 0.5 mg/kg/24 hr, or 15 mg/M²/24 hr; divide into 3–4 doses (O, SC, IM, or IV) **Contraindications and caution:** See above
Carbinoxamine maleate, NF (Clistin) *Available as:* Tablets (scored): 4 mg Tablets (prolonged action): 8 and 12 mg Elixir: 4 mg/5 ml	Dose: 0.4 mg/kg/24 hr, or 12 mg/M²/24 hr; divide into 3–4 doses (O) **Contraindications and caution:** See above
Chlorcyclizine hydrochloride, NF (Perazil) *Available as:* Tablets (plain): 25 and 50 mg Tablets (coated): 25 and 50 mg	Dose: 1.5 mg/kg/24 hr, or 45 mg/M²/24 hr; divide into 2 doses (O) **Contraindications and cautions:** See above
Chlorpheniramine maleate, USP (Chlor-Trimeton, Teldrin, and others) *Available as:* Tablets (scored): 4 mg Capsules (prolonged action): 8 and 12 mg Syrup: 2.5 mg/5 ml Solution: 10 and 100 mg/ml, for injection	Dose: 0.35 mg/kg/24 hr, or 10 mg/M²/24 hr; divided into 4 doses (O or SC); 0.2 mg/kg, or 6 mg/M², as single dose (prolonged action) (O) **Contraindications and cautions:** See above
Cyclizine and cyclizine lactate, NF, and cyclizine hydrochloride (Antivert, Marezine) *Available as:* Tablets (scored): 12.5 and 50 mg Tablets (chewable): 25 mg Suppositories: 50 and 100 mg Solution: 50 mg/ml, for injection	Dose: 3 mg/kg/24 hr, or 100 mg/M²/24 hr, divided into 3 doses (O or IM); rectal dose, double O or IM dose **Contraindications and cautions:** See above

Table continued.

TABLE 30–1 (*Continued*)

DRUG, HOW SUPPLIED	DOSAGE, ROUTES, CONTRAINDICATIONS AND WARNINGS
Cyproheptadine hydrochloride, NF (Periactin hydrochloride) *Available as:* Tablets: 4 mg Syrup: 2 mg/5 ml	Dose: 0.25 mg/kg/24 hr, or 8 mg/M²/24 hr; divide into 3–4 doses (O) **Contraindications and cautions:** See above
Dexbrompheniramine maleate, NF (Disomer) *Available as:* Tablets: 2 mg Tablets (prolonged action): 4 and 6 mg Syrup: 2 mg/5 ml	Dose: 0.17 mg/kg/24 hr, or 5 mg/M²/24 hr; divide into 4 doses (O) **Contraindications and cautions:** See above
Dexchlorpheniramine maleate, NF (Polaramine maleate) *Available as:* Tablets: 2 mg Prolonged action: 4 and 6 mg Syrup: 2 mg/5 ml	Dose: 0.15 mg/kg/24 hr, or 4.5 mg/M²/24 hr; divide into 4 doses (O) **Contraindications and cautions:** See above
Dimenhydrinate, USP (Dramamine) *Available as:* Tablets: 50 mg Suppositories: 100 mg Liquid: 15.6 mg/5 ml Solution: 50 mg/ml, for injection	Dose: 5 mg/kg/24 hr (maximum, 300 mg/24 hr), or 150 mg/M²/24 hr; divide into 4 doses (O, R, or IM) **Contraindications and cautions:** See above
Diphenhydramine hydrochloride, USP (Benadryl hydrochloride) *Available as:* Capsules: 25 and 50 mg Tablets (enteric coated): 50 mg Elixir: 12.5 mg/5 ml Solution: 10 and 50 mg/ml, for injection	Dose: 5 mg/kg/24 hr (maximum, 300 mg/24 hr), or 150 mg/M²/24 hr; divide into 4 doses (O or IM) **Contraindications and cautions:** See above
Doxylamine succinate, NF (Decapryn succinate) *Available as:* Tablets (scored): 12.5 and 25 mg Syrup: 6.25 mg/5 ml	Dose: 2 mg/kg/24 hr, or 60 mg/M²/24 hr; divide into 4–6 doses (O) **Contraindications and cautions:** See above
Methapyrilene fumarate and hydrochloride, NF (Histadyl and many other trade names) *Available as:* Capsules: 25 and 50 mg Syrup: 20 mg/5 ml Solution: 20 mg/ml, for injection	Dose: 5 mg/kg/24 hr (maximum, 300 mg/24 hr), or 150 mg/M²/24 hr; divide into 5 doses (O); 1/4–1/3 oral dose (SC or IM) **Contraindications and cautions:** See above
Methdilazine and methdilazine hydrochloride, NF (Tacaryl and Tacaryl hydrochloride) *Available as:* Hydrochloride: Tablets (scored): 8 mg Syrup: 4 mg/5 ml Base: Tablets (chewable): 3.6 mg	Dose: 0.3 mg/kg/24 hr, or 10 mg/M²/24 hr; divide into 2 doses (O) **Caution:** Phenothiazine derivative; see chlorpromazine hydrochloride

*For individual drugs, see general index. *Consult package inserts.*

Key: M², dose per square meter of body surface; IM, intramuscular; ITh, intrathecal; IV, intravenous; O, oral; R, rectal; SC, subcutaneous; Subl, sublingual; T, topical.

TABLE 30–1 (*Continued*)

DRUG, HOW SUPPLIED	DOSAGE, ROUTES, CONTRAINDICATIONS AND WARNINGS
Promethazine hydrochloride (See Tranquilizers, below)	
Pyrrobutamine phosphate, NF (Pyronil) *Available as:* Tablets (scored): 15 mg	Dose: 0.6 mg/kg/24 hr, or 20 mg/M²/24 hr; divide into 2 doses (O) **Contraindications and cautions:** See above
Trimeprazine tartrate, USP (Temaril) *Available as:* Tablets: 2.5 mg Capsules (prolonged action): 5 mg Syrup: 2.5 mg/5 ml	Dose: Under 2 yr, 3.75 mg/24 hr (maximum); 3–12 yr, 7.5 mg/24 hr, or 6 mg/M²/24 hr; divide into 3 doses (O) **Caution:** Phenothiazine derivative; see chlorpromazine hydrochloride; see above
Tripelennamine citrate and hydrochloride, USP (Pyribenzamine citrate and hydrochloride) *Available as:* Tablets (scored): 50 mg Tablets (coated): 25 mg Tablets (prolonged action): 50 and 100 mg Elixir: 37.5 mg/5 ml Solution: 25 mg/ml, for injection	Dose: 5 mg/kg/24 hr (maximum, 300 mg/24 hr), or 150 mg/M²/24 hr; divide into 4–6 doses/24 hr (O) **Contraindications and cautions:** See above
Triprolidine hydrochloride, NF (Actidil) *Available as:* Tablets (scored): 2.5 mg Syrup: 1.25 mg/5 ml	Dose: Under 2 yr, 1.25 mg/24 hr; over 2 yr, 2.5 mg/24 hr or 4 mg/M²/24 hr; divide into 2–3 doses (O) **Contraindications and cautions:** See above
ANTIHYPERTENSIVES (See Cardiovascular drugs, below)	
ANTIHYPERURICEMICS (See Xanthine oxidase inhibitor, below)	
ANTIMALARIALS (See Antiprotozoan drugs, below, and Section 10)	
ANTI-MOTION SICKNESS DRUGS (See Cyclizine and Dimenhydrinate, above, and Scopolamine, below)	
ANTINEOPLASTICS (See Section 14 for contraindications, caution, and toxicity of individual drugs)	
Adrenal steroids (See Endocrines, below)	
Azathioprine, USP (Imuran) *Available as:* Tablets (scored): 50 mg	Dose: Initial, 3–5 mg/kg/24 hr (O), or 120 mg/M²/24 hr (O), with individualized dosage based on clinical and hematologic response (reduced dosage with impaired renal function or cadaveric kidneys); for maintenance, may reduce to 1–2 mg/kg/24 hr (O), or 45 mg/M²/24 hr (O) **Contraindication:** Hypersensitivity to this drug **Caution:** Toxic; close supervision of patient; bone marrow depression (all elements), decreased clotting; follow with at least weekly Hb, WBC, platelet counts; gastrointestinal symptoms, ulcerations; many other reactions including infection, jaundice
Busulfan, USP (Myleran) *Available as:* Tablets (scored): 2 mg	Dose: 0.06–0.12 mg/kg/24 hr, or 2.3–4.6 mg/M²/24 hr; titrate dosage to yield WBC not less than 10,000/mm³ (chronic myelogenous leukemia)

Table continued.

TABLE 30–1 ***(Continued)***

DRUG, HOW SUPPLIED	DOSAGE, ROUTES, CONTRAINDICATIONS AND WARNINGS*
Chlorambucil, USP (Leukeran) *Available as:* Tablets: 2 mg	Dose: 0.1–0.2 mg/kg, or 4.5 mg/M^2 (O); single daily dose or divided dose
Cyclophosphamide, USP (Cytoxan) *Available as:* Tablets: 50 mg Solution: 100, 200, and 500 mg, for injection	Dose (initial): For *relatively susceptible neoplasms,* 2–3 mg/kg/24 hr, or 60–90 mg/M^2/24 hr; daily O or IV dose for 6 or more days; divide oral doses, or give total of 7 days' dosage (IV) once weekly; subsequent dose regulated by WBC, platelet count, and response; for *relatively resistant neoplasms,* 4–8 mg/kg/24 hr, or 125–250 mg/M^2/24 hr; daily O or IV dose for 6 days; divide oral doses, or give total of 7 days' dosage (IV) once weekly; subsequent dose regulated by WBC, platelet count and response Dose (maintenance): 2–5 mg/kg twice weekly (O), or 50–150 mg/M^2 twice weekly (O) **Caution:** Prolonged use may lead to testicular or ovarian injury, sterility
Cytarabine, USP, cytosine arabinoside (Cytosar) *Available as:* Solution: 20 and 50 mg/ml, for injection	Dose (initial): By direct intravenous injection, 2 mg/kg daily for 10 days; by infusion, 0.5–1 mg/kg in 1–24 hr for 10 days Dose (maintenance): 1 mg/kg twice weekly (SC) **Contraindications:** Known sensitivity to this drug, inadequate marrow reserve; safety in infants not established; teratogenic in animals; weigh benefit against risk for use in pregnancy **Caution:** Highly toxic; constant supervision by physician experienced with cancer chemotherapy; initiate in hospital, follow frequently hematologic, renal and hepatic functions; bone marrow depression (interrupt treatment if platelet count falls to 50,000/mm^3 or less, or PMN 1000/mm^3 or less); reticulocytopenia, purpura, bleeding, thrombophlebitis; gastrointestinal symptoms progressing to ulceration, hemorrhage; fever, rash, cellulitis and pain (injection), infections, conjunctivitis, keratitis, freckling, chest and joint pain, urinary retention, alopecia, neuritis, lethargy, confusion; SGOT rise, uric acid rise; special caution after other cytotoxic drugs or irradiation
Dactinomycin, USP, actinomycin D (Cosmegen) *Available as:* Solution: 0.5 mg, for injection	Dose: 15 μg/kg/24 hr; divide into 4–5 doses (IV); repeat daily dose for 5 days or 2400 μg/M^2 over wk period (IV)
Mechlorethamine hydrochloride, USP, nitrogen mustard (Mustargen) *Available as:* Solution: 10 mg, for injection	Dose: 0.4 mg/kg; single dose (IV) or divide into 2 or more doses with interval of 1–2 days or 1–2 wk; or as 4 daily doses (0.1 mg/kg)
Mercaptopurine, USP, 6-mercaptopurine (Purinethol) *Available as:* Tablets (scored): 50 mg	Dose: 2.5 mg/kg/24 hr, or 70 mg/M^2/24 hr; single dose (O)
Methotrexate, USP (formerly amethopterin) *Available as:* Tablets: 2.5 mg Solution (sodium): 5 and 50 mg, for injection	Dose: 0.12 mg/kg/dose, or 3 mg/M^2/dose; daily dose (O or IM); 0.25–0.5 mg/kg/24 hr (ITh), to be considered as part of total systemic dose
Vinblastine sulfate, USP (Velban) *Available as:* Sterile: 10 mg dry powder (reconstituted, 1 mg/ml)	Dose: 0.1–0.2 mg/kg, or 3–6 mg/M^2; single *weekly* dose (IV); see vincristine

*For individual drugs, see general index. *Consult package inserts.*

Key: M^2, dose per square meter of body surface; IM, intramuscular; ITh, intrathecal; IV, intravenous; O, oral; R, rectal; SC, subcutaneous; Subl, sublingual; T, topical.

TABLE 30–1 *(Continued)*

DRUG, HOW SUPPLIED	DOSAGE, ROUTES, CONTRAINDICATIONS AND WARNINGS
Vincristine sulfate, USP (Oncovin) *Available as:* Solution: 1 and 5 mg, for injection	Dose: 0.05–0.15 mg/kg, or 1.5–4.5 mg/M²; single *weekly* dose; use dry needle technique (IV)
ANTIPROTOZOAN DRUGS (See Section 10 for details)	
Carbarsone, NF *Available as:* Tablets: 0.25 g Capsules: 0.25 g Suppositories (vaginal): 130 mg Vials (powder): 2 g	Dose: For *amebiasis,* 10 mg/kg/24 hr (maximum, 500 mg/24 hr), or 300 mg/M²/24 hr; divide into 2 or 3 doses (O) for 10 days **Contraindications:** Hypersensitivity to arsenic, kidney or liver disease (amebic hepatitis or abscess) **Caution:** Arsenic (cumulative), interrupted therapy; discontinue if the following occur: vomiting, increasing diarrhea, pulmonary congestion, neuritis, dermatitis, pruritus, hepatosplenomegaly, albuminuria; overdose—treat with BAL for arsenic poisoning (See Section 28)
Chloroquine hydrochloride and phosphate salts, USP (Aralen hydrochloride and phosphate, Roquine) (1 mg chloroquine phosphate is equivalent to 0.6 mg base; 1 mg chloroquine hydrochloride is equivalent to 0.8 mg base) *Available as:* Tablets (coated) (phosphate): 250 and 500 mg Solution (hydrochloride): 50 mg/ml	Dose (for amebic hepatitis [base]): *Initial,* 12 mg/kg/24 hr, divided into 2 doses (O) (2 days); for *maintenance,* ½ of above dose/24 hr, given as single dose; for *severe infection and hepatic abscess,* 133–167% of above doses Dose (malaria): oral (see below) **Caution:** Side effects usually reversible, short-term therapy: headache, pruritus, disturbance in visual accommodation; prolonged therapy, high dosage for other diseases: toxicity may be irreversible; ocular, gastrointestinal, dermatologic, neurologic changes, blood dyscrasias

Chloroquine, dose (malaria): oral

Age (yr)	*Initial dose (base)*	*6 hr later*	*Daily dose for next 4 days*
1	150 mg	150 mg	75 mg
2–5	300 mg	150 mg	75 mg
6–10	300 mg	150 mg	150 mg
11–15	450–600 mg	150 mg	150 mg

DRUG, HOW SUPPLIED	DOSAGE, ROUTES, CONTRAINDICATIONS AND WARNINGS
Diiodohydroxyquin, USP (Diodoquin and other trade names) *Available as:* Tablets: 650 mg	Dose: For amebiasis, 30 mg/kg/24 hr (maximum, 1.95 g/24 hr), or 1 g/M²/24 hr; divide into 3 doses (O); administer 21 days **Contraindications:** Liver damage and iodine sensitivity **Caution:** Dermatitis, chills and fever, optic atrophy with long-term administration
Emetine hydrochloride, USP *Available as:* Solution: 30 and 60 mg/ml, for injection	Dose: 1 mg/kg/24 hr (maximum 65 mg/24 hr, or 30 mg/M²/24 hr); divide into 2 doses (deep, SC), for 4–6 days
Quinacrine hydrochloride, USP (Atabrine hydrochloride) *Available as:* Tablets: 100 mg	Dose (giardiasis): 8 mg/kg/24 hr (maximum, 300 mg/24 hr), or 250 mg/M²/24 hr; divide into 3 doses (O); treat for 5 days Dose (tapeworm): 15 mg/kg (maximum, 800 mg), or 0.5 g/M²; divide into 2 doses (O) 1 hr apart; saline purge 2 hr after last dose Dose (antimalarial): See Section 10, Malaria **Caution:** See Section 10, Malaria
Quinine sulfate, USP *Available as:* Capsules: 120, 200, and 300 mg	Dose (antimalarial): See Section 10, Malaria
ANTIPRURITICS	
ANTIHISTAMINICS (See Antihistaminics, above)	
Cholestyramine resin, USP (Cuemid, Questran) *Available as:* Powder: Packets: 9 g (4 g active ingredients)	Dose: 240 mg/kg/24 hr, or 7 g/M²/24 hr, divided into 3 doses (O); give as slurry with water, pulpy fruit juice, applesauce, etc. **Note:** Safe dosage not established for children under 6 yr **Contraindication:** Complete biliary obstruction **Warning:** Supplement vitamins A, D, E and K, owing to impaired absorption

Table continued.

TABLE 30–1 *(Continued)*

DRUG, HOW SUPPLIED	DOSAGE, ROUTES, CONTRAINDICATIONS AND WARNINGS*
	Caution: Increased bleeding (hypoprothrombinemia); this responds to parenteral vitamin K; administer any other drugs 1 hr prior to this drug; may cause hyperchloremic acidosis (prolonged use), constipation, diarrhea, gastrointestinal distress, vomiting, distention, perianal rash, tongue or skin irritation
TRANQUILIZERS (See Tranquilizers, below)	
ANTIPYRETICS (See Analgesics (nonnarcotic) and antipyretics, above)	
ANTISPASMODICS (See Cholinergic blocking agents, below)	
ANTITUBERCULOSIS DRUGS (See Antibiotics and Chemotherapeutics)	
ANTITUSSIVES	
Benzonatate, NF (Tessalon) *Available as:* Capsules: 100 mg	Dose: 8 mg/kg/24 hr, or 250 mg/M^2/24 hr; divide into 3–6 doses (O) **Caution:** Not to be chewed; dermatitis, nasal congestion, constipation, sedation, hypersensitivity
Carbetapentane citrate (Toclase) *Available as:* Syrup: 7.25 mg/5 ml	Dose: Age 2–4 yr, up to 15 mg/24 hr; age 4–12 yr, up to 30 mg/24 hr; over age 12 yr, up to 45–120 mg/24 hr; divide into 3–4 doses (O)
Codeine (See Analgesics, above)	
Dextromethorphan hydrobromide, NF (Methorate hydrobromide, Romilar hydrobromide) *Available as:* Syrup: 15 mg/5 ml	Dose: 1 mg/kg/24 hr, or 30 mg/M^2/24 hr; divide into 3–4 doses (O) **Caution:** Do not mix with penicillins, tetracyclines, salicylates, sodium phenobarbital, iodides; may cause nausea, dizziness
Hydrocodone bitartrate, NF, dihydrocodeinone bitartrate (Dicodid, Hycodan) *Available as:* Tablets: 5 mg Syrup: 5 mg/5 ml	Dose: 0.6 mg/kg/24 hr, or 20 mg/M^2/24 hr; divide into 3–4 doses (O) **Caution:** Addicting
Levopropoxyphene napsylate, NF (Novrad) *Available as:* Capsules: 50 and 100 mg Suspension: 50 mg/5 ml	Dose: 6 mg/kg/24 hr, or 200 mg/M^2/24 hr; divide into 6 doses (O) **Caution:** Rash, drowsiness, jitteriness, dizziness; overdose – muscle tremor, agitation, vomiting, sedation
BARBITURATES (See Sedatives and hypnotics, below)	
BLOOD DERIVATIVES (PROTEINS)	
Albumin, normal serum (human), USP, 25% solution (Albumisol) *Available as:* 25 g albumin/dl	Dose: 2 ml/kg, or 60 ml/M^2 (IV)

*For individual drugs, see general index. *Consult package inserts.*

Key: M^2, dose per square meter of body surface; IM, intramuscular; ITh, intrathecal; IV, intravenous; O, oral; R, rectal; SC, subcutaneous; Subl, sublingual; T, topical.

TABLE 30–1 (*Continued*)

DRUG, HOW SUPPLIED	DOSAGE, ROUTES, CONTRAINDICATIONS AND WARNINGS
Immune serum globulin, USP, gamma globulin *Available as:* Solution (16.5%): 165 mg/ml, for injection	Dose: See index and Sections 9 and 10 **Caution:** IM only
BRONCHODILATORS	
Aminophylline, USP, theophylline with ethylenediamine (85% theophylline) *Available as:* Tablets: 100 and 200 mg Tablets (enteric coated): 100 and 200 mg Tablets (prolonged action); 300 mg Solution: 25 mg/ml (IV), for injection 250 mg/ml (IM), for injection 100 mg/ml (R) Suppositories: 0.125, 0.25, and 0.5 g (R) Rectal solution: 300 and 450 mg	Dose: 12 mg/kg/24 hr, or 0.4 g/M^2/24 hr; divide into 3 doses (IV or IM); rectal dose same as above dose **Caution:** Poisonous by all routes in overdosage; IV dose over 4–5 min or by drip; monitor theophylline plasma levels (5 μg/ml or below) (See Theophylline)
Ephedrine sulfate (See Adrenergics, above)	
Epinephrine hydrochloride (See Adrenergics, above)	
Isoproterenol (See Adrenergics, above)	
Pseudoephedrine hydrochloride, NF (Sudafed) *Available as:* Tablets (scored): 60 mg Tablets (coated): 30 mg Syrup: 30 mg/5 ml	Dose: 4 mg/kg/24 hr, or 125 mg/M^2/24 hr; divide into 4 doses (O) **Caution:** In hypertension
Theophylline, NF (many trade names) *Available as:* Tablets: 100 and 200 mg Elixir: 27 and 50 mg/5 ml Suppositories: 125, 250, and 500 mg	Dose: 10–15 mg/kg/24 hr, or 0.3–0.5 g/M^2/24 hr; divide into 2–3 doses (O) **Caution:** In giving other xanthines (aminophylline, caffeine, theobromine); may be contraindicated in peptic ulcer; care with cardiac, renal or hepatic disease, glaucoma, hyperthyroidism (plasma levels, see aminophylline) **Toxicity:** All routes; irritability and restlessness; hemorrhagic gastritis (vomiting of blood); convulsions, coma, death (cerebral edema)
CALCIUM SALTS	
Calcium chloride, USP (27% Ca) *Available as:* Solution: of desired strength (O) Solution: 100 mg/ml (10%), IV only	Dose: 0.3 g/kg/24 hr, or 8 g/M^2/24 hr; give as 2% solution, divided into 4 doses (every 6 hr) (O); rarely IV **Caution:** Acidifying; give 2–3 days, then change to another calcium salt (newborn); gastric irritation; well diluted and slowly IV; bradycardia, local necrosis with leakage from vein; avoid scalp
Calcium gluceptate, USP (8% Ca) *Available as:* Injection: 22% solution (220 mg/ml), for IV use only; 1 ml = 2 ml of calcium gluconate (10%); 1 ml = 18 mg elemental calcium (0.9 mEq)	Dose: See calcium gluconate; in exchange transfusions in newborns, 0.5 ml after each 100 ml of blood exchanged

Table continued.

TABLE 30–1 (*Continued*)

DRUG, HOW SUPPLIED	DOSAGE, ROUTES, CONTRAINDICATIONS AND WARNINGS*
Calcium gluconate, USP (9% Ca) *Available as:* Powder: (O) Tablets: 0.5 and 1 g Solution: 100 mg/ml (10%), IV only	Dose: 0.5 g/kg/24 hr, or 12 g/M^2/24 hr; divided doses (O or IV diluted and slowly) **Warning:** Not for intramuscular injection in infants and children (abscess formation at site) **Precautions:** Can affect action of digitalis (in digitalized patients may produce arrhythmias) **Adverse reactions:** Bradycardia and local necrosis with leakage from vein; avoid scalp veins as site of injection
Calcium lactate, USP (13% Ca) *Available as:* Powder: (O) Tablets: 0.3 and 0.6 g Wafers: 0.5 and 1 g	Dose: 0.5 g/kg/24 hr, or 12 g/M^2/24 hr; divided doses (O)
CARDIOVASCULAR DRUGS (See also Section 13)	
ANTIARRHYTHMICS	
Procainamide hydrochloride, USP (Pronestyl hydrochloride) *Available as:* Capsules: 0.25, 0.375 and 0.5 g Solution: 100 mg/ml, for injection	Dose: 50 mg/kg/24 hr, or 1.5 g/M^2/24 hr; divide into 4–6 doses/24 hr (O); see Section 13 for IV use **Caution:** Observe for untoward myocardial responses; digitalization reduces these responses; ventricular tachycardia hazardous if myocardium is damaged; danger of emboli with correction of atrial fibrillation; conduction depression in pre-existing A-V conduction disturbances; monitor parenteral use with ECG (discontinue with impending block); stop drug if significant ventricular slowing without gaining regular A-V conduction; signs of overdose with liver and kidney disease; lupus-like syndrome, positive Coombs test, thrombopenia; reversible with discontinuation usually, steroid treatment if not; regular LE test, with maintenance therapy; peripheral dilatation – lowered blood pressure greatest with IV use; hypersensitivity, agranulocytosis (warn of signs) **Contraindications:** Myasthenia gravis, sensitivity to this drug, complete heart block
Propranolol hydrochloride, USP (Inderal) *Available as:* Tablets: 10 and 40 mg Ampules: 1 mg/ml	Doses: Established *for adults only;* oral route preferred Dose (arrhythmias): 10–30 mg (single dose) for adults; 3–4 doses/24 hr (before meals and at bedtime) Dose (hypertrophic aortic stenosis): 20–40 mg (single dose) for adults; 3–4 doses/24 hr (before meals and at bedtime) Dose (pheochromocytoma): Preoperatively, 60 mg/24 hr for adults, in divided doses for 3 days (with alpha-adrenergic blocking agent); in inoperable or metastatic tumor, 30 mg/24 hr, in divided doses Dose (intravenous, with ECG monitoring): 1–3 mg for adults; rate not to exceed 1 mg/min; repeat dose, if needed, after 2 min; no additional dosage within 4 hr; change to oral dosage as soon as possible; for excessive bradycardia, atropine, 0.5–1 mg (IV) **Contraindications:** In bronchial asthma, allergic rhinitis (pollen season), sinus bradycardia, greater than second-degree block, including total heart block, cardiogenic shock, right ventricular hypertension secondary to pulmonary hypertension, congestive heart failure (unless failure is secondary to a tachyarrhythmia treatable with this drug), patients receiving anesthetics producing myocardial depression, and patients on adrenergic-augmenting psychotropic drugs (including MAO inhibitors), and during 2-wk withdrawal periods of such drug **Warning:** *Cardiac failure:* May depress myocardial contractility and precipitate cardiac failure by blocking sympathetic stimulation. *In frank or incipient failure:* Use of this drug should be carried out cautiously,

*For individual drugs, see general index. *Consult package inserts.*

Key: M^2, dose per square meter of body surface; IM, intramuscular; ITh, intrathecal; IV, intravenous; O, oral; R, rectal; SC, subcutaneous; Subl, sublingual; T, topical.

TABLE 30–1 (*Continued*)

DRUG, HOW SUPPLIED	DOSAGE, ROUTES, CONTRAINDICATIONS AND WARNINGS
	preferably with concurrent digitalization. *Patients without history of failure:* With first signs of failure during use of this drug, patients should be fully digitalized and observed closely; (a) if failure progresses, withdraw use of propranolol, (b) if tachyarrhythmia is controlled, maintain on combined dosage, follow closely until threat of failure is over. *Hypoglycemia-prone patients:* This drug may prevent appearance of premonitory signs and symptoms (pulse rate and pulse pressure changes) of acute hypoglycemia; caution in use of this drug in patients subject to hypoglycemia or in diabetics receiving insulin or oral hypoglycemic agents. *In pregnancy:* Use of any drug in pregnancy or women of childbearing potential requires weighing risk to mother and/or fetus against expected therapeutic benefit. (Safe use of this drug in pregnancy has not been established.) **Caution:** Closely observe patients receiving catecholamine-depleting drugs when propranolol use is introduced; use with caution in patients with impaired renal or hepatic failure; may produce hypotension and/or marked bradycardia (vertigo, syncope, orthostatic hypotension), gastrointestinal symptoms, mental depression, rash, paresthesias, fever, sore throat, visual disturbances, hallucinations, respiratory distress and laryngospasm (IV use), elevated BUN (severe heart disease), elevated serum transaminase levels, purpura and alopecia; as with any new drug given over prolonged periods, observe laboratory parameters at regular intervals
Quinidine gluconate and sulfate, USP and other salts *Available as:* Tablets: 200 and 300 mg Tablets (enteric coated): 300 mg Tablets (prolonged action): 300 mg Capsules: 125, 200 and 300 mg Ampules: 80, 120 and 200 mg/ml	Dose: For test dose, 2 mg/kg, or 60 mg/M^2 (O, IV, or IM); for therapeutic dose, 30 mg/kg/24 hr, or 900 mg/M^2/24 hr, divided into 5 doses/24 hr (O, IV, or IM) **Caution:** See text, and package insert
ANTIHYPERTENSIVES AND VASODILATORS (See also Diuretics, below)	
Chlorthalidone (Hygroton) (See Diuretics, below)	
Diazoxide, USP (Hyperstat) *Available as:* Injection: 15 mg/ml	Dose (for hypertension); in adults, 300 mg (20 ml); in children; 5 mg/kg (0.3 ml/kg) or 175 mg/M^2 (12 ml/M^2); give as a single dose; inject (IV only) within 30 seconds (not added to drip); may need second dose in 30 minutes; repeated doses every 4–24 hr according to response; monitor blood pressure **Note:** Sodium and water retention with repeated doses **Contraindications:** Should not be used in the treatment of compensatory hypertension, such as that associated with aortic coarctation or arteriovenous shunt, or in patients hypersensitive to diazoxide or other thiazides, unless the potential benefits outweigh the possible risks. **Warnings:** May produce fetal or neonatal hyperbilirubinemia, thrombocytopenia, altered carbohydrate metabolism; *safety in children has not been* established; hypotension may occasionally result from administration (will usually respond to sympathomimetic agents); hyperglycemia in the majority of patients (usually requires treatment only in patients with diabetes mellitus); hyperglycemia and hyperosmolar coma with transient cataracts developed in one infant and in a few animals receiving repeated daily doses of intravenous or oral diazoxide; diazoxide causes sodium retention, repeated injections may precipitate edema and congestive heart failure (retention responds characteristically to diuretic agents if adequate renal function exists); thiazides may potentiate the antihypertensive, hyperglycemic, and hyperuricemic actions of diazoxide; may displace other substances or drugs which are also bound to protein, such as bilirubin

Table continued.

TABLE 30–1 (*Continued*)

DRUG, HOW SUPPLIED	DOSAGE, ROUTES, CONTRAINDICATIONS AND WARNINGS*
Guanethidine sulfate, USP (Ismelin) *Available as:* Tablets (scored): 10 and 25 mg	Dose: 0.2 mg/kg/24 hr, or 6 mg/M^2/24 hr, as a single dose (O); increase every 7–10 days by above dose as added increment; effective dose may be 5–8 times initial dose **Contraindications:** Monoamine oxidase inhibitors, pheochromocytoma **Caution:** In renal disease with increasing nitrogen retention, encephalopathy, in increased parasympathetic tone (peptic ulcer, etc.), incipient heart failure (edema); discontinue 2 wk before surgery; periodic blood counts and liver function tests; side effect of sympathetic blockage: hypotension, weakness, dizziness, increased bowel activity, bradycardia, urinary incontinence, nasal congestion, many others
Hydralazine hydrochloride, USP (Apresoline hydrochloride) *Available as:* Tablets: 10, 25, 50, and 100 mg Solution: 20 mg/ml, for injection	Dose (oral): Initial, 0.75 mg/kg/24 hr, or 25 mg/M^2/24 hr, divided into 4 doses (O); increase over next 3–4 wk to as much as 10 times above dose if necessary Dose (parenteral, with reserpine): 0.15 mg/kg, or 4 mg/M^2, as a single dose every 12–24 hr (IV or IM) Dose (parenteral, alone): 1.7–3.5 mg/kg/24 hr, or 50–100 mg/M^2/24 hr; divide into 4–6 doses (IV or IM) **Caution:** In reduced renal function; follow blood pressure more closely; cardiovascular, neurologic, gastrointestinal, hematologic (including agranulocytosis and purpura), and skin reactions; lupus-like and arthritis-like reactions
Magnesium sulfate (See Laxatives, below)	
Mecamylamine hydrochloride, NF (Inversine hydrochloride) *Available as:* Tablets: 2.5 and 10 mg	Dose (adult): Initial, 2.5 mg twice daily pc (O); increase 2.5 mg at intervals of 2 or more days to response; average *total* adult dose, 25 mg/24 hr; or 1.5 mg/M^2/24 hr (initial), divided into 2 doses pc (O), with an increase to 15 mg/M^2/24 hr **Caution:** In compromise of renal, cerebral or coronary blood flow; may cause dryness of mouth, blurred vision, diarrhea, constipation (avoid), urinary retention, vomiting, weakness, sedation, syncope, paresthesias, tremor, mental disturbances, postural hypotension
Methyldopa and methyldopate hydrochloride, USP (Aldomet) *Available as:* Tablets: 250 mg Solution: 50 mg/ml, for injection	Dose (oral): 10 mg/kg/24 hr, or 300 mg/M^2/24 hr, divided into 2–3 doses (O); increase or decrease to desired effect; increase at 2-day or more intervals to not more than 65 mg/kg/24 hr, or 2 g/M^2/24 hr Dose (intravenous in crises): 20–40 mg/kg/24 hr, or 0.6–1.2 g/M^2/24 hr, divided into 4 doses (IV); continue same dosage orally when controlled **Contraindications:** Active hepatic disease, pheochromocytoma **Caution:** In hepatic disease (history); may cause sedation, headache, weakness, dizziness, cardiovascular insufficiency, orthostatic hypotension, bradycardia, nasal stuffiness, gastrointestinal symptoms, edema, heart failure, dark urine (in air), psychic changes, fever, abnormal liver function tests, jaundice, BUN rise, hemolytic anemia, positive Coombs test, granulocyte depression, spurious high urinary catecholamines; do hepatic function tests and WBC and differential counts at intervals, first 6 to 8 wk of treatment or with fever (unexplained)
Reserpine, USP Raurine, Reserpoid, Sandril, Serpasil, Serpate, and other trade names) *Available as:* Tablets: 0.1, 0.25, 0.5, 1, 2, 3, 4, and 5 mg Tablets (prolonged action): 0.25 and 0.5 mg	Dose (general): 0.02 mg/kg/24 hr, or 0.6 mg/M^2/24 hr; divide into 1 or 2 doses/24 hr (O) Dose (hypertension): 0.07 mg/kg/dose, or 2 mg/M^2/dose, with hydralazine every 12–24 hr (IM) **Contraindications:** Hypersensitivity to rauwolfia alkaloids; in patients with mental depression (especially with suicidal tendencies), active peptic ulcer, ulcerative colitis, or receiving electroconvulsive therapy **Warnings:** Extreme caution with a history of mental depression (drug-induced depression may persist for several months after drug withdrawal

*For individual drugs, see general index. *Consult package inserts.*

Key: M^2, dose per square meter of body surface; IM, intramuscular; ITh, intrathecal; IV, intravenous; O, oral; R, rectal; SC, subcutaneous; Subl, sublingual; T, topical.

TABLE 30–1 (*Continued*)

DRUG, HOW SUPPLIED	DOSAGE, ROUTES, CONTRAINDICATIONS AND WARNINGS
Elixir: 0.25 and 1.25 mg/5 ml Liquid: 2 mg/ml (dropper bottle) Solution: 2.5 and 5 mg/ml, for injection	and may be severe enough to result in suicide); increased respiratory secretions, nasal congestion, cyanosis, and anorexia may occur in *infants born to reserpine-treated mothers* since this preparation is known to cross the placental barrier, appearing in cord blood and breast milk **Precautions:** With a history of peptic ulcer, ulcerative colitis, or gallstones when biliary colic may be precipitated. Patients on high dosage should be observed carefully at regular intervals to detect possible reactivation of peptic ulcer; when treating hypertensive patients with renal insufficiency since they adjust poorly to lowered blood pressure levels; with digitalis and quinidine since cardiac arrhythmias have occurred with reserpine. Preoperative withdrawal of reserpine does not insure that circulatory instability will not occur. It is important that the anesthesiologist be aware of the patient's drug intake since hypotension has occurred **Adverse reactions:** *Gastrointestinal* (hypersecretion, nausea and vomiting, anorexia and diarrhea); *cardiovascular* (angina-like symptoms, arrhythmias, particularly when used concurrently with digitalis or quinidine, and bradycardia); *neurologic* (drowsiness, depression, nervousness, paradoxical anxiety, nightmares, rare Parkinsonism, dull sensorium, deafness, glaucoma, uveitis, and optic atrophy); *nasal congestion* is a frequent complaint; for *others* see package insert
Thiazides (See Diuretics, below)	
CARDIOTONICS (Digitalis-type preparations; see also Section 13)	Individualize digitalizing and maintenance doses *for each patient*
Deslanoside, desacetyllanatoside C, NF (Cedilanid D) *Available as:* Solution: 0.2 mg/ml, for injection	Dose (digitalizing): In premature and full-term newborn infants, or with reduced renal function or myocarditis, 0.022 mg/kg, or 0.3 mg/M^2; in age range 2 wk to 3 yr, 0.025 mg/kg, or 0.75 mg/M^2; after age 3 yr, 0.0225 mg/kg, or 0.75 mg/M^2; divide into 2–3 doses (IV or IM) with 3–4 hr between doses; in emergency, single dose (IV or IM) **Caution:** Patient should not have had digitalis or long-acting derivatives for 2 wk or more; give slowly, IV; watch ECG, redigitalize with digoxin in 12–24 hr (with care)
Digitalis (leaf), **NF** *Available as:* Tablets: 30, 50, 55, 60, 83, and 100 mg Capsules: 60 and 100 mg Pills: 30, 50, 60, and 100 mg Tincture: 1 ml = 0.1 g Ampules: Variety of preparations	Dose (digitalizing): Under age 1 yr, 0.045 g/kg; 1–2 yr, 0.04 g/kg; over 2 yr, 0.03 g/kg; or 0.75 g/M^2; divide total dose into 3, 4, or more portions with 6 hr or more between doses (O, IV, or IM) Dose (maintenance): Give 1/10 of digitalizing dose daily **Caution:** Patient should not have had digitalis or long-acting derivatives for 2 wk or more; lower dose with renal failure or myocarditis and in premature or full-term infants
Digitoxin, USP (Crystodigin, Digitaline nativelle, Purodigin) *Available as:* Tablets (scored): 0.05, 0.1, 0.15, and 0.2 mg Capsules (in oil): 0.1 and 0.2 mg Solution: 1 mg/ml 0.02 mg/drop Elixir: 0.05 mg/ml Solution: for injection 0.02 mg/ml 0.2 mg/ml	Dose (digitalization): Individualize for each patient; in premature and full-term infants, or with reduced renal function, and myocarditis, 0.022 mg/kg, or 0.3–0.35 mg/M^2; after age 2 wk, and under age 1 yr, 0.045 mg/kg; age 1–2 yr, 0.04 mg/kg; over age 2 yr, 0.03 mg/kg; or 0.75 mg/M^2; divide total dose into 3, 4 or more portions with 6 hr or more between doses (O, IV or IM) Dose (maintenance): Give 1/10 of digitalizing dose daily **Caution:** Patient should not have had digitalis or long-acting derivatives for 2 wk or more
Digoxin, USP (Lanoxin, Saroxin) *Available as:* Tablets (scored): 0.125, 0.25, 0.375, and 0.5 mg Elixir: 0.05 mg/ml (calibrated dropper)	Dose (premature and full-term infants (or in reduced renal function, myocarditis)): Digitalizing dose, 0.03–0.05 mg/kg (IV or IM), or 0.75 mg/M^2 (IV or IM); maintenance dose, 1/10–1/5 of digitalizing dose (O, IV, or IM) Dose (infants age 2 wk to 2 yr): Digitalizing dose (O), 0.06–0.08 mg/kg, or 1.5 mg/M^2; maintenance dose (O), 1/5–1/3 of digitalizing dose; digitalizing dose (IV or IM), 0.04–0.06 mg/kg; maintenance dose (IV or IM), 1/10–1/5 of digitalizing dose

Table continued.

TABLE 30–1 (*Continued*)

DRUG, HOW SUPPLIED	DOSAGE, ROUTES, CONTRAINDICATIONS AND WARNINGS *
Solution: 0.25 mg/ml, for injection Pediatric: 0.1 mg/ml	Dose (children over 2 yr): Digitalizing dose (O), 0.04–0.06 mg/kg, or 1.5 mg/M²; maintenance dose (O), 1/5–1/3 of digitalizing dose; digitalizing dose (IV or IM), 0.02–0.04 mg/kg; maintenance dose (IM or IV), 1/5 of digitalizing dose Regimen: Divide total dose into 3, 4, or more portions with 6 hr or more between doses **Caution:** Patient should not have had digitalis or long-acting derivatives for 2 wk or more; regimens must be individualized, especially in the newborn period
Lanatoside C, (Cedilanid)	Emergency use only: See Section 13
Ouabain, G-strophanthin, USP *Available as:* Solution: 0.25 mg/ml, for injection	Dose: 0.01 mg/kg, or 0.3 mg/M²; 1/2 of dose stat (IV), then fractions of dose every 30 min until response or total dose given (IV); check patient and ECG before each dose; redigitalize with long-acting drug 12 hr after onset of treatment **Caution:** Not to be given if a long-acting digitalis-type of drug given in preceding 2 wk
CATHARTICS (See Laxatives, below)	
CHOLINERGIC BLOCKING AGENTS	
Atropine sulfate, USP *Available as:* Tablets: 0.3, 0.4, and 0.6 mg. Solution: 0.3, 0.4, 0.5, 0.6, 0.8, 1, 1.2, and 2 mg/ml, for injection	Dose: For preanesthetic, see Section 5 Dose: For general use, 0.01 mg/kg/dose (maximum, 0.4 mg), or 0.3 mg/M²/dose; may repeat every 4–6 hr (SC) Antidote: See Section 28 **Contraindications:** Glaucoma, hypersensitivity **Caution:** May cause dry mouth, blurred vision (motor vehicle warning), photophobia, anhidrosis (fever), constipation (completing partial gastrointestinal obstruction), urinary retention, bronchial plugging; major CNS signs (see Section 28); milder CNS signs (dizziness, restlessness, fatigue, tremor); hypersensitivity reactions (rash, exfoliation), leukocytosis **Toxicity:** See Section 28
Belladonna tincture, USP *Available as:* Tincture: About 0.3 mg atropine/ml	Dose: 0.1 ml/kg/24 hr (maximum, 3.5 ml/day), or 2.5 ml/M²/24 hr; divide into 3–4 doses (O) **Contraindications and caution:** See atropine sulfate **Toxicity:** See Section 28
Methantheline bromide, NF (Banthine bromide) *Available as:* Tablets (scored): 50 mg Solution: 50 mg, for injection	Dose: 6 mg/kg/24 hr, or 150 mg/M²/24 hr; divide into 4 doses (O or IM) **Contraindications:** Glaucoma, severe cardiac disease **Caution:** Dry mouth, blurred vision (motor vehicle operation warning), mydriasis, constipation, urinary retention, central nervous stimulation, tachycardia
Methscopolamine bromide, NF, scopolamine methylbromide (Ampyrox, Lescopine bromide, Pamine bromide, Proscomide, Scoline, Tropane) *Available as:* Tablets: 2.5 mg Capsules: 7.5 mg Syrup: 1.25 mg/5 ml Solution: 1 mg/ml, for injection	Dose: 0.2 mg/kg/24 hr, or 6 mg/M²/24 hr; divide into 4 doses pc and hs (O) **Contraindication:** Glaucoma **Caution:** In cardiac disease, pyloric obstruction; may cause dry mouth, blurred vision (motor vehicle operation warning), constipation, dysphagia, urinary retention, dizziness, flushing of skin, nausea

*For individual drugs, see general index. *Consult package inserts.*

Key: M², dose per square meter of body surface; IM, intramuscular; ITh, intrathecal; IV, intravenous; O, oral; R, rectal; SC, subcutaneous; Subl, sublingual; T, topical.

TABLE 30–1 (*Continued*)

DRUG, HOW SUPPLIED	DOSAGE, ROUTES, CONTRAINDICATIONS AND WARNINGS
Oxyphenonium bromide (Antrenyl bromide) *Available as:* Tablets (scored): 5 mg	Dose: 0.8 mg/kg/24 hr, or 25 mg/M^2/24 hr; divide into 4 doses (O); not released for children **Contraindications:** Glaucoma, pyloric obstruction, obstructive uropathy **Caution:** May cause dryness of mouth (motor vehicle operation warning), urinary retention, constipation, weakness, drowsiness, vomiting, tachycardia, skin rash, flushing, urticaria
Propantheline bromide, USP (Pro-Banthine) *Available as:* Tablets (coated): 7.5 and 15 mg prolonged action, 30 mg Sterile: 30 mg	Dose: 1.5 mg/kg/24 hr, or 40 mg/M^2/24 hr (O); divide into 4 doses pc and hs **Contraindications:** See methantheline bromide **Caution:** See methantheline bromide
Scopolamine hydrobromide, USP (hyoscine hydrobromide) *Available as:* Tablets: 0.3, 0.4, 0.6, and 1.2 mg Solution: 0.3, 0.4, 0.5, 0.6, 0.8, and 1 mg/ml, for injection	Dose: 0.006 mg/kg, or 0.20 mg/M^2, as single dose (O or SC) **Contraindications, caution, and toxicity:** See atropine, Section 28
CHOLINERGIC DRUGS (Parasympathomimetics)	
Bethanechol chloride, NF (Urecholine chloride) *Available as:* Tablets: 5, 10, and 25 mg Solution: 5 mg/ml, for injection	Dose: 0.6 mg/kg, or 20 mg/M^2; divide into 3 doses (O); 1/3–1/4 of above dose (SC); avoid IV or IM use Dose (sweat chloride test): To prepare test solution add 1 ml (5 mg) to 3 ml 5% glucose in water; under 1 yr give 0.4 ml (0.5 mg) of test solution; over 1 yr, 0.8 ml (1 mg); administer *intracutaneously;* avoid IV or IM use **Contraindications:** Bronchial asthma, intestinal or bladder neck obstruction **Caution:** Have atropine sulfate syringe immediately available; may cause flushed skin, sweating, asthma, hypotension, circulatory collapse, abdominal cramps, vomiting, diarrhea (bloody), shock, bradycardia, cardiac arrest; avoid IV or IM use **Antidote:** Atropine
Methacholine salts, NF (Mecholyl salts) *Available as:* Tablets (bromide): 0.2 g Sterile (chloride): 25 mg	Dose: Parenterally, 0.1–0.4 mg/kg, or 3–12 mg/M^2, as a single dose (SC); orally, start with 10 times above dose **Contraindications, caution, and toxicity:** See bethanechol above
Pilocarpine hydrochloride *Available as:* Tablets (hypodermic): 15 mg	Dose: 0.1 mg/kg, or 3 mg/M^2, as a single dose (IM or SC) **Contraindications, caution, and toxicity:** See bethanechol, above
CHOLINESTERASE INHIBITORS	
Ambenonium chloride, NF (Mytelase chloride) *Available as:* Tablets: 5, 10, and 25 mg	Dose: Individualize dose; initially, 0.3 mg/kg/24 hr, or 10 mg/M^2/24 hr; for maintenance, increase to 1.5 mg/kg/24 hr, or 50 mg/M^2/24 hr, divided into 3 or 4 doses (O) **Contraindications:** Intestinal or urinary tract obstruction; extreme caution in bronchial asthma **Caution:** May cause muscarinic effects (salivation, sweating, bronchial constriction, vomiting, abdominal cramps, diarrhea, hypotension, etc.), and nicotinic effects (muscle cramps, fasciculations, muscle weakness)
Edrophonium chloride, USP (Tensilon chloride) *Available as:* Solution: 10 mg/ml, for injection	Dose: For myasthenia gravis test, 0.2 mg/kg, or 6 mg/M^2, given as a single dose; give 1/5 of dose slowly IV in 1 min; if tolerated, give remainder; in premature infants, 1 mg single dose (IM or SC) **Warning:** When testing, keep atropine sulfate syringe ready; with caution in bronchial asthma, cardiac dysrhythmias **Caution:** May cause cholinergic reactions (See bethanechol, above)

Table continued.

TABLE 30–1 (*Continued*)

DRUG, HOW SUPPLIED	DOSAGE, ROUTES, CONTRAINDICATIONS AND WARNINGS*
Neostigmine bromide and methylsulfate, USP (Prostigmin bromide and methylsulfate) *Available as:* Tablets: 15 mg Solution, for injection: 0.25 mg/ml (1:4000) 0.5 mg/ml (1:2000) 1 mg/ml (1:1000)	Dose: 2 mg/kg/24 hr, or 60 mg/M²/24 hr; divide into 6–8 doses (O) Dose: For myasthenia gravis test, 0.04 mg/kg/dose (IM), or 1 mg/M²/dose (IM); or 1/2 of above dose (IV) **Contraindications:** As for bethanechol chloride **Caution:** As for bethanechol chloride **Toxicity:** As for bethanecol chloride
Pyridostigmine bromide, USP (Mestinon bromide) *Available as:* Tablets (scored): 60 mg Tablets (prolonged action): 180 mg Syrup: 60 mg/5 ml Injection: 5 mg/ml	Dose: 7 mg/kg/24 hr, or 200 mg/M²/24 hr; divide into 5–6 doses (O) **Contraindications:** See ambenonium **Caution:** Difficulty in differentiation of muscle weakness (including respiratory muscles and death) of cholinergic crisis from overdosage and myasthenic crisis; may cause side effects (see ambenonium), bromide rash **Toxicity:** See bethanechol; atropine may mask signs of overdosage
DECONGESTANTS (NASAL) (See Bronchodilators, above)	
DIAGNOSTIC AGENTS	
Edrophonium chloride (See Cholinesterase inhibitors, above)	
Iodized oil, NF (Descendant Lipiodol) *Available as:* Ampules (40% I): 1, 2, 3, 5, and 10 ml Vials (40% I): 20 ml	Dose: Orally, 40% I; for infants, 5 ml; for weight 10–20 kg, 0.5 ml/kg (maximum, 10 ml) **Caution:** Do not use if dark in color; alters PBI test; iodine sensitivity (urticaria, skin eruptions)
Neostigmine methylsulfate (See Cholinesterase inhibitors, above)	
Phentolamine mesylate, USP; hydrochloride, NF (Regitine mesylate and hydrochloride) *Available as:* Tablets (hydrochloride): 50 mg Solution (mesylate): 5 mg, for injection	Dose (for pheochromocytoma test): In adults, 5 mg; in child, 0.1 mg/kg, or 3 mg/M²; give as single dose (IV) Dose (therapeutic): 5 mg/kg, or 150 mg/M²; divide into 4–6 doses (O) **Caution:** May cause tachycardia, weakness, dizziness, flushing, orthostatic hypotension, nasal stuffiness, gastrointestinal disturbances
DIURETICS	
ACIDIFIERS (See Acidifiers, above)	
ALDOSTERONE INHIBITOR (See Endocrines, below)	
CARBONIC ANHYDRASE INHIBITOR	
Acetazolamide, USP (Diamox) *Available as:* Tablets (scored): 250 mg Syrup: 250 mg/5 ml For injection (sodium): 500 mg	Dose (diuretic): 5 mg/kg/24 hr, or 150 mg/M²/24 hr; single daily dose (O, IM) Dose (epilepsy or glaucoma): 8–30 mg/kg/24 hr, or 300–900 mg/M²/24 hr; divide into 3–4 doses (O) **Contraindications:** With depression of serum Na or K, marked hepatic or kidney disease or dysfunction, adrenal failure, hyperchloremic acidosis **Caution:** Increasing dose may increase drowsiness or paresthesias; may cause sulfonamide-type reactions (fever, rash, crystalluria, renal cal-

*For individual drugs, see general index. *Consult package inserts.*

Key: M², dose per square meter of body surface; IM, intramuscular; ITh, intrathecal; IV, intravenous; O, oral; R, rectal; SC, subcutaneous; Subl, sublingual; T, topical.

TABLE 30–1 (*Continued*)

DRUG, HOW SUPPLIED	DOSAGE, ROUTES, CONTRAINDICATIONS AND WARNINGS
	culus, blood dyscrasias); polyuria, drowsiness, confusion, urticaria, melena, hematuria, glycosuria, hepatic insufficiency, paralysis, convulsions; acidosis (long-term therapy)
MERCURIALS	
Meralluride, NF (Mercuhydrin) *Available as:* Solution (sodium): 130 mg/ml (1 ml contains equivalent of 39 mg Hg and 48 mg theophylline)	Dose: Below 3 kg, 0.125 ml; 3–7 kg, 0.25 ml; 8–15 kg, 0.5 ml; 16–25 kg, 0.75 ml; 26–35 kg, 1 ml; or 1 ml/M² per dose (IM); give once or twice weekly, no more frequently than once daily **Contraindications:** Acute nephritis, intractable oliguria **Caution:** Idiosyncrasy (gastrointestinal disturbances, vertigo, fever, skin reactions); observe for electrolyte imbalance, renal function; use only clean, dry, sterile syringe
Mercaptomerin sodium, USP (Thiomerin sodium) *Available as:* Solution: 125 mg/ml (1 ml equivalent to 40 mg Hg), for injection Syringe (disposable): 125 mg (40 mg Hg) 250 mg (80 mg Hg)	Dose: Same as for meralluride injection **Contraindications:** Nephritis (acute and subacute), ulcerative colitis, dehydration, mercurial sensitivity **Caution:** Maintain sufficient Na intake, instruct patient and/or parents about symptoms of salt depletion; sensitivity may occur (flushed face, fever, chills, gastrointestinal disturbances, skin eruptions, pruritus, urticaria)
THIAZIDES	
Bendroflumethiazide, NF (Naturetin) *Available as:* Tablets: 2.5 and 5 mg	Dose (edema): Initial, up to 0.4 mg/kg, or 12 mg/M², in single or 2 divided doses (O); for maintenance, 1/8–1/4 of above dose, as a single dose (O) Dose (hypertension): Initial, 1/4 to full initial edema dose, given in a single or 2 divided doses (O); for maintenance, 1/8 to 3/4 initial edema dose, given in a single or divided into 2 doses (O) **Contraindications:** In anuria; discontinue if azotemia and oliguria occur during treatment of severe renal disease **Warning:** May precipitate or increase azotemia; avoid cumulation in impaired renal function **Caution:** In hepatic cirrhosis; decrease dose of other antihypertensive drugs; bowel ulcerations (stenosis) associated with thiazides and enteric-coated K salts (care in administration, discontinue with symptoms); observe and test for fluid and electrolyte imbalance (serum and urinary electrolyte determinations) if symptoms suggest (dry mouth, thirst, weakness, muscle pains, hypotension, oliguria, tachycardia, gastrointestinal); avoid hypokalemia and low salt syndrome; hypokalemia may develop with ACTH, steroids or cirrhosis; hypokalemia dangerous with digitalis treatment; discontinue 48 hr before elective surgery; insulin requirements may change; may cause hyperglycemia and glycosuria, blood dyscrasias, jaundice, paresthesias, neonatal thrombocytopenia, glomerulonephritis, pancreatitis, and jaundice (hyperbilirubinemia), weakness, dizziness
Chlorothiazide, NF (Diuril) *Available as:* Tablets (scored): 250 and 500 mg Syrup: 250 mg/5 ml For injection (sodium): 500 mg (IV)	Dose: 20 mg/kg/24 hr, or 600 mg/M²/24 hr; divide into 2 doses (O) **Contraindications and caution:** See bendroflumethiazide
Hydrochlorothiazide, USP (Esidrix, HydroDiuril, Oretic) *Available as:* Tablets (scored): 25 and 50 mg	Dose: 1/10 of chlorothiazide dose **Contraindications and caution:** See bendroflumethiazide
OTHER DIURETICS	
Chlorthalidone, USP (Hygroton) *Available as:*	Dose: Initial, 2 mg/kg, or 60 mg/M², given in single dose, repeat 3 times a week; for maintenance, adjust to need

Table continued.

TABLE 30–1 *(Continued)*

DRUG, HOW SUPPLIED	DOSAGE, ROUTES, CONTRAINDICATIONS AND WARNINGS *
Tablets (scored): 50 and 100 mg	**Contraindications:** Hypersensitivity to this drug, severe renal or hepatic disease **Warning:** Enteric-coated K salts (alone or with thiazide or other diuretics) may be associated with bowel ulcerations **Caution:** Use with care with ganglionic blocking agents, other antihypertensives or curare; periodic BUN, stop drug if rising or if aggravated liver dysfunction; observe for K, Na depletion (muscle weakness, cramps, gastrointestinal symptoms, lethargy, confusion); supply sufficient dietary salt; hypokalemia may develop with ACTH, steroid, digitalis treatment, or cirrhosis; nausea, weakness, headache, dizziness, hypotension, myopia, dysuria, skin reactions, purpura, hyperglycemia, glycosuria, hyperuricemia, blood dyscrasias, pancreatitis, jaundice, paresthesias, necrotizing angiitis may occur
Ethacrynic acid and sodium ethacrynate, USP (Edecrin) *Available as:* Tablets (scored): 25 and 50 mg Solution (sodium): 50 mg, for injection	Dose: For children only; initial, 25 mg, as a single dose (O); for maintenance, increase by 25-mg increments to effect; then maintain on alternate daily schedule, or alternate therapy periods with rest periods **Contraindications:** Anuria, increasing azotemia or oliguria during treatment **Caution:** Follow electrolytes and blood pressure; care in cirrhosis, digitalized patients; weakness, muscle cramps, paresthesias, hyponatremia, hypokalemia, hypotension, shock, hypouricemia, hypoglycemia, gastrointestinal symptoms, jaundice, agranulocytosis, purpura, CNS symptoms, rash may occur; no dose for infants available; similarly, *insufficient pediatric experience precludes recommendation for IV use*
Furosemide, USP (Lasix) *Available as:* Tablets (scored): 40 mg Injection: 10 mg/ml	Dose (adults): initial *oral* dose, 40–80 mg as a single dose, with a second dose in 6–8 hr, and maintenance doses at that interval if response satisfactory; if response not satisfactory, increase dose by 40 mg at 6–8 hr intervals until effect achieved; continue this final (titrated) dose 1–2 times/24 hr (up to 600 mg/24 hr); (40 mg = approximately 0.6 mg/kg or 23 mg/M^2); for *parenteral* administration, proceed as for oral using an initial dose of 20 mg and 20 mg increments at intervals of 2 or more hours; parenteral maintenance 1–2 times/24 hr (IM or IV slowly); replace with oral therapy when practical; for *management of hypertension,* use 40 mg twice daily, reducing dose or discontinuing of other antihypertensives as appropriate, or adding others if necessary Dose (children): No dosage or safety has been established for this drug in children (see Therapeutic Orphans, Section 5) **Contraindications:** In women of childbearing potential except in life threatening situations (balance efficacy against the teratogenic and embryotoxic potential demonstrated in animal studies); in anuria; in hepatic coma and in states of electrolyte depletion, until the basic condition is improved or corrected; in patients with hypersensitivity to this compound; until more experience is accumulated; *children should not be treated* with the drug **Warnings:** Excessive diuresis may result in dehydration and reduction in blood volume, with circulatory collapse and with the possibility of vascular thrombosis and embolism; excessive loss of potassium in patients receiving digitalis glycosides may precipitate digitalis toxicity; care should also be exercised in patients receiving potassium depleting steroids (frequent serum electrolyte, CO_2 and BUN determinations should be performed during the first few months of therapy and periodically thereafter); with hepatic cirrhosis and ascites, initiation of therapy is best carried out in the hospital (see package insert); observe regularly for possible blood dyscrasias, liver damage, or other idiosyncratic reactions **Precautions:** Electrolyte depletion may occur; may potentiate the hypotensive effect of antihypertensive medications; hyperuricemia can occur and gout may rarely be precipitated; reversible elevations of BUN may

*For individual drugs, see general index. *Consult package inserts.*

Key: M^2, dose per square meter of body surface; IM, intramuscular; ITh, intrathecal; IV, intravenous; O, oral; R, rectal; SC, subcutaneous; Subl, sublingual; T, topical.

TABLE 30-1 ***(Continued)***

DRUG, HOW SUPPLIED	DOSAGE, ROUTES, CONTRAINDICATIONS AND WARNINGS
	be seen in association with dehydration; reversible deafness and tinnitus have been reported (transient deafness is more likely to occur in patients with severe impairment of renal function and in patients who are also receiving drugs known to be ototoxic); periodic checks on urine and blood glucose should be made in diabetics and those suspected of latent diabetes; patients receiving high doses of salicylates may experience salicylate toxicity at lower doses because of competitive renal excretory sites; furosemide may enhance the nephrotoxicity of cephaloridine. (they should not be administered simultaneously); advisable to discontinue oral furosemide for one week and parenteral two days prior to any elective surgery. **Adverse Reactions:** Dermatitis, including urticaria and rare cases of exfoliative dermatitis, erythema multiforme pruritus, paresthesia, blurring of vision, postural hypotension, nausea, vomiting, or diarrhea, may occur; anemia, leukopenia, aplastic anemia, and thrombocytopenia (with purpura) may occur (rare cases of agranulocytosis have occurred which responded to treatment); reversible deafness and tinnitus reported when injected at doses exceeding several times the usual therapeutic dose; for other reactions, see package insert; transient pain after intramuscular injection has been reported at the injection site
Glycerin, USP *Available as:* Chemical (USP) *or* Solution (flavored): Osmoglyn (50%)	Dose: 1–1.5 g/kg, or 40 g/M²; single dose (O) in water or milk; repeat in 4–8 hr **Caution:** Nausea, diarrhea, headache; local dental caries (pain)
Mannitol, USP (Osmitrol) *Available as:* Solution (for injection): 50, 100, 150, 200, and 250 mg/ml (5, 10, 15, 20, 25%)	Dose (oliguria, anuria): As a test dose, 0.2 g/kg, or 6 g/M²; single dose, given within 3–5 min (IV) Dose (edema, ascites): As 15–20% solution, 2 g/kg, or 60 g/M²; given over 2–6 hr (IV) Dose (cerebral or ocular): Above dose, in 30–60 min Dose (intoxication): As 5–10% solution, 2 g/kg, or 60 g/M²; continued as needed or until this dose is reached (IV) **Caution:** Circulatory overload, electrolyte imbalance, tremors and convulsions (hyponatremia), headache; nausea, chills, dizziness, tachycardia, intraocular hemorrhage, death in organic CNS disease, pulmonary hypertension; do not mix with infused blood
Spironolactone (Aldactone) (See Endocrines, Aldosterone Inhibitor, below)	
Triamterene, USP (Dyrenium) *Available as:* Capsules: 100 mg	Dose: Initial, 2–4 mg/kg/24 hr (maximum, 300 mg/24 hr), or 60–120 mg/M²/24 hr; divide into 1–2 doses pc every other day (O) **Contraindications:** Severe or progressive kidney disease or dysfunction (except possibly nephrosis), severe hepatic disease, hypersensitivity to this drug, patients with pre-existing hyperkalemia or who develop hyperkalemia while on this drug; avoid potassium supplements (drug or diet) **Warning:** Observe regularly for blood dyscrasias, liver damage, other idiosyncrasies; do periodic BUN and serum K determinations **Caution:** Tends to conserve K, can cause hyperkalemia; withdraw use with elevated serum K; after prolonged use withdraw gradually; may aggravate electrolyte imbalances in heart failure, renal disease, cirrhosis; may cause low salt syndrome with salt restriction, nitrogen retention; observe for hypotension—may potentiate other antihypertensive drugs; may cause gastrointestinal symptoms, weakness, headache, dry mouth, anaphylaxis, photosensitivity, rash
Urea, USP *Available as:* Powder Sterile 16% solution: 40 g/250 ml (Ureaphil) 30% solution (in 10% invert	Dose: As diuretic, 0.8 g/kg/24 hr, or 25 g/M²/24 hr, divided into 3 doses (O) in juice, jelly, jam, etc; for cerebral and ocular use, 1–1.5 g/kg/dose, or 35 g/M²/dose, as solution IV over 30 min **Contraindications:** In severe renal or hepatic dysfunction, marked dehydration, intracranial bleeding **Caution:** May cause headache (relieved by narcotics and phenothiazines)

Table continued.

TABLE 30–1 (*Continued*)

DRUG, HOW SUPPLIED	DOSAGE, ROUTES, CONTRAINDICATIONS AND WARNINGS*
sugar) (Urevert): 40 g/120 ml and 90 g/270 ml	from dehydration, arm pain, phlebitis, skin blebs, slough (local injection sites), thrombosis (*prevent extravasation*); too rapid drip increases reactions – nausea, vomiting, confusion, nervousness, hyperthermia, tachycardia
Xanthines (See Bronchodilators, above)	
EMETICS	
Apomorphine hydrochloride, NF *Available as:* Tablets: 6 mg	Dose: 0.1 mg/kg, or 3 mg/M^2, as a single dose (SC) **Caution:** Do not use solution if green (decomposed)
Ipecac syrup, USP *Available as:* Syrup: 30 ml	Dose: Over 1 yr, 15 ml (O); follow with water; repeat once within 20 min, if needed **Contraindications:** Should not be given to unconscious patients. **Warnings:** Ipecac syrup may not be effective in those cases in which the ingested substance is an antiemetic; can exert a cardiotoxic effect if it is not vomited but is absorbed (recover unvomited doses by lavage); always *order by complete name* – ipecac *syrup* (other preparations, such as fluidextract are highly toxic) **Precautions:** Emesis is not always the proper treatment in cases of potential poisoning; should not be induced when such substances as petroleum distillates, strong alkali, acids, or strychnine are ingested **Note:** This *syrup* is available for over-the-counter sales in 30 ml (1 oz) bottles
ENDOCRINES	
ADRENAL CORTEX – GLUCOCORTICOSTEROIDS AND SYNTHETICS (anti-inflammatory)	*For drugs of this group:* **Contraindications:** In serious fungal, viral or bacterial infections for which adequate therapy is lacking, active tuberculosis (except see Section 10), peptic ulcer, recent intestinal anastomosis **Caution:** Large pharmacologic doses for prolonged periods may be associated with adverse reactions varying with particular drug used; reactions include edema, moon facies, acne, hirsutism, striae, bruising, prominent fat pads, increased appetite, headache, weakness, vertigo; more serious include growth retardation, osteoporosis, myopathy, hyperglycemic effects (increased insulin requirements), reduced resistance to infection, pseudotumor cerebri, papilledema, headache, vomiting, peptic ulcer, adrenal cortical atrophy, increased intravascular clotting, glaucoma, cataracts, CNS stimulation (euphoria, psychotic episodes); with great caution in healed tuberculosis; see individual diseases for uses; may need to give supplemental K and restrict Na
Cortisone acetate, USP (Cortone acetate) *Available as:* Tablets: 5, 10, and 25 mg Sterile suspension: 25 and 50 mg/ml, for injection	Dose: For *physiologic replacement,* 0.7 mg/kg/24 hr, or 20 mg/M^2/24 hr, divided into 3 doses (O), or once daily IM, as 1/3–1/2 of oral dose; for *adrenocortical virilism,* 1.75 mg/kg/24 hr, or 50 mg/M^2/24 hr, divided into 3–4 doses (O), or by an IM dose, the same as oral dose every third day or 1/3–1/2 once daily; for *pharmacologic effect* dose varies with disease; 2.5–10 mg/kg/24 hr, or 75–300 mg/M^2/24 hr, divided into 3–4 doses (O), or by IM dose, 1/3–1/2 of oral dose, every 12–24 hr
Dexamethasone and dexamethasone sodium phosphate, USP (Decadron, Deronil, Dexameth, Gammacorten, Hexadrol) *Available as:* Tablets (scored): 0.25, 0.5, 0.75, and 1.5 mg	Dose: 1/30 of cortisone dose

DRUGS

*For individual drugs, see general index. *Consult package inserts.*

Key: M^2, dose per square meter of body surface; IM, intramuscular; ITh, intrathecal; IV, intravenous; O, oral; R, rectal; SC, subcutaneous; Subl, sublingual; T, topical.

TABLE 30–1 (*Continued*)

DRUG, HOW SUPPLIED	DOSAGE, ROUTES, CONTRAINDICATIONS AND WARNINGS
Elixir: 0.5 mg/5 ml Solution (sodium phosphate): 4 mg/ml, for injection Solution (sodium phosphate): 1 and 4 mg/ml with lidocaine hydrochloride, for injection	
Hydrocortisone and salts, USP (Cortef, Cortril, Hydrocortone) *Available as:* Tablets: 5, 10, and 20 mg Oral suspension: 10 mg/5 ml Retention enema: 100 mg/60 ml Solution, for injection: Acetate, sterile suspension (intra-articular): 12.5, 25, and 50 mg/ml Sodium phosphate (IV, IM): 50 mg/ml Sodium succinate (IV, IM): 100, 250, 500 and 1000 mg	Dose: 4/5 of cortisone dose
Methylprednisolone, NF, and salts, USP (Medrol) *Available as:* Tablets (scored): 2, 4, and 16 mg Capsules (prolonged action): 2 and 4 mg Solution, for injection: Sterile for solution (IV): 40 and 125 mg in 1 or 2 ml Sterile suspension (IM), depot, intralesional: 20 and 40 mg/ml Enema: 40 mg/unit	Dose: 1/6 of cortisone dose
Prednisolone, USP (Delta-Cortef, Hydeltra, Meticortelone, Prednis, Sterane) *Available as:* Tablets (scored): 1, 2.5, and 6 mg Aerosol (T): 16.6 and 50 mg in 50 g	Dose: 1/5 of cortisone dose (O, IM, or IV)
Prednisolone acetate, USP *Available as:* Sterile suspension: 25 mg/ml (IM and intralesional)	Dose: As of prednisolone
Prednisolone butylacetate (Hydeltra-T.B.A.) *Available as:* Sterile suspension: 20 mg/ml (IM and intralesional)	Dose: As of prednisolone
Prednisolone sodium phosphate, USP (Hydeltrasol) *Available as:* Sterile solution: 20 mg/ml (IV, IM)	Dose: As of prednisolone
Prednisolone sodium succinate, NF (Meticortelone soluble) *Available as:* Sterile solution: 50 mg (IV)	Dose: As of prednisolone

Table continued.

TABLE 30-1 (*Continued*)

DRUG, HOW SUPPLIED	DOSAGE, ROUTES, CONTRAINDICATIONS AND WARNINGS*
Prednisone, USP (Deltasone, Deltra, Lisacort, Meticorten, Paracort) *Available as:* Tablets (scored): 1, 2.5, and 5 mg	Dose: Generally, 1/5 of cortisone dose Dose (nephrosis): Initial dose/24 hr for 18 mo–4 yr, 30–40 mg; for 4–10 yr, 60 mg; for older, 80 mg; divide into 4 doses (O) Dose (rheumatic carditis, leukemia, tumors): 2 mg/kg/24 hr, or 60 mg/M^2/24 hr for 2–3 wk, then 1.5 mg/kg/24 hr, or 45 mg/M^2/24 hr for 4–6 wk; divide into 4 doses (O) Dose (tuberculosis): 2 mg/kg/24 hr, or 60 mg/M^2/24 hr, for 2 mo; gradual withdrawal; divide into 4 doses (O)
Triamcinolone, NF, and salts, USP (Aristocort, Kenacort) *Available as:* Tablets (scored): 1, 2, 4, 8, and 16 mg Syrup: 2 and 4 mg/5 ml Sterile suspensions: Acetonide: 10 mg/ml (articular, lesional) 20 mg/ml (articular) 40 mg/ml (IM only) Diacetate: 25 mg/ml (lesional, not turbinates) 40 mg/ml (IM, articular, lesional, R)	Dose: 1/6 of cortisone dose
ADRENAL CORTEX—MINERALOCORTICOIDS	
Desoxycorticosterone acetate, USP, and pivalate (trimethylacetate), **NF** (Cortate, Cortinaq, Decortin, Decosterone, Descotone, Doca acetate, Percorten, Steraq, and others) *Available as:* Tablets (buccal, lingual): 2 and 5 mg Pellets: 75 and 125 mg (implantation) Solution: 5 mg/ml (IM) Sterile suspension (aqueous): 25 mg/ml (IM)	Dose: 1–5 mg/24 hr, or 1.5–2 mg/M^2/24 hr; single dose in oil (IM) **Caution:** Observe for edema, cardiac failure, hypertension, lowered serum K (weakness, ECG changes)
ADRENAL MEDULLA	
Epinephrine hydrochloride (See Adrenergics, above)	
Levarterenol bitartrate (See Adrenergics, above)	
ALDOSTERONE INHIBITOR	
Spironolactone, USP (Aldactone) *Available as:* Tablets: 25 mg	Dose (diagnostic test for primary hyperaldosteronism): 125–375 mg/M^2/24 hr; divided doses (O) Dose (edema and ascites): 3 mg/kg/24 hr, or 60 mg/M^2/24 hr, in divided doses (O); readjust dose after 5th day; may need to triple dose; restrict to 1 mo **Contraindications:** Acute renal insufficiency (lower nephron nephrosis)

*For individual drugs, see general index. *Consult package inserts.*

Key: M^2, dose per square meter of body surface; IM, intramuscular; ITh, intrathecal; IV, intravenous; O, oral; R, rectal; SC, subcutaneous; Subl, sublingual; T, topical.

TABLE 30-1 (*Continued*)

DRUG, HOW SUPPLIED	DOSAGE, ROUTES, CONTRAINDICATIONS AND WARNINGS
	Caution: Judiciously with elevated serum K (K therapy not indicated unless glucocorticoid is given); discontinue drug with hyperkalemia; may cause drowsiness, confusion; rash, androgenic effect, gynecomastia
PANCREAS	
Glucagon, USP (1 unit = 1 mg) *Available as:* Solution: 1 and 10 units, for injection	Dose: 0.025 unit/kg, as single dose (IM or IV); may repeat in 20 min, if needed **Caution:** High doses used for inotropic or chronotropic heart action deliver large doses of phenol
Insulin (See Section 16)	
PITUITARY, ANTERIOR	
Corticotropin, USP, adrenocorticotropic hormone, ACTH (Acthar) (1 unit = 1 mg) *Available as:* Solution (aqueous), for injection: Vials: 10, 20, and 40 units Ampules: 10 units/ml Solution (dry), for injection: 10, 25, and 40 units Gel: Vials: 20, 40, and 80 units/ml Cartridge: 40 units/ml Zinc hydroxide suspension (injection): 20 and 40 units/ml	Dose: For aqueous, 1.6 units/kg/24 hr, or 50 units/M^2/24 hr; divide aqueous preparation into 3–4 doses (IV most effective, or IM or SC); for gel, 0.8 unit/kg/24 hr, or 25 units/M^2/24 hr, as a single dose or divided into 2 doses **Contraindications:** Absolute: acute psychoses, Cushing's syndrome, active tuberculosis or peptic ulcer, congestive heart disease except rheumatic fever **Caution:** Use with greater care in hypertension, diabetes; see also contraindications and caution for glucocorticosteroids
PITUITARY, POSTERIOR	
Posterior pituitary *Available as:* Capsules (powder): 40 mg	Diabetes insipidus: Nasal insufflation prn (T)
Vasopressin injection, USP (Pitressin) *Available as:* Vasopressin injection, aqueous: 20 units/ml Pitressin tannate in oil: 5 units/ml; *shake well*	Dose: Of aqueous, 1–3 ml (SC), divided into 3 doses; of tannate in oil, 0.2 ml/dose (IM), with increase to 1–2 ml, or 0.25–0.5 ml/M^2 (IM); give daily, twice daily or every 2–3 days (prn); titrate dose to effect
THYROID	
Dextrothyroxine sodium, NF (Choloxin) *Available as:* Tablets (scored): 2 and 4 mg	Dose: Initial, 0.05 mg/kg/24 hr, or 1.5 mg/M^2/24 hr, as a single dose (O); increase this dose at monthly intervals to maintenance, recommended to be double initial dose (maximum, 8 times initial dose) **Contraindications:** Euthyroid patients with organic heart disease, hypertensive, hepatic, or renal disease, history of iodism, hyperthyroidism **Caution:** Potentiates coumarin-type anticoagulants, decreases other clotting factors; particular care for surgical and diabetic patients; increases PBI, metabolism, hyperthyroid symptoms and signs, rashes; assess growth; see congenital and acquired hypothyroidism
Levothyroxine sodium, USP (Letter, Levoid, Synthroid sodium) (0.1 mg = 65 mg thyroid, USP) *Available as:* Tablets (scored): 0.025, 0.05, 0.1, 0.15, 0.2, 0.3, and 0.5 mg Solution: 0.1 and 0.5 mg/ml, for injection	Dose: 0.006 mg/kg/24 hr, or 0.15 mg/M^2/24 hr; not less than 0.1 mg/24 hr under 1 yr (cretinism); single dose daily (O) **Contraindications and caution:** See sodium dextrothyroxine

Table continued.

TABLE 30–1 (*Continued*)

DRUG, HOW SUPPLIED	DOSAGE, ROUTES, CONTRAINDICATIONS AND WARNINGS*
Liothyronine sodium, sodium L-triiodothyronine, USP (Cytomel) *Available as:* Tablets: 5, 25, and 50 μg	Dose: Initial, under 7 kg, 2.5 μg/24 hr (O); initial, over 7 kg, 5 μg/24 hr (O); 5 μg increments, at weekly intervals prn (O); for maintenance, 15–20 μg/24 hr (O) **Contraindications and caution:** See sodium dextrothyroxine
Thyroid, USP, desiccated thyroid *Available as:* Tablets (plain or enteric coated): 15, 30, 60, 125, 200, 250, and 300 mg Capsules (in oil): 60, 120, 200, and 300 mg	Dose: 4 mg/kg/24 hr, or 100 mg/M²/24 hr; not less than 60 mg/24 hr under 1 yr (cretinism); single daily dose (O) **Contraindications and caution:** See sodium dextrothyroxine
THYROID INHIBITORS	
Methimazole, USP (Tapazole) *Available as:* Tablets: 5 and 10 mg	Dose: Initial, 0.4 mg/kg/24 hr, or 12 mg/M²/24 hr; for maintenance, ½ initial dose; divide into 3 doses (O) **Contraindications:** Hypersensitivity or idiosyncrasy to this drug **Caution:** Agranulocytosis, pancytopenia, exfoliative dermatitis, hepatitis, neuropathy, CNS stimulation or depression, headache, fever, arthralgia, pruritus, edema, hypothyroidism
Potassium iodide, USP *Available as:* Solution (NF) "saturated"; 1 g/ml	Dose: For thyrotoxicosis, 0.9 ml saturated solution/24 hr (equals 0.9 g KI); divide into 3 doses (O)
Propylthiouracil, USP *Available as:* Tablets: 50 mg	Dose (initial): For 6–10 yr, 50–150 mg/24 hr; for 10 yr and over, 150–300 mg/24 hr, or 150 mg/M²/24 hr; divide into 3 doses every 8 hr (O) Dose (maintenance): 50 mg bid when euthyroid **Contraindication:** Hypersensitivity to this drug **Precautions:** Patients need close surveillance, should report immediately any sore throat, rash, fever, headache or malaise; if such symptoms occur, immediately blood studies for agranulocytosis should be done; mild reactions may respond to temporary discontinuation of medication; for severe reactions, discontinue permanently; severe reactions may follow mild ones **Adverse reactions:** Probably occur in less than 3% of patients; *most commonly reported* are rashes, urticaria, nausea, vomiting, abdominal distress, arthralgia, paresthesias, loss of taste, loss of hair myalgia, headache, drowsiness, neuritis, edema, vertigo, pigmentation, jaundice, sialoadenopathy and lymphadenopathy; *less common* are agranulocytosis, thrombocytopenia, drug fever, a lupus-like syndrome, hepatitis, periarteritis, and hypoprothrombinemia **Note:** About 10% of untreated patients with hyperthyroidism have leukopenia (less than 4000/mm³), often with relative granulocytopenia
ENZYMES	
Pancreatic enzymes (Cotazym, Panteric granules, Viokase), **pancreatin, NF, pancrelipase, NF** *Available as:* Granules: 1 and 4 oz Viokase: Tablets (Pancreatin 4 × NF): 325 mg Powder (Pancreatin 4 × NF) Cotazym: Capsules: 8000 units of lipase, etc.	Dose: *Granules,* ¼–½ tsp with meals (O); *tablets,* 1–2 whole or crushed with meals (O); *powder,* ½ tsp with meals (O); *capsules,* contents of 1–3 with meals (O); *packets,* 1–2 with meals (O); gauge dose by quality of stool **Caution:** Hypersensitivity to hog or beef products

*For individual drugs, see general index. *Consult package inserts.*
Key: M², dose per square meter of body surface; IM, intramuscular; ITh, intrathecal; IV, intravenous; O, oral; R, rectal; SC, subcutaneous; Subl, sublingual; T, topical.

TABLE 30–1 (*Continued*)

DRUG, HOW SUPPLIED	DOSAGE, ROUTES, CONTRAINDICATIONS AND WARNINGS
Packets: 16,000 units of lipase, etc.	
Streptokinase-streptodornase (Varidase) *Available as:* Oral and buccal tablets: 10,000 units of streptokinase and 2500 units of streptodornase Local-topical: Ampules: 100,000 units of streptokinase and 25,000 units of streptodornase IM ampules: 20,000 units of streptokinase and 5000 units of streptodornase	Dose: Buccal tablets, 1–4 daily; topical and local, to be individualized **Contraindications:** Intravenous administration, patients with reduced plasminogen or fibrinogen **Caution:** Allergic and pyrogenic reactions, gastrointestinal symptoms, skin rash, not for use in closed cavities without adequate drainage
GANGLIONIC BLOCKING AGENTS (See Cardiovascular Drugs, Antihypertensives, above)	
HEMATOLOGIC AGENTS (See Section 14)	
IMMUNOSUPPRESSIVE AGENTS (See Antineoplastics, above)	
IRON SALTS AND COMPLEXES (See Section 14) (For Toxicity of iron preparations, see Section 28)	
Iron requirements (elemental Fe)	Dose: For *prophylaxis,* 1 mg/kg/24 hr (single or divided dose); for *treatment,* 6 mg/kg/24 hr; divide into 3 doses
Ferrocholinate, iron choline citrate (Chel-Iron, Ferrolip) (12% Fe) *Available as:* Tablets: 333 mg (40 mg Fe) Syrup: 166 mg (20 mg Fe)/5 ml 417 mg (50 mg Fe)/5 ml Drops (Pediatric): 25 mg Fe/ml	**Caution:** Less reliable than ferrous sulfate
Ferroglycine sulfate complex (Ferronord) (40 mg elemental Fe/tablet or ml) *Available as:* Tablets (enteric coated): 40 mg Fe/tablet Capsules (prolonged action): 75 mg Fe/capsule	**Caution:** Less reliable than ferrous sulfate
Ferrous fumarate, USP (many trade names) (33% Fe) *Available as:* Tablets: 200 mg Tablets (chewable): 200 mg Capsules (prolonged action): 150 mg	
Ferrous gluconate, NF (Fergon, Nionate) (12% Fe) *Available as:* Tablets: 300 mg Elixir: 300 mg/5 ml	

Table continued.

TABLE 30-1 (*Continued*)

DRUG, HOW SUPPLIED	DOSAGE, ROUTES, CONTRAINDICATIONS AND WARNINGS*
Ferrous lactate (Ferro drops) (20% Fe) *Available as:* Drops: 25 mg Fe/ml	
Ferrous sulfate, USP (Feosol) (20% Fe) *Available as:* Tablets (plain and enteric coated) and capsules: 200 mg (40 mg Fe) 300 mg (60 mg Fe) Capsules (prolonged action): 225 mg (45 mg Fe) Syrup (NF): 200 mg (40 mg Fe)/5 ml Elixir (Feosol): 220 mg (44 mg Fe)/5 ml Fer-in-Sol: Drops: 75 mg (15 mg Fe)/0.6 ml 125 mg (25 mg Fe)/ml Syrup: 150 mg (30 mg Fe)/5 ml Capsules: 60 mg Fe	
Iron dextran injection, USP (Imferon) (2% Fe) *Available as:* Solution: Equivalent to 50 mg Fe/ml, for injection	Dose: Surface area in $M^2 \times 55 \times (13.5 -$ patient's Hb in g/dl$) =$ mg Fe needed (formula useful under age 3–4 yr); or wt (kg) $\times$ (13.5 – patient's Hb in g/dl) $\times 2.5 =$ mg Fe needed; or wt (lb) $\times$ (13.5 – patient's Hb in g/dl) = mg Fe needed; add 10–50% to above for stores **Contraindications:** Hypersensitivity to this drug, in all anemias except iron deficiency **Warning:** Has been associated with fatal reactions, allergic and anaphylactic **Caution:** Do not give if sensitive to test dose (0.5 ml); inject only IM by Z technique; may stain skin or cause urticaria, arthralgia, lymphadenopathy, nausea, headache, fever
OTHER HEMATOLOGIC AGENTS	
Aminocaproic acid, NF (Amicar) *Available as:* Tablets: 500 mg Syrup: 1.25 g/5 ml Solution: 250 mg/ml, for injection	Dose: Initial, 100 mg/kg, or 3 g/M^2, as a single dose (O) or by infusion (IV) slowly; for maintenance, 1/3 of above dose hourly to achieve plasma level of 13 mg/dl, not more than 18 g/M^2/24 hr **Contraindications:** Active intravascular clotting **Side effects:** Gastrointestinal symptoms, nasal and ocular suffusion, tinnitus, headache, rash; hypotension, bradycardia and/or arrhythmia by rapid infusion
Cyanocobalamin (vitamin B_{12}) (See Section 3)	
Folic acid (See Section 3)	
Vitamin C (See Section 3)	
HORMONES (See Endocrines, above)	
HYPERTENSIVES (See Adrenergics, above)	

*For individual drugs, see general index. *Consult package inserts.*

Key: M^2, dose per square meter of body surface; IM, intramuscular; ITh, intrathecal; IV, intravenous; O, oral; R, rectal; SC, subcutaneous; Subl, sublingual; T, topical.

TABLE 30–1 (*Continued*)

DRUG, HOW SUPPLIED	DOSAGE, ROUTES, CONTRAINDICATIONS AND WARNINGS
HYPNOTICS (See Sedatives and hypnotics, below)	
IMMUNIZING AGENTS (See Section 4)	
IMMUNOSUPPRESSIVE AGENTS (See Antineoplastics, above)	
IRON PREPARATIONS (See Hematologic agents, above)	
LAXATIVES (See also Stool softeners, below)	
Bisacodyl, USP (Dulcolax) *Available as:* Tablets (enteric coated): 5 mg Suppositories: 10 mg	Dose: 0.3 mg/kg, or 8 mg/M², as a single dose (O) 6 hr before desired action or procedure (swallow whole); for *bowel preparation,* add rectal dose 2 hr before procedure (under age 2 yr, 5 mg (R); over age 2 yr, 10 mg (R)) **Caution:** Usual laxative precautions; avoid rectal use – rectal fissures and ulcerations; avoid chewing tablets
Cascara sagrada, aromatic fluidextract, USP *Available as:* Aromatic fluidextract (liquid)	Dose: Infants, 1–2 ml/dose; children, 2–8 ml/dose, or 5 ml/M²/dose; increase prn for effect (O)
Castor oil, USP *Available as:* Oil or tasteless emulsion	Dose: Infants, 1–5 ml/dose (O); children, 5–15 ml/dose (O), or 15 ml/M²/dose (O)
Magnesium citrate solution, NF *Available as:* Solution: 200 ml	Dose: 4 ml/kg/dose, or 120 ml/M²/dose; flavored solution ready for use (O)
Magnesium sulfate, USP (Epsom salt) *Available as:* Crystals Solution: 100, 250, and 500 mg/ml (10, 25, and 50%), for injection	Dose (cathartic): 0.25 g/kg/dose (O), or 8.0 g/M²/dose (O) Dose (hypertension): *Intramuscular,* using *50% solution,* 0.2 ml/kg/dose, or 5 ml/M²/dose; repeat every 4–6 hr prn (IM); *intravenous,* using *1% solution* (10 mg/ml), to maximum of 100 mg/kg/dose (10 ml/kg/dose), or 3 g/M²/dose (300 ml/M²/dose), slowly (IV); check blood pressure carefully Dose (hypomagnesemia): 0.2 mEq/kg of 25% solution (0.1 ml/kg) every 6 hr for 3–4 doses **Caution:** Respiratory depression; keep calcium gluconate available for use (IV)
Milk of magnesia, USP, magnesium hydroxide suspension *Available as:* USP magma (milk): Contains 8% magnesium hydroxide	Dose: 0.5 ml/kg/dose (O), or 15 ml/M²/dose (O)
Phenolphthalein, NF (many trade names) *Available as:* Various solid and liquid preparations	Dose: 1 mg/kg/dose (O), or 30 mg/M²/dose (O)
Senna, NF *Available as:* NF monographs: powder, fluidextract, and syrup	Dose: As *powder,* 40 mg/kg/dose, or 1.2 g/M²/dose; as *fluidextract,* 0.04 ml/kg/dose, or 1.2 ml/M²/dose; as *syrup,* 0.15 ml/kg/dose, or 4.5 ml/M²/dose; syrup is flavored ready for use (O); fluidextract and powder to be mixed with hospital or household flavors
Sodium phosphate, NF (dihydrogen sodium phosphate) *Available as:* NF chemical	Dose: 80 mg/kg/dose, or 2.5 g/M²/dose; dilute in flavored vehicle (O)

Table continued.

TABLE 30–1 (*Continued*)

DRUG, HOW SUPPLIED	DOSAGE, ROUTES, CONTRAINDICATIONS AND WARNINGS*
Sodium sulfate (Glauber's salt) *Available as:* NF XII chemical	Dose: 0.3 g/kg/dose, or 9 g/M²/dose; dilute in flavored vehicle (O)
MUSCLE RELAXANTS (See also Tranquilizers, below)	
Carisoprodol (Rela, Soma) **Note:** Not recommended for children under 5 yr of age *Available as:* Tablets (coated): 350 mg Capsules: 250 mg	Dose: 25 mg/kg/24 hr, or 0.75 g/M²/24 hr; divide into 4 doses (O) **Contraindications:** Hypersensitivity or idiosyncrasy to drug; porphyria **Caution:** With sensitivity to similar drugs (meprobamate), may cause weakness, dizziness, ataxia, tremor, agitation, headache, gastrointestinal symptoms, respiratory depression, flushed face, eosinophilia, pancytopenia, leukopenia, allergic reactions
Chlorzoxazone (Paraflex) *Available as:* Tablets (scored): 250 mg	Dose: 20 mg/kg/24 hr, or 0.6 g/M²/24 hr; divide into 3–4 doses (O) **Caution:** In patients with known drug allergies, observe for liver damage (withdraw use); may cause gastrointestinal symptoms, drowsiness, dizziness, overstimulation, rashes, petechiae, ecchymoses, angioedema, anaphylaxis
Dantrolene sodium (Dantrium) *Available as:* Capsules: 25 and 100 mg	Dose (adults with spasticity): Initial week, 50 mg/24 hr, divided into 2 doses (O); increase by weekly increments if needed for response to 100, 200, 300, 400 and rarely 800 mg/24 hr; divided into 4 doses (O) Dose (children): Initial week, 2 mg/kg/24 hr, divided into 2 doses (O); increase by weekly increments for response to 4, 8, 12 mg/kg/24 hr (not more than 400 mg/24 hr); divided into 4 doses (O) **Contraindications:** Where spasticity is utilized to sustain upright posture and balance in locomotion or whenever spasticity is utilized to obtain or maintain increased function **Warnings:** Long-term safety and efficacy in humans not established; chronic studies in animals showed growth or weight depression and signs of hepatopathy and possible occlusion nephropathy, all of which were reversible upon cessation of treatment, and an increased incidence of benign and malignant mammary tumors and an increase in the incidence of hepatic lymphangiomas and hepatic angiosarcomas; carcinogenicity in humans cannot be excluded; *use with caution in patients with preexisting liver disease;* safety in children *under the age of* 5 years has not been established **Precautions:** With caution with impaired pulmonary function, particularly those with obstructive pulmonary disease, with severely impaired cardiac function or with impaired hepatic function; caution against driving a motor vehicle or participating in hazardous occupations while taking; caution in the concomitant administration of tranquilizing agents or in exposure to sunlight **Adverse Reactions:** The most frequent are drowsiness, dizziness, weakness, general malaise, fatigue, and diarrhea; for other side effects, see package insert
Diazepam (Valium) (See Tranquilizers, below)	
Mephenesin (Tolserol and many others) **and mephenesin carbamate** (Tolseram) *Available as:* Tablets: 0.25 and 0.5 g Capsules: 0.25 g Elixir: 0.5 g/5 ml Solution: 20 mg/ml, for injection	Dose: 175 mg/kg/24 hr, or 5 g/M²/24 hr, divided into 3–5 doses (O); for *intravenous* use (2% solution), 1–3 ml/kg, or 30–90 ml/M², as a single dose (IV) slowly injected or by slow drip **Caution:** May cause weakness, nystagmus, paresthesias, euphoria, diplopia, muscular incoordination, hemolysis, hemoglobinuria, blurred vision, hypotension; avoid with renal impairment

*For individual drugs, see general index. *Consult package inserts.*

Key: M², dose per square meter of body surface; IM, intramuscular; ITh, intrathecal; IV, intravenous; O, oral; R, rectal; SC, subcutaneous; Subl, sublingual; T, topical.

TABLE 30–1 (*Continued*)

DRUG, HOW SUPPLIED	DOSAGE, ROUTES, CONTRAINDICATIONS AND WARNINGS
Carbamate: Tablets: 0.5 g Oral suspension: 1 g/5 ml	
Methocarbamol, NF (Robaxin) *Available as:* Tablets (scored): 500 and 750 mg Solution: 100 mg/ml, for injection	Dose: Usual dose, 60 mg/kg/24 hr, or 2 g/M^2/24 hr; divide into 4 doses (O, IV, or IM) **Contraindications:** Hypersensitivity to this drug; renal disease if by injection (vehicle) **Caution:** Inject slowly IV (1.8 ml/M^2/min), special caution in epilepsy; avoid extravasation; tetanus, not more than 18 ml (100 mg/ml)/M^2/24 hr for 3 consecutive days; may cause dizziness, drowsiness, gastrointestinal symptoms, skin rash, conjunctivitis, nasal congestion, fainting, collapse **Note:** Except for treatment of tetanus, not recommended for children under 12 yr of age
Neostigmine (Prostigmin) (See Cholinesterase inhibitors, above)	
PARASITICIDES (See Anthelmintics, above)	
PARASYMPATHOLYTICS (See Cholinergic blocking agents, above)	
PARASYMPATHOMIMETICS (See Cholinergics, above)	
RENAL TUBULAR DEPRESSANTS (For Xanthine oxidase inhibitors, see below)	
Probenecid, USP (Benemid) *Available as:* Tablets: 0.5 g (See also p. 1732)	Dose: Initial, 25 mg/kg, or 0.7 g/M^2; for maintenance, 40 mg/kg/24 hr, or 1.2 g/M^2/24 hr; divided into 4 doses (O) **Contraindications:** In children under 2 yr, patients with hypersensitivity to this drug, those with blood dyscrasias or uric acid kidney stones **Caution:** Determine sulfonamide levels when used with sulfonamides; urinary copper-reducing substance; may cause headache, gastrointestinal symptoms, increased urinary frequency, flushing, dizziness, anaphylactoid reactions, hemolytic anemia, aplastic anemia, nephrotic syndrome, hepatic necrosis
SEDATIVES AND HYPNOTICS (See also Anticonvulsants, above)	
BARBITURATES	
Amobarbital, NF, and amobarbital sodium, USP (Amytal and sodium Amytal) *Available as:* Amobarbital: Powder: 1/2 and 4 oz Tablets: 15, 30, 50, and 100 mg Elixir: 22 and 44 mg/5 ml Amobarbital sodium: Powder: 1/2 oz Capsules: 60 and 200 mg Suppositories: 0.2 g Sterile (injection): 60, 125, 250, 500 mg, and 1 g	Dose: For *sedation,* 2 mg/kg/24 hr, or 70 mg/M^2/24 hr, divided into 4 doses (O or R); as *anticonvulsant,* 3–5 mg/kg/dose (IM), or 125 mg/M^2/dose (IM); see below for IV use as anticonvulsant **Contraindications:** In severe hepatic dysfunction, porphyria, hypersensitivity to barbituric acid derivatives, uncontrolled pain **Caution:** Idiosyncrasy (excitement, pain, hangover, prolonged action); in respiratory depression; may cause rash, gastrointestinal symptoms, vertigo; IV rate must not exceed 1 ml/min (0.6 ml/M^2/min) (10% solution) **Toxicity:** From too rapid injection or overdosage; see Section 28, Barbiturates, and Anticonvulsants, above, for phenobarbital
Butabarbital sodium, NF (Butisol sodium and many others)	Same as amobarbital **Contraindications, caution, and toxicity:** See amobarbital

Table continued.

TABLE 30–1 (*Continued*)

DRUG, HOW SUPPLIED	DOSAGE, ROUTES, CONTRAINDICATIONS AND WARNINGS*
Available as: Tablets (scored): 15, 30, 50, and 100 mg Capsules: 15, 30, 50, and 100 mg Elixir: 30 mg/5 ml Solution: 125 mg/ml, for injection	
Pentobarbital sodium, USP (Napental, Nembutal sodium, Pental) *Available as:* Capsules: 30, 50, and 100 mg Capsules (prolonged action): 50 and 100 mg Elixir: 20 mg/5 ml Solution: 50 mg/ml, for injection Suppositories: 30, 60, 120, and 200 mg	Same as amobarbital (As preanesthetic, see Section 5) **Contraindications, caution, and toxicity:** See amobarbital
Phenobarbital (See Anticonvulsants, above)	
Secobarbital and secobarbital sodium, USP (Seconal and Seconal sodium) *Available as:* Tablets (coated): 50 and 100 mg Tablets (enteric coated): 50 and 100 mg Capsules: 30, 50, and 100 mg Suppositories: 30, 60, 125 and 200 mg Elixir: 22 mg/5 ml Sterile (injection): 50 mg/ml Tubex (disposable): 50 and 100 mg	Same as amobarbital
NONBARBITURATES	
Chloral hydrate, USP (Noctec, Somnos, and many other trade names) *Available as:* Oral use: In solution Rectal use: In cottonseed oil Suppositories: 0.5 g Capsules: 250 and 500 mg Syrup: 250 and 500 mg/5 ml Elixir: 267 mg/5 ml	Dose: As hypnotic, 50 mg/kg/24 hr (maximum 1 g/dose), or 1.5 g/M^2/24 hr, divided into 3–4 doses (O or R); as sedative, 1/2 of hypnotic dose **Contraindications:** Marked hepatic or renal impairment, hypersensitivity or idiosyncrasy **Caution:** Avoid large doses in cardiac disease; may cause gastric irritation, excitement, delirium **Warning:** May be habit forming **Precautions:** Sedative action potentiated by concomitant administration of alcohol; do not use large doses in patients with severe heart disease **Adverse reactions:** Gastric irritation; rarely, excitement and delirium or tolerance and addiction
Paraldehyde, USP *Available as:* USP (liquid) (dark bottles) Capsules: 1 g Sterile (injection): 2, 5, and 10 ml	Dose (sedative): 0.15 ml/kg/dose, or 6 ml/M^2/dose (O, R, IM); *oral,* with flavor (iced), or *rectal,* with equal parts of cottonseed oil, or *IV,* in 5% solution in saline or glucose water Dose (hypnotic and anticonvulsant): May double sedative dose (O and R) **Caution:** Use fresh supply, discard bottles opened *more than* 24 hr; avoid in hepatic and pulmonary disease; avoid plastic syringes or containers (use glass); *avoid IV use* (pulmonary hemorrhage and edema, heart failure); oral route irritating (dilute well, may flavor with sweet orange peel tincture) **Overdose:** Respiratory and cardiac depression

*For individual drugs, see general index. *Consult package inserts.*

Key: M^2, dose per square meter of body surface; IM, intramuscular; ITh, intrathecal; IV, intravenous; O, oral; R, rectal; SC, subcutaneous; Subl, sublingual; T, topical.

TABLE 30–1 (*Continued*)

DRUG, HOW SUPPLIED	DOSAGE, ROUTES, CONTRAINDICATIONS AND WARNINGS
STEROIDS (ADRENAL CORTICAL) (See Endocrines, above)	
STIMULANTS (CENTRAL NERVOUS SYSTEM) (See also Analeptics and Adrenergics, above)	
Aminophylline (See Bronchodilators, above)	
Amphetamine sulfate (See Adrenergics, above)	
Dextroamphetamine sulfate (See Adrenergics, above)	
Dyphylline (See Bronchodilators, above)	
Ephedrine sulfate (See Adrenergics, above)	
Methylphenidate (See Analeptics, above)	
Oxytriphylline (See Bronchodilators, above)	
Theophylline (See Bronchodilators, above)	
STOOL SOFTENERS	
Dioctyl sodium sulfosuccinate, USP (Aquatyl, Colace, Doxinate) *Available as:* Tablets: 50, 60, 100, and 125 mg Capsules: 20, 50, 60, 100, and 240 mg Solution: 10 and 50 mg/ml Syrup: 20 mg/5 ml Suppositories: 100 mg	Dose: 5 mg/kg/24 hr, or 150 mg/M^2/24 hr, divided into 3–4 doses (O); as an enema, add 50–100 mg to enema (R)
Poloxalkol (Magcyl, Polykol) *Available as:* Capsule: 250 mg Solution: 250 mg and 1 g/5 ml (dropper)	Dose: Under age 3 yr, 100–200 mg; over age 3 yr, 200 mg; give as single dose 1–3 times/24 hr (O)
SULFONAMIDES (See Antibiotics and chemotherapeutics, above)	
SYMPATHOLYTICS (See Andrenergic blocking agents, above)	
SYMPATHOMIMETICS (See Adrenergics, above)	
TRANQUILIZERS	
Acetophenazine maleate, NF (Tindal) *Available as:* Tablets (coated): 20 mg	Dose: 0.8–1.6 mg/kg/24 hr (maximum, 80 mg/24 hr); or 25–50 mg/M^2/24 hr; divide into 3 doses (O) **Contraindications and caution:** See chlorpromazine hydrochloride; acetophenazine maleate is a piperazine-type phenothiazine **Toxicity:** See chlorpromazine

Table continued.

DRUGS

TABLE 30–1 (*Continued*)

DRUG, HOW SUPPLIED	DOSAGE, ROUTES, CONTRAINDICATIONS AND WARNINGS*
Chlordiazepoxide hydrochloride, USP (Librium) **and chlordiazepoxide, NF** *Available as:* Tablets: 5, 10, and 25 mg Capsules: 5, 10, and 25 mg Sterile (injection): 50 mg/ml	Dose: For children over 6 yr, 0.5 mg/kg/24 hr, or 15 mg/M²/24 hr; divide into 3–4 doses (O or IM) **Caution:** *Injection:* keep under observation for 3 hr (preferably in bed); do not permit vehicle operation; avoid in coma or shock. *Oral and injection:* Avoid concomitant use of other psychotropic drugs; special care with MAO inhibitors or phenothiazine use, with renal or hepatic impairment, and in emotional depression; may cause excitement, stimulation (hyperactive children and psychiatric patients), drowsiness, ataxia, confusion, syncope, skin eruptions, edema, gastrointestinal symptoms, blood dyscrasias, jaundice and hepatic dysfunction, changes in EEG patterns; with protracted treatment, do periodic blood counts and liver function tests; *not indicated for children under 6 yr*
Chlormezanone (Trancopal) *Available as:* Tablets (scored): 100 and 200 mg	Dose: 12 mg/kg/24 hr, or 350 mg/M²/24 hr; divide into 3–4 doses (O) **Caution:** May cause rash, flush, dizziness, drowsiness, weakness, cholestatic jaundice (reversible)
Chlorpromazine hydrochloride, USP (Thorazine hydrochloride) *Available as:* Tablets: 10, 25, 50, 100, and 200 mg Capsules (prolonged action): 30, 75, 150, 200, and 300 mg Syrup (store in dark bottle): 10 mg/5 ml Oral concentrate: 30 mg/ml Solution: 25 mg/ml, for injection Suppositories: 25 and 100 mg	Dose (in *general use*): 2 mg/kg/24 hr, or 60 mg/M²/24 hr; divided into 4–6 doses (O) Dose (chorea): Initially 50 mg, increased 12.5 mg/dose every 6–8 hr for control (O); for maintenance, usual dose is 300–400 mg/24 hr for 10–14 days, reduced by 12.5 mg as possible (O) **Contraindications:** Hypersensitivity to phenothiazines, in bone marrow depression, psychic depression or depression by CNS drugs (barbiturates, narcotics, analgesics, antihistamines, alcohol) **Cautions for phenothiazine drugs:** Extrapyramidal symptoms often with phenothiazines (especially in children); dimethylaminopropyl derivatives (chlorpromazine [Thorazine], promazine [Sparine], and triflupromazine [Vesprin]) more likely to give parkinsonian symptoms (tremors, postural abnormalities, mask facies, salivation, akinesia, rigidity, shuffling gait); piperazine derivatives (acetophenazine [Tindal], carphenazine]Proketazine], fluphenazine [Permitil, Prolixin], perphenazine [Trilafon], prochlorperazine [Compazine], thiopropazate [Dartal], and trifluoperazine [Stelazine]) more likely to give dyskinetic symptoms (especially in children), oculogyric crisis, torticollis, hyperextension of neck and trunk, mask facies, protrusion of tongue, perioral spasms, sweating, pallor, fever, catatonic positions while conscious; symptoms resemble tetanus; use cautiously with convulsive history, grand or petit mal, may precipitate grand mal convulsions; may cause skin reactions, cholestatic jaundice, blood dyscrasias (most common with dimethylaminopropyl and piperidyl groups); incidences of leukopenia, granulocytopenia and agranulocytosis, purpura, and pancytopenia are low but mortality rate high; discontinue drug with symptoms, do appropriate blood tests and counts, discontinue with bilirubinuria or jaundice; avoid use in liver disease; may cause drowsiness (motor vehicle), dizziness, fatigue, sedation, potentiation of CNS depressants (reduce dosage); antiemetics may obscure nausea or vomiting of organic diseases; adrenergic blocking action may cause hypotension (orthostatic) (epinephrine contraindicated in treatment of hypotension), potentiation of antihypertensives, may alter ECG (resembling hypopotassemia or quinidine) (caution in heart disease); anticholinergic action (intraocular tension rise, flushed face, heat prostration); photosensitivity, skin pigmentation, ocular pigmentation and cataracts, dry mouth, urinary retention, constipation, melanosis of internal organs may occur; chlorpromazine is a dimethylaminopropyl phenothiazine
Diazepam, USP (Valium) *Available as:* Tablets (scored): 2, 5, and 10 mg Solution: 5 mg/ml, for injection	Dose: *Orally,* 0.12–0.8 mg/kg/24 hr, or 3.5–24 mg/M²/24 hr, divided into 3–4 doses (O); *parenterally,* 0.04–0.2 mg/kg, or 1.2–6 mg/M², as a single dose IM (deep, slowly) or IV (slowly), may repeat in 2–4 hr (not more than 18 mg/M² in 8 hr period)

*For individual drugs, see general index. *Consult package inserts.*

Key: M², dose per square meter of body surface; IM, intramuscular; ITh, intrathecal; IV, intravenous; O, oral; R, rectal; SC, subcutaneous; Subl, sublingual; T, topical.

TABLE 30–1 (*Continued*)

DRUG, HOW SUPPLIED	DOSAGE, ROUTES, CONTRAINDICATIONS AND WARNINGS
	Note: *Tablets* not to be used in infants under 6 mo; safety and efficacy of *injectable* diazepam not yet established for children under 12 yr **Contraindications:** *In infants;* in patients with a known hypersensitivity to this drug; acute narrow angle glaucoma; in open angle glaucoma unless patients are receiving appropriate therapy. **Warnings:** *When used intravenously the solution should be injected slowly, directly into the vein, taking at least one minute for each 5 mg (1 ml) given. Do not mix or dilute with other solutions or drugs;* extreme care must be used particularly in IV use; cardiac arrest may occur (resuscitative equipment should be available; when used with a narcotic analgesic, the dosage of the narcotic should be reduced by at least one-third and administered in small increments; injectable diazepam should not be administered to patients in shock, coma, or in acute alcoholic intoxication; patients should be cautioned against engaging in hazardous occupations requiring complete mental alertness, such as operating machinery or driving a motor vehicle; withdrawal symptoms (similar in character to those noted with barbiturates and alcohol) have occurred following abrupt discontinuance (see package insert) **Precautions:** May potentiate the action of phenothiazines, narcotics, barbiturates, MAO inhibitors and other antidepressants; usual precautions in treating patients with impaired hepatic function should be observed; caution should be exercised in the administration to patients with compromised kidney function; injectable diazepam has produced hypotension or muscular weakness in some patients particularly when used with narcotics, barbiturates or alcohol **Adverse Reactions:** Most commonly reported are drowsiness, fatigue and ataxia and venous thrombosis and phlebitis at the site of injection; for less frequently reported reactions see package insert
Hydroxyzine hydrochloride, NF (Atarax) *Available as:* Tablets: 10, 25, 50, and 100 mg Syrup: 10 mg/5 ml Solution: 25 and 50 mg/ml, for injection **Hydroxyzine pamoate, NF** (Vistaril) *Available as:* Capsules: 25, 50, and 100 mg Oral suspension: 25 mg/5 ml Solution: 25 and 50 mg/ml, for injection	Dose: 2 mg/kg/24 hr, or 60 mg/M²/24 hr; divide into 4 doses (O) Dose (preoperative): ½ of above dose (IM) Dose (antiemetic): Under 6 yr, 50 mg/24 hr; over 6 yr, 50–100 mg/24 hr, or 45–225 mg/M²/24 hr; divide into 4 doses (O); as a preoperative and postoperative antiemetic, 1 mg/kg, or 30 mg/M², as a single dose (IM) **Contraindications:** Hypersensitivity to this drug; do not inject subcutaneously or intra-arterially **Caution:** May potentiate barbiturates and meperidine (Demerol); reduce dosage of hydroxyzine when used with CNS depressants; may cause drowsiness (vehicle operation), dry mouth, tremor, convulsions
Imipramine hydrochloride, USP (Tofranil) **Note:** Not presently recommended for use in children under 6 yr of age or in conditions other than enuresis *Available as:* Tablets: 10, 25, and 50 mg Solution: 12.5 mg/ml, for injection	Dose (as *tranquilizer*): In *hospitalized adults,* 100 mg/24 hr, initially, in divided doses (O); increase to 200 mg/24 hr (O), as required, in divided doses; if no response in 2 weeks, increase to 250–300 mg/24 hr (O), in divided doses; in *ambulatory adults* (as out-patients), ¾ of above dose, initially, with maintenance at 50–150 mg/24 hr (O), in divided doses, not to exceed 200 mg/24 hr; in *adolescents,* 30–40 mg/24 hr, initially, in divided doses (O), not to exceed 100 mg/24 hr Dose (for *enuresis*): In *children aged 6 yr and older,* 25 mg (O) 1 hr before bedtime, initially; if response not satisfactory, increase to 50 mg (under 12 yr) or 75 mg (over 12 yr), orally; in early night bedwetters, divide into 2 doses, afternoon and bedtime (O); reduce dose gradually **Contraindications:** Concomitant use of monoamine oxidase inhibiting compounds (hyperpyrexic crises or convulsions may occur, sometimes fatal [see package insert]); known sensitivity to this drug contraindicates its use (possible cross-sensitivity to other dibenzazepines. **Warnings:** Extreme caution in *cardiovascular disease* (see package insert), in *glaucoma* (owing to anticholinergic properties), in *hyperthyroidism,* in patients with *seizure disorders* (lowers convulsive threshold), in patients receiving *guanethidine or similar agents* (imipramine may block effects); in *treatment of enuresis in children,* rule out masked genitourinary disease before using imipramine; safety in long-term use in children has not been established; after a favorable response, consider a trial of a

Table continued.

TABLE 30–1 (*Continued*)

DRUG, HOW SUPPLIED	DOSAGE, ROUTES, CONTRAINDICATIONS AND WARNINGS*
	drug-free period; imipramine may impair mental or physical abilities required for potentially hazardous tasks **Precautions:** Consider possibility of suicide in depressed patients; hypomanic or manic episodes may occur; discontinue prior to elective surgery; monitor clinical state and dosage carefully when used with anticholinergic or sympathomimetic drugs; alcohol exaggerates effects; see also package insert **Adverse reactions:** *Cardiovascular* (hypotension, hypertension, tachycardia, others [see package insert]); *neurologic* (paresthesias, incoordination, ataxia, neuropathy, seizures, others [see package insert]); *anticholinergic* (dry mouth, blurred vision, constipation, ileus, urinary retention, others [see package insert]); *allergic* (rashes, photosensitization [avoid sunlight], drug fever, others [see package insert]); *hematologic* (blood dyscrasias, including agranulocytosis [see package insert]); *gastrointestinal* (nausea, vomiting, anorexia, diarrhea, others [see package insert]); *endocrine* (gynecomastia, galactorrhea, hyperglycemia, hypoglycemia, others [see package insert]); *others* (including jaundice [see package insert] **Note:** In enuretic children imipramine has most commonly produced nervousness, sleep disorders, tiredness, and mild gastrointestinal effects as adverse reactions; these are usually transient; constipation, convulsions, emotional disturbances, syncope and collapse also reported
Meprobamate, USP (Equanil, Miltown, Viobamate) *Available as:* Tablets: 200 and 400 mg Capsules (prolonged action): 200 and 400 mg Oral suspension: 200 mg/5 ml Solution: 80 mg/ml, for injection	Dose: 25 mg/kg/24 hr, or 0.7 g/M^2/24 hr; divide into 2–3 doses/24 hr (O) Dose (tetanus): Initial administration parenteral, to be changed to oral dosage when possible; in infants, 600 mg/24 hr, divided into 4 doses (IM) (not for IV use); in older child, 50–70 mg/kg/24 hr (maximum, 3.2 g/24 hr), or 1.5–2 g/M^2/24 hr, divided into 6–8 doses (IM) (not for IV use) **Contraindications:** Previous allergic or idiosyncratic reactions to this drug **Caution:** Dependency may follow prolonged use; sudden withdrawal may precipitate anxiety, insomnia, vomiting, ataxia, tremors, twitching, convulsions; may cause drowsiness (motor vehicles), grand mal attacks in patients prone to grand or petit mal epilepsy, ataxia, urticaria, rash, bullous dermatitis, nonthrombocytopenic purpura, leukopenia, edema, chills, fever, bronchial spasms, hypotension, anaphylaxis, stomatitis, proctitis, fast EEG activity
Methdilazine and methdilazine hydrochloride, NF (Tacaryl and Tacaryl hydrochloride) hydrochloride) (See Antihistamines, above)	
Perphenazine, NF (Trilafon) *Available as:* Tablets: 2, 4, 8, and 16 mg Tablets (prolonged action): 8 mg Syrup: 2 mg/5 ml Concentrate (graduated dropper): 16 mg/5 ml Solution: 5 mg/ml, for injection	Dose: 1–6 yr, 4 mg/24 hr; 6–12 yr, 6 mg/24 hr; over 12 yr (lower adult dose), 6–12 mg/24 hr; or 7 mg/M^2/24 hr; divide into 3 doses (O); rectal dose (R) is 1/2 oral dose **Contraindications and caution:** See chlorpromazine hydrochloride; perphenazine is a piperazine-type phenothiazine
Prochlorperazine and prochlorperazine edisylate or maleate, USP (Compazine) *Available as:* Tablets: 5, 10, and 25 mg	Dose: 0.4 mg/kg/24 hr, or 10 mg/M^2/24 hr; divide into 3–4 doses (O or R); IM dose is 1/2 oral dose **Note:** Not recommended for use in children under 10 kg **Contraindications and caution:** See chlorpromazine hydrochloride; prochlorperazine is a piperazine-type phenothiazine **Toxicity:** As for chlorpromazine, above

*For individual drugs, see general index. *Consult package inserts.*

Key: M^2, dose per square meter of body surface; IM, intramuscular; ITh, intrathecal; IV, intravenous; O, oral; R, rectal; SC, subcutaneous; Subl, sublingual; T, topical.

DRUGS

TABLE 30–1 (*Continued*)

DRUG, HOW SUPPLIED	DOSAGE, ROUTES, CONTRAINDICATIONS AND WARNINGS
Capsules (prolonged action): 10, 15, 30, and 75 mg Suppositories: 2.5, 5, and 25 mg Syrup: 5 mg/5 ml Solution: 5 mg/ml, for injection Concentrate: 10 mg/ml	
Promethazine hydrochloride, USP (Phenergan hydrochloride) *Available as:* Tablets (scored): 12.5, 25, and 50 mg Syrup: 6.25 mg/5 ml 25 mg/5 ml (Fortis) Solution (for injection): Ampules: 25 mg/ml (IM or IV) Vials: 50 mg/ml (IM only) Suppositories: 25 and 50 mg	Dose: 0.5 mg/kg/dose, or 15 mg/M²/dose (O, R, or IM); as an antihistaminic, full dose at night, 1/4 dose am or prn; for nausea or vomiting, 1/2 to full dose every 4–6 hr; preoperative, full or double dose; for motion sickness, full dose, repeat 12 hr prn **Caution:** Phenothiazine derivative
Reserpine (See Cardiovascular drugs, Antihypertensive, above)	
Thioridazine hydrochloride, USP (Mellaril) **Note:** Not recommended for use in children under 2 yr of age *Available as:* Tablets (coated): 10, 25, 50, 100, and 200 mg Solution (oral concentrate): 30 mg/ml	Dose: 1 mg/kg/24 hr, or 30 mg/M²/24 hr; divide into 3–4 doses (O) **Contraindications and caution:** See chlorpromazine hydrochloride; thioridazine is a piperazine-type phenothiazine less likely to cause extrapyramidal reactions or jaundice
Trimeprazine tartrate (Temaril) (See Antihistamines, above)	
URICOSURICS (See Renal tubular depressants, above)	
URINARY ANTISEPTICS (See Antibiotics and chemotherapeutics, above)	
VASODILATORS (See Cardiovascular drugs, antihypertensives, above)	
VASOPRESSORS (See Adrenergics, above)	
VITAMINS (See Section 3)	
Vitamin D (See Section 3)	
Vitamin K (See also Section 3) Synthetic: Menadiol sodium diphosphate, NF, vitamin K analogue (Kappadione, Synkayvite) *Available as:* Tablets: 5 mg Solution: 1, 2.5, 5, 10, and 37.5 mg, for injection	Dose: For prophylaxis of hemorrhagic disease of newborn, 1 mg (IM) **Caution:** See kernicterus
Menadione sodium bisulfite, NF (Hykinone) (5 mg = 2.6 mg menadione)	Dose: For prophylaxis of hemorrhagic disease of newborn, 1 mg (IM) **Caution:** See kernicterus

Table continued.

DRUGS

TABLE 30–1 (*Continued*)

DRUG, HOW SUPPLIED	DOSAGE, ROUTES, CONTRAINDICATIONS AND WARNINGS*
Available as: Tablets: 5 mg Oral solution: 25 mg/5 ml Solution, for injection: 5 mg/1 ml 10 mg/1 ml 72 mg/10 ml	
Natural K_1: Phytonadione, USP (AquaMephyton, Konakion) *Available as:* Tablets: 5 mg Solution: 2 and 10 mg/ml, for injection	Dose: For prophylaxis of hemorrhagic disease of newborn, 1 mg (IV, IM or SC); for treatment, 5–10 mg (IV, IM or SC); Konakion for IM use only Dose (other prothrombin deficiencies): In infants, 2 mg (O); in older infants and children, 5–10 mg (O); aqueous solutions may be given (IV, IM or SC); Konakion IM only **Contraindications:** Repeated doses in liver disease if responses unsatisfactory **Caution:** Avoid rapid intravenous injection (not to exceed 3 mg/M^2/min or total 5 mg); may cause flushing, alteration of taste, dizziness, weak pulse, sweating, hypotension, cyanosis, pain and swelling at injection site, allergic hypersensitivity, anaphylaxis; dosage guided by prothrombin times; hyperbilirubinemia after 25 mg
XANTHINE OXIDASE INHIBITOR (For Uricosuric probenecid, see Renal tubular depressants, above)	
Allopurinol, USP (Zyloprim) *Available as:* Tablets (scored): 100 and 300 mg	Dose: In hyperuricemia of malignancies, under 6 yr, 150 mg/24 hr, and from 6–10 yr, 300 mg/24 hr; divide into 3 doses (O); after 48 hr evaluate and adjust dose; dosage adjusted by uric acid levels (serum) **Contraindications:** Use in children limited to above; not for use in nursing mothers **Warning:** Hepatotoxicity, rise in serum transaminase or alkaline phosphatase (perform periodic tests); drowsiness, precautions in operating machinery; avoid iron medication or use in relatives of patients with idiopathic hemochromatosis; pregnancy, use if benefit exceeds risk **Caution:** Maintain good urine flow, preferably alkaline; observe carefully in renal disease; adjust dose of mercaptopurine or azathioprine prn; withdraw allopurinol use with abnormalities or reactions, reinstitute smaller dose **Adverse reactions:** Skin rash, exfoliation, urticaria, purpura; fever; gastrointestinal symptoms; leukocytosis, eosinophilia; arthralgia; cataracts (with severe dermatitis)

*For individual drugs, see general index. *Consult package inserts.*

Key: M^2, dose per square meter of body surface; IM, intramuscular; ITh, intrathecal; IV, intravenous; O, oral; R, rectal; SC, subcutaneous; Subl, sublingual; T, topical.

TABLES OF NORMAL LABORATORY VALUES*[1]

TABLE 30–2 CHEMISTRY

DETERMINATION	SPECIMEN	AGE/SEX[2]	NORMAL VALUE[3]		
	(serum or plasma unless otherwise indicated)				
Acetone					
qualitative			Negative		
quantitative			0.3–2.0 mg/dl		
Albumin (see Electrophoresis, protein)					
Aldolase[4] (fructose-1, 6-diphosphate, 37 °C)		Infant	1.5–18.8 IU/l		
		Child	2.3–13.5 IU/l		
		Thereafter	2.3–11.3 IU/l		
Alpha-1-antitrypsin			0.8–1.6 mg inhibition/dl		
Amino acids (maximum normal levels)			Neonatal (μm/dl)	Child (μm/dl)	Thereafter (μm/dl)
alanine			52	41	67
α-amino-n-butyric acid			7	3	4
arginine			12	12	20
aspartic acid			2	2	5
citrulline			4	3	6
cystine			8	8	19
glutamic acid			26	20	25
glutamine			210	75	61
glycine			52	52	56
histidine			13	12	12
isoleucine			12	8	10
leucine			22	12	18
lysine			35	30	27
methionine			8	5	4
ornithine			22	15	13
phenylalanine			20	12	12
proline			48	40	44
serine			30	24	19
taurine			22	22	20
threonine			34	32	25
tryptophan			7	7	7
tyrosine			21	15	9
valine			35	35	32
Ammonia	whole blood	Premature/jaundiced infant	100–200 μg/dl		
		Newborn	90–150 μg/dl		
		Child	40– 80 μg/dl		
		Thereafter	20–120 μg/dl		
Amylase[4] (starch, 37 °C)		Newborn	0–2500 IU/l		
		Infant/child	160–3700 IU/l		
		Thereafter	1200–3200 IU/l		
Ascorbic acid			0.5–1.5 mg/dl		

*Footnotes for Tables 30–2 to 30–9 will be found at end of Table 30–9.

Table continued.

TABLE 30–2 CHEMISTRY (*Continued*)

DETERMINATION	SPECIMEN	AGE/SEX	NORMAL VALUE
Bilirubin, total			Premature/Full Term
		Cord	< 2 / < 2 mg/dl
		0–1 day	< 8 / < 6 mg/dl
		1–2 day (See pp.	<12 / < 8 mg/dl
		3–5 day 375–381)	<16 / <12 mg/dl
		Thereafter	< 2 / < 1 mg/dl
Bilirubin, direct			0–1 mg/dl
Bromsulphalein, 5 mg/kg (BSP)			<5% at 45 min
Calcium, total		Newborn	3.7–7.0 mEq/l (For
		Infant	5.2–6.0 mEq/l conversion
		Child	5.0–5.7 mEq/l see Table
		Thereafter	4.5–5.7 mEq/l 30–11)
Calcium, ionized			2.1–2.6 mEq/l
Carbon dioxide content (CO_2)	venous (arterial 2 mEq/l less)	Cord	14–22 mEq/l
		Newborn	19–27 mEq/l
		Infant	20–28 mEq/l
		Child	18–27 mEq/l
		Thereafter	23–29 mEq/l
Carbon dioxide, partial pressure (pCO_2)	whole blood, arterial		35–45 mm Hg
	whole blood, venous		40–50 mm Hg
Carboxyhemoglobin	whole blood		<5%
Carotene		Infant	0– 40 μg/dl
		Child	40–130 μg/dl
		Thereafter	50–300 μg/dl
Ceruloplasmin (p-phenylenediamine dihydrochloride, 37°C)		Newborn–6 mo	1–30 mg/dl
		6 mo–1 yr	15–50 mg/dl
		1–12 yr	30–65 mg/dl
		Thereafter	22–50 mg/dl
Chloride		Cord	96–104 mEq/l
		Newborn	93–112 mEq/l
		Infant	95–110 mEq/l
		Child	101–108 mEq/l
		Thereafter	98–108 mEq/l
Cholesterol, total		Cord	45–100 mg/dl
		Newborn	45–170 mg/dl
		Infant	70–175 mg/dl
		Child	120–240 mg/dl
		Thereafter	150–250 mg/dl
Cholesterol, esters		Newborn	42–71% of total
		Child	55–65% of total
		Thereafter	70–78% of total
Copper		Newborn	20– 70 μg/dl
		Infant/child	30–150 μg/dl
		Child/adolescent	90–240 μg/dl
		Thereafter	70–120 μg/dl
Cortisol			
AM specimen			15–25 μg/dl
PM specimen			5–10 μg/dl

*Footnotes for Tables 30–2 to 30–9 will be found at end of Table 30–9.

TABLE 30–2 CHEMISTRY (*Continued*)

DETERMINATION	SPECIMEN	AGE/SEX	NORMAL VALUE
Creatine		Male	0.2–0.6 mg/dl
		Female	0.6–1.0 mg/dl
Creatine phosphokinase (CPK) (creatine phosphate, 30°C)		Newborn	10–300 IU/l
		Thereafter	
		Male	0– 70 IU/l
		Female	0– 50 IU/l
Creatinine			0.3–1.1 mg/dl
Creatinine clearance (endogenous)[5]	serum and urine	Newborn	40– 65 ml/min/1.73 M^2
		Child	
		Male	98–150 ml/min/1.73 M^2
		Female	95–123 ml/min/1.73 M^2
		Thereafter	
		Male	91–119 ml/min/1.73 M^2
		Female	77–113 ml/min/1.73 M^2

Electrophoresis, protein (cellulose acetate) (see protein)

	Total Protein	Albumin	α_1-glob	α_2-glob	β-glob	γ-glob	Units
Premature	4.3–7.6	3.1–4.2	0.1–0.5	0.3–0.7	0.3–1.2	0.3–1.4	g/dl
Newborn	4.6–7.4	3.6–5.4	0.1–0.3	0.3–0.5	0.2–0.6	0.2–1.2	g/dl
Infant	6.1–6.7	4.4–5.3	0.2–0.4	0.5–0.8	0.5–0.8	0.3–0.7	g/dl
Thereafter	6.2–8.1	4.0–5.8	0.1–0.3	0.4–1.0	0.5–0.9	0.3–1.0	g/dl

DETERMINATION	SPECIMEN	AGE/SEX	NORMAL VALUE
Fatty acids, free			0.4–0.9 mEq/l
Fibrinogen		Newborn	150–300 mg/dl
		Thereafter	200–400 mg/dl
Folate			5–20 ng/dl
Galactose		Newborn/Infant	0–20 mg/dl
Globulins (see Electrophoresis, protein)			
Glucose, fasting (FBS)		Premature	20– 60 mg/dl
		Newborn	30– 80 mg/dl
		Child	60–100 mg/dl
		Thereafter	70–110 mg/dl
Haptoglobin (as hemoglobin-binding capacity)		Neonatal	0– 20 mg/dl
		Thereafter	20–200 mg/dl
Hemoglobin	serum		<5 mg/dl
Immunoglobulin levels[6]	serum		

	γ^G mg/dl	γ^M mg/dl	γ^A mg/dl	Total γ mg/dl
Newborn	645–1,244	5– 30	0– 11	660–1,439
1–3 mo	272– 762	16– 67	6– 56	324– 699
4–6 mo	206–1,125	10– 83	8– 93	228–1,232
7–12 mo	279–1,533	22–147	16– 98	327–1,687
13–25 mo	258–1,393	14–114	19–119	398–1,586
25–36 mo	419–1,274	28–113	19–235	499–1,418
3–5 yr	569–1,597	22–100	55–152	730–1,771
6–8 yr	559–1,492	27–118	54–221	640–1,725
9–11 yr	779–1,456	35–132	12–208	966–1,639
12–16 yr	726–1,085	35– 72	70–229	833–1,284
Adult	569–1,919	47–147	61–330	730–2,365

Table continued.

TABLE 30-2 CHEMISTRY (*Continued*)

DETERMINATION	SPECIMEN	AGE/SEX[2]	NORMAL VALUE[3]
Iodine, total serum organic (PBI)		Newborn 6 wk–16 yr Thereafter	4–14 μg/dl 5– 9 μg/dl 4– 8 μg/dl
Iodine, butanol extractable (BEI)		Newborn 6 wk–16 yr Thereafter	3–13 μg/dl 4– 8 μg/dl 3.2–6.4 μg/dl
Iodine, T_3 (Triosorb) normal hyperthyroidism hypothyroidism			 25–35% >35% <25%
Iodine, T_4-by-column (thyroxine)		Newborn Thereafter	3–12 μg/dl 3.4–6.2 μg/dl
Iodine, T_4/comp. protein bind. (thyroxine)		Newborn Thereafter	3–12 μg/dl 3– 7 μg/dl
Iron		Newborn 4 mo–2 yr Thereafter	100–200 μg/dl 40–100 μg/dl 85–150 μg/dl
Iron-binding capacity (IBC)		Newborn 4 mo–2 yr Thereafter	60–175 μg/dl 100–400 μg/dl 350–450 μg/dl
Lactic acid	whole blood, venous		5–20 mg/dl
Lactic dehydrogenase (LDH)[4] (pyruvate, 30°C)		Newborn Thereafter Male Female	300–1500 IU/l 50– 150 IU/l 40– 140 IU/l
Lead, normal abnormal, nontoxic toxic	whole blood, venous		0–40 μg/dl 40–80 μg/dl >80 μg/dl
Lipase[4] (olive oil, 37°C)		Infant Thereafter	9–105 IU/l 20–136 IU/l
Lipids, total		Newborn-2 yr 2 yr–14 yr Thereafter	170– 450 mg/dl 490–1000 mg/dl 400– 800 mg/dl

Lipoproteins

	Total	Alpha	Beta	Chylo	Units
Newborn	170– 440	70–180	50–160	50–110	mg/dl
Infant	240– 800	70–280	120–450	50–250	mg/dl
Thereafter	500–1100	150–330	225–540	100–270	mg/dl

DETERMINATION	SPECIMEN	AGE/SEX	NORMAL VALUE
Magnesium		Newborn Infant Thereafter	1.4–2.9 mEq/l 1.2–2.7 mEq/l 1.2–2.6 mEq/l
Malic dehydrogenase (MDH)[4] (oxalacetic acid, 37°C)		Cord Thereafter	41–68 IU/l 32–48 IU/l
Methemoglobin	whole blood		0.0–0.3 gm/dl
Osmolality			270–285 mOsm/l

*Footnotes for Tables 30-2 to 30-9 will be found at end of Table 30-9.

TABLE 30-2 CHEMISTRY (*Continued*)

DETERMINATION	SPECIMEN	AGE/SEX	NORMAL VALUE
Oxygen, partial pressure (PO_2)	whole blood, arterial		75–100 mm Hg
	whole blood, venous		20– 50 mm Hg
Oxygen, % saturation	whole blood, arterial	Newborn	40–95%
		Thereafter	95–98%
	whole blood, venous	Newborn	30–80%
		Thereafter	35–85%
pH (37°C)[7]	whole blood, arterial	Premature (cord)	7.15–7.35
		Premature (48 hr)	7.35–7.50
		Newborn	7.27–7.47
		Thereafter	7.35–7.45
Phenylalanine			0.5–2.0 mg/dl
Phosphatase, acid[4] (phenylphosphate, 37°C)		Newborn–2 wk	10.4–16.4 IU/l
		2 wk–13 yr	8.6–12.6 IU/l
		Thereafter	
		Male	0.5–11.0 IU/l
		Female	0.2– 9.5 IU/l
Phosphatase, alkaline[4] (p-nitrophenylphosphate, AMP buffer, 37°C, Auto-Analyzer)		Newborn	50–275 IU/l
		Infant	100–330 IU/l
		Child	90–230 IU/l
		Adolescent	100–250 IU/l
		Thereafter	30– 90 IU/l
Phosphorus		Newborn	3.5–8.6 mg/dl
		Infant	4.5–6.7 mg/dl
		Child	4.5–5.5 mg/dl
		Thereafter	2.5–4.8 mg/dl
Phospholipids (lipids P × 25)		Newborn	75–170 mg/dl
		Infant	100–275 mg/dl
		Child	180–295 mg/dl
		Thereafter	150–380 mg/dl
Potassium		Premature (cord)	5.0–10.2 mEq/l
		Premature (48 hr)	3.0– 6.0 mEq/l
		Newborn (cord)	5.6–12.0 mEq/l
		Newborn	5.0– 7.7 mEq/l
		Infant	4.1– 5.3 mEq/l
		Child	3.5– 4.7 mEq/l
		Thereafter	3.4– 5.6 mEq/l
Protein, total		Premature	4.3–7.6 gm/dl
		Newborn	4.6–7.6 gm/dl
		Child	6.2–8.1 gm/dl
		Thereafter	5.5–7.8 gm/dl
Sodium		Premature (cord)	116–140 mEq/l
		Premature (48 hr)	128–148 mEq/l
		Newborn (cord)	126–166 mEq/l
		Newborn	139–162 mEq/l
		Infant	139–146 mEq/l
		Child	138–145 mEq/l
		Thereafter	135–151 mEq/l
Thiamine	whole blood		5.5–9.5 μg/dl
Transaminases[4]			
Glutamic oxalacetic (GOT)		Newborn/infant	5–70 IU/l

Table continued.

TABLE 30–2 CHEMISTRY (*Continued*)

DETERMINATION	SPECIMEN	AGE/SEX	NORMAL VALUE[3]
(aspartate, 30°C)		Thereafter	5–20 IU/l
Glutamic pyruvic (GPT)		Newborn/infant	5–50 IU/l
(alanine, 30°C)		Thereafter	5–30 IU/l
Transferrin			0.2–0.3 gm/dl
Triglycerides		Newborn/infant	5– 40 mg/dl
		Thereafter	10–190 mg/dl
Urea nitrogen (BUN)		Newborn/infant	5–15 mg/dl
		Thereafter	10–20 mg/dl
Uric acid		Child	2.0–5.5 mg/dl
		Thereafter	
		Male	2.1–7.7 mg/dl
		Female	1.8–6.6 mg/dl
Vitamin A			16–60 μg/dl
Vitamin B_{12}			100–700 pg/ml
Vitamin E (tocopherols)			0.5–1.5 mg/dl

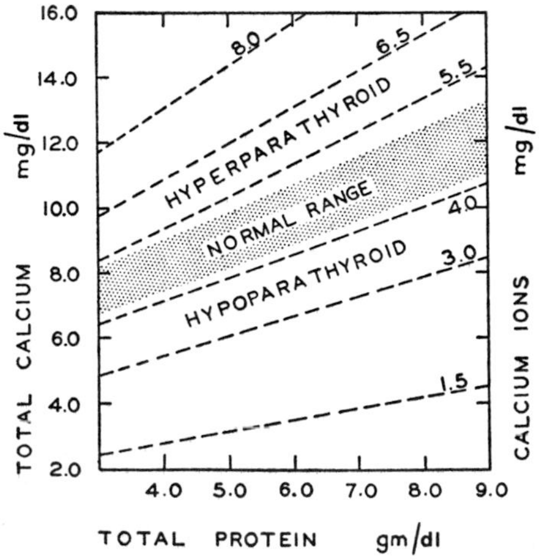

Figure 30–3 *Nomogram for estimation of serum ionized calcium from total calcium and total protein values. Modified by Lytt I. Gardner from the McLean-Hastings data* (J. Biol. Chem., *Vol. 108).*

TABLE 30-3 SPECIAL CHEMISTRY

DETERMINATION	SPECIMEN	AGE/SEX	NORMAL VALUE
(urine unless otherwise indicated)			
Aldosterone			2–26 μg/24 hr
Ammonia		Infant	10–50 mEq/24 hr
		Child	15–50 mEq/24 hr
		Thereafter	20–70 mEq/24 hr
Amylase[4]		Neonatal	0–1000 IU/hr
		Thereafter	700–5200 IU/hr
Calcium			2.5–20 mEq/24 hr
Catecholamines	Norepinephrine	Epinephrine	Units
Newborn	2– 4	0– 1	μg/24 hr
Neonatal	2– 12	1– 2	μg/24 hr
Infant	3– 60	1–15	μg/24 hr
Child	20– 70	1–15	μg/24 hr
Adolescent	30– 80	5–15	μg/24 hr
Adult	40–100	5–15	μg/24 hr
Chloride		Infant	2– 10 mEq/24 hr
		Child	15– 40 mEq/24 hr
		Thereafter	150–250 mEq/24 hr
Chloride	sweat		
Normal			0– 30 mEq/l
Marginal (i.c., asthma, Addison's disease, malnutrition, etc.)			30– 70 mEq/l
Cystic fibrosis			70–200 mEq/l
Creatinine		Infant	8–20 mg/kg/24 hr
		Child	8–22 mg/kg/24 hr
		Adolescent	8–30 mg/kg/24 hr
		Thereafter	14–26 mg/kg/24 hr
Fat, fecal	feces		<5 gm/24 hr
5-Hydroxyindoleacetic acid (5-HIAA)			0–10 mg/dl
17-Ketogenic steroids (17-KGS)		0–2 yr	2– 4 mg/24 hr
		2–6 yr	3– 6 mg/24 hr
		6–10 yr	6– 8 mg/24 hr
		10–14 yr	8–14 mg/24 hr
		Adult: Male	10–20 mg/24 hr
		Female	6–17 mg/24 hr
17-Ketosteroids (17-KS)		0–14 days	0.5– 2.5 mg/24 hr
		14 da–2 yr	0– 0.5 mg/24 hr
		2–6 yr	0– 2.0 mg/24 hr
		6–8 yr	0– 2.5 mg/24 hr
		8–10 yr	0.7– 4.0 mg/24 hr
		10–12 yr: Male	0.7– 6.0 mg/24 hr
		Female	0.7– 5.0 mg/24 hr
		12–14 yr: Male	1.3–10.0 mg/24 hr
		Female	1.3– 8.5 mg/24 hr
		14–16 yr: Male	2.5–13.0 mg/24 hr
		Female	2.5–11.0 mg/24 hr
		Adult: Male	9.0–22.0 mg/24 hr
		Female	6.0–15.0 mg/24 hr

*Footnotes for Tables 30–2 to 30–9 will be found at end of Table 30–9.

Table continued.

TABLE 30-3 SPECIAL CHEMISTRY (*Continued*)

DETERMINATION	SPECIMEN	AGE/SEX	NORMAL VALUE			
			Normal	Abnormal, nontoxic	Toxic	Units
Lead and metabolites						
Lead	whole blood		0– 40	40– 80	> 80	μg/dl
Lead	urine		0– 80	80–150	>150	μg/dl
Coproporphyrin	urine		0–150	150–500	>500	μg/dl
δ-Aminolevulinic acid (ALA)	urine		0.1–0.6	0.6–2.0	>2.0	μg/dl
Lipase[4] (olive oil, 37°C)	duodenal drainage (intestinal juice)		8–35 IU/ml			
Phosphorus			0.7–1.1 g/24 hr			
Pituitary gonadotropins (FSH)		Child	0 mouse u			
		Female				
		Premenopausal	25–40 mouse u			
		Pregnant	2,000–50,000 mouse u			
		Postmenopausal	20–50 mouse u			
		Male	0–20 mouse u			
Porphyrins						
Porphobilinogen			0 μg/24 hr			
Uroporphyrin			0– 30 μg/24 hr			
Coproporphyrin		Male	130–248 μg/24 hr			
		Female	92–176 μg/24 hr			
Potassium			25–100 mEq/24 hr			
Pregnanetriol		Newborn	0 mg/24 hr			
		Infant	0 –0.2 mg/24 hr			
		Child	0.3–1.1 mg/24 hr			
		Thereafter	0.5–4.0 mg/24 hr			
Protein, total (albumin)			2– 8 mg/dl			
			10–100 mg/24 hr			
Sodium		Child	40–180 mEq/24 hr			
		Thereafter	80–220 mEq/24 hr			
Titratable acidity[8]	gastric juice					
Basal acid output (BAO)			0– 6 mEq/hr			
Maximal histamine stimulation acid output (MAO)		Male	10–35 mEq/hr			
		Female	5–30 mEq/hr			
Trypsin (N-benzoyl-arginine ethyl ester, 25°C)	duodenal drainage (intestinal juice)		160–180 μg/ml			
Urobilinogen			<3 mg/24 hr			
Vanilmandelic acid (VMA)		Newborn	0–1 mg/24 hr			
		Neonatal	0–1 mg/24 hr			
		Infant	0–2 mg/24 hr			
		Child	1–5 mg/24 hr			
		Adolescent	1–5 mg/24 hr			
		Thereafter	2–7 mg/24 hr			
Xylose absorption			<20% retention of dose in 5 hr			

*Footnotes for Tables 30-2 to 30-9 will be found at end of Table 30-9.

TABLE 30-4 CEREBROSPINAL FLUID

DETERMINATION	AGE/SEX	NORMAL VALUE	
Calcium		2–3 mEq/l	
Cell count		wbc's/mm³	rbc's/mm³
	Premature	0–18	0–500
	Newborn	0–15	0–500
	Infant	0– 8	0– 10
	Thereafter	0– 5	0– 10
Chloride	Neonatal	108–122 mEq/l	
	Thereafter	112–130 mEq/l	
Glucose[9]	Newborn	20–40 mg/dl	
	Infant/child	70–90 mg/dl	
	Thereafter	50–80 mg/dl	
Lactic dehydrogenase (LDH)[4] (pyruvate, 30°C)	Newborn	5–80 IU/l	
	Thereafter	5–30 IU/l	
Magnesium		2.8–3.3 mg/dl	
Pandy's test (for excess globulins)		Negative	
pH (37°C)		7.33–7.42	
Phosphorus, inorganic		1.5–3.0 mg/dl	
Potassium		2.8–4.1 mEq/l	
Protein, total	Newborn–1 mo	20–120 mg/dl	
	Thereafter	15– 45 mg/dl	
Albumin		52%	
$Alpha_1$		5%	
$Alpha_2$		14%	
Beta		10%	
Gamma		19%	
Sodium		130–165 mEq/l	
Specific gravity		1.007–1.009	
Transaminase[4] Glutamic oxalacetic (GOT) (aspartate, 30°C)		2–10 IU/l	

*Footnotes for Tables 30–2 to 30–9 will be found at end of Table 30–9.

TABLE 30–5 HEMATOLOGY

DETERMINATION	AGE/SEX	NORMAL VALUE
(whole blood unless otherwise indicated)		(see footnotes 1–4)
Hematocrit (PCV)	Newborn	44–64%
	Neonatal	35–49%
	Infant	30–40%
	Child	31–43%
	Thereafter: Male	40–54%
	Female	37–47%
Hemoglobin[10]	Newborn	14–24 gm/dl
	Neonatal	11–20 gm/dl
	Infant	10–15 gm/dl
	Child	11–16 gm/dl
	Thereafter: Male	14–18 gm/dl
	Female	12–16 gm/dl
Hemoglobin, fetal (Hb F)	Newborn	40–70% of total
	Neonatal	20–40% of total
	Infant	2–10% of total
	Thereafter	1– 2% of total
Nucleated RBC's	Cord	250–500/mm^3
	Day 1	200–300/mm^3
	Day 2	20– 30/mm^3
	Thereafter	0
Osmotic fragility		0.44–0.40% NaCl
50% hemolysis		0.5 –1.5% NaCl
Platelet count	Premature	100–300 000/mm^3
	Newborn	140–300 000/mm^3
	Neonatal	150–390 000/mm^3
	Infant	200–473 000/mm^3
	Thereafter	150–450 000/mm^3
Red blood cell count (RBC)	Newborn	4.8–7.1 mil/mm^3
	Neonatal	4.1–6.4 mil/mm^3
	Infant/child	3.8–5.5 mil/mm^3
	Thereafter: Male	4.6–6.2 mil/mm^3
	Female	4.2–5.4 mil/mm^3

*Footnotes for Tables 30–2 to 30–9 will be found at end of Table 30–9.

TABLE 30–5 HEMATOLOGY (*Continued*)

DETERMINATION	AGE/SEX	NORMAL VALUE
Blood indices		
MCH	Newborn	32– 34 μμg
	Thereafter	27– 31 μμg
MCV	Newborn	96–108 μ^3
	Thereafter	82– 91 μ^3
MCHC	Newborn	32– 33%
	Thereafter	32– 36%
Reticulocyte count	Newborn	2.5–6.5% total RBC
	Neonatal	0.1–1.5% total RBC
	Infant	0.5–3.1% total RBC
	Thereafter	0–2.0% total RBC
Sedimentation rate (ESR) (uncorrected)	Newborn	0– 2 mm/hr
	Neonatal/puberty	3–13 mm/hr
	Adult: Male	10–15 mm/hr
	Female	15–25 mm/hr
White blood cell count (WBC)[11]	Newborn, total	9,000–30,000/mm^3
	% neutrophiles	≃61%
	% lymphocytes	≃31%
	1 wk, total	5,000–21,000/mm^3
	% neutrophiles	≃45%
	% lymphocytes	≃41%
	4 wk, total	5,000–19,500/mm^3
	% neutrophiles	≃35%
	% lymphocytes	≃56%
	6–12 mo, total	6,000–17,500/mm^3
	% neutrophiles	≃32%
	% lymphocytes	≃61%
	2 yr, total	6,200–17,000/mm^3
	% neutrophiles	≃33%
	% lymphocytes	≃59%
	Thereafter, total	5,000–10,000/mm^3
	% neutrophiles	≃60%
	% lymphocytes	≃30%

*Footnotes for Tables 30–2 to 30–9 will be found at end of Table 30–9.

TABLE 30–6 COAGULATION[12]

DETERMINATION	SPECIMEN	AGE/SEX	NORMAL VALUE
	(anticoagulants and collection instructions vary for individual laboratories)		
Activated clotting time (ACT)	plasma		<2.16 min
Bleeding time (Ivy)	whole blood	Premature Newborn Thereafter	1–8 min 1–5 min 1–6 min
Clot retraction	whole blood		Complete at 4 hr
Clotting time 2 tubes 3 tubes	whole blood		 5– 8 min 5–15 min
Fibrinogen	plasma	Newborn Thereafter	150–300 mg/dl 200–400 mg/dl
Fibrinolysin (plasminogen)	plasma		Lysis of clot
Partial thromboplastin time (PTT)[13]	plasma	Premature Newborn Thereafter	<120 sec < 90 sec < 60 sec
Prothrombin time, one stage (PT)[13]	plasma	Premature Newborn/neonatal Thereafter	12–21 sec 12–20 sec 12–14 sec
Thromboplastin generation test (TGT)[13]	plasma	Premature Newborn Thereafter	8–24 sec at 6 min tube 8–20 sec at 6 min tube 8–16 sec at 6 min tube

*Footnotes for Tables 30–2 to 30–9 will be found at end of Table 30–9.

TABLE 30–7 SEROLOGY

DETERMINATION	SPECIMEN	VALUE
	(serum unless otherwise indicated)	
Alpha-1-fetoprotein		None detected
Antistreptolysin 0 titer (ASO)		
Normal		12– 100 Todd units
Recent Strep. infection[14]		200–2500 Todd units
Antihyaluronidase titer (AHT)		< 1:256
Colloidal gold curve	CSF	
Normal		Flat curve (1,1,1,1,0,0,0,0,0,0,0)
CNS syphilis, multiple sclerosis		First zone curve (5,5,5,5,4,3,2,1,1,0,0)
Abnormal spinal fluid		Mid zone curve (0,1,2,3,3,3,2,1,0,0,0)
Acute purulent meningitis		End zone curve (0,0,0,1,1,2,3,3,3,3,0)
Cold agglutinins		0–1:32
C-reactive protein (CRP)		None detected
Febrile agglutinins		
Typhoid O		0–1:40[15]
Typhoid H		0–1:20[15]
Brucella		0–1:20
Rickettsia (Proteus OX 19)		0–1:40
Tularemia		0–1:40
Hepatitis associated (Australia) antigen		None detected
Heterophile antibody		
Mono "spot" test		Negative
Thyroid autoantibodies		
Thyroglobulin antibody (tanned red cell method)		0–1:32

*Footnotes for Tables 30–2 to 30–9 will be found at end of Table 30–9.

TABLE 30-8 URINALYSIS

DETERMINATION	AGE/SEX	NORMAL VALUE		
Addis count				
Leukocytes		<1,000,000/12 hrs		
Erythrocytes		< 250,000/12 hrs		
Casts		< 5,000/12 hrs		
Protein		< 20 mg/12 hrs		
Colony count, colonies/ml urine (fresh specimen)		Clean catch,[16] midstream	Catheterization	Suprapubic bladder puncture
	Infant/child	< 1,000	<100	0
	Thereafter	<10,000	<100	0
Gastric analysis/Diagnex Blue titration		>0.6 mg Azure A excreted		
Microscopic				
Leukocytes		0–4 per high-power field		
Erythrocytes		rare per high-power field		
Casts		rare per high-power field		
Osmolality	Premature/newborn	100– 600 mOsm/l		
	Thereafter	50–1400 mOsm/l		
pH	Newborn/neonatal	5 –7		
	Thereafter	4.5–8		
Specific gravity	Newborn/infant	1.001–1.020		
	Thereafter	1.001–1.030		
Volume	Newborn	30– 300 ml/24 hr		
	Neonatal	250– 450 ml/24 hr		
	Infant	400– 600 ml/24 hr		
	Child	500–1000 ml/24 hr		
	Adolescent	500–1500 ml/24 hr		
	Adult	500–2000 ml/24 hr		

*Footnotes for Tables 30–2 to 30–9 will be found at end of Table 30–9.

TABLE 30-9 RADIOISOTOPIC PROCEDURES

DETERMINATION	SPECIMEN	NORMAL VALUE
^{51}Chromium		
Cell survival (T/2)	whole blood	25–35 days 1/2–time
Red cell mass	whole blood	28–32 ml/kg
^{51}Chromium-albumin		
Normal	urine	10–15% of dose in 72 hr
Exudative enteropathy	urine	6–12% of dose in 72 hr
Normal	stool	0– 1% of dose in 72 hr
Exudative enteropathy	stool	2–20% of dose in 72 hr
Iodine (^{131}I) uptake	neck scan	6–17% of dose in 6 hr
	neck scan	10–30% of dose in 24 hr
Rose bengal-^{131}I		
Normal	urine	5–30% of dose in 72 hr
Hepatocellular obstruction	urine	10–20% of dose in 72 hr
Biliary obstruction	urine	15–25% of dose in 72 hr
Normal	stool	40–70% of dose in 72 hr
Hepatocellular obstruction	stool	10–50% of dose in 72 hr
Biliary obstruction	stool	0– 5% of dose in 72 hr

*Footnotes for Tables 30–2 to 30–9 will be found at end of Table 30–9.

FOOTNOTES

[1]Delineation of normal values for laboratory tests depends inevitably on the population sampled, upon the physiologic state at the time of sampling, and upon manner of sample collection, analytic technique and statistical methods employed for setting the numerical ranges. Laboratory values in well infants and children have not been extensively and systematically evaluated for most currently used methods. The following lists of normal values are based on the experience in the Clinical Laboratories, University of Kentucky Medical Center, Lexington. They have proved useful in caring for sick infants and children.

[2]Age ranges are defined as follows:

Premature	birth–1 mo
Newborn	birth–1 wk
Neonatal	1 wk–1 mo
Infant	1 mo–2 yr
Child	2 yr–puberty
Adolescent	puberty–adult
Adult	>18 yr

[3]The Systeme International d'Unites (SI) is becoming the approved means of expressing information in all branches of science and technology, including medicine, and represents international agreement as to conventional nomenclature of units of measurement. Changes to units which would involve an alteration in the numerical value of results (such as occurred when mEq/l replaced mg/100 ml for electrolytes) are not proposed now. SI has six basic units: meter, kilogram, second, ampere, kelvin and candela, supplemented by the radian, steradian and the mole. All other units are derived from these. Decimal multiples and submultiples of units are formed by the use of prefixes as shown:

DECIMAL MULTIPLES AND SUBMULTIPLES

Multiple	*Prefix*	*Symbol*	*Submultiple*	*Prefix*	*Symbol*
10^{12}	tera	T	10^{-1}	deci	d
10^{9}	giga	G	10^{-2}	centi	c
10^{6}	mega	M	10^{-3}	milli	m
10^{3}	kilo	k	10^{-6}	micro	μ
10^{2}	hecto	h	10^{-9}	nano	n
10	deca	da	10^{-12}	pico	p

(e.g., 25 mg/100 ml or mg% becomes 25 mg/dl)

[4]An international unit (IU) equals 1 μmole of substrate transformed or of product formed per minute. Units can be expressed per milliliter or per liter. Temperature of the reaction should be stated.

FACTORS FOR CONVERSION OF CONVENTIONAL UNITS TO INTERNATIONAL UNITS (μmoles/min/liter) FOR ENZYMES OF CURRENT DIAGNOSTIC SIGNIFICANCE

Enzyme	*Conventional Units*	*To Obtain IU Multiply by Factor Listed*
Aldolase	Sibley and Lehninger	0.75
Amylase	Somogyi	2.0
Lactic dehydrogenase	Optical density	0.5
Lipase	Bunch and Emerson	208
Malic dehydrogenase	Optical density	0.5
Phosphatase, acid	King-Armstrong	1.8
	Bodansky	5.4
	Bessey-Lowry	16.6
Phosphatase, alkaline	King-Armstrong	7.1
	Bodansky	5.4
	Bessey-Lowry	16.6
Transaminases	Optical density	0.5

[5]Endogenous creatinine clearance is expressed in ml per minute and is corrected to average adult surface area of 1.73 M^2:

$$\frac{UV}{P} \times \frac{1.73}{A} = \text{ml/min}$$

where U = urine creatinine in mg/ml
P = plasma or serum creatinine in mg/ml
V = urine volume in ml/min
A = estimated surface area in meter^2

Footnotes continued.

FOOTNOTES (*Continued*)

[6]Adapted from Stiehm and Fudenberg: Pediatrics *37*:715, 1966.
[7]Arterial blood is approximately 0.03 pH units greater than circulating venous blood.
[8]At birth the neonate usually has gastric acidity similar to that of adults. Within a few days after birth, however, and for several weeks thereafter, the ability to secrete acid may become impaired. The response to histamine stimulation in older children (when corrected for body weight or surface area) closely resembles that in adults.
[9]Glucose levels in CSF vary with those of serum glucose. CSF value is approximately one half to two thirds the serum glucose level.
[10]During the neonatal period, hemoglobin measurements from capillary blood are 2–3 gm/dl greater than those in blood obtained by venipuncture.
[11]Eosinophilia (up to 20 per cent of white blood cell count) may occur normally in infancy.
[12]Coagulation factors (I to XIV) are low in the newly born, rising to adult levels during the first months of life.
[13]Moderate deficiency of coagulation factors dependent upon vitamin K (II, prothrombin; VII, proconvertin; IX, plasma thromboplastin component; X, Stuart-Prower factor) occurs during the first days of life. Values return to near-normal levels within 1 week. This deficiency may account for prolonged PTT, PT and TGT during this period.
[14]Convalescent specimen should be examined to demonstrate rise in titer.
[15]May be higher in individuals who have received typhoid vaccine.
[16]Pure cultures with colony counts >100,000 are considered diagnostic in adults, whereas colony counts of >10,000 are usually considered diagnostic in children. Intermediate counts must be interpreted relative to the clinical situation. For females, the physician must be aware of the cleanliness and care used in collecting the specimen. Urine obtained by means of a plastic collection device or by voiding into a container without prior preparation of the patient is usually contaminated, and has limited usefulness in evaluating the possibility of urinary tract infection.

C. Charlton Mabry

CONVERSION TABLES

TABLE 30–10 METHOD FOR CONVERSION OF MILLIGRAMS TO MILLIEQUIVALENTS PER LITER (or to Millimoles per Liter)

mg = milligrams   ml = milliliter
gm = grams   1 ml = 1.000027 cc
dl = deciliter = 100 ml

$$\text{mEq/l (milliequivalents per liter)} = \frac{\text{mg per liter}}{\text{equivalent weight}}$$

$$\text{equivalent weight} = \frac{\text{atomic weight}}{\text{valence of element}}$$

For example: A sample of blood serum contains 10 mg of Ca in 1 dl (100 ml). The valence of Ca is 2, and the atomic weight is 40. The equivalent weight of Ca is therefore 40 ÷ 2, or 20. The milliequivalents of Ca per liter are 10 (mg/dl) × 10 (dl/l) ÷ 20, or 5 milliequivalents per liter.

$$\text{mM/l (millimoles per liter)} = \frac{\text{mg/liter}}{\text{molecular weight}}$$

Vol. % (volumes per cent) = mM/liter × 2.24 for a gas whose properties approach that of an ideal gas, such as oxygen or nitrogen.

For carbon dioxide the factor is 2.226.

TABLE 30–11 FACTORS FOR CONVERSION OF CONCENTRATION EXPRESSED IN MILLIEQUIVALENTS PER LITER TO MILLIGRAMS PER DECILITER (100 ml), AND VICE VERSA, FOR COMMON IONS THAT OCCUR IN PHYSIOLOGIC SOLUTIONS

ELEMENT OR RADICAL	mEq PER LITER	to	Mg PER DL	Mg PER DL	to	mEq PER LITER
Sodium	1		2.30	1		0.4348
Potassium	1		3.91	1		0.2558
Calcium	1		2.005	1		0.4988
Magnesium	1		1.215	1		0.8230
Chloride	1		3.55	1		0.2817
Bicarbonate (HCO_3)	1		6.1	1		0.1639
Phosphorus valence 1	1		3.10	1		0.3226
Phosphorus valence 1.8	1		1.72	1		0.5814
Sulfur valence 2	1		1.60	1		0.625

Example: To convert milliequivalents of magnesium per liter to milligrams per deciliter (100 ml), multiply by the factor 1.215.

To convert milligrams of potassium per deciliter (100 ml) to milliequivalents per liter, multiply by the factor 0.2558.

TABLE 30–12 MILLIEQUIVALENTS AND MILLIGRAMS OF CATIONS AND ANIONS PRESENT IN A MILLIMOLE OF SALTS COMMONLY USED IN PHYSIOLOGIC SOLUTIONS

SALT	mM PER LITER	Mg PER LITER	CATION	ANION	mEq CATION PER LITER	Mg CATION PER LITER	mEq ANION PER LITER	Mg ANION PER LITER
Sodium chloride (NaCl)	1	58.5	Na^+	Cl^-	1	23.0	1	35.5
Potassium chloride (KCl)	1	74.6	K^+	Cl^-	1	39.1	1	35.5
Sodium bicarbonate ($NaHCO_3$)	1	84.0	Na^+	HCO_3^-	1	23.0	1	61.0
Sodium lactate ($CH_3CHOHCOONa$)	1	112.0	Na^+	Lactate$^-$	1	23.0	1	89.0
Potassium phosphate (K_2HPO_4) dibasic	1	174.2	K^+	HPO_4^{--}	2	78.2	1	96.0
Potassium phosphate (KH_2PO_4) monobasic	1	136.1	K^+	$H_2PO_4^-$	1	39.1	1	97.0
Calcium chloride anhydrous ($CaCl_2$)	1	111.0	Ca^{++}	Cl^-	2	40.0	2	71.0
Calcium chloride dihydrate ($CaCl_2.2H_2O$)	1	147.0	Ca^{++}	Cl^-	2	40.0	2	71.0
Magnesium chloride anhydrous ($MgCl_2$)	1	95.2	Mg^{++}	Cl^-	2	24.3	2	71.0
Magnesium chloride hexahydrate ($MgCl_2.6H_2O$)	1	203.3	Mg^{++}	Cl^-	2	24.3	2	71.0
Ammonium chloride (NH_4Cl)	1	53.5	NH_4^+	Cl^-	1	18.0	1	35.5

MILLIOSMOLAL AND MILLIOSMOLAR SOLUTIONS

The total osmotic pressure of a solution is dependent on the number of particles in the solution, regardless of their charge, size or shape. In principle, one mole of an ideal substance, assumed to be a nonelectrolyte, dissolved in a kilogram of water will lower the freezing point of the solvent (water) by 1.8557° C. Such a solution would have 1 osmole in a kilogram of water. One milliosmole is equal to one thousandth of an osmole. The osmometer used in the clinical laboratory measures the freezing point by determining the resistance of a glass-enclosed metallic probe at the freezing point of the specimen. The electrical resistance is proportional to the temperature. In this instrument the osmolality of serum, urine or other biological fluids is determined by comparing their freezing points with that of a carefully prepared sodium chloride solution of known osmotic pressure. The lowering of the freezing point is proportional to the mole fraction (gram-mole of solute per kg. of solvent), and gives the milliosm*olal* concentration, which is slightly different from the milliosm*olar* concentration, which represents milliosmoles of solute per liter of solution. For dilute solutions these two values approach each other and are often used without distinction. Osmolality should be the preferred term, because that is what is measured by the osmometer.

In studying osmotic pressure relations in solution it is useful to express the concentration in terms of ionic concentrations. The term "milliosmolar" supplements the term "millimolar" in appreciation of the additive osmotic effect of the ions.

For example: A millimolar solution of glucose (180 mg/l) is also a milliosmolar solution (1 milliosmole/l), because the number of osmotically active particles is not increased in solution, through ionization. On the other hand, owing to the complete ionization of sodium chloride in solution, a millimolar solution of sodium chloride (58.5 mg/liter) contains 1 chemical milliequivalent of sodium ions and 1 milliequivalent of chloride ions. The milliosmolar concentration is 2 milliosmoles per liter, because 1 chemical milliequivalent of sodium or of chloride ions is equal to 1 milliosmole of sodium or of chloride ions, respectively.

A milliequivalent equals a milliosmole for all univalent ions. The chemical milliequivalence of a divalent ion is twice the milliosmolar value. In a millimolar solution of calcium chloride ($CaCl_2$), for example, there are 2 chemical milliequivalents of calcium ions, but only 1 milliosmole of calcium ions. The millimolar solution of calcium chloride contains 2 chemical milliequivalents of chloride ions or 2 milliosmoles of chloride ions per liter. Accordingly, a millimolar solution of calcium chloride contains 3 milliosmoles per liter, because this salt ionizes into 1 calcium ion and 2 chloride ions.

In blood serum containing 10 mg of calcium per dl (100 ml), there are 5 chemical milliequivalents of calcium per liter, but only 2.5 milliosmoles of calcium per liter. The average normal total ionic concentration of blood serum is 290 milliosmoles; cation concentration 151, anion concentration 139. In blood serum the portion of milliosmoles accounted for by glucose or urea (3 to 6 milliosmoles) or by protein (30 milliosmoles) is small compared to the osmolal effect of the electrolytes. The osmotic pressure of the blood serum of infants and children is comparable to that of adults.

HOWARD W. ROBINSON*
VICTOR C. VAUGHAN III

*Deceased.

Conversion of Apothecary's Measures to Metric Equivalents

TABLE 30-13

Weights

Apothecary	*Metric* Approximate		More Nearly Accurate
1 grain	60 mg	0.06 gm	0.06479 gm
2 grains	120 mg	0.12 gm	
3 grains	180 mg	0.2 gm	
5 grains	300 mg	0.3 gm	
15 grains	1000 mg	1.0 gm	
60 grains or 1 dram		4.0 gm	3.888 gm
240 grains or 4 drams, ½ oz.		15.0 gm	
480 grains or 8 drams, 1 oz.		30.0 gm	31.103 gm 31.103 gm (Troy) 28.350 gm (Avoir.)
12 oz or 1 pound		360.0 gm	373.24177 gm
12 oz or 1 pound		360.0 gm	373.24177 gm (Troy)
16 oz or 1 pound		480.0 gm	453.592 gm (Avoir.)
¾ grain		45 mg	
½ grain		30 mg	
⅜ grain		23 mg	
¼ grain		15 mg	
⅙ grain		10 mg	
⅛ grain		8 mg	
1/10 grain		6 mg	
1/16 grain		4 mg	
1/32 grain		2 mg	
1/64 grain		1 mg	
1/100 grain		0.6 mg	
1/250 grain		0.25 mg	
1/300 grain		0.2 mg	
1/1000 grain		0.06 mg	

Liquid Measures

1 minim		0.06 ml	0.06161 ml
3 minims		0.2 ml	
15 minims		1.0 ml	0.92415 ml *
60 minims, 1 fl. dram		4.0 ml	3.6967 ml
480 minims	1 fl oz	30.0 ml	29.5737 ml
	16 fl oz or 1 pt	500.0 ml	473.179 ml
	32 fl oz or 1 qt	1000.0 ml	946.358 ml

*1 ml is equal to 16.23 minims.

Quantity of drug prescribed in grams per 2 ounces (60 ml) gives dose in grains per dram.

TABLE 30-14 EQUIVALENT TEMPERATURE READINGS (CENTIGRADE AND FAHRENHEIT)*

°C	°F	°C	°F	°C	°F	°C	°F
0	32.0	37.2	99	39.2	102.6	41.2	106.2
20	68.0	37.4	99.3	39.4	102.9	41.4	106.5
30	86.0	37.6	99.7	39.6	103.3	41.6	106.9
31	87.8	37.8	100.1	39.8	103.7	41.8	107.2
32	89.6	38.0	100.4	40.0	104	42	107.6
33	91.4	38.2	100.8	40.2	104.4	43	109.4
34	93.2	38.4	101.2	40.4	104.7	44	111.2
35	95.0	38.6	101.5	40.6	105.1	100	212
36	96.8	38.8	101.8	40.8	105.4		
37	98.6	39.0	102.2	41.0	105.8		

*To convert Centigrade readings to Fahrenheit, multiply by 1.8 and add 32. To convert Fahrenheit readings to Centigrade, subtract 32 and divide by 1.8.

TABLE 30–15 COMPOSITION OF COMMONLY USED ORAL AND PARENTERAL SOLUTIONS

FLUID	CHO Gm/dl	Prot* Gm/dl	Calories per l	Na (mEq/l)	K (mEq/l)	Cl (mEq/l)	HCO_3† (mEq/l)	Ca (mEq/l)	P‡ (mEq/l)	Mg (mEq/l)
Oral										
Apple juice	11.9	0.1	480	0.4	26			3	4.5	
Coca-Cola	10.9		435	0.4	12		13.4			
Ginger ale	9.0		360	3.5	0.1		3.6			
Grape juice	16.6	0.2	672	0.4	30		32			
Grapefruit juice (canned, sugar added)	17.8	0.6	736	0.2	35			6.5		
Lytren	7.0		280	25	25	30	36	4	5	4
Milk	4.9	3.5	670	22	36	28	30	60	54	
Orange juice	10.4	0.7	444	0.2	49		50			
Pedialyte	5.0		200	30	20	30	28	4		4
Pepsi-Cola	12.0		480	6.5	0.8		7.3			
Pineapple juice (canned)	13.5	0.4	556	0.2	38			7.5	9	
Prune juice	19	0.4	776	0.9	60			7	20	
Root beer				3.5	0.1					
Seven-Up	8.0		320	7.5	0.2			0.3		
Tomato juice (canned, salted)	4.3		172	100	59	150	10	3	18	
Parenteral										
CHO§ in H_2O	5–10		200–400							
Isotonic saline	0–5		0–200	154		154				
½ Isotonic saline	2.5–5		100–200	77		77				
3% (M/2) saline				500		500				
5% Saline				850		850				
2% Ammonium chloride						400				
M/6 Sodium lactate				167			167			
5% Sodium bicarbonate				595			595			

Ringer's lactate	0–10		0–400	130	4	109	28	3	
Darrow's KNL				121	35	103	53		
Modified Butler's 1	5–10		200–400	25	20	22	23		3
Modified Butler's 2	5–10		200–400	58	25	51	25		13
Talbot's	5–10		200–400	40	35	40	20		15
Ordway's	3.5–10		140–400	26	27	53			
Gastric replacement	0–10		0–400	63	17	150			
Intestinal replacement	5–10		200–400	80	36	64	60	5	
Amigen	5–10	5	345–515	30	15	22		5	30
Amigen, dextrose and Ringer's lactate	3.3	3.3	230	65	10	51	10	5	20
Amigen, dextrose and alcohol	5–12	5	670–800	30	15	22		5	30
Dextran 6%	0–5		0–200						
Dextran 6% in saline				154		154			
Plasmanate		5		110	2	50	50		
Blood¶		3		95	4	50	40		2
Protein hydrolysate 5%	5.0	37–40	340	35	19	20		5	30

Available Additives

Glucose 50%	0.5 gm per ml
Sodium chloride	2.5 or 4.0 mEq per ml
Sodium lactate	4.0 mEq per ml
Sodium bicarbonate	9.0 mEq per ml
Potassium chloride	1.0 or 2.0 mEq per ml
Potassium phosphate	3.0 mEq per ml
Potassium acetate	4.0 mEq per ml
Calcium gluconate 10%	9.3 mg calcium per ml
Calcium chloride 10%	36.0 mg calcium per ml
Ammonium chloride	4.0 mEq per ml
Magnesium sulfate ($MgSO_4 \cdot 7\ H_2O$) 50%	4.0 mEq per ml

*Protein or amino acid equivalent.
†Actual or potential bicarbonate, such as acetate, lactate, citrate.
‡Calculated according to valence of 1.8.
§Glucose (dextrose, fructose or invert sugar)
¶Red cell contents not included in calculations.
Also available Mannitol 5%, 10%, 15% and 20%.

Reference: Church, C. F., and Church, H. N.: Food Values of Portions Commonly Used (Bowes and Church). 11th ed. Philadelphia, J. B. Lippincott Co., 1970.

FOOD VALUES

TABLE 30–16 FOOD COMPOSITION TABLE FOR SHORT METHOD OF DIETARY ANALYSIS

FOOD AND APPROXIMATE MEASURE	WEIGHT GM	FOOD ENERGY CAL	PRO-TEIN GM	FAT GM	CARBO-HY-DRATE GM	CAL-CIUM MG	IRON MG	VITA-MIN A VALUE I U	THIA-MINE MG	RIBO-FLAVIN MG	NIACIN MG	ASCOR-BIC ACID MG
Milk, cheese, cream; related products												
Cheese: blue, cheddar (1 cu in , 17 gm).												
cheddar process (1 oz). Swiss (1 oz)	30	105	6	9	1	165	0.2	345	0.01	0.12	Trace	0
cottage (from skim) creamed (1/2 c)	115	120	16	5	3	105	0.4	190	0.04	0.28	0.1	0
Cream: half-and-half (cream and milk) (2 tbsp)	30	40	1	4	2	30	Trace	145	0.01	0.04	Trace	Trace
For light whipping add 1 pat butter												
Milk: whole (3.5% fat) (1 c)	245	160	9	9	12	285	0.1	350	0.08	0.42	0.1	2
fluid, nonfat (skim) and buttermilk (from skim)	245	90	9	Trace	13	300	Trace	–	0.10	0.44	0.2	2
milk beverage (1 c): cocoa, chocolate drink made with skim milk. For malted milk add 4 tbsp half-and-half (270 gm)	245	210	8	8	26	280	0.6	300	0.09	0.43	0.3	Trace
milk desserts, custard (1 c) 248 gm , ice cream (8 fl oz) 142 gm.		290	8	17	29	210	0.4	785	0.07	0.34	0.1	1
cornstarch pudding (248 gm), ice milk (1 c) 187 gm		280	9	10	40	290	0.1	390	0.08	0.41	0.3	2
White sauce, med (1/2 c)	130	215	5	16	12	150	0.2	610	0.06	0.22	0.3	Trace
Egg: 1 large	50	80	6	6	Trace	25	1.2	590	0.06	0.15	Trace	0
Meat, poultry, fish, shellfish, related products												
Beef, lamb, veal: lean and fat, cooked, inc. corned beef (3 oz) (all cuts)	85	245	22	16	0	10	2.9	25	0.06	0.19	4.2	0
lean only, cooked; dried beef (2+ oz) (all cuts)	65	140	20	5	0	10	2.4	10	0.05	0.16	3.4	0
Beef, relatively fat, such as steak and rib, cooked (3 oz)	85	350	18	30	0	10	2.4	60	0.05	0.14	3.5	0
Liver: beef, fried (2 oz)	55	130	15	6	3	5	5.0	30,280	0.15	2.37	9.4	15
Pork, lean and fat, cooked (3 oz) (all cuts)	85	325	20	24	0	10	2.6	0	0.62	0.20	4.2	0
lean only, cooked (2+ oz) (all cuts)	60	150	18	8	0	5	2.2	0	0.57	0.19	3.2	0
ham, light cure, lean and fat, roasted (3 oz)	85	245	18	19	0	10	2.2	0	0.40	0.16	3.1	0
Luncheon meats: bologna (2 sl), pork sausage, cooked (2 oz), frankfurter (1), bacon, broiled or fried crisp (3 sl)		185	9	16	–	5	1.3	–	0.21	0.12	1.7	0
Poultry												
chicken: flesh only, broiled (3 oz)	85	115	20	3	0	10	1.4	80	0.05	0.16	7.4	0
fried (2+ oz)	75	170	24	6	1	10	1.6	85	0.05	0.23	8.3	0
turkey, light and dark, roasted (3 oz)	85	160	27	5	0	–	1.5	–	0.03	0.15	6.5	0
Fish and shellfish												
salmon (3 oz) (canned)	85	130	17	5	0	165	0.7	60	0.03	0.16	6.8	0
fish sticks, breaded, cooked (3-4)	75	130	13	7	5	10	0.3	–	0.03	0.05	1.2	0
mackerel, halibut, cooked	85	175	19	10	0	10	0.8	515	0.08	0.15	6.8	0
bluefish, haddock, herring, perch, shad, cooked (tuna canned in oil, 20 gm)	85	160	19	8	2	20	1.0	60	0.06	0.11	4.4	0

clams, canned: crab meat, canned; lobster; oyster, raw; scallop; shrimp, canned	85	75	14	1	2	65	2.5	65	0.10	0.08	1.5	0
Mature dry beans and peas, nuts, peanuts, related products												
Beans: white with pork and tomato, canned (1 c)	260	320	16	7	50	140	4.7	340	0.20	0.08	1.5	5
red (128 gm). Lima (96 gm), cowpeas (125 gm), cooked (1/2 c)		125	8	–	25	35	2.5	5	0.13	0.06	0.7	–
Nuts: almonds (12), cashews (8), peanuts (1 tbsp), peanut butter (1 tbsp), pecans (12), English walnuts (2 tbsp), coconut (1/4 c)	15	95	3	8	4	15	0.5	5	0.05	0.04	0.9	–
Vegetables and vegetable products												
Asparagus, cooked, cut spears (2/3 c)	115	25	3	Trace	4	25	0.7	1055	0.19	0.20	1.6	30
Beans: green (1/2 c) cooked 60 gm ; canned 120 gm		15	1	Trace	3	30	0.4	340	0.04	0.06	0.3	8
Lima, immature, cooked (1/2 c)	80	90	6	1	16	40	2.0	225	0.14	0.08	1.0	14
Broccoli spears, cooked (2/3 c)	100	25	3	Trace	4	90	0.8	2500	0.09	0.20	0.8	90
Brussels sprouts, cooked (2/3 c)	85	30	3	Trace	5	30	1.0	450	0.07	0.12	0.7	75
Cabbage (110 gm); cauliflower, cooked (80 gm); and sauerkraut, canned (150 mg) (reduced ascorbic acid value by one-third for kraut) (2/3 c)		20	1	Trace	4	35	0.5	80	0.05	0.05	0.3	37
Carrots, cooked (2/3 c)	95	30	1	Trace	7	30	0.6	10,145	0.05	0.05	0.5	6
Corn, 1 ear, cooked (140 gm); canned (130 gm) (1/2 c)		75	2	Trace	18	5	0.4	315	0.06	0.06	1.1	6
Leafy greens: collards (125 gm), dandelions (120 gm), kale (75 gm), mustard (95 gm), spinach (120 gm), turnip (100 gm cooked, 150 gm canned) (2/3 c cooked and canned) (reduce ascorbic acid one-half for canned)		30	3	Trace	5	175	1.8	8570	0.11	0.18	0.8	45
Peas, green (1/2 c)	80	60	4	1	10	20	1.4	430	0.22	0.09	1.8	16
Potatoes, baked, boiled (100 gm), 10 pc. French fried (55 gm) (for fried, add 1 tbsp cooking oil)		85	3	Trace	30	10	0.7	Trace	0.08	0.04	1.5	16
Pumpkin, canned (1/2 c)	115	40	1	1	9	30	0.5	7295	0.03	0.06	0.6	6
Squash, winter, canned (1/2 c)	100	65	2	1	16	30	0.8	4305	0.05	0.14	0.7	14
Sweet potato, canned (1/2 c)	110	120	2	–	27	25	0.8	8500	0.05	0.05	0.7	15
Tomato, 1 raw, 2/3 c canned, 2/3 c juice	150	35	2	Trace	7	14	0.8	1350	0.10	0.06	1.0	29
Tomato catsup (2 tbsp)	35	30	1	Trace	8	10	0.2	480	0.04	0.02	0.6	6
Other, cooked (beets, mushrooms, onions, turnips) (1/2 c)	95	25	1	–	5	20	0.5	15	0.02	0.10	0.7	7
Other commonly served raw, cabbage (1/2 c , 50 gm), celery (3 sm stalks, 40 gm), cucumber (1/4 med , 50 gm), green pepper (1/2, 30 gm), radishes (5, 40 gm)		10	Trace	Trace	2	15	0.3	100	0.03	0.03	0.2	20
carrots, raw (1/2 carrot)	25	10	Trace	Trace	2	10	0.2	2750	0.02	0.02	0.2	2
lettuce leaves (2 lg)	50	10	1	Trace	2	34	0.7	950	0.03	0.04	0.2	9
Fruits and fruit products												
Cantaloupe (1/2 med)	385	60	1	Trace	14	25	0.8	6540	0.08	0.06	1.2	63
Citrus and strawberries: orange (1), grapefruit (1/2), juice (1/2 c), strawberries (1/2 c), lemon (1), tangerine (1)		50	1	–	13	25	0.4	165	0.08	0.03	0.3	55
Yellow, fresh: apricots (3), peach (2 med).; canned fruit and juice (1/2 c) or dried, cooked, unsweetened: apricot, peaches (1/2 c)		85	–	–	22	10	1.1	1005	0.01	0.05	1.0	5

Table continued.

TABLE 30–16 FOOD COMPOSITION TABLE FOR SHORT METHOD OF DIETARY ANALYSIS (*Continued*)

FOOD AND APPROXIMATE MEASURE	WEIGHT GM	FOOD ENERGY CAL	PROTEIN GM	FAT GM	CARBOHYDRATE GM	CALCIUM MG	IRON MG	VITAMIN A VALUE IU	THIAMINE MG	RIBOFLAVIN MG	NIACIN MG	ASCORBIC ACID MG
Other, dried: dates, pitted (4), figs (2), raisins (1/4 c)	40	120	1	–	31	35	1.4	20	0.04	0.04	0.5	–
Other, fresh: apple (1), banana (1), figs (3), pear (1)		80	–	–	21	15	0.5	140	0.04	0.03	0.2	6
Fruit pie: to 1 serving fruit add 1 tbsp flour, 2 tbsp sugar, 1 tbsp fat												
Grain products												
Enriched and whole grain: bread (1 sl, 23 gm), biscuit (1/2), cooked cereals (1/2 c), prepared cereals (1 oz) Graham crackers (2 lg), macaroni, noodles, spaghetti (1/2 c, cooked), pancake (1, 27 gm), roll (1/2), waffle (1/2, 38 gm)		65	2	1	16	20	0.6	10	0.09	0.05	0.7	–
Unenriched: bread (1 sl, 23 gm), cooked cereal (1/2 c), macaroni, noodles, spaghetti (1/2 c), popcorn (1/2 c), pretzel sticks, small (15), roll (1/2)		65	2	1	16	10	0.3	5	0.02	0.02	0.3	–
Desserts												
Cake, plain (1 pc), doughnut (1). For iced cake or doughnut add value for sugar (1 tbsp). For chocolate cake add chocolate (30 gm)	45	145	2	5	24	30	0.4	65	0.02	0.05	0.2	–
Cookies, plain (1)	25	120	1	5	18	10	0.2	20	0.01	0.01	0.1	–
Pie crust, single crust (1/7 shell)	20	95	1	6	8	3	0.3	0	0.04	0.03	0.3	–
Flour, white, enriched (1 tbsp)	7	25	1	Trace	5	1	0.2	0	0.03	0.02	0.2	0
Fats and Oils												
Butter, margarine (1 pat, 1/2 tbsp)	7	50	Trace	6	Trace	1	0	230	–	–	–	–
Fats and oils, cooking (1 tbsp). French dressing (2 tbsp)	14	125	0	14	0	0	0	0	0	0	0	0
Salad dressings, mayonnaise type (1 tbsp)	15	80	Trace	9	1	2	0.1	45	Trace	Trace	Trace	0
Sugars, sweets												
Candy, plain (1/2 oz), jam and jelly (1 tbsp), syrup (1 tbsp), gelatin dessert, plain (1/2 c.), beverages, carbonated (1 c)		60	0	0	14	3	0.1	Trace	Trace	Trace	Trace	Trace
Chocolate fudge (1 oz), chocolate syrup (3 tbsp)		125	1	2	30	15	0.6	10	Trace	0.02	0.1	Trace
Molasses (1 tbsp), caramel (1/2 oz)		40	Trace	Trace	8	20	0.3	Trace	Trace	Trace	Trace	Trace
Sugar (1 tbsp)	12	45	0	0	12	0	Trace	0	0	0	0	0
Miscellaneous												
Chocolate, bitter (1 oz)	30	145	3	15	8	20	1.9	20	0.01	0.07	0.4	0
Sherbert (1/2 c)	96	130	1	1	30	15	Trace	55	0.01	0.03	Trace	2
Soups: bean, pea (green) (1 c)		150	7	4	22	50	1.6	495	0.09	0.06	1.0	4
noodle, beef, chicken (1 c)		65	4	2	7	10	0.7	50	0.03	0.04	0.9	Trace
clam chowder, minestrone, tomato, vegetable (1 c)		90	3	2	14	25	0.9	1880	0.05	0.04	1.1	3

[illegible] M. E. Principles of Nutrition. 2nd ed. New York, John Wiley & Sons, Inc., 1965, pp. 528–33.

TABLE 30–17 NUTRITIVE VALUE OF BABY FOODS (PER 100 GRAMS EDIBLE PORTION—ABOUT 7 TABLESPOONS)

FOOD	ENERGY CALORIES	PROTEIN GM	FAT GM	CARBO-HYDRATE GM	CALCIUM MG	IRON MG	VITAMIN A VALUE IU	THIAMINE MG	RIBO-FLAVIN MG	NIACIN MG	ASCORBIC ACID MG
Cereals, precooked, dry and other products											
Barley, added nutrients	348	13.4	1.2	73.6	736	53.2	(0)	3.71	1.20	32.2	0
High protein, added nutrients	357	35.2	3.7	48.1	815	63.1	—	3.67	1.15	24.0	0
Mixed, added nutrients	368	15.2	2.9	70.6	820	56.4	—	3.15	1.35	22.3	0
Oatmeal, added nutrients	375	16.5	5.5	66.0	757	48.2	(0)	2.58	1.05	21.3	0
Rice, added nutrients	371	6.6	1.6	80.0	858	50.2	(0)	2.56	1.24	19.7	0
Dinners, canned											
Cereal, vegetable, meat mixtures (approx. 2–4% protein)											
Beef noodle dinner	48	2.8	1.1	6.8	12	0.5	620	0.02	0.05	0.5	2
Cereal, egg yolk and bacon	82	2.9	4.9	6.6	29	0.8	520	0.05	0.06	0.4	
Chicken noodle dinner	49	2.1	1.3	7.2	27	0.3	800	0.03	0.06	0.4	1
Macaroni, tomatoes, meat and cereal	67	2.6	2.0	9.6	21	0.5	500	0.14	0.12	1.0	1
Split peas, vegetables and ham or bacon	80	4.0	2.1	11.2	29	0.7	600	0.08	0.05	0.5	1
Vegetables and bacon, with cereal	68	1.7	2.9	8.7	17	0.6	2200	0.07	0.05	0.6	1
Vegetables and beef, with cereal	56	2.7	1.6	7.6	17	0.8	2800	0.03	0.04	0.9	1
Vegetables and chicken, with cereal	52	2.1	1.4	7.7	33	0.4	1000	0.03	0.04	0.5	Trace
Vegetables and ham, with cereal	64	2.8	2.2	8.3	25	0.3	1000	0.08	0.05	0.5	3
Vegetables and lamb, with cereal	58	2.2	2.0	7.7	23	0.7	2200	0.03	0.05	0.7	1
Vegetables and liver, with cereal	47	3.1	0.4	7.8	17	2.7	4700	0.04	0.37	1.6	3
Vegetables and liver, with bacon and cereal	57	2.4	1.9	7.5	11	2.6	4600	0.03	0.33	1.3	2
Vegetables and turkey, with cereal	44	2.1	0.8	7.2	22	0.3	400	0.01	0.03	0.4	1
Meat or poultry (approx. 6–8% protein)											
Beef with vegetables	87	7.4	3.7	6.0	13	1.2	1100	0.07	0.17	1.6	2
Chicken with vegetables	100	7.4	4.6	7.2	22	0.9	1000	0.09	0.15	1.6	2
Turkey with vegetables	86	6.7	3.2	7.6	38	0.6	1000	0.13	0.13	1.8	2
Veal with vegetables	63	7.1	1.6	5.1	11	0.8	800	0.08	0.15	2.0	2
Fruits and fruit products with or without thickening, canned											
Applesauce	72	0.2	0.2	18.6	4	0.4	40	0.01	0.02	0.1	Trace

Table continued.

TABLE 30–17 NUTRITIVE VALUE OF BABY FOODS (PER 100 GRAMS EDIBLE PORTION—ABOUT 7 TABLESPOONS) (*Continued*)

FOOD	ENERGY CALORIES	PROTEIN GM	FAT GM	CARBO-HYDRATE GM	CALCIUM MG	IRON MG	VITAMIN A VALUE I U	THIAMINE MG	RIBO-FLAVIN MG	NIACIN MG	ASCORBIC ACID MG
Applesauce and apricots	86	0.3	0.1	22.6	4	0.3	600	0.01	0.02	0.1	2
Bananas (with tapioca or cornstarch, added ascorbic acid), strained	84	0.4	0.2	21.6	13	0.2	70	0.02	0.02	0.2	35
Bananas and pineapple (with tapioca or cornstarch)	80	0.4	0.1	20.7	20	0.2	30	0.01	0.01	0.1	2
Fruit dessert with tapioca (apricot, pineapple or orange)	84	0.3	0.3	21.5	15	0.4	450	0.02	0.01	0.2	4
Peaches	81	0.6	0.2	20.7	6	0.3	500	0.01	0.02	0.7	3
Pears	66	0.3	0.1	17.1	7	0.2	30	0.02	0.02	0.2	2
Pears and pineapple	69	0.4	0.2	17.6	7	0.2	20	0.03	0.02	0.2	2
Plums with tapioca, strained	94	0.4	0.2	24.3	5	0.4	250	0.01	0.02	0.2	2
Prunes with tapioca	86	0.3	0.2	22.4	7	0.9	400	0.02	0.06	0.4	4
Meats, poultry and eggs; canned											
Beef:											
Strained	99	14.7	4.0	(0)	8	2.0	—	0.01	0.16	3.5	0
Junior	118	19.3	3.9	(0)	8	2.5	—	0.02	0.20	4.3	0
Chicken	127	13.7	7.6	(0)	—	1.9	—	0.02	0.16	3.5	0
Egg yolks, strained	210	10.0	18.4	0.2	81	3.0	1900	0.12	0.22	Trace	Trace
Lamb:											
Strained	107	14.6	4.9	(0)	9	2.1	—	0.02	0.17	3.3	—
Junior	121	17.5	5.1	(0)	13	2.7	—	0.02	0.21	4.1	—
Liver, strained	97	14.1	3.4	1.5	6	5.6	24,000	0.05	2.00	7.6	10
Liver and bacon, strained	123	13.7	6.6	1.3	6	4.2	22,000	0.05	1.99	7.8	7
Pork:											
Strained	118	15.4	5.8	(0)	8	1.5	—	0.19	0.20	2.7	—
Junior	134	18.6	6.0	(0)	8	1.2	—	0.23	0.23	2.8	—
Veal:											
Strained	91	15.5	2.7	(0)	10	1.7	—	0.03	0.20	4.3	—
Junior	107	18.8	3.0	(0)	8	1.6	—	0.03	0.22	6.0	—
Vegetables, canned:											
Beans, green	22	1.4	0.1	5.1	33	1.1	400	0.02	0.06	0.3	3
Beets, strained	37	1.4	0.1	8.3	18	0.7	20	0.02	0.03	0.1	3
Carrots	29	0.7	0.1	6.8	23	0.5	13,000	0.02	0.03	0.4	3
Mixed vegetables, including vegetable soup	37	1.6	0.3	8.5	22	0.9	4700	0.05	0.04	0.6	2
Peas, strained	54	4.2	0.2	9.3	11	1.2	500	0.08	0.09	1.2	10
Spinach, creamed	43	2.3	0.7	7.5	64	0.6	5000	0.02	0.13	0.3	6
Squash	25	0.7	0.1	6.2	24	0.4	2400	0.02	0.04	0.3	8
Sweet potatoes	67	1.0	0.2	15.5	16	0.4	4900	0.04	0.03	0.4	8
Tomato soup, strained	54	1.9	0.1	13.5	24	0.4	1000	0.05	0.12	0.7	3

[illegible] Therapeutic Nutrition, 13th ed. New York, The Macmillan Company, 1967.

THE DENVER DEVELOPMENTAL SCREENING TEST

The Denver Developmental Screening Test (DDST) offers a simple and effective way of assessing the developmental status of children during the first six years of life. Abbreviated instructions follow:

The Denver Developmental Screening Test (DDST), a device for detecting developmental delays in infancy and the preschool years, has been standardized on a large cross section of the Denver child population. The test is administered with ease and speed and lends itself to serial evaluations on the same test sheet.

Test Materials. Skein of red wool; box of raisins; rattle with a narrow handle; small clear glass bottle with 5/8 in. opening; bell; tennis ball; test form; pencil; 8 one-inch cubical colored (red, blue, yellow, green) blocks.

General Instructions. The mother should be told that this is a developmental screening device to obtain an estimate of the child's level of development and that it is not expected that the child will be able to perform each of the test items. This test relies on observations of what the child can do and on report by a parent who knows the child. Direct observation should be used whenever possible. Since the test requires active participation by the child, every effort should be made to put the child at ease. The younger child may be tested while sitting on the mother's lap. This should be done in such a way that he can comfortably reach the test materials on the table. The test should be administered before any frightening or painful procedures. One may start by laying out one or two test materials in front of the child while asking the mother whether he performs some of the personal-social items. It is best to administer the first few test items well below the child's age level in order to assure him an initial successful experience. To avoid distractions it is best to remove all test materials from the table except those required for the test that is being administered.

Steps in Administering the Test

1. Draw a vertical line on the examination sheet through the four sectors (Personal-Social, Fine Motor-Adaptive, Language, and Gross Motor) to represent the child's chronologic age. Place the date of the examination at the top of the age line. For children who were born prematurely, subtract the number of months of prematurity from the chronologic age.

2. The items to be administered are those through which the child's chronologic age line passes, unless there are obvious deviations. In each sector one should establish the area in which the child passes all the items and the point at which he fails all the items.

3. In the event that a child refuses to do some of the items requested by the examiner, it is suggested that the parent administer the item, provided she does so in the prescribed manner.

4. If a child passes an item, a large letter "P" is written on the bar. "F" designates a failure, and "R" designates a refusal.

5. Note how the child adjusted to the examination (i.e., his cooperation, attention span, self-confidence) and how he related to his mother, the examiner and the test materials.

6. Ask the parent if the child's performance was typical of his performance at other times.

7. To retest the child on the same form, use a different color pencil for the scoring and age line.

8. Instructions for administering footnoted items are on the back of the test form.

Interpretations. The test items are placed into four categories: Personal-Social, Fine Motor-Adaptive, Language, and Gross Motor. Each of the test items is designated by a bar which is so located under the age scale as to indicate clearly the ages at which 25, 50, 75 and 90 per cent of the standardization population could perform the particular test item. The left end of the bar designates the age at which 25 per cent of the standardization population could perform the item; the hatch mark at the top of the bar 50 per cent; the left end of the shaded area 75 per cent, and the right end of the bar the age at which 90 per cent of the standardization population could perform the item. (See below.)

Failure to perform an item passed by 90 per cent of children of the same age should be considered a "delay." Such a failure may be emphasized by coloring the right end of the bar of the failed item. Performances are scored as *abnormal* if two or more sectors have two or more delays, *or* if one sector has two or more delays and one other sector has one delay and in the same sector the age line does not intersect one item that is passed; as *questionable* if any one sector has two or more delays, or if one or more sectors have one delay *and* in the same sectors the age line does not intersect an item that is passed; as *untestable* if refusals occur in numbers large enough to cause the test to be questionable or abnormal if the refusals were scored as failures; and as *normal* if the performance is not abnormal, questionable or untestable.

DENVER DEVELOPMENTAL SCREENING TEST

STO.=STOMACH
SIT=SITTING

PERCENT OF CHILDREN PASSING

25 50 75 90 — R, 1,2,3, etc. TEST ITEM

R=may pass by report
1,2,3, etc. refer to footnotes on back of form

Date
Name
Birthdate
Hosp. No.

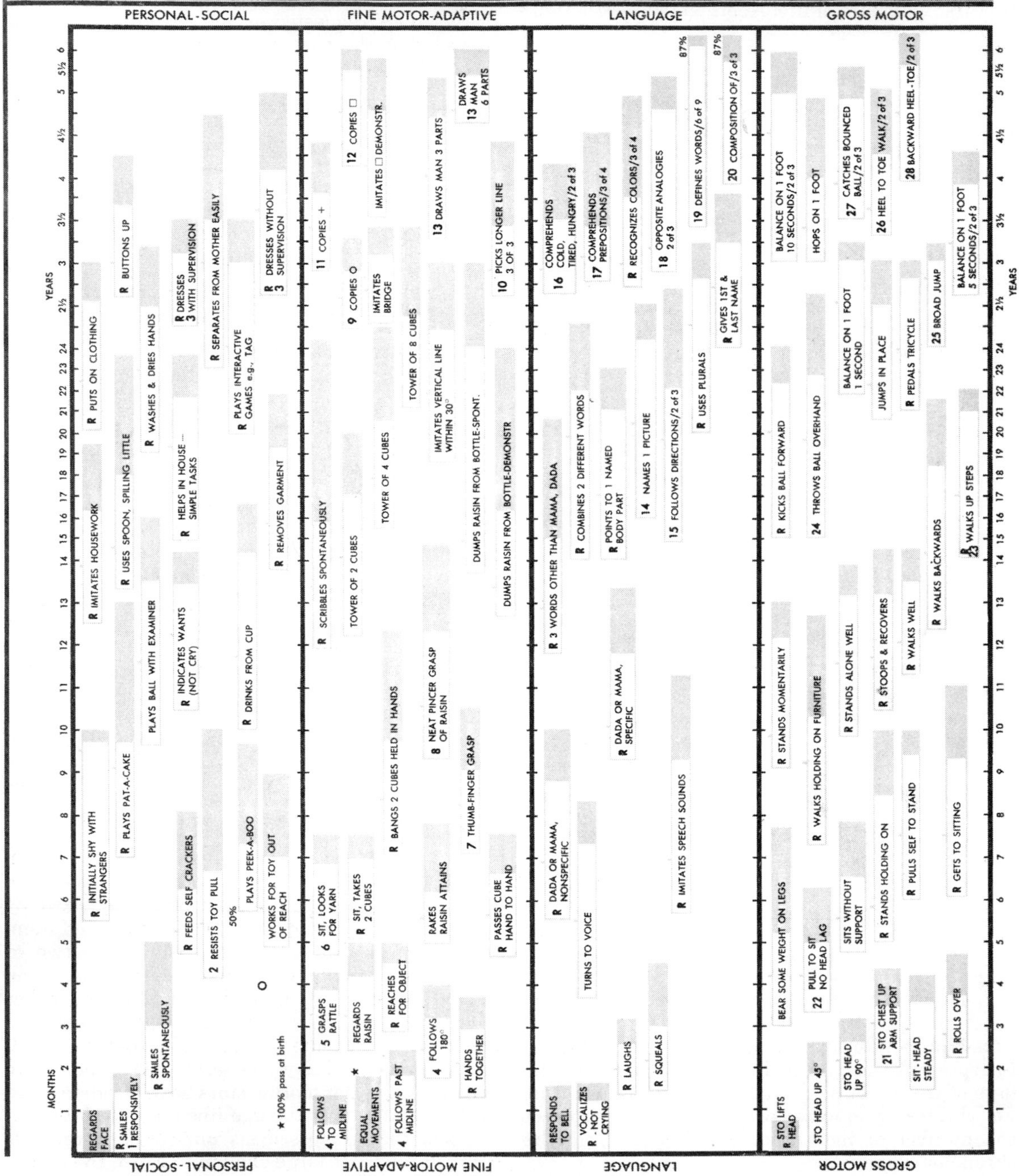

DATE
NAME
DIRECTIONS BIRTHDATE
HOSP. NO.

1. Try to get child to smile by smiling, talking or waving to him. Do not touch him.
2. When child is playing with toy, pull it away from him. Pass if he resists.
3. Child does not have to be able to tie shoes or button in the back.
4. Move yarn slowly in an arc from one side to the other, about 6" above child's face. Pass if eyes follow 90° to midline. (Past midline; 180°)
5. Pass if child grasps rattle when it is touched to the backs or tips of fingers.
6. Pass if child continues to look where yarn disappeared or tries to see where it went. Yarn should be dropped quickly from sight from tester's hand without arm movement.
7. Pass if child picks up raisin with any part of thumb and a finger.
8. Pass if child picks up raisin with the ends of thumb and index finger using an over hand approach.

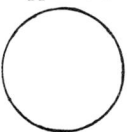

9. Pass any enclosed form. Fail continuous round motions.
10. Which line is longer? (Not bigger.) Turn paper upside down and repeat. (3/3 or 5/6)
11. Pass any crossing lines.
12. Have child copy first. If failed, demonstrate

When giving items 9, 11 and 12, do not name the forms. Do not demonstrate 9 and 11.

13. When scoring, each pair (2 arms, 2 legs, etc.) counts as one part.
14. Point to picture and have child name it. (No credit is given for sounds only.)

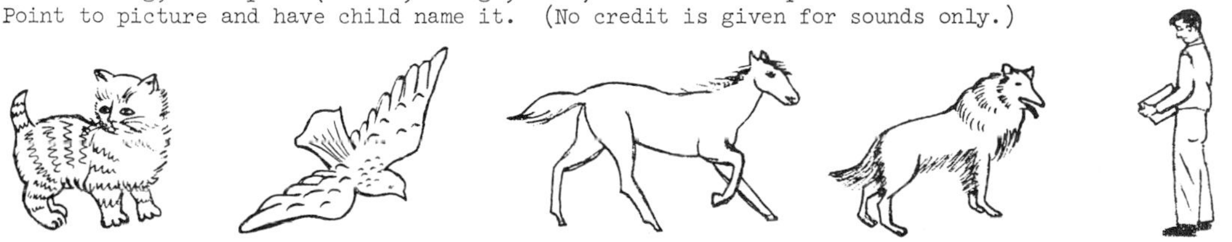

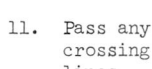

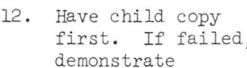

15. Tell child to: Give block to Mommie; put block on table; put block on floor. Pass 2 of 3. (Do not help child by pointing, moving head or eyes.)
16. Ask child: What do you do when you are cold? ..hungry? ..tired? Pass 2 of 3.
17. Tell child to: Put block <u>on</u> table; <u>under</u> table; <u>in front</u> of chair, <u>behind</u> chair. Pass 3 of 4. (Do not help child by pointing, moving head or eyes.)
18. Ask child: If fire is hot, ice is ?; Mother is a woman, Dad is a ?; a horse is big, a mouse is ?. Pass 2 of 3.
19. Ask child: What is a ball? ..lake? ..desk? ..house? ..banana? ..curtain? ..ceiling? ..hedge? ..pavement? Pass if defined in terms of use, shape, what it is made of or general category (such as banana is fruit, not just yellow). Pass 6 of 9.
20. Ask child: What is a spoon made of? ..a shoe made of? ..a door made of? (No other objects may be substituted.) Pass 3 of 3.
21. When placed on stomach, child lifts chest off table with support of forearms and/or hands.
22. When child is on back, grasp his hands and pull him to sitting. Pass if head does not hang back.
23. Child may use wall or rail only, not person. May not crawl.
24. Child must throw ball overhand 3 feet to within arm's reach of tester.
25. Child must perform standing broad jump over width of test sheet. (8-1/2 inches)
26. Tell child to walk forward, heel within 1 inch of toe. Tester may demonstrate. Child must walk 4 consecutive steps, 2 out of 3 trials.
27. Bounce ball to child who should stand 3 feet away from tester. Child must catch ball with hands, not arms, 2 out of 3 trials.
28. Tell child to walk backward, toe within 1 inch of heel. Tester may demonstrate. Child must walk 4 consecutive steps, 2 out of 3 trials.

<u>DATE AND BEHAVIORAL OBSERVATIONS</u> (how child feels at time of test, relation to tester, attention span, verbal behavior, self-confidence, etc,):

Developmental delays may be due to:

1. The unwillingness of the child to use his ability
    a. Owing to temporary factors, such as fatigue, illness, hospitalization, separation from the parent, fear, etc.
    b. General unwillingness to do most things that are asked of him—such a condition may be just as detrimental as an inability to perform
2. An inability to perform the item because of
    a. general retardation
    b. pathologic factors such as deafness or neurologic impairment
    c. familial pattern of slow development in one or more areas

If unexplained developmental delays appear to be valid reflections of a child's abilities, he should be rescreened a month later. If the delays persist he should be further evaluated with more detailed diagnostic studies.

Caution. The DDST is *not* an intelligence test. It is intended as a screening instrument for use in clinical practice to note whether the development of a particular child is within the normal range.

These abbreviated instructions are amplified in the manual.

The test form and footnoted instructions are given on pages 1810 and 1811. The form is copyrighted. Forms, kits, manuals and instructional films may be purchased through LADOCA Project and Publishing Foundation, Inc., East 51st Avenue and Lincoln Street, Denver, Colorado 80216.

We are indebted to the authors for permission to include the test in this volume.

Frankenburg, W. K., and Dodds, J. B.: The Denver Developmental Screening Test. J. Pediatr. *71*:181, 1967.

Frankenburg, W. K., Goldstein, A. D. and Camp, B. W.: The Revised Denver Developmental Screening Test: Its accuracy as a screening instrument. J. Pediatr. *79*:988, 1971.

INDEX